This book is due for return on or before the last date shown below.

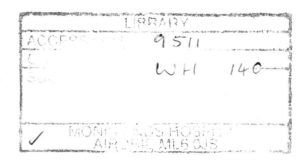

NEOPLASTIC DISEASES OF THE BLOOD
Fourth Edition

In the fourth edition of this classic work on malignant blood cancers, Drs. Peter H. Wiernik, John M. Goldman, Janice P. Dutcher, and Robert A. Kyle, and more than 100 international leaders in the field provide a comprehensive text on the diagnosis and treatment of all hematologic malignancies, both common and rare. The sixty-two chapters are divided into sections on Chronic Leukemias and Related Disorders, Acute Leukemias, Myeloma and Related Disorders, Lymphomas, and Supportive Care, with a devoted editor for each section. This extensively revised and updated edition reflects the tremendous progress in the science and treatment of hematologic malignancies during the eight years since the third edition in 1995. Revisions and new chapters include coverage of stem cell transplantation, molecular genetics, monoclonal antibodies, and other new treatment modalities. This comprehensive treatise on the laboratory and clinical aspects of all hematologic neoplasms includes up-to-date treatment recommendations and thorough discussions of etiology, pathogenesis, and clinical aspects. Written by authors involved first-hand in the clinical and research data presented here, this encyclopedic text is an essential reference for all hematologists and oncologists.

Praise for previous editions:

"No other current text covers the spectrum of hematologic neoplasia as comprehensively."

—*Journal of the American Medical Association*

". . . one of the best (if not the best) general reference sources on the clinical aspects of hematologic neoplastic diseases."

—*New England Journal of Medicine*

". . . this compendium will be an excellent reference source for physicians who are interested in neoplastic hematologic diseases."

—*Mayo Clinic Proceedings*

"Those with a . . . specific interest in the hematologic malignancies will wish to have their own personal copies."

—*Annals of Internal Medicine*

NEOPLASTIC DISEASES OF THE BLOOD

FOURTH EDITION

Edited by

PETER H. WIERNIK, M.D.

Professor of Medicine and Radiation Oncology, New York
Medical College, Valhalla, New York; Director, Our Lady of Mercy
Cancer Center, Bronx, New York

JOHN M. GOLDMAN, D.M.

Professor, Department of Haemotology, Imperial College
London, Hammersmith Hospital, London, England

JANICE P. DUTCHER, M.D.

Professor of Medicine, New York Medical College, Valhalla, New
York; Associate Director for Clinical Affairs, Our Lady of Mercy
Cancer Center, Bronx, New York

ROBERT A. KYLE, M.D.

Professor, Departments of Medicine and Laboratory Medicine,
Mayo Medical School; Consultant, Division of Hematology and
Internal Medicine, Mayo Clinic and Mayo Foundation, Rochester,
Minnesota

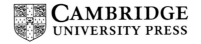

CAMBRIDGE
UNIVERSITY PRESS

PUBLISHED BY THE PRESS SYNDICATE OF THE UNIVERSITY OF CAMBRIDGE
The Pitt Building, Trumpington Street, Cambridge, United Kingdom

CAMBRIDGE UNIVERSITY PRESS
The Edinburgh Building, Cambridge CB2 2RU, UK
40 West 20th Street, New York, NY 10011-4211, USA
477 Williamstown Road, Port Melbourne, VIC 3207, Australia
Ruiz de Alarcón 13, 28014 Madrid, Spain
Dock House, The Waterfront, Cape Town 8001, South Africa

http://www.cambridge.org

First published 2003

Printed in the United States of America

Typefaces Minion 9.5/11.5 pt. and ITC Symbol   *System* QuarkXPress™   [HT]

A catalog record for this book is available from the British Library.

Library of Congress Cataloging-in-Publication Data

Neoplastic diseases of the blood / edited by Peter H. Wiernik . . . [et. al.] – 4th ed.
    p.   cm.
  Includes bibliographical references and index.
  ISBN 0 521 79136 7 (hardback)
    1. Leukemia. 2. Multiple myeloma. 3. Lymphomas. I. Wiernik, Peter H.
    [DNLM: 1. Leukemia. 2. Lymphoma. 3. Multiple Myeloma. WH 250 N438 2003]
  RC643 N46 2003
  616.99′419—dc21

                                                              2002031555

ISBN 0 521 79136 7   hardback

The editors dedicate the fourth edition of this work to our families, to the hundreds of fellows we have trained, and to the thousands of patients we have had the privilege to care for over the decades.

Contents

Contributors

Alan C. Aisenberg, MD, PhD, Professor, Department of Medicine, Harvard Medical School; Physician, Department of Hematology/Oncology, Massachusetts General Hospital, Boston, Massachusetts

Elias J. Anaissie, MD, Professor of Medicine, Arkansas Cancer Research Center, University of Arkansas for Medical Sciences, Little Rock, Arkansas

Claudio Anasetti, MD, Professor of Medicine, Division of Clinical Research, Fred Hutchinson Cancer Research Center, Department of Medicine, Division of Oncology, University of Washington, Seattle, Washington

Kenneth C. Anderson, MD, Professor of Medicine, Department of Adult Oncology, Dana-Farber Cancer Institute; Harvard Medical School, Boston, Massachusetts

Robert J. Arceci, MD, PhD, Director of Pediatric Oncology, King Fahd Professor of Pediatric Oncology, Johns Hopkins Oncology Center, Johns Hopkins University School of Medicine, Baltimore, Maryland

James O. Armitage, MD, Professor and Chairman, Department of Internal Medicine, University of Nebraska College of Medicine, Omaha, Nebraska

Monica Balzarotti, MD, Associate Director, Department of Medical Oncology and Hematology, Instituto Clinico Humanitas, Rozzano (Milano), Italy

Dalsu Baris, MD, PhD, Occupational Epidemiology Branch, National Cancer Institute, Bethesda, Maryland

Anthony Bench, PhD, Department of Haematology, University of Cambridge, Wellcome Trust Centre for Molecular Mechanisms in Disease, Cambridge Institute for Medical Research, Cambridge, England

John M. Bennett, MD, Professor, Department of Medicine, Pathology, and Laboratory Medicine, University of Rochester School of Medicine and Dentistry; Attending Physician, Department of Medicine, Medical Oncology Unit, Strong Memorial Hospital, Rochester, New York

Daniel E. Bergsagel, CM, MD, D.Phil, Professor of Medicine, University of Toronto; Consultant Physician, Ontario Cancer Institute/Princess Margaret Hospital, Toronto, Ontario, Canada

P. Leif Bergsagel, MD, Associate Professor of Medicine, Division of Hematology-Oncology, New York Presbyterian Hospital/Cornell University, New York, New York

Philip J. Bierman, MD, Associate Professor, Section of Oncology and Hematology, Department of Internal Medicine, University of Nebraska College of Medicine, Omaha, Nebraska

Clara D. Bloomfield, MD, William G. Pace III Professor of Cancer Research; Director, The Ohio State University Comprehensive Cancer Center; Deputy Director, Arthur G. James Cancer Hospital and Richard J. Solove Research Institute, Columbus, Ohio

Linda M. Brown, MPH, DrPH, Chief Health Services Officer; Assistant Chief, Biostatistics Branch, Division of Cancer Epidemiology and Genetics, National Cancer Institute, Bethesda, Maryland

Ray Cartwright, PhD, Leukaemia Research Fund Centre for Clinical Epidemiology at the University of Leeds, Institute of Epidemiology, Leeds, United Kingdom

Januario E. Castro, MD, Hematology/Oncology Division, University of California San Diego, San Diego, California

Dharminder Chauhan, PhD, Department of Adult Oncology, Dana-Farber Cancer Institute; Harvard Medical School, Boston, Massachusetts

David Choi, MD, PhD, Resident, Department of Neurology, Beth Israel, New England Deaconess Medical Center, Boston, Massachusetts

Richard J. Creger, PharmD, Comprehensive Cancer Center of the University Hospitals of Cleveland, Case Western Reserve University, Cleveland, Ohio

H. Joachim Deeg, MD, Professor, Department of Medicine, University of Washington School of Medicine; Clinical Research Division, Fred Hutchinson Cancer Research Center, Seattle, Washington

Thomas G. DeLoughery, MD, Assistant Professor, Departments of Medicine and Pathology, Oregon Health Sciences University School of Medicine, Portland, Oregon

Susan S. Devesa, PhD, Chief, Descriptive Studies Section, Biostatistics Branch, Division of Cancer Etiology, National Cancer Institute, National Institutes of Health, Bethesda, Maryland

Gordon Dewald, PhD, Professor of Laboratory Medicine and Medical Genetics, Mayo Clinic, Rochester, Minnesota

Maria Cecilia Dignani, MD, University of Arkansas for Medical Sciences, Little Rock, Arkansas

Meletios A. Dimopoulos, MD, Associate Professor of Medical Oncology, University of Athens School of Medicine, Athens, Greece

Angela Dispenzieri, MD, Assistant Professor of Medicine, Mayo Medical School; Consultant, Division of Hematology, Mayo Clinic, Rochester, Minnesota

Barbara K. Dunn, PhD, MD, Medical Officer, Division of Cancer Prevention, National Cancer Institute, Frederick, Maryland

Janice P. Dutcher, MD, Associate Director for Clinical Affairs, Our Lady of Mercy Cancer Center; Professor of Medicine, New York Medical College, Bronx, New York

Stefan Faderl, MD, Assistant Professor, Department of Leukemia, The University of Texas M.D. Anderson Cancer Center, Houston, Texas

Rafael Fonseca, MD, Associate Professor of Medicine, Department of Internal Medicine, Division of Hematology, Mayo Clinic, Rochester, Minnesota

Emil J. Freireich, MD, DSc (Hon.), Special Medical Education Programs, The University of Texas M.D. Anderson Cancer Center, Houston, Texas

Robert E. Gallagher, MD, Professor, Departments of Medicine and Oncology, Albert Einstein College of Medicine of Yeshiva University; Attending Physician, Department of Oncology, Montefiore Medical Center, Bronx, New York

Morie A. Gertz, MD, Consultant, Division of Hematology and Internal Medicine, Mayo Clinic and Mayo Foundation; Professor of Medicine, Mayo Medical School, Rochester, Minnesota

John Gibson, MB, BS, FRACP, FRCPA, Associate Professor, Department of Medicine, University of Sidney; Senior Haematologist, Institute of Haematology, Royal Prince Alfred Hospital, Sydney, Australia

Nicola Gökbuget, MD, Department of Medicine (Haematology and Oncology) of the Johann Wolfgang-Goethe-University Frankfurt/Main, Germany

John M. Goldman, DM, Professor, Department of Haematology, Imperial College London, Hammersmith Hospital, London, England

Myrtle Y. Gordon, PhD, DSc, Professor, Department of Haematology, Imperial College London, Hammersmith Hospital, London, England

N. Claude Gorin, MD, Professor of Hematology, Service des Maladies du Sang, Unite de Therapie Cellulaire, Hôpital Saint Antoine, Paris, France

Anthony R. Green, PhD, Department of Haematology, University of Cambridge, Wellcome Trust Centre for Molecular Mechanisms of Disease, Cambridge Institute for Medical Research, Cambridge, England

Philip R. Greipp, MD, Professor, Departments of Medicine and Laboratory Medicine, Mayo Medical School; Consultant, Division of Hematology and Internal Medicine and Division of Hematopathology, Mayo Clinic and Mayo Foundation, Rochester, Minnesota

Seymour Grufferman, MD, Professor and Chairman, Department of Family Medicine and Clinical Epidemiology, University of Pittsburgh School of Medicine, Pittsburgh, Pennsylvania

John A. Hansen, MD, Division of Clinical Research, Fred Hutchinson Cancer Research Center, Seattle, Washington

Shelley Heimfeld, PhD, Clinical Research Division, Fred Hutchinson Cancer Research Center, Seattle, Washington

Dieter Hoelzer, MD, Professor, Department of Internal Medicine; Chief, Department of Hematology, University Hospital, Frankfurt, Germany

James F. Holland, MD, Distinguished Professor, Department of Neoplastic Diseases, Mount Sinai School of Medicine of the City University of New York; Director Emeritus, The Gerald H. Ruttenberg Cancer Center, Mount Sinai Hospital, New York, New York

Jimmie C. Holland, MD, Chairman, Department of Psychiatry and Behavioral Sciences, Wayne E. Chapman Chair of Psychiatric Oncology, Sloan-Kettering Cancer Center, New York, New York

Brian J. P. Huntly, PhD, Department of Haematology, University of Cambridge, Wellcome Trust Centre for Molecular Mechanisms in Disease, Cambridge Institute for Medical Research, Cambridge, England

Elaine S. Jaffe, MD, Chief, Hematopathology Section, Laboratory of Pathology, National Cancer Institute, National Institutes of Health, Bethesda, Maryland

Douglas E. Joshua, MS, BS, DPHIL (OXON), FRACP, FRCPA, Clinical Professor, Department of Medicine, University of Sydney; Director, Institute of Haematology, Royal Prince Alfred Hospital, Sydney, Australia

Hagop M. Kantarjian, MD, Professor, Department of Leukemia, The University of Texas M.D. Anderson Cancer Center, Houston, Texas

Jerry A. Katzmann, PhD, Consultant, Department of Laboratory Medicine and Psychology, Association Professor of Laboratory Medicine Mayo Medical, Mayo Clinic and Mayo Foundation, Rochester, Minnesota

Michael J. Keating, MB, BS, Doctor Kenneth B. McCredie Chair in Clinical Leukemia Research, and Professor, Department of Hematology, University of Texas M.D. Anderson Cancer Center, Houston, Texas

Karen E. King, MD, Fellow, Division of Transfusion Medicine, Department of Pathology, The Johns Hopkins University School of Medicine and the Johns Hopkins Hospital, Baltimore, Maryland

Thomas J. Kipps, MD, PhD, Professor, Department of Medicine, University of California San Diego, La Jolla, California

H. Phillip Koeffler, MD, Professor of Medicine, Division of Hematology/Oncology, Cedars-Sinai Medical Center, UCLA School of Medicine, Los Angeles, California

W. Michael Kuehl, MD, Genetics Department, Medical Branch, National Cancer Institute, Bethesda, Maryland

Joanne Kurtzberg, MD, Professor of Pediatrics; Director, Pediatric BMT Program, Duke University Medical Center, Durham, North Carolina

Robert A. Kyle, MD, Consultant, Division of Hematology and Internal Medicine, Mayo Clinic and Mayo Foundation; Professor of Medicine and of Laboratory Medicine, Mayo Medical School, Rochester, Minnesota

Hillard M. Lazarus, MD, FACP, Professor of Medicine, Director, Bone Marrow Transplantation Program, Comprehensive Cancer Center of the University Hospitals of Cleveland, Case Western Reserve University, Cleveland, Ohio

Helen Leather, BPharm, BCPS, Clinical Pharmacy Specialist, Shands Hospital at the University of Florida, Gainesville, Florida

Mark Litzow, MD, Assistant Professor of Medicine, Mayo Clinic, Rochester, Minnesota

Dan L. Longo, MD, Scientific Directory, National Institute on Aging, Baltimore, Maryland

John A. Lust, MD, PhD, Professor, Department of Medicine, Mayo Medical School; Consultant, Division of Hematology and Internal Medicine, Mayo Clinic and Mayo Foundation, Rochester, Minnesota

Tahsine H. Mahfouz, MD, University of Arkansas for Medical Sciences, Little Rock, Arkansas

Paul J. Martin, MD, Fred Hutchinson Cancer Research Center, Seattle, Washington

Susan M. McKenna, MD, Assistant Professor, Division of Pediatrics, Department of Medicine, University of Southern California School of Medicine; Head, Division of Pediatric Oncology, Department of Health Services, Los Angeles County-University of Southern California Medical Center, Los Angeles, California

L. Jeffrey Medeiros, MD, Chief, Lymphoma Section; Professor, Department of Hematopathology, Division of Pathology and Laboratory Medicine, The University of Texas M.D. Anderson Cancer Center, Houston, Texas

Nancy Price Mendenhall, MD, Rodney R. Million Professor of Radiation Oncology, Chairman, Department of Radiation Oncology, University of Florida, Shands Cancer Center, Gainesville, Florida

Maria Messinezy, FRCPath, FRCP, Department of Haematology, Guy's, King's and St. Thomas' School of Medicine, St. Thomas' Hospital, London, England

Carole B. Miller, MD, St. Agnes Healthcare, Baltimore, Maryland

Kenneth B. Miller, MD, Associate Professor of Medicine, Director of Bone Marrow Transplantation, Tufts-New England Medical Center, Boston, Massachusetts

Sandra E. Mitchell, MD, Assistant Professor, Department of Radiation Oncology, University of Florida Health Science Center, Gainesville, Florida

Krzysztof Mrózek, MB, MRCPI, Professor of Medicine, Director, Bone Marrow Transplantation Program, Ohio State University Comprehensive Cancer Center, Columbus, Ohio

Paul M. Ness, MD, Associate Professor, Division of Transfusion Medicine, Department of Pathology, The John Hopkins University School of Medicine; Director, Blood Bank, The Johns Hopkins Hospital, Baltimore, Maryland

Annette J. Neylon, MD, Blood Transfusion Centre, Newcastle Upon Tyne, United Kingdom

Stephen G. O'Brien, PhD, Royal Victoria Infirmary, Newcastle Upon Tyne, United Kingdom

Susan O'Brien, MD, Associate Professor, Department of Leukemia, University of Texas M.D. Anderson Cancer Center, Houston, Texas

Paul V. O'Donnell, MD, PhD, Associate Professor, Fred Hutchinson Cancer Research Center, University of Washington School of Medicine

David G. Oscier, MA, FRCP, FRCPath, Consultant Haematologist, Royal Bournemouth Hospital; Honorary Clinical Senior Lecturer, Southampton University, United Kingdom

Howard Ozer, MD, Eason Chair and Chief, Hematology/Oncology Section, University of Oklahoma Health Sciences Center; Director, Oklahoma University Cancer Center, Oklahoma City, Oklahoma

Elisabeth Paietta, PhD, Professor of Medicine, Our Lady of Mercy Medical Center, New York Medical College, Valhalla, New York; Director, Clinical Immunology and Stem Cell Laboratory, Our Lady of Mercy Cancer Center, Bronx, New York

Rupesh Parikh, MD, Hematology-Oncology Section, Kaiser Permanente, Fontana, California

Dorothy J. Park, MD, PhD, Assistant Professor, Division of Hematology/Oncology, Cedars-Sinai Medical Center, UCLA School of Medicine, Los Angeles, California

Thomas C. Pearson, MD, Department of Haematology, Guy's, King's, and St. Thomas' School of Medicine, St Thomas' Hospital, London, England

Effie W. Petersdorf, MD, Fred Hutchinson Cancer Center, Seattle, Washington

Bernard J. Poiesz, MD, Professor, Departments of Medicine and Microbiology, Upstate Medical University, State University of New York; Head, Division of Hematology/Oncology, Syracuse, New York

Michael J. Poiesz, BA, Research Assistant, Upstate Medical University, State University of New York; Division of Hematology/Oncology, Syracuse, New York

Waldemar Pruzanski, MD, Professor of Medicine; Director, Immunology Diagnostic and Research Center; Director, Clinical Immunology and Allergy; Director, Inflammation Research Group, University of Toronto; Head, Division of Immunology, The Wellesley Hospital, Toronto, Ontario, Canada

S. Vincent Rajkumar, MD, Associate Professor of Medicine, Mayo Medical School, Mayo Clinic, Rochester, Minnesota

John T. Reilly, MD, Department of Haematology, Royal Hallamshire Hospital, Sheffield, United Kingdom

Julie A Ross, PhD, Division of Pediatric Epidemiology and Clinical Research, University of Minnesota Cancer Center, Minneapolis, Minnesota

Andrew J. Roth, MD, Assistant Professor, Department of Psychiatry, Cornell University Medical College; Assistant Attending Psychiatrist, Psychiatry Service, Memorial Sloan-Kettering Cancer Center, New York, New York

Matt Rowley, PhD, Department of Genetics, Cell Biology, and Development, The University of Minnesota, Minneapolis, Minnesota

Armando Santoro, MD, Director, Department of Medical Oncology and Hematology, Istituto Clinico Humanitas, Rozzano (Milano), Italy

Alan Saven, MD, Division of Hematology/Oncology, Scripps Clinic, Ida M. and Cecil H. Green Cancer Center Division, The Scripps Cancer Center, La Jolla, California

Charles A. Schiffer, MD, Karmanos Cancer Institute, Wayne State University School of Medicine, Detroit, Michigan

Arthur T. Skarin, MD, Associate Professor, Department of Medicine, Harvard Medical School; Director, Hematology Laboratory, Division of Medical Oncology, Department of Medicine, Dana-Farber Cancer Institute, Boston, Massachusetts

Richard M. Stone, MD, Assistant Professor, Department of Medicine, Harvard Medical School; Associate Physician, Division of Medical Oncology, Department of Medicine, Dana-Farber Cancer Institute, Boston, Massachusetts

Martin S. Tallman, MD, Associate Professor of Medicine, Director, Leukemia Program, Robert H. Lurie Comprehensive Cancer Center of Northwestern University, Chicago, Illinois

Moshe Talpaz, MD, Professor and Chairman, Department of Bioimmunotherapy, The University of Texas M.D. Anderson Cancer Center, Houston, Texas

Nizar Tannir, MD, FACP, Department of Leukemia The University of Texas M.D. Anderson Cancer Center, Houston, Texas

Nukhet N. Tuzuner, MD, Professor, Department of Pathology, Istanbul University Carrahpasa Medical Faculty, Istanbul, Turkey

Brian Van Ness, PhD, Professor and Head, Department of Genetics, Cell Biology, and Development, University of Minnesota, Minneapolis, Minnesota

Julie M. Vose, MD, Associate Professor, Section of Oncology and Hematology, Department of Internal Medicine, University of Nebraska College of Medicine, Omaha, Nebraska

Dietlind Wahner-Roedler, MD, Consultant, Division of Area General Internal Medicine, Mayo Clinic and Mayo Foundation; Assistant Professor of Medicine, Mayo Medical School, Rochester, Minnesota

Howard J. Weinstein, MD, Associate Professor, Division of Hematology-Oncology, Department of Pediatrics, Harvard Medical School; Dana-Farber Cancer Institute, Children's Hospital, Boston, Massachusetts

Sheila Weitzman, MD, ChB, FRCP, FCP(SA), The Hospital for Sick Children, Toronto, Ontario, Canada

Peter H. Wiernik, MD, Professor of Medicine and Radiation Oncology, New York Medical College; Director, Comprehensive Cancer Center, Our Lady of Mercy Medical Center, New York Medical College, Bronx, New York

John R. Wingard, MD, Professor of Medicine, University of Florida School of Medicine; Director, Bone Marrow Transplant Program, University of Florida College of Medicine, Gainesville, Florida

Preface

The fourth edition of *Neoplastic Diseases of the Blood* is long overdue, as evidenced by the tremendous progress made in our understanding of the nature of hematologic malignancies and their treatment since the third edition appeared in 1995. The fourth edition is current and up to date, draws heavily on recent references, and is designed, as were the previous editions, to be a readable encyclopedic resource for established hematologists and oncologists as well as for Fellows in those disciplines. Six new chapters are included in this edition, and all other chapters have been extensively revised and updated. The new chapters concern the epidemiology of chronic leukemias, molecular biology and cytogenetics of chronic myeloid leukemia, myelodysplastic syndromes, cytokines and signal transduction in multiple myeloma, umbilical cord stem cell transplantation, and HLA typing in hematopoietic cell transplantation. Some 112 authors from 4 continents, more than 50 new to this edition, have contributed their expertise to this work. This edition is divided into the same five sections found in earlier editions, each the primary responsibility of an editor: Chronic Leukemias and Related Disorders (John M. Goldman), Acute Leukemia (Peter H. Wiernik), Myeloma and Related Disorders (Robert A. Kyle), Lymphoma (Peter H. Wiernik), and Supportive Care (Janice P. Dutcher). Dr. Goldman is a new editor for this edition, and those of us who have served as editors previously are delighted to have him join us.

Our sincere hope is that patients with hematologic malignancies will benefit directly from this new edition. That hope is what drives us to take on and complete the huge task that is the creation of this book.

We wish to thank the publisher, Cambridge University Press, for assisting us in every way possible through all phases of the development of the book. Special thanks to Heidi Steinmetz Lovette, Editor, Medicine, and Dr. Richard Barling, Director, Medical and Professional Publishing, for guidance and support. Both were instrumental in bringing this project to completion.

Peter H. Wiernik, MD
John M. Goldman, MD
Janice P. Dutcher, MD
Robert A. Kyle, MD

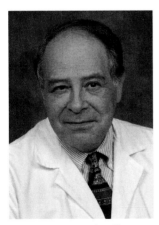

Peter H. Wiernik

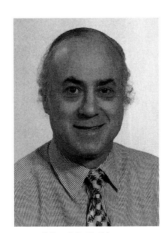

John M. Goldman

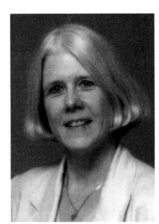

Janice P. Dutcher

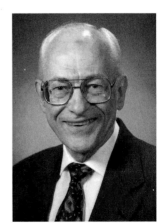

Robert A. Kyle

Chronic Leukemias and Related Disorders

1

A History of the Chronic Leukemias

John M. Goldman and Myrtle Y. Gordon

Although chronic myeloid leukemia (CML) and chronic lymphocytic leukemia (CLL) can be grouped together for some purposes, they differ in many ways, CML being a disease with well-defined progressive stages (chronic phase; acceleration; transformation) occurring in middle life, whereas CLL is a relatively indolent disease involving mainly the elderly. Whereas CML has well characterized molecular features, which can reasonably be assumed to be related to its pathogenesis, the cause of CLL is virtually unknown. The observations that have led to our current state of knowledge and ability to treat patients are the subject of this chapter (Table 1–1). Recent reviews on the history of CML have also been provided by Piller in 1997[1] and Geary in 2000.[2]

DEFINITIONS, CLASSIFICATION, AND CHARACTERIZATION

The recognition that the leukemias are an extremely heterogeneous group of diseases has developed progressively since the condition was first described and owes much to technological development over the past 150 years or so. Thus, the distinctions between the chronic and acute and between the myeloid and lymphoid leukemias did not emerge for some time. The postmortem characteristics of the blood first attracted the attention of the early observers of leukemia. According to Gunz and Henderson,[3] the first accurate description of leukemia was probably made by Velpeau in 1827,[4] although it is likely that leukemia had been seen as early as 1811.[5] This was followed by the observations of Donne[6] and of Craigie.[7] Nevertheless, the recognition of leukemia as a distinct entity is attributed to the virtually simultaneous reports of Bennett in Scotland[8] and Virchow in Germany[9] in 1845. These classic cases involved John Meredith, a 28-year-old slater from Edinburgh and Marie Straide, a 50-year-old cook, in Berlin. Both patients had been unwell for 1.5 to 2 years and their condition had progressively worsened, with increasing weakness, bleeding, and other problems. In both cases the remarkable features at autopsy were the large size of the spleen and the consistency of the blood, in particular the white cell content. Virchow used the term "weisses Blut" to describe the predominance of white cells in the blood and later, in 1847, proposed the term "Leukaemie." Bennett sug-

gested "leucocythaemia." The first diagnosis of leukemia in a living patient was made by Fuller in 1846,[10] by which time Virchow had documented a further nine cases. The first reported case of leukemia in America was in a 17-year-old seaman in Philadelphia in 1852;[11] this was followed by several case reports, mainly from the Boston area.

Early attempts to distinguish different forms of leukemia included Virchow's distinction between splenic and lymphatic leukemias, each of which was associated with particular types of white blood cells.[12] This division is broadly equivalent to myeloid and lymphoid leukemias, with the important observation by Neumann in 1870[13] that the cells responsible for the so-called splenic leukemia were actually made in the bone marrow. Until 1889, when Ebstein first used the term "acute leukemia" on clinical grounds,[14] the disease was considered to be a chronic one. Ebstein also recognized the difference between *de novo* acute leukemia and "acutization" of the chronic disease. It rapidly became apparent that a diagnosis of acute leukemia carried an implication of very short-term survival, whereas patients with chronic leukemia could survive for a little while longer.

The next contribution to the description of the leukemias was provided by Ehrlich in Germany, who developed methods for staining blood cells in 1891.[15] This revealed immediately the differences in morphology between granulocytes and lymphocytes, a distinction that had previously been based only on microscopic examination of unstained granular and agranular cells with different nuclear shapes. Although these early studies provided the foundation for the morphological classification of the myeloid and lymphoid leukemias, they did not permit the discrimination of T cells and B cells. This information was not available until the 1960s.

Table 1–1. Milestones in the History of Chronic Leukemia

1845	Recognition of leukemia as a disease entity (probably CML)
1846	First diagnosis of leukemia in a live patient
1865	First therapy of CML: Fowler's solution
1891	Development of methods for staining blood cells
1895	Discovery of X-irradiation
1924	Recognition of CLL as a distinct clinical entity
1934	Malignant nature of leukemia established experimentally
1946	First effective chemotherapy for leukemia—nitrogen mustard
1960	Identification of the Philadelphia chromosome (22q⁻)
1966	Realization that CLL is a disease of cell accumulation
1966	Introduction of leukapheresis in the treatment of CML
1973	Recognition of the reciprocal nature of the (9;22) translocation
1978	Introduction of autografting for CML
1982	First routine use of allografting for CML
1984	First description of the BCR gene in CML
1990	Demonstration that the *BCR-ABL* gene could cause a CML-like disease in mice.
1999	Introduction of the ABL tyrosine kinase inhibitor into clinical practice as treatment for CML

Abbreviations: CML, chronic myeloid leukemia; CLL, chronic lymphocytic leukemia.

The first person to appreciate the role of the bone marrow may possibly have been William Shakespeare, when he wrote "Thy bone is marrowless, thy blood is cold." In 1878 Neumann realized that the leukemias originated in the bone marrow[16] and added myelogenous leukemias to the splenic and lymphatic leukemias described by Virchow. Ehrlich[15] identified a primitive cell type that he thought was ancestral to the lymphoid and myeloid cell lineages, and thereby probably made the first reference to the concept of a hemopoietic stem cell. The view that there are distinct hemopoietic cell lineages was later supported by Naegeli in 1900,[17] when he distinguished between myeloblasts and lymphoblasts.

During the late nineteenth and early twentieth centuries, many new terms were conjured up to describe a variety of leukemias, and there was some confusion over the relationship between different types of lymphoid neoplasm. However, Turk in 1903 recognized that there was a close connection between lymphoid leukemias and lymphomas (lymphosarcomata) and grouped together the chronic and acute leukemias and the lymphomas as the "lymphomatoses,"[18] a term that is roughly equivalent in meaning to the modern "lymphoproliferative disorders." Until the 1930s, however, there was controversy about the relationship between leukemia in particular and cancer in general. The malignant nature of the leukemias was only established when the disease was induced in rodents by the intramedullary injection of tar and other chemical carcinogens.[19,20] Descriptions of leukemic cells increased in sophistication with the development of special stains and phenotypic markers. The development of these tools led to the detailed definition of the chronic myeloid and lymphoid leukemias and to the description of the various types of transformation or "blast crisis" that ensue in CML. Nevertheless, the divisions made early on between myeloid and lymphoid and between chronic and acute leukemias were remarkably similar then to those used today.

The study of cytogenetics developed during the 1950s, and in 1956 the number of human chromosomes in each normal cell was established as 46. The discovery of the Philadelphia (Ph) chromosome in 1960 by Nowell and Hungerford[21] provided a marker that proved to be pathognomonic for the disease and heralded a new era. With this marker, it was possible to demonstrate that CML is a clonal disorder originating in a hemopoietic stem cell. Moreover, the development of clonogenic assays for hemopoietic progenitor cells in the 1970s enabled Fialkow and colleagues[22] to demonstrate the clonal origin of leukemic progenitor cells from different lineages by study of individuals who were heterozygous for the isoenzymes of glucose-6-phosphate dehydrogenase (G6PD).

During the 1970s much attention was paid to the kinetics of leukemic cells, and it was generally concluded that the proliferating granulocytic compartment divides less actively in CML bone marrow than in normal bone marrow. A variety of indices were established to describe granulopoiesis in CML, and the likelihood that there was an element of residual regulation of granulopoiesis became appreciated.[23,24]

De Klein et al.[25] found that the Ph translocation involved the movement of the normal human counterpart of the murine *v-abl* oncogene from chromosome 9 to chromosome 22, and one year later the reciprocal translocation of genetic material from chromosome 22 to chromosome 9 was identified.[26] The translocation results in the formation of a fusion gene, *BCR/ABL,* on chromosome 22. Because of variability in the breakpoints in the *BCR* gene and the relative constancy of the ABL breakpoint, exon 2 of the *ABL* gene can be linked upstream to exon 2 of BCR (b2a2 junction) or to exon 3 of BCR (b3a2 junction). Both rearrangements result in the production of hybrid messenger RNA and a hybrid BCR/ABL p210 protein tyrosine kinase.[27] With today's molecular technology, it is possible to detect very small numbers of cells expressing the *BCR/ABL* gene using the polymerase chain reaction (PCR),[28] and this has obvious implications for the monitoring of disease and the management of patients. However, the biological effects of p210 expression in CML remain an enigma and a major challenge to cell and molecular biologists.

Chronic lymphocytic leukemia is an acquired B-cell disorder whose clonal origin can now be demonstrated by detecting unique rearrangements of immunoglobulin genes by Southern blot hybridization. The recognition of CLL as a distinct clinical entity can be dated back to the turn of the century. Several authors provided case reports and clinical data that distinguished CLL from lymphoma. Osler in his text *The Principles and Practice of Medicine*[29] recounted his experience of the disease at the Johns Hopkins Hospital in Baltimore, where CLL accounted for 22 percent of all leukemias and survival times of 3 to 11 years were noted. In 1924, Minot and Isaacs[30] published the first comprehensive clinical report on a series of 80 patients, which according to one author,[31] marked the formal emergence of CLL as a distinct and well described clinical entity.

There followed 50 years of definition and clinical description of CLL, which assisted clinical hematologists in their diagnosis, understanding, and treatment of the disease. Some of the most important contributions of this era were made by Galton in 1966[32] and Dameshek in 1967,[33] who realized that CLL is a disease of cell accumulation as a result of a reduced cell death rate, rather than a proliferative disease.[34] This reduction in cell death rate is thought to be due to suppression of apoptotic mechanisms[35] and may be associated with dysfunction of the p53 gene. The tumor suppressor gene BCL-2 also is known to inhibit apoptosis, and small lymphocytic malignancies, including CLL, express moderately high levels of the corresponding bcl-2 protein.[36]

It was not until 1972 that the presence of immunoglobulins on the surface of CLL cells was first demonstrated, thus confirming CLL as a disease of B lymphocytes.[37,38] Thereafter the development of methods for detailed immunological phenotyping led to an accurate description of the phenotype of CLL cells, which are arrested at an intermediate stage of B-cell differentiation.[39,40] Cytogenetic studies revealed that there is no "marker" abnormality in CLL equivalent to the Ph chromosome in CML, but several structural chromosome abnormalities occur consistently in varying proportions of cases. It is now widely recognized that there is an inverse correlation between the extent of chromosome abnormalities and survival in CLL.[31]

The precise etiology of CLL remains uncertain but studies identifying a tendency for CLL to occur in families suggest that there is a genetic disposition, which is expressed only under certain environmental conditions but which is not associated with any discernible pattern of inheritance.[41] It is interesting to note parenthetically that CLL, although relatively common in the Western world, is rare in the Orient.

TREATMENT

Chronic Myeloid Leukemia

Fowler's solution, a 1 percent solution of arsenic trioxide, was probably the first agent to show any beneficial effect in the treatment of CML.[42] It had been introduced in 1786 as a general tonic for people and their animals and had been noted for its beneficial effect on the general health of horses. Lissauer's patient apparently was moribund before receiving Fowler's solution but subsequently became well and remained so for some months.[42] Arsenic was used in the treatment of CML for some 30 years, and appropriate doses were found to control fever, reduce the white cell count, reduce the size of the spleen, relieve pruritis, and considerably improve anemia.[43]

Roentgen's discovery of X-rays in 1895 led to their enthusiastic use in the treatment of leukemias and lymphomas. Direction of X-rays against large spleens in CML resulted in a reduction in splenomegaly, with associated improvements in the blood picture and the patient's general state of health.[44,45] It was recommended at this stage that arsenic should not be given concurrently with X-irradiation but could be used as intermittent therapy.

Remissions induced by X-ray therapy of chronic leukemias were often complete, and although relapse inevitably occurred and life was not prolonged, the patient's quality of life was improved.[46,47] Internal irradiation with radioactive phosphorus also brought about satisfactory clinical and hematological remissions[48] but was not as effective as external X-rays in reducing organomegaly.[49] It soon became apparent that X-irradiation was toxic to normal cells as well as to leukemic cells and that fibrosis could be induced by overtreatment. More optimistically, it was realized that sublethal doses of X-irradiation resulted in reversible marrow hypocellularity, with a return to normal counts within a few weeks.

With the advent of cytotoxic drugs, the role of ionizing radiation in the treatment of CML diminished in the 1960s, before which time it had been the treatment of choice. It became restricted to the treatment of splenomegaly in patients with special features, such as women who are pregnant at the time of diagnosis.[50] The major place for ionizing radiation in the modern treatment of CML consists of myeloablation and immunosuppression prior to autologous or allogeneic transplantation.

The role of surgery in the management of CML is also limited. At one time it was suggested as treatment for distressing priapism.[51] The first splenectomy was carried out in 1866 with fatal results — the patient died as a result of postoperative hemorrhage.[52] Later attempts at splenectomy were also complicated by high rates of mortality, and this situation persisted at least until 1966.[53] Today, the mortality of the procedure in CML is much lower, but the indications for splenectomy remain controversial.

Modern chemotherapy had its origins in secret research on agents for use in chemical warfare. Thus, the first chemotherapeutic agent to be used in the treatment of leukemia was mustard gas or nitrogen mustard (HN2). The fact that it caused profound myelosuppression provided the rationale for its use in the treatment of leukemia.[54,55] Importantly, it was found that patients who were or who became resistant to X-ray therapy could still respond to nitrogen mustard. Blood transfusion was performed without success in the 19th century[56] and did not become a safe procedure until after the discovery of the human blood groups by Landsteiner in 1900. Antibiotics other than the sulfonamides were not available until the late 1940s, and bone marrow examination became more widespread around this time. Consequently, more patients with nonspecific febrile disorders survived, and the number of cases diagnosed as leukemia increased rapidly.

The early experience with chemotherapy led to a search for new agents with increased specificity and lower toxicity. Urethane was used in the treatment of CML and in the maintenance of X-ray-induced remission in the 1940s,[57] but by 1953 busulfan had been introduced[58,59] and rapidly became the treatment of choice for CML. Dibromomannitol, first investigated in 1961,[60] became an alternative for patients in chronic phase who ceased to respond to busulfan. Hydroxyurea was first used in the 1960s and replaced busulfan as the first-line cytotoxic drug for newly diagnosed patients. Hydroxyurea was succeeded by interferon alpha.[61,62] The latest development in the systemic treatment of CML has been contributed by the results obtained from treating patients with imatinib mesylate (previously STI571), a selective inhibitor of ABL tyrosine kinases, which is currently in clinical trials.[63]

The feasibility of leukapheresis as a method of tumor debulking in CML was established in the 1960s and was dependent on the development of continuous-flow blood cell separators.[64,65] Today, there is probably little benefit in the long-term repeated leukapheresis of patients with CML, but the procedure is valuable for producing a rapid initial reduction in the white cell count and as a means for collecting large numbers of cells for use in autografting (see below).

Conventional doses of chemotherapy did not produce substantial increases in patient survival or delay the onset of acute transformation. Buckner et al.[66] and Goldman et al.[67] developed the concept that chronic-phase cells could be harvested at diagnosis, cryopreserved and stored in liquid nitrogen, and used as an autograft when the patient began to show signs of transformation. This was based on the hope that infusion of cells harvested at diagnosis would reinstate chronic-phase hemopoiesis for a period equivalent to the length of the first chronic phase. The Hammersmith experience of autografting chronic-phase CML patients with unmanipulated peripheral blood cells was updated in 1994 by Hoyle et al.[68] This report summarizes a nonrandomized study but does indicate that blood cell autografting may prolong life for many patients and may be the treatment of choice for younger patients who do not have a suitable donor for allogeneic transplantation. It may be possible further to improve the results of peripheral blood autografting by using the strategy first reported by Carella et al.[69,70] who demonstrated that recovery from chemotherapy was associated with the preferential release of Ph-negative, presumably normal, cells into the bloodstream and that these cells could be collected in sufficient numbers for reinfusion into the patient at a later date. In the light of the knowledge that normal stem cells coexist with leukemic stem cells in the marrow of CML patients and that CML stem cells survive poorly in culture, Barnett et al.[71] cultured patient's marrow in vitro prior to autografting in the hope that the normal cells would become relatively enriched. Other potential approaches to purging marrow for autografting include the use of antisense reagents designed to suppress the expression of p210 protein tyrosine kinase.[72]

At present, allogeneic transplantation is the only curative treatment for CML. According to Piller,[5] administration of bone marrow to patients was first advocated by Thomas Fraser in 1894,[73] who recommended that they eat bone marrow in sandwiches or in glycerine flavored with port wine to improve the taste, but it is likely that sporadic attempts at bone marrow transplantation were made earlier. It was not until the understanding of human histocompatibility systems developed further and tissue matching became feasible that allogeneic bone marrow transplantation became a practical option for the treatment of any hematological or nonhematological disease. In this regard, the use of T-cell depletion as a means of reducing graft-versus-host disease (GvHD) confirmed that allogeneic T cells also have graft-versus-leukemia (GvL) activity.[74] This has renewed enthusiasm for the immunotherapy of CML, which is manifest in the use of donor lymphocyte infusion[75] and in efforts to raise cytotoxic T-cell clones restricted to killing cells expressing particular leukemia-associated antigens.[76]

Chronic Lymphocytic Leukemia

The early histories of treating CML and CLL have much in common owing to the limited therapy available and the inability to distinguish the diseases with any degree of accuracy. In the 1940s and 1950s, Osgood[77–79] tested the hypothesis that whole-body external irradiation or administration of radioactive phosphorus could be used in a titratable manner to control the leukocyte count at a level below 30×10^9/L. He claimed that this strategy was effective in patients with slowly progressing disease and that it could increase the chance of survival to 20 years. However, his results were not confirmed in later randomized trials comparing irradiation with chlorambucil and other alkylating agents.[80,81]

Progress in the clinical management of patients with CLL has relied on improved understanding of the different types of disease and improved prognosis. In the past, diseases diagnosed as CLL would have included a mixture of T- and B-cell leukemias, hairy-cell leukemia, and a variety of other conditions associated with lymphocytosis. In contrast, the cells can now be identified accurately by cellular morphology, immunophenotype, and other features,[82] so that subtypes of disease can be grouped together and clinical trials can be designed. In the future, expression profiling may allow further subgrouping of CLL, as it has done for non-Hodgkin's lymphoma.

It has been recognized for many years that cases of CLL have variable clinical courses.[33] This wide range in survival times for patients with CLL, from a few years to more than a decade, made therapeutic decisions difficult, particularly because some patients remained well even if they were not treated. This led to the development of staging systems, based on prognostic indicators and other criteria, to facilitate the choice of therapy for individual patients. The long list of prognostic indicators in CLL now includes age, sex, lymphocyte doubling time, cell morphology, bone marrow involvement, immunophenotype, and cytogenetic abnormalities.[82]

Long-term low-dose treatment with chlorambucil has been a mainstay of CLL therapy and regulates the size of the malignant B-cell clone without major fluctuations in the blood count. The slowly progressing nature of the disease and its occurrence in the elderly has meant that experimental approaches to improve disease control and attempt to achieve a cure are attempted only in the rare cases of patients less than 50 years old or those with progressive disease who become cytopenic.

Progress has been due to several large studies[83–85] and to the introduction of more specific drugs. It is now clear that treatment of stage 0 nonprogressing disease is not indicated and can be harmful. Patients who are resistant to chlorambucil may benefit from the cyclophosphamide-doxorubicin-vincristine-prednisone (CHOP) drug regimen, and fludarabine and 2'-deoxycoformycin seem to have better selectivity of action than other drugs.[86,87] Fludarabine has become acceptable as first-line therapy for symptomatic untreated CLL patients following the results of phase III trials.[88] Monoclonal antibodies such as Campath 1-H (anti-CD52) and rituximab (a chimeric IDEC-CD2B8 monoclonal antibody, which binds to CD20 expressed on B lymphocytes) have also been used to treat CLL.[88–90] Bone marrow transplantation can be curative,[91] but most patients are above the upper age limit for this procedure. However, research is now being carried out into nonmyeloablative conditioning regimens for transplantation, although evidence of efficacy remains confined to small series or case reports.

ACKNOWLEDGMENT

We thank Dr. Amin Rahemtulla for his advice during the preparation of this manuscript.

REFERENCES

1. Piller GJ: John Hughes Bennett: His life and identification of leukaemia. Proc R Coll Physicians Edinb, 1997.
2. Geary CG: The story of chronic myeloid leukaemia. Br J Haematol 110:2, 2000.
3. Gunz FW, Henderson ED: Leukemia, 4th Ed. Grune & Stratton, New York, 1983.
4. Velpeau A: Sur la resorption du puseat sur l'altération du sang dans les maladies clinique de persection nenemant. Premier observation. Rev Med 2:216, 1827.
5. Piller G: The history of leukemia: A personal perspective. Blood Cells 19:521, 1993.
6. Donne A: De l'origine des globules du sang, de leur mode de formation, de leur fin. C R Acad Sci 14:366, 1842.
7. Craigie D: Case of disease of the spleen in which death took place consequent on the presence of purulent matter in the blood. Edinb Med Surg J 64:400, 1845.

8. Bennett JH: Case of hypertrophy of the spleen and liver in which death took place from suppuration of the blood. Edinb Med Surg J 64:413, 1845.

9. Virchow R: Weisses Blut und Milztumoren. Med Z 15:157, 1846.

10. Fuller H: Particulars of a case in which enormous enlargement of the spleen and liver, together with dilatation of all vessels in the body were found coincident with a peculiarly altered condition of the blood. Lancet ii:43, 1846.

11. Wood GB: Trans Coll Physicians Philadelphia p. 265. 1850–52.

12. Virchow R: Zur pathologischen Physiologie des Bluts: Die Bedeutung der milz- und Lymph-Drusen-Krankheiten fur die Blutmischung (Leukaemia). Virchows Arch 5:43, 1853.

13. Neumann E: Ein Fall von Leukamie mit Erkrankung des Knochenmarkes. Arch Heilk 11:1, 1870.

14. Ebstein W: Ueber die acute Leukamie und Pseudoleukamie. Deut Arch Klin Med 44:343, 1889.

15. Ehrlich P: Parbenanalytische Untersuchungen zur Histologie und Klinik des Blutes. Hirschwald, Berlin, 1891.

16. Neumann E: Uber myelogene Leukamie. Berliner Klin Wochenschr 15:69, 1878.

17. Naegeli O: Uber rothes Knochenmark und Myeloblasten. Deut Med Wochenschr 18:287, 1900.

18. Turk W: Ein System der Lymphomatosen. Wien Klin Wochenschr 16:1073, 1903.

19. Bernard J: L'erythro-leucemie experimentale provoquée par les injections intramedullaires du goudron. Sang 8:28, 1934.

20. Storti E: Modifications morphologiques du sang et des organes hematopoietiques provoquées chez le rat blanc par injections intramedullaires de 1–2 benzopyrene. Sang 11:7, 1937.

21. Nowell PC, Hungerford DA: A minute chromosome in human granulocytic leukemia. Science 132:1497, 1960.

22. Fialkow PJ, Martin PJ, Najfeld V, Penfold GK, Jacobson RJ, Hansen JA: Evidence for a multistep pathogenesis of chronic myelogenous leukemia. Blood 58:159, 1981.

23. Stryckmans PA, Debusscher L, Collard E: Cell kinetics in chronic granulocytic leukaemia (CGL). Clin Haematol 6:21, 1977.

24. Pederson B: Kinetics and cell function. In Shaw MT (ed.): Chronic Granulocytic Leukaemia, p. 93. Praeger, Eastbourne UK, 1982.

25. De Klein A, van Kessel A, Grosveld G, Bartram CR, Hagemeijer A, Bootsma D, Spurr NK, Heisterkamp N, Groffen J, Stephenson JR: A cellular oncogene is translocated to the Philadelphia chromosome in chronic myelocytic leukaemia. Nature 300:765, 1982.

26. Groffen J, Heisterkamp N, Stephenson JR, van Kessel A, de Klein A, Grosveld G, Bootsma D: c-sis is translocated from chromosome 22 to chromosome 9 in chronic myelocytic leukemia. J Exp Med 158:9, 1983.

27. Ben-Neriah Y, Daley GQ, Mes-Masson A-M, Witte ON, Baltimore D: The chronic myelogenous leukemia specific p210 protein is the product of the bcr/abl hybrid gene. Science 223:212, 1986.

28. Lee M-S, Stass SA: Detection of chimeric bcr-abl mRNA and minimal residual disease by polymerase chain reaction. Hematology 13:241, 1991.

29. Osler W: Leukaemia. In The Principles and Practice of Medicine, 7th ed, p. 731. D. Appleton, New York, 1909.

30. Minot B, Isaacs R: Lymphatic leukemia: Age, incidence, duration and benefit derived from irradiation. Boston Med Surg J 191:1, 1924.

31. Rai KR: Progress in chronic lymphocytic leukaemia: A historical perspective. Baillieres Clin Haematol 6:757, 1993.

32. Galton DAG: The pathogenesis of chronic lymphocytic leukaemia. Can Med Assoc J 94:1005, 1966.

33. Dameshek W: Chronic lymphocytic leukemia — an accumulative disease of immunologically incompetent lymphocytes. Blood 29:566, 1967.

34. Dormer P, Theml H, Lau B: Chronic lymphocytic leukaemia: A proliferative or accumulative disorder? Leuk Res 7:1, 1983.

35. Hockenberry DM, Oltvai ZN, Yin X-M, Milliman CC, Korsmeyer SJ: Bcl-2 functions in an antioxidant pathway to prevent apoptosis. Cell 75:241, 1993f.

36. Zutter M, Hockenburg D, Silverman KA, Korsemeyer SJ: Immunolocalisation of the Bcl-2 protein within hematopoietic neoplasms. Blood 78:1062, 1991.

37. Aisenberg AC, Bloch KJ: Immunoglobulins on the surface of neoplastic lymphocytes. N Engl J Med 287:272, 1972.

38. Preud'homme JL, Seligmann M: Surface bound immunoglobulins as a cell marker in human lymphoproliferative disease. Blood 40:777, 1972.

39. Giesler CH, Larsen JK, Hansen NE, Hansen MM, Christensen BE, Lund B, Nielson H, Plesner T, Thorling K, Andersen E, Andersen PK: Prognostic importance of flow cytometric immunophenotyping of 540 consecutive patients with B-cell chronic lymphocytic leukemia. Blood 78:1795, 1991.

40. Freedman AS, Nadler LM: Immunological markers in B-cell chronic lymphocytic leukemia. In Cheson B (ed.): Chronic Lymphocytic Leukemia: Scientific Advances and Clinical Developments, p. 1. Marcel Dekker, New York, 1993.

41. Sweet DL, Golomb HM, Ultman JE: The clinical features of chronic lymphocytic leukaemia. Clin Haematol 6:185, 1977.

42. Lissauer H: Zwei Falle von Leukaemie. Berl Klin Wochenschr 2:403, 1865.

43. Forkner CE: Leukaemia and Allied Disorders, 1st ed. Macmillan, New York, 1938.

44. Pusey WA: Report of cases treated with Roentgen rays. JAMA 38:911, 1902.

45. Senn N: Case of splenomedullary leukaemia successfully treated by the use of Roentgen ray. Med Rec (N Y) 64:281, 1903.

46. Minot GR, Buckman TE, Isaacs R: Chronic myelogenous leukaemia: Age incidence, duration and benefit derived from irradiation. JAMA 82:1489, 1924.

47. Hoffman WJ, Carver LF: Chronic myelogenous leukaemia: Value of irradiation and its effect on duration of life. JAMA 97:836, 1931.

48. Lawrence JH, Scott KG, Tuttle WL: Studies on leukaemia with the aid of radioactive phosphorus. Int Clin 3:33, 1939.

49. Reinhard EH, Moore CV, Bierbaum OS, Moore S: Radioactive phosphorus as a therapeutic agent. A review of the literature and analysis of the results of treatment of 155 patients with various blood dyscrasias, lymphomas and other malignant neoplastic diseases. J Lab Clin Med 31:107, 1946.

50. Richards HGH, Spiers ASD: Chronic granulocytic leukaemia in pregnancy. B J Radiol 48:261, 1975.

51. Whitby LEH, Britton CJC: Disorders of the Blood: Diagnosis, Pathology, Treatment, Technique, 6th ed. J and A Churchill Ltd., London, 1950.

52. Bryant T: Case of excision of the spleen for enlargement of the organ, attended with leukocythaemia. Guy's Hosp Rep 12:444, 1866.

53. Wolf JD, Silver RT, Coleman M: Splenectomy in chronic myeloid leukemia. Ann Intern Med 89:684, 1978.

54. Jacobson LO, Spurr CL, Barron ESG, Lushbaugh C, Dick GF: Nitrogen mustard therapy. JAMA 132:263, 1946.

55. Goodman LS, Wintrobe MM, Dameshek W, Goodman MJ, Gilman A, McLennan MT: Nitrogen mustard therapy. JAMA 132:126, 1946.

56. Editorial: Transfusion of blood in leukaemia. Br Med J 1:593 and 2:16, 1873.

57. Dameshek W, Gunz F: Leukemia, 2nd ed. Grune & Stratton, New York, 1964.

58. Galton DAG: Myleran in chronic myeloid leukaemia. Lancet i:208, 1953.

59. Haddow A, Timmis GM: Myleran in chronic myeloid leukaemia: Chemical composition and biological function. Lancet i:207, 1953.

60. Institorisz L, Horvath IP, Csanyi E: Study on the distribution and metabolism of ^{82}Br-labelled dibromomannitol in normal and tumour bearing rats. Neoplasma 11:245, 1964.

61. Talpaz M, McCredie KB, Malvigit GM, Gutterman JU: Leukocyte interferon-induced myeloid cytoreduction in chronic myelogenous leukaemia. BMJ 1:201, 1983.

62. Ozer H: Biotherapy of chronic myelogenous leukemia with interferon. Semin Oncol 16:14, 1988.

63. Druker BJ, Tamura S, Buchdunger E et al: Effects of a selective inhibitor of the Abl tyrosine kinase on the growth of bcr-positive cells. Nat Med 2:574, 1996.

64. Morse EE, Carbone PP, Frieriech EJ, Bronson W, Kliman A: Repeated leukapheresis of patients with chronic myelocytic leukemia. Transfusion 6:175, 1966.

65. Buckner CD, Graw RG, Risel RJ, Henderson ES, Perry S: Leukapheresis by continuous flow centrifugation (CFC) in patients with chronic myelocytic leukemia (CML). Blood 33:353, 1969.

66. Buckner CD, Stewart P, Clift RA, Fefer A, Neiman PE, Singer J, Storb R, Thomas ED: Treatment of blastic transformation of chronic granulocytic leukemia by chemotherapy, total body irradiation and infusion of cryopreserved autologous marrow. Exp Hematol 6:96, 1978.

67. Goldman JM, Catovsky D, Hows J, Spiers ASD, Galton DAG: Cryopreserved peripheral blood cells functioning as autografts in patients with chronic granulocytic leukaemia. BMJ i:1310, 1979.

68. Hoyle C, Gray R, Goldman JM: Autografting for patients with CML in chronic phase: An update. Br J Haematol 86:76, 1994.

69. Carella AM, Pollicardo N, Pungolino E, Raffo MR, Podesta M, Ferrero R, Pierluigi D, Nati S, Congui A: Mobilization of cytogenetically normal blood progenitors by intensive chemotherapy for chronic myeloid and acute lymphoblastic leukemia. Leuk Lymphoma 9:477, 1993.

70. Carella AM, Podesta M, Frassoni F, Raffo MR, Pollicardo N, Pungolini E, Vimercati R, Sessarego M, Parodi C, Rabitti C, Ferrero R, Benvenuto F, Figaro O, Carlier P, Lavcasic G, Valbonesi M, Vitale V, Giordano D, Pierluigi D, Nati S, Guerracio A, Rosso C, Saglio G: Collection of normal blood repopulating cells during early hemopoietic recovery after intensive conventional chemotherapy in chronic myelogenous leukemia. Bone Marrow Transplant 12:267, 1993.

71. Barnett MJ, Eaves CJ, Phillips GL, Gascoigne RD, Hogge DE, Horseman DE, Humphries RK, Klingeman HG, Lansdorp PM, Nantel SH, Reece DE, Shepherd JD, Spinelli JJ, Sutherland HJ, Eaves AC: Autografting with cultured marrow in chronic myeloid leukemia: Results of a pilot study. Blood 84:724, 1994.

72. Kirkland MA, O'Brien SG, Goldman JM: Antisense therapeutics in haematological malignancies. Br J Haematol 87:447, 1994.

73. Fraser TR: Bone marrow in the treatment of pernicious anaemia. BMJ 1:1172, 1984.

74. Apperley JF, Mauro FR, Goldman JM, Gregory W, Arthur CK, Hows J, Arcese W, Papa G, Mandelli F, Wardle D, Gravett P, Franklin IM, Bandini G, Ricci P, Tura S, Iacone A, Torlontano G, Heit W, Champlin R, Gale RP: Bone marrow transplantation for chronic myeloid leukaemia in first chronic phase: Importance of graft-versus-leukaemia effect. Br J Haematol 69:239, 1988.

75. Mackinnon S: Donor leukocyte infusions. Baillieres Clin Haematol 10:357, 1997.

76. Gao L, Ballantuono I, Elsasser A, Marley SB, Gordon MY, Goldman JM, Stauss HJ: Selective elimination of CD34+ progenitor cells by cytotoxic T lymphocytes specific for WT1. Blood 95:2198, 2000.

77. Osgood EE: Titrated, regularly spaced radioactive phosphorus or spray roentgen therapy of leukemias. Arch Intern Med 87:329, 1951.

78. Osgood EE, Koler RD: The results of the 15-year program of treatment of chronic leukemias with titrated regularly spaced total-body irradiation with phosphorus 32 or X-ray. Proceedings of the Sixth International Congress of the International Society of Hematology (Boston, 1956) p. 44, 1958.

79. Osgood EE: Treatment of chronic leukemias. J Nucl Med 5:139, 1964.

80. Huguley CM: Long-term study of chronic lymphocytic leukemia: Interim report after 45 months. Cancer Chemother Rep 16:241, 1962.

81. Rubin P, Bennett JM, Begg C, Bozdech MJ, Silber R: The comparison of total body irradiation vs chlorambucil and prednisone for remission induction of active chronic lymphocytic leukaemia: An ECOG study. Part 1: Total body irradiation. Response and toxicity. Int J Radiat Oncol Biol Phys 7:1623, 1981.

82. Zweibel JA, Cheson BD: Chronic lymphocytic leukemia: Staging and prognostic factors. Semin Oncol 25:42, 1998.

83. French Co-operative Group on Chronic Lymphocytic Leukaemia: Effectiveness of 'CHOP' regimen in advanced untreated chronic lymphocytic leukaemia. Lancet 1:1346, 1988.

84. French Co-operative Group on Chronic Lymphocytic Leukemia: Effects of chlorambucil and initial treatment decision in initial forms of chronic lymphocytic leukemia (stage A): Results of a randomised clinical trial on 612 patients. Blood 75:1414, 1990.

85. Catovsky D, Fooks J, Richards S: Prognostic factors in chronic lymphocytic leukemia: The importance of age, sex and response to treatment in survival. Br J Haematol 72:141, 1989.

86. Keating MJ, Kantarjian H, Talpaz M, Redman J, Koller C, Barlogie B, Velasquez W, Plunkett W, Friereich EJ, McCredie KB: Fludarabine: A new agent with major activity against chronic lymphocytic leukemia. Blood 74:19, 1989.

87. Smyth JF, Prentice HG, Proctor S, Hoffbrand AV: Deoxycoformycin in the treatment of leukemias and lymphomas. Ann N Y Acad Sci 451:123, 1985.

88. Byrd JC, Rai KR, Sausville EA, Grever MA: Old and new therapies in chronic lymphocytic leukemia: Now is the time for reassessment of therapeutic goals. Semin Oncol 25:65, 1998.

89. Osterborg A, Dyer MJS, Bunjes D, Pangalis GA, Bastion Y, Catovsky D, Mellstedt H: Phase II multicenter study of human CD52 antibody in previously treated chronic lymphocytic leukemia. European Study Group of CAMPATH-1H Treatment in Chronic Lymphocytic Leukemia. J Clin Oncol 15:1567, 1997.

90. Winkler U, Jensen M, Manzke O, Schultz H, Diehl V, Engert A: Cytokine-release syndrome in patients with B cell chronic lymphocytic leukemia with high lymphocyte counts after treatment with anti-CD20 monoclonal antibody (Rituximab, IDEC-CD2B8). Blood 94:2217, 1999.

91. Michallet M, Corront B, Molina L et al: Allogeneic bone marrow transplantation in chronic lymphocytic leukemia: 17 cases. Report of the EBMT. Leuk Lymphoma 5(Suppl. 1):127, 1991.

2

Epidemiology of the Chronic Leukemias

Ray Cartwright

CHRONIC LYMPHOCYTIC LEUKEMIA

The epidemiology of chronic lymphocytic leukemia (CLL) is hampered by two features of the condition. First, it is often found as a chance diagnosis and this in turn can be a reflection of medical care in a particular area, rather than a true representation of the totality of the disease. Second, in both descriptive and analytic epidemiological studies little attention is given to the quality of diagnostic definitions. Most epidemiological studies do not attempt to distinguish B-cell disease and most will include prolymphocytic leukemias and possibly lymphocytic lymphomas as part of what they term "CLL."

There have been no large-scale comprehensive and diagnostically sound epidemiological studies of CLL published in the past decade.

Descriptive Epidemiology

Table 2–1 gives comparable age-standardized incidence rates from cancer registries covering registration periods around 1990.[1] Even bearing in mind the caveats in the introduction, it seems clear that the condition is roughly twice as common in men and that rates vary considerably throughout the world.

The only reported exception to the male preponderance is from West Africa, where CLL in women aged 35 to 50 appears to be more common and that may be, in fact, prolymphocytic leukemia (PLL).[2]

The highest rates of CLL occur in Europe and in European populations in North America and Australasia. Lower rates occur in Polynesia, sub-Saharan Africa, and South and East Asia. The lowest recorded rates come from Japan. The Japanese data are likely to be accurate, being based on sound recording protocols. This 30-fold variation in national rates has led to many investigations as to the genetic basis of risk (see later).

Table 2–2 gives the typical European age and sex profile.[3] The number of cases under the age of 30 is very low (and unreliable) whereas there is an 80-fold increase in males in incidence from the 30 to 34 year age group to the 75 to 79 year age group. The equivalent change in Japan is roughly sixfold, with the rates for the 30 to 34 year age band being similar between Asia and Europe but a smaller rise with age occurs in Japan compared with the massive increase in Europe.

Some African populations have a slight age-specific peak in the middle years (35 to 50), possibly due to the PLL cases noted above.[2]

The concept of a genetic basis of risk is reinforced by the observation that Japanese migrants to the United States and their descendants retain low rates.[4] Studies of CLL subtypes in Japan suggest relatively few have the "typical" disease (with 90 percent small lymphocytes), only 7 in a series of 41, the rest being a variety of conditions, particularly large and prolymphocytic cell types.[5]

There is some evidence that CLL declined in incidence in the United States in both White and Black populations[6] between 1973 and 1990. The decline is modest and may reflect diagnostic changes rather than any fundamental change. A similar study in the United Kingdom shows very little change in incidence from 1984 to 1989.[7]

CLL has not shown any evidence of close case aggregation or clustering,[8] but some evidence of heterogeneity of geographic distribution was uncovered in a study of U.K. cases from 1984 to 1988.[3] This observation may well reflect the difficulties in achieving a uniform standard of case ascertainment even in developed countries.

Analytic Epidemiology

Studies have concentrated on genetic and immune dysfunctional aspects of risk, with some attention given to lifestyles and occupations as other possible causes. However, in certain ways the most remarkable issues surrounding CLL concern the lack of

Table 2–1. Age-Standardized World Incidence Rates of Chronic Lymphocytic Leukemia (CLL) and Chronic Myeloid Leukemia (CML)[a]

Country	CLL		CML	
	Male	Female	Male	Female
Harare, Zimbabwe, Africa	(1.7)	(1.3)	1.5	(1.3)
Cali, Colombia	0.5	(0.2)	0.8	0.8
Canada	3.7	1.8	1.4	0.8
U.S. SEER Whites	3.4	1.6	1.4	0.9
U.S. SEER Blacks	2.7	1.6	1.6	1.0
Shanghai, China	0.2	0.1	0.7	0.4
Bombay, India	0.6	0.3	0.9	0.6
Osaka, Japan	0.1	0.0	0.9	0.4
Israel Jews	2.1	1.1	0.8	0.5
Denmark	3.4	1.5	1.1	0.6
Turin, Italy	2.2	0.9	1.5	0.6
The Netherlands	2.2	1.0	0.9	0.5
Tarragona, Spain	2.4	0.9	1.1	0.7
England and Wales, U.K.	2.3	1.1	1.1	0.7
New South Wales, Australia	2.8	1.4	1.7	0.8
Non-Maori, New Zealand	3.0	1.5	1.4	0.9
Maori, New Zealand	(1.6)	(0.8)	2.2	(0.7)

[a] Cases per 100,000 per year.
Note: Results in parentheses are based on small numbers.
(From Parkin et al.[1])

Table 2–2. Chronic Lymphocytic Leukemia (CLL) and Chronic Myeloid Leukemia (CML): Age-Specific Incidence Rates[a]

Age Band	CLL Male	CLL Female	CML Male	CML Female
0–4	0	0.04	0.29	0.09
5–9	0	0.04	0.04	0.13
10–14	0.12	0	0.08	0
15–19	0.07	0.03	0.16	0.21
20–24	0.10	0.10	0.57	0.10
25–29	0.14	0.18	0.60	0.22
30–34	0.51	0.28	0.66	0.56
35–39	0.64	0.39	0.60	0.43
40–44	2.18	0.37	1.17	0.86
45–49	3.32	2.41	0.97	0.93
50–54	6.46	3.79	1.72	1.42
55–59	9.91	5.02	1.75	1.46
60–64	17.67	7.82	2.37	1.92
65–69	20.75	12.58	2.31	1.91
70–74	27.0	14.80	3.4	1.56
75–79	41.09	18.92	4.69	1.87
Total case numbers	2040	1300	387	291

[a] Cases per 100,000 per year. 1984–1989, parts of U.K. Based on special registration collections.
(From Cartwright et al.[3])

clear associations with exposures that commonly cause many other different types of cancer. These include exposures to ionizing irradiation, for example, from the Life Span Study of Japanese A-bomb survivors[9] and from radiotherapy survivor cohorts.[10,11] Also, but slightly less clearly, there is little support for an association between cigarette smoking and CLL. Some case control studies report a risk[12] and others do not;[13] likewise cohort studies also give mixed results, suggesting that a causal link is unlikely. Doll and Peto,[14] in the U.K. cohort that follows medical practitioners, show no risk. Similarly, although benzene is a well-accepted leukemogen there is little evidence of a link with CLL.[15]

Genetics

The role genetics has to play in the etiology of CLL has been explored for many years. McGavran[16] reported a multiple case family and Dameshek et al.[17] recorded CLL in twin brothers aged 56. Since then numerous studies have been undertaken, and some suggest about 5 percent of CLL patients have blood relatives also with CLL.[18,19] Case-control studies have consistently found links in blood relatives of between two- and four-fold.[13,20–22] There is also some support from cohort studies.[23] There is some evidence linking familial CLL with the VH locus.[24]

These studies together with strong evidence of ethnic differences, especially when present after migration, are powerful suggestions that CLL pathogenesis is driven by genetic influences.

Immune Impairment

Links between genetic involvements and immune dysfunction have also been carefully pursued. One study shows that CLL patients had significant excesses of a variety of second malignancies.[25] Further studies suggest that direct therapy-related acute leukemia in CLL patients was rare (3 cases out of 1374 CLL cases over 21 years).[26,27] Once acquired, however, CLL patients undoubtedly display impaired immunity with high risk of infection.[28]

There is no compelling evidence linking CLL with HTLV-I or II infection or with human immunodeficiency virus (HIV) or in those people who are immunosuppressed after organ transplantation. There is weak evidence in a Swedish study to suggest pregnancy confers a protective effect on CLL.[29]

A variety of prior medical conditions have been reported to be in excess in CLL patients. These include scarlet fever, chronic ear infection, and bronchitis;[13] psoriasis;[30] and rheumatoid arthritis, appendectomy, and chronic infections other than TB.[31] However, there is little consistency among these studies; much of the results are based on small case numbers and all these results must be regarded as unreliable.

Sunlight has strong immunosuppressive properties to lymphocytes circulating in the capillaries[32] and a link has been established in Sweden between malignant melanoma and squamous cell cancer of the skin and CLL.[33] Melanoma patients in Denmark have a twofold risk of subsequent CLL.[34]

Occupations

Two Swedish studies suggest a risk of CLL from occupational (not residential) exposure to magnetic fields.[35,36] A third study of Swedish railway workers also found a risk.[37] However, there is little support from other studies apart from one small study from New Zealand,[38] and these results cannot be thought of as conclusive. Most studies in this area fail to distinguish CLL as a specific subtype of leukemia and when they do so, they are negative (see, e.g., Ref. 39).

Other occupational groups considered as potential risk sources for CLL include farming and agriculture, and chemical industry exposure especially the petrochemical industry.

There are many studies showing weak links between various farming activities and lymphomas (usually non-Hodgkin's lymphoma [NHL]); some of these studies include CLL as a separate subtype.[40–42] Suspicions have been centered on pesticide exposures but no conclusive etiologic links exist.

Certain studies have shown an association between CLL and chemical industries generally,[43] with some suspicion directed toward the petrol refinery industry. This suggestion is undoubtedly due to the known links between certain other leukemia types and benzene exposure. However, a large combined analysis of 19 studies shows no relation between CLL mortality and occupational risk in the petrochemical industry in the United States and United Kingdom.[44] The same result holds true for a study of incident cases in the United Kingdom,[45] as did a more recent follow-up of the U.S. industry cohort.[46]

Other occupational studies have examined large registers by record linkage to reveal possible risk exposures. These studies find occasional matches, for example, in the furniture and printing industries.[47] Likewise some case control studies find unexpected results such as dust exposure[48] and coal mining.[49] Such observations are very likely to be chance findings.

Other Risks

Past hair dye use was not associated with CLL risk in one small study[50] and a cohort study.[51]

Conclusions

The most likely risk factors for CLL revolve around genetic effects and possibly related immune dysfunction. There is far less evidence for any significant environmental contribution from either traditional sources of cancer risk such as radiation, benzene, and cigarette smoking or indeed any other source.

CHRONIC MYELOID LEUKEMIA

The epidemiology of chronic myeloid leukemia (CML) could not present more contrast with that of CLL. The study of CML suffers less from problems of case ascertainment and diagnosis; its descriptive epidemiology is quite different and it shares little in common with the etiology of CLL.

Descriptive Epidemiology

CML is a rare disease, roughly half more common in males than females. It remarkably shows little variation worldwide. Table 2–1 shows that for most countries male standardized rates are around 1 per 100,000 per year and females roughly 0.6/0.7. There is a suggestion that African and U.S. Blacks have slightly higher rates. New Zealand Maoris show the highest rates but based on small case numbers. This might be in line with the parallel observation that they also have the highest rates worldwide of acute myeloid leukemia.[1]

Table 2–2 shows the age-specific incidence for the United Kingdom, but is typical of many countries. The condition is found at all ages but it is very rare under the age of 40; thereafter, rates increase from roughly 1 per 100,000 per year for both sexes to a maximum of 4 for males and 2 for females. This very slight increase with age is in contrast to most other leukemias.

The lack of major variations in ethnic rates is coupled with the lack of any local geographic variation in the United Kingdom[3] and with little evidence of case clustering with the exception of one study from Israel.[8] Two studies suggest a decline in incidence in recent years in the United States[6] and in the United Kingdom.[7] There is no evidence of seasonality of occurrence.

The descriptive epidemiology affords little by way of clues to help understand the etiology of the condition.

Analytic Epidemiology

The main problem in determining the epidemiology of CML lies in its rarity; thus many published studies have inadequate case numbers to allow true confidence in the power of the observations reported. Nevertheless, due to consistency between studies more is probably known of the causes of CML than CLL.

Ionizing Irradiation and Chemotherapy

There is substantial evidence that high doses of ionizing irradiation lead to increased risk of CML (and certain other leukemias). The best evidence arises from the Japanese A-bomb survivor cohorts. CML (with acute myelocytic leukemia [AML] and acute lymphocytic leukemia [ALL]) were the earliest malignancies to appear, with CML rates peaking 5 years after the explosion in the younger exposed age groups and some years later in older (over 15) exposed persons. Most of the leukemic excess was over by 1980 and no risk was seen in those exposed in utero or their children. No risk was seen in exposures under 0.4 Gy and thereafter there is a dose-response in risk up to about 4 Gy.[9,52,53]

Slightly lower risks of CML were seen in patients treated for ankylosing spondylitis either by external beam therapy[54] or radium-224.[55] Other case series treated with radiation also occasionally show excess of CML, for example, those treated for cervix cancer[10] or for benign uterine bleeding.[56] Most other therapy-related cohorts are too small to be likely to reveal a risk of CML after follow-up. Similarly CML is very rarely reported as a secondary outcome of chemotherapy for primary cancers. This does not preclude CML as a possible outcome, but if it is the risk is very low.[57]

There is controversy regarding the effects of ionizing irradiation at lower doses, but generally speaking there is little firm and repeatable data. CML appears along with other leukemias in numerous case reports and studies of low-dose exposure either medically or environmentally, but never dominates any study nor is it alone responsible for any statistically significant excesses in such studies.

Nonionizing Irradiation

The numerous studies on leukemia risks associated with magnetic fields occasionally note CML. Most domestic exposure studies are generally negative for a CML risk with a few exceptions (e.g., Ref. 58). This is generally also true of occupational exposure to electromagnetic fields. Like CLL, CML is often pooled as "leukemia" in many exposure group studies of nonionizing irradiation.

Cigarette Smoking

Myeloid leukemias generally are associated with a risk of cigarette smoking; this is seen in several cohorts including the U.S. veteran study.[59] In some studies CML has been separately identified as having an associated risk.[12] Smoking also appears to be associated with a shortened time to blast crisis.[60]

Occupations

CML is regularly reported among those heavily exposed to benzene, together with the acute leukemias. The majority of studies in this area have pooled CML with various AML types as "myeloid" leukemias and have assumed the risks are equal. For the heavily exposed cohorts this could well be true, with risks varying from threefold to 25-fold and showing a crude dose-response relationship with little statistically significant risk being seen in those exposed to less than 10 parts per million for less than 5 years.[61–65]

More recent studies of occupationally exposed workers show far less risk. A large combined analysis of 19 studies show no risk for CML in petroleum workers,[44] no doubt associated with better occupational hygiene and lower exposure levels.

There is no evidence to link CML risk with other solvents such as xylene or toluene.

Other reports of occupational exposure risks associated with CML are not consistent. These include one case of a nurse handling chemotherapeutic agents,[66] two cases linked to high exposure of the pesticide alachlor,[67] and weak links with farming,[68,69] with working in the beverage industry,[47] and with welders.[70]

Other Causes

Apart from some reported links between CML and neurofibromatosis[71] and weaker links with Poland syndrome,[72] there is little to suggest a major genetic association with respect to susceptibility.

Some studies have suggested an association with a past diagnosis of rheumatoid arthritis, appendectomies, and with salicylate use.[31] Another study shows past angina and drugs used for cardiac problems were associated with CML.[73]

A suggested link in children treated with growth hormone has not been seen in an overview study.[74] Hair dye use was not associated with CML risk in a large cohort study[51] or case-control study.[75] Viruses have not been implicated in the pathogenesis of CML, including most recently, the human herpes virus-6.[76]

Conclusion

There is good evidence that common carcinogens (radiation, solvents, and cigarette smoking) are linked to the pathogenesis of CML. Little else appears to confer any notable risks. It is not known to what extent these risks account for the totality of the disease but it is likely much of the etiology of CML remains mysterious. The relative stability of the rates worldwide and its rarity could suggest that chance mutational/cytogenetic events have a major role to play.

HAIRY CELL LEUKEMIA

Pathogenically akin to CLL, hairy cell leukemia (HCL) has had little attention from epidemiologists, not least due to its rarity.

Descriptive Epidemiology

Table 2–3 gives results of age-standardized incidence rates from the same countries shown in Table 2–1. With male rates varying between 1 and 4 per million per year and females stable at about 1, this very rare condition gives few clues as to its possible etiology. It increases in incidence with age as is shown in Table 2–4, so that by the age group 75 to 79 male U.K. incidence is 1.5 per 100,000 per year and female incidence is 0.6.[77] There is no evidence that the condition has changed in incidence between 1984 and 1993.[7]

Little else is known of its descriptive epidemiology.

Table 2–3. Age-Standardized World Incidence Rates of Hairy Cell Leukemia[a]

	Male	Female
Zimbabwe, Africa	–	–
Cali, Colombia	(0.1)	–
Canada	0.4	0.1
U.S. SEER Whites	0.4	0.1
U.S. SEER Blacks	(0.1)	–
Shanghai, China	–	–
Bombay, India	–	–
Osaka, Japan	–	–
Israel Jews	0.5	0.1
Denmark	0.2	0.1
Turin, Italy	0.3	0.1
The Netherlands	0.3	0.1
Tarragona, Spain	–	(0.1)
England and Wales, U.K.	0.2	0.1
New South Wales, Australia	0.3	0.1
Non-Maori, New Zealand	0.2	(0.1)
Maori, New Zealand	(0.4)	–

[a] Cases per 100,000 per year.
Note: Results in parentheses based on small numbers.
(From Parkin et al.[1])

Analytic Epidemiology

The first study of HCL suggested (with very few cases) a link with solvent exposure.[78] Subsequent studies found no such links.[77,79] A related study found risks associated with chemical exposure.[80] No association has been found with cigarette smokers.[77,80] A new occupational risk noted by a French study was an association with farming,[81] which was not clearly seen in other studies.

A Scandinavian study examined risks associated with past medical history and reported a risk of past ingestion of non-steroidal analgesics, based on six cases.[82]

Summary

No real light on HCL is shed by these articles. The links with agriculture and lack of links with cigarette smoking are akin to that seen in CLL. No studies have reported on aspects of genetics of HCL in terms of family histories. This approach, by analogy with CLL, may be more revealing.

PRIMARY POLYCYTHEMIA

Descriptive Epidemiology

Primary polycythemia (PP) has not been routinely recorded as a "malignant condition" in many cancer registries and much of its descriptive epidemiology is based on special surveys, some of which inevitably rely on very small case numbers.

One such study from Malmo suggests a crude incidence rate of 5 per 100,000 per year with roughly equal distribution

Table 2–4. Rare Chronic Leukemias: Crude Incidence Rates from Special Survey 1984–1993 (unpublished data)[a]

Age Groups	HCL		ET		PP		MF	
	Male	Female	Male	Female	Male	Female	Male	Female
0–4	0	0	0	0	0	0	.2	0
5–9	0	0	0	0	0	0	.2	.2
10–14	0	0	0	0	.2	0	0	0
15–19	0	0	.2	0	0	0	0	0
20–24	0	.2	0	.8	.9	.2	.2	.2
25–29	.6	0	1.5	1.0	1.7	.6	.2	0
30–34	.6	.6	.8	2.5	1.0	.6	0	0
35–39	1.6	1.0	1.6	3.9	2.7	2.1	.6	.4
40–44	1.7	.2	1.5	4.7	3.6	3.0	.6	.9
45–49	4.1	1.9	2.4	6.3	6.2	4.6	1.4	1.0
50–54	6.9	2.1	9.2	5.8	10.8	6.8	3.4	3.4
55–59	6.2	3.1	6.8	9.6	14.3	8.6	7.8	2.9
60–64	7.1	2.5	10.9	12.9	23.9	14.9	10.1	7.0
65–69	11.9	4.4	18.4	17.4	32.4	16.3	25.7	10.4
70–79	9.6	3.8	27.2	27.1	37.2	29.1	29.1	16.7
80–84	15.0	4.6	45.1	43.6	39.4	29.2	40.4	19.9
85 +	11.3	4.9	39.7	37.6	39.7	26.7	30.3	10.9
Total case numbers	229	112	415	650	598	544	380	281

Abbreviations: HCL, hairy cell leukemia; ET, essential thrombocythemia; PP, primary polycythemia; MF, myelofibrosis.
[a] Cases per million per year.
Special Survey Data; see Cartwright et al.[3]

between the sexes and a very marked increase in incidence from 1950 to 1984.[83] Earlier studies have reported much lower rates, for example, 0.81 in the United Kingdom,[84] with much depending on the completeness of ascertainment and diagnostic definition. Table 2–4 shows the U.K. rates increase with age but are generally far lower than the Swedish study.

The incidence of this condition appears to be declining.[7] Most studies show a male predominance of the condition.

Analytic Epidemiology

No systematic or large studies have been undertaken on the possible etiological links in PP.

There are strong indications that a familial tendency exists,[85] as does ethnic variation with lower rates in Japan[86] and in U.S. Blacks[87] than in European populations.

There are weak suggestions that previous malignancies, previous medical irradiation, and having been a frequent blood donor in the past may be risk factors.[88]

These observations should be treated with caution but there is some indication that risk factors might be similar to those of CML. This hypothesis, however, would require rigorous testing.

ESSENTIAL THROMBOCYTHEMIA

Descriptive Epidemiology

Very little is known about this condition. Table 2–4 gives an indication of its rarity. The outstanding unusual feature of essential thrombocythemia is the marked female excess.

Analytic Epidemiology

No recent publications exist in this area. Nothing is known of the etiology of this condition.

MYELOFIBROSIS

Descriptive Epidemiology

Table 2–4 shows that the condition is somewhat rarer than polycythemia.

Analytic Epidemiology

Nothing is known of the etiology of this condition.

REFERENCES

1. Parkin DM, Whelan SL, Ferlay J, Ragmand L, Young J (eds.): Cancer Incidence in Five Continents, Volume VII. IARC Sci. Publ., 1997.
2. Fleming AF: Chronic lymphocytic leukaemia in tropical Africa. Leuk Lymph 1:169–173, 1990.
3. Cartwright RA, Alexander FE, McKinney PA, Ricketts TJ: Leukaemia and Lymphoma: An Atlas of Distribution Within Areas of England and Wales 1984–1988. Leukaemia Research Fund, London, 1990.
4. Haenszel W, Kurihara M: Studies of Japanese migrants. I: Mortality from cancer and other diseases among Japanese in the US. JNCI 40:43–68, 1968.
5. Kobayashi T, Kita K, Ohno T, Shirakawa S: Chronic lymphocytic leukaemia in Japan. Jap J Clin Haematol 31:554–563, 1990.

6. Groves FD, Linet MS, Devesa SS: Pattern of occurrence of the leukaemias. Eur J Cancer 31A:941–949, 1995.

7. Cartwright RA, Gilman E, Gurney K: Time trends in incidence of haematological malignancy and related conditions. Br J Haematol 106:281–295, 1999.

8. Chen R, Iscovich J, Goldbourt U: Clustering of leukemia cases in a city in Israel. Stat Med 10:1873–1877, 1997.

9. Preston DL, Kusumi S, Tomonaga M: Cancer incidence in A-bomb survivors III: Leukaemia, lymphoma and multiple myeloma 1950–1987. Radiat Res 137(Suppl. 2):68–97, 1994.

10. Boice JD, Blettner M, Kleinerman RA: Radiation dose and leukaemia risk in patients treated for cancer of the cervix. JNCI 79:1295–1311, 1987.

11. Hall P, Boice J, Berg G: Leukaemia incidence after I^{131} exposure. Lancet 340:1–4, 1992.

12. Brown LM, Gibson R, Blair A: Smoking and risk of leukemia. Am J Epidemiol 135:763–768, 1992.

13. Cartwright RA, Bernard SM, Bird CI, Darwin C: Chronic lymphocytic leukaemia: Case control epidemiology study in York. Br J Cancer 56:79–82, 1987.

14. Doll R, Peto R: Mortality in relation to smoking. 20 years observation in male British doctors. BMJ 2:1525–1536, 1976.

15. Monographs on the evaluation of carcinogenic risks to humans—an updating of IARC monograph 1–45, Suppl 7. IARC Sci. Publ. 1987.

16. McGavran CW: 3 cases of leukemia in one family. Am J Med Sci 164:545–552, 1922.

17. Dameshek W, Savitz H-A, Anbor B: Chronic lymphatic leukemia in twin brothers aged 56. JAMA 92:1348–1349, 1929.

18. Eriksson M, Bergström I: Familial malignant blood disease in the country of Jämtland, Sweden. Eur J Haematol 38:241–245, 1987.

19. Yuille M, Matutes E, Marossy A: Familial chronic lymphocytic leukaemia: A survey and review of published studies. Br J Haematol 109:794–799, 2000.

20. Linet MS, van Notta M, Brookmeyer R, Khoury M: Familial cancer history and chronic lymphocytic leukaemia—a population-based case-control study. Am J Epidemiol 130:655–664, 1989.

21. Pottern L, Linet M, Blair A, Dich F: Familial cancers associated with subtypes of leukaemia and non-Hodgkin's lymphoma. Leuk Res 15:305–314, 1991.

22. Radovanovic Z, Markovi-Denis L, Jakovic S: Cancer mortality of family members of patients with chronic lymphocytic leukaemia. Eur J Epidemiol 10:211–213, 1994.

23. Goldgar D, Easton D, Cannar-Albright L, Skolnich M: Systematic population based assessment of cancer risk in first degree relatives of cancer probands. JNCI 86:1600–1608, 1994.

24. Catovsky D: The search for genetic links in chronic lymphocytic leukaemia. Hematol Cell Ther 39(Suppl. 1):S5–11, 1997.

25. Travis L, Curtis R, Hankey B, Fraumeni J: Second cancers in patients with chronic lymphocytic leukaemia. JNCI 84:1422–1427, 1992.

26. Robertson L, Estey E, Kantorijian M, Koller C, O'Brien S: Therapy related leukemia and myelodysplastic syndrome in chronic lymphocytic leukemia. Leukemia 8:2047–2051, 1994.

27. Cheson B, Venor D, Barrett J, Freidlin B: Second malignancy as a consequence of nucleoside analog therapy for chronic lymphocytic leukemia. J Clin Oncol 17:7454–7460, 1999.

28. Molica S: Infections in chronic lymphocytic leukemia: Risk factors and impact on survival and treatment. Leuk Lymph 13:203–214, 1994.

29. Adami H-O, Tsaik S, Lambe M, Hsiek C, Adami J: Pregnancy and risk of non-Hodgkin's lymphoma: A prospective study. Int J Cancer 70:155–158, 1997.

30. Linet MS, Cartwright RA: Chronic lymphocytic leukaemia: Epidemiology and etiotopic findings. Nouv Rev Fr Hematol 30:353–357, 1988.

31. Zheng W, Linet MS, Shu X, Par R, Gao Y, Fraumeni J: Prior medical conditions and the risk of adult leukaemia in Shanghai. Cancer Causes Control 4:361–368, 1993.

32. Cartwright RA, McNally R, Staines A: The increasing incidence of non-Hodgkin's lymphoma (NHL): The possible role of sunlight. Leuk Lymph 14:387–394, 1994.

33. Adami J, Frisch M, Yuen J, Glimelius B, Melbye M: Evidence of an association between non-Hodgkin's lymphoma and skin cancer. BMJ 310:1491–1495, 1995.

34. Swerdlow A, Storm H, Sasieni P: Risk of second primary malignancy in patients with cutaneous and ocular melanoma in Denmark 1943–1989. Int J Cancer 61:773–779, 1995.

35. Floderus B, Persson T, Stenlund C, Wennberg A, Ost A, Knave B: Occupational exposure to electromagnetic fields in relation to leukaemia and brain tumours: A case-control study in Sweden. Cancer Causes Control 4:465–476, 1993.

36. Feychting M, Forssen U, Floderus B: Occupational and residential magnetic field exposure and leukaemia and CNS tumours. Epidemiology 8:384–389, 1997.

37. Floderus B, Tornqvist S, Stenlund C: Incidence of selected cancers in Swedish railway workers 1961–1979. Cancer Causes Control 5:189–194, 1994.

38. Pearce N, Reif J, Fraser J: Case-control study in cancer in New Zealand electrical workers. Int J Epidemiol 18:55–59, 1989.

39. Guensel P, Nicolas J, Imernon E, Chevalier A, Goldberg M: Exposure to 50HZ electrical fields and incidence of leukemia, brain tumours and other cancers among French electrical utility workers. Am J Epidemiol 144:1107–1121, 1996.

40. Blair A, White D: Leukemia cell type and agricultural practices in Nebraska. Arch Environ Health 40:211–214, 1985.

41. Gilbert HS: Familial myeloproliferative disease. Balliere's Clin Haematol 11:849–858, 1998.

42. Amadori D, Nanni O, Falcini F, Saragoni A, Tilson V: Chronic lymphocytic leukaemias and non-Hodgkin's lymphomas by histological type in farming–animal breeding work. Occup Environ Med 52:374–379, 1995.

43. Malone KE, Koepsell T, Daling J, Weiss N, Morris P: Chronic lymphocytic leukemia in relation to chemical exposures. Am J Epidemiol 130:1152–1158, 1989.

44. Raabe GK, Wang O: Leukaemia mortality by cell type in petroleum workers with potential exposure to benzene. Environ Health Perspect 104:1381–1392, 1996.

45. Rushton L, Romaniuk H: A case-control study to investigate the risk of leukaemia associated with exposure to benzene in petroleum marketing and distribution workers in the UK. Occup Environ Med 54:152–166, 1997.

46. Heubner W, Chen V, Friedlander B, Wu X, Jorgensen G: Incidence of lympho haemopoietic malignancies in a petrochemical industry cohort 1983–1994 follow-up. Occup Environ Med 57:605–614, 2000.

47. Linet M, Malker H, McLaughlin J, Weiner J, Stone B, Blot W: Leukemia and occupation in Sweden—a registry based analysis. Am J Ind Med 14:319–330, 1988.

48. Markovic-Denic L, Jankovic S, Mainkovic J, Radovanovic Z: Brick mortar exposure and chronic lymphocytic leukemia. Neoplasma 42:79–81, 1995.

49. Gilman PA, Ames RG, McCawley M: Leukemia risk among US white male coal miners. A case-control study. J Occup Med 27:669–671, 1985.

50. Zahm SH, Weisenburger D, Babbitt P, Saal R, Vaught J, Blair A: Use of hair colouring products and the risk of lymphoma, multiple myeloma and chronic lymphocytic leukemia. Am J Public Health 82:990–997, 1992.

51. Grodstein F, Hennekens C, Colditz G: A prospective study of permanent hairdye use and hemopoietic cancer. JNCI 86:1466–1470, 1994.

52. Finch S: Leukemia and lymphoma in atomic bomb survivors. In Boice JD, Fraumeni JF (eds.): Radiation Carcinogenesis: Epidemiology and Biological Significance, pp. 37–44. Raven Press, New York, 1984.

53. United Nations Scientific Committee on the Effects of Ionising Radiation Genetic and Somatic Effects, UN, New York, 1986.

54. Darby S, Doll R, Gill S: Long-term mortality after a single treatment course with x-rays in patients treated for ankylosing spondylitis. Br J Cancer 55:179–190, 1987.

55. Speiss H, Mags C, Chmelvsky D: Malignancies in patients injected with radium 224. In Taglon G, May C. (eds.): Risk for Radium and Thorotrast, pp. 7–12. British Institute Radiology, London, 1989, Report 21.

56. Inskip P, Manson R, Wavnor J, Stovall M: Leukaemia following radiotherapy for uterine bleeding. Radiat Res 122:107–119, 1990.

57. Aguiar RC: Therapy related chronic myeloid leukemia: An epidemiological, clinical and pathogenetic appraisal. Leuk Lymph 29:17–26, 1998.

58. Feytching M, Ahlbom A: Magnetic fields, leukaemia and CNS tumours in Swedish adults residing near high voltage power lines. Epidemiology 5:501–509, 1994.

59. McLaughlin J, Hrubec Z, Linet M: Cigarette smoking and leukemia. JNCI 81:1261–1263, 1989.

60. Herr R, Ferguson J, Myers N, Rovira D, Robinson W: Cigarette smoking, blast crisis and survival in chronic myeloid leukemia. Am J Hematol 34:1–4, 1990.

61. Vigliani E: Leukemia associated with benzene exposure. Ann N Y Acad Sci 271:143–151, 1976.

62. Aksoy M: Leukemia in workers due to occupational exposure to benzene. New Istanbul Cont Clin Sci 12:3–14, 1977.

63. Infante P, Rinsky R, Wagner J, Young R: Leukaemia in benzene workers. Lancet 2:76–78, 1977.

64. Ott M, Townsend J, Fishbeck W, Langner R: Mortality in individuals occupationally exposed to benzene. Arch Environ Health 33:3–9, 1978.

65. Rinsky R, Young R, Smith A: Leukemia in benzene workers. Am J Ind Med 2:217–245, 1981.

66. Skov T, Maarup B, Olsen J, Rorth M: Leukaemia and reproductive outcome amongst nurses handling antineoplastic drugs. Br J Ind Med 49:855–861, 1992.

67. Leet T, Acquavella J, Lynch C, Anne M, Weiss N: Cancer incidence among alachlor manufacturing workers. Am J Ind Med 30:380–386, 1996.

68. Kelleher C, Newell J, MacDonagh-White C, MacHale E, Egon E: Incidence and occupational patterns of leukaemias, lymphomas, and testicular tumours in Western Ireland over an 11 year period. J Epidemiol Comm Health 52:651–656, 1998.

69. Blair A, White D: Death certificate study of leukemia among farmers of Wisconsin. JNCI 66:1027–1030, 1981.

70. Preston-Martin S, Peters J: Prior employment as a welder associated with the development of chronic myeloid leukaemia. Br J Cancer 58:105–108, 1988.

71. Matsui I, Tanimura M, Kobayashi N: Neurofibromatosis type I and childhood cancer. Cancer 72:2746–2754, 1993.

72. Costa R, Afonso E, Benedito M: Poland's syndrome associated with chronic granuloyctic leukemia. Sangre (Barc) 36:417–418, 1991.

73. McKinney PA, Roberts BE, O'Brien C, Bird CC, Richards IDG, Alexander FE, Cartwright RA: Chronic myeloid leukaemia in Yorkshire: A case-control study. Acta Haematol 83:35–38, 1990.

74. Shalet SM: Leukaemia in children treated with growth hormone. J Paediatr Endocrinol 6:109–111, 1993.

75. Mele A, Szklo M, Visangi G: Hairdye use and other risk factors for leukemia and pre-leukemia. Am J Epidemiol 139:609–619, 1994.

76. Gentile G, Mele A, Ragara G, Faggiori A: Human herpes virus-6 seroprevalence and leukaemias: A case-control study. Br J Cancer 80:1103–1106, 1999.

77. Staines A, Cartwright RA: Hairy cell leukaemia descriptive epidemiology and a case-control study. Br J Haematol 85:714–717, 1993.

78. Oleske D, Golomb H, Faber M, Levy P: A case-control enquiry into the etiology of hairy cell leukaemia. Am J Epidemiol 121:675–683, 1985.

79. Clavel J, Corso F, Limasset J, Mandereau L, Roach P: Hairy cell leukaemia and occupational exposure to benzene. Occup Environ Med 53:533–539, 1996.

80. Clavel J, Mandereau L, Cordier S, Le Goasta C, Hemon D: Hairy cell leukaemia, occupation and smoking. Br J Haematol 91:154–161, 1995.

81. Clavel J, Hemon D, Mandereau L, Delemotte B, Severi F: Farming pesticide use and hairy cell leukaemia. Scand J Work Environ Health 22:285–293, 1996.

82. Nordstrom M, Hardell L, Fredrikson M: Previous medical history and medication as risk factors for hairy cell leukaemia. Oncol Rep 6:415–419, 1999.

83. Berglund S, Zettervall O: Incidence of polycythemia vera in a defined population. Eur J Haematol 48:20–26, 1992.

84. Prochazka A, Markowe H: The epidemiology of polycythaemia rubra vera in England and Wales 1968–1982. Br J Cancer 53:59–64, 1986.

85. Miller R, Purvis J, Weich J: Familial polycythaemia vera. Clev Clin J Med 56:813–818, 1989.

86. Kurita S: Epidemiological study of polycythaemia vera in Japan. Acta Haematol Japan 37:793–795, 1974.

87. Modan B: Polycythaemia: A review of epidemiological and clinical aspects. J Chronic Dis 18:605–645, 1965.

88. Najean Y, Rain J, Billotey C: Epidemiological data in polycythaemia vera: A study of 842 cases. Hematol Cell Ther 40:159–165, 1998.

3

Pathology and Morphology of Chronic Leukemias and Related Disorders

Richard M. Stone and Arthur T. Skarin

The chronic leukemias, chronic myeloid leukemia (CML) and chronic lymphocytic leukemia (CLL), are hematopoietic malignancies with a relatively indolent clinical course. However, these diseases represent examples of different pathophysiological entities: CML is a myeloproliferative disorder (MPD) whereas CLL falls in the spectrum of chronic lymphoproliferative disease with circulating neoplastic cells. This chapter emphasizes the pathological findings in CML, CLL, and related entities. Indolent lymphoproliferative neoplasms in which a leukemic phase is infrequent are covered in Sections IV (non-Hodgkin's lymphoma) and III (multiple myeloma). Molecular biological, immunobiological, and clinical aspects of the chronic leukemias are discussed in Chapters 4 through 9.

BONE MARROW STEM CELL DISORDERS: MYELOPROLIFERATIVE DISORDERS AND MYELODYSPLASTIC SYNDROMES

Overview and History

The MPDs are a group of clonal bone marrow stem cell disorders characterized by the proliferation of differentiated hematopoietic cells resulting in excess production of red cells, platelets, and/or white cells. Other features typical of the MPDs include (a) propensity to exhibit extramedullary hematopoiesis; (b) reactive proliferation of bone marrow fibroblasts; (c) tendency to transform to acute leukemia; and (d) absence of significant dysplasia in blood or bone marrow cells. Except for CML, objectively definable by the translocation between the *bcr* gene on chromosome 22 and the *abl* gene on chromosome 9,[1] the other MPDs are syndromes characterized by a stereotypical, but often overlapping, set of pathological and clinical features.

The term *myeloproliferative disorder* was first applied in 1951 by Dameshek who referred to a group of diseases that included CML, polycythemia vera (PCV), agnogenic myeloid metaplasia (AMM), essential (idiopathic) thrombocythemia (ET), and the diGuglielmo-erythroleukemia syndrome.[2] He postulated that these disorders were closely related because all manifestations could be explained by neoplastic proliferation of pluripotent bone marrow stem cell or its progeny. In 1971, Ward and Block[3] suggested that CML and erythroleukemia behaved in a similar fashion to acute myeloid leukemia (AML), and should be con-

sidered distinct from AMM, PCV, and ET, each characterized by a benign proliferation of hematopoietic cells. In the French-American-British (FAB) classification schema, erythroleukemia is considered to be an AML subtype[4] (defined by the finding of ≥ 30 percent myeloblasts among nonerythroid cells in marrows displaying ≥ 50 percent erythroblasts). The FAB classification of acute leukemia itself may be supplanted by the proposed WHO scheme in which the inherent molecular, cytogenetic, and biological aspects of the diseases are emphasized.[5] The MPDs are distinct from myelodysplastic syndromes (MDS), which typically also present with hypercellular marrows; however, MDS are characterized by dysplastic maturation of hematopoietic cells and peripheral cytopenias.[6] MDS subgroups have been delineated by an FAB classification scheme as well as by the more biologically based WHO format.[5,7] However, one such entity, chronic myelomonocytic leukemia, might better be classified as an MPD due to the frequency of leukocytosis (with an elevated monocyte count) especially if the white blood cell count is elevated.[9,10] The Polycythemia Vera Study Group (PVSG) has promulgated useful guidelines[11] for the classification of PCV, AMM, and ET. Increased molecular biological understanding of the pathophysiology of these diseases will allow a more biologically based classification system, potentially supplementing the morphological and clinical analysis currently of primary importance for diagnosis and classification of the (non-CML) MPDs.

Pathophysiology

Most cases of MPD are now understood to be neoplasms, insofar as mature blood cells from patients with these disorders have been shown to arise from a single bone marrow stem cell. Although clonal derivation is a unifying pathophysiological theme, there are marked variations in the clinicopathological features of each of the MPDs. The evidence for clonal origin of the MPD is derived from several lines of evidence. The clinical observation that stable phase CML can transform into an acute leukemia with either myeloid, lymphoid, basophilic, megakaryoblastic, or eosinophilic features suggested that this entity is a neoplasm derived from a multipotent hematopoietic stem cell.[12] Specific documentation that mature cells from different lineages in patients with CML were all descended from early stem cells was first proved by Fialkow et al.[13] who studied women with CML who happened to be heterozygotes for the A/B forms of the glucose-6-phosphate dehydrogenase (G6PD) isoenzyme. Neutrophils obtained from normal females who are G6PD heterozygotes will be as likely to express the A as the B form due to random X-chromosome linked inactivation of one of the G6PD alleles in the heterogeneous population of bone marrow stem cells. However, if a single bone marrow stem cell undergoes malignant degeneration, the number of neutrophils having either A or B isoenzyme expression (depending on the particular inactivation event in the original stem cell) will be greatly expanded. Therefore, examination of the neutrophils from a patient with CML who is a G6PD heterozygote will show expression of virtually all A (or B) type of G6PD isoenzyme.

The clonal nature of CML can also be documented by means of detecting evidence for the *bcr-abl* translocation in mature cells. Routine karyotypic analysis, which can be used to define the characteristic translocation between the long arm of chromosome 9 and the long arm of chromosome 22 (i.e., the Philadelphia chromosome) requires metaphases and therefore cannot be used in mature nondividing cells such as neutrophils. However, it is now routinely possible to isolate granulocytes, obtain DNA, and document the rearrangement of the *bcr* or *abl* gene by Southern blotting techniques.[14] Alternatively, the translocation can be sensitively detected by the use of the so-called reverse polymerase chain reaction. In this technique, RNA is isolated from neutrophils and cDNA is created by means of the enzyme reverse transcriptase.[15] A standard polymerase chain reaction is then done, using a *bcr* and an *abl* primer, with amplification occurring only if a *bcr-abl* fusion transcript is present.

Because MPDs other than CML are not currently characterized by a specific chromosomal abnormality, and since it is rare to encounter a female heterozygous for G6PD isoenzyme, other techniques are required to prove clonality in PCV, AMM, and ET. The use of X-linked-restriction fragment length polymorphisms (RFLP) has enabled cells from virtually every female with an MPD to be informative. For example, the human androgen receptor gene, encoded on the X chromosome, is polymorphic in 90 percent of females.[16] By using the appropriate restriction enzymes, and taking advantage of the fact that certain restriction enzymes will only cut in the absence of X-chromosome inactivation, it has been possible to prove a clonal origin of mature cells in the vast majority of patients with all of the MPDs,[17,18] supplementing data derived previously from the rare female G6PD heterozygote.[19] Clonality in PCV has also been assessed by detecting karyotypic abnormalities in mature cells via fluorescent in situ chromosomal hybridization.[20]

Although neutrophils, red cells, and platelets have been shown to be clonally derived, other cell types involved in the pathogenesis of the MPD may proliferate in reactive fashion in response to growth factors elaborated by the neoplastic cells. The marrow-derived fibroblasts in the MPD appear to be only indirectly involved in the neoplastic process. Various studies used to assign clonality, as indicated above, have been used to show that marrow fibroblasts in patients with MPD have a primarily mesenchymal origin, rather than being descended from hematopoietic stem cells.[21,22] Platelet-derived growth factor (PDGF),[23] tumor growth factor beta (TGF-β),[24] and other cytokines have been implicated as substances that may be fibroblast mitogens. Megakaryocytes, which are also increased in the marrows from many patients with MPD, may also, in some cases, proliferate in a reactive fashion. If fibrosis overwhelms the marrow, patients may display hematopoiesis in nonmarrow sites such as the spleen, liver,[25] lung,[26] brain,[27] paraspinal areas,[28] breast,[29] and kidney.[30] However, the signals responsible for the development of extramedullary hematopoietic cells are poorly understood.[31]

The precise molecular pathophysiology of the myeloproliferative disorders PCV, AMM, and ET remains elusive. However, cloning the genes at the CML t(9;22) breakpoint had led to the generally accepted theory that the dysregulated tyrosine kinase activity of bcr-abl fusion protein leads to overabundant proliferation and hence to clinical disease.[32,33] While a description of the relevance of bcr-abl can be found in Chapter 4, this is of critical importance given the ability of an oral administered drug inhibiting c-abl activity to cause remission in patients with CML, even in those with advanced disease.[34] Chronic myelomonocytic leukemia, the disease subtype within the FAB classification scheme but with features of an MPD, is occasionally associated with chromosomal translocation involving fusion into another tyrosine kinase, also in the c-abl family, platelet-derived growth factor receptor β on chromosome 5. Patients with the t(5;12)[35] (producing the TEL-PDGFR), or t(5;7)[36] (HIP-PDGFR fusion) are rare, but are thought to have dysregulated tyrosine kinase function with consequences similar to those noted in CML. Without guiding chromosomal translocations, understanding the pathophysiology of AMM, ET, and PCV has been more elusive. However, abnormalities of the erythropoietin receptor[37] in PCV and the thrombopoietin receptor, c-mpl,[38] in ET are being intensely studied.

Classification

Given currently available knowledge of the pathophysiology of hematological neoplasms, the MPDs are best classified under the rubric of myeloid neoplasms (Table 3–1). The bone marrow stem cell disorders can also be characterized according to the degree of cellular proliferation and whether there is increased production of mature or immature cells. It is also helpful to consider the balance that must exist between proliferation and differentiation in the stem cell compartment for hematopoiesis to continue unabated. If maturation is impaired, it is possible that self-renewal will take precedence and result in an increased percentage of immature nonfunctional stem cells. The expansion of the immature compartment may result in (a) the lack of mature progeny able to carry out the routine functional duties of the blood system; (b) an inability of residual normal clones to find space for growth; and (c) the elaboration of peptides or other factors that have a deleterious effect on the growth of residual normal clones. If the number of immature bone marrow cells, or blasts, exceeds 20 to 30 percent of the total number of bone marrow cells in a bone marrow aspirate, then the patient is considered to have acute leukemia[5,39] (Chapter 25). Aplastic anemia and paroxysmal nocturnal hemoglobinuria are believed to represent, at least in some cases, a relatively complete failure of bone marrow stem cell function resulting in variable degrees of bone marrow hypoplasia.[40,41] Myelodysplastic syndromes, which share the propensity of the MPD to transform into AML, are considered under a separate nosology.[5–7] The MDS refer to a heterogeneous group of disorders characterized by ineffective and abnormal hematopoiesis with variable degrees of cytopenias. MDS, formerly termed dysmyelopoietic syndrome, refractory dysmyelopoietic anemia, smoldering leukemia, or pre-leukemia, have also been shown to originate from a multipotent hematopoietic stem cell precursor with the potential for differentiation.[42] While pathology and histologic classification are useful, (Table 3–2) prognosis in MDS is determined by clinical features such as the number of cytopenias, the degree of marrow infiltration by blasts, and the cytogenetics.[43]

Table 3–1. WHO Classification of Myeloid Neoplasms

Myeloproliferative diseases (overproliferation)
    Chronic myelogenous leukemia, Philadelphia chromosome
        positive [t(9;22)(q34;q11), *BCR/ABL*]
    Chronic neutrophilic leukemia
    Chronic neutrophilic leukemia/hypereosinophilic syndrome
    Chronic idiopathic myelofibrosis
    Polycythemia vera
    Essential thrombocythemia
    Myeloproliferative disease, unclassified
Myelodysplastic/myeloproliferative diseases (overlap)
    Chronic myelomonocytic leukemia
    Atypical chronic myelogenous leukemia
    Juvenile myelomonocytic leukemia
Myelodysplastic syndromes (impaired maturation)
    Refractory anemia
        With ringed sideroblasts
        Without ringed sideroblasts
    Refractory cytopenia (myelodysplastic syndrome) with
        multilineage dysplasia
    Refractory anemia (myelodysplastic syndrome) with excess
        blasts (5–20 percent marrow blasts)
    5q- syndrome
    Myelodysplastic syndrome (unclassified)
Acute myeloid leukemias (both overproliferation and impaired
    maturation)

(From Harris et al.,[5] with permission).

Table 3–2. FAB Classification of the Myelodysplastic Syndromes

Type	Peripheral Blood		Bone Marrow	Dysplasia
RA	—		—	+
RARS	—		Ringed sideroblasts > 15 percent of nucleated cells	+
CMML	0–5 percent blasts with monocytes > 1 × 10³/μl	*and*	< 20 percent blasts	+
RAEB	1–4 percent blasts	*or*	6–20 percent blasts	+
RAEB-T	5–29 percent blasts	*or*	20–29 percent blasts	+

	Red Cell	Megakaryocytic	Granulocytic
Blood	Macrocytes Dimorphism Normoblasts	Giant platelets Platelet fragment	Pelger cells Bilobed neutrophils Hypogranularity
Marrow	Megaloblasts Dyserythropoiesis Cytoplasmic Vacuolization	1–2 small round nuclei	Promyelocytes with sparse granules Nuclear-cyto plasmic dysynergy

International Prognostic Scoring System for Myelodysplastic Syndromes

Variable	Score Value				
	0	0.5	1.0	1.5	2.0
Marrow blasts	< 5	5–10	–	11–20	21–30
Karyotype	Good	Int.	Poor		
Cytopenias	0/1		2/3		

RA = refractory anemia; RACS = refractory anemia with ringed sideroblasts; RAEB = refractory anemia with excess blasts in transformation; CMML = chronic myelomonocytic leukemia.

The MPDs, in contrast, represent an increased production of mature cells. As indicated above, except for CML, these diseases are best grouped according to clinical features, generally pertaining to the degree of cellular proliferation among the several cell lines (Table 3–3). The particular features of each of the MPDs will be discussed subsequently. Another unifying feature of the bone marrow stem cell disorders in general and the MPDs in particular, is the increased propensity of these conditions to transform to acute leukemia (Plate 3–1A). For example, virtually all patients with CML who do not undergo an allogeneic bone marrow transplant will eventually undergo a blastic transformation.[12] However, the likelihood of the conversion to acute leukemia is 10 percent or less in the other MPDs,[44–46] but may be potentiated by the use of therapeutic agents that are mutagenic, such as chlorambucil.[47]

Reactive Fibrosis

The MPDs, characterized by expansion of some or all hematopoietic cell lines, are also associated with reactive proliferation of mesenchymal cells, including fibroblasts and osteoblasts. Proliferation of fibroblasts leads to increased reticulin fibers, collagen, and fibrous tissue deposition in the medullary cavity (myelofibrosis) whereas osteoblastic proliferation results in bone (osteoid) deposition in the bone marrow (osteosclerosis or osteomyelosclerosis). Reactive myelofibrosis has also been noted in non-MPD diseases, including autoimmune conditions,[48] hairy cell leukemia,[49] acute leukemia,[50] especially acute megakaryoblastic leukemia (FAB M7),[51] malig-

nant lymphoma,[52] multiple myeloma,[53] and metastatic non-hematopoietic tumors,[54] especially breast,[55] stomach, prostate, melanoma, and lung cancer.[56] Secondary fibroblastic proliferation associated with malignancy may be extensive enough to mimic the severe fibrosis seen in the MPD agnogenic myeloid metaplasia.[54] In cases of secondary or reactive fibrosis, successful therapy directed against the underlying disease may result in complete resolution of the reticulin deposition and fibrosis.[55] The source of fibroblast mitogens may be the malignant cells themselves,[56] or may occur indirectly[24] due to activation of macrophages, platelets, or other non-neoplastic cells, which may then elaborate peptides or other fibrogenic substances such as TGF-β or PDGF.

Bone marrow fibrosis may sometimes be associated with bone marrow necrosis, believed to result from vascular occlusion of small vessels caused by crowding, vascular obstruction,

Table 3–3. Characteristic Laboratory Findings in Selected MPD Compared with Leukemoid Reaction

	PCV[a]	AMM	CML	ET	Leukemoid Reaction
Anemia	–	+ +	+	±	–
Nucleated RBCs in PB	±	+ +	±	±	–
Smear: tear drop RBCs	–	+ +	–	–	–
Smear: giant platelets	+	+	+	+ +	–
Basophilia	±	+	+ +	±	–
Toxic granulation	–	–	–	–	+
Platelets	often ↑	↑nl, or ↓	often ↑	always ↑	nl (rarely ↑)
LAP	↑	↑nl, or ↓	↓ or absent	nl or ↑	↑
Serum B12	↑	↑	↑	nl or ↑	nl
Uric acid	↑	↑	↑	nl or ↑	nl

Abbreviations: MPD, myeloproliferative disorder; PCV, polycythemia vera; AMM, agnogenic myeloid metaplasia; CML, chronic myelocytic leukemia; ET, essential thrombocythemia; RBCs, red blood cells; LAP, leukocyte alkaline phosphatase.
[a] Findings in late phase vary considerably.
Symbols: —, not present; +, common; + +, very common; ±, variable; ↑, increased; nl, normal; ↓, decreased.

or by tumor necrosis factor production by the malignant clone.[57,58] This process may be associated with systemic illness, bone pain, and a leukoerythroblastic blood reaction. The manifestations of bone marrow fibrosis include variable numbers of nucleated red blood cells and an elevation of the white blood count with a left shift in the granulocytic series potentially including the presence of small numbers of myeloblasts. Polychromasia, basophilic stippling, anisocytosis, and poikilocytosis are characteristically noted in red blood cells. Tear-shaped erythrocytes may be the most striking abnormality in the peripheral blood in early cases. Leukoerythroblastosis is characteristic of myelofibrosis and other marrow infiltrative processes such as osteosclerosis, osteopetrosis (marble bone disease), granulomatous accumulation, or metastatic malignancy and can occur in illnesses that result in stimulation of marrow cells, such as infection, anoxia, hemolysis, and bleeding.[57]

CHRONIC MYELOCYTIC LEUKEMIA

CML is a myeloproliferative disorder in which the crucial pathophysiological event is the fusion of the *bcr* gene on chromosome 22 and the *abl* gene on chromosome 9.[14] The molecular biological details and cell biological consequences of this rearrangement are discussed in Chapter 20. The diagnosis of CML is confirmed when bone marrow or peripheral blood cells are determined to have a Philadelphia chromosome (i.e., a translocation between the long arm of chromosome 9 and the short arm of chromosome 22) by either molecular or karyotypic analysis. Although Philadelphia chromosome-negative CML was considered a distinct pathophysiological entity,[59] if patients do not evidence such a translocation by any method, they do not have CML. Although the Philadelphia chromosome is considered diagnostic of CML, this translocation has also been noted in patients with disorders clinically consistent with essential thrombocytopenia or other MPDs.[61,62] Very rarely patients who present with apparent AML may be found to have a Philadelphia translocation. It is very difficult to dis-

tinguish such patients from those who have had an occult chronic phase of CML in transformation. Cells from approximately 25 percent of adults and 5 percent of children with acute lymphoblastic leukemia have Philadelphia chromosome on cytogenetic analysis.[62] However, molecular analysis reveals that the vast majority of children with Philadelphia-positive ALL and about half the adults with this entity have a different molecular form of the bcr-abl fusion protein than do those with CML (190 kd rather than the typical p210).[63] Those ALL patients whose cells express the p210 bcr-abl fusion protein may have had an occult chronic phase that underwent a lymphoid blast crisis.

The clinical course of CML can be divided into a chronic indolent stable phase, an accelerated phase, and a blastic crisis.[32,64] Most patients with CML are diagnosed in the chronic or indolent phase,[32,65] which is characterized by granulocytic hyperplasia, basophilic, and possibly eosinophilic infiltration in the bone marrow and concomitant elevation of the white count with a differential characterized by a left shift with bands, metamyelocytes, myelocytes, and promyelocytes, and occasional blasts including basophilia and eosinophilia. An elevated white blood cell (WBC) count may be ascribed to either chronic phase CML or a leukemoid reaction due to an inflammatory or infectious process. However, the leukocyte alkaline phosphatase (LAP) score may help to distinguish between these two entities. A low LAP score is found in over 90 percent of patients with CML, but should be elevated in those with a leukemoid reaction. In later phases of the disease, or after treatment, the LAP score may be elevated. Nonetheless, any patient with a persistent leukocytosis and a left-shifted differential should undergo cytogenetic or molecular analysis to exclude the presence of a bcr-abl fusion protein. Any patient whose marrow or blood cells are proven to harbor a t(9;22) by cytogenetic, fluorescent in situ hybridization (FISH), or molecular analysis (whether clinical disease features are typical of CML or any other MPD) should be considered a candidate for therapy known to be useful in CML, especially oral agents that inhibit the c-abl tyrosine kinase.

Bone Marrow

Patients with chronic phase CML generally have hypercellular bone marrows with 0 to 10 percent fat. However, despite this elevated cellularity, bone marrow is usually easily aspirated. Thinning of the bony cortex and localized erosions of trabeculae may occur. The myeloid–erythroid ratio increases to 10–50:1 compared with the normal ratio of 2.5:1. The granulocyte series reveals all stages of development, but generally suggests less maturity than does a simultaneous peripheral blood smear. Mitotic figures are increased four to five times above that of normal marrow. Significant quantities of basophils and eosinophils are usually found. The marrow may be enriched in megakaryocytes, including some with immature or atypical features, such as hypolobation. Evidence of dysplasia, such as coarsely granulated basophils or hypolobated (Pelger-Huet cells) neutrophils is rare (Plate 3–1C–E).

Presumably due to the rapid proliferation and excessive cell death in the marrow with accumulation of membrane contents, lipid-laden benign histiocytes resembling Gaucher cells may become prominent. In addition, well-granulated sea-blue histiocytes can also be observed[66] (Plate 3–1F). The morphologic appearance of these reactive reticuloendothelial cells results from phagocytosis of cellular debris, which consists of glucocerebrosidase and normal constituents of granulocyte and erythroid cell membranes.[67,68]

Myelofibrosis has been reported to accompany the granulocytic hyperplasia of CML in 6 to 22 percent of patients, more commonly late in the course of this disease.[64,69] The occurrence of myelofibrosis has been associated with elevation of the LAP score, imminent blastic transformation, and poor prognosis.[70] Occasionally, totally fibrotic marrows, indistinguishable from advanced agnogenic myeloid metaplasia, may be observed.[61]

Peripheral Blood

Patients with CML generally present with marked elevations of the WBC count. The mean WBC count varies between 200 and 250×10^9/L with a range of 25 to 750×10^9/L.[32,65] If untreated, the WBC count tends to rise over the course of time; however, cyclic variations in the WBC count have also been reported.[71] Such cycles are usually 50 to 70 days in length, probably reflecting a periodicity in granulocyte production.

In stable phase CML, the peripheral blood smear reflects all stages of granulocyte development, including early forms. However, myeloblasts and promyelocytes generally account for less than 10 percent of the cells. Eosinophils and basophils are usually present. The degree of basophilia is inversely related to prognosis and if the percentage of basophils in the peripheral differential exceeds 20 percent, a blast crisis is imminent[72] (Plate 3–1G). A progressive increase in eosinophils may also be a poor prognostic sign, heralding the emergence of an accelerated course.[73] Circulating normoblasts may be present. Thrombocytosis (platelet count greater than 450×10^9/L) occurs in 50 percent of patients at presentation, with an additional 15 percent developing elevated platelet counts during the course of the disease.[74] Levels greater than 1000×10^9/L are noted in about 25 percent of patients with CML.[74] Thrombocytosis,

probably reflective of an increased disease burden, is also inversely related to prognosis.[75]

Reticuloendothelial System

Extensive myeloid metaplasia occurs in the splenic red pulp. Histological sections of the spleen may yield findings similar to those noted in the bone marrow, especially granulocytic predominance. Splenic infarcts and fibrosis may develop. Granulocytic cells may invade the portal tracts in the liver and occasionally extend to the sinusoids. Lymphadenopathy is rare in CML, unless a blastic transformation is ongoing.

Bone

Bone lesions are uncommon in CML, having been reported in only six patients (3 percent of a series of 205 patients at the NCI).[76] In one half of cases, bone involvement occurred during the blastic phase of CML. The bone lesions of CML are painful, tend to occur at the end of long bones, and display osteolytic features on radiographic examinations. In rare cases, symptomatic lytic bone lesions have preceded the diagnosis of CML and/or simulated a primary bone tumor.[77,78] Multiple lytic bone lesions that have suggested multiple myeloma may also occur and even be associated with hypercalcemia.[79] Hypercalcemia without apparent bone destruction has been reported in association with the accelerated phase of CML.[80] If a patient does have a bone lesion, it generally is a myeloblastoma, recognizable with the use of appropriate histochemical stains, cytogenetic studies, or ultrastructural analysis.

Miscellaneous Sites of Involvement

Skin lesions are rare in CML and when present, tend to be nodular.[81] Multiple hemorrhagic soft tissue nodules have been reported in approximately 2 percent of patients with CML at presentation.[82] Biopsy of these nodules has revealed extramedullary hematopoiesis associated with hemorrhage and necrosis. Meningeal involvement in the terminal blastic phase of CML is uncommon, but is even more atypical in chronic phase CML.[82] Rapidly progressive pulmonary infiltrates due to granulocytic infiltration may occasionally occur.[83]

Leukostasis

Although it is not unusual for a patient with stable phase CML to have white counts exceeding 200×10^9/L, leukostatic complications, typically seen in patients with AML,[84,85] are rare, although ischemic digital necrosis, priapism, papilledema, and deafness have been reported.[86] The relatively mature white cells seen in patients with CML are apparently not as able to clump together as are myeloblasts obtained from certain patients with AML.

Accelerated Phase of CML

The accelerated phase of CML may occur at any time during the natural history of this disease, although this phenomenon generally is seen within 30 to 36 months after the initial diagnosis.[12,32] This phase, which develops in about one-half of patients, may be heralded by progressive splenomegaly and leukostasis, and a demonstration that the patient has become refractory to previously effective chemotherapy.[87] The peripheral blood may show erythroid abnormalities such as marked aniso- and poikilocytosis with circulating myeloblasts and a leukoerythroblastic blood picture. Basophils and eosinophils may increase and thrombocytosis may worsen. A bone marrow biopsy performed at this time is likely to show myelofibrosis; cytogenetic studies may reveal chromosomal abnormalities such as new clonal abnormalities and aneuploidy.[88] Features that have suggested entry into an accelerated phase (associated with a median survival of less than 18 months) have included peripheral blood or bone marrow blasts exceeding 15 percent of the nucleated differential, blasts and promyelocytes greater than 30 percent of the differential, or basophils greater than 20 percent of the differential; platelets less than 100×10^9/L; unexplained decrease in hemoglobin (less than 7 g/dl); and extramedullary disease.[88]

Blastic Transformation

Blastic transformation, also called acute blast crisis or terminal phase, occurs in virtually all (nontransplanted) patients with CML, either following an accelerated phase or acutely during the course of stable phase CML.[32,65] Most accept the definition of blast crisis as the development of greater than or equal to 30 percent blasts in the marrow or the peripheral blood.[89] In the blast crisis stage, progressive anemia and thrombocytopenia occur with death usually due to bleeding or infection. Leukemic involvement of most organs is evident at autopsy. The median survival of those who develop a blast crisis is only about 6 months.

Extramedullary blast transformation can result in localized tumor masses, which may be found incidentally or cause serious symptoms. Deposits of immature myeloid cells, formerly called granulocytic sarcoma or chloroma, are now most appropriately termed myeloblastoma. Myeloblastomas may be localized or widespread and occur anywhere in the body. Lymph nodes are the most commonly involved, with nodal infiltration preceding marrow transformation by months or years.[90] Other locations of extramedullary blasts deposition in patients with CML include skin, subcutaneous tissues, breasts, bone, and pleural cavity. The incidence of myeloblastoma may be as high as 5 percent in CML (in contrast to 2.5 percent of AML).[91]

Meningeal leukemia may rarely be the first manifestation of blastic transformation, although it more commonly occurs after systemic blast crisis.[91,92] In an NCI series of 101 patients with CML in blastic phase, 7 subsequently developed meningeal leukemia.[91] All seven patients had a cerebrospinal fluid (CSF) pleocytosis (including myeloblasts) and associated neurological features including headaches and cranial nerve palsies.

Localized blastic transformation may also occur within the marrow (intramedullary myeloblastoma), usually involving the bones of the face and cranium. While they may be nonpigmented, green masses may adhere to the sutures, invade the dura, and fill the orbits, oral nasal sinuses, and mastoids. The green color is derived from the abundance of peroxidase enzyme in the myeloblast. Upon exposure to air, the green color rapidly fades and assumes a dirty yellow tinge. In addition to the facial bones, localized blastic transformation may occur in the sternum, ribs, vertebrae, and pelvis (Plates 3–1H–J).

Morphologic Types of Blastic Transformation

As discussed earlier, CML originates in a pluripotent hematopoietic stem cell. Support for this hypothesis was initially derived from the observation that blastic transformation could result in a leukemic syndrome from one of virtually any hematopoietic lineage. Immature cells in patients having undergone blast transformation have included undifferentiated blasts, myeloblasts, promyelocytes, myelomonoblasts, monoblasts, erythroblasts, megakaryoblasts, or lymphoblasts (Table 3–4).[93] Although morphology alone may be suggestive, the use of histochemical, ultrastructural, enzymatic, or immunologic studies allows for accurate classification of the precise subtype of blastic transformation. It is particularly important to exclude lymphoblastic blast crisis, due to the alternative and potentially less toxic therapeutic approach for patients with this type of disorder. The frequency of the phenotypic subgroups of blast crisis in 275 patients, reported by Greaves,[93] is noted in Table 3–4. Approximately two-thirds of patients transform into a disease that represents acute myeloid leukemia, with Auer rod–containing blasts. Azurophilic cytoplasmic granules have been noted in immature cells obtained from patients with an apparent promyelocytic transformation.[93] Serum lysozyme elevations may occur in patients with leukemias that resemble acute monocytic or acute myelomonocytic leukemia.[94] Demonstration of myeloperoxidase at the ultrastructural level may be a clue to the identity of myeloblasts, which may otherwise be classified as undifferentiated blasts or lymphoblasts by routine light microscopy in histochemical stains.[95] The use of cell surface marker studies and molecular biologic techniques now allow for more likely identification of the cell of origin. In the rare patient whose CML

Table 3–4. Morphological and Phenotypic Subgroups of Blastic Crisis in Philadelphia-Positive CML

	No. (%)
Nonlymphocytic (myelocytic or M type)	174 (63)
Rare variants	
Megakaryoblastic	4
Erythroblastic	4
Monoblastic	2
Lymphocytic (L type)	88 (32)
ALL (CD10 +/−)	76
Null ALL	12
T-ALL	0
B-ALL	0
Mixed L + M type	13 (5)
Total	275 (100)

Abbreviations: CML, chronic myelocytic leukemia; ALL, acute lymphocytic leukemia.
(Data from Greaves.[93])

undergoes erythroblastic transformation, morphological features resemble those of erythroleukemia (DiGingIielmo syndrome) although multinucleated and bizarre erythroblasts are not as common as in patients with M6 AML.[96] Erythroblastic transformation can be confirmed by the demonstration of coarse periodic acid-Schiff (PAS) positive granules on histochemical examination or the presence of red cell membrane (e.g., glycophorin) antigens on immunophenotypic analysis.[97] Patients with megakaryoblastic transformation of CML[98,99] may exhibit cells that display megakaryoblasts with a high nuclear to cytoplastic ratio, a round nucleus with one or two nucleoli, and basophilic cytoplasm often containing vacuoles but no granules. Micromegakaryoblasts, characterized by smaller size and prominent cytoplasmic blasts may also be observed. Giant dysplastic platelet and megakaryocytic fragments are sometimes present in the peripheral blood. Because the morphological assessment of patients with acute megakaryoblastic leukemia has been difficult, the demonstration of platelet peroxidase granules on ultrastructural analysis or platelet-specific glycoprotein antigens on immunophenotypic studies may be helpful.[51]

Approximately one-third of patients with blastic transformation show a predominance of lymphoblasts in the peripheral blood and bone marrow.[100] Patients with lymphoblastic transformation have a higher number of blasts, decreased marrow megakaryocytes, and more profound thrombocytopenia, and somewhat less severe anemia than patients with a myeloblastic transformation.[94] Fever, malaise, and splenomegaly may be seen in all patients with blastic transformation and do not appear to be more likely in individuals with a lymphoblastic crisis. Extramedullary lymphoblastic transformation may also occur, especially in soft tissues, lymph nodes, and meninges. Patients with lymphoblastic crisis may live longer than patients with a myeloblastic crisis (6 months vs. 3 months median survival) and are more likely to respond to chemotherapeutic regimens containing vincristine and prednisone.[101]

Variants of CML

There are several disease entities that resemble CML but lack the Philadelphia chromosome or molecular evidence for *bcr-abl* translocation. Patients who are Philadelphia chromosome negative, but *bcr-abl* translocation positive appear to have a similar natural history to those who are Philadelphia chromosome positive.[102] The term *chronic neutrophilic leukemia*, sometimes characterized as Philadelphia-negative CML, has been used to describe those with an elevated white count with a majority of mature neutrophils with no evidence of a Philadelphia translocation.[103] A variant t(9;22) detectable only by molecular methods has recently been described in such patients.[104] It is very important to rule out a leukemoid reaction, especially when an abdominal mass is present that may simulate splenomegaly.

Chronic eosinophilic leukemia, characterized by eosinophilic leukocytosis, the presence of immature eosinophils and myeloblasts, anemia, thrombocytopenia, or thrombocytosis may exhibit cytogenetic abnormalities other than the Philadelphia chromosome.[105] Hepatosplenomegaly lymphadenopathy,

and male predominance (77 percent) have been noted in this entity, which carries a poor prognosis. It is important to distinguish chronic eosinophilic leukemia from the idiopathic hypereosinophilic syndrome as well as reactive eosinophilic leukemoid reactions (e.g., caused by underlying cancer or parasitic infection).[106] Eosinophilic leukemia may present as a chronic myeloproliferative disorder sharing many features of CML, including terminal blast crisis.[107] Eosinophilia and lymphoblastic lymphoma may coexist in patients with a t(8;13), which represents a rearrangement of the fibroblast growth factor gene.[108]

Chronic myelomonocytic leukemia (CMML)[8-10] is characterized by splenomegaly, anemia, thrombocytopenia, leukocytosis (including monocyte and granulocyte cells in all stages of development) and increased blood and urine lysozyme levels. The FAB classification system considers CMML as a myelodysplastic syndrome characterized by the presence of monocytosis (greater than 1000×10^9/L) and myelodysplastic features in the bone marrow that cannot be infiltrated with greater than 20 to 30 percent blasts. The WHO proposal classifies CMML as an overlap syndrome between MDS and MPD[5] (Table 3–1).

Juvenile chronic myelocytic leukemia (JCML) is a rare childhood malignancy characterized by leukocytosis, monocytosis, anemia with ineffective erythropoiesis, hepatosplenomegaly, marrow myeloid hyperplasia with less than 50 percent blasts, and the absence of the Philadelphia chromosome. Cells from patients with JCML seem to be exquisitely sensitive to granulocyte-macrophage colony-stimulating factor (GM-CSF),[109] which suggests a primary pathogenic role for autocrine or paracrine growth factor stimulation as the primary etiologic event in this syndrome. This condition is a clonal disorder[110] that can respond to retinoic acid.[111]

ESSENTIAL THROMBOCYTHEMIA

Essential thrombocythemia (ET) is a clonal disorder[19] characterized by panmyelosis of the bone marrow with a predominance of megakaryocytes resulting in marked thrombocytosis.[112-114] Megakaryocyte progenitors may be hypersensitive to thrombopoietin. The platelet count usually exceeds 10^6/μl. Mild leukocytosis (20 to 30,000/μl) is often present, but the red cell mass is normal (unless iron deficiency occurs due to bleeding) and must be so to distinguish this entity from polycythemia vera. Bone marrow reticulin may be mildly increased, but an excessive degree of fibrosis excludes ET and suggests the entity of agnogenic myeloid metaplasia with myelofibrosis. Although the bone marrow examination is not diagnostic, clusters of atypical and dysplastic megakaryocytes are generally noted[115] (Plate 3–1K). These cells may contain cytoplasmic blebs and may also be observed in the peripheral blood. Large aggregates of platelets including giant and bizarre forms are seen in peripheral blood (Plate 3–1L). The Polycythemia Vera Study Group has established specific criteria for the diagnosis of ET, which have included the absence of overt fibrosis, the absence of the Philadelphia chromosome, a normal red cell mass, and the absence of any explanation for secondary thrombocytosis.[116]

Both bleeding and clotting diathesis have been reported in patients with ET.[117,118] Such problems are believed to be due to associated platelet functional abnormalities rather than to the absolute magnitude of the thrombocytosis, which does not bear a direct relationship to the severity of clinical problems.[119,120] Splenomegaly is unusual: Although transition to acute leukemia is not unknown, the incidence is enhanced by the use of cytotoxic therapeutic agents.[121,122] The clinical course is quite protracted in most patients with an 80 percent survival at 8 years.[123]

AGNOGENIC MYELOID METAPLASIA-MYELOFIBROSIS

Agnogenic myeloid metaplasia-myelofibrosis has been described by at least 37 different names, such as idiopathic myelofibrosis with myeloid metaplasia.[124,125] Patients with this entity generally present with anemia, massive splenomegaly, and nucleated and tear-drop red cell forms in the peripheral blood. Basophilia and an elevation of the white count with a left shift are not uncommon although as the disease progresses, leukopenia may supervene.[126] Early in the disease (before marrow fibrosis occurs) the marrow may be simply hypercellular and the disease unclassifiable. The platelet count may be high, normal, or decreased. Serum B12 and B12 binding proteins tend to be elevated as is the uric acid level, each suggestive of a significant degree of cell turnover.

The bone marrow aspiration in patients with agnogenic myeloid metaplasia-myelofibrosis is frequently unsatisfactory, due either to profound hypercellularity (early disease) or to the fibrous tissue itself, which may be hard and difficult to penetrate. As such, a bone marrow biopsy is required for accurate diagnosis. Several patterns of findings on bone marrow biopsy examination may be noted. Early in the disease, panhyperplasia is common. Clusters of megakaryocytes, erythroblasts, and granulocytic hyperplasia with normal maturation are present. Small mononuclear megakaryocytes have been observed that may be confused with atypical lymphocytes but can be defined due to characteristic demarcation membranes and bullseye granules. Even in this early stage, a minimal increase in reticulum fibers can be demonstrated on silver staining. However, collagen fibers, detectable by the Mallory reagent, are not increased. Such findings are typical of all the myeloproliferative disorders and do not definitively indicate agnogenic myeloid metaplasia-myelofibrosis. In more advanced cases, myeloid atrophy and fibrosis ensue.[128,129] The marrow cavity becomes fibrotic with small areas of hyperplastic hematopoietic tissue arising above the amorphous background substance, which contains reticulin fibers, collagen fibers, plasma cells, and other residual stromal cells. Endothelial cell proliferation due to angiogenic factors has been noted to accompany the progressive fibrosis.[130] Erythroid progenitors tend to become quite sparse.[131] The cellularity is predominantly megakaryocytic. Fat spaces are usually absent and most patients do not have an increase in bone trabeculae. The most advanced stage of myelofibrosis is defined by myelosclerosis in which bone trabeculae occupy 30 percent or more of the biopsy section leaving minimal residual foci of myeloid tissue (composed mainly of megakaryocytes). The noncellular marrow consists of myelofibrotic areas with increased reticulum and myelosclerotic tissue composed of collagenous fibers. This mesenchymally derived tissue is usually adjacent to bone trabeculae, which may be broad, irregular, and contain thickened osteoid seams (Plates 3–1M,N). Despite the presence of new bone formation, osteoblasts and osteoclasts are usually not present.

The degree of bone marrow fibrosis also correlates with the degree of bone marrow osteosclerosis, suggesting that osteosclerosis and megakaryocyte hyperplasia may both have a common origin, potentially due to a factor secreted by the malignant stem cell in this disease. Deposition of extensive amounts of endothelially produced fibronectin, laminin, and collagen type 4 suggests that endothelial cell proliferation as well as fibroblastic proliferation occur.[129] Precisely what cytokines are responsible for the fibroblastic, endothelial, and osteoblastic proliferation in agnogenic myeloid metaplasia remains speculative.

Extramedullary hematopoiesis causing splenomegaly is the hallmark of even moderately advanced AMM. Circulating clonally derived progenitor cells accumulate in splenic cords. Progressive splenomegaly may lead to a huge abdominal mass. The average spleen weight in patients with advanced myeloid metaplasia is 1.5 to 3 kg. Splenic infarcts result in a thickened and scarred capsule. Microscopically, extramedullary hematopoiesis, which involves the red pulp, is always present. A mild to moderate fibrosis of the red pulp may occur with disease progression. The lymphatic follicles in the white pulp usually become atrophic but are uninvolved by myeloid metaplasia. The splenic histopathology at the time of removal for intractable syndromes may have prognostic value; those with a nodular pattern of extramedullary hematopoiesis (EMH) live longer than those with diffuse EMH or primary immature cells.[132,133]

Hepatic myeloid metaplasia (extramedullary hematopoiesis) also commonly occurs in patients with agnogenic myeloid metaplasia-myelofibrosis and may occupy up to 30 percent of the hepatic lobule[134] (Plate 3–1O–Q). The basic liver architecture is preserved, but erythroblasts and megakaryocytes occupy the hepatic sinusoids and granulocytic precursors reside in the portal tracts. This distribution mimics normal mammalian embryotic hematopoiesis. As the disease progresses, the hematopoiesis becomes more immature but neoplastic invasion of the liver does not occur. Hepatic fibrosis is generally minimal, although patients with portal hypertension and cirrhosis have been described.[134,135] Such severe complications may be due to postsinusoidal obstruction (Budd-Chiari syndrome), presinusoidal thrombotic obstruction, or sinusoidal obstruction secondary to EMH coupled with a high portal blood flow.[135]

Patients with agnogenic myeloid metaplasia-myelofibrosis may exhibit EMH in nonreticuloendothelial sites. Areas of myeloid metaplasia consist of two to three committed cell lines (usually erythroid and megakaryocytic) and do not destroy or invade adjacent structures. With lymph node invasion, the architecture remains intact and the cortical follicles are not destroyed.

A leukoerythroblastic blood picture, possibly including up to 10 percent myeloblasts at diagnosis is typically noted.[136] Basophils may be increased. Tear-drop-shaped red cells are the hallmark of this disease (Plates 3–1R,S). Although the degree of bone marrow dysplasia is often minimal, in contrast to the low leukocyte alkaline phosphatase score in CML, the LAP score in agnogenic myeloid metaplasia is usually increased as it is in PCV and ET.

Cytogenetic abnormalities occur in approximately one-third of cases.[137,138] 20q- deletion, interstitial 13q- deletion, and acquired trisomy 20 are the most common abnormalities. Patients with abnormal karyotypes have a significantly shorter survival than those with a normal cytogenetic study (median of 30 months vs. greater than 6 years).[137] Evolution to more complex karyotypic findings may accompany clinical progression.[138] Transition to acute leukemia occurs in less than 10 percent of cases,[139] with some of these patients being previously exposed to alkylating agents.

POLYCYTHEMIA VERA

Polycythemia vera (PCV) is a well-recognized clinical and pathological entity characterized by trilineage hyperplasia of the bone marrow with increased numbers of circulating erythrocytes, granulocytes, and platelets.[140] Splenomegaly is almost always present, but hepatomegaly is less common, although both organs display EMH. PCV is an acquired monoclonal disorder of a pluripotent stem cell resulting in expansion of committed stem cell pools, most prominently the erythroid series.[140,141] Erythroid progenitors proliferate independently, without requiring extrinsic erythropoietin.[142] Cellular maturation is not significantly impaired and the mature peripheral blood cells function normally. The essential feature in the diagnosis of PCV is an (erythropoietin-independent) elevation of the red cell mass without an explanation for secondary erythrocytosis.[143] Bone marrow findings in PCV are not required for diagnosis and are highly variable. More than 90 percent of those with PCV exhibit hypercellular marrows and most have a moderate increase in bone marrow megakaryocytes.[144] Reticulin content is usually normal or slightly increased. Only 5 percent of patients have stainable marrow iron stores, consistent with the iron depletion that typically characterizes this disease.

Patients with PCV may enter a so-called stable phase, during which normal peripheral blood counts are maintained without any specific therapy. During the stable phase, the bone marrow is gradually replaced by progressive fibrosis, and in some cases, a decrease in the proliferative capacity of the residual marrow occurs. Progressive splenomegaly, along with the appearance of anemia, and a leukoerythroblastic blood picture, including the presence of tear-drop red cell forms signify the evolution of PCV into the late (or spent) phase.[145] At this time the bone marrow biopsy will reveal extensive myelofibrosis. The spent phase, which occurs in approximately 10 percent of patients with PCV, develops after mean elapsed time of 7.5 years (range 39 to 144 months) after diagnosis.[145] Occasionally, patients may initially present for evaluation during this spent phase and may

be diagnosed erroneously as agnogenic myeloid metaplasia unless a history of previous increase in the hematocrit or chronic iron deficiency anemia is obtained. Although prior exposure to therapeutic radiation may be a predisposing factor for post-polycythemic myeloid metaplasia, untreated patients have also developed this complication.

Transition to acute leukemia occurs in approximately 10 percent of patients with PCV.[46] Most patients who transform to acute leukemia have received either chlorambucil or P[32] therapy.[146,147] However, there have been documented cases of patients treated with a phlebotomy alone who developed AML.[146,147] The incidence of leukemia in those patients with post-polycythemic myeloid metaplasia was higher than in those without the spent phase, especially when myelosuppressive therapy had been used. As in many cases of post-therapy AML, myelodysplasia may also precede the transformation to acute leukemia[147,148] especially in patients who have received prior alkylating agent, P[32], or even hydroxyurea therapy.[148] Rare cases of transformation to non-Hodgkin's lymphoma[149] and acute lymphoblastic leukemia have been described,[150,151] although more commonly patients with AML following PCV have blasts that bear biphenotypic markers, consistent with derivation from a pluripotent stem cell.[151]

CHRONIC LYMPHOPROLIFERATIVE LEUKEMIAS

The clinical, laboratory, and immunological features of the lymphoproliferative disorders are covered in detail in Chapters 6–8. In this section, certain pathological and morphological findings are reviewed and correlated to clinical parameters when applicable. The WHO classification system (Table 3–5) has defined subgroups based on our biological understanding of the entity. This chapter includes those entities with a prominent leukemic phase.

Chronic Lymphocytic Leukemia

CLL represents a monoclonal proliferation of mature-appearing B lymphocytes, although approximately 5 percent of patients have a T-cell variant.[152–155] Patients with B-cell CLL present with generalized lymphadenopathy, splenomegaly, and/or slowly progressive lymphocytosis. Although lymphocyte counts in patients with CLL may exceed 200,000/µl, in contrast to the "sticky" myeloblasts in AML, leukostatic syndromes (cerebral or lung involvement) are rare.[156] An absolute lymphocyte count of greater than 10,000/µl is required for the diagnosis of CLL. However, it may be possible to suggest the diagnosis of CLL in patients with lower lymphocyte counts, if immunophenotypic analysis documents the presence of cells that have a characteristic surface marker profile.[157] Such immunophenotypic characteristics detailed in Chapter 6 include the presence of B-cell markers, including weak surface immunoglobulin expression with co-expression of the T1 or CD5 nominal T-cell antigen.[158] Fairly specific for the diagnosis of CLL, CD5 expression is also seen on cells from patients with intermediate lymphoma (mantle cell lymphoma). Mantle cell lymphoma is typ-

Table 3–5. WHO Classification System

B-cell neoplasms
  Precursor B-Cell neoplasm
    Precursor B-lymphoblastic leukemia/lymphoma (precursor B-cell acute lymphoblastic leukemia)
  Mature (peripheral) B-cell neoplasms[a]
    B-cell chronic lymphocytic leukemia/small lymphocytic lymphoma
    B-cell prolymphocytic leukemia
    Lymphoplasmacytic lymphoma
    Splenic marginal zone B-cell lymphoma (+/− villous lymphocytes)
    Hairy cell leukemia
    Plasma cell myeloma/plasmacytoma
    Extranodal marginal zone B-cell lymphoma of MALT type
    Nodal marginal zone B-cell lymphoma (+/− monocytoid B cells)
    Follicular lymphoma
    Mantle-cell lymphoma
    Diffuse large B-cell lymphoma
      Mediastinal large B-cell lymphoma
      Primary effusion lymphoma
    Burkitt's lymphoma/Burkitt cell lymphoma
T-cell and NK-cell neoplasms
  Precursor T-cell neoplasm
    Precursor T-lymphoblastic lymphoma/leukemia (precursor T-cell acute lymphoblastic leukemia)
  Mature (peripheral) T-cell neoplasms[a]
    T-cell prolymphocytic leukemia
    T-cell granular lymphocytic leukemia
    Aggressive NK-cell lymphoma
    Adult T-cell lymphoma/leukemia (HTLV1 +)
    Extranodal NK/T-cell lymphoma, nasal type
    Enteropathy-type T-cell lymphoma
    Hepatosplenic gamma-delta T-cell lymphoma
    Subcutaneous panniculitis-like T-cell lymphoma
    Mycosis fungoides/Sézary syndrome
    Anaplastic large cell lymphoma, T/null cell, primary cutaneous type
    Peripheral T-cell lymphoma, not otherwise characterized
    Angioimmunoblastic T-cell lymphoma
    Anaplastic large-cell lymphoma, T/null cell, primary systemic type

Abbreviations: HTLV1 +, human T-cell leukemia virus; MALT, mucosa-associated lymphoid tissue; NK, natural killer.

Note: Only major categories are included. Subtypes and variants will be discussed in the WHO book[2] and are listed in Tables 7 through 16. Common entities are shown in boldface type.

[a] B- and T-/NK-cell neoplasms are grouped according to major clinical presentations (predominantly disseminated/leukemic, primary extranodal, predominantly nodal).

ically CD23 negative, which is positive in CLL. The lack of expression of CD79b and CD22 also distinguishes CLL from other indolent β-cell neoplasms.[159]

Cytogenetic abnormalities, usually trisomy 12, occur in 40 percent of patients with CLL.[160] Patients whose cells carry additional chromosomal abnormalities have a worse prognosis than those who have trisomy 12 as the sole cytogenetic abnormality.[161,162] Atypical morphology and p53 mutations also augur for a worse prognosis.[152] The low proliferative index character-

istic of CLL cells reduces the rate of successful metaphase spreads required for cytogenetic analysis. However, the technique of FISH allows detection of cytogenetic abnormalities in cells from approximately twice as many CLL patients as noted by cytogenetic studies.[163,164] Loss of the 11q23 region (including the ataxia telangiectasia gene) is noted in 20 percent by FISH analysis.[165] Lymphocytes from 50 percent of CLL patients fail to express the tumor suppressor gene, retinoblastoma,[166] which may correlate with 13q14 abnormalities,[167] a common genetic abnormality in CLL. Neoangiogenesis in marrow from CLL may also play a pathophysiological role.[168]

The bone marrow is involved in virtually all patients with CLL. Such involvement varies from focal lymphocytic infiltration to extensive marrow replacement in advanced disease (Plate 3–2A–C). Some investigators have suggested a correlation between specific bone marrow patterns[169] and clinical outcome, whereas others have not found such an association. Patients with diffuse involvement of the bone marrow by neoplastic lymphocytes are more likely to have a worse prognosis than those who present with nodular involvement. Those with a mixture of diffuse and nodular infiltration have an intermediate prognosis. These patterns of bone marrow involvement in CLL may add prognostic information to the commonly used clinical staging systems.[170,171] However, pathogenic and clinical staging are not independent in that those with higher stage involvement have a greater degree of marrow involvement compared with those with lower stage involvement.

Most lymphoid cells infiltrating the marrows of patients with CLL are small lymphocytes, but occasionally large and immature lymphocytes may be present as well. Neoplastic lymphocytic infiltrates may be confused with normal lymphoid follicles, which are generally located adjacent to bone trabeculae and are especially common in elderly patients. Marrow fibrosis is quite rare.[172] Reed-Sternberg-like cells (perhaps activated B cells) have been occasionally noted.[173,174]

Approximately 25 percent of those with CLL will experience an autoimmune hemolytic anemia at some point during their clinical course.[154,175] In such patients, erythroid hyperplasia may be a prominent histological finding on bone marrow examination.

Peripheral blood findings include the presence of numerous small lymphocytes with clumped nuclear chromatin. Smudge cells (lymphocytes damaged during smear preparation) may be evident, as well as occasional medium-size atypical lymphoid cells and rare blastlike cells. Although most of the small lymphocytes appear morphologically normal, occasional cytoplasmic clear spaces, granules, or inclusions (thought to represent endoplasmic reticulum) may be noted.[176] The nuclear envelopes and cisternae of the rough endoplasmic reticulum may contain monoclonal immunoglobulin molecules.[177]

The most common physical finding in patients with CLL is lymphadenopathy, which may include extensive involvement in one or more lymph node sites. The lymph nodes tend to be soft, painless, discrete, and rubbery; however, as the disease progresses, coalescence and attachment to surrounding tissues may result in large fixed masses. Despite the size of such prominent tumors, they arise solely from lymphocytic infiltration within the capsule. The normal lymph node architecture is diffusely replaced by leukemic lymphocytes (Plate 3–2D). The invasive cells in patients with small lymphocytic lymphoma are immunologically and morphologically identical to CLL cells.[178] A variable number of large, more immature-appearing cells may be mixed with the predominant population of small mature cells in lymph nodes.[179] Only about 10 percent of patients can be shown to have marked numbers of immature or blastic lymphoid cells in involved lymph nodes: It is possible that clonal evolution of these immature cells may result in acute leukemia or lymphomatous transformation of CLL into a more aggressive entity.

The spleen, occasionally weighing more than 1 kg in advanced cases, is almost always enlarged in patients with CLL. In contrast to CML, splenic infarction is rarely noted. Microscopic findings in the spleen in patients with CLL are similar to those present in lymph nodes. Normal architecture is replaced by a monotonous infiltrate of small lymphocytes. Iron pigment may be prominent because of chronic hemolysis. The liver may be slightly enlarged as a result of lymphocytic infiltration of periportal tracts and occasional nodular masses that encroach on the parenchyma. Unlike CML, hepatic sinusoids are rarely infiltrated. Almost any other organ or site (particularly the gastrointestinal tract or kidney)[180] may be infiltrated by lymphocytes although diffuse involvement is uncommon. Central nervous system (CNS) involvement,[181] including leptomeningeal spiral,[182] is rare. Exaggerated reactions to insect bites have been reported in patients with CLL; however, clinical pathological examination of such alledged lesions typically reveals no evidence of a bite.[183]

That there are rare cases of "true" T-cell CLL that behave in an indolent fashion similar to their B-cell counterparts is debatable. In fact, the WHO system (Table 3–5) does not include T-cell CLL but rather several T-cell neoplasms that may be confused with CLL, including adult T-cell leukemia or lymphoma (ATCLL), which occurs in those infected with the HTLV-1 retrovirus (endemic in the southern Japanese island of Kyushu and in the Caribbean).[184,185] Patients with ATCLL tend to present with lymphadenopathy, hypercalcemia, and leukocytosis. Lymph node biopsies and examination of the peripheral blood smear reveals pleomorphic large cells that have immunophenotypic characteristics of the CD8 T-cell subset. Skin lesions, a predilection for CNS involvement, neutropenia, and marrow involvement are also common in this aggressive disease. Morphologically, peripheral T cells from such patients may have a convoluted cerebriform nuclear appearance and scant cytoplasm (Plate 3–2E, F).[185] Occasional cells have a more immature nucleus with a nucleolus and basophilic cytoplasm, resembling prolymphocytes.

Other T-cell chronic leukemias include T-cell granular lymphocytic leukemia, formerly called T-cell lymphocytosis and cytopenia, characterized by an indolent clinical course in most patients, granulocyte or erythrocyte aplasia in the marrow, and a strong association with rheumatoid arthritis.[186–190] The lymphocytes display a characteristic immunophenotype: CD8 (suppressor cell) positive; weak (or **no**) positivity for CD5, Leu-7, and Fc receptors. Importantly, such patients also have CD56

positivity, which is associated with the natural killer (NK) cell phenotype. The morphological hallmark of cells from patients with this disorder are their large size and the presence of acid phosphatase positive azurophilic granules.[187,188] Marrow findings may include nonparatrabecular lymphoid infiltrates, lymphadenopathy is rare, and red pulp cord and sinus infiltrates in the spleen.[191] This so-called large granular lymphocytic leukemia (LGL) has been defined as a T-cell neoplasm.[192] Most patients with this entity have a relatively benign clinical course, although fatal blastic transformation has been described.[193] The CD8+ entity, which is an indolent proliferative process, is generally readily distinguished from an aggressive rapidly fatal disease, termed NK-cell leukemia.[193,194]

Patients with CLL may develop (or "transform" to) a more aggressive clinical entity. Transformation of CLL to a malignant large cell lymphoma,[195,196] called Richter's syndrome, is discussed in Chapter 6. Development of prolymphocytic leukemia during the course of CLL has also been reported (see below). Rarely, CLL may transform into an acute leukemia, with one case of simultaneous CLL and AML having been reported.[197] Moreover, it is also possible for the CLL cells to clonally evolve into a disease resembling ALL.

Prolymphocytic Leukemia

Prolymphocytic leukemia (PLL), once thought to be a variant of CLL,[198] is now a well-characterized clinicopathological entity characterized by specific morphological, immunophenotypic, and histological criteria.[199,200] The relative frequency of PLL among patients with chronic lymphoproliferative disorders at one large center was 10 percent compared with 80 percent for CLL and 10 percent for hairy cell leukemia.[201] B-cell PLL accounts for approximately 80 percent of cases with the more aggressive T-cell PLL accounting for the remainder. PLL is clinically distinct from CLL on the basis of prominent splenomegaly, minimal adenopathy, and extreme leukocytosis with about 50 percent of patients displaying thrombocytopenia, consistent with advanced stage disease (Plate 3–2G,H).

The prolymphocyte is larger than the typical mature lymphocyte of CLL, contains more cytoplasm, and has a prominent nucleolus; however, in contrast to a lymphoblast, nuclear chromatin is relatively condensed (Plate 3–2I). Ultrastructural features include scarce polyribosomes and lysosomes, poorly developed Golgi apparatus, and short segments of rough endoplasmic reticulum.[200] Morphologic variants such as cells with nuclear clefting and intermediate forms with a size between PLL cells and CLL cells may account for up to 20 percent of the WBC differential.[199] Patients with between 10 and 55 percent circulating prolymphocytes have intermediate features between CLL and PLL.[202] PLL may be immunophenotypically distinguished from CLL due to a more intense staining for surface IgM and IgD and inability to form rosettes with mouse blood cells.[201] Importantly, the CD5 antigen, characteristic of CLL cells, is not expressed on PLL cells. The alpha-naphthyl acetate esterase (ANAE; nonspecific esterase) stain is strongly positive in T-cell PLL; the acid phosphatase reaction tends to be stronger in T-cell PLL then in B-cell PLL.[199,203]

Table 3–6. Features of Hairy-Cell Leukemia and Similar Disorders

	Hairy-Cell Leukemia	Chronic Lymphocytic Leukemia	B-Cell Promyelocytic Leukemia	Splenic Lymphoma with Villous Lymphocytes	Hairy-Cell Leukemia Variant
M:F ratio	4:1	1.5:1	1.5:1	2:1	4:1
Palpable splenomegaly	75–90%	>50%	>90%	80%	>90%
Palpable lymphadenopathy	5%	70%	30%	25%	<5%
Pattern of marrow involvement	Patchy or diffuse	Nodular and/or interstitial or diffuse	Nodular and/or patchy, diffuse; diffuse	Nodular, or diffuse; occasionally no detectable infiltration	Patchy or interstitial
Pattern of splenic involvement	Red pulp	White pulp	White pulp	White pulp	Red pulp
Mean WBC ($\times 10^9$/L)	5	112	175	17	88
Tartrate-resistant acid phosphatase	±	–	±	–	+
Immunophenotype					
CD5	–	+	±	±	–
CD11c	+	–	–	±	NI
CD19	+	+	+	+	+
CD25	+	–	–	±	–
sIg	μ, δ, α, γ (moderate)	μ, δ (weak)	μ, δ (strong)	μ, δ, α, γ (moderate)	γ (moderate)
FMC7	+	–	+	+/–	+/–

Note: +, Positive in most cases; –, negative in most cases; ±, some cases positive; NI, no information available. (Data from Greaves.[93])

Cells from patients with T-cell PLL often contain large electron-dense granules. T-cell PLL cells are generally CD4+ and CD8–; however, other patterns may exist in about one-third of patients.[204] Inversion in the long arm of chromosome 14 and trisomy of the long arm of chromosome 8 have been reported in at least one-half of the cases of T-cell PLL.[205] Whether a human lymphotrophic retrovirus is involved in the pathogenesis of T-PLL is controversial.[206]

The higher density of surface immunoglobulins and pattern of heavy chain overexpression suggests that the prolymphocyte is immunologically more mature than the B lymphocyte of CLL. Therefore, the word "prolymphocyte" is misleading. About one-third of patients with PLL display circulating monoclonal immunoglobulin compared to about 5 percent in those with CLL.[201] Despite the apparent derivation from a more mature B cell, the clinical course in patients with B-cell PLL is much more aggressive than observed in patients with typical CLL.[199] Some cases of apparent B-cell PLL exhibit the t(11;14)(q13;q32) cytogenetic abnormality typical of mantle cell lymphoma.[207]

Prolymphocytic transformation may rarely occur in patients with CLL. Careful observation of blood smears from patients with CLL suggest that many do contain at least some prolymphocytes.[201] Prolymphocytic transformation is arbitrarily defined as the presence of more than 55 percent prolymphocytes in the blood. Spleens from patients with PLL are infiltrated with neoplastic lymphoid cells that replace both the red and white pulp (both diffuse and nodular areas).[208] The bone marrow usually shows a diffuse and nodular pattern of involvement with almost total replacement of normal marrow elements. A pseudonodular pattern may be noted in lymph nodes and is associated with almost complete obliteration of architecture. The liver and almost every other organ, including the heart,[209] may also be diffusely infiltrated with neoplastic prolymphocytes in advanced cases.[208]

Hairy Cell Leukemia

Formerly called leukemic reticuloendotheliosis,[210–215] hairy cell leukemia is a well-characterized clinico-pathologic entity for which several successful treatment strategies exist. This disorder was first recognized by Rosenthal and colleagues[212] as well as Bouroncle and co-workers[210] in the 1950s, but was first characterized as hairy cell leukemia after Schrek and Donnelly[213] described the hairy villous cytoplasmic projections of the leukemic cells viewed under phase microscopy in 1966.

Hairy cell leukemia is characterized by chronic anemia or pancytopenia, with variable numbers of hairy cells in the peripheral blood, progressive splenomegaly, slight hepatomegaly, and minimal or no lymphadenopathy.[214] Hairy cells are clonal late B cells, displaying certain immunological features of activation (strong expression of surface immunoglobulin, light chain restricted, CD22, CD25, CD7 and CD40 ligand, CD110).[215] Unusual infections, such as atypical mycobacterial dissemination, may occur.[216] The differential diagnosis of this condition includes malignant lymphoma, CLL, myelofibrosis, acute monocytic leukemia, or idiopathic hypersplenism. Wright-stained hairy cells have an agranular clay-blue cytoplasm and are slightly larger than mature lymphocytes. The cell border is irregular and serrated due to characteristic "hair" cytoplasmic projections or filamentous villi. In some cells, only scant or disrupted cytoplasm is present (Plate 3–2J). The nucleus may be eccentric and is usually round but may be oval or indented with a distinct nuclear membrane. The chromatin is delicate and lacy, rather than clumped as in mature lymphocytes. Single

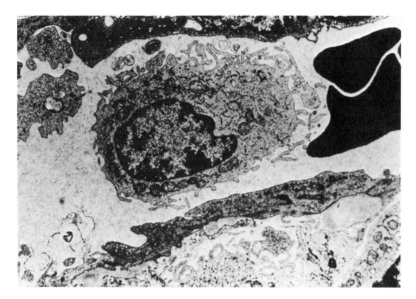

Figure 3–1. Ultrastructural features of a hairy cell within splenic sinusoid. Note typical multiple filamentous cytoplasmic projections. Characteristic ribosome-lamella complexes are not readily seen at this magnification (× 9000).

nucleoli are occasionally evident. An uncommon prolymphocytic variant is characterized by large hairy cells (12 to 30 mm) containing round central nuclei, with condensed chromatin and a single prominent small- to medium-sized nucleolus in approximately 90 percent of cells.[217] The morphology of hairy cells may also be readily visualized by the use of supravital stains or phase microscopy. The most characteristic ultrastructural findings are pseudopods and long cytoplasmic microvilli on the cell surface that measure less than 4 μm in length[218] (Figure 3–1). In addition to several cellular organelles, a distinctive ribosomal-lamellar complex may be noted.[219]

A positive tartrate-resistant acid phosphatase (TRAP) reaction probably also reflective of B-cell activation, historically was a useful confirmatory cytochemical test for the diagnosis of hairy cell leukemia.[220] While hairy cells in the vast majority of cases show a positive TRAP stain (Plate 3–2K), the proportion of positive cells is variable and, in rare patients, may be negative.[220,221] Patients with lymphocytic lymphoma, T-cell CLL, PLL, and Sézary syndrome may also be TRAP positive.[221–223] Because of these limitations, the diagnosis of hairy cell leukemia now rests in the characteristic morphology on trephine biology, typical immunophenotypic pattern (B cells that are CD22+, CD25+, and CD11c+), and characteristic immunocytochemical stains (e.g., DBA44).[224] High levels of cyclin D1 expression, noted in patients with mantle cell lymphoma [with a t(11;14)(q13;q32)] cytogenetic translocation have also been noted in marrows from hairy cell leukemia patients.[225]

The expression of B-cell activation antigens on the surface of hairy cells has taken on a new importance given the availability of monoclonal antibodies with therapeutic utility. An anti-CD25 monoclonal antibody fused to a truncated form of pseudomonas exotoxin may have such a role.[226] Recently a report described responses in a hairy cell leukemia patient failing nucleoside analogue therapy treated with a toxin-linked anti-CD22 antibody.[227]

Attempts at bone marrow aspiration are usually unsuccessful because of marked increase in the reticulum fibers. Diagnostic bone marrow biopsies from patients with hairy cell leukemia reveal diffuse bone marrow involvement (although patchy distribution is also rarely possible) and a hypercellular marrow often diffusely infiltrated with hairy cells (Plate 3–2L,M). It is presumed that hairy cells either directly or indirectly suppress normal hematopoiesis.[228] The mechanism of fibrosis in hairy cell leukemia is likely a reaction to certain surface characteristics and secreted products (e.g., fibronectin) of the malignant cell.[214] Cells derived from patients with hairy cell leukemia were shown to produce basic fibroblast growth factor,[229] which could be a survival and pro-fibrotic factor.

Marked splenomegaly eventually develops in most patients, with 50 percent weighing greater than 1 kg. The cut surface of the spleen is firm, red, and may display old infarctions. The splenic white pulp is conspicuous and gross tumor nodules are not present. Hairy cells infiltrate the red pulp, with the extensive involvement resulting in marked widening of the pulp cords. A reactive proliferation of ellipsoidal histiocytes also occurs in the red pulp, and reticulum fibers are increased. Such phagocytic cells are partly responsible for the secondary hypersplenism that occurs due to extension of the red pulp.[230] The red pulp encroaches on the white pulp, usually resulting in reduction in the diameter of the Malpighian corpuscles, which eventually consist of small lymphocytes, devoid of reaction centers. Formation of characteristic sinuslike structures (or blood lakes) with hairy cells arranged in a luminal side has been described. Those blood lakes may be seen grossly (Plate 3–2N,O). The white pulp eventually atrophies. Morphologically, hairy cells appear to have indistinct nucleoli and no mitosis. Ultrastructural studies suggest that hairy cells adhere to many cell surfaces and structures within the spleen.[230,231] Collections of hairy cells within the subendothelial lymphatic sinuses and cords may impede splenic blood flow, resulting in sinus dilation with formation of abnormal sinuses and blood-filled spaces.[201,231]

Involvement of the liver by hairy cell leukemia is not usually a clinical problem (Plate 3–2P), although sensitive techniques may identify hairy cells in liver biopsy specimens.[232] Abnormal liver function tests are more likely to be associated with other diseases rather than direct hairy cell infiltration of the liver.[232]

Hairy Cell Leukemia: Closely Related Entities

The mature-appearing lymphocytes of CLL may occasionally be confused with hairy cells, but are usually readily distinguished on the basis of morphology, immunophenotype (CD5 positivity and weak surface immunoglobulin staining), and cytochemistry (TRAP-negative) (Table 3–6). A hairy cell leukemia variant has been described[217] in which the white count tends to be higher than in the typical disease, although almost all other features tend to be similar. In addition, the interleukin-2 receptor (CD25) is not expressed as commonly in the variant as it tends to be in straightforward cases. The clinical course of hairy cell leukemia variant tends to be aggressive.

Splenic lymphoma with villous lymphocytes[233] is similar to hairy cell leukemia with prominent splenomegaly, but lymphadenopathy is more common and bone marrow infiltration is less striking than in hairy cell leukemia. The malignant lymphocytes have thin, short, and unevenly distributed villi. The immunophenotypic features are variable with occasional CD5 positivity as in CLL and CD25 expression in hairy cell leukemia.[234] The more clinically aggressive behavior of splenic lymphoma with villous lymphocytes may be accounted for, in some patients, by abnormalities of the p53 tumor suppressor gene,[235] which occurs in about 20 percent. Lymphadenopathy is also common in monocytoid B-cell lymphoma, characterized by CD5+ small lymphocytes without projections and rare bone marrow involvement.[236,237]

Sézary Syndrome

Sézary syndrome is one of several closely related clinicopathological entities referred to as cutaneous T-cell lymphoma (CTCL).[238–242] The most commonly occurring entity, mycosis fungoides, is characterized by chronic, slowly progressive cutaneous lesions (plaques and nodules) with eventual adenopathy, bone marrow involvement, and systemic disease.[243,244] These disorders are caused by the proliferation of mature T cells (CD4 or helper cell phenotype positive) that have a high affinity for the skin.[245] Sézary syndrome refers to one phase of CTCL characterized by intense erythroderma, extreme pruritus, adenopathy, splenomegaly, and a leukemic blood picture.[239,240] Clonal cytogenetic abnormalities and rearrangements of the T-cell antigen receptor gene have confirmed the monoclonal proliferation of these disorders.

Morphologically, Sézary cells are either small (approximately 8 μm) or larger (approximately 15 to 20 μm), the latter reportedly reflecting a block in the cell cycle between G1 and S phase.[239] Sézary cells contain a hyperchromatic convoluted or cerebriform nucleus, which is more serpentine than the convoluted nuclei in T-cell lymphoblastic lymphoma (Plate 3–2Q). Similar-appearing peripheral T cells with cerebriform nuclear contours may rarely be found in patients with non-Hodgkin's lymphoma of the diffuse mixed cell type,[246] although they generally are pathognomonic for CTCL. Sézary cells have also been observed in the skin and blood of patients with a number of benign dermatoses, including erythrodermic eczema, psoriasis, lichen planus, and actinic reticuloid.[247] However, while Sézary cells are CD4+, in chronic actinic dermatitis the cells are immunophenotypically suppressor cells (CD8+). A case of pseudo-Sézary syndrome has been reported in a patient with the acquired immunodeficiency syndrome.[248] Intense erythroid skin infiltration developed as a result of skin infiltration by large atypical lymphoid cells, although Sézary-like cells appeared in the blood. CD8+ and T-cell receptor gene rearrangements were not present, suggesting that this was a polyclonal reaction.[248]

The marked nuclear irregularity of Sézary cells is well seen on ultrastructural analysis.[239,249] Cytogenetic studies have shown serial changes over time from hypo- or pseudodiploidy to hyperdiploidy, near-tetraploidy that correlates with the appearance of large Sézary cells, poor prognosis, and short survival.[250] The WBC count in patients with Sézary syndrome may range from 8.0 to several hundred $\times 10^9$/L with all the cells being neoplastic T cells.[239] Higher leukocyte counts occur in patients with nodal and visceral involvement, but do not bear a relationship to the stage of cutaneous disease. The proliferation of hairy cells may involve constitutive interleukin (IL)-2 receptor alpha expression on the basis of STAT3 (intracellular signaling enzyme) activation.[251] Moreover, sensitive detection techniques can delineate small numbers of Sézary-type cells in the peripheral blood of some patients with early stage mycosis fungoides.[240,252]

Histopathologically, patients with CTCL typically display epidermal involvement with T lymphocytes that may form small clusters of neoplastic and reactive cells called Pautrier's microabscesses.[239,242] Patients whose cutaneous lesions display a predominance of immature cells appear to have a worse prognosis than those with more well-differentiated cells,[253] although clinical stage (e.g., nodal or visceral involvement) is probably a more important factor.

Lymph node biopsy may reveal dermatopathic lymphadenopathy or a variable degree of involvement by malignant convoluted T cells.[254,255] The T-cell zones (paracortical areas) are preferentially infiltrated, but early involvement is not associated with destruction of lymph node architecture.[255] Infiltration of the spleen is also typical and involves the periarteriolar sheets and red pulp.[242] Although not often recognized during life, autopsy studies document the involvement of visceral organs in most patients with CTCL.[256] Pulmonary involvement has been reported, even when the skin eruption has improved.[257] The cellular composition of such involvement closely resembles the cutaneous lesions, although there is a preservation of parenchymal tissue, despite heavy infiltration with the neoplastic T cells.[244] Portal areas may be involved, as in Hodgkin's disease, or the hepatic parenchyma may be infiltrated, as in myeloid leukemia and malignant histiocytosis. The extensive lesions found in autopsy studies are not surprising, in view of prospective staging studies indicating a high frequency of generally asymptomatic extracutaneous dissemination occurring early in the course of disease.[243,244]

Transition of patients with Sézary syndrome into a more aggressive phase of the disease, including a change in morphology (transformation to a large cell lymphoma) of the malignant cells has been reported.[258,259] The large cells express helper T-cell markers suggesting direct evolution from the preceding Sézary cells. This transformation event is more likely in patients with advanced CTCL and carries with it a poor prognosis.[260] The development of a malignant B-cell disorder (plasma cell myeloma) has been reported in a patient with long-standing CTCL.[261] In this case it was postulated that sustained helper cell T-cell activity caused polyclonal plasma cell proliferation with eventual emergence of a monoclonal plasma cell population. There is also a slight increased risk of other malignancies, particularly lung and colon cancer, in patients with long-standing CTCL.[262,263]

REFERENCES

1. Stam K, Heisterkamp N, Grosveld G, et al: Evidence of a new chimeric bcr/c-abl mRNA in patients with chronic myelocytic leukemia and the Philadelphia chromosome. N Engl J Med 313:1429–1433, 1985.

2. Dameshek W: Foreword and a proposal for considering paroxysmal nocturnal hemoglobinuria (PNH) as a "candidate" myeloproliferative disorder. Blood 33:263, 1969.

3. Ward HP, Block MH: The natural history of agnogenic myeloid metaplasia (AMM) and a critical evaluation of its relationship with the myeloproliferative syndrome. Medicine (Baltimore) 50:357, 1971.

4. Bennett JM, Catovsky D, Daniel MT, et al: Proposed revised criteria for the classification of acute myeloid leukemia. Ann Intern Med 103:626–629, 1985.

5. Harris NL, Jaffe ES, Diebold J, et al: World Health Organization Classification of Neoplastic Diseases of the Hematopoietic and Lymphoid Tissues: Report of the Clinical Advisory Committee Meeting—Airlie House, Virginia. JCO 17:3835–3849, 1999.

6. Heany ML, Golde DW: Myelodysplasia. N Engl J Med 340:1649–1660, 1999.

7. Bennett JM, Catovsky D, Daniel MT, et al: Proposals for the classification of myelodysplastic syndromes. Br J Haematol 51:189, 1982.

8. Storniolo AM, Moloney WC, Rosenthal DS, et al: Chronic myelomonocytic leukemia. Leukemia 4:766–770, 1990.

9. Bain RJ: Leuk Lymph 34:443–449, 1999.

10. Germing U, Gattermann N, Minning H: Increasing incidence of myelodysplastic syndromes: Real or ficticious? Leuk Res 22:871–878, 1999.

11. Berk PD, Goldberg JD, Donovan PB, et al: Therapeutic recommendations based on polycythemia vera study group protocols. Semin Oncol 23:132, 1986.

12. Marks SM, McCaffrey R, Rosenthal DS, et al: Blastic transformation in chronic myelogenous leukemia: Experience with 50 patients. Medical Pediatr Oncol 4:159–167, 1978.

13. Fialkow PJ, Jacobson RJ, Papayannopoulou T: Chronic myelocytic leukemia: Clonal origin in a stem cell common to the granulocyte, erythrocyte, platelet and monocyte/macrophage. Ann J Med 63:125, 1977.

14. Groffen J, Stephenson JR, Heisterkamp N, et al: Philadelphia chromosomal breakpoints are clustered within a limited region, bcr, on chromosome 22. Cell 36:93, 1984.

15. Lee MS, Chang KS, Freireich EJ, et al: Detection of minimal chain reaction BCR/ABL transcripts by a modified polymerase chain reaction. Blood 72:893, 1988.

16. Busque L, Zhu J, DeHart D, et al: An expression based clonality assay at the human androgen receptor locus (HUMARA) on chromosome X. Nucleic Acid Res 22:697, 1994.

17. Adamson JW, Fialkow PS, Murphy S, et al: Polycythemia vera: Stem cell and probable clonal origin of the disease. N Engl J Med 295:913, 1976.

18. Kreipe H, Jaquet K, Felgner J, et al: Clonal granulocytes and bone marrow cells in the cellular phase of agnogenic myeloid metaplasia. Blood 78:1814–1817, 1991.

19. Fialkow PJ, Faguet GB, Jacobson RJ, et al: Evidence that essential thrombocythemia is a clonal disorder with origin in a multipotent stem cell. Blood 58:916, 1981.

20. Price CM, Kanfer EJ, Colman SM, et al: Simultaneous genotypic and immunophenotypic analysis of interphase cells using dual-color fluorescence: A demonstration of lineage involvement in polycythemia vera. Blood 80:1033–1038, 1992.

21. Jacobson RJ, Salo A, Fialkow PJ: Agnogenic myeloid metaplasia: A clonal proliferation of hematopoietic stem cells with secondary myelofibrosis. Blood 51:189, 1978.

22. Groopman J: The pathogenesis of myelofibrosis in myeloproliferative disorders. Ann Intern Med 92:857, 1980.

23. Castro-Malaspina H, Rabellino EM, Yen A, et al: Human megakaryocyte stimulation of proliferation in bone marrow fibroblasts. Blood 57:781, 1981.

24. Le Bousse-Kerdiles MC, Souyri M, Smadja-Joffe F, et al: Enhanced hematopoietic growth factor production in an experimental myeloproliferative syndrome. Blood 79:3179–3187, 1992.

25. Liote F, Yeni P, Teillet-Thiebaud F, et al: Ascites revealing peritoneal and hepatic extramedullary hematopoiesis with peliosis in agnogenic myeloid metaplasia: Case report and review of the literature. Am J Med 90:111–117, 1991.

26. Asakura S, Colby TV: Agnogenic myeloid metaplasia with extramedullary hematopoiesis and fibrosis in the lung. Chest 105:1866–1868, 1994.

27. Koch BL, Bisset GS, Bisset RR, et al: Intracranial extramedullary hematopoiesis: MR findings with pathologic correlation. Am J Roentgenol 162:1419–1420, 1994.

28. Glew RH, Haese WH, McIntyre PA: Myeloid metaplasia with myelofibrosis: The clinical spectrum of extramedullary hematopoiesis and tumor formation. Johns Hopkins Med J 132:253, 1973.

29. Zonderland HM, Michiels JJ, Kate RJ: Case report: Mammographic and sonographic demonstration of extramedullary haematopoiesis of the breast. Clin Radiol 44:64–65, 1991.

30. Tuite MJ, Weiss SL: Ultrasound and computed tomographic appearance of extramedullary hematopoiesis encasing the renal pelvis. J Clin Ultrasound 19:238–240, 1991.

31. Smith BD, Moliterno AR: Biology and management of idiopathic myelofibrosis. Curr Opin Oncol 13:91–94, 2001.

32. Sawyers CL: Chronic myeloid leukemia. N Engl J Med 340:1330, 1999.

33. Tomasson MH, Williams IR, Li S, et al: Induction of myeloproliferation disease in mice does not require granulocyte-macrophage colony stimulating factor or interleukin-3. Blood 97:1435, 2001.

34. Druker BJ, Sawyers CL, Kanterjian H, et al: Activity of a specific inhibition of the bcr-abl tyrosine kinase in the blast crisis of chronic myeloid leukemia and acute lymphoblastic leukemia with the Philadelphia chromosome. N Engl J Med 34:1038, 2001.

35. Golub TR, Barker G, Lovett M, Gilliland DG: Fusion of PDGF receptor beta to a novel ets-like gene, tel, in chronic myelomonocytic leukemia with t(5;12) chromosomal translocation. Cell 77:307, 1994.

36. Ross TS, Bernard O, Berger R, Gilliland DG: Fusion of Huntington interacting protein 1 to platelet-derived growth factor beta receptor in chronic myelomonocytic leukemia with t(5;7) (q33;q11,2). Blood 91:4419, 1998.

37. Hinshelwood S, Bench AJ, Green AR: Pathogenesis of polycythemia vera. Blood Rev 11:224, 1997.

38. Taskin AL, Covedic JPL, Dusanter-Fourt I, et al: Autonomous megakaryocytic growth in essential thrombocytopenia and ideopathic myelofibrosis is not related to a c-mpl mutation or to an autocrine stimulation by mpl. Blood 89:125, 1999.

39. Cheson BD, Cassileth PA, Head DR, et al: Report of the National Cancer Institute-sponsored workshop on definitions of diagnosis and response in acute myeloid leukemia. J Clin Oncol 8:813–819, 1990.

40. Appelbaum FR, Fefer A: The pathogenesis of aplastic anemia. Semin Hematol 18:241, 1981.

41. Rosse WF, Parker CJ: Paroxysmal nocturnal hemoglobinurea. Clin Haematol 14:105, 1985.

42. Janssen JWG, Buschle M, Layton M, et al: Clonal analysis of myelodysplastic syndromes: Evidence of multipotent stem cell origin. Blood 73:248, 1989.

43. Greenberg P, Cox C, Le Bean MM, et al: International scoring system for evaluating prognosis in myelodysplastic syndromes. Blood 89:2079, 1997.

44. Kimura A, et al: Blastic transformation in essential thrombocythemia. Cancer 65:1538–1544, 1990.

45. Meytes D, Katz D, Ramot B: Preleukemia and leukemia in polycythemia vera. Blood 47:237, 1976.

46. Rosenthal DS, Maloney WC: Occurrence of acute leukemia in the myeloproliferative disorders. Br J Hematol 36:373, 1977.

47. Berk PD, Goldberg JD, Silverstein MN, et al: Increased incidence of acute leukemia in polycythemia vera associated with chlorambucil therapy. N Engl J Med 304:441, 1981.

48. Paquette RL, Meshkinpour A, Rosen PJ: Autoimmune myelofibrosis. A steroid-responsive cause of bone marrow fibrosis associated with systemic lupus erythematosus. Medicine (Baltimore) 73:145–152, 1994.

49. Golomb HM, Catovsky D, Golde DW: Hairy cell leukemia. Ann Intern Med 89:677, 1978.

50. Manoharan A, Horsley R, Pitney WR: The reticulin content of bone marrow in acute leukaemia in adults. Br J Haematol 43:185, 1979.

51. San Miguel S, Gonzalez M, Canizo MC, et al: Leukemias with megakaryoblastic involvement: Clinical, hematologic, and immunologic characteristics. Blood 72:402–407, 1988.

52. Rubins JM: The role of myelofibrosis in malignant leukoerythroblastosis. Cancer 51:308, 1983.

53. Coughlin C, Greenwald WS, Schraft WC, et al: Myelofibrosis associated with multiple myeloma. Arch Intern Med 138:590, 1978.

54. Kiely JM, Silverstein MN: Metastatic carcinoma simulating agnogenic myeloid metaplasia and myelofibrosis. Cancer 24:1041, 1969.

55. Kiang DR, McKenna RW, Kennedy BJ: Reversal of myelofibrosis in advanced breast cancer. Am J Med 64:173, 1978.

56. Newcom SR, O'Rourke L: Oat-cell carcinoma with fibrosis. Cancer 49:2358, 1982.

57. Janssens AM, Offner FC, Van Hove WZ: Bone marrow necrosis. Cancer 88:1769, 2000.

58. Majumdar G, Phillips JK, Pearson TC: Massive bone marrow necrosis and postnecrotic myelofibrosis in a patient with primary thrombocythaemia. J Clin Pathol 47:674–676, 1994.

59. Kurzrock R, Bueso-Ramos CE, Kantarjian et al: BCR rearrangement-negative chronic myelogenous leukemia revisited. J Clin Oncol 19:2915, 2001.

60. Stoll DB, Peterson P, Exten R, et al: Clinical presentation and natural history of patients with essential thrombocythemia and the Philadelphia chromosome. Am J Hematol 27:77–83, 1988.

61. Nowell PC, Kant JA, Finan JB, et al: Marrow fibrosis associated with a Philadelphia chromosome. Cancer Genet Cytogenet 59:89–92, 1992.

62. Pui CH, Evans WE: Acute lymphoblastic leukemia. N Engl J Med 339:605, 1998.

63. Kantarjian HM, Talpaz M, Dhingra K, et al: Significance of the p210 versus p190 molecular abnormalities in adults with Philadelphia chromosome positive acute leukemia. Blood 78:2411–2418, 1991.

64. Maloney WC: Natural history of chronic granulocytic leukaemia. Clin Haematol 6:41–53, 1977.

65. Silver RT: Chronic myeloid leukemia: A perspective of the clinical and biologic issues of the chronic phase. Hem Onc Clin N Am 4:319, 1990.

66. Dosik H, Rosner F, Sawitsky A: Acquired lipidosis: Gaucher-like cells and "blue-cells" in chronic granulocytic leukemia. Semin Hematol 9:309, 1972.

67. Peters SP, Lee RE, Glew RH: Gaucher's disease, a review. Medicine (Baltimore) 56:425, 1977.

68. Silverstein MN, Ellefson RD: The syndrome of the sea-blue histiocyte. Semin Hematol 9:299, 1972.

69. Gralnick HR, Harbor J, Vogel C: Myelofibrosis in chronic granulocytic leukemia. Blood 37:152, 1971.

70. Buyssens N, Bourgeois NH: Chronic myelocytic leukemia versus idiopathic myelofibrosis. Cancer 40:1548, 1977.

71. Morley AA, Baikie AG, Galton D: Cyclical leucocytosis as evidence of retention of normal homeostatic control in chronic granulocytic leukemia. Lancet 2:1320, 1967.

72. Denburg JA, Wilson WEC, Bienstock J: Basophil production in myeloproliferative disorders: increases during acute blastic transformation of chronic myeloid leukemia. Blood 60:113, 1982.

73. Theologides A: Unfavorable signs in patients with chronic myelocytic leukemia. Ann Intern Med 76:95, 1972.

74. Mason JE, DeVita VT, Canellos GP: Thrombocytosis in chronic granulocytic leukemia: Incidence and clinical significance. Blood 44:483, 1974.

75. Sokal JE, Cox EB, Baccarani M, et al: Prognostic discrimination in "good-risk" chronic granulocytic leukemia. Blood 63:789–799, 1984.

76. Chabner BA, Haskell CM, Canellos GP: Destructive bone lesions in chronic granulocytic leukemia. Medicine (Baltimore) 48:401, 1969.

77. Campbell EJ, Maldonado W, Suhrland G: Painful lytic bone lesion in an adult with chronic myelogenous leukemia. Cancer 35:1354, 1975.

78. Longo DL, Whang-Peng J, Jaffe E, et al: Myeloproliferative syndromes: A unique presentation of chronic myelogenous leukemia (CML) as a primary tumor of bone. Blood 52:793, 1978.

79. Joyner MV, Dujardin P, Cassuto JP, et al: Hypercalcemia as complication of accelerated chronic granulocytic leukaemia. BMJ 2:1060, 1977.

80. Walter RM, Greenberg BR: Hypercalcemia in the accelerated phase of chronic myelogenous leukemia. Cancer 46:1174, 1980.

81. Barton JC, Conrad ME, Poon MC: Pseudochloroma: Extramedullary hematopoietic nodules in chronic myelogenous leukemia. Ann Intern Med 91:735, 1979.

82. Meyer RJ, Cuttner J: Central nervous system involvement at presentation in the chronic phase of chronic myelogenous leukemia in childhood. Cancer 42:305, 1978.

83. Taryle DA, Sahn SA: Rapidly progressive pulmonary infiltrates in chronic myelogenous leukemia. JAMA 242:1525, 1979.

84. McKee LC, Collins RD: Intravascular leukocyte thrombi and aggregates as a cause of morbidity and mortality in leukemia. Medicine (Baltimore) 53:463, 1974.

85. Thompson DS, Golstone EH, Parry HF, et al: Leukostasis in chronic myeloid leukaemia. BMJ 2:202, 1978.

86. Hild DH, Myers TJ: Hyperviscosity in chronic granulocytic leukemia. Cancer 46:1418, 1980.

87. Faderl S, Talpaz M, Estrov Z, et al: Chronic myelogenous leukemia: Biology and therapy. Ann Int Med 131:207, 1999.

88. Kantarjian HM, Dixon D, Keating M, et al: Characteristics of accelerated disease in chronic myelogenous leukemia. Cancer 61:1441, 1988.

89. Karanas A, Silver RT: Characteristics of the terminal phase of chronic granulocytic leukemia. Blood 32:445, 1968.

90. Woodson DL, Bennett EE, Sears DA: Extramedullary myeloblastic transformation of chronic myelocytic leukemia. Arch Intern Med 134:523, 1974.

91. Kwaan HC, Pierre RV, Long DL: Meningeal involvement as first manifestation of acute myeloblastic transformation in chronic granulocytic leukemia. Blood 33:348, 1969.

92. Schwartz JH, Canellos GP, Young RC, et al: Meningeal leukemia in the blastic phase of chronic granulocytic leukemia. Am J Med 59:819, 1975.

93. Greaves MF: 'Target cells', differentiation and clonal evolution in chronic granulocytic leukaemia: A 'model' for understanding the biology of malignancy. In Shaw M (ed.): Chronic Granulocytic Leukemia, p. 15. Praeger, East Sussex, 1982.

94. Skarin AT, Matsuo Y, Moloney WC: Muramidase in myeloproliferative disorders terminating in acute leukemia. Cancer 29:1336, 1972.

95. Weiselberg L, Teichberg S, Vinciguerra V, et al: Electron microscope cytochemical analysis of chronic myelocytic leukemia: A case report. Cancer 47:533, 1981.

96. Rosenthal S, Canellos GP, Gralnick HR: Erythroblastic transformation of chronic granulocytic leukemia. Am J Med 63:116, 1977.

97. Griffin JD, Todd RFI, Ritz J, et al: Differentiation patterns in the blastic phase of chronic myeloid leukemia. Blood 61:85, 1983.

98. Travis WD, Li C, Banks PM, et al: Megakaryoblastic transformation of chronic granulocytic leukemia. Cancer 60:193, 1987.

99. Williams WC, Weiss GB: Megakaryoblastic transformation of chronic myelogenous leukemia. Cancer 49:921, 1982.

100. Rosenthal S, Canellos GP, DeVita VT: Characteristics of blast crisis in chronic granulocytic leukemia. Blood 49:705, 1977.

101. Marks SM, Baltimore D, McCaffrey R: Terminal transferase as a predictor of initial responsiveness to vincristine-prednisone in blastic chronic myelogenous leukemia. N Engl J Med 298:812, 1978.

102. Ganesan TA, Rassool F, Guo A-P, et al: Rearrangement of the bcr gene in Philadelphia chromosome-negative chronic myeloid leukemia. Blood 68:957, 1986.

103. You W, Weisbrot IM: Chronic neutrophilic leukemia. J Clin Pathol 72:233, 1979.

104. Pane F, Frigeri F, Sinlona M et al. Neutrophilic chronic myeloid leukemia: A distinct disease with a specific molecular marker (BCR/ABL with C3/A2 junction). Blood 88:2410, 1996.

105. Benvenisti DS, Ultmann JE: Eosinophilic leukemia. Ann Intern Med 71:731, 1969.

106. Weller PF, Bubley GJ: The idiopathic hypereosinophilic syndrome. Blood 83:2759–2779, 1994.

107. Ellman L, Hammond D, Atkins L: Eosinophilia, chloromas and a chromosome abnormality in a patient with a myeloproliferative syndrome. Cancer 43:2410, 1979.

108. Xiao S, Nalabolu SR, Aster JC, et al: FGFR1 is fused with a novel zinc-finger gene, ZNF198, in the t(8;13) leukemia/lymphoma syndrome. Nature Genet 84:84–87, 1998.

109. Gualtieri RJ, Emanuel PD, Zuckerman KS, et al. Granulocyte-macrophage colony-stimulating factor is an endogenous regulator of cell proliferation in juvenile chronic myelogenous leukemia. Blood 74:2360, 1989.

110. Busque L, Gilliland DG, Prchal JT, et al: Clonality in juvenile chronic myelogenous leukemia. Blood 85:21–30, 1995.

111. Emanuel PD, Snyder PC, Wiley T, et al: Inhibition of juvenile myelomonocytic leukemia cell growth in vitro by farnesyltransferase inhibitors. Blood 95:639–645, 2000.

112. Dudley JM, Messinezy M, Eridani S, et al: Primary thrombocythaemia: Diagnostic criteria and a simple scoring system for positive diagnosis. Br J Haematol 71:331–335, 1989.

113. Hehlmann R, Jahn M, Baumann B, et al: Essential thrombocythemia: Clinical characteristics and course of 61 cases. Cancer 61:2487–2496, 1988.

114. Tefferi A, Hoagland HC: Issues in the diagnosis and management of essential thrombocythemia. Mayo Clin Proc 69:651–655, 1994.

115. Buss DH, O'Connor ML, Woodruft RD, et al: Bone marrow and peripheral blood findings in patients with extreme thrombocytosis. A report of 63 cases. Arch Pathol Lab Med 115:475–480, 1991.

116. Murphy S, Ikand H, Rosenthal D, et al: Essential thrombocythemia: An interim report from the polycythemia vera study group. Semin Hematol 23:177, 1986.

117. Kaywin P, McDonough M, Insel PA, et al: Platelet function in essential thrombocythemia: Decreased epinephrine responsiveness associated with a deficiency of platelet α-adrenergic receptors. N Engl J Med 299:505, 1978.

118. Schafer AI: Bleeding and thrombosis in the myeloproliferative disorders. Blood 64:1–12, 1984.

119. Barbui T, Cortelazzo S, Viero P, et al: Thrombohaemorrhagic complications in 101 cases of myeloproliferative disorders: Relationship to platelet number and function. Eur J Cancer Clin Oncol 19:1593–1599, 1983.

120. Cortelazzo S, Viero P, Finazzi G, et al: Incidence and risk factors for thrombotic complications in a historical cohort of 100 patients with essential thrombocythemia. J Clin Oncol 8:556–562, 1990.

121. Raman SBK, Mahmood A, Slyck EJV, et al: Essential thrombocythemia with transition into acute leukemia. Ann N Y Acad Sci 370:145, 1981.

122. Sedlacek SM, Curtis JL, Weintraub J, et al: Essential thrombocythemia and leukemic transformation. Medicine 65:353, 1986.

124. Bellucci S, Janvier M, Tobelem G, et al: Essential thrombocythemias. Cancer 58:2440, 1986.

125. Smith RE, Chelmowski MK, Szabo EJ, et al: Myelofibrosis: A concise review of clinical and pathologic features and treatment. Am J Hematol 29:174, 1988.

126. Weinstein IM: Idiopathic myelofibrosis: Historical review, diagnosis, and management. Blood Rev 5:98–104, 1991.

127. Lazlo J: Myeloproliferative disorders: Myelofibrosis, myelosclerosis, extramedullary hematopoiesis, undifferentiated MPD, and hemorrhagic thromocythaemia. Semin Hematol 12:75, 1975.

128. Thiele J, et al: Clinical and morphological criteria for the diagnosis of prefibrotic myelofibrosis. Ann Hematol 80:160, 2001.

129. Thiele J, Chen VS, Kvasnicka HM, et al: Evolution of fibro-osteosclerotic bone marrow lesions in primary (idiopathic) osteomyelofibrosis—a histomorphometric study on sequential trephine biopsies. Leuk Lymph 14:163–169, 1994.

130. Thiele J, Rompcik V, Wagner S, et al: Vascular architecture and collagen type IV in primary myelofibrosis and polycythaemia vera: An immunomorphometric study on trephine biopsies of the bone marrow. Br J Haematol 80:227–234, 1992.

131. Patton WN, Bunce CM, Larkins S, et al: Defective erythropoiesis in primary myelofibrosis associated with a chromosome 11 abnormality. Br J Cancer 64:128–31, 1991.

132. Wilkens BS, Green A, Wild AE, Jones OB: Extramedullary hematopoiesis in fetal and adult human spleen: A quantitative immunohistological study. Histopathology 24:241, 1994.

132. Mesa RA, Li C-Y, Schroeder G, Tefferi A: Clinical correlations of splenic histopathology and splenic karyotype in myelofibrosis with myeloid metaplasia. Blood 97:3665, 2001.

133. Silverstein MN, Wollaeger EE, Baggenstoss AH: Gastrointestinal and abdominal manifestations of agnogenic myeloid metaplasia. Arch Intern Med 131:532, 1973.

134. Rosenbaum DL, Murphy GW, Swisher SN: Hemodynamic studies of the portal circulation in myeloid metaplasia. Am J Med 41:360, 1966.

135. Rosenthal DS, Moloney WC: Myeloid metaplasia: A study of 98 cases. Postgrad Med 45:136, 1969.

136. Demory JL, Dupriez B, Fenaux P, et al: Cytogenetic studies and their prognostic significance in agnogenic myeloid metaplasia: A report on 47 cases. Blood 72:1988.

137. Trautmann U, Rubbert A, Gramatzki M, et al: Multiple chromosomal changes and karyotypic evolution in a patient with myelofibrosis. Cancer Genet Cytogenet 61:6–10, 1992.

138. Tasaka T, Nagai M, Murao S, et al: CD7, CD34-positive stem cell leukemia arising in agnogenic myeloid metaplasia. Am J Hematol 44:53–57, 1993.

139. Tefferi A, Solberg A, Silverstein MN: A clinical update: Polycythemia vera and essential thrombocytopenia. Am J Med 109:141, 2000.

140. Murphy S: Polycythemia vera. Dis Month 38:153–212, 1992.

141. Fisher MJ, Prchal JF, Prchal JT, et al: Anti-erythropoietin (EPO) receptor monoclonal antibodies distinguish EPO-dependent and EPO-independent erythroid progenitors in polycythemia vera. Blood 84:1994.

142. Berlin NI: Diagnosis and classification of the polycythemias. Semin Oncol 12:339, 1975.

144. Ellis JT, Silver RT, Coleman M, et al: The bone marrow in polycythemia vera. Semin Hematol 12:433, 1975.

145. Ellis JT, Peterson P, Geller SA, et al: Studies of the bone marrow in polycythemia vera and the evolution of myelofibrosis and second hematologic malignancies. Semin Hematol 23:144, 1986.

146. Nielsen B, Thiede T, Carlsson M, et al: Myelodysplastic syndrome in polycythaemia vera. Br J Haematol 55:193, 1983.

147. Shamdas GJ, Spier DM, List AP: Myelodysplastic transformation of polycythemia vera: Case report and review of the literature. Am J Hematol 37:45, 1991.

148. Holcombe RF, Treseler PA, Rosenthal DS: Chronic myelomonocytic leukemia transformation in polycythemia vera. Leukemia 5:606–610, 1991.

149. Schlaifer D, Dasiugue N, Brousset P, et al: B-cell lymphoma following polycythemia vera: Evidence for the involvement of two different clones. Leukemia 8:895–896, 1994.

150. Neilson JR, Patton WN, Williams MD, et al: Polycythaemia rubra vera transforming to acute lymphoblastic leukaemia with a common immunophenotype. J Clin Pathol 47:471, 1994.

151. Hernandez JM, Oriao A, Gonzalez M, et al: Immunophenotypic characterization of acute leukaemia after polycythemia vera. J Clin Pathol 46:668–671, 1993.

152. Oscier D: Chronic lymphocytic leukemia. Br J Haematol 105(Suppl. 1):1, 1999.

153. Caligarris-Cappio F, Hamblin TJ: B-cell chronic lymphocytic leukemia: A bird of a different feather. J Clin Oncol 17:1, 1999.

154. Byrd JC, Flinn IW, Grever MH: Chronic lymphocytic leukemia. Semin Hematol 25, 1998.

155. Faguet GB: Chronic lymphocytic leukemia: An updated review. J Clin Oncol 12:1974–1990, 1994.

156. Baer M, Stein RS, Dessypris EN, et al: Chronic lymphocytic leukemia with hyperleukocytosis. Cancer 56:2865, 1985.

157. Rudders RA, Howard JP: Clinical and cell surface marker characterization of the early phase of chronic lymphocytic leukemia. Blood 52:25, 1978.

158. Dighiero G, Travade P, Chevret S, et al: B-cell chronic lymphocytic leukemia: Present status and future directions. Blood 78:1901–1914, 1991.

159. Moreau EJ, Matutes E, A-Hern RP, et al: Improvement of the chronic lymphocytic leukaemia scoring system with the monoclonal antibody SN8 (CD79b). Hematopathology 108:378–382, 1997.

160. Knuutila S, Elonen E, Teerenhavi L, et al: Trisomy 12 in B cells of patients with B-cell chronic lymphocytic leukemia. N Engl J Med 314:865, 1986.

161. Juliusson G, Ost RA, Friberg K, et al: Prognostic information from cytogenetic analysis in chronic B-lymphocytic leukemia and leukemic immunocytoma. Blood 65:134, 1985.

162. Han T, Ozer H, Sadamori N, et al: Prognostic importance of cytogenetic abnormalities in patients with chronic lymphocytic leukemia. N Engl J Med 310:288, 1984.

163. Escudier SM, Pereira-Leahy JM, Drach JW, et al: Fluorescent in situ hybridization and cytogenetic studies of trisomy 12 in chronic lymphocytic leukemia. Blood 81:2702–2707, 1993.

164. Que TH, Marco JG, Ellis J, et al: Trisomy 12 in chronic lymphocytic leukemia detected by fluorescence in situ hybridization: analysis by stage, immunophenotype, and morphology. Blood 82:571–575, 1993.

165. Stankovic T, Weber P, Stewart G, et al: Inactivation of ataxia telangiectasia mutated gene in B-cell chronic lymphocytic leukemia. Lancet 353:26–30, 1999.

166. Kornblau SM, Chen N, Giglio AD, et al: Retinoblastoma protein expression is frequently altered in chronic lymphocytic leukemia. Cancer Res 54:242–246, 1994.

167. Oscier DG: Cytogenetic and molecular abnormalities in chronic lymphocytic leukaemia. Blood Rev 8:88–97, 1994.

168. Aguayo A, O'Brien S, Keating M, et al: Clinical relevance of intracellular vascular endothelial growth factor levels in B-cell chronic lymphocytic leukemia. Blood 96:768–770, 2000.

169. Zengin N, Kars A, Sungur A, et al: The significance of the bone marrow biopsy pattern in chronic lymphocytic leukemia: A prognostic dilemma. Am J Hematol 62:208–211, 1999.

170. Rai K, Sawitsky A, Cronkite E, et al: Clinical staging of chronic lymphocytic leukemia. Blood 46:219, 1975.

171. Binet JL, Auguier A, Dighiero C, et al: A new prognostic classification of chronic lymphocytic leukemia derived from a multi-variate survival analysis. Cancer 48:198, 1981.

172. Nieto LH, Raya Sanchez JM, Arguelles HA, et al: A case of chronic lymphocytic leukemia overwhelmed by rapidly progressive idiopathic myelofibrosis. Haematologica 85:973–977, 2000.

173. Tsang WY, Chan JK, Sing C: The nature of Reed-Sternberg-like cells in chronic lymphocytic leukemia. Am J Clin Pathol 99:317–323, 1993.

174. Momose H, Jaffe BS, Shin SS, et al: Chronic lymphocytic leukemia/small lymphocytic lymphoma with Reed-Sternberg-like cells and possible transformation to Hodgkin's disease. Mediation by Epstein-Barr virus. Am J Surg Pathol 16:859–867, 1992.

175. Kipps TJ, Carson DA: Autoantibodies in chronic lymphocytic leukemia and related systemic autoimmune diseases. Blood 81:2475–2487, 1993.

176. Stefani S, Chandra S, Schrek R, et al: Endoplasmic reticulum-associated structures in lymphocytes from patients with chronic lymphocytic leukemia. Blood 50:125, 1977.

177. Ottolander GJD, Brederoo P, Schuurman RKB, et al: Intracellular immunoglobulin G "pseudocrystals" in a patient with chronic B-cell leukemia. Cancer 58:43, 1986.

178. Batata A, Shen B: Relationship between chronic lymphocytic leukemia and small lymphocytic lymphoma. A comparative study of membrane phenotypes in 270 cases. Cancer 70:625, 1992.

179. Dick FR, Maca RD: The lymph node in chronic lymphocytic leukemia. Cancer 41:283, 1978.

180. Phillips JK, Bass PS, Majumdar G, et al: Renal failure caused by leukaemic infiltration in chronic lymphocytic leukaemia. J Clin Pathol 46:1131, 1993.

181. Garofalo M Jr, Muralo R, Halperin I, et al: Chronic lymphocytic leukemia with hypothalamic invasion. Cancer 64:1714, 1989.

182. Morrison C, Shah S, Flinn IW: Leptomeningeal involvement in chronic lymphocytic leukemia. Cancer Practice 6:223, 1998.

183. Barzilai A, Shapiro D, Goldberg I, et al: Insect bite-like reaction in patients with hematologic malignant neoplasms. Arch Dermatol 135:1503–1507, 1999.

184. Uchiyama T, Yodoi J, Sagama K, et al: Adult T-cell leukemia. Clinical and hematologic features of 16 cases. Blood 50:481, 1977.

185. Tobinai K: Adult T-cell leukemia-lymphoma. In Abeloff MD, Armitage JO, Lichter AS, Niederhuber JE (eds.): Clinical Oncology. Churchill Livingston, New York, 2000.

186. Newland AC, Catowsky DL, Linch D, et al: Chronic T-cell lymphocytosis: A review of 21 cases. Br J Haematol 58:433, 1981.

187. Merle-Beral H, Boucheix C, Karry S, et al: A chronic lymphocytic leukemia with large granular lymphocytes. Cancer 59:1296, 1987.

188. Chan W, Link S, Mawle A, et al: Heterogeneity of large granular lymphocyte proliferations: Delineation of two major subtypes. Blood 68:1142, 1986.

189. Loughran TP Jr: Clonal disease of large granular lymphocytes. Blood 82:1, 1993.

190. Semenzato G, Zambello R, Starkebaum G: The lymphoproliferative disease of granular lymphocytes: Updated criteria for diagnosis. Blood 89:256, 1997.

191. Agnarsson BA, Loughran TP Jr, Starkebaum G, Kadin ME: The pathology of large granular lymphocyte leukemia. Human Pathol 20:643–651, 1989.

192. Berliner N, Duby AD, Linch DC, et al: T cell receptor gene rearrangements define a monoclonal T cell proliferation in patients with T cell lymphocytosis and cytopenia. Blood 67:914, 1986.

193. Ohno Y, Amakaw R, Rukuhara S, et al: Acute transformation of chronic large granular lymphocyte leukemia associated with additional chromosome abnormality. Cancer 64:63, 1989.

194. Alvarez-Larran A, Villamor N, Hernandez-Bolida JC, et al. Ablastic natural killer cell leukemia/lymphoma presenting as overt leukemia. Clinical Lymphoma 2:178, 2001.

195. Traweek ST, Liu J, Johnson RM, et al: High-grade transformation of chronic lymphocytic leukemia and low-grade non-Hodgkin's lymphoma. Genotypic confirmation of clonal identity. Am J Clin Pathol 100:519–526, 1993.

196. Kroft SH, Dawson DB, McKenna RW: Large cell lymphoma transformation of chronic lymphocytic leukemia/small lymphocytic lymphoma. A flow cytometric analysis of seven cases. Am J Clin Pathol 115:385–395, 2001.

197. Conlan MG, Mosher DF: Concomitant chronic lymphocytic leukemia, acute myeloid leukemia, and thrombosis with protein C deficiency. Cancer 63:1398, 1989.

198. Galton DAG, Goldman JM, Wiltshaw E, et al: Prolymphocytic leukaemia. Br J Haematol 27:7, 1974.

199. Costello C, Catovsky D, O'Brien M, et al: Prolymphocytic leukaemia. An ultrastructural study of 22 cases. Br J Haematol 44:389, 1980.

200. Kjeldsberg CR, Bearman RM, Rappaport H: Prolymphocytic leukemia. Am J Clin Pathol 73:150, 1980.

201. Catovsky D: Prolymphocytic and hairy cell leukemias. In Henderson TALES (ed.): Leukemia, p. 639. WB Saunders, Philadelphia, 1990.

202. Melo JV, Catovsky D, Galton DAG: The relationship between chronic lymphocytic leukaemia and prolymphocytic leukaemia. Br J Haematol 63:377–387, 1986.

203. Tsai L-MC, Tsai C-C, Hyde TPL, et al: T-cell prolymphocytic leukemia with helper-cell phenotype and a review of the literature. Cancer 54:463–470, 1984.

204. Kluin-Nelemans HC, Gmelig-Meyling FHJ, Kootte AMM, et al: T-cell prolymphocytic leukemia with an unusual phenotype [CD4+ CD8+]. Cancer 60:794–803, 1987.

205. Brito-Babapulle V, Pomfret M, Matutes E, et al: Cytogenetic studies on prolymphocytic leukemia. II. T cell prolymphocytic leukemia. Blood 70:926, 1987.

206. Kojima K, Hara M, Sawada T, et al: Human T-lymphotropic virus type I provirus and T-cell prolymphocytic leukemia. Leuk Lymph 38:381–386, 2000.

207. Schlette E, Bueso-Ramos C, Giles F, et al: Mature B-cell leukemias with more than 55% prolymphocytes. A heterogeneous group that includes an unusual variant of mantle cell lymphoma. Am J Clin Pathol 115:571–581, 2001.

208. Bearman RM, Pangalis GA, Rappaport H: Prolymphocytic leukemia. Cancer 42:2360, 1978.

209. Perry DJ, McCormick D, Veasey S, et al: Right heart obstruction due to intracavitary prolymphocytic leukemia. Am J Med 81:131–134, 1986.

210. Bouroncle BA, Wiseman BK, Doan CA: Leukemic reticuloendotheliosis. Blood 13:609, 1958.

211. Seshadri RS, Brown EJ, Zipursky A: Leukemic reticuloendotheliosis: A failure of monocyte production. N Engl J Med 295:181–184, 1976.

212. Rosenthal RL, Steiner GC, Golub BSL: Hairy cell leukemia: Historical aspects and bone involvement. Mt Sinai J Med (N Y), 46:237, 1979.

213. Schrek R, Donnelly WJ: "Hairy" cells in blood in lymphoreticular neoplastic disease and "flagellated" cells of normal lymph nodes. Blood 27:199, 1966.

214. Pettitt AR, Zugel M, Cawley JC: Hairy cell leukemia: Biology and management. Br J Haematol 106:2, 1999.

215. Burthen J, Zuzel M, Cawley JC: What is the nature of the hairy cell and why should we be interested? Br J Haematol 97:511, 1997.

216. Bennett C, Vardiman J, Golomb H: Disseminated atypical mycobacterial infection in patients with hairy cell leukemia. Am J Med 80:891–896, 1986.

217. Catovsky D, O'Brien M, Melo JV, et al: Hairy cell leukemia (HCL) variant: An intermediate disease between HCL and B prolymphocytic leukemia. Semin Oncol 11:362, 1984.

218. Katayama I, Li CY, Yam LT: Ultrastructural characterization of the "hairy cells" of leukemic reticuloendotheliosis. Am J Pathol 67:361, 1972.

219. Katayama I, Schneider GB: Further ultrastructural characterization of hairy cells of leukemic reticuloendotheliosis. Am J Pathol 86:163, 1977.

220. Variakojis D, Vardiman JW, Golomb HM: Cytochemistry of hairy cells. Cancer 45:72, 1980.

221. Neirnan RS, Sullivan AL, Jaffee R: Malignant lymphoma simulating reticuloendotheliosis. Cancer 43:329, 1979.

222. Palutke M, Tabaczka P, Mirchanadani I, et al: Lymphocytic lymphoma simulating hairy cell leukemia: A consideration of reliable and unreliable diagnostic features. Cancer 48:2047, 1981.

223. Katayama I, Aiba M: Tartrate-resistant acid phosphatase reaction. Am J Clin Pathol 73:143, 1980.

224. Hounieu H, Chittal SM, Saati T, et al: Hairy cell leukemia. Diagnosis of bone marrow involvement in paraffin-embedded sections with monoclonal antibody DBA.44. Am J Clin Pathol 98:26–33, 1982.

225. Miranda RN, Briggs RC, Kinney MC, et al: Immunohistochemical detection of cyclin D1 using optimized conditions is highly specific for mantle cell lymphoma and hairy cell leukemia. Mod Pathol 13:1308–1314, 2000.

226. Robbins DH, Margulies I, Stetler-Stevenson M, Kreitman RJ: Hairy cell leukemia, a B-cell neoplasm that is particularly sensitive to the cytotoxic effect of anti-Tac(Fv)-PE38 (LMB-2). Clin Cancer Res 6:693–700, 2000.

227. Kreitman RJ, Wilson WH, Bergeron K, et al: Efficacy of the anti-CD22 recombinant immunotoxin BL22 in chemotherapy-resistance hairy-cell leukemia. N Engl J Med 345:241, 2001.

228. Brearley RL, Chapman RM, Brozovic B: Hairy-cell leukemia presenting as aplastic anemia. Ann Intern Med 91:228, 1979.

229. Gruber G, Schwarzmeier JD, Shehata M, et al: Basic fibroblast growth factor is expressed by CD19/CD11c-positive cells in hairy cell leukemia. Blood 94:1077–1085, 1999.

230. Burke JS, MacKay B, Rappaport H: Hairy cell leukemia (leukemic reticuloendotheliosis). II. Ultrastructure of the spleen. Cancer 37:2267, 1976.

231. Pilon VA, Davey FR, Gordon GB, et al: Splenic alterations in hairy cell leukemia: An electron microscopic study. Cancer 49:1617, 1982.

232. Yam LT, Janckila AJ, Chan CH, et al: Hepatic involvement in hairy cell leukemia. Cancer 51:1497, 1983.

233. Isaacson PG, Matutes E, et al: The histopathology of splenic lymphoma with villous lymphocytes. Blood 84:3828–3834, 1994.

234. Matutes E, Morilla R, Owusu-Ankomah K, et al: The immunophenotype of splenic lymphoma with villous lymphocytes and its relevance to the differential diagnosis with other B-cell disorders. Blood 83:1558–1562, 1994.

235. Gruszka-Westwood AM, Hamoudi RA, Matutes E, et al: P53 abnormalities in splenic lymphoma with villous lymphocytes. Blood 97:3552–3558, 2001.

236. Traweek ST: Monocytoid B-cell lymphoma. The biologic and clinical implications of peripheral blood involvement. Am J Clin Pathol 97:591–598, 1992.

237. Traweek ST, Sheibani K, Winberg CD, et al: Monocytoid B-cell lymphoma: Its evolution and relationship to other low-grade B-cell neoplasms. Blood 73:573–578, 1989.

238. Sézary A: Une nouvelle reticulose cutanee: La reticulose maligne leucemique a histiomonocytes monstreu et a forme d'erythrodermie oedemateuse et pigmentree. Ann Dermatol Venereol 9:5, 1949.

239. Lutzner M, Edelson R, Schein P, et al: Cutaneous T-cell lymphomas: The Sézary syndome, mycosis fungoides, and related disorders. Ann Intern Med 83:534, 1975.

240. Schein PS, MacDonald JS, Edelson R: Cutaneous T-cell lymphoma. Cancer 38:1859, 1976.

241. Glusac EJ, Shapiro PE, McNiff JM: Cutaneous T-cell lymphoma. Refinement in the application of controversial histologic criteria. Dermatol Clin 17:601–614, 1999.

242. Kim YH, Hoppe RT: Mycosis fungoides and the Sézary syndrome. Semin Oncol 26:276–289, 1999.

243. Huberman MS, Bunn PAJ, Matthews MJ, et al: Hepatic involvement in the cutaneous T-cell lymphomas. Cancer 45:1683, 1980.

244. Rappaport H, Thomas LB: Mycosis fungoides: The pathology of extracutaneous involvement. Cancer 34:1198, 1974.

245. Miller RA, Coleman CN, Fawcett HD, et al: Sézary syndrome: A model for migration of T lymphocytes to skin. N Engl J Med 303:89, 1980.

246. Weisenburger DD, Nathwani BN, Forman SJ, et al: Non-cutaneous peripheral T-cell lymphoma histologically resembling mycosis fungoides. Cancer 49:1839, 1982.

247. Chu AC, Morris JF: Sézary cell morphology induced in peripheral blood lymphocytes: Re-evaluation. Blood 73:1603, 1989.

248. Janier M, Katlama C, Flageul B, et al: The pseudo-Sézary syndrome with CD8 phenotype in a patient with the acquired immunodeficiency syndrome (AIDS). Ann Int Med 110:738, 1989.

249. McNutt NS, Crain WR: Quantitative electron microscopic comparison of lymphocyte nuclear contours in mycosis fungoides and in benign infiltrates in skin. Cancer 47:698, 1981.

250. Whang-Peng J, Bunn PA, Knusten T, et al: Clinical implications of cytogenetic studies in cutaneous T-cell lymphoma (CTCL). Cancer 50:1539, 1982.

251. Erikson KW, Kaltoft K, Mikkelsen G, et al: Constitutive STAT3-activation in Sézary syndrome: Tyrphostin AG490 inhibits STAT3-activation, interleukin-2 receptor expression and growth of leukemic Sézary cells. Leukemia 15:787–793, 2001.

252. Delfau-Larue MH, Laroche L, Wechsler J, et al: Diagnostic value of dominant T-cell clones in peripheral blood in 363 patients presenting consecutively with a clinical suspicion of cutaneous lymphoma. Blood 96:2987–2992, 2000.

253. Vonderheid EC, Tam DW, Johnson WC, et al: Prognostic significance of cytomorphology in the cutaneous T-cell lymphomas. Cancer 47:119, 1981.

254. Colby TV, Burke JS, Hoppe RT: Lymph node biopsy in mycosis fungoides. Cancer 47:351, 1981.

255. Scheffer E, Meijer CJLM, Vloten WAV: Dermatopathic lymphadenopathy and lymph node involvement in mycosis fungoides. Cancer 45:137, 1980.

256. Epstein EH, Levine DL, Groff JD, et al: Mycosis fungoides: Survival, prognostic features, response to therapy, and autopsy findings. Medicine (Baltimore) 51:61, 1972.

257. Sawamura D, Harada K, Aizu T, Umeki K: Sézary syndrome with acute progressive pulmonary infiltration after improvement of skin eruption. Dermatology 202:273–274, 2001.

258. Lawrence EC, Broder S, Jaffe ES, et al: Evolution of lymphoma with helper T-cell characteristics in Sézary syndrome. Blood 52:481, 1978.

259. Schwarzmeier JD, Paietta E, Radaszkiewicz T, et al: Proliferation kinetics of Sézary cells. Blood 57:1049, 1981.

260. Diamandidou E, Colome-Grimmer M, Fayad L, Duvie M, Kurzrock R: Transformation of mycosis fungoides/Sézary syndrome: Clinical characteristics and prognosis. Blood 92:1150–1159, 1998.

261. Bryant E, Ronan SG, and Iossifides, IA. Plasma cell myeloma in a patient with a cutaneous T-cell lymphoma. Cancer 50:2122, 1982.

262. Kantor AF, Curtis RE, Vonderheid EC, et al: Risk of second malignancy after cutaneous T-cell lymphoma. Cancer 63:1612, 1989.

263. Carisbrick JJ, Child FJ, Evans AV, et al: Secondary malignant neoplasms in 71 patients with Sézary syndrome. Arch Dermat 135:1381–1385, 1999.

4

Molecular Biology and Cytogenetics of Chronic Myeloid Leukemia

Stefan Faderl, Moshe Talpaz, and
Hagop M. Kantarjian

Chronic myeloid leukemia (CML) is the best studied of a group of myeloproliferative disorders that result from clonal expansion of primitive hematopoietic progenitor cells. Although, in CML, proliferation of cells of the myeloid compartment predominates, monocytic, erythroid, megakaryocytic, and lymphoid lineages can be involved as well.[1] Almost universally, CML is characterized by a specific chromosomal abnormality called the Philadelphia chromosome.[2] It results from a reciprocal translocation between the long arms of chromosomes 9 and 22 thereby generating the chimeric *BCR-ABL* gene that in turn is transcribed into BCR-ABL fusion proteins whose increased tyrosine kinase activity appears to be central to the molecular and clinical manifestations of CML. CML is unique in that a detailed description of these cytogenetic-molecular events can be linked to the pathogenesis of the disease and to the clinical progression from a chronic, indolent disease stage to a blastic phase paradigmatically reflecting the multistep process of cancer progression. CML has thus become a model for cancerogenesis and disease evolution and has established the use of molecular markers for diagnosis and as targets for novel therapeutic strategies. This chapter provides a concise summary of our current knowledge of the molecular biology and cytogenetics of CML.

CLINICAL SYNOPSIS

CML occurs with an incidence of 1 to 2 cases per 100,000 population and comprises 15 percent of adult leukemias. Its median age at presentation is 45 to 55 years although some series report a median age of 60 years and older.[3] Presently almost half the patients are diagnosed by routine laboratory tests and are asymptomatic at presentation.

CML is typically a triphasic disease. Most patients are diagnosed in the chronic phase. This disease stage is also referred to as indolent or benign and is characterized by excessive proliferation of myeloid progenitor cells in various stages of maturation, their premature release into the peripheral blood, and their tendency to home to extramedullary locations. Despite expansion of the myeloid progenitor stem cell pool, maturation and terminal differentiation of the stem cells are maintained and the disease burden can easily be controlled for months to years by

agents such as hydroxyurea and busulfan or other nontoxic therapies. However, after a median interval of 3 to 4 years, CML invariably progresses into an accelerated phase followed after 3 to 12 months by a blastic phase of short duration in which the blast cells have become resistant to most treatments and patients inevitably succumb to their disease. In one-fourth of patients, blast metamorphosis develops without an intervening accelerated course. Whereas definitions of accelerated phase vary, a rapid increase in peripheral blood and/or bone marrow immature myeloid progenitor cells, the presence of extramedullary blastic infiltrates, and the occurrence of additional cytogenetic-molecular markers (clonal evolution) are usually grave signs of disease progression.[3,4]

The blastic clone expresses lymphoid markers in one-third of the patients and is characterized as myeloblastic or undifferentiated in the remaining two-thirds. Patients whose blasts resemble acute lymphoblastic leukemia (ALL) cells may respond to ALL-type therapy and usually have a better prognosis than patients with acute myeloid or undifferentiated types of leukemia.[5]

CYTOGENETIC-MOLECULAR EVENTS

The Philadelphia Chromosome (Ph)

Working in Philadelphia in 1960, Nowell and Hungerford discovered a "minute chromosome," an abnormal G-group chromosome, in bone marrow cells from two patients with CML.[2] They were the first to identify a chromosomal abnormality that is consistently associated with a human malignancy. Approximately a decade later it was recognized that the "Philadelphia chromosome" is in fact a shortened chromosome 22 and that it is an acquired lesion of the leukemic clone as nonhematopoietic tissues such as bone marrow fibroblasts have a normal karyotype in patients with CML.[1,6,7] In 1973, Rowley et al.[8] found that the abnormality was a reciprocal translocation of segments between chromosomes 9 and 22, hence termed t(9;22). The exact breakpoints of the translocation have been identified as t(9;22)(q34.1;q11.21) using cell synchronization and high-resolution banding techniques (Figure 4–1).[9] Work in the 1980s and 1990s unraveled many of the molecular defects underlying the cytogenetic events illuminating the role of specific *BCR* and *ABL* sequences and the oncogenic potential of the chimeric BCR-ABL products.[10–15]

The Ph is the hallmark of CML where it is observed in almost 95 percent of the patients. It is, however, not specific for CML as it occurs in up to 5 percent of children and 15 to 30 percent of adults with ALL and in a small percentage of patients with acute myeloid leukemia (AML) in whom no evidence of a preceding CML phase is found.[16] Although the Ph in the acute leukemias is cytogenetically identical to that in CML, the molecular rearrangements are frequently different and the prognosis of Ph-positive acute leukemias is remarkably poor when compared to acute leukemias that do not demonstrate the Ph.

Soon after the identification of t(9;22), complex Ph translocations have been recognized that may involve up to five chro-

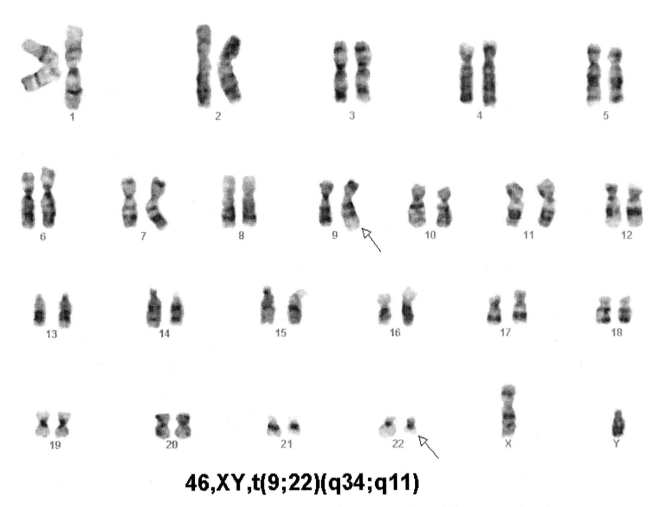

46,XY,t(9;22)(q34;q11)

Figure 4–1. The Philadelphia chromosome is a shortened chromosome 22 that results from a reciprocal translocation between the long arms of chromosomes 9 and 22 (arrows). G banding of metaphase spreads. (Courtesy of Dr. A. Glassman, Cytogenetics Laboratory, The University of Texas M.D. Anderson Cancer Center.)

mosomes, always including 22 and 9.[17] Variant translocations demonstrate involvement of chromosome 22 and a chromosome other than 9 or vice versa.[18,19]

The *BCR-ABL* Rearrangement

The Ph reciprocal translocation between the long arms of chromosomes 9 and 22 transposes the large 3′ segment of *ABL* from chromosome 9q34 to the 5′ part of *BCR* on chromosome 22q11 in a head-to-tail fashion, thus generating a hybrid *BCR-ABL* gene that is then transcribed into a chimeric BCR-ABL mRNA (Figure 4–2).[20]

The *ABL* (Abelson leukemia virus) gene is the protooncogene homologue of the viral transforming *V-ABL* gene that causes nonthymic pre-B-cell lymphomas in mice infected with the Abelson murine leukemia virus (A-MuLV).[21] *ABL* is highly conserved in evolution and is found in virtually every vertebrate genome. It is located on 9q34, spans 230 kilobases (kb), and contains 11 exons that are oriented with their 5′-terminus toward the centromere. The gene has two distinct 5′ exons,

alternative exons 1b and 1a, of which exon 1b is separated by an intron of around 200 kb in the 5′ direction of exons 1a and 2 to 11 (also referred to as a2 to a11) (Figure 4–2). Splicing either 5′ sequence to the common set of the ten 3′ exons creates two major ABL mRNAs of 6 kb and 7 kb, respectively (Table 4–1).[22] Breaks in the *ABL* gene occur at variable sites in the long intron between exons 1b and 1a (i.e., usually 5′ of *ABL* exon 2). Deletions of exon 2 and in-frame joining at the mRNA level of *BCR* sequences to *ABL* exon 3 have been described in CML but are rare.

In contrast, the breakpoint locations on chromosome 22q11 are rather restricted to a narrow sequence that occupies the central portion of the *BCR* (breakpoint cluster region) gene (previously also referred to as *PHL*). The *BCR* gene spans at least 90 kb and is normally transcribed into two mRNA molecules of 4.5 kb and 6.7 kb, respectively (Table 4–1). During the *BCR-ABL* translocation, *ABL* exons 2 to 11 are transposed into the major breakpoint cluster region (M-bcr) of *BCR* between exons 12 to 16 (also referred to as b1 to b5) which extends over 5.8 kb. The breakpoints are located either 5′ on *BCR* between

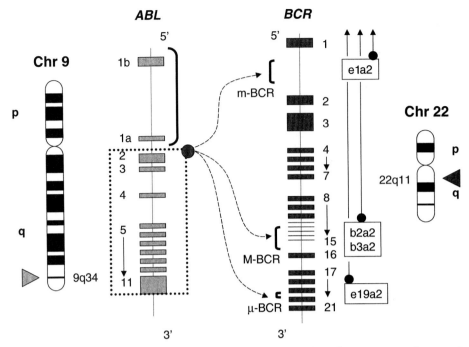

Figure 4–2. Translocation t(9;22)(q34;q11) transposes *ABL* exons a2 to a11 from chromosome 9q34 into one of several breakpoint cluster regions (BCR) on chromosome 22q11. In most cases of patients with CML, the *ABL* exons are transposed into the major (M–) BCR resulting in a b2a2 or b3a3 fusion gene, a chimeric mRNA, and a fusion protein of 210 kd, called p210^BCR-ABL. More frequently in Philadelphia chromosome-positive acute lymphoblastic leukemia (ALL) are the *ABL* exons fused to *BCR* exon e2 creating an e2a2 fusion gene that eventually is translated into a shorter protein of 190 kd, termed p190^BCR-ABL. A third locus of transposition is μ-BCR, which generates an e19a2 fusion and the largest fusion protein, p230^BCR-ABL.

exons b2 and b3 or 3′ between exons b3 and b4. A *BCR-ABL* fusion gene is thus created with either a b2a2 or b3a2 junction.[23] The chimeric 8.5 kb mRNA is translated into a fusion protein of 210 kd (p210^BCR-ABL). In most cases, CML cells demonstrate either b2a2 or b3a2 transcripts, but in a small percentage both fusion proteins are expressed by alternative splicing events. Comparing the 5′ with the 3′ M-bcr breakpoint locations, no differences in response to treatment, prognosis, or clinical features exist except for a higher platelet count in patients with the b3a2 transcripts.[23]

Table 4–1. Characteristics of ABL, BCR, and BCR-ABL

	DNA	RNA	Protein
ABL	Location: chromosome 9q34 Size: 230 kb, contains 11 exons Other: oriented with 5′-end toward the centromere 　2 alternative first exons (1a and 1b)	6-kb (exons 1a to 11) mRNA 7-kb (exons 1b to 11, skipping exon 1a and separating intron to exon 2) mRNA All transcripts share common set of 3′ exons	145-kd protein (p145^ABL)
BCR	Location: chromosome 22q11 Size: 130 kb, contains 21 exons Other: oriented with 5′-end toward the centromere 　5.8-kb segment in central portion includes 5 small exons (1 to 5)	4-kb mRNA (detected in some RNA samples from KG1 cells, lacks sequences from central segment of gene) 4.5-kb mRNA 6.7-kb mRNA	160-kd protein (p160^BCR) 190-kd protein (p190^BCR) also detected by immune complex assays. Predicted amino acid sequence of cDNA would predict a protein of 142 kd
BCR-ABL	Location: chromosome 22q11 *ABL* exons 2 to 11 are transposed into 　M-*BCR* (b2a2 or b3a2 junction) 　m-*BCR* (e1a2 junction) 　μ-*BCR* (e19a2 junction)	8.5-kb mRNA 7-kb mRNA ?	210-kd protein (p210^BCR-ABL) 190-kd protein (p190^BCR-ABL) 230-kd protein (p230^BCR-ABL)

In rare cases of CML, but in about 50 percent of adult Ph-positive ALL and in 80 percent of childhood Ph-positive ALL, the breakpoint on chromosome 22 is located 5′ of M-bcr within a long intron segment between alternative exon e2′ and e2 called the minor breakpoint cluster region (m-bcr) (Figure 4–2).[24] Splicing out exons e1′ and e2′ results in an e1a2 junction BCR-ABL transcript that is translated into a smaller BCR-ABL fusion protein of 190 kd (p190[BCR-ABL]).[25,26] Both p210[BCR-ABL] and p190[BCR-ABL] display increased and constitutive tyrosine phosphokinase activity compared to the normal ABL protein p145[ABL]. A third breakpoint location (μ-bcr) within *BCR* has been identified that is located 3′ from M-bcr between exons e19 and e20 generating a fusion transcript with an e19a2 junction. The translation product is a protein of 230 kd (p230[BCR-ABL]) (Figure 4–2).[27,28] Consistent but low-level coexpression of p190[BCR-ABL] with p210[BCR-ABL] has been demonstrated in most patients with CML in chronic phase.[29] If present in comparable levels to p210[BCR-ABL], p190[BCR-ABL] disease may be characterized by a prominent monocytic component,[30,31] whereas the subgroup of patients who expressed p230[BCR-ABL] has been associated with the neutrophilic leukemia variant, a lower white blood cell count than usually observed, and a slower progression to blast crisis (Table 4–1).[27]

About two-thirds of patients with CML express the reciprocal *ABL-BCR* fusion gene on the derivative chromosome 9q+. The 5′ part of *ABL* exon 1b is fused to the 3′ tail of *BCR* exons b3 or b4. No pathogenetic role has been ascribed to ABL-BCR. Earlier reports of a correlation of ABL-BCR expression with a better response to treatment with interferon-alpha have not been confirmed.[32]

The Oncogenic Potential of *BCR-ABL*

Most of our understanding of the transforming capabilities of *BCR-ABL* has been generated from in vitro assays using factor-dependent hematopoietic cell lines or fibroblasts. However, the in vitro models have limitations; they frequently provide contradictory results and they do not provide the means to further study the pathogenetic mechanisms that are linked to the expression of BCR-ABL. Lacking functional assays using human cells has led to the development of murine CML models to recapitulate the manifestations of the disease.

In vivo animal systems include the use of transgenic mice and retroviral transduction models.[33,34] In a transgenic mouse model, Hariharan and colleagues explored the biological effects of the *BCR-v-ABL* gene that they introduced into the mouse germ line under the control of the immunoglobulin heavy chain enhancer elements or a retroviral long terminal repeat of the myeloproliferative sarcoma virus.[35] Although the transgenic mice develop multiple hematologic neoplasms, they are rarely myeloid and do not recapitulate the characteristics of chronic phase CML in humans. Expression of p190[BCR-ABL] DNA generated myeloid and lymphoid acute leukemias supporting the evidence of a causative relationship between Ph and human leukemias. However, most of the transgenic mice in these models fail to recapitulate a myeloproliferative disease state and are therefore unsuitable to be used as models for human CML.[36,37]

Recently, expression in the progeny of transgenic mice of p210[BCR-ABL] driven by the promoter of the *TEC* gene was demonstrated to generate a myeloproliferative disorder resembling CML.[38] However, the penetrance of this event is undetermined and the latency period of the disease was greater than 1 year.

A more successful approach in recapitulating human CML has been expression of p210[BCR-ABL] in murine bone marrow cells by retroviral transduction.[39–42] In these models, infection of murine bone marrow cells with a retrovirus encoding p210[BCR-ABL] and subsequent transplantation into lethally irradiated syngeneic recipients caused a syndrome that closely resembled the chronic phase of human CML. The mice developed high white blood cell counts, splenomegaly, and extramedullary hematopoiesis, and, in some instances, showed progression from chronic to blastic phase. Limitations of these models include difficulties in generating high-titer BCR-ABL expressing retroviruses, a low incidence of the myeloproliferative disease in transplant recipients, and a low frequency of serial transfer of the myeloproliferative disease. Recently, several investigators have described a new murine CML model in which p210[BCR-ABL] was expressed in bone marrow cells of mice by retrovirus transduction using a murine stem cell vector (MSCV). This model was able to induce a myeloproliferative disease resembling human CML in all mice with a short latency period of 3 to 4 weeks, thus providing a useful CML animal model for future studies.[43,44]

Although it has been suggested that the acquisition of Ph may not be the first clonal event in CML leukemogenesis and that the Ph-positive clone, at least in some cases, may arise by subclone formation, the fact that virtually all patients in chronic phase are Ph-positive and the combined data from animal experiments lend significant weight to the pathogenetic role of *BCR-ABL* as central mediators of myeloid proliferation and transformation in CML.

The Signaling Pathways of BCR-ABL

The transforming capacity of BCR-ABL is largely based on its ability to associate and interact with numerous proteins that connect it to various pathways of intracellular signaling. To understand the structural characteristics of BCR-ABL that facilitate these types of interactions, it is first necessary to dissect the functional sequences of the ABL and BCR proteins, respectively, and then to analyze their contribution to the transformed phenotype in the chimeric protein.

ABL encodes a 145-kd protein (p145[ABL]) that functions as a nonreceptor tyrosine phosphokinase.[45] ABL is primarily located in the nucleus but also found in the cytoplasm where it can also be associated with adhesion molecules. Its ubiquitous expression and the rigorous control of its tyrosine kinase activity hint at an important role in cellular biology.[46] *ABL* knockout mice have a high incidence of neonatal death, have defects in B- and T-cell development, are more susceptible to infections, and show numerous developmental abnormalities of various organ systems.[47–49] The ABL protein appears to be involved in signal transduction and regulation of cell growth, as overexpression of

ABL results in growth arrest of cells during G1 possibly through direct interaction with the p53 and the retinoblastoma tumor suppressor products.[46] It has also been suggested that ABL is activated in the stress response to DNA damaging agents regulating induction of the SEK1/stress-activated protein kinase pathway.[50,51] The N-terminal segment of ABL has structural similarity to C-SRC. It contains three SRC homology (SH) domains, SH1 to SH3, the catalytic domain, and a myristoylation sequence facilitating cytoplasmic localization. The C-terminal segment of ABL includes a DNA-binding domain, nuclear localization signals, and a binding site for actin (Figure 4–3). SH2 and SH3 regulate the tyrosine kinase function of ABL. SH2 attaches to tyrosine phosphorylated proteins that are targets for ABL kinase activity through three conserved arginine residues.[52,53] Defects in the functional integrity of SH2 cause a decrease in phosphotyrosine binding and a decrease in the transforming capabilities of ABL. Conversely, exchanging the SH2 domain by SH2 domains from other proteins maintains the transforming activities of ABL, but changes the cellular target proteins of tyrosine phosphorylation. SH3 has been ascribed negative regulatory activity on the tyrosine kinase function of ABL and may possibly interact with cellular inhibitors.[54,55] Mutational analysis of ABL has demonstrated that deletion of SH3 facilitates the transforming activity of ABL even in the absence of BCR or GAG sequences.[56]

An example of structural alterations of ABL that facilitate its transformation into a protein with leukemogenic potential comes from murine leukemias. The Abelson murine leukemia virus (A-MuLV) is a replication defective virus that in vivo induces primarily nonthymic pre-B-cell lymphomas in susceptible mice.[21] A-MuLV is a fusion product of viral *GAG* sequences and a viral homologue of cellular *ABL. GAG-ABL* encodes a GAG-ABL protein of 160 kd (p160$^{GAG-ABL}$) and, by internal in-frame deletion, a second smaller protein of 120 kd (p120$^{GAG-ABL}$).[57] In either case, GAG is attached to the N-terminus of ABL from which the SH3 domain has been lost (Figure 4–3). Furthermore, the GAG sequences enhance the stability of the GAG-ABL fusion protein thus facilitating their transformation.[58] These events lead to localization of the fusion molecule to the cytoplasm and increased phosphotyrosine kinase activity, a mechanism that appears also at the core of BCR-ABL transforming activities.

The *BCR* gene codes for two proteins of 160 kd and 190 kd, respectively.[59,60] Although the role of the BCR proteins is still largely unknown, several multifunctional domains of BCR have been identified. The N-terminal coiled-coil motif contains a 63 amino acid sequence, common to both p210$^{BCR-ABL}$ and p190$^{BCR-ABL}$, that seems to be crucial for enhancing F-actin binding and tyrosine kinase activity of ABL.[61] The N-terminal portion of BCR itself possesses serine/threonine kinase activity

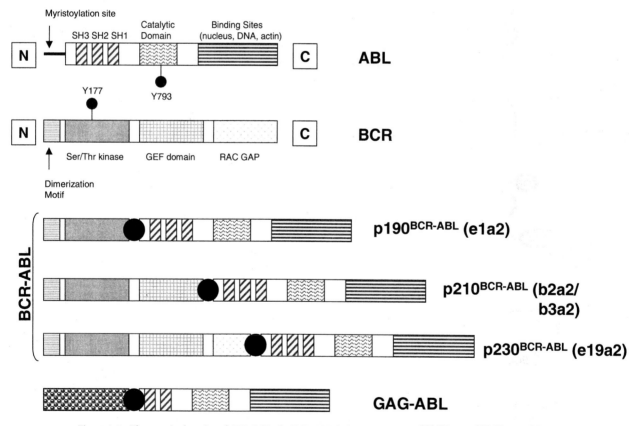

Figure 4–3. The protein domains of ABL, BCR, the BCR-ABL fusion proteins p190$^{BCR-ABL}$, p210$^{BCR-ABL}$, p230$^{BCR-ABL}$, and GAG-ABL from the Abelson murine leukemia virus (AMuLV). Note that the BCR-ABL proteins contain the SH3 domain of ABL that is missing in GAG-ABL.

and contains tyrosine residue 177 (Y177), which is phosphorylated by the ABL tyrosine kinase and serves as a docking site for various adapter proteins (see below).[62] The central portion of BCR is occupied by *DBL* protooncogene-like sequences. DBL catalyzes the exchange of guanine nucleotides on the RAS-related molecule Cdc42Hs and is also referred to as GDP-GTP exchange factor (GEF).[63,64] The C-terminus of BCR contains sequences homologous to the catalytic domains of GTPase activating proteins (GAP) of the GTP protein binding family p21rho and p21 rac (Figure 4–3). Members of this family control the rate of GTP hydrolysis of active RAS proteins to their inactive GDP-bound form thus creating a connection to downstream intracellular signaling pathways.[65]

What determines the transforming activity of ABL in the BCR-ABL fusion? ABL can be activated by itself through internal deletions and point mutations, or by fusion with GAG. In the case of BCR-ABL, however, the SH3 domain is retained. It has been suggested that parts of BCR, by steric hindrance through binding of the first exon of BCR to the SH2 domain of ABL, may interfere with the adjacent SH3 regulatory domain thereby constitutively enhancing the ABL tyrosine phosphokinase activity. In addition, alterations of the N-terminus of ABL

that redistribute its location from the nucleus into the cytoplasm and enhance its F-actin binding capacity contribute to the transforming characteristics of BCR-ABL.[66,67]

The functional domains of BCR-ABL facilitate a multitude of interactions with other cytoplasmic proteins, referred to as adapter proteins, that link BCR-ABL to downstream intracellular signaling pathways. These connections influence expression of gene complexes that generate the phenotypic manifestations of CML that are expressed in altered regulations of cell cycle, programmed cell death (apoptosis), and adhesion (Figure 4–4). An ever-increasing number of proteins is being identified that are complexed with BCR-ABL or represent substrates for tyrosine phosphorylation by BCR-ABL. These include RAS,[68] the phosphatidylinositol-3-kinase (PI3-kinase),[69,70] proteins of the JAK/STAT pathway,[71] NFκB,[72] Src kinases (Hck and Lyn),[73] JUN,[74] MYC, and focal adhesion kinases (FAK).[75]

Involvement of RAS proteins has been determined as a major signaling pathway of BCR-ABL. RAS is a G-protein that occupies a key role in signal transduction, proliferation, and malignant transformation. In the active, GTP-bound state, RAS proteins link signals of activated growth factor receptors to downstream mitogenic effectors.[76] The state of activity of RAS

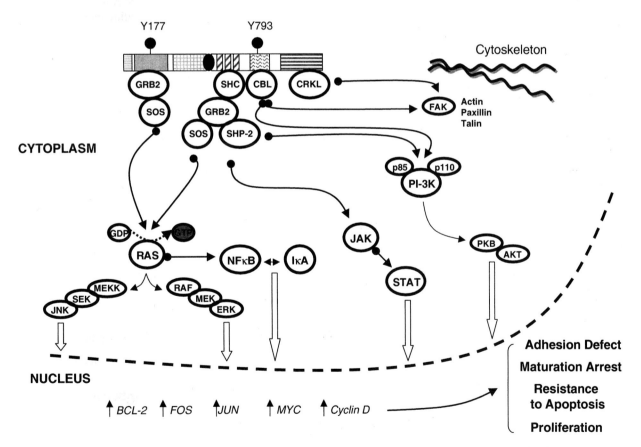

Figure 4–4. Through its tyrosine kinase activity, BCR-ABL can attach to numerous adapter proteins. On phosphorylation, these in turn connect BCR-ABL to downstream protein kinases and enzymes that further transmit the "message" of BCR-ABL to the nucleus. The most important of these downstream effectors are RAS, the JAK/STAT system, and the PI-3K. The signaling network activates the transcription and expression of genes that impact proliferation and differentation of the cell, its regulation of apoptosis, and adhesion to the microenvironment.

is regulated by GTPase-activating proteins (GAPs) and guanine nucleotide exchange factors (GEFs). GAPs enhance the rate of GTP hydrolysis to GDP and negatively regulate RAS function, whereas GEFs induce exchange of GDP for GTP on RAS and act as activators.[77] Evidence for a role of RAS in BCR-ABL signaling is derived from the observation in murine myeloid cells that activated RAS is constitutively elevated, and the fact that dominant negative RAS mutants in RAT-1 fibroblast cells completely block transformation by BCR-ABL.[78,79] BCR-ABL is linked to RAS through several adapter proteins such as GRB2, SHC, CRKL, and CBL. GRB2 is linked with its SH2 domain to the conserved tyrosine residue Y177 within the first exon of BCR in the BCR-ABL molecule.[80] The importance of this association for the activation of RAS is evident from the observation that mutant forms of GRB2 reverse BCR-ABL-induced transformation.[81] Binding of GRB2 to BCR-ABL activates a further adapter protein, SOS ("son-of-sevenless"), which in turn recruits RAS. CRKL, an adapter protein that is tyrosine-phosphorylated only in Ph-positive cells, is the most prominent phosphoprotein in CML cells. It binds to proline-rich sequences of BCR-ABL and activates RAS through its ability to bind to SOS and another CRK SH3-binding guanine nucleotide-releasing protein termed C3G.[82,83] Signaling downstream of RAS is less well characterized. One major path appears to involve association with RAF1 and subsequent activation of MEK kinase and extracellular signal-regulated kinase (ERK). A second pathway involves MEK kinases (MEKK) and the JUN kinase (JNK) pathway, also referred to as stress-activated protein kinase (SAPK) pathway.[84]

Alternatively, RAS can be activated by inhibiting its negative regulator RAS GAP. Recently, another BCR-ABL adapter protein has been identified called p62dok. Hematopoietic progenitor cells isolated from patients with CML in the chronic phase contain constitutively tyrosine-phosphorylated p62dok protein. Under these conditions, p62dok associates with RAS GAP thus inhibiting its activity.[85] p62dok was found to form complexes with the SH2 domain-containing phosphatidylinositol polyphosphate 5-phosphatase SHIP1 in hematopoietic cells expressing BCR-ABL, suggesting more complex interactions of these proteins in BCR-ABL transformed hematopoietic progenitor cells.[86] Other instances where negative regulatory pathways may be antagonized by the activity of p210[BCR-ABL] include protein-tyrosine phosphatase-1B (PTP-1B), which counteracts signaling of p210[BCR-ABL] and the ABL-interactor molecule (ABI-1).[87,88]

A second major pathway of BCR-ABL signaling involves PI3-kinase. PI3-kinase can be activated upon stimulation with multiple growth factors. It is composed of an 85-kd (p85) regulatory subunit that acts as an adapter sequence through its SH2 and SH3 domains, and a 110-kd (p110) catalytic sequence that is responsible for its enzymatic activity.[89] PI3-kinase may be linked to BCR-ABL through CBL (casitas B-lineage lymphoma protein), a protooncogene product that is tyrosine-phosphorylated in BCR-ABL expressing cells. Through interaction of PI3-kinase protein kinase B (PKB) and AKT, BCR-ABL is directly linked to regulatory elements of apoptosis favoring expression of antiapoptotic effects mediated by BCL-XL and BCL-2.[90] It has also been suggested that BCR-ABL positive cells are able to downregulate cyclin-dependent kinase inhibitor p27, thus interfering with the regulation of the cell cycle protein and promoting a proliferative and antiapoptotic phenotype of the CML cells.[91,92]

Constitutive activation of JAK/STAT proteins has been reported in cell lines and samples from patients expressing BCR-ABL.[93,94] STAT proteins (signal transducers and activators of transcription) link cytokine receptor stimulation to gene transcription. Once tyrosine phosphorylated by JAK family kinases, STAT proteins dimerize, translocate to the nucleus, and bind to specific DNA elements.[93,94] Constitutive tyrosine phosphorylation and activation of STAT1, 5, and 6 have been demonstrated in CML cells. Although the significance of STAT activation in CML is still unclear and differences in activation of specific STAT proteins seem to exist in p190[BCR-ABL] and p210[BCR-ABL]-containing cells, it has been suggested that they may represent another link to induce antiapoptotic mechanisms and growth-factor independent growth.[95–99]

Another important target of p210[BCR-ABL] signaling in CML is MYC, a transcription factor involved in cell cycle regulation. Evidence for a role of MYC stems from experiments that demonstrated high levels of MYC RNA in p210[BCR-ABL] transformed cells, facilitation of transformation by overexpression of MYC, and blocking of transformation by expression of a mutant, dominant negative form of MYC.[100]

CRKL seems to establish a link between p210[BCR-ABL] and focal adhesion molecules such as FAK, actin, and paxillin.[101,102] Recently, NFκB has been implicated in signaling pathways of p210[BCR-ABL]. NFκB is a transcription factor that translocates to the nucleus upon activation by growth-factor or cytokine stimulation. Transcription of NFκB has been identified as an inhibitor of apoptosis, but its regulation is complex and it may also be activated in cells undergoing apoptosis in response to serum starvation.[103] It has been suggested that BCR-ABL activates NFκB-dependent transcription. Activation is dependent on tyrosine phosphorylation of NFκB and is partially RAS-dependent. Although NFκB does not appear to be necessary to enable BCR-ABL to protect cytokine-dependent 32D myeloid cells from apoptosis induced by cytokine deprivation or DNA damage, it is nevertheless required for BCR-ABL mediated tumorigenicity in nude mice and for transformation of primary bone marrow cells.[104]

The activity of p210[BCR-ABL] generates activation or suppression of a set of target genes that confer the malignant phenotype on the Ph-positive cell. Some of the early genes identified have been *FOS*, *JUN*, and *MYC*. However, most of the data on altered gene expression through activation of p210[BCR-ABL] are derived from cell lines transformed by ectopic expression of p210[BCR-ABL] rather than acquiring the translocation naturally. Many target genes remain unidentified to date.[105]

THE BIOLOGICAL EFFECTS OF BCR-ABL

Exactly how the molecular abnormalities are linked to the biological behavior of the Ph-positive cells and how they determine the leukemic phenotype, is still poorly understood. Our current knowledge suggests that the increased tyrosine phosphokinase activity of the BCR-ABL proteins activates multiple intracellular signaling pathways that regulate cellular proliferation, apoptosis, cellular differentiation and maturation, as well as interactions with the microenvironment. Inappropriate or untimely activation of one or several of these pathways will eventually tilt the tightly knit balance between these processes. Although much evidence has been accumulated to support involvement of any of these cellular events, their relative contribution to the generation of CML in chronic phase and subsequent changes that take place in the course of transformation remain largely elusive.

One of the most characteristic features of CML is the disorderly expansion of myeloid cells. The normal lineage apportionment is unbalanced in CML in favor of increased granulopoiesis and thrombopoiesis. Expansion of these compartments suggests unregulated proliferation of the leukemic cells, increased self-renewal and life span of the Ph-positive progenitor cells, and a decreased fraction of apoptotic cells in the Ph-positive cell pool. However, cytokinetic studies of CML progenitors have shown that CML progenitors have lower mitotic indices and the same DNA synthesis time as the normal progenitors, resulting in a lower fraction of cells that are actively synthesizing DNA and subsequently longer generation times.[106] In vitro clonogenic assays have also demonstrated that CML progenitor cells are less capable of producing large colonies compared to normal progenitor cells.[107] Eaves and colleagues suggest that "long term culture initiating cells" (LTCIC) of CML progenitors are the leukemic counterpart to LTCIC of normal progenitor cells.[108] They have observed that CML LTCIC differ in two important aspects: CML LTCIC have reduced self-renewal capacity and are therefore outgrown by their normal counterparts. However, by virtue of a deregulated cell cycle status, more CML progenitors are in cycle compared to the rather quiescent population of normal early progenitors. At some stage along the evolution of CML, the defects of cell cycle regulation will dominate the behavior of the CML cells and endow the leukemic progenitors with a growth advantage. Subtle morphological abnormalities of CML cells such as nuclear-cytoplasmic asynchrony, an increase in dysplastic changes, and the presence of chimeric basophil/eosinophil granules are a morphologic correlate to the disordered balance of self-renewal, proliferation, differentiation, and maturation.[109] Clarkson and Strife have suggested that although CML cells contain the capacity for complete maturation, maturation is delayed and shifted from the early stem cell compartment to a more committed progenitor cell compartment thus greatly increasing the myeloid cell mass.[110] Defects in adhesion molecules or receptors (see below) facilitate release of early myeloid cells in the peripheral blood resulting in the characteristic maturational left shift of CML. Even a small increase in the probability of self-renewal in this stage may then disproportionately increase myeloid mass further.[111] Dowding and colleagues[112] calculated that an increase in the probability of self-renewal from 0.5 to only 0.55 will result in a doubling of the stem cell pool after eight stem cell division cycles. With a disproportionate shift of CML progenitors into later maturational compartments, the

CML cells may also become less responsive to growth regulatory signals from either cytokines or from the bone marrow microenvironment. Furthermore, factors to curtail cell production at high cell densities may be abrogated and facilitate the acquisition by the CML progenitor cells of a continuous growth advantage over their normal counterparts.[111]

In addition, BCR-ABL expressing leukemia cells are highly resistant to apoptosis and this mechanism has been suggested as an important aspect in the pathogenesis of CML.[113,114] The abrogation of apoptosis resistance by a combination of mutations in the SH2 domain, GRB2 binding site, and an autophosphorylation site (Y793F) of BCR-ABL lends evidence to the central role of the BCR-ABL protein.[115] Hematopoietic progenitor cells or cell lines that express p210[BCR-ABL] can thus escape growth factor dependency and withstand the damaging effects of exposure to cytotoxic drugs and irradiation.[116,117] In contrast, BCR-ABL cannot suppress apoptosis triggered by the activity of cytotoxic T cells, natural killer cells, and lymphocyte-activated killer cells.[118,119] The detailed antiapoptotic pathways triggered by BCR-ABL have not been elucidated. They appear to involve RAS, the JAK/STAT pathways, and possibly NFκB and PI3-kinase. Pathways through PI3-kinase and activation of STAT may act by enhancing the expression of the antiapoptotic protein BCL-XL. Horita and colleagues[99] demonstrated that interleukin-3-independent expression of BCL-XL is induced by BCR-ABL by activation of STAT5.[99] Conversely, inhibition of the kinase activity of BCR-ABL in BCR-ABL-positive cell lines and CML progenitor cell samples from patients could reverse the antiapoptotic activity by suppressing the capacity of STAT5 to interact with the BCL-XL promoter. de Groot and colleagues[98] have shown that activation of STAT5 in BCR-ABL transformed cells not only activates the BCL-XL gene product, but also targets the cell cycle regulator cyclin D1.[98] The promoters of both cyclin D1 and BCL-XL products contain STAT binding sites to which STAT5 constitutively binds in BCR-ABL transformed cells. BCR-ABL expressing cells have also been shown to block release of mitochondrial cytochrome C and thus inhibit activation of caspase 3 independent from proteins of the BCL-2 family.[120] Further inhibition of apoptotic pathways may also play a role in the evolution of CML to blast phase. After inhibition of the BCR-ABL kinase, expression of BCL-XL is downregulated more rapidly in chronic phase than blast phase CML cells. Furthermore, CML cells from patients in blast crisis are more refractory to apoptosis mediated by FAS than are CML cells from patients in chronic phase.[121]

Stimulation by cytokines and expression of distinct cytokine profiles provide CML progenitor cells with a distinct growth advantage over normal bone marrow cells. Aberrant growth factor production is especially evident in the more advanced stages of CML.[122] CML cells from patients in myeloid or undifferentiated blast crisis that are cultured on a marrow-adherent layer proliferate continuously and exhibit constitutive growth factor expression [interleukin (IL)-1β, IL-6, granulocyte-macrophage colony stimulating factor (GM-CSF)]. Furthermore, experiments showing that progenitor cells from patients with interferon-resistant disease have a reduced response to exogenous growth factors and a relatively autonomous growth pattern in colony assays, support the significance of autocrine/paracrine pathways in CML.[123] Estrov and colleagues[124] were the first to recognize the role of IL-1β as a growth-promoting cytokine in CML. IL-1β synergizes with growth factors either through upregulation of growth factor receptors or production and release of various other cytokines by the hematopoietic stroma or accessory cells. Marrow cells from patients with transformed CML produce high levels of IL-1β. Inhibition of IL-1β by either IL-1 receptor antagonist or soluble IL-1 receptors suppresses CML colony formation. These results suggest that autocrine/paracrine production of growth factors such as IL-1β alters the relation of the leukemic cells to the adjacent microenvironment and thus influences the proliferative and differentiation state of the leukemic cells. The BCR-ABL proteins also appear to bind directly to growth factor receptors and to activate them by tyrosine phosphorylation. The activated receptors such as IL-3R and c-KIT then recruit further downstream signaling pathways contributing to the deregulation of cellular pathways in CML.[125,126]

Adhesion defects of hematopoietic progenitor cells to bone marrow stromal elements have been implicated in the pathogenesis of the manifestations of CML.[127] It may be responsible for inappropriate release of immature precursors into the circulation, evasion of growth-regulatory mechanisms, and subsequently disinhibition of hematopoietic progenitor cell proliferation. Normal hematopoietic progenitor cells adhere to adhesive ligands of extracellular matrix components such as fibronectin receptors (α4, α5, β1 integrins), heparin sulfate or thrombospondin, or immobilized and secreted growth-regulating cytokines. The interactions are mediated by cell surface receptors on hematopoietic progenitors including the cell surface proteoglycan CD44, or the selectins, phosphatidylinositol-linked lymphocyte-associated antigen 3 (LFA 3). Especially β1-integrin-dependent interactions are crucial for the localization, regulation of adhesion, and migration of hematopoietic progenitors. Integrins are cell surface glycoproteins that consist of an a- and b-subunit. Whereas the a-chain determines ligand specificity, the b-chain initiates signal transduction pathways on binding to the ligand.[127] This process generates the recruitment of cytoskeletal adhesion proteins such as actin, talin, paxillin, and FAK. The next step is the activation of adapter proteins and finally of the RAS/MAPK pathway.[128] In a series of in vivo experiments, antibodies against α4β1-integrins inhibited homing and engraftment, and caused premature release of myeloid precursors and stem cells (reviewed in Ref. 129). In contrast to normal stem cells, Ph-positive precursors from the marrow of patients with chronic phase CML adhered significantly less to the feeder layer of marrow stromal cells. Ph-positive progenitors may fail to adhere to the bone marrow stroma through a functional defect of fibronectin receptors and subsequent signaling pathways without changes in receptor expression.[130] Verfaillie and colleagues[131] studied β1-integrin-cytoskeletal interactions in CML and normal CD34-positive primary hematopoietic progenitors, and in BCR-ABL-transfected and mock-transfected MO7e cells. Whereas in normal cells antibody-mediated cross-linking of β1-integrins redistributes them into caps through a process requiring receptor-cytoskeletal interactions, BCR-ABL-expressing cells show significantly impaired β1-integrin capping. Defective β1-integrin capping, increased actin polymerization, and altered actin cytoskeletal organization eventually result in integrin-defective adhesion and disinhibition of proliferation of CML cells. Defective cytoadhesion of CML cells has been restored by preincubation of Ph-positive cells with antisense oligonucleotides against p210[BCR-ABL], tyrosine kinase inhibitors targeted against the BCR-ABL tyrosine kinase, and by incubation with interferon-alpha.[129]

THE CYTOGENETIC-MOLECULAR EVENTS OF TRANSFORMATION

Almost invariably the indolent chronic phase of CML transforms into the blast phase. This transformation is often heralded by refractoriness to treatment, leukocytosis with increases in peripheral blood and bone marrow blasts, basophilia, increases or decreases of platelet counts unrelated to therapy, or clinical signs and symptoms such as unexplained fevers, splenomegaly, extramedullary disease, weight loss, and bone and joint pains. The cytogenetic-molecular events that underlie these changes are being unraveled at an astounding pace and will provide us with more effective therapeutic means to treat these conditions that still bear a dismal prognosis.

The Ph translocation is the predominant cytogenetic abnormality during chronic phase. Other cytogenetic abnormalities are present in less than 10 to 20 percent of patients.[11,132] Clonal evolution, that is, the acquisition of additional karyotype changes, occurs in 50 to 80 percent of patients who progress to the transformed stages. These abnormalities frequently precede the hematological and clinical manifestations of transformed CML. Only about 20 percent of patients progress to blast phase without signs of clonal evolution. Clonal evolution and its accompanying molecular events are probably facilitated by increasing genetic instability in a largely expanded mass of myeloid progenitor cells and is eventually responsible for uncoupling maturation from proliferation in the CML cells.[133]

Several cytogenetic abnormalities predominate in CML evolution.[134] Some include monosomies of chromosomes 7, 17, and Y, trisomy 17 and 21, and translocation t(3;21)(q26;q22). More frequently observed are trisomy 8, isochromosome i(17q), trisomy 19, and an additional Ph chromosome (double Ph). Trisomy 8 is the most common cytogenetic abnormality of transformed CML and predominates in myeloid blast phase. It sometimes occurs in combination with isochromosome i(17q), trisomy 19, and the double Ph. Like trisomy 8, i(17q) occurs almost exclusively in myeloid-type blast phase. It is associated with trisomy 8 and trisomy 19, but not the double Ph.[5,11,34,132]

Multiple molecular abnormalities occur during progression of CML. These involve p53 (chromosome 17p13), RB1 (13q14), MYC (8q24), p16[INK4a]/p14[ARF] (9p21), RAS, and the AML-EVI1 fusion protein resulting from translocation t(3;21)(q26;q22).[135–139] Deregulations of molecular pathways of apoptosis and the significance of telomere length and telomerase activity are being recognized as important components of transformation. Loss of function of *p53* has been associated with suppression of apoptosis and progression into blastic phase. Skorski and colleagues[140] injected immunodeficient mice with p210[BCR-ABL]-positive, *p53*-negative cells and produced the phenotype of a highly aggressive, poorly differentiated acute leukemia. In contrast, injection of p210[BCR-ABL]-positive, *p53*-positive bone marrow cells caused tissue infiltrates with a more differentiated phenotype and clinically less aggressive disease.[140] Honda and colleagues,[141] by cross-mating p210[BCR-ABL] transgenic mice with *p53*-heterozygous mice, demonstrated that mice that expressed BCR-ABL and lacked one allele for *p53* had rapid proliferation of blast cells and died in a short period of time. Interestingly, they also found that the residual normal *p53* allele was frequently and preferentially lost in the leukemic cells, suggesting that certain mechanisms in BCR-ABL expressing cells facilitate the loss of the normal *p53* allele. Whereas abnormalities of *p53* appear to occur predominantly during myeloid transformation, abnormalities of *RB1* are more frequently associated with the development of a lymphoid blast phase. Although this association is weaker than it is between *p53* and myeloid transformation, distinct molecular pathways may exist that selectively involve lymphoid or myeloid transformation.

Telomere shortening has been associated with disease evolution in CML. Telomeres constitute the terminal chromosome sequences whose progressive shortening is thought to be important in the regulation of cellular senescence. Through inherent inadequacies of the cellular replicative apparatus, telomeres continuously shorten during a cell's life span. In contrast, upregulation of telomerase activity in neoplastic cells may maintain an inappropriate telomere length and endow cancer cells with a prolonged life span and the possibility of repeated cell divisions.[142] Normal telomere length at the time of diagnosis of patients with chronic phase CML was associated with lower frequency of transformation and a significantly higher incidence of cytogenetic responses and a favorable prognosis to interferon-alpha therapy.[143] Furthermore, CML patients in blast phase were found to have a significant increase of telomerase activity compared to patients in chronic phase CML.[144] Boultwood and colleagues[145] showed that age-adjusted telomere repeat array (TRA) reduction correlated significantly with time from diagnosis to acceleration. Patients with shortened telomeres entered the accelerated phase more rapidly thus providing a means to select patients with high risk of disease transformation in CML. The fact that cells from patients in transformed phases of CML have significantly shorter telomere lengths than patients in chronic phase or cytogenetic remission, also suggests that Ph-positive stem cells cycle more actively than their counterparts in normal individuals.[146]

BCR-ABL IN DIAGNOSIS AND MONITORING OF MINIMAL RESIDUAL DISEASE

Cytogenetic studies detect the Ph translocation in more than 90 percent of patients with CML in chronic phase. However, the sensitivity of cytogenetic analysis is low (1 to 5 percent) due to the limited number of metaphases that are examined (usually 20 to 25). Cytogenetic analysis is nevertheless pivotal in two areas: 1. at diagnosis where almost 100 percent of CML progenitor cells in a sample express the Ph translocation; and 2. for the identification of additional karyotype abnormalities in the course of the disease (clonal evolution). Several molecular techniques have been developed that allow a more precise assessment of measuring subclinical disease and are therefore more suitable to monitor the levels of residual disease during therapy and their impact on disease relapse. Molecular studies are also pivotal at diagnosis in the 10 percent of patients who will not show a Ph chromosome by cytogenetic analysis. About two-thirds of these patients will be positive for *BCR-ABL* by either Southern blotting or polymerase chain reaction (PCR) and their clinical course and prognosis is identical to patients who are Ph-positive.

Fluorescence in situ hybridization (FISH) and PCR have become the two most important molecular tools that are used to monitor the response of patients under treatment. FISH detects specific DNA target sequences with fluorescent-color-tagged probes on interphase (nondividing) cells (interphase FISH, or I-FISH) and/or metaphase (dividing) cells (hypermetaphase FISH, or H-FISH). In both cases, FISH permits analysis of a large number of cells (> 500) in a timely and efficient manner. Further advantages are that FISH can assess the status of *BCR-ABL* involvement in various cell lineages as much as in single cells, and that the results of FISH are easily quantifiable. I-FISH can be done on peripheral blood samples, but false-positive results occur in up to 10 percent of the patients. In contrast, no false-positive results are observed with H-FISH, but H-FISH cannot be done on peripheral blood.[147–149] FISH techniques that use double-color probes have been introduced for the diagnosis and monitoring of Ph-positive leukemias. Although initial results are promising in view of its superior sensitivity and specificity, not enough data are available to validate its impact in the clinical practice.[150]

Most centers use PCR or one of its variants as their method of choice to detect residual disease on a molecular level. PCR has an unsurpassed sensitivity and can identify one malignant cell among 10^4 to 10^6 normal cells. PCR depends on recognition of a specific primer sequence followed by a target sequence of variable length that is exponentially amplified in a multistep, temperature-regulated reaction cycle. The target sequence may be a leukemia-specific cytogenetic abnormality such as the Ph translocation, or a clone-specific sequence of rearranged immunoglobulin or T-cell receptor genes. In many chromosomal translocations, breakpoints vary or occur within large intronic DNA sequences. In these cases, fusion mRNA (made up entirely of transcribed coding exons) is incubated with the enzyme reverse transcriptase (RT), and the resulting cDNA is amplified by PCR (RT-PCR).[151,152]

Cytogenetic remissions can be achieved by allogeneic stem cell transplantation in 50 to 80 percent of patients with CML in chronic phase, and in about 30 to 40 percent of patients who have been treated with interferon-alpha. Using PCR, *BCR-ABL* transcripts can still be detected in up to 30 percent of patients who are in a complete cytogenetic remission after stem cell transplantation and in almost 100 percent of patients who are treated with interferon-alpha.[153] However, Kurzrock and colleagues[154] have demonstrated that these patients may become PCR-negative if followed long enough.

Many studies have used PCR assays to detect residual disease and have correlated these findings with the outcome of stem cell transplantation and treatment with interferon-alpha. Some observations have emerged from these trials. Qualitative measurements, especially at single time points, are not suitable to predict relapse. Most studies have demonstrated a high incidence of PCR positivity up to 6 months after transplant without evidence of cytogenetic or hematologic relapse.[155–157] In a multivariate analysis of 346 patients with CML who underwent allogeneic stem cell transplantation and were monitored by PCR, detection of *BCR-ABL* at 6 to 12 months after the transplant was associated with relapse.[158] Serial and quantitative evaluations of the expression of *BCR-ABL* suggest that a consistent evolution pattern exists prior to relapse in that rising or persistently high levels of residual disease precede clinical relapse, whereas stable, low, or falling levels predict continued remission.[159]

Molecular diagnosis and monitoring in CML has also illuminated important biological aspects of residual disease and interactions between host and leukemic cells. The observation that patients who are in long-term clinical remission can still harbor *BCR-ABL* transcripts and not relapse offers several possibilities. A specific genetic abnormality may characterize the leukemic cells, but may not be more than a marker that by itself is not able to confer the residual CML cell with the leukemic phenotype. Residual clones of leukemic cells may also establish subclones that have lost the original molecular markers and thus evade detection by PCR or FISH. Tumor cells may survive in a state of tumor dormancy during which the disease burden is either so small or certain host immune mechanisms are so efficient that the residual cells are unable to establish the clinical manifestations of the disease. It should be emphasized, therefore, that a positive PCR reaction does not always equal relapse, and a negative PCR reaction is not always absence of any disease. Therefore, at least in some cases, cure can be understood as "functional" rather than "molecular", that is, the absence of all evidence of disease.[160]

In addition to biological characteristics of the disease, PCR is still faced with technical challenges that may lead to both false-negative and false-positive results (contamination of the samples, discrepancy of results between different laboratories, sensitivity too high). End-point measurements (analysis of the reaction product after amplification is completed) are commonly used for quantification. These measurements are based on multiple dilutions or coamplification of standards (internal or external to the reaction system) and are cumbersome, error prone, and technically demanding. Real-time PCR is a more recent kinetic quantification technique in which the data are acquired during the actual amplification process in a closed system by using fluorogenic probes or intercalating dyes. The kinetic PCR quantification method is more efficient, accurate, and less time-consuming than end-point PCR quantification.[161]

Molecular analysis by PCR has become a cornerstone technique for the diagnosis and monitoring of the response during therapy in patients with CML. Its future impact on clinical decision making for these patients will depend largely on the reproducibility of the results from PCR assays and its correlation to clinical response.[160]

PHILADELPHIA CHROMOSOME-NEGATIVE CML

In 5 to 10 percent of patients with the clinical picture of CML, no Ph can be demonstrated by cytogenetic analysis.[162] However, one-third of these patients have rearrangements of *BCR-ABL* that can be detected by molecular studies such as Southern blotting, FISH, or PCR. Patients with Ph-negative, *BCR-ABL*-positive CML have similar characteristics, clinical course, and outcome compared with Ph-positive patients.[163] The remaining two-thirds of Ph-negative cases have no detectable *BCR-ABL* rearrangements and comprise a spectrum of heterogeneous disorders including chronic myelomonocytic leukemia (CMML), other myelodysplastic syndromes with a myeloproliferative component, and "atypical" CML.[164] Guidelines to distinguish CML, atypical CML, and CMML on the basis of morphological characteristics have been proposed.[165] It should be emphasized, however, that some of the Ph-negative patients may carry variants of the BCR-ABL mRNA transcript that may evade detection by using molecular probes for rearrangements of the M-BCR or m-BCR region only.[166] Hochhaus and colleagues[167] used multiplex RT-PCR and demonstrated the presence of an e6a2 BCR-ABL transcript when analyzing the sequence of the fusion region of the amplified cDNA fragment. This finding could be confirmed by Southern blotting when using a specific probe for intron 6 of the *BCR* gene, whereas Southern blotting with conventional probes for M-BCR were negative.

Compared with *BCR-ABL*-negative CML and CMML, patients with Ph-negative and *BCR-ABL*-positive CML and Ph-positive CML are younger, have a higher white blood cell count at presentation, a higher incidence of thrombocytosis and peripheral blood and bone marrow basophilia, and a lower incidence of anemia, thrombocytopenia, bone marrow blast percentage, and peripheral blood and bone marrow monocytosis.[162,168] Patients with *BCR-ABL*-negative CML respond poorly to therapy and have significantly worse survival rates, with a prognosis that is intermediate between Ph-positive CML and CMML. Only 25 to 50 percent of these patients transform into blastic phase. Most develop an increasing leukemic cell burden, organomegaly, and extramedullary infiltrates, culminating into bone marrow failure and eventually death of the patient.[162,163]

MOLECULAR PATHOGENESIS AS GUIDE FOR NOVEL THERAPIES

Formation of the *BCR-ABL* gene and its chimeric protein is at the core of the pathogenesis of CML. The interaction of BCR-ABL with other cellular proteins and the elements of multiple and complex signaling pathways are increasingly recognized

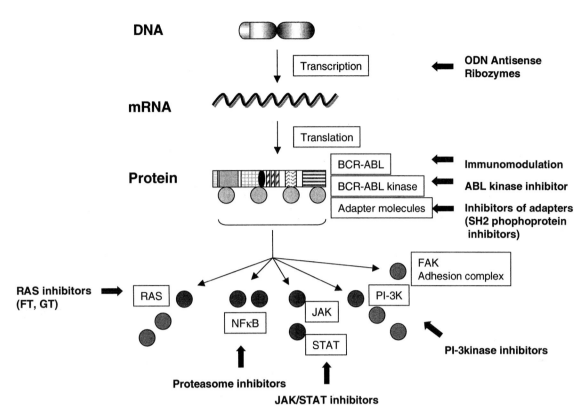

Figure 4–5. The dissection of the BCR-ABL signaling cascade has provided many new targets for therapeutic intervention at almost every level of the pathogenesis of CML. Most promising are the the BCR-ABL tyrosine kinase inhibitors such as STI-571 that are currently used in clinical trials in patients with CML.

as potential targets for novel therapeutic agents (Figure 4–5).[169] Most prominent among these agents are tyrosine kinase inhibitors with an exceptional affinity for ABL. Imatinib merylate (formerly known as STI-571 or CGP57148B), a small 2-phenylaminopyridimine compound, has been identified as the most promising member of these small molecules.[170] It also inhibits the kinase activity of c-KIT and PDGFR, but none of more than 50 other kinases including serine/threonine kinases that have been screened.[171] STI-571 binds to the ATP-binding loop of the ABL protein. This sequence of ABL, like in many other kinases, must have a phosphate group added before it can phosphorylate other proteins. This process changes the conformation of ABL to open it up so that it can bind ATP and the target protein. Although the "active" conformation of this sequence is almost identical in other kinases, imatinib locks ABL in its inactive conformational state that differs among kinases and best explains the specificity of imatinib.[172] This mode of action serves as an example of how enzyme inhibitors can be identified that are specific for their target and can thus be used to knock out part of a specific signal transduction pathway that contributes to the leukemic phenotype. Many peptides, small molecules, and other agents are being identified with the potential to inhibit the chain of transforming events

of *BCR-ABL* at virtually every level from transcription to activation of intracellular signaling pathways.[173–175] However, a great amount of redundancy exists within the *BCR-ABL* signaling network, and additional hits are operative in transformation of the disease, so that inhibition of a single pathway may only have limited efficacy in abrogating leukemogenesis.

CONCLUSION

CML is one of the most extensively studied human malignancies. It is the only neoplasm in which a single genetic event has been linked to the pathogenesis of the disease. CML is also a model for the multistep process of cancer progression in that clonal evolution accompanied by additional molecular hits precedes the clinical manifestations of CML transformation. The dissection of the signaling pathways and its molecular constituents has sparked a surge in the identification of new agents that act at specific sites in this network. Some of these drugs have already shown promising clinical activity. As this field will undoubtedly expand, new lessons are also learned to benefit patients with many other malignant and nonmalignant diseases. The paradigm of *BCR-ABL* is a powerful accolade to the contributions of basic science in cancer medicine.

REFERENCES

1. Fialkow PJ, Jacobson RJ, Papayannopoulou T: Chronic myelocytic leukemia. Clonal origin in a stem cell common to the granulocyte, erythrocyte, platelet, and monocyte/macrophage. Am J Med 63:125–130, 1977.
2. Nowell PC, Hungerford DA: A minute chromosome in human chronic granulocytic leukemia. Science 132:1497–1501, 1960.
3. Kantarjian HM, Deisseroth A, Kurzrock R, et al. Chronic myelogenous leukemia: A concise update. Blood 82:691–703, 1993.
4. Sokal JE, Baccarani M, Russo D: Staging and prognosis in chronic myelogenous leukemia. Semin Hematol 25:49–61, 1988.
5. Derderian PM, Kantarjian HM, Talpaz M, et al: Chronic myelogenous leukemia in the lymphoid blastic phase: Characteristics, treatment, responses, and prognosis. Am J Med 94:69–74, 1993.
6. Caspersson T, Gahrton G, Lindsten J, Zech L: Identification of the Philadelphia chromosome as a number 22 by quinacrine mustard fluorescence analysis. Exp Cell Res 63:238–240, 1970.
7. Maniatis AK, Amsel S, Mitus WJ, Coleman N: Chromosome pattern of bone marrow fibroblasts in patients with chronic granulocytic leukaemia. Nature 222:1278–1279, 1969.
8. Rowley JD: A new consistent chromosomal abnormality in chronic myelogenous leukaemia identified by quinacrine fluorescence and Giemsa staining. Nature 243:290–293, 1970.
9. Prakash O, Yunis JJ: High resolution chromosomes of the t(9;22) positive leukemias. Cancer Genet Cytogenet 11:361–367, 1984.
10. de Klein A, Van Kessel AG, Grosveld G, et al: A cellular oncogene is translocated to the Philadelphia chromosome in chronic myelocytic leukemia. Nature 300:765–767, 1982.
11. Heisterkamp N, Groffen J, Stephenson JR: Chromosomal localization of human cellular homologues of two viral oncogenes. Nature 299:747–749, 1982.
12. Heisterkamp N, Stephenson JR, Groffen J, et al: Localization of the c-abl oncogene adjacent to a translocation break point in chronic myelocytic leukaemia. Nature 306:239–242, 1983.
13. Bartram CR, de Klein A, Hagemeijer A, et al: Translocation of the c-abl oncogene correlates with the presence of a Philadelphia chromosome in chronic myelocytic lelukemia. Nature 306:277–280, 1983.
14. Groffen J, Stephenson JR, Heisterkamp N, et al: Philadelphia chromosomal breakpoints are clustered within a limited region, bcr, on chromosome 22. Cell 36:93–99, 1984.
15. Shtivelman E, Lifshitz B, Gale RP: Fused transcript of abl and bcr genes in chronic myelogenous leukaemia. Nature 315:550–554, 1985.
16. Specchia G, Mininni D, Guerrasio A, et al: Ph positive acute lymphoblastic leukemia in adults: Molecular and clinical studies. Leuk Lymphoma 18:37–42, 1995.
17. Mitelman F: The cytogenetic scenario of chronic myeloid leukemia. Leuk Lymphoma 11(Suppl. 1):11–15, 1993.
18. Sonta SI, Sandberg AA: Chromosomes and causation of human cancer and leukemia. XXIV. Unusual and complex Ph1 translocations and their clinical significance. Blood 50:691–697, 1977.
19. Sandberg AA: Chromosomes and causation of human cancer and leukemia: XL. The Ph¹ and other translocations in CML. Cancer 46:2221–2226, 1980.
20. Faderl S, Talpaz M, Estrov Z, et al: The biology of chronic myelogenous leukemia. N Engl J Med 341:164–172, 1999.
21. Abelson HT, Rabstein LS: Lymphosarcoma: Virus-induced thymic-independent disease in mice. Cancer Res 30:2213–2222, 1970.
22. Shtivelman E, Lifshitz B, Gale RP, et al: Alternative splicing of RNAs transcribed from the human abl gene and from the bcr-abl fused gene. Cell 47:277–284, 1985.

23. Melo JV: The molecular biology of chronic myeloid leukaemia. Leukemia 10:751–756, 1996.
24. Hermans A, Heisterkamp N, Van Linden M, et al: Unique fusion of bcr and c-abl genes in Philadelphia chromosome positive acute lymphoblastic leukaemia. Cell 51:33–40, 1987.
25. Kurzrock R, Shtalrid M, Gutterman JU, et al: Molecular analysis of chromosome 22 breakpoints in adult Philadelphia-positive acute lymphoblastic leukaemia. Br J Haematol 67:55–59, 1987.
26. Kurzrock R, Shtalrid M, Romero R, et al: A novel c-abl protein product in Philadelphia-positive acute lymphoblastic leukaemia. Nature 325:631–635, 1987.
27. Pane F, Frigeri F, Sindona M, et al: Neutrophilic-chronic myeloid leukemia: A distinct disease with a specific molecular marker (BCR/ABL with C3A2 junction). Blood 88:2410–2414, 1996.
28. Saglio G, Guerrasio A, Rosso C, et al: New type of BCR/ABL junction in Philadelphia chromosome-positive chronic myelogenous leukaemia. Blood 76:1819–1823, 1990.
29. van Rhee F, Hochhaus A, Lin F, et al: p190 BCR-ABL mRNA is expressed at low levels in p210-positive chronic myeloid and acute lymphoblastic leukemias. Blood 87:5213–5217, 1996.
30. Melo JV, Myint H, Galton DAG, et al: p190 BCR-ABL chronic myeloid leukemia: The missing link with chronic myelomonocytic leukemia? Leukemia 8:208–211, 1994.
31. Ravandi F, Cortes J, Albitar M, et al: Chronic myelogenous leukaemia with p185(BLR/ABL) expression: Characteristics and clinical significance. Br J Haematol 107:581–586, 1999.
32. Melo J, Hochhaus A, Yan X-H, et al: Lack of correlation between ABL-BCR expression and response to interferon-α in chronic myeloid leukaemia. Br J Haematol 92:684–686, 1996.
33. Adams JM, Cory S: Transgenic models of tumor development. Science 254:1161–1167, 1991.
34. Daley GQ: Animal models of BCR/ABL-induced leukemias. Leuk Lymphoma 11(Suppl. 1):57–60, 1993.
35. Hariharan IK, Harris AW, Crawford M, et al: A bcr-v-abl oncogene induces lymphomas in transgenic mice. Mol Cell Biol 9:2798–2805, 1989.
36. Heisterkamp N, Jenster G, ten Hoove J, et al: Acute leukemia in bcr/abl transgenic mice. Nature 344:251–253, 1990.
37. Honda H, Fujii T, Takatoku M, et al: Expression of p210bcr/abl by metallothionein promoter induced T-cell leukemia in transgenic mice. Blood 85:2853–2861, 1995.
38. Honda H, Oda H, Suzuki T, et al: Development of acute lymphoblastic leukemia and myeloproliferative disorder in transgenic mice expressing p210(bcr/abl): A novel transgenic model for human Ph1-positive leukemias. Blood 91:2067–2075, 1998.
39. Daley GQ, Van Etten RA, Baltimore D: Induction of chronic myelogenous leukemia in mice by the P210bcr/abl gene of the Philadelphia chromosome. Science 247:824–830, 1990.
40. Kelliher MA, McLaughlin J, Witte ON, Rosenberg N: Induction of a chronic myelogenous leukemia-like syndrome in mice with v-abl and BCR/ABL. Proc Natl Acad Sci USA 87:6649–6653, 1990.
41. Elefanty AG, Cory S: Hematologic disease induced in BALB/c mice by a bcr-abl retrovirus is influenced by the infection conditions. Mol Cell Biol 12:1755–1763, 1992.
42. Gishizky M, Johnson-White J, Witte ON: Efficient transplantation of BCR-ABL-induced chronic myelogenous lelukemia-like syndrome in mice. Proc Natl Acad Sci USA 90:3755–3759, 1993.
43. Pear WS, Miller JP, Lanwei X, et al: Efficient and rapid induction of a chronic myelogenous leukemia-like myeloproliferative disease in mice receiving P210 bcr/abl-transduced bone marrow. Blood 92:3780–3792, 1998.
44. Zhang X, Ren R: Bcr-Abl efficiently induces a myeloproliferative disease and production of excess interleukin-3 and granulocyte

macrophage colony-stimulating factor in mice: A novel model for chronic myelogenous leukemia. Blood 92:3829–3840, 1998.

45. Konopka JB, Witte ON: Detection of c-abl tyrosine kinase activity in vitro permits direct comparison of normal and altered gene products. Mol Cell Biol 5:1116–1123, 1985.

46. Wen ST, Jackson PK, Van Etten RA: The cytostatic function of c-Abl is controlled by multiple nuclear localization signals and requires the p53 and Rb tumor suppressor gene products. EMBO J 15:583–590, 1996.

47. Tybulewicz VL, Crawford CE, Jackson PK, et al: Neonatal lethality and lymphopenia in mice with a homozygous disruption of the c-abl protooncogene. Cell 65:1153–1163, 1991.

48. Schwarzberg PL, Stall AM, Hardin JD, et al: Mice homozygous for the ablm1 mutation show poor viability and depletion of selected B and T cell populations. Cell 65:1165–1175, 1991.

49. Hardin JD, Boast S, Schwartzberg PL, et al: Bone marrow B lymphocyte development in c-abl deficient mice. Cell Immunol 165:44–54, 1995.

50. Kharbanda S, Ren R, Pandey P, et al: Activation of the c-Ab I tyrosine kinase in the stress response to DNA-damaging agents. Nature 376:785–788, 1995.

51. Kharbanda S, Pandey P, Ren R, et al: C-Abl activation regulates induction of the SEK1/stress-activated protein kinase pathway in the cellular response to 1-beta-D-arabinosylfuranosylcytosine. J Biol Chem 270:30278–30281, 1995.

52. Wang JYJ: Abl tyrosine kinase in signal transduction and cell-cycle regulation. Curr Opin Genet Dev 3:35–43, 1993.

53. Chung S-W, Daniel R, Wong BY, Wong PC: The ABL genes in normal and abnormal cell development. Crit Rev Oncogen 7:33–48, 1996.

54. Pendergast AM, Muller AJ, Havlik MH, et al: Evidence for regulation of the ABL tyrosine kinase by a cellular inhibitor. Proc Natl Acad Sci USA 88:5927–5931, 1991.

55. Sawyers CL: The bcr-abl gene in chronic myelogenous leukemia. Cancer Surv 15:37–51, 1992.

56. Van Etten RA, Debnath J, Zhou H, Casanovas JM: Introduction of a loss-of-function point mutation from the SH3 region of the Caenorhabditis elegans sem-5 gene activates the transforming ability of c-abl in vivo and abolishes binding of proline-rich ligands in vitro. Oncogene 10:1977–1988, 1995.

57. Whitlock CA, Witte ON: The complexity of virus-cell interactions in Abelson virus infection of lymphoid and other hematopoietic cells. Adv Immunol 37:37–98, 1985.

58. Prywes R, Foulkes G, Baltimore D: The minimum transforming gene of v-abl is the segment encoding protein tyrosine kinase. J Virol 54:114–122, 1985.

59. Ben-Neriah Y, Daley GQ, Mes-Masson A-M, et al: The chronic myelogenous leukemia-specific P210 protein is the product of the bcrlabl hybrid gene. Science 233:212–214, 1986.

60. Stam K, Heisterkamp N, Reynolds FH Jr, Groffen J: Evidence that the Ph1 gene encodes a 160,000-dalton phosphoprotein with associated kinase activity. Mol Cell Biol 7:1955–1960, 1987.

61. McWhirter JR, Galasso DL, Wang JY: A coiled-coil oligomerization domain of bcr is essential for the transforming function of bcr-abl oncoproteins. Mol Cell Biol 13:7587–7595, 1993.

62. Reuter GW, Fu H, Cripe L, et al: Association of the protein kinases c-bcr and bcr-abl with proteins of the 14–3–3 family. Science 266:129–133, 1994.

63. Deikman D, Brill S, Garrett MD, et al: Bcr encodes a GTPase-activating protein for p21 rac. Nature 351:400–402, 1991.

64. Ron D, Zannini M, Lewis M, et al: A region of proto-dbl essential for its transforming activity shows sequence similarity to a yeast cell cycle gene, CDC24, and the human breakpoint cluster gene, bcr. New Biol 3:372–379, 1991.

65. Macara IG, Lounsbury KM, Richards SA, et al: The Ras superfamily of GTPases. FASEB J 10:625–630, 1996.

66. McWhirter JR, Wang JYJ: Activation of tyrosine kinase and microfilament-binding function of c-abl by bcr sequences in bcr/abl fusion proteins. Mol Cell Biol 11:1553–1565, 1991.

67. Heisterkamp N, Voncken JW, Senadheera D, et al: Reduced oncogenicity of p190 Bcr/Abl F-actin-binding domain mutants. Blood 96:2226–2231, 2000.

68. Puil L, Liu J, Gish G, et al: Bcr-Abl oncoprotein binds directly to activators of the Ras signaling pathways. EMBO J 13:764–773, 1994.

69. Skorski T, Kanakaraj P, Nieberowska-Skorska M, et al: Phosphatidylinositol-3 kinase activity is regulated by BCR/ABL and is required for the growth of Philadelphia chromosome-positive cells. Blood 86:726–736, 1995.

70. Harrison-Findik D, Susa M, Vartikovski L: Association of phosphatidyl 3-kinase with SHC in chronic myelogenous leukemia. Oncogene 10:1385–1391, 1995.

71. Ilaria RLJ, Van Etten RA: P210 and p190 (BCR/ABL) induce the tyrosine phosphorylation and DNA binding activity of multiple specific STAT family members. J Biol Chem 271:31704–31710, 1996.

72. Reuther JY, Reuther GW, Cortez D, et al: A requirement for NF-kB activation in Bcr-Abl mediated transformation. Genes Devel 12:968–981, 1997.

73. Warmuth M, Bergmann M, Priess A, et al: The Src family kinase Hck interacts with Bcr-Abl by a kinase-independent mechanism and phosphorylates the Grb2-binding site of Bcr. J Biol Chem 272:33260–33270, 1997.

74. Raitano AB, Halpern JR, Hambuch TM, Sawyers CL: The Bcr-Abl leukemia oncogene activates Jun kinase and requires Jun for transformation. Proc Natl Acad Sci USA 92:11746–11750, 1995.

75. Gotoh A, Myazawa K, Ohyashiki K, et al: Tyrosine phosphorylation and activation of focal adhesion kinase (p125FAK) by BCR-ABL oncoprotein. Exp Hematol 23:1153–1159, 1995.

76. Sawyers CL, McLaughlin J, Witte ON: Genetic requirement for ras in the transformation of fibroblasts and hematopoietic cells by the bcr-abl oncogene. J Exp Med 181:307–313, 1995.

77. Gibbs JB, Marshall MS, Skolnick EM, et al: Modulation of guanine nucleotides bound to Ras in NIH3T3 cells by oncogenes, growth factors, and the GTPase activating protein (GAP). J Biol Chem 265:20437–20442, 1990.

78. Mandanas RA, Leibowitz DS, Gharebaghi K, et al: Role of p21 RAS in p210 bcr-abl transformation of murine myeloid cells. Blood 82:1838–1847, 1993.

79. Satoh T, Nakafuku M, Kaziro V: Function of Ras as a molecular switch in signal transduction. J Biol Chem 267:24149–24152, 1992.

80. Tauchi T, Boswell HS, Leibowitz D, Broxmeyer HE: Coupling between p210bcr-abl and Shc and Grb2 adapter proteins in hematopoietic cells permits growth factor receptor-independent link to Ras activation pathway. J Exp Med 179:167–175, 1994.

81. Gishizky ML, Cortez D, Pendergast AM: Mutant forms of growth factor-binding protein-2 reverse BCR-ABL-induced transformation. Proc Natl Acad Sci USA 92:10889–10893, 1995.

82. Tanaka S, Ouchi T, Hanafusa H: Downstream of Crk adaptor signaling pathway: Activation of Jun kinase by v-Crk through the guanine nucleotide exchange protein C3G. Proc Natl Acad Sci USA 94:2356–2361, 1997.

83. Shi CS, Tuscano J, Kehrl JH: Adaptor proteins CRK and CRKL associate with the serine/threonine protein kinase GCKR promoting GCKR and SAPK activation. Blood 95:776–782, 2000.

84. Marais R, Marshall CJ: Control of the ERK MAP kinase cascade by Ras and Raf. In Parker P, Pawson T (eds.): Cell Signaling, pp. 101–125. Cold Spring Harbor Laboratory Press, Cold Spring Harbor, 1996.

85. Kashige N, Carpino N, Kobahashi R: Tyrosine phosphorylation of p62dok by p210bcr-abl inhibits RasGAP activity. Proc Natl Acad Sci USA 97:2093–2098, 2000.

86. Dunant NM, Wisniewski D, Strife A, et al: The phosphatidylinositol polyphosphatase 5-phosphatase SHIP1 associates with the dok1 phosphoprotein in Bcr-Abl transformed cells. Cell Signal 12:317–326, 2000.

87. La Montagne KR Jr, Flint AJ, Franza BR Jr, et al: Protein tyrosine phophatase 1B anatagonizes signaling by oncoprotein kinase p210 bcr-abl in vivo. Mol Cell Biol 18:2965–2975, 1998.

88. Dai Z, Quackenbush RC, Courtney KD, et al: Oncogenic Abl and Src kinase elicit the ubiquitin-dependent degradation of target proteins through a Ras-independent pathway. Genes Dev 12:1415–1424, 1998.

89. Skorski T, Bellacosa A, Nieberowska-Skorska M, et al: Transformation of hematopoietic cells by BCR/ABL requires activation of a Pl-3k/Akt-dependent pathway. EMBO J 16:6151–6161, 1997.

90. Neshat MS, Raitano AB, Wang HG, et al: The survival function of the Bcr-Abl oncogene is mediated by Bad-dependent and -independent pathways: Roles for phosphatidylinositol 3-kinase and Raf. Mol Cell Biol 20:1179–1186, 2000.

91. Jonuleit T, van der Kuip H, Miething C, et al: Bcr-Abl kinase down-regulates cyclin-dependent kinase inhibitor p27 in human and murine cell lines. Blood 96:1933–1939, 2000.

92. Gesbert F, Sellers WR, Signoretti S, et al: BCR/ABL regulates expression of the cyclin dependent kinase inhibitor p27Kip1 through the PI3K/AKT pathway. J Biol Chem (in press).

93. Danial NN, Rothman P: JAK-STAT signaling activated by Abl oncogenes. Oncogene 19:2523–2531, 2000.

94. Lin TS, Mahajan S, Frank DA: STAT signaling in the pathogenesis and treatment of leukemias. Oncogene 19:2496–2504, 2000.

95. Sexl V, Piekorz R, Moriggl R, et al: Stat5alb contribute to interleukin 7-induced B-cell precursor expansion, but *abl* and *bcr/abl*-induced transformation are independent of Stat 5. Blood 96:2277–2283, 2000.

96. Gesbert F, Griffin JD: Bcr/Abl activates transcription of the *Bcl-X* gene through STAT5. Blood 96:2269–2276, 2000.

97. Nieborowska-Skorska M, Slupianek A, Skorski T: Progressive changes in the leukemogenic signaling in BCR/ABL-transformed cells. Oncogene 19:4117–4124, 2000.

98. de Groot RP, Raaijmakers JA, Lammers JW, Koenderman L: STAT5-dependent cyclin D1 and Bcl-xL expression in Bcr-Abl-transformed cells. Mol Cell Biol Res Commun 3:299–305, 2000.

99. Horita M, Andreu EJ, Benito A, et al: Blockade of the Bcr-Abl kinase activity induces apoptosis of chronic myelogenous leukemia cells by suppressing signal transducer and activator of transcription 5-dependent expression of Bcl-xL. J Exp Med 191:977–984, 2000.

100. Sawyers CL, Callahan W, Witte ON: Dominant negative MYC blocks transformation by ABL oncogenes. Cell 70:901–910, 1992.

101. Oda T, Heaney C, Hagopian JR, et al: Crkl is the major tyrosine-phosphorylated protein in neutrophils from patients with chronic myelogenous leukemia. J Biol Chem 269:22925–22928, 1994.

102. ten Hoeve J, Arlinghaus RB, Guo JQ, et al: Tryosine phosphorylation of CRKL in Philadelphia+ leukemia. Blood 84:1731–1736, 1994.

103. Hamdane M, David-Cordonnier MH, D'Halluin JC: Activation of p65 NF-kappaB protein by p210BCR-ABL in a myeloid cell line (p210BCR-ABL activates p65 NF-kappaB). Oncogene 15:2267–2275, 1997.

104. Reuther JY, Reuther GW, Cortez D, et al: A requirement for NF-kappaB activation in Bcr-Abl-mediated transformation. Genes Dev 12:968–981, 1998.

105. Deininger MWN, Vieira S, Mendiola R, et al: *BCR-ABL* tyrosine kinase activity regulates the expression of multiple genes implicated in the pathogenesis of chronic myeloid leukemia. Cancer Res 60:2049–2055, 2000.

106. Ogawa M, Fried J, Sakai Y, et al: Studies of cellular proliferation in human leukemias. VI. The proliferative activity, generation time, and emergence time of neutrophilic granulocytes in chronic granulocytic leukemia. Cancer 25:1031–1049, 1970.

107. Strife A, Perez A, Lambek C, et al: Characterization of lineage-negative blast subpopulations derived from normal and chronic myelogenous leukemia bone marrows and determination of their responsiveness to human c-kit ligand. Cancer Res 53:401–409, 1993.

108. Eaves C, Udomaski C, Cashman J, et al: The biology of normal and neoplastic stem cells in CML. Leuk Lymphoma 11(Suppl. 1):245–253, 1993.

109. Clarkson B, Strife A, Perez A, et al: Integration of molecular and biological abnormalities in quest for selective treatment of chronic myelogenous leukemia (CML). Leuk Lymphoma 11(Suppl. 1):81–100, 1993.

110. Strife A, Lambek C, Wisniewski D, et al: Discordant maturation as the primary biological defect in chronic myelogenous leukemia. Cancer Res 48:1035–1041, 1988.

111. Clarkson BD, Strife A, Wisniewski D, et al: New understanding of the pathogenesis of CML: A prototype of early neoplasia. Leukemia 11:1404–1428, 1997.

112. Dowding CR, Gordon MY, Goldman JM: Primitive progenitor cells in the blood of patients with chronic granulocytic leukemia. Int J Cell Cloning 4:331–340, 1986.

113. McMahon A, Bissonnette R, Schmitt M, et al: Bcr-Abl maintains resistance of chronic myelogenous leukemia cells to apoptotic cell death. Blood 83:1179–1187, 1994.

114. Bedi A, Barber JP, Bedi GC, et al: Bcr-Abl mediated inhibition of apoptosis with delay of G2/M transition after DNA damage: A mechanism of resistance to multiple cancer agents. Blood 86:1148–1158, 1995.

115. Corez D, Kadlec L, Pendergast AM: Structural and signaling requirements for BCR-ABL-mediated transformation and inhibition of apoptosis. Mol Cell Biol 15:5531–5541, 1995.

116. Sirard C, Laneuville P, Dick JE: Expression of *bcr-abl* abrogates factor-dependent growth of human hematopoietic MO7e cells by an autocrine mechanism. Blood 83:1575–1585, 1994.

117. Chapman RC, Whetton AD, Chresta CM, Dive C: Characterization of drug resistance mediated via the suppression of apoptosis by Abelson protein tyrosine kinase. Mol Pharmacol 48:334–343, 1995.

118. Fuchs EJ, Bedi A, Jones RJ, Hess AD: Cytotoxic T cells overcome BCR-ABL-mediated resistance to apoptosis. Cancer Res 55:463–466, 1995.

119. Roger R, Issaad D, Pallardy M, et al: BCR-ABL does not prevent apoptotic death induced by human natural killer or lymphokine-activated killer cells. Blood 87:1113–1122, 1996.

120. Amarante-Mendes GP, Naekyung Kim C, Liu L, et al: Bcr-Abl exerts its antiapoptotic effect against diverse apoptotic stimuli through blockage of mitochondrial relase of cytochrome c and activation of caspase-3. Blood 91:1700–1705, 1998.

121. Selleri C, Maciejewski JP: The role of FAS-mediated apoptosis in chronic myelogenous leukemia. Leuk Lymphoma 37:283–297, 2000.

122. Wetzler M, Kurzrock R, Lowe DG, et al: Alteration in bone marrow adherent layer growth factor expression: A novel mechanism of chronic myelogenous leukemia progression. Blood 78:2400–2406, 1991.

123. Wetzler M, Kurzrock R, Estrov Z, et al: Altered levels of interleukin-1j3 and interleukin-1 receptor antagonist in chronic myelogenous leukemia: Clinical and prognostic correlates. Blood 84:3142–3147, 1994.

124. Estrov Z, Kurzrock R, Wetzler M, et al: Suppression of chronic myelogenous leukemia colony growth by interleukin-1 (IL-1) receptor antagonist and soluble IL-1 receptors: A novel application for inhibitors of IL-1 activity. Blood 78:1476–1484, 1991.

125. Hallek M, Danhauser-Riedl S, Herbst R, et al: Interaction of the receptor tyrosine kinase p145c-kit with the p210bcr/abl kinase in myeloid cells. Br J Haematol 94:5–16, 1996.

126. Wilson-Rawls J, Liu J, Laneuville P, Arlinghaus RB: P210 Bcr-Abl interacts with the interleukin-3 beta c subunit and constitutively activates Jak2. Leukemia 11(Suppl. 3):428–431, 1997.

127. Verfaillie CM, Hurley R, Zhao RCH, et al: Pathophysiology of CML: Do defects in integrin function contribute to the premature circulation and massive expansion of the BCR/ABL positive clone? J Lab Clin Med 129:584–591, 1997.

128. Schlaepfer DD, Hanks SK, Hunter T, van der Geer P: Integrin-mediated signal transduction linked to ras pathway by GRB2 binding to focal adhesion kinase. Nature 372:786–789, 1994.

129. Verfaillie CM: Biology of chronic myelogenous leukemia. Hematol Oncol Clin North Am 12:1–29, 1998.

130. Verfaillie CM, McCarthy JB, McClave PB: Mechanisms underlying abnormal trafficking of malignant progenitors in chronic myelogenous leukaemia. Decreased adhesion of the basement membrane components laminin and collagen type IV. J Clin Invest 90:1232–1241, 1992.

131. Bhatia R, Munthe HA, Verfaillie CM: Role of abnormal integrin-cytoskeletal interactions in impaired integrin function in chronic myelogenous leukemia hematopoietic progenitors. Exp Hematol 27:1384–1396, 1999.

132. Bernstein R: Cytogenetics of chronic myelogenous leukemia. Semin Hematol 25:20–34, 1988.

133. Gordon MY: Cell biology of CML—a model linking the chronic and terminal phases. Leuk Lymphoma 11(Suppl. 1):93–100, 1993.

134. Kantarjian HM, Keating MJ, Talpaz M, et al: Chronic myelogenous leukemia in blast crisis. Analysis of 242 patients. Am J Med 83:445–454, 1987.

135. Ahuja H, Bar-Eli M, Advani SH, et al: Alterations in the p53 gene and the clonal evolution of the blast crisis of chronic myelocytic leukemia. Proc Natl Acad Sci USA 86:6783–6787, 1989.

136. Marasca R, Luppi M, Barozzi P, et al: P53 gene mutations in chronic myelogenous leukemia medullary and extramedullary blast crisis. Leuk Lymphoma 24:175–182, 1996.

137. Ishikura H, Yufu Y, Yamashita S, et al: Biphenotypic blast crisis of chronic myelogenous leukemia: Abnormalities of p53 and retinoblastoma genes. Leuk Lymphoma 25:573–578, 1997.

138. Sill H, Goldman J, Cross NCP: Homozygous deletion of the p16 tumor-suppressor gene are associated with lymphoid transformation of chronic myeloid leukemia. Blood 85:2013–2016, 1995.

139. Serra A, Gottardi E, della Ragione F, et al: Involvement of the cyclin-dependent kinase-4 inhibitor (CDKN2) gene in the pathogenesis of lymphoid blast crisis of chronic myelogenous leukaemia. Br J Haematol 91:625–629, 1995.

140. Skorski T, Nieborowska-Skorska M, Wlodarski P, et al: Blastic transformation of p53-deficient bone marrow cells by p21 obcr/abl tyrosine kinase. Proc Natl Acad Sci USA 93:13137–13142, 1996.

141. Honda H, Ushijima T, Wakazono K, et al: Acquired loss of p53 induces transformation in p210(bcr/abl)-expressing hematopoietic cells: A transgenic study for blast crisis of human CML. Blood 95:1144–1150, 2000.

142. Ohyashiki K, Ohyashiki JH: Telomere dynamics and cytogenetic changes in human hematologic neoplasias: A working hypothesis. Cancer Genet Cytogenet 94:67–72, 1997.

143. Iwama H, Ohyashiki K, Ohyashiki JH, et al: The relationship between telomere length and therapy-associated cytogenetic response in patients with chronic myeloid leukemia. Cancer 79:1552–1560, 1997.

144. Ohyashiki K, Ohyashiki JH, Iwama H, et al: Telomerase activity and cytogenetic changes in chronic myeloid leukemia with disease progression. Leukemia 11:190–194, 1997.

145. Boultwood J, Peniket A, Watkins F, et al: Telomere length shortening in chronic myelogenous leukemia is associated with reduced time to accelerated phase. Blood 96:358–361, 2000.

146. Brummendorf TH, Holyoake TL, Rufer N, et al: Prognostic implications of differences in telomere length between normal and malignant cells from patients with chronic myeloid leukemia measured by flow cytometry. Blood 95:1883–1890, 2000.

147. Seong D, Kantarjian H, Ro J: Hypermetaphase fluorescence in situ hybridization for quantitative monitoring of Philadelphia chromosome-positive cells in patients with chronic myelogenous leukemia during treatment. Blood 86:2343–2349, 1995.

148. Nolte M, Werner M, Ewig M, et al: Fluorescence in situ hybridization (FISH) is a reliable diagnostic tool for detection of the 9;22 translocation. Leuk Lymphoma 22:287–294, 1996.

149. Muhlmann J, Thaler J, Hilbe W, et al: Fluorescence in situ hybridization (FISH) on peripheral blood smears for monitoring Philadelphia chromosome-positive chronic myeloid leukemia (CML) during interferon treatment: A new strategy for remission assessment. Genes Chromosomes Cancer 21:90–100, 1998.

150. Dewald GW, Wyatt WA, Juneau AL, et al: Highly sensitive fluorescence in situ hybridization method to detect double BCR/ABL fusion and monitor response to therapy in chronic myeloid leukemia. Blood 91:3357–3365, 1998.

151. Sklar J: Polymerase chain reaction: The molecular microscope of residual disease. J Clin Oncol 9:1521–1524, 1996.

152. Bartram CR: Detection of minimal residual leukemia by the polymerase chain reaction: Potential implications for therapy. Clin Chim Acta 217:75–83, 1993.

153. Hochhaus A, Lint F, Reiter A, et al: Variable numbers of BCR-ABL transcripts persist in CML patients who achieve complete cytogenetic remission with interferon-α. Br J Haematol 91:126–131, 1995.

154. Kurzrock R, Estrov Z, Kantarjian H, Talpaz M: Conversion of interferon-induced, long-term cytogenetic remission in chronic myelogenous leukemia. J Clin Oncol 16:1526–1531, 1998.

155. Gaiger A, Lion T, Kahls P, et al: Frequent detection of BCR-ABL specific mRNA in patients with chronic myeloid leukemia (CML) following allogeneic and syngeneic bone marrow transplantation (BMT). Leukemia 7:1766–1772, 1993.

156. Lin F, van Rhee F, Goldman JM, Cross NCP: Kinetics of increasing BCR-ABL transcript numbers in chronic myeloid leukemia patients who relapse after bone marrow transplantation. Blood 87:4473–4478, 1996.

157. Hochhaus A, Lin F, Reiter A, et al: Quantification of residual disease in chronic myelogenous leukemia patients on interferon-α therapy by competitive polymerase chain reaction. Blood 87:1549–1555, 1996.

158. Radich JP, Gehly G, Gooley T, et al: Polymerase chain reaction detection of the BCR-ABL fusion transcript after allogeneic mar-

row transplantation for chronic myeloid leukemia: Results and implications in 346 patients. Blood 85:2632–2638, 1995.

159. Serrano J, Roman J, Sanchez J, et al: Molecular analysis of lineage-specific chimerism and minimal residual disease by RT-PCR of p210(BCR-ABL) and p190(BCR-ABL) after allogeneic bone marrow transplantation for chronic myeloid leukemia: Increasing mixed myeloid chimerism and p190(BCR-ABL) detection precede cytogenetic relapse. Blood 95:2659–2665, 2000.

160. Faderl S, Talpaz M, Kantarjian HM, Estrov Z: Should polymerase chain reaction analysis to detect residual disease in patients with chronic myeloid leukemia be used in clinical decision making? Blood 93:2755–2759, 1999.

161. Heid CA, Stevens J, Livak KJ, Williams PM: Real time quantitative PCR. Genome Res 6:986–994, 1996.

162. Kantarjian H, Kurzrock R, Talpaz M: Philadelphia chromosome-negative chronic myelogenous leukemia and chronic myelomonocytic leukemia. Hematol Oncol Clin North Am 4:389–404, 1990.

163. Cortes J, Talpaz M, O'Brien S, et al: Philadelphia chromosome negative chronic myelogenous leukemia with rearrangement of the breakpoint cluster region: Long-term follow-up results. Cancer 75:464–470, 1995.

164. Costello R, Lafage M, Toiron Y, et al: Philadelphia chromosome-negative chronic myeloid leukaemia: A report of 14 new cases. Br J Haematol 90:346–352, 1995.

165. Bennett JM, Catovsky D, Daniel MT, et al: The chronic myeloid leukaemias: Guidelines for distinguishing chronic granulocytic, atypical chronic myeloid, and chronic myelomonocytic leukemia. Proposals by the French-American-British Cooperative Leukaemia Group. Br J Haematol 87:746–754, 1994.

166. Melo JV: BCR-ABL gene variants. Baillieres Clin Haematol 10:203–222, 1997.

167. Hochhaus A, Reiter A, Skladny H, et al: A novel BCR-ABL fusion gene (e6a2) in a patient with Philadelphia chromosome-negative chronic myelogenous leukemia. Blood 88:2236–2240, 1996.

168. Costello R, Sainty D, Lafage-Pochitaloff M, Gabert J: Clinical and biological aspects of Philadelphia-negative/BCR-negative chronic myeloid leukemia. Leuk Lymphoma 25:225–232, 1997.

169. Faderl S, Kantarjian HM, Talpaz M, O'Brien S: New treatment approaches for chronic myelogenous leukemia. Semin Oncol 27:578–586, 2000.

170. Buchdunger E, Zimmermann J, Mett H, et al: Inhibition of the Abl protein-tyrosine kinase in vitro and in vivo by a 2-phenylaminopyrimidine derivative. Cancer Res 56:100–104, 1996.

171. Druker BJ, Lydon NB: Lessons learned from the development of an Abl tyrosine kinase inhibitor for chronic myelogenous leukemia. J Clin Invest 105:3–7, 2000.

172. Schindler T, Bormann W, Pellicena P, et al: Structural mechanisms for STI-571 inhibition of Abelson tyrosine kinase. Science 289:1938–1942, 2000.

173. Agarwal N, Gewirtz AM: Oligonucleotide therapeutics for hematologic disorders. Biochim Biophys Acta 1489:85–96, 1999.

174. Kardinal C, Konkol B, Schulz A, et al: Cell-penetrating SH3 domain blocker peptides inhibit proliferation of primary blast cells from CML patients. FASEB J 14:1529–1538, 2000.

175. Clark RE, Dodi IA, Hill SC, et al: Direct evidence that leukemic cells present HLA-associated immunogenic peptides derived from the BCR-ABL b3a2 fusion protein. Blood 98:2887–2893, 2001.

5

Diagnosis and Treatment of Chronic Myeloid Leukemia

Annette J. Neylon and Stephen G. O'Brien

The diagnosis of chronic myeloid leukemia (CML) usually presenbuts few problems. In contrast, knowing how to counsel a newly diagnosed patient and planning therapeutic strategy presents many difficulties. Is the patient suitable for an allograft?; should "mini-grafting" be considered?; will they tolerate interferon (IFN)-alpha?; should imatinib (Glivec, Gleevec—formerly ST1571 or CGP57184) be used and can a supply be secured? Even if one is fully informed of current developments, the answers to these questions are not always clear as there have been very significant therapeutic innovations in CML in the past 2 to 3 years. In parallel with these developments has been the Internet information "explosion" that we have witnessed in recent times. The Internet has introduced a new dimension to therapeutic decision making for both patients and their doctors. Patients increasingly have strong views on how they should be treated, often fueled by the Internet, and this can introduce inappropriate pressure to adopt unproven treatments (see end of chapter for some useful Website addresses).

In this chapter, we will review some of the essentials of diagnosis, which will be mostly self-evident to practising hematologists. The main focus will be on available treatment options, the results to date using these various options, and guidance on therapeutic strategy. However, if the reader will forgive a crude paraphrase, there are at least three things about which we can be sure: death, taxes, and that the options for the treatment of CML will change again in the next year.

DIAGNOSIS

Definition, Diagnostic Criteria, and Differential Diagnosis

CML is a clonal myeloproliferative expansion of transformed primitive hematopoietic progenitor cells involving myeloid, monocytic, erythroid, megakaryocytic, B-lymphoid, and occasionally T-lymphoid lineages.[1] Since the 1960s when Nowell and Hungerford[2] described the specific karyotypic abnormality—the Philadelphia (Ph) chromosome—there has been rapid progress in our understanding of pathogenesis, providing us with the means to easily diagnose and monitor the disease.

The detection of *BCR-ABL*, the fusion gene involving the breakpoint cluster region and the cellular oncogene, *ABL*, is the pathognomonic feature of most cases of CML (see comments below on "atypical" CML). Few conditions demonstrate overlapping features, the most common being a "leukemoid reaction" usually in response to severe infection. In this situation however, the presence of splenomegaly and a low leukocyte alkaline phosphatase (LAP) score suggest CML. The presence of the characteristic Ph chromosome will allow the distinction of CML from such disorders as primary proliferative polycythemia, idiopathic myelofibrosis, and primary thrombocythemia, which can occasionally have a somewhat confusing clinical presentation. The detection of *BCR-ABL* in a peripheral blood sample by reverse-transcriptase polymerase chain reaction (RT-PCR) techniques will give the definitive answer, but one should be aware that approximately 5 percent of CML cases are negative for the Ph chromosome.[3,4] Among such Ph-negative patients there is a preponderance of males and older patients, with lower leukocyte counts and thrombocytopenia being more typical of this subgroup. In those patients who are negative for the Ph chromosome, 2.5 percent are also *BCR-ABL* negative and the prognosis is poorer in these patients.[5] Specific mention should be made of those patients apparently with primary thrombocythemia in whom the Ph chromosome is detectable. Such patients should be considered to have CML in a less typical form and thus managed in a similar way. It is therefore implicit that patients with apparent primary thrombocytosis should be tested for the Ph translocation and/or *BCR-ABL* by RT-PCR.

Investigation of a Suspected Case of CML

The specifics of the investigation of a newly presenting patient with CML are detailed in Table 5–1. In the presenting history it may be helpful to elucidate certain features. These include the presence of night sweats or bone pain as they may indicate transforming disease. Symptoms suggestive of hyperviscosity such as headaches, confusion, and visual disturbances are important to identify. It may be helpful to determine exposure to potential mutagens. Allaying fears that the disease may be inherited is important, along with establishing whether the patient has any siblings and hence potential for allografting. Examination should particularly focus on retinal examination and lymph node areas, and include documenting the size of the spleen and liver.

The "gold standard" diagnostic test is the detection of the Ph chromosome and/or the *BCR-ABL* fusion gene. A full blood count and film review are critical in establishing the prognostic score (see later), and the number of blasts, basophils, and eosinophils should be particularly noted for use in calculating a prognostic score.[6] If leukapheresis is considered appropriate, urgent human immunodeficiency virus (HIV) and hepatitis B and C serology will be required prior to the procedure. Before performing the bone marrow examination it may be worthwhile to consider a sample for one of the many research groups interested in CML. Details of morphology and cytogenetics should be recorded. Immunophenotyping will only be relevant to classify blast crisis. The trephine biopsy should be assessed for cellularity and degree of fibrosis.

Table 5-1. Investigations To Be Performed in Suspected Cases of CML

Mandatory
- FBC and blood film
- Biochemistry screen including urate
- Blood group/save serum
- Coagulation screen
- Bone marrow aspirate for:
  Morphology
  Cytogenetics (Fluorescent in situ hybridisation[FISH] if metaphase cultures fail)
  Sample for immunophenotyping (take an EDTA sample but only process if blast crisis is evident morphologically)
  Samples stored for research purposes if appropriate locally or for mailing to research group. (Often in 20 ml container with preservative-free heparin [PFH])
- Bone marrow trephine
  Assess cellularity
  Degree of fibrosis

Consider
- Urgent HIV, Hepatitis B and Hepatitis C serology if leukopheresis being considered
- CMV serology if allograft being considered
- HLA type patient and sibling if allograft being considered
- Peripheral blood leukocyte alkaline phosphatase (LAP) score and possibly peripheral blood *BCR-ABL* RT-PCR if marrow aspirate unavailable/inappropriate (LAP score is obsolete in many labs now).
- RT-PCR (useful to define breakpoint for future monitoring)

Table 5-2. Clinical Presentation of 430 Patients Referred to the Hammersmith Hospital for Consideration of Transplantation from 1981

- 80% of patients are symptomatic at time of presentation
- 20% of patients may have the diagnosis of CML made incidentally on routine FBC
- 93% of patients present with chronic phase disease
- Thrombosis and leukostasis are rare even with very high platelet/white cell counts
- Median FBC values are as follows (range):
  WBC $174 (5.0 - 850.0) \times 10^9$/L
  Hb $10.3 (4.9\text{-}16.6)$ g/dl
  Plt $430 (17\text{-}3182) \times 10^9$/L
- 19% of patients present with a WBC $> 350 \times 10^9$/L
- 25% of patients present with platelets $> 1 \times 10^{12}$ /L

Ten Most Common Symptoms at Presentation	
Fatigue and lethargy	33.5%
Bleeding	21.3%
Weight loss	20.0%
Splenic discomfort	18.6%
Abdominal mass or fullness	14.8%
Sweats	14.6%
Bone pain	7.4%
Infection	6.2%
Headache	5.8%
Dyspnea	4.5%

The Commonest Examination Findings	
Spleen palpable (overall)	75.8%
1-10 cm	36.9%
> 10cm	38.9%
Spleen not palpable	24.2%
Purpura	15.8%
Palpable liver	2.2%

(Data from Savage[7])

Consideration should be given to determining the cytomegalovirus (CMV) status of the patient, both for the initial blood product provision and for assessing potential for an allograft. Equally, HLA-typing of the patient and his or her siblings should be performed at an early stage to enable further planning of therapeutic strategy. The peripheral blood LAP score or even *BCR-ABL* RT-PCR may be helpful if the marrow aspirate is unavailable or inappropriate.

Modes of Presentation

Savage et al.[7] described a series of 430 consecutive cases presenting to one center for consideration of allogeneic transplant. Although this group of patients is preselected, the data are the first to describe the presenting features of such a large group of CML patients. Their data are summarized in Table 5–2. Up to 20 percent of patients were asymptomatic and were diagnosed when a blood sample was taken for other reasons. Some cases had been diagnosed incidentally during pregnancy, while donating blood, or undergoing routine surgery.

Of those presenting with symptoms, the ten most commonly recorded are shown in Table 5–2. In retrospect the patient may be able to describe fatigue, weakness, or a sense of fullness in the left upper quadrant with early satiety after meals. Other symptoms including visual disturbance, weakness, arthralgia, cough, malaise, dizziness, nausea/vomiting, ankle edema, priapism, and mental changes occur in less than 5 percent of cases. Thrombocytosis may occur with a count above 1×10^{12}/L in 25 percent of cases, although there does not appear to be a correlation between bleeding and level of thrombocytosis. Splenomegaly and purpura were the most common physical signs at presentation, at 40 and 16 percent, respectively. The authors also described greater leukocytosis and splenomegaly in males and younger patients.

Phases of Disease

Some 93 percent of patients present in chronic phase,[7] that is, there are less than 5 percent blasts in the bone marrow. It is possible to have a marginal excess of blasts at presentation but after starting treatment it becomes clear the patient is in chronic phase. The duration of chronic phase is usually between 3 and 8 years, with the median duration 4 to 5 years in most series but patients can present in blast crisis or, alternatively, not progress for 15 years (see section on interferon therapy later). The disease then inevitably progresses from this 'benign' stage to the accelerated phase and ultimately blast crisis. At this stage the disease is relatively resistant to treatment and thus rapidly fatal.

The definition of *accelerated phase* is vague but accepted clinical practice follows the criteria laid out in Table 5–3.[8,9] Clinical features may signal the progression to accelerated phase with pyrexia, night sweats, weight loss, and increasing splenomegaly being typical occurrences. Laboratory features may also be indicative of "acceleration," with anemia, increasing basophils or eosinophils, thrombocytopenia, or increasing proportion of blasts being the most common findings. The appearance of hyposegmented neutrophils (i.e., with the Pelger-Huet anomaly) is also recognized.[10] In detailed analysis of the erythroid series it may be possible to detect a slight increase in hemoglobin F,[11] although this is more typical of the CML of childhood.

The definition of *blast crisis* is based on the presence of more than 30 percent blasts in the peripheral blood or bone marrow, or the demonstration of extramedullary infiltration of blast cells. In two-thirds of cases the blasts are myeloid with one-third lymphoid. Caution is required as the morphological features may be misleading and immunophenotyping is therefore recommended in all cases. Lymphoid transformation carries a marginally better prognosis than myeloid, although both are usually fatal despite intensive treatment and have a median survival from diagnosis of blast crisis of only 3 to 6 months. It is difficult to distinguish those patients presenting with Ph-positive acute myelocytic leukemia (AML) or acute lymphocytic leukemia (ALL) from those with blast crisis of CML. Some clinicians hold that the presence of massive splenomegaly is more in keeping with pre-existing CML whereas others believe the presence of p190[BCR-ABL] suggests de novo ALL and p210[BCR-ABL] might suggest pre-existing CML. It is possible, in both children and adults with CML, to develop blast transformation with mixed lineages, that is, both lymphoid and myeloid surface markers detectable on the same cells[12] or some blasts with either lymphoid or myeloid characteristics.[13] T-lymphoid blast transformation is rare but there are several cases showing both the *BCR-ABL* fusion gene and T-cell receptor (TCR) gene rearrangements.[14]

Cytogenetic and molecular changes are well recognized in 50 to 80 percent of patients during transformation to accelerated or blast phase. Minor cytogenetic changes include monosomies of chromosomes 7 and 17, and loss of the Y chromosome;[15] trisomies of chromosomes 17 and 21; and translocations of chromosome 3 with chromosome 21, t(3;21)(q26;q22).[16] Major cytogenetic changes include trisomy 8, isochromosome i(17q), trisomy 19, and a double Ph chromosome.[16–18]

Alterations in p53 on the long arm of chromosome 17 by deletion, rearrangement, or mutation of sequences, occurring predominantly with myeloid blast crisis, have been distinguished in up to 30 percent of CML patients entering the blast phase.[19,20] Even before their clinical manifestations it may be possible to detect these cytogenetic changes in the bone marrow, extramedullary masses, or splenectomy specimens.[3,21,22]

Clinical signs of blastic transformation may be due to the rapid exponential rise in blasts in the peripheral blood. The most significant areas compromised are the cerebral and respiratory circulations, resulting in multifocal bleeding, dyspnea, and hypoxemia.[23,24] Tumors due to the deposition of blast cells, otherwise known as chloromas granulocytic sarcomas, may be visible before the detection of blasts in the peripheral blood.[25] It is important to distinguish such tumors from undifferentiated carcinomas and diffuse large cell non-Hodgkin's lymphoma, which may require immnuohistochemical staining. Commonly the tumors are detected in lymph nodes, cutaneous tissue, or as lucent bone deposits on x-ray. Meningeal deposition may result in cord compression but has also been noted in patients who have achieved remission from blast transformation.[26]

Prognostic Scores

Prognostic models aim to categorize patients into different risk groups at diagnosis, which is particularly important in the analysis of trial data. These scores all require examination of the first blood film that is made on the newly diagnosed patient but regrettably the subsequent loss of this blood film is the most common reason for an incomplete score. Prognostic scores have traditionally been utilized in the context of analyzing large clinical trials and thus they should be applied to the individual patient with some caution. Small variations in the parameters described can make a significant difference to the final score; accurate determination of these parameters is therefore crucial. The details of the more commonly used systems are described in Table 5–4.

Tura et al.,[27] and subsequently in 1982 Cervantes and Rozman,[28] devised scoring systems based on easily recordable parameters to categorize CML patients into three groups or stages. These were then applied to obtain the likely survival times

---

Table 5–3. The Criteria Used in Defining Phases of Disease in CML

Criteria for accelerated phase commonly used in clinical practice:
- WBC difficult to control with IFN and/or hydroxyurea in terms of dose required or shortening of intervals between course.
- Rapid doubling of WBC (< 5 days).
- > 10% blasts in blood or marrow
- > 20% blasts or promyelocytes in blood or marrow
- > 20% basophils/eosinophils
- Anemia and/or thrombocytopenia non-responsive to IFN and/or hydroxyurea.
- Persistent thrombocytosis (> 600 x 10^9/L)
- Additional chromosomal changes*
- Increasing splenomegaly unresponsive to treatment
- Unexplained fevers and bone pains
- Development of myelofibrosis or chloromas.
- * *This is the subject of ongoing debate, and some study protocols do not formally recognize this as a feature of accelerated phase disease.*

Criteria for accelerated phase derived from multivariate analysis:
- Peripheral blasts plus peripheral blasts > 15%
- promyelocytes > 30%
- Peripheral basophils > 20%
- Thrombocytopenia (< 100 ×10^9/L) unrelated to therapy
- Cytogenetic clonal evolution

Criteria for Blast Crisis:
- > 30% blasts in peripheral blood and/or marrow
- Extramedullary infiltrate of blast cells

Table 5–4. The Prognostic Scores Commonly Used in CML

Sokal score (1984) (Sokal, Cox et al.[6])
- Criteria required at presentation (prior to treatment):
  1. Age
  2. Spleen size (cm below costal margin measured clinically with a tape)
  3. Platelet count prior to any treatment
  4. Blast percentage in peripheral blood (preferably 500 cells, but at least 200)
- Formula: Exp[0.0116(age − 43.4) + 0.0345(spleen − 7.51)
    + 0.188 (platelets/700) 2 − 0.563)
    + 0.0887 (% blasts − 2.1)]
  Good prognosis < 0.8
  Moderate prognosis 0.8 − 1.2
  Poor prognosis > 1.2
- An on-line calculator is available at: http://www.ncl.ac.uk/cml

Hasford score (1998) (Hasford, Pfirrmann et al.[29])
- The 'Hasford' score is a more recent and refined, prognostic index
- Data analysed on 1573 patients
- Criteria required at presentation (prior to treatment):
  1. Age
  2. Spleen size (cm below costal margin measured clinically with a tape)
  3. Platelet count prior to any treatment
  4. Blast percentage in peripheral blood (preferably 500 cells, but at least 200)
  5. Eosinophil percentage in peripheral blood (same no. of cells counted)
  6. Basophil percentage in peripheral blood (same no. of cells counted)
- Formula: (0.6666 × age [0 when < 50 years; otherwise 1]
    + 0.0420 × spleen size [cm from costal margin]
    + 1.0956 × platelet count [0 when platelets < 1500; otherwise 1]
    + 0.0584 × blasts [%]
    + 0.0413 × eosinophils [%]
    + 0.2039 × basophils [0 when basophils < 3%; otherwise 1]
  multiplied by 1000
- Interpretation:
- Low risk ≤ 780   median survival 100 months
- Intermediate risk > 780 < 1480   median survival 69 months
- High risk > 1480   median survival 45 months
- An on-line calculator is available at: http://www.pharmacoepi.de/cmlscore.html

Gratwohl's system (1998) (Gratwohl, Hermans et al.[31])
- Criteria based on pre-transplant risk factors:
  1. Histocompatibility (0 if HLA identical sibling; 1 if matched unrelated donor)
  2. Stage of disease at time of transplant (0 if 1st chronic phase; 1 if accelerated phase; 2 if blast crisis or second or later chronic phase)
  3. Age of donor and recipient (0 if < 20 years; 1 if 20-40 years; 2 if > 40 years)
  4. Sex of donor and recipient (0 for all except 1 for male recipient/female donor)
  5. Time from diagnosis to transplant (0 if < 12 months; 1 if > 12 months)
- Interpretation:

Score	5 year survival (%)	Risk of transplant-related mortality (%)
0	72	20
1	70	23
2	62	31
3	48	46
4	40	51
5	18	71
6	22	73

for each stage, which differed significantly according to stage. The later models, such as the system devised by Sokal et al. in 1984,[6,8] are based on multivariate analyses and the hazard ratio, derived using regression calculations. The Sokal model is the most extensively used in clinical research and is widely applied.

Hasford et al.[29] devised a system based on a German trial population,[30] which also includes the percentage of peripheral eosinophils and basophils. Patients can thus be stratified based on the presence or absence of these factors into three risk groups with significantly different outcomes.

Gratwohl et al.[31] devised a simple system based on five main factors following analysis of 3142 patients allografted for CML between 1989 and 1997. These factors can be used for risk assessment to assist in the counseling of patients prior to allografting.

TREATMENT

Although there is considerable optimism that the new drug imatinib (Glivec, imatinib mesylate) may be as good as, if not better than, IFN in extending chronic phase, the only established "curative" therapy (by which is implied disease-free survival for at least 5 years) in 2003 is allogeneic transplantation. However, despite the extended availability of allografting to older individuals through the development of attenuated conditioning regimens—so-called mini-transplant—the majority of CML patients do not have a transplant option, as shown in Figure 5–1. One has to remember that CML is predominantly a disease of older people, the median age at presentation being 60 years,[32] and therefore it is likely that allografting will never be an option for all patients. The development of innovative drug treatments is clearly the way forward to help the majority of patients.

Immediate Management of Newly Diagnosed Patient

The immediate management of a newly presenting patient with possible CML involves the initial history taking and investigation described in the previous sections. The next stage is to control any immediate life-threatening complications such as leukostasis, hemorrhage, or infection, before appropriate antileukemic chemotherapy once the diagnosis is secure. Tumor lysis syndrome is a relatively rare but nonetheless recognized complication and it is prudent to commence allopurinol 300 mg daily by mouth and encourage plentiful oral fluid intake. Once the leukocyte count has fallen below 30×10^9/L allopurinol should no longer be required unless the patient has a history of gout or continues to be hyperuricemic. On some occasions it may be necessary to reduce the leukocyte load more urgently, especially if there is evidence of leukostasis causing the clinical manifestations previously described. This may be achieved by the introduction of large doses of hydroxyurea, in the order of 3.0 to 6.0 g daily, and/or by leukapheresis. Leukapheresis may also considered as the treatment of choice during pregnancy.[33,34] If any form of transplant procedure (autograft or allograft) is a possible future option then leukapheresis with cryopreservation of peripheral blood stem cells is preferable prior to initiating any form of treatment. In centers where the facility of leukapheresis is not immediately available it is possible to perform the procedure at a later date having discontinued the hydroxyurea treatment allowing the leukocytes to climb above 30×10^9/L.

Prior to the initiation of antileukemic therapy it is important to discuss frankly, and document, the implications for future fertility with the patient and possibly his or her partner. It is possible to arrange cryopreservation of spermatocytes and possibly oocytes/ovarian slices and this is preferably done in liason with a center specializing in fertility medicine.

Hydroxyurea, in doses of 2.0 to 3.0 g/day, is usually the agent of first choice.[35,36] This dose is reduced once the white cell count is reduced below 30×10^9/L. Alternative chemotherapeutic agents such as busulfan are no longer routinely used as first line due to their potential for mutagenicity and the number of studies showing benefit of hydroxyurea in patient survival.[37–40] For details of mechanisms of actions see the following section on established drug treatments.

At this stage it is important to establish the CMV status of the patient, if there is the potential for a future allograft.

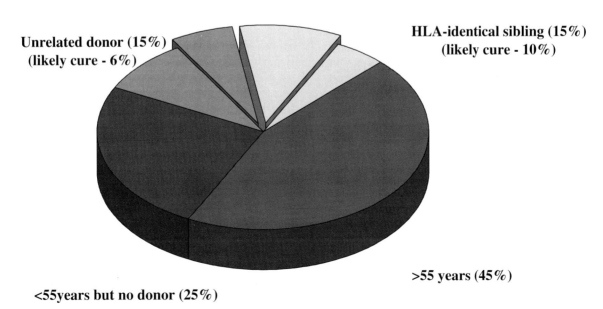

Figure 5–1. An estimate of donor availability and probability of cure as a percentage of all patients with CML assuming that the median age is 50 years and the average number of siblings in a family is two.

Although unusual, if blood products are required in the meantime CMV-negative products should be administered until the CMV status is available. HLA typing of patient and sibling(s), and later unrelated donor panels if appropriate, should be performed if transplant is being considered.

Once these steps have been taken one should move on to strategy. Occasionally CML patients with a modestly elevated white cell count that was discovered incidentally may not require intervention with chemotherapy at presentation but can be closely monitored. The diagnosis of CML represents a time of stress and anguish for the patients and their family. Written and Web-based counseling materials and self-help groups can be of great help (see Appendix).

Management Strategy

It is easy for patients with CML to "drift" in their management, as they are often not unwell when they present, and therefore there may be no immediate impetus to discuss management strategy. There are a number of key issues to address soon after diagnosis in order to plan effectively and in a logical manner. A number of individual therapeutic options are described below but a crucial initial consideration is whether a given patient is suitable for a clinical trial—most are. We have attempted to define a strategy to adopt with newly presenting CML patients; however, the scheme shown in Figure 5–2 is not applicable under all circumstances and is only a guide to decision making.

The first consideration is to determine whether allogeneic transplantation is a viable option and this predominantly depends on the patient's age, general health, and the availability of a donor. Within the first 2 to 3 months of diagnosis it should become clear if a sibling donor is identified. If no potential HLA-identical sibling donors are available, the next step involves searching national and international bone marrow panels. Cord bank panels are also worth considering although the cell dose available may be limited. If the searches prove fruitful the patient must be very carefully and repeatedly counseled about the potential risks and benefits.

If allografting is not immediately appropriate the next key decision is whether to use imatinib or IFN-alpha. Whether to

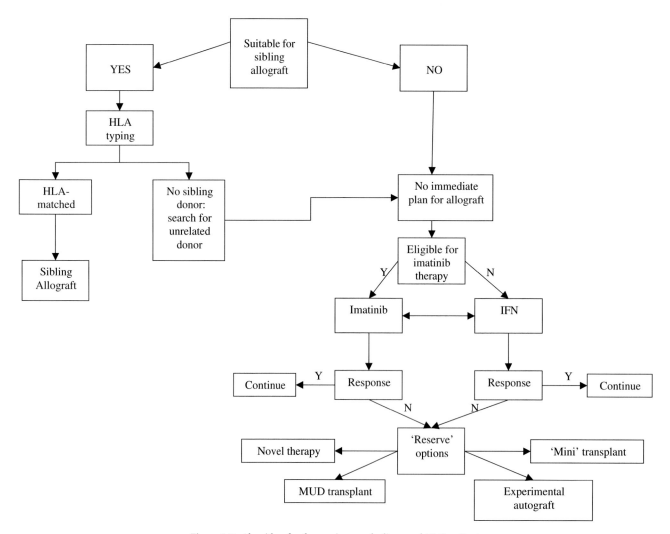

Figure 5–2. Algorithm for therapy in a newly diagnosed CML patient.

perform an "up front" allograft is the key decision and due to the lack of long-term data with imatinib it is difficult to know how best to advise patients. However, many patients are now voting with their feet and choosing a trial of imatinib before considering allografting. Defining "response" to these nontransplant agents is important and a strategy for the evaluation of the degree and duration of cytogenetic and molecular responses must be devised. We propose a scheme in Table 5–5 for the rational use of these relatively expensive techniques. When monitoring CML interphase fluorescent in situ hybridization (FISH) techniques using DNA probes homologous to *BCR* and *ABL* are arguably the most representative investigations, but conventional G-banding on at least 30 metaphases will suffice if FISH is unavailable. Quantitative (including real time) RT-PCR should generally be undertaken if FISH positivity is at or below the false-positive level, which is around 6 percent FISH-positive interphase cells unless dual-probe, dual-fusion technology is used. RT-PCR has an established role following allogeneic bone marrow transplantation[41] and peripheral blood is as good as marrow. There may be protocol requirements and local preferences or differences in availability, which may dictate techniques and frequency of testing and it is important to recognize that the complexity of these tests dictates that stringent validation criteria must be established.

Because some studies have suggested a survival advantage due to IFN regardless of cytogenetic response, it could be argued that regular marrow cytogenetics are unnecessary. However, this contention remains somewhat controversial and monitoring every 6 months seems to be a reasonable policy. Analysis at 3, 6, 9, 12, 18, and 24 months is recommended post-transplant and yearly thereafter until 5 years. Thus, intervention with donor lymphocyte infusions (DLI) can be considered at the earliest recurrence of *BCR-ABL* positivity by RT-PCR. After 5 years monitoring should be at the patient's and clinician's discretion. For other patients, especially older individuals and those on hydroxyurea alone, it would seem reasonable to examine the bone marrow only on clinical suspicion of transforming disease.

Established Drug Treatments in Common Use

Hydroxyurea

Since its introduction in 1972[42] this agent has been the "workhorse" therapy for CML.[35–39] It is highly effective in controlling the hematological aspects of this disorder[43] but does not produce any meaningful cytogenetic responses, even at high dose. It has the advantage of relatively few side effects.

The recently published report by the CML Trialists' Collaborative Group[44] based on meta-analysis of 812 patients shows no statistical significance between hydroxyurea and busulfan but survival is better with hydroxyurea than with busulfan (53.6 percent vs. 45.1 percent) at 4 years.

IFN-alpha

Since the first reports of its activity in CML in 1983,[45,46] IFN-alpha has been widely investigated both as a single agent and in combination. There are no convincing data that there are significant differences between Roferon (Roche) and Intron A (Schering Plough). Both products now come in a pen device similar to those used for delivering insulin. The precise mechanism of action is unclear although many possible mechanisms have been proposed.[47–51]

Most, but not all, prospective randomized trials comparing interferon with conventional maintenance chemotherapy (usually hydroxyurea or busulfan) have shown a survival advantage of interferon,[52–60] leading to the recommendation that IFN-based regimens should be considered in all newly presenting CML patients.[61] A meta-analysis of seven randomized trials by the CML Trialists' Collaborative Group[62] demonstrated a statistically significant survival advantage of IFN over either hydroxyurea or busulfan. Table 5–6 details the 11 trials identified, with data available from 7 of those (Figure 5–3). The 5-year survival rates were 57 percent with IFN compared to 42 percent with either chemotherapy drug. IFN may be expected to increase life expectancy by a median of 20 months.

Hematological and cytogenetic response to IFN was defined by the Houston group.[64,65] A complete hematological response requires the normalization of the leukocyte count to less than 10×10^9/L with the disappearance of immature myeloid cells, normalization of the platelet count to less than 450×10^9/L, along with the disappearance of all signs and symptoms of disease. Cytogenetic response is usually classified according to the proportion of Ph-positive cells. No response is when all metaphases remain Ph-positive; minor response is when 35 to 95 percent of metaphases are Ph-positive; partial response when Ph positivity persists in 1 to 34 percent of metaphases; and complete cytogenetic response occurs when 100 percent of metaphases are negative for the Ph chromosome on at least one karyotypic examina-

Table 5–5. The Role and Relevance of Cytogenetic G-banding, Interphase FISH and BCR-ABL RT-PCR in the Diagnosis and Management of CML in Different Phases

	Conventional G-Banding (at least 30 metaphases)	Interphase Fluorescent in situ hybridization	Quantitative (including 'real time') reverse transcriptase -PCR
Establishing diagnosis	Yes	If G-banding fails	If all others fail or quick answer essential
Monitoring IFN or imatinib therapy	If FISH unavailable or in conjuction with FISH	Yes	If FISH negative or below 'false positive' level
Monitoring post–stem cell transplantation	If FISH unavailable or in conjuction with FISH	Yes	Yes
Transforming disease	Yes (?additional abnormalities)	Not essential	Not helpful

Table 5–6. All Relevant Randomized Trials that Began Before 1990: Interferon-alpha versus Busulfan or Hydroxyurea[a]

Study	Induction Treatment	IFN-alpha	IFN-alpha Target WBC	Additional Therapy if Necessary	Alternative Treatment	Chemotherapy Target WBC	Ph-negative Patients Eligible	No. of Patients	No. of Deaths	Median Years Follow-up of Survivors
Trials that are available										
Italian-CML-86[56]	IFN-alpha	9MU/d		HU or Bu if WBC >30	HU	<30	No	322	198	9
German-CML-1 (Hehlmann, Heimpel et al.[30])	IFN-alpha	5MU/m2/d	2-4	Nil	Bu HU	<20 5-15	Yes	603	329	3
MRC-CML-3 (Allan, Richards et al.[63])	Chemotherapy	3MU/d	2-5	HU or Bu if WBC >30	Bu	4-20 or <30 HU	Yes 4-20	590	331	4
Benelux[58]	Chemotherapy	3MU x 5/w	<10	HU to keep WBC <10	HU	<10	No	197	72	4
Pessac (Broustet, Reiffers et al.[53])	IFN-alpha	4MU/m2/d		Nil	HU	4-10	Yes	22	10	6
EORTC-06887	Chemotherapy	5MU/d	<10	A-BMT if complete cytogenetic response	HU	<15	Yes	78	20	2
Japan (Ohnishi, Ohno et al.[57])	IFN-alpha	9MU/d	5	Nil	Bu	5	No	170	60	4
Trials that are not published										
Washington (Jacobson and St Germain 1991)	IFN-alpha	4MU/m2/d			HU			18		
Schering-plough	IFN-alpha	4MU/m2/d	<15		HU	4-10		133		
MEX-INC-CML	IFN-alpha	5MU/m2/d	<20		Bu	<20		30		
Castilla-Leon (Moro, Gil et al.[52])	Chemotherapy	2MU/d	<10	HU to keep WBC <10	HU	5-10		26		

[a] (Reproduced with permission[62].)

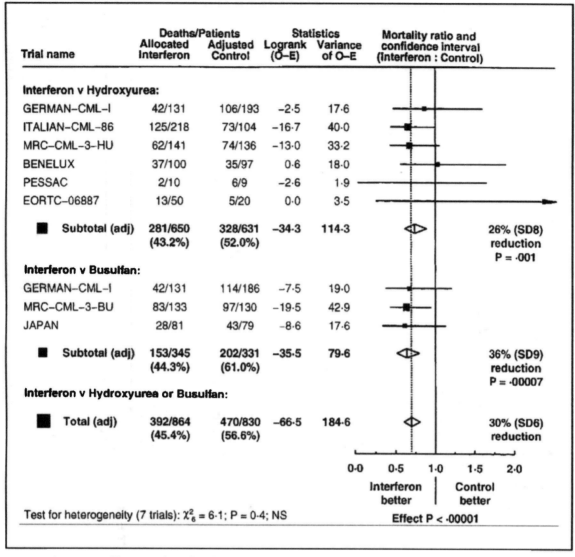

Figure 5–3. Odds ratio analysis of randomized trials of interferon-alpha versus control (HU or Bu) in Ph-positive CML: Combination of evidence from seven trials (1997). (Reproduced with permission[62].)

tion. Complete and partial responses can be grouped together under the category "major" cytogenetic response. There is evidence[56,66] to suggest that attaining cytogenetic response to IFN results in prolonged survival, although survival in all groups treated with IFN is increased. Factors such as attainment of hematological and cytogenetic response as early as 3 months[60] from the start of treatment have been shown to identify those patients who will not respond to IFN and may be better managed with other therapeutic modalities. From the UK MRC CML V Study, it would appear that "low dose" IFN is as effective as standard/high dose Interferon and it is associated with fewer side effects.

Russo et al.[67] showed that significant proportions of CML patients treated with IFN develop neutralizing antibodies (22 percent of all patients treated) and that these are associated with a loss of efficacy of IFN-alpha, resulting in fewer hematological or cytogenetic responses. The median time to development of

these antibodies is 12 months from commencing treatment. Changing these patients to treatment with lymphoblastoid IFN (now discontinued) may restore hematological response but is not likely to achieve a cytogetic response.

The adverse effects of IFN include "acute" fevers, chills and malaise, arthralgia, and myalgia whereas chronic toxicity includes autoimmune-type phenomena, hypothyroidism, Raynaud's phenomenon, connective tissue disorder, and neuropsychiatric disorders.[45,68] Patients commonly feel very tired and depressed. Elevations of liver enzymes and triglycerides are common.

Interferon With and Without Cytarabine

Cytarabine has long been known for its antileukemic properties and its efficacy when given subcutaneously in reducing the number of Ph-positive cells in the bone marrow.[69,70] After a pilot study,[71] Guilhot et al.[72,73] have now reported data from a multicenter randomized trial comparing IFN + Ara-C with IFN alone. They reported a statistically significant increase in the rate of major cytogenetic response (41 percent vs. 24 percent) and improved survival (85.7 percent vs. 79.1 percent) in chronic phase CML patients treated with the combination. The group has also demonstrated the cost-effectiveness of this regimen.[74] The main problem was discontinuation of the combined therapy due to side effects. Other groups of investigators have also demonstrated the efficacy of this regimen[75] but other studies have failed to confirm a survival advantage.

Cytarabine has also been formulated for use as an oral prodrug (YNK01). Preliminary studies with this agent in combination with IFN are promising,[76,77] with comparable hematological and cytogenetic responses to parenteral cytarabine and IFN. Kuhr and colleagues[78] have reported on the efficacy of YNK01 in advanced CML. This may prove a significant step forward for those patients without a transplant option.

Interferon Prior to Allografting

Concerns were raised in 1995 by reports suggesting that the use of IFN prior to allogeneic transplant was detrimental to outcome. Subsequent studies have either supported[79–81] or refuted[82,83] the initial observation. A recent analysis of 873 patients undergoing sibling allograft procedures by the International Bone Marrow Registry[84] has confirmed that a short course (median 2 months) does not appear to affect outcome. Reassuringly, an analysis of 152 transplanted patients by the German CML Study Group suggests that if IFN is stopped at least 3 months prior to an allograft there is no adverse effect.[85]

Newer Drug Treatments

Imatinib (Glivec®, Imatinib Mesylate)

The tyrosine kinase activity of the *BCR-ABL* oncogene is required for transformation of hematopoietic cells in CML.[86,87] The tyrosine kinase inhibitor imatinib inhibits BCR-ABL, TEL-ABL, and v-ABL kinase activity and inhibits growth and viability of cells transformed by any of these ABL oncogenes.[88] imatinib is a 2′-phenylaminopyrimidine compound designed to inhibit the binding of the SH1 tyrosine kinase of ABL to the phosphate donor ATP. This activity prevents the downstream phosphorylation of the signal transduction proteins involved in leukemogenesis. For example, the SH2-containing inositol-5-phosphatase SHIP is a protein that has been shown to regulate hematopoiesis in mice. Targeted disruption of the SHIP gene results in a myelodysplastic syndrome characterized by a dramatic increase in granulocyte-macrophage progenitor cells in the marrow and spleen. imatinib rapidly causes re-expression of SHIP, thereby indicating BCR-ABL is directly but reversibly a regulator of the expression of SHIP protein. The estimated half-life of SHIP protein was reduced from 18 hours to less than 3 hours, although this was suggested to occur via more than one mechanism.[89]

The agent was developed by Lydon and Druker[88,90] in collaboration with Ciba Geigy (now Novartis) in the early 1990s. The compound was designed to act by inhibiting the tyrosine kinase activity of the BCR-ABL, but it was also found to inhibit the tyrosine kinase coded by PDGF-r and c-KIT. imatinib appears to selectively inhibit cells expressing p210$^{BCR-ABL}$ protein tyrosine kinase.[88,91–94] The compound entered clinical use in June 1998; the first patient in the United Kingdom was started on the drug in September 1999. By 1999 it had become clear that imatinib was active in controlling the hematological and clinical features of CML, with high bioavailability as an oral compound. Clinical results of a Phase I study presented at the meeting of the American Society of Hematology in New Orleans (December 1999)[95,96] revealed that at a dosage level of over 300 mg/day by mouth the drug was able to restore the leukocyte count to normal in all of 31 patients with IFN-resistant CML still in chronic phase. Some degree of Philadelphia negativity was seen in 9 (45 percent) of 20 patients treated for 5 months or longer. Three patients achieved 100 percent Ph negativity. The drug is also active in control of the blast cell count in patients in transformation.[97] Patients with myeloid transformation responded well and some remain without evidence of advanced phase disease. Patients with lymphoid transformation also responded well but the majority relapsed within 6 months.

All of the Phase I/II studies have now been published.[97–100] These studies confirm the remarkable efficacy of imatinib, particularly in chronic phase patients. The 110 Study[98] demonstrated a major cytogenetic response rate in late chronic phase patients of 60% (46% being complete cytogenetic responders). Subsequently a Phase III prospective randomized trial was conducted in 1106 patients (the so called IRIS or 0106 Study). Five hundred fifty-three of these patients were randomized to receive interferon and Ara-C as per the previous French regimen,[72] and 553 patients received imatinib at 400 mg daily. The rate of major cytogenetic response on the interferon and Ara-C arm was 34.7% and in patients receiving imatinib was 87.1%. Fourteen and one-half percent of patients receiving interferon and low dose Ara-C achieved a complete cytogenetic response as opposed to 76.2% of patients in the imatinib arm. These differences are highly statistically significant and in terms of side effect profile, tolerability, and quality of life measures, there again were major and significant differences in favor of imatinib.[101] In light of these data, it has been suggested by some authorities that imatinib should be considered first line therapy for all CML patients, but as discussed elsewhere in this chapter, it would seem that allografting may still be appropriate as up-front therapy for certain selected patients.

The drug is well tolerated but imatinib causes some nausea and vomiting, occasional muscle and joint aches, occasional rashes and in some cases swelling of the face and other tissues with weight gain. Derangement of liver function tests occasionally occurs and caution is required with concomitant hepatotoxic drugs such as paracetamol. In general, however, the drug seems to be relatively free of side effects.

Recent reports have detailed potential resistance to this agent.[102,103] Gorre and colleagues recently determined the re-establishment of BCR-ABL kinase activity in 11 relapsed patients; they were able to show a single point mutation occurred in the majority of cases resulting in the replacement of threonine[315] by isoleucine.[105] It has previously been demonstrated that this threonine moiety is important in binding imatinib,[106] and the mutation appears to hinder this interaction with BCR-ABL. However, it is reported that a combination of other chemotherapeutic agents with imatinib may overcome this resistance, as they potentiate the action of imatinib.[107] One of the mechanisms by which IFN augments the apoptotic effect of imatinib in blast crisis was described recently,[108] hence suggesting therapeutic potential.

Combination therapies with imatinib are being explored but at the time of writing there are no published clinical data although in vitro results suggest that synergistic effects may be observed.[107] The UK PISCES Study, the first pilot study of imatinib in combination with interferon, will be published later in 2003.

With only 3 years of experience at the time of writing, it is too early to say whether imatinib "cures" patients or even produces improvement in survival compared to IFN-based regimens. The ongoing 0106 study is attempting to address the survival question in a direct comparison between imatinib monotherapy and IFN plus Ara-C. Many patients wish to cross over from IFN to imatinib in this study and it is uncertain whether the study will have sufficient power to address the survival question. Whether the patients are cured must, one suspects, depend on whether their disease is completely eradicated; so far there have been a minority of patients—perhaps 8–10%—who have been rendered genuinely RT PCR negative for BCR/ABL, but these are still fairly immature data and we need to await the accumulation of more results.

Polyethylene Glycol-IFN

The addition of a polyethylene glycol (PEG) moiety to IFN has been shown to considerably prolong its half-life allowing the administration of PEG-IFN to be given once weekly. The results of a Phase I study of PEG-IFN in 27 patients with chronic phase CML have been reported. Not only are the recognized side effects reduced, also the number of patients attaining hematological remission is increased to 50 percent of patients. Encouragingly, included in those achieving hematological remission were 4 out of 13 patients who had previously been described as resistant to IFN.[109,110] A comparative study of Intron A versus PEG Intron is ongoing but as yet data are unavailable. There is also a study comparing Roferon with PEG Roferon (Pegasys) in progress.

Preliminary results with PEG-IFN are promising but further investigations are required to validate its role in this disease. If it can be shown to be as effective in terms of cytogenetic response rates with a similar or even more favorable side effect profile, PEG-IFN could potentially replace conventional IFN in due course because of its convenience as a once weekly injection.

Farnesyltransferase Inhibitors

Farnesyl transferase inhibitors (FTIs) have been designed to block Ras-mediated signaling, but they also have effects on other farnesylated polypeptide targets. Studies of the FTI compound SCH66336, which inhibits BCR-ABL transformation, have shown selective inhibition of hematopoietic colony formation of primary human CML cells.[111] Mice treated with SCH66336 survived disease-free for more than 1 year when injected intravenously with BCR-ABL-BaF3 cells, in contrast to those mice untreated who died within 4 weeks. A Phase I

study[112] of the FTI drug R115777 in 35 adults with refractory or relapsed acute leukemias reports clinical response in ten (29 percent) including two complete remissions. There is interest in combining an FTI drug with imatinib, as the difference in their targets and mechanism of action may allow enhanced performance without additional toxicity.

Homoharringtonine

Homoharringtonine (HHT) is a novel plant cephalotaxine alkaloid with potent activity in myelosuppression. It is derived from the *Cephalotaxus fortuneii* tree. The team from MD Anderson[113] reported in 1995 its efficacy as an antileukemic agent in CML, and demonstrated its low toxicity by continuous infusion. They report on 71 patients in late chronic phase CML treated with a median of six courses. A total of 72 percent achieved complete hematological remission with 9 percent attaining partial hematological remission. Some 31 percent developed cytogenetic response, with 15 percent major and 7 percent complete. The main side effect of treatment was fever. Because its use as a single agent reported no major toxicity problems, it has been looked at in combination with other treatment modalities. It has been found to exert a synergistic effect with IFN-alpha,[114] Ara-C, and as triple therapy. The triple therapy has demonstrated its efficacy in blast phase of CML also.[115] HHT given sequentially with IFN has been investigated in early chronic phase CML.[114] This agent has also been used in myelodysplastic syndromes and myelodysplasia evolving to acute myeloid leukemia[116] and more recently as a Phase II trial in the treatment of bowel cancer.[117]

5-Aza-2′-Deoxycytidine (Decitabine)

Decitabine is a potent hypomethylating cytidine analogue. Encouraging results have been obtained in accelerated and blast phases of CML with response rates of 53 and 26 percent, respectively.[118] Patients treated with decitabine showed a trend toward better survival which was most pronounced in older patients.[119] The drug affects cells specifically in S phase and it has a short plasma half-life; therefore the antileukemic activity is dependent on the dosing schedule. The use of decitabine may be limited in those patients who have already received cytarabine nucleoside analogs as it employs the same enzymes for metabolism and hence may provoke drug resistance. Granulocytopenia is the major toxic effect, with reported median time to recovery of granulocytes $>0.5 \times 10^9$/L at 48 days. Current clinical trials are examining its role in combination with busulfan and cyclophosphamide as part of a preparatory regimen for allogeneic stem cell transplant. In addition it is being investigated with daunorubicin as first-line treatment of acute myeloid leukemia, in Phase II studies on metastatic lung disease patients, and in hormone-independent metastatic prostate cancer.

Antisense Oligonucleotides/Ribozymes

These synthetic nucleic acid molecules in theory should be able to block *BCR-ABL* gene expression in a highly specific manner; however, in practice there have been difficulties with nonspecific toxicity and poor cellular uptake. Some small clinical pilot studies have been performed[120,121] but these molecules appear too large and fragile to become viable pharmaceuticals at the present time.[122]

Hematopoietic Stem Cell Transplantation

Allografting

As detailed previously in Figure 5–1, allogeneic transplant is only an option for the minority of CML patients and may offer long-term disease-free survival in only 15 percent of patients. If clinicians and their patients require comparative evidence of the benefit of stem cell transplantation from randomized controlled studies to determine treatment strategy, they will be disappointed as such evidence is lacking. However, we know that allografting "cures" patients.[123] Allografting is associated with transplant-related mortality and complications, making the benefits equivocal especially in the short term. The individual needs to weigh the immediate high risk against the potential increase in life expectancy. Younger patients are most likely to benefit and those within 1 or 2 years of diagnosis.

The Fred Hutchinson Cancer Center in Seattle has the largest single appreciable institution experience and reports a survival rate of 70 percent at 10 years.[124] Data on 5725 patients undergoing bone marrow transplantation in chronic phase have been analyzed by the International Bone Marrow Transplant Registry (IBMTR) according to donor type; their results are detailed in Figure 5–4. For a number of years unrelated donors have been used with success in transplantation.

Molecular HLA typing has had an important role in distinguishing different HLA antigens but the increased precision decreases the chance of finding a suitably matched donor for an individual patient. A recent review of 1423 patients with CML undergoing unrelated donor transplant facilitated by the National Marrow Donor Program[125] has reported 63 percent 3-year disease-free survival in those patients less than 35 years of age, in chronic phase, and transplanted within a year of diagnosis. They reported failure of engraftment in 9.9 percent, with late graft failure in a further 6.6 percent. Grade III to IV graft-versus-host disease (GVHD) developed in 33 percent with extensive chronic GVHD in 60 percent at 2 years. It is hoped that in the next decade improvements in conditioning regimens, GVHD prophylaxis, and supportive care will result in better outcome.

The importance of the graft-versus-leukemia (GVL) must be considered when attempting to reduce transplant-related mortality and complications.[126,127] A lesson was learned from the 1980s vogue for T-cell depleted transplants, when relapse rates reached 60 percent.[128] Further evidence for the importance of GVL has arisen from the encouraging data available on donor lymphocyte infusions (DLI) inducing complete remissions without chemotherapy or radiotherapy in patients relapsing after allograft.[129–132]

Relapse and Donor Lymphocyte Infusions

In patients who relapse postallograft, best results are achieved by treating at the earliest possible stage (i.e., at the point of "molecular relapse"). It is important to recognize there can be

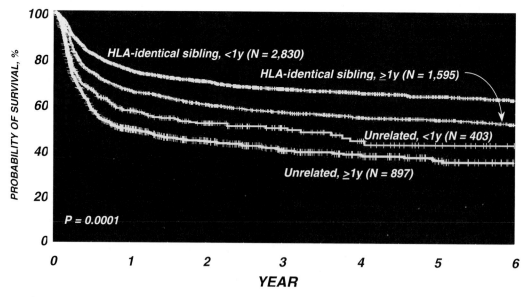

Figure 5–4. Probability of survival after 5,725 allogeneic bone marrow transplants for CML in chronic phase by donor type and disease duration, 1991-1997. The data presented here was obtained from the statistical center of the International Bone Marrow Transplant Registry and Autologous Blood Marrow and Transport Registry. The analysis has not been approved by The Advisory Committee of the IBMTR and ABMTR.

transient BCR-ABL positivity in the first year post-transplant in patients who are ultimately destined *not* to relapse. Two consecutive samples with increasing numbers of BCR-ABL transcripts are ideally required. Options for treatment are the withdrawal of immunosuppression (i.e., stop cyclosporin), consideration of IFN, donor lymphocyte infusions, or contemplation of a second allograft procedure. Chemotherapeutic methods are now a viable option with the advent of imatinib, but hydroxyurea or other forms of chemotherapy have been shown to be unsatisfactory.

DLI therapy has had a major impact on the treatment of relapse postallograft in CML, more so than in other hematological malignancies. DLI therapy relies on exploiting the GVL effect of the original transplant to "mop up" small amounts of recurrent disease, and hence is most effective when performed in the earliest stage of relapse. The two major side effects are GVHD and marrow aplasia, but no pretreatment parameters can reliably predict which patients may suffer these complications. The typical schedule of escalating dose given every 3 months until recurrent disease is eradicated is described in Table 5–7.

"Mini" Transplants

Over the past 3 to 4 years there has been a vogue for nonmyeloablative stem cell transplants (NSTs), so-called mini-transplants, the intention of which is to minimize the morbidity and mortality of the transplant-conditioning regimen so that the procedure might be available to older patients.[133–135] NSTs are based on the hypothesis that transient immunosuppression allows eradication of disease by alloreactive immune cells over time, and hence continuous cell-mediated immunotherapy with donor cells.[136] It is hypothesized that NST can induce transient mixed chimerism that may protect from severe GVHD. One of the earliest regimens from Seattle[137] was to use only minimal immunosuppression [200 cGy-one fraction and oral mycophenolate mofetil (Cellsept)]. Thereafter donor lymphocyte infusions are used to alter the ratio of donor/recipient chimerism in order to eradicate host leukemia.[138] Although the toxicity profile of such procedures has been impressive,[139] there have been considerable problems with failed engraftment, and immunosuppression is being increased. It is suggested that NSTs are not sufficiently cytoreductive in patients with advanced malignancy.[140,141] A number of regimens contain fludarabine and/or Campath, but as yet there are no clear data to suggest the superiority of any one particular regimen. For the moment, "mini-allografts" must be considered as experimental and should not replace conventional allografting for good-risk young patients with CML.

Autografting

Autografting may provide an improvement on the survival benefits seen with IFN-alpha but it is, however, unlikely to provide a cure. Autografting aims to exploit the observation that normal and leukemic cells coexist in many patients during the early stages of the disease and biological advantage is given to normal cells over their leukemic counterparts. Mobilization using a variety of techniques has been described, resulting in Ph-negative progenitor cells.[142] These cells can be used fresh or cryopreserved and used in autografting at a later date. The reason why predominantly Ph-negative progenitors should be released first into the circulation at the beginning of regeneration after chemotherapy with or without granulocyte colony-stimulating factor (G-CSF) is currently poorly understood.

Attempts at in vitro purging have employed such techniques as short-term marrow culture,[143] use of anti-sense oligonucleotides, photodynamic purging,[144] and IFN purging.[145] There is no evidence at present that purged marrow attains better results than unmanipulated autologous marrow.

Although initial data appeared promising, there is no compelling evidence that autografts performed using mobilized stem cells have advantage over any other type of autograft. McGlave et al.[146] conducted an overview analysis of 142 patients autografted during chronic phase in eight major transplant centers. The 4-year survival was in the order of 60 percent but this does not appear borne out with the progress of time. They demonstrated that although age of the patient affected outcome, neither source of stem cells nor use of ex vivo purging influenced survival. Caution should be exercised in the interpretation of these studies as the population is highly selected.

At what stage should patients be autografted? Some of the mobilization studies suggest that outcome is better in those patients treated in the first year[147] and should be considered in those under 60 to 65 years of age. The choice of cytoreduction technique is not generally agreed. The advent of imatinib has shifted emphasis away from autografting and the future of the procedure seems destined to be interwoven with imatinib in new studies.

Trials and Tribulations

Finally, a word about clinical trials. Only a minority of CML patients participate in clinical trials and therapeutic progress is therefore hampered as a result. Almost all patients with the disease could be entered into trials and the most common reason that clinicians do not enter patients is that they do not have enough time and the process is too cumbersome. Investigators must take some responsibility for this in the practical design of trials but many difficulties can be overcome using modern technology and particularly the Internet. The first imatinib and IFN combination study, PISCES, has been conducted in this way

Table 5–7. Donor Lymphocyte Infusion: Escalating Doses Usually Given at Three Month Intervals

Cell dose	Sibling donor (CD3 + cells/kg)	Unrelated donor (CD3 + cells/kg)
First dose	10^7	10^6
Second dose	5×10^7	10^7
Third dose	10^8	5×10^7
Fourth dose	$> 10^8$	10^8

(http://www.pisces-project.org) and the forthcoming SPIRIT trial (imatinib vs. imatinib plus IFN vs. imatinib plus Ara-C) will be conducted across hundreds of centers over three continents using Web technology. All hematologists have a responsibility to improve therapy for their patients and in closing we would encourage you when faced with a new (or existing) CML patient to ask "Can I put this patient in a clinical trial?" Given the remarkable therapeutic advances in CML over the past few years, participation in such trials may offer patients access to some of the most technologically advanced and successful treatments developed by modern medicine. One day it may even be possible to cure CML using drugs alone but we are not there yet.

REFERENCES

1. Fialkow PJ, Jacobson RJ, Papayannopoulou T: Chronic myelocytic leukemia: Clonal origin in a stem cell common to the granulocyte, erythrocyte, platelet and monocyte/macrophage. Am J Med 63:125–130, 1977.

2. Nowell PC, Hungerford DA: A minute chromosome in human chronic granulocytic leukemia. Science 132:1497, 1960.

3. Whang-Peng J, et al: Clinical implications of cytogenetic variants in chronic myelocytic leukemia (CML). Blood 32:755–766, 1968.

4. Ezdinli EZ, et al: Philadelphia-chromosome-positive and -negative chronic myelocytic leukemia. Ann Intern Med 72:175–182, 1970.

5. Kurzrock R, et al: BCR rearrangement-negative chronic myelogenous leukemia revisited. J Clin Oncol 19:2915–2926, 2001.

6. Sokal JE, et al: Prognostic discrimination in "good-risk" chronic granulocytic leukemia. Blood 63:789–799, 1984.

7. Savage DG, Szydlo RM, Goldman JM: Clinical features at diagnosis in 430 patients with chronic myeloid leukaemia seen at a referral centre over a 16-year period. Br J Haematol 96:111–116, 1997.

8. Sokal JE, et al: Staging and prognosis in chronic myelogenous leukemia. Semin Hematol 25:49–61, 1988.

9. Kantarjian HM, et al: Characteristics of accelerated disease in chronic myelogenous leukemia. Cancer 61:1441–1446, 1988.

10. Darte JM, Dacie JV, McSorley JGA: Pelger-like leucocytes in chronic myeloid leukemia. Acta Haematol 12:117–124, 1954.

11. Lie-Injo LE, Tarail R: Carbonic anhydrase deficiency with persistence of foetal haemoglobin: A new syndrome. Nature 211:47–49, 1966.

12. Shumak KH, et al: Myeloblastic and lymphoblastic markers in acute undifferentiated leukemia and chronic myelogenous leukemia in blast crisis. Cancer Res 40:4048–4052, 1980.

13. Forman EN, et al: Ph1-positive childhood leukemias: Spectrum of lymphoid-myeloid expressions. Blood 49:549–558, 1977.

14. Chan LC, et al: Clonal rearrangement and expression of the T cell receptor beta gene and involvement of the breakpoint cluster region in blast crisis of CGL. Blood 67:533–536, 1986.

15. Speed DE, Lawler SD: Chronic granulocytic leukemia: The chromosomes and the disease. Lancet i:403–408, 1964.

16. Mitelman F: The cytogenetic scenario of chronic myeloid leukemia. Leuk Lymphoma 11(Suppl. 1):11–15, 1993.

17. Derderian PM, et al: Chronic myelogenous leukemia in the lymphoid blastic phase: Characteristics, treatment response, and prognosis. Am J Med 94:69–74, 1993.

18. Kantarjian HM, et al: Chronic myelogenous leukemia in blast crisis. Analysis of 242 patients. Am J Med 83:445–454, 1987.

19. Stuppia L, et al: p53 loss and point mutations are associated with suppression of apoptosis and progression of CML into myeloid blastic crisis. Cancer Genet Cytogenet 98:28–35, 1997.

20. Ahuja H, et al: Alterations in the p53 gene and the clonal evolution of the blast crisis of chronic myelocytic leukemia. Proc Natl Acad Sci USA 86:6783–6787, 1989.

21. Mitelman F, Brandt L, Nilsson PG: Cytogenetic evidence for splenic origin of blastic transformation in chronic myeloid leukemia. Scand J Haematol 13:87–92, 1974.

22. Stoll C, Oberling F, Flori E: Chromosome analysis of spleen and/or lymph nodes of patients with chronic myeloid leukemia (CML). Blood 52:828–838, 1978.

23. Freireich EJ, Thomas LB, et al: A distinctive type of intracerebral haemorrhage associated with blast crisis in patients with leukemia. Cancer 13:146, 1960.

24. Vernant JP, et al: Respiratory distress of hyperleukocytic granulocytic leukemias. Cancer 44:264–268, 1979.

25. Neiman RS, et al: Granulocytic sarcoma: A clinicopathologic study of 61 biopsied cases. Cancer 48:1426–1437, 1981.

26. Schwartz JH, et al: Meningeal leukemia in the blastic phase of chronic granulocytic leukemia. Am J Med 59:819–828, 1975.

27. Tura S, Baccarani M, Corbelli G: Staging of chronic myeloid leukemia. Br J Haematol 47:105–119, 1981.

28. Cervantes F, Rozman C: A multivariate analysis of prognostic factors in chronic myeloid leukemia. Blood 60:1298–1304, 1982.

29. Hasford J, et al: A new prognostic score for survival of patients with chronic myeloid leukemia treated with interferon alfa. Writing Committee for the Collaborative CML Prognostic Factors Project Group. J Natl Cancer Inst 90:850–858, 1998.

30. Hehlmann R, et al: Randomized comparison of interferon-alpha with busulfan and hydroxyurea in chronic myelogenous leukemia. The German CML Study Group. Blood 84:4064–4077, 1994.

31. Gratwohl A, et al: Risk assessment for patients with chronic myeloid leukemia before allogeneic blood or marrow transplantation. Chronic Leukaemia Working Party of the European Group for Blood and Marrow Transplantation. Lancet 352:1087–1092, 1998.

32. Thomas MJ, et al: Validation of the Hasford score in a demographic study in chronic granulocytic leukemia. J Clin Pathol 54:491–493, 2001.

33. Caplan SN, Coco FV, Berkman EM: Management of chronic myelocytic leukemia in pregnancy by cell pheresis. Transfusion 18:120–124, 1978.

34. Fitzgerald D, Rowe JM, Heal J: Leukapheresis for control of chronic myelogenous leukemia during pregnancy. Am J Hematol 22:213–218, 1986.

35. Kennedy BJ: Hydroxyurea therapy in chronic myelogenous leukemia. Cancer 29:1052–1056, 1972.

36. Kolitz JE, et al: A phase II pilot trial of high-dose hydroxyurea in chronic myelogenous leukemia. Semin Oncol 19(Suppl. 9):27–33, 1992.

37. Rushing D, et al: Hydroxyurea versus busulfan in the treatment of chronic myelogenous leukemia. Am J Clin Oncol 5:307–313, 1982.

38. Bolin RW, et al: Busulfan versus hydroxyurea in long-term therapy of chronic myelogenous leukemia. Cancer 50:1683–1686, 1982.

39. Kennedy BJ: The evolution of hydroxyurea therapy in chronic myelogenous leukemia. Semin Oncol 19(Suppl. 9):21–26, 1992.

40. Hehlmann R, et al: Randomized comparison of busulfan and hydroxyurea in chronic myelogenous leukemia: Prolongation of survival by hydroxyurea. The German CML Study Group. Blood 82:398–407, 1993.

41. Schoch C, et al: Proposal for an efficient schedule for genetic diagnostics in chronic myeloid leukemia. In 42nd Annual meeting of the American Society for Haematology. San Francisco, CA, 2000.

42. Tura S: New trends in the management of chronic myeloid leukemia. Haematologica 57:741–752, 1972.

43. Schwarzenberg L, et al: Chemotherapy with hydroxyurea, leucopheresis and splenectomy in the treatment of chronic myeloid leukemia at the problastic phase. Haematologica 57:601–611, 1972.

44. Chronic Myeloid Leukemia Trialists' Collaborative Group: Hydroxyurea versus busulphan for chronic myeloid leukemia: An individual patient data meta-analysis of three randomized trials. Br J Haematol 110:573–576, 2000.

45. Talpaz M, et al: Clinical investigation of human alpha interferon in chronic myelogenous leukemia. Blood 69:1280–1288, 1987.

46. Pfeffer LM, et al: Biological properties of recombinant alpha-interferons: 40th anniversary of the discovery of interferons. Cancer Res 58:2489–2499, 1998.

47. Gordon MY, et al: Altered adhesive interactions with marrow stroma of haematopoietic progenitor cells in chronic myeloid leukemia. Nature 328:342–344, 1987.

48. Bhatia R, McCarthy JB, Verfaillie CM: Interferon-alpha restores normal beta 1 integrin-mediated inhibition of hematopoietic progenitor proliferation by the marrow microenvironment in chronic myelogenous leukemia. Blood 87:3883–3891, 1996.

49. Cornelissen JJ, et al: An in vitro model for cytogenetic conversion in CML. Interferon-alpha preferentially inhibits the outgrowth of malignant stem cells preserved in long-term culture. J Clin Invest 102:976–983, 1988.

50. Gordon MY, et al: Treatment with interferon-alpha preferentially reduces the capacity for amplification of granulocyte-macrophage progenitors (CFU-GM) from patients with chronic myeloid leukemia but spares normal CFU-GM. J Clin Invest 102:710–715, 1988.

51. Guilhot F, Lacotte-Thierry L: Interferon-alpha: Mechanisms of action in chronic myelogenous leukemia in chronic phase. Hematol Cell Ther 40:237–239, 1998.

52. Moro M, et al: The treatment of chronic myelogenous leukemia with interferon alfa-2b plus hydroxyurea versus hydroxyurea alone. Haematologica 76(Suppl. 4):117, 1991.

53. Broustet A, et al: Hydroxyurea versus interferon alfa-2b in chronic myelogenous leukemia: Preliminary results of an open French multicentre randomized study. Eur J Cancer 27(Suppl. 4):S18–21, 1991.

54. The Italian Cooperative Study Group on Chronic Myeloid Leukemia: A prospective comparison of alpha-IFN and conventional chemotherapy in Ph+ chronic myeloid leukemia. Clinical and cytogenetic results at 2 years in 322 patients. Haematologica 77:204–214, 1992.

55. The Italian Cooperative Study Group on Chronic Myeloid Leukemia: Treatment of Ph-positive chronic myeloid leukemia with alpha-interferon (ROFERON-A). The Italian Cooperative Study Group experience. Leuk Lymphoma 11(Suppl. 1):153–157, 1993.

56. The Italian Cooperative Study Group on Chronic Myeloid Leukemia: Interferon alfa-2a as compared with conventional chemotherapy for the treatment of chronic myeloid leukemia. N Engl J Med 330:820–825, 1994.

57. Ohnishi K, et al: A randomized trial comparing interferon-alpha with busulfan for newly diagnosed chronic myelogenous leukemia in chronic phase. Blood 86:906–916, 1995.

58. The Benelux CML Study Group: Low-dose interferon-alpha 2b combined with hydroxyurea versus hydroxyurea alone for chronic myelogenous leukemia. Bone Marrow Transplant 17(Suppl. 3):S19–20, 1996.

59. The Benelux CML Study Group: Randomized study on hydroxyurea alone versus hydroxyurea combined with low-dose inter-feron-alpha 2b for chronic myeloid leukemia [see comments]. Blood 91:2713–2721, 1998.

60. Mahon FX, et al: Response at three months is a good predictive factor for newly diagnosed chronic myeloid leukemia patients treated by recombinant interferon-alpha. Blood 92:4059–4065, 1998.

61. Silver RT, et al: An evidence-based analysis of the effect of busulfan, hydroxyurea, interferon, and allogeneic bone marrow transplantation in treating the chronic phase of chronic myeloid leukemia: Developed for the American Society of Hematology. Blood 94:1517–1536, 1999.

62. Chronic Myeloid Leukemia Trialists' Collaborative Group: Interferon alfa versus chemotherapy for chronic myeloid leukemia: A meta-analysis of seven randomized trials: J Natl Cancer Inst 89:1616–1620, 1997.

63. Allan NC, Richards SM, Shepherd PC: UK Medical Research Council randomised, multicentre trial of interferon-alpha n1 for chronic myeloid leukaemia: Improved survival irrespective of cytogenetic response. The UK Medical Research Council's Working Parties for Therapeutic Trials in Adult Leukemia. Lancet 345:1392–1397, 1995.

64. Talpaz M, et al: Chronic myelogenous leukaemia: Haematological remissions with alpha interferon. Br J Haematol 64:87–95, 1986.

65. Talpaz M, et al: Hematologic remission and cytogenetic improvement induced by recombinant human interferon alpha A in chronic myelogenous leukemia. N Engl J Med 314:1065–1069, 1986.

66. Kantarjian HM, et al: Prolonged survival in chronic myelogenous leukemia after cytogenetic response to interferon-alpha therapy. Ann Intern Med 122:254–261, 1995.

67. Russo D, et al: Neutralizing anti-interferon-alpha antibodies and response to treatment in patients with Ph+ chronic myeloid leukemia sequentially treated with recombinant (alpha 2a) and lymphoblastoid interferon-alpha. Br J Haematol 94:300–305, 1996.

68. Wandl UB, et al: Lupus-like autoimmune disease induced by interferon therapy for myeloproliferative disorders. Clin Immunol Immunopathol 65:70–74, 1992.

69. Sokal JE, Gockerman JP, Bigner SH: Evidence for a selective antileukemic effect of cytosine arabinoside in chronic granulocytic leukaemia. Leuk Res 12:453–458, 1988.

70. Robertson MJ, et al: Hematologic remission and cytogenetic improvement after treatment of stable-phase chronic myelogenous leukemia with continuous infusion of low-dose cytarabine. Am J Hematol 43:95–102, 1993.

71. Guilhot F, et al: The treatment of chronic myelogenous leukemia by interferon and cytosine-arabinoside: Rationale and design of the French trials. French CML Study Group. Bone Marrow Transplant 17(Suppl. 3):S29–31, 1996.

72. Guilhot F, et al: Interferon alfa-2b combined with cytarabine versus interferon alone in chronic myelogenous leukemia. French Chronic Myeloid Leukemia Study Group. N Engl J Med 337:223–229, 1997.

73. Guilhot F, et al: Significant survival improvement with a combination of interferon alpha2b and cytarabine in chronic myeloid leukemia. Update of a randomised trial. Proceedings of American Society of Clinical Oncology, 1999.

74. Beck JR, et al: Cytarabine added to interferon improves the cost-effectiveness of initial therapy for patients with early chronic phase chronic myelogenous leukemia. Leuk Lymphoma 41:117–124, 2001.

75. Kantarjian HM, et al: Treatment of Philadelphia chromosome-positive early chronic phase chronic myelogenous leukemia with

daily doses of interferon alpha and low-dose cytarabine. J Clin Oncol 17:284–292, 1999.

76. Mollee P, et al: A phase II study of interferon alpha (IFN) and intermittent oral cytarabine (YNK01) in the treatment of newly diagnosed chronic myeloid leukemia (CML). Blood 96:545a (Abstract), 2000.

77. Kalmantis T, et al: Preliminary report on the CML-GIII-1/97 protocol for the treatment of chronic myelogenous leukemia (CML) and the per os Ara-C derivative YNK01 plus hyroxyurea (HU). Blood 96:737a (Abstract), 2000.

78. Kuhr T, et al: Treatment of patients with advanced chronic myelogenous leukemia with interferon-alpha-2b and continuous oral cytarabine ocfosfate (YNK01): A pilot study. Leuk Res 24:583–587, 2000.

79. Giralt SA, et al: Effect of prior interferon alfa therapy on the outcome of allogeneic bone marrow transplantation for chronic myelogenous leukemia. J Clin Oncol 11:1055–1061, 1993.

80. Zuffa E, et al: Prior treatment with alpha-interferon does not adversely affect the outcome of allogeneic BMT in chronic phase chronic myeloid leukemia. Haematologica 83:231–236, 1998.

81. Tomas JF, et al: Absence of influence of prior treatment with interferon on the outcome of allogeneic bone marrow transplantation for chronic myeloid leukemia. Bone Marrow Transplant 22:47–51, 1998.

82. Beelen DW, et al: Prolonged administration of interferon-alpha in patients with chronic-phase Philadelphia chromosome-positive chronic myelogenous leukemia before allogeneic bone marrow transplantation may adversely affect transplant outcome. Blood 85:2981–2990, 1995.

83. Morton AJ, et al: Association between pretransplant interferon-alpha and outcome after unrelated donor marrow transplantation for chronic myelogenous leukemia in chronic phase. Blood 92:394–401, 1998.

84. Giralt S, et al: Effect of short-term interferon therapy on the outcome of subsequent HLA-identical sibling bone marrow transplantation for chronic myelogenous leukemia: An analysis from the international bone marrow transplant registry. Blood 95:410–415, 2000.

85. Hehlmann R, et al: Interferon-alpha before allogeneic bone marrow transplantation in chronic myelogenous leukemia does not affect outcome adversely, provided it is discontinued at least 90 days before the procedure. Blood 94:3668–3677, 1999.

86. Lugo TG, et al: Tyrosine kinase activity and transformation potency of bcr-abl oncogene products. Science 247:1079–1082, 1990.

87. Oda T, et al: The SH2 domain of ABL is not required for factor-independent growth induced by BCR-ABL in a murine myeloid cell line. Leukemia 9:295–301, 1995.

88. Druker BJ, et al: Effects of a selective inhibitor of the Abl tyrosine kinase on the growth of Bcr-Abl positive cells. Nat Med 2:561–566, 1996.

89. Sattler M, et al: BCR/ABL directly inhibits expression of SHIP, an SH2-containing polyinositol-5-phosphatase involved in the regulation of hematopoiesis. Mol Cell Biol 19:7473–7480, 1999.

90. Druker BJ, Lydon NB: Lessons learned from the development of an abl tyrosine kinase inhibitor for chronic myelogenous leukemia. J Clin Invest 105:3–7, 2000.

91. Carroll M, et al: CGP 57148, a tyrosine kinase inhibitor, inhibits the growth of cells expressing BCR-ABL, TEL-ABL, and TEL-PDGFR fusion proteins. Blood 90:4947–4952, 1997.

92. Deininger MW, et al: The tyrosine kinase inhibitor CGP57148B selectively inhibits the growth of BCR-ABL-positive cells. Blood 90:3691–3698, 1997.

93. Beran M, et al: Selective inhibition of cell proliferation and BCR-ABL phosphorylation in acute lymphoblastic leukemia cells expressing Mr 190,000 BCR-ABL protein by a tyrosine kinase inhibitor (CGP-57148). Clin Cancer Res 4:1661–1672, 1998.

94. Gambacorti-Passerini C, et al: Inhibition of the ABL kinase activity blocks the proliferation of BCR/ABL+ leukemic cells and induces apoptosis. Blood Cells Mol Dis 23:380–394, 1997.

95. Druker BJ, et al: Efficacy and safety of a specific inhibitor of the BCR-ABL tyrosine kinase in chronic myeloid leukemia. N Engl J Med 344:1031–1037, 2001.

96. Druker BJ, et al: Activity of a specific inhibitor of the BCR-ABL tyrosine kinase in the blast crisis of chronic myeloid leukemia and acute lymphoblastic leukemia with the Philadelphia chromosome. N Engl J Med 344:1038–1042, 2001.

97. Talpaz, M, Silver, RT, Druker, BJ, et al. Imatinib induces durable hematologic and cytogenetic responses in patients with accelerated phase chronic myeloid leukemia: Results of a phase 2 study. Blood, 99:1928–1937, 2002.

98. Kantarjian, H, Sawyers, C, Hochhaus, A, et al. Hematologic and cytogenetic responses to imatinib mesylate in chronic myelogenous leukemia. N Engl J Med 346:645–652, 2002.

99. Sawyers, CL, Hochhaus, A, Feldman, E, et al. Imatinib induces hematologic and cytogenetic responses in patients with chronic myelogenous leukemia in myeloid blast crisis: Results of a phase II study. Blood 99:3530–3539, 2002.

100. Ottmann, OG, Druker, BJ, Sawyers, CL, et al. A phase 2 study of imatinib in patients with relapsed or refractory Philadelphia chromosome-positive acute lymphoid leukemias. Blood, 100:1965–19671, 2002.

101. O'Brien, SG, Guilhot F, Larson, RA, et al. The IRIS study: International randomized study of interferon and low-dose Ara-C versus ST1571 [imatinib] in patients with newly-diagnosed chronic phase myeloid leukemia. N Engl J Med, 348:994–1004, 2003.

102. Weisberg E, Griffin JD: Mechanism of resistance to the ABL tyrosine kinase inhibitor STI571 in BCR/ABL-transformed hematopoietic cell lines. Blood 95:3498–3505, 2000.

103. le Coutre P, et al: Induction of resistance to the Abelson inhibitor STI571 in human leukemic cells through gene amplification. Blood 95:1758–1766, 2000.

104. Gorre ME, et al: Clinical resistance to STI-571 cancer therapy caused by BCR-ABL gene mutation or amplification. Science 21:21, 2001.

105. Marx J: Cancer research. Why some leukemia cells resist STI-571. Science 292:2231–2233, 2001.

106. Schindler T, et al: Structural mechanism for STI-571 inhibition of Abelson tyrosine kinase. Science 289:1938–1942, 2000.

107. Thiesing JT, et al: Efficacy of STI571, an abl tyrosine kinase inhibitor, in conjunction with other antileukemic agents against bcr-abl-positive cells. Blood 96:3195–3199, 2000.

108. Barteneva N, et al: Interferon-alpha augments the apoptotic effect of STI571 in Ph+– blastic crisis cell lines by inducing TRAIL and FAS (CD95/AP01). Blood 96:345a (Abstract), 2000.

109. Talpaz M, et al: Updated phase I study of polyethylene glycol formulation of interferon alpha-2b (PEG-Intron; Schering 54031) in Philadelphia chromosome-positive chronic myelogenous leukemia. Blood 96:736a (Abstract), 2000.

110. Talpaz M, et al: PEG-interferon alpha-2a (Pegasys™) with or without cytarabine in patients with relapsed or refractory chronic phase CML. Blood 96:736a (Abstract), 2000.

111. Peters DG, et al: Activity of the farnesyl protein transferase inhibitor SCH66336 against BCR/ABL-induced murine leukemia and primary cells from patients with chronic myeloid leukemia. Blood 97:1404–1412, 2001.

112. Karp JE, et al: Clinical and biologic activity of the farnesyltransferase inhibitor R115777 in adults with refractory and relapsed acute leukemias: A phase 1 clinical-laboratory correlative trial. Blood 97:3361–3369, 2001.

113. O'Brien S, et al: Homoharringtonine therapy induces responses in patients with chronic myelogenous leukemia in late chronic phase. Blood 86:3322–3326, 1995.

114. O'Brien S, et al: Sequential homoharringtonine and interferon-alpha in the treatment of early chronic phase chronic myelogenous leukemia. Blood 93:4149–4153, 1999.

115. Visani G, et al: Effects of homoharringtonine alone and in combination with alpha interferon and cytosine arabinoside on 'in vitro' growth and induction of apoptosis in chronic myeloid leukemia and normal hematopoietic progenitors. Leukemia 11:624–628, 1997.

116. Feldman EJ, et al: Homoharringtonine in patients with myelodysplastic syndrome (MDS) and MDS evolving to acute myeloid leukemia. Leukemia 10:40–42, 1996.

117. Witte RS, et al: A phase II trial of homoharringtonine and caracemide in the treatment of patients with advanced large bowel cancer. Invest New Drugs 17:173–177, 1999.

118. Kantarjian HM, et al: Results of decitabine therapy in the accelerated and blastic phases of chronic myelogenous leukemia. Leukemia 11:1617–1620, 1997.

119. Sacchi S, et al: Chronic myelogenous leukemia in nonlymphoid blastic phase: Analysis of the results of first salvage therapy with three different treatment approaches for 162 patients. Cancer 86:2632–2641, 1999.

120. Szczylik C, et al: Selective inhibition of leukemia cell proliferation by BCR-ABL antisense oligodeoxynucleotides. Science 253:562–565, 1991.

121. De Lord C, et al: Human Philadelphia chromosome-positive chronic myeloid leukemia: A potential model for antisense therapy. Exp Hematol 21:826–828, 1993.

122. Stein CA, Cheng YC: Antisense oligonucleotides as therapeutic agents—is the bullet really magical? Science 261:1004–1012, 1993.

123. Goldman JM: Management of chronic myeloid leukemia. Scand J Haematol 37:269–279, 1986.

124. Clift RA, Anasetti C: Allografting for chronic myeloid leukemia. Baillieres Clin Haematol 10:319–336, 1997.

125. McGlave PB, et al: Unrelated donor marrow transplantation for chronic myelogenous leukemia: 9 years' experience of the National Marrow Donor Program. Blood 95:2219–2225, 2000.

126. Horowitz MM, et al: Graft-versus-leukemia reactions after bone marrow transplantation. Blood 75:555–562, 1990.

127. Antin JH: Graft-versus-leukemia: No longer an epiphenomenon [editorial]. Blood 82:2273–2277, 1993.

128. Goldman JM, et al: Bone marrow transplantation for chronic myelogenous leukemia in chronic phase. Increased risk for relapse associated with T-cell depletion. Ann Intern Med 108:806–814, 1988.

129. Kolb HJ, et al: Donor leukocyte transfusions for treatment of recurrent chronic myelogenous leukemia in marrow transplant patients. Blood 76:2462–2465, 1990.

130. Cullis JO, et al: Donor leukocyte infusions for chronic myeloid leukemia in relapse after allogeneic bone marrow transplantation. Blood 79:1379–1381, 1992.

131. Drobyski WR, et al: Salvage immunotherapy using donor leukocyte infusions as treatment for relapsed chronic myelogenous leukemia after allogeneic bone marrow transplantation: Efficacy and toxicity of a defined T-cell dose. Blood 82:2310–2318, 1993.

132. Porter DL, et al: Induction of graft-versus-host disease as immunotherapy for relapsed chronic myeloid leukemia. N Engl J Med 330:100–106, 1994.

133. Lalancette M, et al: The importance of patient selection in non-myeloablative stem cell transplant for acute and chronic leukemia, myelodysplastic syndrome, and myeloma. Blood 96:199a (Abstract), 2000.

134. Lalancette M, et al: Favourable outcome of non-myeloablative stem cell transplant for chronic myeloid leukemia (CML) in first chronic phase: A retrospective study of the European group for Blood and Marrow Transplantation (EBMT). Blood 96:545a (Abstract), 2000.

135. Sloand E, et al: Non-myeloablative peripheral blood stem cell transplantation for chronic myelogenous leukemia. Blood 96:783a (Abstract), 2000.

136. Pugatsch T, et al: Kinetics of engraftment post non-myeloablative stem cell transplantation (full donor chimerism). Blood 96:172a (Abstract), 2000.

137. Sandmaier B, et al: Induction of molecular remissions in chronic myelogenous leukemia (CML) with non-myeloablative HLA-identical sibling allografts. Blood 96:201a (Abstract), 2000.

138. Slavin S, et al: Non-myeloablative allogeneic stem cell transplantation for the treatment of patients with chronic myeloid leukemia. Blood 96:203a (Abstract), 2000.

139. Reddy V, et al: GvHD and CMV antigenaemia after allogeneic peripheral blood stem cell transplantation: Comparison between myeloablative and non-myeloablative (mini) conditioning regimens. Blood 96:191a (Abstract), 2000.

140. Uberti J, et al: Lower intensity of preparative regimen for allogeneic stem cell transplantation from related donor in patients with advanced hematological malignancy is associated with poor outcome. Blood 96:201a (Abstract), 2000.

141. Rezvani K, et al: Non-myeloablative stem cell transplant in AML, ALL, and MDS: Disappointing outcome for patients with advanced phase disease. Blood 96:479a (Abstract), 2000.

142. Olavarria E, et al: Collection of Ph-negative progenitor cells from interferon responsive patients with chronic myeloid leukemia: Effect of granulocyte-colony-stimulating factor mobilization. Haematologica 85:647–652, 2000.

143. Barnett MJ, et al: Autografting with cultured marrow in chronic myeloid leukemia: Results of a pilot study [see comments]. Blood 84:724–732, 1994.

144. Roy D, et al: Phase I study of autologous progenitor cell transplantation (PCT) purged with a photodynamic approach for patients with chronic myeloid leukemia (CML). Blood 96:583a (Abstract), 2000.

145. O'Brien S, et al: The effect of long-term marrow culture on the nonadherent Philadelphia chromosome-positive clone in chronic myelogenous leukemia: Preliminary observations. Hematol Pathol 1:167–172, 1987.

146. McGlave PB, et al: Autologous transplants for chronic myelogenous leukaemia: Results from eight transplant groups. Lancet 343:1486–1488, 1994.

147. Carella AM, et al: High-dose chemo-radiotherapy followed by autologous Philadelphia chromosome-negative blood progenitor cell transplantation in patients with chronic myelogenous leukemia. Bone Marrow Transplant 17:201–205, 1996.

6

Molecular Biology and Cytogenetics of Chronic Lymphocytic Leukemia

David G. Oscier

Early cytogenetic studies in chronic lymphocytic leukemia (CLL), performed in the 1960s and 1970s, failed to detect clonal cytogenetic abnormalities. This inauspicious start to the investigation of genetic abnormalities in CLL was the consequence of the low spontaneous mitotic rate in CLL and the use of the T-cell mitogen phytohemaglutinin to obtain analyzable metaphases. With the discovery of polyclonal B-cell mitogens, the first cytogenetic abnormality in CLL, trisomy 12, was discovered in 1980.[1,116] Subsequent studies have shown clonal cytogenetic abnormalities in approximately 50 percent of cases of CLL.[2] The most frequent abnormalities are structural abnormalities of chromosome 13q14 and trisomy of chromosome 12, occurring in 10 to 20 percent of cases. Abnormalities of chromosomes 6q, 11q, 14q, and 17p are each found in less than 5 percent of cases. In patients with a cytogenetic abnormality, 50 percent have a single abnormality, 25 percent have two abnormalities, and the remainder have a complex karyotype. The results obtained using different B-cell mitogens, such as tetradecanoyl phorbol acetate (TPA) or the Epstein-Barr virus (EBV), have been comparable, although a recent study in which CLL cells were incubated with a variety of different mitogenic combinations, including TPA, interleukin 2, tumor necrosis factor alpha, and *Staphylococcus aureus* Cowan 1, demonstrated cytogenetic abnormalities in 80 percent of cases.[3] Although cytogenetic analysis has the advantage of being a global technique, small deletions are not detectable and the mitogens employed stimulate normal T cells as well as leukemic B cells. Studies that have combined cytogenetic analysis with immunophenotyping of single cells have clearly shown that the normal mitoses in CLL are frequently derived from the normal T-cell population.[4]

These problems were overcome with the introduction of interphase fluorescent in situ hybridization (FISH) using either centromeric probes specific for individual chromosomes or locus-specific probes cloned into yeast artificial chromosome (YAC), P1-derived artificial chromosome (PAC), or bacterial artificial chromosome (BAC) vectors. By using combinations of these probes selected to detect the most frequent known abnormalities in CLL, genetic abnormalities can be found in 80 percent of cases of CLL. Comparative genomic hybridization (CGH) is a further FISH technique, which enables a global screen for genetic gains, amplifications, and losses of tumor

DNA. Gains of genetic material on chromosomes 4q and 8q have been identified that would not have been predicted from cytogenetic studies.[5,6] The sensitivity of CGH will be greatly enhanced once metaphase chromosomes are replaced as targets by microarrayed DNA fragments.[7]

Molecular techniques, including Southern analysis and microsatellite analysis, to detect loss of heterozygosity have also been employed in CLL. In general the concordance between the techniques described above is high, although both interphase and metaphase FISH show that the complexity of genetic abnormalities, including the presence of multiple subclones, is greater than can be detected from cytogenetic or microsatellite analysis.[8] Although global studies of gene expression are in their infancy, DNA microarray studies are being performed in CLL and differences in gene expression between CLL and other B-cell malignancies and between different subsets of CLL have been identified.[9] Proteomic analysis has also shown differences in protein expression between patients with stable or progressive disease.[10]

The purpose of this chapter is to review the known genetic and epigenetic abnormalities in CLL and to assess their clinical significance in the light of recent data. These show that patients with CLL can be subdivided into two groups with widely differing survivals, depending on the presence or absence of mutations in the immunoglobulin heavy-chain variable-region genes.

CHROMOSOME 13q14

Structural abnormalities involving chromosome 13q14 were first noted to be a recurring cytogenetic abnormality in CLL in 1987.[11] Subsequent larger cytogenetic studies have shown that abnormalities of 13q14 are found in approximately 20 percent of patients, whereas with use of more sensitive techniques, the incidence of loss is 30 to 60 percent. Two-thirds of patients have a deletion usually involving (13)(q14q22) or (13)(q12q14), and the remainder have a translocation involving q14. The translocations involve a wide variety of different partner chromosomes (Figure 6–1) and are frequently complex. FISH analysis of metaphases with 13q14 translocations invariably show that the translocations are accompanied by genetic loss with variable proximal and distal breakpoints.[12]

When 13q abnormalities in CLL were first identified, the only known gene assigned to this region was the retinoblastoma gene *(RB1)*. Loss of RBI was subsequently identified by both Southern and FISH analysis in patients with CLL, including those with a normal karyotype.[13] However, no evidence of *RB1* gene mutations or low or absent retinoblastoma protein expression was found in cases of heterozygous *RB1* loss.[14] In addition, genetic loss at more telomeric loci within 13q14 was identified both at a higher frequency than *RB1* loss and in cases in which the *RB1* locus was intact (Table 6–1). In contrast to other regions of chromosomal deletion found in CLL, homozygous loss at 13q14 is a frequent finding, occurring in 10 to 20 percent of cases, which strongly suggests that one or

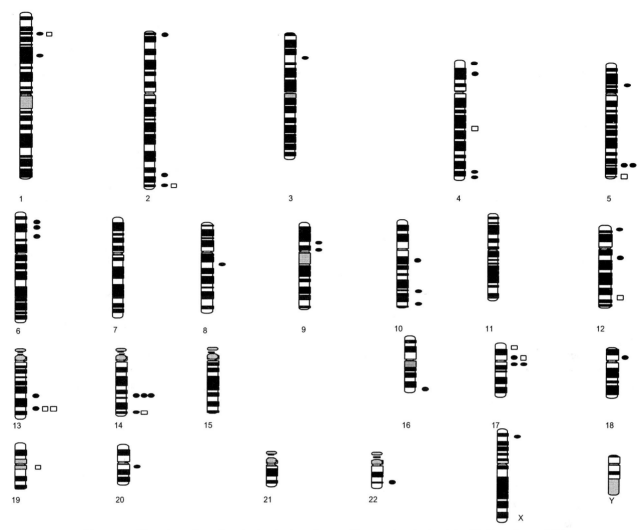

Figure 6–1. The reciprocal translocation breakpoints of cases with a translocation involving 13q14 are shown. Solid circles indicate those cases in which the translocation was clonal and open squares indicate cases with a 13q14 translocation as a single-cell abnormality.

more genes that are important in the pathogenesis of CLL lie within this region.

Several groups of investigators have constructed detailed physical maps of 13q14 and have performed deletion mapping using either FISH, Southern, or microsatellite analysis.[112–115] A number of overlapping regions of minimal genetic loss have been identified, and these are shown in Figure 6–2. One possible explanation for the differing regions of loss is the presence of a large gene, with several splice forms, covering a large genomic region. Another is that chromosome inversion may accompany genomic deletion in a proportion of cases. This would account for the discontinuous regions of loss that we and others have reported. Finally, more than one gene may be implicated. A 10-kb region of minimal loss close to D13S319 encompasses exons of two separate transcripts termed *LEU1* and *LEU2*.[15] The *RFP2* gene is located 50 kb centromeric to the minimally deleted region on chromosome 13 and encodes a 407-amino-acid ring-finger protein, which shares

homology with a number of transcription factors, including *BRCA2*.[16] Sequence analysis of the corresponding mouse genomic region has revealed strong identity between the human and mouse *LEU2* and *RFP2* genes.[17] Although *LEU1*, *LEU2*, and *RFP2* may be considered strong candidate genes, no mutations have been found in these genes in patients with heterozygous loss in this region, nor have mutations been discovered in a 347-kb region of loss encompassing the above three genes.[18] Significant hypermethylation close to *LEU2* occurs in patients with heterozygous loss of *LEU2*, as compared with patients' cases with homozygous retention of this region, suggesting that loss of function of *LEU2* or a neighboring gene may be important in CLL.[19]

Using interphase FISH, Garcio-Marco et al.[20] found loss at 13q12 encompassing *BRCA2*, in 80 percent of patients with CLL, but other studies employing FISH or Southern blotting were unable to confirm the very high incidence of genetic loss at this locus.[21]

Table 6–1. Genetic Loss at Chromosome 13q14 in Chronic Lymphocytic Leukemia

| Study | No. of Patients | Methods | Percent Heterozygous Loss | | | | Percent Homozygous Loss (Any locus) |
			RB1	D13S19	D13S218	D13S25	
Liu et al.[87]	27	SB	30				
Stilgenbauer et al.[88]	35	FISH	31				
Brown et al.[89]	10[a]	SB	40			90	40
Liu et al.[14]	31[a]	SB				45	28
Chapman et al.[90]	68[a]	SB				75	50
Stilgenbauer et al.[91]	85	FISH	35		24		
Newcomb et al.[92]	140	PCR					
Liu et al.[93]	75	SB;PCR		44			13
Corcoran et al.[94]	229	SB		41			10

[a] Includes patients known to have cytogenetic abnormalities of 13q14.

TRISOMY 12

Trisomy 12 is by far the most frequent numerical chromosome abnormality in CLL. By means of restriction fragment length polymorphism studies, the additional chromosome 12 has been shown to derive from duplication of one chromosome 12 with retention of the other homologue rather than from triplication of a single homologue.[22] The incidence of trisomy 12 in studies which have used both cytogenetic and interphase FISH analysis is shown in Table 6–2. The wide variation in incidence may in part reflect the extent to which studies include patients with atypical lymphocyte morphology, which, as discussed later, is strongly associated with trisomy 12.

The genetic consequence of trisomy 12 is unknown. Clues to the identity of the key gene or genes on chromosome 12 may come from the investigation of rare cases with translocations, duplications, or genomic amplifications involving chromosome 12. Two cases in which CLL had transformed to diffuse large-cell lymphoma were shown to have translocations involving 12p13 and 12q13, respectively. In the first case there was disruption of the cyclin D2 promoter.[23] In the second the translocation occurred within the *HMGI-C* gene which encodes a high-mobility group protein known to be overexpressed in a variety of malignancies.[24] Dysregulation of the chondroitin 4–0-sulfotransferase 1 gene has been reported in a single case of CLL with t(12;14)(q23; q32).[25] In a study of duplications result-ing in partial trisomy 12 in patients with low-grade B-cell malignancies, a duplicated region between q13 and q22 was identified in patients with CLL.[26] This region includes the *MDM2* gene, the possible significance of which in CLL is discussed below.

Patients with hereditary papillary renal carcinoma have germ-line mutations of the *MET* oncogene on chromosome 7q31, frequently accompanied by trisomy 7. The duplicated chromosome 7 always carries the *MET* mutation. If trisomy 12 in CLL results in a gene dosage effect, the gene that is implicated may also be abnormal.[27]

DELETION OF 11q

Using a panel of YAC probes spanning 11q14 to q23, Stilgenbauer et al.[28] investigated 38 patients with CLL who had cytogenetic deletions of chromosome 11q. A commonly deleted region of between 2 and 3 Mb at 11q22.3 to q23.1 was identified. In two additional cases with 11q translocations, the translocation breakpoints were localized to the commonly deleted region. In a subsequent larger interphase FISH study, 43 of 214 patients were found to have heterozygous loss of a YAC within the minimally deleted region.[29] This high incidence of loss contrasts with previous cytogenetic studies in which 11q22

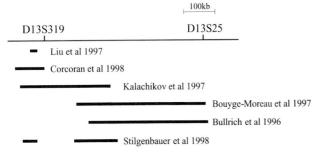

Figure 6–2. The solid bars indicate the minimum regions of genetic loss detected by FISH, microsatellite, or Southern analysis.

Table 6–2. Incidence of Trisomy 12 in Chronic Lymphocytic Leukemia

Study	No. of Patients	+12 by Cytogenetics (%)	+12 by FISH (%)
Perez-Losada[117]	13	0	15
Anastasi et al.[95]	40	18	30
Que et al.[96]	118	9	14
Escudier et al.[97]	117	13	35
Dohner et al.[98]	42	10	14
Criel et al.[99]	111	12	14

to 23 abnormalities were found in less than 5 percent of cases. The minimally deleted region contains a number of candidate tumor suppressor genes, including *RDX*, which has homology to the neurofibromatosis type 2 gene *(NF2 71); PPP2RIB*, a phosphatase which is mutated in sporadic cases of lung and colon cancer; and *ATM*, which is mutated in ataxia telangectasia. The *ATM* gene encodes a 350-kd protein, which has roles in stress response, cell cycle regulation, and DNA repair. Patients with ataxia telangiectasia are prone to a variety of T- and B-cell tumors, although rarely CLL.

Mutation of the *PPP2RIB* gene or loss of phosphatase activity has not been found in cases of CLL with deletion of one copy of the *PPP2RIB* gene.[30] In contrast two studies have shown reduced expression of the ATM protein in 34 and 40 percent of cases of CLL, respectively.[31] Several groups have identified mutations within the *ATM* gene, particularly in patients with 11q23 deletions.[32,33] In two studies germ-line *ATM* mutations were found, raising the possibility that carriers of *ATM* mutations may be at risk of developing CLL. Schaffner et al.[34] detected *ATM* mutations in only 5 of 22 patients with 11q deletions. Although the whole of the *ATM* gene was not analyzed, cases of mantle-cell lymphoma with deletion of 11q all involved mutation of the remaining *ATM* allele, which suggests that other genes situated in 11q may be important in CLL.[35]

THE *p53* PATHWAY

Chromosomal deletions or translocations involving chromosome 17p are found in 1 to 5 percent of patients with CLL. In a recent study using FISH, 10 out of 14 patients with 17p translocations were shown to have dicentric rearrangements[36] (Figure 6–3). The *p53* gene is located at 17p13, and numerous studies (Table 6–3) using a variety of techniques (including single-strand confirmation polymorphism analysis, genomic sequencing, FISH, and p53 protein expression using immunocytochemistry or flow cytometry) have shown *p53* mutation or deletion in 7 to 30 percent of patients with CLL. The varying incidence is partly technical but largely reflects the clinical stage of the patients being studied. Patients with deletion of 17p13 frequently have a mutation of the remaining allele. Mutations of the *p53* gene are usually missense mutations involving exons 4 to 8, although rarely genomic deletions have been identified.[37]

The *p53* gene encodes a DNA-binding protein that induces the expression of genes such as *p21*, involved in cell cycle arrest, and *BAX*, which is proapoptotic. The regulation of functional *p53* protein is complex and is shown in a highly simplified form in Figure 6–4. Failure to upregulate *p21* expression following *in vitro* irradiation appears to identify cases with either *p53* or *ATM* mutations.[38] The *p53* gene induces the expression of *MDM2*, which inactivates *p53* in a variety of ways including

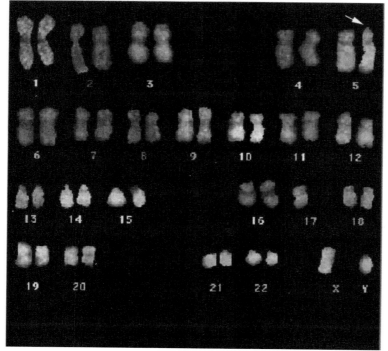
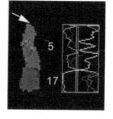

Figure 6–3. FISH can be used to define chromosome rearrangements. (A) An example of a 24-color metaphase FISH karyotype is shown. Conventional cytogenetic analysis revealed that this CLL patient had an abnormal chromosome 5 and loss of one chromosome 17. M-FISH defined this as a derived chromosome 5, resulting from a translocation between chromosomes 5 and 17. The image to the right shows the der(5) pseudocolored to highlight the translocation. Chromosome 5 is colored green, and chromosome 17 is blue. *(continues)*

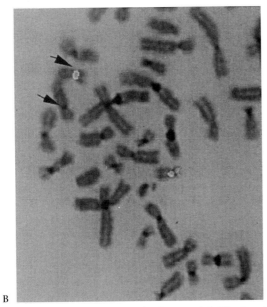

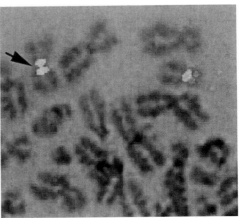

B

C

Figure 6–3. *(continued)* **(B)** Subsequent hybridization with probes specific for chromosome 17 centromere (green) and *p53* (red) shows the rearrangement to be more complex. The der(5) is a dicentric chromosome with an inactive centromere (centromeres indicated with arrows); *p53* has been lost as a result of the rearrangement. **(C)** Although not found as frequently in CLL as in some other hematologic malignancies, a dicentric isochromosome for the long arm of chromosome 17 also results in the loss of *p53* in this CLL patient. In the partial metaphase shown, two separate centromere signals, but no *p53* signal, are visible on the isochromosome to the left, whereas both can be seen on the normal chromosome 17 to the right.

proteoasomic degradation. Overexpression of *MDM2* mRNA and/or protein in CLL has been shown in several studies.[39–41] However, neither the mechanism of overexpression nor the clinical significance is understood. *MDM2* function is also inhibited by the *ARF* tumor suppressor gene encoded at the *p16/ARF* locus on chromosome 9p21. Loss of *ARF* function enables *MDM2* to inhibit *p53*, but the role of this pathway in CLL has yet to be established.

Table 6–3. p53 Mutation or Deletion in Chronic Lymphocytic Leukemia

Study	No. of Patients	Method	Percent Mutation or Loss
Gaidano et al.[100]	40	SSCP/PCR	15
Fenaux et al.[104]	39	SSCP/PCR	10
El Rouby et al.[76]	53	SSCP/PCR	15
Dohner et al.[98]	16	FISH	25
Gardiner et al.[102]	20	SSCP/PCR	35
Lens et al.[79]	32	17p LOH, Immuno-cytochemistry, p53 sequence	30
Cordone et al.[103]	181	Immunocyto-chemistry P53 sequence	15
Dohner et al.[81]	325	FISH	7

IMMUNOGLOBULIN GENE TRANSLOCATIONS

Chromosomal translocations involving the immunoglobulin loci are both frequent and critical to the pathogenesis of many chronic lymphoproliferative disorders but are rare in CLL. The incidence of rearrangement involving the *BCL2* locus is shown in Table 6–4. Initial studies noted a high incidence of translocation involving the immunoglobulin light-chain loci, but in our own series (unpublished) 10 of 13 cases had t(14:18)(q32q21) translocations. The breakpoints within the *BCL2* locus are variable but frequently involve the 5′ variable cluster region. Expression of BCL2 protein is high in these cases; however it is not clear whether the level of expression differs from that found in the majority of cases of CLL that express BCL2 protein in the absence of *BCL2* gene rearrangements. Many cases of immunoglobulin gene/*BCL2* rearrangements are accompanied by trisomy 12, and the *BCL2* rearrangement may be the primary or secondary cytogenetic abnormality.

Translocations involving the immunoglobulin heavy-chain locus on chromosome 14q32 and the *BCL3* gene on 19q13 are found in less than 0.5 percent of patients. The breakpoints in the immunoglobulin heavy-chain gene are usually in the switch region upstream of C-alpha 1 or C-alpha 2.[42] The *BCL3* breakpoints are variable but all result in overexpression of the BCL3 protein, which is an I-κB-like protein. Most cases involve complex cytogenetic abnormalities including trisomy 12.[43,44]

The t(2;14)(p13;q32) is a rare recurring translocation in B-cell malignancies and has been studied molecularly in four clinically aggressive cases of CLL. A zinc-finger gene *(BC211A)* is

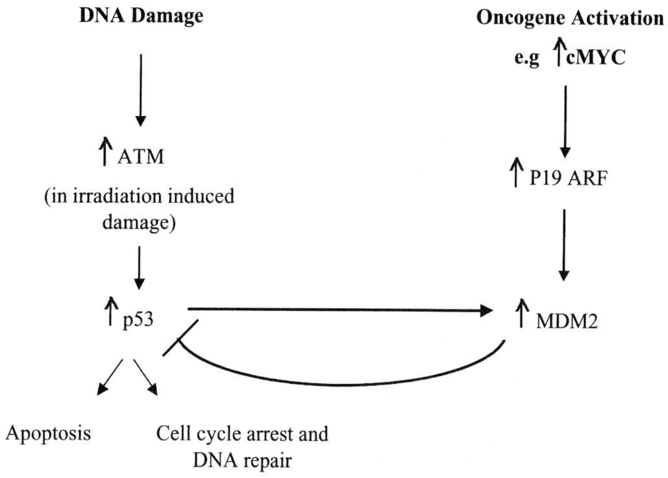

Figure 6–4. Expression of p53 protein following DNA damage results in upregulation of a large number of genes, including P21 and BAX, leading to cell cycle arrest or apoptosis.

juxtaposed to the immunoglobulin heavy-chain locus; *BC211A* interacts with *BCL6*. Both are transcriptional repressors.[45]

The existence of the t(11;14) translocation in CLL is controversial. In almost all reported cases, lymphocyte morphology is atypical and the immunophenotype is more consistent with mantle-cell lymphoma than with CLL.

DELETION OF 6q

Structural abnormalities of chromosome 6 predominantly involve the long arm and comprise deletions affecting bands q21, q23, q25 to 27, or more rarely, translocations that also involve a variety of breakpoints.

The incidence of chromosome 6q deletions was 6 percent in a cytogenetic analysis of 662 cases and 7 percent in a FISH analysis of 285 patients using a YAC probe mapping to band 6q21.[46] Merup et al.[8] observed a minimally deleted region between the microsatellite markers D6S283 and D6S270, which includes the candidate gene *TLX*, a member of the nuclear steroid receptor superfamily.

MUTATION OF THE *CD79B* GENE

The B-cell antigen receptor (BCR) comprises surface immunoglobulin and heterodimers of two accessory proteins, CD79A and CD79B. The BCR mediates signal transduction fol-

lowing cross-linking of surface immunoglobulin, and a functional BCR is essential for B-cell development and the survival of peripheral B cells.

Patients with CLL have reduced or absent expression of the extracellular domain of CD79B. Two groups of investigators have identified mutations in a subset of CLL cases in either exon 4 or 5 of the *CD79B* gene, which encode the transmembrane and cytoplasmic domains of CD79B protein, respectively.[47,48] Transfection of mutant *CD79B* genes into Jurket T cells resulted in either a failure of CD79B cells surface expression or impaired signal transduction.[49] The pattern of *CD79B* mutations in CLL is similar to that seen in immunoglobulin V genes, and it has been suggested that *CD79B* mutations arise through somatic hypermutation. However, these results remain controversial, and other data have suggested that *CD79B* mutations are polymorphisms and that alternative splicing of the *CD79B* gene can result in loss of exon 3, which encodes the extracellular domain.[50] Alternatively spliced variants may be found in normal as well as in malignant B cells, and it remains to be seen whether *CD79B* mutations are transforming events in CLL or whether loss of surface membrane CD79B expression is a secondary phenomenon, possibly arising because CLL cells no longer require a functional BCR for cell survival.

EPIGENETIC ABNORMALITIES

Abnormalities of DNA methylation are common in malignancy and comprise both global hypomethylation and hypermethylation of CpG islands, resulting in loss of gene expression. Global hypomethylation has been found in patients with CLL, including those with early disease.[51,52] A single study demonstrated hypomethylation of the promoter region of the *BCL2* gene, but although this study has been quoted as an explanation for elevated BCL2 protein levels in CLL, the extent of hypomethylation did not correlate with BCL2 expression.[53] No systematic study of DNA hypermethylation in CLL has been performed. As already discussed, we have found specific hypermethylation in close proximity to the *LEU2* gene on 13q14. In another study, hypermethylation of the M27 beta locus on the X chromosome

Table 6–4. *BCL2* Rearrangements in Chronic Lymphocytic Leukemia

Study	Incidence	MBR/mcr	vcr
Adachi et al.[104]	3/32	0	3
Raghoebier et al.[105]	3/44	1	2
Dyer et al.[106]	7/170	3	4
Merup et al.[107]	11/96	2	9

Abbreviations: MBR, major breakpoint region; mcr, minor cluster region; vcr, variable cluster region.

was found in 38 percent of patients with CLL but not in normal controls.[54]

Telomeres are essential for both the function and stability of normal chromosomes. Repeated cell division results in telomere shortening in cells that lack telomerase. Several studies have documented increased telomerase activity and reduced telomere length in advanced CLL as compared with patients with stage A disease (Table 6–5). Both the biological significance and the clinical importance of these findings remain uncertain. Preliminary data using flow FISH have shown that the mean telomere length in cases with unmutated VH genes is significantly shorter than in cases with mutated VH genes despite the unmutated group having higher telomerase activity.[55]

LEUKEMOGENESIS AND GENETIC INSTABILITY IN CHRONIC LYMPHOCYTIC LEUKEMIA

Clonal CD5-positive B-cell populations can be found in more than 80 percent of old mice[56] and in 3 percent of healthy people over the age of 60 if sensitive molecular or FISH techniques are employed.[57] Nothing is known of the genetic abnormalities in these clonal populations. Patients discovered on a routine blood test to have a slight lymphocytosis with morphological and immunophenotypic features of CLL may have stable disease for prolonged periods. Our own cytogenetic FISH and molecular data (unpublished) on this benign subgroup of stage A patients have shown that heterozygous or homozygous loss of chromosome 13q14 is the only consistent genetic abnormality, identifiable in 70 percent of cases. These data suggest that genetic loss at 13q14 is an early event in CLL and may be associated with prolonged lymphocyte survival, possibly due to resistance to apoptosis. Further ongoing studies to determine

the initiating events in leukemogenesis include the investigation of cases of familial CLL,[58–60] mutational analysis of candidate genes such as CD79B (as discussed above), and global gene expression studies using subtractive hybridization techniques or cDNA arrays.[61]

In most human tumors, genetic abnormalities accumulate during the course of the disease and contribute to disease progression and drug resistance.

Sequential cytogenetic and interphase FISH studies have demonstrated clonal evolution in 10 to 20 percent of cases[13,62] and confirmed that deletions of chromosomes 6q, 11q, and 17p are the most frequent secondary abnormalities.[63,64] Trisomy 12 is almost invariably a primary cytogenetic abnormality in CLL, but interphase FISH has shown that only part of the leukemic clone carries the additional copy of chromosome 12.[65] In patients with CLL who develop a diffuse large-cell lymphoma (Richter syndrome), the new clone may be either derived from the CLL clone or unrelated. In those cases in which the large-cell lymphoma is clonally related to CLL, studies on small numbers of patients have not shown a consistent transforming event.[66]

The mechanisms responsible for both genomic abnormalities and genetic instability in CLL are poorly understood. Both *p53* and *ATM* mutations are associated with genomic instability, but these mutations are usually late events in CLL. Trinucleotide repeat sequences have been found close to the chromosome breakpoints in cases with deletion of 11q, and these may be responsible for increased chromosome fragility.[67] Microsatellite instability appears to be rare in CLL.[68] In experimental studies telomere shortening correlates with genomic instability, including the formation of dicentric chromosomes, but the significance of shortened telomeres in advanced CLL is unclear.

THE CLINICAL SIGNIFICANCE OF GENETIC ABNORMALITIES IN CHRONIC LYMPHOCYTIC LEUKEMIA

Interpretation of the clinical significance of genetic abnormalities is dependent on a number of variables. These include the techniques used to identify the abnormality and whether analysis is univariate or multivariate, with account taken of known prognostic factors such as clinical stage, lymphocyte doubling time, B2 microglobulin, and most recently, VH gene status. A further problem is the choice of outcome measure, which may be time to disease progression, time to first treatment, or overall survival. The last would seem to be the most significant, but many patients with CLL are elderly and die of unrelated causes. A particular problem in CLL concerns patients with stage A disease whose date of diagnosis depends on the timing of a routine blood count performed for an incidental reason. Studies that include a large percentage of patients with stage A disease have a median follow-up time of less than 5 years and that use time to progression or treatment as an endpoint are difficult to interpret.

Data from the first and second International Working Party on Chromosomes in CLL, which included large numbers of patients with prolonged follow-up periods, found the median survival of patients with a normal karyotype to be 15 years,

Table 6–5. Telomere Length and Telomerase Activity in Chronic Lymphocytic Leukemia

Study	No. of Patients	Telomer Length	Telomerase Activity
Counter et al.[108]	20	↑ In Rai stage 0–II rather than stage III, IV	↓ In Rai stage 0–II rather than stage III, IV
Bechter et al.[109]	58	↑ In Binet stage A rather than stage C	↓ In Binet stage A rather than stage C
Trentin et al.[110]	15	—	↓ In stable rather than progressive disease
Tsilika et al.[111]	17	↑ In Rai stage 0–II rather than stage III, IV.	—
Damle et al.[55]	66	↑ In cases with mutated VH genes	↓ In cases with mutated VH genes

compared with 7.7 years for patients with a clonal abnormality. Patients with complex karyotypic abnormalities had a poorer survival time than patients with either a normal karyotype or a single abnormality. When patients with single abnormalities only were studied, those with trisomy 12 had a poorer prognosis than patients with abnormalities of chromosome 13 or those with a normal karyotype.[69,70] Subsequent cytogenetic and interphase FISH studies have confirmed the association between abnormalities of chromosome 13q14 and prolonged survival.[71] However, the influence of trisomy 12 on survival remains controversial. Criel et al.[72] found trisomy 12 to be an adverse prognostic factor only in patients with typical lymphocyte morphology. In a multivariate analysis that included both trisomy 12 and lymphocyte morphology, only lymphocyte morphology retained prognostic significance.[73]

In 1997 two studies[29,74] reported that deletion of 11q22–23 was associated with rapid disease progression and poor survival. In addition, patients with 11q deletions presented at a younger age and with more advanced disease, particularly with bulky lymphadenopathy. Of particular interest was the finding that the poor survival of patients with 11q deletion was confined to patients less than 55 years of age. The explanation for the impact of age on survival is unclear because in general younger patients with CLL do not have a more aggressive disease than elderly patients.

In the CLL3 trial of the German CLL Study Group, which is investigating the role of autologous stem cell transplantation, del (11q23) was associated with molecular evidence of persistent disease in 38 percent of patients postautograft compared with only 6 percent of patients without an abnormality of chromosome 11q ($p < .014$).[75]

El Roubey et al.[76] first demonstrated that $p53$ mutations in CLL were associated with poor clinical outcome. Many subsequent studies have confirmed the association between $p53$ loss and/or mutation with advanced clinical stage, an increase in circulating prolymphocytes, rapid disease progression, a poor response to therapy with alkylating agents and purine analogues, and short survival.[77–79] A German multicenter randomized trial of fludarabine versus fludarabine plus epirubicin treatment demonstrated an overall response rate of 81 percent. In patients with del (17)(p13) detected by interphase FISH, the response rate was 25 percent compared with 87 percent without this abnormality ($p < .001$)[80] Pettit et al.[38] showed in vitro that CLL cells with a $p53$ mutation and spleen cells from $p53$ knockout mice were only partially resistant to purine analogue-induced killing. They postulated that in vivo drug resistance to purine analogues was more likely to be due to development of additional genetic abnormalities as a consequence of the genomic instability associated with $p53$ mutation than to a direct consequence of $p53$ dysfunction.

Patients with chromosome 6q deletions have a higher white cell count and more extensive lymphadenopathy than patients without 6q deletions, but there is no impact on either treatment-free or overall survival.[46]

The results of the most comprehensive study of genetic abnormalities in 325 cases of CLL analyzed by interphase FISH for deletions of 6q, 11q, 13q, and 17p, trisomies of 3q, 8q, and

Table 6–6. Incidence and Clinical Significance of Genetic Abnormalities in Chronic Lymphocytic Leukemia

Genetic Abnormality	Incidence (percent)	Median Survival (months)	Median Treatment-Free Survival (months)
del 13q	55	133[a]	92
del 11q	18	79	13
trisomy 12q	16	114	33
del 17p	7	32	9
No abnormality	18	111	49

[a]For patients with del 13q as the sole genetic abnormality
From Dohner et al[80].

12q, and translocations involving 14q32 are shown in Table 6–6. In a multivariate study both 11q and 17p deletions were independent prognostic factors.[81]

THE RELATIONSHIP BETWEEN GENETIC ABNORMALITIES AND IMMUNOGLOBULIN VH GENE MUTATIONS

Two recent studies have shown that the mutational status of the variable region of the immunoglobulin gene is a powerful prognostic indicator in CLL. Patients with unmutated VH genes have a significantly poorer survival than those with VH gene mutations.[82,83] Preliminary data from our own group and from Germany in over 400 patients with CLL show a significant association between unmutated VH genes and deletions of 11q23 and 17p, whereas cases with mutated VH genes are associated with a normal karyotype or deletions of 13q14.[84,85]

For patients with either trisomy 12 or deletion of 13q14, survival is significantly prolonged when there is mutation of VH genes than when they remain unmutated. Our own data demonstrated a median survival of 95 months for patients with trisomy 12 and unmutated VH genes, whereas the median survival

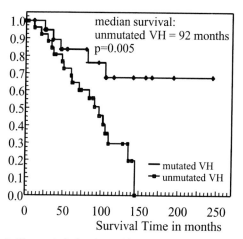

Figure 6–5. The survival of patients with trisomy 12 is dependent on VH gene status. The median survival of cases with mutated VH gene has not been reached.

has not been reached for patients with VH gene mutations ($p = .005$)[86] (Figure 6–5).

Within the subgroup of patients with unmutated VH genes, chromosome abnormalities retain prognostic significance. The median survival of germline cases is approximately 30 months for patients with del (17p13), 70 months for patients with del (11q23), and 90 months for patients with neither of these abnormalities. The prognostic significance of deletions of chromosomes 11q and 17q is also evident in germline cases with Binet stage A disease.[85]

These data, based on relatively small numbers of cases, demonstrate that the adverse prognostic significance of trisomy 12 is entirely due to its association with unmutated VH genes, whereas del (11q23) and del (17p13) appear to be independent prognostic factors.

CONCLUSION

The combination of cytogenetic analysis, interphase FISH, and CGH has identified genetic abnormalities in over 80 percent of cases of CLL. The incidence of abnormalities is highest in patients with advanced disease, whereas deletion of chromosome 13q14 is the only consistent abnormality in patients with a stable mild lymphocytosis, a condition analogous to a monoclonal gammopathy of undetermined significance.

Deletions of chromosome 17p and 11q occur mainly in patients with unmutated VH genes and are independent adverse prognostic factors. Deletions of chromosome 13q and trisomy 12 do not have independent prognostic significance, and the apparently poorer survival of patients with trisomy 12 reflects the association between trisomy 12 and unmutated VH genes. Despite intensive study, the genetic consequences of the common cytogenetic deletions and of trisomy 12 in CLL remain unknown. Although translocations involving chromosome 13q14 are common, they are accompanied by large genetic deletions, which complicate their molecular analysis. Translocations involving the immunoglobulin gene loci are rare in CLL and result in overexpression of the *BCL2*, *BCL3*, and *BCL11* genes.

Concurrently with the investigation of genetic abnormalities, there has been enormous recent progress in elucidating the pathways responsible for apoptosis, cell cycle control, and signal transduction in both normal and malignant B cells. Based on current progress of the human genome sequencing project and of global gene expression analysis, it is reasonable to anticipate that both the key genetic abnormalities and their role in the pathogenesis of CLL will soon be discovered.

REFERENCES

1. Gahrton G, Robert KH, Frinerg K, Zech L, Bird AG: Extra chromosome 12 in chronic lymphocytic leukemia. Lancet 146–147, 1980.
2. Oscier D: Cytogenetic and molecular abnormalities in chronic lymphocytic leukaemia. Blood Rev 8:88–97, 1994.
3. Larramendy ML, Slitonen SM, Zhu A, Hurme M, Vilpo L, Vilpo JA, Knuutila S: Optimized mitogen stimulation induces proliferation of neoplastic B cells in chronic lymphocytic leukemia: Significance for cytogenetic analysis. Cytogenet Cell Genet 82:215–221, 1998.
4. Knuutila S, Elonen E, Teerenhovi L, Rossi L, Leskinen R, Bloomfield CD, de la Chapelle A: Trisomy 12 in B cells of patients with B-cell chronic lymphocytic leukemia. N Engl J Med 314:865–869, 1986.
5. Bentz M, Huck K, du Manoir S, Joos S, Werner CA, Fischer K, Dohner H, Lichter P: Comparative genomic hybridization in chronic B-cell leukemias shows a high incidence of chromosomal gains and losses. Blood 85:3610–3618, 1995.
6. O'Connor SJM, Su'ut L, Morgan GJ, Jack AS: The relationship between typical and atypical B-cell chronic lymphocytic leukemia. A comparative genomic hybridization based study. Am J Clin Pathol 114:448–458, 2000.
7. Lichter P, Joos S, Bentz M, Lampel S: Comparative genomic hybridization: Uses and limitations. Semin Haematol 37(4):348–357, 2000.
8. Merup M, Moreno TC, Heyman M, Ronnberg K, Grander D, Detlofsson R, Rasool O, Liu Y, Soderhall S, Juliusson G, Gahrton G, Einhorn S: 6q deletions in acute lymphoblastic leukemia and non-Hodgkin's lymphomas. Blood 91:3397–3400, 1998.
9. Stratowa C, Loffler G, Lichter P, Stilgenbauer S, Haberl P, Schweifer N, Dohner H, Wilgenbus KK: cDNA microarray gene expression analysis of B-cell chronic lymphocytic leukemia proposes potential new prognostic markers involved in lymphocytic trafficking. Int J Cancer 91(4):474–480, 2001.
10. Voss T, Ahorn H, Haberl P, Dohner H, Wilgenbus K. Correlation of clinical data with proteomics profiles in 24 patients with B-cell chronic lymphocytic leukemia. Int J Cancer 91(2):180–186, 2001.
11. Fitchett M, Griffiths MJ, Oscier DG, Johnson S, Seabright M: Chromosome abnormalities involving band 13q14 in hematologic malignancies. Cancer Genet Cytogenet 24:143–150, 1987.
12. Gardiner AC, Corcoran MM, Oscier DG: Cytogenetic, fluorescence in situ hybridisation, and clinical evaluation of translocations with concomitant deletion at 13q14 in chronic lymphocytic leukaemia. Genes Chromosom Cancer 20:73–81, 1997.
13. Oscier D, Chapman R, Fitchett M, Cowell J: Deletion of a retinoblastoma gene in B cell chronic lymphocytic leukaemia. Blood 76:241a, 1990.
14. Liu Y, Szekely L, Grander D, Soderhall S, Juliusson G, Gahrton G, Linder S, Einhorn S: Chronic lymphocytic leukemia cells with allelic deletions at 13q14 commonly have one intact RB1 gene: Evidence for a role of an adjacent locus. Proc Natl Acad Sci USA 90:8697–8701, 1993.
15. Liu Y, Corcoran M, Rasool O, Ivanova G, Ibbotson R, Grander D, Iyengar A, Baranova A, Kashuba V, Merup M, Wu X, Gardiner A, Mullenbach R, Poltaraus A, Hultstrom AL, Juliusson G, Chapman R, Tiller M, Cotter F, Gahrton G, Yankovsky N, Zabarovsky E, Einhorn S, Oscier D: Cloning of two candidate tumor suppressor genes within a 10 kb region on chromosome 13q14 frequently deleted in chronic lymphocytic leukemia. Oncogene 15:2463–2473, 1997.
16. Kapanadze B, Kashuba V, Baranova A, Rasool O, van Everdink W, Liu Y, Syomov, Corcoran M, Poltaraus A, Brodyansky V, Syomova N, Kazakov A, Ibbotson R, van den Berg A, Gizatullin R, Fedorova L, Sulimova G, Zelenin A Deaven L, Lehrach H, Grander D, Buy C, Oscier D, Zabarovsky ER, Yankovsky N, Einhorn S: A cosmid and cDNA fine physical map of a human chromosome 13q14 region frequently lost in B-cell chronic lymphocytic leukemia and identification of a new putative tumour suppressor gene, Leu 5 FEBS 426:266–270, 1998.
17. Kapanadze B, Makeevaa N, Corcoran MM, Jareborg N, Hammarsund M, Baranova A, Zabarovsky E, Vorontcova O, Merup M,

Jansson O, Gahrton G, Oscier DG, Einhorn S, Grander D, Sangfelt O: Comparative sequence analysis of a region on human chromosome 13q14, frequently deleted in B-cell chronic lymphocytic leukemia and its homologous region on mouse chromosome 14. Blood 96(Suppl. 1):703a, 2000.

18. Migliazza A, Bosch F, Komatsu H, Cayanis E, Martinotti S, Toniato E, Guccione E, Qu X, Chien M, Murty VVV, Gaidano G, Inghirami G, Zhang P, Fischer S, Kalachikov SM, Russo J, Edelman I, Efstratiadis A Dalla-Favera R: Nucleotide sequence, transcription map, and mutation analysis of the 13q14 chromosomal region deleted in B-cell chronic lymphocytic leukaemia. Blood 97:2098–2104, 2001.

19. Corcoran MM, Sangfelt O, Kapanadze B, Makeevaa N, Ibbotson RE, Baranova A, Barovsky E, Merup M, Jansson O, Gahrton G, Einhorn S, Grander D, Oscier DG: Characterisation of a candidate tumor suppressor gene LEU2B located at 13q14.3 in chronic lymphocytic leukemia. Blood 96:702a, 2000.

20. Garcia-Marco JA, Caldas C, Price CM, Wiedemann LM, Ashworth A, Catovsky D: Frequent somatic deletion of the 13q12.3 locus encompassing BRCA2 in chronic lymphocytic leukemia. Blood 88:1568–1575, 1996.

21. Panayiotidis P, Ganeshaguru K, Rowntree C, Jabbar SA, Hoffbrand AV, Foroni L: Lack of clonal BCRA2 gene deletion on chromosome 13 in chronic lymphocytic leukaemia. Br J Haematol 4:844–847, 1997.

22. Einhorn S, Burvall K, Juliusson G, Gahrton G, Meeker T: Molecular analyses of chromosome 12 in chronic lymphocytic leukemia. Leukemia 3:871–874, 1989.

23. Quian L, Gong J, Liu J, Broome JD, Koduru PRK: Cyclin D2 promoter disrupted by t(12;22)(p13;q11.2) during transformation of chronic lymphocytic leukaemia to non Hodgkin's lymphoma. Br J Haematol 106:477–485, 1999.

24. Santulli B, Kazmierczak B, Napolitano R, Caliendo I, Chiappetta G, Rippe V, Bullerdiek J, Fusco A: A 12q13 translocation involving the HMG1-C gene in Richter transformation of a chronic lymphocytic leukemia. Cancer Genet Cytogenet 119:70–73, 2000.

25. Schmidt HH, Dyomin V, Palanisamy N, Nanjangud G, Pirc-Danoewinata H, Haas OA, Chaganti RSK: Dysregulation of the chrondroitin 4–0 sulfotransferase 1, (C4ST-1) gene by a t(12;14)(q23;q32) in a case of B-cell chronic lymphocytic leukemia (B-CLL). Blood 96(Suppl. 2):161b, 2000.

26. Dierlamm J, Wlodarska I, Michaux L, Vermeesch JR, Meeus P, Stul M, Verhoef G, Thomas J, Delannoy A, Louwagie A, Cassiman JJ, Mecucci C, Hagemeijer A, Van den Berghe H: Identified different types of duplications in 12q13–15 as the commonly involved segment B-cell lymphoproliferative malignancies characterized by partial trisomy 12. Genes Chromosom Cancer 20:155–166, 1997.

27. Zhuang Z, Park WS, Pack S, Schmidt L, Vortmeyer AO, Pak E, Pham T, Weil RJ, Candidus S, Lubensky IA, Linehan WM, Zbar B, Weirich G: Trisomy 7-harbouring non-random duplication of the mutant MET allele in hereditary papillary carcinomas. Nat Genet 20:66–69, 1998.

28. Stilgenbauer S, Liebisch P, James MR, Schroder M, Schlegelberger B, Fischer K, Bentz M, Lichter P, Dohner H: Molecular cytogenetic delineation of a novel critical genomic region in chromosome bands 11q22.3–923.1 in lymphoproliferative disorders. Proc Natl Acad Sci USA 93:11837–11841, 1996.

29. Dohner H, Stilgenbauer S, James M, Benner A, Weilguni T, Bentz M, Fischer K, Hunstein W, Lichter P: 11q deletions identify a new subset of B-cell chronic lymphocytic leukemia characterized by extensive nodal involvement and inferior prognosis. Blood 89:2516–2522, 1997.

30. Schaffner C, Scheuermann M, Kalla J, Dohner H, Stilgenbauer S, Lichter P: Analysis of PPP2R1B, a candidate tumor suppressor gene at 11q22-q23, in B-CLL. Blood 96(Suppl. 2):175b, 2000.

31. Starostick P, Manshouri T, O'Brien S, Freireich E, Kantarjian H, Haidar M, Lerner S, Keating M, Albitar M: Deficiency of the ATM protein expression defines an aggressive subgroup of B cell chronic lymphocytic leukemia. Cancer Res 20:2552–4557, 1998.

32. Bullrich F, Rasio D, Kitada S, Starostik P, Kipps T, Keating M, Albitar M, Reed JC, Croce CM: ATM mutations in B-cell chronic lymphocytic leukemia. Cancer Res 59:24, 1999.

33. Stankovic T, Weber P, Stewart G, Bedenham T, Murray J, Byrd PJ, Moss PAH, Taylor AMR: Inactivation of ataxia telangiectasia mutated gene in B-cell chronic lymphocytic leukaemia. Lancet 353:26–29, 1999.

34. Schaffner C, Stilgenbauer S, Rappold GA, Dohner H, Lichter P: Somatic ATM mutations indicate a pathogenic role of ATM in B-cell chronic lymphocytic leukaemia. Blood 94:748–753, 1999.

35. Zhu Y, Monni O, El-Rifai W, Siitonen SM, Vilpo L, Vilpo J, Knuutila S: Discontinuous deletions at 11q23 in B cell chronic lymphocytic leukemia. Leukemia 13:708–712, 1999.

36. Callet-Bauchu E, Salles G, Gazzo S, Poncet C, Morel D, Pages J, Coiffier B, Coeur P, Felman P: Translocations involving the short arm of chromosome 17 in chronic B-lymphoid disorders: Frequent occurrence of dicentric rearrangements and possible association with adverse outcome. Leukemia 13:460–468, 1999.

37. Gandini D, Aguiari GL, Cuneo A, Piva R, Castoldi GL, Del Senno L: Novel small deletions of the p53 gene in late-stage B-cell chronic lymphocytic leukemia. Br J Haematol 88:881–885, 1994.

38. Pettitt AR, Sherrington PD, Cawley JC: The effect of p53 dysfunction on purine analogue cytotoxicity in chronic lymphocytic leukaemia. Br J Haematol 106:1049–1051, 1999.

39. Bueso-Ramos CE, Yang Y, deLeon E, McCown P, Stass SA, Albitar M: The human MDM-2 oncogene is overexpressed in leukemias. Blood 82:2617–2623, 1993.

40. Huang YQ, Raphael B, Buchbinder A, Li JJ, Zhang WG, Friedman-Kien AE: Rearrangement and expression of MDM$_2$ oncogene in chronic lymphocytic leukemia. Am J Hematol 47:139–141, 1994.

41. Watanabe T, Hotta T, Ichikawa A, Kinoshita T, Nagai H, Uchida T, Murate T, Saito H: The MDM2 oncogene overexpression in chronic lymphocytic leukemia and low-grade lymphoma of B-cell origin. Blood 84:3158–3165, 1994.

42. Ohno H, Doi S, Yabumoto K, Fukuhara S, McKeithan TW: Molecular characterization of the t(14;19)(q32;q13) translocation in chronic lymphocytic leukemia. Leukemia 7:2057–2063, 1993.

43. Michaux L, Dierlamm J, Wlodarska I, Bours V, Van den Berghe H, Hagemeijer A: t(14;19)/BCL3 rearrangements in lymphoproliferative disorders: A review of 23 cases. Cancer Genet Cytogenet 94:36–43, 1997.

44. McKeithan TW, Takimoto GS, Ohno H, Bjorling VS, Morgan R, Hecht BK, Dube I, Sandberg AA, Rowley JD: BCL3I rearrangements and t(14;19) in chronic lymphocytic leukemia and other B-cell malignancies: A molecular and cytogenetic study. Genes Chromosom Cancer 20:64–72, 1997.

45. Sonoki T, Satterwhite E, Willis TG, Siebert R, Nowak R, Arriola EL, Liu H, Harder L, Gesk S, Steinemann D, Oscier DG, Schelgelberger B, Tucker PW, Dyer MJS: The BCL11 gene family: Deregulated expression of BCL11A in lymphoma. Blood 96(Suppl. 1):542a, 2000.

46. Stilgenbauer S, Bullinger L, Benner A, Wildenberger K, Bentz M, Dohner K, Ho AD, Lichter P, Dohner H: Incidence and clinical significance of 6q deletions in B cell chronic lymphocytic leukemia. Leukemia 13:1331–1334, 1999.

47. Thompson AA, Talley JA, Do HN, Kagan HL, Kunkel L, Berenson J, Cooper MD, Saxon A, Wall R: Aberrations of the B-cell receptor B29 (CD79b) gene in chronic lymphocytic leukemia. Blood 90:1387–1394. 1997.

48. Payelle-Brogard B, Magnac C, Mauro F, Mandelli F, Dighiero G: Analysis of the B-cell receptor B29 (CD79b) gene in familial chronic lymphocytic leukemia. Blood 94:3516–3522, 1999.

49. Gordon MS, Kato RM, Lansigan F, Thompson AA, Wall R, Rawlings D: Aberrant B cell receptor signaling from B29 (Igβ, CD79b) gene mutations of chronic lymphocytic leukemia B cells. Proc Natl Acad Sci U S A 97:5504–5509, 2000.

50. Alfarano A, Indraccolo S, Circosta P, Minuzzo S, Vallario A, Zamarchi R, Fregonese A, Calderazzo F, Faldella A, Aragno M, Camaschella C, Amadori A, Caligaris Cappio F: An alternatively spliced form of CD79b gene may account for altered B-cell receptor expression in B-chronic lymphocytic leukemia. Blood 93:2327–2335, 1999.

51. Wahlfors J, Hiltunen H, Heinonen K, Hamalainen E, Alhonen L, Janne J: Genomic hypomethylation in human chronic lymphocytic leukemia. Blood 80:2074–2080, 1992.

52. De Capoa A, Grappelli C, Febbo FR, Spano A, Niveleau A, Cafolla A, Cordone I, Foa R: Methylation levels of normal and chronic lymphocytic leukemia B lymphocytes: Computer assisted quantitative analysis of anti-5 methylcytosine antibody binding to individual nuclei. Cytometry 36:157–159, 1999.

53. Hanada M, Delia D, Aiello A, Stadtmauer E, Reed JC: bcl-2 gene hypomethylation and high-level expression in B-cell chronic lymphocytic leukemia. Blood 82:1820–1828, 1993.

54. Crossen PE, Morrison MJ: Hypermethylation of the M27 beta (DXS255) locus in chronic B-cell leukaemia. Br J Haematol 100:191–193, 1998.

55. Damle RN, Batliwalla FM, Albesionao E, Valetto A, Allen SL, Schulman P, Vinciguerra V, Rai K, Ferrarini M, Gregersen PK, Chiorazzi N: Telomere length analysis suggests distinct replicative histories of B-CLL subgroups. Blood 96(suppl. 1):836a, 2000.

56. LeMaoult J, Manavalan JS, Dyal R, Szabo P, Nikolic-Zugic J, Weksler ME: Cellular basis of B cell clonal populations in old mice. J Immunol 162:6384–6391, 1999.

57. Green MJ, Kuzmicki A, Rawstron AC, Kennedy B, Evans PA, Richards SJ, Jack AS, Hillmen P: Clonal B cells with a CLL phenotype are frequently detectable in normal individuals. Blood 96(Suppl. 1):368a, 2000.

58. Bevan S, Catovsky D, Marossy A, Matutes E, Popat S, Antonovic P, Bell A, Berrebi A, Gaminara EJ, Quabeck K, Ribeiro I, Mauro FR, Stark P, Sykes H, van Dongen J, Wimperis J, Wright S, Yuille MR, Houlston RS: Linkage analysis for *ATM* in familial B cell chronic lymphocytic leukaemia. Leukemia 13:1497–1500, 1999.

59. Bevan S, Catovsky D, Matutes E, Antonovic P, Auger MJ, Ben-Bessat I, Bell A, Berrebi A, Gaminara EJ, Junior ME, Mauro FR, Quabeck K, Rassam SMB, Reid C, Ribeiro I, Stark P, van Dongen JJM, Wimperis J, Wright S, Marossy A, Yuille MR, Houlston RS: Linkage analysis for major histocompatibility complex-related susceptibility in familial chronic lymphocytic leukemia. Blood 96:3982–3984, 2000.

60. Yuille MR, Matutes E, Marossy A, Hilditch B, Catovsky D, Houlston RS: Familial chronic lymphocytic leukaemia: a survey and review of published studies. Br J Haematology 109:794–799, 2000.

61. Alizadeh AA, Eisen MB, Davis RE, Ma C, Lossos IS, Rosenwald A, Boldrick JC, Sabet H, Tran T, Yu X, Powell JI, Yang L, Marti GE, Moore T, Hudson J, Lu L, Lewis DB, Ribshirani R, Sherlock G, Chan WC, Greiner TC, Weisenburger DD, Armitage JO, Warnke R, Levy R, Wilson W, Grever MR, Byrd JC, Botstein D, Brown PO, Staudt LM: Distinct types of diffuse large B-cell lymphoma identified by gene expression profiling. Nature 403:503–511, 2000.

62. Juliusson G, Friberg K, Gahrton G: Consistency of chromosomal aberrations in chronic B-lymphocytic leukemia. Cancer 62:500–506, 1988.

63. Fegan C, Robinson H, Thompson P, Whittaker JA, White D: Karyotypic evolution in CLL: Identification of a new sub-group of patients with deletions of 11q and advanced or progressive disease. Leukemia 9:2003–2008, 1995.

64. Finn WG, Kay NE, Kroft SH, Church S, Peterson LC: Secondary abnormalities of chromosome 6q in B-cell chronic lymphocytic leukemia: A sequential study of karyotypic instability in 51 patients. Am J Haematol 59:223–229, 1998.

65. Garcia-Marco J, Matutes E, Morilla R, Ellis J, Oscier D, Fantes J, Catovsky D, Price CM: Trisomy 12 in B-cell chronic lymphocytic leukaemia: Assessment of lineage restriction by simultaneous analysis of immunophenotype and genotype in interphase cells by fluorescence in situ hybridization. Br J Haematol 87:44–50, 1994.

66. Matolcsy A, Inghirami G, Knowles DM: Molecular genetic demonstration of the diverse evolution of Richter's syndrome (chronic lymphocytic leukemia and subsequent large cell lymphoma). Blood 83:1363–1372, 1994.

67. Auer RL, Jones C, Mullenbach RA, Syndercombe-Court D, Milligan DW, Fegan C, Cotter FE: Role for CCG-trinucleotide repeats in the pathogenesis of chronic lymphocytic leukemia. Blood 97:509–515, 2001.

68. Gartenhaus R, Johns MM, Wang P, Rai K, Sidransky D: Mutator phenotype in a subset of chronic lymphocytic leukemia. Blood 87:38–41, 1996.

69. Juliusson G, Oscier DG, Fitchett M, Ross FM, Stockdill G, Mackie MJ, Parker AC, Castoldi GL, Cuneo A, Knuutila S, Elonen E, Gahrton G: Prognostic subgroups in B-cell chronic lymphocytic leukemia defined by specific chromosomal abnormalities. N Engl J Med 323:720–724, 1990.

70. Juliusson G, Gahrton G, Oscier D, Fitchett M, Ross F, Brito-Babapulle V, Catovsky D, Knuutila S, Elonen E, Lechleitner M, Tanzer J, Schoenwald M, Castoldi GL, Cuneo A, Nowell P, Peterson L, Kay N: Cytogenetic findings and survival in B-cell chronic lymphocytic leukemia. Second IWCCLL compilation of data on 662 patients. Leuk Lymphoma (Suppl):21–25, 1991.

71. Hogan WJ, Tefferi A, Borell TJ, Jenkins R, Li CY, Witzig TE: Prognostic relevance of monosomy at the 13q14 locus detected by fluorescence in situ hybridization in B cell chronic lymphocytic leukemia. Cancer Genet Cytogenet 110:77–81, 1999.

72. Criel A, Verhoef G, Vlietinck R, Mecucci C, Billiet J, Michaux L, Meeus P, Louwagie A, Can Orshoven A, Van Hoof A, Boogaerts M, Van den Berghe H, de Wolf-Peeters C: Further characterization of morphologically defined typical and atypical CLL: A clinical, immunopnenotypic, cytogenetic and prognostic study on 390 cases. Br J Haematol 97:383–391, 1995.

73. Oscier DG, Matutes E, Copplestone A, Pickering RM, Chapman R, Gillingham R, Catovsky D, Hamblin TJ: Atypical lymphocyte morphology: An adverse prognostic factor for disease progression in stage A CLL independent of trisomy 12. Br J Haematol 98:934–939, 1997.

74. Neilson JR, Auer R, White D, Bienz N, Waters JJ, Whittaker JA, Milligan DW, Fegan CD: Deletions at 11q identify a subset of patients with typical CLL who show consistent disease in progression and reduced survival. Leukemia 11:1929–1932, 1997.

75. Stilgenbauer S, von Neuhoff N, Bullinger L, Krober A, Lichter P, Dreger P, Dohner H: Deletion 11q23 identifies B-CLL patients at high risk for molecular disease persistence after high dose therapy and autografting. Blood 96(Suppl. 1):715a, 2000.

76. El Rouby S, Thomas A, Costin D, Rosenberg CR, Potmesil M, Silber R, Newcomb E: p53 gene mutation in B-cell chronic lympho-

cytic leukemia is associated with drug resistance and is independent of MDR1/MDR3 gene expression. Blood 82:3452–3459, 1993.

77. Wattel E, Preudhomme C, Hecquet B, Vanrumbeke M, Quesnel B, Dervite I, Morel P, Fenaux P: p53 mutations are associated with resistance to chemotherapy and short survival in hematologic malignancies. Blood 84:3148–3157, 1994.

78. Dohner H, Fischer K, Bentz M, Hansen K, Benner A, Cabot G, Diehl D, Schlenk R, Coy J, Stilgenbauer S, Volkmann M, Galle PR, Poustka A, Hunstein W, Lichter P: p53 gene deletion predicts for poor survival and non-response to therapy with purine analogs in chronic B-cell leukemias. Blood 85:1580–1589, 1995.

79. Lens D, Dyer MJS, Garcia-Marco JM, De Schouwer PJJC, Hamoudi RA, Jones D, Farahat N, Matutes E, Catovsky D: p53 abnormalities in CLL are associated with excess of prolymphocytes and poor prognosis. Br J Haematol 99:848–857, 1997.

80. Dohner H, Stilgenbauer S, Benner A, Leupolt E, Krober A, Bullinger L, Dohner K, Bentz M, Lichter P: Genomic aberrations and survival in chronic lymphocytic leukemia. N Engl J Med 343:1910–1916, 2000.

81. Stilgenbauer S, Rummel M, Bullinger L, Krober A, Lichter P, Bergmann L, Dohner H: Genetic aberrations in a prospective randomized B-cell trial: Deletion 17q13 (p53) predicts for nonresponse to fludarabine. Blood 96(Suppl. 1):515a, 2000.

82. Hamblin TJ, Davis Z, Gardiner A, Oscier DG, Stevenson FK: Unmutated Ig VH genes are associated with a more aggressive form of chronic lymphocytic leukemia. Blood 94:1848–1854, 1999.

83. Damle RN, Wasil T, Fais F, Ghiotto F, Valetto A, Allen SL, Buchbinder A, Budman D, Dittmar K, Kolitz J, Lichtman SM, Schulman P, Vinciguerra VP, Rai KR, Ferrarini M, Chiorazzi N: Ig V gene mutation status and CD38 expression as novel prognostic indicators in chronic lymphocytic leukemia. Blood 94:1840–1847, 1999.

84. Oscier DG, Gardiner A, Mould S, Glide S, Davis Z, Corcoran M, Ibbotson R, Orchard JA, Copplestone JA, Stevenson FK, Hamblin TJ: The mutational status of immunoglobulin V genes is the most important prognostic factor in B-CLL. Blood 96(Suppl. 1):366a, 2000.

85. Krober A, Seiler T, Leupolt E, Dohner H, Stilgenbauer S: IgVH mutated and unmutated B-CLL tumors show distinct genetic aberration patterns. Blood 96(suppl. 1):835a, 2000.

86. Gardiner AC, Mould SJ, Glide S, Davis ZA, Orchard JA, Chapman RC, Copplestone AA, Hamblin TJ, Oscier DG: VH gene status but not additional cytogenetic abnormalities predicts clinical outcome with CLL and trisomy 12. Blood 96:715a, 2000.

87. Liu Y, Grander D, Soderhall S, Juliusson G, Gahrton G, Einhorn S: Retinoblastoma gene deletions in B-cell chronic lymphocytic leukemia. Genes Chromosomes Cancer 4:250–256, 1992.

88. Stilgenbauer S, Dohner H, Bulgay-Morschel M, Weitz S, Bentz M, Lichter P: High frequency of monoallelic retinoblastoma gene deletion in B-cell chronic lymphoid leukemia shown by interphase cytogenetics. Blood 81:2118–2124, 1993.

89. Brown AG, Ross FM, Dunne EM, Steel CM, Weir-Thompson EM: Evidence for a new tumour suppressor locus (DBM) in human B-cell neoplasia telomeric to the retinoblastoma gene. Nat Gen 3:67–72, 1993.

90. Chapman RM, Corcoran MM, Gardiner A, Hawthorn LA, Cowell JK, Oscier DG: Frequent homozygous deletions of the D13S25 locus in chromosome region 13q14 defines the location of a gene critical in leukaemogenesis in chronic B-cell lymphocytic leukaemia. Oncogene 9:1289–1293, 1994.

91. Stilgenbauer S, Leupolt E, Ohl S, Weib G, Schroder M, Fischer K, Bentz M, Lichter P, Dohner H: Heterogeneity of deletions involving RB-1 and the D13S25 locus in B-cell chronic lymphocytic leukemia revealed by fluorescence in situ hybridization. Cancer Res 55:3475–3477, 1995.

92. Newcomb EW, Thomas A, Selkirk A, Lee SY, Potmesil M: Frequent homozygous deletions of D13S218 on 13q14 in B-cell chronic lymphocytic leukemia independent of disease stage and retinoblastoma gene inactivation. Cancer Res 55:2044–2047, 1995.

93. Liu Y, Hermanson M, Grander D, Merup M, Wu X, Heyman M, Rasool O, Juilusson G, Gahrton G, Detlofsson R, Nikforova N, Buys C, Soderhall S, Yankovsky N, Zabarovsky F, Einhorn S: 13q deletions in lymphoid malignancies. Blood 86:1911–1915, 1995.

94. Corcoran MM, Rasool O, Liu Y, Iyengar A, Grander D, Ibbotson RE, Merup M, Wu S, Brodyansky V, Gardiner AC, Juliusson G, Chapman RM, Ivanova G, Tiller M, Gahrton G, Yankovsky N, Zabarovsky E, Oscier DG, Einhorn S: Detailed molecular delineation of 13q14.3 loss in B-cell chronic lymphocytic leukemia. Blood 91:1–10, 1998.

95. Anastasi J, LeBeau MM, Vardiman JW, Fernald AA, Larson RA, Rowley JD: Detection of trisomy 12 in chronic lymphocytic leukemia by fluorescence in situ hybridization to interphase cells: A simple and sensitive method. Blood 79:1796–1801, 1992.

96. Que TH, Garcia-Marco J, Ellis J, Matutes E, Brito Babapulle V, Boyle S, Catovsky D: Trisomy 12 in chronic lymphocytic leukemia detected by fluorescence in situ hybridization: Analysis by stage, immunophenotype and morphology. Blood 82:571–575, 1993.

97. Escudier SM, Pereira-Leahy JM, Drach JW, Weier HU, Goodacre AM, Cork MA, Trujillo JM, Keating MJ, Andreeff M: Fluorescent in situ hybridization and cytogenetic studies of trisomy 12 in chronic lymphocytic leukemia. Blood 81:1702–2707, 1993.

98. Dohner H, Pohl S, Bulgay-Morschel M, Stilgenbauer S, Bentz M, Lichter P: Trisomy 12 in chronic lymphoid leukemias — a metaphase and interphase cytogenetic analysis. Leukemia 7:516–520, 1993.

99. Criel A, Wlodarska I, Meeus P, Stul M, Louwagie A, Van Hoof A, Hidajat M, Mecucci C, Van den Berghe H: Trisomy 12 is uncommon in typical chronic lymphocytic leukaemias. Br J Haematol 87:523–528, 1994.

100. Gaidano G, Ballerini P, Gong JZ, Inghirami G, Neri A, Newcomb EW, Macgrath IT, Knowles DM, Dalla Favera R: p53 mutations in human lymphoid malignancies: Association with Burkitt lymphoma and chronic lymphocytic leukemia. Proc Natl Acad Sci USA 88:5413–5417, 1991.

101. Fenaux P, Preudhomme C, Lai JL, Quiquandon I, Jonveaux P, Vanrumbeke M, Sartiaux C, Morel P, Loucheux-Lefebvre MH, Bauters F, Berger R, Kerckaert JP: Mutations of the p53 gene in B-cell chronic lymphocytic leukemia: A report on 39 cases with cytogenetic analysis. Leukemia 6:246–250, 1992.

102. Gardiner AC, Corcoran MM, Oscier DG: Cytogenetic, fluorescence in situ hybridisation, and clinical evaluation of translocations with concomitant deletion at 13q14 in chronic lymphocytic leukaemia. Genes Chromosom Cancer 20:73–81, 1997.

103. Cordone I, Masi S, Mauro FR, Soddu S, Morsilli O, Valentini T, Vegna ML, Guglielmi C, Mancini F, Giuliacci S, Sacchi A, Mandelli F, Foa R: p53 expression in B-cell chronic lymphocytic leukemia: A marker of disease progression and poor prognosis. Blood 91:4342–4349, 1998.

104. Adachi M, Tefferi A, Greipp PR, Kipps TJ, Tsujimoto Y: Preferential linkage of BCL-2 to immunoglobulin light chain gene in chronic lymphocytic leukemia. J Exp Med 171:559–564, 1990.

105. Raghoebier S, van Krieken JHJM, Kluin-Nelemans JC, Gillis A, van Ommen GJB, Ginsberg AM, Raffeld M, Kuin PhM: Oncogene rearrangements in chronic B-cell leukemia. Blood 77:1560–1564, 1991.

106. Dyer M, Zani VJ, Lu WZ, O'Byrne A, Mould S, Chapman R, Heward J, Kayano H, Jadayel D, Matutes E, Catovsky D, Oscier

DG: BCL2 translocations in leukemias of mature B cells. Blood 83:3682–3688, 1994.

107. Merup M, Spasokoukoyskaja T, Einhorn S, Smith CIE, Gahrton G, Juliusson G: BCL2 rearrangements with breakpoints in both vcr and mbr in non-Hodgkin's lymphomas and chronic lymphocytic leukaemia. Br J Haematol 92:647–652, 1996.

108. Counter CM, Gupta J, Harley CB, Leber B, Bacchetti S: Telomerase activity in normal leukocytes and in hematologic malignancies. Blood 85:2315–2320, 1995.

109. Bechter OE, Eisterer WPG, Hilbe W, Kuhr T, Thaler J: Telomere length and telomerase activity predict survival in patients with B cell chronic lymphocytic leukemia. Cancer Res 21:4918–4922, 1998.

110. Trentin L, Ballon G, Ometto L, Perin A, Basso U, Chieco-Bianchi L, Semenzato G, de Rossi A: Telomerase activity in chronic lymphoproliferative disorders of B-cell linage. Br J Haematol 106:662–668, 1999.

111. Tsilika A, Pappa V, Chalevalakis G, Tafas T, Economopoulos T, Papageorgiou E, Tsirigotis P, Dervenoulas J, Pappa M, Raptis S: Telomere length in peripheral blood cells from patients with B-cell chronic lymphocytic leukemia (B-CLL). EHA Barcelona, 1999.

112. Bouyge-Moreau I, Rondeau G, Avet-Loiseau H, Andre MT, Bezieau S, Cherel M, Saleun S, Cadoret E, Shaikh T, de Angelis MM, Arcot S, Batzer M, Moisan JP, Devilder MC: Construction of a 780-kb PAC, BAC, and cosmid contig encompassing the minimal critical deletion involved in B cell chronic lymphocytic leukemia at 13q14.3. Genomics 46:183–190, 1997.

113. Bullrich F, Veronese ML, Kitada S, Jurlander J, Caliguiri MA, Reed JC, Croce CM: Minimal region of loss at 13q14 in B-cell chronic lymphocytic leukemia. Blood 88:3109–3115, 1996.

114. Kalachikov S, Migliazza A, Cayanis E, Fracchiolla NS, Bonaldo MF, Lawton L, Jelenc P, Ye X, Qu X, Chien M, Hauptschein R, Gaidano G, Vitolo U, Saglio G, Resegotti L, Brodjansky V, Yankovsky N, Zhang P, Soares MB, Russo J, Edelman IS, Efstratiadis A, Dalla Favera R, Fischer SG: Cloning and gene mapping of the chromosome 13q14 region deleted in chronic lymphocytic leukemia. Genomics 42:369–377, 1997.

115. Stilgenbauer S, Nickolenko J, Wilhelm J, Wolf S, Weitz S, Dohner K, Boehm T, Dohner H, Lichter P: Expressed sequences as candidates for a novel tumor suppressor gene at band 13q14 in B-cell chronic lymphocytic leukemia and mantle cell lymphoma. Oncogene 14:1891–1897, 1998.

116. Hurley JN, Man Fu S, Kunkel HG, Chaganti RSK, German J: Chromosome abnormalities of leukaemic B lymphocytes in chronic lymphocytic leukaemia. Nature 283:76–78, 1980.

117. Perez-Losada A, Wessman M, Tiainen M, Hopman AHN, Williard HF, Sole F, Caballin MR, Woessner S, Knuutila S: Trisomy 12 in chronic lymphocytic leukemia: An interphase cytogenetic study. Blood 78:775–779, 1991.

7

Diagnosis and Treatment of Chronic Lymphocytic Leukemia

Nizar Tannir, Michael Keating, and
Susan O'Brien

Chronic lymphocytic leukemia (CLL) is a lymphoproliferative disorder (LPD) characterized by a progressive accumulation of small mature-appearing, long-lived, and functionally defective lymphocytes in the blood and bone marrow, lymph nodes, and spleen. It is the commonest leukemia in the Western world and accounts for 30 percent of all adult leukemias. About 95 percent of CLL cases are of B-cell phenotype.[1–3] In Asian countries such as China and Japan CLL represents only 5 percent of all leukemias with the T-cell phenotype predominating.[4,5] These geographic and ethnic differences in incidence are most likely the result of genetic rather than environmental factors, as it has been observed that Japanese who settled in Hawaii do not have a higher incidence of CLL than native Japanese.[6,7] Also, CLL is the only leukemia not associated with exposure to radiation.[8] Population studies have not shown any evidence linking CLL to known occupational or environmental risk factors.[9–11] Among leukemias, CLL has the strongest familial aggregation, with a two- to sevenfold higher prevalence among family clusters than in the general population.[12–14] About 8,000 new cases are diagnosed in the United States each year, with a median age of 65 years and a male/female ratio 1.3:1.[15,16] The incidence of CLL among Blacks is nearly equal to that among Whites.[17]

The exact cause of CLL is still unknown, as is the precise cell of origin. The normal counterpart of the typical CLL cell is the CD5+ B lymphocyte, which is present in the mantle zone of the secondary lymphoid follicle and in the peripheral blood in small numbers.[18] The CD5 + B cells are the predominant B-cell population in fetal spleen and peripheral blood, and they also constitute 10 to 25 percent of normal adult B cells. These cells produce polyspecific antibodies, including autoreactive antibodies. The CLL lymphocytes express very low amounts of surface immunoglobulins (sIg). Such low amounts of sIgs are only observed in normal B lymphocytes that have been rendered anergic by interaction with self-antigen. It has been hypothesized that B-CLL is a malignancy of a marginal zone-based subpopulation of anergic self-reactive CD5+ B cells, which produce polyreactive natural autoantibodies.[18,19]

DIAGNOSIS OF CLL

Two CLL working groups, the International Workshop on CLL (IWCLL) and the National Cancer Institute Working Group (NCIWG) have summarized the diagnostic criteria for CLL.[20,21] The IWCLL proposed the following criteria:

1. A sustained peripheral blood lymphocyte count above 10 $\times 10^9$ /L, with most of the cells being mature-appearing lymphocytes
2. A bone marrow aspirate showing more than 30 percent lymphocytes
3. Peripheral blood lymphocytes identified as monoclonal B cells

The diagnosis of CLL is established if either criteria 1 and 2 or 3 apply. If the peripheral blood lymphocyte count is below 10 $\times 10^9$/L, then both criteria 2 and 3 must apply.

The NCIWG criteria are similar to those proposed by the IWCLL:

1. A peripheral blood lymphocyte count above 5×10^9/L, with less than 55 percent of the cells being atypical or immature lymphoid cells. The cells should be monoclonal B lymphocytes having B-cell surface antigens (CD19, CD20, CD23) and a low density of surface immunoglobulin (IgM or IgD), with either kappa or lambda light chains, and should be CD5-positive.
2. Fewer than 30 percent of marrow nucleated cells should be lymphocytes.

The IWCLL addressed the minimum diagnostic requirements for CLL that can be applied universally, whereas the NCIWG concentrated on criteria of eligibility to enroll patients in prospective studies. For these purposes, the NCIWG required immunophenotyping. Thus, these criteria accept a lower threshold lymphocyte count of more than 5×10^9/L to diagnose B-cell CLL, whereas for clinical applications of minimum diagnostic criteria, particularly in countries where immunophenotyping is not available, the IWCLL recommends a threshold lymphocyte count of $>10 \times 10^9$/L. With the use of immunophenotying, a bone marrow examination is not required to make the diagnosis of CLL but, as discussed below, it provides prognostic information.

Several B-cell malignancies in which there are increased numbers of small lymphoid cells in the peripheral blood have overlapping clinical manifestations and should be differentiated from CLL. The three disorders most likely to be confused with CLL are prolymphocytic leukemia (PLL), the leukemic phase of non-Hodgkin's lymphoma (usually mantle-cell lymphoma, follicular lymphoma, or splenic lymphoma with circulating villous lymphocytes), and hairy cell leukemia. Immunophenotyping is helpful in differentiating these disorders (Table 7–1).

CLINICAL MANIFESTATIONS

With the use of routine screening, the number of patients with CLL who are asymptomatic at diagnosis has increased to about 40 percent.[1,2] The diagnosis is often incidental and detected during a routine examination or during preoperative evaluation. About 60 percent of patients with CLL present with various symptomatology, including constitutional symptoms. When constitutional symptomatologies are present, the most

Table 7-1. Phenotype of B-cell Lymphoid Leukemias

Type of Leukemia	CD5	CD10	CD19	CD23	FMC7	CD11C	CD22	CD103	SIG	CD79b
CLL	+	−	+	+	+/−	+/−	−	−	+	−
PLL	+/−	−	+	+/−	+	−	−	−	+ +	+
HCL	−	−	+	+	+	+	+	+	+ +	?
SLVL (SMZL)	+/−	−	+	+/−	+	+/−	+	−	+ +	+/−
MCL	+	+/−	+	−	+	−	+/−	−	+ +	+
FL	−	+	+	−	+	−	?	−	+ +	?

Abbreviations: CLL, chronic lymphocytic leukemia; PLL, prolymphocytic leukemia; HCL, hairy cell leukemia; SLVL (SMZL), splenic lymphoma with villous lymphocytes.

common complaint that leads to medical attention is fatigue or malaise. Less often, enlarged lymph nodes or the development of an infection is the initial complaint. Bacterial infections, often pneumonia, are common. Occasionally, infections secondary to opportunistic organisms or herpes zoster virus develop. An exaggerated reaction to insect bites is also common. Weight loss is noted by some patients, but is rarely severe. In contrast to lymphomas and Hodgkin's disease, fever in the absence of infection is rare in CLL. The lymph nodes, when enlarged, are usually discrete, freely movable, and nontender. Painful enlarged nodes usually indicate a superimposed infection or Richter's transformation. Enlargement of the cervical nodes occurs more commonly than axillary or inguinal adenopathy. Hepatomegaly may be noted at the time of diagnosis in about 20 percent of patients. Skin involvement occurs in less than 5 percent of cases. In contrast to lymphomas, gastrointestinal involvement is rare, as is leptomeningeal leukemia.

LABORATORY FINDINGS

Lymphocytosis may be severe but in contrast to acute leukemia, symptoms of leukostasis are uncommon in CLL. The lymphocyte count increases over time, but periodic fluctuations in the lymphocyte counts of untreated patients may occur, and in some patients the lymphocyte counts may remain stable for a long time.[22] In most patients the lymphocytes are small and mature, but there may be a variation in cell morphology, with some lymphocytes being larger or atypical, whereas others may be plasmacytomoid, cleaved, or prolymphocytes.

The French-American-British (FAB) classification system divides patients with CLL into three groups depending on the percentage of abnormal cells.[23] In typical CLL, more than 90 percent of the cells are small; in CLL/PLL, 11 to 54 percent of the cells are prolymphocytes; and in atypical CLL, there is heterogeneous morphology but less than 10 percent of the cells are prolymphocytes. Ruptured lymphocytes or "smudge" cells are commonly seen in the peripheral smear. Three types of lymphoid infiltration of the marrow are recognized in trephine biopsy specimens: nodular, interstitial, and diffuse. Patients with diffuse infiltration tend to have advanced disease and worse outcome. For prognostic purposes, nodular and interstitial patterns may be grouped together as nondiffuse and are associated with less advanced disease and better outcome.[24–26]

Less commonly, anemia and thrombocytopenia may be present at diagnosis. Hemoglobin below 11.0 g/dL or platelets below 100×10^9/L are noted at diagnosis in about 20 percent of patients. A positive direct antiglobulin test (DAT) is seen in about 25 percent of cases, but overt autoimmune hemolytic anemia occurs less frequently. The incidence of a positive DAT (Coombs) increases significantly with disease stage.[27,28] Autoimmune thrombocytopenia is diagnosed by a low platelet count with the bone marrow showing adequate numbers of megakaryocytes. Neutropenia may also be encountered.[29] These cytopenias may occur as a result of bone marrow failure due to "packed" marrow by CLL, as a result of an immune-mediated process, or as a result of hypersplenism. Hypogammaglobulinemia occurs in about 50 percent of patients with CLL. At diagnosis, it may be noted in 8 percent of patients, but its incidence increases significantly (up to 65 percent) with disease progression.[27] Usually, all three immunoglobulin classes (IgG, IgA, and IgM) are decreased, but in some patients only one or two may be low. The IgM and IgA levels are decreased to a greater extent than the IgG levels. Significant hypogammaglobulinemia and neutropenia result in increased susceptibility of patients with CLL to major bacterial infections.

IMMUNOPHENOTYPING

Clonality of CLL is confirmed by restricted light chain (kappa or lambda) expression on the cell surface,[1,18] the presence of unique idiotypic specificities on the immunoglobulins produced by CLL cells,[30] by immunoglobulin gene rearrangement analysis, and at times by detection of a specific cytogenetic abnormality.[31] Using sensitive techniques, monoclonal proteins can be detected in the serum of many patients,[32–34] although only 10 to 20 percent produce large enough quantities of monoclonal proteins to be detected by routine serum electrophoresis. The CLL cells express the B-cell markers CD19, CD20, CD21, and CD23; most CLL cells are also positive for Ia (DR and DC), Fc receptors, and have receptors for mouse erythrocytes.[35–37] Some surface markers that are usually found on normal B cells, including CD22, are found infrequently on CLL cells. The hallmark of CLL is coexpression of a common T-cell marker, CD5. Another disease entity in which B lymphocytes also express CD5 is mantle-cell lymphoma. Caution must be taken to differentiate CLL from the leukemic phase of mantle-cell lymphoma because the prognosis and treatment of these diseases are quite different. Use of antibody to the cell-surface antigen CD23 is most useful because this antigen is found on CLL lymphocytes but not on mantle cells. Rearrangements of immunoglobulin heavy- and light-chain genes are readily demonstrated in patients with CLL.[38] In addition, almost 25 percent of patients with CLL have rearrangements of the T-cell receptor β gene.[39,40]

IMMUNE ABNORMALITIES

Early in the disease, the absolute number of T cells may be increased with inversion of the T-helper to T-suppressor cell ratio.[41–43] The CD4/CD8 ratio may continue to drop with disease progression or after successful therapy with nucleoside analogues. Additionally, a decreased proportion of cells express the CD3 antigen. The T cells may respond normally to mitogens, such as phytohemagglutinin, in vitro and produce interleukin-2 and gamma-interferon,[44] but their reactivity to allogeneic and autologous B cells is impaired.[45,46] Functional studies of the T cells have sometimes shown decreased T-helper functions.[41,45,47] Spontaneous and antibody-dependent cytotoxicity are decreased, which suggests an abnormality in the large granular lymphocyte population, including natural killer (NK) cells.[48] The etiology of these disturbances is not clear. One possibility is that T- and NK-cell functions may be suppressed by factors produced by CLL B cells.[49] The pathogenesis of hypogammaglobulinemia in CLL is poorly understood. However, impaired B-cell function, as well as regulatory abnormalities of T cells, including the reversal of normal helper/suppressor cell ratios, may play a role. Furthermore, CLL-derived NK cells have been shown to suppress immunoglobulin secretion by normal B cells in vitro.[50]

AUTOIMMUNE COMPLICATIONS OF CLL

When autoantibodies are present, they are preferentially targeted against blood cells; this results in autoimmune hemolytic anemia (AIHA), immune-mediated thrombocytopenia (ITP), immune-mediated granulocytopenia (IG), and pure red cell aplasia (PRCA)[51]; PRCA, ITP, and IG as complications of CLL occur less frequently than AIHA.[52] The presence of either thrombocytopenia or anemia, irrespective of the presence of autoantibody, carries a poor prognosis. Several factors suggest that antibodies against blood cell antigens are not produced by the leukemia clone.[53] These autoantibodies are polyclonal and are usually IgG.[19] Furthermore, the severity of the autoimmune phenomenon does not correlate with the severity of CLL, and autoimmune complications may develop in patients whose disease is responding to therapy.[54,55] Rarely, CLL is associated with other autoimmune disorders such as rheumatoid arthritis, Hashimoto's/Graves disease, and systemic lupus erythematosus; these disorders have been found to be more frequent in first-degree relatives of patients with CLL.

STAGING

The natural history of CLL is extremely variable, with survival times ranging from 2 to over 20 years from initial diagnosis. In 1975, Rai et al.[56] proposed a staging system consisting of five stages (Rai 0 to IV) based on Dameshek's proposed model of orderly disease progression in CLL.[57] The Rai stages were found to correlate with prognosis and were confirmed in numerous independent populations. This staging system is applicable to newly diagnosed and to previously treated patients, although the latter group has a less favorable prognosis. The Rai staging system was later modified[58] into a three-stage system: low risk (Rai 0), intermediate risk (Rai I, II), and high risk (Rai III, IV). The actuarial survival curves according to the clinical stage at the time of diagnosis are shown in Figure 7–1. A similar staging system was developed in Europe by Binet et al.[59]; Binet stage C corresponds to the high-risk group (Rai stages III and IV), whereas Binet stages A and B correspond to the low- and intermediate-risk

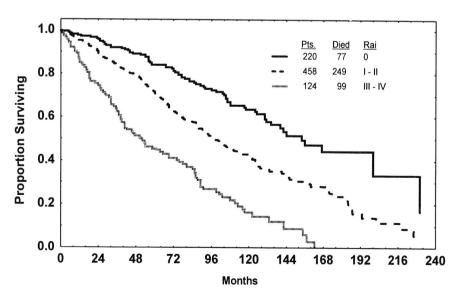

Pts.	Died	Rai
220	77	0
458	249	I - II
124	99	III - IV

Figure 7–1. Actual survival curves by Rai stage.

Table 7–2. Staging Systems for Chronic Lymphocytic Leukemia

The Rai Staging System

Original Five-Stage System	Modified Three-Stage System	Clinical Features	Median Survival (yr)
0	Low risk	lymphocytosis	12.5
I	Intermediate risk	lymphadenopathy	7
II		splenomegaly, ± hepatomegaly	
III	High risk	anemia < 11.0 g/dl	1.5
IV		thrombocytopenia < 100 × 10⁹/L	

The Binet Staging System

Stage	Clinical Features	Median Survival (yr)
A	Less than 3 areas of clinical adenopathy, no anemia or thrombocytopenia	12
B	Three or more involved node areas; no anemia or thrombocytopenia	7
C	Hb < 10g/dl and/or platelets < 100 × 10⁹/L	2

The five lymphoid areas are (1) cervical lymph nodes, (2) axillary lymph nodes, (3) inguinofemoral lymph nodes, (4) spleen, and (5) liver.

groups (Rai stages 0–II) (Table 7–2). The three-stage modified Rai system remains the most widely used system in the United States, whereas the Binet system is commonly used in Europe.

Although many patients in the high-risk group (Rai stages III and IV; Binet stage C) have a progressive clinical course, the course of the disease is not uniform in the other risk groups. Patients in the low- and intermediate-risk groups (Rai stages 0–II, Binet stages A and B) may have an indolent disease course, which spans several years or even decades, or the course may be progressive and associated with a short survival time. Thus, identification of prognostic factors within early-stage disease is important. Several prognostic factors have been found to be associated with inferior survival in CLL.[60,61] These include a short lymphocyte doubling time (less than 12 months),[62] a diffuse pattern of bone marrow infiltration,[25,26] advanced age and male gender,[61] abnormal karyotype,[63–66] high serum levels of β_2-microglobulin,[67,68] soluble CD23,[69,70] and a CLL-PLL category.[71,72] Newer prognostic factors in CLL include the mutational status of Ig genes and CD38 expression on CLL lymphocytes.[73,74] A recent report suggested that IgV gene mutations within CLL lymphocytes correlates with a significantly longer survival.[73] Although controversial, some investigators have suggested that mutated IgV genes correlate with low expression (less than 30 percent) of CD38 on CLL lymphocytes. Although this correlation may not be exact, data examining CD38 expression on CLL lymphocytes clearly show a strong correlation between increased expression and inferior survival.

In the low-risk group, several investigators have defined a "smoldering" group whose disease is unlikely to progress. Investigators from Spain noted that patients with low absolute lym-

phocyte counts (below 30 × 10⁹/L), hemoglobin above 12g/dL, and a bone marrow biopsy showing a nondiffuse (interstitial or nodular) pattern of lymphoid infiltration had a survival similar to those of age- and sex-matched control subjects.[75] Similarly, investigators from France found that patients with Binet stage A disease with hemoglobin above 12 g/dL and blood lymphocytosis below 30 × 10⁹/L had a survival time equal to that of an age- and sex-matched French population.[76]

TREATMENT

The first decision to be made in CLL is whether the patient requires treatment at the time of initial diagnosis. This cautionary approach is based on the older age of the patient, the heterogeneity of the disease course, and lack of evidence that early treatment affects long-term survival. Given these vagaries, the NCIWG has devised guidelines for the initiation of treatment for CLL.[77,78] These include constitutional symptoms, progressive bone marrow failure, AIHA and ITP poorly responsive to corticosteroid therapy, massive or progressive lymphadenopathy or splenomegaly; progressive lymphocytosis, or a doubling time less than 6 months. Hypogammaglobulinemia or the development of a monoclonal protein alone are not sufficient criteria to initiate therapy. Response criteria guidelines have also been established by this group (Table 7–3).

Chemotherapy

For several decades, the backbone of chemotherapy in CLL has been either of two alkylating agents, chlorambucil (CLB) and cyclophosphamide (CTX), with or without the addition of corticosteroids. Both agents are rapidly absorbed from the gastrointestinal tract and can be administered orally.[79,80] Doses

Table 7–3. National Cancer Institute Working Group Response Criteria for Chronic Lymphocytic Leukemia

Parameter	CR[a]	PR[a]
Lymphocytes	≤ 4.0 × 10⁹/L	≥ 50 percent ↓
Lymph nodes (liver, spleen)	No palpable disease	≥ 50 percent ↓
Neutrophils	≥ 1.5 × 10⁹/L	≥ 1.5 × 10⁹/L or ≥ 50% improvement
Platelets	> 100 × 10⁹/L	> 100 × 10⁹/L or ≥ 50% improvement
Hemoglobin	> 11.0 g/dl (untransfused)	> 11.0 g/dl or ≥ 50% improvement
Bone marrow	< 30 percent lymphocytes, no nodules	± nodules
Symptomatology	None	Variable

Abbreviations: CR, complete remission; PR, partial remission. Duration of CR or PR: ≥ 2 months.
[a] Less than 30 percent lymphocytes in marrow with residual nodules = nPR.

and schedules of CLB vary significantly. Commonly used schedules include a daily dose of 0.08 mg/kg (4 to 8 mg total dose per day), or an intermittently pulsed schedule of 0.5 mg/kg (30 to 40 mg in a single day) given every 3 to 4 weeks, or 0.3mg/kg (15 to 20 mg/m^2) given every 2 weeks.[80,81] The dose is adjusted to avoid myelosuppression, which is more common with the daily schedule. Chlorambucil is administered for several weeks until a maximal clinical response is reached. Maintenance chemotherapy is usually not given, but CLB may be restarted if disease recurrence is noted. A proportion of patients may achieve a second and third response after retreatment with CLB. Cyclophosphamide is less likely to cause thrombocytopenia than CLB but is equally effective. It usually is given at a daily dose of 1 to 2 mg/kg. Overall, the response rate with either CLB or CTX is about 40 to 60 percent with about a 3 to 5 percent complete response (CR) rate.

Corticosteroids

Prednisone has been administered as a single agent, usually at a dose of 20 to 100 mg daily, with gradual tapering.[82,83] With prednisone given alone, one-third of patients experience a decrease in the size of lymph nodes or spleen. An increase in the absolute lymphocyte count may be observed in the first 4 weeks due to a shift of lymphocytes from lymph nodes and bone marrow into the blood. Anemia and thrombocytopenia improve in about two-thirds of patients. At present, the major indication for prednisone in CLL is the treatment of AIHA and ITP.

Chlorambucil With or Without Prednisone Regimens

In an attempt to improve response rates, alkylating agents have been combined with steroids. The only study to show improvement in CR and overall response (OR) rate of CLB and prednisone over CLB alone was by Han et al. in 1973.[84] Higher OR and CR rates were obtained with CLB plus prednisone than with CLB alone (87 and 20 percent versus 45 and 9 percent, respectively), but there was no difference in median survival. The number of patients treated was very small, and none of the differences were statistically significant. Sawitsky et al.[85] compared the monthly administration of CLB plus prednisone with daily CLB plus prednisone or prednisone alone and reported 47 percent OR (CR 8 percent), 38 percent OR (CR 3 percent), and 11 percent OR (CR 0 percent), respectively. However, no difference in survival was noted. Jaksic et al.[86] designed a regimen of daily high-dose CLB (15 mg/day until CR or toxicity) versus CLB 75 mg given once weekly for 6 weeks combined with prednisone. A significantly higher response rate was noted for the continuous CLB arm versus the intermittent CLB plus prednisone arm (70 versus 31 percent respectively). A survival advantage was noted for patients who received continuous CLB. The cumulative dose for the continuous CLB arm was five to six times that for the intermittent CLB plus prednisone arm. A number of single-arm studies using CLB plus prednisone have been reported, with about 10 percent of patients achieving a CR and 50 percent a partial response (PR). However, the definition of response has been variable.

Two clinical trials conducted by the French Cooperative Group on CLL in patients with Binet stage A disease compared immediate treatment with CLB (first trial) or CLB plus prednisone (second trial) versus delayed treatment until evidence of progression was noted.[76] Patients on the delayed treatment arm had a somewhat superior survival compared with those on the immediate treatment group arm owing to higher incidence of second malignancies with prolonged CLB exposure.

Chlorambucil With or Without Prednisone Versus Other Regimens

Nonrandomized trials initially reported excellent responses with use of intermittent CTX, vincristine, and prednisone (CVP or COP) in patients with advanced CLL,[87,88] with 44 percent of patients achieving a CR. However, the French Cooperative Group on CLL conducted a randomized study in patients with Binet stage B disease comparing CLB with COP and reported no difference in survival or rate of disease progression to a more advanced stage between the two groups.[89] Similarly, the Eastern Cooperative Oncology Group (ECOG) compared CLB and prednisone versus CVP and reported no difference in CR rate, duration of response, or survival between the two arms.[90] In another trial conducted by the French Cooperative Group on CLL in patients with Binet stage C disease,[91] the COP regimen was compared with a French CHOP regimen adding doxorubicin 25 mg/m^2 on day 1 to COP. The overall survival was significantly superior for the CHOP group. In both groups, CTX was given daily by mouth for 5 days. This study was well conducted, but skepticism was generated by the fact that the median survival in the control COP arm was inferior to that for CVP in the ECOG study (2 years versus 4 years), a median survival time for the CHOP arm being 4 years. In addition, no difference in response or survival was observed in Binet stage B patients treated with CHOP versus CLB and prednisone. Jaksic et al.[92] compared CHOP with high-dose CLB and noted a higher response rate for high-dose CLB (89 percent) than for CHOP (70 percent). Survival was also superior for the CLB-treated group.

Purine Analogues

Several purine analogues have demonstrated major clinical activity in indolent lymphoid malignancies. Fludarabine monophosphate (Fludara), 2-chlorodeoxyadenosine (Cladribine) and deoxycoformycin (Pentostatin) are all active in the treatment of CLL and low-grade lymphomas.

In an initial phase II study with fludarabine given at 20 mg/m^2 daily for 5 days, 54 percent of patients showed clinical improvement.[93] Keating et al. administered fludarabine 30 mg/m^2 daily for 5 days and reported a response rate of 59 percent in 68 previously treated patients, with 15 percent achieving CR.[94] A subsequent study from the same group used the identical dose of fludarabine with prednisone in 101 previously treated patients with CLL.[95] The overall response rate was 55 percent, similar to that obtained with fludarabine alone. The addition of prednisone was associated with an increased incidence of *Pneumocystis carinii* and *Listeria monocytogenes* infections.[95,96] An alternative schedule of fludarabine, using a bolus injection of 20 mg/m^2 followed by a continuous infusion of 30 mg/m^2/day, produced inferior results as compared with the standard 5-day regimen.[97] Whether this was due to the continuous infusion schedule, smaller total dose delivered, or differences in patient population is unclear. In an attempt to reduce toxicity, fludarabine was administered at 30 mg/m² daily for 3 days every 4 weeks.[98] As compared with the standard 5-day treatment schedule, the OR and CR rates were lower (46 and 10 percent, respectively), but there was also a reduction in the infection rate.

Subsequent studies have evaluated fludarabine in a 5-day schedule in previously untreated patients.[95,99] In a series of 35 patients, 26 (74 percent) achieved a CR, although 13 of these had persistent nodules in the bone marrow (nPR). The OR rate was 81 percent.[99] The overall response rate to fludarabine plus prednisone in untreated patients was 79 percent, with 30 percent CR and 37 percent nPR.[95]

2-Chlorodeoxyadenosine (2-CdA) has also been evaluated in CLL and has similar antitumor activity but may be more likely to produce thrombocytopenia.[100–102] Studies with 2-CdA have produced variable response rates ranging from 48 to 72 percent and CR rates of 4 to 39 percent in previously treated patients. In previously untreated patients, data is limited; about 80 percent of patients respond and half of these achieve CR.[102,103] Like fludarabine, 2-CdA is immunosuppressive, with infections being the major toxicity. Although initial studies suggested that patients resistant to fludarabine might respond to 2-CdA, this expectation has not been confirmed.[104,105] In a clinical trial of 28 patients who had disease resistant to fludarabine, only 2 patients had a PR with 2-CdA.[105] Thus, patients with CLL whose disease is resistant to one of these two nucleoside analogues should not be treated with the other.

2-Deoxycoformycin has been less extensively evaluated in CLL.[106–108] The response rate for Pentostatin is approximately 16 to 35 percent, with CR rare. In 13 previously untreated patients, 6 PRs were noted.

Comparative Studies

A randomized multinational phase III trial was conducted in Europe comparing six cycles of fludarabine given at the standard dose and schedule (25 mg/m²/day on days 1 to 5 every 4 weeks) with six cycles of CAP (cyclophosphamide 750 mg/m² on day 1, doxorubicin 50 mg/m² on day 1, and prednisone 40 mg/m² on days 1 to 5 every 3 weeks) in 100 untreated and 96 treated patients with Binet stage B or C CLL.[109] In previously treated patients, a statistically significant higher response rate was observed with fludarabine (48 percent, 13 percent CR) than with CAP (27 percent, 6 percent CR), but there was no improvement in median remission duration or survival between the two groups. In untreated patients, the responses with fludarabine (71 percent, 23 percent CR) were somewhat better than those with CAP (60 percent, 17 percent CR), and the duration of response was significantly longer with fludarabine ($p<.001$). There was also a trend toward longer survival in patients treated with fludarabine ($p=.087$).

Recently, fludarabine was compared with CLB in previously untreated patients with CLL.[110] This intergroup trial enrolled 395 patients, who received fludarabine 25 mg/m² daily for 5 days every 4 weeks or CLB as a single dose of 40 mg/m² every 4 weeks. The duration of treatment in both arms was 12 months.

A third arm administering fludarabine 20 mg/m² daily for 5 days plus CLB at 20 mg/m² on day 1 every 4 weeks was closed early because of toxicity. Crossover was permitted for nonresponse or early relapse. The OR rate with fludarabine was 63 percent with a 20 percent CR rate, whereas the response rate with CLB was 37 percent with a 4 percent CR rate. In addition, a longer duration of response and an improved progression-free survival was noted in patients treated with fludarabine. Half of the patients who failed to respond to CLB responded to fludarabine, in contrast to a 7 percent PR rate with CLB in patients who failed to respond to fludarabine. The incidence of neutropenia, thrombocytopenia, and infections was similar.

Recently 2-CdA was also compared with CLB in previously untreated patients with CLL. Robak et al. randomized 229 patients to 2CdA plus prednisone versus CLB plus prednisone.[111] The CR and OR rates were significantly higher in the group of patients treated with 2-CdA plus prednisone (47 and 87 percent, respectively) than in the group of patients treated with CLB plus prednisone (12 and 57 percent, respectively). Although progression-free survival was significantly longer in the 2-CdA-treated group, overall survival at 2 years was similar in the two arms.

After initial treatment with fludarabine, patients with CLL can achieve a meaningful response to retreatment with fludarabine given at relapse, particularly if their prior response was CR or nPR (72 percent OR rate with 40 percent CR rate for 25 patients with prior CR versus 70 percent OR rate with 13 percent CR rate for 23 patients with prior nPR).[112,113] An oral formulation of fludarabine is currently being evaluated.[114]

Although response rates with fludarabine are high, particularly in previously untreated patients, residual disease is usually detectable, and all patients will relapse.[115] Thus, methods to improve on the single-agent efficacy are needed. One approach is the use of fludarabine and alkylating agents. DNA cross-links formed after exposure of cells to activated CTX are rapidly removed *in vitro*, with most cross-links no longer detectable after 6 hours. Exposure of CLL lymphocytes to small doses of fludarabine prevents repair of alkylator-induced DNA damage by inhibiting DNA repair enzymes.[116,117]

Flinn et al. administered fludarabine 20 mg/m² for 5 days together with CTX 600 mg/m² on day 1 to 60 previously untreated patients with low-grade lymphoma or CLL.[118] The overall response rate in the 17 patients with CLL was 100 percent with 47 percent CR. The use of growth factor support and prophylactic antibiotics resulted in a low incidence of myelosuppression and infections.

O'Brien et al. used fludarabine 30 mg/m² and CTX 300 mg/m², both given for 3 days, to treat 128 patients with CLL.[119] Patients refractory to fludarabine had a response rate of 38 percent, whereas all other patients had a response rate of over 80 percent. The comparative effectiveness of fludarabine versus fludarabine plus CTX is being evaluated in randomized trials by ECOG and the German CLL Study Group.

Biological Therapies

Interferon alpha (IFN-A) may decrease the lymphocyte count in patients with early-stage disease, but it is ineffective in advanced disease.[120–122] It has been given as maintenance therapy in patients who responded to CLB or fludarabine but has had no impact on time to progression or on survival.[123–125]

Monoclonal antibodies are an exciting new therapeutic modality in lymphoid malignancies. Rituximab is a humanized monoclonal antibody, which binds the B-cell antigen CD20. Given at doses of 375 mg/m^2/week for 4 weeks, Rituximab resulted in a 58 percent OR rate in follicular lymphomas but produced only a 12 percent response rate in small lymphocytic lymphoma (SLL).[126] Winkler et al. treated 10 patients with CLL with the standard dose, but only 1 of these responded.[127] Two groups have explored escalated doses of Rituximab in the treatment of CLL. Byrd et al. administered the standard 375 mg/m^2 dose thrice weekly for 4 weeks and reported a 45 percent response rate in 33 patients with SLL/CLL.[128] In a dose escalation trial of 40 patients with previously treated CLL, O'Brien et al. administered Rituximab 375 mg/m^2 the first week and then increased the dose from 500 mg to 2,250 mg/m^2 weekly for 3 weeks. The overall response rate in CLL was 36 percent, and a dose response was observed.[129] Trials combining Rituximab with chemotherapy are ongoing in CLL.[130]

Campath-IH, another humanized monoclonal antibody, binds to CD52, a panlymphocyte antigen present on both B and T lymphocytes.[131] Campath-IH has been evaluated in a number of trials, producing responses rates in previously treated CLL of 33 to 42 percent.[132,133] A recent pivotal trial in fludarabine-refractory patients produced a response rate of 33 percent.[134] Campath-IH was particularly effective in clearing the blood, bone marrow, and spleen of CLL and less effective at bulky lymph nodes sites. Campath-IH is an immunosuppressive antibody, which may be associated with a significant number of infections and viral reactivation. Thus, all patients receiving this antibody should receive prophylaxis against PCP and herpes. The Oncology Drug Advisory Committee recently recommended to the FDA that this antibody be approved for the treatment of patients with CLL refractory to fludarabine.

Transplantation

Allogeneic bone marrow transplantation (allo-BMT) has not been extensively explored in patients with CLL because of the significant toxicity associated with this approach in a population of elderly patients. Nonetheless, several studies have reported on the feasibility of allo-BMT and autologous marrow transplantation (auto-BMT) in CLL. The largest published series reported on 54 patients younger than 60 years who received transplants at 30 centers worldwide between 1984 and 1992.[135] The median age was 41 years. Although a variety of conditioning regimens were used, the majority of the patients received CTX and total body irradiation followed by HLA-matched marrows from siblings. Of these patients 30 died; 24 were alive, all except one in CR. About half of the deaths were due to graft-versus-host disease (GVHD). The 3-year probability of survival was 46 percent, with a projected survival at 5 years of 30 to 40 percent. Of 27 evaluable patients, 16 developed chronic GVHD. In single institution studies, the incidence of GVHD was lower.[136,137] One hypothesis to explain this is the more extensive use of fludarabine in the United States, resulting

in immunosuppression of the recipient and inability to elicit a graft versus host effect. Auto-BMT has been performed in several studies.[136–138] The procedure appears to be safe, with a lower relapse rate in patients who receive their transplant in first remission as an intensification procedure than in patients who receive their transplant as a salvage regimen for active disease. Recently, allogeneic minitransplantation, which employs nonmyeloablative regimens and relies on harnessing the graft-versus-leukemia effect, has expanded the option of transplantation to patients up to age 70 years. A pilot study demonstrated that engraftment occurs; transplant patients who had sensitive disease had a better outcome than those who had resistant disease.[139] With the recognition that 60 percent of CLL patients younger than 55 years eventually develop progressive disease and have a median survival probability of only 5 years after therapy,[140] innovative therapies with curative intent, including the use of transplantation, will play an increasing role in the future.

Splenectomy

Splenectomy may be of benefit in patients with CLL under several circumstances: steroid-refractory immune thrombocytopenia or hemolytic anemia, hypersplenism with cytopenias unresponsive to chemotherapy, and symptomatically enlarged spleens.[141–147] The two largest series describing splenectomy in patients with CLL are from single institutions; investigators from the Mayo Clinic reported 50 patients who underwent splenectomy over a 16-year period.[148] Despite a performance status of 2 or higher in one-third of the patients, the operative mortality was only 4 percent.[148] Most patients (94 percent) had Rai stage III or IV disease with extensive marrow involvement, massive splenomegaly, and refractory cytopenias.[148] Significant hematologic responses were noted; 77 percent of anemic patients improved their hemoglobin by at least 3 g/dL or to over 11 g/dL. Similarly, 70 percent of thrombocytopenic patients achieved a platelet count of more than 100×10^9/L. These responses were durable, lasting more than 1 year in more than 80 percent of patients.[148] There was no association between spleen size or degree of marrow infiltration and response to splenectomy.

In the largest series published to date, investigators at the University of Texas, M. D. Anderson Cancer Center (MDACC) reported their 21-year experience with 55 patients.[149] These patients were compared with a group of 55 patients treated with fludarabine who were matched for baseline characteristics. The hematologic benefits of splenectomy were significant. Of the splenectomized patients, 81 percent had an increase in the platelet count to at least 50×10^9/L at 1 month. Similarly, 59 percent of neutropenic patients achieved a neutrophil increment of 1.0×10^9/L, and 38 percent of patients had an increase in their hemoglobin of at least 3 g/dL. Most patients received chemotherapy following the surgery, and this precluded an analysis of response duration. The authors noted that the hematologic improvements resulted in an increased tolerance to subsequent chemotherapy. Despite this fact and the use of a group of matched controls, they did not show a benefit in the overall survival for splenectomized patients (2-year actuarial survival rate of 50 ± 7 percent versus 46 ± 7 percent in the controls).[149]

Splenic Irradiation and Radiation Therapy

Splenic irradiation may be an alternative to splenectomy when the risks associated with this procedure are unacceptable.[150–157] Retrospective series have reported good results in relieving pain and reducing spleen size but less consistent effects on cytopenias. Side effects included gastrointestinal toxicity and worsening of cytopenia, with several patients developing marked thrombocytopenia and leukopenia in some series.[150–157]

Autoimmune Complications

When present in patients with CLL, autoantibodies are usually targeted against hematopoietic cells.[158] Autoimmune hemolytic anemia (AIHA), immune thrombocytopenia (IT), immune neutropenia, pure red cell aplasia (PRCA), and aplastic anemia[159–160] have all been reported with CLL. The incidence of autoantibodies ranges from 10 to 75 percent[161,162]; the likelihood of a positive Coombs test increases with disease stage.[161]

The treatment for patients with autoimmune cytopenias and CLL is usually oral corticosteroids (prednisone, 60 to 100 mg/day), with three-quarters of patients responding. Alternatives for patients who fail to respond to steroids include intravenous immunoglobulin (IVIG) or splenectomy. Less than 1 percent of these patients develop PRCA,[159] characterized by anemia, absence of reticulocytes, and a marrow failing to demonstrate mature erythroblasts. Cyclosporine has demonstrated activity in this setting, even in patients resistant to conventional therapy.[163] Recently, CSA has been used to treat AIHA and IT associated with CLL.[164] At doses of 300 mg daily, the response rate is 81 percent (13/16); responses were seen in patients failing corticosteroid therapy. Toxicity was minimal, and tumor responses were also noted.

TRANSFORMATION

Most patients with CLL demonstrate a stable histology throughout their clinical course; however, a minority may show evolution to more aggressive disease forms, including Richter's syndrome, prolymphocytoid transformation, and rarely, acute leukemia.[165]

Richter's transformation occurs in 5 to 10 percent of CLL cases and represents a change to a large-cell lymphoma (LCL) histology.[166] Robertson et al.[167] described 39 CLL patients in whom LCL developed. This represented 3 percent of patients enrolled in a computer-based registry at MDACC between 1972 and 1992.[167] Patients in whom LCL was noted included patients in all Rai stages and in 10 patients in remission after fludarabine therapy. The incidence of transformation after fludarabine or 2-CdA therapy was not significantly increased over that in patients treated with alkylating agents. Systemic symptoms and progressive lymphadenopathy were seen in most patients. Extranodal involvement and paraproteinemia were seen in 41

percent and 44 percent, respectively. The most frequent laboratory abnormality was elevation of lactate dehydrogenase (LDH); 82 percent of patients had a value more than twice normal. Only 8 percent of patients with CLL seen at MDACC had this level of LDH elevation. As seen in other studies, median survival was short (5 months), although patients responding to chemotherapy lived longer.[168–171]

The development of acute leukemia or multiple myeloma in patients with CLL is a rare phenomenon, occurring in less than 1 percent of cases and has not been well characterized.[165,172] Isolated cases of CLL transformation into small noncleaved cell lymphoma,[173] lymphoblastic lymphoma,[174] hairy cell leukemia,[175] and Hodgkin's disease[176] have been reported.

SECOND TUMORS

Patients with CLL have an increased incidence of nonhematologic neoplasms, particularly lung cancer.[177–179] In a review by Lee et al.,[180] 25 percent of patients with CLL had second primary tumors, mostly skin cancers, and 7 percent of patients died of complications from these other malignancies rather than from CLL. Results of a randomized trial suggest that long-term treatment with chlorambucil may increase the susceptibility of patients to epithelial tumors.[76] Recently, long-term data for over 200 patients treated on National Cancer Institute Group C protocols with nucleoside analogues were examined, and the number of observed and expected second tumors was compared.[181] Patients included those with CLL treated with fludarabine and patients with hairy cell leukemia treated with 2-deoxycoformycin or 2-CdA. The most common second cancer found in patients with CLL was lung cancer. As compared with age-adjusted 1994 Surveillance and Epidemiology End Results rates for the general population, the observed/expected frequency for patients treated with fludarabine was 1.65 (95 percent confidence interval, 1.04 to 2.47). This increased rate, however, was consistent with the risk associated with the disease alone, and the authors concluded that despite their immunosuppressive properties, nucleoside analogues were not associated with an increased risk of second malignancies.

REFERENCES

1. Dighiero G, Travade P, Chevret S et al: The French Cooperative Group on CLL. B-cell chronic lymphocytic leukemia: Present status and future directions. Blood 78:1901–1914, 1991.
2. O'Brien S, delGiglio A, Keating M: Advances in the biology and treatment of B-cell chronic lymphocytic leukemia. Blood 85:307–318, 1995.
3. Rozman C, Montserrat E: Chronic lymphocytic leukemia. N Engl J Med 333:1052–1057, 1995.
4. Hoyer JD, Ross CW, Li C-Y et al: True T-cell chronic lymphocytic leukemia: A morphologic and immunophenotypic study of 25 cases. Blood 86:1163–1169, 1996.
5. Barliner NT: Gamma lymphocytosis and T cell chronic leukemias. Hematol Oncol Clin North Am 4:473–487, 1990.
6. Haenszel W, Kurihara M: Studies of Japanese migrants. I. Mortality from cancer and other diseases among Japanese in the United States. J Natl Cancer Inst 40:43–68, 1968.

7. Yanagihara ET, Blaisdell RK, Hayashi T, Lukes RJ: Malignant lymphoma in Hawaii-Japanese: A retrospective morphologic survey. Hematol Oncol 7:219–232, 1989.

8. Preston DL, Kusumi S, Tomonoga M et al: Cancer incidence in atomic bomb survivors. Part III. Leukemia, lymphoma and multiple myeloma. Radiat Res 137 (Suppl 2):S68–97, 1994.

9. Arp EW, Wolf PH, Checkoway H: Lymphocytic leukemia and exposure to benzene and other solvents in the rubber industry. J Occup Med 25:598–602, 1983.

10. Blair A, White D: Leukemia cell types and agricultural practices in Nebraska. Arch Environ Health 40:211–214, 1985.

11. Brandt L: Environmental factors and leukemia. Med Oncol Tumor Pharmacother 2:7–10, 1985.

12. Conley CL et al: Genetic factors predisposing to chronic lymphocytic leukemia and autoimmune disease. Medicine (Baltimore) 5:323–334, 1980.

13. Gunz FW et al: Familial leukemia: A study of 909 families. Scand J Haematol 15:117–131, 1975.

14. Linet MS et al: Familial cancer history and chronic lymphocytic leukemia. Am J Epidemiol 130:655–664, 1989.

15. Landis SH, Murray T, Bolden S, Wingo PA: Cancer Statistics 2000: CA Cancer J Clin 50:7, 2000.

16. Landis SH, Murray T, Bolden S, Wingo PA: Cancer statistics 1999. CA Cancer J Clin 49:8–31, 1999.

17. Fleming AF: The epidemiology of lymphomas and leukemias in Africa: An overview. Leuk Res 9:735–740, 1985.

18. Caligaris-Cappio F: B-chronic lymphocytic leukemia: A malignancy of anti-self B cells. Blood 87:2615–2620, 1996.

19. Kipps TJ, Carson DA: Autoantibodies in chronic lymphocytic leukemia and related systemic autoimmune disease. Blood 81:2475–2487, 1993.

20. International Workshop on Chronic Lymphocytic Leukemia: Chronic lymphocytic leukemia: Recommendations for diagnosis, staging and response criteria. Ann Intern Med 110:236–238, 1989.

21. Cheson BD, Bennett JM, Grever M et al: National Cancer Institute-sponsored Working Group guidelines for chronic lymphocytic leukemia: Revised guidelines for diagnosis and treatment. Blood 87:4990–4997, 1996.

22. Gray JL et al: Bone marrow and peripheral blood lymphocytosis in the prognosis of chronic lymphocytic leukemia. Cancer 33:1169–1178, 1974.

23. Bennett JM, Catovsky D, Daniel MT et al: Proposals for the classification of chronic (mature) B and T lymphoid leukemias. J Clin Pathol 42:567–584, 1989.

24. Lipshutz MD, Mir R, Rai KR, Sawitsky A: Bone marrow biopsy and clinical staging in chronic lymphocytic leukemia. Cancer 46:1422–1427, 1980.

25. Pangalis GA, Boussiotis VA, Kittas C: B chronic lymphocytic leukemia. Disease progression in 150 untreated stage A and B patients as predicted by bone marrow pattern. Nouv Rev Fr Hematol 30:373–375, 1988.

26. Rozman C, Montserrat E, Rodriquez-Fernandez JM et al: Bone marrow histologic pattern, the best single prognostic parameter in chronic lymphocytic leukemia: A multivariate survival analysis of 329 cases. Blood 64:642–648, 1984.

27. Pangalis GA, Angelopoulou MK, Vassilakopoulos TP, Siakantaris MP, Kittas C: B-chronic lymphocytic leukemia, small lymphocytic lymphoma, and lymphoplasmacytic lymphoma, including Waldenstrom's macroglobulinemia: A clinical, morphologic, and biologic spectrum of similar disorders. Semin Hematol 36:104–114, 1999.

28. De Rossi G, Granati L, Girelli G et al: Incidence and prognostic significance of autoantibodies against erythrocytes and platelets in chronic lymphocytic leukemia (CLL). Nouv Rev Fr Hematol 30:403–406, 1988.

29. Rustagi P et al: Antigranulocyte antibodies in CLL and other chronic lymphoproliferative disorders. Blood 62(Suppl. 1):106, 1983.

30. Giardina SL et al: The generation of monoclonal anti-idiotypic antibodies to human B-cell derived leukemias and lymphomas. J Immunol 135:653–658, 1985.

31. Oscier D, Fitchett M, Herbert T, Lambert R: Karyotypic evolution in B-cell chronic lymphocytic leukemia. Genes Chromosom Cancer 3:16–20, 1991.

32. Beaume A, Brizard A, Dreyfus B et al: High incidence of serum monoclonal Igs detected by a sensitive immunoblotting technique in B-cell lymphocytic leukemia: Blood 84:1216–1219, 1994.

33. Deegan MT et al: High incidence of monoclonal proteins in the serum and urine of chronic lymphocytic leukemia patients. Blood 64:1207–1211, 1984.

34. Qian GX et al: Circulating monoclonal IgM proteins in B cell chronic lymphocytic leukemia. J Immunol 133:3396–3400, 1984.

35. Geisler CH, Larsen JK, Hansen NE et al: Prognostic importance of flow cytometric immunophenotyping of 540 consecutive patients with B-cell chronic lymphocytic leukemia. Blood 78:1795–1802, 1991.

36. Harris NL, Jaffe ES, Stein H et al: A revised European-American classification of lymphoid neoplasms: A proposal from the International Lymphoma Study Group. Blood 84:1361–1392, 1994.

37. Ikematsu W, Ikematsu H, Okamura S et al: Surface phenotype and Ig heavy-chain gene usage in chronic B-cell leukemias: Expression of myelomonocytic surface markers in CD5-chronic B-cell leukemia. Blood 83:2602–2610, 1994.

38. Rechavi G et al: Immunoglobulin heavy chain rearrangements in chronic lymphocytic leukemia: Correlation with clinical stage. Br J Haematol 72:524–529, 1989.

39. Perl A et al: Rearrangement of the T-cell receptor alpha, beta and gamma chain genes in chronic lymphocytic leukemia. Leuk Res 14:131–137, 1990.

40. Norton JD et al: Rearrangement and expression of T cell antigen receptor genes in B cell chronic lymphocytic leukemia. Blood 71:178–185, 1988.

41. Kay NE: Abnormal T cell subpopulation function in CLL: Excessive suppressor and deficient helper activity with respect to B cell proliferation. Blood 57:418–420, 1981.

42. Platsoucas CD et al: Abnormal T lymphocyte subpopulations in patients with B cell CLL. J Immunol 129:2305–2312, 1982.

43. Catovsky D et al: Increase in T lymphocytes in B-cell CLL. Br J Haematol 47:539–544, 1981.

44. Rossi JF et al: Production of B-cell growth factor interleukin 2 and gamma interferon by peripheral blood lymphocytes from patients with chronic lymphocytic leukemia of B cell type. Am J Hematol 29:183–188, 1988.

45. Han T, Dadly B: In vitro functional studies of mononuclear cells in patients with CLL. Cancer 43:109–117, 1979.

46. Han T et al: Lack of autologous mixed lymphocyte reaction in patients with CLL. Blood 60:1075–1081, 1982.

47. Lauria F et al: T cell functional abnormality in B-CLL: Evidence of a defect of the T helper subset. Br J Haematol 54:277–283, 1983.

48. Ziegler HW et al: Deficiency of natural killer cell activity in patients with CLL. Int J Cancer 27:321–327, 1981.

49. Burton JD et al: Malignant chronic lymphocytic leukemia B cells elaborate soluble factors that down regulate T cell and NK function. Am J Hematol 30:61–67, 1989.

50. Kay NE, Perri RT: Evidence that large granular lymphocytes from B-CLL patients downregulate B cell immunoglobulin synthesis. Blood 73:1016–1019, 1989.

51. Pritsch O, Maloum K, Dighiero G: Basic biology of autoimmune phenomena in chronic lymphocytic leukemia. Semin Oncol 25:34–41, 1998.

52. Diehl LF, Ketchum LH: Autoimmune disease and chronic lymphocytic leukemia: Autoimmune hemolytic anemia, pure red cell aplasia, and autoimmune thrombocytopenia. Semin Oncol 24:80–97, 1998.

53. Hamblin TJ, Oscier DJ, Young BJ: Autoimmunity in chronic lymphocytic leukaemia. J Clin Pathol 39:713–716, 1986.

54. DiRaimondo F, Giustolisi R, Cacciola E et al: Autoimmune hemolytic anemia in chronic lymphocytic leukemia patients treated with fludarabine. Leuk Lymphoma 11:63–68, 1993.

55. Myint H, Copplestone JA, Orchard J et al: Fludarabine-related autoimmune hemolytic anemia in patients with chronic lymphocytic leukemia. Br J Haematol 91:342–344, 1995.

56. Rai KR, Sawitsky A, Cronkite EP et al: Clinical staging of chronic lymphocytic leukaemia. Blood 46:219–234, 1975.

57. Dameshek W: Chronic lymphocytic leukemia: An accumulative disease of immunologically incompetent lymphocytes. Blood 29:566–584, 1967.

58. Rai KR: A critical analysis of staging in CLL. In Gale RP, Rai KR (eds): Chronic Lymphocytic Leukemia: Recent Progress and Future Direction. UCLA Symposia on Molecular and Cellular Biology, New Series, Vol.59, p. 253. Liss, New York, 1987.

59. Binet J-L, Auquier A, Dighiero G et al: A new prognostic classification of chronic lymphocytic leukemia derived from a multivariate survival analysis. Cancer 48:198–206, 1981.

60. Rai KR, Montserrat E: Prognostic factors in chronic lymphocytic leukemia. Semin Hematol 24:252–256, 1987.

61. Zwiebel JA, Cheson BD: Chronic lymphocytic leukemia: Staging and prognostic factors. Semin Oncol 25:42–59, 1998.

62. Montserrat E et al: Lymphocyte doubling time in chronic lymphocytic leukaemia. Analysis of its prognostic significance. Br J Haematol 62:567–575, 1986.

63. Geisler C, Philip P, Hansen M: B-cell chronic lymphocytic leukemia: Clonal chromosome abnormalities and prognosis in 89 cases. Eur J Haematol 43:397–403, 1989.

64. Oscier DG, Stevens H, Hamblin TJ et al: Correlation of chromosome abnormalities with laboratory features and clinical course in B-cell chronic lymphocytic leukaemia. Br J Haematol 76:352–358, 1990.

65. Juliusson G, Oscier DG, Fitchett M et al: Prognostic subgroups in B-cell chronic lymphocytic leukemia defined by specific chromosome abnormalities. N Engl J Med 323:720–724, 1990.

66. Han T, Henderson ES, Emrich LJ, Sandberg AA: Prognostic significance of karyotypic abnormalities in B-cell chronic lymphocytic leukemia: An update. Semin Hematol 24:257–263, 1987.

67. Di Giovanni S, Valentini G, Carducci P, Giallonardo P: Beta-2-microglobulin is a reliable tumor marker in chronic lymphocytic leukemia. Acta Haematol 81:181–185, 1989.

68. Keating MJ, Lerner S, Kantarjian H et al: The serum beta 2-microglobulin (beta2M) level is more powerful than stage in predicting response and survival in chronic lymphocytic leukemia (CLL). 86:606a, 1995.

69. Sarfati M, Chevret S, Chastang C et al: Prognostic importance of serum soluble CD23 level in chronic lymphocytic leukemia. Blood 88:4259–4264, 1996.

70. Knauf WU, Langenmayer I, Ehlers B et al: Serum levels of soluble CD23, but not soluble CD25, predict disease progression in early stage B-cell chronic lymphocytic leukemia. Leuk Lymphoma 27:523–532, 1997.

71. Vallespi T et al: Chronic lymphocytic leukaemia: Prognostic value of lymphocyte morphological subtypes. A multivariate survival analysis in 146 patients. Br J Haematol 77:478–485, 1991.

72. Peterson L et al: Morphology of chronic lymphocytic leukemia and its relationship to survival. Am J Med 59:316–324, 1975.

73. Damle RN, Wasil T, Fais F et al: IgV gene mutation status and CD38 expression as novel prognostic indicators in chronic lymphocytic leukemia. Blood 94:1840–1847, 1999.

74. Naylor M, Capra JD: Mutational status of Ig V_H genes provide clinically valuable information in B-cell chronic lymphocytic leukemia. Blood 94:1837–1839, 1999.

75. Montserrat E, Rozman C: Chronic lymphocytic leukemia: Prognostic factors and natural history. Bailliere Clin Hematol 6:849–866, 1993.

76. Dighiero G, Maloum K, Desablens B et al: Chlorambucil in indolent chronic lymphocytic leukemia. N Engl J Med 338:1506–1514, 1998.

77. Cheson BD, Bennett JM, Rai KR et al: Guidelines for clinical protocols for chronic lymphocytic leukemia (CLL). Recommendations of the NCI-sponsored Working Group. Am J Hematol 29:152–163, 1988.

78. Cheson BC, Bennett JM, Grever M et al: National Cancer Institute-sponsored Working Group guidelines for chronic lymphocytic leukemia: Revised guidelines for diagnosis and treatment. Blood 87:4990–4997, 1998.

79. Colvin M: A review of the pharmacology and clinical use of cyclophosphamide. In Pinedo HM (ed.): Clinical Pharmacology of Antineoplastic Drugs, p. 245. Elsevier-North Holland, Amsterdam, Netherlands.

80. Ezdinli EZ, Stutzman L: Chlorambucil therapy for lymphomas and chronic lymphocytic leukemia. JAMA 191:444, 1965.

81. Knospe WH, Loeb V Jr, Huguley CM Jr: Bi-weekly chlorambucil treatment of chronic lymphocytic leukemia. Cancer 33:555–562, 1974.

82. Ezdinli EZ, Stutzman L, W. Aungst C et al: Corticosteroid therapy for lymphomas and chronic lymphocytic leukemia. Cancer 23:900–909, 1969.

83. Galton DAG, Wiltshaw E, Szur L, et al: The use of chlorambucil and steroids in the treatment of chronic lymphocytic leukaemia. Br J Haematol 7:73, 1961.

84. Han T et al: Chlorambucil vs combined chlorambucil-corticosteroid therapy in chronic lymphocytic leukemia. Cancer 31:502–508, 1973.

85. Sawitsky A, Rai KR, Glidewell O, Silver RT, and participating members of CALGB (Cancer and Leukemia Group B): Comparison of daily versus intermittent chlorambucil and prednisone therapy in the treatment of patients with chronic lymphocytic leukemia. Blood 50:1049–1059, 1977.

86. Jaksic B, Brugiatelli M: High-dose continuous chlorambucil vs intermittent chlorambucil plus prednisone for treatment of B-CLL. IGCI CLL-01 trial. Nouv Rev Fr Hematol 30:437–442, 1988.

87. Liepman M, Votaw ML: Treatment of chronic lymphocytic leukemia with COP chemotherapy. Cancer 41:1664–1669, 1978.

88. Oken MM, Kaplan ME: Combination chemotherapy with cyclophosphamide, vincristine and prednisone in the treatment of refractory CLL. Cancer Treat Rep 63:441–447, 1979.

89. French Cooperative Group on Chronic Lymphocytic Leukemia: A randomized clinical trial of chlorambucil versus COP in Binet stage B chronic lymphocytic leukemia. Blood 75:1422–1425, 1990.

90. Raphael B, Andersen JW, Silber R et al: Comparison of chlorambucil and prednisone versus cyclophosphamide, vincristine, and prednisone as initial treatment for chronic lymphocytic leukemia: Long-term follow-up of an Eastern Cooperative Oncology Group randomized clinical trial. J Clin Oncol 9:770–776, 1991.

91. French Cooperative Group on Chronic Lymphocytic Leukemia: Long-term results of the CHOP regimen in stage C chronic lymphocytic leukemia. Br J Haematol 73:334–340, 1989.

92. Jaksic B, Brugiatelli M, Krc I, et al: High dose chlorambucil versus Binet's modified cyclophosphamide, doxorubicin, vincristine, and prednisone regimen in the treatment of patients with advanced B-cell chronic lymphocytic leukemia: Results of an international multicentric randomized trial. Cancer 79:2107–2114, 1997.

93. Grever MR, Kopecky KJ, Coltman CA et al: Fludarabine monophosphate: A potentially useful agent in chronic lymphocytic leukemia. Nouv Rev Fr Hematol 30:457–459, 1988.

94. Keating MJ, Kantarjian H, Talpaz M et al: Fludarabine: A new agent with major activity against chronic lymphocytic leukemia. Blood 74:19–25, 1989.

95. O'Brien S, Kantarjian H, Beran M et al: Results of fludarabine and prednisone therapy in 264 patients with chronic lymphocytic leukemia with multivariate analysis derived prognostic model for response to treatment. Blood 82:1695–1700, 1993.

96. Cheson B: Infectious and immunosuppressive complications of purine analog therapy. J Clin Oncol 13:2431–2448, 1995.

97. Puccio CA, Mittelman A, Lichtman SM et al: A loading dose continuous infusion schedule of fludarabine phosphate in chronic lymphocytic leukemia. J Clin Oncol 9:1562–1569, 1991.

98. Robertson LE, O'Brien S, Kantarjian H et al: A 3-day schedule of fludarabine in previously treated chronic lymphocytic leukemia. Leukemia 9:1444–1449, 1995.

99. Keating MJ, Kantarjian H, O'Brien S et al: Fludarabine: A new agent with marked cytoreductive activity in untreated chronic lymphocytic leukemia. J Clin Oncol 9:44–49, 1991.

100. Saven A, Carrera CJ, Carson DA, Beutler E, Piro LD: 2-Chlorodeoxyadenosine treatment of refractory chronic lymphocytic leukemia. Leuk Lymphoma 5:133–138, 1991.

101. Juliusson G, Liliemark J: High complete remission rate from 2-chloro-2-deoxyadenosine in previously treated patients with B-cell chronic lymphocytic leukemia. J Clin Oncol 11:679–689, 1993.

102. Robak T, Blasinka-Morawiec M, Krykowski E et al: Intermittent 2-hour intravenous infusions of 2-chlorodeoxyadenosine in the treatment of 110 patients with refractory or previously untreated B-cell chronic lymphocytic leukemia. Leuk Lymphoma 22:509–514, 1996.

103. Saven A, Lemon RH, Kasty M et al: 2-Chlorodeoxyadenosine activity in patients with untreated chronic lymphocytic leukemia. J Clin Oncol 13:570–575, 1995.

104. Juliusson G, Elmhorn-Rosenborg A, Liliemark J: Response to 2-chlorodeoxyadenosine in patients with B-cell chronic lymphocytic leukemia resistant to fludarabine. N Engl J Med 327:1056–1061, 1992.

105. O'Brien S, Kantarjian H, Estey E et al: Lack of effect of 2-chlorodeoxyadenosine therapy in patients with chronic lymphocytic leukemia refractory to fludarabine therapy. N Engl J Med 330:319–322, 1994.

106. Dillman RO, Mick R, McIntyre OR: Pentostatin in chronic lymphocytic leukemia: A phase II trial of Cancer and Leukemia Group B. J Clin Oncol 7:433–438, 1989.

107. Ho AD, Thaler J, Stryckmans P et al: Pentostatin in refractory chronic lymphocytic leukemia: A phase II trial of the European Organization for Research and Treatment of Cancer. J Natl Cancer Inst 82:1416–1420, 1990.

108. Johnson SA, Catovsky D, Child JA, Newland AC, Milligan DW, Janmohamed R: Phase I/II evaluation of Pentostatin (2′-deoxycoformycin) in a five day schedule for the treatment of relapsed/refractory B-cell chronic lymphocytic leukaemia. Invest New Drugs 16:155–160, 1998.

109. The French Cooperative Group on CLL, Johnson S, Smith AG, Löffler H et al: Multicenter prospective randomized trial of fludarabine versus cyclophosphamide, doxorubicin, and prednisone (CAP) for treatment of advanced stage chronic lymphocytic leukaemia. Lancet 347:1432–1438, 1996.

110. Rai KR, Peterson B, Elias I et al: A randomized comparison of fludarabine and chlorambucil for patients with previously untreated chronic lymphocytic leukemia: A CALGB, SWOG, CTG/NCI-C and ECOG Intergroup Study. N Engl J Med. 343:1750–1757, 2000.

111. Robak T, Blonski JZ, Kasznicki M et al: Cladribine with prednisone versus chlorambucil with prednisone as first-line therapy in chronic lymphocytic leukemia: Report of a prospective, randomized, multicenter trial. Blood 96:2723–2729, 2000.

112. Keating MJ, O'Brien S, Lerner S, Koller C, Beran M et al: Long-term follow-up of patients with chronic lymphocytic leukemia (CLL) receiving fludarabine regimens as initial therapy. Blood 92:1165–1171, 1998.

113. Thomas D, O'Brien S, Kantarjian H, Giles FJ, Lerner S, Keating MJ: Outcome in 203 patients (pts) with relapsed or refractory B-cell chronic lymphocytic leukemia (CLL) with salvage therapy (RX): Retreatment with fludarabine (FLU). Blood 92(Suppl. 1):102a (abstr. 419), 1998.

114. Boogaerts MA, Van Hoof A, Catovsky D, Kovacs M et al: Treatment of alkylator resistant chronic lymphocytic leukemia with oral fludarabine phosphate. Blood 11(4):abstr #3113, 1999.

115. Robertson LE, Hu Y, Butler JJ et al: Response assessment in chronic lymphocytic leukemia after fludarabine plus prednisone: Clinical, pathologic, immunophenotypic, and molecular analysis. Blood 80:29–36, 1992.

116. Bellosillo B, Villamor N, Colomer D, Montserrat E et al: In vitro evaluation of fludarabine in combination with cyclophosphamide and/or mitoxantrone in B-cell chronic lymphocytic leukemia. Blood 94:2836–2843, 1999.

117. Koehl L, Nowak B, Van Haperen R, Kornhuber B et al: Synergistic cytotoxicity using cyclophosphamide and nucleoside analogs. In Hiddeman W, Buechner T, Wormann B, Ritter J, Creutzig U, Keating MJ, and Plunkett W (eds): Acute Leukemias VII: Experimental Approaches and Novel Therapies, pp. 549–555. Springer-Verlag, Berlin, 1997.

118. Flinn IW, Byrd JC, Morrison C, Jamison J et al: Fludarabine and cyclophosphamide with filgrastim support in patients with previously untreated indolent lymphoid malignancies. Blood 96:71–75, 2000.

119. O'Brien S, Kantarjian HM, Cortes J, Beran M et al: Results of the fludarabine and cyclophosphamide combination regimen in chronic lymphocytic leukemia. J Clin Oncol 19:1414–1420, 2001.

120. Zeigler-Heitbrock HWL, Schlag R, Flieger D, Thiel E: Favorable response of early stage B-CLL patients to treatment with IFN-α_2. Blood 73:1426–1430, 1989.

121. McSweeney EN, Giles FJ, Worman CP et al: Recombinant interferon alfa 2a in the treatment of patients with early stage B chronic lymphocytic leukemia. Br J Haematol 85:77–83, 1993.

122. Foon KA, Bottino GC, Abrams PG et al: Phase II trial of recombinant leukocyte A interferon in patients with advanced chronic lymphocytic leukemia. Am J Med 78:216–220, 1985.

123. Montserrat E, Villamor N, Urbrano-Ispizua A et al: Treatment of early stage-B chronic lymphocytic leukemia with alpha-2B inter-

feron after chlorambucil reduction of the tumoral mass. Ann Hematol 63:15–19, 1991.

124. O'Brien S, Kantarjian H, Beran M et al: Interferon maintenance therapy for patients with chronic lymphocytic leukemia in remission after fludarabine therapy. Blood 86:1296–1300, 1995.

125. Zinzani PL, Bendandi M, Magagnoli M, Rondelli D et al: Results of a fludarabine induction and α-interferon maintenance protocol in pretreated patients with chronic lymphocytic leukemia and low-grade non-Hodgkin's lymphoma. Eur J Haematol 59:82–88, 1997.

126. McLaughlin P, Grillo-Lopez J, Link BK et al: Rituximab chimeric anti-CD20 monoclonal antibody therapy for relapsed indolent lymphoma: Half of patients respond to a four-dose treatment program. J Clin Oncol 16:2825–2833, 1998.

127. Winkler U, Jenson M, Manzke O, Schulz H, Diehl V, Engert A: Cytokine-release syndrome in patients with B-cell chronic lymphocytic leukemia and high lymphocyte counts after treatment with an anti-CD20 monoclonal antibody (Rituximab, IDEC-C2B8). Blood 94:2217–2224, 1999.

128. Byrd JC, Murphy T, Lucas MS, Howard R et al: Thrice weekly Rituximab demonstrates significant activity in chronic lymphocytic leukemia. Blood 96:abstr. #3615, 2000.

129. O'Brien S, Kantarjan H. Thomas DA et al: Rituximab dose-escalation trial in chronic lymphocytic leukemia (CLL). J Clin Oncol 19(8):2165–2170, 2001.

130. Keating MJ, O'Brien S, Lerner S, Giles F et al: Combination chemo-antibody therapy with fludarabine (F), cyclophosphamide (C) and Rituximab achieves a high CR rate in previously untreated chronic lymphocytic leukemia (CLL). Blood 96:abstr. #2214.

131. Riechmann L, Clark M, Waedmann H et al: Reshaping human antibodies for therapy. Nature 332:323–327, 1988.

132. Osterborg A, Dyer MJS, Bunjes D, Pangalis GA et al: Phase II multicenter study of human CD52 antibody in previously treated chronic lymphocytic leukemia. J Clin Oncol 15:1567–1574, 1997.

133. Rai K, Mercier RJ, Cooper MR, Freter CB et al: Campath-1H is an effective salvage therapy for fludarabine failing CLL patients, results of a Phase II trial. Blood 96:abstr. #703.

134. Keating M, Rai K, Flinn I et al: Multicenter study of Campath-IH in patients with chronic lymphocytic leukemia (B-CLL) refractory to fludarabine. Blood 94(10):75a, 1999.

135. Michallet M, Archimbaud E, Bandini G et al: HLA-identical sibling bone marrow transplantation in younger patients with chronic lymphocytic leukemia. Ann Intern Med 124:311–315, 1996.

136. Rabinowe SN, Soiffer RJ, Gribben JG et al: Autologous and allogeneic bone marrow transplant for poor prognosis patients with B-cell chronic lymphocytic leukemia. Blood 82:1366–1376, 1993.

137. Khouri IF, Keating MJ, Vriesendorp H et al: Autologous and allogeneic bone marrow transplantation for chronic lymphocytic leukemia: Preliminary results. J Clin Oncol 12:748–758, 1994.

138. Sutton L, Malourn K, Gonzalez H, Zouabi H et al: Autologous hematopoietic stem cell transplantation as salvage treatment for advanced B cell chronic lymphocytic leukemia. Leukemia 12:1699–1707, 1998.

139. Khouri IF, Keating M, Korbling M et al: Transplant-Lite: Induction of graft-versus-malignancy using fludarabine-based non-ablative chemotherapy and allogeneic blood progenitor-cell transplantation as treatment for lymphoid malignancies. J Clin Oncol 16, 2817, 1998.

140. Mauro FR, Foa R, Giannarelli D et al: Clinical characteristics and outcome of young chronic lymphocytic leukemia patients: A single institution study of 204 cases. Blood 94:448–454, 1999.

141. Delpero JR, Houvenaeghel G, Gastaut JA et al: Splenectomy for hypersplenism in chronic lymphocytic leukaemia and malignant non-Hodgkin's lymphomas. Br J Surg 77:443, 1990.

142. Ferrant A, Michaux JL, Sokal G: Splenectomy in advanced chronic lymphocytic leukemia. Cancer 58:2130, 1986.

143. Stein RS, Weikert D, Reynolds V et al: Splenectomy for end-stage chronic lymphocytic leukemia. Cancer 59:1815, 1987.

144. Thiruvengadam R, Piedmonte M, Barcos M et al: Splenectomy in advanced chronic lymphocytic leukemia. Leukemia 4:758, 1990.

145. Pegourie B, Sotto J, Hollard D et al: Splenectomy during chronic lymphocytic leukemia. Cancer 59:1626, 1987.

146. Gallhofer G, Melo JV, Spencer J, Catovsky D: Splenectomy in advanced chronic lymphocytic leukaemia. Acta Haematol 77:78, 1987.

147. Majumdar G, Singh AK: Role of splenectomy in chronic lymphocytic leukaemia with massive splenomegaly and cytopenia. Leuk Lymphoma 7:131, 1992.

148. Neal TF Jr, Tefferi A, Witzig TE et al: Splenectomy in advanced chronic lymphocytic leukemia: A single institution experience with 50 patients. Am J Med 93:435–440, 1992.

149. Seymour JF, Cusack JD, Lerner SA et al: Case/control study of the role of splenectomy in chronic lymphocytic leukemia. J Clin Oncol 15:52–60, 1997.

150. Byhardt RW, Brace KC, Wiernik PH: The role of splenic irradiation in chronic lymphocytic leukemia. Cancer 35:1621–1625, 1975.

151. Guiney MJ, Liew KH, Quong GG et al: A study of splenic irradiation in chronic lymphocytic leukemia. Int J Radiat Oncol Biol Phys 16:225–229, 1989.

152. De Rossi G, Biagini C, Lopez M et al: Treatment by splenic irradiation in 22 chronic lymphocytic leukemia patients. Tumori 68:511–514, 1982.

153. Johnson RE: Role of radiation therapy in management of adult leukemia. Cancer 39:852–855, 1977.

154. Johnson RE, Kagan AR, Gralnick HR et al: Radiation-induced remissions in chronic lymphocytic leukemia. Cancer 20:1382–1387, 1967.

155. Aabo K, Walbom-Jorgensen S: Spleen irradiation in chronic lymphocytic leukemia (CLL): Palliation in patients unfit for splenectomy. Am J Hematol 19, 177–180, 1985.

156. Roncadin M, Arcicasa M, Trovo MG et al: Splenic irradiation in chronic lymphocytic leukemia. A 10-year experience at a single institution. Cancer 60:2624–2628, 1987.

157. Chisesi T, Capnist G, Dal Fior S: Splenic irradiation in chronic lymphocytic leukemia. Eur J Haematol 46:202–204, 1991.

158. Hamblin TJ, Oscier DG, Young BJ: Autoimmunity in chronic lymphocytic leukaemia. J Clin Pathol 39:713, 1986.

159. Chikkappa G, Zarrabi MH, Tsan MF: Pure red-cell aplasia in patients with chronic lymphocytic leukaemia. *Medicine (Baltimore)* 65:339, 1986.

160. Singal R, Winfield DA, Greaves M: Bone marrow aplasia in B cell chronic lymphocytic leukemia: Successful treatment with antithymocyte globulin. J Clin Pathol 44:954, 1991.

161. De Rossi G, Granati L, Girelli G et al: Incidence and prognostic significance of autoantibodies against erythrocytes and platelets in chronic lymphocytic leukemia (CLL). Nouv Rev Fr Hematol 30:403, 1998.

162. De Rossi G, Granati L, Girelli G et al: Prognostic value of autoantibodies against erythrocytes and platelets in chronic lymphocytic leukemia (CLL). Tumori 77:100, 1991.

163. Tura S, Finelli C, Bandini G et al: Cyclosporin A in the treatment of CLL associated PRCA and bone marrow hypoplasia. Nouv Rev Fr Hematol 30:479, 1988.

164. Cortes J, O'Brien S, Kantarjian H, Giles FJ, Keating M: Treatment of anemia and/or thrombocytopenia associated with chronic lymphocytic leukemia with cyclosporin A. Blood 92(Suppl 1):104a (abstr. #425), 1998.

165. Foon KA, Gale RP: Clinical transformation of chronic lymphocytic leukemia. Nouv Rev Fr Hematol 30:385, 1988.

166. Giles FJ, O'Brien S, Keating M: Chronic lymphocytic leukemia in (Richter's) transformation. Semin Oncol 25:117–125, 1998.

167. Robertson LE, Pugh W, O'Brien S et al: Richter's syndrome: A report on 39 patients. J Clin Oncol 11:1985, 1993.

168. Foucar K, Rydell RE: Richter's syndrome in chronic lymphocytic leukemia. Cancer 46:118, 1990.

169. Long JC, Aisenberg AC: Richter's syndrome. A terminal complication of chronic lymphocytic leukemia with distinct clinicopathologic features. Am J Clin Pathol 63:766, 1975.

170. Armitage JO, Dick FR, Corder MP: Diffuse histocytic lymphoma complicating chronic lymphocytic leukemia. Cancer 41:422, 1978.

171. Trump DL, Mann RB, Phelps R et al: Richter's syndrome: Diffuse histiocytic lymphoma in patients with chronic lymphocytic leukemia. Am J Med 68:539, 1980.

172. Zarrabi M, Grunwald HW, Rosner F: Chronic lymphocytic leukemia terminating in acute leukemia. Arch Intern Med 137:1059, 1977.

173. Litz CE, Arthur DC, Gajl-Peczalska KJ et al: Transformation of chronic lymphocytic leukemia to small non-cleaved cell lymphoma: A cytogenetic, immunological, and molecular study. Leukemia 5:972, 1991.

174. Pistoia V, Roncella S, Di Celle PF et al: Emergence of a B-cell lymphoblastic lymphoma in a patient with B-cell chronic lymphocytic leukemia: Evidence for the single-cell origin of the two tumors. Blood 78:797, 1991.

175. Duchayne E, Delsol G, Kuhlein E et al: Hairy cell transformation of a B-cell chronic lymphocytic leukemia: A morphological, cytochemical phenotypic and molecular study. Leukemia 5:150, 1991.

176. Fayad L, Robertson LE, O'Brien S, Manning JT et al: Hodgkin's disease variant of Richter's syndrome: Experience at a single institution. Leuk Lymphoma 23:333–337, 1996.

177. Berg JW: The incidence of multiple primary cancers. 1. Development of further cancers in patients with lymphomas, leukemias, and myeloma. J Natl Cancer Inst 38:741, 1967.

178. Pottern LM, Linet M, Blair A et al: Familial cancers associated with subtypes of leukemia and non-Hodgkin's lymphoma. Leuk Res 15:305, 1991.

179. Travis LB, Curtis RE, Hankey BF et al: Second cancers in patients with chronic lymphocytic leukemia. J Natl Cancer Inst 84:1422, 1992.

180. Lee JS, Dixon DO, Kantarjian HM et al: Prognosis of chronic lymphocytic leukemia: A multivariate regression analysis of 325 untreated patients. Blood 69:929, 1987.

181. Cheson BD, Vena DA, Barrett J, Freidlin B: Second malignancies as a consequence of nucleoside analog therapy for chronic lymphoid leukemias. J Clin Oncol 17:2454, 1999.

8

Diagnosis and Treatment of Hairy Cell Leukemia

Alan Saven

Hairy cell leukemia (HCL) is a rare chronic lymphoproliferative disorder, which is characterized by circulating B lymphocytes displaying prominent cytoplasmic projections and infiltrating the bone marrow and spleen. Afflicted individuals are often elderly men who present with pancytopenia, splenomegaly, or recurrent severe infections. This disorder was first described as a distinct clinicopathologic entity in 1958 by Bouroncle et al.,[1] who referred to the disorder as "leukemic reticuloendotheliosis." The descriptive term "hairy cell leukemia" was coined by Schrek and Donnelly in 1966.[2] During the past decade and a half the successful introduction of three effective systemic therapies—alpha-interferon, Pentostatin (2′-deoxycoformycin; dCF) and cladribine (2-chlorodeoxyadenosine; 2-CdA)—has dramatically and favorably altered the treatment options and prognosis for patients with this disease.

EPIDEMIOLOGY, ETIOLOGY, AND PATHOGENESIS

The precise incidence of HCL is unknown, but it is thought to account for 2 to 3 percent of all adult leukemias in the United States, with 600 new patients being diagnosed annually. The disease is particularly rare in Orientals and Blacks. It is predominantly a disease of middle-aged men with a median age at presentation of 52 years. There is a 4:1 male predominance, with Ashkenazi Jewish men being more frequently affected. The cause of HCL is unknown. Familial cases have been described.[3] Early investigators described an association with HTLV-II, but later showed it was not directly related to the disease process.[4] Prior exposure to radiation and organic solvents has been suggested to be more frequent among HCL patients.[5,6]

When cytogenetic analyses were performed in 30 patients with HCL, chromosome 5 was involved in clonal aberrations in 12 patients (40 percent) most commonly as trisomy 5 or pericentric inversions and interstitial deletions involving band 5q13.[7] Hairy cell leukemia has been well characterized as a clonal B-cell disorder. The normal function and precise site of origin in the lymphocytic ontogeny of the hairy cell remains unknown but is believed to occur late in lymphocyte development, before the plasma cell.[8] Macrophage colony-stimulating factor (M-CSF) induces hairy cell motility,[9] and a specific integrin receptor, $\alpha_v\beta_3$, has been identified that is responsible for their motility.[10]

HISTOPATHOLOGY

Peripheral Blood and Bone Marrow

Hairy cells are mononuclear cells with nuclei that are eccentric or central.[11] Nuclear morphology is variable, the nuclei being round, ovoid, reniform, or convoluted (Figure 8–1A). The cells with round and ovoid nuclei are the smallest, those with convoluted nuclei are intermediate in size, and those with indented nuclei are largest, often with nucleoli. Nuclear forms tend to have a fine reticular chromatin pattern. Hairy cells have variable amounts of cytoplasm, which is blue-gray in appearance, exhibiting thin cytoplasmic projections. Rarely, granules or broad-shaped inclusions can be seen in the cytoplasm, which correspond to the ribosomal lamellar complex seen on electron microscopy.[12] The peripheral blood usually demonstrates pancytopenia; the leukopenia is associated with severe monocytopenia in 80 percent of patients.[11]

Because of marrow reticulin fibrosis, the marrow is frequently difficult or impossible to aspirate.[13–15] Occasional cases will, however, reveal typical hairy cells on the aspirated sample and/or on touch preparation of the marrow core biopsy. The hairy cells in the marrow aspirate tend to have a slightly coarser reticular chromatin staining pattern than those found in the peripheral blood. The marrow biopsy specimens usually demonstrate hairy cell infiltrates, which in some patients may be patchy and difficult to discern. The most subtle pattern of HCL infiltration to appreciate is that of a hypocellular marrow with scant infiltration by hairy cells admixed with residual hematopoietic tissue.[11,13–15]

Marrow involvement may be diffuse or focal. The hairy cells have monotonous round, oval, or spindle-shaped nuclei, which are separated by abundant quantities of pale-staining cytoplasm in a fine fibrillar network. This separation of individual hairy cells is characteristic and referred to as the "fried-egg" appearance (Figure 8–2). Fibroblast infiltration has never been noted in the marrow, and it has been demonstrated that hairy cells synthesize and assemble a fibronectin matrix, which is likely responsible for the marrow fibrosis so characteristic of the disease.[16] The pale and delicate network of fibrils between individual hairy cells is usually recognizable but is often better appreciated with the periodic acid–Schiff stain. Among the hairy cells are varying numbers of small lymphocytes, plasma cells, mast cells, and extravasated red blood cells. Cells with round or ovoid nuclei predominate at higher magnification. Occasionally, dilated sinuses with extravasated erythrocytes, similar to the red blood cell lakes seen in the spleen, are present. Rarely, hairy cells may have a peritrabecular distribution.

Spleen and Other Sites

The spleen is usually enlarged with a median weight of 1,300 g.[17] When sectioned, the spleen has a dark red, smooth surface. On light microscopy the hairy cells involve the splenic red pulp, and later the white pulp atrophies and is replaced. Initial HCL involvement is by the focal infiltration of trabeculae and subendothelial infiltrates within trabecular veins.[18] Red cell lakes,

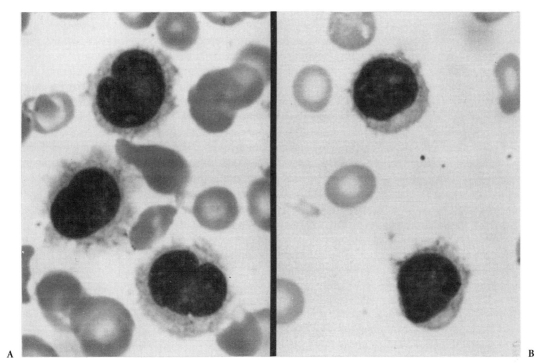

A   B

Figure 8–1. Peripheral blood smears from patients with hairy cell leukemia (**A**) and splenic lymphoma with circulating villous lymphocytes (**B**). The hairy cells are small to medium in size, have ovoid or reniform nuclei with finely clumped chromatin, and demonstrate abundant, frayed gray-blue cytoplasm. In comparison, the circulating villous lymphocytes have increased nuclear to cytoplasmic ratios, round nuclei with coarse chromatin, and basophilic cytoplasm with short, often polar, projections (Wright's stain, × 1,500).

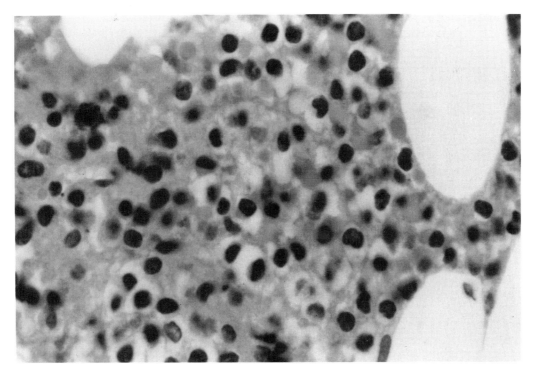

Figure 8–2. Hairy cell leukemia in the bone marrow, characterized by well-spaced lymphocytes with a "fried egg" appearance due to the distinct round to oval nuclei, which are centrally placed within a pale-staining cytoplasmic domain. Extravasated red cells are frequently seen within the infiltrate, along with a background of reticulin fibrosis (× 60).

which are blood-filled spaces lined by hairy cells that have disrupted the normal sinus architecture,[19] are a characteristic but not pathognomonic feature. Cases with splenic but not bone marrow involvement have been described, suggesting a splenic origin for the disease.[20]

Hepatic infiltration is both sinusoidal and portal.[21] Lymph node involvement is marked by both sinusoidal and interstitial involvement.[22] Bony infiltration can progress from the medullary cavity to the cortex, resulting in osteolytic lesions.[23]

Cytochemistry

Hairy cell cytoplasm usually stains strongly for tartrate-resistant acid phosphatase (TRAP). Isoenzyme 5 acid phosphatase present in the hairy cell cytoplasm resists decoloration with tartrate.[24,25] Hairy cells exhibit a range of staining from weak to strongly positive; typical cells stain with moderate intensity (Figure 8–3). A TRAP stain that involves at least two cells with more than 40 granules or with numerous granules obscuring the nucleus is usually diagnostic. When strongly positive TRAP-staining cells with morphology typical of hairy cells are identified, they are highly specific for HCL. In almost 90 percent of cases, TRAP staining of peripheral blood buffy-coat smears is positive.[24] Normal neutrophils and platelets contain acid phosphatases but are not resistant to tartrate and are therefore TRAP stain-negative. Moderate to weak TRAP staining may occur in other diseases, including prolymphocytic leukemia and the non-Hodgkin's lymphomas.

Electron Microscopy

Electron microscopy may help in the differential diagnosis of HCL from other disorders displaying cells with fine filamentous cytoplasmic projections, appearing as ridges or villi.[26] In hairy cells, electron microscopy shows circumferential cytoplasmic projections with fewer and blunter microvilli, as compared with splenic lymphoma with villous lymphocytes in which the projections tend to be polarized at one end of the cell[27,28] (Figure 8–4). Under electron microscopy, ribosomal lamellar complexes appear as membranous structures composed of concentric rings of lamellae lined by ribosomes.[24] Ribosomal lamellar complexes are seen in 50 percent of HCL cases, but because they may be seen in other lymphoid malignancies, they are not specific for HCL.[29]

Immunophenotypic Profile

Hairy cells, being mature B cells, express single or multiple immunoglobulin heavy chains with monotypic light chains.[8,30–34] Hairy cells express the pan B-cell antigens CD19, CD20, and CD22 but not CD21, an antigen lost in the later stages of B-cell ontogeny. They also express PCA-1, an early plasma cell antigen, on their surface. When a panel of multiple monoclonal antibodies was applied to peripheral blood or bone marrow specimens by two-color flow cytometry, a characteristic profile emerged.[35] This pattern was best appreciated by the pan B-cell markers CD11c, CD25, and CD103 (Bly-7).[36] CD11c stains very potently, with an intensity much greater than seen in chronic lymphocytic leukemia and other chronic lymphopro-

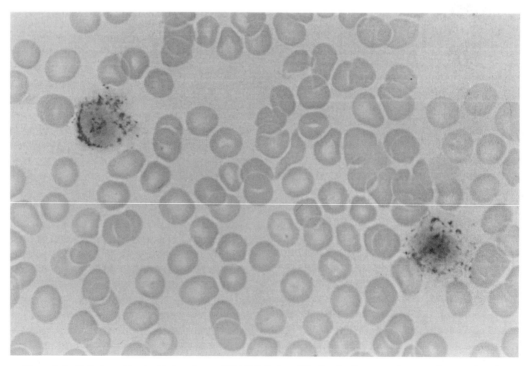

Figure 8–3. Tartrate-resistant acid phosphatase (TRAP) in hairy cell leukemia, demonstrating granular cytoplasmic staining (× 100).

liferative disorders.[37] The staining of CD11 is 30-fold higher than that of chronic lymphocytic leukemia, which therefore aids in its differentiation.

Hairy cell leukemia was the first B-cell lymphoproliferative disorder identified that expressed CD25 (an interleukin-2 [IL-2] receptor). Serum levels of soluble IL-2 receptors are elevated in HCL patients and correlate with disease activity following treatment.[38] CD103 (Bly-7) has the greatest sensitivity and specificity for HCL. This monoclonal antibody is against an antigen associated with the subunit of the B7 integrin, thought to be involved in the process of lymphocyte homing and adhesion.[39] CD22 is also expressed more intensely in HCL than in other B-cell chronic lymphoproliferative disorders; CD22 stains 50 times more intensely in HCL than in chronic lymphocytic leukemia, in which there is only weak expression of CD22.[35] In 26 percent of cases there is weak expression of CD10 (the CALLA antigen), and in 5 percent of cases there is weak expression of CD5; CD5 is the anomalous T-cell antigen strongly expressed on chronic lymphocytic leukemia cells.[35] Peripheral blood flow cytometry revealed that 92 percent of 161 patients with HCL had identifiable circulating hairy cells, in some patients representing less than 1 percent of lymphocytes; this compares with a thorough morphologic evaluation of the peripheral blood, which revealed hairy cells in 80 percent of patients.[35]

Immunohistochemistry

Immunohistochemistry performed on bone marrow biopsy samples may aid in the diagnosis of HCL and is also useful for evaluating minimal residual disease after effective systemic therapies. Hairy cells stain with CD20 (L26) (Figure 8–5) and DBA.44;[40] L26 staining is membranous and accentuates the ruffled abundant cytoplasm, whereas DBA.44, an undefined antigen, stains in both a cytoplasmic granular and a membranous pattern. DBA.44 is again not specific for HCL, because 30 percent of low-grade lymphomas also stain positively with this stain.

CLINICAL MANIFESTATIONS

About 25 percent of patients present with fatigue, 25 percent with repeated infections, and 25 percent with splenomegaly, which in a minority of patients may be massive, or with cytopenias[41] (Table 8–1). In 102 newly diagnosed HCL patients, 86 had anemia, 84 thrombocytopenia, and 78 neutropenia.[42] Splenomegaly was present in 93 patients. Hepatomegaly is present in 20 percent of patients. Although peripheral adenopathy is rarely found clinically, less than 10 percent of patients have peripheral lymphadenopathy larger than 2 cm; now with the frequent use of computed tomographic (CT) scans in the initial evaluation, internal lymphadenopathy is increasingly recognized. Of 43 consecutive patients studied with CT scans, 6 (14 percent) had significant internal adenopathy; 3 had massive abdominal adenopathy (larger than 10 cm), and 1 had bulky adenopathy (5 to 10 cm).[43] Hairy cell leukemia is typically associated with leukopenia, but up to 20 percent of patients may develop a leukemic phase,[44] and 10 percent may present without discernible circulating hairy cells on light microscopy. Other laboratory findings may include liver function test

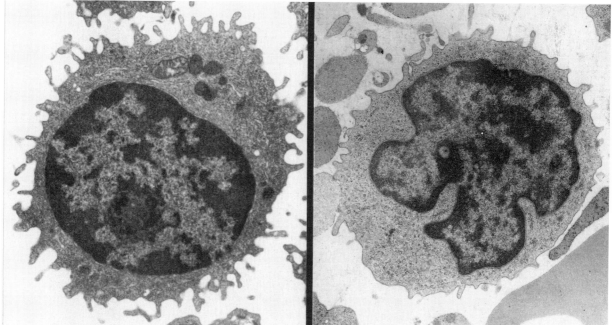

A   B

Figure 8–4. Transmission electron micrographs of peripheral blood comparing the lymphocytes from hairy cell leukemia (**A**) and splenic lymphoma with circulating villous lymphocytes (**B**). The hairy cell has a higher density of more elongated and evenly distributed cytoplasmic projections, compared with the fewer numbers of shorter and less uniformly distributed surface projections of the circulating villous lymphocyte (× 7,000).

Table 8–1. Clinical Stigmata of Hairy Cell Leukemia

Clinical Evaluation
Common
   Splenomegaly (90 percent)
   Circulating hairy cells (90 percent)
   Pancytopenia (70 percent)
   Infection (70 percent)
      Bacterial, fungal and viral infections
      Unique susceptibility to atypical mycobacteria
Less Common
   Hepatomegaly (35 percent)
   Lymphadenopathy (25 percent)
   Osteolytic lesions, autoimmune disease, vasculitis—very rare
Bone Marrow Examination
   Positive staining for tartrate-resistant acid phosphatase (TRAP)
   Dry tap; reticular fibrosis
   Diffusely infiltrating mononuclear cells separated by clear
      cytoplasms giving bone marrow a "fried egg" appearance

---

abnormalities in 19 percent, azotemia in 27 percent, and hypergammaglobulinemia, which may rarely be monoclonal, in 18 percent. Hypogammaglobulinemia, unlike in chronic lymphocytic leukemia, is rare.

Patients with HCL are susceptible to both gram-positive and gram-negative bacterial infections as well as to atypical mycobacterial disease, particularly *Mycobacterium kansasii*. The frequency of infection appears to correlate not with prior splenectomy or previous systemic therapy but with the degree of neutropenia and monocytopenia. Nonpyogenic infections with *Aspergillus*, *Histoplasma*, *Cryptococcus*, and *Pneumocystis carinii* occur with greater frequency among HCL patients. During the follow-up of 127 patients with HCL, 47 had culture-proven infections, 40 had clinically significant infectious episodes without positive culture documentation, and 40 had no infectious complications.[45]

Rarely, HCL may occur in association with immunologic disorders such as polyarthritis nodosa and leukocytoclastic vasculitis. Skin infiltration has been described.[46,47] Bone involvement may present with diffuse osteoporosis or, more commonly, as lytic lesions involving the axial skeleton, particularly the femoral heads.[23,48] Patients with skeletal complications tend to have higher tumor burdens and marrows more diffusely infiltrated by HCL. Patients with chylous and serous ascites, and even pleural effusions, have also been reported.[49,50]

In a series of 116 patients with HCL followed for over two decades, several unusual presentations and complications were encountered, including spontaneous rupture of the spleen, massive splenomegaly from hairy cell infiltration with normal blood counts and bone marrow evaluations, spinal cord compression with paralysis, protein-losing enteropathy from hairy cell infiltration of the bowel, and esophageal perforation with a fistulous tract.[51]

DISORDERS TO BE DISTINGUISHED FROM HAIRY CELL LEUKEMIA

The differential diagnosis of HCL includes other low-grade B-cell lymphoproliferative disorders, such as hairy cell leukemia-variant (HCL-V), chronic lymphocytic leukemia, splenic lymphoma with circulating villous lymphocytes, marginal zone lymphoma of the spleen, and monocytoid B-cell lymphoma[52] (Table 8–2).

Hairy cell leukemia-variant[28] represents a hybrid between prolymphocytic leukemia and HCL; the nucleus more closely resembles a prolymphocyte and the cytoplasm a hairy cell. Afflicted individuals present with massive splenomegaly, and in the leukemia phase, TRAP staining is either negative or weakly positive. In contrast to the flow cytometry results in HCL, the cells in HCL-V are usually CD25-negative and CD103 (Bly-7)-negative. Distinction from HCL is based on nuclear morphol-

---

Table 8–2. Differential Diagnosis of Hairy Cell Leukemia

Parameters	HCL	HCL Variant	Splenic Lymphoma with Villous Lymphocytes	Monocytoid B-Cell Lymphoma/ Marginal Zone Lymphoma
Peripheral blood				
Morphology				
Nuclear shape	Ovoid, reniform	Round	Round	Irregular
Chromatin	Reticular ± nucleolus	Coarse with central nucleolus	Coarse ± nucleolus	Coarse
Cytoplasm	Blue-gray, abundant	Blue-gray, abundant	Basophilic, scant to moderate	Pale, abundant
Monocytopenia	+	−	−	−
TRAP stain	+ + +	±	±	±
Aspirable bone marrow	−	+	+	+
Splenic involvement	Red pulp	Red pulp	White pulp	White pulp
Flow cytometry				
CD22	+ + +	+ +	+ +	+ +
CD11c	+ + +	+ +	+	±
CD25	+ +	−	±	±
CD103 (Bly-7)	+ +	±	−	−

Abbreviations: HCL, hairy cell leukemia; TRAP, tartrate-resistant acid phosphatase.

ogy, the leukemic presentation, the lack of monocytopenia, the aspirable bone marrow, and the morphologic appearance of the cells in the bone marrow biopsy. There is a blastic variant of HCL in which patients have massive splenomegaly, peripheral lymphadenopathy, and pancytopenia.[53] These cells, interestingly, stain positively with the TRAP stain and negatively with myeloperoxidase.

Splenic lymphoma with circulating villous lymphocytes can be difficult to distinguish from HCL, but the cells have more basophilic cytoplasm and the cytoplasmic projections tend to be polar and more subtle in the majority of circulating lymphocytes (Figures 8–1 and 8–4). Circulating plasmacytoid cells are frequently noted.[27] TRAP staining is negative or very weak. Immunophenotyping identifies cells with strong staining for CD11c, but are CD103 (Bly-7)-negative. The bone marrow typically is only minimally involved, with the lymphocytes appearing as small and round and having plasmacytoid features. Peripheral monocytopenia is usually absent. Sections of spleen show predominantly white pulp involvement.

Marginal zone lymphoma/monocytoid B-cell lymphoma involving the spleen can have histopathologic characteristics that may be confused with HCL[54] but are TRAP stain-negative. Strong staining for CD11c and Bly-7 suggests HCL rather than these splenic lymphomas. Aplastic anemia needs to be differentiated from pancytopenia due to the hypoplastic variant of HCL, especially when there is no associated splenomegaly. Bilateral bone marrow examinations with special stains or even diagnostic splenectomy may be necessary in selected patients to make the appropriate diagnosis. Hairy cell leukemia must also be differentiated from mast cell disease, which can mimic HCL, especially when there are infiltrates composed of spindle-shaped cells. Mast cells contain metachromatic granules with the Giemsa stain, and the granules are also positive for chloroacetate esterase.[55] Immunohistochemistry demonstrates positive staining with KPI (CDBP), a marker of macrophages, and negative staining with CD20 (L26). Hairy cell leukemia also needs to be considered in the differential diagnosis of any disorder that results in cytopenias and splenomegaly, for example, myelofibrosis.

MANAGEMENT

Treatment Indications

Ninety percent of patients with HCL will require treatment at presentation or during the course of their disease. Some patients, usually elderly men with smaller spleens, normal blood counts, and a lower HCL burden, may be observed for protracted intervals. Standard hematologic parameters for starting treatment in HCL include anemia (hemoglobin below 8 to 10 g/dL), thrombocytopenia (platelet count below 50 to 100×10^9/L), or neutropenia (absolute neutrophil count below 0.5 to 1.0×10^9/L), especially when associated with recurrent serious infections. Less common indications for initiating treatment include leukocytosis with a high proportion of hairy cells, symptomatic splenomegaly, bulky or painful lymphadenopathy, vasculitis, and bony involvement (Table 8–3).

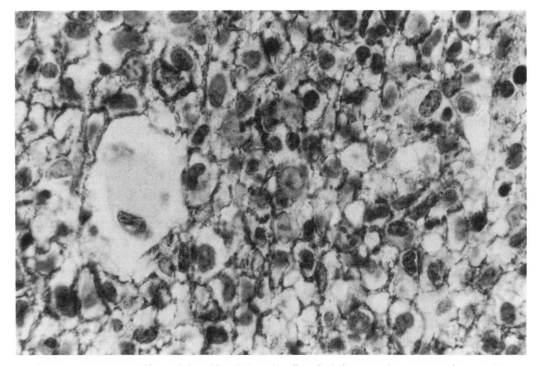

Figure 8–5. Immunoperoxidase staining with anti-CD20 (B-cell marker), demonstrating strong membrane positivity and highlighting the relatively large cytoplasmic domain of the neoplastic cells (× 60).

Table 8–3. Treatment Indications for Hairy Cell Leukemia

Hematologic Parameters
    Hemoglobin < 8–10 g/dL
    Platelets < 50–100 × 10⁹/L
    Absolute neutrophil count < 0.5–1.0 × 10⁹/L
Less Common Indications
    Severe infections
    Leukocytosis with high proportion of hairy cells
    Symptomatic splenomegaly
    Bulky lymphadenopathy
    Vasculitis
    Bony involvement

Given that there are now systemic agents that regularly induce complete remissions in most patients with HCL and in view of the present risks of blood transfusion support, the treatment indications for patients with HCL, especially those who have never received blood products, may need to be relaxed.

First-Line Therapies for Hairy Cell Leukemia and Their Complications

Splenectomy

Splenectomy was the first standard treatment modality regularly employed in the treatment of HCL because it rapidly corrects peripheral cytopenias. In 90 percent of patients, at least one hematologic parameter will be improved, and 40 to 60 percent will have normalization of blood counts.[56,57] Thrombocytopenia reverses in 75 percent of patients and usually within days of splenectomy. Responses to splenectomy cannot be reliably predicted. Splenic size alone is not always predictive of response to splenectomy.[17] Red blood cell pooling in the spleen is greater in HCL than in other lymphoproliferative disorders with comparable splenomegaly, which probably accounts for the inconsistent relationship between splenic weight and response to splenectomy.[58] Patients with only focal involvement of the marrow by HCL respond more favorably to splenectomy regardless of the degree of splenomegaly. Splenectomy has been implicated in the development of second hematologic malignancies, which occur with increased frequency, in patients with HCL.[22,59] Splenectomy is now less commonly employed as a primary treatment in HCL since the introduction of several systemic agents with major activity in the treatment of HCL. Fifty percent of splenectomized patients will require systemic therapy at a median of 8.3 months.[60] The present indications for the up-front use of splenectomy are active and uncontrolled infections and thrombocytopenic bleeding.

Interferon

In 1984 Quesada and colleagues first reported the successful use of partially purified alpha (leukocyte) human interferon in seven patients with HCL. All seven had normalization of their peripheral blood counts and three had eradication of hairy cells from their marrow.[61] In 1986 the use of recombinant alpha-2b interferon (Intron A; Schering Corp., Kenilworth, NJ), at 2 million units/m² for 12 months was reported in 64 HCL patients.[62]

Of those 64 patients, 3 (5 percent) achieved a complete response and 45 (70 percent) a partial response. The same multicenter study was updated in 1990 with 195 patients accrued,[63] and the results were comparable with those previously reported.[63,64] Twelve months of alpha-interferon therapy is optimal because a longer duration of treatment does not increase response rates or lower relapse rates but does increase toxicity.[65,66] The median time to normalization of the platelet count is 2 months; that to a normal hemoglobin concentration is 3 months; and that for neutrophil recovery is 5 months. Median time to treatment failure after discontinuation of interferon therapy is 18 to 25 months.[67] Interferon reinstitution at the time of relapse results in a 77 percent response rate.[68] Recombinant alpha-2a interferon (Roferon; Hoffmann-La Roche, Nutley, NJ), has a cysteine residue and alpha-2b interferon has an arginine residue at position 23; these gave similar response rates when administered to 30 patients with HCL.[48] The presence of splenomegaly does not adversely affect response rates to interferon therapy. Some patients who develop loss of clinical responsiveness to recombinant alpha-2a interferon and have both neutralizing and binding antibodies respond to treatment with natural alpha-interferon therapy.[69]

When the results of five large studies with interferon are combined, the overall response rate is 65 percent, of which 10 percent are complete and 55 percent partial responses (Table 8–4). These results should be interpreted cautiously given the different methods, indications, and types of interferon administered.

The most common side effect of interferon is a flu-like syndrome consisting of fever, myalgia, and malaise. Acetaminophen often ameliorates these symptoms, and tachyphylaxis frequently develops over time. Macular-papular rashes, injection site erythema, mild nausea, and diarrhea are common toxicities. Rarely, central and peripheral nervous system complaints, hepatitis, alopecia, small joint arthritis, and decreased libido have been documented.

The mechanisms by which interferon induces remissions in HCL are poorly understood. Interferon does stimulate natural killer cell activity, which is known to be suppressed in HCL.[70,71] Alpha-interferon is also known to have a growth-inhibitory effect on lymphoma cell lines and to stimulate differentiation in leukemic cell lines.[72,73] It has also been shown that during alpha-interferon administration there is induction of CD11a

Table 8–4. Alpha-Interferon Treatment in Hairy Cell Leukemia

Reference	No. of Patients	Response (percent)			
		Complete	Partial	Minor	None
124	30	9	17	4	0
125	14	1	12	0	1
126	25	7	6	12	0
127	195	7	152	10	26
128	152	16	42	0	94
Total	416	40 (10 percent)	229 (55 percent)	26 (6 percent)	121 (29 percent)

and CD54, leukocyte adhesion molecules, which is accompanied by enhanced susceptibility to lysis by cytotoxic T lymphocytes.[74]

The standard dose recommendation for alpha-2b interferon therapy is 2 million units/m^2, administered subcutaneously three times per week for 12 months, and that for alpha-2a interferon is 3 million units subcutaneously daily for 6 months and then decreased to three times per week for an additional 6 months.

Purine Nucleoside Analogues

In 1972 Giblett et al. made the seminal observation that one-third of children with severe combined immunodeficiency syndrome (SCID) were deficient in the purine catabolic enzyme adenosine deaminase.[75] Adenosine deaminase catalyzes the irreversible deamination of adenosine to inosine and of 2'-deoxyadenosine to 2'-deoxyinosine. Cohen and associates reported that the intracellular accumulation of deoxyadenosine triphosphate was responsible for this lymphopenia.[76] Later, Carson et al. found 2-chlorodeoxyadenosine, a chlorine-substituted purine deoxynucleoside, to be the most potent among a panel of substituted purine analogues screened for in vitro toxicity toward an L1210 murine leukemia.[77] This enhanced insight into the biochemical pathways of adenosine metabolism provided the rational basis for the clinical development of the three newer purine analogues that mimic this experiment of nature. 2'-Deoxycoformycin (dCF) irreversibly binds to adenosine deaminase, and fludarabine and 2-chlorodeoxyadenosine (2-CdA) resist deamination in the purine salvage pathway. 2'-Deoxycoformycin and 2-chlorodeoxyadenosine have been demonstrated to have major activity in a variety of indolent lymphoid malignancies, but their action is most profound in the treatment of HCL. Fludarabine, although more fully evaluated in other lymphoproliferative disorders, has been administered to only a few patients with HCL.

2'-Deoxycoformycin 2'-Deoxycoformycin (dCF, Pentostatin, Nipent; SuperGen, Pleasanton, CA) is a natural product isolated from the cultured broth of *Streptomyces antibioticus.* In 1983 dCF was first shown to have activity in a single patient with HCL.[78] The successful administration of low-dose dCF, 5 mg/m^2 for 2 to 3 days, then weekly for 15 to 16 doses, was reported in 1984.[79]

The Eastern Cooperative Oncology Group (ECOG) treated patients with dCF administered at 5 mg/m^2 for 2 days every other week until complete remission was achieved.[80] Of 27 evaluable patients with HCL, there were 16 (59 percent) complete responders, 10 (37 percent) partial responders, and 1 nonresponder. When this study was updated with 50 patients accrued, 32 (64 percent) of patients achieved a complete remission and 10 (20 percent) of patients a partial remission.[80]

The encouraging high overall response rates and complete remissions seen with dCF prompted the National Cancer Institute to organize a prospective, randomized, intergroup study of dCF versus interferon alfa-2a in previously untreated HCL patients.[81] Patients were randomized to either interferon alpha-2a at 3 million units subcutaneously three times per week or dCF at 4 mg/m^2

intravenously every 2 weeks. Patients who did not respond after 6 months to initial treatment were crossed over. Among interferon patients, 17 of 159 (11 percent) achieved a complete response and 60 of 159 (38 percent) had either a complete or partial response. Among dCF patients, 121 of 154 (79 percent) achieved responses, of which 117 (76 percent) were complete. Of patients who progressed on interferon and who were then treated with dCF, 66 percent achieved a complete response and 9 percent a partial response. No patients who had progressed on dCF responded to interferon. The difference in overall survival between the two groups was not statistically significant, which likely reflects the crossover study design. These results indicate that dCF is substantially more active than interferon when administered as first-line therapy to patients with HCL.

2'-Deoxycoformycin-induced toxicities include fever, nausea, vomiting, photosensitivity, and keratoconjunctivitis.[79,82] Severe myelosuppression may occur soon after the initiation of dCF therapy, especially in those patients with preexisting marrow compromise.[80,83] Patients with satisfactory pretreatment hematologic parameters tend to have less myelosuppression following dCF administration. Serious infections, including disseminated herpes zoster, *Escherichia coli, Haemophilus influenzae,* pneumococcal, and fungal infections (fatal in some patients), were observed early on following the initiation of dCF.[82] In patients with active and uncontrolled infections, a poor performance status, or impaired renal function, dCF is best avoided.[84] 2'-Deoxycoformycin is a potently immunosuppressive agent.[85] During dCF therapy and for at least 14 months following its administration, CD4 and CD8 lymphocytes may decrease to levels below 200 cells per microliter. Low doses of dCF also cause severe immunosuppression.[86] CD4 cells were reduced from a pretreatment median of 669 per microliter to a posttreatment median of 155 per microliter. Despite the severity and duration of the immunosuppression, no significantly increased frequency of either late opportunistic infections or secondary malignancies has been reported thus far. This risk will be clarified with longer follow-up times and larger numbers of patients.

When the results of six studies are combined, the overall response rate is 86 percent, of which 72 percent are complete and 14 percent partial responses (Table 8–5). The standard dose of dCF for patients with HCL is 4 mg per square meter of body surface area every other week for 3 to 6 months until maximum response is obtained.

2-Chlorodeoxyadenosine 2-Chlorodeoxyadenosine (2-CdA, Cladribine, Leustatin; OrthoBiotech, Raritan, NJ) is the chlorinated derivative of 2'-deoxyadenosine and is phosphorylated to its putative active form by deoxycytidine kinase. It is unique among other more conventional antimetabolites in that it is toxic to both dividing and resting lymphocytes, which likely accounts for its major activity in the treatment of indolent lymphoproliferative disorders.[87,88]

In 1990 investigators from Scripps Clinic reported on 12 HCL patients treated with a single 7-day course of 2-CdA at 0.1 mg/kg/day by continuous intravenous infusion.[89] Of those 12 patients, 11 achieved a complete response and 1 a partial response. In 1998 Saven et al. reported the long-term follow-up

Table 8–5. 2′-Deoxycoformycin (dCF), 2-Chlorodeoxyadenosine (2-CdA), and Fludarabine Treatment in Hairy Cell Leukemia

Reference	No. of Patients	Response (percent)		
		Complete	Partial	None
dCF				
80	50	32	10	8
129	23	20	1	2
130	33	11	15	7
131	66	37	15	14
81	154	117	4	33
94	165	135	25	5
	491	352 (72 percent)	70 (14 percent)	69 (14 percent)
2-CdA				
90	349	319	22	8
132	46	36	5	5
133	16	12	0	4
92	49	37	12	0
91	50	40	9	1
94	45	38	7	0
	555	482 (87 percent)	55 (10 percent)	18 (3 percent)
Fludarabine				
101	3	0	2 (67 percent)	1 (33 percent)

of 349 evaluable HCL patients treated with 2-CdA[90]: 319 (81 percent) achieved a complete response and 22 (7 percent) a partial response, with an overall median response follow-up duration of 52 months.[90] Ninety patients (26 percent) relapsed at a median of 29 months. The time to treatment failure rate for all 341 responders was 19 percent at 48 months, 16 percent for complete responders, and 54 percent for partial responders. The overall survival rate was 96 percent at 48 months.

Other investigators have reported similar results (Table 8–5). Tallman et al. reported on 50 HCL patients treated with 2-CdA;[91] 40 (80 percent) achieved a complete response and 9 (18 percent) a partial response. Seven patients relapsed at a median of 24 months. The overall survival rate was 86 percent at 4 years. Hoffman et al. reported on 49 HCL patients treated with 2-CdA,[92] of whom 37 (76 percent) achieved a complete response and 12 (24 percent) a partial response. At a median follow-up of 55 months, the relapse-free survival was 80 percent and the overall survival was 95 percent. A CD25-negative phenotype predicted a poorer response to 2-CdA. A large trial from the National Cancer Institute Group C protocol involving 861 evaluable patients demonstrated an overall response rate of 87 percent, but only 50 percent were complete responses.[93] Overall survival was 86 percent at 48 months, and progression-free survival was 76 percent. 2-Chlorodeoxyadenosine was administered as in other reported series, and the response criteria were identical. In the National Cancer Institute study, however, central pathology review was not performed. It is therefore possi-

ble that some patients had atypical forms of HCL or other low-grade B-cell lymphoproliferative disorders that are less susceptible to 2-CdA treatment.

There has not been a prospective trial of dCF versus 2-CdA in the treatment of HCL. A retrospective analysis of 165 HCL patients treated with dCF and 45 HCL patients treated with 2-CdA was performed by Dearden et al.[94] The response rates were the same in the two groups: 82 percent complete and 15 percent partial responses for dCF, and 84 percent complete and 16 percent partial responses for 2-CdA. Relapse rates were 24 percent for dCF and 29 percent for 2-CdA after median follow-up periods of 71 and 45 months, respectively. The 5-year survival for all patients was 97 percent.

Neutropenic fever was the principal acute toxicity occurring in 42 percent of HCL patients treated in the Scripps Clinic series.[90] The onset of fever was related to the disappearance of hairy cells and appeared most marked in the patients with the greatest pretreatment HCL burden, manifested principally as splenomegaly. At Scripps Clinic, 45 of 358 patients (13 percent) had documented acute infections; oral herpes simplex was cultured from 5 patients and the most common bacterial infection was staphylococcal (10 patients were bacteremic and 23 grew staphylococci from their catheter tip or from the skin of associated cellulitis). Dermatomal herpes zoster was the most frequent late infection.

Like dCF, 2-CdA is also immunosuppressive. When serial flow cytometry was performed on 68 patients with HCL undergoing 2-CdA treatment, the median lymphocyte counts decreased from 2,000 to 300 per microliter.[95] The initial decrease of CD8 cells was greater than that of CD4 cells; median nadir values of CD4 and CD8 cells were 128 and 78 per microliter. Recovery was quicker for CD8 cells, leading to normalization in 3 months, whereas CD4 cells required 1 to 2 years to enter the normal range. In a separate study there was a tendency toward restoration of T-cell subsets between 6 and 12 months,[96] whereas other studies have shown more prolonged CD4 lymphocytopenia.[97] Of 40 patients treated with a single cycle of 2-CdA, the median pretreatment CD4 count decreased from 743 to 139 per microliter and remained significantly lower than baseline at a median of 23 months after therapy. The median time to attain a normal CD4 count, above 365 per microliter, was 40 months. Only a single opportunistic infection, *Candida septicemia,* and no second malignancies were observed during this period.

When the results of six studies are combined, the overall response rate is 97 percent, of which 87 percent are complete and 10 percent are partial (Table 8–5). Given the complete and long-lasting remissions, as well as the favorable toxicity profile, that follow a single 7-day course of 2-CdA administered at 0.1 mg/kg/day by continuous intravenous infusion, 2-CdA has emerged as the treatment of choice for patients with HCL.

Fludarabine Fludarabine, although rigorously evaluated in patients with chronic lymphocytic leukemia,[98,99] has only been evaluated in small numbers of patients with HCL. Although results have been less dramatic than with the other nucleoside analogues discussed, some patients with HCL-V did achieve partial responses[100–102] (Table 8–5).

Salvage Treatment of Relapsed or Refractory Hairy Cell Leukemia

Relapses After Primary Interferon Therapy

In the Intergroup study, when patients with HCL who relapsed after primary interferon treatment were retreated again with interferon, 13 percent achieved complete responses and 18 percent partial responses.[81] In this study, when patients refractory to interferon were crossed over to dCF, 66 percent achieved a complete response and 9 percent a partial response. In the Scripps Clinic report, responses to 2-CdA were independent of prior interferon therapy.[90] In the National Cancer Institute Group C protocol of 429 HCL patients who had relapsed following interferon therapy, 86 percent achieved a response with 2-CdA treatment, which was not significantly different from the response rate of previously untreated HCL patients on the same protocol.[93] These results suggest that HCL patients who relapse after interferon therapy should be treated with a purine nucleoside analogue.

Relapses After Primary Purine Nucleoside Analogue Therapy

In the Intergroup study, four of the nine HCL patients (44 percent) who relapsed following primary dCF therapy achieved a complete response to a second induction therapy with dCF.[81] Of five patients resistant (three patients) or intolerant (two patients) to dCF who were treated with 2-CdA, four patients achieved a complete response, which suggests a possible lack of cross-resistance in HCL between these two agents despite structural and mechanistic similarities.[103] The National Cancer Institute Group C protocol treated 68 patients with 2-CdA who had relapsed following dCF therapy; the overall response rate was 79 percent.[93]

In the Scripps Clinic series of 53 evaluable patients treated with second courses of cladribine at first relapse, 33 (62 percent) achieved complete responses and 14 (26 percent) had partial responses, which suggests that patients who relapse can be successfully retreated with 2-CdA.[90] 2'-Deoxycoformycin may represent a reasonable therapeutic alternative for HCL patients who relapse after 2-CdA therapy, but response rate and duration data in substantial numbers of patients are lacking. Of three patients who relapsed following treatment with 2-CdA, two responded to interferon but then progressed within months of interferon discontinuation.[104] For selected HCL patients refractory to purine analogues, splenectomy remains an option.

Alternative Therapeutic Strategies in Purine Nucleoside Analogue Refractory Hairy Cell Leukemia

Chlorambucil,[105] androgens,[106] and lithium[107] are rarely used today and are now principally of historic interest only.

Kreitman et al. have reported on a novel recombinant immunotoxin administered to patients with refractory HCL.[108] This toxin targets CD25-expressing lymphoid malignancies through the Fc portion of anti-CD25 fused to the truncated portion of the *Pseudomonas* exotoxin. Of four patients, one achieved a complete response and three had at least 98 percent clearing of circulating hairy cells. Thomas et al. have reported on the administration of rituximab, the anti-CD20 monoclonal antibody (Rituxan; IDEC Pharmaceuticals, San Diego, CA) to refractory HCL patients.[109] Four of five patients achieved responses, two being complete responses. Toxicity was mild and limited to rigors.

Second Malignancies Following Systemic Treatment of Hairy Cell Leukemia

One study has now documented an unexpected high incidence of second neoplasms in patients after treatment of HCL with alpha-2b interferon.[110] Of 69 patients followed for a median of 91 months, 13 patients (19 percent) developed a second neoplasm, of which 6 were of hematopoietic origin and 7 were adenocarcinomas. The median survival after diagnosis of the second neoplasm was only 8.8 months.

Saven et al. reported on 358 HCL patients treated with 2-CdA of whom 27 (23 males) developed second malignancies.[90] The majority of these second neoplasms were melanoma and adenocarcinomas of the prostate, colon, and stomach. The observed-to-expected ratio of second cancers was 1.88 (95 percent, confidence interval 1.24 to 2.74). Kurzrock et al. reported that 26 of 350 HCL patients developed second malignancies.[111] There was no excess cancer risk observed in HCL patients treated with purine nucleoside analogues, but a higher incidence of lymphoma and myeloma was noted. Other investigators did not demonstrate an increased incidence of second malignancies in HCL patients similarly treated.[112]

Finally, Au et al. reported on the relative risk of second malignancies in 117 HCL patients compared with an age-matched cohort; 36 percent of patients developed a second cancer and 5 percent had two or more malignancies.[113] Also, 10 percent of patients had been diagnosed with cancer before the diagnosis of HCL was established. The increased relative risk of malignancy in the HCL group slowly decreased to baseline over time, which suggests that hairy cell burden, rather than treatment, contributed to this occurrence.

Curative Potential of Purine Nucleoside Analogues in Hairy Cell Leukemia

Hairy cells exhibit cytoplasmic reactivity against anti-CD22, CD25, CD103, DBA.44, and kappa or lambda monoclonals.[114] Twenty-five to fifty percent of patients in morphologic complete remission after 2-CdA have minimal residual disease detected by immunohistochemical stains on marrow biopsies.[115,116] Wheaton et al. reported on bone marrow results in 39 HCL patients in apparent morphologic complete remission, 5 of whom (13 percent) had minimal residual disease based on immunohistochemistry.[117] Forty percent with detectable minimal residual disease went on to relapse, compared with 7 percent of those without detectable disease. When evaluated by the polymerase chain reaction and clone-specific probes derived from the immunoglobulin heavy-chain genes, all seven patients in apparent complete remission following 2-CdA showed detectable minimal residual disease.[118] Also, although in the

Table 8–6. Features of Alpha-Interferon (α-IFN), 2'-Deoxycoformycin (dCF), and 2-Chlorodeoxyadenosine (2-CdA) Treatment in Hairy Cell Leukemia

	α-IFN	dCF	2-CdA
Approved indication	Untreated HCL	IFN-refractory HCL	Both
Synthesis	Recombinant technology	Complex	Simple
Route of administration	Subcutaneous	Intravenous bolus	Intravenous infusion
Recommended dose	2 million U/m^2, 3 times per week	4 mg/m^2 every other week	0.1 mg/kg/day for 1 week
Duration of treatment	12 months	3 to 6 months	1 week
Major toxicities	Influenza-like syndrome	Nausea, early infections, immunosuppression	Culture-negative fever, immunosuppression
Responses	10 percent CRs, 55 percent PRs	72 percent CRs, 14 percent PRs	87 percent CRs, 10 percent PRs

Abbreviations: HCL, hairy cell leukemia; CR, complete response; PR, partial response.

Scripps Clinic study the time to treatment failure rate for complete responders was 16.3 percent at 4 years, there was no obvious plateau on the time to treatment failure curve.[90] Thus, it is unclear what proportion of patients, if any, will be cured.

Granulocyte Colony-Stimulating Factor (G-CSF)

The granulocyte colony-stimulating factor abrogates the early myelosuppressive effects of interferon[119] and reverses neutropenia in some HCL patients. It does have a role in the initial treatment of actively infected HCL patients. Of four patients with HCL treated with G-CSF at 1 to 6 μg/kg daily for 6 weeks, three had normalization of their absolute neutrophil counts in 1 to 2 weeks.[119] A single patient with HCL and a history of cutaneous vasculitis developed acute neutrophilic dermatosis (Sweet's syndrome) following the administration of G-CSF.

Thirty-five patients with HCL who received G-CSF before and after 2-CdA were compared with one hundred five historic control subjects treated with 2-CdA alone.[120] The G-CSF regularly increased the absolute neutrophil count in patients with HCL and shortened the duration of severe neutropenia after 2-CdA. Nevertheless, the percentage of febrile patients, number of febrile days, and frequency of admissions for antibiotics were not statistically different in the two groups. Accordingly, the routine adjunctive use of G-CSF with 2-CdA in the treatment of HCL cannot be recommended.

Conclusions and Treatment Considerations

The approach to treatment of HCL has undergone a revolution over the last decade. The rarity of HCL belies its importance as the prototype indolent lymphoid malignancy that is sensitive to biological response modifiers (alpha-interferon) and the purine nucleoside analogues (dCF and 2-CdA) (Table 8–6). Since there are now multiple effective treatment options available to patients with HCL, the treatment indications and management guidelines for patients with HCL are in transition.

2-Chlorodeoxyadenosine has emerged as the treatment of choice given that the vast majority of patients achieved a complete and long-lasting remission following only a single course of therapy. The optimum route of administration and method of 2-CdA delivery remain to be defined. The successful administration of subcutaneous[121] and oral 2-CdA[122] has been reported, as well as a weekly intravenous administration method.[123] These newer schemas of drug administration must be evaluated in large numbers of HCL patients with longer follow-up periods before they supersede the standard 7-day continuous intravenous infusion method.

Both dCF and 2-CdA are potently immunosuppressive and should be avoided in actively infected patients, especially those with opportunistic infections, who require a thorough evaluation to identify the causative agent and then the rapid institution of antimicrobials. Depending on the patient's condition, alpha-interferon or splenectomy may be more appropriate treatment options in these infected patients.

Significant numbers of patients in morphologic complete remission still have residual hairy cells in their bone marrows on immunohistochemical evaluations. This may identify a group of patients at higher risk of relapse, but it remains to be proved whether treatment directed at eliminating this minimal residual disease will have a favorable influence on relapse rates or survivals. It should be remembered that repetition of the primary successful treatment induces second responses in the majority of relapsed patients. At present, our recommendation is that relapsing patients be retreated when their blood counts are at levels similar to those indicating need of therapy initially.

Before the successful introduction of effective systemic therapies in HCL, the median survival for patients was only 53 months.[44] The development of the newer purine analogues exemplifies the model of rational drug design and seems destined to improve survival for patients with this disease. Biologic therapy with monoclonal antibodies directed at antigens expressed on the surface of hairy cells represents an additional therapeutic strategy offering new hope in the salvage treatment of HCL patients who have previously failed purine nucleoside analogues.

ACKNOWLEDGMENT

The author gratefully acknowledges the assistance of Kelly Bethel, M.D., Department of Pathology, Scripps Clinic, for her review and analysis of the pathology materials.

REFERENCES

1. Bouroncle BA, Wiseman BK, Doan CA: Leukemic reticuloen-dotheliosis. Blood 13:609–630, 1959.

2. Schrek R, Donnelly J: Hairy cells in blood lymphoreticular neo-plastic disease and "flagellated" cells of normal lymph nodes. Blood 27:199, 1966.

3. Wylis RF, Greene MH, Palretke M, Khilanani P, Tabaczka P, Swiderski G: Hairy cell leukemia in three siblings: An apparent HLA-linked disease. Cancer 49:538–542, 1982.

4. Wachsman W, Golde DW, Chen IS: Hairy cell leukemia and human T cell leukemia virus. Semin Oncol 11:446–450, 1984.

5. Oleske D, Golomb HM, Farber MD, Levy PS: A case-control inquiry into the etiology of hairy cell leukemia. Am J Epidemiol 121:675–683, 1985.

6. Stewart DJ, Keating MJ: Radiation exposure as a possible etiologic factor in hairy cell leukemia. Cancer 46:1577–1580, 1980.

7. Haglund U, Juliusson G, Stellan B, Gahrton G: Hairy cell leukemia is characterized by clonal chromosome abnormalities clustered to specific regions. Blood 83:2637–2645, 1994.

8. Korsmeyer SJ, Greene WC, Cossman J, Hsu SM, Jensen JP, Neckers LM, Marshall SL, Bakhshi A, Depper JM, Leonard WJ, Jaffe ES, Waldmann TA: Rearrangement and expression of immunoglobulin genes and expression of Tac antigen in hairy cell leukemia. Proc Natl Acad Sci USA 80:4522, 1983.

9. Burthem J, Baker PK, Hunt JA, Cawley JC: The function of c-fms in hairy-cell leukemia: Macrophage colony-stimulating factor stimulates hairy-cell movement. Blood 83:1381–1389, 1994.

10. Burthem J, Baker PK, Cawley JC: Hairy cell interactions with extracellular matrix: Expression of specific integrin receptors and their role in the cell's response to specific adhesive proteins. Blood 84:873–882, 1994.

11. Bartl R, Frisch B, Hill W: Bone marrow histology in hairy cell leukemia. Am J Clin Pathol 79:531–545, 1983.

12. Katayama I: Bone marrow in hairy cell leukemia. Hematol Oncol Clin North Am 2:585–602, 1988.

13. Burke JS: The value of the bone-marrow biopsy in the diagnosis of hairy cell leukaemia. J Clin Pathol 70:876–884, 1978.

14. Naeim F, Jacobs AD: Bone marrow changes in patients with hairy cell leukemia treated by recombinant alpha-2 interferon. Hum Pathol 16:1200–1205, 1985.

15. Ratain MJ, Golomb HM, Bardawil RG: Durability of responses to interferon alfa-2b in advanced hairy cell leukemia. Blood 69:872–877, 1987.

16. Burthem J, Cawley JC: The bone marrow fibrosis of hairy-cell leukemia is caused by the synthesis and assembly of a fibronectin matrix by the hairy cells. Blood 83:497–504, 1994.

17. Golomb HM, Vardiman JW: Response to splenectomy in 65 patients with hairy cell leukemia: An evaluation of spleen weight and bone marrow involvement. Blood 61:349–352, 1983.

18. Burke JS, Sheibani K, Winberg CD, Rappaport H: Recognition of hairy cell leukemia in a spleen of normal weight: The contribution of immunologic studies. Am J Clin Pathol 87:276–281, 1987.

19. Nanba K, Soban EJ, Bowling MC, Berard CW: Splenic pseudosinuses and hepatic angiomatous lesions: Distinctive features of hairy cell leukemia. Am J Clin Pathol 67:415–426, 1977.

20. Ng JP, Hogg RB, Cumming RL: Primary splenic hairy cell leukemia: A case report and review of the literature. Eur J Haematol 39:349–352, 1987.

21. Roquet ML, Zafrani ES, Farcet JP: Histopathological lesions of the liver in hairy cell leukemia: A report of 14 cases. Hepatology 5:496–500, 1985.

22. Vardiman JW, Golomb HM: Autopsy findings in hairy cell leukemia. Semin Oncol 11:370–380, 1984.

23. Lembersky BC, Ratain MJ, Golomb HM: Skeletal complications in hairy cell leukemia: Diagnosis and therapy. J Clin Oncol 6:1280–1284, 1988.

24. Yam LT, Janckila AJ, Li CY, Lam WKW: Cytochemistry of tartrate-resistant acid phosphatase: Fifteen years' experience. Leukemia 1:285–288, 1987.

25. Li CY, Yam LT, Lam KW: Studies of acid phosphatase isoenzymes in human leukocytes: Demonstration of isoenzyme specificity. J Histochem Cytochem 18:901–910, 1970.

26. Katayama I, Li CY, Yam LT: Ultrastructural characteristics of the "hairy cells" of leukemic reticuloendotheliosis. Am J Pathol 361:370, 1972.

27. Melo JV, Robinson DS, Gregory C, Catovsky D: Splenic B cell lymphoma with "villous" lymphocytes in the peripheral blood: A disorder distinct from hairy cell leukaemia. Leukemia 1:294–299, 1987.

28. Catovsky D, O'Brien M, Melo JV, Wardle J, Brozovic M: Hairy cell leukemia variant: An intermediate disease between hairy cell leukemia and B prolymphocytic leukemia. Semin Oncol 11:362–369, 1984.

29. Brunning RD, Parkin J: Ribosome-lamella complexes in neoplastic hematopoietic cells. Am J Pathol 79:565–578, 1975.

30. Hsu S, Yang K, Jaffe ES: Hairy cell leukemia: A B-cell neoplasm with a unique antigenic phenotype. Am J Clin Pathol 80:421–428, 1983.

31. Melo JV, San Miguel JF, Moss VE, Catovsky D: The membrane phenotype of hairy cell leukemia: A study with monoclonal antibodies. Semin Oncol 11:381, 1984.

32. Anderson KC, Boyd AW, Fisher DC, Leslie D, Schlossman SF, Nadler LF: Hairy cell leukemia: A tumor of pre-plasma cells. Blood 65:620–629, 1985.

33. Falini B, Pulford K, Erber WN, Posnett DN et al: Use of a panel of monoclonal antibodies for the diagnosis of hairy cell leukemia: An immunocytochemical study of 36 cases. Histopathology 10:671, 1986.

34. Falini B, Schwarting R, Erber W, Posnett DN, Martelli MF, Grignani F, Zuccaccia M, Gatter KC, Cernetti C, Stein H, Mason DY: The differential diagnosis of hairy cell leukemia with a panel of monoclonal antibodies. Am J Clin Pathol 83:289–300, 1985.

35. Robbins BA, Ellison DJ, Spinosa JC, Carey CA, Lukes RJ, Poppema S, Saven A, Piro LD: Diagnostic application of two-color flow cytometry in 161 cases of hairy cell leukemia. Blood 82:1277–1287, 1993.

36. Visser L, Shaw A, Slupsky J, Vos H, Poppema S: Monoclonal antibodies reactive with hairy cell leukemia. Blood 74:320–325, 1989.

37. Hanson CA, Gribbin TE, Schnitzer B, Schlegelmilch JA, Mitchell BS, Stoolman LM: CD11c (LEU-M5) expression characterizes a B-cell chronic lymphoproliferative disorder with features of both chronic lymphocytic leukemia and hairy cell leukemia. Blood 76:2360–2367, 1990.

38. Steis RG, Marcon L, Clark J, Urba W, Longo DL, Nelson DL, Maluish AE: Serum soluble IL-2 receptor as a tumor marker in patients with hairy cell leukemia. Blood 77:1304–1309, 1988.

39. Micklem KJ, Dong Y, Willis A, Pulford KA, Visser L, Dürkop H, Poppema S, Stein H, Mason DY: HML-1 antigen on mucosa-associated T cells, activated cells, and hairy leukemic cells is a new integrin containing the b7 subunit. Am J Clin Pathol 139:1297–1301, 1991.

40. Hounieu H, Chittal SM, al Saati T, De Mascarel A, Sabattini E, Pileri S, Falini B, Ralfkiaer E, Le Tourneau A, Selves J, Voigt JJ, Laurent G, Diebold J, Delsol G: Hairy cell leukemia. Diagnosis of bone marrow involvement in paraffin-embedded sections with monoclonal antibody DBA.44. Am J Clin Pathol 98:26–33, 1992.

41. Flandrin G, Sigaux F, Sebahoun G, Bouffette P: Hairy cell leukemia: Clinical presentation and follow-up of 211 patients. Semin Oncol 11:458–471, 1984.

42. Turner A, Kjeldsberg CR: Hairy cell leukemia: A review. Medicine (Baltimore) 57:477–499, 1978.

43. Hakimian D, Tallman MS, Hogan DK, Rademaker AW, Rose E, Nemcel AA Jr: Prospective evaluation of internal adenopathy in a cohort of 43 patients with hairy cell leukemia. J Clin Oncol 12:268–272, 1994.

44. Golomb HM, Catovsky D, Golde DW: Hairy cell leukemia. A clinical review based on 71 cases. Ann Intern Med 89 (Part 1):677–683, 1978.

45. Golomb HM, Hadad LJ: Infectious complications in 127 patients with hairy cell leukemia. Am J Hematol 16:393, 1984.

46. Dorsey JK, Penick GD: The association of hairy cell leukemia with unusual immunologic disorders. Arch Intern Med 142:902–903, 1982.

47. Eklon KB, Hughes GRV, Catovsky D: Hairy cell leukaemia with polyarteritis nodosa. Lancet 2:280, 1979.

48. Quesada JR, Keating MJ, Libshitz HI, Llamas L: Bone involvement in hairy cell leukemia. Am J Med 74:228, 1983.

49. Davies GE, Wiernik PH: Hairy cell leukemia with chylous ascites. JAMA 238:1541, 1977.

50. Krause JR, Dekker A: Hairy cell leukemia (leukemic reticuloendotheliosis) in serous effusions. Acta Cytol 22:80, 1978.

51. Bouroncle BA: Unusual presentations and complications of hairy cell leukemia. Leukemia 1:288–293, 1987.

52. Harris NL, Jaffe E, Stein H, Banks PM, Chan JKC, Cleary ML: A revised European-American classification of lymphoid neoplasms: A proposal from the International Lymphoma Study Group. Blood 84:1361–1392, 1994.

53. Diez-Martin JL, Li CY, Banks PM: Blastic variant of hairy cell leukemia. Am J Clin Pathol 87:576–583, 1987.

54. Sheibani K, Burke JS, Swartz WG: Monocytoid B-cell lymphoma: Clinicopathologic study of 21 cases of a unique type of low-grade lymphoma. Cancer 62:1531–1538, 1988.

55. Burke JS, Rappaport H: The differential diagnosis of hairy cell leukemia in bone marrow and spleen. Semin Oncol 11:334–346, 1984.

56. Mintz U, Golomb HM: Splenectomy as initial therapy in twenty-six patients with leukemic reticuloendotheliosis (hairy cell leukemia). Cancer Res 39:2366–2370, 1979.

57. Jansen J, Hermans J: Splenectomy in hairy cell leukemia: A retrospective multicenter analysis. Cancer 47:2066–2076, 1981.

58. Lewis SM, Catovsky D, Hows JM, Ardalan B: Splenic red cell pooling in hairy cell leukaemia. Br J Haematol 35:351–357, 1977.

59. Arnalich F, Camacho, Jimenez C: Occurrence of immunoblastic B-cell lymphoma in hairy cell leukemia. Cancer 59:1161–1164, 1987.

60. Golde DW: Therapy of hairy cell leukemia. N Engl J Med 307:495–496, 1982.

61. Quesada JR, Reuben J, Manning JT, Hersh EM, Gutterman JU: Alpha-interferon for induction of remission in hairy cell leukemia. N Engl J Med 310:15–18, 1984.

62. Golomb HM, Jacobs A, Fefer A, Ozer H, Thompson J, Portlock C, Ratain M, Golde D, Vardiman J, Burke JS, Brady J, Bonnem E, Spiegel R: Alpha-2 interferon therapy of hairy cell leukemia: A multicenter study of 64 patients. J Clin Oncol 4:900–905, 1986.

63. Golomb HM, Fefer A, Golde DW, Ozer H, Portlock C, Silber R, Rappeport J, Ratain MJ, Thompson J, Bonnem E, Spiegel RJ, Tensen L, Burke JS, Vardiman JW: Report of a multiinstitutional study of 193 patients with hairy cell leukemia treated with interferon alfa-2b. Semin Oncol 15(Suppl. 5):7–9, 1988.

64. Golomb HM, Fefer A, Golde DW, Ozer H, Portlock C, Rappeport J, Ratain MJ, Thompson J, Bonnem EM, Spiegel RJ, Tensen L, Burke JS, Vardiman JW: Sequential evaluation of alpha-2b interferon treatment in 128 patients with hairy cell leukemia. Semin Oncol 14 (Suppl. 2):13–17, 1987.

65. Golomb HM, Ratain MJ, Fefer A, Thompson J, Golde DW, Ozer H, Portlock C, Silber R, Rappeport J, Bonnem E, Spiegel R, Tensen L, Burke JS, Vardiman JW. Randomized study of the duration of treatment with interferon alfa-2b in patients with hairy cell leukemia. J Natl Cancer Inst 80:369–373, 1988.

66. Berman E, Heller G, Kempin S, Gee T, Tran L, Clarkson B: Incidence of response and long-term follow-up in patients with hairy cell leukemia with recombinant alpha-2a. Blood 75:839–845, 1990.

67. Ratain MJ, Golomb HM, Vardiman JW, Westbrook CA, Barker C, Hooberman A, Bitter MA, Daly K: Relapse after interferon alpha-2b therapy for hairy cell leukemia: Analysis of diagnostic variables. J Clin Oncol 6:1714–1721, 1988.

68. Ratain MJ, Golomb HM, Vardiman JW: Interferon alpha-2b therapy for hairy cell leukemia in 69 patients. A 6-year update. Blood 74:76 (Abstr.), 1989.

69. Von Wussow P, Pralle H, Hochkeppel H, Jakschies D, Sonnen S, Schmidt H, Müller-Rosenau D, Franke M, Haferlach T, Zwinger T, Rapp U, Deicher H: Effective natural interferon-α therapy in recombinant-α-resistant patients with hairy cell leukemia. Blood 78:38–43, 1991.

70. Ruco LP, Procapio A, Maccallini V, Calogero A, Uccini S, Annino L, Mandelli F, Baroni CD: Severe deficiency of natural killer activity in the peripheral blood of patients with hairy cell leukemia. Blood 61:1132, 1983.

71. Lee SH, Kelley S, Chin H, Stebbing N: Stimulation of natural killer cell activity and inhibition of proliferation of various leukemic cells by purified human leukocyte interferon subtypes. Cancer Res 42:1312, 1982.

72. Lieberman D, Voloch Z, Aviv H, Nudel U, Revel M: Effects of interferon on hemoglobin synthesis and leukemia virus production in Friend cells. Mol Biol Rep 1:447–451, 1974.

73. Taylor-Papadimitriou J: Effects of interferons on cell growth and function, in Gresser I (ed): Interferon 1980, pp. 13–46. Academic Press, New York, 1980.

74. Jansen JH, Van der Harst D, Wientjens GJHM, Kooy-Winkelaar YMC, Brand A, Willemze R, Kluin-Nelemans HC: Induction of CD11a/leukocyte function antigen-1 and CD54/intercellular adhesion molecule-1 on hairy cell leukemia cells is accompanied by enhanced susceptibility to T-cell but not lymphokine-activated killer cell cytotoxicity. Blood 80:478–483, 1992.

75. Giblett ER, Anderson JE, Cohen F, Pollara B, Meuwissen HJ: Adenosine deaminase deficiency in two patients with severely impaired cellular immunity. Lancet 2:1067–1069, 1972.

76. Cohen A, Hirshhorn R, Horowitz SD, Rubinstein A, Polmar SH, Hong R, Martin DW Jr: Deoxyadenosine triphosphate as a potentially toxic metabolite in adenosine deaminase deficiency. Proc Natl Acad Sci USA 75:472–476, 1978.

77. Carson DA, Wasson DB, Kaye J, Ullman B, Martin DW Jr, Robins RK, Montgomery JA: Deoxycytidine kinase-mediated toxicity of deoxyadenosine analogs toward malignant human lymphoblasts *in vitro* and toward murine L1210 leukemia *in vivo*. Proc Natl Acad Sci U S A 77:6865–6869, 1980.

78. Stewart DJ, Benjamin RS, McCredie KB, Murphy S, Keating M: The effectiveness of rubidazone in hairy cell leukemia (leukemic reticuloendotheliosis). Blood 54:298–303, 1979.

79. Spiers ASD, Parekh SJ, Bishop MB: Hairy cell leukemia: Induction of complete remission with pentostatin (2′-deoxycoformycin). J Clin Oncol 2:1336–1342, 1984.

80. Cassileth PA, Cheuvant B, Spiers ASD, Harrington DP, Cummings FJ, Neiman RS, Bennett JM, O'Connell MJ: Pentostatin induces durable remissions in hairy cell leukemia. J Clin Oncol 9:243–246, 1991.

81. Grever M, Kopecky K, Foucar MK, Head D, Bennett JM, Hutchison RE, Corbett WEN, Cassileth PA, Habermann T, Golomb H, Rai K, Eisenhauer E, Appelbaum F, Cheson BD: Randomized comparison of pentostatin versus interferon alfa-2a in previously untreated patients with hairy cell leukemia: An intergroup study. J Clin Oncol 13:974–982, 1995.

82. Johnston JB, Glazer RI, Pugh L, Israels LG: The treatment of hairy cell leukaemia with 2'-deoxycoformycin. Br J Haematol 63:525–534, 1986.

83. Ho AD, Thaler J, Stryckmans P, Coiffier B, Luciani M: Pentostatin in refractory chronic lymphocytic leukemia: A phase II trial of the European Organization for Research and Treatment of Cancer. J Natl Cancer Inst 82:1416–1420, 1990.

84. Spiers ASD, Moore D, Cassileth PA, Harrington DP, Cummings FJ, Neiman RS, Bennett JM, O'Connell MJ: Remissions in hairy cell leukemia with pentostatin (2'-deoxycoformycin). N Engl J Med 316:825–830, 1987.

85. Urba WJ, Baseler MW, Kopp WC, Steis RG, Clark JW, Smith JW, II, Coggin DL, Longo DL: Deoxycoformycin-induced immunosuppression in patients with hairy cell leukemia. Blood 73:38–46, 1989.

86. Kuzel TM, Hurria A, Samuelson E, Tallman MS, Roenigk HH Jr, Rademaker AW, Rosen ST: Phase II trial of 2-chlorodeoxyadenosine for the treatment of cutaneous T-cell lymphomas. Blood 87:906–911, 1996.

87. Seto S, Carrera CJ, Kubota M, Wasson DB, Carson DA: Mechanism of deoxyadenosine and 2-chlorodeoxyadenosine toxicity to nondividing human lymphocytes. J Clin Invest 75:377–383, 1985.

88. Saven A, Piro L: Newer purine analogues for treatment of hairy cell leukemia. N Engl J Med 330:691–697, 1994.

89. Piro LD, Carrera CJ, Carson DA, Beutler E: Lasting remissions in hairy cell leukemia induced by a single infusion of 2-chlorodeoxyadenosine. N Engl J Med 322:1117–1121, 1990.

90. Saven A, Burian C, Koziol JA, Piro LD: Long-term follow-up of patients with hairy cell leukemia after cladribine treatment. Blood 92:1918–1926, 1998.

91. Tallman MS, Hakimian D, Rademaker AW, Zanzig C, Wollins E, Rose E, Peterson LC: Relapse of hairy cell leukemia after 2-chlorodeoxyadenosine: Long-term follow-up of the Northwestern University experience. Blood 88:1954–1959, 1996.

92. Hoffman MA, Janson D, Rose E, Rai KR: Treatment of hairy cell leukemia with cladribine: Response, toxicity and long-term follow-up. J Clin Oncol 15:1138–1142, 1997.

93. Cheson BD, Vena DA, Montello MJ, Barrett JA, Damasio E, Tallman M, Annino L, Connors J, Coiffier B, Lauria F: Treatment of hairy cell leukemia with 2-chlorodeoxyadenosine via the Group C Protocol Mechanism of the National Cancer Institute: A report of 979 patients. J Clin Oncol 16:3007–3015, 1986.

94. Dearden CE, Matutes E, Hilditch BL, Swansbury GJ, Catovsky D: Long-term follow-up of patients with hairy cell leukaemia after treatment with pentostatin or cladribine. Br J Haematol 106:515–519, 1999.

95. Juliusson G, Lenkei R, Liliemark J: Flow cytometry of blood and bone marrow cells from patients with hairy cell leukemia: Phenotype of hairy cells and lymphocyte subsets after treatment with 2-chlorodeoxyadenosine. Blood 83:3672–3681, 1994.

96. Carrera CJ, Piro LD, Saven A, Cox K, Beutler E, Carson DA, Kipps TJ: Restoration of lymphocyte subsets following 2-chlorodeoxyadenosine remission induction in hairy cell leukemia. Blood 76(Suppl. 1):260a, (abstr.), 1990.

97. Seymour JF, Kurzrock R, Freireich EJ, Estey EH: 2-Chlorodeoxyadenosine induces durable remissions and prolonged suppression of CD4+ lymphocyte counts in patients with hairy cell leukemia. Blood 83:2906–2911, 1994.

98. Keating MJ, Kantarjian H, Talpaz M, Redman J, Koller C, Barlogie B, Velasquez W, Plunkett W, Freireich EJ, McCreadie KB: Fludarabine: A new agent with major activity against chronic lymphocytic leukemia. Blood 74:19–25, 1989.

99. Keating MJ, Kantarjian H, O'Brien S, Koller C, Talpaz M, Schachner J, Childs CC, Freireich EJ, McCredie KB: Fludarabine: A new agent with marked cytoreductive activity in untreated chronic lymphocytic leukemia. J Clin Oncol 9:44–49, 1991.

100. Kantarjian HM, Redman J, Keating MJ: Fludarabine phosphate therapy in other lymphoid malignancies. Semin Oncol 17(Suppl. 8):66–70, 1990.

101. Kantarjian HM, Schachner J, Keating MJ: Fludarabine therapy in hairy cell leukemia. Cancer 67:1291–1293, 1991.

102. Kraut E, Chun H: Fludarabine phosphate in refractory hairy cell leukemia. Am J Hematol 37:59–60, 1991.

103. Saven A, Piro LD: 2-Chlorodeoxyadenosine-induced complete remissions in patients with hairy cell leukemia resistant or intolerant to 2'-deoxycoformycin. Ann Intern Med 119:278–283, 1993.

104. Seymour JF, Estey EH, Keating MJ, Kurzrock R: Response to interferon-a in patients with hairy cell leukemia relapsing after treatment with 2-chlorodeoxyadenosine. Leukemia 9:929–932, 1995.

105. Golomb HM: Progress report on chlorambucil therapy in postsplenectomy patients with progressive hairy cell leukemia. Blood 57:464–467, 1981.

106. Lusch CJ, Ramsey HE, Katayama I: Leukemic reticuloendoteliosis: Report of a case with peripheral blood remission on androgen therapy. Cancer 41:1964–1966, 1978.

107. Blum SF: Lithium in hairy cell leukemia. N Engl J Med 303:464–465, 1983.

108. Kreitman RS, Wilson WH, Robbins D, Margulies I, Stetler-Stevenson M, Waldmann TA, Pastan I: Responses in refractory hairy cell leukemia to a recombinant immunotoxin. Blood 94:3340–3348, 1999.

109. Thomas DA, O'Brien S, Cortes J, Giles FJ, Koller C, Estey E, Kurzrock R, Faderl S, Pierce S, Keating MJ, Kantarjian H: Pilot study of rituximab in refractory or relapsed hairy cell leukemia (HCL). Blood 94:705a (abstr.), 2000.

110. Kampmeier P, Spielberger R, Dickstein J, Mick R, Golomb H, Vardiman JW: Increased incidence of second neoplasms in patients treated with interferon α-2b for hairy cell leukemia: A clinicopathologic assessment. Blood 83:2931–2938, 1994.

111. Kurzrock R, Strom SS, Estey E, O'Brien S, Keating MJ, Jiang H, Adams T, Talpaz M: Second cancer risk in hairy cell leukemia: Analysis of 350 patients. J Clin Oncol 15:1803–1810, 1997.

112. Cheson BD, Vena DA, Barrett J, Freidlin B: Second malignancies as a consequence of nucleoside analog therapy for chronic lymphoid leukemias. J Clin Oncol 17:2454–2460, 1999.

113. Au WY, Klasa RJ, Gallagher R, Le N, Gascoyne RD, Connors JM: Second malignancies in patients with hairy cell leukemia in British Columbia: A 20-year experience. Blood 92:1160–1164, 1998.

114. Cordone I, Annino L, Masi S, Pescarmona E, Rahimi S, Ferrari A, Giubilei E, Pignoloni P, Faraggiana T, Mandelli F: Diagnostic relevance of peripheral blood immunocytochemistry in hairy cell leukemia. J Clin Pathol 48:955–960, 1995.

115. Ellison DJ, Sharpe RW, Robbins BA, Spinosa JC, Leopard JD, Saven A, Piro LD: Immunomorphologic analysis of bone marrow biopsies after treatment with 2-chlorodeoxyadenosine for hairy cell leukemia. Blood 84:4310–4315, 1994.

116. Hakimian D, Tallman MS, Kiley C, Peterson LA: Detection of minimal residual disease by immunostaining of bone marrow biopsies after 2-chlorodeoxyadenosine for hairy cell leukemia. Blood 82:1798–1802, 1993.

117. Wheaton S, Tallman MS, Hakimian D: Minimal residual disease may predict bone marrow relapse in patients with hairy cell leukemia treated with 2-chlorodeoxyadenosine. Blood 87:1556–1560, 1996.

118. Filleul B, Delannoy A, Ferrant A, Zenebergh A, Van Daele S, Bosly A, Doven C, Mineur P, Glorieux P, Driesschaert P, Sokal G, Martiat P, Michaux JL: A single course of 2-chlorodeoxyadenosine does not eradicate leukemic cells in hairy cell patients in complete remission. Leukemia 8:1153–1156, 1994.

119. Glaspy JA, Baldwin GC, Robertson PA, Souza L, Vincent M, Ambersley J, Golde DW: Therapy for neutropenia in hairy cell leukemia with recombinant human granulocyte colony-stimulating factor. Ann Intern Med 109:789–795, 1988.

120. Saven A, Burian C, Adusumalli J, Koziol JA: Filgrastim for cladribine-induced neutropenic fever in patients with hairy cell leukemia. Blood 93:2471–2477, 1999.

121. Juliusson G, Heldal D, Hippe E, Hedenus M, Malm C, Wallman K, Stolt CM, Evensen SA, Albertioni F, Tjonnfjord G, Lenkei R, Liliemark J: Subcutaneous injections of 2-chlorodeoxyadenosine for symptomatic hairy cell leukemia. J Clin Oncol 13:989–995, 1995.

122. Liliemark J, Albertioni F, Hassan M, Pettersson B, Juliusson G: On the bioavailability of oral and subcutaneous 2-chloro-2′-deoxyadenosine in humans: Alternative routes of administration. J Clin Oncol 10:1514–1518, 1992.

123. Lauria F, Bocchia M, Marotta G, Raspadori D, Zinzani PL, Rondelli D: Weekly administration of 2-chlorodeoxyadenosine in patients with hairy cell leukemia: A new treatment schedule effective and safer in preventing infectious complications (Letter). Blood 89:1838–1839, 1998.

124. Quesada JR, Gutterman J, Hersh EM: Treatment of hairy cell leukemia with alpha interferons. Cancer 57:1678–1680, 1986.

125. Foon KA, Maluish AE, Abrams PG, Wrightington S, Stevenson HC, Alarif A, Fer MF, Overton WR, Poole M, Schnipper EF, Jaffe ES, Herberman RB: Recombinant leukocyte alpha interferon therapy for advanced hairy cell leukemia. Therapeutic and immunologic results. Am J Med 80:351–356, 1986.

126. Rai K, Mick R, Ozer H, Silver R, Papish S, Bloomfield C: Alpha-interferon therapy in untreated active hairy cell leukemia: A Cancer and Leukemia Group B (CALGB) study. Proc Am Soc Clin Oncol 6:159 (abstr.), 1987.

127. Golomb H, Fefer A, Golde D, Ozer H, Portlock C, Silber R, Rappeport J, Ratain M, Thompson J, Bonnem E, Spiegel R, Tensen L, Burke J, Vardiman J: Update of a multi-institutional study of 195 patients (pts) with hairy cell leukemia (HCL) treated with interferon alfa-2b (IFN). Proc Am Soc Clin Oncol 6:215 (abstr.), 1990.

128. Grever M, Kopecky K, Head D: A randomized comparison of deoxycoformycin (DCF) versus alpha-2a interferon (IFN) in previously untreated patients with hairy cell leukemia (HCL): An NCI-sponsored Intergroup Study (SWOG, ECOG, CALGB, NCIC, CTG). Proc Am Soc Clin Oncol 11:868 (abstr.), 1992.

129. Kraut EH, Bouroncle BA, Grever MR: Pentostatin in the treatment of advanced hairy cell leukemia. J Clin Oncol 7:168–172, 1989.

130. Ho AD, Thaler J, Mandelli F, Lauria F, Zittoun R, Willemze R, McVie G, Marmont AM, Prummer O, Stryckmans P, Witt B, Sucia S, Solbu G, de Witte T, Bödewadt-Radzun S: Response to pentostatin in hairy cell leukemia refractory to interferon-alpha. J Clin Oncol 7:1533–1538, 1989.

131. Grem J, King S, Cheson B, Leyland-Jones B, Wittes R: Pentostatin in hairy cell leukemia: Treatment by the special exception mechanism. J Natl Cancer Inst 81:448–453, 1989.

132. Estey EM, Kurzrock R, Kantarjian HM, O'Brien S, McCredie K, Beran M, Koller C, Keating MJ, Hirsch-Ginsberg C, Huy YO, Stass S, Freireich E: Treatment of hairy cell leukemia with 2-chlorodeoxyadenosine (2-CdA). Blood 79:882–887, 1992.

133. Juliusson G, Liliemark J: Rapid recovery from cytopenia in hairy cell leukemia after treatment with 2-chloro-2′-deoxyadenosine (CdA): Relation to opportunistic infections. Blood 79:888–894, 1992.

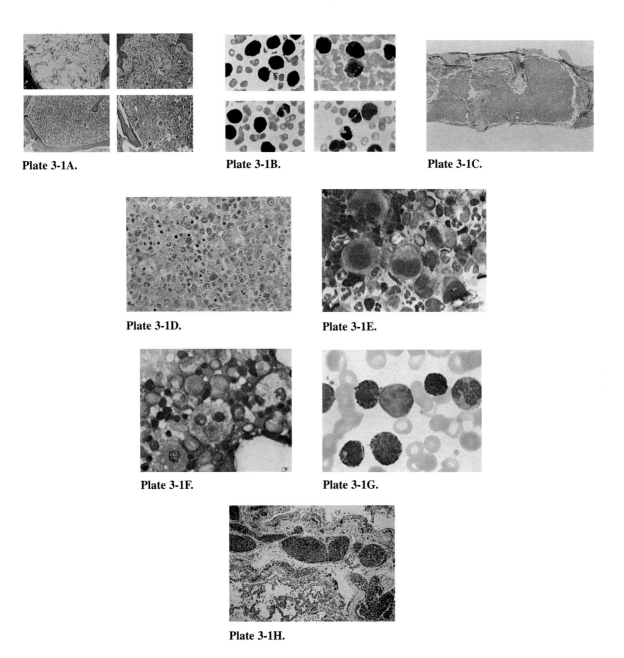

Plate 3-1A.

Plate 3-1B.

Plate 3-1C.

Plate 3-1D.

Plate 3-1E.

Plate 3-1F.

Plate 3-1G.

Plate 3-1H.

Plate 3-1. **(A)** Bone marrow biopsies in three disorders that may terminate in acute leukemia *(lower left panel)*. Marrow in *upper right panel* shows extensive replacement by fibrous tissue (diagnosis: myelofibrosis), while marrow in *lower right panel* shows marked trilineage hypercellularity caused by polycythemia vera. For comparison purposes, marrow from a case of aplastic anemia, which is replaced by fat, is shown in the *upper left panel*. (Hematoxylin and eosin [H&E] stain × 40.) **(B)** Leukocyte alkaline phosphatase stain in MPD, showing marked activity in every neutrophil *(upper left panel)* in a patient with polycythemia vera; moderate increased activity in myelofibrosis with myeloid metaplasia *(upper right panel);* and reactive leukemoid reaction *(lower left panel)* and absent activity in chronic myelocytic leukemia *(lower right panel)*. (Kaplow method, × 1,000.) **(C)** Low-power view of bone marrow needle biopsy from a patient with CML, revealing characteristic hypercellularity, with only 1 to 2 percent fat. Normal marrow should contain 50 to 60 percent fat. (H&E stain, × 25.) **(D)** High-power view of Plate C showing predominance of myeloid cells of varying maturity, including numerous eosinophils. Basophils are not easily seen. (H&E stain, × 100.) **(E)** Bone marrow smear from patient with CML, showing increased numbers of megakaryocytes, including atypical and immature forms. (Wright-Giemsa stain, × 400.) **(F)** Bone marrow smear from patient with CML, showing increased storage cells, including sea-blue histiocytes. (Wright-Giemsa stain, × 400.) **(G)** PB smear in a patient with CML, showing increased basophils (15 percent of differential count). (Wright-Giemsa stain, × 1,000.) **(H)** Section of lung in patient with CML in an accelerated phase (WBC 400,000/mm³), showing marked pulmonary leukostasis, which was fatal. (H&E stain, × 40.) *(Plate continues.)*

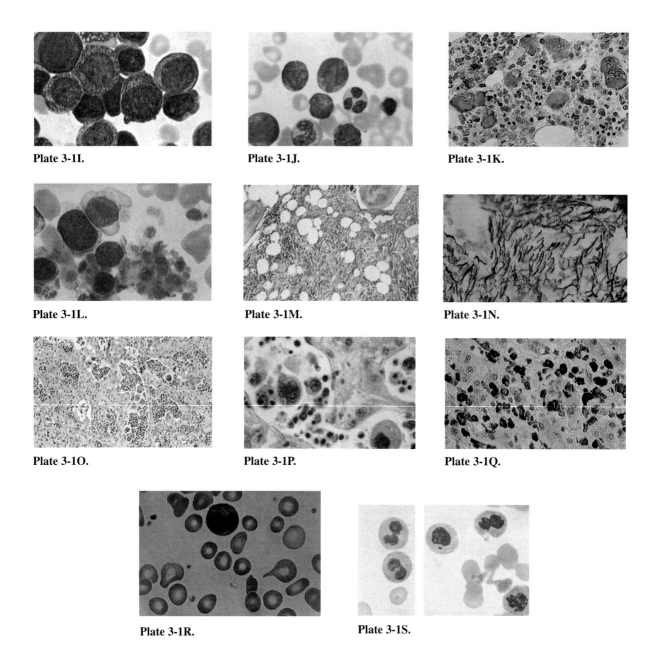

Plate 3-1I.

Plate 3-1J.

Plate 3-1K.

Plate 3-1L.

Plate 3-1M.

Plate 3-1N.

Plate 3-1O.

Plate 3-1P.

Plate 3-1Q.

Plate 3-1R.

Plate 3-1S.

Plate 3-1. *(Continued).* **(I)** PB smear of patient in Plate O, showing left shift in myeloid series. (Wright-Giemsa stain, × 1,000.) **(J)** PB smear from a patient with CML in early blastic crisis. Note four myeloblasts, band, poly, basophil, and nucleated RBC. (Wright-Giemsa stain, × 1,000.) **(K)** Bone marrow section from a patient with ET, showing increased megakaryocytes. (Wright-Giemsa stain, ×400.) **(L)** PB smear from patient with ET, showing circulating megakaryocytic fragments along with large atypical platelets. (Wright-Giemsa stain, ×1,000.) **(M)** Bone marrow biopsy of a patient with myelofibrosis (AMM), showing marked increase in fibrous tissue (blue-staining collagen) with residual marrow elements (red-staining). (Trichrome stain, × 100.) **(N)** Bone marrow biopsy from patient in Plate M, showing marked increase in primitive collagen fibers. (Reticulum stain, × 1,000.) **(O)** Liver biopsy from a patient with myelofibrosis (AMM), showing extramedullary hematopoiesis. Numerous megakaryocytes, erythroid, and some myeloid cells are evident within hepatic sinusoids. (H&E stain, × 100.) **(P)** High-power view of Plate (O) showing several megakaryocytes and other marrow elements in hepatic sinusoids. (H&E stain, ×1,000.) **(Q)** Liver biopsy from patient in Plate (O) stained with immunoperoxidase to lysozyme showing the presence of myeloid cells. (×400.) **(R)** Peripheral blood (PB) smear from a patient with myelofibrosis showing characteristic teardrop-shaped RBCs. (Wright-Giemsa stain, × 1,000.) **(S)** PB smear from a patient with MPD, showing acquired Pelger-Huët defect, characterized by hyposegmentation of nuclei of polys.

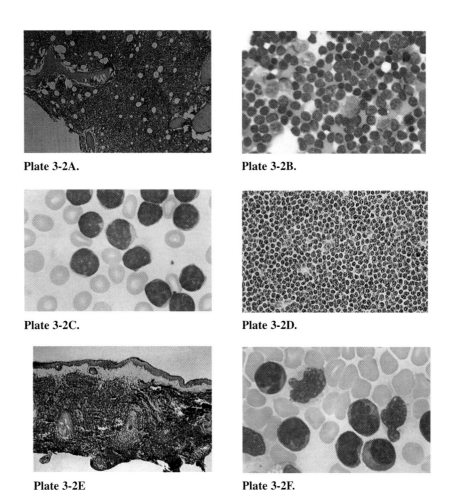

Plate 3-2A.

Plate 3-2B.

Plate 3-2C.

Plate 3-2D.

Plate 3-2E

Plate 3-2F.

Plate 3-2. (A) Bone marrow biopsy from patient with CLL, showing extensive replacement by small, well differentiated lymphocytes. (H&E stain, ×40.) **(B)** Bone marrow aspiration smear from a patient with CLL, showing a predominance of small, mature lymphocytes. Note dark-staining, clumped nuclear chromatin. (Wright-Giemsa stain, ×450.) **(C)** PB smear from patient in Plate B, showing a monotonous population of well differentiated lymphocytes. Cells have a rim of light blue-staining cytoplasm. (Wright-Giemsa stain, ×1,000.) **(D)** Lymph node biopsy from patient with CLL, showing extensive replacement by small, well differentiated lymphocytes. (H&E stain, ×400.) **(E)** Skin biopsy from patient with CLL, T-cell type, showing strong extensive infiltration by small lymphocytes. (H&E stain, × 40.) **(F)** PB smear from patient in Plate E, showing small, mature-appearing lymphocytes, but with irregularly shaped nuclei, having many nuclear indentations or convolutions. (Wright-Giemsa stain, ×1,000.) *(Plate continues.)*

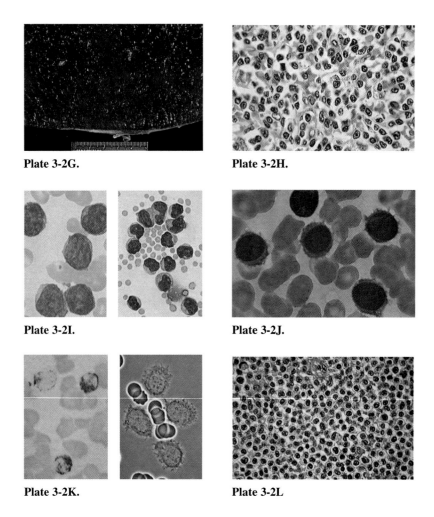

Plate 3-2G.

Plate 3-2H.

Plate 3-2I.

Plate 3-2J.

Plate 3-2K.

Plate 3-2L

Plate 3-2. *(Continued).* **(G)** Low-power view of cut section of spleen removed from a patient with prolymphocytic leukemia, showing extensive nodular infiltrates. **(H)** Section of spleen from patient in Plate G, showing infiltration by medium-sized, moderately immature lymphoid cells, some with prominent nucleoli. (H&E stain, × 400.) **(I)** Touch preparation of spleen from patient in Plate G *(right panel)* showing medium sized lymphoid cells with rather abundant cytoplasm, condensed nuclear chromatin, and a prominent nucleolus. (× 400.) *Left side* of panel shows same cells in the peripheral blood. (Wright-Giemsa stain, × 1,000.) **(J)** PB smear from patient with hairy cell leukemia, showing characteristic filamentous or hairy cytoplasmic projections. Only scant cytoplasm is present in the cells from this patient. (Wright-Giemsa stain, × 1,000.) **(K)** Hairy cells showing a positive stain for tartrate-resistant acid phosphatase *(left panel)* and in vivo appearance as seen by phase microscopy *(right panel)*. (× 1,000.) **(L)** Bone marrow biopsy from patient with hairy cell leukemia, showing extensive involvement by hairy cells. *(Plate continues.)*

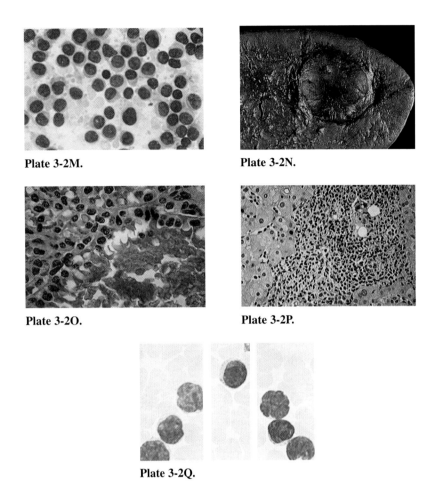

Plate 3-2M.

Plate 3-2N.

Plate 3-2O.

Plate 3-2P.

Plate 3-2Q.

Plate 3-2. *(Continued).* **(M)** Bone marrow aspiration smear from patient in Plate L, showing numerous hairy cells, characterized by round to oval or bean-shaped nucleus, some with nucleoli, and average amount of cytoplasm. Nuclei appear to be eccentric, mainly artifactual. Fragments of cytoplasm are seen in the background. Hairy projections are not easily seen in bone marrow smears. (Wright-Giemsa stain, × 450.) **(N)** Closeup photograph of cut section of spleen from a patient with hairy cell leukemia, showing a prominent blood lake. **(O)** Microscopic section of the edge of a splenic blood lake from Plate N, showing a lake of RBCs contained by lining cells that are neoplastic hairy cells. Normally, splenic sinuses are lined by endothelial cells. Numerous background hairy cells are also noted throughout the red pulp. (H&E stain, × 1,000.) **(P)** Liver biopsy from a patient with hairy cell leukemia, showing striking periportal as well as sinusoidal infiltration by neoplastic cells. (H&E stain, × 400.) **(Q)** PB smear from a patient with Sézary syndrome showing small lymphoid cells with characteristic irregular or convoluted nuclear appearance. (Wright-Giemsa stain, × 1,000.)

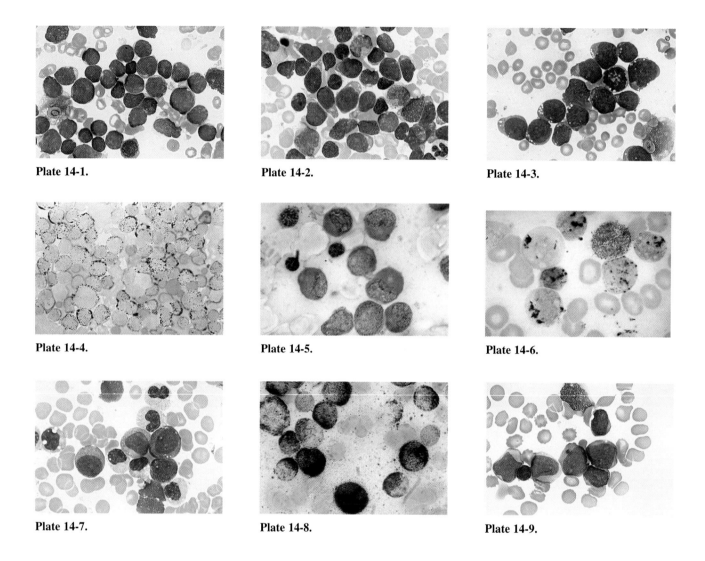

Plate 14-1. Plate 14-2. Plate 14-3.

Plate 14-4. Plate 14-5. Plate 14-6.

Plate 14-7. Plate 14-8. Plate 14-9.

Plate 14–1. Acute lymphocytic leukemia (ALL)(FAB L1): Agranular blasts with high nuclear/cytoplasmic ratio, regular nuclear membrane, and rare nucleoli. MGG stain. (Courtesy of Jean-E. Goasguen.)

Plate 14-2. ALL(FAB L2): More cytoplasm than L1 blasts and prominent nucleoli. MGG stain. (Courtesy of Jean-E. Goasguen.)

Plate 14-3. ALL(FAB L3): Blasts with oval nuclei, finely dispersed chromatin, and basophilic/vacuolated cytoplasm (Burkitt cells). MGG stain. (Courtesy of Jean-E. Goasguen.)

Plate 14-4. ALL: PAS reaction in lymphoblasts. Note the blocklike and ring appearance.

Plate 14-5. PAS reaction in myeloblasts and promyelocytes. Note the blush and finely granular activity.

Plate 14-6. Acid phosphatase reaction in "T"-lymphoblasts. Note the focal or paranuclear reaction.

Plate 14-7. Type I, II, and III blasts and a promyelocyte from a case of MDS. MGG stain. (Courtesy of Jean-E. Goasguen.)

Plate 14-8. Double esterase reaction: Myeloblasts are brick red and monocytic precursors are black. Case of myelomonocytic leukemia (FAB M4).

Plate 14-9. FAB M1: Myeloblasts with less than 10 percent maturation of granulocytic precursors. One blast has an Auer body. MGG stain. (Courtesy of Jean-E. Goasguen.)

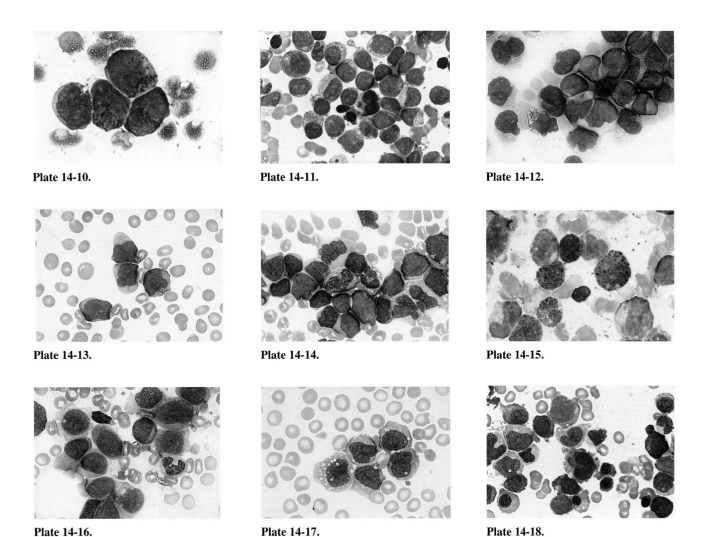

Plate 14-10. **Plate 14-11.** **Plate 14-12.**

Plate 14-13. **Plate 14-14.** **Plate 14-15.**

Plate 14-16. **Plate 14-17.** **Plate 14-18.**

Plate 14-10. FAB M1: Myeloperoxidase stain with black staining granules in a case of AML.

Plate 14-11. FAB M2: Blasts with significant maturation of abnormal granulocytes at the promyelocytic cell and beyond. W-G stain.

Plate 14-12. FAB M3: Hypergranular promyelocytes. Note bundles of Auer rods or faggots and bilobed nuclei. MGG stain. (Courtesy of Jean-E. Goasguen.)

Plate 14-13. FAB M3 variant: Only occasional blasts have visible granules but prominent bilobed and reniform nuclei resemble monoblasts. MGG stain. (Courtesy of Jean-E. Goasguen.)

Plate 14-14. FAB M4 (myelomonocytic leukemia). Both myeloblasts and monoblasts/promonocytes are present. MGG stain. (Courtesy of Jean-E. Goasguen.)

Plate 14-15. FAB M4eo (myelomonocytic leukemia with abnormal eosinophilic granules). Note the magenta staining granules in the myelocyte (exaggerated or prominent primary granules). MGG stain. (Courtesy of Jean-E. Goasguen.)

Plate 14-16. FAB M5a (acute monoblastic leukemia). Numerous blasts that are large with a low N/C. Azurophilic granules are rare. MGG stain. (Courtesy of Jean-E. Goasguen.)

Plate 14-17. FAB M5b (acute monocytic leukemia). More than 20 percent of the monocytic population are promonocytes. There is more abundant cytoplasm, often with a dusting of fine azurophilic granules. MGG stain. (Courtesy of Jean-E. Goasguen.)

Plate 14-18. FAB M6a (acute erythroleukemia). Micromegakaryoblast surrounded by megaloblastic erythroid precursors and myeloblasts. MGG stain.

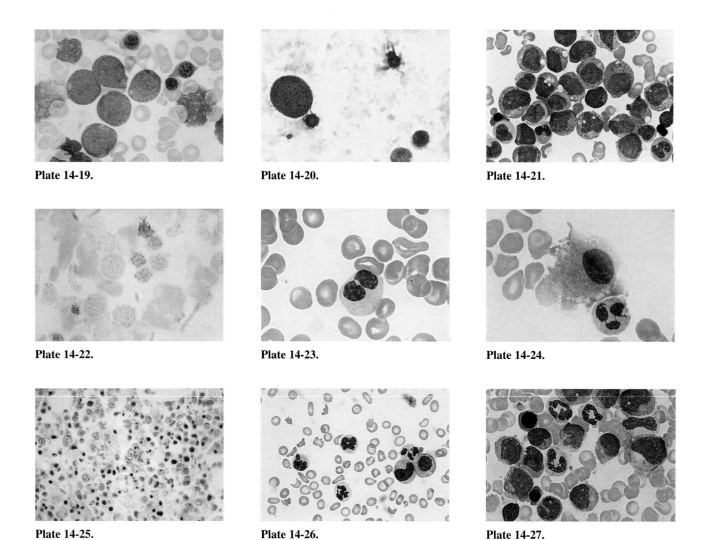

Plate 14-19.

Plate 14-20.

Plate 14-21.

Plate 14-22.

Plate 14-23.

Plate 14-24.

Plate 14-25.

Plate 14-26.

Plate 14-27.

Plate 14-19. FAB M6b: Absence of myeloblasts with exclusive erythroid precursors and increased numbers of erythroblasts. W-G stain.

Plate 14-20. FAB M7 (acute megakaryocytic leukemia). Platelets and one blast stained for CD41. APAPP procedure.

Plate 14-21. FAB M2: Case with t(8;21). Note thin Auer rod. MGG stain.

Plate 14-22. Myelodysplastic syndromes (MDS). Several ringed sideroblasts. Prussian blue reaction.

Plate 14-23. MDS: Dysgranulopoiesis with a pseudo-Pelger-Huet neutrophil that is hypogranular with hypercondensed nuclear chromatin. MGG stain. (Courtesy of Jean-E. Goasguen.)

Plate 14-24. MDS: Dysmegakaryopoiesis, mononuclear megakaryocyte. MGG stain. (Courtesy of Jean-E. Goasguen.)

Plate 14-25. MDS: Abnormal localization of immature precursors (ALIP). Cluster of 5 blasts. H&E stain. (Courtesy of G. Mufti.)

Plate 14-26. MDS: Macrocytosis and variation in size and shape of erythrocytes. Hypogranular neutrophils. Case of refractory anemia with trilineage dysplasia. Peripheral blood. MGG stain. (Courtesy of Jean-E. Goasguen.)

Plate 14-27. MDS (CMML): Monocytic precursors and dysplastic granulocytes. MGG stain. (Courtesy of Jean-E. Goasguen.)

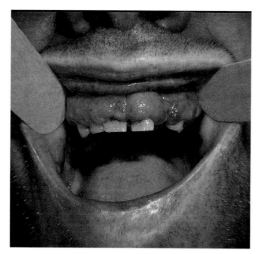

Plate 20-1.

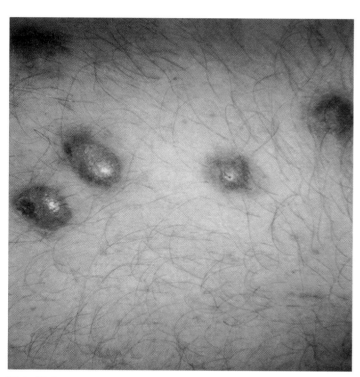

Plate 20-2.

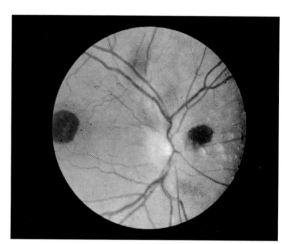

Plate 20-3.

Plate 20-1. Gingival hypertrophy in a patient with FAB M5 subtype of AML. Leukemic infiltration is the cause.

Plate 20-2. Leukemia cutis in a patient with FAB M4 subtype of AML. The raised papules are due to leukemic infiltration of all layers of the corium.

Plate 20-3. Fundic hemorrhage in a thrombocytopenic patient with AML.

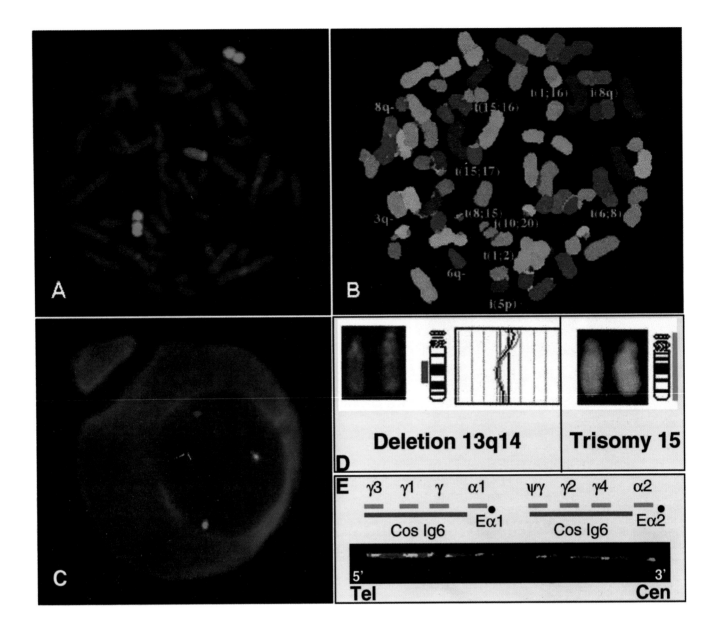

Plate 28-1. Advanced molecular cytogenetic methods. Picture **(A)** shows a metaphase as would be seen for conventional cytogenetic (CC) methods. In addition there is hybridization with whole chromosomal paint for chromosomes 14 (red) and 16 (green), showing a t(14;16)(q32;q23) (chromosome with both colors). **(B)** Results of metaphase SKY of a MM tumor(?) after hybridization and computer reconstruction that identifies each chromosome with a different color. Multiple structural and numerical abnormalities can be readily observed. **(C)** Interphase in situ hybridization experiment coupled with the immunofluorescent detection of the clonal PC by an AMCA (blue) labeled monoclonal antibody (cIg-FISH). The antibody is directed against the kappa or lambda light chain according to the light chain restriction of the clone. The probes shown are for the variable (VH) and constant region (CH) of the IgH locus and are directly labeled. The pattern shows segregation of signals from one of the pairs, indicative of a translocation. **(D)** Results of a CGH experiment for the detection of both loss and gain of material at 13q14 and of chromosome 15 respectively. **(E)** Germline configuration of the IgH constant region as seen by DNA fiber-FISH. The contig of probes used allows for the location of breakpoints when the bar code is disrupted. (Figure B is reproduced with permission from Rao et al.,[43] and Figure D is reproduced with permission from Cigudosa et al.[45]).

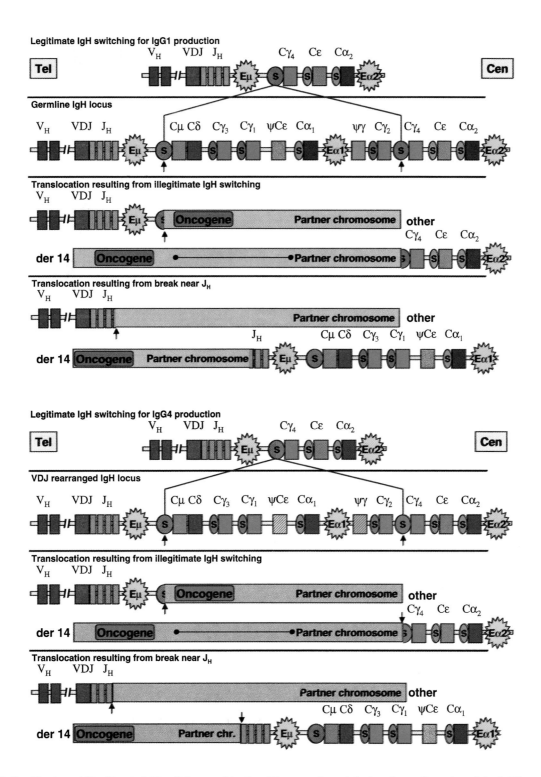

Plate 28-2. Legitimate and illegitimate IgH switch recombination. The second panel depicts the configuration of the IgH locus after VDJ recombination. The upper panel shows the IgH locus after isotype class switching from a IgM to an IgG4 immunoglobulin. The intervening fragment is excised and lost from the cell, while telomeric switch μ sequences are joined with centromeric switch γ4 sequences. Panels 3 and 4 show illegitimate IgH rearrangements resulting in a chromosomal translocation at the IgH locus as a result of rare errors in IgH switching and somatic hypermutation, respectively. In the former case, the breaks in the switch regions (vertical arrows) are the same as for legitimate IgH switching, including loss of the intervening fragment but joining of the two ends to the ends of another chromosome instead of to each other. The boxes indicate coding regions, and the associated circles represent switch regions. The yellow stars depict the intronic μ (Eμ) enhancer and the two 3′ α enhancers (Eα). The arrowhead indicates a potential break that might occur during somatic hypermutation.

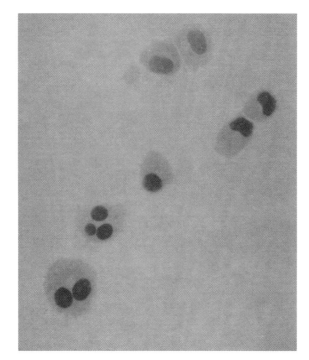

Plate 32-1.

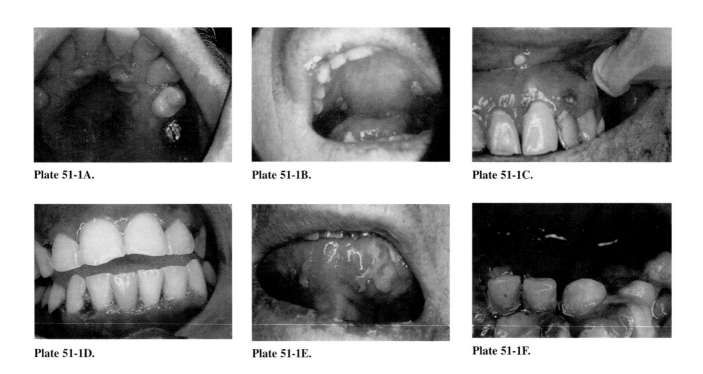

Plate 51-1A.   **Plate 51-1B.**   **Plate 51-1C.**

Plate 51-1D.   **Plate 51-1E.**   **Plate 51-1F.**

Plate 32-1.   Cytospin preparation from the cerebrospinal fluid (CSF) of a patient with meningeal myelomatosis. The CSF cell count was 8 cells/μl.

Plate 51-1.   **(A)** Multiple hard palate ulcerations secondary to HSV. **(B)** Intraoral white plaques often assumed to be secondary to mucocutaneous candidiasis. These are secondary to HSV. **(C & D)** Intraoral infection with gingival ulcerations and gingival papillae necrosis. Pearly margins are characteristic. These are secondary to HSV. **(E)** Diffuse mucosal disruption compatible with chemotherapy or radiation-induced mucositis. This process was due to HSV. **(F)** Patient with AML presenting with gingival hyperplasia and secondary infection with bacteria, *Candida,* and HSV.

9

The Pathogenesis, Diagnosis, and Treatment of Polycythemia Vera

Brian J.P. Huntly, Anthony Bench, and
Anthony R. Green

Polycythaemia vera (PV) was first described in 1892 by Vazquez,[1] in a case report of a patient with ruddy cyanosis, splenomegaly, and an increased red cell count not associated with a congenital form of heart disease. A decade later in 1903 it was defined more clearly by Osler[2] and the disease then became known as Vasquez-Osler disease until this eponymous term was superseded by PV. Along with essential thrombocythemia (ET) and idiopathic myelofibrosis (IMF) it is one of the chronic myeloproliferative disorders (MPDs)(see separate chapters), an overlapping spectrum of preleukemic disorders believed to result from acquired genetic changes in the hematopoietic stem cell compartment. These changes lead to perturbed stem cell function with overproduction of mature cells within one or more of the myeloid lineages and a variable predisposition to acute leukemia. The MPDs were first grouped together, along with chronic myelocytic leukemia (CML), by Dameshek in his seminal paper of 1951.[3] CML is now considered to be a pathogenetically distinct entity, but shares several features with the other MPDs.

EPIDEMIOLOGY

The reported incidence of PV varies from as low as 0.2 cases per million in Japan[4] to around 20 cases per million in Minnesota,[5] with most reports suggesting an incidence of between 5 and 10 cases per million population per year.[6–8] Because the disease is chronic, its prevalence is considerably higher. The wide variation in disease incidence may be explained by a differing predisposition toward PV among certain racial and ethnic backgrounds, with Ashkenazi Jews residing in the United States and Israel having a fourfold increase in incidence by comparison with the remainder of the population[7–9] and African Americans affected less frequently than the remainder of the population of the United States.[10,11] An increased incidence of PV has been reported following exposure to ionizing radiation, with survivors of the atomic bomb detonation in Hiroshima having a higher incidence compared with the rest of the Japanese population,[12] and U.S. military personnel involved with the detonation of an atomic device having a 20-fold incidence compared with the general population.[13] The sex incidence is roughly equivalent with slight male predominance. PV occurs mainly in late middle age and the elderly. In a large retrospective study from the Gruppo Italiano Studio Policitemia[14] involving more than 1000 patients the median age at diagnosis was 60 years. Younger patients are seen, however, with 7 percent presenting before age 40 in this study.

CLINICAL FEATURES AND NATURAL HISTORY

Thrombosis is the major cause of morbidity and mortality in untreated PV. The increased risk of thrombosis relates to the hemorheological effects of the erythrocytosis and may be further exacerbated by accompanying thrombocythemia and possibly by abnormal platelet function. In a large retrospective study of over 1000 patients, 20 percent of patients presented with a thrombotic complication, with arterial and venous events comprising two-thirds and one-third of these thromboses, respectively.[14] Twenty-one percent of these thromboses proved to be fatal. There is an increased risk of thrombosis in treated patients also with an incidence of 3.4 percent per year in the above study,[14] and thrombosis remains the most common cause of mortality in PV. The patients in this study were treated heterogeneously with venesection and myelosuppression and, as is discussed later, the ongoing thrombotic risk relates to treatment modality. Less commonly patients may also present with hemorrhagic complications such as significant gastrointestinal, uterine, or cerebral bleeding.[14] Hemorrhage may also occur with follow-up of treated patients, accounting for 2.6 percent of deaths in the above Italian study[14] and 6.8 percent of recorded fatalities in the Polycythaemia Vera Study Group PVSG-01 protocol.[15] This hemorrhagic tendency may be exacerbated by higher doses of antiaggregating agents as was suggested in the PVSG-05 trial (see below).[16]

Patients with PV are often plethoric and may complain of pruritus, which is classically related to bathing or showering in warm water (aquagenic pruritus) and may be intractable. They may also describe headaches and blurred vision, night sweats, and gout, attributable to hyperviscosity, hypervolemia, and hypermetabolism. Splenomegaly is present in around two-thirds of PV patients at diagnosis and its prevalence increases with disease duration.[17] However, in most cases the diagnosis of PV is first suspected following an abnormal full blood count performed to investigate nonspecific or unrelated symptoms.

There is variable risk of disease transformation to acute myeloid leukemia (AML) or post polycythemic myelofibrosis, also described as the "spent" phase of polycythemia. The percentage of patients progressing to a myelofibrotic state is reported to be around 10 percent at 12.5 years follow-up[4] and as high as 25 to 40 percent at 20 years depending on treatment.[18,19] There is an increased risk of development of AML in patients who have developed marrow fibrosis. This overall risk of leukemic transformation also relates to previous treatment modalities with reports of the incidence varying between 1.5 percent, for patients treated only with phlebotomy, to 14 percent, for patients treated with chlorambucil, after almost 20 years of maximal follow-up.[15] The figure of 1.5 percent probably underestimates the inherent tendency of this disease to transform into AML since the phlebotomy patients represented a selected subgroup with less aggressive disease.[20] The incidence of AML in patients treated with hydroxyurea is between 5 and 10 percent at 9 to 10 years of follow-up.[9,18,21]

In the absence of treatment PV is a fatal disease. Cheivitz and Theide[22] found a median survival of less than 2 years in symptomatic patients who received no treatment. This compares with a median survival of between 9 and 15 years quoted for treated patients.[14,15] In older patients there is controversy over the effect of the disease on life expectancy. Some have found that this does not differ from an age-matched control population[23,24] whereas in one large study the age- and sex-standardized mortality rate was 1.7 times that of the normal control population.[14] In younger patients with PV, however, although the median survival is significantly longer than older patients,[23,25] their survival is significantly less than an age- and sex-matched normal population ($p < .01$).[25] In one study of PV patients less than 50 years of age the observed mortality rate was 4.1 times that of the normal age- and sex-matched population.[25]

PATHOGENESIS OF PV

PV is thought to result from the clonal expansion of a single transformed multipotent stem cell. Progenitors from patients with PV demonstrate abnormal growth responses to several growth factors, suggesting the presence of a defect in a signaling pathway common to different growth factors. PV is also associated with nonrandom cytogenetic abnormalities, the chromosomal location of these changes suggesting the position of genes important to the pathogenesis of the disease. The identification of causal genes may provide much needed diagnostic markers for the disease, allow specific therapy of the molecular and cellular defects, and provide insights into fundamental issues of stem cell behavior.

Clonality

X-chromosome inactivation studies have played a pivotal role in establishing the current concepts of the pathogenesis of many hematological malignancies. These assays provide a means of assessing clonality without any requirement for tumor-specific genetic or cytogenetic markers (reviewed in ref. 26). In the female embryo each cell randomly inactivates one X-chromosome and the progeny of each cell inherits this pattern. As the inactivation is a random process, adult females are therefore mosaic with respect to this pattern of X-chromosome inactivation. Assessment of X-chromosome inactivation requires an ability to distinguish different X-linked alleles, so the various assays are based on polymorphic X-linked genes. It is also necessary to determine which X-chromosome is active. This can be achieved by monitoring expression at the RNA or protein level, or by using DNA methylation as a surrogate marker for the levels of gene activity.

The original studies of clonality in PV used a rare polymorphism of the G6PD gene that gives rise to identifiably different proteins. In two patients erythrocytes, platelets, granulocytes, and bone marrow buffy coat all showed predominant expression of one allele, whereas both alleles were expressed in skin fibroblasts.[27] These data were interpreted as showing that PV results from transformation and subsequent clonal expansion of a multipotent hematopoietic stem cell. Subsequent studies using a variety of molecular methods have extended and confirmed clonality in larger numbers of PV patients.[28–31] In order to distinguish a true clonal pattern in myeloid cells from extreme lyonization, the X-chromosome inactivation patterns in T cells have been concurrently examined alongside granulocytes or unfractionated bone marrow[28,30,31] and the finding of skewed X-inactivation in granulocytes in the presence of a balanced pattern in T cells was felt to indicate a clonal disorder.

Approximately 90 percent of PV patients have a clonal pattern of X-inactivation.[32] Since a clonal pattern of X-inactivation was reported to be rare in normal young females, it was hoped that X-inactivation patterns could be used as a diagnostic tool in the context of PV and the other MPDs. However, it was subsequently demonstrated that X-inactivation patterns become skewed with increasing age (acquired skewing), and 25 to 50 percent of hematologically normal women have "clonal" granulocytes and polyclonal T cells.[33,34] There are several possible explanations for this observation. First, an acquired mutation could lead to clonal expansion as part of a neoplastic process. It is unlikely, however, that such a large proportion of hematologically normal elderly females have a clonal hematological malignancy. Second, it has been suggested that stem cell depletion may occur with age but elderly mice have an increased number of stem cells.[35] Instead current evidence favors a third explanation that entails selection for stem cells whose active X-chromosome is of one parental type. This concept is supported by twin studies[36,37] and by the pattern of skewing observed in elderly cats.[38] These data suggest the existence of one or more X-linked genes, which regulate stem cell kinetics.

Whatever the mechanism, the phenomenon of acquired skewing has important clinical and practical implications. First, the determination of clonality is clearly not a useful diagnostic tool in elderly women. Second, the data raise questions about the dogma that clonal hematopoiesis in patients with PV necessarily reflects the transformation of a multipotent stem cell.

PV Progenitors and Signal Transduction

In 1974 Prchal and Axelrad[39] reported the key observation that cultures of PV bone marrow cells yielded in vitro erythroid colonies even when no exogenous erythropoietin was added to the culture media. These have been termed endogenous erythroid colonies (EEC) or erythropoietin-independent burst forming unit erythroid (BFU-E) but the mechanisms responsible for their formation remain obscure. Growth of BFU-E in the absence of added erythropoietin may reflect complete independence of this cytokine[40] or hypersensitivity to trace amounts present in the culture reagents.[41] In serum-free systems erythropoietin-independent colonies are seen in normal individuals, raising the possibility that BFU-E from PV patients have a reduced sensitivity to an inhibitory factor present in serum.[42] In spite of this biological complexity two conclusions can be drawn from recent studies of PV progenitors. First, erythroid progenitors have been shown to be hypersensitive to several different growth factors including SCF, interleukin (IL)-3, GM-CSF, and IGF-1.[43–45] Second, myeloid progenitors (CFU-Meg and CFU-GM) also show abnormal patterns of growth.[43,46,47] These findings are consistent with a model in which the acquired genetic lesion in PV is not restricted to the erythropoietin-signaling pathway and affects progenitors committed to multiple lineages (Figure 9–1).

A number of signal transduction molecules have been studied as potential PV target genes. Initial attention focused on the erythropoietin receptor (Epo-R). Experimentally induced mutations in the Epo-R result in hypersensitivity to, or independence of, exogenous erythropoietin. Truncation of the cytoplasmic domain of the Epo-R, leading to hypersensitivity to Epo, has been found in primary familial polycythemia[48] and confirmed in several other cases of congenital polycythemia, occasionally occurring sporadically.[49–51] Several groups have therefore looked at the integrity of the Epo-R gene in bone marrow cells from PV patients but none have detected mutations.[52,53] Decreased expression of a shortened Epo-R isoform encoded by an alternate transcript has been implicated in PV[54] but similar alternate splicing events in solid tumors have not been shown to play a causal role in tumor pathogenesis.[55]

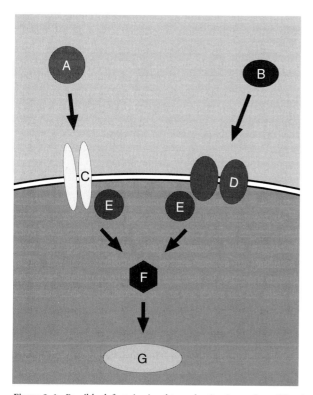

Figure 9–1. Possible defects in signal transduction in myeloproliferative disorder (MPD). Progenitor cells from patients are hypersensitive to a number of cytokines (**A** and **B**) such as EPO, which act through specific receptor molecules (**C** and **D**). There may be a defect in a common receptor component (**E**), a common signalling intermediate (**F**), or a common effector molecule (**G**) such as a transcription factor. (From Hinshelwood et al.,[32] with permission.)

The reported hypersensitivity of PV progenitor cells to multiple cytokines raised the possibility of a defect in a downstream signaling pathway common to multiple different cytokine receptors (Figure 9–1). The tyrosine phosphatase SHP-1 (also known as HCP) was considered a prime candidate as it inhibits signaling from Epo-R and other cytokine receptors, and hematopoietic progenitors carrying a null mutation in SHP-1 are hypersensitive to cytokines. However, SHP-1 protein expression was normal in granulocytes from PV patients and complete nucleotide sequencing of the SHP-1 coding region and promoter in eight patients showed no mutations.[56] These results do not exclude a role for other inhibitory phosphatases and a novel protein with increased phosphatase activity has been reported in PV progenitors.[57]

In addition to the Epo-R, a number of other cytokine receptors have been studied. Axelrad and co-workers have looked at tyrosine phosphorylation of the IGF-1 receptor subunit in the peripheral blood mononuclear cells from PV patients. They detected a higher basal level of phosphorylation of this receptor and enhanced downstream signaling as judged by increased tyrosine phosphorylation following stimulation with IGF-1.[58] The thrombopoietin receptor c-mpl, present on mutilineage progenitors as well as megakaryocytes and platelets is also an attractive candidate. Spivak and others have reported a reduced expression of c-mpl on platelets and megakaryocytes from patients with PV.[59] This finding may distinguish PV from secondary polycythemia[60,61] but not other MPDs.[62,63] A report has suggested that a marked heterogeneity exists in c-mpl protein levels in PV and this question currently limits its use as a diagnostic test.[64] An increase in certain splice variants and glycosylated forms of the c-mpl receptor have also been found with the degree of glycosylation suggested to correlate with the duration of disease and, possibly, with progression to myelofibrosis.[65,66]

It has also been suggested that reduced apoptosis may be important in PV since an increase in Bcl-x_L was reported in erythroid cells from PV patients.[67] However, as with other reports of genes differentially expressed in normal and PV cells, such as the uPAR receptor superfamily member PRV-1,[68] the pathogenetic significance of these observations remains unclear.

Cytogenetic Abnormalities in PV

Unlike CML there is no pathognomonic chromosomal abnormality associated with any of the MPDs. However, a number of nonrandom chromosomal abnormalities have been documented (see Table 9–1). Cytogenetic abnormalities are present in 20 percent of patients at diagnosis, this number increasing to over 80 percent for patients with more than 10 years follow-up.[32,69] Approximately 85 percent of patients whose disease progresses to myelofibrosis and/or acute leukemia show an abnormal karyotype. In one study of 104 patients, although the number of patients with a cytogenetic abnormality at diagnosis was small, the median survival of this group was significantly less than that for patients with a normal karyotype, suggesting that an abnormal karyotype is a poor prognostic indicator.[70] The incidence of chromosomal abnormalities is also greater in patients receiving myelosuppressive therapy (45 percent) than

Table 9–1. Summary of Karyotypic Abnormalities Identified by G-Banding in PV

Abnormality	Number of Occurrences of Abnormality	Percentage of All Patients
Deletion of 20q	45	8.4
Deletion of 13q	16	3.0
Trisomy 8	37	6.9
Trisomy 9	35	6.6
Trisomy of 1q	19	3.6
Deletion of 7q or monosomy 7	5	0.9
Deletion of 5q or monosomy 5	17	3.2
Total number of patients with one or more abnormality	180	33.7
Total patients	534	

(From Bench et al.,[69] and references therein, with permission.)

in untreated patients (17 percent),[32] although it is not known whether this reflects the leukemogenic effects of the treatment regimens themselves or may indicate that patients whose disease is progressive (and therefore requiring more aggressive therapy) are more likely to develop cytogenetic changes.

Some chromosomal changes, such as deletions or monosomies of chromosomes 5 and 7, are almost invariably seen after exposure to myelosuppressive therapy and frequently as part of a complex karyotype. It is therefore unlikely that these chromosomes contain genes involved in the etiology of the MPDs. By contrast, deletions of part of the long arm of chromosome 20 (del 20q) and 13 (del 13q), trisomies of chromosomes 8 and 9, and duplication of the long arm of chromosome 1 have all been seen in untreated patients and are frequently present as sole abnormalities. They are likely, therefore, to mark the site of genes that play an early role in the pathogenesis of the MPDs.

Deletions of Chromosome 20

After t(9;22), del(20q) was the most common sole structural chromosomal abnormality observed in a series of almost 3000 consecutive bone marrow samples analyzed by G-banding at the Mayo clinic,[71] and is the most common cytogenetic abnormality in PV. 20q deletions occur in approximately 8 percent of patients with PV (Table 9–1) but also occur in other MPDs, in 4 percent of patients with myelodysplastic syndromes (MDS), and in 1 to 2 percent of patients with AML.[72] Loss of loci on 20q has also been demonstrated in the transition from chronic phase to blast crisis in 5 of 17 CML patients[73] but deletions of 20q are rarely seen in lymphoid malignancies. Thus a pattern of disease association suggests that the deleted region of chromosome 20 marks the site of one or more genes, loss or inactivation of which perturb the regulation of hematopoietic progenitors. The finding of 20q deletions at diagnosis and as a sole abnormality suggests that, in at least some cases, it plays an early role in disease pathogenesis.

In patients with PV the presence of a 20q deletion does not appear to influence survival, although the number of patients studied is small.[74–76] The 20q deletion can arise in a very early progenitor with both lymphoid and myeloid potential,[77,78] and the deletions can often be detected in mature peripheral blood granulocytes.[79] Molecular analysis of the 20q deletions has been undertaken to identify critical target genes. Fluorescence in situ hybridization (FISH), microsatellite polymerase chain reaction (PCR), and Southern blotting have demonstrated heterogeneity of both the centromeric and telomeric breakpoints[77,80,81] implying that the commonly deleted region (CDR) contains one or more tumor suppressor genes. Physical maps of this region of chromosome 20, in the form of yeast artificial chromosome (YAC) or P1-derived/bacterial artificial chromosome (PAC/BAC) maps[82,83] have been constructed to facilitate gene identification. As 20q deletions occur in a number of myeloid disorders it has been necessary to construct disease specific maps. The most recent MPD CDR spans a distance of 2.7 Mb and overlaps with the CDR generated in MDS/AML of 2.6 Mb, giving a combined "myeloid" CDR of 1.7 Mb[84] (Figure 9–2). Five genes and 11 unique expressed sequence tags (ESTs) are present in this overlap region. A separate CDR of 250 kb, containing five characterized genes, four predicted genes, and nine single ESTs, has been constructed using information from unbalanced translocations involving loss of 20q sequences from two non-MPD patients, one with MDS the other AML[85] (Figure 9–2). Expression profiling of the genes in CD34+ cells has been used to prioritize the MPD CDR for mutational analysis, and candidates from both regions are currently undergoing mutational analysis to identify any tumor suppressor gene.

Analysis of other structural chromosomal abnormalities in PV and the MPDs are at a less advanced stage. A common deleted region has been constructed for 13q deletions in all myeloid disorders[86] and specifically for IMF.[87] This region involves the minimally deleted region also seen in chronic lymphocytic leukemia (CLL) and other low-grade lymphoproliferative disorders although it is not clear whether the same tumor suppressor gene(s) are affected in myeloid and lymphoid disorders.

DIAGNOSIS

The Classification and Differential Diagnosis of Erythrocytoses

The term erythrocytosis has descriptive merit for the nonspecific observation of an increased proportion of red cells in the peripheral blood, and will be used in this differential diagnostic section. Using this term rather than polycythemia avoids the incorrect assumption that "polycythemia" equates with PV. Erythrocytosis defines the pathological change precisely and falls into line with other descriptive terms such as leukocytosis and thrombocytosis. It is more appropriate to define an erythrocytosis in terms of the hematocrit (Hct) rather than the hemoglobin (Hb) value since in the erythrocytoses iron deficiency may occur and then the Hct may be disproportionately higher than the Hb value.[88] The Hct is therefore the best indicator of erythrocytosis available from automated cell counts and, although

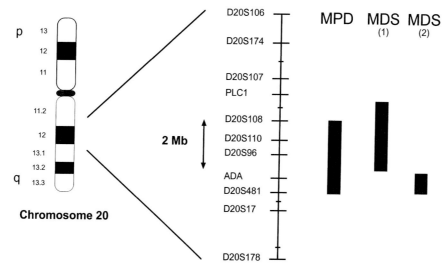

Figure 9–2. Summary of common deleted regions (CDRs) on 20q for myeloproliferative disorders (MPD) and myelodysplastic syndromes (MDS). The MPD CDR is bordered by D20S108 and D20S481. Two distinct CDRs for MDS/AML have been published. MDS CDR (1) is flanked by PACs 620E11 and 196H17. MDS CDR (2) is flanked by PACs 29M7 and 179M20 and includes patients with MDS and AML. (From Bench et al.,[136] with permission.)

the upper limit of normal will vary between laboratories it will be around 0.51 for males and 0.48 for females.[89] However, patients should not be further investigated until a minimum of two separate blood counts have been performed and both have shown a raised Hct. Patients with a raised Hct should be further investigated for an absolute erythrocytosis by measurement of their red cell mass (RCM). However, males and females with Hct values above 0.6 and 0.56 respectively, can be assumed to have an absolute erythrocytosis.[90]

Red Cell Mass: Demonstration of an Absolute Erythrocytosis

A diagnosis of an absolute erythrocytosis can only be made when an individual's RCM measurement is more than 25 percent above their mean predicted value. The RCM result and predicted values should be expressed in terms of the patient's surface area rather than body weight. As fat is relatively avascular, results expressed in terms of total body weight lack precision in the obese patient. Using surface area to calculate the predicted RCM, 98 percent of males and 99 percent of females fell within ± 25 percent of the mean value.[91] Should a patient's RCM fall within the reference range the term *apparent erythrocytosis* should be applied.

The Absolute Erythrocytoses

The initial investigation and classification of the absolute erythrocytoses is given in Figure 9–3. In the primary erythrocytoses it is erythropoiesis itself that is defective, whereas in secondary erythrocytoses intrinsically normal erythropoiesis is increased as a response to physiologically or pathologically increased erythropoietin secretion. The only acquired primary type is the clonal myeloproliferative disorder PV, whereas the only congenital primary type described so far is a mutation of the Epo receptor, which may be due to familial or spontaneous

mutation (see pathogenesis section). The causes of congenital and acquired secondary erythrocytoses are shown in Table 9–2. The term *idiopathic erythrocytosis* is used for the heterogeneous group of patients who cannot, at initial investigation, be defined as either primary or secondary erythrocytosis. Either of these diagnoses may become apparent with time, however.

The Laboratory and Clinical Investigation of an Absolute Erythrocytosis

The starting points in the further investigation of an absolute erythrocytosis are a knowledge of the causes of secondary erythrocytoses and the diagnostic criteria for PV (Tables 9–2 and 9–3, respectively). No single marker for the diagnosis of PV has, as yet, been identified. Currently patients must satisfy a number of diagnostic criteria and are said to have PV if they exceed a combination of "A" (major) and "B" (minor) criteria. Recent modifications to the PVSG, criteria have improved their sensitivity[92] and are shown in Table 9–3. The modifications to the PVSG criteria add the demonstration of clonal hematopoiesis by detection of a karyotypic abnormality to the major criteria and replace leukocyte alkaline phosphatase (LAP) score and serum B12/unbound B12 binding capacity (UB12BC) with new minor criteria. These include radiological evidence of splenomegaly and the demonstration of either a reduced serum Epo level[93] or evidence of endogenous erythroid colony growth in clonogenic assays in the absence of Epo stimulation.[42] The reasons for these substitutions are that LAP scores show poor inter- and intralaboratory reproducibility and that B12 assays are inaccurate at high levels, and few laboratories measure UB12BC.

The investigations may be undertaken in two stages (see Table 9–4). The first stage tests are mainly a battery of relatively simple tests to rule out secondary causes whereas the second stage tests are either more specialized, or are specific diagnostic criteria for PV.

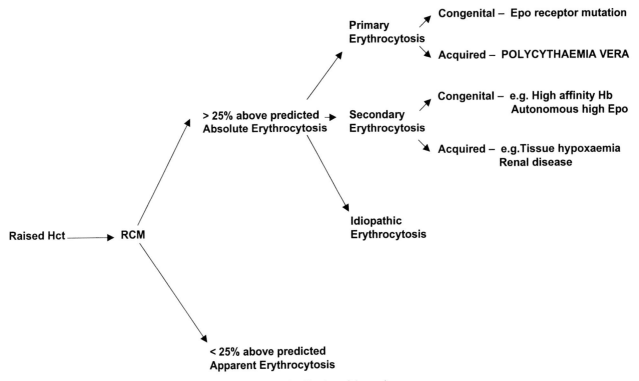

Figure 9–3. Classification of the erythrocytoses.

Full Blood Count

A raised neutrophil and platelet count supports a diagnosis of PV, although it should be remembered that smokers have higher neutrophil counts than nonsmokers do. The red cell indices may be suggestive of iron deficiency, which is common in PV. An eosinophilia and/or basophilia are occasionally found in PV but are only supportive of this diagnosis.

Ferritin, B12, and Folate

Low ferritin levels are more common in PV than secondary erythrocytoses. Serum levels of B12 may be raised in PV due to the release of transcobalamin from an increased granulocyte mass. Folate deficiency has been reported in PV.

Renal and Liver Function Tests and Serum Uric Acid

Any renal impairment may suggest renal causes of secondary erythrocytosis. Cirrhosis and excessive alcohol consumption causing impaired liver function may result in an absolute erythrocytosis due to associated hypoxemia, diminished Epo

Table 9–2. Common Causes of Secondary Polycythemia

Congenital	Mutant high-affinity Hb
	Autonomous high Epo production
Acquired	Arterial hypoxemia
	High altitude
	Cyanotic congenital heart disease
	Chronic lung disease
	Renal lesions
	Renal tumors/cysts
	Diffuse parenchymal disease
	Renal artery stenosis
	Hepatic lesions
	Hepatoma
	Cirrhosis
	Miscellaneous tumors
	Cerebellar hemangioma
	Uterine fibroids
	Endocrine lesions
	Adrenal tumors/androgen therapy

(From Pearson et al.,[88] with permission.)

Table 9–3. Proposed Modified Criteria for the Diagnosis of Polycythemia Vera[a]

A1 Raised red cell mass ($>25\%$ above normal predicted value)	B1 Thrombocytosis (platelet count $> 400 \times 10^9$/L)
A2 Absence of cause of secondary polycythemia	B2 Neutrophil leukocytosis (neutrophil count $> 10 \times 10^9$/L)
A3 Palpable splenomegaly	B3 Splenomegaly demonstrated on isotope/ultrasound scanning
A4 Acquired cytogenetic abnormality	B4 Characteristic BFU-E growth or reduced serum erythropoietin

Abbreviation: BFU-E, Burst-forming unit erythroid.
[a] A1 + A2 + A3 or A4 establishes PV. A1 + A2 + two of B criteria establishes PV.
(From Pearson and Messinezy,[92] with permission.)

Table 9–4. Suggested Stages of Investigation in Patients with a Demonstrated Absolute Erythrocytosis[a]

Stage 1	Stage 2
FBC	Bone marrow aspirate/trephine
Arterial O_2 saturation	Bone marrow karyotype
Ferritin	BFU-E
B12 and folate	Serum Epo estimation
Urea and creatinine	Lung function tests*
Liver function tests	Echocardiogram*
Uric acid	Sleep studies*
Chest x-ray	O_2 dissociation curve (P_{50})*
Abdominal ultrasound	Epo receptor mutation analysis*

Abbreviations: FBC, full blood count; BFU-E, burst forming unit erythroid.
[a] Stage 1 investigations are more general, inexpensive tests aimed at picking up secondary causes. Stage 2 investigations are more specific tests either specifically aimed at proving or disproving a diagnosis of PV, or * may be suggested by the results of stage 1 tests and/or the patient history.
(From Pearson et al.,[88] with permission.)

catabolism, or an increased basal hepatic production of Epo.[94] Patients with PV, like other MPDs, often manifest clinical gout and a raised serum uric acid is common at presentation.

Abdominal Ultrasound

This investigation is essential in all patients. Relevant renal and hepatic pathology can be assessed as can splenic size. Simple renal cysts are common and increase with patient age, but unlike polycystic kidneys, are uncommon causes of erythrocytosis. Hydronephrosis and benign and malignant renal and hepatic tumors can also be ruled out on ultrasound. Further computed tomography (CT) scanning or arteriography may be necessary to define any abnormality found. Palpable splenomegaly in the absence of hepatic pathology is a reliable major criterion of PV, but splenic enlargement occurs before it is clinically palpable. Scanning techniques have shown that two-thirds of all patients with PV have splenic enlargement at diagnosis,[17,95] and radiological evidence of splenomegaly is therefore a minor diagnostic criterion for PV.

Arterial Oxygen Saturation/Measurement of Tissue Oxygenation

Low tissue oxygenation caused by any cardiorespiratory defect will result in an overproduction of erythropoietin and a consequent erythrocytosis. Pulse oximetry is the most convenient measure of arterial oxygen saturation. The oxygen saturation level should be 92 percent or greater; any less has been taken to indicate a causal relationship with an absolute erythrocytosis.[96] Nocturnal arterial desaturation with normal daytime values, however, were observed in 20 percent of patients who would otherwise have been classified as idiopathic erythrocytosis[88] and symptoms that suggest the sleep-apnea syndrome such as daytime somnolence, excessive snoring, and waking unrefreshed should prompt sleep studies. A chest x-ray should be performed routinely to look for parenchymal lung abnormali-

ties. Occasionally pulmonary function tests and an echocardiogram may be necessary to further investigate respiratory or cardiac problems.

Bone Marrow Aspirate, Trephine, and Karyotype

A marrow examination should be performed in every patient with an absolute erythrocytosis, except where the cause is obviously secondary. Characteristic changes can be seen in both the morphology[97] and histology (most recently reviewed Ref. 98). The marrows are often hypercellular with all three cell lineages prominent, megakaryocytes are pleomorphic and may display clustering and increased ploidy, and iron stores are classically absent. The reticulin should be normal or only moderately raised. As the interpretation of bone marrow morphology and histology are subjective and may vary between individuals looking at the same sample, marrow morphology and histology are used only in a confirmatory diagnostic capacity, and do not currently form part of the formal diagnostic criteria for PV.

An acquired abnormality of the marrow karyotype confirms the presence of clonal hematopoiesis, and as such is a major diagnostic criterion for PV. The specific chromosomal abnormalities and their significance are discussed in more detail in the previous pathogenesis section.

Erythropoietin-Independent BFU-E

As discussed in detail in the previous section on pathogenesis, clonogenic assays of purified progenitor cells from patients with PV have shown that their BFU-E are more sensitive than normal to a whole range of growth factors and may grow in serum containing medium without exogenous Epo. Unfortunately these culture techniques are laborious, poorly standardized, expensive, and not generally available outside the setting of research. The linked diagnostic criterion of low serum Epo can be more readily and cheaply demonstrated than the finding of erythropoietin-independent BFU-E.

Serum Epo

In PV, Epo levels are characteristically reduced and remain below the lower level of the normal range in the majority of patients following the normalization of their Hb and Hct. In secondary erythrocytosis due to tissue hypoxemia Epo levels are usually raised. In the rare recessive or dominant erythrocytoses due to an autonomous high Epo production[99–102] different Epo patterns are seen. Some are associated with raised Epo levels irrespective of the Hct, whereas some only have a raised Epo level following Hb reduction to within the normal range.

Other Investigations

Should none of the above tests suggest a diagnosis of either PV or a secondary erythrocytosis then further more specialized tests may be undertaken. An oxygen dissociation curve can be performed to measure the P_{50} and identify patients with a high affinity hemoglobin. Any abnormality should prompt further investigations to identify the Hb, including Hb electrophoresis and direct sequencing. The Epo receptor gene may be assessed for truncating mutations (see pathogenesis) if this facility exists. The current limitation of using X-chromosome inactivation patterns in elderly women has been discussed previously. However, it may have a place in supporting a diagnosis of PV in young women. Similarly platelet and megakaryocyte Tpo levels may have a place in the differentiation of PV from secondary erythrocytoses, but until methodologies are standardized this is also currently only a research tool.

TREATMENT OF PV

Aims of Treatment

Without treatment the median survival of patients with PV is less than 2 years[22] but with adequate treatment the life expectancy of elderly patients may be similar to age- and sex-matched contemporaries.[23,24] However, the overall mortality of younger patients (<50 years old) is significantly different from that of age- and sex-matched controls.[25] In older patients the main cause of death continues to be thrombosis[14] while in younger patients the main cause of death appears to be progression to acute leukemia.[25] Adequate treatment therefore requires correction of the thrombotic tendency by control of the hematocrit and platelet count if raised, possibly along with antiplatelet therapy, especially in the elderly who may have concomitant vascular problems. Current practice suggests that the hematocrit should be less than 0.45 and

that the platelet count should ideally be within the normal range, especially in elderly patients, those with a previous history of thrombosis, or those with other concomitant vascular risk factors. Certain treatment modalities have been associated with an increased risk of progression to AML and a myelofibrotic phase of PV (see below). The treatment modality chosen should reflect this concern over the leukemogenic potential of certain agents and should take into account the age (and therefore likely duration of treatment) of the patient. The treatment of pregnant patients will be considered separately.

Evidence from Trials Conducted in PV

The therapeutic recommendations in PV are based on a few randomized clinical trials, along with certain prospective and retrospective studies that described the natural history of the disease and evaluated the response to different therapies. These trials are summarized in Table 9–5 and their results and relevance are described in more detail in the separate treatment sections.

Phlebotomy

Phlebotomy reduces the hematocrit by the direct removal of blood and, by inducing iatrogenic iron deficiency, controls erythrocyte overproduction without affecting platelet and white cell counts. The PVSG-01 trial was performed over 20 years ago and randomized 431 patients to phlebotomy or myelosuppres-

Table 9–5. Summary of the Major Trials Conducted in Polycythemia Vera.

Study	Patients and Follow-Up		Treatment and Main Results			p Value
Cytoreduction						
PVSG-01 * [103]	431 patients		[32]P	Phlebotomy	Chlorambucil	
	18 years (maximum)	Median survival	11.8 years	13.9 years	8.9 years	.02
		Thrombosis	30%	33%	25%	.08
		Acute leukemia	10%	1.5%	13%	<.0012
EORTC * [137]	293 patients		[32]P	Busulfan		
	8 years (median)	10-year survival	55%	70%		.02
		Vascular deaths	18%	5%		n.r.
Najean et al. * [19]	461 patients		[32]P	[32]P + hydroxyurea		
	16 years (maximum)	Median survival	10.9 years	9.3 years		n.s.
	Age > 65					
Najean et al * [18]	292 patients		Hydroxyurea	Pipobroman		
	16 years (maximum)	14-year survival	70%	70%		n.s.
	Age < 65	Myelofibrosis	17%	2.1%		.03
PVSG-08 [15]	51 patients		Hydroxyurea	Phlebotomy (PVSG-01)		
	15 years (maximum)	Thrombosis	10%	33%		.009
		Acute leukemia	5.9%	1.5%		n.s.
		Myelofibrosis	8%	11%		n.s.
Antiplatelet therapy						
PVSG-05 [16]	166 patients		ASA (900 mg)	[32]P		
	1.6 years (median)	Thrombosis	8%	2%		n.r.
		Hemorrhage	7%	0%		.02
GISP [14]	112 patients		ASA (40 mg)	Placebo		
	1.4 years (median)	Thrombosis	5%	7.7%		n.s.
		Hemorrhage	1.7%	1.9%		n.s.

Note: * Denotes a randomized trial; n.s., nonsignificant; n.r., not reported. ASA, Acetyl salicylic acid.

sion with either radioactive phosphorus (^{32}P) or the alkylating agent chlorambucil. The median survival of the phlebotomy arm (13.9 years) was superior to that of either the ^{32}P arm (11.8 years) or the chlorambucil arm (8.9 years) ($p = .02$).[103] However, there was a markedly increased risk of thrombosis in the phlebotomy arm, particularly within the first 3 years and in patients with previous thrombosis or advanced age ($p = .015$). There was also a startling difference in the quoted incidence of acute leukemia between the randomization arms. After follow-up of between 13 and 15 years, the incidence of leukemia in the phlebotomy arm was only 1.5 percent, whereas it was 10 percent for ^{32}P and 13 percent for chlorambucil ($p = .0045$). The incidence of lymphomas and solid organ tumors was also increased for the two myelosuppressive arms.

The results of this study need to be interpreted with caution, however. The higher thrombosis rate with phlebotomy was thought likely to be due to the uncontrolled thrombocythemia in some patients receiving treatment with phlebotomy alone. This may have been compounded by the initial target hematocrit of 0.52, which was subsequently reduced following the description of the influence of the hematocrit on blood flow and thrombosis.[104,105] After the target hematocrit was reset at 0.45 the rate of thrombosis was the same in all three arms. The incidence of leukemia in the phlebotomy arm is also potentially misleading. Any patient requiring myelosuppression (90 percent of patients by 10 years included in the PVSG-01 study by Najean and Rain[18]) was censored from the analysis and so the AML incidence of 1.5 percent refers to a selected subgroup of patients with relatively benign disease.[20]

There has also been concern over an increased incidence of myelofibrosis in PV patients treated with phlebotomy alone, possibly due to the release of fibrogenic cytokines from elevated platelet and megakaryocyte numbers. In one study[19] the actuarial risk of developing myelofibrosis was higher in patients treated with phlebotomy alone than in patients treated initially with ^{32}P (some of whom later received hydroxyurea). Similar observations have been reported by another group[106] but not by the PVSG.[107]

Thus, although phlebotomy is the initial therapy of choice for patients with PV, additional myelosuppression is necessary in most patients at some time during the course of the disease.

Cytoreductive Therapy

Over time cytoreductive therapy is required in most patients with PV. The PVSG-01 trial raised grave concerns over the increased incidence of acute leukemia with either chlorambucil or ^{32}P, and these agents are seldom used now. However, since ^{32}P and busulfan (an alkylating agent similar to chlorambucil) are given intermittently, they can be useful in the elderly, where regular clinic attendance or drug compliance may be a problem. The main goal in the treatment of PV following the initial findings of the PVSG has been to find a cytoreductive agent that is both safe and well tolerated.

Hydroxyurea

Hydroxyurea (HU) is a potent inhibitor of the enzyme ribonucleotide diphosphate reductase and prevents DNA synthesis. This drug was first used in the PVSG-08 trial, initiated in 1977,

to find a safer agent to prevent the early thrombosis associated with phlebotomy alone. Fifty-one patients were enrolled into this study, all receiving HU and its efficacy and safety were compared retrospectively to the 194 patients previously enrolled into the PVSG-01 phlebotomy arm.[21] Following the first 7 years of follow-up, there was a marked reduction in the number of thrombotic events (PVSG-08, 9.8 percent vs. PVSG-01, 32.8 percent, $p = .009$) in the HU-treated patients.[108] These results were updated with longer follow-up (a median of 8.6 years and maximum follow-up of over 15 years) for the development of acute leukemia and myelofibrosis. The incidence of acute leukemia was low in patients treated with HU at 5.9 percent and did not differ significantly from those treated with phlebotomy alone in PVSG-01 (1.5 percent, $p = .18$) nor did the incidence of myelofibrosis (PVSG-08, 7.8 percent vs. PVSG-01, 11.2 percent, $p = .28$).[15] More recently HU has been compared with the agent pipobroman, which has a structure similar to alkylating agents but acts more like an antimetabolite. This randomized study of 269 patients less than 65 years old observed no difference in overall survival, rate of thrombotic complications, and actuarial incidence of progression to leukemia.[18] The efficacy with which HU reduces thrombotic complications in PV has been confirmed in further studies.[9,18,109]

HU is tolerated extremely well by most patients, with gastrointestinal upset the most commonly reported side effect. Occasionally it can cause skin ulceration, classically of the ankles over the malleoli, with biopsy showing a nonspecific, usually leukocytoclastic vasculitis. HU does not damage DNA in the manner of alkylating agents or ^{32}P, but may interfere with effective DNA repair and, accordingly, there is legitimate concern over its leukemogenic potential. HU is increasingly used in patients with sickle cell disease (SCD), where it increases the proportion of HbF within circulating erythrocytes and ameliorates this disorder. Use in young patients for a disorder without intrinsic malignant potential has prompted a recent review of its mutagenic and carcinogenic potential.[110] Acquired mutations were measured in the peripheral blood mononuclear cells of adults with MPD and SCD treated with HU, from children with SCD treated with HU, and from normal age-matched, untreated controls. In adult patients there was a low mutation rate that was no different from that observed in controls.

A number of studies of MPD patients have raised the possibility that treatment with HU results in a 5 to 10 percent risk of leukemic transformation. However, these studies were small, nonrandomized, or included patients who had received HU together with other cytotoxic agents. Najean and Rain[18] reported an actuarial risk of acute leukemia of 5 percent after 10 years of follow-up and 10 percent after 13 years of follow-up in patients treated with HU, but the latter figure is subject to very wide confidence intervals since only 15 percent of patients remained under observation at 13 years. A study of 201 patients with ET who had received HU alone reported a 3.5 percent risk of leukemic transformation after a median follow-up of over 8 years.[111] There is therefore no evidence to suggest that treatment with HU alone results in a significant increase in leukemic transformation, but anxieties over the theoretical possibility have prompted the evaluation of other agents felt to be less genotoxic.

Interferon-Alpha

The exact mechanism of action of interferon-alpha is unknown but a general antiproliferative action is supported by the reduction in circulating CFU-GM and BFU-E[112] and occasional in vivo cytopenias observed following the introduction of this agent. Interferon also inhibits megakaryopoiesis and antagonizes platelet-derived growth factor, one of the fibrogenic paracrine factors secreted by platelets and megakaryocytes implicated in the pathogenesis of myelofibrosis.[113] It has also been shown to prolong survival in patients with chronic myeloid leukemia by comparison with HU,[114,115] with the degree of survival advantage correlating with its ability to restore normal (Philadelphia-negative) hematopoiesis. Interferon has been shown to control the hematocrit in 60 to 70 percent of patients within the first 6 to 12 months[116] and has been shown to control the associated thrombocytosis, leukocytosis, and splenomegaly in the majority of patients where these occur.[116–118] It appears to be particularly effective for the treatment of PV associated pruritus.[117] Interferon is not thought to be leukemogenic and theoretically may decrease or delay the development of myelofibrosis, but this remains unproven in a randomized trial. Unfortunately interferon is associated with significant side effects, causing treatment withdrawal in up to one-third of all patients.[116,119,120]

Anagrelide

Anagrelide is an oral imidazoquinazolin derivative that can be used to control the platelet count in patients with an MPD, including PV.[121] Its mechanism of action is unclear but it appears to reduce the platelet count by suppressing the maturation of megakaryocytes and also suppresses the Hb levels by 1 to 2 g/L in a proportion of patients with ET. It has no effect on the peripheral leukocyte count. Reported side effects of anagrelide relate to its inhibition of phosphodiesterase and consequent positive inotropic and vasodilator effects with transient headache, palpitations, and fluid retention being common.

Antiplatelet Therapy

In the 1970s following the results of their 01 trial, the PVSG studied whether the addition of antiplatelet agents would reduce the excess thrombotic risk seen in patients treated with phlebotomy alone. This trial (PVSG-05) randomized patients to receive either ^{32}P or phlebotomy and antiplatelet therapy (900 mg aspirin/day and 75 mg pipyridamole/day). However patients in the phlebotomy/antiplatelet arm did not show a reduced rate of thrombosis and yet exhibited a significant increase in the risk of major hemorrhage.

It has subsequently been shown in other patients with vascular disorders that lower doses of aspirin (75 to 325 mg) are equally effective in the prevention of vascular events, with doses throughout this range being equally effective prophylaxis and the lower doses being better tolerated.[122] It therefore seems reasonable to give low-dose aspirin (75 mg) to most PV patients in the absence of overriding contraindications.

Pregnancy and Fertility

The natural physiological changes in pregnancy, such as hemodilution and a mild thrombocytopenia may help to ameliorate the thrombotic diathesis that is present in patients with PV.[123] Pregnancy itself, however, is a physiological hypercoagulable state, with an increase in procoagulant clotting factors (e.g. factor VII, factor VIII, and fibrinogen) and a decrease in natural anticoagulants (e.g., free protein S), occurring from about the third month of pregnancy.[124]

Effects of Cytoreductive Therapy on Fertility and the Fetus

Gonadal suppression resulting in amenorrhea or azoospermia may occur in patients taking cytoreductive agents. High doses of HU, busulfan, and interferon-alpha have been shown to be harmful to spermatogenesis in experimental animals and busulfan has resulted in ovarian failure in older patients.[125] However, fertility has been retained in patients treated with HU and interferon-alpha[126,127] Anagrelide has no effect on fertility in male rats but in female rats, at high dosage, it disrupted implantation and retarded or blocked parturition. Five women have, however, become pregnant on anagrelide therapy. Treatment was stopped as soon as the pregnancy was detected and all five patients delivered normal babies.[125]

The use of cytoreductive therapy in pregnant patients with an MPD is associated with an increased risk of spontaneous abortion, congenital malformation, premature delivery, and intrauterine growth retardation[128] (recently reviewed in Ref. 125). Fetal malformations and fetal loss have been reported with busulfan and HU taken in the first trimester and teratogenicity has been demonstrated in animals treated with HU.[129] Interferon-alpha has been increasingly used in patients with MPD. There have been no reports of adverse effects on the fetus, and successful pregnancies have been reported.[130,131] Interferon-alpha does not appear to cross the placenta to any significant extent;[132] however, teratogenic or other adverse effects cannot be entirely ruled out and it should be used with caution. As many of the agents used to treat PV are excreted in human breast milk a decision should be made whether to discontinue breastfeeding or discontinue the drug, weighing the importance of the drug to the mother.

Outcome of Pregnancies in PV

Only 18 pregnancies have been reported in patients with PV thus far (reviewed in Ref. 125). Two-thirds of these pregnancies were successful, resulting in a live birth. The remaining one-third of pregnancies resulted in fetal loss and the rate of fetal wastage is therefore much higher in patients with PV when compared to the general population. There was also a higher incidence of pregnancy-associated hypertension and two postpartum hemorrhages occurred but thrombosis was not seen in any of the pregnancies.

Management of PV in Pregnancy

To decrease the thrombohemorrhagic complications the Hct should be maintained below 0.45, by phlebotomy if possible. Close monitoring of the Hct and platelet count should be performed on a monthly basis. Low-dose aspirin (75 mg) appears to improve the outcome for pregnant patients with ET[133,134] and should also be given in PV. Cytoreductive agents should be avoided if possible, especially in the first trimester, but if cytoreduction is essential interferon-alpha is the drug of choice. Around 20 percent of all pregnancies result in a cesarean section and both morbidity and mortality are increased in patients with PV who undergo other forms of sugery with an uncontrolled Hct. Control of the Hct prior to surgical delivery is therefore important.

For patients with previous fetal loss or those at high risk of thrombosis, low-molecular weight heparin has been reported to be useful in patients with ET.[135] Anticoagulation should be continued for 6 weeks postpartum and it is important to watch for rebound increases in the Hct and platelet count in this period.

REFERENCES

1. Vazquez M: Concerning a special form of cyanosis with accompanying excessive and persistent hyperglobulia. Compt Rend Soc Biol 44:384–388, 1892.

2. Osler W: Chronic cyanosis, with polycythaemia and enlarged spleen: A new clinical entity. Am J Med Sci 126:187–201, 1903.

3. Dameshek W: Some speculations on the myeloproliferative syndromes. Blood 6:372–375, 1951.

4. Berlin N: Classification of the polycythaemias and initial clinical features in polycythaemia vera. In Wasserman L, Berk P, Berlin N (eds.): Polycythaemia Vera and the Myeloproliferative Disorders, pp. 22–30. W.B. Saunders, Philadelphia, 1995.

5. Mesa R, Tefferri A, et al: The incidence and epidemiology of essential thrombocythemia and agnogenic myeloid metaplasia: An Olmstead County study. Blood 90(Suppl. 1):347a, 1997.

6. Prochazka AV, Markawe HLJ: The epidemiology of polycythaemia rubra vera in England and Wales 1968–1982. Br J Cancer 53:59–64, 1986.

7. Modan B: An epidemiological study of polycythemia vera. Blood 26:657–667, 1965.

8. Modan B, Kallner H, et al: A note on the increased risk of polycythemia vera in Jews. Blood 37:172–179, 1971.

9. Tatarsky I, Sharon R: Management of polycythemia vera with hydroxyurea. Semin Hematol 34:24–28, 1997.

10. Reznikoff P, Foot N, et al: Etiological and pathologic factors in polycythemia vera. Am J Med Sci 189:753–759, 1935.

11. Damon A, Holub D: Host factors in polycythemia vera. Ann Intern Med 49:43–60, 1958.

12. Committee for the Compilation of Materials on Damage Caused by the Atomic Bombs in Hiroshima and Nagasaki. Hiroshima and Nagasaki: The Physical, Medical and Social Effects of the Atomic Bombings. Basic Books, New York, 1981.

13. Caldwell G, Kelley D, et al: Polycythemia vera among participants of a nuclear weapons test. JAMA 252:662–664, 1984.

14. Gruppo Italiano Studio Policitaemia. Polycythaemia vera: The natural history of 1213 patients followed for 20 years. Ann Intern Med 123:656–664, 1995.

15. Berk P, Wasserman L, et al: Treatment of polycythemia vera: A summary of clinical trials conducted by the polycythemia vera study group. In Wasserman L, Berk P, Berlin N (eds.): Polycythemia Vera and the Myeloproliferative Disorders, pp. 166–194. W.B. Saunders, Philadelphia, 1995.

16. Tartaglia A, Goldberg J, et al: Adverse effects of antiaggregating platelet therapy in the treatment of polycythemia vera. Semin Hematol 23:172–176, 1986.

17. Westin J, Lanner L-O, et al: Spleen size in polycythaemia. Act Med Scand 191:263–271, 1972.

18. Najean Y, Rain J-D: Treatment of polycythemia vera: The use of hydroxyurea and pipobroman in 292 patients under the age of 65 years. Blood 90:3370–3377, 1997.

19. Najean Y, Rain J-D: The very long-term evolution of polycythemia vera: An analysis of 318 patients initially treated by phlebotomy or 32P between 1969 and 1981. Semin Hematol 34:6–16, 1997.

20. Pearson T, Green A, et al: Leukemic transformation in polycythemia vera. Blood 92:1837–1838, 1998.

21. Fruchtman S, Mack K, et al: From efficacy to safety: A polycythemia vera study group report on hydroxyurea in patients with polycythemia vera. Semin Hematol 34:17–23, 1997.

22. Cheivitz E, Theide T: Complications and causes of death in polycythaemia vera. Act Med Scand 172:513–523, 1962.

23. Rozman C, Giralt M, et al: Life expectancy of patients with chronic nonleukaemic myeloproliferative disorders. Cancer 67:2658–2663, 1991.

24. Hoffman R, Wasserman L: Natural history and management of polycythaemia vera. Adv Int Med 24:255–285, 1979.

25. Finazzi G, Marchiloi R, et al: Life expectancy and causes of death in 252 patients with polycythemia vera below 50 years of age. Blood 96:740a, 2000.

26. Gale R: Evaluation of clonality in myeloid stem-cell disorders. Semin Hematol 36:361–372, 1999.

27. Adamson JW, Fialkow PJ, et al: Polycythemia vera: Stem cell and probable clonal origin of the disease. N Engl J Med 295:913–916, 1976.

28. Anger B, Janssen JWG, et al: Clonal analysis of chronic myeloproliferative disorders using X-linked DNA polymorphisms. Leukemia 4:258–261, 1990.

29. Lucas GS, Padua RA, et al: The application of X-chromosome gene probes to the diagnosis of myeloproliferative disease. Br J Haematol 72:530–533, 1989.

30. Gilliland DG, Blanchard KL, et al: Clonality in myeloproliferative disorders: Analysis by means of the polymerase chain reaction. 88:6848–6852, 1991.

31. Asimakopoulos FA, Gilbert JGR, et al: Interstitial deletion constitutes the major mechanism for loss of heterozygosity on chromosome 20q in polycythemia vera. Blood 88:2690–2698, 1996.

32. Hinshelwood S, Bench AJ, et al: Pathogenesis of polycythaemia vera. Blood Rev 11:224–232, 1997.

33. Champion KM, Gilbert JGR, et al: Clonal haemopoiesis in normal elderly women: Implications for the myeloproliferative disorders and myelodysplastic syndromes. Br J Haematol 97:920–926, 1997.

34. Gale RE, Fielding AK, et al: Acquired skewing of X-chromosome inactivation patterns in myeloid cells of the elderly suggests stochastic clonal loss with age. Br J Haematol 98:512–519, 1997.

35. Morrison SJ, Wandycz AM, et al: The aging of hematopoietic stem cells. Nat Med 2:1011–1016, 1996.

36. Christensen K, Kristiansen M, et al: X-linked genetic factors regulate stem-cell kinetics in females. Blood 95:2449–2451, 2000.

37. Vickers M, McLeod E, et al: Assessment of mechanism of acquired skewed X inactivation by analysis of twins. Blood 97:1274–1281, 2001.

38. Abkowitz JL, Taboada M, et al: An X chromosome gene regulates hematopoietic stem cell kinetics. Proc Natl Acad Sci USA 95:3862–3866, 1998.

39. Prchel JF, Axelrad AA: Bone marrow responses in polycythemia vera. N Engl J Med 290:1382(letter), 1974.

40. Fisher MJ, Prchal JF, et al: Anti-erythropoietin (EPO) receptor monoclonal antibodies distinguish EPO-dependent and EPO-

independent erythroid progenitors in polycythemia vera. Blood 84:1982–1991, 1994.

41. Eaves CJ, Eaves AC: Erythropoietin (Ep) dose-response curves for three classes of erythroid progenitors in normal human marrow and in patients with polycythemia vera. Blood 52:1196–1199, 1978.

42. Dudley JM, Westwood N, et al: Primary polycythaemia: Positive diagnosis using the differential response of primitive and mature erythroid progenitors to erythropoietin, interleukin-3 and alpha interferon. Br J Haematol 75:188–194, 1990.

43. Dai CH, Krantz SB: et al: Polycythemia vera II. Hypersensitivity of bone marrow erythroid, granulocyte-macrophage and megakaryocyte progenitor cells to interleukin-3 and granulocyte-macrophage colony-stimulating factor. Blood 80:891–899, 1992.

44. Dai CH, Krantz SB, et al: Polycythaemia vera III. Burst-forming units-erythroid (BFU-E) response to stem cell factor and c-kit receptor expression. Br J Haematol 86:12–21, 1994.

45. Correa PN, Eskinazi D, et al: Circulating erythroid progenitors in polycythemia vera are hypersensitive to insulin-like growth factor-1 in vitro: Studies in an improved serum-free medium. Blood 83:99–112, 1994.

46. Kobayashi S, Teramura M, et al: Circulating megakaryocyte progenitors in myeloproliferative disorders are hypersensitive to interleukin-3. Br J Haematol 83:539–544, 1993.

47. Li Y, Hetet G, et al: Spontaneous megakaryocyte colony formation in myeloproliferative disorders is not neutralizable by antibodies against IL3, IL6 and GM-CSF. Br J Haematol 87:471–476, 1994.

48. de La Chapelle A, Traskelin AL, et al: Truncated erythropoietin receptor causes dominantly inherited benign human erythrocytosis. Proc Natl Acad Sci USA 90:4495–4499, 1993.

49. Kralovics R, Indrak K, et al: Two new EPO receptor mutations: Truncated EPO receptors are most frequently associated with primary familial and congenital polycythemias. Blood 90:2057–2061, 1997.

50. Prchal JT, Sokol L: "Benign erythrocytosis" and other familial and congenital polycythemias. Eur J Haematol 57:263–268, 1996.

51. Percy MJ, McMullin MF, et al: Erythrocytosis due to a mutation in the erythropoietin receptor gene. Br J Haematol 100:407–410, 1998.

52. Le Couedic J-P, Mitjavila M-T, et al: Missense mutation of the erythropoietin receptor is a rare event in human erythroid malignancies. Blood 87:1502–1511, 1996.

53. Hess G, Rose P, et al: Molecular analysis of erythropoietin receptor system in patients with polycythaemia vera. Br J Haematol 88:794–802, 1994.

54. Chiba S, Takahashi T, et al: Selective expression of mRNA coding for the truncated form of erythropoietin receptor in hematopoietic cells and its decrease in patients with polycythemia. Blood 90:97–104, 1997.

55. Haber D, Harlow E: Tumour suppressor genes: Evolving definitions in the genomic age. Nat Genet 16:320–322, 1997.

56. Asimakopoulos FA, Hinshelwood S, et al: The gene encoding hematopoietic cell phosphatase (SHP-1) is structurally and transcriptionally intact in polycythemia vera. Oncogene 14:1215–1222, 1997.

57. Sui X, Krantz SB, et al: Identification of increased protein tyrosine phosphatase activity in polycythemia vera erythroid progenitor cells. Blood 90:651–657, 1997.

58. Mirza AM, Correa PN, et al: Increased basal and induced tyrosine phosphorylation of the insulin-like growth-factor-I receptor-beta subunit in circulating mononuclear-cells of patients with polycythemia-vera. Blood 86:877–882, 1995.

59. Moliterno AR, Hankins WD, et al: Impaired expression of the thrombopoietin receptor by platelets from patients with polycythemia vera. N Engl J Med 338:572–580, 1998.

60. Westwood N, Raj K, et al: Platelet expression of mpl is diminished in reactive thrombocytosis and myeloproliferative disorders but is normal in secondary erythrocytosis. Blood 94(Suppl. 1):112a, 1999.

61. Tefferi A, Yoon S-Y, et al: Immunohistochemical staining for megakaryocyte c-mpl may complement morphological distinction between polycythaemia vera and secondary erythrocytosis. Blood 96:771–772, 2000.

62. Horikawa Y, Matsumura I, et al: Markedly reduced expression of platelet c-mpl receptor in essential thrombocythaemia. Blood 90:4031–4038, 1997.

63. Harrison C, Gale R, et al: Platelet c-mpl expression is dysregulated in patients with essential thrombocythaemia but is not of diagnostic value. Br J Haematol 107:139–147, 1999.

64. Le Blanc K, Andersson P, et al: Marked heterogeneity in protein levels and functional integrity of the thrombopoietin receptor c-mpl in polycythaemia vera. Br J Haematol 108:80–85, 2000.

65. Moliterno A, Williams D, et al: An increase in mpl splice variants in polycythaemia vera platelets. Blood 94(Suppl. 1):112a, 1999.

66. Moliterno A, Spivak J: Posttranslational processing of the thrombopoietin receptor is impaired in polycythemia vera. Blood 94:2555–2561, 1999.

67. Silva M, Richard C, et al: Expression of Bcl-x$_L$ in erythroid precursors from patients with polycythaemia vera. N Engl J Med 338:564–571, 1998.

68. Temerinac S, Klippel S, et al: Cloning of PRV-1, a novel member of the uPAR receptor superfamily, which is overexpressed in polycythaemia rubra vera. Blood 95:2569–2576, 2000.

69. Bench AJ, Nacheva EP, et al: Molecular genetics and cytogenetics of myeloproliferative disorders. In Green AR, Pearson TC (eds.): Myeloproliferative Disorders, pp. 819–848. Baillière Tindall, London, UK, 1999.

70. Diez-Martin JL, Graham DL, et al: Chromosome studies in 104 patients with polycythemia vera. Mayo Clin Proc 66:287–299, 1991.

71. Dewald GW, Schad CR, et al: Frequency and photographs of HGM11 chromosome anomalies in bone marrow samples from 3,996 patients with malignant hematologic neoplasms. Cancer Genet Cytogenet 68:60–69, 1993.

72. Asimakopoulos FA, Green AR: Deletions of chromosome 20q and the pathogenesis of myeloproliferative disorders. Br J Haematol 95:219–226, 1996.

73. Mori N, Morosetti R, et al: Allotype analysis in the evolution of chronic myelocytic leukemia. Blood 90:2010–2014, 1997.

74. Aatola M, Armstrong E, et al: Clinical significance of the del 20(q) chromosome in haematologic disorders. Cancer Genet Cytogenet 62:75–80, 1992.

75. Davis MP, Dewald GW, et al: Haematologic manifestations associated with deletions of the long arm of chromosome 20. Cancer Genet Cytogenet 12:63–71, 1984.

76. Campbell LJ, Garson OM: The prognostic significance of deletion of the long arm of chromosome 20 in myeloid disorders. Leukemia 8:67–71, 1984.

77. Hollings PE: Molecular heterogeneity at the breakpoints of smaller 20q deletions. Genes Chrom Cancer 11:21–28, 1994.

78. White NJ, Nacheva E, et al: Deletion of chromosome 20q in myelodysplasia occurring in multipotent precursor of both myeloid cells and B cells. Blood 83:2809–2816, 1994.

79. Asimakopoulos FA, Holloway TL, et al: Detection of chromosome 20q deletions in bone marrow metaphases but not peripheral blood granulocytes in patients with myeloproliferative disorders or myelodysplastic syndromes. Blood 87:1561–1570, 1996.

80. Roulston D, Espinosa R III, et al: Molecular genetics of myeloid leukemia: Identification of the commonly deleted segment of chromosome 20. Blood 82:3424–3429, 1993.

81. Asimakopoulos FA, White NJ, et al: Molecular analysis of chromosome 20q deletions associated with myeloproliferative disorders and myelodyslastic syndromes. Blood 84:3086–3094, 1994.

82. Bench AJ, Aldred MA, et al: A detailed physical and transcriptional map of the region of chromosome 20 that is deleted in myeloproliferative disorders and refinement of the common deleted region. Genomics 49:351–362, 1998.

83. Wang PW, Iannantuoni K, et al: Refinement of the common deleted segment in myeloid leukemias with a del(20q). Gene Chromosom Cancer 21:75–81, 1998.

84. Bench A, Nacheva E, et al: Chromosome 20 deletions in myeloid malignancies: Reduction of the common deleted region, generation of a PAC contig and identification of candidate genes. Oncogene 19:3902–3913, 2000.

85. Wang P, Eisenbart J, et al: Refinement of the smallest commonly deleted segment of chromosome 20 in malignant myeloid diseases and development of a PAC-based physical and transcription map. Genomics 67:28–39, 2000.

86. La Starza R, Wlodarska I, et al: Molecular delineation of 13q deletion boundaries in 20 patients with myeloid malignancies. Blood 91:231–237, 1998.

87. Gardiner A, Corcoran M, et al: An analysis of chromosome 13q14 deletions in myelofibrosis using FISH and Southern-based hybridisation. Blood 90(Suppl. 1):292b, 1997.

88. Pearson T, Messinezy M, et al: A polycythaemia vera update: Diagnosis, pathobiology, and treatment. In Schectner G, Berliner N, Telen M (eds.): Hematology 2000, pp. 51–56. American Society of Hematology, San Francisco, 2000.

89. Williams W, Nelson D, et al: Examination of the blood. In Williams W, Beutler E, Erslev A, Lichtman M (eds.): Haematology, pp. 9–23, McGraw-Hill, New York, 1990.

90. Pearson T: Apparent polycythaemia. Blood Rev 5:205–213, 1991.

91. Pearson T, Guthrie D, et al: Interpretation of measured red cell mass and plasma volume in adults: Expert Panel on Radionuclides of the International Council for Standards in Haematology. Br J Haematol 89:748–756, 1995.

92. Pearson TC, Messinezy M: The diagnostic criteria of polycythaemia rubra vera. Leuk Lymphoma 22:87–93, 1996.

93. Najean Y, Schlageter M, et al: Radioimmunoassay of immunoreactive erythropoietin as a clinical tool for the classification of polycythaemias. Nouv Rev Fr Hematol 32:237–240, 1990.

94. Wolfe J, Tashkin D, et al: Hypoxemia of cirrhosis: Detection of small abnormal pulmonary vascular channels by a quantitative radionuclide method. Am J Med 635:746, 1977.

95. Messinezy M, MacDonald L, et al: Spleen sizing by ultrasound in polycythaemia and thrombocythaemia: Comparison with SPECT. Br J Haematol 98:103–107, 1997.

96. Berlin N: Diagnosis and classification of polycythaemia. Semin Hematol 12:339–351, 1975.

97. Michiels J, Juvonen E: Proposal for revised diagnostic criteria of essential thrombocythaemia and polycythaemia by the thrombocythaemia vera study group. Semin Thromb Hemost 23:339–347, 1997.

98. Georgii A, Buesche G, et al: The histopathology of chronic myeloproliferative diseases. In Green AR, Pearson TC (eds.): Myeloproliferative Disorders, pp. 721–749. Baillière Tindall, London, 1999.

99. Cazzola M, Guamone R, et al: Congenital erythropoietin-dependent erythrocytosis responsive to theophylline therapy. Blood 91:360–361, 1998.

100. Manglani M, DeGroff C, et al: Congenital erythrocytosis with elevated erythropoietin level: An incorrectly set "erythrostat"? J Pediatr Hematol Oncol 20:560–562, 1998.

101. Walterspiel JN, Buchanan GR et al: Erythropoictin-induced congenital erythrocytosis: Treatment with myelosuppressive agent and hookworm infestation. J Pediatr 107:575–577, 1985.

102. Borgna-Pignatti C, Liberato N, et al: Regulation of erythropoietin production in a case of congenital erythropoietin-dependent pure erythrocytosis. Am J Hematol 46:348–353, 1994.

103. Berk P, Goldberg J, et al: Therapeutic recommendations in polycythaemia vera based upon Polycythaemia Vera Study Group protocols. Semin Hematol 23:132–143, 1986.

104. Thomas DJ, du Boulay GH et al: Cerebral blood flow in polycthoemia. Lancet 2:161–163, 1977.

105. Pearson T, Wetherley-Mein G: Vascular occlusive episodes and venous haematocrit in primary proliferative polycythaemia. Lancet 2:1219–1222, 1978.

106. Nand S, Messmore H, et al: Leukemic transformation in PV: Analysis of risk factors. Am J Hematol 34:32–36, 1990.

107. Landaw S: Acute leukemia in polycythemia vera. Semin Hematol 23:156–165, 1986.

108. Kaplan M, Mack K, et al: Long term management of polycythaemia vera with hydroxyurea: A progress report. Semin Hematol 23:167–171, 1986.

109. West W: Hydroxyurea in the treatment of polycythemia vera: A prospective study of 100 patients over a 20 year period. South Med J 80:323–327, 1987.

110. Hanft V, Fruchtman S, et al: Acquired DNA mutations associated with in vivo hydroxyurea exposure. Blood 95:3589–3593, 2000.

111. Sterkers Y, Preudhomme C, et al: Acute myeloid leukaemia and myelodysplastic syndromes following essential thrombocythaemia treated with hydroxyurea: High proportion of cases with 17p deletions. Blood 91:616–622, 1998.

112. Castello G, Lerza L, et al: The in vitro and in vivo effect of recombinant interferon α–2a on circulating haemopoietic progenitors in polycythemia vera. Br J Haematol 87:621–623, 1994.

113. Ganser A, Carlo-Stella C, et al: Effects of interferons α and γ on human bone marrow-derived megakaryocytic progenitors. Blood 70:1173–1179, 1987.

114. The Italian Cooperative Study Group on Chronic Myeloid Leukemia. Interferon-alpha 2a as compared with conventional chemotherapy for the treatment of chronic myeloid leukemia. N Engl J Med 330:820–825, 1994.

115. Allan N, Richards S, et al: UK Medical Research Council randomised multicentre trial of interferon-alpha for chronic myeloid leukemia: Improved survival irrespective of cytogenetic response. Lancet 345:1392–1397, 1995.

116. Silver R: Interferon-α: Effects of long-term treatment for polycythemia vera. Semin Hematol 34:40–50, 1997.

117. Taylor P, Dolan G, et al: Efficacy of recombinant interferon alpha (rIFN-α) in polycythemia vera: A study of 17 patients and an analysis of published data. Br J Haematol 92:55–59, 1996.

118. Elliot M, Tefferi A: Interferon-α therapy in polycythaemia vera and essential thrombocythaemia. Semin Thromb Hemost 23:463–472, 1997.

119. Reilly J, Vellenga E, et al: Interferon treatment in polycythemia vera. Leuk Lymphoma 22(Suppl. 1): 143–148, 1996.

120. Silver R: Interferon-α 2b: A new treatment for polycythemia vera. Ann Int Med 119:1091–1092, 1993.

121. Anagrelide Study Group: Anagrelide: A therapy for thrombocythemic states: Experience in 577 patients. Am J Med 92:69–76, 1992.

122. Antiplatelet Trialists' Collaboration. Collaborative overview of randomised trials of anti-platelet therapy—I. Prevention of death, myocardial infarction and stroke by prolonged antiplatelet therapy in various categories of patient. BMJ 308:81–106, 1994.

123. Ferguson J, Ueland K, et al: Polycythaemia vera and pregnancy. Obstet Gynaecol 62:16–20, 1983.

124. Wright S, Tuddenham E: Myeloproliferative and metabolic causes. In Meade T (ed.): Thrombophilia, pp. 591–635. Balliere Tindall, London, 1994.

125. Greisshammer M, Bergmann L, et al: Fertility, pregnancy and the management of myeloproliferative disorders. In Green A, Pearson T (eds.): Myeloproliferative disorders. Baillière Tindall, London, 1988.

126. Delmer A, Rio B, et al: Pregnancy during myelosuppressive treatment for chronic myelogenous leukaemia. Br J Haematol 82:783–784, 1992.

127. Creagh M, Toh C: Experience with hydroxyurea in the management of essential thrombocythaemia and pregnancy. Br J Haematol 93(Suppl. 1):16, 1996.

128. Doll D, Ringenberg Q, et al: Antineoplastic agents and pregnancy. Semin Oncol 16:337–346, 1989.

129. Chaube S, Simmel E, et al: Hydroxyurea, a teratogenic chemical. 4:10, 1963.

130. Delage R, Demers C, et al: Treatment of essential thrombocythaemia during pregnancy with interferon alpha. Obstet Gynecol 87:814–817, 1996.

131. Diez-Martin J, Banas M, et al: Childbearing age patients with essential thrombocythaemia: Should they be placed on interferon. Am J Hematol 52:331–332, 1996.

132. Haggstrom J, Adriansson M, et al: Two cases of CML treated with alpha-interferon during second and third trimester of pregnancy with analysis of the drug in the new-born immediately postpartum. Eur J Haematol 56:101–102, 1996.

133. Zahner J, Wehmeien A, et al: Schwangerschaft bei essentieller thrombozythaime. Manifestationzeitpunkt und risken fur mutter und kind. Deut Med Wokenschrift 120:1517–1523, 1995.

134. Greisshammer M, Bangerter M, et al: Aspirin in essential thrombocythaemia: Status quo and quo vadis. Semin Thromb Hemost 23:371–377, 1996.

135. Hunt B, Doughty H, et al: Thromboprophylaxis with low-molecular weight heparin (Fragmin) in high risk pregnancies. Thromb Hemost 77:39–43, 1997.

136. Bench AJ, et al: Myeloproliferative disorders. In Buckle, Henry (eds.): Cytogenetics in Haemotology. Baillière Tindall, London, in press.

137. Haanen C, Mathe G et al: Treatment of polycythaemia vera by radiophosphorus or busulphan: A randomized clinical trial. Br J Cancer 44:75–80, 1981.

10

The Diagnosis and Treatment of Essential Thrombocythemia and Chronic Idiopathic Myelofibrosis

John T. Reilly, Maria Messinezy, and Thomas C. Pearson

ESSENTIAL THROMBOCYTHEMIA

Essential thrombocythemia (ET) was regarded as a disease of the elderly with a median age of presentation of 60 years. However, increasingly more young patients, particularly women, are being found to have ET. Classically, it is a clonal disorder originating in a multipotent stem cell. However, definite clonal hemopoiesis has been shown in only half of young female ET patients.[1] "Nonclonal" ET patients are either at an early stage of evolution of classical ET or other mechanisms are involved. A few families with thrombocytosis have been described. Some of these show high thrombopoietin (TPO) production due to one of several different mutations in the TPO gene. This indicates that other mechanisms causing excessive megakaryopoiesis occur and still others have yet to be discovered.

Thrombocytoses can be divided into primary, in which megakaryopoiesis is abnormal, and secondary, in which megakaryopoiesis is normal. Primary causes are ET, polycythemia vera (PV), chronic myeloid leukemia (CML), chronic idiopathic myelofibrosis (CIMF), and myelodysplasia (MDS). Secondary causes include the commonly encountered acquired type; the causes of which are listed in Table 10–1, and the rare familial congenital type with high TPO production.

The Diagnosis of Essential Thrombocythemia

As shown in Table 10–2, the diagnostic criteria of ET are mostly designed to exclude other disease processes. Essential thrombo-

Table 10–1. Causes of Secondary Acquired Thrombocytosis

Acute hemorrhage
Malignant disease (e.g., carcinoma, Hodgkin's and non-Hodgkin's lymphoma)
Chronic inflammatory disorders (e.g., rheumatoid arthritis, ulcerative colitis)
Acute inflammation
Postoperation
Splenectomy and hyposplenism
Marrow recovery from drug suppression, or response to hematinic following deficiency
Iron deficiency

Table 10–2. The Diagnostic Criteria of Essential Thrombocythemia

1. Platelet count above 600×10^9/L (trial); above 400×10^9/L (clinical)
2. No cause of a secondary "reactive" thrombocytosis
3. Normal red cell mass if hematocrit above 51 percent in males, above 47 percent in females, and in those with high normal hematocrit and demonstrable splenomegaly
4. Stainable iron in marrow or normal serum ferritin or normal red cell mean corpuscular volume (if measurement suggests iron deficiency, polycythemia vera cannot be excluded unless a trial of iron therapy fails to increase the red cell mass into the erythrocytotic range)
5. No Philadelphia chromosome or bcr/abl gene rearrangement
6. No histological evidence to support polycythemia vera or chronic idiopathic myelofibrosis
7. No cytogenetic or morphological evidence of a myelodysplastic syndrome

cythemia will remain a heterogenous disease until a specific diagnostic marker is established.[1]

Platelet Count

The normal reference range extends to 400×10^9/L. For clinical trials of ET, counts over 600×10^9/L have been used as an inclusion criterion. However, patients who eventually are shown clearly to have ET can present with thrombotic complications with normal counts.[2] Thus, in clinical practice a count over 400×10^9/L may be taken as the initial diagnostic criterion for ET. Detailed investigation is warranted in patients with persisting thrombocytosis without obvious cause, notably where establishment of a diagnosis of ET would alter clinical management.

Clinical Features and Exclusion of Secondary Thrombocytosis

Vascular occlusion occurs much more commonly in ET than in secondary thrombocytoses (ST). This is particularly true of vasomotor symptoms, such as erythromelalgia and microvascular occlusion. Palpable splenomegaly can be found in ET, but a diagnosis of PV or CIMF should be considered when there is significant splenomegaly. Splenomegaly, demonstrated only by using scanning techniques, occurs in up to a third of ET patients[3] and has a supporting diagnostic role.

The possibility of a familial thrombocytosis is worth exploring in young patients. The majority of the other causes of ST are established by the patient's history and appropriate investigation. Generally, nonspecific markers of a "reactive" state, notably a raised erythrocyte sedimentation rate and C-reactive protein but also serum IL-6 and plasma fibrinogen, are useful.[4]

Qualitative Platelet Changes and Thrombopoietin Levels

A large number of qualitative platelet abnormalities have been described in ET.[5] These include platelet size heterogeneity, reflected in a raised PDW, a storage pool deficiency, reduced aggregation to various agonists, particularly epinephrine, spontaneous platelet aggregation, and defects in arachidonic acid metabolism. These are also found in other myeloproliferative disorders but only occasionally in ST.

Plasma TPO levels are normal or raised and platelet expression of the TPO receptor, c-mpl, is normal or reduced in ET and ST.[6] Therefore, these measurements have no diagnostic value.

Hematopoietic Progenitor Culture Studies

The growth from peripheral blood of so-called endogenous erythroid colonies, BFU-E growing in serum-containing medium without additional erythropoietin, is found in 60 to 70 percent of ET patients.[7] Endogenous megakaryocytic colonies may also be found in ET patients, but there is disagreement on whether this finding is useful in separating ET from ST.[5]

Clonality Markers

The marrow karyotype is nearly always normal in ET. The 1 to 2 percent of ET patients who have variable karyotypic abnormalities might represent a subgroup with a poorer prognosis.[8] The use of X chromosome-linked probes to establish clonality has limitations in female patients over 60 years, 25 to 30 percent of whom have apparent clonal granulocytes.[9,10] In younger patients, only half can be shown to have clonal hemopoiesis, as discussed earlier, but this finding carries diagnostic significance.

Marrow Histology

Marrow histology is useful in the separation of acquired ST, in which the megakaryocyte morphology is normal, from ET and in distinguishing the various MPDs[11,12] (Table 10–3). The key features in support of ET are the normal cellularity and granulopoiesis and the megakaryocyte morphology.

Exclusion of Polycythemia Vera

The hallmark of PV is a raised red cell mass (RCM), which should be measured in patients with high normal or raised hematocrit values (Table 10–2). Judicious iron therapy may be used in those presenting with iron deficiency to see if the hematocrit rises to an abnormally high value. Plasma erythropoietin levels are reduced, as in PV, in up to half of ET patients.[13] In approximately 5 to 10 percent of ET patients, ET transforms to PV in 5 to 10 years after diagnosis.

Exclusion of Chronic Myeloid Leukemia

Occasional patients with chronic myeloid leukemia (CML) show predominantly a thrombocytosis with little or no leukocytosis. Basophilia and/or left shift in granulocytes supports CML rather than ET. Generally, the finding of the ph[1] chromosome establishes CML. Very rarely, the marrow karyotype is normal but bcr/abl fusion can be shown.

Exclusion of Chronic Idiopathic Myelofibrosis

Differentiation of ET from CIMF can occasionally present difficulties, since CIMF may present in a cellular phase with thrombocytosis and ET may undergo myelofibrotic transformation. Features that support CIMF are splenomegaly, typically larger than seen in ET, and peripheral blood leukoerythroblastic change and teardrop poikilocytosis. Marrow histology holds a key diagnostic position in distinguishing the cellular phase of CIMF from ET (Table 10–3). Currently, there is not total agreement on the differentiation of ET from a prefibrotic form of CIMF, but a small proportion of patients diagnosed with ET on other grounds do have the changes as given in Table 10–3 of an early form of CIMF. This may have significance in their disease evolution.

Exclusion of Myelodysplastic Syndromes

A few patients with MDS present with a thrombocytosis. Trilineage dysplasia is the hallmark of MDS. Megakaryocytic hyperplasia, sometimes with marked reticulin increase, may be observed in some MDS patients, but the megakaryocytic dysplasia with small, hypolobulated forms are quite distinct from the changes seen in ET.[14] Cytogenetic abnormalities occur in 30

Table 10–3. Typical Marrow Histological Findings in the Myeloproliferative Disorders

Diagnosis	Cellularity	Erythropoiesis	Iron Stores	Granulopoiesis	Megakaryopoiesis	Reticulin
Essential thrombocythemia	Normal	Normal	Present	Normal	Markedly increased in clusters. Megakaryocytes typically large with abundant cytoplasm and increased nuclear ploidy. No dysmegakaryopoiesis	Normal or modest increase
Polycythemia vera	Increased	Increased	Absent	Increased	Increased, with clustered small to large megakaryocytes with no dysmegakaryopoiesis	Normal or moderate increase
Chronic myeloid leukemia	Increased	Decreased	Present	Markedly Increased	Increased, with small megakaryocytes with reduced ploidy	Normal or moderate increase
Chronic idiopathic myelofibrosis. (in cellular phase)	Increased	Normal or reduced	Present	Increased	Increased with clusters. Small to large megakaryocytes but without very large forms seen in ET and with dysmegakaryopoiesis	Normal (prefibrotic form) to markedly increased

to 50 percent of MDS patients. Patients with the 5q syndrome commonly have a thrombocytosis, but this can also be seen in patients with normal cytogenetics.[14,15]

Treatment of Essential Thrombocythemia

The aim of treatment, as with all diseases, is to reduce morbidity and mortality. Symptoms are present in 30 to 50 percent of patients at diagnosis. An increased incidence of thrombosis in small and (less often) in large vessels and of hemorrhage is well established in ET, particularly in older patients, who form the majority. There is also a small but definite risk of transformation to myelofibrosis and to acute leukemia. Whether transformation is influenced by treatment has not been established by prospective studies. Myelosuppressive (cytoreductive) treatment does decrease the thrombotic risk in older patients and in younger patients who have already experienced a thrombotic event (see below). It has been difficult to establish any improvement in survival, which anyway only becomes somewhat curtailed after many years. The existence of a group of younger patients with ET, (mentioned above), possibly having a rather different natural history and disease process, has been a focus of recent attention. There is particular anxiety about the potential risks of the prolonged use of cytoreductive agents if they were used routinely in this age group. No treatment that eradicates the abnormal clone is currently available.

Antiaggregating Agents

Microvascular occlusion, resulting in symptoms such as painful digits leading to gangrene, transient ischemic attacks, migraine, and erythromelalgia is definitely improved by aspirin.[16] A maintenance dose of 75 mg is usually sufficient and reduces the risk of peptic ulceration associated with larger doses, although it also increases the risk of hemorrhage, particularly at platelet counts above $1,000 \times 10^9$/L. In the occasional patient who has side effects, aspirin may be replaced by dipyridamole, clopidogrel, or newer antiaggregating agents. Whether aspirin reduces the incidence of major vascular occlusion is uncertain. In younger patients who have not had a thrombotic event or other risk factors for thrombosis (hypertension, diabetes, consistently very high platelet counts) treatment of ET by aspirin alone is almost universally accepted.

Cytoreductive Agents

The value of platelet count reduction in ET depends on the estimated risk of major thrombotic or hemorrhagic complications in the untreated patient. The parameters that separate patients into different risk categories are still somewhat uncertain, but there is widespread agreement that older patients with higher platelet counts (rather arbitrary values of 60 years and above 1,000 or $1,500 \times 10^9$/L may be taken), or other thrombotic risk factors as above (particularly a previous ischemic event or thrombosis) would benefit from a cytoreductive agent.[17] Disagreement mainly occurs in the management of young and middle-aged patients, in whom the need for prospective trials is particularly strong. The risk of thrombotic problems in young

untreated patients is uncertain, although there is growing recognition that it may not be negligible.

Hydroxyurea   Hydroxyurea slows DNA synthesis and repair by inhibiting ribonucleotide reductase, which results in reduction of red cells and white cells as well as platelets. It is the most extensively used myelosuppressive agent in the treatment of ET as well as other myeloproliferative disorders. It has to be taken regularly by mouth, and there is a risk of rebound rise of the platelet count if it is stopped suddenly. It can be difficult to maintain a platelet count steadily below the usual target of 400×10^9/L in some patients, and there is sometimes an unacceptable degree of macrocytic anemia or neutropenia. Mild gastrointestinal and cutaneous side effects are not usually a problem, although troublesome leg ulceration can occur and is a contraindication to hydroxyurea use. It is still uncertain whether hydroxyurea increases the background risk of transformation to acute leukemia, a feature of particular relevance in young patients with potentially prolonged exposure. Sterkers et al.[18] in a retrospective study found an incidence of 3.5 percent of acute leukemia or myelodysplasia in patients with ET treated with hydroxyurea alone at a mean follow-up time of 98 months. A decreased risk of myelofibrotic transformation in patients taking hydroxyurea has not yet been established in ET but is a possibility, particularly in those who have histological changes of the so-called prefibrotic myelofibrosis group. Cortelazzo et al.[19] have demonstrated a significant decrease of thrombotic episodes in "high-risk" patients treated with hydroxyurea and compared these patients prospectively with a randomized control group who had no myelosuppression. They observed a 3.6 percent incidence of thrombotic episodes in treated versus 24 percent in untreated patients over a median follow-up period of 27 months. The ability of other platelet-lowering agents (discussed below) to achieve clinical benefit is presumed but has not yet been demonstrated. The use of an untreated "high-risk" control group of patients would now be difficult to justify in prospective trials.

Alpha-interferon   The attraction of a presumed nonleukemogenic agent with the potential to eradicate an abnormal hemopoietic clone has led to the use of α-interferon especially in the young. It can successfully reduce the platelet count, and a maintenance dose of approximately 9 milliunits/week is required.[20] Very occasionally, short remissions occur without the requirement for α-interferon therapy. However, the persistence of nonspecific side effects, rather than the inconvenience of subcutaneous injections, means that more than half of the patients cannot sustain treatment in the long term, thus delaying knowledge of any crucial effects on the progression of ET.

Anagrelide   The oral agent anagrelide was unexpectedly found to specifically reduce platelet counts by inhibiting megakaryocyte platelet budding and is active in 95 percent of patients. It is not expected to have neoplastic potential. Its convenience and probable long-term advantages are now becoming attractive, especially for younger patients. Its use in older patients with ischemic heart disease or cardiac failure is discouraged. Other side effects caused by the drug's vasodilatory action (headaches, diarrhea) and positive inotropic action (palpitations) are usually transient.[21] However, some 20 percent of patients do not tolerate the drug. The results of prospective randomized studies comparing anagrelide with hydroxyurea in terms of thrombotic risk and marrow transformation are awaited.

Busulfan   Suspicion of the potential long-term side effects of all alkylating agents, as well as the risk of prolonged bone marrow suppression, means that busulfan is no longer favored for the treatment of ET, although it has some specific effect on proliferating megakaryocytes. However, it has been successfully and conveniently used in surprisingly small intermittent doses by some centers.[22] Its use is now mainly confined to elderly patients. A recent study suggesting an increased risk of second malignancies after sequential use of busulfan and hydroxyurea strikes a further warning note.[23]

Future Directions

Important future aims in the management of ET are to identify further parameters (e.g., clonality and histological evidence of prefibrotic myelofibrosis) that may predict vascular and disease transformation risks. This would help direct appropriate treatment with the lowest cost/benefit ratio in what is clearly a heterogenous disease.[1] The potential of bone marrow transplantation in ET has not yet been assessed. In any event it would only be considered in the few younger patients who have thrombotic events in spite of optimal traditional treatment.

Pregnancy Effects

Pregnancy is often associated with a spontaneous fall in the platelet count, sometimes to normal levels. Nevertheless, there is an increased first-trimester spontaneous abortion rate (35 percent) and also a higher risk of intrauterine death, growth retardation, and premature delivery (presumably associated with placental vascular occlusion), so that the live birth rate in ET patients may only be a little over 50 percent.[24] Low-dose aspirin is widely recommended. Current or previous thrombotic or hemorrhagic complications or a platelet count above $1,000 \times 10^9/L$ would point toward the use of α-interferon as a cytoreductive agent (hydroxyurea and anagrelide are contraindicated in pregnancy). Additional use of low molecular weight heparin, particularly in those with a previous thrombosis, is an option. Patients are at thrombotic risk particularly in the puerperium, when the use of aspirin, low molecular weight heparin, and possibly cytoreduction should be considered. Further retrospective and particularly prospective studies in pregnant patients with ET are needed.

Acute Management of Essential Thrombocythemia

Patients presenting with ET-related hemorrhage may paradoxically need platelet transfusion to increase the number of normally functioning platelets. Platelet apheresis to reduce the platelet count rapidly while the response to hydroxyurea is awaited has sometimes been used for both persisting hemorrhage and evolving thrombosis. Early use of aspirin (300 mg) in ischemic or thrombotic situations is recommended, and anticoagulation with heparin or warfarin can be considered. Some

bleeding patients with ET have an acquired von Willebrand's disease. The use of desmopressin and von Willebrand's factor concentrate is an option in this situation.

CHRONIC IDIOPATHIC MYELOFIBROSIS

Chronic idiopathic myelofibrosis (CIMF), also known as agnogenic myeloid metaplasia, is a chronic stem cell disorder distinguished by bone marrow fibrosis, extramedullary hematopoiesis, splenomegaly, and a leukoerythroblastic blood picture.

Hematological Features and Diagnosis

Barosi and colleagues[25] have published diagnostic criteria for CIMF (Table 10–4). There is a progressive change in the marrow histology over time. Initially, there is a proliferative phase, in which the marrow is hypercellular, all hemopoietic elements are retained, and the increased fibrous tissue consists of increased coarse reticulin in parallel bundles (Table 10–3). Finally, an osteomyelosclerotic stage is reached, in which there is replacement with highly vascular fibrous tissue containing new bone and markedly dysplastic megakaryocytes. As a result of these marrow changes, the peripheral blood findings are variable, although leukoerythroblastic change is typical. Anemia develops over time. Thrombocytosis may be present initially but can develop later in some patients. The white count is variable. Often pancytopenia with the presence of a small percentage of blast cells eventually occurs. There is progressive splenic and often hepatic enlargement, and myeloid metaplasia in other organs may occasionally be found late in the disease process. Transformation to acute myeloblastic leukemia occurs in approximately 20 percent of patients.

The differential diagnosis encompasses the many causes of secondary bone marrow fibrosis (Table 10–5). Whereas

---

Table 10–4. The Italian Criteria for the Diagnosis of Chronic Idiopathic Myelofibrosis

Necessary criteria
   Necessary criteria
   Absence of Philadelphia chromosome or bcr-abl
      rearrangement in peripheral blood cells
Optional criteria
   Splenomegaly
   Anisopoikilocytosis with tear-drop erythrocytes
   Presence of circulating immature myeloid cells
   Presence of circulating erythroblasts
   Presence of clusters of megakaryocytes and
      dysmegakaryopoiesis in bone marrow sections
   Myeloid metaplasia

Adapted from those given by the Italian Cooperative Study Group on Myelofibrosis with Myeloid Metaplasia.
Diagnosis of idiopathic myelofibrosis is acceptable if the following combinations are present: the two necessary criteria plus any other two optional criteria when splenomegaly is present; the two necessary criteria plus any other four criteria when splenomegaly is absent. Based on the publication of Barosi et al.[25]

Table 10–5. Conditions Associated with Bone Marrow Fibrosis

Malignant	Nonmalignant
Chronic idiopathic myelofibrosis	Infections (e.g., tuberculosis, visceral leishmaniasis, histoplasmosis, HIV)
Other chronic myeloproliferative disorders (e.g., PV, CML, ET)	Renal osteodystrophy
Acute megakaryoblastic leukemia (Acute myelofibrosis)	Vitamin D deficiency
Myelodysplastic syndromes	Hypothyroidism
Acute myeloid leukemia	Hyperthyroidism
Acute lymphoblastic leukemia	Gray platelet syndrome
	Systemic lupus erythematosis
Hairy cell leukemia	Scleroderma
Hodgkin's disease	Radiation exposure
Non-Hodgkin's lymphoma	Benzene exposure
Multiple myeloma	Gaucher's disease
Systemic mastocytosis	Osteopetrosis
Metastatic carcinoma (e.g., breast, prostate, stomach)	

Abbreviations: PV, polycythemia vera; CML, chronic myelocytic leukemia; ET, essential thrombocythemia.

increased fibrosis can occur in PV, ET, and chronic myelocytic leukemia, myelofibrotic transformations of these conditions can also occur with features resembling CIMF. Myelofibrosis associated with primary myelodysplastic syndromes can cause diagnostic difficulties[14] and should be suspected if granulopoiesis and erythropoiesis are dysplastic. Thiele and colleagues[12] have also emphasized the existence of a prefibrotic stage of myelofibrosis that is characterized by a hypercellular marrow containing increased numbers of dysplastic megakaryocytes. This challenging view, which has been discussed earlier, if confirmed could necessitate a reevaluation of published data.

Pathogenesis

The recent advances in our understanding of the nature and pathogenesis of CIMF have recently been reviewed.[26] The characteristic extracellular matrix is composed of a variety of interstitial and basement membrane glycoproteins, including collagen types I, III, IV, V, and VI, fibronectin, vitronectin, laminin, and tenascin, as well as a marked neovascularization. In contrast to the clonal hematopoiesis, the increased stromal tissue is a reactive, or secondary phenomenon, resulting from the inappropriate release of megakaryocyte or platelet-derived growth factors, including PDGF, TGF-β, bFGF, and calmodulin, and monocytic cytokines. Circulating hematopoietic precursors, including pluripotent (CFU-GM) and lineage-restricted progenitor cells (CFU-GEMM, CFU-MK, and BFU-E), are increased up to 160 times their concentrations in control blood. Cytogenetic studies have highlighted three chromosomal abnormalities, namely del(13q), del(20q), and partial trisomy 1q, which account for 70 percent of all abnormalities at diagnosis, and suggest that in many patients gene loss and/or inactivation may be an important pathogenetic mechanism.

Prognosis

The overall median survival is approximately 4 years, although individual survival may range from 1 to over 30 years. Several useful prognostic schemes have been reported that allow high-risk patients to be identified. The Lille scoring system (Table 10–6), based on two adverse prognostic factors, namely hemoglobin below 10g/dL and white cell count below 4 or above 30 × 10⁹/L, is able to separate patients into three groups with low-, intermediate-, and high-risk disease.[27] The Sheffield scheme (Table 10–7), by combining hemoglobin level, age, and karyotype, identifies patients with median survival times that vary from 180 months (good risk) to 16 months (poor risk).[28] These studies, however, included very few young patients, a fact that could limit their value when used to identify cases suitable for high-dose procedures. This criticism has been partly addressed by Cervantes and colleagues,[29] who reported the outcome of 116 patients aged 55 years or younger at presentation. Survival was substantially longer than that reported for CIMF overall, with a median survival exceeding 10.5 years. Two risk groups were identified based on the presence of constitutional symptoms (fever, sweats, weight loss), a hemoglobin value of 10g/dL or lower and a blast cell count of 1 percent or higher in the peripheral blood. The median survival of patients with no, or only one, bad prognostic factor approached 15 years, whereas the minority of patients with two or three adverse factors survived for a median of less than 3 years. The relatively benign course of CIMF presenting in infancy has also been stressed[30] and further emphasizes the need for caution when selecting patients for transplantation (as discussed below). The main causes of death in CIMF are infection, heart failure, thrombohemorrhagic events, and leukemic transformation. The last, which occurs in approximately 20 percent of patients, is associated with increasing cytogenetic abnormalities and responds poorly to therapy.

Treatment

The majority of patients with CIMF remain incurable, and management is aimed at amelioration of symptoms and improvement in quality of life. Therapeutic options include blood transfusions and androgens for anemia, chemotherapy

Table 10–6. The Lille Scoring System for Predicting Survival in Chronic Idiopathic Myelofibrosis

Number of Adverse Prognostic Factors	Risk Group	Cases (%)	Median Survival (months)
0	Low	47	93
1	Intermediate	45	26
2	High	8	13

Adverse prognostic factors: hemoglobin below 10g/dL; white blood count below 4 or above 30 × 10⁹/L.
(Based on Dupriez et al.[27])

Table 10–7. The Sheffield Scheme for Predicting Survival in Chronic Idiopathic Myelofibrosis

Age (yr)	Hb (g/dL)	Karyotype	Median Survival (months) (95 percent confidence interval)
< 68	< 10	N	54 (46–62)
		A	22 (14–30)
	> 10	N	180 (6–354)
		A	72 (32–112)
> 68	< 10	N	44 (31–57)
		A	16 (5–27)
	> 10	N	70 (61–79)
		A	78 (26–130)

Demonstrating median survival times in months with associated 95% confidence intervals: N = normal, A = abnormal.
(Based on Reilly et al.[28])

for control of thrombocytosis, leukocytosis, and/or hypercatabolic symptoms, and splenectomy or splenic irradiation for symptomatic splenomegaly. However, these conventional therapies have not been demonstrated to significantly influence the natural history of the disease, and as a result, asymptomatic individuals may not require intervention and should merely be observed at periodic intervals. In contrast, young patients with a poor prognosis should be identified and be considered for allogeneic bone marrow transplantation.

Treatment of Anemia

Anemia is a common finding in patients with CIMF and is frequently multifactorial. Iron deficiency, ineffective erythropoiesis, red cell sequestration, hemodilution due to plasma volume expansion consequent on splenomegaly, and hemolysis are major mechanisms, whereas folate and/or vitamin B12 deficiency is uncommon. Androgen therapy improves marrow function in approximately 40 percent of patients, with optimal responses occurring in individuals with normal karyotypes and lack of massive splenomegaly. Oxymetholone is the drug of choice and should be prescribed for at least 3 to 6 months to identify responsive patients. Careful monitoring of liver function and periodic ultrasound imaging is recommended to detect liver damage or the development of hepatic tumors. Danazol, a synthetic steroid derived from ethisterone, has been used successfully in some patients and may also reduce the degree of thrombocytopenia. A number of patients with normochromic normocytic anemia have a reduced red cell survival and may respond to prednisolone or low-dose dexamethasone.

Chemotherapy

Cytotoxic chemotherapy has a definite role in the management of patients with CIMF. Hydroxyurea is the drug of choice and is used for the control of leukocytosis, thrombocytosis, hepatosplenomegaly, or constitutional symptoms, and in some cases may lead to an increase in hemoglobin concentration. Oral chemotherapy can also be used in individuals who develop compensatory hepatic myeloid metaplasia following splenectomy and may reduce the degree of bone marrow fibrosis. Responses, however, are short-lived, lasting a median of only 4.5 months, and hematological toxicity is not uncommon and frequently necessitates cessation of therapy.

Bone Marrow Transplantation

Allogeneic bone marrow transplantation (BMT) has recently been shown to be a promising therapeutic approach, which results in complete hematological remission in the majority of cases and long-term survival in a substantial number of patients.[31] The 5-year overall survival of 54 percent for individuals receiving an unmanipulated HLA-matched related graft is particularly encouraging. Splenectomy before transplantation may reduce the risk of delayed engraftment and is recommended in patients with marked splenomegaly. Nevertheless, treatment failure occurs in approximately one quarter of cases and is associated with older age, presence of an abnormal karyotype, and the absence of grade II to IV acute graft-versus-host disease. It would seem reasonable, therefore, to offer allogeneic BMT to young patients with a poor life expectancy (as defined above), although the timing of BMT in patients with a favorable prognosis remains a dilemma. Donor lymphocyte infusions have been reported to induce remission of relapsed disease following allogeneic BMT,[32] a finding that supports the concept of a "graft-versus-myelofibrosis" effect. The latter observation also provides a basis for designing new therapeutic strategies such as the nonmyeloablative or "mini" transplant approach, which could extend the upper age limit for transplantation. Autologous BMT, despite the reinfusion of clonal peripheral blood stem cells, can reduce marrow fibrosis, restore hematopoiesis, and result in an overall improvement in quality of life.[33] Although this is not a curative procedure, we would suggest that peripheral stem cells be harvested at diagnosis and that an autologous BMT be considered in those individuals with advancing disease in whom an allo-BMT is not feasible.

Splenectomy

The indications for splenectomy are now well established and include massive splenomegaly, recurrent splenic infarctions, hypersplenism requiring frequent blood transfusions, severe thrombocytopenia, and portal hypertension. Perioperative bleeding, infection, and thrombosis result in a surgery-related mortality of approximately 10 percent and a surgery-related morbidity rate of over 30 percent.[34] Compensatory hepatic myeloid metaplasia, leading to rapid hepatic enlargement, is a well-recognized complication, as is an enhanced leukemic transformation rate. The importance of the commonly associated coagulopathy should not be underestimated, with 15 percent of patients exhibiting laboratory evidence of disseminated intravascular coagulation.

Splenic Irradiation

Splenic irradiation should be considered as an alternative to splenectomy in patients who are unfit for surgery. Responses are transient, although some patients may experience prolonged relief, and life-threatening cytopenias may be an unpredictable complication.[35] Radiotherapy, however, remains the treatment of choice for peritoneal and pleural extramedullary hematopoiesis, as well as for involvement of vital organs, including the central nervous system.

Experimental Therapies

Bone marrow transplantation is the only therapeutic modality that has been shown to prolong survival. As a result, a number of alternative therapies have been investigated, including vitamin D analogues, alpha interferon, erythropoietin, 2-chlorodeoxyadenosine, etidronate, anagrelide, perfenidone, and suramin. Unfortunately, these agents have not been documented to have a significant clinical benefit.[36] Interest, however, has been shown recently in the antiangiogenic agent thalidomide, as CMIF is characterized by a marked neovascularization.[37] Side effects are a significant problem and include somnolence, paresthesia, and abdominal discomfort. Thalidomide appears effective in reducing splenomegaly and improving anemia in patients who can tolerate the drug. Platelet counts can increase, and the drug should be used with caution in patients with thrombocythemia.[38]

REFERENCES

1. Nimer SD: Essential thrombocythaemia: Another "heterogenous disease" better understood. Blood 93:415–416, 1999.
2. Lengfelder E, Hochhaus A, Kronawitter U, Höche D, Queisser W, Jahn-Elder M, Burkhardt R, Reiter A, Ansari H, Hehlmann R: Should a platelet limit of 600×10^9/L be used as a diagnostic criterion in essential thrombocythaemia? An analysis of the natural course including early stages. Br J Haematol 100:15–23, 1998.
3. Messinezy M, MacDonald LM, Nunan TO, Westwood NB, Chinn S, Pearson TC: Spleen sizing by ultrasound in polycythaemia and thrombocythaemia: Comparison with SPECT. Br J Haematol 98:103–107, 1997.
4. Messinezy M, Westwood N, Sawyer B, Grace R, Holland LJ, Lawrie AS, Pearson TC: Primary thrombocythaemia: A composite approach to diagnosis. Clin Lab Haematol 16:139–148, 1994.
5. Brière J, Kiladjian J-J, Peynaud-Debayle E: Megakaryocytes and platelets in myeloproliferative disorders. Baillieres Clin Haematol 10:65–88, 1997.
6. Harrison CN, Gale RE, Pezella F, Mire-Sluis A, Machin SJ, Linch DC: Platelet c-mpl expression is dysregulated in patients with essential thrombocythaemia but this is not of diagnostic value. Br J Haematol 107: 139–147, 1999.
7. Westwood NB, Pearson TC: Diagnostic applications of haemopoietic progenitor culture techniques in polycythaemias and thrombocythaemias. Leuk Lymphoma. 22(Suppl 1):95–103, 1996.
8. Murphy S, Peterson P, Iland H, Laszlo J: Experience of the Polycythemia Vera Study Group with essential thrombocythemia: A final report on diagnostic criteria, survival, and leukemic transition by treatment. Semin Hematol 34:29–39, 1997.
9. Champion KM, Gilbert JGR, Asimakopoulos FA, Hinshelwood S, Green AR: Clonal haemopoiesis in normal elderly women: Implications for the myeloproliferative disorders and myelodysplastic syndromes. Br J Haematol 75:920–926, 1997.
10. Gale RE, Fielding AK, Harrison CN, Linch DC: Acquired skewing of X-chromosome inactivation patterns in myeloid cells of the eld-

11. erly suggests stochastic clonal loss with age. Br J Haematol 98:512–519, 1997.
11. Georgii A, Buesche G, Kreft A: The histopathology of chronic myeloproliferative diseases. Baillieres Clin Haematol 11:721–749, 1998.
12. Thiele J, Kvasnicka HM, Zankovich R, Diehl V: Relevance of bone marrow features in the differential diagnosis between essential thrombocythemia and early stage idiopathic myelofibrosis. Haematologica 85:1126–1134, 2000.
13. Carneskog J, Kutti J, Wadenvik H, Lundberg P-A, Lindstedt G: Plasma erythropoietin by high-detectability immunoradiometric assay in untreated and treated patients with polycythaemia vera and essential thrombocythaemia. Eur J Haematol 60:278–282, 1998.
14. Pagliuca A, Layton DM, Manoharan A, Gordon S, Green PJ, Mufti GF: Myelofibrosis in primary myelodysplastic syndromes: A clinico-morphological study of 10 cases. Br J Haematol 71:499–504, 1989.
15. Boultwood J, Lewis S, Wainscoat JS: The 5q– syndrome. Blood 84:3253–3260, 1994.
16. Van Genderen PJJ, Mulder PGH, Waleboer M, van de Moesdijk D, Michiels JJ: Prevention and treatment of thrombotic complications in essential thrombocythaemia: Efficacy and safety of aspirin. Br J Haematol 97:179–184, 1997.
17. Barbui T, Finazzi G, Dupuy E, Kiladjian J-J, Brière J: Treatment strategies in essential thrombocythemia. A critical appraisal of various experiences in different centres. Leuk Lymphoma 22(Suppl. 1):149–160, 1996.
18. Sterkers Y, Preudhomme C, Laï J-L, Demory J-L, Caulier M-T, Wattel E, Bordessoule D, Bauters F, Fenaux P: Acute myeloid leukemia and myelodysplastic syndromes following essential thrombocythemia treated with hydroxyurea: High proportion of cases with 17p deletion. Blood 91:616–622, 1998.
19. Cortelazzo S, Finazzi G, Ruggeri M, Vestri O, Galli M, Rodeghiero F, Barbui T: Hydroxyurea for patients with essential thrombocythemia and a high risk of thrombosis. N Engl J Med 332:1132–1136, 1995.
20. Lengfelder E, Griesshammer M, Hehlmann R: Interferon-alpha in the treatment of essential thrombocythemia. Leuk Lymphoma 22 (Suppl. 1):135–142, 1996.
21. Silverstein MN, Petrone ME, Petitt RM, Dement MP, Vukovich RA: The safety profile of anagrelide for treatment of thrombocythemia. Blood. 88:583a, 1996.
22. Van de Pette JEW, Prochazka AV, Pearson TC, Singh AK, Dickson ER, Wetherley-Mein G: Primary thrombocythaemia treated with busulphan. Br J Haematol, 62:229–237, 1986.
23. Finazzi G, Ruggeri M, Rodeghiero F, Barbui T: Second malignancies in patients with essential thrombocythaemia treated with busulphan and hydroxyurea: Long term follow up of a randomized clinical trial. Br J Haematol 110:577–583, 2000.
24. Griesshammer M, Heimpel H, Pearson TC: Essential thrombocythaemia and pregnancy. Leuk Lymphoma 22(Suppl. 1):57–63, 1996.
25. Barosi G, Ambrosetti A, Finelli C, Grossi A, Leoni P, Liberato NL, Petti MC, Pogliani E, Ricetti M, Rupoli S, Visani G, Tura S: The Italian consensus conference on diagnostic criteria for myelofibrosis with myeloid metaplasia. Br J Haematol 104:730–737, 1999.
26. Reilly JT: Pathogenesis of idiopathic myelofibrosis: A review. Hematology 3:205–213, 1998.
27. Dupriez B, Morel P, Demory JL, Lai JL, Simon M, Plantier I, Bauters F: Prognostic factors in agnogenic myeloid metaplasia: A report on 195 cases with a new scoring system. Blood 88:1013–1018, 1996.

28. Reilly JT, Snowden JA, Spearing RL, Fitzgerald PM, Jones N, Watmore A, Potter A: Cytogenetic abnormalities and their prognostic significance in idiopathic myelofibrosis: A study of 106 cases. Br J Haematol 98:96–102, 1997.

29. Cervantes F, Barosi G, Demory J-L, Reilly JT, Guarnone R, Dupriez B, Pereira A, Montserrat E: Myelofibrosis with myeloid metaplasia in young individuals: Disease characteristics, prognostic factors and identification of risk-groups. Br J Haematol 102:684–690, 1998.

30. Altura RA, Head DR, Wang WC: Long-term survival of infants with idiopathic myelofibrosis. Br J Haematol 109:459–462, 2000.

31. Guardiola P, Anderson JE, Bandini G, Cervantes F, Runde V, Arcesse W, Bacigalupo A, Przepiorka D, O'Donnell MR, Polchi P, Buzyn A, Sutton L, Cazals-Hatem D, Sale G, de Witte T, Deeg J, Gluckman E: Allogeneic stem cell transplantation for agnogenic myeloid metaplasia: A European group for blood and marrow transplantation, Société Française de Greffe de Moelle, Gruppo Italiano per il Trapianto del Midollo Osseo, and Fred Hutchinson Cancer Center Collaborative Study. Blood 93:2831–2838, 1999.

32. Byrne JL, Beshti H, Clark D, Ellis I, Haynes AP, Das Gupta E, Russell NH: Induction of remission after donor leucocyte infusion for the treatment of relapsed chronic idiopathic myelofibrosis following allogeneic transplantation: Evidence for a 'graft vs. myelofibrosis' effect. Br J Haematol 108:430–433, 2000.

33. Anderson JE, Deeg HJ, Tefferi A, Craig F, Guardiola P, Gazitt Y, Razvilla B, Alsina M, Callander N, Freytes C, Tsai T: Effective treatment of myelofibrosis by autologous peripheral blood stem cell transplantation. Blood 94:396a, 1999.

34. Tefferi A, Mesa RA, Nagorney DM, Schroeder G, Silverstein MN: Splenectomy in myelofibrosis with myeloid metaplasia: A single institution experience with 223 patients. Blood 95:2226–2233, 2000.

35. Elliot MA, Tefferi A: Splenic irradiation in myelofibrosis with myloid metaplasia: A review. Blood Rev 13:163–170, 1999.

36. Reilly JT: Pathogenesis and management of idiopathic myelofibrosis. Ballieres Clin Haematol 11:751–767, 1999.

37. Reilly JT, Nash JRG, Mackie MJ, McVerry BA: Endothelial cell proliferation in myelofibrosis. Br J Haematol 60:625–630, 1985.

38. Barosi G, Grossi A, Comotti B, Marchetti M: Thalidomide in patients with myelofibrosis with myeloid metaplasia. Blood 96:746a, 2000.

Acute Leukemias

11

Historical Perspectives on Acute Leukemias

James F. Holland

Although the history of acute leukemia begins with the description of the several diseases subsumed by this rubric[1–6] and includes vivid accounts of the inexorability of their natural history, a glimmer of hope attended the description of spontaneous remissions from staphylococcal infection.[7] Attempts at inducing viral infections to cause leukopenia[8] and efforts at cross-transfusion[9] paralleled early drug trials in their lack of success. Exchange blood transfusions caused the first deliberate remissions in the autumn of 1947.[10]

Granulocytopenia in rats was inducible by dietary deficiency and sulfonamides and preventable by the *Lactobacillus casei factor*,[11] which was subsequently shown to be folic (pteroylglutamic) acid.[12]

After failure to demonstrate impressive clinical effects with 4-hydroxylpteroylglutamate derivatives,[13] Farber and colleagues[14] were given the opportunity to test the new 4-aminopteroylglutamic acid antagonist synthesized by Subbarow, aminopterin, shortly after its antimetabolite[15] and antitumor effects had been demonstrated in the laboratory.[16] Temporary regressions of acute lymphocytic leukemia (ALL) of children were widely confirmed,[17] although similar results could not be produced in adults.

The deliberate synthesis of analogs of purines led to 8-azaguanine, 2,6-diaminopurine, and 6-mercaptopurine,[18] and this latter was active in children even when resistance to aminopterin had developed.[19] Nearly simultaneously, adrenocorticotropic hormone and Kendall's compound E, cortisone, were recognized to produce rapid temporary benefit in acute leukemia of childhood.[20]

The quality of experimental systems kept pace with these newly discovered and exciting phenomena. Law et al.[21] produced the transplantable L-1210 leukemia, which was destined to become an indispensable tool in leukemia research. Three critical phenomena were then noted: 1. that resistance to antileukemic agents can occur;[22,23] 2. that independent sensitivities to a purine analogue and a folic acid antagonist were potentiated when the drugs were used simultaneously in combination in mice and led to survival without evidence of disease (cures) when the animals were sacrificed 3 months later;[24] and 3. using the Luria-Delbruck fluctuation test, that resistance depended on pre-existence of cells within the population that were inherently refractory to drug effect.[25]

Goldin and co-workers[26,27] made the critical discoveries that L-1210 leukemia cells could be influenced in their responsiveness to folic acid antagonists by many factors intrinsic to the host, and also by tumor size, the dose of drug, and the schedule by which the drug was given. In addition, Goldin et al.[28] and Burchenal et al.[29] reported that folic acid could mitigate the toxicity of the antifols if given before treatment, but not after, whereas citrovorum factor, the reduced metabolic derivative of folate, was capable of selectively rescuing the host even when given after the antagonist.[30,31] Goldin et al.[32] also showed a superior therapeutic index for amethopterin (methotrexate) compared to aminopterin.

In the first pilot clinical trial at the National Cancer Institute (NCI) beginning in 1953, Holland and co-workers[35] combined 6-mercaptopurine and methotrexate for the treatment of ALL and acute myelocytic leukemia (AML). Upon the arrival of Zubrod and subsequently of Frei, this experience was translated into a comparative study, which imperfectly mimicked the Law and Goldin observations; it compared 6-mercaptopurine and methotrexate given daily with 6-mercaptopurine given daily and methotrexate given twice weekly.[33] This collaborative undertaking between the NCI and Roswell Park Memorial Institute, where Holland had transferred, was the first prospective interinstitutional clinical trial in American cancer research and eventually gave rise to the Acute Leukemia Group B (ALGB). Differences in remission duration did not occur on the two combination arms, which differed only in methotrexate schedule. This led to the second study of what was to be a long and productive series: sequential methotrexate and 6-mercaptopurine, either drug first, versus the combination.[34] The latter study provided clinical evidence of the superiority of combination chemotherapy. A taxonomy of marrow and hematologic changes was promulgated to allow classification of therapeutic responses.[35]

One critical conceptual study was reported in this same early period: the demonstration that antileukemic effectiveness could be recognized despite the clinical absence of disease. After steroid-induced remission, 6-mercaptopurine significantly prolonged remission duration compared with a placebo. This successful therapy of occult micrometastatic tumor underlies much of modern day chemotherapy.[36]

Goldin's observations on intermittency of methotrexate dose were pursued in pilot fashion by Freireich et al. and in a systematic way in the ALGB by Selawry and co-workers.[37] As predicted from the Goldin murine experiments, daily methotrexate and intermittent drug were equally effective in advanced leukemia (at presentation), but when patients induced into remission were randomized a second time, those receiving the twice-weekly methotrexate had appreciably longer remission durations.[37] Vincristine had recently been recognized as an important inducing agent,[38] and vincristine and prednisone in combination were adopted to induce a much higher proportion of children into remission. After induction, twice-weekly methotrexate, which allowed a substantially higher drug dose, was significantly more effective than daily methotrexate and produced remissions that were four times as long.[39] Late effects, which altered the natural history of the disease, accompanied the long remissions, including central nervous system (CNS) leukemia and methotrexate toxic effects on lung, liver, and bones of children. Whiteside and co-workers[40] introduced the intrathecal use of methotrexate, and it was soon adopted as a prophylactic measure.[41]

In a classic monograph, Skipper et al.[42] elaborated on the importance of tumor size and drug dose. From a series of model experiments, they formulated a mathematical model for tumor eradication dependent on logarithmic cell killing. This model has had profound impact on the design of therapy for nearly four decades.

The NCI group, on recognition of the independent effects of vincristine, prednisone, methotrexate, and 6-mercaptopurine, administered all four drugs simultaneously (VAMP) in repetitive courses. This combination administration led to exceptionally long unmaintained remission times.[43] The ALGB studied induction with vincristine and prednisone followed by three intensive courses of 6-mercaptopurine or methotrexate or cyclophosphamide or the sequence of the three drugs, one course of each, followed in a random subset by carmustine (BCNU).[44,45] Of the single drugs, methotrexate provided the longest guarantee time until relapses began, although the four-drug sequence was also impressively active. Based on mathematical models derived from this early experience, a longer series (over 8 months) of methotrexate courses was undertaken, with and without vincristine and prednisone reinforcement interposed between the courses.[46] These patients were also observed unmaintained. They constitute the first evidence of curability of the disease in a controlled study, with some 25 percent of those reaching remission enjoying disease eradication in follow-up exceeding 10 years.[47] Much of the Skipper-Schabel-Wilcox mathematical model[42] was thus translatable to clinical terms.

The recognized value of cranial radiotherapy for manifest clinical CNS disease led to trials in prophylaxis.[48] After showing that craniospinal irradiation produced excessive immunodepression, cranial irradiation with intrathecal methotrexate to eradicate cells in the spinal canal became widely accepted. The latter was the standard therapy until late adverse effects on the brain were recognized. Haghbin and colleagues,[49] using more intensive chemotherapy, never found it desirable or necessary to irradiate the brain.

Simultaneously with the development of intensive chemotherapy, techniques of support became critical to avoid interim mortality from bleeding and infection before remission could be achieved. Platelet transfusion and granulocyte transfusion, facilitated by development of the blood centrifuge,[50–52] had recognizable impact on survival during the phase of marrow aplasia. The galaxy of new and powerful antibiotics similarly played a role, whereas protective isolation, prophylactic nonabsorbable antibiotics, and prophylactic systemic antibiotics were more controversial.[53]

Maintenance chemotherapy was also under study during all this time. Pilot experience with vincristine and steroid induction, followed by 6-mercaptopurine and methotrexate in combination, with reinforcement pulses of vincristine and prednisone, was exceptionally promising in the data of Bernard.[54]

The program was translated into the ALGB where similar excellent results were found.[46]

In independent studies, Condit and Eliel[55] had investigated spaced high doses of methotrexate. Later, Djerassi[56] pioneered intensive methotrexate dosing with citrovorum rescue, proving the relevance of Goldin's observations for humans.

Since 1968, 6-mercaptopurine and methotrexate have been the usual maintenance agents in standard-risk childhood ALL. In one study, vincristine and prednisone were continued as maintenance drugs after inducing remission because of their superlative early killing activity. Early relapse occurred in all patients (ALGB, unpublished data) however – a phenomenon that demonstrated the necessity for either greater cell kill, as in the VAMP regimen (which has been abandoned), or of staged cell killing, in which remission with vincristine and prednisone is achieved before the intensive administration of additional cytotoxic chemotherapy.

Asparaginase was introduced following its recognition by Kidd[57] and elucidation by Broome[58] as an enzyme in guinea pig serum capable of causing regression of mouse lymphocytic leukemia. After discovery in and purification from *Escherichia coli*,[59] and after demonstrated activity in human ALL[60] and occasionally in AML,[61] it was found to be complexly interactive with other antileukemic agents and best administered after vincristine and prednisone.[62] Others have administered it successfully on a continuing basis throughout early remission.

Daunorubicin was shown by Tan et al.[63] and by the ALGB to be of value in relapsed ALL patients[64]; after these findings, it was advanced to earlier first line incorporation in induction schemas, particularly for patients at high risk.

The composite of these systematic investigations evolved by 1976 into a highly useful regimen.[65] It included vincristine, prednisone, asparaginase, intensive intermediate-dose methotrexate (to obtain marrow, testicular, and CNS concentrations higher than ordinary) with citrovorum reversal, and maintenance of 6-mercaptopurine plus methotrexate with vincristine and prednisone reinforcement. Alternative approaches, making use of rotational sequential doublets of active agents, led to equally impressive results in standard-risk patients.[66] Survival data for successive studies continued to improve (Fig. 11–1).

The subclassification of patients with ALL into those with cells bearing common antigen and those with T antigen facilitated the identification of patients at high risk. Those with T-cell disease, older age, higher counts, or age below 1 year are in a high-risk category. An intensive treatment program by Riehm and co-workers[67] achieved remission without relapse in an impressive proportion of high-risk children.

In the early years, patients with AML were treated similarly to those with ALL, and their outcome was unimpressive. 6-Mercaptopurine exhibited low activity and was the only drug of importance[68] until activity was recognized for methylglyoxal bis(guanylhydrazone).[69] This polyamine analogue had an extremely narrow therapeutic index but was of heuristic significance after 10 years of purine analogues without other success. Daunorubicin was rapidly found to be active in patients with AML, as well as those with ALL.[70] About the same time, cyto-

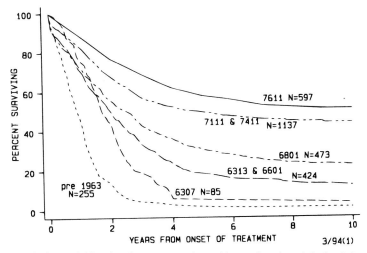

Figure 11–1. Survival of 2971 children less than 20 years of age with acute lymphocytic leukemia in successive studies of the Cancer and Leukemia Group B. All patients who entered are reported. All pre-1963 studies used antimetabolites or steroids for induction and antimetabolite maintenance. The studies in the 1960s used vincristine and prednisone, sometimes with an anthracycline, for induction, with antimetabolite, anthracycline, or alkylating agent intensification, if any, and antimetabolite maintenance. The studies of the 1970s used vincristine, prednisone, and asparaginase for induction, and various antimetabolite regimens for maintenance. Antibiotics and other supportive care measures also improved during this 25-year experience.

sine arabinoside (ara-C) was deliberately synthesized and found to induce remissions of AML.[71]

Ara-C and thioguanine were found to be therapeutically synergistic with decreased toxicity in mouse leukemia experiments.[72] Their use clinically in anecdotal experience and prospective trial was superior to ara-C alone.[73] Murine results also indicated synergy of ara-C plus cyclophosphamide, ara-C plus CCNU (lomustine), and ara-C plus daunorubicin. In prospective trial, 5 days of ara-C at 100 mg/m²/day and 2 days of daunorubicin were found slightly superior to the other regimens and thus were adopted for study in the ALGB.[73] This regimen ordinarily required two courses for induction. Considerations of insufficient reduction in marrow cellularity after a single course led to an exploration of 7 days of ara-C at 100 mg/m²/day by continuous infusion and 3 days of daunorubicin at 45 mg/m²/day. The pilot trial was highly favorable,[74] and a prospective comparison of the seven and three versus five and two regimen established the superiority of the more intensive treatment.[75] Analysis showed that approximately 15 percent of all patients who entered the protocol (about 25 percent of those who reached complete remission) did not fail. Thus cure of AML would appear to have been demonstrated.[47] No advantage was then found for the addition of thioguanine to ara-C and daunorubicin, nor to the prolongation of ara-C beyond 7 days. Similarly doxorubicin is not superior to daunorubicin.[76] The dose of daunorubicin above the age of 60 was shown to be excessive, and 30 mg/m²/day × 3 with the 7 days of ara-C was less toxic and thus more effective.[76] Other single hospital investigators have reported higher induction frequencies, which more likely represent the nature of their patients and support systems than major chemotherapeutic differences from the results of group studies.

Three other topics concerning acute leukemia therapy merit mention.

The nearly universal lymphocytic leukemia in the inbred strain of AKR mice was thought to be genetic by Jacob Furth, its discoverer. Ludwig Gross[77] proved, however, that the leukemia was due to a virus. This demonstrated in mammals what had been known since Ellerman and Bang showed in 1908 that leukemia in chickens, was of viral origin.[77a] That Rous had also found virally induced sarcoma in birds[78] and Shope a viral papilloma in rabbits[79] apparently did not seem relevant, and Gross's findings were received with skepticism, if not ridicule. Friend and Rauscher soon discovered murine leukemias caused by different viruses. A major effort to discover human leukemia viruses in the 1960s was unsuccessful with the techniques of the time, but the discovery of the Epstein-Barr virus in association with Burkitt's tumor[80] and its subsequent acceptance as the causal factor of infectious mononucleosis[81] kept alive the credibility of viral etiology of human hematopoietic diseases. The monumental discovery by Gallo and co-workers[82] of a retrovirus in human T-cell leukemia (HTLV-I) galvanized the field, suggesting, as it does, that other leukemias might be related to viral induction. This would provide an additional target for therapy since prophylaxis against such a rare disease would be extremely difficult.[83]

Considerable data in mice indicate that specific and nonspecific immunization can prevent or participate in the therapeutic control of transplanted and spontaneous neoplasms. Mathe et al.[84] first reported a major beneficial effect of bacillus Calmette-Guérin (BCG) together with irradiated leukemic cells in children with ALL, an observation that has not been duplicated by others using somewhat different protocols. The children who benefitted may have been a particularly responsive immunologic subset. Since no additional relapses occurred in 15 years of observation after abbreviated chemotherapy, however, credence must still attend these observations. BCG was touted in AML based on uncontrolled studies,[85] but prospective controlled trials were nonconfirmatory. Myeloblasts treated with neuraminidase inoculated intradermally in controlled prospective trials showed prolongation of remission.[86]

Bone marrow transplantation has proved of interest in ALL in children after the first relapse and in AML in young adults.[87] Since the transplantation age limit appears to be approximately 50, and most AML occurs after that age, the technique may be limited to a young subset. This group also does the best in chemotherapeutic response, although one controlled trial by Appelbaum and colleagues[88] suggested a benefit for transplantation. Other similar studies also indicate a slight advantage. The antileukemic effectiveness of lethal total body irradiation preceded by high-dose cyclophosphamide requires marrow rescue. An extension of donor histocompatibility beyond leukocyte antigen-identical siblings may be possible by techniques of eliminating lymphocytes that lead to graft-versus-host disease. A recent demonstration that consolidation therapy with repeated courses of high-dose cytarabine after daunorubicin and cytarabine induction led to unmaintained remission duration in patients under age 60 essentially equivalent to results after allogeneic transplant reopens the risk-benefit assessment of early marrow transplants and raises the possibility of chemotherapeutic cures of acute myelocytic leukemia as a realistic goal.[89]

The lessons of history point the way to the future, and the slow but steady advance of progress in the half-century since the introduction of successful chemotherapy for ALL augurs well for eventual success.

ACKNOWLEDGMENTS

This work was supported in part by the T.J. Martell Foundation for Leukemia, Cancer and AIDS Research.

REFERENCES

1. Freidreich N: Ein neuer Fall von Leukamie. Arch Pathol Anat 12:37, 1857.
2. Ebstein W: Uber die acute Leukamie und Pseudoleukamie. Dtsch Arch Klin Med 44:343, 1888–9.
3. Fraenkel A: Ueber acute Leukamie. Dtsch Med Wochenschr 21:639, 663, 676, 699, 712, 1895.
4. Di Guglielmo G: Un caso di eritroleucemia. Folia Med 13:386, 1917.
5. Reschad H, Schilling V: Ueber eine neue Leukämie durch echte Uebergangsformen (Splenozytenleukämie) und ihre Bedeutung fur die Selbststandigkeit dieser Zellen. Munch Med Wochenschr 60:1981, 1913.
6. Naegeli O: Ueber rothes Knockenmark und Myeloblasten. Dtsch Med Wochenschr 26:287, 1900.
7. Diamond LK, Luhby LA: Pattern of "spontaneous" remissions in leukemia of childhood observed in 26 of 300 cases (abstracted). Am J Med 10:238, 1951.
8. Bierman HR, Crile DM, Dod KS et al: Remissions in leukemia of childhood following acute infectious disease; staphylococcus, streptococcus, varicella and feline panleukopenia. Cancer 6:591, 1953.
9. Bierman HR, Byron RL, Kelly KH et al: Studies on cross circulation in man. I. Methods and clinical changes. Blood 6:487, 1951.
10. Bessis M, Bernard J: A propos du traitement de la leucémie aigue par exsanguino-transfusion. Bull Acad Med 131:615, 1947.
11. Kornberg A, Daft FS, Sebrell WH: Dietary granulocytopenia in rats corrected by crystalline L. casei factor. Proc Soc Exp Biol Med 58:46, 1945.
12. Angier RB et al: The structure and synthesis of the liver L. casei factor. Science 103:667, 1946.
13. Farber S, Cutler EC, Hawkins JW et al: The action of pteroylglutamic congutates on man. Science 106:619, 1947.
14. Farber S, Diamond LK, Mercer RD et al: Temporary remissions in acute leukemia in children produced by folic acid antagonist 4-aminopteroyl-glutamic acid (aminopterin). N Engl J Med 238:787, 1948.
15. Seeger DR, Smith JM Jr, Hultiquist ME: Antagonist for pteroylglutamic acid. J Am Chem Soc 69:2567, 1947.
16. Franklin AL, Stokstad ELR, Jukes TH: Observations on the effect of 4-amino-pterogylglutamic acid on mice. Proc Soc Exp Biol Med 67:398, 1948.
17. Proceedings of the Second Conference on Folic Acid Antagonists in the Treatment of Leukemia. Blood 7:97, 1952.
18. Hitchings GH, Elion GB, Falco EA et al: Studies on analogs of purines and pyrimidines. Ann N Y Acad Sci 52:1318, 1950.
19. Burchenal JH, Murphy ML, Ellison RR et al: Clinical evaluation of a new antimetabolite, 6-mercaptopurine, in the treatment of leukemia and allied diseases. Blood 8:965, 1953.
20. Pearson OH, Eliel LP, Talbot TR Jr et al: The use of ACTH and cortisone in acute leukemia. Blood 5:786, 1950.
21. Law LW, Dunn TB, Boyle PJ et al: Observations on the effects of a folic acid antagonist on transplantable lymphoid leukemias in mice. J Natl Cancer Inst 10:179, 1949.
22. Law LW: Resistance in leukemic cells to an adenine antagonist, 6-mercaptopurine. Proc Soc Exp Biol Med 84:409, 1953.
23. Burchenal JH, Robinson E, Johnston SF, Kushida MN: The induction of resistance to 4-amino-N10-methyl-pteroyl-glutamic acid in a strain of transmitted mouse leukemia. Science 111:116, 1950.
24. Law LW: Effects of combinations of antileukemic agents on an acute lymphocytic leukemia of mice. Cancer Res 12:87, 1952.
25. Law LW: Origin of the resistance of leukemic cells to folic acid antagonists. Nature 169:628, 1952.
26. Goldin A, Venditti JM, Humphreys SR, Mantel N: Influence of concentration of leukemic inoculum on the effectiveness of treatment. Science 123:840, 1956.
27. Goldin A, Venditti JM, Humphreys SR, Mantel N: Modification of treatment schedules in the management of advanced mouse leukemia with amethopterin. J Natl Cancer Inst 17:203, 1956.
28. Goldin A, Goldberg B, Ortega LG, Schoenbach EB: Reversal of aminopterin-induced inhibition of sarcoma 180 by folic acid. Cancer 2:87, 1949.
29. Burchenal JH, Kushida MN, Johnston SF, Cremer MA: Prevention of chemotherapeutic effects of 4-amino-N10-methyl-pteroyl-glutamic acid on mouse leukemia by pteroylglutamic acid. Proc Soc Exp Biol Med 71:559, 1949.
30. Goldin A, Mantel N, Greenhouse SW et al: Estimation of the antileukemic potency of the antimetabolite aminopterin administered alone and in combination with citrovorum factor or folic acid. Cancer Res 13:843, 1953.
31. Goldin A, Venditti JM, Humphreys SR et al: Factors influencing the specificity of action of an antileukemic agent (aminopterin). Multiple treatment schedules plus delayed administration of citrovorum factor. Cancer Res 15:57, 1955.
32. Goldin A, Venditti JM, Humphreys SR et al: A quantitative comparison of the anti-leukemic effectiveness of two folic acid antagonists. J Natl Cancer Inst 15:1657, 1955.

33. Frei E III, Holland JF, Schneiderman M et al: A comparative study of two regimens of combination chemotherapy in acute leukemia. Blood 13:1126, 1958.

34. Frei E III, Freireich EJ, Gehan E et al: Studies of sequential and combination antimetabolite therapy in acute leukemia: 6-mercaptopurine and methotrexate (from the Acute Leukemia Group B). Blood 18:431, 1961.

35. Holland JF, Frei E III, Burchenal JH: Criteria for the evaluation of response to therapy of acute leukemia. In Proceedings of the Fourth Congress of the International Society of Hematology, p. 213, Boston, 1956.

36. Freireich EJ, Gehan E, Frei E III et al: The effect of 6-mercaptopurine on the duration of steroid-induced remissions in acute leukemia. A model for evaluation of other potentially useful therapy. Blood 21:699, 1963.

37. Selawry OS, Holland JF, Burgert O, Glidewell O: Relation of methotrexate dose schedule to stage of disease in children with acute lymphocytic leukemia. Cancer Chem Separ 6:127, 1968.

38. Karon MR, Freireich EJ, Frci E III: A preliminary report on vincristine sulfate. A new active agent for the treatment of acute leukemia. Pediatrics 30:791, 1962.

39. Selawry OS, Hananian J, Wolman IJ et al: New treatment schedule with improved survival in childhood. Intermittent parenteral vs daily oral administration of methotrexate for maintenance of induced remission. JAMA 194:75, 1965.

40. Whiteside JA, Philips FS, Dargeon HW, Burchenal JH: Intrathecal amethopterin in neurological manifestations of leukemia. Arch Intern Med 101:279, 1958.

41. Frei E III, Karon M, Levin RH et al: The effectiveness of combinations of antileukemic agents in inducing and maintaining remission in children with acute leukemia. Blood 26:642, 1965.

42. Skipper HE, Schabel F, Wilcox WS: Experimental evaluation of potential anticancer agents: On the criteria and kinetics associated with "curability" of experimental leukemias. Cancer Chemother Rep 35:1964.

43. Freireich EJ, Karon M, Frei E III: Quadruple combination chemotherapy (VAMP) for acute lymphocytic leukemia of childhood. Proc Am Assoc Cancer Res 5:20, 1964.

44. Holland JF: Intensive high dose treatment of children in complete remission of acute lymphocytic leukemia. In Burchenal JH, Burkitt DP (eds.): Treatment of Burkitt's Tumor. UICC Monograph Series, Vol 8, p. 163. Springer-Verlag, Berlin, 1967.

45. Holland JF: Clinical studies of unmaintained remissions in acute lymphocytic leukemia. In Frei E III (ed.): The Proliferation and Spread of Neoplastic Cells, p. 453. Williams & Wilkins, Philadelphia, 1968.

46. Holland JF, Glidewell OJ: Chemotherapy of acute lymphocytic leukemia of childhood. Cancer 30:1480, 1972.

47. Holland JF: Karnofsky Memorial Lecture. Breaking the Cure Barrier. J Clin Oncol 1:75, 1983.

48. Aur RJA, Hustu HO, Verzosa MS et al: Comparison of two methods of preventing central nervous system leukemia. Blood 42:349, 1973.

49. Haghbin M, Tan CTC, Clarkson BD et al: Treatment of acute lymphocytic leukemia in children with "prophylactic" intrathecal methotrexate and intensive system chemotherapy. Cancer Res 35:807, 1975.

50. Freireich EJ et al: A comparative study of the effect of transfusion of fresh and preserved whole blood on bleeding in patients with acute leukemia. N Engl J Med 260:6, 1959.

51. Freireich EJ, Levin RH, Whang J et al: The functions and fate of transfused leukocytes from donors with chronic myelocytic leukemia in leukopenic recipients. Ann N Y Acad Sci 113:1081, 1964.

52. Freireich EJ, Judson G, Levin RH: Separation and collection of leukocytes. Cancer Res 25:1516, 1965.

53. Yates JW, Holland JF: A controlled study of isolation and endogenous microbial suppression in acute myelocytic leukemia patients. Cancer 32:1490, 1973.

54. Bernard J: Acute leukemia treatment. Cancer Res 27: 2565, 1967.

55. Condit PT, Eliel LP: Effects of the large infrequent doses of amethopterin on acute leukemia in children. JAMA 172:451, 1960.

56. Djerassi L: Methotrexate infusions and intensive supportive care in the management of children with acute lymphocytic leukemia: Follow-up report. Cancer Res 27:2564, 1967.

57. Kidd JG: Regression of transplanted lymphomas induced in vivo by means of normal guinea pig serum. I J Exp Med 98:565, 1953.

58. Broome JD: Evidence that the L-asparaginasc activity of guinea pig serum is responsible for its antilymphoma effects. Nature 191:1114, 1961.

59. Mashburn LT, Wriston JC Jr: Tumor inhibitory effect of L-asparaginase from *Escherichia coli*. Arch Biochem 105:451, 1964.

60. Oettgen HF, Old LJ, Boysc EA et al: Inhibition of leukemias in a man by L-asparaginase. Cancer Res 27: 2619, 1967.

61. Ohnuma T, Holland JF, Nagel G, St. Arncault G: Effects of L-asparaginase in acute myelocytic leukemia. JAMA 210:1919, 1969.

62. Jones BJ, Holland JF, Glidewell O et al: Optimal use of L-asparaginase (NSC-109229) in acute lymphocytic leukemia. Med Pediatr Oncol 3:387, 1977.

63. Tan C, Hosaka H, Kov-Ping Y et al: Daunomycin, an antitumor antibiotic in the treatment of neoplastic disease: Clinical evaluation with special reference to childhood leukemia. Cancer 20:333, 1967.

64. Jones B, Cuttner J, Levy RN et al: Daunorubicin (NSC 83142) versus daunorubicin plus prednisone (NSC 10023) versus daunorubicin plus vincristine (NSC 678574) plus prednisone in advanced childhood acute lymphocytic leukemia. Cancer Chemother Rep 56:729, 1972.

65. Freeman AI, Weinberg V, Brecher ML et al: Comparison of intermediate-dose methotrexate with cranial irradiation for the post-induction treatment of acute lymphocytic leukemia in children. N Engl J Med 308: 477, 1983.

66. Hagbin M, Tan CT, Clarkson BD et al: Treatment of acute lymphoblastic leukemia in children with "prophylactic" intrathecal methotrexate and intensive chemotherapy. Cancer Res 35:807, 1975.

67. Riehm HI, Gadner HI, Henz GI, Langermann HIJ, Odenwald E: The Berlin Childhood acute lymphoblastic leukemia therapy study, 1970–1976. Am J Pediatr Hematol Oncol 2:299, 1980.

68. Miner RW (ed.): 6-Mercaptopurine. Ann N Y Acad Sci 60:183, 1954.

69. Freireich EJ, Frei E III, Karon M: Methylglyoxal-bisguanylhydrazone: A new agent active against acute myelocytic leukemia. Cancer Chemother Rep 16:183, 1962.

70. Weil M, Glidewell OJ, Jacquillat C et al: Daunorubicin in the therapy of acute granulocytic leukemia. Cancer Res 33:921, 1973.

71. Ellison RR, Holland JF, Weil M et al: Arabinosyl cytosine: A useful agent in the treatment of acute leukemia in adults. Blood 32:507, 1968.

72. Burchenal JH, Dollinger MR: Cytosine arabinoside (NSC 63878) in combination with 6-mercaptopurine (NSC 755), methotrexate (NSC 740) or fluorouracil (NSC 19893) in L1210 mouse leukemia. Cancer Chemother Rep 51:435, 1967.

73. Carcy RW, Ribas-Mundo M, Ellison RR et al: Comparative study of cytosine arabinoside therapy alone and combined with thioguanine, mercaptopurine, or daunorubicin in acute myelocytic leukemia. Cancer 36(5):1560, 1975.

74. Yates JW, Wallace HJ Jr, Ellison RR, Holland JF: Cytosine arabinoside (NSC 63878) and daunorubicin (NSC 83142) therapy in acute non-lymphocytic leukemia. Cancer Chemother Rep 57:485, 1973.

75. Rai KR, Holland JF, Glidewell OJ et al: Treatment of acute myelocytic leukemia: A study by Cancer and Leukemia Group B. Blood 58:1203, 1981.

76. Yates J, Glidewell O, Wiernik P et al: Cytosine arabinoside with daunorubicin or Adriamycin for therapy of acute myelocytic leukemia. A CALGB study. Blood 60:454, 1982.

77. Gross L: "Spontaneous" leukemia developing in C3H mice following inoculation in infancy with AK-leukemic extracts or AK embryos. Proc Soc Exp Biol Med 76:27, 1951.

77a. Ellerman V, Bang O: Experimentelle Leukämie bei Hühnern. Centralbl. J. Bakt. Abt I (orig) 46:595–609, 1908.

78. Rous P: A sarcoma of the fowl transmissible by an agent separable from the tumor cells. J Exp Med 13:397, 1911.

79. Shope RE: A filtrable virus causing tumor-like conditions in rabbits and its relationship to virus myxomatosum. J Exp Med 56:803, 1932.

80. Epstein MA, Achong BG, Barr YM: Virus particles in cultured lymphoblasts from Burkitt's lymphoma. Lancet 1:702, 1964.

81. Henle G, Henle W, Diehl V: Relation of Burkitt's tumor-associated herpes-type virus to infectious mononucleosis. Proc Natl Acad Sci USA 59:94, 1968.

82. Poiesz BF, Ruscetti FW, Gazdar AF et al: Detection and isolation of type-C retrovirus particles from fresh and cultured lymphocytes of a patient with cutaneous T-cell lymphoma. Proc Natl Acad Sci USA 77:7415, 1980.

83. Holland JF: Immunological control of human leukemia: Discussion. Cancer Res 36:657, 1976.

84. Mathe G, Amiel JL, Schwarzenberg L et al: Active immunotherapy for acute lymphoblastic leukemia. Lancet 1:697, 1969.

85. Gutterman JU, Rodrigucz V, Mavligit G et al: Chemoimmunotherapy of adult acute leukemia. Prolongation of remission in myeloblastic leukemia with BCG. Lancet 1:1405, 1974.

86. Silver RT, Young RC, Holland JF: Some new aspects of modern cancer chemotherapy. Am J Med 63:772, 1977.

87. Thomas ED, Buckner CD, Clift RA et al: Marrow transplantation for acute nonlymphoblastic leukemia in first remission. N Engl J Med 301:597, 1979.

88. Appelbaum FR et al: A prospective study of the value of maintenance therapy of bone marrow transplantation in adult acute nonlymphoblastic leukemia, abstracted. Blood(Suppl. 1) 60:163a, 1982.

89. Mayer RJ et al: Intensive postremission chemotherapy in adults with acute myeloid leukemia. New Engl J Med 331:896, 1994.

12

Human T-Cell Lymphoma/Leukemia Virus – Associated T-Cell Lymphoma and Leukemia

Bernard J. Poiesz, Michael J. Poiesz, and David Choi

The human T-cell lymphoma/leukemia viruses types 1 and 2 (HTLV-1; HTLV-2) belong to a group of primate T-cell lymphoma/leukemia viruses (PTLV) which, together with bovine leukemia virus (BLV), comprise an oncogenic genus of retroviruses (Figure 12–1). Both viruses are transmitted perinatally, sexually, and by blood transfusions and the sharing of needles during intravenous drug abuse. Both viruses can infect all subsets of human lymphocytes and cause polyclonal, oligoclonal,

and monoclonal T-cell lymphocytoses with HTLV-1 being skewed toward CD4+ lymphocytoses and HTLV-2 toward CD8+ lymphocytoses. HTLV-1 has been clearly established as the etiologic agent of intermediate to high-grade CD4+ T-cell non-Hodgkin's lymphoma and leukemia, whereas HTLV-2 has been increasingly associated with rare CD8+ T-lymphocytic malignancies. The discovery of HTLV-1 fulfilled the long search for a pathogenic human retrovirus and the understanding of its mechanisms of pathogenesis serves as a model for understanding human neoplasia.

THE DISCOVERY OF HTLV-1

By the 1970s it had been well established that retroviruses were a common cause of malignancies among animals. Their distinct life cycle (Figure 12–2), which had been shown to depend on a unique RNA-dependent DNA polymerase termed reverse transcriptase (Figure 12–3), had also been fully dissected. Early work in animal retroviruses had revealed that most cells were latently infected but, when induced into the cell cycle, the viral DNA became transcriptionally active. These observations led to an intense effort at the Laboratory of Tumor Cell Biology of the National Cancer Institute (NCI) to identify growth factors capable of sustaining hematopoietic cellular proliferation and to screen such cell cultures for the presence of retroviral reverse transcriptase activity. In 1978 those efforts bore fruit when it was demonstrated that the neoplastic cells from patients with T-lymphocyte malignancies could be induced to grow in the presence of the cytokine interleukin-2 (IL-2) and that some of these cultures expressed retrovirus particles (Figure 12–4) containing a unique reverse transcriptase activity.[1–3] The subsequent purification and characterization of the virions in these cultures and epidemiologic studies verified that HTLV-1 was a unique

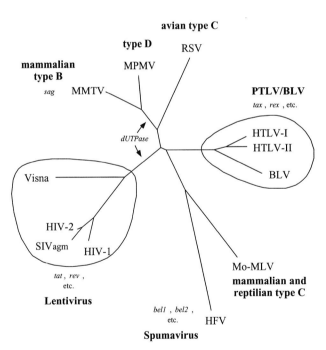

Figure 12–1. Phylogram showing the genetic relationship of the *pol* genes of the seven geni of exogenous retroviruses. The branch lengths are shown to scale and unique gene products are as indicated. MMTV, mouse mammary tumor virus; MPMV, Mason-Pfizer monkey virus; RSV, Rous sarcoma virus; Mo-MLV, Moloney murine leukemia virus; HFV, human foamy virus; SIVagm, simian immunodeficiency virus African green. The lentiviruses, PTLV/BLV, and spumaviruses are complex retroviruses because of the noted additional regulatory proteins encoded in their genomes. The other viruses are referred to as simple viruses because they lack such genes. Both the lentiviruses and the spumaviruses are cytopathic to the host cell, while all of the other geni transform the host cell.

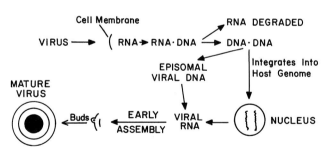

Figure 12–2. Drawing of the life cycle of a retrovirus. The virus binds to a specific cell surface receptor and enters the cell via direct fusion or endocytosis. Its single-stranded RNA is copied into an RNA/DNA hybrid via reverse transcription. The RNA is degraded by Rnase-H and the reverse transcriptase copies the single-stranded DNA into a double-stranded species that ultimately integrates into the host genome as proviral DNA. It can also exist as a circularized nonintegrated episomal form. The proviral DNA replicates with host genomic DNA during cell division. It can remain latent for prolonged periods of time or be transcribed into RNA resulting in the production of viral proteins and genomic RNA that assemble at the cell surface, and bud out of the cell as virions, which "mature" extracellularly to complete the life cycle.

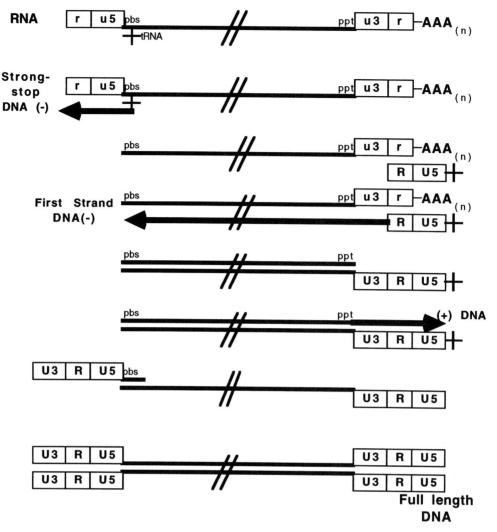

Figure 12–3. Schematic of reverse transcription of retroviral RNA into double-stranded DNA. RNA sequences are shown in small letters and DNA as capital letters. The (+) strand viral genomic RNA contains repetitive sequences (r) at its termini. These are internally flanked by regulatory sequences U5 and U3 at the 5′ and 3′ ends, respectively. These regions are in turn flanked by sequences termed the primer binding site (pbs), which is annealed to a cellular transfer RNA (tRNA) and a polypurine tract (ppt). Initial reverse transcription of (−) strand DNA is primed by the tRNA, proceeds to the 5′ terminus of the genomic RNA, and stops. After Rnase-H degradation of its complementary RNA, this small piece of (−) strand "strong stop" DNA "jumps" to anneal its R sequences to the complementary r sequence of the 3′ terminus of the genomic RNA. First strand (−) DNA synthesis is then primed by this translocated "strong stop" DNA and terminates at the complementary pbs. Studies in our laboratory indicate that the HIVs and HTLVs synthesize "strong stop" DNA at approximately the same efficiency, but that the HIV produces first-strand DNA about 1000-fold greater than HTLV. This difference could explain the marked disparity between both their in vitro and in vivo replication rates. Rnase-H degradation next proceeds (3′ to 5′) up the ppt of the (+) strand RNA. The residual (+) strand RNA then primes initial (+) strand "strong stop" DNA synthesis, which involves copying the still attached tRNA annealing sequences. The remaining (+) strand genomic RNA and the tRNA are then degraded by Rnase-H and the (+) strand "strong stop" DNA "jumps" to anneal to the complementary pbs sequences on the previously synthesized first (−) strand DNA. DNA synthesis then proceeds on both strands to their respective termini. As can be seen, this sequence (of RNA- and DNA-dependent DNA synthesis, RNA degradation of RNA/DNA hybrids, and intramolecular "jumps") results in the production of a larger double-stranded DNA that contains repetitive U3-R-U5 sequences (long terminal repeats or LTR) at both ends. The LTR sequences are important for directing proviral DNA integration and for regulating viral RNA transcription and processing.

human retrovirus.[2–8] The subsequent association of HTLV-1 with a subset of mature CD4+ T-cell malignancies, which were especially prevalent in Southern Japan and the Caribbean, established the fact that HTLV-1 was pathogenic in humans.[9,10]

A few years later, the related virus HTLV-2 was isolated from the cultured T cells of another patient who in retrospect suffered from both hairy cell B-cell leukemia and CD8+ large granular lymphocytic (LGL) leukemia.[11] Parenthetically it should be

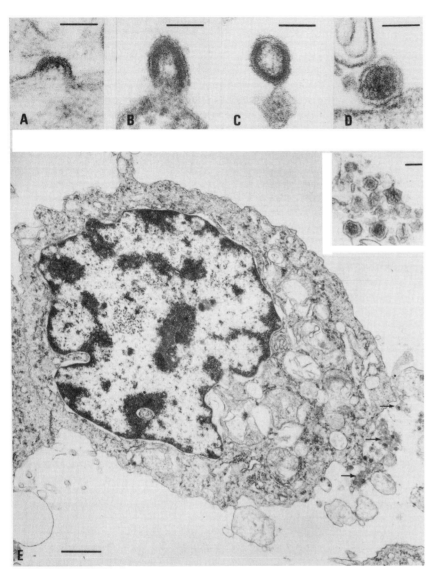

Figure 12–4. Electron micrograph of a cultured neoplastic ATL cell and HTLV-I virions (arrows) (**E**). Virions are 100 nm in diameter. (**A, B**): Early and late budding virions, respectively; (**C, D**): Immature and mature extracellular virions, respectively. Mature virions shown an electron-dense core surrounded by an outer envelope. Accompanying schematic (**F**) illustrates the various viral components within the virion. MA, matrix; CA, capsid; NC, nucleocapsid; PR, protease; IN, integrase; RT, reverse transcriptase; SU, surface; TM, transmembrane.

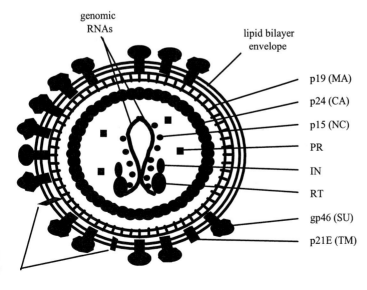

noted that the strategies proven successful for the discovery of HTLV-1 and HTLV-2 became especially useful in the early 1980s in the identification of the much more pathogenic human immunodeficiency virus (HIV).

PHYLOGENY AND EPIDEMIOLOGY OF HTLV-1 AND HTLV-2

Phylogenetic analyses of BLV, HTLV-1, HTLV-2 and simian T-cell lymphoma/leukemia virus strains from around the world indicate that the PTLV diverged from BLV approximately 60,000 to 100,000 years ago.[12] The PTLV are endemic to many, but not all, species of Old World primates including humans. It is clear that many incidences of cross-species transmissions have occurred over many thousands of years and PTLV strains are grouped more by geographic origin than by host species. The PTLV can be taxonomically divided into three major subsets (Figure 12–5). The PTLV-1 have two major subgroups (African and Asian/Austronesian), which differ by about 15

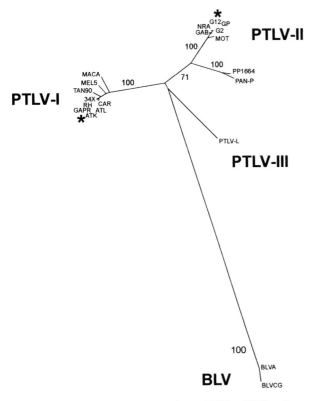

percent at the DNA level. Introduction into humans from other primates occurred at least twice in Africa and Austronesia. Hence, HTLV-1 is endemic in sub-Saharan Africa and throughout Australia and Melanesia. HTLV-1 has been disseminated throughout the world over the past 500 years via European exploration, the slave trade, blood product transfusion, intravenous drug use, and increased travel; it is now endemic in the Caribbean; Latin America; major cities throughout India, Europe, and the United States (particularly on the southern and eastern coasts and Hawaii); Iran; and Southern Japan.[12]

The PTLV-2 can be divided into two major groups, African and Paleo-Amerindian. The African subset has been found in pygmy chimps and isolated groups of human pygmies.[13,14] Very little epidemiological investigation work has been done in these individuals and it is unclear as to whether they suffer from any clinical ailments. There is no evidence that these unique strains have disseminated out of very isolated parts of Africa. HTLV-2 is endemic to Paleo-Amerindians of the New World, being found in Indians of the American Southwest and Florida, Central America, and South America. By the same mechanisms described for HTLV-1, this virus has been disseminated worldwide.

The PTLV-3 consists of a few strains identified in Eritrean baboons whose ancient geographic range extended from the steppes of Central Asia to the Rift Valley in Africa.[15] No other primate has been shown to harbor this strain nor are there any known disease associations, although, again, very little work has been done in this area.

Epidemiological data indicate that the PTLV is transmitted in utero to a very small degree, but at a rate of 10 to 30 percent via breastfeeding. The virus is also transmitted via sexual intercourse, with male to female infection occurring much more effectively than the opposite. The virus is also spread via intravenous drug abuse and the transfusion of cellular but not plasma products. There are no reported incidences of infection occurring via needle stick or other laboratory or clinical work-related injuries.[12,16]

Effective blood donor screening and public health policies (e.g., the use of condoms and bottle-feeding introduced in Japan over the past one to two decades) have had a significant impact on the dissemination of HTLV in certain endemic areas. In the United States all blood and organ donations are screened for HTLV-1 and HTLV-2. It is probably remiss that all pregnant women are not, in that preventing perinatal infection would probably have the most significant impact on preventing HTLV-associated diseases.

Figure 12–5. The complete genomes of many PTLV and BLV strains as analyzed by the neighbor-joining method. The relative distance of all branches are as indicated and the boot-strap values (>70 percent is considered statistically significant) for several of the branches are shown. The tree was rooted to the two BLV strains. The asterisks indicate the location of the PTLV-1 and PTLV-2 strains utilized to make antigens for most clinical HTLV serological assays. The PTLV-1 strains are divided into Asian/Austronesian (MACA and MEL5) and African (all others) subgroups. The PTLV-2 are divided into African (Pan-P and PP1664) and Paleo-Amerindian (all others) subgroups. The PTLV-L, found in Eritrean baboons, forms a unique subgroup, PTLV-3, not yet detected in humans.

DETECTION AND CHARACTERIZATION TECHNIQUES

The diagnosis of HTLV infection is usually performed by detecting antibodies to HTLV-1 and/or 2 antigens using a screening enzyme immunosorbent assay (EIA) and a confirmatory Western blot. According to U.S. Public Health Service criteria, a confirmed positive finding involves reactivity to the GAG p24 and ENV gp46 proteins.[17] Antigen preparations are usually made of purified virions supplemented with recombinant ENV peptides. Some, but not all, serologic assays allow for type-specific discrimination between HTLV-1 and HTLV-2 infection.[18] However, unlike HIV infection, a significant minority of seronegative or seroindeterminate HTLV-1- and HTLV-2-infected individuals exist, partly because of the predominant use of HTLV-1 antigens to screen for both HTLV-1 and HTLV-2 antibodies.[19,20] Because the two viruses are 40 percent divergent, complete sero-cross-reactivity is not found. Also, as described below, because of the low replication rate of HTLV, seroconversion can often take up to 2 years compared with 3 to 6 months that is almost absolutely the case for HIV.[20] Finally, persistent HTLV-1 seronegative T-cell lymphoma/leukemia patients have been described whose malignant cells contain defective HTLV-1 nucleic acid (vide infra).[21,22]

Currently, the most sensitive and specific assay to detect the HTLV viruses is the DNA-dependent polymerase chain reaction (PCR), which is available in a variety of non-FDA licensed research formats by which samples can be amplified and detected in under 6 hours.[21,23] The use of primers and probes in the HTLV *pol*, Tax, and LTR (vide infra) region of the HTLV genome allows for 100 percent detection of all members of PTLV. The assay can be used on fresh, frozen, or formalin (but not B5) fixed cells or tissue samples. The amplified DNA can be subsequently sequenced for phylogenetic comparisons. It should be noted that, unlike the case for HIV, because of its low replication rate, RNA-directed PCR is a relatively insensitive means of detecting HTLV infection.[24]

THE LIFE CYCLE AND MOLECULAR BIOLOGY OF HTLV-1 AND HTLV-2

HTLV-1 and HTLV-2 are genomically and structurally typical of type C oncornaviruses (Figures 12–4 and 12–6). The integrated proviral DNA contains redundant long terminal repeat (LTR) sequences that contain enhancer and promoter elements for viral RNA transcription, the RNA transcriptional start and polyadenylation sites, and, at the 3′ end of the transcribed RNA, a stem-loop structure termed the Rex Response Element (RRE). Like all retroviruses the HTLV contain genes, termed *gag, pol,* and *env,* that encode for critical structural and functional proteins. However, as the case with other complex retroviruses (e.g., the lentiviruses and foamy viruses) the PTLV/BLV genus also contains genes for proteins that regulate viral expression. Also, as is the case with other retroviruses, HTLV-1 and 2 have evolved to make maximal use of their approximately 9-kb genome by employing multiple RNA splicing patterns of their primary RNA transcript and differential and shifting start sites for protein translation.[25]

The life cycle of a typical retrovirus is shown in Figure 12–2. Like all retroviruses HTLV replication is thought to be initiated by the binding of the surface envelope protein gp46 to a specific cell surface receptor. Studies indicate that HTLV-1 and HTLV-2 share the same cell surface receptor, which differs from that of BLV and HIV.[26,27] HTLV receptor(s) have not been definitively established, although two candidate molecules have been identified that may play this role. One is a 71-kd heat-shock-like

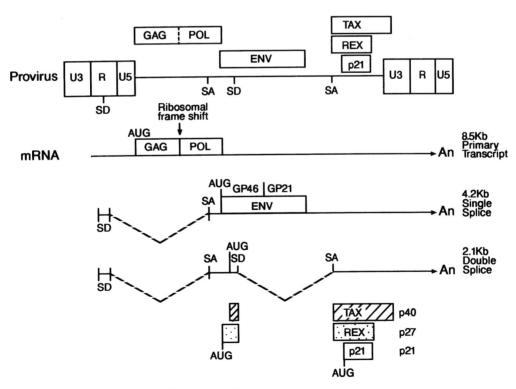

Figure 12–6. Organization of the HTLV proviral DNA and the major cognate polyproteins and cleaved structural, functional, and regulatory proteins. Each gene and protein is discussed in the text.

protein, while the other is a 32-kd protein encoded on the distal arm of chromosome 17q.[28–30] Both viruses can infect many different hematopoietic, epithelial, and mesenchymal cell types in vitro, but analyses indicate that, in vivo, most HTLV-1 or HTLV-2 DNA is found in CD4+ or CD8+ T lymphocytes, respectively.[31]

HTLV virions or purified HTLV surface envelope proteins have been shown to activate human T lymphocytes. Our own data demonstrated that a monoclonal antibody directed against the 32-kd putative HTLV cell surface receptor also activated human T lymphocytes (Choi et al., in preparation). Because activation of target host cells facilitates retroviral reverse transcription and subsequent viral integration of double-stranded DNA into host cellular DNA, it would seem that HTLV has evolved to exploit a heretofore undescribed T-cell activation cascade, in part perhaps explaining its T-cell tropism.

Despite this advantage, however, comparative in vitro experiments indicate that cell-free HTLV virions replicate a thousandfold less efficiently than HIV virions.[32] Our own experiments indicate that HTLV virions contain considerably less surface envelope protein per virion. Also, relative to HIV, HTLV reverse transcription is less robust, with the major difference observed in vitro being the "jump" from minus stranded "strong stop" DNA to plus strand first strand DNA synthesis (Choi et al., in preparation) (Figure 12–3). All of the above may explain the lack of clinical evidence for in vivo HTLV cell-free viral transmission.[16]

Relative to HIV, HTLV reverse transcription is considerably less error prone due to the greater fidelity of its RNA-dependent DNA polymerase.[33,34] There are no known "hot spots" for proviral DNA integration and there are no recognizable oncogenes associated with the HTLV-1 genome.[7,9,16] Most infected cells contain only one integrated copy of viral DNA, which can be on any human chromosome with seemingly random or chaotic flanking host cellular DNA sequences. However, cultured human cells and some fresh tumor specimens have been shown to contain multiple HTLV integrants. Also, defective copies of HTLV have been identified in vivo and in vitro wherein either whole or portions of genes (e.g., *pol*) are missing from the proviral DNA or stop codon mutations result in aborted translation of viral proteins.[22] It is speculated that the presence of defective copies of HTLV could convey a worse clinical prognosis in that, while such genomes would still retain the genes that encode the transforming properties of the virus (vide infra), they would not express all of the major immunogenic epitopes of the virus and thereby escape immune surveillance.

The *gag* gene of the HTLV encodes for three primary proteins (for simplicity we will use the terminology for HTLV-1 although there are subtle size differences between HTLV-1 and HTLV-2 proteins) (Figures 12–4 and 12–6). The p19 protein, which is myristoylated at its amino terminus, anchors the organizing virus replication complex at the interior of the cell surface and facilitates budding of virus particles. The p24 protein forms a capsid in the interior of the virion, which surrounds and protects the ribonucleoprotein complex, which is organized into a preferred three-dimensional structure in part by the *gag* p15 nucleobinding protein.

A translational frameshift allows for the pro-pol polyprotein to also be translated off of the primary RNA transcript (Figure 12–6). The aspartate protease protein functions to cleave the initial *gag* polyprotein into its individual structural components leading to virus maturation and infectivity. The *pol* protein contains the RNA-dependent DNA polymerase and RNAse-H activity critical for reverse transcription and the integrase activity.

The envelope protein is translated as a polyprotein off of the singly spliced RNA message (Figure 12–6). The polyprotein is cleaved into the individual glycosylated surface protein gp46 and the transmembrane protein gp21. While the surface gp46 determines tropism by its binding to the cell surface receptor, the transmembrane gp21 facilitates entry into the target cell via either direct fusion and/or endocytosis.

The multiply spliced RNAs encode for two (and possibly more) key regulatory proteins, Tax and Rex, which modulate HTLV RNA expression and splicing, respectively[7,35,36] (Figure 12–6). Upstream from its TATAA box promoter sequence, the HTLV LTR region contains three 21-bp imperfect repeats that indirectly interact with the Tax protein to *trans*-activate HTLV RNA transcription[37–39] (Figure 12–7). These TAX responsive elements (TRE) have homology to the human cyclic AMP response element (CRE) sequence and TAX activation of viral RNA transcription has been shown to be mediated indirectly by its interaction with cellular CRE binding protein (CREB) (Figure 12–7). Early in HTLV infection most viral RNA is multiply spliced.[40] As more TAX protein is produced, more multiply spliced RNA is produced, eventually leading to increased production of REX protein.

REX is a phosphoprotein localized specifically in the nucleoli of HTLV-infected cells. REX is required for the production of two incompletely spliced viral mRNAs that encode either GAG, POL, or ENV products.[41] REX function depends on the presence of a 5′ splice donor (SD) signal in the beginning of ENV mRNA and in the 5′ LTR for the GAG/POL mRNA as well as the RRE. The 5′ SD seems to destabilize the mRNA in the absence of REX. REX interacts with the RRE to suppress splicing directly or by accelerated transport of the viral RNA into the cytoplasm, either by interference with the splicosome complex, opening specialized RNA transport, or possibly by stabilizing target RNA molecules (or both). REX may also have a second function in addition to regulation of spliced mRNA. At high concentrations of REX a down-regulation or inhibition of TAX-mediated *trans*-activation occurs, providing further regulatory control of virus expression and possibly secondary effects on cellular RNAs.[42]

There are three growth phases in the life cycle of HTLV. In the early phase, the 5′ LTR supports low-level transcription and, because the production of REX is low, the fully spliced regulatory mRNAs are primarily produced. In the mid-phase, increased levels of TAX stimulate overall viral RNA transcription, while REX retards the RNA splicing such that all the viral structural and functional proteins are produced. In the late phase the increased production of REX decreases the production of TAX and REX and decreases the *trans*-activation of

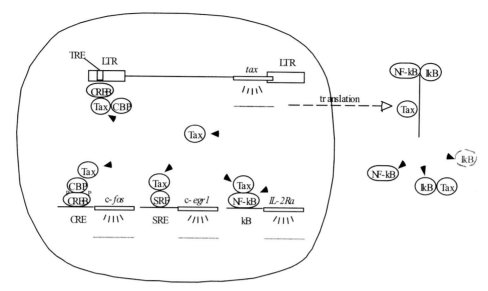

Figure 12–7. Tax mediated *trans*-activation of viral transcripts and host cellular genes. Tax in concert with CBP facilitates the binding of CREB to the TRE located in the HTLV LTR resulting in a marked increase of viral RNA transcription. Similarly, Tax can *trans*-activate a number of cellular genes (e.g., c-fos, c-erg-1, or IL-2R-α) via its interaction with a number of cellular transcription factors (e.g., CREB, serum responsive factor [SRE], or NF-kB). Tax also affects NF-kB regulated transcription in a less direct manner. IkB binds to NF-kB dimers in the cytoplasm and prevents their nuclear localization. Inhibitor of kB kinases (IKKs) phosphorylate IkB causing it to dissociate. NF-kB can then migrate to the nucleus and activate transcription of cellular genes while IkB is degraded via the proteosome pathway. HTLV Tax is known to stimulate the activation of NF-kB at several levels in this pathway. Tax acts to free NF-kB from cytoplasmic constraints by causing its dissociation via the activation of IKKs and by acting as a molecular chaperone for proteolytic degradation due to its ability to physically associate with both the phosphorylated form of IkB and the proteosome. By this mechanism, Tax would be able to guide IkB to the proteosome to promote its degradation and prevent further association with other cytoplasmic NF-kB dimers. Tax also enhances the *trans*-activating capabilities of NF-kB by stimulating its dimerization.

overall viral RNA transcription. Hence, it is the constant interplay of TAX and REX in concert with host cellular factors that influences the levels of HTLV proteins and virions being expressed at any given time and presumably influences the development of disease.

In vitro and in vivo studies indicate that HTLV RNA and proteins are expressed at much lower levels than HIV. This is explained in part by the more varied and robust repertoire of enhancer elements located in the HIV LTR. However, HTLV-infected cells have also been found to harbor natural anti-sense RNA molecules and to make predominantly multiply spliced rather than singly and unspliced viral mRNAs.[40] These observed differences in infection and expression rates make teleological sense given the difference in biological activity of the two viruses. HTLV, which transforms its host cell, expands its genome by increasing the number of host cells containing integrated proviral DNA.[43] Its low expression rate and high degree of latency decrease the probability of immunologic destruction. Hence, it has a low mutation rate.[12] HIV, which ultimately destroys its host cell, requires much higher levels of infectivity, expression, and mutation in order to avoid immunologic inactivation and infect new host cells. The evolution of these biologic properties explains the different clinical effects (oncogenesis for HTLV, cytopenia for HIV) of these two T-lymphotropic viruses.

THE PATHOGENESIS OF HTLV-ASSOCIATED T-CELL LYMPHOMA AND LEUKEMIA

Unlike other oncornaviruses, the BLV/PTLV have not been shown to transduce cellular oncogenes, or rely on insertional mutagenesis (i.e., promoter or enhancer insertion) to transform infected cells. Instead, they induce oncogenesis in a manner more similar to the DNA tumor viruses (e.g., papillomaviruses, adenovirus, SV-40) in that viral regulatory proteins interact with host mechanisms to result in deregulation of the normal cell cycle constraints. The viral protein Tax, in addition to *trans*-activating viral RNA transcription, has been shown, in vitro, to *trans*-activate a number of cellular genes, among them potent T-cell growth factors and antiapoptotic factors. Tax can also act as a *trans*-suppressor by competing with host transcription factors for necessary DNA-binding proteins. Tax has also been shown to promote cellular mutations by inhibiting base excision repair.[44] HTLV-infected cells also upregulate the expression of ATL-derived factor (ADF), a human homologue to *Escherichia coli* thioredoxin, which has the ability to act as an autocrine growth factor, activate host transcription factors, and protect against apoptosis, all by modulating the redox state of the cell.

Activation of protooncogenes by Tax and ADF would promote cell cycle progression in infected cells and, ultimately, transformation. Protection from apoptosis stimulated by these same factors would allow infected cells to elude immune surveillance and protect against DNA damage mediated apoptosis triggered by the accumulation of cellular mutations. These mutations could contribute to tumorogenesis if they activate protooncogenes or deactivate tumor suppressor genes. The *trans*-activation of cellular genes also accounts for many of the paraneoplastic conditions associated with HTLV-1.

Development of HTLV-associated adult T-cell lymphoma/leukemia (ATL) is seemingly controlled by the infected individual's genetic predisposition. If the individual can mount a strong antiviral CTL response, his or her immune system will eliminate cells as they are being transformed, putting that individual at low risk for developing ATL, but increasing the risk for autoimmune diseases that have also been associated with HTLV. Those who cannot mount such a strong CTL response to the virus will not clear transformed cells with the same efficiency, and are therefore at a much greater risk of developing ATL.

The Effects of Tax

Tax mediates its potent *trans*-activating potentials not by binding directly to DNA, but by activating and recruiting host transcription factors (Figure 12–7). Because of this, Tax is capable of *trans*-activating a wide variety of cellular genes in addition to the HTLV provirus. The hyperexpression of these cellular genes can have profound effects on the cell, including promotion of the cell cycle and protection from apoptosis. Tax is able to mediate these effects through direct and indirect interaction with normal T-cell signaling cascades and regulatory mechanisms of cell activation, growth, and apoptosis.

Tax *Trans*-Activation of Nuclear Factor kB

Nuclear factor kB (NF-kB) is an important rapid response transcription factor that is common to all cell types[45] (Figure 12–7). NF-kB related proteins dimerize in the cytoplasm but are inhibited from translocating into the nucleus by the inhibi-

tion of kB (IkB) protein, which binds to the dimer and masks its nuclear localization sequence (NLS). Certain stimuli can activate inhibitor of kB kinases (IKKs). These kinases phosphorylate IkB causing it to dissociate from NF-kB. At this point, NF-kB can migrate to the nucleus and *trans*-activate a number of cellular genes. The phosphorylated form of IkB is susceptible to polyubiquination, which targets it to the proteosome for degradation.

HTLV Tax is known to stimulate the activation of NF-kB at several levels in this pathway (Figure 12–7). Tax acts to free NF-kB from cytoplasmic constraints by causing its dissociation via the activation of IKKs and, presumably, by acting as a molecular chaperone due to its ability to bind both the phosphorylated form of IkB and the proteosome.[46,47] By this mechanism, Tax would be able to guide IkB to the proteosome to promote its degradation and prevent further association with other cytoplasmic NF-kB dimers. Tax also enhances the *trans*-activating capabilities of NF-kB by stimulating dimerization and strengthening the binding of NF-kB to promoter elements.[48]

Tax Manipulation of Antigen-Dependent T-Cell Activation

CD4+ T cells become activated when they recognize antigenic peptide fragments in concert with major histocompatibility complex (MHC) molecules expressed on antigen-presenting cells (APCs).[49] APCs must also express the costimulatory molecule B7, which binds to CD28 on the T-cell surface, to transduce a strong activation signal. Cell surface recognition events trigger a signaling cascade via the TCR and B7, the ultimate result of which is to produce nuclear activators that can *trans*-activate the IL-2 gene.[50] Tax has the ability to bypass the dependence on antigen recognition and activate this pathway, resulting in constitutive expression of IL-2.

HTLV-infected cells are anergic in the sense that they are unresponsive to antigen recognition. Expression of Rex inhibits the splicing of transcripts of the Src and Syk family kinases, resulting in the expression of FynB and Lyn rather than Lyk and Fyn.[51]

Figure 12–8. The effect of HTLV-1 accessory proteins on the antigen-dependent T-cell activation pathway. T-cell activation is triggered by antigen and co-stimulatory molecule recognition. These events trigger two pathways that result in the synthesis of nuclear activators responsible for the expression of the IL-2 gene. The calcium-dependent pathway involves production of inositol tris-phosphate (IP3), which opens calcium gated ion channels, resulting in a considerable calcium influx. Calcium ions bind to calmodulin, rendering it capable of activating calcineurin, which subsequently turns on the nuclear factor of activated T cells (NF-AT), a potent transcriptional activator. The calcium-independent pathway relies on recruitment of a small G protein (Ras), which activates a MAP kinase cascade and, along with a similar cascade transduced through the co-stimulatory molecule CD28, results in the synthesis of AP-1, another potent transcriptional activator.

HTLV-1-infected T cells are rendered anergic by the activity of the Rex protein, a known inhibitor of mRNA splicing. The presence of Rex inhibits the splicing of transcripts of the Src and Syk family kinases, resulting in the expression of FynB and Lyn rather than Lyk and Fyn (1). FynB and Lyn are far less active in the cell than the normal proteins, and do not respond well to receptor aggregation. Along with Tax-mediated *trans*-suppression of Zap-70, and *trans*-activation of Syk (2), antigen recognition is decoupled with cell activation. The ultimate end of the pathway, the transcription of IL-2, can occur constitutively through the Tax-mediated activation of calcineurin (3), a serine/threonine phosphatase, which dephosphorylates NF-AT, which can then migrate to the nucleus, bind to the IL-2 enhancer, and activate transcription of the IL-2 growth factor. Tax can also *trans*-activate the gene for c-Fos (4), resulting in greater amounts of AP-1, another activator of IL-2 transcription. (Adapted from Schwartz,[50] with permission.)

FynB and Lyn are far less active in the cell than the normal proteins, and do not respond well to receptor aggregation. Along with Tax-mediated *trans*-suppression of Zap-70, and *trans*-activation of Syk, antigen recognition is decoupled with cell activation.[51]

Constitutive expression of IL-2 in HTLV-1-infected cells occurs through the Tax-mediated activation of calcineurin, a serine/threonine phosphatase. Tax has been shown to activate calcineurin resulting in constitutive dephosphorylation and consequent activation of the nuclear factor of activated T cells (NF-AT).[52] Activated NF-AT translocates to the nucleus where it binds to CD29 response elements and acts as a potent stimulator of IL-2 production.[53] Tax can also activate IL-2 production by stimulating the transcription of AP-1 substituent and increasing the DNA binding capabilities of AP-1.[54,55] The effects of Tax on antigen-dependent T-cell activation are summarized in Figure 12–8.

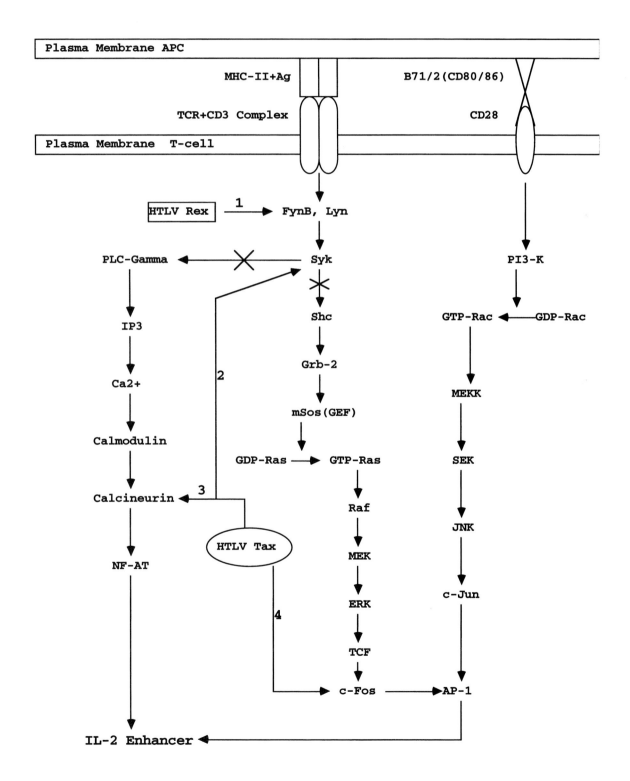

Tax Manipulation of the JAK/STAT Pathway of Clonal Expansion

Extracellular binding of a variety of the type 1 and type 2 cytokines by cell surface cytokine receptors results in receptor oligomerization and activation of the intracellular JAK/STAT pathway.[56] The JAK/STAT pathway is an intracellular signaling cascade that results in the translocation of activated transcription factors to the nucleus where they can recognize response elements associated with the stimulating cytokine. IL-2 response genes are associated with cell cycle progression and proliferation.

HTLV Tax has the ability to activate NF-kB, NF-AT, and AP-1 (by mechanisms previously discussed), which act together to *trans*-activate genes for IL-2 and the IL-2 receptor-alpha chain, among others. This results in high surface expression of the IL-2 receptor and, presumably, a high extracellular concentration of IL-2, which can act as an autocrine factor.[57–59] Tax has also been shown to induce the expression of STAT 1 and STAT 5, which would provide a high concentration of intracellular mediators of the IL-2 response signaling cascade.[60] In HTLV-infected T cells, this pathway would be hyperactive, and would stimulate the cell to proceed through the cell cycle and proliferate in the absence of either direct or indirect antigenic stimulation. The effects of Tax on the JAK/STAT pathway in T cells are summarized in Figure 12–9.

There is some debate over whether or not this autocrine mechanism is necessary for the development of ATL.[61] There have been studies that have shown that some HTLV transformed cells are IL-2 independent.[43,62–64] Although the autocrine mechanism may not be required for chronic leukemogenesis, it is considered to be an important mechanism for initiating the production of leukemic clones and initial lymphocyte transformation. But it must be acknowledged that some mature ATL cell lines produce little IL-2, so the traditional, ligand-mediated, autocrine mechanism of T cell growth is unlikely to stimulate further clonal expansion in these cells. However, we cannot rule out the dysregulation of the JAK/STAT pathway due to mutations in associated proteins in cells of this stage. Quite possibly, the progression of ATL cells through many rounds of division would confer such mutations that would constitutively activate the JAK/STAT pathway in the absence of IL-2. Such abnormalities would most likely be in the genes for JAK 1/3 or STAT 3/5, or the IL-2R-beta chain. If a mutation were to occur that would render any of these gene products unable to be dephosphorylated after the specific tyrosine residues had been phosphorylated, that would constitutively activate this pathway, and incessantly drive the cell through the cell cycle.

IL-2 independent ATL cells expressed constitutive basal phosphorylation of JAK 3 and, usually, STAT 3 and STAT 5, but IL-2 dependent ATL cells do not.[65] IL-2 dependent ATL cells only expressed phosphorylation of JAK 3 and STAT 5 upon addition of IL-2. This observation points to the dependence on accessory mutations in specific protooncogenes in the development of some, but not all, cases of ATL, and explains the discrepancy between IL-2 dependent and IL-2 independent ATL cells.

Tax Inhibition of Rb-Mediated Tumor Suppression

The retinoblastoma (Rb) protein plays an important role in the regulation of the cell cycle.[66] Rb sequesters the transcription factor E2F-1 in the cytoplasm by physically associating with it and masking its nuclear localization sequence (NLS). In the event of cell division, the cyclin-dependent kinase CDK4 phosphorylates Rb, causing it to undergo a conformational change that prevents it from binding to E2F-1. At this point E2F-1 is capable of migrating to the nucleus and activating transcription. During interphase, high concentrations of the cyclin-dependent kinase inhibitor p16ink4a (and other members of the same family) prevent the phosphorylation of Rb and promote cell cycle arrest by inhibiting the activity of CDK4.[67]

HTLV Tax can physically associate with p16ink4a and prevent it from inhibiting CDK4.[68,69] In the presence of Tax there is no mechanism to prevent the phosphorylation of Rb. This results in constitutive activation of E2F-1, and the breakdown of tumor suppression. The effects of Tax on Rb are summarized in Figure 12–10.

Tax-Mediated Inhibition of p53 Mediated Cell Cycle Arrest and Apoptosis

The p53 protein is perhaps the principal cell cycle regulator.[70,71] If there are recognizable mutations after S phase, the concentration of p53 in the nucleus will increase. p53 and the CREB-binding protein (CBP) form a dimer capable of binding to the enhancers of p53 responsive genes. This results in the synthesis of the cyclin-dependent kinase inhibitor p21, cell surface receptor Fas, and the cytoplasmic protein Bax. The presence of p21 results in cell cycle arrest, permitting time for DNA repair so that the mutations do not become permanently etched in the genome. If the damage is irreparable, the increasing levels of Fas surface expression and cytoplasmic Bax renders the cell vulnerable to apoptotic signaling and, ultimately, induces apoptosis.

In order to mediate its *trans*-activating properties, Tax must associate with CBP.[72,73] Tax acts as a competitive inhibitor of the p53/CBP binding event by binding to the same protein folding domain of CBP as p53.[74–76] The effects of Tax on the p53 pathway of tumor suppression are summarized in Figure 12–11. The presence of Tax *trans*-suppresses p53 responsive genes, and protects the cell from both cell cycle arrest and p53 induced apoptosis.

Protection From Receptor-Mediated Apoptotic Signaling

Apoptosis can be triggered by various receptor ligand interactions and intracellular events.[77–82] Trimerization of cell surface tumor necrosis factor receptor (TNFR) and Fas are the two principal mechanisms by which lymphocytes induce apoptosis in immune responses to intracellular pathogens and tumor surveillance. Recognition of TNF and FasL, respectively, by these cell surface complexes can trigger a caspase cascade that results in the cleavage of death substrates and, ultimately, nuclear fragmentation and partitioning of the cell into apoptotic bodies. There are a few interesting characteristics of each of the mechanisms. The TNFR can also trigger a signaling cascade that results in activation of transcription factors (such as NF-kB and

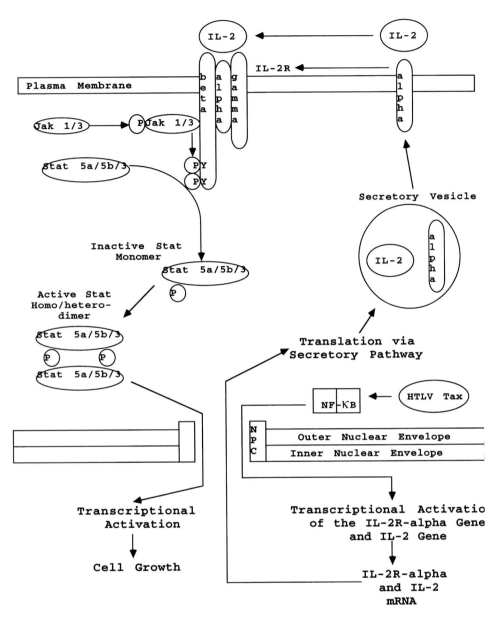

Figure 12–9. Tax mediates constitutive activation of IL-2 signaling pathways. HTLV Tax has the ability to activate NF-kB, which *trans*-activates genes for IL-2 and the IL-2 receptor-alpha chain. In HTLV-infected cells these two proteins are hyperexpressed, causing high surface expression of the IL-2 receptor and a high extracellular concentration of IL-2, which can act as an autocrine factor. IL-2 binding to its cognate receptor transduces a signaling pathway, involving recruitment and phosphorylation of specific members of the Janus family tyrosine kinases (JAKs), and subsequent phosphorylation of specific members of the signal transducers and activators of transcription (STATs) family of transcription factors. This pathway results in the formation of active STAT homo- and heterodimers that can activate the transcription of the IL-2 response genes, which are responsible for cell cycle progression and growth. In HTLV-infected T cells, this pathway would be hyperactive, and would stimulate the cell to proceed through the cell cycle and proliferate in the absence of either direct or indirect antigenic stimulation. (Adapted from Leonard and O'Shea,[56] with permission.)

AP-1) that cause cell cycle progression. Fas can trigger two separate pro-apoptotic cascades each of which result in the activation of caspase 3, the principal effector caspase, and cell death.

Tax activates IKKs and promotes the dissociation and degradation of IkB and *trans*-activates the cJun gene.[46,47] Tax has also been shown to *trans*-activate the XIAP gene, which is an activated caspase 3 inhibitor, and presumably *trans*-activates a FLICE inhibitory protein (FLIP) preventing the activation of caspase 8.[83] Tax inhibits the mitochondria-associated apoptotic pathway by *trans*-suppressing Bax and *trans*-activating the Bcl-Xl gene via NF-kB activation, increasing the Bcl-Xl:Bax ratio.[84,85] This prevents the dissociation of Apaf-1, a necessary substituent of the active caspase 9 complex, from the mitochondrial membrane resulting in protection from apoptosis.

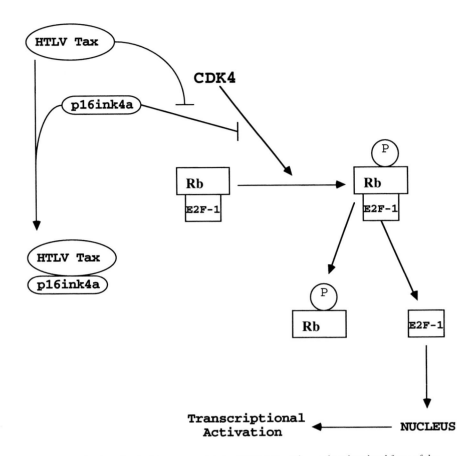

Figure 12–10. Inactivation of retinoblastoma protein by HTLV-1 Tax. The unphosphorylated form of the retinoblastoma (Rb) protein is a tumor suppressor that sequesters E2F-1, a transcriptional activator responsible for cell cycle progression, in the cytoplasm. The ability of Rb to act as a tumor suppressor is dependent on the cyclin-dependent kinase inhibitor p16ink4a (and members of the same family). This inhibitor prevents the phosphorylation of Rb by inhibiting the activity of CDK4, a cyclin-dependent kinase. HTLV Tax can physically associate with p16ink4a and prevent it from inhibiting CDK4. In the presence of Tax there is no mechanism to prevent the phosphorylation of Rb. In its constitutively phosphorylated form, Rb cannot sequester E2F-1, resulting in the unchecked activation of E2F-1, and the breakdown of tumor suppression.

The effects of Tax on the TNF-induced and Fas-induced apoptotic pathways are summarized in Figures 12–12 and 12–13, respectively.

Tax Increases Frequency of Mutation

There have been several studies that have shown that the expression of Tax in HTLV-1-infected cells increases the frequency of mutations in the cellular genome.[86,87] This is presumably mediated by two separate mechanisms, the first of which is dependent on the *trans*-activation of the proliferating cell nuclear antigen (PCNA).[88] PCNA has also been implicated as a necessary factor in both nucleotide excision repair (NER) and mismatch repair (MMR) and also in increasing the processivity of DNA polymerase-delta, an enzyme involved in DNA replication and repair.[89,90] DNA-polymerase-delta mediated repair has been shown to play a role in both NER and MMR. PCNA interacts with the cyclin-dependent kinase inhibitor p21 in the presence of DNA damage to block PCNA-dependent DNA replication without dampening PCNA-dependent DNA repair.[91,92] Excess

PCNA can overcome this competitive inhibition. The second mechanism is mediated by Tax *trans*-suppression of DNA-polymerase-beta.[93] DNA-polymerase-beta has been shown to play an important role in base excision repair (BER). Together, these effects would induce the DNA replicative machinery to proceed even in the presence of DNA damage, increasing the frequency of cellular mutations.

HTLV Modulation of Redox Control

ATL-derived factor (ADF) was first described as an IL-2R-alpha chain-inducing factor.[94] Further experiments determined that ADF was homologous to the bacterial reducing enzyme thioredoxin.[95] Thioredoxin acts as a proton donor to ribonucleotide reductase, a necessary enzyme in the process of DNA replication.[96] Human thioredoxin/ADF is highly expressed in HTLV-1-infected cells.[95,97]

ADF has been shown to enhance the DNA binding of transcription factors AP-1 and NF-kB.[98–101] The reduction of transcription factors allows them to form active DNA-binding

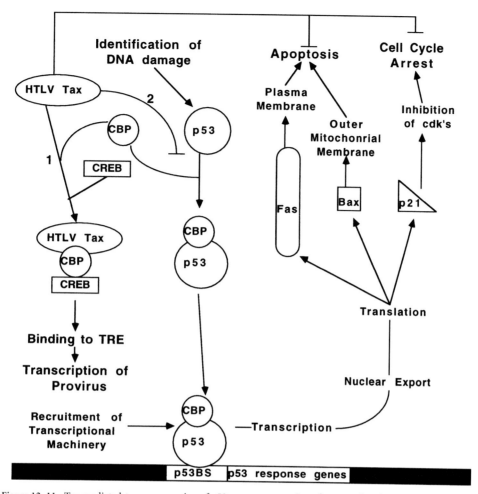

Figure 12–11. Tax-mediated *trans*-suppression of p53 response genes. In order to mediate its *trans*-activating properties, Tax must associate with the cyclic AMP response element binding protein (CREB)-binding protein (CBP) (1). This interaction is required for Tax to augment the binding of CREB to the Tax response element (TRE) in U3 of the proviral LTR, which *trans*-activates viral RNA transcription. CBP also co-activates the tumor suppressor p53 mediated activation (via its binding site) of genes such as Fas (a cell surface receptor that can transduce apoptotic signals [vide infra]), Bax (a cytoplasmic protein responsible for the induction of specific apoptotic events [vide infra]), and p21 (a cyclin-dependent kinase inhibitor). Tax acts as a competitive inhibitor of the p53/CBP binding event (2) by binding to the same protein-folding domain as p53. The presence of Tax *trans*-suppresses p53 response genes, and protects the cell from both cell cycle arrest and p53-induced apoptosis.

configurations so that they can interact with promoter elements to initiate transcription.

ADF also exhibits cytoprotective effects. Although the precise mechanisms are unknown, hyperexpression of ADF has shown protective effects against TNFR-mediated apoptosis and Fas-mediated apoptosis.[102,103] ADF has also been shown to be a potent co-stimulator of cytokine expression, most notably the expression of IL-2 in Molt-4 cells.[104]

HTLV-1 infection can apparently disrupt the normal cellular redox status such that the intracellular environment becomes more reducing. This has multiple effects that could result or aid in carcinogenesis. ADF is required to reduce transcription factors so that they can bind to promoter elements. This activity would explain the stimulation of cytokine production in ADF expressing cells, especially the expression of IL-2 in Molt-4 cells (a CD4+ T-cell line) since IL-2 expression can be initiated by both AP-1

and NF-kB. ADF alone could conceivably act as an activator of growth due to these capabilities, causing manipulation of cellular signaling pathways and mechanisms of growth already discussed.

The cytoprotective effects of ADF could also prove to be important in carcinogenesis by providing an alternate mechanism of avoiding immune surveillance or assisting an already existing one mediated by Tax. In any event, ADF alone seems to be able to protect cells against mechanisms of cytotoxicity.

Development of ATL

The ability of HTLV-1 to transform human T cells is seemingly dependent on the interaction of viral proteins on host cell mechanisms of cell cycle regulation. The development of ATL, however, is probably also dependent on the infected individual's ability to mount a strong immune response to the virus. Manns

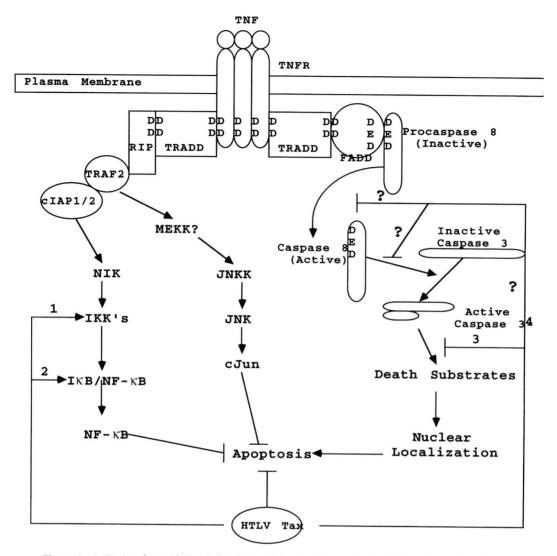

Figure 12–12. Tax interferes with TNF-induced intracellular signaling events. The TNF receptor can transduce several signaling cascades that result either in apoptosis or cell growth and, therefore, protection from apoptosis. The apoptotic signal is delivered through a caspase cascade (initiated by the activation of caspase 8 through recruitment to the cell membrane and subsequent activation of caspase 3) that results in the cleavage of death substrates, which, upon nuclear localization, initiate apoptotic events. The protective events triggered by receptor recognition are mediated through a kinase cascade that results in the activation of *trans*-activators of transcription, among them NF-kB and cJun. These *trans*-activators promote cell growth and serve to activate anti-apoptotic genes. Tax affects these pathways by activating the transcriptional activators NF-kB and cJun by various mechanisms and inhibiting several steps in the caspase cascade. Tax activates IKKs (1) and promotes the dissociation and degradation of IkB (2), and *trans*-activates the cJun gene (not shown). Tax has also been shown to *trans*-activate genes that serve as activated caspase 3 inhibitors (3), and presumably *trans*-activates proteins that could inhibit the caspase cascade at the level of caspase 8 (4), although the exact step that is blocked remains unclear. (Adapted from Screaton and Xu,[82] with permission.)

et al.,[105] in a population study, indicated that certain MHC class II antigens confer susceptibility to the development of either ATL or HTLV-associated myelopathy/tropical spastic paraparesis (HAM/TSP). They showed that 42 percent of HTLV-1 positive individuals expressed the HLA-DR15 allele, as opposed to 4.8 percent of HTLV-1 negative individuals. In addition, 78 percent of positive individuals expressed the HLA-DQ1 allele, as opposed to 53 percent of negative individuals. There were no alleles expressed by negative individuals in greater frequency

than positive individuals that proved to be statistically significant, indicating that there are no alleles among these two loci that would confer absolute resistance to HTLV-1 infection.

The investigators did not find any significant difference between the HLA make-up of ATL patients and asymptomatic carriers with regards to type 2 loci. They did, however, find a significant difference in allelic frequencies between the previous two groups and patients who developed HAM/TSP. There were two DRB1 alleles with higher frequency among the asympto-

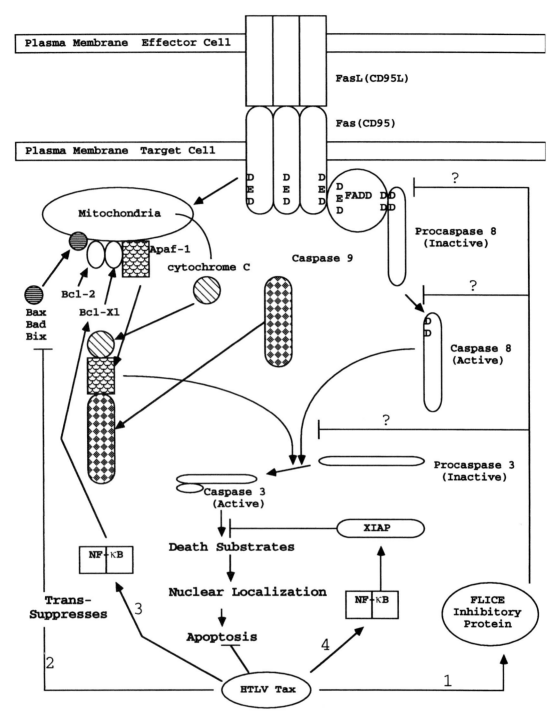

Figure 12–13. Tax interferes with Fas/FasL mediated intracellular signaling. Fas surface receptors can mediate apoptosis through two different caspase cascades. The first involves the activation of caspase 8 by molecules that associate with the receptor (similar to the TNF-induced pathway). The second pathway involves the activation of caspase 9 and is dependent on the release of cytochrome C and Apaf-1 from mitochondria (an event mediated by Bax, Bix, and Bad, which act as competitors for members of the Bcl family of anti-apoptotic molecules). Both of these pathways result in the activation of caspase 3 and the cleavage of death substrates that directly mediate apoptotic events. Tax inhibits the first pathway at the level of caspase 8, presumably by *trans*-activating the FLICE inhibitory protein (1), although the exact step that is inhibited is unknown. Tax inhibits the second pathway by *trans*-suppressing Bax (2) and *trans*-activating the Bcl-Xl gene via NF-κB activation, increasing the Bcl-Xl:Bax ratio. This prevents the dissociation of Apaf-1, a necessary substituent of the active caspase 9 complex, resulting in protection from apoptosis. Tax can inhibit both pathways by *trans*-activating XIAP, which can act as a caspase 3 inhibitor, via NF-κB activation (4). (Adapted from Scaffidi et al.,[81] with permission.)

matic carriers and ATL patients. These were DRB1*1501 and DRB1*1101. One DQB1 allele had significantly greater frequency. This was DQB1*0602. There was no allele that conferred significantly increased susceptibility to HAM/TSP.

In another report, HLA class I alleles, A36 and B18, were found to be increased among patients with ATL compared with HTLV-1 asymptomatics.[106] It is important to note that ATL and HAM/TSP diseases very rarely appear in the same person, and the prevalence of each disease in patients suffering from the other is the same as that of the entire HTLV-1 infected population. Hence, it would seem that the pathogenesis of these two diseases are independent of each other. Since the difference between ATL patients and HAM/TSP patients is in allelic frequencies of certain class II antigens, the basis of that predisposition seems to be immunological.

In vivo experiments with euthymic rats inoculated with HTLV-1-infected cells have shown that suppression of the cell-mediated response by co-stimulatory blockade with monoclonal antibodies (mAbs) to both CD80 and CD86 confers susceptibility to developing tumors.[107] Other experiments with nude rats showed that tumor development can be suppressed by transferring splenic T cells from immunized rats.[108] Immunization in cynomolgus monkeys has shown to provide protective immunity against HTLV-1 infection, presumably by stimulating a strong cell-mediated response to viral antigens.[109]

The induction of apoptosis of infected cells is important to controlling tumor development, considering that several cases of spontaneous regression of ATL have been directly linked to high peripheral cytotoxic activity.[110,111] There have also been studies suggesting the importance of a humoral response to viral envelope glycoproteins to the development of ATL.[112] Individuals with ATL express low antibody titers to envelope glycoproteins when compared with asymptomatic carriers and patients who develop HAM/TSP. Taken together, these results strongly suggest that immunocompetent individuals will be able to control an HTLV infection through CTL attack and induction of apoptosis of infected cells and neutralization of circulating virions through an antibody response. This will prevent both the widespread dissemination of the virus and the expansion of malignant clones in the periphery, and decrease the possibility of developing ATL.

HTLV-1-specific, HLA class I-restricted CD8+ CTLs can be found in HAM/TSP patients and asymptomatic HTLV-1 carriers but are barely detectable in ATL patients.[112–116] This difference can potentially be explained in the differences in class I and class II allelic frequencies among the different clinical states. Among the class II antigens, asymptomatic carriers and ATL patients have similar allelic frequencies, and have significantly higher frequencies than HAM/TSP patients at these loci. This suggests that the MHC-II mechanism of antigen presentation may have an effect on the proliferative response to HTLV-1 antigens. Perhaps the epitopes presented on DRB1*1501, DRB1*1101, and DQB1*0602 are not very immunogenic, and do not stimulate a strong CD4+ proliferative response. The alleles expressed by HAM/TSP patients, however, are able to express the immunodominant epitopes to HTLV-1, and are therefore able to stimulate a strong proliferative response in HTLV-1-specific CD4+ T cells.

The difference between ATL patients and asymptomatic carriers seems to rely on class I restriction. Perhaps the A36 and B18 class I antigens, expressed at a higher frequency among ATL patients, do not mediate strong specific lysis, and the alleles expressed by asymptomatic carriers do. Therefore, despite the weak proliferative response among the asymptomatic carriers, these individuals are able to lyse infected cells efficiently before they develop a malignant clone. ATL patients do not seem to possess this ability.

The difference in numbers of virus-specific CTLs in asymptomatic carriers and ATL patients, despite a predicted similarity in the proliferative response, could be due to this difference in CTL cytotoxicity between the two clinical states. CTLs that cannot mediate specific lysis of infected cells will be eliminated due to Tax-induced apoptosis. Expression of Tax *trans*-activates the gene for Fas-ligand (CD95L).[117] An infected cell will express high surface levels of Fas-ligand. Infected cells have shown the ability to, in vitro, induce T-cell death by apoptosis.[117] Since activated CTLs express Fas, HTLV-1-infected cells will induce apoptosis in antigen-recognizing cells. In ATL patients with CTLs that cannot mediate effective lysis, the virus-specific CTLs would be eliminated at a higher rate than in asymptomatic carriers.

Certain immunological characteristics of the infected individual determine whether HTLV-1 infection will result in the development of ATL. Individuals who can mount a strong immune response, most importantly a strong cell-mediated response, are able to clear infected and transformed cells and are at a decreased risk of developing ATL, although they seem to be at a higher risk for developing autoimmune neurological diseases. In the presence of weak CTL responses, HTLV-1 transformed cells will develop into malignant clones that will go on to cause disease symptoms.

CLINICOPATHOLOGICAL FEATURES OF ATL

ATL was the name given by Japanese investigators to the first human malignancy known to be induced by a retrovirus. ATL patients usually have antibodies against HTLV-1 as well as clonally rearranged T-antigen receptor V-β and V-γ genes and monoclonally integrated proviral HTLV-1 DNA in their mature malignant T lymphocytes. ATL patients have increased numbers of either circulating or tissue-associated lymphocytes with convoluted or "flowered" nuclei, or both. The surface phenotype of the malignant cell is usually CD3+, CD4+, CD7–, CD8–, CD30+, CD25+, and TdT–. Occasional tumors will be CD4+, CD8+, (double positive) or will lack CD4 and CD8 altogether (double negative). Fresh peripheral blood ATL cells secrete high levels of transforming growth factor β1 (TGF-β1) but low levels of IL-2, IL-4, IL-5, and γ-interferon, suggesting that they function (either before or after HTLV-1 infection) as immunological suppressors of normal T- and B-lymphocyte proliferation and function.[118]

Clinically ATL is characterized by 1. adult age of onset; 2. ATL cells with typical morphology; 3. cutaneous involvement (25 to 50 percent); 4. high propensity for parenchymal organ and central nervous system (CNS) involvement (with some patients presenting with primary CNS lymphoma); 5. hypercalcemia usually with concomitant lytic bone disease; 6. impaired immunoglobulin and T-cell immune responses with over 50 percent of patients presenting with or developing opportunistic infections; and 7. geographic or familial associations. Lymphomas are usually deemed to be of the diffuse intermediate or high grade of mixed, lymphoblastic, or immunoblastic morphology.[12] Many patients present with eosinophilia and, in the past, ATL cases were often misdiagnosed as Hodgkin's disease or Wegener's granulomatosis because of the marked proliferation of other hematopoietic cells in biopsy specimens due to release of cytokines by the virally infected cells and the formation of virally induced multinucleated syncytial cells that look like Reed-Sternberg cells or a common midline nasopharyngeal location.[21,119] Most experienced hematopathologists and clinicians can now make a clear distinction among these various entities. The term ATL is actually a misnomer, because ATL has been diagnosed in children as young as 14 months. Also, the disease clinically overlaps with other mature T-cell neoplasms (e.g., cutaneous T-cell lymphomas and peripheral T-cell lymphomas) that are HTLV-1 negative. We consider that a more appropriate term might be HTLV-1-associated T-cell lymphoma/leukemia (HATL) and that the disease be virologically defined, preferably by molecular techniques and certainly in therapeutic clinical trials.

Only a small fraction (estimates range from 0.1 to 3 percent) of HTLV-1-infected patients progress from polyclonal to oligoclonal to monoclonal leukemia proliferation over their lifetime. This figure approaches 10 percent in patients infected perinatally, and no transfusion-acquired cases of HATL have been reported. The disease usually takes three to four decades to manifest after infection. Four clinical presentations of HATL have been described.[120] Acute or prototypic HATL patients present with the common abnormalities listed above. Elevated lactate dehydrogenase (LDH), serum calcium, and bilirubin and high leukemic cell counts are associated with a poor prognosis, and most patients do not survive beyond 1 to 2 years. Smoldering HATL is characterized by a waxing and waning of symptoms over many years. Patients have a low percentage (0.5 to 3 percent) of leukemic cells in their peripheral blood and minimal lymphadenopathy, liver, spleen, and bone marrow involvement. Chronic HATL patients have increased numbers of circulating HTLV-1-infected lymphocytes and slight parenchymal organ involvement. Survival time is midway between the acute and smoldering forms. Eventually, most chronic and smoldering forms evolve into the acute form, which carries a poor prognosis. Lymphoma-type HATL is characterized by a lack of obvious leukemia, marked lymphadenopathy with an intermediate- or high-grade histology, elevated LDH and calcium, and poor survival.[12] It would seem probable that more scientific or molecularly defined grading and staging systems will emerge for HATL as the use of novel clinical treatment increases.

TREATMENT OF HATL

Few large-scale randomized trials have been published regarding the treatment of HATL.[121–124] The standard of care today involves a regimen of chemotherapy indicated for non-Hodgkin's lymphoma (e.g., cyclophosphamide, doxorubicin, vincristine, and prednisone [CHOP]).[16,121–124] Single agent low-dose etoposide and irinotecan hydrochloride have also shown efficacy.[125,126] Median survival with standard dose chemotherapy is usually less than 2 years. Even if induction is successful, complete durable remissions are rare. This lack of sustained efficacy is due in part to the expression of multidrug-resistance-protein (MRP) and lung-resistance-protein (LRP) in HTLV-1-infected cells.[127] MRP belongs to the ATP binding cassette superfamily of transporter proteins, which interacts directly or indirectly with various drugs and actively effects their efflux from human cells.[128] LRP functions as a bidirectional nucleocytoplasmic transporter of molecules and particles.[128] These factors decrease the efficacy of chemotherapeutic agents. Few trials of high-dose chemotherapy with bone marrow or peripheral blood stem cell rescue have been reported, but one report suggests that allogeneic bone marrow transplantation following high-dose chemotherapy regimens can result in prolonged disease-free intervals in HATL.[129]

Despite the poor track record of standard chemotherapies noted above, several palliative treatments can be used to ameliorate symptoms associated with HATL. For example, external beam radiation or orthopedic procedures can be used to treat lytic bone lesions. Biphosphonates can be used to treat hypercalcemia. Topical steroids or cytotoxic agents, electron beam radiation, and/or psoralen plus ultraviolet light (plus/minus interferon-alpha) can all be used to treat skin lesions with modest response rates.[121,123]

A number of novel treatments have demonstrated in vitro and in vivo activity against HTLV-1 transformed cells. Both interferon-alpha and -beta have anti-HTLV effects that are due to direct cytopathicity and/or augmented immune responses.[130] Interferon-alpha has also shown some success clinically when used with zidovudine (AZT), or in vitro against HTLV-1-infected CD4+ cell lines when used with arsenic trioxide.[131,132] Arsenic trioxide has been shown to inhibit growth of leukemic cells by itself, but its effects synergize with those of interferon-alpha to induce cell cycle arrest and apoptosis of leukemic cells.[133] Other agents such as green tea polyphenols have been shown to induce apoptosis in HATL leukemic cells in vitro; ubenimex (Bestatin), has been shown to have clinical activity in chronic HATL.[134,135]

Perhaps some of the most promising specific therapies for HATL involve those directed at surface molecules hyperexpressed in HTLV-infected cells. These have involved using either murine or chimeric monoclonal antibodies directed against either the IL-2 (anti-Tac) or the IL-15 receptors, which are hyperexpressed and functional on HTLV-1-infected cells due to HTLV Tax induced trans-activation.[136,137] Approaches taken included direct binding of the antibodies and allowing for antibody-dependent cell-mediated cytotoxicity and/or complement fixation and activation to occur, or coupling the antibody with Pseudomonas exotoxin, Diphtheria endotoxin, or the radioisotope, Yttrium-90, to deliver a cytotoxic effect specifically to the HTLV-1-infected cells.[138–140] Alternatively, other investigators have developed fusion proteins with IL-2 and either Pseudomonas exotoxin or *Diphtheria* endotoxin to achieve the same effects via the binding of the chimeric ligand to the overexpressed IL-2 receptor.[141]

Given the limited effectiveness of conventional therapies on the overall survival of HATL patients, the obvious question is whether some of the more aggressive (stem cell transplant) or novel (IL-2 receptor mediated) treatments noted above should be employed earlier in the course of HTLV-1-induced leukemogenesis. Certainly, since only a minority of carriers will ever develop HATL, it would be unwise to treat all asymptomatic carriers of HTLV-1. Further, our own in vitro data indicate that, as opposed to its effects on cultured HATL leukemic cells, treatment of peripheral blood mononuclear cell cultures from asymptomatic HTLV-1 carriers with IL-2 *Diphtheria* toxin fusion protein results in increased HTLV-1 DNA content in the cultures over time, presumably because uninfected, anti-HTLV-1, activated, cytotoxic, IL-2 receptor positive T cells are being killed by the agent (Poiesz et al., in preparation). Theoretically, chronic in vivo use of such an agent in HTLV-1 carriers could result in an increased incidence of HATL. However, it would seem possible to episodically monitor the peripheral blood of HTLV-1-infected individuals for clonal expansion of virally infected cells, either by performing PCR for T-cell receptor Vβ or Vγ gene rearrangements or HTLV-1 integration sites.[16] Prospective national or international clinical trials could determine whether such clonal expansion predicts for the ultimate development of HATL and, if so, whether therapeutic intervention at such an early stage could significantly alter the natural history of this almost uniformly fatal disease. Also, preliminary data indicate that, because of its low replication rate and marked conservation of antigenic epitopes, passive and active immunization with neutralizing antibodies of HTLV vaccines would be highly effective in preventing the spread of HTLV infection.

TSP/HAM AND OTHER HTLV-1 ASSOCIATED DISEASES

HTLV-1 is now clearly associated with a variety of inflammatory diseases including a neurological syndrome termed tropical spastic paraparesis/HTLV-1 associated myelopathy (TSP/HAM), polymyositis, polyarthritis, and uveitis.[142–145] TSP/HAM is characterized by the presence of spastic paraparesis of the lower extremities, variable impairment of superficial and deep sensation, and bladder and bowel hyperspasticity. HTLV-1 infection of the cerebrospinal fluid has been documented. Histopathological studies on the CNS of affected patients have demonstrated marked chronic inflammatory reactions with lymphocytic infiltration, perivascular cuffing, and demyelination in the spinal cord, and (to a lesser extent) the brain. HTLV-1 associated polymyositis, uveitis, and polyarthritis show similar histopathological features (intense lymphocytic infiltration and destruction of surrounding tissue). All of the above patients characteristically have evidence of hyperexpression of HTLV-1, particularly at the site of organ involvement, and much higher levels of anti-HTLV-1 humoral and cell-mediated cytotoxic responses relative to asymptomatic carriers.

Epidemiologically, the pathogenesis of these diseases seems to be independent of the development of HATL. Except for synovial cells in arthritis patients, no clear evidence shows that these "autoimmune-like" diseases are caused by direct infection of neuronal, muscle, or ocular tissue by HTLV-1. Rather, it would seem that they are caused by direct toxic effects of HTLV-1, viral proteins, or induced host cytokines or by a more specific or cross-reactive immune response. Some treatment successes have been seen. Danazol produces a high rate of palliation of variable duration in TSP/HAM, and most patients with the other "autoimmune" HTLV-1-associated diseases respond to low-dose steroids.

HTLV-2-INDUCED DISEASES

Long-term epidemiological studies in endemic populations have clearly established that HTLV-2 is much less pathogenic in humans than HTLV-1.[146] Nevertheless, HTLV-2 has clearly been shown to be associated with clonal T-cell lymphocytoses and has been detected in patients with unusual T-cell neoplasias.[5,147–150] It was first isolated from a cell line derived from the spleen of a patient thought to have T-cell hairy cell leukemia.[5] Four years later, a second isolate was obtained from another patient with CD8+ T-cell leukemia and B-cell hairy cell leukemia; the HTLV-2 was monoclonally integrated in the CD8+ leukemia cells but not the B-lymphocytic hairy cells.[148] In retrospect, both the patients probably suffered from CD8+ large granular T-lymphocytic (LGL) leukemia. Since then, several groups have identified similar CD8+, CD3+ HTLV-2-infected LGL patients. However, in larger series it is clear that HTLV-2 infection is only rarely associated with this disease.[149,150] Also, several HIV-1 and HTLV-2 co-infected patients with a generalized severely pruritic erythrodermatitis have been identified.[151–153] Histopathologically, the skin biopsies of these patients have been interpreted as cutaneous T-cell lymphoma (CTCL) and, when examined, the abnormal cells have been shown to be clonal, HTLV-2-infected, CD8+ T lymphocytes. It is unknown whether the natural history of HTLV-2-associated CD8+, T-cell LGL leukemia or CD8+ CTCL differs from that of the HTLV-2 negative forms of these diseases, but patients with both these rare HTLV-associated neoplasms have responded to the conventional treatments usually employed in their viral negative counterparts.

HTLV-2 infection has now been noted in an increasing number of patients with a chronic neurodegenerative disorder.[154] This disease is similar to HTLV-1-induced TSP/HAM in that patients have motor deficits, spasticity, and urinary infrequency, albeit to a milder degree. However, in addition, prominent ataxia and altered mental states were present in the HTLV-2-infected patients. These patients also respond to Danazol. HTLV-2 infection has also been associated with an increased susceptibility to cutaneous bacterial infections and immunoglobulin deficiencies. Further studies will be required to define the diseases associated with HTLV-2.

REFERENCES

1. Poiesz BJ, Ruscetti FW, Mier JW, Woods AM, Gallo RC: T-cell lines established from human T-lymphocytic neoplasias by direct response to T-cell growth factor. Proc Natl Acad Sci USA 77:6815, 1980.

2. Poiesz BJ, Ruscetti FW, Gazdar AF, Bunn PA, Minna JD, Gallo RC: Detection and isolation of type C retrovirus particles from fresh and cultured lymphocytes of a patient with cutaneous T-cell lymphoma. Proc Natl Acad Sci USA 77:7415, 1980.

3. Poiesz BJ, Ruscetti FW, Reitz MS, Kalyanaraman VS, Gallo RC: Isolation of a new type C retrovirus (HTLV) in primary uncultured cells of a patient with Sezary T-cell leukaemia. Nature 294:268, 1981.

4. Reitz MS Jr, Poiesz BJ, Ruscetti FW, Gallo RC: Characterization and distribution of nucleic acid sequences of a novel type C retrovirus isolated from neoplastic human T lymphocytes. Proc Natl Acad Sci USA 78:1887, 1981.

5. Kalyanaraman VS, Sarngadharan MG, Poiesz B, Ruscetti FW, Gallo RC: Immunological properties of a type C retrovirus isolated from cultured T-lymphoma cells and comparison to other mammalian retroviruses. J Virol 38:906, 1981.

6. Rho HM, Poiesz B, Ruscetti FW, Gallo RC: Characterization of the reverse transcriptase from a new retrovirus (HTLV) produced by a human cutaneous T-cell lymphoma cell line. Virology 112:355, 1981.

7. Seiki M, Hattori S, Hirayami Y et al: Human adult T-cell leukemia virus: Complete nucleotide sequence of the provirus genome integrated in leukemia cell DNA. Proc Natl Acad Sci USA 80:3618, 1983.

8. Posner LE, Robert-Guroff M, Kalyanaraman VS, Poiesz BJ, Ruscetti FW, Fossieck B et al: Natural antibodies to the human T-cell lymphoma virus in patients with cutaneous T-cell lymphomas. J Exp Med 154:333, 1981.

9. Yoshida M, Miyoski I, Hinuma Y: Isolation and characterization of retrovirus (ATLV) from cell lines of human adult T-cell leukemia and its implication in the diseases. Proc Natl Acad Sci 79:2031, 1982.

10. Blattner WA, Kalyanaraman VS, Robert-Guroff M, Lister TA, Galton DAG, Sarin PS et al: The human type C retrovirus, HTLV, in blacks from the Caribbean region, and relationship to adult T-cell leukemia/lymphoma. Int J Cancer 30:257, 1982.

11. Kalyanaraman VS, Sarngadharan MG, Robert-Guroff M, Miyoshi I, Golde D, Gallo RC: A new subtype of human T-cell leukemia virus (HTLV-II) associated with a T-cell variant of hairy cell leukemia. Science 218:571, 1982.

12. Poiesz BJ, Sherman M, Saksena N et al: The biology and epidemiology of the human T-cell lymphoma/leukemia viruses. In Neu HC, Levy J, Weiss R (eds.): Frontiers of Infectious Diseases. Focus on HIV, p. 189. Churchill Livingstone, London, 1993.

13. Digilio L, Gire A, Cho N et al: The simian T-lymphotropic/leukemia virus from Pan paniscus belongs to the type 2 family and infects Asian macaques. J Virol 71:3684, 1997.

14. Salemi M, Lewis M, Egan JF, Hall WW, Desmyter J, Vandamme AM: Different population dynamics of human T-cell lymphotropic virus type II in intravenous drug users compared with endemically infected tribes. Proc Natl Acad Sci USA: 96:13253, 1999.

15. Goulau P, Van Brussel M, Vandamme AM et al: A primate T-lymphotropic virus, PTLV-I, different from human T-lymphotropic viruses type I and II, in a wild-caught baboon (Papio hamadryas). Proc Natl Acad Sci USA 91:2848, 1994.

16. Poiesz BJ, Papsidero LD, Ehrlich G, Sherman M, Dube S, Poiesz M et al: Prevalence of HTLV-I associated T-cell lymphoma. Am J Hematol 66:32, 2001.

17. Anderson DW, Epstein JS, Lee TH, Lairmore MD, Saxinger C, Kalyanaraman VS et al: Serological confirmation of human T-lymphotropic virus type I infection in healthy blood and plasma donors. Blood 74:2585, 1989.

18. Lipka JJ, Miyoshi I, Hadlock KG, Reyes GR, Chow TP, Blattner WA et al: Segregation of human T cell lymphotropic virus type I and II infections by antibody reactivity to unique viral epitopes. J Infect Dis 165:268, 1992.

19. Ehrlich GD, Glaser JB, Abbott MA, Slamon DJ, Keith D, Sliwkowski M et al: Detection of anti-HTLV-I Tax antibodies in HTLV-I enzyme-linked immunosorbent assay-negative individuals. Blood 74:1066, 1989.

20. Poiesz BJ, Dube S, Choi D, Esteban E, Ferrer J, Leon-Pomte M et al: Comparative performances of an HTLV-I/II EIA and other serological and PCR assays on samples from persons at risk for HTLV-II infection. Transfusion 40:924, 2000.

21. Duggan DB, Ehrlich G, Davey FP et al: HTLV-I induced lymphoma mimicking Hodgkin's disease: Diagnosis by polymerase chain reaction amplification of specific HTLV-I sequences in tumor DNA. Blood 74:1027, 1988.

22. Hall WW, Liu CR, Schneewind O, Takahashi H, Kaplan MH, Roupe G, Vahlne A: Deleted HTLV-I provirus in blood and cutaneous lesions of patients with mycosis fungoides. Science 253:317, 1991.

23. Dyster LM, Poiesz BJ, Abbot TL et al: Evaluation of enzyme oligonucleotide assays for the specific detection of HIV-1, HTLV-I, and HTLV-II DNA following gene amplification. J Clin Microbiol 32:547, 1994.

24. Dube DK, Dube S, Erensoy S, Jones B, Bryz-Gornia V, Spicer T et al: Serological and nucleic acid analyses for HIV and HTLV infection on archival human plasma samples from Zaire. Virology 202:379, 1994.

25. Sherman MP, Dube S, Dube D, Poiesz BJ: Virally induced T-cell malignancies and associated diseases. In Rich CRA (ed.): Clinical Immunology: Principles and Practice. Mosby-Year Book, St. Louis, 1995.

26. Weiss RA, Clapham P, Nagy K, Hoshino H: Envelope properties of human T-cell leukemia viruses. Curr Top Microbiol Immunol 115:235, 1985.

27. Kirchbaum-Stenger K, Poiesz BJ, Ehrlich G, Gavalchin J, Davis BH, Moore J: Specific adsorption of HTLV-I to various target human and animal cells. Blood 70:1303, 1987.

28. Gavalchin J, Fan N, Lane MJ, Papsidero L, Poiesz BJ: Identification of a putative cellular receptor for HTLV-I by a monoclonal antibody, Mab 34-23. Virology 194:1, 1994.

29. Sagara Y, Ishida C, Inoue Y, Shiraki H, Maeda Y: 71-kilodalton heat shock cognate protein acts as a cellular receptor for syncytium formation induced by human T-cell lymphotropic virus type 1. J Virol 72:535, 1998.

30. Gavalchin J, Fan N, Waterbury PG, Corbett E, Faldasz BD, Peshick SM et al: Regional localization of the putative cell surface receptor for HTLV-I to human chromosome 17q23.2–17q25.3. Virology 212:196, 1995.

31. Yoshida M: Tenth anniversary perspectives on AIDS. Host-HTLV type I interaction at the molecular level. AIDS Res Hum Retroviruses 10:1193, 1994.

32. Fan N, Gavalchin J, Paul B, Wells TH, Lane MJ, Poiesz BJ: Infection of peripheral blood mononuclear cells and cell lines by cell free human T-cell lymphoma/leukemia virus type I. J Clin Microbiol 30:905, 1992.

33. Preston BD, Poiesz BJ, Loeb LA: Fidelity of HIV-1 reverse transcriptase. Science 242:1168, 1988.

34. Temin HM: Retrovirus variation and reverse transcription: Abnormal strand transfers result in retrovirus genetic variation. Proc Natl Acad Sci 90:6900, 1993.

35. Shimotohno K, Takahashi Y, Shimizu N, Gojobori T, Golde DW, Chen IS et al: Complete nucleotide sequence of an infectious clone of human T-cell leukemia virus type II: An open reading frame for the protease gene. Proc Natl Acad Sci USA 82:3101, 1985.

36. Seiki M, Inoue J, Hidaka M, Yoshida M: Two cis-acting elements responsible for post-transcriptional trans-regulation of gene expression of human T-cell leukemia virus type I. Proc Natl Acad Sci USA 85:7124, 1988.

37. Sodroski JG, Rosen CA, Haseltine WA: Trans-acting transcriptional activation of the long terminal repeat of human T lymphotropic viruses in infected cells. Science 225:381, 1984.

38. Felber BK, Paskalis H, Kleinman-Ewing C, Wong-Staal F, Pavlakis GN: The pX protein of HTLV-I is a transcriptional activator of its long terminal repeats. Science 229:675, 1985.

39. Shimotokono K, Takano M, Terewchi T et al: Requirements of multiple copies of a 21-nucleotide sequence in the U3 region of human T-cell leukemia virus type I and type II long terminal repeats for trans-acting activation of transcription. Proc Natl Acad Sci USA 83:8112, 1986.

40. Dube S, Paul B, Bryz-Gornia V et al: Use of PCR in detection of antisense transcripts in HTLV-I-infected patients and human T-cell lines. In Sarkar G (ed.): Methods in Neurosciences, Vol. 26, PCR in Neuroscience, p. 381. Academic Press, New York, 1995.

41. Hidaka M, Inoue J, Yoshida M, Seiki M: Post-transcriptional regulator (rex) of HTLV-1 initiates expression of viral structural proteins but suppresses expression of regulatory proteins. EMBO J 7:519, 1988.

42. Rimsky L, Dodon MD, Dixon EP, Greene WC: Trans-dominant inactivation of HTLV-I and HIV-1 gene expression by mutation of the HTLV-I Rex transactivator. Nature 341:453, 1989.

43. Graziano SL, Lehr B, Merl SA, Moor JL, Hallinan EJ, Hubbel C et al: A quantitative assay for HTLV-I transformation. Cancer Res 47:2468, 1987.

44. Jeang KT, Widen SG, Semmes OJ 4th, Wilson SH: HTLV-I transactivator protein, tax, is a trans-repressor of the human beta-polymerase gene. Science 247:1082, 1990.

45. Lee JI, Burckart GJ: Nuclear factor kappa B: Important transcription factor and therapeutic target. J Clin Pharmacol 38:981, 1998.

46. Hiscott J, Beauparlant P, Crepieux P, DeLuca C, Kwon H, Lin R, Petropoulos L: Cellular and viral protein interactions regulating I kappa B alpha activity during human retrovirus infection. J Leukoc Biol 62:82, 1997.

47. Li XK, Murphy KM, Palka KT, Surabhi RM, Gaynor RB: The human T-cell leukemia virus type-1 Tax protein regulates the activity of the IkB kinase complex. J Biol Chem 274:34417, 1999.

48. Petropoulos L, Lin R, Hiscott J: Human T cell leukemia virus type 1 tax protein increases NF-kappa B dimer formation and antagonizes the inhibitory activity of the I kappa B alpha protein. Virology 225:52, 1996.

49. Judd BA, Koretzky GA: Antigen specific T lymphocyte activation. Rev Immunogenet 2:164, 2000.

50. Schwartz RH: T-cell clonal anergy. Curr Opin Immunol 9:351, 1997.

51. Weil R, Levraud JP, Dodon MD, Bessia C, Hazan U, Kourilsky P, Israel A: Altered expression of tyrosine kinases of the Src and Syk families in human T-cell leukemia virus type I-infected T-cell lines. J Virol 73:3709, 1999.

52. Good L, Maggirwar SB, Harhaj EW, Sun SC: Constitutive dephosphorylation and activation of a member of the nuclear factor of activated T cells, NF-AT1, in Tax-expressing and type I human T-cell leukemia virus-infected human T cells. J Biol Chem 272:1425, 1997.

53. Good L, Maggirwar SB, Sun SC: Activation of the IL-2 gene promoter by HTLV-I tax involves induction of NF-AT complexes bound to the CD28-responsive element. EMBO J 15:3744, 1996.

54. Fujii M, Iwai K, Oie M, Fukushi M, Yamamoto N, Kannagi M, Mori N: Activation of oncogenic transcription factor AP-1 in T cells infected with human T cell leukemia virus type 1. AIDS Res Hum Retroviruses 16:1603, 2000.

55. Iwai K, Mori N, Oie M, Yamamoto N, Fujii M: Human T-cell leukemia virus type 1 tax protein activates transcription through AP-1 site by inducing DNA binding activity in T cells. Virology 279:38, 2001.

56. Leonard WJ, O'Shea JJ: Jaks and STATs: Biological implications. Annu Rev Immunol 16:293, 1990.

57. Sugamura K, Fujii M, Sakitani M, Kobayashi N, Nakai S, Hatanaka M, Hinuma Y: Human retrovirus-induced IL-2 receptors and their possible role in transduction of continuous cell growth signal. Princess Takamatsu Symp 15:269, 1984.

58. Uchiyama T, Wano Y, Tsudo M, Umadome H, Hori T, Tamori S et al: Abnormal expression of interleukin-2 receptor (Tac antigen) in adult T-cell leukemia. Princess Takamatsu Symp 15:253, 1984.

59. Himes SR, Katsikeros R, Shannon MF: Costimulation of cytokine gene expression in T cells by the human T leukemia/lymphotropic virus type 1 trans activator Tax. J Virol 70:4001, 1996.

60. Nakamura N, Fujii M, Tsukahara T, Arai M, Ohashi T, Wakao H et al: Human T-cell leukemia virus type 1 Tax protein induces the expression of STAT1 and STAT5 genes in T-cells. Oncogene 18:2667, 1999.

61. Arima N: Autonomous and interleukin-2-responsive growth of leukemic cells in adult T-cell leukemia (ATL): A review of the clinical significance and molecular basis of ATL cell growth. Leuk Lymphoma 26:479, 1997.

62. Hollsberg P, Wucherpfennig KW, Ausubel LJ, Calvo V, Bierer BE, Hafler DA: Characterization of HTLV-I in vivo infected T cell clones. IL-2-independent growth of nontransformed T cells. J Immunol 148:3256, 1992.

63. Akagi T, Shimotohno K: Proliferative response of Tax1-transduced primary human T cells to anti-CD3 antibody stimulation by an interleukin-2-independent pathway. J Virol 67:1211, 1993.

64. Yang YC, Hung TP, Wang CH, Lin MT, Hsu TY, Chen JY et al: Establishment and characterization of an HTLV-I cell line from a Taiwanese patient with HTLV-I-associated myelopathy. J Neurol Sci 120:46, 1993.

65. Zhang Q, Lee B, Koreck M, Li G, Weyland C, Eck S et al: Differences in phosphorylation of the IL-2R associated JAK/STAT proteins between HTLV-I(+) IL-2-independent and IL-2-dependent cell lines and uncultured leukemic cells from patients with adult T-cell lymphoma/leukemia. Leuk Res 23:373, 1999.

66. Stiegler P, Kasten M, Giordano A: The RB family of cell cycle regulatory factors. J Cell Biochem 30–31(Suppl):30, 1998.

67. Shapiro GI, Edwards CD, Rollins BJ: The physiology of p16(INK4A)-mediated G1 proliferative arrest. Cell Biochem Biophys 33:189, 2000.

68. Suzuki T, Kitao S, Matsushime H, Yoshida M: HTLV-1 Tax protein interacts with cyclin-dependent kinase inhibitor p16-ink4a and counteracts its inhibitory activity towards CDK4. EMBO J 15:1607, 1999.

69. Suzuki T, Narita T, Uchida-Toita M, Yoshida M: Down-regulation of the INK4 family of cyclin-dependent kinase inhibitors by tax protein of HTLV-1 through two distinct mechanisms. Virology 259:384, 1999.

70. Ewen ME, Miller SJ: p53 and translational control. Biochim Biophys Acta 1242:181, 1996.

71. Wang XW, Harris CC: p53 tumor-suppressor gene: Clues to molecular carcinogenesis. J Cell Physiol 173:247, 1997.

72. Yin MJ, Gaynor RB: HTLV-1 21 bp repeat sequences facilitate stable association between Tax and CREB to increase CREB binding affinity. J Mol Biol 264:20, 1996.

73. Harrod R, Tang Y, Nicot C, Lu HS, Vassilev A, Nakatani Y, Giam CZ: An exposed KID-like domain in human T-cell lymphotropic virus type 1 Tax is responsible for the recruitment of coactivators CBP/p300. Mol Cell Biol 18:5052, 1998.

74. Suzuki T, Uchida-Toita M, Yoshida M: Tax protein of HTLV-1 inhibits CBP/p300-mediated transcription by interfering with recruitment of CBP/p300 onto DNA element of E-box or p53 binding site. Oncogene 18:4137, 1999.

75. Van Orden K, Giebler HA, Lemasson I, Gonzales M, Nyborg JK: Binding of p53 to the KIX domain of CREB binding protein. A potential link to human T-cell leukemia virus, type I-associated leukemogenesis. J Biol Chem 274:26321, 1999.

76. Ariumi Y, Kaida A, Lin JY, Hirota M, Masui O, Yamaoka S et al: HTLV-1 tax oncoprotein represses the p53-mediated trans-activation function through coactivator CBP sequestration. Oncogene 19:1491, 2000.

77. Wong B, Choi Y: Pathways leading to cell death in T cells. Curr Opin Immunol 9:358, 1997.

78. Baker SJ, Reddy EP: Modulation of life and death by the TNF receptor superfamily. Oncogene 17:3261, 1998.

79. Chao DT, Korsmeyer SJ: BCL-2 family: Regulators of cell death. Annu Rev Immunol 16:395, 1998.

80. Malek NP, Pluempe J, Kubicka S, Manns MP, Trautwein C: Molecular mechanisms of TNF receptor-mediated signaling. Recent Results Cancer Res 147:97, 1998.

81. Scaffidi C, Kirchhoff S, Krammer PH, Peter ME: Apoptosis signaling in lymphocytes. Curr Opin Immunol 11:277, 1999.

82. Screaton G, Xu XN: T cell life and death signaling via TNF-receptor family members. Curr Opin Immunol 12:316, 2000.

83. Kawakami A, Nakashima T, Sakai H, Urayama S, Yamasaki S, Hida A et al: Inhibition of caspase cascade by HTLV-I tax through induction of NF-kappa B nuclear translocation. Blood 94:3847, 1999.

84. Brauweiler A, Garrus JE, Reed JC, Nyborg JK: Repression of bax gene expression by the HTLV-1 Tax protein: Implications for suppression of apoptosis in virally infected cells. Virology 231:135, 1997.

85. Tsurakahara T, Kannagi M, Ohashi T, Kato H, Arai M, Nunez G et al: Induction of Bcl-x(L) expression by human T-cell leukemia virus type 1 Tax through NF-kappa B in apoptosis-resistant T-cell transfectants with Tax. J Virol 73:7981, 1999.

86. Miyake H, Suzuki T, Hirai H, Yoshida M: Trans-activator Tax of human T-cell leukemia virus type 1 enhances mutation frequency of the cellular genome. Virology 253:155, 1999.

87. Philpott SM, Buehring GC: Defective DNA repair in cells with human T-cell leukemia/bovine leukemia viruses: Role of tax gene. J Natl Cancer Inst 91(11):933, 1999.

88. Kao SY, Marriott SJ: Disruption of nucleotide excision repair by the human T-cell leukemia virus type 1 Tax protein. J Virol 73:4299, 1999.

89. Kelman Z: PCNA: structure, functions and interactions. Oncogene 14(6):629, 1997.

90. Wood RD, Shivji MK: Which DNA polymerases are used for DNA-repair in eukaryotes? Carcinogenesis 18:605, 1997.

91. Saggioro D, Majone F, Forino M, Turchetto L, Leszl A, Chieco-Bianchi L: Tax protein of human T-lymphotropic virus type I triggers DNA damage. Leuk Lymphoma 12:281, 1994.

92. Waga S, Hannon GJ, Beach D, Stillman B: The p21 inhibitor of cyclin-dependent kinases controls DNA replication by interaction with PCNA. Nature 369:574, 1994.

93. Jeang KT, Widen SG, Semmes OJ 4th, Wilson SH: HTLV-I trans-activator protein, tax, is a trans-repressor of the human beta-polymerase gene. Science 247:1082, 1990.

94. Teshigawara K, Maeda M, Nishino K, Nikaido T, Uchiyama T, Tsudo M et al: Adult T leukemia cells produce a lymphokine that augments interleukin 2 receptor expression. J Mol Cell Immunol 2:17, 1985.

95. Tagaya Y, Maeda Y, Mitsui A, Konodo N, Matsui H, Hamuro J et al: ATL-derived factor (ADF), an IL-2 receptor/Tac-inducer homologous to thioredoxin; possible involvement of dithiol reduction in the IL-2 receptor induction. EMBO J 8:757, 1989.

96. Laurent TC, Moore EC, Reichard P: Enzymatic synthesis of deoxyribonucleotides. IV. Isolation and characterization of thioredoxin, the hydrogen donor from Escherichia coli B. J Biol Chem 239:3436, 1964.

97. Yodoi J, Tursz T: ADF, a growth-promoting factor derived from adult T cell leukemia and homologous to thioredoxin: Involvement in lymphocyte immortalization by HTLV-I and EBV. Adv Cancer Res 57:381, 1991.

98. Abate C, Patel L, Rauscher FJ 3rd, Curran T: Redox regulation of fos and jun DNA-binding activity in vitro. Science 249:1157, 1991.

99. Xanthoudakis S, Curran T: Identification and characterization of Ref-1, a nuclear protein that facilitates AP-1 DNA-binding activity. EMBO J 11:653, 1992.

100. Seki S, Akiyama K, Watanabe S, Hatsushika M, Ikeda S, Tsutsui K: cDNA and deduced amino acid sequence of a mouse DNA repair enzyme (APEX nuclease) with significant homology to Escherichia coli exonuclease III. J Biol Chem 266:20797, 1991.

101. Matthews JR, Wakasugi N, Virelizier JL, Yodoi J, Hay RT: Thioredoxin regulates the DNA binding activity of NF-kappa B by reduction of a disulfide bond involving cysteine 62. Nucleic Acids Res 20:3821, 1992.

102. Matsuda M, Masutani H, Nakamura H, Miyajima S, Yamauchi A, Yonehara S et al: Protective activity of adult T cell leukemia-derived factor (ADF) against necrosis factor-dependent cytotoxicity on U937 cells. J Immunol 147:3837, 1991.

103. Nakamura H, Matsuda M, Furuke K, Kitaoka Y, Iwata S, Toda K et al: Adult T cell leukemia-derived factor/human thioredoxin protects endothelial F-2 cell injury caused by activated neutrophils or hydrogen. Immunol Lett 42:75, 1994.

104. Schenk H, Vogt M, Droge W, Schulze-Osthoff K: Thioredoxin as a potent costimulus of cytokine expression. J Immunol 156:765, 1996.

105. Manns A, Hanchard B, Morgan OS, Wilks R, Cranston B, Nam JM et al: Human leukocyte antigen class II alleles associated with human T-cell lymphotropic virus type I infection and adult T-cell leukemia/lymphoma in a Black population. J Natl Cancer Inst 90:617, 1998.

106. White JD, Johnson JA, Nam JM, Cranston B, Hanchard B, Waldmann TA, Manns A: Distribution of human leukocyte antigens in a population of black patients with human T-cell lymphotrophic virus type I-associated adult T-cell leukemia/lymphoma. Cancer Epidemiol Biomarkers Prev 5:873, 1996.

107. Hanabuchi S, Ohashi T, Koya Y, Kato H, Takemura F, Hirokawa K et al: Development of human T-cell leukemia virus type 1-transformed tumors in rats following suppression of T-cell immunity by CD80 and CD86 blockade. J Virol 74:428, 2000.

108. Ohashi T, Hanabuchi S, Kato H, Koya Y, Takemura F, Hirokawa K et al: Induction of adult T-cell leukemia-like lymphoproliferative

disease and its inhibition by adoptive immunotherapy in T-cell-deficient nude rats inoculated with syngeneic human T-cell leukemia virus type 1-immortalized cells. J Virol 73:6031, 1999.

109. Ibuki K, Funahashi SI, Yamamoto H, Nakamura M, Igarashi T, Miura T et al: Long-term persistence of protective immunity in cynomolgus monkeys immunized with a recombinant vaccinia virus expressing the human T cell leukaemia virus type I envelope gene. J Gen Virol 78:147, 1997.

110. Jinnohara T, Tsujisaki M, Sasaki S, Hinoda Y, Imai K: Cytotoxic activity in a case of adult T-cell leukemia/lymphoma with spontaneous regression. Int J Hematol 65:293, 1997.

111. Matsushita K, Arima N, Fujiwara H, Hidaka S, Ohtsubo H, Arimura K et al: Spontaneous regression associated with apoptosis in a patient with acute-type adult T-cell leukemia. Am J Hematol 61:144, 1999.

112. Astier-Gin T, Portail JP, Londos-Gagliardi D, Moynet D, Blanchard S, Dalibart R et al: Neutralizing activity and antibody reactivity toward immunogenic regions of the human T cell leukemia virus type I surface glycoprotein in sera of infected patients with different clinical states. J Infect Dis 175:716, 1997.

113. Mitsuya H, Matis LA, Megson M, Bunn PA, Murray C, Mann DL et al: Generation of an HLA-restricted cytotoxic T cell line reactive against cultured tumor cells from a patient infected with human T cell leukemia/lymphoma virus. J Exp Med 158:994, 1983.

114. Kannagi M, Sugamura K, Kinoshita K, Uchino H, Hinuma Y: Specific cytolysis of fresh tumor cells by an autologous killer T cell line derived from an adult T cell leukemia/lymphoma patient. J Immunol 133:1037, 1984.

115. Jacobson S, Shida H, McFarlin DE, Fauci AS, Koenig S: Circulating CD8+ cytotoxic T lymphocytes specific for HTLV-I pX in patients with HTLV-I associated neurological disease. Nature 348:245, 1990.

116. Kannagi M, Matsushita S, Harada S: Expression of the target antigen for cytotoxic T lymphocytes on adult T-cell-leukemia cells. Int J Cancer 54:582, 1993.

117. Chen X, Zachar V, Zdravkovic M, Guo M, Ebbesen P, Liu X: Role of the Fas/Fas ligand pathway in apoptotic cell death induced by the human T cell lymphotropic virus type I Tax transactivator. J Gen Virol 78:3277, 1997.

118. Tendler CL, Burton JD, Jaffe J, Danielpour D, Charley M, McLoy JP et al: Abnormal cytokine expression in Sézary and adult T-cell leukemia cells correlates with the functional diversity between these T-cell malignancies. Cancer Res 54:4430, 1994.

119. Ehrlich GD, Darey F, Kirchner J et al: A polyclonal CD4+ and CD8+ lymphocytosis in a patient doubly infected with HTLV-I and HIV-I: A clinical and molecular analysis. Am J Hematol 30:128, 1989.

120. Shimoyama M: Diagnostic criteria and classification of clinical subtypes of adult T-cell leukemia/lymphoma: A report from the lymphoma study group (1984–87). Br J Hematol 79:428, 1991.

121. Bann PA Jr, Schecter GP, Jaffe E et al: Clinical course of retrovirus associated adult T-cell lymphoma in the United States. N Engl J Med 309:257, 1983.

122. Shimoyama M, Ota K, Kikuchi M et al: Chemotherapeutic results and prognostic factors of patients with advanced non-Hodgkin's lymphoma treated with VEPA or VEPA-M. J Clin Oncol 6:128, 1988.

123. Shimoyama M: Treatment of patients with adult T-cell leukemia-lymphoma: An overview. Gann Monogy Cancer Res 39:43, 1992.

124. Hanada S, Utsunomiya A, Suzuki S, Uozumi K, Makino T, Arima T: Treatment for adult T-cell leukemia. Cancer Chemother Pharmacol 40(Suppl):S47, 1997.

125. Kojima H, Hori M, Shibuya A, Nagasawa T, Miwa M, Abe T: Successful treatment of a patient with adult T-cell leukemia by daily

oral administration of low-dose etoposide. Decrease in the amount of HTLV-I proviral DNA revealed by the polymerase chain reaction method. Cancer 72:3614, 1993.

126. Tsuda H, Takatsuki K, Ohno R, Masaoka T, Okada K, Shirakawa S et al: Treatment of adult T-cell leukaemia-lymphoma with irinotecan hydrochloride (CPT-11). CPT-11 Study Group on Hematological Malignancy. Br J Cancer 70:771, 1994.

127. Ikeda K, Oka M, Yamada Y, Soda H, Fukuda M, Kinoshita A et al: Adult T-cell leukemia cells over-express the multidrug-resistance-protein (MRP) and lung-resistance-protein (LRP) genes. Int J Cancer 82:599, 1999.

128. Loe DW, Deeley RG, Cole SP: Biology of the multidrug resistance-associated protein, MRP. Eur J Cancer 32A:945, 1996.

129. Borg A, Yin JAL, Johnson PE, Tosswill J, Saunders M, Morris D: Successful treatment of HTLV-1-associated adult T-cell leukemia lymphoma by allogenic bone marrow transplantation. Br J Hematol 94:713, 1996.

130. Tamura K, Makino S, Araki Y et al: Recombinant interferon-β and gamma in the treatment of adult T-cell leukemia. Cancer 59:1059, 1987.

131. Bazarbachi A, Nasr R, El-Sabban ME, Mahe A, Mahieux R, Gessain A et al: Evidence against a direct cytotoxic effect of alpha interferon and zidovudine in HTLV-I associated adult T cell leukemia/lymphoma. Leukemia 14:716, 2000.

132. Bazarbachi A, El-Sabban ME, Nasr R, Quignon F, Awaraji C, Kersual J et al: Arsenic trioxide and interferon-alpha synergize to induce cell cycle arrest and apoptosis in human T-cell lymphotropic virus type I-transformed cells. Blood 93:278, 1999.

133. Ishitsuka K, Hanada S, Suzuki S, Utsunomiya A, Chyuman Y, Takeuchi S et al: Arsenic trioxide inhibits growth of human T-cell leukaemia virus type I infected T-cell lines more effectively than retinoic acids. Br J Haematol 103:721, 1998.

134. Li HC, Yashiki S, Sonoda J, Lou H, Ghosh SK, Byrnes JJ et al: Green tea polyphenols induce apoptosis in vitro in peripheral blood T lymphocytes of adult T-cell leukemia patients. Jpn J Cancer Res 91:34, 2000.

135. Okamura T, Shibuya T, Harada M, Niho Y: Successful treatment of chronic adult T-cell leukemia with ubenimex. Acta Haematol 87:94, 1992.

136. Waldmann TA, White JD, Goldman CK, Top L, Grant A, Bamford R et al: The interleukin-2 receptor: A target for monoclonal antibody treatment of T-cell lymphotrophic virus I-induced adult T-cell leukemia. Blood 82:1701, 1993.

137. Waldmann TA: The promiscuous IL-2/IL-15 receptor: A target for immunotherapy of HTLV-I-associated disorders. J Acquir Immun Defic Synd Hum Retroviruses 13(Suppl 1): S179, 1996.

138. Kreitman RJ, Schneider WP, Queen C, Tsudo M, Fitzgerald DJ, Waldmann TA, Pastan I: Mik-beta 1(Fv)-PE40, a recombinant immunotoxin cytotoxic toward cells bearing the beta-chain of the IL-2 receptor. J Immunol 149:2810, 1992.

139. Kreitman RJ, Chaudhary VK, Waldmann TA, Hanchard B, Cranston B, FitzGerald DJ, Pastan I: Cytotoxic activities of recombinant immunotoxins composed of Pseudomonas toxin or diphtheria toxin toward lymphocytes from patients with adult T-cell leukemia. Leukemia 7:553, 1993.

140. Waldmann TA, White JD, Carrasquillo JA, Reynolds JC, Paik CH, Gansow OA et al: Radioimmunotherapy of interleukin-2R alpha-expressing adult T-cell leukemia with Yttrium-90-labeled anti-Tac. Blood 86:4063, 1995.

141. Nichols J, Foss F, Kugel TM et al: Interleukin-2 fusion protein: An investigational therapy for interleukin-2 receptor expressing malignancies. Eur J Cancer 33:34, 1997.

142. Bhagavati S, Ehrlich G, Kula R et al: Detection of human T-cell lymphoma/leukemia virus type I (HTLV-I) in the spinal fluid and blood of cases of chronic progressive myelopathy and a clinical radiological and electrophysiological profile of HTLV-I associated myelopathy. N Engl J Med 318:1141, 1988.

143. Kitajima I, Yamamoto K, Sato K et al: Detection of human T-cell lymphotropic virus type I expression in synovial cells in chronic inflammatory arthropathy. J Clin Invest 88:1315, 1991.

144. Mochizuki M, Watanabe T, Yamaguchi K et al: HTLV-I uveitis: A distinct clinical entity caused by HTLV-I. Jpn J Cancer Res 83:236, 1992.

145. Harrington WJ Jr, Ucar A, Gill B et al: Clinical spectrum of HTLV-I in South Florida. J Acquir Immun Defic Synd Hum Retroviruses 8:466, 1995.

146. Ferrer JF, Esteban E, Dube S et al: Endemic infection with the human T lymphotropic virus type II B in Argentinean and Paraguayan Indians. Distribution by ethnicity and molecular virus characterization. J Infect Dis 174:944, 1996.

147. Love J, Marchiole CC, Dube S et al: Expansion of clonotypic T-cell populations in the peripheral blood of asymptomatic Gran Chaco Amerindians infected with HTLV-IIB. J Acquir Immun Defic Synd Hum Retroviruses 18:178, 1998.

148. Rosenblatt JD, Giorgie JV, Golde DW et al: Integrated human T-cell leukemia virus II genome in CD8+ T-cells from a patient with "atypical" hairy cell leukemia: Evidence for distinct T- and B-cell lymphoproliferative disorders. Blood 71:363, 1988.

149. Loughran TP Jr, Coyle T, Sherman M et al: Detection of human T-cell leukemia/lymphoma virus type II in a patient with LGL leukemia. Blood 80:1116, 1992.

150. Loughran TP Jr, Sherman MP, Ruscetti FW et al: Prototypical HTLV-I/II infection is rare in LGL leukemia. Leuk Res 18:423, 1994.

151. Ehrlich G, Glaser J, La Vigne K, Quan D, Mildvan D, Sninsky J et al: Prevalence of human T-cell leukemia/lymphoma virus type II infection among high-risk individuals: Type specific identification of HTLVs by polymerase chain reaction. Blood 74:1658, 1989.

152. Kaplan MH, Hall WW, Suin M et al: Syndrome of severe skin disease, eosinophilia, and dermatopathic lymphadenopathy in patients with HTLV-II complicating human immunodeficiency virus infection. Am J Med 91:300, 1991.

153. Poiesz B, Dube D, Dube S et al: HTLV-II-associated cutaneous T-cell lymphoma in a patient with HIV-I infection. N Engl J Med 342:930, 2000.

154. Harrington WJ Jr, Sheremata W, Hjille B et al: Spastic ataxia associated with human T-cell lymphotropic virus type II infection. Ann Neurol 33:411, 1993.

13

Epidemiology and Hereditary Aspects of Acute Leukemia

Julie A. Ross

Leukemias (all types) account for less than 3 percent of the worldwide cancer burden.[1] In the United States, acute lymphoblastic leukemia (ALL) and acute myeloid leukemia (AML) comprise approximately 1 percent of all newly diagnosed malignancies and 1.5 percent of all cancer deaths each year.[2] Although ALL can be diagnosed at any age, it is typically more common in childhood. In contrast, the incidence of AML is higher in adults, increasing notably with age.[3] Five-year survival rates for childhood ALL have increased dramatically over the past 50 years, rising from about 5 percent in the 1960s to nearly 75 percent in the 1990s.[2,4–7] Although children diagnosed with AML do not fare as well, their 5-year survival rates have increased from about 2 percent to about 40 percent during this same time period. In contrast, adults diagnosed with either ALL or AML have generally poor survival rates. For example, adults diagnosed with either ALL or AML between 45 and 54 years of age experience 5-year survival rates of about 1 percent and 19 percent, respectively.[3]

Major advances in molecular biology and immunology have increased our understanding of the malignant processes that occur during hematopoietic cell transformation. With the exception of a few established associations, however, little is known about the causes of acute leukemia. This paucity of knowledge may partly be attributable to small studies that lack statistical power to adequately explore differences and inadequate characterization of leukemia type. These factors can also make it difficult to make direct comparisons between studies. For example, historically, epidemiological studies did not uniformly address differences between acute and chronic forms of leukemia or between lymphoid and myeloid lineages. Even with the introduction of more recent classifications schemes, such as the French-American-British (FAB) system, it is becoming increasingly apparent that even these distinctions may be inadequate. Further subgroups (such as children with hyperdiploidy ALL and adults with promyelocytic leukemia) are being defined by their responses to therapy. Hence, it is possible that these subgroups may also be defined by different etiologies. Although there are some similarities among risk factors associated with childhood and adult leukemia, there are enough differences overall in both molecular characteristics (e.g., cytogenetics) and prognostic factors to suggest that the cause(s) may not be the same. This chapter reviews the current knowledge regarding the etiology of childhood and adult acute leukemia.

ACUTE LEUKEMIA IN CHILDREN

Descriptive Data

Incidence

Leukemia is the most common malignancy diagnosed in childhood, comprising approximately 30 percent of all diagnoses under the age of 15 years.[7] About 3000 children under the age of 20 years will develop leukemia each year in the United States. There are some notable international differences in the incidence of childhood acute leukemia. For childhood ALL, the highest incidence rates occur in Costa Rica, Denmark, Sweden, U.S. Whites, New Zealand (non-Maori), and Los Angeles Hispanics; lowest rates occur in India, Israel, China, and Africa.[8] For childhood AML, the highest rates occur in Costa Rica, Denmark, Japan, and Australia; lowest rates occur in Kuwait, Scotland, and Thailand. Although there is some difficulty in directly comparing international incidence rates as there may be differences in case ascertainment and/or coding practices, these observations can help in hypothesis generation.

For most of the developed world, there is a pronounced age peak in childhood ALL that occurs between the ages of 2 and 5, which became apparent in non-Hispanic White children in the 1930s; it is absent in many developing countries.[8–11] In the United States, the age peak was not noted in Black children until the 1960s.[12] Importantly, the incidence rate of childhood ALL in Black children is consistently about half the rate in White children. Higher socioeconomic status (e.g., income, education) has been associated with an increased risk of childhood ALL in several studies.[13] This observation, coupled with the lack of a childhood age peak in developing countries, has led to the speculation that factors associated with modernization may account for the peak.[14,15] In contrast to childhood ALL, childhood AML peaks in infancy, and then decreases until about the age of 4, where the incidence remains relatively constant throughout childhood.[7] There is about a threefold excess risk of AML in Whites during the first few years of life compared to Blacks; however, Black children have slightly higher rates of childhood AML after the age of 3.

Trends

Recent data from the United States suggest a modest increase in the incidence of childhood leukemia during the period of 1975 to 1995, which was largely due to an inexplicable increase during the period 1983 to 1984.[16] Rates have decreased slightly since 1989. Site-specific analyses suggest a slight increase in the incidence of childhood ALL over the past few decades.[7,17] Gurney et al.[17] reported an average annual percentage change (AAPC) of 1.6 percent (95 percent confidence interval [CI] = 0.2 to 2.3) for ALL during the period 1974 and 1991, which was most notable in the youngest age group (diagnosed < 2 years of age). They also noted a striking decreasing trend for leukemias classified as "other" during this same time period (AAPC = −5.0 percent, 95 percent CI = −6.9 to −2.9). Increasing ALL incidence has also been reported in the North Western Regional Health Authority area of England between 1954 and 1988.[18] However, no increased trend has been observed in Germany.[19] A recent report from the Manchester

Children's Tumour Registry suggests an annual increase of approximately 3 percent in the incidence of pre-B-cell ALL during the period 1980 to 1998.[20] Diagnostic coding changes in part may explain some of the increases observed, but it is possible that other factors either artifactual or real (e.g., changes in the environment) could be important. Thus, ongoing surveillance and monitoring of childhood leukemia trends is important. In contrast to ALL, there has been little fluctuation in AML incidence rates during the past few decades, remaining generally around 5 to 8 cases per million children.[7]

Below are described some of the risk factors that have been investigated with respect to childhood acute leukemia. More recent studies are highlighted.

Parental Factors

Reproductive History

Several studies have explored associations between prior maternal fetal loss (miscarriage, stillbirth) and risk of childhood leukemia.[13,21,22] Although there is some suggestion that a history of fetal loss may be associated with an increased risk, the data are not entirely consistent.[21–26] An association with prior fetal loss could indicate either a chronic environmental exposure and/or some type of genetic susceptibility that results in a spectrum of effects – from nonviability to damage to a single cell lineage.

Cigarette Smoking

Although a few past studies suggested an association with maternal smoking during pregnancy, the majority of studies (many of them sufficiently large enough with adequate statistical power) have not found an association.[24,26–33] By and large, it can be concluded that maternal smoking during pregnancy is a negligible risk factor for childhood leukemia. In contrast, the data concerning paternal smoking are less conclusive. There have been at least three studies that have suggested a positive association with paternal smoking around the time of pregnancy and childhood acute leukemia, although one very large study of over 1800 children with ALL and 500 children with AML reported no association.[32–35] It is difficult to understand the underlying biology that would explain a more powerful association with paternal smoking than maternal smoking, although it is possible that germ cell mutations that would develop before conception might explain this association. With the exception of identified genetic syndromes, however, no studies to date have suggested that childhood leukemia is the result of a parental germ cell mutation.

Alcohol Drinking

Studies that have examined childhood leukemia overall and maternal alcohol consumption during pregnancy have generally reported no association.[24,36] More recent studies, however, that have evaluated more homogeneous subgroups (ALL versus AML) or age at diagnosis, have reported an increased risk (approximately twofold) for children diagnosed with AML at younger ages.[31,32,37] Although these studies provide some pre-liminary evidence that maternal alcohol consumption during pregnancy may be a risk factor for younger age AML, further studies are necessary. This is a good example of how studies that include stratification of cases on leukemia subtype are particularly powerful (provided they have a sufficient number of cases), as they may reveal an association that would be masked in an overall analysis.

Occupational Exposures

There have been a number of studies that have examined maternal and paternal occupational exposures and risk of childhood acute leukemia.[13,38] Although there is a suggestion of some positive associations with parental pesticide, radiation, and solvent exposure (especially with AML), the data are inconsistent. This may reflect the difficulty in measuring the exposure, which often relies on the recall of respondents reviewing a list of specific substances. Current studies are utilizing occupational modules that have been developed by industrial hygienists, which may help in elucidating the role of specific occupational exposures in the development of leukemia in children.

Other Parental Factors

Limited data have been published on diet as a risk factor for childhood leukemia. One study reported an association between parental or child consumption of hot dogs and ALL.[39] One very preliminary study suggested a positive association between maternal consumption of foods that inhibit DNA topoisomerase II and infant AML.[40] Other reported associations include maternal marijuana use during pregnancy,[41] birth order (first born at higher risk) and advanced maternal age,[13] and certain medications used either by the mother[41] or the child.[42] By and large, however, these associations have been either inconsistent, or evaluated in only one study.

Child Exposures and Characteristics

Prior Chemotherapy

An increased risk of secondary AML has been associated with the use of alkylating agents as well as epipodophyllotoxins in children treated for a primary malignancy. Estimates suggest about a 5 percent increased risk of developing AML within a 5-year period.[43] Secondary AML associated with epipodophyllotoxin therapies occurs earlier (usually within the first 2 years following therapy) and is often associated with cytogenetic abnormalities involving the MLL gene at 11q23. In contrast, leukemias following alkylating therapies typically occur several years later, and are often associated with losses of chromosomes 5 and/or 7.[43] These observations can help in developing hypotheses for future studies that investigate de novo leukemia (see Chromosomal Abnormalities below).

Birth Weight

Several studies have reported an association between high birth weight (>4000 g) and childhood leukemia, particularly ALL.[22,44] These positive associations are most consistent for younger children with leukemia. Several theories have been advanced including 1. higher levels of specific growth factors associated with high birth weight may act as promoters; 2. a larger organ mass could contribute to a larger number of susceptible cells; and 3. other exposures (e.g., x-rays, medications) might increase during pregnancy, due to the large size of the unborn child. Given that this is one of the more consistent risk factors for childhood ALL, further investigation is warranted.

X-Rays

Prenatal exposure to diagnostic x-rays is one of the few accepted risk factors for both childhood AML and ALL, with an estimated relative risk of approximately 1.5.[13] No elevated risk of leukemia, however, has been observed for children who were exposed in utero to atomic bomb radiation.[45] Postnatal diagnostic radiation has not been associated with an increased risk of childhood leukemia. However, therapeutic radiation for conditions such as tinea capitis and thymus enlargement are associated with an increased risk.[13]

Radon

Radioactive decay of uranium from the Earth's crust results in radon particles, which has been associated with an increased risk of lung cancer in miners.[46–49] Several ecological studies have demonstrated an increased risk of leukemia in areas with high levels of radon.[50–52] One of the difficulties in interpreting these types of ecological comparisons is the lack of data regarding individual exposure. Two recent case-control studies of childhood leukemia have focused specifically on indoor radon exposure and risk of either ALL or AML. Lubin et al.[53] found no association with indoor radon levels and risk of childhood ALL. Radon exposure was measured by detectors placed in the home(s) where the child resided at least 70 percent of the time, or greater than 5 years prior to diagnosis (or from birth for cases less than 5 years of age). Steinbuch et al.,[49] in a study of childhood AML (173 cases, 254 controls), also found no overall association with indoor radon levels.[49] However, there was an increased risk observed (p trend = .07) for children diagnosed at 2 years of age or greater (odds ratio [OR] = 1.62, 95 percent CI = 1.0 to 2.7; OR = 1.59, 95 percent CI = 0.8–3.2; for radon concentrations of 37–100, and >100 Bq m^{-3}, respectively). Although the authors speculate that this finding may be due to chance, it raises the possibility that there may exist a subset of children who are vulnerable to higher doses of indoor radon.

Residential Magnetic Fields

Nearly 25 years ago, Wertheimer and Leeper[54] published a controversial report suggesting an association between electrical wiring configurations and childhood cancer. Since that time, there have been a number of studies that have examined low-frequency electromagnetic fields (EMFs) and childhood cancer (particularly leukemia and brain tumors) with inconclusive results.[13] One difficulty in interpreting earlier studies is the lack of direct measurement of EMFs. Typically, EMF exposure was estimated through wire codes or distance to power lines, which can lead to substantial misclassification. More recent studies, however, have obtained direct field measurements of EMFs, and

a few smaller studies have reported some positive associations.[55–57] However, the largest studies conducted to date in the United Kingdom, the United States, and Canada have not found an increased risk of childhood leukemia associated with low-level exposure to EMFs.[58–60] Nevertheless, comprehensive reviews and meta-analyses of studies still conclude that there may exist a weak link between EMFs and childhood leukemia.[61,62] In particular, concerns with more recent studies include 1. the fact that transient measures of magnetic fields have not been incorporated (including the rapid changes in magnetic fields that occur when appliances are used, as well as transient changes in distribution lines), and 2. that there is a low frequency of children in the high-exposure categories.

Infectious Etiology

Specific viruses can cause leukemia in animals (feline leukemia virus, bovine leukemia virus), and the human T-cell lymphotropic virus type 1 (HTLV-1) retrovirus is associated with the development of a rare type of adult leukemia (T cell). Although there is currently no biological evidence that viruses play a role in childhood leukemia, there are several intriguing hypotheses based on observations and associations that merit further research.[14,15,63] Two major hypotheses with respect to infectious exposures and childhood leukemia attempt to explain the age peak of ALL in children 2 to 5 years of age.[14,15] The first theory suggests a two-hit model of leukemogenesis: The first event occurs in utero when immature B cells are rapidly dividing; the second genetic event occurs in the first few years of life, and is strongly influenced by the timing of exposure to infectious agents.[14] In contrast, the second theory suggests that childhood leukemia is a rare response to direct viral exposures and that leukemia clusters occur when herd immunity is deregulated by population mixing.[15] Although there have been some indirect studies (cluster, ecological) that provide some support to the latter hypothesis, these associations could also be explained by other factors including chance.[64,65] Findings from recent case-control studies that have investigated patterns of infection and access to day care, which may be a surrogate indicator of the timing of exposure to infectious agents, have been inconsistent; one small study reported an association with timing of day care, where early day care conferred a modest protective effect.[66] However, a recent study of over 1800 cases of childhood ALL found no association with the timing of day care.[67]

Other

A few recent associations include potential protective effects for breastfeeding and risk of ALL and AML, infant vaccination with Haemophilus influenzae type b (Hib) vaccine and ALL, and allergic disorders and ALL.[68–70] These findings need to be confirmed in other studies. Finally, in reviewing putative risk factors, it is important to comment on exposures that are unlikely to be important in the development of childhood acute leukemia. A number of studies have explored prenatal ultrasound, and it can generally be concluded that there is no association.[13,71] Moreover, from a recent review of the published evidence, it is likely that intramuscular vitamin K administration is not an important risk factor for childhood leukemia.[72]

Hereditary and Genetic Aspects

Genetic Syndromes

The proportion of childhood leukemia due to inherited genetic mutations is quite small, with estimates ranging from 2 to 5 percent.[73–75] Down syndrome is the most common genetic syndrome associated with childhood acute leukemia, with afflicted children experiencing nearly a 20-fold increased risk of developing either ALL or AML.[76] Intriguingly, there are reports of as high as a 600-fold increased risk for one particular subtype of myeloid leukemia (AML-M7).[77] It is unknown why children with Down syndrome are at such an increased risk. Several research groups are focusing attention on genes on chromosome 21, given that one of the most common *acquired* abnormalities present in the leukemia cells of children without Down syndrome is an extra copy of chromosome 21.[78–80] Other syndromes associated with childhood leukemia include Bloom syndrome, ataxia telangiectasia, Shwachman syndrome, and neurofibromatosis 1.[81–84]

Familial Patterns of Inheritance

There have been a few reports in the literature of a familial aggregation of childhood leukemia, although this is quite rare.[74] Moreover, these associations cannot rule out shared environmental factors. One notable exception to these rare familial patterns is the risk of leukemia in twins, particularly monozygotic. The risk of leukemia in the unaffected twin is highest in infancy, and decreases with age.[85] Molecular studies suggest that this high concordance is due to shared placental circulation, where the affected twin's leukemia cells migrate to the other twin.[86] Studies of twin infants with leukemia have demonstrated identical rearrangements of chromosomes in their leukemia cells, with no evidence of these rearrangements in parental or remission blood, suggesting that the leukemia took place in utero.[86,87] Finally, in a study of a common chromosomal translocation found in childhood ALL (TEL-AML1), the translocation was found in blood spots collected at birth of children who developed leukemia later in childhood, suggesting that the translocation is insufficient for clinical leukemia and that a postnatal event is also required.[88] These molecular studies have important significance for pinpointing the timing of when the initiating event may have occurred.

Chromosomal Abnormalities

Somatic chromosomal abnormalities are commonly found in childhood acute leukemias. An extra copy of chromosome 21 is the most common numerical change in childhood ALL, followed by an extra X chromosome.[89] Hyperdiploidy, with more than 50 chromosomes per cell, has been found in the leukemia cells of between 25 and 30 percent of children with ALL, low hyperdiploidy (or 47 to 50 chromosomes per cell) is found in about 10 to 15 percent, pseudodiploidy (with a normal copy number but with numerical or structural rearrangements) is found in about

40 percent, diploidy (no detectable abnormalities) in about 10 to 15 percent, and hypoploidy (<46 chromosomes per cell) in about 7 to 8 percent.[90] Interestingly, hyperdiploidy in childhood ALL confers a significant survival advantage, compared to an intermediate prognosis with low hyperdiploidy, and a relatively poor prognosis with hypodiploidy.[91–93] The vast majority of children with B-cell ALL have the translocation t(8;14)(q24.1;q32) in their leukemia cells.[90] Other common translocations observed in childhood ALL include t(9;22) (3 to 5 percent), t(1;19) (5 to 6 percent), and rearrangements involving 11q23 (5 percent).[94] Although the latter translocations, involving a gene, *MLL*, at chromosome band 11q23, are infrequently found overall in childhood ALL, reports suggest nearly 80 percent of infants with ALL have 11q23 translocations.[95] Most recently, cryptic (not seen on conventional karyotyping) rearrangements of the *TEL* gene on chromosome 12 and the *AML-1* gene on chromosome 21 have been described.[96]

Nearly 80 percent of children with AML demonstrate chromosomal abnormalities using conventional techniques.[97] Common numerical cytogenetic abnormalities in childhood AML include trisomy 8 (3 percent), monosomy 7, and loss of an X chromosome.[89] One of the more common translocations involved in AML-M2 is t(8;21)(q22;q22), which is associated with a favorable outcome.[98] For AML-M3, t(15;17)(q22;q12–21) is reported in more than 90 percent of patients.[99] Inversion 16 is found in up to 10 percent of children with AML-M4. Finally, rearrangements involving the *MLL* gene at chromosome band 11q23 are also found in childhood AML, with 15 percent of cases demonstrating some involvement of the gene. Interestingly, infants with AML have the highest proportion of 11q23 rearrangements, with estimates suggesting nearly 60 percent of affected cases.[95] Similar *MLL* abnormalities have also been reported in children and adults who develop secondary AML associated with chemotherapies that inhibit DNA topoisomerase II, including the epipodophyllotoxins.[43] It has been proposed that de novo leukemias may develop from exposure to environmental inhibitors of DNA topoisomerase II.[100,101] As noted above, there is some preliminary evidence that maternal exposure to DNA topoisomerase II inhibitors (which can be found in diet and medications) may be associated with an increased risk of infant AML.[40] Further studies of this nature are warranted.

Genetic Susceptibility Genes

A relatively new area of cancer genetics has emerged, involving exploring the question of genetic susceptibility (i.e., given the same level of exposure, why are only certain individuals at risk?). Several genes important in the detoxification of chemical carcinogens are polymorphic in the population, with certain variants resulting in a reduced capacity to metabolize carcinogens; these individuals may be at a higher risk of developing cancer.[102] Recent studies have explored whether the germline absence of certain genes (e.g., glutathione-S transferase M1, T1), as well as possession of genes that may provide less capability of detoxification (e.g., slow *N*-acetyltransferase-2 (NAT2) genotype, GSTPi valine variant), may be important risk factors for childhood acute leukemia. Davies et al.,[103] in a molecular study of 232 White children with AML, found an overrepresentation of the GSTM1 null genotype among cases with M3 (82 percent) and M4 (72 percent) myeloid leukemia when compared to population controls (47 percent). Another study by Krajinovic et al.[104] of 176 children with ALL reported a higher frequency of the NAT2 slow acetylation genotype when compared to 306 healthy controls (OR = 1.5, 95 percent CI = 1.0 to 2.2). This same group had previously reported a higher frequency of the GSTM1 null genotype and CYP1A1*2A genotype among cases compared with controls.[105] Infante-Rivard et al.[106] recently explored gene-environment interactions in 123 children with ALL and found a statistically significant interaction between specific pesticide exposures and the CYP1A1m1 and CYP1A1m2 genotypes. These explorations of gene-gene and gene-environment interactions may be very important. One of the difficulties in conducting these studies, however, is the potential lack of statistical power due to diminishing numbers of cases in stratified cells. With the additional power of meta-analyses (statistically combining results of studies on the same topic), characterization of genotypes that may be important in the development of childhood leukemia is possible.

ACUTE LEUKEMIA IN ADULTS

Descriptive Data

Incidence

In contrast to children, leukemia accounts for a very small proportion of malignancy in adults, where epithelial cancers of the prostate, breast, lung, and colon predominate. AML is much more common in adults than ALL, with the incidence rising from about 1 case/100,000 under the age of 50, to nearly 10 cases/100,000 over the age of 80 years.[3] In contrast, the incidence of ALL is typically less than 2 cases/million under the age of 50, rising to about 2 cases/100,000. Internationally, the incidence patterns of adult AML are somewhat similar to the patterns observed in children with highest rates observed in New Zealand (non-Maori), Denmark, Australia, and U.S. Whites; lowest rates are seen in India, China, and Colombia.[1] For adult ALL, highest rates are reported in Australia, New Zealand (non-Maori), and Spain; low rates are found in U.S. Blacks, Israel (Jews), and India.

Described below are some of the more common risk factors that have been explored with respect to adult leukemia.

Occupational Exposures

Some of the most intensive epidemiological studies of adult leukemias have focused on specific occupations and occupational exposures. In particular, benzene is considered an established risk factor for adult AML.

Benzene Workers

Since the first case report, benzene has been extensively described as a known leukemogen for AML in several case-control and cohort studies of occupationally exposed workers in the shoe, rubber, leather, and chemical manufacturing industries.[107,108] There is strong evidence of a dose-response effect; workers with higher or longer exposure to benzene are at the highest risk of developing AML.[109] In one of the most recent cohort studies of approximately 75,000 Chinese workers exposed to benzene from 1972 through 1987, individuals exposed to average levels less than 10 parts per million had a relative risk (compared to unexposed workers) for AML of 3.2 (95 percent CI = 1.0 to 10.1), whereas workers exposed to levels of 25 ppm or higher had a relative risk of 7.1 (95 percent CI = 2.1 to 23.7).[110] Other occupational groups that have had higher rates of AML include painters, petroleum refinery workers, and pressmen, all of which could be related to benzene exposure since it is found in most of the products used by these groups.[108] The observed relative risks in these studies range from about a fourfold increased risk to nearly tenfold. It is important to note, however, that these occupational groups likely account for a very small proportion of the adult AML cases. Epidemiologists often use a formula to calculate the population attributable risk to describe the contribution of a particular exposure to the risk of a specific disease.[111] This formula is based on estimates of the relative risk associated with the exposure and the proportion of the population likely exposed. Assuming that less than 1 percent of individuals work in occupations that include exposure to benzene,[112] and given relative risks of between 4 and 10, the population attributable risk of benzene to leukemia development would be between 3 and 8 percent.

Other Occupations

The risk of leukemia has been explored in other industries that may have potential low-dose benzene and other solvent exposure including diesel exhaust workers, gas station attendants, pilots, dry cleaners, chemists, furniture manufacturers, embalmers, painters, auto manufacturing machinists, auto mechanics, professional drivers, and seamen on tankers.[113–122] Although several of these studies found an increased risk of leukemia overall, AML, or AML mortality, others have found no increased risk. It is important to note that many of these studies observed small numbers of leukemia deaths among these workers and compared this number to the number of deaths that would be expected in the general population. In many instances, other factors that may also be associated with an increased risk (i.e., smoking) were not controlled for.

A number of studies have demonstrated positive associations between leukemia and farming, while other studies have found no elevated risk.[108] However, an increased risk of leukemia has also been reported with exposure to certain chemicals used in farming including crop and animal insecticides, herbicides, and fertilizers.[123–125]

Other occupations potentially associated with an increased risk of leukemia include veterinarians and abattoir workers (both of which could be consistent with a viral etiology), nurses, barbers and hairdressers, and firefighters.[108,126,127] With the exception of occupational exposure to benzene, however, the majority of these associations have either been observed in only a limited number of studies, or have been inconsistent among studies.

Chemical and Environmental Exposures

Chemotherapy

As with children, there is a notable increased risk of secondary AML (although ALL has sometimes occurred) following chemotherapy for a primary malignancy. In particular, alkylating agents have been linked with a 10- to 300-fold increased risk of AML among patients treated for Hodgkin's disease, with an increased risk observed for at least 10 years following treatment.[128,129]

Pollutants and EMFs

A few studies have shown associations between acute leukemia and proximity to sources of pollutants, including one study that showed an elevated risk of leukemia among males (but not females) in an area surrounding a chemical plant explosion in Italy.[130–132] By and large, adult leukemia has not been associated with low-voltage EMFs, although one study from Sweden reported a nonsignificant increased risk of AML among adults who resided in homes with the highest magnetic field levels.[108,133]

Ionizing Radiation

In addition to benzene, exposure to ionizing radiation is also considered an established risk factor for adult acute leukemia. Much of what we have learned about the effects of radiation on hematopoietic neoplasms comes from studies of atomic bomb survivors. In an evaluation of leukemia mortality among survivors of Nagasaki and Hiroshima, the highest risk for AML appears to be among individuals exposed to radiation aged 45 years or greater, while ALL risk appears higher in those exposed under the age of 30.[134,135] Occupational exposure to ionizing radiation has also been explored with radium workers and early cohorts of radiologists demonstrating elevated risks of leukemia.[108] Moreover, patients irradiated for benign conditions including menorrhagia, peptic ulcer, or ankylosing spondylitis have been reported to be at an increased risk of leukemia.[136–139] Leukemia risk following radiation fallout from nuclear plants is less conclusive. Earlier studies reported excess risk among nuclear workers, but more recent studies have been inconsistent.[108]

Smoking

Cigarette smoking, which exposes a smoker to benzene and radioactive compounds, has been linked with acute leukemia in adults. Several studies have suggested a small but consistent increased risk of acute leukemia among smokers. In a meta-analysis of studies published through 1992, the estimated relative risk for all leukemia was 1.1 (95 percent CI = 1.0 to 1.2) and 1.3 (95 percent CI = 1.2 to 1.6) for case-control and cohort studies, respectively.[140] Of these studies, the most striking association has been with AML, with risk estimates approaching 1.2. Less conclusive evidence exists regarding risk of ALL; however, one recent study reported a risk estimate of about 1.3 (95 percent CI = 0.8 to 2.2).[140] One difficulty may be the smaller number of adult ALL cases, which would reduce the power to detect statistically significant differences.

Hair Dye

Since the early 1990s, the International Agency for Research on Cancer (IARC) began to evaluate the possible carcinogenicity of hair dye use. These investigations were partly based on epidemiological studies that suggested an increased risk of bladder cancer among hairdressers and barbers.[141] A review of studies published through 1994 suggested no or weak evidence of hair dye use and several types of cancers.[142] The one exception was hematopoietic neoplasms, where it was concluded the data were inconclusive. Correa et al.[143] recently reviewed the literature from 1966 through 1996 regarding the potential relationship between hair dye use and the leukemias. In their review, they included 18 epidemiological studies that explored personal hair dye use and hematopoietic neoplasms, including 14 case-control studies and four cohort studies. In general, most of the individual studies did not report statistically significant associations, with the exception of one study (published in abstract form) that reported an association between ever use of hair dyes and development of acute leukemia (OR = 1.5, 95 percent CI = 1.1 to 2.1).[144] One of the difficulties in interpreting these studies, which Correa et al. nicely raise in their review, is the potential problem with small numbers. For example, if the focus of the study is on dark permanent dyes (which contain the highest amount of colorant), and assuming that 10 percent of the population is exposed, epidemiological studies would have to include over 300 subjects in order to have sufficient power to detect a statistically significant association. It is also important to note that several studies have not adequately addressed for potential confounding by other variables including cigarette smoking.

Viruses

Viruses are known leukemogens for hematopoietic cancers in several animal species.[145] One definitive association that has been established in humans is viral infection with HTLV-1 and the development of a very rare type of leukemia (T-cell ALL).[146] The virus is endemic in parts of the Carribean, Japan, and Central Africa, with a reported seroprevalence of 30 percent or higher.[147] The lifetime risk of an HTLV-1-infected individual developing T-cell ALL is estimated to be between 3 and 5 percent.[148] Moreover, earlier infection with the virus appears to be predictive of risk. Other viruses that have been explored with respect to acute leukemia include bovine leukemia, feline leukemia, Epstein-Barr, and hepatitis B, with largely negative results.[108]

Hereditary and Genetic Aspects

Familial Patterns and Associations

Although there are several case reports of more than one case of leukemia occurring in the same family, these associations could either reflect similar environmental influences, or shared genetic factors.[73,149,150] As with childhood leukemia, however, these familial associations only account for a very small proportion of cases. In contrast to twin studies in children, studies in adults do not show any concordance for the development of leukemia.[151] Interestingly, one report found an increased risk of leukemia among parents of children with Down syndrome.[152]

Finally, a recent report suggested that although the risk of leukemia in individuals with Down syndrome is highest in childhood, there is an elevated risk throughout life.[153]

Chromosomal Abnormalities

As in children, somatic genetic abnormalities are commonly found in adult leukemias. About 50 percent of adult AML cases demonstrate an abnormal karyotype using standard methods.[89,154] With the addition of molecular techniques—including reverse transcriptase polymerase chain reaction (RT-PCR)—the percentage is likely higher. Chromosomal abnormalities that are frequently found in adult AML include loss or deletion of chromosomes 5 and/or 7, addition of chromosome 8, t(9;22), and translocations involving the *MLL* gene at 11q23. Specific chromosomal abnormalities and translocations are also associated with certain FAB groups including t(15;17)(q22;q11) in AML-M3, t(8;21)(q22;q22) in AML-M2, and inversion 16 in AML-M4.[154] Interestingly, several of these abnormalities are associated with prognosis: monosomy 7, found in about 3 percent of AML is typically associated with a poor prognosis, whereas t(15;17) is associated with a better response to therapy.[155] Using cytogenetics and fluorescent in situ hybridization (FISH), somatic chromosomal abnormalities are found in about 70 percent of ALL patients. About 10 percent of adults have high hyperdiploidy, with t(9;22) being the most common chromosomal rearrangement found. Other chromosomal abnormalities found in adult ALL include translocations involving 11q23 (3 to 10 percent of patients), deletion of 6q, and addition of chromosome 12. FAB-associated karyotypes include t(9;22) observed in approximately 20 to 30 percent of pre-B-cell ALL (L1 and L2), t(14q11) in T-cell ALL, and t(1;19) in pre-B-cell ALL.

It is important to note that losses of chromosomes 5 and 7 are often found in treatment-related leukemias.[156] Thus, it is possible that de novo patients could be subclassified based on their karyotype and exposures (e.g., occupational exposure to benzene). Three recent studies have found that exposures to pesticides, smoking, and/or solvents may be more often associated with AML demonstrating chromosomal loss of 5 and/or 7, whereas one study did not.[157–160]

More recent genetic abnormalities that have been explored with respect to adult leukemia include mutations in the ras family of protooncogenes, including N ras, K ras, and H ras. Ras gene products are important in cell signaling and transduction.[161] Mutations in specific areas of these ras genes (particularly N- or K-ras at codons 12, 13, or 61) have been found in about 30 percent of patients with AML and myelodysplastic syndrome.[162–164] Interestingly, in animal studies, these ras mutations appear more frequently in chemically induced tumors.[165] In one small study of 62 patients with AML, ras mutations were found significantly more often among patients who reported employment that involved exposure to chemicals compared to patients who reported no such occupational exposures.[166]

Genetic Susceptibility Genes

As with childhood leukemia, genetic susceptibility genes have been recently explored in adult leukemia. In a study of 557 adults with leukemia and 952 age-, sex-, and geographically matched controls, Rollinson et al.[167] reported a higher frequency of the GST-T1 null genotype among cases (19 percent) than among controls 14 percent (OR = 1.45, 95 percent CI = 1.09 to 1.93); this association was most striking for ALL (OR = 3.28, 95 percent CI = 1.31 to 8.26). The authors found no statistically significant associations between overall leukemia (or subtypes) with the GSTM1 null genotype nor the GSTPi valine variant. Lemos et al.[168] found an increase in the proportion of the NAT2 fast acetylator genotype among adults with leukemia ($n = 64$) compared with controls ($n = 128$). Upon further analyses, however, the highest proportion of fast acetylators was among adults with CLL. Finally, in a recent study by Skibola et al.[169] of 308 adults with acute leukemia and 491 age- and sex-matched controls, there was a decreased proportion of one of the 5′-methylenetetrahydrofolate reductase (MTHFR) genotypes among cases with ALL, but not AML. The MTHFR gene is important in folate metabolism and the authors speculate that folate inadequacy may play a key role in ALL development.

Other Associations

Few studies have explored associations between diet and adult leukemia. An ecological study of international data demonstrated some positive correlations between energy intake and leukemia incidence, particularly with lymphoid leukemia. A case-control study of 119 patients in Poland suggested an increased risk of leukemia associated with consumption of poultry and milk, and a decreased risk with vegetable intake.[170,171] In a study from China, no association was found with antioxidant supplements and leukemia risk.[172] Finally, in contrast to childhood leukemia, there is little evidence that alcohol consumption is a risk factor for adult leukemia.[173]

SUMMARY

There is still a general lack of knowledge regarding the etiology of acute leukemia; however, recent progress has been made. First, molecularly defined subgroups have been identified, which likely have different etiologies (e.g., infants with leukemia, adults with APL, and children with hyperdiploidy ALL). Second, direct measures of exposure have been incorporated in several recent studies (e.g., EMFs, radon), which can help reduce bias. Lastly, collection of biological specimens has provided preliminary evidence that genetic susceptibility may be important. Future epidemiological studies that build upon this recent progress should help lead us to a better understanding of the etiology of acute leukemia.

REFERENCES

1. Parkin DM, Whelan SL, Ferlay J, Raymond L, Young J (eds.): Cancer Incidence in Five Continents, Vol. VII, IARC Scientific Pub. No. 143. International Agency for Research on Cancer, Lyon, France, 1997.
2. Greenlee RT, Murray T, Bolden S, Wingo PA: Cancer Statistics, 2000. CA Cancer J Clin 50:7–33, 2000.

3. Kosary CL, Gloeckler Ries LA, Miller BA, Hankey BF, Harras A, Edwards BK (eds.): SEER Cancer Statistics Review, 1973–1992: Tables and Graphs, NIH Pub. No. 96-2789. National Cancer Institute, Bethesda, MD, 1995.

4. Birch JM, Marsden HB, Morris Jones PH et al: Improvements in survival from childhood cancer: Results of a population-based survey over 30 years. BMJ 296:1372–1376, 1988.

5. Stiller CA, Bunch KJ: Trends in survival for childhood cancer in Britain diagnosed 1971–85. Br J Cancer 62:806–815, 1990.

6. Miller BA, Linet MS, Cheson BD: Leukemias. In Miller BA, Ries LAG, Hankey BH et al. (eds.): Cancer Statistics Review 1973–1990, NIH Pub. No. 93-2789, pp. XIII.1–23. National Cancer Institute, Bethesda, 1993.

7. Smith MA, Gloeckler Ries LA, Gurney JG, Ross JA: Leukemia. In Ries LAG, Smith MA, Gurney JG, Linet M, Tamra T, Young JL, Bunin GR (eds.): Cancer Incidence and Survival Among Children and Adolescents: United States SEER Program 1975–1995, NIH Pub. No. 99-4649, pp. 17–34. National Cancer Institute, SEER Program, Bethesda, MD, 1999.

8. Parkin DM, Kramárová E, Draper GJ, Masuyer E, Michaelis J, Neglia J (eds.): International Incidence of Childhood Cancer, Vol. II, IARC Scientific Pub. No. 144. International Agency for Research on Cancer, Lyon, France, 1998.

9. Court-Brown WM, Doll R: Leukemia in childhood and young adult life. BMJ 1:981–988, 1961.

10. Edington GM, Hendrickse M: Incidence and frequency of lymphoreticular tumors in Ibadan and the western state of Nigeria. J Natl Cancer Inst 50:1623–1631.

11. Amsel S, Nabembezi JS: Two-year survey of hematologic malignancies in Uganda. J Natl Cancer Inst 52:13997–14001, 1974.

12. Pierce MI, Borges WH, Heyn R, Wolff JA, Gilbert ES: Epidemiological factors and survival experience in 177 children with acute leukemia: Treated by members of Children's Study Group A between 1957 and 1964. Cancer 23:1296–1304, 1969.

13. Ross JA, Davies SM, Potter JD, Robison LL: Epidemiology of childhood leukemia with a focus on infants. Epidemiol Rev 16:243–272, 1994.

14. Greaves MF: Speculations on the cause of childhood acute lymphoblastic leukemia. Leukemia 2:120–125, 1986.

15. Kinlen KL: Evidence for an infectious cause of childhood leukaemia: Comparison of a Scottish new town with nuclear reprocessing sites in Britain. Lancet 2:1323–1327, 1988.

16. Linet MS, Ries LAG, Smith MA, Tarone RE, Devesa SS: Recent trends in childhood cancer incidence and mortality in the United States. J Natl Cancer Inst 91:1051–1058, 1999.

17. Gurney JG, Davis S, Severson RK, Fang J-Y, Ross JA, Robison LL: Trends in cancer incidence among children in the U.S. Cancer 78:532–541, 1996.

18. Blair V, Birch JM: Patterns and temporal trends in the incidence of malignant disease in children: I. Leukemia and lymphoma. Eur J Cancer 30A:1490–1498, 1994.

19. Kaatsch P, Haaf G, Michaelis J: Childhood malignancies in Germany—methods and results of a nationwide registry. Eur J Cancer 31A:993–999, 1995.

20. McNally RJQ, Birch JM, Taylor M, Eden OB: Incidence of childhood precursor B-cell acute lymphoblastic leukaemia in northwest England. Lancet 356:485–486, 2000.

21. Ross JA, Potter JD, Shu X-O, Reaman GH, Lampkin B, Robison LL: Evaluating the relationships among maternal reproductive history, birth characteristics, and infant leukemia: A report from the Children's Cancer Group. Ann Epidemiol 7:172–179, 1997.

22. Yeazel MW, Ross JA, Buckley JD, Woods WG, Ruccione K, Robison LL: High birthweight and risk of specific childhood cancers: A report from the Children's Cancer Group. J Pediatr 131:671–677, 1997.

23. Gibson RW, Bross IDJ, Graham S, Lilienfeld AM, Schuman LM, Levin ML et al: Leukemia in children exposed to multiple risk factors. N Engl J Med 279:906–909, 1968.

24. Van Steensel-Moll HA, Valkenburg HA, Vandenbroucke JP, van Zanen GE: Are maternal fertility problems related to childhood leukemia? Int J Epidemiol 14:555–559, 1985.

25. Kaye SA, Robison LL, Smithson WA, Gunderson P, King FL, Neglia JP: Maternal reproductive history and birth characteristics in childhood acute lymphoblastic leukemia. Cancer 68:1351–1355, 1991.

26. Shu XO, Gao YT, Brinton LA, Linet MS, Tu JT, Zheng W, Fraumeni JF: A population-based case-control study of childhood leukemia in Shanghai. Cancer 62:635–644, 1988.

27. Neutel CI, Buck C: Effect of smoking during pregnancy on the risk of cancer in children. J Natl Cancer Inst 47:59–63, 1971.

28. John EM, Savitz DA, Sandler DP: Prenatal exposure to parents' smoking and childhood cancer. Am J Epidemiol 133:123–132, 1991.

29. Stjernfeldt M, Berglund K, Lindsten J et al: Maternal smoking and irradiation during pregnancy as risk factors for childhood leukemia. Cancer Detect Prev 16:129–135, 1992.

30. Pershagen G, Ericson A, Otterblad-Olausson P: Maternal smoking in pregnancy: Does it increase the risk of childhood cancer? Int J Epidemiol 21:1–5, 1992.

31. Severson RK, Buckley JD, Woods WG, Benjamin D, Robison LL: Cigarette smoking and alcohol consumption of parents of children with acute myeloid leukemia: An analysis within morphologic subgroups—a report from the Children's Cancer Group. Cancer Epidemiol Biomarkers Prev 2:433–439, 1993.

32. Shu X-O, Ross JA, Pendergrass TW, Reaman GH, Lampkin B, Robison LL: Parental alcohol consumption, cigarette smoking, and risk of infant leukemia: A Childrens Cancer Group study. J Natl Cancer Inst 88:24–31, 1996.

33. Brondum J, Shu X-O, Steinbuch M, Severson RK, Potter JD, Robison LL: Parental cigarette smoking and the risk of acute leukemia in children. Cancer 85:1380–1388, 1999.

34. Ji BT, Shu XO, Linet MS et al: Paternal cigarette smoking and the risk of childhood cancer among offspring of non-smoking mothers. J Natl Cancer Inst 89:238–244, 1997.

35. Sorahan T, Prior P, Lancashire RJ et al: Childhood cancer and parental use of tobacco: Deaths from 1971 to 1976. Br J Cancer 76:1525–1531, 1997.

36. McKinney PA, Cartwright RA, Saiu JM, Mann JR, Stiller CA, Draper GJ et al: The inter-regional epidemiological study of childhood cancer (IRESCC): A case control study of aetiological factors in leukaemia and lymphoma [published erratum appears in Arch Dis Child 62:644, 1987]. Arch Dis Child 62:279–287, 1987.

37. Van Duijn CM, van Steensel-Moll HA, Coebergh JW, van Zanen GE: Risk factors for childhood acute non-lymphocytic leukemia: An association with maternal alcohol consumption during pregnancy? Cancer Epidemiol Biomarkers Prev 3:457–460, 1994.

38. Shu XO, Stewart P, Wen W-Q, Han D, Potter JD, Buckley JD et al: Parental occupational exposure to hydrocarbons and risk of acute lymphocytic leukemia in offspring. Cancer Epidemiol Biomarkers Prev 8:783–791, 1999.

39. Peters JM, Preston-Martin S, London SJ, Bowman JD, Buckley JD, Thomas DC: Processed meats and risk of childhood leukemia (California, USA). Cancer Causes Control 5:195–202, 1994.

40. Ross JA, Potter JD, Reaman GH, Pendergrass TW, Robison LL: Maternal exposure to potential DNA topoisomerase II inhibitors

and infant leukemia: A report from the Children's Cancer Group. Cancer Causes Control 7:581–590, 1996.

41. Robison LL, Buckley JD, Daigle AE, Benjamin D, Wells R, Arthur DC, Hammond GD: Maternal drug use and risk of childhood acute nonlymphoblastic leukemia: An epidemiologic investigation implicating marijuana. Cancer 63:1904–1911, 1989.

42. Shu XO, Gao YT, Linet MS, Brinton LA, Gao RN, Jin F, Fraumeni JF Jr: Chloramphenicol use and childhood leukaemia in Shanghai. Lancet 2:934–937, 1987.

43. Felix CA: Chemotherapy-related second cancers. In Neugut AI, Meadows AT, Robinson E (eds.): Multiple Primary Cancers, pp. 137–164. Lippincott Williams & Wilkins, Philadelphia, 1999.

44. Ross JA, Perentesis JP, Robison LL, Davies SM: Big babies and infant leukemia: A role for insulin-like growth factor-1? Cancer Causes Control 7:500–506, 1996.

45. Yoshimoto Y: Cancer risk among children of atomic bomb survivors. A review of RERF epidemiologic studies. JAMA 264:596–600, 1990.

46. National Research Council: Committee on the Biological Effects of Ionizing Radiation (BEIR IV): Health Risks of Radon and Other Internally Deposited Alpha-emitters. National Academy Press, Washington, DC, 1988.

47. Samet JM: Radon and lung cancer. J Natl Cancer Inst 81:745–757, 1989.

48. Lubin JH, Boice JD, Edling C, Hornung RW, Howe GR, Kunz E et al: Lung cancer in radon-exposed miners and estimation of risk from indoor exposure. J Natl Cancer Inst 87:817–827, 1995.

49. Steinbuch M, Weinberg CR, Buckley JD, Robison LL, Sandler DP: Indoor residential radon exposure and risk of childhood acute myeloid leukaemia. Br J Cancer 81:900–906, 1999.

50. Lucie NP: Radon and leukaemia (letter). Lancet ii:99–100, 1989.

51. Alexander FE, McKinney PA, Cartwright RA: Radon and leukaemia (letter). Lancet 335:1336–1337, 1990.

52. Henshaw DL, Eatough JP, Richardson RB: Radon as a causative factor in induction of myeloid leukaemia and other cancers. Lancet 335:1008–1012, 1990.

53. Lubin JH, Linet MS, Boice JD Jr, Buckley J, Conrath SM, Hatch EE et al: Case-control study of childhood acute lymphoblastic leukemia and residential radon exposure. J Natl Cancer Inst 90:294–300, 1998.

54. Wertheimer N, Leeper E: Electrical wiring configurations and childhood cancer. Am J Epidemiol 109:273–284, 1979.

55. Michaelis J, Shüz J, Meinert R et al: Combined risk estimates for two German population-based case-control studies on residential magnetic fields and childhood acute leukemia. Epidemiology 9:92–94, 1997.

56. Dockerty JD, Elwood JM, Skegg DCG, Herbison GP: Electromagnetic field exposures and childhood cancers in New Zealand. Cancer Causes Control 9:299–309, 1998.

57. Green LM, Miller AB, Agnew DA, Greenberg ML, Li J, Villeneuve PJ, Tibshirani R: Childhood leukemia and personal monitoring of residential exposures to electric and magnetic fields in Ontario, Canada. Cancer Causes Control 10:233–243, 1999.

58. UK Childhood Cancer Study Investigators: Exposure to power-frequency magnetic fields and the risk of childhood cancer. Lancet 354:1925–1931, 1999.

59. Linet MS, Hatch EE, Kleinerman RA, Robison LL, Kaune WT, Friedman DR et al: Residential exposure to magnetic fields and acute lymphoblastic leukemia in children. N Engl J Med 337:1–7, 1997.

60. McBride ML, Gallagher RP, Thériault G et al: Power-frequency electric and magnetic fields and risk of childhood leukemia in Canada. Am J Epidemiol 149:831–842, 1999.

61. Portier CJ, Wolf MS: National Institute of Environmental Health Sciences Working Group Report. Assessment of health effects from exposure to power-line frequency electric and magnetic fields, NIH publication no. 98-3981. NIEHS, Research Triangle Park.

62. Repacholi MH, Ahlbom A: Link between electromagnetic fields and childhood cancer unresolved. Lancet 354:1918–1919, 1999.

63. Smith M: Considerations on a possible viral etiology for B-precursor acute lymphoblastic leukemia of childhood. J Immunother 20:89–100, 1997.

64. Alexander FE, Boyle P, Carli PM, Coebergh JW, Draper GJ, Ekbom A et al: Spatial temporal patterns in childhood leukaemia: Further evidence for an infectious origin. Br J Cancer 77:812–817, 1998.

65. Alexander FE, Boyle P, Carli PM, Coebergh JW, Draper GJ, Ekbom A et al: Spatial clustering of childhood leukaemia: Summary results from the EUROCLUS project. Br J Cancer 77:818–824, 1998.

66. Petridou E, Kassimos D, Kalmanti M, Kosmidis H, Haidas S, Flyzani V et al: Age of exposure to infections and risk of childhood leukaemia. BMJ 307:774, 1993.

67. Neglia JP, Linet MS, Shu XO, Severson RK, Potter JD, Mertens AC et al: Patterns of infection and day care utilization and risk of childhood acute lymphoblastic leukaemia. Br J Cancer 82:234–240, 2000.

68. Shu XO, Linet MS, Steinbuch M, Wen WQ, Buckley JD, Neglia JP et al: Breast-feeding and risk of childhood acute leukemia. J Natl Cancer Inst 91:1765–1772, 1999.

69. Groves FD, Gridley G, Wacholder S, Shu XO, Robison LL, Neglia JP, Linet MS: Infant vaccinations and risk of childhood acute lymphoblastic leukemia in the USA. Br J Cancer 81:175–178, 1999.

70. Wen W, Shu XO, Linet MS, Neglia JP, Potter JD, Trigg ME, Robison LL: Allergic disorders and the risk of childhood acute lymphoblastic leukemia (United States). Cancer Causes Control 11:303–307, 2000.

71. Naumburg E, Bellocc R, Cnattingius S, Hall P, Ekbom A: Prenatal ultrasound examinations and risk of childhood leukemia: Case-control study. BMJ 320:282–283, 2000.

72. Ross JA, Davies SM: Vitamin K prophylaxis and childhood cancer. Med Ped Oncol 34:434–437, 2000.

73. Gunz FW, Veale AMO: Leukemia in close relatives—accident or predisposition? J Natl Cancer Inst 42:517–524, 1969.

74. Gunz FW, Gunz JP, Veale AMO, Chapman CJ, Houston IB: Familial leukaemia: A study of 909 families. Scand J Haematol 15:117, 1975.

75. Narod S, Stiller C, Lenoir G: An estimate of the heritable fraction of childhood cancer. Br J Cancer 63:993, 1991.

76. Robison LL, Nesbit ME, Sather HN, Level C, Shahidi N, Kennedy A, Hammond D: Down syndrome and acute leukemia in children: A 10-year retrospective survey from Childrens Cancer Study Group. J Pediatrics 105:235–242, 1984.

77. Zipursky A, Thorner P, De Harven E, Christensen H, Doyle J: Myelodysplasia and acute megakaryoblastic leukemia in Down's syndrome. Leuk Res 18:163–171, 1994.

78. Rogan PK, Close P, Blouin JL, Seip JR, Gannutz L, Ladda RL, Antonarakis SE: Duplication and loss of chromosome 21 in two children with Down syndrome and acute leukemia. Am J Med Genet 59:174–181, 1995.

79. Tanaka T, Tanaka K, Ogawa S et al: An acute myeloid leukemia gene, AML1, regulates hematopoietic myeloid cell differentiation and transcriptional activation antagonistically by two alternative spliced forms. EMBO J 14:341–350, 1995.

80. Fourth International Workshop on Chromosomes in Leukemia 1982: Overview of association between chromosome pattern and

cell morphology, age, sex, and race. Cancer Genet Cytogenet 11:265, 1984.

81. German J, Bloom D, Passarge E: Bloom's syndrome. VII. Progress report for 1978. Clin Genet 15:361–367, 1979.

82. Hecht F, Hecht B: Cancer in ataxia-telangiectasia patients. Cancer 46:9, 1990.

83. Woods WG, Roloff JS, Lukens JN, Krivit W: The occurrence of leukemia in patients with Shwachman syndrome. J Pediatr 99:425–428, 1981.

84. Shannon KM, Watterson J, Johnson P et al: Monosomy 7 myeloproliferative disease in children with neurofibromatosis, type 1: Epidemiology and molecular analysis. Blood 79:1311, 1992.

85. Strong LC: Genetics, etiology and epidemiology of childhood cancer. In Sutow WW, Fernbach DJ, Vietti TJ (eds.): Clinical Pediatric Oncology, 3rd ed, pp. 14–41. C.V. Mosby, St. Louis, MO, 1984.

86. Ford AM, Ridge SA, Cabrera ME, Mahmoud H, Steel CM, Chan LC, Greaves M: In utero rearrangements in the trithorax-related oncogene in infant leukemias. Nature 363:358–360, 1993.

87. Gale KB, Ford AM, Repp R, Borkhardt A, Keller C, Eden OB, Greaves MF: Backtracking leukemia to birth: Identification of clonotypic gene fusion sequences in neonatal blood spots. Proc Natl Acad Sci USA 94:13950–13954, 1997.

88. Wiemels JL, Cazzaniga G, Daniotti M, Eden OB, Addison GM, Masera G et al: Prenatal origin of acute lymphoblastic leukaemia in children. Lancet 354:1499–1503, 1999.

89. Perkins D, Brennan S, Carstairs K, Bailey D, Pantalony D, Poon A et al: Regional cancer cytogenetics: A report on 1,143 diagnostic cases. Cancer Genet Cytogenet 96:64–80.

90. Third International Workshop on Chromosomes in Leukaemia 1980: Clinical significance of chromosomal abnormalities in acute lymphoblastic leukaemia. Cancer Genet Cytogenet 4:111–137, 1981.

91. Bloomfield CD, Secker-Walker LM, Goldman AI et al: Six-year follow-up of the significance of karyotype in acute lymphoblastic leukemia. From the Sixth International Workshop on Chromosomes in Leukemia 1987. Cancer Genet Cytogenet 40:171–185, 1989.

92. Williams DL, Raimondi SC, Pui CH et al: Evolving chromosome patterns and new cytogenetic concepts in childhood acute lymphoblastic leukemia. In Gale RP, Hoelzer D (eds.): Acute Lymphoblastic Leukemia: UCLA Symposia on Molecular and Cellular Biology, new series, Vol. 108, pp. 91–100. Wiley-Liss, New York, 1990.

93. Rivera GK, Raimondi SC, Hancock ML et al: Improved outcome in childhood acute lymphoblastic leukaemia with reinforced early treatment and rotational combination chemotherapy. Lancet 337:61–66, 1991.

94. Raimondi SC: Cytogenetics of acute leukemias. In Pui CH (ed.): Childhood Leukemias, pp. 168–196. Cambridge University Press, Cambridge, UK, 1999.

95. Cimino G, Lo Coco F, Biondi A et al: *ALL-1* gene at chromosome 11q23 is consistently altered in acute leukemia of early infancy. Blood 82:544–546, 1993.

96. Shurtleff SA, Buijs A, Behm FG, Rubnitz JE, Raimondi SC, Hancock ML et al: TEL/AML1 fusion resulting from a cryptic t(12;21) is the most common genetic lesion in pediatric ALL and defines a subgroup of patients with an excellent prognosis. Leukemia 9:1985–1989, 1995.

97. Woods WG, Nesbit ME, Buckley J, Lampkin BC, McCreadie S, Kim TH et al: Correlation of chromosome abnormalities with patient characteristics, histologic subtype, and induction success in children with acute nonlymphoblastic leukemia. J Clin Oncol 3:3–11, 1985.

98. Groupe Francais de Cytogenetique Hematologique (GFHC): Acute myelogenous leukemia with an 8;21 translocation: A report on 148 cases from the Groupe Francais de Cytogenetique Hematologique. Cancer Genet Cytogenet 44:169–179, 1990.

99. Grignani F, Fagioli M, Alcalay M et al: Acute promyelocytic leukemia: From genetics to treatment. Blood 83:10–25, 1994.

100. Ross JA, Potter JD, Robison LL: Infant leukemia, topoisomerase II inhibitors, and the *MLL* gene. J Natl Cancer Inst 86:1678–1680, 1994.

101. Greaves MF: Aetiology of acute leukaemia. Lancet 349:344–349, 1997.

102. Perera FP: Molecular epidemiology: On the path to prevention? [Review]. J Natl Cancer Inst 92:602–612, 2000.

103. Davies SM, Robison LL, Buckley JD, Radloff GA, Ross JA, Perentesis JP: Glutathione S-transferase polymorphisms in children with myeloid leukemia: A Children's Cancer Group study. Cancer Epidemiol Biomark Prev 9:563–566, 2000.

104. Krajinovic M, Richer C, Sinnett H, Labuda D, Sinnett D: Genetic polymorphisms of N-acetyltransferases 1 and 2 and gene-gene interaction in the susceptibility to childhood acute lymphoblastic leukemia. Cancer Epidemiol Biomark Prev 9:557–562, 2000.

105. Krajinovic M, Labuda D, Richer C, Karimi S, Sinnett D: Susceptibility to childhood acute lymphoblastic leukemia: Influence of CYP1A1, CYP2D6, GSTM1 and GSTT1 genetic polymorphisms. Blood 93:1496–1501, 1999.

106. Infante-Rivard C, Labuda D, Krajinovic M, Sinnett D: Risk of childhood leukemia associated with exposure to pesticides and with gene polymorphisms. Epidemiology 10:481–487, 1999.

107. Delore P, Borgomano C: Leukemia aigue un cour de l'intoxication benzenique, sur l'origine toxique de certains leukemies aigues et leurs relations avec les anemies graves. J Med Lyon 9:227–233, 1928.

108. Linet MS, Cartwright RA: The leukemias. In Schottenfeld D, Fraumeni JF Jr. (eds.): Cancer Epidemiology and Prevention, 2nd ed., pp. 841–892. Oxford University Press, New York, 1996.

109. Austin H, Delzell E, Cole P: Benzene and leukemia. A review of the literature and a risk assessment. Am J Epidemiol 127:419–439, 1988.

110. Hayes RB, Yin SN, Dosemeci M, Li GL, Wacholder S, Travis LB et al: Benzene and the dose-related incidence of hematologic neoplasms in China. J Natl Cancer Inst 89:1065–1071, 1997.

111. Hennekens CH, Buring JE: In Mayrent SL (ed.): Measures of disease frequency and associations. Epidemiology in Medicine, Little, Brown and Company, Boston, MA, 1987, 92–93.

112. Wallace LA: Major sources of benzene exposure. Environ Health Perspect 82:165–169, 1989.

113. Blair A, Decoufle P, Grauman DJ: Causes of death among laundry and drycleaning workers. Am J Public Health 69:508–511, 1979.

114. Katz RM, Jowet D: Female laundry and dry cleaning workers in Wisconsin: A mortality analysis. Am J Public Health 71:305–307, 1981.

115. Wong O, Morgan RW, Kheifets L et al: Mortality among members of a heavy construction equipment operators union with parental exposure to diesel exhaust emissions. Br J Ind Med 42:435–448, 1985.

116. Miller BA, Silverman DT, Hoover RN et al: Cancer risk among artistic painters. Am J Ind Med 9:281–287, 1986.

117. Schwartz E: Proportionate mortality ratio analysis of automobile mechanics and gasoline service station workers in New Hampshire. Am J Ind Med 12:91–99, 1987.

118. Lindquist R, Nilsson B, Eklund G et al: Acute leukemia in professional drivers exposed to gasoline and diesel. Eur J Haematol 47:98–102, 1991.

119. Hunter WJ, Henman BA, Bartlett DM et al: Mortality of professional chemists in England and Wales, 1965–1989. Am J Ind Med 23:615–627, 1993.

120. Jakobsson R, Ahlbom A, Bellander T et al: Acute myeloid leukemia among petrol station attendants. Arch Environ Health 48:255–259, 1993.

121. Band PR, Le ND, Fang R et al: Cohort study of Air Canada pilots: Mortality, cancer incidence and leukemia risk. Am J Epidemiol 145:137–143, 1996.

122. Nilsson RI, Nordlinder R, Hörte L-G, Järvholm B: Leukaemia, lymphoma, and multiple myeloma in seamen on tankers. Occup Environ Med 55:517–521, 1998.

123. Blair A, Malker H, Cantor KP et al: Cancer among farmers. A review. Scand J Work Environ Health 11:397–407, 1985.

124. Brown LM, Blair A, Gibson R, Everett GD, Cantor KP, Schuman LM et al: Pesticide exposures and other risk factors for leukemia among men in Iowa and Minnesota. Cancer Res 50:6585–6591, 1990.

125. Blair A, Zahm SH: Agricultural exposures and cancer. Environ Health Perspect 103:205–208, 1995.

126. Blair A, Hayes HM Jr: Mortality patterns among United States veterinarians 1947–1977: An expanded study. Int J Epidemiol 2:391–397, 1982.

127. Pearce NE, Smith AH, Reif JS: Increased risks of soft tissue sarcoma, malignant lymphoma, and acute myeloid leukemia in abattoir workers. Am J Ind Med 14:63–72, 1988.

128. Travis LB, Curtis RE, Stovall M, Holowaty EJ, van Leeuwen FE, Glimelius B et al: Risk of leukemia following treatment for non-Hodgkin's lymphoma. J Natl Cancer Inst 86:145–147, 1994.

129. Van Leeuwen FE, Chorus AMJ, Van den Belt-Dusebout AN, Hagenbeek A, Noyon R, van Kerkhoff EHM et al: Leukemia risk following Hodgkin's disease: Relation to relative dose of alkylating agents, treatment with teniposide combinations, number of episodes of chemotherapy, and bone marrow damage. J Clin Oncol 12:1063–1073, 1994.

130. Bertazzi PA, Zocchetti C, Pesatori AC et al: Ten-year mortality study of the population involved in the Seveso incident in 1976. Am J Epidemiol 129:1187–1200, 1989.

131. Linos A, Blair A, Gibson RW et al: Leukemia and non-Hodgkin's lymphoma and residential proximity to industrial plants. Arch Environ Health 46:70–74, 1991.

132. Shore DL, Sandler DP, Davey FR et al: Acute leukemia and residential proximity to potential sources of environmental pollutants. Arch Environ Health 48:414–420, 1993.

133. Feychting M, Ahlbom A: Magnetic fields and cancer in children residing near Swedish high voltage power lines. Am J Epidemiol 138:467–481, 1993.

134. Matsuo T, Tomonaga M, Bennett JM et al: Reclassification of leukemia among A-bomb survivors in Nagasaki using French-American-British (FAB) classification for acute leukemia. Jpn J Clin Oncol 18:91–96, 1988.

135. Shimizu Y, Kato H, Schull W et al: Studies of the mortality of A-bomb survivors. Mortality, 1950–1985. Part 1. Comparison of the risk coefficients for site-specific cancer mortality based on DS86 and T65DR shielded kerma and organ doses. Radiat Res 118:502–524, 1989.

136. Sandler DP, Collman GW: Cytogenetic and environmental factors in the etiology of the acute leukemias in adults. Am J Epidemiol 126:1017–1032, 1987.

137. Cartwright RA, Darwin C, McKinney PA et al: Acute myeloid leukemia in adults: A case-control study in Yorkshire. Leukemia 2:687–690, 1988.

138. Inskip PD, Kleinerman RA, Stovall M et al: Leukemia, lymphoma, and multiple myeloma after pelvic radiotherapy for benign disease. Radiat Res 135:108–124, 1993.

139. Griem MI, Kleinerman RA, Boice JD et al: Cancer following radiotherapy for peptic ulcer. J Natl Cancer Inst 86:842–849, 1994.

140. Kane EV, Roman E, Cartwright R, Parker J, Morgan G: Tobacco and the risk of acute leukaemia in adults. Br J Cancer 81:1228–1233, 1999.

141. International Agency for Research on Cancer: Occupational exposures of hair dressers and barbers and personal use of hair dyes, cosmetic colourants, industrial dyestuffs and aromatic amines. IARC Monogr Eval Carcinog Risks Hum 57:102–148, 1993.

142. La Vecchia C, Tavani A: Epidemiological evidence on hair dyes and the risk of cancer in humans. Eur J Cancer Prevent 4:31–43, 1995.

143. Correa A, Mohan A, Jackson L, Perry H, Helzlsouer K: Use of hair dyes, hematopoietic neoplasms, and lymphomas: A literature review. I. Leukemias and myelodysplastic syndromes. Cancer Invest 18:366–380, 2000.

144. Sandler DP, Shore DL, Bloomfield CD: Hair dye use and leukemia. Am J Epidemiol 138:636–637, 1993.

145. Gross L: Viral etiology of cancer and leukemia: A look into the past, present, and future—GHA Clowes Memorial Lecture. Cancer Res 38:485–493, 1978.

146. Tajima K, and the T- and B-Cell Malignancy Study Group and Co-Authors: The 4th nationwide study of adult T-cell leukemia/lymphoma (ATL) in Japan: Estimates of risk of ATL and its geographical and clinical features. Int J Cancer 45:237–243, 1990.

147. Tajima K, Cartier L: Epidemiological features of HTLV-I and adult T cell leukemia. Intervirology 38:238–246, 1995.

148. Murphy EL, Hanchard B, Figueroa J, Gibbs WN, Lofters WS, Campbell M et al: Modelling the risk of adult T-cell leukemia/lymphoma in persons infected with human T-lymphotropic virus type I. Int J Cancer 43:250–253, 1989.

149. Pottern LM, Linet M, Blair A, Dick F, Burmeister LF, Gibson R et al: Familial cancers associated with subtypes of leukemia and non-Hodgkin's lymphoma. Leuk Res 15:305–314, 1991.

150. Cuttner J: Increased incidence of hematology malignancies in first-degree relatives of patients with chronic lymphocytic leukemia. Cancer Invest 10:103–109, 1992.

151. Harnden DG: Inherited factors in leukemia and lymphoma. Leuk Res 9:705–707, 1985.

152. Miller RW: Relation between cancer and congenital defects: An epidemiologic evaluation. J Natl Cancer Inst 40:1079–1085, 1968.

153. Hasle H, Clemmensen IH, Mikkelsen M: Risk of leukaemia and solid tumours in individuals with Down's syndrome. Lancet 355:165–169, 2000.

154. Glassman AB: Chromosomal abnormalities in acute leukemias. Clin Lab Med 20:39–48, 2000.

155. Rowley JD: Seminars from the University of Minnesota. Chromosome translocations: Dangerous liaisons. J Lab Clin Med 132:244, 1998.

156. Heim S, Mitelman F: Cytogenetic analysis in the diagnosis of acute leukemia. Cancer 70:1701–1709, 1992.

157. Cuneo A, Fagioli F, Pazzi I et al: Morphologic, immunologic and cytogenetic studies in acute myeloid leukemia following occupational exposure to pesticides and organic solvents. Leuk Res 16:789–796, 1992.

158. Fagioli F, Cuneo A, Piva N et al: Distinct cytogenetic and clinico-pathologic features in acute myeloid leukemia after occupational exposure to pesticides and organic solvents. Cancer 70:77–85, 1992.

159. Sandler DP, Shore DL, Anderson JR, Davey FR, Arthur D, Mayer RJ: Cigarette smoking and risk of acute leukemia: Associations

with morphology and cytogenetic abnormalities in bone marrow. J Natl Cancer Inst 85:1994–2003, 1993.

160. Ciccone G, Mirabelli D, Levis A et al: Myeloid leukemias and myelodysplastic syndromes: Chemical exposure, histologic subtype and cytogenetics in a case-control study. Cancer Genet Cytogenet 68:135–139, 1993.

161. McCormick F: Activators and effectors of ras p21 protein. Curr Opin Genet Devel 4:71–76, 1994.

162. Vogelstein B, Civin CI, Preisinger AC, Krischer JP, Steuber P, Ravindranath Y et al: RAS gene mutations in childhood acute myeloid leukemia: A Pediatric Oncology Group study. Genes Chromosom Cancer 2:159–162, 1990.

163. Lubbert M, Oster W, McCormick F, Mertelsmann R, Herrmann F: Clonal analysis of n-ras gene activation in acute myeloid leukemia. Recent Results Cancer Res 131:315–327, 1993.

164. Neubauer A, Dodge RK, George SL, Davey FR, Silver RT, Schiffer CA et al: Prognostic importance of mutations in the ras proto-oncogenes in de novo acute myeloid leukemia. Blood 83:1603–1611, 1994.

165. Mangues R, Pellicer A: ras activation in experimental carcinogenesis. Semin Cancer Biol 3:229–239, 1992.

166. Taylor JA, Sandler DP, Bloomfield CD, Shore DL, Ball ED, Neubauer A et al: ras oncogene activation and occupational exposures in acute myeloid leukemia. J Natl Cancer Inst 84:1626–1632, 1992.

167. Rollinson S, Roddam P, Kane E, Roman E, Cartwright R, Jack A, Morgan GJ: Polymorphic variation within the glutathione S-transferase genes and risk of adult acute leukaemia. Carcinogenesis 21:43–47, 2000.

168. Lemos MC, Cabrita FJ, Silva HA, Vivan M, Plácido F, Regateiro FJ: Genetic polymorphism of CYP2D6, GSTM1 and NAT2 and susceptibility to haematological neoplasias. Carcinogenesis 20:1225–1229, 1999.

169. Skibola CF, Smith MT, Kane E, Roman E, Rollinson S, Cartwright RA, Morgan G: Polymorphisms in the methylenetetrahydrofolate reductase gene are associated with susceptibility to acute leukemia in adults. Proc Natl Acad Sci USA 96:12810–12815, 1999.

170. Hursting SD, Margolin BH, Switzer BR: Diet and human leukemia: An analysis of international data. Prev Med 22:409–422, 1993.

171. Kwiatkowski A: Dietary and other environmental risk factors in acute leukaemias: A case-control study of 119 patients. Eur J Cancer Prev 2:139–146, 1993.

172. Shu XO, Zheng W, Blot WJ et al: Dietary factors and risk of adult leukemia. Am J Epidemiol 138:635–636, 1993.

173. Brown LM, Gibson R, Burmeister LF, Schuman LM, Everett GD, Blair A: Alcohol consumption and risk of leukemia, non-Hodgkin's lymphoma, and multiple myeloma. Leuk Res 16:979–984, 1992.

14

Classification of the Acute Leukemias: Cytochemical and Morphological Considerations

Nukhet N. Tuzuner and John M. Bennett

The acute leukemias are a heterogeneous group of neoplasms affecting uncommitted or partially committed hematopoietic stem cells. The origin of the malignant neoplasm is almost invariably within the marrow. Replacement of the marrow pulp or the repression of normal hematopoietic cells results in variable degrees of anemia, neutropenia, and thrombocytopenia.

Historically, the term "acute" implied not only a poorly differentiated blast population, but also a clinical syndrome that led to a rapidly fatal outcome. Since it is apparent that, with modern chemotherapy, including bone marrow transplantation (BMT), patients with acute leukemia of several morphological types can enjoy complete remission (CR), and indeed cure, the term acute should be maintained only for nosological reasons.

Traditionally, morphology and cytochemistry identified the different involved lineages. During the past 15 years, major advances in our knowledge of the nature of acute leukemia consequent to the application of the techniques of immunology, cytogenetics, and molecular genetics have taken place. The demonstration of membrane and cytoplasmic antigens or enzymes by immunological or immunocytochemical methods and detection of the recurring chromosomal abnormalities either by conventional cytogenetic or molecular methods provide supplementary arguments for accurate classification.

Identification of subclasses of acute leukemia is important for three reasons. First, some leukemias have clinical features that influence the therapeutic approaches. Second, differences in response rate and survival are observed in the treatment of acute leukemias. Third, classification greatly facilitates communication and cooperation around the world, and comparisons of results are possible only through reproducible definitions of acute leukemias.

Examination of both peripheral blood and bone marrow smears is necessary for the diagnosis and classification of the acute leukemias. If the peripheral blast count is 20 percent or more peripheral blood samples may be adequate for morphological and immunological diagnosis. However, bone marrow aspirates will be needed to determine the leukemia cell karyotype.[1]

There are three instances in which the diagnosis of acute leukemia can be made on the basis of histological material. The first occurs when there is an abundance of reticulin in the bone marrow, resulting in a so-called dry-tap.[2] Although bone marrow fibrosis can be present in any of the acute leukemias it is most commonly associated with acute megakaryoblastic leukemia. The second example is hypocellullar (hypoplastic) acute leukemia in which bone marrow aspirations from several sites and biopsy from one site are necessary for diagnosis.[3] The third example is that of an uncommon localized extramedullary mass of cells of the granulocytic-monocytic series (granulocytic sarcomas).[4] These tumors can be seen in an established diagnosis of acute myeloblastic leukemia (AML), either at presentation or as the first manifestation of relapse. In all three instances, although touch preparation smears may be helpful, well-prepared hematoxylin and eosin (H & E) stains and cell lineage specific antibodies (MPO, CD68, factor VIII, CD79a, CD3, CD1a, CD20) that can be applied to paraffin-embedded material that identify cell surface or cytoplasmic antigens[5–7] can often establish the diagnosis.

DIAGNOSIS OF ACUTE LEUKEMIAS

Morphologic examination of the Romanowsky-stained bone marrow and peripheral blood smears as well as cytochemical stains is the method used to identify subtypes of acute leukemia. The initial intent was to separate acute lymphoblastic leukemia (ALL) and AML into easily identifiable cell types. An essential cytochemical stain is one that demonstrates myeloperoxidase (MPO), an enzyme restricted to the primary granules of the granulocytes and monocytes.[8] Acute leukemias are traditionally classified by a combination of morphologic and cytochemical features on the basis of criteria of the French-American-British (FAB) Cooperative Group. However, the addition of acute megakaryoblastic leukemia[9] and the minimally differentiated acute myeloid leukemia[10] went beyond morphology and cytochemistry to include cell phenotype. The distribution of the FAB cell types is indicated in Table 14–1. At diagnosis, mor-

Table 14–1. Classification of the Acute Leukemias

Morphological Type	Subtypes (Common Terms)
Lymphocytic	ALL (FAB)
	Precursor-B ALL (L1–L2)
	T-ALL (L1–L2)
	B-ALL (L3)
Myelocytic	AML
	Myeloblastic without maturation (M0)
	Myeloblastic with minimal maturation (M1)
	Myeloblastic with significant maturation (M2)
	Hypergranular promyelocytic (M3)
	Hypogranular promyelocytic (M3v)
Myelomonocytic	Myelomonocytic (M4)
Monocytic	Poorly differentiated (M5a)
	Differentiated (M5b)
Erythroid	Myeloblast rich (M6A)
	Proerythroblast rich (M6B)
Megakaryocyte	Acute megakaryoblastic leukemia (M7)
Mast cell	Acute mast cell leukemia
Undifferentiated	Acute undifferentiated leukemia
	Acute biphenotypic leukemias

phological definition must be complemented by immunophenotyping and cytogenetics.

Recently, genetic features (cytogenetic and molecular genetic) as well as history of myelodysplasia and prior therapy have been shown to have a significant impact on the clinical behavior of acute leukemias. The major limitations of the FAB classification of the acute leukemias is the absence of cytogenetics and molecular genetic features, many of which were identified after the descriptions of the various FAB subtypes were described. The recently published WHO classification (11) combines the morphocytochemical features with pertinent chromosomal and molecular associations. These features are summarized in Tables 14-2 and 14-3. It is recommended that the reader turn to specific chapters in the extensive WHO publication for more in-depth information.

ACUTE LYMPHOBLASTIC LEUKEMIAS

ALL is the most common malignancy in children and accounts for approximately 80 percent of childhood leukemia.[12,13] ALL seems to be a heterogeneous group of disorders with subgroups that have distinct clinical and prognostic features. It derives from the clonal proliferation of lymphoid progenitors in the bone marrow. The consequence of bone marrow infiltration is various cytopenias in the peripheral blood and is associated with the appearance of peripheral blast cells. In some instances, leukemic cells are not seen in the peripheral blood. Thus, examination of the bone marrow is certainly necessary to confirm the diagnosis. Since the central nervous system (CNS) is infiltrated at diagnosis in 5 percent of patients, examination of the cerebrospinal fluid (CSF) by cytocentrifuge is also necessary.

Morphologic Classification

The FAB group in 1976[14] proposed a uniform classification system for ALL. Three subtypes of ALL are distinguished on the basis of cell size, nuclear shape, number and prominence of nucleoli, and the relative amount of cytoplasm. L1 defines a uniform population of small blast cells with high nuclear/cytoplasmic (N/C) ratio, a small inconspicuous nucleolus, and a regular nucleus (Plate 14–1), whereas L2 is designated as moderate to large cells with irregular nuclear membrane, one or

more nucleoli, more cytoplasm, and lower N/C ratio (Plate 14–2). A rare type seen in approximately equal percentages in children and adults (about 3 percent), referred to as L3, is morphologically identical to the cell characteristics of Burkitt's lymphoma. The cells are large and homogeneous with round to oval nuclei. The chromatin is finely dispersed with prominent nucleoli. The cytoplasm is intensely basophilic with or without vacuoles (Plate 14–3). Modifications for the assessment of lymphoblasts were introduced to improve reproducibility and interobserver concordance.[15] A simplified scoring system is given in Table 14–4. In this system, the sum may vary from +2 to −4. A total score of 0 to +2 defines L1, while a score of −1 to −4 establishes L2.

The relative frequency of the ALL morphologic subtypes varies with age. In children, approximately 80 percent have L1 morphology. In contrast more than 60 percent of adults are classified as L2. In earlier studies it was shown that L1 morphology was associated with a better event-free survival and induction rate than L2.[16] However, classification of ALL using

---

Table 14–3. Proposed WHO Classification of Acute Myeloid Leukemias (AML)

Acute myeloid leukemias with recurrent cytogenetic translocations
  AML with t(8;21)(q22;q22), AML1/ETO
  Acute promyelocytic leukemia [AML with
    t(15;17)(q22;q11–12) and variants], PML/RARα
  AML with abnormal marrow eosinophils [inv(16)(p13q22) or
    t(16;16)(p13;q11)], CBFb/MYH11
  AML with 11q23 (MLL) abnormalities
Acute myeloid leukemia with multilineage dysplasia
  With prior myelodysplastic syndrome
  Without prior myelodysplastic syndrome
Therapy-related acute myeloid leukemia
  Alkylating-agent–related
  Epipodophyllotoxin related (some may be lymphoid)
Acute myeloid leukemia not otherwise categorized
  AML without maturation (FAB M0)
  AML with minimal maturation (FAB M1)
  AML with maturation (FAB M2)
  Acute myelomonocytic leukemia (FAB M4)
  Acute monocytic leukemia (FAB M5)
  Acute erythroid leukemia (FAB M6)
  Acute megakaryocytic leukemia (FAB M7)
  Acute basophilic leukemia (FAB M2Baso)
Acute biphenotypic leukemia

Table 14–2. Proposed WHO Classification of Acute Lymphoblastic Leukemias

Precursor B-cell acute lymphoblastic leukemia (cytogenetic
  subgroups)
    t(9;22)(a34;q11); BCR/ABL
    t(v;11q23);MLL rearranged
    t(1;19)(q23;p13) PBX/E2A
    t(12;21)(p12;q22) ETV/CBFα
Precursor T-cell acute lymphoblastic leukemia
Burkitt cell leukemia

Table 14–4. Simplified Scoring System for FAB L1 and L2

Criteria	Score
High N/C ratio ≥ 75 percent of cells	+
Low N/C ratio ≥ 25 percent of cells	−
0–1 Nucleoli (small)	+
Irregular nuclear membrane ≥ 25 percent of cells	−
Large cells ≥ 50 percent of cells	−
Scoring range: +2 to −4 (L1: 0–+2; L2: −1–4)	−

Abbreviations: N/C, nuclear/cytoplasmic (ratio).

FAB criteria into L1 and L2 types is becoming less relevant because of a poor correlation with immunological and genetic findings and the lack of consistent prognostic significance.[17,18] Nonetheless, hematopathologists and hematologists should be aware of morphological variability in ALL blasts.[19,20] The recent WHO classification[11] has proposed to combine L1 and L2 subgroups into one group. FAB-L3, however, remains a clinically important ALL type, which is associated with *MYC* gene disregulation and mature B-cell phenotype.[21,22]

Cytochemistry

By standard definition, the peroxidase reaction is totally negative in leukemic lymphoblasts. Sudan Black B (SBB) stain is also negative. However, it has been suggested that SBB is less specific than MPO because positive reactions have been reported in ALL.[23] It should be remembered that in case of negative MPO or SBB reaction, megakaryocytic, erythroid, some monocytic, and AML MO subtype as well as lymphoid lineage should be considered in the differential, pending the results of flow cytometry.

The periodic acid-Schiff (PAS) reaction is useful in supporting the diagnosis of ALL (Table 14–5), but its importance has declined, as immunophenotyping has become more important for this purpose. Although blocklike PAS positivity is considered characteristic of ALL only 15 percent of cases have this type PAS reaction[14] (Plate 14–4). It should be noted that blocklike PAS positivity can be seen in monoblasts in monoblastic leukemia and in erythroblasts in erythroleukemia.[24] Moreover, fine granular activity in blocks of PAS material can be identified in all AML cell types (Plate 14–5). PAS stain is therefore a poor discriminator of various cell types, but it may be useful as a part of battery of stains, particularly when many of the reactions are negative or nonspecific.

A strong focal (paranuclear) acid phosphatase (ACP) activity (Plate 14–6) or a strong focal ANAE activity greater than 75 percent of blasts are characteristic of T-ALL.[25] However, it should be remembered that a localized ACP and α-naphthyl acetate esterase (ANAE) reaction is also a feature of AML:M7 and M6.

Immunohistochemistry

Indirect immunoperoxidase and indirect alkaline phosphatase anti-alkaline phosphatase (APAAP) techniques are applied to fixed cells in blood and bone marrow smears, cytospin preparations,[26] or to paraffin-embedded material.[5,7] These methods permit the detection of surface antigens (i.e., CD19, CD20, CD3, CD1a, CD10), cytoplasmic antigens (CD79a, MPO, or cytoplasmic μ chain), and nuclear antigens (e.g., TdT).

Immunophenotyping

Flow cytometry immunophenotyping has a well-established role in the diagnosis and classification of ALL. It is used to distinguish ALL from minimally differentiated AML and to classify ALL into T-cell, B-cell, and various precursor B-cell immunological subtypes, which have prognostic and therapeutic implications.[27] Mature B-cell ALL has characteristic morphological, immunophenotypic, karyotypic, and clinical features, while precursor B-cell and T-cell ALLs are morphologically indistinguishable. Precursor B-cell ALL is an umbrella term that covers leukemias of immature B cells, at different maturational stages, often termed pro-B-cell ALL, early-pre-B-cell ALL, and pre-B-cell ALL.[28,29]

T-ALL is simply classified into T stem cell leukemia and common T-ALL.[29] Numerous efforts to correlate clinical outcome in T-cell ALL with the stage of maturation have yielded inconsistent results,[12,13] suggesting a minor influence of T-cell maturation on treatment responsiveness.[17,30]

Cytogenetic Subgroups of Precursor B-Cell ALL

Close association of specific chromosomal abnormalities with ALL subtypes is apparent. Although detailed cytogenetics is covered in another chapter, the contribution of cytogenetics to the classification of the ALL is briefly summarized (see Table 14–2).

The t(9;22) Translocation

The Philadelphia (Ph) chromosome, a cytogenetic abnormality that is characterized by deletion or translocation of 22q11, was first described in cases of chronic myeloid leukemia (CML), but is now known to occur in 2 to 5 percent of all cases of childhood and 16 to 25 percent of adult ALL.[31,32] In ALL the Ph chromosome arises most often through a t(9;22), with translocation of the c-abl protooncogene on chromosome 9 to either of two breakpoint regions within the *BCR* gene on chromosome 22, which results in production of either a 210-kd or 190-kd fusion protein with tyrosine kinase activity. Presence of a Ph chromosome appears to be an adverse risk factor for both children and adults with ALL[33,34] despite the fact that it is associated with unfavorable presenting features, such as high leukocyte count, older age, organomegaly, and FAB L2 morphology. Almost all cases had immature B-progenitor (CD10+ CD19+ CD34+) immunophenotype. Myeloid markers were present in 24 to 65 percent of Ph+ ALL cases.[35,36] Patients with Ph+ ALL are considered as suitable candidates for innovative and intensified strategies.[37]

Table 14–5. Reaction of Acute Leukemic Cells to Cytochemical Stains

Stain	AML (M1–M3)	AMML (M4)	AmoL (M5)	ALL (L1–L2)
PAS	±	+	+ +	+ +
Acid phosphatase	–	±	+ +	+ + +
Peroxidase	+	+	±	–
Chloroacetate esterase	+	+	–	–
α-Naphthyl acetate esterase	±	+	+ +	+ + + +

Abbreviations: PAS, periodic Acid–Schiff; –, absent; ± occasional activity; +, moderate activity; + +, strong activity; + + +, focally strong activity in T cells; + + + +, focally strong activity at acid pH in T cells.

The t(4;11) Translocation

The MLL gene, located at chromosome 11, band q23 is frequently disrupted by a variety of chromosomal rearrangements that occur in ALL and in a subset of de novo and secondary AMLs. The most common translocation involving 11q23 is translocation t(4;11)(q21;q23).[38] It is observed in more than 60 percent of infants with ALL, 2 percent of children with ALL, and 3 to 6 percent of adults with ALL.[35] It is invariably associated with young age (under 2 years), female sex, high white blood cell (WBC) counts, organomegaly, and CNS involvement.[39–41]

The morphology of the blasts can be either L1 or L2. Immunophenotype is of the early pre-B or pre-B-cell type with rearrangements of the Ig heavy chain (IgH) genes and is variably CD10–. Blast cells frequently express myeloid (CDw65, CD15) antigens. These observations suggest that the cell of origin in these leukemias is an early B-cell progenitor with the capacity to differentiate both lymphoid and myeloid lineages.[34] The clinical outcome for both adults and children with the t(4;11) translocation is poor.[34,39]

The t(1;19) Translocation

This translocation results in the E2A/PBX fusion. A strong association exists between t(1;19) and pre-B-ALL especially in children,[42] where the translocation is present in 25 to 30 percent of cases.[34,43] Presence of t(1;19) identifies a subgroup of pre-B-cell ALL patients who are at risk for early relapse with standard therapy.[44,45] However, it has been reported that patients with unbalanced der(19)t(1;19) translocations had significantly improved outcomes compared with those with balanced t(1;19).[46]

The t(12;21) Translocation

Before the availability of molecular methods such as fluorescent in situ hybridization (FISH) and reverse transcriptase polymerase chain reaction (RT-PCR) to detect t(12;21), it was thought to be of no significant prognostic value. However, in several studies the application of these molecular techniques have shown TEL/AML1 fusion transcripts in up to 27 percent of children with B-lineage ALL. Thus it becomes the most common fusion gene in pediatric ALL.[47–50] The TEL/AML1 rearrangement conferred an exceptionally good outcome in childhood B-precursor ALL and provided prognostic information independent of the risk factors at presentation.[49,51,52]

ACUTE MYELOBLASTIC LEUKEMIAS

AMLs result from a neoplastic transformation of a single pluripotential hematopoietic stem cell. Evidence to support this statement is morphological,[53] immunological,[54] and chromosomal[55] as well as from in vitro cell culture studies. These studies have demonstrated trilineage dysplastic features or myeloid antigen expressions in AML, monocytic, and erythroid precursors in cultures, and elaboration of colony-stimulating factors (CSFs) from monocytes.

Four major types of AML have long been recognized: acute myeloid, acute myelomonocytic, acute monocytic, and acute erythroleukemia. Despite these subtype definitions, Auer rods are the only consistent neoplastic marker demonstrating that a blast is myeloid and of leukemic origin. Auer rods are abnormal azurophilic crystalline-like granules that represent the coalescence of primary lysosomal granules of myeloid precursors, as documented by cytochemical and ultrastructural studies.[56,57]

Morphologic Classification

Morphological classification of AML was proposed by the FAB Cooperative Group in 1976,[14] based on the morphological and cytochemical features of the blast cells. The original proposal was revised and expanded in 1985.[58] Although widely accepted, the FAB classification of AML has been the subject of recent suggestions for revision.[11,59] The FAB criteria identify two clinically significant types of AML: acute promyelocytic leukemia (M3) and acute myelomonocytic leukemia with abnormal eosinophils (M4eos); however, the remaining AML subtypes appear to be a cytogenetically and immunologically heterogeneous group of diseases. Cytogenetic evaluation of AML identifies numerous prognostically significant types of AML. These genetic abnormalities however, do not precisely correlate with FAB categories. Although morphologic subtyping is inadequate as a sole criteria in the classification of AML it should continue to serve as a template from which to build other more clinically and relevant categories.

The recently proposed WHO classification of acute myeloid leukemias is summarized in Table 14–4, which recognizes distinct entities defined by a combination of morphology and cytogenetic abnormalities. According to the WHO proposals AMLs can be divided into three groups: 1. chromosomal abnormalities associated with recurrent translocations [i.e., t(15;17), t(8;21), inv(16)] that are commonly seen in children and young adults; 2. chromosomal abnormalities similar to those which are associated with myelodysplastic syndromes (MDS) (complex chromosomal abnormalities with mainly loss of genetic material). These leukemias are associated with multilineage dysplasia of bone marrow cells. 3. AML cases without having chromosomal abnormalities or multilineage dysplasia.

The FAB standard in the diagnosis of AML has been 30 percent or more blast cells out of all nucleated cells. However, the WHO morphology committee[11] recommended lowering the threshold for the diagnosis of AML from 30 to 20 percent by emphasizing that the survival of patients with 20 to 30 percent blasts have a prognosis similar to that of patients with greater than 30 percent blasts. It is also known that the 30 percent blast threshold is ineffective to separate MDS and *low blast count AML* cases that have cytogenetic abnormalities associated with de novo AML and absence of dysplasia.[60] Differentiation of low blast cell count AML from MDS is based on cytogenetic data. Moreover, in 1989, Cason et al.[61] proposed the term *peripheral acute leukemia* for patients with peripheral blast counts of 30 percent or more and bone marrow blast counts of less than 30 percent whose clinical and cytogenetic characteristics are compatible with de novo AML. This was incorporated into acute leukemia classification by the National Cancer Institute Sponsored Workshop[62] in 1990.

Blast Cell Characteristics

The FAB classification accepts two types of blasts: *type I* blasts are myeloblasts with open chromatin, distinct nucleoli, and immature cytoplasm without granules. *Type II* blasts are similar to type I, except that they contain up to 20 delicate cytoplasmic azurophilic granules or Auer rods, or both. The introduction of *type III* blasts (>20 granules) permits a more accurate assignment of cases with AML and MDS/RAEB (Plate 14–7).[63]

Cytochemistry *(see Table 14–5)*

Myeloperoxidase and Sudan Black B

An essential cytochemical stain is one that demonstrates the presence of MPO, an enzyme restricted to the primary granules of granulocytes and monocytes.[8] This enzyme can be identified by performing a benzidine-based peroxidase reaction or SBB staining or by diaminobenzidine reaction (DAB). The benzidine method is the best available method against which other methods should be compared. However, because of the concern for its potential carcinogenicity, it should not be adopted as the universal reference method.[64]

The SBB reaction, a general stain for intracellular lipids, can be used in the same way. This stain is present in both primary and secondary granules. Sudanophilia and MPO activity are closely parallel.[65]

Specific and Nonspecific Esterases

The chloroacetate esterase reaction can also be used to identify myeloid lineage. Although it is less sensitive than either MPO or SBB in detecting myeloid differentiation, it can be useful, when combined with ANAE in double esterase stain, in confirming a monocytic component. Because ANAE is positive both in neutrophils and in monocytes, inhibition by NAF in monocytes should used to identify these cells (Plate 14–8).[64,65]

Periodic Acid-Schiff Reaction

All glycogen-containing cells as well as neutrophils and granulocytes at all stages of maturation stain with this reaction. Our experience in more than 200 patients has shown that fine granular PAS reactions can be identified in all AML subtypes, ranging from 60 percent in AML (M1 to M3) and 80 percent in AML M5. Moreover, the latter often demonstrates a blocklike reaction pattern characteristic of ALL (J.M. Bennett, unpublished observations). The blocklike pattern of PAS reactivity is seen in erythroid precursors of erythroleukemia.

Electron Microscopy

Although immunophenotyping studies have largely replaced ultrastructural analysis, electron microscopy (EM) still provides valuable information to demonstrate either MPO or platelet peroxidase (PPO). These ultrastructural studies are useful in the confirmation of myeloid (MO) or megakaryocytic (M7) origin of blasts. MPO can be demonstrated by electron microscopy in blast cells that previously had negative results (less than 3 percent positive blasts) by conventional criteria. Although immunophenotyping studies have largely replaced ultrastructural analysis, it is still useful to define the myeloid component in biphenotypic leukemias.[66,67] In megakaryoblasts, the PPO reaction is localized exclusively on the nuclear membrane and the endoplasmic reticulum, whereas in myeloblasts it occurs in the Golgi area and cytoplasmic granules.

Immunohistochemistry

Although flow cytometry is the method of choice for immunophenotyping, immunohistological examination of bone marrow sections has been proposed as an alternative method.[68] Its advantages include identification of morphological features, the possibility of retrospective analysis, and in the situation where peripheral blood or marrow smears are inadequate for study such as bone marrow fibrosis or hypocellular acute leukemia. Paraffin reactive antibodies (i.e., CD34, MPO, CD68, antihemoglobin, and factor VIII-related antigen) can successfully be used to subclassify AML.[6]

Immunophenotyping

AMLs are defined immunologically by the expression of two or more of the following myelomonocytic markers: anti-MPO, CD13, CD33, CDw65, and CD117. Anti-MPO is the most specific marker for the myeloid lineage.[69] Correlation of the immunological profiles with the various AML subtypes according to the FAB classification is suboptimal.[70] However acute myeloblastic leukemia without maturation (M0), acute megakaryoblastic leukemia (M7), and acute erythroleukemia (M6) could be unequivocally defined by the immunophenotype.[28,71] Immunophenotyping of AMLs also identifies aberrant expression of lymphoid antigens in some cases. The significance of this expression is controversial.[70,72,73]

In a recent experience with 382 adult de novo AML patients from ECOG studies, 95 patients were identified with a unique antigen profile characterized by high expression of CD11b. Those patients had a low response rate (54 percent) when compared with AmoL (82 percent) or AML overall (68 percent), independent of age, cytogenetic abnormalities, and p-glycoprotein expression.[74]

MORPHOLOGIC SUBTYPES OF AML

Acute Myeloblastic Leukemia Without Cytologic Maturation (M0)

AML M0 is a rare form of acute myeloid leukemia comprising approximately 2 to 3 percent of AMLs. In 1991 the FAB group criteria[10] for AML M0 included less than 3 percent blasts that were positive for MPO, SBB, or both and expression of myeloid associated markers such as CD13 or CD33 with the absence of lymphoid antigens except for TdT.[72] Morphologically, blasts are large with open chromatin and prominent single or multiple nucleoli. The N/C ratio is low. Cytoplasm is moderately basophilic. Azurophilic granules or Auer rods are not seen. The diagnosis of AML M0 cannot be made on morphological grounds alone and always requires confirmation by immunological techniques. Application of immunohistochemical stain for myeloperoxidase to the paraffin-embedded bone marrow sections is also useful for confirming myeloid lineage. Some phenotypic differences are found between adult and pediatric AML M0 cases. Adult AML M0 is associated with an immature stem cell profile (TdT, CD34, CD13, and CD33),[75–77] in contrast with pediatric AML M0, which usually lacked TdT or CD34 but expressed CD33 with weak or negative CD13.[78] Co-expression of the CD7 was observed in both groups. AML M0 was characterized by more frequent occurrence of complex karyotypes and abnormalities of chromosome 5 and/or 7.[76,77] The concurrent expression of factors having a negative prognostic impact such as CD7, GP170 (mdr phenotype), complex karyotype, and age over 60 years contributes to the very unfavorable prognosis for AML M0.[77,79]

Acute Myeloblastic Leukemia With Minimal Differentiation (M1)

Poorly differentiated myeloblasts are the predominant nonerythroid cell type (type I and type II). Rarely, a case of M1 may present with the majority of blasts being type III. Auer rods may present consistent with the diagnosis (Plate 14–9). More than 3 percent of these blast cells are MPO or SBB positive by conventional cytochemistry (Plate 14–10). The low percentage of MPO-positive (3 to 10 percent) M1 cases may constitute up to 25 percent of all M1 cases.[80] In such cases M1 should be differentiated from ALL L2, acute megakaryoblastic leukemia, and acute monoblastic leukemia without differentiation (M5a). Cytochemical stains and immunophenotyping are necessary for the differential diagnosis. Immunophenotyping to confirm the myeloid nature of blasts is recommended.

Acute Myeloblastic Leukemia With Significant Maturation (M2)

The defining characteristic that separates M2 from M1 is clear evidence of significant differentiation in all cells beyond the promyelocyte stage (Plate 14–11). The sum of the blast cells (type I + type II +, and type III) is greater than 30 percent but less than 90 percent, and generally there is a large predominance of type II blasts. Monocytic precursors cannot exceed 20 percent. Increased numbers of eosinophilic precursors (M2Eo) as well as pseudo-Pelger-Hüet cells and hypogranular neutrophils may be seen. The MPO and SBB reactions are strongly positive. However, M2 cases with a partial MPO deficiency in the granulocytic precursors and mature granulocytes have been reported.[81] M2 may be associated with basophilia and this rare form must be separated from CGL blast crisis.[82] M2Eo should be separated from the more common M4Eo.

Acute Promyelocytic Leukemia (M3)

Acute promyelocytic leukemia (APL) accounts for about 10 percent of cases in adult and for 4 to 8 percent in children.[83] Typical APL is characterized by the presence of hypergranular blast cells, which have the appearance of abnormal promyelocytes. The cytoplasm is dense with coarse dark-staining granules that often obscure the nucleus. The nuclear border is generally irregular and has a folded or reniform appearance (Plate 14–12). Cells contain bundles of delicate needlelike Auer rods, giving a meshwork appearance (so-called faggots), found in some of the leukemic promyelocytes. These abnormal promyelocytes are strongly positive for the MPO, SBB, and CAE reactions. The bundles of Auer rods are recognized easily with the CAE stain. Leukemic blast cells express myeloid antigens with the absence of HLA-DR and CD34.[84] In contrast to other AML subtypes, dysplastic features of the myeloid series associated with leukemic proliferation are not seen.

The FAB classification recognizes a variant of APL (FAB M3v),[85] characterized by bilobate cells or by cells with reniform nucleus and cytoplasm with minimal or no granulations (Plate 14–13). Typical M3 cells are infrequent in the bone marrow. M3v has the same clinical, cytogenetic, and immunological features as hypergranular APL. Since M3v is easily confused with monocytic leukemia special attention should be given to differentiate these cases from M4 and M5b subtypes.

In the recently developed treatment strategies for patients with APL the detection of the t(15;17) or the PML/RARα rearrangement is critical. In the absence of either the likelihood of a response to all-trans-retinoic acid (ATRA) is remote.[86] The t(11;17) and t(5;17) may present with a morphology that can be confused with classical M3 with t(15;17). Recently the FAB group has reviewed 32 cases of APL and variant forms. By utilizing published criteria the ability to make a correct diagnosis by morphology with molecular genetic confirmation and to eliminate cases that did not have the PML/RARα rearrangement was found to be excellent.[87] Similar results have also been presented.[88]

Acute Myelomonocytic Leukemia (M4)

M4 accounts for 20 to 30 percent of adult and 20 percent of childhood AML cases, depending on the application of esterase staining with fluoride inhibition. Its diagnosis and separation from M2 and M5 require assessment of both peripheral blood and bone marrow smears.[89] In bone marrow both granulocytic and monocytic precursors exist in varying proportions (Plate 14–14). The blast cells (types I, II, III) are greater than 30 percent or more, but less than 80 percent, of the nonerythroid cells. The marrow monocytic component must account for 20 percent or more of the nonerythroid nucleated cells but cannot exceed 80 percent (otherwise, the diagnosis is M5). Auer rods are occasionally present. When these findings are present with a peripheral blood monocytosis of 5000/mm^3 or greater, the diagnosis of M4 is not in question. If the peripheral monocytosis is less than 5000/mm^3 a diagnosis of M4 can still be made if the presence of a significant monocytic component (>20 percent) is confirmed by cytochemical stain (e.g., double esterase reaction with NaF or other esterase combinations). Cytochemical stains are also necessary for confirming the diagnosis of M4 in the presence of hypogranular neutrophils that resemble monocytes. Dysplastic features involving granulocytic, erythroid, and megakaryocytic lineages can be identified in approximately 20 percent of patients. Monocytic component can be identified by immunophenotyping using CD14, CD11c, CD11b, and CD68 in conjunction with other granulocyte-restricted antibodies.[70]

A small percentage of patients (about 5 percent) with M4 are characterized by myelomonocytic bone marrow infiltration with abnormal eosinophils (M4Eo). These eosinophils have large basophilic granules and demonstrate CAE and PAS positivity. Often the nuclei have pseudo-Pelger features (Plate 14–15).

Acute Monocytic Leukemia (M5a and M5b)

Acute monocytic leukemia (AMoL) accounts for about 10 percent of the AML and is clonally expressed in cells committed to differentiation to monocytic pathways.[90] AMoL is divided into two morphological subtypes: M5a and M5b.

M5a, or the poorly differentiated subtype, is frequently observed in children; it can be confused with the ALL L3 type. In the bone marrow 80 percent or more of all monocytic cells are monoblasts. Blast cells display abundant deep basophilic cytoplasm, which is often vacuolated and has no or few azurophilic granules and no Auer rods. The nuclei are round to oval, with one or more prominent nucleoli (Plate 14–16). Since the peroxidase reaction may be negative in 40 to 50 percent of such cases and the PAS reaction is often strongly positive with a blocklike pattern, it is very useful to use nonspecific esterase (NSE) staining differential diagnosis. This stain will be strongly positive in more than 90 percent of cases. Occasionally the SBB reaction will be positive in the absence of a peroxidase reaction.

M5b, or the well-differentiated subtype, is defined by the presence of 20 percent or more of abnormal cells being promonocytes with twisted or folded nuclei, gray-blue cytoplasm, and scattered azurophilic granules (Plate 14–17). Rarely, a few cells will contain Auer rods. The percentage of mature monocytes is often much higher in the blood than in the bone marrow. Monocytes with dysplastic features involving the other lineages can also be seen and have an adverse prognostic effect.

Acute Erythroleukemia (M6)

Erythroleukemia accounts for 4 to 5 percent of de novo and 10 to 20 percent of therapy-induced AML (t-AML). In 1976 the FAB cooperative group included erythroleukemia with the classification system of AML as M6 and agreed on a quantitative standard to be used in the diagnosis.[14] The standards were revised in 1985.[58] The proposed criteria for the diagnosis of M6 are different from those used for the other types of AML. A minimum of 30 percent blasts among the nonerythroid cells (NECs) and more than 50 percent erythroid precursors with dysplastic features are necessary for diagnosis (Plate 14–18). Ringed sideroblasts are present. The erythroid proliferation is often megaloblastoid. PAS stain can demonstrate diffuse or blue staining of the cytoplasm. Despite the FAB classification M6 remained a point of controversy. Several studies argued for the evaluation of pronormoblasts in the diagnosis of M6.[91] In 1992, Kowal-Vern and collegues[92] proposed that erythroleukemia with greater than or equal to 30 percent pronormoblasts be incorporated into the FAB classification since its behavior is more consistent with AML than an MDS. As defined by the WHO,[93] there are two types of acute erythroid leukemia. The first type called "erythroid/myeloid" (FAB-M6a) is defined as having ≥ 50 percent erythroid precursors in the bone marrow aspirate and ≥ 20 percent myeloblasts based on the nonerythroid rich leukemia (FAB-M6b) with > 80 percent of the marrow composed of immature cells of the erythroid lineage (proerythroblasts and basophilic erythroblasts) with no evidence of a significant or recognizable myeloblastic component[94] (Plate 14-19). Recent studies revealed that calculating the proerythroblasts as a component of total bone marrow erythroid cells provides a complementary method for delineating the three subsets.[95] Recent studies have also suggested that pure erythroid malignancies such as Di Guglielmo disease (DG), which was defined as more than 30 percent proerythroblasts in the absence of myeloblasts should be included in M6 since both M6 and DG shared some clinical and laboratory features, cytogenetic patterns, and poor prognosis.[96] A review of cytogenetic analysis were similar[96,97] in two respects: two-thirds of studied cases had complex chromosomal abnormalities involving three or more chromosomes and abnormalities involving chromosome 5 and/or 7 occurred in approximately 50 percent of patients.

Acute Megakaryoblastic Leukemia (M7)

Acute megakaryoblastic leukemia (AMkL) is a rare form of AML. It occurs particularly in infants/children younger than 2 years and in adults older than 50 years and represents 10 percent of childhood AML and 0.5 to 1 percent of adult AML.[98,99] AMkL is a heterogeneous disease, comprising at least three entities: M7 with t(1;22)(p13;q13), M7 in Down syndrome (DS), both found in infants and young children, and M7 without DS and without t(1;22), the latter having a typical AML age distribution increasing with age.[100]

In contrast to other types of AML, bone marrow biopsy is invaluable in helping establish the diagnosis of AMkL. The reason is that in only a few cases does the bone marrow aspirate show more than 30 percent of blast cells. By contrast, the bone marrow biopsy may show many clusters of micromegakaryoblasts. This is associated with an increase in reticulum formation and a corresponding decrease in normal hematopoietic precursors. In the peripheral blood, circulating small blast cells resembling either type I blasts or L2 cells can be found. The morphology of the blast cells reveals cells that are very pleomorphic; they may vary from very small with dense nuclear chromatin to somewhat larger with a fine reticulated nuclear chromatin and one or three prominent nucleoli. Cytoplasmic blebs or actual platelet shedding may be found surrounding some blasts. Standard cytochemistry can be helpful but is not specific. The blasts are MPO or SBB negative and the ANAE reaction shows distinct localized positivity, compared with the more diffuse staining in monocytes. PAS and ACP reactions can be positive and show a localized pattern reaction. Thus, the diagnosis of AMkL must be confirmed by immunological and electron microscopic cytochemistry studies. According to the EGIL recommendations[101] the immunophenotypic characterization of megakaryoblasts relied on the negativity of lymphoid antigens together with either the positivity of two megakaryocytic markers or the expression of one megakaryocytic marker associated with CD36 positivity. The PPO reaction by electron microscopic cytochemistry has been found to be more sensitive than monoclonal antibodies (mAbs) directed against platelet glycoprotein IIb/IIIa (CD41) (Plate 14–20).[102] However, PPO is also positive in immature erythroblasts. Recent studies have also suggested a close relationship between the erythroid and megakaryocytic lineages since M6 and M7 leukemias expressed mRNAs for alpha-globin, gpIIb, erythropoietin receptor, and thrombopoietin receptor but not for MPO.[103] These findings support the idea of a common ancestry.[104]

It should be noted that the diagnosis of AMkL might be difficult when criteria cannot be reached. Myelofibrosis and fibrosis of other organs involved in the malignant process together with the prominent organomegaly have mimicked a solid tumor. In a recent report of 39 cases of AMkL from a t(1;22) study group such misdiagnoses have reached up to 18 percent of cases.[105]

Marrow fibrosis is one of the characteristics of AMkL.[106] Abnormal platelets are postulated to release platelet-derived growth factor (PDGF) from α-granules, in turn stimulating the bone marrow fibroblasts and producing fibrosis. The presence of c-SIS mRNA that encodes a chain of PDGF has been demonstrated in M7 cells.

Prognosis of M7 with DS is good; however, it is worse in M7 with t(1;22) and in other M7 subtypes. Therefore BMT is indicated in those cases except in DS.[105]

ACUTE MYELOID LEUKEMIAS WITH RECURRENT CYTOGENETIC ABNORMALITIES

The combined used of FAB morphology and cytogenetic analysis has identified a number of AML subgroups with distinct biological characteristics.[71,107] The contribution of cytogenetics to the classification of AML and acute myeloid leukemias with recurrent cytogenetic abnormalities is briefly discussed below.

The t(8;21) AML1(CBFa)/ETO Translocation

The genes affected by this translocation are the *AML1* gene on chromosome 21 and ETO on chromosome 8. They are consequently fused in the der(8) chromosome to produce a novel chimeric gene. AML1 is a subunit of a multicomponent transcription factor complex known as core binding factor (CBF). CBF-α normally increases the DNA binding affinity of AML1. Thus, the fusion with chromosome 8 appears to disrupt AML1 function.[108,109] Since the breakpoints occurring during the t(8;21) are highly conserved within the single intron of both genes, it is possible to detect this translocation by molecular techniques.

The t(8;21) is found in approximately 7 to 12 percent of AML overall and 20 to 25 percent of AML M2. Although more than 90 percent of t(8;21) have been described in AML M2, this cytogenetic abnormality has also been identified in 6 percent of AML M1 and rarely in AML M4.[110] Its incidence is higher in children[107] and it is often associated with chloromas.[110] An eosinophilic component at least 5 percent is seen in about one-third of patients. Although previous reports had shown characteristic morphological features of t(8;21) positive leukemic blasts[111–113] (Plate 14–21), in recent studies, the cases with t(8;21) morphology did not correspond preferentially to those with a t(8;21) as opposed to an AML/ETO fusion transcript.[108–114]

The t(15;17)(PML/RARα) Translocation

The highly specific t(15;17) translocation is present in at least 90 percent of all acute myelocytic leukemia (APL) cases. Using molecular techniques, virtually 100 percent of APL have the t(15;17). This translocation fuses the *PML* gene of the chromosome 15 to the retinoic acid receptor-α. *(RARα)* gene, producing chimeric *PML/RARα* gene.[115] This fusion confers the exquisite sensitivity of this tumor to differentiation by ATRA.[116] Treatment of APL with ATRA has become a mainstay of therapy for APL. For these reasons, accurate diagnosis of APL is critical.

In a small number of APL patients two other novel translocations [e.g., a fusion product between a novel zinc finger gene and retinoic acid receptor with the t(11;17)(q23;q21)[117] and a different translocation t(5;17)(q32;q12)] associated with the *NPM/RARα* fusion gene[118] were also described. Morphological features in those patients are intermediate between M2 and classic M3 and they do not respond to ATRA.

Structural Abnormalities Involving Chromosome 16

Several groups have observed a strong correlation between structural rearrangements of chromosome 16 and acute myelomonocytic leukemia with eosinophilia (M4Eo).[119–121] Deletions—del(16)(q22)—and inversions—inv(16)(p13;q22)—involving the long arm of the chromosome appear to produce the same clinical features. The eosinophils account for 5 percent or more of the nonerythroid cells. They are reactive to CAE and PAS, contrary to normal eosinophils. In addition to M4Eo structural abnormalities involving chromosome 16 have been demonstrated in cases of M2, M5, and in blast crisis of CML.[121] Patients with chromosome 16 abnormalities tend to respond to chemotherapy better, experience relatively long remissions, and have a better prognosis.[71,107,121,122]

Structural Abnormalities Involving Chromosome 11

Structural lesions involving chromosome 11 band 23 are seen in approximately 14 to 18 percent of childhood[107] and 5 percent of adult AML cases and 85 percent of secondary leukemias that occur in patients treated with topoisomerase II inhibitors,[123] and rarely in patients with MDS.[124] A number of different partners for the balanced 11q23 translocations have been identified, and the most common translocations include t(4;11)(q21;q23), t(9;11)(p22;q23), and t(11;19)(q23;p13). In de novo AML, leukemic blasts containing 11q23 translocations generally have monocytic features and are subclassified as FAB M4 or M5.[125] In infant AML, rearrangements of 11q23 occur in 40 to 45 percent of cases and are strongly associated with the M4/M5 subtypes, high WBC counts, and poor prognosis.[126,127] However, recent studies indicate that MLL/11q23 rearrangements lacked prognostic significance in infant AML,[128,129] whereas the presence of t(9;11) conferred a favorable outcome. In adult cases of de novo AML 11q23 rearrangements have been reported in 23 percent of cases of M4 and M5 subtypes but were not associated with specific clinical or prognostic factors.[130] 11q23 rearrangements have also been observed in biphenotypic leukemias.

Acute Myeloid Leukemia With Multilineage Dysplasia With or Without Prior MDS and Prior Therapy

Ten to 15 percent of cases of de novo AML show marked dysplastic features involving erythroid, granulocytic, and megakaryocytic lineages.[131,132] Such cases have been designated as de novo AML with trilineage myelodysplasia (AML/TMDS) by Brito-Babapulle and co-workers.[133] AML/TMDS is often preceded by a hypoproliferative state and characterized by a relatively lower percentage of blasts in the bone marrow and a poorer response to aggressive chemotherapy compared with typical de novo AML. AML/TMDS could be seen in all FAB types predominantly in M2 and M6 subtypes and was absent in M3. AML/TMDS cases had myelodysplastic remission marrow that predicts a poorer prognosis and early leukemic relapse.[134]

It is known that alkylating agents and topoisomerase II inhibitors can cause distinct forms of therapy-related leukemia and MDS. Alkylating agents–related leukemias are very similar to post-MDS leukemias, being characterized by a long latency period, a preleukemic phase, trilineage dysplasia, and frequent cytogenetic abnormalities involving chromosomes 5 and 7.[135,136] In contrast to the myeloid leukemias induced by alkylating agents, topoisomerase II inhibitor-related AML has a short latency period (median 30 to 34 months), lacks a myelodysplastic phase, and is characterized by a predominance of myelomonoblastic or monoblastic morphological features, as well as balanced chromosomal translocations, generally involving the 11q23 region.[137,138]

The spectrum of cytogenetic abnormalities in AML/TMDS particularly in the elderly shows marked similarities with AML arising in patients with a history of MDS and alkylating-agent–related AML as well as in MDS not associated with prior therapy. Complex karyotypes were most frequent, whereas single abnormalities were rare, and chromosomes 5, 7, and 8 were most frequently involved.[132,139,140] These findings have suggested that all of these disorders may reflect similar genetic damage, which may be either environmental or iatrogenic.[141] There was also a consensus that the presence of multilineage dysplasia at the time of diagnosis of AML, a history of an MDS, or prior alkylating agent therapy were all adverse prognostic factors that may reflect a common pathogenesis.[131,132,142,143] Therefore, the WHO morphology committee[11] recently

included these above features in the classification of AML. Topoisomerase II inhibitors related leukemias are also recognized in the recent WHO classification as distinct from alkylating-agent–related secondary leukemias.

Hypocellular Acute Myeloid Leukemia

Hypocellular AML is a diagnostic dilemma. It does not fit the FAB classification of acute leukemia and often is mistaken for myelodysplasia or even aplastic anemia.[144,145] In general these patients are elderly, most having long-standing hematological complaints before diagnosis and lacking physical findings. Most of them are leukopenic or pancytopenic and have few blasts in the peripheral blood. The bone marrow is hypocellular, with more than 30 percent poorly differentiated type I blasts. The incidence of hypocellular leukemia is reported to be 8 to 14 percent.[144–147] According to most investigators, a case of acute leukemia is considered hypocellular when the bone marrow cellularity is less than 30 percent.[146,147] However, since most patients are elderly and have low cellularity because of age, the cutoff value of bone marrow cellularity is controversial. In a study conducted in our laboratory,[146] bone marrow cellularity of 40 percent would seem to present the upper limit to include such cases into hypocellular AML for clinical comparisons. Recent studies[146,147] revealed that hypocellular AML was a distinct subtype of AML characterized by slow but distinct proliferation of immature blasts. Although most cases had blasts with low or negative MPO activity, immunophenotyping of blast cells showed expression of myeloid antigens. Dysplastic changes were present. In one study[147] karyotyping revealed nonrandom chromosome abnormalities that are considerably different from those seen in MDS.

Evaluation of Remission

In a patient treated with acute leukemia, CR is considered when peripheral blood cell counts approach the normal range, and the bone marrow is normocellular and shows orderly maturation of hematopoietic cells with less than 5 percent blast cells. The criteria for morphological remission of less than 5 percent bone marrow blasts are arbitrary. The leukemic blasts in AML M3 or ALL L3, or blasts containing Auer rods can be readily identified, even when present in small numbers. Persistence of dysplastic hematopoiesis in a patient who might otherwise fulfill the criteria for CR results in a much higher relapse rate.

The current technology is redefining remission. The presence of leukemic blast cells at a level typically under detectable with conventional morphological evaluation is referred to as *minimal residual disease*. The presence of increased precursor B cells or hematogones in the bone marrow of patients with treated precursor B-ALL may pose a diagnostic dilemma with regard to differentiating hematogones from residual or recurrent leukemia. Differentiating hematogones from leukemic B cells can be challenging, given their morphological similarities[148] and often-identical immunological profiles.[149] In distinguishing hematogones from leukemic blast cells in a patient with precursor B-ALL who is in morphological remission, using markers of clonality such as PCR for IgH and TCR gene rearrangements[150–152] and frequently occurring specific translocations[153,154] or deletions have been suggested. The role of FISH is also being explored. Although a positive result may indicate the presence of a small population of clonal cells, whether it necessarily reflects an increased predilection for subsequent morphological relapse is uncertain.

MYELODYSPLASTIC SYNDROME

MDS is a clonal multipotent hematopoietic stem cell disorder characterized by both clinically and morphologically ineffective hematopoiesis. Clinically, MDS represents a condition of bone marrow failure, usually of the elderly (primary MDS), or of patients previously exposed to prior chemotherapy, or radiation, or both (secondary MDS). The correlation of the biology of this clonal disorder with its clinical presentation of cytopenias is varied, ranging from an incidental mild anemia stable for years to a rapidly evolving leukemia.

Clonality of MDS was first verified by glucose 6-phosphatase-dehydrogenase (G6PD) isoenzyme studies.[155] Furthermore, several studies using X-linked restriction fragment length polymorphism (LFRP)[156] demonstrated that MDS arises from a multipotent stem cell with the potential for both myeloid and lymphoid differentiation.

Bone marrow failure in MDS is a result of ineffective hematopoiesis rather than a lack of hematopoietic activity. Recent studies implicate extensive apoptosis as the explanation of the paradoxical observation of marrow hyperplasia but peripheral cytopenia.[157] High levels of TNF-α were found to correlate with high levels of apoptosis.[158] Both precursor and terminally differentiated cells in MDS often have functional defects (i.e., decreased sensitivity to erythropoietin in red cell precursors, decreased MPO, and microbicidal activity in neutrophils, and functional defects in platelets). Among these, neutropenia or neutrophil dysfunction accounts for the primary clinical manifestation of MDS in terms of an increased risk for infection, which is the leading cause of death in MDS.

Certain chromosomal abnormalities are common in MDS, especially loss or gain of all or parts of chromosomes 5, 7, 8, and 20.[159] Recently, a number of MDS cases associated with 11q23 abnormalities have been reported.[124]

By definition MDS is characterized by hypercellular marrow with bi- or trilineage dyplasia. Single line dysplasia of the erythroid, granulocytic, or megakaryocytic precursors has become recognized with increased frequency and is captured in the WHO proposals and listed under MDS, Unclassified, when the blast percentage is less than 5. The bone marrow cellularity at diagnosis was assessed in different stem cell disorders by our group.[160] The estimation of bone marrow cellularity for each group was used both with and without age adjustment, based on normal marrow biopsies. The age-corrected data disclosed that all patients with chronic myeloproliferative disorders (CMPD), 63 percent of patients with AML and only 35 percent of patients with MDS had hypercellular bone marrow according to their age. Our study suggests that in terms of bone mar-

row cellularity, MDS is quite different from AML and CMPDs, and appears to have a different proliferative capacity.

Diagnosis and Classification of MDS

The diagnosis is essentially one of exclusion in first ruling out other disorders that can also cause peripheral blood/bone marrow dysplasia and cytopenias.

The diagnosis of MDS requires minimal descriptions described by the FAB Cooperative group.[8,58,161] Five categories were described on the basis of morphological criteria. With the exception of refractory anemia with ringed sideroblasts (RARS) and chronic myelomonocytic leukemia (CMML), the principal distinction among the subgroups is the percentage of blasts in the bone marrow and peripheral blood. A diagnosis of AML required the presence of more than 30 percent blasts in the bone marrow. In recent years it has been noted that this classification system is sometimes clinically inconsistent.[11,162] Major confusions therefore arise: 1. The use of 30 percent blasts in the bone marrow as the dividing line between AML and MDS is biologically inconsistent and therapeutically confusing, 2. CMML is a separate entity and is related more closely to CMPDs than to the myelodysplasia; and 3. cases with significant trilineage dysplasia but less than 5 percent blasts that have a worse prognosis similar to RAEB are not recognized in the FAB schema. Therefore, the committee of the WHO[11] recommended the following proposals to clarify the discussions mentioned above: 1. Lowering the cutoff value of bone marrow blasts for the diagnosis of AML from 30 to 20 percent, and eliminating the category of refractory anemia excess blasts in transformation (RAEB-T); 2. forming a separate category of myeloid neoplasms (myeloproliferative/myelodysplastic) to contain those cases that are inherently proliferative but show dysplastic features including juvenile myelomonocytic leukemia (JMML), CMML, and atypical chronic myeloid leukemia (aCML); and 3. considering the severe multilineage dysplasia without increasing marrow blasts as a separate entity. The FAB classification and proposed WHO classification of MDS are given in Tables 14–6 and 14–7, respectively.

Predicting overall survival as well as the risk of AML transformation has been improved by the recent development of a scoring system (International Prognostic Scoring System)[163] that incorporates three laboratory variables: percentage of bone marrow blasts, degree of cytopenias, and presence of chromosomal abnormalities. Advanced age and male sex also adversely affected survival. Isolated loss of the Y, 5q, or 20q chromosomes and normal karyotype were associated with a better prognosis (median survival 5.7 years), whereas abnormalities of chromo-

---

Table 14–6. FAB Classification of Myelodysplastic Syndromes (MDS)

Refractory anemia (RA)
Refractory anemia with ringed sideroblasts (RARS)
Refractory anemia with excess blasts (RAEB)
Chronic myelomonocytic leukemia (CMML)
Refractory anemia with excess blasts in transformation (RAEB-T)

Table 14–7. Proposed WHO Classification of Myelodysplastic Syndromes (MDS)

Refractory anemia or refractory cytopenia
    Without ringed sideroblasts
    With ringed sideroblasts
Refractory cytopenia with multilineage dysplasia (RCMD)
Refractory anemia with excess blasts (RAEB); RAEB-I (5–10 percent blasts); RAEB-II (11–20 percent blasts)
5q– syndrome
Unclassifiable MDS
Myelodysplastic/myeloproliferative diseases
    Chronic myelomonocytic leukemia
    Atypical chronic myeloid leukemia (aCML)
    Juvenile myelomonocytic leukemia (JMML)

some 7 or complex cytogenetic changes with three or more abnormalities were associated with a worse prognosis (median 0.4 years). Management of MDS patients can now be based on the patient's respective prognostic subgrouping.

Morphologic Characteristics of Dysplasia

The following discussion highlights the morphologic features used to define MDS.[164–166] In general, these features should be present in at least 10 percent or greater of cells of the respective lineage under consideration.

Dyserythropoiesis (DysE)

Morphological bone marrow DysE may include the presence of ringed sideroblasts, multinuclear fragments, bizarre nuclear shapes, internuclear bridging, mitosis, abnormal intensity of the chromatin or fine chromatin with asynchronous cytoplasm, and abnormal cytoplasmic features (intense basophilia, Howell-Jolly bodies, ghosted cytoplasm). Marked macrocytosis (at least 100 fmoles/L), basophilic stippling, anisocytosis, and poikilocytosis may be observed in the peripheral blood. Quantitative changes include the presence of ringed sideroblasts (exceeding 15 percent of all nucleated erythroid cells) and a number of megaloblastic erythroid precursors.

Normal marrow can have occasional erythroblasts, typically with fewer than five granules. *Pathologic sideroblasts* have five or more granules and are termed *ringed sideroblasts* if the granules cover more than one-third of the nuclear rim (Plate 14–22). Ringed sideroblasts and increased iron stores can be found in any of the MDS, but they are characteristic of RARS.

Dysgranulopoiesis (DysG)

The most common findings are hypogranulation and hyposegmentation of the polymorphonuclear leukocytes (PMLs) with excessive chromatin condensation (pseudo-Pelger-Hüet anomaly) (Plate 14–23). These are seen most easily in the peripheral blood film. In addition, nuclear sticks can be noted particularly in cases of therapy-related MDS. Hypogranulation of the myeloid precursors as well as PMLs is also noted in bone marrow smears.

Dysmegakaryopoiesis (DysM)

Qualitative changes are more common in DysM because the number of megakaryocytes is usually normal, although hypoplasia or hyperplasia can occasionally be seen. In the peripheral blood, large hypo- or hypergranular platelets can be found. In the bone marrow, morphological abnormalities of the megakaryocytic precursors can be seen in half of the patients. Commonly there are micromegakaryocytes (dwarf forms) (Plate 14–24), megakaryocytes with multiple small round, and separate nuclei, and large mononuclear forms.

Bone Marrow Histology

MDS is characterized by architectural disorganization. Therefore, a bone marrow biopsy provides useful information on cellularity, relative proportions of three hematopoietic cell lines, architectural disorganization, and increase in the reticulin fibers. Architectural disorganization affects the spatial localization of the hematopoietic cells so that erythroblasts and megakaryoblasts are found at the trabecular surface. Moreover, small clusters of blast cells may be identified in central marrow regions referred to as abnormal localization of immature precursors (ALIP) (Plate 14–25). Tricot et al.[167] showed that patients presenting with ALIP experienced early leukemic transformation and short survival irrespective of FAB type. Prognostic significance of ALIP was also confirmed by several other studies.[168] However, it is difficult to distinguish ALIP from immature aggregates of normal marrow precursor cells on H & E or Giemsa-stained sections. However, immunohistochemistry can easily be confirmed by both the presence and lineage of these immature cells.[169]

Morphologic Subtypes

Refractory Anemia (RA)

Anemia is the main manifestation (hemoglobin below 11 g/dl with a low reticulocyte count) with variable dyserythropoiesis alone or accompanied by DysG and DysM (Table 14–7). However, the first hematological manifestation could be thrombocytopenia alone or more rarely neutropenia alone. Therefore, this type might be more appropriately termed refractory cytopenias (RC). Granulocytopenia or thrombocytopenia or both may be minimal or absent. Blast cells are not present in the peripheral blood (less than 1 percent) and less than 5 percent in the bone marrow. Ringed sideroblasts should be less than 15 percent. The WHO committee[11] has proposed to separate refractory cytopenia patients into two categories: RC with minimal dysplasia and RC with the multilineage dysplasia, a distinct subset with an unfavorable outcome.

Refractory Anemia With Ringed Sideroblasts

The morphologic features of RARS are similar to those of RA, except that there are more than 15 percent ringed sideroblasts in the bone marrow. Macrocytosis and dysmorphic red cells are present in the peripheral blood (Plate 14–26). In pure RARS DysG and DysM are absent or reveal only occasional individual cell dysplasia (less than 10 percent). These cases are characterized by very low risk of progression to AML. In the dysplastic form of sideroblastic anemia, iron overload is associated with marrow dysplasia; those cases are associated with leukemic progression and shorter overall survival.

In the recent WHO proposal of MDS, RA and RARS are defined as disorders involving only the erythroid line[11] as defined above.

Refractory Cytopenia With Multilineage Dysplasia (RCMD)

In 1996 Rosati et al.[170] reviewed 60 patients for whom the original diagnosis was RA, RARS, unclassifiable, or RAEB, and identified 18 cases characterized by multilineage dysplasia, but with an insufficient number of bone marrow blast cells to meet the FAB criteria for RAEB. This subset of MDS, named refractory cytopenia with multilineage dysplasia (RCMD), had a short survival time (24 months), more similar to that of RAEB (18 months) than RA/RARS (107 months). After this publication, several studies confirmed the previously reported findings.[171,172] Therefore, it is incorporated as a new subgroup of MDS classification.[11]

Refractory Anemia With Excess of Blasts

Conspicuous morphological changes are present, associated with variable cytopenia affecting two or more of the hematopoietic lines. Occasional blasts may be present in the peripheral blood but are always less than 5 percent. Blasts (type I+II+III) range from greater than 5 percent but less than 20 percent in the bone marrow (Plate 14–27). The presence of ALIP in the bone marrow biopsy has been reported to be an adverse prognostic factor.[168]

In the new WHO proposal of MDS, RAEB remains unchanged, but separation of RAEB into two groups has been recommended: RAEB I with less than 10 percent blasts in the bone marrow and RAEB II with 10 to 20 percent blasts in the bone marrow.

Refractory Anemia With Excess Blasts in Transformation

This subclass of MDS is identical to RAEB except for a higher percentage of bone marrow blasts (21 to 30 percent). However, the WHO morphology committee has decided to drop RAEB-T from the classification by lowering the threshold of bone marrow blasts diagnostic of AML from 30 to 20 percent. Further refinement may be necessary because of studies that indicate that the survival of patients with 11 to 20 percent blasts is similar to RAEB-T.

The −5q Syndrome

Among the patients with MDS/RA, those with an isolated deletion of the long arm of chromosome 5 (del 5q or −5q) represent a unique clinical presentation.[173,174] Anemia is the first manifestation, neutropenia if present is mild, and the platelet count is often high. There is marked female predominance. Small mononuclear megakaryocytes with single eccentric nucleus and many granulations are strongly correlated with −5q syndrome.[175]

It is important to distinguish between an isolated deletion in 5q and one that is part of a more complex cytogenetic abnormality, since patients with other chromosomal abnormalities in addition to −5q usually have rapid leukemic progression.

Hypocellular MDS

Hypocellular MDS accounts for less than 10 to 15 percent of all cases.[176,177] According to our experience,[160] hypocellularity is a more common feature of MDS than AML, even after age adjustment based on normal biopsy. To recognize the clinical and morphological features of these patients, we consider bone marrow cellularity of 30 percent the upper limit, to include such cases in hypocellular MDS.

The clinical findings and the morphological features of the bone marrow may be difficult to distinguish from those associated with aplastic anemia.[178] The finding of cytogenetic abnormalities that are typical of MDS permits an accurate diagnosis. However, CD34 and PCNA immunostaining can be of practical value in the absence of cytogenetic data.[179] The diagnostic criteria for hypocellular MDS must be met for FAB criteria. Most cases fall into the categories of RA and RAEB. The natural history of hypocellular MDS seems to be similar to that of normocellular and hypocellular MDS.[180,181]

Myelodysplastic/Myeloproliferative Diseases

The WHO classification[11] recommends that a separate category be formed to include disorders that have both myelodysplastic and myeloproliferative features, including CMML, JMML, and aCML. These disorders have many common features including abnormalities of both granulocytic and monocytic lines and a relatively aggressive course.

Chronic Myelomonocytic Leukemia

The inclusion of CMML into MDS was long debated. It has been recognized that CMML has both myelodysplastic and myeloproliferative features. Patients with myelodysplastic features present with low or normal leukocyte count, multilineage dysplasia, no organomegaly, but with peripheral monocytosis. Bone marrow morphology resembles MDS/RA or MDS/RAEB with monocytosis. However, patients with myeloproliferative features have marked leukocytosis, monocytosis, organomegaly, and skin infiltrations. Whether dysplastic or proliferative CMML represents a different phase of a single disease or are distinct entities remains unclear. The FAB criteria for the diagnosis of CMML is the presence of peripheral absolute monocytosis higher than $1 \times 10^9/L$. Peripheral blood and bone marrow smears show trilineage dysplasia and monocytosis associated with blast cells (Plate 14–27).

Atypical Chronic Myeloid Leukemia (aCML)

This disease predominantly involves the neutrophilic series as in CML but lacks Ph1 chromosome or bcr/abl translocation.[182] aCML has dysplastic and proliferative features as well as an increased monocyte count. Its prognosis is significantly worse than Ph1+ CML. According to recently developed FAB criteria CML, aCML, and CMML can be distinguished from each other by employing five quantitative (WBC count, percentage of immature granulocytes, percentage of monocytes and basophils in peripheral blood, and percentage of erythroid precursors in bone marrow) and one qualitative (granulocytic dysplasia) parameters.[183]

Juvenile Myelomonocytic Leukemia

JMML is a separate disorder seen in children and adolescents and distinct from adult CMML. Young patient age (median 1.8 years), predominant hepatosplenomegaly, frequent skin involvement, leukocytosis, monocytosis, and presence of immature precursors in peripheral blood characterize JMML. Fourteen percent of patients are known to have neurofibromatosis type I by clinical criteria. The JMML cells demonstrate hypersensitivity to GM-CSF in in vitro dose-response assays. Although 65 percent of patients with JMML have a normal karyotype, 25 percent show monosomy 7 and 10 percent complex chromosomal abnormalities.[184,185]

MDS in Children

MDS in childhood accounts for less than 10 percent of all malignancies in this age group,[186] and very heterogeneous disease. It may develop de novo or after chemotherapy or radiation therapy. Constitutional conditions such as Down syndrome are present in one-third of children with MDS.[187] The classification of MDS in childhood using FAB criteria has been the subject of some controversy.[188] The frequency of FAB subtypes of MDS in childhood differs from those observed in adults. Approximately 50 percent of children with de novo MDS have chromosomal abnormalities, with monosomy 7 (−7) or partial deletion of the long arm of chromosome 7 seen in 30 to 40 percent of cases (H. Hasle, personal communication). Monosomy 7 is found in all MDS subgroups. In addition hematological features of some nonclonal disorders such as mitochondriopathies may be indistinguishable from the true clonal MDS/RARS.[185,188]

Therapy-Related MDS

Therapy-related MDS (t-MDS) and AML (t-AML), have become among the most feared long-term complications of cancer therapy. The incidence of t-MDS and t-AML is increasing because of the widespread and successful use of chemoradiotherapy[135] and high-dose therapy with autologous stem cell transplantation (ASCT).[189]

In contrast to primary MDS, most cases of t-MDS are difficult to classify according to FAB criteria. The bone marrow is often hypocellular and fibrotic and severe dysplastic changes are observed. In such cases bone marrow biopsy is important in establishing the diagnosis.[190] Chromosomal abnormalities are found in 76 to 97 percent of cases.[161] Deletions or loss of chromosomes 7 and 5 are commonly associated with exposure to alkylating agents and also seen in t-MDS/AML following ASCT,[135,161,189] and balanced translocations involving chromosome bands 11q23 can occur after treatment with DNA topoisomerase II inhibitors.[123,191] It was thought that t-MDS was clinically separate from primary MDS; however, cytogenetic stratification suggests that the clinical course is more dependent on specific cytogenetic abnormalities than on the presence or absence of a history of toxic exposure.[25,82,83] It is well known that patients with t-MDS are more likely to have karyotypic abnormalities that are associated with poor prognosis.[136,163]

REFERENCES

1. Weinkauff R, Estery EH, Starostik P et al: Use of peripheral blasts vs bone marrow blasts for diagnosis of acute leukemia. Am J Clin Pathol 111:733, 1999.
2. Manohoran A, Horsley R, Ptiney WR: The reticulin content of bone marrow in acute leukemia in adults. Br J Haematol 43:185, 1979.
3. Islam A: A proposal for classification of acute myeloid leukemia on plastic embedded bone marrow biopsy sections. Leuk Res 17:421, 1993.
4. Neiman RS, Barcos M, Berard C et al: Granulocytic sarcoma. Cancer 48:1426, 1976.
5. Chang SS, Li CY: Useful panel of antibodies for the classification of acute leukemia by immunohistological methods in bone marrow trephine biopsy specimens. Am J Clin Pathol 107:410, 1997.
6. Manaloor EJ, Neiman RS, Heilman DK et al: Immunohistochemistry can be used to subtype acute myeloid leukemia in routinely processed bone marrow biopsy specimens. Am J Clin Pathol 113:814, 2000.
7. Pileri SA, Ascani S, Milani M et al: Acute leukemia immunophenotyping in bone marrow routine sections. Br J Haematol 105:394, 1999.
8. Bennett JM, Reed CE: Acute leukemia: Cytochemical applications. Blood Cells 1:101, 1975.
9. Bennett JM, Catovsky D, Daniel M et al: Characterization of megakaryoblastic leukemia. Ann Intern Med 103:460, 1985.
10. Bennett JM, Catovsky D, Daniel MT et al: Proposal for the recognition of minimally differentiated acute myeloid leukemia (AML MO). Br J Haematol 78:325, 1991.
11. Jaffe ES, Harris NL, Stein H, Vardiman JW (Eds.). World Health Organization classification of tumours: Pathology and genetics of tumours of haematopoietic and lymphoid tissues. IARC Press, 2001.
12. Pui CH: Childhood leukemias: N Engl J Med 332:1618, 1995.
13. Cortes JE, Kantarjian HM: Acute lymphoblastic leukemia. A comprehensive review with emphasis on biology and therapy. Cancer 76:2393, 1995.
14. Bennett JM, Catovsky D, Daniel MT et al: Proposal for classification of acute leukemias. Br J Haematol 33:451, 1976.
15. Bennett JM, Catovsky D, Daniel MT et al: The morphologic classification of acute lymphoblastic leukemia: Concordance among observers and clinical correlations. Br J Haematol 47:553, 1981.
16. Miller DR, Krailo M, Bayer WA et al: Prognostic implication of blast cell morphology in childhood acute lymphoblastic leukemia: A report from Children's Cancer Study Group. Cancer Treat Rep 69:1211, 1985.
17. Pui CH, Campana D, Crist WM: Toward a clinically useful classification of the acute leukemias. Leukemia 9:2154, 1995.
18. Khalidi HS, Chang K, Medeiros LJ et al: Acute lymphoblastic leukemia. Survey of immunophenotype, French American British classification, frequency of myeloid antigen expression, and karyotypic abnormalities in 210 pediatric and adult cases. Am J Clin Pathol 111:467, 1999.
19. Head DR, Behm FG: Acute lymphoblastic leukemia and the lymphoblastic lymphomas of childhood. Semin Diagn Pathol 12:325, 1995.

20. Jaffe ES, Harris NL, Chan JKC et al: Society for Hematopathology program. Am J Surg Pathol 21:114, 1997.

21. Dalla-Favera R, Gregni M, Erikson J et al: Human c-myc onc gene is located on the region of chromosome 8 that is translocated in Burkitt's lynphoma cells. Proc Natl Acad Sci USA 79:7824, 1982.

22. Berger R, Bernheim A: Cytogenetic studies on Burkitt's lymphoma-leukemia. Cancer Genet Cytogenet 7:231, 1982.

23. Tricot G, Broeckaert-van Orsheron A, Van Hoof A et al: Sudan Black B positivity in acute lymphoblastic leukemia. Br J Hamatol 51:615, 1982.

24. Bain B, Catovsky D: Current concerns in hematology, 2. Classification of acute leukemia. J Clin Pathol 43:882, 1990.

25. Catovsky D, Cherchi M, Graves MF et al: Acid phosphatase reaction in acute lymphoblastic leukemia. Lancet 1:749, 1978.

26. Cordel JL, Fallini B, Erber WT et al: Immunoenzymatic labelling of monoclonal antibodies using immunocomplexes of alkaline phosphatase and monoclonal alkaline phosphatase (APAAP complexes). J Histochem Cytochem 32:219, 1984.

27. Borowitz MJ: Immunologic markers in childhood lymphoblastic leukemia. Hematol Oncol Clin North Am 4:743, 1990.

28. Bene MC, Castoldi G, Knapp W et al: Proposals for the immunological classification of acute leukemias. European Group for the Immunological Characterization of Leukemias. Leukemia 9:1783, 1995.

29. Del Vecchio I, Noto RD, Pardo CL et al: Immunological classification of acute leukemias: Comments on the EGIL proposals. Leukemia 10:1832, 1996.

30. Pui CH, Behm FG, Crist WM: Clinical and biologic relevance of immunologic marker studies in childhood acute lymphoblastic leukemia. Blood 82:343, 1993.

31. Rowley J: Ph-positive leukemia, including chronic myeloid leukemia. Clin Haematol 9:55, 1980.

32. Riberio RC, Abromowitch M, Raimondi SC et al: Clinical and biologic hallmarks of the Philadelphia chromosome in childhood acute lymphoblastic leukemia. Blood 70:948, 1987.

33. Uckun F, Nachman JB, Sather HN et al: Clinical significance of Philadelphia chromosome positive pediatric acute lymphoblastic leukemia in the context of contemporary intensive therapies. Cancer 83:2030, 1998.

34. Faderi S, Kantarjian HM, Talpaz M, Estrov Z: Clinical significance of cytogenetic abnormalities in adult acute lymphoblastic leukemia. Blood 91:3995, 1998.

35. Groupe Francis de Cytogénétique Hématologique: Cytogenetic abnormalities in adult lymphoblastic leukemia: Correlations with hematologic findings and outcome. A collaborative study of the Groupe Francis de Cytgénétique Hématologique. Blood 87:3135, 1996.

36. Specchia G, Mininni A, Guerrasio A et al: Ph positive acute lymphoblastic leukemia in adults: Molecular and clinical studies. Leuk Lymphoma 18:37, 1995.

37. Arico M, Valsecchi MG, Camitta B et al: Outcome of treatment in children with Philadelphia chromosome-positive acute lymphoblastic leukemia. N Engl J Med 342:998, 2000.

38. Zieman-van der Poel S, McCabe NR, Gill HJ et al: Identification of a gene, MLL, that spans the breakpoint in 11q23 translocations associated with human leukemias. Proc Natl Acad Sci USA 88:10735, 1991.

39. Heerema NA, Sather HN, Ge J et al: Cytogenetic studies of infant acute lymphoblastic leukemia: Poor prognosis in infants with t(4;11)—a report of the Children's Cancer Group. Leukemia 13:679, 1999.

40. Copelan EA, McGuire EA: The biology and treatment of acute lymphoblastic leukemia in adults. Blood 85:1151, 1995.

41. Janssen JWG, Ludwig WD, Borkhardt A et al: Pre-pre-B acute lymphoblastic leukemia: High frequency of alternatively spliced ALL1-AF4 transcripts and absence of minimal residual disease during complete remission. Blood 84:3835, 1994.

42. Carroll AJ, Crist WM, Parmley RT et al: Pre-B cell leukemia associated with chromosome translocation 1;19. Blood 63:721, 1984.

43. Pui CH, Crist WM, Look T: Biology and clinical significance of cytogenetic abnormalities in childhood acute lymphoblastic leukemia. Blood 76:1449, 1990.

44. Crist WM, Carroll AJ, Shuster JJ et al: Poor prognosis of children with pre-B acute lymphoblastic leukemia is associated with the t(1;19)(q23;p13). A Pediatric Oncology Group Study. Blood 76:117, 1990.

45. Privitera E, Luciano A, Ronchetti D et al: Molecular variants of the 1;19 chromosomal translocation in pediatric acute lymphoblastic leukemia. Leukemia 8:554, 1994.

46. Uckun F, Sensel M, Sather HN et al: Clinical significance of translocation t(1;19) in childhood acute lymphoblastic leukemia in the contex of contemporary therapies: A report from the Children's Cancer Group. J Clin Oncol 16:527, 1998.

47. Golup TR, Barker GF, Stegmaier K et al: The TEL gene contributes to the pathogenesis of myeloid and lymphoid leukemias by diverse molecular genetic mechanisms. Curr Top Microbiol Immunol 220:67, 1997.

48. Romana SP, Poirel H, Le Coniat M et al: High frequency of t(12;21) in childhood B-lineage acute lymphoblastic leukemia. Blood 86:4263, 1995.

49. Borkhardt A, Cazzaniga G, Viehmann S et al: "Associazione Italiana Ematologica Oncologia Pediatrica" and the "Berlin-Frankfurt-Münster" study group: Incidence and clinical relevance of TEL/AML1 fusion genes in children with acute lymphoblastic leukemia enrolled in the German and Italian multicenter therapy trials. Blood 90:571, 1997.

50. Shurtleff SA, Buijs A, Behm FG et al: TEL/AML1 fusion resulting from a cryptic t(12;21) is the most commmon genetic lesion in pediatric ALL and defines a subgroup of patients with an excellent prognosis. Leukemia 9:1985, 1995.

51. Rubnitz JE, Shuster JJ, Land JV et al: Case control study suggests a favorable impact of TEL rearrangement in patients with B-lineage acute lymphoblastic leukemia treated with antimetabolite-based therapy: A Pediatric Oncology Group Study. Blood 89:1143, 1997.

52. McLean T, Ringold S, Neuberg D et al: TEL/AML1 dimerizes and is associated with a favorable outcome in childhood acute lymphoblastic leukemia. Blood 88:4252, 1996.

53. Morley A, Higgs D: Abnormal differentiation of leukemic cells in vitro. Cancer 33:716, 1974.

54. Drexler HG, Thiel E, Ludwig WD: Acute myeloid leukemias expressing lymphoid associated antigens: Diagnostic incidence and prognostic significance. Leukemia 7:489, 1993.

55. Jensen MK, Killman SA: Additional incidence for chromosomal abnormalities in erythroid precursors in acute leukemia. Acta Med Scand 189:97, 1971.

56. Ackerman GA: Microscopic and histochemical study on the Auer bodies in leukemic cells. Blood 5:847, 1950.

57. Bainon DF, Friedlander LM, Shohet SB: Abnormalities in granule formations in acute myelogenous leukemia. Blood 49:639, 1977.

58. Bennett JM, Catovsky D, Daniel MT et al: Proposed revised criteria for classification of acute myeloid leukemia. Ann Intern Med 103:626, 1985.

59. Head DR: Revised classification of acute myeloid leukemias. Leukemia 10:1826, 1996.

60. Chan GCF, Wang W, Raimondi S et al: Myelodysplastic syndrome in children: Differentiation from acute myeloid leukemia with a low blast count. Leukemia 11:206, 1997.

61. Cason JD, Trujillo JM, Estey EH et al: Peripheral acute leukemia: High peripheral but low marrow blast count. Blood 74:1758, 1989.

62. Cheson BD, Cassileth A, Head DR et al: Report of National Cancer Institute Sponsored Workshop on definitions and diagnosis and response in acute myeloid leukemia. J Clin Oncol 8:813, 1990.

63. Goasguen JE, Bennett JM, Cox C et al: Prognostic implication and characterization of blast cell population in myelodysplastic syndrome. Leukemia 15:1159, 1991.

64. Bennett JM, Castoldi D, Catovsky D et al: Recommended methods for cytological procedures in hematology. Clin Lab Hematol 7:55, 1985.

65. Goasguen JE, Bennett JM: Classification of acute leukemia. Clin Lab Med 10:661, 1990.

66. Van Wering ER, Brederoo P, Staalduien GJ et al: Contribution of electron microscopy to the classification of minimally differentiated acute leukemia in children. Recent Results Cancer Res 13:177, 1993.

67. Van Wering ER, Brederoo P, van-Dijik-de Leeuw JHS: Electron microscopy: Contribution to further classification of acute unclassifiable childhood leukemia. Blut 60:291, 1990.

68. Chuang SS, Li CY: Useful panel of antibodies for the classification of acute leukemia by immunohistochemical method in bone marrow trephine biopsy specimens. Am J Clin Pathol 107:410, 1997.

69. Buccheri V: The role of anti-myeloperoxidase antibody in the diagnosis and classification of acute leukemia: A comparison with light and electron microscopy cytochemistry. Br J Haematol 80:62, 1992.

70. Khalidi HS, Medeiros LJ, Chang KL et al: The immunophenotype of adult acute myeloid leukemia: High frequency of lymphoid antigen expression and comparison of immunophenotype, French-American-British classification and karyotypic abnormalities. Am J Clin Pathol 109:211–220, 1998.

71. Barnard DR, Kalousek DK, Wiersma SR et al: Morphologic, immunologic, and cytogenetic classification of acute myeloid leukemia and myelodysplastic syndrome in childhood: A report from The Childrens Cancer Group. Leukemia 10:5, 1996.

72. Drexler HG, Thiel E, Ludwig WD et al: Acute myeloid leukemias expressing lymphoid associated antigens: Diagnostic incidence and prognostic significance. Leukemia 7:489, 1993.

73. Launder TM, Bray RA, Stempora L et al: Lymphoid-associated antigen expression by acute myeloid leukemias. Am J Clin Pathol 106:1826, 1996.

74. Paietta E, Andersen J, Yunis J et al: Acute myeloid leukemia expressing the leukocyte integrin CD11b—a new leukemic syndrome with poor prognosis: Result of an ECOG database analysis. Eastern Cooperative Oncology Group 100:265, 1998.

75. Cohen P, Hoyer J, Curtin P et al: Acute myeloid leukemia with mimimal differentiation: Multiparameter study. Am J Clin Pathol 109:32, 1998.

76. Venditti A, Del Poete G, Buccisiano F et al: Minimally differentiated acute myeloid leukemia (AML-MO): Comparison of 25 cases with other French-American-British subtypes. Blood 89:621–629, 1997.

77. Amadori S, Venditti A, Del Poeta G et al: Minimally differentiated acute myeloid leukemia (AML-MO): A distinct clinico-biologic entity with poor prognosis. Ann Hematol 72:208, 1996.

78. Kotylo PK, Seo IS, Smith FO et al: Flow cytometric immunophenotypic characterization of pediatric and adult minimally differentiated acute myeloid leukemia (AML-MO). Am J Clin Pathol 113:193, 2000.

79. Cunero A, Ferrant A, Michaux JL et al: Cytogenetic profile of minimally differentiated (FAB-MO) acute myeloid leukemia: Correlation with clinicobiologic findings. Blood 85:3688, 1995.

80. Matsuo T, Cox C, Bennett JM: Prognostic significance of myeloperoxidase positivity of blast cells in acute myeloid leukemia without maturation (FAB M1). Hematol Pathol 3:153, 1989.

81. Loeffler H: Morphologic basis for the MIC classification in acute myeloid leukemia. Recent results. Cancer Res 131:339, 1993.

82. Catovsky D, Matutes E, Buccheri V et al: Classification of acute leukemia for the 1990's. Ann Hematol 62:16, 1991.

83. Carter M, Kalwinsky DR, Dahl GV et al: Childhood acute promyelocytic leukemia: A rare variant of non lymphoid leukemia with distinctive clinical and biologic features. Leukemia 4:298, 1989.

84. San Miguel JF, Gonzales M, Canizo MC et al: Surface marker analysis in acute myeloid leukemia and correlation with FAB classification. Br J Haematol 64:547, 1986.

85. Bennett JM, Catovsky D, Daniel MT et al: A variant form of hypergranular acute promyelocytic leukemia (M3). French-American-British (FAB) Classfication. Br J Haematol 64:547, 1986.

86. Tallman MS, Andersen JW, Schiffer CA et al: All-trans-retinoic acid in acute promyelocytic leukemia. N Engl J Med 337:1021, 1997.

87. Bennett JM, Catovsky D, Daniel M-T et al: Hypergranular promyelocytic leukemia: Correlation between morphology and chromosomal translocation including t(15;17) and t(11;17). Leukemia 14:1197, 2000.

88. Sainty D, Liso V, Canta-Rajuoldi A. et al: Morphological presentation of acute promyelocytic leukemia (APL) lacking the classical t(15;17) with special reference to a series of nine cases with t(15;17). Blood 92(Suppl. 1):60:3a, 1998.

89. Argyle JC, Benjamin DR, Lampkin B et al: Inter-observer variability and problems in the use of FAB classification. Cancer 63:295, 1989.

90. Ferraris AM, Broccia G, Meloni T et al: Clonal origin of cells restricted to onocytic differentiation in acute nonlymphocytic leukemia. Blood 64:817, 1984.

91. Cuneo A, Van Orshoven A, Michaux JL et al: Morphologic, immunologic and cytogenetic studies in erythroleukemia: Evidence for multilineage involvement and identification of two distinct cytogenetic-clinicopathological types. Br J Haematol 75:346, 1990.

92. Kowal-Vern A, Cotelingam J, Schumacher HR et al: The prognostic significance of proerythroblasts in acute erythroleukemia. Am J Clin Pathol 98:34, 1992.

93. Jaffe ES, Harris NL, Stein H, Vardiman JW (Eds.). World Health Organization classification of tumours: Pathology and genetics of tumours of haematopoietic and lymphoid tissues. Brunning RD, Matutes E, Flandrin G, 97–99. IARC Press, 2001.

94. Garand R, Duchayne E, Blanchard D et al: Minimally differentiated erythroleukaemia (AML M6 'varient'): A rare subset of AML distinct from AML M6. Br J Haematol 90:868, 1995.

95. Kowal-Vern A, Mazzella FM, Cotelingam JD et al: Diagnosis and characterization of acute erythroleukemia subsets by determining the percentages of myeloblasts and proerythroblasts in 69 cases. Am J Hematol 65:5, 2000.

96. Goldberg SL, Noel P, Klumpp TR, Dewald GW: The erythroid leukemias: A comparative study of erythroleukemia (FAB M6) and Di Guglielmo disease. Am J Clin Oncol 21:42, 1998.

97. Davey FR, Abraham N Jr, Brunetto VL et al: Morphologic characteristics of erythroleukemia (acute myeloid leukemia; FAB M6): A CALGB study. Am J Hematol 49:29, 1995.

98. Gassman W, Löffler H: Acute megakaryoblastic leukemia. Leuk Lymphoma 18(Suppl. 1):69, 1995.

99. Ribero RC, Olieria MSP, Fairclough D et al: Acute megakaryoblastic leukemia in children and adolescents: A retrospective analysis of 24 cases. Leuk Lymphoma 10:299, 1993.

100. Lu G, Altman AJ, Benn PA et al: Review of the cytogenetic changes in acute megakaryoblastic leukemia: One disease or several? Cancer Genet Cytogenet 67:81, 1993.

101. Garand R, Robillard N: Immunophenotypic characterization of acute leukemias and chronic lymphoproliferative disorders: Practical recommendations and classifications. Hematol Cell Ther 38:471, 1996.

102. Breton-Goruis J, Vanhaeke D, Pryzwansky KB: Simultaneous detection of membrane markers with monoclonal antibodies and peroxidatic activities in leukemia: Ultrastructural analysis using a new method of fixation preserving the platelet peroxidase. Br J Haematol 58:447, 1984.

103. Linari S, Vannucchi AM, Ciolli S et al: Coexpression of erythroid and megakaryocytic genes in acute erythroblastic (FAB M6) and megakaryoblastic (FAB M7) leukemias. Br J Haematol 102:1335, 1998.

104. Paoletti F, Vannucchi AM, Mocali AM et al: Identification and conditions for selective expression of megakaryocytic markers in Friend erythroleukemia cells. Blood 86:2624, 1995.

105. Bernstein J, Dastugue N, Haas OA et al: Nineteen cases of the t(1;22)(p13;q13) acute megakaryoblastic leukemia of infants/children and review of 39 cases: Report from a t(1;22) study group. Leukemia 14:216, 2000.

106. Imbert N, Nguyen D, Sultan C: Myelodysplastic syndromes (MDS) and acute myeloid leukemias (AML) with myelofibrosis. Leuk Res 16:51, 1992.

107. Raimondi SC, Chang MN, Ravindranath Y et al: Chromosomal abnormalities in 478 children with acute myeloid leukemia: Clinical characteristics and treatment outcome in a cooperative Pediatric Oncology Group Study—POG 8821. Blood 94:3707, 1999.

108. Andrieu V, Radford-Weiss I, Troussard X et al: Molecular detection of t(8;21)/AML1-ETO in AML M1/M2: correlation with cytogenetics, morphology and immunophenotype. Br J Haematol 92:855, 1996.

109. Nucifora G, Rowley JD: AML1 and the 8;21 and 3;21 translocations in acute and chronic myeloid leukemia. Blood 86:1, 1995.

110. Groupe Français de Cytogénétique (GFHC): Acute myelogenous leukemia with an 8;21 translocation. A report on 148 cases from the Groupe Français de Cytogénétique Hématologique. Cancer Genet Cytogenet 44:169, 1990.

111. Berger R, Bernheim A, Daniel M et al: Cytologic characterization and significance of normal karyotypes in t(8;21) acute myeloblastic leukemia. Blood 59:171, 1982.

112. Swirsky DM, Li YS, Matthews JG et al: 8;21 translocation in acute granulocytic leukemia: Cytological, cytochemical and clinical features. Br J Haematol 56:199, 1984.

113. Nucifora G, Dickstein JI, Torbenson V et al: Correlation between cell morphology and expression of the AML1/eto chimeric transcript in patients with acute myeloid leukemia without the t(8;21). Leukemia 8:1533, 1994.

114. Haferlach T, Bennett JM, Loffler H et al: Acute myeloid leukemia with translocation (8;21). Cytomorphology, dysplasia and prognostic factors in 41 cases. AML Cooperative group and ECOG. Leuk Lymphoma 23:227, 1996.

115. Chang KS, Stass SA, Chu DT et al: Characterization of a fusion cDNA(RARA7myl) transcribed from the t(15;17) translocation breakpoint in acute promyelocytic leukemia. Mol Cell Biol 12:800, 1992.

116. Chomienne C, Ballerini P, Balitrand N et al: All-trans-retinoic acid in acute promyelocytic leukemias, II: In vitro studies: structure-function relationship. Blood 76:1710, 1990.

117. Chen Z, Brand N, Chen A et al: A fusion between a novel Kruppel-like zinc finger gene and the retinoic acid receptor-α locus due to a variant t(11;17) translocation associated with acute promyelocytic leukemia. EMBO J 12:1161, 1993.

118. Gorey SJ, Locker J, Oliveri DR et al: A nonclassical translocation involving 17q12(RARA) in a patient with atypical features. Leukemia 8:1350, 1994.

119. Arthur DC, Bloomfield CD: Partial deletion of the long arm of chromosome 6 and bone marrow eosinophilia in acute nonlymphocytic leukemia: A new association. Blood 61:994, 1983.

120. Second MIC Cooperative Study Group: Morphologic, immunologic annd cytogenetic classification of acute myeloid leukemias. Br J Haematol 68:487, 1988.

121. Liu PP, Hajra A, Wijmenga C, Collins FS: Molecular pathogenesis of chromosome 16 inversion in the M4Eo subtype acute myeloid leukemia. Blood 85:2289, 1995.

122. Haferlack T, Gassmann W, Loffler H et al: Clinical aspects of acute myeloid leukemias of the FAB types M3 and M4Eo. The AML Cooperative Group. Ann Hematol 66:165, 1993.

123. Pui CH, Relling MV: Topoisomerase II inhibitor-related acute myeloid leukemia. Br J Haematol 109:13, 2000.

124. Bain BJ, Moorman AV, Johansson B et al: Myelodysplastic syndromes associated with 11q23 abnormalities. Leukemia 12:834, 1998.

125. Sorensen PHB: Molecular rearrangements of the MLL gene are present in most cases of infant acute myeloid leukemia and are strongly correlated with monocytic or myelomonocytic phenotypes. J Clin Invest 93:429, 1994.

126. Rubnitz JE, Behm FG, Downing JR: 11q23 rearrangements in acute leukemia. Leukemia 10:74, 1996.

127. Pui CH, Kane JR, Crist WM et al: Biology and treatment of infant leukemia. Leukemia 9:762, 1994.

128. Stake N, Maseki N, Nishiyama M et al: Chromosome abnormalities and MLL rearrangements in acute myeloid leukemia of infants. Leukemia 13:1013, 1999.

129. Pui CH, Raimondi SC, Srivastava DK et al: Prognostic factors in infants with acute myeloid leukemia. Leukemia 14:684, 2000.

130. Brower M et al: Prevalence and clinical correlations of MLL gene rearrangements in AML-M4/M5. Blood 84:3776, 1994.

131. Tamura S, Kanamaru A: De-novo acute myeloid leukemia with trilineage myelodysplasia (AML/TMDS) and myelodysplastic remission marrow (AML/MRM). Leuk Lymphoma 16:263, 1995.

132. Lima CS, Vassalo J, Metze-Lorand Y, Bachelli AP, Souza CA: The significance of trilineage myelodysplasia in de novo acute myeloblastic leukemia: Clinical and laboratory features. Hematologica 28:85, 1997.

133. Brito-Babapulle F, Catovsky D, Galton DAG et al: Clinical and laboratory features of de novo acute myeloid leukemia with trilineage myelodysplasia. Br J Haematol 66:445, 1987.

134. Tamura S, Takemoto Y, Wada H et al: Significance of trilineage myelodysplasia in de novo acute myeloid leukemia during remission rather than diagnosis. Br J Haematol 101:743, 1998.

135. Leone G, Mele L, Pulsoni Aequitani F, Pagano L: The incidence of secondary leukemias. Hematologica 84:937, 1999.

136. Taketema K, Seto M, Uike N et al: Therapy related leukemia and myelodysplastic syndrome: A large-scale Japanese study of clinical and cytogenetic features as well as prognostic factors. Int J Hematol 71:144, 2000.

137. Pedersen-Bjergaard J, Sigsgaard TC et al: Acute monocytic or myelomonocytic leukemia with balanced chromosome translocations to band 11q23 after therapy with 4-epi-doxorubicin-cis-platin or cyclophosphamide for breast cancer. J Clin Oncol 10:1444, 1992.

138. Pui CH, Relling MV, Rivera GK et al: Epipodophyllotoxin-related acute myeloid leukemia: A study of 35 cases. Leukemia 9:1990, 1995.

139. Rossi G, Pelizzari AM, Bellotti D, Tonelli M, Barlati S: Cytogenetic analogy between myelodysplastic syndrome and acute myeloid leukemia of elderly patients. Leukemia 14:636, 2000.

140. Tamura S, Takemoto Y, Hashimato-Tamonaki T et al: Cytogenetic analysis of de novo acute myeloid leukemia with trilineage myelodysplasia in comparison with myelodysplastic syndrome evolving to acute myeloid leukemia. Int J Oncol 12:1259, 1998.

141. Leith CP, Kopecky KJ, Godwin J et al: Acute myeloid leukemia in elderly: Assessment of multidrug resistance (MDR1) and cytogenetics distinguishes biologic subgroups with remarkably distinct responses to standard chemotherapy. A Southwest Oncology Group Study. Blood 89:3323, 1997.

142. Gahn B, Haase D, Unterhalt M et al: De novo AML with dysplastic hematopoiesis: Cytogenetic and prognostic significance. Leukemia 10:946, 1996.

143. Meckenstock G, Aul C, Hildebrandt B et al: Dyshematopoiesis in de novo acute myeloid leukemia: Cell biological features and prognostic significance. Leuk Lymphoma 29:523, 1998 (erratum 31:623).

144. Needleman SW, Burns P, Dick FR et al: Hypoplastic acute leukemia. Cancer 48:1410, 1981.

145. Gladson CL, Neim F: Hypocellular marrow with increased blasts. Am J Hematol 21:15, 1986.

146. Tuzuner N, Cox C, Rowe J, Bennett JM: Hypocellular acute leukemia: The Rochester (New York) experience. J Hem Pathol 9:195, 1995.

147. Nagai K, Kohno T, Chen Y et al: Diagnostic criteria for hypocellular acute leukemia: A clinical entity distinct from overt leukemia and myelodysplastic syndrome. Leuk Res 20:563, 1996.

148. Davis RE, Longacre TA, Cornbleet PJ: Hematogones in the bone marrow of adults: Immunophenotypic features, clinical setting and differential diagnosis. Am J Clin Pathol 102:202, 1994.

149. Muehleck SD, McKenna RW, Gale PF et al: Terminal deoxynucleotidyl transferase (TdT)-positive cells in bone marrow in the absence of hematologic malignancy. Am J Clin Pathol 79:277, 1983.

150. Sioutas N, Bagg A, Michaud GY et al: Polymerase chain reaction versus Southern blot hybridization: Detection of immunoglobulin heavy chain rearrangements. Diag Mol Pathol 4:8, 1994.

151. Steenbergen EJ, Verhagen OJHM, van Leeuwen EF et al: Prolonged persistence of PCR-detectable minimal residual disease after diagnosis or first relapse predicts poor outcome in childhood B-precursor acute lymphoblastic leukemia. Leukemia 9:1726, 1995.

152. Kallakury BVS, Hartmann D-P, Cossman J, Gootenberg JE, Bagg A: Posttherapy surveillance of B cell acute lymphoblastic leukemia. Value of polymerase chain reaction and limitations of flow cytometry. Am J Clin Pathol 111:759, 1999.

153. Anastasi J, Vardiman JW, Rudinsky R et al: Direct correlation of cytogenetic findings with cell morphology using in-situ hybridization: An analysis of suspicious cells in bone marrow specimens of two patients completing therapy of acute lymphoblastic leukemia. Blood 77:2456, 1991.

154. Potter MN, Steward CG, Oakhill A: The significance of detection of minimal residual disease in childhood acute lymphoblastic leukemia. Br J Haematol 83:412, 1993.

155. Raskind WH, Tirumali N, Jacobson R et al: Evidence for a multistep pathogenesis of myelodysplastic syndrome. Blood 63:1318, 1984.

156. Turhan AG, Humpheries RK, Phillips GL et al: Clonal hematopoiesis demonstrated by X-linked DNA polymorphism after allogeneic bone marrow transplantation. N Engl J Med 320:1655, 1989.

157. Rajapaska R, Ginzton N, Rott LS, Greenberg PL. Altered oncoprotein expression and apoptosis in myelodysplastic syndrome marrow cells. Blood 88:4275, 1996.

158. Raza A, Mundle S, Shetty V et al: Novel insights into the biology of myelodysplastic syndromes: Excessive apoptosis and the role of cytokines. Int J Hematol 63:265, 1996.

159. Pedersen-Bjergaard J, Rowley JD: The balanced and unbalanced chromosome aberrations of acute myeloid leukemia may develop in different ways and may contribute differently to malignant transformation. Blood 83:2780, 1994.

160. Tuzuner N, Cox C, Rowe J, Bennett JM: Bone marrow cellularity in myeloid stem cell disorders: Impact of age correction. Leuk Res 18:559, 1994.

161. Bennett JM, Catovsky D, Daniel MT et al: Proposals for the classification of myelodysplastic syndrome. Br J Haematol 51:189, 1982.

162. Heaney ML, Golde DW: Myelodysplasia. N Engl J Med 340:1649, 1999.

163. Greenberg P, Cox C, LeBeau MM et al: International Scoring System for evaluating prognosis in myelodysplastic syndromes. Blood 89:2079, 1997 (Erratum, Blood 91:1100).

164. Goasguen JE, Bennett JM: Classification and morphologic features of myelodysplastic syndromes. Semin Oncol 19:4, 1992.

165. Kouides PA, Bennett JM: Morphology and classification of myelodysplastic syndromes. Hematol Oncol Clin North Am 6:485, 1992.

166. Bennett JM: The classification and management of the myelodysplastic syndromes: Areas of controversy. Hematol Rev 7:189, 1993.

167. Tricot G, Wolf-Peters CD, Vlietinck R et al: Bone marrow histology in myelodysplastic syndromes: II. Prognostic value of abnormal localization of immature precursors in MDS. Br J Haematol 59:659, 1984.

168. Tricot GJ: Prognostic factors in myelodysplastic syndromes. Leuk Res 19:109, 1992.

169. Mangi MH, Mufti GJ: Primary myelodysplastic syndromes: Diagnostic and prognostic significance of immunohistochemical assessment of bone marrow biopsies. Blood 79:198, 1992.

170. Rosati S, Mick R, Xu F et al: Refractory cytopenia with multilineage dysplasia: Further characterization of an "unclassifiable" myelodysplastic syndrome. Leukemia 10:20, 1996.

171. Matsua A, Jinnai I, Yagasaki F et al: Refractory anemia with severe dysplasia: Clinical significance of morphological features in refractory anemia. Leukemia 12:482, 1998.

172. Balduini CL, Guarnone R, Pecci A, Centenera E, Ascari E: Multilineage dysplasia without increased blasts identifies a poor prognosis subset of myelodysplastic syndromes. Leukemia 12:1655, 1998.

173. Van den Berghe H, Cassiman JJ, David G et al: Distinct hematological disorder with deletion of long arm of no.5 chromosome. Nature 251:437, 1974.

174. Boultwood J, Lewis S, Wainscoat JS: The −5q syndrome. Blood 84:3253, 1994.

175. Thide T, Engquist L, Billstrom R: Application of megakaryocyte morphology in diagnosis of −5q syndrome. Eur J Hematol 41:434, 1988.

176. Nand S, Godwin JE: Hypoplastic myelodysplastic syndrome. Cancer 62:958, 1988.

177. Maschek H, Kaloutsi V, Rodriguez-Kaiser M et al: Hypoplastic myelodysplastic syndrome: Incidence, morphology, cytogenetics amd prognosis. Ann Hematol 66:117, 1993.

178. Appelbaum FR, Barral J, Storb R et al: Clonal cytogenetic abnormalities in patients with otherwise typical aplastic anemia. Exp Hematol 15:1134, 1987.

179. Orazi A, Albitar M, Heerema NA et al: Hypocellular myelodys-plastic syndromes can be distinguished from acquired aplastic anemia by CD34 and PCNA immunostaining of bone marrow biopsy specimens. Am J Clin Pathol 107:268, 1997.

180. Yoshida Y, Oguma H, Maekawa T: Refractory myelodysplastic anemias with hypocellular marrow. J Clin Pathol 41:763, 1988.

181. Tuzuner N, Cox C, Rowe J, Bennett JM: Hypocellular myelodys-plastic syndrome. Br J Haematol 91:612, 1995.

182. Martiat P, Michaux JL, Rodhain J et al: Philadelphia negative (Ph–) chronic myeloid leukemia (CML): Comparison with Ph+ CML and chronic myelomonocytic leukemia. Blood 78:205, 1991.

183. Bennett JM, Catovsky D, Daniel MT et al: Chronic myeloid leukemias: Guidelines for distinguishing chronic granulocytic, atypical chronic myeloid and chronic myelomonocytic leukemia. Proposals by the French-American-British group. Br J Haematol 87:176, 1994.

184. Hasle H, Arico M, Basso G et al: Myelodysplastic syndrome, juve-nile myelomonocytic leukemia, and acute myeloid leukemia asso-ciated with complete or partial monosomy 7. Leukemia 13:376, 1999.

185. Neimeyer CM: Myelodysplastic syndrome in childhood. Leuk Res 23(Suppl. 1):S3, 1999.

186. Hassle H, Jacobsen BB, Pederson NT: Myelodysplastic syndromes in childhood: A population based study of nine cases. Br J Haematol 81:495, 1992.

187. Creutzig U, Ritter J, Vormoor J et al: Myelodysplasia and acute myelogenous leukemia in Down's syndrome. A report of 40 children of the AML-BFM Study group. Leukemia 10:1677, 1996.

188. Meunier BB, Mielot F, Tchernia G et al: Myelodysplastic syn-dromes in childhood: Report of 49 patients from French multi-centre study. Br J Haematol 92:344, 1996.

189. Pedersen-Bjergaard J, Anderson MK, Christiansen D: Therapy-related acute myeloid leukemia and myelodysplasia after high-dose chemotherapy and autologous stem cell transplantation. Blood 95:3273, 2000.

190. Orazi A, Cattoretti G, Saligo D et al: Therapy related myelodys-plastic syndromes. FAB classification, bone marrow histology and immunohistology in the prognostic assessment. Leukemia 7:838, 1993.

191. Pedersen-Bjergaard J, Pedersen M, Roulston D, Philip P: Different genetic pathways in leukemogenesis for patients presenting with therapy-related myelodysplasia and therapy-related acute myeloid leukemia. Blood 86:3542, 1995.

15

Immunobiology of Acute Leukemia

Elisabeth Paietta

Acute leukemias are commonly defined as the expansion of immature cells that are derived from a single transformed hematopoietic progenitor cell. Rather than undergoing normal differentiation and/or normal programmed cell death (apoptosis), leukemic cells engage in abnormal, uncontrolled, and therefore, indefinite proliferation. If leukemic cells had arrested somewhere along the normal hematopoietic pathway, the immunophenotypes of the acute leukemias would mirror variable stages of normal differentiation. In fact, the immunophenotypes of most acute leukemia blasts resemble to a large degree phenotypes found among normal myeloid or lymphoid progenitor cells. However, in most cases immunophenotypic features can be recognized that distinguish the leukemic cells from normal hematopoietic cells. For instance, the European BIO-MED-1 Concerted Action, initiated to improve and standardize the flow cytometric detection of minimal residual disease in acute leukemia, demonstrated that virtually all immunophenotypes of T-lineage acute lymphoblastic leukemia (ALL) fell outside of defined normal T-cell subsets in bone marrow, into areas of flow cytometric plots where no normal cells are found.[1]

Genotypic alterations associated with or responsible for the development of acute leukemia may affect the overall phenotype of the transformed cells. This may explain the occurrence of unique antigens or antigen patterns in leukemia subtypes characterized by particular cytogenetic abnormalities.[2] Examples are the frequent finding of the T-cell antigen CD2 on leukemic myeloblasts containing an inverted chromosome 16 or the combined expression of the B-lymphoid antigen CD19 and the natural killer (NK) cell antigen CD56 on leukemic myeloblasts containing an (8;21) translocation.

It is correct to state that antigens expressed by leukemic cells are the same as those that are expressed by normal hematopoietic cells. To date, there is no knowledge of leukemia-specific antigens, with the exception of proteins that are encoded by novel fusion genes as a result of leukemia-specific chromosomal aberrations,[3] to which, however, diagnostic antibodies are not readily available. In acute promyelocytic leukemia (APL), antibodies to the PML protein, which is the product of one of the two genes involved in the PML/RARα fusion, are useful diagnostic tools owing to the unique abnormal distribution of anti-PML labeling in cells that bear the t(15;17).[4,5]

Of greatest clinical significance is the finding that in most patients the particular combination of antigens expressed by the leukemic cells may be rare or may never be seen in normal hematopoietic tissues. The more sophisticated immunophenotypic analyses have become, the more apparent it is that leukemic cells differ from normal hematopoietic cells and that leukemia categorization cannot be based solely on presumed normal counterparts. Of course, it is still valid to group the acute leukemias according to the major hematopoietic cell lineages (T-lymphoid, B-lymphoid, myeloid) and to distinguish between precursor and more mature subtypes based on the hierarchy of antigen expression observed in normal hematopoiesis. However, refined, clinically relevant subgrouping focuses increasingly on prognostically significant and/or therapy-determining features. The World Health Organization (WHO) classification of neoplastic diseases of the hematopoietic and lymphoid tissues clearly reflects this tendency by recognizing cytogenetic/molecular categories in the new nomenclature of the acute leukemias.[6] It has become one of the major goals of leukemia immunobiology to identify antigens that can serve as surrogate markers of specific cytogenetic/molecular aberrations. The other major goal is to recognize leukemia-associated phenotypes that allow for the detection of immunologic residual disease. Monitoring of minimal residual disease has added a new dimension to leukemia immunophenotyping in addition to diagnosis and prognosis.

IMMUNOPHENOTYPING VERSUS MORPHOLOGY

There is a strong tendency to divide diseases into subtypes that share clinical, biological, and hopefully, prognostic features that can predict success if a uniform treatment approach is taken. In the acute leukemias, the first comprehensive classification scheme was based on the site of origin, that is, myeloblastic leukemia was considered to be that which arises from the bone marrow whereas the lymphoblastic leukemias were considered to originate in lymphoid tissue.[7]

Relatively precise criteria for the differentiation of acute lymphoid from acute myeloid leukemia (AML) were brought forward by a consortium of French, American, and British (FAB) investigators, who relied on morphological and cytochemical cell characteristics.[8] That leukemias comprise a group of diseases much more diverse than represented in the FAB classification scheme is suggested by its insignificant influence on prognosis in both ALL and AML, with the exception of FAB-M3. The clinical importance of the APL subtype FAB-M3 and its hypogranular variant M3v as a morphologic diagnosis is related to two facts: 1. that this diagnosis requires immediate intervention owing to the existing coagulopathy; and 2. that there exists a phenotype-specific therapy, namely, all-trans retinoic acid (ATRA). However, even in the case of FAB-M3, immunophenotypic, cytogenetic, and molecular tests are essential to recognize APL-like phenotypes that lack sensitivity to ATRA.[9] The subclasses FAB-M6 and M7, the acute erythroid and megakaryocytic leukemias, respectively, usually cannot be identified with certainty without immunologic cell marker studies. The FAB-M0 subtype, the AML type that remains unclassified by standard cytological examination,[10] represents a phenotypically and genotypically very heterogeneous group, which awaits further subclassification based on immunophenotypic and/or genetic findings.

Irrespective of FAB subtype, multilineage dysmyelopoiesis presents a highly unfavorable parameter in AML,[11] enough to warrant its own subclass (AML with multilineage dysplasia).[6] The morphologic subclassification of ALL into L1, L2, and L3 was recently found to be no longer relevant.[6]

Diagnoses based on morphology cannot be easily interchanged with immunophenotypic findings, since with the exception of FAB-M3, morphologic subclasses do not relate to specific immunophenotypes. Neither morphology nor cytochemistry can predict the expression of antigens different from those expected to be present on cells of a particular cell lineage, that is, the expression of myeloid antigens by leukemic cells with characteristics of a lymphoid FAB subtype and vice versa. There are rare examples of antigens correlating with particular morphologic features. For instance, in APL, CD34 and CD2 expression is uncommon but when present corresponds to M3v morphology.[12–14] Low expression of CD65$_s$ (defined as 20 percent or less of positive blast cells) in otherwise unequivocal AML shows significant association with immature morphologic FAB classes M0 and M1.[15]

IMMUNOLOGIC FINDINGS AS SURROGATE MARKERS FOR CYTOGENETIC—MOLECULAR ABNORMALITIES

Specific associations between particular antigen expression patterns and cytogenetic—molecular abnormalities have been established. In increasing instances immunophenotypic findings can be used as surrogate markers for genetic aberrations.[2,3] This is important given the prognostic significance of many of the known cytogenetic abnormalities and their molecular equivalents. In cases in which cytogenetic analysis cannot be performed, is unsuccessful (for example, when a bone marrow aspirate could not be obtained), or yields a normal result, particular immunophenotypic findings may predict the presence of certain genetic abnormalities. This may prompt targeted molecular testing or may even be used as diagnostic evidence if molecular testing is unavailable.

For example, in a patient with differentiated AML, immunologic analysis may demonstrate combined expression of CD19 (a B cell–associated antigen) and CD56 (an NK cell marker) on otherwise typical myeloblasts. This antigen pattern is unequivocally associated with the chromosomal (8;21) translocation.[16] In particular, the combination CD19–CD34 accurately predicts t(8;21) AML.[17] Furthermore, blasts containing t(8;21) show low expression of the integrin CD11a,[2] a finding otherwise reserved for APL cells among the myeloid leukemias.[18] Another example is the expression of the interleukin-2 receptor α chain, CD25, by leukemic lymphoblasts containing the Philadelphia chromosome and its molecular equivalent, the BCR/ABL fusion transcript.[19] It is not uncommon in ALL to find BCR/ABL transcripts in patients with an apparently normal karyotype. In view of the strong negative prognostic impact of BCR/ABL transcripts in ALL, including the CD25 antibody in the biologic characterization of ALL can yield a quick and cost-effective indicator of this clinically important genetic abnormality. Borowitz et al.[20] and De Zen et al[21] have suggested that the surface antigen phenotype, in particular the low expression of CD20, in childhood B-precursor ALL can predict the TEL/AML1 rearrangement. The cryptic (12;21)(p13;q22) translocation that results in the TEL-AML1 fusion gene is found in approximately 25 percent of childhood ALL and carries a favorable prognosis. Incidence, outcome, and immunophenotypic data in adult ALL are too limited to permit similar conclusions.

ANTIGENS AS PREDICTORS OF PROGNOSIS

Reports on the prognostic significance of single antigens have to be viewed with caution if they are based on small numbers of patients, if they are unconfirmed, if data are not reported on gated blast cells, or if arbitrary cutoff points of antigen expression were used to determine positivity. To date, few antigens are unequivocally associated with clinical response.

CD56, the neural cell adhesion molecule, is an indicator of poor treatment outcome, particularly short remission duration, both in APL[22,23] and in AML with t(8;21).[24] Acute myeloid leukemia expressing the immature monocytic antigen and integrin CD11b was postulated to represent a new leukemic syndrome based on a large database analysis of the Eastern Cooperative Oncology Group (ECOG).[25] The result of this prognosis-driven retrospective analysis supported previous suggestions of CD11b as a marker for shortened survival in AML.[26–29] Whether this negative effect on outcome seen with CD56 as well as CD11b is related to their function as adhesion molecules is currently unclear. Obviously, it is of great interest when the clinical significance of an antigen finds an explanation in its biologic properties. This may be the case with CD10 and its favorable prognostic implications when expressed in both pediatric and adult T-lineage ALL.[30,31] In normal lymphopoiesis, CD10 marks T cells induced to undergo apoptosis.[32,33]

Two examples of antigens whose prognostic significance had to be reconsidered based on larger data files or methodology of analysis are the stem cell growth factor receptor, c-kit or CD117, and the T cell–associated antigen, CD7. Both were initially reported to confer poor prognosis in AML. For CD117, increasing the number of patients analyzed demonstrated its broad spectrum of expression in AML subtypes irrespective of the level of myeloid differentiation, its characteristic occurrence in APL, its absence in acute monocytic leukemia, its exceedingly rare incidence in ALL, and its value for monitoring minimal residual disease; however, this did not confirm any prognostic impact.[2,34–39]

In the case of CD7, several reports have suggested the unfavorable outcome of patients with CD7+ AML when compared with CD7– AML patients, although other studies have argued against this. All of these studies arbitrarily used 20 percent positive blast cells as the definition of CD7+ AML. In a retrospective analysis, Kornblau et al.[40] found more than 10.5 percent of CD7+ myeloblasts to produce the largest survival difference between CD7+ and CD7− AML according to this criterion. However, there was no statistically significant survival difference between the two groups. That antigens may have a pivotal role in predicting certain clinical behavior, thereby indirectly affecting prognosis, is only starting to be appreciated. Expression of CD13, an aminopeptidase, has been linked to the development of the retinoic acid syndrome (RAS) in APL patients treated with ATRA.[41] Another postulated culprit in the development of RAS in response to ATRA or arsenic trioxide is CD38, an ectoenzyme involved in the metabolism of NAD+.[42] Both agents are potent inducers of CD38, which, through interplay with its ligand CD31 expressed by endothelial cells, may alter the propensity of the leukemic promyelocytes to adhere to the vessel walls as well as to initiate cytokine release. The increased incidence of granulocytic sarcomas in AML with the 8;21 translocation[43] may be related to the expression of the neural cell–adhesion molecule CD56.[44]

ANTIGENS AND THERAPY

There are two aspects to antigens and antibodies and their usefulness in therapy. First, antibodies to carefully selected antigens expressed by the leukemic cells are used for ex vivo purification of autologous bone marrow grafts or for in vivo treatment. Second, therapy may be determined by the specific phenotype of the leukemic cell population. In this case, we speak about phenotype-specific therapy.

The choice of antibodies for bone marrow purging focuses on attacking the leukemic clonogenic cells while sparing the pluripotent hematopoietic stem cells. Some candidate reagents for the elimination of residual blast cells in autologous marrow grafts have been CD33 and CD65$_s$ antibodies in AML, CD7 in T-cell lymphoblastic leukemia, and CD10 (CALLA) and CD52 (CAMPATH) in B-cell lymphoblastic leukemia.[45–49]

In vivo therapy with monoclonal antibodies aims at a specific antigen, which otherwise may be a part of very diverse immunophenotypes. Clinical trials with humanized CD33 monoclonal antibody linked to a cell toxin, such as calicheamicin, constitute one promising ongoing example for that kind of therapeutic approach.[50,51] A major requirement for the success of antigen-targeted therapy is exact knowledge of antigen distribution in normal tissues and of the kind of antigen response to antibody binding. Whereas CD33 is rapidly internalized after antibody binding, which makes this antigen an ideal candidate for conjugation with intracellularly active cytotoxic agents,[52] CD20 antigen, another target of antibody therapy,[53] does not modulate or internalize. The effectiveness of rituximab, a chimeric monoclonal antibody to the CD20 antigen in the chronic lymphoid malignancies tested predominantly to date, results from various mechanisms of action, including activation of the complement cascade, apoptosis, and recruitment of cytotoxic T cells.[53]

The ultimate goal of immunophenotyping is the establishment of phenotypes or phenotypic characteristics with known therapeutic sensitivity. The best, and currently the only, example for phenotype-specific therapy is given by APL with its characteristic immunophenotype[54] and exquisite response to ATRA.[9]

As we learn more about possible physiological consequences of hematopoietic antigen expression, our approach to the overall classification of leukemias may change. Rather than delineating lineage- or maturation-related phenotypes, the power of immunophenotyping may lie in the characterization of functional leukemia subsets, defined by the expression of molecules with specific functional significance, such as adhesion molecules, cytokine receptors, or surface enzymes. This is already suggested by evidence that the presence of a single functional antigen across FAB or immunophenotypic subtypes may guide therapeutic modalities. For instance, the demonstration of P-glycoprotein (Pgp), a unidirectional membrane drug-efflux pump, which is one potential mediator of multidrug resistance (MDR), has led to the identification of Pgp inhibitors such as cyclosporin and their inclusion in clinical trials.[55] Immunophenotyping may indeed provide important information on potential targets for future therapeutic strategies. Once recognized, the disruption of cell regulatory processes due to the presence or overexpression of certain antigens may lead to rational drug design aimed at modulating the activity of such target molecules, as is already being attempted in the case of Pgp.

THE DEVELOPMENT OF IMMUNOPHENOTYPING

Characterization of antigens as a means of leukemia subtyping began in the early 1980s with a limited number of polyclonal antisera that allowed a distinction between T and non-T ALL.[56,57] Following the introduction of monoclonal antibody technology,[58] the first such antibodies that could be widely produced and that found their way into the clinical laboratory were directed against lymphoid antigens, thereby providing an early glimpse at the tremendous immunophenotypic diversity of ALL, which had not been appreciated by conventional morphology and cytochemistry. Perhaps because the generation of antimyeloid antibodies did not proceed as rapidly as that of antilymphoid antibodies or because cytology appeared to be more informative in AML than in ALL, routine immunophenotyping for AML is a much more recent event. A series of seven International Workshops and Conferences on Human Leukocyte Differentiation Antigens ensured that the plethora of emerging antibodies was carefully characterized in terms of specificities and tissue distribution and segregated into clusters of designation (CD).[59–64] The CDw designation (w standing for workshop) is sometimes given to antibodies whose reactivity has not been completely defined or to those of which only a limited number (sometimes only one) seem to form that cluster. During the latest of these workshops held in Harrogate, England, in June 2000,[65] the number of CDs defined increased to a total of 247, now also including cluster assignments for cytokine and growth factor receptors as well as endothelial cell molecules. This latter development reflects our growing understanding that antigens, aside from being essential for the differential diagnosis of leukemias, may be key regulators in signaling pathways determining cell proliferation, differentiation, survival, or programmed cell death.

CLASSIFICATION SCHEMES BASED ON IMMUNOPHENOTYPING

Analogously to the morphology–cytochemistry-based leukemia classification (FAB) system, early immunophenotype-based classification schemes attempted to fit leukemic immunophenotypes into established stages of normal hematopoietic differentiation. Such an approach ignores the fact that phenotypic alterations are due to underlying molecular, disease-specific aberrations. This explains its limited usefulness, which is restricted to diagnosis, and in fact, its counterproductivity concerning the progress of immunophenotyping beyond mere diagnostic goals toward the recognition of prognostic phenotypes, which in turn may lead to phenotype-specific therapies.

Heterogeneity of antigen expression in the acute leukemias offers the valuable opportunity to discover associations of particular antigen profiles either with cytogenetic–molecular aberrations that carry prognostic significance or with clinical outcome independent of other biologic parameters. In both AML and the ALL, cytogenetic–molecular categories are now being recognized as distinct disease entities, such as AML with t(8;21) or ALL with t(9;22).[6] This emphasizes the importance of recognizing associations between immunophenotypic features and

such molecularly defined leukemia subtypes, since immunophenotyping can be performed more rapidly, at lower cost, and at more clinical leukemia laboratories as compared with molecular analyses.

When establishing new leukemia subclasses on the basis of antigen expression patterns alone, one should strive to unravel clinical relevance. Major efforts have been made to formulate a minimal panel of antibodies that will suffice to provide an informative immunophenotype and allow for standardized diagnostic interpretations. In fact, three antibody combinations can reliably discern the lineage trait (T versus B lymphoid versus myeloid) of a blast cell population (see below). If the goal is to describe novel leukemia subtypes or to discover prognostic markers, however, much more elaborate antibody panels must be tested.

HEMATOPOIETIC CELL LINEAGE–SPECIFIC MARKERS

Most of the antigens expressed by leukemic cells are lineage-associated, but few are lineage-specific. As a general rule, the most immature and the most mature markers of a given cell lineage are specific for that lineage. Figure 15–1 illustrates that the three antigens specific for the T- and B-lymphoid and the myeloid lineages are intracytoplasmic CD3, intracytoplasmic CD22, and intracytoplasmic myeloperoxidase protein, respectively. This conclusion is based on experience in leukemia

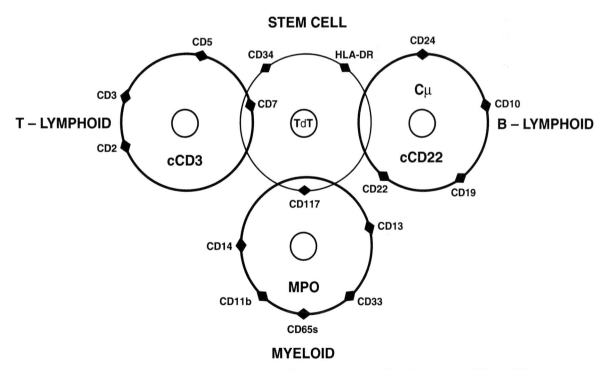

Figure 15–1. Antigenic overlap between the major cell lineages. Lineage-specific antigens are in bold letters. This figure also represents the minimal panel of antibodies and antigens that needs to be tested in a new case of acute leukemia.

immunophenotyping rather than on the fact that these antigens are the first to appear in normal immature cells committed to their cell lineage. In fact, there do exist immature AML cases that lack myeloperoxidase by antibody staining but do express surface CD33 and/or CD13 and lack any evidence of lymphoid, megakaryocytic, or erythroid differentiation. The intracellular localization of these crucial antigens is unfortunate because their detection by flow cytometry requires technical skill and experience. In fact, routine clinical laboratories may shy away from testing intracellular antigens by flow cytometry. Aside from choosing optimal fixation and permeabilization media,[66–68] it is essential that data reflect gated blast cells. Following fixation and permeabilization, scattergram characteristics (size and granularity) of cells change, which makes cell populations collapse. Without the surface marker staining the leukemic cell population, blast cells can often no longer be separated from residual normal bone marrow or peripheral blood cell components. This may lead to the occasional misleading report of myeloperoxidase protein expression in ALL. The other pitfall in the interpretation of immunophenotypic myeloperoxidase detection in a case of presumed ALL results from the use of morphology as the gold standard in assigning lineage affiliation to a leukemic blast cell population. It cannot be emphasized enough that, although viewed together, neither morphology nor immunophenotyping forms the basis of the other's interpretation.

The proposed specificity of cytoplasmic CD79a for B-cell-related ALL requires some discussion. The CD79a (mb-1) polypeptide appears in the cytoplasm early during B-cell differentiation. Together with the later-appearing CD79b, it eventually associates in the B-cell membrane with immunoglobulin and has been assumed to be restricted to B cells, whether normal or neoplastic.[69,70] Given its primary usefulness as an intracellular marker in characterizing B-lineage ALL, antibodies to CD79a were initially produced to intracellular epitopes of the molecule (clones HM47, JCB117). Recently, the diagnostic value of CD79a received an interesting boost when a new antibody to a cell surface epitope of CD79a, clone ZL7.4, was found to distinguish between B-cell chronic lymphocytic leukemia (surface CD79a-negative) and mantle cell lymphoma,[71] as well as B-cell prolymphocytic leukemia and hairy cell leukemia (all surface CD79a-positive). Surprisingly, clone ZL7.4 reacts with intracellular structures in selected cases of AML, particularly of the immunophenotypically undifferentiated subtype (Paietta E, unpublished observation). Further studies are needed to explain this puzzling observation. The occasional observation of CD79a in the cytoplasm of T-ALLs[72,73] and AML,[74,75] particularly APL,[75] even when using antibodies to intracellular CD79a epitopes, further confuses the lineage specificity of this antigen.

The more immature a leukemia subtype, the more the laboratory investigator or pathologist will have to rely on the detection of lineage-specific antigens, because other lineage-associated antigens, which usually assist in establishing the immunophenotypic diagnosis, are absent or sparse. The more mature a leukemia immunophenotype, the more easily the affiliation with a certain cell lineage is established. Therefore, lineage-specific mature antigens are less important in establishing lineage affiliation in the mature subtypes of acute leukemia, where they allow, however, for determining the level of blast cell differentiation. For instance, a leukemic blast cell mature enough to express B-cell-specific surface immunoglobulins will certainly express a series of B-lineage-associated cell surface markers (e.g., CD19, CD22, CD24), which will leave no doubt about lineage affiliation. However, the finding of monoclonal surface immunoglobulin will confirm the diagnosis of mature B-ALL, which has prognostic implications. In the case of T-ALL, the detection of surface T-cell receptor proteins will establish a mature subtype of the disease, and the lineage affiliation will be supported by the presence of additional T-cell markers. As a word of caution, only the expression of immunoglobulins and T-cell receptor proteins, but not immunoglobulin or T-cell receptor gene rearrangements, should be considered specific for their respective cell lineages. For the myeloid lineage, the most mature antigen is lactoferrin, which however is too mature to be found in a leukemic myeloblasts. All cell surface myeloid antigens have been seen on leukemic lymphoblasts and therefore cannot be considered specific for myeloid lineage.

The presence of one of the lineage-specific antigens determines lineage affiliation. It is astonishing and concerning that these antigens were not considered essential in a recent consensus meeting on optimal reagents for acute leukemia immunophenotyping.[76] A blast cell population negative for any of the discussed lineage-specific antigens may fall into one of four categories: true lineage-negative acute leukemia, which is extremely rare; acute monocytic leukemia (AMOL), which is usually myeloperoxidase-negative; acute megakaryocytic leukemia (AMegL); and acute erythroleukemia (AEL). In each of these instances, comprehensive testing will yield the appropriate immunophenotypic diagnosis.

Antigens not established as lineage-specific are considered lineage-associated, and they represent the majority. A selection of antibodies and antigens tested routinely in acute leukemias is compiled in Table 15–1. Calling them lineage-associated means that although they occur predominantly in their respective cell lineage during normal hematopoiesis, they may be found on other cell lineages. They may appear transiently outside their predominant cell lineage during normal development (e.g., CD10 during normal T-cell differentiation) or on leukemic blast cells of another cell lineage (e.g., CD10 on T lymphoblasts). Another example would be CD24. The presence of this antigen supports the diagnosis of B-lineage disease if this diagnosis is suggested by other immunophenotypic parameters. However, CD24 is also extremely valuable in determining the immature state of a given myeloid population because it is expressed by cells at and beyond the promyelocyte stage but not by more immature myeloid cells. In summary, lineage-associated antigens must be considered supportive but not determinant. Along the same line, their expression across lineages is common, as will be discussed in the next section.

Table 15–1. Antibodies (CDs) and Antigens to be Included in Testing Panels for Leukemia Immunophenotyping Arranged According to Lineage Affiliation

Uncommitted	Myeloid/ Monocytic	Lymphoid	Erythroid/ Megakaryocytic
CD133	Myeloperoxidase	Cytoplasmic	CD71
CD135	CD33	CD22	Glycophorin
CD34	CD13	Cytoplasmic	Blood group H
CD117	CD65(s)	CD79a	antigen
HLA-DR	CD15(s)	CD19	CD41
TdT	CD11b	CD10	CD61
CD38	CD11c	CD24	CD9
CD45	CD64	CD20	CD42
Activation	CD35	Surface	CD36
antigens	CD16	CD22	CD62P
(e.g., CD25)	Lactoferrin	Cytoplasmic	
Adhesion	CD68	+ surface μ	
molecules	CD14	Surface κ	
(e.g., CD56,		+ λ	
CD11a)		Cytoplasmic	
Multidrug		CD3	
resistance		CD5	
mediators		CD7	
		CD2	
		CD1	
		CD4 + CD8	
		Surface CD3	
		TCRα/β + TCRγ/δ	

EXPRESSION OF LINEAGE-FOREIGN ANTIGENS IN ACUTE LEUKEMIA

Before an antigen expression pattern should be considered biphenotypic, the first and foremost prerequisite is that lineage affiliation be based on the overall immunophenotypic findings and not on morphology. The WHO classification proposal still includes the subtype "Acute leukemia, biphenotypic"[77,78] and has adopted the EGIL (European Group for the Immunological Characterization of Leukemias) guidelines for their immunologic definition.[79] Their scoring system ignores the fact that the majority of antigens are no longer understood as lineage-specific. As a result, if it is applied verbatim, scores high enough to qualify as biphenotypic leukemia are easily reached, particularly in ALL. To further complicate EGIL criteria, arbitrary cutoff points of 20 percent for most antigens and of 10 percent for myeloperoxidase, CD3, CD79a, and TdT are suggested to define the positivity of a leukemic cell population for a given antigen. This recommendation is of greatest concern,[80] particularly because there is no emphasis on gating procedures, which would ensure that antigen expression data refer exclusively to the blast cell population.

The immunophenotypic criteria for defining leukemic entities coexpressing myeloid and lymphoid antigens recently set forth by Campana and Behm[81] represent more closely our current understanding of leukemia immunobiology. Immunodiagnosis is based on the finding of defined immature (myeloperoxidase, cytoplasmic CD3, or cytoplasmic CD22) or

mature (cytoplasmic or surface immunoglobulin, surface CD3) lineage-specific antigens. In the presence of a lineage-determinant antigen, expression of two or more antigens from another lineage does not alter the basic immunodiagnosis. Given that the prognostic significance of lineage-foreign antigen expression in the adult acute leukemias has yet to be determined, it is best to describe leukemias according to the observed pattern of antigen expression (e.g., CD7+ AML, CD33+, CD13+ Early Pre-B ALL), so that retrospective outcome analyses can eventually be performed. The term "true mixed-lineage" or "bilineage" leukemia must be reserved for those rare cases that concomitantly express lineage-specific antigens from more than one cell lineage, more commonly in distinct leukemic subpopulations. In several such cases, cytogenetic or molecular studies have provided evidence for a common leukemic progenitor cell for both the myeloid and lymphoid component (identical cytogenetic abnormalities or gene rearrangements). Whether or not there are prognostic implications associated with this type of antigen presentation per se is unclear. However, certain genetic defects with well-established prognostic significance that affect stem cells with multipotent differentiation capabilities, such as t(4;11) or t(9;22), may have an increased tendency to present as bilineage leukemias.[82]

METHODS OF DESCRIBING ANTIGEN EXPRESSION

Antigen expression can be characterized according to antigen density, which is described by terms such as bright versus dim staining of antibodies or low versus high antigen expression. These descriptions relate to the intensity with which a fluorescence-conjugated antibody stains a given cell. Fluorescence intensity can be helpful diagnostically when the same antigen is expressed on contaminating normal and leukemic cells with differential density and gating procedures are inefficient in selecting the leukemic cell population. For instance, CD45 fluorescence intensity of staining is characteristically low on myeloid precursor cells, lower than on normal lymphocytes or more mature myeloid cells, which allows their separation in a flow differential.[83] Alternatively, fluorescence intensity may vary among various leukemia subtypes. For instance, staining with antibody to the uncommitted cell marker, terminal transferase (TdT), in leukemic myeloblasts is significantly weaker than TdT staining in leukemic lymphoblasts.[84] Furthermore, abnormally high or low expression of an antigen by a leukemic cell when compared with its normal counterpart can provide a leukemia-specific immunologic fingerprint exploitable for the monitoring of minimal residual disease.[85] If fluorescence intensity is the interpretation of choice, antibody reactivity will be interpreted as negative, dimly positive, moderately positive, brightly positive, or indeterminate.

Particularly for multicenter studies that require comparison of fluorescence intensity data from several laboratories, the use of microbead calibration standards, which provide a reliable quantitative assessment of antigen density, is currently recommended. Flow cytometry data are expressed in the form of molecular equivalents of soluble fluorochrome (MESF), which are calculated from the peak fluorescence of cells with given antibodies relative to that of a set of four or five microbead standards with different titers of MESF units.[86]

Other clinical laboratories describe the percentages of blast cells positive for the various antigens, which are calculated from the proportion of cells that stain with a given antibody with greater intensity than the brightest cells of the negative control or of nonstaining cells present in the cell population. To date, it has been accepted strategy to define antigen positivity of a leukemia population based on arbitrary cutoff levels for antibody staining cells, which range from 1 to 50 percent. Within a given study, the same cutoff level applies to all antigens tested. Recently, a biologically and clinically more meaningful approach has been recommended, which involves the retrospective determination of cutoff points defining the level of antibody staining blast cells that distinguishes between responding and nonresponding patients. Such response-driven cutoff points can then be tested for their validity in a prospective fashion.[40,80,87,88]

Thus, for both methods of antibody binding analysis, strategies to interpret the findings, that is, to define the level of brightness of staining or the cutoff level of percentage of staining cells that defines positivity, are variable and open to ongoing discussion. Either method has apparent flaws, which can affect the results of statistical analyses and the overall usefulness of immunophenotyping for the biologic characterization of leukemia subsets.

Whatever the method of data interpretation, it is absolutely essential that antibody binding be reported exclusively for the leukemic cell population, with exclusion of contaminating normal cells.[89] The physician faced with interpreting an immunophenotype should pay particular attention to any indication that the data refer to either total white cells, total mononuclear cells, or blast cells. Provided that the abnormal cell population was identified and antigen characteristics of that gated population are exclusively reported, the choice between using qualitative (positive or negative based on fluorescence intensity) or quantitative descriptors of antibody binding (percentage of staining cells) becomes less significant. Gating on blast cells can be accomplished by clustering cell components based on CD45 fluorescence intensity combined with scatter characteristics, provided the leukemic blasts express CD45 (a considerable fraction of ALL are partially or completely CD45 negative). Alternatively, blasts cells are selected from a heterogeneous population of normal and abnormal cells with the help of an antibody that recognizes an antigen expressed by the leukemic cells in multicolor flow cytometry.[89] Care must be taken to use an antibody that will distinguish between normal and abnormal cells of the same lineage. For instance, in the case of a T-cell ALL, CD7 would equally recognize both contaminating normal lymphocytes and the blast cells. Figure 15–2 demonstrates that both methods yield equivalent results, although occasionally gating based on a leukemic cell–associated antigen produces a clearer representation of the blast cell population. We recommend pretesting leukemic specimens with limited

antibody panels to determine the ideal antibody for the separation of blast cells (e.g., CD34, CD117, HLA-DR), which will subsequently be added to every antibody tube in the full testing panel (Paietta E, unpublished).

PREFERRED TISSUES AND METHODOLOGIES FOR IMMUNOPHENOTYPING

Multiparameter flow cytometry[90,91] is the favored methodology when establishing a leukemia immunophenotype from anticoagulated peripheral blood or bone marrow aspirate (Figure 15–2). This technique incorporates structural cell characteristics, such as size and granularity, as well as antigenic characteristics, whereby most commonly two to four antigens are captured simultaneously by using various fluorochromes (fluorescein isothiocyanate [FITC], phycoerythrin [PE], etc.) The choice of antibodies and thus the size of antibody panels will vary with the suspected disease, the state of disease (presentation versus remission), and the purpose of the typing. If the purpose is solely to establish a diagnosis, the panel could be stripped to the bare minimum of lineage-specific antigens (myeloperoxidase, cytoplasmic CD3, cytoplasmic CD22). Given that clinically important subtypes would be missed when testing is extremely limited, a minimum antibody panel should be developed in any clinical flow cytometry laboratory that ensures that established prognostic leukemia subtypes are detected (CD11b+ AML, intracytoplasmic mu chain+ Pre-B ALL, etc.) It is recommended to streamline the choice of antibodies. In order to obtain an indication for the lineage association of a leukemic cell population (lymphoid versus myeloid) and to select a marker most suitable as a gating antibody to be added to each test tube, we pretest every leukemia patient on whom no previous immunophenotype information is available. Pretesting is done with a small series of antibody combinations: CD45/CD14, CD33/CD34, CD13/CD115, HLA-DR/CD11b, CD10/CD19, CD7/CD2, CD3/CD5. With the number of available antibodies and their potential diagnostic and prognostic significance continuously increasing, strategies for targeted testing are cost-efficient without compromising the quality of the analysis.

Comparative immunophenotypic analyses in peripheral blood and bone marrow have not shown significant differences in antigen profiles.[92] Staining whole blood or bone marrow is preferred over isolating mononuclear cells in order to avoid selective loss of cell populations and potential effects on antibody binding.[93,94] The results of antibody binding have been found to vary with cell manipulations, such as density gradient centrifugation or preincubation at 37°C, in neutrophils owing to the presence of intracellular storage pools of many of the myelomonocytic antigens (CD35, CD16, etc.).[94] In either case, the white cell count should be adjusted to the amounts of antibody added and antibodies should be incubated with the cells in the presence of human AB serum to block Fc receptors. Removal of erythroid cells is accomplished by erythrocyte lysis, preferably after staining with antibodies directed to surface antigens.

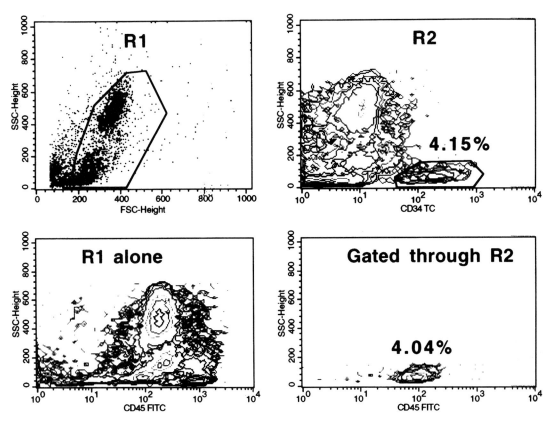

Figure 15–2. Selection of leukemic blast cells by flow cytometry. Cells of interest are selected based on particular criteria. Blasts typically express low side-scatter, dim CD45, and/or specific surface markers (e.g., CD34). This figure demonstrates how gating on the specific marker selects the precise population, which otherwise might be difficult to discern from neighboring cell clusters, as pictured in the "R1 alone" plot.

For body fluids other than peripheral blood or bone marrow, such as peritoneal or pleural effusions or cerebrospinal fluid, addition of anticoagulants is not necessary. Biopsies from lymph nodes, skin, or soft tissue tumors should be collected in tissue culture medium (e.g., RPMI 1640), and cell suspensions should be prepared by mechanical disruption of the tissue. The viability of the white cells in a specimen should be checked to ensure adequate quality of the sample.

Immunohistochemical evaluation of slide preparations (e.g., bone marrow core biopsies or granulocytic sarcoma sections) in acute leukemia is less informative if a distinction between normal and leukemic cells cannot be made and/or the cellular localization of antigens is equivocal because of inferior morphology after freezing or fixation.[95,96] In contrast to the situation with lymphomas, preserving the tissue architecture is of no concern in the immunophenotypic diagnosis of the acute leukemias. Furthermore, if formaldehyde-fixed sections are tested, fewer antibodies are available because of the fixation.[97]

WHEN TO PERFORM IMMUNOPHENOTYPING

Serial immunophenotyping in a patient diagnosed with acute leukemia is essential for monitoring the clinical course of the disease. Based on the diagnostic immunophenotype, a patient-specific immunologic fingerprint is available, which allows for monitoring minimal residual disease (MRD) or for detecting early relapse. Immunophenotyping at the time of a clinically suspected relapse should be as extensive as at the time of initial presentation to address any phenotype switch, as may occur in treatment-related secondary leukemia.

Relapse

The immunologic fingerprint established at the time of presentation may be found to have undergone slight or significant changes when a patient is retested at the time of relapse. In the majority of cases, however, the overall immunophenotypic interpretation will remain the same. A trend toward the development of a less or more mature phenotype may be observed, as reflected by a decrease or increase in the expression of selected maturation antigens (e.g., CD15 in AML or CD10 and CD20 in ALL).[98–101]

Figure 15–3 gives three examples of changes in antigen expression patterns from our experience. In the patient with differentiated AML at presentation, initial diagnosis was based on the expression of CD65s in 60 percent of blast cells positive for myeloperoxidase (partially), CD33, and CD13, which is above our threshold level for this marker in the distinction between differentiated and undifferentiated AML.[2] At the time

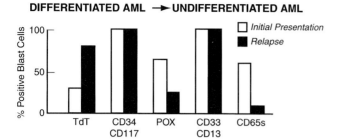

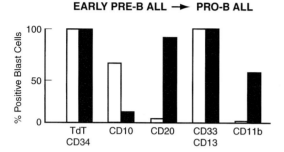

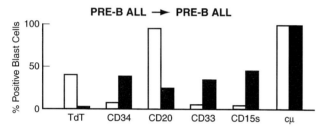

Figure 15–3. Changes in antigen expression between initial diagnosis and relapse. Examples from three patients.

of relapse, significant changes in antigen expression involved an increase in TdT and a decrease in myeloperoxidase and CD65ₛ, indicating development of less differentiated disease. In the patient with initially early Pre-B ALL, diagnosis was based on CD10 expression on 70 percent of blasts cells. At the time of relapse, following the established diagnostic criterion of using 20 percent of CD10-positive lymphoblasts as the threshold level,[2] the patient's diagnosis was consistent with Pro-B ALL despite the observed increase in CD20 expression. In terms of foreign antigen expression, CD33 and CD13 levels remained unchanged although a considerable fraction of relapse blasts expressed CD11b. In the third patient, changes in antigen expression at relapse did not warrant a change in diagnosis because expression of intracytoplasmic mu chains, the diagnostic parameter, remained the same. Important in this case is the loss of TdT because measuring TdT-expressing cells in the cerebrospinal fluid of patients with ALL is a convenient way of monitoring meningeal disease. In each of these patients, some of the changes later seen in relapse were already observed following initiation of chemotherapy during monitoring of residual disease. The lesson to learn from these three cases is that it is extremely important to study leukemic patients serially because this allows for the detection of early changes in the immunophenotype as they may occur in response to therapy.

Furthermore, changes in antigen expression at relapse are often predictable from the antigen constellation at presentation, for example, moderate expression levels of antigens that are subsequently almost or completely lost.

The overall stability of expression patterns of lineage-foreign antigens, that is, myeloid antigen expression in ALL or lymphoid antigen expression in AML, has not yet been established, mainly because of a lack of comprehensive, technically adequate studies. Some data suggest significant changes in the level of "aberrant" antigen expression in most patients with either AML or ALL studied at relapse when compared with their initial diagnoses.[102] The two ALL patients represented in Figure 15–3 demonstrate a robustness in foreign antigen expression, which in our experience is not uncommon. To account for all possible changes, even a complete lineage switch such as may occur in secondary AML following treatment with topoisomerase II targeting reagents of ALL,[103] immunophenotyping at the time of morphologically suspected or established relapse must be as comprehensive as that performed at the time of initial presentation.

Minimal Residual Disease

If the specific antigen profile or immunologic fingerprint of a leukemic cell population in an individual patient was established at the time of presentation, disease activity can be monitored by serial immunophenotyping. The complexity of most leukemia antigen profiles facilitates the recognition of low-level disease in predominantly normal hematopoiesis. One caveat to keep in mind when acute leukemias are monitored is the appearance of increased normal precursor cells in recovering bone marrow after chemotherapy. These cells may be mistaken for persistent leukemia, particularly in ALL due to increased TdT and CD10 expression,[104] if the leukemic immunophenotype resembled that of normal precursor cells. In such cases, the detail and sophistication of immunophenotypic analysis executed at diagnosis will prove valuable and reveal crucial differences between rare leukemic cells and normal regeneration. Normal CD34-positive cell populations present in remission bone marrows usually consist of both lymphoid, generally B-lymphoid, and myeloid precursor cells. Typically, the lymphoid precursors express CD19, CD10, and TdT but lack myeloid antigens. The myeloid CD34-positive fraction expresses CD117 and early myeloid antigens. Importantly, CD65ₛ[45] and CD15[105,106] antigens expressed on the majority of AMLs are absent from normal myeloid bone marrow precursors.

It is unnecessary to recommend antibody panels directed solely at detecting relapse or minimal residual disease (MRD).[100,107,108] Patient-specific antibody combinations should be custom-designed based on the immunophenotype presentation, which should be tested preferably when material is limited, for example, immediately after chemotherapy or consolidation treatment. Either aberrant light scattering characteristics or qualitatively abnormal antigen expression patterns provide useful means for monitoring of MRD or early recurrence.[107,109] The incidence of leukemia-associated immunophenotypes is high, both in ALL and AML.[110,111] The more comprehensive the antibody panel, the higher the incidence of leukemia-associated immunophenotypes. I recommend that testing panels for AML and ALL differ only in terms of surface and cytoplasmic immunoglobulin detection, which can be reserved for the ALL.

Even with the most sophisticated flow cytometric analyses, we must admit to the limitations of immunologically determined MRD in terms of sensitivity, which is clearly inferior to the level achieved by molecular techniques. However, several studies have suggested significant correlations between immunologic MRD status in remission tissues[107,109–111] as well as stem cell collections[112] and clinical outcome. Thus, the lesser sensitivity may not represent a negative aspect but rather be an advantage. Whether molecular remission by quantitative polymerase chain reaction analysis of somatic receptor gene rearrangements or leukemia-specific hybrid genes is the clinically significant goal that treatment must aim for or whether immunologic remission is sufficient for long-term disease-free survival or even cure is still a matter of great controversy.

HEMATOPOIETIC ANTIGENS USEFUL IN ACUTE LEUKEMIA IMMUNOPHENOTYPING

Even though antigen expression patterns in acute leukemia in most cases do not reflect differentiation stages of normal hematopoiesis, antigens expressed by normal and transformed hematopoietic cells are identical. Furthermore, conventional leukemia classification systems that are based on morphology or immunophenotype refer largely to maturation stages observed during normal hematopoiesis.

Lineage-Uncommitted Antigens

Many lineage-uncommitted antigens are stem cell antigens, which in normal hematopoiesis mark cells with self-renewal capacity and differentiation potential along more than one cell lineage. During normal hematopoiesis, their expression diminishes parallel to progressive maturation. When present on leukemic blast cells, they may suggest a less differentiated phenotype. Although their expression in leukemia does not support a particular lineage affiliation, some of these antigens demonstrate lineage preferences, for example, CD117. Because of their paucity in normal bone marrow and particularly peripheral blood, they are extremely useful in the monitoring of residual disease. Typical representatives are CD133 (the earliest of all known hematopoietic antigens and essential for bone marrow engraftment), CD34, HLA-DR, CD117 (c-kit), and CD90 (Thy-1), as well as the diagnostically less commonly used CD135 (FLT-3), CD115 (FMS), and CD105 (endoglin).[64,113–121]

CD133 is a transmembrane cell surface glycoprotein with homology to mouse prominin.[122,123] Its distribution is limited to bone marrow. Normal circulating peripheral blood components[116] and nonhematopoietic tissues fail to express the CD133 antigen, although CD133 transcripts were detected in some organs.[123] A small portion of CD133+ bone marrow progenitor cells express CD135, HLA-DR, CD45, CD38[low] but lack CD34, CD117, and any evidence of lineage affiliation (lin–),[124] which supports the concept that CD133+ cells give rise to

CD34+ cells[121] and that only CD34+/CD133+ cells have repopulating capability, whereas CD34+/CD133– cells do not.[116,119,125] Furthermore, CD133+ progenitor cells exhibited potential to differentiate into endothelial cells.[126,127] Although CD133+, CD34+ bone marrow cells appear to be enriched predominantly among primitive, multilineage, and myeloid progenitor cells,[124] they also contain a minor population of erythroid burst-forming units[116] as well as CD19+ or CD10+ B-lymphoid precursor cells.[128] Because of its relatively recent discovery, the literature on CD133 expression in acute leukemia is somewhat contradictory, probably because most data are based on small numbers of patients. Snell et al.[129] in 1998 suggested that CD133 could not be found in ALL. Since then, others have demonstrated CD133 in three of six patients with early Pre-B ALL, one patient tested with Pro-B-ALL, and one of two patients with T-ALL.[128] In our experience in 155 patients with ALL, CD133 was expressed strongly and on more than 95 percent of blast cells in 71 percent of patients with Pro-B ALL, in 22 percent of patients with Early Pre-B ALL (with weak intensity in another patient), and in 7 percent of patients with Pre-B or mature B-ALL (all with weak fluorescence intensity). Among 25 patients with T-ALL, only two demonstrated weak staining with CD133 on ALL blast cells (Paietta E, unpublished observation). Summarized data in AML suggest that CD133 expression is independent of FAB subtype, surface antigen expression pattern, cytogenetics, or age and without prognostic significance.[128,130–132] In our experience, APL cells are consistently negative for CD133.[18] Despite a close correlation between CD133 and CD34 in most studies, CD133 can be seen on blast cells lacking the CD34 antigen,[133,134] particularly in undifferentiated, Pro-B ALL (8 of 15 CD133+ patients were CD34[low/–]) (Paietta E, unpublished observation).

CD34+ progenitors represent a heterogenous population of cells, the majority of which are already committed to the lymphoid, myeloid, erythroid, or megakaryocytic cell lineage, as demonstrated by the expression of lineage-committed antigens (lin) together with the major histocompatibility complex (MHC) class II molecule HLA-DR and the CD38 antigen. Less than 1 percent of CD34+ cells are CD38[low/–]HLA-DR–lin–[135,136] but express CD133, CD90, CD117, and CD135 as well as CD164, the last representing a new mucin-like molecule with negative regulatory function on CD34+ cell proliferation.[137] These progenitors with the morphology of primitive blast cells differ from their descendants, the clonogenic cells, such as the multilineage progenitors CFU-GEMM (granulocyte-erythroid-macrophage-megakaryocyte CFU and CFU-Mix) and the lineage-committed BFU-E (erythroid burst-forming units), BFU-MK (megakaryocyte burst-forming unit), and CFU-GM (granulocyte-monocyte CFU), by their relative insensitivity to chemotherapy.[136] The dull staining of stem cells with rhodamine[123] reflects the presence of high levels of P-glycoprotein, the multidrug resistance (MDR) -mediating drug pump, causing increased cellular efflux of the dye.[138] Analogous to this situation is the significant correlation between CD34 expression in AML and P-glycoprotein function.[138,139]

In children[140] and adults,[141,142] CD34+ B-lineage ALL is more likely to have an Early Pre-B (CD10+cμ–) or Pro-B

(CD19+CD10–) ALL immunophenotype. In pediatric B-cell ALL, CD34 correlates with good prognostic factors, such as hyperdiploidy and low incidence of central nervous system disease, whereas Early Pre-B ALL in adults is often associated with poor prognostic factors, such as older age and the Philadelphia chromosome (Ph).[142,143] In Ph-negative adult ALL, CD34 has no prognostic impact.[142] It should be mentioned, however, that CD34 determination is not part of many large clinical trials in adult ALL. CD34 is also common on the cμ+sμ+ blasts in transitional Pre-B-ALL, a subtype with better prognosis than Pre-B ALL in general.[145] In pediatric T-cell ALL, CD34 correlates with central nervous system disease and other poor prognostic features.[140]

In pediatric as well as adult AML, the prognostic significance of CD34 ranges from irrelevant to predictive for failure to respond or decreased disease-free and overall survival. Such marked discrepancies reflect either differences in data interpretation, in particular, wide-ranging arbitrary cutoff points in the determination of CD34 positivity of a given leukemic cell population, or heterogeneity in patient populations. In fact, CD34 expression in AML is associated with a variety of poor-risk features, such as an immature phenotype,[15,146,147] functional P-glycoprotein,[139,148] and a higher incidence of chromosome 5 and 7 abnormalities.[139,149,150] There is indication that only patients whose blast cells stain brightly for CD34 have a poor prognosis, whereas dim CD34 staining is prognostically equivalent to CD34 negativity.[151] CD34 staining intensity varies dramatically depending on the fluorochrome used (PE-conjugated CD34 antibodies stain more strongly than FITC conjugates). Furthermore, there are three epitopes contained in the CD34 molecule (classes I, II, and III), whose distribution varies with the stage of cell maturation,[152,153] making the choice of antibody crucial. Intracellular stores of CD34 release protein to the cell surface on extracellular stimulation.[154] This provides an additional source of antigen staining for those laboratories choosing to fix the cells prior to antibody addition. All of these variables contribute to the fact that the prognostic significance of CD34, as a single antigen, is undetermined.

Aside from hematopoietic progenitor cells, the sialomucin CD34 is also expressed on endothelial cells, where it mediates binding of CD62L (L-selectin) on circulating leukocytes.[136,155] A soluble form of CD34 is released from CD34+ cultured cells, and the same may occur during maturation in vivo.[156]

A small fraction of CD133+CD34+CD38^low normal hematopoietic stem cells with long-term repopulating potential express CD90 (Thy-1),[64,157,158] a member of the immunoglobulin superfamily, which is preferentially expressed on endothelial cells. Other human CD90+ hematopoietic tissues include a small percentage of fetal thymocytes and less than 1 percent of CD3+CD4+ circulating T lymphocytes.[64] Expression of CD90 in AML is rare,[159] and its frequency in ALL is poorly documented. Lamkin et al[160] reported in childhood B-lineage ALL a CD34+Thy-1^low phenotype in 65 percent of 49 children tested. To the contrary, we have observed among 230 adult patients with ALL only one case of Early Pre-B ALL with CD90+CD34+CD133– blast cells, one case of undifferentiated Pro-B ALL with CD90^lowCD34^lowCD133+ blast cells, and one case of Pre-B ALL with CD90^lowCD34–CD133– blast cells (Paietta E, unpublished observation). Aside from demonstrating a low incidence of CD90 in adult ALL (1.3 percent), our findings also suggest discordance in the expression pattern of stem cell antigens in acute leukemia.

Among normal mononuclear bone marrow cells, approximately two-thirds of CD34+ precursor cells express CD117 (c-kit), the stem cell factor or mast cell growth factor or steel factor receptor.[161] Human CD117+CD34+lin– stem cells are capable of reconstituting hematopoiesis.[162] Human precursors of all hematopoietic cell lineages exhibit CD117, with its density of expression being correlated with the stage of maturation. Among terminally differentiated hematopoietic cells, mast cells retain CD117 expression, as does a small fraction of natural killer cells expressing high levels of CD56.[161,163] In contrast to this broad distribution of CD117 among normal precursor cells, among the acute leukemias it is preferentially expressed in AML.[34–39] CD117 positivity in the absence of CD34 and HLA-DR expression is a typical feature of APL.[35,164] In non-APL AML, CD117 is more common in phenotypes without a monocytic component[35,38,39] and may be present in the absence of CD34.[165] There are no proven associations between CD117 expression in non-APL AML and cytogenetic abnormalities or outcome in adult or pediatric AML.[35–39,166] Detection of CD117 in ALL is controversial but appears to be rare and restricted to T-lineage ALL when the largest existing studies are considered[36,37,167–169] (Paietta E, unpublished observation).

CD109, another marker of hematopoietic stem cells, is also expressed on activated T lymphocytes, activated platelets, and endothelial cells.[64,170] In combination with CD34, it is a marker of megakaryocytic precursor cells. Data in acute leukemia are sparse, with some indication that CD109 may be found in T-lineage ALL as well as in megakaryoblastic leukemia.[64]

CD105 (endoglin) expression on circulating CD133+ CD34+CD117+CD90+CD38^low/– primitive progenitor cells marks a subset with potential of generating megakaryocytic precursors.[171] As a component of the receptor for transforming growth factor β1 (TGF-β1), it may be involved in the autocrine control of megakaryocytopoiesis by TGF-β1. It is predominantly expressed by endothelial cells, and within the hematopoietic system it is found on early B cells in fetal bone marrow and a fraction of activated monocytes. A study on 318 patients with a variety of hematologic malignancies found CD105 expression in the majority of early B-lineage but not T-lineage ALL cases and in all types of AML cases except APL.[172]

HLA-DR is another marker used to aid in the characterization of hematopoietic stem cells. The CD34++HLA-DR+CD38^low/–lin– fetal and adult bone marrow cells contain uncommitted hematopoietic progenitor cells and give rise to each of the hematopoietic cell lineages in the presence of hematopoietic growth factors.[114] Along the myeloid lineage, its expression decreases with maturation, whereas it is present on the surface of both immature and mature monocytic cells. HLA-DR is expressed through all developmental stages of B lymphocytes and is only lost at the stage of the terminally differentiated plasma cell. During T-lymphopoiesis, HLA-DR is transiently expressed in the thymus and lost with differentiation. Occurrence of HLA-DR in AML and ALL follows the normal distribution. In T-ALL, HLA-DR expression by a subgroup of cases no longer appears of any clinical concern.

Differential expression of CD45 isoforms, derivatives of mRNA splice variants for the leukocyte common antigen complex, a family of transmembrane-type protein tyrosine phosphatases,[64] have been used to segregate early from committed lymphoid and myeloid CD34+ progenitor cells.[173–175] Precursors to CFU-Mix are included in the CD34+CD45RO+ CD45RA–CD90+CD38[low]CD117[low]rhodamine123[dull] cell population,[113] whereas CD34+CD45RA++ cells represent progenitors of the granulocyte–monocyte lineage, and CD34+ CD45RA[low]CD71+ progenitors give rise to BFU-E.[174,176] Evidence for the granulomonocyte committment of CD34+HLA-DR+++CD45RA++ cells is the intracytoplasmic expression of the myeloid-specific myeloperoxidase protein and the surface expression of the myeloid antigens CD33[177] and CD64.[178] Various mature leukocyte subpopulations express characteristic CD45 isoforms or combinations thereof.[64] Using antibodies that bind to all CD45 isoforms, CD45 is ubiquitously found on blast cells from all AML subtypes. Caldwell et al.[179] demonstrated that whereas normal myeloid stages predominantly express isoform CD45RO on the cell surface, most cases of AML express CD45RA, with or without CD45RO. In pediatric as well as adult ALL, 15 to 20 percent of B-lineage ALL cases lack CD45 expression. Absent CD45 expression in childhood ALL correlates with favorable outcome in association with chromosomal hyperdiploidy.[180] The intensity level of CD45 staining appeared as an independent prognostic parameter in a large study of children with B-precursor ALL, with patients having bright CD45 faring the worst.[181]

Stages of progressive differentiation that have lost the ability to sustain prolonged hematopoiesis are associated with a decrease in stem-cell antigen expression concomitant with bright expression of CD38 and lineage-associated markers such as CD33 (myeloid lineage), CD71 (erythroid lineage), or early lymphoid antigens.[114,182] Whereas CD38– cells have the characteristics of primitive blasts, CD38+ cells are blasts with differentiation features of multiple-cell lineages. Thus, the CD38 antigen is a marker for multilineage commitment of bone marrow progenitor cells. It is ubiquitously expressed on more differentiated cell types and is inducible by lymphocyte activation.[64] Expression of CD38 is ubiquitous in both ALL and AML. Low expression or lack of CD38 is a characteristic feature of the leukemic lymphocytes of B-cell chronic lymphocytic leukemia.[2]

Parallel with CD38, the CD7 T-cell molecule is increasingly expressed as another early marker of multipotent commitment.[183] This concept is compatible with the finding of CD34+CD7+CD19+ cells, hypothetically derived from CD34+CD7+CD19– progenitors, which may represent uncommitted (dual T- and B-lineage) lymphoid precursors,[184,185] analogous to the CD34+CD19+ and CD10+ bilineage progenitors that express the T-cell antigen CD2 during fetal hematopoiesis.[186] Gore et al.[187] and Dworzak et al.[188] convincingly demonstrated the existence of CD34+lin– or cytoplasmic CD79a+ cells that expressed the DNA polymerase terminal deoxynucleotidyl transferase (TdT) in adult and pediatric bone marrow. Some CD34+TdT+CD79a+CD7+ cells coexpressed CD33 but not myeloperoxidase or intracytoplasmic CD3,[188] which confirms previous data of CD7 expression on CD34+ myeloid precursor cells in normal bone marrow.[189] Therefore, cross-lineage antigen expression is a well-recognized phenomenon not only in malignant but also in normal hematopoiesis.

Antigens Associated with the Myeloid Lineage

The distribution of myeloid antigens during normal myelopoiesis is tabulated in Table 15–2. The antigens CD34, CD117, and HLA-DR were added to illustrate those stages that

Table 15–2. Antigen Profiles of Normal Myeloid Cells at Various Stages of Differentiation

CFU-GM	Myeloblast	Promyelocyte	Myelocyte/ Metamyelocyte	Granulocyte	Monocyte
CD34	CD34				
CD117	CD117				
HLA-DR	HLA-DR				HLA-DR
MPO	MPO	MPO	MPO	MPO	MPO[low]
CD33	CD33	CD33	CD33	CD33	CD33±
CD13	CD13	CD13	CD13	CD13	CD13
	CD65[(s)]	CD65[(s)]	CD65[(s)]	CD65[(s)]	CD65[(s)] + +
		CD15[(s)]	CD15[(s)]	CD15[(s)]	CD15[(s)]
			CD11b	CD11b	CD11b
		CD24	CD24	CD24	
	CD64	CD64	CD64		CD64
(CD68)	CD68	CD68	CD68±	CD68±	CD68 + +
				CD35	CD35
			CD16±	CD16	
			CD11c±	CD11c	CD11c
				CD10	CD14
			LF	LF	

Abbreviations: MPO, myeloperoxidase; LF, lactoferrin; CFU-GM, granulocyte-macrophage colony-forming unit.

express these stem cell antigens during normal hematopoiesis. The myeloperoxidase (MPO) protein is first detectable at the stage of granulocyte-macrophage colony-forming units (CFU-GM).[177] As discussed earlier, combinations of MPO with intracytoplasmic CD3 or intracytoplasmic CD22 provide information on specific lineage affiliation. The combination of MPO and lactoferrin (LF) distinguishes between immature and mature myeloid stages because LF-containing secondary (specific) granules are first observed at the myelocyte stage and are absent from monocytes.[190] The antigens CD33 and CD13 can be found on lineage-uncommitted, CD34+CD38− precursor cells.[179] Their early appearance, prior to myeloid commitment, corresponds to the immunophenotype of the most immature subtype of AML, characterized by expression of CD33 and CD13 in the absence of other myeloid markers, including myeloperoxidase.[15,191] It also explains the frequent finding of these two antigens on the surface of leukemic lymphoblasts.[192–194] Commitment to the myeloid lineage is signified by high expression of CD33 on CD34+CD38+ progenitor cells, but this antigen is also present on a fraction of CFU-GEMM and BFU-E;[64] CD33, a member of the sialoadhesin family, is expressed throughout myelomonocytic maturation, including macrophages.[64] Although not detected on mature erythroid cells, platelets, or normal lymphocytes, CD33 can be induced on CD4+ and CD8+ peripheral blood T lymphocytes by activation with anti-CD3 antibody plus IL-2.[195] The CD33 antigen is not found in nonhematopoietic tissues,[64] which makes it an ideal candidate in the use of antibodies for the therapeutic purposes. On the contrary, CD13, the aminopeptidase N, has extensive nonhematopoietic distribution,[196] similar to that of the neutral endopeptidase CD10.[64] The cleavage of amino acid residues from peptide or protein substrates by these membrane-associated enzymes may result in reduced cellular responses, particularly important in immune function, inflammation, and tumor cell invasion. CD65 and CD65$_s$ are structurally related carbohydrate antigens of unknown function which are absent from CFU-GEMM or BFU-E and appear at the late CFU-GM and the myeloblast stage.[45,64] Expression of these (sialo)fucooligosaccharide sequences by gangliosides[64,197] is determined by the Lewis fucosyltransferase and may contribute to E-selectin (CD62E)-dependent or P-selectin (CD62P)-dependent cell adhesion.[64,198] Whereas binding of the prototype CD65$_s$ antibody, VIM-2, to both granulocytes and monocytes is neuraminidase-sensitive, CD65 antibodies, such as VIM-8 and VIM-11, bind predominantly to cells of the myeloid rather than the monocytic lineage and the binding is enhanced by neuraminidase treatment.[64] CD65$_s$ is found on leukemic lymphoblasts from a significant percentage of pediatric[194] and adult patients[199] (Paietta E, unpublished observation) with CD10− Pro-B (Pre-Pre-B) ALL. Concomitant expression of CD33, CD13, and CD65/CD65$_s$ in a case of acute leukemia strongly supports the diagnosis of AML.

The first specific marker for granulomonocytic commitment is CD64 (FcγR), a receptor for the IgFc fragment, which is expressed on early, CD34+ myeloid progenitors and remains throughout the maturation of these cells, with downregulation during terminal granulocyte maturation and complete loss in segmented neutrophils.[94,178]

The promyelocyte stage is characterized by the loss of CD34 and HLA-DR and the appearance of CD15–CD15$_s$ and CD24, all evidence of progressive myeloid maturation. The CD15 cluster comprises another family of fucosylated oligosaccharide epitopes having in common fucose that is α-(1,3)- [Lewis X, Le^x determinant, type 2 chain structure and its α-(1,2)- (Le^y) derivative], or α-(1,4)- (Le^a, type 2 chain structure) linked to penultimate or internal N-acetylglucosamine.[200] These carbohydrate determinants can be contained in glycoproteins or glycolipids and can be nonsialylated, sialylated (sialyl Le^x, sialyl Le^a), or sulfated.[63,64] Sialylated and sulfated Le^x structures are ligands for E- (CD62E) and P-selectin (CD62P). Most antibodies distinguish between sialylated and asialo-CD15 epitopes as well as between Le^a and Le^x. Whereas sialyl Le^a is not expressed on the surface of leukocytes, Le^x-structures are expressed to a variable degree on granulocytes (Le^x and sialyl-Le^x positive), monocytes (predominantly sialyl-Le^x positive), and myeloid leukemic cells (Le^x and/or sialyl-Le^x positive).[63,64,201,202] Evidence for the presence of sialyl Le^x through neuraminidase treatment exists for a subset of natural killer (NK) cells, peripheral blood lymphocytes, and lymphoid leukemias.[64] In normal bone marrow, an inverse relationship exists between the expression of CD15 and CD34,[203] which is consistent with the absence of CD15 from most normal CFU-GMs and myeloblasts[63,64] and its appearance from the promyelocyte stage onward,[204] regulated by developmental changes in the relative levels of 3′- and 6′-sialyltransferases and 3-fucosyltransferases.[205] Anchorage proteins for the CD15 oligosaccharide may possess sialyl-[206] or fucosyltransferase activity.[63] Antibodies to sialyl Le^x have been assigned a separate cluster, CD15$_s$.[63,64] The differential expression of CD15–CD15$_s$ antigens by normal and leukemic promyelocytes[54] is extremely helpful in the evaluation of remission bone marrows in patients with the diagnosis of APL. Aside from contributing to leukocyte and tumor cell adhesion as surface-localized molecules, CD15 antigens are also contained in intracellular secondary granules, from where they are transported to the surface upon granulocyte activation to suppress neutrophil bactericidal activity. A soluble form of CD15 is found in serum, and CD15 structures are widely distributed among normal and malignant nonhematopoietic tissues.[63,64]

CD24, a glycosyl phosphatidylinositol (GPI)-anchored antigen, is homologous to mouse heat-stable antigen (HSA) and expressed throughout B-cell development, where it is downregulated at the plasma cell level.[64] During human myelopoiesis, CD24 is expressed at the metamyelocyte–myelocyte stage and persists until the mature granulocyte; most AML populations are CD24-negative. Whereas normal monocytes lack this antigen, it is generally found on leukemic monocytes.[207,208] This antigen is a valuable, though underappreciated, tool for differentiation between normal and leukemic hematopoiesis.

CD11b (Mac-1) is a marker for mature granulomonocytic cells.[64] Although weak staining of some CD34+ bone marrow progenitor cells by CD11b antibody has been reported,[209] expression of this antigen clearly begins at the early myelocyte stage.[94] CD11b and CD11c represent integrin α subunits, which covalently associate with the β$_2$ (CD18) subunits.[210] Both these integrins are transported to the surface of neutrophils and monocytes from intracellular storage pools to mediate the adhesion of these cells to unactivated (involving ICAM-1) and stimulated endothelial cells, respectively.[64] The CD11b antigen is expressed on neutrophilic, eosinophilic, and basophilic cells.[211] Furthermore, it is found on a subset of lymphocytes as well as NK cells.[64,94] In monocytic development CD11b appears earlier than CD14.[212] CD11b+ AML has been identified as a leukemic syndrome with poor prognosis.[25] Although first detected at the myelocyte stage as well, CD11c/CD18 (also called p150,95) appears before CD11b during monocytic differentiation.[94] The majority of peripheral blood granulocytes express CD11c. Interestingly, some undifferentiated AMLs, without displaying other evidence of monocytic differentiation, strongly express CD11c (Paietta et al., unpublished observation). The combined expression of CD11b and CD11c was associated with early death in patients with or without AML-M5 leukemia.[213]

The latest antigens to appear in the myeloid series are CD35 and then CD16. The CD35 antigen, the receptor for C3b/C4b, which is involved in the regulation of complement activation, is expressed on less than 5 percent of metamyelocytes and myelocytes, the majority of neutrophils and monocytes, and a subset of lymphocytes.[64,94] CD16 (FcγRIII) appears at the band stage of myeloid maturation. This antigen is the low-affinity receptor for immunoglobulin G (IgG) and is involved in antibody-dependent cellular cytotoxicity (ADCC) and the regulation of NK cell activity.[64] It is expressed on the majority of NK cells, granulocytes (except eosinophils),[211] monocytes, macrophages, and a subset of T lymphocytes. In one study of adult AML, CD16 was associated with extramedullary disease.[214] A significant fraction of mature neutrophils express CD10.[64]

CD14 is considered a monocyte-specific antigen, expressed on mature monocytes and macrophages but not monocyte precursors. It is weakly expressed on unstimulated granulocytes and is absent from myeloid cells of earlier maturation stage.[62] CD14 is a GPI-anchored surface protein that also exists as a soluble form, lacking the GPI anchor, in plasma and urine and functions as a receptor for lipopolysaccharides (endotoxin).[64] A CD14– subset of normal peripheral blood monocytes with strong expression of CD16 (FcγRIII) shows reduced adherence and phagocytic ability.[215] In AML, CD14 expression is predominantly found in morphologically monocytic leukemia and appears to be associated with shorter survival.[214,216,217] The triple antibody combination, CD13+CD14+CD66, proved to facilitate the distinction among immature myeloid, monocytic, and mature myeloid cells in normal and leukemic bone marrow.[218]

Another monocytic marker is CD68, a hematopoietic mucin-like molecule with homology to lysosomal–plasma membrane shuttling proteins (lamp-1 and lamp-2) of unknown function.[64] Accordingly, CD68 is located predominantly in endosome- or lysosome-like intracellular structures but can be detected in small amounts on the surface of monocytes, neutrophils, and basophils. A few circulating NK cells and a considerable portion of CD19+ B lymphocytes express CD68. Also, CD68 can be found in a sizable fraction of CD34+ bone marrow progenitor cells with granulomonocytic potential.[219]

During further myeloid differentiation, CD68 is strongly expressed in the MPO+LF–CD14– cell population, which contains myeloblasts, promyelocytes, and promonocytes. Like MPO, CD68 molecules have been localized in primary (azurophil) but not secondary neutrophil granules. Downregulation of CD68 occurs in parallel with lactoferrin (LF) expression. Circulating CD14+ monocytes show strongest CD68 expression. Data on CD68 expression in AML vary; in addition to myeloid and megakaryocytic leukemias, B-lineage ALLs have been reported to weakly express CD68.[219]

Mast Cells, Basophils, and Eosinophils

Mast cells, basophils, eosinophils, monocytes, and neutrophils all originate from a CD34+CD117+ cell. Although mast cells were reported to arise separately from a CD34+CD117+CD13+ precursor subset,[220] a recently identified antibody, 97A6, labels distinct CD34+CD117+ bone marrow progenitors that give rise to both mast cells and basophils. Cultured CD34+97A6+ precursors also yield eosinophil and multilineage (basophil-eosinophil-macrophage-neutrophil) colonies; however, only mast cells and basophils react with the 97A6 antibody among all hematopoietic or nonhematopoietic cell types.[221] Both cell types share metachromatic staining properties and express high-affinity surface receptors for the Fc portion of IgE (FcεRI), but differ in tissue distribution, granular contents, morphology, immunophenotype, and production, as well as dependence on growth factors.[222–227] Mast cells are found throughout connective tissues and mucosal surfaces of various organs, where they demonstrate tissue-specific biological features and characteristic antigen profiles, whereas basophils are circulating granulocytes. Both cell types express the panleukocyte antigens CD45, CD33, CD68 (in cytoplasmic granules), and CD9, a molecule of platelets, B cells, and monocytes. Both cell types lack HLA-DR, lymphoid antigens, and CD34. Mast cells express CD14, react with antibodies typical for late-stage macrophage differentiation, and express ICAM-1 (CD54).

Mast cells express c-kit (CD117), and their growth and development require stem cell factor. In contrast, CD117 is lost from basophils during cell maturation. Basophils, on the other hand, express CD123 (interleukin[IL]-3Rα), and IL-3 is their major growth and differentiation factor. Furthermore, basophils differ from mast cells and eosinophils by their expression of Bsp-1, CD26 (dipeptidylpeptidase IV), and CDw17 (lactosylceramide). Basophils express CD11b/CD18, and the nerve growth factor receptor homologue CD40, CD15$_s$ and the T-cell activation antigens CD38 and CD25.

Eosinophils express both CD25 and CD122 (forming a high-affinity IL-2 receptor), are weakly CD4+ and similar to monocytes,[228] and express several adhesive structures, including HLA-DR; the β$_2$ integrins CD11a and CD11b; two CD49/CD29 β$_1$ integrins (VLA-4 and VLA-6); CD44; three members of the Ig gene superfamily, namely CD50 (ICAM-3), CD58 (LFA-3), and CD31 (PECAM-1); and CD43, in addition to complement regulatory proteins [CD35 (CR1, C3b receptor), CD46 (membrane cofactor protein, MCP), CD55 (decay-accelerating factor, DAF), and CD59 (MAC inhibitor)]; and the myeloid antigens CD13,

CD65, and CD15.[63] In their secondary granules eosinophils contain multiple cytokines, such as granulocyte macrophage-colony-stimulating factor, IL-2, IL-6, IL-5, tumor necrosis factor (TNF)-α, nerve growth factor, and stem cell factor.[229]

Commitment to the Erythroid Lineage

Commitment to the erythroid lineage is marked by the appearance of CD71 (transferrin receptor), which increases gradually during maturation paralleled by a decrease in CD38.[230] Although expressed on BFU-E, CD34 and the myeloid antigen CD33 are absent from immediate BFU-E descendants, which continue to be HLA-DR+CD71+ and express transiently the CD41a/CD61 platelet glycoprotein (GP) IIb/IIIa complex.[231] Expression of glycophorin by CD34+CD41+ precursor cells distinguishes erythroid from megakaryocytic precursor cells.[232] Another erythroid progenitor cell antigen that is shared with the megakaryocytic lineage is CD36, the thrombospondin receptor or GPIV.[231,233] CD36 is lost from erythroid cells at the reticulocyte stage concomitantly with the loss of fibronectin receptors, decreased attachment to bone marrow stromal cells, and migration of mature cells to the peripheral blood, whereas in megakaryocytic and monocytic cells, CD36 is a marker of maturation.[233] HLA-DR is lost early, before the appearance of erythroid morphologic characteristics, whereas CD71 and CD36 slowly decrease with maturation. Differentiation from proerythroblasts to basophilic, polychromatophilic, and orthochromatic erythroblasts and finally to erythrocytes is characterized by acquisition of the red cell membrane components glycophorin A, band 3, and the blood group ABH antigen sialoglycoproteins and also of the structural cytoplasmic proteins, hemoglobin and spectrin.[234]

Commitment to the Megakaryocytic Lineage

The most primitive megakaryocytic precursors, the burst-forming units of megakaryocytes (BFU-MK), express CD34 and CD109[170] and are resistant to 5-fluorouracil treatment, in contrast to the more differentiated still CD34+HLA-DR+ megakaryocyte colony-forming units (CFU-MK).[235] Mpl, the product of the gene encoding the thrombopoietic receptor, and GPIIb (CD41) are first expressed in CD34+ precursor cells together with CD9, a member of the tetraspanin superfamily,[236] with GPIIb (CD41) and CD9 being weakly expressed even on bipotent BFU-E/MK.[231,232,236,237] The low expression of CD41 by some CFU-GEMM[235] and the finding that CD34+CD41+ bone marrow cells contain not only megakaryocytic but also erythroid and myeloid progenitors[232] support the concept that this antigen is present on a fraction of multipotent progenitors, as demonstrated in the avian hematopoietic system.[238] This would explain the finding of CD41/CD61 on monocytic CD14+ cells[239] and on metamyelocytes–myelocytes during the chronic phase of some patients with chronic myeloid leukemia and myelodysplasia (Paietta E, unpublished observation). Although CD9 is lost upon erythroid differentiation, its expression is upregulated with increasing megakaryocytic differentiation.[236] The CD34+GPIIb/IIIa+ (CD41/CD61; integrin $\alpha_{IIb}\beta_3$) bone marrow cells give rise to CD34–GPIIb/IIIa+ cells, with an inverse relationship between GPIIb/IIIa and CD34 expression.[240] GPIIb-IIIa functions as the platelet receptor for fibrinogen and von Willebrand factor (vWF). Another vWF receptor, the GPIbαβ-V-IX complex, which in contrast to GPIIb is very specific for platelets, appears later during megakaryocytopoiesis.[241] In culture, dissociated expression of GPIb-IX (CD42bc/CD42a) and GPV (CD42d) can be observed.[241] The CD34+GPIIb/GPIIa+ promegakaryoblast, a transitional stage between clonal progenitors and morphologically recognizable megakaryocytic cells, contains platelet peroxidase and immature α-granules and stains with antibodies to vWF and factor VIII.[240,242] CD34 is lost from the polyploid megakaryoblast concomitantly with the appearance of the GPIb-V-IX complex (CD42), of mature α granules in the cytoplasm,[240] and of CD36 (GPIV, GPIIIb), the platelet collagen and thrombospondin receptor.[233] Although an early differentiation marker in erythropoiesis, CD36 is a late feature in megakaryopoiesis. Signal transduction via CD36 results in platelet activation. First evidence for megakaryocyte maturation is the formation of demarcation membranes preceding the appearance of α-granules.[240] Alpha granules contain P-selectin (CD62P), also called PADGEM (platelet activation–dependent granule–external membrane protein) or GMP-140 (granule membrane protein-140), as well as GPIIa (CD31),[242] also termed PECAM-1 (platelet–endothelial cell adhesion molecule), a member of the Ig gene superfamily.[210] On appropriate activation, these adhesion molecules are mobilized to the external plasma membrane. The receptor for thrombopoietin, c-mpl, clearly appears on late megakaryocytic progenitors and persists until the platelet stage.[243] Although CD41/CD61, CD42, and CD51 (α-chain of the vitronectin receptor noncovalently associated with CD61, the β_3 chain of the vitronectin receptor), do not react with granulocytes or monocytes, CD31 is expressed by monocytes, neutrophils, and a subset of lymphocytes.[210] Alpha granules also contain fibrinogen, thrombospondin, and TGF-β,[244] and the dense granules are storage pools for serotonin, calcium, and dense granular membrane proteins.[242] The lysosomal granules contain CD63, which is translocated to the surface membrane on thrombin stimulation, and the lysosomal–plasma membrane shuttling proteins (lamp-1 and lamp-2, CD107a, CD107b). Platelets lack protein synthesis, and proteins expressed on the membrane on activation are released from intracellular storage sites. Megakaryocytes and platelets have pronounced migratory and adhesive capabilities related to the variety of adhesion molecules expressed by these cells, as indicated above. GPIIb/IIIa, the major platelet integrin, is the receptor for RGD-containing glycoproteins such as fibrinogen, vWF, and fibronectin. Other integrins involved in platelet adhesion and aggregation are VLA-2 (CD49b/CD29), VLA-5 (CD49e/CD29), and VLA-6 (CD49f/CD29).[62–64]

Commitment to the Lymphoid Lineage

Models of lymphoid cell development have long been based on phenotypic features of leukemic lymphoblasts.[245–247] Janossy et al.[248] detected normal bone marrow cells that exhibited antigenic similarities with ALL blasts, and multiparameter flow cytometry and cell sorting have subsequently identified normal transitional stages in lymphopoiesis. Particularly for B-lymphopoiesis, these analyses have corrected previously accepted diagrams of antigen expression. Multiparameter and quantitative flow cytometry suggest that leukemic immunophenotypes do not represent malignant counterparts of normal hematopoietic precursor stages. Rather than attempting to provide a complete summary of lymphoid antigens, the description in this section will be limited to antigens of apparent significance in acute leukemia diagnosis, prognosis, or treatment. For the same reason, the dendritic cell lineage will not be discussed in detail.

A Common Precursor Cell for B, T, Natural Killer and Dendritic Cells and Possibly Myeloid Cells

CD34+CD10+CD45RA+ bone marrow progenitors lacking any other lineage-affiliated markers are capable of developing into B, T, NK, and lymphoid dendritic cells (DC).[249] Thus, CD10 is the earliest B lineage-affiliated antigen to appear at this level of nonlineage commitment and is lost during B lymphopoiesis as cells acquire surface immunoglobulins (Ig). It is lost immediately if differentiation occurs along T- and NK-cell lineages. The CD10 antigen can be found in a substantial fraction of T- ALL cases, in which it confers improved disease-free survival,[30,31] as well as in rare cases of CD56+ NK-ALL with T- or B-lineage marker expression.[250] CD34+CD127(IL-7 receptor)+TdT+CD10+ lymphoid progenitors, expressing the genes for recombinase-activating gene (RAG)-1 and CD79b, were demonstrated to give rise to CD19+ early B-lymphocytes.[251] Another study described CD34+ bone marrow cells expressing the CXCR4 chemokine receptor for stromal cell-derived factor-1, which developed into cells of the B- and T-lineages but not into cells of the myeloid–erythroid lineages.[252] Miller et al.[253] described a possibly even more primitive cell of CD34+ lin–CD38– phenotype, which, when cultured on murine fetal liver cells and supported by a mixture of cytokines, developed into B, NK, DC, or myeloid cells.

Developmental Hierarchy of Antigens Expressed During B-Lymphopoiesis and Their Putative Physiologic Function

The common lymphoid progenitor cell identified by the above studies may be promoted to differentiate into early B cells (CD19– but showing Ig heavy-chain gene rearrangements and containing cytoplasmic CD79a and VpreB protein)[188,254–256] or T/NK/DC trilineage cells.[185] That CD10 precedes the expression of CD19 during normal lymphopoiesis stands in contrast to established stages of B-lineage ALL, in which the most immature subtype expresses CD19 and lacks CD10 (Pro-B ALL or Pre-Pre-B ALL), and where CD10 expression is invariably associated with expression of CD19.

The majority of normal human Pro-B cells express CD34, TdT, CD10, and CD19 and have undergone Ig heavy-chain gene rearrangements (VDJ$_H$.). Only a small fraction of Pro-B cells contain cytoplasmic μ heavy chains (HC).[185] Following functional VDJ$_H$ rearrangement, Pro-B cells differentiate into Pre-B cells, characterized by loss of CD34 and TdT and acquisition of

cytoplasmic μHC. A fraction of Pre-B cells express cell surface μHC associated with surrogate light chains (ψLCs) and the CD79a/b (Igα/Igβ) heterodimer, termed the Pre-B-cell receptor (Pre-BCR). The ψLC consists of two proteins, VpreB and λ5. For an expanded discussion of the Pre-BCR and its related structures, the reader is referred to the review by LeBien.[185] Pre-B cells undergo immunoglobulin light-chain gene rearrangements, whereby κ rearrangement precedes λ rearrangements, yielding this stage of immature B cells which express cell surface μ heavy chains associated with κ- or λ-like chains (the B-cell receptor or BCR).[185]

In terms of B-lineage antigenic determinants, B-lymphoid maturation is characterized by the cytoplasmic expression of CD22 in CD34+TdT+CD10+ cells, followed by membrane CD19 and CD22.[186] In contrast, among leukemic phenotypes intracytoplasmic CD22 in the absence of CD10 and CD19 characterizes the most immature subtype of B-lineage ALL. The finding of surface CD22 on a subpopulation of CD34+CD19– normal immature bone marrow cells[257] further contradicts earlier models of B-lineage differentiation, which suggested membrane CD19 as the earliest and CD22 as a late lineage differentiation antigen.[60] Within normal CD19+ precursor cells, the most immature subpopulation typically lacks CD20 and demonstrates dim CD45 expression. With progressive maturation, both CD20 and CD45 are upregulated parallel with surface Ig expression,[186,257,258] which supports evidence that the tyrosine phosphatase activity of CD45 is involved in the regulation of surface Ig-mediated signal transduction.[64] Although expression of CD19 is assumed to characterize cells irrevocably committed to the B-cell lineage, CD19+CD2+[256] and CD19+CD7+ or CD19+CD7+CD10+[184] normal marrow precursors have been identified. Although the correct placement of these phenotypes along the lymphoid development continuum is unclear, they may provide cells of origin for similar antigen profiles on ALL blasts.

Insights into current models of human B-cell development, such as the necessary interactions of lymphoid precursors with stromal–accessory cells and the role of various cytokines, have been reviewed by LeBien.[185] In terms of known physiologic functions of B-lineage differentiation antigens, CD10 is identical to the human cell surface neutral endopeptidase (zinc metalloprotease) with widespread distribution on fibroblasts, mature granulocytes, bone marrow stromal cells, brush border epithelium, etc.[64] CD19, a member of the Ig gene superfamily, has an extensive cytoplasmic domain with homology to the int-1 oncogene and Epstein-Barr virus (EBV)-encoded proteins, which predestines this antigen for its proposed function in regulating and selectively inhibiting B-cell responses to surface Ig signaling.[62,64] CD22 is a member of the Ig superfamily with homology to myelin-associated glycoprotein, a neural adhesion molecule,[62] which has tyrosine kinase activity and acts as adhesive receptor and signaling molecule.[64]

Acquisition of CD24 and subsequently CD40 provides further evidence for B-cell differentiation.[256] CD24 associates with protein tyrosine kinases and modulates the responses of B-lymphoid cells to activation signals;[64] it is expressed by mature myeloid cells, both in bone marrow and peripheral blood,[62] whereas leukemic myeloid cells are typically CD24-negative.[207,208] The majority of B-lineage ALL cell populations express CD24. It is noteworthy that failure to express CD24 confers radiation resistance to primary clonogenic blasts from children with B-lineage ALL.[259] Although CD40 expression has been reported on CD34+ precursor cells,[64] it is generally absent from CD10− leukemic lymphoblasts and detected predominantly on blast cells of more mature phenotypes (Paietta E, unpublished observation). CD40 protein, which shares structural similarities with the nerve growth factor receptor, shows broad tissue distribution and acts as a costimulatory molecule supporting the survival of B cells.[64,256] Through association with a calcium channel, CD20 appears to regulate transmembrane calcium fluxes, which are necessary for cell cycle progression.[62–64]

Maturation of B cells is paralleled by decreased adhesiveness to bone marrow–derived fibroblasts due to loss of very late antigen-4 (VLA-4) (CD49d/CD29) integrin and its interaction with VCAM-1 (CD106) on bone marrow stromal cells, whereas other adhesion molecules, such as CD11a/CD18, CD44 and CD54, are increasingly expressed,[260] which suggests profound changes in the interactions between the developing B cell and its microenvironment.[185]

Antigen-Specific Receptors of Lymphocytes

The ability of mature lymphoid cells to recognize a multitude of antigens, which constitutes a functional immune system, is mediated by a diversity of cell surface receptors, namely surface-bound Ig on B cells and the T-cell receptors (TCRs) on T cells. The specificity of antigen recognition is generated by rearrangements of separate Ig and TCR gene segments. Recombination events include a variable (V), a diversity (D) (in the case of Ig heavy chains and TCR-β and -δ chains), and a joining (J) gene segment, which encode the antigen-recognizing amino terminal part of antigen receptor chains. During the rearrangement process, nucleotides can be randomly deleted from the germline gene segments or inserted, probably through the activity of TdT polymerase, at the V-D and D-J junctions corresponding to the complementarity-determining region 3 (CDR3), which is of major importance in antigen recognition. Two recombination activation genes, RAG-1 and RAG-2, are absolutely essential for V(D)J joining both at the Ig and TCR loci. The junctional diversification of the genes creates a unique DNA sequence, which is specific for an individual lymphocyte and its progeny and therefore provides a clone-specific genetic marker, which is exploitable for the detection of monoclonality as well as for the monitoring of minimal residual disease in ALL.[261–265]

The B-cell Antigen Receptor Complex

The B-cell antigen receptor complex consists of the membrane Ig glycoprotein and a heterodimer of nonvariant transmembrane proteins, referred to as Igα (CD79a) and Igβ (CD79b). The Igs are tetramers constituted by pairs of disulfide-linked heavy (H) and light (L) chains. In normal B-cell precursors, production of Igα and Igβ molecules precedes IgH gene rearrangement. Appearance of cytoplasmic μHC without LC

characterizes the Pre-B differentiation stage (see above). A small fraction of μ chains does surface at the cell membrane of Pre-B cells after interaction with a pseudo- or surrogate LC chain complex (ψLC), consisting of two proteins, VpreB and λ5, and association with Igα and Igβ, forming the Pre-B cell receptor (Pre-BCR), which appears to be essential for the further advancement of B-cell maturation.[256,264] This differentiation stage can be termed transitional Pre-B cell. Subsequently, IgL κ chain genes rearrange, leading to surface expression (s) of HC and LC together to form the B-cell receptor (BCR), first IgM/κ (immature B cell) and subsequently coexpression of IgM/κ and IgD/κ chains with identical variable domains on the majority of mature, resting circulating B cells. If the κ rearrangement is not functional, the Igλ genes will rearrange and IgH/λ chains will be expressed on the cell membrane, which in humans is the case in about 10 to 30 percent of mature B cells. Each lymphocyte will only express either κ or λ LC, and monoclonality of a given B-cell population for IgLC expression suggests a malignant process. Deduced from the reactivity pattern of antibodies to distinct epitopes of the Pre-BCR, a novel classification system for B-lineage ALL has been proposed based on the intracytoplasmic expression of surrogate light chains, μH chains, Pre-BCRs, and light chains.[266]

The T-cell Receptor Complex

Two types of T-cell receptor (TCR) are expressed on mature T lymphocytes, either a heterodimer composed of α- and β-chain glycoprotein subunits (majority of T cells) or of γ and δ chains (less than 1 to 20 percent of T cells), which can be distinguished with specific antibodies. Clonotypic TCR chains associate noncovalently with multiple signal-transducing subunits, including the CD3γ, CD3δ, and CD3ε molecules and members of the ζ family of proteins, the last being essential for efficient surface expression of the TCR and CD3 components.[267] Typically, CD3,γ/δ T lymphocytes lack both CD4 and CD8 expression, whereas virtually all CD3,α/β T cells express either CD4 or CD8. During early T-cell development, TCR-δ genes rearrange first at the stage of CD34+CD2+CD5+CD1a-immature thymocytes preceded by the expression of intranuclear TdT and the synthesis of cCD3, immediately followed by TCR-γ1 and -γ2 and in most cells TCR-β gene rearrangements in CD34+CD2+ CD5+CD1a+ cells.[268] Transcription of functional TCR-δ and TCR-γ arrests the expression of TCR-α, whereas unproductive rearrangement of δ and/or γ genes and deletion of TCR-δ allows the rearrangement and transcription of the TCR-α genes. Successful rearrangement of TCR-α and -β genes gives rise to TCR-α/β, which will assemble a CD3,α/β antigen receptor complex that will be expressed in the plasma membrane, analogous to the CD3,γ/δ complex. Although no other pairwise combinations of TCR chains have been seen on the surface of normal T cells, CD3,α/β cells may contain functional or sterile γ or δ transcripts in their cytoplasm. In leukemia, expression of TCR-β glycoprotein in the cytoplasm of CD3,γ/δ cells and membrane appearance of a β/δ receptor have been observed.[261] Contrary to the high frequency of cross-lineage somatic gene rearrangements seen in ALL, TCR gene rearrangements are not seen in normal B-cell precursors.[269] This finding demonstrates the danger in extrapolating data from leukemic cells to explain phenomena occurring during normal hematopoiesis.

Chromosomal aberrations in leukemias that involve Ig or TCR loci are highly predictive of the immunophenotype. The IgH locus is at 14q32, Igκ maps to 2p12, IgΛ to 22q11, TCR-α and δ genes are located on chromosome 14q11, the TCR-β genes on chromosome 7q35, and the TCR-γ genes on chromosome 7p14.

Developmental Hierarchy of Antigens Expressed During T/Natural Killer Cell Development and Their Putative Physiologic Function

The thymus is believed to play a central role in the development of the T cell. However, it is well accepted that thymic precursors are derived from bone marrow, because pluripotent stem cells of the CD34+CD38– phenotype have not been identified in fetal or pediatric thymuses.[270–273] The earliest thymic CD34[high]CD45RA+CD90+ precursors cells have the ability to differentiate into various lineages, including T cells, dendritic cells (DCs), and NK cells. Even the CD34+CD2+CD5+ thymic precursor population still contains T/NK differentiation potential. Sequential developmental stages demonstrate populations differing in the intensity of CD33 and CD7 expression, despite similar CD2, CD5, and CD38 expression.[272–274] The study by Márquez et al.[274] suggests that upregulation of CD44 and CD13 on CD34+CD5+CD33[low] thymic precursors cells is the necessary step common to both NK cells and DC to diverge from the T-cell lineage. CD1a expression characterizes the earliest committed T-cell progenitors in the thymus. Although these cells express intracytoplasmic CD3, they still lack surface CD4 and CD8 expression. Subsequently they acquire CD4 before CD8.[272]

The CD34+TdT+CD7+CD2– brightly expressing CD62L (LECAM-1) population in fetal and adult bone marrow contains precursors to CFU-TL (T-lymphocyte CFU)[187,270] and NK cells.[275] Subsequent events include the appearance of CD2 and CD5, followed by cCD3 in CD34+ precursor cells. Differentiation of T cells is characterized by the transient expression of CD1a; a brief early upregulation of CD10 on CD34+ progenitors just before the surface expression of the CD3/TCR complex, which is analogous to its upregulation and subsequent loss at the time of sIgH expression during B-cell differentiation; and the loss of CD34 concomitant with the appearance of CD4 and CD8 and prior to the acquisition of sCD3. With the development from double CD4+/CD8+ immature to single-positive (CD4+ or CD8+) mature T cells and their export into the peripheral blood, the CD38 antigen is lost, as seen during B-cell differentiation, and adhesion molecules involved in T-cell homing such as CD62L and CD44, are upregulated.[270] Usually 95 percent or more of mature, circulating T lymphocytes express CD3, TCRα/β, and 5 percent or less express CD3, TCRγ/δ. Typically, the majority of γδ cells lack CD4, CD8, and often CD5. In contrast, the rare subtype of TCRγδ+ T-ALL displays heterogeneity in terms of its T-lineage antigen expression patterns.[276,277]

The CD34+CD7+ and CD34+CD7+CD2+ bone marrow precursor cells represent direct intermediates in NK cell development.[275] Subsequent differentiation along the NK-cell lineage results in expression of CD16 and CD56. Although adult

NK cells do not rearrange TCR genes and do not express TCR proteins in their cytoplasm or their cell surface, NK cells from fetal liver and cord blood have been found to express CD3,δ and CD3,ε proteins in the cytoplasm.[278] Data on clonal TCR gene rearrangements in lymphoid NK-cell leukemia are inconsistent.[250]

With respect to putative or established physiologic functions of T-cell and NK-cell antigens, the reader is referred to the Proceedings of the Leucocyte Typing Conferences II to VII.[60–65] CD1 proteins comprise different isotypes (CD1a, 1b, 1c, 1d, 1e) with unique properties in the immune system, related to but distinct from those of major histocompatibility complex–encoded molecules.[279] Rather than presenting peptide fragments of antigens, CD1 proteins allow T cells, particularly of the rare CD4–CD8– phenotype, to respond to lipids and glycolipids. CD1a characterizes the cortical thymocyte stage of T-lineage ALL, which in adults and children has improved event-free survival when compared with other T-ALL subgroups.[31,280]

For its function as the mediator of adhesion, CD2 was initially called the sheep red blood cell receptor. The prototype ligand for CD2 is the leukocyte-function-antigen (LFA)-3 or CD58; more recently identified ligands include other GPI-linked structures, namely CD48 (BLAST-1) and CD59, as well as CD15. Expression of CD2 is not limited to T-lymphocytes, in that it is found on a portion of immature and mature B-lymphocytes as well as NK-cells. In acute leukemia, absence of CD2 is a frequent occurrence in T-ALL and associated with decreased survival.[281,282] CD2 expression in B-lineage ALL, in the absence of any other T-cell markers, occurs in less than 5 percent of all ALL cases and may be associated with favorable clinical features, at least in children.[283]

The CD7 antigen is a member of the Ig supergene family involved in T-cell activation and cellular adhesion. In accordance with its features as a hematopoietic stem cell marker,[183,184,189] CD7 is expressed on the leukemic lymphoblasts from the vast majority of T-lineage ALL cases, in a substantial fraction of AML cases, and rarely in B-lineage ALL. A small subset of normal human blood T lymphocytes has been demonstrated to lack CD7. These CD3+CD4+CD7– lymphocytes have been discussed as the normal counterpart to the malignant cells in cutaneous T-cell lymphoma, such as Sézary syndrome.[284,285]

DIFFERENTIAL IMMUNODIAGNOSIS OF THE ACUTE LEUKEMIAS

In ALL, the markers with the most reliable specificity are cytoplasmic CD3 (cCD3) for early T-cell ALL and cytoplasmic CD22 (cCD22) for early B-cell ALL, whereas antigens such as TdT, HLA-DR, CD2, CD7, CD19 and CD10, although informative and complementary for both diagnosis and prognosis, are not restricted to ALL. Somatic antigen receptor proteins also provide specific lineage assignment in that TCR protein expression is restricted to T-lineage ALL and μH chains and LC are confined to B-lineage ALL and should be included in any primary acute leukemia immunophenotyping panel. Whereas protein expression is lineage-specific, TCR and Ig chain gene rearrangements occur across lineage borders[286–289] and can be observed in AML, although rarely.[290]

In AML, intracytoplasmic myeloperoxidase (MPO) protein can be detected by antibody staining in leukemic cells that are negative for MPO by cytochemistry, which suggests the presence of a precursor MPO form lacking enzyme activity.[291,292] Myeloperoxidase activity can be detected ultrastructurally in blasts lacking the enzyme by light microscopic cytochemistry,[293–295] which has prognostic significance inasmuch as such patients do poorly when treated with ALL treatment regimens.[295] This observation is consistent with the proposed role of MPO as a mediator of the resistance of MPO-positive AML to vincristine by catalyzing the oxidative degradation of the drug.[296] Reports on MPO protein detection in ALL[297,298] must be viewed with caution and should only be considered if optimal fixation–permeabilization media were used and, most importantly, if data refer unequivocally and exclusively to gated lymphoblasts. Expression of MPO protein is specific for AML, whereas MPO gene expression, albeit at low levels, is observed in some cases of ALL, frequently in association with the Philadelphia chromosome.[299,300] Myeloperoxidase gene expression has been detected in rare cases of CD7+CD5±CD2– T-ALL, together with the finding of CD3ε or CD3δ mRNA in these lymphoblasts.[301] Lack of or decreased levels of immunologically detectable MPO protein in cases of immature AML or acute monocytic leukemia (AMOL)[292,294] are due to differential regulation of MPO gene transcription.[302]

It is mandatory to test leukemic cells for at least three myeloid surface antigens, CD33, CD13, and CD65 or CD65$_s$ as this trio will identify more than 90 percent of AMLs.[303–305] In combination, these antigens are not expressed in ALL[199,306] (Paietta E, unpublished observation) and cells with lymphoid morphology that express all three myeloid antigens should be tested carefully to rule out AML. In fact, reports of CD33+CD13+CD65$_s$+ triple-positive ALL usually base the diagnosis of ALL on FAB criteria, lack MPO determination by flow, and/or use a 20 percent or lower arbitrary cutoff point to establish myeloid antigen positivity, although they neglect to gate strictly on blast cells, thereby allowing for the contamination of their observations with normal myeloid cells.

Provided that sufficient material is available, there should not be a difference in the composition and the size of antibody panels used to test AML versus ALL. The risk of rendering an immunodiagnosis from limited marker panels lies in the commonly observed coexpression of two lymphoid- or myeloid-associated antigens by blast cells from the opposite cell lineage and the finding that several antigens, particularly those expressed early in hematopoiesis, may be expressed by leukemias of all cell lineages (e.g., TdT, CD33, CD13, CD7, CD10).

An ongoing problem in clinically interfaced laboratory studies in leukemia is that investigators first define leukemia subtypes by strict FAB rules (for instance, more than 3 percent MPO-positive blast cells define AML) and subsequently study their immunophenotype. In other words, a classification system based on imprecise morphologic criteria subject to interpreta-

tion is correlated with the expression of cell characteristics that at the time the FAB system was designed were not taken into consideration and in many instances were not even known yet. As a result, the literature is replete with morphologically defined leukemia subtypes, which, when examined carefully, are immunophenotypically unequivocally committed to a cell lineage that contradicts the morphologic diagnosis. In extreme cases, even the diagnostic power of proven lineage-specific markers, such as cCD3, is ignored in favor of FAB criteria.[307,308] The error in this approach is that a classification system with known prognostic limitations distorts valuable immunophenotypic and clinically relevant information that would be provided by those cases if they were identified by their antigenic features. That this is in fact the case is best demonstrated by clinical results in patients who fail induction treatment that would be appropriate for the diagnosis suggested by morphology but who subsequently respond to therapy for the opposite cell lineage in agreement with the immunophenotypic information.[307]

Undifferentiated (Lin–) Acute Leukemia

Immunologically undifferentiated (lin–) acute leukemias are currently characterized as CD34+TdT±HLA–DR+CD7±, lacking intracytoplasmic and membrane lymphoid or myeloid antigens, including CD117.[309] These cases must not be confused with leukemias classified as FAB AML-M0, which, although morphologically and cytochemically undifferentiated, by definition[10,310] express at least one myeloid lineage–affiliated antigen (e.g., CD33, CD13, CD14), have variable antigenic profiles that frequently include stem cell features, and account for 2 to 7 percent of AML cases. Lin– acute leukemia must also not be mistaken for Null-ALL, the most immature B-cell precursor ALL, which expresses CD19 and/or cCD22 but lacks CD10. True lin– leukemia is exceedingly rare when all currently available tools for immunophenotyping are applied. Campana et al. reported an incidence of less than 1 percent among 750 cases of acute leukemia.[311] However, even this figure may be an overestimation in that MPO protein was detectable in three of the seven cases, albeit in a small percentage of cells possibly reflecting normal myeloid precursor cells. In my laboratory's unpublished experience, we have never seen a case of acute leukemia in which lineage affiliation could not be deduced from the antigen expression pattern. The detection of somatic gene rearrangements in MPO antibody-negative cells[311] or the induction of myeloid antigens by in vitro culture[309,312] can help in the lineage assignment of leukemic phenotypes in question.

Subclassification of Acute Lymphocytic Leukemia

Commonly used subclassifications of T- and B-lineage ALL were determined years ago based on prevailing information on presumed normal maturation stages of lymphopoiesis. More recent insights into normal hematopoietic differentiation stages have revealed that most established ALL classification systems do not reflect normal lymphoid development.

B-Lineage ALL Subtypes

Although the nomenclature for B-lineage ALL subtypes varies among published reports, the major subtypes and their characteristic antigenic features show enough overlap and inherent heterogeneity to justify a coherent presentation (Table 15–3).

The most immature subtype of B-lineage ALL (termed *Pro-B, Pre-Pre-B, CD10– Early Pre-B, Null-Cell, Early-Early-B, early B-precursor ALL, or B1 Subtype*) is recognized as such on the basis of cytoplasmic CD22 (cCD22) and/or cytoplasmic CD79a and/or surface CD19 expression in the absence of other lymphoid or myeloid antigens. Both cCD22+CD19– and cCD22–CD19+ cases have been seen. Typically, these cells are CD34+ HLA–DR+CD117– and often express CD133 (Paietta E, unpublished observation); CD24 may or may not be found. Approximately 10 percent of adult ALL patients present with this immunophenotype. In children, there is the preponderance of this immature leukemia in infants, with the incidence higher the younger the age.[313,314] This is the immunophenotype associated with the (4;11)(q21;q23) cytogenetic abnormality or with the presence of MLL-AF4 transcripts, the molecular consequence of this translocation.[199,313–317] Expression of the myeloid antigens CD65$_{(s)}$ and/or CD15$_{(s)}$ is much more common in this subtype than in more mature B-lineage ALL, whereas the incidence of CD33 and/or CD13 expression is lower.[194,199,318] In terms of outcome, the prognosis of adult patients with this immunophenotype appears to have improved with intensification of therapy.[199,317] In infants, event-free survival of CD10– ALL is significantly worse than that of CD10+ ALL,[314,319] possibly owing to an observed resistance of CD10– B-cell precursor cells to prednisone and L-asparaginase.[314] In children, absence of CD10 is commonly associated with poor prognostic features, such as hyperleukocytosis and pseudodiploidy. However, the poor prognostic impact of CD10 negativity is lost when infants are excluded from the analysis.[320]

Early Pre-B ALL, also termed CD10– Early Pre-B or Common ALL or ALL of B2 Subtype, is characterized by the expression of CD10 in the absence of cytoplasmic or surface immunoglobulin HC or LC expression. The intracellular presence of surrogate LCs (λ5/VpreB) has been documented for this maturation stage.[266] This is the most common immunophenotype in children over the age of 1 year and in adults. CD10+ CD34+ B-lineage ALL is the typical immunophenotype associated with the Philadelphia chromosome (Ph), t(9;22)(q34;q11), and its molecular equivalent, the BCR/ABL fusion transcripts, found in less than 5 percent of children but in up to 25 percent of adults and associated with a poor prognosis.[317,321,322] Expression of CD25, the α chain of the IL-2 receptor, can serve as a surrogate marker for BCR/ABL transcription in Ph+ ALL.[19] In children, CD10 and CD34 are otherwise often accompanied by good prognostic features, such as hyperdiploidy, low incidence of cerebrospinal involvement, and lower leukocyte counts at presentation.[30,140,322] Acute lymphocytic leukemia with TEL/AML1 rearrangement, which results from a cryptic (12;21)(p12;q22) translocation, expresses CD10.[20] In fact, lymphoblasts containing t(12;21) express CD10 with higher fluorescence intensity than is found in t(12;21)-negative cases.[21] High-level expression of CD10 combined with low-level expression of CD20, CD45, and CD34 may thus provide a surrogate marker profile for this genotype.[20,21] Although infrequent in adults,[323,324] TEL/AML1 positivity is the most common molecular finding in children with ALL[325] and is associated with favorable outcome.[324,326] In adults, the CD10+, cytoplasmic HC– immunophenotype carries a superior prognosis among B-lineage ALL subtypes in most studies. CD2+CD19+CD10+ ALL may be related to a normal bipotential lymphoid precursor, which seems to be programmed more toward the B- than the T-cell lineage, as evidenced by in vitro differentiation to the stage of Pre-B cells[283] and by clinical features (e.g., lack of mediasti-

Table 15–3. Subclassification of B-Lineage ALL

SL+		HC+		LC+
Pro-B Pre-Pre B CD10– Early Pre-B Early-Early B B1 Subtype	Null Cell Early Pre-B CD10+ Early Pre-B Common ALL B2 Subtype	Pre-B	Transitional Pre-B ALL ———— B3 Subtype ————	Mature B-ALL
CD34	CD34	(CD34)		
TdT	TdT	TdT	(TdT)	
HLA-DR	HLA-DR	HLA-DR	HLA-DR	HLA-DR
cCD22	cCD22	CD19	CD19	CD19
cCD79a	CD19	CD24	CD24	CD24
(CD19)	CD24	CD10	CD10	CD10
(CD24)	**CD10**	CD20	CD20	CD20
	(CD20)	sCD22	sCD22	CD22
		cμ	**cμ**	**sμ**
			sμ	**sLC**

Parentheses mark variable antigen expression; ALL, acute lymphocytic leukemia; SL, surrogate light chains; HC, immunoglobulin heavy chain; μ, mu heavy chain; LC, immunoglobulin light chain; c, cytoplasmic; s, surface. Bolded antigens characterize subgroups.

nal mass, low white blood cell count).[327] Pediatric ALL patients with this immunophenotype have good clinical outcomes.[283]

The *Pre-B ALL* stage is characterized by the presence of intracytoplasmic μHC in the absence of LC. This immunophenotype is associated with unfavorable features, such as higher leukocyte counts at presentation, higher serum lactic dehydrogenase (LDH) levels, hepatomegaly, and above all the (1;19)(q23;p13) translocation, which results in in the creation of the *E2A/PBX1* fusion gene.[322,328] Lymphoblasts containing this translocation often lack CD34 expression. Monoclonal antibodies specific to the E2A/PBX-encoded chimeric protein have been developed and used to distinguish t(1;19)-positive from t(1;19)-negative leukemia.[329] Pre-B ALL with or without t(1;19) has been associated with poor outcome in some clinical studies but not others and may have benefited from improved therapies.[320,322,328,330]

Transitional Pre-B ALL has been identified in a small subset of children or adults with ALL.[320,322] This recently established subtype of B-lineage ALL demonstrates both intracytoplasmic and surface μHC but not LCs. It represents an intermediate stage between Pre-B and mature B-ALL. Its distinction from mature B ALL is important, since transitional Pre-B ALL carries an excellent prognosis.[320,322]

CD10-negative and CD10-positive Early Pre-B, Pre-B and transitional Pre-B ALL all express TdT. Immunofluorescent TdT determination on cytospin preparations is an easy and reliable tool for monitoring central nervous system (CNS) leukemia in TdT+ ALL subtypes.[331–333]

Mature B-ALL is uncommon. It shares its morphology (FAB L3), immunophenotype, clinical presentation (bulky extramedullary disease, lymphadenopathy, CNS involvement), and cytogenetic abnormalities with Burkitt's lymphoma. In the prototype (8;14)(q24;q32) translocation, the c-myc protooncogene is translocated from chromosome 8 onto chromosome 14 and brought under the transcriptional control of the IgHC locus. The variant translocations, t(2;8)(p12;q24) and t(8;22)(q24;q11), result in the positioning of portions of the κ

(2p12) or λ (22q11) IgLC gene into the vicinity of the c-myc locus on chromosome 8. In either case, regulation of c-myc expression seems affected.[334] Mature B lymphoblasts usually lack TdT and CD34 and demonstrate surface μHC associated with monoclonal LC expression. In most studies, patients with mature B-ALL still experience a reduced remission rate and shorter survival.[322,335,336]

Myeloid Antigen Expression in B- and T-ALL

Myeloid antigen expression can be seen in all subtypes of ALL, although it is usually absent in mature B-ALL. $CD65_{(s)}$ together with $CD15_{(s)}$ is more common in the CD10– subtype, whereas CD33 and/or CD13 is more common in CD10+ B-lineage ALL. In children, the expression of myeloid antigens when compared with myeloid antigen–negative ALL lacks prognostic significance.[193,194] In adults, studies on large cohorts of homogenously treated patients with a comprehensive panel of myeloid antigens have not yet been analyzed; however, ECOG has recently initiated an interim analysis of study E2993 on over 300 patients with adult ALL, so that relevant data may soon be available. It is important to note that the incidence of myeloid antigen expression in ALL is quite high, above 50 percent in CD10– B-lineage ALL[199] and about 30 percent in CD10+ Early Pre-B ALL or T-lineage ALL,[194] provided that a comprehensive panel of myeloid antibodies is tested: CD33, CD13, $CD65_{(s)}$, $CD15_{(s)}$, CD11b, and CD14.

T-Lineage ALL Subtypes

The incidence of T-lineage ALL is lower in children (about 15 percent) than in adults (20 to 25 percent). Nowadays, patients with T-cell ALL fare better than those with B-cell ALL.[31,317,322,336–340] The use of cytosine arabinoside and cyclophosphamide may account for improved treatment results in T-ALL, owing to the the ability of T lymphoblasts to accumulate high levels of cytosine arabinoside triphosphate.[341] Subgroups of T-lineage ALL are commonly defined based on the number of T markers present (maturational stage) and the selective expression of antigens such as CD1 and CD10 (Table 15–4). Significant associations between cytogenetic abnormalities and immunophenotypic T-lineage characteristics or outcome are less pronounced in T-lineage than in B-lineage ALL.[334,340,342,343]

Pro-T, Pro-Thymocyte T, Pre-T, or *stage T_{IA} ALL* represents the most immature stage of T-lineage ALL and is characterized by the absence of CD2. The diagnosis of T-lineage ALL derives from the presence of intracytoplasmic CD3 (cCD3) and surface expression of CD7, with or without CD5. This subgroup has shorter disease-free and overall survival when compared with patients with more mature T-lineage ALL.[281,282,317,339,340] CD2-negative T-ALL may be associated with a mediastinal mass and lymphadenopathy in adults,[281] although unfavorable presenting features were not seen at an increased frequency in children.[340] However, after adjusting for

Table 15–4. Subclassification of T-Lineage ALL

Stage T$_{IA}$	Stage T$_{IB}$	Stage T$_{II}$	Stage T$_{III}$
		Pre-T	T
ProT		Immature T	Mature T
Pre-T	Early T	Cortical T	Late T
Early Thymocyte		Common Thymocyte	MedullaryThymocyte
TdT	TdT	TdT	(TdT)
cCD3	cCD3	cCD3	CD5
CD5	CD5	CD5	CD7
CD7	CD7	CD7	CD2
	CD2	CD2	**CD4 or 8**
	(CD10)	**CD1**	**sCD3**
		CD4 + 8	**(TCR)**
		(CD10)	

Parentheses mark variable antigen expression; ALL, acute lymphoblastic leukemia; c, cytoplasmic; s, surface; TCR, T-cell receptor proteins. Bolded antigens characterize subgroups.

known risk criteria, CD2 negativity still remained a prognostic factor for event–free survival in T-lineage ALL.[282]

The *Immature, Early Thymocyte, Early T ALL, stage T_{IB} ALL*, is characterized by the expression of CD2 in addition to CD5 and CD7. The CD2+CD10– T-ALL subtype correlates with disruption of the *TAL-1*, also termed *SCL*, gene, which occurs in a large percentage of patients with T-ALL.[344,345]

The *Cortical T, Common Thymocyte, or stage T_{II} ALL* demonstrates expression of the thymocyte marker CD1. With respect to membrane CD3, CD4, and CD8 expression, there is large variability within this subtype. CD1 positivity carried prognostic significance for survival in some clinical trials.[31,280] CD10 can be frequently found on the surface of lymphoblasts from this T-ALL subtype and confers a favorable prognosis in children[30] as well as adults.[31,346] Although the biologic basis for this observation is unclear, it is of interest that in normal lymphopoiesis CD10 marks T lymphocytes destined for apoptosis[32,33] Expression of CD34 in T-lineage ALL, which occurs much less frequently than in B-lineage ALL, correlates with CD10 negativity and CNS disease at presentation[140,347] and with delayed achievement of complete remission.[347] HLA-DR, another stem-cell antigen, can be detected in fewer than 20 percent of T-ALL cases. There exist conflicting conclusions regarding its prognostic significance.[31,346]

Mature T, Late T, Medullary Thymocyte, T or stage T_{III} ALL may lack TdT expression. Typically, CD3 and TCR proteins are present in the cell membrane, whereas in earlier stages TCR proteins may be found in the cytoplasm. The bulk of membrane CD3-positive T-ALLs are positive for either CD4 or CD8 and express the classical TCR-α/β, reflecting the maturation stage of the majority of circulating T cells and mature thymocytes. *TCRγδ+ T-cell ALL*, which may or may not be doubly negative for CD4 and CD8, occurs in approximately 10 percent of T-lineage ALL or about half of CD3,TCR+ T-ALL cases.[276,277,348–350] Thus, in T-ALL expressing TCR proteins, the TCRγδ is used much more frequently than by thymocytes or circulating T cells. TCRγδ+ T-ALL appears as a distinct subgroup in children, with better event-free survival when compared with TCRαβ+ disease.[276]

CD117-positive Acute Lymphocytic Leukemia

Although CD117 has a higher specificity in the recognition of AML than have CD33 and CD13, its expression is not exclusively seen on myeloid leukemic cells. Approximately 2 percent of adult ALL expressed CD117 on 100 percent of lymphoblasts in ECOG study E2993 (Paietta E, unpublished observation). These ALLs were of very immature T-cell phenotype, expressing intracytoplasmic, but not membrane CD3, TdT, CD2, and CD7 in the absence of CD5 and usually without CD4 or CD8. Other recent, acceptably large studies have reported an incidence of 3 to 10 percent, predominantly in immature T-cell phenotypes and rarely in B-lineage ALL,[37,168,169,351] with variable levels of CD117 expression. High levels of CD117 are found in CD3-CD4-CD8 triple-negative thymocytes[352,353] that have not yet rearranged their TCR genes,[353] which is reminiscent of the predominant antigen profile of CD117+ ALL. Among myeloid antigens tested, CD13 is correlated with CD117 expression in ALL[354] in the absence of MPO, CD33, CD65s, CD15, and

CD11b. Coexpression of CD34 and CD117 in ALL is not universal, occurring only in approximately half of cases.[169] Given its low frequency, the prognostic significance of CD117+ ALL is not yet established.

CD56 + (Natural Killer Cell) Acute Lymphocytic Leukemia

CD56-positive or NK cell ALL is a rare disease entity. In a recent ECOG database analysis, it accounted for 3 percent of adult ALL.[250] In contrast with other reports reviewed in this paper,[250] CD56+ ALL patients identified by ECOG expressed this NK-cell antigen on at least 90 percent of gated lymphoblasts, thus leaving no doubt regarding the suitability of this immunodiagnosis. The majority of CD56+ ALL cases present with a T-lineage immunophenotype, which is in line with the common developmental pathway of T lymphocytes and NK cells.[271–273,275,278] However, the ECOG analysis unexpectedly revealed CD56 expression in two patients with unequivocal B-lineage ALL.[250] Expression of B-lineage antigen in NK/T leukemia or lymphoma is an uncommon observation.[355,356] A developmental link between NK and B cells has recently been established.[253]

P-Glycoprotein Expression in Acute Lymphocytic Leukemia

Contrary to the association of CD34 with functionally active P-glycoprotein, (Pgp), the product of the MDR-1 gene, in AML,[139,357–359] there exists no apparent correlation between MDR-1 gene transcription and CD34 in adult ALL[360] (Paietta E, unpublished observation). The frequency of functionally active Pgp in ALL appears low.[359,360] The clinical significance of MDR in ALL is unclear, based on small studies and equivocal technologies.[142,360–364] P-Glycoprotein in ALL may be associated with other poor prognostic features, such as high white blood cell count, FAB L3, and a mature B-cell phenotype.[362]

Subclassification of Acute Myeloid Leukemia

In the minds of several investigators, immunophenotyping of AML is still at best complementary to morphologic evaluation. This is a serious mistake. Certain AML subtypes can only be diagnosed with certainty when detailed immunophenotyping is applied; for example, in minimally differentiated AML and within morphologically defined subgroups, immunophenotyping has provided subclassifications, that are prognostically relevant, as in the case of NK-AML with the morphology of hypogranular APL (FAB-M3v). The WHO classification suggested that, as in ALL, certain cytogenetic—molecular categories be recognized as distinct subtypes in AML.[77,78] Surrogate antigen markers already exist for some of these subtypes, for example, CD19/CD56 for t(8;21) leukemia. That the myeloid leukemic immunophenotype may deviate from that of its presumed normal counterstage, despite indistinguishable morphological features, is best exemplified in APL (see below). Phenotypic differences between normal and leukemic cells of similar morphologic appearance are helpful in the immunologic evaluation of remission bone marrows and the detection of residual disease.

Poorly or Minimally Differentiated Acute Myeloid Leukemia

According to the National Cancer Institute workshop on AML definition[310] and the FAB criteria on AML-M0,[10] FAB-M0, the AML subtype with the least morphologic differentiation, is diagnosed on the basis of ultrastructural evidence of MPO and/or blast cell reactivity with at least one "lineage-specific" myeloid antigen (e.g., CD33, CD13) in the absence of the lymphoid markers. Immunophenotypic profiles found in the literature to describe minimally differentiated AML reflect antigen expression patterns established in morphologically defined FAB-M0 leukemia.[147,191,365–367] As a result, minimally differentiated AML, as an immunophenotypic subgroup, represents a heterogeneous accumulation of immature leukemias. Unfortunately, a proposal by Stasi and Amadori[146] of new diagnostic criteria for this AML type does not include a change in this basically misleading approach.

We have taken the opposite approach by establishing the morphology of patients with immunophenotypically defined minimally differentiated AML, defined by low expression of CD65$_s$ (30 percent or less of blast cells).[15] The FAB subtypes within this immunologically homogeneous group differed markedly, with a high percentage of FAB-M0 and M1 accounting, however, for only about 60 percent of cases. It is a misconception that MPO invariably detects the earliest stages of AML.[368] In agreement with Storr et al.,[292] we have found MPO expression in significantly fewer blast cells from patients with minimally differentiated than from those with differentiated AML and have, in fact, seen examples of unequivocally myeloid leukemias lacking MPO and expressing solely CD33 and/or CD13.[15] In AML, intracytoplasmic[369,370] or membrane CD13[15] appears to represent one of the earliest or the earliest sign of myeloid differentiation. Minimally differentiated myeloblasts correspond to the level of early CFU-GM and accordingly lack more mature myeloid antigens (CD65$_{(s)}$, CD15$_{(s)}$) but frequently express stem cell features. If CD11b is present, the diagnosis of CD11b+ AML must be considered.[25] In MPO^{low}/– minimally differentiated AML, it is important to exclude megakaryocytic or erythroid leukemias.

Low and/or absent CD34 and/or HLA-DR and/or CD13 antigen despite CD33 expression should be explored further to exclude immature acute basophilic or mast-cell leukemia. The blasts may express variable MPO activity, and basophilic or mast-cell granulation by light microscopy is commonly absent.[371]

Given that data reported are derived from heterogeneous groups of leukemias, including obvious cases of ALL,[372] the prognosis of minimally differentiated AML is difficult to evaluate from the literature. The unfavorable outcome observed in some studies may be related to older age,[15] frequent expression of Pgp,[373] a high incidence of unfavorable cytogenetics, such as complex abnormalities and chromosome 5 or 7 aberrations,[374,375] or simply the high degree of immunologically defined blast cell immaturity.[303]

Differentiated Acute Myeloid Leukemia (Not Further Characterized)

The immunophenotype of differentiated leukemic myeloblasts in principle corresponds to that of normal myeloblasts that express the immature markers CD34, CD117, and HLA-DR in addition to membrane CD33, CD13, and invariably CD65$_{(s)}$. At the same time, these leukemic cells show evidence of advanced myeloid maturation, such as positivity for CD64 and occasionally CD15, whereas CD11b (a marker of myelocytes and metamyelocytes as well as immature monocytes) and CD14 (a marker of mature monocytes) are absent. The level of maturation is an important prognostic indicator in AML.[303,305]

Acute Myeloid Leukemia with t(8;21)(q22:q22)

Acute myeloid leukemia with t(8;21)(q22;q22), resulting in AML1/ETO fusion gene transcription, is now recognized as a distinct disease entity based on its prognostic implications[77,78] The classical immunophenotype of t(8;21) AML is rather unique, enabling diagnosis of this subtype even in the absence of cytogenetic–molecular information. These myeloblasts invariably express CD34 and commonly express CD19 and/or CD56.[16,17,376,377] The combination of CD19 and CD34 is the most predictive one for t(8;21) AML;[17] however, CD19 status does not appear to affect outcome in this AML subgroup.[378] The increased frequency of extramedullary disease in t(8;21) AML may be related to the expression of CD56, the neural cell adhesion molecule.[43,44] Expression of CD56 has been correlated with short remission duration and short survival in t(8;21) AML.[24] Another adhesion molecule, the integrin CD11a, is characteristically absent from t(8;21) myeloblasts.[18]

Acute Promyelocytic Leukemia

The immunophenotype of APL is unique and closely correlated with FAB-M3 and the cytogenetic hallmark of the disease, t(15;17)(q22;q11.2) and its molecular consequence, transcription of the PML/RARα fusion gene. Antigenic features of APL cells that correspond to those of normal promyelocytes are low expression of CD34, HLA-DR, the myelomonocytic antigens CD11b and CD14, and CD25.[54] Atypical for promyelocytes is the predominant expression of CD15,[54] and the coexpression of the monocyte–macrophage-associated antigens CD68 and CD9.[379] Inconsistency in the literature data on CD15 expression by APL cells results from the variable reactivity patterns of the numerous available CD15 antibodies with the CD15$_s$ molecule.[54,380] In the absence of CD34 and CD133, CD117 is a hallmark of APL, and CD117 is the ideal gating antibody for APL testing panels.[18] A diagnostic finding is the absence of the leukocyte adhesion molecule CD11a on leukemic promyelocytes,[18,381] which is otherwise ubiquitously found on the surface of myeloid leukemic cells with the exception of t(8;21) AML.[18] Whenever present, CD34 and CD2 expression correlate with M3v morphology.[12–14] Associations between immunophenotype, in particular CD2, and certain PML/RARα transcript forms[382,383] and outcome[383] have been suggested by some studies but not confirmed by others.[54,384–386]

The antigen profile of APL cells is similar to that of basophils (CD34–HLA-DR–CD15$_s$+CD14–CD68+CD9+) which has prompted the hypothesis that APL cells may be derived from a basophil precursor cell.[379] As is consistent with this idea, the presence of increased basophils in the bone marrow of some patients with APL,[222] the existence of a rare hyperbasophilic form of APL,[387,388] and the development of basophilia during induction therapy with ATRA,[389] may reflect spontaneous or ATRA-induced terminal differentiation of the leukemic cells into basophils. On the other hand, APL cells and basophils differ immunophenotypically in that basophils express CD11b and CD25 but lack CD117.[222,223]

A lack of CD38[379] in APL cells is not consistently observed. However, upregulation of CD38 expression by ATRA or arsenic trioxide may be the link between these two agents in the induction of the retinoic acid syndrome.[42] The other potential culprit in the development of the syndrome is the aminopeptidase CD13.[41] Expression of CD56 on the leukemic promyelocytes confers poor outcome in terms of overall survival[22,23] and possibly achievement of complete remission.[22]

Acute promyelocytic leukemia cells characteristically express low levels of Pgp, at the mRNA level,[390,391] the protein as well as the functional level.[390,392] Lung resistance-related protein (LRP) and multidrug resistance-associated protein (MRP1) similarly show low expression in APL.[392]

Like normal myeloid precursors and most AML cells, APL cells are CD45RA-positive with low CD45R0 expression.[63,381] In vitro treatment with ATRA decreases CD45RA while increasing the expression of CD45R0,[63,381] which is consistent with progressive myeloid maturation.[179] Further immunologic evidence for a differentiative process in vitro[381] and in vivo[393] is the ATRA-induced expression of CD11b on the previously CD11b-negative APL cells, a marker of mature granulomonocytic cells. Persistent absence of CD11a from these ATRA-induced CD15+ (no longer CD15s+)CD11b+ cells reflects incomplete differentiation.[381] The term "intermediate cells" characterizes a stage during ATRA-induced differentiation at which the leukemic cells, which have lost their promyelocytic appearance, show strong staining for both CD33 and the mature myeloid antigen CD16.[394] This staining pattern is not seen with normal CD16+ granulocytes, which weakly stain for CD33.[62] Immunologically normal CD33^{low}CD16+ granulocytes, which appear subsequently when ATRA-treated APL patients achieve remission, represent the matured progeny of the leukemic clone as suggested by the presence of Auer rods and the demonstration of the t(15;17) in these cells.[394]

Recently, a rare variant of the APL immunophenotype has been recognized, which differs from classical APL only in the positive expression of CD11a and which lacks the (15;17) translocation.[18] Given the exquisite sensitivity of APL to ATRA, it is essential to make every effort to correctly diagnose this disease.

CD56-Positive (Natural Killer) Acute Myeloid Leukemia

CD56+ or NK cell AML is immunophenotypically very similar to CD56+ APL and demonstrates M3v morphology but lacks the t(15;17).[395] The distinction between these two rare AML subtypes (4 to 6 percent of AML cases) is clinically important in that, at least in vitro, myeloid/NK leukemia lacks responsiveness to ATRA[395,396] and can follow an aggressive clinical course, which correlates with the level of NK cell–mediated cytotoxic function attributable to the coexpression of CD56 and CD11a by the blasts.[395] Expression of CD11a and of asialo-CD15 are reliable indicators of NK-AML in the distinction of NK-AML from APL.[18]

Acute Myelomonocytic (AMML) and Monocytic (AMOL) Leukemia

The two most informative markers for a monocytic component within a leukemia cell population are CD11b and CD14. Although CD14-positive leukemias are virtually always CD11b-positive, CD11b positivity does not predict for CD14 expression. CD11b+HLA-DR+CD14– leukemic cells may represent CD11b+ AML (see below); CD11b+HLA-DR–CD14– cells in all likelihood reflect normal maturing myeloid cells. Thus, combined testing for CD11b and HLA-DR will resolve this question. Occasionally, a CD11b+HLA-DR+ but CD14– and a CD14+ leukemic component can be observed side by side within the same leukemia cell population. Whether a minor CD14+ CD11b+HLA-DR+ cell component in a myeloblastic leukemia represents residual normal or leukemic monocytes may be difficult to establish because a major portion of acute monocytic leukemia (AMOL) cells lack CD34[151,159,304] (Paietta et al., unpublished). Lack of MPO expression is another feature typical of many cases of AMOL.[292,294] In such cases, differential expression of the CD24 antigen by normal and malignant myelomonocytic cells can be useful. Normal mature myeloid cells are CD24-positive,[62] whereas normal mature monocytes lack this antigen.[207,208] The opposite is true for their leukemic counterparts in that the majority of AML cells lack CD24 and some AMOL are CD24-positive[207,208] (Paietta et al., unpublished)

Inv(16)(p13q22) Acute Myeloid Leukemia

The WHO classification considers inv(16)(p13q22) AML with CBFβ/MYH11 fusion transcripts as a distinct entity.[77,78] This leukemia subtype typically occurs in association with bone marrow eosinophilia and often with myelomonocytic features. Expression of the T-cell antigen CD2 has been previously suggested as a surrogate marker for the inv(16) aberration.[397] However, CD2 expression in inv(16) AML is highly correlated with expression of the myelomonocytic antigens CD11b and CD14 and the same is true for AMLs lacking inv(16).[398]

CD11b-Positive Acute Myeloid Leukemia

Several studies had suggested the integrin CD11b as a marker of shortened survival in AML,[26–29] when ECOG initiated a retrospective outcome-driven database analysis on CD11b-positive AML.[25] Expression of CD11b by 32 percent or more of blast cells was the statistically defined cutoff point that distinguished between responders and treatment failures. CD11b-positive myeloblasts characteristically express HLA-DR, are frequently CD117-positive, with or without concomitant expression of CD34, and lack CD14. Whereas CD33 and CD13 are invariably present, low or lacking expression of CD65$_{(s)}$ can be noted in some instances. In terms of clinical response, CD11b-positive AML shows a significantly lower response rate than other AML subtypes. Similarly, Del Poeta et al.[399] confirmed an independent negative effect of CD11b on complete remission rate, which, however, was confined to the AML group over the age of 60 years.

Acute Myeloid Leukemia with 11q23 Aberrations

Although leukemias with 11q23 or MLL gene rearrangements are clinically and biologically highly heterogeneous, they are considered one category in the WHO classification.[77,78] Aside from t(4;11), which is predominantly found in ALL, as discussed above, most translocations involving 11q23 occur in both AML and ALL, with predominance toward myeloid lineage.[400] Multiparameter flow cytometry of de novo t(11q23) adult AML demonstrated no difference in antigen distribution when compared with cases of equal morphology but lacking t(11q23), in particular no increase in lymphoid antigen expression.[401,402] In the search for a surrogate marker for MLL gene rearrangements, monoclonal antibody 7.1 specific to the NG2 antigen, a member of the chondroitin sulfate proteoglycan family, has been tested for its reactivity in t(11q23) leukemias. Although 100 percent specificity for leukemic cells with MLL rearrangements has been generally observed,[403–406] sensitivity, particularly in AML, is unconvincingly low (50 to 75 percent).[403,404,406]

Philadelphia Chromosome–Positive Acute Myeloid Leukemia

The incidence of Ph-positive AML is less than 1 percent.[407] The morphology is predominantly immature (FAB M0, M1), and expression of stem cell antigens, such as CD34, CD117, HLA-DR, and TdT, is common. Antigenic evidence of myeloid maturation (e.g., expression of CD65$_s$) may be absent. Expression of one or more lymphoid antigens or the presence of a distinct lymphoid leukemia component is a frequent finding.

Expression of Drug Resistance–Mediating Proteins in Acute Myeloid Leukemia

Acute myeloid leukemia patients with blast cells positive for P-glycoprotein (Pgp) and CD34 represent a subgroup with a particularly poor prognosis for remission achievement[139,217,357,358,408–410] and survival.[217,357,408] Given that CD34 is a surrogate marker for classic Pgp drug efflux activity, for example, as measured flow cytometrically by monitoring rhodamine[123] efflux,[139,357–359,411] these studies correlate functional Pgp with outcome. In contrast, studies basing their outcome correlations merely on Pgp protein or MDR1 gene mRNA analysis collect no information regarding drug efflux activity mediated by Pgp. This may in part explain the divergent data regarding Pgp and its prognostic significance in AML.[412] Other contributing factors are technical pitfalls, such as the use of arbitrary cutoff points of Pgp expression as criteria to define Pgp status[87] and the unwise choice of anti-Pgp antibodies, in particular, the choice of antibodies to intracellular Pgp epitopes[87,413] or of antibodies known to exhibit cross-reactivity with non-Pgp molecules.[414,415] Furthermore, the Pgp protein is posttranslationally modified through glycosylation or phosphorylation, the extent of which may differ in various hematopoietic tissues[413,416] and which can interfere with antibody recognition and Pgp function.[413,416,417] P-glycoprotein is virtually absent in APL,[390,418,419] which may contribute to the exquisite therapeutic sensitivity of this AML subtype. On the other hand, ATRA-resistant APL patients have been found to express Pgp.[420]

Although Pgp expression in normal bone marrow is low,[421] substantial Pgp protein expression can be found in mature hematopoietic cells, following the order CD56+ NK-cells > CD8+ T-cells > B- and CD4+ T cells > monocytes.[422–424] Granulocytes contain MDR1 mRNA but lack both Pgp protein expression and function.[424] These cells often contaminate leukemic bone marrow or peripheral blood specimens and must be excluded during flow cytometric Pgp analysis by gating on the blast cells. The presence of nonleukemic cells presents a problem for MDR1 mRNA analysis because RNA is usually isolated from the total mononuclear cell fraction. Early reports correlating MDR1 mRNA levels with outcome in AML, which were generated before information on Pgp expression in normal cells was available, therefore, have to be viewed with caution. The first International Workshop on MDR Detection Methods, has issued recommendations for standardizing MDR determinations and defining a clinically relevant MDR status.[87]

Recent data implicating Pgp in a drug efflux–independent role in the regulation of cell death or apoptosis shed a completely new light on a potential association between Pgp and outcome in AML.[425,426]

Alternative drug efflux mechanisms must be considered in AML, for instance, the multidrug resistance–associated protein 1 (MRP1), the lung resistance–related protein (LRP), and the breast cancer resistance or mitoxantrone resistance protein (BCRP/MXR).[412] The genes encoding MRP1 and LRP are both located on the short arm of chromosome 16,[427] and deletion of one MRP1 allele has been observed in some patients with inv(16)(p13q22).[428,429] As for Pgp, functional assays using flow cytometry is the preferred method for establishing resistance mediated by these alternative proteins. Multidrug resistance protein (MRP) functional activity is best measured with calcein AM,[430,431] whereas rhodamine[123] is not efficiently transported by MRP.[430] Intracellular daunorubicin accumulation is often used as a collective measure of drug efflux mechanisms in leukemic cells when Pgp, MRP, and LRP are simultaneously evaluated. It is of note in terms of antigenic associations that unlike Pgp expression, MRP1 expression may be more frequent in CD34-negative than in CD34-positive AML.[432] Expression of MRP and LRP protein is found in normal bone marrow and peripheral blood leukocytes.[433–436] Regarding the clinical significance of MRP1 and LRP, the reader is referred to the literature to form an opinion from the multitude of conflicting data.[412,434,436–443]

Immunophenotyping of Acute Erythroid and Megakaryocytic Leukemia

There exists considerable overlap between the erythroid and megakaryocytic lineage at the gene as well as the protein level, both during normal development and in leukemic disorders.[231–233,236,237,444,445] In terms of their immunophenotypic diagnosis, the lack of MPO expression by blast cells is the first indication of acute erythroid (AEL) or acute megakaryocytic leukemia (AMegL).

Acute Erythroid Leukemia

The majority of patients with AEL lack CD34 and HLA-DR expression.[446] Despite the finding of glycophorin A as early as at the level of BFU-E,[232] blasts in a fraction of AEL fail to react with antibodies to this most specific erythroid marker[447,448] (Paietta E, unpublished observation). CD36 antibodies (to platelet glycoprotein IV), although strongly reactive with AEL cells[446] will also stain megakaryocytic cells.[233] The same is true for antibodies to blood group H antigen, the precursor structure of ABO blood group substances.[449] Both these antigens, however, identify early stages of erythroid maturation, thereby increasing the odds of identifying a case of AEL. Blood group H antigen has also been demonstrated on leukemic blasts from patients with acute or chronic myelogenous leukemia.[450] Myeloblasts and erythroblasts that are positive for blood group H antigen are distinguishable based on the myeloid antigens MPO or CD33, CD13, CD15, which are never, or rarely and selectively, expressed on erythroblasts, respectively.[446] This differentiation is important because myeloblasts may constitute a significant component of the leukemic cell population in AEL.

Acute Megakaryocytic Leukemia

Antibodies to platelet-specific glycoproteins (GPIIb/IIIa [CD41/CD61], GPIb-GPIX [CD42], GPIV [CD36, GPIIIb]) are most valuable in characterizing MPO– acute leukemia as AMegL. If platelet peroxidase (PPO) activity, the enzymatic marker of megakaryocytic precursor cells,[242] is detected by electron microscopy in more cells than are recognized as megakaryocytic by platelet GP expression,[297] two explanations may apply. Either this finding reflects the appearance of PPO activity before platelet-specific GP during megakaryocytopoiesis,[451] or it represents staining of PPO-like activity transiently present during early stages of normal and leukemic erythropoiesis.[446] Therefore, surface marker analysis with platelet GP-specific antibodies is essential in the diagnosis of AMegL. The expression of GPIIIa or GPIIb/GPIIIa on CFU-MK,[235,240] which lack PPO activity,[242] implies that platelet GP analysis may not only be methodologically easier but also more specific and more sensitive than PPO studies. False-positive staining of AML blast cells with antiplatelet antibodies is due to the adhesion of platelets, possibly mediated by CD15, the ligand for P-selectin (CD62P) expressed on the cell surface of activated platelets[452] (Paietta et al., unpublished). The platelet GPs CD41 and CD36 are expressed during erythropoiesis, but CD41 and to a lesser degree CD36 are restricted to early, HLA-DR+CD34– erythroid precursors, usually expressing CD71.[231] In AMegL, CD41 is commonly associated with CD34, whereas CD36 is a late differentiation marker of CD34– megakaryocytic cells that also express CD42.[233] The differential expression of CD41 (immature and mature) and CD42 (mature) on megakaryocytic cells is used to distinguish between promegakaryocytic CD41+ and megakaryoblastic CD41+CD42+ AMegL.[453] The AMegL cells commonly express HLA-DR,[453,454] CD34,[454,455] and the early megakaryocytic antigens CD105 and CD109 (Paietta E, unpublished observation), suggesting their derivation from the promegakaryoblast or CFU-MK stage,[240] which is consistent with their undifferentiated lymphoid-like appearance.[242] Staining of subsets of cells in AMegL for the myeloid antigens CD33, CD13, or CD11b may represent a myeloblast component, particularly in cases in which megakaryocytic blasts account for less than 50 percent of leukemic cells, or may reflect coexpression of platelet and myeloid antigens by the megakaryocytic blasts.[454,455] The immunologic detection of micromegakaryocytes in the peripheral blood of patients with myelofibrosis is indicative of AMegL,[455,456] since megakaryoblasts produce and secrete an active form of transforming growth factor (TGF)-β, which promotes the synthesis of collagen in bone marrow fibroblasts.[456]

Expression of c-mpl, the thrombopoietin receptor, does not predict for AMegL[457,458] (Paietta E, unpublished observation); this is comparable to the finding that it does not predict for commitment to the megakaryocytic lineage during normal hematopoiesis.[232] Favorable cytogenetics in AML appear to correlate with lower levels of c-mpl protein.[458] Inferior treatment responses have been seen in AML patients expressing c-mpl mRNA.[457,459,460]

The vast information provided today on detailed phenotypic profiles of leukemic cells using a multiparameter technological approach offers a chance to challenge conventional viewpoints on leukemogenesis by gaining novel insights into the origin and behavior of these malignant cells. As a result, our perspectives on the significance of characterizing acute leukemias according to immunobiological features may shift from the mere search for malignancy-associated qualitative phenotypic alterations to recognizing immunophenotyping as an essential source of information regarding the disruption of the specific regulatory circuits of cell proliferation and differentiation that lead to leukemia.

REFERENCES

1. Porwit-MacDonald A, Björklund E, Lucio P et al: BIOMED-1 Concerted Action report: Flow cytometric characterization of CD7+ subsets in normal bone marrow and as a basis for the diagnosis and follow-up of T cell acute lymphoblastic leukemia (T-ALL). Leukemia 14:816–825, 2000.

2. Paietta E: Immunophenotyping of adult leukemia. In Steele GD Jr, Phillips TL, Chabner BA, Gansler TS (eds): American Cancer Society Atlas of Clinical Oncology. Series Volume, Wiernik PH (ed): Adult Leukemias BC Decker, Hamilton, Ont., 2001 (in press).

3. Paietta E, Papenhausen P: Cytogenetic alterations and related molecular consequences in adult leukemia. In Steele GD Jr, Phillips TL, Chabner BA, Gansler TS (eds): American Cancer Society Atlas of Clinical Oncology Series Volume, Adult Leukemias Wiernik PH (ed.): BC Decker, Hamilton, Ont. 2001 (in press)

4. Dyck JA, Warrell RP Jr, Evans RM et al: Rapid diagnosis of acute promyelocytic leukemia by immunohistochemical localization of PML/RARα protein. Blood 86:862, 1995.

5. Falini B, Flenghi L, Fagioli M et al: Immunocytochemical diagnosis of the acute promyelocytic leukemia (M3) with the monoclonal antibody PG-M3 (anti-PML). Blood 90:4046, 1997.

6. Harris NL, Jaffe ES, Diebold J et al: World Health Organization classification of neoplastic diseases of the hematopoietic and lymphoid tissues: Report of the clinical advisory committee meeting (Airlie House, Virginia, November 1997). J Clin Oncol 17:3835, 1999.

7. Forkner CE: Leukemia and Allied Disorders. Macmillan, New York, 1938.

8. Bennett JM, Catovsky D, Daniel MT et al: Proposed revised criteria for the classification of acute myeloid leukemia. Ann Intern Med 103:620, 1985.

9. Melnick A, Licht JD: Deconstructing a disease: RARα, its fusion partners, and their roles in the pathogenesis of acute promyelocytic leukemia. Blood 93:3167, 1999.

10. Bennett JM, Catovsky D, Daniel MT et al: Proposal for the recognition of minimally differentiated acute myeloid leukemia. Br J Haematol 78:325, 1991.

11. Goasguen JE, Matsuo T, Cox C et al: Evaluation of the dysmyelopoiesis in 336 patients with de novo acute myeloid leukemia: Major importance of dysgranulopoiesis for remission and survival. Leukemia 6:520, 1992.

12. Exner M, Thalhammer R, Kapiotis S et al: The "typical" immunophenotype of acute promyelocytic leukemia (APL-M3): Does it prove true for M3-variant? Cytometry 42:106, 2000.

13. Sainty D, Liso V, Cantù-Rajnoldi A et al: A new morphologic classification system for acute promyelocytic leukemia distinguishes cases with underlying PLZF/RARA gene rearrangements. Blood 96:1287, 2000.

14. Specchia G, Mestice A, Carluccio P et al: Biological features of CD34+ CD2+ acute promyelocytic leukemia (APL). Blood 96:115a, #495, 2000.

15. Paietta E, Neuberg D, Bennett JM et al: Novel definition of undifferentiated (UNDIF) acute myeloid leukemia (AML) by low expression of the CD65s carbohydrate molecule: Analysis of 996 patients from the ECOG database. Blood (Suppl 1):220b, #3723, 1997.

16. Hurwitz CA, Raimondi SC, Head D et al: Distinctive immunophenotypic features of t(8;21)(q22;q22) acute myeloblastic leukemia in children. Blood 80:3182, 1992.

17. Ferrara F, Di Noto R, Annunziata M et al: Immunophenotypic analysis enables the correct prediction of t(8;21) in acute myeloid leukemia. Br J Haematol 102:444, 1998.

18. Paietta E: Immunophenotyping and P-glycoprotein in APL. In Advances in Blood Disorders, Series Volume: Tallman MS, Avvisati G (eds.) APL: Towards the Curability of Acute Myeloid Leukemia. (in press)

19. Paietta E, Racevskis J, Neuberg D et al: Expression of CD25 (interleukin-2 receptor α chain) in adult acute lymphoblastic leukemia predicts for the presence of BCR/ABL fusion transcripts: Results of a preliminary laboratory analysis of ECOG/MRC Intergroup Study E2993. Leukemia. 11:1887, 1997.

20. Borowitz MJ, Rubnitz J, Nash M et al: Surface antigen phenotype can predict TEL-AML1 rearrangement in childhood B-precursor ALL: A Pediatric Oncology Group study. Leukemia 12:1764, 1998.

21. De Zen L, Orfao A, Cazzaniga G et al: Quantitative multiparametric immunophenotyping in acute lymphoblastic leukemia: Correlation with specific genotype I ETV6/AML1 ALLs identification. Leukemia 14:1225, 2000.

22. Murray CK, Estey E, Paietta E et al: CD56 expression in acute promyelocytic leukemia: A possible indicator of poor treatment outcome? J Clin Oncol 17:293, 1999.

23. Ferrara F, Morabito F, Martino B et al: CD56 expression is an indicator of poor clinical outcome in patients with acute promyelocytic leukemia treated with simultaneous all-trans retinoic acid and chemotherapy. J Clin Oncol 18:1295, 2000.

24. Baer MR, Stewart CC, Lawrence D et al: Expression of the neural cell adhesion molecule CD56 is associated with short remission duration and survival in acute myeloid leukemia with t(8;21)(q22;q22). Blood 90:1643, 1997.

25. Paietta E, Andersen J, Yunis J et al: Acute myeloid leukemia expressing the leucocyte integrin CD11b—a new leukemic syndrome with poor prognosis: Result of an ECOG database analysis. Br J Haematol 100:265, 1998.

26. Tucker J, Dorey E, Gregory WM et al: Immunophenotype of blast cells in acute myeloid leukemia may be a useful predictive factor for outcome. Hematol Oncol 8:47, 1990.

27. Bradstock K, Matthews J, Benson E et al: Prognostic value of immunophenotyping in acute myeloid leukemia. Blood 84:1220, 1994.

28. Vidriales MB, Orfao A, López-Berges MC et al: Prognostic value of S-phase cells in AML patients. Br J Haematol 89:342, 1995.

29. Repp RP, Schaekel U, Soucek S et al: Immunophenotyping is an independent factor for risk stratification in AML. Proc Am Soc Clin Oncol 20:282a, #1126, 2001.

30. Pui C-H, Rivera GK, Hancock ML et al: Clinical significance of CD10 expression in childhood acute lymphoblastic leukemia. Leukemia 7:35, 1993.

31. Boucheix C, David, B, Sebban C et al: Immunophenotype of adult acute lymphoblastic leukemia, clinical parameters, and outcome: An analysis of a prospective trial including 562 tested patients (LALA87). Blood 84:1603, 1994.

32. Cutrona G, Leanza N, Ulivi M et al: Expression of CD10 by human T-cells that undergo apoptosis both in vitro and in vivo. Blood 94:3067, 1999.

33. Bladon J, Taylor P: The expression of CD10 by apoptotic lymphocytes is preceded by a pronounced externalization of phosphatidylserine. (Letter) Blood :96:4009, 2000.

34. Macedo A, Orfao A, Martínez A et al: Immunophenotype of c-kit cells in normal human bone marrow: Implications for the detection of minimal residual disease in AML. Br J Haematol 89:338, 1995.

35. Di Noto R, Lo Pardo C, Schiavone EM et al: Stem cell factor receptor (c-kit, CD117) is expressed on blast cells from most immature types of acute myeloid malignancies but is also a characteristic of a subset of acute promyelocytic leukemia. Br J Haematol 92:562, 1996.

36. Valverde LR, Matutes E, Farahat N et al: C-kit receptor (CD117) expression in acute leukemia. Ann Hematol 72:11, 1996.

37. Bene MC, Bernier M, Casasnovas RO et al: The reliability and specificity of c-kit for the diagnosis of acute myeloid leukemias and undifferentiated leukemias. Blood 92:596, 1998.

38. Nomdedéu JF, Mateu R, Altès A et al: Enhanced myeloid specificity of CD117 compared with CD13 and CD33. Leuk Res 23:341, 1999.

39. Schwartz S, Heinecke A, Zimmermann M et al: Expression of the c-kit receptor (CD117) is the feature of almost all subtypes of de novo acute myeloblastic leukemia (AML), including cytogenetically good-risk AML, and lacks prognostic significance. Leuk Lymphoma 34:85, 1999.

40. Kornblau SM, Thall P, Huh YO et al: Analysis of CD7 expression in acute myelogenous leukemia: Martingale residual plots com-

bined with "optimal" cutpoint analysis reveals absence of prognostic significance. Leukemia 9:1735, 1995.

41. Vahdat L, Maslak P, Miller WH Jr et al: Early mortality and the retinoic acid syndrome in acute promyelocytic leukemia: Impact of leukocytosis, low-dose chemotherapy, PMN/RAR-α isoform, and CD13 expression in patients treated with all-trans retinoic acid. Blood 84:3843, 1994.

42. Deaglio S, Mehta K, Malavasi F: Human CD38: A (r)evolutionary story of enzymes and receptors. Leuk Res 25:1, 2001.

43. Tallman MS, Hakimian D, Shaw JM et al: Granulocytic sarcoma is associated with the 8;21 translocation in acute myeloid leukemia. J Clin Oncol 11:690, 1993.

44. Krishnan K, Ross CW, Adams PT et al: Neural cell-adhesion molecule (CD-56)-positive, t(8;21) acute myeloid leukemia (AML, M-2) and granulocytic sarcoma. Ann Hematol 69:321, 1994.

45. Delwel R, Bot F, Knapp W et al: Vim-2, candidate monoclonal antibody for purging autologous marrow grafts in acute myeloblastic leukemia. Bone Marrow Transplantation 2:149, 1987.

46. Preijers FWMB, De Witte T, Wessels JMC et al: Autologous transplantation of bone marrow purged in vitro with anti-CD7-(WT1-) ricin A immunotoxin in T-cell lymphoblastic leukemia and lymphoma. Blood 74:1152, 1989.

47. Robertson MJ, Soiffer RJ, Freedman AS et al: Human bone marrow depleted of CD33-positive cells mediates delayed but durable reconstitution of hematopoiesis: Clinical trial of MY9 monoclonal antibody-purged autografts for the treatment of acute myeloid leukemia. Blood 79:2229, 1992.

48. Grossbard ML, Press OW, Appelbaum FR et al: Monoclonal antibody-based therapies of leukemia and lymphoma. Blood 80:863, 1992.

49. Selvaggi KJ, Wilson LE, Mills LE et al: Improved outcome for high-risk acute myeloid leukemia patients using autologous bone marrow transplantation and monoclonal antibody-purged bone marrow. Blood 83:1698, 1994.

50. Sievers EL, Larson RA, Estey E et al: Preliminary results of the efficacy and safety of gemtuzumab ozogamicin in patients with AML in first relapse. Pr Am Soc Clin Oncol 18:21a, 1999.

51. Stadtmauer EA, Larson RA, Sievers EL et al: An updated report of the efficacy and safety of gemtuzumab ozogamicin in 188 patients with acute myeloid leukemia in first relapse. Proc Am Soc Clin Oncol 20:301a, #1203, 2001.

52. Naito K, Takeshita A, Shigeno K et al: Calicheamycin-conjugated humanized anti-CD33 monoclonal antibody (gemtuzumab zogamicin, CMA-676) shows cytocidal effect on CD33-positive leukemia cell lines, but is inactive on P-glycoprotein-expressing sublines. Leukemia 14:1436, 2000.

53. Hainsworth JD: Monoclonal antibody therapy in lymphoid malignancies. Oncologist 5:376, 2000.

54. Paietta E, Andersen J, Gallagher R et al: The immunophenotype of acute promyelocytic leukemia (APL): An ECOG study. Leukemia 8:1108, 199.

55. Sonneveld P: Multidrug resistance in hematological malignancies. J Intern Med 247:521, 2000.

56. Greaves M: Clincal applications of cell surface markers. Prog Haematol 9:255, 1975.

57. Rodt H, Netzel B, Thiel E et al: Classification of leukemic cells with T- and O-ALL-specific antisera. In Thierfelder S, Rodt H, Thiel E (eds): Immunological Diagnosis of Leukemias and Lymphomas. p. 87. Springer Verlag, Berlin, 1977.

58. Köhler G, Milstein C: Continuous cultures of fused cells secreting antibody of predefined specificity. Nature 256:495, 1975.

59. Bernard A, Boumsell L, Dausset J et al: Leucocyte Typing: Human Leucocyte Differentiation Antigens Detected by Monoclonal Antibodies. Springer-Verlag, Berlin, 1984.

60. Reinherz EL, Haynes BF, Nadler LM et al: Leucocyte Typing II. Springer-Verlag, New York, 1986.

61. McMichaels AJ, Beverly PCL, Cobbold S et al: Leucocyte Typing III: White Cell Differentiation Antigens. Oxford University Press, Oxford, 1987.

62. Knapp W, Dorken B, Gilks WR et al: Leucocyte Typing IV: White Cell Differentiation Antigens. Oxford University Press, Oxford, 1989.

63. Schlossman SF, Boumsell L, Gilks W et al: Leucocyte Typing V: White Cell Differentiation Antigens. Oxford University Press, Oxford, 1994.

64. Kishimoto T, Kikutani H, von dem Borne AEGK et al: Leucocyte Typing VI: White Cell Differentiation Antigens. Garland Publishing, New York, 1998.

65. Mason D, Anolré P, Bensussan A et al: Leucocyte Typing VII. White Cell Differentiation Antigen. Oxford University Press, 2002.

66. Lanza F, Latorraca A, Moretti S et al: Comparative analysis of different permeabilization methods for the flow cytometry measurement of cytoplasmic myeloperoxidase and lysozyme in normal and leukemic cells. Cytometry 30:134, 1997.

67. Kappelmayer J, Gratama JW, Karászi E et al: Flow cytometric detection of intracellular myeloperoxidase, CD3 and CD79a. Interaction between monoclonal antibody clones, fluorochromes and sample preparation protocols. J Immunol Methods 242:53, 2000.

68. Koester SK, Bolton WE: Intracellular markers. J Immunol Methods 243:99, 2000.

69. Mason DY, Cordell JL, Tse AGD et al: The IgM-associated protein mb-1 as a marker of normal and neoplastic B cells. J Immunol 147:2474, 1991.

70. Verschuren MCM, Comans-Bitter WM, Kapteijn CAC et al: Transcription and protein expression of mb-1 and B29 genes in human hematopoietic malignancies and cell lines. Leukemia 7:1939, 1993.

71. Bell PB, Rooney N, Bosanquet AG: CD79a detected by ZL74 separates chronic lymphocytic leukemia from mantle cell lymphoma in the leukemic phase. Cytometry 38:102, 1999.

72. Lai R, Juco J, Lee SF et al: Flow cytometric detection of CD79a expression in T-cell acute lymphoblastic leukemia. Am J Clin Pathol 113:823, 2000.

73. Pilozzi E, Pulford K, Jones M et al: C-expression of CD79a (JCB117) and CD3 by lymphoblastic lymphoma. J Pathol 186:140, 1998.

74. Buccheri V, Mihaljevi B, Matutes E et al: mb-1: A new marker for B-lineage lymphoblastic leukemia. Blood 82:853, 1993.

75. Arber DA, Jenskins KA, Slovak ML: CD79α expression in acute myeloid leukemia. High frequency of expression in acute promyelocytic leukemia. Am J Pathol 149:1105, 1996.

76. Braylan RC, Orfao A, Borowitz MJ et al: Optimal number of reagents to evaluate hematolymphoid neoplasias: Results of an international consensus meeting. Cytometry 46:23, 2001.

77. Bennett JM: World Health Organization classification of the acute leukemias and myelodysplastic syndrome. Int J Hematol 72:131, 2000.

78. Jaffe ES, Harris NL, Stein H, Vardiman JW (eds.): WHO Classification of Tumors: Pathology and Genetic Series: Hematopoietic and Lymphoid Neoplasms. IARC Press, Washington, Lyon, 2001.

79. Bene AC, Castoldi G, Knapp W et al: Proposals for the immunologic classification of acute leukemias. Leukemia 9:1783, 1995.

80. Paietta E, Andersen J, Wiernik PH: A new approach to analyzing the utility of immunophenotyping for predicting clinical outcome in acute leukemia. Leukemia 10:1, 1996.

81. Campana D, Behm FG: Immunophenotyping of leukemia. J Immunol Methods 243:59, 2000.

82. Willman CL: Acute leukemias: The paradigm for the integration of new technologies in diagnosis and classification. Mod Pathol 12:218, 1999.

83. Stelzer GT, Shults KE, Loken MR: CD45 gating for routine flow cytometric analysis of human bone marrow specimens. Ann N Y Acad Sci 677:265, 1993.

84. Paietta E, Racevskis J, Bennett JM, Wiernik PH: Differential expression of terminal transferase (TdT) in acute lymphocytic leukemia expressing myeloid antigens and TdT positive acute myeloid leukemia as compared to myeloid antigen negative acute lymphocytic leukemia. Br J Haematol 84:416, 1993.

85. Terstappen LWMM, Safford M, Könemann S et al: Flow cytometric characterization of acute myeloid leukemia. Part II Phenotypic heterogeneity at diagnosis. Leukemia 5:757, 1991.

86. Stelzer GT, Marti G, Hurley A et al: US–Canadian consensus recommendations on the immunophenotypic analysis of hematological neoplasia by flow cytometry: Standardization and validation of laboratory procedures. Cytometry 30:214, 1997.

87. Beck WT, Grogan T, Willman C et al: The St. Jude workshop on methods to detect P-glycoprotein-associated multidrug resistance: Findings and consensus recommendations. Cancer Res 56:3010, 1996.

88. Cualing H, Kothari R, Balachander T: Immunophenotypic diagnosis of acute leukemia by using decision tree induction. Lab Invest 79:205, 1999.

89. Borowitz MJ, Bray R, Gascoyne R et al: US-Canadian consensus recommendations on the immunophenotypic analysis of hematologic neoplasia by flow cytometry: Data analysis and interpretation. Cytometry 30:236, 1997.

90. Willman CL, Stewart CC: General principles of multiparameter flow cytometric analysis: Applications of flow cytometry in the diagnostic pathology laboratory. Semin Diagn Pathol 6:3, 1989.

91. Jennings CD, Foon KA: Recent advances in flow cytometry: Application to the diagnosis of hematologic malignancy. Blood 90:2863, 1997.

92. Weinkauff R, Estey EH, Starostik P et al: Use of peripheral blood blasts vs bone marrow blasts for diagnosis of acute leukemia. Am J Clin Pathol 111:733, 1999.

93. Islam D, Lindberg AA, Christensson B: Peripheral blood cell preparation influences the level of expression of leukocyte cell surface markers as assessed with quantitative multicolor flow cytometry. Cytometry 22:128, 1995.

94. Elghetany MT: Surface marker abnormalities in the myelodysplastic syndromes. Haematologica 83:1104, 1998.

95. Nagai K, Sohda H, Kuriyama K et al: Usefulness of immunocytochemistry for phenotypical analysis of acute leukemia; improved fixation procedure and comparative study with flow cytometry. Leuk Lymphoma 16:319, 1995.

96. Arber DA, Jenkins KA: Paraffin section immunophenotyping of acute leukemias in bone marrow specimens. Am J Clin Pathol 106:462, 1996.

97. Juneja S, Trute L, Westerman D et al: Paraffin section immunotyping in leukemias. Br J Haematol 109:267, 2000.

98. Thomas X, Campos L, Archimbaud E et al: Surface marker expression in acute myeloid leukemia at first relapse. Br J Haematol 81:40, 1992.

99. Chucrallah AE, Stass SA, Huh YO et al: Adult acute lymphoblastic leukemia at relapse. Cancer 76:985, 1995.

100. Guglielmi C, Cordone I, Boecklin F et al: Immunophenotype of adult and childhood acute lymphoblastic leukemia: Changes at first relapse and clinico-prognostic implications. Leukemia 11:1501, 1997.

101. Stewart CC: Monitoring minimal residual disease in AML. Cytotherapy 1:341, 1999.

102. Oelschlägel U, Nowak R, Schaub A et al: Shift of aberrant antigen expression at relapse or at treatment failure in acute leukemia. Cytometry 42:247, 2000.

103. Thirman MJ, Larson RA: Therapy-related myeloid leukemia. Hematol Oncol Clin North Am 10:293, 1996.

104. Van Wering ER, Van der Linden-Schrever BEM, Szczepanski T et al: Regenerating normal B-cell precursors during and after treatment of acute lymphoblastic leukemia: Implications for monitoring of minimal residual disease. Br J Haematol 110:139, 2000.

105. Macedo A, Orfao A, Martinez A et al: Immunophenotype of c-kit cells in normal human bone marrow: Implications for detection of minimal residual disease in AML. Br J Haematol 89:338, 1995.

106. Nakamura K, Ogata K, An E et al: Flow cytometric assessment of CD15+CD117+ cells for the detection of minimal residual disease in adult acute myeloid leukemia. Br J Haematol 108:710, 2000.

107. Campana D, Coustan-Smith E: Detection of minimal residual disease in acute leukemia by flow cytometry. Cytometry 38:139, 1999.

108. Plata E, Choremi-Papadopoulou H, Viglis V et al: Flow-cytometric detection of minimal residual disease with atypical antigen combinations in patients with de novo acute myeloid leukemia. Ann Hematol 79:543, 2000.

109. San Miguel JF, Martinez A, Macedo A et al: Immunophenotyping investigation of minimal residual disease is a useful approach for predicting relapse in acute myeloid leukemia patients. Blood 90:2465, 1997.

110. Yin JA, Tobal K: Detection of minimal residual disease in acute myeloid leukemia: Methodologies, clinical and biological significance. Br J Haematol 106:578, 1999.

111. Griesinger F, Pirò-Noack M, Kaib N et al: Leukemia-associated immunophenotypes (LAIP) are observed in 90% of adult and childhood lymphoblastic leukemia: Detection in remission marrow predicts outcome. Br J Haematol 105:241, 1999.

112. Reichle A, Rothe G, Krause S et al: Transplant characteristics: Minimal residual disease and impaired megakaryocytic colony growth as sensitive parameters for predicting relapse in acute myeloid leukemia. Leukemia 13:1227, 1999.

113. Craig W, Kay R, Cutler RL et al: Expression of Thy-1 on human hematopoietic progenitor cells. J Exp Med 177:1331, 1993.

114. Huang S, Terstappen LWMM: Lymphoid and myeloid differentiation of single human CD34+, HLA-DR+, CD38– hematopoietic stem cells. Blood 83:1515, 1994.

115. Broudy VC: Stem cell factor and hematopoiesis. Blood 90:1345, 1997.

116. Yin AH, Miraglia S, Zanjani ED et al: AC133, a novel marker for human hematopoietic stem and progenitor cells. Blood 90:5002, 1997.

117. Rappold I, Ziegler BL, Köhler I et al: Functional and phenotypic characterization of cord blood and bone marrow subsets expressing FLT3 (CD135) receptor tyrosine kinase. Blood 90:111, 1997.

118. Ratajczak MZ, Pletcher CH, Marlicz W et al: CD34+, kit+, rhodamine123^{low} phenotype identifies a marrow cell population highly enriched for human hematopoietic stem cells. Leukemia 12:942, 1998.

119. De Wynter EA, Buck D, Hart C et al: CD34+AC133+ cells isolated from cord blood are highly enriched in long-term culture-initiating cells, NOD/SCID-repopulating cells and dendritic cell progenitors. Stem Cells 16:387, 1998.

120. Pierelli L, Scambia G, Bonanno G et al: CD34+/CD105+ cells are enriched in primitive circulating progenitors residing in the G0 phase of the cell cycle and contain all bone marrow and cord blood CD34+/CD38$^{low/-}$ precursors. Br J Haematol 108:610, 2000.

121. Gallacher L, Murdoch B, Wu DM et al: Isolation and characterization of human CD34–Lin– hematopoietic stem cells using cell surface markers AC133 and CD7. Blood 95:2813, 2000.

122. Corbeil D, Röper K, Weigmann A et al: AC133 hematopoietic stem cell antigen: Human homologue of mouse kidney prominin or distinct member of a novel protein family? (Letter). Blood 91:2625, 1998.

123. Miraglia S, Godfrey W, Buck D: A response to AC133 hematopoietic stem cell antigen: Human homologue of mouse kidney prominin or distinct member of a novel protein family? (Letter). Blood 91:4390, 1998.

124. Bühring H-J, Seiffert M, Bock TA et al: Expression of novel surface antigens on early hematopoietic cells. Ann N Y Acad Sci 872:25, 1999.

125. Vavrova J, Filip S, Vokurkova D et al: Ex vivo expansion of CD34+/AC133+ -selected autologous peripheral blood progenitor cells (PBPC) in high-risk breast cancer patients receiving intensive chemotherapy. Hematol Cell Ther 41:105, 1999.

126. Peichev M, Naiyer AJ, Pereira D et al: Expression of VEGFR-2 and AC133 by circulating human CD34+ cells identifies a population of functional endothelial precursors. Blood 95:952, 2000.

127. Gehling UM, Ergun S, Schumacher U et al: In vitro differentiation of endothelial cells from AC133-positive progenitor cells. Blood 95:3106, 2000.

128. Bühring H-J, Seiffert M, Marxer A et al: AC133 antigen expression is not restricted to acute myeloid leukemia blasts but is also found on acute lymphoid leukemia blasts and on a subset of CD34+ B-cell precursors. (Letter). Blood 94:832, 1999.

129. Snell V, Jackson E, Buck D et al: Expression of AC133 antigen in leukemic and normal progenitors. Blood 92:119a, 1998.

130. Horn P, Tesch H, Staib P et al: Expression of AC133, a novel hematopoietic precursor antigen, on the acute myeloid leukemia cells. (Letter). Blood 93:1435, 1999.

131. Vercauteren SM, Sutherland HJ: Significance of AC133 expression on NOD/SCID engrafting ability and clinical outcome in acute myeloid leukemia (AML). Blood 96:106a, 454, 2000.

132. Fauth F, Weidmann E, Martin H et al: AC133 expression of acute myeloid leukemia blasts: Correlation to FAB and to CD34 expression and possible implications for peripheral blood progenitor cell purging in AML. Leuk Res 25:191, 2001.

133. Kratz-Albers K, Zühlsdorf M, Leo R et al: Expression of AC133, a novel stem cell marker, on human leukemic blasts lacking CD34 antigen and on a human CD34+ leukemic cell line: MUTZ-2. (Letter). Blood 92:4485, 1998.

134. Ebener U, Brinkmann A, Zotova V et al: Expression of AC133 vs. CD34 in acute childhood leukemias. Klin Padiatr 212:90, 2000.

135. Terstappen LWMM, Huang S, Safford M et al: Sequential generations of hematopoietic colonies derived from single nonlineage-committed CD34+ CD38– progenitor cells. Blood 77:1218, 1991.

136. Krause DS, Fackler MJ, Civin IC et al: CD34: Structure, biology, and clinical utility. Blood 87:1, 1996.

137. Watt SM, Bühring H-J, Rappold I et al: CD164, a novel sialomucin on CD34+ and erythroid subsets, is located on human chromosome 6q21. Blood 92:849, 1998.

138. Chaudhary PM, Roninson IB: Expression and activity of P-glycoprotein, a multidrug efflux pump, in human hematopoietic stem cells. Cell 66:85, 1991.

139. Paietta E: Classical multidrug resistance in acute myeloid leukemia. Med Oncol 14:53, 1997.

140. Pui C-H, Hancock ML, Head DR et al: Clinical significance of CD34 expression in childhood acute lymphoblastic leukemia. Blood 82:889, 1993.

141. van't Veer MB, van Putten WLJ, Verdonck LF et al: Acute lymphoblastic leukemia in adults: Immunological subtypes and clinical features at presentation. Ann Hematol 66:277, 1993.

142. Preti A, Kantarjian HM: Management of adult acute lymphocytic leukemia: Present issues and key challenges. J Clin Oncol 12:1312, 1994.

143. Lestingi TM, Hooberman AL: Philadelphia chromosome-positive acute lymphoblastic leukemia. Hematol Oncol Clin North Am 7:161, 1993.

144. Preti HA, O'Brien S, Giralt S et al: Philadelphia-chromosome positive adult acute lymphocytic leukemia: Characteristics, treatment results, and prognosis in 41 patients. Am J Med 97:60, 1994.

145. Koehler M, Behm FG, Shuster J et al: Transitional Pre-B-cell acute lymphoblastic leukemia of childhood is associated with favorable prognostic clinical features and an excellent outcome: A Pediatric Oncology Group study. Leukemia 7:2064, 1993.

146. Stasi R, Amadori S: AML-M0: A review of laboratory features and proposal of new diagnostic criteria. Blood Cells Mol Dis 25:120, 1999.

147. Kotylo PK, Seo I-S, Smith FO et al: Flow cytometric immunophenotypic characterization of pediatric and adult minimally differentiated acute myeloid leukemia (AML-M0). Am J Clin Pathol 113:193, 2000.

148. Campos L, Guyotat D, Archimbaud E et al: Clinical significance of multidrug resistance P-glycoprotein expression on acute nonlymphoblastic leukemia cells at diagnosis. Blood 79:473, 1992.

149. Geller RB, Zahurak M, Hurwitz CA et al: Prognostic importance of immunophenotyping in adults with acute myelocytic leukemia: The significance of the stem-cell glycoprotein CD34 (My10). Br J Haematol 76:340, 1990.

150. Sperling C, Büchner T, Sauerland C et al: CD34 expression in de novo acute myeloid leukemia. Br J Haematol 85:635, 1993.

151. Lanza F, Rigolin GM, Moretti S et al: Prognostic value of immunophenotypic characteristics of blast cells in acute myeloid leukemia. Leuk Lymphoma 13:81, 1994.

152. Serke S, Huhn D: Expression of class I, II, and III epitopes of the CD34 antigen by normal and leukemic hematopoietic cells. Cytometry 26:154, 1996.

153. Steen R, Egeland T: CD34 molecule epitope distribution on cells of hematopoietic origin. Leuk Lymphoma 30:23, 1998.

154. Fackler MJ, Civin CI, May WS: Up-regulation of transmembrane CD34 is associated with protein kinase C-mediated hyperphosphorylation of CD34. J Biol Chem 267:17540, 1992.

155. Spertini O, Cordey A-S, Monai N et al: P-selectin glycoprotein 1 is a ligand for L-selectin on neutrophils, monocytes, and CD34+ hematopoietic progenitor cells. J Cell Biol 135:523, 1996.

156. Fernandez M, Simon V, Minguell JJ: Production of soluble CD34 by human myeloid cells. Br J Haematol 111:426, 2000.

157. Murray L, Chen B, Galy A et al: Enrichment of human hematopoietic progenitor stem cell activity in the CD34+Thy-1+Lin– subpopulation from mobilized peripheral blood. Blood 85:368, 1995.

158. Humeau L, Bardin F, Maroc C et al: Phenotypic, molecular, and functional characterization of human peripheral blood CD34+Thy-1+ cells. Blood 87:949, 1996.

159. Geller RB, Bray RA: CD34 expression on acute myelocytic leukemia cells. (Commentary). Leuk Res 21:387, 1997.

160. Lamkin T, Brooks J, Annett G et al: Immunophenotypic differences between putative hematopoietic stem cells and childhood B-cell precursor acute lymphoblastic leukemia cells. Leukemia 8:1871, 1994.

161. Broudy VC: Stem cell factor and hematopoiesis. Blood 90:1345, 1997.

162. Ratajczak MZ, Pletcher CH, Marlicz W et al: CD34+, kit+, rhodamine 123^{low} phenotype identifies a marrow cell population highly enriched for human hematopoietic stem cells. Leukemia 12:942, 1998.

163. Escribano L, Ocqueteau M, Almeida J et al: Expression of the c-kit (CD117) molecule and normal and malignant hematopoiesis. Leuk Lymphoma 30:459, 1998.

164. Paietta E: Immunophenotypic peculiarities of APL. Proc 2nd Int Symp on Acute Promyelocytic Leukemia—A Curable Disease. p. 10, 1997.

165. Wells SJ, Bray RA, Stempora LL et al: CD117/CD34 expression in leukemic blasts. Am J Clin Pathol 106:192, 1996.

166. Smith FO, Broudy VC, Zsebo KM et al: Cell surface expression of c-kit receptors by childhood acute myeloid leukemia blasts is not of prognostic value: A report from the Childrens Cancer Group. Blood 84:847, 1994.

167. Sykora KW, Tomeczkowski J, Reiter A: C-kit receptors in childhood malignant lymphoblastic cells. Leuk Lymphoma 25:201, 1997.

168. Baersch G, Baumann M, Ritter J et al: Expression of AC133 and CD117 on candidate normal stem cell populations in childhood B-cell precursor acute lymphoblastic leukemia. Br J Haematol 107:572, 1999.

169. Uçkan D, Hiçsönmez G, Yetgin S et al: CD34/CD117 co-expression in childhood acute leukemia. Leuk Res 24:201, 2000.

170. Murray LJ, Bruno E, Uchida N et al: CD109 is expressed on a subpopulation of CD34+ cells enriched in hematopoietic stem and progenitor cells. Exp Hematol 27:1282, 1999.

171. Pierelli L, Scambia G, Bonanno G et al: CD34+/CD105+ cells are enriched in primitive circulating progenitors residing in the G0 phase of the cell cycle and contain all the bone marrow and cord blood CD34+/CD38$^{low/-}$ precursors. Br J Haematol 108:610, 2000.

172. Lo Pardo C, Altomonte M, Boccuni P et al: CD105 Workshop: Expression of CD105 on acute leukemia blast cells: Application for minimal residual disease detection. In Kishimoto T, Kikutani H, von dem Borne AEGK et al. (eds.): Leucocyte Typing VI: White Cell Differentiation Antigens, p. 711. Garland Publishing, New York, London, 1998.

173. Lansdorp PM, Sutherland HJ, Eaves CJ: Selective expression of CD45 isoforms on functional subpopulations of CD34+ hematopoietic cells from human bone marrow. J Exp Med 172:363, 1990.

174. Fritsch G, Buchinger P, Printz D et al: Rapid discrimination of early CD34+ myeloid progenitors using CD45-RA analysis. Blood 81:2301, 1993.

175. Galy AHM, Cen D, Travis M et al: Delineation of T-progenitor cell activity within the CD34+ compartment of adult bone marrow. Blood 85:2770, 1995.

176. Lansdorp PM, Dragowska W: Long-term erythropoiesis from constant numbers of CD34+ cells in serum-free cultures initiated with highly purified progenitor cells from human bone marrow. J Exp Med 175:1501, 1992.

177. Strobl H, Takimoto M, Majdic O et al: Myeloperoxidase expression in CD34+ normal human hematopoeitic cells. Blood 82:2069, 1993.

178. Olweus J, Lund-Johansen F, Terstappen LWMM: CD64/FcγRI is a specific granulomonocytic lineage marker on CD34+ hematopoietic progenitor cells. Blood 85:2402, 1995.

179. Caldwell CW, Patterson WP, Toalson BD et al: Surface and cytoplasmic expression of CD45 antigen isoforms in normal and malignant cell differentiation. Am J Clin Pathol 95:180, 1991.

180. Behm FG, Raimondi SC, Schell MJ et al: Lack of CD45 antigen on blast cells in childhood acute lymphoblastic leukemia is associated with chromosomal hyperdiploidy and other favorable prognostic features. Blood 79:1011, 1992.

181. Borowitz MJ, Shuster J, Carroll AJ et al: Prognostic significance of fluorescence intensity of surface marker expression in childhood B-precursor acute lymphoblastic leukemia. A Pediatric Oncology Group Study. Blood 89:3960, 1997.

182. DiGiusto D, Chen S, Combs J et al: Human fetal bone marrow early progenitors for T, B, and myeloid cells are found exclusively in the population expressing high levels of CD34. Blood 84:421, 1994.

183. Barcena A, Muench MO, Roncarolo MG et al: Tracing the expression of CD7 and other antigens during T- and myeloid-cell differentiation in the human fetal liver and thymus. Leuk Lymphoma 17:1, 1995.

184. Grümayer ER, Griesinger F, Hummell DS et al: Identification of novel B-lineage cells in human fetal bone marrow that coexpress CD7. Blood 77:64, 1991.

185. LeBien TW: Fates of human B-cell precursors. Blood 96:9, 2000.

186. Uckan FM: Regulation of human B-cell ontogeny. Blood 76:1908, 1990.

187. Gore SD, Kastan MB, Civin CI: Normal human bone marrow precursors that express terminal deoxynucleotidyl transferase include T-cell precursors and possible lymphoid stem cells. Blood 77:1681, 1991.

188. Dworzak MN, Fritsch G, Fröschl G et al: Four-color flow cytometric investigation of terminal deoxynucleotidyl transferase-positive lymphoid precursors in pediatric bone marrow: CD79a expression precedes CD19 in early B-cell ontogeny. Blood 92:3203, 1998.

189. Chabannon C, Wood P, Torok-Storb B: Expression of CD7 on normal human myeloid progenitors. J Immunol 149:2110, 1992.

190. Knapp W, Strobl H, Majdic O: Flow cytometric analysis of cell-surface and intracellular antigens in leukemia diagnosis. Cytometry 18:187, 1994.

191. Villamor N, Zarco M-A, Rozman M et al: Acute myeloblastic leukemia with minimal myeloid differentiation: Phenotypical and ultrastructural characteristics. Leukemia 12:1071, 1998.

192. Lauria F, Raspadori D, Martinelli G et al: Increased expression of myeloid antigen markers in adult acute lymphoblastic leukemia patients: Diagnostic and prognostic implications. Br J Haematol 87:286, 1994.

193. Uckun FM, Sather HN, Gaynon PS et al: Clinical features and treatment outcome of children with myeloid antigen positive acute lymphoblastic leukemia: A report from the Children's Cancer Group. Blood 90:28, 1997.

194. Putti MC, Rondelli R, Cocito MG et al: Expression of myeloid markers lacks prognostic impact in children treated for acute lymphoblastic leukemia: Italian experience in AIEOP–ALL 88–91 studies. Blood 92:795, 1998.

195. Nakamura Y, Noma M, Kidokoro M et al: Expression of CD33 antigen on normal human activated T lymphocytes. Blood 83:1442, 1994.

196. Bordessoule D, Jones M, Gatter KC, Mason DY: Immunohistological patterns of myeloid antigens: Tissue distribution of CD13, CD14, CD16, CD31, CD36, CD65, CD66 and CD67. Br J Haematol 83:370, 1993.

197. Macher BA, Buehler J, Scudder P et al: A novel carbohydrate, differentiation antigen on fucogangliosides of human myeloid cells recognized by monoclonal antibody VIM-2. J Biol Chem 263:10186, 1988.

198. Lowe JB, Kukowska-Latallo JF, Nair RP et al: Molecular cloning of a human fucosyltransferase gene that determines expression of

the Lewis x and VIM-2 epitopes but not ELAM-1-dependent cell adhesion. J Biol Chem 266:17467, 1991.

199. Ludwig W-D, Rieder H, Bartram CR et al: Immunophenotypic and genotypic features, clinical characteristics, and treatment outcome of adult Pro-B acute lymphoblastic leukemia: Results of the German multicenter trials GMALL 03/87 and 04/89. Blood 92:1898, 1998.

200. Hakomori S: Le^x and related structures as adhesion molecules. Histochem J 24:771, 1992.

201. Bevilacqua MP, Nelson RM: Selectins. J Clin Invest 91:379, 1993.

202. Muroi K, Suda T, Nojiri H et al: Reactivity profiles of leukemic myeloblasts with monoclonal antibodies directed to sialosyl-Le^x and other lacto-series type 2 chain antigens: Absence of reactivity with normal hematopoietic progenitor cells. Blood 79:713, 1992.

203. Majdic O, Liszka K, Lutz D, Knapp W: Myeloid differentiation antigen defined by a monoclonal antibody. Blood 58:1127, 1981.

204. Civin CI, Mirro J, Banquerigo ML: My-1, a new myeloid-specific antigen identified by a mouse monoclonal antibody. Blood 57:842, 1981.

205. Skacel PO, Edwards AJ, Harrison CT, Watkins WM: Enzymic control of the expression of the X determinant (CD15) in human myeloid cells during maturation: The regulatory role of 6'-sialyltransferase. Blood 78:1452, 1991.

206. Paietta E, Stockert RJ, Morell AG et al: Unique antigen of cultured Hodgkin's cells. A putative sialyltransferase. J Clin Invest 78:349, 1986.

207. Abramson CS, Kersey JH, LeBien TW: A monoclonal antibody (BA-1) reactive with cells of human B lymphocyte lineage. J Immunol 126:83, 1981.

208. Raife TJ, Lager DJ, Kemp JD, Dick FR: Expression of CD24 (BA-1) predicts monocytic lineage in acute myeloid leukemia. Am J Clin Pathol 101:296, 1994.

209. Louache F, Debili N, Marandin A et al: Expression of CD4 by human hematopoietic progenitors. Blood 84:3344, 1994.

210. Carlos TM, Harlan JM: Leukocyte-endothelial adhesion molecules. Blood 84:2068, 1994.

211. Terstappen LWMM, Safford M, Loken MR: Flow cytometric analysis of human bone marrow. III. Neutrophil maturation. Leukemia 4:657, 1990.

212. Terstappen LWMM, Loken MR: Myeloid cell differentiation in normal bone marrow and acute myeloid leukemia assessed by multidimensional flow cytometry. Anal Cell Pathol 2:229, 1990.

213. Tucker J, Dorey E, Gregory WM et al: Immunophenotype of blast cells in acute myeloid leukemia may be a useful predictive factor for outcome. Hematol Oncol 8:47, 1990.

214. Solary E, Casasnovas R-O, Campos L et al: Surface markers in adult acute myeloblastic leukemia: Correlation of CD19+, CD34+ and CD14+/DR- phenotypes with shorter survival. Leukemia 6:393, 1992.

215. Passlick B, Flieger D, Ziegler-Heitbrock HWL: Identification and characterization of a novel monocyte subpopulation in human peripheral blood. Blood 74:2527, 1989.

216. Kristensen JS, Hokland P: Monoclonal antibodies in myeloid diseases: Prognostic use in acute myeloid leukemia. Leuk Res 15:693, 1991.

217. Del Poeta G, Stasi R, Venditti A et al: Prognostic value of cell marker analysis in de novo acute myeloid leukemia. Leukemia 8:388, 1994.

218. Bonde J, Meyer K, Kjærvig Broe M et al: Improved flow cytometric identification of myelopoiesis by the simultaneous labeling with CD13, CD14 and CD66 monoclonal antibodies. Br J Haematol 92:269, 1996.

219. Strobl H, Scheinecker C, Csmarits B et al: Flow cytometric analysis of intracellular CD68 molecule expression in normal and malignant hemopoiesis. Br J Haematol 90:774, 1995.

220. Kirshenbaum AS, Goff JP, Semere T et al: Demonstration that human mast cells arise from a progenitor cell population that is CD34+, c-kit+, and expresses aminopeptidase N (CD13). Blood 94:2333, 1999.

221. Bühring HJ, Simmons PJ, Pudney M et al: The monoclonal antibody 97A6 defines a novel surface antigen expressed on human basophils and their multipotent and unipotent progenitors. Blood 94:2343, 1999.

222. Denburg JA: Basophil and mast cell lineages in vitro and in vivo. Blood 79:846, 1992.

223. Valent P: The phenotype of human eosinophils, basophils, and mast cells. J Allergy Clin Immunol 94:1177, 1994.

224. Füreder W, Agis H, Willheim M et al: Differential expression of complement receptors on human basophils and mast cells. J Immunol 155:3152, 1995.

225. Agis H, Beil WJ, Bankl HC et al: Mast cell-lineage versus basophil lineage involvement in myeloproliferative and myelodysplastic syndromes: Diagnostic role of cell immunophenotyping. Leuk Lymphoma 22:187, 1996.

226. Falcone FH, Haas H, Gibbs BF: The human basophil: A new appreciation of its role in immune responses. Blood 96:4028, 2000.

227. Sperr W, Horny H-P, Lechner K et al: Clinical and biologic diversity of leukemias occurring in patients with mastocytosis. Leuk Lymphoma 37:473, 2000.

228. Rand TH, Silberstein DS, Kornfeld H, Weller PF: Human eosinophils express functional interleukin 2 receptors. J Clin Invest 88:825, 1991.

229. Hartman M-L, Piliponsky AM, Temkin V et al: Human peripheral blood eosinophils express the stem cell factor. Blood 97:1086, 2001.

230. Civin CI, Strauss LC, Brovall C et al: Antigenic analysis of hematopoiesis. III. A hematopoietic progenitor cell surface antigen defined by a monoclonal antibody raised against KG-1a cells. J Immunol 133:157, 1984.

231. Okumura N, Tsuji K, Nakahata T: Changes in cell surface antigen expressions during proliferation and differentiation of human erythroid progenitors. Blood 80:642, 1992.

232. Basch RS, Zhang X-M, Dolzhanskiy A et al: Expression of CD41 and c-mpl does not indicate commitment to the megakaryocytic lineage during hematopoietic development. Br J Haematol 105:1044, 1999.

233. Greenwalt DE, Lipsky RH, Ockenhouse CF et al: Membrane glycoprotein CD36: A review of its roles in adherence, signal transduction, and transfusion medicine. Blood 80:1105, 1992.

234. Telen MJ: Erythrocyte blood group antigens: Not so simple after all. Blood 85:299, 1995.

235. Hoffman R: Regulation of megakaryocytopoiesis. Blood 74:1196, 1989.

236. Clay D, Rubinstein E, Mishal Z et al: CD9 and megakaryocyte differentiation. Blood 97:1982, 2001.

237. Debili N, Coulombel L, Croisille L et al: Characterization of a bipotent erythromegakaryocytic progenitor in human bone marrow. Blood 88:1284, 1996.

238. Ody C, Vaigot P, Quere P et al: Glycoprotein IIb-IIIa is expressed on avian multi-lineage hematopoietic progenitor cells. Blood 93:2898, 1999.

239. Law HKW, Bol SJL, Palatsides M et al: Analysis of human megakaryocytic cells using dual-color immunofluorescence labeling. Cytometry 41:308, 2000.

240. Debili N, Issaad C, Massé J-M, et al: Expression of CD34 and platelet glycoproteins during human megakaryocytic differentiation. Blood 80:3022, 1992.

241. Lepage A, Leboeuf M, Cazenave J-P et al: The $\alpha_{IIb}\beta_3$ integrin and GPIb-V-IX complex identify distinct stages in the maturation of CD34+ cord blood to cells to megakaryocytes. Blood 96:4169, 2000.

242. Breton-Gorius J, Vainchenker W: Expression of platelet proteins during the in vitro and in vivo differentiation of megakaryocytes and morphological aspects of their maturation. Semin Hematol 23:43, 1986.

243. Debili N, Wendling F, Cosman D et al: The mpl receptor is expressed in the megakaryocytic lineage from late progenitors to platelets. Blood 85:391, 1995.

244. Fava RA, Casey TT, Wilcox J et al: Synthesis of transforming growth factor-β1 by megakaryocytes and its localization to megakaryocytes and platelet α-granules. Blood 76:1946, 1990.

245. Seligmann M, Vogler LB, Pred'Homme JL et al: Immunological phenotypes of human leukemias of the B-cell lineage. Blood Cells 7:237, 1981.

246. Nadler LM, Korsmeyer SJ, Anderson KC et al: B cell origin of non-T cell acute lymphoblastic leukemia. A model for discrete stages of neoplastic and normal pre-B cell differentiation. J Clin Invest 74:332, 1984.

247. Brown G, Bunce CM, Howie AJ, Lord JM: Stochastic or ordered lineage commitment during hemopoiesis. Leukemia 1:150, 1987.

248. Janossy G, Bollum FJ, Bradstock KF et al: Terminal transferase-positive human bone marrow cells exhibit the antigenic phenotype of common acute lymphoblastic leukemia. J Immunol 123:1525, 1979.

249. Galy A, Travis M, Cen D et al: Human T, B, natural killer, and dendritic cells arise from a common bone marrow progenitor cell subset. Immunity 3:459, 1995.

250. Paietta E, Neuberg D, Richards S et al: Rare adult acute lymphocytic leukemia with CD56 expression in the ECOG experience shows unexpected phenotypic and genotypic heterogeneity. Am J Hematol 66:189, 2001.

251. Ryan DH, Nuccie BL, Ritterman I et al: Expression of interleukin-7 receptor by lineage-negative human bone marrow progenitors with enhanced lymphoid proliferative potential and B-lineage differentiation capacity. Blood 89:929, 1997.

252. Ishii T, Nishihara M, Ma F et al: Expression of stromal cell-derived factor-1/pre-B cell growth-stimulating factor receptor, CXC chemokine receptor 4, on CD34+ human bone marrow cells is a phenotypic alteration for committed lymphoid progenitors. J Immunol 163:3612, 1999.

253. Miller JS, McCullar V, Punzel M et al: Single adult human CD34+/Lin–/CD38– progenitors give rise to natural killer cells, B-lineage cells, dendritic cells, and myeloid cells. Blood 93:96, 1999.

254. Bertrand FE III, Billips LG, Burrows PD et al: Ig D_H gene segment transcription and rearrangement before surface expression of the pan-B-cell marker CD19 in normal human bone marrow. Blood 90:736, 1997.

255. Davi F, Faili A, Gritti C et al: Early onset of immunoglobulin heavy chain gene rearrangements in normal human bone marrow CD34+ cells. Blood 90:4014, 1997.

256. Wang Y-H, Nomura J, Faye-Petersen OM et al: Surrogate light chain production during B-cell differentiation: Differential intracellular versus cell surface expression. J Immunol 161:1132, 1998.

257. Lúcio P, Parreira A, van den Beemd MWM et al: Flow cytometric analysis of normal B-cell differentiation: A frame of reference for the detection of minimal residual disease in precursor-B-ALL. Leukemia 13:419, 1999.

258. Chang KL, Arber DA, Weiss LM: CD20: A review. App Immunohistochem 4:1, 1996.

259. Uckun FM, Song CW: Lack of CD24 antigen expression in B-lineage acute lymphoblastic leukemia is associated with intrinsic radiation resistance of primary clonogenic blasts. Blood 81:1323, 1993.

260. Ryan DH, Nuccie BL, Abboud CN, Winslow JM: Vascular cell adhesion molecule-1 and the integrin VLA-4 mediate adhesion of human B cell precursors to cultured bone marrow adherent cells. J Clin Invest 88:995, 1991.

261. Van Dongen JJM, Wolvers-Tettero ILM: Analysis of immunoglobulin and T cell receptor genes. Part I: Basic and technical aspects. Clin Chim Acta 198:1, 1991.

262. Lieber MR: Site-specific recombination in the immune system. FASEB J 5:2934, 1991.

263. Sklar J, Longtine J: The clinical significance of antigen receptor gene rearrangements in lymphoid neoplasia. Cancer 70 (suppl.):1710, 1992.

264. van Noesel CJM, van Lier RAW: Architecture of the human B-cell antigen receptor. Blood 82:363, 1993.

265. Nemazee D, Weigert M: Revising B cell receptors. J Exp Med 191:1813, 2000.

266. Tsuganezawa K, Kiyokawa N, Matsuo Y et al: Flow cytometric diagnosis of the cell lineage and developmental stage of acute lymphoblastic leukemia by novel monoclonal antibodies specific to human pre-B-cell receptor. Blood 92:4317, 1998.

267. Orloff DG, Ra C, Frank SJ et al: Family of disulphide-linked dimers containing the ζ and η chains of the T-cell receptor and the γ chain of Fc receptors. Nature 347:189, 1990.

268. Blom B, Verschuren MCM, Heemskerk MHM et al: TCR gene rearrangements and expression of the pre-T cell receptor complex during human T-cell differentiation. Blood 93:3033, 1999.

269. LeBien TW, Elstrom RL, Moseley M et al: Analysis of immunoglobulin and T-cell receptor gene rearrangements in human fetal bone marrow B lineage cells. Blood 76:1196, 1990.

270. Terstappen LWMM, Huang S, Picker LJ: Flow cytometric assessment of human T-cell differentiation in thymus and bone marrow. Blood 79:666, 1992.

271. Sánchez MJ, Muench MO, Roncarolo MG et al: Identification of a common T/natural killer cell progenitor in human fetal thymus. J Exp Med 180:569, 1994.

272. Spits H, Lanier LL, Philips JH: Development of human T and natural killer cells. Blood 85:2654, 1995.

273. Res P, Martinez-Cáceres E, Jaleco AC et al: CD34+/CD38^{dim} cells in the human thymus can differentiate into T, natural killer, and dendritic cells but are distinct from pluripotent stem cells. Blood 87:5196, 1996.

274. Márquez C, Trigueros C, Franco JM et al: Identification of a common developmental pathway for thymic natural killer cells and dendritic cells. Blood 91:2760, 1998.

275. Miller JS, Alley KA, McGlave P: Differentiation of natural killer (NK) cells from human primitive marrow progenitors in a stroma-based long-term culture system: Identification of a CD34+7+ NK progenitor. Blood 83:2594, 1994.

276. Schott G, Sperling C, Schrappe M et al: Immunophenotypic and clinical features of T-cell receptor $\gamma\delta$+ T-lineage acute lymphoblastic leukemia. Br J Haematol 101:753, 1998.

277. Langerak AW, Wolvers-Tettero ILM, van den Beemd MWM et al: Immunophenotypic and immunogenotypic characteristics of TCR$\gamma\delta$+ T cell acute lymphoblastic leukemia. Leukemia 13:206, 1999.

278. Phillips JH, Hori T, Nagler A et al: Ontogeny of human natural killer (NK) cells: Fetal NK cells mediate cytolytic function and express cytoplasmic CD3ε,δ proteins. J Exp Med 175:1055, 1992.

279. Bendelac A: CD1: Presenting unusual antigens to unusual T lymphocytes. Science 269:185, 1995.

280. Niehues T, Kapaun P, Harms DO et al: A classification based on T-cell selection-related phenotypes identifies a subgroup of childhood T-ALL with favorable outcome in the COALL studies. Leukemia 13:614, 1999.

281. Thiel E, Kranz BR, Raghavachar A et al: Prethymic phenotype and genotype of pre-T (CD7+/ER−)-cell leukemia and its clinical significance within adult acute lymphoblastic leukemia. Blood 73:1247, 1989.

282. Uckun FM, Steinharz PG, Sather H et al: CD2 antigen expression on leukemic cells as a predictor of event-free survival after chemotherapy for T-lineage acute lymphoblastic leukemia: A Children's Cancer Group Study. Blood 88:4288, 1996.

283. Uckun FM, Gaynon P, Sather H et al: Clinical features and treatment outcome of children with biphenotypic CD2+CD19+ acute lymphoblastic leukemia: A Children's Cancer Group Study. Blood 89:2488, 1997.

284. Legac E, Autran B, Merle-Beral H et al: CD4+CD7−CD57+ T cells: A new T-lymphocyte subset expanded during human immunodeficiency virus infection. Blood 79:1746, 1992.

285. Reinhold U, Abken H, Kukel S et al: CD7− T cells represent a subset of normal human blood lymphocytes. J Immunol 150:2081, 1993.

286. Hara J, Benedict SH, Champagne E et al: Relationship between rearrangement and transcription of the T-cell receptor α, β, and γ genes in B-precursor acute lymphoblastic leukemia. Blood 73:500, 1989.

287. Nosaka T, Kita K, Miwa H et al: Cross-lineage gene rearrangements in human leukemic B-precursor cells occur frequently with V-DJ rearrangements of IgH genes. Blood 74:361, 1989.

288. Dyer MJS: T-cell receptor δ/α rearrangements in lymphoid neoplasms. Blood 74:1073, 1989.

289. Sigaux F: The V(D)J recombination in acute lymphoid leukemias: A short review. Leuk Lymphoma 13:53, 1994.

290. Paietta E, Van Ness B, Bennett J et al: Lymphoid lineage-associated features in acute myeloid leukemia: Phenotypic and genotypic correlations. Br J Haematol 82:324, 1992.

291. Van der Schoot CE, Daams GM, Pinkster J et al: Monoclonal antibodies against myeloperoxidase are valuable immunological reagents for the diagnosis of acute myeloid leukemia. Br J Haematol 74:173, 1990.

292. Storr J, Dolan G, Coustan-Smith E et al: Value of monoclonal anti-myeloperoxidase (MPO7) for diagnosing acute leukemia. J Clin Pathol 43:847, 1990.

293. Kantarjian HM, Hirsch-Ginsberg C, Yee G et al: Mixed-lineage leukemia revisited: Acute lymphocytic leukemia with myeloperoxidase-positive blasts by electron microscopy. Blood 76:808, 1990.

294. Austin GE, Chan WC, Zhao W, Racine M: Myeloperoxidase gene expression in normal granulopoiesis and acute leukemia. Leuk Lymphoma 15:209, 1994.

295. Heil G, Gunsilius E, Raghavachar A et al: Ultrastructural demonstration of peroxidase expression in acute unclassified leukemias: Correlation to immunophenotype and treatment outcome. Blood 77:1305, 1991.

296. Schlaifer D, Cooper MR, Attal M et al: Myeloperoxidase: An enzyme involved in intrinsic vincristine resistance in human myeloblastic leukemia. Blood 81:482, 1993.

297. Buccheri V, Shetty V, Yoshida N et al: The role of an anti-myeloperoxidase antibody in the diagnosis and classification of acute leukemia: A comparison with light and electron microscopy cytochemistry. Br J Haematol 80:62, 1992.

298. Vela JA, Delgado I, Oña F: Myeloperoxidase detection by three-color flow cytometry in acute lymphoblastic leukemia. Am J Clin Pathol 112:122, 1999.

299. Crisan D, Topalovski M, O'Malley B: Myeloperoxidase mRNA analysis in acute lymphoblastic leukemia. Diagn Mol Pathol 5:236, 1996.

300. Serrano J, Lo Coco F, Sprovieri T et al: Myeloperoxidase gene expression in non-infant pro-B acute lymphoblastic leukemia with or without ALL1/AF4 transcript. Br J Haematol 111:1065, 2000.

301. Yoneda N, Tatsumi E, Teshigawara K et al: Lineage determination of CD7+ CD5− CD2− and CD7+ CD5+ CD2− lymphoblasts: Studies on phenotype, genotype, and gene expression of myeloperoxidase, CD3ε, and CD3δ. Am J Hematol 45:310, 1994.

302. Lübbert M, Oster W, Ludwig W-D et al: A switch toward demethylation is associated with the expression of myeloperoxidase in acute myeloblastic and promyelocytic leukemias. Blood 80:2066, 1992.

303. Paietta E, Andersen J, Rowe J et al: Myeloid maturation of blast cells determines response in adult de novo acute myeloid leukemia (AML): Results of a response-driven antigen expression analysis in 382 Eastern Cooperative Oncology Group (ECOG) patients. Proc Am Soc Clin Oncol 14:86, #47, 1995.

304. Ludwig W-D, Thiel E: Routine immunophenotyping of acute leukemias Beut (Letter). 60:48, 1990.

305. Legrand O, Perrot J-Y, Baudard M et al: The immunophenotype of 177 adults with acute myeloid leukemia: Proposal of a prognostic score. Blood 96:870, 2000.

306. Ludwig W-D, Reiter A, Löffler H et al: Immunophenotypic features of childhood and adult acute lymphoblastic leukemia (ALL): Experience of the German multicentre trials ALL-BFM and GMALL. Leuk Lymphoma 13:71, 1994.

307. Cross AH, Goorha R, Nuss R et al: Acute myeloid leukemia with T-lymphoid features: A distinct clinical and biological entity. Blood 72:579, 1988.

308. Del Vecchio L, Finizio O, Lo Pardo C et al: Co-ordinate expression of T-cell antigens on acute myelogenous leukemia and of myeloid antigens on T-acute lymphoblastic leukemia. Speculation on a highly balanced bilinearity. Leukemia 5:815, 1991.

309. Bernier M, Massy M, Deleeuw N et al: Immunological definition of acute minimally differentiated myeloid leukemia (M0) and acute undifferentiated leukemia (AUL). Leuk Lymphoma 18:13, 1995.

310. Cheson BD, Cassileth PA, Head DR et al: Report of the National Cancer Institute-sponsored workshop on definitions of diagnosis and response in acute myeloid leukemia. J Clin Oncol 8:813, 1990.

311. Campana D, Hansen-Hagge TE, Matutes E et al: Phenotypic, genotypic, cytochemical, and ultrastructural characterization of acute undifferentiated leukemia. Leukemia 4:620, 1990.

312. Van der Schoot CE, Visser FJ, Tetteroo PAT, von dem Borne AEGKr: In-vitro differentiation of cells of patients with acute undifferentiated leukemia. Br J Haematol 71:351, 1989.

313. Heerema NA, Sather HN, Ge J et al: Cytogenetic studies of infant acute lymphoblastic leukemia: Poor prognosis of infants with t(4;11) – a report of the Children's Cancer Group. Leukemia 13:679, 1999.

314. Biondi A, Cimino G, Pui C-H: Biological and therapeutic aspects of infant leukemia. Blood 96:24, 2000.

315. Griesinger F, Elfers H, Ludwig W-D et al: Detection of HRX-FEL fusion transcripts in pre-pre-B-ALL with and without cytogenetic demonstration of t(4;11). Leukemia 8:542, 1994.

316. Uckun FM, Herman-Hatten K, Crotty M-L et al: Clinical significance of MLL-AF4 fusion transcript expression in the absence of

a cytogenetically detectable t(4;11)(q21;q23) chromosomal translocation. Blood 92:810, 1998.

317. Czuczman MS, Dodge RK, Stewart CC et al: Value of immunophenptype in intensively treated adult acute lymphoblastic leukemia: Cancer and Leukemia Group B Study 8364. Blood 93:3931, 1999.

318. Borowitz MJ, Carroll AJ, Shuster JJ et al: Use of clinical and laboratory features to define prognostic subgroups in B-precursor acute lymphoblastic leukemia: Experience of the Pediatric Oncology Group. In Ludwig W-D, Thiel E (eds.): Recent Results in Cancer Research. Recent Advances in Cell Biology of Acute Leukemia, p. 257. Springer Verlag, Berlin, 1993.

319. Basso G, Rondelli R, Covezzoli A et al: The role of immunophenotype in acute lymphoblastic leukemia of infant age. Leuk Lymphoma 15:51, 1994.

320. Pui C-H, Behm FG, Crist WM: Clinical and biologic relevance of immunologic marker studies in childhood acute lymphoblastic leukemia. Blood 82:343, 1993.

321. Crist W, Carroll A, Shuster J et al: Philadelphia chromosome positive childhood acute lymphoblastic leukemia: Clinical and cytogenetic characteristics and treatment outcome. A Pediatric Oncology Group Study. Blood 76:489, 1990.

322. Cortes JE, Kantarjian HM: Acute lymphoblastic leukemia. Cancer 76:2393, 1995.

323. Aguiar RCT, Sohal J, van Rhee F et al: TEL-AML1 fusion in acute lymphoblastic leukemia of adults. Br J Haematol 95:673, 1996.

324. McLean TW, Ringold S, Neuberg D et al: TEL/AML-1 dimerizes and is associated with a favorable outcome in childhood acute lymphoblastic leukemia. Blood 88:4252, 1996.

325. Codrington R, O'Connor HE, Jalali GR et al: Analysis of ETV6/AML1 abnormalities in acute lymphoblastic leukemia: Incidence, alternative spliced forms and minimal residual disease value. Br J Haematol 111:1071, 2000.

326. Rubnitz JE, Pui C-H, Downing JR: The role of TEL fusion genes in pediatric leukemias. Leukemia 13:6–13, 1999.

327. Lenormand B, Vannier JP, Bene MC et al: CD2+ CD19+ acute lymphoblastic leukemia in 16 children and adults: Clinical and biological features. Br J Haematol 83:580, 1993.

328. Hunger SP: Chromosomal translocations involving the E2A gene in acute lymphoblastic leukemia: Clinical features and molecular pathogenesis. Blood 87:1211, 1996.

329. Sang B-C, Shi L, Dias P et al: Monoclonal antibodies specific to the acute lymphoblastic leukemia t(1;19)-associated E2A/pbx1 chimeric protein: Characterization and diagnostic utility. Blood 89:2909, 1997.

330. Gaynon PS, Crotty ML, Sather HN et al: Expression of BCR-ABL, E2A-PBX1, and MLL-AF4 fusion transcripts in newly diagnosed children with acute lymphoblastic leukemia: A Children's Cancer Group initiative. Leuk Lymphoma 26:57, 1997.

331. Hooijkaas H, Hählen K, Adriaansen HJ et al: Terminal deoxynucleotidyl transferase (TdT)-positive cells in cerebrospinal fluid and development of overt CNS leukemia: a 5-year follow-up study in 113 children with a TdT-positive leukemia or non-Hodgkin's lymphoma. Blood 74:416, 1989.

332. Homans AC, Barker BE, Forman EN et al: Immunophenotypic characteristics of cerebrospinal fluid cells in children with acute lymphoblastic leukemia at diagnoses. Blood 76:1807, 1990.

333. Subirá D, Castañon S, Román A et al: Flow cytometry and the study of central nervous disease in patients with acute leukemia. Br J Haematol 112:381, 2001.

334. Faderl S, Kantarjian HM, Talpaz M et al: Clinical significance of cytogenetic abnormalities in adult acute lymphoblastic leukemia. Blood 91:3995, 1998.

335. Davey FR, Lawrence D, MacCallum J et al: Morphologic characteristics of acute lymphoblastic leukemia (ALL) with abnormalities of chromosome 8, band q24. Am J Hematol 40:183, 1992.

336. Levitt L, Lin R: Biology and treatment of adult acute lymphoblastic leukemia. West J Med 164:143, 1996.

337. Hoelzer D, Thiel E, Löffler H et al: Prognostic factors in a multicenter study for treatment of acute lymphoblastic leukemia in adults. Blood 71:123, 1988.

338. Reiter A, Schrappe M, Ludwig W-D et al: Chemotherapy in 998 unselected childhood acute lymphoblastic leukemia patients. Results and conclusions of the multicenter trial ALL-BFM 86. Blood 84:3122, 1994.

339. Copelan EA, McGuire EA: The biology and treatment of acute lymphoblastic leukemia in adults. Blood 85:1151, 1995.

340. Uckun FM, Sensel MG, Sun L et al: Biology and treatment of childhood T-lineage acute lymphoblastic leukemia. Blood 91:735, 1998.

341. Plunkett W, Liliemark JO, Estey E et al: Saturation of ara-CTP accumulation during high-dose ara-C therapy: Pharmacologic rationale for intermediate-dose ara-C. Semin Oncol 14 (Suppl 1):159, 1987.

342. Heerema NA, Sather HN, Sensel MG et al: Frequency and clinical significance of cytogenetic abnormalities in pediatric T-lineage acute lymphoblastic leukemia: A report from the Children's Cancer Group. J Clin Oncol 16:1270, 1998.

343. Schneider NR, Carroll AJ, Shuster JJ et al: New recurring cytogenetic abnormalities and association of blast cell karyotypes with prognosis in childhood T-cell acute lymphoblastic leukemia: a Pediatric Oncology Group report of 343 cases. Blood 96:2543, 2000.

344. Bash RO, Crist WM, Shuster JJ et al: Clinical features and outcome of T-cell acute lymphoblastic leukemia in childhood with respect to alterations at the TAL1 locus: A Pediatric Oncology Group study. Blood 81:2110, 1993.

345. Begley CG, Green AR: The SCL gene: From case report to critical hematopoietic regulator. Blood 93:2760, 1999.

346. Garand R, Vannier JP, Béné MC et al: Comparison of outcome, clinical, laboratory, and immunological features in 164 children and adults with T-ALL. Leukemia 4:739, 1990.

347. Thomas X, Archimbaud E, Charrin C et al: CD34 expression is associated with major adverse prognostic factors in adult acute lymphoblastic leukemia. Leukemia 9:249, 1995.

348. Gouttefangeas C, Bensussan A, Boumsell L: Study of the CD3-associated T-cell receptors reveals further differences between T-cell acute lymphoblastic lymphoma and leukemia. Blood 75:931, 1990.

349. Campana D, van Dongen JJM, Mehta A et al: Stages of T-cell receptor protein expression in T-cell acute lymphoblastic leukemia. Blood 77:1546, 1991.

350. Alfsen GC, Beiske K, Holte H et al: T-cell receptor γδ+/CD3+4–8– T-cell acute lymphoblastic leukemias: A distinct subgroup of leukemias in children. A report of five cases. Blood 77:2023, 1991.

351. Sperling SC, Schwartz S, Büchner T et al: Expression of the stem cell factor receptor c-kit (CD117) in acute leukemias. Haematologica 82:617, 1997.

352. DeCastro CM, Denning SM, Langdon S et al: The c-kit proto-oncogene receptor is expressed on a subset of human CD3–CD4–CD8– (triple-negative) thymocytes. Exp Hematol 22:1025, 1994.

353. Godfrey DI, Kennedy J, Mombaerts P et al: Onset of TCR-beta gene rearrangement and role of TCR-beta expression during CD3–CD4–CD8–thymocyte differentiation. J Immunol 152:4783, 1994.

354. Nishii K, Kita K, Miwa H et al: c-kit expression in CD7-positive acute lymphoblastic leukemia: Close correlation with expression of myeloid-associated antigen CD13. Leukemia 6:662, 1992.

355. Ino T, Tsuzuki M, Okamoto H et al: Acute leukemia with the phenotype of a natural killer/T cell bipotential precursor. Ann Hematol 78:43, 1999.

356. Gloeckner-Hofmann K, Ottesen K, Schmidt S et al: T-cell/natural killer cell lymphoblastic lymphoma with an unusual coexpression of B-cell antigens. Ann Hematol 79:635, 2000.

357. Campos L, Guyotat D, Archimbaud E et al: Clinical significance of multidrug resistance P-glycoprotein expression on acute nonlymphoblastic leukemia cells at diagnosis. Blood 79:473, 1992.

358. te Boekhorst PAW, de Leeuw K, Schoester M et al: Predominance of functional multidrug resistance (MDR-1) phenotype in CD34+ acute myeloid leukemia cells. Blood 82:3157, 1993.

359. Ludescher C, Eisterer W, Hilbe W et al: Low frequency of activity of P-glycoprotein (P-170) in acute lymphoblastic leukemia compared to acute myeloid leukemia. Leukemia 9:350, 1995.

360. Tafuri A, Sommaggio A, Burba L et al: Prognostic value of rhodamine-efflux and MDR-1/P-170 expression in childhood acute leukemia. Leuk Res 19:927, 1995.

361. Goasguen JE, Dossot J-M, Fardel O et al: Expression of the multidrug resistance-associated P-glycoprotein (P-170) in 59 cases of de novo acute lymphoblastic leukemia: Prognostic implications. Blood 81:2394, 1993.

362. Savignano C, Geromin A, Michieli M et al: The expression of the multidrug resistance related glycoprotein in adult acute lymphoblastic leukemia. Haematologica 78:261, 1993.

363. Brophy NA, Marie JP, Rojas VA et al: Mdr1 gene expression in childhood acute lymphoblastic leukemias and lymphomas: A critical evaluation by four techniques. Leukemia 8:327, 1994.

364. Dhooge C, De Moerloose B, Laureys G et al: P-glycoprotein is an independent prognostic factor predicting relapse in childhood acute lymphoblastic leukemia: Results of a 6-year prospective study. Br J Haematol 105:676, 1999.

365. Segeren CM, de Jong-Gerrits GCMM, van't Veer MB et al: AML-MO: Clinical entity or waste basket for immature blastic leukemias? A description of 14 patients. Ann Hematol 70:297, 1995.

366. Venditti A, Del Poeta G, Buccisano F et al: Minimally differentiated acute myeloid leukemia (AML-MO): comparison of 25 cases with other French-American-British subtypes. Blood 89:621, 1997.

367. Cascavilla N, Melillo L, D' Arena G et al: Minimally differentiated acute myeloid leukemia (AML-MO): clinico-biological findings of 29 cases. Leuk Lymphoma 37:105, 2000.

368. Praxedes MK, Zimermnan de Oliveira L, da Veiga Pereira W et al: Monoclonal antibody anti-MPO is useful in recognizing minimally differentiated acute myeloid leukemia. Leuk Lymphoma 12:233, 1994.

369. Pombo de Oliveira P, Matutes E, Rani S et al: Early expression of MCS2 (CD13) in the cytoplasm of blast cells from acute myeloid leukemia. Acta Haematol 80:61, 1988.

370. Urbano-Ispizua A, Matutes E, Villamor N et al: The value of detecting surface and cytoplasmic antigens in acute myeloid leukemia. Br J Haematol 81:178, 1992.

371. Dick FR: Evolution of the French-American-British (FAB) proposals. Is there a place for acute basophilic leukemia? Am J Clin Pathol 96:153, 1991.

372. van't Veer MB: The diagnosis of acute leukemia with undifferentiated or minimally differentiated blasts. Ann Hematol 64:161, 1992.

373. Stasi R, Del Poeta G, Venditti A et al: Analysis of treatment failure in patients with minimally differentiated acute myeloid leukemia (AML-M0). Blood 83:1619, 1994.

374. Cuneo A, Ferrant A, Michaux JL et al: Cytogenetic profile of minimally differentiated (FAB M0) acute myeloid leukemia: Correlation with clinicobiologic findings. Blood 85:3688, 1995.

375. Amadori S, Venditti A, Del Poeta G et al: Minimally differentiated acute myeloid leukemia (AML-M0): A distinct clinico-biologic entity with poor prognosis. Ann Hematol 72:208, 1996.

376. Paietta E, Wiernik PH, Andersen J: Immunophenotypic features of t(8;21)(q22;q22) acute myeloid leukemia in adults. Blood 81:1975, 1993.

377. Paietta E, Andersen J, Yunis J et al: Expression of the multidrug-resistance gene product, P-glycoprotein, in adult acute myeloid leukemia: Association with stem cell antigen CD34 and specific cytogenetic abnormalities. In Abraham NG, Asano S, Brittinger G, Maestroni GJM, Shadduck RK (eds.): Molecular Biology of Hematopoiesis, Vol 5, pp. 201–206, Plenum, New York, 1996.

378. Rege K, Swansbury GJ, Atra AA et al: Disease features in acute myeloid leukemia with t(8;21)(q22;q22). Influence of age, secondary karyotype abnormalities, CD19 status, and extramedullary leukemia on survival. Leuk Lymphoma 40:67, 2000.

379. Erber WN, Asbahr H, Rule SA, Scott CS: Unique immunophenotype of acute promyelocytic leukemia as defined by CD9 and CD68 antibodies. Br J Haematol 88:101, 1994.

380. Ball ED, Schwarz LM, Bloomfield CD: Expression of the CD15 antigen on normal and leukemic myeloid cells: Effects of neuraminidase and variable detection with a panel of monoclonal antibodies. Mol Immunol 28:951, 1991.

381. Di Noto R, Schiavone EM, Ferrara F et al: Expression and ATRA-driven modulation of adhesion molecules in acute promyelocytic leukemia. Leukemia 8:1900, 1994.

382. Claxton DF, Reading CL, Nagarajan L et al: Correlation of CD2 expression with PML gene breakpoints in patients with acute promyelocytic leukemia. Blood 80:582, 1992.

383. Guglielmi C, Martelli MP, Diverio D et al: Immunophenotype of adult and childhood acute promyelocytic leukemia: Correlation with morphology, type of PML gene breakpoint and clinical outcome. A cooperative Italian study on 196 cases. Br J Haematol 102:1035, 1998.

384. Maslak P, Miller WH Jr, Heller G et al: CD2 expression and PML/RAR-α transcripts in acute promyelocytic leukemia. (Letter). Blood 81:1666, 1993.

385. Biondi A, Luciano A, Bassan R et al: CD2 expression in acute promyelocytic leukemia is associated with microgranular morphology (FAM M3v) but not with any PML gene breakpoint. Leukemia 9:1461, 1995.

386. Gallagher RE, Willman CL, Slack JL et al: Association of PML/RARα fusion mRNA type with pretreatment characteristics but not treatment outcome in acute promyelocytic leukemia: An intergroup molecular study. Blood 90:1656, 1997.

387. Tallman MS, Hakimian D, Snower D et al: Basophilic differentiation in acute promyelocytic leukemia. Leukemia 7:521, 1993.

388. Castoldi GL, Liso V, Specchia G, Tomasi P: Acute promyelocytic leukemia: Morphological aspects. Leukemia 8:1441, 1994.

389. Koike T, Tatewaki W, Aoki A et al: Severe symptoms of hyperhistaminemia after the treatment of acute promyelocytic leukemia with tretinoin (all-trans retinoic acid). N Engl J Med 327:385, 1992.

390. Paietta E, Andersen J, Racevskis J et al: Significantly lower P-glycoprotein expression in acute promyelocytic leukemia than in other types of acute myeloid leukemia: Immunological, molecular and functional analyses. Leukemia 8:968, 1994.

391. Drach D, Zhao S, Drach J et al: Low incidence of MDR1 expression in acute promyelocytic leukemia. Br J Haematol 90:369, 1995.

392. Michieli M, Damiani D, Ermacora A et al: P-glycoprotein (PGP), lung resistance-related protein (LRP) and multidrug resistance-associated protein (MRP) expression in acute promyelocytic leukemia. Br J Haematol 108:703, 2000.

393. Drach J, Lopez-Berestein G, McQueen T et al: Induction of differentiation in myeloid leukemia cell lines and acute promyelocytic leukemia cells by liposomal all-*trans*-retinoic acid. Cancer Res 53:2100, 1993.

394. Warrell RP, Frankel SR, Miller WH Jr et al: Differentiation therapy of acute promyelocytic leukemia with tretinoin (all-*trans*-retinoic acid). N Engl J Med 324:1385, 1991.

395. Scott AA, Head DR, Kopecky KJ et al: HLA-DR–, CD33+, CD56+, CD16– myeloid/natural killer cell acute leukemia: A previously unrecognized form of acute leukemia potentially misdiagnosed as French-American-British acute myeloid leukemia-M3. Blood 84:244, 1994.

396. Paietta E, Gallagher RE, Wiernik PH: Myeloid/natural killer cell acute leukemia: A previously unrecognized form of acute leukemia potentially misdiagnosed as FAB-M3 acute myeloid leukemia. (Letter). Blood 84:2824, 1994.

397. Adriaansen HJ, te Boekhorst PAW, Hagemeijer AM et al: Acute myeloid leukemia M4 with bone marrow eosinophilia (M4Eo) and inv(16)(p13q22) exhibits a specific immunophenotype with CD2 expression. Blood 81:3043, 1993.

398. Paietta E, Wiernik PH, Andersen J et al: Acute myeloid leukemia M4 with bone marrow eosinophilia (M4Eo) and inv(16)(p13q22) exhibits a specific immunophenotype with CD2 expression. (Letter). Blood 82:2595, 1993.

399. Del Poeta G, Venditti A, Buccisano F et al: Expression of leukocyte integrin CD11b is associated with drug resistance in elderly acute myeloid leukemia (AML). Blood 92(Suppl 1): #2499, 606a, 1998.

400. DiMartino JF, Cleary ML: MLL rearrangements in hematological malignancies: Lessons from clinical and biological studies. Br J Haematol 106:614, 1999.

401. Baer MR, Stewart CC, Lawrence D et al: Acute myeloid leukemia with 11q23 translocations: Myelomonocytic immunophenotype by multiparameter flow cytometry. Leukemia 12:317, 1998.

402. Tien H-F, Hsiao C-H, Tang J-L et al: Characterization of acute myeloid leukemia with MLL rearrangements – no increase in the incidence of coexpression of lymphoid-associated antigens of leukemic blasts. Leukemia 14:1025, 2000.

403. Smith FO, Rauch C, Williams DE et al: The human homologue of rat NG2, a chondroitin sulfate proteoglycan, is not expressed on the cell surface of normal hematopoietic cells but is expressed by acute myeloid leukemia blasts from poor-prognosis patients with abnormalities of chromosome band 11q23. Blood 87:1123, 1996.

404. Behm FG, Smith FO, Raimondi SC et al: Human homologue of the rat chondroitin sulfate proteoglycan, NG2, detected by monoclonal antibody 7.1, identifies childhood acute lymphoblastic leukemias with t(4;11)(q21;q23) or t(11;19)(q23;p13) and MLL gene rearrangements. Blood 87:1134, 1996.

405. Hilden JM, Smith FO, Frestedt JL et al: MLL gene rearrangement, cytogenetic 11q23 abnormalities, and expression of the NG2 molecule in infant acute myeloid leukemia. Blood 89:3801, 1997.

406. Wuchter C, Harbott J, Schoch C et al: Detection of acute leukemia cells with mixed lineage leukemia (MLL) gene rearrangements by flow cytometry using monoclonal antibody 7.1. Leukemia 14:1232, 2000.

407. Paietta E, Racevskis, J, Bennett JM et al: Biologic heterogeneity in Philadelphia chromosome-positive acute leukemia with myeloid morphology: the Eastern Cooperative Oncology Group experience. Leukemia 12:1881, 1998.

408. Lamy T, Goasguen JE, Mordelet E et al: P-glycoprotein (P-170) and CD34 expression in adult acute myeloid leukemia (AML). Leukemia 8:1879, 1994.

409. Samdani A, Vijapurkar U, Grimm MA et al: Cytogenetics and P-glycoprotein (Pgp) are independent predictors of treatment outcome in acute myeloid leukemia (AML). Leuk Res 20:175, 1996.

410. Schaich M, Illmer T, Harbich E et al: A multivariate analysis of the impact of MDR1, MRP and LRP resistance gene expression on treatment response in adult acute myeloid leukemia. Blood 92 (Suppl 1):#2497, 605a, 1998.

411. Paietta E, Andersen J, Racevskis J et al: Modulation of multidrug resistance in de novo adult acute myeloid leukemia: Variable efficacy of reverting agents in vitro. Blood Rev 9:47, 1995.

412. Sonneveld P: Multidrug resistance in haematological malignancies. J Intern Med 247:521, 2000.

413. Broxterman HJ, Lankelman J, Pinedo HM: How to probe clinical tumour samples for P-glycoprotein and multidrug resistance-associated protein. Eur J Cancer 32A:1024, 1996.

414. Thiebaut F, Tsuruo T, Hamada H et al: Immunohistochemical localization in normal tissues of different epitopes in the multidrug transport protein P170: Evidence for localization in brain capillaries and crossreactivity of one antibody with a muscle protein. J Histochem Cytochem 37:159, 1989.

415. Rao VV, Anthony DC, Piwnica-Worms D: Multidrug resistance P-glycoprotein monoclonal antibody JSB-1 crossreacts with pyruvate carboxylase. J Histochem Cytochem 43:1187, 1995.

416. Cumber PM, Jacobs A, Hoy T et al: Expression of the multiple drug resistance gene (mdr-1) and epitope masking in chronic lymphatic leukemia. Br J Haematol 76:226, 1990.

417. Hait WN, Aftab DT: Rational design and pre-clinical pharmacology of drugs for reversing multidrug resistance. Biochem Pharmacol 43:103, 1992.

418. Takeshita A, Shinjo K, Ohnishi K et al: Expression of multidrug resistance P-glycoprotein in myeloid progenitor cells of different phenotype: Comparison between normal bone marrow cells and leukemia cells. Br J Haematol 93:18, 1996.

419. Martinez A, San Miguel JF, Valverde B et al: Functional expression of MDR-1 in acute myeloid leukemia: Correlation with the clinical-biological, immunophenotypical, and prognostic disease characteristics. Ann Hematol 75:81, 1997.

420. Kizaki M, Ueno H, Yamazoe Y et al: Mechanisms of retinoid resistance: Possible role of cytochrome P450 and P-glycoprotein. Blood 87:725, 1996.

421. Marie J-P, Brophy NA, Ehsan MN et al: Expression of multidrug resistance gene mdr1 mRNA in a subset of normal bone marrow cells. Br J Haematol 81:145, 1992.

422. Chaudhary PM, Mechetner EB, Roninson IB: Expression and activity of the multidrug resistance P-glycoprotein in human peripheral blood lymphocytes. Blood 80:2735, 1992.

423. Drach D, Zhao S, Drach J et al: Subpopulations of normal peripheral blood and bone marrow cells express a functional multidrug resistant phenotype. Blood 80:2729, 1992.

424. Klimecki WT, Futscher BW, Grogan TM, Dalton WS: P-glycoprotein expression and function in circulating blood cells from normal volunteers. Blood 83:2451, 1994.

425. Pallis M, Russell NH: P-glycoprotein plays a drug-efflux-independent role in augmenting cell survival in acute myeloblastic leukemia and is associated with modulation of a sphingomyelin-ceramide apoptotic pathway. Blood 95:2897, 2000.

426. Johnstone RW, Ruefli AA, Tainton KM et al: A role for P-glycoprotein in regulating cell death. Leuk Lymphoma 38:1, 2000.

427. Slovak M, Ho JP, Cole SPC et al: The LRP gene encoding a major vault protein associated with drug resistance maps proximal to

MRP on chromosome 16: Evidence that chromosome breakage plays a key role in MRP or LRP gene amplification. Cancer Res 55:4214, 1995.

428. Kuss BJ, Deeley RG, Cole SPC et al: The biological significance of the multidrug resistance gene MRP in inversion 16 leukemias. Leuk Lymphoma 20:357, 1996.

429. Van der Kolk DM, Vellenga E, van der Veen AY et al: Deletion of the multidrug resistance protein MRP1 gene in acute myeloid leukemia: The impact on MRP activity. Blood 95:3514, 2000.

430. Feller N, Kuiper CM, Lankelma J et al: Functional detection of MDR1/P170 and MRP/P190-mediated multidrug resistance in tumor cells by flow cytometry. Br J Cancer 72:543, 1995.

431. Olson DP, Taylor BJ, Ivy SP: Detection of MRP functional activity: Calcein AM but not BCECF AM as a multidrug resistance-related protein (MRP1) substrate. Cytometry 46:106, 2001.

432. Legrand O, Simonin G, Perrot JV et al: Pgp and MRP activities using calcein-AM are prognostic factors in adult acute myeloid leukemia patients. Blood 91:4480, 1998.

433. Legrand O, Perrot J-Y, Tang RP et al: Expression of the multidrug resistance-associated protein (MRP) mRNA and protein in normal peripheral blood and bone marrow hematopoietic cells. Br J Haematol 94:23, 1996.

434. List A: Role of multidrug resistance and its pharmacological modulation in acute myeloid leukemia. Leukemia 10:937, 1996.

435. Izquierdo MA, Scheffer GL, Flens MJ et al: Major vault protein LRP-related multidrug resistance. Eur J Cancer 32A:979, 1996.

436. Damiani D, Michieli M, Ermacora A et al: P-glycoprotein (Pgp), and not lung resistance-related protein (LRP), is a negative prognostic factor in secondary leukemias. Haematologica 83:290, 1998.

437. McKenna SL, Padua RA: Multidrug resistance in leukemia. Br J Haematol 96:659, 1997.

438. Smeets MEP, Raymakers RAP, Vierwinden G et al: Idarubicin DNA intercalation is reduced by MRP1 and not Pgp. Leukemia 13:1390, 1999.

439. Broxterman HJ, Sonneveld P, Pieters R et al: Do P-glycoprotein and major vault protein (MVP/LRP) expression correlate with in vitro daunorubicin resistance in acute myeloid leukemia? Leukemia 13:258, 1999.

440. Legrand O, Zittoun R, Marie J-P: Role of MRP1 in multidrug resistance in acute myeloid leukemia. Leukemia 13:578, 1999.

441. Michieli M, Damiani D, Ermacora A et al: P-glycoprotein, lung resistance-related protein and multidrug resistance associated protein in de novo acute non-lymphocytic leukemias: Biological and clinical implications. Br J Haematol 104:328, 1999.

442. Filipits M, Stranzl T, Pohl G et al: Drug resistance factors in acute myeloid leukemia: a comparative analysis. Leukemia 14:68, 2000.

443. Borg AG, Burgess R, Green LM et al: P-glycoprotein and multidrug resistance-associated protein, but not lung resistance protein, lower the intracellular daunorubicin accumulation in acute myeloid leukemia cells. Br J Haematol 108:48, 2000.

444. Ito E, Kasai M, Toki T et al: Expression of erythroid-specific genes in megakaryoblastic disorders. Leuk Lymphoma 23:545, 1996.

445. Linari S, Vannucchi AM, Ciolli S et al: Coexpression of erythroid and megakaryocytic genes in acute erythroblastic (FABM6) and megakaryoblastic (FABM7) leukemias. Br J Haematol 102:1335, 1998.

446. Breton-Gorius J, Villeval JL, Mitjavila MT et al: Phenotypes and ultrastructure of blasts from acute erythroblastic leukemia. In Grignani F, Martelli MF, Mason DY (eds): Genotypic, Phenotypic and Functional Aspects of Haematopoiesis, p. 87. Raven Press, New York, 1987.

447. Garand R, Duchayne E, Blanchard D et al: Minimally differentiated erythroleukemia (AML M6 'variant'): A rare subset of AML distinct from AML M6. Br J Haematol 90:868, 1995.

448. Davey FR, Abraham N Jr, Brunetto VL et al: Morphologic characteristics of erythroleukemia (acute myeloid leukemia; FAB-M6): A CALGB study. Am J Hematol 49:29, 1995.

449. Dunstan RA, Simpson MB, Knowles RW et al: The origin of ABH antigens on human platelets. Blood 65:615, 1985.

450. Schwarzinger I, Valent P, Köller U et al: Prognostic significance of surface marker expression on blasts of patients with de novo acute myeloblastic leukemia. J Clin Oncol 8:423, 1990.

451. Breton-Gorius J, van Haeke D, Pryzwansky KB et al: Simultaneous detection of membrane markers with monoclonal antibodies and method of fixation preserving the platelet peroxidase. Br J Haematol 58:447, 1984.

452. Betz SA, Foucar K, Head DR et al: False-positive flow cytometric platelet glycoprotein IIb/IIIa expression in myeloid leukemias secondary to platelet adherence to blasts. Blood 79:2399, 1992.

453. Imamura N, Kajihara H, Kuramoto A: Flow cytometric analysis of peroxidase negative acute leukemias by monoclonal antibodies – II. Acute megakaryoblastic and acute promegakaryocytic leukemia. Leuk Res 12:279, 1988.

454. Yumura-Yagi K, Hara J, Kurahashi H et al: Mixed phenotype of blasts in acute megakaryocytic leukemia and transient abnormal myelopoiesis in Down's syndrome. Br J Haematol 81:520, 1992.

455. Cuneo A, Mecucci C, Kerim S et al: Multipotent stem cell involvement in megakaryoblastic leukemia: Cytologic and cytogenetic evidence in 15 patients. Blood 74:1781, 1989.

456. Terui T, Niitsu Y, Mahara K et al: The production of transforming growth factor-β in acute megakaryoblastic leukemia and its possible implications for myelofibrosis. Blood 75:1540, 1990.

457. Wetzler M, Baer MR: Thrombopoietin receptor in acute myeloid leukemia. Leuk Res 23:191, 1999.

458. Albitar M, Manshouri T, Kantarjian H et al: Correlation between lower c-mpl protein expression and favorable cytogenetic groups in acute myeloid leukemia. Leuk Res 23:63, 1999.

459. Bouscary D, Prudhomme C, Quesnel B et al: c-mpl expression in hematologic disorders. Leuk Lymphoma 17:19, 1995.

460. Schröder JK, Kolkenbrock S, Tins J et al: Analysis of thrombopoietin receptor (c-mpl) mRNA expression in de novo acute myeloid leukemia. Leuk Res 24:401, 2000.

16

Cytogenetics of Acute Leukemia

Gordon Dewald and Mark Litzow

By using chromosome nonbanding techniques, the correct chromosome number of humans was reported in 1956.[1] Over the next few years, the association of trisomy 21 with Down syndrome, 45,X with Turner syndrome, and 47,XXY with Klinefelter syndrome was reported.[2–4] In 1960, an abnormal small chromosome 22 (subsequently known as the Philadelphia chromosome) was identified in cells from patients with chronic myeloid leukemia (CML).[5] These discoveries and some others collectively mark the birth of the prebanding era of clinical cytogenetics.

A variety of chromosome banding techniques were discovered in the late 1960s and early 1970s that made it possible to accurately identify each chromosome in the human karyotype.[6] Thus, identification of specific chromosomes involved in aneuploid conditions became possible. Moreover, with these new chromosome-staining methods it became possible to subdivide chromosomes into individual bands, each with a characteristic location, size, and staining intensity. Thus, it became possible to recognize more than 400 chromosome bands in the human karyotype and to detect subtle structural abnormalities. In 1972 chromosome banding techniques were used to discover that the Philadelphia chromosome was actually part of a translocation between chromosomes 9 and 22.[7] Subsequently, other recurring chromosomal translocations were reported in acute leukemia, including t(8;21)(q22;q22) in 1973,[8] t(15;17)(q22;q11–12) in 1977,[9] t(9;11)(p21;q23) in 1982,[10] and inv(16)(p13q22) in 1983.[11,12] The correlation of these chromosomal abnormalities with clinicopathologic observations led to the recognition that acute leukemia is not one homogeneous disease but is rather a heterogeneous group that can be subclassified into distinct disorders.[13]

In the mid 1980s, the 9;22 translocation in CML was shown to be associated with the fusion of DNA of the Ableson (ABL) oncogene on the long arm of chromosome 9 and the breakpoint cluster region (BCR) on chromosome 22.[14] Subsequent studies showed that this DNA fusion produces a BCR/ABL mRNA transcript,[15] which in turn produces a BCR/ABL protein with malignant potential.[16,17] These cytogenetic and molecular genetic discoveries arguably mark the birth of molecular genetics in hematologic disorders and have been the prototype for studies of other chromosomal abnormalities in human leukemias and cancer.[18]

Today, many physicians use cytogenetic studies to help classify acute leukemia into subtypes that are associated with specific chromosome abnormalities, to obtain information on prognosis, and to help make appropriate decisions about treatments.[18] Moreover, cytogenetic studies on specimens collected after treatment are often useful to assess response to treatment and to monitor remission. As adjunct procedures, the applications of fluorescence in situ hybridization (FISH) with chromosome-specific DNA probes and of the reverse transcriptase polymerase chain reaction (RT-PCR) significantly enhance the utility of genetic testing in hematologic malignancies. Cytogenetic studies are done on mitotic (proliferating) cells. The FISH technique readily permits analysis of large numbers of proliferating and nonproliferating (interphase nuclei) cells and is useful to establish the percentage of neoplastic cells before and after therapy, whereas RT-PCR is particularly useful to detect very low levels of disease.

This chapter summarizes the most common chromosome abnormalities in acute leukemia and emphasizes their significance in clinical practice. Today it is difficult to separate the various genetic testing methods and to know when in the course of disease they should be used. Thus, various genetic testing strategies used to evaluate patients with acute leukemia before and after treatment are discussed in the context of their applications in clinical practice.

GENETIC TESTING STRATEGIES FOR HEMATOLOGIC MALIGNANCIES

The central genetic dogma for some hematologic malignancies suggests that certain structural chromosome abnormalities result in fusion of an oncogene and a promotor gene, which in turn produces a specific mRNA, which then produces a protein product with malignant potential. Most of these chromosome abnormalities can be detected by cytogenetic studies. At the DNA level, the fusion of genes associated with these chromosome abnormalities can be detected by FISH, Southern blot analysis, and/or PCR. At the RNA level, the messenger RNA transcript of these genes can be detected by RT-PCR. At the protein level, the chimeric gene product can be detected by Western blot. Each of these methods can be used to quantify tumor burden, but they are associated with varying degrees of accuracy, cost, and turnaround time. Because laboratories and personnel at different institutions vary, genetic testing strategies will not be identical among institutions.

Conventional Cytogenetic Studies

Conventional chromosome studies are the standard method to study proliferating cells in acute leukemia. Cytogenetic methods are relatively standard and available the world over.[18] Generally, cytogenetic studies are based on analysis of up to 25 metaphases and can be used to detect most chromosome abnormalities and determine the percentage of proliferating neoplastic cells. To accurately quantitate proliferating disease, it is important to randomly select metaphases because bias can influence the percentage of normal and abnormal metaphases.[19] Quantitative cytogenetic studies do not usually detect certain cryptic chromosomes such as t(12;21) associated with pre-B-cell acute lymphoblastic lymphoma. Conventional chromosome studies are particularly valuable when a specific hematologic diagnosis or classification is not apparent by morphologic criteria. Cytogenetics studies are important screening methods to detect chromosome abnormalities, but the technique is limited by the need for mitotic neoplastic cells, takes 2 to 3 days to perform, and is relatively expensive.

Fluorescence in situ Hybridization with Chromosome-Specific DNA Probes

Fluorescence in situ hybridization is rapidly becoming part of clinical practice in the work-up of patients with hematologic malignancies. Probes for FISH are classified by where they hybridize. Some hybridize to specific centromeres[20,21] and others to specific gene loci.[22–26] Some probes hybridize to unique DNA sequences over the length of each chromosome, producing a paintlike pattern for each chromosome.[27] Still other probes hybridize to chromosome-specific telomere regions.[28] DNA probes can be used individually or in combinations and can be labeled with different colored fluors.

The advantages of FISH are significant. Many DNA probes can be purchased, but "home-brew" probes are easy to make. Commercial probes are usually preferred to avoid the rigorous quality control needed with making home-brew probes. Both nonproliferating and proliferating cells can be studied by FISH. Most FISH tests cost approximately half as much as a complete chromosome study. Because FISH can be performed overnight, it is particularly useful in urgent medical conditions. By using FISH, it is easy to analyze large numbers of cells, and the results are reproducible.

Moreover, FISH can be performed on various types of specimens. Fixed-cell pellets left over from cytogenetic studies on bone marrow or blood are very suitable for FISH.[22,25,29] In addition, FISH works well with bone marrow or peripheral blood smears, touch preparations, and paraffin-embedded tissues,[22,30,24] and it is particularly useful to detect genetic abnormalities when results of cytogenetic studies are inconclusive, for example, in the absence of metaphases or when the results are normal because of cryptic or masked translocations.

A good FISH strategy to detect aneuploidy and deletions uses a probe of one color for the centromere and a probe of another color for an interstitial site on the same chromosome.[18] The most common colors of fluors are red and green. This FISH strategy produces two red and two green signals in interphase cells. False positive signal patterns are obtained when signals overlap, when any probe fails to hybridize, or when crosshybridization occurs. It is important to establish the normal range and to gain experience with FISH in untreated patients before using this method in clinical practice. This method can detect neoplastic clones in which more than 3 percent of cells are trisomy, more than 5 percent of cells are monosomy, or more than 7 percent of cells have deletions.

Several FISH strategies can detect fusion of loci associated with chromosome translocations and inversions. These include S-FISH, which produces a single fusion signal;[31] ES-FISH, which produces a fusion signal and an extra signal; D-FISH, which produces double or two fusion signals;[25] and BAP-FISH, which shows two fused signals in a normal cell, but in which one separates or breaks apart in cells with a translocation or inversion.[18] The sensitivity of these methods varies significantly. For example, in 500 nuclei, more than 1 percent of neoplastic cells can be detected by

D-FISH, 3 percent by ES-FISH, 3 percent by BAP-FISH, and 10 percent by S-FISH.[18] The sensitivity of D-FISH studies can be increased to 0.079 percent by analyzing 6,000 nuclei.

In BAP-FISH the probes hybridize to a specific region on only one chromosome. The probes are so designed that a red signal occurs on one side of the breakpoint and a green signal on the other side. In a fluorescent microscope, red and green signals merge to form a yellow fusion signal. The reciprocal translocation causes the fusion signal to "break apart" and form a red signal on one chromosome and a green signal on the other chromosome. In interphase, one red, one green, and one yellow signal are observed.

The D-FISH method uses red and green probes that hybridize to different loci.[25] The hybridization sites span the breakpoint on each chromosome. The reciprocal translocation produces adjacent red and green hybridization sites on each abnormal chromosome. Thus in interphase, one red, one green, and two yellow signals are observed.

The ES-FISH strategy also uses red and green probes that hybridize to different loci. The hybridization site spans the breakpoint on one of the chromosomes, the hybridization site of the other chromosome being relegated to one side of the breakpoint. The reciprocal translocation produces a yellow fusion signal on one abnormal chromosome and a small residual red signal on the other abnormal chromosome. In interphase, two red, one green, and one yellow signal are observed.

With S-FISH also, red and green probes that hybridize to different loci are used.[31] The green hybridization site occurs on one side of the breakpoint on one chromosome, and the red hybridization site occurs on the other side of the breakpoint on the other chromosome. The reciprocal translocation produces a yellow fusion signal on one of the abnormal chromosomes. In interphase, one red, one green, and one yellow signal are observed.

Multiple probes can be applied to any specimen as a "panel FISH test." For example, a set of probes for chromosomes 5, 7, 8, 11, 13, and 20 allows detection of common abnormalities in myelodysplasia.[28]

For metaphase, whole chromosome paints can be used to identify most major structural anomalies.[27] However, this method allows analysis of only a few chromosomes at a time. Moreover, the method is expensive and does not appear to reveal chromosome abnormalities frequently enough to make its use practical in routine clinical practice. A variant of whole chromosome paints is called *multicolor FISH* because it paints each of the 24 sets of human chromosomes a different color. This method is particularly useful to accurately characterize chromosome abnormalities in metaphases with complex karyotypes.[32]

Polymerase Chain Reaction Studies

Polymerase chain reactions can be used to amplify DNA fragments if the flanking sequences are known. Thus, if the breakpoints for a given gene are clustered within a small area, PCR can be used to detect the mutation in the genome. If the breakpoints associated with a specific chromosome abnormality are spread over a large area of DNA, then RT-PCR can be used to amplify the gene transcript or mRNA.

In RT-PCR, the RNA sequences are converted into complementary DNA (cDNA), which is then amplified by PCR. The analytical sensitivity of most RT-PCR tests is very high and can detect one neoplastic cell in 10^4 to 10^6 cells. Thus, these methods are particularly useful to study miniscule amounts of residual disease.[33]

Although RT-PCR may produce a qualitative result, that is, positive or negative, quantitative RT-PCR methods are available,[34,35] which can be used to distinguish between stable remission and impending relapse. Quantitative RT-PCR can be performed either by a competitive technique or by the cycle–cycle technique.[36,37]

The RT-PCR is significantly reduced by RNA degradation and inefficiency in the reverse transcription of mRNA to the cDNA step. Moreover, RT-PCR generates a very large number of copies of the amplified gene, which can lead to contamination among specimens. The cost of performing RT-PCR is somewhat less than that of FISH, but RT-PCR is not useful for detecting many chromosome abnormalities such as numeric anomalies and deletions.

ROLE OF CYTOGENETICS IN THE CLASSIFICATION OF ACUTE LEUKEMIA

Among children with acute leukemia, 85 percent have acute lymphoblastic leukemia (ALL), and 15 percent have acute myeloid leukemia (AML). Among adults with acute leukemia, 20 percent have ALL and 80 percent have AML. The yearly incidence of AML is 1.2 per 100,000 (children), 3.5 per 100,000 (age 50), 15 per 100,000 (age 70), and 35 per 100,000 (age 90). The yearly incidence of ALL is 9.8 per 100,000 in children and 12.8 per 100,000 in adults. Patients with AML, particularly those over the age of 55, often have chromosome abnormalities that are similar to those associated with myelodysplastic syndromes, and indeed, AML in elderly individuals often evolves from a prior myelodysplastic syndrome. In contrast, patients with AML who are less than 55 years of age more often have chromosome abnormalities that are associated with *de novo* AML.

Classification Schemes of Acute Leukemia

Prior to 1976, the acute leukemias were not classified on a consistent basis from institution to institution. In 1976, a group of French, American, and British (FAB) pathologists defined acute leukemia as a hematologic malignancy involving 30 percent or more blasts in a diagnostic bone marrow aspirate and biopsy.[38] Based on morphologic and cytochemical criteria, the acute leukemias were initially divided into six types of AML (termed M1 to M6) and three kinds of ALL (termed L1 to L3). Subsequently, two additional subtypes of AML, M7 and M0, were described[39,40] (Table 16–1). Hematologic malignancies involving less than 30 percent blasts were classified as myelodysplastic syndromes by the FAB group.[41]

The development of technologies using monoclonal antibodies made it possible to subclassify hematologic malignancies

Table 16–1. FAB Classification System for Acute Leukemias[38–40]

Acute Myeloid Leukemia[a]

FAB Subtype	Frequency in Children, Percent	Frequency in Adults, Percent	
M0	< 5	2–3	Agranular myeloblasts; < 3 percent blasts reactive to myeloid antigens
M1	11	20	Lack of maturation beyond the blast stage; ≥3 percent blasts reactive to myeloid antigens
M2	32	25–30	Maturation to the progranulocyte stage or beyond
M3	8	8–15	Abnormal (hypogranular or hypergranular) progranulocytes that display bundles of Auer rods
M4	24	20–25	Blasts with both monocytic and granulocytic characteristics. Monocytes exceed 20 percent of the nucleated cell population
M5a	11	5	Monoblastic cells > 50 percent monocytic differentiation
M5b			Monocytic cells > 50 percent monocytic differentiation
M6	5	5	Erythrocytic cells predominantly erythroid
M7	9	1–2	Megakaryocytic cells predominately megakaryocytes

Acute Lymphocytic Leukemia[b]

FAB Subtype	Frequency in Children, Percent	Frequency in Adults, Percent	
L1	80	30	Small blasts, regular nuclear outline, few or no visible nucleoli, scant cytoplasm
L2	15–20	65–70	Larger blasts (×2 small lymphocyte), irregular or cleft nucleoli, one or more prominent nucleoli, variable to abundant cytoplasm
L3	3	3	Burkitt's type, large cells, dense chromatin, round or oval nucleus, moderately abundant cytoplasm, deeply basophilic cytoplasm with prominent vacuoles

[a] Acute myeloid leukemia is classified into eight categories on the basis of cell morphology.
[b] Acute lymphocytic leukemia is classified into three categories on the basis of cell morphology.
Abbreviation: FAB, French-American-British.

based on expression of certain cell surface and cytoplasmic antigens identified by immunohistochemical or flow cytometry. These monoclonal antibody-based technologies combined with cytogenetic studies permitted identification of new subtypes of acute leukemia. In addition, studies of genes associated with these chromosome abnormalities have elucidated the pathogenesis of certain types of acute leukemia and resulted in molecular genetic and FISH techniques that can help classify patients into appropriate cytogenetic subtypes.

Based on these various methods and others, a working group of the World Health Organization published a classification scheme intended to define disease entities that could be recognized by pathologists and have relevance in clinical practice.[42] Several important cytogenetic categories were included in this classification scheme (Table 16–2). This revised classification is expected to provide more uniform diagnoses, produce better correlations with patient prognosis, and result in more reliable therapeutic decisions. However, the scheme has been criticized for its reclassification of certain subtypes of myelodysplastic syndromes.[43]

Cytogenetic abnormalities at diagnosis appear to be powerful predictors of patient outcome in AML, but they may not be as useful for predicting disease progression for myelodysplasia.[44] Nevertheless, certain chromosomal abnormalities tend to be associated with *de novo* AML, especially among patients under 55 years of age. Other chromosome abnormalities associated with different forms of AML are more frequently seen in elderly patients with a history of prior myelodysplastic syndrome or following chemotherapy for another malignancy or inflammatory disorder.

Cytogenetics and Molecular Genetics

Certain chromosome abnormalities are strongly associated with *de novo* acute leukemia, for example, t(15;17), t(8;21), t(12;21) and inv(16). Patients with these chromosome abnormalities are generally younger than 55 years of age and their prognosis with current forms of therapy for acute leukemia is better than that of other patients with acute leukemia. The heterodimeric transcription factor known as *core binding factor* (CBF) is involved in each of these chromosome anomalies. The alpha component of this dimeric transcription factor is encoded by a gene on chromosome 21 at band q22, and the beta component is encoded by a gene on the long arm of chromosome 16 at band 22. This transcription factor plays a critical role in the transcriptional activation of multiple genes that are important in hematopoietic development, including genes for myeloperoxidase, *IL-3*, *MCSF* receptor, and GM-CSF.[45]

Approximately 15 percent of adult patients with AML have a t(8;21), which makes it one of the most frequent cytogenetic abnormalities in this form of acute leukemia. This translocation fuses the *CBFα* gene (also known as AML1) on chromosome 21 with the *ETO* gene on chromosome 8. The mechanism of leukemic transformation by the *CBFα/ETO* fusion protein is unclear but may represent a dominant inhibitory activity of transcriptional activation by *CBFα* (AML1).

The inv(16) anomaly results in fusion of the *CBFβ* subunit at 16q22 and the smooth muscle myosin heavy-chain gene *(SMMHC)* at 16p13. This fusion protein may function in a fashion similar to that of *AML1/ETO* and acts as a dominant negative inhibitor of wild-type AML1 function.

More recently, the *TEL/AML1* fusion protein has been associated with t(12;21) and identified in approximately 25 percent of patients with pediatric ALL which makes it the most common gene rearrangement in a childhood cancer.[46] The *TEL/AML1* fusion is a consequence of a cryptic translocation between chromosomes 12 and 21 and is not easily detected by standard cytogenetics.

The t(15;17) is strongly associated with acute promyelocytic leukemia (FAB subtype M3). This translocation fuses a promyelocytic leukemia *(PML)* gene on chromosome 15 with the retinoic acid receptor alpha *(RARα)* gene on chromosome 17. The *RARα* gene is involved in all cases of AML-M3, but rare variants of this type of leukemia involve fusion of other genes with RARα, such as the *TLZF* gene on chromosome 11 and the *MNPM* gene on chromosome 5. This translocation appears to function as a dominant negative inhibitor of wild-type *RARα* function.[47]

Table 16–2. Proposed WHO Classification of Acute Leukemia[42]

Acute myeloid leukemias (AMLs)
  AMLs with recurrent cytogenetic translocations
    AML with t(8;21)(q22;q22), *AML1(CBFα)/ETO*
    Acute promyelocytic leukemia (AML with
      t(15;17)(q22;q11–12) and variants, *PML/RARα*)
    AML with abnormal bone marrow eosinophils
      (inv(16)(p13q22) or t(16;16)(p13;q11), *CBFβ/MYH11X*)
    AML with 11q23 *(MLL)* abnormalities
  AML with multilineage dysplasia
    With prior myelodysplastic syndrome
    Without prior myelodysplastic syndrome
  AML and myelodysplastic syndromes, therapy-related
    Alkylating agent-related
    Epipodophyllotoxin-related (some may be lymphoid)
    Other types
  AML not otherwise categorized
    AML minimally differentiated
    AML without maturation
    AML with maturation
    Acute myelomonocytic leukemia
    Acute monocytic leukemia
    Acute erythroid leukemia
    Acute megakaryocytic leukemia
    Acute basophilic leukemia
    Acute panmyelosis with myelofibrosis
Acute biphenotypic leukemias
Acute lymphoid leukemia
  Precursor B-cell acute lymphoblastic leukemia (cytogenetic
    subgroups)
    t(9;22)(a34;q11); *BCR/ABL*
    t(v;11q23); MLL rearranged
    t(1;19)(q23;p13) *E2A/PBX1*
    t(12;21)(p12;q22) *ETV/CBF-α*
  Precursor T-cell acute lymphoblastic leukemia
  Burkitt-cell leukemia

FREQUENCY OF CHROMOSOME ABNORMALITIES IN ACUTE LEUKEMIA

Prior to 1985, 43 specific chromosome abnormalities were associated with hematologic disorders. In 1985 the frequency of each of these abnormalities was calculated from data on 748 predominantly adult patients with an abnormal clone seen at one institution.[48] Collectively, these 748 patients had 1,352 chromosome abnormalities. The 43 recognized chromosome abnormalities were seen in 61 percent of the patients. The remaining 39 percent of the patients had other chromosome abnormalities that were not yet associated with any specific hematologic disorder.

The most common specific chromosome abnormality was the Ph-chromosome, followed by +8, −Y, 5q−, −7, 20q−, and +21. The most common trisomy was trisomy 8, followed by trisomy of chromosomes 21, 19, 9, 11, and 7. Loss of the Y chromosome was the most common monosomy followed by monosomy of chromosomes 7, 5, and X. The most common deletion was 5q−, followed by 20q−, 7q−, 6q−, 13q−, 11q−, 9q−, and 16q−. The most common translocation was t(9;22), followed by t(8;21), t(1;7), t(8;14), t(9;11), t(4;11), and t(14;18). Isochromosomes, inversions, duplications, haploidy, and polyploidy were infrequent.

Since 1985, many other chromosome abnormalities associated with hematologic disorders have been reported.[49] Many of the newly discovered chromosome abnormalities were either relatively rare or cryptic in nature. Eventually, the clinical disorder(s) associated with each specific chromosome abnormality will be correlated. Currently, physicians and cytogeneticists who interpret chromosome abnormalities need to correlate the cytogenetic results with the clinical scenario of the patient.

Several important international attempts have been made to review the cytogenetic literature in order to correlate chromosome abnormalities with specific hematologic disorders.[50–52] Most recently, breakpoints for 1,803 structural abnormalities, including 215 balanced and 1,588 unbalanced anomalies associated with hematologic disorders and solid tumors were summarized.[52] Similar information is also available on the Internet

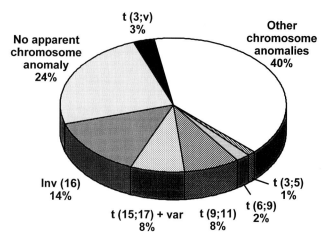

Figure 16–1. Frequency of different translocations in children and young adults with AML.[53–55]

at the site for the Atlas of Genetics and Cytogenetics in Oncology and Haematology (Atlas Genet Cytogenet Oncol Haematol, 1998, URL www.infobiogen.fr/services/chromcancer).

Fifty-five of the more common chromosome abnormalities associated with acute leukemia are summarized in Table 16–3. These abnormalities are found in each cell of the neoplastic disorder and thought to be the primary genetic event of the hematologic disorder. The abnormal clones in many patients contain subclones and multiple secondary anomalies in addition to the primary anomalies. These secondary anomalies form subclones and are less characterized than the primary anomalies, but they no doubt contribute to progression of disease and to resistance of treatment.[18]

The frequency of some well-known chromosome abnormalities in acute leukemia have been estimated for children and young adults (Figures 16–1 and 16–2).[53–56] In these age groups, more than 40 percent of patients with AML and more than 25 percent of patients with ALL do not have any of the so-called well-known chromosome abnormalities. Moreover, older patients with AML that evolves from myelodysplastic syn-

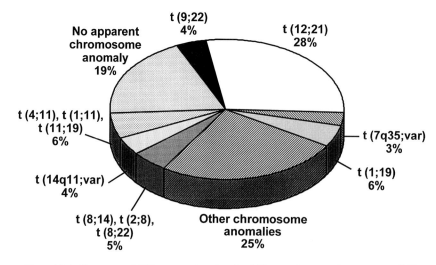

Figure 16–2. Frequency of different translocations in children and young adults with ALL.[53–55]

Table 16–3. Common Chromosome Abnormalities in Acute Leukemia

	Anomaly	Genes	Associated Disorders
AML	+8		ALL, AML, CLD, MPD, MDS, PV
	del(5)(q13;q33)		AML,MDS, MPD, 5q– syn
	del(7)(q22;q34)		AML, CLD, CMD, MDS, NHL
	del(9)(p21)		ALL, AML, CLD, NHL
	del(12)(p12)		ALL, AML-M2, AML-M4, MDS, NHL
	inv(3)(q21;q26)	*Ribophorin I, EVII*	AML-M4, AML-M6, CML Ph +, MDS
	inv(16)(p13;q22)	*MYH11, CBFβ*	AML-M4Eo
	t(1;3)(p36;q21)		AML-M1, AML-M4, MDS
	t(1;11)(p32;q23)	*TAL1, MLL*	ALL, AML
	t(1;11)(q21;q23)	*AFIρ, MLL*	AML-M4, AML-M5
	t(1;17)(p36;q21)	*?, RARα*	AML-M3
	t(1;22)(p13;q13)		AML-M7
	t(3;3)(q21;q26)	*Ribophorin I, EVII*	AML, MDS
	t(3;5)(q21;q31)	*MLF1, NPM*	AML-M6
	t(3;5)(q25;q34)		AML
	t(3;21)(q26;q22)	*EAP, AML1*	AML, CML Ph +, MDS
	t(4;11)(q21;q23)	*AF-4, MLL*	ALL, AML
	t(5;17)(p23;q11–12)	*NPM, RARα*	AML-M3
	t(6;9)(p23;q34)	*DEK, CAN*	AML-M1, AML-M2, AML-M4, MDS
	t(6;11)(q27;q23)	*AF6, MLL*	AML-M4, AML-M5
	t(7;11)(p15;p15)	*HOXA9, NUP98*	AML, AML-M2
	t(8;16)(p11;p13)	*MOZ, CBP*	AML-M4, AML-M5
	t(8;21)(q22;q22)	*ETO, AML1*	AML-M2, AML-M4, MDS
	t(9;11)(p22;q23)	*AF-9, MLL*	ALL, AML-M5, MDS, t-MDS
	t(9;22)(q34;q11)	*ABL, BCR*	ALL, AML-M1, AML-M2, CML, MPD
	t(10;11)(p13;q23)	*AF10, MLL*	AML-M4, AML-M5
	t(11;17)(q23;q21)	*PLZF, RARα*	AML-M3
	t(11;17)(q23;q21)	*MLL, AF17*	AML-M4, AML-M5
	t(11;19)(q23;p13)	*MLL, ENL*	ALL, AML-M4, AML-M5, t-AML
	t(15;17)(q22;q21)	*PML, RARα*	AML-M3, CML Ph +
	t(16;16)(p13;q22)	*MYH11, CBFβ*	AML-M4Eo, MDS
	t(16;21)(q24;q22)	*MTG16, AML-M2*	AML-M2, AML-M4, childhood AML
	t(16;21)(q24;q22)	*FUS, ERG*	AML-M1, AML-M2
ALL	del(12)(p12)		ALL, AML-M2, AML-M4, MDS, NHL
	t(1;11)(p32;q23)	*AFIρ, MLL*	ALL, AML
	t(1;14)(p32;q11)	*TAL1, TCRαδ*	T-ALL
	t(1;19)(q23;p13)	*PBX1, E2A*	Pre-B-ALL
	t(2;8)(p12;q24)	*Igκ, c-MYC*	ALL-L3, BL, NHL
	t(4;11)(q21;q23)	*AF-4, MLL*	ALL, AML
	t(5;14)(q31;q32)	*IL3, IgH*	ALL
	t(7;9)(q35;q32)	*TCRβ, TAL2*	T-ALL
	t(7;19)(q35;p13)	*TCRβ, LY1*	T-ALL
	t(8;14)(q11;q32)	*?, IgH*	ALL
	t(8;14)(q24;q32)	*c-MYC, IgH*	ALL-L3, BL, MM, NHL
	t(8;14)(q24;q11)	*c-MYC, TCRαδ*	T-ALL
	t(8;22)(q24;q11)	*c-MYC, Igλ*	ALL-L3, BL
	t(9;11)(p22;q23)	*AF-9, MLL*	ALL, AML-M5, MDS, t-MDS
	t(9;22)(q34;q11)	*ABL, BCR*	ALL, AML-M1, AML-M2, CML, MPD
	t(10;14)(q24;q11)	*HOX11, TCRαδ*	T-ALL
	t(11;14)(p13;q11)	*Rhom2, TCRαδ*	T-ALL, NHL
	t(11;19)(q23;p13)	*MLL, ENL*	ALL, AML-M4, AML-M5, t-AML
	t(12;21)(p13;q22)	*TEL, AML1*	ALL
	t(14;22)(q32;q11)	*IgH, BCR*	ALL
	t(17;19)(q21–22;p13)	*HLF, E2A*	ALL
	t(X;11)(q13;q23)	*AFX1, MLL*	T-ALL

ALL, acute lymphocytic leukemia; AML, acute myeloid leukemia; AMM, agnogenic myeloid metaplasia; BL, Burkitt's lymphoma; CLD, chronic lymphoproliferative disorder, CLL, chronic lymphocytic leukemia; CML Ph +, chronic myeloid leukemia with Philadelphia chromosome; CMML, chronic myelomonocytic leukemia; MDS, myelodysplastic syndrome; MM, multiple myeloma; MPD, myeloproliferative disorder; NHL, Non-Hodgkin lymphoma; pre-B-ALL, precursor B-cell acute lymphocytic leukemia; PLL, prolymphocytic leukemia; PV, polycythemia vera; RARS, refractory anemia with ringed sideroblasts; t-AML, therapy-related acute myeloid leukemia; t-MDS, therapy-related myelodysplastic syndrome; 5q– syn, 5q– syndrome.

dromes or myeloproliferative disorders are not included in these figures.

The risk of a myelodysplastic syndrome evolving to AML varies considerably, depending on underlying characteristics of the myelodysplastic syndrome. The most important prognostic variables include the percentage of bone marrow blasts, the results of cytogenetic studies of bone marrow, and the number of cytopenias that a patient experiences. If the patient is in a low-risk prognostic group, the risk of progressing to AML can be less than 20 percent at 5 years. By comparison, patients with increasing numbers of adverse risk factors have a risk of progressing to AML that can approach 100 percent by 5 years.[44]

Patients whose AML arises from prior chemotherapy or radiotherapy appear to constitute 10 to 15 percent of all patients presenting with AML.[57] Patients with myeloproliferative disorders have a lower risk of progressing to AML, but this varies depending on the type of myeloproliferative disorder and the patient's prior therapy.[58] In clinical practice, these lesser known chromosome abnormalities can be detected by conventional chromosome studies.

SPECIFIC CHROMOSOME ABNORMALITIES IN ACUTE LEUKEMIA

This section provides the frequency, prognosis, cytogenetic breakpoints and variants, availability of FISH tests, and possible molecular testing for 21 chromosome abnormalities that are relatively common in acute leukemia[59–69] (Table 16–3). These abnormalities are organized by cytogenetic order, beginning with abnormalities of chromosome 1 and proceeding systematically through chromosome 22.

t(1;14)(p32;q11)

- Specific for T-ALL in 10 to 30 percent of patients
- Often young males with mediastinal mass
- Positive cerebrospinal fluid and high white count common
- 1p32 breakpoint in *TAL1;* 14q11 breakpoint in *TCR α or δ* (T-cell receptor genes)
- Commercial FISH strategy not available, but it is possible to detect *TAL1/TCRαδ* fusion
- Defined gene breakpoints amenable to Southern blot or RT-PCR analysis

t(1;19)(q23;p13)

- 30 percent of children with pre-B-cell ALL
- Low leukocyte count
- Cytogenetic variant: t(17;19)(q21–22;p13)
- Poor to intermediate prognostic significance
- 1q23 breakpoint in *PBX1;* 19p13 breakpoint in *E2A*
- Commercial FISH strategy not available, but home-brew methods have been reported
- Defined gene breakpoints amenable to Southern blot or RT-PCR analysis

t(1;22)(p13;q13)

- Specific for AML-M7 in 25 to 35 percent of patients
- Found predominantly in infants
- Associated with organomegaly due to leukemic infiltration
- Poor prognostic significance
- Commercial FISH strategy not available
- Gene breakpoints undefined, so molecular tests not available

inv(3)(q21q26)

- AML-M2, M4, and M6; 2 percent of patients with AML
- Frequently associated with thrombocytosis (rare in other forms of AML)
- Poor prognostic significance
- Cytogenetic variants include t(3;3)(q21;q26) and ins(3;3)(q26;q21q26)
- 3q21 breakpoint in *ribophorin;* 3q26 breakpoint in *EVI1*
- Commercial FISH strategy not available, but home-brew methods have been reported
- Defined gene breakpoints amenable to Southern blot or RT-PCR analysis

t(3;5)(q25.1;q34)

- Associated with AML-M6
- Young age
- 3q25.1 breakpoint in *MLF1;* 5q34 breakpoint in *NPM*
- Commercial FISH strategy not available, but possible to detect *MLF1/NPM* fusion
- Defined gene breakpoints amenable to Southern blot or RT-PCR analysis.

t(3;21)(q26;q22)

- AML, myelodysplastic syndromes, and secondary anomaly in CML
- 3q26 breakpoint undefined (candidate genes *EVI1, EAP,* or *MDS1*); 21q22 breakpoint in AML1
- Commercial FISH strategy is available to detect breaking apart of *AML1* locus
- Gene breakpoints undefined so molecular tests not available

del(5)(q13q33)

- 10 percent of patients with AML; usually previous myelodysplastic syndromes
- Poor prognostic significance
- "5q– syndrome" accounts for one-third of patients with a 5q– chromosome
    Subset of young women with 5q– as sole abnormality
    Small megakaryocytes and abnormal erythropoiesis
    Good prognosis
    Chromosome evolution and progression to AML uncommon

- Two-thirds patients with 5q– have various myelodysplastic syndrome subtypes

    50 percent patients have additional chromosome abnormalities with associated worse prognosis

    Common variants include del(5)(q31q35) and del(5)(q22q33)

    Breakpoint at 5q33 occurs in 70 percent of patients

    Most patients lack 5q31; candidate genes include *EGR1*, *CSF1R*, and *IRF1*

    Commercial FISH strategy available to detect loss of *EGR1* and *CSF1R*

    Molecular strategy not applicable

t(6;9)(p23;q34)

- 1 to 2 percent of patients with AML (AML-M2, M4, and rarely, M1); refractory anemia with excess blasts
- May be associated with bone marrow basophilia
- Disease onset at age 20 to 40 years
- Poor to intermediate prognostic significance
- 6p23 breakpoint in *DEK*; 9q34 breakpoint in *CAN*
- Commercial FISH strategy not available, but possible to detect *DEK/CAN* fusion
- Defined gene breakpoints amenable to Southern blot or RT-PCR analysis

t(8;16)(p11;p13)

- Associated with AML-M4 and M5b
- Found mainly in infants and children
- Associated with disseminated intravascular coagulation and erythrophagocytosis
- Poor prognostic significance
- Commercial FISH strategy not available
- Gene breakpoints undefined, so molecular tests not available

t(8;21)(q22;q22)

- 5 to 10 percent of AML; 10 to 30 percent of AML-M2; 7 percent of AML-M4; 20 percent of childhood AML
- Disease onset at age 25 to 30 years
- Generally good prognostic factor, although long-term survival in children is poor
- 70 percent of males have associated loss of the Y chromosome (likely no prognostic importance)
- 60 percent of females have associated loss of the X chromosome (likely no prognostic importance)
- t(16;21)(q24;q22) may be a rare variant
- 8q22 breakpoint in *ETO*; 21q22 breakpoint in *AML1*
- Commercial FISH strategy available to detect fusion of *ETO* and *AML1*
- Defined gene breakpoints amenable to Southern blot or RT-PCR analysis

t(9;22)(q34;q11.2)

- Philadelphia chromosome (Ph)
- 5 percent of children with ALL; 25 to 35 percent of adults with ALL (usually L2); 1 percent of AML-M1

- Poor prognostic significance
- 50 percent of adult ALL and nearly 100 percent of childhood ALL patients have fusion gene e1a2

t(10;14)(q24;q11)

- 1 to 3 percent of patients with T-cell ALL
- 10q24 breakpoint in *HOX11*; 14q11 breakpoint in *TCRαδ* (T-cell receptor αδ)
- Commercial FISH strategy not available, but possible to detect *HOX11/TCRαδ* fusion
- Defined gene breakpoints are amenable to Southern blot or RT-PCR analysis

t(11;var)(q23;var)

- Group of translocations with breakpoint at 11q23 and various partner chromosomes
- Mostly children and young adults
- 70 percent of children less than 1 year old with acute leukemia; 3 percent of patients with therapy-related AML
- Prognostic significance is poor in ALL and intermediate in AML
- t(4;11)(q21;q23) occurs in 5 to 8 percent of children with ALL who are less than 1 year of age
- t(9;11)(p21;q23) or t(11;19)(q23;p13) occurs in 35 percent of patients with AML-M5 and 50 percent of patients with AML-M5a
- t(10;11)(p13;q23) occurs in 30 percent of patients with AML-M4 or -M5
- t(X;11)(q13;q23) in T-cell ALL
- Over 30 different chromosome partners described
- 11q23 breakpoint in *MLL* (mixed-lineage leukemia gene)
- 1p32 breakpoint in *AF1P*;4q21 in *AF4*; 9p21 in *AF9*; 10p13 in *AF10*; 19p13.1 in *ELL*; 19p13.3 in *ENL*; Xq13 in *AFX1*
- Tandem duplications of exons 2 to 6 in *MLL* account for 10 percent of cytogenetically normal AML
- Commercial FISH strategy available to detect breaking apart of *MLL* gene
- Breakpoints in *MLL* cluster in an 8.3-kb region detected by Southern blot or RT-PCR analysis

del(12)(p12)

- Two percent of patients with AML, most have M2 or M4
- Associated with basophilia
- Poor prognostic significance
- Frequently associated with monosomy 7
- Gene at 12p13.1 breakpoint is unknown, but *TEL* or *KIP1* (p27 protein) frequently lost
- Commercial FISH strategy available to detect loss of *TEL1*
- Gene breakpoints undefined, so molecular tests are not available

t(12;21)(p13;q22)

- 25 percent of children with ALL; 3 percent of adults with ALL

- Good prognostic significance
- Difficult to detect by conventional cytogenetic studies
- Often an unbalanced translocation with loss of abnormal chromosome 12
- 12p13 breakpoint in *TEL;*21q22 breakpoint in *AML1*
- Commercial FISH strategy available to detect fusion of *TEL* and *AML1*
- Defined gene breakpoints amenable to Southern blot or RT-PCR analysis

t(15;17)(q22;q21)

- Specific for AML-M3, also known as acute promyelocytic leukemia (APL)
- Accounts for up to 30 to 40 percent of AML in certain ethnic groups
- 20 percent of patients have a hypogranular or microgranular variant (M3v)
- Median age of onset 38 years
- Patients frequently present with disseminated intravascular coagulation (DIC)
- Good prognostic significance; responds to all-trans-retinoic acid treatment
- One percent of patients have cryptic translocations or variants
- Most common variants include t(11;17)(q23;q21), t(5;17)(q32;q21), t(1;17)(p36;q21)
- 15q22 breakpoint in *PML* (also known as *MYL*); 17q21 breakpoint in *RARα* (retinoic acid receptor alpha)
- Commercial FISH strategy available to detect *PML/RARα* fusion
- Defined gene breakpoints amenable to Southern blot or RT-PCR analysis

inv(16)(p13q22)

- This anomaly or a variant occurs in all patients with AML-M4Eo
- 25 percent of patients with AML-M4; 6 percent of patients with AML
- Clinically associated with bone marrow eosinophilia, lymphadenopathy, and hepatomegaly
- Good prognostic significance
- Most common cytogenetic variant is t(16;16)(p13;q22)
- del(16)(q22) linked with AML-M4Eo, but clinical phenotype may differ
- 16p13 breakpoint in *MYH11;* 16q22 breakpoint in *CBFβ* (also known as *PEBP2B*)
- Commercial FISH strategy is available to detect breaking apart of *CBFβ* locus
- Defined gene breakpoints amenable to Southern blot or RT-PCR analysis

Hyperdiploidy without Apparent Structural Anomalies

- 25 to 30 percent of children with ALL, often non-T-cell, non-B-cell

- Neoplastic clones usually have 50 to 60 chromosomes
- Most common trisomies include +4, +6, +10, +14, +17, +18, +20, +21, +X
- Trisomy 21 or tetrasomy 21 occurs in nearly 100 percent of patients
- Good prognostic significance, especially when +4 and +10 are involved
- Commercial FISH strategy available, with centromere-specific probes being used to detect aneuploidy
- Molecular strategy not applicable

Near Haploidy

- 1 percent of children with ALL
- Neoplastic clones with 26 to 36 chromosomes
- Diploid copies of chromosomes 10, 14, 18, 21, and X or Y are common
- Poor prognostic significance
- Commercial FISH strategy available, centromere-specific probes being used to detect aneuploidy
- Molecular strategy not applicable

THERAPY-RELATED SPECIFIC CHROMOSOME ABNORMALITY IN LEUKEMIA AND THERAPY-RELATED MYELODYSPLASIA

At least three cytogenetic categories of therapy-related leukemia may exist:[60,63,70–72] 1. hypodiploid with abnormalities of chromosomes 5 and/or 7; 2. der(1;7) translocations; and 3. t(11;var)(q23;var). In a consecutive series of 3,976 patients with hematologic disorders seen at the Mayo Clinic, 121 were hypodiploid with abnormalities of chromosomes 5 and/or 7; 39 had der(1;7) translocations; and 29 had t(11;var)(q23;var). The same chromosome abnormalities have been associated with patients who have acute leukemia and a history of exposure to environmental carcinogens. Therapy-related leukemia represents approximately 10 to 20 percent of patients with AML. Chromosomally abnormal clones can be identified in 90 percent of patients with therapy-related myelodysplasia (t-MDS) or acute myeloid leukemia (t-AML). Features of the three cytogenetic categories of therapy-related leukemia are summarized as follows:

Hypodiploid and Abnormalities of Chromosomes 5 and 7

- Modal number of chromosomes less than 46
- Associated with prior treatment with alkylating chemotherapeutic agents or radiation
- Time from treatment to bone marrow dysfunction 2 to 5 years
- Patients usually present with myelodysplastic syndromes
- 50 percent of patients with t-MDS progress to AML in 6 months
- Poor prognostic significance
- Critical region most likely in 5q31, 7q11–q21, and/or 7q31–q36

- FISH strategy available to detect structural and numeric anomalies of chromosomes 5 and 7
- Molecular strategy not applicable

der(1;7)(q10;p10)

- Unbalanced translocation, with loss of the chromosome 7q arm and three copies of the chromosome 1q arm
- 70 percent of patients have a therapy-related hematologic disorder
- Associated with prior treatment with alkylating chemotherapeutic agents or radiation
- Time from treatment to bone marrow dysfunction 2 to 5 years
- Patients usually present with myelodysplastic syndromes and rarely progress to AML
- Pathogenesis may be related to loss of tumor suppressor genes on the chromosome 7q arm
- Commercial FISH strategy available to detect loss of chromosome 7q arm and fusion of the centromeres of chromosome 1 and 7
- Molecular strategy not applicable

t(11;var)(q23;var)

- Translocations with breakpoints at 11q23 and various partner chromosomes
- Due to topoisomerase II inhibitor chemotherapy such as doxorubicin and etoposide
- No myelodysplastic syndrome prodrome
- AML develops 1 to 2 years following treatment
- Favorable response to subsequent chemotherapy
- Most common translocations t(9;11)(p21;q23) and t(10;11)(p13;q23)
- 11q23 breakpoint in *MLL* (mixed-lineage leukemia gene)

CYTOGENETICS AND TREATMENT DECISIONS

Diagnosis

The importance of using cytogenetic and molecular genetic tests to make accurate diagnoses and using precise quantification of disease to monitor response to therapy has been most thoroughly demonstrated for CML. In this disease, both the FISH and PCR techniques permit the diagnosis of patients in whom the *BCR/ABL* translocation is masked and not apparent by conventional cytogenetics.[19] The crucial importance of this distinction therapeutically is evidenced by the fact that allogeneic blood and bone marrow transplant has an established role in the curative therapy of CML whereas its role in other myeloproliferative disorders is less well defined.[73] Additionally, detection of *BCR/ABL* in blood and bone marrow in the post-transplant period is crucial to allow early application of donor lymphocyte therapy. This form of therapy has been shown to be most effective if applied at the time of molecular or cytogenetic relapse as compared with hematologic relapse.[74]

Monitoring Therapy

Detection of *BCR/ABL* in CML is also crucial for the monitoring of medical therapy because achievement of a complete or major cytogenetic remission following therapy with alpha-interferon has been shown to be associated with improved disease control and prolonged progression free-survival.[75–78] Detection of *BCR/ABL* will continue to be increasingly important in the monitoring of therapy of CML, especially with the development of new treatments such as specific BCR/ABL tyrosine kinase inhibitor STI571 (Imatinib, mesylate, Gleevec®).[79] This new and exciting oral agent is currently undergoing clinical testing and has become established as the first line treatment for CML.[80]

Although a diagnosis of acute leukemia can usually be made on the basis of morphologic and cytologic characteristics, including immunophenotyping by histochemical or flow cytometric techniques, it is essential that every patient have conventional cytogenetic evaluation performed on their initial diagnostic bone marrow. If the clinical or morphologic features of a particular patient suggest certain subtypes of acute leukemia, for example, acute promyelocytic leukemia, then FISH or PCR assays for a particular translocation or deletion may be appropriate. Additionally, FISH or PCR assays may be important at diagnosis to establish a baseline value, which can then be compared with posttherapy results.

Cytogenetics and Prognosis

Acute myeloid leukemia can be grouped into three broad cytogenetic risk categories. One subset of patients with de novo AML (generally younger individuals) have translocations involving one of the subunits of the core binding factor (alpha or beta) or translocations involving the retinoic acid receptor alpha. These patients generally have a good response to chemotherapy and a favorable remission duration.

A second group of patients with AML have a poor prognosis. This group includes those patients with an antecedent myelodysplastic syndrome, patients with AML arising from chemical exposure, and many de novo cases among elderly individuals. The presence of multilineage dysplasia in these cases suggests that a stem cell or early progenitor cell is mutated to trigger the onset of the disease.

The third cytogenetic risk group contains a large number of patients with AML who have normal cytogenetics or cytogenetic abnormalities that are rare in occurrence. In these cases, the natural history of the disease is less clear but is generally associated with an intermediate or poorer prognosis. It is likely that many patients with normal cytogenetics will, with further technological advances and discoveries, turn out to have recurring molecular and/or chromosomal abnormalities that will allow their disease to be better characterized. Already, a subset of these patients have been found with a tandem duplication of the long arm of chromosome 11, a finding not generally detected by routine cytogenetic analysis.[81] More recently, at least two kinds of patients with AML with normal cytogenetics were found to have point mutations or internal tandem duplications of the *flt3* gene. These *flt3* mutations are important genetic anomalies in AML and appear to confer a poor prognosis.[82,83]

At least two clinical trials have attempted to define different chromosome abnormalities as favorable, intermediate, or unfavorable when found in patients with untreated AML. In one clinical trial,[84] the favorable risk group included patients with either inv(16), t(16;16), del(16q) or t(15;17), or t(8;21) with or without other chromosome abnormalities. The intermediate group included either normal karyotype, 11q23 abnormalities, and +8, del(9q), del(7q), +21, +22 and all other chromosome abnormalities. The unfavorable risk group included either del(5q), −5, −7, abnormal (3q), complex karyotypes (five or more chromosome abnormalities), t(9;22), or t(6;9).

In a more recent clinical trial,[85] the favorable group of chromosome abnormalities included either inv(16), t(16;16), del(16q), or t(15;17), with or without other chromosome abnormalities, or t(8;21) without either del(9q), or part of a complex karyotype. The intermediate risk category included either +8, −Y, +6, del(12p) or normal karyotype. The unfavorable risk category included one or more of −5/del(5q), −7/del(7q), inv(3q), t(3;3); abnormal 11q, 20q or 21q, del(9q), t(6;9), t(9;22); abnormal 17p, or complex karyotype defined as three or more abnormalities. These studies clearly illustrate the value of using cytogenetic risk categories to treat patients with AML.

Certain chromosome abnormalities are associated with myelodysplastic syndromes or AML arising from chemotherapy or radiotherapy or from environmental or occupational exposure such as exposure to pesticides containing arsenic, organic solvents, petroleum, or benzene. These forms of AML in elderly individuals share similar morphologic and cytogenetic characteristics of secondary AML and myelodysplasia. The most common clonal chromosome abnormalities in these patients involve chromosomes 5, 7, 8, 11, 13, and 17. The karyotype of the neoplastic clone in these patients usually involve a complex karyotype (three or more chromosome abnormalities). These elderly patients with AML have a poor response to chemotherapy similar to the response to therapy-related leukemia or AML arising from an antecedent myelodysplastic syndrome. Some patients with hematologic malignancies have two or more cytogenetic clones. This is particularly common in therapy-related leukemia, in which cells with one karyotype reflect the original disease and cells with another karyotype are associated with therapy-related leukemia.

In ALL, cytogenetic and molecular abnormalities can be detected in nearly all patients. Thus, genetic testing is frequently helpful to assess prognosis and to make therapeutic decisions at diagnosis and at relapse. The following chromosome abnormalities have been linked with particular prognoses and are listed in order of worsening event-free survival: hyperdiploidy greater than 50 (DNA index >1.16), t(12;21), t(1;19); near haploidy, t(9;22); and various translocations involving 11q23 rearrangements of MLL. Cytogenetic abnormalities in patients with ALL vary significantly by age. Adults with ALL rarely have t(12;21) or t(1;19), whereas t(9;22) is rare in children but is present in up to 25 percent of adults with ALL. Many patients with adult ALL also have deletions of various tumor suppressor and cell cycle regulatory genes, such as p15, p16, p53, and the Rb[1] gene.[86]

Need for Accurate Genetic Diagnosis

In most series, the observation of additional cytogenetic abnormalities with favorable cytogenetic subtypes did not change the clinical outcome. The importance of defining a patient's cytogenetic subtype at diagnosis results from our nascent abilities to provide specific therapies for certain cytogenetic subtypes of AML (e.g., acute promyelocytic leukemia) and our ability to alter the intensity of postremission therapy based on cytogenetic subtype of AML. Additionally, cytogenetic or molecular techniques can be used to monitor the quality of remission posttransplant and allow the clinician to intervene earlier in the course of relapse at the time of a molecular relapse rather than waiting until morphologic relapse has occurred.

Acute myeloid leukemia M3 or acute promyelocytic leukemia is currently the best example of acute leukemia to illustrate the relationship between an accurate cytogenetic or molecular diagnosis and selection of an appropriate initial and subsequent treatment. In cases morphologically suspected to represent AML-M3, FISH, PCR, or cytogenetic studies should be performed to confirm the diagnosis and to help guide therapy. Cases that morphologically resemble AML-M3 but lack rearrangement of the RARα gene may represent other subtypes of leukemia, such as AML expressing a natural killer cell phenotype.[87] Some cases of AML-M3 have variant translocations such as t(11;17), t(5;17), and others. The AML-M3 associated with t(11;17) (q23;q21) is resistant to therapy with all-trans retinoic acid (ATRA), and characterization of this subtype of AML-M3 is important in order to avoid inappropriate therapy.

Monitoring of PML/RARα fusion or expression following completion of therapy in patients with AML-M3 is useful to look for relapse. It has been shown that patients with persistent PML/RARα expression or fusion by molecular or cytogenetic techniques have a poor prognosis. Early studies using only ATRA to treat AML-M3 demonstrated that patients with persistent disease have a high risk of relapse.[88,89] As a consequence, a combination of ATRA and chemotherapy has been used to successfully cure a significant proportion of patients with AML-M3.[90] In this treatment setting, persistence of PML/RARα fusion transcripts was also highly predictive of relapse.[91] Unfortunately, some patients with AML-M3 who become negative for PML/RARα by FISH or nested RT-PCR techniques still relapse following completion of therapy.

The results of one recent clinical trial indicated that patients with AML-M3 who undergo surveillance bone marrows every 3 months and who show recurrent PCR positivity have a high risk of relapse.[92] In approximately 70 percent of patients who relapse, the relapses are successfully predicted by this technique; most of the time relapse occurs within the first 6 months following the end of therapy. Another clinical trial demonstrated that patients with AML-M3 who relapse following initial therapy with ATRA and chemotherapy have only a 65 percent chance of achieving a second remission and achieve a two-year survival of only 44 percent.[86] Combining the results of these two clinical trials would suggest that treatment at the time of molecular relapse can increase chances of an improved outcome as compared with waiting until frank hematologic relapse occurs.[47]

One clinical trial established that the majority of patients with AML-M3 also express reciprocal RARα/PML fusion transcripts and attempted to determine if measuring this molecular parameter could enhance the sensitivity of the method to detect minimal residual disease.[93] In fact, this assay did detect residual disease in an additional 20 percent of patients who otherwise appeared to be in morphologic remission. However, the majority of patients who relapsed had negative PCR assays for either transcript at the end of treatment, which suggests that there was less than one AML-M3 cell in 10^5 marrow cells.

An alternative approach has been to perform molecular assays at different stages following induction and consolidation chemotherapy. The results suggest that the detection of *PML/RARα* transcripts at any stage following induction or during consolidation is associated with an increased risk of relapse. It appears that the most predictive time for determining relapse is following the third course of chemotherapy, when the presence of a positive PCR assay predicted a significantly increased risk of relapse (57 versus 27 percent, $p = .006$). This finding also was associated with a poorer overall survival (57 versus 89 percent, $p = .02$) at 3 years in comparison with patients who had no evidence of minimal residual disease by PCR.[93] This outcome appeared to be independent of other prognostic factors and suggests that molecular monitoring could identify groups of patients at high risk of relapse and help determine whether additional consolidation therapy, including blood and marrow transplantation, in first remission might be of benefit.

The role of monitoring *PML/RARα* following blood and marrow transplant has also been studied. In one investigation of 15 patients who underwent autologous bone marrow transplant, the PCR status immediately preceding transplant was found to be a key indicator of subsequent relapse-free survival.[94] Patients who were PCR-positive pretransplant ultimately relapsed. By comparison, seven of eight patients testing PCR-negative pretransplant maintained long-term remission.

Both t(8;21) and inv(16) produce abnormal core binding factor alpha and beta subunits, and patients with these chromosome abnormalities have a favorable prognosis when high-dose cytosine arabinoside is incorporated into consolidation therapy. Thus, it is important to accurately identify patients with these subtypes of AML.[95]

In one investigation, a series of patients with AML who achieved remission with standard chemotherapy were randomly assigned to receive consolidation chemotherapy with high, standard, or intermediate doses of cytarabine.[96] Each patient was categorized into one of three cytogenetic groups, t(8;21) or inv(16), normal cytogenetic results, or chromosome abnormalities other than t(8;21) or inv(16). Univariate analysis demonstrated that a higher cytarabine dose was associated with a longer duration of complete remission, especially in patients with t(8;21) or inv(16). Of patients with t(8;21) or inv(16) who received 3 g/m^2 cytarabine, 78 percent maintained a long complete remission. By comparison, only 57 percent of patients receiving 400 mg/m^2 cytarabine and 16 percent of patients receiving 100 mg/m^2 cytarabine maintained complete remission. In the multivariate analysis of data from this study, the dose of cytarabine remained the most significant prognostic factor for long-term continuous complete remission.[96]

In another study, 50 patients with AML and t(8;21) were treated in four successive Cancer and Leukemia Group B (CALGB) trials.[97] The outcome of these patients was established retrospectively for patients who received one cycle of high-dose cytarabine compared with patients who received three or more cycles of high-dose cytarabine. Among patients who received only one course of high-dose cytarabine, 62 percent relapsed compared with 19 percent of patients who received three or more cycles. Nearly 59 percent of patients who received only one cycle of cytarabine died of AML compared to 24 percent of patients who received three or more cycles of high-dose cytarabine. These results further emphasize the importance of accurately identifying the correct subtypes of AML based on a combination of morphology, immunophenotyping, cytogenetics, and molecular studies in order to provide the most effective and least toxic therapy for individual patients. The ability to cure a significant proportion of patients with certain subtypes of AML without having to resort to the toxicity of blood and marrow transplant is an obvious benefit to these patients.

Using molecular genetic methods to monitor patients with a t(8;21) translocation following therapy has led to some conflicting results and emphasizes certain difficulties that still occur with these assays. Several studies have shown that *AML1/ETO* transcripts can be detected in patients who remain in long-term remission of their leukemia following therapy, regardless of whether the treatment is chemotherapy or autologous or allogeneic bone marrow transplant.[98–100] Other studies have demonstrated the absence of *AML1/ETO* transcripts in a significant proportion of patients in long-term remission of their disease.[101,102] The reason for these conflicting data is unclear but may be related to different methodologies with varying sensitivities.[103] The presence of residual *AML1/ETO* transcripts following apparently successful therapy may indicate that the presence of *AML1/ETO* is necessary but not sufficient for the presence of clinically significant leukemia. Additional studies have suggested that quantitation of *AML1/ETO* transcripts may help distinguish patients who are at risk of relapse from those who have stable disease.[104] For example, increasing quantities of *AML1/ETO* transcripts may predict relapse, whereas low and stable levels of *AML1/ETO* transcripts may be associated with continued remission.

Reports on the use of cytogenetic or molecular assays to monitor patients with inv(16) and *CBFβ/MYH11* fusion gene are limited to several small case series of five or fewer patients, and the results are mixed. Some patients remain persistently positive for *CBFB/MYH11* transcripts even in hematologic remission.[103] These data suggest that quantitative assays may be more useful to predict relapse in this subset of patients.

In ALL, specific chromosomal abnormalities can be found in the leukemic cells of up to 60 to 75 percent of patients. These genetic abnormalities include deletions, translocations, and hyperdiploidy or hypodiploidy. Many of these chromosomal abnormalities are powerful predictors of patient prognosis and, in conjunction with other disease characteristics, can allow an accurate risk assessment of patient outcome. For example, 70 to 80 percent of children under 1 year of age generally have a poor prognosis, especially when the *MLL* gene is abnormal.[105,106] Rearrangements of *MLL* and the presence of a Ph-chromosome or *BCR/ABL* gene rearrangement are associated with a poor prognosis and are common in patients with ALL.[107,108] In contrast, patients with hyperdiploidy (more than 50 chromosomes per cell) and rearrangements involving *TEL/AML1* associated with t(12;21)(p13;q22) or *E2A/EBX1* associated with t(1;19)(q23;p13) have more favorable prognoses.[109,110] These abnormalities are more common in children 1 to 9 years of age and tend to be associated with other good prognostic factors (e.g., hyperdiploidy is often associated with a low leukocyte count).

Favorable cytogenetic subgroups of ALL are less common in adults than in childhood ALL. This is in part related to the observation that the presence of the *BCR/ABL* fusion gene in ALL is much more common in adults than in children. This genetic abnormality is associated with a poor prognosis in both adults and children with ALL.

Although cytogenetic abnormalities can help predict a patient's prognosis, their predictive value is not perfect, because up to 20 percent of children with hyperdiploidy or the *TEL/AML1* fusion eventually experience disease relapse. Other clinical markers of risk assessment, such as the rate of clearance of leukemic cells from the blood or bone marrow during the early phase of therapy, can help predict which patients will have a better and which a poorer prognosis.[86]

The use of FISH or PCR to monitor patients for minimal residual disease is becoming more common.[111] It appears that patients who achieve a leukemic state involving less than 0.01 percent of bone marrow cells as determined by molecular or immunologic techniques have a better clinical outcome than those who achieve a morphologic remission. However, the presence of specific genetic abnormalities detected by molecular techniques is not always predictive of the outcome of treatment.[112] Nevertheless, the use of molecular techniques is becoming increasingly sophisticated. For example, the ability to quantitate the amount of disease will undoubtedly improve the potential to direct the intensity of therapy based on the quantity of disease present at various time points of therapy.

COST-EFFECTIVE TESTING STRATEGIES FOR ACUTE LEUKEMIA

Treatment protocols for hematologic disorders require testing procedures that can quantify tumor burden before and after therapy to assess responsiveness to therapy. This can be done by using various genetic tests, including quantitative cytogenetic studies, FISH, and RT-PCR (for more information on these methods, see the section on genetic testing strategies earlier in this chapter). No single genetic testing procedure fulfills all the needs of clinical care for patients with acute leukemia. Thus, it is important to use combinations of testing methods that are both accurate and cost-effective for each clinical situation. Testing strategies need to be adjusted over time as methodologies improve or change. Thus, the effort to develop enhanced genetic testing methods should be part of a continuous quality improvement program. Moreover, the availability of and experience with different genetic tests varies among institutions. Thus, different institutions may employ varying genetic testing strategies for hematologic malignancies.

Many chromosome abnormalities associated with acute leukemia cannot be detected by current FISH or RT-PCR methods either because it is technically not possible or because suitable probes or primers have not yet been developed. For patients with these abnormalities, conventional chromosome studies are the sole method of detecting them. Some chromosome abnormalities associated with acute leukemia can be detected by cytogenetics, FISH, and PCR. In these cases, the genetic test of choice should be selected according to cost, turnaround time, and clinical situation, that is, at the time of diagnosis versus quantitation of residual disease following therapy. Since all genetic tests are relatively expensive and genetic laboratories are busy, it is not reasonable to routinely perform all available genetic tests. General genetic testing strategies for acute leukemia are shown in Figure 16–3 and 16–4.

At diagnosis of acute leukemia, quantitative cytogenetic studies are useful to establish the presence and kind of chromosome abnormalities as well as the percentage of mitotic neoplastic cells. If a FISH test is available to detect the primary chromosome abnormality, this test can be performed on bone marrow and blood at diagnosis, when it also serves to establish a benchmark for percentage of neoplastic cells. After treatment, quantitative cytogenetic studies and/or FISH can be used to establish the percentage of neoplastic cells and help assess the effectiveness of therapy. If the percentage of neoplastic cells by FISH is less than the sensitivity of the test, then more sensitive procedures such as RT-PCR should be employed. For acute leukemia, this kind of approach is useful for t(8;21), t(9;22), t(11;var), inv(16), −5/5q−, −7/7q− and some others (for more details on available genetic tests see earlier section on specific chromosome abnormalities in acute leukemia).

For some hematologic malignancies, the primary chromosome abnormality is difficult to detect. The 15;17 translocation associated with AML-M3 is an example of this kind of cytogenetic problem. If AML-M3 is strongly suspected, the initial genetic study could be FISH or RT-PCR to detect PML/RARα fusion (Figure 16–3). An ES-FISH test is available to detect cells with *PML/RARα* when these cells exceed 3 percent of all cells. Most untreated patients with AML-M3 have 50 to 91 percent of

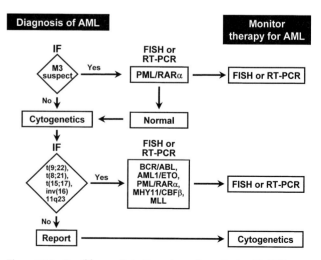

Figure 16–3. Possible genetic testing scheme for patients with AML at diagnosis and for monitoring therapy.

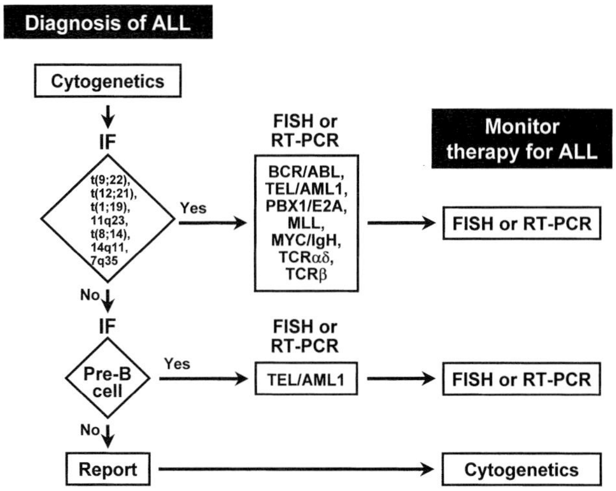

Figure 16–4. Possible genetic testing scheme for patients with ALL at diagnosis and for monitoring therapy.

cells with *PML/RARα* fusion in their bone marrow. Moreover, rare patients with AML-M3 have a translocation other than 15;17 (for more details, see t(15;17) in section on specific chromosome abnormalities in acute leukemia). This FISH test can usually detect these variants as the hybridization site for *RARα* breaks apart, but no *PML/RARα* fusion is observed. This FISH test is particularly valuable because it can be performed overnight and applied to cells prepared for standard cytogenetic studies. Thus, if the results of this FISH test are normal, conventional cytogenetic studies can then be performed to assess the entire karyotype of the abnormal clone to look for other chromosome abnormalities. If AML-M3 is not initially suspected, cytogenetic studies do not reveal a 15;17 translocation and morphology studies strongly suggest AML-M3, then FISH or RT-PCR studies for *PML/RARα* should be performed. A FISH test for *PML/RARα* can be performed on leftover cells from cytogenetic studies or on unstained blood or bone marrow aspirate smears.

The 12;21 translocation associated with pre-B-ALL is very difficult to detect by conventional cytogenetic studies because the band pattern of the chromatin that is exchanged between chromosomes 12 and 21 is nearly identical. Thus, when ALL is suspected and the results of chromosome studies are normal, then a FISH or PCR test for *TEL/AML1* fusion is important to properly classify this hematologic malignancy. Nevertheless, the initial genetic test at diagnosis of ALL should be cytogenetic studies, as this method detects a wide variety of abnormalities (Figure 16–4). If the cytogenetic result is abnormal but no well-known chromosome abnormality associated with ALL is detected, then it is useful to perform a FISH or RT-PCR test for *TEL/AML1* fusion, as patients with such karyotypes often harbor a 12;21 translocation.

Cytogenetic studies are valuable to assess the effectiveness of therapy. For acute leukemia, patients have predominantly cells with normal chromosomes in remission. When the disease of these patients relapses, the cells with the original chromosome abnormalities are observed. The sensitivity of conventional cyto-

genetic studies is sometimes underestimated. Because cytogenetic studies focus on mitotic cells, they sometimes detect one or two abnormal metaphases even when other genetic tests are normal. Moreover, cytogenetic studies can detect chromosome abnormalities associated with therapy-related leukemia. Nevertheless, if a good FISH or RT-PCR test is available to quantify disease, these are the genetic tests of choice to monitor remission because they are less expensive and more sensitive. If therapy-related leukemia is suspected, it is useful to perform a cytogenetic study.

Because the tumor burden following bone marrow transplantation is very small, the best genetic method to monitor disease may be RT-PCR. This method has proved particularly useful to detect *PML/RARα* fusion in the period following bone marrow transplantation and is useful to detect relapse of disease. Also, FISH can be used to monitor the tumor burden after bone marrow transplantation; various FISH strategies are available to monitor patients posttransplant. Probes for the X and Y chromosome can be used for opposite-sex bone marrow transplantation,[21] the XY and XX nuclei being easy to detect by the red and green signals. This method can detect less than 0.3 percent XY cells in females and less than 0.6 percent XX cells in males. This method defines the ratio of host versus donor cells but does not directly establish the percentage of neoplastic cells, which, however, can be determined by an appropriate FISH test, if one is available, for any given patient with a hematologic malignancy. Depending on the FISH test used, these methods can detect disease when it exceeds 1 to 3 percent of all cells.

FISH and RT-PCR both require prior knowledge of the primary genetic abnormality for any given patient and do not detect other abnormalities. To overcome this weakness, some investigators have begun to use panel FISH tests or multiplexed RT-PCR for hematologic disorders. For ALL, a panel FISH test to detect t(9;22), t(12;21), t(1;19), t(8;14), and hyperdiploidy may be useful. For AML, a panel FISH test to detect t(9;22), t(8;21), t(15;17), t(11;var), inv(16) and common abnormalities of chromosomes 5 and 7 may be useful. Given the karyotype diversity of acute leukemia, these methods are not generally substitutes for cytogenetic studies at diagnosis. Nevertheless, these methods hold promise, because evidence is emerging to suggest that multiplex RT-PCR and panel FISH testing may detect neoplastic clones in a few patients with acute leukemia when the results of cytogenetic studies are normal, not possible, or too complex to reveal a classical chromosome abnormality.

REFERENCES

1. Tjio J, Levan A: The chromosome number in man. Hereditas 42:1–6, 1956.
2. Lejeune J, Gautier M, Turpin R: Etude des chromosomes somatiques de neuf enfants mongoliens. C R Acad Sci III 248:1721–1722, 1959.
3. Jacobs P, Strong J: A case of human intersexuality having a possible XXY sex-determining mechanism. Nature 183:302–303, 1959.
4. Ford C, Jones K, Polani P et al: A sex-chromosome anomaly in a case of gonadal dysgenesis (Turner's syndrome). Lancet i:711–713, 1959.
5. Nowell P, Hungerford D: A minute chromosome in human chronic granulocytic leukemia. Science 132:1497, 1960.

6. Dewald G: Modern methods of chromosome analysis and their application in clinical practice. Clin Lab Ann 2:1–29, 1983.

7. Rowley J: A new consistent chromosomal abnormality in chronic myelogenous leukemia identified by quinacrine fluorescence and Giemsa staining. Nature 243:290–293, 1973.

8. Rowley J: Identification of a translocation with quinacrine fluorescence in a patient with acute leukemia. Ann Genet 16:109, 1973.

9. Rowley J, Golomb H, Vardiman J et al: Further evidence for a non-random abnormality in acute promyelocytic leukemia. Int J Cancer 20:869–872, 1977.

10. Hagemeijer A, Hahlen K, Sizoo, W et al: Translocation (9;11)(p21;q23) in three cases of acute monoblastic leukemia. Cancer Genet Cytogenet 5:95–105, 1982.

11. Le Beau M, Larson R, Bitter M et al: Association of an inversion of chromosome 16 with abnormal marrow eosinophils in acute myelomonocytic leukemia. N Engl J Med 309:630–636, 1983.

12. Koeffler H: Syndromes of acute nonlymphocytic leukemia. Ann Intern Med 107:748–758, 1987.

13. Fourth International Workshop on Chromosomes in Leukemia: A prospective study of acute nonlymphocytic leukemia. Cancer Genet Cytogenet 11:249–360, 1984.

14. Westbrook C, Rubin C, Carrino J et al: Long-range mapping of the Philadelphia chromosome by pulsed-field gel electrophoresis. Blood 71:697–702, 1988.

15. Gale R, Canaani E: An 8-kilobase abl RNA transcript in chronic myelogenous leukemia. Proc Natl Acad Sci USA 81:5648–5652, 1984.

16. Canaani E, Gale R, Steiner-Saltz D et al: Altered transcription of an oncogene in chronic myeloid leukaemia. Lancet 1:593–595, 1984.

17. Stam K, Heisterkamp N, Reynolds FJ et al: Evidence that the phl gene encodes a 160,000-dalton phosphoprotein with associated kinase activity. Mol Cell Biol 7:1955–1960, 1987.

18. Dewald G, Ketterling R, Wyatt W et al: Cytogenetic studies in neoplastic hematologic disorders. In McClatchey K (ed.): Clinical Laboratory Medicine, 2nd ed. Lippincott Williams & Wilkens, Baltimore, pp 658–685, 2002.

19. Dewald GW, Juneau AL, Schad CR et al: Cytogenetic and molecular genetic methods for diagnosis and treatment response in chronic granulocytic leukemia. Cancer Genet Cytogenet 94:59–66, 1997.

20. Jenkins R, LeBeau M, Kraker W et al: Fluorescence in situ hybridization; a sensitive method for trisomy 8 detection in bone marrow specimens. Blood 79:3307–3315, 1992.

21. Dewald GW, Schad CR, Christensen ER et al: Fluorescence in situ hybridization with X and Y chromosome probes for cytogenetic studies on bone marrow cells after opposite sex transplantation. Bone Marrow Transplant 12:149–154, 1993.

22. Schad CR, Hanson CA, Paietta E et al: Efficacy of fluorescence in situ hybridization for detecting PML/RARA gene fusion in treated and untreated acute promyelocytic leukemia. Mayo Clin Proc 69:1047–1053, 1994.

23. Juneau AL, Kaehler M, Christensen ER et al: Detection of RB1 deletions by fluorescence in situ hybridization in malignant hematologic disorders. Cancer Genet Cytogenet 103:117–123, 1998.

24. Remstein E, Kurtin P, Buno I et al: Diagnostic utility of fluorescence in situ hybridization in mantle cell lymphoma. Br J Haematol 110:856–862, 2000.

25. Dewald GW, Wyatt WA, Juneau AL et al: Highly sensitive fluorescence in situ hybridization method to detect double BCR/ABL fusion and monitor response to therapy in chronic myeloid leukemia. Blood 91:3357–3365, 1998.

26. Dewald G, Wyatt W, Silver R: Atypical BCR and ABL D-FISH patterns in chronic myeloid leukemia and their possible role in therapy. Leuk Lymphoma 34:481–491, 1999.

27. Jalal S, Law M, Dewald G: Atlas of Whole Chromosome Paint Probes: Normal Patterns and Utility for Abnormal Cases. Mayo Foundation for Medical Education and Research. Rochester, MN, 1996.

28. Knight S, Lese C, Precht K et al: An optimized set of human telomere clones for studying telomere integrity and architecture. Am J Hum Genet 67:820–332, 2000.

29. Buno I, Wyatt WA, Zinsmeister AR et al: A special fluorescent in situ hybridization technique to study peripheral blood and assess the effectiveness of interferon therapy in chronic myeloid leukemia. Blood 92:2315–2321, 1998.

30. Jenkins RB, Kimmel DW, Moertel CA et al: A cytogenetic study of 53 human gliomas. Cancer Genet Cytogenet 39:253–279, 1989.

31. Dewald GW, Schad CR, Christensen ER et al: The application of fluorescent in situ hybridization to detect Mbcr/abl fusion in variant Ph chromosomes in CML and ALL. Cancer Genet Cytogenet 71:7–14, 1993.

32. Jalal S: Detection of diagnostically critical, often hidden, anomalies in complex karyotypes of hematologic disorders by M-FISH analysis. Br J Haematol 112:975–980, 2001.

33. Liu Yin J, Tobal K: Detection of minimal residual disease in acute myeloid leukaemia: Methodologies, clinical and biological significance. Br J Haematol 106:578–590, 1999.

34. Cross N, Feng L, Chase A et al: Competitive polymerase chain reaction to estimate the number of BCR-ABL transcripts in chronic myeloid leukemia patients after bone marrow transplantation. Blood 82:1929–1936, 1993.

35. Tobal K, Liu Yin J: Monitoring of minimal residual disease by quantitative reverse transcriptase polymerase chain reaction for AML-MTG8 transcripts in AML-M2 with t(8;21). Blood 88:3704–3709, 1996.

36. Higuchi R, Dollinger G, Walsh P et al: Simultaneous amplification and detection of specific DNA sequences. Biotechnology 10:413–417, 1992.

37. Higuchi R, Fockler C, Dollinger G et al: Kinetic PCR analysis: Real-time monitoring of DNA amplication reactions. Biotechnology 11:1026–1030, 1993.

38. Bennett J, Catovsky D, Daniel M et al: Proposals for the classification of the acute leukaemias. French-American-British (FAB) Cooperative Group. Br J Haematol 33:451–458, 1976.

39. Bennett J, Catovsky D, Daniel M et al: Proposed revised criteria for the classification of acute myeloid leukemia. A report of the French-American-British Cooperative Group. Ann Intern Med 103:620–625, 1985.

40. Bennett J, Catovsky D, Daniel M et al: Proposal for the recognition of minimally differentiated acute myeloid leukaemia (AML-MO). Br J Haematol 78:325–329, 1991.

41. Bennett J, Catovsky D, Daniel M et al: Proposals for the classification of the myelodysplastic syndromes. Br J Haematol 51:189–199, 1982.

42. Harris N, Jaffe E, Diebold J et al: World Health Organization classification of neoplastic diseases of the hematopoietic and lymphoid tissues: Report of the clinical advisory committee meeting, Airlie House, Virginia, November 1997. J Clin Oncol 17:3835–3849, 1999.

43. Greenberg P, Anderson J, de Witte T et al: International MDS Study Group. Problematic WHO reclassification of myelodysplastic syndromes (letter). J Clin Oncol 18:3447–3452, 2000.

44. Greenberg P, Cox C, LeBeau M et al: International scoring system for evaluating prognosis in myelodysplastic syndrome. Blood 89:2079–2088, 1997.

45. Marcucci G, Caligiuri M, Bloomfield C: Molecular and clinical advances in core binding factor primary acute myeloid leukemia: A paradigm for translational research in malignant hematology. Cancer Invest 18:768–780, 2000.

46. Shurtleff S, Buijs A, Behm F et al: TEL/AML1 fusion resulting from a cryptic t(12;21) is the most common genetic lesion in pediatric ALL and defines a subgroup of patients with an excellent prognosis. Leukemia 9:1985–1989, 1995.

47. Grimwade D, Howe K, Langabeer S et al: Minimal residual disease detection in acute promyelocytic leukemia by reverse-transcriptase PCR: Evaluation of PML-RAR alpha and RAR alpha-PML assessment in patients who ultimately relapse. Leukemia 10:61–66, 1996.

48. Dewald GW, Schad CR, Lilla VC et al: Frequency and photographs of HGM11 chromosome anomalies in bone marrow samples from 3,996 patients with malignant hematologic neoplasms. Cancer Genet Cytogenet 68:60–69, 1993.

49. Mitelman F: Catalog of Chromosome Aberrations in Cancer, 4th ed. Alan R. Liss, New York, 1991.

50. Mitelman F, Kaneko Y, Trent J: Report of the committee on chromosome changes in neoplasia. Cytogenet Cell Genet 58:1053–1079, 1991.

51. Mitelman F, Kaneko Y, Berger R: Report of the committee on chromosome changes changes in neoplasia. In Cuticchia A, Chipperfield M, Foster P (eds.): Human Gene Mapping 1995: A Compendium. p. 1332–1350. Johns Hopkins University Press, Baltimore, 1996.

52. Mitelman F, Mertens F, Johansson B: A breakpoint map of recurrent chromosomal rearrangements in human neoplasia. Nat Genet 15(special issue):417–474, 1997.

53. Wilman C: Acute leukemia: A paradigm for the integration of new technologies in diagnosis and classification. Mod Pathol 12:218–228, 1999.

54. Raimondi S, Chang M, Ravindranath Y et al: Chromosomal abnormalities in 478 children with acute myeloid leukemia: Clinical characteristics and treatment outcome in a Cooperative Pediatric Oncology Group Study POG 8821. Blood 94:3707–3716, 1999.

55. Faderl S, Kantarjian H, Talpaz M et al: Clinical significance of cytogenetic abnormalities in adult acute lymphoblastic leukemia. Blood 91:3995–4019, 1998.

56. Rubnitz J, Look A: Molecular genetics of childhood leukemia. J Pediatr Hematol Oncol 20:1–11, 1998.

57. Kantarjian H, Keating M: Therapy-related leukemia and myelodysplastic syndrome. Semin Oncol 14:435, 1987.

58. Bloomfield C, Brunning R: Acute leukemia as a terminal event in leukemia hematopoietic disorders. Semin Oncol 3:297, 1976.

59. Drexler H, Borkhardt A, Janssen J: Detection of chromosomal translocations in leukemia-lymphoma cells by polymerase chain reaction. Leuk Lymphoma 19:359–380, 1995.

60. Brunning R, McKenna R: Tumors of the bone marrow. In Atlas of Tumor Pathology. Armed Forces Institute of Pathology, Washington, D.C., 1994.

61. McCarthy K: Molecular diagnosis of lymphomas and associated diseases. Cancer Metastasis Rev 16:109–125, 1997.

62. Block A: Cancer Cytogenetics. In Gersen S, Keagle M (eds.): The Principles of Clinical Cytogenetics. pp. 345–420. Humana Press, Totowa, NJ, 1999.

63. Roulston D, Le Beau M: Cytogenetic analysis of hematologic malignant diseases. In M. J. Barch TK, J. Spurbeck (eds.): The AGT Cytogenetics Laboratory Manual, 3rd ed. pp. 352–372. Lippincott-Raven, Philadelphia, 1997.

64. Chessells J, Swansbury G, Reeves B et al: Cytogenetics and prognosis in childhood lymphoblastic leukaemia: Results of MRC UKALL X. Br J Haematol 99:93–100, 1997.

65. Lu G, Altman A, Benn P: Review of the cytogenetic changes in acute megakaryoblastic leukemia: One disease or several? Cancer Genet Cytogenet 67:81–89, 1993.

66. Barnard D, Kalousek D, Wiersma S et al: Morphologic, immunologic, and cytogenetic classification of acute myeloid leukemia and myelodysplastic syndrome in childhood: A report from the Childrens Cancer Group. Leukemia 10:5–12, 1996.

67. Harrison C, Secker-Walker L: The importance of cytogenetics and associated molecular techniques in the management of patients with leukemia. Clin Oncol (R Coll Radiol) 10:255–261, 1998.

68. Gilliland DG: Molecular genetics of human leukemia. Leukemia 12:S7–S12, 1998.

69. Johansson B, Mertens F, Mitelman F: Secondary chromosomal abnormalities in acute leukemias. Leukemia 8:953–962, 1994.

70. Vallespi T, Imbert M, Mecucci C et al: Diagnosis, classification, and cytogenetics of myelodysplastic syndromes. Haematologica 83:258–275, 1998.

71. Giles F, Koeffler H: Secondary myelodysplastic syndromes and leukemias. Curr Opin Hematol 1:256–260, 1994.

72. Thirman M, Larson J: Therapy-related myeloid leukemia (Review). Hematol Oncol Clin North Am 10:293–320, 1996.

73. Tefferi A, Litzow MR, Noel P et al: Chronic granulocytic leukemia: Recent information on pathogenesis, diagnosis, and disease monitoring. Mayo Clin Proc 72:445–452, 1997.

74. Van Rhee F, Lin F, Cullis J et al: Relapse of chronic myeloid leukemia after allogeneic bone marrow transplant: The case for giving donor leukocyte transfusions before the onset of hematologic relapse. Blood 83:3377–3383, 1994.

75. Talpaz M, Kantarjian H, Kurzrock R, Trujillo JM, Gutterman JU. Interferon-alpha produces sustained cytogenetic responses in chronic myelogenous leukemia. Philadelphia chromosome-positive patients. Annals of Internal Medicine 114:532–538, 1991.

76. Leukemia. ICSGoCM. Interferon alfa-2a as compared with conventional chemotherapy for the treatment of chronic myeloid leukemia. N Engl J Med 330:820–825, 1994.

77. Kloke O, Niederle N, Qiu JY et al. Impact of interferon alpha-induced cytogenetic improvement on survival in chronic myelogenous leukaemia. Br J Haematol 83:399–403, 1993.

78. Allan NC, Richards SM, Sherpherd PC. UK Medical Research Council randomised, multicentre trial of interferon-alpha n1 for chronic myeloid leukaemia: Improved survival irrespective of cytogenetic response. The UK Medical Research Council's Working Parties for Therapeutic Trials in Adult Leukaemia. Lancet 345:1392–397, 1995.

79. Thiesing J, Ohno-Jones S, Kolibaba K et al: Efficacy of STI571, an Abl tyrosine kinase inhibitor, in conjunction with other antileukemic agents against Bcr-Abl-positive cells. Blood 96:3195–3199, 2000.

80. Druker B. STI1571 (Gleevec/Glivec, imatinib) versus interferon (IFN) + cytarabine as initial therapy for patients with CML: Results of a randomized study. For the IRIS (International Randomized IFN vs. STI1571) Study Group, Oregon Health & Science University, Portland, OR. Proceedings of ASCO 21:1A, 2002.

81. Schnittger S, Kinkelin U, Schoch C et al: Screening for MLL tandem duplication in 387 unselected patients with AML identify a prognostically unfavorable subset of AML. Leukemia 14:796–804, 2000.

82. Schnittger S, Schoch C, Dugas M, et al. Analysis of FLT3 length mutations in 1003 patients with acute myeloid leukemia: Correlation to cytogenetics, FAB subtype, and prognosis in the AMLCG study and usefulness as a marker for the detection of minimal residual disease. Blood 100:59–66, 2002.

83. Kottaridis PD, Gale RE, Frew ME et al. The presence of a FLT3 internal tandem duplication in patients with acute myeloid leukemia (AML) adds important prognostic information to cyto-

genetic risk group and response to the first cycle of chemotherapy: Analysis of 854 patients from the United Kingdom Medical Research Council AML 10 and 12 trials. Blood 98:1752–1759, 2001.

84. Grimwade D, Walker H, Oliver F et al: The importance of diagnostic cytogenetics on outcome in AML: Analysis of 1,612 patients entered into the MRC AML 10 trial. The Medical Research Council Adult and Children's Leukaemia Working Parties. Blood 92:2322–2333, 1998.

85. Slovak M, Kopecky K, Cassileth P et al: Karyotypic analysis predicts outcome of preremission and postremission therapy in adult acute myeloid leukemia: A Southwest Oncology Group/Eastern Cooperative Oncology Group study. Blood 96:4075–4083, 2000.

86. Pui C, Evans W: Acute lymphoblastic leukemia. N Engl J Med 339:605–615, 1998.

87. Scott A, Head D, Kopecky K et al: HLA-DR-, CD33+, CD56+, CD16- myeloid/natural killer cell acute leukemia: A previously unrecognized form of acute leukemia potentially misdiagnosed as French-American-British acute myeloid leukemia-M3. Blood 84:244–255, 1994.

88. Huang M, Yu-Chen Y, Shu-Rong C et al: Use of all-trans retinoic acid in the treatment of acute promyelocytic leukemia. Blood 72:567–572, 1988.

89. Castaigne S, Chomienne C, Daniel M et al: All-trans retinoic acid as a differentiation therapy for acute promyelocytic leukemia. Clinical results. Blood 76:1704–1709, 1990.

90. Fenaux P, Le Deley M, Castaigne S et al: Effect of all transretinoic acid in newly diagnosed acute promyelocytic leukemia. Results of a multicenter randomized trial. European APL 91 Group. Blood 82:3241–3249, 1993.

91. Lo Coco F, Diverio D, Pandolfi P et al: Molecular evaluation of residual disease as a predictor of relapse in acute promyelocytic leukaemia. Lancet 340:1437–1438, 1992.

92. Diverio D, Rossi V, Avvisati G et al: Early detection of relapse by prospective reverse transcriptase–polymerase chain reaction analysis of the PML/RARα fusion gene in patients with acute promyelocytic leukemia enrolled in the GIMEMA–AIEOP multicenter "AIDA" trial. Blood 92:784–789, 1998.

93. Burnett A, Grimwade D, Solomon E et al: Presenting white blood cell count and kinetics of molecular remission predict prognosis in acute promyelocytic leukemia treated with all-trans retinoic acid: Result of the Randomized MRC Trial. Blood 93:4131–4143, 1999.

94. Meloni G, Diverio D, Vignetti M et al: Autologous bone marrow transplantation for acute promyelocytic leukemia in second remission: Prognostic relevance of pretransplant minimal residual disease assessment by reverse-transcription polymerase chain reaction of the PML/RARα fusion gene. Blood 90:1321–1325, 1997.

95. Bloomfield C, Lawrence D, Byrd J et al: Frequency of prolonged remission duration after high-dose cytarabine intensification in acute myeloid leukemia varies by cytogenetic subtype. Cancer Res 58:4173–4179, 1998.

96. Mayer R, Davis R, Schiffer C et al: Intensive postremission chemotherapy in adults with acute myeloid leukemia. Cancer and Leukemia Group B. N Engl J Med 331:896–903, 1994.

97. Byrd J, Dodge R, Carroll A et al: Patients with t(8;21)(q22;q22) and acute myeloid leukemia have superior failure-free and overall survival when repetitive cycles of high-dose cytarabine are administered. J Clin Oncol 17:3767–3775, 1999.

98. Nucifora G, Larson R, Rowley J: Persistence of the 8;21 translocation in patients with acute myeloid leuekmia type M2 in long-term remission. Blood 82:712–715, 1993.

99. Kusec R, Laczika K, Knobl P et al: AML1/ETO fusion mRNA can be detected in remission blood samples of all patients with t(8;21) acute myeloid leukemia after chemotherapy or autologous bone marrow transplantation. Leukemia 8:735–739, 1994.

100. Jurlander J, Caligiuri M, Ruutu T et al: Persistence of the AML1/ETO fusion transcript in patients treated with allogeneic bone marrow transplantation for t(8;21) leukemia. Blood 88:2183–2191, 1996.

101. Kwong Y, Chan V, Wong K et al: Use of polymerase chain reaction in the detection of AML1/ETO fusion transcript in t(8;21). Cancer 75:821–825, 1995.

102. Satake N, Maseki N, Kozu T et al: Disappearance of AML1-MTG8 (ETO) fusion transcript in acute myeloid leukaemia patients with t(8;21) in long-term remission. Br J Haematol 91:892–898, 1995.

103. Yin J, Tobal K: Detection of minimal residual disease in acute myeloid leukaemia: Methodologies, clinical and biological significance. Br J Haematol 106:578–590, 1999.

104. Tobal K, Liu Yin J: Monitoring of minimal residual disease by quantitative reverse transcriptase polymerase chain reaction for AML-MTG8 transcripts in AML-M2 with t(8;21). Blood 88:3704–3709, 1996.

105. Pui C-H, Frankel L, Carroll A et al: Clinical characteristics and treatment outcome of childhood acute lymphoblastic leukemia with the t(4;11)(q21;q23): A collaborative study of 40 cases. Blood 77:440–447, 1991.

106. Behm F, Raimondi S, Frestedt J et al: Rearrangement of the MLL gene confers a poor prognosis in childhood acute lymphoblastic leukemia, regardless of presenting age. Blood 87:2870–2877, 1996.

107. Groupe Français de Cytogénétique Hématologique: Cytogenetic abnormalities in adult acute lymphoblastic leukemia: Correlations with hematologic findings and outcome. A collaborative study of the Groupe Français de Cytogénétique Hématologique. Blood 87:3135, 1996.

108. Wetzler M, Dodge R, Krzysztof M et al: Prospective karyotype analysis in adult acute lymphoblastic leukemia: The cancer and leukemia group B experience. Blood 93:3983–3993, 1999.

109. Rubnitz J, Downing J, Pui C-H et al: TEL gene rearrangement in acute lymphoblastic leukemia: A new genetic marker with prognostic significance. J Clin Oncol 15:1150–1157, 1997.

110. Borkhardt A, Cazzaniga G, Viehmann S et al: Incidence and clinical relevance of TEL/AML1 fusion genes in children with acute lymphoblastic leukemia enrolled in the German and Italian multicenter therapy trials. Blood 90:571–577, 1997.

111. Campana D, Pui C-H: Detection of minimal residual disease in acute leukemia: Methodologic advances and clinical significance. Blood 85:1416–1434, 1995.

112. Hunger S, Fall M, Camitta B et al: E2A-PBX1 chimeric transcript status at end of consolidation is not predictive of treatment outcome in childhood acute lymphoblastic leukemias with a t(1;19)(q23;p13): A Pediatric Oncology Group Study. Blood 91:1021–1028, 1998.

17

Diagnosis and Treatment of Childhood Acute Lymphoblastic Leukemia

Susan M. McKenna

DEFINITION AND HISTORY

Leukemia, a cancer of the blood-forming cells thought to arise in the bone marrow, was first described as an independent clinical entity by Bennett[1] in 1845 and by Virchow[2] in 1847. Ehrlich[3] in 1891 described techniques for cell staining that resulted in improved ability to understand the pathogenesis of leukemia and to help in differentiating it from other, nonmalignant conditions of the blood. The advent of cytochemistry aided in defining the lineage of the malignant cell, separating acute leukemias of lymphoid origin from those of myeloid and monocytoid origins. The employment of clinical features of the child presenting with leukemia, as well as the results of recent immunologic and cytogenetic studies to further define the origin of the lymphoblast cell involved in the leukemic process, has refined our ability to predict outcome with modern chemotherapeutic regimens.

The fatal prognosis for a child presenting with acute lymphoblastic leukemia (ALL) remained unchanged until 1948, when Farber et al. described an approximate 20 percent remission induction rate obtained by using the folic acid antagonist aminopterin.[4] In the following decade, steroids, 6-mercaptopurine (6-MP) and cyclophosphamide (Cytoxan) proved effective in treating ALL. In the 1960s vincristine, daunorubicin, doxorubicin, cytosine arabinoside (ara-C), and L-asparaginase (L-asp) were synthesized and shown to have antileukemic effects as well.

Treatment with single agents was effective for short periods of time in some patients. Significant changes in survival were not seen, however, until combinations of agents were implemented in treatment protocols. A second significant factor in improving the outcome of children with ALL was the institution of prophylactic treatment of the central nervous system (CNS).[5] Further improvement in survival continued during the 1970s with intensification of treatment programs and aggressive supportive care. Since the last decade of the twentieth century, children with ALL have had a 95 percent chance of achieving remission. The long-term survival and cure rates for children with ALL are significantly better than 50 percent in most cases, and in certain good prognostic groups is at least 85 percent.[6–9]

INCIDENCE

Cancer is the second most common cause of death in children under the age of 15 years, accounting for approximately 2.5 deaths per 100,000 children per year (10.6 percent of all deaths). Only accidental causes exceed the rate of mortality due to cancer (39.8 percent).[10] Approximately 7000 new cases of cancer are diagnosed annually, of which one-third will be leukemia, the most frequent childhood malignancy. Of childhood cancer deaths, 30 percent occur in patients with acute leukemia,[10,11] and 80 percent of the childhood leukemias occurring before age 15 are ALL.

Acute lymphoblastic leukemia occurs in approximately twice as many white as nonwhite children. The peak incidence of ALL in white children occurs between the ages of 3 and 4 with slightly more boys affected than girls.[12] Following puberty, the incidence of ALL decreases, whereas that of acute nonlymphocytic forms (ANLL) increases.[13–15] In nonwhite children, the incidence occurs at a relatively constant rate until age 20.[12]

ETIOLOGY

The precise etiology of leukemia in humans is still not clear, but mounting circumstantial evidence incriminates interactions of viruses as causative agents, as well as chromosomal alterations and/or environmental influences. Retroviruses (RNA viruses) can cause leukemias and lymphomas in animal species,[16] including avian leukosis[17] and murine leukemia,[18] as well as leukemia in cats, cattle, and gibbons.[19] These retroviruses are transmitted as exogenous infections and are not transmitted in the germ line (endogenous). In endemic areas, the feline leukemia virus causes spontaneous leukemia in a significant number of pet cats.[20–22] In humans, failure to find "viral footprints" by using known retroviral probes does not rule out a new subclass of retrovirus as the etiologic agent in human leukemia.[19] A retrovirus has been implicated in human T-cell leukemia and lymphoma.[19] This virus, human T-cell leukemia virus (HTLV), is similar to the bovine leukemia virus in that the tumor cells were first cultured in vitro before the virus could be isolated. Since then, HTLV has been demonstrated in cultured T cells from many patients worldwide. It appears to be an exogenous or infectious human virus because sequences from HTLV are not present in healthy donors.[33] Antibodies to HTLV have been found in the United States and Europe but have been detected in a higher proportion of Japanese and West Indian patients, in whom T-cell leukemia occurs in an endemic pattern.[19] Only one case of HTLV-associated T-cell leukemia has been reported in a child.[24]

Certain groups are well documented to have a greater than normal risk of developing acute leukemia. Many of these risk factors are associated with genetic abnormalities and often alterations of DNA repair mechanisms, which leads to speculation about the role of these chromosomal changes in the etiology of leukemia. In 30 percent of patients with Fanconi's anemia, leukemia or preleukemia will develop.[25] Patients with Bloom's syndrome have a 12 percent chance of developing leukemia.[31]

Ataxia–telangiectasia has been associated with malignancies of the lymphoreticular system, including ALL.[27–29] Children with trisomy 21 are at increased risk of developing leukemia (approximately 1 percent).[26] In addition, certain congenital disorders that are not associated with chromosomal findings have an increased association with ALL. These include Poland's syndrome[29,30] (absence of the pectoralis major muscle), Schwachman's syndrome[31] (pancreatic enzyme deficiency and neutropenia), and Rubinstein-Taybi syndrome[32] (retarded osseous maturation). Neurofibromatosis has also been associated with an increased incidence of acute leukemia.[33]

Although the observed chromosomal changes in leukemia clones were first linked to prognosis, some are now being studied as possible leukemogenic events.[34–36] In Burkitt's lymphoma and B-cell leukemia, the t(8;14) translocation, fusing the c-myc oncogene with genes encoding immunoglobulins (Igs), may deregulate cell proliferation.[37] Both myeloid and lymphoid leukemias with translocation of 11q23 have been shown to have breakpoints clustering in the area of the HXR gene, which encodes proteins that mediate DNA interactions. Fusion proteins derived from several of the 11q23 translocations seem to function as altered transcription factors.[35,36] Similar chimeric transcription factors have been identified following t(1;19).[34]

Considerable attention has been focused on the role of p53, the so-called tumor suppressor gene. Alterations of the gene have been described in a large variety of tumors.[38] In its physiologic role, p53 is thought to be involved in cellular differentiation, DNA repair, and apoptosis (programmed cell death). Of de novo cases of common childhood ALL, 2 to 3 percent are found to have mutations of p53; this proportion is even higher among cases of relapse and treatment-related second malignancies.[39,40] Although some of the chromosomal deviations catalogued may be initiating events, most appear not to be. If a model similar to Knudson's[41] two-hit hypothesis is invoked, it appears that some of the alterations may predispose to abnormal cellular responses following other stimuli, such as viral infection or exposure to environmental toxins.

In 1999 Sun et al. published two reports that describe the presence of abnormal isoforms of the Ikaros gene in leukemia cells of a small group of children with ALL.[42,43] The normal Ikaros gene codes for DNA binding, "zinc finger" proteins. In mice Ikaros is essential for normal lymphocyte development. Ikaros-deficient mice not only lack normal lymphoid tissue and lymphocyte precursors but also develop an aggressive lymphoblastic leukemia 3 to 6 months after birth. Ikaros is thought to regulate both development and maturation of lymphocytes and to suppress leukemogenesis. The presence of Ikaros isoforms that lack DNA binding or have abnormal binding in the blasts of children with ALL was hypothesized to lead to dysregulation of normal lymphocyte differentiation by impairing expression of necessary regulatory proteins. Such a maturation arrest may predispose precursor cells to second hits and leukemic transformation. Sun and colleagues also hypothesize that overexpression of abnormal Ikaros isoforms may also lead to inactivation of tumor suppressor genes.[42,43]

Immunodeficiency states, both congenital and acquired, have been associated with an increased risk of leukemia. Children with congenital immunodeficiency states, including Wiskott–Aldrich syndrome, ataxia–telangiectasia, and hypogammaglobulinemia have an increased risk for leukemia.[30] Drug-induced immunosuppression to prevent rejection of renal transplants also has been associated with an increased incidence of lymphoreticular cancer.[44]

Siblings of children with leukemia have a fourfold higher risk than the population at large for developing leukemia. The identical twin of a child with ALL has approximately a 20 percent chance of developing leukemia. This frequently occurs within 6 months of diagnosis of the affected twin.[45] Nonconstitutional rearrangement of the HXR (MLL) gene has been reported in monozygotic twins.[46] The hypothesis of in utero transfer of malignant cells is supported by dichorionic/diplacental[47] twins with MLL gene rearrangements and by monozygotic twins with comigration of identical 11q23 rearrangements and oligoclonal heavy-chain immunoglobulin gene rearrangements.[48]

Exposure to radiation of various types predisposes to the development of acute leukemia. In individuals exposed to the atomic bomb blasts in Japan, both ALL and ANLL were seen, depending on age at exposure.[49–52] The threshold dose for leukemogenesis in humans appears to be in the range of 50 to 100 Gy.[53–55] An increased risk of leukemia has been observed following fetal exposure to radiation, especially when the exposure occurred in the first trimester.[56,57] The lay press has also raised many questions about the leukemogenic effect of exposure to high-voltage transmission lines and household magnetic fields. As reviewed by Michaelson,[58] however, the data cited previously had many deficiencies and left the questions unanswered. The National Institutes of Health (NIH) and Children's Cancer Group (CCG), reporting results of their combined studies, found no increased incidence of ALL in children living near high-voltage power lines or low-frequency magnetic fields.[59,60]

CLINICAL PRESENTATION

The history in most cases suggests an acute onset, with symptoms present for only a few days to few weeks. Only rarely are complaints noted for months. In general, children with ALL present with the symptoms of bone marrow failure due to replacement of normal precursor blood cells by leukemic cells. This results in the typical findings of fever, pallor, petechiae, and bruising. Fever, the most common feature, is present in approximately 60 percent of patients. In many cases, fever may be due to the leukemia per se. Freeman et al.[61] reported that 70 percent of patients became afebrile within 72 hours of starting induction therapy without antibiotics. Nevertheless, because many patients are neutropenic and the function of circulating neutrophils may be abnormal, it is common to administer antibiotics in all febrile patients until culture results are available. In a study of 100 children receiving induction therapy, Hughes and Smith[62] documented sepsis or meningitis in 7, moderate infections (pneumonia, urinary tract infections, cellulitis, etc.) in 9, and mild infections in 35. The mortality rate in their study was 4 percent. The use of more intense therapy during induction did not appear to increase the mortality rate, reported as 3.5 percent in another study of children with high-risk features.[63,64] Leukemic infiltration of the liver, spleen, or lymph nodes may cause hepatomegaly, splenomegaly, or lymphadenopathy. Bone and joint pain, often with a limp, may result from the presence of leukemic infiltrates in these areas. Back pain, an uncommon complaint in children, may result from vertebral compression fractures secondary to bone demineralization and/or leukemic infiltrates.[65] Even more rare are cutaneous, nontender nodules, especially of the face or scalp. These occurred in 1.6 percent of 1359 children with ALL in one European study.[66]

Many of the presenting features of ALL are nonspecific findings common to other childhood illnesses, which must be considered in the differential diagnosis. Epstein-Barr virus and cytomegalovirus infections can present with similar complaints of fever, anorexia, malaise, lymphadenopathy, hepatomegaly, or splenomegaly. Ecchymoses, petechiae, and rarely, hemorrhage, are clinically indistinguishable from the findings of idiopathic thrombocytopenic purpura. Juvenile rheumatoid arthritis often presents with a similar clinical picture, and rarely, leukemic infiltration of bone or joints may mimic lesions of osteomyelitis or primary bone tumors. Other childhood malignancies may present with metastatic bone marrow disease, including lymphoma, neuroblastoma, rhabdomyosarcoma, Ewing's sarcoma, and retinoblastoma.

Lymphocytosis may be associated with pertussis, parapertussis, or acute infectious lymphocytosis. The leukemoid reaction, especially in infants with trisomy 21, may be clinically impossible to differentiate from leukemia. Although the most frequent cause of eosinophilia in children is parasitic infestation, symptomatic hypereosinophilia in association with ALL has been reported.[66–70] In rare instances, the hypereosinophilia preceded the presentation of ALL by months.

Children with pancytopenia may have aplastic anemia. The preleukemic syndrome with cytopenias and marrow hypoplasia is more frequently associated with adult ANLL but has been reported in children, both those with ANLL and those with ALL.[71,72] The preleukemia associated with ALL may exist for several months before lymphoblasts appear. Erythroid and/or myeloid hypoplasia occur in both pre-ANLL and pre-ALL; ineffective megakaryocyte production usually precedes ANLL.

Laboratory studies may help to confirm the impressions gained from a thorough history and complete physical examination. The complete blood count may reveal abnormalities of one or more cell lines. Blood chemistries help to define involvement of the kidneys or liver. Chest radiographs are important in evaluating the presence of mediastinal widening, typically present in T-cell leukemias. The definitive diagnostic test is examination of the bone marrow aspirate and biopsy sample, usually by microscopic morphology, immunohistochemical staining, immunophenotyping, and cytogenetic analysis. The technical advances that allow more precise definition of the cell's origin through immunophenotyping have caused some to question the future role of both morphologic classification and immunohistochemistry.

Central nervous system (CNS) and testicular involvement at onset are rare, but every child must be evaluated for these possibilities. Leukemia of the CNS is present at diagnosis in less than 5 percent of children.[73] The most frequent signs and symptoms are those of increased intracranial pressure, including vomiting, headache, papilledema, and lethargy. Rarely, CNS disease may include ocular findings, including leukemic infiltration of the anterior chamber, retinal hemorrhage and/or detachment, and optic nerve infiltration. Evaluation of the cerebrospinal fluid (CSF) for the presence of lymphoblasts is an essential part of the diagnostic work-up, and must include cytocentrifuge analysis as well as routine cell count and chemistries. Central nervous system leukemia is defined as five or more white blood cells (WBCs) per microliter on the CSF count, with the presence of blasts on the cytocentrifuge preparation. The fate of children with fewer than five WBCs in the CSF but with blasts present is unclear. The Children's Cancer Group reported in 1994 that such children were at no increased risk of CNS relapse.[74] A report from St. Jude's Children's Research Hospital in 1993, with follow-up data reported in 1998, however, disputes that finding.[75,76]

Although overt testicular disease (typically, painless testicular swelling) is equally infrequent, as many as 25 percent of boys may be found to have occult disease on biopsy at the time of diagnosis.[77] Despite this fact, with the use of newer, more aggressive treatment protocols, testicular biopsy is not routinely performed.[78,79]

DIAGNOSTIC CLASSIFICATION

Acute lymphoblastic leukemia is diagnosed when more than 25 percent of the cells in the bone marrow are lymphoblasts. In general, the diagnosis of ALL is readily established in the child who presents with anemia, thrombocytopenia, and hepatosplenomegaly and has typical lymphoblasts in the peripheral blood and bone marrow. The clinical association of high WBC count, mediastinal mass, marked adenopathy, and hepatosplenomegaly in adolescent boys with T-cell leukemia has been well reported.[13,14,80] Most B-cell leukemias are easily classified by their characteristic basophilic cytoplasm with vacuoles, giving the classic "starry sky" appearance. The majority of leukemias, however, are only defined by the cumulative results of several different diagnostic tests. Special stains (e.g., periodic acid–Schiff [PAS], peroxidase, Sudan black, and nonspecific esterase) and cell markers may help confirm this diagnosis.[81] Methods to identify discrete classes of lymphoblasts have developed significantly beyond Ehrlich's first staining techniques.

Morphology

The French-American-British (FAB) classification has subdivided ALL into three morphologic types[82,83]; L1 (84 percent) is the most common type seen in childhood ALL; L3 (1 to 2 percent) has Burkitt's-like, mature B-cell morphology; and L2 (14 percent) has somewhat larger cells than L1. Special stains aid in distinguishing ALL from ANLL and its variants. Lymphoblasts are negative for the following stains: peroxidase, Sudan black, naphthol chloracetate esterase, and usually, α-naphthyl acetate esterase.[84] In contrast, they are generally positive for PAS, frequently with coarse granules seen in the cytoplasm. Catovsky[85] noted that acid phosphatase is positive in blasts of T-cell ALL and may be useful in separating this subgroup from other types of ALL.

Immunophenotype

The immunologic separation of ALL into several phenotypic classes[86–92] was a major advance in diagnosis and has led to the development of specific treatment for different classes.[93] Monoclonal antibodies (mAbs) developed against various ALL classes mirror those associated with normal cells and suggest that malignant clones can develop at essentially all stages of cellular differentiation.[87,94] As discussed in detail by Greaves et al.,[95] it is unclear whether the association of a specific phenotype represents malignant transformation of a normal cell at that stage of differentiation. It could also represent transformation of a precursor cell that alters further differentiation or possibly transformation of a completely different cell line with aberrant expression of surface antigens. Lymphoblasts with surface immunoglobulin (sIg) characteristic of mature (differentiated) B cells account for only 1 to 2 percent of lymphoblastic leukemias. Early techniques identified T-cell lymphoblasts by their ability to form erythrocyte rosettes with sheep red blood cell (RBC) antisera. Newer monoclonal antibody techniques confirm T-cell phenotype in approximately 20 percent of cases of ALL.[80,96,97]

The remaining 80 percent of cases were first described as null cell leukemias, lacking either B-cell or T-cell surface markers. Refinement of techniques has since identified cytoplasmic Ig in approximately 20 percent of these, placing them in a classification of early (Pre-) B-cell differentiation.[98] Most cells lacking B-cell or T-cell surface characteristics express the antigen CD10 (formerly termed common-ALL antigen or CALLA).[93,99] Lymphoblasts may show dual cell-surface markers in 5 to 10 percent of childhood ALL cases.[100,101] Various hypotheses have been formulated in an effort to explain this phenomenon, including aberrant gene expression, malignant transformation of a pluripotent stem cell with differentiation along both pathways as the clone develops, or malignant transformation of a progenitor capable of expressing both lymphoid and myeloid antigens.[102–106]

The CD34 antigen is a transmembrane sialoglycoprotein expressed by several cell types, including myeloid and lymphoid progenitors. A recent study has found CD34 antigen in approximately 70 percent of ALL cases. In early Pre-B ALL, 83 percent of cells were positive, as were 61 percent of those in Pre-B ALL, and 46 percent of those in T-cell ALL.[107]

Even more specific delineation of cell phenotype is possible by genetic analysis of immunoglobulin (Ig) rearrangement[108,109] or T-cell receptor genes.[110,111] The multiplicity of immunologic responses appears to be possible by rearrangements of genes coding for heavy and light chains, and the order in which they occur is associated with differentiation of the cell. Concurrent expression of surface Ig evolves. Approximately 40 percent of non-B, non-T-cell lymphoblasts reveal light-chain rearrangements, marking them as Pre-B-cell clones. Cells in which only heavy-chain genes are rearranged are the least mature, and express only those surface antigens characteristic of early development. Cytoplasmic Ig is detected in only 25 percent of these cells.[108,109] Similar changes occur in T-cell receptor genes, allowing further subclassification by differentiation stages.[111,112] Steenberger et al. have shown that ongoing gene rearrangement can occur after malignant transformation, giving the casual appearance of polyclonal origins.[113]

Terminal deoxynucleotidyl transferase (TdT)[114] is an intracellular enzyme, which is generally not detected in mature lymphocytes.[115] It is found in most patients with ALL, excluding those with the B-cell subtype, and may serve to detect early relapse or residual leukemic cells.[116–119] However, approximately 5 percent of ANLL may be TdT-positive.[120,121]

Improved techniques in cytogenetics have led to more extensive analysis of chromosomal changes in malignant cell lines. Abnormalities, in either chromosome number or structure, may be found in as many as 90 percent of cases of childhood ALL.[122–124] Changes in the number of chromosomes are frequent, most often diploidy or hyperdiploidy. The most frequent structural abnormalities are translocations, present in approximately 40 percent of cases.[125–127] These are usually seen in conjunction with pseudodiploid clones. Translocations result in dysregulation of normal cellular proteins or in fusion genes, with production of novel chimeric proteins. The most common translocations associated with childhood ALL are listed in Table 17–1.

The persistent finding of t(8;14)(q24;q32) in B-cell leukemias and the less frequent variants t(2;8)(p11–13;q24) and t(8;22)(q24;q11) suggests that this disease is a disseminated form of Burkitt's lymphoma.[128] In each, the *c-myc* oncogene is brought into proximity with genes coding for portions of Igs. The normal *c-myc* product is a nuclear protein active in directing cell proliferation, which in the translocated species may undergo deregulation of its expression.[129]

Originally thought to be pathognomonic of chronic myelocytic leukemia (CML), t(9;22) can be identified in approximately 4 percent of childhood leukemias.[129–131] Although the t(9;22) translocations in ALL and CML are cytogenetically indistinguishable and both involve translocation of the chromosome 9 *c-abl* gene, the breakpoints on chromosome 22 are

Table 17–1. Translocations Common in Childhood ALL

Translocation	FAB	Phenotype
t(8;14)(q24;q32)	L3	B-cell, SIg +
t(2;8)(p11–13;q24)	L3	B-cell, SIg +
t(8;22)(q24;q11)	L3	B-cell, SIg +
t(1;19)(q23;p13)	L1, L2	Pre-B-cell, CIg +
t(4;11)(q21;q23)	L1, L2	early Pre-B-cell
t(9;22)	L1, L2	early Pre-B, Pre-B, or T-cell
t(7;9)	L1, L2	T-cell
t(11;14)(p13;q13)	L1, L2	T-cell
t(11;19)(q23;p13.3)	L1, L2	Pre-B or T-cell
t(12;21)	L1, L2	Pre-B-cell

FAB, French-American-British classification.

different. The t(9;22) ALL immunophenotype may be seen in early B-cell, Pre-B-cell, and T-cell leukemia.

More common, occurring in approximately 30 percent of Pre-B ALL, is t(1;19).[126,129,131,132] Lymphoblasts with t(1;19) express cytoplasmic Ig, but not sIg. Only 1 of 1000 pediatric cases of ALL involves t(12;21) as determined by routine chromosomal banding techniques. The resulting fusion protein, TEL-AML1, however, can be detected in nearly 25 percent of cases of precursor B-cell ALL by molecular techniques.[133,134] The t(4;11)(q21;q23) translocation is also associated with B-cell precursor lymphoblasts.[135,136] These cells express HLA-DR antigens and have heavy-chain Ig gene rearrangement. In vitro, these cells can be induced to express monocytic features, leading to speculation that they possess dual capacity for differentiation.

Lymphoblasts with T-cell immunophenotypes are associated with both t(11;14) and t(7;9).[126,127,129] The breakpoint on chromosome 14 involves the α-chain locus of the T-cell receptor gene; that on chromosome 9, the T-cell receptor β-chain. Deletions of the p21–22 region of chromosome 9 have been reported in association with methylthioadenosine phosphorylase (MTAase) deficiency,[137,138] often with a concomitant loss of α- and β-interferon (IFN) genes. T-cell ALL is also associated with t(8;12)(q13;p13).[139] It is not clear whether the loss of IFN genes or other closely associated genes is critical, but it is hypothesized that tumor-suppressor activity is dysfunctional. MTAase is active in purine salvage; its deficiency may have important therapeutic implications; MTAase deficiency may be present without chromosomal abnormalities[140] and has also been reported in ANLL and a few solid tumors.[141] It appears to have increased frequency in T-cell disease[138] and in one report was associated with lymphomatous presentation of T-cell ALL.[139]

PROGNOSTIC FACTORS

A number of studies have tested the prognostic significance of various features present at diagnosis. These include age, WBC count, race, immunophenotype, hemoglobin, FAB classification, sex, hepatosplenomegaly, lymphadenopathy, platelet count, the presence of CNS disease, Ig levels, cytogenetic abnormalities, and time to achieve a remission marrow after start of induction chemotherapy.[142–146] Many of the purported prognostic features are interdependent. Infants with ALL usually present with marked leukocytosis (WBC of 100,000/mm³ or greater) and marked hepatosplenomegaly. Unlike their teenage counterparts, however, they rarely have mediastinal masses, have very early B-cell phenotypes rather than T-cell markers, and are CALLA-negative.[147–152] Chromosomal alterations of 11q23 with the *MLL-ENL* fusion gene are frequent in such cases.[153–154] Therefore, it is important to establish independent prognostic variables by multivariate analysis. It should also be emphasized that successful therapy may override prognostic features, and that the better the treatment, the less relevant certain prognostic features become.

Also, the prognostic features noted at presentation lose their significance to predict cure after $1\frac{1}{2}$ to 2 years of sustained clinical remission (CR). One exception to this is male sex, which imparts a higher chance of relapse after discontinuation of chemotherapy.[155–157] Whether the prognostic role of race can be influenced by intense therapy is unclear. Early reports showed that the prognosis for black children with ALL was not as good as that for white children[158] when these black children were classified within the same prognostic subgroups. However, Falletta and colleagues[159] indicated that there was a high incidence of Pre-B ALL and T-cell ALL in black children, which may have accounted, at least in part, for the worse prognosis. St. Jude's evaluated the response to treatment of children with cancer in each of two time intervals, 1962 to 1983 and 1984 to 1992. In the earlier time interval, black children had a 37 percent chance of survival versus 50 percent for white children. The later groups had equal survival, which was attributed to improved access and more effective treatment.[160] A later report by the Pediatric Oncology Group (POG), however, compared outcomes for African-American and Hispanic versus white children with ALL of the same risk groups, treated on the same protocols. Although the overall survival of African-American children was improved as compared with historic control subjects, there was still a significantly worse outcome for African-American and Hispanic children. The authors hypothesized that this difference may be related to as yet undetermined biologic characteristics of the disease but may also be related to interracial differences in drug metabolism.[161]

Two features, age and WBC count, remain important prognostic variables.[155] The best survival rates are observed in children between the ages of 1 and 9 years, with WBCs of less than 5,000/mm³. Children under 1 year of age have a worse prognosis, with survival rates less than 50 percent. Teenagers also have a worse prognosis.[144,157,162–164] A significant trend in outcome is directly related to levels of WBCs at presentation. Skipper et al.[165] first showed that the ability to cure L1210 leukemia in the mouse model depended on the leukemic burden. Goldie and Coldman[166] developed the mathematical model, indicating that resistant clones increased in direct proportion with the number of cancer cells present. Thus, a large cancer burden at presentation as reflected by a high blast count, hepatosplenomegaly, and perhaps adenopathy is associated with a poor prognosis.

For years it was stated that patients with L1 morphology had the best prognosis, those with L3 the worst, and those with L2 had an intermediate outlook. Although L3 morphology is generally associated with a Burkitt's or B-cell leukemia, the L1 and L2 morphology exhibit no correlation with immunophenotype.[14,93] Until recently the poor prognosis of B-cell leukemia, both in initial response to induction therapy and in long-term survival, was accepted. A poor prognosis associated with the presence of 10 percent L2 lymphoblasts was shown in several studies.[144,167,168] In a series of 3500 patients with ALL, the CCG demonstrated that patients with 10 percent or more L2 cells had lower survival rates than patients with predominantly L1 morphology. Other studies have found that although the remission induction rate of patients with L2 morphology was worse, the overall survival was not significantly different after other independent factors were taken into consideration. Unlike the CCG study, data from St. Jude's failed to identify L2 morphology as an independent prognostic variable, except in T-cell ALL.[104,169]

The presence of T- or mature B-cell markers on lymphoblasts worsens prognosis, although not all studies confirm them as independent variables.[143,144,170,171] Henze et al.[172] failed to show any prognostic significance of cell surface markers, possibly reflecting an example of effective therapy overcoming prognostic variables. A study by the POG identified the T-cell immunophenotype as an independent prognostic variable in that the induction rate for patients with T-cell ALL was worse and the duration of remission shorter.[173] A later POG study argued that the prognostic indicators found significant in precursor B-cell ALL were not predicated on the response in T-cell ALL. They concluded that with appropriate therapy, the outcome in T-cell ALL was best correlated with the maturity or differentiation stage of the T cell.[174]

Investigators have also delineated a worse prognosis among patients with Pre-B immunophenotype as compared with patients with early Pre B-cell ALL.[175–178] This group does, however, have a significantly better prognosis than does B-cell leukemia. It should be noted that the induction rate for patients with Pre-B-cell leukemia is the same as for the early Pre B-cell group, but the duration of remission is shorter. There was also a higher incidence of CNS relapse.[178,179] Patients with early pre B-cell ALL that is CALLA-positive and IA-positive have been reported to have a better prognosis.[93,171] CD34 antigen positivity is associated with a favorable prognosis in Pre B-cell ALL.[180]

Concern exists over the 30 percent of children with apparently good prognostic features, including Pre-B-cell immunophenotype, low WBC count and favorable age, who nevertheless relapse or never achieve remission. A British study of ALL patients with such characteristics looked at Ig or *TCR* gene clonal diversity. Relapse occurred in 13 of 20 (65 percent) of the patients found to have clonal diversity, but in only 7 of 36 (19 percent) of those without clonal diversity. Additionally, the diversity was found to have changing patterns between disease presentation and relapse, suggesting a possible role of changing phenotype in tumor progression or the development of drug resistance.[181]

Conflicting reports suggest that the prognosis in leukemias with both myeloid and lymphoid morphology is worse or unchanged from that in other cases of ALL with matched characteristics. Myeloid antigen-positive ALL is often found in children less than 1 year of age with elevated peripheral WBC counts and/or chromosomal translocation, all of which are associated with poor outcomes.[181–184]

The chromosomal abnormalities seen in as many as 90 percent of ALL cell lines appear to have prognostic significance. Thirty percent of lymphoblasts demonstrate hyperdiploidy (more than 50 chromosomes), which is associated with the best prognosis.[129,185–189] The finding of trisomy 21 in malignant clones of patients with ALL who have no constitutional chromosomal changes is associated with a good outcome.[190] Similarly, the presence of t(12;21) or the *TEL-AML1* fusion gene imparts more than 90 percent EFS.[132,191,192] In contrast, hypodiploidy has been associated with a poor prognosis,[187,193,194] as has near haploidy. The latter is typically seen in adolescent girls with high WBC counts at the time of diagnosis.[195,196]

The poor prognosis of patients with pseudodiploid chromosome numbers may be related to the presence of translocations.

Early treatment failures are associated with t(8;14), t(9;22), and t(4;11) and provide further evidence for activation of oncogenes and subsequent involvement of gene products in resistant leukemias.[35,125,126,129,136] Alternations of 11q23 are frequently associated with ALL in early infancy and with a poor prognosis.[136,152,154,197–199] This translocation is also frequently seen in secondary leukemias following topoisomerase therapy.[39,199,200] In 1999 St. Jude Children's Research Center reported on 3578 patients with ALL, of whom 35 had t(11;19). Of the 35, 13 were infants; only 2 of the 13 infants had a CR, compared with 6 of 11 older children.[153] Again, as is the case with the prognostic importance of immunophenotype, better therapy may eliminate the influence of cytogenetic changes.[201]

Emerging as one of the most important prognostic features is the early reduction of disease. Various groups have studied the outcome of ALL patients and observed lower rates of survival in children with persistent circulating blasts after 7 days of induction[202] or prephase single-agent treatment with prednisone[203] or with more than 25 percent marrow blasts on bone marrow aspiration at day 7 or 14.[204–207] Children with persistent marrow disease on day 28 of therapy have the worst prognosis, with fewer than 20 percent of these achieving remission or maintaining long-term survival.[208] Similarly, polymerase chain reaction (PCR) techniques have been employed to determine response and predict risk of relapse. Traditionally, remission was judged by the microscopic finding of no more than 5 percent bone marrow blasts. However, PCR allows detection of minute numbers of cells, referred to as minimal residual disease. Several groups have studied the significance of this, with reports of 23 to 60 percent of patients having minimal residual disease at the end of therapy. Higher levels of detectable disease and longer persistence of minimal disease are significant but not absolute predictors of relapse.[209–213]

TREATMENT

Principles of Chemotherapy

Cancer may arise when a single normal cell transforms into a cancer cell, either by spontaneous mutation or following induction with chemicals, viruses, or radiation.[214] By the time a lesion measures 1 cm in diameter, it has undergone approximately 30 doublings.[215] Therefore, although a diagnosis of cancer may be made at an early clinical stage, essentially all tumors are recognized relatively late in their biological growth cycle. At late stages, relatively few doublings have a dramatic impact on total leukemic burden. The increasing doubling time, which occurs as a cancer grows in size, is due to a lengthening of the generation time of dividing tumor cells.[216,217] With increasing cancer size, there is a progressively larger proportion of the viable cell population entering a nonproliferative state (G_0).[214]

Skipper et al.[165] were the first to demonstrate that chemotherapeutic kill of tumor cells followed first-order kinetics; that is, a constant percentage, rather than a constant number of cells is killed by a given therapeutic maneuver. For example, a child with advanced ALL harbors approximately 10^{12} (or about 1 kg) leukemic cells. A drug capable of killing 99.99 percent of these cells would reduce this burden to 10^8 cells, resulting in a CR. Without further treatment, the remaining 10^8 cells could obviously continue dividing and cause a relapse. Unfortunately, cure most likely requires total eradication of leukemic cells, because in experimental models, a single cancer cell injected into a susceptible host can kill that animal.[218,219]

The cell cycle is defined as the interval between the mitosis and the midpoint of the subsequent mitosis in one or both daughter cells. The cycle is subdivided into four phases. The G_1 is the first phase, during which cells synthesize RNA, enzymes, and proteins in preparation for DNA synthesis. This phase is the most variable in time; slowly growing populations contain cells that have long G_1 periods.[220] The S phase is the period during which the DNA replicates and chromosomal proteins are laid down on the newly synthesized DNA. During this phase, several critical enzymes, including thymidine kinase,[221] DNA polymerase,[222] dihydrofolate reductase,[223] and ribonucleotide reductase[224] are synthesized. The G_2 phase is the interval between the completion of DNA synthesis and mitosis. In this period, the substrates necessary for the two daughter cells are produced. The M phase is the period of mitosis. In any tumor cell population, some cells are cycling continuously while others may be in the G_0 or resting state. Cells in the G_0 phase, although not actively proliferating, have the potential to reenter the proliferating pool and cell cycle. To be effective, certain agents such as the antimetabolites require cells to be in cycle, whereas other agents (e.g., alkylating agents) may destroy cells whether or not they are passing through the cell cycle.

Phases of Therapy

The use of multiple effective agents given in combination, as well as the treatment of subclinical CNS leukemia (CNS prophylaxis) has greatly improved the prognosis for a child with ALL. Therapy of ALL was initially separated into two phases, induction and maintenance. Maintenance therapy was instituted because patients who achieved CR and received no further therapy relapsed within a few months.[225] The so-called standard therapy, against which effects of new treatment protocols must be measured, includes induction with prednisone (PRED), vincristine (VCR), and L-asparaginase (L-asp); a consolidation phase with prophylactic CNS irradiation; and finally

a maintenance phase with methotrexate and 6-mercaptopurine. The most common chemotherapeutic agents used in the treatment of ALL are listed in Tables 17–2, 17–3, and 17–4.

As improved techniques have facilitated the identification of lymphoblasts and distinguished groups with distinct prognoses, it has also become apparent that a standard therapy for all subclasses of ALL is no longer appropriate. Many studies have focused on improvement of survival in high-risk groups by intensification of therapy. Conversely, other studies attempt to reduce the potential toxicities from aggressive therapy in the best prognostic groups without sacrificing long-term survival.

Induction

The induction phase aims to destroy as many leukemic cells as possible, converting florid disease into CR, in which the disease is microscopically undetectable.[226,227] During this time, the leukemic cell burden declines from approximately 10^{11} or 10^{12} to approximately 10^8 cells. The induction rate in childhood ALL using PRED and VCR is over 85 percent.[228–230] Jones et al.[230] showed that adding L-asp to PRED and VCR induction improved the duration of CR but did not improve the induction rate. However, Ortega et al.[231] achieved an overall induction rate of 93 percent using the same combination. Although the benefit of adding anthracyclines to induction therapy was initially debated, later studies suggest that addition of daunomycin to the standard three-drug regimen improves long-term survival, especially in patients with poor prognostic features.[232–237] With standard therapy, the induction remission rates for children with high-risk features have been significantly worse than those for children with good prognoses.[238,239] According to a CCG study for high-risk patients (CCG-106),[237] remission induction rates of 99 and 94 percent were achieved on the two intensified induction arms, versus 84 percent on the standard treatment arm. Because of the cardiotoxicity of anthracyclines, most centers now reserve four-drug induction for patients in higher-risk groups.

The time required to achieve remission appears to have prognostic significance for overall survival. Treatment protocols have been designed to allow more flexibility in directing maximal intensity of therapy when needed while (hopefully) reduc-

Table 17–2. Chemotherapeutic Agents Used in Induction

Agent	Mechanism of Action	Side Effects and Toxicity
Prednisone	Lympholytic agent G_1-S delay	Increased appetite and weight gain; cushingoid appearance; hypertension; diabetes mellitus; behavior changes; increased susceptibility to infection; gastritis or gastrointestinal ulcers
L-Asparaginase	G_1-S delay	Hypersensitivity reaction; diabetes mellitus; pancreatitis; hepatotoxicity; anorexia; nausea/vomiting
Vincristine	Inhibitor of mitotic spindle formation	Peripheral neuropathy; ileus; local irritation if extravasates; alopecia; syndrome of inappropriate antidiuretic hormone (rare)
Daunorubicin	DNA intercalation	Myelosuppression; mucositis; anorexia; nausea/vomiting; red coloration of urine; cellulitis/necrosis if extravasates; arrhythmia (acute); progressive cardiomyopathy (late effects)

Table 17–3. Chemotherapeutic Agents Used in Consolidation

Agent	Mechanism of Action	Side Effects and Toxicity
Methotrexate (intrathecal)	Dihydrofolate reductase inhibition	Myelosuppression; nausea/vomiting; leukoencephalopathy (late)
Irradiation (gamma)	Oxygen radical-induced cytotoxicity	Tissue necrosis; myelosuppression; alopecia; bone growth arrest; encephalopathy; memory deficit or learning disability (late effect)
Cyclophosphamide	Alkylating agent	Myelosuppression; anorexia; nausea/vomiting; alopecia; hemorrhagic cystitis; bladder fibrosis (late); sterility
Cytosine arabinoside	Pyrimidine antagonist	Myelosuppression; mucositis; anorexia; nausea/vomiting; fever; diarrhea (rare); hepatotoxicity; alopecia

ing unnecessary toxicities to children at lower risk of recurrent disease.[203,204,208,211]

Intensification

The intensification, consolidation, or sanctuary phase, administered soon after a patient achieves remission, attempts to further reduce the systemic leukemic burden while simultaneously eradicating disease in so-called pharmacologic sanctuary sites, including the CNS and testes. The additional effect of "early intensive consolidation" therapy continues to be debated. Two early studies used consolidation therapy.[233,236] However, since these were single-arm studies, the effect could not be assessed. A series of subsequent studies demonstrated improved survival rates in high-risk patients with the use of intensified therapy during the consolidation phase.[3,63,240–243] A recent study that further intensified the BFM regimen with protracted use of high-dose L-asp failed to show an advantage.[244]

Whether the risk of greater morbidity from intensified therapy is balanced by greatly improved survival in children with low-risk ALL is yet undetermined. A study of intermediate-dose methotrexate and cytosine arabinoside demonstrated outcomes similar to those seen in protocols that used drugs with higher potential for toxicity.[245] Another study found intermediate dose intravenous methotrexate alone superior to the same methotrexate dose plus either L-asp or ara-C.[246] Recently there has been a report of improved outcome in patients who received reduced doses of both anthracycline and cranial radiation.[6] As noted previously, low-risk patients with a slow initial response to treatment have a worse outcome. More intense postinduction therapy in this group results in improved survival.[204]

As chemotherapeutic regimens allowed children to survive for longer periods, the incidence of overt CNS disease rose markedly. Evans reported a change in incidence from 4 percent in 1947 to 40 percent in 1960.[247,248] St. Jude Children's Research Center was the first to study radiotherapy as a means of preventing leukemic proliferation in the CNS, after reporting CNS disease in 59 to 67 percent of ALL patients who received no prophylactic therapy. A series of studies led to the use of 2400 cGy to the craniospinal axis, with a reduction in CNS relapse to only 4 percent.[228,249–251] This has remained the standard against which all other treatment modalities are evaluated. A study by POG, which delayed CNS treatment to week 9, emphasized the need for appropriate timing of CNS therapy. Thirty-three percent of the patients in their study had CNS relapse before reaching the ninth week.[252] Delivery of craniospinal radiation, however, requires precisely detailed technique. Extension of radiation fields to include the spinal axis also increases the myelotoxicity, with the risk of delay in systemic treatment.

Several other centers later tested the prophylactic effects of intrathecal methotrexate (MTX) plus cranial radiation.[135,232,253–257] Recalculation of MTX doses by Bleyer et al.,[258] based on age-specific CSF volumes rather than surface area, led to improved results. A later CCG study demonstrated that 1800 cGy cranial radiation used with intrathecal MTX was as effective as 2400 cGy craniospinal or 2400 cGy cranial radiation with intrathecal MTX.[259] The ALL-BFM 90 study cited previously demonstrated equal efficacy with 1200 cGy.[6]

Efforts continue in an attempt to eliminate the risk of CNS relapse, while at the same time minimizing the risk of CNS toxicity, especially in the very young child with an immature nervous system. A joint study by the CCG and the Pediatric Branch of the National Cancer Institute showed that continuous 24-hour infusion of high-dose methotrexate was as effective as 2400 cGy cranial radiation plus intrathecal MTX in treating the CNS.[260] A later study confirmed that finding.[261] Reports from

Table 17–4. Chemotherapeutic Agents Used in Maintenance

Agent	Mechanism of Action	Side Effects and Toxicity
6-Mercaptopurine	DNA and RNA synthesis inhibitor (purine analogue)	Myelosuppression; hepatotoxicity; mucositis (rare); nausea/vomiting (rare)
Methotrexate	Dihydrofolate reductase inhibitor	Myelosuppression; megaloblastosis; hepatotoxicity; mucositis; anorexia; nausea/vomiting (rare)
Vincristine	See Table 17–2	See Table 17–2
Prednisone	See Table 17–2	See Table 17–2

several studies now also show improved survival and decreased CNS relapse by using intensified regimens of intrathecal therapy without radiation.[261–263]

Maintenance

The clinical impetus for the concept of maintenance therapy came when patients with ALL were randomized to either receive or not receive maintenance therapy following induction.[264] Those patients who received 6-mercaptopurine following induction did considerably better, and it became common practice to add maintenance therapy. Several centers have studied combinations of drugs during the maintenance phase.[232,234,237,251,265–269] The standard regimen derived from these studies is daily 6-MP, weekly or twice weekly MTX, and monthly pulses of VCR and PRED. Central nervous system treatment continues for most patients as well, with intrathecal MTX every 3 months.

A series of studies in Germany (BFM) added a second intense phase of therapy before maintenance[234,235,270] in an attempt to eradicate the small but persistent leukemia burden.[271] The survival rate in these studies was 65 percent, even within groups of patients with high-risk features. Subsequent studies have confirmed that even patients with the least favorable prognostic characteristics have survival rates as high as 70 percent following intensified therapy.[63,232,272,273] A later study by the BFM group failed to show greater survival after a third phase of intensified therapy,[274] although Chessells et al. cited benefit.[275] Historically, fewer than 20 percent of infants with ALL have achieved long-term survival. A POG study attempted unsuccessfully to improve on that rate with alternating pairs of aggressive chemotherapeutic agents.[276] Two sequential studies by the CCG used intensive systemic therapy to prevent CNS disease and showed modest increases in overall survival rates to 33 and 39 percent, respectively.[261]

A major goal of treatment programs now must be to maximize long-term survival while minimizing treatment-related toxicity, both acute and chronic. Whether therapy for groups of children with the most favorable prognostic signs can safely be reduced is under investigation. At least one study by the BFM group suggests more intensive therapy is beneficial even in these children.[270] Unanswered is the question of why therapy fails in 15 to 20 percent of children with "good risk" ALL. Application of new technologies to better define differences among groups of patients who are phenotypically similar may allow continued refinement of treatment plans. The possibility that cells develop resistance has also been considered. A Dutch study in 1994 measured differing resistance to various chemotherapeutic agents in children with low-risk versus high-risk ALL. This study also demonstrated greater resistance to multiple drugs in cells from relapsed patients.[277] In the case of steroid resistance, higher-dose dexamethasone was later shown to overcome the resistance.[278]

Another explanation may be inadequate drug levels, either from variable absorption or from lack of compliance. Evening administration of 6-mercaptopurine and methotrexate, with or without concomitant food intake, has been shown to be more effective in one study.[279] Studies measuring red blood cell folate and methotrexate levels following oral or intramuscular administration have shown significantly higher levels associated with the latter.[280] Low-risk ALL patients treated in one study with predominantly parenterally administered therapy achieved higher blood levels of 6-mercaptopurine and methotrexate and showed a 94 percent survival rate.[265] High-risk patients treated on the same protocol also had an improved survival rate.[281] Other studies have shown no benefit from intravenous 6-mercaptopurine.[282,283]

As technology improves, so may the clinical and economic feasibility of measuring individual intracellular drug levels, thus allowing tailored doses based on patient-specific metabolism. Evans et al. showed improved survival in children who had doses modified to account for individual clearance rates.[284] Similarly, greater understanding of drug metabolism within cell types may improve treatment design. Folate antagonists are widely used in the treatment of ALL. Conversion of both natural folates and folate antagonists (e.g., methotrexate) requires activity of folylpolyglutamate synthetase (FPSG), which is constitutively expressed in lymphoblasts, as well as in their normal counterparts, at a level higher than that seen in myeloid cells. Expression of FPSG is increased in ALL blasts after exposure to methotrexate, and intracellular accumulation of the active metabolite can be measured. The increase seen in pre-B ALL is significantly greater than that seen in T-cell ALL. This may in part be responsible for the improved outcome of those patients receiving treatment by current protocols, which frequently use repeated doses of methotrexate.[285]

An unresolved issue is the optimal length of treatment. Early studies showed that 5 years of maintenance therapy were as effective as 7 years,[286] later studies showed that 3 years were as effective as 5 years.[287–289] More intense therapy reported in newer studies may prove that even shorter periods of treatment are effective. Reports by the German cooperative group BFM[290] and the French group FSOP (French Pediatric Oncology Society) showed significantly improved survival in children with B-cell leukemia following 4 to 6 months of intensive treatment. Given the poor prognosis of patients with specific chromosme translocations, including the Philadelphia positive (t9;22), some groups recommend bone marrow transplantation early in first remission.[292,293]

Drug Interactions

It was observed at the Sidney Farber Cancer Institute that an average of 5.6 noncancer drugs per patient were administered on any one day.[294] Up to 60 percent of nonchemotherapeutic drugs can influence the action or toxicity of chemotherapeutic agents. For example, methotrexate, which like many chemotherapeutic agents only exerts its anticancer effect when it is in its free form, is 60 percent bound to albumin. Weak acids such as aspirin can free MTX from its binding sites, thus increasing its bioavailability.[268]

Microsomal enzymes of the liver may be induced by barbiturates, antidepressants, and anticoagulants. This may decrease the toxicity and interfere with the action of chemotherapeutic drugs that depend on activation or protein binding in the liver, as well as of those excreted by the liver. Two examples of such drugs are the anthracycline antibiotics and cyclophosphamide. In contrast, drugs that inhibit microsomal enzyme induction, such as allopurinol and phenylbutazone, will increase the toxicity of the above chemotherapeutic drugs. Drugs that alter renal function, such as diuretics, aminoglycoside antibiotics, and probenecid may increase the toxicity of chemotherapeutic drugs such as MTX that are excreted primarily by the kidneys.[294]

One of the principal causes of the failure of cancers to respond to chemotherapy is drug resistance.[295] When a cancer is large enough to be diagnosed, clones resistant to any single agent are already present. These resistant clones grow freely as the sensitive cells are eliminated.[296] Thus, the tumor will regrow from cells of the resistant clone. Goldie and Coldman[166] developed a mathematical model relating tumor size to the spontaneous mutation rate of tumor cells, demonstrating that the probability of resistant clones increases in parallel fashion with the size of the tumor. Additionally, P-glycoprotein encoded by the multidrug resistance (MDR1) gene has been shown to be expressed in some leukemias.[297]

Since resistance to a chemotherapeutic agent may be induced when tumor cells are exposed to low concentrations of drugs for prolonged periods of time,[298] intermittent high-dose therapy is likely to be more effective. Indeed, Skipper[299] and Goldin[300] have shown that intermittent high-dose therapy, given at a maximally tolerated dose and repeated when toxicity has subsided, forms the basis for the optimal schedule of treatment. The problem of emerging resistant cell lines may best be avoided by alternating cycles of different effective agents that are not cross-resistant.

When phase-specific agents such as antimetabolites are used, the duration of exposure of the tumor cell is as important as the peak drug levels achieved. Maintaining prolonged therapeutic levels results in maximum cell kill as tumor cells cycle through the particular phase affected by agents.

Supportive Care

More intensive treatment regimens have made anticipatory supportive care an essential part of therapeutic programs for children with ALL. Careful attention to fluid and electrolyte balance is essential. Administration of bicarbonate to alkalize the urine and of allopurinol to block uric acid formation from rapid tumor lysis helps to prevent uric acid nephropathy and the complications of renal failure. Patients with signs of renal compromise before starting treatment should be evaluated by renal ultrasound examination. The presence of renal enlargement suggests leukemic infiltration of the kidneys. Low-dose radiation to the kidneys will reduce the tumor burden and usually lead to improved renal function. With careful attention to fluid management and electrolyte replacement, tumor lysis syndrome can usually be managed without the need for dialysis.

Two conditions, hyperleukocytosis and the tumor lysis syndrome, represent true emergencies in the initial management of a child with ALL.[301–304] Hyperleukocytosis is defined as a white blood cell count greater than 100,000/mm³ and is associated with an increased risk for hemorrhage (especially intracranial

hemorrhage) or thrombosis. The tumor lysis syndrome associated with hyperuricemia, hyperphosphatemia, hyperkalemia, and hypocalcemia is most commonly seen in patients with hyperleukocytosis. The presence of massive extramedullary leukemia or a rapid rate of cell division, as in T- or B-ALL, may also increase the risk of developing tumor lysis syndrome. The complications of tumor lysis syndrome are frequently avoided by decreasing the leukocyte count prior to initiation of full therapy. Various methods have been employed to decrease the number of circulating lymphoblasts and thus reduce the risk of complications from hyperleukocytosis.[301,303–305] Not uncommonly, hydration alone for 12 to 24 hours will decrease the cell count sufficiently to allow safe institution of induction chemotherapy. If further reduction is necessary, leukophoresis or, in small children, exchange transfusion, is currently recommended.

Use of prophylactic platelet transfusions has significantly reduced mortality due to severe hemorrhage, especially intracerebral hemorrhage. Administration of empiric antibiotics to febrile, neutropenic patients has been another major factor responsible for improved survival during induction therapy.[14,306] Recombinant bone marrow growth factors, such as granulocyte colony-stimulating factor (G-CSF), granulocyte-macrophage colony-stimulating factor (GM-CSF), and interleukin 3(IL3), have been used to enhance bone marrow recovery following intensive myelosuppressive chemotherapy.[307] At least one group, however, found that use of G-CSF did not significantly reduce the number of patients hospitalized with fever and neutropenia, decrease the number of serious infections, or change survival.[308] Growth factors have also been used to mobilize bone marrow stem cells into the peripheral blood of allogeneic donors. There they can be harvested and administered to patients to speed recovery following mylosuppressive chemotherapy.[309]

Beyond the initial phase of remission induction, the risk of opportunistic infections continues.[306] Prophylactic use of trimethoprim–sulfamethoxazole to prevent *Pneumocystis carinii* pneumonia, once a significant cause of mortality in patients receiving immunosuppressive chemotherapy, is widely accepted and has essentially eliminated the incidence of this infection.[310,311] Most centers also suspend immunizations with live-virus vaccines. Administration of varicella zoster immune globulin within 72 to 96 hours of exposure to chickenpox is recommended for immunosuppressed patients, and gamma-globulin is often employed as prophylaxis against measles in exposed, susceptible patients. The antiviral agent acyclovir is generally employed in cases of actual varicella infection, herpes simplex, or herpes zoster infections.

It was noted earlier that arthralgia and/or arthritis may be presenting symptoms. These usually resolve quickly after initiation of treatment and reduction of intramedullary pressure. Prednisone, even as a single agent, is very effective in reducing tumor burden. As is seen in other chronic illnesses treated with long-term steroids, the risk of bone complications is increased in children receiving therapy for ALL. During the 1990s dexamethasone was introduced in several treatment protocols. Its longer half-life and increased CNS penetration were hypothesized to afford an increase in treatment efficacy. An increase in fractures (especially in boys 9 to 18 years old)[312] and in osteonecrosis[313,314] has been attributed to its use.

Inherent in the long-term treatment of a child with ALL is appreciation of the psychological stress imposed not only on the patient but also on the family. In essence the family becomes the patient, as with any chronic illness. In most treatment centers the care of children with ALL is approached by a multidisciplinary team composed of physicians, nurses, social workers, and often psychologists and play therapists. The concept of informed consent connotes more than merely obtaining permission to treat. Involvement of parents in decision making and in the child's care helps to foster confidence in the treatment team and enhances compliance with the therapy. When developmentally appropriate, the child should also be included in the care plan and allowed to maintain some control over events in his or her life.

TREATMENT OF RELAPSE

Following cessation of therapy, the overall relapse rate is approximately 20 percent.[315–317] Relapse occurs most frequently in the year following diagnosis and becomes progressively less common until the fourth year, after which it is very rare. However, late relapses, occurring up to 9 or 10 years after diagnosis, have been reported.[318] Three-fourths of the relapses occur in the bone marrow.[315,319] Relapse after therapy is higher in boys than in girls, in part because of testicular disease. The long-term disease-free survival rate for children being retreated after cessation of therapy is 20 to 40 percent. The salvage rate is higher in patients who have only extramedullary relapse[320] and in those who relapse more than 6 months after discontinuing treatment.[321–323]

Bone marrow relapse while receiving chemotherapy has a poor outcome with few survivors.[321,322] Successful HLA-matched sibling bone marrow transplantation offers the best chance for cure.[227,324–327] Nonetheless, this group of patients still has a high reinduction remission rate of approximately 70 percent when treated with prednisone, vincristine, and L-asparaginase.[328–330] Addition of DNM has improved reinduction rates to 90 percent.[331,332] Although readily induced, remission in these cases is usually short-lived.[333–335] In the most promising results, a median hematologic remission duration of approximately 1 year was obtained with a modified Capizzi regimen of vincristine, methotrexate, and L-asparaginase.[336] The use of high-dose ara-C followed by L-asparaginase as both induction and maintenance in this group of patients has also met with some success.[337] Central nervous system prophylaxis is a necessary part of treatment for relapsed ALL.[338–340]

Central Nervous System Relapse

Until recently, very few children with ALL who developed CNS leukemia were cured. The duration of CNS remission lasted only 3 to 5 months regardless of whether chemotherapy and radiation (usually less than 1000 cGy) or intrathecal antifolates were used.[341–345] Sullivan et al.[346] demonstrated that triple intrathecal therapy (methotrexate, ara-C, and hydrocortisone), when given as maintenance following initial clearing of the CSF, resulted in significant prolongation of CNS remission.

Several investigators have shown that a proportion of patients may be cured following an isolated CNS relapse.[347,348] Land[349] and Frankel[350] have observed salvage rates of over 50 percent. In these two studies, systemic reintensification used new drugs as well as specific CNS therapy. More recent studies also using intensive systemic and intrathecal therapy but delaying cranial–spinal radiation have shown improved results as well.[351,352] Children who relapsed more than 18 months after first remission were shown to have a greater than 80 percent survival rate, whereas those who relapsed early had a 46 percent 4-year event-free survival.[352] The outcome for patients who have previously received intensive chemotherapy and cranial radiation is very poor.[351,353]

Testicular Relapse

Testicular relapse may occur as an isolated event or in conjunction with bone marrow and/or CNS relapse. Patients with T-cell ALL or a high white blood cell count are more likely to experience a testicular relapse. One study found that 15 percent of boys successfully completing maintenance therapy showed occult leukemic disease on routine testicular biopsy.[354] Thus, some have suggested that all males undergo testicular biopsy on completion of maintenance. Others question the efficacy of this invasive procedure in view of the high rate of false-negative testicular biopsies.[355–357] The type of systemic therapy may influence the incidence of testicular relapse, and successful therapy may obviate the need for testicular biopsy. The use of intermediate-dose systemic methotrexate significantly reduced the frequency of testicular involvement in at least one study.[358]

The advantage of detecting occult disease is also questionable. In a series of CCG studies, testicular biopsy was routinely performed at the completion of maintenance. The overall survival rate of those patients with occult testicular leukemia (10 percent) was 65 ± 14 percent.[359] This is equivalent to the survival rate cited by earlier studies of patients with overt testicular relapse.[360] Bowman pointed out that patients with an isolated testicular relapse during therapy had a poor prognosis, in contrast to patients who relapsed after completing therapy. Isolated testicular relapse is often followed by bone marrow relapse because these patients usually have occult residual or recurrent leukemia beyond the testes.[361] Therapy should be designed accordingly. Systemic therapy, in addition to testicular radiation, has demonstrated substantial salvage from isolated testicular relapse.[362]

Bone Marrow Transplantation

Jacobson[363] and Lorenz et al.[364] first demonstrated that lethally irradiated mice could be rescued by intravenous infusion of bone marrow. This led to the use of bone marrow transplantation (BMT) as a therapeutic modality. Preparative regimens have used total body irradiation and chemotherapeutic drugs at extremely high doses.[365,366] Initially, end-stage patients were studied. As a result, allogeneic grafts were successful in only 13 percent of patients. Following this, patients with ALL in the second or subsequent complete remission received transplants, with 7 of 22 patients surviving.[367]

Johnson et al.[368] compared BMT with chemotherapy for children with ALL in the second or subsequent remission. They observed that 9 of 24 patients who received BMT in remission remained in CR, in contrast to 1 of 21 who received conventional chemotherapy. The benefit of BMT for children with relapse of ALL less than 36 months from diagnosis has been reiterated in data reported by other groups.[327,369] The benefit of BMT for children in later relapse or without a matched sibling donor is less clear.[322] One group concluded in 1995 that there was no improvement in survival[322] but reversed that opinion in a review published in 2000.[370] A series of reports from England argue that there is little benefit of BMT for any patient.[371] There are major complications associated with allogeneic bone marrow transplants, including recurrent leukemia, seen more commonly in patients with ALL than in those with ANLL; opportunistic infections; interstitial pneumonia; failure of donor marrow to engraft; and graft-versus-host disease (GVHD).[366,372]

LATE TOXICITIES

With most children now being cured of leukemia, the long-term effects of therapy must be assessed. Central nervous system toxicity, reproductive capabilities, and potential damage to the heart, liver, lungs, and kidneys need careful evaluation. Because radiation therapy and alkylating agents are carcinogens and because having one cancer predisposes an individual to a second primary, the risk of a second cancer must be considered as well.

Central nervous system, toxicity, in particular, has been of great concern. Although some reports suggest that chemotherapy and radiation do not interfere with CNS function,[353,373,374] others have shown adverse effects.[375–381] Moss et al. compared the IQs of children with ALL treated with chemotherapy and radiation plus repetitive intrathecal chemotherapy with those of their siblings and showed a significant mean drop in IQ of approximately 12 points in the patient group.[382] Comparing test results of children with ALL 1 month after diagnosis and 1 to 3 years later, Meadows et al. found significant declines in IQ and impairment in neuropsychological function.[378] Therapy for all children included cranial radiation (2400 cGy) and six doses of intrathecal methotrexate. The decline in scores was most pronounced in children younger than 6 years of age at diagnosis. In contrast, children in a comparison group, who received intrathecal methotrexate but no cranial radiation showed no changes in test scores. In Japan, 55 survivors who received 2400 cGy CNS radiotherapy plus intrathecal methotrexate continued to show a decline in IQ scores 10 years after treatment.[383] Those children who survive following a second course of cranial radiation have a high risk of significant intellectual impairment.[384]

An NIH study of 32 children who had received prophylactic CNS radiotherapy (2400 cGy) identified a number of intracranial abnormalities on computed tomography (CT) scans.[385] A later study correlated impairment of neuropyschologic function with abnormalities on CT scan in the same children.[386] The same group also showed that intracranial calcifications could develop 5 to 7 years after initiation of therapy.[387] Follow-up evaluation of 23 of these patients who had abnormal CT findings showed most significant deficits in verbal memory and verbal learning.[388] Similar CT scan abnormalities have been reported in 19 children treated in Argentina with 2400 cGy cranial radiation plus intrathecal methotrexate. Impaired neuropsychologic function was measured in eight of these children, but not in children who received only intrathecal therapy.[389]

Protection from neuropsychologic morbidity by exclusive use of parenteral therapy has not been observed, however, by all researchers.[390] Mulhern et al. showed no difference in neuropsychologic ability of children treated with 1800 cGy plus intrathecal methotrexate versus those treated with intrathecal therapy and high-dose intravenous methotrexate.[391,392] Their initial study also failed to show heightened impairment of function in younger children. They did, however, identify subtle differences in behavior of all treated children as compared with normal control subjects. An increased risk of impairment in girls was also found.[391] Waber et al. reported similar findings of increased neurotoxicity in girls only, following a single intensive dose of methotrexate intravenously in addition to intrathecal methotrexate.[393]

A subsequent analysis by Mulhern et al. compared neuropsychological function of children treated as infants for ALL versus a group treated as infants for Wilms' (kidney) tumor. At a global performance level, no significant differences were observed. Survivors of ALL, however, had measurable decreases in IQ, visual memory, and auditory memory, as well as decreased mathematical ability. Children in the ALL group more often received special educational intervention.[394] This contrasts again with data from the CCG in 1999, which reported no differences in neurodevelopmental indices of infants treated with intensified intravenous and intrathecal therapy as compared with age-based population standards.[395]

Another concern is the effect of therapy on growth. Children treated with cranial radiation in doses of 3000 to 5500 cGy for malignant brain tumors are known to have both growth hormone deficiency and growth failure. Whether the lower doses of radiation used to treat ALL have similar effects is debated. Children who received cranial–spinal radiation appear to have significantly reduced growth. The contribution of growth hormone deficiency secondary to cranial radiation in relation to the decrease in spinal epiphyseal growth centers is unclear.[396] Reduced levels of growth hormone have been measured in some patients following cranial radiation with 2400 cGy but without concomitant decreases in growth.[397] A study at the NIH, however, showed that children treated with 2400 cGy of cranial radiation had reduced 24-hour secretion of growth hormone and diminished diurnal variation, associated with decreased height.[398] Costin confirmed growth hormone deficiency in most of 16 long-term survivors who had received either 1800 or 2400 cGy and showed that all of these experienced a significantly higher rate of height increase after growth hormone replacement.[399] Another study evaluated 80 children with a mean survival of 7.9 years.[400] Whereas linear growth was markedly decreased in only a few children, obesity was a more common problem. Of even greater concern was the finding that 12 of the 80 had a head circumference less than the third percentile. The finding of increased obesity in survivors was confirmed in later studies.[401,402] Growth hormone deficiency has also been associated with decreased bone density in young adults as late as 11 years after they received cranial radiation.[403]

Intensification of treatment protocols to improve survival in patients at high risk of treatment failure may also increase the incidence of treatment toxicity.[404] Addition of anthracyclines to treatment protocols for ALL may have improved survival rates from leukemia but has also increased the risk of cardiac dysfunction in later life.[405] Although the doses of anthracyclines commonly used in ALL are far below known cardiotoxic levels, long-term effects remain to be determined. Two small studies in Boston[406] and Pavia, Italy[407] showed no overt cardiac dysfunction or pulmonary impairment. Children who received high-dose anthracyclines did show lower ventricular shortening fractions than children who received lower doses, but overt cardiac function was still within normal limits.[406]

Alkylating agents are associated with sterility in certain circumstances, as well as with an increased risk of second malignancy.[408] The doses used to treat ALL, however, are usually well below the known toxic doses. Germ cell dysfunction is found in more than half of males who receive testicular radiation and a smaller number of those whose testes are in the scatter field of spinal axis radiation.[409] Female survivors who received cranial–spinal radiation may have some ovarian dysfunction, although in a study of 40 patients none had complete dysfunction.[410] Topoisomerase II inhibitors also have a well-established association with secondary acute myelogenous leukemia.[411] An increased frequency of brain tumors has been reported,[412,413] especially when radiotherapy was preceded by intensive doses of systemic antimetabolites.[412] Patients with decreased thiopurine methlytransferase activity were found to be at particular risk.[412] Children who received higher doses of radiotherapy to treat overt CNS leukemia also had higher rates of secondary malignant brain tumor.[413] The Dana Farber Cancer Institute however, demonstrated that the risk of relapse is ten times greater than the risk of a second malignant tumor.[414] Two recent studies confirm that although 5-year survivors of childhood cancer have a higher risk of death than other young adults, the majority die from disease recurrence.[415,416]

The possible effect on the offspring of these patients is uncertain. The risk of teratogenic effects is rarely a concern within the pediatric population but in adults has been shown to be limited following the first trimester. The risk of oncogenesis to children unborn and more specifically, those not yet conceived, has not been widely studied. Reports of normal children with no increase in the incidence of malignancy are reassuring.[417,418] Included among these is a report from the Nordic Society of Pediatric Hematology/Oncology, which followed 5847 offspring of 14,652 survivors of childhood cancer (including 2232 leukemia survivors), diagnosed in the 1940s and 1950s.[417]

The treatment of children with ALL has been enormously successful in the last two decades. A major focus of both basic and clinical research has been the identification of biologically distinct subgroups with differing responses to so-called standard therapy. A second goal has been the development of treatment plans for specific subgroups to attempt to maximize survival rates. As larger numbers of long-term survivors are followed, the details of late effects to patients and their children will become apparent. The goals of the next decade will naturally include improvement of survival rates in children who now have a high risk of treatment failure. It is imperative, however, that these goals also continue to include efforts to reduce the physical toxicities and psychological stresses suffered by these children.

REFERENCES

1. Bennett JM: Case of hypertrophy of the spleen and liver in which death took place from suppuration of the blood. Edinburgh Med Soc J 64:413, 1845.
2. Virchow R: Weisses Blut and Milztumoren. Med Z 16:9, 1847.
3. Ehrlich P: Farbenanalytische Untersuchungen zur Histologie und Klinik des Blutes. A. Hirschwald, Berlin, 1891.
4. Farber S, Diamond LK, Mercer RD et al: Temporary remission in acute leukemia in children produced by folic acid antagonist, 4-aminopteroyl-glutamic acid (aminopterin). N Engl J Med 238:787, 1948.
5. Reiselbach RE, Morse EE, Rall DP et al: Intrathecal aminopterin therapy of meningeal leukemia. Arch Intern Med 1211:620, 1963.
6. Schrappe M, Reiter A, Ludwig W-D et al: Improved outcome in childhood acute lymphoblastic leukemia despite reduced use of anthracyclines and cranial radiotherapy: Results of trial ALL-BFM 90. Blood 95:3310–3322, 2000.
7. Chessells JM, Bailey C, Richards SM: Intensification of treatment and survival in all children with lymphoblastic leukaemia: Results of UK Medical Research Council trial UKALL X. Lancet 345:143–148, 1995.
8. Schrappe M, Reiter A, Zimmermann M et al: Long-term results of four consecutive trials in childhood ALL performed by the ALL-BFM (Berlin-Frankfurt-Münster). Study Group from 1981 to 1995. Leukemia 14:2205–2222, 2000.
9. Silverman LB, Declerck L, Gelber RD et al: Results of Dana-Farber Cancer Institute consortium protocols for children with newly diagnosed acute lymphoblastic leukemia (1981–1995). Leukemia 14:2247–2256, 2000.
10. Greenlee RT, Hill-Harmon MB, Murray T, Thum M: Cancer statistics 2001. Cancer J Clinicians 51:15–36, 2001.
11. Neglia JP, Robison LL: Epidemiology of the childhood acute leukemias. Pediatr Clin North Am 35:675, 1988.
12. Miller RW, Dalager NA: U.S. childhood cancer death by cell type. J Pediatr 85:64, 1060–1068, 1974.
13. Miller DR: Hematologic malignancies: Leukemia and lymphoma. In Miller DR and Baehner RL (eds.): Blood Diseases of Infancy and Childhood, pp. 604. CV Mosby, St. Louis, 1989.
14. Poplack DG, Reaman G: Acute lymphoblastic leukemia in childhood. Pediatr Clin North Am 35:903, 1988.
15. Nader LM, Korameyer SJ, Anderson KC et al: B-cell origin of non-T-cell acute lymphoblastic leukemia. J Clin Invest 74:332, 1984.
16. Henze G, Langerman HJ, Ritter J et al: Treatment strategy for different risk groups in childhood acute lymphoblastic leukemia: A report from the BFM group. In Neth R et al (eds.): Modern Trends in Human Leukemia, Vol. 4, pp. 87. Springer-Verlag, Berlin, 1981.

17. Ellermann V, Bang O: Experimentelle Leukamie bei Huhnen. Centr Bakteriol Abt I Orig 46:595, 1908.

18. Gross L: "Spontaneous" leukemia developing in C3H mice following inoculation in infancy, with AK-leukemic extracts, or AK-embryos. Proc Soc Exp Biol Med 76:27, 1951.

19. Gallo RC, Wong-Staal F: Retroviruses as etiologic agents of some animal and human leukemias and lymphomas and as tools for elucidating the molecular mechanism of leukemogenesis. Blood 60:545, 1982.

20. Essex M: Horizontally and vertically transmitted oncornaviruses of cats. Adv Cancer Res 21:175, 1975.

21. Hardy WD Jr, Old LJ, Hess PW et al: Horizontal transmission of feline leukemia virus. Nature 244:266, 1973.

22. Jarrett WFH, Crawford ER, Martin WB et al: A virus-like particle associated with leukemia (lymphosarcoma). Nature 202:567, 1964.

23. Reitz MS, Poiesz BJ, Ruscetti FW et al: Characterization and distribution of nucleic acid sequences of a novel type C retrovirus isolated from neoplastic human T lymphocytes. Proc Natl Acad Sci U S A 78:1887, 1981.

24. Ratner L, Poiesz BJ: Leukemias associated with human T-cell lymphotrophic virus type I in a non-endemic region. Medicine (Baltimore) 67:401, 1988.

25. Schaison G, Leverger G, Yildiz I et al: Follow-up of Fanconi's anemia (FA) high frequency of acute leukemia. Proc ASCO (abstr) 1:136, 1982.

26. Miller RW: Persons with exceptionally high risk of leukemia. Cancer Res 27:2420, 1967.

27. Hecht F, McCaw BK, Koler RD: Ataxia telangiectasia clonal growth of translocation lymphocytes. N Engl J Med 289:286, 1973.

28. Miller RW: Epidemiology of leukemia. In Neth R, Callo RC, Hufschneider PH, Mannweiler K (eds.): Modern Trends in Human Leukemia, Vol. 3, pp. 3. Springer-Verlag, New York, 1979.

29. Peterson RDA, Cooper MD, Good RA: Lymphoid tissue abnormalities with ataxia telangiectasia. Am J Med 41:342, 1966.

30. Miller RW: Relation between cancer and congenital defects: An epidemiologic evaluation. J Natl Cancer Inst 40:1079–1085, 1968.

31. Nesbit M, Robison LL, Littman PH et al: Presymptomatic central nervous system therapy in previously untreated childhood acute lymphoblastic leukemia: Comparison of 1800 rad and 2400 rad. A report for Children's Cancer Study Group. Lancet 1:461, 1981.

32. Jonas DM, Helbros DC, Albumin AR: Rubinstein-Taybi syndrome and acute leukemia. J Pediatr 92:851, 1978.

33. Bader JL, Miller RW: Neurofibromatosis and childhood leukemia. J Pediatr 92:925, 1978.

34. Privitera E, Kamps MP, Hayashi Y et al: Different consequences of the 1;19 chromosomal translocation in childhood B-cell precursor acute lymphoblastic leukemia. Blood 79:1781, 1992.

35. Rubnitz JE, Link MP, Shuster JJ et al: Frequency and prognostic significance of HRX rearrangements in infant acute lymphoblastic leukemia: A Pediatric Oncology Group study. Blood 84:570, 1994.

36. Rubnitz JE, Morrissey JJ, Savage PA, Cleary ML: ENL, the gene fused with HRX in t(11;19) leukemias, encodes a nuclear protein with transcriptional activation potential in lymphoid and myeloid cells. Blood 84:1747, 1994.

37. Look AT: The cytogenetics of childhood leukemia: Clinical and biologic implications. Pediatr Clin North Am 35:723, 1988.

38. Prokocimer M, Rotter V: Structure and function of p53 in normal cells and their aberrations in cancer cells: Projection on the hematologic cell lineages. Blood 84:2391–2411, 1994.

39. Hsiao MH, Yu AL, Yeargin J et al: Nonhereditary p53 mutations in T-cell acute lymphoblastic leukemia are associated with the relapse phase. Blood 83:2922, 1994.

40. Imamura J, Miyoshi I, Koeffler HP: p53 in hematologic malignancies. Blood 84:2412, 1994.

41. Knudson AG: Mutation and cancer: Statistical study of retinoblastoma. Proc Natl Acad Sci U S A 68:820, 1971.

42. Sun L, Heerema N, Crotty L et al: Expression of dominant-negative and mutant isoforms of the antileukemic transcription factor Ikaros in infant acute lymphoblastic leukemia. PNAS Online 96:680–685, 1999.

43. Sun L, Goodman PA, Wood CM et al: Expression of aberrantly spliced oncogenic Ikaros isoforms in childhood acute lymphoblastic leukemia. J Clin Oncol 17:3753–3766, 1999.

44. Penn I: Second malignant neoplasms associated with immunosuppression medications. Cancer 37:1024, 1976.

45. MacMahon B, Levy MA: Prenatal origin of childhood leukemia. Evidence from twins. N Engl J Med 270:1082, 1964.

46. Ford AM, Ridge SA, Cabrera ME et al: In utero rearrangements in the trithorax-related oncogene in infant leukemias. Nature 363:358, 1993.

47. Super HJG, Rothberg PG, Kobayshi H et al: Clonal, nonconstitutional rearrangements of the MLL gene in infant twins with acute lymphoblastic leukemia: In utero chromosome rearrangement of 11q23. Blood 83:641, 1994.

48. Mahmoud HH, Ridge SA, Behm FG et al: Intrauterine monoclonal origin of neonatal concordant acute lymphoblastic leukemia in monozygotic twins. Med Pediatr Oncol 24:77–81, 1995.

49. Bizzerozzero OJ Jr, Johnson KG, Ciocco A: Radiation-related leukemia in Hiroshima and Nagasaki. 1946–64. I. Distribution, incidence and appearance in time. N Engl J Med 274:1095, 1966.

50. Folley JH, Borges W, Yamawaki T: Incidence of leukemia in the survivors of the atomic bomb in Hiroshima and Nagasaki, Japan. Am J Med 13:311, 1962.

51. Moloney WC: Leukemia in survivors of atomic bombing. N Engl J Med 253:88, 1955.

52. Morgan KZ: Radiation-induced health effects. Science 195:344, 1977.

53. Cronkite EP, Maloney W, Bond VP: Radiation leukemiogenesis. An analysis of the problem. Am J Med 28:673, 1960.

54. Lewis EB: Leukemia and ionizing radiation. Science 125:965, 1984.

55. Upton AC: The dose-response relation in radiation-induced cancer. Cancer Res 21:717, 1961.

56. National Academy of Sciences: Biological effects of atomic radiation. National Research Council, Washington, DC, 1980.

57. Schull WJ, Kato H: Malignancies and exposure of the young to ionizing radiation. Cancer Bull 34(3):84, 1982.

58. Michaelson SM: Household magnetic fields and childhood leukemia: A critical analysis. Pediatrics 88:3, 1991.

59. Kleinerman RA, Kaune WT, Hatch WW et al: Are children living near high-voltage power lines at increased risk of acute lymphoblastic leukemia? Am J Epidemiol 151:512–515, 2000.

60. Auvinen A, Linet MS, Hatch EE et al: Extremely low-frequency magnetic fields and childhood acute lymphoblastic leukemia: An exploratory analysis of alternative exposure metrics. Am J Epidemiol 152:20–31, 2000.

61. Freeman AI, Pantazopoulos N, de Castro L et al: Infections in children with acute leukemia. Med Pediatr Oncol 1:167, 1975.

62. Hughes WT, Smith DR: Infection during induction of remission in acute lymphoblastic leukemia. Cancer 31:1008, 1973.

63. Gaynon PS, Bleyer WA, Albo VC et al: Intensive therapy for children with acute lymphoblastic leukemia and unfavorable presenting features: Early conclusions of study CCG-106 by the Childrens Cancer Study Group. Lancet 2:921, 1988.

64. Tuten HR, Gabos PG, Kumar SJ, Harter GD: The limping child: A manifestation of acute leukemia. J Pediatr Orthop 18:625–629, 1998.

65. Scully RE (ed.): Case records of the Massachusetts General Hospital Case 32-200. N Engl J Med 343:1168–1176, 2000.

66. Millot F, Robert A, Bertrand Y et al: Cutaneous involvement in children with acute lymphoblastic leukemia or lymphoblastic lymphoma. Pediatrics 100:60–64, 1997.

67. Catovsky D, Bernasconi C, Verdonck PJ: The association of eosinophilia with lymphoblastic leukaemia or lymphoma: A study of seven patients. Br J Haematol 45:523, 1980.

68. Gaynon PS, Gonzalez-Crussi F: Exaggerated eosinophilia and acute lymphoid leukemia. Am J Pediatr Hematol Oncol 4:334, 1984.

69. Hogan TF, Koss W, Murgo AJ et al: Acute lymphoblastic leukemia with chromosomal 5;14 translocation and hypereosinophilia: Case report and literature review. J Clin Oncol 5:382, 1987.

70. Nelken RP, Stockman JA: The hypereosinophilic syndrome in association with acute lymphoblastic leukemia. J Pediatr 89:771, 1976.

71. Breatnach F, Chessels JM, Graves MF: The aplastic presentation of childhood leukaemia: A feature of common ALL. Br J Haematol 49:387, 1981.

72. Sills RH, Stockman JA: Preleukemic states in children with acute lymphoblastic leukemia. Cancer 48:110, 1981.

73. Miller DR, Sandford L, Albo V et al: Prognostic factors and therapy in acute lymphoblastic leukemia of childhood: CCG-141. Cancer 51:1041, 1983.

74. Tubergen DG, Cullen JW, Boyett JM et al: Blasts in CSF with a normal cell count do not justify alteration of therapy for acute lymphoblastic leukemia in remission: A Childrens Cancer Group study. J Clin Oncol 12:273–278, 1994.

75. Mahmoud HH, Rivera GK, Hancock ML et al: Low leukocyte counts with blast cells in cerebrospinal fluid of children with newly diagnosed acute lymphoblastic leukemia. N Engl J Med 329:314–319, 1993.

76. Pui C-H, Mahmoud HH, Rivera GK et al: Early intensification of intrathecal chemotherapy virtually eliminates central nervous system relapse in children with acute lymphoblastic leukemia. Blood 92:411–415, 1998.

77. Eden OB, Innes EM: Testicular infiltration in acute lymphoblastic leukemia. Arch Dis Child 53:841, 1978.

78. Hudson MM, Frankel LS, Mullins J et al: Diagnostic value of surgical testicular biopsy after therapy for acute lymphocytic leukemia. J Pediatr 107:50, 1985.

79. Pui C-H, Bowman WP, Abramowich M et al: Elective testicular biopsy during chemotherapy for childhood leukaemia is of no clinical value. Lancet 2:410, 1985.

80. Reinherz EL, Nadler LM, Sallas SE et al: Subset derivation of T-cell acute lymphoblastic leukemia in man. J Clin Invest 64:392–397, 1979.

81. Fledges AJ, Aur RJA, Verzosa MS et al: Periodic acid-Schiff reaction, a useful index of duration of complete remission in acute childhood leukemia. Acta Haematol 52:8, 1974.

82. Bennett JM, Catovsky D, Daniel MT et al: Proposals for the classification of the acute leukemias. Br J Haematol 33:451, 1976.

83. Bennett JM, Catovsky D, Daniel MT et al: The morphological classification of acute lymphoblastic leukemia: Concordance among observers and clinical correlations. Br J Haematol 47:553, 1981.

84. Shaw M: The cytochemistry of acute leukemia: A diagnostic and prognostic evaluation. Semin Oncol 3:219–228, 1976.

85. Catovsky D: T-cell origin of acid-phosphatase positive lymphoblasts. Lancet 2:236, 1975.

86. Dow LW, Martin P, Moohr J et al: Evidence for clonal development of childhood acute lymphoblastic leukemia. Blood 66:902, 1985.

87. Foon KA, Todd RF: Immunologic classification of leukemia and lymphoma. Blood 68:1, 1986.

88. Li C-Y: Immunocytochemical techniques for identifying leukemias. Mayo Clin Proc 59:185, 1984.

89. McKenna RW, Kerset JH, Brynes RK et al: Cytochemistry profiles in acute lymphoblastic leukemia. Am J Pediatr Hematol Oncol 1:263, 1979.

90. Raghavachar A, Bartram CR, Ganser A et al: Acute undifferentiated leukemia: Implications for cellular origin and clonality suggested by analysis of surface markers and immunoglobulin gene rearrangement. Blood 68:658, 1986.

91. Vogler LB, Crist W, Bockman D et al: Pre-B leukemia: A new phenotype of childhood lymphoblastic leukemia. N Engl J Med 298:872, 1978.

92. McGregor AM: Monoclonal antibodies; production and use. British Medical Journal 283:1143, 1981.

93. Greaves MF, Janossy G, Peto J et al: Immunologically defined subclasses of acute lymphoblastic leukaemia in children: Their relationship to presentation features and prognosis. Br J Haematol 48:179, 1981.

94. Dow LW, Martin P, Moohr J et al: Evidence for clonal development of childhood acute lymphoblastic leukemia. Blood 66:902, 1985.

95. Greaves MF, Brown G, Rapson NT et al: Antisera to acute lymphoblastic leukemia cells. Clin Immunol Immunopathol 4:67, 1975.

96. Roper M, Crist W, Metzgar R et al: Monoclonal antibody characterization of surface antigens in childhood T-cell lymphoid malignancies. Blood 61:830, 1983.

97. Sondel PM, Borcherding W, Shahidi NT et al: Recategorizing childhood acute lymphoblastic leukemia with monoclonal antibodies to human T-cells. Blood 57:1135, 1981.

98. Vogler LB, Crist W, Bockman D et al: Pre-B leukemia: a new phenotype of childhood lymphoblastic leukemia. N Engl J Med 298:872, 1978.

99. Ritz J, Pesando JM, Notis-McConarty J et al: A monoclonal antibody to human acute lymphoblastic leukaemia antigen. Nature 283:583, 1980.

100. Altman AJ: Clinical features and biological implications of acute mixed lineage (hybrid) leukemias. Am J Pediatr Hematol/Oncol 12:123, 1990.

101. Drexler HG, Ludwig WD: Incidence and clinical relevance of myeloid antigen-positive acute lymphoblastic leukemia. Recent results. Cancer Res 131:53, 1993.

102. Barrett SG, Schwade JG, Ranken R et al: Lymphoblasts with both T and B markers in childhood leukemia and lymphoma. Blood 50:71, 1977.

103. Mirro J, Zipf TF, Pui C-H et al: Acute mixed lineage leukemia: Clinicopathologic correlation and prognostic significance. Blood 66:1115, 1985.

104. Pui C-H, Behm FG, Crist WM: Clinical and biologic relevance of immunologic marker studies in childhood acute lymphoblastic leukemia. Blood 82:343, 1993.

105. Roberts GT, El Badawi SB, Sackey K et al: Lineage ambiguity in acute leukemia. Cancer 58:1473, 1986.
106. Stass SA, Mirro J: Lineage heterogeneity in acute leukaemia: Acute mixed-lineage leukaemia and lineage switch. Clin Haematol 15:811–827, 1986.
107. Pui C-H, Raimondi SC, Head DR et al: Characterization of childhood acute leukemia with multiple myeloid and lymphoid markers at diagnosis and at relapse. Blood 78:1327, 1991.
108. Raghavachar A, Thiel E, Hansen-Hagge TE et al: Rearrangement of T cell receptor beta, gamma and delta gene loci in human pre-T cell acute lymphoblastic leukemia. Leukemia 3:413–418, 1989.
109. Waldmann TA, Korsmeyer SJ, Bakhshi A et al: Immunoglobin genes and the c-myc oncogene. In Waldmann TA (moderator): Molecular Genetic Analysis of Human Lymphoid Neoplasms. Ann Intern Med 102:497, 1985.
110. Felix CA, Reaman GH, Korsmeyer SJ et al: Immunoglobin and T cell receptor gene configuration in acute lymphoblastic leukemia of infancy. Blood 70:536, 1987.
111. Kitchingman GR, Rovigatti U, Mauer AM et al: Rearrangement of immunoglobulin heavy chain genes in T-cell acute lymphoblastic leukemia. Blood 65:725, 1985.
112. Yokota S, Hansen-Hagge TE, Bartram CR: T-cell receptor delta gene recombination in common acute lymphoblastic leukemia: Preferential usage of V delta 2 and frequent involvement of the J alpha cluster. Blood 77:141–148, 1991.
113. Steenbergen EJ, Verhagen OJ, van Leeuwen EF et al: Distinct ongoing Ig heavy chain rearrangement processes in childhood B-precursor acute lymphoblastic leukemia. Blood 82:581–589, 1993.
114. Coleman MS, Greenwood MF, Hutton JJ et al: Serial observations on terminal deoxynucleotidyl transferase and lymphoblast surface markers in acute lymphoblastic leukemia. Cancer Res 36:120, 1976.
115. Bollman EJ: Terminal deoxynucleotidyl transferase as a hematopoietic cell marker. Blood 54:1203, 1979.
116. Froehlich TW, Buchanan GR, Cornet JAM et al: Terminal deoxynucleotidyl transferase containing cells in peripheral blood: Implications for the surveillance of patients with lymphoblastic leukemia or lymphoma in remission. Blood 58:214, 1981.
117. Hecht T, Forman SJ, Winkler US et al: Histochemical demonstration of terminal deoxynucleotidyl transferase in leukemia. Blood 58:856, 1981.
118. Kalwinsky DK, Weathered WH, Dahl GV et al: Clinical utility of initial terminal deoxynucleotidyl transferase determinations in childhood acute leukemias. Cancer Res 41:2877, 1981.
119. McCaffrey R, Lilliquist A, Sallan S et al: Clinical utility of leukemia cell terminal transferase measurements. Cancer Res 41:4814, 1981.
120. McCaffrey R, Smoler DF, Baltimore D: Terminal deoxynucleotidyl transferase in a case of childhood acute lymphoblastic leukemia. Proc Natl Acad Sci U S A 70:512, 1973.
121. Srivastava BIS, Khan SA, Minowada J et al: High terminal deoxynucleotidyl transferase activity in pediatric patients with acute lymphocytic and acute myelocytic leukemia. Int J Cancer 22:4, 1978.
122. Bloomfield CD, Goldman AI, Berger AR: Chromosomal abnormalities identify high-risk and low-risk patients with acute lymphoblastic leukemia. Blood 67:415, 1986.
123. Lonsdale D, Gejan EA, Fernbach DJ et al: Interrupted vs continued maintenance therapy in childhood acute leukemia. Cancer 36:341, 1975.
124. Raimondi SC: Current status of cytogenetic research in childhood acute lymphoblastic leukemia. Blood 81:2237, 1993.
125. Wiliams DL, Harber J, Murphy SB: Chromosomal translocations play a unique role in influencing prognosis in childhood acute lymphoblastic leukemia. Blood 68:205, 1986.
126. Williams DL, Look AT, Melvian SL et al: New chromosomal translocations correlate with specific immunophenotypes of childhood acute lymphoblastic leukemia. Cell 36:101, 1984.
127. Wright JJ, Poplack DG, Bakhshi A: Gene rearrangements as markers of clonal variation and minimal residual disease in acute lymphoblastic leukemia. J Clin Oncol 5:735–741, 1987.
128. Berger P, Bernheim JC, Brouet JC et al: t18;14 translocation in a Burkitt's type lymphoblastic leukemia (L₃). Br J Haematol 43:87, 1979.
129. Look AT: The cytogenetics of childhood leukemia: Clinical and biologic implications. Pediatr Clin North Am 35:723, 1988.
130. Ribeiro RC, Abromowitch M, Raimondi SC et al: Clinical and biologic hallmarks of the Philadelphia chromosome in childhood acute lymphoblastic leukemia. Blood 70:948, 1987.
131. Secker-Walker LM, Summersgill BM, Swansbury GJ et al: Philadelphia positive blast crises masquerading as acute lymphoblastic leukemia in children. Lancet 2:1405, 1976.
132. Rubnitz JE, Crist WM: Molecular genetics of childhood cancer: Implications for pathogenesis, diagnosis and treatment. Pediatrics 100:101–108, 1997.
133. Takahashi Y, Horibe K, Kiyoi H et al: Prognostic significance of TEL/AML1 fusion transcript in childhood B-precursor acute lymphoblastic leukemia. J Pediatr Hematol/Oncol 20:190–195, 1998.
134. Maloney KW, McGavran L, Murphy JR et al: TEL-AML1 fusion identifies a subset of children with standard risk acute lymphoblastic leukemia who have an excellent prognosis when treated with therapy that includes a single delayed intensification. Leukemia 13:1708–1712, 1999.
135. Stong RC, Korsmeyer SJ, Parkin JL et al: Human acute leukemia cell line with the t(4;11) chromosomal rearrangement exhibits B lineage and monocytic characteristics. Blood 65:21, 1985.
136. Chen CS, Sorensen PHB, Domer PH et al: Molecular rearrangements on chromosome 11q23 predominate in infant acute lymphoblastic leukemia and are associated with specific biologic variables and poor outcome. Blood 81:2386, 1993.
137. Chilcote RR, Brown E, Rowley JD: Lymphoblastic leukemia with lymphomatous features associated with abnormalities of the short arm of chromosome 9. N Engl J Med 313:286, 1985.
138. Diaz MO, Ziemin S, Le Beau MM et al: Homozygous deletion of the alpha- and beta 1-interferon genes in human leukemia and derived cell lines. Proc Natl Acad Sci U S A 85:5259, 1988.
139. Schneider NR, Carroll AJ, Shuster JJ et al: New recurring cytogenetic abnormalities and association of blast cell karyotypes with prognosis in childhood T-cell acute lymphoblastic leukemia: A Pediatric Oncology Group report of 343 cases. Blood 96:2543–2549, 2000.
140. Traweek ST, Riscoe MK, Ferro AJ et al: Methylthioadenosine phosphorylase deficiency in acute leukemia: Pathologic, cytogenetic and clinical features. Blood 71:1568, 1988.
141. Fitchen JH, Riscoe MK, Dana BW et al: Methioadenosine phosphorylase deficiency in human leukemia and solid tumors. Cancer Res 46:5409, 1986.
142. George SI, Fernbach DJ, Vietti TJ et al: Factors influencing survival in pediatric acute leukemia. The SWOG experience, 1958–1970. Cancer 32:1542, 1973.
143. Miller DR, Leikin S, Albo V et al: Prognostic factors and therapy in acute lymphoblastic leukemia of childhood: CCG-141: A report from Children's Cancer Study Group. Cancer 51:1041, 1983.

144. Miller DR, Leikin S, Albo V et al: Intensive therapy and prognostic factors in acute lymphoblastic leukemia of childhood CCG 141. In Neth R et al. (eds.): Modern Trends in Human Leukemia, Vol. 4, p. 77. Springer-Verlag, Berlin, 1981.

145. Miller DR, Leikin S, Albo V et al: The use of prognostic factors in improving the design and efficacy of clinical trials in childhood leukemia. Cancer Treat Rep 64:381, 1980.

146. Miller DR, Coccia PF, Bleyer WA et al: Early response to induction therapy as a predictor of disease-free survival and late recurrence of childhood acute lymphoblastic leukemia: A report from the Children's Cancer Study Group. J Clin Oncol 7:1807, 1989.

147. Crist W, Pullen J, Boyett J et al: Clinical and biologic features predict a poor prognosis in acute lymphoid leukemias in infants: A Pediatric Oncology Group Study. Blood 67:135, 1986.

148. Dinndorf PA, Reaman GH: Acute lymphoblastic leukemia in infants: Evidence for B-cell origin of disease by use of monoclonal antibody phenotyping. Blood 68:975, 1986.

149. Hammond D, Sather H, Nesbit M et al: Analysis of prognostic factors in acute lymphoblastic leukemia. Med Pediatr Oncol 14:124, 1986.

150. Leiper AD, Chessells J: Acute lymphoblastic leukaemia under 2 years. Arch Dis Child 61:1007, 1986.

151. Leverger G, Bancillon A, Schaison G et al: Acute lymphoblastic leukemia in very young children: Diagnostic and therapeutic aspects of 43 cases. Am J Pediatr Hematol Oncol 8:213, 1986.

152. Reaman G, Zeltzer P, Bleyer WA et al: Acute lymphoblastic leukemia in infants less than one year of age: A cumulative experience of the Childrens Cancer Study Group. J Clin Oncol 3:1513, 1985.

153. Rubnitz JE, Camitta BM, Mahmoud H et al: Childhood acute lymphoblastic leukemia with the MLL-ENL fusion and t(11;19)(q23;p13.3) translocation. J Clin Oncol 17:191–196, 1999.

154. Uckun FM, Downing JR, Chelstron LM et al: Human t(4;11) (q21;q23) acute lymphoblastic leukemia in mice with severe combined immunodeficiency. Blood 84:859, 1994.

155. Sather H, Coccia P, Nesbit M et al: Disappearance of the predictive value of prognostic variables in childhood acute lymphoblastic leukemia. Cancer 48:370, 1981.

156. Shuster JJ, Wacker P, Pullen J et al: Prognostic significance of sex in childhood B-precursor acute lymphoblastic leukemia: A Pediatric Oncology Group study. J Clin Oncol 16:2854–2863, 1998.

157. Pui C-H, Boyett JM, Relling MV et al: Sex differences in prognosis for children with acute lymphoblastic leukemia. J Clin Oncol 17:818–824, 1999.

158. Walters TR, Bushmore M, Simone J: Poor prognosis in Negro children with acute lymphoblastic leukemia. Cancer 29:210, 1972.

159. Falletta J, Boyett J, Pullen DJ: Clinical and phenotype features of childhood acute lymphocytic leukemia (ALL) by race and Spanish origin. Proceedings of the International Workshop on the Influence of the Environment on Leukemia and Lymphoma Subtypes. Raven Press, New York, 1982.

160. Pui C-H, Boyett JM, Hancock ML et al: Outcome of treatment for childhood cancer in black as compared with white children: The St. Jude's Research Hospital experience, 1962 through 1992. JAMA 273:633–637, 2000.

161. Pollock BH, DeBraun MR, Camitta BM et al: Racial differences in the survival of childhood B-precursor acute lymphoblastic leukemia: A Pediatric Oncology Group study. J Clin Oncol 18:813–823, 2000.

162. Pui C-H, Evans WE: Acute lymphoblastic leukemia in infants. J Clin Oncol 17:438, 1999.

163. Biondi A, Cimino G, Pieters R, Pui C-H: Biological and therapeutic aspects of infant leukemia. Blood 96:24–33, 2000.

164. Reaman GH, Sposto R, Sensel MG et al: Treatment outcome and prognostic factors for infants with acute lymphoblastic leukemia treated on two consecutive trials of the Children's Cancer Group. J Clin Oncol 17:445, 1999.

165. Skipper HE, Schabel FM Jr, Wilcox WS: Experimental evaluation of potential anti-cancer agents. XIII. On the criteria and kinetics associated with "curability" of experimental leukemia. Cancer Chemother Rep 35:3, 1964.

166. Goldie JH, Coldman AJ: A mathematical model for relating the drug sensitivity of tumors at their spontaneous mutation rate. Cancer Treat Rep 63:1727, 1979.

167. Lilleyman JS, Hann IM, Stevens RF et al: French American British (FAB) morphology classification of childhood lymphoblastic leukemia and its clinical importance. J Clin Pathol 39:998, 1986.

168. Miller DR, Krailo M, Bleyer WA et al: Prognostic implications of blast cell morphology in childhood acute lymphoblastic leukemia: A report from the Children's Cancer Study Group. Cancer Treat Rep 69:1211, 1985.

169. Kalwinsky DK, Robertson P, Dahl G et al: Clinical relevance of lymphoblast biological features in children with acute lymphoblastic leukemia. J Clin Oncol 3:477, 1985.

170. Chessels JM, Hardisty RM, Rapson NT et al: Acute lymphoblastic leukemia in children: Classification and prognosis. Lancet 2:1307, 1977.

171. Sallan SE, Ritz J, Pesando J et al: Cell surface antigens: Prognostic implications in childhood acute lymphoblastic leukemia. Blood 55:395, 1980.

172. Henze G, Rüdiger F, Hartman R et al: Six-year experience with a comprehensive approach to the treatment of recurrent childhood acute lymphoblastic leukemia (ALL-REZ BFM 85). A relapse study of the BFM group. Blood 78:1166, 1991.

173. Pullen DJ, Crist WM, Falletta JM et al: A Pediatric Oncology Group classification protocol for acute lymphocytic leukemia (AlinC 13): Immunologic phenotypes and correlation with treatment results. In Murphy S, Gilbert J (eds.): Leukemia Research: Advances in Cell Biology and Treatment, p. 221. Elsevier North Holland, Excerpta Medica, New York, 1983.

174. Pullen J, Shuster JJ, Link M et al: Significance of commonly used prognostic factors differs for children with T cell acute lymphocytic leukemia (ALL), as compared to those with B-precursor ALL. A Pediatric Oncology Group (POG) study. Leukemia 13:1696–1707, 1999.

175. Boyett J, Pullen J, Crist W et al: Immune phenotype as an independent prognostic factor within non-B acute lymphocytic leukemia (ALL): Initial WBC is not prognostic within Pre-B ALL. Blood 60:121a, 1982.

176. Crist W, Boyett J, Jackson J et al: Prognostic importance of the pre-B cell immunophenotype and other presenting features in B-lineage childhood acute lymphoblastic leukemia: A Pediatric Oncology Group study. Blood 74:1252, 1989.

177. Crist W, Boyett J, Roper M et al: Pre-B cell leukemia responds poorly to treatment: A Pediatric Oncology Group study. Blood 63:407, 1984.

178. Roper M, Crist W, Ragab A et al: Pre-B leukemia differs in its response to therapy. Presented at American Society of Hematology. (Abstr.) Blood 58:150a, 1981.

179. Volger LB, Crist W, Sarrif AM et al: An analysis of clinical and laboratory features of acute lymphocytic leukemias with emphasis on 35 children with pre-B leukemia. Blood 58:135, 1981.

180. Pui C-H, Hancock ML, Head DR et al: Clinical significance of CD34 expression in childhood acute lymphoblastic leukemia. Blood 82:889, 1993.

181. Green E, McConville CM, Powell JE et al: Clonal diversity of Ig and T-cell-receptor gene rearrangements identifies a subset of childhood B-precursor acute lymphoblastic leukemia with increased risk of relapse. Blood 92:952–958, 1998.

182. Altman AJ: Clinical features and biological implications of acute mixed lineage (hybrid) leukemias. Am J Pediatr Hematol Oncol 12:123, 1990.

183. Pui C-H, Raimondi SC, Head DR et al: Characterization of childhood acute leukemia with multiple myeloid and lymphoid markers at diagnosis and at relapse. Blood 78:1327, 1991.

184. Weirsma S, Ortega J, Sobel E, Weinberg K: Clinical importance of myeloid antigen expression in acute lymphoblastic leukemia of childhood. N Engl J Med 324:800, 1991.

185. Look AT, Robertson PK, Williams DL et al: Prognostic importance of blast cell DNA content in childhood acute lymphoblastic leukemia. Blood 65:1079, 1985.

186. Morse AG, Odom LF, Tubergen D et al: Prognosis in acute lymphoblastic leukemia of childhood as determined by cytogenetic studies at diagnosis. Med Pediatr Oncol 11:310, 1983.

187. Sandberg AA: The Chromosomes in Human Cancer and Leukemia. Elsevier North Holland, New York, 1980.

188. Third International Workshop on Chromosomes in Leukemia, Lund, Sweden, July 21–25, Cancer Genet Cytogen 4:95, 1980.

189. Trueworthy R, Shuster J, Look T et al: Ploidy of lymphoblasts is the strongest predictor of treatment outcome in B-progenitor cell acute lymphoblastic leukemia of childhood: A Pediatric Oncology Group study. J Clin Oncol 10:606, 1992.

190. Watson MS, Carroll AJ, Shuster JJ et al: Trisomy 21 in childhood lymphoblastic leukemia: A Pediatric Oncology Group study (8602). Blood 82:3098, 1993.

191. Takahashi Y, Horibe K, Kiyoi H et al: Prognostic significance of TEL/AML1 fusion transcript in childhood B-precursor acute lymphoblastic leukemia. J Pediatr Hematol Oncol 20:190–195, 1998.

192. Maloney KW, McGavran L, Murphy JR et al: TEL-AML1 fusion identifies a subset of children with standard risk acute lymphoblastic leukemia who have an excellent prognosis when treated with therapy that includes a single delayed intensification. Leukemia 13:1708–1712, 1999.

193. Brodeur GM, Williams DL, Look AT et al: Near-haploid acute lymphoblastic leukemia. A unique subgroup with a poor prognosis. Blood 58:14, 1981.

194. Rowley JD: Chromosomes in leukemia and lymphoma. Semin Hematol 15:301, 1978.

195. Oshimura M, Freeman AI, Sandberg AA: Chromosomes and causation of human cancer and leukemia XXXIII. Near-haploidy in acute leukemia. Cancer 40:1143, 1977.

196. Whang-Peng J, Knutesen T, Ziegler J: Cytogenetics studies in acute lymphocytic leukemia: Special emphasis on long-term survival. Med Pediatr Oncol 2:233, 1976.

197. Pui C-H, Behm FG, Downing JR et al: 11q23/MLL rearrangement confers a poor prognosis in infants with acute lymphoblastic leukemia. J Clin Oncol 12:909, 1994.

198. Heerema NA, Arthur DC, Sather H et al: Cytogenetic features of infants less than 12 months of age at diagnosis of acute lymphoblastic leukemia: Impact of the 11q23 breakpoint on outcome: A report of the Childrens Cancer Group. Blood 83:2274, 1994.

199. Rowley JD: Chromosome translocations: Dangerous liaisons. J Lab Clin Med 132:244–250, 1998.

200. Hunger SP, Tkachuk DC, Amylon MD et al: HRX involvement in de novo and secondary leukemias with diverse chromosome 11q23 abnormalities. Blood 81:3197, 1993.

201. Fletcher JA, Kimball VM, Lynch E et al: Prognostic implications of cytogenetic studies in an intensively treated group of children with acute lymphoblastic leukemia. Blood 74:2130, 1989.

202. Gajjar A, Ribeiro R, Hancock ML et al: Persistence of circulating blasts after 1 week of multiagent chemotherapy confers a poor prognosis in childhood acute lymphoblastic leukemia. Blood 80:1292–1295, 1995.

203. Schrappe M, Aricò M, Harbott J et al: Philadelphia chromosome-positive (Ph+) childhood acute lymphoblastic leukemia: Good initial steroid response allows early prediction of a favorable treatment outcome. Blood 92:2730–2741, 1998.

204. Nachman JB, Sather HN, Sensel MG et al: Augmented post-induction therapy for children with high-risk acute lymphoblastic leukemia and slow response to initial therapy. N Engl J Med 338:1663–1671, 1998.

205. Gaynon PS, Desai AA, Bostrom BC et al: Early response to therapy and outcome in childhood acute lymphoblastic leukemia. Cancer 80:1717–1726, 1997.

206. Steinherz PG, Gaynon PS, Breneman JC et al: Cytoreduction and prognosis in acute lymphoblastic leukemia – the importance of early marrow response: Report from the Childrens Cancer Group. J Clin Oncol 14:389–398, 1996.

207. Gaynon PS, Bleyer WA, Steinherz PG et al: Day 7 marrow response and outcome for children with acute lymphoblastic leukemia and unfavorable presenting features. Med Pediatr Oncol 18:273–279, 1990.

208. Silverman LB, Gelber RD, Young ML et al: Induction failure in acute lymphoblastic leukemia of childhood. Cancer 85:1395–1404, 1999.

209. Ciudad J, San Miguel JF, López-Berges MC: Prognostic value of immunophenotypic detection of minimal residual disease in acute lymphoblastic leukemia. J Clin Oncol 16:3774–3781, 1999.

210. Van Dongen JJM, Seriu T, Panzer-Grumayer ER et al: Prognostic value of minimal residual disease in acute lymphoblastic leukaemia in childhood. Lancet 352:1731–1738, 1998.

211. Cave H, van der Werff ten Bosch J, Suciu S et al: Clinical significance of minimal residual disease in childhood acute lymphoblastic leukemia. N Engl J Med 339:591–598, 1998.

212. Coustan-Smith E, Behm FG, Sanchez J et al: Immunological detection of minimal residual disease in children with acute lymphoblastic leukaemia. Lancet 351:550–554, 1998.

213. Goulden NJ, Knechtli CJ, Garland RJ et al: Minimal residual disease analysis for the prediction of relapse in children with standard-risk acute lymphoblastic leukaemia. Br J Haematol 100:235–244, 1998.

214. Schabel FM Jr: Concept for systemic treatment of micrometastasis. Cancer 35:15, 1975.

215. Silver RT, Young RC, Holland JF: Some new aspects of modern cancer chemotherapy. Am J Med 63:772, 1977.

216. Schabel FM Jr: The use of tumor growth kinetics in planning "curative" chemotherapy of advanced solid tumors. Cancer Res 29:2384, 1966.

217. Skipper HE, Schabel FM Jr: Quantitative and cytokinetic studies in experimental tumor models. In Holland J, Frei E (eds.): Cancer Medicine, pp. 629. Lea & Febiger, Philadelphia, 1973.

218. Ishibachi K: Studies on the number of cells necessary for the transplantation of Yoshida sarcoma. Gann 41:1, 1950.

219. Schabel FM Jr: Concept and practice of total tumor cell kill. In Clark RL et al. (eds): Oncology Proceedings of the Tenth International Cancer Congress, Vol. 2. Experimental Cancer Therapy, p. 35. Year Book Medical Publishers, Chicago, 1970.

220. Baserga R: The cell cycle. N Engl J Med 304:453, 1981.

221. Brent TP, Butler JAV, Crathorn AR: Variations in phosphokinase activities during the cell cycle in synchronous populations of HeLa cells. Nature 207:176, 1965.

222. Spadari S, Weissbach A: The interrelationship between DNA synthesis and various DNA polymerase activities in synchronized HeLa cells. J Mol Biol 86:11, 1974.

223. Johnson LF, Fuhrman CL, Wiedmemann LM: Regulation of dihydrofolate reductase gene expression in mouse fibroblasts during the transition from the resting to growing state. J Cell Physiol 97:397, 1978.

224. Larson A: Ribonucleotide reductase from regenerating rat liver. Eur J Biochem 11:113, 1969.

225. Freireich E, Gehan E, Frei E III et al: Effects of mercaptopurine (6-MP) on duration of steroid induced remission. Blood 21:699, 1963.

226. Aur RJA, Simone JV, Hustu HO et al: Central nervous system therapy and combination chemotherapy in childhood lymphocytic leukemia. Blood 37:236, 1971.

227. Aur RJA, Verzosa MS, Hustu HO et al: Response to combination therapy after relapse in childhood acute lymphocytic leukemia. Cancer 30:334, 1972.

228. Aur RJA, Simone JV, Hustu HO et al: Central nervous system therapy and combination chemotherapy in childhood lymphocytic leukemia. Blood 37:272, 1971.

229. Hyman CB, Bogle JM, Brubaker CA et al: Central nervous system involvement by leukemia in children, II. Therapy with intrathecal methotrexate. Blood 25:13, 1965.

230. Jones B, Holland JF, Glidewell O et al: Optimal use of L-asparaginase (NSC-1009229) in acute lymphocytic leukemia. Med Pediatr Oncol 3:387, 1977.

231. Ortega JA, Nesbit ME, Donaldson MH et al: L-asparaginase, vincristine and prednisone for induction of first remission in acute lymphocytic leukemia. Cancer Res 37:535, 1977.

232. Clavell LA, Gelber RD, Cohen HJ et al: Four agent induction and intensive asparaginase therapy for treatment of childhood acute lymphoblastic leukemia. N Engl J Med 315:657, 1986.

233. Haghbin M: Chemotherapy of acute lymphoblastic leukemia in children. Am J Hematol 1:201, 1976.

234. Riehm H, Gadner H, Henze G et al: Acute lymphoblastic leukemia: Treatment results in three BFM studies (1970–1981). In Murphy SB, Gilbert J (eds): Leukemia Research: Advances in Cell Biology and Treatment, p. 252. Elsevier North Holland, New York, 1983.

235. Riehm H, Gadner H, Henze G et al: The Berlin childhood acute lymphoblastic leukemia therapy study, 1970–1976. Am J Pediatr Hematol Oncol 2:4, 1980.

236. Sallan SE, Camitta BM, Cassady JR et al: Intermittent combination chemotherapy with Adriamycin for childhood acute lymphoblastic leukemia. Clinical results. Blood 51:425, 1978.

237. Steinherz PG, Gaynon P, Miller DR et al: Improved disease-free survival of children with acute lymphoblastic leukemia at high risk for early relapse with the New York regimen–a new intensive therapy protocol: A report from the Childrens Cancer Study Group. Journal of Clinical Oncology 4:744, 1986.

238. Bowman WP: Childhood acute lymphocytic leukemia: Progress and problems in treatment. Can Med Assoc J 124:129, 1981.

239. Freeman AI, Weinberg V, Brecher ML et al: Comparison of intensification treatments: Intermediate dose methotrexate (IDM) with cranial radiation (CRT) for the treatment of acute lymphocytic leukemia in children: A report for Cancer and Leukemia Group. N Engl J Med 308:477, 1983.

240. Reaman GH, Ladisch S, Echelberger C, Poplack DG: Improved treatment results in the management of single and multiple relapses of acute lymphoblastic leukemia. Cancer 45:3090, 1980.

241. Gaynon PS, Bleyer WA, Steinherz PG: Modified BFM therapy for children with previously untreated acute lymphoblastic leukemia and unfavorable prognostic features: Report of the Childrens Cancer Study Group study CCG-193P. Am J Pediatr Hematol Oncol 10:42, 1988.

242. Pinkerton CR, Bowman A, Hotzel H, Chessells JM: Intensive consolidation chemotherapy for acute lymphoblastic leukaemia (UKALL X pilot study). Arch Dis Child 62:12, 1987.

243. Schorin MA, Blattner S, Gelber RD et al: Treatment of childhood acute lymphoblastic leukemia: Results of Dana-Farber Cancer Institute/Children's Hospital acute lymphoblastic leukemia consortium protocol 85-01. J Clin Oncol 12:740, 1994.

244. Rizzari C, Valsecchi MG, Aricò M et al: Effect of protracted high-dose L-asparaginase given as a second exposure in a Berlin-Frankfurt-Münster-based treatment: Results of the randomized 9102 intermediate-risk childhood acute lymphoblastic leukemia study – a report from the Associazione Italiana Ematologia Oncologia Pediatrica. J Clin Oncol 19:1297–1303, 2001.

245. Land VJ, Shuster JJ, Crist WM et al: Comparison of two schedules of intermediate-dose methotrexate and cytarabine consolidation therapy for childhood B-precursor cell acute lymphoblastic leukemia: A Pediatric Oncology Group study. J Clin Oncol 12:1939, 1994.

246. Harris MB, Shuster JJ, Pullen DJ et al: Consolidation therapy with antimetabolite-based therapy in standard-risk acute lymphocytic leukemia of childhood: A Pediatric Oncology Group study. J Clin Oncol 16:2840–2847, 1998.

247. Evans AE, D'Angio GJ, Mitus A: Central nervous system complications of children with acute leukemia: An evaluation of treatment methods. J Pediatr 65:94, 1964.

248. Evans AE, Gilbert ES, Zandstra A: The increasing incidence of central nervous system leukemia in children (Children's Cancer Study Group A). Cancer 26:404, 1970.

249. Aur RJA, Simone JV, Hustu HO et al: A comparative study of central nervous system irradiation and intensive chemotherapy early in remission of childhood acute lymphocytic leukemia. Cancer 29:381, 1972.

250. Aur RJA, Hustu HO, Verzosa MS et al: Comparison of two methods of preventing central nervous system leukemia. Blood 42:349, 1973.

251. Aur RJA, Simone JV, Hustu HO et al: Multiple combination therapy for childhood acute lymphocytic leukemia (abstr). Blood 52:238, 1978.

252. Crist W, Boyett L, Frankel R et al: Extended triple intrathecal chemotherapy (TIC) is highly effective and superior to brief TIC and intermediated dose MTX as CNS prophlylaxis in non-T, non-B ALL: A Pediatric Oncology Group study. Med Pediatr Oncol 16:387, 1988.

253. Holland JF, Glidewell OJ: Oncologist reply. Survival expectancy in acute lymphocytic leukemia. N Engl J Med 287:769, 1972.

254. Pinkel D, Woo S: Prevention and treatment of meningeal leukemia in children. Blood 84:355, 1994.

255. Inati A, Sallan SE, Cassady JR et al: Efficacy and morbidity of central system "prophylaxis" in childhood acute lymphoblastic leukemia: Eight years experience with cranial irradiation and intrathecal methotrexate. Blood 61:297, 1983.

256. Komp DM, Fernandez CH, Falletta JM et al: CNS prophylaxis in acute lymphoblastic leukemia. Comparison of two methods. A Southwest Oncology Group study. Cancer 50:1031, 1982.

257. Sullivan MP, Chen T, Dyment PG et al: Equivalence of intrathecal chemotherapy and radiotherapy as central nervous system prophylaxis in children with acute lymphatic leukemia: a Pediatric Oncology Group study. Blood 60:948, 1982.

258. Bleyer WA, Coccia PF, Sather HN et al: Reduction in central nervous system leukemia with a pharmacokinetically derived intrathecal methotrexate dosage regimen. J Clin Oncol 1:317, 1983.

259. Nesbit M, Robinson LL, Littman PH et al: Presymptomatic central nervous system therapy in previously untreated childhood acute lymphoblastic leukemia: Comparison of 1800 rad and 2400 rad. A report for Children's Cancer Study Group. Lancet 1:461, 1981.

260. Poplack DG, Reaman GH, Bleyer WA et al: Central nervous system preventive therapy with high-dose methotrexate in acute lymphoblastic leukemia: A preliminary report (abstr.). Proc Am Soc Clin Oncol 3:204, 1984.

261. Reaman GH, Sposto R, Sensel MG et al: Treatment outcome and prognostic factors for infants with acute lymphoblastic leukemia treated on two consecutive trials of the Children's Cancer Group. J Clin Oncol 17:445–455, 1999.

262. Nachman J, Sather HN, Cherlow JM et al: Response of children with high-risk acute lymphoblastic leukemia treated with and without cranial irradiation: A report from the Children's Cancer Group. J Clin Oncol 16:920–930, 1998.

263. Pui C-H, Mahmoud HH, Rivera GK et al: Early intensification of intrathecal chemotherapy virtually eliminates central nervous system relapse in children with acute lymphoblastic leukemia. Blood 92:411–415, 1998.

264. Freireich E, Gehan E, Frei E III et al: Effects of mercaptopurine (6-MP) on duration of steroid induced remission. Blood 21:699, 1963.

265. Camitta B, Leventhal B, Lauer S et al: Intermediate-dose intravenous methotrexate and mercaptopurine therapy for non-T, non-B acute lymphocytic leukemia of childhood: A Pediatric Oncology Group study. J Clin Oncol 7:1539, 1989.

266. Pinkerton CR, Bowman A, Hotzel H, Chessells JM: Intensive consolidation chemotherapy for acute lymphoblastic leukaemia (UKALL X pilot study). Arch Dis Child 62:12, 1987.

267. Krivit W, Gilchrist G, Beatty EC: The need for chemotherapy after prolonged complete remission in acute leukemia of childhood. J Pediatr 76:138, 1970.

268. Frei E III, Sallan SE: Acute lymphoblastic leukemia: Treatment. Cancer 42:828, 1978.

269. Land VJ, Thomas PRM, Boyett JM et al: Comparison of maintenance treatment regimens for first central nervous system relapse in children with acute lymphoblastic leukemia: A Pediatric Oncology Group study. Cancer 56:81, 1985.

270. Riehm H, Gadner H, Henze G et al: Results and significances of 6 randomized trials in 4 consecutive ALL-BFM studies. Hamatol Bluttransfusion 33:439, 1990.

271. Norton L, Simon RL: Tumor size, sensitivity to therapy and design of treatment schedules. Cancer Treat Rep 61:1307, 1977.

272. Rivera GK, Pinkel D, Simone JV et al: Treatment of acute lymphoblastic leukemia: 30 years' experience at St. Jude Children's Research Hospital. N Engl J Med 329:1290, 1993.

273. Schorin MA, Blattner S, Gelber RD et al: Treatment of childhood acute lymphoblastic leukemia: Results of Dana-Farber Cancer Institute/Children's Hospital acute lymphoblastic leukemia consortium protocol 85–01. J Clin Oncol 12:740, 1994.

274. Reiter A, Schrappe M, Ludwig WD et al: Chemotherapy in 998 unselected childhood acute lymphoblastic leukemia patients. Results and conclusions of the multicenter trial ALL-BFM 86. Blood 84:3122, 1994.

275. Chessells JM, Bailey C, Richards SM: Intensification of treatment and survival in all children with lymphoblastic leukaemia: Results of UK Medical Research Council trial UKALL X. Lancet 345:143–148, 1995.

276. Lauer SJ, Camitta BM, Leventhal BG et al: Intensive alternating drug pairs after remission induction for treatment of infants with acute lymphoblastic leukemia: A Pediatric Oncology Group pilot study. J Pediatr Hematol Oncol 20:229–233, 1998.

277. Pieters R, Kaspers GJL, Klumper E, Veerman AJP: Clinical relevance of in vitro drug resistance testing in childhood acute lymphoblastic leukemia: The state of the art. Med Pediatr Oncol 22:299–308, 1994.

278. Schwartz CL, Thompson EB, Gelber RD et al: Improved response with higher corticosteroid dose in children with acute lymphoblastic leukemia. J Clin Oncol 19:1040–1046, 2001.

279. Schmiegelow K, Glomstein A, Kristinsson J et al: Impact of morning versus evening schedule for oral methotrexate and 6-mercaptopurine on relapse risk for children with acute lymphoblastic leukemia. J Pediatr Hematol Oncol 19:102–109, 1997.

280. Kamen BA, Holcenberg JS, Turo K, Whitehead M: Methotrexate and folate content of erythrocytes in patients receiving oral vs intramuscular therapy with methotrexate. J Pediatr 104:131, 1984.

281. Camitta B, Mahoney D, Leventhal B et al: Intensive intravenous methotrexate and mercaptopurine treatment of higher-risk non-T, non-B acute lymphocytic leukemia: A Pediatric Oncology Group study. J Clin Oncol 12:1383, 1994.

282. Bostrom B, Gaynon PS, Sather S et al: Dexamethasone (DEX) decreases central nervous system (CNS) relapse and improved event-free survival (EFS) in lower risk acute lymphoblastic leukemia (ALL). Proc Am Soc Clin Oncol 17:527a, 1998.

283. Mahoney DH, Shuster J, Nitschke R et al: Intemediate-dose intravenous methotrexate with intravenous mercaptopurine is superior to repetitive low-dose oral methotrexate with intravenous mercaptopurine for children with lower-risk B-lineage acute lymphoblastic leukemia: A Pediatric Oncology Group phase III trial. J Clin Oncol 16:246–254, 1998.

284. Evans WE, Relling MV, Rodman JH et al: Conventional compared with individualized chemotherapy for childhood acute lymphoblastic leukemia. N Engl J Med 338:499–505, 1998.

285. Barredo JC, Synold TW, Laver J et al: Differences in constitutive and postmethotrexate folylpolyglutamate synthetase activity in B-lineage and T-lineage leukemia. Blood 84:564, 1994.

286. Jones B, Holland JF, Glidewell O et al: Optimal use of L-asparaginase (NSC-1009229) in acute lymphocytic leukemia. Med Pediatr Oncol 3:387, 1977.

287. Miller DR, Leiken S, Albo V et al: Three versus five years of maintenance therapy are equivalent in childhood acute lymphoblastic leukemia: A report from the Childrens Cancer Study Group. J Clin Oncol 7:316, 1989.

288. Nesbit M, Robinson L, Ortega J et al: A randomized study of the duration of chemotherapy for children with acute lymphoblastic leukemia. Blood 52(Suppl. I):266, 1978.

289. Nesbit M, Sather HN, Robinson LL et al: Randomized study of 3 versus 5 years of chemotherapy in childhood acute lymphoblastic leukemia. J Clin Oncol 1:308, 1983.

290. Reiter A: Therapy of B-cell acute lymphoblastic leukemia in childhood: The BFM experience. Baillieres Clin Haemat 7:321, 1994.

291. Patte C, Michon J, Frappaz D et al: Therapy of Burkitt and other B-cell acute lymphoblastic leukemia and lymphoma: Experience with the LMB protocols of the SFOP (French Paediatric Oncology Society) in children and adults. Baillieres Clin Haematol 7:339, 1994.

292. Marks DI, Bird JM, Cornish JM et al: Unrelated donor bone marrow transplantation for children and adolescents with Philadelphia-positive acute lymphoblastic leukemia. J Clin Oncol 16:931–936, 1998.

293. Aricò M, Valsecchi MG, Camitta B et al: Outcome of treatment in children with Philadelphia chromosome-positive acute lymphoblastic leukemia. N Engl J Med 342:998–1006, 2000.

294. Frei E III: In Pharmacology of Cancer, Achievements, Challenges and Prospects for the 1980's, p. 31. Grune & Stratton, New York, 1981.

295. Brockman RW: Resistance to therapeutic agents. In Burchenal JH, Oettgen H (eds): Cancer Achievements, Challenges and Prospects for the 1980's, Vol. 2, p. 55. Grune & Stratton, New York, 1981.

296. Skipper HE: Reasons for success and failure in treatment of murine leukemias with the drugs now employed in treating human leukemias. In Cancer Chemotherapy, Vol. 1. University Microfilms International, Ann Arbor, MI, 1978.

297. Miwa H, Kita K, Nishii K et al: Expression of MDRI gene in acute leukemia cells: Association with CD7 acute myeloblastic leukemia/acute lymphoblastic leukemia. Blood 82:3445, 1993.

298. Bertino JR: Toward improved selectivity in cancer chemotherapy. The Peshard and Hinda Rosenthal Foundation Award Lecture. Cancer Res 39:293, 1979.

299. Skipper HE: Concurrent comparisons of some 2-, 3-, and 4-drug combinations delivered simultaneously and sequentially (L1210 and P388 leukemia systems). In Cancer Chemotherapy. Vol. 9. University Microfilms International, Ann Arbor, MI, 1980.

300. Goldin A, Venditti J, Humphreys S et al: Modification of treatment schedules in the management of advanced mouse leukemia with amethopterin. J Natl Cancer Inst 17:203, 1956.

301. Dearth JC, Fountain KS, Smithson WA et al: Extreme leukemic leukocytosis (blast crisis) in childhood. Mayo Clin Proc 53:207, 1978.

302. Mauer HS, Steinherz PG, Gaynon PS et al: The effect of initial management of hyperleukocytosis on early complications and outcome of children with acute lymphoblastic leukemia J Clin Oncol 6:1425–1432, 1988.

303. Bunin NJ, Pui C-H: Differing complications of hyperleukocytosis in children with acute lymphoblastic or acute nonlymphoblastic leukemia. J Clin Oncol 3:1590, 1985.

304. Lichtman MA, Rowe JM: Hyperleukocytic leukemias: Rheological, clinical, and therapeutic considerations. Blood 60:279, 1982.

305. Mauer HS, Steinherz PG, Gaynon PS et al: The effect of initial management of hyperleukocytosis on early complications and outcome of children with acute lymphoblastic leukemia. J Clin Oncol 6:1425, 1988.

306. Albano EA, Pizzo PA: Infectious complications in childhood acute leukemia. Pediatr Clin North Am 35:873, 1988.

307. Ohno R, Tomonaga M, Kobayashi T et al: Effect of granulocyte colony-stimulating factor after intensive induction therapy in relapsed or refractory acute leukemia. N Engl J Med 323:871, 1990.

308. Pui C-H, Boyett JM, Hughes WT et al: Human granulocyte colony-stimulating factor after induction chemotherapy in children with acute lymphoblastic leukemia. N Engl J Med 336:1781–1787, 1997.

309. Weaver CH, Buckner CD, Longin K et al: Syngeneic transplantation with peripheral blood mononuclear cells collected after the administration of recombinant human granulocyte colony-stimulating factor. Blood 82:1981, 1993.

310. Hughes WT, McNabb PC, Makres TD, Feldman S: Efficacy of trimethoprim and sulfamethoxazole in the prevention and treatment of *Pneumocystis carinii* pneumonitis. Antimicrob Agents Chemother 5:289, 1974.

311. Masur H: Prevention and treatment of pneumocystis pneumonia. N Engl J Med 327:1853, 1992.

312. Strauss AJ, Su JT, Dalton VMK et al: Bony morbidity in children treated for acute lymphoblastic leukemia. J Clin Oncol 19:3066–3072, 2001.

313. Muttano LA Jr, Sather HN, Trigg ME et al: Osteonecrosis during the treatment of childhood acute lymphoblastic leukemia: A prospective MRI study. J Clin Oncol 18:3262–3272, 2000.

314. Ojala AE, Paakko E, Lanning P, Lanning M: Osteonecrosis during treatment of childhood acute lymphoblastic leukemia: A prospective MRI study. Med Pediatr Oncol 32:11–17, 1999.

315. George S, Aur RJA, Mauer AM et al: A reappraisal of the results of stopping therapy in childhood leukemia. N Engl J Med 300:269, 1979.

316. Johansen OJ, Moe PJ: Relapse rate after cessation of therapy in childhood leukemia. A follow-up report on 277 cases from the five Nordic countries. Acta Paediatr Scand 69:663, 1980.

317. Land VJ, Askin AH, Ragab A et al: Late overt or occult testicular leukemia–incidence and prognosis (abstr.). Proc Am Soc Clin Oncol 20:378, 1979.

318. Schweinle JE, Alperin JB: Central nervous system recurrence ten years after remission of acute lymphoblastic leukemia. Cancer 45:16–18, 1980.

319. Baum E, Sather H, Nachman J et al: Relapse rates following cessation of chemotherapy during complete remission of acute lymphocytic leukemia. Med Pediatr Oncol 7:25, 1976.

320. Rivera G, Aur RJA, Dahl GV et al: Second cessation of therapy in childhood lymphocytic leukemia. Blood 53:1114, 1979.

321. Gaynon PS, Qu RP, Chappell RJ et al: Survival after relapse in childhood acute lymphoblastic leukemia. Impact of site and time to first relapse – the Children's Cancer Group experience. Cancer 82:1387–1395, 1998.

322. Uderzo C, Valsecchi MG, Bacigalupo A et al: Treatment of childhood acute lymphoblastic leukemia in second remission with allogeneic bone marrow transplantation and chemotherapy: Ten-year experience of the Italian Bone Marrow Transplantation Group and the Italian Pediatric Hematology Oncology Association. J Clin Oncol 13:352–358, 1995.

323. Miniero R, Saracco P, Pastore G et al: Relapse after first cessation of therapy in childhood acute lymphoblastic leukemia: A 10-year follow-up study. Med Pediatr Oncol 24:71–76, 1995.

324. Butturini A, Bortin MM, Rivera GK, Gale RP: Which treatment for childhood acute lymphoblastic leukemia in second remission? Lancet 1:429, 1987.

325. Kersey JH, Weisdorf D, Nesbit ME et al: Comparison of autologous and allogeneic bone marrow transplantation for treatment of high-risk refractory acute lymphoblastic leukemia. N Engl J Med 317:461, 1987.

326. Thomas ED, Sanders JE, Flournoy N et al: Marrow transplantation for patients with acute lymphoblastic leukemia in remission. Blood 54:468, 1979.

327. Boulad F, Steinherz P, Reyes B et al: Allogeneic bone marrow transplantation versus chemotherapy for the treatment of childhood acute lymphoblastic leukemia in second remission: A single-institution study. J Clin Oncol 17:197, 1999.

328. Woods WG, Nesbit ME, Ramsay NK et al: Intensive therapy followed by bone marrow transplantation for patients with acute lymphocytic leukemia in second or subsequent remission: Determination of prognostic factors. Blood 61:1182, 1983.

329. Sutow WW, Garcia F, Starling KA et al: L-Asparaginase in children with advanced leukemia. Cancer 28:819, 1971.

330. Kung FH, Nyhan WL, Cuttner J et al: Vincristine, prednisone and L-asparaginase in the induction of remission in children with acute lymphoblastic leukemia following relapse. Cancer 41:428, 1978.

331. Reaman GH, Ladisch S, Echelberger C, Poplack DG: Improved treatment results in the management of single and multiple relapses of acute lymphoblastic leukemia. Cancer 45:3090, 1980.

332. Rivera G, Buchanan G, Boyett JM et al: Intensive retreatment of childhood acute lymphoblastic leukemia in first bone marrow relapse. N Engl J Med 315:273, 1986.

333. Kearney PJ, Baumer JH, Howlett BC: Marrow relapse on maintenance chemotherapy in childhood acute lymphoblastic leukemia. Br J Cancer 40:890, 1979.

334. Chessells JM, Cornbleet M: Combination chemotherapy for bone marrow relapse in childhood lymphoblastic leukemia (ALL). Med Pediatr Oncol 6:359, 1979.

335. Rivera G, Murphy SB, Aur RJA et al: Recurrent childhood lymphocytic leukemia. Clinical and cytokinetic studies of cytosine arabinoside and methotrexate for maintenance of second hematologic remission. Cancer 42:2521, 1978.

336. Baum E, Nachman J, Ramsay N et al: Prolonged second remissions in childhood acute lymphocytic leukemia: A report from the Childrens Cancer Study Group. Med Pediatr Oncol 11:1, 1983.

337. Capizzi RL, Poole M, Cooper MR et al: Treatment of poor risk acute leukemia with sequential high-dose ARA-C and asparaginase. Blood 63:694, 1984.

338. Bührer C, Hartmana R, Fengler R et al: Importance of effective central nervous system therapy in isolated bone marrow relapse of childhood lymphoblastic leukemia. Blood 83:3468, 1994.

339. Henze G, Rüdiger F, Hartman R et al: Six-year experience with a comprehensive approach to the treatment of recurrent childhood acute lymphoblastic leukemia (ALL-REZ BFM 85). A relapse study of the BFM group. Blood 78:1166, 1991.

340. Rivera G, George SL, Bowman WP et al: Second central nervous system prophylaxis in children with acute lymphoblastic leukemia who relapse after elective cessation of therapy. J Clin Oncol 1:471, 1983.

341. Reiselbach RE, Morse EE, Rall DP et al: Intrathecal aminopterin therapy of meningeal leukemia. Arch Intern Med 1211:620, 1963.

342. Haghbin M, Zuelzer WW: A long-term study of cerebrospinal leukemia. J Pediatr 67:23, 1965.

343. Hustu HO, Aur RJA, Verzosa MS et al: Prevention of central nervous system leukemia by irradiation. Cancer 32:585, 1973.

344. Shaw RK, Moore EW, Freireich EJ et al: Meningeal leukemia: A syndrome resulting from increased intracranial pressure in patients with acute leukemia. Neurology 10:823, 1960.

345. Whiteside JA, Philips FS, Dargeon HW et al: Intrathecal aminopterin in neurological manifestations of leukemia. Arch Intern Med 101:279, 1958.

346. Sullivan MP, Moon TE, Trueworthy R et al: Combination intrathecal therapy for meningeal leukemia: Two vs three drugs. Blood 50:471, 1977.

347. Wells RJ, Weetman RM, Baehner RL: The impact of isolated central nervous system relapse following initial complete remission in childhood acute lymphoblastic leukemia. J Pediatr 97:429, 1980.

348. Willoughby MLN: Treatment of overt meningeal leukemia in children: Results of second MRC meningeal leukemia trial. BMJ 1:864, 1976.

349. Land VJ, Thomas PRM, Boyett JM et al: Comparison of maintenance treatment regimens for first central nervous system relapse in children with acute lymphoblastic leukemia: A Pediatric Oncology Group study. Cancer 56:81, 1985.

350. Frankel LD, Hockenberry MJ, Johnston DA: The curative potential of central nervous system (CNS) relapse in childhood acute lymphocytic leukemia (ALL) (abstr.) Proc Am Soc Clin Oncol 1:124, 1982.

351. Ribeiro RC, Rivera GK, Hudson M et al: An intensive re-treatment protocol for children with an isolated CNS relapse of acute lymphoblastic leukemia. J Clin Oncol 13:333–338, 1995.

352. Ritchey AK, Pollock BH, Lauer SJ et al: Improved survival of children with isolated CNS relapse of acute lymphoblastic leukemia: A Pediatric Oncology Group study. J Clin Oncol 17:3745–3752, 1999.

353. Eiser C, Lansdown R: Retrospective study of intellectual development in children treated for acute lymphoblastic leukemia. Arch Dis Child 52:525, 1977.

354. Eden OB, Innes EM: Testicular infiltration in acute lymphoblastic leukemia. Arch Dis Child 53:841, 1978.

355. Hudson MM, Frankel LS, Mullins J et al: Diagnostic value of surgical testicular biopsy after therapy for acute lymphocytic leukemia. J Pediatr 107:50, 1985.

356. Pui C-H, Bowman WP, Abramowich M et al: Elective testicular biopsy during chemotherapy for childhood leukaemia is of no clinical value. Lancet 2:410, 1985.

357. Tiedemann K, Chessells JM, Sandland RM: Isolated testicular relapse in boys with acute lymphoblastic leukemia: Treatment and outcome. BMJ 285:1614, 1982.

358. Freeman AI, Weinberg V, Brecher ML et al: Comparison of intensification treatments: Intermediate dose methotrexate (IDM) with cranial radiation (CRT) for the treatment of acute lymphocytic leukemia in children: A report for Cancer and Leukemia Group. N Engl J Med 308:477, 1983.

359. Nachman J, Palmer NF, Sather HN et al: Open-wedge testicular biopsy in childhood acute lymphoblastic leukemia after two years of maintenance therapy: Diagnostic accuracy and influence on outcome – a report from Children's Cancer Study Group. Blood 75:1051, 1990.

360. Bowman WP, Aur RJ, Hustu HO, Rivera G: Isolated testicular relapse in acute lymphocytic leukemia of childhood: Categories and influence on survival. J Clin Oncol 2:924, 1984.

361. Baum E, Nesbit M Jr, Tilford D et al: Extent of disease in pediatric patients with acute lymphocytic leukemia experiencing isolated testicular relapse (abstr.). Proc Am Soc Clin Oncol 20:435, 1979.

362. Askin FB, Land VJ, Sullivan MP et al: Occult testicular leukemia: Testicular biopsy at three years continuous complete remission of childhood leukemia. A Southwest Oncology Group study. Cancer 47:470, 1981.

363. Jacobson IO: Evidence for a humoral factor (or factors) concerned in recovery from radiation injury. A review. Cancer Res 12:315, 1952.

364. Lorenz F, Uphoff D, Reid TR et al: Modification of irradiation injury in mice and guinea pigs by bone marrow injections. J Natl Cancer Inst 12:197, 1951.

365. Thomas ED, Storb R, Clift RA et al: Bone marrow transplantation. N Engl J Med 292:832, 1975.

366. Thomas ED: The use and potential of bone marrow allograft and whole-body irradiation in the treatment of leukemia. Cancer 50:1449, 1982.

367. Thomas ED, Sanders JE, Flournoy N et al: Marrow transplantation for patients with acute lymphoblastic leukemia in remission. Blood 54:468, 1979.

368. Johnson FL, Thomas ED, Clark BS et al: A comparison of marrow transplantation with chemotherapy for children with acute lymphoblastic leukemia in second or subsequent remission. N Engl J Med 305:846, 1981.

369. Barrett AJ, Horowitz MM, Pollock BH et al: Bone marrow transplants from HLA identical siblings as compared with chemotherapy for children with acute lymphoblastic leukemia in second remission. N Engl J Med 331:1253, 1994.

370. Uderzo C, Dini G, Locatelli F et al: Treatment of childhood acute lymphoblastic leukemia after the first relapse: Curative strategies. Haematologica 85:47–53s, 2000.

371. Wheeler K, Richards S, Chessells JM: Comparison of bone marrow transplant and chemotherapy for relapsed childhood acute lymphocytic leukemia – the MRC UKALL X experience. Br J Haematol 101:94, 1988.

372. Sullivan KM, Shulman HM, Storb R et al: Chronic graft-versus-host disease in 52 patients. Adverse natural course and successful treatment with combination immunosuppression. Blood 57:267, 1981.

373. Obetz SW, Smithson WA, Groover RV et al: Neuropsychologic follow-up study of children with acute lymphocytic leukemia. A preliminary report. Am J Pediatr Hematol Oncol 1(3):94, 1980.

374. Soni SS, Marten GW, Pitner SE et al: Effects of central nervous system irradiation on neuropsychologic functioning of children with acute lymphocytic leukemia. N Engl J Med 293:113, 1975.

375. Barr RD, Furlong W, Dawson S et al: An assessment of global health status in survivors of acute lymphoblastic leukemia in childhood. J Pediatr Hematol Oncol 15:284, 1993.

376. Eiser C: Effects of chronic illness on intellectual development: A comparison of normal children with those treated for childhood leukaemia and solid tumors. Arch Dis Child 55:766, 1980.

377. Gluch RA, Baron IS, Brailler DR et al: Follow-up of central nervous system (CNS) prophylaxis in acute lymphocytic leukemia (ALL) (abstr.). Pediatr Res 14:534, 1980.

378. Meadows AT, Massari DJ, Fergusson J et al: Declines in IQ scores and cognitive dysfunctions in children with acute lymphoblastic leukemia treated with cranial irradiation. Lancet 2:1015, 1981.

379. Moss HA, Nannis ED, Poplack DG: The effects of prophylactic treatment of the central nervous system on the intellectual functioning of children with acute lymphocytic leukemia. Am J Med 71:47, 1981.

380. Pavlovsky S, Fishman N, Arizaga R et al: Neuropsychological study in patients with ALL. Am J Pediatr Hematol Oncol 5:79, 1983.

381. Rowland J, Glidwell O, Sibley JR et al., for Cancer and Leukemia Group B: Effect of cranial radiation (CRT) on neuropsychologic function in children with acute lymphocytic leukemia (ALL). (abstr.). Proc Am Soc Clin Oncol 1:123, 1982.

382. Moss HA, Nannis ED, Poplack DG: The effects of prophylactic treatment of the central nervous system on the intellectual functioning of children with acute lymphocytic leukemia. Am J Med 71:47, 1981.

383. Kato M, Azuma E, Ido M et al: Ten-year survey of the intellectual deficits in children with acute lymphoblastic leukemia receiving chemoimmunotherapy. Med Pediatr Oncol 21:435–440, 1993.

384. Longeway K, Mulhern R, Crisco J et al: Treatment of meningeal relapse in childhood acute lymphoblastic leukemia: II. A prospective study of intellectual loss specific to CNS relapse and therapy. Am J Pediatr Hematol Oncol 12:45–50, 1990.

385. Peylan-Ramu N, Poplack DG, Pizzo PA et al: Abnormal computed tomography (CT) scans in children with acute lymphocytic leukemia (ALL) following CNS prophylaxis. N Engl J Med 298:815, 1978.

386. Brouwers P, Riccardi R, Fedio P, Poplack DG: Long-term neuropsychologic sequelae of childhood leukemia: Correlation with CT brain scan abnormalities. J Pediatr 106:723, 1985.

387. Riccardi R, Brouwers P, Chiro G, Poplack DG: Abnormal computed tomography brain scans in children with acute lymphoblastic leukemia: Serial long-term follow-up. J Clin Oncol 3:12, 1985.

388. Brouwers P, Poplack D: Memory and learning sequelae in long-term survivors of acute lymphoblastic leukemia: Association with attention deficits. Am J Pediatr Hematol Oncol 12:174, 1990.

389. Pavlovsky S, Fishman N, Arizaga R et al: Neuropsychological study in patients with ALL. Am J Pediatr Hematol Oncol 5:79, 1983.

390. Ochs J, Mulhern R, Fariclough D et al: Comparison of neuropsychologic functioning and clinical indicators of neurotoxicity in long-term survivors of childhood leukemia given cranial radiation or parenteral methotreaxate: A prospective study. J Clin Oncol 9:145, 1991.

391. Mulhern RK, Fairclough D, Ochs J: A prospective comparison of neuropsychologic performance of children surviving leukemia

who received 18-Gy, 24-Gy, or no cranial irradiation. J Clin Oncol 9:1348, 1991.

392. Mulhern RK, Wasserman AL, Fairclough D, Ochs J: Memory function in disease-free survivors of childhood acute lymphocytic leukemia given CNS prophylaxis with or without 1800 cGy cranial irradiation. J Clin Oncol 6:315, 1988.

393. Waber DP, Tarbell NJ, Kahn CM et al: The relationship of sex and treatment modality to neuropsychologic outcome in childhood acute lymphoblastic leukemia. J Clin Oncol 10:810, 1992.

394. Mulhern RK, Kovar E, Langston J et al: Long-term survivors of leukemia treated in infancy: Factors associated with neuropsychologic status. J Clin Oncol 10:1095, 1992.

395. Kaleita TA, Reaman GH, MacLean WE et al: Neurodevelopmental outcome of infants with acute lymphoblastic leukemia. A Children's Cancer Group report. Cancer 85:1859–1865, 1999.

396. Griffin NK, Wadsworth J: Effect of treatment of malignant disease on growth in children. Arch Dis Child 55:600, 1980.

397. Voorhess ML, Brecher ML, MacGillivray MH et al: Effect of different forms of central nervous system (CNS) prophylaxis on pituitary function of children with acute lymphocytic leukemia (ALL). Proc Am Soc Clin Oncol 22:397, 1981.

398. Blatt J, Bercu BB, Gillin C et al: Reduced pulsatile growth hormone secretion in children after therapy for acute lymphoblastic leukemia. J Pediatr 104:182, 1984.

399. Costin G: Effects of low-dose cranial radiation on growth hormone secretory dynamics and hypothalamic-pituitary function. Am J Dis Child 142:847, 1988.

400. Dacou-Voutetakis C, Kitra V, Grafakos S et al: Auxologic data and hormonal profile in long-term survivors of childhood acute lymphoid leukemia. Am J Pediatr Hematol Oncol 15:277, 1993.

401. Halton JM, Atkinson SA, Barr RD: Growth and body composition in response to chemotherapy in children with acute lymphoblastic leukemia. Int J Cancer Supplement 11:81–84, 1998.

402. Talvensaari KK, Knip M, Lanning P, Lanning M: Clinical characteristics and factors affecting growth in long-term survivors of cancer. Med Pediatr Oncol 26:166–172, 1996.

403. Nysom K, Holm K, Michaelsen KF et al: Bone mass after treatment for acute lymphoblastic leukemia in childhood. J Clin Oncol 16:3752–3760, 1998.

404. Pui C-H, Dodge RK, Look AT et al: Risk of adverse events in children completing treatment for acute lymphoblastic leukemia: St. Jude total therapy studies VIII, IX, and X. J Clin Oncol 9:1341, 1991.

405. Lipshultz SE, Colan SD, Gelber RD et al: Late cardiac effects of doxorubicin therapy for acute lymphoblastic leukemia in childhood. N Engl J Med 324:808, 1991.

406. Turner-Gomes SO, Lands LC, Halton J et al: Cardiorespiratory status after treatment for acute lymphoblastic leukemia. Med Pediatr Oncol 26:160–165, 1996.

407. Fulgoni P, Zoia MC, Corsico A et al: Lung function in survivors of childhood acute lymphoblastic leukemia. Chest 116:1163–1167, 1999.

408. Hoover R, Fraumeni JF Jr: Drug-induced cancer. Cancer 47:1071, 1981.

409. Sklar CA, Robison LL, Nesbit ME et al: Effects of radiation on testicular function in long-term survivors of childhood acute lymphoblastic leukemia: A report from the Childrens Cancer Study Group. J Clin Oncol 8:1981, 1990.

410. Wallace WHB, Shalet SM, Tetlow LJ, Morris-Jones PH: Ovarian function following the treatment of childhood acute lymphoblastic leukaemia. Med Pediatr Oncol 21:333–339, 1993.

411. Sandoval C, Pui C-H, Bowman LC et al: Secondary acute myeloid leukemia in children previously treated with alkylating agents,

intercalating topoisomerase II inhibitors, and irradiation. J Clin Oncol 11:1039, 1993.

412. Relling MV, Rubnitz JE, Rivera GK et al: High incidence of secondary brain tumours after radiotherapy and antimetabolites. Lancet 354:34–39, 1999.

413. Walter AW, Hancock ML, Pui C-H et al: Secondary brain tumors in children treated for acute lymphoblastic leukemia at St. Jude Children's Research Hospital. J Clin Oncol 16:3761–3767, 1998.

414. Dalton VMK, Gelber RD, Li F et al: Second malignancies in patients treated for childhood acute lymphoblastic leukemia. J Clin Oncol 16:2848–2853, 1998.

415. Mertens AC, Yasui Y, Neglia JP et al: Late mortality experience in five-year survivors of childhood and adolescent cancer: The Childhood Cancer Survivor study. J Clin Oncol 19:3163–3172, 2001.

416. Möller TR, Garwicz S, Barlow L et al: Decreasing late mortality among five-year survivors of cancer in childhood and adolescence: A population-based study in the Nordic countries. J Clin Oncol 19:3173–3181, 2001.

417. Sankila R, Olsen JH, Anderson H: Risk of cancer among offspring of childhood-cancer survivors. N Engl J Med 338:1339–1344, 1998.

418. Kenney LB, Nicholson HS, Brasseux CY et al: Birth defects in offspring of adult survivors of childhood acute lymphoblastic leukemia: A Children's Cancer Group/National Institutes of Health report. Cancer 78:169–176, 1996.

18

Diagnosis and Treatment of Adult Acute Lymphoblastic Leukemia

Dieter Hoelzer and Nicola Gökbuget

Acute lymphoblastic leukemia (ALL) is the most frequent neoplastic disease in childhood and accounts for about 20 percent of the acute leukemias in adults. An early peak of ALL incidence occurs at the age of 4 to 5 years. About one-quarter of patients with ALL are aged 15 years or more. It is relatively infrequent in younger adults but the incidence seems to increase in adults aged over 50.[115] The median age of patients in most adult ALL studies ranges from 25 to 39 years.

In the past decades substantial progress has been made in the treatment of ALL mainly based on intensive chemotherapy regimens and improved supportive care. With contemporary regimens complete remission (CR) rates of 80 percent and cure rates of 30 to 40 percent can be achieved.[121] This applies particularly for the formerly poor prognostic subgroups of T-ALL and mature B-ALL with cure rates greater than 50 percent in contemporary trials. The results in children are even more impressive; CR rates approach 95 percent and long-term leukemia free survival (LFS) is about 70 percent.[198,221]

The differences in terms of LFS rates between children and adults have several reasons. Overall outcome in ALL decreases continuously with increasing age. The incidence of poor prognostic subgroups such as Ph/BCR-ABL positive ALL (>40 percent in patients >50 years versus 3 percent in children), early T-ALL (6 percent in adults versus 1 percent in children), and pro B-ALL (11 vs. 1 percent) is significantly higher in older patients. In addition unfavorable drug pharmacokinetics (e.g., for methotrexate), higher incidence of drug resistance, and lower tolerance to chemotherapy have to be considered. Thus lower dose intensity can be applied in adults due to hematological and nonhematological toxicities.

Therefore options for further dose intensification are limited in adult ALL. Beside optimization of current chemotherapy regimens, stem cell transplantation (SCT) and supportive care new treatment options are urgently required. These include risk-adapted treatment regimens, individualized treatment based on evaluation of minimal residual disease (MRD), antibody treatment, and new molecular treatment approaches such as tyrosine kinase inhibitors.[121]

CLINICAL FEATURES

The clinical presentation of adult ALL is almost always acute and the patient usually has symptoms of only a few weeks' duration. Patients show a rapid decline in general condition and feel generally ill. In rare cases, ALL may also develop from a transient preceding pancytopenia.

Most of the symptoms of adult patients with ALL are nonspecific and are not usually severe. The patients may complain of progressive malaise with lethargy, fatigue, and occasionally weight loss. They may also complain of fever and night sweats in the absence of clinical infection. In older patients complications of anemia such as dyspnea, angina, and dizziness may dominate the clinical picture. Adult ALL patients may have minor arthralgias and bone pain but much less frequently than in children. One-third of the patients have infections or fever. As infections, hemorrhages are also less frequent than in acute myeloid leukemia (AML). There may be a history of some easy bruising and mucosal hemorrhage. In a series of 1273 consecutive ALL patients (15 to 65 years) treated in the German Multicenter Trials for Adult ALL (GMALL) one-third had some signs of minor bleeding tendency such as petechiae. Fever or infections had the same frequency. A few patients may present with neurological symptoms such as headache, alteration of mental function, or cranial nerve palsies due to leukemic infiltration.

An outline of the clinical approach to a patient with adult ALL is given in Table 18–1. Physical examination will show some degree of organomegaly in most adult patients with ALL: lymphadenopathy, usually cervical, is present in about half of the patients (57 percent) and palpable splenomegaly (56 percent) or hepatomegaly (47 percent) also in about half. A thymic mass can be found from chest roentgenograms or computer tomograms in 15 percent of all adult ALL patients. The majority of these patients have a T-cell ALL, but patients with other subtypes may occasionally also present with a mediastinal mass. Massive thymic enlargement can cause dyspnea, especially when associated with large pleural effusions. Some patients with mediastinal enlargement have pericardial effusions as well.

Presentation with clinically detectable signs related to leukemic infiltration of the central nervous system (CNS) occurs in about 5 to 10 percent of adult ALL patients (summarized in Ref. 103). Risk factors for CNS involvement include a high initial white blood cell (WBC) count, T-cell phenotype, and L3 or Burkitt morphology. CNS involvement may manifest as raised intercranial pressure with headache and papilledema without focal neurological signs or, rarely, as cranial nerve palsies, the sixth and seventh cranial nerves being most frequently involved. Careful examination of the ocular fundus must be made for leukemic infiltration as well as for hemorrhages due to thrombocytopenia.

Virtually any organ can be involved by infiltration of leukemic cells. The presence of bone lesions could be found in the above-mentioned ALL series in only 1.2 percent. Also the initial involvement of the testis was very rare (0.3 percent). Other leukemic infiltrations were observed in the retina (0.9 percent), skin (0.9 percent), tonsils (0.5 percent), lung (0.5 per-

Table 18–1. Adult ALL: Clinical Approach and Laboratory Investigation

Complete medical history, including
    Past medical history, especially heart, lung, liver or renal disease, and diabetes mellitus
    Family history
    Occupational history
Complete physical examination, with special attention to
    Lymphadenopathy and hepatosplenomegaly
    Temperature
    Potential sites of infection including lungs, oropharynx, and perineum
    Signs of abnormal hemorrhage
    Optic fundi
    Full neurological examination including the cranial and peripheral nerves
Diagnostic hematological studies
    Full blood examination including hemoglobin, platelet count, and white blood cell count (total and differential)
    Bone marrow aspirate and trephine biopsy
    Wright's stain and FAB
    Cytochemical stains
    Immunological markers: T-cell, B-cell, immunological subtypes
    Enzyme markers: TdT
    Cytogenetic analysis
    Molecular analysis, for diagnosis and follow-up of disease after therapy
Biochemical studies
    Including renal and hepatic function, serum uric acid, serum electrolytes including calcium and phosphate, blood glucose, and serum LDH
Coagulation studies
    Including prothrombin ratio, partial thromboplastin time, fibrinogen, and ATP III
Cardiac assessment
    Including electrocardiograph: echocardiogram and other noninvasive tests of myocardial function if indicated
Chest roentgenogram: PA and lateral
Computer tomograph, if mediastinal lymph nodes, tumor or abdominal masses are suspected
Serological studies
    ABO and Rh blood group
    HLA typing
Microbiological studies
    Culture from any infected site or lesion
    Surveillance cultures
    Serum for antibody titers, CMV, EBV, HIV, candida, aspergillosis
CSF examination
    Examination for cell count and cytocentrifuge preparation for morphology and, if necessary, immunophenotyping

Abbreviations: FAB, French-American-British; HLA, human leukocyte antigen; PA, posterior-anterior; TdT, terminal deoxynucleotidyl transferase; CMV, cytomegalovirus; EBV, Epstein-Barr virus; HIV, human immunodeficiency virus.

cent) and kidney (0.5 percent). These organ manifestations present a typical clinical pattern of non-Hodgkin's lymphoma (NHL). They occur more frequently in mature B-cell ALL (32 percent).

DIAGNOSTIC PROCEDURES

The diagnosis of ALL is made by examination of the peripheral blood and bone marrow. Other investigations also need to be performed to further categorize and subclassify the disease and in preparation for therapy. These include cytochemical stains, immunological markers, enzyme markers, cytogenetic analysis, and molecular genetic methods.

Peripheral Blood

Peripheral blood examination characteristically shows anemia, thrombocytopenia, and neutropenia (Table 18–2) although the total WBC count is variable. The reduction in the level of hemoglobin is mild to moderate, but nearly one-third of the patients have a hemoglobin level below 8 g/dl. Although clinical bleeding due to thrombocytopenia is not very common, about half of the patients have a platelet count below 50×10^9/L. The proportion (30 percent) of adult ALL patients having had some history of hemorrhage corresponds well with the 30 percent of patients with a platelet count below 25×10^9/L. The proportion of patients with a granulocyte count below 0.5×10^9/L, usually associated with high risk of infection, was only one-fifth in this series. Only a small minority of patients had clotting defects and of these 5 percent had an initially decreased fibrinogen level, which might be of relevance if an immediate L-asparaginase treatment is anticipated. The WBC count was reduced in 27 percent, normal or modestly elevated in 60 percent, and 16 percent had a marked leukocytosis (WBC count $>100 \times 10^9$/L) at presentation. However, even in the cases where the WBC count was reduced or normal, characteristic lymphoblasts could be identified on a well-stained blood smear in more than 90 percent (Table 18–2).

Bone Marrow

Bone marrow examination provides further material for diagnostic assessment including morphology, cytochemical stains, immunological markers, and cytogenetic and molecular analysis. Smears of the bone marrow aspirate show markedly hypercellular particles. The majority of cells present are leukemic lymphoblasts. A total of 97 percent of the adult ALL patients had a bone marrow infiltration with leukemic lymphoblasts above 50 percent (Table 18–2). The normal hematopoietic elements are greatly reduced or absent but, in contrast to AML, they have essentially normal morphology. The trephine biopsy of the bone marrow will further demonstrate marked hypercellularity with replacement of fat spaces and normal marrow elements by infiltration with leukemic cells. A slight increase in marrow reticulin is seen in a small proportion of patients with ALL but much less commonly than with AML. If an adequate bone marrow aspiration is available it remains open whether an additional biopsy should be done. In our hands a biopsy was necessary when aspiration was not possible due to heavily packed leukemic cells or increased reticulin fibers, which was the case in 16 percent of patients.

Table 18–2. Laboratory Findings at Diagnosis of Adult ALL in 1273 Patients

Laboratory Finding	Percent
Total leukocytes ($\times 10^9$/L)	
< 5	27
5–10	14
10–50	31
50–100	12
> 100	16
Granulocytes ($\times 10^9$/L)	
< 0.5	22
0.5–1.0	14
1.0–1.5	9
> 1.5	55
Hemoglobin (g/dL)	
< 6	8
6–8	20
8–10	26
10–12	24
> 12	22
Thrombocytes ($\times 10^9$/L)	
< 25	30
25–50	22
50–150	33
> 150	16
Fibrinogen (mg/dL)	
< 100	5
> 100	95
Leukemic blast cells in PB	
Present	92
Absent	8
Leukemic blast cells in BM	
< 50%	4
51–90%	25
> 90%	71

Data from unpublished GMALL studies.

Laboratory Investigations

The laboratory investigations that should be performed at the time of diagnosis (Table 18–1) will serve as a baseline for subsequent studies during the induction period, and may also document metabolic abnormalities that require correction before the start of treatment or modification of drug dosage. Renal impairment, hyperuricemia, and electrolyte imbalance should be corrected if possible before treatment is begun. Serum lactic dehydrogenase (LDH) levels are markedly elevated in most patients with ALL. Fasting or random estimations of blood glucose should be made, especially if L-asparaginase is to be included in the treatment protocol. A full hemostatic profile should be performed to detect the very occasional adult ALL patients with disseminated intravascular coagulation or with an incidental clotting abnormality related to pre-existing liver disease or liver infiltration. Besides cultures from any clinically infected site, surveillance cultures from the nose, throat, axillae, groin, vagina, perianal area, and of sputum and urine are taken to detect clinically occult infec-

tion and to provide useful information about microbiological etiology if septicemia or severe infection subsequently develops. An aliquot of serum should be stored that can be used to provide baseline antibody titers in the assessment of infection during the induction phase. In patients with a past medical history of heart disease and in elderly patients where treatment with an anthracycline is anticipated, an echocardiogram with myocardial function, including the ejection fraction, should be carried out.

Cerebrospinal Fluid

The examination of the cerebrospinal fluid (CSF) is an essential diagnostic procedure in ALL to exclude or confirm initial CNS disease. There are different opinions as to when the first lumbar puncture should be done. One procedure is to delay the examination until remission is achieved, in order to avoid seeding of the CNS by circulating leukemic blast cells from the peripheral blood, and not to deliver intrathecal chemotherapy at the time of first lumbar puncture in case a second diagnostic test is required. On the other hand, early recognition of CNS disease is clinically important because more aggressive CNS therapy is required for such patients. Since in a small percentage (2 to 3 percent) CNS involvement in the absence of clinical signs can only be substantiated by microscopic examination of CSF, other clinicians have preferred to make the lumbar puncture as soon as possible. This procedure is restricted to patients with an adequate platelet count ($>20 \times 10^9$/L), an absence of manifest clinical hemorrhages, and without a high WBC count. For safety reasons such patients should receive intrathecal methotrexate at the first lumbar puncture. Clearly this procedure necessitates an atraumatic lumbar puncture since in childhood ALL blood contamination of the CSF was associated with a higher relapse risk.

DIFFERENTIAL DIAGNOSIS

Difficulty is rarely experienced in establishing the diagnosis of ALL. Viral infection may cause lymphadenopathy and hepatosplenomegaly with lymphocytosis in the blood and bone marrow and, although the distinction can usually be made on clinical and morphological grounds, the results of viral antibody titers, lymphocyte surface markers, and cytogenetic analyses may be required. The leukemic phase of non-Hodgkin's lymphoma can mostly be recognized by clinical and morphological features, by the type and pattern of immunological cell surface markers, and by the degree and distribution of bone marrow infiltration. In the rare cases with a low bone marrow infiltration an arbitrary distinction between ALL and NHL is usually chosen according to the degree of infiltration, above or below 25 percent. With more advanced immunological marker application, mixed leukemias having myeloid as well as lymphoid surface markers are diagnosed which might be allocated to a treatment strategy for either ALL or AML.

CLASSIFICATION

There is a wide heterogeneity within ALL. Therefore accurate morphological classification, determination of the immunological phenotype, and cytogenetic analysis, which are of prognostic and therapeutic relevance, should be performed in every case of ALL. In addition, molecular analyses are part of standard diagnosis in ALL. In all patients material from the time point of diagnosis should be stored in order to identify individual markers for detection of minimal residual disease.

Morphology

Bone marrow aspirates and blood smears are stained with Wright's or Wright's-Giemsa stain and the blast cells are classified according to the French-American-British (FAB) classification.[24] The FAB classification is discussed in Chapter 14. The reproducibility of the system has been improved by the addition of a scoring system and the classification is more reliably made on bone marrow preparations than on peripheral blood smears. In adults there is a significantly lower incidence of the L1 type (28 percent) and higher incidence of the L2 type (66 percent) than in children (82 and 17 percent, respectively). The L3 FAB subtype is characteristic for mature B-ALL, which is important to identify since different treatment approaches are used in this subset.[158] Occasionally the discrimination of an L1 type from an M1 or a poorly differentiated M5 type is difficult but the distinction is ensured by cytochemistry and phenotyping.

Cytochemistry

The cytochemical stains to discriminate between AML and ALL are Sudan black, myeloperoxidase, and chloracetate or nonspecific esterase. These reactions are negative in ALL, negativity being usually defined as less than 3 percent of leukemic blast cells positive. Cytochemical stains to confirm ALL are periodic acid-Schiff (PAS) and acid phosphatase.[158] The PAS stain will show coarse granules or block positivity in at least some cells of most patients with adult ALL of the L1 or L2 type, the incidence of positivity being approximately 60 to 70 percent in both groups.[158] The acid phosphatase reaction is positive in 20 to 30 percent of all ALL being more specific for T-ALL. About 70 percent of patients with T-ALL will show strong and localized paranuclear staining with acid phosphatase. PAS or acid phosphatase reactivity is, however, not restricted to ALL and since it can be positive in some cases (M5) of AML the additional reactions for peroxidase and acetate esterase must be negative.

Immunophenotyping

The main aim of immunophenotyping of leukemic blast cells is to distinguish between AML and within the acute lymphoblastic leukemia between B- or T-lineage ALL by using monoclonal antibodies to pan-B (CD19), pan-T (CD7), and pan-myeloid surface antigens (CD13, CD33, CDw65).[23,84,107,160] To detect early lymphoid or myeloid differentiation, lineage-specific markers which are first exhibited in the cytoplasm (cy) of B- (cyCD22), T-cell (cyCD3), and myeloid precursor cells (myeloperoxidase) are used. To define further maturational stages within the B- and T-cell lineages, markers more specific for particular maturational stages are used; for B-lineage CD20, cy immunoglobulin μ heavy chain (cyIgM) and surface immunoglobulin (sIg), and for T-lineage CD1, CD2, CD4, CD8, and surface sCD3. The maturation stages are not identified by the presence or absence of a single antigen but by a pattern of antigen expression.

With the availability of more specific monoclonal antibodies 98 to 99 percent of the acute leukemias can now be reliably classified by immunological marker analysis. In addition, ALL can be subdivided according to various maturational stages of B or T lineage, whereby it is assumed that they are in differentiation arrest corresponding to normal maturational stages. Immunological classification of ALL subtypes is summarized in Table 18–3.

B-Lineage ALL

With the analysis of CD10 (the common ALL antigen), cyIgM and sIg, the B-lineage ALL can be subdivided into three subgroups of B-cell-precursor ALL and the more mature B-ALL. Pro-B-ALL (also termed Pre-Pre-B-ALL, Null-ALL, CD10 negative ALL) is the most immature subtype of the B-ALL lineage. This subtype is characterized by the expression of CD19, cyCD22, and mostly CD24, while CD10, cyIgM, and SIg are negative. Common ALL, the major immunological subtype in childhood as well as in adult ALL, is characterized by the expression of CD10 in combination with CD19, cy or sCD22, and CD24. Common ALL blast cells do not carry markers of relatively mature B cells such as cyIgM or sIg. Pre-B-ALL is characterized by the expression of cyIgM, being negative in common ALL but otherwise identical with all other markers, such as CD19, cy or sCD22, CD24, and only very rarely CD10 may be absent in this subtype. In most adult clinical studies Pre-B-ALL is included in the common ALL category. The distinction between these three subgroups of B-precursor-ALL has been somewhat arbitrary due to the different cut-off points applied. In most studies common ALL is defined by surface antigen expression of CD10 on 20 percent or more of leukemic cells and the diagnosis of pre-B-ALL by cyIgM in 10 percent or more of blast cells. Virtually all B-precursor-ALLs are positive for HLA-DR and TdT.

Leukemic blast cells in mature B-ALL express sIg and B-cell antigens including CD19, CD20, CD22, CD24, and usually CD10. In contrast to the B-precursor-ALLs leukemic cells in B-ALL are mostly negative for TdT. Most B-ALLs can be identified morphologically as L3 FAB subtype. However, also FAB L1 subtypes may be associated with the monoclonal sIg positivity.

T-Lineage ALL

There are different suggestions about how T-lineage ALL should be subclassified.[23,61,199] Early T-ALL is characterized by expression of cyCD3 with no additional differentiation markers.[235] CD2 is generally negative. In cases positive for CD2 but negative for CD4, CD8, sCD3, and CD1a, an early T-ALL is present as well. Cortical T-ALL, also referred to as thymic T-ALL, is characterized by expression of CD1 in combination with CD7, CD5,

Table 18–3. Immunological, Morphological, Cytogenetic, and Molecular Characterization of ALL[a]

Subtypes	Marker	Incidence (percent)	FAB Subtype	Frequent Cytogenetic Aberrations	Fusion Transcripts
B-lineage ALL	HLA-DR +, TdT +, CD19 + and/or CD79a + and/or CD22 +	76			
Pro-B-ALL	No additional differentiation markers	12	L1, L2	t(4;11)(q21;q23)	ALL1-AF4
Common ALL	CD10 +	49	L1, L2	t(9;22)(q34;q11) del(6q)	BCR-ABL
Pre-B-ALL	CD10±, cyIg +	11	L1, L2	t(9;22)(q34;q11) t(1;19)(q23;p13)	BCR-ABL E2A-PBX1
Mature B-ALL	CD10 ±, sIg +	4	L3	t(8;14)(q24;q32) t(2;8)(p12;q24) t(8;22)(q24;q11)	
T-lineage ALL	cyCD3 or sCD3	23			
Early T-ALL	No additional differentiation markers, mostly CD2–	6	L1, L2	t/del(9p)	
Cortical T-ALL	CD1a +, sCD3±	12		t(8;14)(q24;q11)	
Mature T-ALL	sCD3 +, CD1a–	5		t(10;14)(q24;q11) t(11;14)(p13;q11)	

[a] N = 946 adult ALL patients.[160]

and CD2, and sometimes also sCD3, CD4, and CD8. Mature T-ALL is characterized by positivity for sCD3, CD7, CD5, and CD2 while CD1 is negative. CD4 and CD8 are present in most cases.

Null or Unclassified ALL

The subset previously defined as null or unclassified ALL comprised a very heterogeneous group of immunophenotypes, such as CD10 negative, non-T-, non-B-ALLs and acute leukemias positive for TdT and HLA-DR but lacking B-, T-, and myeloid-lineage-associated markers. Most of these null-ALL cases, which constituted more than 20 percent in most adult ALL series, can now with more specific immunophenotyping be defined as immature Pro-B-ALL characterized by the combined expression of early B-cell antigens (e.g., CD19, CD24) and rearrangement of Ig heavy-chain genes. Probably also some immature AML and pre-T-ALLs were included. Since lineage commitment of leukemic cells can now be established in more than 98 percent of cases, the term null ALL need no longer be used.

Myeloid Antigen positive ALL (My+ ALL)

Immunophenotyping has shown the existence of acute leukemia cases in which the blast cells express markers supposedly specific for or associated with another cell lineage.[23,66] A variety of terms have been used to refer to these acute leukemias as hybrid-, biphenotypic-, and mixed-lineage leukemia. The myeloid-antigen-associated monoclonal antibodies that are used for the detection of My+ ALL are CD13, CD14, CD15, CD33, and CDw65. The reported frequencies of My+ ALL differ widely, ranging from 5 to 46 percent depending on the definition and an approximate figure for adult My+ ALL may be 18 percent. Commonly a case is considered as My+ ALL if 20 percent or more of the blast cells are reactive with the myeloid-lineage-associated monoclonal antibodies. The incidence of My+

ALL is higher in B-lineage than in T-lineage ALL and is characteristic for immature subtypes such as Pro-B- and early T-ALL.

Frequency and Clinical Features of Immunological Subtypes

The frequency of immunological subtypes in adult ALL shows distinct differences from that in childhood ALL.[160] Approximately 84 percent of the children have a B-precursor ALL and common ALL is, with 63 percent, the most frequent subtype, whereas this subtype is only observed in one-half of adult ALL patients. There is a significantly higher proportion of the Pro-B-ALL, with 12 percent in adults compared to only 5 percent in children. Mature B-ALL is rare in both childhood and adult ALL. Adult T-ALL, with 23 percent, has a twofold higher incidence in adults than the 13 percent observed in children. As in the B-lineage the most immature form, Pre-T-ALL, has a higher incidence in adults compared to children.

The clinical features of the immunological subtypes of ALL are quite distinct. The immature Pro-B-ALL has a peak in infants less than 1 year old and is associated with high leukocyte count, massive hepatosplenomegaly, CNS disease, myeloid co-expression, and approximately 70 percent of the patients show t(4;11). Nearly one-half of the patients with c-ALL or Pre-B-ALL show t(9;22) and the incidence increases with age. Mature B-ALL is characterized by frequent abdominal tumor masses, often kidney involvement, an increased incidence of CNS leukemia, and a male preponderance. T-ALL is associated with mediastinal masses in nearly half the patients, occasionally associated with pleural and pericardial effusions, an increased incidence of organomegaly, a higher incidence of CNS disease, a high WBC count, and male prevalence. The major clinical differences between immunological subtypes of adult ALL are summarized in Table 18–4.

Table 18–4. Characteristics of Immunological Subtypes of Adult ALL

Subgroup	Clinical/Laboratory Characteristics	Relapse Kinetics and Localization
B-Lineage		
Pro-B-ALL	t(4;11)/*ALL1-AF4* (70 percent)	Mainly BM (> 90 percent)
	High WBC (> 100/ml) (26 percent)	
	Frequently myeloid coexpression (> 50 percent)	
c-ALL/Pre-B-ALL	Higher age (24 percent > 50 years)	Mainly BM (> 90 percent)
	Ph/*BCR-ABL* (40–50 percent)	Prolonged relapse kinetics (up to 5–7 years)
	m-BCR (70 percent), M-BCR (30 percent)	
B-ALL	Higher age (27 percent > 50 years)	Frequent CNS (10 percent)
	Frequent organ involvement (32 percent)	Short relapse kinetics (up to 1–1 $\frac{1}{2}$ years)
	Frequent CNS involvement (13 percent)	
T-Lineage	Younger age (90 percent < 50 years)	Frequent CNS (10 percent)
	Frequent mediastinal tumors (60 percent)	Extramedullary (6 percent)
	Frequent CNS involvement (8 percent)	Intermediate relapse kinetics (up to 3–4 years)
	High WBC (> 50/ml) (46 percent)	

Data based on German multicenter trials of adult ALL.

Cytogenetic Analysis

Cytogenetic analysis should be performed in all cases of adult ALL since chromosome abnormalities are independent prognostic variables for the outcome (overview in Ref. 77 and in Chapter 16). Since chromosomal aberrations are correlated to immunological subtype and clinical features (Table 18–3) they also provide additional information for diagnostic confirmation.

Clonal chromosomal aberrations are identified by banding techniques in 62 to 85 percent of adult ALL patients.[46,224,255] The most frequent numerical chromosomal aberrations are hypodiploid karyotype with less than 46 chromosomes (4 to 8 percent), hyperdiploid karyotype with 47 to 50 chromosomes (7 to 15 percent), or greater than 50 chromosomes (7 to 8 percent). The most frequent structural aberration is the translocation t(9;22)/Philadelphia chromosome (Ph+ ALL) which is detected in 20 to 30 percent of adult ALL patients compared to 3 to 5 percent in childhood ALL. Other translocations occur less frequently and are mostly associated with distinct immunological subtypes such as (4; 11) (3 to 4 percent) in Pro-B-ALL, t(8;14) (5 percent) in mature B-ALL, t(1;19) (2 to 3 percent) in pre-B-ALL, and t(10;14) (3 percent), 9p– (5 to 15 percent), 6q– (4 to 6 percent), and 12p aberrations (4 to 5 percent) mainly in T-ALL.[46,224,255]

By giving careful attention to the collection of the bone marrow, to rapid transport, and to preservation, the successful analysis of marrow cells can be increased and the identification of clonal abnormalities was possible in more than 90 percent[260] of children with ALL.

Molecular Genetics

With molecular analysis (polymerase chain reaction [PCR]) additional cases of clonal aberrations can be identified. PCR analysis for *BCR-ABL* and *ALL1-AF4* is part of standard diagnosis in adult ALL. The translocation t(9;22) leads to a break within the breakpoint cluster region *(BCR)* gene on chromo-

some 22 and transfer of the *ABL* protooncogene from chromosome 9 to a position adjacent to the truncated *BCR* gene, forming a chimeric *bcr-abl* gene. In one-third of the *BCR-ABL* positive patients a 210-kd BCR-ABL protein is expressed similar to CML with two different breakpoints (b3a2, b2a2). In two-thirds the translocation results in expression of a 190-kd BCR-ABL protein with the breakpoint e1a2, which is specific for ALL. The *abl* gene encodes a protein with tyrosine kinase activity and is physiologically involved in signal transduction and control of cell proliferation. The fusion protein BCR-ABL shows increased tyrosine kinase activity and leads by interaction with other mediators of signal transduction (RAS, MYC, CYCLIN D1, STAT5) to complex disturbances of signal transduction and cell cycle regulation. In *bcr-abl* positive cell lines an inhibition of apoptosis was also observed and *bcr-abl* positive cells show decreased cell adhesion (overview in Refs. 37 and 49).

In the t(4;11) translocation the mll gene (synonyms: *MLL, hrx, all-1*) on chromosome 11 is fused with the *af4-* gene on chromosome 4 leading to a fusion gene named *all1-af4*.

Detection of Minimal Residual Disease

Conventional microscopic evaluation of bone marrow smears has a detection limit of 1 to 5 percent. With new methods for detection of MRD residual blast cells can be detected and measured quantitatively below this level with a sensitivity of 10^4 to 10^6. With these methods individual follow-up analyses can be performed in patients with clinical and morphological CR. ALL is an "ideal" disease for detection of MRD since more than 90 percent of the patients show individual clonal markers. Most experience has been accumulated with MRD detection by flow cytometry and PCR (overviews in Refs. 38 and 86).

MRD detection by flow cytometry targets individual leukemia-specific combinations of surface antigens and reaches a sensitivity of 10^4. PCR detection may target leukemia-specific fusion genes such as *bcr-abl* or *mll-af4*, which may be detected in 30 to 40 percent of adult ALL cases. A more widespread applicability is reached with detection of clonal rearrangements of immunoglobulin heavy chain (IgH) or T-cell receptor (TCR-β, -δ, -γ) gene rearrangements. This method reaches a sensitivity of 10^4 to 10^6 and combinations of two or more target structures can be identified in more than 80 percent of ALL patients. To an increasing extent semi-automatized methods for quantitative PCR detection (real-time PCR) are applied since they provide results rapidly with high sensitivity.

SUPPORTIVE CARE

The management of adult patients undergoing induction therapy for ALL requires intensive treatment of initial complications and supportive care to prevent and manage the infectious, hemorrhagic, metabolic, and psychological problems that may arise.

Metabolic Abnormalities

A few general measures can be started at once. Sufficient fluid intake to guarantee urine production of at least 100 ml/hour throughout induction therapy reduces the risk of uric acid formation. This may require parenteral fluid administration when the patient's oral intake is inadequate because of nausea or difficulty in swallowing. If the venous system does not offer an easy approach, access by catheter or port is advantageous when anticipating a longer period of induction therapy or when part of the therapy will be carried out on an outpatient basis.

Hyperuricemia is frequently present at diagnosis; it may worsen following the initiation of chemotherapy and, if not treated, can lead to renal failure. Adequate doses of allopurinol (300 to 600 mg/day) should be given and the urine alkalinized before chemotherapy. Allopurinol has to be reduced when 6-mercaptopurine is given.

In patients presenting with renal impairment an attempt must be made to re-establish renal function before chemotherapy is started.[161] Renal failure is often observed in patients with Burkitt's lymphoma or B-ALL with abdominal tumor masses and can be resolved by a gentle pretreatment with cyclophosphamide (C) combined with prednisone (P) or dexamethasone (DX) alone.

The acute tumor lysis syndrome is most frequently seen in patients with B-ALL or T-ALL but may also occur in other subtypes with high WBC count or large tumor mass.[55,183] Massive and rapid tumor cell lysis leads to hyperkalemia, hyperphosphatemia, hyperuricemia, and hypocalcemia, which can largely be prevented by the C + P treatment in B-ALL or by a gentle therapy with steroids, vincristine (V), or C in the other subtypes.

Infections

The problem of infection is fully discussed in Chapters 49–51. Approximately one-third of adult ALL patients present with infections, which are a major problem in the management of the disease. Fever or infection at the time of admission is mainly caused by severe granulocytopenia, especially if the granulocyte count is less than 5×10^9/L but may also be due to immunological deficiency (e.g., CD4 lymphopenia) or mucosal lesions. Combination chemotherapy causes additional hematological toxicity and at least 50 percent of adults undergoing induction treatment will experience severe or life-threatening infections. Whereas formerly gram-negative microorganisms were the leading cause of febrile neutropenia, in the last decade the incidence of infections with gram-positive bacteria has increased – especially those due to more frequent use of indwelling catheters. Fungal infections also occur more frequently.[173]

Much attention has been paid to prophylactic measures against infection. They include oral hygiene using antiseptic soaps and mouthwashes and disinfection of the anogenital region. Other precautions include reverse protective isolation and air filtration, if available, which can reduce especially the risk of Aspergillus infections. Simple precautions that can always be carried out are: no live plants in the room, no humidifiers, no i.m./s.c. injections if avoidable, no uncooked vegetables, no unpeeled fruits, no visitors having any kind of infection.

Prophylactic medication includes agents against bacterial and fungal infection. For antibacterial prophylaxis, mostly co-trimoxazole or fluorocinolones, both mainly directed against gram-negative organisms, have been used.[204] Co-trimoxazole additionally reduces the incidence of Pneumocystis carinii pneumonia, which occurs in about 20 percent of patients without prophylaxis.[128] Gastrointestinal decontamination with nonabsorbable antibiotics seems of reasonable benefit.

Whereas antifungal prophylaxis with oral amphotericin B solution or triazoles may successfully reduce Candida colonization and prevent local Candida infections, the prophylactic procedures for reducing systemic mycoses are disappointing. Fluconazole has been reported to reduce only systemic Candida albicans infections in bone marrow transplant patients, but increases of C. non-albicans, especially C. krusei, have been found. Due to its high lethality, Aspergillus infection is particularly feared. Attempts to prevent aspergilloses have included prophylaxis with itraconazole, intravenous low-dose amphotericin B, liposomal amphotericin B, and inhalation with aerosolized amphotericin B, but in randomized studies no benefit could be shown.[243] Viral prophylaxis (e.g., against herpes simplex virus) for selected patient populations may be considered.

The diagnostic procedures in febrile neutropenia include physical examination; cultures of blood, urine, sputum, and other sites of suspected infection; and imaging procedures such as chest x-ray or abdominal ultrasound. The high-resolution computed tomography of the lungs is especially important for the early diagnosis of Aspergillus pneumonia. With bronchoalveolar lavage also fungal pneumonias may be microbiologically proven. Increasingly PCR methods are applied for earlier detection of fungal infections.

The standard treatment of febrile neutropenia is the empirical administration of broad-spectrum antibiotics without waiting for microbiological results. As initial therapy, combinations of beta-lactam antibiotics plus aminoglycosides have been the "gold standard," but monotherapy with carbapenems or cephalosporins of class 3 and 3a has been suggested to be equally effective.[200] Considering the increasing problems due to systemic fungal infections, empirical antimycotic treatment for persisting fever despite adequate antibacterial therapy in patients with pulmonary infiltration has been introduced.[230] Standard antifungal therapy is conventional amphotericin B, which may be combined with 5-flucytosine. Other formulations of amphotericin B such as liposomal amphotericin B, the colloidal dispersion or the lipid complex, have been introduced to reduce amphotericin B toxicity.[117] In patients with severe infections empirical broad-spectrum antibiotics should be given immediately, even before the results of cultures are available.

Hematopoietic Growth Factors

The use of hematopoietic growth factors (HPGFs) such as colony-stimulating factor–granulocyte (G-CSF) and colony-stimulating factor–granulocyte/macrophage (GM-CSF), is a valuable component of supportive therapy during the treatment of ALL. There is no indication that these CSFs stimulate leukemic cell growth in a clinically significant manner. The majority of clinical trials demonstrate that the prophylactic administration of G-CSF significantly accelerates neutrophil recovery[93,135,147,188,216] and several prospective randomized studies also showed that this is associated with a substantially reduced incidence and duration of febrile neutropenia and of severe infections.[93,147,188] The enhanced marrow recovery allows closer adherence to the dose and schedule of chemotherapeutic regimens. However it still remains open whether the increased dose intensity translates into an improved LFS.

The advantage of G-CSF administration is particularly evident in patients at high risk for prolonged granulocytopenia. Furthermore, scheduling appears to be important. When CSFs are first given at the end of a 4-week chemotherapy regimen potential benefits are limited. Therefore it is noteworthy that G-CSF may be given in parallel with chemotherapy without aggravating the myelotoxicity of these specific regimens.[93,147,188] and that this scheduling is an important determinant of the clinical efficacy.

Hemorrhage

Hemorrhage is discussed in Chapters 53 and 61. The thrombocytopenia present in one-third of the patients at diagnosis will worsen following chemotherapy, requiring transfusion of platelet concentrates. Platelet transfusions should be given for bleeding and to prevent bleeding when platelet counts are below 20×10^9/L especially during febrile periods, which interfere with platelet function. Most often 4 to 8 platelet packs are given daily until bleeding stops and HLA-matched platelets from plateletpheresis are given to patients who become refractory to random donor platelets. When a long induction period is anticipated and there is a likelihood that a patient will need frequent platelet transfusions it might be preferable to start with HLA-matched platelets immediately, if this is logistically possible (technical facilities, costs), to avoid refractoriness to random platelets.

L-asparaginase treatment leads to a decrease in fibrinogen, which should be substituted if levels fall below about 100 mg/dl. Also, in those few patients with initially decreased fibrinogen level L-asparaginase treatment can be started if the fibrinogen is substituted and the levels closely followed. In some adult ALL patients during induction therapy antithrombin III levels decrease, thereby increasing the risk of thromboembolic events; in this case antithrombin III should be substituted or fresh frozen plasma given.

CHEMOTHERAPY

The approach to therapy of adult ALL has evolved along similar lines to that successfully employed in childhood ALL. An induction therapy is followed by a postremission or consolidation therapy. Whereas the induction phase of therapy is usually well defined, the postremission therapy may consist of consolidation, intensification, maintenance, and in addition there is a CNS therapy during induction and maintenance treatment. SCT is also an important part of consolidation therapy of adult ALL.

Initial Treatment in Highly Leukemic Patients

In patients with a large leukemic cell burden, that is, a high WBC count and/or massive organomegaly, cell reduction with a cautious preinduction therapy is recommended. Patients with high WBC count ($>100 \times 10^9$/L), where hyperviscosity due to leukostasis with cerebral impairment may occur, were successfully managed with leukopheresis.[113,153] However, such technical facilities may not be available and these patients can also be managed with a gentle chemotherapy consisting of V or C and P or DX in nearly all cases without complications. For patients with mature B-ALL and high tumor burden a preinduction therapy with P or DX and C is recommended (e.g., C, 200 mg/m^2 and P, 60 mg/m^2, each days 1 to 5). Thus leukapheresis in adult ALL might not be necessary except on very rare occasions such as leukemia during pregnancy.

Remission Induction

A number of drugs including V, P, daunorubicin (D), L-asparaginase (A), and adriamycin (AD) were shown during the 1960s and early 1970s to have activity against adult ALL producing as single agents CR rates of 25 to 50 percent. The combination of V + P improved the response rate to about 40 to 60 percent in adult ALL, which is clearly inferior to the results in childhood ALL where 70 to 90 percent achieve CR. In adult ALL series using V + P for induction the median remission durations were only 3 to 12 months despite additional consolidation and maintenance therapy.

An increase in CR rate by the addition of D to the standard V + P ± A therapy was shown in several series and convincingly achieved in a randomized trial.[99] In most trials D is administered for 2 to 3 days at a dose level from 30 to 60 mg/m^2. There is some evidence that dose intensity of anthracyclines may contribute to remission quality.[20]

A does improve remission quality and thereby the length of remission in childhood ALL.[54,213] A randomised study in adult ALL has shown no advantage for CR rate but a longer LFS when A was added.[180] PEG-L-A is a new A preparation replacing approximately 2 weeks of treatment with conventional A due to its prolonged half-life. However experience is still scarce and results of prospective studies are awaited.

Dexamethasone (DX) is currently evaluated as an alternative to P in childhood and adult ALL. DX shows a higher antileukemic activity.[141] DX also has a longer half-life in the CSF compared to P.[12] In a randomized study in childhood ALL comparing DX and P during induction therapy, the rate of CNS relapses was significantly lower with DX (14 vs. 26 percent).[133] There is, however, also evidence that the extensive use of DX may increase the risk of severe septicemias and fungal infections.[129] This problem and the known risk of bone marrow necrosis may be overcome by the shorter application compared to earlier trials.

The addition of other agents such as cytarabine (AC), 6-mercaptopurine (MP), methotrexate (MTX) to V and P in induction probably does not increase the CR rate substantially but may affect remission quality. The addition of C led to an improved outcome for patients with T-ALL.[22,124] Overall the highest remission rates have been achieved with multidrug induction regimens including six to eight different cytostatic drugs (Table 18–5).

High-Dose Treatment in Induction Therapy

Several attempts have been made to include high-dose chemotherapy – particularly high-dose AC (HdAC) – in induction therapy. This approach has been followed either by up-front application – before conventional induction – or after conventional induction (Table 18–6). CR rates ranged between 67 and 100 percent in small studies and were generally not superior to intensive multidrug induction regimens without HdAC with some exceptions.[137] Furthermore it remains open whether HdAC may contribute to improved remission quality and for which subtypes of ALL it may be beneficial.

A large number of different drug combinations have been employed in adult ALL and the published results of larger studies with more than 100 patients, most of them prospective national trials published after 1990, are summarized in Table 18–5. The CR rates ranged from 64 to 85 percent and the weighted mean for more than 6000 adult ALL patients is 78 percent.

Definition of Complete Remission

CR is defined[114] as a state in which there is no clinical or laboratory manifestation of leukemia: the peripheral blood count and bone marrow appearances are within normal limits except for abnormalities attributable to chemotherapy; the marrow blast cell count is less than 5 percent; also examination of the CSF shows no blast cells. CR includes also the disappearance of organomegalies, but it should be noted that the persistence of splenomegaly is not always due to leukemic infiltration.[90] Definition of complete remission may be revised when evaluation of MRD provides new parameters (see Prognostic Factors Minimal Residual Disease).

Remission Duration and LFS

The median remission duration in the studies listed in Table 18–5 is 2 years with a wide range from 11 to 32 months. Approximately one-third of adult ALL patients are disease free at 4 to 18 years and these patients may be cured. But there is also a substantial variation in LFS ranging from 18 to 40 percent or greater. Remission duration and LFS are, as discussed before, clearly dependent on a variety of prognostic factors.

Failure to Respond to Induction Therapy

Ten to 20 percent of adult ALL patients do not achieve a CR in contrast to less than 5 percent of children with ALL. Furthermore about 5 to 10 percent of the adult patients will die during the first 8 weeks after diagnosis and initiation of therapy. Mortality during induction is age dependent and increases from less than 3 percent in children to 20 percent or more in adults over 60 years.[118,193] In two-thirds of these patients the cause of death is infection, whereby fungal infection increases with the duration of neutropenia and use of antibiotics. For the patients refractory to induction therapy alternative chemotherapy, possibly incorporating newer agents, should be considered (see Relapsed ALL). When at least a good partial remission is achieved, allogeneic SCT is also a therapeutic option with survival rates of approximately 15 to 30 percent.

Postremission Therapy

When in ALL CR is achieved treatment has to be continued because a high percentage of patients show MRD after induction therapy. Continuation or postremission therapy consists of intensification or consolidation and maintenance. Consolidation/intensification refers either to high-dose therapy, the use of multiple new agents, or less often, readministration of the induction regimen. SCT is also included in postremission therapy in many trials. Maintenance is usually a less intensive therapy. In most studies that involve repeated consolidation cycles over the entire treatment period it is difficult to analyze critically the effect of the different treatment phases on outcome.

Earlier randomized trials comparing consolidation therapy versus none showed an advantage for either median remission duration[212] or LFS[81] as demonstrated in Table 18–7. Also a recently published randomized study by the British Medical Research Council demonstrated a reduction of relapse risk in patients receiving early (week 5) and late (week 20) intensification cycles (37 percent LFS) versus those without (28 percent).[69] In a similar study conducted in childhood ALL there was a significant advantage for patients with early and late intensification (71 percent) compared to those without (57 percent).[47]

Other randomized studies showed no benefit of intensified versus a moderate consolidation therapy. When the European Organisation for Treatment of Cancer (EORTC) leukemia group randomized patients to receive or not the 3 months consolidation with MTX, cytarabine, and thioguanine both groups had the LFS of 40 percent in spite of a considerably longer median remission duration for the group given longer consolidation.[226] This shows the difficulty in assessing the efficacy of specific consolidation elements. Also a Cancer and Leukemia Group B (CALGB) randomized study showed no advantage for two consolidation courses, comprising the AML regimens "7+3" (cytarabine × 7 + D × 3) and "5+2," over two courses of mercaptopurine and MTX with identical continuous CR (CCR) rates of 29 percent at 9 years for the standard and intensive

Table 18–5. Results of Chemotherapy in Adult ALL in Recent Large Studies[a]

Group	Year	Ref.	N	Median Age	Induction	Consolidation	Maintenance	CR (percent)	mrd (months)	DFS/CCR (percent)	at (year)
MDACC	1990	138	105	30	V,AD,DX,C	MTX,A,AD,HdAC,V,P	IdM,D,MP,P,C,BC,VP	84	22	34	5
MSKCC	1990	52	199	25	V,P[D,A,AD,C]	AC,TG,A,V,P,MTX,C,BCNU	ActD,BC,V,P,AD,MTX,MP,C	82	28	33	18
GATLA	1991	156	145	29	V,P,D,A,C,AC,MP	AD,V,DX,A,AC,C,MP	MP,MTX,V,P,	78	28	34	6
JALSG	1991	241	117	38	V,P,AD,C	VP,MI + other	MP,MTX,A + other	81		30	4
CALGB 8011	1991	71	277	33	V,P,A,D	[AC,D],MTX,MP	V,P,MP,MTX	64	21	29	9
CALGB 8513	1992	60	164	32	V,P,Mi/D,HdM	V,P,D/Mi,HdM,AC,MP,A	none	64	11	18	3
EORTC	1992	226	106	27	V,P,AD,(HdAC)	A,HdC,(MTX,TG,AC)	V,P,MTX,AD,BC,C,MP,MTX	74	32	40	8
L + B + V	1992	15	212	27	V,P,AD,A,(HdC/HdAC)	V,P,AD,A,(HdC/HdAC)	MP,MTX,C	71	23	32	10
GMALL 01	1993	127	368	25	V,P,A,D,C,AC,MTX,MP	V,DX,AD,AC,C,TG	MP,MTX	74	24	35	10
GMALL 02	1993	127	562	28	V,P,A,D,C,AC,MTX,MP	V,DX,AD,AC,C,TG,VM	MP,MTX	75	27	39	7
CALGB 8811	1992	218	165	32	V,P,D,A,C	V,P,D,MTX,Mi,AC,MP,A	MP,MTX	85	19	26	6
FGTALL	1993	82	572		V,P,D/R,C,(AM,AC)	AD,AC,A	MP,MTX,V,C,PAD,AC	76	23	32	4
UK ALL IX	1993	68	266		V,P,A,IdM/D		V,P,MP,MTX,AC	68	29	22	8
USCF	1991	154	109		V,P,A,D	V,P,A,D,IdM,VM,AC	MTX,MP	88		42	5
FGTALL	1995	11	135	31	V,P,A,D;C,AC,MP	HdM,AC,allo/auto SCT	[IL-2]	93		44	3
CALGB 8811	1995	146	197	32	V,P,A,D,C	C,MP,AC,V,A,MTX,AD,DX,TG	MP,MTX,V,P	85	32	30	5
GIMEMA 0183	1996	164	358	31	V,P,A,D	V,IdM,IdAC,P,VM	MP,MTX,V,P[A,ARAC,VM,IdAC]	79	20	25	10
GIMEMA 0288	1996	165	767	28	V,P,A,D,C[HdAC,Mi]	V,HdM,IdAC,DX,VM	MP,MTX,V,P,[AC,Mi,VM,HDAC,HdM,DX]	82	28	34	6
HOVON	1997	63	130	35	V,P,D,A	HdAC,AM,Mi,VP	—	73		22	5
SAKK	1997	252	140	31	V,P,D,M,A, HdAC,VP	allo/auto SCT; > 50 years: HdC [AC,VP,D,TG]		69		21	5
MRC XA	1997	69	618	15	V,P,A,D		MP,MTX,V,P	82		28	5
Pethema	1998	202	108	28	V,P,D,A,C	HdM,V,D,P,A,C,VM,AC	MP,MTX [VD,P,Mi,A,C,VM,AC]	86		41	4
CALGB 9111	1998	147	198	35	C,D,V,P,A	C,MP,AC,V,A,MTX,AD,DX,TG,P	MP,MTX,V,P	85		40	3
Swedish ALL	1999	112	120	44	HdAC,C,D,V,BM	AM,HdAC,V,BM,C,D,VP ± SCT	nr	85		36	3
MDACC	2000	137	204	39	V,AD,DX,C	HdM,HdAC,P	MTX,MP,V,P	91		38	5
Lombardia 8/96	2001	21	121	35	I,V,A,P [C]	I,V,C,VM,HdAC,HdM,DX (risk adapted) ± SCT	MP, MTX	84	25	49	3
			6463	30[b]				78[b]	25[b]	32[b]	

Abbreviations: [ ] with or without; / or; AC, cytarabine; AD, adriamycin; AM, amsacrine; A, asparaginase; BC, BCNU; BM, betamethasone; C, cyclophosphamide; D, daunorubicin; DX, dexamethasone; HdAC, high-dose cytarabine; I, idarubicin; IdAC, intermediate-dose cytarabine; IL-2, interleukin-2; MTX, methotrexate; IdM, intermediate-dose methotrexate; HdM, high-dose methotrexate; MP, mercaptopurine; Mi, Miantrone; P, prednisone; R, rubidazone; TG, thioguanine; V, vincristine; VD, vindesine; VM, VM26 (teniposide); VP, VP16 (etoposide); mrd, median remission duration.
[a] > 100 patients; [b] weighted mean.

Table 18–6. High-Dose Cytosine Arabinoside in Induction/Consolidation Therapy of de novo Adult ALL

Author	Year	Ref.	Induction	CR rate (percent)	Consolidation	N	Mrd (months)	CCR/LFS (percent)/(years)
Boogaerts	1987	31	V, P, C, A	82	HdAC 3 g/m^2 × 8	78	8–26.5	
Willemze	1988	258	HdAC 1 g/m^2 × 12 V, P, AD	100	HdAC 3 g/m^2 × 8 V, P, AD	6	24	5/6
Kantarjian	1990	138	V, AD, DX, C	84	HdAC 3 g/m^2 × 6 V, P	63 HR 25 SR	13	27/4 years 73/4 years
Arlin	1991	7	HdAC 3 g/m^2 × 5 Mi, V, P	100	V, P, A	11	1 + to 11 +	9/11/1.5 years
Stryckmans	1992	226	HdAC 2.5 g/m^2 × 1 V, P, AD	74	A, C, ± (MTX, TG, AC)	56	25	27/5 years
Bassan	1992	15	HdAC 2 g/m^2 × 12 V, P, AD, A	67	V, AD	22 HR 36 All	(26) 25	
Cassileth	1992	43	HdAC 3 g/m^2 × 12	69	V, P, AD, C, MTX, A	89	10	13
Hoelzer	1992	126	V, P, D, A, C, AC, MP	76	HdAC 3 g/m^2 × 8 Mi	81 HR	21	43/4 years
Wernli	1994	253	V, D, IdM, A, P	78	HdAC 3 g/m^2 × 12 VP, ± SCT	140	32	21/EFS
Willemze	1995	259	HdAC 2 g/m^2 × 12 VP, AM, P	72	HdAC 3 g/m^2 × 8 V, AM, P	26 HR	24	35/5 years
Attal	1995	11	V, P, A, D, C, AC, MP	93	HdAC 4 g/m^2 × 2 HdM ± SCT	135	n.r.	44/3 years
Mandelli	1996	165	V, P, A, D, [C] [HdAC 1 g/m^2 × 4, Mi]^1	82	V, HdM, AC, DX, VM	767	28	34/6 years
Kaufmann	1996	142	HdAC 2–4 g/m^2 × 3 V, P, D	69	SCT or maintenance (MP, C, MTX, V, P)	43	n.r.	n.r.
			HdAC 2 g/m^2 × 3 VP, A, V, P, D	77	SCT or maintenance (MP, C, MTX, V, P)	42	n.r.	n.r.
Weiss	1996	248	HdAC 3 g/m^2 × 5 Mi	84	V, P, MTX, A, AC, VP	37	17	(38)/5 years
Dekker	1997	63	V, P, D, A	73	HdAC 2 g/m^2 × 12 AM, Mi, VP ± SCT	130	n.r.	22/OS
Linker	1997	155	D, V, P, A	92	HdAC 2 g/m^2 × 4 VP, D, MTX, MP	62	n.r.	47/5 years
Daenen	1998	62	[AC, VP], V, P, AD	88	T-ALL: HdAC 2 g/m^2 × 8, VP All: 0.7 g/m^2 × 4, A	66	n.r.	(45)/10 years
Todeschini	1998	240	V, P, D, A	93	HdAC 2 g/m^2 × 4, VP V, D, P, C, MP, M	60	34	55/5 years
Hallbook	1999	112	HdAC 3 g/m^2 × 3 C, D, V, BM	85	HdAC 3 g/m^2 × 4 AM, V, BM, C, D, VP	120	n.r.	36/3 years
Ifrah	1999	131	HdAC 1 g/m^2 × 6 I, P	72	HdAC 1 g/m^2 × 10 P, Mi, VP ± SCT	64	n.r.	24/OS
Kantarjian	2000	137	V, AD, DX, C	91	HdAC 3 g/m^2 × 4 HdM, P	204	33	36/5 years

Abbreviations: ( ) estimate from published remission duration curve; SR, standard risk; HR, high risk; OS, overall survival. For abbreviations of drug names, see Table 18–5.

treatment groups.[71] The possible advantage of the intensified consolidation therapy may be outweighed by the intensified maintenance therapy used in these protocols.

In a large randomized trial conducted by the Italian GIMEMA group comparing conventional versus intensified consolidation no advantage for intensified treatment could be demonstrated (34 percent overall LFS at 5 years[164]). In this study, however, all patients had received an early intensification before randomization. A recent randomized trial also did not show any benefit in LFS for patients with late intensification (45 percent) compared to those without (55 percent).[202] The latter

protocol had overall a higher dose intensity. The great discrepancy between LFS for patients without late intensification – 28 percent in one trial[69] compared to 55 percent in the other[202] – may, however also be due to the question whether intent-to-treat analysis was performed or whether only patients who actually received late intensification (excluding early relapses) were analyzed.

Thus, although randomized trials show no clear advantage in favor of consolidation therapy, results from large prospective multicenter trials indicate that in most studies the improved LFS is due to the addition of intensive consolidation without

Table 18–7. Randomized Studies of Consolidation and Maintenance Therapy in Adult ALL

Group	Year	Ref.	N	CR Rate (percent)		Consolidation	Maintenance	Duration	mrd (months)	CCR (percent/years)
GATLA	1974	212	112	76	R	A	MTX, MP, D/AD, V, P		20	
						none			13	
FGTALL	1987	81	146	73	R	A, AD, AC	MTX, MP, (V,C,P or AD, AC)	2 years		38/3
						none		2 years		0/3
CALGB	1991	71	277	64	R	DA(7 + 3), DA(5 + 2)	V, P, MTX, MP	3 years		29/9
						MTX, MP				29/9
EORTC	1992	226	100	74	R	MTX, TG, AC, A, C	V, P, AD/BC, MP, MTX, ActD	3 years	45	40/5
						A, C			24	40/7
CALGB	1991	60	164	64	R	D	None	8 months	12	18/3
						Mi			11	18/3
GIMEMA 0183	1996	165	358	79		Both arms: V, P, HdMTX, ARAC, MTX, MP, A	MTX, MP, P, V	12 months		27/10
					R	P, V, D, A, VM, AC	P, A, V, MTX, AC, VM, AC, D, MP	14 months	17	28/10
GIMEMA 0288	1996	164	767	86		Both arms: V, AC, HDM, DX, VM	MP, MTX, V, P	24 months (post intens.)		
					R	C, AC, V, D, P, MT, VM, HDM, DX			24	34/6 (no diff)
						None				
UKALL XA	1997	69	618	82		None	V, P, MP, MTX		n.r.	28
					R	V, D, VP, AC, TG (week 5)				34
						V, D, VP, AC, TG (week 20)				25
						V, D, VP, AC, TG (week 5 and 20)				37
Pethema	1998	202	110	86		Both arms: V, D, DX, A, C, VM, AC	MP, MTX	24 months	34	
					R	VD, Mi, P, A, C, VM, AC (month 11)				45
						None				55

For abbreviations of drug names, see Table 18–5. R, Randomization; ActD, actinomycin D.

high-dose schedules. In the GMALL, a different approach was used for consolidation; a regimen nearly identical to the induction therapy was given after 3 months. This "reinduction" included V, DX, AD, AC, CP, and TG and led to a MRD of 24 months and a survival rate at 10 years of 35 percent.[125,127] That this type of consolidation may be important is evident from two consecutive protocols of the Argentine Group for Treatment of Acute Leukemia (GATLA). The addition of the previous consolidation therapy in the second study, but also extension of the induction regimen from 4 to 8 weeks, improved the 5-year sur-

vival rate from 22 to 35 percent.[156] Also several other trials demonstrated an improved LFS by adding intensive consolidation without high-dose schedules.[53,92,81,130,166]

High-Dose Chemotherapy in Consolidation

High-dose chemotherapy – either HdAC or HdMTX – during consolidation has been mainly used to overcome drug resistance and to achieve therapeutic drug levels in the CSF. Although there is great experience with HdAC it still remains uncertain what dose and schedule is optimal in ALL. HdAC has been included in several trials in adult de novo ALL during induction, as part of consolidation therapy, or both (Table 18–6). Overall the results for the LFS range between 13 and 55 percent and are not superior to trials without HdAC.[15,43,52,62,63,112,131,138,226,240,259] Superior results were only described from smaller trials. Thus a high CR rate (88 percent) and LFS (45 percent at 10 years) was reported with a regimen including pretreatment with AC and etoposide followed by conventional induction and intensive rotational consolidation/maintenance chemotherapy over a total treatment period of 3 years.[62] With a regimen including high doses of D during induction, followed by HdAC in postremission and intensified maintenance for a total duration of 3 years, the LFS was 55 percent at 5 years.[240]

It is an important question whether specific subgroups of ALL may profit from an HdAC treatment; thus HdAC may have a role in the treatment of mature B-ALL,[192] pro-B-ALL,[159] and is also active in the treatment of overt CNS leukemia.[178] For other adult poor risk groups such as late responders, Ph+ ALL, or pre T-ALL the value of HdAC remains open.

The use of HdMTX has been extensively studied for the treatment of childhood ALL and to a lesser extent in adult ALL (reviewed in Ref. 97). HdMTX appears to be effective in preventing systemic and testicular relapses[87] and at higher doses treatment of CNS relapse.[13] In adult ALL studies HdMTX was used at dose levels ranging from 0.5 g/m^2 to 3 g/m^2. In these studies there is wide variation in outcome from 13 to 57 percent and again it is difficult to deduce what the contribution of HdMTX might be.[48,59,72,75,154,166,202,256] Most favorable results were again achieved in small studies with HdMTX as part of intensive multidrug consolidation regimens with LFS rates of 42 to 57 percent.[72,75,154]

With respect to the effectivity of HdMTX in subgroups of ALL it is established that it contributed significantly to the impressive improvement of cure rates for mature B-ALL. For other subtypes results from childhood ALL indicate effects in standard risk B-precursor ALL[162] but also in T-ALL.[220] For adult ALL this question remains open so far.

The use of HdAC as well as HdMTX as consolidation therapy was reported from six trials with LFS rates ranging between 21 and 47 percent.[11,137,155,164,165,253] The repeated application of treatment cycles including intensive D, A, HdAC, and HdMTX led to a high CR rate (92 percent) and improved LFS (47 percent at 5 years) as well, which was particularly evident in B-lineage ALL.[155] Overall there is some evidence that the inclusion of HdAC and HdMTX as part of multidrug consolidation treatment may improve overall results in adult ALL.

Maintenance Therapy

Maintenance therapy usually includes 6-mercaptopurine (MP) and MTX for a total duration of 2 years, a strategy transferred from childhood ALL. In many series it is combined with other drugs on a cyclic basis – mostly V and P (Table 18–7). There are, however, very few randomized trials giving information on the overall value of maintenance, the optimal drug combination, and the dosage and duration of treatment. One large multicenter study addressing this question in a randomized comparison

failed to demonstrate a benefit in terms of LFS for intensified (28 percent) versus conventional (27 percent) maintenance.[164] The duration of maintenance for 12 or 14 months in this study was probably too short to answer this question.

In contrast to reinforced maintenance, there were attempts to omit maintenance altogether after intensive induction and consolidation therapy. Overall these studies yielded inferior results despite intensive induction and the application of HdAC,[63,259] HdMTX,[60] or both[253] unless patients were referred to an early SCT. On the other hand, no large trial demonstrated a clear advantage for patients treated with intensive maintenance therapy.

With regard to subtypes of ALL it is established that maintenance therapy is not required in mature B-ALL. It remains open whether this also applies to other subtypes with rapid disease proliferation such as T-ALL. For common ALL it seems that in studies with intensive induction and consolidation therapy patients might benefit from reinforced maintenance when compared to those with a similarly intensive induction and consolidation but with a conventional approach using MTX and MP only. This might be explained by the low proliferation rate of common ALL blasts, which may prevent total eradication even during intensive induction and consolidation. Since the major aim of maintenance therapy is the eradication of residual disease, the upcoming evaluation of MRD will hopefully provide rational criteria for the decision on subgroup-specific indications, and intensity and duration of maintenance therapy in ALL.

Central Nervous System Therapy

Prophylactic CNS Therapy

Without some form of prophylactic CNS therapy around 30 percent (Table 18–8) of adults with ALL will develop overt CNS leukemia.[57,187] If only patients surviving more than 12 months were analyzed the rate of CNS recurrence even reached 50 percent.[149] In the only randomized prospective trial of prophylactic CNS therapy[257] a higher incidence of CNS relapse was seen in the group not receiving CNS therapy although no effect was detected on remission duration and survival. The importance of prophylactic CNS therapy is that CNS leukemia is more easily prevented than treated and that, once CNS leukemia has developed, it is generally followed by systemic relapse shortly after.

Several treatment options are available for prevention of CNS relapse: intrathecal (i.th.) therapy, cranial irradiation (CRT), and systemic high dose chemotherapy (overviews in Refs. 28 and 102). I.th. therapy is usually based on MTX as single drug but combinations with AC and/or steroids are used in some studies. The route of application is generally lumbar puncture. CRT (18 to 24 Gy in 12 fractions over 16 days) may be administered early during remission or delayed during consolidation with or without parallel i.th. therapy. Systemic HD chemotherapy may comprise HdAC or HdMTX since both drugs reach cytotoxic drug levels in the CSF and showed effectivity in overt CNS leukemia.

Various combinations of these approaches have been used in adult ALL trials but the issue of CNS prophylaxis has not been

Table 18–8. Rate of Isolated CNS and Combined CNS/BMT Relapses in Relation to CNS Prophylaxis in Adult ALL

	Intrathecal Therapy	Cranial Irradiation	High-Dose Chemotherapy	No. of Studies	No. of Patients	CNS Prophylaxis	Percent CNS Relapse Rates[a] (range)
Without CNS prophylaxis				2	107	None	31[a] (30–32)
One modality	X			3	440	IT-MTX, OM-MTX (± IT-DX)	13[a] (8–19)
			X	2	167	HdAC, HdMTX	14[a] (10–16)
Two Modalities	X	X		11	2215	24 Gy + IT-MTX (± IT-DX)	12[a] (5–26)
	X		X	11	1597	HdAC, HdMTX, IT-MTX (± IT-P, AC)	8 (0–12)
Three Modalities	X	X	X	7	662	HdAC, HdMTX, IT-MTX, 24 Gy	5 (0–12)

Abbreviations: OM, via Ommaya reservoir. For abbreviations of drug names, see Table 18–5.
[a] Weighted mean of CNS and combined CNS and BM relapses in relation to CR patients.

addressed prospectively. For analysis of published trials it has to be considered that most authors only report the frequency of isolated CNS relapses. However, in a significant proportion of adult ALL patients combined CNS and bone marrow relapses occur. Overall there is evidence that CNS relapse rates decrease with increasing intensity of prophylaxis and with the number of applied modalities (Table 18–8).

With i.th. therapy only CNS relapse rates of 8 to 19 percent have been reported.[51,130,156] There was, however, a wide variability of frequency and total number of i.th. applications. Particularly the early onset of i.th. therapy appears to be important.

The combination of i.th. therapy and CRT yielded CNS relapse rates of 5 to 26 percent. There is some evidence that early CRT after remission induction is superior to delayed CRT during consolidation treatment since trials with delayed CRT reported a higher CNS relapse rate of 12 to 26 percent.[71,114,146] A similar observation has been made in the GMALL trials.[96] High-dose chemotherapy (HDT) as sole CNS-directed treatment was used in only a few studies and apparently does not provide sufficient prophylaxis, with CNS relapse rates of 10 and 16 percent in two studies.[57,256] HDT, however, shows beneficial effects if combined with other modalities. Thus HDT combined with i.th. therapy led to CNS relapse rates of 0 to 12 percent and even lower CNS relapse rates were reported if in addition CRT was administered. The efficacy of intensified CNS prophylaxis was also demonstrated in a retrospective analysis from the M.D. Anderson Cancer Center, where the lowest CNS relapse rate (2 percent) was achieved in a recent trial with early HDT and i.th. therapy for all patients.[57] In recent series with combined modality CNS prophylaxis the CNS relapse rate was generally 5 percent or lower.[19,69,137,202,240]

The incidence of CNS relapse is influenced by several risk factors and ranged in a retrospective analysis between 4 and 54 percent after 1 year according to differing risk groups.[139] These risk factors include biological features such as immunophenotype (T-ALL, B-ALL), extreme leukocytosis, high leukemia cell proliferation rate, high serum LDH levels, and extramedullary organ involvement. Risk-adapted CNS prophylaxis may be based on these features.[57] This approach is, however, in contrast to childhood ALL, not widely used in adults, which may be due to the lower toxicity of CNS prophylaxis in adult patients.

Therapy of Established CNS Disease

About 5 to 10 percent of adult ALL patients present with manifestations of CNS leukemia. The incidence is correlated to the immunological subtype and is higher in T-ALL and mature B-ALL. Treatment of overt CNS leukemia is usually undertaken with either i.th. MTX alone, in combination with AC or hydrocortisone or with CRT. I.th. MTX is administered 2 to 3 times per week and continued over 2 or 3 weeks until two consecutive CSF examinations show no evidence of leukemic infiltration. Following the establishment of a remission there is some evidence that continued maintenance i.th. chemotherapy at less frequent intervals is beneficial in prolonging the duration of CNS remission. When adult ALL patients with CNS leukemia at diagnosis are treated adequately they have no inferior outcome with regard to LFS or CNS relapse rate.

Complications of CNS Therapy

The complications and toxicity of CNS therapy have been reviewed elsewhere.[28,196] In childhood ALL with a high rate of long-term survivors the side effects of CNS directed treatment have been investigated extensively and range from subclinical neurological sequelae to encephalopathy, neuropsychological and growth impairment, endocrine dysregulation, and brain tumors.[184] In adult ALL the neurological side effects particularly of CRT appear to be far less pronounced. Ten years after five applications of i.th. MTX and CRT in 17 long-term survivors of ALL only subclinical neurological sequelae were detected. Neurological symptoms and moderate brain atrophy were more pronounced in patients older than 30 years. Nevertheless all patients have been fully rehabilitated and returned to their normal occupational activities.[242]

CRT in adults rarely produces the somnolence syndrome found in children, which is due to a transient radiation encephalopathy and is generally self-limiting. Craniospinal irradiation may produce profound and prolonged bone marrow suppression, which may severely limit continued systemic therapy. I.th. chemotherapy may occasionally be complicated by infective meningitis, and the implantation of Ommaya reservoirs may be complicated by infection and hemorrhage. I.th.

MTX frequently causes meningeal irritation and chemical arachnoiditis, as may i.th. AC. The severity of the symptoms is variable and includes backache, headache, vomiting, fever, and leg pain. Steroids (either oral DX or intrathecal hydrocortisone) will largely prevent these symptoms. Care should be taken to use preservative-free MTX in Elliot's B solution or lactated Ringer's solution, as the use of other preparations may be responsible for some cases of arachnoiditis. More serious forms of MTX toxicity such as permanent disablement or even fatal leukoencephalopathy occur rarely.[83] The risk increases with intensity of CNS-directed treatment and particularly with the number of combined treatment modalities.[29,95] Thus in the GMALL studies leukoencephalopathy mainly ocurred in patients with intensively retreated CNS relapse.[100]

STEM CELL TRANSPLANTATION

SCT is an integral part of treatment strategy for adult ALL. Bone marrow and to an increasing extent peripheral blood are used as stem cell source. Which of the different SCT modalities, allogeneic (allo) SCT from sibling or matched unrelated donor (MUD), autologous (auto) SCT, or non-myeloablative SCT (NMSCT), is indicated, in which stage of the disease, and which might be superior is still a matter of controversy.

Allogeneic SCT

Adult ALL patients transplanted in first remission achieve an average survival of 50 percent (21 to 71 percent) at 5 years (Table 18–9). Thus overall survival after allo SCT is better than that achieved by chemotherapy. However, the results are influenced by selection of patients for SCT. The survival for similarly defined cohorts of first CR patients, adjusted for differences in the disease characteristics and the time to transplant, receiving either SCT (collected by the IBMTR) or chemotherapy (GMALL trials) were not significantly different with an LFS of

Table 18–9. Results of Stem Cell Transplantation in Adult ALL

	N	Percent Relapse Incidence	Percent LFS (range)
Allogeneic[a]			
CR1	1100	24	50 (21–71)
CR2	1019	48	34 (13–60)
Relapsed/refractory	216	75	18 (8–33)
Autologous[a]			
CR1	1369	51	42 (15–60)
CR2	258	70	24 (20–27)
Unrelated[56]			
CR1	64	9	32
CR2/3	16	8	17
Relapsed/refractory	47	31	5

[a] Summarized data (weighted means) from published studies.

38 percent for chemotherapy and 44 percent for SCT.[263] A similar comparison of IBMTR data and chemotherapy results of the Japan Adult Leukemia Study Group (JALSG) revealed a superior LFS for SCT only in patients younger than 30 years whereas in older patients no difference was detected – mainly due to the higher transplant-related mortality (TRM).[185] These studies and others have also shown that risk factors for relapse in first CR after chemotherapy or allo SCT are similar.

Evidence in favor of allo SCT – at least in subgroups of adult ALL – comes from randomized studies. Randomization is biological in these studies, which generally means that patients with a sibling donor receive allo SCT whereas others are treated with chemotherapy or auto SCT – sometimes compared in a randomized fashion (Table 18–10). In the first trial focusing on this issue allo SCT was scheduled for all patients below 40 years with sibling donor whereas the remaining patients were randomized (control group) to receive either auto SCT or chemotherapy.[82] The survival after allo SCT was significantly superior (46 percent) compared to the control group (31 percent). The advantage was, however, only evident in high risk (HR) patients with a survival of 37 percent after SCT compared to 15 percent in the control group. In standard risk (SR) ALL no significant difference was observed (46 vs. 42 percent).[80] In the ongoing ECOG/MRC trial a similar comparison is performed. In a preliminary analysis the LFS after 3 years was 58 percent for patients who actually received allo SCT compared to 39 percent for the control group. Allo SCT yielded superior LFS for HR (57 vs. 32 percent) and for SR (71 vs. 54 percent) ALL patients less than 60 years.[207] For this study an intent-to-treat analysis is awaited.

Allo SCT in second remission of adult ALL gives survival rates of 13 to 60 percent at 3 years or longer (Table 18–9) and it is undoubtedly superior to chemotherapy alone where the survival rate at 5 years is only 5 percent. Transplants in advanced, either refractory or relapsed ALL, result in 8 to 33 percent LFS at 3 years (Table 18–9). These results are clearly superior to those reported with chemotherapy where there are virtually no cures at this stage of the disease.

Beside reduction of TRM the still high relapse rate is the major problem in allo SCT. New approaches include the use of donor leukocyte infusions (DLI), new conditioning regimens, and exploration of non-myeloablative transplantation.

Graft-versus-leukemia (GvL) effects are less pronounced in ALL compared to AML or CML. There is, however, a lower relapse rate in patients with acute or chronic graft-versus-host disease (GvHD) compared to those without, indicating that GvL effects have a role in ALL as well.[203] In single patients with relapse after allo SCT, remission was achieved with DLI or interruption of GvHD prophylaxis. Overall DLI may be not be used in patients with overt relapse but preferably in patients with residual disease after allo SCT.

NMSCT is another approach to utilize GvL effects in ALL and may be a treatment alternative for older HR patients and for patients with contraindications for allo SCT such as fungal infection. In a pilot study of the GMALL group five of ten patients (mainly with Ph+ ALL) survived after primary NMSCT compared to 1 of 11 patients with NMSCT after

Table 18–10. Randomized Studies of Stem Cell Transplantation (SCT) in Adult ALL

Author	Year	N	CR Rate (percent)	Comparison	LFS (percent)	Subgroup Analysis (percent)	
					Overall: 27, 10 years	*High risk*	*Low risk*
Thiebaut et al.[234]	1993	572	76	Allo SCT for all pts with donor	46	44	49
				Auto SCT vs. chemo (control) (remaining pts incl. pts > 50 yrs)	34 vs. 29	10 vs. 16	49 vs. 40
Attal et al.[11]	1995	135	93	Allo SCT for all pts with donor	Overall: 38, 3 years 68		
				Auto SCT in remaining pts	26		
					Overall: n.r.	*High risk*	*Low risk*
Rowe et al.[207]	1999	920	89	Allo SCT for all pts with donor	58, 3 years	57	71
				Auto SCT vs chemo in remaining pts	39, 3 years	32	54

Abbreviations: allo, allogeneic; auto, autologous; chemo, chemotherapy; pts, patients.

relapse. Whether or not NMSCT offers a new option in the treatment of adult ALL remains to be answered in prospective studies.

The optimal conditioning regimens in ALL are still not defined. Further intensification of chemotherapy is limited due to the already high TRM. Targeted therapy with radiolabeled antibodies may be an alternative. In several studies antibodies such as anti-CD33, anti-CD45, anti-CD164b, and anti-CD22 have been conjugated to radioemitters such as ^{131}I, ^{99}Tc, and ^{90}Y in order to achieve an additional irradiation dose in the hematopoietic tissue. This treatment may be used as intensification before conventional conditioning regimens for allo SCT in ALL. Preliminary experience indicated that there is no excessive organ toxicity.[36] For this issue also further studies in larger patient cohorts are warranted.

Autologous SCT

Only one-third of potential transplant candidates will have an HLA-identical sibling donor. Furthermore older patients (>55 years) are generally not considered eligible for allo SCT. Therefore auto SCT is still of importance for the treatment of ALL particularly for HR patients. Auto SCT in first CR yields LFS rates of 42 percent with a wide range of 15 to 60 percent (Table 18–9). There is apparently no significant difference in LFS whether peripheral blood (PBSCT) (41 percent) or bone marrow (35 percent) is used as stem cell source. The differences in outcome in published studies may be related to several other factors (e.g., risk factors, median age, time point of auto SCT, previous chemotherapy, and transplantation-associated features such as purging or maintenance therapy after auto SCT).

Randomized comparisons of auto SCT and chemotherapy generally did not show an advantage for auto SCT (Table 18–10). In the above-mentioned French study the LFS after auto SCT was 34 percent compared to 29 percent for chemotherapy.[234] On the other hand an Italian trial reported an LFS of 36 percent for auto SCT compared to 17 percent for patients with chemotherapy alone.[19] In this study chemotherapy results were inferior compared to the majority of adult ALL trials.

Whereas TRM after auto SCT is low (<10 percent) the high relapse rate (51 percent) remains the major problem. Purging of bone marrow or peripheral blood controlled by measurement of MRD in the graft is one attempt to reduce tumor load and thereby the relapse risk. Two recent trials indicate a benefit of purging. In one study residual blasts in the graft could be reduced by median 1 log by purging, and a higher LFS (87 percent) was observed for patients with an MRD level less than 5 percent in the graft compared to those greater than 5 percent.[175] In another trial the LFS at 3 years was 52 percent for purged auto SCT compared to 13 percent for unpurged.[106] Similar findings with a reduction of MRD by 2–3 log were reported for Ph+ ALL.[10] Other attempts to improve outcome of auto SCT are intensified preparative regimens including double transplantation and maintenance therapy after auto SCT probably adjusted to MRD status.

AutoSCT in second remission ALL gives a survival rate of 24 percent (20 to 27 percent) (Table 18–9); these results also are more promising than those achieved in second remission ALL treated with chemotherapy.

Matched Unrelated SCT

For younger patients MUD SCT is increasingly employed if no sibling donor is available. From a recent retrospective analysis from 47 centers an LFS rate of 32 percent at 4 years was reported for 64 adult HR patients transplanted in CR1. MUD SCT had a strong antileukemic effect with a low relapse mortality of 9 percent probably due to more pronounced GvL effects. This was, however, outweighed by a high TRM (54 percent).[56] Despite this, MUD is a therapeutic option for adult HR patients in CR1. The major problem is the reduction of TRM. In the above-mentioned report Karnofsky index greater than 90 percent; HLA matching for A, B, and DRB1; CMV seronegativity; and shorter interval from diagnosis to SCT were associated with lower TRM.

In CR2/3 and in relapsed/refractory ALL the LFS was 17 percent and 5 percent, respectively, with TRM of 75 percent and 64 percent and still low relapse rates of 8 percent and 31 percent, respectively.[56]

Which SCT Modality in Which Disease Status?

There is agreement that allo or auto SCT is superior to chemotherapy for ALL in second remission or with advanced ALL. SCT may even be attempted in beginning relapse, partial remission, or aplasia. However, it is still controversial which adult ALL patients in first remission should have an SCT: none, HR only, or all, and whether it should be allo or auto SCT.

In HR patients there is evidence that allo SCT is superior to chemotherapy alone although optimal induction and consolidation before SCT, conditioning regimens, and age limits remain to be defined. In SR patients with cure rates greater than 50 percent after chemotherapy the decision is less clear and results of prospective trials have to be awaited. For evaluation of beneficial effects of allo SCT quality of life after transplantation has to be considered. Auto SCT offers the chance of shortened treatment and has a low TRM. Comparisons of auto SCT and chemotherapy are, however, not conclusive and particularly results for risk groups are lacking. Ongoing studies will hopefully help to answer this question. For patients with very high risk of relapse (i.e., Ph+ ALL) any type of SCT appears superior to chemotherapy with long-term LFS less than 10 percent.

PROGNOSTIC FACTORS

ALL is not a uniform disease but characterized by subgroups with different biological and clinical features and cure rates. For various parameters prognostic value for either the achievement of remission or for remission duration have been established in adult ALL.[92,125] At the present time the following are the most important prognostic features: age, initial WBC count, immunophenotype, abnormal cytogenetics or molecular genetics, and to an increasing extent response criteria such as time to achieve CR and MRD.

Morphology

Correlation of the L1 versus the L2 FAB morphology of ALL blast cells is not predictive for achievement of remission or survival. The L3 subtype is important for immediate suspicion of a mature B-ALL subtype and allocation for specific treatment but since the diagnosis of B-ALL requires confirmation by pheno-

typing, L3 morphology alone is no longer used as a prognostic parameter.

Immune Phenotype

There have been several reports on the role of immunophenotype as an independent prognostic variable.[61,91,107,110] However, with change in treatment strategies and improved results (e.g., for T-ALL and mature B-ALL, which formerly had a poor outcome) the prognostic impact of the immune phenotype has changed. Furthermore, other prognostic variables (e.g., Ph/BCR-ABL positive ALL in common ALL and Pre-B-ALL), influence the prognostic significance of the immune phenotype itself. Therefore, in recent trials there is a tendency not to use the immune phenotype as a prognostic factor but rather to adjust the treatment regimens to the subtypes. Table 18–11 summarizes the results for a large number of adult patients with different immunological subtypes of ALL collected from published studies.

T-ALL

T-ALL formerly had a poor outcome in children as well as in adults with CR rates of about 70 percent, an MRD of less than 10 months, and survival rates below 10 percent. Results for adult T-ALL have now improved to CR rates of greater than 80 percent and LFS of 46 percent (Table 18–11). Sufficient in vivo and in vitro evidence has accumulated that CP and AC, in addition to the usual cytostatic drugs for ALL, are mainly responsible for this improvement. The inclusion of AC and CP pulses during continuation therapy was beneficial in childhood T-ALL.[148] Also in adult ALL the combination of AC and CP added to the conventional drugs improved CR rate and LFS in T-ALL.[52,124] An increased CR rate and LFS for T-ALL was also observed in a CALGB study by adding CP to the conventional induction with V, P, DNR, and A[218] and in an Italian study by addition of a pre-phase treatment with CP.[22] In childhood ALL HDMTX,[78,219] HDAC,[6] and A[3] contributed to a better outcome of T-ALL. For adult T-ALL the possible benefit of these approaches remains open. In adult T-ALL very favorable results have also been reported for allo SCT.[11,207]

Within T-ALL several prognostic factors are of relevance. An increased WBC count – probably with a higher cut-point ($>100,000/\mu L$) compared to B-precursor ALL ($30,000/\mu L$) –

Table 18–11. Outcome of Immunological Subtypes in Adult ALL According to Treatment

Subtype	No. of Studies	No. of Patients	CR Rate (percent)	mrd (months)	LFS (percent)
Pro B-ALL	7	287	75 (71–85)		34 (10–55)
Pre-B/c-ALL	16	1497	82 (65–92)	22 (17–36)	34 (15–68)
B-ALL					
Conventional therapy	9	63	44 (0–67)		< 10
Short, intensive therapy	8	148	75 (62–81)		54 (20–71)
T-ALL					
Without AraC/C	5	58	72 (40–89)	9 (3–12)	< 10
With AraC/C	16	807	85 (61–97)	25 (11–NR)	46 (25–68)

Summarized data (weighted means) from published studies.

and late achievement of CR confer poorer prognosis. However these factors may be outweighed by the prognostic impact of immunological subtype. Thus the immature subtype early T-ALL (cyCD3+, CD2−) has probably a poorer prognosis.[42,235] In the GMALL trials the CR rates (90 vs. 71 percent) and the LFS (55 vs. 15 percent) were inferior for early T-ALL compared to thymic or mature T-ALL.[120] Recent data also indicate that mature T-ALL (sCD3+, CD1−) may be associated with poorer outcome. This was observed by the GMALL study group but also in childhood ALL.[199]

For optimal treatment of T-ALL some subgroup-specific issues have to be considered. Thus T-ALL patients often present with high WBC count, mediastinal tumor, and bear a higher risk of CNS relapse. Therefore, intensive CNS prophylaxis is mandatory. Mediastinal tumors mostly respond very well to chemotherapy and it remains open whether additional mediastinal irradiation (MRT) is required. In two earlier trials MRT was successfully administered after initial cell reduction by chemotherapy.[124] With more intensive chemotherapy the additional MRT increases toxicity, particularly neutropenia. Therefore, MRT should probably be restricted to patients with residual tumors after induction therapy. In order to avoid excessive hematological toxicity it should be directed to the remaining tumor mass and not to the initially involved field.

In recent studies the latest relapses for T-ALL occur at approximately 3 to 4 years. The optimal duration of treatment for T-ALL is as yet undefined as is also the value of a conventional maintenance therapy with MP and MTX, with or without reinforcements.

Common/Pre-B-ALL

Common ALL and Pre-B-ALL show no differences in terms of clinical characteristics and outcome. The LFS for this subtype has not changed very much in recent years and ranges between 25 and 35 percent with a few exceptions (Table 18–11). Patients relapse in most studies over a period of up to 5 to 6 years and a long follow-up is required to estimate cure rates. Prolonged and intensified maintenance may therefore have a role in this subtype. In childhood ALL favorable results were achieved with intensive use of HDMTX. It remains open whether this is feasible in adult ALL and leads to a similar improvement. There is also one study indicating that higher doses of an anthracycline (daunorubicin), given early in induction and reaching a certain cumulative amount may also improve the outcome for adult common ALL.[239]

Within common/Pre-B-ALL prognostic factors (WBC count, time to CR, cytogenetics, molecular genetics) help to identify patients with high risk of relapse being candidates for SCT in CR1. However, also patients without conventional risk factors show a continuous relapse rate and no significant improvement of overall results. Therefore, the evaluation of MRD seems to be of particular interest and in future trials treatment decisions may be based on MRD results.

Pro-B-ALL

Pro-B-ALL was formerly associated with unfavorable prognosis. In recent studies prognosis seems to be improved by intensive chemotherapy with an LFS approaching 50 percent in some studies (Table 18–11). HDAC and even more allo SCT appear to be efficient strategies.[159]

Mature B-ALL

In earlier studies, CR rates for adult B-ALL were low and LFS poor. In nine studies (Table 18–11) with a total of 63 patients the weighted mean CR rate was 44 percent and most patients relapsed rapidly, reflected by the median remission duration of 11 months and the very low survival rate.

Outcome was significantly improved with new strategies derived from childhood ALL studies in B-ALL and Burkitt's lymphoma.[179,222] In childhood B-ALL CR rates reach 81 to 96 percent and LFS rates of up to 78 percent are reported.[192,201] The drugs responsible for the improvement are fractionated CP in moderate doses, HDMTX (0.5 to 8 g/m^2), and HDAC. In the Berlin-Frankfurt-Münster (BFM) protocols, CR rates of 91 to 93 percent were obtained with moderate doses of CP or ifosphamide and HDMTX (0.5 to 5 g/m^2) but without HDAC.[201] In addition to CP, HDMTX, or HDAC, the regimens contain the cytostatic drugs ADM, AC, VM26, V, P, DNR, and VP16. When these childhood B-ALL protocols were transferred to adult patients with B-ALL, the results were also substantially improved. The CR rates now approach 70 percent and long-term survival rates of 40 to 50 percent or even higher can be achieved in adult B-ALL (Table 18–11).[122,150,236] Maintenance treatment has been omitted in B-ALL studies since relapses occur almost exclusively within the first year.

B-ALL has a higher CNS involvement rate at diagnosis and relapses often occur in the CNS. Therefore, effective measures against CNS disease, such as HDMTX and HDAC as well as i.th. therapy, are an important component of treatment regimens. The role of prophylactic CRT for prophylaxis of CNS and systemic relapse remains to be established.

Cytogenetics and Molecular Genetics

Chromosomal abnormalities and molecular aberrations are correlated with outcome in ALL independent of other features. The most important aberration for clinical practice is Ph/BCR-ABL positive (Ph+) ALL. For other aberrations such as t(4;11), 7−, 9+, and hypodiploid karyotype inferior outcome has been reported by single studies.[46,224,255] On the other hand, hyperdiploid karyotype (without additional structural aberrations) and the TEL-AML1 aberration was associated with better outcome in childhood ALL. In adults the incidence of these aberrations is low and a prognostic impact could not be demonstrated so far. Furthermore, several aberrations are associated with distinct subtypes such as t(10;14) in T-ALL and t(4;11) in Pro-B-ALL and outcome may be related to the subtype rather to the cytogenetic aberrations. Also t(8;14) in mature B-ALL has lost its prognostic impact with improved results in patients with mature B-ALL and Burkitt's lymphoma. In addition, outcome for specific aberrations shows a large variability in published studies, indicating that treatment procedure has an important role. Therefore, definitions of prognostic factors according to cytogenetics results in larger uniformly treated patient cohorts are awaited.

The prognostic value of molecular aberrations remains open as well since it was only evaluated retrospectively in small cohorts. This applies for homozygotous deletions of the *p16* tumor suppressor gene, which is detected in 20 to 40 percent of adult and childhood ALL.[76,172,210] and mutations of the tumor suppressor gene *p53*, which have an incidence less than 10 percent in ALL and may have prognostic impact in T-ALL.[65]

Philadelphia Chromosome/*BCR-ABL*-Positive ALL

Ph/*BCR-ABL*-positive (Ph+) ALL is the subgroup of ALL having the worst prognosis in children as well as in adults. In 21 studies with a total of 721 patients the weighted mean CR rate was 69 percent (Table 18–12). The median remission duration in all series is short (5 to 44 months) and the survival rate, from 0 to 30 percent at 2 to 5 years, is extremely poor in all reports. This unsatisfactory outcome for Ph+ ALL is the major challenge in adult ALL where Ph+ ALL constitutes 20 to 30 percent of de novo ALL and more than 50 percent of all relapsed patients.

Although the CR rate appears to be increasing in recent trials there is no significant improvement by conventional chemotherapy even if cycles with HDAC or HDMTX are included. The approach to use biological response modifiers, such as α-interferon or interleukin-2, was initially encouraging[111,186] but has not fulfilled its promise. The overall outcome in terms of median remission duration may show a slight improvement due to the more frequent incorporation of SCT in all ongoing studies for this subgroup.

The main option for treatment of Ph+ ALL is SCT. From the latest series with 33, 17, and 24 patients, respectively, LFS rates of 38, 46, and 65 percent were reported.[14,45,225] In multicenter studies results of allo SCT appear to be somewhat lower. The results for auto SCT are inferior but it has to be considered that the patient population is generally older. The largest series with 23 patients showed an LFS of 25 percent at more than 2 years.[169] In this study it could also be demonstrated that purging with immunomagnetic beads and antibodies reduced the tumor load in stem cell grafts by 2 to 3 logs. Furthermore it was shown that the content of *bcr-abl* positive cells is significantly lower in peripheral stem cell compared to bone marrow grafts.[10] As discussed previously MUD SCT is a valuable treatment option for Ph+ ALL patients without a sibling donor.

Abl-tyrosine kinase inhibitor STI571. The *BCR-ABL* fusion gene leads to an upregulation of tyrosine kinase (TK) activity, which plays a crucial role in pathogenesis and disease progression of *BCR-ABL*-positive leukemias. With a selective inhibitor of the Abl-tyrosine kinase (STI571) cellular proliferation of *BCR-ABL*-positive CML and ALL cells can be inhibited selectively.[67] Promising results have also been achieved in a Phase II study in heavily pretreated patients with relapsed or refractory Ph+ ALL with hematological response in 19 out of 32 patients.[189] Clinical responses were correlated to MRD levels in bone marrow and peripheral blood.[217] Thus quantitative PCR provides an option for continuous monitoring of the therapeutic effects of STI571. Oral treatment with STI571 is also generally well tolerated and feasible in elderly patients. Based on these promising results Phase II studies in patients with de novo Ph+ ALL have been started. Several approaches such as treatment with STI571 in patients with MRD after induction therapy or after BMT or parallel to induction chemotherapy will be evaluated. This new treatment option may contribute to an improved outcome in elderly Ph/*BCR-ABL*+ ALL patients not eligible for

Table 18–12. Treatment Results for Adult Ph/*bcr-abl* Positive ALL

Author	Year	Ref.	N	CR rate (percent)	mrd (months)	3-year Survival (percent)
Gaynor	1988	92	18	72	7	0
Bloomfield	1990	30	18	44	10	< 10
Ohyashiki et al.	1991	186	7	71	9	n.r.
Cuttner	1991	60	12	75	10	
Secker-Walker	1991	223	22	64	7	15
Linker	1991	154	10	70	11	0
Westbrook	1992	254	17	71	10	n.r.
Götz	1992	105	25	76	9	6
Cassileth et al.	1992	43	12	58	5	n.r.
Hoelzer	1993	127	103	75	9	10
Mandelli	1993	163	29	76	11	16
Preti	1994	197	41	56		10
Stryckmans et al.	1994	228	19	68		16
Fière	1993	82	58	57		11
Scherrer et al.	1994	215	7	86	18	0
Larson et al.	1995	146	30	70	9	0
Charrin et al.	1996	46	127	59	5	0
Stryckmans et al.	1997	229	125	78		30
Annino et al.	1998	4	12	100	44	n.r.
Faderl et al.	1998	77	29	90	11	n.r.
Weighted mean			721	69	7	11

SCT but also to a reduced relapse rate after SCT in younger patients.

Advanced Age

Treatment results in elderly patients with ALL are worse with regard to a lower CR rate, shorter remission duration, and survival.[118,193] There is no definite age limit but in most studies ALL patients above 50 or 60 years fare worse. Although in children the CR rate approaches 95 percent, there is a continuous decline in CR rate from 80 to 90 percent for adolescents, down to CR rates of 60 to 35 percent or even less for patients older than 60 years.

The median survival time in older ALL patients is 3 to 14 months[16,64,79,151,232] with an LFS less than 10 percent.[64,71] There are several reasons that may account for this. Increased hematological and nonhematological toxicity (e.g., hepato- and cardiotoxicity) results in a higher morbidity and mortality during induction therapy. The death rate during induction therapy for elderly patients reaches 20 to 30 percent.[151] Incomplete drug administration and extended intervals between cycles of therapy may lead to inferior long-term results. For example, in an early GMALL trial the median remission duration for patients receiving only two-thirds of the proposed treatment was 8.7 months compared to 14.8 months for patients who received the full treatment.[123] There is a higher frequency of adverse biological features in adults; thus the incidence of Ph+ ALL patients increases from 3 percent in children to 20 to 30 percent in patients above 50 years.[223] The incidence of unfavorable immunophenotypes such as early T-ALL and Pro-B-ALL is also higher in older patients.[104] There is, however, no good evidence that within an identical biological subtype of ALL the leukemic blast cells in elderly ALL patients are more resistant than in younger patients.

The optimal treatment for older ALL patients remains to be defined. Palliative treatment only yields a short survival.[119] Mild induction therapy (V, P) yielded a remission rate of 53 percent in a retrospective analysis compared to 77 percent with more intensive chemotherapy (V,P,A,D). Survival after 3 years was less than 10 percent for both treatment arms.[79] However, few studies have evaluated treatment of elderly ALL patients prospectively. In one study with a moderate induction and outpatient postremission therapy only 3 of 22 patients older than 60 years achieved long-term survival. Median survival was significantly higher in CR patients (12 months) compared to patients with treatment failure (1 month).[16] In four consecutive GMALL studies continuous remission rate for older ALL patients (50 to 65 years) could be improved from 19 to 32 percent after 6 years. There was a beneficial effect of mild consolidation therapy with VM26 and AC but not of high-dose consolidation therapy with HdAC (1 g/m²).[119] In patients older than 65 years the CR rate was 50 percent with a survival of CR patients of 22 percent (median 17 months) after 2 years. There was a significantly better outcome for patients with common/Pre-B-ALL with WBC count less than 30,000 or Pro-B-ALL compared to common/pre-B-ALL with WBC count greater than 30,000 or Ph/*BCR-ABL*.[101]

Considering the poor results for elderly ALL patients, intensification of induction and consolidation therapy must be carefully weighed against the possible disadvantages of toxicity, mortality, and quality of life. The attempt to achieve a remission should be made whenever possible. Particularly in older patients with good clinical condition a curative approach should be followed with dose-reduced regimens omitting drugs such as A, prolonged steroid treatment, and others known to have increased toxicity in older patients. Results indicate that prognostic factors are also valid in the older patient population. Since an improvement is not possible by intensification of chemotherapy, other nonchemotherapy approaches such as antibody treatment, NMSCT, or STI571 are of particular interest.

WBC Count

A high WBC count at presentation adversely influenced the CR rate in only a few studies. It has, however, an adverse impact on remission duration in the majority of trials. Fewer long-term survivors are found among patients with a markedly elevated WBC count at diagnosis.[18,63,71,82,125,146,147,215] The limits are set continuously from a WBC count of 10 to 100×10^9/L. In recent adult series, the critical level was 25 to 35×10^9/L, a limit similar to that in childhood ALL. In T-ALL the prognostic value of increased WBC count and the relevant cut-point is not clear.

Response to Treatment

The time to achieve CR is inversely related to remission duration. In childhood ALL even prednisone response on day 7 is an important predictor for LFS.[221] Adult ALL patients not remitting within 4 or 5 weeks also fare poorly. In the first GMALL study, the median remission duration was 31 months in the 220 patients achieving CR within 4 weeks, compared with only 10 months in 52 patients requiring more than 4 weeks.[123] There was a clear difference in long-term outcome with CCR rates of 42 percent and 23 percent, respectively. Similar observations have been reported by others.

Minimal Residual Disease

With molecular methods for evaluation of MRD (see CLASSIFICATION, Detection of Minimal Residual Disease) it is now possible not only to perform quantitative evaluation of response but also MRD follow-up analysis after achievement of CR and to evaluate thereby individual response to chemotherapy. Mainly in childhood ALL it was demonstrated that MRD level after induction therapy but also during course of chemotherapy is a strong and independent predictor of relapse risk. The majority of MRD analyses were based on measurement of IgH and TCR rearrangements[44,191,244] but similar results were reported with a somewhat lower sensitivity for flow cytometry analysis of MRD.[50,58,108] The few results of MRD evaluation in adult ALL generally confirm those in childhood ALL.[34,35,85,168]

In the future MRD evaluation may have several consequences for treatment and risk stratification in adult ALL (Table 18–13).

Table 18–13. Prognostic Value of MRD at Different Time Points

Time Point	MRD Level	Relapse Risk (percent)
After induction	High ($> 10^{-3}$)	High (50–90)
	Negative ($< 10^{-4}$)	Low (~ 10)
	Intermediate (10^{-4}–10^{-3})	Open
During consoli-dation (1st year)	Continuously high ($> 10^{-4}$)	High (> 70)
	Decreasing/negative ($< 10^{-4}$)	Low (~ 10?)
	Fluctuating	Open
	Increase by 2 log	Beginning relapse?

Redefinition of Complete Remission

In addition to conventional cytological criteria molecular remission status can be assessed. Nearly 50 percent of ALL patients remain MRD positive after induction therapy despite clinical and cytological CR and in nearly all patients with Ph+ ALL the BCR-ABL transcript remains detectable. Prospective studies are now required to assess whether patients with molecular failure need early intensification (e.g., by SCT) and which cut-points of MRD are relevant.

Risk Classification

The individual course of MRD is a new, important prognostic factor. Essentially two features can be considered for risk stratification according to MRD:

MRD after induction therapy. High MRD levels after induction therapy are associated with poor prognosis since a stable remission is not achieved. The relapse risk for patients with MRD greater than 10^{-3} ranges between 55 and 93 percent.[33,34,44,132,244,247]

On the other hand in MRD negative patients or patients with low MRD ($< 10^{-3}$ to 10^{-5}) a low relapse risk can be expected. In childhood ALL around 10 percent of patients relapse although MRD is not detected.[44,109,132,244] Since these were mainly retrospective analyses they apply to patients in whom standard chemotherapy was continued. So far no outcome data are available for MRD negative patients in whom treatment was stopped. The consequences of intermediate MRD levels after induction therapy are less clear and need to be defined in prospective studies.

Course of MRD during postremission period. There is sufficient evidence that the predictive value of MRD even increases at later time points. Thus relapse patients generally showed continuously high MRD levels ($>10^{-3}$ to 10^{-4}) during consolidation and maintenance therapy.[44,58,85,181,182,244] If MRD analysis is performed regularly a rapid increase of MRD may herald relapse.

In contrast patients with continuous complete remission show a continuous decrease of MRD and achieve negative MRD status.[44,244] The MRD status at 12 months appeared to be highly discriminative with a relapse rate of 9 percent in MRD negative compared to 86 percent in MRD positive childhood ALL patients.[244] In adult ALL a lower rate of molecular remission, a

generally higher MRD level, slower decrease, and a higher overall relapse rate can be expected.

In one study in adult ALL no relation between relapse risk and MRD level was demonstrated for time points during the first 2 months after diagnosis. Prognostic significance increased at later time points and was highest after 12 to 24 months.[168] A GMALL pilot study demonstrated that the predictive value of MRD in adult ALL is higher if several time points are combined. MRD levels greater than 10^{-4} at 1 or more time points after induction therapy were associated with a significantly higher relapse rate of 73 percent compared to 13 percent in patients with MRD less than 10^{-4} at all time points.[35]

There are, however, exceptions for example, patients with detectable MRD remaining in long-term remission and patients without detectable MRD relapsing (e.g., due to clonal evolution of leukemic blasts, insufficient sensitivity, or extramedullary relapse localization). Repeated confirmation of negative results, analysis of a second marker, and a sufficient sensitivity level ($<10^{-4}$) is therefore required. Furthermore, the ideal time point and the most predictive MRD level remain to be defined and it is open whether subgroup-specific differences have to be taken into account. MRD-based risk factors will most probably be included in risk models based on "conventional" prognostic factors.

MRD Adapted Treatment

New treatment regimens could be based on MRD and lead to individual treatment decisions. Patients with repeatedly negative MRD results have a high probability of cure and treatment could be stopped (e.g., after 1 year) in order to avoid undue toxicity and discomfort. In patients with persisting MRD despite intensive induction and consolidation therapy further treatment (e.g. SCT) or experimental treatment approaches could be considered. Further prospective studies are required in adult ALL to define comprehensive criteria for MRD-based treatment decisions.

Evaluation of Single Treatment Elements

MRD may serve for evaluation of effectivity of single treatment elements such as new consolidation cycles, SCT, purging, etc. As described before purging efficacy in bcr-abl-positive ALL has already been evaluated by quantitative PCR measurement of bcr-abl transcripts.[10] It was also demonstrated that the MRD level before and after SCT is associated with relapse risk.[144] Consolidation cycles, immunotherapy, or DLI are interesting options for MRD evaluation as well.

Other Prognostic Factors

For several other features poor prognostic impact has been reported, such as high LDH, organ involvement at presentation such as extensive lymphadenopathy, hepatomegaly, splenomegaly, CNS leukemia or mediastinal involvement, the number of immature cells in the peripheral blood, low platelet count at diagnosis, elevated serum glutamic oxalacetic transaminase levels, weight loss, and male gender. It remains open whether these features still have prognostic relevance with con-

Table 18–14. Adverse Prognostic Factors In Adult ALL

High white blood cell count	• > 30,000/μl in B-precursor ALL
Immunological subtype	• Pro B-ALL • Early T-ALL, mature T-ALL
Karyotype/molecular genetics	• t(9;22)/*BCR-ABL* • t(4;11)/*ALL1-AF4*
Treatment response	• Achievement of CR > 2 to 4 weeks • High level and course of MRD after induction therapy

temporary treatment regimens and furthermore in which subtypes they may have a role. This applies also for the prognostic impact of myeloid antigen expression particularly since it is often associated with specific subtypes such as immature Pro-B and T-ALL or Ph+ ALL.

Stratification Into Risk Groups

Prognostic factors for remission duration can identify standard-risk and high-risk patients in adult ALL. In the majority of adult ALL trials there is agreement on the following poor risk features: age, time to achieve CR, initial WBC count, cytogenetic and molecular aberrations (Ph/BCR-ABL, t(4;11)/ALL1-AF4). Immunophenotypes such as Pro-B-ALL and early T-ALL and MRD have recently emerged as prognostic features. Table 18–14 summarizes the current risk model of the GMALL trials.

Standard-risk patients without any adverse features have an LFS of more than 50 percent beyond 5 years compared to less than 30 percent for high-risk patients. In several study groups prognostic factors are used for allocation of patients to risk-group-specific regimens (e.g., short intensive treatment protocols for mature B-ALL) and development of new subgroup-adjusted treatment regimens. Furthermore, decisions on treatment intensity – particularly indications for SCT – are often based on risk stratification.

RELAPSED ALL

Relapse Time and Sites

More than half the adult patients with ALL will relapse despite treatment. The overall relapse rate is highest within the first 2 years and continues thereafter with a lower probability. Relapse patterns seem to depend on immunophenotype. The relapse probability becomes very low for common ALL after 5 to 6 years, for T-ALL after 3 to 4 years, and for B-ALL after 1 year.

Approximately 80 percent of all relapses occur in the bone marrow and the remainder in extramedullary sites, predominantly the CNS. Other extramedullary relapses, such as in lymph nodes, skin, or other organ sites, comprise less than 3 to 5 percent in adult ALL series. Relapses in the mediastinum are rare, even in those patients with initial mediastinal involvement. Testicular relapse rate in adult ALL (<1 percent) could be underestimated since it might not be as carefully and closely controlled as in male children. Patients with isolated extramedullary relapse are at high risk for subsequent hematological relapse and require local treatment followed by systemic reinduction therapy.

Therapy of Relapsed and Resistant Leukemia

Patients who fail to achieve CR and those who subsequently relapse have been treated with a wide variety of different protocols (Table 18–15) (summarized in Refs. 17 and 250). Repetition of initially effective induction therapy (e.g., with V,P,D,A) is still an option particularly for patients with late relapse and yielded remission rates of 52 percent (29 to 69 percent) (Table 18–15). In earlier studies the sequential administration of HdMTX and A was based on pharmacological studies demonstrating both synergism between the two drugs and modulation of MTX toxicity by A. The relatively high CR rate of 56 percent (33 to 80 percent) indicates that pretreatment may have been less intensive formerly. Other combinations of two drugs such as VM26 or VP16 yielded CR rates less than 30 percent.

The most frequent drug in the treatment of refractory or relapsed adult ALL is HdAC alone or in combination with A, m-AMSA, idarubicin, Miantrone, or recently fludarabine (Table 18–15). With these combinations remission rates around 50 to 60 percent were achieved. Again wide variations reflect the intensity of pretreatment and patient selection. Thus for selection of salvage therapy beside pretreatment, duration of previous remission, age, and further treatment options (e.g., donor availability) should be considered.

Overall the median remission duration after any of these treatments is only 2 to 6 months and long-term LFS is only obtained in less than 5 percent. In relapsed ALL SCT offers the only chance of cure with LFS rates of 34 percent for allo SCT in second CR, 24 percent for auto, and 17 percent in a small group of MUD SCT (Table 18–9). Also for SCT new treatment options are required to reduce the high relapse rate after SCT in second CR.

FUTURE PROSPECTS

Future improvement of treatment results in adult ALL may in part be achieved by optimization of conventional treatment approaches such as chemotherapy, SCT, and supportive care. This includes evaluation of new prognostic factors such as MRD. More importantly, however, new approaches are required for further development of individualized, subgroup-specific treatment for ALL.[121] The following options may be included in this concept.

Subgroup-Adjusted Treatment

Major improvement has already been achieved with treatment concepts adjusted to subtypes of ALL such as T-ALL and mature B-ALL. Further refinement by inclusion of additional drugs with specific activity seems possible such as HDAC in Pro-B-ALL; HdMTX and MP in B-precursor ALL; C, AC, and

Table 18–15. Results of Combination Chemotherapy for Refractory/Relapsed Adult ALL

Author	Year	Ref.	Drugs	N	CR Rate (percent)	Median Remission Duration (months)
Conventional induction						
Woodruff	1979	261	V,P,D,A	23	69	2
Elias	1979	70	V,P,D	10	50	3.8
Bostrum	1987	32	V,P,D,A	40	65	6
Paciucci	1987	190	V,P,Mi	14	57	5.5
Gaynor	1988	92	L2–L17	73	52	n.r.
Kantarjian	1990	138	V, AD, DX	64	38	2
Thomas	1997	237	I,IFO,DX	24	29	n.r.
Koller	1997	145	V,AD,DX,C	66	44	12
Freund	1997	88	VD,D,P,A	67	67	7
				381	52	
VM + other						
Carella	1984	41	VM, AC	12	42	n.r.
Sanz	1986	214	VM, AC	19	42	n.r.
Ryan	1987	211	VM, IFO	48	16	n.r.
				79	26	
VP + other						
Morra	1984	177	VP, AC	15	27	4.5
Rowe	1989	206	VP, ACL	12	25	n.r.
Bernasconi	1989	26	VP, AC	18	33	4.5
				45	29	
MTX/A						
Capizzi	1977	39	MTX,A	10	80	
Lobel	1979	157	MTX,A	2	33	7
Yap	1981	262	MTX,A	26	58	4.3
				48	56	
MTX/A ± other						
Yap	1981	262	MTX,A,IFO	11	55	3.5 +
Esterhay	1982	74	MTX,A,V,DX	14	70	7.5
Terebelo	1986	233	MTX,A,V,P	36	25	5
Aguaya	1999	1	MTX, PEG-A, V, P	32	22	4
				93	34	
HDAC/A						
Jones	1977	134	HdAC,A	5	20	n.r.
Amadori	1984	2	HdAC,A	10	30	4.5
Capizzi	1984	40	HdAC,A	10	30	8
Wells	1985	251	HdAC,A	22	45	2
				47	36	
HDAC/AMSA±other						
Zittoun	1985	264	HdAC, AM	14	21	
Peters	1987	194	HdAC, AM,P,VP	13	77	
Arlin	1988	9	HdAC, AM	40	72	4
Stryckmans	1987	227	HdAC, AM	4	50	n.r.
Marit	1990	167	HdAC, AM	7	43	2
				78	60	
HDAC/Ida						
Berman	1989	25	HdAC,I	11	18	
Petti	1989	195	HdAC,I	32	50	
Arcese	1991	5	HdAC,I	168	64	2.5
Giona	1992	94	HdAC,I	61	51	4
Freund	1997	88	HdAC,I	27	44	n.r.
Weiss	1998	249	HdAC,I	18	44	
				317	56	
HDAC + VP ± other						
Gore	1989	98	HdAC,VP	18	56	3.5
Milpied	1990	174	HdAC,VP,Mi,P	43	70	3
Bigman	1993	27	HdAC, VP, Mi	17	76	n.r.
Mazza	1996	171	HdAC, VP, Mi	38	17	2
				116	51	

(continued)

Table 18–15. *(Continued)*

Author	Year	Ref.	Drugs	N	CR Rate (percent)	Median Remission Duration (months)
HDAC + other						
Arlin	1991	8	HdAC,Mi,V,P,A	10	80	3
Freund	1991	89	HdAC,VD,D,A,VP	56	60	3
Martino	1999	170	IdAC,VD,Mi,C,P,MTX	45	74	4.6
				111	68	
HDAC + Mi						
Hiddemann	1990	116	HdAC,Mi	24	50	3.5
Lejeune	1990	152	HdAC,Mi	20	50	6
Rozmylowicz	1990	208	HdAC,Mi	18	33	3
Rubio-Borja	1992	209	HdAC,Mi	27	63	3.5
Kantarjian	1992	136	HdAC,Mi	34	36	7
Weiss	1996	248	HdAC,HdMi	37	84	n.r.
Kern	1997	143	sHdAC,Mi	4	75	n.r.
Koller	1997	145	HdAC, Mi	63	38	7
Thomas	1999	238	HdAC,Mi	20	55	7
Rosen	2000	205	HdAC, Mi	31	23	n.r.
				278	48	
HDAC/Flu±other						
Suki	1993	231	FLU, HdAC	30	30	n.r.
Visani	1996	246	FLU, HdAC	13	67	n.r.
Montillo	1997	176	FLU, HdAC	12	83	n.r.
Koller	1997	145	FLU,HdAC,Mi	5	40	
Virchis	1999	245	FLU, HdAC	7	43	n.r.
Virchis	1999	245	FLU, HdAC, IDA	20	55	n.r.
				87	50	

For abbreviations of drug names, see Table 18–5. IFO, ifosfamide; PEG-A, polyethylene-glycol-conjugated A; ACL, aclacinomycin.

A in T-ALL; and HdAC together with HdMTX in mature B-ALL.

Treatment Regimens Adapted to MRD

Evaluation of MRD offers the possibility to evaluate treatment response in individual patients independent of predefined "conventional" prognostic factors. Thereby treatment intensity and duration may be adapted to individual course of disease avoiding undue toxicity in patients with good response and offering optimal treatment intensity to patients with poor response.

Stem Cell Transplantation

Age limits and indications for SCT are extended continuously. Improvement of antileukemic activity of conditioning regimens as well as approaches for induction of GvL effects such as DLI and minitransplants may be promising.

Molecular Targeting

Molecular targeting with STI571 has been successfully developed for treatment of CML and Ph+ ALL. It cannot be expected that single drug treatment yields optimal results. Ongoing studies evaluate the combination of STI571 with chemotherapy (parallel or cyclic) in Ph+ ALL patients in first CR and in the future new combination regimens (e.g., with farnesyl transferase inhibitors) may be developed.

Drug Resistance

Data on mechanisms and modulation of drug resistance in adult ALL are still scarce. Although resistance to important antileukemic drugs – as measured by in vitro assays – is clearly associated with inferior outcome,[140] these findings are not translated in therapeutic procedures. Drug resistance profiles may be included in prognostic models in the future and may also serve for selection of active cytostatic drugs in relapse treatment.

The data on the role of multidrug resistance measured by expression of MDR-1, MRP, and others are inconclusive in ALL. However, a recent report based on 279 prospectively studied adult ALL patients indicated that MDR1 overexpression is found in 25 percent of the cases and that it was associated with a lower remission rate and shorter LFS. Thus it seems reasonable to evaluate drugs circumventing MDR such as idarubicin and to explore drug resistance modifiers such as PSC833.

Drug Pharmacokinetics

Evaluation of pharmacokinetics and pharmacogenomics of cytostatic drugs in adult ALL may contribute to the development of individualized treatment strategies with higher efficacy and lower toxicity.

Immunotherapy

Immunotherapy with monoclonal antibodies directed to ALL-specific surface antigens offers new treatment options with low toxicity and acts specifically in subtypes of ALL. Thus more than 70 percent of patients with mature B-ALL are CD20-positive. Treatment with anti-CD20 may therefore be included in treatment of mature B-ALL and Burkitt's lymphoma. Also other subtypes of ALL express a variety of antigens such as CD22, CD52, CD3, CD19, and others that may be targeted by specific antibodies. Immunotherapy is particularly promising if administered in combination with chemotherapy (e.g., in mature B-ALL) in CR patients with persistent MRD, in elderly patients with limited tolerance to chemotherapy, and finally in patients who are not eligible for intensive chemotherapy (e.g., due to previous complications).

REFERENCES

1. Aguayo A, Cortes J, Thomas D, Pierce S, Keating M, Kantarjian H: Combination therapy with methotrexate, vincristine, polyethylene-glycol conjugated-asparaginase, and prednisone in the treatment of patients with refractory or recurrent acute lymphoblastic leukemia. Cancer 86:1203–1209, 1999.

2. Amadori S, Papa G, Avvisati G, Fenu S, Monarca B, Petti MC et al: Sequential combination of high dose ARA-C (HiDAC) and asparaginase (ASP) for the treatment of advanced acute leukemia and lymphoma. Leuk Res 8:729–735, 1984.

3. Amylon MD, Shuster J, Pullen J, Berard C, Link MP, Wharam M et al: Intensive high-dose asparaginase consolidation improves survival for pediatric patients with T cell acute lymphoblastic leukemia and advanced stage lymphoblastic lymphoma: A Pediatric Oncology Group study. Leukemia 13:335–342, 1999.

4. Annino L, Elia M, Lamanda A et al: Clinical relevance of BCR/ABL and ALL1/AF4 molecular markers in adult acute lymphoblastic leukaemia (ALL). A retrospective study. Br J Haematol 102:(Abstract), 1998.

5. Arcese W, Meloni G, Giona F et al: Idarubicin plus ARA-C followed by allogeneic or autologous bone marrow transplantation in advanced acute lymphoblastic leukemia in adults. Bone Marrow Transplant 2:38a, 1991.

6. Arico M, Basso G, Mandelli F, Rizzari C, Colella R, Barisone E et al: Good steroid response in vivo predicts a favourable outcome in children with T-cell acute lymphoblastic leukemia. Cancer 75:1684–1693, 1995.

7. Arlin Z, Feldman E, Finger LR et al: Short course high dose mitoxantrone with high dose cytarabine is effective therapy for adult lymphoblastic leukemia. Leukemia 5:712, 1991.

8. Arlin Z, Feldman E, Mittelman A, Ahmed T, Cook P, Puccio C et al: High dose short course mitoxantrone (M) with high dose cytarabine (HiDac) is safe effective therapy for acute lymphoblastic leukemia (ALL). Proc ASCO 10:223, 1991.

9. Arlin ZA, Feldman E, Kempin S, Ahmed T, Mittelman A, Savona S et al: Amsacrine with high-dose cytarabine is highly effective therapy for refractory and relapsed acute lymphoblastic leukemia in adults. Blood 72:433–435, 1988.

10. Atta J, Fauth F, Keysen M, Petershofen E, Weber C, Lippok G, Hoelzer D, Martin H: Purging in BCR-ABL-positive acute lymphoblastic leukemia using immunomagnetic beads: Comparison of residual leukemia and purging efficiency in bone marrow vs peripheral blood stem cells by semiquantitative polymerase chain reaction. Bone Marrow Transplant 25:97–104, 2000.

11. Attal M, Blaise D, Marit G, Payen C, Michallet M, Vernant J-P et al: Consolidation treatment of adult acute lymphoblastic leukemia: A prospective, randomized trial comparing allogeneic versus autologous bone marrow transplantation and testing the impact of recombinant interleukin-2 after autologous bone marrow transplantation. Blood 86:1619–1628, 1995.

12. Balis FM, Lester CM, Chrousos GP et al: Differences in cerebrospinal fluid penetration of corticosteroids: Possible relationship to the prevention of meningeal leukemia. J Clin Oncol 5:202–207, 1987.

13. Balis FM, Savitch JL, Bleyer WA et al: Remission induction of meningeal leukemia with high-dose intravenous methotrexate. J Clin Oncol 3:485, 1985.

14. Barrett AJ, Horowitz MM, Ash RC, Atkinson K, Gale RP, Goldman JM et al: Bone marrow transplantation for Philadelphia chromosome-positive acute lymphoblastic leukemia. Blood 79(11):3067–3070, 1992.

15. Bassan R, Battista R, Rohatiner AZS, Love S, Carter M, Buelli M et al: Treatment of adult acute lymphoblastic leukaemia (ALL) over a 16 year period. Leukemia 6(Suppl. 2):186–190, 1992.

16. Bassan R, Di Bona E, Lerede T, Pogliani E, Rossi G, D'Emilio A et al: Age-adapted moderate-dose induction and flexible outpatient postremission therapy for elderly patients with acute lymphoblastic leukemia. Leuk Lymphoma 22:295–301, 1996.

17. Bassan R, Lerede T, Barbui T: Strategies for the treatment of recurrent acute lymphoblastic leukemia in adults. Haematologica 81:20–36, 1996.

18. Bassan R, Lerede T, Di Bona E, Rambaldi A, Rossi G, Pogliani E et al: Induction-consolidation with an idarubicin-containing regimen, unpurged marrow autograft, and post-graft chemotherapy in adult acute lymphoblastic leukaemia. Br J Haematol 104:755–762, 1999.

19. Bassan R, Lerede T, Di Bona E, Rambaldi A, Rossi G, Pogliani E et al: Induction-consolidation with an idarubicin-containing regimen, unpurged marrow autograft, and post-graft chemotherapy in adult acute lymphoblastic leukaemia. Br J Haematol 104:755–762, 1999.

20. Bassan R, Lerede T, Rambaldi A, DiBona E, Rossi G, Pogliani E et al: The role of anthracyclines in adult acute lymphoblastic leukaemia. Leukemia 10(Suppl. 2):58–61, 1996.

21. Bassan R, Pogliani E, Casula P, Rossi G, Fabris P, Morandi S et al: Risk-oriented postremission strategies in adult acute lymphoblastic leukemia: Prospective confirmation of anthracycline activity in standard-risk class and role of hematopoietic stem cell transplants in high-risk groups. Hematol J 2:117–126, 2001.

22. Bassan R, Pogliani E, Lerede T, Fabris P, Rossi G, Morandi S et al: Fractionated cyclophosphamide added to the IVAP regimen (idarubicin-vincristine-L-asparaginase-prednisone) could lower the risk of primary refractory disease in T-lineage but not B-lineage acute lymphoblastic leukemia: First results from a phase II clinical study. Haematologica 84:1088–1093, 1999.

23. Bene MC, Castoldi G, Knapp W, Ludwig W-D, Matutes E, Orfao A, van't Veer MB: Proposal for the immunological classification of acute leukemias. Leukemia 9:1783–1786, 1995.

24. Bennett JM, Catovsky D, Daniel MT, Flandrin G, Galton DAG, Gralnick HR, Sultan C: Proposals for the classification of the acute leukaemias. Br J Haematol 33:451, 1976.

25. Berman E, Raymond V, Gee T, Kempin SJ, Gulati S, Andreeff M et al: Idarubicin in acute leukemia: Results of studies at Memorial Sloan-Kettering Cancer Center. Semin Oncol 16:30–34, 1989.

26. Bernasconi C: Etoposide: Fifteen years experience. Bone Marrow Transplant 4 (Suppl. 1):52–55, 1989.

27. Bigman K, Arlin Z, Ahmed T, Baskind P, Seiter K, Cook P et al: A phase I-II trial of etoposide (VP-16), high dose cytarabine (HiDAc) and high dose mitoxantrone (MX) in the treatment of acute myeloid leukemia (AML), acute lymphocytic leukemia (ALL) and blastic chronic myelogenous leukemia (BLCML). Proc ASCO 12:304, 1993.

28. Bleyer WA: Central nervous system leukemia. In Henderson ES et al. (eds.): Leukemia, pp. 733–768. W.B. Saunders Company, Philadelphia, 1990.

29. Bleyer WA, Poplack DG: Prophylaxis and treatment of leukemia in the central nervous system and other sanctuaries. Semin Oncol 12:131–148, 1985.

30. Bloomfield CD, Wurster-Hill D, Peng G et al: Prognostic significance of the Philadelphia chromosome in adult acute lymphoblastic leukemia. In Gale RP et al. (ed.): Acute Lymphoblastic Leukemia, pp. 101–109. Alan R. Liss, New York, 1990.

31. Boogaerts M, Emonds MP, Kennes C et al: Intensive consolidation and maintenance therapy for acute lymphoblastic leukemia in adults. 4th International Symposium Therapy of Acute Leukemias, Rome, Italy, p. 442.

32. Bostrum B, Woods WG, Nesbit ME et al: Successful reinduction of patients with acute lymphoblastic leukemia who relapse following bone marrow transplantation. J Clin Oncol 5:376, 1987.

33. Brisco MJ, Condon J, Hughes E, Neoh S-H, Sykes PJ, Seshadri R et al: Outcome prediction in childhood acute lymphoblastic leukaemia by molecular quantification of residual disease at the end of induction. Lancet 343:196–200, 1994.

34. Brisco MJ, Hughes E, Neoh SH, Sykes PJ, Bradstock K, Enno A et al: Relationship between minimal residual disease and outcome in adult acute lymphoblastic leukemia. Blood 87:5251–5256, 1996.

35. Brueggemann M, Droese J, Scheuring U, Gökbuget N, Hoelzer D, Nakao M et al: Minimal residual disease in adult patients with acute lymphoblastic leukemia during the first year of therapy predicts clinical outcome. Hematol J 1:700a, 2001.

36. Bunjes D, Duncker C, Seitz U, Karakas T, Träger H, Stefanic M et al: Intensification of the conditioning regimen for high-risk leukaemia with a 188Re-labelled anti-CD 164b monoclonal antibody: Results of feasibility study. Blood 92:4471a, 1998.

37. Butturini A, Arlinghaus RB, Gale RP: BCR/ABL and leukemia. Leuk Res 20:523–529, 1996.

38. Campana D: Immunophenotypic analysis in the monitoring of minimal residual disease. Rev Clin Exp Hematol 1:42–56, 1997.

39. Capizzi RL, Keiser LW, Sartorelli AC: Combination chemotherapy—theory and practice. Semin Oncol 4:227–253, 1977.

40. Capizzi RL, Poole M, Cooper MR, Richards F, Stuart JJ, Jackson DV Jr et al: Treatment of poor risk acute leukemia with sequential high-dose ARA-C and asparaginase. Blood 63:694–700, 1984.

41. Carella AM, Santini G, Martinengo M, Giordano D, Nati S, Congiu A et al: VM-26 and cytarabine combination chemotherapy in refractory or relapsed adult acute lymphoblastic leukemia. Haematologica 69:747–751, 1984.

42. Cascavilla N, Musto P, D'Arena G, Ladogana S, Melillo L, Carella AM et al: Are "early" and "late" T-acute lymphoblastic leukemias different diseases? A single center study of 34 patients. Leuk Lymphoma 21:437–442, 1996.

43. Cassileth PA, Andersen JW, Bennett JM, Hagland HC, Mazza JJ, O'Connell MC et al: Adult acute lymphocytic leukemia: The Eastern Cooperative Oncology Group experience. Leukemia 6(Suppl. 2P):178–181, 1992.

44. Cavé H, Van der Werff ten Bosch J, Suciu S, Guidal C, Waterkeyn C, Otten J et al., and for the European Organization for Research and Treatment of Cancer-Childhood Leukemia Cooperative Group: Clinical significance of minimal residual disease in childhood acute lymphoblastic leukemia. N Engl J Med 339:591–598, 1998.

45. Chao NJ, Blume KG, Forman SJ, Snyder DS: Long-term follow-up of allogeneic bone marrow recipients for Philadelphia chromosome-positive acute lymphoblastic leukemia. N Engl J Med 332:3353–3354, 1995.

46. Charrin C: Cytogenetic abnormalities in adult acute lymphoblastic leukemia: Correlations with hematologic findings and outcome. A collaborative study of the Groupe Francais de Cytogénétique Hématologique. Blood 87:3135–3142, 1996.

47. Chessels JM, Bailey C, Richards SM, for the Medical Research Council Working Party on Childhood Leukaemia: Intensification of treatment and survival in all children with lymphoblastic leukemia: Results of UK Medical Research Council trial UKALL X. Lancet 345:143, 1995.

48. Chiu EKW, Chan LC, Liang R, Lie A, Kwong YL, Todd D, Chan TK: Poor outcome of intensive chemotherapy for adult lymphoblastic leukemia: A possible dose effect. Leukemia 8:1469–1473, 1994.

49. Chopra R, Pu QQ, Elefanty AG: Biology of BCR-ABL. Blood Rev 13:211–229, 1999.

50. Ciudad J, San Miguel JF, López-Berges MC, Vidriales B, Valverde B, Ocqueteau M et al: Prognostic value of immunophenotypic detection of minimal residual disease in acute lymphoblastic leukemia. J Clin Oncol 16:3774–3781, 1998.

51. Clarkson B, Ellis S, Little C et al: Acute lymphoblastic leukemia in adults. Sem Oncol 12:160, 1984.

52. Clarkson B, Gaynor J, Little C, Berman E, Kempin S, Andreef M et al: Importance of long-term follow-up in evaluating treatment regimens for adults with acute lymphoblastic leukemia. Haematol Blood Trans 33:397, 1990.

53. Clarkson BD, Gee T, Mertelsmann R et al: Current status of treatment of acute leukemia in adults: An overview of the Memorial experience and review of literature. CCR Crit Rev Oncol Hematol 4:221, 1986.

54. Clavell L, Gelber R, Cohen H et al: Four agent induction and intensive asparaginase therapy for treatment of childhood acute lymphoblastic leukemia. N Engl J Med 315:657–663, 1986.

55. Cohen LF, Balow JE, Magrath IT, Poplack DG, Ziegler JL: Acute tumor lysis syndrome. A review of 37 patients with Burkitt's lymphoma. Am J Med 68:486–491, 1980.

56. Cornelissen JJ, Carston M, Kollman C, King R, Dekker AW, Lowenberg B, Anasetti C: Unrelated marrow transplantation for adult patients with poor-risk acute lymphoblastic leukemia: Strong graft-versus-leukemia effect and risk factors determining outcome. Blood 97:1572–1577, 2001.

57. Cortes J, O'Brien SM, Pierce S, Keating MJ, Freireich EJ, Kantarjian HM: The value of high-dose systemic chemotherapy and intrathecal therapy for central nervous system prophylaxis in different risk groups of adult acute lymphoblastic leukemia. Blood 86:2091–2097, 1995.

58. Coustan-Smith E, Behm FG, Sanchez J, Boyett JM, Hancock ML, Raimondi SC et al: Immunological detection of minimal residual disease in children with acute lymphoblastic leukaemia [see comments]. Lancet 351:550–554, 1998.

59. Cuttner J: Leukemia, 1992.

60. Cuttner J, Mick R, Budman DR, Mayer RJ, Lee EJ, Henderson ES et al: Phase III trial of brief intensive treatment of adult acute lymphocytic leukemia comparing daunorubicin and mitoxantrone: A CALGB study. Leukemia 5(5):425–431, 1991.

61. Czuczman MS, Dodge RK, Stewart CC, Frankel SR, Davey FR, Powell BL et al: Value of immunophenotype in intensively treated

adult acute lymphoblastic leukemia: Cancer and Leukemia Group B study 8364. Blood 93:3931–3939, 1999.

62. Daenen S, van Imhoff GW, van den Berg E, de Kam PJ, Haaxma-Reiche H, Vellenga E et al: Improved outcome of adult acute lymphoblastic leukaemia by moderately intensified chemotherapy which includes a 'pre-induction' course for rapid tumour reduction: Preliminary results on 66 patients. Br J Haematol 100:273–282, 1998.

63. Dekker AW, van't Veer MB, Sizoo W, Haak HL, van der Lelie J, Ossenkoppele G et al., for the Dutch Hemato-Oncology Research Group: Intensive postremission chemotherapy without maintenance therapy in adults with acute lymphoblastic leukemia. J Clin Oncol 15:476–482, 1997.

64. Delannoy A, Ferrant A, Bosly A et al: Acute lymphoblastic leukemia in the elderly. Eur J Haematol 45:90, 1990.

65. Diccianni MB, Yu J, Hsiao M, Mukherjee S, Shao LE, Yu AL: Clinical significance of p53 mutations in relapsed T-cell acute lymphoblastic leukemia. Blood 84:3105–3112, 1994.

66. Drexler HG, Ludwig WD: Incidence and clinical relevance of myeloid antigen-positive acute lymphoblastic leukemia. Recent Res Cancer Res 131:53, 1993.

67. Druker BJ, Sawyers C, Kantarjian H, Resta DJ, Fernandes Reese S, Ford JM et al: Activity of a specific inhibitor of the BCR-ABL tyrosine kinase in the blast crisis of chronic myeloid leukemia and acute lymphoblastic leukemia with the Philadelphia chromosome. N Engl J Med 344:1038–1042, 2001.

68. Durrant IJ: Results of Medical Research Council trial UKALL IX in acute lymphoblastic leukaemia in adults: Report from the Medical Research Council Working Party on Adult Leukaemia. Br J Haematol 85:84–92, 1993.

69. Durrant IJ, Prentice HG, Richards SM: Intensification of treatment for adults with acute lymphoblastic leukaemia: Results of U.K. Medical Research Council randomized trial UKALL XA. Br J Haematol 99:84–92, 1997.

70. Elias L, Shaw MT, Raab SO: Reinduction therapy for adult acute leukemia with adriamycin, vincristine, and prednisone: A Southwest Oncology Group study. Cancer Treat Rep 63:1413–1415, 1979.

71. Ellison RR, Mick R, Cuttner J, Schiffer CA, Silver RT, Henderson ES et al: The effects of postinduction intensification treatment with cytarabine and daunorubicin in adult acute lymphocytic leukemia: A prospective randomized clinical trial by cancer and leukemia Group B. J Clin Oncol 9:2002–2015, 1991.

72. Elonen E, Almqvist A, Hänninen A, Jansson S-E, Järventie G, Koistinen P et al: Intensive treatment of acute lymphatic leukaemia in adults: ALL86 protocol. Haematologica, 76(Suppl. 4):133, 1991.

73. Elonen E for the Finnish Leukaemia Group: Long-term survival in acute lymphoblastic leukaemia in adults. A prospective study of 51 patients. Eur J Haematol 48:75–82, 1992.

74. Esterhay RJ Jr, Wiernik PH, Grove WR, Markus SD, Wesley MN: Moderate dose methotrexate, vincristine, asparaginase, and dexamethasone for treatment of adult acute lymphocytic leukemia. Blood 59:334–345, 1982.

75. Evensen SA, Brinch L, Tjonnfjord G, Stavem P, Wisloff F: Estimated 8-year survival of more than 40% in a population-based study of 79 adult patients with acute lymphoblastic leukaemia. Br J Haematol 88:88–93, 1994.

76. Faderl S, Kantarjian HM, Manshouri T, Chan CY, Pierce S, Hays KJ et al: The prognostic significance of p16INK4a/p14ARF and p15INK4b deletions in adult acute lymphoblastic leukemia. Clin Cancer Res 5:1855–1861, 1999.

77. Faderl S, Kantarjian HM, Talpaz M, Estrov Z: Clinical significance of cytogenetic abnormalities in adult acute lymphoblastic leukemia. Blood 91:3995–4019, 1998.

78. Feickert HJ, Bettoni C, Schrappe M, Reiter A, Ludwig W-D, Bode U et al: Event-free survival of children with T-cell acute lymphoblastic leukemia after introduction of high dose methotrexate in multicenter trial ALL-BFM 86. Proc ASCO 12:317, 1993.

79. Ferrari A, Annino L, Crescenzi S, Romani C, Mandelli F: Acute lymphoblastic leukemia in the elderly: Results of two different treatment approaches in 49 patients during a 25-year period. Leukemia 9:1643–1647, 1995.

80. Fiere D: Long term results of a prospective Belgium French protocol of treatment for adult acute lymphoblastic leukemia (ALL): LALA87 study. Ann Hematol 78:32a, 1999.

81. Fiere D, Extra JM, David B et al: Treatment of 218 adult acute lymphoblastic leukemias. Semin Oncol 24:64, 1987.

82. Fière D, Lepage E, Sebban C, Boucheix C, Gisselbrecht C, Vernant J-P et al: Adult acute lymphoblastic leukemia: A multicentric randomized trial testing bone marrow transplantation as postremission therapy. J Clin Oncol 11:1990–2001, 1993.

83. Filley CM, Kleinschmidt-DeMasters BK: Toxic leukoencephalopathy. N Engl J Med 345:425–432, 2001.

84. Foon KA, Todd FR: Immunologic classification of leukemia and lymphoma. Blood 68:1, 1986.

85. Foroni L, Coyle LA, Papaioannou M, Yaxley JC, Cole-Sinclair MF, Chim JS: Molecular detection of minimal residual disease in adult and childhood acute lymphoblastic leukaemia reveals differences in treatment response. Leukemia 11:1732–1741, 1997.

86. Foroni L, Harrison CJ, Hoffbrand AV, Potter MN: Investigation of minimal residual disease in childhood and adult acute lymphoblastic leukaemia by molecular analysis. Br J Haematol 105:7–24, 1999.

87. Freeman AI, Weinberg V, Brecher ML et al: Comparison of intermediate methotrexate with cranial irradiation for the post-induction treatment of acute lymphocytic leukemia in children. N Engl J Med 308:477, 1983.

88. Freund M, Heil G, Arnold R, Balleisen L, Bartram C, Büchner T et al: Treatment of relapsed ALL—studies of the German ALL Cooperative Group. Ann Hematol 74:A15, 1997.

89. Freund M, Link H, Diedrich H, LeBlanc S, Wilke HJ, Poliwoda H: High-dose ara-C and etoposide in refractory or relapsing acute leukemia. Cancer Chemother Pharmacol 28:487–490, 1991.

90. Friedman A, Schauer P, Mertelsmann R, Cirrincione C, Thaler H, Dufour P et al: The significance of splenomegaly in 101 adults with acute lymphoblastic leukemia (ALL) at presentation and during remission. Blood 57:798–801, 1981.

91. Garand R, Vannier JP, Béné MC, Faure G, Favre M, Bernard A, and Groupe d'Etude Immunologique des Leucémies: Comparison of outcome, clinical, laboratory, and immunological features in 164 children and adults with T-ALL. Leukemia 4:739–744, 1990.

92. Gaynor J, Chapman D, Little C, McKenzie S, Miller W, Andreef M et al: A cause-specific hazard rate analysis of prognostic factors among 199 adults with acute lymphoblastic leukemia: The Memorial Hospital Experience since 1969. J Clin Oncol 6(6):1014–1030, 1988.

93. Geissler K, Koller E, Hubmann E, Niederwieser D, Hinterberger W, Geissler D et al: Granulocyte colony-stimulating factor as an adjunct to induction chemotherapy for adult acute lymphoblastic leukemia—a randomized phase-III study. Blood 90:590–596, 1997.

94. Giona F, Annino L, Rondelli R, Arcese W, Meloni G, Testi AM et al: Treatment of adults with acute lymphoblastic leukaemia in first bone marrow relapse. Br J Haematol 97:896–903, 1997.

95. Glass JP, Lee YY, Bruner J, Fields WS: Treatment related leukoencephalopathy. A study of three cases and literature review. Medicine 65:154, 1986.

96. Goekbuget N, Aguion-Freire E, Diedrich H, Digel W, Faak T, Kasper C et al: Characteristics and outcome of CNS relapse in patients with acute lymphoblastic leukemia (ALL). Blood 94:1287a, 1999.

97. Goekbuget N, Hoelzer D: High-dose methotrexate in the treatment of adult acute lymphoblastic leukemia. Ann Hematol 72:194–201, 1996.

98. Gore MJML, Powles R, Lakhani A et al: Treatment of relapsed and refractory acute leukemia with high-dose cytosine arabinoside and etoposide. Cancer Chemother Pharmacol 23:373–376, 1989.

99. Gottlieb AJ, Weinberg V, Ellison RR et al: Efficacy of daunorubicin in the therapy of adult acute lymphocytic leukemia: A prospective randomised trial by the Cancer and Leukemia Group B. Blood 64:267–274, 1984.

100. Gökbuget N, Arnold R, Büchner T, Freund M, Gassmann W, Heil G et al: Akute lymphatische Leukämie des Erwachsenen. Praxis 88:407–420, 1999.

101. Gökbuget N, de Wit M, Gerhardt A, Lipp Th, Schwartz S et al: Results of a shortened, dose reduced treatment protocol in elderly patients with acute lymphoblastic leukemia (ALL). Blood 96:3104a, 2000.

102. Gökbuget N, Hoelzer D: Akute lymphatische Leukämie des Erwachsenen. Onkologe 4:778–790, 1998.

103. Gökbuget N, Hoelzer D: Meningeosis leukaemica in adult acute lymphoblastic leukaemia. J Neurol Oncol 38:167–180, 1998.

104. Gökbuget N, Hoelzer D, Arnold R, Böhme A, Bartram CR, Freund M et al: Subtypes and treatment outcome in adult acute lymphoblastic leukemia (ALL) <> 55 yrs. Hematol J 1:694a, 2001.

105. Götz G, Weh HJ, Walter TA, Kuse R, Kolbe K, Dölken G et al: Clinical and prognostic significance of the Philadelphia chromosome in adult patients with acute lymphoblastic leukemia. Ann Hematol 64:97–100, 1992.

106. Granena A, Castellsague X, Badell I, Ferra C, Ortega J, Brunet S et al: Autologous bone marrow transplantation for high risk acute lymphoblastic leukemia: Clinical relevance of ex vivo bone marrow purging with monoclonal antibodies and complement. Bone Marrow Transplant 24:621–627, 1999.

107. Greaves MF, Lister TA: Prognostic importance of immunologic markers in adults with acute lymphoblastic leukemia. N Engl J Med 119:304, 1981.

108. Griesinger F, Pirò-Noack M, Kaib N, Falk M, Renziehausen A et al: Leukaemia-associated immunophenotypes (LAIP) are observed in 90% of adult and childhood acute lymphoblastic leukaemia: Detection in remission marrow predicts outcome. Br J Haematol 105:241–255, 1999.

109. Gruhn B, Hongeng S, Yi H, Hancock ML, Rubnitz JE, Neale GA, Kitchingman GR: Minimal residual disease after intensive induction therapy in childhood acute lymphoblastic leukemia predicts outcome. Leukemia 12:675–681, 1998.

110. Guglielmi C, Vegna ML, Annino L, Specchia G, Del Vecchio L, Ciolli S et al., for the GIMEMA Group: Clinical relevance of immunophenotype in adult acute lymphoblastic leukaemia (ALL): An Italian collaborative study on 701 cases of the GIMEMA ALL 0288 randomized clinical trial. Br J Haematol 93(S2):57, 1996.

111. Haas OA, Mor W, Gadner H, Bartram CR: Treatment of Ph-positive acute lymphoblastic leukemia with α-interferon. Leukemia 2:555, 1988.

112. Hallbook H, Simonsson B, Bjorkholm M, Braide I, Carneskog J, Grimfors G et al: High dose ara-c as upfront therapy for adult

113. Harousseau JL, Tobelem G, Schaison G, Chastang C, Auclerc MF, Weil M et al: High risk acute lymphocytic leukemia: A study of 141 cases with initial white blood cell counts over 100,000/cu mm. Cancer 46:1996–2003, 1980.

114. Henderson ES, Scharlau C, Cooper MR, Haurani FI, Silver RT, Brunner K et al: Combination chemotherapy and radiotherapy for acute lymphocytic leukemia in adults: Results of CALGB protocol 7113. Leuk Res 3:395–407, 1979.

115. Hernandez JA, Land KJ, McKenna RW: Leukemias, myeloma, and other lymphoreticular neoplasms. Cancer 75:381–394, 1995.

116. Hiddemann W, Büchner T, Heil G, Schumacher K, Diedrich H, Maschmeyer G et al: Treatment of refractory acute lymphoblastic leukemia in adults with high-dose cytosine arabinoside and mitoxantrone (HAM). Leukemia 4:637–640, 1990.

117. Hiemenz JW, Walsh TJ: Lipid formulations of amphotericin B: Recent progress and future directions. Clin Infect Dis 22:133–144, 1996.

118. Hoelzer D: Which factors influence the different outcome of therapy in adults and children with ALL? Bone Marrow Transplant 4(Suppl. 1):98–100, 1989.

119. Hoelzer D: Aggressive chemotherapy of ALL in elderly patients. Hematol Oncol 11(Suppl. 1):12–14, 1993.

120. Hoelzer D, Arnold R, Freund M, Gassmann W, Gökbuget N, Heil G et al: Characteristics, outcome and risk factors in adult T-lineage acute lymphoblastic leukemia (ALL). Blood 94:2926a, 1999.

121. Hoelzer D, Gökbuget N: New approaches in acute lymphoblastic leukemia in adults: Where do we go? Semin Oncol 27:540–559, 2000.

122. Hoelzer D, Ludwig W-D, Thiel E, Gaßmann W, Löffler H, Fonatsch C et al: Improved outcome in adult B-cell acute lymphoblastic leukemia. Blood 87:495–508, 1996.

123. Hoelzer D, Thiel E, Löffler H, Bodenstein H, Plaumann L, Büchner T, Urbanitz D: Intensified therapy in acute lymphoblastic and acute undifferentiated leukemia in adults. Blood 64:38–47, 1984.

124. Hoelzer D, Thiel E, Löffler H, Büchner T, Freund M, Ganser A et al: Intensified chemotherapy and mediastinal irradiation in adult T-cell acute lymphoblastic leukemia. In Gale RP et al. (ed): Acute Lymphoblastic Leukemia, pp. 221–229. Alan R. Liss, Inc., New York.

125. Hoelzer D, Thiel E, Löffler H, Büchner T, Ganser A, Heil G et al: Prognostic factors in a multicenter study for treament of acute lymphoblastic leukemia in adults. Blood 71:123–131, 1988.

126. Hoelzer D, Thiel E, Ludwig WD, Loffler H, Buchner T, Freund M et al: The German multicentre trials for treatment of acute lymphoblastic leukemia in adults. The German Adult ALL Study Group. Leukemia 6(Suppl. 2):175–177, 1992.

127. Hoelzer D, Thiel E, Ludwig WD, Loffler H, Buchner T, Freund M et al: Follow-up of the first two successive German multicentre trials for adult ALL (01/81 and 02/84). German Adult ALL Study Group. Leukemia 7(Suppl. 2):S130–134, 1993.

128. Hughes WT, Rivera GK, Schell MJ et al: Successful intermittent chemoprophylaxis for Pneumocystis carinii pneumonitis. N Engl J Med 316:1627–1632, 1987.

129. Hurwitz CA, Silverman LB, Schorin MA, Clavell LA, Dalton VK, Glick KM et al: Substituting dexamethasone for prednisone complicates remission induction in children with acute lymphoblastic leukemia. Cancer 88:1964–1969, 2000.

130. Hussein KK, Dahlberg S, Head D, Waddell CC, Dabich L, Weick JK et al: Treatment of acute lymphoblastic leukemia in adults with intensive induction, consolidation and maintenance chemotherapy. Blood 73(1):57–63, 1989.

131. Ifrah N, Witz F, Jouet JP, Francois S, Lamy T, Linassier C et al: Intensive short term therapy with granulocyte-macrophage-

colony stimulating factor support, similar to therapy for acute myeloblastic leukemia, does not improve overall results for adults with acute lymphoblastic leukemia. GOELAMS Group. Cancer 86:1496–1505, 1999.

132. Jacquy C, Delepaut B, Van Daele S, Vaerman JL, Zenebergh A, Brichard B et al: A prospective study of minimal residual disease in childhood B-lineage acute lymphoblastic leukaemia: MRD level at the end of induction is a strong predictive factor of relapse. Br J Haematol 98:140–146, 1997.

133. Jones B, Freeman AI, Shuster JJ, Jacquillat C, Weil M, Pochedly C et al: Lower incidence of meningeal leukemia when prednisone is replaced by dexamethasone in the treatment of acute lymphocytic leukemia. Med Pedatr Oncol 19:269–275, 1991.

134. Jones B, Holland JF, Glidewell O, Jacquillat C, Weil M, Pochedly C et al: Optimal use of L-asparaginase (NSC-109229) in acute lymphocytic leukemia. Med Pediatr Oncol 3:387–400, 1977.

135. Kantarjian HM, Estey E, O'Brien S, Anaissie E, Beran M, Pierce S et al: Granulocyte-stimulating factor supportive treatment following intensive chemotherapy in acute lymphocytic leukemia first remission. Cancer 72:2950–2955, 1993.

136. Kantarjian HM, Estey EH, O'Brien S, Anaissie E, Beran M, Riso MB et al: Intensive chemotherapy with mitoxantrone and high-dose cytosine arabinoside followed by granulocyte-macrophage colony-stimulaing factor in the treatment of patients with acute lymphocytic leukemia. Blood 79:876–881, 1992.

137. Kantarjian HM, O'Brien S, Smith TL, Cortes J, Giles FJ, Beran M et al: Results of treatment with hyper-CVAD, a dose-intensive regimen, in adult acute lymphocytic leukemia. J Clin Oncol 18:547–561, 2000.

138. Kantarjian HM, Walters RS, Keating MJ, Smith TL, O'Brien S, Estey EH et al: Results of the vincristine, doxorubicin, and dexamethasone regimen in adults with standard- and high-risk acute lymphocytic leukemia. J Clin Oncol 8:994–1004, 1990.

139. Kantarjian HM, Walters RS, Smith TL, Keating MJ, Barlogie B, McCredie KB, Freireich EJ: Identification of risk groups for development of central nervous system leukemia in adults with acute lymphocytic leukemia. Blood 72(5):1784–1789, 1988.

140. Kaspers GJ, Veerman AJ, Pieters R, Van ZI, Hahlen K, van WE: Drug combination testing in acute lymphoblastic leukemia using the MTT assay. Leuk Res 19:175–181, 1995.

141. Kaspers GJ, Veerman AJ, Popp-Snijders C, Lomecky M, van Zantwijk CH, Swinkels LM et al: Comparison of the antileukemic activity in vitro of dexamethasone and prednisolone in childhood acute lymphoblastic leukemia. Med Pediatr Oncol 27:114–121, 1996.

142. Kaufmann SH, Karp JE, Burke PJ, Gore SD: Addition of etoposide to initial therapy of adult acute lymphoblastic leukemia: A combined clinical and laboratory study. Leuk Lymphoma 23:71–83, 1996.

143. Kern W, Schleyer E, Unterhalt M, Wörmann B, Büchner T, Hiddemann W: High antileukemia activity of sequential high dose cytosine arabinoside and mitoxantrone in patients with refractory acute leukemias. Cancer 79:59–68, 1997.

144. Knechtli CJC, Goulden NJ, Hancock JP, Grandage VLG, Harris EL, Garland RJ et al: Minimal residual disease status before allogeneic bone marrow transplantation is an important determinant of successful outcome for children and adolescents with acute lymphoblastic leukemia. Blood 92:4072–4079, 1998.

145. Koller CA, Kantarjian HM, Thomas D, O'Brien S, Rios MB, Kornblau S et al: The hyper-CVAD regimen improves outcome in relapsed acute lymphoblastic leukemia. Leukemia 11:2039–2044, 1997.

146. Larson RA, Dodge RK, Burns CP, Lee EJ, Stone RM, Schulman P et al: A five-drug remission induction regimen with intensive consolidation for adults with acute lymphoblastic leukemia: Cancer and Leukemia Group B study 8811. Blood 85:2025–2037, 1995.

147. Larson RA, Dodge RK, Linker CA, Stone RM, Powell BL, Lee EJ et al: A randomized controlled trial of filgrastim during remission induction and consolidation chemotherapy for adults with acute lymphoblastic leukemia: CALGB study 9111. Blood 92:1556–1564, 1998.

148. Lauer SJ, Pinkel D, Buchanan GR, Sartain P, Cornet JM, Krance R, Borella LD: Cytosine arabinoside/cyclophosphamide pulses during continuation therapy for childhood acute lymphoblastic leukemia. Cancer 60:2366–2371, 1987.

149. Law IP, Blom J: Adult acute leukemia: Frequency of central system involvement in long term survivors. Cancer 40:1304–1306, 1977.

150. Lee EJ, Pettoni GR, Freter CE, Johnson JL, Schiffer CA, Peterson BA, for Cancer and Leukemia Group B: Brief duration high intensity chemotherapy (CT) for patients (pts) with small non-cleaved lymphoma (IWF J) and FAB L3 acute lymphocytic leukemia (L3) in adults: Preliminary results of CALGB 9251. Proc Am Soc Clin Oncol 16:24a, 1997.

151. Legrand O, Marie J-P, Marjanovic Z, Cadiou M, Blanc C, Ramond S et al: Prognostic factors in elderly acute lymphoblastic leukaemia. Br J Haematol 97:596–602, 1997.

152. Lejeune C, Tubiana N, Gastaut JA, Maraninchi D, Richard B, Launay MC et al: High-dose cytosine arabinoside and mitoxantrone in previously-treated acute leukemia patients. Eur J Haematol 44:240–243, 1990.

153. Lichtman MA, Rowe JM: Hyperleukocytic leukemias: Rheological, clinical, and therapeutic considerations. Blood 60:279–283, 1982.

154. Linker CA, Levitt LJ, O'Donnell M, Forman SJ, Ries CA: Treatment of adult acute lymphoblastic leukemia with intensive cyclical chemotherapy: A follow-up report. Blood 78:2814–2822, 1991.

155. Linker CA, Ries CA, Damon LE, Rugo HS: Intensified and shortened chemotherapy for adult acute lymphoblastic leukemia. Blood 90:1485a, 1997.

156. Lluesma-Gonalons M, Pavlovsky S, Santarelli MT, Eppinger-Heft M, Bavea ED, Corrado C et al: Improved results of an intensified therapy in adult acute lymphocytic leukemia. Ann Oncology 2:33–39, 1991.

157. Lobel JS, O'Brien RT, Mclntosh S, Aspnes GT, Capizzi RL: Methotrexate and asparaginase combination chemotherapy in refractory acute lymphoblastic leukemia of childhood. Cancer 43:1089–1094, 1979.

158. Löffler H, Gassmann W: Morphology and cytochemistry of acute lymphoblastic leukemia. Bailliere's Clin Haematol 7(2):263, 1994.

159. Ludwig W-D, Rieder H, Bartram CR, Heinze B, Schwartz S, Gassmann W et al: Immunophenotypic and genotypic features, clinical characteristics, and treatment outcome of adult pro-B acute lymphoblastic leukemia: Results of the German multicenter trials GMALL 03/87 and 04/89. Blood 92:1898–1909, 1998.

160. Ludwig WD, Raghavachar A, Thiel E: Immunophenotypic classification of acute lymphoblastic leukemia. Bailliere's Clin Haematol 7(2):235, 1994.

161. Lundberg WB, Cadman ED, Finch SC, Capizzi RL: Renal failure secondary to leukemic infiltration of the kidneys. Am J Med 62:636, 1977.

162. Mahoney DH Jr, Shuster JJ, Nitschke R, Lauer S, Steuber CP, Camitta B: Intensification with intermediate-dose intravenous methotrexate is effective therapy for children with lower-risk B-precursor acute lymphoblastic leukemia: A Pediatric Oncology Group study. J Clin Oncol 18:1285–1294, 2000.

163. Mandelli F, Annino L, Ciolli S, Fabbiano F, Fanin R, Fioritoni G et al., for the GIMEMA Group: Philadelphia chromosome (Ph 1)

positive acute lymphoblastic leukemia (ALL) in adults: Interim results of GIMEMA ALL 0288 pilot study. Blood 82(Suppl. 1):58a, 1993.

164. Mandelli F, Annino L, Rotoli B: The GIMEMA ALL 0183 trial: Analysis of 10-year follow-up. Br J Haematol 92:665–672, 1996.

165. Mandelli F, Annino L, Vegna ML, Ferrari A, Ciolli S, Chierichini A et al: Adult acute lymphoblastic leukemia (ALL): Results of the Gimema ALL 0288 trial. Br J Haematol 93(S2):144, 1996.

166. Marcus RE, Catovsky D, Johnson SA, Gregory WM, Talavera JG, Goldman JM, Galton DA: Adult acute lymphoblastic leukaemia: A study of prognostic features and response to treatment over a ten year period. Br J Cancer 53:175–180, 1986.

167. Marit G, Cony P, Duclos F, Puntous M, Broustet A, Reiffers J: Treatment of relapsed or refractory acute leukemia: Comparison of two different regimens. Hamatol Bluttransfus 33:614–618, 1990.

168. Mortuza FY, Papaioannou M, Moreira IM et al. Minimal residual disease tests provide an independent predictor of clinical outcome in adult acute lymphoblastic leukemia. J Clin Oncol. 20:1094–1104, 2002.

169. Martin H, Fauth F, Atta J, Klein SA, Wassmann B, Hermann S, Hoelzer D: Single versus double autologous BMT/PBSCT in patients with BCR-ABL-positive acute lymphoblastic leukemia. Blood 94:2588a, 1999.

170. Martino R, Bellido M, Brunet S, Altes A, Sureda A, Guardia R et al: Intensive salvage chemotherapy for primary refractory or first relapsed adult acute lymphoblastic leukemia: Results of a prospective trial. Haematologica 84:505–510, 1999.

171. Mazza JJ, Leong T, Rowe JM, Wiernik PH, Cassileth PA: Treatment of adult patients with acute lymphocytic leukemia in relapse. Leuk Lymphoma 20:317–319, 1996.

172. Meckenstock G, Heyll A, Schneider EM, Hildebrandt B, Runde V, Aul C et al: Acute leukemia coexpressing myeloid, B- and T-lineage associated markers: Multiparameter analysis of criteria defining lineage commitment and maturational stage in a case of undifferentiated leukemia. Leukemia 9:260–264, 1995.

173. Meunier F: Targeting fungi: A challenge. Am J Med 99:60–67, 1995.

174. Milpied N, Gisselbrecht C, Harousseau J-L, Sebban C, Witz J-L, Troussard X et al: Successful treatment of adult acute lymphoblastic leukemia after relapse with prednisone, intermediate-dose cytarabine, mitoxantrone, and etoposide (PAME) chemotherapy. Cancer 66:627–631, 1990.

175. Mizuta S, Ito Y, Kohno A, Kiyoi H, Miyamura K, Tanimoto M et al: Accurate quantitation of residual tumor burden at bone marrow harvest predicts timing of subsequent relapse in patients with common ALL treated by autologous bone marrow transplantation. Nagoya BMT Group. Bone Marrow Transplant 24:777–784, 1999.

176. Montillo M, Tedeschi A, Centuriono R, Leoni P: Treatment of relapsed adult acute lymphoblastic leukemia with fludarabine and cytosine arabinoside followed by granulocyte colony-stimulating factor (FLAG-GCSF). Leuk Lymphoma 25:579–582, 1997.

177. Morra E, Lazzarino M, Alessandrino EP, Inverardi D, Canevari A, Bernasconi C: VP 16-213 and cytosine-arabinoside combination chemotherapy for refractory acute lymphoblastic leukemia in adults. Eur J Cancer Clin Oncol 20:1471–1475, 1984.

178. Morra E, Lazzarino M, Inverdadi D, Brusamolino E, Orlandi E, Canevari A et al: Systemic high-dose Ara-C for the treatment of meningeal leukemia in adult acute lymphoblastic leukemia and non-Hodgkin's lymphoma. J Clin Oncol 4:1207–1211, 1986.

179. Murphy SB, Bowman WP, Abromowitch M, Mirro J, Ochs J, Rivera G et al: Results of treatment of advanced-stage Burkitt's

lymphoma and B cell (SIg+) acute lymphoblastic leukemia with high-dose fractionated cyclophosphamide and coordinated high-dose methotrexate and cytarabine. J Clin Oncol 4:1732–1739, 1986.

180. Nagura E: Nation-wide randomized comparative study of doxorubicin, vincristine and prednisolone combination therapy with and without L-asparaginase for adult acute lymphoblastic leukemia. Cancer Chemother Pharmacol 33:359–365, 1994.

181. Neale GAM, Menarguez J, Kitchingman GR, Fitzgerald TJ, Koehler M, Mirro J, Goorha RM: Detection of minimal residual disease in T-cell acute lymphoblastic leukemia using polymerase chain reaction predicts impending relapse. Blood 78:739–747, 1991.

182. Nizet Y, Martiat P, Vaerman JL, Philippe M, Wildmann C, Staelens JP et al: Follow-up of residual disease (MRD) in B lineage acute leukaemias using a simplified PCR strategy: Evolution of MRD rather than its detection is correlated with clinical outcome. Br J Haematol 79:205–210, 1991.

183. O'Regan S, Carson S, Chesney RW, Drummond KN: Electrolyte and acid-base disturbances in the management of leukemia. Blood 49:345–353, 1977.

184. Ochs J, Mulhern R: Long-term sequelae of therapy for childhood acute lymphoblastic leukemia. Bailliere's Clin Haematol 7(2):365, 1994.

185. Oh H, Gale RP, Zhang M-J, Passweg JR, Ino T, Murakami H: Chemotherapy vs HLA-identical sibling bone marrow transplants for adults with acute lymphoblastic leukemia in first remission. Bone Marrow Transplant 22:243–257, 1998.

186. Ohyashiki K, Ohyashiki JH, Tauchi T, Fujieda H, Hojo H, Ohtaka M et al: Treatment of Philadelphia chromosome-positive acute lymphoblastic leukemia: A pilot study which raises important questions. Leukemia 5:611–614, 1991.

187. Omura GA, Moffitt S, Vogler WR, Salter MM: Combination chemotherapy of adult acute lymphoblastic leukemia with randomized central nervous prophylaxis. Blood 55:199, 1980.

188. Ottmann OG, Hoelzer D, Gracien E, Ganser A, Kelly K, Reutzel R et al: Concomitant granulocyte colony-stimulating factor and induction chemoradiotherapy in adult acute lymphoblastic leukemia: A randomized phase III trial. Blood 86:444–450, 1995.

189. Ottmann OG, Sawyers C, Druker B, Reiffers J, Goldman JM, O'Brien SG et al., and The International STI571 Study Group: A phase II study to determine the safety and anti-leukemic effects of STI571 in adult patients with Philadelphia-chromosome positive acute leukemias. Blood 96:828a(Abstract), 2000.

190. Paciucci PA, Keaveney C, Cuttner J, Holland JF: Mitoxantrone, vincristine and prednisone in adults with relapsed or refractory acute lymphocytic leukemia and terminal deoxynucleotidyl transferase positive blastic phase chronic myelocytic leukemia. Cancer Res 47:5234, 1987.

191. Panzer-Grumayer ER, Schneider M, Panzer S, Fasching K, Gadner H: Rapid molecular response during early induction chemotherapy predicts a good outcome in childhood acute lymphoblastic leukemia. Blood 95:790–794, 2000.

192. Patte C, Michon J, Frappaz D, Leverger G, Rubie H, Soussain C, Pico JL: Therapy of Burkitt and other B-cell acute lymphoblastic leukaemia and lymphoma: Experience with the LMB protocols of the SFOP (French Paediatric Oncology Society) in children and adults. Bailliere's Clin Haematol 7(2):339, 1994.

193. Perentesis JP: Why is age such an important independent prognostic factor in acute lymphoblastic leukemia? Leukemia 11:4–7, 1997.

194. Peters WG, Willemze R, Colly LP: Intermediate and high-dose cytosine arabinoside-containing regimens for induction and con-

solidation therapy for patients with acute lymphoblastic leukemia and lymphoblastic non-Hodgkin's lymphoma: The Leyden experience and review of the literature. Semin Oncol 14:86–91, 1987.

195. Petti MC, Mandelli F: Idarubicin in acute leukemias: Experience of the Italian Cooperative Group GIMEMA. Semin Oncol 16:10–15, 1989.

196. Pochedly C: Neurotoxicity due to CNS therapy for leukemia. Med Pediatr Oncol 3:101–115, 1977.

197. Preti HA, O'Brien S, Giralt S, Beran M, Pierce S, Kantarjian HM: Philadelphia-chromosome-positive adult acute lymphocytic leukemia: Characteristics, treatment results, and prognosis in 41 patients. Am J Med 97:60–65, 1994.

198. Pui CH: Acute lymphoblastic leukemia in children. Curr Opin Oncol 12:3–12, 2000.

199. Pullen J, Shuster JJ, Link M, Borowitz M, Amylon M, Carroll AJ et al: Significance of commonly used prognostic factors differs for children with T cell acute lymphocytic leukemia (ALL), as compared to those with B-precursor ALL. A Pediatric Oncology Group (POG) study. Leukemia 13:1696–1707, 1999.

200. Ramphal R, Gucalp R, Rotstein C et al: Clinical experience with single agent and combination regimens in the management of infection in the febrile neutropenic patient. Am J Med 100:83–89, 1996.

201. Reiter A, Schrappe M, Tiemann M, Ludwig WD, Yakisan E, Zimmermann M et al: Improved treatment results in childhood B-cell neoplasms with tailored intensification of therapy: A report of the Berlin-Frankfurt-Munster Group Trial NHL-BFM 90. Blood 94:3294–3306, 1999.

202. Ribera JM, Ortega JJ, Oriol A, Fontanillas M, Hernádez-Rivas JM, Brunet S et al., and members of the PETHEMA Cooperative Group: Late intensification chemotherapy has not improved the results of intensive chemotherapy in adult aucte lymphoblastic leukemia. Results of a prospective multicenter trial (PETHEMA ALL-89). Haematologica 83:222, 1998.

203. Ringden O, Labopin M, Gluckman E et al., for the Acute Leukemia Working Party of the European Group for Blood and Bone Marrow Transplantation: Graft-versus-leukemia effect in allogeneic marrow transplant recipients with acute leukemia is maintained using cyclosporin A combined with methotrexate as prophylaxis. Bone Marrow Transplant 18:921–929, 1996.

204. Rogers TR: Prevention of infection during neutropenia. Br J Haematol 79:544–549, 1991.

205. Rosen PJ, Rankin C, Head DR, Boldt DH, Luthardt FW, Norwood T et al: A phase II study of high dose ARA-C and mitoxantrone for treatment of relapsed or refractory adult acute lymphoblastic leukemia. Leuk Res 24:183–187, 2000.

206. Rowe JM, Chang AY, Bennett JM: Treatment of refractory acute leukaemia with aclacinomycin A. Bone Marrow Transplant 4(Suppl. 3):47–48, 1989.

207. Rowe JM, Richards S, Wiernik PH, Franklin IM, Burnett AK, Lazarus HM et al: Allogeneic bone marrow transplantation (BMT) for adults with acute lymphoblastic leukemia (ALL) in first complete remission (CR): Early results from the international ALL trial (MRC UKALL/ECOG E2993). Blood 94:732a, 1999.

208. Rozmylowicz T, Palynyczko G, Mazur J et al: Mitoxantrone in treatment of refractory acute leukemias. Blood 76:315a(Abstract), 1990.

209. Rubio-Borja ME, Gonzalez-Llaven J, Sanchez-Cortes E, Ovilla-Martinez R: Relapsed or refractory adult acute leukemia: Results of reinduction with high dose Ara-C/mitoxantrone vs high dose Ara-C/etoposide. Blood 80:458a, 1992.

210. Rubnitz JE, Behm FG, Pui C-H, Evans WE, Relling MV, Raimondi SC et al: Genetic studies of childhood acute lymphoblastic

leukemia with emphasis on p16, MLL, and ETV6 gene abnormalities: Results of St. Jude Total Therapy Study XII. Leukemia 15:1201–1206, 1997.

211. Ryan DH, Kopecky KJ, Head D, Gumbart CN, Grever MR, Karanes C et al: Phase II evaluation of teniposide and ifosfamide in refractory adult acute lymphocytic leukemia: A Southwest Oncology Group Study. Cancer Treat Rep 71:713–716, 1987.

212. Sackmann-Muriel F, Pavlovsky S, Penalver JA et al: Evaluation of induction of remission, intensification and central nervous system prophylactic treatment in acute lymphoblastic leukemia. Cancer 34:418, 1974.

213. Sallan S, Hitchcock-Bryan S, Gelber R et al: Influence of intensive asparaginase in the treatment of childhood non-T-cell acute lymphoblastic leukemia. Cancer Res 43:5601–5607, 1983.

214. Sanz GF, Sanz MA, Rafecas FJ, Martinez JA, Martin-Aragones G, Marty ML: Teniposide and cytarabine combination chemotherapy in the treatment of relapsed adolescent and adult acute lymphoblastic leukemia. Cancer Treat Rep 70:1321–1323, 1986.

215. Scherrer R, Bettelheim P, Geissler K, Jäger U, Knöbl P, Kyrle PA: High efficiency of the German multicenter ALL (GMALL) protocol for treatment of adult acute lymphoblastic leukemia (ALL)—a single institution study. Ann Hematol 69:181–188, 1994.

216. Scherrer R, Geissler K, Kyrle PA, Gisslinger H, Jäger U, Bettelheim P et al: Granulocyte colony-stimulating factor (G-CSF) as an adjunct to induction chemotherapy of adult acute lymphoblastic leukemia (ALL). Ann Hematol 66:283–289, 1993.

217. Scheuring U, Wassmann B, Pfeiffer H, Capdeville R, Petershofen E, Gschaidmeier H et al: Minimal residual disease (MRD) analysis of BCR-ABL positive acute lymphocytic leukemia (ALL) patients during STI571 kinase inhibitor therapy. Blood 96:465a, 2000.

218. Schiffer CA, Larson RA, Bloomfield CD: Cancer and leukemia group B (CALGB) studies in adult acute lymphocytic leukemia. Leukemia 6(Suppl. 2):171–174, 1992.

219. Schorin MA, Blattner S, Gelber RD, Tarbell NJ, Donnelly M, Dalton V et al: Treatment of childhood acute lymphoblastic leukemia: Results of Dana-Farber Cancer Institute/Children's Hospital acute lymphoblastic leukemia consortium protocol 85-01. J Clin Oncol 12:740–747, 1994.

220. Schrappe M, Reiter A, Ludwig WD, Harbott J, Zimmermann M, Hiddemann W et al: Improved outcome in childhood acute lymphoblastic leukemia despite reduced use of anthracyclines and cranial radiotherapy: Results of trial ALL-BFM 90. German-Austrian-Swiss ALL-BFM Study Group. Blood 95:3310–3322, 2000.

221. Schrappe M, Reiter A, Ludwig WD, Harbott J, Zimmermann M, Hiddemann W et al: Improved outcome in childhood acute lymphoblastic leukemia despite reduced use of anthracyclines and cranial radiotherapy: Results of trial ALL-BFM 90. German-Austrian-Swiss ALL-BFM Study Group. Blood 95:3310–3322, 2000.

222. Schwenn MR, Blattner SR, Lynch E, Weinstein HJ: Hi-COM: A 2-month intensive chemotherapy regimen for children with stage III and IV Burkitt's lymphoma and B-cell acute lymphoblastic leukemia. J Clin Oncol 9:133, 1991.

223. Secker-Walker LM, Craig JM, Hawkins JM, Hoffbrand AV: Philadelphia positive acute lymphoblastic leukemia in adults: Age distribution, BCR breakpoint and prognostic significance. Leukemia 5:196–199, 1991.

224. Secker-Walker LM, Prentice HG, Durrant J, Richards S, Hall E, Harrison G: Cytogenetics adds independent prognostic information in adults with acute lymphoblastic leukaemia on MRC trial UKALL XA. Br J Haematol 96:601–610, 1997.

225. Snyder DS, Nademanee AP, O'Donnell MR, Parker PM, Stein AS, Margolin K et al: Long-term follow-up of 23 patients with

Philadelphia chromosome-positive acute lymphoblastic leukemia treated with allogeneic bone marrow transplant in first complete remission. Leukemia 13:2053–2058, 1999.

226. Stryckmans P, de Witte T, Marie JP, Fillet G, Peetermans M, Bury J et al: Therapy of adult ALL: Overview of 2 successive EORTC studies: (ALL-2 & ALL-3). Leukemia 6(Suppl. 2):199–203, 1992.

227. Stryckmans P, Marie JP, Suciu S, Solbu G, Debusscher L, Bury J et al: Therapy for adolescent and adult acute lymphoblastic leukemia: Randomization of induction and consolidation therapies (preliminary results of EORTC Study 58791). In Buechnert et al (eds.): Haematology and Blood Transfusion. Acute Leukemias, Springer-Verlag, Berlin, Heidelberg, 1987.

228. Stryckmans P, Muus P, Marie JP, Fillet G, Labar B, Peetermans M et al: Adult Ph+ acute lymphoblastic leukemia in ALL-3 EORTC study. Blood 84(Suppl. 1):144a, 1994.

229. Stryckmans P, Suciu S, Annino L et al: Molecular evaluation of consolidation therapy and early allograft or autograft for BCR-ABL-positive adult acute lymphoblastic leukemia patients: A pilot study of EIGLE (European Intergroup of GIMEMA, French LALA and EORTC). Blood 90:(Abstract), 1997.

230. Sugar AM: Empiric treatment of fungal infections in the neutropenic host. Arch Intern Med 150:2258–2264, 1990.

231. Suki S, Kantarjian H, Gandhi V, Estey E, O'Brien S, Beran M et al: Fludarabine and cytosine arabinoside in the treatment of refractory or relapsed acute lymphocytic leukemia. Cancer 72:2155–2160, 1993.

232. Taylor PR, Reid MM, Bown N, Hamilton PJ, Proctor SJ: Acute lymphoblastic leukemia in patients aged 60 years and over: A population-based study on incidence and outcome. Blood 80(7):1813–1817, 1992.

233. Terebelo HR, Anderson K, Wiernik PH, Cuttner J, Cooper RM, Faso L, Berenberg JL: Therapy of refractory adult acute lymphoblastic leukemia with vincristine and prednisone plus tandem methotrexate and L-asparaginase. Results of a Cancer and Leukemia Group B Study. Am J Clin Oncol 9:411–415, 1986.

234. Thiebaut A, Vernant JP, Degos L, Huguet FR, Reiffers J, Sebban C et al: Adult acute lymphocytic leukemia study testing chemotherapy and autologous and allogeneic transplantation. A follow-up report of the French protocol LALA 87. Hematol Oncol Clin North Am 14:1353–1366, 2000.

235. Thiel E, Kranz BR, Raghavachar A, Bartram CR, Löffler H, Messerer D et al: Prethymic phenotype and genotype of pre-T(CD+/ER−)-cell leukemia and its clinical significance within adult acute lymphoblastic leukemia. Blood 73:1247–1258, 1989.

236. Thomas DA, Cortes J, O'Brien S, Pierce S, Faderl S, Albitar M et al: Hyper-CVAD program in Burkitt's-type adult acute lymphoblastic leukemia. J Clin Oncol 17:2461–2470, 1999.

237. Thomas X, Bauduer F, Brion A, Maloisel F, Fenaux P, Rossi JF et al: Idarubicin and ifosfamide in the treatment of refractory and relapsed acute lymphoblastic leukemia (ALL). Ann Hematol 74:A42, 1997.

238. Thomas X, Bouheddou N, Fiere D: High-dose cytarabine (HD-AraC) combined to mitoxantrone (MIT) in the treatment of refractory and relapsed acute lymphoblastic leukemia. Ann Hematol 78:S41(Abstract), 1999.

239. Todeschini G, Tecchio C, Meneghini V, Pizzolo G, Ambrosetti A, Veneri D et al: High dose daunorubicin (DNM) in induction of adult ALL patients. Preliminary results of a pilot protocol (ALLVR589). Blood 84(Suppl. 1):44a, 1994.

240. Todeschini G, Tecchio C, Meneghini V, Pizzolo G, Veneri D, Zanotti R et al: Estimated 6-year event-free survival of 55% in 60 consecutive adult acute lymphoblastic leukemia patients treated with an intensive phase II protocol based on high induction dose of daunorubicin. Leukemia 12:144–149, 1998.

241. Tomonaga M, Omine M, Morishima Y, Hirano M, Imai K, Hiraoka A, Asoh N: Individualized induction therapy followed by intensive consolidation and maintenance including asparaginase in adult ALL:JALSG-ALL87 study. Haematologica 76(Suppl. 4):68, 1991.

242. Tucker J, Prior PF, Green CR, Ede GMV, Stevenson JF, Gawler J et al: Minimal neuropsychological sequelae following prophylactic treatment of the central nervous system in adult leukaemia and lymphoma. Br J Cancer 60:775–780, 1989.

243. Uzun O, Anaissie EJ: Antifungal prophylaxis in patients with hematologic malignancies: A reappraisal. Blood 86:2063–2072, 1995.

244. van Dongen JJ, Seriu T, Panzer-Grümayer ER, Biondi A, Pongers-Willemse MJ et al: Prognostic value of minimal residual disease in acute lymphoblastic leukemia in childhood. Lancet 352:1731–1738, 1998.

245. Virchis AE, Koh MBC, Rankin P, Hoffbrand AV, Mehta AB, Potter MN, Prentice HG: Fludarabine, ARA-C, G-CSF+/− Idarubicine in the treatment of high risk acute leukemia and MDS. Blood 94:1328a(Abstract), 1999.

246. Visani G, Tosi P, Zinzani PL, Manfroi S, Ottaviani E, Cenacchi A et al: FLAG (fludarabine, cytarabine, G-CSF) as a second line therapy for acute lymphoblastic leukemia with myeloid antigen expression: In vitro and in vivo effects. Eur J Haematol 56:308–312, 1996.

247. Wasserman R, Galili N, Ito Y, Silber JH, Reichard BA, Shane S et al: Residual disease at the end of induction therapy as a predictor of relapse during therapy in childhood B-lineage acute lymphoblastic leukemia. J Clin Oncol 10:1879–1888, 1992.

248. Weiss M, Maslak P, Feldman E, Berman E, Bertino J, Gee T et al: Cytarabine with high-dose mitoxantrone induces rapid complete remission in adult acute lymphoblastic leukemia without the use of vincristine or prednisone. J Clin Oncol 14:2480–2485, 1996.

249. Weiss MA, Drullinsky P, Maslak P, Scheinberg D, Golde DW: A phase I trial of a single high dose of idarubicin combined with high-dose cytarabine as induction therapy in relapsed or refractory adult patients with acute lymphoblastic leukemia. Leukemia 12:865–868, 1998.

250. Welborn JL: Impact of reinduction regimens for relapsed and refractory acute lymphoblastic leukemia in adults. Am J Hematol 45:341–344, 1994.

251. Wells RJ, Feusner J, Devney R, Woods WG, Provisor AJ, Cairo MS et al: Sequential high-dose cytosine arabinoside-asparaginase treatment in advanced childhood leukemia. J Clin Oncol 3:998–1004, 1985.

252. Wernli M, Abt A, Bargetzi M, Fey MF, Tobler A, von Rohr A et al., for the Swiss Group of Clinical Cancer Research SAKK: A new therapeutic strategy in adult acute lymphoblastic leukemia: Intensive induction/consolidation, early transplant, maintenance-type therapy in relapse only. Proc Am Soc Clin Oncol 16:6a, 1997.

253. Wernli M, Tichelli A, von Fliedner V, Brun del Re G, Chapuis B, Fey MF et al: Intensive induction/consolidation therapy without maintenance in adult acute lymphoblastic leukaemia: A pilot assessment. Br J Haematol 87:39–43, 1994.

254. Westbrook CA, Hooberman AL, Spino C, Dodge RK, Larson RA, Davey F et al: Clinical significance of the BCR-ABL fusion gene in adult acute lymphoblastic leukemia: A Cancer and Leukemia Group B study (8762). Blood 80:2983–2990, 1992.

255. Wetzler M, Dodge RK, Mrozek K, Carroll AJ, Tantravahi R, Block AMW et al: Prospective karyotype analysis in adult acute lym-

phoblastic leukemia: The Cancer and Leukemia Group B experience. Blood 93:3983–3993, 1999.

256. Wiernik PH, Dutcher JP, Paietta E, Gucalp R, Markus S, Weinberg V et al: Long-term follow-up of treatment and potential cure of adult acute lymphocytic leukemia with MOAD: A non-anthracycline containing regimen. Leukemia 7:1236–1241, 1993.

257. Willemze R, Drenthe-Schonk AM, van Rossum J et al: Treatment of acute lymphoblastic leukemia in adolescents and adults. Scand J Haematol 24:(Abstract), 1980.

258. Willemze R, Jager U, Jehn U, Stryckmans P, Bury J, Suciu S et al: Intermediate and high dose Ara-C and m-AMSA for remission induction and consolidation treatment of patients with acute myeloid leukemia: An EORTC Leukemia Cooperative Group phase II study. Eur J Cancer Clin Oncol 24:1721–1725, 1988.

259. Willemze R, Zijlmans JMJM, den Ottolander GJ, Kluin-Nelemans JC, Falkenberg JHF, Starrenburg CWJ et al: High-dose Ara-C for remission induction and consolidation of previously untreated adults with ALL or lymphoblastic lymphoma. Ann Hematol 70:71–74, 1995.

260. Williams DL, Raimondi SC, Rivera G et al: Presence of clonal chromosome abnormalities in virtually all cases of acute lymphoblastic leukemia. N Engl J Med 313:640, 1985.

261. Woodruff RK, Lister TA, Paxton AM, Whitehouse JM, Malpas JS: Combination chemotherapy for haematological relapse in adult acute lymphoblastic leukaemia (ALL). Am J Hematol 4:173–177, 1978.

262. Yap BS, McCredie KB, Keating MJ, Bodey GP, Freireich EJ: Asparaginase and methotrexate combination chemotherapy in relapsed acute lymphoblastic leukemia in adults. Cancer Treat Rep 65(Suppl)1:83–87, 1981.

263. Zhang MJ, Hoelzer D, Horowitz MM, Gale RP, Messerer D, Klein JP et al: Long-term follow-up of adults with acute lymphoblastic leukemia in first remission treated with chemotherapy or bone marrow transplantation. The Acute Lymphoblastic Leukemia Working Committee. Ann Intern Med 123:428–431, 1995.

264. Zittoun R, Rio B, Marie JP, Blanc CM: Combination of AMSA-high dose cytosine arabinoside in acute leukemia. Presse Med 14:1417–1420, 1985.

19

Diagnosis and Treatment of Childhood Acute Myelogenous Leukemia

Howard J. Weinstein

Acute myelogenous leukemia (AML) accounts for 15 to 20 percent of the acute leukemias in children and 80 percent of acute leukemia in adults.[1,2] Recent advances in our understanding of stem cell physiology and the molecular basis of AML have elucidated the heterogeneity of AML and are beginning to identify novel targets for therapy.[3,4] The improvement in overall survival for children and young adults with AML can be attributed to better supportive care and advances in the application of chemotherapy and bone marrow transplantation. Although AML in children and young adults has many similarities, there are important differences that will be emphasized in this chapter.

EPIDEMIOLOGY

Approximately 400 of the 2600 new cases of childhood leukemia per year in the United States are diagnosed as AML.[2] Geographic variations in the incidence and subtypes of leukemia have been observed in children. For example, in several African countries, the incidence of AML is higher than that of acute lymphoblastic leukemia (ALL) in children, and orbital myeloblastomas (chloromas) are quite common.[5,6] The frequency of leukemia in patients under 15 years of age increases rapidly after birth and peaks before 5 years of age. Acute lymphoblastic leukemia accounts for this early age peak.

In contrast to ALL, the annual incidence of AML is quite constant from birth throughout the first 10 years. A slight peak in late adolescence occurs, and the incidence remains nearly constant to age 55, after which it rises progressively. The ALL/AML case ratio in children under 15 years old is 4:1, approximately the reverse of the ratio in adults.

The cause of AML is unknown and the vast majority of children newly diagnosed with AML have no known predisposition. Familial cases of AML are quite rare, and the increased concordance of leukemia (about 15 percent) in monozygotic twins appears be a consequence of placental metastasis of leukemia from one twin to the other rather than a genetic predisposition.[7,8]

There are several genetic disorders that are associated with an increased risk for AML. These include Down syndrome, congenital bone marrow failure syndromes (Diamond-Blackfan anemia and Kostmann's agranulocytosis), Fanconi's anemia,

and neurofibromatosis type 1.[9–12] Since the advent of G-CSF, children with Kostmann's agranulocytosis[10] are surviving into late childhood and have been noted to have as high as a 10 to 15 percent risk of developing AML. Children with neurofibromatosis type 1 are predisposed to peripheral nerve sheath tumors, gliomas, and leukemias, particularly myelodysplastic syndromes and juvenile myelomonocytic leukemia.[12] The *NF1* gene appears to function as a tumor suppressor because of homozygous mutations of the *NF1* gene in leukemic blasts from children with *NF1* and AML.[13]

Children with Down syndrome (trisomy 21) have a greater than 15-fold increased risk of leukemia during the first decade of life.[14] Interestingly, before 3 years of age, the predominant leukemia seen in these children is AML (FAB M7), but thereafter the ratio of ALL to AML follows the usual childhood distribution.

In addition to an increased risk of developing acute leukemia, children with Down syndrome or trisomy 21 mosaicism may present with a leukemia-like syndrome as neonates.[15] This unique clinical-pathologic entity has been referred to as transient leukemia or transient myeloproliferative syndrome (TMS), and it cannot be readily distinguished from congenital leukemia. The incidence of this syndrome is not known. Interestingly, the blasts from neonates with TMS are often clonal in origin and have morphologic, ultrastructural, and immunophenotypic features characteristic of megakaryoblasts and erythroblasts.[16] In contrast to congenital leukemia, TMS spontaneously resolves within 2 to 3 months without chemotherapy. However, as many as 20 to 30 percent of infants with a prior history of TMS eventually develop AML (usually FAB M7) by 2 to 3 years of age.[15]

Children, like adults, are susceptible to both radiation- and chemotherapy (alkylating agent and topoisomerase-2 inhibitors)-related AML.[17,18] The secondary AML cases after treatment with topoisomerase inhibitors such as etoposide are usually of the FAB M4 or M5 subtypes and have chromosomal translocations involving 11q23 with rearrangement of the *MLL* gene.[19] Identical chromosomal abnormalities of 11q23 have been associated with precursor B ALL in very young children[13] and de novo AML of the FAB M4 and M5 subtypes.[20–22]

CLONALITY AND CELL OF ORIGIN

In contrast to normal blood cells, blasts from patients with AML are clonally derived.[23] The clonal origin of AML has been demonstrated by (1) cytogenetic analysis of AML cells;[24] (2) studies of female patients heterozygous for glucose 6-phosphate dehydrogenase (G6PD) isoenzymes;[25] and (3) studies of restriction fragment length polymorphisms (RFLPs) of X chromosome genes.[26] Cytogenetic studies have identified a clonal chromosomal abnormality in the spontaneous dividing bone marrow cells of more than 70 percent of children with AML.[24,27] During remission, the bone marrow karyotype returns to normal and the same clone is detected at relapse, suggesting that the leukemic clone was suppressed, not eradicated, by chemotherapy. In very rare situations, persistent clonal hematopoiesis has been documented in complete remission.[23] The significance of this observation has not been determined.

The initial transforming event in AML may occur at any point during the maturation of the pluripotent or myeloid stem.[28,29] Chromosome and G6PD isoenzyme studies have indicated that AML is heterogeneous with respect to the cell of origin but most likely does not originate at the level of the pluripotent stem cell.[25] In some patients with AML, the clonal marker is expressed in both erythroid and granulocytic cells, suggesting involvement of a less committed progenitor. In other patients, the clonal marker is expressed in cells restricted to the granulocytic lineage, suggesting involvement of a more committed progenitor (granulocyte-macrophage colony-forming unit [CFU-GM]). The limited data suggest that the latter situation is representative of AML in children and young adults, whereas in older adults with AML, especially those with an antecedent hematologic disorder, the leukemia may be expressed in both red blood cells and granulocytes.[25]

CLASSIFICATION

Acute myelogenous leukemia has long been recognized to be morphologically heterogeneous but only recently have these observations been extended to a molecular genetic level. Multiple methods are available for characterizing AML.[30–33] These include standard morphologic interpretation of Romanowsky-stained specimens in conjunction with cytochemistry, karyotyping, immunophenotyping, in vitro cell growth, and molecular genetics.

By using the French-American-British (FAB) classification, cases of AML have been subdivided into seven major groups (M0 to M7).[30,31] Table 19–1 presents an approximate distribution of FAB subtypes of AML for patients less than 21 years of age. Of note is that 80 percent of children less than 2 years of age with AML have either the M4 or M5 FAB subtype.[34,35] These young children with AML are more likely to have myeloblastomas (especially leukemia cutis), high leukocyte counts, and a higher incidence of central nervous system (CNS) leukemia than older children with AML.

These are several interesting features of FAB M7 leukemia in children.[36] Almost one-half of cases occur in children younger than 3 years of age, whereas only 18 percent of cases of AML occur in this age group. As discussed by Zipursky et al.[14] AML M7 is the most common leukemia seen in children with Down syndrome.[14] Finally, M7 AML in young children has been associated with discrete lytic bone lesions.

IMMUNOPHENOTYPE ANALYSIS IN AML

In less than 20 percent of cases of AML, morphology and cytochemistry are inconclusive or insufficient to distinguish AML and ALL.[37] By using a combination of monoclonal antibodies recognizing B-cell, T-cell, and myeloid antigens, it is possible to diagnose most of these difficult cases.[38] Confirmation of the rare cases of M0 AML in children and adults requires immunophenotyping or flow cytometric or ultrastructural peroxidase studies. Adult AML-M0 has been associated with an immature myeloid profile (CD34+, terminal deoxynucleotidyl transferase (Tdt) +, CD13+, and CD33+), in contrast to pediatric AML-M0, which usually lacks Tdt or CD34 but expresses bright CD33 with weak or negative CD13.[39] Coexpression of CD7 is observed in both adult and pediatric M0 cases. The M7

Table 19–1. FAB Subtypes of AML and Their Associated Chromosomal Abnormalities and Clinical Features

FAB Subtype	Proportion of Cases (Percent)	Chromosomal Abnormality	Clinical or Laboratory Features
M0	2	del(5), del(7)	Blasts express CD33; minimally differentiated
M1	10–18	—	—
M2	27–29	t(8;21) (q22;q22) t(6;9) (p23;q34)	Myeloblastomas (especially orbital); favorable prognosis
M3	5–10	t(15;17) (q22;q21)	Disseminated intravascular coagulation; favorable prognosis with ATRA and chemotherapy
M4eo		inv(16) (p13;q22) or t(16;16) (p13;q22)	CNS leukemia, eosinophilia; favorable prognosis
M4	16–25	t(9;11) (p22;q23) t(11;19) (q23;p13.1) t(10;11) (p12;q23)	Infants and children under 2 yr, extramedullary leukemia
M5	13–22	t(9;11) (p22;q23) t(11;19) (q23;p13.1) t(10;11) (p12;q23)	Infants and children under 2 yr, extramedullary leukemia, secondary leukemia after exposure to epipodophyllotoxins
M6	1–3	—	—
M7	4–8	t(1;22) (p13;q13)	Infant onset (under 1 year), Down syndrome
All types		+8	Prior myelodysplastic syndrome
		−5 or del(5) (q11–q35)	Rare; prior myelodysplastic syndrome
		−7 or del(7) (q22–q36)	Rare: prior myelodysplastic syndrome

Abbreviations: FAB, French-American-British; AML, acute myelogenous leukemia; ATRA, all-*trans*-retinoic acid.

FAB subtype also may be suspected based on morphology or histochemistry, but it needs to be confirmed by either ultrastructural histochemistry (platelet peroxidase) or immunophenotypic analysis (identification of platelet or megakaryocytic antigens).[32] Flow cytometric analyses in AML may also be useful for detecting minimal residual disease after induction or consolidation chemotherapy.[1]

HYBRID OR ACUTE MIXED-LINEAGE LEUKEMIAS

Approximately 5 to 15 percent of cases of acute leukemia have morphologic, cytochemical, immunophenotypic, or genetic evidence of more than one hematopoietic lineage.[40–42] In these hybrid or acute mixed-lineage leukemias, individual blasts may express features of more than one lineage, or there may be two distinct populations of blasts. The pathogenesis of these hybrid leukemias remains poorly understood.

In a study from St. Jude Children's Research Hospital, blasts from approximately 17 percent of children with AML coexpressed at least two lymphoid-associated antigens,[42] T lineage–associated antigens being identified in 14 of 16 lymphoid-positive AML cases. The lymphoid-positive AML cases were typically FAB M1 or M2, with low levels of myeloperoxidase (MPO) reactivity. In many cases, two populations of blasts (large MPO-positive or small blasts) were evident. Several patients with T cell–positive AML who had a poor response to myeloid induction therapy subsequently responded to an ALL induction regimen. Mixed-lineage expression in AML, however, lacked prognostic significance. In a Pediatric Oncology Group study, approximately 60 percent of patients with AML expressed at least one lymphoid-associated antigen, most commonly CD4, CD7, or CD19.[41] Once again, such expression did not correlate with an unfavorable prognosis. Because the clinical and therapeutic implications of these findings are unclear, patients with AML whose blasts express lymphoid markers should continue to be treated according to AML protocols.

CHROMOSOMAL CHANGES

Studies using techniques of short-term culture, cell synchronization, and quianacrine or Giemsa banding now identify clonal chromosomal abnormalities in most children with AML.[27] As in adult AML, many of the chromosomal abnormalities correlate with specific FAB subtypes of AML (Table 19–1). In children with AML, monosomies or deletions of chromosomes 5 and/or 7 are less commonly observed than in older patients. A unique chromosomal translocation t(1;22)(p13;q13) has been described in infants with the FAB M7 subtype of AML.[43] In this report, all children were under 1 year of age at diagnosis, and none had Down syndrome. To date, this translocation has not been detected in other FAB subtypes of AML or in ALL.

Approximately 70 percent of cases of the FAB M4 and M5 subtypes of AML in infants and young children are associated with chromosome 11q23 translocations, including t(1;11), t(9;11), t(10;11), and rearrangements of the *MLL (All-1, HRX)* gene.[21,35] Rearrangements of *MLL* genes are also identified in children, especially infants, with precursor B-ALL and often are the result of a t(4;11) translocation. As in adult AML, favorable-prognosis karyotypes include inv(16)/t(16;16) and t(8;21).[27] (see section on prognostic factors below).

CLINICAL AND LABORATORY MANIFESTATIONS

The signs and symptoms of the child presenting with AML reflect the degree of bone marrow infiltration with leukemic cells as well as the extent of extramedullary spread. Acute myelogenous leukemia is, rarely, diagnosed as an incidental finding on a routine blood count in an asymptomatic child. Most children present with pallor, fatigue, bleeding, or fever as manifestations of their underlying anemia, thrombocytopenia, and neutropenia (Table 19–2). Lymphadenopathy, bone pain, and arthralgias are presenting features in less than 20 percent of children with AML and are more commonly observed in children with ALL.[44] Approximately 50 percent of children with AML have hepatomegaly or splenomegaly (more than 5 cm below the costal margin in 10 to 30 percent of cases). Infants with AML are more likely to have organomegaly, leukemic cutis, CNS leukemia, and high presenting leukocyte counts as compared with older children with AML.[35]

Table 19–2. Presenting Clinical and Laboratory Features in Children with Acute Myelogenous Leukemia (AML-BFM-83 Study)

Feature	Number of Patients
Sex (M/F)	96/77
Age (yr)	
< 2	31
2 to 9	68
= 10	74
Leukocyte count (× 10^9/μL)	
< 20	83
20–100	60
> 100	30
Hemoglobin	
= 8 g/dL	80
> 8 g/dL	89
Platelets (× 10^9/μL)	
= 50	91
> 50	81
Liver (cm)	
= 5	148
> 5	24
Spleen (cm)	
= 5	150
> 5	24
CNS	
Absent	153
Present	9

(Data from Creutzig et al.[87])

The anemia associated with both ALL and AML is usually normocytic, with occasional teardrop and nucleated red blood cells observed on peripheral smear. Initial hemoglobin levels ranged from 2.7 to 14.3 g/dl (median, 7 g/dl) in one large series of children with AML.[44]

Bleeding in a child with newly diagnosed AML is usually due to thrombocytopenia with or without disseminated intravascular coagulation. As in adults, most thrombocytopenic bleeding occurs when the platelet count is less than 20,000/μl. Approximately 50 percent of children with AML present with platelet counts of less than 50,000/μl. Disseminated intravascular coagulation is usually associated with acute promyelocytic leukemia (FAB M3), but the FAB M4 and M5 subtypes of AML in children have been associated with coagulation abnormalities and early death from hemorrhagic complications.[45]

Initial leukocyte counts in most children with AML are less than 50,000/μl. However, 20 percent will have white blood cell counts greater than 100,000/μl at diagnosis (Table 19–2) Leukostasis or intravascular clumping of blasts leading to hemorrhage and infarction can lead to life-threatening complications in children with AML, especially when the leukocyte count is in excess of 200,000/μl.[46] Leukostasis often manifests as somnolence, seizures, stroke, or tachypnea with hypoxemia.

DIFFERENTIAL DIAGNOSIS

A careful history and physical examination, as well as an examination of peripheral blood and bone marrow, result in a straightforward diagnosis of AML in approximately 90 percent of cases. However, for the difficult cases other diagnoses must be systemically excluded. Some of these include chronic myeloproliferative disorders, myelodysplastic syndromes, aplastic anemia, and overwhelming infections that result in leukemoid reactions or neutropenia.

As previously mentioned, newborns with Down syndrome or trisomy 21 mosaicism may show a transient proliferation of blast cells.[14,15,47] This so-called transient myeloproliferative syndrome is often clinically and hematologically indistinguishable from congenital AML.

EXTRAMEDULLARY LEUKEMIA

Infants with AML have a propensity for extramedullary dissemination of disease. In a review of AML in 29 infants at St. Jude Children's Research Hospital, 13 were found to have leukemia cutis, and 11 presented with central nervous system (CNS) leukemia.[48] The subcutaneous chloromas and leukemia cutis are bluish to slate gray in color, may appear in all sites, and are palpated as rubbery nodules of the deep skin. It has been postulated that a more intense blood supply present in neonatal skin and the propensity for monocytes to migrate to extramedullary sites may account in part for the high frequency of leukemia cutis seen in neonates and infants with AML.

Approximately 5 to 15 percent of children with AML have blasts detected in cerebrospinal fluid (CSF) at diagnosis,[49,50] but most of these children are asymptomatic. The clinical manifestations of CNS leukemia reflect leukemic infiltration of the leptomeninges and may include signs and symptoms of increased intracranial pressure, as well as isolated cranial nerve palsies (most common is palsy of the cranial nerve VII). Testicular involvement is extraordinarily rare in children with AML and, like CNS leukemia, is associated with the M4 and M5 FAB subtypes.[51]

Chloromas or myeloblastomas are seen in fewer than 5 percent of children with AML.[6,51] As in adults, chloromas may appear simultaneously with bone marrow infiltration or may present as the initial clinical manifestation of leukemia weeks to months before overt bone marrow disease can be detected. Chloromas in children are frequently seen in the bones and soft tissues of the head and neck (often orbits), skin, and epidural areas.[52]

TREATMENT

The prognosis for children with AML has gradually improved during the past 25 years.[50,53–59] The likelihood of achieving a complete remission (CR) is about 80 percent. Fifty percent of the complete responders who are given intensive postremission chemotherapy remain in remission for 5 or more years after diagnosis.[57–59] Data from several but not all pediatric AML clinical trials show a disease-free survival advantage for allogeneic bone marrow transplantation from an HLA-matched family member as compared with chemotherapy.[57,60,61] Five-year overall survival rates are now approaching 50 percent. Most children with newly diagnosed or suspected leukemia are referred to a tertiary care center staffed by pediatric hematologists-oncologists. The majority of children with AML are treated according to cooperative group clinical trials, such as those by the Pediatric Oncology Group, Children's Cancer Group, Berlin-Frankfurt-Münster Group, and the UK Medical Research Council (UKAML).[57,59–61]

During the immediate hours after diagnosis, prompt recognition and treatment of life-threatening complications is necessary. The most likely oncologic emergencies in this setting include leukostasis, sepsis, hemorrhage, and mass effect from myeloblastomas (e.g., spinal cord compression).

In one large series of children with AML, 10 percent of patients died as a result of hemorrhage, leukostasis, or both before or during the first 12 days of therapy.[45,62] Most of these early deaths were due to intracerebral hemorrhage, and the major risk factors were hyperleukocytosis, coagulopathy, and acute monocytic leukemia. Hyperleukocytosis was defined as a white blood cell count greater than 100×10^6/L. Leukapheresis (or exchange transfusion in very young infants) is well tolerated and very effective in transiently lowering the white blood cell count.[63] Hydroxyurea is often given in this setting after vigorous hydration, alkalinization of the urine with intravenous sodium bicarbonate, and administration of allopurinol.[64] The tumor lysis syndrome (hyperkalemia, hyperphosphatemia, hypocalcemia, and hyperuricemia) is more common in children with ALL than in those with AML.[46]

REMISSION INDUCTION

Once the patient is stabilized, remission induction therapy should begin without delay. Most pediatric AML remission induction protocols employ a 7- to 10-day course of cytosine arabinoside (ara-C), plus 2 to 3 days of doxorubicin, daunorubicin or mitoxantrone, with or without thioguanine or etoposide.[56–61] Approximately 75 to 85 percent of children with AML achieve CR using current protocols. For children under 1 year of age or who have a body surface area of less than 0.6 m², drug doses should be calculated on a milligram per kilogram (mg/kg) basis, rather than on a milligram per square meter (mg/m²) basis, to avoid excessive toxicity.

Because of the narrow therapeutic index for ara-C and the anthracyclines, one can expect 2 to 3 weeks of pancytopenia before there is evidence of bone marrow recovery. Therefore, the remission induction period is associated with considerable morbidity and mortality.[57,59]

Approximately 5 to 10 percent of children die during induction therapy as a result of either direct leukemic causes, infection, or hemorrhage. Chemotherapy-induced gastrointestinal toxicity contributes to the risk of bacterial or fungal sepsis.[65,66] The most severe manifestation of gastrointestinal toxicity has been referred to as enterocolitis or typhlitis.[67] Severe neutropenia coupled with chemotherapy-induced mucosal damage to the distal ileum and proximal colon are thought to be predisposing factors. Typhlitis is characterized by right lower quadrant abdominal pain with or without rebound tenderness. In severe cases, there may be vomiting, ileus, abdominal distention, fever, and septic shock. The relative lack of gas from the right lower quadrant and minimal distention of the small bowel may be seen on plain abdominal radiographs. Abdominal ultrasound and CT scans may reveal thickening of the wall of the cecum. The management of a child with typhlitis should include bowel rest, intravenous fluids, broad-spectrum antibiotics, and appropriate blood components. Surgery is reserved for intestinal perforation, abdominal wall fasciitis, or massive bleeding. In the differential diagnosis of typhlitis, one must also consider common surgical conditions of childhood, including appendicitis or intussusception. Typhlitis is less common with remission induction regimens using daunorubicin rather than doxorubicin combined with ara-C.[68]

Central Nervous System Prophylaxis

Central nervous system prophylaxis became an integral component of ALL therapy when CNS sequestration of leukemic cells became evident, and the pattern of systemic relapse after the appearance of CNS disease strongly suggested that the recurrence was due to reseeding of leukemic cells from the CNS to the bone marrow.[1] The introduction of this phase of therapy unequivocally increased the number of long-term disease-free survivors of ALL and constituted a major therapeutic advance. Without CNS-directed therapy, the incidence of isolated CNS relapse during hematologic remission in children with AML is approximately 20 percent.[49,50] Children with the M4 and M5 subtypes of AML have the highest risk of CNS relapse.[43]

Intrathecal methotrexate[54] or cytosine arabinoside[60] or cranial irradiation plus intrathecal methotrexate[58] have all been used to reduce the risk of CNS relapse in children with AML. It has yet to be demonstrated in a prospective randomized, clinical trial, however, that CNS prophylaxis improves disease-free survival in children with AML. The only data supporting the use of CNS prophylaxis in AML derive from Berlin-Frankfurt-Münster protocols.[58,69]

About 10 to 15 percent of children with AML have blasts in the CSF at diagnosis. Interestingly, this finding does not appear to have an adverse impact on overall survival.[50,70] Overt CNS leukemia has been treated with weekly intrathecal methotrexate or ara-C until the CSF is clear of blasts. This is often followed by CNS irradiation given toward the end of systemic chemotherapy.

Postremission Therapy

Successful remission induction therapy reduces the leukemic burden by two to four orders of magnitude. Therefore, additional therapy is necessary to achieve prolonged remission durations in both children and adults with AML. The intensity and duration of postremission chemotherapy, as well as the role of bone marrow transplantation in first remission, remain controversial. Pediatric AML studies initiated during the 1970s and early 1980s tested whether modestly myelosuppressive combination (maintenance) chemotherapy,[53,71] nonspecific immunotherapeutic agents (e.g., bacillus Calmette-Guérin [BCG]),[72] or splenectomy[73] would prolong remission duration. Disease-free survival rates with these approaches were less than 30 percent at 5 years, and there was no obvious benefit for splenectomy or adjuvant BCG.

Because of these disappointing results, other treatment approaches were explored, including intensification/consolidation chemotherapy and allogeneic bone marrow transplantation early in first remission.[50,74,75] Intensification chemotherapy was based on the steep dose-response curve for many of the chemotherapeutic agents such as ara-C. Other strategies included the use of sequential non-cross-resistant drug combinations in an effort to circumvent the problem of acquired drug resistance.[50] Although these strategies were explored in nonrandomized clinical trials, the overall results suggested a benefit for this approach.

During the 1980s, it became apparent that high doses of ara-C could produce remissions in patients with AML who were refractory to conventional-dose ara-C.[76] These exciting results led to the use of high-dose ara-C as consolidation therapy during first remission.[54] An important Cancer and Leukemia Group B (CALGB) protocol for adults with AML randomly assigned patients to receive four courses of ara-C at one of three doses: 100 mg/m² for 5 days, 400 mg/m² for 5 days, or 3 g/m² on days 1, 3, and 5. The probability of remaining in remission for patients under 60 years of age was 44 percent in the 3 g/m² group, which was significantly different from the 24 percent for the 100 mg/m² group and 29 percent for the 400 mg/m² group.[77] Based on these results as well as the previously mentioned studies, one or more courses of high-dose ara-C were included in the consolidation phase of many pediatric AML protocols (Table 19–3). Pediatric AML studies have not shown a benefit for maintenance chemotherapy given after consolidation chemotherapy.[71]

ACUTE PROMYELOCYTIC LEUKEMIA

The biology and molecular genetics of acute promyelocytic leukemia (FAB M3) are identical in children and adults.[62,78] The International Cooperative Group ATRA (all-*trans*-retinoic acid) trials have included both children and adults with M3 AML.[79] The combined use of ATRA, anthracyclines, and ara-C is recommended for remission induction.[80] All-trans-retinoic acid is associated with a respiratory distress/capillary leak syndrome and pseudotumor cerebri. Pseudotumor cerebri appears to occur more often in children than adults but usually abates within a week after withdrawal of ATRA. The drug can usually be safely restarted at a reduced dose. Recent data also indicate a role for ATRA maintenance.[80] Arsenic trioxide is very active as a single agent in both children and adults with relapsed APL.[81,82] The potential benefit of consolidation with arsenic is currently being tested in a combined pediatric and adult cooperative group trial.

During the mid-1970s, allogeneic bone marrow transplants (allo-BMT) from histocompatible family donors were first evaluated in children and young adults with AML in first remission.[74,75] About 25 percent of potential transplant candidates were eligible by virtue of having an HLA-identical family donor. The early data were quite encouraging, with 5-year disease-free survival rates of 50 to 70 percent compared with less than 30 percent for chemotherapy. These results were also obtained in a very selected group of patients. The relapse rate of AML after allo-BMT was lower than that after chemotherapy (20 versus 60 percent), but the difference in leukemia-free survival was less dramatic because of fatal post-BMT complications from graft-versus-host-disease and infections.

The CCG was one of the first groups to prospectively compare the outcome of chemotherapy and allo-BMT and avoid the bias of patient selection.[83] When the data were analyzed on the basis of intent to transplant (HLA-identical donor available), a statistically significant disease-free survival advantage was found for transplant compared with chemotherapy (48 versus 36 percent). Similar results have been reported in other recent studies (Table 19–3). With continued improvement in the outcome after intensive chemotherapy, however, other studies have not demonstrated a statistically significant disease-free or overall survival advantage for allo-BMT as compared with chemotherapy.[59] Based on the available data, allo-BMT should be seriously considered for children with AML in first remission who have an HLA-matched sibling donor and high-risk features (see discussion of prognostic factors, below). For children with "favorable" prognostic features such as inv16 and t(8;21), an alternative strategy would be to reserve transplantation for second remission. Of patients with AML who received transplants in early relapse or second remission, 30 to 40 percent appear to be long-term leukemia-free survivors.[84]

Because of the promising results of autologous marrow transplantation (ABMT) in patients with AML in second remission,[85] randomized clinical trials comparing ABMT with chemotherapy in children with AML in first remission were initiated.[59–61] In several studies, marrow was purged with either 4-hydroperoxycyclophosphamide or mafosfamide. The results of the Italian,[61] Pediatric Oncology Group,[61] and Children's Cancer Group[57] studies do not show a disease free survival advantage for ABMT over chemotherapy.

PROGNOSTIC FACTORS

The prognostic significance of several pretreatment- and therapy-related factors have been evaluated in children with AML.[86–88] Some factors appear to influence the CR rate, whereas others appear to influence remission duration (Table 19–4). A high leukocyte count (greater than $100,000/\mu L$) and monosomy 7 have been associated with lower CR rates.[70] The lower CR rates associated with hyperleukocytosis are in part explained by early death from intracranial hemorrhage (leukostasis). In several studies, FAB M4 and M5, high leukocyte counts and age under 2 years were found to have an adverse impact on remission duration.[86,88] Other investigators, however, have not confirmed these findings.[57,58] In a BFM study,[87] the presence of Auer rods in the FAB M1 subtype was associated with a higher remission induction rate and with longer remission duration.

Certain chromosomal abnormalities have influenced both CR rates and disease-free survival. For example, −7/7q− has been associated with both low CR rates and high relapse rates. As in adult AML studies,[89] t(8;21) and inv16/del(16q22) have been associated with favorable outcomes in terms of remission induction rates and disease-free survival.[27] The use of blast cell

Table 19–3. Prospective Comparisons of Disease-Free Survival (DFS) Following Allogeneic and Autologous Bone Marrow Transplantation (BMT) and Postremission Chemotherapy

Study	Allo-BMT (percent)	Auto-BMT (percent)	Chemo-therapy (percent)	Overall EFS (percent)
POG-8821[60]	52[a]	38	36	34
CCG-2891[57]	55[a]	42	47	42[d]
AIEOP/LAM 87[61]	51[a]	21	27	25
MRC AML 10[59]	67	68[b]	46	48
AML BFM 93[58]	64[c]	—	62	51

[a] Statistically significant DFS and survival advantage for allo BMT.
[b] Statistically significant DFS but not survival advantage for auto BMT.
[c] High-risk patients only.
[d] Intensive timing arm of study.
Abbreviations: POG, Pediatric Oncology Group; CCG, Children's Cancer Group; AIEOP/LAM – Associazone Italiana Emetologia ed Oncologia Pediatrica/Leucemia Acuta Mieloide; MRC, Medical Research Council; BFM, Berlin-Frankfurt-Münster Group; EFS, event-free survival from diagnosis.

Table 19–4. Adverse Prognostic Factors in Childhood Acute Myelogenous Leukemia (AML)

Complete Remission Rate	Remission Duration
WBC count above 100 × 10⁹/L	WBC count > 100 × 10⁹/L
FAB M1 without Auer rods	FAB M1 without Auer rods
Monosomy 7 (7q–)	Monosomy 7 (7q–)
Secondary AML or prior MDS	Secondary AML or prior MDS
	11q23 translocations – controversial
	FAB M5 – controversial
	Courses to CR (greater than 1)

Abbreviations: CR, complete remission; MDS, myelodysplastic syndrome; WBC, white blood cell; FAB, French-American-British.

immunophenotype has not been predictive of outcome for children with AML.[40–42] Interestingly, children with Down syndrome and AML have a very favorable prognosis.[90,91] In some studies, increased expression of the multidrug resistance 1(mdr 1)-encoded P-glycoprotein has been identified as an adverse prognostic factor in adults with AML.[92] These observations have not been confirmed in pediatric AML studies.[93] Newer molecular probes are expected ultimately to prove useful in identifying novel, therapeutic targets as well as providing prognostic information.

MANAGEMENT OF RELAPSE

Management of children with relapsed AML is a major challenge. The response to secondary therapy is very dependent on the timing of the relapse. Children who relapse while receiving chemotherapy or during the first year and a half of remission have a lower likelihood of achieving a second remission compared with those patients who relapse later.[94] A variety of different reinduction regimens have been used in children with refractory AML, including high-dose ara-C with or without L-asparaginase[95] or mitoxantrone,[96] etoposide (VP-16), and amsacrine with or without azacytidine,[97] etoposide and mitoxantrone with cyclosporine,[98] and 2-chlorodeoxyadenosine.[99] The second CR rates are about 30 to 50 percent the above regimens. Unfortunately, the durations of second remission are brief, especially for patients with short first remissions.

For these reasons, bone marrow transplantation is recommended for patients who achieve a second remission.[84] Currently, the survival rate after either allogeneic or autologous transplantation for children with AML in second remission is about 30 percent. The use of transplants (marrow or cord blood) from unrelated donors has largely replaced the use of autologous marrow.[100] The option of an immediate marrow transplant after relapse is attractive because of the low second remission rates, but the logistics of such an approach are problematic. Newer approaches for treating relapsed or refractory AML include the use of monoclonal antibodies (e.g., Mylotarg; anti-CD33 toxin conjugate)[101] and drugs such as cyclosporine that are capable of reversing the multidrug resistance phenotype in vitro.[98]

SUPPORTIVE CARE

General principles of supportive care in children with AML include replenishment of deficient blood components; prompt recognition and treatment of metabolic, nutritional, and infectious complications; placement of central venous access devices; and psychosocial intervention and support.

Relapsed leukemia remains the primary cause of death in children with AML, but infections continue to cause morbidity and mortality. Susceptibility to bacterial and fungal infection is the result of neutropenia caused initially by bone marrow replacement with leukemia and later by chemotherapy-induced bone marrow suppression, cellular and humoral immunosuppression, breakdown of skin and gastrointestinal barriers from therapy, and the use of central venous access devices.[65,66] Children receiving high dose ara-C are at particular risk for alpha-hemolytic streptococcal infection.[102] As the intensity of AML therapy has increased, so has the rate of invasive fungal disease.

The empirical use of broad-spectrum antibiotics and amphotericin B or fluconazole in febrile neutropenic patients, the prophylactic use of trimethoprim-sulfamethoxazole to prevent *Pneumocystis carinii* pneumonia, and the use of acyclovir in children with herpes zoster virus or varicella zoster virus infections have contributed significantly to the improved outlook in childhood acute leukemia.[65,66] Oral nonabsorbable antibiotics and protected environments (i.e., laminar airflow) have not been advocated. The use of hematopoietic growth factors (e.g., granulocyte- and granulocyte-macrophage-colony-stimulating factors [G-CSF and GM-CSF]) has not been shown to increase remission rates or overall survival in children with AML.[57]

Hemorrhagic deaths have generally been preventable with the liberal use of platelet concentrates, particularly in patients with platelet counts below 10 to 20,000 per cubic mm. Alloimmunization to random platelet concentrates is a potential problem, especially for children with AML who require frequent blood component support. HLA-matched platelets may be effective when patients become refractory to random donor platelet concentrates. All blood products should be leuko-depleted and irradiated.[103]

CONSEQUENCES OF SURVIVAL

With an increasing number of children with AML surviving disease-free for long periods, attention has been drawn to late effects of leukemia and its treatment, including the risk of second neoplasms.[104,105] Growth and development and sexual maturation have generally been normal in both boys and girls who have completed chemotherapy for AML, but the reproductive capacity of successfully treated patients needs to be established. Gonadal failure and short stature are more commonly observed after BMT.[106] Late cardiotoxic effects of anthracyclines are a potential problem, and children should be monitored with echocardiagrams on a regular basis (e.g., every other year).[107] Current studies are addressing quality-of-life issues, as they will undoubtedly have an impact on the selection of treatment options (e.g., marrow transplantation versus chemotherapy in first remission).[108]

For an increasing proportion of children with AML, their disease has become a long-term problem. Patients and their families must be counseled in these terms. The effects of leukemia on parents and siblings of the affected child have taught us that the impact of this disease is shared by the entire family.

REFERENCES

1. Pui C-H: Childhood leukemias. N Engl J Med 332:1617–30, 1995.
2. American Cancer Society: Cancer Factors and Figures in 1994. p. 14, American Cancer Society, Atlanta.
3. Tenen D, Hrumas R, Licht J et al: Transcription factors, normal myeloid development, and leukemia. Blood 90:489–519, 1997.
4. Rubnitz JE, Look AT: Molecular genetics of childhood leukemias. J Pediatr Hematol Oncol 20(1):1–11, 1998.
5. Cavdar A, Arcasoy A, Babacan E et al. Ocular granulocytic sarcoma (chloroma) with acute myelomonocytic leukemia in Turkish children. Cancer 41:1606–9, 1978.
6. Schwyzer R, Sherman GG, Cohn RJ et al: Granulocytic sarcoma in children with acute myeloblastic leukemia and t(8;21). Med (Pediatr Oncol) 31(3):144–9, 1998.
7. Greaves M: A natural history for pediatric acute leukemia. Blood 82:1043–51, 1993.
8. Richkind KE, Loew T, Meisner L et al: Identical cytogenetic clones and clonal evolution in pediatric monozygotic twins with acute myeloid leukemia: presymptomatic disease detection by interphase fluorescence in situ hybridization and review of the literature. J Pediatr Hematol Oncol 20:264–7, 1998.
9. Li FP, Bader JL: Epidemiology of cancer in childhood. In Nathan DG, Oski FA (eds.): Hematology of infancy and childhood, 4th ed., pp. 1102–1119. WB Saunders, Philadelphia, 1993.
10. Rosen RB, Kang SJA: Congenital agranulocytosis terminating in acute myelomonocytic leukemia. J Pediatr 94:406–8, 1979.
11. Wasser J, Yolken R, Miller D et al: Congenital hypoplastic anemia (Diamond-Blackfan syndrome) terminating in acute myelogenous leukemia. Blood 51:991–5, 1978.
12. Korf BR: Malignancy in neurofibromatosis type 1. The Oncol 5:477–85, 2000.
13. Shannon K, O'Connell P, Martin G et al: Loss of the normal NF1 allele from the bone marrow of children with type 1 neurofibromatosis and malignant myeloid disorders. N Engl J Med 330:597–601, 1994.
14. Zipursky A, Poon A, Doyle J: Leukemia in Down syndrome: A review. Pediatr Hematol Oncol 9:139–49, 1992.
15. Homans AC, Verissimo AM, Vlacha V: Transient abnormal myelopoiesis of infancy associated with trisomy 21. Am J Pediatr Hematol Oncol 15:392–9, 1993.
16. Kurahashi H, Hara J, Yumura-Yagi K et al: Monoclonal nature of transient, abnormal myelopoiesis in Down's syndrome. Blood 77:1161–3, 1991.
17. Shimizu Y, Schull WJ, Kato H: Cancer risk among atomic bomb survivors: the RERF Life Span Study. JAMA 264:601–4, 1990.
18. Tucker MA, Meadows AT, Boice JD et al: Leukemia after therapy with alkylating agents for childhood cancer. J Natl Cancer Inst 78:459–64, 1987.
19. Pui C-H, Ribeiro RC, Hancock ML et al: Acute myeloid leukemia in children treated with epipodophyllotoxins for acute lymphoblastic leukemia. N Engl J Med 325:1682–7, 1991.
20. Pui C-H, Raimondi SC, Murphy SB et al: An analysis of leukemic cell chromosomal features in infants. Blood 69:1289–93, 1987.
21. Thirman MJ, Gill HJ, Burnett RC et al: Rearrangement of the MLL gene in acute lymphoblastic and acute myeloid leukemias with 11q23 chromosomal translocations. N Engl J Med 329:909–14, 1993.
22. Sorensen P, Chen CS, Smith FO et al: Molecular rearrangements of the MLL gene are present in most cases of infant acute myeloid leukemia and are strongly correlated with monocytic or myelomonocytic phenotypes. J Clin Invest 93:429–37, 1991.
23. Busque L, Gilliland DG: Clonal evolution in acute myeloid leukemia. Blood 82:337–42, 1993.
24. Rowley JD: Recurring chromosome abnormalities in leukemia and lymphoma. Semin Hematol 27:122–36, 1990.
25. Fialkow PJ, Singer JW, Raskind W et al: Clonal development, stem-cell differentiation, and clinical remissions in acute nonlymphocytic leukemia. N Engl J Med 317:468–73, 1987.
26. Vogelstein B, Fearon ER, Hamilton SR et al: Use of restriction fragment length polymorphisms to determine the clonal origin of human tumors. Science 227:642–5, 1985.
27. Raimondi SC, Chang MN, Ravindranath Y et al: Chromosomal abnormalities in 478 children with acute myeloid leukemia: Clinical characteristics and treatment outcome in a cooperative Pediatric Oncology Group study—POG 8821. Blood 94:3707–16, 1999.
28. Griffin JD, Lowenberg B: Clonogenic cells in acute myeloblastic leukemia. Blood 68:1185–95, 1986.
29. Bonnet D, Dick J: Human acute myeloid leukemia is organized as a hierarchy that originates from a primitive hematopoietic cell. Nat Med 3:730–7, 1997.
30. Behm FG. Diagnosis of childhood acute myeloid leukemia. Clin Lab Med 19(1):187–237, 1999.
31. Bennett JM, Catovsky D, Daniel MT et al: Proposed revised criteria for the classification of acute myeloid leukemia. Ann Intern Med 103:620–5, 1985.
32. Bennett JM, Catovsky D, Daniel M et al: Criteria for the diagnosis of acute leukemia of megakaryocyte lineage (M7). Ann Intern Med 103:460–2, 1985.
33. Bennett JM, Catovsky D, Daniel MT et al: Proposal for the recognition of minimally differentiated acute myeloid leukaemia (AML-M0). Br J Haematol 78:325–9, 1991.
34. Creutzig U, Schaaff A, Ritter J et al: Acute myelogenous leukemia in children under 2 years of age: Studies and treatment results in 23 children in the AML therapy study BFM-78. Klin Paediatr 196:130–4, 1984.
35. Pui C-H, Raimondi SC, Srivastava DK et al: Prognostic factors in infants with acute myeloid leukemia. Leukemia 14:684–7, 2000.
36. Windebank KP, Tefferi A, Smithson WA et al: Acute megakaryocytic leukemia (M7) in children. Mayo Clin Proc 64:1339, 1989.
37. Chan LC, Pegram SM, Greaves MF: Contribution of immunophenotype to the classification and differential diagnosis of acute leukemia. Lancet 1:475–9, 1985.
38. Cheson B, Cassileth P, Head D et al: Report of the National Cancer Institute-sponsored workshop on definitions of diagnosis and response in acute myeloid leukemia. J Clin Oncol 8:813–9, 1990.
39. Kotylo PK, Seo I-S, Smith FO et al: Flow cytometric immunophenotypic characterization of pediatric and adult minimally differentiated acute myeloid leukemia (AML-M0). Am J Clin Pathol 113:193–200, 2000.
40. Creutzig U, Harbott J, Sperling C et al: Clinical significance of surface antigen expression in children with acute myeloid leukemia: Results of study AML-BFM-87. Blood 86:3097–108, 1995.

41. Kuerbitz S, Civin C, Krischer J et al: Expression of myeloid-associated and lymphoid-associated cell-surface antigens in acute myeloid leukemia of childhood: A Pediatric Oncology Group study. J Clin Oncol 10:1419–29, 1992.

42. Pui C-H, Raimondi SC, Head D et al: Characterization of childhood acute leukemia with multiple myeloid and lymphoid markers at diagnosis and relapse. Blood 78:1327–37, 1991.

43. Carroll A, Civin C, Schneider N et al: The t(1;22) (p13,q13) is nonrandom and restricted to infants with acute megakaryoblastic leukemia: A Pediatric Oncology Group study. Blood 78:748–52, 1991.

44. Choi S, Simon JV: Acute nonlymphocytic leukemia in 171 children. Med Pediatr Oncol 2:119–46, 1976.

45. Creutzig U, Ritter J, Budde M et al: Early deaths due to hemorrhage and leukostasis in childhood acute myelogenous leukemia. Cancer 60:3071–9, 1987.

46. Bunin NJ, Pui COH: Differing complications of hyperleukocytosis in children with acute lymphoblastic or acute non-lymphoblastic leukemia. J Clin Oncol 3:1590–5, 1985.

47. Hayashi Y, Eguchi M, Sugita K et al: Cytogenetic findings and clinical features in acute leukemia and transient myeloproliferative disorder in Down's syndrome. Blood 72:15–23, 1988.

48. Pui C-H, Kalwinsky D, Schell M et al: Acute nonlymphoblastic leukemia in infants: Clinical presentation and outcome. J Clin Oncol 6:1008–13, 1988.

49. Pui C-H, Dahl GV, Kalwinsky DK et al: Central nervous system leukemia in children with acute nonlymphoblastic leukemia. Blood 66:1062–7, 1985.

50. Weinstein HJ, Mayer RJ, Rosenthal DS et al: Chemotherapy for acute myelogenous leukemia in children and adults: VAPA update. Blood 62:315–9, 1983.

51. Chessells JM, O'Callaghan U, Hardisty RM: Acute myeloid leukemia in childhood: Clinical features and prognosis. Br J Haematol 6:555–64, 1986.

52. Shome DK, Gupta NK, Prajapati N et al: Orbital granulocytic sarcomas (myeloid sarcomas) in acute non-lymphocytic leukemia. Cancer 70:2298–301, 1992.

53. Buckley J, Chard R, Baehner R et al: Improvement in outcome for children with acute nonlymphocytic leukemia. Cancer 63:1457–65, 1989.

54. Ravindranath Y, Steuber CP, Krischer J et al: High dose cytarabine for intensification of early therapy of childhood acute myeloid leukemia: A Pediatric Oncology Group study. J Clin Oncol 9:572–80, 1991.

55. Wells R, Woods W, Lampkin B et al: Impact of high dose cytarabine and asparaginase intensification on childhood acute myeloid leukemia: A report from the Children's Cancer Group. J Clin Oncol 11:538–45, 1993.

56. Lie SO, Jonmundsson G, Mellander L et al: A population-based study of 272 children with acute myeloid leukaemia treated on two consecutive protocols with different intensity: Best outcome in girls, infants and children with Down's syndrome. Br J Haematol 4:82–8, 1996.

57. Woods WG, Neudorf S, Gold S et al: A comparison of allogeneic bone marrow transplantation, autologous bone marrow transplantation, and aggressive chemotherapy in children with acute myeloid leukemia in remission: A report from the Children's Cancer Group. Blood 97:56–62, 2001.

58. Creutzig U, Ritter J, Zimmermann M et al: Improved treatment results in high-risk pediatric acute myeloid leukemia patients after intensification with high-dose cytarabine and mitoxantrone: Results of study acute myeloid leukemia – Berlin-Frankfurt-Münster 93. J Clin Oncol 19:2705–13, 2001.

59. Stevens RF, Hann IM, Wheatley K et al: Marked improvements in outcome with chemotherapy alone in paediatric acute myeloid leukaemia: Results of the United Kingdom Medical Research Council's 10th AML trial. Br J Haematol 101:130–40, 1998.

60. Ravindranath Y, Yeager A, Chang M et al: Autologous bone marrow transplantation versus intensive consolidation chemotherapy for acute myeloid leukemia in childhood. N Engl J Med 334:1428–34, 1996.

61. Amadori S, Testi AM, Arico M et al: Prospective comparative study of bone marrow transplantation and postremission chemotherapy for childhood acute myelogenous leukemia. J Clin Oncol 11:1046–54, 1993.

62. Lemons R, Keller S, Gietzen D et al: Acute promyelocytic leukemia. J Pediatr Hematol Oncol 17:198–210, 1995.

63. Cuttner J, Holland J, Norton L: Therapeutic leukapheresis for hyperleukocytosis in acute myelocytic leukemia. Med Pediatr Oncol 11:76–8, 1983.

64. Grund F, Armitage J, Burns C: Hydroxyurea in the prevention of the effects of leukostasis in acute leukemia. Arch Intern Med 137:1246–7, 1977.

65. Pizzo PA, Robichaud KJ, Gill FA et al: Empiric antibiotic and antifungal therapy for cancer patients with prolonged fever and granulocytopenia. Am J Med 72:101–11, 1982.

66. Pizzo PA: Management of fever in patients with cancer and treatment-induced neutropenia. N Engl J Med 328:1323–32, 1993.

67. Shamberger RC, Weinstein HJ, Delorey MJ et al: The medical and surgical management of typhlitis in children with acute nonlymphocytic (myelogenous) leukemia. Cancer 57:603–9, 1986.

68. Buckley JD, Lampkin BC, Nesbit ME et al: Remission induction in children with acute non-lymphocytic leukemia using cytosine arabinoside and doxorubicin or daunorubicin: A report from the Children's Cancer Study Group. Med Pediatr Oncol 17:382–90, 1989.

69. Creutzig U, Ritter J, Zimmermann M et al: Does cranial irradiation reduce the risk for bone marrow relapse in acute myelogenous leukemia? Unexpected results of the childhood acute myelogenous leukemia study BFM-87. J Clin Oncol 11:279–86, 1993.

70. Woods W, Kobrinsky N, Buckley J et al: Timed-sequential induction therapy improves post-remission outcome in acute myeloid leukemia: A report from the Children's Cancer Group. Blood 87:4979–89, 1996.

71. Boulad F, Kernan N: Treatment of childhood acute nonlymphoblastic leukemia: A review. Cancer Invest 11:534–53, 1993.

72. Baehner RL, Bernstein ID, Sather H et al: Improved remission induction rate with D-ZAPO but unimproved remission duration with addition of immunotherapy to chemotherapy in previously untreated children with ANLL. Med Pediatr Oncol 7:127, 1979.

73. Dahl GW, Kalwinsky DK, Murphy S et al: Cytokinetically based induction therapy and splenectomy for childhood acute nonlymphocytic leukemia. Blood 60:856, 1982.

74. Clift RA, Buckner CD, Thomas ED et al: The treatment of acute non-lymphoblastic leukemia by allogeneic marrow transplantation. Bone Marrow Transplant 2:243–58, 1987.

75. Brochstein JA, Kernan NA, Groshen S et al: Allogeneic bone marrow transplantation after hyperfractionated total-body irradiation and cyclophosphamide in children with acute leukemia. N Engl J Med 317:1618–24, 1987.

76. Herzig RH, Lazarus HM, Wolff SM et al: High-dose cytosine arabinoside therapy with and without anthracycline antibiotics for remission reinduction of acute nonlymphoblastic leukemia. J Clin Oncol 3:992–7, 1985.

77. Mayer R, Davis R, Schiffer C et al: Intensive postremission chemotherapy in adults with acute myeloid leukemia. N Engl J Med 331:896–903, 1994.

78. Kantarjian H, Keating M, Walters R et al: Acute promyelocytic leukemia. Am J Med 80:789–97, 1986.

79. Tallman M, Anderson J, Schiffer C et al: All-trans-retinoic acid in acute promyelocytic leukemia. N Engl J Med 337:1021–8, 1997.

80. Fenaux P, Chomienne C, Deglos L: All-trans retinoic acid and chemotherapy in the treatment of acute promyelocytic leukemia (review). Semin Hematol 38(1):13–25, 2001.

81. Shen ZX, Chen GQ, Ni JL et al: Use of arsenic trioxide (As_2O_3) in the treatment of acute promyelocytic leukemia (APL): II. Clinical efficacy and pharmacokinetics in relapsed patients. Blood 89:3354–60, 1997.

82. Soignet S, Maslak P, Wang ZG et al: Complete remission after treatment of acute promyelocytic leukemia with arsenic trioxide. N Engl J Med 339:1341–8, 1998.

83. Nesbit M, Buckley J, Feig S et al: Chemotherapy for induction of remission of childhood acute myeloid leukemia followed by marrow transplantation or multiagent chemotherapy. A report from the Children's Cancer Group. J Clin Oncol 12:127–35, 1994.

84. Abella E, Ravindranath Y: Therapy for childhood acute myeloid leukemia: Role of allogeneic bone marrow transplantation. Curr Oncol Rep 2:529–38, 2000.

85. Yeager AM, Kaizer H, Santos GW et al: Autologous bone marrow transplantations in patients with acute non-lymphocytic leukemia, using ex vivo marrow treated with 4-hydroperoxycyclophosphamide. N Engl J Med 315:141–7, 1986.

86. Grier HE, Gelber RD, Camitta BM et al: Prognostic factors in childhood acute myelogenous leukemia. J Clin Oncol 5:1026–32, 1987.

87. Creutzig U, Ritter J, Schellong G: Identification of two risk groups in childhood acute myelogenous leukemia after therapy intensification in study AML-BFM-83 as compared with study AML-BFM-78. Blood 75:1932–40, 1990.

88. Chang M, Raimondi SC, Ravindranath Y et al: Prognostic factors in children and adolescents with acute myeloid leukemia (excluding children with Down syndrome and acute promyelocytic leukemia): Univariate and recursive partitioning analysis of patients treated on Pediatric Oncology Group (POG) Study 8821. Leukemia 14:1201–7, 2000.

89. Keating MJ, Smith TL, Kantarjian H et al: Cytogenetic pattern in acute myelogenous leukemia. A major reproducible determinant of outcome. Leukemia 2:403, 1988.

90. Ravindranath Y, Abella E, Krischer J et al: Acute myeloid leukemia (AML) in Down's syndrome is highly responsive to chemotherapy: Experience on Pediatric Oncology Group AML Study 8498. Blood 80:2210–14, 1992.

91. Taub JW, Huang X, Matherly LH et al: Expression of chromosome 21-localized genes in acute myeloid leukemia: Differences between Down syndrome and non-Down syndrome blast cells and relationship to in vitro sensitivity to cytosine arabinoside and daunorubicin. Blood 94:1393–400, 1999.

92. Marie JP, Zittoun R, Sikic BI: Multidrug resistance (MDR1) gene expression in adult acute leukemia: Correlation with treatment outcome and in vitro drug sensitivity. Blood 78:586–92, 1991.

93. Sievers EL, Smith FO, Woods WG et al: Cell surface expression of the multidrug resistance P-glycoprotein (P-170) as detected by monoclonal antibody MRK-16 in pediatric acute myeloid leukemia fails to define a poor prognostic group: A report from the Children's Cancer Group. Leukemia 9:2042–8, 1995.

94. Stahnke K, Boos J, Bender-Götze C et al: Duration of first remission predicts remission rates and long-term survival in children with relapsed acute myelogenous leukemia. Leukemia 12:1534–8, 1998.

95. Wells RJ, Feusner J, Devney R et al: Sequential high-dose cytosine arabinoside – asparaginase treatment in advanced childhood leukemia. J Clin Oncol 3:998, 1985.

96. Wells RJ, Gold SH, Krill CE et al: Cytosine arabinoside and mitoxantrone induction chemotherapy followed by bone marrow transplantation or chemotherapy for relapsed or refractory pediatric acute myeloid leukemia. Leukemia 8:1626–30, 1994.

97. Steuber P, Krischer J, Holbrook T et al: Therapy of refractory or recurrent childhood AML using amsacrine and etoposide with or without 5-azacytidine: A Pediatric Oncology Group randomized phase 2 study. J Clin Oncol 14:1521–5, 1996.

98. Dahl GV, Lacayo NJ, Brophy N et al: Mitoxantrone, etoposide, and cyclosporine therapy in pediatric patients with recurrent or refractory acute myeloid leukemia. J Clin Oncol 18:1867–75, 2000.

99. Santana V, Mirro J, Kearns C et al: 2-Chlorodeoxyadenosine produces a high rate of complete hematologic remission in relapsed acute myeloid leukemia. J Clin Oncol 10:364–70, 1992.

100. Rubinstein P, Carrier C, Scaradavou A et al: Outcomes among 562 recipients of placental-blood transplants from unrelated donors. N Engl J Med 339:1565–77, 1998.

101. Sievers EL: Clinical studies of new "biologic" approaches to therapy of acute myeloid leukemia with monoclonal antibodies and immunoconjugates. (review). Curr Opin Oncol 2(1):30–5, 2000.

102. Gamis AS, Howells WB, DeSwarte-Wallace J et al: Alpha hemolytic streptococcal infection during intensive treatment for acute myeloid leukemia: A report from the Children's Cancer Group Study CCG-2891. J Clin Oncol 18:1845–55, 2000.

103. Anderson KC, Weinstein HJ: Irradiation of blood components to prevent graft-vs-host disease. In Kurtz SR, Baldwin ML and Sirchia G (eds.): Controversies in Transfusion Medicine: Immune Complications and Cytomegalovirus Transmission. pp. 57–80. American Association of Blood Banks, Arlington, VA, 1990.

104. Liesner RJ, Leiper AD, Hann IM et al: Late effects of intensive treatment for acute myeloid leukemia and myelodysplasia in childhood. J Clin Oncol 12:916–924, 1994.

105. Leung W, Hudson MM, Strickland DK et al: Late effects of treatment in survivors of childhood acute myeloid leukemia. J Clin Oncol 18(18):3273–9, 2000.

106. Sanders JE, Pritchard S, Mahoney P et al: Growth and development following marrow transplantation for leukemia. Blood 68:1129–35, 1986.

107. Lipshultz S, Lipsitz S, Mone S et al: Female sex and higher drug dose as risk factors for late cardiotoxic effects of doxorubicin therapy for childhood cancer. N Engl J Med 332:1738–43, 1995.

108. Parsons SK, Gelber S, Cole BF et al: Quality-adjusted survival after treatment for acute myeloid leukemia in childhood: a Q-TWiST analysis of the Pediatric Oncology Group Study 8821. J Clin Oncol 17:2144–52, 1999.

20

Diagnosis and Treatment of Adult Acute Myeloid Leukemia Other Than Acute Promyelocytic Leukemia

Peter H. Wiernik

Acute myeloid leukemia (AML) includes all acute leukemias characterized by cells of other than lymphoid origin. AML subgroups with special clinical features have been defined by morphologic, immunologic, and cytogenetic techniques as discussed in Chapters 14, 15, and 16, respectively. All subtypes other than acute progranulocytic leukemia (APL) will be discussed in this chapter and APL is discussed in Chapter 21.

From a patient management point of view, the most serious pathologic consequence of AML is pancytopenia, rather than the production of leukemic cells. Therefore, management of AML requires prophylaxis and treatment of life-threatening complications of the absence of normal blood elements as well as eradication of the neoplastic clone from which the leukemic cells are derived. Prevention and treatment of the challenges to health posed by pancytopenia are discussed in the section: Supportive Care. The pathogenesis, clinical manifestations, and specific treatment for AML are discussed in this chapter and in Chapter 21. It will be evident from those chapters and those on supportive care that the management of a patient with AML is complicated and must be provided by a coordinated team of health care professionals thoroughly versed in the clinical nuances and complications of the disease, treatment of the disease, and the impact of this catastrophic illness on patient, family, and society if optimal results are to be achieved. Such care is usually available only at major institutions and it is strongly recommended that, in general, the patient with AML be referred to such an institution immediately after the diagnosis is made. Some patients may not wish to be treated with curative intent and therefore need not be referred.

CLINICAL FEATURES OF AML AT PRESENTATION

AML is diagnosed primarily in adults, although it can occur at any age. The median age at diagnosis in most large series is in the fifth or sixth decade, and the sexes have an approximately equal incidence. There is usually only a vague history of lethargy or lassitude prior to diagnosis, but approximately one-fourth of patients present with a serious infection of soft tissue or the lower respiratory tract associated on occasion with septicemia. Most patients have petechiae as evidence of intracutaneous capillary bleeding but rarely more serious bleeding may

be present initially. Lymphadenopathy is unusual in AML and splenomegaly is found in less than 25 percent of patients. If hepatomegaly is present it is almost always due to a cause other than AML in a de novo patient. Gingival hypertrophy (Plate 20–1) is found in approximately half of patients with acute monocytic (FAB M5) or myelomonocytic (FAB M4) subtypes of AML. With one exception, those patients have the highest incidence of all forms of extramedullary infiltration including leukemia cutis, and central nervous system disease. The exception is granulocytic sarcoma, which in some series is more common in patients with the M2 subtype of AML who demonstrate the t(8;21) cytogenetic abnormality. Perirectal lesions such as fissures or abscesses[1] may be present initially or during severe granulocytopenia at any time, especially in patients with M4 and M5 subtypes.

An elevated white blood cell (WBC) count is found in approximately one-third of patients with AML at diagnosis, and an equal number of patients have a normal WBC count or leukopenia. Hyperleukocytosis (WBC count >100,000 cells/μl) is uncommon, but may require special therapeutic interventions when present (see below).

Blast forms are present in the peripheral blood of 85 percent of patients with AML before treatment. Therefore, about 15 percent of patients will not have a firm diagnosis made by examination of peripheral blood alone. The absolute granulocyte count is reduced in virtually all patients with AML and is less than 500 cells/μl in approximately half of patients on the first examination. Thrombocytopenia is virtually universal and as many as one-third of patients will present with a platelet count less than 20,000/μl and they are candidates for immediate prophylactic platelet transfusion. Moderate anemia is the rule, but severe anemia may be found in patients with active bleeding other than petechial.

All patients with AML require bone marrow aspiration and biopsy. A biopsy is necessary to determine marrow cellularity. While the marrow is usually markedly hypercellular in de novo patients it may be hypocellular, especially in older patients, patients with secondary AML after treatment of another neoplasm with chemotherapy or radiotherapy, or in patients who have developed AML after certain nonmalignant hematologic entities such as paroxysmal nocturnal hemoglobinuria.[2] Obviously, the marrow specimen must be obtained from a previously unirradiated site. It is important to assess marrow cellularity before and after treatment so that meaningful comparisons can be made. The pretreatment and subsequent marrow aspirates should be examined for morphology, histochemical reactions, immunophenotype, and karyotype as discussed in other chapters in this section. Marrow aspirates submitted for immunological and cytogenetic studies must be collected in heparin or acid citrate dextrose (ACD).

Leukemic blast cells account for at least one-half of marrow nucleated elements in approximately 75 percent of AML patients at presentation. In elderly patients the leukemic cells may be less numerous. In some patients with peripheral blood findings suggestive of acute leukemia, the marrow may contain many fewer blasts. Usually, a diagnosis of acute leukemia is not made unless blasts account for at least 30 percent of the marrow nucleated elements. Serial examinations in some patients will be necessary to determine the correct diagnosis and the rate of progression of the marrow infiltration. The number of marrow blasts may increase slowly in some patients over several months or longer. It may be possible to withhold chemotherapy temporarily in some patients under those circumstances, especially elderly patients, as long as they are clinically well and the blood platelet and granulocyte counts are not dangerously low (<20,000/µl and <1,000/µl, respectively).

The marrow aspirate may reveal other abnormalities in addition to leukemic cell infiltration. In patients with the M4 subtype relative erythroid hyperplasia is often present, despite anemia. There may be increased numbers of eosinophil precursors, especially in the M4E variant. Megakaryocytes are usually reduced in number except in secondary leukemia developing in a patient with polycythemia vera or primary thrombocytosis. Patients with the M7 subtype may have morphologically recognizable megakaryocytosis, but more often cell surface immunological or electron microscopic studies will be necessary to establish the lineage of the leukemic cells. Bone marrow necrosis may be evident prior to therapy,[3] or discovered after therapy,[4] especially in septic patients, and myelofibrosis may be detected in secondary leukemia or the FAB M7 subtype. Both marrow necrosis and myelofibrosis impair prognosis.

A minimal or moderate elevation in serum uric acid concentration is found in 50 percent of patients with AML. Serum lactate dehydrogenase levels may be elevated, especially in M4 or M5 subtypes, but usually to a lesser degree than in patients with acute lymphocytic leukemia (ALL). Lysozyme (muramidase) is elevated in the serum[5] and urine of patients with M4 and M5 subtypes. As is the case with serum uric acid, levels of lysozyme directly reflect the body burden of tumor. Serial determinations of lysozyme may aid in evaluating response to therapy in patients with initial elevations.[6]

AML is not simply a disease of the bone marrow and blood. Dysfunction of a number of organs may result directly from leukemic infiltration or indirectly from other consequences of the disease, and may dominate the clinical picture. Petechiae resulting from capillary hemorrhage secondary to thrombocytopenia are the most common skin and mucous membrane lesions. They tend to occur on dependent or traumatized areas of the body surface and may become confluent over some areas, especially in obese patients. Petechiae also occur on the surface and in the parenchyma of internal organs, but such lesions are usually clinically silent. Painless, nontender, small, raised nodules of leukemic cells may be palpable on the skin (leukemia cutis) of a small minority of patients with AML, especially those with M4 or M5 subtypes.[7,8] Such lesions are usually pink in color and not pruritic (Plate 20–2). On rare occasion, leukemia cutis may be evident before bone marrow or other evidence of the disease is discovered,[7] or it may be the first sign of relapse. Leukemia cutis has rarely been noted solely around central venous catheter exit sites.[9,10] Leukemia cutis does not alter prognosis, but can be disturbing to the patient or even grossly disfiguring.[11] The lesions usually involve the entire corium, and the cells comprising them may have a different phenotype than the leukemic marrow cells.[7] The discordance may be due to par-

tial differentiation of the skin lesion cells into macrophages.[7] The lesions almost always respond to systemic chemotherapy rapidly, even if a complete remission is not ultimately obtained.

Rarely, a patient, especially a young patient, with AML will present with or develop a large subcutaneous or other mass of leukemic cells termed a granulocytic sarcoma. On occasion, there is no other evidence of acute leukemia.[12] Such lesions may also arise from subperiosteal areas of bone, particularly ribs, sternum, and orbit.[13] Although granulocytic sarcoma of bone is rare, other bone lesions such as metaphyseal lines that occur frequently in children with acute leukemia are even rarer in adults.

Granulocytic sarcomas may occur in ovary,[14] uterus,[15] breast,[16] cranial or spinal dura[17] (Fig. 20–1), gastrointestinal tract,[18] lung,[19] mediastinum,[20] prostate,[21] and other organs and may present diagnostic difficulties in the absence of the usual manifestations of AML.[12] Such lesions may present as primary tumors of the organs involved, or suggest the diagnosis of lymphoma, plasmacytoma, or eosinophilic granuloma. Typical AML may be discovered simultaneously, later, or never. A Wright-stained touch preparation of the lesion may help immeasurably in establishing the correct diagnosis. Immunohistochemical studies of fixed tissue may also be helpful in addition to routine histological studies.[22,23] When isolated granulocytic sarcomas occur without other evidence of AML, radiotherapy or surgery may be indicated. Although there is some evidence that treatment of an isolated granulocytic sarcoma with systemic chemotherapy will prevent the later occurrence of typical AML,[24] this is not always true and it is best to withhold systemic therapy until frank leukemia develops unless the granulocytic sarcoma cannot be treated locally.

Granulocytic sarcomas may occur more frequently in patients with M2 AML and t(8;21),[17,25,26] but it is clear that they also occur in patients with other cytogenetic abnormalities.[27] Their increased frequency as paraspinal tumors with t(8;21) may be related to the co-expression of a neural cell-adhesion molecule (CD56) expressed by leukemic cells with that karyotype.[28]

Acute febrile neutrophilic dermatosis (Sweet syndrome) is a rare skin disorder that occurs in AML and other neoplasms more frequently than expected, for unknown reasons. The syndrome is characterized by fever, multiple painful papular and erythematous cutaneous eruptions, and a dense dermal infiltrate of mature granulocytes.[29,30] A rapid response to glucocorticoids is usually obtained.

Fundic hemorrhage (Plate 20–3) due to thrombocytopenia or leukemic infiltration of the retina may be found in patients of all ages with acute leukemia,[31] including adults with AML.[32] Retinal leukemic infiltration is uncommon, is essentially confined to those patients with extreme hyperleukocytosis (blood blast count >200,000/µl, and is seen as one or more Roth-like spots with surrounding hemorrhage upon fundoscopic examination. Such lesions should be immediately irradiated if sight in the affected eye is to be preserved, but hemorrhage alone responds to successful platelet transfusion.[32] Other fundoscopic findings, such as cotton-wool spots; central vein obstruction; and vitreous, choroidal, or macular hemorrhage are occasionally found.[31,32] Certain treatments, such as high-dose cytara-

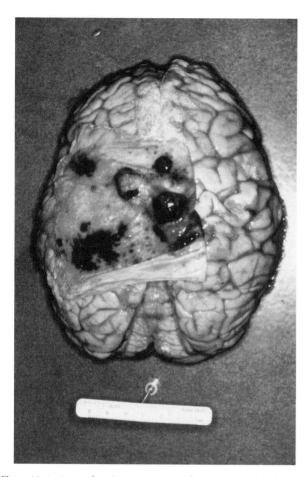

Figure 20–1. A granulocytic sarcoma arising from the dura of the brain in a patient with FAB M2 subtype of AML with t(8;21) karyotype. The dura has been retracted to expose several dark nodules of tumor, which were dark green, due to myeloperoxidase contained in the cytoplasmic granules of the myeloid blast cells.

bine, may cause conjunctival and corneal pathology that results in impaired visual acuity.[33] The lesions resolve and normal visual acuity returns after discontinuation of the drug, and the problem can be prevented or attenuated with glucocorticoid ophthalmic drops administered during cytarabine treatment in most patients.

Pulmonary dysfunction in patients with AML usually results from infection, which is discussed in Chapter 51. A rare patient may develop dyspnea with or without an asthma-like syndrome due to pulmonary capillary leukostasis.[34] Such patients often have high blood blast counts[35,36] and usually have the M3, M4, or M5 subtype of AML, but the frequency of this syndrome in patients with moderate degrees of leukocytosis may be underestimated.[34] The chest radiograph may be normal, show a ground-glass appearance suggestive of hemorrhage, or reveal diffuse alveolar consolidations.[37] This complication is frequently not recognized premortem, especially in patients with unrevealing chest radiographs.[38] Therefore, a therapeutic trial of bilateral low-dose whole lung irradiation should be considered in an AML patient who has inexplicably developed pro-

gressively deteriorating pulmonary function.[39–41] Severe and often fatal bilateral pulmonary hemorrhage may occur in end-stage patients who are thrombocytopenic and refractory to platelet transfusion, or in patients with a coagulopathy. This problem rarely arises during initial treatment. Although such hemorrhage has usually been ascribed to severe thrombocytopenia it may occur after successful platelet transfusion and other evidence suggests that its cause may be multifactorial. Diffuse alveolar cell damage may precede the hemorrhage, and cytoplasmic swelling and bleb formation have been noted in both capillary endothelial and alveolar lining cells in such patients.[42] While it is possible that these histologic changes represent toxic effects of extravascular blood, similar changes have resulted from cytarabine administration[43] or sepsis.[44]

Heart conduction defects, murmurs, pericarditis, and congestive heart failure secondary to leukemic infiltration have been reported in AML.[45–47] Rarely, leukemic cardiac infiltration may occur in the absence of other evidence of AML.[48] These lesions are quite responsive to radiotherapy, which should be considered when leukemic infiltration cannot be ruled out as the etiology of such complications.

It is important to have a dentist examine a patient with AML prior to therapy. Periodontal infections are common when AML is diagnosed and they may result in septicemia in a granulocytopenic patient. Dental extractions may be required[49] before initiation of chemotherapy but often dental infections can be managed medically without interruption of leukemia treatment.[50] Other problems experienced by patients with AML in the region of the head and neck include leukemic infiltration of or hemorrhage into oropharyngeal structures that results in dysphagia or obstruction.[51,52] Leukemic infiltration of the inner, middle, and external ear has also been reported.[53]

As noted above, perirectal abscess and rectal fissure may develop in AML patients with the M4 or M5 subtypes. A small mucosal tear exquisitely painful on defecation or examination associated with fever may be the only indication of this potentially serious problem in a granulocytopenic patient, since infiltration and inflammation are often minimal.[54] Such lesions are usually the result of infection with gram-negative organisms, and bacteremia is frequent if proper treatment is delayed.

Necrotizing enterocolitis, or typhlitis, previously thought to occur primarily in children with acute leukemia, is described with increasing frequency in adults with AML who have been treated intensively.[55] Common symptoms include abdominal pain and distention with or without lower gastrointestinal bleeding. Abdominal radiographs may show only a nonspecific bowel gas pattern or lesions as serious as pneumatosis intestinalis, usually in the right colon. The lesions consist of mucosal ulcerations with inflammatory or leukemic infiltrates and usually involve the cecum but may also involve the ileum or the ascending colon. Bacteremia or fungemia frequently accompanies these lesions. Medical management may suffice[56] but surgery, which is usually successful when appropriate supportive care is available, may be required in some cases.[57]

Renal dysfunction secondary to leukemic infiltration of the kidney or urate nephropathy are uncommon in adults with AML. Leukemic infiltration of the prostate[58] may obstruct the flow of urine and may rarely require irradiation. In most instances, however, induction chemotherapy will completely resolve the problem. Rarely, prostatic infiltration may be the first and only evidence of AML. Under no circumstances should a urinary catheter remain in place in a granulocytopenic AML patient.

Testicular relapse is common in ALL, especially in children, and has also been reported in adults with AML.[59] Postrelapse survival is frequently quite short in most such patients.

Potassium wasting and other evidence of renal tubular dysfunction may occur in patients with the M4 and M5 subtypes who excrete lysozyme (muramidase), which is toxic to the proximal renal tubular epithelium.[6] The problem resolves with reduction of the tumor cell mass with chemotherapy. Lactic acidosis is a rare but difficult problem in AML.[60] Patients usually have large, vacuolated leukemic cells that may be difficult to fully classify. The etiology of the acidosis is obscure. Most patients have poorly controlled disease, and many have significant hepatic leukemic infiltration. The acidosis may require phenomenal quantities of alkali for control even after a partial remission of the leukemia is obtained.

Patients with AML may develop hypercalcemia,[61] but hypocalcemia is more common. The latter may be a result of increased endogenous phosphorus production secondary to destruction of leukemic cells by either ineffective leukopoiesis, chemotherapy, or both but septicemia and nephrotoxic antibiotics are frequently contributing factors.[62] On rare occasion, hypocalcemia and hypophosphatemia may result from accelerated bone formation stimulated by leukemic cells.[63]

Patients with AML subtypes M4 and M5 often present with hypocholesterolemia, which is thought to be due to increased low-density lipoprotein catabolism by mature monocytic phagocytes. Levels return to normal with remission, and fall again with relapse of the leukemia.[64]

Rarely, an AML patient presents with a markedly elevated peripheral blood blast cell count (>200,000 blasts/μl). This is a medical emergency since such a patient has approximately a 25 percent chance of a fatal intracerebral hemorrhage within a day or two.[65–67] This potential catastrophe is the result of intracerebral leukostasis secondary to increased blood viscosity. The hyperviscous blood causes sludging of blast cells at the low-pressure venous end of the capillary bed, which leads to plugging and eventual rupture of the vessel. The bleeding that then occurs would go unnoticed in most organs, but not in the brain. Those patients who undergo induction therapy with hyperleukocytosis are at extreme risk of tumor lysis syndrome, which can be fatal even if recognized early.[68] Therefore, prophylactic emergency treatment directed at rapidly lowering the blood blast count and destroying established intracerebral foci of leukemic cells must be initiated at once (see below).

Many patients with AML are anergic to a battery of intradermal skin tests. This finding is of little clinical significance today since modern therapy has eliminated cutaneous anergy as a poor prognostic factor in AML. Some AML patients have decreased serum concentration of IgG and increased IgM concentration of unknown significance at presentation. Immunoglobulin levels usually normalize during induction therapy. On rare occasions, a serum paraprotein is present initially, which disappears after chemotherapy.[69,70] Most patients with AML have a normal ability to raise a secondary antibody response.[71,72]

DIAGNOSIS OF AML

A thorough evaluation of a patient suspected of having AML must be conducted in a systematic fashion. A complete history should be taken with emphasis on exposure to medications, chemicals, and radiation, and the presence or absence of other diseases associated with an increased incidence of AML, including other neoplasms. A thorough family history should be taken, since a surprisingly high number of patients with AML have a history of hematologic disorders in the family.

A complete physical examination is essential. If the patient is febrile, a thorough search for a focus of infection (periodontal disease, hemorrhoids, sinusitis, otitis, pharyngitis, pneumonia, abscess) must be made. The presence or absence of lymphadenopathy, splenomegaly, optic fundus pathology, central nervous system (CNS) leukemia including cranial nerve palsy, and bleeding must be established. Granulocytopenic patients should not routinely undergo digital rectal examination.

Required peripheral blood studies include hematocrit, WBC count, platelet count, and differential WBC count. The peripheral blood smear should be examined by an oncologist or hematologist with experience in hematologic malignancies. A bone marrow biopsy and aspiration should be obtained from the posterior iliac crest with a Jamshidi needle or similar instrument. If it is impossible to obtain a posterior iliac crest aspirate, an attempt to obtain one from the sternum just under the ridge of the sternal angle with an Illinois or similar needle should be made. It is important to learn to perform these procedures properly from someone with experience. The biopsy is necessary to determine marrow cellularity and to assess the extent of the leukemic infiltrate. The aspirate should be examined after thin air-dried preparations are made, preferably on cover slips. No anticoagulant should be added to the aspirate obtained for routine staining and histochemistry, since some anticoagulants cause morphologic abnormalities in the leukemic cells, such as vacuolization, which may lead to diagnostic confusion. Aspirate smears should be stained with Wright's stain and a battery of histochemical reactions as detailed in Chapter 14. Such stains facilitate differentiation among the various AML subgroups, and between AML and ALL, and are required for proper French-American-British (FAB) classification. An iron stain should also be obtained on the biopsy to assess iron stores, and on the aspirate to identify sideroblasts found commonly in secondary AML after treatment for Hodgkin's disease or multiple myeloma, and ringed sideroblasts that may be found in erythroleukemia (FAB M6).

An aspirate anticoagulated with heparin or ACD should be sent for immunophenotypic and cytogenetic studies. The importance of these studies in the diagnosis of AML is detailed in Chapters 15 and 16, respectively.

Certain blood chemistry studies are required for proper assessment of the patient. Serum electrolytes, uric acid, lactate dehydrogenase, creatinine, lysozyme, and blood urea nitrogen should be determined. Routine coagulation studies and a plasma fibrinogen concentration are especially important in a patient suspected of having the M3 subtype of AML. Since hypogranular variants of that subtype exist, it is important to study all patients initially. It should be remembered that some antibiotics commonly used in leukemia patients may cause abnormalities of coagulation unless vitamin K is administered prophylactically.

It is only necessary to examine the cerebrospinal fluid (CSF) routinely in asymptomatic AML patients with the M4E subtype. A lumbar puncture should only be performed in thrombocytopenic patients after a successful platelet transfusion has elevated the platelet count to 75,000/µl or more and in patients with a coagulopathy only after the plasma fibrinogen level has risen above 100 mg percent. Only 25 gauge needles should be used. The CSF obtained should be studied for routine parameters and, in addition, a cytocentrifuged specimen should be studied after staining with Wright's stain. Some training is required to accurately assess such specimens. Occasionally ependymal and other cells will be seen that may be mistaken for leukemic cells by the untrained observer. An elevated β_2-microglobulin CSF concentration may suggest occult CNS leukemia.

A posteroanterior and lateral chest radiograph should be obtained primarily as a baseline in an asymptomatic patient. Rarely, a mediastinal mass will be observed. This finding may confuse the observer unless one is aware of this rare manifestation of granulocytic sarcoma in AML.[20]

Finally, the patient's blood should be typed and at least two packed red cell units cross-matched with the patient's blood should be available at all times. If the patient has circulating lymphocytes the HLA type should be determined so that this information is available if bone marrow transplantation is contemplated in the future or if HLA-compatible platelet transfusions become necessary. At the same time, family members who may agree to donate platelets, granulocytes, or bone marrow to the patient should be HLA typed also.

PREPARATION FOR INDUCTION THERAPY

It is usually not necessary or wise to begin induction chemotherapy immediately upon the diagnosis of AML. It is best to spend a day or two diagnosing the leukemic disorder precisely and resolving whatever medical emergencies are evident or developing.

Thrombocytopenic hemorrhage is more easily prevented than treated. Therefore, an AML patient with a platelet count less than 15,000 to 20,000/µl is a candidate for prophylactic platelet transfusion, which is discussed fully in Chapter 55. Prophylactic platelet transfusion has virtually eliminated hemorrhage as a cause of death during induction therapy. Platelet transfusion should not be given to a patient with a coagulopathy until heparin therapy is begun, or the coagulopathy may be aggravated.

An AML patient with a serious, uncontrolled infection at the time induction therapy is begun has a greatly reduced chance of remission. Therefore, documented or suspected infection should be under treatment and showing clear evidence of resolution before the institution of chemotherapy whenever possible. It is especially important not to begin chemotherapy until infection is controlled if the patient has circulating granulocytes. If absolute granulocytopenia exists in an infected patient, chemotherapy and antibacterial antibiotic therapy should be started simultaneously. Empiric broad-spectrum antibiotic therapy should be instituted immediately in a febrile granulocytopenic AML patient.[73] It should be remembered that fever may be the only clue to a serious infection in such a patient since the usual signs and symptoms of infection, which are largely due to granulocytic infiltration of infected tissues, may be absent.

The prophylaxis of intracerebral hemorrhage secondary to hyperblastosis[74] usually consists of emergency irradiation to the entire cranium with 600 cGy in a single dose and the administration of oral hydroxyurea (3 g/m² given daily for 2 days). The former will resolve already established intracerebral foci of leukemia, and the latter will rapidly reduce the blood blast count and thereby reduce blood viscosity, which is necessary to prevent reformation of intracapillary collections of blasts. Emergency leukapheresis has also been reported to be effective in this setting.[75] The procedure requires the availability of a blood cell separator and has not been demonstrated to be more effective than simple hydroxyurea administration. Management of hyperblastosis solely with hydration, urinary alkalinization, and allopurinol has been reported to be effective in infants[76] but is not recommended for adults.

Urate nephropathy is unusual in AML, except in patients with hyperleukocytosis. However, it is prudent to begin allopurinol (300 mg orally, daily for 1 or 2 days) before induction therapy and equally prudent to discontinue the drug after the marrow has become hypocellular following chemotherapy. Unnecessary prolongation of allopurinol administration may result in cutaneous eruption, which occurs with about 20 percent of prolonged courses of the agent. Patients who present with elevated serum uric acid concentration and an unusually large tumor load due to hyperleukocytosis or granulocytic sarcoma will require double or triple the usual allopurinol dose initially, or treatment with recombinant urate oxidase.[77]

Infection prevention methods should be instituted before induction therapy. The patient should be placed in strict reverse isolation in a meticulously cleaned room with air supplied only through high-efficiency particulate (HEPA) air filtration systems. Certain patients, primarily elderly patients undergoing reinduction therapy, are at increased risk of infection and may benefit from the use of special patient isolators with HEPA filters. Patients treated in such isolators acquire fewer new potential pathogens and experience fewer bacterial infections and essentially no fungal pneumonias compared with patients treated in a clean, standard environment.

A triple lumen Hickman catheter or similar device should be installed prior to treatment to facilitate blood drawing and intravenous therapy. If at all possible, the catheter should be placed at a time when the patient has circulating granulocytes, and use of the catheter should be restricted to personnel who have been specifically trained in the proper use and care of such devices.

Special consideration needs to be given to the pregnant patient with AML. Commonly administered induction agents can be given with relative safety to mother and fetus during the third and probably the second trimester.[78,79] Children born to mothers undergoing induction therapy for AML during those trimesters have experienced only minor problems at birth and after long-term follow-up.[78–80] Induction therapy during the first trimester is very likely to result in abortion.[79] It may therefore be prudent to induce abortion under controlled circumstances prior to therapy in such cases. Rarely, spontaneous temporary remission of untreated AML may occur after cesarean section,[16] or other event, usually a pyogenic infection.[81]

CHEMOTHERAPY FOR AML

Chemotherapy for AML is usually administered in two stages, induction therapy followed by consolidation therapy. Allogeneic or autologous bone marrow transplantation may follow consolidation therapy in some circumstances, or consolidation therapy may be followed by or replaced by long-term maintenance therapy in other circumstances. The purpose of induction therapy is to achieve complete clinical and hematological remission, which is defined as the absence of all clinical evidence of leukemia as well as a normocellular marrow devoid of leukemic cells and with normal trilineage hematopoiesis. Peripheral blood counts and the differential WBC count are within the normal range in patients in complete remission. The purpose of postremission therapy is to reduce the body burden of subclinical leukemia to, theoretically, zero. There is overwhelming evidence to support the concept of postremission therapy in that in virtually all studies in which outcome with and without postremission therapy has been prospectively compared, disease-free and overall survival is greater in patients who continue treatment while in complete remission. Furthermore, most available data demonstrate a dose-response relationship for postremission therapy so that, in general, cure rates are higher with postremission dose intense regimens than with regimens of lesser dose intensity. While there is no question that intensive postremission therapy is currently necessary in order to achieve optimal results, some studies have suggested that intensification of induction therapy may improve disease-free and overall survival despite no improvement in remission rate.[82]

Although there is little evidence that the major FAB subtypes respond differently to standard induction therapy for AML, the development of all-*trans* retinoic acid therapy for the M3 subtype suggests that more subtype-specific therapy for AML may be developed in the future, and that remission induction by mechanisms other than leukemia cell kill may be possible. There is already evidence that some dose-intense postremission regimens may be more beneficial in certain subtypes of AML than in others.[83]

There is no need for CNS prophylaxis in adult AML. The frequency of overt CNS leukemia is less than 1 to 2 percent, and cytarabine is virtually always used during induction therapy in intravenous doses that result in therapeutic CSF levels.

Results of induction therapy vary inversely with age and vary with cytogenetic characteristics of the patient, as well as with many other factors. A favorable abnormal karyotype [inv(16), t(8;21) or t(15;17)] has a major positive impact on outcome of treatment, compared with other abnormalities or a normal karyotype.[83] In general, approximately 70 percent of unselected patients with de novo AML will achieve complete remission after one course of induction therapy. At least 25 percent, and perhaps as many as 40 percent of complete responders will be cured after appropriate postremission therapy. In a number of studies long-term results are significantly better in women.[84]

When to Begin Treatment

It should be emphasized that some patients with AML do not require immediate treatment. Such patients are usually elderly, have slowly progressive disease as judged by serial blood and marrow examinations, and usually have a history of one or more cytopenias. Some such patients may have been previously given a diagnosis of myelodysplastic syndrome. In such patients chemotherapy must be instituted before dangerous levels of cytopenia occur if not present initially, but not before progressive deterioration of normal blood counts is documented. Elderly patients and others with smoldering AML respond less well to induction therapy than others, and attention to these details will allow an occasional patient with AML to defer chemotherapy for weeks or months. Unfortunately, most patients will experience daily deterioration of hematological parameters after diagnosis and require therapy within a few days. In those patients it is important to begin treatment once the progressive nature of the disease is established, before infection due to granulocytopenia occurs.

Induction Therapy

The standard induction regimen for adults with AML for decades has been the two-drug combination of daunorubicin and cytarabine, and complete response rates on the order of 65 percent have regularly been reported with that combination[85–89] in unselected patients. Patients over the age of 60 years usually have a lower response rate. The administration of yeast-derived recombinant human granulocyte-macrophage colony-stimulating factor (rhGM-CSF) to elderly patients after induction therapy has rendered the marrow hypoplastic and until peripheral granulocyte count recovery has occurred may improve outcome in elderly patients. In a prospective, randomized ECOG study elderly patients treated with a standard induction regimen plus GM-CSF had a higher response rate, lower rate of infection, and lower death rate.[90] A similar study utilizing an investigational GM-CSF derived from *Escherichia coli* showed no advantage for the growth factor.[91] The ECOG study demonstrated that GM-CSF does not stimulate leukemia when used after marrow hypoplasia occurs, since patients receiving the growth factor did not have shorter disease-free or overall survival.[90] However, priming with GM-CSF before induction therapy may be harmful in some patients[92] and priming with GM-CSF[93] or G-CSF[94] does not improve the efficacy of induction therapy.

A commonly used induction regimen is a continuous intravenous 7-day infusion of cytarabine given at the rate of 100 mg/m²/day, plus daunorubicin given as 3 daily bolus injections of 45 mg/m² each, beginning on the first day of treatment. There is no evidence that increasing the dose of daunorubicin by as much as one-third[84,95] or that double[96] or larger doses of cytarabine[97] improve outcome. The addition of etoposide to the regimen improved disease-free and overall survival without improving the response rate, especially in patients less than 50 years of age in one study[82] but not in others.[98,99]

In three randomized, prospective large studies the combination of mitoxantrone and cytarabine was compared with daunorubicin and cytarabine for induction therapy in adults with AML.[100–102] The standard dose and schedule of cytarabine was employed and mitoxantrone 12 mg/m² given daily for 3 days was substituted for daunorubicin in one arm of each study. No significant difference in outcome with respect to complete response rate, disease-free or overall survival, or toxicity was observed in any of the studies.

Daunorubicin and cytarabine were prospectively compared in five major randomized studies with an identical regimen except for the substitution of idarubicin for daunorubicin.[102–106] There were no significant differences in toxicity between the two treatments in any of the studies. In three of the studies[103–105] the complete response rate was superior with idarubicin plus cytarabine and the differences were significant for patients under the age of 60 years, and disease-free and overall survival were significantly greater in idarubicin-treated patients in two of the studies.[103,104] The idarubicin–cytarabine regimen was significantly more effective in remission induction in patients with hyperleukocytosis than the daunorubicin–cytarabine regimen in the two studies in which that question was examined.[103,104] In an Italian study for patients over the age of 55 years no difference in response rate or duration, or survival was noted between the two treatments, but a significantly greater number of complete responders achieved remission with one course of idarubicin and cytarabine than with daunorubicin and cytarabine.[106] In the ECOG study[102] of 349 patients over the age of 55 years the complete response rates were 40, 43, and 43 percent with the daunorubicin, idarubicin, and mitoxantrone regimens, respectively, but the differences were not significant. The median disease-free survival was 5.7, 9.7, and 6.9 months, respectively, but again the differences were not significant. For patients under the age of 70 years the differences in complete response rates were greater (46, 53, and 52 percent, respectively) but the differences were still not significant. These data strongly suggest that idarubicin is a more effective anthracycline than daunorubicin in the treatment of adult AML, especially in younger patients, and this fact was confirmed by a meta-analysis of 1052 patients randomized to receive daunorubicin or idarubicin with cytarabine.[107] These clinical observations are consistent with the more favorable clinical pharmacokinetics of idarubicin[108] compared with those of daunorubicin, and with the observation that the intracellular

accumulation of idarubicin is decreased to a much lesser degree by P-glycoprotein than is that of daunorubicin.[109] Many investigators interpret currently available data to suggest that idarubicin should replace daunorubicin in the treatment of adults with AML, and an appropriate treatment regimen is detailed in Table 20–1.

Toxicity of Induction Therapy

Virtually all patients treated with the regimen recommended in Table 20–1 will develop total capital alopecia, which is often more disconcerting to young men than to others. Attempts to prevent alopecia with scalp tourniquets or hypothermia caps are ill-advised during leukemia treatment since the scalp may become a pharmacologic sanctuary when such methods are employed.

Moderately severe nausea and vomiting accompanies induction therapy in approximately 80 percent of patients not premedicated with antiemetics. Older patients tend to have a lower incidence of emesis, perhaps due to poorer blood supply to the chemoreceptor trigger zone of the brain. Modern antiemetics, such as ondansetron[110] and granisetron[111] usually completely eliminate nausea and vomiting during induction therapy. It is not necessary to include dexamethasone in the antiemetic regimen, and it may indeed be unwise to do so since glucocorticoids inhibit anthracycline reductase activity, which may result in decreased anthracycline effectiveness.

Stomatitis, esophagitis, and diarrhea are usually only of grade 1 to 2 intensity and can be expected in approximately 65, 15, and 80 percent of patients, respectively.[104] Oral mucosal ulceration is usually well managed with viscous xylocaine or a paste of gelatin, pectin, and carboxymethyl cellulose. Hepatic toxicity manifested by serum liver enzyme elevations occurs in half of patients and is usually unaccompanied by clinically significant hepatic dysfunction and virtually always resolves with the completion of induction therapy.

Patients with significant impairment of hepatic excretory function (serum alkaline phosphatase activity or serum total bilirubin > twice the upper limit of normal) require a 50 percent reduction in daily anthracycline dose in order to avoid excessive bone marrow toxicity. These agents are partially metabolized and excreted by the liver, and the suggested dosage reduction will result in near normal pharmacokinetics of them

---

Table 20–1. A Standard Remission Induction Regimen for Adult AML

A. Idarubicin (12 mg/m²) is given daily on each of the first 3 days of treatment. The drug is given as an injection over 10 to 15 minutes into a central venous catheter. Severe paravenous tissue damage may result from extravasation.

B. Cytosine arabinoside is given as a continuous 7-day intravenous infusion at the rate of 100 mg/m²/day beginning on the first day of idarubicin administration. The infusion must be controlled by an electronic device to ensure the proper rate of administration.

in the setting of significant hepatic dysfunction and yield results comparable to those obtained with standard doses in patients with normal liver function.

A generalized mild to moderate erythroderma may result from cytarabine or idarubicin treatment, and a unique cutaneous eruption has been reported after etoposide administration.[112]

Profound bone marrow hypoplasia and pancytopenia are expected and desirable after induction therapy since, except in patients with the M3 subtype, complete remission is virtually never achieved without these results of therapy. Pancytopenic patients will require platelet transfusion and, very likely, packed red cell transfusion until the bone marrow recovers, usually in 3 to 4 weeks after the end of treatment. Transfusion support is discussed in Chapters 54 and 55.

Response to Induction Therapy

Approximately 90 percent of patients who achieve complete remission will do so within the month after completion of the first induction course. Another 10 percent of patients who ultimately obtain a complete remission will require a second induction course to do so. The second course should be given in the same doses and schedule as the first. While it has been demonstrated that some patients will achieve a complete remission only after a third induction course of the same treatment, it is generally agreed that failure after two courses indicates significant resistance to the regimen, and subsequent remission induction attempts should utilize different drugs with incomplete cross-resistance to those used initially. Patients who fail induction therapy with two courses of idarubicin and cytarabine may be candidates for regimens employing mitoxantrone,[113] carboplatin,[114] 2-chlorodeoxyadenosine,[115] fludarabine,[116] high-dose cytarabine,[117] CD33-calicheamicin immunoconjugate,[118] or bone marrow transplantation, all of which are discussed below. Unfortunately, patients who fail initial therapy are not likely to subsequently do well, and at the present time it is difficult to recommend a standard approach to such patients.[119]

Often the first sign of complete remission after induction therapy is a spontaneous rise in the platelet count. If the marrow aspirate demonstrates repopulation with normal elements at that time, and leukemic cells are rare, blood counts should be observed until they are normal. At that time another marrow aspirate should be examined to diagnose complete remission or persistent leukemia. No additional induction therapy is necessary if the former pertains, whereas the second induction course should be administered if less than complete marrow remission has been achieved. If residual leukemia without any evidence of maturation in the granulocyte series appears to be present in the first postinduction marrow aspirate, another aspirate should be examined several days later, before reinstituting induction therapy. This is necessary because a marrow recovering from anthracycline drug administration may appear hypocellular and frankly leukemic, but normalize without further therapy. Indeed, an occasional blast may even be found in the blood after anthracycline therapy in a patient who subsequently manifests complete remission without further therapy. In such patients the platelet count may begin to rise, followed within a week by a rise in the granulocyte count. Progressive improvement in both to normal levels as indicated by daily blood counts is usually a harbinger of complete remission. A transient platelet count elevation, often without a concomitant rise in granulocyte count, usually indicates an incomplete response to induction therapy. This must be confirmed by bone marrow examination when the progressive platelet count improvement levels off or reverses. Almost always the marrow examination will confirm an incomplete response in that situation. However, rarely the marrow examination may lead to confusion due to the presence of a megaloblastic maturation arrest in the granulocyte and erythroid series and no evidence of leukemia. In such cases the patient may be folate depleted, especially if significant mucous membrane toxicity occurred during treatment. Such patients may have a dramatic response to daily physiologic doses of parenteral folate, with morphologically normal marrow and normal blood counts evident 10 to 14 days after initiation of folate therapy. In other cases, all criteria for the diagnosis of complete remission may be present except for the continuation of significant thrombocytopenia and a continuing need for platelet transfusion despite an adequate number of megakaryocytes in the marrow. Most such patients will respond with a normal platelet count to daily, oral low-dose cyclosporin A administration (100 to 200 mg/day) for unknown reasons.[120] In such patients, cyclosporin A may need to be continued indefinitely.

Many prognostic factors influence induction therapy results. There is an inverse relationship between time to achieve complete remission after one course of chemotherapy, and disease-free and overall survival in patients with AML.[121] The patient's age has the most consistent influence on results. Elderly patients, especially those older than 70 years, are less likely to withstand the severity of treatment.[122,123] It is not entirely clear why this is so, but other coincidental medical problems such as cardiopulmonary disease common in the elderly may make them less likely to sustain treatment without intolerable toxicity. Poor marrow reserve usually found in the aged may delay or disallow bone marrow recovery after treatment and facilitate infectious complications. In addition, poor-prognosis karyotypes are more frequent in the elderly whereas good-prognosis karyotypes are more frequent in young adults.[122] For these reasons and others, some have advocated less intensive therapy for elderly patients.[124] Others disagree.[125] Clearly, elderly patients require the maximum in supportive care if intensive treatment is to be given. When intensive treatment is given in a setting of maximum supportive care it is likely to be successful in elderly patients and is likely to yield more benefit than less aggressive therapy without additional significant toxicity.[125–127] Although in many studies remission duration in the elderly treated with standard induction regimens has been poor,[122] remission duration and survival have been prolonged in others.[127] Elevated blood urea nitrogen concentration, poor performance status, high peripheral blood blast count, and hepatomegaly have been reported to be particularly poor prognostic factors for survival in the elderly with AML.[128]

Patients with secondary AML, discussed in Chapter 22, and AML developing after a preleukemic phase or myelodysplastic syndrome[129] have a poorer response rate, response duration, and survival than do patients with de novo AML.

The bone marrow and blood become normal morphologically and the quantities of various cellular elements normalize absolutely and relative to each other in the majority of patients when complete remission is achieved. Some complete responders, however, manifest myelodysplastic changes permanently after stem cell damage from chemotherapy but produce normal blood cells in normal numbers.[130,131] Remission is usually explained by the premise that chemotherapy kills most of the abnormal cells and allows residual normal stem cells to repopulate the marrow and function normally. However, some evidence suggests that remission may result from maturation and differentiation of leukemia cells induced by standard chemotherapy.[132–134] Rarely, patients in remission are noted to have Auer rods in otherwise normal granulocytes[134,135] and some patients have been noted to degranulate mature granulocytes before other evidence of relapse is apparent. In addition, the normal leukocytes of some patients in remission express reverse transcriptase activity characteristic of leukemic cells and uncharacteristic of normal leukocytes.[136] These observations, together with the fact that a large number of agents, including many chemotherapeutic agents, are known to cause differentiation and maturation of leukemic cells in vitro,[137,138] suggest that remission does not necessarily derive from the cytotoxicity of induction therapy alone.

POSTREMISSION THERAPY

It is now universally agreed that postremission therapy prolongs complete remission and enhances the cure rate in AML. From the mid-1960s until recently, myriad maintenance regimens were tested. These regimens were usually given for a finite period each month, were usually less intensive than induction regimens, and usually consisted of multiple drugs most of which were not given during the induction phase of treatment. These treatments may have had a minimal favorable effect on remission duration,[139] but were largely unsuccessful. The value of such treatments became even more doubtful when it was demonstrated that the frequency of their administration had no effect on remission duration.[85] Furthermore, some studies during that period suggested that remission duration was not adversely affected by omitting maintenance therapy altogether.[140,141] Confusion was further compounded by the fact that most studies initiated after 1979 gave better remission duration results than previous studies irrespective of postremission therapy schemes. Most of those studies have employed an intensive induction regimen with an anthracycline and cytosine arabinoside in a schedule and doses similar to the treatment in Table 20–1. Not only have those studies resulted in superior response rates and durations compared with previous ones, but the number of disease-free long-term survivors resulting from them was significantly greater.[85,87] These observations suggest that the efficacy of induction chemotherapy is one important determinant of remission duration. This concept is further supported by several idarubicin studies.[103–105] Such has also proved to be the case in other highly treatable hematologic

neoplasms such as advanced Hodgkin's disease and other lymphomas. Some biochemical substantiation of that contention has been offered by Rustum and Preisler,[142] who found that patients with the longest remission durations were those whose pretreatment leukemic cells best activated cytosine arabinoside to cytosine arabinoside triphosphate and retained the activated compound longest intracellularly.

More recently, it has been suggested that postremission schemes as described above are ineffective not because the concept of postremission therapy is wrong, but because the treatments were less intensive than necessary for optimal results. Therefore, a number of studies employing postremission schemes for a finite period that were at least as intensive as induction therapy were instituted.[87,95,143–147] The results of such studies have been very impressive. Median durations of complete remission on the order of 18 to 24 months have been obtained and 20 to 45 percent or more of complete responders so treated have remained disease-free for up to 15 years[148] after achieving complete remission. The intensive postremission programs, in general, produce results superior to those obtained with previously employed lower dose postremission therapy.

Four types of successful postremission therapy have emerged from studies conducted over the last 20 years. Consolidation therapy, which is usually given as one or more courses of high-dose cytarabine with or without other agents, has become a standard form of treatment.[95,143,145,149] Such programs appear to be most effective when the dose of cytarabine is greater than 400 mg/m^2 given every 12 hours, and doses of 3 g/m^2 are commonly employed on that schedule.[143] However, the optimal dose between 400 mg/m^2 and 3 g/m^2 on such schedules remains to be determined. This is important, since cytarabine toxicity escalates steeply above doses of 500 mg/m^2 given twice daily.[97] Treatment with a high-dose consolidation program is outlined as option I in Table 20–2. Other, more complicated regimens have been studied,[144,150] but results are similar or inferior to those obtained with the regimen in that table.

High-dose cytarabine-based consolidation programs that employ cytarabine doses of 3 g/m^2 are toxic and associated with a death rate during remission of 10 to 20 percent. Patients with hepatic or renal dysfunction and older patients tolerate this treatment especially poorly. Older patients are especially prone to severe neurotoxicity from this treatment.[143,151] Whether cytarabine 3 g/m^2 in multiple doses is more effective than lower doses as consolidation therapy is the subject of much debate.[152] Others have employed half that dose without apparent loss of efficacy,[90] although the two doses have never been prospectively compared. Neither GM-CSF[90] nor G-CSF[153] has been particularly useful during the consolidation phase of treatment.

A less toxic but effective approach to postremission therapy utilizes conventional doses of cytarabine and 6-thioguanine given on an open-ended schedule until marrow hypoplasia is achieved[87] and is summarized as option II in Table 20–2. This treatment is associated with only a 1 percent death in remission rate and can safely be given to patients up to the age of 75 years. Long-term results are excellent, but this approach has also never been prospectively compared with a high-dose cytarabine-based regimen.

Table 20–2. Postremission Therapy Options for Adult AML Patients in First Remission

I. High-dose consolidation therapy of short duration
Example: adapted from Mayer et al.[143]
Regimen: Cytarabine, 3 g/m² is given as a 3-hour infusion every 12 hours on days 1, 3, and 5 for a total of 6 doses per course, beginning within 1 month of complete remission. Courses are repeated every 28 to 35 days, depending on marrow recovery. A total of 4 courses are given.
Comment: This regimen resulted in a 44 percent projected disease-free survival at 5 years for patients 60 years of age or less.[143] Results were significantly poorer and toxicity was prohibitive in older patients. Toxicity was substantial in patients over the age of 45 years. Therefore, the regimen may only be generally applicable to patients less than 45 years old. Serious neurotoxicity (usually cerebellar ataxia) occurred in 12 percent of patients and was permanent in 40 percent of patients who experienced it. Other serious toxicity included confluent maculopapular rash and desquamation, conjunctivitis, pulmonary fibrosis, and gastrointestinal tract ulceration. Treatment-related death occurred in 5 percent of patients.
II. Intensive recurring regimen given on an open schedule for 3 years.
Example: Dutcher et al.[87]
Regimen: Cytarabine, 100 mg/m² as an i.v. bolus and oral 6-thioguanine, 100 mg/m² are both given every 12 hours until severe marrow hypoplasia is achieved. The treatment is given every 3 months for 3 years beginning 1 month after complete remission is established.
Comment: Approximately 10 days of treatment are required to achieve marrow hypoplasia with the first several courses, but only 5 to 7 days of treatment are necessary after 12 to 18 months. Results are equal in younger and older patients up to age 75. Toxicity is virtually limited to the bone marrow, and only 1 percent drug-related deaths during remission have been noted in recent years. An observed 20 percent disease-free survival at 15 years has been reported.[148]
III. Allogeneic bone marrow transplantation
Examples: Young et al.,[154] Clift et al.,[155] Bortin et al.,[156] Zittoun et al.,[157] Cassileth et al.[162]
Regimens: The patient's marrow is ablated with high doses of chemotherapy (usually alkylating agents) with or without total body irradiation. In some studies ablation with irradiation + alkylating agent resulted in superior relapse rate, disease-free, and overall survival compared with alkylating agent ablation only.[158] Marrow from an HLA-identical sibling whose lymphocytes do not react in vitro with those of the recipient is preferable.
Comment: The probability of disease-free survival at 5 years has been estimated to be 45 to 60 percent, and treatment-related death rates in remission have been reported to be 25 to 40 percent in various studies. Results vary inversely with age, and patients over the age of 45 years rarely do well. For logistical and other reasons, approximately half of patients for which this therapy is planned never receive it.[160]
IV. Autologous bone marrow transplantation
Examples: Gorin et al.,[164] Körbling et al.,[165] Zittoun et al.,[157] Cassileth et al.[162]
Regimens: Preparation of the patient is similar to that for allogeneic transplantation. Marrow must be harvested from the patient after complete remission is achieved and before high-dose chemotherapy. Some investigators purge the harvested marrow in vitro with mafosfamide or etoposide, but it is unclear whether this reduces the likelihood of relapse. Some evidence suggests that autologous marrow transplantation may be replaced in the future by peripheral stem cell harvest and reinfusion.
Comment: Long-term disease-free survival comparable to that obtained with allogeneic marrow transplantation has been reported by various authors. Autologous transplantation is much safer that allogeneic transplantation, with only 3 to 5 percent treatment-related deaths during remission observed with the former. Autologous marrow transplantation may, therefore, be preferable for older patients (up to age 60 years). The relative merits of both types of marrow transplantation and other high-dose cytarabine-based postremission options are currently being prospectively evaluated by several large cooperative group studies.

Allogeneic bone marrow transplantation is described as option III in Table 20–2. Best results have been reported in young patients, and most reported series are heavily weighted with patients younger than 30 years. Preparative regimens usually consist of alkylating agents such as busulfan and cyclophosphamide, or busulfan and total body irradiation. The latter was more effective than the former with respect to relapse rate, disease-free, and overall survival in the only prospective randomized study of patients with AML.[158] With currently available techniques, patients under the age of 60 years, who have an HLA-compatible sibling donor whose blood lymphocytes do not react with those of the potential recipient in mixed lymphocyte culture, are considered optimal candidates for the procedure. Postremission consolidation therapy with high-dose cytarabine before allogeneic marrow transplantation for AML in first complete remission does not improve outcome compared with proceeding directly to transplantation after recovery from induction therapy.[159] Allogeneic transplants are more successful when the donor is less than 40 years old.[163] Thus, only 20 percent or less of patients with AML who achieve complete remission can be considered optimal candidates for allogeneic marrow transplantation using a sibling donor at this time, and only a minority of them actually are transplanted due to logistical and other problems.[160]

Allogeneic bone marrow transplantation utilizing an HLA-matched unrelated donor has been studied in patients who do not have a sibling donor. In one study of 161 patients[161] leukemia-free survival at 5 years was 50 ± 12 percent for patients transplanted during first complete remission, and the relapse rate was 19 percent after a median post-transplant follow-up of 2.9 years. There was a direct relationship between the duration of leukemia-free survival and the dose of marrow cells infused. These results closely approach those obtained with sibling allografts and represent significant improvement in the efficacy of this procedure.

Autologous bone marrow transplantation, option IV in Table 20–2, has been developed more recently than allogeneic transplantation as a postremission option for AML, and in some studies,[157,162] but not all,[166,167] results have been equivalent to those obtained with allogeneic transplantation. Others have suggested that autologous[168] or allogeneic[169,170] peripheral blood stem cell reinfusion may be a highly effective method for supporting high-dose postremission therapy in AML, but further studies will be required to determine whether this method is valid. Marrow recovery seems to be more rapid after transplantation with allogeneic peripheral blood stem cells compared with marrow cells.[169,170] Autologous bone marrow transplantation with[171,172] and without[157,166] ex vivo purging appears to yield similar results.

Disease-free and overall survival for AML patients transplanted during first remission have been reported by innumerable investigators from around the world. The 5-year disease-free survival rate projected from actuarial analysis in most studies has ranged from 30 to 50 percent, and relapse rates of 15 to 25 percent have been reported. Occasionally, relapses are extramedullary,[173] late,[174] and possibly due to induction of leukemia in the graft.[175] Most adult long-term survivors of marrow transplantation have been reasonably, if not entirely, well. In one large study, patients with no recurrence of leukemia at 2 years had an overall 82 percent chance of being alive in complete remission at 9 years following transplantation regardless of the type of transplant. Patients allografted, however, experienced a lower frequency of late relapse than patients autografted.[176] Females had a lower relapse rate than males, an observation also reported after chemotherapy alone.[84] In another large similar study[177] of patients who were free of AML 2 years after allogeneic transplantation, mortality remained higher than in the normal population through the ninth year post-transplantation. Recurrent leukemia was the major cause of death.

There is no doubt that both allogeneic and autologous bone marrow transplantation can cure AML. The question is the relative frequency of cure from these and other methods. In an effort to answer the question, a number of prospective studies were performed in which allogeneic or autologous bone marrow transplantation and intensive consolidation chemotherapy alone were compared.[95,145,157,162,167,178–180] The results have been quite similar in most of these trials. Allogeneic bone marrow transplantation results in fewer leukemic relapses than consolidation chemotherapy alone, but overall survival of the two groups of patients is similar, and results with autologous transplantation are often in the middle.[157] The high death rate during remission after allogeneic transplantation is primarily due to acute graft-versus-host disease (GvHD). Unfortunately, treatments that reduce the incidence of acute or chronic GvHD, with the possible exception of thalidomide,[181] usually lead to an increased incidence of leukemic relapse,[182] since the undesired GvHD effect cannot yet be separated from the desired graft versus leukemia effect of allogeneic transplantation.[183] Some data suggest that patients with favorable cytogenetics have longer disease-free survival after either autologous or allogeneic bone marrow transplantation than with consolidation chemotherapy alone[184,185] and that patients with unfavorable cytogenetics fare best with allogeneic bone marrow transplantation, but these data need to be confirmed in a larger series.

TREATMENT OF REFRACTORY AND RELAPSED AML

Although significant improvement has been made in the therapy of AML and the number of potentially cured patients has increased in recent years, most patients still relapse after complete remission and ultimately die of their disease. However, many relapsed patients respond to reinduction therapy with durable remissions and some of them, especially those with favorable cytogenetics such as inv(16), appear to be cured after obtaining a second complete remission. Complete responses are much more common in patients who have relapsed after an initial complete response than in patients who were refractory to initial therapy,[186] and more common as well as more durable in patients whose first remission was longer than 1 year. Relapsed and refractory AML patients should generally undergo reinduction therapy. It may not only be of benefit to the patient, but new potentially therapeutic interventions can be tested in such patients first and, if successful, introduced subsequently into the initial management of future patients with the disease.

New agents with major activity against relapsed or refractory AML continue to be identified. Azacytidine continues to be studied in pediatric AML patients, but interest in that agent in the treatment of adult AML has declined, despite its significant activity in Phase II studies.[187] Amsacrine[188] and homoharringtonine,[189] other agents with significant Phase II activity, have also been largely discarded, primarily because of toxicity. New anthracycline agents with significant activity in AML include esorubicin,[190] a doxorubicin analog that appears to have activity comparable to that of the parent compound but no advantage over it. Taxol, despite initial suggestions to the contrary,[191] appears to be essentially inactive in AML. Topotecan, a topoisomerase I inhibitor, has recently been reported to be active in refractory AML,[192] and further study of that agent may be productive.[193]

Carboplatin was first reported by Lee et al.[194] to have antileukemic activity, and at least 9 additional Phase II studies (summarized by Delmer et al.[195]) have confirmed complete and partial response rates on the order of 30 percent in relapsed AML, but disappointing activity in refractory disease. Since the mechanism of action of this agent is different from that of standard antileukemic agents and its spectrum of toxicity is different, it is an ideal drug to study in combination with drugs with established activity against AML.

Impressive activity of 2-chlorodeoxyadenosine in AML has been reported, when given as a 5-day continuous intravenous infusion at high dose.[196,197] Other studies have been disappointing.[198] The agent appears to be more productive of complete responses in children, and may be prohibitively neurotoxic in adults.

High-dose cytarabine, alone or in combination with other agents, has been extensively studied as induction therapy for relapsed or refractory patients with AML. In the first major study of this approach,[199] cytarabine alone, given at a dose of 3 g/m^2 every 12 hours for 6 days, yielded a 50 percent complete response rate and a median response duration of approximately 4 months in a small group of previously treated patients. Building on this lead, numerous investigations of drug combinations including high-dose cytarabine were explored. Capizzi et al.[200] reported that L-asparaginase and high-dose cytarabine were synergistic in the treatment of poor-prognosis AML patients, but activity greater than that expected from high-dose cytarabine alone has not been observed.[201] A regimen of high-dose cytarabine, 3 g/m^2 every 12 hours for 4 days, and mitoxantrone, 12 mg/m^2/day on days 3 to 5 or longer, yielded a 53 percent complete response rate in poor prognosis patients in a study by Hiddemann et al.,[202] and this regimen has become popular, especially in Europe. Unfortunately, response duration was no better than might be expected from high-dose cytarabine alone. Minor variations in dose and schedule of that regimen have reduced toxicity and preserved efficacy.[203] Although this regimen is clearly productive of complete remissions in the majority of AML patients in first relapse, it is not clear that it is more effective than standard-dose cytarabine and mitoxantrone, which, in at least one study, yielded a 63 percent complete response rate in patients in first relapse.[204] Both regimens give poor results in refractory patients.[203,204]

A number of other cytarabine-based regimens have been explored in poor-prognosis AML. Archimbaud et al.[205] used mitoxantrone, 12 mg/m^2/day on days 1 to 3; etoposide, 200 mg/m^2/day as a continuous infusion on days 8 to 10; and cytarabine, 500 mg/m^2/day also as a continuous infusion on days 1 to 3 and 8 to 10; in 72 patients aged less than 60 years. Complete remission occurred in 45 percent of refractory patients (defined as those with no response to prior therapy, or in early first relapse, or multiply relapsed patients) and in 81 percent of patients in late relapse. The median duration of aplasia with this treatment was 30 days and sepsis occurred in 57 percent of those treated. Severe gastrointestinal toxicity was common as well. Although the median survival of patients after induction with this regimen and additional postremission therapy was short (7 months), 21 percent of patients were projected to survive disease-free for almost 4 years, and one-quarter of patients not transplanted in remission had a remission with this approach that was longer than their previous remission. These results are impressive, but in a subsequent study led by the same authors,[206] rhGM-CSF (E. coli) administration failed to improve the median duration of granulocytopenia or the sepsis rate. Approximately 20 percent of patients treated in first relapse are long-term disease-free survivors with this approach.[207]

The combination of fludarabine, cytarabine, and G-CSF has been found to be quite active in poor-prognosis AML. The combination of nucleosides results in enhanced intracellular accumulation of Ara-CTP, the intracellularly active form of cytarabine, and in increased DNA damage. G-CSF was thought to enhance the cytotoxicity of cytarabine by recruiting cells into the S-phase of the cell cycle and render them more sensitive to cycle-specific drugs,[116,208] but it does not appear to do this sufficiently to improve clinical results.[209] Results appear to be excellent with this regimen, with or without G-CSF, although it is quite toxic. Opportunistic infections with unusual organisms and rare but severe neurotoxicity[210] detract from its clinical usage in its present form.

Mitoxantrone as a single agent has been studied in various doses and schedules, including continuous infusion schedules, in relapsed and refractory patients, and complete remissions have been recorded.[211] Mitoxantrone plus etoposide regimens have also been productive.[212]

Based on observations that the anthracycline, aclacinomycin A (aclarubicin), is at least as active in newly diagnosed patients with AML as daunorubicin,[213] that agent has been tested alone[214] and in combination with etoposide[215] in poor-prognosis AML with results comparable to those of studies with more extensively explored agents, but without any obvious advantage over them.

Selective ablation of the leukemic clone in AML may be possible with an anti-CD33 calicheamicin immunoconjugate (Myelotarg), since CD33 is expressed by most AML cells but not by normal hematopoietic stem cells.[216] A complete response was recently reported in 30 percent of 142 elderly patients with AML in first relapse with that agent.[217] Further investigation of that agent is warranted.

It seems clear from the foregoing that no combination regimen is superior to high-dose cytarabine alone for reinduction therapy of AML or for induction of refractory patients, and that high-dose cytarabine may not be superior to lower doses of that agent in either setting. The relative merits of such treatments are difficult to evaluate because most studies of second-line regimens are small, are not randomized, define refractory disease variously, and do not analyze for the influence of important prognostic factors such as cytogenetics. There is no doubt, however, that some cytarabine-based regimens can cure a small fraction (perhaps 5 percent) of relapsed patients. Those patients are usually young, have had durable previous remissions, and have favorable cytogenetics, such as inv(16) as the only chromosomal abnormality.

Second remissions are usually only of several months duration, but with many current regimens, 10 to 20 percent of patients enjoy second remissions of substantial duration. There are few data on post second remission therapy that suggest that one treatment is superior to another. Robles et al.[218] recently demonstrated that low-dose cytarabine, 10 mg/m^2 given subcutaneously every 12 hours until relapse, may have resulted in a second remission duration longer than that expected from no maintenance therapy. If these data can be confirmed, postremission cytarabine will be the first agent demonstrated to prolong second remission. A surprising finding in that study was the fact that 18 percent of patients in the control group also had second remissions longer than the first,[219] which suggests that reinduction therapy was more effective antileukemic therapy than initial induction and postremission therapy in that group. Therefore, it is essential to perform prospectively controlled post second remission studies if new active therapies are to be identified, rather than simply to determine "inversion" rates from uncontrolled studies.

There has been interest in low-dose interleukin-2 (IL-2) as a possibly effective post second remission therapy for AML patients, generated by two Phase II studies of the agent in that setting.[220,221] These studies were initiated following the observation that high-dose IL-2 could induce complete remission in some patients with minimal residual disease.[222,223] Recent results in relapsed and refractory patients have been disappointing.[224] There is no doubt that bone marrow transplantation can cure some patients with relapsed and even refractory AML.[225–228] However, it has been suggested by some that a bone marrow preparative regimen without stem cell support may yield results equivalent to those reported after transplantation.[229] In a study by Forman et al.,[225] 12 adults with AML who failed induction therapy were treated with an allogeneic transplant from a matched sibling and 75 percent achieved a complete remission. One-third of the complete responders relapsed and two-thirds (ages 20 to 29) remain in continuous complete remission for approximately 18 to 108 months. In a larger Seattle study[226] that included some older patients, allogeneic transplantation was tested in AML patients in untreated first relapse and the 5-year disease-free survival was projected to be 23 percent. Only 1 of 10 patients with AML given an allogeneic transplant in second complete remission in another study[227] survived in long-term complete remission.

Autologous bone marrow transplantation for patients in first relapse or in second complete remission was studied by Petersen et al.[228] In all patients, marrow was harvested and cryopreserved during first complete remission. The actuarial probabilities of relapse-free survival at 2 years for patients transplanted in first relapse (21 patients) or second remission (26 patients) were 45 and 32 percent, respectively. The outcome in patients who were in first relapse was comparable to that of other studies in which remission was induced prior to transplantation, which suggests that there is no clinical disadvantage in proceeding directly to autologous transplantation upon the diagnosis of relapse. Early data from the same institution suggested that the addition of IL-2 to the management of autologous transplant patients in first relapse or later stages may improve outcome.[230] However, recent data suggest no benefit for IL-2 for patients in first remission after autologous marrow transplantation.[231,232]

The complete response data of Brown et al.,[229] derived from a study of a regimen similar to a popular regimen for autologous marrow transplantation but used without transplantation in AML patients resistant to conventional therapy, compare very favorably to the above referenced and to other transplant studies. A complete response was obtained in 42 percent of 40 resistant AML patients, including 6 of 20 resistant to high-dose cytarabine. However, the longest complete response duration at the time of their report was only 1 year, and all except 1 patient had relapsed. All of these reports taken together suggest that cure of relapsed or refractory AML is more likely to be obtained by allogeneic marrow transplant-based regimens than by other methods. Large, prospective, and randomized trials will be necessary to properly assess the relative merits of these and other approaches.

Relapse after allogeneic bone marrow transplantation is infrequently treated successfully. Giralt et al.[233] demonstrated that administration of filgrastim (rhG-CSF) may stimulate residual donor cells in AML patients who relapse after allogeneic transplantation without stimulating the leukemic clone and thereby re-establish complete remission. Follow-up was less than 1 year, but this observation is exciting and potentially important.

Infusion of lymphocytes from the original marrow donor is highly effective in treating chronic myelocytic leukemia patients who relapse after allogeneic marrow transplantation, but donor lymphocyte infusions are less effective in treating post-transplant relapsed patients with AML.[234] The major problem with this form of treatment is the frequent induction of serious GvHD, which can be fatal.[235] However, such infusions can be successful, even for relapse after unrelated donor marrow transplantation.[234] Porter et al.[236] treated 23 patients with AML who relapsed after an unrelated donor marrow transplantation and 42 percent obtained a complete response with an estimated 1 year disease-free survival rate of 23 percent. Donor lymphocyte infusions may also be able to eradicate persistent disease after allogeneic hematopoietic cell transplantation.[237]

CENTRAL NERVOUS SYSTEM LEUKEMIA

The diagnosis and treatment of CNS leukemia is discussed earlier in this chapter. CNS leukemia is an uncommon type of relapse in adults with AML, the incidence of which has decreased since the common usage of infusional cytarabine in induction regimens due to the attainment of therapeutic levels of cytarabine in the CSF with such induction therapy. Nevertheless, about 1 to 2 percent of patients who relapse will have CNS leukemia with or without marrow evidence of relapse. These are usually young patients. Intracerebral leukemia is much less common in AML than in ALL, and virtually all adults with AML with CNS leukemia demonstrate meningeal leukemia, cranial nerve palsy, or both. For reasons that are not understood, patients with AML usually have longer remissions of CNS leukemia after treatment than do patients with ALL.[238] As is the case in ALL, rapid attainment of remission of meningeal leukemia, long duration of initial marrow remission, and the absence of cranial nerve palsy are favorable factors for CNS leukemia remission duration after treatment.[236]

FUTURE DIRECTIONS

New growth factors developed to stimulate platelet production in patients with hematologic malignancies have recently entered clinical trial. Pegylated recombinant human megakaryocyte growth and development factor (PEG-rHuMGDF) was found to stimulate megakaryocytopoiesis in the marrow of some patients with AML in vitro by Liu et al.[239] Two randomized, double-blind placebo-controlled clinical trials have been conducted to date with that agent in patients with AML.[240,241] Archimbaud et al.[240] studied several different doses and schedules of the agent given after the completion of induction chemotherapy. There was no evidence for stimulation of leukemia and no adverse events related to the growth factor. Biological activity was observed that was directly dose related, but there was no effect on the median time to transfusion-independent platelet recovery. Virtually identical results were reported by Schiffer et al.[241] Thus, although biologically active and safe, PEG-rHuMGDF appears to be clinically disappointing in the doses and schedules studied. Studies of this agent administered before and during induction therapy should be conducted before drawing final conclusions about its clinical usefulness. Recombinant thrombopoietin was shown to facilitate proliferation of CD7+ leukemic myeloblasts,[242] a fact that may dampen further development of that agent for support of patients with AML.

Currently there is considerable interest in developing molecular tests for minimal residual disease in patients with AML who have achieved complete hematologic remission, and testing whether or not additional treatment for patients with detectable residual disease is beneficial for them. Most studies have been in patients with acute promyelocytic leukemia (discussed in Chapter 21) but a growing body of information is currently being developed for patients with t(8;21) as well. Tobal et al.[243] developed a sensitive reverse-transcriptase polymerase chain reaction (RT-PCR) to assay for AML1-MTG8 transcripts from the fusion gene created by t(8;21). They found that levels as high as 1×10^2 molecules/μg of RNA in peripheral blood were associated with durable clinical remissions, but patients with higher levels of the transcript relapsed within 6 months. Similar results have recently been reported by others.[244–247] It remains to be determined, however, that clinical intervention with currently available agents based on RT-PCR results obtained during clinical remission will alter the course of t(8;21)-positive AML.

REFERENCES

1. Grewal H, Guillem JG, Quan SHQ et al: Anorectal disease in neutropenic leukemic patients. Dis Colon Rectum 37:1095, 1994.
2. Devine DV, Gluck WL, Rosse W et al: Acute myeloblastic leukemia in paroxysmal nocturnal hemoglobinuria. J Clin Invest 79:314, 1987.
3. Kiraly JF III, Wheby MS: Bone marrow necrosis. Am J Med 60:361, 1976.
4. Cassileth PA, Brooks SJ: The prognostic significance of myelonecrosis after induction therapy in acute leukemia. Cancer 60:2363, 1987.
5. Resnitzky P, Shaft D: Distinct lysozyme content in different subtypes of acute myeloid leukaemic cells: An ultrastructural immunogold study. Br J Haematol 88:357, 1994.
6. Wiernik PH, Serpick AA: Clinical significance of serum and urinary muramidase activity in leukemia and other hematologic malignancies. Am J Med 46:330, 1969.
7. Kaiserling E, Horny H-P, Geerts M-L et al: Skin involvement in myelogenous leukemia: Morphologic and immunophenotypic heterogeneity of skin infiltrates. Modern Pathol 7:771, 1994.
8. Sepp N, Radaszkiewicz T, Meijer CJLM et al: Specific skin manifestations in acute leukemia with monocytic differentiation. Cancer 71:124, 1993.
9. Baden TJ, Gammon WR: Leukemia cutis in acute myelomonocytic leukemia. Preferential localization in a recent Hickman catheter scar. Arch Dermatol 123:88, 1987.
10. Harakati MS: Cutaneous granulocytic sarcoma at the exit site of Hickman indwelling venous catheter. Int J Hematol 57:39, 1993.
11. Schiffer CA, Sanel FT, Steckmiller BK et al: Functional and morphologic characteristics of the leukemia cells of a patient with acute monocytic leukemia: Correlation with clinical features. Blood 46:17, 1975.
12. Sreejith G, Gangadharan VP, Elizabath KA et al: Primary granulocytic sarcoma of the ovary. Am J Clin Oncol 23:239, 2000.
13. Cavdar AO, Babacan E, Gözdasoglu S et al: High-risk subgroup of acute myelomonocytic leukemia (AMML) with orbito-ocular granulocytic sarcoma (OOGS) in Turkish children. Retrospective analysis of clinical, hematological, ultrastructural and therapeutic findings of thirty-three OOGS. Acta Haematol 81:80, 1989.
14. Lane DM, Birdwell RL: Ovarian leukemia detected by pelvic sonography. Cancer 58:2338, 1986.
15. Harris NL, Scully RE: Malignant lymphoma and granulocytic sarcoma of the uterus and vagina. Cancer 53:2530, 1984.
16. Antunez de Mayolo J, Ahn YS, Temple JD et al: Spontaneous remission of acute leukemia after the termination of pregnancy. Cancer 63:1621, 1989.
17. Wodzinski MA, Collin R, Winfield DA et al: Epidural granulocytic sarcoma in acute myeloid leukemia with 8;21 translocation. Cancer 62:1299, 1988.
18. Rottenberg GT, Thomas BM: Case report: Granulocytic sarcoma of the small bowel—A rare presentation of leukaemia. Clin Radiol 49:501, 1994.
19. Wong KF, Chan JKC, Chan JCW et al: Acute myeloid leukemia presenting as granulocytic sarcoma of the lung. Am J Hematol 43:77, 1993.
20. McCluggage WG, Boyd HK, Jones FG et al: Mediastinal granulocytic sarcoma: A report of two cases. Arch Pathol Lab Med 122:545, 1998.
21. Thalhammer F, Gisslinger H, Chott A et al: Granulocytic sarcoma of the prostate as the first manifestation of a late relapse of acute myelogenous leukemia. Acta Hematol 68:97, 1994.
22. Hudock J, Chatten J, Miettinen M: Immunohistochemical evaluation of myeloid leukemia infiltrates (granulocytic sarcomas) in formaldehyde-fixed, paraffin-embedded tissue. Am J Clin Pathol 102:55, 1994.
23. Goldstein NS, Ritter JH, Argenyi ZB et al: Granulocytic sarcoma. Int J Surg Pathol 2:177, 1995.
24. Byrd JC, Edenfield J, Shields DJ, Dawson NA: Extramedullary myeloid cell tumors in acute nonlymphocytic leukemia: A clinical review. J Clin Oncol 13:1800, 1995.
25. Abe R, Umezu H, Uchida T et al: Myeloblastoma with an 8;21 chromosome translocation in acute myeloblastic leukemia. Cancer 58:1260, 1986.
26. Tallman MS, Hakimian D, Shaw JM et al: Granulocytic sarcoma is associated with the 8;21 translocation in acute myeloid leukemia. J Clin Oncol 11:690, 1993.
27. Heimann P, Vamos E, Ferster A et al: Granulocytic sarcoma showing chromosomal changes other than the t(8;21). Cancer Genet Cytogenet 74:59, 1994.
28. Krishnan K, Ross CW, Adams PT et al: Neural cell-adhesion molecule (CD 56)-positive, t(8;21) acute myeloid leukemia (AML, M-2) and granulocytic sarcoma. Ann Hematol 69:321, 1994.
29. Soppi E, Nousiainen T, Seppa A, Lahtinen R: Acute febrile neutrophilic dermatosis (Sweet's syndrome) in association with myelodysplastic syndromes: A report of three cases and a review of the literature. Br J Haematol 73:43, 1989.
30. Cohen PR, Talpaz M, Kurzock R: Malignancy associated Sweet's syndrome: Review of the world literature. J Clin Oncol 6:1887, 1988.

31. Schachat AP, Markowitz JA, Guyer DR et al: Ophthalmic manifestations of leukemia. Arch Ophthalmol 107:697, 1989.

32. Karesh JW, Goldman EJ, Reck K et al: A prospective ophthalmic evaluation of patients with acute myeloid leukemia: Correlation of ocular and hematologic findings. J Clin Oncol 7:1528, 1989.

33. Ritch PS, Hansen RM, Heuer DK: Ocular toxicity from high-dose cytosine arabinoside. Cancer 51:430, 1983.

34. Soares FA, Landell GAM, Cardoso MCM: Pulmonary leukostasis without hyperleukocytosis: A clinicopathologic study of 16 cases. Am J Hematol 40:28, 1992.

35. Dombret H, Hunault M, Faucher C et al: Acute lysis pneumopathy after chemotherapy for acute myelomonocytic leukemia with abnormal marrow eosinophils. Cancer 69:1356, 1992.

36. Wurthner JU, Kohler G, Behringer D et al: Leukostasis followed by hemorrhage complicating the initiation of chemotherapy in patients with acute myeloid leukemia and hyperleukocytosis. Cancer 85:368, 1999.

37. van Buchem MA, Wondergem JH, Kool LJS et al: Pulmonary leukostasis: Radiologic-pathologic study. Radiology 165:739, 1987.

38. Doran HM, Sheppard MN, Collins PW et al: Pathology of the lung in leukaemia and lymphoma: A study of 87 autopsies. Histopathology 18:211, 1991.

39. Mangal AK, Growe GH: Extensive pulmonary infiltration by leukemic blast cells treated with irradiation. Can Med Assn J 128:424, 1983.

40. Von Eyben FE, Siddiqui MZ, Spanos G: High-voltage irradiation and hydroxyurea for pulmonary leukostasis in acute myelomonocytic leukemia. Acta Haematol 77:180, 1987.

41. Flasshove M, Schuette J, Sauerwein W et al: Pulmonary and cerebral irradiation for hyperleukocytosis in acute myelomonocytic leukemia. Leukemia 8:1792, 1994.

42. Smith LJ, Katzenstein ALA: Pathogenesis of massive pulmonary hemorrhage in acute leukemia. Arch Intern Med 142:2149, 1982.

43. Andersson BS, Luna MA, Yee C et al: Fatal pulmonary failure complicating high-dose cytosine arabinoside therapy in acute leukemia. Cancer 65:1079, 1990.

44. Vansteenkiste JF, Boogaerts MA: Adult respiratory distress syndrome in neutropenic leukemia patients. Blut 58:287, 1989.

45. Wiernik PH, Sutherland JC, Steckmiller BK et al: Clinically significant cardiac infiltration in acute leukemia, lymphocytic lymphoma and plasma cell myeloma. Med Pediatr Oncol 2:75, 1976.

46. McAdams HP, Schaefer PS, Ghaed VN: Leukemic infiltrates of the heart: CT findings. J Comput Assist Tomogr 13:525, 1989.

47. Allen DC, Alderdice JM, Morton P et al: Pathology of the heart and conduction system in lymphoma and leukaemia. J Clin Pathol 40:746, 1987.

48. Foucar K, Foucar E, Willman C et al: Nonleukemic granulocytic sarcoma of the heart: A report of a fatal case. Am J Hematol 25:325, 1987.

49. Williford SK, Salisbury PL III, Peacock JE Jr et al: The safety of dental extractions in patients with hematologic malignancies. J Clin Oncol 7:798, 1989.

50. Toljanic JA, Bedard J-F, Larson RA, Fox JP: A prospective pilot study to evaluate a new dental assessment and treatment paradigm for patients scheduled to undergo intensive chemotherapy for cancer. Cancer 85:1843, 1999.

51. Sklansky BD, Jafek BW, Wiernik PH: Otolaryngologic manifestations of acute leukemia. Laryngoscope 84:210, 1974.

52. Fulp SR, Nestok BR, Powell BL et al: Leukemic infiltration of the esophagus. Cancer 71:112, 1993.

53. Almadori G, Del Ninno M, Cadoni G et al: Facial nerve paralysis in acute otomastoiditis as presenting symptom of FAB M2, T8;21 leukemic relapse. Case report and review of the literature. Int J Pediatr Otorhinolaryngol 36:45, 1996.

54. Schimpff SC, Wiernik PH, Block JB: Rectal abscesses in cancer patients. Lancet 2:844, 1972.

55. Cartoni C, Dragoni F, Micozzi A et al: Neutropenic enterocolitis in patients with acute leukemia: Prognostic significance of bowel wall thickening detected by ultrasonography. J Clin Oncol 19:756, 2001.

56. O'Brien S, Kantarjian HM, Anaissie E et al: Successful medical management of neutropenic enterocolitis in adults with acute leukemia. Southern Med J 80:1233, 1987.

57. Bishop JF, Schiffer CA, Aisner J et al: Surgery in acute leukemia: A review of 167 operations in thrombocytopenic patients. Am J Hematol 26:147, 1987.

58. Thalhammer F, Gisslinger H, Chott A et al: Granulocytic sarcoma of the prostate as the first manifestation of a late relapse of acute myelogenous leukemia. Ann Hematol 68:97, 1994.

59. Ferry JA, Snigley JR, Young RH: Granulocytic sarcoma of the testis: A report of two cases of a neoplasm prone to misinterpretation. Mod Pathol 10:320, 1997.

60. Wainer RA, Wiernik PH, Thompson WL: Metabolic and therapeutic studies of a patient with acute leukemia and severe lactic acidosis of prolonged duration. Am J Med 55:255, 1973.

61. Gewirtz AM, Stewart AF, Vignery A et al: Hypercalcemia complicating acute myelogenous leukemia: A syndrome of multiple aetiologies. Br J Haematol 54:133, 1983.

62. Koeppler H, Pflueger KH, Knapp W et al: Establishment of three permanent human leukaemia cell lines producing immunoreactive calcitonin. Br J Haematol 65:405, 1987.

63. Schenkein DP, O'Neill C, Shapiro J et al: Accelerated bone formation causing profound hypocalcemia in acute leukemia. Ann Intern Med 105:375, 1986.

64. Budd D, Ginsberg H: Hypocholesterolemia and acute myelogenous leukemia. Cancer 58:1361, 1986.

65. Fritz RD, Forkner Jr CD, Freireich EJ: The association of fatal intracranial hemorrhage and "blastic crisis" in patients with acute leukemia. N Engl J Med 261:59, 1959.

66. Dutcher JP, Schiffer CA, Wiernik PH: Hyperleukocytosis in adult acute nonlymphocytic leukemia: Impact on remission rate and duration, and survival. J Clin Oncol 5:1364, 1987.

67. van Buchem MA, te Velde J, Willemze R et al: Leucostasis, an underestimated cause of death in leukaemia. Blut 56:39, 1988.

68. Ventura GJ, Hestar JP, Smith TL et al: Acute myeloblastic leukemia with hyperleukocytosis: Risk factors for early mortality in induction. Am J Hematol 27:34, 1988.

69. VanCamp B, Reynaerts PH, Naets JP et al: Transient IgA1-paraprotein during treatment of acute myelomonocytic leukemia. Blood 55:21, 1980.

70. Atkins H, Drouin J, Izahuirre CA et al: Acute promyelocytic leukemia associated with a paraprotein that reacts with leukemic cells. Cancer 63:1750, 1989.

71. Schiffer CA, Lichtenfeld JL, Wiernik PH et al: Antibody response in patients with acute nonlymphocytic leukemia. Cancer 37:2177, 1976.

72. Spickermann D, Gause A, Pfreundschuh M et al: Impaired antibody levels to tetanus toxoid and pneumococcal polysaccharides in acute leukemias. Leuk Lymphoma 16:89, 1994.

73. Furno P, Dionisi MS, Bucaneve G et al: Ceftriaxone versus beta-lactams with antipseudomonal activity for empirical, combined antibiotic therapy in febrile neutropenia: A meta-analysis. Support Care Cancer 8:293, 2000.

74. Lichtman MA, Rowe JM: Hyperleukocytic leukemias: Rheological, clinical, and therapeutic considerations. Blood 60:279, 1982.

75. Cuttner J, Holland JF, Norton L et al: Therapeutic leukapheresis for hyperleukocytosis in acute myelocytic leukemia. Med Pediatr Oncol 11:76, 1983.

76. Nelson SC, Bruggers CS, Kurtzberg J et al: Management of leukemic hyperleukocytosis with hydration, urinary alkalinization, and allopurinol. Am J Pediatr Hematol Oncol 15:351, 1993.

77. Pui CH, Mahmoud HH, Wiley JM et al: Recombinant urate oxidase for the prophylaxis or treatment of hyperuricemia in patients with leukemia or lymphoma. J Clin Oncol 19:697, 2001.

78. Reynoso EE, Sheperd FA, Messner HA et al: Acute leukemia during pregnancy: The Toronto Leukemia Study Group experience with long-term follow-up of children exposed in utero to chemotherapeutic agents. J Clin Oncol 5:1098, 1987.

79. Feliu J, Juarez S, Ordonez A et al: Acute leukemia and pregnancy. Cancer 61:580, 1988.

80. Aviles A, Niz J: Long-term follow-up of children born to mothers with acute leukemia during pregnancy. Med Pediatr Oncol 16:3, 1988.

81. Sanz GF, Sanz MA: Remision completa espontanea en leucemia mieloblastica aguda. Rev Clin Espanola 178:229, 1986.

82. Bishop JF, Lowenthal RM, Joshua D et al: Etoposide in acute non-lymphocytic leukemia. Blood 75:27, 1990.

83. Byrd JC, Dodge RK, Carroll A et al: Patients with t(8;21)(q22;q22) and acute myeloid leukemia have superior failure-free and overall survival when repetitive cycles of high-dose cytarabine are administered. J Clin Oncol 17:3767, 1999.

84. Schiller G, Gajewski J, Territo M et al: Long-term outcome of high-dose cytarabine-based consolidation chemotherapy for adults with acute myelogenous leukemia. Blood 80:2977, 1992.

85. Yates G, Glidewell OH, Wiernik PH et al: Cytosine arabinoside with daunorubicin or adriamycin for therapy of acute myelocytic leukemia. A CALGB study. Blood 60:454, 1982.

86. Van Sloten K, Wiernik PH, Schimpff SC: Evaluation of levamisole as an adjuvant to chemotherapy for treatment of acute nonlymphocytic leukemia. Cancer 51:1576, 1983.

87. Dutcher JP, Wiernik PH, Markus S et al: Intensive maintenance therapy improves survival in adult acute nonlymphocytic leukemia: An eight-year follow-up. Leukemia 2:413, 1988.

88. Rai KR, Holland JF, Glidewell OH et al: Treatment of acute myelocytic leukemia: A study by Cancer and Leukemia Group B. Blood 58:1203, 1981.

89. Preisler H, Davis RB, Kirshner J et al: Comparison of three remission induction regimens and two postinduction strategies for the treatment of acute nonlymphocytic leukemia: A Cancer and Acute Leukemia Group B study. Blood 69:1441, 1987.

90. Rowe JM, Andersen JW, Mazza JJ et al: A randomized placebo-controlled phase III study of granulocyte macrophage colony-stimulating factor in adult patients (>55 to 70 years of age) with acute myelogenous leukemia: A study of the Eastern Cooperative Oncology Group (E1490). Blood 86:457, 1995.

91. Stone RM, Berg DT, George SL et al: Granulocyte-macrophage colony-stimulating factor after initial chemotherapy for elderly patients with primary acute myelogenous leukemia. Cancer and Leukemia Group B. N Engl J Med 332:1671, 1995.

92. Einzig AI, Dutcher JP, Wiernik PH: Life-threatening hyperleukocytosis and pulmonary compromise after priming with recombinant human granulocyte-macrophage colony- stimulating factor in a patient with acute myelomonocytic leukemia. J Clin Oncol 13:304, 1995.

93. Estey E, Thall PF, Kantarjian H et al: Treatment of newly diagnosed acute myelogenous leukemia with granulocyte-macrophage colony-stimulating factor (GM-CSF) before and during continuous-infusion high-dose ara-C + daunorubicin: Comparison to patients treated without GM-CSF. Blood 79:2246, 1992.

94. Ohno R, Naoe T, Kanamaru A et al: A double-blind controlled study of granulocyte colony-stimulating factor started two days before induction chemotherapy in refractory acute myeloid leukemia. Blood 83:2086, 1994.

95. Cassileth PA, Lynch E, Hines JD et al: Varying intensity of postremission therapy in acute myeloid leukemia. Blood 79:1924, 1992.

96. Dillman RO, Davus RB, Green MR et al: A comparative study of two different doses of cytarabine for acute myeloid leukemia: A phase III trial of Cancer and Leukemia Group B. Blood 78:2520, 1991.

97. Weick JK, Kopecky KJ, Appelbaum FR et al: A randomized investigation of high-dose versus standard-dose cytosine arabinoside with daunorubicin in patients with previously untreated acute myeloid leukemia: A Southwest Oncology Group study. Blood 88:2841, 1996.

98. Hann IM, Stevens RF, Goldstone AH et al: Randomized comparison of DAT versus ADE as induction chemotherapy in children and younger adults with acute myeloid leukaemia. Results of the Medical Research Council's 10th AML trial (MRC AML10). Adult and childhood leukaemia working parties of the Medical Research Council. Blood 89:2311, 1997.

99. Miyawaki S, Tanimoto M, Kobayashi T et al: No beneficial effect from addition of etoposide to daunorubicin, cytarabine, and 6-mercaptopurine in individualized induction therapy of acute myeloid leukemia: The JALSG-AML92 study. Japan Adult Leukemia Study Group. Int J Hematol 70:97, 1999.

100. Arlin Z, Case DC Jr, Moore J et al: Randomized multicenter trial of cytosine arabinoside with mitoxantrone or daunorubicin in previously untreated adult patients with acute nonlymphocytic leukemia (ANLL). Leukemia 4:177, 1990.

101. Pavlovsky S, Gonzalez Llaven J, Garcia Martinez MA et al: A randomized study of mitoxantrone plus cytarabine versus daunomycin plus cytarabine in the treatment of previously untreated adult patients with acute nonlymphocytic leukemia. Ann Hematol 69:11, 1994.

102. Rowe JM, Neuberg D, Friedenberg W et al: A phase III study of daunorubicin vs idarubicin vs mitoxantrone for older adult patients (>55 yrs) with acute myelogenous leukemia (AML): A study of the Eastern Cooperative Oncology Group (E3993). Blood 92(Suppl. 1):2517a, 1998.

103. Berman E, Heller G, Santorsa J et al: Results of a randomized trial comparing idarubicin and cytosine arabinoside with daunorubicin and cytosine arabinoside in adult patients with newly diagnosed acute myelogenous leukemia. Blood 77:1666, 1991.

104. Wiernik PH, Banks PLC, Case DC Jr et al: Cytarabine plus idarubicin or daunorubicin as induction and consolidation therapy for previously untreated adult patients with acute myeloid leukemia. Blood 79:313, 1992.

105. Vogler WR, Velez-Garcia E, Weiner RS et al: A phase III trial comparing idarubicin and daunorubicin in combination with cytarabine in acute myelogenous leukemia: A Southeastern Cancer Study Group study. J Clin Oncol 10:1, 1992.

106. Mandelli F, Petti MC, Ardia A et al: A randomised clinical trial comparing idarubicin and cytarabine to daunorubicin and cytarabine in the treatment of acute non-lymphoid leukaemia. Eur J Cancer 27:750, 1991.

107. AML Collaborative Group: A systematic collaborative overview of randomized trials comparing idarubicin with daunorubicin (or

other anthracyclines) as induction therapy for acute myeloid leukaemia. Br J Haematol 103:100, 1998.

108. Robert J, Rigal-Huguet F, Hurteloup P: Comparative pharmacokinetic study of idarubicin and daunorubicin in leukemia patients. Hematol Oncol 10:111, 1992.

109. Berman E, McBride M: Comparative cellular pharmacology of daunorubicin and idarubicin in human multidrug-resistant leukemia cells. Blood 79:3267, 1992.

110. Carden PA, Mitchell SL, Waters KD et al: Prevention of cyclophosphamide/cytarabine- induced emesis with ondansetron in children with leukemia. J Clin Oncol 8:1531, 1990.

111. Italian Group for Antiemetic Research: Dexamethasone, granisetron, or both for the prevention of nausea and vomiting during chemotherapy for cancer. N Engl J Med 332:1, 1995.

112. Yokel BK, Friedman KJ, Farmer ER et al: Cutaneous pathology following etoposide therapy. J Cutan Pathol 14:326, 1987.

113. Bezwoda WR, Bernasconi C, Hutchinson RM et al: Mitoxantrone for refractory and relapsed acute leukemia. Cancer 66:418, 1990.

114. Vogler WR, Harrington DP, Winton EF et al: Phase II clinical trial of carboplatin in relapsed and refractory leukemia. Leukemia 6:1072, 1992.

115. Santana VM, Mirro J Jr, Kearns C et al: 2-chlorodeoxyadenosine produces a high rate of complete hematologic remission in relapsed acute myeloid leukemia. J Clin Oncol 10:364, 1992.

116. Gandhi V, Estey E, Keating MJ et al: Fludarabine potentiates metabolism of cytarabine in patients with acute myelogenous leukemia during therapy. J Clin Oncol 11:116, 1993.

117. Schiller G: Treatment of resistant acute myeloid leukemia. Blood Rev 5:220, 1991.

118. van Der Velden VH, te Marvelde JG, Hoogeveen PG et al: Targeting of the CD33-calicheamicin immunoconjugate Mylotarg (CMA-676) in acute myeloid leukemia: In vivo and in vitro saturation and internalization by leukemic and normal myeloid cells. Blood 97:3197, 2001.

119. Welborn JL, Lewis JP, Meyers FJ: Impact of reinduction regimens on the clinical course of adult acute nonlymphocytic leukemia. Leukemia 2:711, 1988.

120. Novik Y, Oleksowicz L, Wiernik PH: Therapeutic effect of cyclosporin A in thrombocytopenia after myeloablative chemotherapy in acute myeloid leukaemia. Med Oncol 14:43, 1997.

121. Estey EH, Shen Y, Thall PF: Effect of time to complete remission on subsequent survival and disease-free survival time in AML, RAEB-t, and RAEB. Blood 95:72, 2000.

122. Estey EH: How I treat older patients with AML. Blood 96:1670, 2000.

123. Whitely R, Hannah P, Holmes F: Survival in acute leukemia in elderly patients. J Am Geriatr Soc 38:527, 1990.

124. Kanamori H, Maruta A, Miyashita H et al: Low-dose cytosine arabinoside for treating hypocellular acute leukemia in the elderly. Am J Hematol 39:52, 1992.

125. Yin JAL, Johnson PRE, Davies JM et al: Mitozantrone and cytosine arabinoside as first-line therapy in elderly patients with acute myeloid leukemia. Br J Haematol 79:415, 1991.

126. Sebban C, Archimbaud E, Coiffier B et al: Treatment of acute myeloid leukemia in elderly patients. A retrospective study. Cancer 61:227, 1988.

127. Lowenberg B, Zittoun R, Kerkhofs H et al: On the value of intensive remission-induction chemotherapy in elderly patients of 65+ years with acute myeloid leukemia: A randomized phase III study of the European Organization for Research and Treatment of Cancer Leukemia Group. J Clin Oncol 7:1268, 1989.

128. Johnson PRE, Hunt LP, Yin JAL: Prognostic factors in elderly patients with acute myeloid leukaemia: Development of a model to predict survival. Br J Haematol 85:300, 1993.

129. Gajewski JL, Ho WG, Nimer SD et al: Efficacy of intensive chemotherapy for acute myelogenous leukemia associated with a preleukemic syndrome. J Clin Oncol 7:1637, 1989.

130. Chang J, Geary CG, Testa NG: Long-term bone marrow damage after chemotherapy for acute myeloid leukaemia does not improve with time. Br J Haematol 75:68, 1990.

131. Tamura S, Kanamaru A: De-novo acute myeloid leukemia with trilineage myelodysplasia (AML/TMDS) and myelodysplastic remission marrow (AML/MRM). Leuk Lymphoma 16:263, 1995.

132. Fearon ER, Burke PJ, Schiffer CA et al: Differentiation of leukemia cells to polymorphonuclear leukocytes in patients with acute nonlymphocytic leukemia. N Engl J Med 315:15, 1986.

133. Fialkow PJ, Singer JW, Raskind WH et al: Clonal development, stem-cell differentiation, and clinical remissions in acute nonlymphocytic leukemia. N Engl J Med 317:468, 1987.

134. Huang C, Deng M, Guo R et al: A study of the induction of differentiation of human leukemic cells by harringtonine combined with cytarabine. Leukemia 2:518, 1988.

135. Davies AR: Auer bodies in mature neutrophils. JAMA 202:895, 1968.

136. Viola MV, Frazier M, Wiernik PH et al: Reverse transcriptase in leukocytes of leukemic patients in remission. N Engl J Med 294:75, 1976.

137. Koeffler HP: Review: Induction of differentiation of human acute myelogenous leukemic cells: Therapeutic implications. Blood 62:709, 1983.

138. Schwartz EL, Wiernik PH: Differentiation of leukemic cells by chemotherapeutic agents. J Clin Pharmacol 28:779, 1988.

139. Preisler HD, Anderson K, Rai K et al: The frequency of long-term remission in patients with acute myelogenous leukemia treated with conventional maintenance chemotherapy: A study of 760 patients with a minimal follow-up time of 6 years. Br J Haematol 71:189, 1989.

140. Embury SH, Elias L, Heller PM et al: Remission maintenance therapy in acute myelogenous leukemia. West J Med 126:267, 1977.

141. Vaughan WP, Karp JE, Burke PJ: Long chemotherapy-free remissions after single-cycle timed sequential chemotherapy for acute myelocytic leukemia. Cancer 45:859, 1980.

142. Rustum YM, Preisler HD: Correlation between leukemic cell retention of 1-β-D-arabinofuranosyl-cytosine 5′-triphosphate and response to therapy. Cancer Res 39:42, 1979.

143. Mayer RJ, Davis RB, Schiffer CA et al: Intensive postremission chemotherapy in adults with acute myeloid leukemia. N Engl J Med 331:896, 1994.

144. Zittoun R, Jehn U, Fiere D et al: Alternative v repeated postremission treatment in adult acute myelogenous leukemia: A randomized phase III study (AML6) of the EORTC Leukemia Cooperative Group. Blood 73:896, 1989.

145. Schiller GJ, Nimer SD, Territo MC et al: Bone marrow transplantation versus high-dose cytarabine-based consolidation chemotherapy for acute myelogenous leukemia in first remission. J Clin Oncol 10:41, 1992.

146. Harousseau JL, Milpied N, Briere J et al: Double intensive consolidation chemotherapy in adult acute myeloid leukemia. J Clin Oncol 9:1432, 1991.

147. Giordano M, Riccardi A, Girino M et al: Postremission chemotherapy in adult acute nonlymphoblastic leukemia including intensive or non-intensive consolidation therapy. Eur J Cancer 27:437, 1991.

148. Dutcher JP, Wiernik PH, Markus S et al: 15-year follow-up of adult patients with acute myeloid leukemia: Study BCRC 7802: Proc XXV Cong Intl Soc Hematol, abstract #48, 1994.

149. Ranson MR, Scarffe JH, Morgenstern GR et al: Post consolidation therapy for adult patients with acute myeloid leukaemia. Br J Haematol 79:162, 1991.

150. Tallman MS, Appelbaum FR, Amos D et al: Evaluation of intensive postremission chemotherapy for adults with acute nonlymphocytic leukemia using high-dose cytosine arabinoside with L-asparaginase and amsacrine with etoposide. J Clin Oncol 5:918, 1987.

151. Rubin EH, Andersen JW, Berg DT et al: Risk factors for high-dose cytarabine neurotoxicity: An analysis of a Cancer and Leukemia Group B trial in patients with acute myeloid leukemia. J Clin Oncol 10:948, 1992.

152. Berman E: Chemotherapy in acute myelogenous leukemia: High dose, higher expectations? J Clin Oncol 13:1, 1995.

153. Harousseau JL, Witz B, Lioure B et al: Granulocyte colony-stimulating factor after intensive consolidation chemotherapy in acute myeloid leukemia: Results of a randomized trial of the Groupie Oust-Est Leukemias Agues Myeloblastics. J Clin Oncol 18:780, 2000.

154. Young JW, Papadopoulos EB, Cunningham I et al: T-cell-depleted allogeneic bone marrow transplantation in adults with acute non-lymphocytic leukemia in first remission. Blood 79:3380, 1992.

155. Clift RA, Buckner CD, Appelbaum FR et al: Allogeneic marrow transplantation in patients with acute myeloid leukemia in first remission: A randomized trial of two irradiation regimens. Blood 76:1867, 1990.

156. Bortin MM, Horowitz MM, Rowlings PA et al: 1993 progress report from the International Bone Marrow Transplant Registry. Bone Marrow Transplant 12:97, 1993.

157. Zittoun RA, Mandelli F, Willemze R et al: Autologous or allogeneic bone marrow transplantation compared with intensive chemotherapy in acute myelogenous leukemia. N Engl J Med 332:217, 1995.

158. Blaise D, Maraninchi D, Michallet M et al: Long-term follow-up of a randomized trial comparing the combination of cyclophosphamide with total body irradiation or busulfan as conditioning regimen for patients receiving HLA-identical marrow grafts for acute myeloblastic leukemia in first complete remission. Blood 97:3669, 2001.

159. Tallman MS, Rowlings PA, Milone G et al: Effect of postremission chemotherapy before human leukocyte antigen-identical sibling transplantation for acute myelogenous leukemia in first complete remission. Blood 96:1254, 2000.

160. Berman E, Little C, Gee T et al: Reasons that patients with acute myelogenous leukemia do not undergo allogeneic bone marrow transplantation. N Engl J Med 326:156, 1992.

161. Sierra J, Storer B, Hansen JA et al: Unrelated donor marrow transplantation for acute myeloid leukemia: An update of the Seattle experience. Bone Marrow Transplant 26:397, 2000.

162. Cassileth PA, Harrington DP, Appelbaum FR et al: Chemotherapy compared with autologous or allogeneic bone marrow transplantation in the management of acute myeloid leukemia in first remission. N Engl Med 339:1649, 1998.

163. Zwann FE, Herman J: Report of the E.M.B.T. leukemia working party. Exp Hematol 11:3, 1983.

164. Gorin NC, Labopin M, Meloni G et al: Autologous bone marrow transplantation for acute myeloblastic leukemia in Europe: Further evidence of the role of marrow purging by mafosfamide. Leukemia 5:896, 1991.

165. Körbling M, Hunstein W, Fliedner TM et al: Disease-free survival after autologous bone marrow transplantation in patients with acute myelogenous leukemia. Blood 74:1898, 1989.

166. Reiffers J, Gaspard MH, Maraninchi D et al: Comparison of allogeneic or autologous bone marrow transplantation and chemotherapy in patients with acute myeloid leukaemia in first remission: A prospective controlled trial. Br J Haematol 72:57, 1989.

167. Woods WG, Neudorf S, Gold S et al: A comparison of allogeneic bone marrow transplantation, autologous bone marrow transplantation, and aggressive chemotherapy in children with acute myeloid leukemia in remission. Blood 97:56, 2001.

168. Reiffers J, Stoppa AM, Attal M et al: Autologous stem cell transplantation versus chemotherapy for adult patients with acute myeloid leukemia in first remission: The BGMT group experience. Nouv Rev Fr 35:17, 1993.

169. Blaise D, Kuentz M, Fortanier C et al: Randomized trial of bone marrow versus lenograstim-primed blood cell allogeneic transplantation in patients with early-stage leukemia: a report from the Societe Francaise de Greffe de Moelle. J Clin Oncol 18:537, 2000

170. Champlin RE, Schmitz N, Horowitz MM et al: Blood stem cells compared with bone marrow as a source of hematopoietic cells for allogeneic transplantation. IBMTR histocompatibility and stem cell sources working committee and the European group for blood and marrow transplantation (EBMT). Blood 95:3702, 2000

171. Chao NJ, Stein AS, Long GD et al: Busulfan/etoposide--initial experience with a new preparatory regimen for autologous bone marrow transplantation in patients with acute nonlymphocytic leukemia. Blood 81:319, 1993

172. Laporte JP, Douay L, Lopez M et al: One hundred twenty-five adult patients with primary acute leukemia autografted with marrow purged by mafosfamide: a 10-year single institution experience. Blood 84:3810, 1994

173. To LB, Chin DKF, Blumberg PA et al: Central nervous system relapse after bone marrow transplantation for acute myeloid leukemia. Cancer 52:2236, 1983

174. Witherspoon R, Flournoy N, Thomas ED et al: Recurrence of acute leukemia more than two years after allogeneic marrow grafting. Exp Hematol 14:178, 1986

175. Stein J, Zimmerman PA, Kochera M et al: Origin of leukemic relapse after bone marrow transplantation: comparison of cytogenetic and molecular analyses. Blood 73:2033, 1989

176. Frassoni F, Labopin M, Gluckman E et al: Are patients with acute leukemia, alive and well 2 years post bone marrow transplantation cured? A European survey. Leukemia 8:924, 1994

177. Socie G, Stone JV, Wingard JR et al: Long-term survival and late deaths after allogeneic bone marrow transplantation. N Engl J Med 341:14, 1999

178. Conde E, Iriondo A, Rayon C et al: Allogeneic bone marrow transplantation versus intensification chemotherapy for acute myelogenous leukaemia in first remission: a prospective controlled trial. Br J Haematol 68:219, 1988

179. Zander AR, Keating M, Dicke C et al: A comparison of marrow transplantation with chemotherapy for adults with acute leukemia of poor prognosis in first complete remission. J Clin Oncol 6:1548, 1988

180. Appelbaum FR, Fisher LD, Thomas ED et al: Chemotherapy v marrow transplantation for adults with acute nonlymphocytic leukemia: a five-year follow-up. Blood 72:179, 1988

181. Vogelsang GB, Farmer ER, Hess AD et al: Thalidomide for the treatment of chronic graft-versus-host disease. N Engl J Med 326:1055, 1992

182. Bäckman L, Ringden O, Tollemar J et al: An increased risk of relapse in cyclosporin-treated compared with methotrexate-treated patients: long-term follow-up of a randomized trial. Bone Marrow Transplant 3:463, 1988

183. Storb R, Deeg HJ, Pepe M et al: Methotrexate and cyclosporine versus cyclosporine alone for prophylaxis of graft-versus-host dis-

ease in patients given HLA-identical marrow grafts for leukemia: long-term follow-up of a controlled trial. Blood 73:1729, 1989

184. Slovak ML, Kopecky KJ, Cassileth PA et al: Karyotypic analysis predicts outcome of preremission and postremission therapy in adult acute myeloid leukemia: a Southwest Oncology Group/Eastern Cooperative Oncology Group study. Blood 96:4075, 2000

185. Linker CA, Ries CA, Damon LE et al: Autologous bone marrow transplantation for acute myeloid leukemia using busulfan plus etoposide as a preparative regimen. Blood 81:311, 1993

186. Smits P, Schoots L, de Pauw BE et al: Prognostic factors in adult patients with acute leukemia at first relapse. Cancer 59:1631, 1987

187. Levi JA, Wiernik PH: A comparative clinical trial of 5-azacytidine and guanazole in previously treated adults with acute non-lymphocytic leukemia. Cancer 38:36, 1976

188. Griffin JD, Maguire ME, Mayer RJ: Amsacrine in refractory acute leukemia. Cancer Treat Rep 69:787, 1985

189. Kantarjian HM, Keating MJ, Walters RS et al: Phase II study of low-dose continuous infusion homoharringtonine in refractory acute myelogenous leukemia. Cancer 63:813, 1989

190. Dutcher JP, Riggs CE, Strauman JJ et al: A phase I-II trial of 4'-deoxydoxorubicin (esorubicin) in refractory or relapsed acute leukemia. Clin Pharmacol Ther 45:424, 1989

191. Rowinsky EK, Burke PJ, Karp JE et al: Phase I and pharmacodynamic study of taxol in refractory acute leukemias. Cancer Res 49:4640, 1989

192. Rowinsky EK, Adjei A, Donehower RC et al: Phase I and pharmacodynamic study of the topoisomerase I-inhibitor topotecan in patients with refractory acute leukemia. J Clin Oncol 12:2193, 1994

193. Cortes J, Estey E, Beran M et al: Cyclophosphamide, Ara-C and topotecan (CAT) for patients with refractory or relapsed acute leukemia. Leuk Lymphoma 36:479, 2000

194. Lee EJ, Egorin MJ, Van Echo DA et al: Phase I and pharmacokinetic trial of carboplatin in refractory adult leukemia. J Natl Cancer Inst 80:131, 1988

195. Delmer A, Bauduer F, Vekhoff A et al: Evaluation of carboplatin as a single agent in highly refractory acute myeloid leukemia. Leukemia & Lymphoma 15:311, 1994

196. Santana VM, Hurwitz CA, Blakley RL et al: Complete hematologic remissions induced by 2-chlorodeoxyadenosine in children with newly diagnosed acute myeloid leukemia. Blood 84:1237, 1994

197. Vahdat L, Wong ET, Wile MJ et al: Therapeutic and neurotoxic effects of 2-chlorodeoxyadenosine in adults with acute myeloid leukemia. Blood 84:3429, 1994

198. Gordon MS, Young ML, Tallman MS et al: Phase II trial of 2-chlorodeoxyadenosine in patients with relapsed/refractory acute myeloid leukemia: a study of the Eastern Cooperative Oncology Group (ECOG), E9995. Leuk Res 24:871, 2000

199. Herzig RH, Wolff SN, Lazarus HM et al: High-dose cytosine arabinoside therapy for refractory leukemia. Blood 62:361, 1983

200. Capizzi RL, Davis R, Powell B et al: Synergy between high-dose cytarabine and asparaginase in the treatment of adults with refractory and relapsed acute myelogenous leukemia: a Cancer and Leukemia Group B study. J Clin Oncol 6:499, 1988

201. Evans C, Winkelstein A, Rosenfeld CS et al: High-dose cytosine arabinoside and L-asparaginase therapy for poor-risk adult nonlymphocytic leukemia. Cancer 65:2624, 1990

202. Hiddemann W, Kreutzmann H, Straif K et al: High-dose cytosine arabinoside and mitoxantrone: a highly effective regimen in refractory acute myeloid leukemia. Blood 69:744, 1987

203. Reece DE, Elmongy MB, Barnett MJ et al: Chemotherapy with high-dose cytosine arabinoside and mitoxantrone for poor-prognosis myeloid leukemias. Cancer Invest 11:509, 1993

204. Paciucci PA, Dutcher JP, Cuttner J et al: Mitoxantrone and Ara-C in previously treated patients with acute myelogenous leukemia. Leukemia 1:565, 1987

205. Archimbaud E, Leblond V, Michallet M et al: Intensive sequential chemotherapy with mitoxantrone and continuous infusion etoposide and cytarabine for previously treated acute myelogenous leukemia. Blood 77:1894, 1991

206. Archimbaud E, Fenaux P, Reiffers J et al: Granulocyte-macrophage colony-stimulating factor in association to timed-sequential chemotherapy with mitoxantrone, etoposide, and cytarabine for refractory acute myelogenous leukemia. Leukemia 7:372, 1993

207. Archimbaud E, Thomas X, Leblond V et al: Timed sequential chemotherapy for previously treated patients with acute myeloid leukemia: long-term follow-up of the etoposide, mitoxantrone, and cytarabine-86 trial. J Clin Oncol 13:11, 1995

208. Tosi P, Visani G, Ottaviani E et al: Fludarabine + Ara-C + G-CSF: cytotoxic effect and induction of apoptosis on fresh acute myeloid leukemia cells. Leukemia 8:2076, 1994

209. Estey E, Thall P, Andreeff M et al: Use of granulocyte colony-stimulating factor before, during, and after fludarabine plus cytarabine induction therapy of newly diagnosed acute myelogenous leukemia or myelodysplastic syndromes: comparison with fludarabine plus cytarabine without granulocyte colony-stimulating factor. J Clin Oncol 12:671, 1994

210. Kornblau SM, Cortes-Franco J, Estey E: Neurotoxicity associated with fludarabine and cytosine arabinoside chemotherapy for acute leukemia and myelodysplasia. Leukemia 7:378, 1993

211. Kaminer LS, Choi KE, Daley KM et al: Continuous infusion mitoxantrone in relapsed acute nonlymphocytic leukemia. Cancer 65:2619, 1990

212. Ho AD, Lipp T, Ehninger G et al: Combination of mitoxantrone and etopside in refractory acute myelogenous leukemia-an active and well-tolerated regimen. J Clin Oncol 6:213, 1988

213. Hansen OP, Pedersen-Bjergaard J, Ellegaard J et al: Aclarubicin plus cytosine arabinoside versus daunorubicin plus cytosine arabinoside in previously untreated patients with acute myeloid leukemia: a Danish national phase III trial. Leukemia 5:510, 1991

214. Sato S, Sakashita A, Ishiyama T et al: Possible differentiation treatment with aclacinomycin A in acute myelomonocytic leukemia refractory to conventional chemotherapy. Anticancer Res 12:371, 1992

215. Rowe JM, Chang AYC, Bennett JM: Aclacinomycin A and etoposide (VP-16-213): an effective regimen in previously treated patients with refractory acute myelogenous leukemia. Blood 71:992,1988

216. Sievers EL, Appelbaum FR, Spielberger RT et al: Selective ablation of acute myeloid leukemia using antibody-targeted chemotherapy: A phase I study of an anti-CD33 calicheamicin immunoconjugate. Blood 93:3678, 1999

217. Sievers EL, Larson RA, Stadtmauer EA et al: Efficacy and safety of gemtuzumab ozogamicin in patients with CD33-positive acute myeloid leukemia in first relapse. J Clin Oncol 19:3244, 2001

218. Robles C, Kim KM, Oken MM et al: Low-dose cytarabine maintenance therapy vs observation after remission induction in advanced acute myeloid leukemia: an Eastern Cooperative Oncology Group Trial (E5483). Leukemia 14:1349, 2000

219. Lee S, Tallman MS, Oken MM et al: Duration of second complete remission compared with first complete remission in patients with acute myeloid leukemia. Eastern Cooperative Oncology Group. Leukemia 14:1345, 2000

220. Wiernik PH, Dutcher JP, Todd M et al: Polyethylene glycolated interleukin-2 as maintenance therapy for acute myelogenous leukemia in second remission. Am J Hematol 47:41, 1994

221. Bergmann L, Heil G, Kolbe K et al: Interleukin-2 bolus infusion as late consolidation therapy in 2nd remission of acute myeloblastic leukemia. Leukemia & Lymphoma 16:271, 1995

222. Foa R, Meloni G, Tosti S et al: Treatment of acute myeloid leukaemia patients with recombinant interleukin 2: a pilot study. Br J Haematol 77:491, 1991

223. Meloni G, Foa R, Vignetti M et al: Interleukin-2 may induce prolonged remissions in advanced acute myelogenous leukemia. Blood 84:2158, 1994

224. Maraninchi D, Vey N, Viens P et al: A phase II study of interleukin-2 in 49 patients with relapsed or refractory acute leukemia. Leuk Lymphoma 31:343, 1998

225. Forman SJ, Schmidt GM, Nademanee AP et al: Allogeneic bone marrow transplantation as therapy for primary induction failure for patients with acute leukemia. J Clin Oncol 9:1570, 1991

226. Clift RA, Buckner CD, Appelbaum FR et al: Allogeneic marrow transplantation during untreated first relapse of acute myeloid leukemia. J Clin Oncol 10:1723, 1992

227. Blume KG, Kopecky KJ, Henslee-Downey JP et al: A prospective randomized comparison of total body irradiation-etoposide versus busulfan-cyclophosphamide as preparatory regimens for bone marrow transplantation in patients with leukemia who were not in first remission: a Southwest Oncology Group study. Blood 81:2187, 1993

228. Petersen FB, Lynch MHE, Clift RA et al: Autologous marrow transplantation for patients with acute myeloid leukemia in untreated first relapse or in second complete remission. J Clin Oncol 11:1353, 1993

229. Brown RA, Herzig RH, Wolff SN et al: High-dose etoposide and cyclophosphamide without bone marrow transplantation for resistant hematologic malignancy. Blood 76:473, 1990

230. Fefer A, Benyunes MC, Massumoto C et al: Interleukin-2 therapy after autologous bone marrow transplantation for hematologic malignancies. Semin Oncol 20 (suppl 9):41, 1993

231. Blaise D, Attal M, Pico JL et al: The use of a sequential high dose recombinant interleukin 2 regimen after autologous bone marrow transplantation does not improve the disease free survival of patients with acute leukemia transplanted in first complete remission. Leuk Lymphoma 25:469, 1997

232. Blaise D, Attal M, Reiffers J et al: Randomized study of recombinant interleukin-2 after autologous bone marrow transplantation for acute leukemia in first complete remission. Eur Cytokine Netw 11:91, 2000

233. Giralt S, Escudier S, Kantarjian H et al: Preliminary results of treatment with filgrastim for relapse of leukemia and myelodysplasia after allogeneic bone marrow transplantation. N Engl J Med 329:757, 1993

234. Dazzi F, Goldman J: Donor lymphocyte infusions. Curr Opin Hematol 6:394, 1999

235. Imoto S, Muryama T, Gomyo H et al: Long-term molecular remission induced by donor lymphocyte infusions for recurrent acute myeloblastic leukemia after allogeneic bone marrow transplantation. Bone Marrow Transplant 26:809, 2000

236. Porter DL, Collins RH Jr, Hardy C et al: Treatment of relapsed leukemia after unrelated donor marrow transplantation with unrelated donor leukocyte infusions. Blood 95:1214, 2000

237. McSweeney PA, Niederwieser D, Shizuru JA et al: Hematopoietic cell transplantation in older patients with hematologic malignancies: replacing high-dose cytotoxic therapy with graft-versus-tumor effects. Blood 97:3390, 2001

238. Stewart DJ, Smith TL, Keating MJ et al: Remission from central nervous system involvement in adults with acute leukemia. Cancer 56:632, 1985

239. Liu YJA, Adams JA, Brereton ML et al: Magakaryocytopoiesis in vitro in myelodysplastic syndromes and acute myeloid leukaemia: effect of pegylated recombinant human megakaryocyte growth and development factor in combination with other growth factors. Br J Haematol 108:743, 2000

240. Archimbaud E, Ottmann OG, Yin JA et al: A randomized, double-blind, placebo-controlled study with pegylated recombinant human megakaryocyte growth and development factor (PEG-rHuMGDF) as an adjunct to chemotherapy for adults with de novo acute myeloid leukemia. Blood 94:3694, 1999

241. Schiffer CA, Miller K, larson RA et al: A double-blind, placebo-controlled trial of pegylated recombinant human megakaryocyte growth and development factor as an adjunct to induction and consolidation therapy for patients with acute myeloid leukemia. Blood 95:2530, 2000

242. Tokunaga Y, Miyamoto T, Gondo H et al: Effect of thrombopoietin on acute myelogenous leukemia blasts. Leuk Lymphoma 37:27, 2000

243. Tobal K, Newton J, Macheta M et al: Molecular quantitation of minimal residual disease in acute myeloid leukemia with t(8;21) can identify patients in durable remission and predict clinical relapse. Blood 95:815, 2000

244. Wattjes MP, Krauter J, Nagel S et al: Comparison of nested competitive RT-PCR and real-time RT-PCR for the detection and quantification of AML1/MTG8 fusion transcripts in t(8;21) positive acute myelogenous leukemia. Leukemia 14:329, 2000

245. Sugimoto T, Das H, Imoto S et al: Quantitation of minimal residual disease in t(8;21)-positive acute myelogenous leukemia patients using real-time quantitative RT-PCR. Am J Hematol 64:101, 2000

246. Fujimaki S, Funato T, Harigae H et al: A quantitative reverse transcriptase polymerase chain reaction method for the detection of leukaemic cells with t(8;21) in peripheral blood. Eur J Haematol 64:252, 2000

247. Morschhauser F, Cayuela JM, Martini S et al: Evaluation of minimal residual disease using reverse-transcription polymerase chain reaction in t(8;21) acute myeloid leukemia: a multicenter study of 51 patients. J Clin Oncol 18:788, 2000

21

Acute Promyelocytic Leukemia

Peter H. Wiernik, Robert E. Gallagher, and
Martin S. Tallman

Overall Perspective

Perhaps more is known about the molecular biology of APL, both in terms of genetic mechanism and potential for tumor cell specific therapy, than for any other specific type of human cancer. The historical background underlying this statement derives from two independent lines of investigation. One is genetic in nature, beginning with the discovery in 1977 that the APL phenotype of AML is consistently associated with a reciprocal translocation between chromosomes 15 and 17.[18] The second is biological, stemming from the finding in 1981 that APL cells are unique in their property of undergoing terminal differentiation after exposure in short-term tissue culture to supraphysiological concentrations of the naturally occurring metabolite of vitamin A, ATRA.[19] The clinical relevance of the in vitro findings was demonstrated in 1988 when Chinese investigators reported that ATRA produces complete remissions in a high percentage of APL patients.[20] In 1990, there was a remarkable confluence of these two investigative lines with the discovery that the t(15;17) consistently produced breakage of the retinoic acid receptor-alpha (RARα) gene on chromosome band 17q11-21.[21–23] This seminal discovery provided instant access to a wealth of molecular information that had been developed related to the RARα gene since its discovery in 1987,[24,25] which, as a ligand-dependent nuclear transcription factor that mediates cellular responses to ATRA, had obvious implications for the selective action of ATRA in APL cells. The following year, the fusion partner of the RARα gene from chromosome 15 was identified and was originally called myl but subsequently renamed PML (for ProMyeLocytes or ProMyelocytic Leukemia).[26–28] Thus, the two hybrid gene products that result from the reciprocal t(15;17) in APL are PML-RARα and RARα-PML (Figure 21–1).

Acute promyelocytic leukemia (APL) is designated M3 in the French-American-British (FAB) classification. Because of its unique clinical features and unique response to certain differentiation inducing agents, and because of our advanced understanding of the molecular biology of this leukemia, APL deserves to be presented and discussed in detail, apart from the other acute myeloid leukemias.

APL was first described by Hillestad in 1957.[1,2] He described three patients with the characteristic morphology of hypergranular APL, hypofibrinogenemia, and a hemorrhagic diathesis.[1] Caen et al.[3] established that the hemorrhagic syndrome was directly related to the proliferation of the leukemic cells in APL, and Bernard et al.[4] provided a precise description of the disease in a presentation that included 20 patients. Bernard et al.[5] subsequently discovered the unusual sensitivity of this AML variant to daunorubicin. Rowley et al. in 1976–1977 described the balanced cytogenetic translocation (15;17) in APL[6,7] and found it to be present in virtually every patient (Figure 21–1).[8] Kantarjian et al.[9] reported that chemotherapy could induce complete remissions in APL without inducing marrow hypoplasia and that remission was often the result of a gradual morphologic evolution, an observation later confirmed by Stone et al.[10] who suggested that the mechanism of remission in APL may be leukemic cell differentiation. Breitman et al.[11] demonstrated that maturation and differentiation of leukemic cells thought to be human APL cells (HL-60 cell line) could be accomplished in vitro by several agents including retinoids. Huang et al.[12] reported the first large series of APL patients treated with oral all-*trans* retinoic acid (ATRA) and demonstrated a phenomenally high rate of relatively brief complete remissions. Fenaux and collegues[13] treated APL with ATRA and standard chemotherapy, and reported results superior to those obtained with either treatment alone, and more recently, arsenic trioxide was identified as an agent with major activity in APL.[14] Coincident with these treatment advances, there has been an explosion of knowledge of APL at the molecular level. All of these events taken together have fostered speculation that APL may be the most likely acute myeloid leukemia variant to be routinely cured in the near future.[15,16] For a more detailed history of APL, the reader is referred to Bernard.[17]

In the intervening years, four alternative fusion gene partners of RARα have been discovered in rare cases of APL, each associated with a unique chromosome translocation (Table 21–1 and see below).[29–32] All of the fusion proteins include the same amino-truncated portion of RARα. This points out the central role of RARα in the pathogenesis of APL and, paradoxically, in the response of APL to ATRA. The involvement of the *PML* gene in greater than 99 percent of APL cases implies that it also contributes some essential function to pathogenesis, which has gained support from a variety of findings. Although the alternative fusion genes, generically referred to as *X-RARα*s, are rare and, hence are of limited clinical impact, they have provided very useful information about molecular mechanisms of APL and about the effect of therapeutic agents on APL cells. The variable formation and expression of the reciprocal translocation fusion genes, *RARα-Xs*, has provided further insights into the disturbances of molecular pathways in APL. Studies of the relationship of PML-RARα to APL cell pathology and drug response were markedly abetted by the establishment of the fusion gene-positive APL cell line NB4 in 1991.[33] More recently, the development of transgenic mice bearing the fusion genes has provided resources for evaluating the role of the different fusion genes in APL pathogenesis and models for evalu-

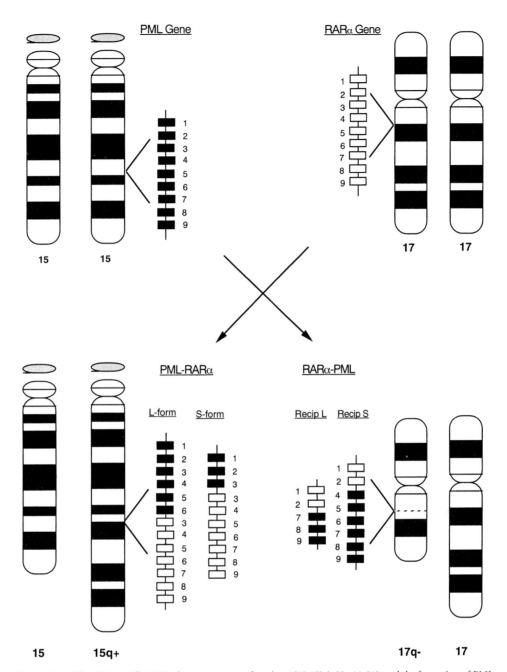

Figure 21–1. The APL-specific 15/17 chromosome translocation, t(15;17) (q22;q11-21), and the formation of PML-RARα and its reciprocal (recip) product RARα-PML. Vertical chains of boxes represent the nine exons of both the *PML* and *RARα* genes (filled boxes, PML; empty boxes, RARα). The S and L forms of PML-RARα are formed by break sites in PML introns 3 or 6, respectively, whereas RARα is uniformly broken in intron 2.

ating treatment (reviewed in Ref. 34). Important conclusions from the transgenic mouse studies are that the fusion genes are insufficient as single genetic lesions to produce APL, implying the requirement of complementary mutations. In some instances, co-expression of the X-RARα and RARα-X translocation products may complement one another in disease pathogenesis. Finally, in clinical trial application, the APL-specific *PML-RARα* fusion gene has provided a means for monitoring residual disease post-therapy,[35,36] and the finding of mutations in the *PML-RARα* gene of a significant fraction of patients who

relapse from ATRA-containing therapy has provided further evidence of the essential role of *PML-RARα* as an ATRA therapeutic target.[37] Detailed reviews of the molecular biology of APL are available.[38,39]

RARα and the Essentials of Nuclear Receptor Function

RARα is a member of the steroid/thyroid hormone receptor gene superfamily, which encodes proteins that function as *trans*-acting, ligand-dependent regulators of gene transcription

Table 21−1. Retinoic Acid Receptor-Alpha Fusion Genes Generated by Alternative Chromosome 17q11-21 Translocations in APL

Fusion Gene	Karyotype	Frequency	ATRA Response	Reciprocal Product	References
PML-RARα	t(15;17)(q22;q11-21)	> 99 percent	Yes	Yes (75 percent)	26−28,169,186
PLZF-RARα	t(11;17)(q23;q11-21)	~ 20 cases	No	Yes	29
NPM-RARα	t(5;17)(q32;q11-21)	3 cases	Yes	Yes	30
NuMA-RARα	t(11;17)(q13;q11-21)	1 case	Yes	No	31
STAT5b-RARα	t(17;17)(q11-21;q11-21)	1 case	No?	No	32

(reviewed in Ref. 40). In order to perform this common function, these proteins contain two essential domains, a DNA binding domain (DBD) near the amino terminus and a ligand binding domain (LBD) near the carboxy terminus (Figure 21–2). The DBD, which contains two characteristic zinc finger motifs, serves to bind the proteins to specific oligonucleotide sequences, hormone response elements (HREs), in the promoter region of select genes, many of which have central effects on cell and tissue growth, differentiation, and homeostasis. RARs, which include separate genes for RARβ and RARγ in addition to RARα, belong to one major branch of the steroid/hormone receptor superfamily, along with the thyroid hormone receptors and vitamin D3 receptor. These nuclear receptors have the common property of residing in the nucleus in a bound state to their respective HREs, consisting of two direct repeats of the hexanucleotide (A/G)G(G/T) TCA (Figures 21–2 and 21–3A). These receptors also share the property of binding to HREs as a heterodimer with common adapter proteins called retinoid X receptors (Figures 21–2 and 21–3A), of which there are also three different genes (RXR-α, β, and γ).

The discriminator for HRE specificity is the number of nucleotides between the two direct repeats, which is two or five retinoic acid response elements (RAREs), three for vitamin D3 RE (VDRE), and four for thyroid hormone RE (TREs). Additionally, HRE spacers with one nucleotide have specificity for RXR homodimers or, in some cases, may heterodimerize with RAR in reverse polarity.[41] Through expression of different combinations of RAR/RXR heterodimers, variations in RAREs, competition between nuclear receptors and alternative transcription factors for limiting quantities of RXRs and differences in retinoid ligand utilization, the retinoid receptor system can generate enormous heterogeneity that has been related to the discriminatory, instructive role of retinoids in different tissues and cells types during development (reviewed in Ref. 40).

In addition to the DBD and LBD domains, respectively designated as the C and E regions, there are three other subregions of RARα (Figure 21–2). The A-region, which constitutes the amino-terminus of the RARα-X fusion proteins, has autonomous, ligand-independent transcriptional activation function (AF-1) that is regulated by phosphorylation of a spe-

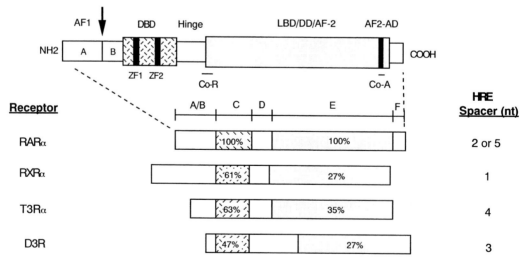

Figure 21–2. Structure of RARα and its homology to related members of the RAR-RXR-T3R-D3R branch of the steroid-thyroid hormone receptor gene superfamily. AF1, activation function 1 (ligand-independent) domain; DBD, DNA binding domain; LBD/DD/AF2, overlapping ligand binding, dimerization, and activator function 2 (ligand-dependent) domains; ZF1 and ZF2, zinc fingers 1 and 2; AF2-AD/Co-A, AF2 activation core domain containing consensus sequence for binding coactivators (Co-A); Co-R, co-repressor binding region. A through F indicate standardly recognized regions/domains of these proteins. Vertical arrow indicates the universal break site in RARα between the A and B domains that occurs in formation of the various fusion proteins. Percentage numbers indicate the degree of amino acid sequence homology of the DNA binding (C-regions) and ligand binding (E-regions) of each receptor protein to RARα. HRE, hormone response element; the numbers beneath indicate the number of nucleotides (nt) between the two one-half site direct repeats, PuG(G/T)TCA.

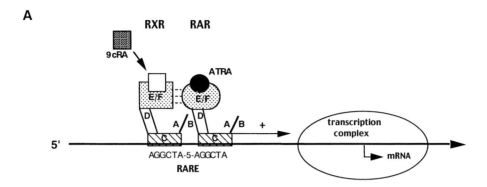

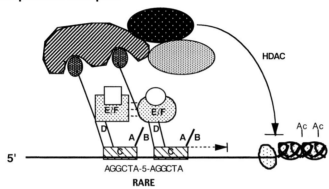

Figure 21–3. Model for regulation of an ATRA-responsive gene promoters. **(A)** Formation of RAR-RXR heterodimer on retinoic acid response element (RARE). The diagram shows RXR bound to the upstream RARE half-site and RAR bound to the downstream half-site, the two separated by a 5 nucleotide spacer and with noncovalent bonding (dotted lines) between apposed portions of the E-domains of the two proteins. All-*trans* RA (ATRA) has already bound to RAR, which produces steric changes in RXR, which then becomes permissive for binding its specific ligand, 9-*cis* RA. **(B)** Formation of co-repressor complex in the absence of ligand binding. Specific peptide motifs in the proximal portion of the E/LBD-region and distal D/hinge-region (Co-R Box) interact with complementary motifs in nuclear receptor co-repressor proteins (N-CoR or SMRT), which, in turn, bind to a common adaptor protein mSin3 that forms a complex with further interacting proteins with histone deacetylase activity (HDAC). Removal of negatively charged acetyl residues (Ac) from core histones leads to tighter interaction of these proteins with the negatively charged DNA helix producing condensed heterochromatin, blocking transcriptional activity. *(continued)*

cific serine residue.[42] The D-region serves a rotational or "hinge" function related to heterodimer formation on HREs, and at its carboxy-terminus. It contains a conserved motif, called the Co-R Box, important for interaction with co-repressor proteins (see below).[41] The function of the F-region, which is unique to RARs, is unknown.

The E-region of RAR has multiple functions in addition to serving as the LBD. This region has now been analyzed by many different methods, including extensive site-directed mutagenesis studies and crystallographic analysis of purified LBD in the presence and absence of ligand.[40,43] Such analysis has defined the three-dimensional structure of the region to consist of 12 α-helices and 2 β-strands linked by a series of angled loops. From this conformational model, it has been determined that key amino acids from many components of the LBD contribute to the formation of a binding pocket for ATRA, while those from a more restricted area stabilize a RAR:RXR dimerization interface through specific noncovalent bond interactions. The presence of ATRA in the binding pocket produces an overall tight-

ening of the three-dimensional structure, a very prominent feature of which is a closing of the 12th, carboxy-terminal α-helix over the opening to the occupied binding site. The latter movement (schematically illustrated in Figures 21–3B and C), which has been likened to the springing of a mousetrap, has been correlated with the acquisition of the capacity of a highly conserved 7 amino acid long stretch in α-helix 12, called the AF-2 activation domain (AF-2 AD), to interact with crucial coactivator (Co-A) proteins (Figure 21–3C). This interaction is mandatory for activation of the transcription complex, since mutations that prevent AF-2 AD/coactivator interactions completely eliminate transcriptional activation by RARE-bound RARs.[40,44] Another consequence of the ligand-induced conformational change of the LBD of RARs is ejection of co-repressor proteins from binding sites from the Co-R Box sequences in the hinge-proximal LBD region of the RAR component of the RARE-bound RXR:RAR dimer.[41] The binding of these co-repressors in the absence of ligand is functionally active, reducing promoter-driven transcription below basal levels. Thus, the essence of

C. p160 Coactivator complex

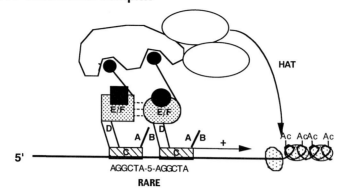

D. Multi-component transcription activation complexes

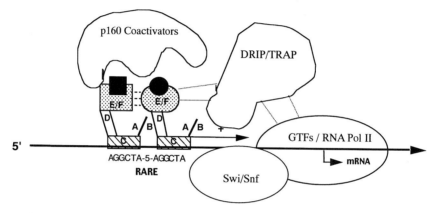

Figure 21–3. *(Continued)* (C) Formation of co-activator complex. Ligand binding produces a conformational shift in the RAR and RXR proteins, such that the twelfth, carboxy-terminal α-helix swings over the bound ligand. This shift helps to discharge co-repressor proteins and brings peptide motifs in the AF-2 activator domain (AF-2 AD) core sequence (Co-A) into contact with complementary motifs in co-activator proteins of the p160 class, which, in turn, interact with other proteins, including a CREB-binding protein (CBP/p300) group. CBP contains target sites for many transcriptional regulatory signals and, additionally, interacts with other proteins that have histone acetyl transferase (HAT) activity and proteins of the basal transcriptional apparatus, including RNA polymerase II. The acetylation of core histones loosens the chromatin structure, allowing access of transcription factors to promoter sites and fostering transcriptional activity. (D) Two additional multiprotein complexes complement the p160 co-activators to enhance access and functional activity of general transcription factors (GTFs) to transcribe RNA from active promoter sites, the DRIP/TRAP and Swi/Snf complexes.

RARα function as a transcriptional regulator is embodied in the E-region, which serves as a sensitive switch to either repress or activate RARE-containing gene promoters in the absence or presence of ATRA, respectively.

In the past 5 years, there has been astonishing progress in identifying the detailed molecular mechanisms by which nuclear receptor proteins and their associated co-repressor and co-activator complexes regulate gene transcription.[40,45,46] For RAR/RXRs, four separate protein complexes, each consisting of at least 14 individual proteins (R. Evans, American Society of Hematology meeting, 12/2000), have been defined that can regulate the general transcriptional apparatus containing RNA polymerase II on RARE-containing gene promoters (Figure 21–3D). For two of these complexes, the co-repressor and co-activator complexes, a primary functional element is the regulation of the level of acetylation of histones, the primary structural components of nucleosomal chromatin (Figures 21–3B and C).

Co-repressors accomplish this by recruiting members of the histone deacetylase (HDAC) enzyme family.[47] Conversely, co-activators either contain endogenous histone acetylase (HAT) enzyme activity or recruit auxiliary proteins with this activity.[48] Deacetylated histones maintain nuclear chromatin in a condensed, inactive state, while acetylated histones have just the opposite effect. These antagonistic processes are in a dynamic state such that histone remodeling can be rapidly modified by ATRA-RAR interactions on RARE-containing gene promoters. Ongoing investigations continue to provide revelations about the specificity of acetylation of amino acid residues in the lysine-rich tails of histone,[49] about the interaction of these events with the alternative transcriptional control system involving DNA and histone methylation by specific methyltransferases,[50,51] and about the role of acetylation of alternative transcription complex proteins during the transcriptional activation response.[52] A third transcription complex involved in transcriptional activation of

RARE-regulated promoters is the so-called DRIP/TRAP complex.[53] This complex, like the HAT co-activator system, interacts directly with the AF-2 region of nuclear receptors in a ligand-dependent manner and is also directly linked to RNA pol II. Although required for the activational transcription response, the relationship of the DRIP/TRAP complex to the HAT co-activator complex is unclear. A fourth complex, or more accurately an example of several complexes, involved in transcriptional activation is the Swi/Snf (acronyms from yeast genetic terminology) family of ATP-dependent "chromatin remodeling machines."[54] These complexes act in concert with acetylated lysines to promote chromatin alterations required for transcriptional activation. Although any of the four complexes (in addition to the receptor itself) could, theoretically, be the target of therapeutic manipulation, interest has focused on stimulation of histone acetylation through the discovery of several types of compounds that inhibit histone deacetylase activity.[55,56]

Molecular Dissection of PML-RARα-Positive APL

Structure and Function of PML

The *PML* gene belongs to a large gene family that has a variety of associated functions, most related to DNA replication-repair and transcriptional regulation.[26,27,57,58] The core region of the encoded PML protein has a characteristic tripartite structure consisting of a particular cysteine/histidine-rich (Cys3HisCys4) cluster called the RING motif, followed by two alternative cysteine/histidine clusters called B-boxes, followed, in turn, by an α-helical coiled-coil domain (Figure 21–4B).[59] This tripartite structure is shared by eight other genes of this protein subfamily, two members of which in addition to PML, the ret finger protein[60] and T18/TIF1,[61] can form oncogenic hybrid proteins as the result of tumor-associated chromosome translocations. All three of the cysteine/histidine clusters bind to zinc ions (zinc fingers).[59,62] Although many zinc finger proteins function by binding to specific nucleotide sequences in DNA, no such sequences have been found for PML, and current evidence indicates that the RING domain functions through protein-protein

interactions. These interactions are likely importantly facilitated by hydrophobic amino acid heptad repeats in the coiled-coil region, which serves as a critical interface for the formation of PML homodimers and of heterodimers with PML-RARα in APL cells.[57,63,64]

PML is expressed in a wide variety of cell types, in most at low levels.[65–67] In hematopoietic cells, PML is most highly expressed in immature myeloid cells, where it appears to be important for terminal differentiation, since PML knock-out (PML–/PML–) mice have reduced numbers of circulating granulocytes and monocytes associated with diminished responsiveness of myeloid progenitors to retinoic acid–induced clonogenic activity.[68] A notable feature of PML expression is its localization to the nucleus, where it is associated with organelles called nuclear bodies (NBs; also referred to as promyelocytic oncogenic domains, PODs, or as nuclear domain 10, ND 10) that form part of the nuclear matrix.[57,69–72] From recent studies using cells derived from PML–/PML– mice (reviewed in Refs. 73 and 74), it has been determined that PML expression is central to both NB structure and function. PML NBs contain over 20 proteins, many of which are displaced from their normal location in PML NBs in the absence of PML.[38] A minority of the PML NB proteins have been demonstrated to directly interact with PML, importantly including a ubiquitin-related enzyme, SUMO-1 (small ubiquitin-related modifier; also called sentrin, PIC1 or UBL-1), which produces post-translational modification of PML required for the recruitment of other PML NB proteins.[75,76]

PML is a multifunctional protein affecting fundamental cell processes, such as proliferation, apoptosis, and differentiation (reviewed in Ref. 68). Initial reports indicated that overexpression of PML by transfection in a variety of cell types, including in the APL cell line NB4, produces potent growth inhibition.[65,77,78] Conversely, there is reduced sensitivity of various types of cells derived from PML–/PML– cells, including hematopoietic progenitors, to growth arrest under some conditions.[68] For example, the well-characterized senescence response of murine embryo fibroblasts (MEFs) to expression of oncogenic ras, accompanied by G1 cell cycle arrest, requires

A PML Gene Structure and Breakpoint Cluster Regions

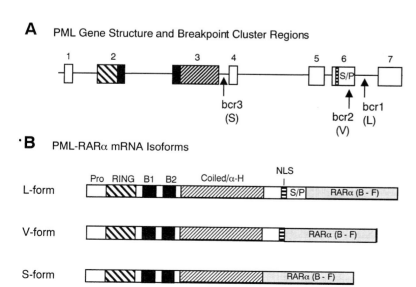

B PML-RARα mRNA Isoforms

Figure 21–4. Formation and structure of PML-RARα mRNA isoforms. (A) DNA level diagram is limited to the portion of the 5′-region of the PML locus involved in the formation of PML-RARα mRNA. Boxes, numbered exons; lines, introns. Arrows indicate breakpoint cluster region (bcr) sites of DNA breakage resulting in the formation of S-, V-, and L-form types of PML-RARα mRNA. (B) PML-RARα isoforms produced by the fusion of the three types of 5′-PML regions linked to the common RARa segment (regions B to F; see Figure 21–2). The variable filled rectangles in the PML portion indicate the mRNA coding regions for the proline-rich (Pro), RING, two B-box (B1&2), and coiled-coiled/alpha-helical domains. NLS indicates a nuclear localizing sequence in PML exon 6 and S/P indicates a serine/proline-rich segment.

increased PML expression and is defective in PML–/PML– MEF cells.[79,80]

A second function of PML is as a mediator of multiple apoptotic pathways, including Fas- and caspase-mediated DNA-damage pathways after a variety of apoptogenic stimuli, as demonstrated using PML–/PML– cells,[81] and, when overexpressed, caspase-independent pathways.[82] The Fas-mediated pathway has been demonstrated to involve the recruitment to NBs and binding to PML of the chromatin-binding protein Daxx.[75,83] Whether PML activation results in cell growth arrest or apoptotic response may depend on the status of the p14/p19 ARF/mdm2/p53 pathway.[80]

The biological effects of PML are at least partially related to its function as a transcriptional cofactor. Since there is no evidence that PML interacts directly with DNA, this appears to occur through interactions with recruited proteins that have direct or indirect transcriptional regulatory activity. Both transcriptional repressor and activator activities have been described.[80,84–87] The net cell biological effect of even the activational activities, however, appears to be primarily inhibitory, since PML-mediated activation of retinoid receptors,[86] p53[63], or GATA-2[70] all result in decreased cell proliferation. Conversely, the increased proliferative capacity of PML–/PML– progenitor myeloid cells was associated with the inability of ATRA-liganded RAR/RXR to activate transcription of the RARE-containing cyclin-dependent kinase inhibitor gene *p21WAF1/CIP1* in the absence of PML co-activator activity, which could contribute to the expansion of a prematurely arrested leukemic clone.[68]

The in vivo relevance of the above findings is indicated by observations that PML–/PML– mice have about twice the incidence of skin papillomas and lymphomas, many of high grade, after treatment with a chemical mutagen[68] and that APL develops much more rapidly in transgenic PML-RARα PML–/PML– mice than PML+/PML+ mice, while heterozygotes (PML+/PML–) have an intermediate course.[88] All of the above activities, as well as additional activities related to DNA stability[89] and cytokine-mediated antiviral activity (reviewed in Ref. 38), are likely contributory to the function of PML as a tumor suppressor with the capability of inhibiting the transforming activities of oncogenes.[77] A recent study indicated that PML-RARα transgenic mice with an inactivating mutation in the RARα region develop leukemia whereas RARα transgenic mice with the same mutation did not develop leukemia.[90] This indicates that the PML domain plays an indispensable role in the development of PML-RARα leukemogenesis but leaves open the question of whether this is due to a unique positive action of the PML component of PML-RARα, especially in the context of APL cells in which there is haploinsufficiency of normal PML, as well as RARα, as a result of the t(15;17) (see below).

Structure and Expression of PML-RARα

The *PML-RARα* fusion gene derives in each APL case from breakage of the *PML* gene on chromosome 15 in one of three breakpoint cluster regions (bcrs) and from breakage of the *RARα* gene on chromosome 17 in randomly distributed sites throughout the second intron (Figure 21–4; reviewed in Ref. 91). PML-RARα bcr1 cases result from genomic DNA breaks in PML intron 6, producing, after mRNA processing, the long(L)-form PML-RARα fusion transcript. In bcr3 cases the breaksite occurs in PML intron 3, producing the short(S)-form of PML-RARα mRNA. Compared to L-form mRNA, the S-form transcript lacks PML exons 4 to 6, which primarily encode a proline/serine-rich region with several potential phosphorylation sites. Exon 6 also contains the PML nuclear localizing sequence (NLS) and an important proteolytic site (see below). In bcr2 cases, the PML breaksite occurs in or near the 3′-end of PML exon 6, which results in deletion of variable amounts of coding sequence from the resultant variable(V)-form PML-RARα fusion transcript. Frequently, additional nucleotides derived from RARα intron 2 are incorporated at the end of the deleted PML 6 exon, which preserves the translational open reading frame (ORF) in all PML-RARα V-form cases (reviewed in Ref. 92). Among 221 PML-RARα-positive adult cases, the frequency of L-, S-, and V-form fusion transcripts were 55, 37, and 8 percent, respectively.[91] In pediatric cases, there is a higher frequency of V-form cases, up to 27 percent, and a proportionate reduction in S-form- cases.[93,94]

A remarkable feature of PML-RARα in APL cells is that by immunocytochemistry it is primarily expressed in myriad tiny speckles in the nucleus (~100 microspeckles/nucleus). Deletion analysis has demonstrated that this distribution requires the RING domain and to a lesser extent the coiled-coil domain of the PML region of the molecule.[64] Notably, the high-level expression of PML-RARα delocalizes normal PML from PML NBs through the formation of PML-RARα:PML heterodimers, involving the interaction of the homologous coiled-coil regions of these proteins. A number of other PML-RARα interacting proteins, including RARα, RXRα, PLZF, co-repressor proteins, and a variety of other proteins normally associated with PML NBs are also recruited to the microspeckles. Treatment of APL cells with either ATRA or arsenic trioxide (ATO) results in dissolution of the microspeckles and re-establishment of PML NBs. It should be noted that most studies have been performed with the NB4 APL cell culture line, which contains the L-form of PML-RARα.[26,33] In fresh APL blasts, particularly with the S-form of PML-RARα that lacks the PML NLS, more PML-RARα is localized in the cytoplasm, but, nevertheless, the treatment reversible relationship to PML NB disaggregation appears to pertain.[57,69]

Role of PML-RARα in Leukemogenesis

The functions embodied in PML-RARα are the primary driving factors in the development and specification of the APL subtype of AML. This conclusion recently gained strong support from the successful transduction of multipotential human hematopoietic progenitor/stem cells (HSC) with PML-RARα, which has been difficult to accomplish because of the toxic nature of this gene product in hematopoietic cells.[95] In these experiments, it was demonstrated that expression of PML-RARα co-opted the differentiation program of the HSC, rapidly committing the transduced cells to differentiate almost exclusively along the neutrophilic granulocyte pathway, which could not be deterred by treatment with hematopoietic growth factors (HGFs), culminating in a maturation arrest of the HSC at the promyelocyte stage. These results are consistent with other basic investigations demonstrating that the intrinsic expression pattern of certain potent transcription factors can be the primary driving element in hematopoietic cell differentiation and take precedence over the potential lineage instructive effects of HGFs (reviewed in Ref. 96).

The primary pathogenetic role of PML-RARα in APL is also strongly supported by experiments in transgenic mice.[97–99] In these mice the *PML-RARα* transgene is regulated from random genomic integration sites by the promoter region of either the *MRP8* or *cathepsin G* genes, which are normally expressed only in subterminally differentiated neutrophilic granulocytes. The leukemias develop in a proportion of the founder transgenic mice after a latency period of 6 to 12 months, indicating that other somatic genetic alterations are required for leukemia to develop. Although the phenotype of the transgenic leukemias are not faithful replicas of APL, they do have sufficient features of the disease, including responsiveness to ATRA to certify the specific oncogenic role of PML-RARα. Future murine models in which the transgene for PML-RARα is "knocked in" to appropriate somatic hematopoietic progenitors may provide more exact phenocopies of the human disease.[34]

The most essential molecular mechanism by which the PML-RARα oncoprotein has been experimentally linked to the APL phenotype is by recruiting abnormal quantities of tightly bound co-repressor proteins to RARE-regulated gene promoters.[95,100,101] This primarily occurs through binding of the co-repressor complex to the LBD of the RARα-region of PML-RARα, which maintains genes required for terminal neutrophilic differentiation in a transcriptionally inactive state, at least partly due to associated HDAC activity (Figure 21–3B). Thus, it is notable that overexpression of normal RARα in murine bone marrow progenitors can produce a differentiation arrest at the promyelocyte stage and cell immortalization in vitro.[102,103] However, this promyelocytic transformation can be overcome by low, physiologic concentrations of ATRA (< 10 nM), consistent with the relatively loose association of the co-repressor complex with normal RARα, in contrast to the high, pharmacological ATRA concentrations (≥ 100 nM) required to accomplish this for PML-RARα (Figures 21–5A and B).[104–107] A recent study indicates that physiologic ATRA concentrations, acting through RARα, have a dual effect on normal hematopoiesis, delaying the differentiation of primitive cells, as well as stimulating terminal granulocyte/monocyte differentiation.[108] These observations suggest that PML-RARα has the potential to interfere with earlier stages of RARα-modulated hematopoietic differentiation,[95] although polymorphic genetic marker studies indicate that the PML-RARα transformed APL clone(s) does not involve multipotential HSCs as in other types of AML.[109]

The PML region of PML-RARα is primarily responsible for generating the high density of co-repressors recruited to RARE-containing gene promoters by forming multimeric/oligomeric complexes.[100,101,110,111] The base interaction is between the

A. Normal RARα

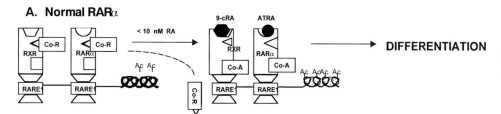

B. Fusion Gene Type 1 Homodimers: PML-RARα, NPM-RARα, NuMA-RARα

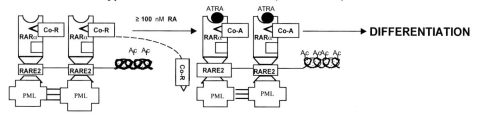

C. Fusion Gene Type 2 Homodimers: PLZF-RARα, possibly STAT5b-RARα

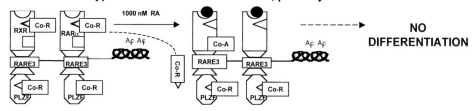

Figure 21–5. Differentiation response of normal RARα/RXR heterodimers and sensitive (Type 1) or insensitive (Type 2) *X-RARα* fusion gene homodimers following transcriptional activation by variable concentrations of ATRA.

PML coiled-coil regions of two PML-RARα molecules, which then recruit further PML-RARα molecules. Recombinant studies demonstrated that the coiled-coil region alone or other dimerization interfaces linked to RARα can serve equally well for recruiting co-repressors and effecting transcriptional silencing.[100,101] In fact, a common property of four alternative amino-terminal fusion partners of RARα (see below) is the formation of oligomeric complexes of the fusion genes (reviewed in Ref. 101).

A possible alternative explanation for PML-RARα specifying the APL phenotype is altered transcriptional regulation of PML-RARα vis-a-vis normal RARα on RA-regulated gene promoters (reviewed in Ref. 90). This possibility appears to have been excluded, however, since PML-RARα with a RARα-region mutation that inactivates RA transcriptional regulation was, nonetheless, leukemogenic.[90] In this study, normal RARα with the same mutation was not leukemogenic. Further studies are required to determine if the contribution of the PML component of the mutant PML-RAR can be accounted for by quantitative differences in co-repressor binding or whether RARα-independent PML-specified activities are involved (see PML section). Notably, the leukemias that developed in the mutant PML-RARα transgenic mice were more differentiated than those in wild-type PML-RARα-induced leukemias, suggesting that under natural conditions (i.e., in subpharmacological ATRA concentrations in vivo) PML-RARα transcriptional regulation may have a suppressive effect on terminal neutrophilic differentiation.[90] Thus, although excessive co-repressor density on RARE-regulated gene promoters appears to be the major driving force in PML-RARα-induced APL, altered RARα-independent PML-specific dysfunction could have a significant secondary role.

A final potential element in APL pathogenesis related to the t(15;17) is the reciprocal RARα-PML fusion protein. Clearly, it is not required, since it is present in only approximately 75 percent of APL cases, and, further, the presence, absence, or variable expression of RARα-PML is not associated with any significant phenotypic or clinical differences (reviewed in Ref. 112). The theoretical basis for a possible biological effect is the ligand-independent co-activator activity that resides in the amino-terminus of RARα (see RARα section). A cathepsin G-promoted *RARα-PML* transgene alone was not leukemogenic in mice, but transgenic mice expressing both PML-RARα and RARα-PML had an increased incidence than those expressing PML-RARα alone.[113] A caveat to this study is that an S-form *RARα-PML* transgene was utilized with an L-form PML-RARα transgene (duplicated PML exon 4 to 6 information). Overall, the data suggest that *RARα-PML* has, at best, a minor effect on APL pathogenesis, although further genetic studies are in progress.[34]

Role of PML-RARα in the Response to Treatment

Both ATRA and ATO, two agents that have selectively potent therapeutic effects in APL compared to other types of leukemia, have the common property of inducing proteolytic degradation of PML-RARα in NB4 APL cultured cells.[114,115] The simplest and most direct explanation for the therapeutic effect of these agents is that by removing the dominant-negative suppressor effect of PML-RARα, normal RARα and PML (produced by the nontranslocated gene loci) can re-establish physiological pathways leading to granulocyte terminal differentiation and/or apoptosis.[114,116,117] Although this may provide a partial explanation, the experimental details indicate that the molecular response is more complex, as well as different, for the two agents.

Following exposure to ATRA, initial reduction in the expression level of L-form PML-RARα in NB4 cells has been noted as early as 1 hour postexposure.[118] Much greater reduction occurs after 6 to 12 hours, accompanied by the appearance of a proteolytic fragment, called dPML-RARα, between 12 to 24 hours.[114,116,118,119] After a variable time (48 to >96 hours in different laboratories) continuing proteolysis results in the virtual disappearance of PML-RARα and dPML-RARα, and, subsequently, there is also a reduction in normal RARα protein, associated with changes in phosphorylation.[118,120] During this process, there is no change in PML-RARα mRNA levels, while the RARα transcript is unchanged or increased.[118,120] The degradation of PML-RARα has been demonstrated to involve activities of both the proteosome and caspase pathways, although neither is sufficient for complete degradation.[114,116,118,121] The primary site of caspase proteolysis resides in PML exon 6 of PML-RARα.[118,121] On the other hand, the degradation of PML-RARα by the proteosome primarily depends on RARα structure, since mutations in the DNA binding domain and certain areas of the LBD prevented this activity.[118] The latter activity may be the source of the dPML-RARα fragment, since size analysis of the amino-truncated protein suggests that it lacks only the PML RING + B box structures.[119] S-form PML-RARα lacks PML exon 6 containing the caspase-sensitive cut site, and, based on a study of transfected human erythroleukemia cells, is modestly resistant to ATRA-induced proteolysis.[122]

The relationship of PML-RARα proteolysis to the differentiation response of APL cells to ATRA is poorly understood. In contrast to the hypothesis that PML-RARα hydrolysis unblocks the dominant negative effect on normal RARα, several studies suggest that at least the initial response to ATRA involves direct, positive transcriptional regulation by intact PML-RARα. These studies include the demonstration that transfection of PML-RARα into non-APL myeloid leukemia cell lines increases the differentiation response to ATRA and depends on the functional integrity of the PML-RARα fusion protein,[64,123] that sensitivity to ATRA is partially restored by increasing PML-RARα protein expression in an NB4 subline in which resistance to ATRA is correlated with excess PML-RARα catabolism by a hyperactive proteosome,[124] and that inhibition of caspase activity is associated with increased sensitivity to ATRA-induced differentiation.[121] Studies of gene expression profiles in APL cells indicate that following ATRA exposure there is a succession of gene activation/deactivation events involving genes associated with a wide variety of biological activities.[125,126] However, the temporal and, more importantly, the cause-and-effect relationship of the coincident changes in PML-RARα and RARα to these gene modulation events remains to be determined.[118,119,126]

The role of PML-RARα in the selective response of APL to ATO is controversial. This is partly related to the complex, concentration-dependent biological effects of ATO on APL cells. A consensus, primarily based on experiments with NB4 cells, is that at relatively high concentrations ($\geq$ 1 μM), ATO produces predominant apoptosis, while at low concentrations ($\leq$ 0.5 μM), it has a predominant, albeit modest, differentiation-inducing effect.[115,127–129] In ATO-treated patients, signs of both apoptosis and partial differentiation of APL cells can be detected in the bone marrow after some delay (2 to 3 weeks).[127,130] Another aspect of the controversy is that in the 1 to 5 μM range, ATO can produce apoptosis in vitro in many other types of neoplastic hematopoietic cells, including non-APL myeloid leukemias, acute lymphocytic leukemias, and multiple myeloma.[131–133] Important elements in determining this PML-RARα-independent apoptotic response include the redox state of the leukemic cells and the status of cytokine-mediated signal transduction pathways affecting cell viability and growth.[129,134–136] Taking such factors into account, APL cells may not have much greater in vitro sensitivity to ATO-induced apoptosis than other types of leukemia cells.[119] Nevertheless, the much greater clinical efficacy of ATO in the treatment of APL compared to other forms of leukemia, implies selective biological effects related to APL-specific PML-RARα protein.

In several reports, the biological activity of ATO in NB4 cells, including ATRA-resistant sublines, as well as in fresh APL cells, has been linked to the degradation of PML-RARα.[115,117,119,128,137] This process differs from that following ATRA exposure in several respects: It occurs more rapidly (complete within 6 to 12 hours), it is not associated with the generation of a proteolytic fragment(s), and it is associated with the more rapid reformation of PML NBs that are fewer in number but larger in size. This process has been attributed to ATO-induced changes in the PML region of PML-RARα, since targeting of normal PML to NBs followed by degradation and accompanied by apoptosis was found in non-APL cells.[117] The critical role of PML in NB recruitment was subsequently shown to involve and, in fact, to require post-translational modification by SUMO-1 (see PML section).[76,120,137] However, in contrast to earlier studies, two studies found that recruitment of hypersumoylated PML to NB after ATO exposure produced protein stabilization rather than degradation.[137,138] Divergent results were observed related to PML-RARα: Although hypersumoylation of the fusion protein was noted following ATO exposure, in one report this was quickly followed by degradation,[137] while in the other, undegraded hypersumoylated PML-RARα was stoichiometrically recovered as heterogeneous, high molecular mass forms.[138] The reasons for these experimental variations is unclear but may be related to the performance of transfection assays in different cell types. Sumoylation has been determined to be a very dynamic, reversible process, and the presence of varying quantities of sumoylating or desumoylating enzymes in different target cell types might affect results.

The above account does not permit a definitive conclusion about how PML-RARα is related to the selective sensitivity of APL to ATO. This may be primarily passive by the degradative removal of the anti-apoptotic activity of PML-RARα,[123,129,139] relieving the sequestration of normal PML with pro-apoptotic

activity.[81,82] Similarly, the degradation of PML-RARα may foster APL cell terminal differentiation by removing the dominant-negative suppressive effect of PML-RARα on normal RARα, which, being relatively resistant to ATO-induced degradation, may then be able to respond to physiological concentrations of ATRA.[117,119,137,140] On the other hand, if sumoylation were to stabilize PML-RARα, there is the possibility that it could play a positive role in either the apoptotic or differentiative response of APL cells to ATO.[138]

Role of PML-RARα in Acquired Resistance to Treatment

Unfortunately, from the initial clinical studies of ATRA as a single agent in APL, there is no record of studies of PML-RARα at the time of relapse on continuous treatment. More recent studies of relapse cases after combined ATRA plus chemotherapy-induced remissions have, however, detected missense mutations in the LBD of the RARα region of PML-RARα.[37,141–144] In relapse cases from a Phase III study of previously untreated APL, which included a randomization arm to chemotherapy only versus three alternative arms with different sequences of combined ATRA/chemotherapy (INT0129),[145] PML-RARα mutations were only detected in cases that had received ATRA.[37] In a subsequent study of multiple-relapse cases after two or more remission induction regimens with ATRA-containing therapy, a higher incidence of PML-RARα missense mutations was found compared to first relapse cases (75 vs. 25 percent).[144] Analyses of these mutations indicate that they are inactivating in nature.[142,144,146] These results establish missense mutations of PML-RARα as a significant mechanism of clinical ATRA resistance that can develop after combined ATRA chemotherapy. However, since it occurs in only a minority of first-relapse cases, while APL cells from a majority of these cases already have demonstrable resistance to ATRA-induced differentiation in vitro,[37] further studies are required to assess the importance of these mutations relative to other possible cellular resistance mechanisms. In favor of a primary pathological role is the analogous location and effect of these mutations to naturally occurring mutations in the closely related thyroid hormone receptor, which have been demonstrated to be causative in the more-studied "resistance to thyroid hormone syndrome."[144,146,147] Possible alternative mechanisms of APL cellular and systemic ATRA resistance have been reviewed elsewhere.[148,149] An additional consideration is that alternative differentiation/cell death pathways utilizing alternative retinoid ligands in an RAR-independent manner likely are functional in APL cells.[150]

Alternative RARα Fusion Genes

Four other RARα fusion gene partners have been discovered in association with APL: *PLZF* (promyelocytic leukemia zinc finger)[29], *NPM* (NucleoPhosMin)[30], *NuMA* (nuclear mitotic apparatus)[31], and *STAT5b* (signal transduction and transcription factor 5b)[32] (Table 21–1 and Figure 21–6). These alternative fusion genes are rare, and, thus, have limited clinical application. They have, however, provided very useful information about molecular mechanisms involved in APL and about the effect of therapeutic agents on APL cells. In all cases, the coding exons for the B to F regions of RARα are fused to a 5′ segment of the alternative fusion partner. As for PML, a critical function of each alternative partner gene is that it provides an anchor for the formation of dimeric and multimeric X-RARα complexes, which, in turn, recruit excess amounts of co-repressor proteins that, as described for PML-RARα, can interfere with the regulation of ATRA-response genes.

PLZF-RARα APL

PLZF-RARα-positive APL is distinguished by the lack of response to ATRA (Table 21–1 and Figure 21–5C).[151,152] Detailed molecular studies have disclosed that the primary reason for the ATRA-insensitivity of PLZF-RARα is an amino-terminal structure of PLZF, called the POZ- (Poxvirus and Zinc finger) or BTB- (Broad Complex-tramtrac-Bric-a-brac) domain (Figure 21–6) (reviewed in Ref. 38). The POZ-domain can bind the same nuclear co-repressor protein as RARα but in a non-ATRA-dependent manner.[104–107] Thus, treatment of PLZF-RARα-positive APL cells may lead to the displacement of co-repressors from the RARα-region binding site and, perhaps, even the recruitment of some co-activator proteins, but it does not successfully displace co-repressors from the PLZF-region POZ-domain (Figure 21–5C). A number of other molecular factors may also contribute to the poor RA response of PLZF-RARα APL cells. These include the sequestration of RXR,[153] loss of association of PLZF-RARα with a carboxy-situated binding component, possibly PML (see below),[154,155] and the limited positive transactivation activity of PLZF-RARα on RARE-regulated genes.[38] Notably, the differentiation block

imposed on APL cells by PLZF-RARα can be at least partially overcome by treatment with HDAC inhibitors, which bypass the blocked RA receptor pathway.[105–107] This activity remains strictly ATRA dependent, implying that ATRA produces some essential change in PLZF-RARα/RARα that allows activation of specific ATRA-response genes, although no details about how this occurs have been forthcoming. Also of note, ATRA produces degradation of PLZF-RARα despite its inability to induce APL cell differentiation,[155,156] suggesting that other molecular factors contribute to ATRA insensitivity.

There is additional evidence that the cellular dysfunctions engendered by PLZF-RARα are not sufficient to account for the properties of PLZF-RARα-harboring APL cells. For example, the introduction of PLZF-RARα into normal progenitor bone marrow cells by retroviral infection was reported to produce continuous replication of primitive hematopoietic cells that can be induced to differentiate by a relatively low ATRA concentration (10^{-7} M).[103] Further, in transgenic mice (TM), PLZF-RARα induced a form of chronic myeloid leukemia, which was resistant to ATRA treatment in vivo.[104] These TM leukemic cells, however, remained sensitive to ATRA ex vivo. An additional factor in PLZF-RARα APL that has been postulated to account for such differences is the reciprocal t(11;17) product RARα-PML, which is present in all cases of PLZF-RARα-positive APL.[38,157] This postulate is strongly supported by data in the TM model in which double transformation with both PLZF-RARα and RARα-PLZF produced an acute leukemia phenotypically more similar to the human form with APL cells highly resistant to ATRA.[158]

Structural and functional considerations of PLZF provide additional support for the contribution of RARα-PLZF to PLZF-RARα APL. PLZF belongs to a gene family homologous to the Drosophila gene *Krüppel* that characteristically contains nine zinc fingers near the carboxy-terminus (Figure 21–6). These zinc fingers interact with a DNA response element as part of the essential function of PLZF as a transcription factor.[153,159] In PLZF-RARα only two (occasionally three) of the zinc fingers are included in the fusion gene (Figure 21–6). Thus, seven (or six) of the zinc fingers are incorporated into the reciprocal RARα-PLZF fusion gene resulting from the t(11;17).[29,152] Notably, RARα-PLZF was found to activate PLZF-regulated promoters, whereas PLZF suppresses transcription from these promoters.[159] By this transcriptional effect, PLZF can repress cell proliferation.[38] This occurs, at least partially, by inhibiting the cyclin *A2* gene that, in combination with CDK2, regulates progression from the G1 to the S phase of the cell cycle.[160] Furthermore, PLZF is most strongly expressed in progenitor hematopoietic cells and is down-regulated during spontaneous and ATRA-induced differentiation.[29,161] From these observations, it has been hypothesized that PLZF has an important function in preserving the reservoir of hematopoietic stem cells, and that, in this context, the opposing transcriptional activity of RARα-PLZF complements PLZF-RARα in leukemogenesis by augmenting cell proliferation and inhibiting the antiproliferative effect of ATRA associated with differentiation.[38]

Additionally, PLZF interacts via its first two zinc fingers with PML, and PML-RARα recruits PLZF to its microparticulate

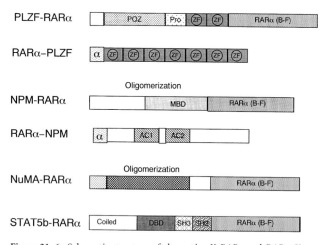

Figure 21–6. Schematic structure of alternative *X-RARα* and *RARα-X* fusion genes. Note that all 4 X-RARα fusion partners have protein interaction/oligomerization domains at the amino-terminus: PLZF, POZ domain; NPM, an alpha helical oligomerization domain, including a metal binding domain (MBD); NuMA, an extended alpha helical oligomerization domain; and STAT5b a coiled-coiled interaction domain. Other abbreviations: ZF, zinc finger; AC, acidic cluster; DBD, DNA binding domain. See text and references for additional information.

nuclear pattern in PML-RARα-positive APL.[138] Conversely, PLZF-RARα-positive APL, which has a distinct microparticulate pattern, does not recruit PML from coexisting NBs. This has suggested that interference with the normal function of PLZF could be an important component of PML-RARα APL as well as PLZF-RARα APL.[38,155]

NPM-RARα APL

Like PML and PLZF, NPM is a complex multifunctional nuclear matrix phosphoprotein (reviewed in Ref. 38). It is most prominently localized in the nucleolus, where it has a key role in ribonucleoprotein processing. Its expression level changes as a function of cell growth and differentiation, and it may have a regulatory role in these processes through binding to the transcription factor Yin Yang 1 and interferon response factor-1. The carboxy-situated NPM domains coding for these functions, as well as nuclear and nucleolar localizing sequences, are incorporated in the RARα-NPM fusion gene product resulting from the reciprocal t(5;17).[30,38] Since RARα-NPM mRNA is expressed in the cognate APL cells,[30,162] this raises the possibility that this reciprocal fusion gene product might have an active role in the leukemic process analogous to that described above for RARα-PLZF.

The *NPM-RARα* fusion gene incorporates the oligomerization domain of NPM, which is likely crucial for the formation of NPM-RARα homodimers or oligomers analogous to the function of other X-RARαs (Figure 21–6).[30,163] Likely, it is also related to the displacement of normal NPM from its nucleolar location to a disperse nuclear pattern observed for NPM-RARα in the associated APL cells.[162] Notably, NPM-RARα displaces PLZF but not PML from a normal nuclear distribution to a microparticulate pattern.[162] Since this same phenomenon has been noted in APL cells harboring PLZF-RARα and NuMa-RARα, this further implicates an essential role of PLZF rather than PML in the APL phenotype. NPM-RARα APL cells, however, behave very similarly to PML-RARα APL cells in their positive differentiation response to ATRA[164] and in the failure of the NPM moiety to bind co-repressors (Figure 21–5B).[163] NPM-RARα formed heterodimers with RXRs that bound to DNA up to tenfold more avidly than NPM-RARα homodimers, suggesting that RXR sequestration might have a particularly important role in this form of APL.[163] Otherwise, the RARα-region receptor function of NPM-RARα behaved very similarly to that of PML-RARα, including the heterogeneity of ATRA transcriptional activation of a variety of RARE-containing gene promoters and dominant-negative inhibition of normal RARα transcription in transfection/reporter assays, the retarded dissociation of co-repressor by ATRA, and the recruitment of co-activator by ATRA.[163] Interestingly, in these comparative studies of NPM-RARα with RARα and PML-RARα, it was noted that after ATRA exposure the two fusion genes bound co-activator with two- to threefold higher affinity than normal RARα even though the co-repressor protein was incompletely dissociated. As suggested, this observation could be importantly related to the apparent requirement of ATRA for HDAC inhibitor activity and for the restriction of such activity to RARE-containing gene promoters.[163]

NuMA-RARα and STAT5b-RARα APL

Only limited molecular information is available from the single case reports of these two APL-associated fusion genes.[31,32] In common with other X-RARα APLs, the amino-situated components of both NuMA and STAT5b fusion proteins contain oligomerization domains that promote protein-protein interactions (Figure 21–6). Although no data are available regarding the transcriptional function of these two fusion genes, they presumably alter the receptor function of the RARα receptor component similar to that of other X-RARα proteins. In neither case was the reciprocal RARα-X mRNA detectable in the patient's APL cells, and, in the STAT5b-RARα case, this was related to deletion of the STAT5b carboxy-encoding genomic information. Like cases of NPM-RARα APL, the NuMA-RARα case occurred in a pediatric patient,[31,165] whereas the STAT5b-RARα case occurred in an elderly adult.[32,166] The NuMa-RARα case was ATRA sensitive, whereas the STAT5b-RARα case was ATRA resistant (Table 21–1). This could be related to the markedly different nature of the NuMA and STAT5b proteins. NuMA is an abundant, ubiquitously expressed protein that is a structural component of the nuclear matrix during interphase and that plays an important role in nuclear reformation after mitosis (reviewed in Ref. 38). STAT5b is an essential component of the janus kinase (JAK)-STAT signaling pathway utilized by a diversity of extracellular cytokines (reviewed in Ref. 32). In its latent state STAT5b is a cytoplasmic protein but, following JAK-directed phosphorylation, the coiled-coil domain becomes accessible to form homo- or heterodimers with other STAT molecules, which move to the cell nucleus. The NuMA-RARα protein does not displace PML from NBs in APL cells, while this information was not reported for STAT5b-RARα. It was suggested that the ATRA-insensitivity of STAT5b-RARα might be due to sequestration of co-factors for RARα function by the STAT5b coiled-coil domain.[32] However, notably, the leukemic cells with an APL phenotype (M3 variant) formed only a minority of the bone marrow blasts,[32] raising the possibility that ATRA-insensitivity might have been due to leukemic chimerism with a predominant M1 phenotype. Clearly, more information about the function of both NuMA-RARα and STAT5b-RARα would be of interest.

MOLECULAR BIOLOGY OF APL IN CLINICAL TRIALS

PML-RARα/RARα-PML as Pretreatment Prognostic Markers

The differences in PML coding information in the L and S isoforms of PML-RARα are associated with some differences in retinoid binding characteristics,[167] nuclear localization,[57] and transactivation activity in recombinant RARE-reporter vector assays.[25–27,57] Additionally, APL cells with V-form PML-RARα were noted to have reduced in vitro sensitivity to ATRA-induced differentiation.[168] From such data, a logical hypothesis was that PML-RARα type might be associated with differences in clinical outcome and provide a pretreatment diagnostic marker. Early Phase II-type studies with relatively small numbers of patients, in fact, suggested that S-form APL cases had a poorer prognosis than those with L-form PML-RARα.[169–171] However, in an analysis of over 200 uniformly treated patients registered to the first North American intergroup Phase III APL trial (INT0129),[145] no differences were found between S- and L-form cases, if it was taken into account that the S-form is more frequently associated with an increased white blood cell count, increased circulating leukemic promyeloblasts, and the M3 variant phenotype, all of which are independently associated with poorer clinical outcome.[91] These conclusions have been confirmed in other large Phase III trials.[36,172,173] Since only 18 V-form cases were included in trial INT0129, there was insufficient statistical power to determine if the rather high 61 percent treatment failure rate and 50 percent death rate of these cases differed from that of S- and L-form cases.[92] In a separate study of the INT0129 cases, it was demonstrated that the reciprocal RARα-PML fusion gene, which is expressed in about 75 percent of cases and which has different subtypes, was related neither to clinical outcome nor to other pretreatment hematologic parameters.[112] It thus appears that the effectiveness of combined ATRA–chemotherapy overcomes the relatively minor biological differences related to PML-RARα/RARα-PML subtype. To date, no alternative molecular prognostic marker has been identified, but this would be of great value both to discriminate the minority of patients destined to relapse (~30 percent), who need more or alternative treatment, from the majority, some of whom may be overtreated on current regimens with the attendant risk of long-term drug-related adverse consequences.

PML-RARα as a Post-treatment Residual Disease Indicator

Since the *PML-RARα* fusion gene produces mRNA transcripts that are completely specific for clonally expanded APL cells, it can be used as a means for monitoring the presence of these cells as a subpopulation amongst a predominant population of normal cells. The method employed is reverse-transcriptase polymerase chain reaction (RT-PCR), which is rendered APL-specific by amplifying a segment of the mRNA transcript that crosses the fusion point between PML and RARα sequences in PML-RARα. This is a GC-rich region of the transcript with some redundancy, which has posed rather low limits on the level of sensitivity that can be routinely achieved with the amplification of this fusion gene segment in comparison to that of other leukemia-specific fusion gene transcripts (e.g., BCR-ABL in chronic myelogenous leukemia). In most studies that have been conducted in association with clinical trials, the level of sensitivity has been in the detection range of 1 APL cell in 10^3 to 10^4 (referred to as the reciprocal, 10^{-3}–10^{-4}) normal hematopoietic cells from bone marrow or peripheral blood.[174,175] However, by using appropriate primers and adjusting the amplification conditions, including the use of real-time RT-PCR, it has been possible to achieve sensitivity levels up to 10^{-6}.[91,176,177] As a monitoring tool, this brings the potential for detecting minimal residual disease (MRD) in APL patients after the induction of total clinical and hematological remission to a level up to 10,000-fold higher than the 10^{-2} level that can be achieved by cytologic bone marrow examination and cytogenetic techniques.

A summary of results from several laboratories of MRD tests at the 10^{-3}–10^{-4} sensitivity level after the completion of various types of induction/consolidation regimens with ATRA and chemotherapy showed that 36 of 122 patients were positive and 86 of 122 were negative for PML-RARα mRNA.[178] Within the first 6-month follow-up period, relapse occurred in 27 of the positive cases (75 percent) but in only 5 of the negative cases (6 percent)($p < .001$). This provided strong evidence that MRD in the 10- to 100-fold lower range than detectable by standard hematological techniques was associated with a very high probability of early relapse. Subsequently, evidence was provided that lower levels of MRD, either detected by using higher sensitivity assays for PML-RARα or for the reciprocal RARα-PML mRNA, can be detected in some APL cases during long-term remissions.[179–181] Based on this information, the 10^{-4} level RT-PCR assay at the postconsolidation therapy checkpoint in combination with serial monitoring in the postconsolidation follow-up period was adopted by the Italian group (GIMEMA) for further evaluation.[178] By this method only 4 percent of 324 cases were PML-RARα-positive post–consolidation therapy.[35] Since this was used as an indication for further, more intensive therapy, including allogeneic bone marrow transplant, the spontaneous relapse rate of these positive cases is not known. Using a similar assay, a British group similarly found that only 7 of 76 (9 percent) of postconsolidation patients were PML-RARα-positive.[36] Four of these cases (57 percent) relapsed without further treatment in a 3-year period. Of the majority PML-RARα-negative postconsolidation cases, 28 of 163 (17 percent)[35] and 19 of 69 (27 percent)[36] cases subsequently relapsed, respectively, with 18 and 36 months of follow-up. Although these relapse rates were significantly lower than those in patients with PML-RARα-positive assays after consolidation therapy, the 10^{-4} sensitivity assay failed to identify a numerically greater number of PML-RARα-negative cases who were destined to relapse. In the Italian study, 17 of 28 of these cases converted to a PML-RARα-positive assay status prior to clinical relapse by serial MRD monitoring in the follow-up postconsolidation period. Using a criterion of two successive positive assays,[31] such RT-PCR assay conversion patients were treated with salvage therapy prior to clinical relapse.[182] Twelve of these patients (86 percent) achieved a second clinical and molecular remission, and this has been sustained in 10 of 12 patients. Compared to a historical control group in which the same salvage therapy was not administered until the time of relapse, disease-free survival was significantly better (92 percent vs. 44 percent 2-year disease-free survival; $p < .05$).[182] This suggests that the administration of salvage therapy based on molecular relapse data may give superior outcome results compared to waiting for clinical relapse; however, confirmation of these results with larger case numbers and, ideally, under more controlled conditions, is required.

The results developed with the 10^{-4} sensitivity RT-PCR assay poses the obvious question of whether or not a more sensitive and quantitative assay would be more efficacious in predicting relapse, particularly in cases with less abundant MRD that are PML-RARα-negative. An additional major technical shortcoming of the widely used, manual RT-PCR assay is that sensitivity is determined by reference to an external standard with only a crude estimation of the sensitivity in the actual test samples by the ability to detect an alternative transcript using the same RNA preparation. In the alternative real-time RT-PCR procedure, it is possible to both achieve much higher sensitivity for the detection of PML-RARα and to accurately determine the sensitivity in each test assay by concurrently measuring the expression level of a constantly expressed housekeeping gene control.[177,183] Further, by normalizing the expression level of PML-RARα mRNA to that of the housekeeping gene control, an accurate quantitative value, adjusted for variations in the actual amount of transcribed RNA, can be determined for each sample, rather than simply assigning a positive or negative designation to each sample as in the manual assay.

In an initial application of the real-time RT-PCR procedure to clinical trial material (INT0129), the normalized expression level of PML-RARα mRNA was found to vary over a greater than 10^9-fold range in different APL cases from prior to therapy to the lowest detectable level of MRD during clinical remission.[184] Based on the internal, housekeeping gene control, the assays with a sensitivity of less than 10^{-4} were excluded from analysis, while evaluable samples varied in sensitivity from $\geq 10^{-4}$ to greater than 10^{-6}. This more sensitive assay yielded a much higher percentage of PML-RARα-positive cases at the post–consolidation therapy checkpoint (38 percent) than the established manual assay (4 to 9 percent). With ≥ 5 years of follow-up, 11 of 20 (55 percent) of these PML-RARα-positive cases relapsed. Conversely, 45 percent of PML-RARα-positive cases continued in remission despite the presence of MRD after consolidation therapy. This is consistent with previous reports of persistent positivity for PML-RARα mRNA[180,181] and other leukemia-specific fusion genes[185] in long-term remission cases. When the INT0129 cases were stratified based on the quantitative level of PML-RARα, it was found that cases with an expression level of $\geq 10^{-8}$ relative to the housekeeping gene control were at the greatest risk of relapse (hazard ratio = 2.82; $p = .037$). These data suggest that it will be possible to define a quantitative cut-off level under the highly standardizable conditions of real-time RT-PCR to identify a subgroup of patients with a sufficiently critical level of MRD at the postconsolidation checkpoint to support implementation of additional, more-intensive therapy. On the other hand, 34 percent of patients who were PML-RARα-negative after consolidation therapy at the higher level of sensitivity ($\geq 10^{-4}$ to 10^{-6}) subsequently relapsed (Gallagher et al., unpublished data). These data indicate that quantitative real-time assays at the postconsolidation checkpoint will not eliminate the need for continued MRD monitoring in the follow-up period to try to identify patients with either low-level PML-RARα-positive or PML-RARα-negative status who will subsequently relapse. The data also indicate that relapse can occur from very low or undetectable levels of MRD, and the follow-up period data from this study suggest that this may occur rather precipitously in some cases. Although this may be a limitation of the application of this methodology in a small fraction of APL cases, the data suggest that adequately spaced monitoring in the follow-up period may discriminate cases with a high versus low probability of relapse in the presence or absence of detectable MRD.

CLINICAL FEATURES

Virtually all of the features described under this heading in the previous chapter apply to APL also, unless specifically indicated otherwise. Only differences in the clinical aspects of APL compared with other FAB types will be discussed here.

APL accounts for about 10 percent of adults diagnosed with AML, and the incidence appears to be approximately constant with respect to age,[187] an observation not previously reported for any other neoplasm. The incidence in children is usually reported to be less,[188] although the incidence of APL in children diagnosed with AML and living in Italy seems to be about twice that of children living in Germany or the United States.[189] When Latinos develop AML they are significantly more likely to develop APL than another AML subtype,[190–192] and an investigation of the Eastern Cooperative Oncology Group databases for leukemia studies E2491 and E3489 reveals that more APL patients are Latinos than are other AML patients ($p = .005$).[193] There is no difference in incidence between the sexes[194] and the median age of patients with APL appears to be about 15 years younger than that of patients with other forms of AML (43 years vs. 59 years, $p < .00001$).[195] Curiously, increasing body mass index was strongly associated with a diagnosis of APL among patients with AML ($p = .0003$) in one study.[191] Some epidemiological studies have implicated exposure to electromagnetic fields[195] and radon exposure[194] in the etiology of APL.

The most significant clinical feature of APL is a hemorrhagic diathesis manifested by ecchymoses, intracranial hemorrhage, or orificial bleeding, some evidence of which is present at diagnosis in the majority of patients.[196,197] Sudden blindness due to sinus vein thrombosis has been reported[198] and other large vessel thromboses have been reported as well,[199] although hemorrhage is much more common than thrombosis in APL. The most frequently documented laboratory evidence of the bleeding diathesis includes hypofibrinogenemia, increased fibrin degradation products in the serum, a prolonged prothrombin time, and, of course, thrombocytopenia.[196,197,200] The potential for bleeding is exacerbated by cytotoxic chemotherapy.[197,201] The diagnosis and treatment of this important manifestation of APL is fully discussed below.

The diagnostic hallmark of APL is the balanced cytogenetic translocation (15;17)(q22;q11.2–12)[202] that has been discussed in detail in Chapter 16. However, approximately one-third of patients have additional cytogenetic abnormalities, most frequently trisomy 8.[203–205] The influence, if any, of additional cytogenetic abnormalities on the course of APL is presently unclear, but important data have recently appeared. In a study of 47 APL patients, 17 with additional cytogenetic aberrations, Schoch et al.[206] found no influence of such abnormalities on prognosis. Some of their patients were treated with ATRA, others with chemotherapy. In a larger study of 161 patients treated with chemotherapy alone, Slack et al.[207] found that secondary cytogenetic changes were associated with significantly longer complete remission and event-free survival. They concluded that additional cytogenetic changes do not impair prognosis of patients with APL. Pantic et al.[208] studied 43 APL patients treated with ATRA alone and found additional cytogenetic changes in 33 percent. The complete remission and early death rates were significantly different between those patients with and without additional abnormalities (76 vs. 36 percent, $p = .0148$; 24 vs. 64 percent, $p = .0141$, respectively). They concluded that patients treated with ATRA who have additional cytogenetic abnormalities have a more aggressive disease than those with only t(15;17). De Botton et al.[204] studied 292 patients treated with ATRA and chemotherapy. Additional cytogenetic abnormalities were present in 26 percent of cases and there was no difference in outcome between patients with and without additional cytogenetic aberrations. Others have reported similar results in patients treated with ATRA and anthracyclines together.[205]

The Eastern Cooperative Oncology Group and the Southwest Oncology Group[209] recently reported on 156 patients with APL, 29 percent of whom had additional cytogenetic changes and were significantly older than those without them. In patients with t(15;17) only, DFS ($p = .007$) and, perhaps, overall survival ($p = .057$) were longer when treated with ATRA alone than with chemotherapy alone. However, in patients with additional cytogenetic changes, no such differences were observed. They concluded that additonal cytogenetic changes may render patients less sensitive to ATRA, as suggested by the data of Pantic et al.[208] Consistent with these observations, Xu et al.[205] after a study of 284 patients with APL recently reported that relapse-free and overall survival are significantly poorer in patients with complex karyotypes compared with patients with only t(15;17).

Rarely, APL patients present with t(11;17)[210] as the only cytogenetic abnormality, and such patients are usually refractory to ATRA treatment. Jansen et al.[211] induced a complete molecular remission in such a patient with the combination of ATRA plus G-CSF after demonstrating the efficacy of that regimen in vitro. This approach deserves further study.

The immunophenotype of APL cells is unique among the myeloid leukemias, since they are characteristically HLA-DR–, CD34–, p-glycoprotein-negative, and CD33+ although the M3v subtype may be positive for either CD34, p-glycoprotein, or both (see Chapter 15). In addition, certain T-cell antigens, such as CD2, are frequently expressed by the FAB-M3v (microgranular variant) type of APL (see below).[197,212] Rarely, APL cells express CD56, a neural-cell adhesion molecule. Such patients appear to have a poor prognosis for complete response and response duration.[213]

The morphology of the leukemic cells in APL is unique and discussed in Chapter 14. Briefly, three morphological subtypes have been described. In the hypergranular type, which is the most common form of the disease, the cells appear to be abnormal promyelocytes with abundant cytoplasmic granulation that stains purple or pink with routine stains. Auer rods are common, usually multiple, and frequently appear in bundles (haystacks).[214] The nucleus is bilobed, folded or reniform, and suggestive of the nucleus of a monocyte.[197,214] In the M3v type,[215] which accounts for approximately 25 percent of all APL cases,[216,217] cytoplasmic granules are difficult to see with the light microscope and Auer rods are rare. Occasional typical M3 cells are seen in the peripheral blood and are much more

numerous in the bone marrow. The nucleus in M3v appears similar to that of M3. M3v cells are much more commonly CD2+ than are M3 cells.[212,216] The t(15;17) abnormality is always present.[212,216,218] A third, rare form of APL has been designated as the hyperbasophilic microgranular form,[214,219] or M3b[220] by some authors. The cytoplasmic granules are intensely basophilic and prominent cytoplasmic budding is often evident in M3b as well as is in M3v. The morphology of M3b[219] and M3v[200] cells is reminiscent of that of micromegakaryocytes. Cytogenetic and immunophenotypic characteristics are typical for APL, except that in M3b additional cytogenetic abnormalities such as 12p13,[221] which has been described in AML with basophilic differentiation, the M2-baso FAB type[214] may be found. Distinction between M2-baso and M3b can be accomplished by cytogenetic and histochemical studies[200] as well as by immunophenotyping (see Chapter 14). The cytoplasmic granules in M3b[220] and in some cases of M3 APL[222] stain metachromatically with toluidine blue. At least one M3b patient developed hyperhistaminemia after treatment, presumably secondary to release of histamine from the basophilic granules of killed cells.[223] Both M3v and M3b patients seem to have more severe bleeding at diagnosis than M3 patients[216,218,220] despite higher platelet counts,[217] and both are much more common in non-Whites[197,216–218,224–226] and in females.[188,212,216,218]

Histochemically, M3 cells are strongly peroxidase- and Sudan black-positive and, on occasion, strong α-naphthylacetate esterase activity sensitive to sodium fluoride may be demonstrated,[214,227–229] similar to that often observed in FAB-M4 or M5 AML. This finding is not observed in normal promyelocytes. M3v cells are less frequently peroxidase or esterase positive than M3 cells.[217] Complete remission with chemotherapy is less often achieved in M3v than in M3, but remission duration and survival of complete responders are similar in the three types of APL.[217]

Typically, patients with APL present with lower white blood cell counts than do other patients with AML and counts of less than 1000 cells/μl are common.[197,220] Patients with M3v generally present with higher white blood cell counts and leukocytosis is frequent.[188,212] Anemia is common at presentation[197] and may be severe in bleeding patients. Organomegaly, lymphadenopathy, and central nervous system (CNS) leukemia are rare in all forms of APL in the United States,[188,197] but may be more common in other countries for unknown reasons.[220,230] Skin infiltration in APL is rare[201,224] but extramedullary relapse after treatment with chemotherapy or ATRA may occur.[201,231]

Most patients with APL do not have an antecedent hematologic or neoplastic disease. However, secondary APL with the typical t(15;17) has been rarely reported after treatment for other neoplasms, including non-Hodgkin's lymphoma,[232] papillary thyroid carcinoma,[233] and breast cancer. In fact, most reported cases of secondary APL were patients previously treated for breast cancer.[234] This is curious because BRCA1 is located on chromosome 17 near the breakpoint involved in the formation of t(15;17). Secondary APL is more fully discussed in Chapter 22. In addition, karyotypically confirmed promyelocytic blast crisis of chronic myelogenous leukemia (CML) has been occasionally reported,[235–238] and promyelocytic blast crisis of CML with cytogenetic abnormalities other than t(15;17) but involving chromosome 17 has been documented.[239] Rarely, patients with APL relapse with a cytogenetically different AML or myelodysplasia following treatment of the original leukemia.[240–243] All such patients to date have received prior anthracycline therapy.

TREATMENT OF APL

APL patients must be prepared for induction therapy as described for other FAB types in Chapter 20 whenever possible, but time is of the essence in APL more so than in other FAB types in that the diagnosis of APL may be a medical emergency that requires immediate intervention.

Prior to induction therapy, the hemorrhagic diathesis, which clinically or subclinically is present in virtually every patient, must be brought under control. This is especially true if treatment is to be initiated with cytotoxic chemotherapy, since such therapy will exacerbate the bleeding problem, especially in patients with leukocytosis. Specific recommendations for controlling hemorrhage are given below.

Once bleeding has been controlled and the plasma fibrinogen concentration is stable above 100 mg/dl, induction chemotherapy may be initiated. If initial treatment is to be with ATRA, that therapy may be begun immediately upon the diagnosis of APL, usually without other efforts to reverse the hemorrhagic diathesis.[244,245]

Induction Chemotherapy

The response of APL to appropriate induction chemotherapy is unique among the acute leukemias. As initially pointed out by Daly et al.,[196] hematologic recovery from induction chemotherapy in at least 85 percent of patients is accompanied by an increase rather than a decrease of promyelocytes in the bone marrow, which spontaneously mature over several or more weeks in the vast majority of patients. Postinduction chemotherapy bone marrow specimens with increased promyelocytes have frequently been erroneously interpreted as indicative of chemotherapy failure and retreatment has led to the death of many patients. Only a small minority of patients who have survived induction chemotherapy will require a second course. The second course should be withheld in the face of a maturing marrow, especially if accompanied by resolution of the bleeding diathesis and a rising platelet count.

Specific Induction Chemotherapy

Anthracyclines have been the cornerstone of chemotherapy for APL since the landmark observation of Bernard et al. that daunorubicin induced a high percentage of complete responses in this leukemia[5] and that complete responses were of unusually long duration, compared with those in other FAB types. Since that discovery, the most common treatment reported for APL has been the standard daunorubicin and cytarabine regimen

originally described by Yates and colleagues[246] and recommended by them for all FAB types. There is, however, surprisingly little evidence that cytarabine is actually active as an induction agent in APL.[247–249] At least 350 patients with APL treated with daunorubicin alone can be gleaned from the literature, with an overall complete response rate greater than 70 percent.[196,219,230,250–255] This result compares very favorably with the 67 percent complete response rate published since 1990 for 537 patients induced with daunorubicin and cytarabine with or without other chemotherapy.[197,254–261] Larger than standard daunorubicin doses, (i.e., larger than 45 mg/m²/day, daily × 3) have been advocated by some in combination with other agents[249] as superior to standard therapy, but confirmation of that observation will require prospective, controlled trials that have not yet been reported. In one recent study, both high-dose cytarabine and larger than standard daunorubicin doses (60 mg/m², daily × 3) were used in conjunction with ATRA for induction therapy.[262] The results were excellent, but no better than those of many other studies in which standard doses of both agents were used. In a trial of idarubicin and cytarabine compared with historical controls treated with daunorubicin and cytarabine,[263] the former yielded significantly greater disease-free and overall survival compared with the latter. This result may be valid, since the same advantage for idarubicin and cytarabine over standard therapy has been reported for AML in general,[264,265] and others[266] have reported an unusually high complete response rate with idarubicin alone in APL.

ATRA Induction Therapy

Orally administered ATRA induces complete, albeit relatively brief remissions in the vast majority of patients with APL. Unfortunately, relapse usually occurs within months if no postremission therapy is given. Complete remission with ATRA is accomplished by induction of differentiation and maturation of leukemic cells, and not by a cytotoxic mechanism.[267] Isolated reports have suggested that 13-*cis*-retinoic acid may also induce complete remission in APL,[268] but the frequency with which that agent is effective appears to be far below that of ATRA.

Pharmacology of ATRA

ATRA pharmacology has been discussed earlier in this chapter, but certain aspects will be reiterated and expanded upon here. Orally administered ATRA, 45 mg/m², results in a peak plasma concentration in 1 to 2 hours[269] and is rapidly eliminated from humans, with a terminal half-life of approximately 45 minutes after an initial dose.[270,271] Following long-term daily administration of the agent, plasma concentrations of ATRA decrease significantly over time.[271,272] The only known metabolite is 4-oxo-all-*trans* retinoic acid, which is found in plasma and urine, but accounts for only about 10 percent of administered ATRA.[269] ATRA does not enter the cerebrospinal fluid.[269] The mean area under the curve for plasma drug concentration times time for ATRA varies considerably from patient to patient.[200] In contrast, oral 13-*cis*-retinoic acid administration is associated with a long terminal half-life of approximately 17 hours[273] and plasma concentrations do not deteriorate with long-term administration.[274] The pharmacokinetics of ATRA are consistent with a capacity-limited (saturable) elimination process in monkeys[275] and peak plasma concentrations following oral administration to patients at the usual 45 mg/m^2 dose approach the kM for that process.[275] It was suggested that relapse on continuous administration of ATRA may be due to the progressive reduction of plasma concentrations described above to levels below those that effect leukemic cell differentiation, since leukemic cells from patients who relapsed on ATRA usually continued to be sensitive to the agent in vitro at ATRA concentrations that resulted in differentiation initially.[271] However, it is now known that marked decreases in plasma concentration occur within days of initial administration, long before relapse occurs in virtually all patients.[269] Induction of accelerated catabolism by a cytochrome P-450–like enzyme system has been suggested as a mechanism for these peculiar aspects of ATRA catabolism.[269] This suggestion has merit, since inhibitors of oxidation by cytochrome P-450 enzymes such as ketoconazole, fluconazole,[276] and liarozole[277] significantly increase plasma concentrations of ATRA and decrease concentrations of the oxo-metabolite when administered with ATRA. However, it is not yet known whether the co-administration of these agents will prolong the clinical activity of ATRA. A recently offered possible alternative explanation for the accelerated ATRA catabolism observed after its continuous administration is that ATRA administration appears to result in increased levels of plasma lipid hydroperoxides, which accelerate the oxidative catabolism of ATRA in human microsomes in vitro.[278] And, of course, it is quite possible that ATRA blood levels correlate poorly with ATRA activity because they are irrelevant. Intracellular ATRA concentrations may be much more determinant of ATRA activity.[279]

Clinical Results with ATRA

Huang et al.[12] first reported on the clinical usefulness of ATRA in APL in 1988. They treated 16 previously untreated and 8 previously treated patients with oral ATRA, 45 to 100 mg/m^2/day. All patients achieved a hematologic and clinical complete remission without developing bone marrow hypoplasia. Eight patients experienced early relapses within 5 months while still receiving ATRA, but the others remained in remission at the time of their publication for as long as 11+ months. This landmark observation that ATRA could induce remissions in the vast majority of patients with APL presumably by differentiation induction attracted little attention initially in the United States, but French collaborators of the Chinese investigators immediately recognized the importance of this observation and initiated their own trials, which proved to be confirmatory.[280] Chen et al.[281] observed that patients who were induced into remission with ATRA and then maintained with conventional chemotherapy could usually be successfully reinduced into second remission with ATRA after relapse, whereas patients who received both ATRA and chemotherapy as postremission treatment usually could not be induced into second remission with ATRA alone. Based on these observations, they suggested that

ATRA should be discontinued upon the achievement of complete remission.

Subsequent studies by a large number of investigators demonstrated that, while the vast majority of patients with APL achieved complete remission with ATRA, some patients, perhaps 10 to 20 percent, did not respond well. In addition, a serious problem with ATRA therapy, termed the retinoic acid syndrome,[282,283] became evident. This occasionally fatal, rapidly developing pulmonary distress syndrome related to pulmonary leukostasis and usually associated with a rapidly rising peripheral white blood cell count consisting of predominantly maturing cells developed in as many as one-quarter of patients within days or weeks of starting ATRA therapy. This observation, and those of Chen et al.[281] discussed above, led Fenaux et al.[284] to combine ATRA induction therapy with postremission chemotherapy on a flexible schedule. Their plan was to begin treatment with ATRA and switch to anthracycline-based chemotherapy after remission was achieved unless a rising white blood cell count occurred with ATRA (then considered a dangerous harbinger of the ATRA syndrome), in which case chemotherapy was administered early along with ATRA until remission was documented, after which chemotherapy alone was continued. A complete response in 96 percent of patients was achieved with this approach in a pilot study of 26 patients and the actuarial disease-free survival of 87 percent at 18 months was significantly better than the 59 percent rate observed in their previous chemotherapy-alone study.[284] This pilot study led to a larger multi-institutional study in which 101 patients under the age of 65 years were randomized to receive daunorubicin and cytarabine alone, or those drugs preceded by ATRA treatment.[285] Both groups received two courses of daunorubicin and cytarabine as consolidation therapy after complete remission was achieved. The three-drug induction regimen yielded a 91 percent complete response rate and a 9 percent death during induction rate, compared with an 81 percent complete response rate and an 8 percent death during induction rate for the two-drug regimen. Neither of the differences is significant. However, the estimated 4-year event-free survival in the ATRA plus chemotherapy induction group was 63 percent compared with 17 percent in the chemotherapy-alone group, which is a highly statistically significantly different outcome. Overall survival at 4 years for the combined modality and chemotherapy-alone groups was 76 and 49 percent, respectively, which is also a highly significant difference.[286] Therefore, although the addition of ATRA to standard induction chemotherapy did not result in a significantly higher complete response rate or reduced early death rate, disease-free survival of complete responders was predicted to be greatly enhanced. In addition, ATRA therapy rapidly resolved the coagulopathy in most patients, an observation subsequently confirmed by others.[287] This approach to APL treatment was validated by Kanamaru et al.,[288] who obtained results virtually identical to those of Fenaux et al.[285] In that study,[288] approximately 89 percent of 110 patients achieved complete remission with ATRA alone or ATRA and early chemotherapy and 6.3 percent developed the retinoic acid syndrome. With a median follow-up of 21 months, 81 percent of the complete responders were projected to be disease-free at 23 months, which was significantly greater than the disease-free survival rate observed in a prior chemotherapy-alone study. Unlike the study reported by Fenaux et al.,[286] the Japanese study demonstrated a significantly lower early mortality rate than observed in the chemotherapy-alone historical control.[288] Burnett et al.[289] demonstrated that prolonged ATRA administration starting simultaneously with chemotherapy and continuing throughout the induction period until complete response is diagnosed gave superior results compared with a short course of ATRA prior to chemotherapy. Patients in the former group had a significantly higher complete response rate and fewer induction deaths, as well as superior survival at 4 years, compared with those treated with a short course of ATRA.

Recent data suggest that liposomal ATRA given intravenously may be more active than orally administered ATRA.[290,291] When administered every other day at a dose of 90 mg/m^2, blood levels are maintained, rather than observed to decline as is the case with orally administred ATRA. Results are similar with the two formulations, but liposomal ATRA is more likely to yield a molecular remission as determined by PCR than is oral ATRA.[290] It seems clear from the above that therapy with ATRA in conjunction with or followed by induction chemotherapy for AML is superior to either approach alone for initial treatment of APL. The combined approach may not reduce the early death rate associated with APL therapy, however. Furthermore, complete response rates with chemotherapy, ATRA, or a sequential combination of both appear to be quite similar. The major advantage for combined modality treatment with ATRA and chemotherapy is the significantly greater disease-free and overall survival achieved with the combination in virtually all controlled trials.[292] In addition, patients treated with ATRA prior to chemotherapy may have more rapid recovery of the peripheral granulocyte count compared with patients treated with chemotherapy alone.[293]

Questions remain about the optimal use of ATRA in induction with or without chemotherapy in APL, such as optimal ATRA dose,[294] and optimal schedule (should ATRA and chemotherapy be given sequentially or simultaneously?).[295] Furthermore, studies are necessary to determine if reducing ATRA catabolism[276,277] will translate into greater therapeutic efficacy for prolonged ATRA administration. Whether other retinoids[296] are superior to ATRA in the treatment of APL needs to be determined also. Observations on the potentiation of megakaryocytopoiesis by ATRA[128,129] and on the inhibition of marrow angiogenesis by ATRA,[299] require further study as does the recent observation that the tyrosine kinase inhibitor STI571 (Gleevec®)[300] may potentiate the activity of ATRA.

Retinoic Acid Toxicity

The most serious toxicity associated with ATRA therapy is the retinoic acid syndrome,[301] which occurs in 25 percent or more of patients treated with that agent alone.[302] Fever and respiratory distress with or without pulmonary infiltrates on chest x-ray are the hallmarks of the syndrome. Weight gain, pedal edema, pleural and pericardial effusion, and hypotension may also occur. These signs may suddenly appear within days or weeks of ATRA administration, and result in death in as many as one-third of patients without intervention. Autopsy reveals massive pulmonary infiltration with maturing myeloid cells. In most, but not all patients the syndrome is preceded by a rapidly rising white blood cell count. ATRA must be discontinued at once when the onset of the syndrome is first suspected and dexamethasone, 10 mg intravenously every 12 hours should be administered until complete clinical resolution of the syndrome is obtained, usually in several days. Most patients so treated will survive and, once the syndrome has resolved, ATRA therapy can usually be safely reinstituted.[302] The syndrome rarely, if ever, occurs in patients receiving ATRA as postremission therapy.[302]

The pathogenesis of the ATRA syndrome is not entirely known. Expression of CD13 by APL cells obtained at diagnosis significantly correlated with the development of the ATRA syndrome in one study,[282] which is interesting since expression of that antigen (aminopeptidase N) has previously been associated with a poor prognosis in AML[303] and with tumor invasive capacity in some human tumor cell lines.[304] It has been suggested that bestatin,[304] a specific inhibitor of aminopeptidase N, should be tested as a possible prophylactic agent against the ATRA syndrome.[282]

Other toxicities associated with ATRA therapy are usually mild and include dry mucous membranes, bone pain, headache, hypertriglyceridemia, hepatic enzyme elevation, and skin rash, which may rarely evolve into erythema nodosum.[305] Pseudotumor cerebri has been reported with some frequency in children and young adults.[201] Sweet syndrome[306,307] has rarely been reported after ATRA administration, presumably due to a mechanism similar to that of the ATRA syndrome. Occasionally, serious thrombotic episodes may occur with ATRA therapy even when thrombocytopenia is present.[308] ATRA-induced thrombocytosis has also been reported.[309,310]

Postremission Therapy in APL

Maintenance therapy has fallen into disfavor in general in AML although some studies strongly support its use.[311] Methotrexate and 6-mercaptopurine were reported to be particularly useful maintenance agents in APL years ago by Kantarjian et al.[312] The North American Intergroup Study[313,314] conclusively proved the value of postremission ATRA therapy. In that study, 350 patients were randomly assigned to induction therapy with standard doses of daunorubicin and cytarabine, or ATRA. Patients who achieved complete remission received another course of the successful induction regimen followed by a course of high-dose cytarabine plus standard-dose daunorubicin and were then randomized to maintenence therapy with ATRA, 45 mg/m^2 daily orally for a year, or observation. With a median follow-up of more than 6 years, the 5-year disease-free and overall survival rates for all patients induced with ATRA were substantially better than those for patients induced with chemotherapy (64 vs. 30 percent, $p < .0001$; 69 vs. 45 percent, $p = .0001$, respectively) although complete response rates were similar (73 vs. 70 percent, respectively). The 5-year disease-free survival was highest, 74 percent, in the subgroup of patients induced with

ATRA and maintained with ATRA, which compared favorably to the 55 percent disease-free survival rate observed in those induced with ATRA who did not receive postconsolidation ATRA. Furthermore, providing ATRA maintenance to chemotherapy-induced complete responders improved the disease-free survival rate threefold, compared with observation alone. These data strongly indicate the value of ATRA therapy during remission. Equally compelling data on the value of maintenance therapy in APL come from Fenaux et al.[315] In a study of 413 patients, those investigators randomized patients in complete remission to observation, intermittent ATRA (15 days every 3 months for 2 years), 6-mercaptopurine and methotrexate for 2 years, or that therapy plus intermittent ATRA for 2 years. The relapse rate at 2 years was 25 percent for patients who received no ATRA during remission and approximately half that for patients who did, 27 percent for patients who received no chemotherapy and less than half that for patients who did. The highest relapse rate (approximately 30 percent) was in the group that received no maintenance therapy at all. The study, therefore, confirms the value of maintenance therapy in APL with either ATRA or 6-mercaptopurine and methotrexate, and suggests that both are effective alone but not additive. Short-term consolidation therapy with nonanthracycline drugs does not appear to be of value, however.[316] Most investigators recommend that bone marrow transplantation be considered in relapse or second remission in APL, and not be routinely offered in first remission.

Treatment of Relapsed APL

Whether to begin treatment for relapsed APL early (molecular relapse, normal morphology) or late (morphologic relapse) is the subject of much study. No prospective, randomized trials have been reported, but an important historically controlled study suggests a major advantage for treatment of molecular relapse.[317]

The same approach to relapsed AML patients discussed in Chapter 20 applies to patients with relapsed APL. In addition, ATRA and ATRA followed by anthracycline-based chemotherapy are as successful in inducing remission in relapsed patients not previously exposed to ATRA as in previously untreated patients.[318] Patients who have relapsed after receiving ATRA more than a year earlier are likely to respond to retreatment with ATRA, especially liposomal ATRA given intravenously.[291]

9-cis-retinoic acid (9-cisRA) was brought to clinical trial because of its significant activity against APL cell lines in vitro, and the fact that it does not induce its own catabolism to the same degree that ATRA does.[319] In a study in which 9-cisRA was given as a daily oral dose of 30 to 230 mg/m^2, 4 of 12 relapsed APL patients (3 of whom previously received ATRA) achieved complete remission.[320] To date, 9-cisRA does not appear to have any clinical advantage over ATRA. Whether ATRA and 9-cisRA are significantly non-cross-resistant remains to be proven.

Am-80 is a synthetic retinoid that is a more active inducer of differentiation in HL-60 and NB4 cells than is ATRA.[321] Of 24 evaluable patients with relapsed APL after ATRA-induced complete remission treated with Am-80, 6 mg/m^2 orally daily, 58

percent achieved complete remission.[322] Four patients relapsed within 6 months, but long-term responses (>49 months) were also observed. The same group recently updated that study but, curiously, no new patients had been entered in the trial for approximately 3 years.[323]

Other strategies under investigation for the treatment of relapsed patients with APL include the addition of phenylbutyrate, an inhibitor of histone deacetylase to ATRA therapy,[324] and approaches that include allogeneic and autologous stem cell transplantation.[325] New approaches, such as radioimmunotherapy with ^{131}I-anti-CD33 monoclonal antibody as a means of eradicating MRD after induction of second complete clinical remission with ATRA are under investigation.[326]

The most important new development in the treatment of APL in recent years is the reappearance of arsenic trioxide (ATO) as a therapeutic agent. The drug had been used in the late 1800s in the treatment of chronic myelocytic leukemia, with some success.[327] Shen et al.[14,328] first discovered the activity of this agent in APL a few years ago. They administered ATO, 10 mg daily as a continuous intravenous infusion to ten patients who relapsed after ATRA induction and chemotherapy maintenance and achieved a clinical complete remission in 90 percent[14] without significant toxicity. Soignet et al.[329] subsequently treated 12 patients with APL who had relapsed after extensive prior therapy with ATO doses ranging from 0.06 to 0.2 mg/kg/day until bone marrow remission could be documented morphologically. Eleven patients achieved a complete remission after 12 to 39 days of treatment and a total dose of 160 to 515 mg. Eight of 11 patients who initially had a positive RT-PCR assay for the PML-RARα fusion transcript tested negative during remission. Three other patients remained PCR-positive and relapsed early. This is an important observation, since ATRA therapy alone rarely results in a negative test. Side effects were also reported to be minimal in this study.

The Shanghai group[330] more recently reported on 47 relapsed and 11 newly diagnosed patients with APL treated with ATO; 8 of the newly diagnosed patients (73 percent) and 40 of the relapsed patients (85 percent) achieved a complete remission, with a median disease-free survival of 17 months. Patients received a variety of postremission treatments and those that received postremission chemotherapy plus ATO had significantly longer remissions ($p = .01$). Unlike previous studies, however, serious ATO toxicity was reported in this study. Seven cases of significant hepatic toxicity, including two deaths, were observed, and in other recent studies other toxic effects of ATO such as renal failure, cardiac dysfunction, and chronic neuromuscular degeneration have been observed.[331] Furthermore, the frequent occurrence of leukocytosis (58 percent of patients in one study[332]) and the retinoic acid syndrome (31 percent of patients in the same study[332]) after treatment with ATO is now well documented.[332,333]

Of major concern is the recently reported serious cardiac toxicity associated with ATO treatment. Ohnishi et al.[334] treated eight patients with APL with commercially available ATO, 0.15 mg/kg administered as daily 2-hour infusions for a maximum of 60 days. Five patients achieved complete remission. Prolonged QT intervals were observed in all patients during treatment and ventricular premature contractions occurred during 75 percent of treatment courses. Four patients required treatment for unsustained ventricular tachycardia. Unnikrishnan et al.[335] reported three patients who developed torsades de pointes (a form of ventricular tachycardia that has been observed in arsenic poisoning) after treatment with ATO, 10 mg total daily dose as a continuous intravenous infusion. Westervelt et al.[336] reported three sudden deaths among ten patients with relapsed APL who received ATO, 0.1 mg/kg/day intravenously. One of the patients became asystolic and died while being continuously monitored with cardiac telemetry, and the cause of death was unknown in the other two. It seems clear from these reports that the cardiac toxicity of therapeutic doses of ATO is greater than previously appreciated, and that fact must be taken into account in future studies, which must include continuous cardiac monitoring.

In an effort to limit exposure to ATO, Kwong et al.[337] treated eight patients with relapsed APL with ATO, 10 mg daily dose intravenously until remission was achieved and then gave 3 monthly cycles of idarubicin. All patients were in molecular remission after idarubicin treatment, and six have remained so after a median follow-up of 13 months. Jing et al.[338] reported that the combination of ATO and ATRA may be more effective therapy than either drug alone. Others have reported that ATO plus GM-CSF may be more effective therapy than ATO alone.[339] The future of ATO in the treatment of APL may very well reside in combination regimens that limit ATO dose. The current U.S. and Canadian Intergroup study investigates the value of postremission ATO compared with other options.

APL and Pregnancy

The treatment of AML in pregnancy is discussed in general in Chapter 20. Although retinoids are well known to be teratogenic and their use during pregnancy has been advised against,[201] reports of successful use of ATRA during the second and third trimesters in at least 15 patients have appeared[340–343] and in no cases were teratogenic effects observed.[343] Since ATRA rapidly controls the coagulopathy associated with APL, it may be an attractive induction agent for the APL patient in late pregnancy. However, most women with APL treated with standard chemotherapy in late pregnancy have also survived and delivered normal children.[344]

Summary of Treatment Recommendations

Currently available information discussed above suggests that induction therapy for APL with ATRA, 45 mg/m² orally daily, followed by idarubicin, 12 mg/m² alone or with cytarabine, 100 mg/m² daily for 7 days as a continuous intravenous infusion beginning on the second or third day of ATRA treatment is optimal. After complete recovery from induction chemotherapy, at least one consolidation course of idarubicin alone, or combined with cytarabine at the same dose(s) on the same schedule(s) used during induction therapy should be given. ATRA should be continued through consolidation therapy and continued continuously or intermittently for at least 2 years, or

at least 3 months after molecular remission has been demonstrated by PCR performed on two consecutive monthly bone marrow specimens.

THE COAGULOPATHY ASSOCIATED WITH APL

A major feature distinguishing APL from all other subtypes of AML is the very frequent association with a severe life-threatening coagulopathy. The pathogenesis of the coagulopathy is complex and includes disseminated intravascular coagulation (DIC), fibrinolysis, and proteolysis.[345,346] Historically, approximately 10 to 30 percent of patients with APL die of early fatal hemorrhage, often intracerebral hemorrhage.[347–353] This is particularly problematic since several studies have suggested that patients with APL have a relatively favorable prognosis compared to other subtypes of AML once they survive initial induction therapy.[354,355]

In every study to date, successful remission induction with ATRA has been accompanied by rapid resolution of clinical bleeding and generally, of biochemical evidence of the coagulopathy, although elevated plasma levels of sensitive markers of clotting activation may persist.[356–359] Studies of arsenic trioxide in patients with relapsed and refractory APL also show rapid correction of the clotting abnormality.[360,361]

Pathophysiology of the Coagulopathy in APL

Approximately 70 to 80 percent of patients with either previously untreated APL or relapsed disease have either laboratory or clinical evidence of this life-threatening hemorrhagic syndrome.[347–352,361–364] The characteristic pattern of laboratory abnormalities includes thrombocytopenia; prolongations of the prothrombin time (PT), partial thromboplastin time (PTT), and thrombin times; increased levels of fibrin degradation products; and hypofibrinogenemia.[365–368] These findings are consistent with both DIC and hyperfibrinolysis or both. However, patients with APL can have potentially fatal bleeding even in the absence of abnormal PT and PTT. Furthermore, levels of several anticoagulant proteins such as antithrombin III and protein C, often low in the setting of DIC, are usually not decreased in patients with APL.[369] Platelet survival in these patients is normal, reflecting a more complex process than DIC alone.[370]

Several procoagulant mediators have been described in patients with APL (Table 21–2). Tissue factor (TF) is the major procoagulant that initiates blood coagulation in vivo and is the membrane protein reception for factor VII.[371] The resulting factor VIIa activities factors IX and X, which leads to thrombin generation and fibrin formation. The TF gene is expressed in cells from patients with APL.[372–374] A second procoagulant mediator is cancer procoagulant (CP), a protein with properties of a cysteine proteinase enzyme that directly initiates coagulation by activating factor in the absence of factor VII.[375,376] Cells from patient with APL express particularly high levels of CP, which become undetectable when patients are in complete remission.[377] Cytokines such as interleukin-1 (IL-1), tumor

Table 21–2. Procoagulant, Profibrinolytic, and Anticoagulant Mediators in APL

Procoagulant mediators
  Tissue factor
  Cancer procoagulant
  Interleukin-1
  Other cytokines such as TNF and VPF interferon-γ
Profibrinolytic mediators
  Tissue-type plasminogen activator
  Urokinase-type plasminogen activator
  Plasminogen activator inhibitors I and II
Anticoagulant mediators
  Annexin-VIII
  Annexin-II
  Von Willebrand factor

necrosis factor (TNF), and vascular permeability factor (VPF) are indirect procoagulants by initiating coagulation through the induction of TF in endothelial cells and monocytes.[378–381] Interleukin-1 secreted by leukemic cells may induce DIC.[382,383] Cytokines can generate plasminogen activator inhibitors that inhibit vessel wall fibrinolytic activity promoting coagulation.[384,385] Interferon-γ and VPF-like mediators can also induce endothelial cell procoagulant activity.[386,387]

Excessive fibrinolysis is also an important factor in coagulopathy in APL.[388,389] Plasminogen and alpha-2-plasmin inhibitor levels are reduced in patients with APL.[390,391] Furthermore, leukemic promyelocytes release plasminogen activators that cleave plasminogen and initiate fibrinolysis. Circulating tissue-type plasminogen activator can be found in the plasma of some patients with APL.[392] Decreased levels of circulating plasminogen-activator inhibitor type 1 (PAI-1) have been reported in some patients.[392] APL cells contain elastases that inactivate alpha-2-plasmin inhibitor.[393] Annexin-VIII is one of a group of naturally occurring proteins that bind phospholipids and have both anticoagulant and phospholipase-A_2 inhibitory properties.[394] Annexin-VIII gene is expressed in a greater degree in cells from patients with APL compared to cells from patients with other subtypes of AML.[395] Annexin-VIII is highly expressed in the APL cell line NB4 and is significantly reduced after exposure to ATRA. Annexin-II is a cell surface receptor for plasminogen and its activator, tissue plasminogen activator (t-PA), which functions as a t-PA cofactor.[396] Annexin-II is expressed in high levels on leukemic promyelocytes compared to leukemic cells from patients with other subtypes of AML.[397] Recent studies suggest that plasmin- and elastase-induced degradation of von Willebrand factor contributes to the hemostatic defect in APL.[398]

Influence of ATRA on Coagulation Parameters

A number of studies have examined the specific changes in coagulation parameters before and after ATRA. Dombret and colleagues studied a small number of patients with APL treated with ATRA and reported that both DIC and proteolysis improved within 14 days.[356] Although proteolysis appeared to completely resolve, low-grade procoagulant activity persisted, even after patients achieved complete response, particularly in patients who developed hyperleukocytosis during treatment. Markers of thrombin generation such as thrombin-antithrombin complex (TAT), prothrombin fragment 1+2 (F1+2), and D-dimer did not completely normalize. These findings reflect a dissociation between the resolution of proteolysis (fibrinogenolysis) and DIC and may explain sporadic reports of thromboembolic events during treatment with ATRA, particularly when ATRA is combined with antifibrinolytic therapy as prophylaxis against bleeding.[399–401] The down-regulation of the thrombomodulin gene and up-regulation of the TF gene, both induced by tumor necrosis factor-α, in human endothelial cells can be blocked by ATRA potentially counteracting the procoagulant effect of TF.[402] Profound inhibitory effect on the expression of the TF gene with ATRA in NB4 cells has also been reported.[403] Falanga and colleagues[404] have shown reduction in a procoagulant activity of leukemic promyelocytic blasts cells, both TF-like and factor-VII-independent (CP-like), during and after ATRA exposure. In addition, plasma markers of coagulation including D-dimer, TAT, and F1+2, which are elevated prior to ATRA exposure in patients with APL, decreased to normal (D-dimer) or near normal (TAT and F1+2) levels after exposure to ATRA. These findings are consistent with the observations of Dombret and colleagues and reflect the persistent hypercoagulable state.[356] Markers of fibrinolysis such as plasma levels of t-PA activity appear to be unchanged and elastase remains elevated in patients treated with ATRA alone, although elastase levels decreased in patients treated with both chemotherapy and ATRA. De Stefano and colleagues also showed excessive procoagulant activity in leukemic promyelocytic blast cells prior to exposure to ATRA, represented mostly by TF, which in culture was significantly reduced after exposure to ATRA.[404,405] A significant decrease was observed after only 3 days of incubation with ATRA. In contrast, both elastase and tissue plasminogen activator antigen concentration were lower than in control neutrophils, both prior to and with exposure to ATRA. No appreciable amounts of urokinase-type plasminogen activator antigen were detected in leukemic promyelocyte cultures prior to ATRA exposure, but after 9 days of culture with ATRA, increases in urokinase-type plasminogen activator levels were observed. Several studies have demonstrated that retinoic acid stimulates tissue-type plasminogen activator in human endothelial cells, which can initiate the fibrinolytic cascade and counterbalance the effects of other procoagulant mediators.[406,407] Falanga and co-investigators recently reported that treatment of NB4 cells with ATRA resulted in a significantly decreased expression of CP.[408] In addition, a variety of markers of procoagulation decrease rapidly including D-dimer, TAT, and F1+2.

Falanga and colleagues reported that markers of procoagulation decreased rapidly even when ATRA was given concurrently with chemotherapy that in the past has exacerbated clinical bleeding. Tallman and colleagues[409] found that the levels of markers of activation of coagulation including D-dimer, F1+2, TAT, and fibrinopeptide A were markedly elevated prior to exposure to chemotherapy or ATRA, but declined markedly following either treatment strategy. The plasma levels of D-dimer, F1+2, TAT, and fibrinopeptide-A generally decreased more rapidly among patients treated with ATRA compared to chemotherapy. The D-dimer and F1+2 declined to normal levels among ATRA-treated patients whereas only the F1+2 was reduced to normal levels among chemotherapy-treated patients. However, the D-dimer, TAT, and fibrinopeptide A levels remain significantly elevated, well above the upper limit of normal among the chemotherapy-treated patients. Watanabe and colleagues observed that plasma levels of D-dimer, TAT, and plasmin-α_2 plasmin inhibitor complex were elevated prior to treatment and decreased to normal or near normal levels within 7 days of treatment.[357] However, later in the course during ATRA re-elevation in several molecular markers occurred in some patients attributable to cytotoxic chemotherapy and infection in most patients. These studies support the unifying hypothesis that as ATRA induces terminal differentiation of leukemic promyelocytes, markers of both procoagulant activity and fibrinolytic activity decrease with evidence of persistent mild DIC.

Effect of the Improvement in the Bleeding Diathesis on Outcome of APL Patients Treated With ATRA

Nonrandomized and randomized prospective trials have compared the outcome of patients treated with ATRA alone or with chemotherapy.[410–417] In the aggregate experience fatal hemorrhage accounts for 30 to 60 percent of early death in studies evaluating contemporary strategies that include ATRA.[410–417] The first prospective randomized trial (APL91) was designed to compare chemotherapy alone to ATRA followed by chemotherapy in previously untreated patients.[410] The event-free survival at 12 months was significantly better among 54 patients treated with ATRA then among 47 patients receiving daunorubicin and cytosine arabinoside induction therapy (79 vs. 50 percent of patients, respectively). Mortality from induction therapy was not different, but there was a significant difference in the relapse rate. It is important to know that 71 percent of patients randomized to ATRA alone actually received chemotherapy because of a rapidly rising white blood cell count. No difference in complete response rate or early death rate was observed. The majority of early deaths were attributable to hemorrhage. The European APL group conducted a successor trial in which patients were randomized to either sequential ATRA followed by chemotherapy or concurrent ATRA plus chemotherapy. Once again, there was no difference seen in the complete response rate or early death rate and approximately 30 percent of early deaths were due to bleeding.[411] In the North American Intergroup trial, ATRA was compared to standard chemotherapy (daunorubicin plus cytarabine) for induction.[412] There was no difference between the two arms in treatment-related mortality during induction with 24 deaths (14 percent) in the chemotherapy group compared to 19 (11 percent) in the ATRA group ($p = .41$). The incidence of severe hemorrhage was the same in the two groups, although there were fewer infections among patients treated with ATRA than among those receiving chemotherapy; more patients treated with ATRA had serious pulmonary toxic effects than did patients treated with chemotherapy. The Medical Research Council (MRC) in the

United Kingdom conducted a prospective comparative trial in which patients were randomized to a short 5-day preinduction course of ATRA followed by chemotherapy versus an extended course of ATRA administered concurrently with chemotherapy.[413] In this trial, the complete response rate was superior among patients receiving the extended ATRA exposure (ATRA given concurrently with chemotherapy) compared to those receiving the 5-day exposure to ATRA prior to chemotherapy (87 vs. 69 percent, $p = .001$). This benefit was attributable both to a reduction in the early death rate (12 vs. 23 percent, $p = .02$), as well as a reduction in the incidence of resistant disease (2 vs. 9 percent, $p = .03$). In this trial, the 28 percent of patients who presented with a white blood cell count greater than 10,000/μL had an inferior outcome irrespective of the ATRA schedule. Updated results from the AIDA trial conducted by the Italian GIMEMA cooperative group shows that although the early mortality rate is only 7 percent, 59 percent of patients dying early did so because of hemorrhage.[414] In the study conducted by the Japan Adult Leukemia Study Group (JALSG), all patients received ATRA (plus chemotherapy for leukocytosis) until the achievement of complete remission.[415] In this study, 21 patients (11 percent) developed organ bleeding (14 in the central nervous system, 3 in the lung, 2 in the gastrointestinal tract, and 2 in both the central nervous system and gastrointestinal tract), and in fact, 16 of the 196 patients (8 percent) had fatal bleeding. Among the 16 patients with fatal bleeding, 3 had received ATRA alone, 5 ATRA plus additional chemotherapy because of leukocytosis, 7 seven received ATRA and concurrent chemotherapy, and 1 received ATRA plus both concurrent and later chemotherapy. Of the 14 deaths due to hemorrhage 3 died within 48 hours after the start of treatment and another 6 patients died within 6 days. The Spanish PETHEMA group also found that almost one-third of early deaths were due to bleeding in patients treated with ATRA plus idarubicin.[416] The GIMEMA group has retrospectively compared the early death rate from hemorrhage among patients treated with chemotherapy alone (randomized to idarubicin alone or idarubicin with cytarabine) or ATRA plus idarubicin.[417] There was a statistically significant decrease in the number of deaths from all causes within 10 days among patients receiving ATRA (12 [5 percent] vs. 20 [8 percent], $p = .0006$). Furthermore, a similar difference was observed in the number of patients dying early of hemorrhage (8 [1 percent] vs. 15 [6 percent], $p < .0001$). Finally, the numbers of platelet and red blood cell (RBC) transfusions were statistically less among patients receiving ATRA (platelets 22.2 ± 21.3 vs. 39.7 ± 27.3, $p < .0001$). However, among patients dying of hemorrhage within 10 days, 14 of the 15 (93 percent) patients treated with chemotherapy alone sustained a cerebral hemorrhage as did 7 of the 8 (88 percent) patients treated with ATRA plus idarubicin. Although deaths attributable to hemorrhage were reduced with ATRA, cerebral hemorrhage remained a major cause of mortality. The GIMEMA Cooperative group has retrospectively examined the impact of ATRA on bleeding by comparing the impact of ATRA on the coagulopathy and hemorrhagic deaths among patients treated with idarubicin alone or idarubicin plus ATRA. Induction deaths within 10 days among 499 patients treated with ATRA plus idarubicin occurred with an incidence of 3.8 percent compared to 7.3 percent among 123 patients treated with idarubicin alone. However, induction deaths due to hemorrhage occurred in 3 and 4 percent, respectively.

Effect of Arsenic Trioxide on Coagulopathy

Arsenic trioxide induces rapid loss of membrane procoagulant activity and TF mRNA.[418] Preliminary studies have shown that arsenic trioxide also has a beneficial effect on the coagulopathy in APL.[360,361] Since the mechanism of induction of remission of arsenic trioxide appears to be different from that of ATRA, new opportunities are present to explore the pathogenesis of the coagulopathy and the pathophysiologic basis for its improvement.

Excellent reviews of the diagnosis and management of patients with APL have recently appeared.[419–421]

REFERENCES

1. Hillestad L: Acute promyelocytic leukemia. Acta Med Scand 159:189, 1957.
2. Stavem P: Acute hypergranular promyelocytic leukemia. Priority of discovery. Scand J Haematol 20:287, 1978.
3. Caen J, Mathe G, Xuan Chat L, Bernard J: Etude de la fibrinolyse au cours des hémopathies malignes. In Transactions of the 6th Congress of the European Society of Hématology, p. 502. Karger, Based, 1957.
4. Bernard J, Mathe G, Boulay J, Ceoura B: La leucose aiguë à promyélocytes. Etude portant sur 20 observations. J Suisse Med 23:604, 1959.
5. Bernard J, Weil M, Boiron M et al: Acute promyelocytic leukemia. Results of treatment with daunorubicin. Blood 41:489, 1973.
6. Golomb HM, Rowley JD, Vardiman J et al: Partial deletion of long arm of chromosome 7. A specific abnormality in acute promyelocytic leukemia? Arch Intern Med 136:825, 1976.
7. Rowley J, Golomb H, Dougherty C: 15/17 translocation: A consistent chromosomal change in acute promyelocytic leukemia. Lancet 1:549, 1977.
8. Larson RA, Kondo K, Vardiman JW et al: Evidence for a 15;17 translocation in every patient with acute promyelocytic leukemia. Am J Med 76:827, 1984.
9. Kantarjian HM, Keating MJ, Walters RS et al: Acute promyelocytic leukemia. M.D. Anderson Hospital experience. Am J Med 80:789, 1986.
10. Stone RM, Maguire M, Goldberg MA et al: Complete remission in acute promyelocytic leukemia despite persistence of abnormal bone marrow promyelocytes during induction therapy: Experience in 34 patients. Blood 71:690, 1988.
11. Breitman T, Selonick S, Collins S: Induction of differentiation of the human promyelocytic leukemic cell line (HL-60) by retinoic acid. Proc Natl Acad Sci USA 77:2936, 1980.
12. Huang M-E, Ye Y-C, Chen S-R et al: Use of all-trans retinoic acid in the treatment of acute promyelocytic leukemia. Blood 72:567, 1988.
13. Fenaux P, Chastang C, Degos L: Treatment of newly diagnosed acute promyelocytic leukemia (APL) by a combination of all-trans retinoic acid (ATRA) and chemotherapy. Leukemia 8 (Suppl. 2):S42, 1994.
14. Chen GQ, Shi XG, Tang W et al: Use of arsenic trioxide (As2O3) in the treatment of acute promyelocytic leukemia (APL): I. As2O3 exerts dose-dependent dual effects on APL cells. Blood 89:3345, 1997.
15. Wiernik PH: Acute promyelocytic leukemia: Another pseudoleukemia? Blood 76:1675, 1990.
16. Degos L: Is acute promyelocytic leukemia a curable disease? Treatment strategy for a long-term survival. Leukemia 8:S6, 1994.
17. Bernard J: History of promyelocytic leukemia. Leukemia 8(Suppl. 2):S1, 1994.
18. Rowley J, Golomb H, Dougherty C: 15/17 translocation: A consistent chromosomal change in acute promyelocytic leukemia. Lancet 1:549, 1977.
19. Breitman TR, Collins SJ, Keene BR: Terminal differentiation of human promyelocytic leukemic cells in primary culture in response to retinoic acid. Blood 57:1000, 1981.
20. Huang M-E, Ye Y-C, Chen S-R et al: Use of all-trans retinoic acid in the treatment of acute promyelocytic leukemia. Blood 72:567, 1988.
21. Borrow J, Goddard AD, Sheer D, Solomon E: Molecular analysis of acute promyelocytic leukemia breakpoint cluster region on chromosome 17. Science 249:1577, 1990.
22. de The H, Chomienne C, Lanotte M et al: The t(15;17) translocation of acute promyelocytic leukaemia fuses the retinoic acid receptor α gene to a novel transcribed locus. Nature 347:558, 1990.
23. Longo L, Pandolfi P, Biondi A et al: Rearrangements and aberrant expression of the retinoic acid receptor α gene in acute promyelocytic leukemias. J Exp Med 172:1571, 1990.
24. Petkovich M, Brand NJ, Krust A, Chambon P: A human retinoic acid receptor which belongs to the family of nuclear receptors. Nature 330:444, 1987.
25. Giguere V, Segui P, Evans RM: Identification of a receptor for the morphogen retinoic acid. Nature 330:624, 1987.
26. de The H, Lavau C, Marchio A et al: The PML-RARα fusion mRNA generated by the t(15;17) translocation in acute promyelocytic leukemia encodes a functionally altered RAR. Cell 66:675, 1991.
27. Kakizuka A, Miller WH Jr, Umesono K et al: Chromosomal translocation t(15;17) in human acute promyelocytic leukemia fuses RARα with a novel putative transcription factor, PML. Cell 66:663, 1991.
28. Pandolfi P, Grignani F, Alcalay M et al: Structure and origin of the acute promyelocytic leukemia myl/RARα cDNA and characterization of its retinoid-binding and transactivation properties. Oncogene 6:1285, 1991.
29. Chen Z, Brand N, Chen A et al: Fusion between a novel Kruppel-like zinc finger gene and the retinoic acid receptor-α locus due to a variant t(11;17) translocation associated with acute promyelocytic leukemia. EMBO J 12:1161, 1993.
30. Redner RL, Rush EA, Faas S et al: The t(5;17) variant of acute promyelocytic leukemia expresses a nucleophosmin-retinoic acid receptor form. Blood 87:882, 1996.
31. Wells RA, Catzavelos C, Kamel-Reid S: Fusion of retinoic acid receptor α to NuMA, the nuclear mitotic apparatus protein by a variant translocation in acute promyelocytic leukemia. Nat Genet 17:109, 1997.
32. Arnould C, Philippe C, Bourdon V et al: The signal transducer and activator of transcription STAT5b gene is a new partner of retinoic acid receptor α in acute promyelocytic-like leukaemia. Hum Mol Genet 8:1741, 1999.
33. Lanotte M, Martin-Thouvenin B, Najman S et al: NB4, a maturation inducible cell line with t(15;17) marker isolated from a human acute promyelocytic leukemia (M3). Blood 77:1080, 1991.

34. He LZ, Merghoub T, Pandolfi PP: In vivo analysis of the molecular pathogenesis of acute promyelocytic leukemia in the mouse and its therapeutic implications. Oncogene 18:5278, 1999.

35. Diverio D, Rossi V, Avvisati G et al: Early detection of relapse by prospective reverse transcriptase-polymerase chain reaction analysis of the PML/RARα fusion gene in patient with acute promyelocytic leukemia enrolled in the GIMEMA-AIEOP multicenter "AIDA" trial. Blood 92:784, 1998.

36. Burnett AK, Grimwade D, Solomon F et al: Presenting white blood cell count and kinetics of molecular remission predict prognosis in acute promyelocytic leukemia treated with all-trans retinoic acid: Result of the randomized MRC trial. Blood 93:4131, 1999.

37. Ding W, Li YP, Nobile LM et al: Leukemic cellular retinoic acid resistance and missense mutations in the PML-RARα fusion gene after relapse of acute promyelocytic leukemia from treatment with all-trans retinoic acid and intensive chemotherapy. Blood 92:1172, 1998.

38. Melnick A, Licht JD: Deconstructing a disease: RARα, its fusion partners, and their roles in the pathogenesis of acute promyelocytic leukemia. Blood 93:3167, 1999.

39. Slack JL, Gallagher RE: The molecular biology of acute promyelocytic leukemia. Cancer Treat Res 99:75, 1999.

40. Chambon P: A decade of molecular biology of retinoic acid receptors. FASEB J 10:940, 1996.

41. Kurokawa R, Soderstrom M, Horlein A et al: Polarity-specific activities of retinoic acid receptors determined by a co-repressor. Nature 377:451, 1995.

42. Rochette-Egly C, Adam S, Rossignol M et al: Stimulation of RARα activation function AF-1 through binding to the general transcription factor TFIIH and phosphorylation by CDK7. Cell 90:97, 1997.

43. Renaud J-P, Rochel N, Ruff M et al: Crystal structure of the RAR-γ ligand binding domain bound to all-trans retinoic acid. Nature 378:681, 1995.

44. vom Baur E, Zechel C, Heery D et al: Differential ligand-dependent interactions between the AF-2 activating domain of nuclear receptors and the putative transcriptional intermediary factors mSUG and TIF1. EMBO J 15:110, 1996.

45. Collingwood TN, Urnov FD, Wolffe AP: Nuclear receptors: Coactivators, corepressors and chromatin remodeling in the control of transcription. J Mol Endocrinol 23:255, 1999.

46. McKenna NJ, Lanz RB, O'Malley BW: Nuclear receptor coregulators: Cellular and molecular biology. Endocrine Rev 20:321, 1999.

47. Perissi V, Staszewski LM, McInerney EM et al: Molecular determinants of nuclear receptor-corepressor interaction. Genes Dev 13:3198, 1999.

48. Westin S, Rosenfeld MG, Glass CK: Nuclear receptor coactivators. Adv Pharmacol 47:89, 2000.

49. Strahl BD, Allis CD: The language of covalent histone modification. Nature 403:41, 1998.

50. Bird AP, Wolffe AP: Methylation-induced repression-belts, branches and chromatin. Cell 99:451, 1999.

51. Rea S, Eisenhaber F, O'Carroll D et al: Regulation of chromatin structure by site-specific histone H3 methyltransferases. Nature 406:593, 2000.

52. Chen H, Lin RJ, Xie W et al: Regulation of hormone-induced histone hyperacetylation and gene activation via acetylation of an acetylase. Cell 98:675, 1999.

53. Freedman LP: Increasing the complexity of coactivation in nuclear receptor signalling. Cell 97:5, 1999.

54. Cairns BR: Chromatin remodeling machines: Similar motors, ulterior motives. Trends Biochem Sci 23:20, 1998.

55. Yoshida M, Horinouchi S, Beppu T: Trichostatin A and trapoxin: Novel chemical probes for the role of histone acetylation in chromatin structure and function. BioEssays 17:423, 1995.

56. Marks PA, Richon VM, Rifkind RA: Histone deacetylase inhibitors: Inducers of differentiation or apoptosis of transformed cells. J Natl Cancer Inst 92:1210, 2000.

57. Kastner P, Perez A, Lutz Y et al: Structure, localization and transcriptional properties of two classes of retinoic acid receptor α fusion proteins in acute promyelocytic leukemia (APL): Structural similarities with a new family of oncoproteins. EMBO J 11:629, 1992.

58. Lovering R, Hanson I, Borden K et al: Identification and preliminary characterization of a protein motif related to the zinc finger. Proc Natl Acad Sci USA 90:2112, 1993.

59. Borden KLB, Boddy MN, Lally J et al: The solution structure of the RING finger domain from the acute promyelocytic leukaemia proto-oncoprotein PML. EMBO J 14:1532, 1995.

60. Takahashi M, Inaguma Y, Hiai H, Hirose F: Developmentally regulated expression of a human finger containing gene encoded by the 5′ half of the ret transforming gene. Mol Cel Biol 8:1853, 1988.

61. Miki T, Fleming TP, Crescenzi M et al: Development of a highly efficient expression cDNA cloning system: Application to oncogene isolation. Proc Natl Acad Sci USA 88:5167, 1991.

62. Borden KL, Lally JM, Martin SR et al: In vivo and in vitro characterization of the B1 and B2 zinc-binding domains from the acute promyelocytic leukemia protoconcoprotein PML. Proc Natl Acad Sci USA 93:1601, 1996.

63. Perez A, Kastner P, Sethi S et al: PMLRAR homodimers: Distinct DNA binding properties and heterodimeric interactions with RXR. EMBO J 12:3171, 1993.

64. Grignani F, Testa U, Rogaia D et al: Effects on differentiation by the promyelocytic leukemia PML/RARα protein depend on the fusion of the PML protein dimerization and RARa DNA binding domains. EMBO J 15:4949, 1996.

65. Koken MHM, Linares-Cruz G, Quignon F et al: The PML growth suppressor has an altered expression in human oncogenesis. Oncogene 10:1315, 1995.

66. Terris B, Baldin V, Dubois S et al: PML nuclear bodies are general targets for inflammation and cell proliferation. Cancer Res 55:1590, 1995.

67. Flenghi L, Fagioli M, Tomassoni L et al: Characterization of a new monoclonal antibody (PG-M3) directed against the aminoterminal portion of the PML gene product: Immunocytochemical evidence for high expression of PML proteins on activated macrophages, endothelial cells, and epithelia. Blood 85:1871, 1995.

68. Wang ZG, Delva L, Gaboli M et al: Role of PML in cell growth and the retinoic acid pathway. Science 279:1547, 1998.

69. Koken MHM, Puvion-Dutilleul F, Guillemin MC et al: The t(15;17) translocation alters a nuclear body in a retinoic acid-reversible fashion. EMBO J 13:1073, 1994.

70. Dyck JA, Maul GG, Miller WH Jr et al: A novel macromolecular structure is a target of the promyelocyte-retinoic acid receptor oncoprotein. Cell 76:333, 1994.

71. Weis K, Rambaud S, Laqvau C et al: Retinoic acid regulates aberrant nuclear localization of PML-RARα in acute promyelocyte leukemia. Cell 76:345, 1994.

72. Chang K-S, Fan Y-H, Andreeff M et al: The PML gene encodes a phosphoprotein associated with the nuclear matrix. Blood 85:3646, 1995.

73. Ruggero D, Wang ZG, Pandolfi PP: The puzzling multiple lives of PML and its role in the genesis of cancer. Bioessays 22:827, 2000.

74. Maul GG, Negorev D, Bell P, Ishov AM: Review: Properties and assembly mechanisms of ND10, PML bodies, or PODs. J Struct Biol 129:278, 2000.

75. Ishov AM, Sotnikov AG, Negorev D et al: PML is critical for ND10 formation and recruits the PML-interacting protein daxx to this nuclear structure when modified by SUMO-1. J Cell Biol 147:221, 1999.

76. Zhong S, Muller S, Ronchetti S et al: Role of SUMO-1-modified PML in nuclear body formation. Blood 95:2748, 2000.

77. Mu Z-M, Chin K-V, Liu J-H et al: PML, a growth suppressor disrupted in acute promyelocyte leukemia. Mol Cel Biol 14:6858, 1994.

78. Ahn M-J, Nason-Burchenal K, Moasser M, Dmitrovsky E: Growth suppression of acute promyelocytic leukemia cells having increased expression of the non-rearranged alleles: RARα or PML. Oncogene 10:2307, 1995.

79. Ferbeyre G, de Stanchina E, Qjuerido E et al: PML is induced by oncogenic ras and promotes premature senescence. Genes Dev 14:2015, 2000.

80. Pearson M, Carbone R, Sebastiani C et al: PML regulates p53 acetylation and premature senescence induced by oncogenic Ras. Nature 406:207, 2000.

81. Wang ZG, Ruggero D, Ronchetti S et al: Pml is essential for multiple apoptotic pathways. Nat Genet 20:266, 1998.

82. Quignon F, De Bels F, Koken M et al: PML induces a novel caspase-independent death process. Nat Genet 20:259, 1998.

83. Zhong S, Salomoni P, Ronchetti S et al: Promyelocytic leukemia protein (PML) and Daxx participate in a novel nuclear pathway for apoptosis. J Exp Med 191:631, 2000.

84. Vallian S, Chin KV, Chang KS: The promyelocytic leukemia protein interacts with Sp2 and inhibits its transactivation of the epidermal growth factor receptor. Mol Cel Biol 18:7147, 1998.

85. Doucas V, Tini M, Egan DA, Evans RM: Modulation of CREB binding protein function by the promyelocytic (PML) oncoprotein suggests a role for nuclear bodies in hormone signaling. Proc Natl Acad Sci USA 96:2627, 1999.

86. Zhong S, Delva L, Rachez C et al: A RA-dependent, tumour-growth suppressive transcription complex is the target of the PML-RARα and T18 oncoproteins. Nat Genet 23:287, 1999.

87. Tsuzuki S, Towatari M, Saito H, Enver T: Potentiation of GATA-2 activity through interactions with the promyelocytic leukemia protein (PML) and the t(15;17)-generated PML-retinoic acid receptor α oncoprotein. Mol Cel Biol 20:6276, 2000.

88. Wang ZG, Rego E, Peruzzi D et al: Loss of PML function enhances the frequency and onset of APL in PML-RARα transgenic mice. Blood 92(Suppl. 1):479a, 1998.

89. Zhong S, Hu P, Ye TZ et al: A role for PML and the nuclear body in genomic stability. Oncogene 18:7941, 1999.

90. Kogan SC, Hong SH, Shultz DB et al: Leukemia initiated by PML-RARα: The PML domain plays a critical role while retinoic acid-mediated transactivation is dispensable. Blood 95:1541, 2000.

91. Gallagher RE, Willman CL, Slack JL et al: Association of PML-RARα fusion mRNA type with pretreatment hematologic characteristics but no treatment outcome in acute promyelocytic leukemia: An intergroup molecular study. Blood 90:1656, 1997.

92. Slack JL, Willman CL, Andersen JW et al: Molecular analysis and clinical outcome of adult APL patients with the type V PML-RARα isoform: Results from Intergroup protocol 0129. Blood 95:398, 2000.

93. Kane JR, Head DR, Balazs L et al: Molecular analysis of the PML/RAR alpha chimeric gene in pediatric acute promyelocytic leukemia. Leukemia 10:1296, 1996.

94. Guglielmi C, Martelli MP, Diverio D: Immunophenotype of adult and childhood acute promyelocytic leukaemia: Correlation with morphology, type of PML gene breakpoint and clinical outcome: A cooperative Italian study on 196 cases. Br J Haematol 102:1035, 1998.

95. Grignani F, Valtieri M, Gabbianelli M et al: PML/RARα fusion protein expression in normal human hematopoietic progenitors dictates myeloid commitment and the promyelocytic phenotype. Blood 96:1531, 2000.

96. Enver T, Heyworth CM, Dexter TM: Do stem cells play dice? Blood 92:348, 1998.

97. Brown D, Kogan S, Lagasse E et al: A PML-RARα transgene initiates murine acute promyelocytic leukemia. Proc Natl Acad Sci USA 94:2551, 1997.

98. Grisolano JL, Wesselschmidt RL, Pelicci PG, Ley TJ: Altered myeloid development and acute leukemia in transgenic mice expressing PML-RARα under control of cathepsin G regulatory sequences. Blood 89:376, 1997.

99. He LZ, Tribioli C, Rivi R et al: Acute leukemia with promyelocytic features in PML/RARα transgenic mice. Proc Natl Acad Sci USA 94:5302, 1997.

100. Lin RJ, Evans RM: Acquisition of oncogenic potential by RAR chimeras in acute promyelocytic leukemia through formation of homodimers. Mol Cell 5:821, 2000.

101. Minucci S, Maccarana M, Cioce M et al: Oligomerization of RAR and AML1 transcription factors as a novel mechanism of oncogenic activation. Mol Cell 5:811, 2000.

102. Onodera M, Kunisada T, Nishikawa S et al: Overexpression of retinoic acid receptor alpha suppresses myeloid cell differentiation at the promyelocyte stage. Oncogene 11:1291, 1995.

103. Du C, Redner RL, Cooke MP, Lavau C: Overexpression of wild-type retinoic acid receptor alpha (RARα) recapitulates retinoic acid-sensitive transformation of primary myeloid progenitors by acute promyelocytic leukemia RARα-fusion genes. Blood 94:793, 1999.

104. He LZ, Guidez F, Tribioli C et al: Distinct interactions of PML-RARα and PLZF-RARα with co-repressors determine differential responses to RA in APL. Nat Genet 18:126, 1998.

105. Guidez F, Ivins S, Zhu J et al: Reduced retinoic acid-sensitivities of nuclear receptor corepressor binding to PML- and PLZF-RARα underlie molecular pathogenesis and treatment of acute promyelocytic leukemia. Blood 91:2634, 1998.

106. Grignani F, De Matteis S, Nervi C et al: Fusion proteins of the retinoic acid receptor-α recruit histone deacetylase in promyelocytic leukemia. Nature 391:815, 1998.

107. Lin RJ, Nagy L, Inoue S et al: Role of the histone deacetylase complex in acute promyelocytic leukemia. Nature 391:811, 1998.

108. Purton LE, Bernstein ID, Collins SJ: All-trans retinoic acid delays the differentiation of primitive hematopoietic precursors (lin-c-kit+Scal-(+)) while enhancing the terminal maturation of committed granulocyte/monocyte progenitors. Blood 94:483, 1999.

109. Turhan AG, Lemoine FM, Debert C et al: Highly purified primitive hematopoietic stem cells are PML-RARA negative and generate nonclonal progenitors in acute promyelocytic leukemia. Blood 85:2154, 1995.

110. Nervi C, Poindexter EC, Grignani F et al: Characterization of the PML-RARα chimeric product of the acute promyelocytic leukemic-specific t(15;17) translocation. Cancer Res 52:3687, 1992.

111. Jansen JH, Mahfoudi A, Rambaud S et al: Multimeric complexes of the PML-retinoic receptor alpha protein in acute promyelocytic leukemia cells and interference with retinoid and peroxi-

some-proliferator signaling pathways. Proc Natl Acad Sci USA 92:7401, 1995.

112. Li YP, Andersen J, Zelent A et al: RARa1/RARα2-PML mRNA expression in acute promyelocytic leukemia cells: A molecular and laboratory-clinical correlative study. Blood 90:306, 1997.

113. Pollock JL, Grisolano JL, Goda P et al: A bcr-3 isoform of RARalpha-PML potentiates the development of PML-RARalpha-driven acute promyelocytic leukemia. Proc Natl Acad Sci USA 96:15103, 1999.

114. Yoshida H, Kitamura K, Tanaka K et al: Accelerated degradation of PML-retinoic acid receptor α (PML-RARA) oncoprotein by all-trans retinoic acid in acute promyelocytic leukemia: Possible role of the proteasome pathway. Cancer Res 56:2945, 1996.

115. Chen GQ, Zhu J, Shi XG et al: In vitro studies on cellular and molecular mechanisms of arsenic trioxide (As2O3) in the treatment of acute promyelocytic leukemia: As2O3 induces NB4 cell apoptosis with downregulation of bcl-2 expression and alteration of PML-RARα/PML protein localization. Blood 88:1052, 1996.

116. Raelson JV, Nervi C, Rosenauer A et al: The PML/RARα oncoprotein is a direct molecular target of retinoic acid in acute promyelocytic leukemia cells. Blood 88:2826, 1996.

117. Zhu J, Koken MHM, Quignon F et al: Arsenic-induced PML targeting onto nuclear bodies: Implications for the treatment of acute promyelocytic leukemia. Proc Natl Acad Sci USA 94:3978, 1997.

118. Zhu J, Gianni M, Kopf E et al: Retinoic acid induces proteasome-dependent degradaton of retinoic acid receptor α (RARα) and oncogenic RARα fusion proteins. Proc Natl Acad Sci USA 96:14807, 1999.

119. Jing Y, Wang L, Xia L et al: Combined effect of all-trans retinoic acid and arsenic trioxide in acute promyelocytic leukemia cells in vitro and in vivo. Blood 97:264, 2001.

120. Duprez E, Lillehaug JR, Naoe T, Lanotte M: cAMP signalling is decisive for recovery of nuclear bodies (PODs) during maturation of RA-resistant t(15:17) promyelocytic leukemia NB4 cells expressing PML-RARα. Oncogene 12:2451, 1996.

121. Nervi C, Ferrara FF, Fanelli M et al: Caspases mediate retinoic acid-induced degradation of the acute promyelocytic leukemia PML/RARα fusion protein. Blood 92:2244, 1998.

122. Slack JL, Yu M: Constitutive expression of the promyelocytic leukemia-associated oncogene PML-RARα in TF1 cells: Isoform-specific and retinoic acid-dependent effects on growth, bcl-2 expression, and apoptosis. Blood 91:3347, 1998.

123. Grignani F, Ferrucci P, Testa U et al: The acute promyelocytic leukemia-specific PML-RARα fusion protein inhibits differentiation and promotes survival of myeloid precursor cells. Cell 74:423, 1993.

124. Fanelli M, Minucci S, Gelmetti V et al: Constitutive degradation of PML/RARα through the proteosome pathway mediates retinoic acid resistance. Blood 93:1477, 1999.

125. Tamayo P, Slonim D, Mesirov J et al: Interpreting patterns of gene expression with self-organizing maps: Methods and application to hematopoietic differentiation. Proc Natl Acad Sci USA 96:2907, 1999.

126. Liu T-X, Zhang J-W, Tao J et al: Gene expression networks underlying retinoic acid-induced differentiation of acute promyelocytic leukemia cells. Blood 96:1496, 2000.

127. Chen GQ, Shi XG, Tang W et al: Use of arsenic trioxide (As2O3) in the treatment of acute promyelocytic leukemia (APL): I. As2O3 exerts dose-dependent dual effects on APL cells. Blood 89:3345, 1997.

128. Shao W, Fanelli M, Ferrara FF et al: As2O3 induced apoptosis and loss of PML/RARα protein in both retinoid sensitive and resistant APL cells. J Natl Cancer Inst 90:124, 1998.

129. Gianni M, Koken MHM, Chelbi-Alix MK et al: Combined arsenic and retinoic acid treatment enhances differentiation and apoptosis in arsenic persistent NB4 cells. Blood 91:4300, 1998.

130. Soignet SL, Maslak P, Wang ZG et al: Complete remission after treatment of acute promyelocytic leukemia with arsenic trioxide. N Engl J Med 339:1341, 1998.

131. Wang ZG, Rivi R, Delva L et al: Arsenic trioxide and melarsoprol induce programmed cell death in myeloid leukemia cell lines and function in a PML and PML/RARα independent manner. Blood 92:1497, 1998.

132. Zhu X-H, Shen Y-L, Jing Y-K et al: Apoptosis and growth inhibition in malignant lymphocytes after treatment with arsenic trioxide at clinically achievable concentrations. J Natl Cancer Inst 91:772, 1999.

133. Rousselot P, Labaume S, Marolleau J-P et al: Arsenic trioxide and melarsoprol induce apoptosis in plasma cell lines and in plasma cells from myeloma patients. Cancer Res 59:1041, 1999.

134. Jing Y, Dai J, Chalmers-Redman RME et al: Arsenic trioxide selectively induces acute promyelocytic leukemia cell apoptosis via a hydrogen peroxide-dependent pathway. Blood 94:2102, 1999.

135. Kroemer G, de The H: Arsenic trioxide: A novel mitochondriotoxic anticancer agent? J Natl Cancer Inst 91:743, 1999.

136. Gallagher RE: Arsenic—new life for an old potion. N Engl J Med 339:1389, 1998.

137. Muller S, Matunis MJ, Dejean A: Conjugation with the ubiquitin-related modifier SUMO-1 regulates the partitioning of PML within the nucleus. EMBO J 17:61, 1998.

138. Sternsdorf T, Puccetti E, Jensen K et al: PIC-1/SUMO-1 modified PML-retinoic acid receptor α mediates arsenic trioxide-induced apoptosis in acute promyelocytic leukemia. Mol Cel Biol 19:5170, 1999.

139. Nason-Burchenal K, Allopenna J, Bégue A et al: Targeting of PML/RARα is lethal to retinoic acid-resistant promyelocytic leukemia cells. Blood 92:1758, 1998.

140. Cai X, Shen YL, Zhu Q et al: Arsenic trioxide-induced apoptosis and differentiation are associated respectively with mitochondrial transmembrane potential collapse and retinoic acid signaling pathways in acute promyelocytic leukemia. Leukemia 14:262, 2000.

141. Imaizumi M, Suzuki H, Yoshinari M et al: Mutations in the E-domain of RARα portion of the PML/RARa chimeric gene may confer clinical resistance to all-trans retinoic acid in acute promyelocytic leukemia. Blood 92:374, 1998.

142. Takayama N, Kizaki M, Hida T et al: Novel mutation in the PML/RARalpha chimeric gene exhibits dramatically decreased ligand-binding activity and confers acquired resistance to retinoic acid in acute promyelocytic leukemia. Exp Hematol 29:864, 1998.

143. Marasca R, Zucchini P, Galimberti S et al: Missense mutations in the PML/RARα ligand binding domain in ATRA-resistant AS2O3 sensitive relapse acute promyelocytic leukemia. Haematologica 84:963, 1999.

144. Zhou D-C, Kim S, Ding W et al: Frequent mutations in the ligand binding domain of PML-RARα after multiple relapses of acute promyelocytic leukemia: Analysis for functional relationship to response to all-trans retinoic ancid and histone deacetylase inhibitors in vitro and in vivo. Blood 99:1356, 2002.

145. Tallman MS, Andersen JW, Schiffer CA et al: All-trans retinoic acid in acute promyelocytic leukemia. N Engl J Med 337:1021, 1997.

146. Cote S, Zhou D, Bianchini A et al: Altered ligand binding and transcriptional regulation by mutations in the PML/RARα ligand-binding domain arising in retinoic acid-resistant patients with acute promyelocytic leukemia. Blood 96:3200, 2000.

147. Kopp P, Kitajima K, Jameson JL: Syndrome of resistance to thyroid hormone: Insights into thyroid hormone action. Proc Soc Exp Biol Med 211:49, 1996.

148. Warrell RP Jr: Retinoid resistance in acute promyelocytic leukemia: New mechanisms, strategies and implications. Blood 82:1949, 1993.

149. Slack JL, Gallagher RE: The molecular biology of acute promyelocytic leukemia. In Tallman MS, Gordon LJ (eds.): Diagnostic Therapeutic Advances in Hematologic Malignancies, p. 75. Kluwer Academic Publishers, Norwell, MA, 1999.

150. Benoit G, Altucci L, Flexor M et al: RAR-independent RXR signaling induces t(15;17) leukemia cell maturation. EMBO J 18:7011, 1999.

151. Guidez F, Huang W, Tong J-H et al: Poor response to all-trans retinoic acid therapy in a t(11;17) PLZF/RARa patient. Leukemia 8:312, 1994.

152. Licht J, Chomienne C, Goy A et al: Clinical and molecular characterization of a rare syndrome of acute promyelocytic leukemia associated with translocation (11;17). Blood 85:1083, 1995.

153. Licht JD, Shaknovich R, English MA et al: Reduced and altered DNA-binding and transcriptional properties of the PLZF-retinoic acid receptor-α chimera generated in t(11;17)-associated acute promyelocytic leukemia. Oncogene 12:323, 1996.

154. Dong S, Zhu J, Reid A et al: Amino-terminal protein-protein interaction motif (POZ-domain) is responsible for activities of the promyelocytic leukemia zinc finger-retinoic acid receptor-α fusion protein. Proc Natl Acad Sci USA 93:3624, 1996.

155. Koken MHM, Reid A, Quignon F et al: Leukaemia-associated RARα fusion partners, PML and PLZF, heterodimerize and co-localize onto nuclear bodies. Proc Natl Acad Sci USA 94:10255, 1997.

156. Rego EM, He LZ, Warrell Jr RP et al: Retinoic acid (RA) and As2O3 treatment in transgenic models of acute promyelocytic leukemia (APL) unravel the distinct nature of the leukemogenic process induced by the PML-RARalpha and PLZF-RARalpha oncoproteins. Proc Natl Acad Sci USA 97:10173, 2000.

157. Grimwade D, Biondi A, Mozziconacci MJ et al: Characterization of acute promyelocytic leukemia cases lacking the classic t(15;17): Results of the European Working Party. Blood 96:1297, 2000.

158. He L, Bhaumik M, Tribioli C et al: Two critical hits for promyelocytic leukemia. Mol Cell 6:1131, 2000.

159. Li JY, English MA, Ball HJ et al: Sequence-specific DNA binding and transcriptional regulation by the promyelocytic zinc finger protein. J Biol Chem 272:22447, 1997.

160. Yeyati PL, Shaknovich R, Boterashvili B et al: Leukemia translocation protein PLZF inhibits cell growth and expression of cyclin A. Oncogene 18:925, 1999.

161. Reid A, Gould A, Brand N et al: Leukemia translocation gene, PLZF, is expressed with a speckled nuclear pattern in early hematopoietic cells. Blood 86:4544, 1995.

162. Hummel JL, Wells RA, Dube ID et al: Deregulation of NPM and PLZF in a variant t(5;17) case of acute promyelocytic leukemia. Oncogene 18:633, 1999.

163. Redner RL, Chen JD, Rush EA et al: The t(5;17) acute promyelocytic leukemia fusion protein NPM-RAR interacts with co-repressor and co-activator proteins and exhibits both positive and negative transcriptional properties. Blood 95:2683, 2000.

164. Redner RL, Corey SL, Rush EA: Differentiation of t(5;17) variant acute promyelocytic leukemic blasts by all-trans retinoic acid. Leukemia 11:1014, 1997.

165. Wells RA, Hummel JL, De Koven A et al: A new variant translocation in acute promyelocytic leukaemia: Molecular characterization and clinical consideration. Leukemia 10:735, 1996.

166. Jonveaux P, Le Coniat M, Derre J et al: Chromosome microdissection in leukemia: A power tool for the analysis of complex chromosomal rearrangements. Genes Chromosomes Cancer 15:26, 1996.

167. Benedetti L, Levin AA, Scicchitano BM et al: Characterization of the retinoid binding properties of the major fusion products present acute promyelocytic leukemia cells. Blood 90:1175, 1997.

168. Gallagher RE, Li Y-P, Rao S et al: Characterization of acute promyelocytic leukemia cases with PML-RARα break/fusion sites in PML exon 6: Identification of a subgroup with decreased in vitro responsiveness to all-trans-retinoic acid. Blood 86:1540, 1995.

169. Borrow J, Goddard AD, Gibbons B et al: Diagnosis of acute promyelocytic leukaemia by RT-PCR detection of PML-RARA and RARA-PML fusion transcripts. Br J Haematol 82:529, 1992.

170. Huang W, Sun G-L, Li X-S et al: Acute promyelocytic leukemia: Clinical relevance of two major PML-RARα isoforms and detection of minimal residual disease by retrotranscriptase/polymerase chain reaction to predict relapse. Blood 82:1264, 1993.

171. Vahdat L, Maslak P, Miller Jr WH et al: Early mortality and the retinoic acid syndrome in acute promyelocytic leukemia: Impact of leukocytosis, low-dose chemotherapy, PMN/RAR-α isoform, and CD13 expression in patients treated with all-trans retinoic acid. (Review) Blood 84:3843, 1994.

172. Fukutani H, Naoe T, Ohno R et al: Isoforms of PML-retinoic acid alpha fused transcripts affect neither clinical features of acute promyelocytic leukemia nor prognosis after treatment with all-trans retinoic acid. Leukemia 9:1478, 1995.

173. Mandelli F, Diverio D, Avvisati, G et al: Molecular remission in PML/RARα-positive acute promyelocytic leukemia by combined all-trans retinoic acid and idarubicin (AIDA) therapy. Blood 90:1014, 1997.

174. Miller WH Jr, Kakizuka A, Frankel SR et al: Reverse transcription polymerase chain reaction for the rearranged retinoic acid receptor-α clarifies diagnosis and detects minimal residual disease in acute promyelocytic leukemia. Proc Natl Acad Sci USA 89:2694, 1992.

175. Biondi A, Rambaldi A, Pandolfi P et al: Molecular monitoring of myl/retinoic acid-α fusion gene in acute promyelocytic leukemia by polymerase chain reaction. Blood 80:492, 1992.

176. Seale JRC, Varma S, Swirsky DM et al: Quantification of PML-RARα transcripts in acute promyelocytic leukemia: Explanation for the lack of sensitivity of RT-PCR for the detection of minimal residual disease and induction of the leukemia-specific mRNA by alpha interferon. Br J Haematol 95:985, 1996.

177. Slack JL, Bi WB, Livak KJ et al: Pre-clinical validation of a novel, highly sensitive assay to detect PML-RARα mRNA using real-time reverse-transcription-PCR. J Mol Diagn 3:141, 2001.

178. Diverio D, Pandolfi PP, Rossi V et al: Monitoring of treatment outcome in acute promyelocytic leukemia by RT-PCR. Leukemia 8:1105, 1994.

179. Tobal K, Saunders M, Grey M, Yin L: Persistence of RARα-PML fusion mRNA detected by reverse transcriptase polymerase chain reaction in patients with long-term remission of acute promyelocytic leukaemia. Br J Haematol 90:615, 1995.

180. Grimwade D, Howe K, Langabeer S et al: Minimal residual disease detection in acute promyelocytic leukemia by reverse-transcriptase PCR: Evaluation of PML-RARα and RARα-PML assessment in patients who ultimately relapse. Leukemia 10:61, 1996.

181. Tobal K, Lin-Yin JA: RT-PCR method with increased sensitivity shows persistence of PML-RARA fusion transcripts in patients in long-term remission of APL. Leukemia 12:1349, 1998.

182. Lo Coco F, Diverio D, Avvisati G et al: Therapy of molecular relapse in acute promyelocytic leukemia. Blood 94:2225, 1999.

183. Cassinat B, Zassadowski F, Balitrand N et al: Quantitation of minimal residual disease in acute promyelocytic leukemia patients with t(15;17) translocation with real-time RT-PCR. Leukemia 14:324, 2000.

184. Willman CL, Yeap B, Bi W et al: Predictive value of automated, quantitative real-time RT-PCR performed at the end of consolidation of acute promyelocytic leukemia: A SWOG, CALGB and ECOG Intergroup Study (INT-0129). Proc ASCO 19:5a, 2000.

185. Jurlander J, Caligiuri MA, Ruutu T: Persistence of the AML/ETO fusion transcript in patients treated with allogeneic bone marrow transplantation for t(8;21) leukemia. Blood 88:2183, 1996.

186. Alcalay M, Zangrilli D, Fagioli M et al: Expression pattern of the RARα-PML fusion gene in acute promyelocytic leukemia. Proc Natl Acad Sci USA 89:4840, 1992.

187. Vickers M, Jackson G, Taylor P: The incidence of acute promyelocytic leukemia appears constant over most of a human lifespan, implying only one rate limiting mutation. Leukemia 14:722, 2000.

188. Carter M, Kalwinsky DK, Dahl GV et al: Childhood acute promyelocytic leukemia: A rare variant of nonlymphoid leukemia with distinctive clinical and biologic features. Leukemia 3:298, 1989.

189. Biondi A, Rovelli A, Cantù-Rajnoldi A et al: Acute promyelocytic leukemia in children: Experience of the Italian Pediatric Hematology and Oncology Group (AIEOP). Leukemia 8(Suppl. 2):S66, 1994.

190. Malta-Corea A, Pacheco Espinoza C, Cantù-Rajnoldi A et al: Childhood acute promyelocytic leukemia in Nicaragua. Ann Oncol 4:892, 1993.

191. Estey E, Thall P, Kantarjian H et al: Association between increased body mass index and a diagnosis of acute promyelocytic leukemia in patients with acute myeloid leukemia. Leukemia 12:1503, 1997.

192. Douer D, Preston-Martin S, Chang E et al: High frequency of acute promyelocytic leukemia among Latinos with acute myeloid leukemia. Blood 87:308, 1996.

193. Wiernik PH, Andersen JW: Unpublished observations, 1994.

194. Mele A, Stazi MA, Pulsoni A et al: Epidemiology of acute promyelocytic leukemia. Haematologica 80:405, 1995.

195. Pulsoni A, Stazi A, Cotichini R et al: Acute promyelocytic leukemia: Epidemiology and risk factors. A report of the GIMEMA Italian archive of adult acute leukaemia. GIMEMA Cooperative Group. Eur J Haematol 61:327, 1998.

196. Daly PA, Schiffer CA, Wiernik PH: Acute promyelocytic leukemia—Clinical management of 15 patients. Am J Hematol 8:347, 1980.

197. Biondi A, Luciano A, Bassan R et al: CD2 expression in acute promyelocytic leukemia is associated with microgranular morphology (FAB M3v) but not with any PML gene breakpoint. Leukemia 9:1461, 1995.

198. Hazani A, Weidenfeld Y, Tatarsky I, Bental E: Acute promyelocytic leukemia presenting as sudden blindness and sinus vein thrombosis. Am J Hematol 28:56, 1988.

199. Jetha N: Promyelocytic leukemia with multiorgan infarctions and large vessel thrombosis. Arch Pathol Lab Med 105:683, 1981.

200. Hoyle CF, Swirsky DM, Freedman L, Hayhoe FGJ: Beneficial effect of heparin in the management of patients with APL. Br J Haematol 68:283, 1988.

201. Wiernik PH, De Bellis R, Muxi P, Dutcher JP: Extramedullary acute promyelocytic leukemia. Cancer 78:2510, 1996.

202. Lavau C, Dejean A: The t(15;17) translocation in acute promyelocytic leukemia. Leukemia 8(Suppl. 2):S9, 1994.

203. Sessarego M, Fugazza G, Balleari E et al: High frequency of trisomy 8 in acute promyelocytic leukemia: A fluorescence in situ hybridization study. Cancer Genet Cytogenet 97:161, 1997.

204. De Botton S, Chevret S, Sanz M et al: Additional chromosomal abnormalities in patients with acute promyelocytic leukaemia (APL) do not confer poor prognosis: Results of APL 93 trial. Br J Haematol 111:801, 2000.

205. Hernandez JM, Martin G, Gutierrez NC et al: Additional cytogenetic changes do not influence the outcome of patients with newly diagnosed acute promyelocytic leukemia treated with ATRA plus anthracyclin based protocol. A report of the Spanish group PETHEMA. Haematologica 86:807, 2001.

206. Schoch C, Haase D, Haferlach T et al: Incidence and implication of additional chromosome aberrations in acute promyelocytic leukaemia with translocation t(15;17)(q22;q21): A report on 50 patients. Br J Haematol 94:493, 1996.

207. Slack JL, Arthur DC, Lawrence D et al: Secondary cytogenetic changes in acute promyelocytic leukemia—prognostic importance in patients treated with chemotherapy alone and association with the intron 3 breakpoint of the PML gene: A Cancer and Leukemia Group B study. J Clin Oncol 15:1786, 1997.

208. Pantic M, Novak A, Marislavljevic D et al: Additional chromosome aberrations in acute promyelocytic leukemia: Characteristics and prognostic influence. Med Oncol 17:307, 2000.

209. Wiernik PH, Kim H, Gundacker H et al: Prognostic implications of additional cytogenetic aberrations in de novo acute myeloid leukemia (AML) with t(15;17), t(8;21) or inv (16). Blood, in press.

210. Grimwade D, Biondi A, Mozziconacci MJ et al: Characterization of acute promyelocytic leukemia cases lacking the classic 9t(15;17): Results of the European Working Party. Group Francais de Cytogenetique, Groupe de Francais d'Hematologie Cellulaire, UK Cancer Cytogenetics Group and BIOMED 1 European Community-Concerted Action "Molecular Cytogenetic Diagnosis in Haematological Malignancies". Blood 96:1297, 2000.

211. Jansen JH, de Ridder MC, Geertsma WM et al: Complete remission of t(11;17) positive acute promyelocytic leukemia induced by all-trans retinoic acid and granulocyte colony-stimulating factor. Blood 94:39, 1999.

212. Krause JR, Stolc V, Kaplan SS, Penchansky L: Microgranular promyelocytic leukemia: A multiparameter examination. Am J Hematol 30:158, 1989.

213. Murray CK, Estey E, Paietta E et al: CD56 expression in acute promyelocytic leukemia: A possible indicator of poor treatment outcome? J Clin Oncol 17:293, 1999.

214. Castoldi GL, Liso V, Specchia G, Tomasi P: Acute promyelocytic leukemia: Morphological aspects. Leukemia 8(Suppl. 2):S27, 1994.

215. Bennett JM, Catovsky D, Daniel MT et al: A variant form of hypergranular promyelocytic leukemia (M3). French-American-British (FAB) Co-operative Group. Br J Haematol 44:169, 1980.

216. Rovelli A, Biondi A, Cantù Rajnoldi A et al: Microgranular variant of acute promyelocytic leukemia in children. J Clin Oncol 10:1413, 1992.

217. Davey FR, Davis RB, MacCallum JM et al: Morphologic and cytochemical characteristics of acute promyelocytic leukemia. Am J Hematol 30:221, 1989.

218. Golomb HM, Rowley JD, Vardiman JW et al: "Microgranular" acute promyelocytic leukemia: A distinct clinical, ultrastructural, and cytogenetic entity. Blood 55:253, 1980.

219. McKenna RW, Parkin J, Bloomfield CD et al: Acute promyelocytic leukemia: A study of 39 cases with identification of a hyperbasophilic microgranular variant. Br J Haematol 50:201, 1982.

220. Invernizzi R, Iannone AM, Bernuzzi S et al: Acute promyelocytic leukemia: Morphological and clinical features. Haematologica 78:156, 1993.

221. Tallman MS, Hakimian D, Snower D et al: Basophilic differentiation in acute promyelocytic leukemia. Leukemia 7:521, 1993.

222. Erber WN, Asbahr H, Rule SA, Scott CS: Unique immunophenotype of acute promyelocytic leukemia as defined by CD9 and CD68 antibodies. Br J Haematol 88:101, 1994.

223. Koike T, Tatewaki W, Aoki A et al: Brief report: Severe symptoms of hyperhistaminemia after the treatment of acute promyelocytic leukemia with tretinoin (all-trans-retinoic acid). N Engl J Med 327:385, 1992.

224. Gilbert RD, Karabus CD, Mills E: Acute promyelocytic leukemia: A childhood cluster. Cancer 59:933, 1987.

225. Williams CKO, Folani AO, Saditan AAO et al: Childhood acute leukemia in a tropical population. Br J Cancer 42:89, 1982.

226. Scott RM, Mayer RJ: The unique aspects of acute promyelocytic leukemia. J Clin Oncol 8:1913, 1990.

227. Das Gupta A, Sapre RS, Shah AS et al: Cytochemical and immunophenotypic heterogeneity in acute promyelocytic leukemia. Acta Haematol 81:5, 1989.

228. Scott CS, Patel D, Drexler HG et al: Immunophenotypic and enzymatic studies do not support the concept of mixed monocytic-granulocytic differentiation in acute promyelocytic leukemia (M_3): A study of 44 cases. Br J Haematol 71:505, 1989.

229. Drexler HG: Classification of acute myeloid leukemia: A comparison of FAB and immunophenotyping. Leukemia 1:697, 1987.

230. Sanz MA, Jarque I, Martín G et al: Acute promyelocytic leukemia. Therapy results and prognostic factors. Cancer 61:7, 1988.

231. Ko B-S, Tang J-L, Chen Y-C et al: Extramedullary relapse after all-trans retinoic acid treatment in acute promyelocytic leukemia—the occurrence of retinoic acid syndrome is a risk factor. Leukemia 13:1406, 1999.

232. De Renzo A, Santoro LFE, Notaro R et al: Acute promyelocytic leukemia after treatment for non-Hodgkin's lymphoma with drugs targeting topoisomerase II. Am J Hematol 60:300, 1999.

233. Kantarjian HM, Keating MJ, Walters RS et al: The association of specific "favorable" cytogenetic abnormalities with secondary leukemia. Cancer 58:924, 1986.

234. Detourmignies L, Castaigne S, Stoppa AM et al: Therapy-related acute promyelocytic leukemia: A report of 16 cases. J Clin Oncol 10:1430, 1992.

235. Castaigne S, Berger R, Jolly V et al: Promyelocytic blast crisis of chronic myelocytic leukemia with both t(9;22) and t(15;17) in M3 cells. Cancer 54:2409, 1984.

236. Rosenthal NS, Knapp D, Farhi DC: Promyelocytic blast crisis of chronic myelogenous leukemia. A rare subtype associated with disseminated intravascular coagulation. Am J Clin Pathol 103:185, 1995.

237. Misawa S, Lee E, Schiffer CA et al: Association of the translocation (15;17) with malignant proliferation of promyelocytes in acute leukemia and chronic myelogenous leukemia at blast crisis. Blood 67:270, 1986.

238. Hogge DE, Misawa S, Schiffer CA, Testa JR: Promyelocytic blast crisis in chronic granulocytic leukemia with 15;17 translocation. Leuk Res 6:1019, 1984.

239. Wiernik PH, Dutcher JP, Paietta E et al: Treatment of promyelocytic blast crisis of chronic myelogenous leukemia with all trans-retinoic acid. Leukemia 5:504, 1991.

240. Hatzis T, Standen GR, Howell RT et al: Acute promyelocytic leukaemia (M3): Relapse with acute myeloblastic leukemia (M2) and dic(5;17)(q11;p11). Am J Hematol 48:40, 1995.

241. Bseiso AN, Kantarjian H, Estey E: Myelodysplastic syndrome following successful therapy of acute promyelocytic leukemia. Leukemia 11:168, 1977.

242. Felice MS, Rossi J, Gallego M et al: Acute trilineage leukemia with monosomy of chromosome 7 following an acute promyelocytic leukemia. Leuk Lymphoma 34:409, 1999.

243. Zompi S, Legrand O, Bouscany D et al: Therapy-related acute myeloid leukemia after successful therapy for acute promyelocytic leukaemia with t(15;17): A report of two cases and a review of the literature. Br J Haematol 110:610, 2000.

244. Di Bona E, Avvisati G, Castaman G et al: Early haemorrhagic morbidity and mortality during remission induction with or without all-trans retinoic acid in acute promyelocytic leukaemia. Br J Haematol 108:689, 2000.

245. Visani G, Gugliotta L, Tosi P et al: All-trans retinoic acid significantly reduces the incidence of early hemorrhagic death during induction therapy of acute promyelocytic leukemia. Eur J Haematol 64:139, 2000.

246. Yates JW, Wallace J Jr, Ellison RR, Holland JF: Cytosine arabinoside (NSC-63878) and daunorubicin (NSC-83142) therapy in acute nonlymphocytic leukemia. Cancer Chemother Reports 57:485, 1973.

247. Estey E, Thall PF, Pierce S et al: Treatment of newly diagnosed acute promyelocytic leukemia without cytarabine. J Clin Oncol 15:483, 1997.

248. Sanz MA, Guillermo M, Rayon C et al: A modified AIDA protocol with anthracycline-based consolidation results in high antileukemic efficacy and reduced toxicity in newly diagnosed PML/RARα-positive acute promyelocytic leukemia. Blood 94:3015, 1999.

249. Head DR, Kopecky KJ, Weick J et al: Effect of aggressive daunomycin therapy on survival in acute promyelocytic leukemia. Blood 86:1717, 1995.

250. Pallavicini EB, Luliri P, Anselmetti L et al: High-dose daunorubicin (DNR) for induction and treatment of relapse in acute promyelocytic leukemia (APL): Report of 17 cases. Haematologica 73:49, 1988.

251. Carotenuto M, Greco M, Bavaro P et al: Acute promyelocytic leukemia: Results of treatment of 10 cases (Abstr). In Proceedings of the 3rd International Symposium on Therapy of Acute Leukemias, 1982.

252. Salvaneschi L, Lazzarino M, Morra E et al: Survival in adult acute myeloid leukemia under conventional chemotherapy (Abstr). In Proceedings of the 3rd International Symposium on Therapy of Acute Leukemias, 1982.

253. Marty M, Ganem G, Fisher J et al: Leucémie aiguë promyélocytaire: Étude rétrospective de 119 malades traités par daunorubicine. Novu Rev Fr Hématol 26:371, 1984.

254. Mandelli F, Petti MC, Avvisati G et al: GIMEMA experience in the treatment of adult myelogenous. In Gale RP (ed): Acute Myelogenous Leukemia: Progress and Controversies, p. 273. Wiley-Liss, New York, 1990.

255. Petti MC, Avvisati G, Amadori S et al: Acute promyelocytic leukemia: Clinical aspects and results of treatment in 62 patients. Haematologica 72:151, 1987.

256. Bennett JM, Andersen JW, Cassileth PA: Long term survival in acute myeloid leukemia: The Eastern Cooperative Oncology Group. Leuk Res 15:223, 1991.

257. Clarkson B: Retinoic acid in acute promyelocytic leukemia: The promise and the paradox. Cancer Cells 3:211, 1991.

258. Fenaux P, Pollet JP, Vandenbossche-Simon L et al: Treatment of acute promyelocytic leukemia: A report of 70 cases. Leuk Lymphoma 4:239, 1991.

259. Head DR, Kopecky K, Hewlett J et al: Survival with cytotoxic therapy in acute promyelocytic leukemia, a SWOG report. Blood 78:268a, 1991.

260. Thomas X, Archimbaud E, Treille-Ritouet D et al: Prognostic factors in acute promyelocytic leukemia: A retrospective study of 67 cases. Leuk Lymphoma 4:249, 1991.

261. Willemze R, Suciu S, Mandelli F et al: Treatment of patients with acute promyelocytic leukemia. The EORTC-LCG experience. Leukemia 8(Suppl. 2):S48, 1994.

262. Lengfelder E, Reichert A, Schoch C et al: Double induction strategy including high dose cytarabine in combination with all-*trans* retinoic acid: Effects in patients with newly diagnosed acute promyelocytic leukemia. Leukemia 14:1362, 2000.

263. Berman E: A review of idarubicin in acute leukemia. Oncology 7:91, 1993.

264. Berman E, Heller G, Santorsa J et al: Results of a randomized trial comparing idarubicin and cytosine arabinoside with daunorubicin and cytosine arabinoside in adult patients with newly diagnosed acute myelogenous leukemia. Blood 77:1666, 1991.

265. Wiernik PH, Banks PLC, Case DC Jr et al: Cytarabine plus idarubicin or daunorubicin as induction and consolidation therapy for previously untreated adult patients with acute myeloid leukemia. Blood 79:313, 1992.

266. Avvisati G, Mandelli F, Petti MC et al: Idarubicin (4-demethoxy-daunorubicin) as a single agent for remission induction of previously untreated acute promyelocytic leukemia: A pilot study of the Italian cooperative group GIMEMA. Eur J Haematol 44:257, 1990.

267. Tallman MS, Rowe JM: Acute promyelocytic leukemia: A paradigm for differentiation therapy with retinoic acid. Blood Rev 8:70, 1994.

268. Haferlach T, Löffler H, Glass B, Gassmann W: Repeated complete remission in a patient with acute promyelocytic leukemia after treatment with 13-*cis*-retinoic acid first and with all-*trans*-retinoic acid in relapse. Clin Invest 71:774, 1993.

269. Muindi J, Frankel S, Huselton C et al: Clinical pharmacology of oral all-trans retinoic acid with acute promyelocytic leukemia. Cancer Res 52:2138, 1992.

270. Lefebvre P, Thomas G, Gourmel B et al: Pharmacokinetics of oral all-trans retinoic acid with acute promyelocytic leukemia. Leukemia 5:1054, 1991.

271. Muindi J, Frankel S, Miller WH Jr et al: Continuous treatment with all-trans retinoic acid causes a progressive reduction in plasma drug concentrations: Implications for relapse and retinoid "resistance" in patients with acute promyelocytic leukemia. Blood 79:299, 1992.

272. Smith MA, Adamson PC, Balis FM et al: Phase I trial and pharmacokinetic evaluation of all-*trans*-retinoic acid in pediatric patients. J Clin Oncol 10:1666, 1992.

273. Meyskens FL Jr, Goodman GE, Alberts DS: 13-*cis*-retinoic acid: Pharmacology, toxicology and clinical applications for the prevention and treatment of human cancer. Crit Rev Oncol Hematol 3:75, 1985.

274. Brazzell RK, Vane FM, Ehmann CW et al: Pharmacokinetics of isotretinoin during repetitive dosing to patients. Eur J Clin Pharmacol 24:695, 1983.

275. Adamson PC, Balis FM, Smith MA et al: Dose-dependent pharmacokinetics of all-*trans*-retinoic acid. J Natl Cancer Inst 84:1332, 1992.

276. Schwartz EL, Hallam S, Gallagher RE, Wiernik PH: Inhibition of all-trans retinoic acid metabolism by fluconazole in vitro and in patients with acute promyelocytic leukemia. Mol Pharmacol 50:923, 1995.

277. Miller VA, Rigas JR, Muindi JRF et al: Modulation of all-*trans* retinoic acid pharmacokinetics by liarozole. Cancer Chemother Pharmacol 34:522, 1994.

278. Muindi JF, Scher HI, Rigas JR et al: Elevated plasma lipid peroxide content correlates with rapid plasma clearance of all-*trans*-retinoic acid in patients with advanced cancer. Cancer Res 54:2125, 1994.

279. Agadir A, Cornic M, Lefebvre P et al: All-*trans* retinoic acid pharmacokinetics and bioavailability in acute promyelocytic leukemia: Intracellular concentrations and biologic response relationship. J Clin Oncol 13:2517, 1995.

280. Degos L, Chomienne C, Daniel MT et al: All-*trans*-retinoic acid treatment for patients with acute promyelocytic leukemia. In Saurat J-H (ed.): Retinoids: 10 Years On, p. 121. Karger, Basel, 1991.

281. Chen Z-X, Xue Y-Q, Zhang R et al: A clinical and experimental study on all-trans retinoic acid-treated acute promyelocytic leukemia patients. Blood 78:1413, 1991.

282. Vahdat L, Maslak P, Miller Jr W et al: Early mortality and the retinoic acid syndrome in acute promyelocytic leukemia: Impact of leukocytosis, low-dose chemotherapy, PML/RAR-α isoform, and CD13 expression in patients treated with all-*trans* retinoic acid. Blood 84:3843, 1994.

283. Fenaux P, Degos L: Treatment of acute promyelocytic leukemia with all trans retinoic acid. Leuk Res 8:655, 1991.

284. Fenaux P, Castaigne S, Dombret H et al: All-trans retinoic acid followed by intensive chemotherapy gives a high complete remission rate and may prolong remissions in newly diagnosed acute promyelocytic leukemia: A pilot study on 26 cases. Blood 80:2176, 1992.

285. Fenaux P, Le Deley MC, Castaigne S et al: Effect of all trans retinoic acid in newly diagnosed acute promyelocytic leukemia. Results of a multicenter randomized trial. Blood 82:3241, 1993.

286. Fenaux P, Chevret S, Guerci A et al: Long-term follow-up confirms the benefit of all-*trans* retinoic acid in acute promyelocytic leukemia. Leukemia 14:1371, 2000.

287. Kawai Y, Watanabe K, Kizaki M et al: Rapid improvement of coagulopathy by all-*trans* retinoic acid in acute promyelocytic leukemia. Am J Hematol 46:184, 1994.

288. Kanamaru A, Takemoto Y, Tanimoto M et al: All-*trans* retinoic acid for the treatment of newly diagnosed acute promyelocytic leukemia. Blood 85:1202, 1995.

289. Burnett AK, Grimwade D, Solomon E et al: Presenting white blood cell count and kinetics of molecular remission predict prognosis in acute promyelocytic leukemia treated with all-trans retinoic acid: Result of the randomized MRC trial. Blood 93:4131, 1999.

290. Estey E, Koller C, Cortes J et al: Treatment of newly-diagnosed acute promyelocytic leukemia with liposomal all-trans retinoic acid. Leuk Lymphoma 42:309, 2001.

291. Douer D, Estey E, Santillana S et al: Treatment of newly diagnosed and relapsed acute promyelocytic leukemia with intravenous liposomal all-trans retinoic acid. Blood 97:73, 2001.

292. Warrell RP Jr, Maslak P, Eardley A et al: Treatment of acute promyelocytic leukemia with all-trans retinoic acid: An update of the New York experience. Leukemia 8(Suppl. 2):S33, 1994.

293. Visani G, Tosi P, Cenacchi A et al: Pre-treatment with all-trans retinoic acid accelerates polymorphonuclear recovery after chemotherapy in patients with acute promyelocytic leukemia. Leuk Lymphoma 15:143, 1994.

294. Castaigne S, Lefebvre P, Chomienne C et al: Effectiveness and pharmacokinetics of low-dose all-trans retinoic acid (25 mg/m^2) in acute promyelocytic leukemia. Blood 82:3560, 1993.

295. Fenaux P, Chastang C, Chomienne C et al: Treatment of newly diagnosed acute promyelocytic leukemia (APL) by all transretinoic acid (ATRA) combined with chemotherapy: The European experience. Leuk Lymphoma 16:431, 1995.

296. Levin A, Sturzenbecker L, Kazmer S et al: 9-cis retinoic acid stereoisomer binds and activates the nuclear receptor RXRα. Nature 355:359, 1992.

297. Visani G, Zauli G, Ottaviani E et al: All-trans retinoic acid potentiates megakaryocyte colony formation: In vitro and in vivo effects after administration to acute promyelocytic leukemia patients. Leukemia 8:2183, 1994.

298. Visani G, Ottaviani E, Zauli G et al: All-*trans* retinoic acid at low concentration directly stimulates normal adult megakaryocytopoiesis in the presence of thrombopoietin or combined cytokines. Eur J Haematol 63:149, 1999.

299. Kini AR, Peterson LA, Tallman MS, Lingen MW: Angiogenesis in acute promyelocytic leukemia: Induction by vascular endothelial growth factor and inhibition by all-trans retinoic acid. Blood 97:3919, 2001.

300. Gianni M, Kalac Y, Ponzanelli I et al: Tyrosine kinase inhibitor STI571 potentiates the pharmacologic activity of retinoic acid in acute promyelocytic leukemia cells: Effects on the degradation of RARα and PML-RARα. Blood 97:3234, 2001.

301. Frankel SR, Eardley A, Lauwers G et al: The "retinoic acid syndrome" in acute promyelocytic leukemia. Ann Intern Med 117:292, 1992.

302. Tallman MS, Andersen JW, Schiffer CA et al: Clinical description of 44 patients with acute promyelocytic leukemia who developed the retinoic acid syndrome. Blood 95:90, 2000.

303. Griffin JD, Davis R, Nelson DA et al: Use of surface marker anaysis to predict outcome of adult acute myeloblastic leukemia. Blood 68:1232, 1986.

304. Saiki I, Fujii H, Yoneda J et al: Role of aminopeptidase N (CD13) in tumor cell invasion and extracellular matrix degeneration. Intl J Cancer 54:137, 1993.

305. Hakimian D, Tallman MS, Zugerman C et al: Erythema nodosum associated with all-trans retinoic acid in the treatment of acute promyelocytic leukemia. Leukemia 7:758, 1993.

306. Shirono K, Kiyofuji C, Tsuda H: Sweet's syndrome in a patient with acute promyelocytic leukemia during treatment with all-*trans* retinoic acid. Int J Hematol 62:183, 1995.

307. Christ E, Linka A, Jacky E et al: Sweet's syndrome involving the musculoskeletal system during treatment of promyelocytic leukemia with all-*trans* retinoic acid. Leukemia 10:731, 1996.

308. Torromeo C, Latagliata R, Avvisati G et al: Intraventricular thrombosis during all-*trans* retinoic acid treatment in acute promyelocytic leukemia. Leukemia 15:1311, 2000.

309. Losada R, Espinosa E, Hernandez C et al: Thrombocytosis in patients with acute promyelocytic leukaemia during all-*trans* retinoic acid treatment. Br J Haematol 95:704, 1996.

310. Kentos A, Le Moine F, Crenier L et al: All-*trans* retinoic acid induced thrombocytosis in a patient with acute promyelocytic leukaemia. Br J Haematol 97:685, 1997.

311. Dutcher JP, Wiernik PH, Markus S et al: Intensive maintenance therapy improves survival in adult acute nonlymphocytic leukemia: An eight-year follow-up. Leukemia 2:413, 1988.

312. Kantarjian HM, Keating MJ, Walters RS et al: Role of maintenance chemotherapy in acute promyelocytic leukemia. Cancer 59:1258, 1987.

313. Tallman MS, Andersen JW, Schiffer CA et al: All-trans retinoic acid in acute promyelocytic leukemia. N Engl J Med 337:1021, 1997.

314. Tallman MS, Andersen JW, Schiffer CA et al: All-trans retinoic acid in acute promyelocytic leukemia: Long-term outcome results and prognostic factor analysis from the North American Intergroup protocol. Blood 100:4298, 2002.

315. Fenaux P, Chastang C, Chevret S et al: A randomized comparison of all trans retinoic acid (ATRA) followed by chemotherapy and ATRA plus chemotherapy and the role of maintenance therapy in newly diagnosed acute promyelocytic leukemia. Blood 94:1192, 1999.

316. Sanz MA, Lo Coco F, Martin G et al: Definition of relapse risk and role of nonanthracycline drugs for consolidation in patients with acute promyelocytic leukemia: A joint study of the PETHEMA and GIMEMA cooperative groups. Blood 96:1247, 2000.

317. Lo Coco F, Diverio D, Avvisati G et al: Therapy of molecular relapse in acute promyelocytic leukemia. Blood 94:2225, 1999.

318. Cortes JE, Kantarjian H, O'Brien S et al: All-trans retinoic acid followed by chemotherapy for salvage of refractory or relapsed acute promyelocytic leukemia. Cancer 73:2946, 1994.

319. Miller WH Jr, Jakubowski A, Tong WP et al: 9-*cis* retinoic acid induces complete remission but does not reverse clinically acquired retinoid resistance in acute promyelocytic leukemia. Blood 85:3021, 1995.

320. Soignet SL, Benedetti F, Fleishauer A et al: Clinical study of 9-cis retinoic acid (LGD1057) in acute promyelocytic leeukemia. Leukemia 12:15118, 1998.

321. Takeshita A, Shibata Y, Shinjo K et al: Successful treatment of relapse of acute promyelocytic leukemia with a new synthetic retinoid, Am80. Ann Intern Med 124:893, 1996.

322. Tobita T, Takeshita A, Kitamura K et al: Treatment with a new synthetic retinoid, AM80, of acute promyelocytic leukemia relapsed from complete remission induced by all-*trans* retinoic acid. Blood 90:967, 1997.

323. Shinjo K, Takeshita A, Ohnishi K et al: Good prognosis of patients with acute promyelocytic leukemia who achieved second complete remission (CR) with a new retinoid, Am80, after relapse from CR induced by all-trans-retinoic acid. Int J Hematol 72:470, 2000.

324. Warrell RP Jr, He LZ, Richon V et al: Therapeutic targeting of transcription in acute promyelocytic leukemia by use of an inhibitor of histone deacetylase. J Natl Cancer Inst 90:1621, 1998.

325. Thomas X, Dombret H, Cordonnier C et al: Treatment of relapsing acute promyelocytic leukemia by all-*trans* retinoic acid therapy followed by timed sequential chemotherapy and stem cell transplantation. Leukemia 14:1006, 2000.

326. Jurcic JG, DeBlasio T, Dumont L et al: Molecular remission induction with retinoic acid and anti-CD33 monoclonal antibody HuM195 in acute promyelocytic leukemia. Clin Cancer Res 6:372, 2000.

327. Aulde J: A study of the pharmacology and therapeutics of arsenic. N Y Med J 53:390, 1891.

328. Shen ZX, Chen GQ, Ni JH et al: Use of arsenic trioxide (As2O3) in the treatment of acute promyelocytic leukemia (APL): II. Clinical efficacy and pharmacokinetics in relapsed patients. Blood 89:3354, 1997.

329. Soignet SL, Maslak P, Wang Z-G et al: Complete remission after treatment of acute promyelocytic leukemia with arsenic trioxide. N Engl J Med 339:1341, 1998.

330. Niu C, Yan H, Yu T et al: Studies on treatment of acute promyelocytic leukemia with arsenic trioxide: Remission induction, follow-up, and molecular monitoring in 11 newly diagnosed and 47 relapsed acute promyelocytic leukemia patients. Blood 94:3315, 1999.

331. Huang S-Y, Yang C-H, Chen Y-C: Arsenic trioxide therapy for relapsed acute promyelocytic leukemia: An (sic) useful salvage therapy. Leuk Lymphoma 38:283, 2000.

332. Camacho LH, Soignet SL, Chanel S et al: Leukocytosis and the retinoic acid syndrome in patients with acute promyelocytic leukemia treated with arsenic trioxide. J Clin Oncol 18:2620, 2000.

333. Lin C-P, Huang M-J, Chang IY et al: Retinoic acid syndrome induced by arsenic trioxide in treating recurrent all-trans retinoic acid resistant acute promyelocytic leukemia. Leuk Lymphoma 38:195, 2000.

334. Ohnishi K, Yoshida H, Shigeno K et al: Prolongation of the QT interval and ventricular tachycardia in patients treated with

arsenic trioxide for acute promyelocytic leukemia. Ann Intern Med 133:881, 2000.

335. Unnikrishnan D, Dutcher JP, Varshneya N et al: Torsades de pointes in 3 patients with leukemia treated with arsenic trioxide. Blood 97:1514, 2001.

336. Westervelt P, Brown RA, Adkins DR et al: Sudden death among patients with acute promyelocytic leukemia treated with arsenic trioxide. Blood 98:266, 2001.

337. Kwong YL, Au WY, Chim CS et al: Arsenic trioxide- and idarubicin-induced remissions in relapsed acute promyelocytic leukemia: Clinicopathological and molecular features of a pilot study. Am J Hematol 66:274, 2001.

338. Jing Y, Wang L, Xia L et al: Combined effects of all-trans retinoic acid and arsenic trioxide in acute promyelocytic leukemia cells in vitro and in vivo. Blood 97:264, 2001.

339. Muto A, Kizaki M, Kawamura C et al: A novel differentiation-inducing therapy for acute promyelocytic leukemia with a combination of arsenic trioxide and GM-CSF. Leukemia 15:1176, 2001.

340. Stentoft J, Nielsen JL, Hvidman LE: All-trans retinoic acid in acute promyelocytic leukemia in late pregnancy. Leukemia 8:1585, 1994.

341. Harrison P, Chipping P, Fothergill GA: Successful use of all-trans retinoic acid in acute promyelocytic leukaemia presenting during the second trimester of pregnancy. Br J Haematol 86:681, 1994.

342. Lipovsky MM, Biesma DH, Christiaens GCML et al: Successful treatment of acute promyelocytic leukaemia with all-*trans*-retinoic-acid during late pregnancy. Br J Haematol 94:699, 1996.

343. Giagounidis AAN, Beckmann MW, Giagoundidis AS et al: Acute promyelocytic leukemia and pregnancy. Eur J Haematol 64:267, 2000.

344. Hoffman MA, Wiernik PH, Kleiner GJ: Acute promyelocytic leukemia and pregnancy. A case report. Cancer 76:2237, 1995.

345. Tallman MS, Kwaan HC: Reassessing the hemostatic disorder associated with acute promyelocytic leukemia. Blood 79:543, 1992.

346. Barbui T, Finazzi G, Falanga A: The impact of all-trans-retinoic acid on the coagulopathy of acute promyelocytic leukemia. Blood 91:3093, 1998.

347. Gralnick HR, Bagley J, Abrell E: Heparin treatment for the hemorrhagic diathesis of acute promyelocyte leukemia. Am J Med 52:167, 1972.

348. Jones ME, Saleem A: Acute promyelocytic leukemia: A review of the literature. Am J Med 65:673, 1978.

349. Cordonnier C, Vernant JP, Brun B et al: Acute promyelocytic leukemia in 57 previously untreated patients. Cancer 55:18, 1985.

350. Kantarjian HM, Keating MJ, Walters RS et al: Acute promyelocytic leukemia: The MD Anderson Hospital experience. Am J Med 80:789, 1986.

351. Cunningham I, Gee TS, Reich LM et al: Acute promyelocytic leukemia: Treatment results during a decade at Memorial Hospital. Blood 72:1116, 1989.

352. Rodeghiero F, Avvisati G, Castaman G et al: Early deaths and antihemorrhagic treatments in acute promyelocytic leukemia. A GIMEMA retrospective study of 268 consecutive patients. Blood 75:2112, 1990.

353. Head D, Kopecky KJ, Weick J et al: Effect of aggressive daunomycin therapy on survival in acute promyelocytic leukemia. Blood 86:1717, 1995.

354. Goldberg MA, Ginsburg D, Mayer RJ et al: Is heparin administration necessary during induction chemotherapy for patients with acute promyelocytic leukemia? Blood 69:187, 1987.

355. Bennett JM, Young ML, Andersen JW et al: Long-term survival in acute myeloid leukemia: The Eastern Cooperative Oncology Group Experience. Cancer 80:2205, 1997.

356. Dombret H, Scrobohaci ML, Zini JM et al: Coagulation disorders associated with acute promyelocytic leukemia: Corrective effect of all-trans retinoic acid treatment. Leukemia 7:2, 1993.

357. Watanabe R, Murata M, Takayama N et al: Long-term follow-up of hemostatic molecular markers during remission induction therapy with all-trans retinoic acid for acute promyelocytic leukemia. Keio Hematology-Oncology Cooperative Study Group (KHOCS). Thromb Haemost 77:641, 1997.

358. Kawai Y, Watanabe K, Kizaki M et al: Rapid improvement of coagulopathy by all-trans retinoic acid in acute promyelocytic leukemia. Am J Hematol 46:184, 1994.

359. Dombret H, Scrobohaci ML, Daniel MT et al: In vivo thrombin and plasmin activities in patients with acute promyelocytic leukemia (APL): Effect of all-trans retinoic acid (ATRA) therapy. Leukemia 9:19, 1995.

360. Zhang P, Wang Sy, Hu XH: Arsenic trioxide treated 72 cases of acute promyelocytic leukemia. Chin J Hematol 16:26, 1995.

361. Shen ZX, Chen GQ, Ni JH et al: Use of arsenic trioxide (As_2O_3) in the treatment of acute promyelocytic leukemia (APL): II. Clinical efficacy and pharmacokinetics in relapsed patients. Blood 89:3354, 1997.

362. Sanz MA, Jarque I, Martin G et al: Acute promyelocytic leukemia. Therapy results and prognostic factors. Cancer 61:7, 1988.

363. Petti MC, Avvisati G, Amadori S et al: Acute promyelocytic leukemia: Clinical aspects and results of treatment in 62 patients. Haematologica 72:151, 1987.

364. Fenaux P, Pollet JP, Vandenbossche-Simon L et al: Treatment of acute promyelocytic leukemia: A report of 70 cases. Leuk Lymphoma 4:239, 1990.

365. Fenaux P, Tertian G, Castaigne S et al: A randomized trial of amsacrine and rubidazone in 39 patients with acute promyelocytic leukemia. J Clin Oncol 9:1556, 1991.

366. Gralnick HR, Sultan, C: Acute promyelocytic leukemia: Hemorrhagic manifestations and morphologic criteria. Br J Haematol 29:373, 1975.

367. Groopman J, Ellman L: Acute promyelocytic leukemia. Am J Hematol 7:395, 1979.

368. Collins AJ, Bloomfield CD, Peterson BA et al: Acute promyelocytic leukemia: Management of the coagulopathy during daunorubicin-prednisone remission induction. Arch Int Med 138:1677, 1978.

369. Bennett B, Booth NA, Croll A, Dawson AA: The bleeding disorder in acute promyelocytic leukemia: Fibrinolysis due to u-PA rather than defibrination. Br J Haematol 71:511, 1989.

370. Bennett M, Parker AC, Ludlam CA: Platelet and fibrinogen survival in acute promyelocytic leukemia. Br Med J 2:565, 1976.

371. Nemerson Y: Tissue factor and hemostasis. Blood 71:1, 1988.

372. Bauer KA, Conway EM, Bach R et al: Tissue factor gene expression in acute myeloblastic leukemia. Thromb Res 50:425, 1989.

373. Andoh K, Sadakata H, Uchiyama T et al: One-stage method for assay of tissue factor activity of leukemic cells with special reference to disseminated intravascular coagulation. Am J Clin Pathol 93:679, 1990.

374. Kubota T, Andoh T, Sadakata H et al: Tissue factor released from leukemic cells. Thromb Haemost 65:59, 1991.

375. Gordon SG, Franks JJ, Lewis B: Cancer procoagulant A: A factor X activating procoagulant from malignant tissue. Thromb Res 6:127, 1975.

376. Falanga A, Gordon SG: Isolation and characterization of cancer procoagulant A: A cystine proteinase from malignant tissue. Biochem 24:5558, 1985.

377. Donati MB, Falanga A, Consonni R et al: Cancer procoagulant in acute nonlymphoid leukemia: Relationship of enzyme detection to disease activity. Thromb Haemost 64:11, 1990.

378. Bevilacqua MP, Pober JS, Majeau GR et al: Interleukin-1 expression activity of procoagulant activity in human vascular endothelia cells. J Exp Med 160:618, 1984.

379. Bevilacqua MP, Pober JS, Majeau GR et al: Recombinant human tissue necrosis factor induces procoagulant activity in cultured human vascular endothelium. Characterization and comparison with interleukin-1. Proc Natl Acad Sci USA 83:4533, 1986.

380. Nawroth PP, Handley D, Esmon CT, Stern DM: Interleukin-1 induces cell surface anticoagulant activity. Proc Natl Acad Sci USA 83:3460, 1986.

381. Nawroth PP, Stern MD: Modulation of endothelial cell hemostatic properties by tumor necrosis factor. J Exp Med 163:740, 1986.

382. Clauss M, Gerlach M, Gerlach H et al: Vascular permeability factor: A tumor-derived polypeptide that induces endothelial cell and monocyte procoagulant activity and promotes monocyte migration. J Exp Med 172:1535, 1990.

383. Cozzolino F, Torcia M, Miliani A et al: Potential role of interleukin-1 as the trigger for diffuse intravascular coagulation in acute nonlymphoblastic leukemia. Am J Med 84:240, 1988.

384. Emeis JJ, Koastra T: Interleukin-1 and lipopolysaccharides induce an inhibitor of plasminogen activator in vivo and in human cultured endothelial cells. J Exp Med 163:1260, 1986.

385. Nachman RL, Hajjar KA, Silverstein RL, Dinarello CA: Interleukin-1 induces endothelial cell synthesis of plasminogen activator inhibitor. J Exp Med 163:1595, 1996.

386. Miyauchi S, Morohama T, Kyoizumi S et al: Malignant tumor cell lines produce interleukin-1-like factor in vivo. In Vitro Cell Dev Biol 24:753, 1988.

387. Noguchi M, Sakai T, Kisiel W: Identification and partial purification of novel tumor-derived protein that induces tissue factor in cultured human endothelial cells. Biochem Biophys Res Commun 160:222, 1989.

388. Chan TK, Chan GT, Chan V: Hypofibrinogenemia due to increased fibrinolysis in two patients with acute promyelocytic leukemia. Aust NZ J Med 14:245, 1984.

389. Sterrenberg L, Haak HL, Brommer EJP, Nieuwenhuizen W: Evidence of fibrinogen breakdown by leukocyte enzymes in a patient with acute promyelocytic leukemia. Haemostasis 15:126, 1985.

390. Schwartz BS, Williams EC, Conlan MG, Mosher DF: Epsilon-aminocaproic acid in the treatment of patients with acute promyelocytic leukemia and acquired alpha-2-plasmin inhibitor deficiency. Ann Intern Med 105:873, 1986.

391. Velasco F, Torres A, Andres P et al: Changes in plasma levels of protease and fibrinolytic inhibitors induced by treatment of acute promyelocytic leukemia. Thromb Haemost 52:81, 1984.

392. Wilson EL, Jacobs P, Dowdle EB: The secretion of plasminogen activators by human myeloid leukemia cells in vitro. Blood 61:568, 1983.

393. Sakata Y, Murakami T, Noro A et al: The specific activity of plasminogen activator inhibitor-1 in disseminated intravascular coagulation with acute promyelocytic leukemia. Blood 77:1949, 1991.

394. Hirata F, Schiffman E, Venkatasubramanian K et al: A phospholipase A_2 inhibitory protein in rabbit neutrophils induced by glucocorticoids. Proc Natl Acad Sci USA 77:2533, 1980.

395. Chang KS, Wang G, Freireich EJ et al: Specific expression of the annexin VIII gene in acute promyelocytic leukemia. Blood 79:1802, 1992.

396. Hajjar KA, Jacovina AT, Chacko J: An endothelial cell receptor for plasminogen/tissue plasminogen activator. I. Identity with annexin II. J Biol Chem 269:21191, 1994.

397. Menell JS, Cesarman GM, Jacovina AT et al: Annexin II and bleeding in acute promyelocytic leukemia. N Engl J Med 340:994, 1999.

398. Federici AR, Diamico EA: The role of von Willebrand factor in the hemostatic defect of acute promyelocytic leukemia. Leuk Lymphoma 31:491, 1998.

399. Runde V, Aul C, Heyll A, Schneider W: All-trans retinoic acid: Not only a differentiating agent, but also an inducer of thromboembolic events in patients with M_3 leukemia. Blood 79:534, 1992.

400. Escudier SM, Kantarjian HM, Estey EH: Thrombosis in patients with acute promyelocytic leukemia treated with and without all-trans retinoic acid. Leuk Lymphoma 20:435, 1996.

401. Hashimoto S, Koike T, Tatewaki W et al: Fatal thromboembolism in acute promyelocytic leukemia during all-trans retinoic acid therapy combined with antifibrinolytic therapy as prophylaxis of hemorrhage. Leukemia 8:1113, 1994.

402. Ishii H, Horie S, Kizaki K, Kazama M: Retinoic acid counteracts both the down-regulation of thrombomodulin and the induction of tissue factor in cultured human endothelial cells exposed to tumor necrosis factor. Blood 80:2556, 1992.

403. Rickles FR, Hair G, Schmeizel M et al: All-trans-retinoic (ATRA) inhibits the expression of tissue factor in human progranulocytic. (Abstr) Haemost Thromb 69:107, 1993.

404. Falanga A, Iacoviello L, Evangelista V et al: Loss of blast cell procoagulant activity and improvement of hemostatic variables in patients with acute promyelocytic leukemia administered all-trans-retinoic acid. Blood 86:1072, 1995.

405. De Stefano V, Teofili L, Sica S et al: Effect of all-trans retinoic acid on procoagulant and fibrinolytic activities of cultured blast cells from patients with acute promyelocytic leukemia. Blood 86:3535, 1995.

406. Medh R, Santell L, Levin EG: Stimulation of tissue plasminogen activator production by retinoic acid: Synergistic effect on protein kinase c-mediated activation. Blood 80:981, 1992.

407. Lansink M, Kooistra T: Stimulation of tissue-type plasminogen activator expression by retinoic acid in human endothelial cells retinoic acid receptor β2 induction. Blood 88:531, 1996.

408. Falanga A, Consom R, Marchetti M et al: Cancer procoagulant in the human promyelocytic cell line NB4 and its modulation by all-trans retinoic acid. Leukemia 8:156, 1994.

409. Tallman MS, Lefebrvre P, Cohen I et al: Procoagulant, profibrinolytic and proinflammatory mediators in patients with previously untreated acute promyelocytic leukemia (APL). (Abstr) Blood 86:675, 1995.

410. Fenaux P, Le Deley MC, Castaigne S et al: Effect of all-trans retinoic acid in newly diagnosed acute promyelocytic leukemia: Results of a multicenter randomized trial. Blood 82:3241, 1993.

411. Fenaux P, Chastang C, Chevret S et al: A randomized comparison of all trans-retinoic acid (ATRA) followed by chemotherapy and ATRA plus chemotherapy and the role of maintenance therapy in newly diagnosed acute promyelocytic leukemia. The European APL Group. Blood 94:1192, 1999.

412. Tallman MS, Andersen JW, Schiffer CA et al: All-trans retinoic acid in acute promyelocytic leukemia. N Engl J Med 337:1021, 1997.

413. Burnett AK, Goldstone AH, Gray RG, Wheatley K: All trans retinoic acid given concurrently with induction chemotherapy improves the outcome of APL: Results of the UK MRC ATRA trial. (Abstr) Blood 90:1474, 1997.

414. Avvisati G: AIDA Protocol: The Italian way of treating APL. (Abstr) Br J Haematol 102:593a, 1998.

415. Asou N, Adachi K, Tamura J et al: Analysis of prognostic factors in newly diagnosed acute promyelocytic leukemia treated with all-trans retinoic acid and chemotherapy. J Clin Oncol 16:78, 1998.

416. Sanz MA, Martin G, Rayon C et al: A modified AIDA protocol with anthracycline-based consolidation results in high antileukemic efficacy and reduced toxicity in newly diagnosed PML/RAR-alpha-positive acute promyelocytic leukemia. Blood 94:3015, 1999.

417. Di Bona E, Avvisati G, Castaman G et al: Early haemorrhagic morbidity and mortality during remission induction with or without all-trans retinoic acid in acute promyelocytic leukaemia. Br J Haematol 108:689, 2000.

418. Zhu J, Guo WM, Yao YY et al: Tissue factors on acute promyelocytic leukemia and endothelial cells are differently regulated by retinoic acid, arsenic trioxide and chemotherapeutic agents. Leukemia 13:1062, 1999.

419. Slack JL, Rusiniak ME: Current issues in the management of acute promyelocytic leukemia. Ann Hematol 79:227, 2000.

420. Avvisati G, Lo Coco F, Mandelli F: Acute promyelocytic leukemia: Clinical and morphologic features and prognostic factors. Semin Hematol 38:4, 2001.

421. Fenaux P, Chomienne C, Degos L: All-trans retinoic acid and chemotherapy in the treatment of acute promyelocytic leukemia. Semin Hematol 38:13, 2001.

22

Therapy-Related Acute Myelogenous Leukemia

Dorothy J. Park and H. Phillip Koeffler

Therapy-related acute myelogenous leukemia (t-AML) is a recognizable subclass of acute myelogenous leukemia (AML). Features of the syndrome include a preleukemic phase several years after chemotherapy and/or radiation therapy for a primary disease, distinct chromosomal abnormalities in the preleukemic and leukemic cells, and a short survival after the development of leukemia. Therapy-related leukemia has become increasingly common, accounting for 10 to 20 percent of all AMLs. The accelerating incidence can be partly attributed to a variety of factors including longer survival of individuals after successful treatment of their primary malignancy associated with the increasing use of more intensive chemotherapy and/or radiation therapy including hematopoietic stem cell transplantation, frequent use of adjuvant chemotherapy, exposure to various environmental toxins, and greater awareness of this particular diagnosis (Table 22–1). Because of a poor response to therapy, t-AML and therapy-related myelodysplastic syndrome (t-MDS) are among the most feared long-term complications of cancer therapy today.

Nomenclature for the syndrome has not been clearly established. Such terms as therapy- or treatment-related leukemia are descriptive because patients previously received chemo- or radiation therapy, or both, for a primary disease. These terms are restrictive because the leukemia that develops after exposure to either benzene or several other occupational mutagens is very similar, if not identical, to the therapy-related leukemia syndrome. The term secondary leukemia correctly denotes that the disease did not develop spontaneously or de novo. The term is too broad, however, because a number of pathways, including genetic predisposition, probably lead to the development of AML. We favor the term *mutagen-related leukemia* because it accurately reflects the fact that the individuals had prior exposure to a mutagen.

CLINICAL AND LABORATORY FEATURES

Many of the clinical and laboratory features of t-MDS and t-AML are similar to MDS and AML when they occur de novo. Most of these individuals experience various symptoms of bone marrow failure at diagnosis, such as fatigue, weakness, and fever. Nearly all affected individuals show physical signs of anemia, such as pallor and exertional dyspnea. Signs of thrombocytopenia, bruising, and hemorrhage are also relatively common, as are signs of infection. Less frequently, patients may have clinical manifestations of hepatomegaly, splenomegaly, lymphadenopathy, gingival hypertrophy, skin infiltration, and neurological abnormalities.

Preleukemic Phase

A preleukemic or myelodysplastic phase occurs in over 70 percent of patients in whom AML develops following chemotherapy and/or radiation therapy for another disease,[1–9] whereas about 20 percent of patients with de novo AML have a similar preleukemic phase (Table 22–2). Indeed, the data suggest that a preleukemic period can be observed in nearly all patients with therapy-related leukemia when these patients are monitored closely. Exceptions are those individuals in whom t-AML develops after therapy with epipodophyllotoxins (VP16 and VM26) or other DNA-topoisomerase II inhibitors. In these patients, t-AML often develops with no preleukemic phase.[10,11] The mean duration of the preleukemic phase is 11.2 months in typical t-AML. The preleukemic phase in individuals with "de novo" MDS who go on to develop AML is similar, about 14 months.[2,3,9]

The clinical manifestation of the preleukemic phase in t-AML is marked by ineffective hematopoiesis. The bone marrow morphology is characterized by trilineage dysplasia. The degree of dysplasia is usually very prominent. Even in patients with a bone marrow that satisfies French-American-British (FAB) classification criteria for either refractory anemia (RA) or refractory anemia with ringed sideroblasts (RARS), the degree of dysplasia is often closer to the bone marrow of patients with refractory anemia with excess blasts (RAEB) or refractory anemia with excess blasts in transformation (RAEB-t). Therefore, application of the FAB classification to t-MDS has been difficult. Nevertheless, the RAEB and RAEB-t subgroups are more frequent in t-MDS (73 percent) than in de novo MDS (53 percent).[12]

Prominent abnormalities are observed in the red blood cells (RBCs) and their precursors. Most patients show decreased red cell production with low reticulocyte counts.[4] Oval macrocytosis and nucleated red cells are often the earliest recognizable changes observed in the peripheral blood in the preleukemic phase.[13] Macrocytosis after therapy for Hodgkin's disease was

---

Table 22–1. Risk Factors for Mutagen-Related Leukemia

Alkylating agent therapy
DNA-topoisomerase II inhibitor therapy (epipodophyllotoxins and anthracyclines)
Intense therapy
  High doses of chemotherapy for prolonged periods as in therapy for Hodgkin's disease and non-Hodgkin's lymphoma
  Direct correlation between intensity of original therapy and latency period to development of myelodysplasia
High energy β-emitters: ^{32}P for polycythemia rubra vera
Occupational exposure: benzene, xylene

Table 22–2. Comparison of Therapy-Related and De Novo Acute Myelogenous Leukemia

Therapy-Related AML	De Novo AML
1. Frequent preleukemic phase (70 percent)	1. Less frequent preleukemic phase (20 percent)
2. Frequent chromosomal abnormality (80 to 90 percent); especially −5/5q− and/or −7/7q−	2. Chromosomal abnormality less frequent, especially + 8, −7, t(8,21), and t(15,17)
3. Hypodiploid modal number of chromosomes most common; often complex chromosomal abnormalities	3. Diploid or hyperdiploid modal number of chromosomes (95 percent)
4. Refractory to antileukemic therapy (80 percent)	4. Remission induced by antileukemic therapy (75 percent)
5. Short survival after leukemia diagnosis (mean 4 to 6 months)	5. Longer survival after leukemia diagnosis (mean 20 months)

retrospectively found to be associated with a high risk of the development of leukemia.[14] Mild neutropenia is present in 75 percent of the individuals.[4] Neutrophils may be poorly granulated, and their nuclei can be hyposegmented (pseudo-Pelger-Hüet anomaly).[15] Thrombocytopenia occurs in approximately 60 percent of patients,[4] and they may be abnormally large and degranulated. Both the neutrophils and platelets can have a variety of qualitative defects.

The bone marrow is often hypercellular, although hypo- and normocellular marrow can occur. Erythroid hyperplasia, megaloblastoid features, and occasionally ringed sideroblasts dominate the marrow picture.[15–17] Abnormalities of the marrow granulocytic and megakaryocytic series are usually more subtle. Micromegakaryocytes may be seen, particularly with monosomy 7. The percentage of immature granulocytic and megakaryocytic cells may be increased. The primary and specific granules of the granulocyte precursors occasionally are either deficient or abnormally large. Marrow fibrosis often is present during the preleukemic phase.

In summary, the development of unexplained pancytopenia and the finding of karyotypic abnormalities in the marrow cells of patients who received chemotherapy and/or radiation therapy for another disease is pathognomonic of preleukemia. Evolution to overt leukemia is universal if the preleukemic individual survives the complications of hemorrhage and infection. t-MDS can be viewed as an early phase of t-AML in which the malignant hematopoietic clone is established and becomes predominant.

Acute Leukemia Phase

Clinical manifestations of individuals with t-AML are typical of bone marrow failure, and their clinical course is rapidly fatal often from complications of bleeding and infection. The bone marrow morphology of t-AML can be difficult to classify according to FAB criteria for AML, as most of the leukemias demonstrate trilineage involvement and appear to bridge several subtypes. Nevertheless, the blast cells of patients with t-AML most often are myeloblastic in appearance (FAB M1, M2). A lower frequency of acute monocytic forms of leukemia has been reported in several studies (FAB M4, M5) as compared to de novo AML.[8,18]

Auer rods are rarely observed in the blast cells in t-AML, but are seen in blast cells of 35 percent of patients with de novo AML. Many of the blast cells in t-AML lack myeloperoxidase and other granulocyte-specific enzymes. In one series, only one of ten patients with secondary leukemia had more than 10 percent peroxidase-positive blast cells compared with nearly 100 percent peroxidase-positive blast cells in 95 percent of patients with de novo leukemia.[18] In addition, less than 20 percent of the t-AML patients have either greater than or equal to 10 percent naphthol ASD chloroacetate esterase-positive blast cells compared with 47 percent of patients with de novo leukemia. These histochemical data suggest that the leukemic cells from secondary leukemia patients are blocked at an earlier stage of differentiation than the leukemic cells from most de novo leukemia patients.

Karyotypic Abnormalities in t-MDS/t-AML

Clonal chromosomal abnormalities can be detected in the blast cells of 80 to 95 percent of t-MDS/t-AML patients by currently available techniques.[1,5,6,8,19–21] Although the same abnormalities have been reported in primary MDS/AML, their frequency is clearly higher in t-MDS/t-AML (Table 22–2). A hypodiploid modal number of chromosomes occurs most frequently in t-MDS/t-AML patients. Hyperdiploidy, mainly trisomy 8 is rare and is often observed as an inconsistent aberration present in only a subclone of cells.[20] The most common abnormalities are losses of all or part of chromosomes 5 and/or 7, especially in patients previously treated with high doses of alkylating agents.[19,22–24] Review of the literature demonstrates that more than 70 percent of the patients have lost either part or all of chromosome 5 and/or 7 and that these patients have an extremely short survival. In a recently updated series from University of Chicago of 257 patients with t-MDS/t-AML, 94 percent had a clonal abnormality, and 71 percent had abnormalities involving chromosomes 5 and/or 7. Other recurring abnormalities (14.7 percent) included t(11q23), t(3;21), t(8;21), t(21q22), t(15;17), +8, inv(16), −13, del(13q), del(20q), del(11q), +11, +21, and −Y. Although the same recurring chromosome abnormalities occur in de novo AML, their frequency of specific changes is clearly different. Chromosome 5 or 7 abnormalities occur much less frequently (20 percent) in de novo AML.

Chromosomes 5q and 7q probably contain critical myeloid tumor suppressor genes. The breakpoints for the deletions are variable, but a common chromosome region, the so-called critical region, is almost always deleted. The critical region for 7q deletions involves a region at band 7q22 proximally, with the distal breakpoint varying from q32 to q36.[25–27] Potentially important genes have been mapped to 7q, including those for erythropoietin, p glycoprotein/multiple drug resistance-1

(MDR-1), and MDR-3.[28] However, none has yet been shown to be implicated in development of t-MDS/t-AML. Le Beau et al.[29] delineated the critical region for chromosome 5 (i.e., 5q31.1), which includes the early growth response gene (EGR-1).[29] Other important proteins encoded in the region of 5q31 include macrophage colony-stimulating factor (M-CSF), its receptor (FMS or M-CSFR), granulocyte-macrophage colony-stimulating factor (GM-CSF), and interleukins-3, -4, and -5 (IL-3, -4, -5).[19,30-33] The loss or abnormal regulation of these proteins could certainly contribute to hematopoietic dysregulation. However, no evidence implicates these proteins. Although most of the chromosomal abnormalities reported in t-MDS/t-AML are either monosomy 7 and/or 5, or del(7q) and/or del(5q), in recent years recurring unbalanced translocations that also result in loss of the long arm of 7 and/or 5 have been reported with increasing frequency. These include t(1;7)(p11;q11), t(5;7)(q11.2;p11.2), and t(7;17)(p11;p11) for chromosome 7, and t(5;7)(q11.2;p11.2) and t(5;17)(p11;p11) for chromosome 5.[34] While the loss of function of a single gene in each of these relatively large regions is possibly responsible for the development of t-MDS/t-AML, hemizygous loss of the function of several genes in each of these regions could also contribute to the disease phenotype. Another, not mutually exclusive hypothesis is that an unknown initiating abnormality causes genomic instability leading to the deletion and rearrangement of particularly susceptible chromosome regions, such as those on chromosome 5q and 7q. Cytogenetic studies have shown that progressive instability of these regions occurs during disease progression.

A review of 431 cases of secondary leukemia found 16 nonrandom chromosomal changes involving chromosomes 3, 5, 7, 8, 9, 11, 14, 17, and 21. These changes were dependent on the type of primary disease, previous therapy, age, and sex.[35] In another single institution study consisting of 63 patients, additional abnormalities in chromosomes 1, 4, 5, 7, 12, 14, and 18 occurred, with significantly increased frequency of these changes in t-AML as compared to de novo AML.[19]

Abnormalities in chromosome 17, especially translocations involving bands 17p11-p13 and 17q21 are occasionally observed in t-AML, for example, t(15;17)(q22;q11–21).[23,24] Other chromosomes often reported to be abnormal in t-MDS/t-AML are chromosomes 21 and 11, particularly involving balanced translocations of chromosome bands 11q23 and 21q22 in t-AML [i.e., t(4;11), t(6;11), t(9;11), t(11;19), t(3;21), and t(8;21)].[20,34-36] These translocations are associated with previous therapy targeting DNA-topoisomerase II, primarily the epipodophyllotoxins and the anthracyclines. The 11q23 reciprocal translocations and interstitial deletions structurally interrupt a small region of the MLL (also known as HRX, ALL-1, HTRX1) gene that codes for a human homolog of the Drosophila trithorax gene.[37,38] A fragment of the MLL gene translocates to one of at least 30 other chromosomal regions, resulting in the creation of a fusion protein with the partner gene.[39,40]

In addition to balanced translocations involving chromosome bands 11q23 and 21q22, other balanced aberrations such as inv(16), t(8;16), t(15;17), and t(6;9) have been observed in t-AML after previous therapy with drugs targeting DNA topoiso-

merase II (Table 22–3).[20,34] In contrast, the unbalanced rearrangements of the same two bands, 11q23 and 21q22, were most often associated with therapy with alkylating agents alone or in combination with radiation therapy.[36] Translocations to chromosome band 11q23 predominate in children with t-AML after therapy with the epipodophyllotoxins for acute lymphocytic leukemia (ALL).[10] In Chinese patients treated for psoriasis with bimolane, t(15;17) has been frequently reported. Also, therapy with doxorubicin has been associated with an increased incidence of t-AML with balanced translocations at chromosome band 21q22, in particular t(3;21).[20,35]

Chromosome studies have shown that when t-MDS becomes clinically diagnosable, the preleukemic clone represents a majority of the hematopoietic cells.[1,8,19] Additional chromosomal abnormalities occur in the original abnormal clone in 60 to 70 percent of cases as the disease evolves to frank leukemia.[41,42] Karyotypic evolution usually involves further deletions or losses of chromosomes and a change to a lower modal chromosome number; rarely, the evolution is associated with a gain of chromosome 8. Evidence suggests that t-MDS patients who have a mixture of karyotypically normal and abnormal cells (AN) survive longer than those who have only abnormal cells (AA).[43] Most individuals who are AN in the preleukemic phase become AA as the disease progresses.[19]

LATENCY AND RISK OF THERAPY-RELATED LEUKEMIA

The increased incidence of acute leukemia following the treatment of Hodgkin's disease was first observed in the early 1970s. Numerous studies have since clearly shown that chemotherapy or radiation therapy, or both, for the primary disease is strongly linked to an elevated risk of acute leukemia. However, the incidence and risk of t-MDS/t-AML remain difficult to estimate and highly variable between different studies and different primary diseases. This variability is due in part to cohort differences in age, duration, intensity, and the types of treatment, as well as the rigor of the follow-up. Nonetheless, the problem is considerable and is likely to increase, as we are more successful in treating various malignancies.

Median latency to the development of t-MDS/t-AML reported over the last 20 years has been quite consistent among

---

Table 22–3. Features of Therapy-Related Acute Myelogenous Leukemia Associated with Prior Exposure to DNA-Topoisomerase II Inhibitors

Short median latency period (33 months)
Frequently no preleukemic phase; if preleukemic phase, it rapidly evolves to acute leukemia
Morphologic phenotype often M4/M5 by FAB classification
Chromosomal abnormalities usually do not involve chromosome 5 and/or 7, but often occur at chromosome 11q23 or 21q22
Response to cytotoxic therapy similar to de novo AML, according to karyotypic abnormalities

studies, about 4 to 5 years after chemotherapy and/or radiation therapy for a primary disease.[36] The incidence is highest between 24 and 60 months after therapy, declining steadily thereafter.

The risk of developing t-AML depends on the type of treatment. Chemotherapy either with or without radiation therapy carries a higher risk, and radiation therapy alone carries the smallest risk. Total body irradiation is riskier than high dose, limited-field therapy. A positive correlation exists between the intensity of therapy given to an individual or experimental animal and their risk of developing leukemia. An inverse correlation may exist between the amount of therapy given to an individual and their latency period for development of secondary leukemia. For example, those who received the largest amount of alkylating agents[44–47] or etoposide[10,11,48,49] had the greatest risk of t-AML.

Although not the subject of this chapter, the incidence of several nonleukemic neoplasms, such as non-Hodgkin's lymphoma (NHL), breast cancer, lung cancer, and others, is clearly increased in individuals who received therapy for another disease.[50–52] The heavily irradiated survivors of Hiroshima and Nagasaki had an increased incidence of chronic myelogenous leukemia (CML) and ALL, as well as AML.[53] Curiously, only rare reports have associated the development of CML with prior exposure to chemotherapy, benzene, or other industrial toxins. This finding suggests a different pathogenesis of CML

compared with therapy-related leukemia. Likewise, the incidence of solid tumors was not increased in multiple myeloma patients who received alkylating agents.[52] The assessment of risk of leukemia in relationship to type of primary disease is not available. One composite report suggests that the leading disease categories associated with t-AML are Hodgkin's disease, multiple myeloma, NHL, and breast and ovarian cancer (appearing in order of frequency). The risk of leukemia, however, is related more to the type of therapy given for the primary disease than to the category of primary disease.

Hodgkin's Disease

Leukemia that follows treatment of Hodgkin's disease has been the most studied t-MDS/t-AML (Table 22–4).[54–68] The expected occurrence of AML is two to three per year in a general population of 100,000 individuals of all age groups.[69] The actuarial risk of t-MDS/t-AML is 3 to 4 percent at 9 to 10 years after intensive chemotherapy and/or radiation therapy for Hodgkin's disease.[70] This represents about a 100- to 200-fold increase in the ratio of observed to expected frequency of leukemia.[70] Most of these cases occurred within 2 to 10 years following therapy for Hodgkin's disease, with a median latency of 4 to 6 years and a plateau of leukemia incidence after 10 years. In general, most of the studies showed either no or little risk of developing t-MDS/t-AML with radiation therapy alone,

Table 22–4. t-MDS/t-AML Following the Treatment of Hodgkin's Disease

Investigators	No. of Patients	Median Follow-Up (Years)	No. With t-AML	Relative Risk (95 Percent Confidence Interval)	Absolute Risk[a]	Actuarial Risk Percent	Actuarial Risk Years	Median Latency (Range)
Devereux et al. (1990)[62]	2676	NS	17[b]	NS	NS	1.7	15	79.9 months (35–155)
Kaldor et al. (1990)[57,c]	29,552	NS	149[b]	RT 1.0 CT 9.0 (4.1–20) RT + CT 7.7 (3.9–15)	NS	NS		NS
Cimino et al. (1991)[55]	947	10.5	23	NS	NS	2.8 3.6 10.0	10 15 19	58 months (13–209)
Abrahamsen et al. (1993)[59]	1152	8	9	24.3 (11.1–46.2)	10.4	1.5	18	5.8 years
Swerdlow et al. (1993)[60]	2846	6.1	16	16.0 (9.2–26.0)	8.7	NS		NS
Dietrich et al. (1994)[61]	892	NS	8	27.59 (11.91–54)	15	1.7 1.7	10 15	NS
van Leeuwen et al. (1994)[56]	1939	9.2	31[d] (12 MDS)	34.7 (23.6–49.3) 48.2 (34.9–64.9)[e]	18.1	4.0[e]	20	NS
Bhatia et al. (1996)[66]	1380	11.4	26	NS	NS	2.8	14	NS
Mauch et al. (1996)[67]	794	11	8	66.2 (28.1–130.7)	9.3	NS		5 years
Wolden et al. (1998)[68]	694	13.1	8	40.9 (17.7–80.7)	9.3	NS		4.3 years

Abbreviations: NS, not stated; RT, radiation therapy; CT, chemotherapy; MDS, myelodysplasia; t-AML, therapy-related myelogenous leukemia; t-MDS, therapy-related myelodysplasia.
[a] Absolute excess risk per 10,000 person-years.
[b] Includes 4 cases of MDS and 2 cases of ALL.
[c] Case-control study.
[d] Includes 27 cases of t-AML and 4 cases of other types of therapy-related leukemia.
[e] Risks of leukemia when 12 MDS cases are included in analysis.

even though relatively high doses of radiation therapy are used in the treatment of Hodgkin's disease. Chemotherapy alone especially as either combinations containing mechloremethamine, vincristine (Oncovin), procarbazine, and prednisone (MOPP) or MOPP-like regimens, significantly increased the risk of leukemia. Data are unclear if addition of radiation therapy to chemotherapy increases the risk of leukemia. A significantly increased risk ($p < .001$) associated with extended-field radiation therapy and MOPP was reported as compared with supradiaphragmatic irradiation and MOPP (15-year cumulative incidence of 9.0 percent versus 2.2 percent, respectively).[54] Furthermore, an actuarial risk of 1.8 percent at both 10 and 19 years after treatment of Hodgkin's disease with chemotherapy alone, as compared with 3.1 percent and 8.1 percent at 10 and 19 years, respectively, for those that received combined modality therapy (difference, significant at $p = .04$).[55] Another study also found an increased relative risk for combined modality therapy in comparison to chemotherapy alone.[59] The relative risk associated with chemotherapy alone was 22.2 (95 percent confidence interval [CI], 2.7 to 80.3); for combined therapy, it was 53.9 (95 percent CI, 21.7 to 111.0). In contrast, a case control study of 1939 patients found no significant difference in the relative risk of leukemia among patients with Hodgkin's disease who received combined modality therapy as compared with those who received chemotherapy alone ($p = .16$).[56,58]

Most patients with Hodgkin's disease who developed t-AML were treated with an alkylating agent. Treatment with MOPP or MOPP-like regimens either with or without radiation therapy strongly correlated with the development of leukemia. By contrast, chemotherapy with doxorubicin (Adriamycin), bleomycin, vinblastine, and dacarbazine (ABVD) without radiation therapy carried a much lower risk of developing acute leukemia.[55,70–72] Significant reduction in the risk of developing secondary leukemia following the treatment of Hodgkin's disease observed in the 1980s is largely due to the introduction of ABVD regimen in the treatment of Hodgkin's disease.[56]

A correlation exists between the amount of chemotherapy and the risk of developing t-AML in individuals treated for Hodgkin's disease. Also, intensive therapy for Hodgkin's disease decreased the latent period between the diagnosis of Hodgkin's disease and the development of leukemia. Intensive chemotherapy is defined as at least six cycles of MOPP or an equivalent group of drugs; intensive radiation therapy is defined as either at least total nodal or extended-field irradiation. In one series, patients who received intensive chemo- or radiation therapy, or both, had a mean interval from initiation of therapy to diagnosis of leukemia of 3.4 years, which was significantly shorter than the mean interval of 7.6 years in patients who received less intensive therapy.[73] The National Cancer Institute (NCI) has reported that patients receiving salvage chemotherapy for refractory Hodgkin's disease have a 10 percent incidence of AML, compared with 5 percent at 5 years for all Hodgkin's patients treated with combined modality therapy.[42]

Prior studies identified age at diagnosis as a potential risk factor for development of leukemia.[47,74] In one series, the cumulative risk of leukemic complications 9 years after beginning chemotherapy for Hodgkin's disease was 8.6 percent for individuals under 40 years of age compared with 40 percent for those aged 40 years or older. In another series, the actuarial risk of leukemia was 20.7 percent at 7 years after therapy for Hodgkin's disease patients aged 40 years or older and was approximately 6.6 percent at 7 years for all patients.[47] Also, individuals over 50 years of age who were treated for other types of cancer had a higher risk of secondary leukemia with a short latency. One study of 105 cases of t-AML in patients treated for a large variety of cancers found that the time to development of preleukemia was the same for those who had Hodgkin's disease compared to other cancers, which was 57.5 and 76.5 months in individuals over 50 and under 30 years of age, respectively.[75] Paradoxically, several recent large studies in children showed a significant trend of greater risk with younger age at first treatment when the observed risks at various age groups were compared to the expected risks.[59,60]

Since van Leeuwen et al. suggested in 1987 that splenectomy in Hodgkin's disease patients may contribute to the risk of leukemia, many studies reported a similar significantly increased risk.[57,58,61,76] Investigators have suggested that the increased risk may be due to loss of splenic immunosurveillance. Others have reported that splenic irradiation as well as splenectomy are significant risk factors.[61] However, a number of reports also state that splenectomy does not pose a significant risk for development of leukemia.[60,64,65]

Non-Hodgkin's Lymphoma

The risk of therapy-related leukemia in patients treated for NHL has been extensively studied, and Table 22–5 lists some of the recent reports.[77–82] As in Hodgkin's disease, alkylating agents are the major risk factor. Within a cohort study of 11,386 2-year survivors of NHL, 35 patients with t-AML were matched to 140 controls. Investigators concluded that despite the definite excess of t-AML associated with specific therapies, especially with prednimustine, mechlorethamine, procarbazine, and high cumulative doses of chlorambucil, the risk remains small.[77] Of 10,000 NHL patients treated for 6 months with selected regimens including low cumulative doses of cyclophosphamide and followed for 10 years, an excess of four leukemias might be expected. Cyclophosphamide regimens were associated with a small, nonsignificantly increased risk of t-AML (RR = 1.8; 95 percent CI, 0.7 to 4.9). Treatment with epipodophyllotoxins, doxorubicin, or bleomycin was not associated with elevated leukemic risk when adjusted for the effects of alkylating agents. The median cumulative dose of epipodophyllotoxins was relatively small: 453 mg for the leukemic group and 833 mg for the control cohort.[77]

The role of radiation therapy in leukemogenesis in NHL is unclear. In one study, low-dose total body or hemibody irradiation was more leukemogenic than high-dose irradiation.[83] However, conflicting reports exist concerning the risk associated with high-dose irradiation.[36,77]

Multiple Myeloma

Some investigators have suggested that acute leukemia, other than plasma cell leukemia, may be part of the natural history of

Table 22–5. t-MDS/t-AML Following the Treatment of Non-Hodgkin's Lymphoma

Investigators	No. of Patients	Median Follow-Up (Years)	No. With t-AML	Relative Risk (95 Percent Confidence Interval)	Actuarial Risk Percent	Actuarial Risk Years	Median Latency (Range)
Pedersen-Bjergaard et al. (1985)[79]	602	NS	9	76	1.8	4	51 months (26–81)
					6.3	7	
					8.0	9	
Ingram et al. (1987)[80]	261[a]	3–9	6	NS	7.8	7	3 years
Travis et al. (1991)[81]	29,153	3.12	29	2.88 (1.93–4.13)	NS		61 months (2–160)
Travis et al. (1993)[82]	6171	7.4	14	4.83 (2.64–8.10)	NS		7.6 years (2.4–18.2)

Abbreviations: NS, not stated; t-MDS, therapy-related myelodysplasia; t-AML, therapy-related acute myelogenous leukemia.
[a] Includes 166 children with non-Hodgkin's lymphoma and 95 children with T-cell leukemia.

multiple myeloma. However, little evidence exists to support this concept.[36,84] The typical treatment regimen for multiple myeloma includes prolonged use of alkylating drug therapy, such as melphalan, which has been clearly shown to be leukemogenic. The risk of leukemia in multiple myeloma should therefore be considered to result from its therapy. Table 22–6 lists some of the studies that illustrate the leukemogenic risks in patients with multiple myeloma.[50,85,86] All therapies used in these studies included an alkylating agent. The actuarial risk reported in multiple myeloma is as high as 20 percent. Cuzick et al.[85] studied the relationship between the duration and dose of treatment with either melphalan or cyclophosphamide in a total of 648 multiple myeloma patients. Twelve cases of myelodysplasia or acute leukemia were observed in the entire cohort. The duration and cumulative dose of melphalan therapy were the most significant determinant of risk. Cyclophosphamide therapy was not associated with the increased leukemic risk.[85] In another study of 364 multiple myeloma patients, actuarial risk of developing t-AML was 4 percent after 3 years and 19.6 percent after 4.2 years of alkylating drug therapy.[86] No significant difference in risk of leukemia was observed between different alkylators. Another study of 908 myeloma patients receiving alkylating agent therapy found an actuarial risk of 2.8 percent and 10.1 percent after 5 and 10 years, respectively.[50] Seven additional patients developed t-MDS who were not included in the analysis of leukemia risk. Prolonged use of alkylating agents in multiple myeloma poses a clear leukemogenic risk.

Ovarian Cancer

Individuals who have received alkylating agent chemotherapy for ovarian carcinoma are at increased risk of acute leukemia with a cumulative risk of 7 to 10 percent at 5 to 10 years after therapy (Table 22–7).[44,46,87–91] Most of these prior reports studied individuals who received single alkylating agents for prolonged periods. The risk appears to correlate with the type, dose, and duration of alkylating agents used. In one series of 773 ovarian carcinoma patients, 9 of the 10 cases of leukemia developed in patients who received more than 700 mg of melphalan.[46] Among the patients who received only melphalan, the average dose was 1150 mg, and the mean number of cycles of treatment was 21. Two other patients in whom leukemia developed in this study had received more than 2000 mg of chlorambucil. A case-control study identified 101 patients with leukemia among 99,113 survivors of ovarian cancer.[90] Radiation therapy alone did not produce a significant increase in risk, as compared with surgery alone. Chemotherapy alone was associated with a relative risk of 12.0 (95 percent CI, 4.4 to 32; $p < .001$). The addition of radiation therapy to chemotherapy did not produce any additional risk (RR 9.8 [95 percent CI, 3.4 to 28], $p < .41$). Among various alkylating agents, chlorambucil and melphalan were the most leukemogenic, followed by thiotepa, cyclophosphamide, and treosulfan.[90] The frequency of leukemia for individuals who received one of the five agents paralleled the dose of the drug that was given. Patients who received the combination of doxorubicin hydrochloride and cisplatin also showed an increase in leukemogenic risk (RR 6.5).

Table 22–6. Risk of t-MDS/t-AML Following Treatment of Multiple Myeloma

Investigators	No. of Patients	Median Follow-Up	No. With t-AML	Median Latency	Relative Risk	Actuarial Risk Percent	Actuarial Risk Years
Cuzick et al. (1987)[85]	648	97 months	12[a]	85.5 months	NS	10	8
Kyle (1983)[50]	908	NS	17	NS	NS	10.1	10
Bergsagel et al. (1982)[86]	364	NS	14	NS	230	19.6	4.2

Abbreviations: NS, not stated; t-MDS, therapy-related myelodysplasia; t-AML, therapy-related acute myelogenous leukemia.
[a] Includes patients with MDS.

Table 22–7. t-MDS/t-AML Following Therapy for Ovarian Carcinoma

Investigators	No. of Patients	Therapy	Median Follow-Up (Years)	No. With t-MDS/ t-AML	Relative Risk (95 Percent Confidence Interval)	Actuarial Risk Percent	Actuarial Risk Years	Mean Latency (Range)
Reimer et al. (1977)[87]	5455	CT ± RT	NS	13	36.1 (19.2–61.8) 171.4 (88.5–299.5)[a]	NS		41.5 months (30–90)
Pedersen-Bjergaard et al. (1980)[88]	553	Dihydroxybusulfan	NS	7	125	7.6	5	50 months (21–58)
Greene et al. (1986)[89]	3363	No RT or CT (595)	5.7	0	93 (61–136)[b]	0	10	NS
		RT (955)		2		0.1	10	
		CT (1179)		21		8.6	10	
		RT + CT (539)		12		8.3	10	
Kaldor et al. (1990)[90,c]	99,113	Surgery	NS	6	1.0	NS		4–5 years
		RT		15	1.6 (0.51–4.8)			
		CT		41	12.0 (4.4–32)			
		RT + CT		39	9.8 (3.4–28)			
Travis et al. (1999)[91,c]	28,971	RT	NS	1	0.4 (0.04–3.5)	NS		3.3 years
		CT[d]		65	6.5 (2.3–18.5)			
		RT + CT[d]		25	8.1 (2.6–25.6)			

Abbreviations: NS, not stated; RT, radiation therapy; CT, chemotherapy; t-MDS, therapy-related myelodysplasia; t-AML, therapy-related acute myelogenous leukemia.

[a] Relative risk for patients surviving greater than 2 years.
[b] Relative risk among 1794 women who have received chemotherapy.
[c] Case-control study.
[d] Alkylating drugs including platinum derivatives.

Many of the above-mentioned drugs are no longer in common use, and the trend in treatment for ovarian cancer today is toward pulse combination chemotherapy rather than more continuous single-agent therapies. Platinum-based combinations are often used for advanced ovarian cancer. A case-control study of 28,971 women with invasive ovarian cancer receiving alkylating agents including platinum compounds found that 90 patients developed t-MDS/t-AML resulting in a relative risk of 6.5 (95 percent CI, 2.3 to 18.5).[91] If patients received a platinum agent as the principal alkylating drug, the relative risk was 4.0 (95 percent CI, 1.4 to 11.4), which was considerably lower than the risk after treatment with melphalan (RR 20.8; 95 percent CI, 6.3 to 68.3). The relative risk with carboplatin and cisplatin was 6.5 (95 percent CI, 1.2 to 36.6) and 3.3 (95 percent CI, 1.1 to 9.4), respectively. A clear increase in the risk occurred with higher cumulative dose and longer duration of platinum treatment. In addition, added risk occurred when platinum compounds were used in combination with radiation or other alkylating agents such as melphalan. In this series,[91] 42 percent of the women who developed t-MDS/t-AML had early-stage ovarian cancer emphasizing the importance of risk-benefits evaluation of the adjuvant therapies in early-stage disease. Paclitaxel is often used in combination with platinum, but the leukemogenic risk of paclitaxel has not been defined.

Testicular Cancer

Approximately 80 percent of patients with testicular cancer can be cured with combination chemotherapy regimens, even those with an advanced stage of disease. Increasingly, long-term complications of therapy are emerging as an important problem in testicular cancer patients including therapy-related MDS and leukemia, but the overall risk appears to be relatively low (Table 22–8).[92–97] No leukemias have been reported following four cycles of standard dose cisplatin, vinblastine, and bleomycin (PVB) combination chemotherapy, and only one case was reported after prolonged therapy with PVB with a total dose of 1.3 g of cisplatin over 12 months.[98] Other retrospective analyses have also shown no increased risk of t-AML after PVB therapy.[93,96,99,100] In the 1980s, the epipodophyllotoxin derivative etoposide was introduced in the first-line treatment of germ cell tumors resulting in excellent therapeutic outcome in patients with advanced disease.[101] An early report of chemotherapeutic regimens with PEB (etoposide, cisplatin, bleomycin) found a markedly increased risk of AML (RR 336, 95 percent CI, 92 to 861).[96] Since this initial report, several studies have addressed the leukemogenic potential of etoposide containing chemotherapy in germ cell tumors. A cumulative etoposide dose of 2 g/m^2 or less conferred a relatively low incidence of t-AML (approximately 0.5 percent after 5 years).[93–96,102,103] In contrast, a cumulative etoposide dose greater than 2 g/m^2 resulted in an overall incidence of 2 percent (range 0.8 to 8 percent) at 5 years.[96,102–105] The high relative risk in the initial report may have resulted from the very high doses of cisplatin in addition to high cumulative dose of etoposide administered to these individuals.[96] A risk-benefit analysis for germ cell tumor patients estimated that etoposide-containing regimens like PEB

Table 22–8. t-MDS/t-AML Following Testicular Cancer Therapy

Investigators	No. of Patients	Therapy	Median Follow-Up (Years)	No. With t-MDS/ t-AML	Relative Risk (95 Percent Confidence Interval)	Actuarial Risk Percent	Actuarial Risk Years
Pedersen-Bjergaard et al. (1991)[96]	212	Etoposide	NS	5	336 (92–861)	4.7	5.7
	127	No etoposide		0			
Bajorin et al. (1993)[95]	503	Etoposide	NS	6	NS	< 1	
Bokemeyer et al. (1993)[93]	1025	Surgery (22 percent) RT (32.6 percent) CT (40.5 percent) RT + CT (4.8 percent)	5 years (1–20)	0	NS	NS	
Nichols et al. (1993)[94]	538	Etoposide	NS	2	66 (8–238)	NS	
van Leeuwen et al. (1993)[92]	1909	Surgery	7.7 years	0	0	NS	
		RT		3[a]	5.2 (1.1–15.1)		
		CT		1[a]	20.0 (0.51–111)		
		RT + CT		2[a]	66.7 (8.1–241)		

Abbreviations: NS, not stated; t-MDS, therapy-related myelodysplasia; t-AML, therapy-related acute myelogenous leukemia; RT, radiation therapy; CT, chemotherapy.

[a] Includes two cases myelodysplasia, one case acute lymphocytic leukemia, one case acute myelogenous leukemia, one case chronic lymphocytic leukemia, and one case chronic myeloid leukemia.

(compared to PVB) at standard doses can cure approximately 20 additional individuals per every case of t-AML,[106] suggesting that the benefit of standard dose etoposide-containing regimens outweighs the risk of developing t-AML in those with advanced germ cell tumors. However, less aggressive therapies should be considered when the disease has been diagnosed at an earlier stage.

Extragonadal germ cell tumors comprise only 2 to 3 percent of all germ cell tumors. Recently, 635 patients with extragonadal germ cell tumors were analyzed for the incidence of secondary malignancies.[107] Seventeen hematologic disorders were identified among 287 individuals with primary nonseminomatous mediastinal germ cell tumors. None of either 283 individuals with retroperitoneal germ cell tumors or 51 individuals with mediastinal seminomas developed a hematologic disorder. All of the 17 cases showed features that are typical of hematological disorders that are associated with nonseminomatous mediastinal germ cell tumors, such as i(12p), but not typical of t-MDS/t-AML. This study suggests that apart from a recognized occurrence of hematologic malignancies associated with germ cell tumors, the risk of developing therapy-related leukemias appears to be low in those with extragonadal germ cell tumors treated with cisplatin-based chemotherapy (median follow-up of 55 months).[107,108]

Breast Cancer

Increasing numbers of individuals with early-stage breast cancer are receiving adjuvant chemotherapy containing potential leukemogenic agents such as cyclophosphamide and anthracyclines. An increase in the occurrence of t-AML has been recognized in these patients. Leukemogenic potential was higher with regimens that included melphalan compared to cyclophosphamide. Few studies have examined the risk of developing t-AML in individuals receiving current adjuvant regimens. Milan Cancer Institute reported a study of 845 women who were included in two consecutive CMF (cyclophosphamide, methotrexate, and 5-fluorouracil) adjuvant trials.[109] Women were treated either surgery alone or surgery followed by 6 to 12 cycles of CMF. After a median follow-up in excess of 10 years, no cases of t-AML were observed. Similarly, the Eastern Cooperative Oncology Group (ECOG) has reported that the risk of t-MDS/t-AML among 2638 women receiving standard dose cyclophosphamide-containing adjuvant chemotherapy is not much higher than in the general population.[110] The addition of anthracyclines, such as doxorubicin or mitoxantrone either with or without radiation therapy may, however, slightly increase the risks. Fourteen cases of t-AML were observed among 1107 patients who were treated with FAC (5-fluorouracil, doxorubicin, and cyclophosphamide) either with or without other agents in an adjuvant or neoadjuvant setting.[111] The 10-year estimated leukemia rate was 1.5 percent (95 percent CI, 0.7 to 2.9) for all patients, 2.5 percent (95 percent CI, 1.0 to 5.1) for the radiation and chemotherapy group, and 0.5 percent (95 percent CI, 0.1 to 2.4) for the chemotherapy only group. This difference was statistically significant ($p = .01$). Others have also reported that radiation therapy in combination with chemotherapy or treatment with combination chemotherapy regimens containing an anthracycline such as mitoxantrone or 4-epidoxorubicin increased the risk of therapy-related leukemia in breast cancer patients. Although the benefits of adjuvant chemotherapy for early breast cancer are well established, ongoing evaluation of the potential long-term risks of the therapy is important to maximize the good clinical outcome.

Autologous Hematopoietic Stem Cell Transplantation

High-dose therapy (HDT) followed by autologous hematopoietic stem cell transplantation (ASCT) is increasingly used to treat various malignancies including Hodgkin's disease, NHL, germ cell tumor, breast cancer, and multiple myeloma. In the majority of cases, HDT is utilized in an attempt to salvage relapsed or refractory diseases or to consolidate remissions in patients with high risk of recurrence of disease. The short-term treatment-related mortality and morbidity of HDT-ASCT have improved significantly with modern supportive care measures and better patient selection. However, during the last decade, the increasing risk of t-MDS/t-AML following high-dose chemotherapy and ASCT has emerged as one of the most significant long-term toxicities of this treatment. The use of dose-intensive therapy has clearly benefited many patients who were otherwise incurable; however, the risk of t-MDS/t-AML raises a serious concern. Table 22–9 summarizes the data from recently reported studies.[105,112–124] The reported actuarial risk of t-MDS/t-AML varies significantly depending on the series. For example, in a study of 229 breast cancer patients, no cases of t-MDS/t-AML occurred with a median follow-up of 42 months after ASCT.[123] In contrast, HDT-ASCT for 76 Hodgkin's disease and NHL patients was associated with an actuarial risk of 24.3 percent at 43 months.[114] The reason for these variations is a reflection of many differences between these studies, such as the primary diagnoses, the duration and kinds of pretransplant treatments, type of priming to collect the stem cells and conditioning used to treat the cancer, and the duration and methods of follow-up of the patients.

Similar to the results of conventional therapy, increased risk of t-MDS/t-AML with HDT-ASCT correlates with increasing age of the patient and increasing cumulative dose of alkylating agents given before the ASCT. Age at the time of HDT-ASCT was an independent and significant risk factor ($p < .001$) in a study by the EBMTR.[118] Other significant risk factors included a lengthy duration of pretransplant therapy, a prolonged interval from primary diagnosis to ASCT, a number of prior relapses, treatment with an alkylating agent, and chemotherapy with MOPP and with lomustine. A study of HDT-ASCT of HD and NHL patients from New Castle found that the cumulative risk for t-MDS/t-AML was only 1.1 percent at 20 months in the cohort of patients who were predominantly transplanted in first relapse.[125] In contrast, the actuarial risk was 24.3 percent at 43 months among patients who had multiple treatments prior to transplant.[114] The risk of t-MDS/t-AML appears to be relatively low after HDT-ASCT in patients with nonhematologic malignancies such as breast cancer and germ cell tumors.[105,122,123] However, this may reflect the paucity of pretransplant therapy given to many breast cancer patients or the younger age among those with germ cell tumors.

The leukemogenic potential of radiation therapy alone has been controversial. Several studies have shown no increased risks in the setting of conventional treatment. However, in the setting of HDT-ASCT, previous radiation therapy, in particular pelvic radiation, was a significant risk factor ($p = .003$).[126] In

Table 22–9. t-MDS/t-AML Following Autologous Transplantation

Investigators	Primary Diagnosis	No. of Patients	No. with t-MDS/t-AML	Actuarial Risk		Median Latency	
				Percent	Year	Primary Diagnosis	HDT-ASCT
Darrington et al. (1994)[112]	HD	249	6	4	5	80 months	44 months
	NHL	262	6				
Bhatia et al. (1996)[113]	HD	82	4	13.5	6	NS	4 months
	NHL	176	6				
Pedersen-Bjergaard et al. (1997)[114]	HD	27	4	24.5	3.6	16–74 months	4–43 months
	NHL	49	2				
André et al. (1998)[115]	HD	467	8	4.3	5	NS	
Friedberg et al. (1999)[116]	NHL	552	41	19.8	10	NS	47 months
Sobecks et al. (1999)[117]	HD	79	5	NS		5.5 years	1.5 years
	NHL	103	1				
Milligan et al. (1999)[118]	HD	4998	66	4.6	5	NS	
	NHL			3.0	5		
Harrison et al. (1999)[119]	HD	595	8	3.1	5	NS	
Krishnan et al. (2000)[120]	HD	218	11	8.6	6	3.8 years	1.9 years
	NHL	394	11				
Micallef et al. (2000)[121]	NHL	230	27	14.2	5	9.1 years	4.4 years
Laughlin et al. (1998)[122]	Breast cancer	864	5	1.6	4	NS	
Martinez-Climent et al. (2000)[123]	Breast cancer	229	0	0		NS	
Kollmannsberger et al. (1998)[105]	Germ cell tumors	302	6	1.3	4.3	NS	
Govindarajan et al. (1996)[124]	Multiple myeloma	71[a]	0	0		NS	
		117[b]	7	12	4		

Abbreviations: NS, not stated; t-MDS, therapy-related myelodysplasia; t-AML, therapy-related acute myelogenous leukemia; HD, Hodgkin's disease; NHL, non-Hodgkin's lymphoma; HDT-ASCT, high-dose therapy-autologous stem cell transplantation.
[a] Single transplant.
[b] Double tandem transplant.

addition, total body irradiation (TBI) used as part of the conditioning regimen for ASCT appears to increase the risk of t-MDS/t-AML.[112] At Dana Farber Institute, HD/NHL patients transplanted after receiving TBI-containing regimen had a very high cumulative risk of t-MDS/t-AML: 18 percent at 6 years and 19.8 percent at 10 years.[116,126] In contrast, a similar group of patients at the same institution who were treated only with a chemotherapy conditioning regimen had a lower risk of 4.2 percent at 5 years. Multiple transplants in patients with multiple myeloma, HD, or NHL resulted in an enhanced risk.

In general, the overall outcome of ASCT was equivalent between the two sources of hematopoietic stem cells, bone marrow or peripheral blood. However, several recent studies suggested that the risk of t-MDS/t-AML was higher following ASCT using stem cells harvested from peripheral blood (after chemotherapy priming and growth factors) compared to those from the bone marrow.[113,115,120] Whether the differences in risk were due to biological differences of the stem cells themselves, toxicity of the priming used to harvest the stem cells, and/or other unknown factors are not clear.

Clinical presentation of t-MDS/t-AML following HDT-ASCT usually is similar to other precipitating causes of t-MDS/t-AML. However, the bone marrow following HDT-ASCT in some patients can be hypoplastic and fibrotic with a low percentage of blasts despite refractory cytopenias, and the diagnosis according to FAB classification may be difficult. Dysplastic changes are usually observed. Cytogenetic evaluation of the bone marrow may be required for the definitive diagnosis of t-MDS/t-AML in these cases. Similar to most causes of t-MDS/t-AML, cytogenetic abnormalities include loss of chromosome 7, 7q, and/or 5, 5q, or a complex karyotype. The leukemia that develops in those individuals exposed to a DNA topoisomerase II inhibitor such as etoposide prior to ASCT often has a balanced translocation that involves either chromosome 11q23 or 21q22.[120] Some investigators advocate cytogenetic screening of the bone marrow or examining for clonality such as X-chromosome inactivation using the human androgen receptor gene prior to harvesting stem cells for HDT-ASCT especially in heavily pretreated patients to avoid transplanting patients with pre-existing t-MDS.[127]

The latent period to t-MDS/t-AML after HDT-ASCT has been as short as 4 to 8 months, and more than 25 percent of cases occurred within 12 months. In these cases, the malignant clone might have been established by therapy prior to ASCT. The survival of these patients is very poor. Allogeneic bone marrow transplantation in these cases is usually unsuccessful. In summary, the currently available data suggest that many cases of t-MDS/t-AML following HDT-ASCT are due to pre-transplant therapy.

Nonmalignant Hematologic Diseases

Individuals with polycythemia rubra vera (PRV) have an increased incidence of AML as part of the natural history of their disease. However, the risk of AML is greater if the individuals with PRV are treated with chlorambucil or ^{32}P as compared to phlebotomy alone.[45] The Polycythemia Vera Study Group

(PVSG) has found that leukemia developed in 1.5 percent of patients in the phlebotomy treatment group, in 10 percent of the patients in the ^{32}P group, and in 13 percent of the chlorambucil treatment group among 431 previously untreated patients with a maximum follow-up of 18 years (PVSG-01 trial). A large number of individuals withdrew from the phlebotomy alone treatment arm, which probably resulted in the underestimation of the risk of leukemia in the phlebotomy only arm. Recent "intention to treat" analysis revealed a slightly higher incidence of leukemia (3.7 percent)[128] in the phlebotomy only treated patients. The relative risk of leukemia developing in PRV patients was four times greater with daily doses of chlorambucil above 4 mg than with doses of 4 mg or less; and the leukemia risk was five times greater when the drug was given for more than 50 percent of the days of the study compared with 50 percent or less.[45] In search of a less mutagenic agent, PVSG-08 trial evaluated hydroxyurea in the treatment of PRV.[128] Recently updated analysis revealed that the hydroxyurea group (median follow-up of 8.6 years) showed a tendency to the development of more cases of acute leukemia (9.8 percent vs. 3.7 percent in the historical control group of phlebotomy only arm from the PVSG-01 trial). This result, however, is not statistically significant. In another study, a slightly lower incidence of acute leukemia (5.6 percent) were observed in 71 PRV patients treated with hydroxyurea (median and maximum treatment duration of 7.3 and 15 years, respectively).[129] Other studies have also suggested that the therapy with hydroxyurea may increase the tendency of PRV to transform to acute leukemia.[130,131]

SPECIFIC THERAPIES ASSOCIATED WITH THE DEVELOPMENT OF t-MDS/t-AML

Chemotherapeutic Drugs

Alkylating agents have long been among the most frequently used chemotherapeutic agents and have been clearly shown to cause second malignancies, especially leukemias. These agents interact with DNA in a variety of ways: monoadduct formation, inter- and intrastrand cross-links, as well as alkylation of free DNA bases. These actions not only can lead to cell death, but also can cause termination of DNA replication and chromosome loss, leading to mutagenesis and particularly leukemogenesis. Alkylation events can also change the stereometric configuration of DNA bases, causing them to mispair resulting in single base mutations. Many of the alkylating agents have been clearly implicated in leukemogenesis. These include nitrogen mustards, chlorambucil, cyclophosphamide, and melphalan, as well as nitrosoureas (BCNU, CCNU, and methyl CCNU), busulfan, platinum compounds, and the nonclassic alkylating agent, procarbazine. Virtually every alkylating agent has been implicated in the development of leukemia.

Alkylating agents probably are the most potent chemotherapeutic inducers of leukemia; more than 85 percent of patients who developed chemotherapy-related leukemia had received an alkylator.[132] Melphalan, chlorambucil, or cyclophosphamide was the offending agent in nearly 65 percent of patients. Alkylating agents may be associated with varying risks of leukemogenesis. For example, one study compared the rates of mutagen-related leukemia in ovarian cancer patients treated with either melphalan or cyclophosphamide, and found that melphalan may be a more potent leukemogen than cyclophosphamide. This may mean that different mutagenic potentials exist within broad groups of antineoplastic agents.[89]

The nitrosourea compounds including semustine (methyl-CCNU) are mechanistically related to the alkylating agents, and they are leukemogenic in humans. Analysis of nine prospectively controlled trials comparing the combination of methyl-CCNU plus 5-FU with other therapies without methyl-CCNU in the surgical adjuvant treatments of gastric, colon, and rectal cancers (more than 3600 patients) showed that the combined therapy including methyl-CCNU was associated with a greater relative risk of 14.4 and a 6-year actuarial risk of 4 percent of developing preleukemia or t-AML. The absolute risk was 2.3 cases/1000 persons/year. Another chemotherapeutic agent, procarbazine, is often used in combination chemotherapy for Hodgkin's disease. The drug is a strong mutagen and is leukemogenic in monkeys[133] and probably in humans.

Purine and pyrimidine antimetabolites have rarely been associated with the development of leukemia in either humans or experimental animals.[3,134,135] As mentioned above, prolonged treatment with hydroxyurea in PRV patients has been associated with slightly higher incidence of AML. Adriamycin and bleomycin have only rarely been associated with secondary leukemia.[70,136] In a large series of Hodgkin's disease patients, t-AML developed in 17 of 606 patients who received combined chemo- and radiation therapy that included an alkylating agent or procarbazine, or both; no leukemias developed in 84 patients who received radiation therapy and the combination of Adriamycin, bleomycin, vinblastine, and dacarbazine (ABVD).[136] Few cases of t-AML have been reported in patients who have received ABVD in combination with radiation therapy.

Recently, several studies have reported t-AML in patients treated with a cytostatic drug not belonging to the alkylating family of agents. These include drugs targeting DNA-topoisomerase II, such as epipodophyllotoxins (etoposide and teniposide), doxorubicin, 4-epidoxorubicin, mitoxantrone, razoxane, and bimolane. At the molecular level, these compounds act by formation of stabilized topoisomerase II–DNA complexes, which inhibit DNA repair and produce single- and double-strand DNA breaks. These drugs are important components of modern-day chemotherapy regimens for many tumors, such as testicular cancer, ALL, NHL, lung cancer, and many others. Razoxane and bimolane, which have been used in the treatment of psoriasis, have also been demonstrated to be leukemogenic. Those patients in whom t-AML develops after therapy with DNA-topoisomerase II inhibitors often have acute leukemia with no preleukemic phase[10,11] and a short latency period, in contrast to alkylating agent–induced AML.

The predominant chromosomal aberrations associated with t-AML after therapy with DNA-topoisomerase II inhibitors are balanced translocations involving either chromosome 11q23 or 21q22. Less frequently, other balanced aberrations, such as inv(16), t(8;16), t(15;17), and t(6;9) have been observed. The

t(15;17) has been found in patients who were treated in China for psoriasis with bimolane.

The DNA-topoisomerase II inhibitors are increasingly cited as leukemogenic agents, but their precise impact on leukemogenesis requires further study. Therapy-related leukemias observed in these individuals are not restricted to the myeloid lineage, or to the exclusive use of high-dose etoposide. Occasionally, ALL is an observed second malignancy in these patients. The increased leukemic risk may be directly associated with the cumulative exposure to this class of agents.

Carcinogens in our environment including benzene and other chemical solvents, petrol products, and insecticides are leukemogenic.[43,137–139] Humans chronically exposed to benzene have a 5- to 20-fold excess risk of AML compared with nonexposed individuals.[43,139] Most t-AML patients have had contact with benzene for 1 to 15 years with a mean of 9.7 years, and many have 6 months to 6 years of pancytopenia before the development of acute leukemia. Many similarities are shared between the leukemia that develops after benzene exposure and the one that develops after chemotherapy. Both have a similar latent period, a preleukemia phase, a specific karyotypic abnormality, and a failure to respond to leukemic treatment.

Radiation

Ionizing radiation clearly increases the risk of developing AML in humans and experimental animals.[47,53,69,140–144] The incidence of leukemia after 400 cGy or less of radiation exposure from the Hiroshima nuclear explosion was approximately two cases of leukemia/10^6 persons/year/cGy.[53] Nearly the same incidence of leukemia was reported in patients who received 300 to 1500 cGy of spinal irradiation for ankylosing spondylitis. Likewise, increased myelogenous leukemia rates occurred in radiologists who practiced during the early years of clinical radiology before modern safety standards.[140] Low-dose, chronic irradiation induces leukemia in experimental animals. In 50 percent of dogs that received a daily low dose (5 to 10 cGy) of cobalt γ-irradiation, AML developed after about 1000 days of exposure.[143] Single whole body irradiation initiates leukemia in rodents. Myelogenous leukemia developed in 20 percent of mice after a single brief whole body irradiation of 200 cGy.[47] The dose-response relationship was curvilinear; pulse low-dose irradiation (at least 300 cGy) induced significantly fewer cases of leukemia than the 200-cGy dose. Doses of greater than 300 cGy of irradiation produced marrow cell death, probably decreasing the number of cells that would otherwise have undergone malignant transformation.

Even though radiation therapy is leukemogenic,[4,8,73,145] studies in Hodgkin's disease suggest that the incidence of secondary leukemia in patients receiving radiation therapy alone was low compared with those receiving chemotherapy alone.[70,74] In one study, a total of 957 patients received exclusively radiation therapy, and none developed leukemia. By contrast, 542 patients received only chemotherapy, and 12 developed leukemia. A similar finding had been reported in ovarian cancer patients who received either chemo- or radiation therapy.[46] In most studies, the risk of AML in patients with either

Hodgkin's disease or ovarian carcinoma treated exclusively with chemotherapy is not different from that in patients treated with both chemotherapy and radiation therapy.[4,8,46,73,145] The composite data strongly suggest that most secondary leukemias observed in those patients who are treated with combined therapies are attributable to chemotherapy.

In a study of chromosomal abnormalities, only 37 of 344 patients with secondary leukemia had been treated with radiation therapy alone; the incidence of a normal karyotype was higher in patients who received only radiation than in patients who received chemotherapy either with or without radiation therapy (24.3 versus 11.7 percent). Normal karyotype is associated with better response to therapy, but with little improvement in overall survival.[146] Another study of 63 patients with either t-MDS or t-AML found that 11 of 63 had received only radiation, in most cases to ports including the pelvis or spinal bone marrow.[19] In this study, only two patients had a normal karyotype. The low risk of leukemia after currently used high-voltage irradiation may be analogous to the above-mentioned murine model where high-dose irradiation has a lethal effect on marrow cells in contrast to lower-dose exposure, which may be more likely to produce nonlethal marrow cell injury and mutations.

TREATMENT

Although the studies only utilizing modern-day supportive care are extremely limited, in general the median survival of patients with t-AML who are not treated with induction chemotherapy is less than 3 months. Various attempts to improve survival in these patients have failed to change the course of the disease, with deaths due to infection, bleeding, or progression of the acute leukemia. Supportive therapy is, therefore, an important aspect of the medical care of these patients. No significant differences in survival have been shown between those patients who received chemotherapy and supportive care and those who received supportive care alone. Patients with t-MDS/t-AML tend to tolerate further chemotherapy poorly. Most patients have limited hematopoietic reserves as well as co-morbid diseases from the toxicity of prior treatment. Thus, supportive therapy with transfusions of red blood cells and platelets for symptomatic anemia or bleeding complications, or both, is often necessary as well as the treatment with antibiotics for infections. Supportive care alone may well be adequate in either elderly patients or those with significant co-morbid disease. The goal of therapy in these individuals should be to maintain an acceptable quality of life. Clearly, innovative and radically novel approaches to this syndrome are required if these patients are to be cured.

Preleukemic Phase

Generally, no effective drug therapy is available during the preleukemic phase. Folic acid is often given because of the frequent morphologic features of megaloblastic anemia, but the drug is not helpful unless true folate deficiency exists. Similarly, pyridoxine, androgens, or prednisone are occasionally tried, but

are almost never of use.[36] Interferons, both alpha and gamma, have been tried in MDS, but these had no significant responses.[144,147] Vitamin D3 analogues have been shown to inhibit proliferation and induce differentiation of leukemia cells in preclinical studies.[148] However, when 1,25-dihydroxyvitamin D3 was tried in patients with MDS, no objective responses were noted.[149] Retinoids have also been shown to suppress proliferation and induce differentiation of leukemic cell lines and induce complete responses (CR) in patients with acute promyelocytic leukemia (APL).[150,151] Despite encouraging results seen in pilot studies with 13-*cis* retinoic acid in MDS, randomized studies failed to reproduce previously observed response rates.[12,152,153] Sixty-eight patients with MDS including nine t-MDS patients were randomized to receive either 13-*cis* retinoic acid or placebo; no difference in survival was observed.[152] Patients with t-MDS were not analyzed separately. More recently, patients with MDS were treated with all-*trans* retinoic acid, and again no significant responses were observed.[154]

Use of growth factors has not been rigorously studied in patients with t-MDS. However, administration of growth factors can improve cytopenias in patients with MDS. Administration of GM-CSF improved leukopenias and lessened infectious complications; however, the responses have been incomplete.[155–157] Trilineage improvement was rare, and the abnormal clone was not eradicated. In some instances, blast cells have increased, especially in patients with chronic myelomonocytic leukemia (CMML).[158] Granulocyte colony-stimulating factor (G-CSF) also improves neutropenias,[159,160] but it can be dangerous in those individuals with a very low peripheral platelet count because the initial administration of the drug can be associated with a further fall in the platelet count resulting in hemorrhage. Ten to 20 percent of patients with serum erythropoietin (EPO) levels less than 500 u/μl will have an improvement in their anemia if they are treated with recombinant EPO, and up to 40 percent of patients will have improvement of their red cell counts if they receive both EPO and G-CSF.[161] Administration of growth factors in selected, symptomatic patients is clinically useful; however, no evidence is available to show that they improve survival.

Cytotoxic therapy in the preleukemic phase has not been helpful. Low-dose cytosine arabinoside (ara-C) and 5-azacytidine can induce differentiation of leukemic cells; in vivo, these agents probably are cytotoxic and may as well induce differentiation of the abnormal clone of cells. Treatment with low-dose ara-C results in relatively low response rates of 10 to 25 percent in MDS; the median duration of response is short, usually in the range of 3 to 15 months. A meta-analysis of low-dose ara-C therapy showed that 27 of 170 patients (16 percent) achieved CR with a median duration of response of 10.5 months, but achievement of CR did not prolong survival.[162] The median survival for all patients was 3 months. Eight patients in this review had t-MDS; however, these patients were not analyzed separately. In one study, 43 patients with MDS were treated with 5-azacytidine; seven patients had t-MDS.[163] Overall response rate was 49 percent with 12 percent having a complete response rate. The overall median survival was 13.3 months. Further studies are ongoing with this compound and the related 2-deoxy-5-azacytidine (Decitabine).

Induction and Postremission Chemotherapy

The efficacy of various therapeutic modalities of t-MDS/t-AML has been difficult to access because the number of reported cases is small. In addition, data for t-MDS/t-AML have been reported together with secondary leukemias following other hematological disorders such as MDS or de novo MDS and AML, making the evaluation difficult. The overall response rate to standard AML induction chemotherapy (low-dose ara-C and anthracycline) in secondary leukemias in general, is lower than de novo leukemia. The overall complete response rate ranges between 16 and 73 percent and averages about 35 to 40 percent. Some of the studies have suggested that high dose ara-C might provide greater response rates in this high-risk population, but other studies have failed to confirm this observation.[164] For example, in one study at M.D. Anderson, 148 secondary AML patients were treated with either conventional-dose or high-dose ara-C. The complete response rate was similar, 35 percent with conventional-dose ara-C and 38 percent with high-dose ara-C.[12]

Recently, the efficacy and safety of topotecan and high-dose cytarabine with G-CSF were evaluated in advanced MDS.[165] A relatively high CR rate was achieved in MDS patients (61 percent) with a median follow-up of 7 months. Seven percent of the patients died during induction therapy. Treatment was particularly effective in patients with poor prognosis karyotype involving chromosomes 5 and/or 7 and secondary MDS, producing CR rates of 71 and 72 percent, respectively.[165] The topotecan/ara-C regimen may be an active induction regimen in high-risk MDS patients and is associated with a relatively low mortality rate, but longer follow-up is necessary.

Studies have suggested that no significant differences exist in clinical outcome between the therapy-related leukemia and the AML secondary to either prior MDS or myeloproliferative disorders. Rather, the differences in outcome largely depend on the cytogenetic findings similar to the situation with de novo AML.[166] The secondary leukemias with favorable cytogenetic findings, such as t(8;21), t(15;17), inv (16), have a complete response rate essentially the same as de novo AML with the same karyotype.[34,167] Similarly, patients who have secondary AML with unfavorable cytogenetic findings such as deletion of chromosomes 5 or 7 do poorly, similar to de novo AML individuals with the same abnormality. Thus, the rate of remission during induction therapy and the overall survival parallels the cytogenetic findings in secondary AML.

No single form of postremission therapy has been shown to be superior for t-AML. Recent trials with agents that modify multidrug resistance have shown disappointing results.[168] Other approaches have included retinoids, hematopoietic growth factors, 5-azacytidine, low-dose cytosine arabinoside, and hormonal agents, all with no improvement in survival. In general, postremission therapy with high-dose ara-C probably is appropriate in patients with favorable cytogenetic findings except for those t-APL patients with t(15;17). Patients with t-APL should be treated with the combination of all-*trans*-retinoic acid and chemotherapy similar to de novo patients. In contrast, because of their extremely poor outcome, patients with unfavorable cytogenetic findings should be encouraged to enter clinical trials. As part of the discussion of treatment options, t-AML patients with an extremely poor prognosis should probably be offered the spectrum of treatments from supportive care alone to intensive chemotherapy with or without allogeneic hematopoietic stem cell transplantation.

Allogeneic Transplantation

Allogeneic bone marrow transplantation is an effective therapy in selected patients with de novo MDS and AML. One study compared results of allogeneic bone marrow transplantation for 18 t-MDS and 25 primary MDS patients.[169] The actuarial disease-free survival was 24 percent (95 percent CI, 6 to 42) for the t-MDS and 43 percent (95 percent CI, 22 to 64) for the primary MDS with a median follow-up of 3 years. The difference in survival between these small cohorts was not statistically significant ($p = .42$). The transplant-related mortality was high (50 to 60 percent) in both groups. A similar experience was reported from the Fred Hutchinson Cancer Research Center.[170,171] Median survival for allogeneic transplantation for the entire group of individuals with t-MDS ($n = 31$) and t-AML ($n = 39$) as reported by French Society of Bone Marrow Transplantation was 197 days (95 percent CI, 117 to 314 days).[172] At a median follow-up of 7.9 years, 16 patients were alive without evidence of disease, and 54 patients had died, either from relapse or transplant-related complications. The results included an estimated 2-year overall survival of 30 percent (95 percent CI, 19 to 40), an event-free survival of 28 percent (95 percent CI, 18 to 39), and relapse and transplant-related mortality rates of 42 percent (95 percent CI, 26 to 57) and 49 percent (95 percent CI, 36 to 62), respectively. In multivariate analysis, age greater than 37 years was associated with a poor outcome. Several studies showed that cytogenetic prognostic subgroups as defined by the International Prognostic Scoring System (IPSS) paralleled their outcome after BMT in patients with primary MDS as well as t-MDS and t-AML.[173,174] The value of cytoreductive chemotherapy prior to BMT remains to be determined.

Although allogeneic BMT can provide a substantial chance of long-term survival and cure in selected subgroups of patients with t-MDS/t-AML, major limitations of allogeneic BMT are donor availability and patients' age. Alternative treatment strategies include nonmyeloablative allogeneic BMT ("minitransplant") especially for older patients to decrease their treatment-related morbidity and mortality as well as to exploit the benefit of graft-versus-leukemia effect.

FUTURE CLINICAL CONSIDERATIONS

Aggressive chemotherapy and radiation therapy produce prolonged survival of patients with a variety of malignancies including lymphoma, choriocarcinoma, ALL, myeloma, and testicular and possibly ovarian carcinoma. Adjuvant chemotherapy frequently is given to recently diagnosed breast cancer patients without distant metastases and in surgically resected, lymph node–positive colon and rectal cancer patients. Antineoplastic agents are also frequently used for prolonged periods in individuals with nonmalignant diseases. A greater incidence of secondary acute nonlymphocytic leukemia probably will occur as all of these treated patients survive longer. Therapy clearly improves both survival and quality of life but assessment of the risk of secondary leukemia will have to become part of any overall therapeutic plan. Thought should be given to the carcinogenic potential of therapeutic regimens. Alkylating agents, methyl-CCNU, and procarbazine should not be used when less leukemogenic compounds, such as antimetabolites, are equally effective in the treatment of a specific disease. For example, consideration should be given to treatment of essential thrombocythemia in young patients with anegrelide or interferon-alpha instead of alkylating agents or hydroxyurea, and treatment of stage IIIB or IV Hodgkin's disease with ABVD instead of MOPP. Caution must be exercised in giving adjuvant alkylating chemotherapy to patients with a low risk of relapse, such as those with small carcinoma of the breast with negative axillary lymph nodes. Finally, alkylating agents should be given with extreme caution to patients with nonmalignant diseases.

PATHOGENESIS OF t-MDS/t-AML

t-MDS/t-AML is a clonal hematopoietic stem cell disorder characterized by specific chromosomal alterations brought on by exposure to chemo- or radiation therapy, or both. One of the basic hypotheses is that t-AML represents a distinct subgroup of myeloid leukemia that arises from a specific alteration of DNA in a single myeloid pluripotent stem cell. Radiation and mutagenic compounds break chromosomes. If a myeloid progenitor cell in a genetically predisposed individual has a DNA break leading to loss of the critical part of the chromosome, the cell will have a growth advantage and give rise to a clone of transformed cells. These cells probably undergo at least several mutational events resulting in the fully leukemogenic transformation.

Natural History of Primary Disease or Common Etiologic Factors

Perhaps certain diseases have an intrinsic predisposition to leukemic transformation, but before the era of aggressive therapy, these individuals did not live long enough to develop leukemia. Nevertheless, most patients with untreated Hodgkin's disease or ovarian carcinoma do not have an increased frequency of leukemia. The composite of several reports totaling 4591 patients from 1931 to 1970 shows that Hodgkin's disease patients did not develop AML if radiation therapy or chemotherapy was not given.[175–178] Likewise, no increase in the incidence of acute nonlymphocytic leukemia occurred in a group of 13,300 patients with all stages of ovarian cancer, the majority of whom received no chemotherapy.[87] Many of these patients survived for 40 to 50 months. Ovarian cancer patients who received aggressive antineoplastic therapy at the time of diagnosis and developed acute nonlymphocytic leukemia had a median latency of 45 months to development of leukemia. In contrast, untreated individuals with a variety of lymphoproliferative diseases[179–181] or polycythemia rubra vera[45,182] do have a low background incidence of acute nonlymphocytic leukemia.

In one extensive review, 19 of 145 cases of leukemia occurred nearly simultaneously with the diagnosis of multiple myeloma.[180] The data could be consistent with the notion that the same etiological factor caused both neoplasms. Injection of mineral oil into the peritoneal cavity of BALB/c mice can result in development of myelomonocytic leukemia or plasmacytoma.[183] Likewise, intraperitoneal injection of methylcholanthrene into Wistar rats can produce either acute leukemia or breast cancer.[184] In most cases, however, therapy-related leukemia is temporally related to the therapy of the primary neoplasia and not to the development of the primary disease.

Most evidence shows convincingly that leukemic transformation does not occur in the cells of the patient's primary disease. Many patients are in complete remission when secondary leukemia develops, and therapy-related leukemia occurs in some patients who never had a neoplasm, such as those receiving immunosuppressive therapy. Finally, the karyotype of the cells from the primary neoplasm is usually different from the karyotype of the leukemic cells. However, a report described two patients with small cell lung cancer with deletion of chromosome 3(p13;p23). After combined modality therapy, both patients developed M6 AML with the same karyotypic abnormality in the leukemic cells as in their small cell lung cancer, suggesting a common origin for small cell lung cancer and acute nonlymphocytic leukemia in these two patients.[185] Reports of mediastinal germ cell primary tumors associated with AML have also been reported.[108,186–188] The chromosomal abnormality i(12p) is a highly specific marker for a germ cell tumor, and it is also found in some leukemias, especially acute megakaryoblastic subtype. Surprisingly, this rare leukemia often occurs either simultaneously or shortly after the diagnosis of the mediastinal germ cell tumor. Rapid onset of clinical symptoms and the general lack of chromosome 5 or 7 abnormalities are the main features of this syndrome.

Decreased Immunosurveillance

The immune system is frequently impaired by aggressive antineoplastic therapy in patients with malignancy, but immunosuppression probably does not account for the subsequent development of AML. Individuals with congenital or acquired immunodeficiency states have a markedly increased incidence of neoplasms, but most of these are lymphoid. Almost no cases of myeloid leukemia are associated with immunodeficiency.[189,190] Untreated Hodgkin's disease patients have an abnormality of the immune system, especially of the T lymphocytes. This probably does not account for the patient's high risk of secondary leukemia. Before the availability of chemotherapy and radiation therapy, many of these patients survived for a long duration and did not develop leukemia.[191,192] Most cases of AML in patients with Hodgkin's disease have occurred within the past 30 years, suggesting that the increased incidence of AML is secondary to radiation therapy and chemotherapy and not to depression of the immune system.

Alteration of Sequences and/or Control of DNA

The alkylating agents and radiation are strong mutagens in vitro, and their mutagenic activity is closely correlated with both their carcinogenic potency and their cytotoxic potency.[135] By contrast, a number of nonalkylating chemotherapeutic agents, such as the antimetabolites, are cytotoxic but are not potent mutagens. All the alkylating agents have structural similarities. They are all strong electrophilic reactants that bind avidly to nucleophilic sites of DNA.[183,193] The electrophilic reactivity occurs because of the presence of either uncharged or positively charged electron-deficient atoms that react nonenzymatically to form covalent bonds through the sharing of electron pairs of the DNA bases. The alkylation reaction can occur in a number of sites, including all nitrogens and oxygens of the four bases, as well as the phosphodiester bond and the 2′ oxygen of ribose.[194] The DNA repair is least effective for the alkylation of oxygen.[6] The alkylation of the DNA can be mutagenic by altering the tautomeric equilibrium of the base so that it will base pair with an incorrect base during DNA replication. The ability of an alkylating agent to produce alkylation of the oxygen at carbon-6 of guanine in DNA correlates very well with the induction of tumors and may be one of the critical reactions involved in leukemia initiation by these compounds.[6] However, oxygen alkylation may only be a fortuitous indicator of a potent carcinogen, and additional reactions may contribute to leukemogenesis.

X-rays can produce single-chain DNA breaks, which can be repaired by excision followed by new nucleotide synthesis using the undamaged DNA chain as the template. The rate of mutations induced by x-rays increases as the square of the dose. The atomic bombs dropped on Japan produced predominantly x-rays, γ-rays, and electrons, and the incidence of secondary myeloid leukemia in survivors was proportional to the square of the radiation dose that the survivors received.

Alkylating agents and radiation induce a wide range of chromosomal aberrations including breaks, complex rearrangements, and loss of part or all of a chromosome in cells.[195] In one study of 53 women with ovarian cancer, the chromosomes of lymphocytes were examined after the patients received cyclophosphamide or radiation therapy. Of the dividing cells, about 15 percent in the cyclophosphamide-treated group and 30 percent in the radiation therapy group had detectable large chromosomal aberrations compared with less than 2 percent of cells from untreated patients with gynecological neoplasms.[195] In another study of 25 patients with Hodgkin's disease and NHL, the chromosomes of patients who were treated with chemotherapy and radiation therapy were much more susceptible to breaks and gaps induced by 5-bromodeoxyuridine than the chromosomes of control patients. This difference occurred only in bone marrow cells and not in circulating lymphocytes. This may indicate that these individuals have an increased risk of leukemia secondary to increased chromosomal instability.[196]

Various theories have been proposed to explain the molecular pathogenesis of therapy-related myeloid leukemias. Leukemogenesis might occur in part by promotion of expression or by mutation of normal cellular oncogenes. Another possible explanation for leukemogenesis in patients with genetic deletions is the presence of tumor suppressor genes whose products may normally act to suppress uncontrolled cellular proliferation. Human oncogenes implicated in development of leukemia include *MYC*, *RAS*, *FMS*, *MYB*, *MLL*, and *FLT3*.[40,197–200] The mechanism of leukemic induction by oncogenes is not completely understood, but several oncogenes are located at heritable fragile sites that may be associated with breakpoints in hematopoietic stem cells, and this may play a role in leukemic induction.[201]

The *ras* gene family encodes for a group of 21-kd guanosine triphosphate-binding proteins that appear to play a role in signal transduction from membrane receptors. Mutations affecting the regulatory domains of *ras* protooncogenes in particular have been associated with mutagen-induced neoplasia in animal systems and have been extensively evaluated in MDS and AML. Approximately 10 to 20 percent of patients with AML and a similar proportion of patients with MDS exhibit point mutations in either the *N*- or *K-ras* gene.[202] In MDS, the presence of *N-ras* mutations may be associated with a poor prognosis and an increased risk of transformation to acute leukemia.[203] Of 220 evaluable patients, 20 (9 percent) had a point mutation of *N-ras*. The median survival of MDS patients with *N-ras* mutations was 19 ± 7 months compared with 39 ± 14 months for patients without an *N-ras* mutation.[203] Few cases of *ras* mutations have been reported in t-MDS/t-AML; however, larger studies are necessary to evaluate its role in the pathogenesis of t-MDS/t-AML.

Oncogene *c-fms* has also been studied as a possible participant in leukemogenesis. The *c-fms* gene encodes the receptor for M-CSF and possesses ligand-dependent tyrosine kinase activity.[204,205] Mutations of *c-fms* at codon 301 have been associated with transforming activity, and mutations at codon 969 lead to up-regulation of the fms.[206,207] When hematologically normal patients were studied following cytotoxic therapy, 11 out of 70 had a mutation at codon 969, three of whom also had a *ras* mutation, suggesting that point mutations found here may be an early occurrence in therapy-related leukemogenesis.[208,209] *c-fms* is localized to 5q34, but is not rearranged in t-MDS/t-AML.[32,33] Mutations involving *c-fms* are seen in MDS patients in 5 to 15 percent of cases,[210] and these mutations appear to occur more frequently in patients with CMML or M4 type of AML.[211]

An oncogene might be abnormally modulated in several ways. Chemical carcinogens and radiation might induce elevated expression of a cellular oncogene by altering regulatory DNA sequences (by point mutation or DNA modification) and/or by causing chromosomal rearrangements that alter regulation of the cellular oncogene such as in the Philadelphia chromosome. As mentioned earlier, some oncogenes occur at heritable fragile sites that are more susceptible to breakage and rearrangement. Carcinogens might induce mutations of normal structural genes (or cellular homologues of viral oncogenes), which then code for functionally altered proteins such as the activated *ras* genes.

Many cases of t-MDS/t-AML have unbalanced chromosome aberrations with loss of whole or part of chromosomes strongly suggesting the presence of a tumor suppressor gene in this region, and the search for putative tumor suppressor genes is ongoing. For chromosome 5, Le Beau et al. have narrowed down the critical region to 5q31.1.[29] Other genes located on the long arm of chromosome 5 include many growth factor genes including GM-CSF, IL-3, IL-4, IL-5, IL-9, and M-CSF; and the growth factor receptor genes known to be present on the long arm of chromosome 5 include those for M-CSF *(fms)*, platelet-derived growth factor (PDGF), glucocorticoid, alpha1-adrenergic, beta2-adrenergic, and D1-dopamine receptors.[36,212] No evidence exists, however, that abnormalities of these proteins contribute to hematopoietic dysregulation.

The breakpoints for the deletions of 7q are variable, but a common chromosome region, the so-called critical region, is located at band 7q22 proximally and the distal breakpoint varying from q32 to q36. Potentially important genes have been mapped to 7q, including genes for erythropoietin, p glycoprotein 1/multiple drug resistance 1, and p glycoprotein 3. However, none has yet been shown to be involved in the development of t-MDS/t-AML.[25,29,36,212]

In familial MDS with chromosome 7q abnormality (the "monosomy 7 syndrome"), the predisposition locus for development of MDS was mapped to a chromosomal location that is not 7q but to an unidentified location.[213,214] These yet unidentified genetic loci may control predisposition to chromosomal instability leading to secondary losses of specific chromosomal regions such as 5q, 7q, and others, and MDS and leukemia ultimately develop. Familial platelet disorder with leukemia (FPD/AML) is an autosomal-dominant congenital disorder with thrombocytopenia, and the affected individuals have a high likelihood to develop MDS, AML, and more rarely CML.[215,216] The MDS and AML that develop frequently have cytogenetic abnormalities that are common to the classic t-MDS/t-AML (i.e., chromosomes 5q, 7q, and complex abnormalities). The predisposition locus in FPD/AML is *AML1* *(CBFA2)* on chromosome 21q22.[216] This gene is the most frequently disrupted locus associated with acute myeloid leukemias, and includes various reciprocal translocations and inversions, such as t(8;21), inv(16), t(3;21), and t(12;21). In FPD/AML, heterozygous mutations and small deletions of one *AML1* allele were found in these different pedigrees. All the mutations affected the DNA-binding domain of one *AML1* allele, particularly two arginine residues at position 166 and 201.[216] How this results in predilection to AML is unclear. The disrupted *AML1* may be acting in a dominant negative fashion to inhibit the other allele. The hemizygous loss of one *AML1* allele may result in 50 percent decrease in expression of this transcription factor, which may be sufficient to initiate leukemogenesis in affected individuals by unknown mechanisms.

Tumor suppressor genes have been implicated in human tumors such as the *Rb* gene in retinoblastoma and the *p53* gene in a variety of malignancies. Leukemia is included among many types of tumors that are associated with the inherited familial cancer syndrome involving *p53*, which is known as Li-Fraumeni syndrome.[217–220] However, the *p53* gene is infrequently altered in primary MDS and AML, with a frequency of about 5 and 15 percent, respectively.[221–225] The mutational frequency increases to about 50 to 60 percent in MDS and AML samples having 17p monosomy.[224,226] Because chromosome 17 has often been one of the more frequently involved chromosomal abnormalities reported in t-MDS/t-AML, the frequency of *p53* alterations in t-MDS/t-AML may be higher. *p53* alterations seen in MDS are mostly missense point mutations, and these mutations occur in the subtypes of MDS with a prognostically poor FAB classification (e.g., RAEB, RAEB-t, CMML), with a high propensity to evolving into acute leukemia. Mutations of *p53* have not been reported in patients with either RA or RARS. In one study, the presence of *p53* mutation in MDS and AML was found to be a strong indicator for lack of response to chemotherapy and a short survival.[226]

Mutations in the retinoblastoma *(RB)* gene were first described in patients with retinoblastoma.[227,228] However, further studies revealed that *RB* gene abnormalities can be found in many malignancies including leukemia. Frequently, altered *RB* expression occurs in the blast cells of patients with AML, and the reduced expression is associated with a poorer prognosis.[229–231] Specific mutations of the *RB* have been less frequently identified in MDS, and whether alterations in the *RB* gene are more common in t-MDS/t-AML than de novo MDS/AML is not known.

The cyclin-dependent kinase inhibitors including p16 *(MTS1, INK4A)* and p15 *(MTS2, INK4B)* are frequently deleted in ALL.[232] They are also mutated in AML cell lines, but are rarely altered in AML and MDS cells harvested from patients.[233,234] However, *p15INK4B*, but not *p16INK4A* gene, is frequently and selectively hypermethylated in MDS.[235] Sequential analyses have shown that methylation of the *p15INK4B* gene increases with disease evolution toward AML.[236]

The mismatch repair genes play a role in maintaining the genetic stability of DNA. Several highly conserved mismatch repair genes have been found, including *MSH2, MLH1, PMS1,* and *PMS2.* Loss of DNA repair function of these genes may lead to a mutator phenotype, which has been proposed to lead to the accumulation of the mutations in oncogenes or tumor suppressor genes. A consequence of the mutator phenotype is the production of multiple replication errors in simple repetitive DNA sequences, resulting in microsatellite instability (MSI). Although several studies have reported infrequent MSI in MDS and AML,[237,238] one study in therapy-related leukemia observed a high frequency of MSI (94 percent) and p53 mutations (38 percent).[239] Another study has found that in acute leukemia, abnormal expression of MSH2 proteins was found in 32.6 percent of cases, and the abnormal expression was associated with therapy-related leukemia and/or older age of the patient.[240] Loss of heterozygosity (LOH) at the *MSH2* locus was found in 5 of 11 cases studied. In this study, abnormal MSH2 expression was more frequent in cases with *p53* mutation (35.7 vs. 3.4 percent). These results suggest that abnormalities of DNA mismatch repair may play a key role in leukemogenesis, especially in AML in the elderly patients or in t-AML.

Epidemiologic studies have demonstrated associations between MDS and smoking, exposure to chemical compounds (particularly petroleum products, and diesel derivatives, exhausts, organic solvents, fertilizers, and nitro-organic explosives), semi-metals (arsenic and thallium), stone dusts (such as silica), and cereal dusts.[241,242] Leukemogenic susceptibility of an individual may depend on the efficiency of DNA repair processes as well as polymorphisms in the metabolism of mutagenic agents (such as chemotherapy). A complex genetic predisposition to MDS may involve naturally occurring DNA polymorphisms in genes that mediate DNA repair and metabolize environmental carcinogens.

Greater levels of carcinogen activation (or lesser levels of carcinogen detoxification) probably lead to higher levels of DNA adduct formation, greater levels of persistent mutations, and increased risk for leukemic transformation after exposure to cancer therapies. Consequently, some of the studies have focused their attention to the naturally occurring polymorphisms in genes that mediate carcinogen metabolism, such as NAD(P)H:quinone oxdoreductase (NQO1) and glutathione S-transferases (GSTs). NQO1 gene plays a crucial role in detoxifying benzene metabolites. Nonfunctioning C to T polymorphic change at residue 609 of NQO1 gene has been reported to be associated with an increase in incidence of hematologic malignancies in Chinese workers exposed to benzene.[243] Since this report, Larson et al.[244] have studied 104 patients (56 t-AML, 30 primary MDS, 9 de novo AML, and 9 CML) for NQO1 polymorphism. Eleven percent of the t-AML patients were homozygous and 41 percent were heterozygous for the NQO1 polymorphism, which was significantly higher than expected. Of the 45 patients with clonal abnormalities of chromosomes 5 or 7, or both, 16 percent were homozygous for the inactivating polymorphism, 38 percent were heterozygous. Eighty-eight percent (7 of 8) of the nonfunctioning homozygotes had abnormal chromosome 5 and/or 7. Larson et al. reported that the inactivating polymorphism of NQO1 was more frequent in individuals with t-AML having a chormosomal abnormality of chromosome 5 and/or 7, suggesting that these individuals with homozygous or heterozygous inactivating NQO1 polymorphisms may be at higher risk of developing mutagen-related leukemogenesis.[244]

The GSTs are a family of proteins capable of detoxifying a number of carcinogenic electrophiles by catalyzing their conjugation to glutathione.[245] Two of the members of this class, GST mu-1 (GSTM1) and GST theta (GSTT1), are homozygously absent in a significant percentage of the population (approximately 50 percent for GSTM1 and 20 percent for GSTT1). Some of the studies have suggested that the null phenotype in either GSTM1 or GSTT1 is associated with higher incidence of MDS, but others have failed to confirm this association.[246–249] These observations warrant further confirmation in larger studies.

The cytochrome P450 (CYP-450) enzymes are involved in metabolic activation of precarcinogens to reactive metabolites, as well as in the detoxification of natural products. CYP1A1, a member of CYP-450 gene family, has been implicated in the increased susceptibility of cancer.[250,251] Possibly, the combination of high levels of carcinogen-activating enzymes and low levels of detoxifying enzymes might confer an increased susceptibility to mutagen-related leukemia.

Relationship of DNA Alteration to Leukemogenesis

Long Latency

A feature of therapy-induced leukemogenesis is a relatively long latency period between the exposure to the carcinogen and the clinical development of leukemia. Seven years was the mean latency period for development of leukemia for survivors within 1500 m of the atomic bomb blasts at Hiroshima and Nagasaki. Theoretically, only 80 days would be required from neoplastic transformation of a single hematopoietic cell to clinical diagnosis of leukemia if we assume a leukemic cell doubling time of 60 hours, no cell death, and the need for 10^{10} blast cells to diagnose clinically the disease. This is clearly a highly artificial situation that assumes a single step in transformation and immediate full expression of the malignant phenotype.

The explanation for the long latency period in therapy-induced leukemias is unclear. Perhaps irradiation or drugs cause random chromosomal breaks including chromosome 5 and/or 7. A break on chromosome 5 and/or 7 of a pluripotent myeloid stem cell might stimulate expression of the transformed phenotype only after the cell is stimulated to divide, which may be some time after the initial mutagenic event. The initial deletion of chromosome 5 and/or 7 is not enough to cause leukemia, but a further mutation of the myeloid stem cell in the normal allele on chromosome 5 and/or 7 is also needed.[252] The requirement for several nonrandom mutagenic insults to produce leukemic transformation would explain both the long latency period for leukemogenesis and why aggressive or intensive chemotherapy is more leukemogenic than nonaggressive chemotherapy.

Clonality in t-AML

The somatic mutation theory of carcinogenesis is based on a hypothesis that tumors are the result of a monoclonal expansion of a single cell having a selective growth advantage because of acquired somatic mutation(s). Earlier studies using glucose 6-phosphate dehydrogenase (G6PD) isoenzyme markers strongly suggested that the neoplastic cells in AML evolved from a clonal (unicellular) origin.[253–255] This finding might be slightly more surprising in t-AML because many hematopoietic cells are exposed to the carcinogen and either only one cell undergoes a rare and unique transformation or many cells are transformed, but only one clone proliferates to the point of expressing clinical disease. Evidence from clonality studies also suggests that the neoplastic transformation in elderly patients with possible secondary leukemia occurs in the myeloid pluripotent stem cell, whereas neoplastic transformation can occur in a more committed myeloid stem cell in young patients.[253–255] The heterogeneity of stem cell involvement could have prognostic and therapeutic importance and might explain why aggressive therapy of secondary leukemia patients frequently results in death with either marrow aplasia or incomplete elimination of the blast cells.

Clonality of the hematopoiesis can be accessed by several methods, such as cytogenetic analysis, fluorescent in situ hybridization, restriction fragment length polymorphism (RFLP), and X-chromosome inactivation analysis.[256] The most widely used currently are based on Lyon's hypothesis of X-chromosome inactivation, which states that most of the X-chromosome genes are transcribed in each female somatic cell exclusively from the active X-chromosome, which is either maternally or paternally derived.[257] This process, which occurs in early embryogenesis, results in the terminal inactivation of most of the genetic material on the other X-chromosome.

Because it is a random event, normal polyclonal female tissue is mosaic, in contrast to clonal tissue that contains cells bearing the same active X-chromosome. The initial clonality studies in malignancy took advantage of this event by using analysis of isoenzyme expression for *G6PD*.[258] However, the occurrence of this polymorphism in only a minority of those of a single racial group has limited its usefulness.

Second-generation clonality assays have taken advantage of restriction fragment polymorphisms on the X-chromosome and have distinguished active from inactive X-linked alleles on the basis of differences in methylation patterns at the polymorphic locus.[259] X-chromosome polymorphic DNA probes available for methylation analysis include the phosphoglycerate kinase (PGK) gene, the human androgen receptor gene *(HUMARA)*, and hypervariable DXS255 locus (M27β).[259–262] The major limitation of the methylation-based clonality assay is the potential for incomplete (unreliable) methylation patterns of some DNA sequences.[263] The *PGK* and *HPRT* genes have relatively reliable methylation patterns but are limited because of modest informativeness (< 35 percent) in the general female population. On the other hand, the M27β probe is highly informative but has less reliable methylation patterns.[264] The *HUMARA* gene is less well-studied but has high informativeness and appears to have reliable methylation patterns.[263] More recently, expression-based *HUMARA* assays have shown good correlation between methylation patterns and gene expression at this locus.[265,266]

A third type of clonality assessment is based on the detection of a transcriptional polymorphism of the active X chromosome. There is a C/T polymorphism that occurs at the exonic nucleotide no. 1311 of the *G6PD* gene.[267] This technique uses a polymerase chain reaction (PCR)-based gene expression analysis with reverse transcription of *G6PD* mRNA. This assay has the advantages of not depending on methylation patterns and allowing the study of non-nucleated cells such as reticulocytes and platelets, but has the disadvantage of only modest informativeness at the *G6PD* C/T locus.

Several studies have used clonality studies in screening patients who are undergoing high-dose therapy with autologous stem cell transplantation. In one study, *HUMARA* assay was performed on 104 female patients who were undergoing ASCT.[127] Clonal hematopoiesis at the time of ASCT correlated with future development of t-MDS/t-AML. A recent analysis has shown that clonality of normal hematopoietic cells can occur naturally in the elderly and therefore interpretation of clonal results in the elderly population needs to be tempered.

Relationship of Particular Karyotypic Pattern in Acute Leukemia to Age and Occupation

Specific karyotypic abnormalities of the leukemic cells predominate at specific ages of the patient.[268] For instance, loss of chromosome 5 is very rare in children with acute nonlymphocytic leukemia and loss of chromosome 7 is relatively uncommon; on the other hand, the translocation of chromosomal segments between chromosomes 8 and 21 involving *AML1/ETO* in nonlymphocytic leukemia cells is very common in children, but rare in adults. Loss of chromosome 5 and/or 7 more than doubles in individuals over the age of 50 compared with those

under 50 years of age. A gain of chromosome 8 increases with age, but not quite so dramatically. In the few studies in which the occupation of the leukemic patient has been correlated with the karyotype of the leukemic cells, losses of chromosome 5 and/or 7 or gain of chromosome 8 were increased by 50 percent in the occupationally exposed compared with the nonexposed patients.[137,138,268] Patients who worked with chemical solvents, pesticides, or petroleum products were classified as exposed, whereas those who were students, housewives, or white collar workers were classified as nonexposed. The observation that loss of chromosome 5 and/or 7 is rare in children and increases with age and that these same changes are much more common in leukemic patients who are classified as occupationally exposed to mutagenic agents lends support to our hypothesis that these chromosomal aberrations are both particularly sensitive indicators of exposure to mutagens and are probably critical to the development of therapy-related leukemia.

SUMMARY

Therapy-related AML is a recognizable subgroup of AML. The hallmarks of the syndrome are a preleukemic phase occurring several years after chemotherapy or radiation therapy for a primary disease, a distinct chromosomal abnormality in the preleukemic and leukemic clone of cells, evolution to karyotypically more abnormal sublines from the genetically unstable clone, and a brief survival after progression to leukemia. Alkylating agents are the most frequent therapy associated with treatment-related leukemia. Generally, the greater the amount and the longer the duration of alkylating agent chemotherapy given to an individual, the greater the incidence and shorter the latency period for development of leukemia. Patients older than 40 years probably have an increased likelihood of developing therapy-related leukemia. The disease arises from a series of mutations in a single hematopoietic stem cell, and these DNA changes provide a growth advantage to the progeny of the transformed cell. The abnormal clone of cells usually has a hypodiploid modal number of chromosomes and a deletion of part or all of chromosome 5 and/or 7. The study of therapy-induced leukemias is important for the clinician because the syndrome is increasing in frequency and for the basic scientist because it provides an important model of leukemogenesis.

ACKNOWLEDGMENTS

The authors thank the support of NIH, Joseph Troy Fund, Frederick Begell Foundation, C. and H. Koeffler Fund, Lymphoma Foundation of America, and the Horn Foundation. H.P.K. is a member of the Jonsson Cancer Center and holds the Mark Goodson Endowed Chair of Oncology.

REFERENCES

1. Anderson RL, Bagby GC, Richert-Boe K et al: Therapy-related preleukemic syndrome. Cancer 47:1867, 1981.
2. Dreyfus B: Preleukemic states. I. Definition and classification. II. Refractory anemia with an excess of myeloblasts in the bone mar-

row (smoldering acute leukemia). Nouv Rev Fr Hematol Blood Cells 17:33, 1976.

3. Koeffler HP, Golde DW: Human myeloid leukemia cell lines: A review. Blood 56:344, 1980.

4. Pedersen-Bjergaard J, Philip P, Mortensen BT et al: Acute non-lymphocytic leukemia, preleukemia, and acute myeloproliferative syndrome secondary to treatment of other malignant diseases. Clinical and cytogenetic characteristics and results of in vitro culture of bone marrow and HLA typing. Blood 57:712, 1981.

5. Kapadia SB, Krause JR, Ellis LD et al: Induced acute non-lymphocytic leukemia following long-term chemotherapy: A study of 20 cases. Cancer 45:1315, 1980.

6. Papa G, Alimena G, Annino L et al: Acute non lymphoid leukaemia following Hodgkin's disease. Clinical, biological and cytogenetic aspects of 3 cases. Scand J Haematol 23:339, 1979.

7. Rowley JD, Alimena G, Garson OM et al: A collaborative study of the relationship of the morphological type of acute nonlymphocytic leukemia with patient age and karyotype. Blood 59:1013, 1982.

8. Rowley JD, Golomb HM, Vardiman JW: Nonrandom chromosome abnormalities in acute leukemia and dysmyelopoietic syndromes in patients with previously treated malignant disease. Blood 58:759, 1981.

9. Saarni MI, Linman JW: Preleukemia. The hematologic syndrome preceding acute leukemia. Am J Med 55:38, 1973.

10. Pui CH, Behm FG, Raimondi SC et al: Secondary acute myeloid leukemia in children treated for acute lymphoid leukemia. N Engl J Med 321:136, 1989.

11. Ratain MJ, Kaminer LS, Bitran JD et al: Acute nonlymphocytic leukemia following etoposide and cisplatin combination chemotherapy for advanced non-small-cell carcinoma of the lung. Blood 70:1412, 1987.

12. Kantarjian HM, Estey EH, Keating MJ: Treatment of therapy-related leukemia and myelodysplastic syndrome. Hematol Oncol Clin North Am 7:81, 1993.

13. Dohy H, Genot JY, Imbert M et al: Myelodysplasia and leukaemia related to chemotherapy and/or radiotherapy—a haematological study of 13 cases. Value of macrocytosis as an early sign of bone marrow injury. Clin Lab Haematol 2:111, 1980.

14. Ballen KK, Antin JH: Treatment of therapy-related acute myelogenous leukemia and myelodysplastic syndromes. Hematol Oncol Clin North Am 7:477, 1993.

15. Vardiman JW, Golomb HM, Rowley JD, Variakojis D: Acute non-lymphocytic leukemia in malignant lymphoma: A morphologic study. Cancer 42:229, 1978.

16. Khaleeli M, Keane WM, Lee GR: Sideroblastic anemia in multiple myeloma: A preleukemic change. Blood 41:17, 1973.

17. Maldonado JE, Maigne J, Lecoq D: Comparative electron-microscopic study of the erythrocytic line in refractory anemia (preleukemia) and myelomonocytic leukemia. Nouv Rev Fr Hematol Blood Cells 17:167, 1976.

18. Vardiman JW, Coelho A, Golomb HM, Rowley J: Morphologic and cytochemical observations on the overt leukemic phase of therapy-related leukemia. Am J Clin Pathol 79:525, 1983.

19. Le Beau MM, Albain KS, Larson RA et al: Clinical and cytogenetic correlations in 63 patients with therapy-related myelodysplastic syndromes and acute nonlymphocytic leukemia: Further evidence for characteristic abnormalities of chromosomes no. 5 and 7. J Clin Oncol 4:325, 1986.

20. Pedersen-Bjergaard J, Rowley JD: The balanced and the unbalanced chromosome aberrations of acute myeloid leukemia may develop in different ways and may contribute differently to malignant transformation. Blood 83:2780, 1994.

21. Chromosomes in acute non-lymphocytic leukaemia. First International Workshop on Chromosomes in Leukaemia: Br J Haematol 39:311, 1978.

22. Kantarjian HM, Keating MJ, Walters RS et al: Therapy-related leukemia and myelodysplastic syndrome: Clinical, cytogenetic, and prognostic features. J Clin Oncol 4:1748, 1986.

23. Pedersen-Bjergaard J, Philip P, Larsen SO et al: Chromosome aberrations and prognostic factors in therapy-related myelodysplasia and acute nonlymphocytic leukemia. Blood 76:1083, 1990.

24. Johansson B, Mertens F, Heim S et al: Cytogenetics of secondary myelodysplasia (sMDS) and acute nonlymphocytic leukemia (sANLL). Eur J Haematol 47:17, 1991.

25. Kere J, Donis-Keller H, Ruutu T, de la Chapelle A: Chromosome 7 long-arm deletions in myeloid disorders: Terminal DNA sequences are commonly conserved and breakpoints vary. Cytogenet Cell Genet 50:226, 1989.

26. Kere J, Ruutu T, Davies KA et al: Chromosome 7 long arm deletion in myeloid disorders: A narrow breakpoint region in 7q22 defined by molecular mapping. Blood 73:230, 1989.

27. Mitelman F, Kaneko Y, Trent JM: Report of the committee on chromosome changes in neoplasia. Cytogenet Cell Genet 55:358, 1990.

28. Tsui LC, Farrall M, Donis-Keller H: Report of the committee on the genetic constitution of chromosomes 7 and 8. Cytogenet Cell Genet 51:166, 1989.

29. Le Beau MM, Espinosa R, Neuman WL et al: Cytogenetic and molecular delineation of the smallest commonly deleted region of chromosome 5 in malignant myeloid diseases. Proc Natl Acad Sci USA 90:5484, 1993.

30. Le Beau MM, Epstein ND, O'Brien SJ et al: The interleukin 3 gene is located on human chromosome 5 and is deleted in myeloid leukemias with a deletion of 5q. Proc Natl Acad Sci USA 84:5913, 1987.

31. Le Beau MM, Lemons RS, Espinosa R et al: Interleukin-4 and interleukin-5 map to human chromosome 5 in a region encoding growth factors and receptors and are deleted in myeloid leukemias with a del(5q). Blood 73:647, 1989.

32. Nienhuis AW, Bunn HF, Turner PH et al: Expression of the human c-fms proto-oncogene in hematopoietic cells and its deletion in the 5q-syndrome. Cell 42:421, 1985.

33. Le Beau MM, Westbrook CA, Diaz MO et al: Evidence for the involvement of GM-CSF and FMS in the deletion (5q) in myeloid disorders. Science 231:984, 1986.

34. Quesnel B, Kantarjian H, Bjergaard JP et al: Therapy-related acute myeloid leukemia with t(8;21), inv(16), and t(8;16): A report on 25 cases and review of the literature. J Clin Oncol 11:2370, 1993.

35. Pedersen-Bjergaard J, Johansson B, Philip P: Translocation (3;21)(q26;q22) in therapy-related myelodysplasia following drugs targeting DNA-topoisomerase II combined with alkylating agents, and in myeloproliferative disorders undergoing spontaneous leukemic transformation. Cancer Genet Cytogenet 76:50, 1994.

36. Levine EG, Bloomfield CD: Leukemias and myelodysplastic syndromes secondary to drug, radiation, and environmental exposure. Semin Oncol 19:47, 1992.

37. Cimino G, Moir DT, Canaani O et al: Cloning of ALL-1, the locus involved in leukemias with the t(4;11)(q21;q23), t(9;11)(p22;q23), and t(11;19)(q23;p13) chromosome translocations. Cancer Res 51:6712, 1991.

38. Ziemin-van DP, McCabe NR, Gill HJ et al: Identification of a gene, MLL, that spans the breakpoint in 11q23 translocations associated with human leukemias. Proc Natl Acad Sci USA 88:10735, 1991.

39. Dimartino JF, Cleary ML: MLL rearrangements in haematological malignancies: Lessons from clinical and biological studies. Br J Haematol 106:614, 1999.

40. Thirman MJ, Gill HJ, Burnett RC et al: Rearrangement of the MLL gene in acute lymphoblastic and acute myeloid leukemias with 11q23 chromosomal translocations. N Engl J Med 329:909, 1993.

41. Baccarani M, Bosi A, Papa G: Second malignancy in patients treated by Hodgkin's disease. Cancer 46:1735, 1980.

42. Bernstein ML, Vekemans MJ: Chromosomal changes in secondary leukemias of childhood and young adulthood. Crit Rev Oncol Hematol 5:325, 1986.

43. Aksoy M, Erdem S: Followup study on the mortality and the development of leukemia in 44 pancytopenic patients with chronic exposure to benzene. Blood 52:285, 1978.

44. Einhorn N: Acute leukemia after chemotherapy (melphalan). Cancer 41:444, 1978.

45. Berk PD, Goldberg JD, Silverstein MN et al: Increased incidence of acute leukemia in polycythemia vera associated with chlorambucil therapy. N Engl J Med 304:441, 1981.

46. Greene MH, Boice JD, Greer BE et al: Acute nonlymphocytic leukemia after therapy with alkylating agents for ovarian cancer: A study of five randomized clinical trials. N Engl J Med 307:1416, 1982.

47. Coltman CA, Dixon DO: Second malignancies complicating Hodgkin's disease: A Southwest Oncology Group 10-year followup. Cancer Treat Rep 66:1023, 1982.

48. DeVore R, Whitlock J, Hainsworth JD, Johnson DH: Therapy-related acute nonlymphocytic leukemia with monocytic features and rearrangement of chromosome 11q. Ann Intern Med 110:740, 1989.

49. Ratain MJ, Rowley JD: Therapy-related acute myeloid leukemia secondary to inhibitors of topoisomerase II: From the bedside to the target genes. Ann Oncol 3:107, 1992.

50. Kyle RA: Second malignancies associated with chemotherapeutic agents. Semin Oncol 9:131, 1982.

51. Krikorian JG, Burke JS, Rosenberg SA, Kaplan HS: Occurrence of non-Hodgkin's lymphoma after therapy for Hodgkin's disease. N Engl J Med 300:452, 1979.

52. Stegman R, Alexanian R: Solid tumors in multiple myeloma. Ann Intern Med 90:780, 1979.

53. Bizzozero OJ, Johnson KG, Ciocco A: Radiation-related leukemia in Hiroshima and Nagasaki, 1946–1964. I. Distribution, incidence and appearance time. N Engl J Med 274:1095, 1966.

54. Andrieu JM, Ifrah N, Payen C et al: Increased risk of secondary acute nonlymphocytic leukemia after extended-field radiation therapy combined with MOPP chemotherapy for Hodgkin's disease. J Clin Oncol 8:1148, 1990.

55. Cimino G, Papa G, Tura S et al: Second primary cancer following Hodgkin's disease: Updated results of an Italian multicentric study. J Clin Oncol 9:432, 1991.

56. van Leeuwen FE, Klokman WJ, Hagenbeek A et al: Second cancer risk following Hodgkin's disease: A 20-year follow-up study. J Clin Oncol 12:312, 1994.

57. Kaldor JM, Day NE, Clarke EA et al: Leukemia following Hodgkin's disease. N Engl J Med 322:7, 1990.

58. van Leeuwen FE, Chorus AM, van den Belt-Dusebout AW et al: Leukemia risk following Hodgkin's disease: Relation to cumulative dose of alkylating agents, treatment with teniposide combinations, number of episodes of chemotherapy, and bone marrow damage. J Clin Oncol 12:1063, 1994.

59. Abrahamsen JF, Andersen A, Hannisdal E et al: Second malignancies after treatment of Hodgkin's disease: The influence of treatment, follow-up time, and age. J Clin Oncol 11:255, 1993.

60. Swerdlow AJ, Douglas AJ, Vaughan HG et al: Risk of second primary cancer after Hodgkin's disease in patients in the British National Lymphoma Investigation: Relationships to host factors, histology and stage of Hodgkin's disease, and splenectomy. Br J Cancer 68:1006, 1993.

61. Dietrich PY, Henry-Amar M, Cosset JM et al: Second primary cancers in patients continuously disease-free from Hodgkin's disease: A protective role for the spleen? Blood 84:1209, 1994.

62. Devereux S, Selassie TG, Vaughan HG et al: Leukaemia complicating treatment for Hodgkin's disease: The experience of the British National Lymphoma Investigation. BMJ 301:1077, 1990.

63. Tarbell NJ, Gelber RD, Weinstein HJ, Mauch P: Sex differences in risk of second malignant tumours after Hodgkin's disease in childhood. Lancet 341:1428, 1993.

64. Henry-Amar M, Dietrich PY: Acute leukemia after the treatment of Hodgkin's disease. Hematol Oncol Clin North Am 7:369, 1993.

65. Tucker MA, Coleman CN, Cox RS et al: Risk of second cancers after treatment for Hodgkin's disease. N Engl J Med 318:76, 1988.

66. Bhatia S, Robison LL, Oberlin O et al: Breast cancer and other second neoplasms after childhood Hodgkin's disease. N Engl J Med 334:745, 1996.

67. Mauch PM, Kalish LA, Marcus KC et al: Second malignancies after treatment for laparotomy staged IA-IIIB Hodgkin's disease: Long-term analysis of risk factors and outcome. Blood 87:3625, 1996.

68. Wolden SL, Lamborn KR, Cleary SF et al: Second cancers following pediatric Hodgkin's disease. J Clin Oncol 16:536, 1998.

69. Third National Cancer Survey: Incidence data: Natl Cancer Inst Monogr 41:10, 1975.

70. Valagussa P, Santoro A, Fossati BF et al: Absence of treatment-induced second neoplasms after ABVD in Hodgkin's disease. Blood 59:488, 1982.

71. Amadori S, Papa G, Anselmo AP et al: Acute promyelocytic leukemia following ABVD (doxorubicin, bleomycin, vinblastine, and dacarbazine) and radiotherapy for Hodgkin's disease. Cancer Treat Rep 67:603, 1983.

72. Valagussa P, Santoro A, Fossati-Bellani F et al: Second acute leukemia and other malignancies following treatment for Hodgkin's disease. J Clin Oncol 4:830, 1986.

73. Cadman EC, Capizzi RL, Bertino JR: Acute nonlymphocytic leukemia: A delayed complication of Hodgkin's disease therapy: Analysis of 109 cases. Cancer 40:1280, 1977.

74. Pedersen-Bjergaard J, Larsen SO: Incidence of acute nonlymphocytic leukemia, preleukemia, and acute myeloproliferative syndrome up to 10 years after treatment of Hodgkin's disease. N Engl J Med 307:965, 1982.

75. De Gramont A, Louvet C, Krulik M et al: Preleukemic changes in cases of nonlymphocytic leukemia secondary to cytotoxic therapy. Analysis of 105 cases. Cancer 58:630, 1986.

76. van der Velden JWC, van Putten WL, Guinee VF et al: Subsequent development of acute non-lymphocytic leukemia in patients treated for Hodgkin's disease. Int J Cancer 42:252, 1988.

77. Travis LB, Curtis RE, Stovall M et al: Risk of leukemia following treatment for non-Hodgkin's lymphoma. J Natl Cancer Inst 86:1450, 1994.

78. Cimino G, Anselmo AP, Cartoni C et al: Secondary acute non lymphoid leukemia in patients treated for non Hodgkin's lymphoma: No risk of therapy-related ANLL after PROVECIP schedule. Tumori 73:363, 1987.

79. Pedersen-Bjergaard J, Ersboll J, Sorensen HM et al: Risk of acute nonlymphocytic leukemia and preleukemia in patients treated with cyclophosphamide for non-Hodgkin's lymphomas. Comparison with results obtained in patients treated for Hodgkin's disease and ovarian carcinoma with other alkylating agents. Ann Intern Med 103:195, 1985.

80. Ingram L, Mott MG, Mann JR et al: Second malignancies in children treated for non-Hodgkin's lymphoma and T-cell leukaemia with the UKCCSG regimens. Br J Cancer 55:463, 1987.

81. Travis LB, Curtis RE, Boice JD et al: Second cancers following non-Hodgkin's lymphoma. Cancer 67:2002, 1991.

82. Travis LB, Curtis RE, Glimelius B et al: Second cancers among long-term survivors of non-Hodgkin's lymphoma. J Natl Cancer Inst 85:1932, 1993.

83. Greene MH, Young RC, Merrill JM, DeVita VT: Evidence of a treatment dose response in acute nonlymphocytic leukemias which occur after therapy of non-Hodgkin's lymphoma. Cancer Res 43:1891, 1983.

84. Rosner F, Grunwald HW: Simultaneous occurrence of multiple myeloma and acute myeloblastic leukemia: Fact or myth? Am J Med 76:891, 1984.

85. Cuzick J, Erskine S, Edelman D, Galton DA: A comparison of the incidence of the myelodysplastic syndrome and acute myeloid leukaemia following melphalan and cyclophosphamide treatment for myelomatosis. A report to the Medical Research Council's working party on leukaemia in adults. Br J Cancer 55:523, 1987.

86. Bergsagel DE, Bailey AJ, Langley GR et al: The chemotherapy on plasma-cell myeloma and the incidence of acute leukemia. N Engl J Med 301:743, 1979.

87. Reimer RR, Hoover R, Fraumeni JF, Young RC: Acute leukemia after alkylating-agent therapy of ovarian cancer. N Engl J Med 297:177, 1977.

88. Pedersen-Bjergaard J, Nissen NI, Sorensen HM et al: Acute non-lymphocytic leukemia in patients with ovarian carcinoma following long-term treatment with Treosulfan (dihydroxybusulfan). Cancer 45:19, 1980.

89. Greene MH, Harris EL, Gershenson DM et al: Melphalan may be a more potent leukemogen than cyclophosphamide. Ann Intern Med 105:360, 1986.

90. Kaldor JM, Day NE, Pettersson F et al: Leukemia following chemotherapy for ovarian cancer. N Engl J Med 322:1, 1990.

91. Travis LB, Holowaty EJ, Bergfeldt K et al: Risk of leukemia after platinum-based chemotherapy for ovarian cancer. N Engl J Med 340:351, 1999.

92. van Leeuwen FE, Stiggelbout AM, van den Belt-Dusebout AW et al: Second cancer risk following testicular cancer: A follow-up study of 1909 patients. J Clin Oncol 11:415, 1993.

93. Bokemeyer C, Schmoll HJ: Secondary neoplasms following treatment of malignant germ cell tumors. J Clin Oncol 11:1703, 1993.

94. Nichols CR, Breeden ES, Loehrer PJ et al: Secondary leukemia associated with a conventional dose of etoposide: Review of serial germ cell tumor protocols. J Natl Cancer Inst 85:36, 1993.

95. Bajorin DF, Motzer RJ, Rodriguez E et al: Acute nonlymphocytic leukemia in germ cell tumor patients treated with etoposide-containing chemotherapy. J Natl Cancer Inst 85:60, 1993.

96. Pedersen-Bjergaard J, Daugaard G, Hansen SW et al: Increased risk of myelodysplasia and leukaemia after etoposide, cisplatin, and bleomycin for germ-cell tumours. Lancet 338:359, 1991.

97. Redman JR, Vugrin D, Arlin ZA et al: Leukemia following treatment of germ cell tumors in men. J Clin Oncol 2:1080, 1984.

98. Nichols CR, Hoffman R, Einhorn LH et al: Hematologic malignancies associated with primary mediastinal germ-cell tumors. Ann Intern Med 102:603, 1985.

99. Roth BJ, Greist A, Kubilis PS et al: Cisplatin-based combination chemotherapy for disseminated germ cell tumors: Long-term follow-up. J Clin Oncol 6:1239, 1988.

100. van Leeuwen FE, Stiggelbout AM, van den Belt-Dusebout AW et al: Second cancer risk following testicular cancer: A follow-up study of 1909 patients. J Clin Oncol 11:415, 1993.

101. Williams SD, Birch R, Einhorn LH et al: Treatment of disseminated germ-cell tumors with cisplatin, bleomycin, and either vinblastine or etoposide. N Engl J Med 316:1435, 1987.

102. Boshoff C, Begent RH, Oliver RT et al: Secondary tumours following etoposide containing therapy for germ cell cancer. Ann Oncol 6:35, 1995.

103. Smith MA, Rubinstein L, Anderson JR et al: Secondary leukemia or myelodysplastic syndrome after treatment with epipodophyllotoxins. J Clin Oncol 17:569, 1999.

104. Bokemeyer C, Schmoll HJ, Kuczyk MA et al: Risk of secondary leukemia following high cumulative doses of etoposide during chemotherapy for testicular cancer. J Natl Cancer Inst 87:58, 1995.

105. Kollmannsberger C, Beyer J, Droz JP et al: Secondary leukemia following high cumulative doses of etoposide in patients treated for advanced germ cell tumors. J Clin Oncol 16:3386, 1998.

106. Kollmannsberger C, Hartmann JT, Kanz L, Bokemeyer C: Therapy-related malignancies following treatment of germ cell cancer. Int J Cancer 83:860, 1999.

107. Hartmann JT, Nichols CR, Droz JP et al: The relative risk of second nongerminal malignancies in patients with extragonadal germ cell tumors. Cancer 88:2629, 2000.

108. Hartmann JT, Nichols CR, Droz JP et al: Hematologic disorders associated with primary mediastinal nonseminomatous germ cell tumors. J Natl Cancer Inst 92:54, 2000.

109. Valagussa P, Tancini G, Bonadonna G: Second malignancies after CMF for resectable breast cancer. J Clin Oncol 5:1138, 1987.

110. Tallman MS, Gray R, Bennett JM et al: Leukemogenic potential of adjuvant chemotherapy for early-stage breast cancer: The Eastern Cooperative Oncology Group experience. J Clin Oncol 13:1557, 1995.

111. Diamandidou E, Buzdar AU, Smith TL et al: Treatment-related leukemia in breast cancer patients treated with fluorouracil-doxorubicin-cyclophosphamide combination adjuvant chemotherapy: The University of Texas M.D. Anderson Cancer Center experience. J Clin Oncol 14:2722, 1996.

112. Darrington DL, Vose JM, Anderson JR et al: Incidence and characterization of secondary myelodysplastic syndrome and acute myelogenous leukemia following high-dose chemoradiotherapy and autologous stem-cell transplantation for lymphoid malignancies. J Clin Oncol 12:2527, 1994.

113. Bhatia S, Ramsay NK, Steinbuch M et al: Malignant neoplasms following bone marrow transplantation. Blood 87:3633, 1996.

114. Pedersen-Bjergaard J, Pedersen M, Myhre J, Geisler C: High risk of therapy-related leukemia after BEAM chemotherapy and autologous stem cell transplantation for previously treated lymphomas is mainly related to primary chemotherapy and not to the BEAM-transplantation procedure. Leukemia 11:1654, 1997.

115. André M, Henry-Amar M, Blaise D et al: Treatment-related deaths and second cancer risk after autologous stem-cell transplantation for Hodgkin's disease. Blood 92:1933, 1998.

116. Friedberg JW, Neuberg D, Stone RM et al: Outcome in patients with myelodysplastic syndrome after autologous bone marrow transplantation for non-Hodgkin's lymphoma. J Clin Oncol 17:3128, 1999.

117. Sobecks RM, Le Beau MM, Anastasi J, Williams SF: Myelodysplasia and acute leukemia following high-dose chemotherapy and autologous bone marrow or peripheral blood stem cell transplantation. Bone Marrow Transplant 23:1161, 1999.

118. Milligan DW, Ruiz DEM, Kolb HJ et al: Secondary leukaemia and myelodysplasia after autografting for lymphoma: Results from the EBMT. EBMT Lymphoma and Late Effects Working Parties. European Group for Blood and Marrow Transplantation. Br J Haematol 106:1020, 1999.

119. Harrison CN, Gregory W, Hudson GV et al: High-dose BEAM chemotherapy with autologous haemopoietic stem cell transplantation for Hodgkin's disease is unlikely to be associated with a major increased risk of secondary MDS/AML. Br J Cancer 81:476, 1999.

120. Krishnan A, Bhatia S, Slovak ML et al: Predictors of therapy-related leukemia and myelodysplasia following autologous transplantation for lymphoma: An assessment of risk factors. Blood 95:1588, 2000.

121. Micallef IN, Lillington DM, Apostolidis J et al: Therapy-related myelodysplasia and secondary acute myelogenous leukemia after high-dose therapy with autologous hematopoietic progenitor-cell support for lymphoid malignancies. J Clin Oncol 18:947, 2000.

122. Laughlin MJ, McGaughey DS, Crews JR et al: Secondary myelodysplasia and acute leukemia in breast cancer patients after autologous bone marrow transplant. J Clin Oncol 16:1008, 1998.

123. Martinez-Climent JA, Comes AM, Vizcarra E et al: Chromosomal abnormalities in women with breast cancer after autologous stem cell transplantation are infrequent and may not predict development of therapy-related leukemia or myelodysplastic syndrome. Bone Marrow Transplant 25:1203, 2000.

124. Govindarajan R, Jagannath S, Flick JT et al: Preceding standard therapy is the likely cause of MDS after autotransplants for multiple myeloma. Br J Haematol 95:349, 1996.

125. Taylor PR, Jackson GH, Lennard AL et al: Low incidence of myelodysplastic syndrome following transplantation using autologous non-cryopreserved bone marrow. Leukemia 11:1650, 1997.

126. Stone RM, Neuberg D, Soiffer R et al: Myelodysplastic syndrome as a late complication following autologous bone marrow transplantation for non-Hodgkin's lymphoma. J Clin Oncol 12:2535, 1994.

127. Mach-Pascual S, Legare RD, Lu D et al: Predictive value of clonality assays in patients with non-Hodgkin's lymphoma undergoing autologous bone marrow transplant: A single institution study. Blood 91:4496, 1998.

128. Fruchtman SM, Mack K, Kaplan ME et al: From efficacy to safety: A Polycythemia Vera Study group report on hydroxyurea in patients with polycythemia vera. Semin Hematol 34:17, 1997.

129. Tatarsky I, Sharon R: Management of polycythemia vera with hydroxyurea. Semin Hematol 34:24, 1997.

130. Weinfeld A, Swolin B, Westin J: Acute leukaemia after hydroxyurea therapy in polycythaemia vera and allied disorders: Prospective study of efficacy and leukaemogenicity with therapeutic implications. Eur J Haematol 52:134, 1994.

131. Najean Y, Rain JD: Treatment of polycythemia vera: The use of hydroxyurea and pipobroman in 292 patients under the age of 65 years. Blood 90:3370, 1997.

132. Casciato DA, Scott JL: Acute leukemia following prolonged cytotoxic agent therapy. Medicine 58:32, 1979.

133. O'Gara RW, Adamson RH, Kelly MG, Dalgard DW: Neoplasms of the hematopoietic system in nonhuman primates: Report of one spontaneous tumor and two leukemias induced by procarbazine. J Natl Cancer Inst 46:1121, 1971.

134. Vismans JJ, Briet E, Meijer K, den Ottolander GJ: Azathioprine and subacute myelomonocytic leukemia. Acta Med Scand 207:315, 1980.

135. Carver JH, Hatch FT, Branscomb EW: Estimating maximum limits to mutagenic potency from cytotoxic potency. Nature 279:154, 1979.

136. Valagussa P, Santoro A, Kenda R et al: Second malignancies in Hodgkin's disease: A complication of certain forms of treatment. BMJ 280:216, 1980.

137. Brandt L, Nilsson PG, Mitelman F: Occupational exposure to petroleum products in men with acute non-lymphocytic leukaemia. BMJ 1:553, 1978.

138. Mitelman F, Brandt L, Nilsson PG: Relation among occupational exposure to potential mutagenic/carcinogenic agents, clinical findings, and bone marrow chromosomes in acute nonlymphocytic leukemia. Blood 52:1229, 1978.

139. Rinsky RA, Young RJ, Smith AB: Leukemia in benzene workers. Am J Ind Med 2:217, 1981.

140. Ginevan ME: Nonlymphatic leukemias and adult exposure to diagnostic X-rays: The evidence reconsidered. Health Phys 38:129, 1980.

141. Land CE: Estimating cancer risks from low doses of ionizing radiation. Science 209:1197, 1980.

142. Major IR, Mole RH: Myeloid leukaemia in x-ray irradiated CBA mice. Nature 272:455, 1978.

143. Seed TM, Tolle DV, Fritz TE et al: Irradiation-induced erythroleukemia and myelogenous leukemia in the beagle dog: Hematology and ultrastructure. Blood 50:1061, 1977.

144. Elias L, Hoffman R, Boswell S et al: A trial of recombinant alpha 2 interferon in the myelodysplastic syndromes: I. Clinical results. Leukemia 1:105, 1987.

145. Coleman CN, Williams CJ, Flint A et al: Hematologic neoplasia in patients treated for Hodgkin's disease. N Engl J Med 297:1249, 1977.

146. De Braekeleer M: Cytogenetic studies in secondary leukemia: Statistical analysis. Oncology 43:358, 1986.

147. Galvani DW, Nethersell AB, Cawley JC: Alpha-interferon in myelodysplasia; clinical observations and effects on NK cells. Leuk Res 12:257, 1988.

148. Cheson BD: The myelodysplastic syndromes: Current approaches to therapy. Ann Intern Med 112:932, 1990.

149. Koeffler HP, Hirji K, Itri L: 1,25-Dihydroxyvitamin D3: In vivo and in vitro effects on human preleukemic and leukemic cells. Cancer Treat Rep 69:1399, 1985.

150. Huang ME, Ye YC, Chen SR et al: Use of all-trans retinoic acid in the treatment of acute promyelocytic leukemia. Blood 72:567, 1988.

151. Warrell RP, Frankel SR, Miller WH et al: Differentiation therapy of acute promyelocytic leukemia with tretinoin (all-trans-retinoic acid). N Engl J Med 324:1385, 1991.

152. Koeffler HP, Heitjan D, Mertelsmann R et al: Randomized study of 13-cis retinoic acid v placebo in the myelodysplastic disorders. Blood 71:703, 1988.

153. Clark RE, Ismail SA, Jacobs A et al: A randomized trial of 13-cis retinoic acid with or without cytosine arabinoside in patients with the myelodysplastic syndrome. Br J Haematol 66:77, 1987.

154. Kurzrock R, Estey E, Talpaz M: All-trans retinoic acid: Tolerance and biologic effects in myelodysplastic syndrome. J Clin Oncol 11:1489, 1993.

155. Estrov Z, Kurzrock R, Talpaz M et al: Granulocyte-macrophage colony-stimulating factor and interleukin-3 in combination: A potent and consistent myelodysplastic syndrome bone marrow stimulant in vitro. Ann Hematol 63:297, 1991.

156. Willemze R, van der Lely N, Zwierzina H et al: A randomized phase-I/II multicenter study of recombinant human granulocyte-macrophage colony-stimulating factor (GM-CSF) therapy for patients with myelodysplastic syndromes and a relatively low risk of acute leukemia. EORTC Leukemia Cooperative Group. Ann Hematol 64:173, 1992.

157. Ganser A, Seipelt G, Lindemann A et al: Effects of recombinant human interleukin-3 in patients with myelodysplastic syndromes. Blood 76:455, 1990.

158. Ganser A, Volkers B, Greher J et al: Recombinant human granulocyte-macrophage colony-stimulating factor in patients with myelodysplastic syndromes—a phase I/II trial. Blood 73:31, 1989.

159. Negrin RS, Haeuber DH, Nagler A et al: Treatment of myelodysplastic syndromes with recombinant human granulocyte colony-

stimulating factor. A phase I–II trial. Ann Intern Med 110:976, 1989.

160. Vadhan-Raj S, Keating M, LeMaistre A et al: Effects of recombinant human granulocyte-macrophage colony-stimulating factor in patients with myelodysplastic syndromes. N Engl J Med 317:1545, 1987.

161. Hellstrom-Lindberg E, Ahlgren T, Beguin Y et al: Treatment of anemia in myelodysplastic syndromes with granulocyte colony-stimulating factor plus erythropoietin: Results from a randomized phase II study and long-term follow-up of 71 patients. Blood 92:68, 1998.

162. Cheson BD, Jasperse DM, Simon R, Friedman MA: A critical appraisal of low-dose cytosine arabinoside in patients with acute non-lymphocytic leukemia and myelodysplastic syndromes. J Clin Oncol 4:1857, 1986.

163. Silverman LR, Holland JF, Weinberg RS et al: Effects of treatment with 5-azacytidine on the in vivo and in vitro hematopoiesis in patients with myelodysplastic syndromes. Leukemia 7(Suppl. 1):21, 1993.

164. Preisler HD, Early AP, Raza A et al: Therapy of secondary acute non-lymphocytic leukemia with cytarabine. N Engl J Med 308:21, 1983.

165. Beran M, Estey E, O'Brien S et al: Topotecan and cytarabine is an active combination regimen in myelodysplastic syndromes and chronic myelomonocytic leukemia. J Clin Oncol 17:2819, 1999.

166. Estey E, Thall P, Beran M et al: Effect of diagnosis (refractory anemia with excess blasts, refractory anemia with excess blasts in transformation, or acute myeloid leukemia [AML]) on outcome of AML-type chemotherapy. Blood 90:2969, 1997.

167. Fenaux P, Lucidarme D, Lai JL, Bauters F: Favorable cytogenetic abnormalities in secondary leukemia. Cancer 63:2505, 1989.

168. Lee EJ, George SL, Caligiuri M et al: Parallel phase I studies of daunorubicin given with cytarabine and etoposide with or without the multidrug resistance modulator PSC-833 in previously untreated patients 60 years of age or older with acute myeloid leukemia: Results of cancer and leukemia group B study 9420. J Clin Oncol 17:2831, 1999.

169. Ballen KK, Gilliland DG, Guinan EC et al: Bone marrow transplantation for therapy-related myelodysplasia: Comparison with primary myelodysplasia. Bone Marrow Transplant 20:737, 1997.

170. Anderson JE: Bone marrow transplantation for myelodysplasia. Blood Rev 14:63, 2000.

171. Anderson JE, Gooley TA, Schoch G et al: Stem cell transplantation for secondary acute myeloid leukemia: Evaluation of transplantation as initial therapy or following induction chemotherapy. Blood 89:2578, 1997.

172. Yakoub-Agha I, de La Salmoniere P, Ribaud P et al: Allogeneic bone marrow transplantation for therapy-related myelodysplastic syndrome and acute myeloid leukemia: A long-term study of 70 patients—report of the French society of bone marrow transplantation. J Clin Oncol 18:963, 2000.

173. Appelbaum FR, Anderson J: Allogeneic bone marrow transplantation for myelodysplastic syndrome: Outcomes analysis according to IPSS score. Leukemia 12(Suppl. 1):S25, 1998.

174. Deeg HJ, Shulman HM, Anderson JE et al: Allogeneic and syngeneic marrow transplantation for myelodysplastic syndrome in patients 55 to 66 years of age. Blood 95:1188, 2000.

175. Berg JW: The incidence of multiple primary cancers. I. Development of further cancers in patients with lymphomas, leukemias, and myeloma. J Natl Cancer Inst 38:741, 1967.

176. Mathe G, Tubiana M, Calman F et al: [Acute leukemia syndromes (ALS) appearing during the evolution of hematosarcomas and chronic leukemias (clinical analysis)]. Nouv Rev Fr Hematol 7:543, 1967.

177. Newell GR, Krementz ET, Roberts JD, Kinnear BK: Multiple primary neoplasms in blacks compared to whites. I. Further cancers in patients with Hodgkin's disease, leukemia, and myeloma. J Natl Cancer Inst 52:635, 1974.

178. Newman DR, Maldonado JE, Harrison EG et al: Myelomonocytic leukemia in Hodgkin's disease. Cancer 25:128, 1970.

179. Kjeldsberg CR, Nathwani BN, Rappaport H: Acute myeloblastic leukemia developing in patients with mediastinal lymphoblastic lymphoma. Cancer 44:2316, 1979.

180. Rosner F, Grunwald HW: Multiple myeloma and Waldenstrom's macroglobulinemia terminating in acute leukemia. Review with emphasis on karyotypic and ultrastructural abnormalities. N Y State J Med 80:558, 1980.

181. Zech L, Haglund U, Nilsson K, Klein G: Characteristic chromosomal abnormalities in biopsies and lymphoid-cell lines from patients with Burkitt and non-Burkitt lymphomas. Int J Cancer 17:47, 1976.

182. Lundberg WB, Farber LR, Cadman EC, Skeel RT: Spontaneous acute leukemia in polycythemia vera. Ann Intern Med 84:294, 1976.

183. Miller JA: Carcinogenesis by chemicals: An overview—G. H. A. Clowes Memorial Lecture. Cancer Res 30:559, 1970.

184. Carey RW, Holland JF, Sheehe PR, Graham S: Association of cancer of the breast and acute myelocytic leukemia. Cancer 20:1080, 1967.

185. Whang-Peng J, Lee EC, Minna JD et al: Deletion of 3(p14; p23) in secondary erythroleukemia arising in long-term survivors of small cell lung cancer. J Natl Cancer Inst 80:1253, 1988.

186. Ladanyi M, Samaniego F, Reuter VE et al: Cytogenetic and immunohistochemical evidence for the germ cell origin of a subset of acute leukemias associated with mediastinal germ cell tumors. J Natl Cancer Inst 82:221, 1990.

187. Chaganti RS, Ladanyi M, Samaniego F et al: Leukemic differentiation of a mediastinal germ cell tumor. Genes Chromosomes Cancer 1:83, 1989.

188. Nichols CR, Roth BJ, Heerema N et al: Hematologic neoplasia associated with primary mediastinal germ-cell tumors. N Engl J Med 322:1425, 1990.

189. Gatti RA, Good RA: Occurrence of malignancy in immunodeficiency diseases. A literature review. Cancer 28:89, 1971.

190. Keast D: Immunosurveillance and cancer. Lancet 2:710, 1970.

191. Lacher MJ: Long survival in Hodgkin's disease. Ann Intern Med 70:7, 1969.

192. Smetana HF: Hodgkin's disease: A follow-up study of patients surviving more than twenty years after the original diagnosis. J Pathol 98:231, 1969.

193. Miller EC: Some current perspectives on chemical carcinogenesis in humans and experimental animals: Presidential Address. Cancer Res 38:1479, 1978.

194. Singer B: N-nitroso alkylating agents: Formation and persistence of alkyl derivatives in mammalian nucleic acids as contributing factors in carcinogenesis. J Natl Cancer Inst 62:1329, 1979.

195. Schmid E, Bauchinger M: Comparison of the chromosome damage induced by radiation and cytoxan therapy in lymphocytes of patients with gynaecological tumours. Mutat Res 21:271, 1973.

196. Genuardi M, Zollino M, Serra A et al: Long-term cytogenetic effects of antineoplastic treatment in relation to secondary leukemia. Cancer Genet Cytogenet 33:201, 1988.

197. Yunis JJ: The chromosomal basis of human neoplasia. Science 221:227, 1983.

198. Pelicci PG, Lanfrancone L, Brathwaite MD et al: Amplification of the c-myb oncogene in a case of human acute myelogenous leukemia. Science 224:1117, 1984.

199. Blick M, Westin E, Gutterman J et al: Oncogene expression in human leukemia. Blood 64:1234, 1984.

200. Horiike S, Yokota S, Nakao M et al: Tandem duplications of the FLT3 receptor gene are associated with leukemic transformation of myelodysplasia. Leukemia 11:1442, 1997.

201. LeBeau MM, Rowley JD: Heritable fragile sites in cancer. Nature 308:607, 1984.

202. Nakagawa T, Saitoh S, Imoto S et al: Multiple point mutation of N-ras and K-ras oncogenes in myelodysplastic syndrome and acute myelogenous leukemia. Oncology 49:114, 1992.

203. Paquette RL, Landaw EM, Pierre RV et al: N-ras mutations are associated with poor prognosis and increased risk of leukemia in myelodysplastic syndrome. Blood 82:590, 1993.

204. Sherr CJ, Rettenmier CW: The fms gene and the CSF-1 receptor. Cancer Surv 5:221, 1986.

205. Yarden Y, Ullrich A: Growth factor receptor tyrosine kinases. Annu Rev Biochem 57:443, 1988.

206. Roussel MF, Downing JR, Rettenmier CW, Sherr CJ: A point mutation in the extracellular domain of the human CSF-1 receptor (c-fms proto-oncogene product) activates its transforming potential. Cell 55:979, 1988.

207. Woolford J, McAuliffe A, Rohrschneider LR: Activation of the feline c-fms proto-oncogene: Multiple alterations are required to generate a fully transformed phenotype. Cell 55:965, 1988.

208. Taylor C, McGlynn H, Carter G et al: RAS and FMS mutations following cytotoxic therapy for childhood acute lymphoblastic leukaemia. Leukemia 9:466, 1995.

209. Carter G, Ridge S, Padua RA: Genetic lesions in preleukemia. Crit Rev Oncog 3:339, 1992.

210. Ridge SA, Worwood M, Oscier D et al: FMS mutations in myelodysplastic, leukemic, and normal subjects. Proc Natl Acad Sci USA 87:1377, 1990.

211. Tobal K, Pagliuca A, Bhatt B et al: Mutation of the human FMS gene (M-CSF receptor) in myelodysplastic syndromes and acute myeloid leukemia. Leukemia 4:486, 1990.

212. List AF, Jacobs A: Biology and pathogenesis of the myelodysplastic syndromes. Semin Oncol 19:14, 1992.

213. Shannon KM, Turhan AG, Chang SS et al: Familial bone marrow monosomy 7. Evidence that the predisposing locus is not on the long arm of chromosome 7. J Clin Invest 84:984, 1989.

214. Luna-Fineman S, Shannon KM, Lange BJ: Childhood monosomy 7: Epidemiology, biology, and mechanistic implications. Blood 85:1985, 1995.

215. Ho CY, Otterud B, Legare RD et al: Linkage of a familial platelet disorder with a propensity to develop myeloid malignancies to human chromosome 21q22.1–22.2. Blood 87:5218, 1996.

216. Song WJ, Sullivan MG, Legare RD et al: Haploinsufficiency of CBFA2 causes familial thrombocytopenia with propensity to develop acute myelogenous leukaemia. Nat Genet 23:166, 1999.

217. Levine AJ, Momand J, Finlay CA: The p53 tumour suppressor gene. Nature 351:453, 1991.

218. Hollstein M, Sidransky D, Vogelstein B, Harris CC: p53 mutations in human cancers. Science 253:49, 1991.

219. Prokocimer M, Rotter V: Structure and function of p53 in normal cells and their aberrations in cancer cells: Projection on the hematologic cell lineages. Blood 84:2391, 1994.

220. Imamura J, Miyoshi I, Koeffler HP: p53 in hematologic malignancies. Blood 84:2412, 1994.

221. Sugimoto K, Hirano N, Toyoshima H et al: Mutations of the p53 gene in myelodysplastic syndrome (MDS) and MDS-derived leukemia. Blood 81:3022, 1993.

222. Jonveaux P, Fenaux P, Quiquandon I et al: Mutations in the p53 gene in myelodysplastic syndromes. Oncogene 6:2243, 1991.

223. Slingerland JM, Minden MD, Benchimol S: Mutation of the p53 gene in human acute myelogenous leukemia. Blood 77:1500, 1991.

224. Fenaux P, Jonveaux P, Quiquandon I et al: P53 gene mutations in acute myeloid leukemia with 17p monosomy. Blood 78:1652, 1991.

225. Fenaux P, Preudhomme C, Quiquandon I et al: Mutations of the P53 gene in acute myeloid leukaemia. Br J Haematol 80:178, 1992.

226. Wattel E, Preudhomme C, Hecquet B et al: p53 mutations are associated with resistance to chemotherapy and short survival in hematologic malignancies. Blood 84:3148, 1994.

227. Friend SH, Bernards R, Rogelj S et al: A human DNA segment with properties of the gene that predisposes to retinoblastoma and osteosarcoma. Nature 323:643, 1986.

228. Weinberg RA: The Rb gene and the negative regulation of cell growth. Blood 74:529, 1989.

229. Kornblau SM, Xu HJ, Zhang W et al: Levels of retinoblastoma protein expression in newly diagnosed acute myelogenous leukemia. Blood 84:256, 1994.

230. Ahuja HG, Jat PS, Foti A et al: Abnormalities of the retinoblastoma gene in the pathogenesis of acute leukemia. Blood 78:3259, 1991.

231. Kornblau SM, Xu HJ, del Giglio A et al: Clinical implications of decreased retinoblastoma protein expression in acute myelogenous leukemia. Cancer Res 52:4587, 1992.

232. Hebert J, Cayuela JM, Berkeley J, Sigaux F: Candidate tumor-suppressor genes MTS1 (p16INK4A) and MTS2 (p15INK4B) display frequent homozygous deletions in primary cells from T- but not from B-cell lineage acute lymphoblastic leukemias. Blood 84:4038, 1994.

233. Ogawa S, Hirano N, Sato N et al: Homozygous loss of the cyclin-dependent kinase 4-inhibitor (p16) gene in human leukemias. Blood 84:2431, 1994.

234. Cayuela JM, Hebert J, Sigaux F: Homozygous MTS1 (p16INK4A) deletion in primary tumor cells of 163 leukemic patients. Blood 85:854, 1995.

235. Quesnel B, Fenaux P: P15INK4b gene methylation and myelodysplastic syndromes. Leuk Lymphoma 35:437, 1999.

236. Tien HF, Tang JL, Tsay W et al: Methylation of the p15INK4B gene in myelodysplastic syndrome: It can be detected early at diagnosis or during disease progression and is highly associated with leukaemic transformation. Br J Haematol 112:148, 2001.

237. Tasaka T, Lee S, Spira S et al: Microsatellite instability during the progression of acute myelocytic leukaemia. Br J Haematol 98:219, 1997.

238. Rimsza LM, Kopecky KJ, Ruschulte J et al: Microsatellite instability is not a defining genetic feature of acute myeloid leukemogenesis in adults: Results of a retrospective study of 132 patients and review of the literature. Leukemia 14:1044, 2000.

239. Ben-Yehuda D, Krichevsky S, Caspi O et al: Microsatellite instability and p53 mutations in therapy-related leukemia suggest mutator phenotype. Blood 88:4296, 1996.

240. Zhu YM, Das-Gupta EP, Russell NH: Microsatellite instability and p53 mutations are associated with abnormal expression of the MSH2 gene in adult acute leukemia. Blood 94:733, 1999.

241. Nisse C, Lorthois C, Dorp V et al: Exposure to occupational and environmental factors in myelodysplastic syndromes. Preliminary results of a case-control study. Leukemia 9:693, 1995.

242. West RR, Stafford DA, White AD et al: Cytogenetic abnormalities in the myelodysplastic syndromes and occupational or environmental exposure. Blood 95:2093, 2000.

243. Rothman N, Smith MT, Hayes RB et al: Benzene poisoning, a risk factor for hematological malignancy, is associated with the NQO1 609C->T mutation and rapid fractional excretion of chlorzoxazone. Cancer Res 57:2839, 1997.

244. Larson RA, Wang Y, Banerjee M et al: Prevalence of the inactivating 609C->T polymorphism in the NAD(P)H:quinone oxidoreductase (NQO1) gene in patients with primary and therapy-related myeloid leukemia. Blood 94:803, 1999.

245. Hayes JD, Pulford DJ: The glutathione S-transferase supergene family: Regulation of GST and the contribution of the isoenzymes to cancer chemoprotection and drug resistance. Crit Rev Biochem Mol Biol 30:445, 1995.

246. Chen H, Sandler DP, Taylor JA et al: Increased risk for myelodysplastic syndromes in individuals with glutathione transferase theta 1 (GSTT1) gene defect. Lancet 347:295, 1996.

247. Preudhomme C, Nisse C, Hebbar M et al: Glutathione S transferase theta 1 gene defects in myelodysplastic syndromes and their correlation with karyotype and exposure to potential carcinogens. Leukemia 11:1580, 1997.

248. Atoyebi W, Kusec R, Fidler C et al: Glutathione S-transferase gene deletions in myelodysplasia. Lancet 349:1450, 1997.

249. Sasai Y, Horiike S, Misawa S et al: Genotype of glutathione S-transferase and other genetic configurations in myelodysplasia. Leuk Res 23:975, 1999.

250. Alexandrie AK, Sundberg MI, Seidegard J et al: Genetic susceptibility to lung cancer with special emphasis on CYP1A1 and GSTM1: A study on host factors in relation to age at onset, gender and histological cancer types. Carcinogenesis 15:1785, 1994.

251. Kawajiri K, Nakachi K, Imai K et al: The CYP1A1 gene and cancer susceptibility. Crit Rev Oncol Hematol 14:77, 1993.

252. Miller EC, Miller JA: Mechanisms of chemical carcinogenesis. Cancer 47:1055, 1981.

253. Fialkow PJ, Singer JW, Adamson JW et al: Acute nonlymphocytic leukemia: Expression in cells restricted to granulocytic and monocytic differentiation. N Engl J Med 301:1, 1979.

254. Fialkow PJ, Singer JW, Adamson JW et al: Acute nonlymphocytic leukemia: Heterogeneity of stem cell origin. Blood 57:1068, 1981.

255. Wiggans RG, Jacobson RJ, Fialkow PJ et al: Probable clonal origin of acute myeloblastic leukemia following radiation and chemotherapy of colon cancer. Blood 52:659, 1978.

256. Busque L, Gilliland DG, Prchal JT et al: Clonality in juvenile chronic myelogenous leukemia. Blood 85:21, 1995.

257. Lyon MF: The William Allan memorial award address: X-chromosome inactivation and the location and expression of X-linked genes. Am J Hum Genet 42:8, 1988.

258. Beutler E, Collins Z, Irwin LE: Value of genetic variants of glucose-6-phosphate dehydrogenase in tracing the origin of malignant tumors. N Engl J Med 276:389, 1967.

259. Vogelstein B, Fearon ER, Hamilton SR, Feinberg AP: Use of restriction fragment length polymorphisms to determine the clonal origin of human tumors. Science 227:642, 1985.

260. Vogelstein B, Fearon ER, Hamilton SR et al: Clonal analysis using recombinant DNA probes from the X-chromosome. Cancer Res 47:4806, 1987.

261. Allen RC, Zoghbi HY, Moseley AB et al: Methylation of HpaII and HhaI sites near the polymorphic CAG repeat in the human androgen-receptor gene correlates with X chromosome inactivation. Am J Hum Genet 51:1229, 1992.

262. Boyd Y, Fraser NJ: Methylation patterns at the hypervariable X-chromosome locus DXS255 (M27 beta): Correlation with X-inactivation status. Genomics 7:182, 1990.

263. Busque L, Gilliland DG: Clonal evolution in acute myeloid leukemia. Blood 82:337, 1993.

264. Fey MF, Liechti-Gallati S, von Rohr A et al: Clonality and X-inactivation patterns in hematopoietic cell populations detected by the highly informative M27 beta DNA probe. Blood 83:931, 1994.

265. Busque L, Zhu J, DeHart D et al: An expression based clonality assay at the human androgen receptor locus (HUMARA) on chromosome X. Nucleic Acids Res 22:697, 1994.

266. Willman CL, Busque L, Griffith BB et al: Langerhans'-cell histiocytosis (histiocytosis X)—a clonal proliferative disease. N Engl J Med 331:154, 1994.

267. Prchal JT, Guan YL, Prchal JF, Barany F: Transcriptional analysis of the active X-chromosome in normal and clonal hematopoiesis. Blood 81:269, 1993.

268. The Fourth International Workshop on Chromosomes in Leukemia: A prospective study of acute nonlymphocytic leukemia. Cancer Genet Cytogenet 11:249, 1984.

23

Myelodysplastic Syndromes

Kenneth B. Miller

The myelodysplastic syndromes (MDS) are a heterogeneous group of clonal stem cell disorders characterized by impaired proliferation and maturation of hematopoietic progenitor cells resulting in symptomatic anemia, leukopenia, or thrombocytopenia. Morphological and functional abnormalities involving one or more cell lines are common. The clinical course is very variable, ranging from a chronic, stable, mildly symptomatic disorder, to one that rapidly progresses to acute myeloid leukemia. Infections and/or bleeding are the most frequent causes of morbidity and mortality in patients with MDS. MDS shares many clinical, cytogenetic, and laboratory features with aplastic anemia, the myeloproliferative disorders, and the acute leukemias. The classification of MDS remains controversial and attempts to separate it from the myeloproliferative disorders and the acute leukemias. Many patients with MDS present with clinical and laboratory features suggestive of other stem cell disorders and it is important to ascertain if the patient has MDS versus dysplasia associated with another disorder (Figure 23–1). This chapter discusses the pathogenesis, clinical manifestations, classification, prognostic variables, and specific treatments for MDS. The cytogenetic findings are discussed in Chapter 16.

MDS is a progressive clonal disorder and the diagnostic studies and the initial evaluations are similar to those used in other stem cell disorders. However the clinical course, prognosis, and treatment approaches for a patient with one of the MDSs is different from the other stem cell disorders and the acute leukemias. The bone marrow and peripheral blood abnormalities in MDS can be subtle and require the cooperative efforts of pathologists, cytogeneticists, and clinicians to diagnosis, subtype, assign prognosis, and recommend therapy. Treatment should be individualized and based on the patient's MDS subtype, age, coexisting medical disorders, and prognostic variables.

MDS is not a new disease, but only recently has it been assigned a separate classification. Rhodes and Barker in 1938 reported on a group of elderly patients with refractory anemia and morphological abnormalities who were unresponsive to treatment with iron, folic acid, or B12.[1] Further studies identified patients with hypercellular bone marrows, with increased sideroblasts who developed progressive anemia. Crosby et al. applied the term sideroachrestic anemia to a group of elderly patients who presented with chronic cytopenias and terminated in acute leukemia.[2] Patients with MDS were also described as having a smoldering leukemia, preleukemia, and oligoblastic leukemia; these terms reflected that patients did not meet the usual criteria of acute leukemia, greater than 30 percent blast forms, but presented with a hypercellular marrow with increased blast forms and dysplastic changes in one or more cell lines.[3] In MDS, as in acute myeloid leukemia (AML), a malignant transforming event occurs at the level of the myeloid stem cell or pluripotential stem cell.[4,5] Chromosome abnormalities have confirmed the clonality of the oncogenic event and, in part, determine the biology of the disease. While many patients with MDS have features suggestive of an early leukemia, and rapidly evolve into one of the myeloid leukemias, most do not evolve into AML but die as a result of the MDS and its treatment.[6,7] MDS, therefore should not be considered as a primary preleukemic disorder, but as a disease of the pluripotential stem cell that is characterized by a progressive clonal proliferation of abnormal precursors that demonstrate both impaired maturation and proliferation. The separation of AML and MDS continues to be problematic, which is reflected in the classification system, prognostic features, and treatment options.

PATHOGENESIS AND ETIOLOGY

MDS is characterized by ineffective hematopoiesis.[8] The bone marrow is typically hypercellular with an increase in hematopoietic precursors. Apoptosis, programmed cell death, is increased in MDS resulting in an increased rate of progenitor cell division but with an impaired production and release of mature cells.[9] The clonal origin of MDS has been confirmed by isozyme analysis of glucose 6 phosphate dehydrogenase (G6PD) in heterozygous females and more recently by molecular analysis of other loci such as the androgen receptor gene.[10,11] The clonal origin of the abnormal granulocytes and erythroid precursors in MDS has been confirmed.[12] The involvement of lymphoid progenitors is more variable and it remains controversial if B and T lymphocytes are also part of the abnormal clone.[13,14] The appearance of a clonal abnormality appears to be an early event and cytogenetic abnormalities can be demonstrated, in some patients, before any morphological or clinical findings.[15,16] The initial cytogenetic events are part of a multi-

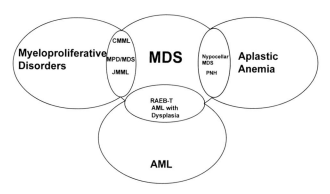

Figure 23–1. Relationship of MDS and other clonal disorders.

step process, which promotes the acquisition of other additional, secondary genetic events.[17] Alterations in the N-*ras* oncogene; the *p53* and *IRF-1* tumor-suppressor genes; the anti-apoptotic *Bcl-2* gene; methylation of specific gene promoters; and the transcription-factor genes are all associated with the stepwise progression of MDS.[18–21]

Genetic, environmental, and exposure factors have been associated with an increased risk for the development of MDS. However, for most patients there is no known etiology. The possibility of an inherited predisposition in patients with MDS is controversial. Inherited constitutional genetic defects have been associated with up to 30 percent of children with MDS and related myeloproliferative disorders.[22] Children with Schwachman-Diamond syndrome, Fanconi anemia, and neurofibromatosis type 1 have constitutional genetic defects that are associated with the increased risk for the development of both MDS and AML.[22,23] Mutations of specific genes mediating DNA repair appear to predispose to the acquisition of secondary cytogenetic abnormalities that can lead to the development of MDS.[23–26]

Mutations resulting in the activation of the *ras* oncogene have been reported in patients with MDS.[27] The frequency of these mutations increases with progression of the disease and the subsequent development of secondary cytogenetic events.[28] The etiological role of N-*ras* mutations in the development of MDS is unclear and these mutations may just reflect the genetic instability of the MDS clone and its propensity to develop random genetic mutations. MDS patients have defects in a number of signal transduction pathways that appear to be related to the evolving ineffective hematopoiesis.[29,30] These acquired abnormalities, however, may contribute to the further dysregulation of progenitor cell cycle kinetics and the maintenance of DNA integrity, which results in progressive genetic instability.

Abnormalities of the bone marrow microenvironment and aberrant cytokine production have also been noted in patients with MDS. Abnormalities in the regulation of tumor necrosis factor alpha (TNF-α), transforming factor–beta, and interleukin 1b have been reported, and may in part support the continued growth and expansion of the abnormal clone.[31]

The bone marrow in MDS has an increase in the number of apoptotic cells.[32] The accelerated apoptosis is most marked in the less proliferative, better prognostic, forms of MDS.[33] The etiological role of apoptosis in MDS, however, remains controversial. Purified CD34+ progenitors from patients with MDS are more resistant to FAS-mediated apoptosis as compared to a similar population of normal control cells.[34] The resistance of precursor MDS cells to apoptosis could be one of the factors that confers a survival advantage to the MDS clone. The lineage committed MDS cells, however, do appear to be more susceptible to apoptosis as they differentiate, which may reflect their disordered, ineffective, and impaired maturation.[35] The increased apoptosis of committed precursors could result in the observed peripheral cytopenias despite the hypercellular bone marrow and increased proliferation of immature precursors.[36,37] The increased apoptosis may also be a secondary event reflecting the impaired maturation and proliferation of the abnormal clone modulated by changes in the bone marrow microenvironment. The overexpression of TNF-α produced by MDS mononuclear cells can inhibit the growth of residual normal hematopoiesis and lead to increased cell death of normal precursors.[38–40]

MDS is associated with a number of immunoregulatory abnormalities including the development of autoantibodies, and monoclonal gammopathies.[41] In subsets of patients with MDS, autoreactive T-cell clones are present that inhibit autologous erythroid and granulocytic colony growth.[42,43] T-cell-mediated suppression of bone marrow growth and maturation appears to be an important process in the hypoplastic variants of MDS, as in patients with aplastic anemia.[44,45] MDS is also associated with a number of other immune-mediated disorders.[41] The immunoregulatory abnormalities may explain the response to immunosuppressive therapy in selected patients with MDS.

Environmental agents have been implicated in the etiology of MDS. Case-controlled studies have demonstrated an association between MDS and cigarette smoking, exposure to benzene, petroleum products, organic solvents, fertilizers, pesticides, and inorganic dusts.[46–50] It remains controversial if there is a defined genetic predisposition in MDS that relates to naturally occurring complex DNA polymorphisms in genes that mediate DNA repair and the metabolism of environmental carcinogens.[51,52] In selected genetically predisposed individuals, MDS may arise as a result of cumulative environmental exposures. Studies have linked the development of MDS and the nonfunction $^{609}C \rightarrow T$ polymorphic allele of the NAD(P)H:quinone oxidoreductase *(NQO1)* gene. These genes appear to play a critical role in detoxifying benzene metabolites. This association is controversial, but may explain the increased incidence of MDS in some patients exposed to organic solvents and benzene-containing compounds.[51,52] Similar controversial results have been noted in the glutathione S-transferase *(GST)* genes that mediate the metabolism of cytotoxic and genotoxic agents.[52–55]

A prior exposure to alkylating agents (cyclophosphamide, chlorambucil, and melphalan) is associated with an increased risk of MDS. The risk is, in part, related to the dose and duration of treatment and generally occurs 3 to 7 years after the exposure. Patients who received combination radiation therapy and chemotherapy are at an increased risk for the development of MDS. Patients with Hodgkin's disease treated with alkylating agent–based chemotherapy and radiation therapy have a 13 percent projected incidence of secondary MDS (t-MDS) at 10 years post-treatment.[56] Total body irradiation, administered as part of the preparative regimen for an autologous stem cell transplantation, is associated with an increased risk for MDS.[57] The combination of high-dose alkylating therapy and total body irradiation was associated with a 10 to 15 percent risk of t-MDS and secondary AML. The chronic exposure to purine analogues and hydroxyurea has been associated with the development of MDS in some series.[58,59] The MDS that occurs after chemotherapy exposure has a very poor prognosis.[59,60] Therapy-related MDS is associated with a high frequency of karyotypic abnormalities involving chromosomes 5 and/or 7.[61]

MDS most commonly affects patients over the age of 50 years with an overall incidence of 3.5 to 12.6/100,000/year.[62] In people over the age of 70 years the incidence is between 15 and

50/100,000/year, a prevalence similar to other common hematological malignancies in this population.[63] However, the overall incidence of MDS may be much higher due to difficulties in diagnosis, classification, and recording. MDS has not been reported as a malignant disorder and therefore the true incidence of MDS may be much higher. There is no clear evidence that the incidence of MDS is increasing, other than that due to the demographics associated with the aging population. The incidence is similar in men and women with the exception of the 5q–, which has a marked female predominance.[64] While the majority of patients with MDS are elderly it can occur in children and young adults.[65] Series of familial MDS with karyotypic abnormalities have been reported.[66,67]

CLASSIFICATION

The classification and diagnosis of MDS is controversial and evolving to include prognostic variables and cytogenetics. The FAB (French-American-British) group was the first to define morphological criteria in the blood and bone marrow for the diagnosis and classification of MDS.[68] The FAB classification is based solely on morphology, and the percentage of blast forms in the blood and bone marrow is useful in categorizing patients and broadly assessing prognosis. The FAB group's classification attempted to separate MDS from AML, other myeloproliferative disorders, and aplastic anemia (Figure 23–2). This classification system, although generally adopted, is sometimes clinically and biologically inconsistent. The separation of MDS from

AML and other clonal disorders is based on an arbitrary number of blast forms. Moreover, many patients with MDS have clinical and laboratory features of AML, aplastic anemia, and myeloproliferative disorders. While the FAB criteria does not apply to all cases it remains a useful and widely accepted classification system for diagnosis of MDS.[61,69–71] The FAB group defined five categories, subtypes of MDS (Table 23–1). The subtypes are based on the morphology, cytochemical stain for iron, percentage monocytes, and the percentage of blast forms in the bone marrow and peripheral blood.

Refractory Anemia

Refractory anemia (RA) constitutes 30 to 40 percent of all cases of MDS. Patients usually present with a macrocytic anemia and a low reticulocyte count. One or more cell lines are usually abnormal. Red cell abnormalities include anisocytosis (abnormalities in size), poikilocytosis (abnormalities in the shape) and basophilic stippling. Patients may be neutropenic and/or thrombocytopenic. Neutrophils may show the pseudo-Pelger-Huet anomaly or hypogranular neutrophils or large agranular platelets. Thrombocytosis is occasionally seen and when present is suggestive of the 5q– chromosomal abnormality. The bone marrow aspirate and biopsy are typically hypercellular for the patient's age with dysplastic erythropoiesis. Bone marrow blasts constitute less than 5 percent of all cells and less than 1 percent of blast forms are in the blood. Ring sideroblasts may be present but do not exceed 15 percent of erythroblasts. A small minority of patients may present with modest hepatosplenomegaly.

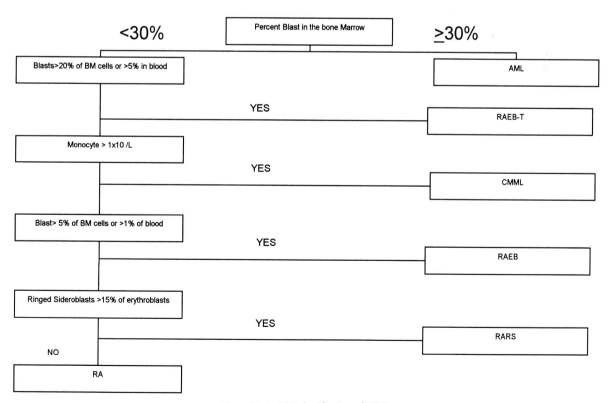

Figure 23–2. FAB classification of MDS.

Table 23–1. MDS Classification

FAB Classification System	WHO Classification System
Myelodysplastic syndromes	**Myelodysplastic syndromes**
Refractory anemia (RA)	Refractory anemia (RA)
Refractory anemia with ringed sideroblasts (RARS)	with ringed sideroblasts (RARS)
	without ringed sideroblasts
Refractory anemia with excess blasts (RAEB)	Refractory cytopenia with multilineage dysplasia (RCMD)
Refractory anemia with excess blasts in transformation (RAEB-T)	Refractory anemia with excess blasts (RAEB)
Chronic myelomonocytic leukemia (CMML)	5q– syndrome
	Myelodysplastic syndrome, unclassifiable
	Myelodysplastic/myeloproliferative diseases
	Chronic myelomonocytic leukemia (CMML)
	Atypical chronic myelogenous leukemia (aCML)
	Juvenile myelomonocytic leukemia leukemia (JMML)
	Acute myeloid leukemia with multilineage dysplasia
	with prior myelodysplastic syndrome
	without prior myelodysplastic syndrome
	Acute myeloid leukemia and MDS therapy related
	Alkylating agent related
	Epipodophyllotoxin related

Refractory Anemia with Ringed Sideroblasts

Refractory anemia with ringed sideroblasts (RARS), also designated primary acquired sideroblastic anemia, constitutes 15 to 25 percent of all MDS cases. Patients usually present with signs and symptoms of anemia. The red cells are usually macrocytic, but can be normocytic or microcytic. Basophilic stippled red cells and Pappenheimer bodies, red cells that contain basophilic iron-containing granules, may be noted on the peripheral blood film. In most patients the findings in RARS are confined to the erythroid lineage. Neutropenia or thrombocytopenia is rare. The bone marrow is typically hypercellular with erythroid hyperplasia and dyserythropoiesis. Erythroblasts may show defective hemoglobinization. On an iron stain ringed sideroblasts are easily identified. Ringed sideroblasts are erythroid precursors with iron staining in the mitochondria forming a necklace at least a third or more around the nucleus. The FAB group initially proposed that ringed sideroblasts account for more than 15 percent of all nucleated cells in the bone marrow.[68] However, it is now generally accepted that the ringed sideroblasts are expressed as a percentage of erythroblasts.[71] There is also an increase in sideroblasts in which iron-containing granules are increased in size and number but do not form a ring. In RARS the siderotic granules often present in early erythroid precursors, from basophilic erythroblasts onwards, whereas in secondary sideroblastic anemia the changes are confined to the more mature erythroid cells. Iron stores are generally increased when a patient presents even in the absence of transfusions. If a patient with RARS becomes iron deficient the percentage of ringed sideroblasts falls or may totally disappear, only to reappear when iron stores are replenished.

Refractory Anemia with Excess Blasts

Refractory anemia with excess blasts (RAEB) constitutes 15 to 25 percent of MDS cases. Patients usually present with signs and symptoms of anemia and thrombocytopenia. Most patients present with involvement of two or more lineages with dysplastic changes in all three lineages with less than 5 percent circulating blast forms. The peripheral smear may have features of either RA or RARS. The bone marrow is usually hypercellular with increased blast forms: greater than 5 percent but less than 20 percent. The blasts are generally small, with scanty cytoplasm, and undifferentiated. Ringed sideroblasts may be present and may exceed 15 percent of erythroblasts. In those cases without 5 percent blasts in the bone marrow the peripheral blood blasts must be greater than 1 percent for the diagnosis of RAEB.

Refractory Anemia with Excess Blasts in Transformation

Refractory anemia with excess blasts in transformation (RAEB-T) constitutes 5 to 10 percent of MDS cases. This category includes patients with 5 percent blasts in the blood and between 21 and 30 percent blasts in the bone marrow. Auer rods may be present (aggregates of lysozymes appearing as thin rods in the cytoplasm of immature myeloid cells). Greater than 50 percent of patients will transform to AML. Hepatomegaly and splenomegaly may be present on physical examination. Trilineage dysplasia is usual and some patients may have a monocytosis but less than 1×10^9/L.

Chronic Myelomonocytic Leukemia

Chronic myelomonocytic leukemia (CMML) comprises 15 percent of MDS cases. CMML has features of both a myeloproliferative disorder and MDS. The peripheral blood demonstrates a monocytosis (>1 × 10⁹/L). Many patients will present with prominent splenomegaly and an elevated total white blood count. The monocytes are often morphologically abnormal with hypersegmented and atypical shaped nuclei. The monocytes may also appear immature with increased cytoplasmic basophilia and prominent cytoplasmic granules. Some promonocytes may be noted but monoblasts are rare. The neutrophil count may also be elevated but is not a diagnostic feature. The bone marrow is hypercellular with prominent promonocytes. Mature monocytes may not be increased. In some cases there may be marked granulocytic hyperplasia and monocytic precursors may represent a minority of the cells. Esterase cytochemistry may be helpful to differentiate promonocytes from promyelocytes. Immunological abnormalities are most common in this subtype; about half the patients demonstrate autoantibodies and 5 to 10 percent will have a monoclonal antibody, or hypergammaglobulinemia and an elevated erythrocyte sedimentation rate.[72] Some patients may present with pleural or pericardial effusions, ascites, or synovitis.[41] Lymphadenopathy, and skin and gum infiltration with monocytes may occur. Hepatomegaly and splenomegaly are more common in this subtype than the other types of MDS. The FAB attempted to distinguish two subgroups of CMML: an MDS type and a myeloproliferative type based on the white blood count, percentage of immature granulocytes, percentage of monocytes and basophils and erythroid precursors in the bone marrow.[73] CMML has many features of both MDS and a myeloproliferative disorder.

The distinction between MDS and AML in some patients is difficult. The World Health Organization (WHO) has recently proposed that 20 percent blasts, rather than the previously accepted 30 percent, should be the dividing line between MDS and AML.[74] The RAEB-T MDS subtype is classified as AML with multilineage dysplasia in the WHO classification. Moreover, elderly patients with AML have many clinical and cytogenetic features of RAEB-T.[75] The WHO has also proposed removing CMML from the MDS classification and placing it into a separate myelodysplastic/myeloproliferative disorders group (Table 23–1).

Subtypes Not Specifically Defined by the FAB Group

Myelodysplastic Syndromes and Myeloproliferative Disorders

The myeloproliferative disorders (MPDs) are clonal stem cell disorders characterized by increased but effective hematopoiesis resulting in an increase in peripheral blood levels of one or more cell lines. The bone marrow is typically hypercellular without dysplasia. Patients usually present with a leukocytosis and hepatosplenomegaly. The myelodysplastic/myeloproliferative subtype is an overlap disorder reflecting that some patients have features of both MDS and MPD. Patients present with a clinical picture that demonstrates both increased proliferation with maturation and dysplastic and ineffective maturation.[74,76] The MDS/MPD category includes patients with juvenile myelomonocytic leukemia, subtypes of chronic myelomonocytic leukemia, and atypical chronic myelogenous leukemia (Philadelphia chromosome negative). The bone marrow and the blood show evidence of both effective, increased hematopoiesis with maturation, and dysplasia or ineffective hematopoiesis. MDS/MPD disorders resemble both a chronic myeloproliferative disorder and a syndrome of ineffective and impaired maturation and function. The MDS/MPD disorders have a variable course but a generally poor prognosis and are associated with an increased incidence of leukemic transformation.[73,76]

5q– Syndrome

The 5q– syndrome is a favorable prognostic subtype of MDS defined by the specific cytogenetic abnormalities, the loss of all or part of the long arm of chromosome 5. The q, long arm, of chromosome 5 contains the genes that encode for a number of growth factors including interleukin (IL)-3, IL-5, IL-9, and granulocyte-macrophage colony-stimulating factor (GM-CSF).[77] How the loss of some of the genes that code for these factors contributes to the development of this syndrome is unclear. The 5q– syndrome is frequently associated with morphological features of RA and to a lesser extent RARS and the other subtypes. A majority of the patients present with a refractory macrocytic anemia, normal or mildly low leukocyte counts, thrombocytosis (a platelet count >400,000 cmm), and less than 5 percent blast forms in the bone marrow. In contrast to the other MDS subtypes, where the mononuclear megakaryocytes are smaller (micromegakaryocytes), in the 5q– syndrome they are bilobed or nonlobulated but of normal size.[78] The 5q– syndrome has a marked female predominance (70 percent), and rarely transforms to AML.[79] A majority of patients have progressive anemia and become red cell transfusion dependent. Particular attention should be paid to managing and preventing iron overload early in the course of the disease which otherwise has a favorable prognosis.

Hypoplastic MDS

Most patients with MDS present with a hypercellular or normal cellular bone marrow with ineffective hematopoiesis. A subset of patients present with a hypocellular bone marrow (less than 15 percent cellularity on bone marrow biopsy) and minimal dysplasia. Hypocellular MDS must be differentiated from aplastic anemia and hypocellular AML.[80] The distinction between these two disorders can be difficult.[80–82] Hypocellular MDS and aplastic anemia may also be pathophysiologically related.[69] The role of the immune suppression of hematopoiesis in both disorders is suggested by their response to immunosuppressive therapy. It is important to distinguish between this MDS variant versus an evolving, or early aplastic anemia. MDS tends to occur in older patients, with a more gradual onset and dysplasia involves more than one cell line. Dysplastic megakaryocytes are also more prominent in MDS than in aplastic anemia. Megaloblastic red cell precursors and paroxysmal nocturnal hemoglobinuria (PNH)-like cells occur in both conditions and are therefore not helpful diagnostic features.[83] A characteristic MDS cytogenetic abnormality sometimes helps to define this disorder (i.e., −5, −7, +8, 20q–). Reflecting the heterogeneity of this subtype the prognosis for patients is controversial. Patients who respond to immunosuppressive therapy remain at risk for the late development of other disorders including AML and PNH.

Pediatric MDS

MDS is uncommon in children and congenital syndromes such as Fanconi anemia and neurofibromatosis should be excluded. Inherited constitutional genetic disorders are found in approximately 30 percent of children with MDS and related myeloproliferative disorders.[23] MDS and acute leukemia are much higher in children with Down syndrome. Abnormalities of chromosome 7, including monosomy 7 and 7q–, are more frequent in pediatric MDS. However, unlike in adult patients, this cytogenetic abnormality is not associated with an adverse prognosis. Moreover, the involvement of chromosome 7 in the monosomy 7 syndrome does not appear to be the primary etiological event.[25,84] The cytogenetic abnormality appears to predispose the patient to other secondary cytogenetic and cellular events. A similar defect has been noted in affected individuals with autosomal dominant congenital thrombocytopenia, which is associated with the development of MDS and AML.[67] These disorders are associated with the loss of function of defined alleles that confer a susceptibility to the acquisition of additional secondary mutations. The rate of progression to AML is high in the pediatric MDS population. Juvenile chronic myelomonocytic leukemia, one of the common pediatric MDS, has features of both MDS and a myeloproliferative disorder.

Myelodysplasia With Bone Marrow Fibrosis

An increase in bone marrow reticulin is noted in up to 25 percent of MDS patients.[85] The majority of these patients have a focal increase in fibrosis and the clinical significance of this finding is unclear.[86] Rarely, less than 1 percent of MDS patients will present with extensive fibrosis and collagen deposition. These patients have features of both a myeloproliferative disorder and MDS. The presence of trilineage dysplasia and the absence of hepatosplenomegaly help to distinguish this disorder from agnogenic myeloid metaplasia and myelofibrosis. It may be difficult to distinguish MDS with marrow fibrosis from an acute megakaryocytic leukemia (AML M7).[87] The bone marrow is usually not aspiratable (dry tap) and morphological findings of dysplasia may be difficult to identify on the biopsy sample. Megakaryoblasts can be identified by staining the marrow biopsy and circulating blast forms with megakaryocytic lineage-specific antigens such as factor VIII or GP IIb/IIIa.[87] MDS with fibrosis is associated with a generally poor prognosis.[88]

Therapy-Related MDS

MDS that occurs following exposure to cytotoxic chemotherapy and/or ionizing radiation is referred to as secondary-therapy–related MDS (t-MDS). Secondary MDS should be considered as entity separate from primary-de novo MDS. The FAB classification, standard prognostic indicators, and approaches to treatment are not applicable in patients with t-MDS. MDS secondary to alkylating agents is associated with deletions or loss of chromosomes 5, 7, and 8, has a latency period of 3 to 7 years, and usually progresses to AML. In contrast the topoisomerase II inhibitors, including the epipodophyllotoxins and anthracyclines, are associated with balanced translocations involving chromosome bands 3q26, 11q23, and 21q22 and a latency period of 18

months to 3 years after exposure.[89] The clinical presentation of these two types of therapy-related disorders is also different. The alkylator-related disorders present initially with a slowly progressive illness with many features of de novo MDS including trilineage dysplasia and pancytopenia.[60] In contrast, the topoisomerase II associated disorders rarely present with features of de novo MDS and rapidly evolves to AML. The prognosis of all t-MDS is very poor. Patients do not respond to the standard treatments for MDS and an allogeneic transplant, if a donor is available, should be considered as the primary therapy for all eligible patients.

CLINICAL AND LABORATORY FEATURES OF MDS

A majority of patients with MDS are asymptomatic at presentation and are usually noted to have an unexplained macrocytic anemia (MCV >102) and an absolute low reticulocyte count. Anemia is the most common presenting abnormality and patients may complain of insidious onset fatigue and progressive dyspnea on exertion. Bone pain and weight loss are uncommon. While patients may be neutropenic and have dysplastic and impaired neutrophil function, infections are unusual at presentation. The physical examination is notable for the lack of adenopathy, cutaneous lesions, prominent splenomegaly, or hepatomegaly, except in CMML. Table 23–2 includes disorders that should be considered in the evaluation of patients with a suspected MDS. The diagnosis of MDS relies largely on the morphological findings in the peripheral blood and the bone marrow. The morphological interpretation of dysplastic changes in

---

Table 23–2. Differential Diagnosis of MDS

Acquired disorders
  Aplastic anemia
  Early AML
  Hypoplastic AML
  Acute myelofibrosis
  Paroxysmal nocturnal hemoglobinemia (PNH)
  Large granular lymphocytic disease
Congenital disorder
  Hereditary sideroblastic anemia
  Congenital dyserythropoietic anemia
  Fanconi anemia
  Schwachman syndrome
Nutritional disorders
  B12 deficiency
  Folate deficiency
Toxins
  Alcohol
  Antimetabolites
  Postchemotherapy
Viral infections
  HIV
  Parvovirus
  Cytomegalovirus
  EBV
Other
  Chronic renal failure
  SLE
  Felty syndrome

the bone marrow can be difficult and is often subjective. Other disorders should be excluded including aplastic anemia, myeloproliferative disorders, nutritional deficiencies, and autoimmune disorders including system lupus erythematosus. Patients infected with human immunodeficiency virus (HIV) can present with anemia, thrombocytopenia, or pancytopenia with dysplastic changes in the bone marrow.[90] AML in elderly patients may also present with progressive pancytopenia with rare circulating blast forms.[75] The differentiation of AML with dysplasia from MDS can be difficult. Patients with acute erythroleukemia (AML M6) may have prominent dysplastic erythroid precursors and may initially be diagnosed with one of the MDSs.[91,92] Patients with hypoplastic AML can also be confused with one of the MDS subtypes.[93] In prospective trials of MDS up to 15 percent of the patients were later reclassified as having AML.[94]

The finding of a clonal cytogenetic abnormality characteristic of MDS is important in establishing the diagnosis and differentiating it from other disorders. The most common cytogenetic abnormalities include gain or loss of all or parts of chromosomes 5, 7, 8, and 20. The use of spectral karyotyping and fluorescence in situ hybridization (FISH) with specific probes are helpful when insufficient material is available or if there are inadequate numbers of dividing cells.[95] The study of interphase cells may be helpful in identifying specific rearrangements not recognized by banding studies alone. FISH appears to be an acceptable alternative to standard chromosomal analysis when karyotyping is not available or unsatisfactory.[96] A major disadvantage of FISH studies is that the analysis is restricted to specific, defined chromosomal abnormalities. The patient's clinical findings and history are helpful in guiding the use of FISH; that is, a patient with MDS and an elevated platelet count should be evaluated for the possibility of –5/del(5q). The diagnosis of MDS may require the collaborative efforts of clinicians, pathologists, and cytogeneticists. Cytogenetics analysis should be a routine part of the evaluation of all patients with MDS. Detectable clonal cytogenetic abnormalities are found in 38 to 78 percent of de novo MDS and greater than 80 percent of t-MDS patients.[97] Cytogenetics are also helpful in evaluating disease progression and prognosis. The acquisition of new cytogenetic abnormalities is generally associated with progression of the disease and a poor prognosis.

Although anemia is the most common presenting laboratory feature in patients with MDS, approximately 50 percent of patients will demonstrate a abnormality of more than one cell line.[98] The white blood count is usually low, but rarely less than 1000 cmm. Patients may be at risk for bacterial infection due to qualitative abnormalities of neutrophil function.[99] Platelet functional abnormalities are associated with increased risk for bleeding even with an adequate platelet count. Iron studies may demonstrate increased iron stores especially in patients with the refractory anemia with ringed sideroblast subtype.

Blood and Bone Marrow Findings

Red Cells/Anemia

Macrocytosis or a macrocytic anemia with a low reticulocyte count are common in MDS and due to ineffective erythropoiesis (Table 23–3). Impaired red cell maturation has been associated with acquired abnormalities of globin chain synthe-

Table 23–3. Hematological Features of MDS	
Blood	**Bone Marrow**
Erythropoiesis	
Macrocytosis	Hyperplasia
Polychromasia	Megaloblastic changes
Anisocytosis	Ringed sideroblasts
Basophilic stippling	Binuclearity
Pappenheimer bodies	Nuclear fragmentation
Poikilocytosis	Macronormoblasts
Myeloid	
Neutropenia	Hyperplasia
Acquired Pelger-Huet anomaly	Hypogranular promyelocytes
Hypersegmented nuclei	ALIP
Agranular	Abnormal shapes
Hypogranular	Increased monocytes
Cytoplasmic vacuolation	Lack of mature neutrophils
Promonocytes	Dysplastic eosinophils
Auer rods	
Hypogranulated eosinophils	
Platelets	
Thrombocytopenia	Mononuclear megakaryocytes
Thrombocytosis	Micromegakaryocytes
Giant platelets	Hypolobulated
Hypogranular platelets	megakaryocytes
Micromegakaryocytes	Multinucleated
	megakaryocytes
	Hypogranular megakaryocytes

sis, and red cell enzymes.[100,101] PNH has been described in the setting of MDS.[102] These patients have many of the typical features of PNH including a defect in the synthesis of the glycosylphosphatidylinositol (GPI)-linked surface protein.[102] On the peripheral blood smear patients may have abnormalities in the size and shape of red cells including basophilic stippling (red cell inclusions composed of ribonucleoprotein and mitochondrial remnants), Pappenheimer bodies, basophilic iron-containing granules peripherally located in red cells, macro-ovalocytes, teardrop forms, and nucleated red cells. The bone marrow may reveal ringed sideroblasts, multinuclear fragments, internuclear bridging, and nuclear cytoplasm asynchrony.

Neutrophils

Qualitative abnormalities of neutrophil function are a common feature of MDS and may explain the increased risk for bacterial infections.[99,103–105] Morphological abnormalities include hypogranular and hyposegmented neutrophils, which are associated with a negative peroxidase reaction and decreased myeloperoxidase activity. The neutrophils are hyposegmented and may be confused with band forms. Nuclear fragmentation and nuclear-cytoplasmic asynchrony in early myeloid precursors may be a prominent feature in the bone marrow. Dysplastic myeloid precursors can be difficult to distinguish from blast forms and therefore the bone marrow should be reviewed by a pathologist experienced in the interpretation of MDS.

Platelets

Thrombocytopenia and abnormal platelet function occur in MDS. Thrombocytopenia is an adverse prognostic feature in

MDS.[106–109] Impaired platelet function explains the spontaneous bruising and bleeding after surgery seen in patients with a normal platelet count.[110] Dysplastic platelets and abnormal megakaryocytes are important diagnostic features and help in distinguishing MDS from other disorders.[111] Giant platelets and megakaryocytic fragments in the peripheral blood film are important diagnostic features in MDS.

Bone Marrow Findings

A bone marrow aspirate and biopsy is essential for diagnosis and to define the MDS subtype. Bone marrow cytogenetics should be performed to assign prognosis and differentiate MDS from other disorders. The bone marrow is usually hypercellular but may be normal or hypocellular for the patient's age. Abnormal distribution of cells is often present; erythroid islands may be absent or very large. Granulocytic precursors may be clustered centrally rather than their normal paratrabecular distribution. This phenomenon has been designated as abnormal localization of immature precursors (ALIP) and is associated with a poorer prognosis.[111] The presence of ALIP can be helpful in distinguishing MDS from other disorders. Micromegakaryoctes, mononuclear megakaryocytes, and hyperlobulated megakaryocytes are important diagnostic features of MDS and are reliable morphological evidence of dysplasia in the bone marrow smear and biopsy. The megakaryocytes may be clustered or adjacent to the bony trabeculum. The 5q– syndrome has mononuclear megakaryocytes that are of normal size but with a single eccentrically placed round nonlobulated nucleus.[77] Megaloblastic changes (nuclear cytoplasm asynchrony) can be seen in the myeloid and erythroid precursors. Dysgranulopoiesis and dyserythropoiesis are more readily noted in the bone marrow smear and not the biopsy. The bone marrow smear is necessary to identify ringed sideroblasts that may not be apparent on the biopsy sample. Immunohistochemistry may be a useful supplement to histology. The use of anti-glycophorin antibodies may be helpful to identify erythroid precursors and differentiate them from ALIP. Antibodies against the von Willebrand factor may recognize small mononuclear megakaryocytes that can be confused with myeloid precursors. A biopsy is necessary to access the degree of reticulin fibrosis and overall bone marrow cellularity.

CLINICAL AND PROGNOSTIC FEATURES

MDS is a heterogeneous group of disorders with a variable clinical course and prognosis. Patients may have a prolonged, asymptomatic, indolent disease that rarely evolves to AML or develop progressive anemia and thrombocytopenia that rapidly evolves to acute leukemia. The currently used FAB criteria were based solely on morphology, and were not developed as a prognostic classification system. However, the designated subtypes are clinically relevant with regards to transformation to AML and survival (Table 23–4). Patients with RAEB and RAEB-T have a median survival of 12 and 5 months, respectively. In contrast, the RA or RARS subtypes have a median survival of 6 and 3 years, respectively, and rarely transform to AML. Despite the historic use of preleukemia to describe MDS only about 30 percent of patients with MDS eventually develop AML. A majority of the patients die as a result of their MDS or concomitant medical illnesses. The percentage of blast forms in the bone marrow is one of the most useful prognostic indicators in MDS. The survival shortens as the percentage of blast forms increases.[110] Patients with complex cytogenetic abnormalities or defects involving chromosome 7 have a poor prognosis, whereas a normal karyotype, 20q– or 5q–, is associated with a more favorable outcome. Each of these factors appears to be independent prognostic variables. In an effort to better assign prognosis the international MDS risk analysis workshop developed the International Prognostic Scoring System (IPSS). The IPSS score addresses clinical features not included in the FAB classification and attempts to define prognosis based on these clinical criteria[7] (Table 23–5). The scoring system assigns a point score for each the following variables: the number of bone marrow blast forms, karyotypic abnormalities, and number of cell lines affected (cytopenias). The combined score determines the overall risk category: low (score 0), intermediate 1 (score 0.5 to 1.0), intermediate 2 (score 1.5 to 2.0), and high (score >2.5) (Table 23–6). The IPSS risk category and score correlates with the overall survival and probability of transformation to AML. The IPSS scoring system supplements the FAB classification system in assigning prognosis and therefore in planning treatment. For instance, patients with RA and less than 5 percent blasts in the bone marrow and favorable cytogenetics (low risk category), have a median survival of greater than 5 years and infrequently evolve to AML. In contrast, patients with a blast count of greater than 11 percent and unfavorable cytogenetics (high risk category) have a

Table 23–4. The Myelodysplastic Syndromes: FAB Classification and Survival

FAB Subtype	Bone Marrow Blasts (Percent)	Blood Blasts (Percent)	Auer Rods	Monocytes > 1 × 10⁹/L	Ring Sideroblast (Percent)	Survival (Median Months)	Transformation to AML (Percent)
RA	< 5	< 1	Absent	No	None	48	10–15
RAR-S	< 5	< 1	Absent	No	> 15	72	5–10
RAEB	5–20	< 5	Absent	No	Rare < 15	12	30–45
RAEB-T	21–30	> 5	Present	No	Rare < 15	6	50–60
CMML	< 20	< 5	Absent	Yes	Rare	30	25–35

Table 23–5. International Prognostic Scoring System for MDS

	Score Value				
Variable	0	0.5	1	1.5	2
Marrow blasts	< 5 percent	5–10 percent		11–20 percent	21–30 percent
Karyotype[a]	Good	Intermediate	Poor		
Cell lines[b]	0–1	2–3			

[a] Good = Normal, −, 5q−, 20q−. Poor = > 3 abnormalities, −7, complex. Intermediate = others.
[b] Neutrophils < 1800 cmm; platelets < 100,000 cmm; hemoglobin < 10 g/dl.

median survival of less than 2 years and frequently progress to AML. While age was not a variable in the IPSS score, in all subgroups patients over the age of 60 had a shorter survival.[7] Other prognostic scoring systems have been proposed: The Spanish system used marrow blasts, age, and platelet count, and the Bournemouth Scoring system used platelet count, marrow blasts, and karyotype.[106–109,112] The IPSS score represents the current standard for assigning prognosis and discriminating among the different subtypes of MDS.

TREATMENT

Treatment should be individualized based on the patient's age, subtype, percentage blasts in the marrow, and cytogenetics. The majority of patients with MDS are elderly and tolerate intensive chemotherapy poorly. Moreover, standard therapies do not result in a cure and their impact on survival for most patients is unclear. Therefore any potential benefits of treatment must be weighed against the side effects and the patient's overall prognosis. The alleviation of disease-related complications and improved quality of life are important goals for most patients. The standard of care for most patients with MDS remains supportive care. Although there are a number of therapeutic options available for MDS patients, none, other than an allogeneic stem cell transplantation, has been shown to be better than supportive therapy with regards to both overall survival and leukemic transformation. The therapeutic options for patients with MDS include the use of hematopoietic growth and trophic factors, immunosuppressive agents, low-intensity cytoreductive chemotherapy, intensive chemotherapy, and stem cell transplantation.

Table 23–6. International Prognostic System: Score, Age, and Survival

Overall Score	Median Survival, Age < 60 Year (Years)	Median Survival, Age > 60 Year (Years)
Low (0)	11.8	4.8
Intermediate 1 (.5–1.0)	5.2	2.7
Intermediate 2 (1.5–2.0)	1.8	1.1
High (> 2.5)	0.4	0.5

(From Greenberg et al.,[7] with permission.)

Guidelines have been recently proposed to standardize the criteria for response in patients with MDS.[113] These guidelines attempted to define acceptable, standard, criteria for complete and partial responses to treatment. Moreover, the response criteria emphasized that the goals of treatment of MDS was to alter the natural history of the disease and alleviate the disease-related complications and improve the quality of life. A majority of patients in most studies demonstrate partial responses. Stable disease or minimal responses are difficult to interpret and make comparisons between trials difficult. In addition, the response rate in some Phase II trials did not translate into prolongation of survival, time to treatment failure, or improvement in the quality of life.

Supportive Therapy

Supportive therapy represents the standard of care for most patients with MDS. Red cell and platelet transfusions are administered for the symptomatic treatment of the anemia and thrombocytopenia. Patients may require multiple transfusions over many years and the potential for iron overload should be addressed early in a patient's course. Chelation therapy with desferrioxamine to prevent progressive iron overload should be considered for stable, good prognosis patients who will receive greater than 20 units of packed red cells.

Platelet dysfunction is common and patients may bleed even with an adequate platelet count. Therefore, platelet support may be required prior to surgery and procedures to prevent excess bleeding. Neutropenia and impaired neutrophil function are common in MDS patients. The use of prophylactic antibiotics, however, is not warranted for most patients.

Trophic Agents

Recombinant Growth Factors

Hematopoietic growth factors have been used with varying degrees of success to treat the cytopenias in MDS. Recombinant human erythropoietin (rHuEPO, EPO), granulocyte colony-stimulating factor (G-CSF), and GM-CSF have a role in managing the anemia and neutropenia in selected patients with MDS. EPO has been studied extensively and approximately 30 percent of anemic patients with MDS will respond to treatment.[114] The best responses to EPO are observed in patients with an endogenous EPO level less than 200 U, and a transfusion requirement of less than 2 units/month.[115] High doses are generally required, 100 to 300 U/kg daily or tiw. In a meta-analysis study the overall response rate to EPO for all subtypes of MDS was 16 percent but varied considerably according to MDS subtype and endogenous EPO level.[115] Patients with RARS responded significantly less well to EPO administered as a single agent, 8 versus 21 percent for RARA and the non-RARS group, respectively. The response rate was 21 and 10 percent for patients with an EPO level below and above 200 U/L. The duration of response was approximately 11 to 24 months and there was no increase in the percentage of patients who received EPO that transformed to AML as compared to historical controls.[116]

The addition of low doses of G-CSF or granulocyte-monocyte colony-stimulating factor (GM-CSF) to EPO appears to increase the red cell response in selected patients. G-CSF and GM-CSF plus EPO may be synergistic to induce erythroid responses in EPO-resistant patients.[117,118] The synergistic effect was most pronounced in patients with the RARS subtype. A predictive model for treatment with EPO and G-CSF demonstrated that patients with an EPO level of less than 100 U/L, and a pretreatment transfusion requirement of less than 2 units/month responded best.[119] All patients should have adequate iron stores documented prior to starting EPO treatment as the failure to respond or loss of response may be a manifestation of depleted iron stores. EPO should be started at a dose of 100 to 150 U/kg administered three times a week and sequentially increased in nonresponders to 300 U/L daily. Low doses of G-CSF (1 μg/kg) with EPO can be added to patients who fail to respond. The mechanism of the response to high doses of EPO is unclear but the growth factors may modulate apoptosis and MDS progenitors and enhance erythropoiesis.[120]

GM-CSF or G-CSF can increase the neutrophil count in most patients with MDS.[121,122] However, the response is not sustained when the growth factor is stopped and some patients developed worsening of their thrombocytopenia.[122] The use of G-CSF did decrease the incidence of serious infections but did not favorably impact survival in a prospective controlled trial.[122] The use of these cytokines did increase the white blood count but did not appear to accelerate the progression to acute leukemia. Although in selected patients with active, serious infections there may be a role for the use of these cytokines in combination with antibiotics, at present there is no evidence to support the general use of either G-CSF or GM-CSF as single-agent therapy for patients with MDS.

Danazol is an attenuated, synthetic androgen that has been used in the treatment of immune-mediated thrombocytopenia (ITP). Danazol may increase the platelet count in low-risk MDS patients who are thrombocytopenic.[123,124] The mechanism of action is unclear, but may reflect that some patients with MDS have immune-mediated thrombocytopenia that responds to the immunoregulatory effects of danazol.[125] Danazol, 200 mg po tid, is generally well tolerated and associated with an increase in platelets in 10 to 46 percent of treated patients.[124,126,127] The duration of response is variable, 2 to 26+ months, and maintained only while the drug is administered. Patients with platelet counts greater than 15,000 cmm appear

to respond best, and the impact on survival or disease progression is unknown.

Amifostine (Ethyol) is a phosphorylated organic thiol that may have trophic effects on myelodysplastic progenitors. Amifostine may protect cells from oxidative stress after exposure to cytokines, suppress cytokine release, and decreases the rate of apoptosis.[128] The overall response rate and duration of response to amifostine in MDS remains to be determined. In the low proliferative MDS subtypes (RA and RA-S) trilineage responses have been observed in selected patients.[129] However, the responses to amifostine were not maintained off therapy and its effect, if any, on overall survival and the duration of the responses are unclear.[130] The combination of amifostine, pentoxifylline, ciprofloxacin, and dexamethasone has been used to optimize a potential anticytokine effect.[131] There were no complete responses in these studies and the duration of response was not sustained. The role of amifostine or other agents to modulate a cytokine response in MDS remains unclear.

Low-Dose Chemotherapy

Potential Differentiating Agents

Cytarabine administered at low doses (low dose ara-C: LoDAC) has been the most extensively used chemotherapy for elderly patients with high-risk, symptomatic MDS.[132] Cytarabine is administered daily by either continuous infusion or bolus subcutaneous injections at doses of 10 to $20/mg^2$ for 14 to 21 days. At low dose cytarabine may induce differentiation.[132] In a prospective controlled trial patients with RAEB and RAEB-T had the highest response rates, 20 to 35 percent (complete remission partial response [CR] + PR). The median duration of response for all subtypes was 8 to 15 months, with a range of 6 to 24 months.[94] The response to LoDAC correlated with its cytoreductive effect on the bone marrow. In a Phase III trial treatment with low-dose cytarabine was not superior to supportive care with regards to overall survival or leukemic transformation.[94] The role of low-dose cytarabine in the treatment of patients with high-risk MDS is controversial. In high-risk patients it remains a widely used treatment that may be effective in inducing transient responses in a subset of patients with progressive disease who are not candidates for more intensive chemotherapy.[133,134]

The DNA hypomethylating agents 5-azacytidine (5-Aza) and 2,5-deoxycytidine have shown therapeutic promise in selected MDS patients. 5-Aza is a pyrimidine analogue that inhibits DNA methyltransferase activity, which leads to hypomethylation of cytosine residues. Low doses of 5-Aza inhibit DNA methyltransferase activity, which leads to hypomethylation of cytosine residues. 5-Aza is administered subcutaneously ($75 g/m^2$/day) for 7 consecutive days each month. The overall response rate was 20 to 66 percent with a complete remission rate of approximately 11 percent. While some patients had a complete clinical response while receiving 5-Aza, the durations of the response were short and not maintained off treatment.[135] Myelosuppression was frequently observed in patients receiving 5-Aza and its role as a differentiating agent in MDS is unclear. Toxicity was less than with standard intensive chemotherapy regimens and hematological responses and improved quality of life in some patients receiving the drug was noted.[136] The impact of treatment on survival was unclear.

Decitibine (2,5-deoxycytidine, DAC) given intravenously over 3 to 4 hours, appears to also have activity in MDS.[137] The overall response rate in MDS was 49 and 64 percent in high-risk patients.[138] The actuarial median survival time was 15 months and myelosuppression was common. Both of these hypomethylating agents, 5-Aza and DAC, appear to alter the natural course of MDS and may be of benefit for selected patients. However, additional studies are needed to define their role in MDS.

The results of treatment with differentiating agents such as the retinoids, phenylbutyrate, vitamin D derivatives, and the interferons have thus far been disappointing.[139–141] The combination of cytotoxic chemotherapy and differentiating agents may have activity in selected patients.[142]

Low doses of chemotherapy may have a supportive role in selected patients with MDS. A number of trials have addressed the use of low doses of oral chemotherapy that was well tolerated and administered over a prolonged period. Low-dose oral etoposide (VP-16) and hydroxyurea were effective in controlling symptoms in patients with CMML.[143,144] The use of steroids alleviated some of the cytokine-mediated symptoms in CMML and produced transient hematological improvements.[145] Low-dose melphalan (2 mg/day until response or progression) has been used in high-risk patients with MDS. The treatment was well tolerated and responses were noted in both hypercellular and hypocellular MDS.[146,147] The overall response rate to a prolonged course of low-dose melphalan in Phase II studies was approximately 40 percent.[147] The response rate was better in patients with a hypocellular bone marrow. The treatment was well tolerated, easily administered, and was not associated with a prolonged period of myelosuppression. The duration of the responses to low-dose melphalan is unclear and additional studies are needed to determine its role in MDS.

Immunosuppressive Therapy

Patients with MDS can present with a number of immunoregulatory abnormalities resulting in immune-mediating pancytopenias that can respond to immunosuppressive therapy.[146] Some patients with hypocellular MDS responded to immunosuppressive regimens used for the treatment of aplastic anemia. In selected patients with hypocellular or normal cellular marrows the responses have been complete and remissions durable.[82] Antithymocyte globulin (ATG) administered at 40 mg/kg/day for 4 days produced responses in 16 of 42 patients.[147] The highest responses were seen in patients with RA (66 percent) although patients with RAEB also responded (32 percent). Trilineage responses were observed in some patients and the median duration of response was 10 months. Responses were more frequent with hypocellular MDS but were even noted in patients with hypercellular marrows. No patients with RARS responded to ATG. Improvement were seen in patients with low-, intermediate-, and high-risk IPSS scores. The responses did not correlate with the loss of a previously noted cytogenetic abnormality, suggesting that the treatment was not affecting the MDS clone. A majority of the patients attained a partial response and treatment did not restore normal hematopoiesis. The mechanism of action is not clear but in vitro studies suggest that the response may be mediated by a loss of cytotoxic T-lymphocyte activity directed against autologous CFU-GM, which correlated with changes in the T-cell receptor profiles.[148] The response to ATG appears greatest in low-risk RA patients. In some patients who initially responded to ATG and then relapsed retreatment was effective.[149] Toxicity of ATG therapy was mainly fevers and rigors associated with the infusions and less than 15 percent of patients developed serum sickness.

Cyclosporin (CSA), another immunosuppressive agent, may also be effective in hypocellular MDS patients. In one study 14 of 17 patients with hypocellular RA treated with CSA at doses of 5 to 6 mg/kg/day responded.[150] The combination of CSA and ATG may enhance the response in selected patients.[82,151]

In the reported studies of ATG and CSA the patients are highly selected and the subset of patients that respond represent a minority of patients with MDS. Many of the patients present with hypocellular marrows (<15 percent cellularity) with minimal dysplasia. The responses of MDS patients to immunosuppressive therapy reflects the heterogeneity of the disorder. The use of immunosuppressive therapy to modulate the abnormal clone represents a potential treatment approach that needs to be further evaluated.

Intensive Chemotherapy

Combination, intensive cytoreductive induction chemotherapy should be considered as a possible therapy for selected younger patients who present with poor prognosis MDS. Selected patients with high-risk features who are younger than 55 years of age are candidates for intensive combination chemotherapy. Newly diagnosed patients with RAEB-T without a prior history of MDS appear to respond to standard AML induction chemotherapy in a similar fashion to de novo AML.[152] However, patients who present with an antecedent or evolving MDS generally respond poorly to intensive AML-type induction chemotherapy. The complete remission rate varies from 13 to 40 percent with an incidence of toxic deaths of 12 to 53 percent.[153–155] Moreover, the role of postinduction chemotherapy is unclear in patients with MDS who respond to treatment.[156] In selected younger patients with MDS intensive chemotherapy including an anthracycline and cytarabine has resulted in complete remission rates of 20 to 60 percent but with a relapse rate of 90 percent.[154,156] The differences noted may be due to patient selection, sample size, and the heterogeneity of MDS. The remission durations are typically 6 to 12 months with only rare instances of prolonged disease-free survival. The poor response of MDS patients to intensive induction chemotherapy reflects the biological differences between de novo AML that occurs in younger patients and MDS. Patients with chromosome abnormalities involving 5 or 7 have a very low response to treatment with short duration of remission that is similar to poor risk de novo AML with similar cytogenetic abnormalities.[152,155] Newer combination chemotherapy regimens such as the addition of topotecan and fludarabine may improve on the initial response rate but do not appear to impact remission duration or more importantly overall survival.[157] Topotecan, a topoisomerase I inhibitor, administered as a single agent or in combination with intermediate cytarabine, has been reported to have activity in the high-risk MDS subtypes.[158,159] The complete response rate is 20 to 30 percent and the median duration of response is 7 months. Topotecan induced severe mucositis in 23 percent of patients and more than 50 percent of patients had documented infections. Topotecan has been combined with intermediate dose cytarabine (1 g/m^2) in high-risk MDS patients.[158] The use of these intensive regimens should be reserved for investigative studies in poor-risk patients with a good performance status who can tolerate intensive chemotherapy.

The use of agents to overcome drug resistance in MDS patients has been controversial. Quinine added to intensive induction appeared to improve the response in patients expressing P-glycoprotein, 18 versus 52 percent for patients treated without or with the addition of quinine.[161–163] These results, however, need to be confirmed in additional larger clinical trials.

Stem Cell Transplantation

Autologous and allogeneic stem cell transplantation have been used in patients with MDS or MDS-AML. The role of autologous transplantation remains controversial. The 3-year disease-free survival in a selected group of patients ranges from 14 to 58 percent.[164,165] All patients were transplanted in first remission and adequate number of stem cells were harvested. The 2-year survival in selected patients reported to the EBMT for patients in first complete remission was 39 percent, with a disease-free survival of 34 percent and a relapse rate of 64 percent.[164] In patients over the age of 40 years the disease-free survival was 25 percent with a transplant-related mortality of 39 percent. Patients younger than 40 years of age, and in first complete remission, had a significantly improved outcome. The transplant-related mortality was high: 39 percent for patients over the age of 40 years and 17 percent for patients less than 40 years of age. The relapse rate is higher than in patients with de novo AML. Larger prospective studies are needed to define the potential role of autologous stem cell transplantation for patients with MDS. These studies did demonstrate that in some patients polyclonal and karyotypically normal progenitors can be harvested from peripheral blood in patients with MDS following intensive induction chemotherapy.[166–168]

Allogeneic stem cell transplantation should be considered for young patients who have an HLA compatible donor. Allogeneic transplantation is at present the only potentially curative therapy for patients with MDS. However, patients with MDS appear to have an increased incidence of transplant-related complications.[169–171] The nonrelapse morbidity and mortality in MDS patients is high and not solely explained by the older age of the patient population.[171] Younger patients with MDS also appear to have an increased incidence of transplant-related complications.[172] Patients with advanced disease and unfavorable cytogenetics have a higher probability of relapse and lower overall survival. The outcome is better for primary than secondary MDS and patients with a lower IPSS score. The probability of survival in a single institution study was 100, 54, 44, and 30 percent for low-risk, intermediate 1 risk, intermediate 2 risk, and high-risk groups, respectively.[171] Moreover, the standard risk factors that predict overall survival in MDS appear to affect the post-transplant outcome.[172] The timing of the transplant remains controversial for good risk patients considering that the incidence of nonrelapse mortality is similar in good and poor risk patients.[171] However, for the younger patient with a good performance status and a suitable HLA matched donor an allogeneic stem cell transplant should be considered as the only potential curative therapy.

FUTURE DIRECTIONS

Advances in treatment will parallel our understanding of the molecular and immunological events involved in development and progression of MDS. The use of cytokines that work on earlier precursors or a combination of cytokines may modulate MDS and normal hematopoiesis.[173,174] Angiogenesis may have a role in pathogenesis for a number of disorders including AML and MDS.[175,176] The role of agents that may effect angiogenesis are being applied to the treatment of MDS patients.[176,177] Arsenic trioxide induces apoptosis by directly influencing the mitochondrial permeability transition pores.[178] Arsenic trioxide–induced apoptosis leads to the disruption of microtubule formation during mitosis resulting in cell death. Arsenic trioxide may have a role in the treatment of selected patients with MDS.[179,180] New therapeutic agents are being developed that attempt to target the molecular events in MDS.[181]

SUMMARY

The myelodysplastic syndromes are a heterogeneous group of disorders with a variable clinical course. The classification system is controversial and attempts to separate MDS from other clonal disorders. The development of a prognostic, risk-based scoring system developed by the International MDS Risk Analysis Workshop has helped in planning therapy. Cytogenetics and percentage of blast cells are an important predictor of outcome. The cellular and molecular events in MDS are poorly understood. An alteration of progenitor cell survival may be one of the underlying mechanisms to explain the ineffective hematopoiesis and cytopenias that are characteristic of MDS.

The treatment of patients with MDS remains problematic; the majority of patients with MDS are elderly and the standard therapies are not curative. Therefore the side effects of any planned treatment must be carefully weighed against any potential benefits and the patient's overall prognosis. Although a number of therapeutic options are available, none, other than allogeneic transplant, has been shown to offer a survival advantage over supportive care alone.

REFERENCES

1. Rhodes CP, Barker WH: Refractory anemia. JAMA 110:794, 1938.

2. Crosby WH, Feinstein FE, Heilmeyer L et al: Hypoplastic-aplastic anemia. Blood 12:193, 1957.

3. Koeffle HP, Golde DW: Human preleukemia. Ann Intern Med 93:347, 1980.

4. Busque L, Gilliland DG: X-inactivation analysis in the 1990s: Promise and potential problems. Leukemia 12:128, 1998.

5. Raskind WH, Steinmann L, Najfeld V: Clonal development of myeloproliferative disorders: Clues to hematopoietic differentiation and multistep pathogenesis of cancer. Leukemia 12:108, 1998.

6. Rossi G, Pelizzari AM, Bellotti D et al: Cytogenetic analogy between myelodysplastic syndrome and acute myeloid leukemia of elderly patients. Leukemia 14:636, 2000.

7. Greenberg P, Cox C, LeBeau MM et al: International scoring system for evaluating prognosis in myelodysplastic syndromes. Blood 91:1100, 1998.

8. Raza A, Alvi S, Broady-Robinson L et al: Cell cycle kinetic studies in 68 patients with myelodysplastic syndromes following intravenous iodo- and/or bromodedeoxyuridine. Exp Hematol 25:530, 1997.

9. Rajapakso R, Gliston N, Rott LS, Greenberg PL: Altered oncoprotein expression and apoptosis in myelodysplastic syndrome marrow cells. Blood 88:4275, 1996.

10. Busque L, Zhu J, Dehart D et al: An expression based clonality assay at the human androgen receptor locus (HUMARA) on chromosome X. Nucl Acids Res 22:697, 1994.

11. Jansen JWG, Buschle M, Layton M et al: Clonal analysis of myelodysplastic syndromes: Evidence of multipotent stem cell origin. Blood 73:248, 1989.

12. Weimar IS, Bourhis J-H, de Gast GC et al: Clonality in myelodysplastic syndromes. Leuk Lymphoma 13:215, 1994.

13. Lawrence HJ, Broudy VC, Magenis RE et al: Cytogenetic evidence for involvement of B lymphocytes in acquired sideroblastic anemia. Blood 70:1003, 1987.

14. Van Kamo H, Fibbe WE, Jansen RP et al: Clonal involvement of granulocytes and monocytes, but not of T and B lymphocytes and natural killer cells in patients with myelodysplasia. Analysis by X-linked restriction fragment polymorphisms and polymerase chain reaction of the phosphoglycerate kinase gene. Blood 80:1774, 1992.

15. Traweek ST, Slovak ML, Nademanee AP et al: Clonal karyotypic hematopoietic cell abnormalities occurring after autologous bone marrow transplantation for Hodgkin's disease and non-Hodgkin's lymphoma. Blood 84:957, 1994.

16. Mecucci M: Molecular features of primary MDS with cytogenetic changes. Leuk Res 22:293, 1998.

17. Johansson B, Mertens F, Mitelman F: Primary versus secondary neoplasia associated chromosomal abnormalities—balanced rearrangements vs. genomic imbalance? Genes Chrom Cancer 16:155, 1996.

18. Williams CL, Sever CE, Pallavicine MG et al: Deletions of IRF-1, mapping to chromosome 5q31.1 in human leukemia and preleukemic myelodysplasia. Science 259:968, 1993.

19. Uchida T, Kinoshitia T, Nagal H et al: Hypomethylation of the p15^{INK4B} gene in myelodysplastic syndromes is frequent and acquired during disease progression. Blood 91:2985, 1998.

20. Bollag G, Clapp DW, Shih S et al: Loss of NFI results in activation of the RAS pathway and leads to aberrant growth in hematopoietic cells. Nat Genet 12:144, 1996.

21. Padua RA, Gunn BA, Al-Shabah A et al: RAS, FMS, and p53 mutations and poor clinical outcome in myelodysplasias. A 10 year follow up. Leukemia 12:887, 1998.

22. Luna-Fineman S, Shannon KM, Atwater SK et al: Myelodysplastic and myeloproliferative disorders of childhood: A study of 167 patients. Blood 93:459, 1999.

23. D'Andrea AD, Grompe M: Molecular biology of Fanconi anemia: Implications for diagnosis and therapy. Blood 90:1725, 1997.

24. Tuncer MA, Pagliuca A, Hisonmez G et al: Primary myelodysplastic syndrome in children: The clinical experience in 33 cases. Br J Haematol 82:347, 1992.

25. Paul B, Reid MM, Davidson EV et al: Familial myelodysplasia: Progressive disease associated with emergence of monosomy 7. Br J Haematol 65:321, 1987.

26. Song W-J, Sullivan MG, Legare RD et al: Haploinsufficiency of CBFA(AML) causes familial thrombocytopenia with propensity to develop acute myelogenous leukemia (FDP/AML). Nat Genet 23:166, 1999.

27. Van Kamp H, de Pijper C, Verlaan-de Vries M et al: Longitudinal analysis of point mutations of the N-ras proto-oncogene in patients with myelodysplasia using archived blood smears. Blood 79:1266, 1992.

28. Hirai H, Okada M, Mizoguchi H et al: Relationship between an activated N-ras oncogene and chromosomal abnormality during leukemic progression from myelodysplastic syndrome. Blood 71:256, 1988.

29. Quesnel B, Guillerm GM, Vereecque R et al: Methylation of the p15^{INK4b} gene in myelodysplastic syndromes is frequent and acquired during disease progression. Blood 91:2985, 1998.

30. Hoefsloot LH, Amelvoort MR, Broeders LCAK et al: Erythropoietin-induced activation of STATs is impaired in the myelodysplastic syndrome. Blood 89:1690, 1997.

31. Rosenfeld C, List A: A hypothesis for the pathogenesis of myelodysplastic syndromes: Implications for new therapies. Leukemia 14:2, 2000.

32. Raza A, Gezer S, Mundle S et al: Apoptosis in bone narrow biopsy samples involving stromal and hematopoietic cells in 50 patients with myelodysplastic syndrome. Blood 86:268, 1995.

33. Parker JE, Fishlock KL, Mijovic A et al: "Low risk" myelodysplastic syndrome is associated with excessive apoptosis and an increased ratio of pr versus anti-apoptotic bcl-2 related proteins. Br J Haematol 103:1075, 1998.

34. Horikawa K, Nakakuma H, Kawaguchi T et al: Apoptosis resistance of blood cells from patients with paroxysmal nocturnal hemoglobinuria, aplastic anemia, and myelodysplastic anemia. Blood 90:2716, 1997.

35. Bouscary D, De Vos J, Guesnu M et al: Pas/Apo 1 (CD95) expression and apoptosis in patients with myelodysplastic syndromes. Leukemia 6:571, 1997.

36. Hatfill SJ, Faster ED, Steyler JG: Apoptotic megakaryocyte dysplasia in myelodysplastic syndrome. Hematol Pathol 8:97, 1993.

37. Clark DM, Lampert I: Apoptosis is a common histopathological finding in myelodysplasia: The correlate of ineffective hematopoiesis. Leuk Lymphoma 2:415, 1990.

38. Kitagawa M, Saito L, Kuwata T et al: Overexpression of tumor necrosis factor (TNF)-alpha and interferon (IFN)-gamma by bone marrow cells from patients with myelodysplastic syndromes. Leukemia 11:2049, 1997.

39. Deeg HJ, Beckham C, Loken MR et al: Negative regulators of hemopoiesis and stroma function in patients with myelodysplastic syndrome. Leuk Lymphoma 37:405, 2000.

40. Verhoef GEG, De Schouwer P, Ceuppens JL, Van Damme J, Goossens W, Boogaerts MA: Measurement of serum cytokine levels in patients with myelodysplastic syndromes. Leukemia 2:1268, 1992.

41. Hamblin TJ: Immunological abnormalities in myelodysplastic syndromes. Semin Hematol 33:150, 1996.

42. Molldrem JJ, Jiang YZ, Steder-Stevenson MA et al: Haematological response of patients with myelodysplastic syndrome to antithymocyte globulin is associated with a loss of lymphocyte-mediated inhibition of CGU-GM and alterations to T-cell receptor V beta profiles. Br J Haematol 102:1314, 1998.

43. Sugarawa T, Endo K, Shishido T et al: T-cell mediated inhibition of erythropoiesis in myelodysplastic syndromes. Am J Hematol 41:304, 1992.

44. Tichelli A, Gratwohl A, Wuersch A et al: Antilymphocyte globulin for myelodysplastic syndrome? Br J Haematol 68:139, 1988.

45. Biesma DH, Van den Tweel JG, Verdonck LF et al: Immunosuppressive therapy for hypoplastic myelodysplastic syndrome. Cancer 79:1548, 1997.

46. Nisse C, Lorthois C, Dorp V et al: Exposure to occupational and environmental factors in myelodysplastic syndromes. Preliminary results of a case control study. Leukemia 9:693, 1995.

47. West RR, Stafford DA, White AD et al: Cytogenetic abnormalities in the myelodysplastic syndromes and occupational or environmental exposure. Blood 95:2093, 2000.

48. Perera FA: Environment and cancer: Who are susceptible? Science 278:1068, 1997.

49. Rothman N, Smith MT, Hayes RB et al: Benzene poisoning, a risk factor for hematological malignancy, is associated with the NQOI 609 C→T mutation and rapid fractional excretion of chloroxazone. Cancer Res 57:2839, 1997.

50. Bjork J, Albin M, Mauritzson N et al: Smoking and myelodysplastic syndromes. Epidemiology 11:285, 2000.

51. Larson RA, Wang Y, Banarjee M et al: Prevalence of the inactivating 609C→T polymorphism in the NAD(P)H:quinone oxidoreductase (NQO1) gene in patients with primary and therapy-related myeloid leukemias. Blood 94:803, 1999.

52. Wiernals JL, Pagnamenta A, Taylor GM et al: A lack of functional NAD(P)H:quinone oxireductase allele is selectively associated with pediatric leukemias that have MLL fusions. Cancer Res 59:4095, 1999.

53. Chan H, Sandier DP, Taylor JA et al: Increased risk for myelodysplastic syndromes in individuals with glutathione transferase theta I (GSTT1) gene defect. Lancet 347:295, 1996.

54. Preudhomme C, Nisse C, Hebbar M et al: Glutathione S transferase theta I gene defects in myelodysplastic syndromes and their correlation with karyotype and exposure to potential carcinogens. Leukemia 11:1580, 1997.

55. Atoyebi W, Kusec R, Fidler C et al: Glutathione S-transferase gene deletions in myelodysplasia. Lancet 349:1450, 1997.

56. Pedersen-Bjergaard J, Larsen SO, Struck J et al: Risk of therapy-related leukemia and preleukemia after Hodgkin's disease. Relation to age, cumulative dose of alkylating agents, and time from chemotherapy. Lancet 2:83, 1987.

57. Stone RM, Neuberg D, Soiffer R et al: Myelodysplastic syndrome as a late complication following autologous bone marrow transplantation for non-Hodgkin's lymphoma. J Clin Oncol 12:2535, 1994.

58. Sterkers Y, Preudhomme C, Lai JL et al: Acute myeloid leukemia and myelodysplastic syndromes following essential thrombocythemia treated with hydroxyurea: High proportion of cases with 17p deletion. Blood 91:616, 1998.

59. Orchard JA, Bolam S, Oscier DG: Association of myelodysplastic changes with purine analogues. Br J Haematol 100:677, 1998.

60. Thirman MJ, Larson RA: Therapy related myeloid leukemia. Hematol Oncol Clin North Am 10:293, 1996.

61. Heaney ML, Golde DW: Myelodysplasia. New Engl J Med 340:1649, 1999.

62. Williamson PJ, Kruge AR, Reynolds PJ et al: Establishing the incidence of myelodysplastic syndrome. Br J Haematol 87:743, 1994.

63. Aul C, Gatterman N, Schneider W: Age related incidence of and other epidemiological aspects of meylodysplastic syndromes. Br J Haematol 82:358, 1992.

64. Pederson B: Anatomy of the 5q– deletion: Different sex ratios and deleted 5q bands in MDS and AML. Leukemia 10:1883, 1996.

65. Tuncer MA, Paliuca A, Hisonmez G et al: Primary myelodysplastic syndrome in children: The clinical experience in 33 cases. Br J Haematol 82:347, 1992.

66. Kumar T, Mandla SG, Greer WL: Familial myelodysplastic syndrome with early age of onset. Am J Hematol 64:53, 2000.

67. Ho CY, Brith O, Legare RD et al: Linkage of a familial platelet disorder with a propensity to develop myeloid malignancies to human chromosome 21q22.1–22.2. Blood 87:5218, 1996.

68. Bennett JM, Catovsky D, Daniel MT et al: Proposals for the classification of the myelodysplastic syndromes. Br J Haematol 51:189, 1982.

69. Barrett J, Saunthararajah Y, Molldrem J: Myelodysplastic syndrome and aplastic anemia: Distinct entities or disease defined by a common pathophysiology. Semin Hematol 37:15, 2000.

70. Verhoef GE, Pittaluga S, De Wolf-Peters C et al: FAB classification of myelodysplastic syndromes: Merits and controversies. Ann Hematol 71:3, 1995.

71. Kouides PA, Bennett JM: Morphology and classification of the myelodysplastic syndromes and their pathological variants. Semin Hematol 33:95, 1996.

72. Tefferi A, Hoagland HC, Therneau TM, Pierre RV: Chronic myelomonocytic leukemia: Natural history and prognostic determinants. Mayo Clin Proc 64:1246, 1989.

73. Bennett JM, Catovsky D, Daniel MT et al: The chronic myeloid leukaemias: Guidelines for distinguishing chronic granulocytic, atypical chronic myeloid, and chronic myelomonocytic leukaemia. Proposals by the French-American-British Cooperative Leukemia Group. Br J Haematol 87:746, 1994.

74. Harris NL, Jaffe ES, Diebold J et al: World Health Organization Classification of the hematologic malignancies report of the Clinical Advisory Committee. Airlie House, Virginia, November 1997. J Clin Oncol 17:3835, 1999.

75. Lancet JE, Willman CL, Bennett JM: Acute myelogenous leukemia in the elderly. Hematol/Oncol Clin North Am 14:251, 2000.

76. Ribera JM, Cervantes F, Rozman C: A multivariate analysis of prognostic factors in chronic myelomonocytic leukemia according to the FAB criteria. Br J Haematol 65:307, 1987.

77. Boultwood J, Lewis S, Wainscoat JS: The 5q– syndrome. Blood 84:3253, 1994.

78. Nimer SD, Golde DW: The 5q– abnormality. Blood 70:1705, 1987.

79. Mathew P, Tefferi A, Dewald GW et al: The 5q– syndrome: A single institution study of 43 consecutive patients. Blood 81:1040, 1993.

80. Fohlmeister I, Fischer R, Modder B et al: Aplastic anemia and the hypocellular myelodysplastic syndrome: Histomorphological, diagnostic, and prognostic features. J Clin Pathol 38:1218, 1985.

81. Jonasova A, Neuwirtova R, Cermak J et al: Cyclosporin A therapy in hypoplastic MDS patients and certain refractory anaemias without hypoplastic bone marrow. Br J Haematol 200:304, 1998.

82. Molldrem JJ, Caples M, Mavroudis D, Plante M, Young NS, Barrett AJ: Antithymocyte globulin for patients with myelodysplastic syndrome. Br J Haematol 99:699, 1997.

83. Young NS, Madejewski J: The pathobiology of acquired aplastic anemia. N Engl J Med 336:1365, 1997.

84. Shannon KM, Turhan AG, Chang SS et al: Familial bone marrow monsomy 7. Evidence that the predisposing locus is not the long arm of chromosome 7. J Clin Invest 89:984, 1989.

85. Lambertenghi-Deliliers G, Orazi A, Luksch R et al: Myelodysplastic syndromes with increased marrow fibrosis; a distinct clincopathological entity. Br J Haematol 78:161, 1991.

86. Maschek H, Georgii A, Kaloutsi V et al: Myelofibrosis in primary myelodysplastic syndromes: A retrospective study of 352 patients. Eur J Haematol 48:208, 1992.

87. Bennett JM, Catovsky D, Daniel MT et al: Criteria for the diagnosis of acute leukemia of megakaryocytic lineage. Ann Intern Med 103:460, 1985.

88. Verhoef GE, De Wolf-Peeters C, Ferrant A et al: Myelodysplastic syndromes with bone marrow fibrosis: A myelodysplastic syndrome with proliferative features. Ann Hematol 63:235, 1991.

89. Pedersen-Bjergaard J, Pedersen M, Roylston D, Phillip P: Different genetic pathways in leukemogenesis for patients presenting with therapy related myelodysplasia and therapy-related acute myeloid leukemia. Blood 86:354, 1995.

90. Bain BJ. The haematological features of HIV infection. Br J Haematol 99:1, 1997.

91. Cuneo A, Van Orshoven A, Michaux JL et al: Morphologic, immunologic and cytogenetic studies in erythroleukaemia: Evidence for multilineage involvement and identification of two distinct cytogenetic-clinicopathological types. Br J Haematol 75:346, 1990.

92. Roggli VL, Saleem A: Erythroleukemia: A study of 15 cases and literature review. Cancer 49:101, 1982.

93. Tuzuner N, Cox C, Rowe J, Bennett JM: Hypocellular acute myeloid leukemia. Hematol Pathol 9:195, 1995.

94. Miller K, Kyungmann K, Morrison FS et al: The evaluation of low dose cytarabine in the treatment of myelodysplastic syndromes: A Phase III intergroup study. Ann Hematol 65:162, 1992.

95. Gozzatti A, Le Beau MM: Fluorescence in situ hybridization: Uses and limitations. Semin Hematol 37:320, 2000.

96. Dewald G, Hicks G, Higgins R et al: Comparison of interphase FISH and metaphase cytogenetics to study myelodysplasia: An Eastern Cooperative Oncology Group (ECOG) study. (Abstr.) Blood 96:148a, 2000.

97. Jotterand M, Parlier V: Diagnostic and prognostic significance of cytogenetics in adult primary myelodysplastic syndromes. Leuk Lymphoma 23:253, 1996.

98. Uneja SK, Imbert M, Jouault H et al: Haematological features of primary myelodysplastic syndromes (PMDS) at initial presentation: A study of 118 cases. J Clin Pathol 36:1129, 1983.

99. Pomeroy C, Oken MM, Rydell RE et al: Infection in the myelodysplastic syndromes. Am J Med 90:338, 1991.

100. Chalevelaski G, Karaoulis S, Yalouris AG et al: Globin chain synthesis in myelodysplastic syndromes. J Clin Pathol 44:134, 1991.

101. Lintula R: Red cell enzymes in myelodysplastic syndromes: A review. Scand J Haematol 36(Suppl. 45):56, 1986.

102. Dunn DE, Tanawattanacharoen P, Boccune P et al: Paroxysmal nocturnal hemoglobinuria in patients with bone marrow failure syndrome. Ann Intern Med 131:401, 1999.

103. Ruutta T: Granulocyte function in the myelodysplastic syndromes. Scand J Haematol 36(Suppl. 45):66, 1986.

104. Boogaerts MA, Nelissen V, Roelant C, Goosens W: Blood neutrophil function in primary myelodysplastic syndromes. Br J Haematol 55:217, 1983.

105. Martin S, Baldock SC, Ghoneim ATM, Child JA: Defective neutrophil function and microbicidal mechanisms in the myelodysplastic syndromes. J Clin Pathol 36:1120, 1983.

106. Mufti GJ, Stevens JR, Oscier DG et al: Myelodysplastic syndromes: A scoring system with prognostic significance. Br J Haematol 59:311, 1985.

107. Sanz GF, Sanz MA: Prognostic factors in myelodysplastic syndromes. Leuk Res 16:77, 1992.

108. Sanz GF, Sanz MA, Vallespi T et al: Two regression models and a scoring system for predicting survival and planning treatment in myelodysplastic syndromes: A multivariate analysis of prognostic factors in 370 patients. Blood 74:395, 1989.

109. Coiffler B, Adeleine P, Viala JJ et al: Dysmyelopoietic syndromes: A search for prognostic factors in 193 patients. Cancer 52:83, 1983.

110. Rasi V, Lintula R: Platelet function in the myelodysplastic syndrome. Scand J Haematol 36:71, 1986.

111. Tricot G, De Wolf Peeters C, Hendrick B, Verwilghen RL: Bone marrow histology in myelodysplastic syndromes. Br J Haematol 56:423, 1984.

112. Sanz G, Sanz M, Greenberg P: Prognaotic factors and scoring systems in myelodysplastic syndromes. Haematologica 83:358, 1998.

113. Cheson BD, Bennett JM, Kantarjian H et al: Report of an international working group to standardize response criteria for myelodysplastic syndromes. Blood 96:3671, 2000.

114. Rose EH, Abels RI, Nelson RA et al: The use of rHuEpo in the treatment of anemia related to myelodysplasia (MDS). Br J Haematol 89:831, 1995.

115. Hellstrom-Lindberg E: Efficacy of erythropoietin in the myelodysplastic syndromes: A meta-analysis of 205 patients from 17 studies. Br J Haematol 89:67, 1995.

116. Miller K: Erythropoietin, with and without granulocyte-colony stimulating factor (G-CSF), in the treatment of myelodysplastic syndrome (MDS) patients. Leuk Res 22:13, 1998.

117. Hellstrom-Lindberg E, Negrin R, Stein R et al: Erythroid response to treatment with G-CSF plus erythropoietin for the anemia of patients with myelodysplastic syndrome: Proposal for a predictive model. Br J Haematol 99:344, 1997.

118. Negrin RS, Stein R, Doherty K et al: Maintenance treatment of the anemia of myelodysplastic syndrome with recombinant human granulocyte colony-stimulating factor and erythropoietin evidence for in vivo synergy. Blood 87:4076, 1996.

119. Remacha AF, Arrizabalaga B, Villegas A et al: Erythropoietin plus granulocyte colony-stimulating factor in the treatment of myelodysplastic syndromes. Identification of a subgroup of responders. The Spanish Erythropathology Group. Haematologica 84:1058, 1999.

120. Hellstrom-Lindberg F, Kanter-Lweensohn L, Ost A: Morphological changes and apoptosis in bone marrow from patients with myelodysplastic syndromes treated with granulocyte-CSF and erythropoietin. Leuk Res 21:415, 1997.

121. Negrin RS, Haeuber DH, Nagler A et al: Treatment of myelodysplastic syndromes with recombinant human granulocyte colony-stimulating factor. Ann Intern Med 23:262, 1989.

122. Greenberg P, Taylor K, Larson R et al: Phase III randomized multicenter trial of G-CSF vs observation for myelodysplastic syndromes. (Abstr.) Blood 78:1658, 1991.

123. Cines D, Cassileth PA, Kiss JE: Danazol therapy for myelodysplasia. Ann Intern Med 103:58, 1985.

124. Chabannon C, Molina L, Pegourie-Bandelier B et al: A review of 76 patients with myelodysplastic syndrome treated with danazol. Cancer 73:3073, 1994.

125. Selleri C, Catalano L, De Rosa G et al: Danazol in vitro effects on human hematopoiesis and in vitro activity in hypoplastic and myelodysplastic disorders. Eur J Haematol 47:197, 1991.

126. Chan G, Di Venuti G, Miller KB: Danazol for the treatment of thrombocytopenia in myelodysplastic syndrome. (Abstr.) 96:147a, 2000.

127. Wattel E, Cambier N, Caulier MT et al: Androgen therapy in myelodysplastic syndromes with thrombocytopenia: A report on 20 cases. Br J Haematol 87:205, 1994.

128. List AF, Heaton R, Glinsmann-Gibson B, Capizzi RL: Amifostine protects primative hematopoietic progenitors against chemotherapy cytotoxicity. Semin Oncol 23:58, 1996.

129. List AF, Brasfield F, Heaton R et al: Stimulation of hematopoiesis by amifostine in patients with myelodysplastic syndrome. Blood 90:3364, 1997.

130. Bowen DT, Denzlinger C, Brugger W et al: Poor response rate to continuous schedule of amifostine therapy for "low/intermediate risk" myelodysplastic patients. Br J Haematol 103:785, 1998.

131. Razz A, Qawi H, Lisak L et al: Patients with myelodysplastic syndromes benefit from palliative therapy with amifostine, pentoxifylline and ciprofloxacin with or without dexamethasone. Blood 95:1580, 2000.

132. Griffin JD. Spriggs D, Wisch J, Kufe DW: Response of preleukemic syndromes with continuous intravenous infusion of low-dose cytosine arabinoside. J Clin Oncol 3:982, 1985.

133. Cheson BD, Simon R: Low-dose ara-C in acute nonlymphocytic leukemia and myelodysplastic syndromes: A review of 20 years experience. Semin Oncol 14:126, 1987.

134. Fukuhara T, Miyake T, Maekawa I et al: Treatment with low dose cytosine arabinoside followed by administration of macrophage colony stimulating factor prolongs the survival of patients with RAEB, RAEB-T, or leukemic phase myelodysplastic syndrome: A pilot study. Int J Hematol 71:366, 2000.

135. Silverman LR, Holland JF, Weinberg RS et al: Effects of treatment with 5-azacytidine on the in vivo and in vitro hematopoiesis in patients with myelodysplastic syndromes. Leukemia 7(Suppl.):21, 1993.

136. Silverman LR, Dermakos ERP, Peterson B et al: A randomized controlled trial of subcutaneous azacytidine (aza c) in patients with the myelodysplastic syndrome: A study of Cancer and Leukemia Group B (CALGB). (Abstr.) Proc Am Soc Clin Oncol 17:14a, 1998.

137. Wihermans PW, Krulder JWM, Hujgens PC, Neve P: Continuous infusion of low dose 5-aza-2-deoxycitidine in elderly patients with high risk myelodysplastic syndrome. Leukemia 11:19, 1997.

138. Wihermans PW, Hubbert M, Verhoef G et al: Low-dose 5-aza-2'-deoxycytidine, a DNA hypomethylating agent, for the treatment of high risk myelodysplastic syndrome. A multicenter phase II study in elderly patients. J Clin Oncol 18:956, 2000.

139. Morosetti R, Koeffler HP: Differentiation therapy in myelodysplastic syndromes. Semin Hematol 33:236, 1996.

140. Mellibovsky L, Diez A, Perez-Vila E et al: Vitamin D treatment in myelodysplastic syndromes. Br J Haematol 100:516, 1998.

141. Petti MC, Lagagliata R, Avvisati G et al: Treatment of high-risk myelodysplastic syndromes with lymphoblastoid alpha-interferon. Br J Haematol 95:364, 1996.

142. Slapak CA, Desforges JF, Fogaren T, Miller KB: Treatment of acute myeloid leukemia in the elderly with low dose cytarabine, hydroxyurea, and calcitriol. Am J Hematol 41:178, 1992.

143. Doll DC, Kasper LM, Taetle R et al: Treatment with low-dose oral etoposidase in patients with myelodysplastic syndromes. Leuk Res 22:7, 1998.

144. Wattel E, Guerci A, Hecquet B et al: A randomized trial of hydroxyurea versus VP 16 in adult chronic myelomonocytic leukemia. Groupe Francais des Myelodysplasies and European CMML Group. Blood 88:2840, 1996.

145. Bagby GC, Gabourel JD, Linman JW: Glucocorticoid therapy in the preleukemic syndrome (hemopoietic dysplasia): Identification of response in patients using in-vitro mechanism. Ann Intern Med 92:55, 1980.

146. Omoto E, Deguchi S, Takaba S et al: Low-dose melphalan for treatment of high-risk myelodysplastic syndromes. Leukemia 10:609, 1996.

147. Denzlinger C, Benz D, Biweb D et al: Low-dose melphalan induces favourable responses in elderly patients with high risk myelodysplastic syndromes or secondary leukemia. Br J Haematol 108:93, 2000.

146. Enright H, Jacobs HS, Vercellotti G et al: Paraneoplastic autoimmune phenomena in patients with myelodysplastic syndromes: Response to immunosuppressive therapy. Br J Haematol 91:403, 1995.

147. Molldrem JJ, Caples M, Mavroudis D et al: Antithymocyte globulin for patients with myelodysplastic syndrome. Br J Haematol 99:705, 1997.

148. Molldrem JJ, Jang YZ, Stetler-Stevenson M et al: Haematological response of patients with myelodysplastic syndrome to antithymocyte globulin is associated with loss of CGU-GM and alterations in T-cell receptor v_b profiles. Br J Haematol 102:1314, 1998.

149. Killick AB, Marsh JC, Cavenagh JD et al: Antithymocyte globulin for the treatment of patients with "low risk" myelodysplastic syndromes. (Abstr.) Blood 94:306a, 1999.

150. Jonasova A, Neuwirtova R, Cermak J et al: Cyclosporin A therapy in hypoplastic MDS patients and certain refractory anaemias without hypoplastic bone marrows. Br J Haematol 200:304, 1998.

151. Biesma DH, van den Tweel JG, Verdonek LE: Immunosuppressive therapy for hypoplastic myelodysplastic syndrome. Cancer 79:1548, 1997.

152. Bernstein SH, Brunetto VL, Davey FR et al: Acute myeloid leukemia-type chemotherapy for newly diagnosed patients without antecedent cytopenias having myelodysplastic syndrome as defined by French-American-British criteria. A Cancer and Leukemia Group B Study. J Clin Oncol 14:2486, 1996.

153. Armitage JO, Dick FR, Needleman SW et al: Effect of chemotherapy for the dysmyelopoietic syndrome. Cancer Treat Rep 65:610, 1981.

154. Wattel E, De Botton S, Luc Lai J et al: Long-term follow-up of de novo myelodysplastic syndromes treated with intensive chemotherapy: Incidence of long-term survivors and outcome of partial responders. Br J Haematol 98:983, 1997.

155. Estey E, Thall P, Beran M et al: Effect of diagnosis (refractory anemia with excess blast, refractory anemia with excess blasts in transformation, or acute myeloid leukemia[AML]) on outcome of AML-type chemotherapy. Blood 90:2969, 1997.

156. de Whitte T, Suciu S, Peetermans M et al: Intensive chemotherapy for poor prognosis myelodysplasia (MDS) and secondary acute myeloid leukemia (sAML) following MDS of more than 6 months duration: A pilot study by the Leukemia Cooperative Group of the European Organisation for Research and Treatment in Cancer (EORTC-LCG). Leukemia 9:1805, 1995.

157. Parker JE, Pagliuca A, Mijovic A et al: Fludarabine, cytarabine, G-CSF and idarubicin (FLAG) for the treatment of poor-risk myelodysplastic syndromes and acute myeloid leukemia. Br J Haematol 99:939, 1997.

158. Estey E: Topotecan for myelodysplastic syndromes. Oncology 12: NCCN Proc 18, 1998.

159. Beran M, Kantarijan H, O'Brien S et al: Topotecan, a topoisomerase I inhibitor, is active in the treatment of myelodysplastic syndromes and chronic myelomonocytic leukemia. Blood 88:2473, 1996.

160. Estey E, Thall P, Wang X: Routine use of fludarabine- or topotecan containing chemotherapy is not indicated in AML, RAEB-T, or RAEB. (Abstr.) Blood 96:2170, 2000.

161. Wattel E, Solary F, Hecquet B et al: Quinine improves the results of intensive chemotherapy in myelodysplastic syndromes expressing P glycoprotein: Results of a randomised study. Br J Haematol 102:1015, 1998.

162. Leith CP, Leith KJ, Kopecky J et al: Acute myeloid leukemia in the elderly: Assessment of multidrug resistance (MDR I) and cytoge-

netics distinguishes biologic subgroups with remarkably distinct responses to standard chemotherapy: A Southwest Oncology Group Study. Blood 89:3323, 1997.

163. Willman CL: The prognostic significance of the expression and function of multidrug resistance transporter proteins in acute myeloid leukemia: Studies of the Southwest Oncology Group Leukemia Research Program. Semin Hematol 34(Suppl. 5):25, 1997.

164. De Witte T, Van Biezen A, Hermans J et al: Autologous bone marrow transplantation for patients with myelodysplastic syndrome (MDS) or acute myeloid leukemia following MDS. Blood 90:3853, 1997.

165. Laporte JP, Isnard F, Lesage S et al: Autologous bone marrow transplantation with marrow purged by mafosfamide in seven patients with myelodysplastic syndromes in transformation. (AML-MDS): A pilot study. Leukemia 7:2030, 1993.

166. Carella AM, Dejana A, Lerna E et al: In vivo mobilization of kary-otypically normal peripheral blood progenitor cells in high-risk MDS, a secondary or therapy-related acute myelogenous leukemia. Br J Haematol 95:127, 1996.

167. Delforge M, Demuynck H, Vanderberghe P et al: Polyclonal prim-itive hematopoietic progenitors can be detected in mobilized peripheral blood from patients with high-risk myelodysplastic syndrome. Blood 86:3660, 1995.

168. Demuynck H, Delforge M, Verhoef GE et al: Feasibility of peripheral blood progenitor cell harvest and transplantation in patients with poor-risk myelodysplastic syndromes. Br J Haematol 92:351, 1996.

169. Anderson JE, Anasetti C, Appelbaum FR et al: Unrelated donor marrow transplantation for myelodysplasia (MDS) and MDS-related acute myeloid leukemia. Br J Haematol 93:59, 1996.

170. Anderson JE, Appelbaum FR, Schoch G et al: Allogeneic trans-plantation for myelodysplastic syndrome with advanced disease morphology: A phase II study of busulfan, cytophosphamide, and total-body irradiation and analysis of prognostic factors. J Clin Oncol 14:220, 1996.

171. Deeg HJ, Shulman HM, Anderson JE et al: Allogeneic and syn-geneic marrow transplantation for myelodysplastic syndrome in patients 55 to 66 years of age. Blood 95:1188, 2000.

172. Nevill TJ, Fung HC, Shepard JD et al: Cytogenetic abnormalities in primary myelodysplastic syndrome are highly predictive of outcome after allogeneic bone marrow transplantation. Blood 92:1910, 1998.

173. Glinsmann-Gibson B, Spier C, Baier M et al: Mast cell growth fac-tor (c-kit ligand) restores growth of multipotent progenitors in myelodysplastic syndrome. Leukemia 8:827, 1994.

174. Tafuri A, Lemoli RM, Petricco MT et al: Thrombopoietin and interleukin 11 have different modulatory effects on cell cycle and programmed cell death in primary acute myeloid leukemia. Exp Hematol 27:1255, 1999.

175. Nara K, Kurokawa H, Tohda S et al: The effect of basic and acidic fibroblast growth (bFGF and aFGF) on the growth of leukemic blast progenitors in acute myelogenous leukemia. Exp Hematol 23:1030, 1995.

176. Dililiers GL, Pruneri GC, Cortelezzi et al: Angiogenesis in myelodysplastic syndromes. Leuk Res 23:S24, 1999.

177. Raza A, Lisak L, Andrews C et al: Thalidomide produces transfu-sion independence in patients with long standing refractory ane-mias and myelodysplastic syndromes (MDS). (Abstr.) Blood 94:661a, 1999.

178. Dai J, Weinberg RS, Waxman S et al: Malignant cells can be sensi-tized to undergo growth inhibiton and apoptosis by arsenic triox-ide through modulation of the glutathione redox system. Blood 93:268, 1999.

179. Donelli A, Chiodino C, Panissidi T et al: Might arsenic trioxide be useful in the treatment of advanced myelodysplastic syndromes? Haematologica 85:1002, 2000.

180. Dutcher JP, Wiernik PH, Novik Y et al: Major hematologic response in a patient with myelodysplasia (MDS) to arsenic triox-ide (ATO). (Abstr.) Blood 96:260b, 2000.

181. Cheson D, Zwiebel JA, Dancey J, Murgo A: Novel therapeutic agents for the treatment of myelodysplastic syndromes. Semin Oncol 27:560, 2000.

Myeloma and Related Disorders

24

History of Multiple Myeloma

Robert A. Kyle

Saturday, Nov. 1st 1845

"Dear Dr. Jones,

The tube contains urine of very high specific gravity. When boiled it becomes slightly opaque. On the addition of nitric acid, it effervesces, assumes a reddish hue, and becomes quite clear; but as it cools, assumes the consistence and appearance which you see. Heat reliquifies it. What is it?"[1]

This cryptic note and a urine sample were sent by a leading physician of London, Dr. Thomas Watson, to Henry Bence Jones, a 31-year-old physician at St. George's Hospital who had already established a reputation as a chemical pathologist.

The patient, Thomas Alexander McBean, was identified by examining the Register of Deaths and searching for males 45 to 47 years old whose name began with M and who died in London on January 1 or 2, 1846.[2] He was seen on October 30, 1845, by Dr. William Macintyre, a 53-year-old Harley Street consultant and physician to the Metropolitan Convalescent Institution and to the Western General Dispensary, St. Marylebone.[2] Mr. McBean, 44 years of age and a highly respectable grocer of "temperate habits and exemplary conduct," had taken a vacation in the country in September 1844 to regain his strength, which he felt had been impaired by work and a family illness. He married early and had numerous offspring. With the exception of two or three severe attacks of "frontal neuralgia," he had enjoyed uninterrupted good health. For a year, his family had noted that he fatigued easily and appeared to stoop while walking. He also had urinary frequency and was concerned that his "body linen was stiffened by his urine" despite the absence of a urethral discharge.

While vaulting out of an underground cavern on his country vacation, he had "instantly felt as if something had snapped or given way within the chest, and for some minutes he lay in intense agony, unable to stir."[3] The pain abated, and he was able to walk to a neighboring inn. Dr. Macintyre subsequently applied a strengthening plaster to the chest because movement of the arms produced chest pain. The application of the plaster and his carefully abstaining from exertion allowed the patient to resume work. Minimal pain and stiffness of the chest persisted but was relieved by the application of a "strengthening plaster to the chest." Three or 4 weeks later, the pain recurred, and the patient was treated by the removal of a pound of blood and the application of leeches. As might be expected, this was followed by considerable weakness for 2 or 3 months.

In the spring of 1845, he had an episode of pleuritic pain in the right side, between the ribs and the hip, which was treated by cupping. Therapeutic bleeding produced much greater weakness than before. Wasting, pallor, and slight puffiness of his face and ankles led to consultation with Dr. Thomas Watson. Steel and quinine therapy resulted in rapid improvement. By the middle of summer, he was able to travel to Scotland, where on the seacoast "he was capable of taking active exercise on foot during the greater part of the day, bounding over the hills, to use his own expression, as nimbly as any of his companions."[3] His appetite became ravenous—he expressed it as being so much so that he dreamed of eating dogs and cats.[1] His recovery was interrupted by an episode of diarrhea, which proved to be obstinate, reducing his strength considerably. In September of 1845, he returned to London in a very debilitated state but free of the excruciating pains that he had experienced during the spring and early part of the summer. In October, lumbar and sciatic pain became severe. Warm baths, Dover's powder (ipecac and opium powder), acetate of ammonia, camphor julep, and compound tincture of camphor did not help.

On October 30, he was seen by Dr. Macintyre who, because edema had been observed 4 months before, personally examined the urine but found no evidence of sugar. The urine specimen was opaque, acid, and of high density, with a specific gravity of 1.035. When heated, the urine was found to "abound in animal matter." With the addition of nitric acid, it became clear, but a precipitate developed after an hour. This precipitate "underwent complete solution on the application of heat, but again consolidated on cooling."[3]

Every movement of McBean's trunk produced excruciating pain. Great care and cautious maneuvering enabled him to "get in and out of bed on all fours." The patient became weaker and was confined to his bed. He developed flatulence and pronounced fullness and hardness in the region of the liver. He had phlegm in his chest and coughed, and he had another episode of diarrhea. On November 15, Dr. Henry Bence Jones saw the patient in consultation and recommended alum as treatment "with the view of checking the exhausting excretion of animal matter." The patient improved and was able to sit up and enjoy his food, but on December 7 "experienced a dreadful aggravation of lumbar pains."[3] He had almost continual pain, became weaker, and died on January 1, 1846, exhausted, in full possession of his mental faculties. The cause of death was listed as "atrophy from albuminuria."[2] Involvement of the bones, aside from pain, was not recognized during the patient's illness.

Postmortem examination revealed emaciation. The ribs, which crumbled under the heel of the scalpel, were soft, brittle, readily broken, and easily cut by the knife. Their interior was filled with a soft "gelatiniform substance of a blood-red colour and unctuous feel." The sternum was soft and fragile and snapped when raised and turned back. The heart and lungs were not remarkable. "The liver was voluminous, but of healthy structure." The kidneys appeared to be normal on both gross and microscopic examination. They (the kidneys) had "proved equal to the novel office assigned them" and had "discharged the task without sustaining, on their part, the slightest danger." The thoracic and lumbar vertebrae had the same changes as found in the ribs and sternum, but the humeri and femurs resisted "all efforts to bend or break them by manual force."[3]

John Dalrymple, surgeon to the Royal Ophthalmic Hospital, Moorfields, examined two lumbar vertebrae and a rib of Mr. McBean. He noted that the lumbar vertebrae were markedly compressed and stated that they "scarcely exceed in thickness the intervertebral substance, and have lost nearly one-third of their normal bulk."[4] The disease appeared to begin in the cancellous bone; it then grew and produced irregularly sized round dark-red projections that were visible through the periosteum. Nucleated cells formed the bulk of the gelatiniform mass that filled the large cancellous cavities. Most of these cells were round or oval and about one-half to two times as large as an average blood cell. The cells contained one or two nuclei, each with a bright, distinct nucleolus. Wood engravings made from the accurate drawings of Mr. Dalrymple are consistent with the appearance of myeloma cells (Figure 24–1).[4] Dalrymple postulated that the nucleated cells had a limited duration of life in mollities ossium and disintegrated and were "carried out of the system by the circulation of the kidneys." Both Dalrymple and Macintyre believed that the disorder was a malignant disease of bone. Bright's disease was considered in the differential diagnosis because of the albuminous matter in the urine, but there was no dropsy. The diarrhea, weakness, emaciation, hepatic enlargement, flatulence, dyspepsia, edema of the ankles, puffiness of the face, and large amounts of Bence Jones proteinuria all suggest the possibility of amyloidosis, in addition to myeloma, but the autopsy findings of a normal heart and kidneys and "voluminous liver of healthy structure" make the presence of amyloidosis unlikely. Because the lardaceous or waxy changes of amyloidosis in the liver were commonly recognized in this era, it is unlikely that amyloidosis would have been overlooked.

Multiple myeloma has most likely been present for centuries. Four cases of possible multiple myeloma in American Indian skeletons from AD 200 to 1300 were reported by Morse et al. in 1974.[5] Lesions were lytic with sharply demarcated borders and no evidence of sclerosis or formation of new bone. One skeleton was that of a 45-year-old man, but the other three were less than 40 years of age, and this casts some doubt on the diagnosis of multiple myeloma. As with many so-called first cases, one can find an earlier example. It is almost certain that 39-year-old Sarah Newbury, the second patient described by Solly in 1844,[6] had multiple myeloma. She had experienced fatigue and, 4 years before her death, was seized with a violent pain in her back when stooping. Rheumatic pains occurred a year later. Pain in her limbs had increased after a fall in February 1842, and she

was confined to her room. Her femurs fractured 2 months later, when her husband lifted her and carried her to her bed. Fractures of the clavicles, right humerus, and right radius and ulna occurred. She was admitted to St. Thomas's Hospital on April 15, 1844, and was treated with an infusion of orange peel and a rhubarb pill when necessary, and an opiate at night if required. Examination of her urine revealed a large quantity of phosphate of lime. Results of examination of the blood were normal. She died suddenly on April 20, 1844, of asphyxia. The thoracic cavity was reduced to 4 inches in its transverse diameter. The right lung was compressed to about one-fourth of its natural size, and the left lung was decreased to one-half the extent of the right lung because of skeletal involvement. Autopsy revealed that the cancellous portion of the sternum (Figure 24–2) had been replaced by a red substance that Macintyre reported was similar to that seen in Mr. McBean. A red matter had replaced much of the femur and ranged from Modena red to a bright scarlet crimson (Figure 24–3). Solly examined the red matter with Mr. Birkett of Guy's Hospital, who described the cells as "very clear, their edge being remarkably distinct, and the clear *oval* outline enclosing *one* bright *central* nucleus, *rarely two, never more.*" Dalrymple noted that the microscopic appearance reported by Mr. Birkett "accords very nearly" with his descrip-

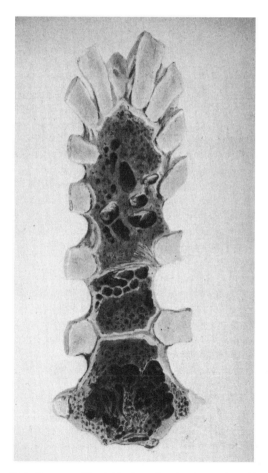

Figure 24–2. Sternum of Sarah Newbury showing destruction of bone. (From Solly,[6] with permission.)

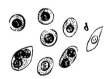

Figure 24–1. Plasma cells (wood engravings made from drawings by Mr. Dalrymple). (From Dalrymple,[4] with permission.)

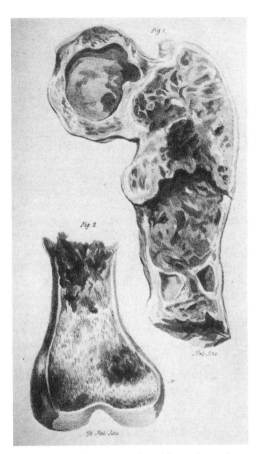

Figure 24–3. Sarah Newbury. Destruction of femurs by myeloma tumor. (From Solly,[6] with permission.)

tion of McBean's marrow. Solly postulated that the process was inflammatory and had begun with an abnormality of the blood vessels, in which the "earthy matter of the bone is absorbed and thrown out by the kidneys in the urine."[6]

Having received specimens of urine from both Watson and Macintyre on November 1, Bence Jones corroborated the finding that the addition of nitric acid produced a precipitate that was redissolved by heat and formed again on cooling. He calculated that the patient excreted more than 60 g/day. Bence Jones concluded that the protein was an oxide of albumin, specifically "hydrated deutoxide of albumen."[7] He postulated that chlorine caused this new protein to form from albumin. Bence Jones calculated that there were 66.97 parts of "hydrated deutoxide of albumen" per 1000 parts of urine and that this amount was equivalent to the proportion of albumin in healthy blood, so that every ounce of urine secreted was equivalent to the protein loss of an equal quantity of blood.[1,7]

Some justification exists for changing the name *multiple myeloma* to *McBean's disease with Macintyre's proteinuria*. Although Macintyre described the heat properties of the urine, Bence Jones emphasized its place in the diagnosis of myeloma, for he said, "I need hardly remark on the importance of seeking for this oxide of albumen in other cases of mollities ossium."[1]

The modest Dr. Macintyre stated that his "share in this part of the inquiry, it must have been seen, was very humble." He went on to say that "I shall be content if I have succeeded in pointing out to future observers, gifted with the requisite qualifications for conducting researches of a higher order, certain definite and distinctive characters by which a peculiar and hitherto unrecorded pathological condition of the urine may be recognised and identified."[3] Macintyre died 7 years after reporting his findings. Thomas Watson later became a baronet and physician-in-ordinary to the queen. He was president of the Royal College of Physicians for 5 years, and his popular book *Principles and Practice of Physic* earned him the title the "British Cicero."

Henry Bence Jones was born on December 31, 1813, at Thorington Hall in Yoxford, Suffolk, England, in a house lent to his family by his maternal grandfather, the Reverend Mr. Bence Sparrow, Rector of Beccles. Mr. Sparrow adopted the name Bence in May 1804 and apparently was known as Bence Bence. The Bences were related to the Winthrops of colonial America, including John Winthrop, first governor of Connecticut.[8] His youngest child, Matilda, married Lieutenant Colonel William Jones, of the Fifth Dragoon Guards, who were active in the Peninsular War at Salamanca.

Bence Jones went to Harrow in 1827 when it was at its lowest state, with fewer than 150 boys. He became a good "cricketer, football, and racquet player, in all games I took immense delight" and became "best player in the school."[9] After tutoring in Euclid, in which he did well, and algebra, in which he did not, he entered Trinity College, Cambridge. He joined the Second Trinity Crew, where he rowed number 5. He attended the Divinity Lectures and obtained a certificate for ordination, but when he took his degree in January 1836, he had resolved not to enter the church.[10]

He considered emigrating to New Zealand and procured the papers, but his father suggested that he study medicine. He entered under Mr. George Badington, surgeon at St. George's Hospital, who introduced him to the apothecary, Mr. Hammerton. Bence Jones prepared medicine in the apothecary shop for 6 months and stated that it "was of the utmost use to me all my life."[9] He became a full-time pupil at St. George's on October 1, 1838, and began attending lectures and the dissecting room. After a short time as a dresser in the surgeons' ward, he returned to the physicians' ward, where he did his utmost to learn about the stethoscope from Dr. Hope, an assistant physician. He developed rheumatic fever in the spring of 1839 and returned home for 6 weeks but "recovered without complications of disease of the heart."

Returning to London in the fall of 1839, Bence Jones enrolled as a private pupil to Prof. Graham of University College at a cost of 50 pounds. Most of the teaching was done by Mr. Fownes. Results of his analysis of a large sulfur-containing cystine calculus became his first paper. He became a licentiate of the College of Physicians in early 1841. On Easter Sunday, 1841, he traveled to Giessen, Germany, to study chemistry with Justus von Liebig. Returning to St. George's on October 1, 1841, he studied in the physicians' wards. After his proposal to his second cousin, Lady Millicent Acheson, some difficulties were overcome by the aid of Lady Noel Byron, and they were married in May 1842.

Bence Jones obtained his M.A. in Cambridge and then began working at St. George's, where his analyses of the calculi in the museum resulted in his second paper. He was asked to give 100 lectures beginning in the fall of 1843 to "six attentive pupils" at Middlesex Hospital because Prof. Fownes was too busy and later said "In preparation for these lectures, I acquired more practical knowledge of chemistry than I could possibly have done in any other way."[9] On December 19, 1845, an Assistant Physicianship vacancy occurred at St. George's and "after a comparatively easy contest, I was appointed to that office."

In May 1846, he became a Full Physician at St. George's Hospital. In 1845, he was elected Fellow of the College of Physicians and in 1846 Fellow of the Royal Society.

Bence Jones was an accomplished physician who acquired a large and remunerative practice. He stated "Each year my practice gradually increased, and I endeavored to let no year pass without doing something original in natural science as applied to medicine."[9] In one year (April 5, 1864, to April 5, 1865), his profits reached £7,400.[11] He specialized in disorders of the genitourinary tract as well as gout and rheumatism.[8] Among his patients was the great naturalist Charles Darwin, whom he had treated with a diet that "half starved him to death."[12] Other patients included the German chemist August Wilhelm Hofmann and the English biologist Thomas Huxley. Hermann von Helmholtz, a physiologist and the inventor of the ophthalmoscope, had a great deal of respect for him. On one occasion, he dined with Dr. Bence Jones and described him as a charming man, simple, harmless, cordial as a child, and extraordinarily kind.

Bence Jones was well acquainted with Florence Nightingale and had a high opinion of her. She regarded him as the best "chemical doctor" in London. He sought her advice about a project that he was considering for reform of nurses' training in the hospitals of London. He served as one of the original members of the Council of the Nightingale Fund. He was also influential in the establishment of the Hospital for Sick Children in Great Ormond Street, on whose board he served.

He was interested in physics and became a friend and physician to Michael Faraday. This friendship resulted in a two-volume biography of the prominent physicist in 1870.

Henry Bence Jones was the first to describe xanthine crystals in the urine.[13] He emphasized the frequency of diabetes in the older population—11 of his 29 patients with diabetes were more than 60 years of age.[14] He noted that sugar was still found in the urine despite the withholding of sugar-containing foods.[15] Bence Jones introduced the use of biochemical tracers. He injected lithium carbonate into guinea pigs and then determined the presence of lithium in vascular tissues, cartilage of the hip joint, and humors of the eye.[10] He also described one of the first pharmacological studies of drug metabolism when he determined the rate of diffusion of quinine into the organs of the guinea pig using a fluorescent method.[16]

He published a series of lectures on the "applications of chemistry and medicine to pathology and therapeutics." He became Secretary of the Royal Institution in 1860 and subsequently wrote a history of the Royal Institution, its founders, and first professors, and served as editor of the *Manual of Chemistry*. He believed that medicine would be better served if medical men spent time acquiring knowledge of chemistry and physics rather than Latin and Greek.

Bence Jones began his laboratory work each day at dawn and spent the afternoons and evenings doing hospital rounds. Medical students did not seek his clerkship, because he was not adept at clinical teaching and had a well-known lack of punctuality. He made his diagnoses quickly and briefly. Irritable in manner and at times impetuous, he was sometimes too quick with criticism for those with opposing views. He was self-reliant and strong-willed. His chief characteristics were scientific truth, accuracy, and a dislike of empiricism. He insisted on the medical facts. His lifelong goal was to improve the chemical training of physicians and to inculcate an attitude of scientific thinking as the basis for diagnosis and treatment. He endeavored to upgrade the requirements for science and to reform the examination system for election to fellowship in the Royal College of Physicians.

In 1861, "Frequent palpitations of the heart led me to examine myself carefully with a flexible stethoscope, and I found chronic rheumatism had done permanent injury to one of the valves."[9] Therefore, he resigned his physicianship at St. George's in early 1862 but ceased to have trouble with his heart, and his practice grew. In early 1866, his health began to fail, and after examining himself he said "I fancied that one side was half full of fluid."[9] After a meeting of the Chemical Section of the British Association Meetings in Nottingham, he returned to Folkstone on September 1 and was "taken dangerously ill." His illness was almost fatal in January 1867, but he slowly recovered. From that time on his energy decreased, and in a letter to John Tyndall, written at Folkstone on August 17, 1870, he stated "I am very lazy and feel unfit for any work and as neither eating, drinking nor sleeping come pleasantly to me I am a useless mortal and had better be helping the worms and the grass to grow faster than they otherwise would do…"[8] In 1870, he went with difficulty to Oxford, where he received the Honorary Degree of Doctor of Civil Letters (DCL). In early 1873, he gave up his practice because of hepatomegaly, ascites, and anasarca. He died at his home at 84 Brook Street in London of congestive heart failure on April 20, 1873, at the age of 59 years and was buried at Kensall Green Cemetery.[11] He was survived by his wife and five of his seven children. His friend and mentor, Liebig, had died a day earlier. The Bence Jones Ward still exists at the new St. George's Hospital in Tooting. It is currently devoted to gynecology patients.

Interestingly, although Bence Jones's obituary described his work on renal stones, diabetes mellitus, and malignant and tuberculous involvement of the kidney—as well as his emphasis on the value of microscopic analysis of the urine—no mention was made of his papers on the unique urinary protein that bears his name.[15]

Henry Bence Jones did not use the hyphen in his name, and it does not appear in any of his more than 40 papers and books; books published during his lifetime enter him under Jones. His descendants now use a hyphen, added a half-century after his death.[17]

A number of other persons were involved in the story of Bence Jones proteinuria. In 1846, J.F. Heller described a protein in the urine that precipitated when warmed a little above 50°C and then disappeared on further heating. Although Heller did not recognize the precipitation of the protein when the urine was cooled, it is nearly certain that this was Bence Jones protein. He distinguished this new protein from albumin and casein.[18] Fleischer[19] was the first to use the term "Bence Jones protein." Kühne[20] described Bence Jones protein in a patient who died in 1869. The urine of Kahler's patient was described in detail by Huppert.[21] In 1898 Bradshaw[22] found that meals had little or no influence on the amount of Bence Jones proteinuria. There was no nocturnal variation, and he believed that the rate of excretion was "pretty constant throughout the 24 hours." Walters[23] made a study of three patients with multiple myeloma and reported that the quantity of Bence Jones proteinuria was independent of the protein intake. He also noted no diurnal variation. In one patient, the intravenous injection of Bence Jones protein appeared to increase the amount of Bence Jones proteinuria. Walters found Bence Jones protein in the blood of one patient and in the bronchial secretions of another. He concluded that Bence Jones protein was of endogenous origin and was probably derived from blood proteins through the action of abnormal cells in the bone marrow.

Two distinct groups of Bence Jones proteins were recognized by Bayne-Jones and Wilson in 1922.[24] They made 12 preparations of Bence Jones proteins from five patients, two of whom had previously been reported on by Walters. Rabbits were immunized by intravenous injection of the Bence Jones protein, and precipitin tests were done with the Bence Jones protein preparations. They concluded that Bence Jones proteins consisted of a group of similar but not identical proteins. In 1956, Korngold and Lipari[25] demonstrated a relationship between Bence Jones protein and the serum proteins of multiple myeloma. As a tribute to Korngold and Lipari, the two major classes of Bence Jones proteins have been designated κ and λ. Using ^{13}C-labeled glycine, Putnam and Hardy[26] demonstrated that syntheses of the abnormal serum globulin and of Bence Jones protein were independent processes. The Bence Jones protein was rapidly excreted and apparently derived directly from the nitrogen pool rather than from the plasma or a tissue protein precursor.

One hundred seventeen years after the description of the unique heat properties, Edelman and Gally[27] demonstrated that the light chains prepared from a serum immunoglobulin G (IgG) myeloma protein and the Bence Jones protein from the same patient's urine had the same amino acid sequence, similar spectrofluorometric behavior, the same molecular weight, identical appearance on chromatography with carboxymethyl-cellulose and on starch gel electrophoresis after reduction and alkylation, and the same ultracentrifugal pattern—as well as the same thermal solubility. The light chains precipitated when heated to between 40°C and 60°C, dissolved on boiling, and reprecipitated when cooled to between 40°C and 60°C. Hilschmann and Craig[28] and Titani et al.[29] showed that Bence Jones proteins were not only related to the light chains of gamma globulin but that each light chain was divided into a "variable" or V region and a "constant" or C region. This accounts for the heterogeneity of normal gamma globulins and for antibody specificity and diversity.

In 1867, Hermann Weber[30] described a 40-year-old man with myeloma who suffered frequent colds in the spring and experienced sternal pain in May. The sternum was tender and then became deformed. The patient also had severe pain in the lumbar region. Movement of his head produced pain in his neck and arms. He died 3 1/2 months after the onset of pain. Postmortem examination revealed that the sternum had been almost entirely replaced by a grayish red substance that had the microscopic appearance of a sarcoma. Two fractures of the sternum were also seen. Several round defects in the skull had been replaced by the same morbid substance as that found in the sternum. Many of the ribs, several vertebrae, and parts of the pelvis were involved. Amyloid was found in the kidneys and spleen. In 1872, William Adams[31] for Dr. Dowse described a patient with "acute rheumatism" characterized by bone pain, fractures, and fever. The left humerus and femur fractured while the body was being placed on the autopsy table. Lardaceous changes were found in the liver and kidneys. The cancellous portions of the bones had been replaced by a homogeneous, soft, gelatinoid substance. When examined microscopically, the substance filling the hollowed bone was shown to consist of small spherical and oval cells that contained one oval nucleus (rarely two), with a bright nucleus.

The term *multiple myeloma* was introduced by von Rustizky in 1873[32] when, during autopsy, he found eight separate tumors of bone marrow and designated them as multiple myelomas. The patient, a 47-year-old man, had presented with a gradually enlarging tumor in the right temple. Subsequently, thickening of the manubrium and seventh rib developed, followed by paraplegia. At autopsy, it was revealed that a fist-sized tumor in the right frontal region extended into the orbit and had produced ophthalmoplegia. Other findings included an apple-sized tumor in the right fifth rib, a tumor in the left seventh rib (producing a fracture), a tumor of the sternum, a tumor of the sixth to the eighth thoracic vertebrae (producing paraplegia), and three tumors of the right humerus. Although von Rustizky's description of the tumor cells is vague, he described round cells whose nucleus was located in the periphery near the cell membrane. The presence of an eccentric nucleus is suggestive of plasma cells. He did not mention albumosurie (Bence Jones protein).

In 1883 Kühne[20] described a 40-year-old man with tenderness of the cervical and thoracic spine and abnormal curvature of the spine. The patient was unable to lie on his back and had to remain on his side. His head was flexed forward. During the last weeks of the patient's life, dysphasia and paralysis of the seventh cranial nerve developed, probably from an extradural plasmacytoma. The patient died on August 27, 1869, 9 months after the onset. There was no autopsy report. His urine precipitated on warming to between 40°C and 50°C and cleared at 100°C. Kühne isolated the protein and found that the carbon, hydrogen, and nitrogen levels were similar to those described by Bence Jones. Kühne attributed any differences to the fact that his preparation was more pure than Bence Jones's preparation. He named the protein "albumosurie."

Little further interest was shown in the disease until 1889, when Otto Kahler[33] described a striking case involving a 46-year-old physician named Dr. Loos. His first symptom, noted in

July 1879, consisted of sudden severe pain in the right upper thorax, which was aggravated by taking a deep breath. Six months later, the pain recurred and became localized to the right third rib, which was tender to pressure. During the next 2 years, intermittent pain, aggravated by exercise, occurred in the ribs, spinal column, left shoulder, upper arm, and right clavicle. Albuminuria was first noticed in September 1881. Skeletal pain, made worse by movement, continued to occur intermittently. Pallor was noted in 1883 and pneumonia developed in February 1884. In December 1885, Dr. Loos was first seen by Kahler, who noted anemia, severe kyphosis, and tenderness of many bones. When Dr. Loos stood, the lower ribs touched the iliac crest. He had recurrent bronchial infections and intermittent hemoptysis. During the following year, kyphosis increased and his height decreased monthly. He became dwarflike. The kyphosis of the upper thoracic spinal column increased, and his chin pressed against the sternum, producing a decubitus ulcer. On August 26, 1887, Dr. Loos died. Autopsy revealed hepatosplenomegaly. The ribs were soft and could be broken with minimal effort. Soft gray-reddish masses were noted in the ribs and thoracic vertebrae. Microscopic examination showed large round cells, consistent with myeloma. Albumosurie was first noted in December 1885. It is interesting to note that the patient had a high fluid intake and took sodium bicarbonate on a regular basis. This regimen may have helped prevent renal failure. Kahler recognized that the urinary protein had the same characteristics that Bence Jones had described. Examination of the urine by Huppert[21] showed that the protein precipitated at 53°C to 59°C, cleared with heating to boiling, and then precipitated during cooling. The patient excreted 6.7 g of the protein daily. It did not contain albumin.[21] It is likely that the 43-year-old engineer reported by Coats[34] as having multiple sarcoma of bone actually had multiple myeloma. A large tumor of the sternum had developed 5 years before, along with tumors in the right clavicle, right humerus, and left hip. The patient had back pain radiating to the lower extremities and experienced weakness of his legs and later a fracture of the right humerus. Postmortem examination revealed multiple tumors and involvement of the ribs and vertebral bodies. Microscopic examination showed round or polygonal cells with oval nuclei constituting more than half the diameter of the cells.

Otto Kahler, born in 1849, was the son of a well-known physician in Prague. He received his M.D. degree from the University of Prague in 1871 and then worked as an assistant in Professor Halla's clinic. During a sabbatical in Paris, he met two French neurologists, Jean Martin Charcot and G.B.A. Duchenne (Duchenne de Boulogne). Kahler became interested in neurology and particularly in anatomy. Kahler contributed to the pathological anatomy of the central nervous system and to the anatomy of tabes dorsalis, localization of partial central occulomotor paralysis, and slow compression of the spinal cord. He became professor of medicine in Prague and, after Halla's resignation, head of the Second Medical Clinic at the German University of Prague. In 1889, Kahler was asked to succeed the famous physician Heinrich Bamberger as professor at the University of Vienna.[35] In his inaugural address on May 13, 1889, Kahler paid tribute to Professor Bamberger and finished his lec-

ture with the statement, "Ars longa, vita brevis" (the art of medicine is long, life is short).[36] Little did he realize that the biopsy of a tumor on his tongue in the summer of 1889 would prove to be malignant. His carcinoma of the tongue recurred the following year. A huge tumor developed, causing paralysis of the vagus nerve and compression of the esophagus and main bronchus. Kahler died on January 24, 1893, shortly after his 44th birthday.[37] His obituaries and eulogies made no mention of his famous case report, but they noted that he was extremely kind to his patients and was an excellent teacher. It is of interest that the landmark contributions by Henry Bence Jones and Otto Kahler were not recognized during their lifetimes.

Probably the first reported case of multiple myeloma in the United States was published by Herrick and Hektoen.[38] A 40-year-old white woman had lumbar pain and a nodule on the lower end of the sternum. At autopsy, multiple nodules attached to the sternum, right clavicle, and ribs were found. The sternum was thickened, irregular, and covered with tumor masses but was soft and flexible. Multiple nodules were found on the ribs, which bent readily without cracking. Two of the dorsal vertebral bodies were largely replaced by soft tumor masses. Fungoid masses were seen in the skull. Microscopic examination revealed round, lymphoid cells with large nuclei.

In 1898, Weber[39] reported a case of multiple myeloma and stated that radiographs would greatly facilitate the diagnosis of such cases. He concluded, after reporting another case, that Bence Jones protein was produced by the bone marrow. He also believed that the presence of Bence Jones protein was of "fatal significance" and nearly always indicated that the patient had multiple myeloma.[40] Weber and Ledingham[41] later suggested that Bence Jones protein came from the cytoplasmic residua of karyolyzed plasma cells. Geschickter and Copeland[42] presented an analysis of all 425 cases reported since 1848. They called attention to six cardinal features of the disease: multiple involvement by tumors of the skeletal trunk, pathological fracture, Bence Jones protein, back pain, anemia, and chronic renal disease. Sternal aspiration of bone marrow, described by Arinkin,[43] greatly increased the antemortem recognition of multiple myeloma. Rosenthal and Vogel[44] reported that only three cases of multiple myeloma had been recognized at the Mt. Sinai Hospital from 1916 to 1935 but that 13 cases were found in the ensuing 2 1/2 years. They attributed this marked increase in recognition to the use of sternal puncture in patients with obscure anemia or skeletal abnormalities and stated that many cases had been missed in the past. They emphasized that hyperproteinemia, positive formol-gel reaction, Bence Jones proteinuria, and abnormal x-rays suggested the diagnosis, which, they said, should be proven by sternal puncture. Bayrd and Heck[45] described 83 patients with histological proof of multiple myeloma who were seen at the Mayo Clinic through December 1945. The duration of survival ranged from 1 to 84 months (median, 15 months).

The term *plasma cell* was coined by Waldeyer in 1875,[46] but his description is not characteristic of plasma cells, and it is most likely that he described tissue mast cells. Plasma cells were described accurately by Ramón y Cajal in 1890,[47] during study of syphilitic condylomas; he stated that the unstained perinuclear area (hof) contained the Golgi apparatus. In 1891, Unna[48] used the term *plasma cell* while describing cells seen in the skin of patients with lupus erythematosus. However, it is not known whether he actually saw plasma cells. In 1895, Marschalkó[49] outlined the essential characteristics of plasma cells, including blocked chromatin, eccentric position of the nucleus, a perinuclear pale area (hof), and a spherical or irregular cytoplasm. In 1900, Wright[50] described a 54-year-old man with multiple myeloma and pointed out that the tumor consisted of plasma cells. Wright emphasized that the neoplasm originated not from red marrow cells collectively but from only one type of cell, the plasma cell. Interestingly, this patient was probably the first in whom radiographs revealed changes in the ribs, thus contributing to the diagnosis.

Although in 1917 Jacobson[51] had reported Bence Jones protein in the serum, it was not until 1928 that Perlzweig et al.[52] reported hyperproteinemia when they described a patient with multiple myeloma who had 9 to 11 g of globulin in his serum. The patient also had Bence Jones proteinuria and probably a small amount of Bence Jones protein in the plasma. Perlzweig and co-workers noted that it was almost impossible to obtain serum from the clotted blood because the clot failed to retract, even on prolonged centrifugation. Cryoglobulinemia was recognized by Wintrobe and Buell in 1933[53] and named *cryoglobulin* by Lerner and Watson in 1947.[54] Lerner and Watson's patient had been previously reported as a case of allergic purpura with hypersensitivity to cold.[55] In 1938, von Bonsdorff et al.[56] described a patient with cryoglobulinemia in which the globulins crystallized after exposure to the cold for 24 hours.

Tiselius's[57] studies of the moving boundary method of electrophoresis led to his doctoral dissertation in 1930. His manuscript describing the apparatus for electrophoresis[57] was not accepted in the chemical publication to which it was sent first because it was too "physical"; and it was subsequently published in the *Transactions of the Faraday Society*.[58] Later that same year, Tiselius described the separation of serum globulins into three components, which he designated α, β, and γ.[59] Two years later, Tiselius and Kabat[60] localized antibody activity to the γ-globulin fraction of the plasma proteins. They noted that antibodies to albumin or *Pneumococcus* type I were found in the area of γ-mobility in rabbit serum, and antibodies to pneumococcal organisms migrated between β and γ in horse serum. Later it was recognized that some antibodies migrate in the fast γ-region and others in the slow and that some sediment in the ultracentrifuge as 7S and others as 19S molecules. The concept of a family of proteins with antibody activity was not proposed until late in the 1950s.[61] Before 1960, the term γ-*globulin* was used for any protein that migrated in the γ-mobility region of the electrophoretic pattern. Now these γ-globulins are referred to as immunoglobulins—IgG, IgA, IgM, IgD, and IgE. Tiselius's moving-boundary electrophoresis apparatus using a U tube soon became commercially available at a cost of $5,000. A. J. Cohn from Harvard University ordered an instrument built in the Uppsala workshop.

In 1939, Longsworth et al.[62] applied electrophoresis to the study of multiple myeloma and demonstrated the tall, narrow-based "church spire" peak. This method was cumbersome and difficult; therefore, it was not readily available until the early 1950s, when filter paper was introduced as a supporting medium (zone electrophoresis). Cellulose acetate has since supplanted filter paper.[63] In 1953, Grabar and Williams[64] described immunoelectrophoresis, which has facilitated the diagnosis of multiple myeloma.

Immunofixation or direct immunoelectrophoresis was reported by Wilson in 1964,[65] when he applied antisera on the surface of the agar immediately after completion of electrophoresis. Immunofixation is useful when the results of immunoelectrophoresis are equivocal.[66] Immunofixation is also helpful in the recognition of small monoclonal light chains when none are found with immunoelectrophoresis.[67] When combined with immunofixation, high-resolution agarose gel electrophoresis is more sensitive than immunoelectrophoresis in detecting small monoclonal proteins.[68]

Monoclonal proteins were considered abnormal because of their homogeneity, which is seen as a localized band or narrow spike with electrophoresis. Kunkel believed that monoclonal proteins were a product of malignant plasma cells and were the equivalent of normal antibodies produced by normal plasma cells. Thus, monoclonal proteins were said to be representative of a heterogeneous population of gamma globulins. He showed that each heavy chain subclass and light chain type in monoclonal proteins had its counterpart among normal immunoglobulins and also among antibodies. After the discovery of the two types of light chains, kappa and lambda, in monoclonal proteins in a ratio of approximately 2:1, the same light chains were detected in essentially the same ratio among normal immunoglobulins. Similarly, the IgG and IgA subclasses and the IgD class were discovered among myeloma proteins and were then found as normal serum components.[69] Even the antigenic determinants ("idiotypic specificities" or "individual antigenics specificities") that are associated with the binding sites were believed to be associated uniquely with myeloma proteins but have been shown to occur among antibodies.[70]

The concept of monoclonal versus polyclonal gammopathies was lucidly presented in the Harvey Lecture series by Waldenström.[71] He clearly described patients with a narrow band of hypergammaglobulinemia as having a monoclonal protein. Although many of these patients had multiple myeloma, others had no evidence of malignancy and were considered as having "essential hypergammaglobulinemia" or benign monoclonal gammopathy. Most physicians now use the term "monoclonal gammopathy of undetermined significance"[72] because in some of these patients multiple myeloma, macroglobulinemia, or a related disorder will eventually develop.[73] Waldenström further correctly regarded the broad band in hypergammaglobulinemia as a polyclonal increase in proteins. This simple distinction is extremely important clinically because patients with a monoclonal gammopathy already have or may develop a neoplastic process, whereas patients with a polyclonal gammopathy have an inflammatory or reactive cause of their hypergammaglobulinemia.[71,74] In 1947, Alwall[75] reported that a patient with typical multiple myeloma had a reduction in globulin from 5.9 to 2.2 g/dl, an increase in hemoglobin from 60 to 87 percent, disappearance of proteinuria, and a reduction in bone marrow plasma cells from 33 to 0 percent when treated with urethane. For almost 20 years, urethane was commonly used for the treatment of myeloma. Holland et al.[76] randomized 83 patients with treated or untreated multiple myeloma to receive urethane or a placebo consisting of cherry- and cola-flavored syrup. No difference was seen in objective improvement or survival of the two treatment groups. In fact, the urethane-treated patients died earlier on the average than those treated with placebo. This difference was ascribed to the increased mortality of urethane-treated patients who were azotemic. The patients with poorer prognostic features had a significantly shorter survival with urethane therapy.

In 1958, Blokhin et al.[77] reported benefit in three of six patients with multiple myeloma who were treated with sarcolysin. Four years later, Bergsagel et al.[78] found significant improvement in 8 of 24 patients with multiple myeloma who were treated with DL-phenylalanine mustard (melphalan, Alkeran). Six other patients obtained improvement in one or more objective factors. In another report, cyclophosphamide-treated patients with myeloma had a median survival of 24.5 months, whereas an ancillary myeloma group had a median survival of 9.5 months.[79] Objective improvement occurred in 81 of 207 patients. Various combinations of alkylating agents have been used for the treatment of multiple myeloma, but no unequivocal evidence shows that they are superior to melphalan and prednisone.[80,81]

ACKNOWLEDGMENT

This work was supported in part by research grant CA-62242 from the National Institutes of Health, U.S. Public Health Service, and by the Toor Myeloma Research Fund.

REFERENCES

1. Bence Jones H: Chemical pathology. Lancet 2:88, 1847.
2. Clamp JR: Some aspects of the first recorded case of multiple myeloma. Lancet 2:1354, 1967.
3. Macintyre W: Case of mollities and fragilitas ossium, accompanied with urine strongly charged with animal matter. Med Chir Trans Lond 33:211, 1850.
4. Dalrymple J: On the microscopical character of mollities ossium. Dublin Q J Med Sci 2:85, 1846.
5. Morse D, Dailey RC, Bunn J: Prehistoric multiple myeloma. Bull N Y Acad Med 50:447, 1974.
6. Solly S: Remarks on the pathology of mollities ossium with cases. Med Chir Trans Lond 27:435, 1844.
7. Bence Jones H: On the new substance occurring in the urine of a patient with mollities ossium. Philos Trans R Soc Lond Biol 55, 1848.
8. Putnam FW: Henry Bence Jones: The best chemical doctor in London. Perspect Biol Med 36:565, 1993.
9. Bence Jones H: An Autobiography (with elucidations at later dates by his son, A.B. Bence-Jones). Crusha & Sons, Ltd. (privately printed), London, 1929.
10. Coley NG: Henry Bence-Jones, M.D., F.R.S. (1813–1873). Notes Rec R Soc Lond 28:31, 1973.
11. Obituary: Henry Bence Jones, M.D., M.A., F.R.C.P., F.R.S. Med Times Gaz 1:505, 1873.
12. Rosenbloom J: An appreciation of Henry Bence Jones, M.D., F.R.S. (1814–1873). Ann Med Hist 2:262, 1919.
13. Bence Jones H: On a deposit of crystallized xanthin in human urine. J Chem Soc Lond 15:78, 1862.
14. Bence Jones H: On intermitting diabetes, and on the diabetes of old age. Med Chir Trans Lond 36:403, 1853.
15. Obituary: Dr. Henry Bence Jones. Lancet 1:614, 1873.
16. Bence Jones H, Dupré A: On a fluorescent substance, resembling quinine, in animals; and on the rate of passage of quinine into the vascular and nonvascular textures of the body. Proc R Soc Lond [Biol] 15:73, 1866.
17. Rosenfeld L: Henry Bence Jones (1813–1873): The best "chemical doctor" in London. Clin Chem 33:1687, 1987.
18. Heller JF: Die mikroskopisch-chemisch-pathologische untersuchung. p. 576. In von Gaal G (ed.): Physikalische Diagnostik und Deren Anwendung in der Medicin, Chirurgie, Oculistik Otiatrik und Geburtshilfe, enthaltend: Inspection, Mensuration, Palpation, Percussion und Auscultation, Nebst Einer Kurzen Diagnose der Krankheiten der Athmungs und Kreislaufsorgane. Braumüller and Seidel, Vienna, 1846.
19. Fleischer R: XXIV. Ueber das Vorkommen des sogenannten Bence Jones' schen Eiweisskörpers im normalen Knochenmark. Arch Pathol Anat Physiol Klin Med 80:482, 1880.
20. Kühne W: Ueber Hemialbumose im Harn. Z Biol 19:209, 1883.
21. Huppert: Ein Fall von Albumosurie. Prager Med Wochenschr XIV:35, 1889.
22. Bradshaw TR: A case of albumosuria in which the albumose was spontaneously precipitated. Med Chir Trans Lond 63:259, 1898.
23. Walters W: Bence-Jones proteinuria: A report of three cases with metabolic studies. JAMA 76:641, 1921.
24. Bayne-Jones S, Wilson DW: Immunological reactions of Bence-Jones proteins. II. Differences between Bence-Jones proteins from various sources. Bull Johns Hopkins Hosp 33:119, 1922.
25. Korngold L, Lipari R: Multiple-myeloma proteins. III. The antigenic relationship of Bence Jones proteins to normal gamma-globulin and multiple-myeloma serum proteins. Cancer 9:262, 1956.
26. Putnam FW, Hardy S: Proteins in multiple myeloma. III. Origin of Bence-Jones protein. J Biol Chem 212:361, 1955.
27. Edelman GM, Gally JA: The nature of Bence-Jones proteins: Chemical similarities to polypeptide chains of myeloma globulins and normal γ-globulins. J Exp Med 116:207, 1962.
28. Hilschmann N, Craig LC: Amino acid sequence studies with Bence Jones proteins. Proc Natl Acad Sci USA 53:1403, 1965.
29. Titani K, Whitley E Jr, Putnam FW: Immunoglobulin structure: Variation in the sequence of Bence Jones proteins. Science 152:1513, 1966.
30. Weber H: Mollities ossium, doubtful whether carcinomatous or syphilitic. Trans Pathol Soc Lond 18:206, 1867.
31. Adams W: Mollities ossium. Trans Pathol Soc Lond 23:186, 1872.
32. von Rustizky J: Multiples myelom. Dtsch Z Chir 3:162, 1873.
33. Kahler O: Zur Symptomatologii des multiplen Myleoms; Beobachtung von Albumosurie. Prag Med Wochenschr 14:45, 1889.
34. Coats J: A case of multiple sarcoma of bone. Glasgow Med J 36:420, 1891.
35. Kraus F: Gedächtnisrede auf Otto Kahler. Wien Klin Wochenschr 27:771, 1904.
36. Sigmund: Zur örtlichen Behandlung: syphilitischer Mund-, Nasen- und Rachenaffektionen. Wien Med Wochenschr 20:781, 1870.
37. Nothnagel: Hofrath Otto Kahler. Wien Klin Wochenschr 6:79, 1893.
38. Herrick JB, Hektoen L: Myeloma: Report of a case. Med News 65:239, 1894.
39. Weber FP: General lymphadenomatosis of bones, one form of "multiple myeloma." J Pathol 5:59, 1898.

40. Weber FP, Hutchison R, Macleod JJR: Multiple myeloma (myelomatosis), with Bence-Jones protein in the urine: (myelopathic albumosuria of Bradshaw, Kahler's disease). Am J Med Sci 126:644, 1903.

41. Weber FP, Ledingham JCG: A note on the histology of a case of myelomatosis (multiple myeloma) with Bence-Jones protein in the urine (myelopathic albumosuria). Proc R Soc Med 2:193, 1909.

42. Geschickter CF, Copeland MM: Multiple myeloma. Arch Surg 16:807, 1928.

43. Arinkin MI: Die intravitale Untersuchungs-methodik des Knochenmarks. Folia Haematol (Leipz) 38:233, 1929.

44. Rosenthal N, Vogel P: Value of the sternal puncture in the diagnosis of multiple myeloma. Mt Sinai J Med (NY) 4:1001, 1938.

45. Bayrd ED, Heck FJ: Multiple myeloma: a review of eighty-three proved cases. JAMA 133:147, 1947.

46. Waldeyer W: Ueber Bindegewebszellen. Arch Mikr Anat 11:176, 1875.

47. Ramón y Cajal S: Estudios histológicos sobre los tumores epiteliales. Rev Trimest Microgr 1:83, 1896.

48. Unna PG: Über plasmazellen, insbesondere beim Lupus. Monatsschr Prakt Dermatol 12:296, 1891.

49. MarschalKó T: Ueber die sogenannten Plasmazellen, ein Beitrag zur Kenntniss der Herkunft der entzündlichen Infiltrationszellen. Arch Dermatolsyph Syph 30:241, 1895.

50. Wright JH: A case of multiple myeloma. Johns Hopkins Hosp Rep 9:359, 1900.

51. Jacobson VC: A case of multiple myelomata with chronic nephritis showing Bence-Jones protein in urine and blood serum. J Urol 1:167, 1917.

52. Perlzweig WA, Delrue G, Geschickter C: Hyperproteinemia associated with multiple myelomas: report of an unusual case. JAMA 90:755, 1928.

53. Wintrobe MM, Buell MV: Hyperproteinemia associated with multiple myeloma: with report of a case in which an extraordinary hyperproteinemia was associated with thrombosis of the retinal veins and symptoms suggesting Raynaud's disease. Bull Johns Hopkins Hosp 52:156, 1933.

54. Lerner AB, Watson CJ: Studies of cryoglobulins. I, Unusual purpura associated with the presence of a high concentration of cryoglobulin (cold precipitable serum globulin). Am J Med Sci 214:410, 1947.

55. Peters GA, Horton BT: Allergic purpura with special reference to hypersensitiveness to cold. Mayo Clin Proc 16:631, 1941.

56. von Bonsdorff B, Groth H, Packalén T: On the presence of a high-molecular crystallizable protein in the blood serum in myeloma. Folia Haematol (Leipz) 59:184, 1938.

57. Tiselius A: Reflections from both sides of the counter. Annu Rev Biochem 37:1, 1968.

58. Tiselius A: A new apparatus for electrophoretic analysis of colloidal mixtures. Trans Faraday Soc 33:524, 1937.

59. Tiselius A: Electrophoresis of serum globulin. II. Electrophoretic analysis of normal and immune sera. Biochem J 31:1464, 1937.

60. Tiselius A, Kabat EA: An electrophoretic study of immune sera and purified antibody preparations. J Exp Med 69:119, 1939.

61. Heremans JF: Immunochemical studies on protein pathology: the immunoglobulin concept. Clin Chim Acta 4:639, 1959.

62. Longsworth LG, Shedlovsky T, MacInnes DA: Electrophoretic patterns of normal and pathological human blood serum and plasma. J Exp Med 70:399, 1939.

63. Kohn J: A cellulose acetate supporting medium for zone electrophoresis. Clin Chim Acta 2:297, 1957.

64. Grabar P, Williams CA: Méthode permettant l'étude conjuguée des propriétés électrophorétiques et immunochimiques d'um mélange de protéines. Application au sérum sanguin. Biochim Biophys Acta 10:193, 1953.

65. Wilson AT: Direct immunoelectrophoresis. J Immunol 92:431, 1964.

66. Ritchie RF, Smith R: Immunofixation. III. Application to the study of monoclonal proteins. Clin Chem 22:1982, 1976.

67. Whicher JT, Hawkins L, Higginson J: Clinical applications of immunofixation: a more sensitive technique for the detection of Bence Jones protein. J Clin Pathol 33:779, 1980.

68. Reichert CM, Everett DF Jr, Nadler PI, Papadopoulos NM: High-resolution zone electrophoresis, combined with immunofixation, in the detection of an occult myeloma paraprotein. Clin Chem 28:2312, 1982.

69. Kunkel HG: The "abnormality" of myeloma proteins. Cancer Res 28:1351, 1968.

70. Natvig JB, Kunkel HG: Human immunoglobulins: Classes, subclasses, genetic variants, and idiotypes. Adv Immunol 16:1, 1973.

71. Waldenström J: Studies on conditions associated with disturbed gamma globulin formation (gammopathies). Harvey Lect 56:211, 1961.

72. Kyle RA: Monoclonal gammopathy of undetermined significance. Natural history of 241 cases. Am J Med 64:814, 1978.

73. Kyle RA: 'Benign' monoclonal gammopathy—after 20 to 35 years of follow-up. Mayo Clin Proc 68:26, 1993.

74. Kyle RA: Multiple myeloma: An odyssey of discovery. Br J Haematol 110:1, 2000.

75. Alwall N: Urethane and stilbamidine in multiple myeloma: Report on two cases. Lancet 2:388, 1947.

76. Holland JF, Hosley H, Scharlau C et al: A controlled trial of urethane treatment in multiple myeloma. Blood 27:328, 1966.

77. Blokhin N, Larionov L, Perevodchikova N et al: Clinical experiences with sarcolysin in neoplastic diseases. Ann NY Acad Sci 68:1128, 1958.

78. Bergsagel DE, Sprague CC, Austin C et al: Evaluation of new chemotherapeutic agents in the treatment of multiple myeloma. IV. L-Phenylalanine mustard (NSC-8806), Cancer Chemother Rep 21:87, 1962.

79. Korst DR, Clifford GO, Fowler WM et al: Multiple myeloma. II. Analysis of cyclophosphamide therapy in 165 patients. JAMA 189:758, 1964.

80. Gregory WM, Richards MA, Malpas JS: Combination chemotherapy versus melphalan and prednisolone in the treatment of multiple myeloma: An overview of published trials. J Clin Oncol 10:334, 1992.

81. Myeloma Trialists' Collaborative Group: Combination chemotherapy versus melphalan plus prednisone as treatment for multiple myeloma: An overview of 6633 patients from 27 randomized trials. J Clin Oncol 16:3832, 1998.

25

Cytokines and Signal Transduction in Multiple Myeloma

Dharminder Chauhan and Kenneth C. Anderson

Multiple myeloma (MM) is a hematological malignancy that will affect 13,700 new individuals in the United States in 2000[1] and account for 2 percent of cancer-related deaths. Despite conventional and high-dose therapies, it remains incurable with a median survival of 3 to 4 years. Novel biologically based treatment approaches to this disease are therefore urgently needed that target mechanisms regulating MM cell growth, survival, and apoptosis.

In MM, tumor cells predominate in the bone marrow (BM) microenvironment due to binding via adhesion molecules on MM cells to both extracellular matrix proteins and bone marrow stromal cells (BMSCs). The interaction between tumor cells and BMSCs not only localizes tumor cells in the BM, but also confers protection against apoptosis and triggers secretion of cytokines mediating autocrine[2,3] and paracrine[4,5] growth and survival of MM cells. Trigger via CD40 on the MM cell surface induces autocrine interleukin (IL)-6-mediated tumor cell growth.[2] In addition, adherence of tumor cells to BMSCs augments paracrine MM cell growth by up-regulating IL-6 transcription and secretion within BMSCs[4,5] and allowing for secretion of cytokines by tumor cells (i.e., transforming growth factor-β), which further enhance IL-6 transcription and secretion in BMSCs.[5,6] This is of central importance since IL-6 is a major growth and survival factor for MM cells, which triggers in vitro proliferation of MM cells and confers resistance to Dex-induced apoptosis.[7–9] Moreover, high serum levels of IL-6 in MM patients can also contribute to chemoresistance.[10] Therefore defining the signaling pathways mediating growth and survival of MM cells may derive new and effective treatment strategies based on targeting novel apoptotic and anti-apoptotic proteins. This chapter focuses on cytokines present within the BM millieu and related signal transduction pathways mediating MM cell growth and survival.

GROWTH AND SURVIVAL SIGNALING PATHWAYS

Cell growth and apoptosis are essential and yet opposing cellular processes, and cross-talk between these signaling pathways regulating growth and survival determines the ultimate fate of the tumor cell. IL-6 is the major growth and survival factor in MM cells, and IL-6-induced signaling pathways are well delin-

eated.[11–15] IL-6 binds to its receptor (IL-6R/gp80), which interacts with the signal transducer gp130. Tyrosine kinases of Janus family JAK1, JAK2, and Tyk2 are constitutively associated with the cytoplasmic domain of gp130. Upon ligand binding, JAK1 and JAK2 are activated by autophosphorylation and further phosphorylate certain tyrosine motifs within the cytoplasmic domain of gp130. These phosphotyrosine motifs represent recruitment sites for protein tyrosine phosphatase SHP2, also known as SH-PTP2,[16,17] as well as transcription factors STAT-1 and STAT-3. After activation, STATs either form homodimers or heterodimers and rapidly translocate to the nucleus where they bind to IL-6 response elements on the promoter of IL-6-induced genes (e.g., acute-phase protein genes). Finally, IL-6 also triggers the Ras-dependent mitogen-activated protein kinase (MAPK) cascade, with sequential activation of Shp2→Grb2→ Sos1→ Ras→ Raf→ MEK→ MAPK. Activation of this cascade leads to activation of transcription factors, such as NF-κB, NF-IL6, and AP-1 complex (Jun/Fos).[12–15] We have demonstrated that IL-6-induced proliferation of MM cells is mediated via the MAPK cascade.[14,15]

Some therapies in MM exert their effects, at least in part, via disruption of the IL-6-dependent MM cell growth pathway. For example, interferon-γ and all-*trans* retinoic acid (ATRA) have been reported to inhibit MM cell growth by down-regulating IL-6R and gp130.[18–21] Our studies have shown that dexamethasone (Dex) induces up-regulation of p21 and growth arrest,[22] as well as down-regulation of growth-related kinases including MAPK and p70^{RSK}.[8,23] Activation of MAPK is a relatively late event during IL-6 signaling, and upstream gp130-associated kinases, such as members of Janus family of kinases (JAK1, JAK2, or JAK3) and STAT family of proteins (STAT-1 and STAT-3) have therefore been examined as potential therapeutic targets. For example, overexpression of dominant negative forms of JAK2 and JAK1 represses signaling via gp130.[11] Alternatively, inhibitory peptides against JAK2 decrease tumor cell growth in acute lymphocytic leukemia and chronic myelocytic leukemia murine models.[24,25] In a similar approach, STAT activation can be inhibited either by using anti-sense oligonucleotides or small inhibitory molecules against STAT.[26,27] For example, blocking STAT-3 using the JAK inhibitor AG490 enhances sensitivity to Fas-mediated apoptosis of an IL-6 dependent MM cell line.[28] Finally, using dominant negative STATs that lack a binding domain but are able to form dimers with endogenous STATs suppresses STAT function and decreases tumor cell growth.[29] Although this dominant negative approach has been useful in delineating the importance of STAT signaling in vitro, it is probably too cumbersome for the clinical setting. In addition, the toxic effects of interfering with this pathway may preclude this approach, since STAT family members regulate many genes controlling normal cellular functions. For example, animals that lack STAT-3 die early in embryogenesis, making it difficult to predict the effects of STAT-3 inhibition after development is completed.[30] Figure 25–1 summarizes the IL-6-dependent MM cell growth signaling cascade and potential targets for novel therapeutics.

Although multiple studies have provided evidence for the role of IL-6 in the growth and survival of MM cells, some tumor

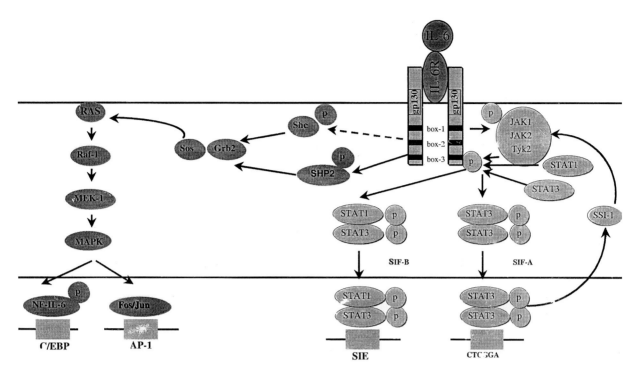

Figure 25–1. IL-6-induced growth signaling cascade in MM cells.

cells grow in an IL-6-independent fashion. There may be genetic abnormalities underlying this growth mechanism, such as Ras mutations; abnormalities of cell cycle regulatory proteins, such as retinoblastoma (Rb), p16, and p21; and intrinsic activation of signaling cascades.[14,15,22,31–34] For example, a lack of Sos-1 activation is associated with the loss of IL-6 responsiveness in MM cells that can grow independently of IL-6.[15]

Role of IL-6 as an Anti-Apoptotic Factor

IL-6 is not only a growth factor, but also an anti-apoptotic agent in MM cells.[8,35,36] Apoptosis of MM cells induced by Fas and γ-irradiation (IR) is associated with activation of various serine/threonine kinases, such as stress-activated protein kinase (SAPK) or c-Jun-N-terminal kinase (JNK) and p38 kinase (Figure 25–2). Retinoblastoma (Rb) protein is one of the downstream targets of SAPK, which suggests that Rb is involved in IR-induced apoptosis.[23] Although IL-6 does not rescue MM cells from IR-induced apoptosis, it protects MM cells against Fas-induced apoptosis via inhibition of the JNK/SAPK pathway.[35,37] Dex-induced apoptosis is not associated with JNK/SAPK and p38 stress kinase activation, but rather is associated with decreased activity of growth-related kinases, such as MAPK and p70^{RSK}.[8] Importantly, IL-6 inhibits both apoptosis and the down-regulation of MAPK triggered by Dex in MM cells.[8]

The induction of apoptosis by various stimuli is associated with activation of downstream effector cysteine proteases (caspases) and cleavage of poly (ADP ribose) polymerase (PARP),[38] DNA-PK,[39] protein kinase C delta (PKC-δ),[40] and other substrates. Caspases are functionally interconnected, since upstream (initiator) caspases cleave and activate downstream (effector) caspases. Activation of other members of the caspase family, in particular CPP32, is a well-characterized biochemical hallmark of apoptosis. In MM cells, we recently demonstrated that three distinct stress agents (i.e., Dex, IR, and Fas), induce cleavage and activation of caspase-3.[8] Therefore, although the upstream signaling pathway for each of these stress agents is distinct, all these pathways converge at the level of caspases (Figure 25–2).

Recent studies have shown that mitochondria play an important role in apoptosis,[41] since various cell death inducers cause a disruption in mitochondrial membrane potential that precedes either apoptosis or cytolysis; and conversely, drugs that stabilize mitochondrial membranes can prevent apoptosis. For example, cyclosporin-A both inhibits mitochondrial membrane permeability and blocks the CD-437-induced apoptosis in MM cells.[42] Importantly, the release of mitochondrial cytochrome-c (cyto-c) apoptogenic protein mediates apoptosis,[43–45] since addition of exogenous cyto-C to cytosolic preparations from growing cells both activates caspases and also induces DNA fragmentation in isolated nuclei.[43] A novel retinoid CD437/AHPN, a retinoic acid receptor (RAR) gamma activator, induces apoptosis in MM cells that involves mitochondria but is independent of the nucleus. Our studies have demonstrated that IR-induced apoptosis of human MM cell lines and patient MM cells, but not apoptosis of these cells triggered by Dex or Fas, is associated with accumulation of cytosolic cyto-C. These data indicate that there are at least two distinct apoptotic signaling cascades in MM cells: one triggered by IR and associated with the release of cyto-C from mitochondria; and another which is independent of cyto-C and triggered by Dex and Fas (Figure 25–2).

Since Dex is a commonly used therapy for MM, our recent studies have attempted to identify proteins mediating Dex-

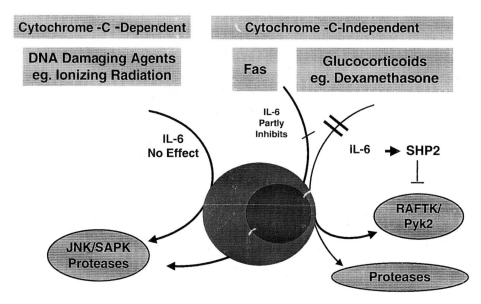

Figure 25–2. Apoptotic and anti-apoptotic signaling cascades in MM cells.

induced apoptosis, as well as mechanisms of resistance to Dex. We demonstrated that Dex-induced apoptosis, in contrast to apoptosis triggered by Fas or IR, is associated with tyrosine phosphorylation and kinase activity of related adhesion focal tyrosine kinase (RAFTK), also known as proline rich tyrosine kinase (Pyk2).[46,47] RAFTK/Pyk2 is a member of the focal adhesion kinase (FAK) subfamily and is activated by tumor necrosis factor (TNF)-α, UV light, and increased intracellular calcium levels. Overexpression of RAFTK in both fibroblastic and epithelial cell lines leads to apoptosis.[48] Our study demonstrates that RAFTK is activated by Dex in MM cells undergoing apoptosis; conversely, Dex failed to activate RAFTK in MM cells that are Dex resistant.[49] Overexpression of wild-type RAFTK in MM cells leads to apoptosis, whereas transient transfection of dominant negative RAFTK blocks apoptosis triggered by Dex, without affecting the apoptotic response to either IR or Fas. These data suggest that Dex-triggered apoptosis is dependent on RAFTK activation, and that induction of apoptosis in response to diverse stress agents can de distinguished by RAFTK-dependent and RAFTK-independent mechanisms. Finally, our results further demonstrate that IL-6, a survival factor for MM cells, inhibits Dex-induced activation of RAFTK and apoptosis. Taken together, these findings demonstrate that apoptotic stimuli utilize two distinct signaling pathways: one pathway is induced by Dex, RAFTK dependent, cytochrome C independent, and inhibited by IL-6; and the other is induced by IR and anti-Fas, RAFTK independent, associated with cytochrome C release, and unaffected by IL-6[49] (Figure 25–2).

The molecular mechanisms by which IL-6 inhibits Dex-induced apoptosis are undefined. IL-6 binds to its receptor (IL-6R/gp80), which interacts with the signal transducer gp130. The cytoplasmic domain of gp130 contains phosphotyrosine motifs for recruitment of a protein tyrosine phosphatase SHP2, also referred to as SH-PTP2.[17,50] SHP2 is widely expressed and is required as a positive (i.e., signal enhancing) component of

growth factor and cytokine signal transduction pathways.[51–53] For example, we and others have demonstrated that IL-6 triggers proliferation of MM cells via the MAPK cascade, which includes SHP2 activation.[14] Moreover, fibroblasts from SHP2 mutant mice exhibit impaired MAPK activation in response to fibroblast growth factor, epidermal growth factor, and insulin-like growth factor.[54,55] Although SHP2 may directly bind and dephosphorylate cytokine receptors or other cytoplasmic protein tyrosine kinases,[50,52,56] its role in regulating apoptotic signaling is at present undefined.

Our recent study suggests that SHP2 mediates the protective effects of IL-6 against Dex-induced apoptosis in MM cells.[57] Specifically, IL-6 activates SHP2 in MM cells, and treatment of MM cells with IL-6 and Dex induces binding of activated SHP2 with RAFTK, resulting in dephosphorylation of RAFTK (Figure 25–3). Importantly, we show that RAFTK is a substrate of SHP2, both in vitro and in vivo. Overexpression of dominant negative SHP2 abrogates the protective effect of IL-6 against Dex-induced apoptosis. Taken together, these findings demonstrate that SHP2 mediates the protective effect of IL-6 against Dex-induced apoptosis in MM cells and further identify both RAFTK/Pyk2 and SHP2 as novel therapeutic targets in MM.

Additional therapeutic targets have been identified in MM cells. For example, constitutive activation of STAT-3 confers resistance to apoptosis in human U266 MM cells,[58] whereas inhibiting its activity can induce apoptosis. A recent report that MM cells selected for resistance to Fas-mediated apoptosis show lack of cross-resistance to cytotoxic drugs both provides evidence for independent mechanisms of caspase activation,[59] and suggests the potential clinical utility of inhibiting survival signaling cascades. Further characterization of growth and survival pathways may therefore provide the framework for treatments based on either the triggering of apoptosis or inhibiting survival signals in tumor cells.

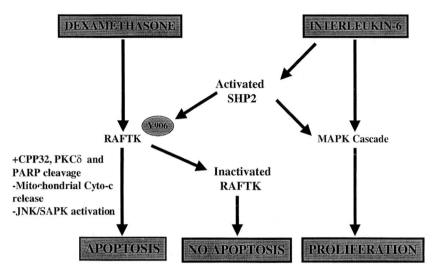

Figure 25–3. SHP2 mediates the protective effect of IL-6 against Dex-induced apoptosis.

Interleukin-6 and Cell Cycle Proteins

Abnormalities in cell cycle regulatory proteins also contribute to MM cell growth. For example, mutations in *RB* gene or abnormalities in RB protein (pRB) have been noted in up to 70 percent of MM patients and 80 percent of MM patient derived cell lines. Both dephosphorylated and phosphorylated pRB are present in MM cells, and the latter predominates.[33] IL-6 further shifts pRB from its dephosphorylated to its phosphorylated form in responsive MM cells, thereby promoting tumor cell growth via two mechanisms: first, by decreasing binding of dephosphorylated pRB to E2F and releasing G1 growth arrest; and second, by up-regulating IL-6 secretion by MM cells and IL-6 mediated autocrine tumor cell growth. Abnormalities in other cell cycle associated proteins also underlie abnormalities in MM cell growth regulation. For example, with progression to PCL, loss of p16 protein is observed due to transcriptional inactivation of *p16* gene by methylation in PCL cells.[34,60] In addition, p21 protein is constitutively expressed in the majority of MM cells independent of the status of p53. Its expression is up-regulated by Dex and down-regulated by IL-6, which also inhibits the increase in p21 triggered by Dex.[22] Furthermore, Dex induces G1 growth arrest in MM cells, whereas IL-6 facilitates G1 to S phase transition and blocks the effect of Dex. The correlation of changes in p21 expression and cell cycle implicates p21 in the coupling of Dex and IL-6 related signals to cell cycle regulation in MM. Finally, murine double minute two (MDM2) is constitutively expressed in MM cells and may enhance cell cycle progression in tumor cells both by activating E2F-1 and by down-regulating wild-type p53 and p21.[32] Overexpression of MDM2 in MM may therefore contribute to both growth and survival of tumor cells, suggesting the potential utility of therapeutic strategies targeting MDM2 in MM.

At present there is also considerable evidence supporting a role for IL-6 in the growth and manifestations of MM in vivo. Elevated IL-6 serum levels in some studies correlate with poor prognosis and higher tumor cell mass.[10,61] In addition, patients with monoclonal gammopathy of undetermined significance (MGUS), indo-

lent MM, or smoldering MM have serum IL-6 levels similar to healthy individuals, in contrast to those patients with fulminating MM or PCL, who have the highest IL-6 levels. Direct measurement of serum IL-6 levels, or of C-reactive protein as a surrogate marker synthesized in the liver in response to IL-6, may also be a prognostic factor in MM.[10] IL-6 serves as an osteoclast activating factor in MM bone disease.[62] Finally, IL-6 transgenic mice develop histopathological changes characteristic of MM kidney.[63]

Several studies suggest potential therapeutic utility of inhibiting IL-6 in MM. Anti-IL-6 monoclonal antibody (m Ab) therapy can transiently reverse disease manifestations in patients with MM,[64] further confirming its in vivo significance in MM. Anti-humanized IL-6R and gp130 antibodies inhibit the growth of IL-6-dependent plasmacytoma cells in vivo.[20] IL-6 fused to pseudomonas exotoxin or diphtheria toxin effectively and selectively kills MM cell lines.[65,66] IL-6 receptor superantagonists, which bind IL-6 but do not trigger via gp 130, block IL-6-dependent MM cell growth.[67–69] Finally, Dex has been shown to inhibit IL-6 and IL-6 receptor gene expression, consistent with another possible mechanism for inhibition of tumor cell growth by corticosteroids.[70] Bisphosphonates may also inhibit IL-6 production from MM BMSCs.[68]

Transforming Growth Factor β

Transforming growth factor β (TGF-β) is secreted by MM cells and can trigger IL-6 production by BMSCs,[6] further augmenting paracrine MM cell growth. TGF-β secreted by MM cells also contributes to the immunodeficiency characteristic of MM by down-regulating B cells, T cells, and natural killer cells, without similarly inhibiting the growth of MM cells themselves.

Interleukin-1

Recombinant IL-1-alpha (α) stimulates MM cells to produce IL-6, which consequently augments proliferation of MM cells.[71] IL-1β mRNA is found within MM cells, and IL-1β mediates bone-resorbing activity in MM.[72] These data suggest a possible

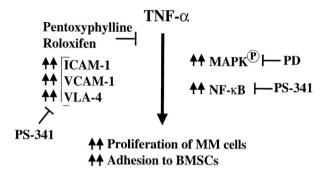

Figure 25–4. TNF-α-induced signaling cascade in MM cells.

therapeutic strategy for IL-1β antagonists in the treatment of lytic bone disease in MM. Serum levels of IL-1β, as well as IL-6, were found to be chronically elevated in patients with polyneuropathy, organomegaly, endocrinopathy, monoclonal protein, and skin changes (POEMS syndrome), consistent with the view that these cytokines may mediate systemic manifestations of this disease.[73] Most recently, it has been suggested that IL-1β present in MGUS cells may identify those patients likely to progress to MM.[74]

Role of TNF-α in the Pathophysiology of MM

The role of TNF-α in the pathophysiology of MM is unclear. We have examined the activity of TNF-α on human MM cell growth and survival[75] (Figure 25–4). TNF-α triggered a modest increment in proliferation, associated with p44/p42 MAPK signaling, in MM cells. The TNF inhibitors pentoxiphylline and roloxifen blocked this increment in proliferation of MM cells, without altering baseline tumor cell growth. Importantly, TNF-α induced ICAM-1, VCAM-1, and MUC-1, but not LFA-1 or VLA-4, expression on human MM cells. Although TNF-α had no effect on proliferation of BMSCs, it also increased VCAM-1 and ICAM-1 expression on BMSCs. Importantly, percent specific binding of MM cells to BMSCs pretreated with TNF-α was two- to fourfold higher than that to nontreated BMSCs; conversely, pretreatment of MM cells with TNF-α similarly augmented their adhesion to BMSCs. This increased adhesion triggered by TNF-α was blocked by Abs to ICAM-1, VCAM-1, and VLA-4. TNF-α also activated NF-κB in MM cells and BMSCs. Importantly, pretreatment of either MM cells or BMSCs with the proteasome inhibitor PS-341 completely abrogates TNF-induced NF-κB activation, induction of ICAM-1 and VCAM-1 on BMSCs, and increased MM cell to BMSC adhesion. Although our data therefore demonstrate only a modest direct effect of TNF-α on MM cell growth, they illustrate the importance of studying MM cell interactions in the BM milieu.[75] Agents that act to inhibit TNF-α may therefore abrogate paracrine tumor cell growth and the survival advantage conferred by MM cell adhesion in the BM microenvironment.

Other Growth Factors

Peripheral blood mononuclear cells isolated from patients with MM cultured with IL-3 and IL-6 for 6 days in vitro give rise to a population of proliferating B cell blasts that differentiate into idiotypic cytoplasmic Ig+ plasma cells.[76] However, the clinical importance of IL-3 in MM remains to be defined. Several reports suggest that the bone-resorbing activity produced by cultured human MM cells can be mostly blocked by neutralizing antibodies to lymphotoxin,[77] suggesting that this factor may be involved in bone disease in vivo. IL-4 inhibits the growth of MM cells in vitro, perhaps by blocking endogenous IL-6 synthesis,[78] although clinical studies to date are negative. Oncostatin M, leukemia inhibitory factor, and ciliary neurotropic factor induce in vitro DNA synthesis by MM and plasmacytoma cells using the common gp130 receptor.[79] Granulocyte-macrophage colony-stimulating factor (GM-CSF) has been reported to enhance the IL-6 responsiveness of MM cells in vitro and has been utilized to facilitate the development of IL-6-dependent human MM lines.[80] IL-11, a factor that can support the growth of IL-6-dependent cell lines and promote B-cell differentiation, cannot augment DNA synthesis by purified MM cells.[81,82] IL-10 is a proliferation factor, but not a differentiation factor, for human MM cells.[83] Insulin-like growth factor (IGF-1) has been shown to augment MM cell growth and survival, and octreotide can inhibit IGF-1 signaling and related tumor cell growth.[84] Macrophage inflammatory protein-1α is a potential osteoclast stimulatory factor in MM.[85] Autocrine growth mediated by IL-15 has been demonstrated in both MM cell lines and patient cells.[86] Hepatocyte growth factor may potentially induce bone resorption in MM.[87] RANK-ligand (RANK-L), expressed by stromal cells, interacts with RANK receptor on osteoclast precursors to induce osteoclastogenesis.[88,89] Osteoprotegerin (OPG), which prevents the interaction of RANK-L with its receptor, can inhibit osteoclastogenesis. Further, transgenic animals that overexpressed OPG developed osteoporosis, thus providing a rationale for using OPG to inhibit the imbalance in bone formation/resorption seen in MM. Finally, long-term engraftment of both MM cell lines and freshly isolated tumor cells from MM patients has been reported in severe combined immunodeficient (SCID) mice and in SCID-hu mice, providing models for studying the role of growth factors in the growth and survival of human MM cells in the human BM milieu in vivo.[90–93]

Angiogenic Factors in MM

Vascular endothelial growth factor (VEGF) is known to play a role in progression of solid tumors. Recent studies demonstrate that MM cells secrete VEGF, which augments IL-6 secretion in BMSCs; conversely, IL-6 augments VEGF secretion from MM cell.[94] (Figure 25–5A). The presence of Flt-1 on some MM cells also suggests autocrine VEGF-mediated MM cell growth[95] (Figure 25–5A). Our studies confirm that VEGF is produced both by MM cells and BMSCs, and that adherence of MM cells to BMSCs triggers increased VEGF secretion. Furthermore, VEGF causes modest increases in tumor cell proliferation.[96] In an effort to identify signaling pathways mediating these effects, we first demonstrated that high-affinity VEGF receptor fms-like tyrosine kinase-1 (Flt-1), but not fetal liver kinase-1 (Flk-1), is

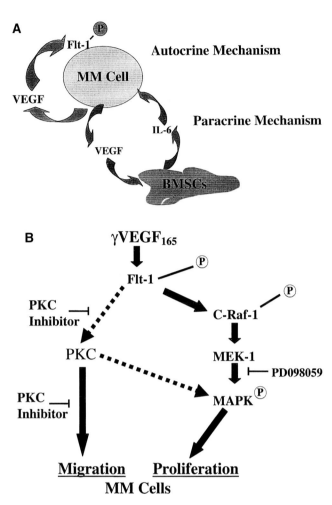

Figure 25–5. (A) Role of vascular endothelial growth factor (VEGF) and interleukin-6 (IL-6) in autocrine and paracrine MM cell growth. (B) VEGF induces MAPK and proliferation as well as PKC signaling and migration in MM cells.

will both enhance our understanding of disease pathogenesis and provide the framework for novel therapeutic strategies.

Serum Cytokine/Receptor Levels

Serum IL-2 levels were significantly higher in MM patients than in normal controls, and higher serum IL-2 levels were associated with a prolonged actuarial survival.[97] Serum IL-6 levels in some studies appear to correlate both with advanced stage of disease and decreased survival.[10, 61] IL-6 stimulates hepatocytes to produce acute phase proteins, such as C-reactive protein (CRP). CRP therefore reflects the IL-6 level and proliferative status of BM plasma cells. Indeed, CRP levels are significantly lower in patients with MGUS than in those with MM, and survival can be correlated with serum CRP level.[98] High levels of serum soluble IL-6 receptor (sIL-6R),[99] hepatocyte growth factor,[100] and syndecan-1,[101] as well as low serum hyaluronate levels,[102] are independent prognostic factors predicting poor outcome.

NOVEL THERAPEUTIC STRATEGIES

In vitro characterization of the mechanisms regulating MM growth and resistance to apoptosis provides the framework for novel therapies to specifically inhibit tumor cell growth and/or trigger apoptosis. Already agents that inhibit signal transduction pathway molecules have shown promise in ongoing clinical trials. These include antibodies and small molecules that inhibit growth factor receptors and their receptor tyrosine kinases; inhibitors of cytoplasmic second messengers such as ras, raf, and MEK; inhibitors of protein trafficking; kinase inhibitors; and inhibitors of protein degradation. For example, early clinical trials targeting IL-6 are evaluating antibodies to IL-6 or IL-6 receptor (IL-6R), IL-6 superantagonists that bind to IL-6R but do not trigger downstream signaling, IL-6 fused to immunotoxins, and ATRA, which down-regulates IL-6R on MM cells.[20] Our recent studies demonstrating obligate activation of RAFTK during Dex-induced apoptosis in MM cells suggest that novel strategies to activate death signaling distal to RAFTK may overcome Dex resistance.[49] Furthermore, the demonstration that the protective effect of IL-6 against Dex-induced apoptosis is mediated by SHP2[57] has provided the framework for development of small molecule SHP2 inhibitor therapies. Further delineation of these pathways will suggest additional strategies to trigger apoptosis, overcome Dex resistance, and inhibit survival signals.[103]

Novel therapies may also be based on inhibiting cell to cell interaction and cytokines in the BM. For example, excess plasma cells specifically adhere both to ECM proteins and BMSCs in the BM millieu.[104] Adhesion molecules not only localize tumor cells within the BM microenvironment, but also have multiple functional sequelae. First, since adherence to BMSCs confers resistance to apoptosis,[105] agents that block adhesion may confer sensitivity to treatment. Second, adherence of MM cells to BMSCs up-regulates NF-kB dependent IL-6 transcription and secretion within BMSCs.[5] Moreover, tumor cell secretion of cytokines, including TGF-β, within the BM

expressed on MM cells (Figure 25–5B). Treatment of MM cell lines and MM patient cells with rVEGF$_{165}$ induces activation of both Flt-1 and c-Raf-1. In contrast, pretreatment with anti-humanVEGF antibody or the MEK-1 inhibitor PD098059 blocked the proliferative effect of VEGF, confirming the involvement of the ERK-2 signaling cascade. Neither of the other prominent MAPK pathways (p38, or SAPK) nor the STAT3 kinase pathway was activated by VEGF in MM cells. The effect of VEGF on tumor cell migration was assayed by measuring the transfilter migration activity of MM and PCL cells seeded on membranes precoated with fibronectin. VEGF induced activation of cell migration in MM cells and PCL cells, which was significantly blocked in the presence of protein kinase C inhibitor bisindoylmaleimide-I-hydrochloride. Taken together these data indicate that VEGF plays a pivotal role in MM patients, not only during BM neo-angiogenesis, but also by triggering proliferation and migration of tumor cells. Further delineation of VEGF-induced signaling mediating these effects milieu further enhances IL-6 transcription and secretion in BMSCs.[6] This is of central importance, since studies have shown that IL-6 is both a growth and survival factor for MM cells.[106] Proteasome inhibitors are novel drugs that inhibit activation of NF-kB,[107] and our recent studies show that they can both directly induce apoptosis of MM cells that are resistant to conventional therapy and also inhibit NF-kB dependent up-regulation of IL-6 in BMSCs triggered by adherence of MM cells to BMSCs.[108] Their acceptable toxicity profile, coupled with responses in MM patients enrolled in Phase I studies, provide a strong rationale for further clinical evaluation in MM.

Our recent studies suggest that both MM cells and BMSCs secrete VEGF, that adhesion of MM cells to BMSCs up-regulates VEGF secretion, and that VEGF triggers low-grade proliferation and migration of MM cells. VEGF-receptor inhibitors may therefore offer therapeutic promise. VEGF may, at least in part, be responsible for increased angiogenesis observed in MM BM. Importantly, thalidomide, based on its anti-angiogenic activity, has already been used very successfully to treat patients with refractory MM.[109] Although thalidomide may be acting in MM as an anti-angiogenic agent, there are multiple other potential mechanisms of action of thalidomide and/or its in vivo metabolites[110] (Figure 25–6). First, thalidomide may have a direct effect on the MM cell and/or BMSC to inhibit their growth and survival. For example, free radical-mediated oxidative DNA damage may play a role in the teratogenicity of thalidomide, and may have direct antitumor effects. Second, adhesion of MM cells to BMSCs both triggers secretion of cytokines, which augment MM cell growth and survival, and confers drug resistance; thalidomide modulates adhesive interactions and thereby may alter tumor cell growth, survival, and

drug resistance. Third, cytokines secreted into the BM microenvironment by MM cells and/or BMSCs, such as IL-6, IL-1β, IL-10, and TNF-α, may augment MM cell growth and survival; and thalidomide may alter their secretion and bioactivity. Finally, thalidomide may be acting against MM via its immunomodulatory effects, such as induction of a Th1 T-cell response with secretion of IFN-γ and IL-2. Understanding which of these mechanisms mediate anti-MM activity will be critical both to optimally define its clinical utility and to derive analogues with enhanced potency and fewer side effects. Already two classes of thalidomide analogues have been reported, including selected cytokine inhibitory drugs (SelCIDs), which are phosphodiesterase 4 inhibitors and inhibit TNF-α but have little effect on T-cell activation, and immunomodulatory drugs (IMiDs), which are not phosphodiesterase 4 inhibitors but do markedly stimulate T-cell proliferation as well as IFN-α and IL-2 secretion,[111] as well as inhibit TNF-α. In recent studies, we have delineated mechanisms of anti-MM activity of thalidomide and the more potent IMiDs.[112] Importantly, these agents act directly to induce apoptosis or G1 growth arrest in MM cell lines and patient MM cells resistant to melphalan, doxorubicin, and Dex. Moreover, thalidomide and the IMiDs enhance the anti-MM activity of Dex, and apoptotic signaling triggered by thalidomide and IMiDs, as with Dex, is associated with activation of RAFTK. Most recent studies suggest that treatment with these drugs may alter MM cell adherence to BMSCs and fibronectin and abrogate the up-regulation of IL-6 and VEGF induced by tumor cell binding. Finally, these drugs appear to up-regulate natural killer cell–mediated killing of autologous MM cells. These studies therefore establish the framework for the development and test-

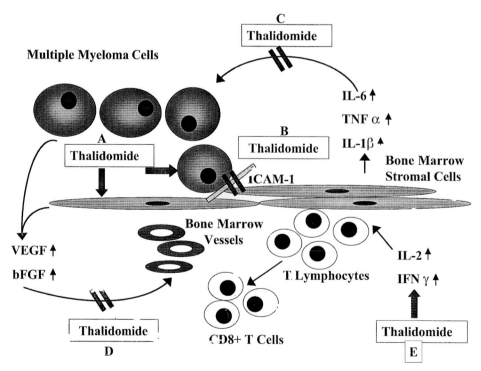

Figure 25–6. Mechanisms of thalidomide's anti-MM activity.

ing of thalidomide and the IMiDs in a new treatment paradigm to target both the tumor cell and the microenvironment, overcome classical drug resistance, and achieve improved outcome.

ACKNOWLEDGMENTS

Supported by NIH CA 78373, The Multiple Myeloma Research Foundation (DC), and The Doris Duke Distinguished Clinical Research Scientist Award (KCA).

REFERENCES

1. Greenlee RT, Murray T, Bolden S et al: Cancer Statistics, 2000. CA Cancer J Clin 50:7–33, 2000.
2. Urashima M, Chauhan D, Uchiyama H et al: CD40 ligand triggered interleukin-6 secretion in multiple myeloma cells. Blood 85:1903–1912, 1996.
3. Anderson KC, Jones RC, Morimoto C et al: Response of purified myeloma cells to hematopoietic growth factors. Blood 73:1915–1924, 1989.
4. Uchiyama H, Barut BA, Mohrbacher AF et al: Adhesion of human myeloma-derived cell lines to bone marrow stromal cells stimulates IL-6 secretion. Blood 82:3712–3720, 1993.
5. Chauhan D, Uchiyama H, Akbarali Y et al: Multiple myeloma cell adhesion-induced interleukin-6 expression in bone marrow stromal cells involves activation of NF-κB. Blood 87:1104–1112, 1996.
6. Urashima M, Ogata A, Chauhan D et al: Transforming growth factor β1: Differential effects on multiple myeloma versus normal B cells. Blood 87:1928–1938, 1996.
7. Anderson K: Advances in the biology of multiple myeloma: Therapeutic applications. Semin Oncol 26:10–22, 1999.
8. Chauhan D, Pandey P, Ogata A et al: Dexamethasone induces apoptosis of multiple myeloma cells in a JNK/SAP kinase independent mechanism. Oncogene 15:837–843, 1997.
9. Lichtenstein A, Tu Y, Fady C et al: Interleukin-6 inhibits apoptosis of malignant plasma cells. Cell Immunol 162:248–255, 1995.
10. Bataille R, Jourdan M, Zhang XG et al: Serum levels of interleukin-6, a potent myeloma cell growth factor, as a reflection of disease severity in plasma cell dyscrasias. J Clin Invest 84:2008–2011, 1989.
11. Heinrich PC, Behrmann I, Muller-Newen G et al: Interleukin-6-type cytokine signaling through the gp130/Jak/STAT pathway. Biochem J 334:297–314, 1998.
12. Kishimoto T, Taga T, Akira S: Cytokine signal transduction. Cell 76:253, 1994.
13. Kishimoto T, Akira S, Narazaki M et al: Interleukin-6 family of cytokines and gp130. Blood 86:1243, 1995.
14. Ogata A, Chauhan D, Teoh G et al: Interleukin-6 triggers cell growth via the ras-dependent mitogen-activated protein kinase cascade. J Immunol 159:2212–2221, 1997.
15. Ogata A, Chauhan D, Urashima M et al: Blockade of mitogen-activated protein kinase cascade signaling in interleukin-6 independent multiple myeloma cells. Clin Can Res 3:1017–1022, 1997.
16. Feng G, Hui C, Pawson T: SH2-containing phosphotyrosine phosphatase as a target of protein-tyrosine kinases. Science 259:1607–1611, 1993.
17. Vogel W, Lammers R, Huang J et al: Activation of a phosphotyrosine phosphatase by tyrosine phosphorylation. Science 259:1611–1614, 1993.
18. Jernberg-Wiiklund H, Petterson M, Nilsson K: Recombinant interferon-gamma inhibits the growth of IL-6 dependent human multiple myeloma cell lines in vitro. Eur J Hematol 46:231–239, 1991.
19. Portier M, Zhang XG, Caron E et al: (1993). Gamma-interferon in multiple myeloma: Inhibition of interleukin 6 dependent myeloma cell growth and downregulation of IL-6 receptor expression in vitro. Blood 81:3076–3082, 1993.
20. Ogata A, Nishimoto N, Shima Y et al: Inhibitory effect of all-trans retinoic acid on the growth of freshly isolated myeloma cells via interference with interleukin-6 signal transduction. Blood 84:3040–3046, 1994.
21. Schwabe M, Brini AT, Bosco MC et al: Disruption by interferon-gamma of autocrine IL-6 growth loop in IL-6 dependent U266 myeloma cells by homologous and heterologous downregulation of the IL-6 receptor alpha and beta chains. J Clin Invest 94:2317–2325, 1994.
22. Urashima M, Teoh G, Chauhan D et al: Interleukin-6 overcomes p21^{WAF1} upregulation and G1 growth arrest induced by dexamethasone and interferon-γ in multiple myeloma cells. Blood 90:279–289, 1997.
23. Chauhan D, Hideshima T, Treon SP et al: Functional interaction between retinoblastoma protein and stress activated protein kinase in multiple myeloma cells. Cancer Res 59:1192–1195, 1999.
24. Meydan N, Grunberger T, Dadi H et al: Inhibition of acute lymphoblastic leukaemia by JAK-2 inhibitor. Nature 379:645–648, 1996.
25. Druker BJ, Tamura S, Buchdunger E et al: Effects of a selective inhibitor of the Abl tyrosine kinase on the growth of Bcr-Abl positive cells. Nat Med 2:561–566, 1996.
26. Marra F, Choudhary GG, Abboud HE: Interferon-gamma mediated activation of STAT-1 regulates growth-induced mitogenesis. J Clin Invest 98:1218–1239, 1996.
27. Frank DA: STAT signaling in the pathogenesis and treatment of cancer. Mol Med 5:432–456, 1999.
28. Carlett-Falcone R, Landowski TH, Oshira MM et al: Constitutive activation of STAT-3 signaling confers resistance to apoptosis in human U266 myeloma cells. Immunity 10:105–115, 1999.
29. Neiborowska-Skaska M, Wasik MA, Slupianek A et al: Signal transducer and activator of transcription (STAT)-5 activation by Bcr-Abl is dependent on intact Src homology (SH3) and SH2 domains of Bcr-Abl, and is required for leukemogenesis. J Exp Med 189:1229–1242, 1999.
30. Takeda K, Noguchi K, Shi W et al: Targeted disruption of the mouse STAT-3 gene leads to early embryonic lethality. Proc Natl Acad Sci 94:3801–3804, 1997.
31. Urashima M, Teoh G, Ogata A et al: Characterization of p16^{INK4A} expression in multiple myeloma and plasma cell leukemia. Clin Can Res 3:2173–2179, 1997.
32. Teoh G, Urashima M, Ogata A et al: MDM2 protein overexpression promotes proliferation and survival of multiple myeloma cells. Blood 90:1982–1992, 1997.
33. Urashima M, Ogata A, Chauhan D et al: Interleukin-6 promotes multiple myeloma cell growth via phosphorylation of retinoblastoma protein. Blood 88:2219–2227, 1996.
34. Urashima M, Teoh G, Ogata A et al: Role of CDK4 and p16^{INK4A} in interleukin-6-mediated growth of multiple myeloma. Leukemia 11:1957–1963, 1997.
35. Chauhan D, Kharbanda S, Ogata A et al: Interleukin-6 inhibits Fas-induced apoptosis and stress-activated protein kinase activation in multiple myeloma cells. Blood 89:227–234, 1997.
36. Chauhan D, Pandey P, Ogata A et al: Cytochrome-c dependent and independent induction of apoptosis in multiple myeloma cells. J Biol Chem 272:29995–29997, 1997.
37. Xu F, Sharma S, Gardner S et al: Interleukin-6 induced inhibition of multiple myeloma cell apoptosis: Support for the hypothesis that protection is mediated via inhibition of the JNK/SAPK pathway. Blood 92:241–251, 1998.

38. Thornberry NA, Lazebnik Y: Caspases: Enemies within. Science 281:1312–1316, 1998.

39. Casiola-Rosen L, Nikolson DW, Chang T et al: Apopain/CPP32 cleaves proteins that are essential for cellular repair—A fundamental principle of apoptotic death. J Exp Med 183:1957–1964, 1996.

40. Emoto Y, Mannome Y, Meinhardt G et al: Proteolytic activation of protein kinase C-Delta by an ICE-like protease in apotic cells. EMBO J 14:6148–6156, 1995.

41. Susin SA, Zamzami N, Kroemer G: Mitochondria as regulators of apoptosis: Doubt no more. Biochem Biophys Acta 1366:151–165, 1998.

42. Marchetti P, Zamzami N, Joseph B et al: The novel retinoid 6-[3-(1-adamantyl)-2-naphtalene carboxylic acid can trigger apoptosis through a mitochondrial pathway independent of the nucleus. Cancer Res 59:6257–6266, 1999.

43. Liu X, Zou H, Slaughter C et al: DFF, a heterodimeric protein that functions downstream of caspase-3 to trigger DNA fragmentation during apoptosis. Cell 89:175–184, 1997.

44. Yang J, Liu X, Balla K et al: Prevention of apoptosis by Bcl-2: Release of cytochrome-c from the mitochondria blocked. Science 275:1129–1132, 1997.

45. Kluck RM, Kashibatta S: A lively meeting of a deathly topic. Apoptosis 2:337–342, 1997.

46. Avraham S, London R, Fu YG et al: Identification and characterization of a novel related adhesion focal tyrosine kinase (RAFTK) from megakaryocytes and brain. J Biol Chem 270:27742–27751, 1995.

47. Lev S, Moreno H, Martinez R et al: Protein tyrosine kinase PYK2 is involved in CA2+-induced regulation of ion channel and MAP kinase functions. Nature 376:737–745, 1995.

48. Xiong WC, Parsons JT: Induction of apoptosis after expression of PYK2, a tyrosine kinase structurally related to focal adhesion kinase. J Cell Biol 139:529–539, 1997.

49. Chauhan D, Hideshima T, Pandey P et al: RAFTK/PYK2-dependent and independent apoptosis in multiple myeloma cells. Oncogene 18:6733–6740, 1999.

50. Feng GS: Shp-2 tyrosine phosphatase: Signaling one cell or many. Exp Cell Res 253:47–54, 1999.

51. Neel BG, Tonks NK: Protein tyrosine phosphatases in signal transduction. Curr Opin Cell Biol 9:193–204, 1997.

52. Streuli M: Protein tyrosine phosphatases in signaling. Curr Opin Cell Biol 8:182–188, 1996.

53. Vanvactor D, O'Reilly AM, Neel BG: Genetic analysis of protein tyrosine phosphatases. Curr Opin Gen Dev 8:112–126, 1998.

54. Saxton TM, Pawson T: Morphogenetic movements at gastrulation require the SH2 tyrosine phosphatase Shp2. Proc Natl Acad Sci 96:3790–3795, 1999.

55. Shi ZQ, Lu W, Feng GS: The SHP-2 tyrosine phosphatase has opposite effects in mediating the activation of extracellular signal-regulated and c-jun NH2-terminal mitogen-activated protein kinases. J Biol Chem 273:4904–4908, 1998.

56. Marengere LEM, Waterhouse P, Duncan GS et al: Regulation of T cell receptor signaling by tyrosine phosphatase SYP association with CTLA-4. Science 272:1170–1173, 1996.

57. Chauhan D, Pandey P, Hideshima T et al: SHP2 mediates the protective effect of interleukin-6 against dexamethasone-induced apoptosis in multiple myeloma cells. J Biol Chem 275:27845–27850, 2000.

58. Catlett-Falcone R, Dalton WS, Jove R: STAT proteins as novel targets for cancer therapy. Signal transducer and activator of transcription. Curr Opin Oncol 11:490–506, 1999.

59. Landowski TH, Shain KH, Oshiro MM et al: Myeloma cells selected for resistance to CD95-mediated apoptosis are not cross-resistant to cytotoxic drugs: Evidence for independent mechanisms of caspase activation. Blood 94:265–274, 1999.

60. Ng MHL, Chung YF, Lo KW et al: Frequent hypermethylation of p16 and p15 genes in multiple myeloma. Blood 87:2500, 1997.

61. Ludwig H, Nachbaur DM, Fritz E et al: Interleukin-6 is a prognostic factor in multiple myeloma. Blood 77:2794–2795, 1991.

62. Barille S, Collette M, Bataille R et al: Myeloma cells upregulate IL-6 but downregulate osteocalcin production by osteoblastic cells through cell to cell contact. Blood 86:3151–3159, 1995.

63. Fattori E, Della Rocca C, Costa P et al: Development of progressive kidney damage and myeloma kidney in interleukin-6 transgenic mice. Blood 83:2570–2579, 1994.

64. Bataille R, Barlogie B, Yang Z et al: Biologic effects of anti-interleukin-6 murine monoclonal antibody in advanced multiple myeloma. Blood 86:685–691, 1995.

65. Chadwick D, Jamal N, Messner HA et al: Differential sensitivity of human myeloma cell lines and bone marrow colony forming cells to a recombinant diphtheria toxin-interleukin-6 fusion protein. Br J Haematol 85:25–36, 1993.

66. Kreitman R, Siegall CB, Fitzgerald DJP et al: Interleukin-6 fused to mutant form of pseudomonas exotoxin kills malignant cells from patients with multiple myeloma. Blood 79:1775–1780, 1992.

67. Ehlers M, de Hon FD, Klasse Bos H et al: Combining two mutations of human interleukin-6 that affect gp 130 activation results in a potent interleukin-6 receptor antagonist on human myeloma cells. J Biol Chem 270:8158–8163, 1995.

68. Savage AD, Belson DJ, Vescio RA et al: Pamidronate reduces IL-6 production by bone marrow stroma from multiple myeloma patients. Blood 88:105a, 1996.

69. Sporeno E, Savino R, Ciapponi L et al: Human interleukin-6 receptor super antagonists with high potency and wide spectrum on multiple myeloma cells. Blood 87:4510–4519, 1996.

70. Klein B, Zhang XG, Lu XY et al: Interleukin-6 in human multiple myeloma. Blood 85:863–872, 1995.

71. Kawano M, Tanaka H, Ishikawa H et al: Interleukin-1 accelerates autocrine growth of myeloma cells through interleukin-6 in human myeloma. Blood 73:2145–2148, 1989.

72. Cozzolino F, Torcia M, Aldinucci D et al: Production of interleukin-1 by bone marrow myeloma cells: Its role in the pathogenesis of lytic bone lesions. Blood 74:380–387, 1989.

73. Gherardi RK, Belec L, Fromont G et al: Elevated levels of interleukin-1β (IL-1β) and IL-6 in serum and increased production of IL-1β mRNA in lymph nodes of patients with polyneuropathy, organomegaly, endocrinopathy, M protein, and skin changes (POEMS) syndrome. Blood 83:2587–2593, 1994.

74. Lacy MQ, Donovan DA, Heimbach JH et al: Comparison of interleukin-1β expression by in situ hybridization in monoclonal gammopathy of undetermined significance and multiple myeloma. Blood 93:300–305, 1999.

75. Hideshima T, Chauhan D, Schlossman R et al: Role of TNF-alpha in the pathophysiology of multiple myeloma (MM). Oncogene 20:4519º4527, 2001.

76. Bergui L, Schena M, Gaidano G et al: Interleukin 3 and interleukin 6 synergistically promote the proliferation and differentiation of malignant plasma cell precursors in multiple myeloma. J Exp Med 170:613–618, 1989.

77. Garrett IR, Durie BGM, Nedwin GE et al: Production of lymphotoxin, a bone resorbing cytokine, by cultured human myeloma cells. N Engl J Med 317:526–532, 1987.

78. Hermann F, Andreff M, Gruss HJ et al: Interleukin 4 inhibits growth of multiple myeloma by suppressing interleukin 6 expression. Blood 78:2070–2078, 1991.

79. Chauhan D, Kharbanda S, Ogata A et al: Oncostatin M induces association of Grb2 with Janus Kinase JAK2 in multiple myeloma cells. J Exp Med 182:1801–1806, 1995.

80. Zhang XG, Bataille R, Jourdan M et al: Granulocyte-macrophage colony-stimulating factor synergizes with interleukin-6 in supporting the proliferation of human myeloma cells. Blood 76:2599, 1990.

81. Anderson KC, Morimoto C, Paul SR et al: Interleukin-11 promotes accessory cell dependent B cell differentiation in man. Blood 80:2797–2804, 1992.

82. Paul SD, Barut BA, Cochran MA et al: Lack of a role of interleukin-11 in the growth of multiple myeloma. Leuk Res 16:247–252, 1992.

83. Lu ZY, Zhang XG, Rodriguez C et al: Interleukin-10 is a proliferation factor but not a differentiation factor for human myeloma cells. Blood 85:2521, 1995.

84. Georgii-Hemming P, Stromberg T, Janson ET et al: The somatostatin analog octreotide inhibits growth of interleukin-6 (IL-6)-dependent and IL-6-independent human multiple myeloma cell lines. Blood 93:1724–1731, 1999.

85. Choi SJ, Cruz JC, Craig F et al: Macrophage inflammatory protein 1-alpha is a potential osteoclast stimulatory factor in multiple myeloma. Blood 96:671–675, 2000.

86. Tinhofer I, Marschitz I, Henn T et al: Expression of functional interleukin-15 receptor and autocrine production of interleukin-15 as mechanisms of tumor propagation in multiple myeloma. Blood 95:610–618, 2000.

87. Borset M, Seidel C, Hjorth-Hansen H et al: The role of hepatocyte growth factor and its receptor c-Met in multiple myeloma and other blood malignancies. Leuk Lymphoma 32:249–256, 1999.

88. Burgess TL, Qian Y, Kaufman S et al: The ligand for osteoprotegrin (OPGL) directly activates mature osteoclasts. J Cell Biol 145:527–538, 1999.

89. Hsu Hst, Lacey DL, Dunstan CR et al: Tumor necrosis factor receptor family member RANK mediates osteoclast differentiation and activation induced by osteoprotegrin ligand. Proc Natl Acad Sci USA 96:3540–3545, 1999.

90. Feo-Zuppardi FJ, Taylor CW, Iwato K et al: Long-term engraftment of fresh human myeloma cells in SCID mice. Blood 80:2843–2850, 1992.

91. Huang Y-W, Richardson JA, Tong AW et al: Disseminated growth of a human multiple myeloma cell line in mice with severe combined immunodeficiency disease. Cancer Res 53:1392–1396, 1993.

92. Urashima M, Chen BP, Chen S et al: The development of a model for the homing of multiple myeloma cells to human bone marrow. Blood 90:754–765, 1997.

93. Yaccoby S, Barlogie B, Epstein J: Primary myeloma cells growing in SCID-hu mice: A model for studying the biology and treatment of myeloma and its manifestations. Blood 92:2908–2913, 1998.

94. Dankar B, Padro T, Leo R et al: Vascular endothelial growth factor and interleukin-6 in paracrine tumor-stromal cell interactions in multiple myeloma. Blood 95:2630–2336, 2000.

95. Bellamy W, Richter L, Frutiger Y et al: Expression of vascular endothelial growth factor and its receptor in hematological malignancies. Cancer Res 59:728–733, 1999.

96. Podar K, Tai YT, Hideshima T et al: Regulation of VEGF-mediated multiple myeloma (MM) cell growth. Blood 98:428–435, 2001.

97. Cimino G, Avvisati G, Amadori S et al: High serum IL-2 levels are predictive of prolonged survival in multiple myeloma. Br J Haematol 75:373–377, 1990.

98. Bataille R, Boccadoro M, Klein B et al: C-reactive protein and β-2 microglobulin produce a simple and powerful myeloma staging system. Blood 80:733–737, 1992.

99. Greipp PR, Gaillard JP, Kalish LA et al: Independent prognostic value for serum soluble interleukin-6 receptor (sIL-6R) in Eastern Cooperative Oncology Group (ECOG) myeloma trial E9487. Proc Am Soc Cliin Oncol 12:404, 1993.

100. Seidel C, Borset M, Turesson I et al: Elevated serum concentrations of hepatocyte growth factor in patients with multiple myeloma. Blood 91:806–812, 1998.

101. Seidel C, Sundan A, Hjorth M et al: Serum syndecan-1: A new independent prognostic marker in multiple myeloma. Blood 95:388–392, 2000.

102. Dahl IMS, Turesson I, Holmberg E et al: Serum hyaluron in patients with multiple myeloma: Correlation with survival and Ig concentration. Blood 93:4144–4148, 1999.

103. Chauhan D, Anderson KC: Apoptosis in multiple myeloma: Therapeutic implications. Apoptosis, 5:47–55, 2001.

104. Teoh G, Anderson KC: Interaction of tumor and host cells with adhesion and extracellular matrix molecules in the development of multiple myeloma. Hematol Oncol Clin N Am 11:27–42, 1997.

105. Damiano JS, Cress AE, Hazlehurst LA et al: Cell adhesion mediated drug resistance (CAM-DR): Role of integrins and resistance to apoptosis in human myeloma cell lines. Blood 93:1658–1667, 1999.

106. Hallek M, Bergsagel PL, Anderson KC: Multiple myeloma: Increasing evidence for a multistep transformation process. Blood 91:3–21, 1998.

107. Dou Q, Li B: Proteasome inhibitors as potential novel anticancer agents. Drug Resist Updates 2:215–223, 1999.

108. Hideshima T, Chauhan D, Shima Y et al: Thalidomide and its analogues overcome drug resistance of human multiple myeloma cells to conventional therapy. Blood 96:2943–2950, 2000.

109. Singhal S, Mehta J, Desikan R et al: Anti-tumor activity of thalidomide in refractory multiple myeloma. N Engl J Med 341:1565–1571, 1999.

110. Raje N, Anderson KC: Thalidomide: A revival story. N Engl J Med 341:1606–1609, 1999.

111. Corral LG, Haslett PAJ, Muller GW et al: Differential cytokine modulation and T cell activation by two distinct classes of thalidomide analogues that are potent inhibitors of TNF-α. J Immunol 163:380–386, 1999.

112. Hideshima T, Richardson P, Chauhan D et al: The proteasome inhibitor PS341 overcomes apoptotic resistance mechanisms in human multiple myeloma cells. Can Res 61:3071–3076, 2001.

26

Epidemiology of Multiple Myeloma

Linda M. Brown, Dalsu Baris,
and Susan S. Devesa

Multiple myeloma, a plasma cell tumor arising in the bone marrow, is a rare cancer with an elusive etiology. In the United States multiple myeloma is estimated to account for approximately 1 percent of all diagnosed cancers and 2 percent of all cancer deaths.[1] According to estimates provided by the American Cancer Society, approximately 5800 men and 5400 women were expected to die from multiple myeloma in the United States during 2000.[1] The lifetime risk of being diagnosed with myeloma in the United States is 0.85 percent for black men, 0.61 percent for white men, 0.99 percent for black women, and 0.50 percent for white women.[2]

DESCRIPTIVE EPIDEMIOLOGY

U.S. Mortality Patterns

Based on data from the National Center for Health Statistics, 1950–1997, age-adjusted mortality rates (using the 1970 U.S. standard) among whites almost tripled, reaching highs of 3.6 per 100,000 and 2.4 per 100,000 among men and women, respectively, in 1995 to 1997 (Figure 26–1). Rates among nonwhites (consisting of the combined group of blacks, Asians and Pacific Islanders, and American Indians and Alaskan Natives) more than quadrupled during this 47-year period, reaching a high of 4.4 per 100,000 among women in 1995 to 1997 and 6.2 per 100,000 among men in 1990 to 1994 before falling to 5.9 in 1995 to 1997. These increases are among the highest observed for any cancer during this time period.[2]

Rates specific for blacks, available since the early 1970s, are higher than rates for all nonwhites combined, and the rates increased more rapidly, with the highest rates for males (7.5 per 100,000) observed in 1990 to 1994 and for females (5.4 per 100,000) in 1995 to 1997.

To evaluate whether the increases in multiple myeloma mortality during the past five decades were confined to certain age groups or specific time periods, rates were examined according to age group and year of birth (Figure 26–2). For all race and sex categories, the increases in mortality occurred primarily among individuals aged 55 years and older, with the most marked changes occurring in the two oldest age groups, 75 to 84 and over 85. The risk of dying from multiple myeloma rose steadily among individuals born in the middle to late 1800s and early

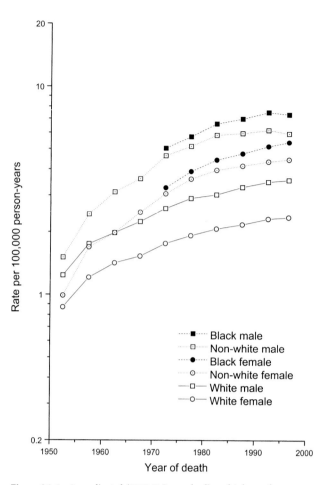

Figure 26–1. Age-adjusted (1970 U.S. standard) multiple myeloma mortality trends in the United States by race and sex, 1950–54 to 1990–94, 1995–97.

1900s, whereas more recent birth cohorts experienced little change in risk. Whether the substantial rises among persons born prior to the early 1900s were due to improving diagnosis or to increasing risk due to environmental exposures is not well understood. It is noteworthy that rates among persons born more recently have not risen in a similar fashion.

U.S. Survival Patterns

Survival data based on follow-up evaluation of newly diagnosed cases since the 1970s are available from the Surveillance, Epidemiology, and End Results (SEER) program.[2] Presented are data from nine SEER population-based cancer registries surveying approximately 10 percent of the U.S. population. Although survival among patients diagnosed with multiple myeloma is poor for all race and sex groups, significant improvements in the 5-year relative survival rates have occurred over the past two decades, from 24.5 percent among patients diagnosed during 1974 to 1976 to 28.5 percent among those diagnosed during 1989 to 1996 (data not shown).[2]

The 5-year relative survival rates by age at diagnosis, race, and sex for patients diagnosed during 1989 to 1996 are pre-

434

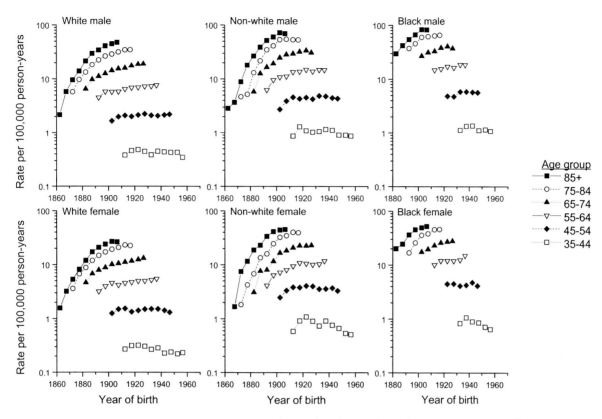

Figure 26–2. Age-specific multiple myeloma mortality trends in the United States by sex, race, age group, and cohort year of birth, 1860 to 1970.

sented in Table 26–1.[2] For all race and sex groups, survival was more favorable among those diagnosed at younger ages than among the elderly. The 5-year relative survival rates for all myeloma patients combined in the age groups under 45, 45 to

Table 26–1. Five-Year Relative Survival Rates (Percent) Among Patients Diagnosed with Multiple Myeloma in the U.S. Nine SEER Areas During 1989 to 1996 by Age at Diagnosis, Sex, and Race[a]

Age at Diagnosis (yr)	Whites		Blacks	
	Males	Females	Males	Females
< 45	42.1	47.7	52.1	49.1
45–54	40.7	41.3	44.1	42.9
55–64	34.8	32.0	37.8	30.1
65–74	25.5	26.8	26.8	24.0
75 +	18.8	17.8	21.1	17.6
All ages	28.8	26.7	34.2	28.0
Under 65	37.2	36.5	42.6	36.7
65 and older	22.9	22.3	25.0	21.2

Source: SEER Cancer Statistics Review 1973 to 1997, National Cancer Institute, 2000.

[a] SEER, National Cancer Institute. Based on data from nine population-based registries in Connecticut, New Mexico, Utah, Iowa, Hawaii, Atlanta, Detroit, Seattle–Puget Sound, and San Francisco–Oakland. Rates are based on follow-up study of patients through 1997.

54, 55 to 64, 65 to 74, and 75 years or older were 47, 42, 33, 27, and 19 percent, respectively, with rates of 37 versus 23 percent among those under versus those older than age 65. Survival rates for all ages combined were higher for blacks than for whites (30.9 versus 27.8 percent) and for males than for females (29.7 versus 27.2 percent).

U.S. Incidence Patterns

In contrast to the notable increases in age-adjusted mortality rates during 1950 to 1997, age-adjusted incidence rates (using the 1970 U.S. standard) rose only modestly in the nine SEER areas during 1973 to 1997 (Figure 26–3). Rates were highest among black men, followed by black women and then white men; they were lowest among white women. Age-adjusted incidence rates among white men peaked at 5.4 per 100,000 in 1988 to 1992 and then declined to 5.1 per 100,000 in 1993 to 1997, whereas rates among black men increased to 11.4 per 100,000 in 1993 to 1997. Rates changed little among white women, but they rose steadily among black women, reaching 8.6 per 100,000 in 1993 to 1997.

Age-specific incidence rates for multiple myeloma for 1973 to 1997 are presented in Figure 26–4. Among white men and black women, incidence rates rose steadily with age, whereas they increased and then decreased for white women and black men aged 85 and older. Rates consistently were higher among blacks than whites and among males than among females.

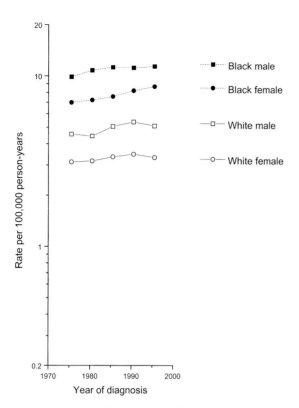

Figure 26–3. Age-adjusted (1970 U.S. standard) multiple myeloma incidence trends in the U.S. nine SEER areas by race and sex, 1973–77 to 1993–97.

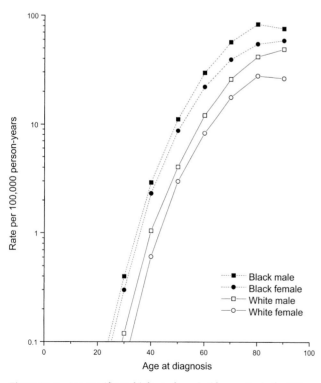

Figure 26–4. Age-specific multiple myeloma incidence rates in the U.S. nine SEER areas by race and sex, 1973 to 1997.

Table 26–2. Age-Adjusted (1970 U.S. Standard) Multiple Myeloma Incidence and Mortality Rates in the U.S. 11 SEER areas by race/ethnicity and sex, 1990–1997[a]

Race/Ethnicity	Incidence Rate per 100,000 Persons[b]		Mortality Rate per 100,000 Persons[c]	
	Males	Females	Males	Females
All races	5.6	3.7	3.8	2.6
White	5.2	3.4	3.5	2.3
White Hispanic	5.2	3.3	3.0	2.1
White Non-Hispanic	5.2	3.4	3.5	2.3
Black	11.2	8.3	7.4	5.2
Asian/Pacific Islander	3.5	2.2	1.8	1.2
American Indian	3.5	2.4	—[d]	—[d]
Hispanic	4.8	3.2	2.8	2.0

Source: SEER Cancer Statistics Review 1973 to 1997, National Cancer Institute, 2000.

[a] Rates per 100,000 person-years, age-adjusted using 1970 U.S. standard.

[b] SEER, National Cancer Institute. Based on data from eleven population-based registries in Connecticut, New Mexico, Utah, Iowa, Hawaii, Atlanta, Detroit, Seattle–Puget Sound, San Francisco–Oakland, San Jose-Montery, and Los Angeles.

[c] Based on data from the National Center for Health Statistics.

[d] Fewer than 25 deaths.

For all races combined and individually, the incidence and mortality rates were higher in males than in females (Table 26–2). The incidence rates for multiple myeloma among males and females combined in the 11 SEER registries were more than twice as high among blacks (9.5 per 100,000) as among whites (4.2 per 100,000). Although the data are based on small numbers, rates among Hispanics were slightly lower than among whites (3.9 per 100,000), whereas rates among Asians/Pacific Islanders (2.8 per 100,000) and American Indians (2.9 per 100,000) were substantially lower than those among whites. In as much as mortality rates for blacks, whites, and Hispanics are about two-thirds of the incidence rates, a similar racial and ethnic pattern is seen. However, mortality rates are lower than expected for Asians and Pacific Islanders (1.4 per 100,000) and higher than expected for American Indians (2.3 per 100,000), presumably owing to better survival among Asians and Pacific Islanders and poorer survival among American Indians.

International Patterns

International differences in multiple myeloma incidence, 1973 to 1977 to 1988 to 1992, as published in Volumes IV through VII of Cancer Incidence in Five Continents, are dramatic.[3–6] Generally increases in age-adjusted rates (world standard) over the two decades were noted for males in the U.S. SEER registry blacks and whites; the Canadian provinces of Quebec and British Columbia; Finland; Denmark; the United Kingdom; Spain; and Osaka and Miyagi, Japan (Figure 26–5A). For most countries, the time trends for females were similar to those for males, with consistent increases apparent in the U.S. SEER registry blacks and whites; British Columbia; Finland; Denmark;

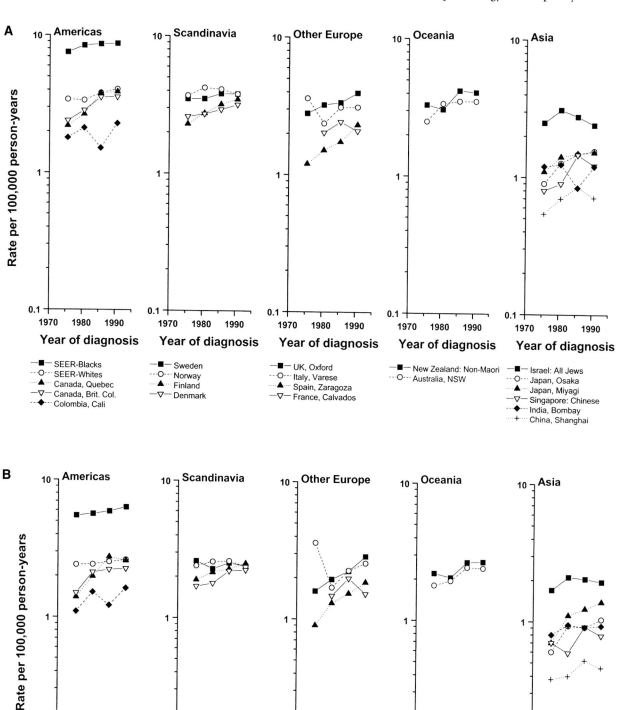

Figure 26–5. International incidence trends in age-adjusted (world standard) multiple myeloma rates by continent, 1973–77 to 1988–92. (A) Males; (B) Females.

the United Kingdom, Spain; and Miyagi, Japan (Figure 26–5B). Among both males and females, substantial increases were apparent in British Columbia, Spain, the United Kingdom, and Miyagi, Japan; less rapid rises occurred in SEER registry blacks and whites, Finland, Denmark, and Australia; and rates changed little in Norway, France, and Israel. Rates among males for the most recent time period, 1988 to 1992, were highest for SEER blacks (8.7 per 100,000), followed by New Zealand non-Maoris and SEER whites, and lowest in Shanghai, China (0.7 per 100,000). Rates were relatively low in Asia, except for Israel. Among females the rates for the time period 1988 to 1992 ranged from 6.3 per 100,000 for SEER blacks to 0.5 per 100,000 in Shanghai, China. In the most recent time period, rates varied more than 12-fold internationally and were higher in men than women in all selected populations; the male/female rate ratio varied from 1.08 in Italy to 1.60 in Norway.

ETIOLOGIC FACTORS

Ionizing Radiation

Most of the data on the effects of ionizing radiation on multiple myeloma risk come from studies of Japanese atomic bomb survivors[7–9] and studies of therapeutically exposed populations.[10–13] However, multiple myeloma also has been associated with lower levels of radiation exposure in several occupational studies.[14–17]

Atomic Bomb Survivors

Investigation of cancer incidence for the years 1950 to 1979[7] and cancer mortality for the years 1950 to 1985[8] among Japanese atomic bomb survivors suggested an increased multiple myeloma risk with increasing radiation dose. However, a more recent analysis of the incidence data for the years 1950 to 1987 yielded an estimated absolute risk of 0.08 cases per 10,000 person-years Sv (95 percent confidence interval less than 0 to 0.3), with no variation by sex, age at exposure, or time since exposure and no evidence of a significant dose–response relationship.[9] The most recent mortality analysis, covering the time period 1950 to 1990, yielded an estimated 0.17 excess risk per 10,000 person-years Sv (95 percent confidence interval, 0.02–0.40) for both sexes combined. Thus, the data available to date provide some support for an association between ionizing radiation from the atomic bombs and risk of multiple myeloma. However, additional years of follow-up evaluation will be required to elucidate the true nature of the association owing to the small number of exposed subjects who develop this cancer.

Diagnostic and Therapeutic X-Rays

Diagnostic x-ray exposure has not been clearly linked with multiple myeloma. Although several epidemiological studies reported no association between exposure to diagnostic x-rays and elevated risk of multiple myeloma,[18–22] other studies noted a positive association.[23,24]

Studies of the effects of therapeutic irradiation on myeloma risk have also been inconsistent. A few case-control interview studies have shown an excess risk of myeloma with radiation therapy[18] whereas others have not.[13,25] Elevated risks of multiple myeloma were reported in follow-up studies of patients receiving x-ray treatment for ankylosing spondylitis,[26,27] cervical cancer,[10] and metropathia hemorrhagica.[11]

Radiation-Related Occupations

Studies of occupationally exposed individuals have provided additional information on ionizing radiation and risk of multiple myeloma. An excess of myeloma deaths among American radiologists was first reported in the early 1960s.[28] More recently, myeloma risk was found to be twice as high among U.S. radiologists exposed to low-dose radiation than among physicians in other specialties[29]; however, no excess of myeloma was reported in a large study of Chinese diagnostic x-ray workers as compared with other medical specialists.[30]

Employment in nuclear facilities and risk of myeloma has been investigated in several cohort studies. Small excesses of myeloma mortality were reported among employees at Sellafield in Britain[14,31,32] and Hanford, in the United States, although the increase seen at Hanford did not reach statistical significance in a later follow-up study.[34] A combined analysis of cancer mortality data for over 95,000 nuclear industry workers employed at U.S. (Hanford), U.K. (Sellafield), and Canadian nuclear plants found an almost twofold significant increase for multiple myeloma.[16] Although a recent nested case-control study of workers employed at Hanford and Savannah River did not demonstrate an association between lifetime cumulative whole-body ionizing radiation dose and multiple myeloma, there was a significant effect of age at exposure, with positive associations between multiple myeloma and doses received at older ages.[17] An apparent trend of increasing risk of myeloma mortality with increasing estimated external radiation dose, noted among workers included in the National Registry for Radiation Workers in the United Kingdom, disappeared after excluding workers monitored for exposure to internal radiation emitters.[35]

Although several follow-up studies evaluated the risk of multiple myeloma mortality among military participants at nuclear weapon sites, the results were inconsistent. Elevated risk of myeloma was observed among military personnel in the United Kingdom[36] but not in New Zealand[37] or the United States.[38]

Residential Exposures

A recent study in Spain reported an excess risk of multiple myeloma mortality in the residential area near a nuclear power plant.[39] However, little evidence of an increased risk of multiple myeloma had been noted in previous investigations of the effect of residential proximity to nuclear facilities.[40–42]

Occupational Exposures

Farming and Other Agricultural Occupations

The majority of epidemiologic studies that evaluated the risk of multiple myeloma among farmers and other agricultural workers have reported positive associations.[43–53] A recent meta-analysis of 32 studies of multiple myeloma and farming published between

1981 and 1996 yielded an overall estimated relative risk of 1.23 (95 percent confidence interval, 1.14–1.32).[54] Exposures commonly experienced by farmers that might contribute to the increased risk of multiple myeloma include grain dusts,[55,56] engine exhausts and fuels,[57] farm animals,[58,59] and pesticides.[43,49,51,60] A number of epidemiologic studies have evaluated use of specific pesticides. Although some studies have noted positive findings with chlorinated phenoxy herbicides,[58] insecticides,[60] or DDT,[58,61] other studies observed no associations with specific pesticides.[47,62]

Metal Workers

Increased myeloma risk has been reported among workers in various metal occupations and industries,[63–67] although there are only limited data for exposure to specific metals.[58,68] Significantly elevated risks have been observed among smelter and metallurgy workers,[65] machinists,[63] nickel refinery workers,[66] and sheet metal workers.[67] In contrast, other studies have reported no notable associations with occupational metal exposures.[69–71]

Rubber Manufacturing

Some epidemiologic studies have suggested an association between multiple myeloma and employment in the rubber manufacturing industry.[19,72–76] However, overall results from a recent review of 12 cohort studies in nine countries, seven industry-based case-control studies, 48 community-based case-control studies in 16 countries, and 23 studies based on administrative data reported no excess risk for multiple myeloma with employment in this industry.[77] In addition, multiple myeloma was not found to occur in excess among workers exposed to styrene or butadiene in the rubber or the reinforced plastics and composites industry.[76,78–80]

Wood Products Workers

Several studies reported associations between myeloma risk and employment in the wood, furniture, and pulp and paper manufacturing industries.[81–84] Other studies showed little or no elevation in myeloma risk among wood product workers,[65,71,85,86] with the possible exception of forestry workers.[58]

Other Industries and Occupational Exposures

An association between multiple myeloma and employment in textile processing has been suggested in a few studies.[67,83,87,88] In contrast, two cohort studies of textile workers revealed no significant increase in deaths due to multiple myeloma.[89,90] Excess risks of myeloma among workers employed in the paint manufacturing industry have been noted in several studies.[64,91–94]

Other occupations linked with elevated risk of multiple myeloma in at least one study include nursing,[95] science technicians,[96] child care workers,[97] female workers exposed to silica,[98] railway carriage construction and repair workers,[99] meatcutters,[100] and firefighters.[49,101]

Specific Occupational Exposures

The relationship between benzene exposure and risk of multiple myeloma remains controversial.[102–104] Although benzene was replaced decades ago by toluene or xylene in most developed countries, it still remains as a low-level contaminant in gasoline, other solvents, and many products used or manufactured by the petroleum industry. Several studies have suggested benzene as a possible etiologic agent for multiple myeloma,[105,106] and one study reported an excess of myeloma among women residing within 7.5 kilometers of a petrochemical plant in South Wales.[107] In other studies, however, either the number of exposed myeloma subjects was too small to yield significantly elevated risk estimates or there was no elevation in risk.[108–113] In addition, no excess risk of myeloma was reported in a recent meta-analysis of data from 22 cohort mortality studies of petroleum workers in the United Kingdom, Canada, the United States, and Australia.[114]

Other Chemical Exposures

Excess myeloma mortality has been reported in some[115,116] but not all[117–119] investigations of chemical workers. Elevated risk of myeloma was linked to high levels of dioxin exposure in a follow-up study among residents of Seveso, Italy,[120] among fishermen residing on the east coast of Sweden,[121] and among verified clusters of multiple myeloma located near dioxin-contaminated bodies of water.[122] Exposure to organic solvents among aircraft maintenance workers and workers in the painting industry has also been linked to excess risk of multiple myeloma.[49,91,94,123,124] A positive association between myeloma and asbestos exposure has been reported in some[20,68,125] but not all[19,49,86,126] studies.

Lifestyle Factors

Cigarette Smoking and Alcohol Consumption

No relation with cigarette smoking has been reported for most epidemiologic studies of multiple myeloma.[19,55,68,88,127–133] However, significantly elevated risks were noted in a cohort of Seventh Day Adventists,[134] among women in the Third National Cancer Survey,[135] and for ex-smokers in a Swedish case-control study.[25] No epidemiologic study has reported a significant association between alcohol consumption and myeloma.[19,55,68,129,136]

Hair Dyes

There is conflicting evidence as to whether personal use of hair dyes increases the risk of developing multiple myeloma. Elevated risks of myeloma have been reported among women and men who used hair dyes in some[137–139] but not all[88,138] case-control studies, with the greatest risk observed among those using permanent hair dyes and dark hair coloring products.[139] No overall increased risk of myeloma among women who used permanent hair dyes was found in the American Cancer Society prospective mortality study; however, an elevated risk was observed among women who used black hair dye for 20 years or more.[140,141] Although the Nurse's Health Study lacked information on color of hair dye used, they found no excess risk of myeloma among women whose natural hair color was dark brown or black.[142] There are also inconsistencies in the epidemiologic literature concerning the relation between multiple myeloma and employment as a hairdresser, beautician, or cosmetologist, with excess risks reported in some studies[88,143,144] but not in others.[83,138,145]

Diet and Nutritional Factors

Only a few epidemiologic studies have investigated the role of dietary or nutritional factors in the etiology of multiple myeloma. Elevated risk of myeloma has been linked with overweight and obesity in two cohorts of outpatients from a health maintenance organization in northern California[146] and in a case-control study conducted in three areas of the United States.[147] Protective effects have been reported in relation to frequent intake of vitamin supplements (especially vitamin C), fish, whole grains, and green vegetables (notably cruciferous vegetables).[147–150] Elevated risks have been reported for sources of animal fat, primarily liver and butter.[150]

Socioeconomic Status

The relation between socioeconomic status (SES) and multiple myeloma, whether measured by occupation, income, or education, has been evaluated in a number of epidemiologic studies. Two recent population-based case-control studies and a nested case-control study reported elevated risks of myeloma associated with lower SES.[19,151,152] In contrast, earlier studies observed either no association or a positive association between myeloma and SES, possibly owing to underascertainment of the disease in lower social class individuals.[81,135,153–156]

Medication Use and Medical Conditions

Medication Use

Although significantly elevated risks of multiple myeloma have been reported with use of laxatives, erythromycin, and mineral oil (in females but not males),[68,157,158] there is little evidence to suggest that any particular over-the-counter or prescription drug plays a important role in the etiology of multiple myeloma.[18,21,157] The assertion that chronic drug ingestion may predispose to myeloma[159] needs confirmation.

Monoclonal Gammopathy of Undetermined Significance

Monoclonal gammopathy of undetermined significance (MGUS) is an asymptomatic disorder characterized by a low proliferation of plasma cells and the presence of a monoclonal protein (M-protein) in the serum of persons without evidence of multiple myeloma, Waldenström's macroglobulinemia, primary amyloidosis, or other lymphoproliferative disorder.[160] It is well known that individuals with MGUS are prone to develop multiple myeloma. In a large Swedish MGUS cohort followed for 15 years, the standardized incidence ratio for myeloma was 34.3 (95 percent confidence interval, 24.8 to 46.2), as compared with the general population.[161] The actuarial probability for malignant transformation in two large series of MGUS patients was 31 percent at 20 years[162] and 40 percent at 25 years.[163] There are currently no clinical or laboratory findings that can predict which MGUS patients will develop a lymphoproliferative malignancy.

Chronic Immune Stimulation

A number of epidemiologic studies have investigated the hypothesis that repeated or chronic stimulation of the immune system may lead to multiple myeloma.[164] Risk of myeloma has been evaluated by assessing past history of individual immune-stimulating medical conditions, by examining categories of immune-stimulating medical conditions, such as autoimmune conditions and allergies, and by classifying medical conditions according to their biologically or immunologically related immune response mechanisms.[164–166] Although some studies have observed elevated risks for specific immune-stimulating medical conditions such as rheumatoid arthritis or for groups of medical conditions such as inflammatory diseases and chronic bacterial illnesses,[18,59,132,165,167,168] others have not.[65,68,166,169–172] Overall, the findings do not support a causal relationship between chronic immune stimulation and myeloma.[164,166,173,174]

Infectious Agents

The role of viruses or other infectious agents in the etiology of multiple myeloma is unclear. It has been suggested that immune-compromised persons may lack the ability to fight off viruses or other infections.[175] Many AIDS-related cancers have been associated with specific human herpesvirus infections,[176] and human herpesvirus 8 (HHV-8) has been detected in Kaposi's sarcoma and primary effusion lymphoma.[177] An increased incidence of myeloma was recently reported among people with AIDS in two large registry-based studies of AIDS,[175,178] and HHV-8 was found in the nonmalignant bone marrow dendritic cells of myeloma patients.[179] However, the role of HHV-8 in the pathophysiology of multiple myeloma is controversial[177] because most investigators have failed to detect a high seroprevalence of HHV-8 antibodies in patients with myeloma.[180–183]

Familial and Genetic Factors

Familial Aggregation of Cancer

An inherited component to multiple myeloma has been suggested by case reports of families with multiple affected members, especially siblings, and by observations that persons with multiple myeloma are more likely than others to have relatives with multiple myeloma or hematolymphoproliferative (HLP) cancer.[184–190] In case-control studies of multiple myeloma, investigators found two- to sixfold excess risks of myeloma among subjects who reported having a first-degree relative with myeloma and twofold excess risks among subjects with a history of HLP cancer in a first degree relative.[184,185,187,189] In the one study that investigated racial differences for myeloma, risk estimates for having a family history of HLP cancer tended to be higher for African Americans than for whites, although the difference in risks was not statistically significant.[185]

Genetic Factors

Although the etiology of multiple myeloma is unknown, there is growing evidence that certain cytokines, including interleukin-6 (IL-6), Il-1β, and IL-10, play an important role in the growth of plasma cells and may be involved in the pathogenesis of myeloma.[191–193] In addition, recent studies have demonstrated that most if not all patients with multiple myeloma exhibit chromosomal abnormalities, but no specific abnormality common to all myeloma patients has been identified.[194] Typical abnormalities include a rearrangement involving the *IGH* gene at 14q32, with reciprocal translocations most often involving 11q13 and 4p16; chromosomal loss, most frequently monosomy 13; and structural rearrangement of chromosome 1.[194–197] Although *p53* gene mutations have been reported among multiple myeloma cell lines,[198,199] they are rarely found in myeloma patients and thus unlikely to play a major role as a tumor suppressor gene in myeloma development.[199–201]

CONCLUSION

Multiple myeloma is an intriguing malignancy. From an epidemiologic perspective, it is the only hematolymphoproliferative cancer, other than chronic myeloid leukemia and peripheral T-cell lymphoma,[202,203] that is characterized by higher incidence rates among blacks than whites. Although many investigators have studied the epidemiology of multiple myeloma, little is known about its etiology or reasons for the black excess in incidence.

The strongest associations have involved exposure to ionizing radiation and organic solvents and chemicals and employment in farming and agricultural occupations. Recent studies suggest that certain lifestyle and genetic factors, particularly low socioeconomic status, overweight and obesity, and familial aggregation of cancer may be linked to excess risk of multiple myeloma. Exposure to cigarette smoking and alcohol use do not appear to be related to myeloma, but the data on personal use of hair dyes remain controversial. Recent attention also has been focused on viruses and other infectious agents, but their role in the etiology of myeloma remains unclear.

There is growing evidence that certain cytokines and chromosomal abnormalities may be involved in the pathogenesis of multiple myeloma. These laboratory-based genetic measures need to be incorporated into future epidemiologic studies to better understand the complex relationships between genetic and environmental/lifestyle factors on the development of multiple myeloma.

REFERENCES

1. Greenlee RT, Murray T, Bolden S et al: Cancer statistics, 2000. CA Cancer J Clin 50:7, 2000.
2. Ries LAG, Eisner MP, Kosary CL et al: SEER Cancer Statistics Review, 1973–1997. National Cancer Institute, Bethesda, MD, 2000.
3. Waterhouse J, Muir CS, Shanmugaratnam K et al: Cancer incidence in five continents, Vol. IV. IARC Scientific Publication, Lyons, France, 1982.
4. Muir C, Waterhouse J, Mack T et al: Cancer incidence in five continents, Vol. V. IARC Scientific Publication, Lyons, France, 1987.
5. Parkin DM, Muir CS, Whelan SL et al: Cancer incidence in five continents, Vol. VI. IARC Scientific Publication, Lyons, France, 1992.
6. Parkin DM, Whelan SL, Ferlay J et al: Cancer incidence in five continents, Vol. VII, p. 1. IARC Scientific Publication, Lyons, France, 1997.
7. Ichimaru M, Ishimaru T, Mikami M et al: Multiple myeloma among atomic bomb survivors in Hiroshima and Nagasaki, 1950–76: Relationship to radiation dose absorbed by marrow. J Natl Cancer Inst 69:323, 1982.
8. Shimizu Y, Kato H, Schull WJ: Studies of the mortality of A-bomb survivors. 9. Mortality, 1950–1985: Part 2. Cancer mortality based on the recently revised doses (DS86). Radiat Res 121:120, 1990.
9. Preston DL, Kusumi S, Tomonaga M et al: Cancer incidence in atomic bomb survivors. Part III. Leukemia, lymphoma and multiple myeloma, 1950–1987. Radiat Res 137:S68–S97, 1994.
10. Boice JD Jr, Day NE, Andersen A et al: Second cancers following radiation treatment for cervical cancer. An international collaboration among cancer registries. J Natl Cancer Inst 74:955, 1985.
11. Darby SC, Reeves G, Key T et al: Mortality in a cohort of women given X-ray therapy for metropathia haemorrhagica. Int J Cancer 56:793, 1994.
12. Boice JD Jr, Engholm G, Kleinerman RA et al: Radiation dose and second cancer risk in patients treated for cancer of the cervix. Radiat Res 116:3, 1988.
13. Inskip PD, Kleinerman RA, Stovall M et al: Leukemia, lymphoma, and multiple myeloma after pelvic radiotherapy for benign disease. Radiat Res 135:108, 1993.
14. Smith PG, Douglas AJ: Mortality of workers at the Sellafield plant of British Nuclear Fuels. BMJ 293:845, 1986.
15. Gilbert ES, Fry SA, Wiggs LD et al: Analyses of combined mortality data on workers at the Hanford Site, Oak Ridge National Laboratory, and Rocky Flats Nuclear Weapons Plant. Radiat Res 120:19, 1989.
16. Cardis E, Gilbert ES, Carpenter L et al: Effects of low doses and low dose rates of external ionizing radiation: Cancer mortality among nuclear industry workers in three countries. Radiat Res 142:117, 1995.
17. Wing S, Richardson D, Wolf S et al: A case control study of multiple myeloma at four nuclear facilities. Ann Epidemiol 10:144, 2000.
18. Eriksson M: Rheumatoid arthritis as a risk factor for multiple myeloma: A case-control study. Eur J Cancer 29A:259, 1993.
19. Boffetta P, Stellman SD, Garfinkel L: A case-control study of multiple myeloma nested in the American Cancer Society prospective study. Int J Cancer 43:554, 1989.
20. Cuzick J, De Stavola B: Multiple myeloma – a case-control study. Br J Cancer 57:516, 1988.
21. Friedman GD: Multiple myeloma: Relation to propoxyphene and other drugs, radiation and occupation. Int J Epidemiol 15:424, 1986.
22. Davis FG, Boice JD, Hrubec Z et al: Cancer mortality in a radiation-exposed cohort of Massachusetts tuberculosis patients. Cancer Res 49:6130, 1989.
23. Boice JD Jr, Morin MM, Glass AG et al: Diagnostic x-ray procedures and risk of leukemia, lymphoma, and multiple myeloma. JAMA 265:1290, 1991.
24. Herrinton LJ, Demers PA, Koepsell TD et al: Epidemiology of the M-component immunoglobulin types of multiple myeloma. Cancer Causes Control 4:83, 1993.
25. Flodin U, Fredriksson M, Persson B: Multiple myeloma and engine exhausts, fresh wood, and creosote: A case-referent study. Am J Ind Med 12:519, 1987.
26. Darby SC, Doll R, Gill SK et al: Long term mortality after a single treatment course with X-rays in patients treated for ankylosing spondylitis. Br J Cancer 55:179, 1987.

27. Weiss HA, Darby SC, Doll R: Cancer mortality following X-ray treatment for ankylosing spondylitis. Int J Cancer 59:327, 1994.

28. Lewis EB: Leukemia, multiple myeloma and aplastic anemia in American radiologists. Science 142:1492, 1963.

29. Matanoski GM, Seltser R, Sartwell PE et al: The current mortality rates of radiologists and other physician specialists: Specific causes of death. Am J Epidemiol 101:199, 1975.

30. Wang JX, Boice JD Jr, Li BX et al: Cancer among medical diagnostic x-ray workers in China. J Natl Cancer Inst 80:344, 1988.

31. Douglas AJ, Omar RZ, Smith PG: Cancer mortality and morbidity among workers at the Sellafield plant of British Nuclear Fuels. Br J Cancer 70:1232, 1994.

32. Omar RZ, Barber JA, Smith PG: Cancer mortality and morbidity among plutonium workers at the Sellafield plant of British Nuclear Fuels. Br J Cancer 79:1288, 1999.

33. Gilbert ES, Petersen GR, Buchanan JA: Mortality of workers at the Hanford site: 1945–1981. Health Phys 56:11, 1989.

34. Gilbert ES, Cragle DL, Wiggs LD: Updated analyses of combined mortality data for workers at the Hanford Site, Oak Ridge National Laboratory, and Rocky Flats Weapons Plant. Radiat Res 136:408, 1993.

35. Muirhead CR, Goodill AA, Haylock RG et al: Occupational radiation exposure and mortality: Second analysis of the National Registry for Radiation Workers. J Radiol Protect 19:3, 1999.

36. Darby SC, Kendall GM, Fell TP et al: A summary of mortality and incidence of cancer in men from the United Kingdom who participated in the United Kingdom's atmospheric nuclear weapon tests and experimental programmes. BMJ 296:332, 1988.

37. Pearce N, Prior I, Methven D et al: Follow up of New Zealand participants in British atmospheric nuclear weapons tests in the Pacific. Br Med J 300:1161, 1990.

38. Caldwell GG, Kelley D, Zack M et al: Mortality and cancer frequency among military nuclear test (Smoky) participants, 1957 through 1979. JAMA 250:620, 1983.

39. Lopez-Abente G, Aragones N, Pollan M et al: Leukemia, lymphomas, and myeloma mortality in the vicinity of nuclear power plants and nuclear fuel facilities in Spain. Cancer Epidemiol Biomarkers Prev 8:925, 1999.

40. Dousset M: Cancer mortality around La Hague nuclear facilities. Health Phys 56:875, 1989.

41. Cook-Mozaffari PJ, Darby SC, Doll R et al: Geographical variation in mortality from leukaemia and other cancers in England and Wales in relation to proximity to nuclear installations, 1969–78. Br J Cancer 59:476, 1989.

42. Jablon S, Hrubec Z, Boice JD et al: Cancer in Populations Living Near Nuclear Facilities. Vol. 1: Report and Summary. NIH Pub. No. 90-874. Washington DC, 1990.

43. Blair A, Zahm SH, Pearce NE et al: Clues to cancer etiology from studies of farmers. Scand J Work Environ Health 18:209, 1992.

44. Blair A, Zahm SH: Agricultural exposures and cancer. Environ Health Perspect 103(Suppl. 8):205, 1995.

45. Franceschi S, Barbone F, Bidoli E et al: Cancer risk in farmers: Results from a multi-site case-control study in north-eastern Italy. Int J Cancer 53:740, 1993.

46. Burmeister LF: Cancer in Iowa farmers: Recent results. Am J Ind Med 18:295, 1990.

47. Brown LM, Burmeister LF, Everett GD et al: Pesticide exposures and multiple myeloma in Iowa men. Cancer Causes Control 4:153, 1993.

48. Viel JF, Richardson ST: Lymphoma, multiple myeloma and leukaemia among French farmers in relation to pesticide exposure. Soc Sci Med 37:771, 1993.

49. Demers PA, Vaughan TL, Koepsell TD et al: A case-control study of multiple myeloma and occupation. Am J Ind Med 23:629, 1993.

50. Wiklund K, Dich J: Cancer risks among male farmers in Sweden. Eur J Cancer Prev 4:81, 1995.

51. Kristensen P, Andersen A, Irgens LM et al: Incidence and risk factors of cancer among men and women in Norwegian agriculture. Scand J Work Environ Health 22:14, 1996.

52. Pukkala E, Notkola V: Cancer incidence among Finnish farmers, 1979–93. Cancer Causes Control 8:25, 1997.

53. Cerhan JR, Cantor KP, Williamson K et al: Cancer mortality among Iowa farmers: Recent results, time trends, and lifestyle factors (United States). Cancer Causes Control 9:311, 1998.

54. Khuder SA, Mutgi AB: Meta-analyses of multiple myeloma and farming. Am J Ind Med 32:510, 1997.

55. Gallagher RP, Spinelli JJ, Elwood JM et al: Allergies and agricultural exposure as risk factors for multiple myeloma. Br J Cancer 48:853, 1983.

56. Alavanja MC, Rush GA, Stewart P et al: Proportionate mortality study of workers in the grain industry. J Natl Cancer Inst 78:247, 1987.

57. Flodin U, Fredriksson M, Persson B: Multiple myeloma and engine exhausts, fresh wood, and creosote: A case-referent study. Am J Ind Med 12:519, 1987.

58. Eriksson M, Karlsson M: Occupational and other environmental factors and multiple myeloma: A population based case-control study. Br J Ind Med 49:95, 1992.

59. Pearce NE, Smith AH, Howard JK et al: Case-control study of multiple myeloma and farming. Br J Cancer 54:493, 1986.

60. Nanni O, Falcini F, Buiatti E et al: Multiple myeloma and work in agriculture: Results of a case-control study in Forli, Italy. Cancer Causes Control 9:277, 1998.

61. Cocco P, Blair A, Congia P et al: Long-term health effects of the occupational exposure to DDT – a preliminary report. Ann N Y Acad Sci 837:246, 1997.

62. Cocco P, Kazerouni N, Zahm SH: Cancer mortality and environmental exposure to DDE in the United States. Environ Health Perspect 108:1, 2000.

63. Gallagher RP, Threlfall WJ: Cancer mortality in metal workers. Can Med Assoc J 129:1191, 1983.

64. Morris PD, Koepsell TD, Daling JR et al: Toxic substance exposure and multiple myeloma: A case-control study. J Natl Cancer Inst 76:987, 1986.

65. McLaughlin JK, Malker HS, Linet MS et al: Multiple myeloma and occupation in Sweden. Arch Environ Health 43:7, 1988.

66. Egedahl RD, Coppock E, Homik R: Mortality experience at a hydrometallurgical nickel refinery in Fort Saskatchewan, Alberta between 1954 and 1984. J Soc Occup Med 41:29, 1991.

67. Fritschi L, Siemiatycki J: Lymphoma, myeloma and occupation: Results of a case-control study. Int J Cancer 67:498, 1996.

68. Linet MS, Harlow SD, McLaughlin JK: A case-control study of multiple myeloma in whites: Chronic antigenic stimulation, occupation, and drug use. Cancer Res 47:2978, 1987.

69. Teta MJ, Ott MG: A mortality study of a research, engineering, and metal fabrication facility in western New York state. Am J Epidemiol 127:540, 1988.

70. Sorahan T, Cooke MA: Cancer mortality in a cohort of United Kingdom steel foundry workers: 1946–85. Br J Ind Med 46:74, 1989.

71. Heineman EF, Olsen JH, Pottern LM et al: Occupational risk factors for multiple myeloma among Danish men. Cancer Causes Control 3:555, 1992.

72. Andjelkovich D, Taulbee J, Blum S: Mortality of female workers in rubber manufacturing plant. J Occup Med 20:409, 1978.

73. Monson RR, Nakano KK: Mortality among rubber workers. II. Other employees. Am J Epidemiol 103:297, 1976.

74. Gustavsson P, Hogstedt C, Holmberg B: Mortality and incidence of cancer among Swedish rubber workers, 1952–1981. Scand J Work Environ Health 12:538, 1986.

75. Delzell E, Monson RR: Mortality among rubber workers: X. Reclaim workers. Am J Ind Med 7:307, 1985.

76. Matanoski G, Elliott E, Tao X et al: Lymphohematopoietic cancers and butadiene and styrene exposure in synthetic rubber manufacture. Ann N Y Acad Sci 837:157, 1997.

77. Kogevinas M, Sala M, Boffetta P et al: Cancer risk in the rubber industry: A review of the recent epidemiological evidence. Occup Environ Med 55:1, 1998.

78. Wong O, Trent LS, Whorton MD: An updated cohort mortality study of workers exposed to styrene in the reinforced plastics and composites industry. Occup Environ Med 51:386, 1994.

79. Divine BJ, Hartman CM: Mortality update of butadiene production workers. Toxicology 113:169, 1996.

80. Sathiakumar N, Delzell E, Hovinga M et al: Mortality from cancer and other causes of death among synthetic rubber workers. Occup Environ Med 55:230, 1998.

81. Blattner WA, Blair A, Mason TJ: Multiple myeloma in the United States, 1950–1975. Cancer 48:2547, 1981.

82. Demers PA, Boffetta P, Kogevinas M et al: Pooled reanalysis of cancer mortality among five cohorts of workers in wood-related industries. Scand J Work Environ Health 21:179, 1995.

83. Pottern LM, Heineman EF, Olsen JH et al: Multiple myeloma among Danish women: Employment history and workplace exposures. Cancer Causes Control 3:427, 1992.

84. Tollerud DJ, Brinton LA, Stone BJ et al: Mortality from multiple myeloma among North Carolina furniture workers. J Natl Cancer Inst 74:799, 1985.

85. Cuzick J, De Stavola BL: Autoimmune disorders and multiple myeloma [letter]. Int J Epidemiol 18:283, 1989.

86. La Vecchia C, Negri E, D'Avanzo B et al: Occupation and lymphoid neoplasms. Br J Cancer 60:385, 1989.

87. Linet MS, McLaughlin JK, Malker HS et al: Occupation and hematopoietic and lymphoproliferative malignancies among women: A linked registry study. J Occup Med 36:1187, 1994.

88. Miligi L, Seniori CA, Crosignani P et al: Occupational, environmental, and life-style factors associated with the risk of hematolymphopoietic malignancies in women. Am J Ind Med 36:60, 1999.

89. Delzell E, Grufferman S: Cancer and other causes of death among female textile workers, 1976–78. J Natl Cancer Inst 71:735, 1983.

90. Dubrow R, Gute DM: Cause-specific mortality among male textile workers in Rhode Island. Am J Ind Med 13:439, 1988.

91. Bethwaite PB, Pearce N, Fraser J: Cancer risks in painters: Study based on the New Zealand Cancer Registry. Br J Ind Med 47:742, 1990.

92. Firth HM, Herbison GP, Cooke KR et al: Male cancer mortality by occupation: 1973–86. N Z Med J 106:328, 1993.

93. Lundberg I: Mortality and cancer incidence among Swedish paint industry workers with long-term exposure to organic solvents. Scand J Work Environ Health 12:108, 1986.

94. Lundberg I, Milatou-Smith R: Mortality and cancer incidence among Swedish paint industry workers with long-term exposure to organic solvents. Scand J Work Environ Health 24:270, 1998.

95. Petralia SA, Dosemeci M, Adams EE et al: Cancer mortality among women employed in health care occupations in 24 U.S. states, 1984–1993. Am J Ind Med 36:159, 1999.

96. Burnett C, Robinson C, Walker J: Cancer mortality in health and science technicians. Am J Ind Med 36:155, 1999.

97. Robinson CF, Walker JT: Cancer mortality among women employed in fast-growing U.S. occupations. Am J Ind Med 36:186, 1999.

98. Fillmore CM, Petralia SA, Dosemeci M: Cancer mortality in women with probable exposure to silica: A death certificate study in 24 states of the U.S. Am J Ind Med 36:122, 1999.

99. Battista G, Belli S, Comba P et al: Mortality due to asbestos-related causes among railway carriage construction and repair workers. Occup Med 49:536, 1999.

100. Metayer C, Johnson ES, Rice JC: Nested case-control study of tumors of the hemopoietic and lymphatic systems among workers in the meat industry. Am J Epidemiol 147:727, 1998.

101. Baris D, Garrity T, Telles JL, Heineman EF, Olshan A, Zahm SH: A cohort mortality study of Philadelphia firefighters. Am J Ind Med 39:463, 2001.

102. Bezabeh S, Engel A, Morris CB et al: Does benzene cause multiple myeloma? An analysis of the published case-control literature. Environ Health Perspect 104(Suppl. 6):1393, 1996.

103. Bergsagel DE, Wong O, Bergsagel PL et al: Benzene and multiple myeloma: Appraisal of the scientific evidence. Blood 94:1174, 1999.

104. Goldstein BD, Shalat SL: The causal relation between benzene exposure and multiple myeloma [letter; comment]. Blood 95:1512, 2000.

105. Decoufle P, Blattner WA, Blair A: Mortality among chemical workers exposed to benzene and other agents. Environ Res 30:16, 1983.

106. Goldstein BD: Is exposure to benzene a cause of human multiple myeloma? Ann N Y Acad Sci 609:225, 1990.

107. Sans S, Elliott P, Kleinschmidt I et al: Cancer incidence and mortality near the Baglan Bay petrochemical works, South Wales. Occup Environ Med 52:217, 1995.

108. Divine BJ, Hartman CM, Wendt JK: Update of the Texaco mortality study 1947–93: Part II. Analyses of specific causes of death for white men employed in refining, research, and petrochemicals. Occup Environ Med 56:174, 1999.

109. Dement JM, Hensley L, Kieding S et al: Proportionate mortality among union members employed at three Texas refineries. Am J Ind Med 33:327, 1998.

110. Raabe GK, Collingwood KS, Wong O: An updated mortality study of workers at a petroleum refinery in Beaumont, Texas. Am J Ind Med 33:61, 1998.

111. Schnatter AR, Armstrong TW, Nicolich MJ et al: Lympho-haematopoietic malignancies and quantitative estimates of exposure to benzene in Canadian petroleum distribution workers. Occup Environ Med 53:773, 1996.

112. Hayes RB, Yin SN, Dosemeci M et al: Benzene and the dose-related incidence of hematologic neoplasms in China. Chinese Academy of Preventive Medicine – National Cancer Institute Benzene Study Group. J Natl Cancer Inst 89:1065, 1997.

113. Lewis RJ, Schnatter AR, Katz AM et al: Updated mortality among diverse operating segments of a petroleum company. Occup Environ Med 57:595, 2000.

114. Wong O, Raabe GK: Multiple myeloma and benzene exposure in a multinational cohort of more than 250,000 petroleum workers. Regul Toxicol Pharmacol 26:188, 1997.

115. Hagmar L, Bellander T, Englander V et al: Mortality and cancer morbidity among workers in a chemical factory. Scand J Work Environ Health 12:545, 1986.

116. Ott MG, Teta MJ, Greenberg HL: Assessment of exposure to chemicals in a complex work environment. Am J Ind Med 16:617, 1989.

117. Burchfiel CM, Cartmill JB, Axe FD et al: General mortality and respiratory cancer among a cohort of male chemical workers in California. Am J Ind Med 22:69, 1992.

118. Bond GG, McLaren EA, Cartmill JB et al: Cause-specific mortality among male-chemical workers. Am J Ind Med 12:353, 1987.

119. Massoudi BL, Talbott EO, Day RD et al: A case-control study of hematopoietic and lymphoid neoplasms: The role of work in the chemical industry. Am J Ind Med 31:21, 1997.

120. Bertazzi PA, Zocchetti C, Guercilena S et al: Dioxin exposure and cancer risk: A 15-year mortality study after the "Seveso accident." Epidemiology 8:646, 1997.

121. Svensson BG, Mikoczy Z, Stromberg U et al: Mortality and cancer incidence among Swedish fishermen with a high dietary intake of persistent organochlorine compounds. Scand J Work Environ Health 21:106, 1995.

122. Schwartz GG: Multiple myeloma: Clusters, clues, and dioxins. Cancer Epidemiol Biomarkers Prev 6:49, 1997.

123. Spirtas R, Stewart PA, Lee JS et al: Retrospective cohort mortality study of workers at an aircraft maintenance facility. I. Epidemiological results. Br J Ind Med 48:515, 1991.

124. Blair A, Hartge P, Stewart PA et al: Mortality and cancer incidence of aircraft maintenance workers exposed to trichloroethylene and other organic solvents and chemicals: Extended follow up. Occup Environ Med 55:161, 1998.

125. Raffn E, Lynge E, Juel K et al: Incidence of cancer and mortality among employees in the asbestos cement industry in Denmark. Br J Ind Med 46:90, 1989.

126. Schwartz DA, Vaughan TL, Heyer NJ et al: B cell neoplasms and occupational asbestos exposure. Am J Ind Med 14:661, 1988.

127. Adami J, Nyren O, Bergstrom R et al: Smoking and the risk of leukemia, lymphoma, and multiple myeloma (Sweden). Cancer Causes Control 9:49, 1998.

128. Brown LM, Everett GD, Gibson R et al: Smoking and risk of non-Hodgkin's lymphoma and multiple myeloma. Cancer Causes Control 3:49, 1992.

129. Brown LM, Pottern LM, Silverman DT et al: Multiple myeloma among blacks and whites in the United States: Role of cigarettes and alcoholic beverages. Cancer Causes Control 8:610, 1997.

130. Brownson RC: Cigarette smoking and risk of myeloma. J Natl Cancer Inst 83:1036, 1991.

131. Friedman GD: Cigarette smoking, leukemia, and multiple myeloma. Ann Epidemiol 3:425, 1993.

132. Gramenzi A, Buttino I, D'Avanzo B et al: Medical history and the risk of multiple myeloma. Br J Cancer 63:769, 1991.

133. Heineman EF, Zahm SH, McLaughlin JK et al: A prospective study of tobacco use and multiple myeloma: Evidence against an association. Cancer Causes Control 3:31, 1992.

134. Mills PK, Newell GR, Beeson WL et al: History of cigarette smoking and risk of leukemia and myeloma: Results from the Adventist health study. J Natl Cancer Inst 82:1832, 1990.

135. Williams RR, Horm JW: Association of cancer sites with tobacco and alcohol consumption and socioeconomic status of patients: Interview study from the Third National Cancer Survey. J Natl Cancer Inst 58:525, 1977.

136. Brown LM, Gibson R, Burmeister LF et al: Alcohol consumption and risk of leukemia, non-Hodgkin's lymphoma, and multiple myeloma. Leuk Res 16:979, 1992.

137. Brown LM, Everett GD, Burmeister LF et al: Hair dye use and multiple myeloma in white men. Am J Public Health 82:1673, 1992.

138. Herrinton LJ, Weiss NS, Koepsell TD et al: Exposure to hair-coloring products and the risk of multiple myeloma. Am J Public Health 84:1142, 1994.

139. Zahm SH, Weisenburger DD, Babbitt PA et al: Use of hair coloring products and the risk of lymphoma, multiple myeloma, and chronic lymphocytic leukemia. Am J Public Health 82:990, 1992.

140. Altekruse SF, Henley SJ, Thun MJ: Deaths from hematopoietic and other cancers in relation to permanent hair dye use in a large prospective study (United States). Cancer Causes Control 10:617, 1999.

141. Thun MJ, Altekruse SF, Namboodiri MM et al: Hair dye use and risk of fatal cancers in U.S. women. J Natl Cancer Inst 86:210, 1994.

142. Grodstein F, Hennekens CH, Colditz GA et al: A prospective study of permanent hair dye use and hematopoietic cancer. J Natl Cancer Inst 86:1466, 1994.

143. Guidotti S, Wright WE, Peters JM: Multiple myeloma in cosmetologists. Am J Ind Med 3:169, 1982.

144. Spinelli JJ, Gallagher RP, Band PR et al: Multiple myeloma, leukemia, and cancer of the ovary in cosmetologists and hairdressers. Am J Ind Med 6:97, 1984.

145. Teta MJ, Walrath J, Meigs JW et al: Cancer incidence among cosmetologists. J Natl Cancer Inst 72:1051, 1984.

146. Friedman GD, Herrinton LJ: Obesity and multiple myeloma. Cancer Causes Control 5:479, 1994.

147. Brown LM, Gridley G, Pottern LM et al: Diet and nutrition as risk factors for multiple myeloma among blacks and whites in the United States. Cancer Causes Control 12:117, 2000.

148. Chatenoud L, Tavani A, La Vecchia C et al: Whole grain food intake and cancer risk. Int J Cancer 77:24, 1998.

149. Fernandez E, Chatenoud L, La Vecchia C et al: Fish consumption and cancer risk. Am J Clin Nutr 70:85, 1999.

150. Tavani A, Pregnolato A, Negri E et al: Diet and risk of lymphoid neoplasms and soft tissue sarcomas. Nutr Cancer 27:256, 1997.

151. Baris D, Brown LM, Silverman DT et al: Socioeconomic status and multiple myeloma among US blacks and whites. Am J Public Health 90:1277, 2000.

152. Koessel SL, Theis MK, Vaughan TL et al: Socioeconomic status and the incidence of multiple myeloma. Epidemiology 7:4, 1996.

153. Johnston JM, Grufferman S, Bourguet CC et al: Socioeconomic status and risk of multiple myeloma. J Epidemiol Community Health 39:175, 1985.

154. Nandakumar A, Armstrong BK, de Klerk NH: Multiple myeloma in western Australia: A case-control study in relation to occupation, father's occupation, socioeconomic status and country of birth. Int J Cancer 37:223, 1986.

155. Vagero D, Persson G: Occurrence of cancer in socioeconomic groups in Sweden. Scand J Soc Med 14:151, 1989.

156. Velez R, Beral V, Cuzick J: Increasing trends of multiple myeloma mortality in England and Wales, 1950–79: Are the changes real? J Natl Cancer Inst 69:387, 1982.

157. Doody MM, Linet MS, Glass AG et al: Risks of non-Hodgkin's lymphoma, multiple myeloma, and leukemia associated with common medications. Epidemiology 7:131, 1996.

158. Selby JV, Friedman GD, Fireman BH: Screening prescription drugs for possible carcinogenicity: Eleven to fifteen years of follow-up. Cancer Res 49:5736, 1989.

159. Malik TQ, Cawley JC, Finn R: The relationship between chronic drug ingestion and multiple myeloma [letter]. Leukemia 9:2158, 1995.

160. Kyle RA, Lust JA: Monoclonal gammopathies of undetermined significance. Semin Hematol 26:176, 1989.

161. Gregersen H, Mellemkjaer L, Salling IJ et al: Cancer risk in patients with monoclonal gammopathy of undetermined significance. Am J Hematol 63:1, 2000.

162. Pasqualetti P, Festuccia V, Collacciani A et al: The natural history of monoclonal gammopathy of undetermined significance. A 5- to 20-year follow-up of 263 cases. Acta Haematol 97:174, 1997.

163. Kyle RA, Rajkumar SV: Monoclonal gammopathies of undetermined significance. Hematol Oncol Clin North Am 13:1181, 1999.

164. Herrinton LJ, Weiss NS, Olshan AF: Multiple myeloma. In Schottenfeld D, Fraumeni JF Jr (eds.): Cancer Epidemiology and Prevention. Oxford University Press, New York, 1996.

165. Bourguet CC, Logue EE: Antigenic stimulation and multiple myeloma. A prospective study. Cancer 72:2148, 1993.

166. Lewis DR, Pottern LM, Brown LM et al: Multiple myeloma among blacks and whites in the United States: The role of chronic antigenic stimulation. Cancer Causes Control 5:529, 1994.

167. Hakulinen T, Isomaki HA, Knekt P: Multiple tumor incidence in patients with rheumatoid arthritis or allied disorders. J Chronic Dis 38:775, 1985.

168. Katusic S, Beard CM, Kurland LT et al: Occurrence of malignant neoplasms in the Rochester, Minnesota, rheumatoid arthritis cohort. Am J Med 78:50, 1985.

169. Cibere J, Sibley J, Haga M: Rheumatoid arthritis and the risk of malignancy. Arthritis Rheum 40:1580, 1997.

170. Cohen HJ, Bernstein RJ, Grufferman S: Role of immune stimulation in the etiology of multiple myeloma: A case control study. Am J Hematol 24:119, 1987.

171. Gridley G, McLaughlin JK, Ekbom A et al: Incidence of cancer among patients with rheumatoid arthritis. J Natl Cancer Inst 85:307, 1993.

172. Mellemkjaer L, Linet MS, Gridley G et al: Rheumatoid arthritis and cancer risk. Eur J Cancer 32A:1753, 1996.

173. Doody MM, Linet MS, Glass AG et al: Leukemia, lymphoma, and multiple myeloma following selected medical conditions. Cancer Causes Control 3:449, 1992.

174. Koepsell TD, Daling JR, Weiss NS et al: Antigenic stimulation and the occurrence of multiple myeloma. Am J Epidemiol 126:1051, 1987.

175. Goedert JJ, Cote TR, Virgo P et al: Spectrum of AIDS-associated malignant disorders. Lancet 351:1833, 1998.

176. Beral V, Newton R: Overview of the Epidemiology of immunodeficiency-associated cancers. J Natl Cancer Inst Monogr 1, 1998.

177. Sjak-Shie NN, Vescio RA, Berenson JR: The role of human herpesvirus-8 in the pathogenesis of multiple myeloma. Hematol Oncol Clin North Am 13:1159, 1999.

178. Grulich AE, Wan X, Law MG et al: Risk of cancer in people with AIDS. AIDS 13:839, 1999.

179. Rettig MB, Ma HJ, Vescio RA et al: Kaposi's sarcoma-associated herpesvirus infection of bone marrow dendritic cells from multiple myeloma patients. Science 276:1851, 1997.

180. Chauhan D, Bharti A, Raje N et al: Detection of Kaposi's sarcoma herpesvirus DNA sequences in multiple myeloma bone marrow stromal cells. Blood 93:1482, 1999.

181. Olsen SJ, Tarte K, Sherman W et al: Evidence against KSHV infection in the pathogenesis of multiple myeloma. Virus Res 57:197, 1998.

182. Rask C, Kelsen J, Olesen G et al: Danish patients with untreated multiple myeloma do not harbour human herpesvirus 8. Br J Haematol 108:96, 2000.

183. Sitas F, Carrara H, Beral V et al: Antibodies against human herpesvirus 8 in black South African patients with cancer. N Engl J Med 340:1863, 1999.

184. Bourguet CC, Grufferman S, Delzell E et al: Multiple myeloma and family history of cancer. A case-control study. Cancer 56:2133, 1985.

185. Brown LM, Linet MS, Greenberg RS et al: Multiple myeloma and family history of cancer among blacks and whites in the U.S. Cancer 85:2385, 1999.

186. Crozes-Bony P, Palazzo E, Meyer O et al: Familial multiple myeloma. Report of a case in a father and daughter. Review of the literature. Rev Rhum Engl Ed 62:439, 1995.

187. Eriksson M, Hallberg B: Familial occurrence of hematologic malignancies and other diseases in multiple myeloma: A case-control study. Cancer Causes Control 3:63, 1992.

188. Grosbois B, Jego P, Attal M et al: Familial multiple myeloma: Report of fifteen families. Br J Haematol 105:768, 1999.

189. Shpilberg O, Modan M, Modan B et al: Familial aggregation of haematological neoplasms: A controlled study. Br J Haematol 87:75, 1994.

190. Shoenfeld Y, Berliner S, Shaklai M et al: Familial multiple myeloma. A review of thirty-seven families. Postgrad Med J 58:12, 1982.

191. Anderson KC, Lust JA: Role of cytokines in multiple myeloma. Semin Hematol 36:14, 1999.

192. Klein B, Lu ZY, Gu ZJ et al: Interleukin-10 and Gp130 cytokines in human multiple myeloma. Leuk Lymphoma 34:63, 1999.

193. Lust JA, Donovan KA: The role of interleukin-1 beta in the pathogenesis of multiple myeloma. Hematol Oncol Clin North Am 13:1117, 1999.

194. Avet-Loiseau H, Li JY, Morineau N et al: Monosomy 13 is associated with the transition of monoclonal gammopathy of undetermined significance to multiple myeloma. Intergroupe Francophone du Myelome. Blood 94:2583, 1999.

195. Calasanz MJ, Cigudosa JC, Odero MD et al: Cytogenetic analysis of 280 patients with multiple myeloma and related disorders: Primary breakpoints and clinical correlations. Genes Chromosom Cancer 18:84, 1997.

196. Sawyer JR, Waldron JA, Jagannath S et al: Cytogenetic findings in 200 patients with multiple myeloma. Cancer Genet Cytogenet 82:41, 1995.

197. Taniwaki M, Nishida K, Takashima T et al: Nonrandom chromosomal rearrangements of 14q32.3 and 19p13.3 and preferential deletion of 1p in 21 patients with multiple myeloma and plasma cell leukemia. Blood 84:2283, 1994.

198. Mazars GR, Portier M, Zhang XG et al: Mutations of the p53 gene in human myeloma cell lines. Oncogene 7:1015, 1992.

199. Ollikainen H, Syrjanen S, Koskela K et al: p53 gene mutations are rare in patients but common in patient-originating cell lines in multiple myeloma. Scand J Clin Lab Invest 57:281, 1997.

200. Avet-Loiseau H, Li JY, Godon C et al: P53 deletion is not a frequent event in multiple myeloma. Br J Haematol 106:717, 1999.

201. Schultheis B, Kramer A, Willer A et al: Analysis of p73 and p53 gene deletions in multiple myeloma. Leukemia 13:2099, 1999.

202. Linet MS, Devesa SS: Epidemiology of leukemia: Overview and patterns of occurrence. In Henderson E, Lister TA, Greaves MF (eds.). Leukemia. WB Saunders, Philadelphia, 2002.

203. Groves FD, Travis LB, Devesa SS: Cancer surveillance series: Non-Hodgkin's lymphoma incidence by histologic subtype in the United States from 1978 through 1995. J Natl Cancer Inst 92:1240, 2000.

27

Immunoglobulins and Laboratory Recognition of Monoclonal Proteins

Robert A. Kyle, Jerry A. Katzmann,
John A. Lust, and Angela Dispenzieri

IMMUNOGLOBULINS

Each monoclonal protein (M protein or myeloma protein) consists of two heavy polypeptide chains of the same class and subclass and two light polypeptide chains of the same type[1] (Table 27–1). Different kinds of monoclonal proteins are designated by capital letters that correspond to the class of their heavy chains, which are designated by Greek letters: γ in immunoglobulin G (IgG), α in immunoglobulin A (IgA), μ in immunoglobulin M (IgM), δ in immunoglobulin D (IgD), and ε in immunoglobulin E (IgE). Their subclasses are IgG1, IgG2, IgG3, IgG4, or IgA1 and IgA2, and their light chain types are kappa (κ) and lambda (λ).

A brief review of the history, structure, properties, and functions of immunoglobulins is necessary for an understanding of the monoclonal proteins.

In 1937, Tiselius,[2] using electrophoretic techniques, separated serum globulins into three components, which he designated α, β, and γ. Interestingly, this paper, which led to his Nobel Prize and later to the presidency of the Nobel Foundation, was rejected initially by *The Biochemical Journal*.[3] Electrophoresis was applied to the study of multiple myeloma by Longsworth et al.,[4] who demonstrated the tall, narrow-based "church-spire" peak. The method was cumbersome and diffi-

cult, so electrophoresis was not readily available until the early 1950s, when filter paper was introduced as a supporting medium (zone electrophoresis). Cellulose acetate then supplanted filter paper[5] and now electrophoresis is performed on agarose gel.

Before 1960, the term γ-globulin was used to designate those proteins that migrated in the γ-mobility region (toward the cathode) of the electrophoretic pattern. The γ-globulin level was increased by immunization and decreased when absorbed by exposure to the specific antigen. Later, it was recognized that some antibodies migrate in the fast γ-region and others in the slow γ-area and that some sediment in the ultracentrifuge as 7S and others as 19S molecules. It was not until late in the 1950s that the concept of a family of proteins with antibody activity was recognized. These proteins are now referred to as *immunoglobulins;* the five groups presently recognized and their properties are listed in Table 27–2.[6]

Immunoglobulin G

In normal serum, three-fourths of the immunoglobulin present is IgG. This class has a molecular weight of 150,000 and a sedimentation coefficient of 6.7S. Its electrophoretic mobility ranges from slow γ (cathodal region) to α_2. Many antibodies to both bacteria and viruses are of the IgG class.

A reducing agent such as mercaptoethanol disrupts the disulfide bonds linking the polypeptide chains of the IgG molecule. If the reduced protein is alkylated with iodoacetamide and is fractionated in the presence of a solvent (e.g., guanidine or urea) that is capable of dissociating noncovalent bonds, two kinds of polypeptide chains can be recovered: heavy (H) and light (L) (Figure 27–1).

Heavy Chains

Both heavy chains of the IgG molecule are of the γ-class, and the two light chains are alike—both κ or both λ. Each heavy chain has a molecular weight of approximately 55,000 and consists of 440 to 450 amino acids. Each has a variable (V_H) region in which many amino acid substitutes make each chain different

---

Table 27–1. Classification of Immunoglobulins of Normal Human Serum

	IgG	IgA	IgM	IgD	IgE
Heavy chain					
Classes	Gamma (γ)	Alpha (α)	Mu (μ)	Delta (δ)	Epsilon (ε)
Subclasses	IgG1, IgG2, IgG3, IgG4	IgA1, IgA2	None	None	None
Light chain types	Kappa, κ	κ	κ	κ	κ
	Lambda, λ	λ	λ	λ	λ
Molecular formula	$\gamma_2\kappa_2$	$\alpha_2\kappa_2$[a]	$(\mu_2\kappa_2)5$	$\delta_2\kappa_2$	$\varepsilon_2\kappa_2$
	$\gamma_2\lambda_2$	$\alpha_2\lambda_2$[a]	$(\mu_2\lambda_2)5$	$\delta_2\lambda_2$	$\varepsilon_2\lambda_2$
Designation	IgG-κ	IgA-κ	IgM-κ	IgD-κ	IgE-κ
	IgG-λ	IgA-λ	IgM-λ	IgD-λ	IgE-λ

[a] May form polymers.
(From Kyle and Bayrd,[1] with permission.)

Table 27-2. Properties of Immunoglobulins of Normal Human Serum

	IgG	IgA	IgM	IgD	IgE
Electrophoretic mobility	$\gamma-\alpha_2$	$\gamma-\beta$	$\gamma-\beta$	$\gamma-\beta$	$\gamma-\beta$
Sedimentation coefficient	6.7S	7–15S[a]	19S	7S	8S
Molecular weight	150,000	160,000–400,000[a]	900,000	180,000	200,000
Carbohydrate (percent)	2.6	5–10	10	10–12	11
T$^{1}/_{2}$, days	23	5.8	5.1	2.8	2.3
Serum concentration, mg/dl	700–1500	60–400	60–300	0–14	0.05
Percentage of total serum immunoglobulin	74	21	5	0.2	0.002
Percentage of total body pool in intravascular space	45	42	76	75	51
Percentage of intravascular pool catabolized per day (normal)	6.7	25	18	37	89
Normal synthetic rate, mg/kg/day	33	24	6.7	0.4	0.02
Fixes complement	IgG1 and IgG3; IgG2 variable	Alternate pathway	Yes	No	No
Crosses placenta	Yes	No	No	No	No

[a] Tends to form polymers of the monomer form.
(Modified from Kyle and Bayrd,[1] with permission.)

from the next, and a constant (C_H) region in which very few amino acid differences are found from one γ-chain to the next. The variable region of the γ-chain consists of approximately 110 amino acid residues, beginning at the amino (NH_2) terminal of the chain. The constant region of the γ-chain consists of 310 to 330 amino acids and contains three *homology regions* or *domains*, designated Cγ1, Cγ2, and Cγ3. Homology region Cγ1 is in the Fd fragment (Figure 27–1) and extends from about amino acid 110 to amino acid 220; Cγ2 and Cγ3 are in the Fc fragment (Figure 27–1), Cγ2 extending from approximately amino acid 220 to amino acid 330 and Cγ3 from there to the COOH terminus.

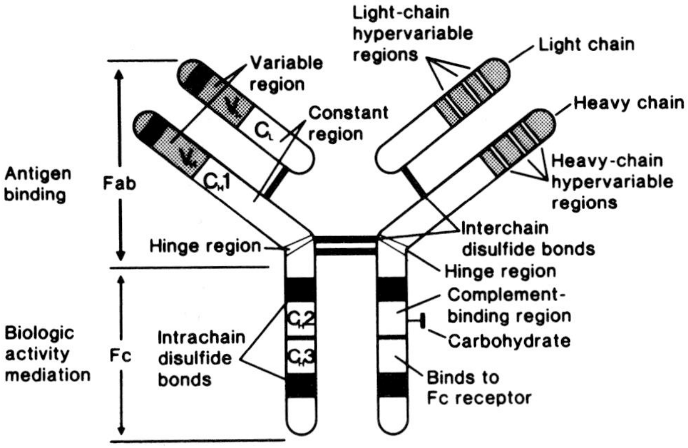

Immunological analysis of myeloma proteins has disclosed four distinct subclasses of γ-heavy chains, designated IgG1, IgG2, IgG3, and IgG4 (Tables 27–3 and 27–4). IgG catabolism is increased at high protein concentrations. At low IgG concentrations, most of the IgG is phagocytized into vesicles, where it is protected from catabolism. When the IgG concentration is high, most IgG molecules will not be bound and will be degraded, the result of which is a high catabolic rate.[7] The average biological half-life of IgG1, IgG2, and IgG4 myeloma proteins injected into patients with malignancies is 21 days, whereas IgG3 has a half-life of 7 to 8 days. This shorter time is probably due to its four-fold longer hinge region, which appears to be easily accessible to proteolytic enzymes. In addition, IgG3 contains a large number of disulfide bonds. A wide angle of 45 to 180 degrees in IgG3 indicates a mobile molecule. Although the hinge region in the IgG3 molecule is four times longer than that in IgG1, it exists in a compact state. In the extended confirmation, the hinge region

Figure 27–1. Schematic representation of immunoglobulin G (IgG) molecule, with cleavage by papain into Fab and Fc fragments. (Modified from Terhorst C, David J: Antigens, antibodies, and T cell receptors. p. 4. In Rubenstein E, Federman DD (eds.): Scientific American Medicine: Immunology 6. Vol. 2. Scientific American, New York, 1990, with permission.)

Table 27-3. Physicochemical Properties of IgG Subclasses

	IgG1	IgG2	IgG3	IgG4
Normal				
Percent IgG	70	20	6	4
mg/dl serum	5.4	2.1	0.58	0.6
Molecular weight of γ-chain	51,600	51,600	59,500	51,600
Isoelectric point	8.3–9.5	7–7.3	8.45–8.95	—
Inter-heavy chain disulfide bonds	2	4	5–13	2
Papain digestion	Sensitive	Resistant	Very sensitive	Resistant
Pepsin digestion	Resistant	Resistant	Sensitive	Sensitive

(Modified from Schur,[22] with permission.)

Table 27–4. Biologic Characteristics of IgG Subclasses

	IgG1	IgG2	IgG3	IgG4
Biologic half-life (days)	21	21	7	21
Human monocyte receptors	Yes	No	Yes	No
Fixation of complement	Yes	Variable	Yes	No
Reaction with staphylococcal A protein	Yes	Yes	No	Yes
Restricted antibody toward: isoagglutinins, Rh, diphtheria or tetanus toxoid, viruses (HIV, CMV)	Yes	No	No	No
Tetanus toxoid, teichoic acid, polysaccharides, lipopolysaccharides	No	Yes	No	No
Rh, viral neutralizing, HIV, CMV	No	No	Yes	No
Circulating anticoagulants, factors VIII and IX, phospholipase A	No	No	No	Yes

Abbreviations: HIV, human immunodeficiency virus; CMV, cytomegalovirus.
(Modified from Reynolds,[11] with permission.)

is 7 to 9 nm and the length of the intact molecule is only 25 nm.[8] IgG3 does not bind staphylococcal protein A except in rare cases.[9] IgG1 and IgG3 fix complement readily via the classic pathway, but IgG2 does so less well.

Although many antigens evoke an antibody response within the IgG subclasses proportional to their distribution in normal serum, others produce antibodies mainly within one subclass. For example, almost all antibodies to factor VIII (found in hemophilic persons, postpartum women, and elderly patients) are of the IgG4 subclass, while without predilection only 3 to 4 percent of the antibodies would be of this subclass.[10] Most antibodies to dextran, levan, and teichoic acid are of the IgG2 subclass. Antibodies developed against polysaccharide antigens are also primarily found in IgG2.[11]

Although it has been reported that the serum antiplatelet antibody was restricted to the IgG3 subclass in idiopathic thrombocytopenic purpura (ITP), all four IgG subclasses were bound to platelets of ITP patients in the same distribution as in normal serum.[12] Presumably, these differences represent nonspecific binding to platelets.

Among a group of patients with selective IgA deficiency, those with reduction of IgG2 had frequent respiratory infections, but those with normal IgG2 levels did not.[13] In 139 patients with isolated IgA deficiency and an increased susceptibility to infection, IgG4 deficiency was more common than in controls. Contrary to the prior study, there was no significant association between IgG subclass deficiency and increased susceptibility to infection.[14] IgG2 subclass deficiency is thought to be most important in protecting against bacterial sepsis.[15] In a series of 22 patients with ataxia-telangiectasia, very low or borderline-low serum IgG2 levels were found in all, and IgG4 was undetectable in 19 of the 22 patients. Nine of the patients with an undetectable or very low IgG2 level had chronic lung disease

or chronic sinusitis, or both.[16] In another series, 4 of 422 unselected patients were found to have an isolated absence of IgG4, as determined by a sensitive radioimmunoassay. All had severe recurrent sinopulmonary infections.[17] Others have suggested that deficiency of IgG3 is becoming more common and is more frequently associated with mild infections.[18] In a group of 89 patients with bronchiectasis, the IgG1, IgG2, and IgG3 levels were increased compared with controls. There was an overall incidence of deficiency of 1 percent for subclasses IgG1, 2, and 3 and 5 percent for IgG4. The authors concluded that IgG subclass deficiency was comparatively rare in bronchiectasis.[19]

We have found that the distribution of IgG subclasses did not differ among patients with multiple myeloma and those with monoclonal gammopathy of undetermined significance (MGUS; benign monoclonal gammopathy).[20] There was also no relationship between clinical and laboratory features in multiple myeloma of different subclass types. Patients with a monoclonal protein of different IgG subclasses have greatly different patterns of suppression. For example, patients with IgG2 monoclonal proteins are more likely to have repressed residual IgG than are patients with IgG3, IgG1, or IgG4.[21]

Radial immunodiffusion in agar with appropriate antisera is commonly used for semiquantitative concentrations of IgG subclasses in sera. However, assay kits based on radial immunodiffusion lack accuracy. Interlaboratory correlation and interbatch reproducibility are poor. In addition, because monoclonal antibody-containing enzyme-linked immunosorbent assays (ELISA) kits may have a higher affinity for λ than for κ, erroneous results are produced.[18] Nephelometry is now commonly used for quantitation of IgG subclasses. These procedures are similar to those used for IgG, IgA, and IgM assays, and they are rapid and reliable. Extensive reviews of IgG subclass deficiency have been published.[22–24]

Light Chains

Historically, the light chains were encountered in 1845, when Macintyre[25] and Henry Bence Jones[26] noted that the urine of a patient with multiple myeloma precipitated when heated, cleared when boiled, and reprecipitated when cooled. In 1962, Edelman and Gally[27] demonstrated that the light chains prepared from a serum IgG myeloma protein and the Bence Jones protein from the same patient's urine not only had the same thermal solubility but also had similar spectrofluorometric behavior, the same molecular weight, identical appearance on chromatography with carboxymethylcellulose and on starch-gel electrophoresis after reduction and alkylation, the same ultracentrifugal pattern, and the same amino acid sequence. Thus, it was found that the urinary proteins that evoked such interest from Macintyre and Bence Jones were the light chain components of the immunoglobulin molecule.

Two distinct groups of Bence Jones proteins (group I and group II) were recognized by Bayne-Jones and Wilson[28] in 1922. In 1956, two major classes of Bence Jones proteins were described by Korngold and Lipari,[29] and these have been designated κ and λ. Approximately two-thirds of serum IgG monoclonal proteins are of the κ-type and the remainder are λ. In patients with Waldenström's macroglobulinemia, approximately 80 percent are κ, but the opposite occurs in IgD myeloma, in which 60 percent are λ.[30]

The light chains (Bence Jones proteins) have a molecular weight of 22,500 and contain 210 to 220 amino acids. Analysis of amino acid sequence in individual light chains has disclosed a constant and a variable domain. The region of the chain from amino acid 107 to the COOH terminus at position 210 to 220 is very similar in chains of the same type (κ or λ) and has been designated as the constant domain (C_L)—although amino acid substitutions have been found at a dozen different positions in the constant region of human λ chains.[31] The region from the NH_2 terminus (position 1) to approximately position 107 has been different in every light chain thus far analyzed, and it is called the variable domain (V_L). The variable half of the light chain contains the unique thermal solubility characteristics of Bence Jones proteins.[32]

The amino acid differences in the constant domain of the light chains can be related to certain allotypic markers. In human κ-chains, if the amino acid leucine is at position 191, the protein is inv(1) or inv(2), whereas if valine is at this position, the light chain is inv(3). Inv(1) has valine at position 153; the others have alanine. Of the White population who have the inv(1) antigen, 98 percent also have the inv(2) antigen. By contrast, no genetic factors have been identified for human λ-chains. The isotypic markers in these chains include Oz(+) if lysine is at position 193 and Oz(−) if arginine is present. Another marker in λ-chains has been designated Kern(+) when glycine is present at position 156 and Kern(−) when serine is there. Another variant, Mcg, has threonine instead of glycine at position 103.[33,34]

Amino acid sequence studies have revealed four basic groups of κ-light chains, designated κI, κII, κIII, and κIV.[35] Their frequencies of occurrence are approximately 60, 10, 28, and 2 percent, respectively, and as expected, these figures reflect the proportion of κI, κII, κIII, and κIV light chains in immunoglobulins of normal serum.[34] In a series of 23 patients with acquired Fanconi syndrome, 96 percent had a monoclonal κ-protein.[36] In another series, eight of nine patients with acquired Fanconi syndrome had κ1-subtype.[37] In light chain deposition disease, the light chain is κ in 90 percent of patients, but the κIV subclass is overrepresented.[38,39] Six subclasses of λ have been reported with the following distribution: λI, 26 percent; λII/λV, 38 percent; λIII, 22 percent; λIV, 3 percent; and λVI, 11 percent.[40] There is a preferential association of λVI subclass with primary systemic amyloidosis (AL).[41] In fact, with rare exceptions, all patients with λVI subclass have amyloidosis.

Ordinarily κ-chains are in the monomeric form (molecular weight 22,500), but they may exist as noncovalently linked dimers or as a mixture of monomers and dimers, whereas λ-proteins occur as dimers (molecular weight 45,000) linked covalently via their penultimate cysteinyl residues.[34] In addition, κ-light chains precipitate maximally over a narrower range of pH than do λ-light chains.[42] Recognition of light chains as κ or λ by monospecific antisera depends on the variable and constant domains as well as the interdomain "switch" region between the variable and the constant regions.[43]

Bence Jones proteins are synthesized de novo in plasma cells and are not degradation products of the complete immunoglobulin in the serum. Putnam and Hardy[44] showed that ^{13}C-labeled

Table 27–5. IgG Light and Heavy Chains

Property	Light	Heavy
Molecular weight	22,500	55,000
Carbohydrate	None	Present
Classes	κ, λ	IgG1, IgG2
		IgG3, IgG4
Allotypes		
Km (1), Km (2), Km (3) [InV]	Cκ	Absent
Isotypes		
Mcg (22 percent)	Cλl	Absent
Kern (18 percent)	CλII	Absent
Oz (25 percent)	CλIII	Absent
Gm markers	Absent	Present
Relationship to Bence Jones protein	Same	Unrelated

glycine is incorporated promptly into Bence Jones protein and cannot be the result of breakdown of serum or other tissue protein. Light chains clearly are catabolized by the kidney. After injection into mice, ^{131}I-labeled Bence Jones proteins of humans were cleared rapidly from the circulation. Ligating and severing the ureters lengthened the disappearance time only slightly, but removal of the kidneys greatly prolonged the survival of light chains, a finding indicating the major role of renal catabolism. Human IgG was not cleared by the kidney in the same experiments.[45] The properties of light and heavy chains are shown in Table 27–5.

Fab and Fc Fragments

Treatment of IgG with a proteolytic enzyme, papain, cleaves it into three pieces: two Fab fragments, so named because they possess antigen-binding activity, and an Fc fragment, because in certain species it can be crystallized (Figures 27–1 and 27–2). Each Fab fragment (molecular weight 52,000) consists of the amino terminal region of a heavy chain and a complete light chain. The hinge region, consisting of 15 amino acid residues between Cγp1 and Cγ2, is a flexible junction between Fab and Fc fragments. This hinge permits the angle between the Fab fragments to vary from a few degrees to almost 180 degrees.

Three regions of "hypervariability" have been identified in V_L: positions 24 to 34, 50 to 56, and 89 to 97.[46] This hypervariability and the existence of similar hypervariable regions in the variable region of the heavy chain (V_H) in positions 30 to 37, 51 to 68, 84 to 91, and 101 to 110 permit the formation of many different antigen-combining sites—each consisting of approximately 30 amino acid residues.[47] These hypervariable regions constitute the antigen binding site, and the three segments are called complementarity-determining regions, or CDRs (CDR1, CDR2, and CDR3).

The Fc fragment (molecular weight 48,000) consists of the C-terminal region of both heavy chains, which are linked to each other by disulfide bonds. Biological activities of the Fc fragment include fixation of complement; passive cutaneous anaphylaxis (PCA); binding with rheumatoid factors; binding with receptors on macrophages, monocytes, neutrophils, and

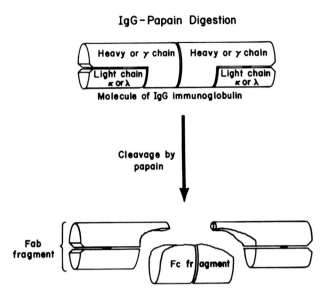

IgG-Papain Digestion

Figure 27–2. Schematic representation of immunoglobulin G (IgG) molecule, showing Fab and Fc fragments. (From Kyle and Bayrd,[1] with permission.)

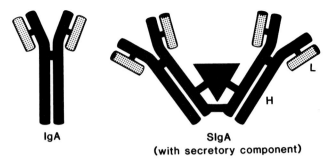

Figure 27–3. Schematic representation of immunoglobulin A (IgA) and secretory IgA (SIgA) molecules (L, light chain; H, heavy chain). (From Kyle et al.,[6] with permission.)

lymphocytes; reaction with staphylococcal A protein; and transfer across the placenta. Isotypic specificity—specificity for γ, α, μ, δ, or ε—resides in the Fc fragment. The Fc piece is devoid of antibody activity.

Gm Factors

The genetic factors associated with IgG are present on the C region of γ-chains and are referred to as *Gm factors* or determinants.[48] If one coats an Rh-positive red cell with an incomplete Rh antibody, the addition of rheumatoid serum (anti-γ-globulin) results in agglutination. Serum that prevents agglutination is called Gm+. By alteration of the coating of the red cell and the agglutinating serum, more than 20 Gm factors can be distinguished. Individual Gm factors are associated with individual subclasses of IgG; numerous Gm determinants are present on IgG1 and IgG3, but few on the other two subclasses.

Immunoglobulin A

Two identical heavy α-chains and two identical light chains (both κ or both λ) form IgA[49] (Figure 27–3). IgA has a molecular weight of 160,000 and a sedimentation coefficient of 7S, but it also has a propensity to form polymers with sedimentation coefficients of 9S to 15S. Concentration of IgA polymers correlates directly with the serum viscosity.[50] Its catabolic rate of 5.8 days (T 1/2) is greater than that of IgG. Aggregated IgA can fix the late components of complement, beginning with C3 (alternate pathway).

There are two subgroups of the α-chain, α1 and α2, and the consequence is IgA1 and IgA2 proteins. Approximately 90 percent of monoclonal IgA proteins are of the IgA1 class. IgA2 molecules are unique among the immunoglobulins in that the light chains are bound to the α-chains by noncovalent forces instead of disulfide bonds. In a series of 20 previously healthy

persons, 1.37 percent of all bone marrow plasma cells stained with IgA. The mean percentage of cells staining was 1.19 percent for IgA1 and 0.19 percent for IgA2. The cells containing IgA1 constituted 85.7 percent of all cells that stained for total IgA. All IgA cells represented mature, normal-appearing plasma cells.[51] Almost 90 percent of all patients with IgA multiple myeloma and nonmyelomatous paraproteins have IgA1. Thus, the distribution of IgA subclasses is the same in both malignant and benign monoclonal gammopathies.[52] The subclasses IgA1 and IgA2 are similar in French and Japanese patients—94.8 percent of the French and 91 percent of the Japanese were IgA1 in one study.[53]

IgA2 has been found in the glomerular deposits of primary IgA nephropathy, in glomerulonephritis accompanying alcoholic cirrhosis, and in nephritis from Henoch-Schönlein purpura, whereas a preponderance of IgA1 is associated with lupus nephritis.[54] In contrast, as recently reported, oversialylation of polymeric IgA1 may play a role in the pathogenesis of IgA nephropathy.[55] IgA deficiency occurs in two-thirds of patients with ataxia-telangiectasia.[56] Patients with IgA monoclonal gammopathies may produce false-positive reactions of IgA anticardiolipin and anti-β2-glycoprotein I antibodies.[57]

The daily production of IgA is approximately that of IgG, but the serum concentration is lower because of the greater catabolism of IgA.[58] Monomeric serum IgA may protect endogenous antigens expressed on various cells and tissues by preventing their interaction with humoral and cellular immune mechanisms that may lead to tissue damage.[59] A major source of monomeric IgA is the bone marrow. Spleen cells also produce predominantly monomeric IgA. Production of IgA begins at 4 weeks after birth and approaches the adult level at 1 year. No significant changes in concentration occur during adulthood. Cunningham-Rundles[60] provided an extensive review of the genetic aspects of IgA deficiency.

Secretory Immunoglobulin A

Secretory IgA (SIgA) (Figure 27–3) is found in high concentration in the secretions of many glands lining the respiratory and gastrointestinal tracts and in tears, colostrum, and urine. SIgA has a sedimentation coefficient of 11S and a molecular weight of 390,000. It is composed of two IgA molecules attached by disulfide bonds to a glycoprotein (molecular weight 60,000 to 80,000) called the *secretory component.* Secretory component increases the resistance of the molecules against digestion by trypsin and pepsin. The secretory component is synthesized in mucosal epithelial cells. In one unusual case, cancer cells from bronchogenic adenocarcinoma produced large amounts of secretory component, resulting in high serum levels of SIgA.[61] Serum IgA does not make a significant contribution to IgA in gastrointestinal fluids.[62]

In both the gastrointestinal and respiratory tracts, dimeric IgA with J chain (described in the next section) is synthesized in plasma cells and secreted, after which it combines with secretory component on the epithelial cell surface. SIgA is then transported through the cytoplasm in endocytic vesicles to the luminal surface.[63]

SIgA exhibits antibacterial and antiviral activity, and evidence indicates the SIgA antibodies are stimulated preferentially by upper respiratory tract infections. SIgA has a neutralizing effect on viral replication.[64]

In secretions, IgA prevents microorganisms and foreign proteins from adhering to and penetrating the mucosal surfaces.[62] SIgA provides the most potent immunoglobulin signal for the degranulation of eosinophils. It may be the principal immunoglobulin that mediates eosinophil effector function at mucosal surfaces.[65]

In contrast to that in serum IgA, approximately 50 percent of SIgA is of the IgA2 subclass. Approximately 95 percent of IgA in secretions is polymeric, whereas 90 percent of serum IgA is monomeric. A patient with no free secretory component in the saliva and chronic intestinal candidiasis has been described.[66]

The intestinal lamina propria cells produce the largest amount of polymeric IgA.[67] In a patient with pronounced serum IgA deficiency, most of the serum IgA was monomeric and from tonsillar IgA-producing cells.[68]

Joining Chains

The joining (J) chain is a nonimmunoglobulin protein with a molecular weight of approximately 15,000.[69] It is bound by disulfide bridges to the Fc portion of the heavy chain and thus forms the dimers or polymers of IgA and the pentamer structure of IgM. It is never found in IgG or in monomers of IgA proteins, and yet J chain is found in cells secreting IgG. Only one J chain is present in each polymer of IgA or pentamer of IgM. The J chain of IgM is identical to that of IgA. The lack of J chain reduces the ability of IgAl to bind secretory component and interferes with the epithelial transport of polymeric IgA.[70]

Immunoglobulin M

A third immunoglobulin, IgM, is composed of subunits linked by disulfide bonds[71,72] (Figure 27–4). The heavy chain (μ) of IgM has a molecular weight of approximately 70,000. Two such heavy chains and two light chains form an IgM subunit, which has a molecular weight of approximately 180,000 to 190,000. Since the molecular weight of IgM is approximately 900,000, it evidently comprises five subunits. The pentamer is assembled in the rough endoplasmic reticulum of plasma cells.[73] The μ-chain

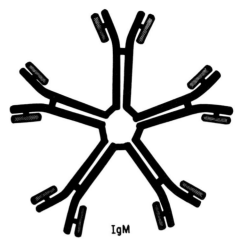

Figure 27–4. Schematic representation of immunoglobulin M (IgM) molecule. (From Kyle et al.,[6] with permission.)

consists of one variable (V_H) domain and four constant (Cμ1, 2, 3, 4) domains. In contrast to IgG, IgM does not have a hinge. V_H and Cμ1 are in the Fd piece, Cμ2 is in the "hinge" region, and Cμ3 and Cμ4 are in the Fc fragment.[74] Although IgM has a sedimentation coefficient of 19S, more rapidly sedimenting molecules of 22S (composed of dimers of the 19S molecule) and 35S may be seen. Low molecular weight IgM (sedimentation coefficient 7S) has been found in patients with various pathologic conditions, including lupus erythematosus, macroglobulinemia, other lymphoproliferative processes, and cirrhosis. Low molecular weight IgM (7S) may be detected by nephelometry or immunoblotting.[75]

J chains identical to those associated with IgA polymers have been isolated from IgM also. These aid in initiating or maintaining the tertiary structure of the molecule. The biologic function of secretory IgM was recently reviewed.[76] Electron microscopy of IgM has shown figures resembling spiders, each with a central ring, where the Fc portions join together, and legs consisting of the Fab fragments. Subclasses of μ-chains have been reported from three laboratories, but they do not correspond, and presently specific subclasses of IgM are not recognized. IgM antibodies are the first produced in a primary immune response, and they avidly fix complement. Cold agglutinins, isoagglutinins, rheumatoid factor, and heterophil and Wasserman antibodies, as well as antibodies to various bacteria, are of the IgM class. Rapid IgM synthesis begins during the first few days of life, and adult serum levels are attained at 1 year. IgM concentrations have been reported to decrease by the sixth decade. Nephelometry frequently overestimates the amount of IgM, when compared with densitometry of serum protein electrophoretograms.[77] Riches et al.[78] reported that 30 percent of IgM samples had a value with nephelometry double that calculated from the densitometer pattern. Consequently, the size of the IgM monoclonal protein should be followed with densitometry rather than nephelometry.

Approximately 80 percent of IgM monoclonal proteins are of the κ-type, in contrast to two-thirds of IgG and IgA monoclonal proteins. Unexpectedly, plasmapheresis may not produce a greater loss of IgM than the lower molecular weight immunoglobulins IgA and IgG. In one report, plasmapheresis consisting of 2 to 3 L was performed in 23 patients. Four patients had a monoclonal protein. The average percentage decrease of IgG was 52 percent, that of IgA was 55 percent, and that of IgM was 51 percent.[79]

Immunoglobulin D

In 1965, Rowe and Fahey[80] found a myeloma protein containing a heavy chain unlike those of the other immunoglobulins. This class, IgD, is present in a trimodal distribution, with modes at approximately 0.25, 5, and 35 IU/ml. The distribution suggests that levels of IgD in normal persons are strongly influenced by inheritance through a monogenic mechanism.[81] Two-dimensional gel electrophoresis has been reported to be of value in the recognition of IgD monoclonal proteins.[82] However, immunofixation is satisfactory for most cases. IgD is rapidly catabolized and has a serum half-life of 2.8 days. The molecules are relatively heat-labile and sensitive to proteases, and they are readily broken down to Fab and Fc fragments. δ-Heavy chains contain three constant domains and a long hinge consisting of 64 amino acid residues. Human IgD has been sequenced.[83] Antigen-combining activity associated with IgD has been reported with thyroglobulin, nuclear antigens, and insulin. Most circulating B lymphocytes bear IgD, together with IgM, on their surface as membrane-bound immunoglobulin. However, the function of serum and B-cell membrane-bound IgD is not known.[84]

About 75 percent of IgD is intravascular, a distribution that may be the result of irregularities in the shape of the molecule. IgD is often found on the surface of lymphocytes.[85]

Most patients with an IgD monoclonal protein will have multiple myeloma or primary amyloidosis. IgD accounts for only 2 percent of patients with multiple myeloma. Incidences of extramedullary plasmacytomas (19 percent), associated amyloidosis (19 percent), frequency of Bence Jones proteinuria (96 percent), and predominance of λ-light chains (60 percent) are greater than those in myeloma associated with IgG or IgA proteins. By contrast, patients with IgD myeloma are more similar to those with light chain (Bence Jones) myeloma.[30] IgD monoclonal proteins have rarely been associated with benign monoclonal gammopathy.[86]

Immunoglobulin E

The fifth class of immunoglobulins, IgE, has been purified from the serum of allergic patients[87] and subsequently identified in multiple myeloma.[88,89] IgE myeloma is rare. Several reviews in the literature identified fewer than 40 cases of IgE myeloma.[90–92] There is a higher frequency of plasma cell leukemia and Bence Jones proteinuria. IgE has a molecular weight of 190,000 and a sedimentation coefficient of 8S. The ε-chain consists of one variable region (V_H) and four constant domains but no hinge region. The combination of a short biologic half-life (2.3 days) and a very low rate of synthesis results in an extremely low serum concentration in normal persons.

IgE mediates the wheal-and-flare reaction associated with reaginic allergies and binds to IgE receptors on basophils or tissue mast cells. IgE is fixed on those cells, and histamine is released when the cell-fixed IgE reacts with the allergen. IgE is often increased in patients with extrinsic asthma and hay fever and in those with parasitic infections.[93]

The discovery of IgE has not made any significant changes in the treatment of allergic diseases.[94] The physiologic contribution of IgE to the maintenance of health remains speculative.[88]

Immunoglobulin Gene Structure and Rearrangement

Molecular cloning of the genes for the immunoglobulin heavy and light chains has shown that their genomic sequences consist of noncontiguous variable, diversity (heavy chain only), joining, and constant region segments.[95–107] Figure 27–5 shows the basic structure of each gene complex and its chromosome location.[95–101,105] During B-cell differentiation, DNA rearrangement occurs, and one of several κ-variable regions (Vκ) combines with a specific joining region (Jκ) segment[96,97,102,107] (Figure 27–6). This rearranged allele that encodes Vκ, Jκ, and the single κ-constant region (Cκ) is now transcribed. The remaining intervening sequences are removed by RNA splicing, and the resultant messenger RNA is translated into the κ-light chain protein. The leader portion of the mRNA is responsible for the transport of the protein through the cell and is later removed. Figure 27–6 shows that both the rearranged variable and joining light chain gene segments encode the variable portion of the light chain protein.[96,97,107]

The κ-light chain gene complex consists of approximately 100 variable region segments, 5 joining segments, and 1 constant κ region[102,103] (Figure 27–5). The λ-gene complex is also composed of many variable region segments (Vλ)[105] but, in contrast to κ, the λ-gene complex exhibits multiple duplicated constant regions (Cλ), each associated with a separate J region (Jλ).[96,106] Furthermore, unlike κ, the human λ-constant gene locus often varies from one individual to another, as evidenced by different restriction fragment length polymorphisms on Southern analysis.[106]

The organization of the heavy chain gene complex is different from that of the light chain genes in that three DNA segments, rather than two, join to code for the variable portion of the rearranged heavy gene.[108–114] Families of diversity segments (D_H) and six joining segments (J_H) are illustrated in Figure 27–5.[111–114] One heavy chain diversity segment combines with one joining segment that ultimately joins with one variable region segment (V_H) during the process of heavy chain gene recombination.[108,109] After the first DNA rearrangement that joins the V_H, D_H, and J_H segments to the heavy chain constant region, a B cell can produce IgM and IgD simultaneously[115–118] (Figure 27–7). Subsequently, a second DNA recombination occurs at one of the switch sites that precede each of the constant region segments and results in an isotype class switch. Figure 27–7 demonstrates that rearrangement of Sμ and Sα and the loss of the intervening heavy chain constant region gene segments result in a class switch from IgM to IgA.[115–118]

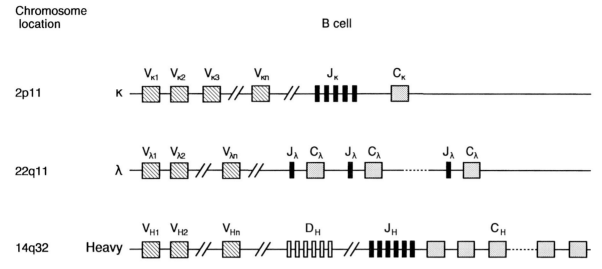

Figure 27–5. Schematic representation of immunoglobulin heavy chain and κ- and λ-light chain loci. The chromosome location of each of the human loci is given at the left. Germline or unrearranged configuration for each gene complex is diagrammed. C, constant; D, diversity; J, joining; V, variable. (Modified from Cossman et al.,[106] with permission.)

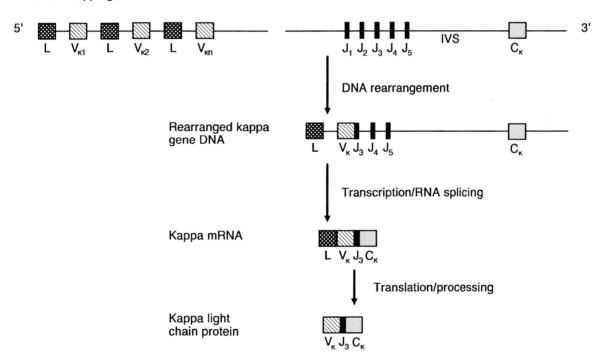

Figure 27–6. Schematic representation of rearrangement of κ-gene locus. During B-cell differentiation, DNA rearrangement takes place and one of several κ-variable regions (V_κ), each accompanied by a leader (L) sequence, combines with one of five joining (J_κ) segments. This rearranged allele that encodes V_κ, J_κ, and a single κ-constant region (C_κ) is transcribed and ultimately translated into the κ-light chain protein. IVS, intervening sequence. (Modified from Korsmeyer SJ, Waldmann TA: Immunoglobulins. II: Gene organization and assembly. p. 43. In Stites DP, Stobo JD, Fudenberg HH, Wells JV (eds.): Basic and Clinical Immunology. 5th Ed. Lange Medical Publications, Los Altos, CA, 1984, with permission.)

In normal B-cell differentiation, immunoglobulin heavy chain genes rearrange at the pre-B stage before κ-genes.[119] The κ-genes rearrange or are deleted before λ-light chain gene rearrangement can occur.[119] The D_H segment accounts for a large portion of the heavy chain's third hypervariable region and is a major component of the resultant antibody's idiotype.[111,112,120] Idiotype refers to the variable region segments of the antibody molecule and relates to the diversity at the antigen binding site. Recent studies demonstrate that myeloma heavy chain VDJ genes contain somatic mutations but show little intraclonal variation. These findings suggest that clonal proliferation takes place in a cell type that has already passed through the phase of somatic hypermutation.[121,122]

The ability of an individual to generate a large immunoglobulin repertoire is now evident from an understanding of the mechanism of gene rearrangement. Antibody diversity may occur through: 1) selection of one of the large number of different variable regions for the heavy and light chain gene complexes; 2) gene rearrangement in which specific variable, joining, and diversity segments recombine to encode a unique variable region domain; and 3) somatic mutation of V genes during B-cell ontogeny.[123,124] Because each lymphocyte produces one type of immunoglobulin, the antigen will select and stimulate the B cells that produce high-affinity antibodies.[123,124]

MONOCLONAL PROTEINS

Relationship to Normal Immunoglobulins

Although monoclonal proteins have long been considered abnormal, studies during the past several years indicated that they are excessive quantities of immunoglobulins that occur normally. The striking feature of monoclonal proteins that led investigators to consider them abnormal is their homogeneity. Whereas normal IgG in human serum is electrophoretically heterogeneous and is distributed from the α_2- to the slow γ-regions, IgG monoclonal proteins are localized sharply in their electrophoretic migration.

Kunkel[125] showed that each heavy chain subclass and light chain type in monoclonal proteins has its counterpart among normal immunoglobulins and also among antibodies. After the discovery of the two types of light chains (κ and λ) in myeloma proteins in a ratio of approximately 2:1, these same light chains were detected in essentially the same ratio among normal immunoglobulins. Similarly, the IgG and IgA subclasses and IgD class were discovered among myeloma proteins and then found as normal serum components. These identifications have gradually weakened the belief that the monoclonal proteins of multiple myeloma and macroglobulinemia are abnormal and have suggested that they represent the overproduction of a nor-

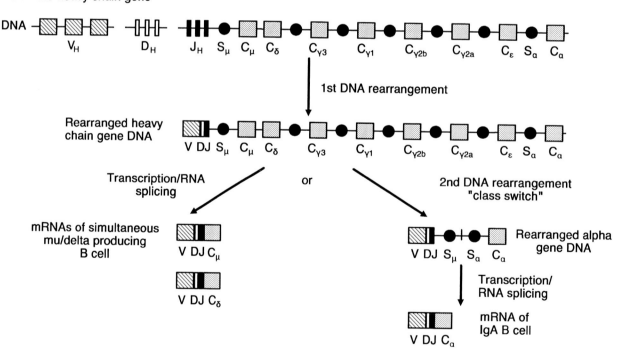

Figure 27–7. Schematic representation of heavy chain gene locus, indicating order of the heavy chain constant region genes. After the initial DNA gene rearrangement, a B cell can simultaneously produce IgM and IgD using different sites of RNA splicing. Alternatively, a second DNA rearrangement may occur at switch sites ($S_\mu S_\alpha$) in which a "class switch" takes place, resulting in IgA production. (Modified from Korsmeyer SJ, Waldmann TA: Immunoglobulins. II: Gene organization and assembly. p. 43. In Stites DP, Stobo JD, Fudenberg HH, Wells JV (eds.): Basic and Clinical Immunology. 5th Ed. Lange Medical Publications, Los Altos, CA, 1984, with permission.)

mal product by a clone of abnormally functioning cells. However, many of the heavy chains found in the heavy chain diseases show significant deletions of amino acids: they are abnormal immunoglobulins.

Even the antigenic determinants ("idiotypic specificities" or "individual antigenic specificities") that are associated with the binding sites were believed to be associated uniquely with myeloma proteins but have been shown to occur among antibodies.[126] Conversely, studies of highly purified antibodies have revealed a homogeneity approaching that seen in monoclonal proteins. In some instances, after primary immunization with a carbohydrate antigen, monoclonal immunoglobulins consisting of a single light chain type and single IgG heavy chain subclass have been seen.[127]

The possibility expressed by Kunkel[125] that myeloma proteins are individual antibodies and are products of the individual plasma cells arising from a single clone of malignant cells has been supported by their antigen-combining activity.[128] Monoclonal antibody activity in humans has been associated with cold agglutinin disease as well as with a wide variety of bacterial antigens including streptolysin O, staphylococcal protein, *Klebsiella* polysaccharides, and *Brucella*.[129] It is almost certain that more human monoclonal proteins will be found to have antibody activity. Indeed, it has been postulated that all myeloma proteins may have such activity.[130]

In this view, as illustrated in Figure 27–8, the normal assortment of IgG molecules comprises minute amounts of homogeneous proteins from many diverse single clones of plasma cells and so is polyclonal. If a single clone escapes the normal controls over its multiplication, it reproduces excessively and synthesizes an excess of protein with a single heavy chain class and subclass and light chain type. More than 50 years ago, Gutman[131] used the term *M component* (or *peak*) in describing a monoclonal protein. This monoclonal protein often is associated with a neoplastic process. Support for the one-cell, one-immunoglobulin concept comes from the studies of the cellular localization of these proteins. Experiments performed with antisera to light chains have shown that nearly all individual plasma cells contain κ- or λ-light chains but not both.

Patterns of Overproduction

Normally, plasma cells produce heavy chains and a slight excess of light chains that spill over into the urine which are catabolized. In IgG myeloma, about three-fourths of patients have an excess of light chains that may be excreted into the urine (Bence Jones proteinuria) or catabolized.[132] A small excess of light chain production could be due to imbalance in translation or transcription within the clone or a possible suppression of heavy chain synthesis in the clone. In other instances, heavy chain is not produced by the plasma cell and only excessive quantities of light chains are detected ("light chain myeloma").[133] Finally, a small proportion of myeloma cells do not secrete either heavy or light chains in detectable amounts, whether because of a simple failure of synthesis or a blocking of secretion, and these are called *nonsecretory*. In heavy chain disease, portions of the heavy chains of IgG, IgA, or IgM are present in serum or urine.

LABORATORY METHODS FOR STUDY OF MONOCLONAL PROTEINS

Analysis of the serum or urine for monoclonal proteins requires a sensitive, rapid, dependable screening method to detect the presence of a monoclonal protein and a specific assay to identify it according to its heavy chain class and light chain type.[134–136] Electrophoresis with high-resolution agarose gel is preferred for screening.[137] After electrophoresis, immunofixation should be used to confirm the presence of a monoclonal protein and to distinguish the immunoglobulin heavy chain class and its light chain type. Immunofixation also should be done if multiple myeloma, macroglobulinemia, primary amyloidosis, or a related disorder is suspected,[136] even if the agarose gel electrophoresis does not show a localized band or spike.

Analysis of Serum for Protein

Electrophoresis

Serum protein electrophoresis should be done when multiple myeloma, macroglobulinemia, or amyloidosis is suspected. In addition, this test is indicated in any case of unexplained weakness or fatigue, anemia, elevation of the erythrocyte sedimenta-

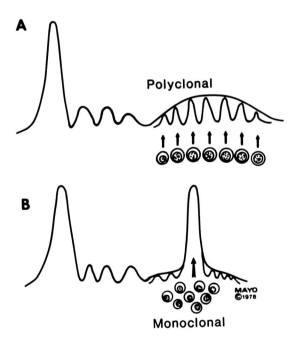

Figure 27–8. Polyclonal and monoclonal electrophoretic patterns. (**A**) Broad outline comprising small peaks of many different homogeneous proteins (each represented here in normal amount, related by *arrow* to its peak), which have been produced by many different plasma cell clones (polyclonal). (**B**) Tall, narrow peak of homogeneous protein (single heavy chain class and subclass and single light chain type), which is excessive output of single clone (monoclonal). (From Kyle and Greipp,[134] with permission.)

tion rate (ESR), back pain, osteoporosis or osteolytic lesions or fracture, immunoglobulin deficiency, hypercalcemia, Bence Jones proteinuria, renal insufficiency, or recurrent infections.[136] Serum protein electrophoresis should also be performed in adults with peripheral neuropathy, carpal tunnel syndrome, refractory congestive heart failure, nephrotic syndrome, orthostatic hypotension, or malabsorption, because a localized band or spike is strongly suggestive of primary amyloidosis.

The constituents of the major components of the serum electrophoretic pattern are listed in Table 27–6. Immunoglobulins (IgG, IgA, IgM, IgD, and IgE) make up the γ-component, but it must be emphasized that they are found in the β–γ and β-regions also and that IgG extends to the α_2-globulin region. Thus an IgG monoclonal protein may be found to range from the slow γ to the α_2-globulin region.

A decrease in albumin and increases in α_1- and α_2-globulins, and occasionally in γ-globulin, are nonspecific features of inflammatory processes (tissue inflammation and destruction) such as infection or metastatic malignancy. Rarely, two albumin bands (bisalbuminemia) may be found. This familial abnormality produces no symptoms.[138]

Hypogammaglobulinemia (γ-globulin less than 0.6 g/dl) is characterized by a definite decrease in the gamma component, and the diagnosis should be confirmed by quantitative determination of the immunoglobulin levels. Hypogammaglobulinemia is seen in about 10 percent of patients with multiple myeloma and most of these also have a large monoclonal protein (Bence Jones) in the urine. Approximately one-fifth of patients with primary systemic amyloidosis have hypogammaglobulinemia.

A large decrease in the α_1-globulin component is usually attributable to a congenital deficiency of α_1-antitrypsin and may be associated with recurrent pulmonary infections and chronic obstructive pulmonary disease.

After electrophoresis, a monoclonal protein (having a single heavy chain class and single light chain type) usually is seen as a narrow peak (like a church spire) in the γ-, β-, or α_2-region of the densitometer tracing or as a dense, discrete band on agarose gel (Figure 27–9). By contrast, an excess of polyclonal immunoglobulins (having one or more heavy chain types with both κ- and λ-light chains) makes a broad-based peak or broad band (Figure 27–10) and usually is limited to the γ-region. In 4 percent of sera, there is an additional monoclonal protein of different immunoglobulin class, and this situation is designated *biclonal gammopathy* (Figure 27–11)[139]

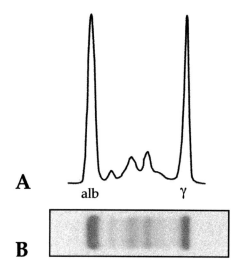

Figure 27–9. (A) Monoclonal pattern of serum protein as traced by densitometer after electrophoresis on agarose gel: tall, narrow-based peak of γ mobility. (B) Monoclonal pattern from electrophoresis of serum on agarose gel (anode on left): dense, localized band representing monclonal protein of γ mobility.

A tall, narrow homogeneous peak or a discrete band (monoclonal protein) is most suggestive of monoclonal gammopathy of undetermined significance, myeloma, or Waldenström's macroglobulinemia, but monoclonal peaks may also occur in amyloidosis and in lymphoma.

Other features may misleadingly suggest a monoclonal protein in the serum. For example, a large, broad peak in the α_2-globulin region may represent free hemoglobin-haptoglobin complexes resulting from hemolysis. The serum is often pink and should suggest the possibility of hemolysis. Another serum sample should be obtained from the patient. Large amounts of transferrin in patients with iron-deficiency anemia may produce a localized band in the β-region. Fibrinogen (in plasma) is seen as a discrete band between the β- and the γ-regions. When a small β–γ band is seen, the specimen should be examined for the presence of a clot. If a clot is not seen, thrombin should be added to the sample; this produces a clot if fibrinogen is present. If the discrete band can no longer be detected when electrophoresis is repeated, the presence of fibrinogen is established.

Table 27–6. Constituents of the Major Components of the Serum Electrophoretic Pattern[a]

+ (Anode) Albumin	α_1-Globulin	α_2-Globulin	β-Globulin	− (Cathode) γ-Globulin
Albumin	α_1-Antitrypsin	α_2-Macroglobulin	β-Lipoprotein	IgG
	α_1-Lipoprotein	α_2-Lipoprotein	Transferrin	IgA
	α_1-Acid glycoprotein	Haptoglobin	Plasminogen	IgM
	(orosomucoid)	Ceruloplasmin	Complement	IgD
		Erythropoietin	Hemopexin	IgE

[a] Immunoglobulins may migrate from the slow γ- to the α_2-globulin area.

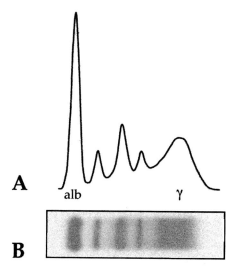

Figure 27–10. (A) Polyclonal pattern from densitometer tracing of agarose gel: broad-based peak of γ mobility. (B) Polyclonal pattern from electrophoresis of agarose gel (anode on left). Band at right is broad and extends throughout the γ area.

Certain other conditions have distinctive electrophoretic patterns. The nephrotic syndrome produces a serum pattern featuring decreased albumin and γ-globulin and increased α_2- and β-globulins (Figure 27–12). The increased α_2 and β-globulin may look like a monoclonal peak of rapid mobility and might be mistaken for a myeloma protein. The urinary pattern consists mainly of albumin (Figure 27–12).

Chronic infections, connective tissue diseases, and chronic liver diseases may be characterized by a large, broad-based polyclonal pattern. This pattern is common in chronic active hepatitis, where the γ-component may be 4 or 5 g/dl or greater. This

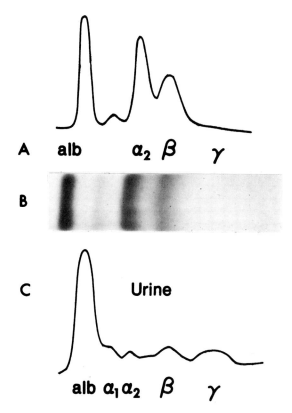

Figure 27–12. Nephrotic syndrome. (A) Serum electrophoretic pattern (densitometer tracing) showing decreased albumin (narrow peak), increased α_2- and β-peaks, and hypogammaglobulinemia. (B) Cellulose acetate tracing. (C) Urine electrophoretic pattern: Most of protein is albumin. (From Kyle and Greipp,[134] with permission.)

large γ-band may be confused with that seen in multiple myeloma or macroglobulinemia. Occasionally, lymphoproliferative processes may have a large polyclonal increase in immunoglobulins. We have seen a number of patients in whom no underlying disease is apparent and in whom the polyclonal increase in immunoglobulins persists for years.

A monoclonal protein may be seen as a rather broad band on the agarose gel or a broad peak in the densitometer tracing and can be mistaken for a polyclonal increase in immunoglobulins. Presumably, this broad band or peak is the result of a complex of monoclonal protein with other plasma components, aggregates of IgG, polymers of IgA, or dimers of IgM. Immunofixation is required for identification.[140]

It must be emphasized that a patient can have a monoclonal protein when the total protein concentration, β- and γ-globulin levels, and quantitative immunoglobulin values are all within normal limits. A small monoclonal peak may be concealed among the β- or γ-components and therefore be missed. Indeed, the agarose gel pattern and densitometer tracing may appear normal even though a monoclonal protein is present (Figure 27–13). A monoclonal light chain (Bence Jones proteinemia) is rarely seen on the cellulose acetate tracing. In a number of cases of IgD myeloma, the monoclonal protein appears small or is not evident at all. Often the monoclonal pro-

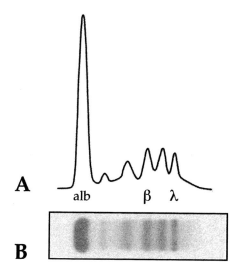

Figure 27–11. (A) Serum protein electrophoresis on agarose gel, showing two γ peaks. (B) Biclonal pattern of electrophoresis of serum on agarose gel (anode at left): two discrete γ bands.

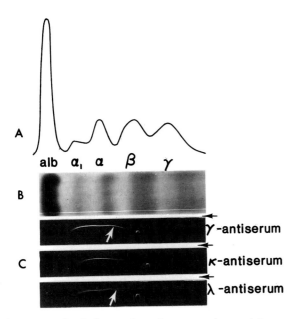

Figure 27–13. Results from analyses of serum samples containing mono-clonal protein (same patient). (**A & B**) Electrophoresis produced normal patterns in densitometer tracing and on cellulose acetate. (**C**) Immuno-electrophoresis produced localized bowing of immunoglobulin G (IgG) (γ) and λ-arcs, indicating IgG λ-protein. (Modified from Kyle and Greipp,[134] with permission.)

tein is not apparent in the heavy chain diseases. In fact, the serum protein electrophoretic pattern is normal in half the cases of α-heavy chain disease, and an unimpressive broad band in the α$_2$- or β-region is the only electrophoretic abnormality among the rest. The characteristic sharp band or peak sugges-tive of a monoclonal protein is never seen. In μ-heavy chain dis-ease, the electrophoretic pattern appears normal except for hypogammaglobulinemia, and a dense band is often not appar-ent. In γ-heavy chain disease, a localized band is usually seen in the β–γ region, but often it is broad, appears heterogeneous, and is more suggestive of a polyclonal than a monoclonal protein. Thus a normal value for the components of the electrophoretic pattern or a normal-appearing or nonspecific pattern may still contain a monoclonal protein, and consequently immunoelec-trophoresis or immunofixation is critical.

Capillary Zone Electrophoresis

Capillary zone electrophoresis also may be used for separation of proteins.[141] Protein is separated by its net charge in a narrow-bore silica capillary. Direct online measurement of protein is done by measurement of peptide bonds at 214 nm. Conse-quently, protein stains are not needed and no point of application artifact exists. In one study, no monoclonal protein detected with agarose electrophoresis was overlooked with capillary zone elec-trophoresis.[142] In another study of 131 serum samples containing a monoclonal protein documented by immunofixation, cellulose acetate electrophoresis detected the abnormality in 83 percent of the samples, agarose gel in 93 percent, and capillary elec-trophoresis in 98 percent.[143] Surprisingly, fibrinogen is not

detectable as a distinct band with capillary electrophoresis. A recently introduced clinical laboratory instrument is the Paragon CZE-2000 Clinical Capillary Electrophoresis System (Beckman Instruments, Brea, CA). This provides automation and rapid turnaround and may be useful to large clinical laboratories.

Immunofixation

Immunofixation is essential for the identification and character-ization of monoclonal proteins. If multiple myeloma, primary amyloidosis, or a related disorder is highly suspected despite normal results of serum protein electrophoresis, immunofixa-tion of the serum is essential. It is helpful for differentiating a monoclonal from a polyclonal increase in immunoglobulins. Monospecific antisera must be used to determine whether the increase of a heavy chain class is associated with an increase in either κ or λ light chains (monoclonal protein) or with an increase of both light chain types (polyclonal protein). Poly-clonal increases of immunoglobulins are usually associated with an inflammatory or reactive process, whereas a monoclonal pro-tein is associated with a neoplastic or potentially neoplastic pro-liferation of plasma cells. Immunofixation is also helpful for the recognition of biclonal gammopathy. It is particularly useful for detecting a small monoclonal protein in patients with primary amyloidosis or a plasmacytoma. It is also helpful for treated myeloma or macroglobulinemia when the M-spike has disap-peared on agarose electrophoresis.

Automated Immunofixation

Immunofixation can be done by several different semiauto-mated techniques. Our laboratory uses the SEBIA HYDRASYS system (SEBIA PN 1210) and HYDRAGEL IF PENTAKIT and

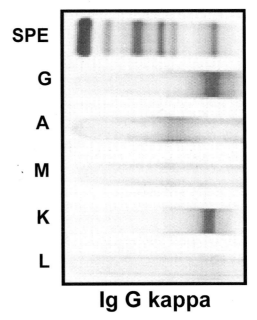

Figure 27–14. Immunofixation of serum with antisera to IgA, IgG, IgM, κ, and λ shows a localized band with IgG and κ antisera, indicating an IgG κ monoclonal protein. SPE, serum protein electrophoresis. (Sebia 4IF.)

4IF KIT (Sebia, Inc., Norcross, GA). The system uses agarose gels and either monospecific antisera (i.e., 4 IF) or a mixture of five specific antisera (i.e., PENTA). The PENTAFIX, using a mixture of γ, α, μ, κ, and λ antisera, can be used as a screen for patients with a normal serum protein electrophoretic pattern. If a band is seen on PENTAFIX, one proceeds with 4IF. In 799 sera for which monoclonal protein studies were requested and in which the agarose electrophoretic pattern appeared normal, 97 had a monoclonal protein on PENTAFIX and were subsequently characterized with 4IF.[144]

A sharp, well-defined band of a single heavy chain class and a single light chain type is seen with a monoclonal protein (Figure 27–14), and broad, diffuse, heavily stained bands with heavy and light chain antisera are characteristic of a polyclonal gammopathy. The presence of a localized band with antisera to IgG or IgA and a corresponding band with either κ or λ antisera is consistent with monoclonal gammopathy of undetermined significance, multiple myeloma, primary amyloidosis, or a related disorder. The presence of a localized band with IgM antisera and a similar localized band with κ or λ antisera is characteristic of monoclonal gammopathy of undetermined significance of the IgM class, Waldenström's macroglobulinemia, or other lymphoproliferative disorders or primary amyoidosis (AL) (Figure 27–15). The presence of a monoclonal IgD or IgE protein is consistent with multiple myeloma or AL.

A biclonal gammopathy has two monoclonal heavy chains and two respective monoclonal light chains (Figure 27–16). A biclonal gammopathy also may consist of two heavy chains of the same class and monoclonal light chains of the same type. In Figure 27–17A, one of the IgM λ monoclonal proteins migrates in the cathodal area and the other IgM λ monoclonal protein migrates in the anodal area. When both IgM κ proteins migrate in either the anodal or the cathodal area, they would most likely represent 7S and 19S molecules from a single IgM κ monoclonal protein (Figure 27–17B).

Occasionally three monoclonal proteins constituting a triclonal gammopathy are seen (Figure 27–18). The identification of a free monoclonal light chain (in the absence of γ, α, μ, δ, or ε heavy chains) is consistent with multiple myeloma, AL, or light chain deposition disease and should be pursued with a 24-hour urine protein study (Figure 27–19).

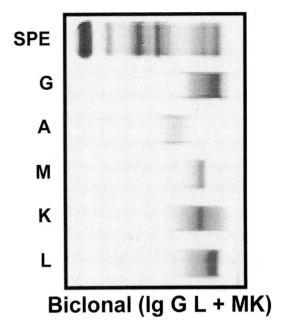

Biclonal (Ig G L + MK)

Figure 27–16. Immunofixation of serum with antisera to IgA, IgG, IgM, κ, and λ shows a discrete IgG band with a similar λ band and a discrete IgM band with a similar κ band, indicating a biclonal gammopathy consisting of IgG λ (G L) and IgM κ (M K) monoclonal proteins. SPE, serum protein electrophoresis. (Sebia 4IF.)

Immunosubtraction

The type of monoclonal protein also can be identified with immunosubtraction. Capillary electrophoresis is performed and then repeated after incubation of the serum with each of the anti-heavy and anti-light chain solid phase antibodies to determine which reagent removes the electrophoretic abnormality (Figure 27–20). This method is rapid and can be automated. However, it is useful only for characterizing monoclonal proteins that can be detected as a spike on capillary zone electrophoresis.

In a prospective study of 1518 serum samples, we compared agarose gel electrophoresis followed by immunofixation with capillary electrophoresis and immunosubtraction. In 215 samples with a monoclonal protein detected by immunofixation, 7 showed no abnormality on serum protein electrophoresis and therefore could not be identified by immunosubtraction. The immunosubtraction procedure worked well, however, with sera containing a discrete monoclonal spike and was simpler to perform than immunofixation or immunoelectrophoresis. It must be emphasized that if there is no spike on the electrophoretic pattern, immunofixation must be used to screen and identify the monoclonal protein. Consequently, if clinical suspicion is high for multiple myeloma, AL, or a related disorder, immunofixation should be performed.

Immunoelectrophoresis

Immunoelectrophoresis has been the standard technique for detection of a monoclonal protein over the years. The antigen-

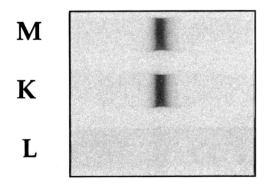

Figure 27–15. Immunofixation of serum with antisera to IgM, κ, and λ shows a discrete IgM band and a similar κ band, indicating an IgM κ monoclonal protein.

A

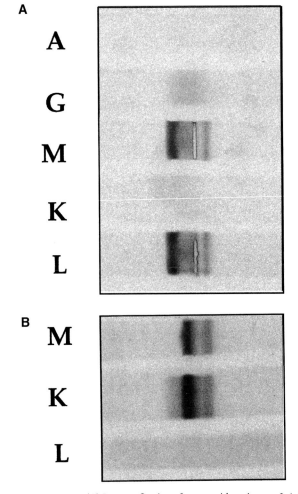

B

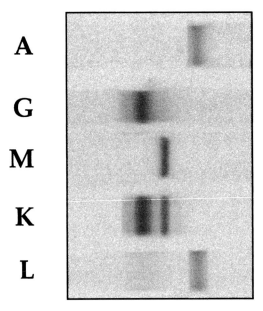

Figure 27–18. Immunofixation of serum with antisera to IgA, IgG, IgM, κ, and λ. There is a discrete IgG band and a similar κ band, a discrete IgM band and a similar κ band, and a discrete IgA band and a similar λ band (triclonal gammopathy: IgG κ, IgM κ, IgA λ).

Figure 27–17. (A) Immunofixation of serum with antisera to IgA, IgG, IgM, κ, and λ. Note a discrete IgM band and a similar λ band migrating in the cathodal area and a small, discrete IgM band and a similar λ band migrating in the anodal area. The site of application of the serum sample is between the two IgM λ monoclonal proteins. (B) Immunofixation of serum with antisera to IgM, κ, and λ. This shows a dense IgM band and a similar κ band at the point of application and a small IgM and a similar κ band in the anodal area, indicating an IgM κ monoclonal protein. The dense band represents 19S IgM κ, and the smaller bands in the anodal area represent 7S IgM κ.

antibody reaction produces a precipitin arc. The procedure is technically easier and less expensive than immunofixation, but it is not as sensitive. In one report, immunofixation detected monoclonal proteins in 15 cases when immunoelectrophoresis failed to recognize them.[145] In fact, most laboratories prefer to perform immunofixation rather than immunoelectrophoresis.

Nephelometry for Detection of Monoclonal Protein

Nephelometry with monospecific κ and λ antisera may be used to detect the light chain type of large monoclonal proteins. However, small monoclonal proteins will have a normal κ:λ ratio and consequently will not be recognized.[146] Although most large monoclonal proteins can be detected, small mono-

clonal proteins will be overlooked.[135,147,148] There also may be a discrepancy in potency between monoclonal light chains from different sources.[149] In addition, nephelometry is of no value in the detection of biclonal or triclonal gammopathies. In summary, we do not advise the use of nephelometry for the identification of monoclonal proteins.

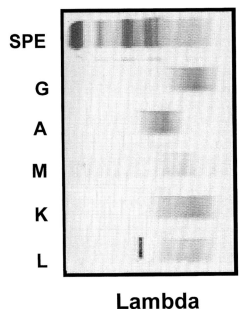

Lambda

Figure 27–19. Immunofixation of serum with antisera to IgG, IgA, IgM, κ, and λ. There is a discrete band with λ antiserum. SPE, serum protein electrophoresis. (Sebia 4IF.)

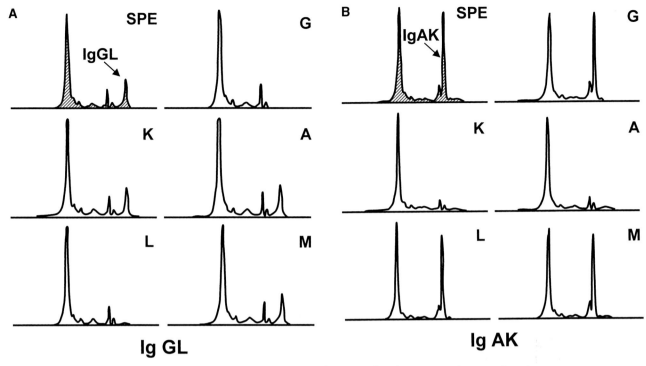

Figure 27–20. Immunosubtraction electropherogram. The two panels each represent an immunosubtraction assay in which six aliquots of serum are electrophoresed by capillary zone electrophoresis (CZE). One aliquot is used for serum protein electrophoresis (SPE) to visualize any abnormality on CZE, and the five other aliquots are electrophoresed after incubation with solid-phase reagents containing anti-γ (G), α (A), μ (M), κ (K), or λ (L) antiserum. The first serum (**A**) sample contains an M-peak in the middle of the gamma fraction. This peak is no longer detected in the CZE patterns after incubation with anti-γ (G) and anti-λ (L). The M-peak is therefore an IgG λ (L) monoclonal protein. The second serum sample (**B**) contains a large M-peak in the β_2 region and a small abnormality in the fast γ region. Both of these abnormalities are removed with antisera to α (A) and κ (K). This serum contains a large IgA κ (K) monoclonal protein in the β_2 region, and the small peak in the fast-γ region presumably is composed of polymers of the monoclonal IgAκ protein.

Practical Approach to Identification of Monoclonal Proteins

We recommend agarose gel electrophoresis as a screening test for the detection of monoclonal proteins. If a large spike is present on the densitometer tracing, we recommend immunosubtraction by capillary electrophoresis. If there is a small spike or if there is no visible spike, we use PENTAFIX for screening. Any abnormality on the PENTAFIX must be characterized with 4IF. If there is a clinical suspicion of myeloma, primary amyloidosis, plasmacytoma, or a related disorder and no spike on agarose gel, we proceed immediately to 4IF.[150]

All patient sera with a monoclonal κ or λ light chain and no abnormality of the IgG, IgA, or IgM heavy chains require screening for IgD and IgE monoclonal proteins. Our practice is to screen the sera by Ouchterlony immunodiffusion with antisera to IgD and IgE against the patient's serum. All sera forming a precipitin band (Figure 27–21) are then studied further by immunofixation with monospecific antisera to IgD, IgE, κ, and λ. Because most sera produce no reaction on immunodiffusion, immunofixation is usually unnecessary.

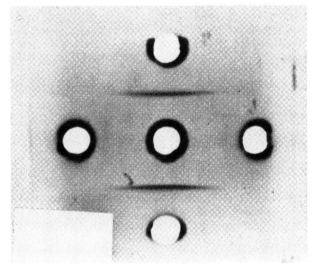

Figure 27–21. Immunodiffusion with antiserum to IgD in the central well and sera of two patients with IgD myeloma in the top and bottom wells. Dense precipitin bands confirm the presence of IgD protein. (From Kyle RA, Bieger RC, Gleich GJ: Diagnosis of syndromes associated with hyperglobulinemia. Med Clin North Am 54:917, 1970. By permission of W.B. Saunders Company.)

Quantitation of Immunoglobulins

Nephelometry is the most practical method for quantitation of immunoglobulins. The antibody to the immunoglobulin is exposed to the serum sample. The antigen-antibody reaction produces an increase in light scatter that is converted to a peak rate signal that is a function of the concentration of the sample immunoglobulin. The peak rate signal for the particular assay is automatically converted to concentration units by the analyzer. The nephelometric technique accurately measures 7S IgM, polymers of IgA, or aggregates of IgG because the method is not affected by molecular size of the antigen.[151] Lipemic sera may produce light scattering and make accurate measurement of immunoglobulins impossible. A fasting specimen may be required. Dust particles or other particulate matter also may alter the results.

Quantitation of immunoglobulins is more useful than immunoelectrophoresis or immunofixation for the detection of hypogammaglobulinemia. Quantitation has been performed by radial immunodiffusion.[152] Low-molecular-weight (7S) IgM produces a spuriously increased value of IgM because its rate of diffusion is greater than that of 19S IgM used as a standard. Similarly, polymeric IgA will produce spuriously low values because the standards consist of 7S IgA. Consequently, radioimmunodiffusion is not recommended.

It must be emphasized that the level of IgM may be 1000 to 2000 mg/dl greater than expected from the monoclonal protein in the densitometer tracing. The IgG and IgA levels also may be spuriously increased.[78] Schreiber et al.[153] also reported that serum samples from normal blood donors gave higher values for immunoglobulins when determined by nephelometry than with agarose gel electrophoresis. Discrepancy also may exist because of κ-light chain antisera of different sources. In one report, the mean κ-value was 26.8 g/L with κ-antisera from Beckman Instruments, Inc. (Brea, CA) and 18.2 g/L with antisera from Kallestad (Austin, TX).[149] In addition, it is well known that antisera may give high results if they contain many antibodies that react with the determinants in a specific monoclonal protein or low results if they contain few such antibodies.

If a monoclonal protein is small, the use of quantitative immunoglobulins includes the amount of polyclonal immunoglobulin. To monitor the size of the monoclonal protein, we recommend that serum protein electrophoresis be used. If the monoclonal protein is large and there is little polyclonal immunoglobulin, nephelometry can be used to monitor the size of the monoclonal protein. Because the results of the two methods are not identical, it should be emphasized that sequential monitoring using different assays is not recommended.[154]

Serum Viscometry

Serum viscometry should be done when there is more than 4 g/dl of IgM monoclonal protein or more than 5 g/dl of IgA or IgG protein and in any patient with oronasal bleeding, blurred vision, or neurological, symptoms suggestive of a hyperviscosity syndrome. The Ostwald-100 viscometer is a satisfactory instrument for this purpose, but a Wells-Brookfield viscometer (Brookfield Engineering Laboratories, Stoughton, MA) is preferred because it is more accurate, requires less serum (approximately 1.0 ml), and can perform at different shear rates and at variable temperatures. In addition, determinations can be made much more rapidly, especially if the viscosity of the serum is high. Symptoms of hyperviscosity are rare unless the value is more than 4 centipoises (cp). Indeed, some patients with a value of 10 cp or more do not have symptoms of hyperviscosity.

Waldenström's macroglobulinemia is the most common cause of hyperviscosity and accounts for more than 80 percent of cases. Multiple myeloma of IgA type or, rarely, IgG may produce hyperviscosity.[155] The signs or symptoms of the hyperviscosity syndrome include segmental dilation of retinal veins and flame-shaped hemorrhages, oronasal bleeding, blurring or loss of vision, headaches, vertigo, nystagmus, decreased hearing, ataxia, paresthesias, diplopia, somnolence, stupor, or coma.[156]

Cryoglobulins

Cryoglobulins are proteins that precipitate when cooled and dissolve when heated (Figure 27–22). Five ml of fresh, centrifuged serum kept at 37°C is placed in a tube and incubated at 0°C (in an ice bath in a cold room) for 24 hours. If a precipitate or gel is seen, the tube is centrifuged and the cryocrit level is read. The precipitate is washed in cold saline and then placed in a 37°C waterbath. Immunofixation or immunoelectrophoresis is performed on the resuspended cryoprecipitate with monospecific antisera to IgG, IgA, IgM, κ, and λ.

Cryoglobulins may be classified as follows: type I (monoclonal—IgG, IgM, IgA, or rarely monoclonal light chains); type II (mixed—two or more immunoglobulins, of which one is

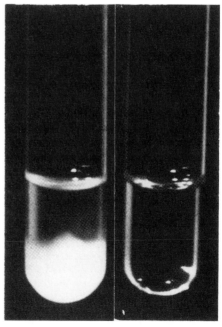

Figure 27–22. Cryoglobulinemia. *(Left)* Precipitate formed on exposure to 0°C. *(Right)* Disappearance of precipitate when heated to 37°C. (From Kyle and Greipp,[134] with permission.)

monoclonal); and type III (polyclonal—in which no monoclonal protein is found).[157]

In most cases, monoclonal cryoglobulins are IgM or IgG, but IgA and Bence Jones cryoglobulins have been reported. Unexpectedly, many patients with large amounts of cryoglobulin are completely asymptomatic, whereas others with small monoclonal cryoglobulins in the range of 1 to 2 g/dl have pain, purpura, Raynaud's phenomenon, cyanosis, and even ulceration and sloughing of skin and subcutaneous tissues on exposure to the cold. The temperature at which the cryoglobulin precipitates is much more important than the amount of protein. We have seen patients in whom the protein produced serious problems by precipitating at 26°C.[158] By contrast, we have been impressed with a number of patients who had 4 to 5 g of a monoclonal IgG or IgM cryoprotein that precipitated at 4°C but no symptoms whatever upon exposure to cold.

Cryoglobulinemia may produce a spurious elevation of the leukocyte count on the model S Coulter counter. It is believed that this may be due to particles formed by combination of the cryoglobulin and fibrinogen.

Most commonly, mixed cryoglobulins (type II) consist of monoclonal IgM and polyclonal IgG, but IgG-IgG and IgA-IgG combinations have been reported.[157] Usually the quantity of the "precipitating protein" is less than 0.2 g/dl, and it may not reach maximum amounts for 7 days, while the serum protein electrophoretic pattern indicates normality or diffuse hypergammaglobulinemia. Patients with mixed cryoglobulinemia frequently have vasculitis, glomerulonephritis, or lymphoproliferative or chronic infectious processes. Hepatic dysfunction and serologic evidence of previous infection with hepatitis B virus is common in some series.[159] Hepatitis C is often associated with mixed cryoglobulinemia (type II).[160]

Pyroglobulins precipitate when heated to 56°C and do not dissolve when cooled. They are usually discovered when serum is inactivated for another laboratory procedure. Pyroglobulins resemble Bence Jones protein in that both precipitate when heated to 60°C, but the two can be distinguished easily by immunofixation with appropriate antisera. In most cases, pyroglobulinemia is associated with multiple myeloma, but it may also occur in macroglobulinemia, lymphoproliferative syndromes, and other neoplastic diseases.[161] Pyroglobulins are usually of the IgG class, but IgM[162,163] and IgA pyroglobulins have been seen.[164,165] IgD pyroglobulins were found in one patient with plasma cell leukemia who also had a λ-monoclonal protein in the urine that showed pyroglobulin properties.[166]

Analysis of Urine for Protein

When patients who have gammopathies are studied, analysis of urine is essential. Sulfosalicylic acid or Exton's test is more reliable for the detection of protein. Sulfosalicylic acid detects albumin and globulin as well as Bence Jones protein, polypeptides, and proteases. False-positive reactions may be induced by penicillin or its derivatives, tolbutamide metabolites, sulfisoxazole metabolites, and certain organic radiographic contrast media.[167] Quantitation of protein may be accomplished by precipitation with trichloroacetic acid, biuret, or dye binding.[168]

Dipstick tests are used in many laboratories to screen for protein. The dipstick is impregnated with a buffered indicator dye that binds to protein in the urine and produces a color change proportional to the amount of protein bound to it. However, the dipsticks are often insensitive to Bence Jones protein and should not be used when a possibility of Bence Jones proteinuria exists.[169,170]

Almost from the time of the discovery of the unique thermal properties of urinary light chains, screening tests for their detection have been in use. All have shortcomings, but the heat test of Putnam et al.[42] is the simplest. Most, but not all, monoclonal light chains in the urine precipitate at 40°C to 60°C, dissolve at 100°C, and reprecipitate on cooling to between 40°C and 60°C. Occasionally, the result of the heat test is positive even though the patient's urine reveals no sharp peak or localized globulin band on electrophoresis and no evidence of a monoclonal light chain on immunoelectrophoresis. Such urine usually produces a broad-based λ-band and normal-appearing κ- and λ-arcs. Presumably, the positive result of the test is due to an excess of polyclonal light chains. Such false-positive results occur most often in cases of renal insufficiency, connective-tissue disease, or malignant disease.[171] However, the Bence Jones heat test results have been negative when urinary electrophoresis has shown a dense globulin band or spike and when immunoelectrophoresis has demonstrated a monoclonal light chain. It is obvious that the heat test for Bence Jones protein has many shortcomings and cannot be recommended. The recognition of Bence Jones proteinuria depends on the demonstration of a monoclonal light chain by electrophoresis and immunofixation of an adequately concentrated urine specimen.

Electrophoresis

First, a 24-hour collection of urine must be made for determination of the total amount of protein excreted per day. The amount of monoclonal protein in the urine is helpful in differentiating between monoclonal gammopathy of undetermined significance and multiple myeloma or other malignant plasma cell proliferative disease. It is most important when following the course of a patient with a monoclonal light chain in the urine because the amount of protein correlates directly with the size of the plasma-cell burden. An aliquot of the 24-hour urine specimen must first be concentrated to approximately 3 g/dl. We prefer the Vivaspin 20 centrifugal concentrator (Vivascience LTD, Stonehouse, GL, UK).

A urinary monoclonal protein is seen as a dense, localized band on the agarose gel strip or a tall, narrow, homogeneous peak on the densitometer tracing (Figure 27–23). Generally, a monoclonal protein in urine produces a wider band than a monoclonal protein in serum, so immunoelectrophoresis or immunofixation must be done. Occasionally two discrete globulin bands may be seen in the agarose gel tracing of the urine. These bands may be a monoclonal light chain plus a monoclonal immunoglobulin fragment from the serum, or they may be monomers and dimers of the monoclonal light chain. Therefore immunofixation with the appropriate heavy and light chain antisera is necessary. Rarely, two monoclonal light chains (κ and λ) have been noted in the urine.[172]

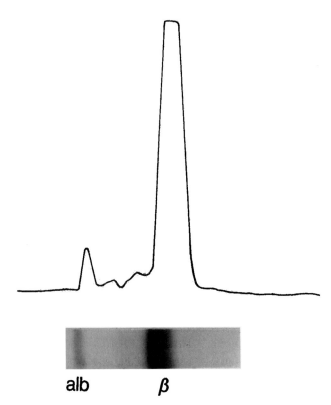

Figure 27–23. Monoclonal urine protein. *(Top)* Densitometer showing a tall, narrow-based peak of β-mobility. *(Bottom)* Cellulose acetate electrophoretic pattern showing a dense band of β-mobility. This is consistent with a monoclonal urine protein (Bence Jones protein). (From Kyle and Garton,[177] with permission.)

A polyclonal increase of light chains is seen as a very broad band extending through most of the λ-region; it has fuzzy, indistinct cathodal and anodal borders. The densitometer tracing is broad based, and immunoelectrophoresis shows both normal-appearing κ-arcs and λ-arcs.

The amount of monoclonal protein is best measured by multiplying the percentage of the M-spike by the total protein in the 24-hour specimen. The amount of urine protein can be expressed as mg/dl or mg/L, but it is much more useful to report the monoclonal protein in grams per 24 hours (g/24 hours) because the patient may be producing 500 to 4000 ml of urine daily. The 24-hour urine specimen requires no preservative and may be kept at room temperature during collection. The normal values for total protein are less than 150 mg/24 hours for males and less than 100 mg/24 hours for females. The total amount of protein in the urine should be measured to ascertain whether a nephrotic syndrome is present (≥ 3 g/24 hours) with a large amount of albumin and small amounts of globulin and to measure the monoclonal light chain (Bence Jones protein).

Immunofixation

Immunofixation is needed for the detection of monoclonal light chains and is more sensitive than immunoelectrophoresis.[173] Immunofixation should be performed in every patient who has a monoclonal protein concentration of more than 1.5 g/dl in the serum or in whom multiple myeloma, macroglobulinemia, primary amyloidosis, or a related disorder is suspected.[136] It is the preferred method for identifying a monoclonal protein in urine and should be performed on the urine of any patient in this group even if the routine urinalysis is negative for protein. Immunofixation of urine also should be done in the evaluation of an older patient with an "idiopathic" nephrotic syndrome. It is not uncommon for the urine osmolality to be normal or increased and the reaction for protein to be negative and yet for immunofixation to detect a localized globulin band consisting of a monoclonal light chain.

The presence of a monoclonal protein is characterized by a discrete band with either κ or λ antisera (Figure 27–24). Two discrete bands with either κ or λ antisera may be found and may be due to the presence of monomers and dimers of the monoclonal light chain (Figure 27–25). A discrete band with heavy chain antisera corresponding to the type of heavy chain in the serum may coincide with one of two light chain bands. Figure 27–26 shows the presence of a monoclonal λ light chain plus an IgG λ fragment.

If the patient has a nephrotic syndrome (a large amount of albumin and a small amount of globulin), the presence of a monoclonal light chain suggests primary amyloidosis[174] or light chain deposition disease. In contrast, a monoclonal protein greater than 1 g/24 hours and a predominance of globulin over albumin suggest myeloma.

Immunofixation establishes the presence or absence of light chains and determines whether they are monoclonal or polyclonal. It is not unusual to have a negative reaction for serum and to find no spike in the urine with electrophoresis or a negative result from immunoelectrophoresis yet find a monoclonal light chain with immunofixation.

Immunofixation of concentrated urine is performed with antisera to κ and λ and the appropriate heavy chain. Theoretically, antisera that recognize only free κ or free λ light chains should be used, rather than light chain antisera that recognize both free light chains and those that are part of an intact immunoglobulin. However, such free light chain antisera are often either nonspecific or not potent enough. In addition, a patient may have an immunoglobulin fragment that free κ or free λ would not recognize. Consequently, it is advisable to use κ and λ antisera that are monospecific and potent and that recognize both free and combined light chains.

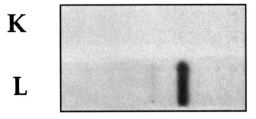

Figure 27–24. Immunofixation of concentrated urine specimen with antisera to κ and λ shows a discrete λ band. This indicates a monoclonal λ light chain.

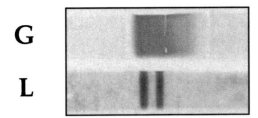

Figure 27–25. Immunofixation of urine with antisera to IgG and λ shows two discrete λ bands. The reaction with IgG is polyclonal. The two discrete bands represent monomers and dimers of the monoclonal λ light chain.

If electrophoresis of the urine reveals a localized globulin band and immunofixation of κ and λ antisera does not demonstrate a monoclonal light chain, one must suspect the possibility of γ-heavy chain disease. Immunofixation then should be done with antisera to IgG (γ heavy chains). Occasionally one sees regularly spaced, faint but discrete multiple bands in the immunofixation pattern. These restrictive bands represent related polyclonal free light chains and are not to be confused with a monoclonal light chain. This has been described as "ladder light chain" or "pseudo-oligoclonal pattern."[175] Free fragments of γ chains may be seen in the immunofixation pattern. These migrate in the α_2-globulin area and should not be confused with γ-heavy chain disease.[176]

Immunofixation is most helpful when a monoclonal light chain occurs in the presence of a polyclonal increase in light chains[177] (Figure 27–27). It is also useful for detecting monoclonal heavy chain (Figure 27–26). It is not uncommon to find a small γ-chain fragment unaccompanied by light chains when they cannot be found in the serum. In γ-heavy chain disease, one always finds a monoclonal heavy chain in the serum. These small free fragments of γ chain should not be confused with γ-heavy chain disease.[176]

Immunoelectrophoresis

Immunoelectrophoresis may be used to identify the heavy chain class and light chain type of a monoclonal protein in the urine. The urine specimen is placed in a well on a microscope slide covered with 1 percent agar and subjected to electrophoresis. The trough, which is cut into the agar before electrophoresis, parallel to the line of migration of the components, is filled with

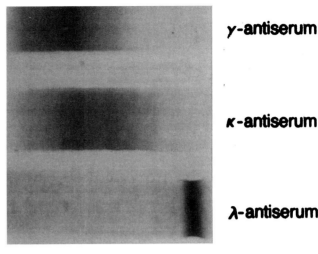

γ-antiserum

κ-antiserum

λ-antiserum

Figure 27–27. Immunofixation of urine. *(Top)* Normal-appearing band with IgG (γ) antiserum. *(Middle)* Normal-appearing band with κ-antiserum. *(Bottom)* Dense, narrow band with λ-antiserum. Patient has monoclonal λ-protein (Bence Jones protein). (From Kyle and Garton,[177] with permission.)

monospecific antisera. Proteins from the electrophoresis sample (antigen) and the antisera (antibodies to κ or λ) are allowed to diffuse toward each other and form a precipitin arc from the antigen-antibody complex. The monoclonal protein forms a locally bowed or restricted arc with κ or λ antisera, whereas a polyclonal increase in light chains causes elongation or fuzziness of both κ and λ arcs. In renal insufficiency, faint, fuzzy, elongated κ and λ arcs are often seen, but if there is underlying myeloma or amyloidosis, an additional bowed or restricted arc with either κ or λ antisera may be seen.

The need for collection of a 24-hour urine specimen cannot be overemphasized. This allows the amount of the monoclonal protein excreted in the urine to be measured, which is an excellent indication of the effect of chemotherapy or evidence of progression of the disease and is also very useful in following the course of a patient with amyloidosis and nephrotic syndrome.[178]

To demonstrate a monoclonal protein in the urine, electrophoresis and either immunofixation or immunoelectrophoresis of an adequately concentrated aliquot from a 24-hour specimen are the appropriate techniques.

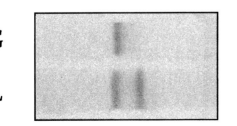

Figure 27–26. Immunofixation of urine with antisera to IgG and λ. There are two λ bands. A discrete IgG band corresponds to one of the λ bands. The findings indicate a λ monoclonal protein plus an IgG λ fragment.

ACKNOWLEDGMENTS

Portions of this chapter and Figures 27–9 through 27–11, 27–14 through 27–20, and 27–24 through 27–26 were published in Kyle RA, Katzmann JA, Lust JA, Dispenzieri A: Immunochemical characterization of immunoglobulins. In Rose NR, Hamilton RG, Detrick B (eds.): Manual of Clinical Laboratory Immunology. 6th ed. Washington DC, ASM Press, 2002. By permission of ASM Press.

This work was supported in part by CA 62242 from the National Cancer Institute.

REFERENCES

1. Kyle RA, Bayrd ED: The Monoclonal Gammopathies: Multiple Myeloma and Related Plasma-Cell Disorders. Charles C Thomas, Springfield, IL, 1976.

2. Tiselius A: Electrophoresis of serum globulin. II. Electrophoretic analysis of normal and immune sera. Biochem J 31:1464, 1937.

3. Putnam FW: From the first to the last of the immunoglobulins: Perspectives and prospects. Clin Physiol Biochem 1:63, 1983.

4. Longsworth LG, Shedlovsky T, MacInnes DA: Electrophoretic patterns of normal and pathological human blood serum and plasma. J Exp Med 70:399, 1939.

5. Kohn J: A cellulose acetate supporting medium for zone electrophoresis. Clin Chim Acta 2:297, 1957.

6. Kyle RA, Bieger RC, Gleich GJ: Diagnosis of syndromes associated with hyperglobulinemia. Med Clin North Am 54:917, 1970.

7. Virella G, Wang A-C: Biosynthesis, metabolism and biological properties of immunoglobulins. Immunol Ser 58:91, 1993.

8. Ryazantsev S, Tishchenko V, Vasiliev V et al: Structure of human myeloma IgG3 Kuc. Eur J Biochem 190:393, 1990.

9. Recht B, Frangione B, Franklin E, van Loghem E: Structural studies of a human γ3 myeloma protein (GOE) that binds staph protein A. J Immunol 127:917, 1981.

10. Shapiro SS: Characterization of factor VIII antibodies. Ann NY Acad Sci 240:350, 1975.

11. Reynolds HY: Immunoglobulin G and its function in the human respiratory tract. Mayo Clin Proc 63:161, 1988.

12. Hymes K, Schur PH, Karpatkin S: Heavy-chain subclass of bound antiplatelet IgG in autoimmune thrombocytopenic purpura. Blood 56:84, 1980.

13. Oxelius VA, Laurell AB, Lindquist B et al: IgG subclasses in selective IgA deficiency: Importance of IgG2-IgA deficiency. N Engl J Med 304:1476, 1981.

14. Aittoniemi J, Koskinen S, Laippala P et al: The significance of IgG subclasses and mannan-binding lectin (MBL) for susceptibility to infection in apparently healthy adults with IgA deficiency. Clin Exp Immunol 116:505, 1999.

15. Jefferis R, Kumararatne DS: Selective IgG subclass deficiency: Quantification and clinical relevance. Clin Exp Immunol 81:357, 1990.

16. Oxelius VA, Berkel AI, Hanson LÅ: IgG2 deficiency in ataxia-telangiectasia. N Engl J Med 306:515, 1982.

17. Beck CS, Heiner DC: Selective immunoglobulin G₄ deficiency and recurrent infections of the respiratory tract. Am Rev Respir Dis 124:94, 1981.

18. Aucouturier P, Mariault M, Lacombe C, Preud'homme J-L: Frequency of selective IgG subclass deficiency: A reappraisal. Clin Immunol Immunopathol 63:289, 1992.

19. Hill SL, Mitchell JL, Burnett D, Stockley RA: IgG subclasses in the serum and sputum from patients with bronchiectasis. Thorax 53:463, 1998.

20. Kyle RA, Gleich GJ: IgG subclasses in monoclonal gammopathy of undetermined significance. J Lab Clin Med 100:806, 1982.

21. Papadea C, Reimer CB, Check IJ: IgG subclass distribution in patients with multiple myeloma or with monoclonal gammopathy of undetermined significance. Ann Clin Lab Sci 19:27, 1989.

22. Schur PH: IgG subclasses—a review. Ann Allergy 58:89, 1987.

23. Smith TF: IgG subclasses. Adv Pediatr 39:101, 1992.

24. Preud'homme J-L, Hanson LÅ: IgG subclass deficiency. Immunodefic Rev 2:129, 1990.

25. Macintyre W: Case of mollities and fragilitas ossium, accompanied with urine strongly charged with animal matter. Med Chir Soc 33:211, 1850.

26. Bence Jones H: Papers on chemical pathology: Prefaced by the Gulstonian lectures, read at the Royal College of Physicians, 1846. Lancet 2:88, 1847.

27. Edelman GM, Gally JA: The nature of Bence-Jones proteins: Chemical similarities to polypeptide chains of myeloma globulins and normal γ-globulins. J Exp Med 116:207, 1962.

28. Bayne-Jones S, Wilson DW: Immunological reactions of Bence-Jones proteins. II. Differences between Bence-Jones proteins from various sources. Bull Johns Hopkins Hosp 33:119, 1922.

29. Korngold L, Lipari R: Multiple-myeloma proteins. III. The antigenic relationship of Bence Jones proteins to normal gamma-globulin and multiple-myeloma serum proteins. Cancer 9:262, 1956.

30. Bladé J, Lust JA, Kyle RA: IgD multiple myeloma: Presenting features, response to therapy, and survival in a series of 53 cases. J Clin Oncol 12:2398, 1994.

31. Lieu TS, Deutsch HF, Tischendorf FW: Human λ-chain sequence variations and serologic associations. Immunochemistry 14:429, 1977.

32. Solomon A, McLaughlin CL: Bence-Jones proteins and light chains of immunoglobulins. I. Formation and characterization of amino-terminal (variant) and carboxyl-terminal (constant) halves. J Biol Chem 244:3393, 1969.

33. Fett JW, Deutsch HF: Primary structure of the Mcg λ chain. Biochemistry 13:4102, 1974.

34. Solomon A: Bence-Jones proteins and light chains of immunoglobulins. N Engl J Med 294:17, 91, 1976.

35. Wang AC, Fudenberg HH, Wells JV, Roelcke D: A new subgroup of the kappa chain variable region associated with anti-Pr cold agglutinins (editorial). Nature New Biol 243:126, 1973.

36. Lacy MQ, Gertz MA: Acquired Fanconi's syndrome associated with monoclonal gammopathies. Hematol Oncol Clin North Am 13:1273, 1999.

37. Messiaen T, Deret S, Mougenot B et al: Adult Fanconi syndrome secondary to light chain gammopathy. Clinicopathologic heterogeneity and unusual features in 11 patients. Medicine (Balt) 79:135, 2000.

38. Ronco PM, Aucouturier P: The molecular bases of plasma cell dyscrasia-related renal diseases. Nephrol Dial Transplant 14(Suppl. 1):4, 1999.

39. Denoroy L, Deret S, Aucouturier P: Overrepresentation of the V kappa IV subgroup in light chain deposition disease. Immunol Lett 42:63, 1994.

40. Solomon A: Light chains of immunoglobulins: Structural-genetic correlates. Blood 68:603, 1986.

41. Solomon A, Kyle RA, Frangione B: Light chain variable region subgroups of monoclonal immunoglobulins in amyloidosis AL. In Glenner GG, Osserman EF, Benditt EP et al (eds.): Amyloidosis, p. 449. Plenum Press, New York, 1986.

42. Putnam FW, Easley CW, Lynn LT et al: The heat precipitation of Bence-Jones proteins. I. Optimum conditions. Arch Biochem Biophys 83:115, 1959.

43. Solomon A: Bence Jones proteins and light chains of immunoglobulins. XIV. Conformational dependency and molecular localization of the kappa (κ) and lambda (λ) antigenic determinants. Scand J Immunol 5:685, 1976.

44. Putnam FW, Hardy S: Proteins in multiple myeloma. III. Origin of Bence-Jones protein. J Biol Chem 212:361, 1955.

45. Wochner RD, Strober W, Waldmann TA: The role of the kidney in the catabolism of Bence Jones proteins and immunoglobulin fragments. J Exp Med 126:207, 1967.

46. Wu TT, Kabat EA: An analysis of the sequences of the variable regions of Bence Jones proteins and myeloma light chains and

their implications for antibody complementarity. J Exp Med 132:211, 1970.

47. Capra JD, Kehoe JM: Hypervariable regions, idiotypy, and the antibody-combining site. Adv Immunol 20:1, 1975.

48. Steinberg AG: Globulin polymorphisms in man. Annu Rev Genet 3:25, 1969.

49. Tomasi TB Jr: Human immunoglobulin A. N Engl J Med 279:1327, 1968.

50. Chandy KG, Stockley RA, Leonard RCF et al: Relationship between serum viscosity and intravascular IgA polymer concentration in IgA myeloma. Clin Exp Immunol 46:653, 1981.

51. Lenormand P, Crocker J: Distribution of IgA₁ and IgA₂ subclasses in normal bone marrow trephines and in trephines infiltrated by IgA producing multiple myeloma. J Clin Pathol 40:200, 1987.

52. Tichý M, Hrncír Z: Distribution of subclasses in a series of 62 sera with IgA paraprotein. Neoplasma 33:507, 1986.

53. Aucouturier P, Musset L, Itoh Y et al: Isotypic and allotypic analysis with monoclonal antibodies and jacalin of 309 serum monoclonal IgA from French and Japanese myeloma patients. Immunol Lett 32:31, 1992.

54. André C, Berthoux FC, André F et al: Prevalence of IgA2 deposits in IgA nephropathies: A clue to their pathogenesis. N Engl J Med 303:1343, 1980.

55. Leung JC, Poon PY, Lai KN: Increased sialylation of polymeric immunoglobulin A₁: Mechanism of selective glomerular deposition in immunoglobulin A nephropathy? J Lab Clin Med 133:152, 1999.

56. Rivat-Peran L, Buriot D, Salier JP et al: Immunoglobulins in ataxia-telangiectasia: Evidence for IgG4 and IgA2 subclass deficiencies. Clin Immunol Immunopathol 20:99, 1981.

57. Bizzaro N, Pasini P, Finco B: False-positive reactions for IgA anti-phospholipid and anti-β₂-glycoprotein I antibodies in patients with IgA monoclonal gammopathy. Clin Chem 45:2007, 1999.

58. Heremans JF: Immunoglobulin A. In Sela M (ed.): The Antigens, p. 395. Vol. 2. Academic Press, San Diego, 1974.

59. Mestecky J, Russell MW, Jackson S, Brown TA: The human IgA system: A reassessment. Clin Immunol Immunopathol 40:105, 1986.

60. Cunningham-Rundles C: Genetic aspects of immunoglobulin A deficiency. Adv Hum Genet 19:235, 1990.

61. Gotoh T, Takishita Y, Doi H, Tsubura E: Secretory-component-producing lung cancer with hypergammaglobulinemia of secretory IgA. Cancer 48:1776, 1981.

62. Conley ME, Delacroix DL: Intravascular and mucosal immunoglobulin A: Two separate but related systems of immune defense? Ann Intern Med 106:892, 1987.

63. Goodman MR, Link DW, Brown WR, Nakane PK: Ultrastructural evidence of transport of secretory IgA across bronchial epithelium. Am Rev Respir Dis 123:115, 1981.

64. DeCoteau WE: The role of secretory IgA in defense of the distal lung. Ann NY Acad Sci 221:214, 1974.

65. Abu-Ghazaleh RI, Fujisawa T, Mestecky J et al: IgA-induced eosinophil degranulation. J Immunol 142:2393, 1989.

66. Strober W, Krakauer R, Klaeveman HL et al: Secretory component deficiency: A disorder of the IgA immune system. N Engl J Med 294:351, 1976.

67. Kutteh WH, Prince SJ, Mestecky J: Tissue origins of human polymeric and monomeric IgA. J Immunol 128:990, 1982.

68. Brandtzaeg P, Guy-Grand D, Griscelli C: Intestinal, salivary, and tonsillar IgA and J-chain production in a patient with severe deficiency of serum IgA. Scand J Immunol 13:313, 1981.

69. Koshland ME: Structure and function of the J chain. Adv Immunol 20:41, 1975.

70. Vaerman JP, Langendries A, Giffroy D et al: Lack of SC/pIgR-mediated epithelial transport of a human polymeric IgA devoid of J chain: In vitro and in vivo studies. Immunology 95:90, 1998.

71. Hayzer DJ, Jaton J-C: Immunoglobulin M (IgM). Methods Enzymol 116:26, 1985.

72. Metzger H: Structure and function of γM macroglobulins. Adv Immunol 12:57, 1970.

73. Tartakoff A, Vassalli P: Plasma cell immunoglobulin M molecules: Their biosynthesis, assembly, and intracellular transport. J Cell Biol 83:284, 1979.

74. Putnam FW, Florent G, Paul C et al: Complete amino acid sequence of the mu heavy chain of a human IgM immunoglobulin. Science 182:287, 1973.

75. Harries R, Beckman I, Roberts-Thomson P: Low molecular weight IgM detection using immunoblotting. J Immunol Methods 88:97, 1986.

76. Reddy PS, Corley RB: The contribution of ER quality control to the biologic functions of secretory IgM. Immunol Today 20:582, 1999.

77. Abu-Farsakh FA, Abu-Farsakh HA: M-component overestimated by laser nephelometry in Waldenström's macroglobulinemia, abstracted. Clin Chem 34:428, 1988.

78. Riches PG, Sheldon J, Smith AM, Hobbs JR: Overestimation of monoclonal immunoglobulin by immunochemical methods. Ann Clin Biochem 28:253, 1991.

79. Filomena CA, Filomena AP, Hudock J, Ballas SK: Evaluation of serum immunoglobulins by protein electrophoresis and rate nephelometry before and after therapeutic plasma exchange. Am J Clin Pathol 98:243, 1992.

80. Rowe DS, Fahey JL: A new class of human immunoglobulins. I. A unique myeloma protein. J Exp Med 121:171, 1965.

81. Dunnette SL, Gleich GJ, Miller RD, Kyle RA: Measurement of IgD by a double antibody radioimmunoassay: Demonstration of an apparent trimodal distribution of IgD levels in normal human sera. J Immunol 119:1727, 1977.

82. Stulík J, Tichý M, Kovárová H: Two-dimensional gel electrophoresis of four serum samples from patients with IgD myeloma. Clin Chim Acta 218:149, 1993.

83. Putnam FW, Takahashi N, Tetaert D et al: The last of the immunoglobulins: Complete amino acid sequence of human IgD. Ann NY Acad Sci 399:41, 1982.

84. Spiegelberg HL: Immunoglobulin D (IgD). Methods Enzymol 116:95, 1985.

85. Van Boxel JA, Paul WE, Terry WD, Green I: IgD-bearing human lymphocytes. J Immunol 109:648, 1972.

86. Bladé J, Kyle RA: IgD monoclonal gammopathy with long-term follow-up. Br J Haematol 88:395, 1994.

87. Ishizaka K, Ishizaka T, Hornbrook MM: Physicochemical properties of reaginic antibody. V. Correlation of reaginic activity with γE-globulin antibody. J Immunol 97:840, 1966.

88. Geha RS: Human IgE. J Allergy Clin Immunol 74:109, 1984.

89. Johansson SGO, Bennich H: Immunological studies of an atypical (myeloma) immunoglobulin. Immunology 13:381, 1967.

90. Invernizzi F, Monti G, Caviglia AG et al: A new case of IgE myeloma. Acta Haematol 85:41, 1991.

91. Macro M, André I, Comby E et al: IgE multiple myeloma. Leuk Lymphoma 32:597, 1999.

92. Kairemo KJ, Lindberg M, Prytz M: IgE myeloma: A case presentation and a review of the literature. Scand J Clin Lab Invest 59:451, 1999.

93. Yunginger JW, Gleich GJ: The impact of the discovery of IgE on the practice of allergy. Pediatr Clin North Am 22:3, 1975.

94. Ishizaka K. Twenty years with IgE: From the identification of IgE to regulatory factors for the IgE response (presidential address). J Immunol 135:1, 1985.

95. Erikson J, Martinis J, Croce CM: Assignment of the genes for human λ immunoglobulin chains to chromosome 22. Nature 294:173, 1981.

96. Honjo T: Immunoglobulin genes. Annu Rev Immunol 1:499, 1983.

97. Seidman JG, Leder P: The arrangement and rearrangement of antibody genes. Nature 276:790, 1978.

98. Hieter PA, Max EE, Seidman JG et al: Cloned human and mouse kappa immunoglobulin constant and J region genes conserve homology in functional segments. Cell 22:197, 1980.

99. Hieter PA, Hollis GF, Korsmeyer SJ et al: Clustered arrangement of immunoglobulin lambda constant region genes in man. Nature 294:536, 1981.

100. Malcolm S, Barton P, Murphy C et al: Localization of human immunoglobulin kappa light chain variable region genes to the short arm of chromosome 2 by in situ hybridization. Proc Natl Acad Sci USA 79:4957, 1982.

101. Kirsch IR, Morton CC, Nakahara K, Leder P: Human immunoglobulin heavy chain genes map to a region of translocations in malignant B lymphocytes. Science 216:301, 1982.

102. Lorenz W, Straubinger B, Zachau HG: Physical map of the human immunoglobulin κ locus and its implications for the mechanisms of Vκ-Jκ rearrangement. Nucleic Acids Res 15:9667, 1987.

103. Pohlenz HD, Straubinger B, Thiebe R et al: The human V kappa locus. Characterization of extended immunoglobulin gene regions by cosmid cloning. J Mol Biol 193:241, 1987.

104. Meindl A, Klobeck HG, Ohnheiser R, Zachau HG: The V kappa gene repertoire in the human germ line. Eur J Immunol 20:1855, 1990.

105. Williams SC, Winter G: Cloning and sequencing of human immunoglobulin V lambda gene segments. Eur J Immunol 23:1456, 1993.

106. Cossman J, Uppenkamp M, Sundeen J et al: Molecular genetics and the diagnosis of lymphoma. Arch Pathol Lab Med 112:117, 1988.

107. Seidman JG, Max EE, Leder P: A κ-immunoglobulin gene is formed by site-specific recombination without further somatic mutation. Nature 280:370, 1979.

108. Early P, Huang H, David M et al: An immunoglobulin heavy chain variable region gene is generated from three segments of DNA: V_H, D, and J_H. Cell 19:981, 1980.

109. Reth MG, Jackson S, Alt FW: VHDJH formation and DJH replacement during pre-B differentiation: Nonrandom usage of gene segments. EMBO J 5:2131, 1986.

110. Berman JE, Mellis SJ, Pollock R et al: Content and organization of the human Ig VH locus: Definition of three new VH families and linkage to the Ig CH locus. EMBO J 7:727, 1988.

111. Siebenlist U, Ravetch JV, Korsmeyer S et al: Human immunoglobulin D segments encoded in tandem multigenic families. Nature 294:631, 1981.

112. Ichihara Y, Matsuoka H, Kurosawa Y: Organization of human immunoglobulin heavy chain diversity gene loci. EMBO J 7:4141, 1988.

113. Ravetch JV, Siebenlist U, Korsmeyer S et al: Structure of the human immunoglobulin mu locus: Characterization of embryonic and rearranged J and D genes. Cell 27:583, 1981.

114. Buluwela L, Albertson DG, Sherrington P et al: The use of chromosomal translocations to study human immunoglobulin gene organization: Mapping DH segments within 35 kb of the C mu gene and identification of a new DH locus. EMBO J 7:2003, 1988.

115. Davis MM, Kim SK, Hood LE: DNA sequences mediating class switching in alpha-immunoglobulins. Science 209:1360, 1980.

116. Kataoka T, Miyata T, Honjo T: Repetitive sequences in class-switch recombination regions of immunoglobulin heavy chain genes. Cell 23:357, 1981.

117. Marcu KB, Lang RB, Stanton LW, Harris LJ: A model for the molecular requirements of immunoglobulin heavy chain class switching. Nature 298:87, 1982.

118. Sakano H, Maki R, Kurosawa Y et al: Two types of somatic recombination are necessary for the generation of complete immunoglobulin heavy-chain genes. Nature 286:676, 1980.

119. Korsmeyer SJ, Hieter PA, Ravetch JV et al: Developmental hierarchy of immunoglobulin gene arrangements in human leukemic pre-B-cells. Proc Natl Acad Sci USA 78:7096, 1981.

120. Kabat EA, Wu TT, Bilofsky H et al: Sequences of Proteins of Immunological Interest. 4th Ed. U.S. Department of Health and Human Services, National Institutes of Health, Washington, DC, 1983.

121. Ralph QM, Brisco MJ, Joshua DE et al: Advancement of multiple myeloma from diagnosis through plateau phase to progression does not involve a new B-cell clone: Evidence from the Ig heavy chain gene. Blood 82:202, 1993.

122. Bakkus MHC, Heirman C, Van Riet I et al: Evidence that multiple myeloma Ig heavy chain VDJ genes contain somatic mutation but show no intraclonal variation. Blood 80:2326, 1992.

123. Seidman JG, Leder A, Nau M et al: Antibody diversity. Science 202:11, 1978.

124. Tonegawa S: Somatic generation of antibody diversity. Nature 302:575, 1983.

125. Kunkel HG: The "abnormality" of myeloma proteins. Cancer Res 28:1351, 1968.

126. Natvig JB, Kunkel HG: Human immunoglobulins: Classes, subclasses, genetic variants, and idiotypes. Adv Immunol 16:1, 1973.

127. Krause RM: The search for antibodies with molecular uniformity. Adv Immunol 12:1, 1970.

128. Potter M: Myeloma proteins (M-component) with antibody-like activity. N Engl J Med 284:831, 1971.

129. Seligmann M, Brouet JC: Antibody activity of human myeloma globulins. Semin Hematol 10:163, 1973.

130. Osterland CK, Espinoza LR: Biological properties of myeloma proteins. Arch Intern Med 135:32, 1975.

131. Gutman AB: The plasma proteins in disease. Adv Protein Chem 4:155, 1948.

132. Buxbaum JN: The biosynthesis, assembly, and secretion of immunoglobulins. Semin Hematol 10:33, 1973.

133. Stone MJ, Frenkel EP: The clinical spectrum of light chain myeloma: A study of 35 patients with special reference to the occurrence of amyloidosis. Am J Med 58:601, 1975.

134. Kyle RA, Greipp PR: The laboratory investigation of monoclonal gammopathies. Mayo Clin Proc 53:719, 1978.

135. Whicher JT, Wallage M, Fifield R: Use of immunoglobulin heavy- and light-chain measurements compared with existing techniques as a means of typing monoclonal immunoglobulins. Clin Chem 33:1771, 1987.

136. Kyle RA: Sequence of testing for monoclonal gammopathies. Arch Pathol Lab Med 123:114, 1999.

137. Reichert CM, Everett DF Jr, Nadler PI, Papadopoulos NM: High-resolution zone electrophoresis, combined with immunofixation, in the detection of an occult myeloma paraprotein. Clin Chem 28:2312, 1982.

138. Pola V, Tichý M: Bisalbuminemia: Critical review and report of a case of an acquired form in a myeloma patient [German]. Folia Haematol Int Mag Klin Morphol Blutforsch 112:208, 1985.

139. Kyle RA, Robinson RA, Katzmann JA: The clinical aspects of biclonal gammopathies: Review of 57 cases. Am J Med 71:999, 1981.

140. Whicher JT, Calvin J, Riches P, Warren C: The laboratory investigation of paraproteinaemia. Ann Clin Biochem 24:119, 1987.

141. Keren DF: Capillary zone electrophoresis in the evaluation of serum protein abnormalities. Am J Clin Pathol 110:248, 1998.

142. Clark R, Katzmann JA, Wiegert E et al: Rapid capillary electrophoretic analysis of human serum proteins: Qualitative comparison with high-throughput agarose gel electrophoresis. J Chromatogr A 744:205, 1996.

143. Katzmann JA, Clark R, Wiegert E et al: Identification of monoclonal proteins in serum: A quantitative comparison of acetate, agarose gel, and capillary electrophoresis. Electrophoresis 18:1775, 1997.

144. Massey MA, Thompson CK, Katzmann JA et al: Pentafix as an efficient screening assay for monoclonal proteins. Clin Chem 46(Suppl.):A170, 2000 (abstract).

145. Duc J, Morel B, Peitrequin R, Frei PC: Identification of monoclonal gammopathies: A comparison of immunofixation, immunoelectrophoresis and measurements of kappa- and lambda-immunoglobulin levels. J Clin Lab Immunol 26:141, 1988.

146. Deegan MJ, Perry M, Hayashi H: A rapid method for identifying the light chain component of a monoclonal protein, abstracted. Blood 66(Suppl. 1):186a, 1985.

147. Keren DF, Warren JS, Lowe JB: Strategy to diagnose monoclonal gammopathies in serum: High-resolution electrophoresis, immunofixation, and κ/λ quantification. Clin Chem 34:2196, 1988.

148. Jones RG, Aguzzi F, Bienvenu J et al: Use of immunoglobulin heavy-chain and light-chain measurements in a multicenter trial to investigate monoclonal components: II. Classification by use of computer-based algorithms. Clin Chem 37:1922, 1991.

149. Bush D, Keren DF: Over- and underestimation of monoclonal gammopathies by quantification of κ- and γ-containing immunoglobulins in serum (editorial). Clin Chem 38:315, 1992.

150. Kyle RA, Katzmann JA, Lust JA, Dispenzieri A: Immunochemical characterization of immunoglobulins, pp 71–91. In Rose NR, Hamilton RG, Detrick B (eds.): Manual of Clinical Laboratory Immunology, 6th Ed. ASM Press, Washington, DC, 2002.

151. Markowitz H, Tschida AR: Automated quantitative immunochemical analysis of human immunoglobulins. Clin Chem 18:1364, 1972.

152. Fahey JL, McKelvey EM: Quantitative determination of serum immunoglobulins in antibody-agar plates. J Immunol 94:84, 1965.

153. Schreiber WE, Chiang E, Tse SSL: Electrophoresis underestimates the concentration of polyclonal immunoglobulins in serum. Am J Clin Pathol 97:610, 1992.

154. Katzmann JA, Massey MA, Greipp PR et al: Artifactually low IgG monoclonal protein (M-spike) quantitation on agarose gel electrophoresis: Comparison of agarose gel electrophoresis, capillary zone electrophoresis, and nephelometry. Clin Chem 46(Suppl.):A169, 2000.

155. Pruzanski W, Watt JG: Serum viscosity and hyperviscosity syndrome in IgG multiple myeloma. Report on 10 patients and a review of the literature. Ann Intern Med 77:853, 1972.

156. Gertz MA, Kyle RA: Hyperviscosity syndrome. J Intens Care Med 10:128, 1995.

157. Brouet JC, Clauvel JP, Danon F et al: Biologic and clinical significance of cryoglobulins: A report of 86 cases. Am J Med 57:775, 1974.

158. Letendre L, Kyle RA: Monoclonal cryoglobulinemia with high thermal insolubility. Mayo Clin Proc 57:629, 1982.

159. Gorevic PD, Kassab HJ, Levo Y et al: Mixed cryoglobulinemia: Clinical aspects and long-term follow-up of 40 patients. Am J Med 69:287, 1980.

160. Dammacco F, Sansonno D: Antibodies to hepatitis C virus in essential mixed cryoglobulinaemia. Clin Exp Immunol 87:352, 1992.

161. Martin WJ, Mathieson DR, Eigler JOC: Pyroglobulinemia: Further observations and review of 20 cases. Proc Staff Meet Mayo Clin 34:95, 1959.

162. Caulin-Glaser T, Prelli F, Franklin EC: Structural studies on an IgM-λ pyroglobulin. J Lab Clin Med 99:845, 1982.

163. Patterson R, Weiszer I, Rambach W et al: Comparative cellular and immunochemical studies of two cases of pyroglobulinemia. Am J Med 44:147, 1968.

164. Invernizzi F, Cattaneo R, Rosso di San Secondo V et al: Pyroglobulinemia: A report of eight patients with associated paraproteinemia. Acta Haematol (Basel) 50:65, 1973.

165. Sugai S: IgA pyroglobulin, hyperviscosity syndrome and coagulation abnormality in a patient with multiple myeloma. Blood 39:224, 1972.

166. Tsuda H, Kishimoto S: IgD-plasma cell leukemia associated with pyroglobulinemia and pyroglobulinuria: New types of pyroglobulin and cytoplasmic fibrils. Acta Haematol (Basel) 67:80, 1982.

167. Line DE, Adler S, Fraley DS, Burns FJ: Massive pseudoproteinuria caused by nafcillin. JAMA 235:1259, 1976.

168. Whicher JT, Calvin J, Riches P, Warren C: The laboratory investigation of paraproteinaemia. Ann Clin Biochem 24:119, 1987.

169. Hinberg IH, Katz L, Waddell L: Sensitivity of in vitro diagnostic dipstick tests to urinary protein. Clin Biochem 11:62, 1978.

170. Scarpioni L, Ballocchi S, Bergonzi G et al: Glomerular and tubular proteinuria in myeloma: Relationship with Bence Jones proteinuria. Contrib Nephrol 26:89, 1981.

171. Perry MC, Kyle RA: The clinical significance of Bence Jones proteinuria. Mayo Clin Proc 50:234, 1975.

172. Dalal FR, Winsten S: Double light-chain disease: A case report. Clin Chem 25:190, 1979.

173. Whicher JT, Hawkins L, Higginson J: Clinical applications of immunofixation: A more sensitive technique for the detection of Bence Jones protein. J Clin Pathol 33:779, 1980.

174. Kyle RA, Gertz MA: Primary systemic amyloidosis: Clinical and laboratory features in 474 cases. Semin Hematol 32:45, 1995.

175. Harrison HH: The "ladder light chain" or "pseudo-oligoclonal" pattern in urinary immunofixation electrophoresis (IFE) studies: A distinctive IFE pattern and an explanatory hypothesis relating it to free polyclonal light chains. Clin Chem 37:1559, 1991.

176. Charles EZ, Valdes AJ: Free fragments of γ chain in the urine: A possible source of confusion with γ heavy-chain disease. Am J Clin Pathol 101:462, 1994.

177. Kyle RA, Garton JP: Laboratory monitoring of myeloma proteins. Semin Oncol 13:310, 1986.

178. McLaughlin P, Alexanian R: Myeloma protein kinetics following chemotherapy. Blood 60:851, 1982.

28

Cytogenetic Abnormalities in the Monoclonal Gammopathies

Rafael Fonseca, P. Leif Bergsagel, and W. Michael Kuehl

Multiple and complex chromosomal abnormalities have been described in multiple myeloma (MM).[1–6] Early studies revealed that both structural and numeric abnormalities were seen when metaphases were analyzed by conventional cytogenetic (CC) methods. Interest in the biologic and prognostic significance of these abnormalities has been rekindled by reports describing their importance for specific abnormalities in the biology of the disease and for establishing patient prognoses.[7,8] In this review we will summarize the current knowledge of chromosomal abnormalities associated with malignant plasma cells (PCs) and their biologic and clinical significance.

CONVENTIONAL CYTOGENETICS

Conventional cytogenetics have demonstrated that abnormal metaphases, including both numerical and structural chromosomal changes, are present in up to 30 percent of patients with MM[1–5] (Figure 28–1). However, the proportion of MM patients with aneuploidy by DNA content analysis was much higher.[9] Subsequent attempts to stimulate clonal plasma cells (PCs) to

proliferate with mitogenic cytokines failed.[10] The prevailing hypothesis among cytogeneticists was that nearly all patients with MM had chromosomally abnormal clones but were not evaluable because of the low mitotic index of the cells or technical limitations. We now know that most, if not all, MM tumors are cytogenetically abnormal. Dewald and colleagues demonstrated that abnormal metaphases were more frequently observed in patients with advanced stages of the disease and that survival was lower in patients with a higher proportion of abnormal metaphases.[1]

Among all reported chromosomal abnormalities a few were recurrent, including numerical abnormalities of chromosomes 3, 7, 9, 11, 15; abnormalities of chromosome 1; deletions of the long arm of chromosome 13; monosomy of chromosome 13; and more importantly, reciprocal translocations (TRXs) involving chromosome 14 in approximately 20 to 40 percent of cases with abnormal metaphases.[1–5] Translocations involving chromosome 14 usually occurred at band q32, the site of the immunoglobulin heavy-chain (IgH) locus as seen in other B-cell neoplastic disorders.[1] The most common translocation partner was chromosome 11, and in most of the other translocations, a 14q32+ chromosome without an identifiable partner chromosome was described.[1,11,12] Partner chromosomes described in balanced TRXs involving 14q32 in other B-cell neoplasias (chromosome 8 at the *c-myc* locus,[13–18] and 18 at the *bcl-2* locus,[19,20]) have seldom been reported. The promiscuity of 14q32 awaited further description.[21–23]

Conventional cytogenetics presents some difficulties in the evaluation of MM.[24] In particular, CC depends on proliferating cells, and in many patients MM PCs divide infrequently.[25] In fact, when abnormal metaphases are observed, it is more likely that they represent the more advanced proliferative fraction of the clone and thus introduce bias. Most metaphases are normal and are thus derived from normal myeloid cells rather than from the malignant clone. It has been suggested that in aneuploid neoplasias, proliferating cells are occasionally less likely to

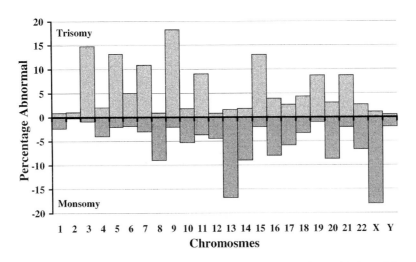

Figure 28–1. Aneuploidy in multiple myeloma from conventional cytogenetics. The graph is formed from composite published data.[1–5] The upper bars depict the percentage of patients with chromosomal trisomy for each of the different 23 chromosomes and the lower bars depict percentage of patients with monosomy.

exhibit metaphase morphology when exposed to tubulin-disrupting agents such as nocodazole or colcemid.[26,27] In addition, some of the prominent cytogenetic abnormalities in MM are cryptic when usual banding techniques are used.[28–30] Karyotypic anomalies in the evaluation of patients with MM and prior alkylator therapy may be present in myeloid cells but not in the MM tumor cells.[31–33] The presence of chromosomal abnormalities in CC may be an important marker of cells with a higher proliferative rate. In fact, by using CC we have shown a striking correlation between the PC proliferative rate as determined by the labeling index and the observation of an abnormal clone.[34]

Since the initial observations by Dewald and colleagues,[1] several investigators have made the important observation that finding abnormal metaphases carries adverse prognostic significance for patients with MM.[1,7] In two reports from the University of Arkansas, three abnormalities associated with an adverse outcome were identified and designated "unfavorable cytogenetics" (TRXs, abnormalities of 11q, and deletions of 13q).[7,8] Both overall survival and event-free survival decrements were associated with the observation of these structural abnormalities as detected by CC.

NOVEL TECHNIQUES

Fluorescent in situ hybridization (FISH) can be used to analyze either metaphase chromosomes (Plate 28–1A) or interphase chromosomes (Plate 28–1C) in infrequently dividing cells to detect specific chromosomal abnormalities. Using FISH we now know that all PC dyscrasias, including monoclonal gammopathy of undetermined significance (MGUS), harbor both numerical[35–38] and structural chromosomal abnormalities.[35,36] The incorporation of simultaneous fluorescent staining of cytoplasmic immunoglobulins and chromosomal DNA (cIg-FISH, FICTION)[39] allows for the precise identification of clonally restricted abnormalities (Plate 28–1C). This is especially important in cases with a low percentage of MM tumor cells because the malignant PC coexists with normal hematopoietic cells in the bone marrow.[40–42] Alternatively, FISH can be performed on cells that have been selected by either flow-cytometric cell sorting or immunomagnetic bead separation.

Specialized FISH techniques include multiple-color FISH (M-FISH, or SKY), used by several groups to further characterize or identify chromosomal abnormalities not previously recognizable by CC of metaphase chromosomes (Plate 28–1B). Metaphase chromosomes are hybridized with DNA whole-chromosome painting probe combinations such that each normal chromosome can be assigned a specific color. Thus, cryptic numerical and structural abnormalities may become apparent and/or more accurately identified. However, this technique is not useful in the evaluation of nonproliferating cells. Rao and colleagues identified recurrent chromosomal abnormalities involving breakpoints in 3q27, 17q24–25, and 20q11.[43] Sawyer and colleagues could identify, among other abnormalities, the t(14;16)(q32;q22–23) as

recurrent in patients with MM, something previously undescribed by CC.[44]

Comparative genomic hybridization (CGH) is a technique devised to detect an abnormal amount of neoplastic DNA of a given region when compared with normal genomic DNA. Normal metaphase chromosomes are hybridized with equimolar concentrations of tumor and normal DNA that have been differentially labeled with two fluorophores. Deviations from the expected mixture fluorescence identify areas of gain or loss of DNA in the tumor sample (Plate 21–1D). It is thus valuable in cases of large chromosomal regions of loss or gain, such as are seen in aneuploidy (monosomy, trisomy), deletions, insertions, unbalanced TRXs, or amplification.[45] However, CGH is not useful for the analysis of balanced structural abnormalities (e.g., 14q32 TRXs in MM). Cigudosa et al. detected multiple recurrent changes, including gain of chromosome 19p and complete or partial deletions of chromosome 13 in MM.[45] Other recurrent changes included gains of 9q, 11q, 12q, 15q, 17q, and 22q and losses of 6q and 16q. Avet-Loiseau et al. identified loss on 13q and 14q and gain on 1q and chromosome 7 as recurrent chromosomal abnormalities. They also identified "hot spots" of sequence loss in 13q12.1-q21, 13q32-q34, 14q11.2-q13, and 14q23-q31.[46]

FISH done on stretched DNA fibers (DNA-fiber-FISH) is a powerful tool (Plate 28–1E) for the analysis of TRX.[47] Such an approach has been used for the study of t(11;14)(q13;q32) in mantle cell lymphoma and MM.[48] This technique is especially useful for the mapping of translocation breakpoints when scattered over several hundred kilobases (kb), as is seen in MM.[48] Vaandrager and colleagues[49] used this technique to define the breakpoints of the MM cell line KMS-12.

SPECIFIC CHROMOSOMAL ABNORMALITIES

Aneuploidy

Multiple myeloma is a disorder characterized by the frequent occurrence of aneuploidy[1–5,35–38,50] (Figure 28–1). When taken as a whole, aneuploidy is the most common chromosomal abnormality in MM.[1–5,35–38,50] It is heterogenous, and no specific numerical abnormality has been identified as constant or indicative of disease progression,[1–5,35–38,50] although Perez-Simon and colleagues reported that trisomy of chromosomes 6, 9, and 17 was associated with improved survival.[51] Hypodiploid MM has been associated with an interior response to therapy and shorter survival.[50] We have also shown that aneuploidy is particularly frequent in MM, with high incidence for chromosomes 7, 11, and 15 (personal communication) (Table 28–1).

Deletions of 13q

The presence of chromosome 13 deletions has been associated, in several studies, with a poor prognosis in MM patients.[7,8,89] The important sites for deletion at 13q have not been established, and there is no proven pathogenetic role for 13q14 dele-

Table 28–1. Percentages of Multiple Myeloma Patients with Aneuploidy as Tested by Fluorescent In Situ Hybridization

Author	n	Newly Diagnosed Patients	1	3	6	7	8	9	11	12	13	15	16	17	18	Xf	Xm	Aneuploidy (percent)
Trisomy																		
Tabernero[38]	52	37	37	31	32	28	8	52	33	3	0	48	ND	22	24	0	6	80
Drach[35]	36	3	36	61	ND	56	17	ND	53	25	ND	ND	25	22	39	11	6	89
Fonseca[9]	55	39	ND	ND	ND	69	ND	81	60	ND	ND	75	ND	ND	42	28	50	100
Mean			37	46	32	51	13	67	49	14	0	62	25	22	35	13	21	
Monosomy																		
Tabernero[38]	52	37	3			ND	5	ND	3	ND	26	ND	ND	ND	6	31	0	
Drach[35]	36	3	11			ND	6	ND	ND	3	ND	ND	6	22	11	42	0	
Fonseca[9]	55	39	ND			23	ND	2	13	ND	ND	15	ND	ND	60	56	0	
Mean			7			23	6	2	8	3	26	15	6	22	26	43	0	

n, number of patients; Xf, chromosome X analysis in females; Xm, chromosome X analysis in males. Aneuploidy refers to the proportion of patients with at least one numerical chromosomal abnormality detected.

a Fonseca, unpublished information.

tion in MM. In a report by the University of Arkansas, the presence of 13q abnormalities as detected by CC was the single most important prognostic indicator.[52] Shaughnessy and colleagues identified a high prevalence of 13q- in the clonal PCs of patients with MM when multiple FISH probes were used.[53] They reported observing complex FISH patterns that were consistent with large deletions of 13q14.[53] A study by Drach and colleagues has confirmed the adverse prognosis associated with deletions of 13q when detected by FISH studies.[54] We have studied a total of 351 patients for deletions of 13q14 and found an abnormality prevalence of 54 percent.[55] In most cases these deletions apparently include sequences telomeric to the 13q14 site, occurring as a consequence of either long deletions of the q arm or monosomy.[53,55] Deletions of 13 were similarly associated with an adverse outcome.

Deletions of 17p13.1

Deletions of the long arm of chromosome 17 at 17p13.1, with resulting loss of the tumor suppressor gene *p53*, have also been observed in 10 to 40 percent of MM cases and are associated with a poor prognosis when detected by FISH.[56] Drach et al. found that patients with deletions of *p53* had a median survival of 13.9 months, compared with 38.7 months for those patients without loss of the *p53* region (*p*<.0001).[56] A striking correlation between *p53* deletions and stage III disease was also observed. However, a more recent report suggested loss of *p53* signals in approximately 10 percent of patients.[57] Similarly, mutations of *p53* have been observed in a fraction of MM patients. They have been observed in approximately 5 percent of early myeloma versus 20 to 40 percent of plasma cell leukemia cases.[58–61] The interaction between these two abnormalities at 17p13.1 has not been systematically evaluated.

Translocations Involving 14q32

An increasing body of evidence suggests that chromosomal translocations, at the immunoglobulin heavy-chain locus at 14q32 are of major significance in the pathogenesis of MM and MGUS.[12,21,22,28,29,62–68] We and others have shown that these TRXs are nearly universal in PC lines[22,64] and are common in MM patient samples. Indeed, using interphase FISH, Nishida et al. reported that 14q32 TRXs are found in 73 percent of patients with MM,[69] Avet-Loiseau et al. found TRXs involving 14q32 in 60 percent of patients,[21] and we have documented immunoglobulin (IgH) TRXs in nearly two-thirds of patients with advanced MM tumors (W. M. Kuehl, unpublished data). We and others have also shown that TRXs are present in MGUS,[66,67] where they may be identified in all of the clonal plasma cells, which indicates that they are likely an initiating oncogenic event that precedes progression to frankly malignant MM.

Immunoglobulin heavy-chain TRXs are promiscuous and involve an ever-increasing number of nonrandom partner chromosomes.[28,29,62,63] These TRXs are thought to occur mostly in the IgH switch regions associated with the nonproductive allele, although they sometimes occur in the JH region, likely as a result of unrepaired double-strand breaks that occur during somatic hypermutation (Plate 28–2). In MM as in other B-cell neoplasias, these TRXs result in the juxtaposition of oncogenes with the powerful enhancer regions of 14q32, mostly the 3' enhancer.[22,70] It is believed IgH TRXs in MM are balanced, whereas TRXs involving other loci usually are not.

The extensive diversity of the nonrandom chromosomal partners is not well understood but likely reflects some combination of the presence of a relevant oncogene near the translocation breakpoint and the inherent chromosomal structure surrounding the translocation breakpoints of the involved genomic loci. For instance, it seems likely that the 16q23 breakpoints result from genomic instability of the fragile site FRA16D.[29,71] Generally, breakpoints in the partner chromosomes are widely scattered, frequently over several hundred kb.[29] Importantly, for all TRXs that have been fully characterized, there is selective dysregulation and overexpression of one or more oncogenes that can be located up to 1 Mb from the translocation breakpoint. It is thought that the dysregulation is mediated by juxtaposition of the oncogene to one or more of the strong IgH enhancers, Eμ, 3' Eα1, 3' Eα2 (Plate 28–2).

The t(11;14)(q13;q32) Translocation

The t(11;14)(q13;q32) translocation was the first well recognized recurrent translocation in MM.[1,5] It is present in approximately 25 percent of human MM cell lines[62] and dysregulates *cyclin D1* and in some cases also a novel putative oncogene *myeov*.[48] Breakpoints in 11q13 are widely scattered and located as far as 330 kb centromeric to *cyclin D1* on 11q13.[49] Similar mechanistic upregulation of *cyclin D1* has also been observed through the switch recombination-mediated excision and insertion of IgH constant and enhancer sequences at 11q13, as is seen in the cell line U266.[72] *Cyclin D1* is overexpressed in a fraction of myeloma patients[73–75] as well, but immunohistochemical methods seem less able to detect the abnormality than cIg-FISH. An alternative is to use a competitive reverse transcriptase polymerase chain reaction (RT-PCR) to compare relative expression of *cyclin D1* and *D3*.[76] This, however, requires a meaningful proportion (more than about 10 percent) of clonal PCs in a studied sample. When interphase FISH techniques are used, the incidence of this translocation is closer to 15 to 20 percent.[21,55,77] We have recently studied a total of 350 patients with newly diagnosed MM by cIg-FISH and found the abnormality in 16 percent of cases.[55] In all those cases in which we could demonstrate the *cyclin D1* upregulation (by immunohistochemistry) we could also detect the t(11;14).[55] This translocation is also seen in the MGUS stage of the disease.[66,67] Although this translocation was initially thought[7,78,79] to be associated with an adverse outcome, recent studies show that, if anything, patients with this abnormality fare equally as well as if not better than others.[90] In fact, we have observed a higher response rate to treatment and longer overall survival time and progression free-time of patients with the t(11;14) than were found in patients without the abnormality, although these findings did not achieve statistical significance.

The t(4;14)(p16.3:q32) Translocation

The t(4;14)(p16.3;q32) translocation also is seen in approximately 25 percent of human MM cell lines.[28,80] It results in the upregulation of the fibroblast growth factor receptor-3 (*FGFR-3*), which is located on der(14).[28] In addition, hybrid mRNA transcripts, including IgH sequences and the novel gene *MMSET (WHSC1)*, which is homologous to the *MLL* gene that is involved in the pathogenesis of leukemia, are produced from der(4). The t(4;14) translocation provides the first example of a translocation that simultaneously dysregulates two putative oncogenes (Plate 28–2) The Ig/*MMSET* transcripts are readily detectable by RT-PCR and provide a useful tool for the detection of the abnormality. The translocation breakpoints at 4p16.3 are dispersed over 200 kb and located centromeric to the *FGFR3* gene[28,63] and within the 5′ introns of *MMSET*. There is selective expression of one *FGFR3* allele in all informative cases, which is consistent with dysregulated expression of *FGFR3* by the TRX. Kinase-activating mutations of *FGFR3*, identical to those causing thanatophoric dwarfism, have also been observed in the *FGFR3* translocated allele.[28,63] It appears that these mutations appear after translocation and are associated with disease progression.[91]

This translocation is found in 15 to 25 percent of MM patients.[21,80–83] It was identified by RT-PCR in 11 of 53 (20 percent),[84] and by using interphase FISH Avet-Loiseau found this translocation in 17 of 141 (12 percent)[21] patients with MM. This translocation has also been observed in MGUS, although at a lower frequency than in MM.[66,67] This translocation is associated with a shorter survival.[90,92]

The t(14;16)(q32;q23) Translocation

The t(14;16)(q32;q23) translocation also has been described in 20 percent of human MM cell lines and in PC leukemia,[21,29] and is seen in about 10 percent of MM samples analyzed by SKY. Although not common and occasionally not detected,[66] it has also been observed in MGUS cases.[66,67] The gene *c-maf* has been shown to have transforming activity in chicken fibroblasts,[85] and is dysregulated by this translocation. Translocations at 16q23 also include variant TRXs involving the lambda chains locus (8226 and XG-6), in which cases the breakpoints are telomeric to *c-maf*. Several factors support the notion that *c-maf* is the important oncogene dysregulated by this translocation: upregulation of *c-maf* is only seen in the cell lines with the t(14;16); informative cells lines (KMS-11 and 8266) only express one allele; and *c-maf* is bracketed by the 16q32 breakpoints of both the IgH and Ig lambda TRXs.[29] Breakpoints in 16q23 can be widely dispersed and go to an unprecedented distance of over 1Mb[29] from the initiation of transcription of *c-maf* without intervening deletions (R. Fonseca, unpublished data). The 16q23 breakpoints in cell lines with this translocation are located in intron 5 (KMS-11) and intron 8 (all other 14q32 TRXs) of the newly described *WWOX* gene, which covers most of the 1-Mb region centromeric to *c-maf*. This translocation is also associated with a short survival.

The t(6;14)(p25;q32) Translocation

The translocation t(6;14)(p25;q32) has also been described in human MM cell lines,[86] and it results in dysregulation of the *MUM1/IRF4* gene. In one study of patient samples using interphase FISH, there was a marked discrepancy between the number of MM tumor cells in the sample and the number of cells noted to harbor the t(6;14) translocation.[87] This may be explained by technical difficulties but might indicate that only a fraction of the MM cells have the translocation. The latter possibility is consistent with the hypothesis that the t(6;14)(p25;q32) translocation may represent a secondary event related to tumor progression.[87]

The t(8;14)(q24;q32) Translocation

Chromosomal TRXs that juxtapose *c-myc* with one of the three Ig loci are an essentially invariant oncogenic event in Burkitt's lymphoma and murine plasmacytoma tumors.[13–18] These reciprocal TRXs appear to occur early in tumorigenesis as a result of errors in IgH switch recombination or somatic hypermutation, and result in dysregulation of the affected *c-myc* allele. The unaffected *c-myc* allele is not expressed, as is consistent with the absence of *c-myc* expression in the normal-cell counterparts of these tumors. The similarities in phenotype of human MM and these tumors prompted numerous attempts to demonstrate Ig TRXs involving *c-myc*, but conventional cytogenetics identified *c-myc*/Ig TRX or *c-myc* amplification in less than 10 percent of MM tumors and cell lines analyzed. Recently, however, through the use of the advanced cytogenetic methods described above, we have shown that more than 90 percent of MM cell lines and nearly 50 percent of advanced primary MM tumors have complex karyotypic abnormalities of the *c-myc* locus.[88] Most but not all *c-myc* karyotypic abnormalities involve juxtaposition to an IgH or IgL locus. In contrast to murine plasmacytoma and Burkitt's lymphoma tumors, we hypothesize that the dysregulation of *c-myc* is a late, progression event mediated by secondary TRXs that do not involve errors in VDJ or IgH switch recombination or in somatic hypermutation. In addition, it seems likely that some of the other 14q32 TRXs (perhaps TRXs involving 6p25) identified in MM result from similar secondary translocation events, although this remains to be firmly established.

Igλ-I Translocations in Multiple Myeloma

Translocations involving the Igλ loci have been described in only a small fraction of MM tumors. For example, the SKY analysis of 50 advanced MM tumors by Sawyer et al. identified about 10 tumors (20 percent) with a translocation near the Igλ locus at 22q11 and perhaps 1 or 2 tumors (less than 4 percent) with a translocation near the Igκ locus at 2p11.[30] Using metaphase FISH analyses, we have found TRXs involving the Igλ locus in about 20 percent of MM cell lines and about 20 percent of advance MM tumors but have detected no Igκ TRXs thus far (M. Kuehl, unpublished data). In addition, we have found Igλ TRXs in about 20 MGUS tumors by interphase FISH analyses.[67]

DONOR CHROMOSOME THEORY

The TRXs in MM are promiscuous and involve a number of partner chromosomes, as described above.[28,29,62,63] They include early, initiating events that are mediated by errors in B cell-specific DNA modification processes and precede clonal expansion (11q13, 4p16, 16q23, and many others) but also late events associated with disease progression that are not mediated by errors in B cell-specific DNA modification processes (e.g., 8q24). At diagnosis the majority of MM patients present with only one 14q32 translocation, so that the donor chromosomes may identify distinct, nonoverlapping molecular subtypes of MM. Each of the donor chromosomes could result in a different phenotypic expression of the disease, such as natural history, biologic features, prognosis, and hopefully, successful therapeutic interventions (donor chromosome theory). It may be that MM is not one disease but rather a group of disorders, each of which is characterized by a different chromosomal abnormality.

ACKNOWLEDGMENT

RF is a Leukemia and Lymphoma Society Translational Research Awardee. RF is also supported by the Mayo Foundation and by the CI-5 Cancer Research Fund Lilly Clinical Investigator Award of the Damon Runyon–Walter Winchell Foundation. This work was also supported in part by Public Health Service grant R01 CA83724-01 from the National Cancer Institute.

REFERENCES

1. Dewald GW, Kyle RA, Hicks GA, Greipp PR: The clinical significance of cytogenetic studies in 100 patients with multiple myeloma, plasma cell leukemia, or amyloidosis. Blood 66:380–90, 1985.
2. Gould J, Alexanian R, Goodacre A, Pathak S, Hecht B, Barlogie B: Plasma cell karyotype in multiple myeloma. Blood 71:453–456, 1988.
3. Lai JL, Zandecki M, Mary JY et al: Improved cytogenetics in multiple myeloma: A study of 151 patients including 117 patients at diagnosis. Blood 85:2490–2497, 1995.
4. Zandecki M: Multiple-Myeloma–almost all patients are cytogenetically abnormal. Br J Haematol 94:217–227, 1996.
5. Sawyer JR, Waldron JA, Jagannath S, Barlogie B: Cytogenetic findings in 200 patients with multiple myeloma. Cancer Genet Cytogenet 82:41–9, 1995.
6. Fonseca R, Coignet LJ, Dewald GW: Cytogenetic abnormalities in multiple myeloma [review]. Hematol Oncol Clin North Am 13:1169–80, 1999.
7. Tricot G, Barlogie B, Jagannath S et al: Poor prognosis in multiple myeloma is associated only with partial or complete deletions of chromosome 13 or abnormalities involving 11q and not with other karyotype abnormalities. Blood 86:4250–6, 1995.
8. Tricot G, Sawyer JR, Jagannath S et al: Unique role of cytogenetics in the prognosis of patients with myeloma receiving high-dose therapy and autotransplants. J Clin Oncol 15:2659–66, 1997.
9. Latreille J, Barlogie B, Johnston D, Drewinko B, Alexanian R: Ploidy and proliferative characteristics in monoclonal gammopathies. Blood 59:43–51, 1982.
10. Lai JL, Zandecki M, Mary JY et al: Improved cytogenetics in multiple myeloma: A study of 151 patients including 117 patients at diagnosis [review]. Blood 85:2490–7, 1995.
11. Fonseca R, Hoyer J, Ahmann G et al: The t(11;14)(q13;q32) is strongly associated with cyclin D1 over-expression in bone marrow plasma cells of multiple myeloma (MM) patients. Blood 92:Abstract 1068, 1998.
12. Fonseca R, Hoyer J, Aguayo P et al: Multiple myeloma and the translocation t(11;14)(q13;q32). Leuk Lymphoma 35:599–605, 1999.
13. Crews S, Barth R, Hood L, Prehn J, Calame K: Mouse c-myc oncogene is located on chromosome 15 and translocated to chromosome 12 in plasmacytomas. Science 218:1319–21, 1982.
14. Stanton LW, Watt R, Marcu KB: Translocation, breakage and truncated transcripts of c-myc oncogene in murine plasmacytomas. Nature 303:401–6, 1983.
15. Keath EJ, Kelekar A, Cole MD: Transcriptional activation of the translocated c-myc oncogene in mouse plasmacytomas: Similar RNA levels in tumor and proliferating normal cells. Cell 37:521–8, 1984.
16. Piccoli SP, Caimi PG, Cole MD: A conserved sequence at c-myc oncogene chromosomal translocation breakpoints in plasmacytomas. Nature 310:327–30, 1984.
17. Erikson J, Miller DA, Miller OJ et al: The c-myc oncogene is translocated to the involved chromosome 12 in mouse plasmacytoma. Proc Natl Acad Sci U S A 82:4212–6, 1985.
18. Adams JM, Harris AW, Pinkert CA et al: The c-myc oncogene driven by immunoglobulin enhancers induces lymphoid malignancy in transgenic mice. Nature 318:533–8, 1985.
19. Levine EG, Arthur DC, Frizzera G, Peterson BA, Hurd DD, Bloomfield CD: There are differences in cytogenetic abnormalities among histologic subtypes of the non-Hodgkin's lymphomas. Blood 66:1414–22, 1985.

20. Yunis JJ, Oken MM, Kaplan ME, Ensrud KM, Howe RR, Theologides A: Distinctive chromosomal abnormalities in histologic subtypes of non-Hodgkin's lymphoma. N Engl J Med 307:1231–6, 1982.

21. Avet-Loiseau H, Li JY, Facon T et al: High incidence of translocations t(11;14)(q13;q32) and t(4;14)(p16;q32). Cancer Res 58:5640–5, 1998.

22. Bergsagel PL, Chesi M, Nardini E, Brents LA, Kirby SL, Kuehl WM: Promiscuous translocations into immunoglobulin heavy chain switch regions in multiple myeloma. Proc Natl Acad Sci U S A 93:13931–6, 1996.

23. Bergsagel PL, Nardini E, Brents L, Chesi M, Kuehl WM: IgH translocations in multiple myeloma: A nearly universal event that rarely involves c-myc. Curr Top Microbiol Immunol 224:283–7, 1997.

24. Van Den Berghe H: Chromosomes in plasma-cell malignancies. [review]. Eur J Haematol Suppl 51:47–51, 1989.

25. Greipp PR, Witzig TE, Gonchoroff NJ et al: Immunofluorescence labeling indices in myeloma and related monoclonal gammopathies. Mayo Clin Proc 62:969–77, 1987.

26. Cahill DP, Lengauer C, Yu J et al: Mutations of mitotic checkpoint genes in human cancers. Nature 392:300–3, 1998.

27. Cahill DP, da Costa LT, Carson-Walter EB, Kinzler KW, Vogelstein B, Lengauer C: Characterization of MAD2B and other mitotic spindle checkpoint genes. Genomics 58:181–7, 1999.

28. Chesi M, Nardini E, Brents LA et al: Frequent translocation t(4;14)(p16.3;q32.3) in multiple myeloma is associated with increased expression and activating mutations of fibroblast growth factor receptor 3. Nat Genet 16:260–4, 1997.

29. Chesi M, Bergsagel PL, Shonukan OO et al: Frequent dysregulation of the c-maf proto-oncogene at 16q23 by translocation to an Ig locus in multiple myeloma. Blood 91:4457–63, 1998.

30. Sawyer JR, Lukacs JL, Munshi N et al: Identification of new non-random translocations in multiple myeloma with multicolor spectral karyotyping. Blood 92:4269–78, 1998.

31. Soenen V, Preudhomme C, Roumier C et al: Myelodysplasia during the course of myeloma. Restriction of 17p deletion and p53 overexpression to myeloid cells. Leukemia 12:238–41, 1998.

32. Schmetzer HM, Mittermuller J, Duell T, Wilmanns W: Development of myeloma and secondary myelodysplastic syndrome from a common clone. Cancer Genet Cytogenet 100:31–5, 1998.

33. Fonseca R, Rajkumar SV, Ahmann GJ et al: FISH demonstrates treatment related chromosome damage in myeloid cells but not plasma cells in primary systemic amyloidosis. Leuk Lymphoma 39:391–5, 2000.

34. Rajkumar SV, Fonseca R, Dewald GW et al. Cytogenetic abnormalities correlate with the plasma cell labeling index and extent of bone marrow involvement in myeloma. Cancer Genet Cytogenet 113:73–77, 1999.

35. Drach J, Schuster J, Nowotny H et al: Multiple myeloma: High incidence of chromosomal aneuploidy as detected by interphase fluorescence in situ hybridization. Cancer Res 55:3854–9, 1995.

36. Fonseca R, Ahmann GJ, Juneau AL et al: Cytogenetic abnormalities in multiple myeloma and related plasma cell disorders; a comparison of conventional cytogenetic analysis to fluorescent in-situ hybridization with simultaneous cytoplasmic immunoglobulin staining (meeting abstract). Blood 90(10):1558a, p. 349, 1997.

37. Zandecki M, Lai JL, Facon T: Multiple myeloma: Almost all patients are cytogenetically abnormal. Br J Haematol 94:217–27, 1996.

38. Tabernero D, San Miguel JF, Garcia-Sanz M et al: Incidence of chromosome numerical changes in multiple myeloma: Fluorescence in situ hybridization analysis using 15 chromosome-specific probes. Am J Pathol 149:153–61, 1996.

39. Ahmann GJ, Jalal SM, Juneau AL et al: A novel three-color, clone-specific fluorescence in situ hybridization procedure for monoclonal gammopathies. Cancer Genet Cytogenet 101:7–11, 1998.

40. Fonseca R, Ahmann GJ, Jalal SM et al: Chromosomal abnormalities in systemic amyloidosis. Br J Haematol 103:704–710, 1998.

41. Drach J, Angerler J, Schuster J et al: Interphase fluorescence in situ hybridization identifies chromosomal abnormalities in plasma cells from patients with monoclonal gammopathy of undetermined significance. Blood 86:3915–21, 1995.

42. Zandecki M, Obein V, Bernardi F et al: Monoclonal gammopathy of undetermined significance: Chromosome changes are a common finding within bone marrow plasma cells. Br J Haematol 90:693–6, 1995.

43. Rao PH, Cigudosa JC, Ning Y et al: Multicolor spectral karyotyping identifies new recurring breakpoints and translocations in multiple myeloma. Blood 92:1743–8, 1998.

44. Sawyer JR, Lukacs JL, Munshi N et al: Identification of new non-random translocations in multiple myeloma with multicolor spectral karyotyping. Blood 92:4269–78, 1998.

45. Cigudosa JC, Rao PH, Calasanz MJ et al: Characterization of non-random chromosomal gains and losses in multiple myeloma by comparative genomic hybridization. Blood 91:3007–10, 1998.

46. Avet-Loiseau H, Andree-Ashley LE, Moore D 2nd et al: Molecular cytogenetic abnormalities in multiple myeloma and plasma cell leukemia measured using comparative genomic hybridization. Genes Chromosom Cancer 19:124–33, 1997.

47. Vaandrager JW, Schuuring E, Zwikstra E et al: Direct visualization of dispersed 11q13 chromosomal translocations in mantle cell lymphoma by multicolor DNA fiber fluorescence in situ hybridization. Blood 88:1177–82, 1996.

48. Janssen JW, Vaandrager JW, Heuser T et al: Concurrent activation of a novel putative transforming gene, myeov, and cyclin D1 in a subset of multiple myeloma cell lines with t(11;14)(q13;q32). Blood 95:2691–8, 2000.

49. Vaandrager JW, Kluin P, Schuuring E: The t(11;14)(q13;q32) in multiple myeloma cell line KMS12 has its 11q13 breakpoint 330 kb centromeric from the cyclin D1 gene [letter]. Blood 89:349–50, 1997.

50. Smadja NV, Bastard C, Brigideau C, Leroux D, Fruchart C: On behalf of the Groupe Français de Cytogénétique Hématologique. Blood 98:229–2238, 2001.

51. Perez-Simon JA, Garcia-Sanz R, Tabernero MD et al: Prognostic value of numerical chromosome aberrations in multiple myeloma: A FISH analysis of 15 different chromosomes. Blood 91:3366–71, 1998.

52. Barlogie B, Sawyer J, Ayers D et al: Chromosome 13 myeloma is a distinct entity with poor prognosis despite tandem autotransplants. Blood 92:Abstract 1059, 1998.

53. Shaughnessy J, Tian E, Sawyer J et al: High incidence of chromosome 13 deletion in multiple myeloma detected by multiprobe interphase FISH. Blood 96:1505–1511, 2000.

54. Drach J, Zojer N, Königsberg R et al: Cytogenetically defined subgroups of patients with multiple myeloma (MM) have significantly different overall survival times. A study based on interphase-FISH analysis. Blood 92:Abstract #2944, 1998.

55. Fonseca R, Harrington D, Oken M et al: Myeloma and the t(11;14)(q13;q32) represents a uniquely defined biological subset of patients. Blood 99:3735–3741, 2002.

56. Drach J, Ackermann J, Fritz E et al: Presence of a p53 gene deletion in patients with multiple myeloma predicts for short survival after conventional-dose chemotherapy. Blood 92:802–9, 1998.

57. Schultheis B, Kramer A, Willer A, Hegenbart U, Goldschmidt H, Hehlmann R: Analysis of p73 and p53 gene deletions in multiple myeloma. Leukemia 13:2099–103, 1999.

58. Mazars GR, Portier M, Zhang XG et al: Mutations of the p53 gene in human myeloma cell lines. Oncogene 7:1015–8, 1992.

59. Corradini P, Inghirami G, Astolfi M et al: Inactivation of tumor suppressor genes, p53 and Rb1, in plasma cell dyscrasias. Leukemia 8:758–67, 1994.

60. Neri A, Baldini L, Trecca D, Cro L, Polli E, Maiolo AT: p53 gene mutations in multiple myeloma are associated with advanced forms of malignancy. Blood 81:128–35, 1993.

61. Preudhomme C, Facon T, Zandecki M et al: Rare occurrence of P53 gene mutations in multiple myeloma. Br J Haematol 81:440–3, 1992.

62. Chesi M, Bergsagel PL, Brents LA, Smith CM, Gerhard DS, Kuehl WM: Dysregulation of cyclin D1 by translocation into an IgH gamma switch region in two multiple myeloma cell lines. Blood 88:674–81, 1996.

63. Chesi M, Nardini E, Lim R, Smith K, Kuehl W, Bergsagel P: The t(4;14) translocation in myeloma dysregulates both FGFR3 and a novel gene, MMSET, resulting in IgH/MMSET hybrid transcripts. Blood 92:3025–34, 1998.

64. Bergsagel PL, Chesi M, Brents LA, Kuehl WM: Translocations into IgH switch regions – the genetic hallmark of multiple myeloma. Blood 86:223–223, 1995.

65. Avet-Loiseau H, Brigaudeau C, Morineau N et al: High incidence of cryptic translocations involving the Ig heavy chain gene in multiple myeloma, as shown by fluorescence in situ hybridization. Genes Chromosom Cancer 24:9–15, 1999.

66. Avet-Loiseau H, Facon T, Daviet A et al: 14q32 translocations and monosomy 13 observed in monoclonal gammopathy of undetermined significance delineate a multistep process for the oncogenesis of multiple myeloma. Intergroupe Francophone du Myelome. Cancer Res 59:4546–50, 1999.

67. Fonseca R, Bailey RJ, Ahmann GJ et al: Genomic abnormalities in monoclonal gammopathy of undetermined significance. Blood 100:1417–1424, 2002.

68. Fonseca R, Dewald G, Coignet L: Cytogenetic abnormalities in multiple myeloma. Hematol Oncol Clin North Am 13:1169–1180, 1999.

69. Nishida K, Taniwaki M, Misawa S, Abe T: Nonrandom rearrangement of chromosome 14 at band q32.33 in human lymphoid malignancies with mature B-cell phenotype. Cancer Res 49:1275–81, 1989.

70. Hallek M, Bergsagel PL: Anderson KC: Multiple myeloma: Increasing evidence for a multistep transformation process [review]. Blood 91:3–21, 1998.

71. Ried K, Finnis M, Hobson L et al: Common chromosomal fragile site FRA16D sequence: Identification of the FOR gene spanning FRA16D and homozygous deletions and translocation breakpoints in cancer cells. Hum Mol Genet 9:1651–1663, 2000.

72. Gabrea A, Bergsagel PL, Chesi M, Shou Y, Kuehl WM: Insertion of excised IgH switch sequences causes overexpression of cyclin D1 in a myeloma tumor cell. Mol Cell 3:119–23, 1999.

73. Hoyer JD, Hanson CA, Fonseca R, Greipp PR, Dewald GW, Kurtin PJ: The (11;14)(q13;q32) translocation in multiple myeloma. A morphologic and immunohistochemical study. Am J Clin Pathol 113:831–7, 2000.

74. Vasef MA, Medeiros LJ, Yospur LS, Sun NC, McCourty A, Brynes RK: Cyclin D1 protein in multiple myeloma and plasmacytoma: An immunohistochemical study using fixed, paraffin-embedded tissue sections. Mod Pathol 10:927–32, 1997.

75. Ronchetti D, Finelli P, Richelda R et al: Molecular analysis of 11q13 breakpoints in multiple myeloma. Blood 93:1330–1337, 1999.

76. Uchimaru K, Taniguchi T, Yoshikawa M et al: Detection of cyclin D1 (bcl-1, PRAD1) overexpression by a simple competitive reverse transcription – polymerase chain reaction assay in t(11;14)(q13;q32)-bearing B-cell malignancies and/or mantle cell lymphoma. Blood 89:965–74, 1997.

77. Pruneri G, Fabris S, Baldini L et al: Immunohistochemical analysis of cyclin D1 shows deregulated expression in multiple myeloma with the t(11;14). Am J Pathol 156:1505–13, 2000.

78. Fonseca R, Witzig TE, Gertz MA et al: Multiple myeloma and the translocation t(11;14)(q13;q32) – a report on 13 cases. Br J Haematol 101:296–301, 1998.

79. Fonseca R, Hoyer JD, Aguayo P et al: Clinical significance of the translocation (11;14)(q13;q32) in multiple myeloma. Leuk Lymphoma 35:599–605, 1999.

80. Richelda R, Ronchetti D, Baldini L et al: A novel chromosomal translocation t(4;14)(p16.3;q32) in multiple myeloma involves the fibroblast growth-factor receptor 3 gene. Blood 90:4062–70, 1997.

81. Nakazawa N, Nishida K, Tamura A et al: Interphase detection of t(4;14)(p16.3;q32.3) by in situ hybridization and FGFR3 overexpression in plasma cell malignancies. Cancer Genet Cytogenet 117:89–96, 2000.

82. Otsuki T, Nakazawa N, Taniwaki M et al: Establishment of a new human myeloma cell line, KMS-18, having t(4;14)(p16.3;q32.3) derived from a case phenotypically transformed from Ig A-lambda to BJP-lambda, and associated with hyperammonemia. Int J Oncol 12:545–52, 1998.

83. Finelli P, Fabris S, Zagano S et al: Detection of t(4;14)(p16.3;q32) chromosomal translocation in multiple myeloma by double-color fluorescent in situ hybridization. Blood 94:724–732, 1999.

84. Malgeri U, Baldini L, Perfetti V et al: Detection of t(4;14)(p16.3;q32) chromosomal translocation in multiple myeloma by reverse transcription – polymerase chain reaction analysis of IGH-MMSET fusion transcripts. Cancer Res 60:4058–61, 2000.

85. Kataoka K, Nishizawa M, Kawai S: Structure–function analysis of the maf oncogene product, a member of the b-Zip protein family. J Virol 67:2133–41, 1993.

86. Iida S, Rao PH, Butler M et al: Deregulation of MUM1/IRF4 by chromosomal translocation in multiple myeloma. Nat Genet 17:226–30, 1997.

87. Yoshida S, Nakazawa N, Iida S et al: Detection of MUM1/IRF4-IgH fusion in multiple myeloma. Leukemia 13:1812–6, 1998.

88. Shou Y, Martelli ML, Gabrea A et al: Diverse karyotypic abnormalities of the c-myc locus associated with c-myc dysregulation and tumor progression in multiple myeloma. Proc Natl Acad Sci U S A 97:228–33, 2000.

89. Facon T, Avet-Louiseau H, Guillerm G et al. Chromosome 13 abnormalities identified by FISH analysis and serum beta-2-microglobulin produce a powerful myeloma staging system for patients receiving high-dose therapy. Blood 97:1566–1571, 2001.

90. Moreau P, Facon T, Leleu X et al. Recurrent 14q32 translocations determine the prognosis of multiple myeloma, especially in patients receiving intensive chemotherapy. Blood 100:1579–83, 2002.

91. Chesi M, Brents LA, Ely SA et al. Activated fibroblast growth factor receptor 3 is an oncogene that contributes to tumor progression in multiple myeloma. Blood 97:729–36, 2001.

92. Fonseca R, Harrington D, Blood E et al. Clinical and biologic implications of recurrent chromosomal abnormalities in myeloma. Blood (in press).

29

Molecular Genetics in Multiple Myeloma and Related Disorders

Matt Rowley and Brian Van Ness

Multiple myeloma (MM) is characterized by the accumulation of clonal plasma cells in the bone marrow. The idea that myeloma results from the transformation of a terminally differentiated B cell is giving way to suggestions that the disease involves earlier lineage cells that differentiate and accumulate at the plasma cell stage. There is considerable genetic heterogeneity associated with MM that can affect disease progression and response to therapy. A number of karyotypic abnormalities have been described that are associated with myeloma (see Chapter 28). In addition, there are point mutations and abnormal gene expression that can differentially alter myeloma cell growth and therapeutic response.

A growing number of studies show the importance of the bone marrow microenvironment in MM. Myeloma cells accumulate in the bone marrow, where there are adhesive and various cytokine interactions. In addition, the myeloma cells are able to alter the marrow microenvironment, which can affect

normal stromal functions such as hematopoiesis. Thus, the genetic abnormalities and cellular interactions can have a significant effect on the myeloma cells and the gene expression patterns of their environment. Mutations can also alter signal transduction pathways and cell cycle regulation, both of which can have an effect on proliferation, apoptosis, and response to therapeutic agents. A better understanding of different genetic changes found to be associated with the myeloma cell will eventually lead to a better understanding of the disease as well as better treatment options. Figure 29–1 summarizes a variety of genetic alterations that influence the initiation and progression of the disease. In this chapter we will discuss the genetic characterization of and abnormalities associated with myeloma and the impact that these abnormalities have on the malignant plasma cell, its environment, and therapeutic response.

IMMUOGLOBULIN RECEPTOR GENE REARRANGEMENTS IN MYELOMA PLASMA CELLS

One of the hallmarks of B-cell development is the rearrangement of immunoglobulin (Ig) gene segments; B cells undergo an ordered rearrangement of heavy- and then light-chain gene segments defining specific stages of development. In the germline, the Ig heavy-chain genes are arranged as discontinuous coding segments referred to as variable (V_H), diversity (D_H), joining (J_H), and constant (C) regions. During B-cell development, one of the D_H segment genes is combined with a J_H segment gene, which is followed by the addition of a V_H segment gene to give the rearranged VDJ sequence. During rearrangement, random nucleotides can be inserted between the rearranged segments by terminal deoxytransferase (TdT). Additionally, nucleotides may

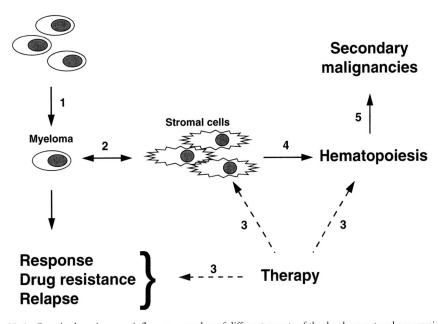

Figure 29–1. Genetic alterations can influence a number of different aspects of the development and progression of multiple myeloma. These alterations can (1) lead to initial transforming events; (2) alter the interactions of the myeloma cell with the environment; (3) alter the response to therapeutic agents; (4) disrupt normal hematopoiesis; and (5) lead to the development of secondary malignancies.

be deleted from the ends of rearranging V_H, D_H, and J_H segments. Each rearrangement results in a unique Ig sequence due to the various combinations of V_H, D_H, and J_H gene segments as well as the random insertion and deletion of nucleotides at the junction. Myeloma cells from most patients have rearranged the Ig genes on both the heavy- and light-chain loci and express a monoclonal protein. Thus, Ig gene rearrangement can serve as a useful molecular marker of clonal B-cell tumors. Recombination of Ig gene segments repositions restriction enzyme recognition sites, which can be characterized by changes on a Southern blot analysis. The detection of clonal Ig gene rearrangements can be applied as a diagnostic test. The relative hybridization intensity of the rearranged band is roughly proportional to the tumor burden. One of the limitations of Southern blot techniques for following clonal B cells is that detection requires 2 to 5 percent clonality in the sample. Below 2 percent, the clonal rearrangement is difficult to detect, which makes the technique impractical for monitoring minimal residual disease.

DETECTION OF MINIMAL RESIDUAL DISEASE

Detection of minimal residual disease has become more important owing to advances in treatment of MM. Several techniques have been described to detect minimal residual disease, including flow cytometry, fluorescent in situ hybridization (FISH), and polymerase chain reaction (PCR). Flow cytometry can be used to measure minimal residual disease by combining light scatter with multiparameter staining to detect tumor-specific patterns.[1–3] Recently, FISH has been used to evaluate minimal residual disease in myeloma patients after high-dose therapy.[4]

Persistence of abnormal plasma cells was detected in 12 of 14 patients using fluorescent probes to follow tumor-specific cytogenetic changes such as deletions and translocations.

Allele-specific oligonucleotide (ASO) PCR is currently the most commonly used technique to follow minimal residual disease.[5–12] Briefly, V- and J-region consensus oligonucleotide primers are designed that recognize highly conserved regions of V and J gene segments. These primers are used to amplify the junctional regions of the rearranged Ig heavy-chain gene from the diagnostic bone marrow of the myeloma patient (Figure 29–2). From the sequence of the amplified product, a tumor-specific ASO primer can be synthesized (based on the highly unique junctional sequences) and used in subsequent PCR reactions to specifically detect the patient's malignant clone. The ASO-PCR technique is highly specific, sensitive enough to detect one malignant cell in a background of 100,000 normal cells, and can be quantitative.[5]

POSSIBLE CLONAL PRECURSORS TO THE MYELOMA PLASMA CELL

In MM, malignant plasma cells are found almost exclusively in the bone marrow and typically express either IgG or IgA. There is some debate, however, about the presence and identity of earlier-lineage cells that are clonally related to the malignancy and their potential as myeloma precursor cells. Several reports have suggested that populations of B cells in various stages of development are clonally related to the myeloma plasma cell.[13–22] Anti-idiotypic antibodies generated to the myeloma monoclonal protein have been shown to cross-react with B cells displaying

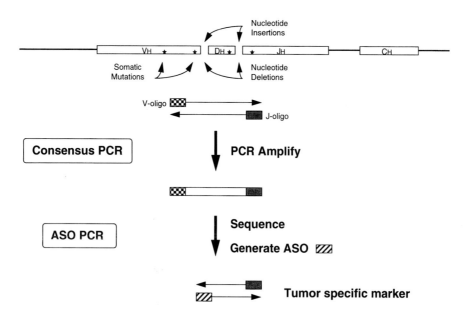

Figure 29–2. ASO-PCR can be used to detect minimal residual disease. Using family-specific primers to the conserved region of the V_H and J_H gene segments, the rearranged allele can be amplified and sequenced, and an ASO can be synthesized. ASO-PCR can subsequently be used to detect tumor-specific DNA sequences, reflecting minimal residual disease.

different isotypes.[13,14] Furthermore, coexpression of early B-cell lineage markers and plasma cell markers has been observed in the malignant population.[15–19] These findings point to the possibility of an oncogenic event affecting B cells early in the differentiation pathway, and that these early B cells may act as precursors to the myeloma plasma cells. During B-cell development, the cells initially express IgM. A number of studies using tumor-specific primers have found evidence for IgM-expressing cells that are clonally related to the malignant myeloma cells.[20–22] Additionally, analysis of V_H gene clones from a number of different myeloma patients shows marked somatic mutation but no intraclonal variation.[23–25] Taken together, these data show that there are postgerminal center B cells representing either memory B cells or plasmablasts that have the potential to differentiate into plasma cells on entering the bone marrow. It has been suggested that the myeloma precursor cell is an IgM-expressing, postgerminal center B cell.[22,26] This cell can undergo isotype switching to either an IgA- or IgG-expressing cell and then migrate through the blood to the bone marrow, where it will be supported by the microenvironment.

THE ROLE OF INTERLEUKIN-6 IN MULTIPLE MYELOMA AND ITS IMPACT ON SIGNALING AND GENE EXPRESSION

During normal B-cell development, interleukin-6 (IL-6) promotes terminal differentiation of mature B-cells to antibody-secreting plasma cells.[27] Although IL-6 stimulates Ig secretion, it does not promote normal B-cell proliferation.[28] In contrast, IL-6 has been shown to be a potent growth factor for myeloma cells. Early work by Potter and Boyce[29] demonstrated that pristane-treated mice developed plasmacytomas, and subsequent work showed that IL-6 served as a potent growth factor in tumor development.[30–32] Transgenic mice carrying the human IL-6 gene fused to an Ig heavy-chain transcriptional enhancer sequence were shown to develop massive plasmacytosis.[33] Moreover, a human myeloma cell line transfected with an IL-6 expression vector was shown to transplant successfully into nude mice as a subcutaneous tumor.[34] The addition of IL-6 in cell culture media augments the clonal proliferation of myeloma cells, whereas anti-IL-6 or antisense IL-6 oligonucleotides inhibit the proliferation of myeloma cell lines.[35] Additionally, mutations that affect IL-6 signal transduction pathways are often associated with myeloma (see below). Thus, IL-6 and its associated signal pathways may be important components in the disease progression.

The source of IL-6 has been the subject of some controversy. Kawano and colleagues[31] have reported that fresh myeloma cells are capable of autocrine IL-6 production and that these cells also express IL-6 receptors. In contrast, Klein et al.[36] have reported that the high level of IL-6 found in the bone marrow of myeloma patients is derived from adherent stromal cells in the marrow. Other studies have shown that bone marrow monocytic and myeloid cells but not all myeloma cells express IL-6 mRNA.[37] Some studies have suggested that IL-1 production by myeloma cells may be responsible for the paracrine

expression of IL-6 by marrow stromal cells.[38] Culture supernatants of plasma cells isolated from all of 12 myeloma patients contained significant levels of IL-1.[39] Thus, it seems likely that both autocrine and paracrine mechanisms play a role in the pathogenesis of myeloma.

GENETIC ABNORMALITIES ASSOCIATED WITH MULTIPLE MYELOMA

There is considerable heterogeneity in genetic alterations associated with MM. Although there are currently no known genetic alterations that are associated with every case of myeloma, there are some genetic abnormalities found in a relatively high percentage of cases. These abnormalities include mutations, deletions, translocations, and aberrant expression of various genes. The genetic alterations can have an effect on many different properties of the myeloma cell. Mutations can affect signal transduction through constitutively activated signaling molecules such as Ras. Mutation or aberrant expression of genes that regulate the cell cycle, such as c-myc or cyclin D1, can lead to uncontrolled proliferation. Changes in expression of Bcl-2 family members can lead to cells that are more resistant to apoptosis. Moreover, changes in any of these pathways and control mechanisms can lead to altered response to therapeutic agents and other outside stimuli.

Genetic Alterations that Affect Signal Transduction

Stimulation of myeloma cells with IL-6 results in the activation of a variety of downstream signal transduction pathways. The JAK/STAT and Ras/MAPK cascades are the best characterized IL-6 signal transduction pathways in myeloma (Figure 29–3). Mutations that affect any part of the pathway can alter the IL-6 response and lead to changes in cell growth and apoptosis.

Interleukin-6 signals through the Ras family of guanosine triphosphate–binding proteins.[40] Mutations in codon 12, 13, or 61 of N- or K-ras lead to a constitutively active Ras protein and have been found in 40 to 50 percent of myeloma cases.[41–44] The introduction of activated ras genes into lymphoblastoid cell lines has been shown to cause tumorigenic conversion and plasmacytoid differentiation, leading to the establishment of cell lines having characteristics of human myeloma cells.[45] This finding suggests that ras oncogenes may contribute to early steps in pathogenesis by leading to the transformation and plasmacytoid differentiation of earlier myeloma precursors. In one report, it was found that ras mutations appeared to be more common in patients with fulminating disease (67 percent) than in patients with less aggressive disease (26 percent).[42] Additionally, longitudinal analyses of patient samples have shown ras mutations in some relapse samples that were not present at the time of the original diagnosis.[44] These findings suggest that ras mutations correlate with more aggressive disease or that mutations in ras may be acquired after the original malignant transformation and may contribute to a more aggressive disease. It has been shown that activating mutations in either N- or K-ras can provide a proliferation signal independent of any additional

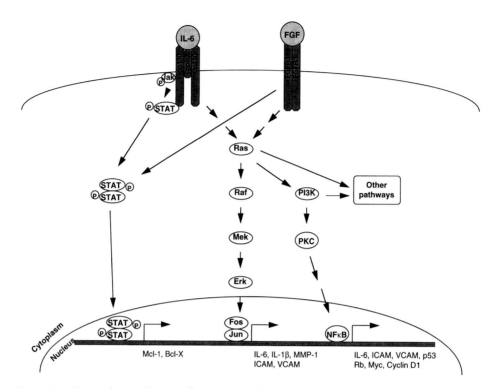

Figure 29–3. Genetic abnormalities can affect signal transduction pathways. Activating mutations in *Ras* can alter signal transduction and lead to changes in transcription factor activation and gene expression. This can provide growth factor independence and also provide protection from apoptosis. Overexpression of the FGF receptor can activate signaling pathways that are similar to IL-6 signaling and lead to cells that are less dependent on IL-6.

IL-6 in a myeloma cell line.[46,47] Thus, *ras* mutations may alleviate IL-6 dependence and alter the growth properties of myeloma cells, possibly making them less dependent on the bone marrow microenvironment. In addition, *ras* mutations have been shown to protect myeloma cell lines from apoptosis induced by chemotherapeutic agents.[48]

The t(4;14)(p16;q32) translocation is found in approximately 15 to 25 percent of MM cases. This translocation results in the deregulated expression of both fibroblast growth factor receptor 3 *(FGFR3)* and the *MMSET* (multiple myeloma SET domain) gene.[49–51] The role of MMSET in myeloma is still unknown. Stimulation of FGFR3 by one of the FGF family members activates signaling pathways that lead to cell growth. Overexpression of a constitutively active form of FGFR3 in an IL-6 dependent murine B-cell line results in IL-6 independence, decreased apoptosis, and enhanced proliferative response to IL-6.[52] Similarly, overexpression of wild-type (wt) FGFR3 also results in enhanced proliferation and survival in the presence of ligand.[52] Signaling through either wt or mutant FGFR3 resulted in increased STAT3 phosphorylation and Bcl-X$_L$ expression. Additionally, expression of FGFR mutants in PC12 cells led to phosphorylation of Shp2, PLC-γ, and MAPK as well as activation of STAT1 and STAT3.[53] Taken together, this suggests that deregulated expression of FGFR3 may lead to additional proliferative or antiapoptotic signals provided by bone marrow stromal cells expressing FGF and that STAT activation is one of the major signaling pathways involved.

Genetic Alterations That Affect Cell Cycle

Genes that control cell cycle are overexpressed or deleted in a number of different cancers, including multiple myeloma. Aberrant expression of cell cycle control genes can alter the regulation of other cell cycle–associated genes and lead to uncontrolled proliferation (Figure 29–4). Approximately 25 to 30 percent of myeloma patients express *cyclin D1*.[54,55] *Cyclin D1* is involved in the regulation of the G$_1$ to S stage of the cell cycle. Expression of *cyclin D1* in MM correlates with greater tumor burden due to elevated proliferation, leading to a poor clinical prognosis.[55–57] *Cyclin D1* can form complexes with cyclin-dependent kinases (cdk) and sequester the cell cycle inhibitors p27^{kip1} and p21$^{cip1/waf1}$.[58] This promotes cell cycle progression by increasing Rb-1 phosphorylation and release of E2F, which activates transcription of cell cycle genes.

Aberrant expression of *c-myc* can also lead to uncontrolled cellular proliferation by inducing the expression of *cyclins D1* and *D2*.[58,59] Translocation of *c-myc* to switch regions of the IgH locus occurs in most murine plasmacytomas.[60] This finding prompted an examination of *c-myc* expression in human myeloma. High levels of *c-myc* expression have been reported in about 25 percent of myeloma patients[61]; however, only rarely has this been the result of a translocation. Recently, it has been shown that the 5′ untranslated region of *c-myc* contains an internal ribosome entry segment (IRES), and that 42 percent of bone marrow samples from myeloma patients con-

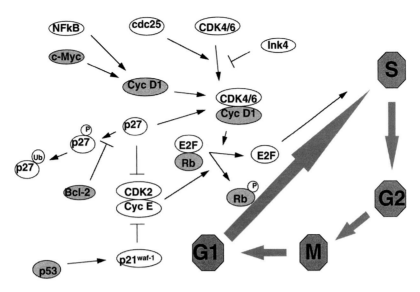

Figure 29–4. A number of genetic abnormalities can alter cell cycle regulation. Genes that are often affected in multiple myeloma are shown in gray. Overexpression of *c-myc* or *cyclin D1* leads to an increase in *cyclin D1* complexed with CDK4 or CDK6, resulting in Rb phosphorylation and release of E2F, which drives transition from the G_1 to the S phase. Mutations in *p53* lead to an increase in *cyclin E* complexed with CDK2, resulting in Rb phosphorylation and E2F release.

tain a mutation in the IRES that leads to overexpression of *c-myc*.[62] In addition, *c-myc* expression has been reported to correlate with the grade of malignancy, type of myeloma, and tumor cell burden.[63]

The retinoblastoma tumor suppressor gene *(Rb-1)* is involved in the control of transition of the cell cycle from the G_1 into the S phase. In addition, *Rb-1* is able to suppress expression of the *IL-6* gene.[64] A number of different types of mutations have been reported that can affect the *Rb-1* gene, including loss of expression, point mutations, and selective loss of exons resulting in nonfunctional proteins.[65] Monoallelic deletions of *Rb-1* are found in 70 to 80 percent of myelomas but appear to have no effect on gene activation or *Rb-1* expression.[66] However, in another study, 35 percent of myeloma patients studied showed a complete loss of Rb-1 protein.[67] Loss of *Rb-1* expression can lead to more aggressive disease via an increase in autocrine IL-6 expression and loss of cell cycle control.

Genetic Alterations That Affect Apoptosis

The role of the Bcl-2 family of proteins in regulating apoptosis has been well established. The Bcl-2 family consists of both antiapoptotic members (Bcl-2, Bcl-X_L, Mcl-1) and proapoptotic members (Bax, Bad, Bcl-X_S). Overexpression of Bcl-2 in transgenic mouse models is able to prolong the life span of primary, as well as secondary, antibody-secreting plasma cells.[68–70] Several reports have shown that Bcl-2 overexpression is common in both MGUS and myeloma,[71,72] suggesting that overexpression of Bcl-2 may be an early event in tumorigenesis of myeloma. Prolonged survival of plasma cells in MGUS may

allow for further genetic changes, which ultimately lead to progression to myeloma.

Interleukin-6 is able to provide protection from apoptosis for myeloma cells in part by upregulating Bcl-X_L and Mcl-1.[73–75] Bcl-X_L and Mcl-1 upregulation can be inhibited by blocking STAT3 activity.[76–78] This suggests that Bcl-X_L and Mcl-1 may play a more prominent role in regulating myeloma cell death than Bcl-2, which appears to be unaffected by IL-6 signaling.

The *p53* tumor suppressor gene is among the most commonly mutated genes in human cancers. Interestingly, *p53* mutations are relatively uncommon in MM. Mutations in *p53* have been reported in 10 to 20 percent of myelomas and appear to be associated with patients who have relapsed or are in terminal stages of the disease.[42,79] Wild-type *p53* has been shown to suppress autocrine IL-6 expression in HeLa cells[80] and recently in a myeloma cell line.[48] This demonstrates that one mechanism by which *p53* mutations can lead to more aggressive disease is by upregulation of IL-6 expression, leading to cells that are less dependent on the bone marrow microenvironment.

THE BONE MARROW MICROENVIRONMENT CAN SUPPORT MYELOMA CELL GROWTH AND SURVIVAL

One of the features of MM is the almost exclusive homing of the malignant plasma cells to the bone marrow. The bone marrow stroma consists of a number of different cell types, which produce adhesion molecules, cytokines, and a meshwork of extracellular matrix proteins. Recently, the bone marrow microenvironment has been shown to play an important role in supporting myeloma cells. Additionally, the bone marrow microenvironment has been shown to change in response to the presence and adhesion of myeloma cells.[81–83]

Adhesion Molecule Interactions

A broad spectrum of adhesion molecules are expressed on myeloma cells, including NCAM (CD56), ICAM-1 (CD54), VLA-4 (CD49d/CD29), LFA-1 (CD11a/CD18), and syndecan-1; NCAM is believed to be an important adhesion molecule, expression of which is associated with MM. Although NCAM is highly expressed on most myeloma plasma cells, it is not found on normal plasma cells or plasma cells isolated from MGUS patients.[84–86] In addition, the progression of MM to plasma cell leukemia (PCL) involves the loss of NCAM expression and mobilization of the plasma cells out of the bone marrow.[87] Together, these data suggest that NCAM plays an important role in adhesion of myeloma cells to the bone marrow microenvironment.

Expression of ICAM also plays an important role in myeloma and homing to the bone marrow. This molecule is found on the surface of both normal plasma cells and myeloma cells.[85] However, ICAM is inducible by IL-1β.[88] Introduction of an IL-1 cDNA into a murine B-cell line leads to increased ICAM expression and homing of the cells to the bone marrow.[89] In addition, pretreatment of SCID mice with anti-ICAM antibodies is able to suppress hind limb paralysis and bone lesions in mice injected with the ARH myeloma cell line.[90]

Several other interactions between myeloma cells and the microenvironment have also been observed. The MM cells can localize to the bone marrow by binding VLA-4 to VCAM-1 or fibronectin and LFA-1 to ICAM-1.[91–93] Several of these interactions have been associated with an induction of IL-6 expression.[92–94] The receptor for hyaluronan (HA)-mediated motility (RHAMM) is overexpressed in myeloma plasma cells as compared with plasma cells from normal donors.[95] Binding of RHAMM to HA may be important for the induction of motility, migration, and spread of the tumor.[96]

Cytokine Interactions

Adhesion of myeloma cells in the bone marrow microenvironment is also able to regulate cytokine secretion by both the stromal cells and the myeloma cells. Interleukin-6 is one of the major growth and survival factors provided by the bone marrow microenvironment. Binding of myeloma cells to stromal cells through VLA-4 and VCAM-1 can induce IL-6 production by the stromal cells.[93] In addition, stimulation of CD40 on the myeloma and stromal cells also upregulates IL-6 expression through the activation of NF-κB.[97–99]

Myeloma cells produce high levels of IL-1β; however, normal plasma cells and plasma cells from MGUS patients do not.[39,100–102] Interleukin-1β acts as a potent osteoclast-activating factor and likely leads to the presence of bone lesions found in myeloma patients. In addition, IL-1β is able to upregulate IL-6 expression by the stromal cells.[38] Secretion of tumor necrosis factor α (TNFα) from the myeloma cells has also been shown to increase IL-6 expression by stromal cells.[103]

The importance of angiogenesis in the formation of solid tumors has been well established. It has been shown that angiogenesis in the bone marrow is higher in patients with active MM than in patients with MGUS or patients with nonactive myeloma.[81,82] In addition, the extent of angiogenesis in the bone marrow of myeloma patients has been shown to correlate with patient survival.[104] Myeloma cell lines and plasma cells from myeloma patients produce vascular endothelial growth factor (VEGF) in response to IL-6.[105,106] This factor stimulates angiogenesis and tumor neovascularization and is able to stimulate bone marrow stromal cells to produce IL-6.[106] The mutual stimulation between VEGF and IL-6 suggests that there may be paracrine interactions between the myeloma and stromal cells in the increase of angiogenesis associated with myeloma.

The bone marrow microenvironment can also play a role in resistance of the myeloma cells to chemotherapy. Adhesion of myeloma cells to fibronectin through VLA-4 was found to confer resistance to both doxorubicin and melphalan.[107] The protection was associated with a G_1 arrest of the cell cycle due to increased levels of p27[kip1].[108] Other studies have shown that stromal cells are able to protect myeloma cells from apoptosis induced by dexamethasone.[109,110] The protection from dexamethasone appears to be a result of IL-6 secretion from the stromal cells because fixed stromal cells were not able to protect from apoptosis induced by dexamethasone.[110]

Human Herpesvirus 8

Recently it has been shown that human herpesvirus 8 (HHV-8) was present in long-term cultures of bone marrow stromal cells from myeloma patients.[111] This virus was of interest because it encodes a viral IL-6 homologue that, although not as potent as human IL-6, is able to stimulate the growth of a human myeloma cell line.[112] The role of HHV-8 in MM currently remains controversial, however, because a number of studies have failed to detect the presence of viral sequences in myeloma patients.[113]

DRUG RESISTANCE IN MYELOMA ASSOCIATED WITH P-gp EXPRESSION

There is a high rate of response to initial treatment for MM. Unfortunately, many patients relapse as a result of developing drug resistance. Resistance in MM typically involves a multidrug resistant (MDR) phenotype, which results in resistance to many different chemotherapeutic agents. One of the better described mechanisms of MDR involves upregulation of the *MDR1* gene, which encodes a transmembrane glycoprotein known as permeability glycoprotein (P-gp).[114] This glycoprotein acts as an ATP-dependent efflux pump and is capable of reducing intracellular levels of drugs, including vincristine, doxorubicin, and dexamethasone.[115] In general, greater expression of P-gp results in a greater level of resistance. Expression of P-gp is generally absent or present at low levels in untreated MM patients. After exposure to VAD (vincristine, doxorubicin, and dexamethasone) treatment, the expression of the MDR1 gene is above background in 75 percent of patients.[116] The expression of P-gp correlates with the dose of treatment received.[116]

DISORDERS RELATED TO MULTIPLE MYELOMA

A related disorder that may represent a preneoplastic state of myeloma is monoclonal gammopathy of undetermined significance (MGUS). Patients with this disorder show evidence of monoclonal serum Ig and elevated plasma cells in the bone marrow, but in contrast to MM patients, they do not have anemia, bone lesions, renal failure, or hypercalcemia.[117] These patients may be followed without treatment for many years without clinical complications, but approximately 25 percent eventually develop MM or a related disorder.[118] This suggests that MGUS may represent a preneoplastic step in the development of myeloma.

The exact mechanism by which MGUS develops into myeloma is unknown. One possible mechanism may be the upregulation of IL-1β in myeloma cells. Abnormal IL-1β expression is common in myeloma cells[100–102]; however, expression of IL-1β is not detected in most MGUS patients.[102] One feature distinguishing between myeloma and MGUS is the development of bone lesions in myeloma that are not present in MGUS patients. Since IL-1β has potent osteoclast-activating factor activity, it may be partially responsible for the bone lesions. The presence of IL-6 may also play a role in the development of myeloma. In one study, significant IL-6 levels were found in 30 of 85 myeloma patients but only 1 of 22 MGUS patients.[119] The development of new genetic abnormalities is also likely to be involved in the transition from MGUS to myeloma. One study showed that although translocations involving the 14q32 (Ig switch) region were observed with a similar incidence in MM and MGUS, a significant difference was found in the incidence of monosomy 13 in MM (40 percent) and MGUS (21 percent).[120] In another study, Ras, p53, or Rb-1 mutations were not detected in an analysis of 15 MGUS samples.[67] There may be a number of different mechanisms by which MGUS may progress to myeloma, including changes in cytokine expression or mutations in oncogenes or tumor suppressor genes. More work is needed to fully characterize this transition.

Some myeloma patients develop plasma cell leukemia (PCL), a condition that is defined by the presence of more than 20 percent of plasma cells in the peripheral blood. The exact mechanism involved in the progression of myeloma to PCL is unknown, but a number of possibilities have been studied. Interleukin-6 can downregulate syndecan-1 and upregulate type 1 collagen.[121,122] In addition, expression of NCAM is also lost on PCL cells.[87] Together, this loss of adhesion can facilitate mobilization of MM cells from the bone marrow and support the development of PCL.

One potential consequence of treatment of MM is the development of secondary malignancies such as acute myeloid leukemia (AML) or myelodysplastic syndrome (MDS). The incidence of secondary AML or MDS in myeloma patients is 10 to 17 percent 4 to 8 years after treatment.[123,124] Use of alkylating agents such as melphalan in the treatment of MM is believed to be one of the causes of secondary malignancies. Hematopoietic stem cells are a target of these drugs and may sustain considerable DNA damage that may not be completely repaired.[125] These abnormal stem cells may have a growth advantage over the normal cells and can lead to development of secondary malignancies.

SUMMARY AND FUTURE DIRECTIONS

Multiple myeloma is a very heterogeneous disease. There are currently no known genetic defects that are associated with all cases of MM. There are, however, a number of genetic abnormalities that are found with high frequency. These defects can have significant effects on disease progression and response to therapeutic agents.

A number of genetic abnormalities can have an effect on cellular control mechanisms. Signal transduction pathways can be altered by mutations in signaling molecules such as Ras or by aberrant expression of the FGF receptor. Both of these can lead to cells that are less dependent on IL-6 for proliferation and survival. Genes that control the cell cycle are also commonly overexpressed (cyclin D1, c-myc) or deleted (Rb-1), leading to uncontrolled proliferation. Genetic alterations in apoptotic genes have also been described in myeloma. Overexpression of Bcl-2 family members can protect the myeloma cells from apoptosis induced by a number of therapeutic agents.

In addition to affecting cellular control mechanisms, genetic abnormalities can have an effect on the interaction of the myeloma cells with the bone marrow microenvironment. Adhesion of the myeloma cells to the bone marrow can alter gene expression pattern in both the myeloma cells and the stromal cells. Adhesion is able to increase the expression of growth and survival factors such as IL-6. In addition, interactions between the myeloma cell and the stromal cells can lead to changes in the bone marrow environment, including increased expression of osteoclast-activating factors and angiogenic factors. This not only affects the myeloma cells but also can alter normal hematopoiesis.

The genetic heterogeneity found associated with myeloma can affect therapeutic response and the development of secondary malignancies. A number of genetic polymorphisms have been described in detoxification genes, including glutathione-S-transferase (GST), N-Acetyl transferase 2 (NAT2), and myeloperoxidase (MPO).[126] These polymorphisms have the potential to be genetic markers for prediction of therapeutic response and development of secondary malignancies. Future studies that correlate gene expression with disease progression and response to therapy may be important in choosing an effective patient-specific therapy.

The development of gene array technology will open up a number of new avenues for genetic research on myeloma. Gene arrays have been used in to reclassify patients with diffuse large B-cell lymphoma (DLBCL) on the basis of gene expression.[127]

The new classifications have correlated with patient survival. Similar classifications based on gene expression may be used in myeloma to try to predict therapeutic response and patient survival. In addition, gene arrays can be used to follow genetic changes associated with disease progression. Cell banks can be set up, with patient samples collected from diagnosis through disease progression and treatment. Gene expression in a single patient can be followed through disease progression and response to therapy to determine which genes are involved in transition from MGUS to MM or from MM to PCL.

REFERENCES

1. Nowak R, Oelschlagel U, Range U et al: Flow cytometric DNA quantification in immunophenotyped cells as a sensitive method for determination of aneuploid multiple myeloma cells in peripheral blood stem cell harvests and bone marrow after therapy. Bone Marrow Transplant 23:895, 1999.

2. Almeida J, Orfao A, Ocqueteau M et al: High-sensitive immunophenotyping and DNA ploidy studies for the investigation of minimal residual disease in multiple myeloma. Br J Haematol 107:121, 1999.

3. Ward MS: The use of flow cytometry in the diagnosis and monitoring of malignant hematological disorders. Pathology 31:382, 1999.

4. Genevieve F, Zandecki M, Lai J-L et al: Evaluation of minimal residual disease by interphase FISH in multiple myeloma: Does complete remission exist? Leukemia 13:641, 1999.

5. Billadeau D, Blackstadt M, Greipp P et al: Analysis of B-lymphoid malignancies using allele-specific polymerase chain reaction: A technique for sequential quantitation of residual disease. Blood 78:3021, 1991.

6. Billadeau D, Quam L, Thomas W et al: Detection and quantitation of malignant cells in the peripheral blood of multiple myeloma patients. Blood 80:1818, 1992.

7. Gerard CJ, Olsson K, Ramanathan R et al: Improved quantitation of minimal residual disease in multiple myeloma using real-time polymerase chain reaction and plasmid-DNA complementary determining region III standards. Cancer Res 58:3957, 1998.

8. Van der Griend R, Verdonck LF, Petersen EJ et al: Donor leukocyte infusions inducing remissions repeatedly in a patient with recurrent multiple myeloma after allogeneic bone marrow transplantation. Bone Marrow Transplant 23:195, 1999.

9. Martinelli G, Terragna C, Zamagni E et al: Molecular remission after allogeneic or autologous transplantation of hematopoietic stem cells for multiple myeloma. J Clin Oncol 18:2273, 2000.

10. Ladetto M, Donovan JW, Harig S et al: Real-time polymerase chain reaction of immunoglobulin rearrangements for quantitative evaluation of minimal residual disease in multiple myeloma. Biol Blood Marrow Transplant 6:241, 2000.

11. Cavo M, Terragna C, Martinelli G et al: Molecular monitoring of minimal residual disease in patients in long-term complete remission after allogeneic stem cell transplantation for multiple myeloma. Blood 96:355, 2000.

12. Martinelli G, Terragna C, Zamagni E et al: Polymerase chain reaction-based detection of minimal residual disease in multiple myeloma patients receiving allogeneic stem cell transplantation. Haematologica 85:930, 2000.

13. Kubagawa H, Vogler LB, Capra JD et al: Studies on the clonal origin of multiple myeloma. Use of individually specific (idiotype) antibodies to trace the oncogenic event to the earliest point of expression in B-cell differentiation. J Exp Med 150:792, 1979.

14. King MA, Nelson DS: Tumor cell heterogeneity in multiple myeloma: Antigenic, morphologic, and functional studies of cells from blood and bone marrow. Blood 73:1925, 1989.

15. Epstein J, Xiao HQ, He XY: Markers of multiple hematopoietic-cell lineages in multiple myeloma. N Engl J Med 322:664, 1990.

16. Grogan TM, Durie BGM, Lomen C et al: Delineation of a novel pre-B cell component in plasma cell myeloma: Immunochemical, immunophenotypic, genotypic, cytologic, cell culture and kinetic features. Blood 70:932, 1987.

17. Grogan TM, Durie BGM, Spier CM et al: Myelomonocytic antigen positive multiple myeloma. Blood 73:763, 1989.

18. Chan CSP, Wormsleym SB, Pierce LE et al: B-cell surface phenotypes of proliferating myeloma cells: Target antigens for immunotherapy. Am J Hematol 33:101, 1990.

19. Epstein J, Barlogie B, Katzmann J, Alexanian R: Phenotypic heterogeneity in aneuploid multiple myeloma indicates pre-B cell involvement. Blood 71:861, 1988.

20. Billadeau D, Ahmann G, Greipp P, Van Ness B: The bone marrow of multiple myeloma patients contains B cell populations at different stages of differentiation that are clonally related to the malignant plasma cell. J Exp Med 178:1023, 1993.

21. Carradini P, Boccadoro M, Voena C, Pileri A: Evidence for a bone marrow B cell transcribing malignant plasma cell VDJ joined to C-mu sequence in IgG and IgA secreting multiple myeloma. J Exp Med 178:1091, 1993.

22. Bakkus MH, Van Reit I, Van Camp B, Theilemans K: Evidence that the clonogenic cell in multiple myeloma originates from a pre-switched but somatically mutated B cell. Br J Haematol 87:68, 1994.

23. Vescio RA, Cao J, Hong CH et al: Myeloma Ig heavy chain V region sequences reveal prior antigenic selection and marked somatic mutation but no intraclonal diversity. J Immunol 155:2487, 1995.

24. Bakkus MHC, Heirman C, Van Riet B et al: Evidence that multiple myeloma Ig heavy chain VDJ genes contain somatic mutations but show no intraclonal variation. Blood 80:2326, 1992.

25. Ralph QM, Brisco MJ, Joshua DE et al: Advancement of multiple myeloma from diagnosis through plateau phase to progression does not involve a new B-cell clone: Evidence from the Ig heavy chain gene. Blood 82:202, 1993.

26. Corradini P, Boccadoro M, Voena C, Pileri A: Evidence for a bone marrow B cell transcribing malignant plasma cell VDJ joined to Cm sequence in immunoglobulin (IgG)- and IgA-secreting multiple myelomas. J Exp Med 178:1091, 1993.

27. Muraguchi A, Hirano T, Tang B et al: The essential role of B cell stimulating factor 2 (BDF-2/IL-6) for the terminal differentiation of B cells. J Exp Med 167:332, 1988.

28. Alderson MR, Oike BL: Recombinant human IL-6 (B cell stimulatory factor 2) enhances immunoglobulin secretion by single murine hapten-specific B cells in the absence of cell division. Int Immunol 1:20, 1989.

29. Potter M, Boyce C: Induction of plasma cell neoplasms in strain BALB/c mice with mineral oil and mineral oil adjuvants. Nature 193:1086, 1962.

30. Nordan RP, Potter M: A macrophage-derived factor required by plasmacytomas for survival and proliferation in vitro. Science 233:556, 1986.

31. Kawano M, Hirano T, Matsuda T et al: Autocrine generation and requirement of BSF-2/IL-6 for human myelomas. Nature 332:83, 1988.

32. Zhang XG, Klein B, Bataille R: Interleukin-6 is a potent myeloma cell growth factor in patients with aggressive multiple myeloma. Blood 74:11, 1989.

33. Suematsu S, Matsuda T, Aozasa K et al: IgG1 plasmacytosis in interleukin-6 transgenic mice. Proc Nat Acad Sci U S A 86:7547, 1989.

34. Okuno Y, Takahasi T, Suzuki A et al: Acquisition of growth auton-omy and tumorgenicity by an interleukin-6 dependent human cell line transfected with interleukin-6 cDNA. Exp Hematol 20:395, 1992.

35. Schwab G, Siegall CB, Aarden LA et al: Characterization of an interleukin-6 mediated autocrine loop in the human multiple myeloma cell line, U266. Blood 77:587, 1991.

36. Klein B, Zhang XG, Jourdan M et al: Paracrine rather than autocrine regulation of myeloma cell growth and differentiation by interleukin-6. Blood 73:517, 1989.

37. Portier M, Rajzbaum G, Zhang XG et al: In vivo interleukin-6 expression in the tumoral environment in multiple myeloma. Eur J Immunol 21:1759, 1991.

38. Carter A, Merchav S, Silvian-Draxler I et al: The role of inter-leukin-1 and tumor necrosis factor-alpha in human multiple myeloma. Br J Haematol 74:424, 1990.

39. Cozzolino F, Torcia M, Aldinucci D et al: Production of inter-leukin-1 by bone marrow myeloma cells. Blood 74:380, 1989.

40. Hirano T, Nakajima K, Masahiko H: Signaling mechanisms through gp130: A model of the cytokine system. Cytokine Growth Factor Rev 8:241, 1997.

41. Neri A, Murphy JP, Cro L et al: Ras oncogene mutation in human multiple myeloma. J Exp Med 170:1715, 1989.

42. Portier M, Moles JP, Mazars GR et al: p53 and RAS gene muta-tions in multiple myeloma. Oncogene 7:2539, 1992.

43. Corradini P, Ladetto M, Voena C et al: Mutational activation of N- and K-ras oncogenes in plasma cell dyscrasias. Blood 81:2708, 1993.

44. Liu P, Quam L, Billadeau D et al: Activating mutations of N- and K-ras in multiple myeloma show distinct clinical associations: Analysis of the Eastern Cooperative Oncology Group phase III trial. Blood 88:2699, 1996.

45. Seremetis S, Inghirami D, Ferrero E et al: Ras oncogenes cause malignant transformation and plasmacytoid differentiation of EBV transfected human B lymphoblasts. Science 243:660, 1989.

46. Billadeau D, Jelinek DF, Shah N et al: Introduction of an activated N-ras oncogene alters the growth characteristics of the interleukin-6 dependent myeloma cell line ANBL6. Cancer Res 55:3640, 1995.

47. Billadeau D, Liu P, Jelinek DF et al: Activating mutations in the N- and K-ras oncogenes differentially affect the growth properties of the IL-6 dependent myeloma cell line ANBL6. Cancer Res 57:2268, 1997.

48. Rowley M, Liu P, Van Ness B: Heterogeneity in therapeutic response of genetically altered myeloma cell lines to IL-6, dexam-ethasone, doxorubicin, and melphalan. Blood 96:3175, 2000.

49. Chesi M, Nardini E, Brents LA et al: Frequent translocation t(4;14)(p16.3;q32.3) in multiple myeloma is associated with increased expression and activating mutations of fibroblast growth factor receptor 3. Nat Genet 16:260, 1997.

50. Richelda R, Ronchetti D, Baldini L et al: A novel chromosomal translocation t(4;14)(p16.3;q32) in multiple myeloma involves the fibroblast growth factor receptor 3 gene. Blood 90:4062, 1997.

51. Chesi M, Nardini E, Lim RS et al: The t(4;14) translocation in myeloma disregulates both FGFR3 and a novel gene, MMSET, resulting in IgH/MMSET hybrid transcripts. Blood 92:3025, 1998.

52. Plowright EE, Li Z, Bersagel PL et al: Ectopic expression of fibro-blast growth factor receptor 3 promotes myeloma cell proliferation and prevents apoptosis. Blood 95:992, 2000.

53. Hart KC, Robertson SC, Kanemitsu MY et al: Transformation and Stat activation by derivatives of FGFR1, FGFR3, and FGFR4. Oncogene 19:3309, 2000.

54. Vasef MA, Madeiros LJ, Yospur LS et al: Cyclin D1 protein in mul-tiple myeloma and plasmacytoma: An immunohistochemical study using fixed, paraffin embedded tissue sections. Mod Pathol 10:927, 1997.

55. Lai R, Medeiros LJ, Wilson CS et al: Expression of the cell cycle related proteins E2F-1, p53, mdm-2, p21waf-1, and Ki-67 in mul-tiple myeloma: Correlation with cyclin D1 immunoreactivity. Mod Pathol 11:642, 1998.

56. Fonseca R, Hoyer JD, Aguayo P et al: Clinical significance of the translocation (11;14)(q13;q32) in multiple myeloma. Leuk Lym-phoma 35:599, 1999.

57. Hoechtlen-Vollmar W, Menzel G, Bartl R et al: Amplification of cyclin D1 gene in multiple myeloma: Clinical and prognostic rel-evance. Br J Haematol 109:30, 2000.

58. Perez-Roger I, Kim S-H, Griffiths B et al: Cyclins D1 and D2 mediate Myc induced proliferation via sequestration of p27^{Kip1} and p21^{Cip1}. EMBO J 18:5310, 1999.

59. Bouchard C, Thieke K, Maier A et al: Direct induction of cyclin D2 by Myc contributes to cell cycle progression and sequestration of p27. EMBO J 18:5321, 1999.

60. Wiener F, Potter M: In Kirsch IR (ed.): The Causes and Conse-quences of Chromosomal Aberrations, pp. 91–124. CRC, New York, 1993.

61. Selvanayagam P, Blick M, Marni F et al: Alteration and abnormal expression of the c-myc oncogene in human multiple myeloma. Blood 71:30, 1988.

62. Chappell SA, LeQuesne JP, Paulin FE et al: A mutation in the c-myc-IRES leads to enhanced internal ribosome entry in multi-ple myeloma: A novel mechanism of oncogene deregulation. Oncogene 19:4437, 2000.

63. Agnantis N, Hadjiyannakis M, Tsenga A et al: Expression of c-myc p62 oncoprotein in multiple myeloma: An immunohistochemical study of 180 cases. Anticancer Res 13:1091, 1993.

64. Ray A, Sassone-Corsi P, Seghal P: A multiple cytokine and second messenger-responsive element in the enhancer of the human interleukin-6 gene: Similarities with c-fos gene regulation. Mol Cell Biol 9:5537, 1989.

65. Lee EY-HP, Huang S, Shew J-Y: Diverse mutations lead to inacti-vation of the retinoblastoma gene. p. 221. In: Molecular Biology of the Retina: Basic and Clinically Relevant Studies. Wiley-Liss, Inc., New York 1991.

66. Juge-Morineau N, Mellerin MP, Francois S et al: High incidence of deletions but infrequent inactivation of the retinoblastoma gene in human myeloma cells. Br J Haematol 91:664, 1995.

67. Corradini P, Inghirami G, Astolfi M et al: Inactivation of tumor suppressor genes, p53 and Rb1, in plasma cell dyscrasias. Leukemia 8:758, 1994.

68. McDonnell TJ, Korsmeyer SJ: Progression from lymphoid hyper-plasia to high grade malignant lymphoma in mice transgenic for the t(14;18). Nature 349:254, 1991.

69. Strasser A, Harris AW, Cory S: Eμ-Bcl-2 transgene facilitates spontaneous transformation of early pre-B and immunoglobu-lin-secreting cells but not T-cells. Oncogene 8:1, 1993.

70. Strasser A, Whittingham S, Vaux DL et al: Enforced Bcl-2 expres-sion in B-lymphoid cells prolongs antibody responses and elicits autoimmune disease. Proc Nat Acad Sci U S A 88:861, 1991.

71. Ladanyi M, Wang S, Niesvizky R et al: Proto-oncogene analysis in multiple myeloma. Am J Pathol 141:949, 1992.

72. Bloem A, Lockhorst H: Bcl-2 antisense therapy in multiple myeloma. Pathol Biol (Paris) 47:216, 1999.

73. Puthier D, Derenne S, Barille S et al: Mcl-1 and Bcl-xL are coregu-lated by IL-6 in human myeloma cells. Br J Haematol 107:392, 1999.

74. Liu P, Oken M, Van Ness B: Interferon-alpha protects myeloma cell lines from dexamethasone-induced apoptosis. Leukemia 13:473, 1999.

75. Schwarze MM, Hawley RG: Prevention of myeloma cell apoptosis by ectopic bcl-2 expression or interleukin 6-mediated up-regula-tion of Bcl-xL. Cancer Res 55:2262, 1995.

76. Catlett-Falcone R, Landowski TH, Oshiro MM et al: Constitutive activation of Stat3 signaling confers resistance to apoptosis in human U266 myeloma cells. Immunity 10:105, 1999.

77. Kawamura C, Kizaki M, Yamato K et al: Bone morphogenetic protein-2 induces apoptosis in human myeloma cells with modulation of STAT3. Blood 96:2005, 2000.

78. Puthier D, Bataille R, Amiot M: IL-6 up-regulates mcl-1 in human myeloma cells through JAK/STAT rather than ras/MAP kinase pathway. Eur J Immunol 29:3945, 1999.

79. Neri A, Baldini L, Trecca D et al: p53 mutations in multiple myeloma are associated with advanced forms of malignancy. Blood 81:128, 1993.

80. Santhanam U, Ray A, Seghal PB: Repression of the interleukin-6 gene promoter by p53 and the retinoblastoma susceptibility gene product. Proc Natl Acad Sci U S A 88:7605, 1991.

81. Vacca A, Ribatti D, Roncali L et al: Bone marrow angiogenesis and progression in multiple myeloma. Br J Haematol 87:503, 1994.

82. Vacca A, Di Loreto M, Ribatti D et al: Bone marrow patients with active multiple myeloma: Angiogenesis and plasma cell adhesion molecules LFA-1, VLA-4, LAM-1, and CD44. Am J Hematol 50:9, 1995.

83. Gregoretti MG, Gottardi D, Ghia P et al: Characterization of bone marrow stromal cells from multiple myeloma. Leuk Res 18:675, 1994.

84. Van Camp B, Durie BG, Spier C et al: Plasma cells in multiple myeloma express a natural killer cell-associated antigen: CD56 (NKH-1; Leu-19). Blood 6:377, 1990.

85. Van Riet I, Van Camp B: The involvement of adhesion molecules in the biology of multiple myeloma. Leuk Lymphoma 9:441, 1993.

86. Sonneveld P, Durie BG, Lokhorst HM et al: Analysis of multidrug-resistance (MDR-1) glycoprotein and CD56 expression to separate monoclonal gammopathy from multiple myeloma. Br J Haematol 83:63, 1993.

87. Smith SR, Auerbach B, Morgan L: Serum neural cell adhesion molecule in multiple myeloma and other plasma cell disorders. Br J Haematol 92:67, 1996.

88. Collins T, Read MA, Neish AS et al: Transcriptional regulation of endothelial cell adhesion molecules: NF-kappa B and cytokine-inducible enhancers. FASEB J 9:899, 1995.

89. Hawley RG, Wang MH, Fonz AZ et al: Association between ICAM-1 expression and metastatic capacity of murine B-cell hybridomas. Clin Exp Metastasis 11:213, 1993.

90. Huang YW, Richardson JA, Vitetta ES: Anti-CD54 (ICAM-1) has antitumor activity in SCID mice with human myeloma cells. Cancer Res 55:610, 1995.

91. Kim I, Uchiyama H, Chauhan D et al: Cell surface expression and functional significance of adhesion molecules on human derived myeloma cell lines. Br J Haematol 87:483, 1994.

92. Uchiyama H, Barut BA, Chauhan D et al: Characterization of adhesion molecules on human myeloma cell lines. Blood 80:2306, 1992.

93. Uchiyama H, Barut BA, Mohrbacher AF et al: Adhesion of human myeloma-derived cell lines to bone marrow stromal cells stimulates interleukin-6 secretion. Blood 82:3712, 1993.

94. Lokhurst HM, Lamme T, de Smet M et al: Primary tumour cells of myeloma patients induces interleukin-6 secretion in long term bone marrow cultures. Blood 84:2269, 1994.

95. Crainie M, Belch AR, Mant MJ, Pilarski LM: Overexpression of the receptor for hyaluronan-mediated motility (RHAMM) characterizes the malignant clone in multiple myeloma: Identification of three distinct RHAMM variants. Blood 93:1684, 1999.

96. Masellis-Smith A, Belch AR, Mant MJ et al: Hyaluronan-dependent motility of B-cells and leukemic plasma cells in blood, but not bone marrow plasma cells, in multiple myeloma: Alternate use of receptor for hyaluronan-mediated motility (RHAMM) and CD44. Blood 87:1891, 1996.

97. Westendorf JJ, Ahmann GJ, Armitage RJ et al: CD40 expression in malignant plasma cells. Role in stimulation of autocrine IL-6 secretion by a human myeloma cell line. J Immunol 152:117, 1994.

98. Urashima M, Chauhan D, Uchiyama H et al: CD40 ligand triggered interleukin-6 secretion in multiple myeloma. Blood 85:1903, 1995.

99. Chauhan D, Uchiyama H, Urashima M et al: Regulation of interleukin 6 in multiple myeloma and bone marrow stromal cells. Stem Cells 13(Suppl. 2):35, 1995.

100. Lichtenstein A, Berenson J, Norman D et al: Production of cytokines by bone marrow cells obtained from patients with multiple myeloma. Blood 74:1266, 1989.

101. Klein B, Lu ZY, Gaillard JP et al: Inhibiting IL-6 in human multiple myeloma. Curr Top Microbiol Immunol 182:237, 1992.

102. Donovan KA, Lacy MQ, Kline MP et al: Contrast in cytokine expression between patients with monoclonal gammopathy of undetermined significance or multiple myeloma. Leukemia 12:593, 1998.

103. Andrews DF, Mochizuki DY et al: Human marrow stroma cells: Response to interleukin-6 (IL-6) and control of IL-6 expression. Blood 74:1929, 1989.

104. Rajkumar SV, Leong T, Roche PC et al: Prognostic value of bone marrow angiogenesis in multiple myeloma. Clin Cancer Res 6:3111, 2000.

105. Bellamy WT, Richter L, Frutiger Y, Grogan TM: Expression of vascular endothelial growth factor and its receptors in hematopoietic malignancies. Cancer Res 59:728, 1999.

106. Dankbar B, Padro T, Leo R et al: Vascular endothelial growth factor and interleukin-6 in paracrine tumor–stromal cell interactions in multiple myeloma. Blood 95:2630, 2000.

107. Damiano JS, Cress AE, Hazlehurst LA et al: Cell adhesion mediated drug resistance (CAM-DR): Role of integrins and resistance to apoptosis in human myeloma cell lines. Blood 93:1658, 1999.

108. Hazlehurst LA, Damiano JS, Buyuksal I et al: Adhesion to fibronectin via beta₁ integrins regulates p27kip1 levels and contributes to cell adhesion mediated drug resistance (CAM-DR). Oncogene 19:4319, 2000.

109. Grigorieva I, Thomas X, Epstein J: The bone marrow stromal environment is a major factor in myeloma cell resistance to dexamethasone. Exp Hematol 26:597, 1998.

110. Wan-Cheung C, Van Ness B: The bone marrow stromal microenvironment influences myeloma therapeutic response in vitro. Leukemia (submitted)

111. Rettig M, Ma H, Vescio R et al: Kaposi's sarcoma-associated herpesvirus infection of bone marrow dendritic cells from myeloma patients. Science 276:1851, 1997.

112. Burger R, Neipel FM, Fleckenstein B et al: Human herpesvirus type 8 interleukin-6 homologue is functionally active on human myeloma cells. Blood 91:1858, 1998.

113. Tarte K, Chang Y, Klein B: Kaposi's sarcoma-associated herpes virus and multiple myeloma: Lack of criteria for causality. Blood 93:3159, 1999.

114. Kartner N, Riordan JR, Ling V: Cell surface P-glycoprotein associated with multidrug resistance in mammalian cell lines. Science 221:1285, 1983.

115. Dalton WS, Jove R: Drug resistance in multiple myeloma: Approaches to circumvention. Semin Oncol 26(5, Suppl. 13):23, 1999.

116. Grogan TM, Spier CM, Salmon SE et al: P-glycoprotein expression in human plasma cell myeloma: Correlation with prior chemotherapy. Blood 81:490, 1993.

117. Kyle RA, Lust JA: Monoclonal gammopathies of undetermined significance. Semin Hematol 26:176, 1989.

118. Kyle RA: Benign monoclonal gammopathy after 10–35 years of follow-up. Mayo Clin Proc 68:26, 1993.

119. Bataille R, Jourdan M, Zhang XG, Klein B: Serum levels of interleukin 6, a potent myeloma cell growth factor, as a reflection of disease severity in plasma cell dyscrasias. Blood 84:2008, 1985.

120. Avet-Loiseau H, Li JY, Morineau N et al: Monosomy 13 is associated with the transition of monoclonal gammopathy of undetermined significance to multiple myeloma. Intergroupe Francophone du Myelome. Blood 94:2583, 1999.

121. Nemunaitis J, Andrews DF, Mochizuki DY et al: Human marrow stromal cells: Response to interleukin-6 (IL-6) and control of IL-6 expression. Blood 74:1929, 1989.

122. Sneed TB, Stanley DJ, Young LA et al: Interleukin-6 regulates expression of the syndecan-1 proteoglycan on B lymphoid cells. Cell Immunol 153:456, 1994.

123. Bergsagel DE, Bailey AJ, Langley AJ et al: The chemotherapy of plasma cell myeloma and the incidence of acute leukemia. N Engl J Med 301:743, 1979.

124. Cuzick J, Erskine S, Edelman D et al: A comparison of the incidence of the myelodysplastic syndrome and acute myeloid leukaemia following melphalan and cyclophosphamide treatment for myelomatosis. Br J Cancer 55:523, 1987.

125. Shulman NL: Therapy related secondary malignancies. Hematol Oncol Clin North Am 7:325, 1993.

126. Evans WE, Relling MV: Pharmacogenomics: Translating functional genomics into rational therapeutics. Science 256:487, 1999.

127. Alizadeh AA, Eisen MB, Davis RE et al: Distinct types of diffuse large B-cell lymphoma identified by gene expression profiling. Nature 403:503, 2000.

30

Staging, Kinetics, and Prognosis in Multiple Myeloma

Philip R. Greipp and Robert A. Kyle

All patients with multiple myeloma (MM) have clonal neoplastic plasma cells in the bone marrow (Figure 30–1), and 98 percent have an identifiable monoclonal immunoglobulin (M-protein) in the serum or urine.[1] Tumor burden is measurable by the level of M-protein and is an important element in staging and prognosis. Ultimately tumor burden is determined by tumor growth. Unchecked growth causes anemia. Cytokines produced by myeloma cells and the microenvironment cause osteoporosis, bone lesions, and fractures.[2] Bone destruction results in hypercalcemia, which along with free nephrotoxic light chains causes kidney failure.[3,4] Myeloma also causes defects in the immune system, with consequent decreased resistance to infection and a weak antitumor response.[5] Chemotherapy often brings about a response and improvement in organ function, but chemotherapy may also weaken the immune system. Ultimately drug resistance develops, chemotherapy is no longer effective, and the patient dies from infection or bleeding.[6] Forecasting these events classically includes variables related to tumor burden, renal insufficiency, and the growth rate of clonal marrow myeloma cells.[7] Immune

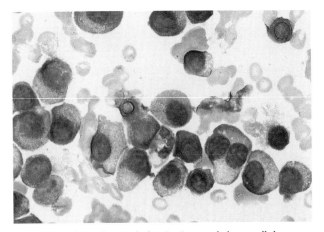

Figure 30–1. Photomicrograph showing increased plasma cells by Wright-Giemsa stain of a bone marrow aspirate in a patient with multiple myeloma. Patients with multiple myeloma have more than 10 percent clonal plasma cells in the marrow.

suppression is also an important predictor of infection and poor survival.[8]

Two percent of patients over age 50 have monoclonal gammopathy of undetermined significance (MGUS), which is the benign counterpart of MM[9] and which can be a prelude to MM. It is characterized by an M-protein in the serum or urine, but at the time of recognition there is no evidence of MM or other serious gammopathy-related disorder. The M-protein may be IgG, IgA, IgM, or rarely, IgD. Patients with MGUS do not have bone marrow suppression, lytic bone lesions, hypercalcemia, renal failure, or susceptibility to infection, and MGUS without conversion to myeloma or another serious disorder is not associated with shortened survival. Standard clinical features do not predict who will develop MM and who will remain stable. This chapter addresses the clinical and biological features that accompany progression of MGUS and MM and examines those variables that may be used for staging or prognosis.

PARADIGM OF MGUS TO MULTIPLE MYELOMA

Of patients with MGUS, nearly 1 percent per year will develop MM[9] (Figure 30–2). It can be difficult to distinguish MGUS from asymptomatic MM, particularly if the level of M-protein and percent marrow plasma cells is higher than expected. We look to clinical and biological differences to assist in the distinction between MGUS and MM. Why does one patient have MGUS or stable MM while another has advanced and progressive MM? Are there clinical and biological features that can allow one to better predict disease behavior? Do these clinical features and biological observations provide ideas about how we might predict an individual patient's disease behavior? What is the underlying biology of MGUS and MM progression in different groups of patients?

The major clinical difference between MGUS and MM is the burden of clonal marrow plasma cells; MGUS always has less than 10 percent marrow plasma cells (PCs), and organ damage is absent.[10] In active MM there is always 10 percent or more clonal marrow PCs, which may be present diffusely or focally in the marrow.[11] In MM the higher the percentage of marrow PCs, the greater the likelihood of organ damage and the worse the prognosis. Some patients with the incidental discovery of an uncomplicated monoclonal gammopathy have a bone marrow performed to rule out early MM. Those patients with 10 percent or more bone marrow PCs are probably best classified as having smoldering MM rather than MGUS.[12] An estimated 20 percent or more of MM patients have smoldering or asymptomatic myeloma.[9,13] They have no significant or progressive organ damage and can remain stable for years. Conversely, up to 10 percent of patients with active MM have organ damage but they have less than 10 percent PCs in a marrow examination due to sampling of patchy marrow involvement and only focal increases in PCs. In such patients the diagnostic criteria for MM necessitate a repeat marrow to demonstrate 10 percent or more marrow PCs. Although a higher percent of PCs is an independent predictor of survival in multivariate statistical analyses,[14] the variability of the measurement seen when the disease is

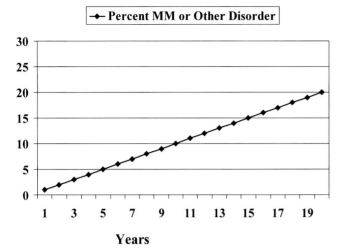

Figure 30–2. Graphic representation of the rate of progression of monoclonal gammopathy of undetermined significance to multiple myeloma or another gammopathy-associated disorder. The rate is a constant 1 percent per year among uncensored patients (Adapted from the data of Kyle and Rajkumar.[9])

patchy or focal in the marrow makes it a suboptimal prognostic factor in MM.

Another clinical feature of MM as compared with MGUS is the level of M-protein. Whether the level of M-protein is high or low is useful but much less useful than percent of PCs for diagnosis and prognosis. Patients with MGUS whose level of serum M-protein is less than 1 g/dl are less likely to progress to MM. Most often the level of M-protein is between 1 and 3 g/dl, and the median is 1.2 g/dl. Many such patients still have less than 10 percent marrow PCs despite the higher level of M-protein and consequently they have a lower likelihood of progressing to MM. Patients with even higher levels of M-protein (3 g/dl or more) are likely to also have 10 percent or more marrow PCs and thereby a higher likelihood of progressing to active MM.[15] We must conclude that the level of serum M-protein used alone is neither diagnostic nor predictive of progression to MM relative to the percent of plasma cells except at the extreme. However, if the level of M-protein increases the follow-up period, there is almost a certainty of progression to MM.[16] Only close follow-up observation of M-protein and hemoglobin level, serum creatinine and calcium level, and bone x-rays will determine when an individual patient with newly diagnosed MGUS progresses to MM.

Clinical features that clearly define active MM include anemia, destructive bone disease, hypercalcemia, and renal insufficiency. Such organ damage is not a feature of MGUS, and its frequency increases in MM as the tumor burden increases. Infection is not increased in MGUS and is an indicator of more advanced myeloma with a high tumor burden. All active MM patients have some component of organ damage.[17] Two of three active myeloma patients have anemia, four of five have destructive bone disease, one of five has hypercalcemia, and one of six has renal insufficiency.

When MM is diagnosed in the asymptomatic phase, there is no anemia, bone disease, hypercalcemia, or renal insufficiency. Prognostication and treatment decisions can be very difficult. Screening electrophoresis is increasing the awareness and recognition of asymptomatic MM. Close follow-up of patients with MGUS and asymptomatic MM involves serial measurement of the serum and urine M-protein levels. Avoiding chemotherapy forestalls complications such as myelodysplastic syndrome and acute leukemia.

An estimated 20 percent of more of MM cases are diagnosed in the asymptomatic phase.[13] On recognition of asymptomatic MM, it is not known whether organ damage is just about to occur or whether the condition is stable. Stable patients have been said to have smoldering MM,[12] stage 1 asymptomatic MM,[18] or indolent MM,[19] each of which represents different categories of asymptomatic MM. Such patients have 10 percent or more PCs, so they fulfill the generally accepted criteria for MM. Even with a high or slowly increasing M-protein level, they can be observed without therapy, sometimes for years. Other asymptomatic MM patients develop minimal organ damage, which can be managed with supportive therapy unless more significant damage threatens. For example, isolated anemia may be manageable with erythropoietin administration, and minimal bone abnormalities may be manageable with intravenous bisphosphonates. In contrast, hypercalcemia, advancing bone destruction, or renal insufficiency is an indication for immediate treatment aimed at producing a prompt response.

In asymptomatic MM, the time to progression cannot be easily predicted. The time to chemotherapy is 17 to 95 months or more (Figure 30–3).[13] Median time to progression is 48 months.[20] Median survival is similar in patients who receive immediate versus delayed chemotherapy for asymptomatic stage 1 MM.[21] Observing these patients closely until they progress and require chemotherapy is a reasonable approach.

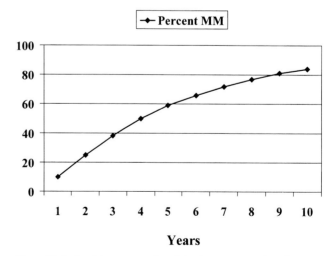

Figure 30–3. Graphic representation of the time to progression of asymptomatic multiple myeloma to active multiple myeloma. The median time to progression to active multiple myeloma is 4 years. (The rate is estimated from the data of Weber et al.[13])

Asymptomatic patients with MM may be candidates for clinical trials using biological therapy to prevent progression, thus delaying the need for chemotherapy and avoiding its complications. Patients with solitary plasmacytoma of bone or extramedullary plasmacytoma who do not have evidence of progression to MM should also be closely followed without treatment.[22] Median time to progression for patients with solitary plasmacytoma of bone is 4 1/2 years.[23] Bone damage may be detected early in some cases by special imaging beyond the standard bone x-rays. Magnetic resonance imaging (MRI) and computed tomography (CT) scanning has diagnostic and prognostic utility and has been reviewed elsewhere.[24] Clinical variables such as a serum M-protein level of 3 g/dl or more, urine Bence Jones protein of 50 mg/dl or more, IgA protein type, and MRI scanning abnormalities are helpful,[13] but they do not adequately differentiate those who will progress from those who will not progress. Some patients progress early with significant bone or renal damage. Patients who progress unexpectedly early during follow-up observation especially point out the need for the development of better prognostication and predictive tests.

Study of the biology of myeloma can yield better tests to distinguish active MM from MGUS and asymptomatic MM and patients. A low marrow plasma cell labeling index (PCLI)[25] (Figure 30–4) or low numbers of circulating myeloma cells clearly support the decision to observe.[26] An increased PCLI and/or increased circulating plasma cells accompany the diagnosis of active MM in 90 percent of cases.[27] We need to develop more practical biological tests to better diagnose MGUS and MM in the future. The following sections focus on those clinical and biologic factors that predict response, progression, and prognosis.

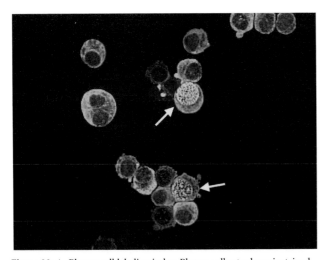

Figure 30–4. Plasma cell labeling index. Plasma cell cytoplasm is stained with fluorescein-conjugated anti-kappa or -lambda light chain. Nuclei incorporating bromodeoxyuridine are labeled with rhodamine-conjugated antibromodeoxyuridine antibody. The plasma cell labeling index (PCLI) is the percent of plasma cells in S-phase of the cell cycle as detected by the bromodeoxyuridine antibody. Arrows point to two labeled monoclonal plasma cells.

CLINICAL CHANGES IN MGUS AND MM PROGRESSION

No single clinical test distinguishes MM from MGUS and smoldering multiple myeloma (SMM).[9] A combination of clinical and laboratory observations is used. All patients with MGUS and SMM are followed with serial M-protein measurement for the development of myeloma or other serious disease.

It is likely that MGUS and MM represent two distinct phases in the same disease course. In a study of MM patients in Olmsted County, Minnesota, 58 percent had a prior MGUS or plasmacytoma.[28] Because of the retrospective nature of the study, some patients with the diagnosis of MM did not have prior electrophoresis to detect MGUS. If all patients with MM had had prior studies to detect an M-protein, most would probably have had prior MGUS. Progression from MGUS to MM or other serious and related diseases occurs in 40 percent of patients with 25 or more years of follow-up observation.[9] The preceding stable phase can be long, with a median duration of 10 years; conversely, the transitional phase to MM during which the M-protein rises and complications develop is often relatively brief, usually less than 6 to 12 months. In most cases the transition from MGUS to MM occurs after a long period of stable M-protein levels.[16] From these observations it is easy to deduce that distinct biological events cause the transition.

There are three patterns of progression from MGUS to MM.[9] In a study of 241 patients with MGUS in which 25 developed MM, nearly 50 percent showed a stable M-protein for 4 to 18 years and then a gradual increase, leading to a clinical diagnosis of myeloma in a median of 3 years. Just over 25 percent of the patients were stable for a time and then showed a rapid rise, leading to clinical myeloma in under a year. The remaining 25 percent of patients had a fluctuating but gradually increasing M-protein level until MM was diagnosed 5 to 29 years later, with a median of 7 years. Thus about 75 percent of patients with MGUS who develop myeloma show a clear transition to progressive MM. One can conclude that MM most commonly arises from a prior MGUS state. The transformation from MGUS to MM is most often a discrete event.

A typical course for active MM is depicted in Figure 30–5. At diagnosis patients receive chemotherapy, and most respond to treatment. This response can be sustained for a significant period in unmaintained remission. This stable remission period is referred to as the plateau phase. Subsequent responses can be achieved, but eventually progression occurs and resistance to therapy develops. It is likely that just as in the transition from MGUS to MM, discrete biological events accompany the clinical changes as MM progresses.

EVENTS DURING MGUS AND MM PROGRESSION

Clinical differences between MGUS and MM are clues to the underlying biological features that differentiate MGUS from MM. The increase in M-protein indicates an increase in clonal marrow PCs and reflects an underlying increase in PC proliferation or a decrease in apoptosis. This increase in clonal plasma

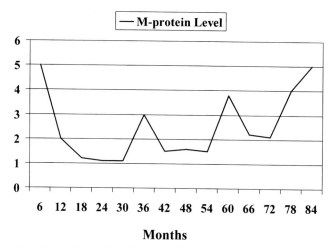

Figure 30–5. The graph depicts a typical course for a myeloma patient over a 7-year time course. The level of M-protein is plotted against time. Regardless of the duration of survival, the characteristic pattern is one of remitting and relapsing disease, with shorter and shorter remissions and more rapid relapses.

recruit osteoblasts and osteoclasts to produce myeloma cell growth factors, so-called paracrine growth regulation.

The development of anemia is a clue to mechanisms underlying bone marrow suppression, including changes in cytokine production by myeloma cells and their microenvironment. Renal failure and underproduction of erythropoietin is a factor. Renal failure is caused by an increase in production of nephrotoxic free light chain.

The occurrence of infection in newly diagnosed MM reflects a defective immune system. There is suppression of normal immunoglobulin production by B cells and their progeny, accompanied by complex changes in regulatory T cells, including loss of or increase in certain types of T cells.

It is clear that MGUS and MM progression are due to alterations in the clonal plasma cells and their interactions with the marrow microenvironment. Alterations in myeloma plasma cell growth are complex and include alterations in cytogenetic, molecular, cell signaling, cytokine, and adhesion molecules that increase myeloma cell growth and survival. Alterations in the microenvironment include changes in stromal cell, osteoblast, osteoclast, vessel endothelial cell, and immune cell interactions. These changes in turn result in activation, adhesion, and cytokine production that fuel myeloma cell proliferation and survival. Changes in these interactions also play a role in the spread of myeloma through the circulation, homing, and adhering myeloma cells to the cytokine-rich bone marrow microenvironment, causing resistance to treatment.

A better understanding of MGUS and MM progression has yielded new targets for therapy. New agents are being developed to block these pathways. Understanding the biological changes

cell growth can be measured by an increase in the PCLI or a decrease in apoptosis that is seen in MM as compared with MGUS (Figure 30–6).

Studies of myeloma bone disease and how the myeloma PC interacts with the bone-forming cells and bone matrix have provided a wealth of knowledge regarding myeloma growth. In contrast to MGUS plasma cells, plasma cells from MM patients

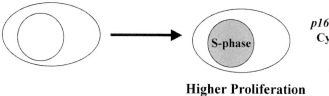

Higher Proliferation

ras **Mutation**
p16 **and** *p15* **Hypermethylation**
Cyclin D1 and D3 Activation
c-myc **Activation**
Autocrine IL-6, sIL-6R,
and VEGF
and Paracrine effects

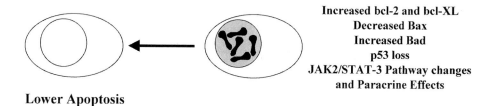

Lower Apoptosis

Increased bcl-2 and bcl-XL
Decreased Bax
Increased Bad
p53 loss
JAK2/STAT-3 Pathway changes
and Paracrine Effects

Figure 30–6. This is a graphic presentation of changes associated with the growth of multiple myeloma. The increase in tumor burden is due to an increase in proliferating cells and a decrease in apoptosis. These changes are characteristic of the progression in monoclonal gammopathy of undetermined significance and multiple myeloma. Known mechanisms for increased proliferation and decreased apoptosis are shown at the right.

that occur as myeloma progresses is improving staging and prognosis and improving our ability to predict outcome.

SPECIFIC PROGRESSION EVENTS IN MGUS AND MM

Overview

Clonal plasma cells of MM and MGUS undergo transforming or progression-related events, which together with events in the microenvironment lead to disease progression. Such events cause the progression from MGUS to MM, progression during the course of myeloma, and resistance to therapy.

The expansion of clonal neoplastic plasma cells is due to an increase in proliferation or a decrease in programmed cell death or both. We measure proliferation changes using the PCLI.[29] Regulatory signals underlie the proliferation. These include hypermethylation of the cyclin-dependent kinase (CDK) pathway regulatory gene $p16$.[30] Hypermethylation of $p16$ is associated with plasmablastic features, and by implication, high proliferative rates. Cell proliferation changes may also be caused by mutation of the ras oncogene.[31] It is controversial whether ras gene mutations and hypermethylation of the cell-cycle regulatory genes $p16$ and $p15$ are early events seen in MGUS or late events occurring in MM.[32] Decrease in apoptosis, or programmed cell death, may be associated with changes in the JAK2 STAT-3 pathways.[6] Mutation of $p53$ is distinctly uncommon, but loss of $p53$ occurs in 10 percent of patients with newly diagnosed MM and is a particularly adverse prognostic factor.[33]

Chromosomal events underlie many of the proliferation and apoptotic changes that cause progression in MGUS and MM. By using florescence in situ hybridization (FISH), the t(11;14) translocation is found in 16 percent of MM patients.[34] The t(11;14) abnormality is predictably associated with overexpression of cyclin D1,[35] which is necessary for the progression of cells from the G1/G0 phase to the DNA synthesis or S-phase of the cell cycle. Yet the t(11;14) translocation appears to be just as frequent in stable MGUS (15 percent of cases) as it is in active MM.[36] The t(11;14) therefore must be an early event. In isolation it is not sufficient to produce active MM. Neither does it predict poorer survival after MM develops.[34] Deletion of chromosome 13 (del 13) is detected by FISH in 54 percent of newly diagnosed MM cases[37] and by conventional cytogenetics (CC) in only 8 to 9 percent of such cases. It is comparatively rare in MGUS.[36] It is likely that multiple transforming events cause MM and that combinations of specific factors may be necessary for disease progression. The complexity of the cytogenetic abnormalities does not reduce the potential importance of single events but stresses the importance of understanding complex interactions. It is hoped that continued study of chromosomal abnormalities will reveal patterns associated with progression to myeloma.

Interleukin-6 (IL-6) is the principal growth and survival factor for myeloma cells; however, C-reactive protein (CRP) is often thought of as a surrogate for IL-6 measurement. We see elevated serum levels of IL-6 and CRP in MM more than in MGUS because of an increase in IL-6 production by marrow stromal cells. In the past, investigators have found that serum IL-6 levels are not useful in discriminating MGUS from early-stage MM. Some investigators have suggested that IL-6 serum levels may be useful for distinguishing smoldering from active and stage 1 from stages 2 and 3 MM.[38] Recent investigations have failed to show discriminatory value for the serum IL-6 levels in MGUS and SMM versus MM or to find a role for these levels in predicting the course of active MM.[39] We conclude that neither CRP not IL-6 level is a very useful diagnostic discriminant, and the eventual role of these measures in prognosis awaits further investigation.

Beta$_2$-microglobulin (β_2-M) is the light chain of the HLA class II histocompatibility complex and is actively shed from myeloma cells. The β_2-M level is increased in half of patients with MM and is rarely increased in MGUS. An elevated value predicts for poorer survival.[40] However, in almost half of the MM cases with elevated β_2-M values, the increase is secondary to renal insufficiency, whereas in other cases it is a reflection of tumor burden, and there are probably other causes of serum β_2-M elevation in MM. The serum β_2-M level is not useful in distinguishing between MGUS and early-stage MM.

Cell adhesion and homing of myeloma cells to the marrow microenvironment is critical to development of MGUS and MM. Studies have shown that circulating clonal plasma cells are increased in MM as compared with MGUS.[27] Early studies suggested that an increased frequency of expression of the neural cell adhesion molecule (NCAM or CD56) on clonal plasma cells is characteristic of MM as compared with MGUS. However, later studies showed that CD56 expression is similar in MGUS and MM owing to CD56-positive clonal plasma cells.[41,42] The interpretation that MM contains more CD56-positive cells than MGUS comes from inclusion of polyclonal CD56-negative plasma cells, which are residual in many MGUS cases. Several investigators have shown that the NCAM expression is decreased in plasma-cell leukemia relative to myeloma.[43] Very late antigen-5 (VLA-5) on clonal plasma cells binds to fibronectin and collagen. Immature proliferating myeloma cells lose such adhesion owing to lost expression of VLA-5.[44] The loss of adhesion markers such as CD56 as cells move from the marrow to the blood suggests that the expression of adhesion markers is dynamic and functional. Both internal cellular and external microenvironment factors play a role in altering myeloma cell adhesion. The role of adhesion markers in myeloma is discussed in the comprehensive review by Witzig.[45]

Bone lesions are unique to MM and are not found in MGUS. Osteoclast activity provides growth factors for myeloma, therefore the mechanisms of bone resorption are critical targets for therapy. Interleukin-1beta (IL-1β) is a principal regulator of osteoclast function, which is expressed in most MM cases and in a minority of MGUS cases, and then only at a low level.[46] Macrophage inflammatory factor-1alpha (MIP-1α) is a potent cytokine, which, together with the receptor activator of nuclear transcription factor-kappaB (NF-κB) and the receptor activator of NF-κB-ligand (RANK-L), potently induces osteoclastic bone resorption.[47,48] Osteoclastic bone destruction then releases growth factors and cytokines from the bone matrix, which stimulate myeloma cell proliferation. A limiting factor in bone resorption is the antiosteoclastic factor osteoprotegerin (OPG), which is decreased in MM but not MGUS.[49] Osteoprotegerin binds to and limits the osteoclastic activation properties of RANK-L. Immunohistochemical studies suggest that RANK-L, also known as tumor necrosis factor-related activation-induced cytokine (TRANCE), is increased in MM as compared with MGUS.[49] There are also interesting interactions between the bone-forming cells and the immune system. By way of example, activated T cells are able to inhibit osteoclast-induced bone resorption in MM.[50] Further study of the pathways of bone destruction will likely yield more information about the growth pathways of myeloma and their prognostic significance.

There are also specific changes in the marrow microenvironment during the progression from MGUS to MM. In active MM the marrow microenvironment shifts its energy to support myeloma cell growth and survival by producing, among other factors, a higher level of IL-6,[51] the major myeloma cell proliferation and survival factor. Microenvironment changes in fibroblasts, osteoblasts, and osteoclasts can clearly be caused by myeloma cell alterations. Collectively these cells and others constitute the stromal cell population that grows out after weeks of culture of primary marrow aspirate material. They do this by a cooperative interaction among myeloma cells and stromal cells. One key example of this interaction is that marrow plasma cell production of IL-1β stimulates these stromal cells to produce IL-6 to support myeloma cell growth and survival.[46,52]

In addition to changes induced by myeloma plasma cells, myeloma cell growth may also be affected by stromal cell alterations that are independent of any stimulus from myeloma cells. The latter are hinted at by the controversial finding that viral infection of dendritic cells containing HHV-8 virus components may provide growth factor and cytokine homologues that may foster myeloma cell growth.[53]

The stromal cell alteration can be induced by injury to the bone. In one case electrical injury to the bone led to localized growth of plasmacytomas specifically in the area of bilateral tibial injuries. Myeloma failed to develop systemically during more than 12 years of follow-up observation.[54] This finding stresses the importance of the marrow microenvironment in the development and progression of MM.

Increased angiogenesis and increased microvessel density in MM bone marrow as compared with MGUS marrow was first shown in a study from Bari, Italy,[55] in which microvessel density was associated with a high PCLI. Our group showed that increased marrow angiogenesis and microvessel density in MM was associated not only with a higher PCLI but also with shorter survival.[56] Angiogenic factors can double as growth factors for myeloma. For instance, marrow myeloma cells proliferate in response to release of vascular endothelial growth factor (VEGF) from bone marrow stroma.[57] This occurs when the integrins VLA-4 and VLA-5 (very late antigens 4 and 5) on myeloma cells adhere to vascular cell adhesion molecule 1 (VCAM-1) on stromal cells, resulting in the release of proliferative cytokines. Comparison of these mechanisms among MGUS and MM patients is needed. Another factor made by myeloma cells is fibroblast growth factor b (bFGF); this factor is also proangiogenic, and bone marrow is the likely source since levels are higher in the bone marrow than in the serum.[58,59]

Morphology

Morphological immaturity and dedifferentiation are common in MM as compared with MGUS (Table 30–1).[25] Greater nucleolar size characterizes MM. In a multicenter trial of 295 MGUS and 266 MM patients, MM differed from MGUS by percentage of bone marrow plasma cells, a shift from plasmacytic toward plasmablastic cytology, an increase in bone marrow cellularity and fibrosis, and a diffuse rather than an interstitial pattern.[60] There is also a concomitant decrease in residual hematopoiesis and an increase in osteoclasts. In a fraction of MM cases plasma cells are mature in appearance.[61] These studies support the notion that MM is characterized by morphological changes in plasma cells but that cytological criteria are inadequate for differentiating MM from MGUS and SMM. It is likely that proliferative differences underlie the morphological changes, and direct measurement of proliferation is preferable to more refined morphologic classification to distinguish MM from MGUS and SMM.

Proliferation

A higher PCLI of 1 percent or more is found in one-third of patients with MM, whereas most patients with MGUS have a PCLI less than or equal to 0.2 percent. The PCLI best discriminates MM from MGUS and SMM[25] and is best performed by immunofluorescence microscopy.[29] Cells are incubated with bromodeoxyuridine (BrDU), which is taken up in the nuclei of replicating cells. The cells are concentrated onto a glass slide using a cytocentrifuge. The slide is stained with antibody to kappa or lambda light chain conjugated with fluorescein. An antibody to BrDU is added along with DNAase, followed by addition of an antimouse immunoglobulin conjugated to rhodamine to recognize S-phase cells. Atypical plasma cell morphology and bright green kappa or lambda immunostaining identify cells belonging to the myeloma clone. Bright orange

Table 30–1. Mean Values for Clinical, Morphologic, and Cell Kinetic Factors in Multiple Myeloma, Monoclonal Gammopathy of Undetermined Significance, and Smoldering Multiple Myeloma

Factor	MM (n = 23)	MGUS (n = 43)	SMM (n = 9)
Serum monoclonal protein (g/dl)	3.2	2.2[d]	3.4
Urine monoclonal protein (g/24 h)	2.9	0.3[b]	0.2
Marrow plasma cells, percent	49	5[a]	17[d]
Marrow lymphocytes, percent	10	15[c]	21[d]
Nucleolar size (μm)	1.6	1.0[a]	1.3
Grade	1.6	1.1[a]	1.3
Asynchrony	0.5	0.3[c]	0.5
Plasma cell labeling index, percent	1	0.1[a]	0.1[b]
Lymphocyte labeling index, percent	0.6	0.1	1.0

P values represent significant difference from MM value (Kruskal-Wallis test; chi-square approximation).
[a] $P < .0001$; [b] $P < .001$; [c] $P < .01$; [d] $P < .05$.
(From Greipp and Kyle,[25] with permission)

nuclear staining identifies cells in S-phase. The PCLI is determined by simply counting the percent of plasma cells in S-phase. The PCLI best discriminates patients with MM from those with MGUS and SMM, as compared with standard clinical, laboratory, and morphologic variables (Table 30–1). All studies to date have confirmed the diagnostic value of the PCLI in discriminating MM from MGUS and SMM.[25,62–68] A summary of these studies is shown in Table 30–2.

Nuclear staining with Ki-67, an index of the growth fraction, can also discriminate between early-stage MM and MGUS.[69] However, we have found the PCLI to be more useful diagnostically. A high PCLI and an abnormal marrow plasma cell κ/λ ratio discriminated MM from SMM in another study; low PCLI and less abnormal plasma cell κ/λ ratios characterized MGUS.[64] Discriminant analysis showed statistically significant differences in plasma cell κ/λ ratio, marrow percent plasma cells, PCLI, CD3, CD4, and CD8 lymphocyte absolute values among patients with MM compared with MGUS.[65] DNA S-phase analysis by flow cytometry has not proved successful in discriminating MGUS from SMM and MM. A DNA S-phase flow cytometry method offers the possibility of greater speed and efficiency in assessing plasma cell proliferation and correlates closely with the slide method results.[70]

Other potentially useful ways to assess myeloma cell proliferation are being examined. Cyclin D1 staining and Ki-67 staining have not gained wide acceptance because they are difficult to perform in MGUS owing to the small percentage of marrow plasma cells. Assays for DNA S-phase using flow cytometry and propidium iodide fluorescence staining techniques are similarly problematic and need to be better optimized and standardized to be used routinely for diagnosis of MM. We have shown a correlation between the PCLI and this method but only when 20 percent or more plasma cells are present.[71] Eventually a more simplified assay for myeloma cell proliferation should prove useful in clinically differentiating MM from MGUS and early asymptomatic MM.

Apoptosis

Assessment of proliferation alone is not sufficient to evaluate myeloma growth. Growth depends on both proliferation and apoptosis of the population of cells being analyzed. Studies of apoptosis have shown decreased apoptosis in MM plasma cells compared with MGUS.[68] In this study the median plasma cell apoptotic indices (PCAIs) for patients with MGUS, SMM, and MM were 5.2, 3.4, and 2.4, respectively. Interleukin-6 from the microenvironment of myeloma cells is probably the major factor contributing to cell survival in MM. Sources include IL-6 produced by stromal cells. Increased CD40 ligand may also contribute to reduced apoptotic rates in MM. Although increase in the antiapoptotic bcl-2 protein is found in the majority of patients with MM,[72,73] recent studies suggest that increases in Bcl-XL may be a more important antiapoptotic factor in increasing myeloma cell survival.[6,74–76] Bcl-XL is an antiapoptotic protein that is tightly regulated by IL-6. Expression of Bcl-XL in MGUS and SMM has been reported to be intermediate between expression in normal plasma cells and myeloma cells. The diagnostic and prognostic usefulness of measures of apoptosis remains to be seen. Low BAX expression identifies a cohort of patients with long survival.[76]

Circulation and Spread

Since the neoplastic clonal plasma cells in MGUS and MM are found at all marrow sites, they must circulate in the peripheral blood. Identifying and quantifying putative precursor B cells has proved elusive. The circulating plasma cells themselves are proliferative and are easier to characterize using cytoplasmic kappa or lambda immunoglobulin staining and surface CD38 and CD138 (syndecan-1) and CD45. The circulating clonal plasma cells are increased in MM but are rare in MGUS and SMM.[27,77,78] In 57 percent of newly diagnosed and 81 percent of

Table 30–2. Diagnostic Value of the Bone Marrow Plasma Cell Labeling Index

Test	Reference	Year	No. of Cases	Mean LI (percent)		Discriminant (percent)	P Value
				MGUS/SMM	MM		
[³H]TdrLI	Greipp and Kyle[25]	1983	75	0.1/0.1	1.0	0.4	< .001[a]
							< .001[b]
[³H]TdrLI	Boccadoro et al.[62]	1984	52	NA	NA	1.0	< .001
BrdUrdLI	Greipp et al.[63]	1987	52	0.3/—	1.4	0.8	< .002
BrdUrdLI	Boccadoro et al.[336]	1987	43	0.3/—	1.4	1.0	.004[c]
BrdUrdLI	Büchi et al.[64]	1990	43	0.6/0.8	2.5	1.0	< .05
BrdUrdLI	Girino et al.[69]	1991	59	0.3/—	1.9	—	< .05
BrdUrdLI	Ahsmann et al.[67]	1992	28	0.4/—	1.4	—	—
BrdUrdLI	Leo et al.[66]	1992	53	0.3/—	1.4	—	—
BrdUrdLI	Büchi et al.[65]	1993	47	0.6/0.8	2.4	1.0	< .05
BrdUrdLI	Witzig et al.[68]	1999	91	NA	NA	1.0	< .001

Abbreviations: BrdUrdLI, bromodeoxyuridine labeling index; [³H]TdrLI, tritiated thymidine labeling index; LI, labeling index; NA, not available.
[a] For differences between MGUS (monoclonal gammopathy of undetermined significance) and MM (multiple myeloma).
[b] For differences between SMM (smoldering multiple myeloma) and MM.
[c] For differences between MGUS and stage I MM (continuous variable).

relapsed MM cases there were more than 3×10^6 monoclonal plasma cells per liter. All MGUS patients had less than 3×10^6 plasma cells per liter. The number of circulating clonotypic plasma cells is a better discriminator of disease activity than the morphologically measured B-cell light-chain κ/λ ratio. Flow cytometric measurement of circulating plasma cells makes this useful diagnostic technique more widely applicable.[79] Chromosome abnormalities by conventional cytogenetics, fluorescent in situ hybridization (FISH), and DNA content aneuploidy are limited to the circulating plasma cells.[80] These studies confirm that circulating plasma cells are part of the neoplastic clone. The precursor neoplastic B cell is rare; it is difficult to identify in the marrow or peripheral blood except by molecular techniques, including polymerase chain reaction (PCR) detection.[78] Southern blot analysis has also shown an increased peripheral blood involvement in MM compared with MGUS.[81] The circulating neoplastic plasma cells from the blood of myeloma patients are not static but contain a proliferative compartment. The median PCLI was 0.2 percent for the 29 patients with MGUS and SMM, 0.8 percent for the 35 patients with new, untreated multiple myeloma (MM), and 1.7 percent for the 41 patients with relapsed MM.[27] Monoclonal cytoplasmic immunoglobulin (cIg)-positive plasma cells obtained from T cell-depleted non-adherent monoclonal cells grew in the presence of IL-3 and IL-6 in 15 of 27 patients with MM compared with none of 3 MGUS patients.[82] Proliferation of peripheral blood clonal plasma cells confirms that they include a growth compartment. That a greater number of such clonal cells are present in MM than in MGUS is not surprising.

In contrast to the high numbers of circulating myeloma plasma cells seen in MM as compared with MGUS, CD5 B lymphocytes are decreased in patients with active MM as compared with MGUS and stable MM.[83] However, the issue of circulating B cells belonging to the neoplastic clone remains controversial. Whereas some have shown reduced numbers of CD19+ B cells in MM,[84] others have reported that late-stage B cells expressing CD19, CD20, PCA-1, and CD45RO are markedly increased in MM and MGUS.[85,86] Investigations have found that some of these cells bear IgH rearrangements the same as the malignant clone.[87] Many other investigators are unable to find an increase in such CD19-positive cells in peripheral blood. Some investigators have shown that CD19-positive B cells infused into NOD-SCID mice produce clonal myeloma-like involvement of the marrow.[88] However, others suggest that normal B cells can also produce such involvement. Such conflicting information is hard to resolve. Whether or not abnormal B cells bearing markers of late-stage B-cell development exist in numbers that are quantifiable and that actually contribute to the growth of the malignant clone needs to be clarified.

Comparing 18 patients with MGUS and 52 patients with MM, Omede et al. found no significant phenotypic differences in the numbers of circulating lymphocytes expressing plasma cell antigens (CD38 and PCA-1).[89] Peripheral blood monoclonal B-cell excess, defined by surface immunoglobulin clonal κ or λ light-chain excess, has been found in MM but not in MGUS.[90] These cells were less often seen in early stage 1 myeloma (one of seven patients) but were common in stage 2 (eight of eight) and stage 3 MM (four of six). Increases in "clonal" B cells in MM were associated with a high labeling index of marrow plasma cells. However, circulating plasma cells may also express surface immunoglobulin. These observations do not prove a role for clonal circulating B cells in the development of MM. Furthermore clonality, as assessed by surface phenotypic changes or light-chain ratios, could be the result of unbalanced T-cell regulation of normal B cells causing changes in the light-chain ratios. Recently, more compelling evidence for the presence of clonal B cells in the peripheral blood has been found by using PCR allele-specific oligonucleotide techniques.[91] Correlation with results of immunofluorescence microscopy suggests that PCR-detectable cells are often mature clonal plasma cells. A small proportion may represent immature clonally related B cells inasmuch as they are smaller by light scatter characteristics and possess $C\mu$ immunoglobulin rearrangements.[92]

Interpretation of the data suggests that a preswitch clonal B cell myeloma cell precursor may be found in myeloma. However, a small number of postswitch B cells mimic preswitch cells by undergoing rearrangements of their immunoglobulin genes.[93] In a study of myeloma isotype-switch variants in the murine 5T myeloma model, it was shown that myeloma IgM and IgA expressing subclones can originate from the IgG-expressing tumor. Because detection of immunoglobulin gene rearrangements is often below the limits of morphologic discrimination of plasma cells from B cells, it is not possible to exclude the possibility that a small number of circulating clonal plasma cells are responsible for molecular detection of clonally rearranged cells. It is also possible that many studies purporting to identify monoclonal B cells in the blood have actually identified circulating plasma cells. Until more definitive evidence that a preswitch B cell is contributing to myeloma growth, it is still reasonable to conclude that the myeloma cell is derived from transforming events in postswitch B cells. Although myeloma plasma cells clearly circulate and proliferate in the blood of myeloma patients and measurement of these cells may be used to differentiate MM from MGUS and early asymptomatic MM, it is premature to conclude that this is true for clonal B cells.

Cytokines and Growth Factors

The search for a growth factor for myeloma cells culminated in the identification of IL-6, formerly known as B-cell growth factor or hybridoma growth factor.[94] Interleukin-6 is likely the central growth factor, essential for myeloma cell proliferation.[95] The source of IL-6 is predominantly macrophages, fibroblasts, osteoblasts, osteoclasts, and monocytes in the bone marrow or blood (paracrine mechanism)[96] (Figure 30–7) and myeloma cells themselves (autocrine mechanism).[97,98] Support for the autocrine mechanism comes from observations that in freshly obtained myeloma cell cultures, anti-IL-6 antibody and anti-IL-6R antibody inhibits growth in the presence or absence of exogenous IL-6.[99] Although pathways independent of IL-6 exist, most myeloma cell lines both secrete and are dependent on IL-6 for their growth. The IL-6 gene was expressed in only 2 of 10 human myeloma cell lines in one study.[100] Using PCR, others have found IL-6 gene expression in 45 percent of

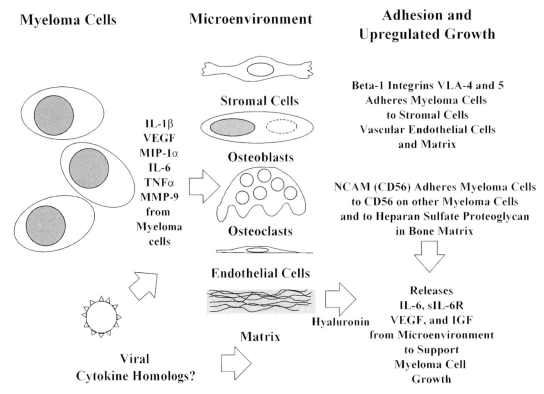

Figure 30–7. Paracrine growth is the dominant growth pattern in multiple myeloma. Myeloma cells secrete factors that release myeloma adhesion and growth factors from the microenvironment. Herpesvirus homologues of growth factors have been found in dendritic cells of patients with monoclonal gammopathy of undetermined significance and multiple myeloma. Their role in myeloma growth is uncertain.

myeloma patients.[101] Although the relative contributions of the autocrine and paracrine IL-6 mechanisms remain controversial, it is likely that in most myeloma patients paracrine mechanisms predominate.

That antibody to IL-6 effectively blocks myeloma cell proliferation in IL-6-dependent cell lines indicates that IL-6 can be a necessary growth factor in myeloma. Patients respond when treated with antibody to IL-6.[102] They have decreases in bone pain, percent marrow plasma cells, PCLI, and M-protein in the serum and urine. Unfortunately, they develop neutralizing antibodies to the mouse immunoglobulin and after only a few weeks the MM progresses.

Interleukin-6 and its cell surface receptor are necessary for myeloma cell growth. They represent a distinct target for treatments aimed at blocking myeloma cell proliferation. One approach is use of antibody to the cell-bound IL-6 receptor; another is the construction of mutant IL-6 receptors that lack the gp130-binding region. These mutant receptors compete for circulating IL-6 but do not bind to myeloma PCs and can be inhibitory for myeloma cell growth.[103] Because the patterns of growth inhibition by various receptor mutants and antibodies differ, combinations may be more effective than a single mutant or receptor antibody.[104] A "humanized " IL-6R monoclonal antibody has been constructed that shows strong antiproliferative and apoptotic activity against myeloma cells.[105]

Uncertainty exists about the significance of serum IL-6 levels because it is not yet clear whether serum or plasma levels

best measure IL-6 and whether special precautions must be taken to ensure accurate testing. Furthermore, serum IL-6 levels may not reflect levels in the marrow close to the sites of plasma cell proliferation. Nevertheless, serum IL-6 levels are more commonly elevated in MM than in MGUS. In one study IL-6 levels were elevated in 42 percent of 47 MM patients and 13 percent of 24 MGUS patients.[106] They were higher in patients with active and advanced-stage disease than in patients with stage 1 MM, MGUS, or plateau-phase MM. Almost identical results were found in another study of 64 patients with MM, 7 with SMM, and 57 with MGUS,[38] in which IL-6 levels were correlated with myeloma cell proliferation rate by using a CD38/Ki-67 assay. On radioimmunoassay, IL-6 levels have been correlated with neopterin, tumor necrosis factor alpha, β_2-M, and hemoglobin levels,[51] and IL-6 levels in MM have also been significantly correlated with bone marrow plasmacytosis, lactate dehydrogenase (LDH), β_2-M, serum calcium, hemoglobin, and features of aggressive disease.[106]

Unexpectedly high serum IL-6 levels were found in 12 patients with MGUS, and 22 with Sjögren's syndrome compared with control subjects, 9 patients with chronic lymphocytic leukemia, and 16 patients with MM.[21] These high results in MGUS compared with MM are not easily explained. The contradictory high results call for circumspection in interpreting these and similar serum cytokine assays to distinguish MM from MGUS.

Myeloma marrow stroma is characterized by increased secretion of IL-6, but MGUS patients and normal subjects have only low-level production.[75,107] Among marrow stromal cells, the osteoblast is an important producer of IL-6. Although osteoclasts derived from monocytes are the important mediators of the lytic bone lesions in myeloma, coincident osteoblastic recruitment is also found, particularly in early MM even before the development of bone lesions. Osteoblast recruitment is not found in MGUS.[108] Stimulated osteoblasts produce large amounts of IL-6, a potent myeloma cell growth factor. Among marrow stromal cells, osteoblasts could play a pivotal role during the transition from MGUS to MM. Interleukin-6 stimulates only the proliferation of already proliferating myeloma cells.[109] There are other cytokines and growth factors produced by stromal cells that maintain myeloma growth.[110] One of these factors is insulin-like growth factor (IGF),[111–117] which can directly stimulate myeloma cell growth and can enhance myeloma cell response to IL-6 without induction of additional IL-6.

Higher proportions of IL-2-secreting cells are seen in MM than in MGUS and stable MM.[118] Serum levels of IL-2 are increased in MM patients compared with control subjects, levels being highest in patients with stable MM.[119] It is attractive to suggest that IL-2 has a role in stabilizing myeloma plasma cell proliferation.

Tumor necrosis factor-alpha (TNF-α) is increased in myeloma. This factor and TNF-related apoptosis-inducing ligand (TRAIL), a member of the TNF family of cytokines, induce myeloma cell apoptosis despite bcl-2 antiapoptotic signals.[120] Elevated TNF-α may have an adverse effect on survival.[121] Serum levels of IL-6, TNF-α, and soluble receptor for interleukin-2 (sIL-2R) are significantly increased in patients with active MM when compared with normal control subjects. Furthermore, MM patients with advanced aggressive disease have significantly higher levels of IL-6, TNF-α, and sIL-2R than those with MM in the plateau phase.[122] Increased TNF-α-induced NF-κB activation and increased myeloma cell-to-stromal cell adhesion via stromal cells expressing VCAM-1 and ICAM-1 have been well documented in MM.[123] The increased adhesion releases more IL-6 from stromal cells and induces myeloma cell proliferation. Interferon gamma has also been examined in MM. Patients with MM were found to produce significantly higher levels of both interferon-gamma and tumor necrosis factor-beta (TNF-β) but lower levels of TNF-α than normal individuals.[124] Interferon-gamma appears to increase the number and activation of CD3-positive T cells. The main mechanism by which CD3+ CD25+ T cells affected plasma cells was by direct cell-to-cell contact rather than via cytokines. However, these cells may show poor killing of myeloma cells in vitro. In contrast, natural killer (NK) cells show increased killing. The importance of this observation is emphasized by studies showing that thalidomide therapy, which downregulates IL-2 and interferon-gamma, increases CD3-negative CD56-positive NK cells in patients responding to therapy.[125]

Tumor necrosis factor-β is produced in abundance by myeloma plasma cells. It inhibits IL-2 responsiveness of T cells, thus contributing to the immune defects of MM,[126] and also inhibits normal bone marrow progenitors.[127]

Interleukin-1β (IL-1β) is a potent bone-resorbing cytokine, which may contribute most to the development of lytic bone disease in MM. Myeloma cells themselves secrete IL-1β.[128] The amounts of IL-1β produced by MM marrow is greater than that produced in MGUS.[129] Expression of the IL-1β gene has been identified in freshly separated myeloma cells.[130] Plasmacytoma cell lines transfected with IL-1α produce metastatic bone lesions in syngeneic mice compared with nontransfected cells, which do not.[131] Also IL-1α induces adhesion molecules such as I-CAM and CD44 on the surface of mouse plasmacytoma cells.[132] Although IL-1β is expressed in more than 95 percent of MM cases, it is expressed in less than 25 percent of MGUS cases and then very weakly.[133] The weight of evidence suggests that IL-1β is a critical early step in the transition from MGUS to MM.[46]

Production of IL-1β by myeloma cells may mark the progression from MGUS to MM.[133] Stromal cells, including marrow macrophages, megakaryocytes, fibroblasts, and osteoblasts produce small amounts of IL-1β in the marrow. In MM patients, IL-1β is a major factor responsible for bone lesions. Although IL-1β does not stimulate myeloma cell proliferation directly, it may by virtue of its effect on stromal cells in the marrow and blood induce production of IL-6.[52] Myeloma cells may thus recruit cells to produce IL-6 for their own growth. Measuring IL-1β expression by plasma cells may provide a much better way to confirm the diagnosis of myeloma in clinical practice and clinical trials. Interleukin-1 receptor antagonists inhibit IL-1-mediated IL-6 production and could be useful in treating MM.[130]

A combination of IL-3 and IL-6 can stimulate the production of proliferating myeloma cells from blood mononuclear cells.[82] A source for IL-3 has not been identified and the findings have not been repeated, so the significance of IL-3 in myeloma is uncertain. Granulocyte colony-stimulating factor (G-CSF) has been reported to exacerbate stable monoclonal gammopathy.[134] Granulocyte monocyte colony-stimulating factor (GM-CSF) has also shown proliferative effects on myeloma cells and has been reported to cause extramedullary progression of MM.[135] Myeloma cell proliferation is stimulated by IL-6, G-CSF, GM-CSF, and IL-3, all members of the cytokine superfamily, through gp130. The relative roles of IL-3, G-CSF, and GM-CSF in myeloma cell proliferation are unknown. Oncostatin M (OSM), leukemia inhibitory factor (LIF), and IL-10 also cause proliferation of an IL-6-secreting and IL-6-dependent cell line through gp 130.[136]

Erythropoietin receptors have been described on myeloma cells, and in several instances a growth factor effect of erythropoietin has been postulated.[137,138] We have seen a patient whose stable myeloma became active after treatment with erythropoietin, as manifested by a significant increase in M-protein. The M-protein level decreased after cessation of erythropoietin.

Hepatocyte growth factor is overexpressed in MM and has prognostic significance.[139] It is produced by mesenchymal cells and reacts with the cellular receptor c-met. It has not been reported in MGUS.

Surprisingly little is known about insulin-like growth factor 1 (IGF-1), known to be an important myeloma cell growth and survival factor produced by marrow stromal cells. Early work suggested that IGF-1 is a growth factor in human MM[117] and that an autocrine IGF-1 growth loop may be operative in promoting growth and survival in some MM cell lines.[116] Also, IGFs may play an important role in multiple myeloma by directly stimulating myeloma cell growth as well as modulating IL-6-driven growth.[115] When bound to its cell surface receptor on myeloma cell lines IGF-1 appears to inhibit apoptosis by increasing expression of Bad. It stimulates growth through the mitogen-activated protein (MAP) kinase pathway. The result of IGF-1 stimulation is a doubling of the rate of tumor growth in an animal model using the SCID mouse and the OPM-2 myeloma cell line.[111] Also, IGF-1 may promote myeloma growth by stimulating chemotaxis and adhesion to marrow stromal cells in a mouse myeloma cell line.[112] Chemotaxis effects of IGF-1 have been demonstrated in another mouse model of myeloma. In a study using purified human myeloma cells, the proliferative and antiapoptotic effects of IL-6 and IL-15 appeared to be stronger than those of IGF-1,[113] which is inhibited by insulin-like growth factor binding protein-4 (IGFBP4). This protein is made by myeloma tumor cells adjacent to bone, and it may inhibit IGF-1-stimulated osteoblast growth and contribute to the decreased bone formation seen in MM.[140] More needs to be learned about the effects of IGF-1 and IL-15 in myeloma.

Because many cytokines and growth factors work in concert, it is likely that the measurement of individual factors or even combinations of factors will not be useful diagnostically or prognostically. However, demonstration of a diagnostic or prognostic consequence of a single new growth factor such as VEGF could have great biological significance and implications for treatment.

Soluble Receptors and Other Soluble Factors

A soluble receptor for interleukin-6 (sIL-6R) has been identified in serum of patients with MM.[141] In vitro, sIL-6R potentiates the myeloma cell growth effect of IL-6. The soluble receptor binds IL-6, and the complex binds to the membrane-bound gp130 molecule on the surface of the myeloma cells. The IL-6 cell signaling pathways are activated, and myeloma cell proliferation results. Myeloma cells secrete a novel sIL-6R.[103] Although this sIL-6R itself does not stimulate myeloma cell growth, it can enhance myeloma cell responsiveness to IL-6 in vitro 10-fold by bringing IL-6 into proximity with the myeloma cell membrane.

Soluble serum IL-6 receptor levels are increased with similar frequency in MGUS and in MM cases, 51 and 44 percent, respectively, but in overt MM increases of 116 percent have been observed.[141] Increases in sIL-6R were independent of PCLI and β_2-M. Remarkably, elevated serum sIL-6R levels are unchanged, even after elimination of myeloma cells by the conditioning treatment used for stem cell transplant. It is apparent that regulatory cells, probably stromal cells rather than myeloma cells, are responsible for this stable production of sIL-6R in MM. The production of sIL-6R is likely an important factor in the development and progression of MM.

Novel studies have shown that sIL-6R may trigger osteoclast formation by enhancing the osteoclast-activating activities of IL-6.[142] Osteoclast formation was also induced by IL-11, OSM, and LIF through gp130, the signal-transducing chain of the cell-bound IL-6R. New evidence indicates that sIL-6R stimulates osteoblast recruitment from stromal cell preparations.[143]

Soluble syndecan has been found at elevated levels in the serum in 79 percent of myeloma patients.[144] Serum syndecan-1

correlated with serum creatinine, 24-hour secretion of urine M-component, soluble IL-6 receptor, C-terminal telopeptide of type I collagen, β_2-M, percentage of plasma cells in the bone marrow, disease stage, and serum M-component concentration. In another study, the presence of increased syndecan-1 in MM was associated with decreased serum matrix metalloproteinase-9 (MMP-9).[145] Both elevated syndecan-1 and decreased MMP-9 were associated with higher marrow plasmacytosis and serum beta-2 microglobulin and paraprotein levels. Soluble NCAM or sCD56 has been shown to be a statistically significant discriminant of MM versus MGUS.[146] Soluble CD16 or soluble heavy-chain FC fragment (sCD16) is decreased in active MM and has been reported to be a discriminant between MM and MGUS evolving to MM versus stable MGUS.[147]

Bone and Stroma Interactions

Myeloma produces characteristic pure lytic bone lesions. There is an uncoupling of the usually tightly regulated balance between osteoclastic and osteoblastic activity. Regardless of the initiating signal, whether IL-1β, IL-6 and sIL-6R, TNFα, MIP-1α, RANK ligand, or PTHrP,[48] the endpoint is myeloma bone destruction. Since the bone microenvironment plays an important role in myeloma propagation, it is reasonable to postulate that markers of bone destruction might be important in staging and prognosis.

Interleukin-1β produced in MM marrow but not in MGUS marrow causes IL-6 release from stromal cells, thereby providing the key growth factor for myeloma cells. Also, IL-1β increases osteoclast precursors and activates osteoclasts, which results in an increased number of osteoclasts in MM but not MGUS.[46]

Vascular endothelial growth factor has important interactions with bone marrow stromal cells. Exposure of stromal and microvascular endothelial cells to recombinant human VEGF induces a time- and dose-dependent increase in IL-6 secretion.[148] Conversely, IL-6 stimulates VEGF expression and secretion in myeloma cell lines and in plasma cells purified from marrow of patients with MM. This mutual stimulation suggests paracrine interactions between myeloma and marrow stromal cells triggered by VEGF and IL-6. Myeloma cells have VEGF receptors on their surface, so VEGF also acts as a growth factor for myeloma cells.[57] Also, VEGF is a potent angiogenic factor. Levels in the marrow supernatant are higher than in the serum.[59]

Macrophage inflammatory protein-1α (MIP-1α) is a recently described osteoclast-activating factor, which has elevated expression by RNAase protection assay in freshly isolated bone marrow from myeloma patients.[149] Levels are not increased in the peripheral blood, however. Recombinant MIP-1α induces osteoclast formation in human bone marrow cultures.[47] Antibody to MIP-1α blocks increased osteoclast formation induced by patient plasma. Further work is needed to determine the relative contribution of MIP-1α to bone destruction in myeloma and its potential application to prognosis.

Matrix metalloproteinases (MMPs) have been studied in MM. One of these, MMP9, a gelatinase, is overexpressed in MM[150] and is not regulated by IL-6 or by other cytokines active in MM. Interleukin-1β and TNF are associated with overexpression of MMP-1, a collagenase.[150] We do not yet know the results in MGUS but one suspects overexpression will be found less frequently in MGUS than MM.

Surface expression of CD138 or syndecan-1 is almost an obligate marker of myeloma cells and is used for enrichment of myeloma cells. Syndecan-1 is the surface receptor for bFGF. Serum levels of syndecan-1 are increased in MM. The role of basic fibroblast growth factor (bFGF) in the growth of myeloma cells is under active investigation, but bFGF is a potent angiogenic factor.[58] Osteoprotegerin (OPG), which is necessary to retain balance between osteoblastic and osteoclastic activity, is reported to be reduced in myeloma patients as compared to control subjects and MGUS patients, which supports its role in myeloma bone disease. It is interesting to note that syndecan-1 binds OPG, which suggests a possible role in myeloma bone disease.[49]

Bone matrix contains hyaluronan (HA), which recently was shown to affect IL-6-induced myeloma cell proliferation.[151] Hyaluronan, a major nonprotein glycosaminoglycan component of the extracellular matrix in the marrow, is a survival and proliferation factor for human myeloma cells. The effect of HA is mainly mediated through a gp80–IL-6 receptor pathway. Hyaluronan probably retains and concentrates IL-6 close to its site of secretion, thus favoring its autocrine activity. In addition, HA-mediated survival and proliferation of myeloma cells is associated with downregulation in the expression of p27(kip1) cyclin-dependent kinase inhibitor and hyperphosphorylation of the retinoblastoma protein (pRb). These data suggest that HA could be an important component in the in vivo physiopathology of the myeloma cell by potentiating autocrine and/or paracrine IL-6 activities. Complex pathways that lead to the same endpoint, destruction of bone and bone matrix, can thus greatly enhance myeloma cell growth and survival.

Cytogenetic Alterations

Although no cytogenetic abnormality as yet identifies which patients with MGUS will go on to develop active MM, it seems likely that FISH-detectable cytogenetic abnormalities will be found that increase the risk of progression of MGUS to active MM. Conventional cytogenetics (CC) is nearly always normal in MGUS because the plasma cells of patients with MGUS are slowly proliferating. They have a very low PCLI and therefore do not yield metaphases in CC, so that CC has no predictive value in true MGUS. It does very insensitively detect chromosomal abnormalities in MM, again because the neoplastic clonal plasma cells are usually very slowly proliferative. Therefore the significance of CC-detected chromosome del 13 abnormalities for prognosis[152] is not clearly different than other CC abnormalities. In a study of 427 patients with newly diagnosed or treated MM who received tandem transplants, abnormal karyotypes were detected in 37 percent, most of whom had been treated for some time before their first autotransplant. In addition to previously recognized unfavorable implications of CC-detected del 13 and 11q abnormalities, the investigators observed that the presence of any translocation likewise portended poor outcome.[153]

Nearly all myeloma patients have abnormal chromosomes by FISH, including deletions, aneuploidy, and translocations. Iden-

tification of the chromosome abnormalities by CC may reflect underlying increased proliferation. In fact, we have shown that CC abnormalities correlate with the PCLI.[154] Fluorescence in situ hybridization probes can be used to identify abnormal chromosome number or aneuploidy in nonproliferating or proliferating interphase plasma cells in MGUS and MM; they can also identify deletions of portions of chromosomes and translocations in MGUS plasma cells. By using FISH it was shown that there are similar degrees of chromosomal aneuploidy in MGUS and MM and that the chromosomes affected are the same. Del 13 is found in MGUS as well as in MM,[155–157] although less frequently.[158] The prognostic significance of del 13 is seen by FISH but less impressively than with CC. Immunoglobulin heavy-chain (IgH) translocations involving chromosome 14 were observed by using FISH, with a similar incidence (60 percent) in MGUS and MM or plasma cell leukemia (PCL); del 13 was present in 40 percent of MM and PCL patients but in only 4 of 19 MGUS individuals. Interestingly, in 20 patients with MM and a previous MGUS history, the incidence of del 13 was 70 percent, versus 31 percent in MM patients without a known history of MGUS. Serial FISH analyses of individuals with MGUS will be needed to determine whether del 13 represents a risk factor for the development of MM.

Translocations into the IgH switch region on chromosome 14 are seen in most patients with active MM.[158] Partners in these translocations cause heavy-chain illegitimate switch region recombinations with chromosome 11, 4, 6, and 16.[159] The most common in MM is the t(11;14) translocation.[34] By increasing *cyclin D1* expression, the t(11;14) translocation regulates the passage of plasma cells into the S-phase of the cell cycle. It is surprising therefore that the t(11;14) translocation is also common in MGUS. *Cyclin D1* expression strongly correlated with the t(11;14) translocation in MM, although MM may be seen without this translocation as well.[35] The other chromosome 14 translocations activate other oncogenes. In cell lines an Ig translocation involving 16q23 is associated with overexpression of *c-maf*; translocations involving 4p16 are associated with overexpression of *FGFR3* and *MMSET;* and translocations involving 6p25 are associated with overexpression of *MUM1* and *cyclin D3*.[160] Mutations of *FGFR3* are graded in terms of their activation capability, which thus suggests that they may play a critical role in the tumor progression of MM patients with t(4;14).[161] In some cases translocations involving 8q24 *(c-myc)* and 21q22 may occur. It remains to be seen whether other translocations such as t(4;14), t(6;14), or t(16;14) are more common in active MM or predict the progression of MGUS to active MM. Small interstitial translocations involving *c-myc* are difficult to detect but have only been seen in MM to date.[162] It would not be surprising to see that increased expression of the *c-myc* oncogene due to translocation plays a role in the progression of MGUS to MM.

Oncogenes

Most single-point mutations of critical oncogenes are activating mutations, that is, they trigger specific pathways of cell signaling that induce growth, production of a growth factor, loss of apoptosis, or expression of a transcription factor. In MM the most frequent mutations involve the *ras* oncogene; K- and N-*ras* mutations have been described in 39 percent of newly diagnosed MM patients.[31] In one study *ras* mutations were found in 3 of 12 MM patients but in none of 3 MGUS patients.[163] In another study, no mutations of N- and K- *ras* were found among 30 patients with MGUS.[164] Mutations in *p53* occurred in 6 of 30 patients with active MM[165]; 4 of the 6 had terminal aggressive-phase MM. No *ras* or *p53* mutations have been described in MGUS to date. It is possible that many *ras* mutations are missed. Use of a PCR restriction fragment length polymorphism (RFLP) technique showed that all of 34 newly diagnosed MM patients had *ras* mutations, which implies that *ras* mutation is a mandatory event in the development of MM.[166] In this study enriched populations of MM cells were used to increase the sensitivity of detection of *ras* mutations. Part of the problem in detecting *ras* mutations in MGUS may lie in the difficulty of detecting mutations in the very small numbers of clonal plasma cells present in the marrow of MGUS patients.

The *p53* tumor suppressor gene is rarely mutated. It is likely that oncogene single-point mutations of *p53* will not be found in many patients with MGUS because they are usually found in patients with aggressive MM who have a very poor prognosis. Deletions of *p53* have been observed to occur in about 10 percent of MM patients but not in MGUS.[33,167] Homozygous deletions or nullisomy has not been observed. The *p53* deletion in MM has been associated with expression of a drug-resistant phenotype caused by expression of lung resistance protein (LRP).[168] Molecular genetic abnormalities of MM are covered in more depth in Chapter 29.

The c-myc protein and c-myc RNA are overexpressed in some MM patients.[169] Overexpression of *c-myc* has not yet been correlated with myeloma cell proliferation. Mechanisms of *c-myc* overexpression are not clear, although cytogenetic translocations may play a role.[162]

The *bcl-2* proto-oncogene is a member of a family of antiapoptotic genes whose regulation controls programmed cell death. Levels of *bcl-2* expression in MM and MGUS are higher than with reactive plasmacytosis.[170] Proliferating plasma cells tend to have lower *bcl-2* expression. On the other hand, *bcl-XL* seems to be the predominant antiapoptotic proto-oncogene in myeloma cell lines.[171] *BAX* expression is increased in MM relative to SMM and MGUS.[76] *BAX* expression was not related to proliferation as assessed by proliferating cell nuclear antigen (PCNA). Multiple myeloma patients with lower *BAX* expression tend to have longer survival. The relative roles of *bcl-2*, *BAX* and *bcl-XL* need to be further assessed, as does their role in clonal plasma cell apoptosis in MGUS and MM.

Cell Signaling

Most of what we know about cell signaling has been learned by the study of cytokine and CD40 ligand stimulation of myeloma cell signaling pathways. We know that IL-6 and sIL-6R without IL-6 signal through gp130 on the myeloma cell surface.[172] We also know that the MAP-K and JAK/STAT pathways are activated by this interaction.[173–175] STAT3, a key molecule involved in IL-6 signaling, is constitutively activated and phosphorylated

in IL-6-independent cell lines as compared with the IL-6-dependent cells. Of upstream signaling pathways, JAK-1 was also constitutively present.[176] Comparisons of signaling pathway activation between MGUS and MM are needed.

ANBL-6, a myeloma cell line that is IL-6-dependent, can be induced to produce autocrine IL-6 using anti-CD40 as an artificial ligand.[177] CD40 expression has been observed on the surface of malignant plasma cell lines and plasma cells from almost all myeloma patients but not normal plasma cells.[178] CD40 ligand stimulation of autocrine IL-6 may be one mechanism whereby myeloma tumor cells are induced to proliferate. Further studies should increase our understanding of the role of CD40 in myeloma.

By using MM cell lines, MM patient cells, and IL-6-dependent B9 cells, it was learned that IL-6 induces phosphorylation of JAK kinases and gp130, regardless of the proliferative response of MM cells to this growth factor. Studies of downstream IL-6 signaling via the STAT3, STAT1, and Ras-dependent mitogen-activated protein kinase (MAPK) cascades showed that IL-6 triggered phosphorylation of STAT1 and/or STAT3 in MM cells independently of their proliferative response to IL-6. In contrast, IL-6 induced phosphorylation of Shc and its association with Sos1, as well as phosphorylation of MAPK, only in MM cells and B9 cells that proliferated in response to IL-6. Moreover, MAPK antisense, but not sense, oligonucleotide inhibited IL-6-induced proliferation of these cells. These data suggest that STAT1 and/or STAT3 activation may occur independently of the proliferative response to IL-6 and that activation of the MAPK cascade is an important distal pathway for IL-6-mediated growth.[175]

Vascular endothelial growth factor is a key factor in myeloma angiogenesis but also possibly in myeloma cell proliferation by an autocrine or paracrine pathway. Myeloma cells express VEGF receptors and VEGF whether measured by immunohistochemistry or mRNA.[148] Thus, an autocrine pathway may be operative. In addition, VEGF is produced by stromal cells in a paracrine pathway. Signaling is via a protein kinase C (PKC)-independent Raf-1-MEK-extracellular signal-regulated protein kinase pathway. Myeloma cell migration is regulated by VEGF via a PKC-dependent pathway.[57] We know that VEGF levels are increased in the serum in MGUS, but expression by MGUS plasma cells has not been reported. Signaling in MGUS has not been reported.

Bone morphogenetic protein-2 (BMP-2) upregulates cyclin-dependent kinase inhibitors p21 and p27 and causes hypophosphorylation of retinoblastoma (Rb) protein. It also induces apoptosis in various human myeloma cells by means of the downregulation of *bcl-XL* and by cell-cycle arrest through the upregulation of *p21(CIP1/WAF1)* and *p27(KIP1)*, and by the hypophosphorylation of *Rb*. The signal transducer and activator of transcription (STAT3) was inactivated immediately after BMP-2 treatment. BMP-2 could be useful as a novel therapeutic agent in the treatment of multiple myeloma by its antitumor effect and also its favorable effects against bone resorption.[179]

In seven myeloma cell lines, the IGF-I receptor (IGF-IR) was found to be expressed and autophosphorylated in response to ligand. Downstream of IGF-IR, insulin receptor substrate 1 was phosphorylated, leading to the activation of phosphatidylinositol-3'-kinase (PI-3K), which in turn regulated two distinct pathways. The first included Akt and Bad, leading to an inhibition of apoptosis; the second included MAPK, resulting in proliferation. Biologic relevance of this pathway was demonstrated by the finding that in vitro IGF-I induced both an antiapoptotic and a proliferative effect. Importantly, in vivo administration of IGF-I to SCID mice inoculated with the OPM-2 line led to approximately twice the growth rate of tumor cells as in control animals. These results suggest that IGF-I activates at least two pathways affecting myeloma cell growth and contributes significantly to expansion of these cells in vivo.[111]

Signal transduction of IL-6-induced gp130 signaling involves the Janus tyrosine kinases (JAK) JAK1, JAK2, and Tyk2 and then the downstream effectors comprising the STAT3 and MAPK pathways. The JAK2 inhibitor tyrophostin AG490 suppresses cell proliferation and induces apoptosis in IL-6-dependent MM cell lines. JAK2 kinase activity, ERK2, and STAT3 phosphorylation were inhibited. These results suggest that the chemical blocking of the gp130 signaling pathway at the JAK level could be a relevant therapeutic.[180]

Analysis of the role of the MAPK and antiviral signaling pathways using two cell lines suggests that the antiviral and growth regulatory effects of IFN-alpha display a differential requirement for activation of the MAPK pathway.[181] The heterogeneity in IFN-alpha-mediated growth effects in myeloma cells correlates with differential induction of cyclin D2 and p19(INK4d) expression.[182] Interleukin-6 protects MM cells against anti-fas-induced apoptosis through its inhibitory effects on JNK/c-jun, but protection against dexamethasone occurs through separate, yet unknown pathways.[183]

Although signaling pathway differences have not been clearly linked to the MGUS-to-myeloma transition or to myeloma progression, it seems likely that knowledge of these events will be important not only to diagnosis but also to development of small molecules directed against specific sensitive signaling pathway targets. The above background should be helpful in guiding future research. A more comprehensive examination of the role of growth factors and growth factor signaling pathways in myeloma is available in the review by Anderson.[184]

Adhesion and Other Cellular Markers

A simplified model of myeloma cell adhesion to bone matrix, vessels, stromal cells, and other myeloma cells is shown in Figure 30–8. By interacting with their microenvironment, myeloma cells are able to recruit their own growth factors by a paracrine pathway (Figure 30–9). A cell-adhesion molecule belonging to the immunoglobulin superfamily CD56 (NCAM) was strongly expressed in most plasma cells in 43 of 55 myeloma patients,[185] and CD56 expression in high density was present in 43 of 57 untreated MM but in none of 23 MGUS patients.[186] In MGUS strong plasma cell CD56 reactivity is found in a subset of plasma cells.[187] A lower percentage of CD56+ plasma cells in MGUS has been explained in one study by the presence of residual normal plasma cells that are CD56 negative.[188] In contrast, the bone marrow of 45 patients with MM and 8 patients with MGUS revealed no differences in the

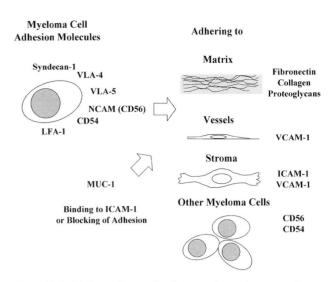

Figure 30–8. Myeloma plasma cells adhere to microenvironment cells. They do this by upregulating surface adhesion molecules, which then bind to matrix components and adhesion partners on bone matrix, stromal cells, blood vessels, and other myeloma cells. This puts myeloma cells in close proximity to elements of the microenvironment that can provide growth and survival factors for myeloma cells.

expression of CD56 in MGUS and MM.[66] CD56 staining failed to differentiate MM from MGUS in yet another study.[66] Our studies were also negative; we found a similar percentage of strongly CD56-positive plasma cells in MM and MGUS cases.[41] It is unlikely that staining of plasma cell CD56 can accurately distinguish between MGUS and MM except in cases in which there are a large number of residual normal plasma cells identified by CD56 negativity. Overexpression of CD56 in marrow versus circulating plasma cells suggests a role for NCAM (CD56) in homing and cell adhesion to the marrow. Adhesion may be a dynamic process that occurs as myeloma plasma cells approach stromal cells in the marrow microenvironment.

Among other plasma cell adhesion molecules, LFA-3 has been studied most. In one study, all MGUS cases were negative for LFA-3, but 12 of 18 myeloma cases and 2 of 10 normal cases were positive for LFA-3.[189] The adhesion markers LFA-1 (CD11a), CD54 (ICAM-1), and CD44 (HCAM) did not distinguish between MM and MGUS. In another study, LFA-1 (CD11a) was increased in active MM but not in MGUS, normal individuals, or MM patients in an inactive phase of their disease.[67] There was a correlation between LFA-1 expression and PCLI. As with CD56, nonconcordant results with other adhesion markers mean that more detailed study is warranted before one can confirm which adhesion marker plays the dominant role in the development of myeloma. Another adhesion molecule affecting myeloma cells, very late antigen-4 (VLA-4), may act to bind myeloma cells to fibronectin in bone marrow.[190] Under certain conditions, upregulation of VLA-4 and a number of other adhesion molecules results in a fivefold increase in IL-6 production by stroma.[123] Blocking VLA-4 and VLA-5 adherence mechanisms inhibits growth. Allowing VLA-4- and VLA-

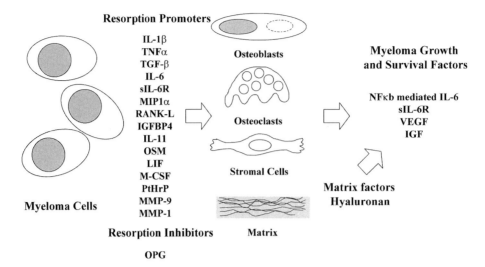

Figure 30–9. After adhering in the microenvironment, myeloma cells induce the production of critical growth and survival factors, including IL-6, sIL-6R, VEGF, and IGF. Release of hyaluronan from the bone matrix can amplify this response.

5-mediated binding also causes drug resistance, which is termed cellular adhesion molecule drug resistance (CAM-DR). Cell–cell contact between marrow stromal cells and myeloma cells via VCAM-1 and alpha(4)beta(1)-integrin enhances production of osteoclast-stimulating activity.[191] VCAM-1 is a very important stromal cell adhesion molecule.[192]

Changes in other cellular markers provide both clues to the factors underlying evolution from MGUS to MM and a challenge to those trying to interpret them. Plasma cell MB-2 antigen expression was higher in marrow biopsies of MM than in those of MGUS.[193] Of 59 biopsy samples from patients with MM, 54 contained high-intensity staining MB-2 plasma cells compared with 3 of 41 biopsy samples from patients with MGUS. Strong MDR-1 expression was found in the plasma cells of 32 of 38 untreated MGUS patients as compared with 33 of 105 patients with untreated stage 1 to stage 3 MM (84 percent versus 32 percent) and in none of 10 normal plasma cell samples.[186] In one study, the MDR-positive cells in MM were limited to the B cells in the blood. These cells were reported to demonstrate extensive and variable DNA hyperdiploidy by DNA stain.[194] If these cells are myeloma precursor cells, they could provide a reservoir of proliferative cells that are resistant to chemotherapy. Other studies in MGUS and MM have been negative or marginally different. Plasma cells from the bone marrow of 45 patients with MM and 8 patients with MGUS showed no differences in the expression of CD38. Coexpression of B-cell antigens CD19 and CD20 and of the myeloid antigen CD33 was uncommon and observed only in MM.[43] Coexpression of the pre-B-cell antigen CD10 and of the monocyte antigen CD14 occurred rarely in MM plasma cells but not at all in MGUS.[66]

One cannot assume that the status of CD45, VLA-5, and other markers are indicators of myeloma cell differentiation. There is conflicting evidence on whether the CD45-positive population contains the proliferative fraction.[195,196] Several studies show the VLA-5-negative population to be the proliferating fraction in MM.[195,197]

Investigators must use caution in interpreting the phenotypic study of plasma cells in patients with MGUS because the residual normal plasma cells are phenotypically different from MGUS and MM cells and can dilute the results, especially in MGUS, where the clonal cells are fewer. At this time we cannot recommend phenotyping to reliably distinguish MM from MGUS. Multiparameter, multistep flow cytometry may help to identify the fraction of plasma cells in MGUS that are abnormal by virtue of the presence of surface CD38 and/or CD138 and CD56 and the absence of CD19.

Angiogenesis

Myeloma cells promote angiogenesis by a number of direct and indirect pathways leading to endothelial cell proliferation (Figure 30–10). An increase in marrow angiogenesis accompanies the progression from MGUS to MM.[198] New blood vessels are often found within aggregates of myeloma cells in the marrow. Known cytokine mechanisms for angiogenesis include vascular endothelial growth factor (VEGF), which is secreted heavily by myeloma plasma cells but less so by MGUS plasma cells because of reduced numbers[199]; VEGF may also contribute to MM cell proliferation because MM cells also express the two high-affinity receptors for VEGF.[200] Another potent vascular growth factor heavily expressed in MM as compared with MGUS is bFGF. Both VEGF and bFGF can be measured in the serum, and levels correlate with diagnosis of MM versus MGUS and are higher in more advanced stages of MM.[58] Increased angiogenesis in MM is closely correlated with cell proliferation and a high PCLI (Figure 30–11). Whether the increased angiogenesis and higher PCLI are causally related or are both coincidental effects of a common factor such as VEGF is not known.

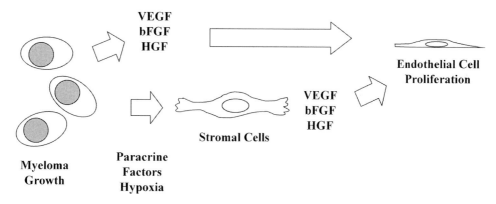

Figure 30–10. Bone marrow angiogenesis is increased in myeloma in association with increased plasma cell growth. The primary angiogenic cytokines are VEGF, bFGF, and HGF. Myeloma cells use both direct and paracrine pathway stimulation of endothelial cell proliferation.

Aquaporin 1 is associated with the blood vessels of myeloma-infiltrated marrow. Higher expression correlates disease progression and angiogenesis grade.[201] There is greater expression of aquaporin 1 in MM than in MGUS. Aquaporin 1 may be a better marker of microvessel density than CD34 or von Willebrand factor staining.[201]

Immune Alterations

Host immunity in myeloma is reduced by a number of factors, including cellular and humoral impairment, in addition to the well-known hypogammaglobulinemia. Myeloma cells produce immunosuppressive agents such as TGF-β, FasL, VEGF, and

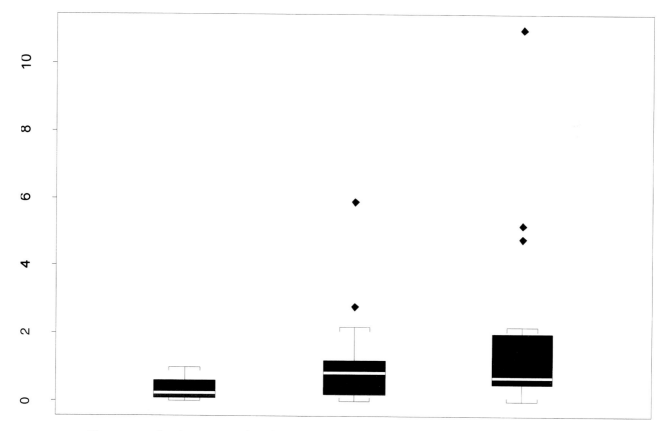

Figure 30–11. There is a strong correlation between the degree of angiogenesis and the plasma cell labeling index (PCLI). Low-, intermediate-, and high-grade angiogenesis are associated with a progressively higher PCLI. The increased PCLI may be due to increased oxygen delivery afforded by the neoangiogenesis. Alternatively, the increased plasma cell and endothelial cell proliferation may be due to a common factor, such as VEGF production by the clonal plasma cells and stromal cells. (Adapted from Rajkumar et al.[56] with permission.)

Muc-1; they also express granzyme B and perforin, normally expressed exclusively by cytotoxic T cells (CTLs) and natural killer (NK) cells.[202] This may be a way for tumor cells to actively kill immune effector cells.

Subsets of T cells are similar in MGUS patients and normal control subjects.[203] Immune defects have been found to be more common in MM than in MGUS, which suggests that immune deregulation may be part of the transition to MM.[204] In the same study, MM patients were characterized by marked shifts toward CD8(+), CD57(+), CD62L(−), CD(16 + 56)(+), and HLA-DR+ T cells, suggesting in vivo immune activation. Half of the MGUS patients had similar profiles to the MM patients, which implies marked heterogeneity among the MGUS and MM groups. One MGUS patient with a T-cell activation profile progressed 13 months later to a stage IA MM and required chemotherapy. Another study documents the increase in activated T cells in MM as compared to MGUS.[205]

In MM, most infections occur within the first 2 or 3 months of treatment,[206] often in older patients with advanced or primarily resistant disease. A combination of neutropenia and a loss of both B-cell and T-cell populations make infection the most common cause of death late in the disease course, usually occurring during more intensive chemotherapy for resistant disease.

Changes in circulating B-cell numbers and their phenotypes reviewed in the preceding paragraphs may reflect underlying regulatory T-cell changes. Proliferation of lymphocytes in response to low concentrations of Fab 2 immunoglobulin fragments of autologous M-components were found in one patient with MGUS and two patients with MM, stage 1, providing evidence for idiotypic reactive T cells in MGUS and MM.[207] Shared immunoglobulin idiotypes have been observed in both MGUS and MM.[208] Normal B-cell κ/Λ ratio is seen in patients with MGUS but is lost as myeloma develops.[90] Normal immunoglobulin production and primary immune responses are decreased in MM. These data support the suggestion that T cells may act as regulatory cells in MGUS, but this regulatory function may be lost on progression to myeloma. The percentage of CD4 cells was reduced and that of CD8 cells expanded during progression of myeloma.[89] Supporting evidence for T-cell abnormalities in MM comes from observations in both MGUS and MM that T cells show selective V-gene segment usage of both CD4+ and CD8+ T cells.[209] Recently a cooperative group study of T-cell immunity in MM has shown that newly diagnosed MM is accompanied by an altered T-cell repertoire characterized in part by expanded T-cell clones.[210] In one study, individual MM patients were found who had expanded T cells with specific TCR V region expression as compared with the control group. Several MM patients had multiple expanded CD4 and/or CD8 subsets based on TCR V region expression.[210] Simple study of the numbers of CD4+ and CD8+ proportions is inadequate to detect T-cell reactions against the malignant clone.

An increased frequency of CD16+/CD3+ peripheral blood mononuclear cells in 7 of 15 patients with MGUS indicated that T lymphocytes with NK-like phenotype are expanded in at least a subset of MGUS patients,[211] but there was no difference in functional NK activity between patients with MGUS and those with MM. In another study, the ability to induce lymphokine-activated killer (LAK) cells was significantly decreased in MM compared with MGUS patients despite an increase in CD8+/CD11b+ cells. Purified CD8+/CD11b+ lymphocytes were purified and were intrinsically unable to generate LAK activity following recombinant IL-2 simulation.[212] These same authors found that anti-CD3 monoclonal antibody could activate T cells from patients with MM, reducing the number of surviving myeloma cells in culture by direct cell-to-cell contact.[124] These activated T cells, which were CD3+ CD25+, had antiplasma plasma cell activity. Anti-idiotype activity has been observed in T cells of patients with MM.[118] This activity can be augmented by immunization techniques.[213,214]

Increase in a novel subset of NK cells was found in 5 of 23 patients with MM and plasmacytoma.[215] As evidence for NK origin, they were positive for CD16 and CD56 and CD2 but were negative for CD3. They expressed low density of CD5 and HLA-DR. Sorted cells were large granular lymphocytes. Natural killer cells have reduced function in MM, particularly in response to interferon.[216] Their activity can be increased during thalidomide treatment.[125] One study revealed no evidence that either the percentage or the absolute number of any subpopulation of the NK cells or CD56+ T cells correlated with disease activity. Their regulatory and prognostic significance is not known.

Taken together, these data suggest complex dysregulation of T-cell effector functions and NK activities in patients with MM. Despite the data suggesting a role for T-cell dysregulation in MM, it is interesting to note lack of impact of human immunodeficiency virus (HIV) on monoclonal gammopathy. Infection with HIV did not predict a higher rate of conversion from MGUS to MM.[217] Eleven HIV-infected patients developed MGUS, all of whom were followed for a mean of 50 months. All had low M-proteins initially; in nine the level was 0.5g/dl or less. Seven showed disappearance of the M-protein, and three of these developed additional M-proteins. Of the four remaining aside from these seven, none developed malignant disease.

Serum Markers

Serum markers are not useful for distinguishing early-stage MM from MGUS, and elevated values contribute little to the diagnosis of advanced stage MM, which has already been easily established. Further, the plethora of serum tests suggests that no single test is very useful. In 684 patients with newly diagnosed monoclonal gammopathy, including 343 with MGUS and 341 with MM, the most useful diagnostic discriminants were bone marrow plasma cells (more than 20 percent), erythrocyte sedimentation rate, percent reduction in normal immunoglobulin, level of serum M-component, and thymidine kinase (TK) levels.[218] Serum osteocalcin is elevated more frequently in MM than in MGUS.[219] Serum neopterin levels helped to discriminate 73 MM patients, 63 at diagnosis, 58 at remission, and 35 at relapse, as compared with 56 patients with MGUS.[220] Statistically significant differences in leukocyte alkaline phosphatase (LAP) scores were seen in 20 patients with MM compared with 18 patients with MGUS.[221] Of 20 patients with MM, 19 had elevated LAP scores. In the MGUS group, only 6 of 18 had elevated LAP scores, but in two of these, a cause other than MGUS was present. Plasma cell cytoplasmic 5′-nucleotidase levels were more often elevated in patients with MM (46.4 percent) than in those with MGUS (15.3 percent) and control subjects (1.2 percent).[222]

Levels of C-reactive protein (CRP) are often elevated in MM. It is an acute-phase reactant produced by hepatic cells in response to IL-6.[223] Because serum levels correlate closely with serum IL-6 levels, CRP has been proposed as a surrogate for IL-6 measurement in patients with myeloma. The assay is cheaper and more widely available than the IL-6 assay and very reproducible. Like other serum markers, CRP does not help to distinguish early-stage MM from MGUS.

Elevated TK levels helped to distinguish patients with stage 1 MM in a study of 149 MM and 97 MGUS patients.[224] In two patients TK levels increased at the time of progression to overt MM. Serum TK levels did not predict transition to MM in four of five patients in another series of 35 patients developing MM during a 4-year period.[225] Elevations greater than 10 mg/L in CRP were found in 27 percent of 51 myeloma patients and in none of 17 MGUS patients.[226] Differences in haptoglobin, ceruloplasmin, transferrin, and α_2-macroglobulin did not predict the development of MM. Serum albumin and hemoglobin values were considered the best differential clinical diagnostic factors in patients with normal renal function in one series.[227] More sensitive and specific serum markers are needed for discrimination of MGUS and MM.

Other Differences

The sensitivity of detecting myeloma bone lesions can be enhanced using CT and MRI[228,229] when standard radiographs are negative. Judicious use of these techniques can increase the accuracy of diagnosis of myeloma.[230] Imaging of bone lesions in MM has been reviewed by Lecouvet et al.[24]

The immunoglobulin class and isotype do not help to distinguish MM from MGUS. Patients with IgD benign monoclonal gammopathy have been described.[231–233] In a series of 128 patients diagnosed with MGUS who were followed over a 20-year period, analysis of different presenting features possibly predicting malignant transformation to MM suggested that the IgA type of MGUS was the only variable associated with a higher probability of such an event.[234] This observation has not been confirmed. Multiple myeloma bone marrow plasma cells express an excess of the same immunoglobulin light-chain isotype as found in the serum or urine in MM. Marrow plasma cells in MGUS are sometimes polyclonal owing to the presence of residual normal plasma cells.[235] In our experience, plasma cells in almost all MGUS patients show predominance of cells with the involved immunoglobulin light chain, with ratios greater than 4:1 in the case of κ and less than 0.5:1 in the case of λ MGUS. Plasma cell light chain ratios do not pick up clonal plasma cells so easily in patients with few clonal plasma cells and low M-proteins because normal background immunoglobulin producing polyclonal plasma cells mask the small number of clonal plasma cells.

Myeloma cell DNA content aneuploidy by flow cytometry is of little help in distinguishing MM from MGUS. In one study aneuploidy was detected in the bone marrow of 25 of 46 MM patients (54 percent) and in one of 15 MGUS patients (7 percent).[236] In our experience, DNA ploidy is as common in MGUS as in MM. ANBL-6, a myeloma cell line, exhibited clonally rearranged immunoglobulin but was composed of both near diploid and near tetraploid populations. Cytogenetic studies showed two aneuploid karyotypes with numerous shared structural abnormalities, including a near-tetraploid and a near-diploid subclone, probably arising during clonal evolution.[237] These studies support observations by Epstein and colleagues suggesting the possible origin of DNA aneuploid myeloma cells from DNA diploid myeloma cells.[238] Chromosome replication checkpoint errors must exist but are as yet undefined.

Many new observations of differences between MGUS and MM have been made; each needs to be evaluated on its own merits and in relation to previously observed differences between MGUS and MM. Single studies involving few patients provide preliminary evidence that can be confirmed in larger, more comprehensive analyses.

SUMMARY OF MECHANISMS OF MGUS AND MM PROGRESSION

We have described differences between clinical and biologic factors observed to be overexpressed in MM as compared with MGUS or more expressed in progressive myeloma. However, serial samples taken during progression from MGUS to MM or during progression of myeloma are more likely to demonstrate key elements in the progression. Such observations are rare in the MGUS to MM paradigm because they require that samples of highly purified clonal plasma cells be obtained from the marrow at the time of diagnosis of MGUS and then again at the time of progression to MM. However, in such patients plasma cell proliferation changes represent a key focus for studying progression. Together with loss of apoptosis, or programmed cell death, a powerful model depicting progression from MGUS to MM or from stable to progressive myeloma can be developed. Acquisition of adhesion markers by neoplastic plasma cells may play a role in homing of myeloma cells to marrow stromal cells. Production of IL-1 by myeloma plasma cells is an early event in MM, which mediates (1) the acquisition of adhesion markers; (2) the development of lytic bone lesions; and (3) the stimulation of paracrine IL-6 from marrow stromal cells, including osteoblasts. Autocrine IL-6 likely follows. Soluble IL-6R production by myeloma cells enhances response of myeloma cells to IL-6. All changes lead to the malignant phenotype, in which a morphologically more immature plasma cell shows increased proliferation and decreased apoptosis. The resulting expansion of clonal plasma cells comes about through greater adhesion to and interaction with stroma and greater production of cytokines by myeloma cells and stroma.

Oncogenes play a critical role in the development and progression of MM. It is likely that *c-myc* resulting from karyotypic changes maintains B-cell clones, and in some patients *ras* mutation and expression plays a role in the transition to MM and its progression by stimulating the mitogen-activated protein

Table 30–3. Criteria for Diagnosis of Monoclonal Gammopathy of Undetermined Significance (MGUS) and Smoldering Multiple Myeloma (SMM) with Use of New Ancillary Tests to Supplement Current Established Methods

MGUS[a]
- Serum monoclonal protein (usually less than 3 g/dl)
- No anemia, renal failure, or hypercalcemia
- Ancillary tests negative[b]
  - Bone lesions absent on radiographic bone survey[c]
  - Bone marrow contains less than 10 percent plasma cells without aggregates on biopsy
  - Bone marrow plasma cell labeling index below 1.0 percent
  - Plasmablasts absent

SMM[a]
- Serum monoclonal protein (usually more than 3 g/dl)
- On biopsy, 10 percent or less of marrow plasma cells or aggregates
- No anemia, renal failure, or hypercalcemia attributable to myeloma
- Ancillary tests negative[b] (as above)

[a] Patients with MGUS and SMM must not have solitary plasmacytoma, amyloidosis, or light-chain deposition disease.

[b] Normal β_2-M value, absence of circulating isotype-specific plasma cells, peripheral blood plasma cell labeling index less than 0.5 percent, light chain isotype suppression, urinary light chains less than 500 mg/24 h, and stable monoclonal protein level in the serum or urine during the follow-up period.

[c] Computed tomography or magnetic resonance imaging may be needed to rule out skeletal lesions.

(MAP) kinase pathway of cell proliferation. Abnormalities of *p16*, especially hypermethylation, also play a role. Later in the course of disease, loss of *rb* or *p53* and additional *ras* overexpression may allow uncontrolled myeloma cell proliferation by increasing expression of autocrine IL-6. Cytogenetic changes underlying these effects have been difficult to elucidate. Simple karyotyping is inadequate because myeloma cells proliferate

Table 30–4. Criteria for Diagnosis of Multiple Myeloma with Use of Supplemental Ancillary Tests for More Difficult Cases[a]

Monoclonal protein present in serum or urine
10 percent or less of marrow plasma cells or aggregates on biopsy or histologic evidence of plasmacytoma
Plus one or more of the following:
- Ancillary findings[b]
- Anemia
- Lytic lesions[c] or osteoporosis and 30 percent or less plasma cells in marrow
- Bone marrow plasma cell labeling index higher than 1 percent
- Renal insufficiency
- Hypercalcemia

[a] Patients with multiple myeloma may have associated amyloidosis or light chain deposition disease.

[b] Increased β_2-M level, peripheral blood B-cell labeling index higher than 0.5, circulating monoclonal isotype-specific plasma cells, and loss of light chain isotype suppression may be included.

[c] Computed tomography or magnetic resonance imaging for suspected skeletal lesions.

slowly and do not produce many metaphases. Fluorescent in situ hybridization techniques to detect interphase translocation are more helpful.

Circulating MM cells likely play a much greater role in the spread of the disease than previously believed. The role of precursor B cells, including those that may circulate in the peripheral blood, is controversial and needs to be better studied. Sensitive and specific molecular, biological, cell culture system, and animal models are needed to determine whether precursor B cells aid in the initiation and development of MM.

Serum markers may obtain an estimate of myeloma activity, but they do not adequately differentiate MGUS from MM. Markers such as neopterin, sIL-6R, soluble CD16 (Fc receptor), soluble syndecan, and soluble CD56 show promise in differentiating MM from MGUS and in detecting myeloma progression.

Simple changes in the percentage of T cells, T-cell subsets, and NK cells are not likely to play a major role in the progression of MGUS to MM. However, detection of activated T cells and spectratyping may be of greater use. The observation that B-cell light-chain isotype ratios shift to favor the malignant clone as patients progress to MM suggests that a functional change in T-cell regulation of B cells operates in MGUS and may be lost in MM. The role of anti-idiotype T cells and T cells with restricted V-region receptor expression is actively being studied. Levels of serum β_2-M,TK,LDH,IL-6, CRP, and albumin are not very helpful in distinguishing early-stage MM from MGUS or in identifying progression.

CLINICALLY DIFFERENTIATING MM FROM MGUS

Standard criteria for differentiating MGUS from MM can be improved. The PCLI and enumeration of circulating monoclonal plasma cells are very helpful ancillary tests. Schemes for more accurate differentiation of MGUS and MM are shown in Tables 30–3 and 30–4. Further investigation is needed to improve diagnostic accuracy. Methods such as measurement of IL-1 production by monoclonal plasma cells could have useful diagnostic value and should be examined.

Myeloma signaling pathways are extremely complex, but the impressive increase in knowledge concerning pathways of growth and apoptosis has led to better understanding of myeloma progression and means to target it, including the *ras* signaling pathway.

Circumspection is necessary when interpreting results of studies comparing MGUS and MM. Conflicting results are caused by (1) differences in patient characteristics, for example, stage and aggressiveness of the myeloma being compared with MGUS; (2) contamination of monoclonal plasma cells by residual normal plasma cells in MGUS; (3) differences in analytic methods and use of bioassay versus enzyme-linked immunosorbent assay (ELISA) for IL-6; (4) misinterpretation of phenotypic and molecular changes; and (5) conclusions based on too few patients. Each investigator interpreting studies needs to consider these pitfalls.

There are major biologic and molecular differences between MM and MGUS, including increased cell proliferation, cytokine changes, cytogenetic abnormalities, oncogene mutations, alteration in oncogene expression, and difference in regulatory cell number and function. We do not know which are the critical molecular differences. Further knowledge may be gained through a prospective serial study in which changes are observed as patients move from MGUS or SMM to MM. We must identify the phenotypic and biologic characteristics of the myeloma precursor cell because they may hold the key to better understanding of differences between MGUS and MM. An elevated PCLI and increased circulating plasma cells predict the development of MM with a high degree of accuracy. These and similar tests are beginning to be more widely available. This is important because no other clinical test predicts which patients with MGUS will eventually develop MM.

CLINICALLY PREDICTING MM SURVIVAL

What controls progression in MM is not easily defined. We know that the median survival of MM patients receiving standard chemotherapy therapy has increased to $3^{1}/_{2}$ years.[11] One out of five patients dies during the first year of treatment; one out of three lives at least 5 years, but only 1 out of 15 lives 10 years or more with standard chemotherapy. For patients who receive an autologous peripheral stem cell transplant (PSCT), the median survival improves to 4 to 5 years in patients who receive a delayed transplant,[239,240] compared with 5.8 years after early tandem transplant and intensive multiagent combination or total chemotherapy.[241] Despite their apparent improvement in survival, even patients who receive transplants relapse in a median of 18 to 22 months and eventually develop chemotherapy resistance regardless of the type of treatment. Better survival after transplantation may be explained in part by selection of good-risk patients whose outcome is superior. Simple eligibility for stem cell transplant (SCT) yields longer survival, the median being 5 years. This stresses the importance of randomized clinical trials to examine the advantages of SCT. One such randomized trial in newly diagnosed MM patients suggests that patients who receive transplants have a median survival about $1^{1}/_{2}$ years longer than those who receive standard chemotherapy.[242] However, in this trial the standard chemotherapy-treated group did unusually poorly. Most believe the survival advantage for SCT may not be that long. In a contrasting study, the median survival after SCT was just over 5 years whether the transplant was performed early or late in the course of the disease. Despite modest but significant improvement in survival, it is disappointing to know that transplantation does not overcome the prognostic impact of factors such as a high β2-M level or a high PCLI. At the time of the writing of this manuscript, we still need to know the proper timing of transplantation and which patients are better served with SCT than with standard treatment.

Maximum treatment response to chemotherapy usually occurs 6 months to a year after starting therapy. In some patients a very slow decrease in M-protein signals a very slow response to treatment, which continues over several years. These patients have better overall survival. Overall survival is similar with simple oral melphalan and prednisone, which pro-

duce a 50 to 60 percent partial response rate (PR), or with combination chemotherapy, which produces a 70 to 75 percent PR rate. Complete response (CR) occurs in less than 10 percent of patients receiving standard chemotherapy, although a CR rate of 17 percent has been observed in a large trial of patients receiving standard therapy plus interferon during induction. In one study the achievement of CR was the strongest predictor of subsequent survival.[243] It is not clear whether the increased survival is because CR patients are more responsive to chemotherapy or whether the dose-intensive therapy really improves outcome. There can be major differences in the frequency of CR, depending on the method of detection of minimal residual disease. Methods include modern immunofixation techniques and assays that detect low levels of free light chains. Two-step multiparameter flow cytometry can detect 1 in 10,000 to 1 in 100,000 myeloma cells in the marrow. Molecular techniques such as PCR can detect minimal residual disease in nearly all patients with MM who are thought to be in CR on the basis of other methods. Standard criteria for clinical CR used by the European Group for Blood and Marrow Transplant[244] include disappearance of the M-protein by immunofixation of the serum and urine, demonstrated twice at least 6 weeks apart, and less than 5 percent plasma cells in the marrow. An estimated 30 percent of patients achieve CR after autologous PSCT. Many patients with no spike in the electrophoretic pattern of the serum or urine will have an M-protein by light chain analysis or by immunofixation, or they will have residual monoclonal plasma cells in the marrow as determined by flow cytometric immunophenotyping. Molecular CR by allele-specific oligonucleotide detection of clonal plasma cells is rarely achieved even after PSCT. In most patients the response is partial, but a stable or plateau state is achieved that in many ways resembles MGUS. Failure to completely eradicate minimal residual disease (MRD) or to maintain the MRD state is the ultimate cause of relapse.

After PR or CR is achieved whether by standard chemotherapy or by PSCT, most patients remain stable for a year or more. In PR patients the stable state is called plateau, which can be defined as a less than 20 percent fluctuation in M-protein after response. Patients achieving a plateau phase live longer than those who do not. Escape from CR or escape from plateau phase heralds relapse. Escape from CR is defined by the reappearance of the M-protein in the serum or urine and indicates "chemical relapse." Chemical relapse is ultimately followed by clinical relapse as the M-protein reaches threshold levels. Clinical relapse is usually manifest by the redevelopment of the patient's original symptoms including anemia, bone pain with lytic lesions, or compression fractures from progressive osteoporosis. Patients who are followed closely enough are generally treated sometime after chemical relapse and before clinical relapse. Survival after relapse averages only 7 to 14 months. Survival after relapse has less to do with response and more to do with differences in the biology of the malignant plasma cells and their microenvironment and ultimately with the almost universal development of resistance to chemotherapy.

Accurate predictive and prognostic models are needed for better management of the worldwide increasing problem of MM, including the nearly 15,000 patients who develop MM each year and the over 11,000 who die of it each year in the United States alone. We need to know the factors that predict progression of MGUS to MM and response of MM to treatment. We need to know the prognostic factors that estimate the likelihood of survival. While prognostic factors are not yet able to predict which patients are better treated with standard chemotherapy and which PSCT, novel new therapy clinical trials may be chosen for those patients with a particularly poor prognosis. With this background we can begin to discuss in detail the factors that govern progression from MGUS to MM and the survival of MM patients.

PROGNOSTIC FACTORS AND THEIR APPLICATION

Why are prognostic factors needed? There is a wide spectrum of disease behavior in MM, with survival varying from months to many years. We are unable to identify the subset of patients who may be curable by more intensive or novel therapy programs, nor are we able to recognize patients who already have just as long expected survival with standard therapy. Similarly, we are still not able to identify the patients who benefit from standard chemotherapy or transplantation versus those who need novel approaches. Prognostic factors are needed for better stratification in myeloma clinical trials and better counseling of patients. Ancillary laboratory studies in clinical trials can identify new prognostic factors. They also have the potential to determine whether a new treatment may be more effective in a selected group of patients defined by such factors. We review here the biological features of MM affecting disease course that may serve as useful prognostic factors.

Patient age, performance status, and socioeconomic status can have a negative impact on survival in patients with MM. Knowledge of a given patient's prognosis has the potential to effect changes in the clinical management of patients. Also, active or passive inclusion or exclusion of patients with different risk characteristics in a clinical trial can significantly change results.[245] Easily available clinical features such as hemoglobin, creatinine, calcium, albumin, immunoglobulin type and level, urine M-protein levels, and bone marrow plasma cell percentage have long been known to predict survival.[246] The predictive value of individual factors varies from study to study, but reproducibility has been improved by combining them into clinical staging systems. Durie-salmon myeloma staging takes into account hemoglobin level, calcium level, serum and urine protein levels, bone lesions, and creatinine.[247] Quantification of bone lesions used in this staging system is not always reliable as a prognostic factor.[248] The staging system itself has occasionally failed to predict survival.

Many biologic features of myeloma and of myeloma regulatory cells and cytokines can now be measured in blood and marrow. As a result, new prognostic factors are being discovered, and others have been proposed and are being tested.

Clinical Staging

The wide variation in myeloma behavior is due to the disease's underlying cytogenetic, molecular genetic and cell kinetic het-erogeneity. Some myeloma patients live only for months and others live for 10 years or more. Such short and long survivals may be observed both in patients treated with standard chemotherapy and in those treated with SCT. Survival differences are predicted poorly by most routinely available clinical laboratory tests. High levels of M-protein and organ damage, including anemia, renal insufficiency, hypercalcemia, and advanced bone disease, reflect greater tumor burden but they are not all independently prognostic. Rather these factors each reflect greater tumor burden. They have been skillfully combined to develop the Durie Salmon staging system, which is a useful way to classify MM patients with low, intermediate, and high tumor burden (Table 30–5). Stage predicts survival only modestly, and it is not an independent risk factor for survival compared with other individual factors such as the serum β_2-M level or even serum creatinine. Neither stage nor any individual clinically available test accurately predicts myeloma response to initial chemotherapy.

It is helpful to better understand tumor burden-based clinical staging before examining the prognostic factors that govern MM progression. Durie Salmon clinical staging was developed in 1975 to provide a practical way to measure MM tumor burden. Tumor burden measurement was first derived scientifically. Knowing the immunoglobulin production by each plasma cell and the half-life of circulating immunoglobulin, it was possible to mathematically derive the total myeloma cell number and tumor burden. The tumor burden could then be correlated with individual clinical laboratory and x-ray features, including levels of hemoglobin, serum calcium, and creatinine, and serum and urine M-protein, and the number and size of bone lesions to define the clinical staging system. Clinical Durie Salmon stage therefore provides a simple and practical estimate of tumor burden. It has become an accepted way to categorize MM. Patients have stage 1, 2, or 3 disease, depending on the degree of anemia, hypercalcemia, levels of M-protein in the serum and urine, or bone lesions. Associations among the elements of staging are common. Patients without or with creatinine of 2 mg/dl or more are designated A or B. More than two-thirds of patients with the B designation have advanced stages of disease (Table 30–5) due to lower levels of hemoglobin, more frequent hypercalcemia, and higher levels of urine M-protein. Simply having a creatinine 2 mg/dl or more is associated with a poor prognosis independently of Durie Salmon stage. There are further limitations to staging. Stage 3 without renal insufficiency, even with hypercalcemia, does not predictably lead to early mortality in MM. It is important for the clinician evaluating patient risk to be aware that patients who are in stage 3 only because they meet the bone lesion criteria do not have a poorer prognosis. In some large series, patients with no bone lesions even have a better prognosis. Patients presenting with renal failure often become symptomatic only after they have achieved a high tumor burden. Most do not have the bone lesions and bone pain that would attract medical attention earlier in the course.

With the growth of understanding of myeloma pathobiology, it is not surprising that the prognostic significance of stage as a predictor of survival has been eclipsed by newer prognostic

Table 30–5. Clinical Staging System for Multiple Myeloma Developed From Correlation of Measured Myeloma Cell Mass With Presenting Clinical Features, Response to Treatment, and Survival

Stage	Criteria	Measured Myeloma Cell Mass (cells X $10^{12}/m^2$)
I	*All* of the following:	
	1. Hemoglobin value above 10 g/dl	
	2. Serum calcium value normal ($\leq$12 mg/dl or less)	
	3. On radiograph, normal bone structure (scale 0) or solitary bone plasmacytoma only	< 0.6 (low)
	4. Low M-component production rates	
	a. IgG value less than 5 g/dl	
	b. IgA value less than 3 g/dl	
	c. Urine light chain M-component on electrophoresis less than 4 g/24 h	
II	Fitting neither stage I nor stage II	0.6–1.20 (intermediate)
III	*One or more* of the following	
	1. Hemoglobin value below 8.5 g/dl	
	2. Serum calcium value above 12 mg/dl	
	3. Advanced lytic bone lesions (scale 3)	> 1.20 (high)
	4. High M-component production rates	
	a. IgG value above 7 g/dl	
	b. IgA value above 5 g/dl	
	c. Urine light chain M-component on electrophoresis above 12 g/24 h	

Subclassification
  A. Relatively normal renal function (serum creatinine value below 2.0 mg/dl)
  B. Abnormal renal function (serum creatinine value at or above 2.0 mg/dl)
Examples
  Stage IA: Low cell mass with normal renal function
  Stage IIIB: High cell mass with abnormal renal function

(From Durie and Salmon,[247] with permission.)

factors based on myeloma biology. Improvement in prognostication beyond clinical staging can be obtained with simple measurement of the serum β_2-M level, which reflects myeloma tumor burden, renal insufficiency, and as yet unknown aspects of myeloma. Myeloma cell proliferation as measured by the bone marrow PCLI has repeatedly been shown to be a most significant and independent prognostic factor for patient survival.

Patients with more rapid growth rate as evidenced by a high PCLI present at a more advanced stage. Patients whose disease is slowly progressive may present at an earlier stage even before symptoms develop because of the widespread use of screening serum protein electrophoresis during the longer preclinical phase of their disease. Patients who are symptomatic early because of localized destructive and painful bone lesions may also present at an early stage. From these observations, it is clear that tumor burden estimation and the kinetics of the myeloma cells can be associated with developments that define important differences in disease behavior in MM.

Myeloma Cell Morphology

Studies performed in 1948[249] showed for the first time that patients with very immature plasma cell morphology had shortened survival. There have been a number of studies, including our own,[61] identifying the prognostic impact of plasmablastic morphology (Figure 30–12). Studies have been done on either aspirate or plastic section biopsy material.[250] Interpretation of morphology is necessarily subjective and reproducibility is limited. Smaller studies have shown that the plasmablastic subset may not be unfavorable unless combined with the larger group with immature morphology.[251] Nevertheless, plasmablastic myeloma has repeatedly proved itself to be a reliable and powerful predictor of poor survival in MM.[252–256] Conversely, mature plasma cell morphology may act as a favorable prognostic factor.[257] Plasmablastic morphology is an independent predictor and is associated with a high PCLI, a higher level of sIL-6R and *ras* mutations. Poor survival in MM may also be related to the degree of marrow infiltration and tumor cell mass (TCM).[258] A classification based on a combination of clinical and histologic parameters has been proposed.[259] Electron microscopy confirms that immature nuclear morphology and nuclear cytoplasmic asynchrony correlate with one another and with poor prognosis.[260,261] Nuclear immaturity and three cytoplasmic abnormalities – scattered pattern of mitochondria, single-sac looplike structures, and numerous intramitochondrial granules – were associated with poor outcome.

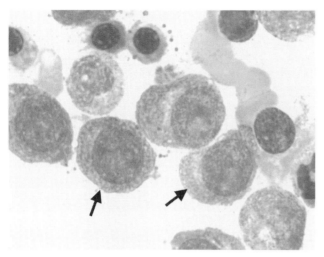

Figure 30–12. Plasmablastic myeloma. Shown by the arrows are two clear-cut plasmablasts. Plasmablasts are characterized by open nuclear chromatin, large nucleoli, and a high nuclear to cytoplasm ratio (greater than 1:1). The presence of just a few plasmablasts reproducibly throughout the marrow is indicative of a very poor prognosis. (Adapted from Greipp et al.[61,255] with permission.)

Immunocytochemical studies applied to marrow biopsies in patients with myeloma have shown that elevated acid phosphatase and β-glucuronidase are associated with poorer survival.[262] Cyclin D1 staining is increased in myeloma in association with the t(11;14) translocation, but this finding does not translate into worse survival for these patients.[35,263] Patients with a higher PCLI have a poor correlation with the t(11;14)

translocation which suggests that there are other mechanisms for increased cyclin D1 expression in MM.

Cell Kinetics

The PCLI is a reproducible and powerful prognostic factor in MM.[264] It is determined by an immunofluorescence slide-based assay.[61] Cells in the DNA S-phase of the cell cycle incorporate bromodeoxyuridine, which can be recognized by using a monoclonal antibody. The S-phase cells are then marked with a second antibody, and plasma cells are recognized by morphology and reactivity with anti-human-immunoglobulin kappa and lambda light chains.[265] The PCLI also provides an index of tumor progression.

An elevated PCLI predicts short remission and survival but does not predict response to therapy. All survival studies done at Mayo Clinic have confirmed the independent prognostic value of the PCLI in multivariate analysis.[40,61,254,266,267] Results of a large clinical trial by the Eastern Cooperative Oncology Group confirm its independent prognostic value in a multi-institutional study.[255,256] All large studies published to date have confirmed the prognostic value of the PCLI (Table 30–6). It is unusual for a prognostic factor to be so reproducible across studies. The PCLI may be an especially important prognostic factor in patients who are rapid responders to chemotherapy. Among rapid responders, those with a PCLI of 2 percent or more survived a median of 16 months, whereas those with a PCLI of less than 2 percent had not reached median survival at 47 months.[268] The shorter survival of rapid responders with high PCLI was due to a shorter remission duration, with a median 12 months. The data strongly support use of the PCLI in clinical practice.

Table 30–6. Prognostic Value of the Plasma Cell Labeling Index (PCLI) in Nine Published Studies

Reference	Year	No. of Cases	PCLI (percent)	Median Survival (mo)	Univariate P Value
Durie et al.[337]	1980	79	≥1	NA	.02
			< 1	NA	
			≥3	NA	.002
Latreille et al.[338]	1982	50	≥1	NA	.04
Montecucco et al.[339]	1986	37	≥2	10	< .01
			< 2	55	
Greipp et al.[266]	1988	100	≥0.4	18	.02
			< 0.4	38	
Boccadoro et al.[289]	1989	65	≥2	16	< .004
		42	< 2	47	
Boccadoro et al.[340]	1991	173	≥2	16.4	< .0001
			< 2	42.4	
Greipp et al.[40]	1993	107	≥1	17	.0004
			< 1	42	
			≥2	15	< .0001
			< 2	40	
Cornelissen et al.[341]	1994	63	≥3	17	.029
			< 3	29	
Greipp et al.[255]	1998	453	≥1	121	< .0001
			< 1	305	

Abbreviation: NA, not available.

Immunocytochemical staining of bone marrow plasma cells using the Ki-67 antibody has been used as a measure of the labeling index.[269] Comparison with bromodeoxyuridine labeling in a small number of patients suggests that a potential advantage for the Ki-67 assay is a wider range of values.[69] In one study an increase in Ki-67 was associated with an increase in p16 and Rb expression.[270] Increased expression of Ki67 also correlated with tumor grade. A disadvantage of the Ki67 assay is the difficulty in recognizing some patients' malignant plasma cells morphologically on immunocytochemical-stained slides. This limits its clinical application, especially when the numbers of plasma cells are few. Nevertheless, Ki-67 staining is biologically relevant, and expression correlates with tumor grade, histological stage, *p21* and *p53* expression, and *Rb* expression. Recently *cyclin D1* gene expression, which is increased in some MM patients, was shown to be an independent predictor of survival in MM.[271] In slightly to intermediately proliferative MM cases, *cyclin D1* is probably upregulated by t(11;14), but an alternative mechanism is more probable in highly proliferative MM.[263] Further development and testing of immunohistochemical techniques are needed before they are adopted for diagnosis and prognosis in MM.

Trendle et al. found that flow cytometric S-phase measurement using propidium iodide immunofluorescence is prognostic and can be more easily performed than the bromodeoxyuridine PCLI method.[71] Others have demonstrated correlation with the PCLI.[43,70] Wider application of flow methods for prognosis awaits a practical method that can measure S-phase in MM and MGUS patients with fewer than 20 percent plasma cells.

Low *BAX* expression identifies a cohort of patients with long survival.[76] Studies suggest that decrease in apoptosis accompanies the progression from MGUS to SMM to MM.[68]

Circulating Myeloma Plasma Cells

Studies suggest that circulating myeloma cells are a subset of neoplastic bone marrow plasma cells and represent an independent, self-replenishing population.[195] Apoptosis studies suggest that the VLA-5-positive population of neoplastic plasma cells is nonproliferating and apoptotic, whereas the VLA-5-negative population is surviving and proliferative. The number of circulating myeloma cells is independently prognostic in newly diagnosed patients. In one study patients with 4 percent or more of circulating PCs had a median survival of 2.4 years versus 4.4 years for those with less than 4 percent of circulating PCs.[272] Circulating clonal plasma cell number also helps to differentiate MGUS and SMM from MM.[27] In SMM patients the median time to progression for patients with abnormal peripheral blood PCs was 0.75 years, compared with 2.5 years for those patients without abnormal peripheral blood PCs.[26]

Beta-2-Microglobulin

Beta-2-microglobulin (β_2-M) is the strongest, most reliable prognostic factor for MM that is routinely available. Elevated β_2-M values predict early death but do not predict response to chemotherapy; normal values predict a long median survival. This value was first shown to be a significant predictor of sur-

vival in France.[273] This finding was confirmed repeatedly, and in 1992 a simple staging system was designed that combined the prognostic utility of the β_2-M and C-reactive protein (CRP) values.[223] There is room for improvement, however. An interesting analysis of β_2-M conducted by the British MRC has shown that if a group of patients survives 2 years, their initial β_2-M level is no longer predictive of outcome.[274] β_2-Microglobulin is most useful when combined with PCLI, since the two factors are independent predictors of survival.[275] Of particular interest is a subset of patients under the age of 65 with low PCLI and low β_2-M who had a long median survival of 6 years (Table 30–7). Patients with low PCLI and β_2-M who respond may receive more benefit that those with a high PCLI and β_2-M, who seem to benefit the least. Only a randomized trial with appropriate prognostic factor correlative studies can answer this important question.

The β_2-M level depends not only on tumor burden but also on a variety of other factors. It is a small molecule, 19 kd molecular weight, and it is readily cleared in the urine, so it is always elevated in renal insufficiency. Formulas to correct the β_2-M level for renal insufficiency have not improved the predictive value of the β_2-M[276]; however, β_2-M level is still a highly significantly prognostic factor in myeloma patients with normal renal function.[266] There is a strong relationship between β_2-M and ICTP, a marker of bone turnover. Thus, β_2-M remains a simple and most useful measure of prognosis in patients with myeloma.

Cytogenetics

Conventional cytogenetics (CC) in MM identify a group of patients with a particularly poor prognosis. The frequency of abnormal karyotypes is low at diagnosis of MM. In several studies, 14 to 39 percent of newly diagnosed untreated myeloma patients had abnormal karyotypes.[277–280] The actual frequency is not clear because the latest of these studies, published in 2000, includes patients who progressed or were resistant to prior single-dose therapy and would be more likely to be selective for CC abnormalities. Furthermore, two reports in the same year from the same group quoted frequencies of 18 percent and 39 percent for newly diagnosed patients. We conclude that the frequency of cytogenetic abnormalities on a single specimen obtained at diagnosis is closer to 18 percent. The frequency of chromosomal abnormalities is close to 100 percent based on current FISH analysis. The reports of 82 percent of normal karyotypes by CC are probably best considered uninformative inasmuch as they probably reflect the karyotypes of normal proliferating myeloid precursor populations. The observed low frequency of abnormal metaphases by CC is due to the very low proliferation rate of myeloma cells in most patients.[154] Wide application of CC is also limited by expense. Five-day culture with IL-4 or unstimulated 72-hour culture yielded 47 percent abnormal metaphases in one study.[281] However, abnormal results were mostly seen in patients with far advanced disease and poor performance status, and with a high S-phase rather than in newly diagnosed patients with better prognoses.[281] Many were relapsing patients. It is not clear how much the prolonged culture and cytokine stimulation helped to increase the frequency of abnormal metaphases. Use of growth factors has not increased the yield of CC consistently enough to warrant its routine use. Hypodiploid karyotypes including del 13 are more often seen in plasma cell leukemia.[282] Patients with CC abnormalities had shorter survival in all studies so far. It is a matter of debate whether del 13 is significantly worse than other chromosomal abnormalities by CC. We need less costly and more informative cytogenetic methods that can identify abnormalities in nonproliferating interphase nuclei in newly diagnosed patients.

Recently FISH chromosome probes have allowed us to detect aneuploidy and translocations in nonproliferating interphase PCs. The term *aneuploidy* covers hypodiploid chromosome abnormalities, including monosomy, and also hyperdiploid chromosome abnormalities, including polysomy. Monosomies of chromosome 5 and 7 are relatively infrequent and have not been well studied. The most common form of monosomy is monoallelic loss of a portion of chromosome 13 (del 13). The prognostic significance of del 13 by FISH is less than that for del 13 by CC. Of 351 patients entered on a large cooperative group trial, 54 percent had del 13 by FISH.[37] The median survival for patients with del 13 was 34.9 months and for those without del 13 it was 51 months. Similar frequency of del 13 and similar survival differences were documented in another study, in which there was a close correlation between del 13 and Ki-67 proliferative index, bone marrow plasma cell percent and high β_2-M.[283]

It is likely that del 13 by FISH is a significant prognostic factor, but its independent prognostic significance is not yet well established. Up to 75 percent of patients with MM have translocations involving the heavy chain gene on chromosome 14. These translocations include "illegitimate switch recombinations" of the variable regions of the immunoglobulin heavy chain gene at 14q32. In one study of the three best characterized 14q32 translocations, there was a tight association of del 13 abnormalities and high β_2-M levels with the unfavorable t(4;14) and t(16;14) translocations.[284] The frequency of high β_2-M or del 13 was half as frequent in patients with the t(11;14) abnormality. This suggests that the poor prognosis associated with del 13 may be due to other nonrandom associated chromosomal abnormalities.

Trisomy is common by FISH and includes chromosomes 3, 6, 9, 11, and 15.[43] In another study, trisomy of chromosome 3, 7, and 11 accounted for over 50 percent of the hyperdiploid cases.[285] Chromosomes 1 and 14 are commonly involved. Trisomies of chromosomes 6, 9, and 17 were associated with prolonged survival.[155]

Much of the prognostic value of abnormal CC results may be due to the higher proliferation rate and therefore more informative karyotypes from the myeloma cell populations in patients with a higher PCLI.[286] Translocations can now be detected by FISH, and preliminary data suggest that the most common translocations and del 13 define prognostically different subsets, which may result in a new molecular genetic classification of myeloma.

The t(8;14) translocation is exceedingly rare in myeloma and in myeloma cell lines. However, other translocations involving *c-myc* associated with disease dysregulation and progression have been described in 50 percent of advanced myeloma cases and most cell lines.[162] It is likely that *c-myc* abnormalities will assume a role in prognosis along with other chromosomal abnormalities.

Oncogenes and Tumor Suppressor Genes

Mutations of *ras* were first observed in fulminating disease[165] and were found early on in 27 percent of newly diagnosed patients.[287] Subsequently, they were demonstrated in 39 percent of newly diagnosed patients in a large clinical trial.[31] Patients with *ras* mutations had a median survival of 2.1 years versus 4 years for patients with wild-type *ras.*

Mutated *p53* is rare in freshly explanted myeloma cells but is common in human myeloma cell lines.[165] Mutated *p53* genes are more common in patients with a terminal phase of myeloma. Deletions of *p53* as seen in FISH analysis are likely to be more important. In one study, 33 percent of patients with newly diagnosed myeloma had deletion of one *p53* gene by FISH.[288] Median survival was 15.9 months for those with a deletion and 38 months for those newly diagnosed patients without a deletion of *p53*. In another study, only 9 percent of newly diagnosed patients had a *p53* deletion.[33] Differences were attributed to a false high detection of deletions due to hybridization efficiency. It is likely that deletions of *p53* will be an important prognostic factor for survival in patients with MM. The retinoblastoma (*Rb*) gene is located on the deleted portion of chromosome 13 detected so frequently in MM. Some phenomenon other than loss of the *Rb* gene is the reason for the poorer survival seen in del 13, perhaps an association with other genetic abnormalities.

Oncoproteins of one kind or another show increased expression in most myelomas. In one study, plasma cells expressing these proteins were 53 percent for *c-myc*, 28 percent for *Rb*, 28 percent for *bcl-2*, 27 percent for *c-fos*, 24 percent for *p53* wild, 22 percent for *p53* mutant, 13 percent for *c-neu*, and 13 percent for pan-*ras*. When a panel of eight antibodies was used, 82 percent of the samples had an increased incidence of expression by at least one oncoprotein or tumor suppressor gene product.[169]

Del 13 was present by FISH in 12 of 23 patients with myeloma; however, a karyotype abnormality of chromosome 13, where rb-1 resides, was found in only 4 of 23 patients.[278] This difference illustrates the potential advantages of FISH over standard karyotyping. Since both *p53* and *Rb* function as transcriptional repressors of IL-6 gene expression,[289] loss of *p53* and *Rb* function could result in increased IL-6 production by myeloma cells (autocrine cell growth). Such patients may be expected to have a high level of proliferation and a poor prognosis.

The *c-myc* gene is often overexpressed in myeloma without evidence of a mutation,[290] but *c-myc* could play a role in early oncogenesis of myeloma. Mutated *c-myc* is rare in human myeloma but is critical to the development of myeloma in mice.

Angiogenesis

Numerous studies have suggested the prognostic significance of increased microvessel density in MM. The first description of increased angiogenesis in MM was a comprehensive study of MM and MGUS, which showed a strong association with diagnosis and with an increase in the S-phase fraction of plasma cells measured by the PCLI.[55] The first large prognostic study was carried out in association with a clinical trial.[56] In that study we confirmed the strong correlation between angiogenesis and the PCLI. Median survivals were 4.4, 4, and 2 years in patients with low, intermediate, and high microvessel density (Figure 30–13). The study included only 74 patients, and we did not see independent prognostic significance for angiogenesis in a model that included PCLI, β2-M and percentage of marrow plasma cells. In another study, angiogenesis failed to predict survival.[291] It is not known whether levels of angiogenic cytokines such as VEGF, bFGF, or HGF are associated with poor survival, but levels are reduced during effective chemotherapy.[58] A study of angiogenic cytokines and their prognostic value is needed.

Cytokines and Soluble Receptors

A French study first showed the correlation between elevated serum IL-6 and severity of MM, the highest levels being seen in plasma cell leukemia or in MM cases with a high PCLI.[292] Serum IL-6 levels correlate directly with bone marrow plasmacytosis, serum lactate dehydrogenase, beta-2-microglobulin, and calcium and inversely with hemoglobin level.[106] Patients with higher-stage MM (stage 2 or 3) and progressive disease show higher serum IL-6 levels than patients with stage 1 MM.[51] Many assays are available, including bioassays, radioimmunoassays, and ELISA. In a recent study, IL-6 was a significant and independent prognostic factor in newly diagnosed MM patients along with sIL-6R, and β₂-M. The prognostic significance of IL-6 levels was shown in another study.[293] Differences among studies are common, however, possibly owing to methodological

considerations.[39] C-reactive protein levels are used as a surrogate for IL-6 measurement, (results are detailed in the discussion of serum markers, below). We also found in a large clinical trial that sIL-6R may be an independent prognostic factor.[255] In some other studies, sIL-6R demonstrated prognostic significance,[294,295] but in yet another study the influence of sIL-6R level on survival was weak.[296]

Elevated IL-2 levels are found in MM, and they suggest a better prognosis.[297] These study results are unconfirmed. If the source of IL-2 is activated T cells, perhaps IL-2 may be used therapeutically to improve duration of remission after standard or myeloablative therapy.[298] It may be better to examine immune cells themselves rather than their serum levels to assess the importance of such T-cell cytokines as IL-2 and interferon-gamma.

Bone Markers

Prognostic significance has been shown for a number of serum markers (Figure 30–14). However one must keep in mind that a single serum marker does not define poor prognosis in myeloma. Only when serum markers are combined with other, independent prognostic factors do we see a major separation of survival curves. We examined the role of serum markers of bone metabolism in 313 MM patients enrolled in a phase 3 trial (E9486), including osteoclastic factors, the C-terminal telopeptide of collagen I (ICTP), tartrate-resistant acid phosphatase (TRAP), osteoblastic factors, bone alkaline phosphatase (BAP), osteocalcin, and C-terminal propeptide of collagen I (PICP).[299] Of these markers, ICTP and BAP correlated with bone pain, bone lesions, and fractures, and ICTP also correlated with creatinine and was significantly associated with survival; however,

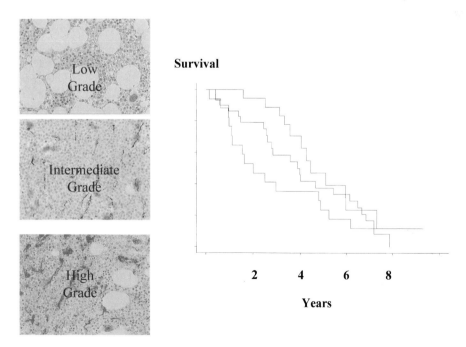

Figure 30–13. Increasing angiogenesis grade is associated with worsening survival. (Adapted from Rajkumar et al.,[56] with permission.)

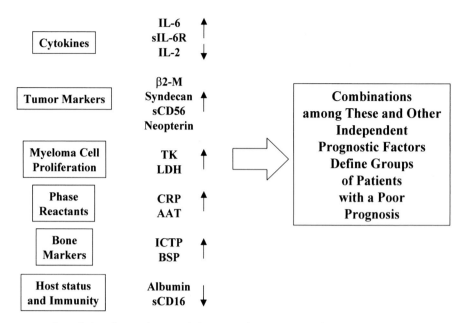

Figure 30–14. Compilation of serum factors with demonstated prognostic significance. Only the beta-2-microglobulin (β_2-M) has constantly demonstrated its independent prognostic value in all studies. Contradictory results for cytokines, thymidine kinase (TK), c-reactive protein (CRP), and albumin have been reported. Confirmatory studies are needed for serum syndecan, bone sialoprotein (BSP), and other prognostic factors. Ideally, these would be made in a setting with multiple serum factors so that their independent prognostic significance could be measured.

ICPT was not significant in a multivariate analysis in our study and another large-group study.[300] Cross-linked N-telopeptides of type I collagen (NTx) can be tested in the serum or urine and seem to constitute the most sensitive indicator of bone turnover.[301] Of all the markers, NTx in urine shows a strong positive correlation with the dynamic histomorphometric indices of bone resorption.[302] A prognostic study of serum or urine NTx needs to be completed.

Serum bone sialoprotein (BSP), a noncollagenous bone matrix component, seems to be a marker of tumor burden and neoplastic bone involvement and a prognostic factor in MM. Its concentrations were measured in 62 patients with newly diagnosed MM, 46 patients with MGUS, 71 patients with untreated benign vertebral osteoporosis (OPO), and 139 healthy adults. In MM patients, serum BSP was higher than in healthy control subjects or in MGUS or OPO patients. Levels of BSP correlated with the bone marrow plasma cells and serum β_2-M. After chemotherapy, BSP reflected the response to treatment and correlated with the change in monoclonal protein ($r = .55$, $P < .001$). Multiple myeloma patients with normal baseline BSP levels survived longer than patients with initially elevated BSP values. Bone sialoprotein was an independent predictor of survival. It should be further studied to assess its relative prognostic value against classical prognostic factors in a larger group of patients with MM.

Other Serum Markers

French investigators first showed that CRP was useful as a univariate prognostic marker in MM.[303] They subsequently showed its independent prognostic significance.[223] Shortly thereafter, the univariate prognostic significance of CRP was established in a group of patients from the Mayo Clinic.[304] However, a multivariate analysis showed that once PCLI and β_2-M were known, CRP no longer provided prognostic information. This failure to demonstrate usefulness in a multivariate analysis may have been due to the relatively small number of patients (107) in the study. In a larger Mayo Clinic study of 234 patients, CRP was not significant in a multivariate model with PCLI and circulating plasma cells and β_2-M.[272] In a preliminary study in ECOG trial E9487, CRP was useful in univariate and multivariate analysis as an independent prognostic factor.[305] In another multivariate model with β_2-M and another acute-phase protein, CRP was not statistically significant as a prognostic factor.[306] Neither has CRP been shown to be useful as a marker of disease status.[307] Apparently, CRP has appreciable variable significance as a prognostic marker in MM.

Lactic dehydrogenase (LDH) elevations identify a group of patients with very poor prognosis.[308] These patients may have very aggressive lymphoma-like disease characterized by tumor masses and retroperitoneal adenopathy with a very short clinical course.[309] In our experience only around 5 percent of newly diagnosed patients with myeloma will have an elevated LDH. This marker may be most useful in documenting the especially poor prognosis of the patient with clinically obvious aggressive disease. Other investigators have found high LDH levels in 11 percent of newly diagnosed MM patients.[309] This higher frequency could be due to differences in study populations.

Serum thymidine kinase (TK) levels have been shown to have prognostic value in myeloma.[307] Elevations of TK were independent of β_2-M levels. However, in another study TK levels were not useful either for diagnosis of MM or for prognosis.[225] In a British Medical Research Council trial, TK proved to be a highly significant prognostic indicator for 270 melphalan-treated patients but had no prognostic significance for 277 patients treated with ABCM (doxorubicin, carmustine, cyclophosphamide, and melphalan).[310] There was a correlation with PCLI, but in our experience TK identifies only a small fraction of the patients with elevated PCLI.[275]

Other serum markers that have provided useful prognostic information in myeloma include neopterin,[220] AAT,[306] type 1 collagen (ICTP),[299,311] and B12 binding protein.[312] A soluble cell adhesion molecule from plasma cells, NCAM or sCD56, is also attractive as a prognostic marker in MM and should be further examined.[313,314] Larger serum proteins such as NCAM and soluble Fc receptor (CD16),[147] are less affected by renal failure and may provide a better marker for myeloma prognosis than β_2-M. Soluble syndecan or CD138 is a very promising prognostic factor. In one study of 138 patients, serum syndecan correlated with serum creatinine and other prognostic factors, including secretion of urine M-component over the course of 24 hours, soluble IL-6 receptor, C-terminal telopeptide of type I collagen, beta-2-microglobulin, percentage of plasma cells in the bone marrow, disease stage, and serum M-component concentration. The median survival of patients with low values was 44 months while the survival of the high group was only 21 months. Serum syndecan was an independent predictor of survival in a multivariate analysis.[144]

Immune Cells

In MM, measurement of T cells, T-cell subsets, and T-cell subset function has been undertaken based on the hypothesis that either by direct contact or through secretion of cytokines, T cells regulate myeloma cell proliferation. One would postulate the association of increased T-helper cells with a worse prognosis and of increased activated T cells with a better prognosis. Paradoxically, however, San Miguel et al. have demonstrated that a loss of CD4 (helper) cells is associated with a worse prognosis.[315] These results were recently confirmed and extended in a large series of patients in a clinical trial.[5] It is likely that a lower number of CD4 or helper T cells reflected an impaired immune system. This observation is supported by the finding in the same study that CD19 B cells could substitute for CD4 T cells in the survival model. The prognostic significance of CD4 T cells is present throughout the course of disease, including after the completion of chemotherapy and at relapse.[8] Increased circulating T cells with activation of plasma cell markers are associated with a worse prognosis.[89] Such activated T cells persist even after chemotherapy.[316] Their prognostic significance is not known. Increased subsets of T cells with restricted T-cell receptor rearrangement were shown to circulate in myeloma.[317] Three patients had expanded predominant T-cell receptor V gene usage, indicated by the reactivity with the limited panel of T-cell repertoire (TCR) monoclonal antibodies, but these "clonal" T cells did not bind the idiotype. The study supports the existence of idiotype-specific T cells in the peripheral blood of patients with monoclonal gammopathy. These cells with restricted TCR expression have been found in patients entering a large myeloma trial.[210] Their prognostic significance is not known. We can conclude that immune cell competence as assessed by the number or CD4+ T cells or CD19+ B cells is an important prognostic variable in MM and that further work is needed to define the role of T-cell subsets in prognosis.

Phenotyping

Phenotypic characterization of myeloma cells using flow cytometry and immunocytochemical staining demonstrate aberrant phenotypes in a varying percentage of patients. Whereas most patients express mature plasma cell antigens such as CD38,[89] some also demonstrate immature lymphocyte antigens such as CD20 and CD10 (CALLA).[66] Results of phenotypic studies of particular antigens have been variable, probably because of small patient numbers and methodological considerations. This is particularly true for CALLA, which in separate studies has identified groups of patients with poor prognosis[318] or good prognosis.[238] Some evidence suggests that myeloma cells expressing surface CD20, a late B cell but pre–plasma cell antigen, or other atypical antigens may identify a group of patients with poor prognosis.[43] Because of the variability of results and outcomes with surface antigen phenotyping, it is likely that molecular phenotyping or genotyping will provide more reliable prognostic value. Surface antigen phenotyping could prove more useful for identifying target antigens for monoclonal antibody therapy such as anti-CD20.[319]

Drug Resistance

One form of drug resistance is marked by multidrug resistance (MDR)-1 expression on plasma cells by immunocytochemistry.[320] This is detected by the presence of P-glycoprotein in the cell membrane of PCs of patients with MM and is associated with a poor prognosis. Drug resistance measured by immunocytochemical detection of lung resistance protein is highly correlated with failure of response to melphalan and poor subsequent survival.[168] Lung resistance protein should be further studied in MM. There is as yet no practical clinical use established for drug resistance markers.

DNA Aneuploidy

Flow cytometric determination of DNA content has demonstrated DNA aneuploidy in the majority of patients with myeloma. An early study suggests no prognostic significance for DNA content measurement.[236] In a still earlier study, hypodiploid DNA content characterized a group of patients with very poor survival and drug-resistant disease.[321] In a later study, near diploid (normal) DNA content identified a group of patients with poor prognosis.[43] We found that whereas hypodiploid myeloma had a worse prognosis,[322] prognostic differences were also observed in the near diploid group, and most of the difference could be described as better prognoses for the clearly hyperdiploid group.[323] The usefulness of DNA content measurement in patients with myeloma is limited because of the small percentage of plasma cells in some patients, usually less than 5 percent, and conflicting evidence demonstrating prognostic significance of diploid or hyperdiploid DNA content.

DNA Array Techniques

Recently, by using Atlas complementary DNA (cDNA) arrays, comprising 268 genes coding for intercellular signaling molecules, genes that are uniquely overexpressed in myeloma cell lines were found to include the oncogenic Tyro3 tyrosine kinase receptor; the heparin-binding epidermal growth factor-like growth factor (HB-EGF), which is an epithelial autocrine tumor growth factor; the thrombin receptor (TR), which is linked to HB-EGF and syndecan-1 processing and to cell invasion; chemokine receptors CCR1 and CCR2; the Wnt pathway frizzled-related protein (FRZB); and the notch receptor ligand Jagged 2. Tyro3, HB-EGF, TR, and FRZB gene expression were also documented in purified primary malignant plasma cells from patients with plasma cell leukemia or MM.[324] Although there are as yet no other publications, it is likely that in the near future we will be seeing reports of the usefulness of DNA array techniques in the classification and prognosis of myeloma.

New Staging Systems

Durie Salmon stage has been the standard of prognosis in MM. For a number of reasons outlined earlier, a new system is needed. Following are some of the new staging systems offered for conventional chemotherapy treated patients. Indeed, in a study of 109 patients studied over a 10-year period, there were no significant differences in survival between stage 2 and 3 patients. Differences in these stages were mostly due to the presence or absence of renal insufficiency.[325] Other deficiencies include the subjectivity of interpretation of the severity of bone lesions and their questionable prognostic value, as well as the limited value of hypercalcemia as a prognostic indicator. Because of these and other deficiencies of Durie Salmon staging, a variety of new clinical staging systems have been developed. In one study, bone marrow plasma cell content more than 30 percent, hemoglobin less than 11.0 g/dl, lytic bone lesions of degree 2 or 3, serum β_2-M levels higher than 678 nmol/L, and the presence of Bence Jones proteinuria were the most important prognostic factors. Based on results of studies by the Mayo Clinic and the ECOG, the combination of PCLI and β_2-M was proposed as the most significant prognostic variable.[7] Later, plasmablastic features were added to the independent prognostic variables (Table 30–7).[255] S-phase PCs, together with β_2-M, age, and performance status were the most important prognostic variables.[326] The combination of del 13 by FISH and β_2-M was recently proposed as the basis of a new staging system.[327] In a study limited to IgG myeloma patients under age 75 years, a new staging system composed of β_2-M and hemoglobin was proposed.[328] Recently, a new staging system relying predominantly on the β_2-M level was proposed using the SWOG myeloma experience.[329] It is not clear which prognostic factor combination will be accepted as the successor to Durie Salmon

Table 30–7. Use of Plasma Cell Labeling Index (PCLI), β_2-Microglobulin (β_2-M), and Plasmablastic Features (PB) to Predict Survival in Myeloma

PCLI > 2%, β_2-M > 4 µg/ml, and PB features	No.	Estimated 5-Year Survival (%)	Median Survival (mo)
PB + high β_2-M + PCLI	16	0	13
PCLI + β_2-M	77	13	27
PCLI only	25	20	30
β_2-M only	192	32	46
0 values high	93	52	66

(Data from Greipp et al.[330])

stage for clinical use. However, plasmablastic features, PCLI, and β_2-M offers dramatically superior separation of survival (Table 30–7).[330]

Prognosis in High-Dose Therapy

All the prognostic factors described above were derived from patients treated with conventional dose chemotherapy. For many patients under age 70, peripheral stem cell transplantation has become a standard of therapy. One has to ask if the same variables that are important prognostic indicators in chemotherapy patients will be prognostic in high-dose therapy (HDT) patients. It is disappointing that the same prognostic factors seem to show up in HDT as in conventional-dose chemotherapy. This means that HDT likely has not overcome the poor prognostic import of these factors. In an early study, renal function, performance status, and LDH were important prognostic factors.[331] In another study, high β_2-M and PCLI were important prognostic factors,[332] and in still another study, β_2-M and CRP were significant factors.[333] In a nonrandomized retrospective study it was suggested that patients with high PCLI benefited from HDT but that patients with high β_2-M did not.[334] Plasmablastic morphology remains a predictor of very poor survival despite HDT,[254] as does conventional cytogenetic determination of abnormal chromosomes, as well as high PCLI.[286] Del 13 and 11q abnormalities have been singled out.[153] Del 13 can be found in only a small proportion of cases. It may be that any chromosome abnormality is significant because it reflects a higher PCLI.[286] While del 13 by FISH and high β_2-M have been associated with a poor prognosis in one series of patients, the follow-up time was short and a large study with a longer follow-up period and assessment of other FISH abnormalities needs to be performed.[327] A high number of circulating monoclonal plasma cells in the blood also remains a predictor of poor survival after HDT.[335]

Future Studies

Newly proposed prognostic factors in myeloma must be regarded as preliminary. Only a minority of studies have sufficient numbers to demonstrate independent risk factors. Only immunocytochemistry to detect the novel drug-resistant lung resistance protein satisfactorily predicts which patients will fail to respond to treatment. This is unfortunate because these high-risk patients may be prime candidates for new investigational therapies.

What is needed is comprehensive studies in association with clinical trials and an international consensus. This would allow comparison of effects of treatment in large numbers of patients, with shorter accrual times for high-risk patients. Standardized treatment regimens allow one to test the hypothesis that a new treatment can alter the course of patients with a particularly unfavorable prognostic factor. This approach augments the yield of the treatment trial at minimal cost if it identifies a superior treatment for a particular subset of patients. We are currently engaged in performing a battery of prognostic studies in a large ECOG conventional-dose chemotherapy trial and in the intergroup HDT trial. In an ECOG phase III trial, preliminary results identify PCLI, β_2-M, percent plasma cells from the PCLI assay but not from the bone marrow aspirate, sIL-6R, and CRP as independent prognostic factors suitable for developing an improved classification system.[305] Plasmablastic morphology is also significant.[255]

When new prognostic factors are examined, they should be demonstrated to be independently prognostic as compared with previous independent prognostic factors. Independent prognostic factors derived from multivariate analysis can potentially be combined to provide better prognostic staging systems. A classification derived in this manner is likely to yield the best distinction between good and poor prognosis groups for stratification in clinical trials and to test new hypotheses about the efficacy of the ability of new, intensive, and biologic treatments to effect outcomes in myeloma patients at higher risk. New prognostic factors should be shown to be reproducible from trial to trial and institution to institution and over time before they are accepted as universal prognostic factors.

Soluble receptors that are measurable in serum are attractive because of their biologic significance and the accessibility of serum. Of these, serum syndecan or CD138 is particularly promising.[144]

Future studies should not just focus on markers that are simply measures of tumor cell mass or cell proliferation. Loss of apoptosis marked by bcl-2 or Bcl-XL expression may provide added prognostic power independent of measures of cell proliferation in tumor mass. Drug-resistant markers such as LRP may prove useful in prognostic studies.[168]

In the future, it is clear that the way will be led by molecular prognostic indicators, including FISH detection of heavy chain illegitimate switch translocations involving chromosome 14, del 13, loss of p53, ras mutations, and c-myc. It is likely that proliferation assays such as the PCLI or new flow-cytometric S-phase methods will likely retain their independent prognostic significance, along with some serum markers such as β_2-M and perhaps a new marker such as serum syndecan.

In conclusion, the best independent prognostic factors available for patients with myeloma at this time include the PCLI and serum β_2-M level along with plasmablastic morphology. Conventional cytogenetic abnormalities also are good prognostic indicators but are present in a minority of patients, and they are likely simple reflections of cell proliferation assays. Chromosomal and molecular abnormalities detected by FISH will likely supplant conventional cytogenetics. Eventually, easier, more widely applicable S-phase assays will replace the PCLI. New technologies such as cDNA array, oncogene expression, and cell signaling assays will improve identification of patients who are more likely to respond to a particular regimen or who might better be treated with investigational therapy. Cytokines and their soluble receptors, serum syndecan, circulating myeloma cells and their precursors, and markers of apoptosis and drug resistance round off the list of prognostic factors that need to be investigated. Meanwhile, an international consensus is needed on a prognostic index in MM that can be universally available and accepted.

ACKNOWLEDGMENT

This work was supported by U.S. Public Health Service Grant CA62242 and Grant CA21115 from the National Cancer Institute.

REFERENCES

1. Kyle RA: Diagnostic criteria of multiple myeloma. Hematol Oncol Clin North Am 6:347–58, 1992.
2. Bataille R, Manolagas SC, Berenson JR: Pathogenesis and management of bone lesions in multiple myeloma. Hematol Oncol Clin North Am 11:349–61, 1997.
3. Clark AD, Shetty A, Soutar R: Renal failure and multiple myeloma: Pathogenesis and treatment of renal failure and management of underlying myeloma [review, 116 refs]. Blood Rev 13:79–90, 1999.
4. Kyle RA: Monoclonal proteins and renal disease. Annu Rev Med 45:71–7, 1994.
5. Kay NE, Leong T, Bone N et al: T-helper phenotypes in the blood of myeloma patients on ECOG phase III trials E9486/E3A93. Br J Haematol 100:459–63, 1998.
6. Dalton WS, Jove R: Drug resistance in multiple myeloma: Approaches to circumvention. Semin Oncol 26:23–7, 1999.
7. Greipp PR: Prognosis in myeloma. Mayo Clin Proc 69:895–902, 1994.
8. Kay NE, Leong TL, Bone N et al: Blood levels of immune cells predict survival in myeloma patients: Results of an Eastern Cooperative Oncology Group phase 3 trial for newly diagnosed multiple myeloma patients. Blood 98:23–8, 2001.
9. Kyle RA, Rajkumar SV: Monoclonal gammopathies of undetermined significance. Hematol Oncol Clin North Am 13:1181–202, 1999.
10. Kyle RA: Monoclonal gammopathy of undetermined significance. Blood Rev 8:135–41, 1994.
11. Oken MM, Leong T, Lenhard RE Jr et al: The addition of interferon or high dose cyclophosphamide to standard chemotherapy in the treatment of patients with multiple myeloma: Phase III Eastern Cooperative Oncology Group Clinical Trial EST 9486. Cancer 86:957–68, 1999.
12. Kyle RA, Greipp PR: Smoldering multiple myeloma. N Engl J Med 302:1347–9, 1980.
13. Weber DM, Dimopoulos MA, Moulopoulos LA et al: Prognostic features of asymptomatic multiple myeloma. Br J Haematol 97:810–4, 1997.
14. Greipp PR: Prognosis in myeloma [Review]. Mayo Clin Proc 69:895–902, 1994.

15. Baldini L, Guffanti A, Cesana BM et al: Role of different hematologic variables in defining the risk of malignant transformation in monoclonal gammopathy. Blood 87:912–8, 1996.

16. Vuckovic J, Ilic A, Knezevic N et al: Prognosis in monoclonal gammopathy of undetermined significance. Br J Haematol 97:649–51, 1997.

17. Kyle RA: Multiple myeloma: review of 869 cases. Mayo Clin Proc 50:29–40, 1975.

18. Alexanian R, Barlogie B, Dixon D: Prognosis of asymptomatic multiple myeloma. Arch Intern Med 148:1963–5, 1988.

19. Alexanian R: Localized and indolent myeloma. Blood 56:521–5, 1980.

20. Facon T, Menard JF, Michaux JL et al: Prognostic factors in low tumour mass asymptomatic multiple myeloma: A report on 91 patients. The Groupe d'Etudes et de Recherche sur le Myelome (GERM). Am J Hematol 48:71–5, 1995.

21. Hjorth M, Hellquist L, Holmberg E et al: Initial versus deferred melphalan-prednisone therapy for asymptomatic multiple myeloma stage I – a randomized study. Myeloma Group of Western Sweden. Eur J Haematol 50:95–102, 1993.

22. Dimopoulos MA, Moulopoulos A, Delasalle K et al: Solitary plasmacytoma of bone and asymptomatic multiple myeloma. Hematol Oncol Clin North Am 6:359–69, 1992.

23. Wiltshaw E: The natural history of extramedullary plasmacytoma and its relation to solitary myeloma of bone and myelomatosis. Medicine (Baltimore) 55:217–38, 1976.

24. Lecouvet FE, Vande Berg BC, Malghem J et al: Magnetic resonance and computed tomography imaging in multiple myeloma. Semin Musculoskelet Radiol 5:43–55, 2001.

25. Greipp PR, Kyle RA: Clinical, morphological, and cell kinetic differences among multiple myeloma, monoclonal gammopathy of undetermined significance, and smoldering multiple myeloma. Blood 62:166–71, 1983.

26. Witzig TE, Kyle RA, O'Fallon WM et al: Detection of peripheral blood plasma cells as a predictor of disease course in patients with smouldering multiple myeloma. Br J Haematol 87:266–72, 1994.

27. Witzig TE, Gonchoroff NJ, Katzmann JA et al: Peripheral blood B cell labeling indices are a measure of disease activity in patients with monoclonal gammopathies. J Clin Oncol 6:1041–6, 1988.

28. Kyle RA, Beard CM, O'Fallon WM et al: Incidence of multiple myeloma in Olmsted County, Minnesota: 1978 through 1990, with a review of the trend since 1945. J Clin Oncol 12:1577–83, 1994.

29. Greipp PR, Witzig TE, Gonchoroff NJ: Immunofluorescent plasma cell labeling indices (LI) using a monoclonal antibody (BU-1). Am J Hematol 20:289–92, 1985.

30. Ng MH, Wong IH, Lo KW: DNA methylation changes and multiple myeloma [review with 62 refs]. Leuk Lymphoma 34:463–72, 1999.

31. Liu P, Leong T, Quam L et al: Activating mutations of N- and K-ras in multiple myeloma show different clinical associations: Analysis of the Eastern Cooperative Oncology Group Phase III Trial. Blood 88:2699–706, 1996.

32. Guillerm G, Gyan E, Wolowiec D et al: p16(INK4a) and p15(INK4b) gene methylations in plasma cells from monoclonal gammopathy of undetermined significance. Blood 98:244–6, 2001.

33. Avet-Loiseau H, Li JY, Godon C et al: P53 deletion is not a frequent event in multiple myeloma. Br J Haematol 106:717–9, 1999.

34. Fonseca R, Harrington D, Oken MM et al: Myeloma (MM) and the t(11;14)(q13;q32); increasing evidence for a biologically distinct subset of patients. Blood 96:547a, 2000.

35. Hoyer JD, Hanson CA, Fonseca R et al: The (11;14)(q13;q32) translocation in multiple myeloma. A morphologic and immunohistochemical study. Am J Clin Pathol 113:831–7, 2000.

36. Avet-Loiseau H, Facon T, Daviet A et al: 14q32 translocations and monosomy 13 observed in monoclonal gammopathy of undetermined significance delineate a multistep process for the oncogenesis of multiple myeloma. Intergroupe Francophone du Myelome. Cancer Res 59:4546–50, 1999.

37. Fonseca R, Oken MM, Harrington D et al: Deletions of chromosome 13 in multiple myeloma identified by interphase FISH usually denote large deletions of the q arm or monosomy. Leukemia 15:981–6, 2001.

38. Thaler J, Fechner F, Herold M et al: Interleukin-6 in multiple myeloma: Correlation with disease activity and Ki-67 proliferation index. Leuk Lymphoma 12:265–71, 1994.

39. Schaar CG, Kaiser U, Snijder S et al: Serum interleukin-6 has no discriminatory role in paraproteinaemia nor a prognostic role in multiple myeloma. Br J Haematol 107:132–8, 1999.

40. Greipp PR, Lust JA, O'Fallon WM et al: Plasma cell labeling index and beta 2-microglobulin predict survival independent of thymidine kinase and C-reactive protein in multiple myeloma [see comments]. Blood 81:3382–7, 1993.

41. Mathew P, Ahmann GJ, Witzig TE et al: Clinicopathological correlates of CD56 expression in multiple myeloma: A unique entity?. Br J Haematol 90:459–61, 1995.

42. Almeida J, Orfao A, Mateo G et al: Immunophenotypic and DNA content characteristics of plasma cells in multiple myeloma and monoclonal gammopathy of undetermined significance. Pathol Biol (Paris) 47:119–27, 1999.

43. Garcia-Sanz R, Orfao A, Gonzalez M et al: Primary plasma cell leukemia: Clinical, immunophenotypic, DNA ploidy, and cytogenetic characteristics [see comments]. Blood 93:1032–7, 1999.

44. Ishikawa H, Kawano MM: Biological significance of heterogeneity in human myeloma cells [review]. Int J Hematol 68:363–370, 1998.

45. Witzig TE: The role of adhesion receptors in the pathogenesis of multiple myeloma. Hematol Oncol Clin North Am 13:1127–43, 1999.

46. Lust JA, Donovan KA: The role of interleukin-1 beta in the pathogenesis of multiple myeloma. Hematol Oncol Clin North Am 13:1117–25, 1999.

47. Han JH, Choi SJ, Kurihara N et al: Macrophage inflammatory protein-1 alpha is an osteoclastogenic factor in myeloma that is independent of receptor activator of nuclear factor κB ligand. Blood 97:3349–53, 2001.

48. Roodman GD: Biology of osteoclast activation in cancer. J Clin Oncol 19:3562–71, 2001.

49. Sordillo EM, Wong BR, Liau DF et al: Multiple myeloma disrupts the TRANCE/OPG cytokine axis. Blood 96:549a, 2000.

50. Choi Y, Woo KM, Ko SH et al: Osteoclastogenesis is enhanced by activated B cells but suppressed by activated CD8(+) T cells. Eur J Immunol 31:2179–88, 2001.

51. Nachbaur DM, Herold M, Maneschg A et al: Serum levels of interleukin-6 in multiple myeloma and other hematological disorders: Correlation with disease activity and other prognostic parameters. Ann Hematol 62:54–8, 1991.

52. Carter A, Merchav S, Silvian-Draxler I et al: The role of interleukin-1 and tumour necrosis factor-alpha in human multiple myeloma. Br J Haematol 74:424–31, 1990.

53. Sjak-Shie NN, Vescio RA, Berenson JR: The role of human herpesvirus-8 in the pathogenesis of multiple myeloma. Hematol Oncol Clin North Am 13:1159–67, 1999.

54. Mongkonsritragoon W, Kyle RA, Shreck RR et al: Primary plasmacytoma at the site of exit wounds after electrical injury. Am J Hematol 58:77–9, 1998.

55. Vacca A, Ribatti D, Roncali L et al: Bone marrow angiogenesis and progression in multiple myeloma. Br J Haematol 87:503–8, 1994.

56. Rajkumar SV, Leong T, Roche PC et al: Prognostic value of bone marrow angiogenesis in multiple myeloma. Clin Cancer Res 6:3111–6, 2000.

57. Podar K, Tai YT, Davies FE et al: Vascular endothelial growth factor triggers signaling cascades mediating multiple myeloma cell growth and migration. Blood 98:428–35, 2001.

58. Sezer O, Jakob C, Eucker J et al: Serum levels of the angiogenic cytokines basic fibroblast growth factor (bFGF), vascular endothelial growth factor (VEGF) and hepatocyte growth factor (HGF) in multiple myeloma. Eur J Haematol 66:83–8, 2001.

59. Di Raimondo F, Azzaro MP, Palumbo G et al: Angiogenic factors in multiple myeloma: Higher levels in bone marrow than in peripheral blood. Haematologica 85:800–5, 2000.

60. Riccardi A, Ucci G, Luoni R et al: Bone marrow biopsy in monoclonal gammopathies: Correlations between pathological findings and clinical data. The Cooperative Group for Study and Treatment of Multiple Myeloma. J Clin Pathol 43:469–75, 1990.

61. Greipp PR, Raymond NM, Kyle RA et al: Multiple myeloma: Significance of plasmablastic subtype in morphological classification. Blood 65:305–10, 1985.

62. Boccadoro M, Gavarotti P, Fossati G et al: Low plasma cell 3(H) thymidine incorporation in monoclonal gammopathy of undetermined significance (MGUS), smouldering myeloma and remission phase myeloma: A reliable indicator of patients not requiring therapy. Br J Haematol 58:689–96, 1984.

63. Greipp PR, Witzig TE, Gonchoroff NJ et al: Immunofluorescence labeling indices in myeloma and related monoclonal gammopathies. Mayo Clin Proc 62:969–77, 1987.

64. Büchi G, Girotto M, Veglio M et al: Kappa/lambda ratio on peripheral blood lymphocytes and bone marrow plasma cell labeling index in monoclonal gammopathies. Haematologica 75:132–6, 1990.

65. Büchi G, Veglio M, Reviglione G et al: The discriminating analysis in the differential diagnosis of monoclonal gammopathies. Pathologica 85:175–81, 1993.

66. Leo R, Boeker M, Peest D et al: Multiparameter analyses of normal and malignant human plasma cells: CD38++, CD56+, CD54+, cIg+ is the common phenotype of myeloma cells. Ann Hematol 64:132–9, 1992.

67. Ahsmann EJ, Lokhorst HM, Dekker AW et al: Lymphocyte function-associated antigen-1 expression on plasma cells correlates with tumor growth in multiple myeloma. Blood 79:2068–75, 1992.

68. Witzig TE, Timm M, Larson D et al: Measurement of apoptosis and proliferation of bone marrow plasma cells in patients with plasma cell proliferative disorders. Br J Haematol 104:131–137, 1999.

69. Girino M, Riccardi A, Luoni R et al: Monoclonal antibody Ki-67 as a marker of proliferative activity in monoclonal gammopathies. Acta Haematol 85:26–30, 1991.

70. Pope B, Brown R, Gibson J et al: The bone marrow plasma cell labeling index by flow cytometry. Cytometry 38:286–92, 1999.

71. Trendle MC, Leong T, Kyle RA et al: Prognostic significance of the S-phase fraction of light-chain-restricted cytoplasmic immunoglobulin (cIg) positive plasma cells in patients with newly diagnosed multiple myeloma enrolled on Eastern Cooperative Oncology Group treatment trial E9486. Am J Hematol 61:232–7, 1999.

72. Ladanyi M, Wang S, Niesvizky R et al: Proto-oncogene analysis in multiple myeloma. Am J Pathol 141:949–53, 1992.

73. Miguel-Garcia A, Orero T, Matutes E et al: Bcl-2 expression in plasma cells from neoplastic gammopathies and reactive plasmacytosis: a comparative study. Haematologica 83:298–304, 1998.

74. Jourdan M, De Vos J, Mechti N et al: Regulation of Bcl-2-family proteins in myeloma cells by three myeloma survival factors: Interleukin-6, interferon-alpha and insulin-like growth factor 1. Cell Death Differ 7:1244–52, 2000.

75. Cheung WC, Van Ness B: The bone marrow stromal microenvironment influences myeloma therapeutic response in vitro. Leukemia 15:264–71, 2001.

76. Renner S, Weisz J, Krajewski S et al: Expression of BAX in plasma cell dyscrasias. Clin Cancer Res 6:2371–80, 2000.

77. Witzig TE, Kyle RA, Greipp PR: Circulating peripheral blood plasma cells in multiple myeloma. Curr Top Microbiol Immunol 182:195–9, 1992.

78. Billadeau D, Van Ness B, Kimlinger T et al: Clonal circulating cells are common in plasma cell proliferative disorders: A comparison of monoclonal gammopathy of undetermined significance, smoldering multiple myeloma, and active myeloma. Blood 88:289–96, 1996.

79. Witzig TE, Meyers C, Therneau T et al: A prospective study of CD38/45 flow cytometry and immunofluorescence microscopy to detect blood plasma cells in patients with plasma cell proliferative disorders. Leuk Lymphoma 38:345–50, 2000.

80. Zandecki M, Bernardi F, Genevieve F et al: Involvement of peripheral blood cells in multiple myeloma: Chromosome changes are the rule within circulating plasma cells but not within B lymphocytes. Leukemia 11:1034–9, 1997.

81. Fend F, Weyrer K, Drach J et al: Immunoglobulin gene rearrangement in plasma cell dyscrasias: Detection of small clonal cell populations in peripheral blood and bone marrow. Leuk Lymphoma 10:223–9, 1993.

82. Goto H, Shimazaki C, Ashihara E et al: Effects of interleukin-3 and interleukin-6 on peripheral blood cells from multiple myeloma patients and their clinical significance. Acta Haematol 88:129–35, 1992.

83. Bataille R, Duperray C, Zhang XG et al: CD5 B lymphocyte antigen in monoclonal gammopathy. Am J Hematol 41:102–6, 1992.

84. Kay NE, Leong T, Kyle RA et al: Circulating blood B cells in multiple myeloma: Analysis and relationship to circulating clonal cells and clinical parameters in a cohort of patients entered on the Eastern Cooperative Oncology Group phase III E9486 clinical trial. Blood 90:340–5, 1997.

85. Jensen GS, Mant MJ, Belch AJ et al: Selective expression of CD45 isoforms defines CALLA+ monoclonal B-lineage cells in peripheral blood from myeloma patients as late stage B cells. Blood 78:711–9, 1991.

86. Jensen GS, Belch AR, Kherani F et al: Restricted expression of immunoglobulin light chain mRNA and of the adhesion molecule CD11b on circulating monoclonal B lineage cells in peripheral blood of myeloma patients. Scand J Immunol 36:843–53, 1992.

87. Bergsagel PL, Smith AM, Szczepek A et al: In multiple myeloma, clonotypic B lymphocytes are detectable among CD19+ peripheral blood cells expressing CD38, CD56, and monotypic Ig light chain [published erratum appears in Blood 1995 Jun 1;85(11):3365]. Blood 85:436–47, 1995.

88. Pilarski LM, Hipperson G, Seeberger K et al: Myeloma progenitors in the blood of patients with aggressive or minimal disease: Engraftment and self-renewal of primary human myeloma in the bone marrow of NOD SCID mice. Blood 95:1056–65, 2000.

89. Omede P, Boccadoro M, Gallone G et al: Multiple myeloma: Increased circulating lymphocytes carrying plasma cell-associated antigens as an indicator of poor survival. Blood 76:1375–9, 1990.

90. Oritani K, Katagiri S, Tominaga N et al: Aberrant expression of immunoglobulin light chain isotype in B lymphocytes from patients with monoclonal gammopathies: Isotypic discordance and clonal B-cell excess. Br J Haematol 75:10–5, 1990.

91. Billadeau D, Quam L, Thomas W et al: Detection and quantitation of malignant cells in the peripheral blood of multiple myeloma patients. Blood 80:1818–24, 1992.

92. Billadeau D, Ahmann G, Greipp P et al: The bone marrow of multiple myeloma patients contains B cell populations at different stages of differentiation that are clonally related to the malignant plasma cell. J Exp Med 178:1023–31, 1993.

93. Bakkus MH, Asosingh K, Vanderkerken K et al: Myeloma isotype-switch variants in the murine 5T myeloma model: Evidence that myeloma IgM and IgA expressing subclones can originate from the IgG expressing tumour. Leukemia 15:1127–32, 2001.

94. Nordan RP, Mock BA, Neckers LM et al: The role of plasmacytoma growth factor in the in vitro responses of murine plasmacytoma cells. Ann N Y Acad Sci 557:200–5, 1989.

95. Klein B: Cytokines, cytokine receptors and oncogenes in human multiple myeloma (Meeting abstract). International Conference on Multiple Myeloma, from Biology to Therapy Current Concepts (October 1994).

96. Klein B, Zhang XG, Jourdan M et al: Paracrine rather than autocrine regulation of myeloma-cell growth and differentiation by interleukin-6. Blood 73:517–26, 1989.

97. Klein B, Bataille R: Cytokine network in human multiple myeloma. Hematol Oncol Clin North Am 6:273–84, 1992.

98. Kawano M, Hirano T, Matsuda T et al: Autocrine generation and requirement of BSF-2/IL-6 for human multiple myelomas. Nature 332:83–5, 1988.

99. Nishimoto N, Ogata A, Shima Y et al: Oncostatin M, leukemia inhibitory factor, and interleukin 6 induce the proliferation of human plasmacytoma cells via the common signal transducer, gp130. J Exp Med 179:1343–7, 1994.

100. Portier M, Zhang XG, Ursule E et al: Cytokine gene expression in human multiple myeloma. Br J Haematol 85:514–20, 1993.

101. Hata H, Xiao H, Petrucci MT et al: Interleukin-6 gene expression in multiple myeloma: A characteristic of immature tumor cells. Blood 81:3357–64, 1993.

102. Bataille R, Barlogie B, Lu ZY et al: Biologic effects of anti-interleukin-6 murine monoclonal antibody in advanced multiple myeloma. Blood 86:685–91, 1995.

103. Lust JA, Jelinek DF, Donovan KA et al: Sequence, expression and function of an mRNA encoding a soluble form of the human interleukin-6 receptor (sIL-6R). Curr Top Microbiol Immunol 194:199–206, 1995.

104. Taetle R, Dos Santos B, Ohsugi Y et al: Effects of combined anti-growth factor receptor treatment on in vitro growth of multiple myeloma. J Natl Cancer Inst 86:450–5, 1994.

105. Sato K, Tsuchiya M, Saldanha J et al: Reshaping a human antibody to inhibit the interleukin 6-dependent tumor cell growth. Cancer Res 53:851–6, 1993.

106. Solary E, Guiguet M, Zeller V et al: Radioimmunoassay for the measurement of serum IL-6 and its correlation with tumour cell mass parameters in multiple myeloma. Am J Hematol 39:163–71, 1992.

107. Merico F, Bergui L, Gregoretti MG et al: Cytokines involved in the progression of multiple myeloma. Clin Exp Immunol 92:27–31, 1993.

108. Bataille R, Chappard D, Marcelli C et al: Recruitment of new osteoblasts and osteoclasts is the earliest critical event in the pathogenesis of human multiple myeloma. J Clin Invest 88:62–6, 1991.

109. Zhang XG, Klein B, Bataille R: Interleukin-6 is a potent myeloma-cell growth factor in patients with aggressive multiple myeloma. Blood 74:11–3, 1989.

110. Van Riet I, De Greef C, Aharchi F et al: Establishment and characterization of a human stroma-dependent myeloma cell line

(MM5.1) and its stroma-independent variant (MM5.2). Leukemia 11:284–93, 1997.

111. Ge NL, Rudikoff S: Insulin-like growth factor I is a dual effector of multiple myeloma cell growth. Blood 96:2856–61, 2000.

112. Asosingh K, Gunthert U, Bakkus MH et al: In vivo induction of insulin-like growth factor-I receptor and CD44v6 confers homing and adhesion to murine multiple myeloma cells. Cancer Res 60:3096–104, 2000.

113. Hjorth-Hansen H, Waage A, Borset M: Interleukin-15 blocks apoptosis and induces proliferation of the human myeloma cell line OH-2 and freshly isolated myeloma cells. Br J Haematol 106:28–34, 1999.

114. Vanderkerken K, Asosingh K, Braet F et al: Insulin-like growth factor-1 acts as a chemoattractant factor for 5T2 multiple myeloma cells. Blood 93:235–41, 1999.

115. Jelinek DF, Witzig TE, Arendt BK: A role for insulin-like growth factor in the regulation of IL-6-responsive human myeloma cell line growth. J Immunol 159:487–96, 1997.

116. Georgii-Hemming P, Wiklund HJ, Ljunggren O et al: Insulin-like growth factor I is a growth and survival factor in human multiple myeloma cell lines. Blood 88:2250–8, 1996.

117. Freund GG, Kulas DT, Way BA et al: Functional insulin and insulin-like growth factor-1 receptors are preferentially expressed in multiple myeloma cell lines as compared to B-lymphoblastoid cell lines. Cancer Res 54:3179–85, 1994.

118. Osterborg A, Yi Q, Bergenbrant S et al: Idiotype-specific T cells in multiple myeloma stage I: An evaluation by four different functional tests. Br J Haematol 89:110–6, 1995.

119. Vacca A, Di Stefano R, Frassanito A et al: A disturbance of the IL-2/IL-2 receptor system parallels the activity of multiple myeloma. Clin Exp Immunol 84:429–34, 1991.

120. Gazitt Y, Shaughnessy P, Montgomery W: Apoptosis-induced by TRAIL and TNF-alpha in human multiple myeloma cells is not blocked by BCL-2. Cytokine 11:1010–9, 1999.

121. Usnarska-Zubkiewicz L: Level of interleukin-6 (IL-6), soluble interleukin-6 receptors (sIL-6R) and tumor necrosis factor alpha (TNF-alpha) in untreated and progressing multiple myeloma (in Polish). Pol Arch Med Wewn 99:30–7, 1998.

122. Filella X, Blade J, Guillermo AL et al: Cytokines (IL-6, TNF-α, IL-lα) and soluble interleukin-2 receptor as serum tumor markers in multiple myeloma. Cancer Detect Prev 20:52–6, 1996.

123. Hideshima T, Chauhan D, Schlossman R et al: The role of tumor necrosis factor alpha in the pathophysiology of human multiple myeloma: Therapeutic applications. Oncogene 20:4519–27, 2001

124. Massaia M, Attisano C, Peola S et al: Rapid generation of antiplasma cell activity in the bone marrow of myeloma patients by CD3-activated T cells. Blood 82:1787–97, 1993.

125. Davies FE, Raje N, Hideshima T et al: Thalidomide and immunomodulatory derivatives augment natural killer cell cytotoxicity in multiple myeloma. Blood 98:210–6, 2001.

126. Cook G, Campbell JD, Carr CE et al: Transforming growth factor beta from multiple myeloma cells inhibits proliferation and IL-2 responsiveness in T lymphocytes. J Leukoc Biol 66:981–8, 1999.

127. Eaves CJ, Cashman JD, Kay RJ et al: Mechanisms that regulate the cell cycle status of very primitive hematopoietic cells in long-term human marrow cultures. II. Analysis of positive and negative regulators produced by stromal cells within the adherent layer. Blood 78:110–7, 1991.

128. Lichtenstein A, Berenson J, Norman D et al: Production of cytokines by bone marrow cells obtained from patients with multiple myeloma. Blood 74:1266–73, 1989.

129. Cozzolino F, Torcia M, Aldinucci D et al: Production of interleukin-1 by bone marrow myeloma cells. Blood 74:380–7, 1989.

130. Costes V, Portier M, Lu ZY et al: Interleukin-1 in multiple myeloma: producer cells and their role in the control of IL-6 production. Br J Haematol 103:1152–60, 1998.

131. Hawley TS, Lach B, Burns BF et al: Expression of retrovirally transduced IL-1 alpha in IL-6-dependent B cells: A murine model of aggressive multiple myeloma. Growth Factors 5:327–38, 1991.

132. Hawley RG, Wang MH, Fong AZ et al: Association between ICAM-1 expression and metastatic capacity of murine B-cell hybridomas. Clin Exp Metastasis 11:213–26, 1993.

133. Lacy MQ, Donovan KA, Heimbach JK et al: Comparison of interleukin-1 beta expression by in situ hybridization in monoclonal gammopathy of undetermined significance and multiple myeloma. Blood 93:300–5, 1999.

134. Sawamura M, Sakura T, Miyawaki S: Exacerbation of monoclonal gammopathy in a patient treated with G-CSF. Ann Intern Med 118:318, 1993.

135. Celsing F, Hast R, Stenke L et al: Extramedullary progression of multiple myeloma following GM-CSF treatment – grounds for caution? Eur J Haematol 49:108, 1992.

136. Juge-Morineau N, Francois S, Puthier D et al: The gp130 family cytokines IL-6, LIF and OSM but not IL-11 can reverse the antiproliferative effect of dexamethasone on human myeloma cells. Br J Haematol 90:707–10, 1995.

137. Gooding RP, Bybee A, Cooke F et al: Phenotypic and molecular analysis of six human cell lines derived from patients with plasma cell dyscrasia. Br J Haematol 106:669–81, 1999.

138. Okuno Y, Takahashi T, Suzuki A et al: Expression of the erythropoietin receptor on a human myeloma cell line. Biochem Biophys Res Commun 170:1128–34, 1990.

139. Borset M, Seidel C, Hjorth-Hansen H et al: The role of hepatocyte growth factor and its receptor c-Met in multiple myeloma and other blood malignancies. Leuk Lymphoma 32:249–256, 1999.

140. Feliers D, Woodruff K, Abboud S: Potential role of insulin-like growth factor binding protein-4 in the uncoupling of bone turnover in multiple myeloma. Br J Haematol 104:715–22, 1999.

141. Gaillard JP, Bataille R, Brailly H et al: Increased and highly stable levels of functional soluble interleukin-6 receptor in sera of patients with monoclonal gammopathy. Eur J Immunol 23:820–4, 1993.

142. Tamura T, Udagawa N, Takahashi N et al: Soluble interleukin-6 receptor triggers osteoclast formation by interleukin 6. Proc Natl Acad Sci U S A 90:11924–8, 1993.

143. Karadag A, Scutt AM, Croucher PI: Human myeloma cells promote the recruitment of osteoblast precursors: Mediation by interleukin-6 and soluble interleukin-6 receptor. J Bone Miner Res 15:1935–43, 2000.

144. Seidel C, Sundan A, Hjorth M et al: Serum syndecan-1: A new independent prognostic marker in multiple myeloma. Blood 95:388–92, 2000.

145. Dhodapkar MV, Kelly T, Theus A et al: Elevated levels of shed syndecan-1 correlate with tumour mass and decreased matrix metalloproteinase-9 activity in the serum of patients with multiple myeloma. Br J Haematol 99:368–71, 1997.

146. Ong F, Kaiser U, Seelen PJ et al: Serum neural cell adhesion molecule differentiates multiple myeloma from paraproteinemias due to other causes. Blood 87:712–6, 1996.

147. Mathiot C, Galon J, Tartour E et al: Soluble CD16 in plasma cell dyscrasias. Leuk Lymphoma 32:467–474, 1999.

148. Dankbar B, Padro T, Leo R et al: Vascular endothelial growth factor and interleukin-6 in paracrine tumor–stromal cell interactions in multiple myeloma. Blood 95:2630–6, 2000.

149. Choi SJ, Cruz JC, Craig F et al: Macrophage inflammatory protein 1-alpha is a potential osteoclast stimulatory factor in multiple myeloma. Blood 96:671–5, 2000.

150. Barille S, Akhoundi C, Collette M et al: Metalloproteinases in multiple myeloma: Production of matrix metalloproteinase-9 (MMP-9), activation of proMMP-2, and induction of MMP-1 by myeloma cells. Blood 90:1649–55, 1997.

151. Vincent T, Jourdan M, Sy MS et al: Hyaluronic acid induces survival and proliferation of human myeloma cells through an interleukin-6-mediated pathway involving the phosphorylation of retinoblastoma protein. J Biol Chem 276:14728–36, 2001.

152. Seong C, Delasalle K, Hayes K et al: Prognostic value of cytogenetics in multiple myeloma. Br J Haematol 101:189–94, 1998.

153. Tricot G, Sawyer JR, Jagannath S et al: Unique role of cytogenetics in the prognosis of patients with myeloma receiving high-dose therapy and autotransplants. J Clin Oncol 15:2659–66, 1997.

154. Rajkumar SV, Fonseca R, Dewald GW et al: Cytogenetic abnormalities correlate with the plasma cell labeling index and extent of bone marrow involvement in myeloma. Cancer Genet Cytogenet 113:73–7, 1999.

155. Perez-Simon JA, Garcia-Sanz R, Tabernero MD et al: Prognostic value of numerical chromosome aberrations in multiple myeloma: A FISH analysis of 15 different chromosomes. Blood 91:3366–71, 1998.

156. Zojer N, Konigsberg R, Ackermann J et al: Deletion of 13q14 remains an independent adverse prognostic variable in multiple myeloma despite its frequent detection by interphase fluorescence in situ hybridization. Multicenter Investigation of Bone Marrow Transplantation for Sickle Cell Disease. Blood 95:1925–30, 2000.

157. Konigsberg R, Ackermann J, Kaufmann H et al: Deletions of chromosome 13q in monoclonal gammopathy of undetermined significance. Leukemia 14:1975–9, 2000.

158. Avet-Loiseau H, Li JY, Morineau N et al: Monosomy 13 is associated with the transition of monoclonal gammopathy of undetermined significance to multiple myeloma. Intergroupe Francophone du Myelome. Blood 94:2583–9, 1999.

159. Chesi M, Kuehl WM, Bergsagel PL: Recurrent immunoglobulin gene translocations identify distinct molecular subtypes of myeloma [Review, 16 refs]. Ann Oncol 11(Suppl. 1):131–5, 2000.

160. Shaughnessy J Jr, Gabrea A, Qi Y et al: Cyclin D3 at 6p21 is dysregulated by recurrent chromosomal translocations to immunoglobulin loci in multiple myeloma. Blood 98:217–23, 2001.

161. Ronchetti D, Greco A, Compasso S et al: Deregulated FGFR3 mutants in multiple myeloma cell lines with t(4;14): Comparative analysis of Y373C, K650E and the novel G384D mutations. Oncogene 20:3553–62, 2001.

162. Shou Y, Martelli ML, Gabrea A et al: Diverse karyotypic abnormalities of the c-myc locus associated with c-myc dysregulation and tumor progression in multiple myeloma. Proc Nat Acad Sci U S A 97:228–33, 2000.

163. Matozaki S, Nakagawa T, Nakao Y et al: RAS gene mutations in multiple myeloma and related monoclonal gammopathies. Kobe J Med Sci 37:35–45, 1991.

164. DuVillard L, Guiguet M, Casasnovas RO et al: Diagnostic value of serum IL-6 level in monoclonal gammopathies [see comments]. Br J Haematol 89:243–9, 1995.

165. Portier M, Moles JP, Mazars GR et al: p53 and RAS gene mutations in multiple myeloma. Oncogene 7:2539–43, 1992.

166. Kalakonda N, Rothwell DG, Scarffe JH et al: Detection of N-Ras codon 61 mutations in subpopulations of tumor cells in multiple myeloma at presentation. Blood 98:1555–60, 2001.

167. Schultheis B, Kramer A, Willer A et al: Analysis of p73 and p53 gene deletions in multiple myeloma. Leukemia 13:2099–103, 1999.

168. Filipits M, Drach J, Pohl G et al: Expression of the lung resistance protein predicts poor outcome in patients with multiple myeloma. Clin Cancer Res 5:2426–2430, 1999.

169. Brown RD, Pope B, Luo XF et al: The oncoprotein phenotype of plasma cells from patients with multiple myeloma. Leuk Lymphoma 16:147–56, 1994.

170. Miguelgarcia A, Orero T, Matutes E et al: Bcl-2 expression in plasma cells from neoplastic gammopathies and reactive plasmacytosis – a comparative study. Haematologica 83:298–304, 1998.

171. Gauthier ER, Piche L, Lemieux G et al: Role of bcl-X(L) in the control of apoptosis in murine myeloma cells. Cancer Res 56:1451–6, 1996.

172. Gaillard JP, Mani JC, Liautard J et al: Interleukin-6 receptor signaling. I. gp80 and gp130 receptor interaction in the absence of interleukin-6. Eur Cytokine Netw 10:43–8, 1999.

173. Gaillard JP, Liautard J, Klein B et al: Major role of the soluble interleukin-6/interleukin-6 receptor complex for the proliferation of interleukin-6-dependent human myeloma cell lines. Eur J Immunol 27:3332–40, 1997.

174. Hallek M, Neumann C, Schaffer M et al: Signal transduction of interleukin-6 involves tyrosine phosphorylation of multiple cytosolic proteins and activation of Src-family kinases Fyn, Hck, and Lyn in multiple myeloma cell lines. Exp Hematol 25:1367–77, 1997.

175. Ogata A, Chauhan D, Teoh G et al: IL-6 triggers cell growth via the Ras-dependent mitogen-activated protein kinase cascade. J Immunol 159:2212–21, 1997.

176. Rawat R, Rainey GJ, Thompson CD et al: Constitutive activation of STAT3 is associated with the acquisition of an interleukin-6-independent phenotype by murine plasmacytomas and hybridomas. Blood 96:3514–21, 2000.

177. Westendorf JJ, Ahmann GJ, Armitage RJ et al: CD40 expression in malignant plasma cells. Role in stimulation of autocrine IL-6 secretion by a human myeloma cell line. J Immunol 152:117–28, 1994.

178. Pellat-Deceunynck C, Bataille R, Puthier D et al: Evolution of plasma cell phenotype during the different phases of malignancy (Meeting abstract). International Conference on Multiple Myeloma, from Biology to Therapy Current Concepts (October 1994).

179. Kawamura C, Kizaki M, Yamato K et al: Bone morphogenetic protein-2 induces apoptosis in human myeloma cells with modulation of STAT3. Blood 96:2005–11, 2000.

180. De Vos J, Jourdan M, Tarte K et al: JAK2 tyrosine kinase inhibitor tyrphostin AG490 downregulates the mitogen-activated protein kinase (MAPK) and signal transducer and activator of transcription (STAT) pathways and induces apoptosis in myeloma cells. Br J Haematol 109:823–8, 2000.

181. Arora T, Floyd-Smith G, Espy MJ et al: Dissociation between IFN-alpha-induced anti-viral and growth signaling pathways. J Immunol 162:3289–97, 1999.

182. Arora T, Jelinek DF: Differential myeloma cell responsiveness to interferon-alpha correlates with differential induction of p19(INK4d) and cyclin D2 expression. J Biol Chem 273:11799–805, 1998.

183. Xu FH, Sharma S, Gardner A et al: Interleukin-6-induced inhibition of multiple myeloma cell apoptosis: Support for the hypothesis that protection is mediated via inhibition of the JNK/SAPK pathway. Blood 92:241–51, 1998.

184. Anderson KC: Novel biologically based therapies for myeloma. Cancer J 7 (Suppl. 1):S19–23, 2001.

185. Van Camp B, Durie BG, Spier C et al: Plasma cells in multiple myeloma express a natural killer cell–associated antigen: CD56 (NKH-1; Leu-19). Blood 76:377–82, 1990.

186. Sonneveld P, Durie BG, Lokhorst HM et al: Analysis of multidrug-resistance (MDR-1) glycoprotein and CD56 expression to separate monoclonal gammopathy from multiple myeloma. Br J Haematol 83:63–7, 1993.

187. Almeida J, Orfao A, Mateo G et al: Immunophenotypic and DNA content characteristics of plasma cells in multiple myeloma and monoclonal gammopathy of undetermined significance [Review, 61 refs]. Pathol Biol (Paris) 47:119–27, 1999.

188. Harada H, Kawano MM, Huang N et al: Phenotypic difference of normal plasma cells from mature myeloma cells. Blood 81:2658–63, 1993.

189. Barker HF, Hamilton MS, Ball J et al: Expression of adhesion molecules LFA-3 and N-CAM on normal and malignant human plasma cells. Br J Haematol 81:331–5, 1992.

190. Uchiyama H, Barut BA, Mohrbacher AF et al: Adhesion of human myeloma-derived cell lines to bone marrow stromal cells stimulates interleukin-6 secretion. Blood 82:3712–20, 1993.

191. Michigami T, Shimizu N, Williams PJ et al: Cell-cell contact between marrow stromal cells and myeloma cells via VCAM-1 and alpha(4)beta(1)-integrin enhances production of osteoclast-stimulating activity. Blood 96:1953–60, 2000.

192. Okada T, Hawley RG, Kodaka M et al: Significance of VLA-4-VCAM-1 interaction and CD44 for transendothelial invasion in a bone marrow metastatic myeloma model. Clin Exp Metastasis 17:623–9, 1999.

193. Dehou MF, Schots R, Lacor P et al: Diagnostic and prognostic value of the MB2 monoclonal antibody in paraffin-embedded bone marrow sections of patients with multiple myeloma and monoclonal gammopathy of undetermined significance. Am J Clin Pathol 94:287–91, 1990.

194. Pilarski LM, Belch AR: Circulating monoclonal B cells expressing P glycoprotein may be a reservoir of multidrug-resistant disease in multiple myeloma. Blood 83:724–36, 1994.

195. Rawstron AC, Barrans SL, Blythe D et al: In multiple myeloma, only a single stage of neoplastic plasma cell differentiation can be identified by VLA-5 and CD45 expression. Br J Haematol 113:794–802, 2001.

196. Joshua D, Petersen A, Brown R et al: The labelling index of primitive plasma cells determines the clinical behaviour of patients with myelomatosis. Br J Haematol 94:76–81, 1996.

197. Kawano MM, Huang N, Harada H et al: Identification of immature and mature myeloma cells in the bone marrow of human myelomas. Blood 82:564–70, 1993.

198. Rajkumar SV, Greipp PR: Angiogenesis in multiple myeloma. Br J Haematol 113:565, 2001.

199. Rajkumar SV, Witzig TE: A review of angiogenesis and antiangiogenic therapy with thalidomide in multiple myeloma. Cancer Treat Rev 26:351–62, 2000.

200. Bellamy WT, Richter L, Frutiger Y et al: Expression of vascular endothelial growth factor and its receptors in hematopoietic malignancies. Cancer Res 59:728–33, 1999.

201. Vacca A, Frigeri A, Ribatti D et al: Microvessel overexpression of aquaporin 1 parallels bone marrow angiogenesis in patients with active multiple myeloma. Br J Haematol 113:415–21, 2001.

202. Xagoraris I, Paterakis G, Zolota B et al: Expression of granzyme B and perforin in multiple myeloma. Acta Haematol 105:125–9, 2001.

203. Cavanna L, Di Stasi M, Fornari F et al: T-cell subsets defined by monoclonal antibodies in monoclonal gammopathy of undetermined significance (MGUS). Tumori 71:543–6, 1985.

204. Vandenhove LE, Meeus P, Derom A et al: Lymphocyte profiles in multiple myeloma and monoclonal gammopathy of undetermined significance – flow-cytometric characterization and analysis in a two-dimensional correlation biplot. Ann Hematol 76:249–256, 1998.

205. Boccadoro M, Omede P, Massaia M et al: Human myeloma: Several subsets of circulating lymphocytes express plasma cell-associated antigens. Eur J Haematol 40:299–304, 1988.

206. Oken MM, Pomeroy C, Weisdorf D et al: Prophylactic antibiotics for the prevention of early infection in multiple myeloma. Am J Med 100:624–8, 1996.

207. Osterborg A, Masucci M, Bergenbrant S et al: Generation of T-cell clones binding F(ab')2 fragments of the idiotypic immunoglobulin in patients with monoclonal gammopathy. Cancer Immunol Immunother 34:157–162, 1991.

208. Berenson JR, Lichtenstein A, Hart S et al: Expression of shared idiotypes by paraproteins from patients with multiple myeloma and monoclonal gammopathy of undetermined significance. Blood 75:2107–11, 1990.

209. Janson CH, Grunewald J, Osterborg A et al: Predominant T cell receptor V gene usage in patients with abnormal clones of B cells. Blood 77:1776–80, 1991.

210. Kay N, Leong T, Kyle RA et al: Altered T cell repertoire usage in CD4 and CD8 subsets of multiple myeloma patients, a study of the Eastern Cooperative Oncology Group (E9487). Leuk Lymphoma 33:127–33, 1999.

211. Famularo G, D'Ambrosio A, Quintieri F et al: Natural killer cell frequency and function in patients with monoclonal gammopathies. J Clin Lab Immunol 37:99–109, 1992.

212. Massaia M, Bianchi A, Dianzani U et al: Defective interleukin-2 induction of lymphokine-activated killer (LAK) activity in peripheral blood T lymphocytes of patients with monoclonal gammopathies. Clin Exp Immunol 79:100–4, 1990.

213. Mellstedt H, Osterborg A: Active idiotype vaccination in multiple myeloma. GM-CSF may be an important adjuvant cytokine. Pathol Biol (Paris) 47:211–5, 1999.

214. Osterborg A, Henriksson L, Mellstedt H: Idiotype immunity (natural and vaccine-induced) in early stage multiple myeloma. Acta Oncol 39:797–800, 2000.

215. Ishiyama T, Watanabe K, Fukuchi K et al: The increase of CD5LOW+NK cells in patients with multiple myeloma and plasmacytoma. Anticancer Res 14:725–30, 1994.

216. Nielsen H, Nielsen HJ, Tvede N et al: Immune dysfunction in multiple myeloma. Reduced natural killer cell activity and increased levels of soluble interleukin-2 receptors. APMIS 99:340–6, 1991.

217. Lefrere JJ, Debbia M, Lambin P: Prospective follow-up of monoclonal gammopathies in HIV-infected individuals. Br J Haematol 84:151–5, 1993.

218. Ucci G, Riccardi A, Luoni R et al: Presenting features of monoclonal gammopathies: An analysis of 684 newly diagnosed cases. Cooperative Group for the Study and Treatment of Multiple Myeloma. J Intern Med 234:165–73, 1993.

219. Williams AT, Shearer MJ, Oyeyi J et al: Serum osteocalcin in the management of myeloma. Eur J Cancer 29A:140–2, 1992.

220. Boccadoro M, Battaglio S, Omede P et al: Increased serum neopterin concentration as indicator of disease severity and poor survival in multiple myeloma. Eur J Haemat 47:305–309, 1991.

221. Majumdar G, Hunt M, Singh AK: Use of leucocyte alkaline phosphatase (LAP) score in differentiating malignant from benign paraproteinaemias. J Clin Pathol 44:606–7, 1991.

222. Majumdar G, Heard SE, Singh AK: Use of cytoplasmic 5'-nucleotidase for differentiating malignant from benign monoclonal gammopathies. J Clin Pathol 43:891–2, 1990.

223. Bataille R, Boccadoro M, Klein B et al: C-Reactive protein and beta-2 microglobulin produce a simple and powerful myeloma staging system. Blood 80:733–7, 1992.

224. Luoni R, Ucci G, Riccardi A et al: Serum thymidine kinase in monoclonal gammopathies. A prospective study. The Cooperative Group for Study and Treatment of Multiple Myeloma. Cancer 69:1368–72, 1992.

225. Back H, Jagenburg R, Rodjer S et al: Serum deoxythymidine kinase: No help in the diagnosis and prognosis of monoclonal gammopathy. Br J Haematol 84:746–8, 1993.

226. Dubost JJ, Ristori JM, Soubrier M et al: Acute phase proteins in monoclonal gammopathies (in French). Pathol Biol (Paris) 39:769–73, 1991.

227. Elias J, Dauth J, Senekal JC et al: Serum beta-2-microglobulin in the differential diagnosis of monoclonal gammopathies. S Afr Med J 79:650–3, 1991.

228. Dimopoulos MA, Moulopoulos A, Smith T et al: Risk of disease progression in asymptomatic multiple myeloma. Am J Med 94:57–61, 1993.

229. Dimopoulos MA, Moulopoulos LA, Datseris I et al: Imaging of myeloma bone disease – implications for staging, prognosis and follow-up. Acta Oncol 39:823–7, 2000.

230. Callander NS, Roodman GD: Myeloma bone disease. Semin Hematol 38:276–85, 2001.

231. O'Connor ML, Rice DT, Buss DH et al: Immunoglobulin D benign monoclonal gammopathy. A case report. Cancer 68:611–6, 1991.

232. Blade J, Kyle RA: IgD monoclonal gammopathy with long-term follow-up. Br J Haematol 88:395–6, 1994.

233. Kinoshita T, Nagai H, Murate T et al: IgD monoclonal gammopathy of undetermined significance. Int J Hematol 65:169–72, 1997.

234. Blade J, Lopez-Guillermo A, Rozman C et al: Malignant transformation and life expectancy in monoclonal gammopathy of undetermined significance. Br J Haematol 81:391–4, 1992.

235. Majumdar G, Grace RJ, Singh AK et al: The value of the bone marrow plasma cell cytoplasmic light chain ratio in differentiating between multiple myeloma and monoclonal gammopathy of undetermined significance. Leuk Lymphoma 8:491–3, 1992.

236. Tienhaara A, Pelliniemi TT: Flow cytometric DNA analysis and clinical correlations in multiple myeloma. Am J Clin Pathol 97:322–30, 1992.

237. Jelinek DF, Ahmann GJ, Greipp PR et al: Coexistence of aneuploid subclones within a myeloma cell line that exhibits clonal immunoglobulin gene rearrangement: Clinical implications. Cancer Res 53:5320–7, 1993.

238. Epstein J, Barlogie B, Katzmann J et al: Phenotypic heterogeneity in aneuploid multiple myeloma indicates pre-B cell involvement. Blood 71:861–5, 1988.

239. Gertz MA, Lacy MQ, Inwards DJ et al: Delayed stem cell transplantation for the management of relapsed or refractory multiple myeloma. Bone Marrow Transplant 26:45–50, 2000.

240. Gertz MA, Lacy MQ, Inwards DJ et al: Early harvest and late transplantation as an effective therapeutic strategy in multiple myeloma. Bone Marrow Transplant 23:221–6, 1999.

241. Barlogie B, Jagannath S, Desikan KR et al: Total therapy with tandem transplants for newly diagnosed multiple myeloma. Blood 93:55–65, 1999.

242. Attal M, Harousseau JL, Stoppa AM et al: A prospective, randomized trial of autologous bone marrow transplantation and chemotherapy in multiple myeloma. Intergroupe Francais du Myelome. N Engl J Med 335:91–7, 1996.

243. Attal M, Harousseau JL: Standard therapy versus autologous transplantation in multiple myeloma. Hematol Oncol Clin North Am 11:133–46, 1997.

244. Blade J, Samson D, Reece D et al: Criteria for evaluating disease response and progression in patients with multiple myeloma treated by high-dose therapy and haemopoietic stem cell trans-

plantation. Myeloma Subcommittee of the EBMT. European Group for Blood and Marrow Transplant. Br J Haematol 102:1115–23, 1998.

245. Hjorth M, Holmberg E, Rodjer S et al: Impact of active and passive exclusions on the results of a clinical trial in multiple myeloma. Br J Haematol 80:55–61, 1992.

246. Diem H, Fateh-Moghadam A, Lamerz R: Prognostic factors in multiple myeloma: Role of beta 2-microglobulin and thymidine kinase. Clin Invest 71:918–23, 1993.

247. Durie BG, Salmon SE: A clinical staging system for multiple myeloma. Correlation of measured myeloma cell mass with presenting clinical features, response to treatment, and survival. Cancer 36:842–54, 1975.

248. Rapoport BL, Falkson HC, Falkson G: Prognostic factors affecting the survival of patients with multiple myeloma. A retrospective analysis of 86 patients. S Afr Med J 79:65–7, 1991.

249. Bayrd ED: The bone marrow on sternal aspiration in multiple myeloma. Blood 3:987, 1948.

250. Bartl R, Frisch B, Fateh MA et al: Histologic classification and staging of multiple myeloma. A retrospective and prospective study of 674 cases. Am J Clin Pathol 87:342–55, 1987.

251. Murakami H, Nemoto K, Sawamura M et al: Prognostic relevance of morphological classification in multiple myeloma. Acta Haematol 87:113–7, 1992.

252. Carter A, Hocherman I, Linn S et al: Prognostic significance of plasma cell morphology in multiple myeloma. Cancer 60:1060–5, 1987.

253. Paule B, Quillard J, Bisson M et al: Prognostic significance of plasma cell morphology in multiple myeloma. Nouv Rev Fr Hematol 30:209–12, 1988.

254. Rajkumar SV, Fonseca R, Lacy MQ et al: Plasmablastic morphology is an independent predictor of poor survival after autologous stem-cell transplantation for multiple myeloma. J Clin Oncol 17:1551–7, 1999.

255. Greipp PR, Leong T, Bennett JM et al: Plasmablastic morphology – an independent prognostic factor with clinical and laboratory correlates: Eastern Cooperative Oncology Group (ECOG) myeloma trial E9486 report by the ECOG Myeloma Laboratory Group. Blood 91:2501–7, 1998.

256. Greipp PR, Bennett JM, Gaillard JP et al: Poor survival in plasmablastic myeloma in Eastern Cooperative Oncology Group study E9487: Cell kinetic, ploidy, biological marker, and clinical correlations (meeting abstract). Proc Annu Meet Am Soc Clin Oncol 14, 1995.

257. Goasguen JE, Zandecki M, Mathiot C et al: Mature plasma cells as indicator of better prognosis in multiple myeloma. New methodology for the assessment of plasma cell morphology [see comments]. Leuk Res 23:1133–40, 1999.

258. Sailer M, Vykoupil KF, Peest D et al: Prognostic relevance of a histologic classification system applied in bone marrow biopsies from patients with multiple myeloma: A histopathological evaluation of biopsies from 153 untreated patients. Eur J Haematol 54:137–46, 1995.

259. Schambeck CM, Bartl R, Hochtlen-Vollmar W et al: Characterization of myeloma cells by means of labeling index, bone marrow histology, and serum beta 2-microglobulin. Am J Clin Pathol 106:64–8, 1996.

260. Kurabayashi H, Kubota K, Shirakura T et al: Electron microscopic analysis of myeloma cells in relation to drug response and prognosis. Ultrastruct Pathol 16:379–83, 1992.

261. Kurabayashi H, Kubota K, Shirakura T et al: Prediction of prognosis by electron microscopic analysis of myeloma cells. Ann Hematol 73:169–73, 1996.

262. Saeed SM, Stock ND, Pohlod R et al: Prognostic correlation of plasma cell acid phosphatase and beta-glucuronidase in multiple myeloma: A Southwest Oncology Group study. Blood 78:3281–7, 1991.

263. Wilson CS, Butch AW, Lai R et al: Cyclin D1 and E2F-1 immunoreactivity in bone marrow biopsy specimens of multiple myeloma: Relationship to proliferative activity, cytogenetic abnormalities and DNA ploidy. Br J Haematol 112:776–82, 2001.

264. Rajkumar SV, Greipp PR: Prognostic factors in multiple myeloma. Hematol Oncol Clin North Am 13:1295–314, xi., 1999.

265. Greipp PR: Advances in the diagnosis and management of myeloma. Semin Hematol 29:24–45, 1992.

266. Greipp PR, Katzmann JA, O'Fallon WM et al: Value of beta 2-microglobulin level and plasma cell labeling indices as prognostic factors in patients with newly diagnosed myeloma. Blood 72:219–23, 1988.

267. Greipp PR, Lust JA, Katzmann JA et al: The role of beta 2-microglobulin, plasma cell labeling index, thymidine kinase and C-reactive protein as prognostic factors in 107 cases of multiple myeloma. Blood 78 (Suppl 1):273a, 1991.

268. Boccadoro M, Marmont F, Tribalto M et al: Early responder myeloma: Kinetic studies identify a patient subgroup characterized by very poor prognosis. J Clin Oncol 7:119–25, 1989.

269. Drach J, Gattringer C, Glassl H et al: The biological and clinical significance of the KI-67 growth fraction in multiple myeloma. Hematol Oncol 10:125–34, 1992.

270. Kanavaros P, Stefanaki K, Vlachonikolis J et al: Immunohistochemical expression of the p53, p21/Waf-1, Rb, p16 and Ki67 proteins in multiple myeloma. Anticancer Res 20:4619–25, 2000.

271. Hoechtlen-Vollmar W, Menzel G, Bartl R et al: Amplification of cyclin D1 gene in multiple myeloma: Clinical and prognostic relevance. Br J Haematol 109:30–8, 2000.

272. Witzig TE, Gertz MA, Lust JA et al: Peripheral blood monoclonal plasma cells as a predictor of survival in patients with multiple myeloma. Blood 88:1780–7, 1996.

273. Bataille R, Magub M, Grenier J et al: Serum beta-2-microglobulin in multiple myeloma: Relation to presenting features and clinical status. Eur J Cancer Clin Oncol 18:59–66, 1982.

274. Cuzick J, De SBL, Cooper EH et al: Long-term prognostic value of serum beta 2 microglobulin in myelomatosis. Br J Haematol 75:506–10, 1990.

275. Greipp PR, Lust JA, O'Fallon WM et al: Plasma cell labeling index and beta 2-microglobulin predict survival independent of thymidine kinase and C-reactive protein in multiple myeloma. Blood 81:3382–7, 1993.

276. Ortega F, Gonzalez M, Moro MJ et al: Prognostic effect of beta 2-microglobulin in multiple myeloma. (in Spanish). [Review, 25 refs] Med Clin (Barc) 99:645–8, 1992.

277. Dewald GW, Kyle RA, Hicks GA et al: The clinical significance of cytogenetic studies in 100 patients with multiple myeloma, plasma cell leukemia, or amyloidosis. Blood 66:380–90, 1985.

278. Tricot G, Barlogie B, Jagannath S et al: Poor prognosis in multiple myeloma is associated only with partial or complete deletions of chromosome 13 or abnormalities involving 11q and not with other karyotype abnormalities. Blood 86:4250–6, 1995.

279. Sawyer JR, Waldron JA, Jagannath S et al: Cytogenetic findings in 200 patients with multiple myeloma. Cancer Genet Cytogenet 82:41–9, 1995.

280. Desikan R, Barlogie B, Sawyer J et al: Results of high-dose therapy for 1000 patients with multiple myeloma: Durable complete remissions and superior survival in the absence of chromosome 13 abnormalities. Blood 95:4008–10, 2000.

281. Gutierrez NC, Hernandez JM, Garcia JL et al: Correlation between cytogenetic abnormalities and disease characteristics in multiple myeloma: Monosomy of chromosome 13 and structural abnormalities of 11q are associated with a high percentage of S-phase plasma cells. Haematologica 85:1146–52, 2000.

282. Avet-Loiseau H, Daviet A, Brigaudeau C et al: Cytogenetic, interphase, and multicolor fluorescence in situ hybridization analyses in primary plasma cell leukemia: A study of 40 patients at diagnosis, on behalf of the Intergroupe Francophone du Myelome and the Groupe Français de Cytogenetique Hematologique. Blood 97:822–5, 2001.

283. Zojer N, Konigsberg R, Ackermann J et al: Deletion of 13q14 remains an independent adverse prognostic variable in multiple myeloma despite its frequent detection by interphase fluorescence in situ hybridization. Blood 95:1925–30, 2000.

284. Avet-Loiseau H: Nonrandom distribution of chromosomal abnormalities and correlation with clinical stage and prognostic presentation: A novel model for oncogenesis of multiple myeloma. Proceedings of the 8th International Multiple Myeloma Workshop: 10–11, 2001.

285. Drach J, Schuster J, Nowotny H et al: Multiple myeloma: High incidence of chromosomal aneuploidy as detected by interphase fluorescence in situ hybridization. Cancer Res 55:3854–9, 1995.

286. Rajkumar S, Fonseca R, Lacy M et al: Abnormal cytogenetics predict poor survival after high-dose therapy and autologous blood cell transplantation in multiple myeloma. Bone Marrow Transplant 24:497–503, 1999.

287. Neri A, Murphy JP, Cro L et al: Ras oncogene mutation in multiple myeloma. J Exp Med 170:1715–25, 1989.

288. Drach J, Ackermann J, Fritz E et al: Presence of a P53 gene deletion in patients with multiple myeloma predicts for short survival after conventional-dose chemotherapy. Blood 92:802–809, 1998.

289. Santhanam U, Ray A, Sehgal PB: Repression of the interleukin-6 gene promoter by p53 and the retinoblastoma susceptibility gene product. Proc Natl Acad Sci U S A 88:7605–9, 1991.

290. Stephenson J, Akdag R, Ozbek N et al: Methylation status within exon 3 of the c-myc gene as a prognostic marker in myeloma and leukaemia. Leuk Res 17:291–3, 1993.

291. Ahn MJ, Park CK, Choi JH et al: Clinical significance of microvessel density in multiple myeloma patients. J Korean Med Sci 16:45–50, 2001.

292. Bataille R, Jourdan M, Zhang XG et al: Serum levels of interleukin-6, a potent myeloma cell growth factor, as a reflect of disease severity in plasma cell dyscrasias. J Clin Invest 84:2008–11, 1989.

293. Pelliniemi TT, Irjala K, Mattila K et al: Immunoreactive interleukin-6 and acute phase proteins as prognostic factors in multiple myeloma. Finnish Leukaemia Group. Blood 85:765–71, 1995.

294. Pulkki K, Pelliniemi TT, Rajamaki A et al: Soluble interleukin-6 receptor as a prognostic factor in multiple myeloma. Finnish Leukaemia Group. Br J Haematol 92:370–4, 1996.

295. Kyrtsonis MC, Dedoussis G, Zervas C et al: Soluble interleukin-6 receptor (sIL-6R), a new prognostic factor in multiple myeloma. Br J Haematol 93:398–400, 1996.

296. Stasi R, Brunetti M, Parma A et al: The prognostic value of soluble interleukin-6 receptor in patients with multiple myeloma. Cancer 82:1860–6, 1998.

297. Cimino G, Amadori S, Cava MC et al: Serum interleukin-2 (IL-2), soluble IL-2 receptors and tumor necrosis factor-alfa levels are significantly increased in acute myeloid leukemia patients. Leukemia 5:32–5, 1991.

298. Gottlieb DJ, Prentice HG, Mehta AB et al: Malignant plasma cells are sensitive to LAK cell lysis: Preclinical and clinical studies of interleukin 2 in the treatment of multiple myeloma. Br J Haematol 75:499–505, 1990.

299. Fonseca R, Trendle MC, Leong T et al: Prognostic value of serum markers of bone metabolism in untreated multiple myeloma patients. Br J Haematol 109:24–9, 2000.

300. Turesson I, Abildgaard N, Ahlgren T et al: Prognostic evaluation in multiple myeloma: An analysis of the impact of new prognostic factors. Br J Haematol 106:1005–12, 1999.

301. Terpos E, Palermos J, Tsionos K et al: Effect of pamidronate administration on markers of bone turnover and disease activity in multiple myeloma. Eur J Haematol 65:331–6, 2000.

302. Abildgaard N, Glerup H, Rungby J et al: Biochemical markers of bone metabolism reflect osteoclastic and osteoblastic activity in multiple myeloma. Eur J Haematol 64:121–9, 2000.

303. Bataille R, Boccadoro M, Klein B et al: C-reactive Protein (CRP): A direct indicator of interleukin-6 (IL-6) and the best prognostic factor in multiple myeloma (MM). Blood 78(Suppl. 1):174a, 1991.

304. Greipp P, Lust J, O'Fallon W et al: Plasma cell labeling index and beta 2-microglobulin predict survival independent of thymidine kinase and C-reactive protein in multiple myeloma. Blood 81:3382–7, 1993.

305. Greipp PR, Gaillard JP, Klein B et al: Independent prognostic value for plasma cell labeling index (PCLI), immunofluorescence microscopy plasma cell percent (IMPCP), beta 2-microglobulin (B2M), soluble interleukin-6 receptor (sIL-6R), and c-reactive protein (CRP) in myeloma trial E9487 (meeting abstract). Blood 84, 1994.

306. Merlini G, Perfetti V, Gobbi PG et al: Acute phase proteins and prognosis in multiple myeloma. Br J Haematol 83:595–601, 1993.

307. Brown RD, Snowdon L, Uhr E et al: C-reactive protein (CRP) levels do not reflect disease status in patients with multiple myeloma. Leuk Lymphoma 9:509–12, 1993.

308. Simonsson B, Brenning G, Kallander C et al: Prognostic value of serum lactic dehydrogenase (S-LDH) in multiple myeloma. Eur J Clin Invest 17:336–9, 1987.

309. Dimopoulos MA, Barlogie B, Smith TL et al: High serum lactate dehydrogenase level as a marker for drug resistance and short survival in multiple myeloma. Ann Intern Med 115:931–935, 1991.

310. Brown RD, Joshua DE, Nelson M et al: Serum thymidine kinase as a prognostic indicator for patients with multiple myeloma: Results from the MRC (UK) V trial. Br J Haematol 84:238–41, 1993.

311. Elomaa I, Virkkunen P, Risteli L et al: Serum concentration of the cross-linked carboxyterminal telopeptide of type I collagen (ICTP) is a useful prognostic indicator in multiple myeloma. Br J Cancer 66:337–41, 1992.

312. Arnalich F, Zamorano AF, Martinez-Hernandez P et al: Additional predictive value of serum unsaturated vitamin B12 proteins in multiple myeloma. J Med 21:277–86, 1990.

313. Kaiser U, Jaques G, Havemann K et al: Serum NCAM: A potential new prognostic marker for multiple myeloma. Blood 83:871–3, 1994.

314. Kaiser U, Oldenburg M, Jaques G et al: Soluble CD56 (NCAM): A new differential-diagnostic and prognostic marker in multiple myeloma. Ann Hematol 73:121–6, 1996.

315. San Miguel JF, Gonzalez M, Gascon A et al: Lymphoid subsets and prognostic factors in multiple myeloma. Cooperative Group for the Study of Monoclonal Gammopathies. Br J Haematol 80:305–9, 1992.

316. Kay NE, Oken MM, Kyle R et al: Sequential phenotyping of myeloma patients on chemotherapy: Persistence of activated T-cells and natural killer cells. Leuk Lymphoma 16:351–4, 1995.

317. Osterborg A, Masucci M, Bergenbrant S et al: Generation of T cell clones binding F(ab′)2 fragments of the idiotypic immunoglobulin in patients with monoclonal gammopathy. Cancer Immunol Immunother 34:157–62, 1991.

318. Durie BG, Grogan TM: CALLA-positive myeloma: An aggressive subtype with poor survival. Blood 66:229–32, 1985.

319. Treon SP, Anderson KC: The use of rituximab in the treatment of malignant and nonmalignant plasma cell disorders. Semin Oncol 27:79–85, 2000.

320. Grogan TM, Spier CM, Salmon SE et al: P-glycoprotein expression in human plasma cell myeloma: Correlation with prior chemotherapy. Blood 81:490–5, 1993.

321. Barlogie B, Alexanian R, Dixon D et al: Prognostic implications of tumor cell DNA and RNA content in multiple myeloma. Blood 66:338–41, 1985.

322. Morgan RJ Jr, Gonchoraff NJ, Katzmann JA, Witzig TE et al: Detection of hypodiploidy using multi-parameter flow cytometric analysis: A prognostic indicator in multiple myeloma. Am J Hematol 30:195–200, 1989.

323. Greipp PR, Trendle MC, Leong T et al: Is flow cytometric DNA content hypodiploidy prognostic in multiple myeloma? Leuk Lymphoma 35:83–89, 1999.

324. De Vos J, Couderc G, Tarte K et al: Identifying intercellular signaling genes expressed in malignant plasma cells by using complementary DNA arrays. Blood 98:771–80, 2001.

325. Spasov E, Goranova V: Prognostic assessment of the Durie and Salmon staging system in patients with multiple myeloma. Folia Med (Plovdiv) 40:121–3, 1998.

326. San Miguel JF, Garcia-Sanz R, Gonzalez M et al: A new staging system for multiple myeloma based on the number of S-phase plasma cells. Blood 85:448–55, 1995.

327. Facon T, Avet-Loiseau H, Guillerm G et al: Chromosome 13 abnormalities identified by FISH analysis and serum beta2-microglobulin produce a powerful myeloma staging system for patients receiving high-dose therapy. Blood 97:1566–71, 2001.

328. Sirohi B, Powles R, Mehta J et al: Complete remission rate and outcome after intensive treatment of 177 patients under 75 years of age with IgG myeloma defining a circumscribed disease entity with a new staging system. Br J Haematol 107:656–66, 1999.

329. Crowley J, Jacobson J, Alexanian R: Standard-dose therapy for multiple myeloma: The Southwest Oncology Group experience. Semin Hematol 38:203–8, 2001.

330. Greipp P, Kyle R, Leong T et al: Redefinition of risk factors in myeloma: Analysis of ECOG phase III trial E9486 with a focus on 5-year survival. Proc 7th International Multiple Myeloma Workshop:43–44, 1999.

338. Latreille J, Barlogie B, Johnston D et al: Ploidy and proliferative characteristics in monoclonal gammopathies. Blood 59:43–51, 1982.

339. Montecucco C, Riccardi A, Ucci G et al: Analysis of human myeloma cell population kinetics. Acta Haematol 75:153–6, 1986.

340. Boccadoro M, Marmont F, Tribalto M et al: Multiple myeloma: VMCP/VBAP alternating combination chemotherapy is not superior to melphalan and prednisone even in high-risk patients. J Clin Oncol 9:444–8, 1991.

341. Cornelissen JJ, Sonneveld P, Schoester M et al: MDR-1 expression and response to vincristine, doxorubicin, and dexamethasone chemotherapy in multiple myeloma refractory to alkylating agents. J Clin Oncol 12:115–9, 1994.

31

Diagnosis and Treatment of Multiple Myeloma

Douglas E. Joshua and John Gibson

Myeloma, the most common plasma cell dyscrasia, is a paradigm of a mature B-cell tumor. The malignant cells have a mature B-cell phenotype and secrete a monoclonal immunoglobulin (Ig). The incidence of myeloma varies from 1 to 2 in 100,000 Orientals, to 4 in 100,000 in American whites, and to almost double that figure in the Afro-American population.[1,2] The disease is sporadic, with only occasional reports of family associations and geographic clusters, and the phenomenon of "anticipation" has been reported in a number of families.[3] Both radiation and benzene exposure have been implicated in its etiology, but whether there is a relationship between benzene and myeloma remains unclear.[4,5] A number of occupational associations (including agriculture and the rubber, wood, leather, and textile manufacturing industries) have also been reported.[6]

CLINICAL MANIFESTATIONS

The clinical manifestations of myeloma are a direct reflection of the disease pathophysiology and can be listed in five categories:

1. Effect of the malignancy on the skeleton, particularly bone destruction
2. Effects of the secreted paraprotein either in the serum or urine (Bence Jones proteinuria)
3. Marrow infiltration leading to bone marrow failure
4. Immunosuppression caused by hypogammaglobulinemia and an associated primary immune deficit (and subsequently the secondary effects of treatment)
5. Renal disease, the etiology of which is multifactorial

Myeloma and the Skeleton

Myeloma usually involves the axial skeleton and proximal ends of the long bones. Lytic bone lesions, detectable radiologically, are often associated with generalized osteolysis, radiologically manifest as osteoporosis. As the disease progresses, both spinal compression due to crush fractures of the vertebral bodies and pathologic fractures of the long bones and ribs may occur. Bone disease is due to tumor infiltration and to uncoupling of the osteoblast–osteoclast nexus with active dissolution of bone.

Bone pain is the most common clinical symptom and is present at the time of diagnosis in more than two-thirds of patients. Common syndromes include back pain due to compression fractures of vertebral bodies or to myeloma infiltration of the vertebrae or pelvic bones and pathological fractures of ribs leading to pleuritic pain. Rib fractures are often precipitated by coughing caused by respiratory tract infections. Loss of height is very common due to compression fractures and the development of a dorsal kyphosis. Spinal cord damage and paraplegia may result from extension of vertebral tumor into the spinal canal. In patients with known myeloma, emergency radiologic localization of the site of the spinal lesion followed by radiotherapy to the lesion is the mainstay of therapy. Surgery is indicated if the diagnosis is doubtful or if the patient fails to respond rapidly to radiation therapy. Computed tomography (CT) scanning or magnetic resonance imaging (MRI) have replaced myelography as the investigation of choice in patients with suspected spinal compression. In addition, MRI is the most sensitive technique for determining lytic lesions and differentiating tumor involvement from osteoporotic crush fractures.[7]

Other bones commonly affected are those of the skull, where punched-out lytic lesions, best seen in a lateral view, are present in over two-thirds of patients (Figure 31–1). Almost any bone of the body can, however, be affected by lytic lesions (Figure 31–2). By contrast, 20 percent of patients present with osteoporosis alone, and a small number can show osteosclerotic changes. Osteosclerotic myeloma has been associated with peripheral nerve lesions, skin changes, and endocrinopathy (the POEMS syndrome – polyneuropathy, organomegaly, endocrinopathy, monoclonal paraprotein, and skin changes).[8] The neurologic findings are usually a predominant motor nerve dysfunction caused by a chronic inflammatory demyelinating polyneuropathy.

Hypercalcemia is a frequent accompaniment of myeloma and is usually but not always associated with extensive bone destruction. It occurs in about one-quarter of patients at diagnosis and more frequently with disease progression. The symptoms of hypercalcemia include nausea, polyuria, thirst, constipation, and clouding of consciousness. Acute hypercalcemia is a medical emergency requiring urgent treatment with hydration and saline diuresis. Glucocorticoids in high doses and bisphosphonates are also frequently required.

Extramedullary plasmacytomas or soft tissue masses may be seen in up to 10 percent of myeloma patients. The most common sites are the pleura, often without adjacent bone destruction, and they occur most often in patients with IgA myeloma. Other sites include the mediastinum and the abdomen. Myeloma may rarely cause pulmonary infiltration.

Effects of Elevated Serum Immunoglobulins

Excessively high Ig levels can produce the clinical syndrome of hyperviscosity, with characteristic clinical features including lassitude, confusion, obtundation, and loss of consciousness. Symptoms usually arise when the relative serum viscosity reaches 5, but this relationship is fairly imprecise. Physical signs

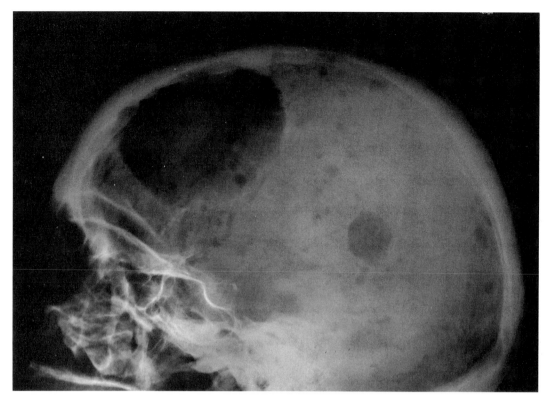

Figure 31–1. Lytic lesions in the skull are characteristic of multiple myeloma. These are often multiple and can be extensive.

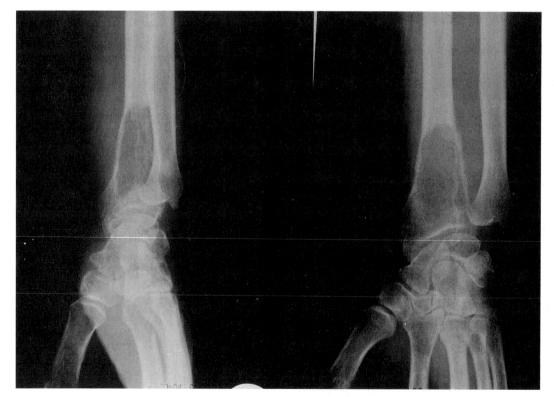

Figure 31–2. Lytic lesions of bone may occur at any site, although they are most common in the axial skeleton. This radiograph shows an expansile lytic lesion in the distal end of the radius.

include sludging of blood flow, visible as segmental dilation of retinal veins and retinal hemorrhages (Figure 31–3). Generalized hemorrhage due to hyperviscosity-associated coagulopathy is also seen. In its severest form the hyperviscosity syndrome is most frequently associated with IgM paraproteins, a reflection of the high molecular weight of this Ig class and its tendency to polymerize as pentamers. Similar effects can also be seen with IgA (dimers) and IgG$_3$ paraproteins. The concentration of IgA polymers has been found to correlate with serum viscosity, and IgA paraproteins are most frequently seen in the hyperviscosity-coagulopathy syndrome.[9]

The antibody activity of monoclonal proteins seen in myeloma has only rarely been identified.[10] Nevertheless, a number of cases have been described in which the antibody activity has led to a specific disease process. These include reactivity against red cells, as in cold hemagglutinin disease, and against factor VIII, leading to acquired hemophilia or von Willebrand's disease.[11] Reactivity against human IgG has been associated with cryoglobulinemia. In addition, antibodies directed against lipoproteins have been associated with hyperlipemia and xanthomata formation.[12] Isolated and interesting cases of proteins binding to transferrin (leading to hemochromatosis), to flavin (leading to pigmentation), and to copper (leading to ocular deposition of copper) have also been described.[13] Finally, rare cases of hypothyroidism associated with antithyroxine antibodies and hypoglycemia due to insulin-binding antibodies have been reported.[14,15]

The monoclonal proteins have also been implicated in the etiology of peripheral neuropathies associated with myeloma, although this can occasionally be due to amyloid deposition.[16] The clinical picture is usually that of a mixed sensorimotor polyneuropathy with distal weakness and loss of proprioception. Histologic examination of affected nerves often shows coexistent demyelination and remyelination. Some IgM paraproteins have been shown to possess antibody activity against a carbohydrate epitope expressed on myelin-associated glycoprotein (MAG), and the destruction of myelin has been shown to depend on the interaction with complement.[17,18] Prognosis of this condition is favorable, frequently with only slow progression.[19] By contrast, less is known about the mechanism of peripheral neuropathies associated with IgG paraproteins, and no putative antigenic determinant has been identified.[20] Severe motor neuropathy has been reported in younger patients with osteosclerotic myeloma in the context of the POEMS syndrome. In a number of cases the neuropathy is the main feature of the underlying monoclonal gammopathy, which can vary from MGUS (most commonly) to overt myeloma. Plasmapheresis is the only therapy shown to be of benefit in controlled studies.[21]

Bone Marrow Failure

Anemia is common in patients with myeloma and may occur independently of leukopenia and thrombocytopenia. The causes of anemia are multiple and include bone marrow infil-

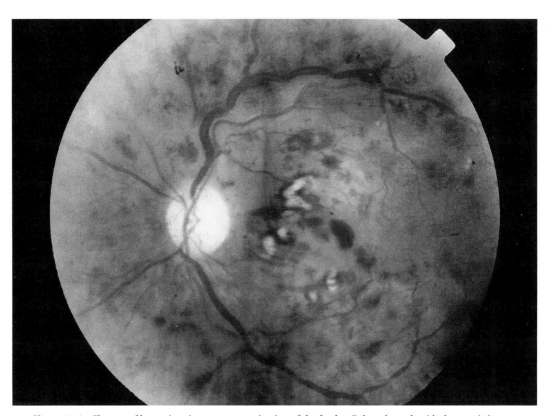

Figure 31–3. Changes of hyperviscosity seen on examination of the fundus. Enlarged vessels with characteristic constrictions and hemorrhages and exudates are prominent.

tration, renal failure, the effects of chemotherapy, and the anemia associated with chronic disease. Both interleukin-6 (IL-6) and IL-1 have been shown to inhibit erythropoiesis, and a number of studies have identified anemia as an important prognostic factor.[22] Leukopenia and thrombocytopenia are attributed to marrow replacement and the myelosuppressive effects of chemotherapy. Paradoxically, some patients may present with or develop thrombocytosis. This phenomenon has been attributed to the thrombopoietic effects of IL-6. High levels of serum Igs cause rouleau formation and the high erythrocyte sedimentation rate that is so characteristic of myeloma.

Although occasional circulating plasma cells can be seen in many patients, plasma cell leukemia is usually deemed to be present when the peripheral blood plasma cell count is more than 2.0×10^9/L. This may occur de novo but more usually occurs in end-stage disease. Sensitive techniques, including flow cytometry, molecular studies, and immunohistochemistry, invariably reveal the presence of circulating malignant cells in the blood, either plasma cells or B cells belonging to the malignant clone, at all stages of the disease.[23–26]

Infections and the Primary Immune Deficit of Myeloma

Recurrent infections, usually caused by highly pathogenic bacteria, are a major cause of both morbidity and mortality. Early studies demonstrated a high incidence of pneumococcal infection, especially pneumonia, and this remains the classic dogma.[27] In recent years, however, the importance of infection with gram-negative organisms has been recognized, and the frequency of these infections may be rising. Data from a number of studies have shown that there is a particular period of high infection risk associated with the introduction of therapy and covering the subsequent 2 to 3 months.[28]

Two main factors have been implicated in the increased susceptibility to infections of myeloma patients. Most patients have marked depression of the synthesis of the normal Ig, and thus serum levels of the residual normal Igs are low. In addition, the primary immune response to external antigens is impaired. The latter is manifested by impaired responses to pneumococcal polysaccharides I and II and is associated with failure of protection by pneumococcal vaccine. The role of high doses of prophylactic intravenous Ig to protect patients during the initial crucial 3 months of therapy has been investigated in a randomized study by the U.K. Medical Research Council (MRC). In this study the frequency and incidence of infection was not altered. In contrast, other studies have reported benefit from prophylactic Ig in chronic lymphocytic leukemia (CLL)[29] and in myeloma during the plateau phase.[30] The use of prophylactic antibiotics for the initial 2 months of therapy, however, was reported to significantly reduce infective incidents.[28]

In general, patients with myeloma have normal or nearly normal cellular immunity at least in the early phases of the disease. Myeloma patients can mount delayed-type hypersensitivity reactions to common antigens and can also be sensitized to new antigens such as 2,4-dinitro-1-fluorobenzene and keyhole limpet hemocyanin. The clinical correlate of these findings is the lack of fungal and viral infections as major clinical problems except in patients receiving high-dose corticosteroids, undergoing bone marrow transplantation, or both. Herpes zoster, however, is frequently encountered.

The mechanism of the immunosuppression has been extensively studied both in the murine plasmacytoma model and in human myeloma. The reduction in polyclonal Igs found in almost all patients with myeloma is due to impaired synthesis. Studies in IgG myeloma have also demonstrated hypercatabolism of residual normal IgG at a rate almost twice that seen in normal subjects. Immunoglobulin G is, however, the only class of Ig that exhibits a direct concentration–hypercatabolism relationship.[31] Patients with IgA myeloma have reduced IgG levels and normal IgG catabolism.

Myeloma and the Kidney

Proteinuria is present to some extent in almost all patients, and 80 percent excrete Bence Jones protein. Renal failure is seen in over one-fourth of cases of myeloma at presentation. The pathogenesis of azotemia is multifactorial, but hypercalcemia and deposition of Bence Jones protein as laminated casts in the proximal convoluted tubules are believed to be major causes. The unique properties of Bence Jones protein that cause nephrotoxicity remain unknown. It has been postulated that nephrotoxicity is related to the isoelectric point of the protein, with cationic chains being more nephrotoxic than anionic chains.[32] This hypothesis has been evaluated by Solomon et al.,[33] who injected mice intraperitoneally with purified Bence Jones protein from 40 patients with myeloma and studied the renal pathology in the mice together with the corresponding human renal biopsy material. This study found no relationship between nephrotoxicity and the isoelectric point, molecular weight, or isotype of the paraprotein. Thus, the specific features responsible for renal toxicity remain unclear. Other important factors that contribute to the renal failure include dehydration, uric acid nephropathy, radiographic contrast medium, infection, and amyloidosis. In addition, it is has recently been recognized the concomitant use of angiotensin-converting enzyme (ACE) inhibitors in myeloma patients is a common cause of renal impairment.[34]

The management of myeloma-associated renal failure has undergone considerable conceptual evolution over the last decade. Prior to the ready availability of dialysis, patients who presented with advanced azotemia had a very poor outlook. Key studies such as those by the MRC (UK), have shown that renal impairment at presentation is often reversible with hydration alone and that reversal does not depend on the need to reduce Bence Jones protein excretion dramatically.[35] Plasmapheresis may also play a role in some patients.[36] In some patients advanced renal failure per se need not necessarily adversely affect the prognosis of the disease in general. In such cases renal disease is an early manifestation of the nephrotoxic potential of Bence Jones protein in patients who may otherwise have a fairly indolent B cell malignancy. Primary renal amyloidosis and light chain deposition disease are extreme examples of this phenomenon.[37] These patients predominantly present with renal failure and have an indolent B-cell disorder that may require no specific chemotherapy. Hemodialysis is appropriate therapy for renal failure even in the event of overt active myeloma.[38–40]

DIAGNOSIS

Clinical Findings

The typical patient with myeloma usually exhibits the combination of lytic bone lesions in association with a monoclonal infiltration of plasma cells in the marrow and a paraprotein or M component either in the serum or in the urine. Many patients, however, do not show all three characteristics. For instance, extensive marrow infiltration with a normal skeletal survey is a not uncommon clinical scenario. In addition a number of patients, the so-called nonsecretors, do not secrete Ig and present with hypogammaglobulinemia. To help resolve confusion regarding the definitive diagnosis of myeloma and its separation from determined monoclonal gammopathy of undetermined significance (MGUS), a variety of authors have suggested diagnostic criteria. One such system is shown in Table 31–1. A particular advantage of this system is the identification of those patients with so-called smoldering myeloma, who do not necessarily need treatment at diagnosis.[41]

Laboratory Findings

Electrophoresis on cellulose acetate has traditionally been used to detect the presence of monoclonal proteins in both serum

---

Table 31–1. Features of MGUS, Smoldering Multiple Myeloma (SMM), and Multiple Myeloma (MM)

MGUS
  Serum monoclonal protein less than 3 g/dl
  Fewer than 10 percent plasma cells in the bone marrow biopsy
  No anemia, renal failure, or hypercalcemia
  Bone lesions absent on radiographic bone survey
  Plasmablasts absent
  Normal β_2-microglobulin levels
  Urinary light chain excretion less than 0.5 g in 24 hours
SMM
  Serum monoclonal protein less than 3 g/dl
  Plasma cells on bone marrow biopsy, 10 percent or less
  No anemia, renal failure, or hypercalcemia attributable to myeloma
  Low or normal β_2-microglobulin
  PCLI < 1%
MM
  M protein present in serum or urine
  ≥ 10% marrow plasma cells or aggregates on biopsy
  Anemia
  Lytic lesions or osteoporosis
  Bone marrow PCLI higher than 1 percent
  Renal insufficiency
  Hypercalcemia

MGUS, monoclonal gammopathy of undetermined significance; PCLI, plasma cell labeling index

---

and urine. The speed of migration of proteins during electrophoresis depends on the size and electric charge at the pH of the buffer. Paraproteins represent a homogeneous population of Ig molecules and are identified as a characteristic narrow band or peak in the γ-, β-, or α-regions of the serum protein electrophoresis. The broad band of polyclonal hypergammaglobulinemia is usually restricted to the γ-region. Serum is preferred to plasma as a source sample, since fibrinogen forms a band in the fast βγ-region.

Precise typing of the monoclonal protein requires immunologic identification to identify the heavy chain class and the light chain isotype. Immunofixation is the recommended method to investigate abnormal bands detected by electrophoresis. This technique, originally described by Wilson,[42] is easier to interpret than immunoelectrophoresis and is also more sensitive, especially when the results of immunoelectrophoresis are equivocal. Immunofixation relies on a combination of protein electrophoresis through cellulose acetate or agarose and subsequent reaction of the separated proteins with a monospecific antibody, resulting in the deposition of an insoluble complex. A monoclonal protein is demonstrated by a localized well-defined band in the heavy or light chain lanes or in both. Bence Jones protein is characterized by demonstration of either κ- or λ-chains in the urine and no corresponding heavy chain reaction (Figure 31–4). Light chain bands can also be seen in serum, especially in cases of renal impairment; they have the same mobility as urinary Bence Jones protein. The presence of light chains in the serum may indicate polymerization of light chains (especially the λ-chains, because of the availability of a penultimate cystine residue).

The presence, type, and amount of monoclonal protein in the serum or urine or in both are important in the differential diagnosis of myeloma. Paraproteins are found in a variety of malignant B-cell disorders such as chronic lymphocytic leukemia and low-grade non-Hodgkin's lymphoma, in addition to myeloma, macroglobulinemia, and amyloidosis. Rarely, they can also be detected in association with a variety of other diseases such as lichen myxedematosis and peripheral neuropathies. A large monoclonal peak (3g/dl) is usually the result of overt multiple myeloma, although it can occur in patients with well differentiated lymphocytic lymphoma or chronic lymphocytic leukemia. The presence of large amounts of Bence Jones protein almost always signifies active myeloma or primary amyloidosis, although rare patients can excrete large amounts of Bence Jones protein and yet have a stable clinical course over many years. Some patients with Bence Jones proteinuria have even been followed for over 18 years before the overt development of multiple myeloma.[43,44] Reduced levels of the residual normal Igs are a sign that a monoclonal protein is more likely to be the result of a malignant process.

A variety of factors may give rise to restricted or spurious bands (or both) on protein electrophoresis. For example, the hemoglobin–haptoglobin complex in hemolyzed serum forms a band between the α_2 and β region, free hemoglobin forms a band in the β region, and large quantities of transferrin in patients with iron deficiency may produce a band in the β region. Patients with light chain disease as well as IgD and IgE

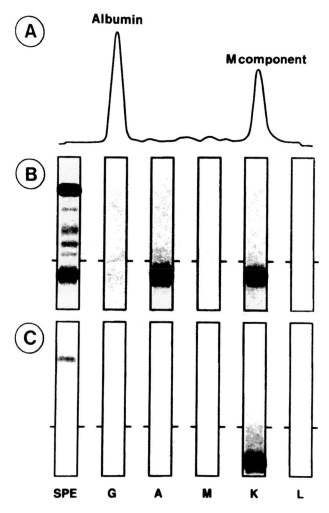

Figure 31–4. Identification of an M component detected (A) on electrophoresis and (B) by immunofixation. The immunoglobulin is identified as IgAK, and free (K) light chains are seen on the urine (C). SPE, nonspecific protein stain; G, IgG; A, IgA; M, IgM; K, κ light chains; L, λ light chains.

monoclonal globulin; (2) plasmacytosis more than 5 percent on either bone marrow aspirate or tissue biopsy; and (3) osteolytic lesions unexplained by other causes.

TUMOR STAGING AND PROGNOSTIC EVALUATION

A number of prognostic factors reflecting various aspects of disease biology have been identified in myeloma. The important prognostic factors so far identified relate to four main variables: the intrinsic proliferative capacity of the myeloma clone; tumor mass (bulk); renal function; and host–tumor interactions[46] (Table 31–2). Despite the predictive value of the recognized prognostic factors, wide variations in survival stress the need for improved prognostic factors to be determined, especially when assessing the need for newer aggressive therapy programs.[47]

Intrinsic Properties of the Malignant Clone

Factors that relate to the intrinsic properties of the malignant clone include the plasma cell labeling index (PCLI), the serum thymidine kinase (STK) level, and the morphologic features of the malignant clone. The PCLI measures plasma cell proliferative activity and is one of the most significant prognostic tools so far identified.[48,49] It can differentiate between MGUS, smoldering myeloma, and active myeloma.[50] Originally measured with tritiated thymidine incorporation, it is more conveniently assessed by incorporation of bromodeoxyuridine which can be identified with a monoclonal antibody.[51] Recent adaptations to flow cytometric methods have improved both the accuracy and usefulness of this test in the routine laboratory.[52]

The PCLI is highly correlated with STK, elevated levels of which have been associated with increased tumor cell proliferation in a wide variety of malignancies.[53] In myeloma, STK is a reliable monitor of loss of plateau phase and development of progressive disease. It is also a prognostic marker for patients

myeloma often do not display a monoclonal peak, or the peak produced may be so small that it is not visualized by standard electrophoresis.[45]

In general, patients with myeloma have a marrow plasmacytosis of more than 10 percent. When assessing patients with low levels of infiltration, it is important to determine whether this proliferation exhibits light chain restriction before a confident diagnosis of multiple myeloma can be made. Increased plasma cell numbers can be seen in the bone marrows of patients with chronic inflammatory and immunologic diseases and in patients who are suffering from human immunodeficiency virus (HIV) infection. Such patients usually have a polyclonal, broad-based elevation of γ-globulins, and their plasma cells express both κ and λ light chains.

A committee of the Chronic Leukemia and Myeloma Task Force of the National Cancer Institute has suggested three minimum criteria for the diagnosis of myeloma: (1) the presence of

Table 31–2. Prognostic Factors in Myeloma

Factors reflecting inherent proliferative capacity of the malignant clone
  Labeling index (LI)
  Serum thymidine kinase (STK)
  Plasma cell morphology of the malignant clone
  Multidrug resistance (MDR) phenotype
  Chromosomal abnormalities
Factors reflecting tumor bulk
  β_2-microglobulin (β_2M)
  Stage (Durie-Salmon and others)
Factors reflecting renal function
  Creatinine
  β_2M
Factors reflecting host–tumor interactions
  C-reactive protein (CRP)
  Interleukin-6 (IL-6) and soluble IL-6 receptor (sIL-6R)
  CD38+ cells
  IL-2 levels

treated with melphalan, although not multiagent protocols.[54] Serum thymidine kinase does not correlate with β_2-microglobulin (β_2M) or serum creatinine and is thus not a measure of tumor bulk. In the absence of PCLI, STK can be combined with β_2M to improve prognostic information.[55]

A number of morphologic features have also been correlated with prognosis. These features include the plasma cell type as well as the associated morphologic features in the surrounding marrow.[56] Cellular grading (plasmablastic versus mature plasma cells) is probably the most important variable and may reflect not only intrinsic malignant potential but also the biosynthetic activity of plasma cells.[57] The role of nucleoli as a prognostic factor in plasma cell morphology remains unclear.

As in acute leukemia, chromosomal abnormalities are proving to play a very important role in predicting prognosis in myeloma. By using sophisticated techniques, cytogenetic abnormalities can be identified in all patients with myeloma. The most adverse prognostic changes are associated with deletions of chromosome 13 and abnormalities of chromosome 11q.[58] Cytogenetic abnormalities are more marked in plasma cell leukemia,[59] and prognostic cytogenetic groups have been determined.[60] Although the biological correlates of these cytogenetic changes remain unknown, mutation in *ras* oncogenes shows varying disease phenotypes and prognoses.[61]

It is possible that multidrug resistance (MDR) may become an important prognostic indicator in myeloma, although its exact significance and independence from other prognostic factors is as yet uncertain. This is further discussed later in connection with new avenues of therapy.

Tumor Mass

The two most widespread methods for assessing myeloma tumor mass are β_2M and the clinical staging systems. β_2M, a low molecular weight protein identical to the light chain of human leukocyte antigen (HLA) class I molecules, is shed into the circulation and is one of the most important prognostic indicators of disease activity.[62,63] Most prognostic information comes from the initial β_2M levels, and is restricted to the first 2 years after diagnosis.[64] A relationship exists between the level of β_2M and the measured myeloma cell mass, but β_2M is not related to the PCLI and is not a proliferative marker.[65] The combination of β_2M level and PCLI is the most powerful prognostic tool so far identified, and patients who have low β_2M levels and low PCLI have an exceptionally good outlook.[55]

The most widely used clinical staging system is the Durie-Salmon three-stage system, which was developed by analysis of presenting clinical features, response to treatment, and survival of a cohort of patients with multiple myeloma in whom indirect measurements of total body myeloma mass had also been made.[66] The three stages, I, II, and III, are subclassified into A and B, depending on the presence or absence of renal failure. The usefulness of this staging system has been confirmed by a number of groups. However, it adds little to prognostic information once the β_2M level and PCLI are known, and in some studies it has been found not to predict prognosis.[55] Durie-Salmon stage IA, however, clearly identifies a group of good-prognosis patients who have smoldering myeloma and who may not require initial therapy. Such patients invariably have low PCLI and β_2M levels. Other staging systems have been proposed and are based on routine diagnostic investigations. These include systems from the Acute Leukemia Group B and the Eastern Cooperative Oncology Group (ECOG),[67] the Southeastern Cancer Study Group,[68] and the U.K. Medical Research Council (MRC).[69] All systems provide similar information.[70]

One difficulty in patient evaluation using such staging systems relates to the assessment of lytic bone lesions. Such lesions per se are often not an adverse prognostic factor and thus may falsely assign patients into late (poor prognosis) stages. Another difficulty relates to assessing response to therapy solely on the basis of changes in paraprotein levels. It is well recognized that in some patients with high M components the levels do not fall with chemotherapy. The inference that lack of response or the high levels themselves are an adverse event representing advanced or progressive disease may be incorrect. Stability of the protein (and attainment of plateau phase) is a much more powerful prognostic feature than "response," as determined by the fall of the paraprotein level.[71,73]

Factors Reflecting Renal Function

Renal failure is common in newly diagnosed myeloma and is more common in patients with light chain disease and in those who have high excretion rates of Bence Jones protein. Most patients with renal failure present with advanced disease (stage III Durie-Salmon), and renal failure is present in approximately 50 percent of patients with hypercalcemia.[38] In most patients with myeloma renal failure is reversible, often within the first 3 months.[35,40] The correction of renal failure depends on the correction of dehydration, hypercalcemia, hyperuricemia, and acidosis. Saline rehydration is the crucial factor, and allopurinol to prevent uric acid nephropathy and treatment of acidosis may help. Renal failure is often precipitated by a pyogenic infection, not necessarily within the renal tract, which should be treated promptly. No difference in therapeutic responses has been noted between patients who have renal failure and patients who do not. This finding has led to a reevaluation of the use of dialysis in patients with myeloma.[39,40] In a number of patients renal failure is the presentation of a very indolent B-cell disease that will either respond well to chemotherapy or not require much chemotherapy. Nevertheless, it is important to commence chemotherapy early in patients who present with renal failure. Melphalan is a poor drug in this situation because it is principally excreted by the kidney and dose adjustment is difficult. Chemotherapy regimes of choice include vincristine, doxorubicin, and dexamethasone (VAD) or vincristine, doxorubicin, and methylprednisolone (VAMP).[74]

Factors Reflecting Tumor–Host Interactions

The central role of IL-6 in the in vitro growth of myeloma cells has been recognized for some years. However, its role and importance in vivo and its role as an independent prognostic indicator remain controversial. Multivariate analyses demonstrating that

IL-6 levels give additional information over that provided by the β_2M level and the PCLI are lacking. In univariate analysis C-reactive protein (CRP) levels do reflect prognosis, although this value is lost in multivariate analysis once the β_2M level and PCLI are known.[55] Similar information appears to be provided by serum levels of lactate dehydrogenase and neopterin.

Soluble IL-6 receptor levels are elevated in myeloma, and high levels are correlated with an adverse prognosis. Levels are not correlated with PCLI, however, and thus are not a reflection of tumor proliferation per se. The explanation for the adverse prognostic effect of the level of the soluble IL-6 receptor is still to be established.

Many investigators have studied the alteration in surface antigen expression of a variety of subtypes of peripheral blood cells and correlated their findings with disease activity in myeloma. For instance, elevated levels of CD38+ cells are correlated with an adverse outcome, and CD38 levels rise with progressive disease.[75] The CD38+ cells are T lymphocytes and thus appear to be a reflection of a host–tumor interaction. Along similar lines, elevated IL-2 levels have been reported to correlate with a favorable outlook, perhaps reflecting lymphokine-activated killer cell activity against the malignant clone.[76] Further reinforcing the role of T-cell immunoregulation of the malignant clone, recent data have documented the presence of T-cell clones in the majority of patients with myeloma and clearly identified their presence as a good prognostic factor.[77]

In summary, myeloma is a complex disease; a variety of interacting factors can affect disease activity and stability. The very strong relationship between PCLI and prognosis must reflect a close relationship between the malignant clone and the plasma cell on which the PCLI is measured. The explanation for the highly significant effect of β_2M levels on prognosis still remains unclear, and it is likely that factors other than tumor bulk are involved.

Development of Leukemia After Myeloma

Among patients with myeloma who have survived for more than 2 years, the incidence of secondary leukemia gradually increases. This complication occurs at a frequency of 50 to 100 times that seen in the normal population and is in the majority of cases thought to be related to the use of alkylating agents, especially melphalan. Cytogenetic studies almost always confirm loss or deletion of the long arm of chromosome 5 or 7, which is consistent with an effect induced by an alkylating agent.[78]

A small number of patients have also been described in whom there was a simultaneous onset of acute leukemia and myeloma or in whom leukemia was not associated with the use of alkylating agents.[78] Such observations have previously been used to support a stem cell origin of myeloma. A recent case report demonstrated the persistence of myeloma in a patient with myeloma and acute promyelocytic leukemia (APML), with a t(15;17) and a *PML-RAR* fusion gene that was lost when remission of the APML was achieved. This indicates different lineages of the two malignancies.[79] Finally, there is no evidence to show that the presence of a paraprotein is related to the presence of underlying solid tumors.[80]

TREATMENT

The treatment of multiple myeloma is complex and requires many patient-specific decisions. Factors such as the patient's general state of health and the presence of disease complications often assume importance equal to that of the chemosensitivity of the tumor. A particular problem is presented by the management of bone disease and measures to prevent the progression of bony destruction. The recent introduction of the bisphosphonates into management protocols represents a major advance in the therapy of this complication and of myeloma in general. Although disease-specific therapy with conventional chemotherapy and radiation therapy has changed little over recent years, the demonstration of the efficacy of high-dose chemotherapeutic approaches with autologous transplantation has dramatically changed the approach to treatment in younger patients. In addition, there has been a reawakening of interest in allogeneic transplantation and much interest in new pharmacologic agents such as thalidomide[81,82] and P-glycoprotein blockers,[83] which are being evaluated as alternatives, adjuncts or both to conventional chemotherapy in an attempt to improve treatment response. Finally, attempts to stimulate a tumor response by a variety of "vaccination" strategies have also been made. In all but a few instances, the results of such new treatment approaches are still preliminary, and as yet it is not possible to draw firm conclusions concerning their ultimate role in the treatment of myeloma.

Like all malignancies that primarily afflict the elderly, measurement of treatment benefit is important in myeloma. Although response is typically measured by the percentage drop in paraprotein level, it has been well documented that monitoring paraprotein levels is of no prognostic value in determining ultimate survival. A major determinant of survival is the introduction and the attainment of a state of disease quiescence called the *plateau* phase. This can be defined as 3 to 6 months of clinical stability, stable paraprotein levels, and transfusion independence. In patients treated with conventional therapy, entry into plateau and the duration of plateau, rather than the amount by which the paraprotein falls, is the major prognostic factor. Patients who attain plateau after chemotherapy or who are in plateau at diagnosis have similar survivals. Such patients fare significantly better than those who fail to attain plateau, irrespective of their initial response to treatment.[71] Little is known about the nature of plateau and the mechanisms that are postulated to be responsible for its existence, but an essential accompaniment is a low proliferative state of the malignant plasma cells. Thus, plateau is always associated with a low PCLI and low and stable levels of other markers of proliferation, such as the STK. Markers of cell death, for example, urinary spermidine, are also low. It is believed that plateau is a state of tumor quiescence in which the malignant clone appears to be "dormant."[84]

A number of patients present in plateau phase. These patients, who have indolent or smoldering myeloma, account for approximately 5 to 10 percent of all myeloma patients and are identified by a lack of symptoms, generally a low paraprotein level (although occasionally it can be quite elevated), a fairly modest marrow infiltration, and minimal or no anemia. Most of these patients will have normal renal function, and lytic bone lesions are infrequent. The β_2M levels and PCLI are invariably low. There is no evidence that the early introduction of chemotherapy affects the ultimate outlook for these patients. When treatment eventually becomes necessary, the response rate is similar to that of patients treated immediately for symptomatic myeloma.[85] In contrast, and as will be more fully discussed below, the concept of plateau phase has less relevance to patients treated with high-dose regimens. In this setting the importance of obtaining a complete remission has been recently confirmed. A complete remission (CR), defined as a normal bone marrow and lack of M component detectable by immunofixation, has been shown to be achievable in more than 30 percent of such patients and is an important feature in determining overall survival.[86,87]

Another group of patients in whom management decisions should be individualized have so-called solitary or localized plasmacytomas of bone or extramedullary plasmacytomas. The outlook for patients who present with true solitary plasmacytomas is superior to that of those who present with disseminated myeloma, even though approximately 60 percent of patients with solitary plasmacytoma will eventually develop dissemination of the disease.[88] Solitary plasmacytomas of bone are best treated with localized radiation therapy, which will usually eradicate tumor within the radiation field. The usual dose is 40 to 50 Gy. A second tumor, a number of years or even decades later, is usual and may occur locally (10 percent of cases) or distally. By contrast, extramedullary plasmacytomas tend to occur in an older population and behave more like lymphomas, with involvement of the upper respiratory or gastrointestinal tracts and adjacent lymph nodes.[89,90] Local irradiation (40 to 50 Gy) is the appropriate management and usually prevents local recurrence. It has not yet been demonstrated that patients with solitary plasmacytomas of bone or extramedullary plasmacytomas benefit directly from adjuvant chemotherapy after local treatment. Local excision of the tumor is rarely advisable, and surgery, other than for diagnostic purposes, is usually not indicated.[91,92] An exception occurs with patients who may require orthopedic procedures to treat spinal cord compression.

MANAGEMENT OF SPECIFIC COMPLICATIONS

Hypercalcemia

Hypercalcemia, a common complication, is found in approximately 25 percent of patients at presentation, and an additional 25 percent will develop it during the course of the disease. It is also a frequent terminal complication. A variety of etiologic factors have been implicated, the most important being the uncoupling of the normal osteoblastic–osteoclastic nexus.[93] Osteoclast overactivity is believed to be caused by cytokines secreted by the tumor cells.[94] Several cytokines, namely lymphotoxin, tumor necrosis factor, insulin-like growth factor, and IL-1β have the ability to enhance bone reabsorption, and these have been called the osteoclast-activating factors (OAFs).[95–98] Osteoclasts are a major source of IL-6, which has been shown to be synergistic with other OAFs in enhancing their lytic activity.[96,99]

The symptoms of hypercalcemia are well described and include polyuria and thirst, constipation, lethargy, clouding of consciousness, nausea, and vomiting. The calcium level should be corrected for the level of serum albumin, since patients with myeloma are commonly hypoalbuminemic. A few patients with paraproteins that bind calcium have been described. Such patients have strikingly high levels of calcium in the absence of symptoms. Measurement of the ionized calcium level reveals the problem.[100]

Patients with significant hypercalcemia are invariably dehydrated and initially should be vigorously rehydrated. Intravenous saline expands the intravascular volume and produces natriuresis, thus accelerating calcium clearance. Natriuresis can be enhanced by the use of a loop diuretic such as furosemide, but thiazides should be avoided. Diuretic therapy alone, without expansion of the intravascular volume, is contraindicated. Corticosteroids also play a major role in the management of this complication. In addition to direct antitumor activity, they also enhance osteoblastic activity. Other possible agents include calcitonin and mithramycin. Calcitonin is a peptide hormone secreted by the parafollicular cells of the thyroid gland, which when used in pharmacologic doses (8 IU per kilogram of body weight) will result in a fall of the serum calcium within 2 to 4 hours. The effect lasts only 48 hours and thus is only a short-term measure. Mithramycin, at an intravenous dose of 25 μg/kg over 2 to 4 hours, lowers calcium within 24 to 48 hours. Thrombocytopenia is an occasional unwanted toxic side effect. Both calcitonin and mithramycin have, however, largely been superseded by bisphosphonates.[101] To date the most widely used agent has been aminohydroxypropylidene phosphate (ADP), or pamidronate, which up until recently was probably the most rapid hypocalcemic agent available. In clinical trials, pamidronate has been shown to be significantly superior to mithramycin, corticosteroids, and calcitonin in the treatment of tumor-induced hypercalcemia.[102] Newer agents such as zolendronate may even be superior to pamidronate. Reduction of serum calcium usually occurs within 24 hours of the initiation of treatment, with normalization of serum levels within 3 to 7 days. The side effects of this drug are generally mild and include fever that may last for up to 48 hours. The usual dose of ADP is a single 30- to 90-mg intravenous infusion over 2 to 4 hours. Although use of these diphosphonates is not necessary in all cases of hypercalcemia, a bisphosphonate is the agent of choice in the initial management of acute hypercalcemia associated with myeloma and other malignancies. New biological recombinant agents such as osteoprotegerin are yet to be evaluated in this clinical setting, but may also, based on recent studies,[103,104] be an effective clinical osteoclast inhibitor.

Hyperviscosity

The clinical manifestations of hyperviscosity are varied, although central nervous system effects with confusion and visual disturbances are most frequent. In addition, especially in patients with IgA myeloma, the hyperviscosity syndrome can be accompanied by a coagulopathy in which the paraprotein interferes with platelet function and thrombin generation.[105,106] Isolated cases of paraproteins with anti-factor VIII activity have also been described. The coagulopathy of the hyperviscosity syndrome cannot be treated with replacement of coagulation factors or platelets and requires plasmapheresis. Hyperviscosity can also aggravate renal failure. Plasma exchange is the management of choice for patients with symptomatic hyperviscosity and can be a life-saving procedure. In general, a 4- to 5-L exchange with normal plasma or albumin replacement is required and is repeated as frequently as indicated by clinical features and measurement of plasma viscosity.[107]

Cryoglobulinemia

Approximately 5 percent of patients with myeloma have paraproteins that form complexes at temperatures below 37°C (i.e., cryoprecipitates). In myeloma this is usually a type I-cryoglobulinemia, in contrast to the mixed polyclonal proliferation seen in autoimmune diseases. Cryoglobulins are usually IgM, IgG_3, or IgA, but occasional cases of cryoglobulinemia with Bence Jones proteins only have been described. Cryoglobulinemia is best treated by treating the underlying disease and by plasmapheresis if necessary. It is important to advise the patient to avoid cold to prevent intravascular precipitation.

Bony Disease

Bone disease, in particular bone destruction and its attendant consequences (pain, disability, hypercalcemia), often constitutes the major symptom complex of multiple myeloma. A number of studies have evaluated agents such as the bisphosphonates, which inhibit bony reabsorption and thus limit these complications. Such trials include studies using either pamidronate, ethidronate, or clodronate. Overall, ethidronate has not been successful in preventing bony progression,[108] although recent large studies using pamidronate or clodronate appear to demonstrate a role for their use as an adjuvant to standard chemotherapy.[109–112] A suggestion has been made that pamidronate itself has an antimyeloma action and may affect survival,[112,113] and the possible use of pamidronate alone as initial therapy for smoldering myeloma has been postulated. A large randomized international study on pamidronate has demonstrated a highly significant reduction in skeletal events in those patients receiving monthly pamidronate at a dose of 90 mg intravenously over 2 hours with minimal side effects.[112] Oral pamidronate is ineffective.[114] Currently bisphosphonate is recommended for the majority of patients with active myeloma.

CHEMOTHERAPY

Single Agents

Melphalan

Initial reports on the use of alkylating agents in myeloma showed that L-phenylalanine mustard (melphalan) could induce remissions in approximately one-third of a group of poor-risk patients.[115] Melphalan is an orally absorbed, stable nitrogen mustard derivative in which the phenylalanine replaces the methyl group of nitrogen mustard. It has a plasma half-life of approximately 90 minutes and is excreted by the kidney. One of the major problems with oral administration of melphalan is variable absorption; its bioavailability ranges between 60 and 100 percent of the oral dose.[116] This often requires biologic determination of the correct dose, as manifested by the onset of mild hematologic toxicity. The MRC and Cancer and Leukemia Group B (CALGB) trials have clearly demonstrated the efficacy of melphalan in patients with untreated myeloma.[117,118] In the MRC trials in particular, its equivalence in nonablative doses to cyclophosphamide was also demonstrated.[119] When given along conventional lines, melphalan can be expected to produce significant objective responses in 40 to 60 percent of patients with newly diagnosed myeloma. The average median remission duration and survival are 2 and 3 years, respectively, with very few patients surviving longer than 10 years and no evidence for cure.

Although a number of intermittent schedules have been proposed, none have clearly been shown to be superior. Commonly used schedules are 0.25 mg/kg/day for 4 days every 6 weeks or 8mg/m² for 4 days every 6 weeks. Even though intermittent melphalan has not been shown to produce improved survival (compared with low-dose continuous melphalan), its ease of use and monitoring and perhaps its lower incidence of hematologic toxicity and acute myeloid leukemia have brought about the almost universal use of intermittent melphalan schedules (first described by Alexanian et al).[120] Because melphalan is excreted by the kidney, its use in patients with renal failure is problematic. Dose adjustments are required and care in prescribing is essential. Melphalan can be given intravenously but this method is usually restricted to high-dose protocols, in which it has proved to be one of the most important conditioning regimens (see below).

Corticosteroids

Since their introduction in 1967 by Salmon et al.[121] for the treatment of myeloma, corticosteroids have remained some of the most active single agents for treatment of this disease.[122] High doses of corticosteroids, either dexamethasone as used in the VAD regime[123] or prednisone as in the doxorubicin (Adriamycin), bleomycin, cyclophosphamide, melphalan, and prednisone (ABCMP) regimen of the MRC studies,[124] are extremely effective in inducing disease responses, even in patients refractory to alkylating agents. It has been suggested that most of the therapeutic effect of VAD may in fact be due to the high doses of dexamethasone.[125] Some of the antimyeloma activity may result from the metabolic effect of glucocorticoids on protein catabolism, but high-dose corticosteroids, in particular, are known to cause tumor lysis. Nevertheless, no randomized trial has conclusively demonstrated that addition of high doses of glucocorticoids to melphalan-based treatments improves survival in patients treated with other effective forms of chemotherapy.

Cyclophosphamide

Cyclophosphamide is a stable, orally absorbed nitrogen mustard derivative with a relatively long plasma half-life. It has equal activity to melphalan in myeloma.[119] The parent compound is not an alkylator but is activated by the hepatic P450 system to 4-hydroxycyclophosphamide, which is catabolized to produce a series of active agents that are subsequently excreted via the kidneys. The advantages of cyclophosphamide include the relative lack of cumulative myeloid and stem cell toxicity and the platelet-sparing effect, which makes it useful in thrombocytopenic patients. Representative schedules for administration of cyclophosphamide as a single agent include 600 mg/m^2 intravenously every second week or 150 mg/m^2 orally for 4 days repeated at 3- to 4-week intervals. The significant complications of cyclophosphamide are myelotoxicity and the production of an irritant agent, acrolein, which can induce a sterile hemorrhagic cystitis. This latter complication can be ameliorated by forcing a fluid diuresis and by giving 2-mercaptoethanol sodium sulfonate (mesna), which detoxifies acrolein in the urine.[126]

More recently, higher doses of cyclophosphamide have been used in a variety of treatment scenarios. Doses of up to 4 to 7 g/m^2, with or without etoposide and hemopoietic colony-stimulating factors (CSFs) have been used in patients with refractory disease.[127] In addition, this approach is used for priming patients prior to peripheral blood stem cell collection, inasmuch as use of cyclophosphamide (with or without CSFs) is not only an efficient means of mobilizing stem cells but also a highly effective antitumor therapy.[128]

Vincristine

Although vincristine is used extensively in multidrug protocols such as vincristine-carmustine-melphalan-cyclophosphamide-prednisone (VBMCP), vincristine-carmustine-doxorubicin-prednisone (VBAP), and VAD, considerable doubt exists about its value as an active agent. The large MRC IV study demonstrated that intermittent vincristine when used as an adjuvant to melphalan and prednisone was no more effective than melphalan and prednisone alone.[129] Toxicity includes a peripheral neuropathy, which may result in irreversible nerve damage. Importantly, the autonomic nervous system can be affected, with resulting constipation and ileus. These effects are exacerbated by concomitant use of narcotic analgesics. Thus, although vincristine is not myelotoxic, there seems to be little point in recommending its routine use.

Interferon-α

The activity of interferon-α (IFN-α) in myeloma was first demonstrated in 1979 when Mellstedt et al.[130] reported the initial experience of IFN therapy in four previously untreated patients who received partially purified human leukocyte IFN. Numerous studies since that time have confirmed the activity of IFN-α in myeloma; overall response rates of 15 to 20 percent have been reported in patients with disease resistant to alkylating agents.[131]

The mechanism of action of IFN-α in myeloma has not been precisely elucidated. A number of studies have shown an in vitro antiproliferative effect on the putative myeloma stem cell,[132] and an effect on the maturation and proliferation of certain myeloma cell lines has also been documented.[133] In addition, it has been postulated that IFN, acting as a biologic response modifier, has in vivo effects on host–tumor immunoregulation, perhaps via activation of natural killer cells. Interferon-α also has in vitro synergism with chemotherapeutic agents, including melphalan, and a number of trials have explored the feasibility of combining IFN with melphalan and prednisone.[134] However, IFN adds to the myelotoxicity of melphalan, and there is little evidence that IFN when used as a coinduction agent adds significantly to the response or survival of myeloma patients. A possible exception is IgA and light chain myeloma, in which IFN has been shown to be of benefit.[135]

The major role of IFN-α may be its ability to prolong the plateau phase after either standard or high-dose chemotherapy.[124,136–138] A meta-analysis by the Myeloma Trialists collaborative group in Oxford, based on the individual data of over 4000 patients from 24 randomized trials, has shown that interferon produced a significant but minor improvement in relapse-free survival and overall survival.[139] A recent overview has suggested that the impact of interferon may be limited to a small but unpredictable cohort of patients.[140]

Combination Therapy

One of the controversial areas in myeloma therapy is the choice of primary chemotherapy. Multidrug combinations, at nonablative doses, are probably not superior to melphalan (with or without prednisone).[141,142] Although intermittent courses of melphalan with or without prednisone have been the standard chemotherapy for myeloma for many years, the difficulty in using this agent and the less than optimal response has led many authors to investigate multiagent combinations in an attempt to improve response rates. A number of studies and controlled trials have been performed to evaluate this issue. Some have shown a significant benefit with the combinations,[143,144] and others have shown no benefit.[145–148] Interpretation of this mass of data is difficult and is burdened by a number of factors. For instance, a variety of drugs, doses, and schedules are employed and not all combinations are equally aggressive; also, many studies have been too small to produce a clear answer. In an attempt to resolve this issue, meta-analyses of many of these trials have been undertaken. In general, such analyses have failed to demonstrate a clear advantage for the various combinations over traditional melphalan therapy, and although increased response rates have been documented, there is no evidence of improvement in survival.[141]

Vincristine-doxorubicin-dexamethasone has also been extensively studied in patients with newly diagnosed myeloma.[123] This combination often produces high-frequency rapid "responses." "Complete" remissions (normal marrow appearance with the absence of a paraprotein on immunofixation) have occurred in approximately 30 percent of patients. However, whereas early remission is an advantage in patients with hypercalcemia and renal failure, neither remission duration nor survival is prolonged by the use of VAD as a first-line agent compared with standard therapies.[149,150] The efficacy of VAD may be primarily due to the intermittent courses of high-dose dexamethasone.[151] The efficacy of vincristine in myeloma is doubtful, and the toxicity of doxorubicin infusion remains a clinical problem. High doses of dexamethasone are useful when radiation therapy is required for pathologic fractures or incipient cord compression. In addition, because of the lack of cumulative stem cell toxicity, VAD and VAD-like protocols such as VAMP and (C)VAMP, in which dexamethasone is replaced by methylprednisolone, are also useful in patients who are being considered for stem cell harvest and high-dose therapy.

RADIATION THERAPY

Radiation therapy plays a crucial palliative or adjuvant role in the management of myeloma. However, with the possible exception of its use in transplantation, radiation therapy per se does not affect the natural history of the disease. Early studies using total body irradiation showed this approach to be impractical; many complications were seen, including radiation pneumonitis. Hemibody irradiation has been applied in a sequential fashion, and although this is certainly technically possible, it has yet to be shown to be of any benefit other than for palliation. Studies evaluating this approach typically delivered 8 Gy to the upper or lower body, which was followed by treatment of the other half of the body 6 to 8 weeks later. Approximately half the patients treated in this way experienced pain relief, but their outlook was extremely poor and no evidence was provided that this approach was better than that achieved with second-line chemotherapy.[152]

The key role of radiation is in alleviating localized bony pain, especially the pain of vertebral column involvement. In addition, radiation of pathologic fractures after fixation and of other lytic lesions, especially in cases of solitary plasmacytoma or extramedullary plasmacytoma, is extremely valuable. Combining standard chemotherapy in nonablative doses with radiation therapy does not seem to be of value. Studies have not shown any real benefit nor has any benefit been demonstrated for radiation therapy in the maintenance of the plateau phase. Its role in transplantation with high-dose melphalan is discussed below.[153]

MAINTENANCE THERAPY

In patients who enter the plateau phase after induction therapy, continuation of the same therapy does not appear to be beneficial. Moreover, continuous alkylating therapy increases the chance of the development of acute myeloid leukemia and other myelodysplasias. In a number of studies of patients who were in plateau or remission 12 months after induction chemotherapy, such patients were randomly assigned to continued treatment with alkylating agents or to no further therapy.[154–156] No significant difference in survival has been demonstrated. Often the duration of "first" remission was longer in those receiving maintenance therapy, but the patients who had not received maintenance therapy had a much higher response to treatment at the time of relapse. Kinetic studies of myeloma cells indicating low proliferative activity in "remission" compared with time of diagnosis provide an explanation for the lack of efficacy of conventional chemotherapy in maintaining the plateau phase.[157] Cases of myeloid leukemia occur after approximately 18 months of therapy with alkylating agents and increase considerably with continual use of this treatment, reaching levels of 15 to 20 percent.[158] Such programs of continual alkylating agent therapy are rarely used today.

Interferon-α has also been extensively used in maintenance therapy. The initial reports from an Italian controlled trial indicated prolongations of plateau phase and of survival. Other controlled trials have also demonstrated prolongation of plateau phase, but prolongation of survival has not been seen,[124,136–138] with the exception of a study from Sweden that showed prolongation of survival in patients with IgA and light chain myeloma who were treated with IFN-α.[159]

Thus, whereas IFN-α as a maintenance treatment appears to increase response duration, no significant survival benefit has been conclusively demonstrated. In addition, IFN-α side effects may interfere with the quality of life of patients, and the routine use of this agent in all patients once the plateau phase is established is still controversial. An alternative role of IFN-α in maintenance therapy has been postulated for patients undergoing bone marrow transplantation, but overview meta-analysis shows marginal efficacy, and the role of IFN is still unclear.[139,140]

TRANSPLANTATION

High-Dose Therapy and Stem Cell Transplantation

Conventional chemotherapy cures few, if any, patients; only a small proportion, probably less than 5 percent, survive for 10 years. In many of the latter patients prolonged survival is likely to be more a function of the indolent nature of the disease than a true therapeutic response. The rationale for the use of high-dose therapy relates not only to the apparent failure of conventional therapy but to the demonstration of a drug–dose relationship, such that the increased dose can lead to an increased response rate and to a prolonged remission. In addition, in some patients undergoing allogeneic transplantation, a graft-versus-myeloma effect is now well recognized and believed to contribute to the overall clinical response.

Historically, the development of high-dose protocols in myeloma rests on two observations. The first was the demonstration of a cohort of long-term survivors in those individuals receiving syngeneic (twin) bone marrow transplants.[160] An interesting observation is that many such patients still demonstrate small paraproteins in either their blood or urine. The other major development was the introduction of high-dose melphalan therapy protocols by McElwain and Powles at the Royal Marsden Hospital in England.[161] Initially melphalan was used at a dose of 140 mg/m² unsupported by stem cell rescue. Dramatic responses were seen in some cases, including some complete clinical remissions, although most patients subsequently relapsed. The use of bone marrow and subsequent blood stem cell rescue has enabled further dose escalations and the use of additional agents in an attempt to increase the efficacy of high-dose therapy by overcoming drug resistance.[162]

Allogeneic Transplantation

It is currently recognized that allogeneic (or syngeneic) transplantation may cure a small number of patients with myeloma. The first group of patients to undergo transplantation in myeloma were those with identical twin donors. A few are currently alive in complete remission many years after transplantation, which suggests that such patients are highly likely to be cured of their disease. High-dose therapy alone, without a graft-versus-myeloma effect and even in patients who were previously resistant to alkylating agents, may therefore result in a cure.[163]

The complete response rates after allogeneic sibling transplantation range from 30 to 75 percent, which exceed those seen with conventional chemotherapy.[164,165] This is even more encouraging when it is realized that many such patients would have failed one or more courses of therapy before undergoing transplantation. Despite these encouraging responses, relapses after bone marrow transplantation still occur in a large number of patients, and it is not yet clear whether a true plateau in survival has been achieved. Prognostic factors for transplantation appear to be the same as those for conventional chemotherapy; despite high response rates, the duration of response and the relative value of transplantation (in terms of both quality of life and cost of therapy compared with conventional treatment or autologous stem cell transplantation) remain to be determined.

The largest reported series of allogeneic transplantation, from the European Bone Marrow Transplant group, includes a large number of transplantation patients from numerous centers followed for up to 7 years.[164] A complete response rate of 43 percent, an overall 5-year survival of 40 percent, and a 30 percent disease-free survival have been recorded. Patients who were sensitive to chemotherapy and who had received only a minimum amount of chemotherapy prior to transplantation fared better than those who had failed multiple regimes. A large number of preparative regimes were used in the cohort, although most of the protocols included cyclophosphamide or melphalan (or both) plus total body irradiation. Data from Seattle, using busulfan and cyclophosphamide as a preparative regime, show similar results, with overall survival at 50 months of approximately 39 percent and disease-free survival of 34 percent.[165] In both these studies transplant-related deaths have been somewhat higher than reported in otherwise good-risk patients with other hematopoietic malignancies. In myeloma, factors such as a poorer clinical state, greater age, and comorbidity illnesses are likely explanations. Other transplant centers have provided similar results,[166] and a number of recent reviews have been published.[167,168]

Currently, the ratio of patients undergoing autologous as opposed to allogeneic stem cell transplantation for myeloma is approximately 3:1 (International Bone Marrow Transplant Registry data). The majority of initial transplantations used allogeneic donors, and the recipients, with the exception of those with identical twin donors, principally had end-stage disease. This, coupled with the average age of most myeloma patients, led to high treatment-related toxicity and high rates of graft-versus-host disease. Thus the application of allogeneic approaches has been limited. Data from the European Blood and Bone Marrow Transplant Group's long-term follow-up study of allogeneic transplantation in myeloma suggest that at 9 years less than 20 percent of patients are alive and many of these still have residual disease.[164] A reawakening interest in allogeneic transplantation has, however, occurred over the last few years. Recent European Group for Blood and Marrow Transplantation (EBMTR) (and other) data have demonstrated a significant reduction in treatment-related toxicity and thus improved survival. Depletion of donor marrow T cells is also increasingly employed to reduce further toxicity from graft-versus-host disease, as is the "mini allograft," in which transplant conditioning is reduced and reliance is placed on immunological effects for the therapeutic response, as it is now clear that immunological factors play a major role in the results of therapy after allogeneic transplantation. A graft-versus-myeloma effect has been demonstrated and the beneficial role of donor lymphocyte infusions has been documented.[169–173]

A recent matched-pair analysis, however, performed by the EBMTR demonstrated a superior survival for patients undergoing autologous transplants compared with those undergoing allogeneic transplants,[174] and although allogeneic transplantation is a major option for younger patients with a suitable compatible donor, the timing of the transplant remains unclear. It is controversial whether allogeneic bone marrow transplantation should be performed at diagnosis, after achievement of the initial plateau, or at the earliest signs of escape from the plateau.

Autologous Transplantation

Autologous transplantation in myeloma was encouraged by the results of treatment with high-dose melphalan alone in the pioneering work by McElwain and colleagues during the 1980s.[161,162] Subsequently a number of investigators have evaluated a variety of autologous transplantation options in myeloma, and it is now widely performed and accepted as the best option for younger patients with myeloma.

Pivotal to the widespread acceptance of autologous transplantation in myeloma was the study by Attal et al.,[175] which demonstrated that a single (bone marrow) transplant was superior to conventional multiagent chemotherapy such as VMCP–VBAP in terms of both overall survival and disease-free survival, which were 28 versus 10 percent and 52 versus 12 percent, respectively. The benefit was most apparent in patients under 60 years of age. Long-term follow-up evaluation of this study has confirmed the initial reports, as have recent data from Scandinavia.[176] The most extensive experience of autologous transplantation comes from Arkansas, where investigators have used an intensive program of debulking therapy and double autologous transplantation followed by maintenance therapy with interferon-α total therapy,[177] and they have delineated prognostic factors, response rates, and total survival rates in patients with myeloma suitable for such aggressive regimes. They have suggested possible cure in the absence of certain adverse prognostic factors, especially deletions of chromosome 13 in tumor cells. Subsequent randomized studies have looked at the issues of one versus two transplants and early versus late transplantation. As yet, both studies show no difference in overall survival in the patient cohorts, although follow-up periods are still relatively short.[178] Randomized studies have also demonstrated the superiority of mobilized blood stem cells over bone marrow-derived cells in terms of speed of hematopoietic recovery, although a survival advantage has not been demonstrated.[179]

Reinfusion of the malignant cells is of course, a conceptual hurdle for all forms of autologous transplantation for malignancy. Sensitive assays have repeatedly detected contamination of marrow and mobilized blood stem cells in myeloma patients. Thus there have been numerous attempts to purge autologous collections of contaminating tumor cells. Although a variety of techniques have been employed, the most frequently used has been positive selection of normal hematopoietic progenitor cells based on their expression of the CD34 antigen. This antigen is believed to be absent from malignant plasma cells, or at least the majority of such cells. Thus, use of a CD34-positive selection procedure will lead to a reduction in contaminating tumor cells. A reproducible reduction of plasma cells by three orders of magnitude has been reported.[180,181]

A large randomized study of CD34-selected versus CD34-unselected single autologous transplants has been recently completed and the preliminary results have been published. Median tumor depletion was greater than three orders of magnitude in the CD34-selected group, and the kinetics of hematopoietic engraftment were equivalent. With short follow-up periods, disease-free and overall survival are, however, equivalent.[182] Elderly patients may also benefit from high-dose therapy but with increased therapy-related morbidity.[183,184] It is also apparent that the benefit of high-dose therapy remains even if the transplant is delayed to a later stage of a patient's illness rather than given at diagnosis.[185]

In summary, the results of current studies permit some conclusions as to the value of high-dose therapy, although it is by no means clear that it should be embarked on at diagnosis in every patient. If a patient has a fully matched compatible sibling and is under the age of 55, allogeneic transplantation at some stage in that patient's disease is appropriate. Whether it should occur at the beginning of the illness or after the plateau phase is unclear. Prognostic factors predicting a poor outlook may be used to determine the time of treatment. With regard to autologous transplantation, it is also not clear whether this procedure should be carried out at the beginning of the disease, at early relapse, or after the establishment of an optimum clinical response. Finally, definitive data are needed to show which is the best preparatory regime prior to allogeneic or autologous transplantation. Nevertheless, autologous transplantation after initial debulking chemotherapy remains the standard of care for young patients with myeloma at present.

NEW AVENUES OF THERAPY

IL-6 Antibodies and Anti-CD20 Antibodies

One novel approach to therapy is the use of monoclonal antibodies against IL-6. Such therapy has been pioneered by French investigators, who have demonstrated that such antibodies can have antitumor and antiproliferative effects on myeloma plasma cells.[186] This therapeutic modality has only been used in patients with end-stage disease, and its role in the maintenance of plateau-phase disease or after bone marrow transplantation (or both) is yet to be determined. Other new avenues of therapy currently being explored include the use of anti-CD20 antibodies. A proportion of myeloma cells are CD20-positive,[187] and humanized anti-CD20 antibodies show a response in a percentage of patients whose cells are CD20-positive. Full clinical evaluation of the role of CD20 antibodies is awaited.

Erythropoietin

Anemia is a very common complication of myeloma and results in considerable impairment in the quality of life. It is often an early symptom and may in fact lead to the diagnosis of myeloma. Alternatively, it can develop as the disease progresses, and a myeloma-associated anemia is observed in about 50 percent of patients. Erythropoietin has been used to ameliorate the anemia and reduce dependence on blood transfusions. It appears to be particularly successful in early-stage disease.[188] High levels of endogenous erythropoietin are predictive of non-responsiveness to external erythropoietin. Sensitivity to erythropoietin is lost when patients are infected or during disease progression and increasing marrow infiltration.

Drug Resistance Development and Reversal

One of the main obstacles to successful chemotherapy is the emergence of drug resistance.[83,189] Although most patients initially respond to chemotherapy, at relapse their disease is frequently refractory not only to the drugs used in the first treatment but to a variety of other drugs. One of the biochemical explanations for this clinical observation of multidrug resistance (MDR), in which the malignant cell actively excludes a variety of substances, including anthracyclines, vinca alkaloids, and epipodophyllotoxins, is the expression of P-glycoprotein. P-glycoprotein is an ADP-dependent, unidirectional drug efflux pump with broad substrate specificity, which reduces the intracellular cytotoxic drug concentration. The de novo expression of P-glycoprotein is rare in myeloma but increases following exposure to drugs such as vincristine and doxorubicin.[190] In drug-resistant myeloma, increased P-glycoprotein expression is almost always present. The circulating clonogenic cell of myeloma may constitutively express P-glycoprotein.[191]

A number of modulators of MDR have been described, including verapamil and cyclosporin.[192,193] Such agents are relatively toxic, however, prompting the search for newer agents with less toxicity, such as the cyclosporin analogue SD2-OSC-833.[194] Addition of these drugs in vitro can lead to restoration of higher intracellular levels of doxorubicin and vincristine in MDR cell lines, and clinical trials have demonstrated the potential of this approach. However, whether these drugs will have any ultimate role is unclear, and initial studies have been disappointing.[193]

Immune-Based Therapies

Several observations suggest that an antitumor response is present in myeloma. Clonal T-cell populations are present in some patients with myeloma, and their presence correlates with a favorable prognosis.[77] Attempts to utilize T-cell responses by vaccination strategies are now being actively developed. Such approaches include protein, peptide, and DNA vaccines[195–198] with dendritic cells,[199] utilizing the myeloma idiotype as the predominant immunogen. The exquisite ability of antigen-primed dendritic cells to stimulate an immune response has also led to an investigation of this approach to vaccination as a means of heightening the immune response to the tumor, in myeloma as well as other malignancies. Clinical results are not yet available and are awaited with interest.

Thalidomide

Thalidomide, an antiangiogenic agent, has been demonstrated to be of value in patients with multiple myeloma. In patients with refractory disease, a 30 percent response has been reported by the group from Arkansas, with responses occurring over a period of 1 to 2 months.[81] The value of this agent as maintenance therapy or for use as a coinduction agent is still not clear, but several studies are addressing this at present. In particular, thalidomide with dexamethasone is effective.[200] Side effects are common and consist of sedation and neuropathy; the latter can be permanent. Cytopenia is, however, unusual and, this makes thalidomide a very useful agent in refractory patients with pancytopenia. Low doses also appear effective.[201]

The development of thalidomide and perhaps more potent antiangiogenic agents and the growing enthusiasm for immune-based therapies signify the development of expanding options for the treatment of multiple myeloma. With conventional therapeutic approaches, the fundamental problem of myeloma therapy remains drug resistance and the inability to eradicate the disease despite initial responses in most patients. It is to be hoped that in the future new techniques will allow improved survival, improved quality of life, and perhaps even cure.

REFERENCES

1. Davis LDH: International trends in cancer mortality in France, West Germany, Italy, Japan, England and Wales, and the USA. Lancet 336:474, 1990.
2. Cuzick J, Velez R, Doll R: International variations and temporal trends in mortality from multiple myeloma. Int J Cancer 32:13, 1983.
3. Deshpande HA, Hu XP, Marino P et al: Anticipation in familial plasma cell dyscrasias. Br J Haematol 103:696, 1998.
4. Cuzick J: Radiation induced myelomatosis. N Engl J Med 304:204, 1981.
5. Bergsagel DE, Wong O, Bergsagel PL et al: Benzene and multiple myeloma: Appraisal of the scientific evidence. Blood 94:1174, 1999.
6. Morris PD, Koeppsell TD, Darling JR et al: Toxic substances and multiple myeloma: A case control study. J Natl Cancer Inst 76:9867, 1986.
7. Mariette X, Zagdanski AM, Guermazi A et al: Prognostic value of vertebral lesions detected by magnetic resonance imaging in patients with stage I multiple myeloma. Br J Haematol 104:723, 1999.
8. Driedger H, Pruzanski W: Plasma cell neoplasia with peripheral polyneuropathy. Medicine (Baltimore) 59:301, 1980.
9. Chandy KG, Stockley RA, Leonard RCF et al: Relationship between serum viscosity and intravascular IgA polymer concentration in IgA myeloma. Clin Exp Immunol 46:653, 1981.
10. Seligmann M, Brouet JC: Antibody activity of human myeloma globulins. Semin Hematol 10:163, 1973.
11. Zettervall O, Nilsson IM: Acquired von Willebrand's disease caused by a monoclonal antibody. Acta Med Scand 204:521, 1978.
12. Farhangi M, Osserman ET: Myeloma with xanthoma to an IgG λ monoclonal antiflavin antibody. N Engl J Med 294:177, 1976.
13. Baker BL, Hultquist DE: A copper binding immunoglobulin from a myeloma patient. J Biol Chem 253:8444, 1978.
14. Trimarchi F, Berrenga S, Fenzi F et al: Immunoglobulin binding of thyroid hormones in a case of Waldenström's macroglobulinaemia. J Clin Endocrinol Metab 52:1045, 1982.
15. Redmon B, Pysdrowski K, Elson M et al: Brief report: Hypoglycemia due to monoclonal insulin binding antibody in multiple myeloma. N Engl J Med 326:994, 1992.
16. Rajani B, Rajani V, Prayson RA: Peripheral nerve amyloidosis in aural nerve biopsies: A clinicopathologic analysis of 13 cases. Arch Pathol Lab Med 124:114, 2000.
17. Hafler DA, Johnson D, Kelly J et al: Monoclonal gammopathy and neuropathy: Myelin-associated glycoprotein reactivity and clinical characteristics. Neurology 36:75, 1986.
18. Monaco S, Bonetti B, Ferrari S et al: Complement-mediated demyelination in patients with IgM monoclonal gammopathy and polyneuropathy. N Engl J Med 332:649, 1990.
19. Nobile Orazio E, Meucci N, Baldini L et al: Long-term prognosis of neuropathy associated with anti-MAG IgM M-proteins and its relationship to immune therapies. Brain 123:710, 2000.
20. Bleasel AF, Hawke S, Pollard J et al: IgG monoclonal paraproteinaemia and peripheral neuropathy. J Neurol Neurosurg Psychiatry 56:52, 1993.
21. Gorson KC: Clinical features, evaluation, and treatment of patients with polyneuropathy associated with monoclonal gammopathy of undetermined significance (MGUS). J Clin Apheresis 14:149, 1999.
22. Hirano T: Biological and clinical apsects of interleukin-6. Immunol Today 11:443, 1990.
23. Van Riet I, Heirman C, Lacor P et al: Detection of monoclonal B lymphocytes and BM in peripheral blood of multiple myeloma patients by immunoglobulin gene rearrangement studies. Br J Haematol 73:289, 1989.
24. Billadeau D, Quam L, Thomas W: Detection and quantitation of malignant cells in the peripheral blood of multiple myeloma patients. Blood 80:1818, 1992.
25. Corradini P, Voema C, Omede P et al: Detection of circulating tumour cells in multiple myeloma by a PCR based method. Leukemia 7:1879, 1993.
26. Brown RD, Luo X-F, Gibson J et al: Longitudinal analysis of circulating myeloma cells detected by allele specific mRNA in situ hybridization. Am J Hematol 58:273, 1998.
27. Fahey JL, Scoggins R, Utz J et al: Infection, antibody response and gamma globulin components in multiple myeloma and macroglobulinaemia. Am J Med 35:698, 1963.
28. Oken MM, Pomeroy C, Weisdorf D et al: Prophylactic antibiotics for the prevention of early infection in multiple myeloma. Am J Med 100:624, 1996.

29. Weeks JC, Tierney MR, Weinstein MC: Cost effectiveness of prophylactic intravenous immune globulin in chronic lymphocytic leukemia. N Engl J Med 325:81, 1991.

30. Chapel HM, Lee M, Hargreaves R et al. for the UK Group for Immunoglobulin Replacement Therapy in Multiple Myeloma: Randomised trial of intravenous immunoglobulin as prophylaxis against infection in plateau phase multiple myeloma. Lancet 343:1059, 1994.

31. Waldmann TA, Strober W: Metabolism of immunoglobulins. Prog Allergy 13:1, 1969.

32. McIntyre OR, Kochwa S, Propert KJ: Prognostic value of light chain isoelectric point (IEP) in multiple myeloma. Proc Am Soc Clin Oncol 7:884A, 1988.

33. Solomon A, Weiss D, Kaltine A: Nephrotoxic potential of Bence Jones proteins. N Engl J Med 324:1845, 1991.

34. Rabb H, Gunasekaran S, Saba SR: Acute renal failure from multiple myeloma precipitated by ACE inhibitors. Am J Kidney Dis 33:E5, 1999.

35. MacLennan ICM, Cooper E, Chapman CE et al: Renal failure in myelomatosis. Eur J Haematol 43:60, 1989.

36. Moist L, Nesrallah G, Kortas C et al: Plasma exchange in rapidly progressive renal failure due to multiple myeloma. A retrospective case series. Am J Nephrol 19:45, 1999.

37. Buxbaum J, Gallo G: Nonamyloidotic monoclonal immunoglobulin deposition disease. Light-chain, heavy-chain, and light- and heavy-chain deposition diseases. Hematol Oncol Clin North Am 13:1235, 1999.

38. Clark AD, Shetty A, Soutar R: Renal failure and multiple myeloma: Pathogenesis and treatment of renal failure and management of underlying myeloma. Blood Rev 13:79, 1999.

39. Sharland A, Snowdon L, Joshua DE et al: Hemodialysis: An appropriate therapy in myeloma-induced renal failure. Am J Kidney Dis 30:786, 1997.

40. Blade J, Fernandez-Llama P, Bosch F et al: Renal failure in multiple myeloma: Presenting features and predictors of outcome in 94 patients from a single institution. Arch Intern Med 158:1889, 1998.

41. Kyle RA, Greipp PR: Smoldering multiple myeloma. N Engl J Med 302:1347, 1980.

42. Wilson AT: Direct immunoelectrophoresis. J Immunol 92:431, 1964.

43. Kyle RA, Maldonado JE, Bayrd ED: Idiopathic Bence Jones proteinuria – a distinct entity? Am J Med 302:1347, 1980.

44. Kyle RA, Greipp PR: Idiopathic Bence Jones proteinuria: Long term follow up in seven patients. N Engl J Med 306:564, 1982.

45. Joshua DE: Immunoglobulins. In Malpas JS, Bergsagel DE, Kyel RA, Anderson KC (eds.): Myeloma Biology and Management. Oxford University Press, Oxford, 1998.

46. Joshua DE, Brown R, Gibson J: Prognostic factors in myeloma: What do they tell us about the pathophysiology of the disease? Leuk Lymphoma 15:375, 1994.

47. Kyle RA: Why better prognostic factors for multiple myeloma are needed. Blood 83:1713, 1994.

48. Greipp PR, Katzman JA, O'Fallon WM et al: Value of β_2-microglobulin level and plasma cell labelling indices as prognostic factors in patients with newly diagnosed myeloma. Blood 72:219, 1988.

49. Boccadoro M, Massaia M, Dianzani U et al: Multiple myeloma: Biological and clinical significance of bone marrow plasma cell labelling index. Haematologica 72:171, 1987.

50. Boccadoro M, Gavarotti P, Foscati G: Low plasma cell ^{3}H thymidine incorporation in monoclonal gammopathy of undetermined significance (MGUS), smouldering myeloma and remission

51. Greipp PR, Witzig TE, Gonchoroff NJ: Immunofluorescent plasma cell labelling indices (LI) using a monoclonal antibody (BU-1). Am J Hematol 20:289, 1985.

52. Pope B, Brown R, Gibson J et al: The bone marrow plasma cell labelling index by flow cytometry. Cytometry 38:286, 1999.

53. Brown RD, Joshua DE, Ioannidis R et al: Serum thymidine kinase as a marker of disease activity in patients with multiple myeloma. Aust N Z J Med 19:226, 1989.

54. Brown RD, Joshua DE, Nelson M et al: Serum thymidine kinase as a prognostic indicator for patients with multiple myeloma: Results from the MRC (UK) V trial. Br J Haematol 84:238, 1992.

55. Greipp PR, Lust JA, O'Fallon WM et al: Plasma cell labelling index and beta 2-microglobulin predict survival independent of thymidine kinase and C-reactive protein in multiple myeloma. Blood 81:3382, 1993.

56. Bartl R, Frisch B, Diem H et al: Histologic, biochemical and clinical parameters for monitoring multiple myeloma. Cancer 68:2241, 1991.

57. Greipp PR, Raymond NM, Kyle RA et al: Multiple myeloma: Significance of plasmablastic subtype in morphological classification. Blood 65:305, 1985.

58. Tricot G, Barlogie B, Jagannath S et al: Poor prognosis in multiple myeloma is associated only with partial or complete deletions of chromosome 13 or abnormalities involving 11q and not with other karyotype abnormalities. Blood 86:4250, 1995.

59. Garcia Sanz R, Orfao A, Gonzalez M et al: Primary plasma cell leukemia: Clinical, immunophenotypic, DNA ploidy, and cytogenetic characteristics. Blood 94:1032, 1999.

60. Smadja NV, Fruchart C, Isnard F et al: Chromosomal analysis in multiple myeloma: Cytogenetic evidence of two different diseases. Leukemia 12:960, 1998.

61. Liu P, Leong T, Quam L et al: Activating mutations of N- and K-ras in multiple myeloma show different clinical associations: Analysis of the Eastern Cooperative Oncology Group Phase III Trial. Blood 88:2699, 1996.

62. Bataille R, Durie BGM, Geriner J: Serum $\beta2$-microglobulin and survival duration in multiple myeloma: A simple, reliable marker for staging. Br J Haematol 55:439, 1983.

63. Durie BGM, Stock-Novack D, Salmon SE: Prognostic value of pre-treatment serum $\beta2$-microglobulin in myeloma. A Southwest Oncology Group study. Blood 75:823, 1990.

64. Cuzick J, Be Stavola BL, Coopert EH et al: Long-term prognostic value of serum $\beta2$-microglobulin in myelomatosis. Br J Haematol 33:101, 1990.

65. Boccadoro M, Durie BGM, Frutiger Y et al: Lack of correlation between plasma cell thymidine labelling index and serum $\beta2$-microglobulin in monoclonal gammopathies. Acta Haematol 78:239, 1987.

66. Durie BG, Salmon SE: A clinical staging system for multiple myeloma: Correlation of measured myeloma cell mass with presenting clinical features, response to treatment and survival. Cancer 36:842, 1975.

67. Costa G, Engle RL Jr, Schilling A et al. for the Acute Leukemia Group B and the Eastern Cooperative Oncology Group: Melphalan and prednisone: An effective combination for the treatment of multiple myeloma. Am J Med 54:589, 1973.

68. Southeastern Cancer Study Group: Treatment of myeloma. Comparison of melphalan, chlorambucil and azathioprine. Arch Intern Med 135:157, 1975.

50. (continued) phase myeloma: A reliable indicator of patients not requiring therapy. Br J Haematol 58:689, 1984.

69. Medical Research Council Working Party on Leukaemia in Adults: Prognostic features in the third MRC myelomatosis trial. Br J Cancer 42:831, 1980.

70. Gassmann W, Pralle H, Haferlach T et al: Staging systems for multiple myeloma: A comparison. Br J Haematol 59:703, 1985.

71. Joshua DE, Snowdon L, Gibson J et al: Multiple myeloma: Plateau phase revisited. Haematol Rev 5:59, 1991.

72. Long term survival in multiple myeloma: A Finnish Leukaemia Group study. Br J Haematol 105:942, 1999.

73. Corso A, Nozza A, Lazzarino M et al: Plateau phase in multiple myeloma: An end-point of cenventional-dose chemotherapy. Haematologica 84:336, 1999.

74. Forgeson GV, Selby P, Lakhani S et al: Infused vincristine and Adriamycin with high dose methyl prednisolone (VAMP) in advanced previously treated multiple myeloma patients. Br J Cancer 58:469, 1988.

75. Joshua DE, Wolf M, Mathews J et al: Peripheral blood lymphocyte surface antigen expression and prognosis in myeloma: Australian Leukaemia Study Group study. Leuk Lymphoma 14:305, 1994.

76. Cimino G, Avvisati G, Amadori S et al: High serum IL-2 levels are predictive of prolonged survival in multiple myeloma. Br J Haematol 75:373, 1990.

77. Brown RD, Yuen E, Nelson M et al: The prognostic significance of T cell receptor beta gene rearrangements and idiotype-reactive T cells in multiple myeloma. Leukemia 11:1312, 1997.

78. Bergsagel D, Bailey A, Langley G: The chemotherapy of plasma cell myeloma and the incidence of acute leukemia. N Engl J Med 301:743, 1979.

79. Dunkley S, Gibson J, IIand H et al: Acute promyelocytic leukaemia complicating multiple myeloma: evidence of different cell lineages. Leuk Lymphoma 35:623, 1999.

80. Talerman A, Haige WG: The frequency of M components in sera of patients with solid malignant neoplasms. Br J Cancer 27:276, 1973.

81. Singhal S, Mehta J, Desikan R et al: Antitumor activity of thalidomide in refractory multiple myeloma. N Engl J Med 341:1606, 1999.

82. Raje N, Anderson K: Thalidomide – a revival story. N Engl J Med 341:1606, 1999.

83. Sonneveld P: Multidrug resistance in haematological malignancies. J Intern Med 247:521, 2000.

84. Joshua DE, Gibson J, Brown RD: Mechanisms of the escape phase of myeloma. Blood Rev 8:13, 1994.

85. Hjorth M, Hellquist L, Holmberg E et al: Initial versus deferred melphalan-prednisone therapy for asymptomatic multiple myeloma stage 1 – a randomized study. Eur J Haematol 50:95, 1993.

86. Barlogie B: Advances in therapy of multiple myeloma: Lessons from acute leukemia. Clin Cancer Res 3:2605, 1997.

87. Tribalto M, Amadori S, Cudillo L et al: Autologous peripheral blood stem cell transplantation as first line treatment of multiple myeloma: An Italian Multicenter Study. Haematologica 85:52, 2000.

88. Bataille R, Sany J: Solitary myeloma: Clinical and prognostic features of a review of 114 cases. Cancer 48:845, 1981.

89. Knowling MA, Hardwood AR, Bergsagel DE: A comparison of extramedullary plasmacytomas with solitary and multiple plasma cell tumours of bone. J Clin Oncol 1:255, 1983.

90. Woodruff RK, Whittle JM, Malpas JS: Solitary plasmacytoma. I. Extramedullary soft tissue plasmacytoma. Cancer 43:2340, 1979.

91. Wak MK, Yun KJ, Omar RA: Extramedullary plasmacytomas of the head and neck. Otolaryngol Head Neck Surg 109:877, 1993.

92. Galieni P, Cavo M, Pulsoni A et al: Clinical outcome of extramedullary plasmacytoma. Haematologica 85:47, 2000.

93. Bataille R, Chappard D, Marcelli C et al: Recruitment of new osteoblasts and osteoclasts is the earliest critical event in the pathogenesis of human multiple myeloma. J Clin Invest 88:62, 1991.

94. Bataille R, Chappard D, Klein B: Mechanisms of bone lesions in multiple myeloma. Hematol Oncol Clin North Am 6:285, 1992.

95. Mundy GR, Luben RA, Raisz LG et al: Bone resorbing activity in supernatants from lymphoid cell lines. N Engl J Med 290:867, 1974.

96. Garrett IR, Durie BGM, Nedwin GE et al: Production of lymphotoxin, a bone-resorbing cytokine, by cultured human myeloma cells. N Engl J Med 317:52, 1987.

97. Feliers D, Woodruff K, Abboud S: Potential role of insulin-like growth factor binding protein-4 in the uncoupling of bone turnover in multiple myeloma. Br J Haematol 104:715, 1999.

98. Sati HI, Greaves M, Apperley JF et al: Expression of interleukin-1 beta and tumour necrosis factor-alpha in plasma cells from patients with multiple myeloma. Br J Haematol 104:350, 1999.

99. Franchimont N, Rydziel S, Canalis E: Transforming growth factor-beta increases interleukin-6 transcripts in osteoblasts. Bone 26:249, 2000.

100. Annesley TM, Burritt MF, Kyle RA: Artifactural hypercalcemia in multiple myeloma. Mayo Clin Proc 57:572, 1982.

101. Diel IJ: Antitumour effects of bisphosphonates: First evidence and possible mechanisms. Drugs 59:391, 2000.

102. Ralston SH, Gardner MD, Dryburgh FJ: Comparison of aminohydroxypropylidene diphosphonate mithramycin and corticosteroids/calcitonin in the treatment of cancer associated hypercalcaemia. Lancet 2:907, 1985.

103. Honore P, Luger NM, Schwei MJ et al: Osteoprotegerin blocks bone cancer-induced skeletal destruction, skeletal pain and pain-related neurochemical reorganization of the spinal cord. Nat Med 6:521, 2000.

104. Capparelli C, Kostenuik PJ, Morony S et al: Osteoprotegerin prevents and reverses hypercalcemia in a murine model of humoral hypercalcemia of malignancy. Cancer Res 60:783, 2000.

105. Perkins H, MacKenzie M, Fudenberg H: Hemostatic defects in dysproteinemias. Blood 35:695, 1970.

106. Robert F, Mignucci M, McCurdy SA et al: Hemostatic abnormalities associated with monoclonal gammopathies. Am J Med Sci 306:359, 1993.

107. Siami GA, Siami FS: Plasmapheresis and paraproteinemia: Cryoprotein-induced diseases, monoclonal gammopathy, Waldenström's macroglobulinemia, hyperviscosity syndrome, multiple myeloma. Ther Apher 3:8, 1999.

108. Daragon A, Humex C, Michot C et al: Treatment of multiple myeloma with etidronate: Results of a multi-centre double-blind study. Groupe d'Etudes et de Recherches sur le Myeloma (Germ). Eur J Med 2:449, 1993.

109. McCloskey EV, MacLennan IC, Drayson MT et al: A randomized trial of the effect of clodronate on skeletal morbidity in multiple myeloma. MRC Working Party on Leukaemia in Adults. Br J Haematol 100:317, 1998.

110. Bruce NJ, McCloskey EV, Kanis JA et al: Economic impact of using clodronate in the management of patients with multiple myeloma. Br J Haematol 104:358, 1999.

111. Berenson JR, Lichtenstein A, Porster L et al: Efficacy of pamidronate in reducing skeletal events in patients with advanced multiple myeloma. Myeloma Aredia Study Group. N Engl J Med 334:488, 1996.

112. Berenson JR, Lichtenstein A, Porter L et al: Long-term pamidronate treatment of advanced multiple myeloma patients reduces skeletal events. Myeloma Aredia Study Group. J Clin Oncol 16:593, 1998.

113. Dhodapkar MV, Singh J, Mehta J et al: Anti-myeloma activity of pamidronate in vivo. Br J Haematol 103:530, 1998.

114. Brincker H, Westin J, Abildgaard N et al: Failure of oral pamidronate to reduce skeletal morbidity in multiple myeloma: A double-blind placebo-controlled trial. Danish-Swedish co-operative study group. Br J Haematol 101:280, 1998.

115. Bergsagel D, Sprague CC, Austin C et al: Evaluation of new chemotherapeutic agents in the treatment of multiple myeloma. IV. L-Phenylalanine mustard (NSC-8806). Cancer Chemother Rep 21:87, 1962.

116. Woodhouse KW, Hamilton P, Lennard A et al: The pharmocokinetics of melphalan in patients with multiple myeloma: An intravenous/oral study using a conventional dose regimen. Eur J Clin Pharmacol 24:283, 1983.

117. Cooper MR, McIntyre OR, Anderson K: Single, sequential, and multiple alkylating agent therapy for multiple myeloma: A CALGB study. J Clin Oncol 4:1331, 1986.

118. Medical Research Council Working Party on Leukaemia in Adults: Treatment comparison in the third MRC myelomatosis trial. Br J Cancer 42:823, 1980.

119. Medical Research Council Working Party for Therapeutic Trials in Leukaemia: Myelomatosis: Comparison of melphalan and cyclophosphamide therapy. BMJ 1:640, 1971.

120. Alexanian R, Haut A, Khan AU et al: Treatment for multiple myeloma: Combination chemotherapy with different melphalan dose regimens. JAMA 208:1680, 1969.

121. Salmon SE, Shadduck RK, Schilling A: Intermittent high dose prednisone (NSC-10023) therapy for multiple myeloma. Cancer Chemother Rep 51:179, 1967.

122. McIntyre OR, Pajak TF, Kyel RA et al: Response and survival in myeloma patients receiving prednisone alone. Med Pediatr Oncol 13:329, 1985.

123. Barlogie B, Smith L, Alexanian R: Effective treatment of advanced multiple myeloma refractory to alkylating agents. N Engl J Med 310:1353, 1984.

124. Drayson MT, Chapman CE, Dunn JA et al: MRC trial of alpha2b-interferon maintenance therapy in first plateau phase of multiple myeloma. MRC Working Party in Leukaemia in Adults. Br J Haematol 101:195, 1998

125. Alexanian R, Dimopoulos MA, Delasalle K et al: Primary dexamethasone treatment of multiple myeloma. Blood 80:887, 1992.

126. Shaw IC, Graham MI: Mesna – a short review. Cancer Treat Rev 14:67, 1987.

127. Dimopoulos MA, Delasalle KB, Champlin R et al: Cyclophosphamide and etoposide therapy with GM-CSF for VAD-resistant multiple myeloma. Br J Haematol 83:240, 1993.

128. Boirin JM, Marit G, Faberes C et al: Collection of peripheral blood stem cells in multiple myeloma following single high dose cyclophosphamide with and without recombinant human granulocyte-macrophage colony stimulating factor (rhGM-CSF). Bone Marrow Transplant 12:49, 1993.

129. MacLennan ICM, Cusick J: Objective evaluation of the role of vincristine in induction and maintenance therapy for myelomatosis. Br J Cancer 52:153, 1985.

130. Mellstedt H, Ahre A, Bjorkholm M et al: Interferon therapy in myelomatosis. Lancet 1:245, 1979.

131. Quesada JR, Alexanian R, Hawkins M et al: Treatment of multiple myeloma with recombinant alpha-interferon. Blood 67:275, 1986.

132. Ludwig H: In vitro inhibitory effect of interferon on multiple myeloma stem cell. Cancer Immunol Immunother 9:139, 1990.

133. Brenning G, Jernberg H, Gidlund M et al: The effect of alpha and gamma-interferon on proliferation and production of IgE and beta 2-microglobulin in the human myeloma cell line U-266 subline. Scand J Haematol 37:280, 1986.

134. Cooper MR, Dear K, McIntyre OR et al: A randomized clinical trial comparing melphalan/prednisone with or without alpha 2b interferon in newly diagnosed multiple myeloma: A CALGB study. J Clin Oncol 11:155, 1993.

135. Osterborg A, Bjorkholm M, Bjoreman M et al: Natural interferon-α in combination with MP vs MP in the treatment of multiple myeloma stages II and III: A randomised study from the Myeloma Group of Central Sweden. Blood 81:1428, 1993.

136. Mandelli F, Avvisati G, Amadori S et al: Maintenance treatment with recombinant interferon alpha 2-b in patients with multiple myeloma responding to conventional induction chemotherapy. N Engl J Med 322:1430, 1990.

137. Joshua DE, Penny R, Matthews JP et al: Australian Leukaemia Study Group Myeloma II: A randomized trial of intensive combination chemotherapy with or without interferon in patients with myeloma. Br J Haematol 97:38, 1997.

138. Joshua DE, MacCallum S, Gibson J: Role of alpha interferon in multiple myeloma. Blood Rev 11:191, 1997.

139. Wheatley K, on behalf of the Myeloma Trialists' Collaborative Group: Which myeloma patients benefit from interferon therapy? An overview of 24 randomised trials with 4000 patients. (Abstr.) Br J Haematol 102:140, 1998.

140. Blade J, Esteve J: Viewpoint on the impact of interferon in the treatment of multiple myeloma: Benefit for a small proportion of patients? Med Oncol 17:77, 2000.

141. Myeloma Trialists' Collaborative Group: Combination chemotherapy versus melphalan plus prednisone as treatment for multiple myeloma: An overview of 6633 patients from 27 randomized trials. J Clin Oncol 16:3832, 1998.

142. Boccadoro M, Pileri A: Standard chemotherapy for myelomatosis: An area of great controversy. Haematol Oncol Clin North Am 6:371, 1992.

143. MacLennan ICM, Chapman C, Dunn J et al: Combined chemotherapy with ABCM versus melphalan for treatment of myelomatosis. Lancet 339:200, 1992.

144. Salmon SE, Haut A, Bonnett JD et al: Alternating combination chemotherapy and levamisole improves survival in multiple myeloma: A Southwest Oncology Group study. J Clin Oncol 1:453, 1983.

145. Pavlovsky S, Saslavsky J, Tezanos et al: A randomized trial of melphalan and prednisone versus melphalan, prednisone, cyclophosphamide, MeCCNU and vincristine in untreated multiple myeloma. J Clin Oncol 2:836, 1984.

146. Peest D, Deicher H, Coldewey R et al: Induction and maintenance therapy in multiple myeloma: A multi-centre trial of MP versus VCMP. Eur J Cancer 24:1061, 1988.

147. Boccadoro M, Marmont F, Tribalto M et al: Multiple myeloma: VMCP/VBAP alternating combination chemotherapy is not superior to melphalan and prednisone even in high risk patients. J Clin Oncol 9:444, 1991.

148. Bladé J, San Miguel JF, Alcalá A et al: Alternating combination VMCP/VBAP chemotherapy versus melphalan and prednisone in the treatment of multiple myeloma: A randomised multicentric study of 487 patients. J Clin Oncol 11:1165, 1993.

149. Samson D, Gaminare E, Newland A: Infusion of vincristine and doxorubicin with oral dexamethasone as first-line therapy for multiple myeloma. Lancet 2:882, 1989.

150. Alexanian R, Barlogie B, Tucker S: VAD-based regimens as primary treatment for multiple myeloma. Am J Hematol 33:86, 1990.

151. Alexanian R, Barlogie B, Dixon D: High-dose glucocorticoid treatment of resistant myeloma. Ann Intern Med 105:8, 1986.

152. Salmon SE, Tesh D, Crowley J: Chemotherapy is superior to sequential hemibody irradiation for remission consolidation in multiple myeloma: A Southwest Oncology Group Study. J Clin Oncol 8:1575, 1990.

153. McIntyre OR, Tefft M, Propert K et al: Melphalan and prednisone plus total bone marrow irradiation as initial treatment for multiple myeloma. Int J Radiat Oncol Biol Phys 15:1007, 1988.

154. Alexanian R, Gehan E, Haut A et al: Unmaintained remissions in multiple myeloma. Blood 51:1005, 1978.

155. Alexanian R, Balcerzak S, Haut A et al: Remission maintenance therapy for multiple myeloma. Arch Intern Med 135:147, 1979.

156. Cohen HJ, Bartulucci A, Forman WB et al. for the Southeastern Cancer Study Group: Consolidation and maintenance therapy in multiple myeloma: Randomised comparison of a new approach to therapy after initial response to treatment. J Clin Oncol 4:888, 1986.

157. Pileri A, Carmagnola A, Boccadoro M: Human myeloma: Kinetics of the remission phase. Acta Haematol 68:237, 1982.

158. Bergsagel DE: Plasma cell neoplasms and acute leukaemia. Clin Haematol 1:221, 1982.

159. Westin J, Cortelezzi A, Hjorth M et al: Interferon therapy during the plateau phase of multiple myeloma: An update of the Swedish Study. Eur J Cancer 27:45, 1991.

160. Bensinger WI, Demirer T, Buckner CD et al: Syngeneic marrow transplantation in patients with multiple myeloma. Bone Marrow Transplant 18:527, 1996.

161. McElwain TJ, Powles RL: High-dose intravenous melphalan for plasma-cell leukaemia and myeloma. Lancet 2:822, 1983.

162. Selby PJ, McElwain TJ, Nandi AC et al: Multiple myeloma treated with high dose intravenous melphalan. Br J Haematol 66:55, 1987.

163. Gahrton G, Svensson H, Bjorkstrand B et al: Syngeneic transplantation in multiple myeloma – a case-matched comparison with autologous and allogeneic transplantation. Bone Marrow Transplant 24:741, 1999.

164. Gahrton G, Tura S, Ljungman P et al: Allogeneic bone marrow transplantation in multiple myeloma. European Group for Bone Marrow Transplantation. N Engl J Med 325:1267, 1991.

165. Bensinger WI, Buckner CD, Clift RA et al: Phase 1 study of busulphan and cyclophosphamide in preparation for allogeneic marrow transplant for patients with multiple myeloma. J Clin Oncol 10:1492, 1992.

166. Kulkarni S, Powles RL, Treleaven JG et al: Impact of previous high-dose therapy on outcome after allografting for multiple myeloma. Bone Marrow Transplant 23:675, 1999.

167. Schlossman RL, Anderson KC: Bone marrow transplantation in multiple myeloma. Curr Opin Oncol 11:102, 1999.

168. Bensinger WI, Buckner D, Gahrton G: Allogeneic stem cell transplantation for multiple myeloma. Hematol Oncol Clin North Am 11:147, 1997.

169. Van der Griend R, Verdonck LF, Petersen EJ et al: Donor leukocyte infusions inducing remissions repeatedly in a patient with recurrent multiple myeloma after allogeneic bone marrow transplantation. Bone Marrow Transplant 23:195, 1999.

170. Keil F, Kalhs P, Chen X et al: Hematopoietic donor chimerism and graft-versus-myeloma effect in relapse of multiple myeloma after allogeneic bone marrow transplantation. Ann Hematol 78:376, 1999.

171. Rondelli D, Bandini G, Cavo M et al: Discrepancy between serological complete remission and concomitant new bone lytic lesions after infusion of escalating low doses of donor lymphocytes in multiple myeloma: A case report. Bone Marrow Transplant 24:685, 1999.

172. Orsini E, Alyea EP, Schlossman R et al: Changes in T cell receptor repertoire associated with graft-versus-tumor effect and graft-versus-host disease in patients with relapsed multiple myeloma after donor lymphocyte infusion. Bone Marrow Transplant 25:623, 2000.

173. Zomas A, Stefanoudaki K, Fifis M et al: Graft-versus-myeloma after donor leukocyte infusion: Maintenance of marrow remission but extramedullary relapse with plasmacytomas. Bone Marrow Transplant 21:1163, 1998.

174. Bjorkstrand BB, Ljungman P, Svensson H et al: Allogeneic bone marrow transplantation versus autologous stem cell transplantation in multiple myeloma: A retrospective case-matched study from the European Group for Blood and Marrow Transplantation. Blood 88:4711, 1996.

175. Attal M, Harousseau JL, Stoppa AM et al: A prospective, randomised trial of autologous bone marrow transplantation and chemotherapy in multiple myeloma. Intergroupe Français du Myélome. N Engl J Med 225:91, 1996.

176. Lenhoff S, Hjorth M, Holmberg E et al. for the Nordic Myeloma Study Group: Impact on survival of high-dose therapy with autologous stem cell support in patients younger than 60 years with newly diagnosed multiple myeloma: A population-based study. Blood 95:7, 2000.

177. Barlogie B, Jagannath S, Desikan KR et al: Total therapy with tandem transplants for newly diagnosed multiple myeloma. Blood 93:55, 1999.

178. Attal M, Payen C, Facon T et al: Single versus double transplant in myeloma: A randomized trial of the "Inter Groupe Français du Myélome" (IFM). (Abstr.) Blood 90:418, 1997.

179. Harousseau JL, Attal M, Divine M et al: Comparison of autologous bone marrow transplantation after first remission induction treatment in multiple myeloma. Bone Marrow Transplant 15:963, 1995.

180. Dyson P, Horvath N, Joshua D et al: CD34+ selection of autologous peripheral blood stem cells for transplantation following sequential cycles of high dose therapy and mobilisation in multiple myeloma. Bone Marrow Transplant 25:1175, 2000.

181. Gupta D, Bybee A, Cooke F et al: CD34+ selected peripheral blood progenitor cell transplantation in patients with multiple myeloma: Tumour cell contamination and outcome. Br J Haematol 204:166, 1999.

182. Vescio R, Schiller G, Stewart AK et al: Multicenter phase III trial to evaluate CD34(+) selected versus unselected autologous peripheral blood progenitor cell transplantation in multiple myeloma. Blood 93:1858, 1999.

183. Palumbo A, Triolo S, Argentino C et al: Dose-intensive melphalan with stem cell support (MEL100) is superior to standard treatment in elderly myeloma patients. Blood 94:1248, 1999.

184. Sirohi B, Powles R, Treleaven J et al: The role of autologous transplantation in patients with multiple myeloma aged 65 years and over. Bone Marrow Transplant 25:533, 2000.

185. Fermand JP, Ravaud P, Chevret S et al: High-dose therapy and autologous peripheral blood stem cell transplantation in multiple myeloma: Up-front or rescue treatment? Results of a multicenter sequential randomized clinical trial. Blood 92:3131, 1998.

186. Klein B: Murine anti-interleukin-6 monoclonal antibody therapy in myeloma. Blood 78:1198, 1991.

187. Pope B, Brown R, Gibson J et al: B7-2-positive myeloma: Incidence, clinical characteristics, prognostic significance, and implications for tumor immunotherapy. Blood 96:1274, 2000.

188. Ludwig H, Fritz E, Kotzmann H et al: Erythropoietin in the treatment of anemia associated with multiple myeloma. N Engl J Med 322:1693, 1993.

189. Vossebeld PJ, Sonneveld P: Reversal of multidrug resistance in hematological malignancies. Blood Rev 13(2):67, 1999.

190. Grogan TM, Spier CM, Salmon SE et al: P-glycoprotein expression in human plasma cell meyloma: Correlation with prior chemotherapy. Blood 81:490, 1993.

191. Pilarski LM, Belch AR: Intrinsic expression of the multidrug transporter, P-glycoprotein 170, in multiple myeloma: Implications for treatment. Leuk Lymphoma 17:367, 1995.

192. Sonneveld P, Durie BGM, Lockhost HM et al: Modulation of multi-drug resistant multiple myeloma by cyclosporin. Lancet 340:255, 1992.

193. Dalton WS, Crowley JJ, Salmon SS et al: A phase III randomized study of oral verapamil as a chemosensitizer to reverse drug resistance in patients with refractory myeloma. A Southwest Oncology Group study. Cancer 75:815, 1995.

194. Sonneveld P, Lokhorst HM, Vossebeld P: Drug resistance in multiple myeloma. Semin Hematol 34(4, Suppl. 5):34, 1997.

195. Massaia M, Borricone P, Battaglio S et al: Idiotype vaccination in human myeloma: Generation of tumor-specific immune responses after high-dose chemotherapy. Blood 94:678, 1999.

196. Wen YJ, Ling M, Bailey-Wood R et al: Idiotypic protein-pulsed adherent peripheral blood mononuclear cell-derived dendritic cells prime immune system in multiple myeloma. Clin Cancer Res 4:957, 1998.

197. Kwak LW, Taub DD, Duffey PL et al: Transfer of myeloma idiotype-specific immunity from an actively immunised marrow donor. Lancet 345:1016, 1995.

198. Stevenson F, Anderson KC: Introduction: Immunotherapy for multiple myeloma: Insights and advances. Semin Hematol 36(1, Suppl. 3):1, 1999.

199. Hajek R, Butch AW: Dendritic cell biology and the application of dendritic cells to immunotherapy of multiple myeloma. Med Oncol 17:2, 2000.

200. Munshi N, Desikan R, Zngari M et al: Chemoangiotherapy with DT-PACE for previously treated multiple myeloma (MM). (Abstr.) Blood 94:730, 1999.

201. Larkin M: Low-dose thalidomide seems to be effective in multiple myeloma. Lancet 354:925, 1999.

32

Syndromes and Special Presentations Associated with Plasma Cell Myeloma

Daniel E. Bergsagel and Waldemar Pruzanski

This chapter presents some of the unusual manifestations of plasma cell neoplasia. How were these topics chosen? In truth, we write about subjects that interest us, and are important, but have somehow escaped the attention of our current collaborators. Our topics are presented within the context of plasma cell neoplasia in general. Extramedullary plasmacytomas and solitary osseous plasmacytomas are compared with plasma cell myeloma. Myelomatous involvement of the central nervous system and the sensorimotor neuropathy associated with plasma cell neoplasia are presented within a classification of all of the neurological complications of these diseases. The Fanconi syndrome, nodular glomerulopathy, and systemic light chain deposition disease are also presented within the context of the other renal manifestations of plasma cell neoplasia. The newly recognized association of chronic neutrophilia and plasma cell neoplasia appears to result from the aberrant production of granulocyte colony-stimulating factor by the monoclonal plasma cells. The unique features of IgD myeloma, IgE myeloma, nonsecretory myeloma, and plasma cell leukemia are emphasized by comparing them with the usual presentation of plasma cell myeloma. A description of the acute terminal phase of the disease concludes the chapter.

EXTRAMEDULLARY PLASMACYTOMAS AND SOLITARY PLASMACYTOMAS OF BONE

Plasma cell tumors may arise in extramedullary sites, especially in the upper respiratory tract, or as solitary or multiple tumors of bone. In a series of 822 patients seen at one institution (Table 32–1) between 1958 and 1980, 25 individuals, or 3 percent, presented as extramedullary plasmacytomas (EMPs), and the same number had solitary osseous plasmacytomas (SOPs). The three presentations occur in distinctive patient groups that have different survival expectations.[6,30,37,46,80,181,184,185]

Solitary Osseous Plasmacytoma

The median age at diagnosis of SOP is 50, 11 years younger than patients with multiple myeloma (MM), and 9 years younger than those with EMP (Table 32–1). The minimum criteria for diagnosis include a solitary bone lesion (composed of plasma cells) on a

Table 32–1. Characteristics of Patients With Plasma Cell Tumors[a]

Variable	Multiple Myeloma	Extramedullary Plasmacytoma	Solitary Osseous Plasmacytoma
Number (% of total)	772 (93.9)	25 (3.0)	25 (3.0)
Male/female ratio	1.06:1	5.25:1	2.13:1
Median age (yr)			
Males	60	64	50
Females	61	55	55
All ages	61	59	50
Median survival (mo)	24.0	100.8	86.4

[a] Numbers of patients seen at the Princess Margaret Hospital between 1958 and 1980. The median survival for multiple myeloma is calculated for 560 previously untreated patients seen between 1967 and 1976.

complete skeletal survey, and a normal marrow aspirate or biopsy. Today, patients thought to have a solitary bone lesion should also be examined with magnetic resonance imaging (MRI). This technique can detect lesions that are not seen on bone radiographs.[111] SOPs usually present with pain at the site of the bone lesion. Some may have neurological dysfunction caused by spinal cord or nerve root compression. In the series shown in Table 32–1, the lesion occurred in the bones of the axial skeleton in 15 of the 25 patients; 3 patients presented with paraplegia. An M protein was present in the serum of two patients, and excreted as a monoclonal light chain in the urine of three. If the SOP is truly solitary, the M protein should disappear following adequate local radiation therapy; this occurred in all of these five patients. In another series it was noted that the likelihood of disappearance of the M protein is greater following radiation therapy if the baseline value is small; the M protein persisted in all patients with baseline serum levels greater than 10 g/L.[45]

Most SOP patients are treated with radiation therapy, using doses of 3500 to 4000 cGy in 15 to 20 fractions. This treatment relieves the bone pain and results in bone healing. In our series,[80] the median time to progression was 6.5 years following radiation therapy (Figure 32–1A). Of the 13 patients who progressed, MM developed in 12, and 1 had another osseous plasmacytoma. The median survival for SOP patients is 7.2 years from the onset of treatment (Figure 32–1B). Most patients die as a result of progression to multiple myeloma.

Patients with SOP appear to have an early form of MM. Like MM, SOP lesions occur mainly in the axial skeleton, and there is minimal male predominance. Patients are about a decade younger than those who present with MM. Progression to MM occurs in the majority of SOP patients, usually within 3 years. However, later relapses have been reported 15 years, or more, after the initial treatment.[180] The risk of progression to MM is much lower if the M protein disappears following radiation therapy. In one large series of 57 patients progression to MM occurred in only 2 of the 11 patients who responded to radiotherapy with disappearance of the M protein.[92]

Extramedullary Plasmacytomas

The median age at diagnosis is 59 for EMP. This tumor occurs 5.25 times more frequently in males (Table 32–1). The usual site of origin is in the mucosa of the oronasopharynx, or the paranasal sinuses (Table 32–2). In one series local lymph nodes were involved in 8 of 25 patients at diagnosis[80]; in 3 of these a primary site was not identified, and the plasmacytoma appeared to be confined to the lymph node. In 3 additional patients the first sign of disease progression occurred in regional lymph nodes. Symptoms at presentation are related to the site, and consist of bleeding from friable tissue, obstruction of nasal passages, or the presence of a mass. In our series of 25 patients a serum M protein was detected in 6, a monoclonal urinary light chain in 2, and amyloid infiltration of the primary tumor, with no evidence of systemic amyloidosis, occurred in 4.[80]

Local irradiation with 3500 to 4000 cGy in 15 to 20 fractions is the usual treatment. The radiation field should include the regional lymph nodes because they are frequently involved at presentation, or as the first site of progression. The response is variable. In some patients the tumor mass and the M protein disappear promptly, while in others they decrease, but do not disappear. Tumor masses with marked amyloid infiltration

rarely regress completely. EMPs appear to remain localized following irradiation. This is illustrated by the persistence of a serum M protein in the serum of two patients following irradiation of nasopharyngeal tumors with 3000 and 3500 cGy. In both patients, the M protein disappeared following the surgical resection of the residual plasmacytoma. This observation suggests that the radiation dose was sufficient to sterilize the myeloma cells, which stopped growing. However, these myeloma cells continued to produce the M protein until they were surgically resected.[80]

EMPs are usually well controlled with local irradiation and salvage resection. In a series of 25 EMP patients, only 5 progressed after local radiation: 1 developed a single bony lesion, 2 progressed to MM, and 2 developed multiple EMP.[80] Since EMP can usually be controlled with local therapy, progression-free survival is excellent, with 70 percent of patients surviving beyond 10 years without progression (Figure 32–1A). Ten-year progression-free survival has been recorded in 68 to 82 percent of EMP patients in five additional series treated with radiotherapy.[46] Most EMP patients die as the result of unrelated causes, rather than from the plasma cell tumor. The overall survival of EMP and SOP patients is very similar, but it should be noted that most SOP patients die as the result of plasma cell neopla-

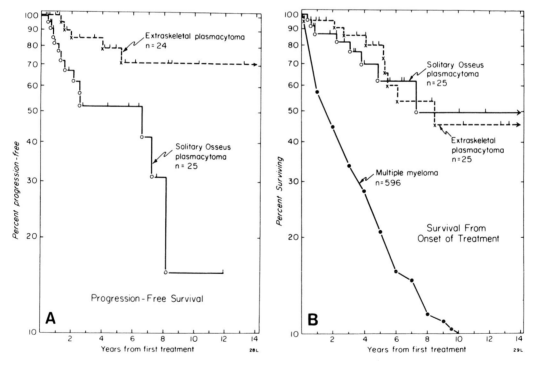

Figure 32–1. (A) Progression-free survival was measured from the onset of a complete response for patients with solitary osseous plasmacytomas and extramedullary plasmacytomas. The end point was the first sign of progression. Patients who died of other causes, with no sign of progression, were removed from the population at risk. Progression-free survival is significantly better for patients with extramedullary plasmacytomas: $p = .02$. (B) Survival from the onset of treatment for previously untreated patients with solitary osseous and extramedullary plasmacytomas seen between 1958 and 1980, and all untreated patients with multiple myeloma seen between 1967 and 1976 at the Princess Margaret Hospital. Death from any cause was used as the end point for these survival curves.

Table 32–2. Sites of Extramedullary Plasmacytomas

Site	n	Percent
Upper air passages (tonsil, palate, nasal sinuses, nasopharynx, nose, orbit)	248	76
Lymph nodes and spleen	18	6
Bronchi and lung	13	4
Skin and subcutaneous	12	3.5
Gastrointestinal tract	10	3
Thyroid	9	3
Testes	3	1
Other	12	3.5
Total	325	100

(Data from Corwin and Lindberg,[37] Knowling et al.,[79] Woodruff et al.,[184,185] and Wiltshaw.[180])

Table 32–3. Neurological Manifestations Associated With Plasma Cell Neoplasia

Complication	Neurologic Manifestations
Hypercalcemia	Lethargy, weakness, confusion, coma
Hyperviscosity	Headache, visual disturbances, retinopathy, obtundation, coma
Spinal cord compression	Paraspinal mass, radicular pain, sensory loss, muscle weakness, loss of bladder control, paraplegia, cranial nerve palsies
Cerebral compression by plasma cell tumors arising in the calvaria	Tumors in the scalp, dysphagia, hemiparesis, increased intracranial pressure, and so forth
Intracranial plasmacytomas	Neurologic manifestations determined by site; usually solitary
Meningeal myelomatosis	Increased intracranial pressure, stiff neck, nerve root palsies, increased plasma cells and M protein in the cerebrospinal fluid
Peripheral neuropathies	Amyloid related (carpal tunnel syndrome; amyloid deposits in nerve fibers or perineural blood vessels)
	Diffuse sensorimotor polyneuropathy with increased cerebrospinal fluid protein; associated with osteosclerotic bone lesions
	Systemic light chain deposition disease
Infections	Bacterial meningitis (e.g., pneumococcal. H. influenzae)
	Viral (herpes zoster; multifocal leukoencephalopathy)

sia, whereas the majority of EMP patients succumb to other causes.

Chemotherapy is useful in the treatment of EMPs that progress and become generalized. Wiltshaw[181] observed complete regressions, including disappearance of the M protein and soft tissue tumors, and healing of bone lesions, in 2 of 20 patients with EMP that had become generalized. The sensitivity to single agents varies; if the tumor fails to respond to one agent, others should be tried.

MYELOMATOUS INVOLVEMENT OF THE CENTRAL NERVOUS SYSTEM

Plasma cell neoplasms cause many neurological complications. For the sake of completeness we have classified these complications and the neurological manifestations they cause in Table 32–3, but only complications 3 to 7 are discussed in this section. The other complications are dealt with in Chapter 30.

Spinal Cord Compression

Spinal cord compression by an extradural plasma cell tumor occurs frequently in myeloma patients. In a series of 114 myeloma patients followed in a hematology clinic in Israel, symptoms and signs of spinal cord compression (SCC) were present at diagnosis in 8, and developed during the course of the disease in 9 additional patients.[21] SCC occurred in 23 of 97 Chinese patients evaluated between 1972 and 1985[182]; 17 presented with this complication and 6 developed it later. Patients with IgA myeloma were at greater risk of developing SCC than those producing other types of M protein. Patients developing SCC presented with higher hemoglobin levels, and were more likely to have hypercalcemia and multiple lytic bone lesions. A French series encountered SCC in 22 of 184 myeloma patients, and emphasized the value of MRI in detecting early cord compression, before the development of motor weakness.[18] We recognized SCC in 66 of 470 myeloma patients (14 percent) during a 5-year period (1976 to 1981) at the Princess Margaret Hospital.

Back pain precedes the diagnosis of SCC in most patients. The occurrence of a paraspinal mass is another useful early warning sign, which may be detected before any signs or symptoms become evident. The plasma cell tumor may originate in a vertebra and invade the spinal canal directly, or it may develop from a vertebra, or a rib, and invade the spinal canal through an intervertebral foramen. Radiographs of the entire vertebral column should be checked carefully for evidence of a paraspinal mass, or vertebral destruction (e.g., loss of a pedicle), as part of the initial evaluation of all patients, and should be repeated if the patient develops unexplained back pain. Episodes of pain that have a radicular distribution and are aggravated by coughing or sneezing suggest the possibility of SCC.

Early diagnosis is the key to successful treatment. The objective is to detect and treat early evidence of SCC before there is any evidence of sensory or motor loss. For this reason, an MRI examination of the spine should be done as soon as there is a suspicion of SCC. MRI can demonstrate early myeloma changes in vertebra that cannot be visualized on plain radiographs, and has detected imminent SCC before symptoms appear.[93] MRI has replaced myelography as the preferred method for investigating patients suspected of having SCC. Cerebrospinal fluid (CSF) should be examined, whenever possible. The most useful tests are a CSF cytospin, in the search for plasma cells, and the total protein. The dura is resistant to invasion and penetration by adjacent tumors, and it is rare to find plasma cells in the CSF of patients with SCC caused by extradural plasma cell tumors. The detection of plasma cells in the CSF indicates that the meninges have been invaded by myeloma cells, usually via the blood stream. CSF protein is usually elevated, but this is rarely helpful in a diagnostic sense. IgG, monomeric IgA, and free κ- and λ-light chain M proteins diffuse freely into the CSF, while polymeric IgA and IgM do not.[177]

These tumors are radiosensitive and are adequately treated with radiation therapy. Surgical decompression is rarely required if the SCC is known to be caused by a plasma cell tumor. We start patients on prednisone, 40 to 100 mg per day, or dexamethasone, 4 mg every 6 hours, as soon as SCC is suspected, and continue this dose during radiation therapy, in order to reduce the risk that irradiation may cause swelling and increased pressure on the spinal cord. The area with SCC is radiated, using generous margins. A tumor dose of 2000 cGy in 5 days with a ^{60}Co source is usually adequate for local control of a plasma cell tumor. The degree of neurological recovery is determined largely by the severity of the defect before treatment. Recovery of sensory loss, bladder control, and muscle strength is expected if the patient retains a flicker of motor function in the lower limbs, such as the ability to move the toes voluntarily, before radiation is started. Recovery is less common if all evidence of motor function is lost. Delayed recovery of spinal cord function has been observed as long as 12 to 18 months after effective treatment of SCC in some patients with severe paraplegia (Simpson, W.K.J., personal communication).

Cranial Plasmacytomas

Cranial plasmacytomas may originate in bone,[67,72,97,109,153] or in extraskeletal tissues such as the dura and meninges.[2,36,81,83,124,146] Cranial plasmacytomas causing neurological signs and symptoms are rare. A review of the literature uncovered 32 cases in 1980.[150] Of these, 16 had other evidence of multiple myeloma, while the remainder appeared to be solitary lesions. The diploë of the cranium is commonly riddled with nodules of myelomatous tissue in patients with multiple myeloma. These rarely cause cerebral compression since the tumors tend to expand through the outer rather than the inner plate of the cranium. When cerebral compression does develop it usually occurs late in the course of the disease.[21,67,72,153] Growing external masses on the cranium usually precede the development of neurological signs by 4 to 6 months. These patients often complain of headaches, and develop papilledema. Focal neurological sympoms such as convulsions, hemiparesis, and cranial nerve palsies precede the development of coma. Plasma cell tumors cause pressure on the dura, but rarely, if ever, invade or penetrate it. The development of neurological signs in a patient with expanding cranial plasma cell tumors should suggest the possibility of cerebral compression.

Patients with solitary cranial plasmacytomas usually present with neurological manifestations. Most solitary intracranial plasmacytomas appear to arise in the dura or pia mater,[2,36,83,124,146] but rare cases such as one arising at the base of the skull in the petrous, have been described.[97] Dural plasmacytomas often present with clinical findings suggestive of a meningioma.[2] The Foster Kennedy syndrome, consisting of an association of anosmia, primary optic atrophy, central scotoma, and contralateral papilledema, has been described in two cases.[36,109] This syndrome is usually produced by olfactory groove or sphenoidal meningiomas. Solitary intracranial lesions are best treated with radiation therapy. Recurrence-free survival 8 and 13 years after treatment suggests that this form of treatment may be curative.[83] Determining whether the plasmacytoma is solitary is important in predicting prognosis. Kohli and Kawazu[81] suggest that a solitary lesion should be strongly suspected in patients with intracranial lesions when M proteins not demonstrable in the serum are present in the CSF.

Meningeal Myelomatosis

Plasma cell tumors originating in bone rarely invade the meninges.[95,151] The route of invasion of the meninges by myeloma cells is believed to be via the blood stream, as in the acute leukemias. Myeloma cells with the proliferative capacity to form a colony have been demonstrated in the blood of myeloma patients.[158] Thus, myeloma cells with the proliferative capacity to initiate metastatic colonies do circulate in the blood of some myeloma patients.

Meningeal myelomatosis develops late in the course of the disease, during a period of rapid growth in patients with aggressive myeloma. Durie et al.[49] found that a small subgroup of patients with both a high myeloma cell mass and a high labeling index (greater than 3 percent) have an increased risk of meningeal relapse. We encountered only 6 patients with meningeal myeloma during the investigation of 470 myeloma patients at the Princess Margaret Hospital between 1976 and 1981.

Meningeal myelomatosis frequently presents with multiple cranial nerve palsies.[183] Confusion, headache, long tract signs, nuchal rigidity, and back pain are frequent presenting features, while others may have no findings suggestive of neurological involvement.

All patients with meningeal involvement have myeloma cells in the CSF.[1] We use this finding as a criterion for diagnosing meningeal myeloma. With the cytospin technique[183] for concentrating and spreading cells from the CSF on a slide, it is possible to detect myeloma cells even when the CSF cell count is low. For example, the cytospin myeloma cells shown in Plate 32–1 were obtained from a patient with a cell CSF count of only 8 cells/ml. CSF protein is usually greatly elevated, and is composed mainly of the M protein.

There are limited treatment options for meningeal myeloma. Intrathecal methotrexate has been unsuccessful.[183] It should be remembered that drugs such as methotrexate and arabinosyl cytosine, which can be administered intrathecally, have not been shown to be effective in the treatment of myeloma.[13] The survival prognosis is short for patients who develop meningeal myeloma. The objective of treatment should be to relieve symptoms, using radiation of the affected local sites to control local symptoms, and a simple regimen such as weekly cyclophosphamide and alternate-day prednisone[13] to control systemic disease.

PLASMA CELL NEOPLASIA WITH PERIPHERAL POLYNEUROPATHY

Peripheral polyneuropathy (PPN) is a rare complication of plasma cell neoplasia, the incidence being 38 of 2714 (1.4 percent) among patients with these diseases.[107] Among 279 patients with PPN of unknown etiology, 28 (10 percent) were found to have an M component.[85] PPN associated with M components comprises a diverse group of disorders,[143] including AL amyloidosis,[74] systemic light chain deposition in the nerves,[127] multiple myeloma, or other plasma cell diseases[107] (Table 32–3). The pathogenesis of PPN is poorly understood; factors such as cytokines, hepatitis C virus, vascular endothelial growth factor, and others may play a role.[143] The clinical picture, radiological manifestations, and laboratory data are quite different for myeloma patients with and without PPN. The PPN may precede, sometimes by many years, may occur simultaneously, or may develop after the diagnosis of plasma cell neoplasia.

Many factors play a role in the pathogenesis of nonamyloid PPN in plasma cell neoplasia. Binding of the M protein to the nerve has been found in some cases,[40,50,89,157] but is not a universal finding. PPN has been induced experimentally in mice by inoculating a plasma cell tumor.[40] Such mice develop loss of myelin sheaths in their nerves, and occasionally axonal degeneration. Of more significance is the fact that mice injected with purified IgG, or its Fab fragment, taken from a patient with plasma cell neoplasia and PPN, developed demyelination and PPN.[16] Indeed, a case of PPN with an IgM/κ M protein with demonstrated antibody activity against peripheral nerve myelin, has been reported.[89] The observation that the manifestations of PPN often improve following the initiation of effective treatment for myeloma[48] suggests that the plasma cell neoplasm in these patients produce a neurotoxic factor. Recent extensive immunological studies have shown that M proteins in PPN, especially of the IgM class, bind to myelin-associated glycoprotein (MAG).[155] Some were also found to have cold agglutinin activity, specifically against the Pr_2 antigen,[179] and react more generally with disialosyl groups on the gangliosides. Anti-MAG antibody has also been detected in the CSF.[20]

Peripheral neuropathy affects males more frequently than females. The age of onset varies from 20 to 82 years. Clinical manifestations of PPN often precede those of the plasma cell neoplasia, or were the dominant subjective complaint. More than 80 percent of patients complained of motor and/or sensory impairment, usually localized first in the lower extremity. Skeletal pain is uncommon. In MM, in general, PPN has been detected in 5 percent of patients.[84] The incidence of lymphadenopathy, splenomegaly, and hepatomegaly is much higher in patients with PPN and osteosclerotic bone lesions than in those with PPN and lytic bone lesions. Myeloma patients who present with demyelinating PPN often have osteosclerotic bone lesions.[88]

The results of laboratory tests in patients with PPN are shown in Table 32–4. In comparison with myeloma in general, PPN patients were less anemic, azotemia and hyperuricemia were uncommon, and hypercalcemia was not observed. The total serum protein was often normal and seldom exceeded 80 g/L. The level of albumin was usually normal as well. M proteins, as detected by serum electrophoresis, were detected in only 56 percent of patients with PPN. Such a low incidence may be explained by the low concentration of M protein in these patients, usually less than 20 g/L. Immunoquantitation often showed normal or slightly reduced normal polyclonal immunoglobulins. Serum immunoelectrophoresis detected M proteins in greater than 80 percent of patients. In almost all of the reported series, IgM M proteins were overrepresented,[20,155] but in some a predominance of IgA was noted.[107] Since the investigation of Bence Jones proteinurea was often incomplete, its incidence cannot be estimated. CSF protein was almost invariably increased. M proteins were detected in the CSF by electro- or immunoelectrophoresis in about half of the patients. The CSF cell count was usually normal, and no plasma cells were detected in the examined specimens. Routine marrow aspirations from radiologically uninvolved regions often showed a normal, or only slightly increased number of plasma cells. However, malignant plasma cells were invariably observed when osteolytic or sclerotic sites were biopsied, or at autopsy. A high incidence of osteosclerotic bone lesions has been noted in patients with PPN; at least 60 percent of these patients have osteosclerotic lesions alone, or in combination with lytic dis-

Table 32–4. Laboratory Data in 82 Patients With Plasma Cell Neoplasia and Peripheral Neuropathy

Finding	PPN Series (%)	Multiple Myeloma in General (%)
Anemia (Hb < 12.0 g/dl)	21/59 (36)	62
Erythrocyte sedimentation rate (> 20 mm/h)	25/59 (42)	90
Azotemia (BUN > 30 mg/dl or creatinine > 1.5 mg/dl)	16/53 (30)	55
Hypercalcemia (> 11.0 mg/dl)	0/49 (0)	30
Proteinuria	18/41 (44)	88
Increased CSF protein (> 50 mg/dl)	55/61 (90)	NR
CSF M component	7/15 (47)	NR
Bone marrow plasmacytosis[a]	71/71 (100)	92
Osteolytic lesions only	20/82 (24)	71
Osteosclerotic lesions only[b]	20/82 (24)	NR
Osteolytic and osteosclerotic lesions[b]	30/82 (37)	NR
Osteoporosis or normal skeleton	12/82 (15)	27

Abbreviations: BUN, blood urea nitrogen; Hg, hemoglobin; NR, not reported; PPN, peripheral neuropathy.

[a] Including biopsy of skeletal lesions and autopsy. In 11 patients no detailed results were reported.

[b] Often solitary lesions were observed.

(Data from Kyle,[34] Drieger and Pruzanski,[48] Kelly et al.,[74] and Pruzanski.[125])

ease. About half of these patients have less than three skeletal lesions, and often only a solitary osteosclerotic focus is found.

Peripheral neuropathy usually presents as progressive, symmetrical, distal-type sensorimotor neuropathy of variable severity.[74,107,127] PPN often presents in the feet and progresses rapidly up the lower extremities. A few patients with pure motor, and a few others with pure sensory PPN have been reported.[74] Occasional patients develop severe ataxia. The mixed type of PPN is often labeled as chronic inflammatory demyelinating polyradiculoneuropathy (CIDP).[22] Pain and autonomic nervous system involvement are not pronounced; when present, these manifestations suggest the presence of systemic amyloidosis (AL). Nerve conduction and electromyographic (EMG) studies have shown reduced motor conduction velocity, prolonged distal motor latencies, fibrillations, low-amplitude muscle action potentials, and low or absent sensory nerve action potentials. Light and electron microscopy show progressive degeneration of both large and small myelinated fibers, with relative preservation of nonmyelinated fibers. Segmental demyelination and axonal degeneration occur in various combinations. Small mononuclear cells may infiltrate the epineurium. The number of denervated Schwann cell clusters per surface of fascicular area has been found to be increased.[65,74] In some cases, immunofluorescence studies showed deposits of M proteins in the perineurium, endoneurium, and blood vessels.[17,39,50]

Most patients were treated with various combinations of radiotherapy, chemotherapy, steroids, intravenous gammaglobulin, and plasmapheresis.[17,20,22,85,107] Improvement in the PPN was observed in about half of the treated patients. Patients with osteolytic, or mixed lytic/sclerotic bone lesions appear to have responded better than those with purely sclerotic lesions, or those with normal skeletons.[48] However, complete or partial remissions of more than 10 years have been observed in the latter group as well.[74,128] Newer approaches to treatment with interferon, rituximab, and high-dose melphalan followed by hematopoietic stem cell transplantation have been introduced.[143] The prognosis for myeloma patients with PPN appears to be better than for those without PPN. In the Mayo clinic series, the 5-year survival of myeloma patients with PPN was 60 percent, compared to 20 percent for those without this complication.[107] The association of PPN with sclerotic bone lesions is of considerable interest.[48,69,105,130,[???]]

An interesting variant of plasma cell neoplasia with PPN has been described in Japan.[4,48,65,110,115,125,129,170] The clinical features include polyneuropathy, organomegaly, endocrinopathy, M protein and skin changes, the POEMS syndrome.[4] These patients present with small M proteins, the bone lesions are frequently sclerotic, and they develop a variety of cutaneous, endocrine, neurologic, and serosal membrane-related manifestations (Table 32–5). Lymph nodes in some patients show a histologic picture similar to that of Castleman disease.[168] A few cases have been complicated by the development of a cardiomyopathy.[64,159] There is a tendency to expand the clinical scope of POEMS syndrome. In some patients a scleroderma-like picture preceded other manifestations of the syndrome.[161] Arterial obliteration and pulmonary hypertension have also

been described.[91,149] Azotemia, leading to renal failure seems to be more frequent than previously reported.[114] The POEMS syndrome is reported less frequently from outside of Japan; however; many of the clinical manifestations in these patients could easily be missed, or considered to be unrelated. The pathogenesis of the POEMS syndrome is still not clear. An increase in circulating interleukin (IL)-6,[53,114] and low IL-6 soluble receptor,[53] have been reported. Of interest is the finding of a marked increase in the circulating vascular endothelial growth factor in POEMS syndrome,[114,148,176] and a decrease in its concentration after effective therapy.[176] The significance of finding human herpesvirus 8 DNA in the tissues of some patients with POEMS syndrome[9] requires further study. In one case, monoclonal IgG bound to neuroendocrine tissue,[129] and in another amorphous,

Table 32–5. Clinical and Laboratory Findings Associated with POEMS Syndrome

Profile/Clinical Manifestations	No. Positive/ No. Evaluable	Percent
Age at onset (yr), mean 46, range 26–80		
Sex M/F, 90/40, ratio 2.3:1		
Serum M component	90/130	69
Bone marrow plasmacytosis	27/121	23
Osteosclerotic or mixed lesions	69/130	53
Hepatomegaly	98/125	78
Splenomegaly	48/121	41
Lymphadenopathy	81/124	65
Peripheral polyneuropathy	130/130	100
Papilledema	69/119	58
Elevated cerebrospinal fluid protein	116/124	94
Dermatologic manifestations		
Hyperpigmentation	118/130	90
Hypertrichosis	85/111	76
Thickening of the skin	73/109	67
Hyperhidrosis	59/105	56
Digital clubbing	56/118	47
Endocrinologic manifestations		
Diabetes or abnormal GTT	38/121	31
Hypogonadism (impotence or amenorrhea)	66/104	63
Gynecomastia	52/90	58
Hypothyroidism	7/27	31
Peripheral edema	107/123	87
Ascites	61/109	56
Pleural and/or pericardial effusions	47/114	41
Polycythemia/thrombocytosis	26/58	45
Rarer manifestations		
White nails		
Galactorrhea		
Arthropathy		
Malabsorption		
Proteinuria		
Raynaud's phenomenon		
Verrucous angiomata		

Abbreviations: GTT, glucose tolerance test; POEMS syndrome, polyneuropathy, organomegaly, endocrinopathy, M protein, and skin changes (also known as Crow-Fucase, or Takatsuki syndrome).
(Data from Drieger and Pruzanski,[48] Kelly et al.,[74] Iwashita et al.,[65] Bardwick et al.,[4] and Viard et al.[170])

nonfibrillar, Congo Red-negative deposits were detected around endoneural blood vessels.[170] The fact that the PPN manifestations usually improve in myeloma patients who respond to antineoplastic therapy strongly suggests that myeloma cells produce a toxic factor responsible for the polyneuropathy.

NEUTROPHILIA AND PLASMA CELL NEOPLASIA

At least 24 patients have been described with the association of a marked neutrophil leukocytosis and a monoclonal gammopathy.[44,63,100,113,162] Additional studies have demonstrated normal karyotypes, with absence of the Ph1 chromosome and no evidence of clonal gene rearrangement of the breakpoint cluster region (bcr); elevated leukocyte alkaline phosphatase scores and serum B12 and frequent hepatosplenomegaly. The monoclonal gammopathy was diagnosed as multiple myeloma in 13, and MGUS in 6 of a reviewed series.[63] The leukocytosis is composed primarily of mature neutrophils; the marrow shows myeloid hyperplasia and a monoclonal increase in plasma cells. Most of these cases have been interpreted as having the association of two diseases: chronic neutrophilic leukemia and either myeloma or MGUS. However, an analysis of the clonality of the neutrophils in one of these cases, using the X-linked probe M27β, demonstrated that the neutrophils were polyclonal.[152] This finding, and the absence of other findings associated with a myeloid malignancy, suggests that the neutrophilia is not a leukemic process, but results from specific stimulation of normal granulopoiesis.

The recent report of a patient with neutrophilia and myeloma, with elevated serum levels of granulocyte colony-stimulating factor (G-CSF), and myeloma cells that stained positively with anti-G-CSF, indicates a plausible mechanism to explain the development of neutrophilia in some myeloma patients.[165] The neutrophilia and hepatosplenomegaly gradually subsided in one patient, without treatment. During a 12-year follow-up of a 30-year-old male with IgG/κ MGUS, the leukocyte count fell progressively from 42.2×10^9/L (91 percent mature neutrophils) to 10.0×10^9/L, as IgG levels slowly increased from 1269.5 to 3000.0 mg/dl.[63] These observations suggest that in this patient the mechanism responsible for increased neutrophil production was not linked to the abnormality causing the progressive growth of the MGUS clone.

The neutrophilia did not progress to frank leukemia in any of the reported patients, and was associated with surprisingly good survival. The median survival of 13 patients with myeloma and neutrophilia was 4 years.[63] Therapy should be directed at controlling the disease manifestations caused by the myelomatosis process. The neutrophilia itself is harmless, and has not required treatment.

RENAL COMPLICATIONS OF PLASMA CELL NEOPLASIA

Renal damage occurs frequently during the course of myeloma. Proteinuria is detected initially in 70 percent of patients by routine urinalysis, while more sensitive techniques, such as immunoelectrophoresis or immunofixation, will detect a monoclonal urinary protein in 80 percent.[86] The excretion of nephrotoxic monoclonal light chains produced by plasma cell tumors is the major factor responsible for the kidney damage, leading to the development of the "myeloma kidney."[8,145] Variants of the renal injury caused by light chains are nodular glomerulopathy, the Fanconi syndrome, and systemic light chain deposition disease.

Several additional factors contribute. Hypercalcemia leading to dehydration and renal tubular damage is a common but reversible cause of azotemia in myeloma patients. Dehydration and infection often lead to renal failure,[33] and nonsteroidal anti-inflammatory drugs may be involved.[35,131,132] The injection of contrast media for intravenous pyelography may lead to acute renal failure, but the risks are minimal if dehydration is avoided.[103] It appears that the use of low osmolality and nonionic contrast media may cause less renal toxicity.[26] Treatment with aminoglycoside antibiotics may be complicated by a rising serum creatinine, or acute renal failure. About 10 percent of myeloma patients develop amyloid deposits that may cause a nephrotic syndrome, renal insufficiency, or both. Patients with a nephrotic syndrome and monoclonal light chains in the urine almost always have AL amyloid deposits in renal glomeruli, or light chain deposition disease (see Chapter 34).

Myeloma Kidney

The myeloma kidney is characterized by slowly progressive tubular failure, obstruction of distal and collecting tubules with large, dense, waxy laminated casts composed of precipitated monoclonal light chains, small amounts of albumin, Tamm-Horsfall protein, fibrinogen, and polyclonal light chains (see Chapters 26 and 30). Studies of myeloma kidneys have shown that tubular basement membranes stain positively with light chain antisera,[94,139] and granular dense deposits are found in this basement membrane by electron microscopy.[139] Glomeruli are either well preserved, or only minimally damaged.[169] Interstitial fibrosis and nephrocalcinosis are also observed.

The mechanism of light chain nephrotoxicity is not clear. Precipitation of light chains within the proximal tubular cells may directly injure these cells and release lysosomal enzymes. Damage to tubular cells by intratubal casts also contributes to the development of renal failure. Some have suggested that light chains with a high isoelectric point promote cast formation and renal failure,[32,104] but others have not been able to confirm this finding.[38,132] Recently investigators have shown that light chain nephrotoxicity and amyloidogenicity is related to the propensity of these components to form high molecular weight aggregates under physiological conditions.[112] The fact that an almost identical pattern of renal injury can be induced in mice and rats by the intraperitoneal injection of human monoclonal light chains provides additional evidence that light chains play an important role in the pathogenesis of renal tubular lesions.[8]

The electrophoresis pattern of the urine protein in myeloma patients provides a useful guide about the site of the renal lesion. When the lesion is mainly tubular, as in the common form of myeloma kidney and the Fanconi syndrome, the urine contains light chains and a small amount of albumin. In these patients, the electrophoresis pattern shows two peaks: a small albumin fraction and a light chain peak in the gamma, beta, or alpha regions. When the major lesion is in the glomerulus, as in patients with AL amyloidosis or nodular glomerulosclerosis, there is a nonspecific loss of all serum proteins (the nephrotic syndrome). As a result, the urine electrophoresis pattern resembles that of serum.

The excretion of monoclonal light chains in the urine can lead to other unusual types of nephropathy, with features that differ from those described above for the myeloma kidney. These include Fanconi syndrome, systemic light chain deposition disease, and nodular glomerulopathy. These will be presented in the following two sections.

Acquired Fanconi Syndrome

In the acquired Fanconi syndrome (FS), crystalline cytoplasmic inclusions composed of monoclonal light chains are usually found in marrow plasma cells and renal tubular cells.[119] The syndrome is characterized by dysfunction of the proximal renal tubules, which results in glucosuria, phosphaturia, aminoaciduria, acidosis, and often osteomalacia. The monoclonal light chain excreted in the urine is almost always type kappa.[96] The glomerular filtration rate and distal tubular functions are usually normal.[7,87]

FS is a rare manifestation of myeloma. The clinical and laboratory features of 30 patients reported to have plasma cell neoplasia (PCN) and the acquired FS are shown in Table 32–6. There were 15 males and 15 females, aged from 34 to 81 years, with a mean of 55 years. In the majority of 19 patients in whom the time relationship was mentioned, FS preceded the diagnosis of a PCN. Both conditions were seldom recognized simultaneously. In one patient, Bence Jones proteinuria was discovered 14 years before the development of FS.

The full criteria for the diagnosis of both FS and a PCN were present in only 9 of the 30 cases. Eleven patients had typical FS, but a diagnosis of myeloma could not be confirmed. The major diagnostic problems were a normal or insufficient marrow aspirate, and/or a lack of skeletal abnormalities. All of the patients, however, had a serum M protein, and/or monoclonal light chain proteinuria. It is probable that all of these patients had myeloma, since a normal marrow differential, especially when the marrow is aspirated only once, and normal skeletal radiographs do not rule out the diagnosis. In addition, some of these patients may have had MGUS.

Most patients complained of skeletal pain, chiefly in the shoulders, ribs, back, pelvis, and legs. Muscular pain, weakness, and extreme fatigue were frequent. A swaying, shuffling or waddling gait, weight loss, hemorrhagic phenomena, frequency, nocturia, and polyuria were common. Physical findings included bony tenderness, muscular weakness, abnormal gait, and occasionally fractures.

The laboratory data for 30 patients with PCN and FS are shown in Table 32–6. In addition, the serum alkaline phosphatase was elevated in 14 of 17 patients (82 percent), and 6 of 17 patients (32 percent) had a diabetic glucose tolerance test. The serum calcium was elevated in 2 of 25 patients. Five of 24 patients were anemic. Radiographs of the skeleton detected abnormalities in 22 of 25 patients: osteoporosis in 12, Milkman fractures in 10, osteomalacia in 10, fractures in 7, and osteolytic lesions in 6.

Histologic examination of the kidney was possible in 16 cases, from biopsies or autopsies. The proximal renal tubules were abnormal in all cases, showing crystals in the cytoplasm of proximal renal tubular cells, prominent atrophy, degeneration of cells, and often intraluminal casts. Intracellular crystals were found in 15 patients. Four patients had crystals in the plasma cells of the bone marrow and various organs. Three others had crystals in plasma cells and proximal renal tubular cells, while four had crystals in proximal renal tubular cells only. Occasionally crystals were noted in liver cells, in macrophages, and in interstitial spaces of the kidney, bone marrow, and lymph nodes. In some patients, the kappa light chains and their V domain fragment have the property of crystallization in vitro,[3,41,106] and kappa light chains have been found in nonamyloid fibrils and cytoplasmic crystals in renal tubular cells of a patient with FS.[119] Some progress has occurred in the investigation of the light chains in the Fanconi syndrome associated with low-mass myeloma. In one series all of the patients had kappa light chains, with crystals in the proximal renal tubules and the bone marrow. In eight of nine investigated cases the light chains were of the V kappa I subgroup, with a hydrophobic residue at position 30. All were resistant to proteolysis with cathepsin B.[106]

Systemic Light Chain Deposition Disease (SLCDD)

In 1976, Randall et al.[127] described a new clinical syndrome characterized by the deposition of light chains in various organs and tissues, resulting in a multisystem disease. Two patients suffered from renal failure, involvement of the liver and spleen, neurologic impairment, and heart disease. One had kappa light chain myeloma. The second had nodular glomerulosclerosis,

Table 32–6. Laboratory Manifestations in 30 Patients With Plasma Cell Neoplasia and Fanconi Syndrome

Finding	Incidence[a]
Hypophosphatemia	25/26 (95)
Hypouricemia	20/22 (91)
Hypopotassemia	19/27 (70)
Hyperchloremia	11/23 (48)
Azotemia	17/25 (68)
Proteinuria	28/28 (100)
Glycosuria	30/30 (100)
Aminoaciduria	28/29 (97)
Serum M component	16/17 (94)
Urinary M components[b]	29/29 (100)
Abnormal bone marrow	26/30 (87)
Osteoporosis	13/26 (50)
Osteolytic lesions	6/26 (23)
Osteomalacia and fractures	17/26 (65)

[a] Number found/number investigated (percent).
[b] Including monoclonal light chains and other M components.
(Data from Pruzanski[125] and Walb et al.[175])

dark brown skin pigmentation, ascites, confusion, grand mal seizures, and hypothyroidism, in addition to the main findings described earlier. More than 75 patients with SLCDD have been reported since the original paper.[24,34,56,61,66,76,78,102,122,123,163] The age of these patients ranges from 35 to 76 years, with a mean of 56 years. Males outnumber females 2.5:1. SLCDD occurs in about 5 percent of myeloma patients; 80 percent have kappa light chains, with overrepresentation of V IV.[75] In the remainder, either lambda light chains, or whole immunoglobulin molecules were deposited. The clinical spectrum ranges from overt myeloma, Waldenström's macroglobulinemia, or other malignant lymphoproliferative process, to MGUS.[34,61]

SLCDD is characterized by the deposition of amorphous eosinophilic material (composed mainly of light chains) along basement membranes, diffuse parenchymal infiltrates, and tumorlike nodules in the kidneys and other organs. The kidneys are affected in all patients. The light chains of granular deposits exhibit amino acid substitutions that arise from somatic mutations and result in increased hydrophobicity and aggregation.[171] An experimental model for the in vivo expression of human kappa light chains in mice showed tissue deposits similar to those observed in patients with SLCDD; these light chains had altered V regions.[75] Extrarenal deposits were found in more than 40 percent of investigated patients. Involvement of the liver, lungs, gastrointestinal tract, heart, blood vessels, muscles, skin, marrow, and other tissues has been recorded. The deposition of both light chains and amyloid fibrils have been observed in a few patients.[66,78] Biosynthetic studies have shown that abnormal light chains, shorter than normal, are produced in SLCDD.[24,123] A low synthetic rate, and an increased affinity of light chains for tissues explain why light chains may not be detected in the serum and urine of some patients with SLCDD. The approach to treatment is the same as for myeloma in general.

The deposition of monoclonal light chains in the renal glomerulus leads to renal insufficiency or the nephrotic syndrome, in which distinctive nodular glomerulosclerosis (NGS) develops. These patients present with renal failure, hypertension, and often congestive heart failure.[55,57,123,139,142,147,174] It should be noted that hypertension rarely complicates the course of the usual form of myeloma with tubular cast formation and the "myeloma kidney." With NGS, the renal disease is usually rapidly progressive. Renal function may stabilize or improve with effective chemotherapy, if the presenting serum creatinine is less than 4.0 mg/dl,[61] and remarkable improvement has been observed in some patients.[57,78]

Histologically NGS presents with glomerular hypercellularity and the formation of amorphous mesangial nodules.[55,142] Laminar deposits can be found along the glomerular and tubular basement membranes,[142] and light chains (usually of kappa type) were detected along the tubular basement membrane by immunofluorescent techniques.[55,57,139,142]

IMMUNOTACTOID SYNDROME

A syndrome known as immunotactoid glomerulopathy (ITG) has been described recently.[27,82,108,188] There seem to be two forms called fibrillary glomerulonephritis (FG) with fibrils 20 nm in diameter, and immunotactoid glomerulopathy (IG) with large microtubular deposits.[77] More than 70 patients with ITG have been reported with proteinuria, and often, hypertension and hematuria. About 40 percent progress to end-stage renal failure. Amyloid fibrils must be distinguished from ITG fibrils, which are larger, and composed of polyclonal IgG, C3, and amyloid P component. These proteins do not stain with Congo Red. IG can be distinguished from amyloid deposits by investigating the concentration of decorin in renal deposits. Decorin accumulates in amyloid, but not in IG deposits.[154] Although both κ- and λ-light chains are usually detected, in one case only κ-light chains, and in another only IgG3-κ were found. ITG has been described primarily as a renal syndrome; however, case reports have described leukocytoclastic vasculitis,[136,137] and alveolar capillary interstitial involvement[101] along with the nephropathy. One patient with IgG-κ MGUS and peripheral neuropathy had immunotactoid-like endoneural deposits, suggesting the possibility that some cases of ITG, or its variants, may be related to monoclonal gammopathies.[108] An association of IG with hepatitis C infection has been suggested, but not proven.[98]

IMMUNOGLOBULIN D MULTIPLE MYELOMA

The incidence of IgD M proteins varies from 0.25 to 4.5 percent among subjects with M components, and from 0.7 to 5.7 percent among patients with myeloma.[31,68] In our series, 25 cases of IgD myeloma were found among 1591 myelomas (1.6 percent), and among 2795 M components (0.9 percent).[68] In a summary of series from other countries, 120 subjects with IgD were detected among 16,719 M components (0.72 percent), and 72 with IgD myeloma among 3832 myeloma patients (1.9 percent).[5,10,23,25,29,31,42,54,58,59,62,68,71,99,116,117,138,160,164,166,172,173,178] The clinical manifestations of IgD myeloma are very similar to those of other myelomas. Some of the distinctive features of IgD myeloma, compared to other myelomas, are shown in Table 32–7.

Of 243 reported patients, 170 (70 percent) were men. Plasma cell leukemia occurred in 12 percent of IgD myeloma patients, at six times the frequency observed in IgG and IgA myeloma. Azotemia complicated the course of IgD myeloma more than twice as frequently as in IgG and IgA myeloma. In striking contrast to IgG and IgA myeloma, where the κ/λ ratio is 2:1, the light chain in 223 of 254 IgD myeloma patients (88 percent) was λ, for a ratio of 1:9. In a few patients, IgD M proteins did not react with antisera to light chains,[5,10,29,116] raising the possibility of heavy-chain disease.[174]

A recent publication, not included in Table 32–7, reviews the presenting features, response to treatment, and survival of 53 patients with IgD myeloma treated at the Mayo Clinic.[19] This study confirms many of the distinctive features of IgD myeloma noted here. In addition, it is noted that IgD myelomas usually present with a small, or invisible, spike on serum electrophoresis, hypogammaglobulinemia, and light chain proteinurea; these cases are easy to confuse with light chain myeloma. The frequency of extraskeletal plasmacytomas in lymph nodes and other tissues (28 percent) and amyloidosis (19 percent), was

Table 32–7. Comparison of Clinical Manifestations of IgD With Other Myelomas

Manifestation	IgD	IgG	IgA	LCD
Mean age at Dx	56	62	64	61
Male/female ratio	2.3:1	1:1	1:1	1:1
Lymphadenopathy, hepatosplenomegaly	50	10	10	20
Plasma cell leukemia (%)	12	2	2	7
Azotemia (%)	70	30	30	57
κ/λ ratio	1:9	2:1	2:1	1.2:1
Median survival (κ) (months)	24	35	22	30
Median survival (λ) (month)	16.1	25	19	10

Abbreviations: Dx, diagnosis; LCD, light chain disease.
(Data from Jancelewicz et al.[68] and Shustik et al.[140])

much higher than in myelomas producing other types of M protein. The overall response rate for 45 assessable patients was 58 percent. IgD myeloma is usually rapidly progressive. Despite the good response rate, the median survival for this group of patients was only 21.4 months, considerably shorter than the median of 31.8 months for IgG myeloma.

IMMUNOGLOBULIN E MULTIPLE MYELOMA

More than 35 cases have been reported since the first patient with IgE myeloma.[51,60,70,90,186] About 75 percent of IgE M proteins have κ-light chains. Although the clinical and laboratory features of IgE myeloma do not differ significantly from other myelomas, it seems that these patients are slightly younger, and the anemia is more marked. Plasma cell leukemia developed in 4 of 20 patients (20 percent) with IgE myeloma, for the highest incidence of plasma cell leukemia among all classes of myeloma. A 14-month remission was achieved in one case of IgE plasma cell leukemia with combination chemotherapy followed by interferon-alpha maintenance.[187]

NONSECRETORY MULTIPLE MYELOMA

An M protein is not found in the serum or urine of about 1 percent of myeloma patients.[126] In these subjects the myeloma cells either do not produce a monoclonal immunoglobulin or light chain (nonproducers), or produce an M protein, but are unable to secrete it (producers-nonsecretors). The myeloma cells also fail to express a surface M protein. In producers-nonsecretors, the cytoplasmic M protein can be demonstrated with immunofluorescent or immunoperoxidase techniques, using antibodies to heavy, light, or J-chains. The most common cytoplasmic monoclonal immunoglobulins are IgG and IgA, but IgM, IgD, and light chains have been reported.[73,120,141] Nonsecretor myeloma cells have been shown to release osteoclast-activating factor, demonstrating that the ability to secrete immunoglobulin and this cytokine are not linked.[167] Clinical features such as osteoporosis, lytic skeletal lesions, hypercalcemia, depressed normal immunoglobulins, and anemia are similar in secretory and nonsecretory myeloma. Renal failure occurs less commonly in the nonsecretors. Some authors suggest that the survival of patients with secretory and nonsecretory myeloma is similar.[28,135] However, in the two largest series of patients with nonsecretory myeloma,[47,144] the nonsecretors lived longer than the secretors, possibly because the nonsecretory disease presents in younger patients at an earlier stage, when the tumor mass is low, and there are fewer renal complications.[144] A cultured B-cell line from a patient with nonsecretory myeloma showed complex chromosomal abnormalities, and produced in vitro abundant quantities of IL-6 and PTH-related protein. Exposure of this cell line to anti-IL-6 antibody inhibited its growth.[118]

ACUTE TERMINAL PHASE

The clinical course of plasma cell myeloma resembles that of chronic myelogenous leukemia (CML) in many ways. Both usually present during the chronic phase of the disease, and frequently respond well initially to treatment with an alkylating agent. There is a progressive increase in the growth rate of the leukemic and myelomatous clones during the course of the disease.[11] Both diseases eventually enter an accelerated phase marked by rapid growth; the formation of soft tissue tumors in the skin, lymph nodes, and the meninges; and the development of marrow failure marked by pancytopenia (with a hypercellular marrow), and an unexplained fever. There is an actuarial risk of 85 percent of developing a terminal blast cell leukemia in chronic myelogenous leukemia, and 25 percent risk in myeloma patients.[12]

The equivalent of the accelerated phase of CML has been termed the acute terminal phase in myeloma.[15] This phase appears when the M protein doubling time shortens to less than 30 days. These patients usually develop a pancytopenia, not caused by treatment, since the marrow is hypercellular. In addition, extramedullary plasmacytomas appear in the subcutaneous tissues, lymph nodes, and meninges. Biopsies of the soft tissue masses may reveal a poorly differentiated tumor resembling an immunoblastic sarcoma.[52,156] An unexplained fever, which appears to be caused by the aggressive tumor, is frequently observed.[15,156] These patients often remain sensitive to chemotherapy, but the regrowth rate after treatment is so rapid that the remissions are very short-lived (kinetic "resistance"). Treatment during the acute terminal phase is unsatisfactory. Even with combination chemotherapy responses are incomplete and short. The persistent pancytopenia makes it difficult to treat these patients aggressively. We often use weekly doses of 300 mg/m^2 cyclophosphamide (oral or iv), and prednisone, 50 to 100 mg on alternate mornings. We emphasize supportive measures, using radiation for painful bony lesions, transfusions for anemia, and antibiotics for infections. Survival is brief after the onset of the acute terminal phase, with a median of about 3 months.[15,156]

The acute terminal phase may also be regarded as a preleukemic stage, for in many an acute leukemia develops as the terminal event.[14] The actuarial risk of developing acute leukemia develops early in the course of myeloma, and increases to 25 percent at 10 years.[15] We believe that acute leukemia is part of the natural history of myeloma because 1. there is an increased incidence of acute leukemia in untreated patients with myeloma, macroglobulinemia, and MGUS; 2. the increased incidence of acute leukemia in treated myeloma patients is not associated with an increased incidence of any other neoplasm (if alkylating agents and radiation act as carcinogens, one would expect to observe an increased incidence of all tumors in treated myeloma patients); and 3. the increased incidence of acute leukemia occurs earlier, and to a greater extent than in other patients, such as Hodgkin's disease or carcinoma of the ovary, who are treated similarly.[12] An alternate hypothesis is that the leukemia is secondary to treatment with alkylating agents. This view is supported by the observation that in a group of myeloma patients who developed acute leukemia, and had chomosome studies, the abnormal karyotypes in most patients were hypodiploid, and involved loss or structural abnormalities of chromosomes 5 or 7.[43] These are the chromosome abnormalities that have been associated with treatment-related leukemia.[121,134]

REFERENCES

1. Afifi AM: Myeloma cells in the cerebrospinal fluid in plasma cell neoplasia. J Neurol Neurosurg Psychiatry 37:1162–1165, 1974.
2. Atweh GF, Jabbour N: Intracranial solitary extraskeletal plasmacytoma resembling meningioma. Arch Neurol 39:57–59, 1982.
3. Aucouturier P, Bauwens M, Khamlichi AA, Denoroy L, Spinelli S, Touchard G et al: Monoclonal Ig L chain and L chain V domain fragment crystallization in myeloma-associated Fanconi's syndrome. J Immunol 150:3561–3568, 1993.
4. Bardwick PA, Zvaifler NJ, Gill GN, Newman D, Greenway GD, Resnick DL: Plasma cell dyscrasia with polyneuropathy, organomegaly, endocrinopathy, M protein and skin changes: The POEMS syndrome. Medicine (Balt) 59:311–322, 1980.
5. Bartoloni C, Flamini G, Logroscino C, Guidi L, Scuderi F, Gambassi G, Terranova T: IgD (kappa) "nonsecretory" multiple myeloma: Report of a case. Blood 56:898–901, 1980.
6. Bataille R, Sany J: Solitary myeloma: Clinical and prognostic features of a review of 114 cases. Cancer 48:845–851, 1981.
7. Bate KL, Clouston D, Packham D, Ratnaike S, Ebeling PR: Lambda light chain induced nephropathy: A rare cause of the Fanconi syndrome and severe osteomalacia. Am J Kidney Dis 32:E3, 1998.
8. Beaufils M, Morel-Morager L: Pathogenesis of renal disease in monoclonal gammopathies: Current concepts. Nephron 20:125–131, 1978.
9. Belec L, Mohamed AS, Authier FJ, Hallouin MC, Soe AM, Cotigny S et al: Human herpesvirus 8 infection in patients with POEMS syndrome-associated multicentric Castleman's disease. Blood 93:3643–3653, 1999.
10. Benjamin D, Joshua H, Djaldetti M, Hazaz B, Pinkhas J: Nonsecretory IgD-kappa multiple myeloma in a patient with Gaucher's disease. Scand J Haematol 22:179–184, 1979.
11. Bergsagel DE: Assessment of the response of mouse and human myeloma to chemotherapy and radiotherapy. In Drewinko B, Humphrey RM (eds.): Growth Kinetics and Biochemical Regulation of Normal and Malignant Cells, pp. 705–717. Williams & Wilkins, Baltimore, 1977.
12. Bergsagel DE: Chemotherapy of myeloma: Drug combinations versus single agents, an overview, and comments on acute leukemia in myeloma. Hematol Oncol 6:159–166, 1988.
13. Bergsagel DE: Chemotherapy of myeloma. In Malpas JS, Bergsagel DE, Kyle RA, Anderson KM (eds.): Myeloma: Biology and Management, pp. 269–302. Oxford University Press, Oxford and New York.
14. Bergsagel DE, Bailey AJ, Langley GR, MacDonald RN, White DF, Miller AB: The chemotherapy of plasma-cell myeloma and the incidence of acute leukemia. N Engl J Med 301:743–748, 1979.
15. Bergsagel DE, Pruzanski W: Treatment of plasma cell myeloma with cytotoxic agents. Arch Intern Med 135:172–176, 1975.
16. Besinger UA, Toyka KV, Anzil AP, Fateh-Mognadam A, Rouscher R, Heininger K: Myeloma neuropathy: Passive transfer from man to mouse. Science 213:1027–1030, 1981.
17. Betourne C, Buge A, Dechy H, Dorra M, Dournon E, Rancurel G: The treatment of peripheral neuropathies in a case of IgA myeloma and one of mixed cryoglobulinaemia. Repeated plasmapheresis (author's transl). Nouv Presse Med 9:1369–1371, 1980.
18. Bisagni-Faure A, Ravaud P, Amor B, Menkes CJ: Myeloma and epidural invasiveness. Clinical and therapeutic aspects (a study of 22 cases). Rev Rhum Mal Osteoartic 58:501–506, 1991.
19. Blade J, Lust JA, Kyle RA: Immunoglobulin-D multiple myeloma—presenting features, therapy, and survival in a series of 53 cases. J Clin Oncol 12:2398–2404, 1994.
20. Bosch EP, Smith BE: Peripheral neuropathies associated with monoclonal proteins. Med Clin North Am 77:125–139, 1993.
21. Brenner B, Carter A, Tatarsky I, Gruszkiewicz J, Peyser E: Incidence, prognostic significance and therapeutic modalities of central nervous system involvement in multiple myeloma. Acta Haematol 68:77–83, 1982.
22. Bromberg MB, Feldman EL, Albers JW: Chronic inflammatory polyradiculoneuropathy: Comparison of patients with and without an associated monoclonal gammopathy. Neurology 42:1157–1163, 1992.
23. Buchi G, Palestro G, Leonardo E, Termine G, Autino R: Monoclonal immunoproliferative disorder of B-lymphocytes IgD/lambda changing from chronic lymphocytic leukaemia to myeloma and plasmacytic leukaemia pattern. Acta Haematol 68:105–108, 1982.
24. Buxbaum JN, Chuba JV, Hellman GC, Solomon A, Gallo GR: Monoclonal immunoglobulin deposition disease: Light chain and light and heavy chain deposition diseases and their relation to light chain amyloidosis. Clinical features, immunopathology, and molecular analysis. Ann Intern Med 112:455–464, 1990.
25. Caggiano V, Nielsen SL, Glassy FJ, Dozier DF Jr: Immunoglobulin D myeloma: Report of a case with unusual neurological complications. West J Med 134:153–158, 1981.
26. Campese VM, Iseki K: Contrast-induced acute renal failure. Adv Exp Med Biol 212:135, 1987.
27. Casanova S, Donini U, Zucchelli P, Mazzucco G, Monga G, Linke RP: Immunohistochemical distinction between amyloidosis and fibrillar glomerulopathy. Am J Clin Pathol 97:787–795, 1992.
28. Cavo M, Galieni P, Gobbi M, Baldrati L, Leardini L, Baccarani M, Tura S: Nonsecretory multiple myeloma. Presenting findings, clinical course and prognosis. Acta Haematol 74:27–30, 1985.
29. Cejka J, Kithier K: IgD myeloma protein with "unreactive" light chain determinants. Clin Chem 25:1495–1498, 1979.
30. Chak LY, Cox RS, Bostwick DG, Hoppe RT: Solitary plasmacytoma of bone: Treatment, progression, and survival. J Clin Oncol 5:1811–1815, 1987.
31. Chernokhvostova EV, Batalova TN, German GP, Andreyeva NE: Immunodiagnosis of IgD multiple myeloma. A report of 17 cases.

Folia Haematol Int Mag Klin Morphol Blutforsch 108:539–552, 1981.

32. Clyne DH, Pesce AJ, Thompson RE: Nephrotoxicity of Bence Jones proteins in the rat. The importance of protein isoelectric point. Kidney Int 16:345–352, 1979.

33. Cohen DJ, Sherman WH, Osserman EF, Appel GB: Acute renal failure in patients with multiple myeloma. Am J Med 76:247–256, 1984.

34. Confalonieri R, Barbiano di Belgiojoso G, Banfi G, Ferrario F, Bertani T, Pozzi C et al: Light chain nephropathy: Histological and clinical aspects in 15 cases. Nephrol Dial Transplant 3:150–156, 1988.

35. Cooper K, Bennett WM: Nephrotoxicity of common drugs used in clinical practice. Arch Intern Med 147:1213–1218, 1987.

36. Coppero JR, Monteiro MLR, Collins J, Uphof D, Bear L: Foster-Kennedy syndrome caused by solitary intracranial plasmacytoma. Surg Neurol 19:267–272, 1983.

37. Corwin J, Lindberg RD: Solitary plasmacytoma of bone vs. extramedullary plasmacytoma and their relationship to multiple myeloma. Cancer 43:1007–1013, 1979.

38. Coward RA, Delamore TW, Mallick NP, Robinson EL: The importance of urinary immunoglobulin light chain isoelectric point (IP) in nephrotoxicity in multiple myeloma. Clin Sci 66:229–232, 1984.

39. Dalakas MC, Engel WK: Polyneuropathy with monoclonal gammopathy: Studies of 11 patients. Ann Neurol 10:45–52, 1981.

40. Dayan AD, Stokes MI: Peripheral neuropathy and experimental myeloma in the mouse. Nat New Biol 236:117–118, 1972.

41. Deret S, Denoroy L, Lamarine M, Vidal R, Mougenot B, Frangione B et al: Kappa light chain-associated Fanconi's syndrome: Molecular analysis of monoclonal immunoglobulin light chains from patients with and without intracellular crystals. Protein Eng 12:363–369, 1999.

42. DeWaal A, Potgieter GM, Visser AE, Heyns AD: IgD myeloma. A report of 4 new cases. S Afr Med J 61:407–410, 1982.

43. Dewald GW, Kyle RA, Hicks GA, Greipp PR: The clinical significance of cytogenetic studies in 100 patients with multiple myeloma, plasma cell leukemia, or amyloidosis. Blood 66:380–390, 1985.

44. Dieguez JC, Fernandes JA, Amian A, Rodriguez JN, Martino ML, Canavate M, Prados D: Chronic neutrophilic leukemia associated with myeloma. Simultaneous presentation. Sangre 37:403–406, 1992.

45. Dimopoulos MA, Goldstein J, Fuller L, Delasalle K, Alexanian R: Curability of solitary bone plasmacytoma. J Clin Oncol 10:587–590, 1992.

46. Dimopoulos MA, Kiamouris C, Moulopoulos LA: Solitary plasmacytoma of bone and extramedullary plasmacytoma. Hematol Oncol Clin North Am 13:1249–1257, 1999.

47. Dreicer R, Alexanian R: Nonsecretory multiple myeloma. Am J Hematol 13:313–318, 1982.

48. Driedger H, Pruzanski W: Plasma cell neoplasia with peripheral polyneuropathy. A study of five cases and a review of the literature. Medicine (Balt) 59:301–310, 1980.

49. Durie BG, Salmon SE, Moon TE: Pretreatment tumor mass, cell kinetics, and prognosis in multiple myeloma. Blood 55:364–372, 1980.

50. Elder G, Dalakas MC, Papadopoulos N, Sever JL: Peripheral neuropathy and light chain myeloma: Case report [letter]. Neurology 37:173–174, 1987.

51. Endo T, Okumura H, Kikuchi K, Munakata J, Otake M, Nomura T, Asakawa H: Immunoglobulin E (IgE) multiple myeloma: A case report and review of the literature. Am J Med 70:1127–1132, 1981.

52. Falini B, De Solas I, Levine AM, Parker JW, Lukes RJ, Taylor CR: Emergence of B-immunoblastic sarcoma in patients with multiple myeloma: A clinicopathologic study of 10 cases. Blood 59:923–933, 1982.

53. Feinberg L, Temple D, de Marchena E, Patarca R, Mitrani A: Soluble immune mediators in POEMS syndrome with pulmonary hypertension: Case report and review of the literature. Crit Rev Oncogen 10:293–302, 1999.

54. Ford HC, Casey BR, Walker S, Mason A: Multiple myeloma with an IgD kappa monoclonal protein. Am J Clin Pathol 74:105–107, 1980.

55. Gallo GR, Feiner HD, Katz LA, Feldman GM, Correa EB, Chuba JV, Buxbaum JN: Nodular glomerulopathy associated with non-amyloidotic kappa light chain deposits and excess immunoglobulin light chain synthesis. Am J Pathol 99:621–644, 1980.

56. Ganeval D, Noel LH, Droz D, Leibowitch J: Systemic lambda light-chain deposition in a patient with myeloma. Br Med J (Clin Res Ed) 282:681–683, 1981.

57. Gipstein RM, Cohen AH, Adams DA, Adams T, Grabie MT: Kappa light chain nephropathy without evidence of myeloma cells. Response to chemotherapy with cessation of maintenance hemodialysis. Am J Nephrol 2:276–281, 1982.

58. Goldfarb SB, Bishop CR: IgD myeloma and acute myelomonocytic leukemia [letter]. Blood 49:489–490, 1977.

59. Gomez EC, Margulies M, Rywlin A, Cabello B, Dominguez C: Cutaneous involvement by IgD myeloma. Arch Dermatol 114:1700–1703, 1978.

60. Hegewisch S, Mainzer K, Braumann D: IgE myelomatosis. Presentation of a new case and summary of literature. Blut 55:55–60, 1987.

61. Heilman RL, Velosa JA, Holley KE, Offord KP, Kyle RA: Long-term follow-up and response to chemotherapy in patients with light-chain deposition disease. Am J Kidney Dis 20:34–41, 1992.

62. Ioachim NJ, McKenna PJ, Halperin I, Chung FJ: IgD myeloma: Immunology and ultrastructure. Ann Clin Lab Sci 8:209–218, 1978.

63. Ito T, Kojima H, Otani K, Komeno T, Mitsuhashi S, Hasegawa Y et al: Chronic neutrophilic leukemia associated with monoclonal gammopathy of undetermined significance. Acta Haematol 95:140–143, 1996.

64. Iwasaki H, Ogawa K, Yoshida H, Takashima F, Shimizu K, Lee JD et al: Crow-Fukase syndrome associated with pulmonary hypertension. Intern Med 32:556–560, 1993.

65. Iwashita H, Ohnishi A, Asada M, Kanazawa Y, Kuroiwa Y: Polyneuropathy, skin hyperpigmentation, edema, and hypertrichosis in localized osteosclerotic myeloma. Neurology 27:675–681, 1977.

66. Jacquot C, Saint-Andre JP, Touchard G, Nochy D, D'Auzac de Lamartinie C, Oriol R et al: Association of systemic light-chain deposition disease and amyloidosis: A report of three patients with renal involvement. Clin Nephrol 24:93–98, 1985.

67. Jakubowski J, Kendall BE, Symon L: Primary plasmacytomas of the cranial vault. Acta Neurochirurg 55:117–134, 1980.

68. Jancelewicz Z, Takatsuki K, Sugai S, Pruzanski W: IgD multiple myeloma. Review of 133 cases. Arch Intern Med 135:87–93, 1975.

69. Jeha MT, Hamblin TJ, Smith JL: Coincident chronic lymphocytic leukemia and osteosclerotic myeloma. Blood 57:617–619, 1981.

70. Johansson SG, Bennich H: Immunological studies of an atypical (myeloma) immunoglobulin. Immunology 13:381–394, 1967.

71. Johnston JB, Weinerman B, Cooney T, Bowman DM, Pettigrew NM, Orr K: IgD kappa plasma cell dyscrasias: Extraosseous manifestations including isolated leptomeningitis. Am J Clin Pathol 77:60–65, 1982.

72. Jordan DR, Drouin J, Berry G, Watson GW: Intracranial plasmacytoma associated with multiple myeloma. Can J Ophthalmol 19:275–278, 1984.

73. Kanoh T, Niwa Y: Nonsecretory IgD (kappa) multiple myeloma. Report of a case and review of the literature. Am J Clin Pathol 88:516–519, 1987.

74. Kelly JJ Jr, Kyle RA, Miles JM, O'Brien PC, Dyck PJ: The spectrum of peripheral neuropathy in myeloma. Neurology 31:24–31, 1981.

75. Khamlichi AA, Rocca A, Touchard G, Aucouturier P, Preudhomme JL, Cogne M: Role of light-chain variable region in myeloma with light-chain deposition disease—evidence from an experimental-model. Blood 86:3655–3659, 1995.

76. Kijner CH, Yousem SA: Systemic light chain deposition disease presenting as multiple pulmonary nodules. A case report and review of the literature. Am J Surg Pathol 12:405–413, 1988.

77. King JA, Culpepper RM, Corey GR, Tucker JA, Lajoie G, Howell DN: Glomerulopathies with fibrillary deposits. Ultrastruct Pathol 24:15–21, 2000.

78. Kirkpatrick CJ, Curry A, Galle J, Melzner I: Systemic kappa light chain deposition and amyloidosis in multiple myeloma: Novel morphological observations. Histopathology 10:1065–1076, 1986.

79. Knowling MA, Harwood AR, Bergsagel DE: Comparison of extramedullary plasmacytomas with solitary and multiple plasma cell tumors of bone. J Clin Oncol 1:255–262, 1983.

80. Knowling MA, Harwood AR, Bergsagel DE: Comparison of extramedullary plasmacytomas with solitary and plasma cell tumors of bone. J Clin Oncol 1:255–262, 1983.

81. Kohli CM, Kawazu T: Solitary intracranial plasmacytoma. Surg Neurol 17:307–312, 1982.

82. Korbet SM, Schwartz MM, Lewis EJ: Immunotactoid glomerulopathy. Am J Kidney Dis 17:247–257, 1991.

83. Krumholz A, Weiss HD, Jiji VH, Bakal D, Kirsh MB: Solitary intracranial plasmacytoma: Two patients with extended follow-up. Ann Neurol 11:529–532, 1982.

84. Kyle RA: Multiple myeloma: Review of 869 cases. Mayo Clin Proc 50:29–40, 1975.

85. Kyle RA: Monoclonal proteins in neuropathy. Neurol Clin 10:713–734, 1992.

86. Kyle RA: Monoclonal proteins and renal disease. Annu Rev Med 45:71–77, 1994.

87. Lacy MQ, Gertz MA: Acquired Fanconi's syndrome associated with monoclonal gammopathies. Hematol Oncol Clin North Am 13:1273–1280, 1999.

88. Lacy MQ, Gertz MA, Hanson CA, Inwards DJ, Kyle RA: Multiple myeloma associated with diffuse osteosclerotic bone lesions: A clinical entity distinct from osteosclerotic myeloma (POEMS syndrome) [Review]. Am J Hematol 56:288–293, 1997.

89. Latov N, Sherman WH, Nemni R, Galassi G, Shyong JS, Penn AS et al: Plasma-cell dyscrasia and peripheral neuropathy with a monoclonal antibody to peripheral-nerve myelin. N Engl J Med 303:618–621, 1980.

90. Lawlor E, Collins DM, O'Connor FB: A case of IgE myeloma. Clin Chem 32:697, 1986.

91. Lesprit P, Godeau B, Authier FJ, Soubrier M, Zuber M, Larroche C et al: Pulmonary hypertension in Poems syndrome—a new feature mediated by cytokines. Am J Resp Crit Care Med 157:907–911, 1998.

92. Liebross RH, Ha CS, Cox JD, Weber D, Delasalle K, Alexanian R: Solitary bone plasmacytoma: Outcome and prognostic factors following radiotherapy. Int J Radiat Oncol Biol Phys 41:1063–1067, 1998.

93. Ludwig H, Fruhwald F, Tscholakoff D, Rasoul S, Neuhold A, Fritz E: Magnetic resonance imaging of the spine in multiple myeloma. Lancet 2:364–366, 1987.

94. Mackenzie MR, Wuepper KE, Jordon C, Fudenberg HH: Rapid renal failure in a case of multiple myeloma: The role of Bence Jones proteins. Clin Exp Immunol 3:593–601, 1968.

95. Maldonado JE, Kyle RA, Ludwig J, Okazaki H: Meningeal myeloma. Arch Intern Med 126:660–663, 1970.

96. Maldonado JE, Velosa JE, Kyle RA, Wagoner RD, Holley KE, Salassa RM: Fanconi syndrome in adults: A manifestation of a latent form of myeloma. Am J Med 58:354–364, 1975.

97. Mancardi GI, Mandybur TI: Solitary intracranial plasmacytoma. Cancer 51:2226–2233, 1983.

98. Markowitz GS, Cheng JT, Colvin RB, Trebbin WM, D'Agati VD: Hepatitis C viral infection is associated with fibrillary glomerulonephritis and immunotactoid glomerulopathy. J Am Soc Nephrol 9:2244–2252, 1998.

99. Mascret B, Blanc AP, Jauffret P, Ratignier A, Garabedian C: IgD myeloma of the leukemic type with myelofibrosis (letter). Nouv Presse Med 10:2907–2908, 1981.

100. Masini L, Salvarani C, Macchioni P, Baldi G, Rossi F, Croci G et al: Chronic neutrophilic leukemia (CNL) with karyotypic abnormalities associated with plasma cell dyscrasia: A case report. Haematologia 77:277–279, 1992.

101. Masson RG, Rennke HG, Gottlieb MN: Pulmonary hemorrhage in a patient with fibrillary glomerulonephritis. N Engl J Med 326:36–39, 1992.

102. McAllister HA Jr, Seger J, Bossart M, Ferrans VJ: Restrictive cardiomyopathy with kappa light chain deposits in myocardium as a complication of multiple myeloma. Histochemical and electron microscopic observations. Arch Pathol Lab Med 112:1151–1154, 1988.

103. McCarthy CS, Becker JA: Multiple myeloma and contrast media. Radiology 183:519–521, 1992.

104. Melcion C, Mougenot B, Badouin B, Ronco P, Moulonguet-Doleris L, Vanhille P et al: Renal failure in myeloma: Relationship with isoelectric point of immunoglobulin light chains. Clin Nephrol 22:138–143, 1984.

105. Menu Y, Dhermy D, Brousse N, Grenier P, Pallardy G, Nahum H: Myeloma condensant. A propos de trois case. Révue de la littérature. Ann Radiol (Paris) 24:265–269, 1981.

106. Messiaen T, Deret S, Mougenot B, Bridoux F, Dequiedt P, Dion JJ et al: Adult Fanconi syndrome secondary to light chain gammopathy. Clinicopathologic heterogeneity and unusual features in 11 patients. Medicine (Balt) 79:135–154, 2000.

107. Miralles GD, O'Fallon JR, Talley NJ: Plasma-cell dyscrasia with polyneuropathy. The spectrum of POEMS syndrome. N Engl J Med 327:1919–1923, 1992.

108. Moorhouse DF, Fox RI, Powell HC: Immunotactoid-like endoneurial deposits in a patient with monoclonal gammopathy of undetermined significance and neuropathy [see comments]. Acta Neuropathol 84:484–494, 1992.

109. Morgan WKC: Foster Kennedy syndrome produced by myelomatous deposits in the skull. BMJ 1:708, 1955.

110. Morrow JS, Schafer EJ, Huston DP, Rosen WS: POEMS syndrome. Studies in a patient with IgG-κ M-protein, but no polyneuropathy. Arch Intern Med 142:1231–1234, 1982.

111. Moulopoulos LA, Moulopoulos MA, Weber D, Fuller L, Libshitz HI, Alexanian R: Magnetic resonance imaging in the staging of solitary plasmacytoma of bone. J Clin Oncol 11:1311–1315, 1993.

112. Myatt EA, Westholm FA, Weiss DT, Solomon A, Schiffer M, Stevens FJ: Pathogenic potential of human monoclonal light chains—relationship of in vitro aggregation to in vivo organ deposition. Proc Nat Acad Sci USA 91:3034–3038, 1994.

113. Nagai M, Oda S, Iwamoto M, Marumoto K, Fujita M, Takahara K: Granulocyte-colony stimulating factor concentrations in a patient

with plasma cell dyscrasia and clinical features of chronic neu-trophilic leukaemia. J Clin Pathol 49:858–860, 1996.

114. Nakamoto Y, Imai H, Yasuda T, Wakui H, Miura AB: A spectrum of clinicopathological features of nephropathy associated with POEMS syndrome. Nephrol Dial Transplant 14:2370–2378, 1999.

115. Nakanishi T, Sobue I, Toyokura Y, Nishitani H, Kuroiwa Y, Satoyoshi E et al: The Crow-Fucase syndrome: A study of 102 cases in Japan. Neurology 34:712–720, 1984.

116. Nelis GF: An unusual case of myeloma. Non-secretory IgD-kappa myeloma with de-differentiation of kappa myeloma evolving from solitary plasmacytoma. Acta Med Scand 211:141–144, 1982.

117. Nestler JE: Immunoglobulin D multiple myeloma with thrombo-cytosis [letter]. Ann Intern Med 94:412, 1981.

118. Ohmori M, Nagai M, Fujita M, Dobashi H, Tasaka T, Yamaoka G et al: A novel mature B-cell line (DOBIL-6) producing both parathyroid hormone-related protein and interleukin-6 from a myeloma patient presenting with hypercalcaemia. Br J Haematol 101:688–693, 1998.

119. Orfila C, Lepert JC, Modesto A et al: Fanconi's syndrome, kappa light-chain myeloma, non-amyloid fibrils and cytoplasmic crys-tals in renal tubular epithelium. Am J Nephrol 11:345, 1991.

120. Ozaki M, Yamanaka H: An unusual case of Bence Jones myeloma with extremely low levels of monoclonal immunoglobulin. Oral Surg Oral Med Oral Pathol 61:498–503, 1986.

121. Pedersen-Bjergaard J, Nissen NI, Sorensen HM, Hou-Jensen K, Larsen MS, Ernst P et al: Acute non-lymphocytic leukemia in patients with ovarian carcinoma following long-term treatment with Treosulfan (= dihydroxybusulfan). Cancer 45:19–29, 1980.

122. Peng SK, French WJ, Cohen AH, Fausel RE: Light chain car-diomyopathy associated with small-vessel disease. Arch Pathol Lab Med 112:844–846, 1988.

123. Preud'Homme JL, Morel-Maroger L, Brouet JC, Mihaesco E, Mery JP, Seligmann M: Synthesis of abnormal heavy and light chains in multiple myeloma with visceral deposition of mono-clonal immunoglobulin. Clin Exp Immunol 42:545–553, 1980.

124. Pritchard PB 3rd, Martinez RA, Hungerford GD, Powers JM, Perot PL Jr: Dural plasmacytoma. Neurosurgery 12:576–579, 1983.

125. Pruzanski W: Unusual manifestations of plasma cell dyscrasia. In Ritzmann SE (ed.): Protein Abnormalities, Vol. 2. Allan R. Liss, New York, 1982.

126. Pruzanski W, Ogryzlo MA: Abnormal proteinuria in malignant diseases. Adv Clin Chem 13:335–382, 1970.

127. Randall RE, Williamson WC Jr, Mullinax F, Tung MY, Still WJ: Manifestations of systemic light chain deposition. Am J Med 60:293–299, 1976.

128. Reitan JB, Pape E, Fossaå SD, Julsrud OJ, Slettnes ON, Solheim OP: Osteosclerotic myeloma with polyneuropathy. Acta Med Scand 208:137–144, 1980.

129. Reulecke M, Dumas M, Meier C: Specific antibody activity against neuroendocrine tissue in a case of POEMS syndrome with IgG gammapathy. Neurology 38:614–616, 1988.

130. Rogers JS 2nd, Spahr J, Judge DM, Varano LA, Eyster ME: IgE myeloma with osteoblastic lesions. Blood 49:295–299, 1977.

131. Rose PE, McGonigle R, Michael J, Broughton BJ: Renal failure and the histopathological features of myeloma kidney reversed by inten-sive chemotherapy and peritoneal dialysis. BMJ 294:411–412, 1987.

132. Rota S, Mougenot B, Boudouin B, De Meyer-Brasseur M, Lemaitre V, Michel C et al: Multiple myeloma and severe renal failure: A clinicopathologic study of outcome and prognosis in 34 patients. Medicine 66:126–137, 1987.

133. Rousseau JJ, Franck G, Grisar T, Reznik M, Heynan G, Salmon J: Ostosclerotic myeloma with polyneuropathy and ectopic secre-tion of calcitonin. Eur J Cancer 14:133–140, 1978.

134. Rowley JD, Golomb HM, Vardiman J, Fukuhara S, Dougherty C, Potter D: Further evidence for a non-random chromosomal abnormality in acute promyelocytic leukemia. Int J Cancer 20:869–872, 1977.

135. Rubio-Felix D, Giralt M, Giraldo MP, Martinez-Penuela JM, Oyarzabal F, Sala F, Raichs A: Nonsecretory multiple myeloma. Cancer 59:1847–1852, 1987.

136. Schaar CG, Kaiser U, Snijder S, Ong F, Hermans J, Franck PF, Kluin-Nelemans JC: Serum interleukin-6 has no discriminatory role in paraproteinaemia nor a prognostic role in multiple myeloma. Br J Haematol 107:132–138, 1999.

137. Schifferli JA, Merot Y, Cruchaud A, Chatelanat F: Immunotactoid glomerulopathy with leucocytoclastic skin vasculitis and hypocom-plementemia: A case report. Clin Nephrol 27:151–155, 1987.

138. Schulman P, Sun T, Sharer L, Hyman P, Vinciguerra V, Feinstein M et al: Meningeal involvement in IgD myeloma with cerebrospinal fluid paraprotein analysis. Cancer 46:152–155, 1980.

139. Seymour AE, Thompson AJ, Smithe PS, Woodroffe AJ, Clarkson AR: Kappa light chain glomerulosclerosis in multiple myeloma. Am J Med 101:557–580, 1980.

140. Shustik C, Bergsagel DE, Pruzanski W: Kappa and lambda light chain disease: Survival rates and clinical manifestations. Blood 48:41–51, 1976.

141. Shustik C, Michel R, Karsh J: Nonsecretory myeloma: A study on hypoimmunoglobulinemia. Acta Haematol 80:153–158, 1988.

142. Silva FG, Meyrier A, Morel-Maroger L, Pirani CL: Proliferative glomerulonephropathy in multiple myeloma. J Pathol 130:229–236, 1980.

143. Simmons Z: Paraproteinemia and neuropathy. Curr Opin Neurol 12:589–595, 1999.

144. Smith DB, Harris M, Gowland E, Chang J, Scarffe JH: Non-secre-tory multiple myeloma: A report of 13 cases with a review of the literature. Hematol Oncol 4:307–313, 1986.

145. Smithline N, Kassirer JP, Cohen JJ: Light-chain nephropathy. Renal tubular dysfunction associated with light chain protein-urea. N Engl J Med 294:71–74, 1976.

146. Soffer D, Siegal T: Solitary dural plasmacytoma with conspicuous cytoplasmic inclusions. Cancer 49:2500–2504, 1982.

147. Solling K, Solling J, Jacobsen NO, Thomsen OF: Nonsecretory myeloma associated with nodular glomerulosclerosis. Acta Med Scand 207:137–143, 1980.

148. Soubrier M, Guillon R, Dubost JJ, Serre AF, Riston JM, Boyer L, Sauvezie B: Arterial obliteration in POEMS syndrome: Possible role of vascular endothelial growth factor. J Rheumatol 25:813–815, 1998.

149. Soubrier MJ, Dubost JJ, Sauvezie B, Arfi S, Audhuy B, Aumaitre O et al: Poems-syndrome—a study of 25 cases and a review of the literature. Am J Med 97:543–553, 1994.

150. Spaar FW: Paraproteinemias and multiple myeloma. In Hand-book of Clinical Neurology, Vol. 39, p. 131. North Holland, Ams-terdam, 1980.

151. Spiers AS, Halpern R, Ross SC, Neiman RS, Harawi S, Zipoli TE: Meningeal myelomatosis. Arch Intern Med 140:256–259, 1980.

152. Standen GR, Steers FJ, Jones L: Clonality of chronic neutrophilic leukaemia associated with myeloma: Analysis using the X-linked probe M27β. J Clin Pathol 46:297–298, 1993.

153. Stark RJ, Henson RA: Cerebral compression by myeloma. J Neu-rol Neurosurg Psychiatry 44:833–836, 1981.

154. Stokes MB, Holler S, Cui Y, Hudkins KL, Eitner F, Fogo A, Alpers CE: Expression of decorin, biglycan, and collagen type I in human renal fibrosing disease. Kidney Int 57:487–498, 2000.

155. Suarez GA, Kelly JJ: Polyneuropathy associated with monoclonal gammopathy of undetermined significance: Further evidence that

IgM-MGUS neuropathies are different than IgG-MGUS. Neurology 43:1304–1308, 1993.

156. Suchman AL, Coleman M, Mouradian JA, Wolf DJ, Saletan S: Aggressive plasma cell myeloma. A terminal phase. Arch Intern Med 141:1315–1320, 1981.

157. Swash M, Perin J, Schwartz MS: Significance of immunoglobulin deposition in peripheral nerves in neuropathies associated with paraproteinaemia. J Neurol Neurosurg Psychiatry 42:179–183, 1979.

158. Takahashi T, Lim B, Jamal N, Tritchler D, Lockwood G, McKinney S et al: Colony growth and self renewal of plasma cell precursors in multiple myeloma. J Clin Oncol 3:1613–1623, 1985.

159. Tanus T, Miller HJ: POEMS syndrome presenting with cardiomegaly and cardiomyopathy. J Int Med 231:445–448, 1992.

160. Toth J: IgD myeloma: A case report [letter]. Can Med Assoc J 116:1235–1236, 1238, 1977.

161. Toussaint P, Sibaud V, Labbe L, Geniaux M: POEMS syndrome revealed by a scleroderma-like skin thickening. Ann Dermatol Venereol 127:73–76, 2000.

162. Troussard X, Lebrun E, Marco M, Gallateau F, Reman O, Leporrier M: Neurophilic leukemia and multiple myeloma. 2 cases (letter). Ann Med Interne 143:136–139, 1992.

163. Tubbs RR, Gephardt GN, McMahon JT, Hall PM, Valenzuela R, Vidt DG: Light chain nephropathy. Am J Med 71:263–269, 1981.

164. Udoji WC, Pemmaraju S: IgD myeloma with myelofibrosis and amyloidosis. Arch Pathol Lab Med 101:10–13, 1977.

165. Usuda H, Naito M, Ohyach K, Iizumi A: A case of multiple myeloma producing granulocyte colony-stimulating factor. Pathol Int 47:866–869, 1997.

166. Valenzuela R, Govindarajan S, Tubbs R, Deodhar S, Bukowski R: IgD myeloma. Report of a case with unusual clinical and immunologic features. Am J Clin Pathol 72:246–250, 1979.

167. Van Slyck EJ, Kleerekoper M, Abraham JP, Deegan MJ: Nonsecretory multiple myeloma with osteoporosis: Immunocytologic and bone resorptive studies. Am J Med Sci 291:347–351, 1986.

168. Vastni PS, Erickson DG, Williams RC Jr, Tung KS: Benign monoclonal gamma-globulinemia and glomerulonephritis. Am J Med 62:324–329, 1977.

169. Verroust P, Mery JP, Morel-Maroger L, Clauvel JP, Richet G, Bouteiller AM, Fumagalli N: Glomerular lesions in monoclonal gammopathies and mixed essential cryoglobulinemias IgG-IgM. Adv Nephrol Necker Hosp 1:161–194, 1971.

170. Viard JP, Lesavre P, Boitard C, Noel LH, Roth A, Said G, Bach JF: POEM syndrome presenting as systemic sclerosis—clinical and pathological study of a case with microangiopathic glomerular lesions. Am J Med 84:524–528, 1988.

171. Vidal R, Goni F, Stevens F, Aucouturier P, Kumar A, Frangione B et al: Somatic mutations of the L12a gene in V-kappa(1) light chain deposition disease: Potential effects on aberrant protein conformation and deposition. Am J Pathol 155:2009–2017, 1999.

172. Vilpo JA, Irjala K: IgD-lambda myeloma with separate heavy- and light-chain M-components. Clin Chem 26:1760–1761, 1980.

173. Vladutiu AO: IgD myeloma or delta heavy-chain disease? [letter]. Clin Chem 26:353–354, 1980.

174. Vladutiu AO, Kohli RK, Prezyna AP: Monoclonal IgE with renal failure. Am J Med 61:957–962, 1976.

175. Walb D, Wohlenberg H, Rumpelt HJ, Schmidt H, Thomas L: Fanconi syndrome in an adult coincident with early myeloma with monoclonal IgG, type kappa, anomaly (author's transl). Dtsch Med Wochenschr 105:1355–1359, 1980.

176. Watanabe O, Maruyama I, Arimura K, Kitajima I, Arimura H, Hanatani M et al: Overproduction of vascular endothelial growth factor/vascular permeability factor is causative in Crow-Fucase (POEMS) syndrome. Muscle Nerve 21:190–197, 1998.

177. Weiss AH, Smith E, Christoff N, Kochwa S: Cerebrospinal fluid paraproteins in multiple myeloma. J Lab Clin Med 66:280–293, 1965.

178. White GC 2nd, Jacobson RJ, Binder RA, Linke RP, Glenner GG: Immunoglobulin D myeloma and amyloidosis: Immunochemical and structural studies of Bence Jones and amyloid fibrillar proteins. Blood 46:713–722, 1975.

179. Willison HJ, Paterson G, Veitch J, Inglis G, Barnett SC: Peripheral neuropathy associated with monoclonal IgM anti-Pr$_2$ cold agglutinins. J Neurol Neurosurg Psychiatry 56:1178–1183, 1993.

180. Wiltshaw E: The natural history of extramedullary plasmacytoma and its relation to solitary myeloma of bone and myelomatosis. Medicine (Balt) 55:217–238, 1976.

181. Wiltshaw E: Chemotherapy in the management of extramedullary plasmacytoma. Cancer Chemother Pharmacol 1:167–175, 1978.

182. Woo E, Yu YL, Ng M, Huang CY, Todd D: Spinal cord compression in multiple myeloma: Who gets it? Aust N Z Med 16:671–675, 1986.

183. Woodruff RK, Ireton HJ: Multiple cranial nerve palsies as the presenting feature of meningeal myelomatosis. Cancer 49:1710–1712, 1982.

184. Woodruff RK, Malpas JS, White FE: Solitary plasmacytoma. II: Solitary plasmacytoma of bone. Cancer 43:2344–2347, 1979.

185. Woodruff RK, Whittle JM, Malpas JS: Solitary plasmacytoma. I: Extramedullary soft tissue plasmacytoma. Cancer 43:2340–2343, 1979.

186. Yamagata N, Shimazaki C, Goto H, Hirata T, Ashihara E, Oku N et al: IgE plasma cell leukemia successfully treated with combination VAD (vincristine, doxorubicin, dexamethasone) and MP (melphalan, prednisolone) followed by interferon-alpha [see comments]. Am J Hematol 45:262–264, 1994.

187. Yamagata N, Shimazaki C, Goto H, Hirata T, Ashihara E, Oku N et al: IgE plasma-cell leukemia successfully treated with combination (vincristine, doxorubicin, dexamethasone) and MP (melphalan, prednisolone) followed by interferon-alpha. Am J Hematol 45:262–264, 1994.

188. Yang GC, Nieto R, Stachura I, Gallo GR: Ultrastructural immunohistochemical localization of polyclonal IgG, C3, and amyloid P component on the Congo Red-negative amyloid-like fibrils of fibrillary glomerulopathy. Am J Pathol 141:409–419, 1992.

33

Waldenström's Macroglobulinemia

Meletios A. Dimopoulos

Waldenström's macroglobulinemia (WM) is a lymphoproliferative disorder characterized by the presence of monoclonal lymphocytes that produce monoclonal immunoglobulin M (IgM). This disease was described in 1944 by Jan Waldenström who reported two patients with oronasal bleeding, mild generalized lymphadenopathy, significant anemia, elevated erythrocyte sedimentation rate, and marked hyperviscosity. Large amounts of a high-molecular-weight globulin were detected in the serum of these patients and their bone marrow aspirate showed increased numbers of lymphocytoid cells.[1] The abnormal serum globulin was subsequently called immunoglobulin M (IgM).

DIFFERENTIAL DIAGNOSIS

The diagnosis of WM is obvious when there is evidence of large amounts of monoclonal IgM, infiltration of the bone marrow by small lymphocytes, plasmacytoid lymphocytes and plasma cells, anemia with or without hepatosplenomegaly, or lymphadenopathy. Elevations of serum monoclonal IgM ranging from 1.0 to 3.0 g/dl have been suggested in order to assign the diagnosis of WM.[2,3] However, Kyle and Garton[4] have shown that all patients with bone marrow lymphoplasmacytic infiltrate associated with a serum monoclonal IgM should be included under the diagnosis of WM regardless of the amount of IgM.

In some persons, a monoclonal IgM of less than 2 g/dl is detected by chance but there are no symptoms or signs of a malignant lymphoproliferative disorder and the bone marrow is normal or reveals a mild lymphocytosis. Such individuals fulfill the diagnostic criteria of monoclonal gammopathy of undetermined significance (MGUS) of IgM type.[4,5] The incidence of IgM MGUS is three to four times higher than that of WM.[4,6] These persons do not require any treatment but they should be followed with serial physical exams, blood counts, biochemical profile, serum protein electrophoreses, and quantitation of serum immunoglobulins. In some of these individuals overt WM or amyloidosis may develop in the future. There are no established parameters at the diagnosis of MGUS that can identify the individuals in whom a malignant condition will develop.

In other individuals, a fortuitous detection of monoclonal IgM triggers further evaluation that reveals an overt lymphoplasmacytic infiltration of the bone marrow. When these patients with WM are asymptomatic, have normal hemoglobin or only mild anemia, significant hepatosplenomegaly or lymphadenopathy is absent, and no other complications of monoclonal IgM are present, they should be followed closely without treatment until there is evidence of disease progression. Several months or years may elapse before treatment is required.[7]

Finally, some patients present with a complication caused by the monoclonal IgM such as cold-agglutinin anemia, cryoglobulinemia, peripheral neuropathy, or amyloidosis but the concentration of IgM is low and there is no evidence of involvement of the bone marrow, of the lymph nodes, or of the spleen. In such patients, the specific property of the IgM caused symptoms before the development of overt WM.[8,9] The treatment of such patients focuses on the management of the IgM-induced disorder and systemic chemotherapy may be of benefit.

INCIDENCE

Waldenström's macroglobulinemia is an infrequent disease affecting approximately 1500 Americans each year. Herrinton and Weiss[10] reported an age-standardized annual incidence rate of 6.1 per million in White men and 2.5 per million in White women. In contrast to multiple myeloma, WM was significantly more common in Whites than in Blacks. Groves et al. found that the age-adjusted incidence rates for WM per 1 million person-years at risk were 3.4 among males and 1.7 among females. The rates increased sharply with age from 0.1 at age less than 45 years to 36.3 at age greater than 75 years for males. The rates for WM were comparable to those for hairy cell leukemia, but considerably lower than those for multiple myeloma or chronic lymphocytic leukemia.[11]

ETIOLOGY

The etiology of WM is unclear. A role of genetic predisposition was suggested 40 years ago when the disease was diagnosed in two brothers and a monoclonal IgM without overt WM was also detected in their mother.[12] Since then several families have been described in which there have been more than one patient in a single family including monozygotic twins.[13–17] Several families of patients with WM have shown multiple immunoglobulin abnormalities and immunologic disorder. Either monoclonal IgM or polyclonal elevation of IgM has been reported.[14] The incidence of antigammaglobulin factor in first-degree relatives of patients may be increased.[18]

There is an increased incidence of WM in patients with abnormal immune function such as those with Sjogren syndrome.[19] Furthermore, in several patients, the monoclonal IgM behaves as an autoantibody against tubulin, actin, myoglobin, and thyroglobulin.[20] It is possible that autoantibody clones are more susceptible to malignant evolution perhaps secondary to continuous stimulation.[21]

The diagnosis of WM in three shoe repairers implied a possible association with exposure to leather, rubber dyes, and paint.[22] However, a survey of workers exposed to benzene and other solvents in China did not reveal any case of WM.[23] In one case-control study patients with WM were slightly better educated, but no significant differences were found for occupational exposure, alcohol or tobacco use, medication history, past medical history, or familiar cancer history.[24] Macroglobulinemia was diagnosed in five young African-Americans who had a history of intravenous heroin abuse.[25]

PATHOLOGY

According to the revised European-American classification of lymphoid neoplasm, WM represents the majority of cases that are included under the diagnosis of lymphoplasmacytoid lymphoma/immunocytoma.[26] This disease always involves the bone marrow. The bone marrow smear typically shows a diffuse proliferation of small lymphocytes, plasmacytoid lymphocytes (cells with abundant basophilic cytoplasm, but lymphocyte-like nuclei), and plasma cells.[26] Mast cells and Dutcher bodies, which represent periodic acid-Schiff (PAS)-positive intranuclear and intracytoplasmic inclusions, are often seen.[27] The extent of marrow infiltration is more adequately assessed with a biopsy. Bartl et al.[28] distinguished three types of bone marrow involvement: lymphoplasmacytoid (47 percent), lymphoplasmacytic (42 percent), and polymorphous (11 percent). Examination of involved lymph nodes under light microscopy shows that the growth pattern is often interfollicular with sparing of the sinuses.[26]

BIOLOGY

Studies using antibodies against both isotype and idiotype of the monoclonal IgM indicated that the malignant cell of origin was a lymphoid cell that had already been committed to its final isotype. The idiotype and isotype of the IgM of bone marrow WM cells were always the same with that expressed in the serum.[29] Thirty years ago, immunofluorescent studies performed on bone marrow and blood smears demonstrated that the overwhelming majority of the bone marrow pleomorphic lymphoid cells were expressing surface IgM. These cells lack intracytoplasmic IgM; the latter was restricted to the plasma cells and to some lymphocytoid plasma cells. It was also found that most lymphocytes circulating in the blood were expressing surface IgM despite the absence of blood lymphocytosis.[30] Such studies indicated that WM is characterized by a continuum of differentiation, starting from small, mature lymphocytes expressing surface immunoglobulin and evolving to terminally differentiated plasma cells that have lost the surface immunoglobulin but still maintained intracytoplasmic immunoglobulin.[31] With the use of flow cytometry it can be demonstrated that the malignant clone in WM expresses several B-cell-associated antigens such as CD19, CD20, and CD22, but the CD23 antigen, which is usually expressed in chronic lymphocytic leukemia, is not expressed in WM. The plasma cells are usually strongly positive for CD38 but the small lymphocytes are usually negative. Negativity for CD5 and CD10 are also characteristic for WM.[26,32–34] By using three-color flow cytometry it has been demonstrated that 86 percent of patients with WM were characterized by a CD19+, CD20+, CD5–, CD10–, CD23– immunophenotype.[35] The use of immunophenotyping may help in the more accurate diagnosis of occasional patients with follicular lymphoma or mantle cell lymphoma who may produce monoclonal IgM.

Abnormal karyotypes have been described in up to 30 percent of patients with WM. The abnormalities usually found involve trisomies or deletions of chromosomes 6, 10, 11, 12, 15, 20, and 21. Structural aberrations involving chromosomes 6q and 11q have been reported.[36] Several patients have complex karyotypes. The translocation t(9;14)(p13;q32) is considered specific for lymphoplasmacytoid lymphomas. In this translocation the PAX-5 gene, which encodes a B-cell-specific transcription factor, is juxtaposed to the IgH locus in 14q32.[37] Using interphase fluorescence in situ hybridization, deletions of the TP53 suppressor gene were detected in 15 percent of patients; this abnormality was associated with shorter survival.[38]

Kaposi's sarcoma-associated herpesvirus (KSHV) is suspected to play a role in the etiology of multiple myeloma through the expression of a viral IL-6.[39] In a preliminary analysis of dendritic cell-enriched peripheral blood mononuclear cells from four patients with WM, KSHV was detected in all samples.[40] Agbalika et al.[41] obtained amplified KSHV sequences from six out of ten WM bone marrow biopsies. However, Brousset et al.[42] performed two rounds of amplification and found that only 1 out of 20 of the DNA samples, obtained from biopsies, had a detectable KSHV sequence. Stone et al. tested samples from 15 patients with WM for antibodies to lytic and latent HHV-8 antigens by indirect immunofluorescence. They found that 27 percent of patients were positive for the lytic antibody but none were positive for the latent antibody.[43] Thus, the role of KSHV in the pathogenesis of WM remains unclear.

CLINICAL AND LABORATORY FEATURES

General Symptoms and Signs

The median age at diagnosis of WM is 65 years. In recent years an increasing number of patients are being diagnosed by chance and are asymptomatic. The clinical manifestations associated with WM are related to direct tumor infiltration and to the amount and specific properties of monoclonal IgM. The malignant cells divide slowly but they can disseminate throughout the lymphoid system and other tissues where B lymphocytes recirculate. However, many complications of this disease are the result of the unique properties of the IgM monoclonal protein itself, including its large size, high carbohydrate content, and capacity to bind to other components of the blood and other tissues. Monoclonal IgM may behave as an autoantibody that can recognize the I antigen on red cells, antigens in the nervous system, the skin, skeletal muscle, etc. Moreover, the IgM can behave as a cryoglobulin or can have cold agglutinin activity.

When the IgM molecules form complexes with each other or with other serum proteins, they may localize in the walls of blood vessels and produce widespread vascular damage affecting several organs including the skin and the glomeruli.

Thus, the clinical manifestations of WM can be variable and depend on which property of IgM predominates in individual patients.[2,3,4,7,44,45] The most common symptoms are weakness and fatigue. Anorexia and weight loss affect one-third of the patients. Symptoms and signs of elevated serum viscosity such as oronasal bleeding, dizziness, and visual disturbances occur in 10 to 30 percent of patients at diagnosis. Hepatomegaly, splenomegaly, and lymphadenopathy occur in 20 to 30 percent of patients each. The incidence of these abnormalities increases if routine computed tomography is being used for the staging of the disease.[46] Symptoms and signs of peripheral neuropathy occur in 5 to 20 percent of patients. In some patients cryoglobulinemia or cold agglutinin disease may predominate.

Laboratory Findings

Anemia is present at diagnosis in the majority of patients with symptomatic WM. Blood smears are usually normochromic and normocytic and rouleau formation is usually found. The anemia is primarily due to bone marrow infiltration but also to a dilutional effect secondary to plasma volume expansion secondary to IgM.[47] In some patients the monoclonal IgM has cold agglutinin activity that may result in cold sensitivity and chronic hemolysis with acute exacerbations related to cold exposure.[48,49] Occasional patients may develop autoimmune hemolytic anemia.

The leukocyte count is usually normal but mild lymphocytosis is not uncommon and monoclonal lymphocytes are detected with flow cytometry in the blood of virtually all patients. Mild thrombocytopenia occurs in one-third of patients but less than 50×10^9/L platelets are seen in fewer than 10 percent of patients at diagnosis. Some patients may present with pancytopenia. Renal and liver function tests are usually normal, hyperuricemia may be present, and hypercalcemia occurs in 4 percent of patients.[4,7]

All patients have a serum monoclonal protein almost always migrating in the gamma area. The amount of serum monoclonal protein is better evaluated from the serum protein electrophoresis strip rather than the nephelometry, which may overestimate the concentration of serum IgM. The presence of an IgM monoclonal protein and its light-chain type must be confirmed by immunofixation. The median serum monoclonal protein for symptomatic WM is 4 g/dl and the κ:λ ratio is approximately 3:1.[4,7] In some patients the IgM may behave as cryoglobulin and has the ability to reversibly precipitate at low temperatures. For proper diagnosis, blood should be collected, and separated at 37°C before refrigeration. The precipitate should be redissolved and then undergo electrophoresis in order to determine the presence of monoclonal and/or polyclonal immunoglobulins.[50] In other patients the IgM may behave as a cold reactive antibody that displays progressively greater affinity for red cells as the temperature approaches 0°C. In such cases, the cold agglutinin titer, assessed at 40°C, is usu-

ally elevated. Most patients present with Bence Jones protein and this abnormality exceeded 500 mg/24 hour in 21 percent of patients.[45] Serum β-2 microglobulin is elevated in many patients.[7] Uninvolved immunoglobulins are depressed in most patients but their reduction is less severe than that in myeloma.[4,7] Cellular immunity appears to be preserved in most patients, although in some studies a decreased CD4:CD8 ratio, mainly from the reduction of CD4 T cells, was found.[7,51]

Hyperviscosity Syndrome

IgM proteins are large, asymmetric molecules that are 80 percent intravascular. Thus an increased concentration of these proteins results in an increased osmotic pressure and this causes an increase of plasma volume.[47,52,53] The circulation becomes slow and the hyperviscosity syndrome occurs. This syndrome occurs in one-third of patients with WM and is characterized by chronic bleeding from the nose, the gums, and less commonly, from the gastointestinal tract. Patients complain of headache, tinnitus, vertigo, impaired hearing, or ataxia. Ocular symptoms include blurring or loss of vision and fundoscopic examination may reveal distended, "sausage-shaped" retinal veins, flame-shaped hemorrhage, or papilledema. If plasma viscosity continues to rise, edema, high output heart failure, somnolence, stupor, and coma may occur.

Most patients develop symptoms when the relative serum or plasma viscosity is more than 4 centipoise (normal values: 1.4 to 1.8), but the symptomatic threshold varies from patient to patient. Virtually all patients with viscosity greater than 8 will have symptoms. Most patients with symptoms of hyperviscosity have a serum monoclonal IgM above 4 g/dl but it appears that interactions of the paraprotein with other plasma proteins and cells are more important for this process than the concentration of IgM.[2,4,5,54]

Neurological Abnormalities

Five to 20 percent of patients with WM present with or develop symptoms and signs suggestive of a peripheral polyneuropathy. This complication has been also described in individuals with monoclonal IgM but without evidence of overt lymphoma. IgM-related polyneuropathy is composed of an immunochemically and clinically heterogeneous group of neuropathies in which the monoclonal IgM appears to be an antibody against various glycoproteins or glycolipids of the peripheral nerve. In roughly one-half of these patients, the monoclonal protein (predominantly IgMk) is directed against carbohydrate epitopes of myelin-associated glycoprotein (MAG).[55,56] The anti-MAG IgM paraproteins coreact with a sulfoglucuronyl glycosphingolipid (SGPG), which is thought to be the most specific antigenic target.[57] MAG-reactive polyneuropathy is predominantly a demyelinating process and exhibits a chronic, slowly progressive course. Foot numbness, paresthesias, imbalance, and gait ataxia are the principal complaints, whereas pain is typically absent. Weakness of the distal leg muscles with variable atrophy occurs later in the course of the disease.[55,56,58,59] Direct immunofluorescence usually shows IgM deposits at the periphery of the myelin sheath and the sural nerve biopsy demonstrates a diminished number of myelinated axons.[60,61]

In the remaining one-half of patients, the peripheral neuropathy is MAG-nonreactive. In such patients, the IgM may react with various gangliosides, with GD1b or GM1 glycolipids, with sulfatides or chondroitin sulfate.[56,59,62,63] In about 30 percent of the patients, IgM does not recognize a known antigen. Patients with MAG-nonreactive polyneuropathies usually have a sensory neuropathy (demyelinating or axonal) but some patients may have a predominantly motor axonal neuropathy. Finally, WM patients may develop a peripheral neuropathy secondary to cryoglobulinemia or to amyloidosis.[64,65] Peripheral nerve dysfunction may also occur as a consequence of direct infiltration of the peripheral nerves by malignant cells.[66] An association of WM with POEMS syndrome has been described.[67]

The central nervous system is rarely involved in WM. The Bing-Neel syndrome, which was described in 1936, consists of headache, vertigo, impaired hearing, ataxia, nystagmus, diplopia, and eventually coma.[68] This syndrome is due to longstanding hyperviscosity that causes altered vascular permeability, permeation of the white matter by IgM, perivascular infiltration of lymphoplasmacytoid cells, and eventually multifocal leukoencephalopathy.[69] Infiltration of meninges and nerve roots by lymphoplasmacytic cells may cause rapidly progressive proximal leg weakness. This complication may respond to a combination of chemotherapy and radiotherapy.[70] Infiltration of the cerebral meninges, simulating meningioma, has been also reported.[71,72]

Bone Involvement

Lytic bone lesions are uncommon and are detected in less than 5 percent of patients with WM.[4,7,73] These patients have typical features of WM and should be treated as WM. A recent report of a patient with macroglobulinemia and osteolytic lesions, who underwent flow cytometric studies, indicated a "hybrid" phenotype with strong expression of CD38, CD20, FMC7 but lack of CD45 and DR.[74]

Amyloidosis

In a large series of patients from the Mayo Clinic, amyloidosis developed in 2 percent of patients with monoclonal IgM. Among those patients, 21 percent had WM. Organs more commonly affected by the amyloid deposition were the heart, the kidneys, the liver, and the lungs. Peripheral and/or autonomic neuropathy was evident at diagnosis in 38 percent of patients.[75] Amyloidosis should be suspected in patients with WM presenting with or developing autonomic neuropathy, albuminuria, heart failure, significant hepatomegaly, or unexplained respiratory symptoms.

Renal Involvement

In contrast to multiple myeloma, renal tubular abnormalities are rare in macroglobulinemia. However, glomerular abnor-malities are more frequently seen in macroglobulinemia than in multiple myeloma. Glomerular changes with large subendothelial deposits or thrombi have been described. Immunofluorescent studies have shown that these deposits contain exclusively IgM.[76] It is thought that these lesions are formed by the passive deposition of circulating IgM, partly as a result of increased serum viscosity. Such patients may present with uremia, dehydration, and nonselective proteinuria. This complication can be completely reversed with plasmapheresis.[77] The low incidence of hypercalcemia and the absence of significant Bence Jones proteinuria explain the rarity of renal tubular cast formation in patients with WM.[4,7] The presence of significant albuminuria is usually related to an underlying amyloid deposition.[75,78] Occasional patients, however, have developed nephritic or nephrotic syndrome because the IgM behaved as an antibody against the glomerular basement membrane and caused an immune-mediated glomerulonephritis.[79–81] Finally, in some patients, a direct infiltration of the kidneys by lymphoplasmacytic cells has caused renal or perirenal masses.[82]

Pulmonary Involvement

Three to five percent of patients with WM present with or develop lung disease. A review of 44 such patients with histologically proven lung involvement showed diffuse pulmonary infiltrates, isolated masses, or pleural effusion. Symptoms included dyspnea, nonproductive cough, and chest pain but some patients were asymptomatic. Endobronchial disease has also been described.[83,84]

Cutaneous Involvement

Monoclonal IgM gammopathy and sometimes overt WM, has been associated with urticarial skin lesions (Schnitzler syndrome).[85] Infiltration of the dermis with malignant cells has caused maculopapular lesions.[86] Firm, translucent, flesh-colored papules and nodules have occasionally been reported. Biopsy and immunohistochemistry have revealed intraepidermal deposits of IgM called *storage papules* without evidence of malignant infiltrate.[87] In one patient with this condition the circulating monoclonal IgM behaved as an antiepidermal basement membrane zone antibody.[88] Finally occasional patients have developed vesiculobullous eruptions consistent with paraneoplastic pemphigus or presented with a skin fragility similar to that seen in epidermolysis bullosa acquisita. Immunofluorescence detected circulating IgM autoantibodies reacting with the basement membrane zone.[89–91]

Involvement of the Gastrointestinal Tract

Involvement of the stomach and the bowel has been reported.[92–94] Occasional patients with macroglobulinemia have developed diarrhea with or without evidence of malabsorption.[94,95] In some of these patients there is deposition of an extracellular amorphous material in the lamina propria of the small intestine that stains positive for PAS but negative for amyloid and consists of monoclonal IgM.[96]

Eye Involvement

Ocular manifestations of WM typically result from the increased serum viscosity and are frequently confined to the retina. Orbital involvement can be caused by lesions involving the retro-orbital lymphoid tissue and lacrimal glands.[97] Infiltration of the conjuctiva and malignant vitreitis have been reported.[98,99]

Abnormalities of Coagulation

Patients with WM have an increased bleeding tendency that is primarily due to the increased serum viscosity. Hyperviscosity reduces blood flow and this causes hypoxia and vascular damage. Several patients have a prolonged bleeding time and decreased platelet adhesiveness.[100] The monoclonal IgM may interact with various clotting factors including fibrinogen, and factor V, VII, and VIII. Thus an increased bleeding tendency may occur. These abnormalities are reversible after the administration of systemic treatment or after plasmapheresis.[101]

Infectious Complications

Patients with WM have impaired humoral immunity due to the reduction of uninvolved immunoglobulins. Furthermore, some studies have indicated impaired cellular immunity, even at diagnosis, mainly from the reduction of CD4+ T cells.[7,51] Recent data suggest that monocyte function is constitutively abnormal in patients with macroglobulinemia and can be further inhibited by high monoclonal protein levels.[102] Thus patients with macroglobulinemia have an increased incidence for infections. This probability is increased when the immunosuppressive and myelosuppressive effects of chemotherapy are added.

TREATMENT

The Decision to Treat

Some patients with overt WM are diagnosed by chance during the investigation of mild anemia, elevated serum protein, or increased erythrocyte sedimentation rate but symptoms attributable to the disease are absent. Such patients with asymptomatic macroglobulinemia should be followed without any treatment until a complication of IgM, worsening anemia, weakness, fever, pruritus, or symptomatic organomegaly become evident. It should be emphasized that several patients with indolent WM have survived for years before initiation of treatment becomes necessary.[7,57]

Response Criteria

The assessment of disease response after systemic treatment has not been prospectively established in WM. Response criteria have been adapted from those used in evaluating patients with multiple myeloma and low-grade lymphoma. Partial response may be defined as a decrease by at least 50 percent of mono-clonal protein concentration in the serum and urine for at least 2 months with more than a 50 percent reduction of tumor infiltrate at all involved sites. Complete response requires the disappearance of the monoclonal protein by immunofixation, resolution of lymphadenopathy and hepatosplenomegaly, and less than 20 percent lymphocytes in the bone marrow.[7]

Plasmapheresis

In several patients symptoms may be due exclusively to hyperviscosity but significant anemia, lymphadenopathy, or splenomegaly are absent. Plasma exchange is an effective means of reducing rapidly the amount of circulating IgM and may be very valuable in patients with elevated serum viscosity causing symptoms.[103] Small reductions in the circulating monoclonal IgM with plasma exchange can dramatically reduce the viscosity and lead to resolution of symptoms.[54] Reduction of IgM by an average of 35 percent resulted in a decrease of plasma viscosity from 5 to 2.1.[104] In some patients a long-term plasmapheresis program has been used in order to delay the administration of cytotoxic treatment.[105] In most patients, however, concomitant institution of chemotherapy is indicated in order to suppress the underlying malignant process. Plasmapheresis has also been used as the primary method of treatment for some patients with predominant symptoms of peripheral polyneuropathy but without other complications of the underlying macroglobulinemia.[106,107]

Alkylating Agents

When cytotoxic therapy is indicated, the standard treatment has been the administration of oral alkylating agents. The agent most commonly used is chlorambucil. Chlorambucil has been administered either on a daily basis at low doses or intermittently at higher doses. At least 50 percent of patients achieve a partial response and patients' median survival is about 5 years.[2,108] The rate of decrease of IgM is slow and several months are required to determine the chemosensitivity of the disease. Kyle et al. randomized 46 patients with previously untreated WM to either chlorambucil 0.1 mg/kg daily continuously or to chlorambucil 0.3 mg/kg daily for 1 week every 6 weeks. The median survival was 5.4 years with no difference in the two regimens. Myelodysplasia or acute leukemia occurred in four patients (9 percent); all four patients were treated with intermittent chlorambucil.[45] There is no evidence that the addition of steroids to chlorambucil improves patients' survival but prednisone may be of benefit in patients with autoimmune hemolytic anemia, cryoglobulinemia, or cold-agglutinin disease.[7] Several Phase II studies have attempted to improve patients' outcome by administering combinations of alkylating agents with or without a vinca alkaloid, an anthracycline, or a nitrosourea. The M2 protocol (BCNU, cyclophosphamide, vincristine, melphalan, and prednisone) has been administered to 33 patients; 82 percent achieved an objective response and the median survival of the whole series was 4.2 years.[109] A combination of melphalan, cyclophosphamide, and prednisone was active in 68 percent of patients.[110] The combination of cyclophosphamide, doxorubicin, vincristine, and prednisone (CHOP) has been administered to a limited number of patients without improved outcome.[7] Although no prospective randomized trials have compared those more complicated regimens to standard chlorambucil, there is no obvious benefit from these combinations.

Nucleoside Analogues

The nucleoside analogues cladribine and fludarabine have been administered to previously untreated patients with WM. Cladribine has been administered either at a dose of 0.1 mg/kg/day for a 7-day continuous infusion or at a dose of 0.15 mg/kg by 2-hour intravenous infusion for 5 consecutive days at monthly intervals. Five series that included a total of 63 patients administered primary therapy with cladribine. Despite some differences in response criteria, 47 patients (75 percent) achieved at least a partial response.[111–115] Using only two courses of cladribine we have noted that the median time to a 50 percent reduction of IgM synthesis was only 1.2 months and even after cladribine was stopped, gradual reduction of abnormal protein was continued in all responding patients.[111] These studies provided limited follow-up data so that the impact of cladribine on patients' survival could not be determined. However, a preliminary report from the MD Anderson Cancer Center indicated that the 58 patients who were treated with cladribine-based regimens had a significantly higher response rate (75 percent) than that observed previously in 115 patients treated with alkylating agent–glucocorticoid programs (55 percent) ($p = .01$). The projected cause-specific median survival with cladribine was 6 years, approximately 1 year longer than that noted previously ($p = .13$).[116] Although primary treatment of WM with cladribine has not been prospectively compared with chlorambucil, because of its rapid cytoreduction, cladribine may be the treatment of choice when a rapid control of the disease is desirable because of hyperviscosity, pancytopenia, or severe peripheral neuropathy.

Fludarabine has also been administered to previously untreated patients with WM. An Intergroup study of the Southwest Oncology Group and the Eastern Cooperative Oncology Group included patients who were treated with fludarabine 30 mg/m[2] iv daily for 5 consecutive days every 4 weeks. At least 50 percent reduction of tumor mass was noted in 33 percent of patients and the median progression-free survival was 42 months.[117] In this study, the response rate obtained with fludarabine appeared inferior to that obtained with either cladribine or chlorambucil. However, a smaller European multicenter Phase II study was recently published that included 20 previously untreated patients with WM who received fludarabine 25 mg/m[2] iv daily for 5 consecutive days every 4 weeks. Objective response was noted in 79 percent of patients and the median time to disease progression was 40 months.[118]

The major adverse effects of cladribine and fludarabine are myelosuppression and immunosuppression. The myelosuppression is usually moderate but with repetitive courses of these agents there is evidence of cumulative and protracted myelotoxicity. Furthermore, the profound and sustained reduction of monocytes and of CD4+ and CD8+ lymphocytes increases substantially the risk for opportunistic infections.[119] Administration of a limited course of nucleoside analogues may be associated with less myelosuppression and immunosuppression without reducing the chance for response.[111]

Fludarabine was the first nucleoside analogue to induce responses in about one-third of patients who had been resistant to previous treatments.[120] These results were subsequently confirmed by other studies.[117,121–123] The recommended dose of fludarabine is 25 to 30 mg/m[2] iv daily for 5 days every 4 weeks. Data on 109 patients from three published series demonstrated an objective response in 31 percent of patients.[121–123] In the largest series published to date, which included primarily patients treated with fludarabine during a refractory relapse phase of their disease, 21 of 71 patients (30 percent) achieved a partial response. Patients' median survival was 23 months; anemia and thrombocytopenia correlated with shorter survival.[123] The preliminary data of the Intergroup trial indicated that 33 percent of patients responded, the median progression-free survival was 27 months, and the median overall survival was 37 months.[117]

Cladribine has also shown activity in previously treated patients with WM.[124] Among 112 patients from five series, 53 patients (47 percent) achieved an objective response.[113–115,125,126] Thus, both fludarabine and cladribine provide an opportunity for response in pretreated patients with macroglobulinemia. The status of the disease at the time of salvage treatment with a nucleoside analogue may be an important factor that predicts the likelihood and durability of the response. An analysis of 46 pretreated patients who received cladribine therapy indicated that patients more likely to benefit are those relapsing from an unmaintained remission and those with primary refractory disease. The response rates for these two groups of patients were 78 and 44 percent, respectively.[125] The duration of primary resistance was also an important parameter. Fifty-seven percent of patients with primary resistance of less than 1 year duration responded to cladribine in contrast to 17 percent of patients with longer duration or primary resistance. Patients who were treated while their disease was relapsing despite salvage therapy (refractory relapse) had a significantly lower response rate (21 percent) and a median survival of 13 months. The median progression-free survival of all responding patients is about 12 months.[125] Prior resistance to fludarabine is also associated with cross-resistance to cladribine. While three of four patients who had previously responded to fludarabine and were relapsing from unmaintained remission achieved a partial response with cladribine, only one of ten patients with disease refractory to fludarabine responded to cladribine.[127]

All the previous data have been accumulated from Phase II studies. The results of a multicenter randomized trial comparing the efficacy of cyclophosphamide, doxorubicin, and prednisone (CAP) to that of fludarabine in 92 patients with WM resistant to first-line therapy (42 patients) or in first relapse (50 patients), were recently reported.[128] A partial response occurred in 11 percent of patients treated with CAP and in 28 percent of patients treated with fludarabine ($p = .019$). The median time to progression of the responding patients and the time to treat-

ment failure for all patients were statistically longer for the fludarabine group. The median survival times of the two arms
were similar and this may be explained by the fact that patients
resistant to one regimen were allowed to cross over to the other
regimen.[128] Thus, both Phase II and Phase III trials indicate that
treatment with a nucleoside analogue may benefit about one-
third of patients with pretreated macroglobulinemia.

Interferons

Interferon-gamma induced a partial response in two of five
patients with WM.[129] Interferon-alpha has been administered
at low doses to some patients with WM. Approximately one-
third of patients have achieved an objective response.[130,131] This
limited experience suggests that interferon-alpha may have a
role in the treatment of WM and prospective studies are needed
to assess its role as a remission maintenance treatment.

High-Dose Therapy

High-dose therapy with autologous bone marrow or blood support is effective in many patients with low-grade lymphoma
and multiple myeloma. Some patients with WM have been
treated with high-dose therapy. Two small series have been published and both have reported an objective response in all
treated patients.[132,133] This preliminary experience suggests that
high-dose therapy can be effective even in patients with resistance to conventional chemotherapy, and needs further investigation in younger patients who present with adverse prognostic
features.

Splenectomy

Some patients with WM resistant to chemotherapy and with
clinically significant splenomegaly have been treated with
splenectomy. This treatment resulted not only in an improvement of cytopenia but also in a major decrease of serum
IgM.[134,135] The role of splenectomy in the management of
macroglobulinemia requires prospective evaluation in the context of a clinical trial.

Monoclonal Antibody Therapy

Rituximab, a chimeric anti-CD20 monoclonal antibody, can
induce objective responses in several patients with previously
treated or untreated low-grade lymphoma. Because the CD20
antigen is expressed on the WM cells, rituximab has been
administered to some patients with this disease. Four weekly
administrations of rituximab at a dose of 375 mg/m^2 iv have
been associated with partial response.[136–138] The time to
response was usually short (approximately 2 months) and the
median time to disease progression was approximately 9
months. A retrospective multicenter study that included 28
patients confirmed activity of rituximab in 28 percent of
patients.[139] Combination of rituximab with chemotherapy may
improve the results of either modality.[138]

Other Treatments

Al-Katib et al. have established a permanent WM cell line, WSV-
WM, which grows as a xenograft in severe combined immune
deficient mice.[140] Using this model they have observed that
bryostatin and auristatin PE were associated with tumor growth
inhibition and tumor cell kill.[141,142] Preliminary evidence suggests that thalidomide may be active in some patients with
macroglobulinemia.[143]

PROGNOSIS AND OUTCOME

In most series the median survival of patients with macroglobulinemia is 5 years. However at least 20 percent of patients survive for more than 10 years and up to one-fifth of patients die
of unrelated causes. In view of the rarity of this disease, relatively few studies have defined prognostic factors. Bartl et al.
reported that the type of bone marrow involvement was of
importance.[28] However, these results were not confirmed by
Andriko et al.[144] In another series, the only parameter predictive for survival was patients' age: the median survival for
patients over 60 years of age was 4 years whereas the median
survival for patients younger than 50 years was 13 years.[7] A retrospective study from a single institution indicated that three
prognostic factors were associated with inferior survival:
advanced age, elevated serum lactate dehydrogenase (LDH),
and presence of lymphadenopathy.[145]

Three large recent studies have performed a multivariate
analysis of prognostic factors in patients with macroglobulinemia. Facon et al. reported that male gender, age older than 60
years, hemoglobin less than than 10 g/dl, and neutrophils less
than 1.7×10^9/L were adverse prognostic factors for survival.[3] A
similar multivariate analysis from Gobbi et al. indicated that age
older than 70 years, hemoglobin less than 9 g/dl, presence of
weight loss, and cryoglobulinemia were associated with shorter
survival.[44] Based on these parameters, the patient population
could be divided into a favorable group with none or only one
negative parameter and an unfavorable group with two or more
negative parameters.[44] A scoring system for WM was described,
based on age (1 point for age ≥65 years, 0 for age <65 years),
albumin (1 for <40 g/dl, 0 for ≥40 g/dl) and the total number of
cytopenias (0 for no cytopenia, 1 for one cytopenia, and 2 for
three cytopenias). The total score (0 to 4) was able to separate
patients in three groups with low (score 0 or 1), intermediate
(score 2), or high (score 3 or 4) risk, which included 27, 27, and
46 percent of patients with a 5-year survival at 86, 61, and 26
percent, respectively.[146]

More recently, Dhodapkar et al.[147] performed a prognostic
factor analysis on 179 patients who were prospectively enrolled
in the Phase II Intergroup trial of fludarabine in WM. Most
patients had not received prior therapy but approximately one-
third of patients were previously treated. A multivariate analysis indicated that low levels of serum β-2 microglobulin (<4
g/L) and high levels of serum IgM (≥4 g/dl) were favorable
prognostic factors for both progression-free survival (PFS) and
overall survival (OS). They defined three risk groups. The low-
risk group was defined by a serum β-2 microglobulin less than

4 g/L, included 67 percent of the total patient population, and had a median PFS of 61 months while the median OS was not reached at the time of the analysis. The intermediate-risk group was defined by a serum β-2 microglobulin less than 4 g/L and serum IgM greater than or equal to 4 g/dL, included 20 percent of the patients, and had a median PFS of 31 months and an overall survival of 42 months. The high-risk group was defined by a serum β-2 microglobulin greater than or equal to 4 g/dl and serum IgM less than 4 g/dl, included 13 percent of the patients and had a median PFS of 7 months and a median OS of 26 months.[147]

Most patients with WM die of progressive disease that has become refractory to treatment. In advanced phases of the disease many patients suffer from the complications of pancytopenia, which is usually due to the heavily infiltrated bone marrow. However, in some patients the cytopenias may be due to the development of myelodysplastic syndrome or acute myeloid leukemia associated with the use of alkylating agents.[148–150] In approximately 5 percent of patients the disease may transform into a diffuse large cell lymphoma (Richter syndrome) characterized by the development of fever, weight loss, rapidly enlarging lymph nodes, extranodal involvement, and reduction of monoclonal protein synthesis. The outcome of these patients is poor.[145,148,151,152]

REFERENCES

1. Waldenstrom J: Incipient myelomatosis or "essential" hyperglobulinemia with fibrinogenopenia—A new syndrome? Acta Med Scand 117:216, 1944.
2. Mackenzie MR, Fudenberg HH: Macroglobulinemia: An analysis of forty patients. Blood 39:874, 1972.
3. Facon T, Brouillard M, Duhamel A et al: Prognostic factors in Waldenstrom's macroglobulinemia: A report of 167 cases. J Clin Oncol 11:1553, 1993.
4. Kyle RA, Garton JP: The spectrum of IgM monoclonal gammopathy in 430. cases. Mayo Clin Proc 62:719, 1987.
5. Krajny M, Pruzanski W: Waldenstrom's macroglobulinemia: Review of 45 cases. Can Med Assoc J 114:899, 1976.
6. Waldenstrom JG: Benign monoclonal gammopathy. Acta Med Scand 216:435, 1984.
7. Dimopoulos MA, Alexanian R: Waldenstrom's macroglobulinemia. Blood 831:1452, 1994.
8. Waldenstrom JG: Macroglobulinemia: A review. Haematologica 71:437, 1986.
9. Dimopoulos MA, Panayiotidis P, Moulopoulos LA et al: Waldenstrom's macroglobulinemia: Clinical features, complications and management. J Clin Oncol 18:214, 2000.
10. Herrinton LJ, Weiss NS: Incidence of Waldenstrom's macroglobulinemia. Blood 82:3148, 1993.
11. Groves FD, Travis LB, Devesa SS et al: Waldenstrom's macroglobulinemia: Incidence patterns in the United States, 1988–1994. Cancer 82:1078, 1998.
12. Massari R, Fine JM, Metais R: Waldenstrom's macroglobulinemia observed in two brothers. Nature 196:176, 1962.
13. Seligmann M: A genetic predisposition to Waldenstrom's macroglobulinaemia. Acta Med Scand 445:10, 1966.
14. Bjornsson OG, Arnason A, Gudmundsson S et al: Macroglobulinaemia in an Icelandic family. Acta Med Scand 203:283, 1978.
15. Fine JM, Mullier JY, Rochu D: Waldenstrom's macroglobulinemia in monozygotic twins. Acta Med Scand 220:369, 1986.
16. Renier G, Ifrah N, Chevalier A et al: Four brothers with Waldenstrom's macroglobulinemia. Cancer 64:1554, 1989.
17. Ogmundosdottir HM, Jahanneson GM, Sveinsdottir S et al: Familial macroglobulinemia: Hyperactive B-cells but normal natural killer function. Scand J Immunol 40:195, 1994.
18. Seligmann M, Danon F, Mihaesco C: Immunoglobulin abnormalities in families of patients with Waldenstrom's macroglobulinemia. Acta Haematol 47:33, 1972.
19. Kassan SS, Thomas TL, Moutsopoulos HM et al: Increased risk of lymphoma in sicca syndrome. Ann Intern Med 89:888, 1978.
20. Dellagi K, Brouet JC, Perreau J et al: Human monoclonal IgM with autoantibody activity against intermediate filaments. Proc Natl Acad Sci U S A 79:446, 1982.
21. James JM, Brouet JC, Orvoenfrija E et al: Waldenstrom's macroglobulinaemia in a bird breeder. Clin Exp Immunol 68:397, 1997.
22. Williamson LM, Greaves M, Waters JR et al: Waldenstrom's macroglobulinemia: Three cases in shoe repairers. BMJ 298:498, 1989.
23. Travis LB, Li CY, Zhang ZN et al: Hematopoietic malignancies and related disorders among benzene-exposed workers in China. Leuk Lymphoma 14:91, 1994.
24. Linet MS, Humphrey RL, Mehl ES et al: A case-control and family study of Waldenstrom's macroglobulinemia. Leukemia 7:1363, 1993.
25. Ahmed S, Shurafa MS, Bishop CR et al: Waldenstrom's macroglobulinemia in young African-American adults. Am J Hematol 60:229, 1999.
26. Harris NL, Jaffe ES, Stein H et al: A revised European-American classification of lymphoid neoplasms: A proposal from the International Lymphoma Study Group. Blood 84:1361, 1994.
27. Dutcher TF, Fahey JL: The histopathology of macroglobulinemia of Waldenstrom. J Natl Cancer Inst 22:887, 1959.
28. Bartl R, Frisch B, Mahl G et al: Bone marrow histology in Waldenstrom's macroglobulinemia. Clinical relevance of subtype recognition. Scand J Haematol 31:359, 1983.
29. Scheidel D, Peest D, Stunkel K et al: Idiotype bearing peripheral blood lymphocytes in human multiple myeloma and Waldenstrom's macroglobulinemia. Scand J Immunol 11:437, 1980.
30. Preud'homme JL, Seligmann M: Immunoglobulins on the surface of lymphoid cells in Waldenstrom's macroglobulinemia. J Clin Invest 51:701, 1972.
31. Petterson D, Mellstedt H, Holon G: Characterization of the monoclonal blood and bone marrow B lymphocytes in Waldenstrom's macroglobulinemia. Scand J Immunol 11:593, 1980.
32. Kucharska-Pulczynska M, Ellegard J, Hokland P: Analysis of leucocyte differentiation antigens in blood and bone marrow from patients with Waldenstrom's macroglobulinemia. Br J Haematol 65:395, 1987.
33. Feiner HD, Rizk CC, Finfer MD et al: IgM monoclonal gammopathy/Waldenstrom's macroglobulinemia: A morphological and immunophenotypic study of the bone marrow. Mod Pathol 3:348, 1990.
34. Jensen GS, Andrews EJ, Mant MJ et al: Transitions in CD45 isoform expression indicate continuous differentiation of a monoclonal CD5+CD11b+ B lineage in Waldenstrom's macroglobulinemia. Am J Hematol 37:20, 1991.
35. Owen RG, Parapia LA, Higginson J et al: Clinicopathological correlates of IgM paraproteinemias. Clin Lymph 1:39, 2000.
36. Louviaux I, Michau L, Hagemeijer A et al: Cytogenetic abnormalities in Waldenstrom's disease: A single center study of 45 cases. Blood 92(Suppl. 1):184b, 1998 (Abstract 3776).

37. Lida S, Rao PH, Nallasivarn P et al: The t(9;14)(p13;q32) chromosomal translocation associated with lymphoplasmacytoid lymphoma involves the PAX-5 gene. Blood 88:4110, 1996.

38. Shaw GR, Kronberger DL: TP53 deletions but not trisomy 12 are adverse in B-cell lymphoproliferative disorders. Cancer Genet Cytogenet 119:146, 2000.

39. Said JW, Retting MR, Heppner K et al: Localization of Kaposi's sarcoma-associated herpesvirus in bone marrow samples from patients with multiple myeloma. Blood 20:4278, 1997.

40. Rettig M, Vescio R, Ma H et al: Detection of Kaposi's sarcoma associated herpesvirus in the dendritic cells of Waldenstrom's macroglobulinemia and primary amyloidosis patients. Blood 90(Suppl. 1): 86a, 1997 (Abstract 374).

41. Agbalika F, Mariette X, Pierre Matolleau JP et al: Detection of human herpesvirus-8 DNA in bone marrow biopsies from patients with multiple myeloma and Waldenstrom's macroglobulinemia. Blood 91:4393, 1998.

42. Brousset P, Theriault C, Roda D et al: Kaposi's sarcoma-associated herpesvirus (KSHV) in bone marrow biopsies of patients with Waldenstrom's macroglobulinemia. Br J Haematol 102:795, 1998.

43. Stone SA, Lennette ET, Newman JT et al: Serologic prevalence of antibody to human herpesvirus type 8 in patients with various monoclonal gammopathies. Leuk Lymphoma 37:197, 2000.

44. Gobbi P, Bettini R, Montecucco C et al: Study of prognosis in Waldenstrom's macroglobulinemia: A proposal for a simple binary classification with clinical and investigational utility. Blood 83:2939, 1994.

45. Kyle RA, Greipp P, Gertz M et al: Waldenstrom's macroglobulinemia: A prospective study comparing daily versus intermittent oral chlorambucil. Br J Haematol 108:737, 2000.

46. Moulopoulos LA, Dimopoulos MA, Varma DG et al: Waldenstrom macroglobulinemia: MR imaging of the spine and computed tomography of the abdomen and pelvis. Radiology 188:669, 1993.

47. Alexanian R: Blood volume in monoclonal gammopathy. Blood 49:301, 1977.

48. Pruzanski W, Shumak H: Biologic activity of cold reactive autoantibodies. N Engl J Med 297:538, 1977.

49. Rose WF, Adams J, Logue G: Hemolysis by complement and cold reactive antibody. Am J Hematol 2:259, 1977.

50. Brouet JC, Clauvel JP, Danon F et al: Biologic and clinical significance of cryoglobulins. Am J Med 57:775, 1974.

51. San Miguel JF, Caballero MD, Gonzales M: T-cell subpopulations in patients with monoclonal gammopathies. Am J Hematol 20:267, 1985.

52. Crawford J, Cox EB, Cohen HJ: Evaluation of hyperviscosity in monoclonal gammopathies. Am J Med 79:13, 1985.

53. MacKenzie MR, Lee TK: Blood viscosity in Waldenstrom macroglobulinemia. Blood 49:507, 1977.

54. Gertz MA, Kyle RA: Hyperviscosity syndrome. J Intens Care Med 10:128, 1995.

55. Dalakas MC, Engle WK: Polyneuropathy with monoclonal gammopathy. Ann Neurol 10:45, 1981.

56. Latov N, Braun PE, Gross RB et al: Plasma cell dyscrasia and peripheral neuropathy: Identification of the myelin antigens that react with human paraproteins. Proc Natl Acad Sci U S A 78:7139, 1981.

57. Ilyas AA, Dalakas MC, Brady RO et al: Sulfated glucuronyl glycolipids reacting with anti-myelin associated glycoprotein monoclonal antibodies including IgM paraproteins in neuropathy species distribution and partial characterization of epitopes. Brain 385:1, 1986.

58. Dellagi K, Dupouey P, Brouet JC et al: Waldenstrom's macroglobulinemia and peripheral neuropathy: A clinical and immunologic study of 25 patients. Blood 62:280, 1983.

59. Nobile-Orazio E, Marmireli P, Baldini L et al: Peripheral neuropathy in macroglobulinemia. Neurology 37:1506, 1987.

60. Mendell JR, Sahhenk Z, Whitaker JN et al: Polyneuropathy and monoclonal gammopathy: Studies on the pathogenetic role of anti-myelin-associated glycoprotein antibody. Ann Neurol 17:243, 1985.

61. Vital A, Vital C, Julien J et al: Polyneuropathy associated with IgM monoclonal gammopathy. Immunological and pathological study in 31 patients. Acta Neuropathol (Berl) 79:160, 1989.

62. Ilyas AA, Li SC, Chou DKH et al: Gangliosides GM2, IV4GAL NaC GM1b and IV4GaL NaC GD1a as antigens for monoclonal immunoglobulin M neuropathy associated with gammopathy. J Biol Chem 263:439, 1988.

63. Nobile-Orazio E, Manfredini E, Carpo M et al: Frequency and clinical correlates of anti-neuronal IgM antibodies in neuropathy associated with IgM monoclonal gammopathy. Ann Neurol 36:416, 1994.

64. Garsia-Bragado F, Fernandez JM, Navarro C et al: Peripheral neuropathy in essential mixed cryoglobulinemia. Arch Neurol 45:1210, 1988.

65. Ropper AH, Gorson KC: Neuropathies associated with paraproteinemia. N Engl J Med 338:1601, 1998.

66. Ince PG, Shaw PJ, Fawsett PR et al: Demyelinating neuropathy due to primary IgM kappa B-cell lymphoma of peripheral nerves. Neurology 37:1231, 1987.

67. Pavord SR, Murphy PT, Mitchell VE: POEMS syndrome and Waldenstrom's macroglobulinemia. J Clin Pathol 49:181, 1996.

68. Bing J, Neel AV: Two cases of hyperglobulinaemia with affection of central nervous system on toxi-infectious basis. Acta Med Scand 88:492, 1936.

69. Scheithauer BW, Rubinstein LJ, Herman MM: Leucoencephalopathy in Waldenstrom's macroglobulinemia. J Neuropathol Exp Neurol 43:408, 1984.

70. Abad S, Zagdanski AM, Brechignac S et al: Neurolymphomatosis in Waldenstrom's macroglobulinemia. Br J Haematol 106:100, 1999.

71. Civit T, Coulbois S, Baylac F et al: Waldenstrom's macroglobulinemia and cerebral lymphoplasmocytic proliferation. Neurochirurgie 43:245, 1997.

72. Richards AI: Response of meningeal Waldenstrom's macroglobulinemia to 2-chlorodeoxyadenosine. J Clin Oncol 13:2476, 1995.

73. Leb L, Grimes E, Balogh K et al: Monoclonal macroglobulinemia with osteolytic lesions. Cancer 39:227, 1977.

74. Haghighi B, Yanagihara R, Cornbleet PJ: IgM myeloma: Case report with immunophenotypic profile. Am J Hematol 59:302, 1998.

75. Gertz MA, Kyle RA, Noel P: Primary systemic amyloidosis: A rare complication of immunoglobulin M monoclonal gammopathies and Waldenstrom's macroglobulinemia. J Clin Oncol 11:914, 1993.

76. Morel L, Basch A, Danon F et al: Pathology of the kidney in Waldenstrom's macroglobulinemia. N Engl J Med 283:123, 1970.

77. Fudenberg HH, Virella G: Multiple myeloma and Waldenstrom's macroglobulinemia: Unusual presentations. Sem Hematol 17:63, 1980.

78. Soetekouw R, Bruijn JA, Hogewind BL et al: A 66-year-old woman with nephrotic syndrome and an IgM monoclonal gammopathy. Ann Hematol 76:227, 1998.

79. Lindstrom FD, Hed J, Enestrom S: Renal pathology of Waldenstrom's macroglobulinemia with monoclonal and glomerular antibodies and nephrotic syndrome. Clin Exp Immunol 41:196, 1980.

80. Meyrier A, Simon P, Mignon F et al: Rapidly progressive glomerulonephritis and monoclonal gammopathies. Nephron 38:156, 1984.

81. Muso E, Tamura I, Yashiro M et al: Waldenstrom's macroglobulinemia associated with amyloidosis and membranous nephropathy. Jpn J Nephrol 35:61, 1993.

82. Moore DF, Moulopoulos LA, Dimopoulos MA: Waldenstrom's macroglobulinemia presenting as renal or perirenal mass: Clinical and radiographic features. Leuk Lymphoma 14:331, 1995.

83. Rausch RG, Herion JC: Pulmonary manifestations of Waldenstrom's macroglobulinemia. Am J Haematol 9:201, 1980.

84. Fadil A, Taylor DE: The lung and Waldenstrom's macroglobulinemia. South Med J 91:681, 1998.

85. Schnitzler L, Schubert B, Boasson M et al: Urticaire chronique, lesions osseuses, macroglobulinemie IgM: Maladie de Waldenstrom? Bull Soc Fr Derm Syph 81:363, 1974.

86. Bergroth V, Reitamo S, Konttinen YT et al: Skin lesions in Waldenstrom's macroglobulinemia. Acta Med Scand 209:129, 1981.

87. Hanke CW, Steck WD, Bergfeld WF et al: Cutaneous macroglobulinosis. Arch Dermatol 116:575, 1980.

88. Cobb MW, Domloge-Hutch N, Frame JN et al: Waldenstrom macroglobulinemia with an IgM-K antiepidermal basement membrane zone antibody. Arch Dermatol 128:372, 1992.

89. Becker LR, Bastian BC, Wesselmann U et al: Paraneoplastic pemphigus treated with dexamethasone/cyclophosphamide pulse therapy. Eur J Dermatol 8:551, 1998.

90. West NY, Fitzpatrick JE, David-Bafar KM et al: Waldenstrom macroglobulinemia-induced bullous dermatosis. Arch Dermatol 134:1127, 1998.

91. Morita E, Horiuchi K, Yamamoto S et al: A case of acquired autoimmune bullous disease associated with IgM macroglobulinaemia. J Dermatol 26:671, 1999.

92. Rosenthal JA, Curran WJ, Schuster SJ: Waldenstrom's macroglobulinemia resulting from localized gastric lymphoplasmacytoid lymphoma. Am J Hematol 58:244, 1998.

93. Veloso FT, Fraga J, Saleifo JV: Macroglobulinemia and small intestinal disease. A case report with review of the literature. J Clin Gastroenterol 10:546, 1988.

94. Yasui O, Tukamoto F, Sasaki N et al: Malignant lymphoma of the transverse colon associated with macroglobulinemia. Am J Gastroenterol 92:2299, 1997.

95. Tait RC, Oagarah PK, Houghton JB et al: Waldenstrom's macroglobulinemia secreting a paraprotein with lupus anticoagulant activity: Possible association with gastrointestinal tract disease and malabsorption. Clin Pathol 46:678, 1993.

96. Pruzanski W, Warren RE, Goldie JH et al: Malabsorption syndrome with infiltration of the intestinal wall by extracellular monoclonal macroglobulin. Am J Med 58:811, 1973.

97. Krishnan K, Adams PT: Bilateral orbital tumors and lacrimal gland involvement in Waldenstrom's macroglobulinemia. Eur J Haematol 55:205, 1995.

98. Klapper SR, Jordan DR, Pelletier C et al: Ptosis in Waldenstrom's macroglobulinemia. Am J Ophthalmol 126:315, 1998.

99. Knox CM, Wong IG, Howes EL et al: Vitreitis and Waldenstrom's macroglobulinemia. Am J Ophthalmol 126:314, 1998.

100. Perkins HA, McKenzie MR, Fudenberg HH: Hemostatic defects in dysproteinemias. Blood 35:695, 1970.

101. Farhangi M, Merlini G: The clinical implications of monoclonal immunoglobulins. Semin Oncol 13:366, 1986.

102. Mainwaring CJ, Williams MA, Singer CR et al: Monocyte dysfunction in patients with multiple myeloma and lymphoplasmacytic disorders is related to serum paraprotein levels. Br J Haematol 105:948, 1999.

103. Schwab PJ, Fahey JL: Treatment of Waldenstrom's macroglobulinemia by plasmapheresis. N Engl J Med 263:574, 1960.

104. Reinhart WH, Lutolf O, Nydegger UR et al: Plasmapheresis for hyperviscosity syndrome in macroglobulinemia Waldenstrom and multiple myeloma. J Lab Clin Med. 119:69, 1992.

105. Buskard NA, Galton DAG, Goldman JM et al: Plasma exchange in the long-term treatment of Waldenstrom's macroglobulinemia. Can Med Assoc J 117:135, 1977.

106. Dalakas MC, Flaum MA, Rick M et al: Treatment of polyneuropathy in Waldenstrom's macroglobulinemia. Role of paraproteinemia and immunological studies. Neurology 33:1406, 1983.

107. Haas DC, Tatum AH: Plasmapheresis alleviates neuropathy accompanying IgM anti-myelin-associated glycoprotein paraproteinemia. Ann Neurol 23:394, 1988.

108. McCallister BD, Bayrd ED, Harrison EG et al: Primary macroglobulinemia. Am J Med 43:394, 1967.

109. Case DC, Ervin TJ, Boyd MA: Long term results and disease characteristics of patients with Waldenstrom's macroglobulinemia treated with the M-2 protocol. Blood 82(Suppl. 1):561a, 1993 (Abstract 2230).

110. Petrucci MT, Avvisati G, Tribalto et al: Waldenstrom's macroglobulinemia: Results of a combined oral treatment in 34 newly diagnosed patients. J Intern Med 226:443, 1989.

111. Dimopoulos MA, Kantarjian H, Weber D et al: Primary therapy of Waldenstrom's macroglobulinemia with 2-chlorodeoxyadenosine. J Clin Oncol 12:2694, 1994.

112. Fridrik MA, Jager G, Baldinger C et al: First-line treatment of Waldenstrom's disease with cladribine. Ann Hematol 74:7, 1997.

113. Hellmann A, Lewandowski K, Zancha JM et al: Treatment of Waldenstrom's macroglobulinemia with 2-chlorodeoxyadenosine. Eur J Haematol 63:35, 1999.

114. Liu F, Burian C, Miller W et al: Bolus administration of cladribine in the treatment of Waldenstrom's macroglobulinemia. Br J Haematol 103:690, 1998.

115. Delannoy A, Van Den Neste E, Michaux JL et al: Cladribine for Waldenstrom's macroglobulinemia. Br J Haemaol 104:933, 1999.

116. Weber D, Delasalle K, Gavino M et al: Primary treatment of Waldenstrom's macroglobulinemia with subcutaneous 2-chlorodeoxyadenosine and oral cyclophosphamide. Blood 90(Suppl. 1): 357a, 1997 (Abstract 1592).

117. Dhodapkar M, Jacobson J, Gertz M et al: Phase II intergroup trial of fludarabine in Waldenstrom's macroglobulinemia: Results of Southwest Oncology Group trial in 220 patients. Blood 90(Suppl. 1):577a, 1997 (Abstract 2571).

118. Foran JM, Rohatiner AZ, Coiffier B et al: Multicenter phase II study of fludarabine phosphate for patients with newly diagnosed lymphoplasmacytoid lymphoma, Waldenstrom's macroglobulinemia, and mantle-cell lymphoma. J Clin Oncol 17:546, 1999.

119. Van Den Neste E, Delannoy A, Vanderscan B et al. Infectious complications after 2-chlorodeoxyadenosine therapy. Eur J Haematol 56:235, 1996.

120. Kantarjian HM, Alexanian R, Koller CA et al: Fludarabine therapy in macroglobulinemic lymphoma. Blood 75:1928, 1990.

121. Dimopoulos MA, O'Brien S, Kantarjian H et al: Fludarabine therapy in Waldenstrom's macroglobulinemia. Am J Med 95:49, 1993.

122. Zinzani PL, Gherlinzoni F, Bendandi M et al: Fludarabine treatment in resistant Waldenstrom's macroglobulinemia. Eur J Haematol 54:120, 199.

123. Leblond V, Ben-Othman T, Deconinck E et al: Activity of fludarabine in previously treated Waldenstrom's macroglobulinemia: A report of 71 cases. Group Cooperatif Macroglobulinemie. J Clin Oncol 16:2060, 1998.

124. Dimopoulos MA, Kantarjian HM, Estey EH et al: Treatment of Waldenstrom's macroglobulinemia with 2-chlorodeoxyadenosine. Ann Intern Med 118:195, 1993.

125. Dimopoulos MA, Weber D, Delasalle KB et al: Treatment of Waldenstrom's macroglobulinemia resistant to standard therapy with 2-chlorodeoxyadenosine: Identification of prognostic factors. Ann Oncol 6:49, 1995.

126. Betticher DC, Schmitz SF, Ratschiller D et al: Cladribine (2-CDA) given as subcutaneous bolus injection is active in pretreated Waldenstrom's macroglobulinaemia. Swiss Group for Clinical Cancer Research. Br J Haematol 99:358, 1997.

127. Dimopoulos MA, Weber DM, Kantarjian H et al: 2-chlorodeoxyadenosine therapy of patients with Waldenstrom macroglobulinemia previously treated with fludarabine. Ann Oncol 5:288, 1994.

128. Leblond V, Levy V, Cazin B et al: Results of multicentric randomized study comparing the efficacy of fludarabine to that of cyclophosphamide, doxorubicin, prednisone in patients in first relapse or primary refractory disease with Waldenstrom's macroglobulinemia. Blood 98:2640,2001.

129. Quesada JR, Alexanian R, Kurzrock R et al: Recombinant interferon gamma in hairy cell leukemia, multiple myeloma, and Waldenstrom's macroglobulinemia. Am J Hematol 29:1, 1988.

130. Rotoli B, De Renzo A, Frigeri F et al: A phase II trial on alpha-interferon effect in patients with monoclonal IgM gammapathy. Leuk Lymphoma 13:463, 1994.

131. Legouffe E, Rossi JF, Laporte JP et al: Treatment of Waldenstrom's macroglobulinemia with very low doses of alpha interferon. Leuk Lymphoma 19:337, 1995.

132. Desikan R, Dhodapkar M, Siegel D et al: High dose therapy with autologous haemopoietic stem cell support for Waldenstrom's macroglobulinemia. Br J Haematol 105:993, 1999.

133. Dreger P, Glass B, Kuse R et al: Myeloablative radiochemotherapy followed by reinfusion of purged autologous stem cells for Waldenstrom's macroglobulinemia. Br J Haematol 106:115, 1999.

134. Humphrey JS, Lockard C: Durable complete remission of macroglobulinemia after splenectomy. Am J Hematol 48:262, 1995.

135. Takemori N, Hira K, Onodera R et al: Durable remission after splenectomy for Waldenstrom's macroglobulinemia with massive splenomegaly in leukemic phase. Leuk Lymphoma 26:387, 1997.

136. Byrd JC, White CA, Link B et al: Rituximab therapy in Waldenstrom's macroglobulinemia: Preliminary evidence of clinical activity. Ann Oncol 10:1525, 1999.

137. Foran JM, Rohatiner AZ, Cunningham D et al: European phase II study of rituximab for patients with newly diagnosed mantle-cell lymphoma and previously treated mantle-cell lymphoma, immunocytoma and small B-cell lymphocytic lymphoma J Clin Oncol 18:317, 2000.

138. Weber DM, Garino M, Huh Y et al: Phenotypic and clinical evidence supports rituximab for Waldenstrom's macroglobulinemia. Blood 94(Suppl. 1):125a, 1999 (Abstract 551).

139. Treon SP, Agus DB, Link B et al: Rituximab is an active agent in Waldenstrom's macroglobulinemia Proc Am Soc Clin Oncol 19:6a, 2000 (Abstract 13).

140. Al-Katib A, Mohammad R, Hamdam M et al: Propagation of Waldenstrom's macroglobulinemia cells in vitro and in severe combined immune deficient mice: Utility as a preclinical drug screening model. Blood 81:3034, 1993.

141. Mohammad RM, Al-Katib A, Pettit GR et al: Successful treatment of human Waldenstrom's macroglobulinemia with combination of biological and chemotherapy agents. Cancer Res 54:165, 1994.

142. Mohammad RM, Limvarapuss C, Wall NR: A new tubulin polymerization inhibitor, auristatin PE, induces tumor regression in a human Waldenstrom's macroglobulinemia xenograft model. Int J Oncol 15:367, 1999.

143. Dimopoulos M, Viniou N, Zomas A et al: Activity of thalidomide in Waldenstrom's macroglobulinemia. J Clin Oncol 19:3596, 2001.

144. Andriko JA, Aguilea NS, Chu WS et al: Waldenstrom's macroglobulinemia: A clinico-pathologic study of 22 cases. Cancer 80:1926, 1997.

145. Kyrtsonis MC, Angelopoulou MK, Siakantaris MD et al: Waldenstrom's macroglobulinemia: Clinical course and prognostic factors in 60 patients. Ann Hematol 80:722, 2000.

146. Morel P, Monconduit M, Jacomy D et al: A new scoring system in Waldenstrom's macroglobulinemia; Description on 232 patients with validation on 167 other patients. Blood 96:852, 2000.

147. Dhodapkar MV, Jacobson J, Gertz M et al: Serum beta 2 microglobulin and IgM identify district prognostic subsets in patients with Waldenstrom's macroglobulinemia. Blood 98:41, 2001.

148. Garcia R, Hernandez JM, Caballero et al: Immunoblastic lymphoma and associated non-lymphoid malignancies following two cases of Waldenstrom's macroglobulinemia. Eur J Haematol 50:299, 1993.

149. Rodriguez JN, Fernandez-Jurado A, Martino ML et al: Waldenstrom's macroglobulinemia complicated with acute myeloid leukemia. Report of a case and review of the literature. Hematologica 83:91, 1998.

150. Rosner F, Grunwald HW: Multiple myeloma and Waldenstrom's macroglobulinemia terminating in acute leukemia. N Y State J Med 80:558, 1980.

151. Leonhard SA, Muhleman AF, Hurtubise PF et al: Emergence of immunoblastic sarcoma in Waldenstrom's macroglobulinemia. Cancer 45:3102, 1980.

152. Hamada T, Ishizuka H, Asai Y et al: A case of anaplastic large cell (ki-1) lymphoma of B-cell phenotype, occuring in Waldenstrom's macroglobulinemia. Pathol Int 49:913, 1999.

34

Heavy-Chain Disease

Dietlind Wahner-Roedler and Robert A. Kyle

The heavy-chain diseases (HCDs) are monoclonal lympho-plasma-cell proliferative disorders involving B cells and are characterized by the synthesis of truncated heavy chains without associated light chains. They have been described for the three main immunoglobulin (Ig) classes. The most frequent is α-HCD; μ-HCD is rare and the incidence of γ-HCD is intermediate. In contrast to γ- and α-HCD, which usually have no detectable monoclonal light chains, light chains that do not assemble with the secreted deleted heavy chains are produced in about two-thirds of cases of μ-HCD. The monoclonal proteins are always present in the serum and often in the urine of patients with γ-HCD, but monoclonal heavy chains are infrequent in the urine in μ-HCD and occur in small amounts in α-HCD. Because the diagnosis depends entirely on immunochemical studies of the serum Igs and can be easily overlooked in serum electrophoretic patterns, the HCDs are currently underdiagnosed. The association of several distinct gene alterations – somatic mutations, deletions, and insertions – accounts for the complex abnormalities of HCD proteins and the usual lack of normal light chains.

γ-HEAVY-CHAIN DISEASE

Since the first report of γ-HCD in 1964,[1] approximately 100 patients with γ-HCD have been described in the literature.[2,3] Although a lymphoma-like illness, with lymphadenopathy, splenomegaly, and hepatomegaly, together with a lympho-plasmacytic proliferation similar to that of Waldenström's macroglobulinemia, has been considered characteristic of γ-HCD, it does not represent a specific pathologic process but is a biochemical expression of a mutant B-cell clone. The "disease" should be considered a serologically determined entity.

Clinical Features

γ-Heavy-chain disease has been described throughout the world, and no epidemiologic pattern has been recognized. No familial cases have been reported. The disease usually involves an older age group; 75 percent of patients are in the sixth decade of life or beyond. However, the disease may occur in children or very young adults and has been noted before the age of 20 years in several patients.[4–9] There is a slight predilection for men.

γ-Heavy-chain disease can present with a great variety of clinical and pathologic features. It has been difficult to integrate these various changes into a unified disease concept. Wester et al.[10] suggested that patients with γ-HCD can be placed into three broad categories on the basis of the underlying pathologic process and its distribution: (1) those with disseminated lymphoproliferative disease, which occurs in approximately two-thirds of patients; (2) those with localized lymphoproliferative disease, occurring in approximately 25 percent (11 percent extramedullary and 14 percent involving the bone marrow only); and (3) those with no apparent proliferative disease. Of the patients with no proliferative disease (approximately 10 percent), many have autoimmune disorders.[10]

Most often, γ-HCD presents as a lymphoproliferative disorder. Lymphadenopathy and constitutional symptoms such as fever, weakness, and fatigue are the most common initial features. Generalized peripheral lymphadenopathy with prominent cervical involvement is present in about 55 percent of patients, and fever is present at the time of diagnosis in 25 percent.[2] Lymphadenopathy obstructing the vena cava has been noted.[5,11] Waxing and waning of lymphadenopathy may occur. Edema of the uvula and palate occurs in about 20 percent of patients, presumably because of lymphatic obstruction due to involvement of Waldeyer's ring lymph nodes. Splenomegaly is present in about 60 percent of patients and ranges from a palpable tip to massive splenomegaly. Isolated splenomegaly may be the presenting feature of γ-HCD.[2] Spontaneous rupture of the spleen has been described.[2] Hepatomegaly is less frequent and occurs in about half of patients.[2]

Several extrahematopoietic organs have been involved by tumors. Skin lesions in general have been noted to be the most frequent extrahematopoietic manifestation.[12] Cutaneous or subcutaneous involvement, featured by an extranodal mass[2,13,14] or skin nodules,[8,11–13,15–20] has been described. Patients have presented with extramedullary plasmacytoma of the thyroid[13,21–24] or with parotid or submandibular swelling.[1,13,25] A patient with dysphagia and hoarseness from an oropharyngeal mass consisting of plasma cells has been described.[26] A 12-year-old Turkish girl presented with malabsorption and marked infiltration of the intestine with lymphoplasmacytoid cells (similar to α-HCD),[4] and a 63-year-old woman with γ-HCD associated with mucosa-associated lymphoid tissue (MALT) lymphoma of the duodenum has been reported in the Japanese literature.[27] In several other cases, the initial symptoms were due to a gastric lymphoid tumor.[28–30]

The occurrence of autoimmune disorders, with or without associated underlying lymphoid proliferation, is frequent in patients with γ-HCD. Rheumatoid arthritis has been reported in about a dozen patients.[2,16,31–42] Rheumatoid arthritis preceded the diagnosis of γ-HCD by as many as 25 years. Two patients with rheumatoid arthritis had only transient monoclonal γ-heavy chains.[33,40] Systemic lupus erythematosus[43] was documented in one case and discoid lupus in another.[21] Vasculitis with or without associated rheumatoid arthritis[2,35,39] and livedoid vasculitis[44] have been reported. Sjögren's syndrome was present in two cases,[45,46] and keratoconjunctivitis sicca, vasculitis, hypocomplementemia, and Coombs-positive hemolytic anemia were noted in another.[47] Two patients with myasthenia gravis have been described[2,21]; peripheral neuropathy has been reported in several patients[2,48,49]; and another patient had a past history of Guillain-Barré syndrome.[13]

Among solid tumors that have been diagnosed in patients with γ-HCD are prostate cancer,[13,48] uterine sarcoma,[2,32] gastric carcinoma,[2] and pancreatic cancer[50]; these are probably fortuitous. A myeloproliferative disorder was documented in three cases.[10,51,52] Herpes zoster involved the eye of one patient[53] and was generalized in another.[54]

Laboratory Findings

Hematologic Abnormalities

Anemia is frequent and ultimately develops in nearly all patients. It is usually normochromic, normocytic, and moderate, except in patients with autoimmune hemolytic anemia. A Coombs-positive autoimmune hemolytic anemia has been reported in several cases[8,13,36,47,55,56] and has sometimes been associated with idiopathic thrombocytopenic purpura (Evans' syndrome).[8,13] The leukocyte count and differential count are usually normal, but both leukopenia and leukocytosis may occur. Lymphocytosis with or without atypical lymphocytes may be present, and an occasional patient presents with chronic lymphocytic leukemia. Plasmacytoid lymphocytes or plasma cells may be found in the peripheral blood, and plasma cell leukemia has been reported in two patients.[9,57] Eosinophilia may occur. Thrombocytopenia due to an autoimmune process, hypersplenism, and, less frequently, bone marrow failure have been reported, but thrombocytosis is not a feature of γ-HCD. The erythrocyte sedimentation rate can range from normal to more than 100 mm in 1 hour.

Bone Marrow Findings

Bone marrow aspirates and biopsy specimens frequently reveal an increase of plasma cells, lymphocytes, or plasmacytoid lymphocytes, which is similar to the bone marrow picture of Waldenström's macroglobulinemia. Typical bone marrow features of multiple myeloma[58,59] or chronic lymphocytic leukemia[2,13] are rare. Marrow changes consistent with a myeloproliferative disorder have been noted in a few patients.[10,51,52] Eosinophilia is rarely found. The presence of mast cells has been mentioned.[60] A marked increase in erythropoiesis is present in patients with hemolytic anemia. In several instances, the bone marrow aspirate and biopsy specimens have been normal.

Other Features

Bone lesions are very rare in γ-HCD; only four cases with skeletal involvement have been reported.[2,17,18,59,61] Hypercalcemia was noted in five patients,[5,13,18,19,62] three of whom had no apparent skeletal involvement. Renal insufficiency is uncommon but may occur in association with hypercalcemia. Lymphoid infiltration involving the kidneys,[13,56] adrenals,[14,63] lungs,[13,20] and the central nervous system[35] has been detected, mainly at postmortem examinations.

Protein Findings

The serum protein electrophoretic pattern is extremely variable. In approximately 40 percent of patients the abnormal protein is not detectable by electrophoresis,[2] and the pattern is normal, shows hypogammaglobulinemia, or shows hypergammaglobulinemia with a polyclonal pattern or an increase in the protein migrating in the β region without a detectable spike. The range of mobility of the γ-HCD protein is wide, but an abnormal band in the $β_1$ or $β_2$ region is the most common pattern. The serum level of the γ-HCD protein is usually less than 1 g/dl, but it can range from unmeasurable levels to 9 g/dl.[2] Analysis of the distribution of the IgG subclasses in γ-HCD shows a lower than expected incidence of IgG_2 HCD protein. The most common subclass is IgG_1, which occurs in 65 percent of cases; IgG_3 has been identified in 27 percent, IgG_4 in 5 percent, and IgG_2 in 3 percent of patients,[2] whereas the normal distribution of IgG subclasses is IgG_1 64 to 70 percent, IgG_2 23 to 28 percent, IgG_3 4 to 7 percent, and IgG_4 3 to 4 percent.[64] IgA and IgM are usually reduced in γ-HCD.

The response to the Bence Jones heat test is in general negative. Two patients with γ-HCD and Bence Jones proteinuria have been described.[36,65] The amount of γ-HCD protein excreted in the urine is less than 1 g in 24 hours in most instances but may reach 20 g in 24 hours. In many cases, careful study of adequately concentrated urine is necessary to detect the γ-HCD protein. The mobility of the monoclonal protein in the urine is the same as that in the serum, with only rare exceptions.[5]

Relatively homogeneous free fragments of γ-chains unaccompanied by light chains may be found during examination of the urine by high-resolution electrophoresis and immunofixation. This urinary protein, which should not be confused with the γ-HCD protein,[66] is similar to the fragment generated by the secondary action of papain on the Fc' fragment. Differentiation from the γ-HCD protein can be accomplished by gel diffusion analysis. From a practical point of view, however, such studies are not required because the γ-HCD protein is always present in the serum and migrates into the β-γ region, whereas the free γ-chain fragments described by Charles and Valdes[66] are found only in the urine and migrate into the $α_2$ region. These fragments are of no known clinical significance. They probably originate from extracellular degradation of the IgG molecule.

Cytogenetic Abnormalities

Cytogenetic abnormalities have been recognized infrequently. They have been reported in 7 of 15 patients, of whom 4 had aneuploidy,[2,13,15,32] and the other 3 had trisomy 7,[20] trisomy 21,[7] and multiple chromosome abnormalities.[2] Three of these patients[2,32] had received prior chemotherapy, which could have been responsible for some of the chromosome abnormalities. No chromosome abnormalities were found in seven other patients.[1,2,25,31,33,67]

Structural Protein Abnormalities

Heavy-chain disease proteins are synthesized as truncated chains. In some cases, an additional limited postsynthetic degradation occurs with removal of the N-terminal sequences, which can be documented in the proliferating cells. Immunochemical studies indicate that the HCD proteins have intact carboxyl-terminal regions. The alterations most often involve the V and the C_H1 domains. The precise boundaries of the deletions vary from one case to another. Structural studies have shown that most γ-HCD proteins are dimers of deleted heavy chains devoid of light chains and consist mainly of the Fc region. The molecular weight of the monomeric γ chain ranges from 27,000 to 49,000. The carbohydrate content of the γ-HCD proteins is high. The length of the γ chain varies from case to case but usually is one-half to three-fourths of the length of its normal counterpart.[68] Often, the deletions are internal, with a portion of the V sequence present at the amino terminus, ruling out postsynthetic degradation. The resumption of the normal sequence occurs precisely at the beginning of a domain. On the basis of their structure, the γ-HCD proteins can be placed into several groups (Figure 34–1):

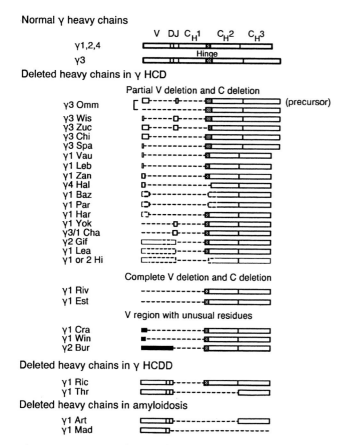

Normal γ heavy chains

Deleted heavy chains in γ HCD

Deleted heavy chains in γ HCDD

Deleted heavy chains in amyloidosis

Figure 34–1. Structure of various deleted γ-heavy chains in γ-heavy-chain disease (γ-HCD), γ-heavy chain deposition disease (γ-HCDD), and amyloidosis compared with that of normal chains. Hatched bars correspond to hinge regions, closed bars indicate unusual sequences, dotted bars indicate regions potentially present but not sequenced, and dotted lines indicate deletions. V, variable region; D, diversity; J, joining; C_H, constant region. Omm,[50,69] Wis,[70,71] Zuc,[72] Chi,[73] Spa,[74] Vau and Leb,[75] Zan,[71] Hal,[76] Baz,[77] Par,[78] Har,[79] Yok,[80] Cha,[81] Gif,[82] Lea,[79] Hi,[83] Riv,[84] Est,[85] Cra,[79,86] Win,[65] Bur,[87] Ric,[88] Thr,[88] Art,[89] Mad.[90] (Modified from Cogné et al.,[95,97] with permission.)

1. Most γ-HCD proteins contain a fragment of a V region. Usually they have a normal V region amino terminus followed by an internal deletion of the V and the entire C_H1 domain. In all HCD proteins with an internal V region deletion, the residues corresponding to the VDJ junction are missing. Some of these proteins contain a portion of this region and are featured by two noncontiguous deletions (γ3 Omm, γ3 Wis, γ3 Zuc). The γ3 Omm protein has been shown to undergo postsynthetic degradation to yield an NH_2-terminal deleted protein.[91]

2. Some γ-HCD proteins lack the entire V and C_H1 domains, with the sequence starting within the hinge region (γ1 Riv, γ1 Est).

3. The third group is characterized by an unusual amino acid sequence preceding the deletion. An abnormal sequence of 10 residues has been found in protein γ1 Cra. The seven N-terminal amino acid residues found in protein γ1 Win are not translated from any of the known immunoglobulin heavy-chain gene sequences.[65] The complete sequence of γ2-HCD Bur has been reported.[87] This mutant is composed of a complete V region, hinge, C_H2, and C_H3 domains. The unique features of this V region are the presence of methionine at position 11, two cysteine residues at positions 50 and 53, and three glycosylation sites.

In most cases of HCD, the association of several distinct gene alterations is responsible for both the complex structural abnormalities found among these proteins and the usual absence of light-chain synthesis. The alterations found in two γ-heavy-chain genes (γ-HCD protein Omm, γ-HCD protein Riv) and in one light-chain gene (κ Riv) include somatic mutations, deletions, and insertions in rearranged V genes. The HCD protein γ3 Omm was found to be the product of two deletions, a splice correction and postsynthetic NH_2 terminal proteolysis.[69] Sequencing of the γ1 Riv gene revealed that it had undergone V_H–J_H and H chain class switch recombinations. However, normal RNA splice sites had been eliminated by a DNA insertion–deletion (V_H acceptor site), mutations (J_H donor site), or a large deletion (C_H1 region). These DNA alterations resulted in aberrant mRNA processing in which the leader region was spliced directly to the hinge region, accounting for the HCD protein[84] (Figure 34–2).

Like genes encoding HCD proteins, the κ chain gene of patient Riv showed deletions, insertions, and a very high rate (25 percent) of somatic mutations in the VJ region. Mutations of spliced sites bounding the $V_{\kappa}J_{\kappa}$ region resulted in exon skipping and splicing of the leader peptide exon onto the C_{κ} exon. A short mRNA was present and coded for a C_{κ} fragment devoid of the V domain.[92]

Usually, γ-HCD cells do not secrete light chains. There are, however, a few cases in which light chains or light-chain fragments were detected as Bence Jones protein in serum and urine by immunofluorescence or internal labeling. In γ-HCD patient Win, λ Bence Jones protein was found in the serum and urine,[65,93] and IgGκ and IgMλ and κ and λ Bence Jones proteins were detected in another patient's serum and urine, respec-

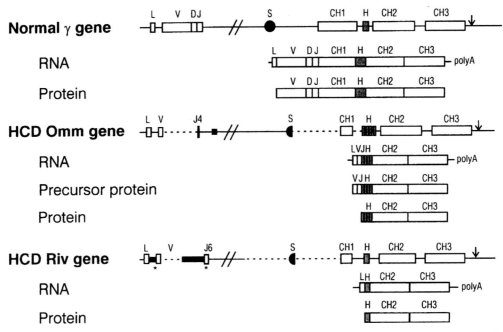

Figure 34–2. Structure of γ-heavy-chain disease (HCD) productive gene, RNA transcript, and protein compared with their normal rearranged counterpart. S, switch region; V, variable region; L, leader; H, hinge; CH, constant region; D, diversity; J, joining. Asterisks indicate altered splice site; solid bars represent insertions in coding (large bar) or noncoding (small bar) regions; dashed lines indicate deletion. (From Fermand and Brouet,[3] with permission.)

tively.[36] In one (patient Mo) of nine patients with γ-HCD, nonsecreted monotypic light chains were found by direct immunofluorescence in the cytoplasm and at the surface of blood and bone marrow cells.[94] Small amounts of a truncated κ chain corresponding to the C domain were found in cytoplasmic extract by internal labeling when studying HCD protein Riv. This light-chain fragment was undetectable by immunofluorescence.[92,95]

Heavy- and light-chain assembly is critical for immunoglobulin secretion, and unless deleted, free heavy chains are not secreted in the absence of light chains. Under these circumstances, entire heavy chains remain associated with a heavy-chain binding protein (BiP) in the lumen of the endoplasmic reticulum and are not secreted.[96] However, truncated heavy chains appear to escape the interaction with BiP and are secreted or expressed at the cell surface in the absence of light chains. Any mutation or deletion impeding the normal folding, assembly, or intracellular transport of immunoglobulin chains could thus select for the various gene alterations seen in HCD to maintain immunoglobulin secretion.[95,97] Although these observations favor a concept in which the light-chain abnormality occurs first, the complexity of the genomic abnormalities described makes a multitude of alterations occurring in the most fragile regions of the Ig genes more likely.

Oncogene activation has been demonstrated in one patient with γ-HCD (patient Omm). DNA from a lymphoid line generated from peripheral blood of the patient transformed NIH/3T3 cells, which produced tumors in white mice. Molecular studies demonstrated an activating N-*ras* 61 mutation, as has been noted in one-third of patients with multiple myeloma.[98]

Lymph Node Pathology

No consistent morphologic pattern corresponds to serologically defined γ-HCD. In 18 (38 percent) of 47 patients in whom lymph nodes were examined, non-Hodgkin's lymphoma was present without any consistent morphologic type. Lymphoplasmacytic proliferation, with or without atypia, was present in 36 percent of cases. Hyperplastic nodes and plasmacytoma each made up 11 percent of the total. There was one case of Hodgkin's disease and one case of "probable Hodgkin's disease."[10] Three additional cases of γ-HCD associated with Hodgkin's disease have been reported.[15,99,100]

Diagnosis

γ-Heavy-chain disease can present with a diversity of clinical features. The diagnosis can be easily overlooked on serum protein electrophoresis because a narrow abnormal band suggestive of a monoclonal protein is seen in less than 50 percent of patients. Proteinuria may not be detectable.

The diagnosis is established by immunofixation or immunoelectrophoresis (Figure 34–3) of the serum and of a concentrated urine specimen using specific antisera combined with immunoselection. A modified immunoselection technique for the diagnosis of heavy-chain disease has been described by Sun et al.[101] Two-dimensional electrophoresis and immunoblotting also have been used for the recognition of γ-HCD.[102,103] Tissot et al.[104] showed that the combination of serum protein agarose electrophoresis and two-dimensional electrophoresis can be used to further characterize abnormal protein bands detected by immunofixation.

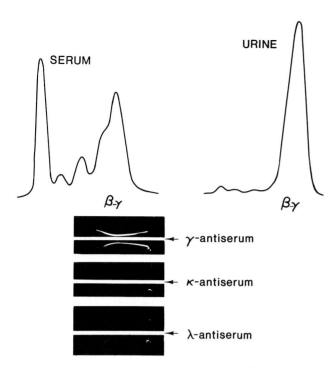

Figure 34–3. *(Top)* Densitometer tracings, with peaks of β–γ mobility in serum and in urine profiles. *(Bottom)* Immunoelectrophoresis. In each tray the top well contained the patient's serum and the bottom well contained concentrated urine. With γ antiserum, both serum and urine formed dense, thick, asymmetric arcs. With κ and with λ antisera, serum and urine formed no visible arcs. This patient has monoclonal γ chain in serum and urine (γ heavy-chain disease). (From Kyle and Greipp,[297] with permission.)

We believe that γ-HCD is underdiagnosed and urge that immunofixation of serum and urine be performed in all cases of lymphoplasma cell proliferative diseases.

Clinical Course

As expected from the diverse picture, the course of γ-HCD varies from an asymptomatic presence of a monoclonal heavy chain in serum or urine to a rapidly progressive downhill course. The presence of a γ-HCD protein by itself does not influence the prognosis. Patients with features of a benign monoclonal gammopathy or monoclonal gammopathy of undetermined significance (MGUS) have remained clinically well during 2 to 7 years of follow-up evaluation.[21,105–107]

Disappearance of the γ-HCD protein also has been reported.[2,24,33,60,108] In one patient, the protein was detected during a recurrent febrile illness but disappeared after a cholecystectomy.[60,108] In another patient, in whom biopsies had shown an invasive plasmacytic proliferation, the monoclonal γ-heavy chain disappeared from the serum 8 months after irradiation for a thyroid mass and cervical lymphadenopathy.[24] In two patients with rheumatoid arthritis, the γ-HCD protein disappeared.[2,33] One of these patients has been followed for more than 10 years, and despite slowly progressive rheumatoid arthri-

tis the γ-HCD protein has not reappeared and an overt lymphoproliferative disorder has not developed.[2]

When an underlying lymphoid malignancy exists, the histopathologic pattern is essential for the determination of prognosis, and it is obvious that patients with an aggressive malignant process will do less well than those with more favorable pathologic findings.

The clinical course may be prolonged. The diagnosis in one case had been preceded 22 years by cervical lymphadenopathy and 17 years by a hemolytic anemia.[8] The median duration of survival in 49 patients for whom some data were available was 12 months (range, 1 to 264 months).[13]

Treatment

Because γ-HCD is a heterogeneous condition that does not really deserve the designation of a disease process and, as suggested by Roda et al.,[15] should rather be named "monoclonal γ-HCD protein associated with…," the choice of therapy should rely entirely on the underlying disorder and the pathologic findings. In an asymptomatic patient with an MGUS, no therapy is indicated. Any associated autoimmune disease should be managed with standard therapy without taking into account the existence of the abnormal monoclonal component. In symptomatic patients with a low-grade lymphoplasmacytic malignancy, a trial of chlorambucil may be beneficial. Melphalan and prednisone can be used if the proliferation is predominantly plasmacytic. We recommend a trial of cyclophosphamide, vincristine, and prednisone for patients with γ-HCD and evidence of a progressive lymphoplasma cell proliferative process or high-grade non-Hodgkin's lymphoma. If there is no response to this regimen, doxorubicin should be added. Agrawal et al.[109] described a patient who achieved a complete remission with disappearance of the heavy chain after six courses of fludarabine. Successful treatment of γ-HCD with low-dose etoposide has been reported in a Japanese patient whose disease was unresponsive to combination chemotherapy.[110]

The amount of serum γ-HCD protein usually parallels the severity of the associated malignant process. Disappearance of the monoclonal component from serum and urine associated with apparent complete remission has been induced by chemotherapy,[2,109] radiation therapy,[2,24] or surgical removal of a localized process.[22,23] In a few instances, however, relapse is not accompanied by reappearance of the pathologic protein.[2] In general, therapeutic responses have been variable and disappointing in that responses often are incomplete or of short duration.

Monoclonal Immunoglobulin and γ-HCD

Biclonal gammopathy is reported to occur in approximately 1 to 3 percent of all patients with serum M components.[111–113] In contrast, the association between γ-HCD and another monoclonal gammopathy is much higher. In a review of 56 cases of γ-HCD, 9 cases of biclonality were identified (16 percent).[13] The average age of 13 patients with biclonal γ-HCD was 56 years, and males predominated 2:1.[114] The associated monoclonal immunoglobulin has been of the IgM[2,29,30,34,57,114–117] or

IgG type.[35,50,118–122] No association between γ-HCD and a monoclonal IgA has yet been described, whereas the IgG–IgA association is the most frequent in series of biclonal gammopathies.[111,123] There was a higher frequency of λ chain expression.[114] All cases except for one[35] were associated with a lymphoplasma proliferative process. The median duration of survival in patients with biclonal disease was 22 months,[114] whereas it was 12 months in patients with γ-HCD alone.[13] One patient described by Lebreton et al.[122] was unique in that the serum contained two deleted γ chains of different subclasses (IgG₁ and IgG₂). One of these persisted without change during the disease, and the level of the other diminished and had disappeared at the time of death. The reason for the relative predilection of γ-HCD to coexist with other unrelated paraproteins remains unclear. Three possible mechanisms have been delineated by bone marrow immunofluorescence studies: (1) double heavy-chain-specific precursor cells develop into two separate cell populations, each secreting different immunoglobulins of the same idiotype; (2) both paraproteins are synthesized simultaneously by cells of a single clone; and (3) rarely, two independent neoplastic cell lines coexist.[123]

γ-Heavy-Chain Deposition Disease

Monoclonal immunoglobulin deposition disease is a well-recognized, pathologically defined entity. Continuous linear deposits of κ or λ immunoglobulin light chains are the immunohistologic hallmark of light-chain deposition disease (LCDD). Some cases of monoclonal immunoglobulin deposition disease have deposits of both light and heavy chains (LHCDD).[124] In 1992 Tubbs et al.[125] described two patients for whom they proposed the term "pseudo-γ heavy chain deposition disease." Both patients presented with acute renal failure. Renal biopsy demonstrated a nodular intercapillary glomerulopathy and continuous electron-dense granular deposits, associated with a linear pattern of IgG₄ heavy-chain deposition in vascular, tubular, and glomerular basement membranes. Light-chain deposits were absent in one patient and were very faint and limited to the glomerular basement membrane in the other. The authors believed that these immunohistologic findings were best explained by a change in the three-dimensional conformational structure of the protein after entrapment and binding to the basement membrane, rendering the light-chain antigenic sites inaccessible to antibody reagent and thereby undetectable. This was the basis for their proposed designation of pseudo-γ heavy chain deposition disease. In view of the subsequent reports describing kidney deposits containing short heavy chains but no detectable light chains, the cases reported by Tubbs et al. are now considered examples of γ-heavy-chain deposition disease (γ-HCDD).[126,127] Thirteen patients with γ-HCDD belonging to the subgroups γ₁ (five patients),[88,128–130] γ₃ (four patients),[41,42,131–133] and γ₄ (four patients)[125–127] have been described. In two other patients with γ-HCDD, the subtype was not determined.[134,135]

In all cases of γ-HCDD in which the constant domains have been studied, the common feature is C_H1 deletion (patient Ric, Figure 34–1).[88] In addition to the C_H1 deletion, absence of the

hinge and CH2 domain have been reported in another patient (patient Thr, Figure 34–1).[88] When the structures of the heavy chains in γ-HCDD and γ-HCD are compared, the variable regions are found to be particularly or entirely deleted in HCD. Thus, failure of tissue deposition of the heavy chains in HCD appears to be caused by the partial or complete deletion of the variable region.

The most common clinical findings in γ-HCDD are nephrotic syndrome, hypertension, microhematuria, and, in some cases, hypocomplementemia. Renal insufficiency is usually present at the time of diagnosis. Beside important renal involvement, there may be heavy-chain deposits in other organs such as skin and skeletal muscle, as described in one case by Rott et al.,[131] and in synovial tissue in a patient with seronegative rheumatoid arthritis, as described by Husby et al.[41,42] The characteristic lesion on renal biopsy is nodular sclerosing glomerulopathy, sometimes with crescents. Immunofluorescence and electron microscopy show heavy-chain deposition in the mesangium and basement membranes of glomeruli, tubules, and blood vessels. Except for the composition of the deposits detected by immunofluorescence, the renal biopsy findings are otherwise indistinguishable from those of LCDD and LHCDD. In contrast to LCDD, in γ-HCDD nodular glomerulosclerosis is a constant feature, hypertension and microhematuria are more frequent, and the hematologic disorder is generally mild. In most cases of γ-HCDD, a monoclonal protein can be documented in the serum, urine, or bone marrow biopsy specimen, although its demonstration may require special studies. Often the monoclonal proteins are detected in only minute quantities in serum or urine, probably in large part because of the avid tissue-binding properties of the heavy chains.

There is no consensus on treatment of γ-HCDD, and in most cases the renal outcome is poor.[133] Moulin et al.[130] suggested that patients older than 60 years with γ-HCDD in association with myeloma (which has been reported in four patients[126,130,133]) should be treated with conventional chemotherapy, but intensive therapy with blood stem-cell autografting should be considered in younger patients. Treatment of nonmyeloma patients should be modulated according to clinical presentation.

Heavy-Chain-Associated Amyloidosis

Eulitz et al.[89] described a patient (Art) with systemic heavy-chain amyloidosis in whom the amyloid component consisted of a short IgG heavy chain. The shortened heavy chain belonged to the γ₁ subclass and contained a normal variable domain directly linked to the third constant domain (Figure 34–1). A second case of heavy-chain-associated amyloidosis (patient Mad) has been reported.[90] Amyloid protein Mad is characterized by the presence of a virtually intact V_H region plus a D segment and lack of the J_H segment and the entire C_H region (Figure 34–1). These data are compatible with the hypothesis that constant-domain deletion in heavy chains may be responsible for free heavy-chain secretion, whereas variable-domain conformational singularities rather than gross structural alterations might promote either HCDD or heavy-chain-associated amyloidosis.[88,136,137] The discovery that certain forms of heavy chains, as well as light chains, can form amyloid provides further information on the chemical basis of amyloidogenicity and the diverse nature of this disease.

α-HEAVY-CHAIN DISEASE

In 1968 Seligmann et al.[138] described an Arab woman with severe malabsorption resulting from a lymphoplasmacytic infiltrate in the small bowel who had a monoclonal α-heavy chain in the serum. Since this first description, more than 400 cases[139] have been reported in the literature, and α-HCD is the most frequent of the HCDs. The disease is defined as a lymphoid proliferation involving the IgA secretory system and producing a homogeneous population of immunoglobulin molecules consisting of incomplete α chains devoid of light chains. The initial benign-appearing antibiotic-responsive immunoproliferative lesions often evolve to fatal, highly malignant lymphoma. α-Heavy-chain disease might be considered a model showing the complex interactions of the environment with genetic factors and the complex infection-immunity–cancer interrelationships originating from the same proliferating clone.

Epidemiology

The syndrome of primary upper small intestinal lymphoma with malabsorption and clubbing of the fingers, which improved with small oral doses of tetracycline, was first described in Peru among poor mestizos.[140,141] Most reports of α-HCD have been of Arab or Jewish patients from the Mediterranean area or from the Middle East, but numerous cases also have been described in inhabitants of Eastern Europe, the Indian subcontinent, the Far East, Central, North, and South America, and sub-Saharan Africa. It is of interest that α-HCD in developed countries often occurs among Third World immigrants and underprivileged native populations. Probably α-HCD will be more frequently detected in the United States in the future because of the migration of Mexican workers.[142] The prevalence is slightly higher in males than females. Unlike multiple myeloma and the other HCDs, α-HCD has a predilection for young adults; most patients are in their twenties or thirties, although α-HCD has also been reported in children[143–148] and in persons in the seventh decade of life.[149] A common denominator for these patients is a low socioeconomic status and substandard hygiene resulting in recurrent infectious diarrhea and chronic parasitic infestation. Geophagia since early infancy was almost constant in subjects at risk in Tunisia.[150]

Pathogenesis

The cause of α-HCD is unknown. Current clinical, histologic, molecular, and immunologic data indicate that the evolutionary cause of α-HCD is a complex, multistep process. The lymphoplasmacytic infiltration of the intestinal mucosa and regional mesenteric lymph nodes is likely a response of the alimentary tract's immune system to protracted luminal antigenic stimulation. The epidemiologic features of the disease strongly suggest that environmental factors operating since early infancy could play a major role in its pathogenesis. No specific microorganism has been found in bacteriologic, virologic, or parasitologic studies.[151] However, the putative agent may be present only at the onset of the disease and absent at the time of diagnosis. Bacterial lipopolysaccharides, dietary lectins,[152–154] enterotoxins of *Vibrio* cholera,[155] oncogenic viruses,[154,156] and asbestosis[157] have been suspected of providing antigenic stimulation that triggers the histoimmunopathologic changes. The Epstein-Barr virus, which has been associated with B-cell lymphoproliferative disorders, was documented to play no role in the induction of B-cell proliferation in immunoproliferative small intestinal disease (IPSID) in eight patients,[158] whereas ultrastructural studies of lymph nodes of another patient with α-HCD described by Arista-Nasr et al.[156] revealed viruses that resembled the Epstein-Barr virus. The influence of environmental factors is supported by a report of spontaneous remission of α-HCD after departure from an endemic area[159] and a decline in the incidence rate of primary small intestinal lymphoma associated with immunoproliferative small intestinal disease among Jews born in Israel compared with Jewish immigrants with a relatively low socioeconomic standard from North Africa and Asia.[160]

The postulated environmental antigenic stimulation might be associated with an underlying immunodeficiency, which could be due to malnutrition, especially in early infancy, or to genetic factors. An increased incidence of immunoglobulin abnormalities has been found in first-degree relatives of patients with α-HCD: 23 of 129 apparently normal family members of 8 patients with α-HCD had abnormal immunoglobulin patterns.[161] In the same families, both patients with α-HCD and normal first-degree relatives had an increase of circulating B lymphocytes and a decrease of T lymphocytes. They also had decreased cellular immunity, as shown by sensitization to dinitrochlorobenzene. Tuberculin skin test reactions were also negative.[162,163]

A genetic element is suggested by the finding that patients with α-HCD have a greater association of the HLA-AW19 and HLA-B12 antigens than do normal blood donors or patients with malabsorption.[164] However, familial α-HCD has not been recognized.

Clinical Features

α-Heavy-chain disease most commonly presents in the "digestive form." Its onset may be gradual or, more often, abrupt. During the early stage, diarrhea can be intermittent; progression of the disease is manifested by sustained chronic diarrhea, with malabsorption, steatorrhea, weight loss, abdominal pain, and vomiting.[165] Patients may present with abdominal surgical emergencies or with chronic small bowel obstruction.[166] "Tumoral" signs are more often observed in the late stages of the disease.[167] Ascites, tetany, or edema may be present. Amenorrhea, alopecia, and growth retardation in children and adolescents correlate with the duration and severity of the malabsorptive process.[168] Clubbing of the fingers appears to be more frequent than in any other intestinal disease.[168] Fever is uncommon. Hepatosplenomegaly and peripheral lymphadenopathy are infrequent findings.[169]

α-Heavy-chain disease may be confined to the respiratory tract, but this respiratory form is rare. Two of the described patients were children, an 8-year-old girl who presented with pulmonary infiltrates, hilar adenopathy, skull lesions, and a pharyngeal tumor[144] and a 3-year-old boy who had recurrent respiratory infections, hypogammaglobulinemia, and an α-HCD fragment.[145] Another patient presented with dyspnea and had diffuse interstitial pulmonary fibrosis, pleural effusion, and mediastinal nodes.[170]

A lymphoma form of α-HCD has been described in three cases from Japan.[171–174] A striking clinical feature in two of these cases was long-standing and recurring skin eruptions, which developed before systemic lymphadenopathy.[171,172] In the third patient, who had a history of rheumatoid arthritis, marked cervical and inguinal lymphadenopathy developed, and α-HCD protein was identified in the serum and urine. Infiltrating malignant cells in the lymph nodes were found to be the site of α-HCD protein synthesis.[173] Neither the gastrointestinal nor the respiratory tract was involved in these patients.

Lymphomatous infiltration of the duodenum, jejunum, nasopharynx, and bone marrow was described in a Mauritanian man with α-HCD.[175] α-Heavy-chain disease has been reported in a patient with a goiter from a plasmacytoma of the thyroid[176] and in a patient with amyloidosis.[177]

Laboratory Findings

Hematologic and Metabolic Abnormalities

Mild to moderate anemia of variable cause is often found. Hypokalemia, hypocalcemia, and hypomagnesemia are common. The serum albumin level is nearly always low. The frequently increased serum alkaline phosphatase value is usually due to an increase in the intestinal isoenzyme fraction.[178] Serum lipid values are low even if steatorrhea is mild. Results of the Schilling test with intrinsic factor are low in two-thirds of patients, and results of the D-xylose test are almost always abnormal. The 24-hour fecal fat excretion ranged between 6 and 15 g in 43 percent and was more than 15 g in 52 percent of patients studied.[165] Heavy parasitic infestation of the intestine is a common occurrence; however, this does not appear to be significantly different from that of the general population living in the same area.

Immunologic Findings

Defects in humoral and delayed immunity have been demonstrated in patients with α-HCD, even in the tumor-free stage.[179] An increase in circulating B lymphocytes and a decrease in T lymphocytes have been reported. Decreased cellular immunity has been demonstrated by negative tuberculin skin tests and failure to be sensitized to dinitrochlorobenzene.[161–163]

Radiographic Findings

Radiographic manifestations of the small intestine include hypertrophic and pseudopolypoid mucosal folds in the duodenum and jejunum, sometimes associated with strictures or filling defects, which suggests extrinsic compression by hypertrophic peripancreatic or mesenteric lymph nodes.[165] Double-contrast studies of the small intestine are helpful in revealing precise mucosal changes.[180]

Endoscopic Findings

Because α-HCD intestinal lesions nearly always affect the duodenum and jejunum, fiberoptic endoscopy with biopsies is a useful tool in the work-up of patients with suspected α-HCD. Five primary endoscopic patterns occurring either alone or in various combinations have been defined. The infiltrated pattern is the most sensitive and specific finding, followed by the nodular pattern. Other primary lesions (ulcerations, mosaic pattern, and mucosal fold thickening alone) are nonsensitive, nonspecific or both.[181]

Protein Findings

Unlike other monoclonal gammopathies, the characteristic sharp spike of a monoclonal protein is not detected on serum protein electrophoresis in α-HCD.[182] In about half of the cases, an abnormal broad band is seen in the α_2- or β-globulin region. This broad band is due to the propensity of α-heavy chains to form polymers. In the remainder of the patients, serum protein electrophoresis shows no evidence of an abnormal protein.

In most patients, the α-HCD protein can be found in the serum, but its concentration is often low.[154] Bence Jones proteinuria has never been documented. The concentration of α-HCD protein in the urine is low. In most cases studied, the α-HCD protein was also found in jejunal secretions when its presence was documented in the serum.[150,183] Interestingly, however, α-HCD protein was found in the intestinal or gastric fluid in two cases in which it was undetectable in the serum and urine.[184,185]

It is unclear whether monomeric or polymeric α-HCD protein is present in external secretions and whether α-HCD protein in jejunal fluid is linked to the secretory component. In several patients with α-HCD, no association was found between the α-HCD protein and the secretory component in the jejunal fluid or in the epithelial cells of the jejunum.[146,178,186] However, these data conflict with another report demonstrating that jejunal fluid from two patients with α-HCD contained secretory component-associated α-HCD protein[187] and with immunofluorescence observations on rectal epithelial cells in an α-HCD case involving the large bowel.[143,188]

The linkage of polymeric α-HCD protein to the secretory component likely depends on balanced synthesis of α-chains and J-chains in the proliferating B cells, giving rise to polymers with the binding site for the secretory component expressed as an epithelial receptor. Insufficient receptor-mediated transport capacity results in passive external transfer of polymers without bound secretory component, along with leakage of serum-derived or locally produced monomeric α-HCD protein. The latter presumably originates from immunocytes with little or no J-chain synthesis.[175]

In all cases studied so far, the α-HCD protein belonged to the α_1 subclass, although 10 percent of normal serum Ig is of the α_2 subclass.

Cytogenetic Abnormalities

Cytogenetic abnormalities have been found in the lymphoid cells of patients with α-HCD. The clonal proliferation in this disease appears to be associated with frequent alterations of chromosome 14 at band q32 resulting from translocations that differ from those observed in the vast majority of other non-Hodgkin's lymphomas.[189] Berger et al.[189] reported abnormal karyotypes in three of four patients, two of whom had not reached the stage of malignant lymphoma. In two instances, a rearrangement of 14q32 resulting from a t(9;14)(p11;q32) and a t(2;14)(p12;q32) translocation was observed. Cloning and sequencing of the der(14) breakpoint of a chromosome translocation involving the 14q32 immunoglobulin locus suggested that the translocation originated from a local pairing of the two chromosomes 9 and 14.[190,191] One case showed complex rearrangements, including t(5;9). No abnormalities were found in the intestinal tumor of the fourth patient with immunoblastic lymphoma. An abnormal chromosome marker (14q+) has been reported in the marrow of a patient with α-HCD.[192]

Structural Protein Abnormalities

Most α-HCD proteins consist of multiple polymers. The molecular weight of the monomeric unit ranges from 29,000 to 34,000, and its length varies from one-half to three-fourths that of a normal α-chain. The shortening results from an internal deletion involving most of V_H and the first constant domain. Sequence data are available for several α-HCD proteins (Def,[193] Ait,[194] Mal,[195] Yao[196]). In all instances, the normal sequence of

the α1 chain constant region resumes at a valine residue in the hinge (Figure 34–4). The NH_2 terminal of protein Def is heterogeneous and, after a short segment corresponding to the variable region, displays a gap that comprises the C_H1 constant domain.[193] Attempts to determine the amino-terminal sequence of protein Ait have been unsuccessful. It has not been established how much of the V region is present in protein Ait. However, molecular weight determinations suggest that the V region is very short, as in protein Def. Studies by Wolfenstein-Todel et al.[193,194] indicate that protein Ait is synthesized as an internally deleted α chain followed by postsynthetic amino-terminal proteolysis. The α-HCD proteins Mal and Yao are devoid of V_H and C_H1 domains. No V-region sequence could be found.[195,196]

In a study of the nucleotide sequence of mRNA Mal[195] and Yao[196] and the nucleotide sequence of α-mRNA for six other α-HCD proteins (Ben, Arf, Mec, Lte, Har, Ayo),[197] all eight mRNAs were found to lack the V_H and C_H1 sequences (Figure 34–5). They contain inframe inserts of unknown origin between the leader peptide and the normal C_H2 and C_H3 coding sequences. These inserts are of variable length and unrelated; thus, it is unlikely that they originate from an infectious agent. The presence of inserted sequences of unknown origin appears to be a common feature of α-HCD-productive mRNA. Because the amino acid sequence of α-HCD proteins begins with the C_H2 domain, the amino-terminal sequence encoded by these inserts most likely is cleaved intracellularly before secretion.[197] In studying the α-HCD protein Ben, Fakhfakh et al.[198] found two molecular species, one starting at the beginning of the hinge region and the other, which was two amino acids shorter, missing the first two amino acids of

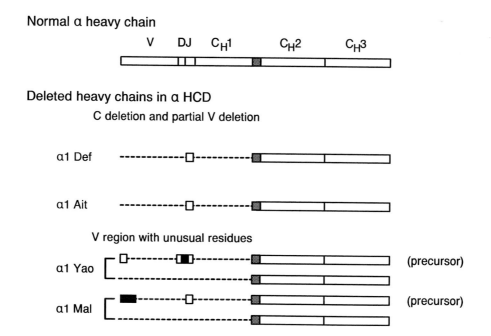

Figure 34–4. Structure of α-heavy-chain disease (HCD) proteins compared with that of normal chain. Hatched bars correspond to hinge regions, closed bars indicate unusual sequences, dotted lines indicate deletions. V, variable region; D, diversity; J, joining; C_H, constant region. α1 Def,[193] α1 Ait,[194] α1 Mal,[195] α1 Yao.[196] (Modified from Cogné et al.,[95,97] with permission.)

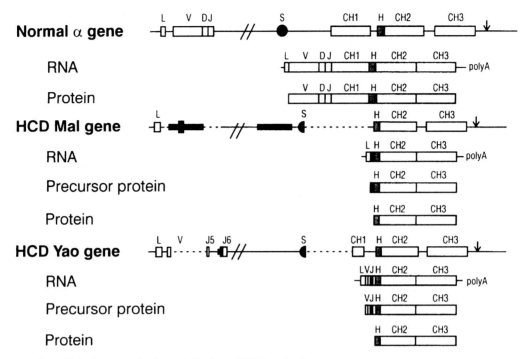

Figure 34–5. Structure of α-heavy-chain disease (HCD) productive gene, RNA transcript, and protein compared with their normal rearranged counterpart. S, switch region; V, variable region; L, leader; H, hinge; CH, constant region; D, diversity; J, joining. Solid bars represent insertions in coding (large bar) or noncoding (small bar) regions; dashed lines indicate deletion. (From Fermand and Brouet,[3] with permission.)

the hinge region. Intracellular cleavage could explain the presence of these two populations of α-HCD proteins; however, a limited postsecretion proteolysis also may be responsible for these findings.

Currently available molecular biologic studies indicate that genomic abnormalities such as multiple deletion–insertion processes, mutations, or duplications that are focused in the V_H–J_H and C_H1 regions are at least partly responsible for the production of α-HCD proteins.[199,200] These proteins are monoclonal even in the early stage of the disease.[201,202] Although nonsecretory α-HCD has been described,[185,201] the molecular basis for nonsecretion is incompletely understood. In a case of nonsecretory α-HCD (α1-Sec), the productive α gene was noted to bear several noncontiguous deletions. Two deletions were accompanied by peculiar insertions containing duplications. One of the deletions located at 3′ to C_H3 eliminated the polyadenylation site of the secreted form of α-mRNA. As a result, only the membrane form of α-mRNA was present in the tumoral plasma cells, thus explaining the nonsecretory phenotype of the disease.[203]

As a means of better understanding the molecular mechanism leading to the loss of light-chain production, a murine cell line model of α-HCD was studied.[204] In this model, the failure of light-chain synthesis was shown to result from a disruption in the normal splicing pattern caused by the insertion of a 358-nucleotide non-Ig sequence into the intron separating the leader exon from V_κ, leading to two mRNAs, neither of which encodes a functional light chain.[204]

Pathology

Enteric disease is the predominant manifestation of α-HCD. In this digestive form of α-HCD, the proliferation involves mainly the whole length or at least the proximal half of the small intestine and the mesenteric lymph nodes. In a few cases, intestinal lesions spare the duodenum and jejunum or are limited to a segment of the latter.[183,205] Gastric and colorectal mucosae that belong to the IgA-secretory system may be involved.[185,206] α-Heavy-chain disease confined to the stomach[184,207,208] or presenting as a colonic mass[209] has been reported. The disease progresses in three histopathologic stages.[210] In stage A, a mature plasmacytic or lymphoplasmacytic infiltration of the mucosal lamina propria is noted. Villous atrophy is variable and inconstant. Stage B is characterized by the presence of atypical plasmacytic or lymphoplasmacytic cells and more or less atypical immunoblast-like cells extending at least to the submucosa. Subtotal or total villous atrophy is present. Stage C corresponds to an immunoblastic lymphoma, either forming discrete ulcerated tumors or extensively infiltrating long segments and invading the whole depth of the intestinal wall.[210,211] Equivalent to the changes described in the small intestine, three histologic stages (A, B, C) corresponding to the cellular type of infiltrate and the degree of the nodal architecture in the mesenteric lymph nodes have been described. Involvement of liver, spleen, and peripheral lymph nodes is uncommon.

The histologic lesions may progress at any given site from stage A to stage B or from stage B to stage C. However, different stages can be found at the same time in different organs or even at different sites of the same organ. This asynchronism is important for staging.

The major lymphoma cell type in patients with α-HCD is immunoblastic lymphoma with various degrees of plasmacytoid differentiation.[150] Although α-HCD associated with multiple polypoid lymphocytic lymphoma of the small intestine is rare, a patient with α-HCD associated with multiple polypoid lymphocytic lymphoma and leukemic manifestation without evidence of bone marrow involvement has been described; the findings suggest that the circulating plasmacytoid lymphocytes originated from the tumor in the small intestine. Cytogenetic analysis showed the same abnormal karyotypes of neoplastic clones in the intestinal tumor cells as in the circulating leukemic cells.[212]

Isaacson et al.[213,214] and Spencer and Isaacson[215] suggested that the histopathologic findings in α-HCD fall into the group of lymphomas arising from mucosa-associated lymphoid tissue (MALT). Histologically, the diagnosis of MALT lymphoma is based on the existence of four elements: centrocyte-like cells, lymphoepithelial lesions, plasma cells, and reactive or residual follicles.[216] Spencer and Isaacson[215] hypothesized that in α-HCD, all large cells sometimes clustering in nodules at stage B are neoplastic follicular center cells, although "often cytologically bizarre." Similarly, the invasion, disruption, and partial destruction of intestinal crypts, sometimes found even at stage A, are part of the "lymphoepithelial lesions" due to centrocytic-like cells of the same clonal origin as plasma cells and are pathognomonic of all gut-associated lymphoid tissue lymphomas. Stage C tumors contain a mixture of the cytologic components.[150,183]

Lavergne et al.[217] described a case of HCD mimicking T-cell lymphoma. A marked predominance of small T cells in the mucosal infiltrate initially masked the underlying plasma cell proliferation, and small T-cell lymphoma was diagnosed before immunoglobulin studies on the plasma cells were performed. The T cells were polyclonal, partially repressed during the follow-up period, and thought to be characteristic centrocyte-like cells.

In a few patients with the typical clinical and pathologic features of α-HCD, another monoclonal Ig (γ-HCD protein),[4,27] a complete monoclonal IgA,[218–221] or a polyclonal expression of IgA was found.[222,223]

There has been some confusion in regard to the terminology of so-called Mediterranean lymphoma. In 1976 the World Health Organization suggested the term *immunoproliferative small intestinal disease* (IPSID).[224] This term should be restricted to small intestinal lesions whose pathology is identical to that of α-HCD at any of its histologic stages irrespective of the type of Ig synthesized by the proliferating cells.[225–227] Because previously used methods to detect the protein were not very sensitive, data regarding the presence of the abnormal protein vary.[228] In the experience of Rambaud et al.,[150] among 19 consecutive patients with the epidemiologic, clinical, and pathologic features of IPSID, 16 had the α-HCD protein in their serum and 1 had it in the jejunal juice only. In one case, immunofluorescence study of the small bowel mucosa showed that most of the infiltrating cells were positive for α chains and negative for other heavy or light chains (nonsecretory).[185] The 19th patient showed a massive infiltration of the small intestine by polyclonal plasma cells.[222]

The pathologic changes in the few cases with the respiratory form of α-HCD are poorly documented. It can be postulated that additional cases of the respiratory form will be described in the future. In a case of "lymph node" form or "lymphoma" form, lymph node biopsy showed diffuse plasmacytic lymphoma.[171]

Persistent ulcerated lesions developed on the gingiva of a patient with a previous history of IPSID. Histologic assessment of a gingival biopsy specimen revealed several features in common with the intestinal lesions of IPSID. In particular, a large plasma cell infiltrate subjacent to the gingival epithelium was noted.[229] There was no mention of the presence of an α-HCD protein.

Diagnosis

Because α-HCD in its intestinal form nearly always affects the duodenum and the jejunum, endoscopy has been advocated as the first diagnostic procedure in the investigation of patients clinically suspected of having α-HCD. Enteric presentation of γ-HCD,[4] monoclonal IgA secretion with a complete molecule,[220] variable immunodeficiency,[230] and acquired immunodeficiency syndrome (AIDS)[231] with clinicopathologic features simulating IPSID must be excluded.

The diagnosis of α-HCD depends on the identification of a free α heavy chain. Several methods may be used to document α-HCD protein in biological fluids.[232] A modified immunoselective technique described by Sun et al.[101] appears to be simple, convenient, and specific.

Synthesis of the α-HCD protein by the proliferating cells has been demonstrated by immunohistochemical or immunocytochemical methods and by biosynthesis studies in vitro. These techniques are not necessary when the α-HCD protein is found in the serum or intestinal fluid, but they are helpful in the recognition of nonsecreting forms of α-HCD.[185,187,201,203,233–236]

The quantity of abnormal α chains in the serum seems to be related to the nature (plasma-cell or immunoblastic type) of cells predominantly present in the intestinal mucosa or the mesenteric lymph nodes. During the course of the disease, the progressive diminution of mature plasma cells and their replacement by immature immunoblasts likely is followed by a progressive decrease in the serum concentration of α-HCD protein.[237] Hyposecretion of α-HCD protein may be found early and during the terminal evolutionary stage of the disease.[238]

Clinical Course and Treatment

The course of α-HCD is variable but generally progressive in the absence of therapy. Spontaneous clinical and immunologic remission in an Italian patient with the digestive form of α-HCD was reported after the patient's departure from Libya.[159] The α-HCD protein disappeared after total thyroidectomy in another patient with α-HCD, who presented with a goiter from an extramedullary plasmacytoma.[239]

In general, treatment depends on knowledge of the extent and histopathologic stage of the disease. Because of the frequent asynchronous histopathologic lesions, staging laparotomy should be performed.[150,240] Supportive therapy with intravenously administered fluids, electrolytes, calcium and magnesium replacement, albumin, and in some cases total parenteral nutrition may be necessary in preparing for staging laparotomy and during the early treatment period. Whether improved diagnostic tools such as computed tomography (CT) or magnetic resonance imaging (MRI) will reduce the need for staging laparotomy remains to be seen. Given the predilection of α-HCD to occur in developing countries, it is unlikely that these diagnostic techniques will be available.

Present therapeutic guidelines are as follows. Patients with stage A lesions limited to the bowel and to mesenteric lymph nodes should be treated initially with oral antibiotics. In case of intestinal bacterial overgrowth, antibiotics selected by the sensitivity pattern should be given. In the absence of a documented parasite and intestinal bacterial overgrowth, tetracycline or metronidazole and ampicillin are good choices. Any documented parasite should be eradicated. Eradication of *Helicobacter pylori* led to complete remission in two patients with α-HCD,[241,242] one of whom was unresponsive to prior combination chemotherapy.[242] A minimum 6-month trial of tetracycline (1 to 2 g/day) is the prerequisite for establishing responsiveness of the lesion,[228,240] although in cases in which complete remission (chemical, immunologic, and histopathologic) is obtained with antibiotics alone, the clinical improvement occurs early. Maintenance antibiotic treatment is unnecessary. Close surveillance for the early detection of overt lymphomatous transformation is advised.[243] The development of abdominal lymphadenopathy and thickening of the small intestinal wall can be monitored by sequential ultrasound examinations.[244] Of interest is the finding of a persistently abnormal α-chain mRNA, despite an apparently complete clinical, pathologic, and immunopathologic remission after tetracycline therapy in one patient. Consistent with this finding was the subsequent rapid recurrence of α-HCD with transformation to immunoblastic lymphoma.[201]

In patients with stage B or C disease, antiparasitic and antibiotic treatments are also useful for improving the malabsorption syndrome. Patients with stage B or C lesions or stage A lesions without marked improvement after a 6-month course of antibiotic treatment should be given chemotherapy. In a prospective randomized study, a doxorubicin-based regimen (CHOP: cyclophosphamide [Cytoxan], doxorubicin hydrochloride [Adriamycin], vincristine [Oncovin], and prednisone) provided a higher response rate than a non-doxorubicin-containing protocol (C-MOPP: cyclophosphamide, vincristine, procarbazine, prednisone) or total abdominal radiation.[245] Similar results were noted in a retrospective study by Salimi and Spinelli.[246] Encouraging results were obtained in a treatment trial of cyclophosphamide, doxorubicin, teniposide, and prednisone with or without alternation with bleomycin, vinblastine, and doxorubicin.[247] Chemotherapy with CEOP-IMVP-Dexa (cyclophosphamide, epidoxorubicin, vincristine, prednisolone, ifosfamide, VP-16, dexamethasone, methotrexate) resulted in a complete remission in a patient with HCD associated with a high-grade malignant non-Hodgkin's lymphoma.[248]

In a prospective study,[247] 20 of 21 Tunisian patients with α-HCD underwent laparotomy and were staged according to the method of Galian et al.[210] Of the 21 patients, 6 were classified as having stage A, 2 as stage B, and 13 as stage C. The six patients with stage A were first treated with antibiotics alone. Two had complete responses persisting 42 and 55 months later, and the four in whom antibiotics failed underwent chemotherapy, with subsequent failures in all four and two deaths. For stages B and C, combination therapy including doxorubicin led to nine complete remissions with one early relapse, and salvage chemotherapy led to one more complete remission. Survival of the total group was 90 percent at 2 years and 67 percent at 3 years. All patients alive beyond 3.5 years were disease-free.

Akbulut et al.[249] reported 5-year treatment results of 23 Turkish patients with IPSID, including 5 with the secretory type. Seven patients had stage A disease and were treated with tetracycline for a median of 7 months, whereas the remaining 16 patients (9 stage B, 7 stage C) received combination chemotherapy (cyclophosphamide, vincristine, procarbazine, and prednisolone [COPP]). The median follow-up was 68 months. In patients with stage A disease, tetracycline yielded a 71 percent complete response and a 43 percent disease-free survival rate. Of the 16 patients (69 percent) with stage B or C disease who received the COPP regimen, 11 achieved complete response and only 2 had a recurrence (disease-free survival rate of 56 percent). The 5-year overall survival rate for the entire group was 70 percent, and the 5-year disease-free survival rate for patients with a complete response was 75 percent. However, the median overall survival rate for three patients with immunoblastic lymphoma was only 7 months.

Price[250] studied 13 patients who had IPSID associated with α-HCD. Six patients, two with high-grade lymphoma and four with low-grade disease, received chemotherapy or radiation therapy or both. One of these patients died at 76 months, and five were alive (3 disease-free) an average of 92 months after presentation. Five patients, all with low-grade disease, received conservative therapy (antibiotics and in some cases prednisone and total parenteral nutrition). All were alive an average of 40 months after presentation. Three of these five patients achieved histologic remission at 5, 27, and 6 months. Two of the five patients had persistent disease at 25 and 20 months, despite good clinical response. Two patients were not treated and died of high-grade lymphoma.

Shih et al.[251] described six patients who had α-HCD with lymphoma, mainly localized in the jejunum and mesenteric nodes. The histologic subtypes were diffuse large cell in two patients, immunoblastic in three, and diffuse-mixed in one. All patients responded poorly to chemotherapy; the median survival was 10.5 months.

Malik et al.[252] studied 12 patients with IPSID, 6 of whom presented with stage A disease. Four responded to antibiotics or steroids. In two patients, stage A disease evolved into stage C. One patient was lost to follow-up evaluation, and one patient is alive with disease. Of three patients who presented with stage B disease, two responded completely to chemotherapy but the third refused treatment and died after 16 months. Three patients with stage C disease at diagnosis received aggressive combination chemotherapy and remained in complete remission with a median follow-up period of 2.2 years.

Preliminary results suggest that flow cytometric analysis of the S-phase fraction may be useful as a prognostic indicator and in the clinical management of patients with IPSID.[253]

When a focal or bulky transmural lymphomatous tumor is found during staging laparotomy, the bowel segment bearing the tumor may be surgically resected to significantly debulk or prevent perforation or occlusion.[228,254] This approach, followed by combination chemotherapy, may induce complete remission.[150] Because most patients are young, those with disseminated stage C disease showing a good response to conventional or salvage chemotherapy could be candidates for autologous bone marrow transplantation.[255]

It is difficult to evaluate the optimal treatment on the basis of the literature, partly because of the small number of cases in any one study, but mainly because of the poor long-term follow-up evaluation in most series. Because of the rarity of the disease, precise therapeutic protocols performed as multicenter studies are needed.

Follow-up evaluation should include periodic search for α-heavy chain protein in serum and urine and if this is negative, in the intestinal juice. Finally, bowel radiography and esophagogastric-duodenal-jejunal endoscopy with multilevel biopsy samples studied by immunohistochemical techniques should be performed. A second-look laparotomy may be necessary for accurate evaluation.[150] Relapses, sometimes after a long disease-free interval, may occur after treatment at any stage of the disease.

Because antibiotic therapy in the early stage of intestinal α-HCD can result in full clinical remission, awareness of the incidence and increased efforts to detect the disease before the lymphomatous phase are of importance.[243,256–258] The disease may well be eradicated without any medical intervention by improving the socioeconomic status of the underprivileged population in underdeveloped countries.[240]

α-Heavy-Chain Deposition Disease

Cheng et al.[259] described a patient who presented with many of the clinicopathologic features common to patients with γ-HCDD, namely, hypertension, progressive renal failure, and nephrotic syndrome, with a renal biopsy showing crescentic nodular glomerulosclerosis and refractile granular electron-dense deposits in the glomerular and tubular basement membranes. The immune deposits stained for α-Ig heavy chain only but not for γ- and μ-Ig heavy chains and light chains and not with anti-α$_1$ and anti-α$_2$ subclass-specific reagents. On the basis of these findings, the authors hypothesized that the abnormally short α-Ig heavy chain may arise from a genetic mutation that deletes the genomic sequences that encode the C$_H$1 and C$_H$2 domains, which would be similar to the findings in patients with γ-HCDD.

μ-HEAVY-CHAIN DISEASE

μ-Heavy-chain disease is rare. It was first found in a patient with chronic lymphocytic leukemia in 1969.[260,261] Since then, only 31 additional cases have been described in the world literature.[262–266]

Clinical Features

Most patients with μ-HCD are older than 40 years. The median age at the time of diagnosis in 27 patients with μ-HCD was 57.5 years (range, 15 to 80 years).[262] Of the 32 reported patients, 17 were male, and 26 were white, 3 were African-American,[267–269] 2 were Asian,[264,270] and 1 was African.[266] An associated lymphoplasma cell proliferative disorder (chronic lymphocytic leukemia, lymphoma, Waldenström's disease, or myeloma) at some time during the disease was noted in 22 of 27 patients.[262] The μ-HCD protein has been described in one patient each with systemic lupus erythematosus,[271] hepatic cirrhosis,[268] hepatosplenomegaly with ascites,[269] pulmonary infection,[272] splenomegaly with pancytopenia,[267] and myelodysplasia.[265] Although most patients with μ-HCD have an associated lymphoproliferative disorder, μ-chain secretion is a rare feature of chronic lymphocytic leukemia. Bonhomme et al.[267] were unable to detect any cases when they screened more than 150 patients with chronic lymphocytic leukemia for this abnormality.

Splenomegaly and hepatomegaly are common in μ-HCD and have been noted in 21 of 22 and 15 of 21 patients, respectively. Peripheral lymphadenopathy is less frequent and has been described in 10 of 25 patients.[262]

Laboratory Findings

Anemia is frequent, but lymphocytosis and thrombocytopenia are uncommon. Examination of the bone marrow usually shows an increase in lymphocytes, plasma cells, or plasmacytoid lymphocytes. Plasmacytosis was noted in 18 of 20 cases; in 13 of these, vacuolated plasma cells were found.[262] Lytic bone lesions are rare, having been described in 3 of 15 patients[262]; osteoporosis has been mentioned in 3 others.[260,261,273,274] Hypogammaglobulinemia has been noted in 10 of 21 patients.[262] Hyperimmunoglobulinemia with a polyclonal immunoglobulin expansion in the γ-globular fraction has been described in one case.[265]

A monoclonal spike on routine serum protein electrophoresis is found in less than half of the patients (8 of 19).[262] Three of the reported 32 patients had a biclonal gammopathy: IgA κ and μ,[275] IgG and μ,[276] and IgGκ and μ.[271] In contrast to γ- and α-HCD, in which there usually is no detectable monoclonal light chain in the serum and urine, the production of light chains (Bence Jones protein) is found in more than half of patients with μ-HCD. Of 22 patients with μ-HCD, 14 had Bence Jones proteinuria; 11 excreted a κ chain and 2 a λ chain, and in 1 patient the type of light chain was not reported.[262] The μ-HCD protein was found in the urine of only two patients.[267,269]

Bence Jones proteinuria may lead to the occurrence of cast nephropathy. Preud'homme et al.[277] described a patient with μ-HCD in whom renal failure developed after a 3-year follow-up period. Kidney biopsy showed numerous tubular eosinophilic casts that stained for κ-chain determinants by immunofluorescence. Hence, this report paradoxically puts μ-HCD in the list of immunoproliferative disorders with light-chain-related visceral complications.

One patient with hyperglobulinemia and anemia was found to have a positive direct antiglobulin test; however, the anemia was not of autoimmune hemolytic origin. The eluate from the patient's red blood cells contained IgG and an immunoglobulin structure that was reactive with anti-IgM in a red blood cell agglutination assay and with anti-μ antiserum in a nephelometric investigation. Whether this IgM on the patient's erythrocytes was pentameric or oligomeric, complete IgM, or the heavy chain could not be determined from these observations.[265]

Structural Protein Abnormalities

The molecular weight of the μ-HCD protein, which has been determined in eight patients, varied between 26,500 and 158,000.[260,261,267,268,270,274,278–280] The higher molecular weights are believed to be due to polymerization of the μ-chain fragments. The μ-heavy-chain fragments from six patients have been subjected to detailed chemical analysis.[263,280–287] Figure 34–6 depicts the structure of these six μ-HCD proteins compared with that of the normal μ-heavy chain. The V_H domain is absent in all cases. The normal sequence begins with C_H1 in three cases, C_H2 in two cases, and C_H3 in one case. The deletion of protein Gli involves the first 130 residues from the amino terminus.[281] Protein Bw is similar to protein Gli. The sequence begins at amino acid position 5 within the first constant region domain. In protein Bur, the normal amino acid sequence resumes at the very beginning of C_H3.

Proteins Bot[282,283] and Dag[284] are similar in that the normal sequence resumes at the beginning of C_H2 but the deleted chain starts with an aberrant amino acid sequence (extra sequence) displaying no known homology with the protein sequences in the databases currently available. The "extra sequence" of protein Dag consists of 17 amino acids. No homology was detected when the extra sequence of protein Bot containing 42 amino acid residues was compared with the extra sequence of protein Dag.

Figure 34–7 depicts the structure of a μ-HCD-productive gene, RNA transcript, and protein compared with their normal rearranged counterpart.

The reasons for the failure to assemble a complete immunoglobulin are not understood. In studying μ-HCD protein Roul under dissociating conditions, Cogné et al.[263] found monomers and covalent dimers of normal-sized κ chains, but no such free light chains could be detected under nondissociating conditions. Because of the lack of the V region, the interaction between the heavy and light chains might be too weak to promote the formation of the disulfide bridge.

Bakhshi et al.[280,288] suggested that a defect at the level of the Ig gene structure–assembly is responsible for the synthesis of the truncated μ-HCD protein Bw by deleting coding information or formation of an aberrant RNA.

Diagnosis

Without a suspicion for the disease, μ-HCD is difficult to diagnose. The finding of Bence Jones proteinuria in a patient with a lymphoproliferative disorder and vacuolated plasma cells in the bone marrow deserves further investigation for possible μ-HCD. Immunofixation or immunoelectrophoresis of both the serum and urine should be performed. When these procedures yield ambiguous results, two-dimensional gel electrophoresis is a useful additional tool.[176]

Clinical Course

The median duration of survival in μ-HCD from the time of diagnosis is 24 months and ranges from less than 1 month to 11 years.[262] This is in contrast to that in Waldenström's macroglobulinemia, in which the median duration of survival is 5 years.[289] Because several of the reported patients had findings consistent with μ-HCD before recognition of the μ-HCD protein, the course is longer than indicated by the reported survival. μ-

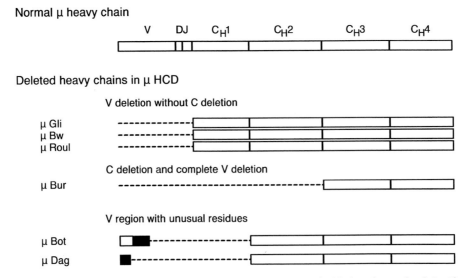

Figure 34–6. Structure of six μ-heavy-chain disease (HCD) proteins compared with that of normal μ chain. Closed bars indicate unusual sequences; dotted lines indicate deletions. V, variable region; D, diversity; J, joining; C_H, constant region. Gli,[281] Bw,[288] Roul,[263] Bur,[285] Bot,[282,283] Dag.[284] (Modified from Cogné et al.,[95,97] with permission.)

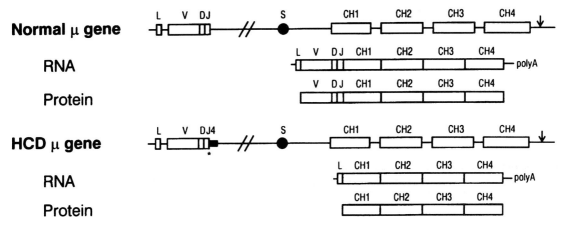

Figure 34–7. Structure of μ heavy-chain disease (HCD) productive gene, RNA transcript, and protein compared with their normal rearranged counterpart. S, switch region; V, variable region; L, leader; CH, constant region; D, diversity; J, joining. Asterisk indicates altered splice site; solid small bar represents insertion in noncoding region. (From Fermand and Brouet,[3] with permission.)

Heavy-chain disease can present as a benign monoclonal gammopathy for years before the development of a lymphoproliferative disorder.[262] In one patient,[279] the hematologic data became normal and the μ-heavy chain disappeared after 2 years without any specific treatment.

Treatment

There is no specific treatment for μ-HCD. Currently, the finding of a μ-HCD protein in the serum of an apparently normal patient should be considered to represent an MGUS and the patient should be followed closely for the development of a symptomatic lymphoplasma-cell proliferative disorder. Once this develops, chemotherapy is necessary. Initially, a combination of cyclophosphamide, vincristine, and prednisone is a reasonable choice. In the event of lack of response, doxorubicin should be added. If the patient presents with a non-lymphoplasma cell proliferative clinical disease, this should be treated according to current standard therapy.

Nonsecretory μ-HCD

Three cases of nonsecretory μ-HCD have been described.[290–292] In a 32-year-old man with follicular center cell lymphoma, immunofluorescence revealed μ chains on the cell surface of proliferative lymphocytes but no detectable light chains. Lysates of lymph node cells incubated with ³H leucine revealed synthesis of μ-chains but no light chains.[290] The labeled μ-chains were not secreted into the culture supernatant. The patient was given chemotherapy.

Immunofluorescence showed only cytoplasmic μ-heavy chains in the bone marrow plasma cells of a 67-year-old woman who presented with lytic bone lesions, anemia, and a serum protein electrophoretic pattern without an M band. Immunoelectrophoresis of serum and urine was negative. The patient was treated with cyclophosphamide and vincristine, and she was still alive and reported to be in satisfactory condition after 16 months.[291]

Similarly, cytoplasmic μ-heavy chains without light chains were detected by immunofluorescence in all bone marrow plasma cells of a 50-year-old man with weight loss, fever, splenomegaly, and 45 percent immature plasma cells in the bone marrow. Immunoelectrophoresis revealed no abnormality in either serum or urine. The patient was treated with melphalan, cyclophosphamide, and prednisone and later with vincristine and doxorubicin. He died 3 ¹/₂ months after diagnosis.[292]

μ-Heavy-Chain Deposition Disease

Liapis et al.[293] described a 68-year-old Greek woman with hypertension, decreased renal clearance, and proteinuria. No abnormal protein was detected in her serum, and Bence Jones protein was not found in her urine. A renal biopsy performed to evaluate the cause of the proteinuria showed nodular glomerulosclerosis. Monotypic μ heavy-chain mesangial deposits without κ or λ chains were identified by immunofluorescence. No evaluation was done to determine whether the deposited μ-heavy chain was normal or deleted. Two years after the diagnosis, the patient had stable renal disease and had not required dialysis.

δ-HEAVY-CHAIN DISEASE

One case of δ-HCD has been described by Vilpo et al.[294] This patient presented with renal insufficiency and features of multiple myeloma. Osteolytic lesions were seen in the skull, and the bone marrow contained abnormal plasma cells. Serum protein electrophoresis revealed a small, localized band migrating between β_2 and γ, which was identified as a tetramer of δ heavy chains. No monoclonal light chains were found. On the basis of molecular weight calculations, the δ chains appeared complete, but a partial deletion could not be excluded. The possibility that the δ-heavy chain represented a degradation product from an intact IgD monoclonal protein could not be excluded. The susceptibility of δ-chains to cleavage has been demonstrated.[295]

Rabhi et al.[296] described a patient with clinical, hematologic, and radiologic features of multiple myeloma in whom spontaneous enzymatic cleavage of IgD myeloma protein simulated δ-HCD. The M component in the serum reacted with IgD antiserum. The failure to react with anti-light-chain antisera, observed by immunoelectrophoresis, immunofixation, and rocket-immunoselection, strongly suggested δ-HCD. However, further analysis by crossed-immunoelectrophoresis demonstrated the presence of a light chain. It then became obvious that the observed pattern was generated by enzymatic cleavage of native IgD myeloma protein.

ACKNOWLEDGMENT

Supported in part by Research Grant CA 62242 from the National Institutes of Health.

REFERENCES

1. Franklin EC, Lowenstein J, Bigelow B, Meltzer M: Heavy chain disease – a new disorder of serum γ-globulins: Report of the first case. Am J Med 37:332, 1964.
2. Fermand JP, Brouet JC, Danon F, Seligmann M: Gamma heavy chain "disease": heterogeneity of the clinicopathologic features. Report of 16 cases and review of the literature. Medicine (Baltimore) 68:321, 1989.
3. Fermand JP, Brouet JC: Heavy-chain diseases. Hematol Oncol Clin North Am 13:1281, 1999.
4. Bender SW, Danon F, Preud'homme JL et al: Gamma heavy chain disease simulating alpha chain disease. Gut 19:1148, 1978.
5. Bloch KJ, Lee L, Mills JA, Haber E: Gamma heavy chain disease – an expanding clinical and laboratory spectrum. Am J Med 55:61, 1973.
6. Dammacco F, Rigoli E, Ferrarese M, Bonomo L: Gamma heavy chain disease in a young girl. Haematologica 61:278, 1976.
7. Pruzanski W, Parr DM, Prchal J, Chan EY: Gamma 3-heavy-chain disease (gamma 3-HCD) in a young patient with Down syndrome. Study of peripheral blood lymphocytes and of susceptibility to infection. Clin Immunol Immunopathol 12:253, 1979.
8. Rabin BS, Moon J: Clinical findings in a case of newly defined gamma heavy chain disease protein. Clin Exp Immunol 14:563, 1973.
9. Woods R, Blumenschein GR, Terry WD: A new type of human gamma heavy chain disease protein: Immunochemical and physical characteristics. Immunochemistry 7:373, 1970.
10. Wester SM, Banks PM, Li CY: The histopathology of gamma heavy-chain disease. Am J Clin Pathol 78:427, 1982.
11. Gallart MT, Canals J, Canadell E et al: A new case of gamma-heavy chain disease. Acta Haematol 59:262, 1978.
12. Lassoued K, Picard C, Danon F et al: Cutaneous manifestations associated with gamma heavy chain disease. Report of an unusual case and review of literature. J Am Acad Dermatol 23:988, 1990.
13. Kyle RA, Greipp PR, Banks PM: The diverse picture of gamma heavy-chain disease. Report of seven cases and review of literature. Mayo Clin Proc 56:439, 1981.
14. Osserman EF, Takatsuki K: Clinical and immunochemical studies of four cases of heavy (Hγ²) chain disease. Am J Med 37:351, 1964.
15. Roda L, David MJ, Biron P et al: Gamma heavy chain disease DUB: Clinical, immunochemical and pathological studies. Haematologica 70:232, 1985.
16. Dickson JR, Harth M, Bell DA et al: Gamma heavy chain disease and rheumatoid arthritis. Semin Arthritis Rheum 18:247, 1989.
17. Kanoh T, Takigawa M, Niwa Y: Cutaneous lesions in gamma heavy-chain disease. Arch Dermatol 124:1538, 1988.
18. Kanoh T, Nakasato H: Osteolytic gamma heavy chain disease. Eur J Haematol 39:60, 1987.
19. Case records of the Massachusetts General Hospital (Case 50-1970). N Engl J Med 283:1332, 1970.
20. O'Conor GT Jr, Wyandt HE, Innes DJ et al: Gamma heavy chain disease: Report of a case associated with trisomy of chromosome 7. Cancer Genet Cytogenet 15:1, 1985.
21. Westin J, Eyrich R, Falsen E et al: Gamma heavy chain disease. Reports of three patients. Acta Med Scand 192:281, 1972.
22. Matsubayashi S, Tamai H, Suzuki T et al: Extramedullary plasmacytoma of the thyroid gland producing gamma heavy chain. Endocrinol Jpn 32:427, 1985.
23. Otto S, Peter I, Vegh S et al: Gamma-chain heavy-chain disease with primary thyroid plasmacytoma. Arch Pathol Lab Med 110:893, 1986.
24. Rouesse J, Gerard-Marchant R, Chevalier A, Seligmann M: Gamma heavy chain disease with thyroid involvement. Rev Eur Etud Clin Biol 17:405, 1972.
25. Faguet GB, Barton BP, Smith LL, Garver FA: Gamma heavy chain disease: Clinical aspects and characterization of a deleted, noncovalently linked gamma 1 heavy chain dimer (BAZ). Blood 49:495, 1977.
26. Blum DJ, Doyle JA, Greipp PR, McDonald TJ: Gamma heavy-chain disease involving upper airway. Otolaryngol Head Neck Surg 93:677, 1985.
27. Ieko M, Kohno M, Ohmoto A et al: Gamma-heavy chain disease associated with MALT lymphoma of the duodenum. Rinsho Ketsueki 39:512, 1998.
28. Papae RJ, Rosenstein RW, Richards F, Yesner R: Gamma heavy chain disease seen initially as gastric neoplasm. Arch Intern Med 138:1151, 1978.
29. Roda L, David MJ, Souche S et al: Gamma 3 heavy chain disease and monoclonal IgMκ in a patient with a gastrointestinal lymphoma. Haematologica 70:115, 1985.
30. Virella G, Monteiro JM, Lopes-Virella MF et al: Asynchronous development of two monoclonal proteins (IgM lambda and delta 1 chains) in a patient with abdominal lymphoma. Cancer 39:2247, 1977.
31. Zawadzki ZA, Benedek TG, Ein D, Easton JM: Rheumatoid arthritis terminating in a heavy-chain disease. Ann Intern Med 70:335, 1969.
32. Loyau G, Barre JP, L'Hirondel JL, Maniece M, Preud'Homme JL: Gamma heavy chain disease. A new case. Nouv Presse Med 4:957, 1975.
33. Gaucher A, Bertrand F, Brouet JC et al: Gamma heavy chain disease associated with rheumatoid arthritis. Spontaneous disappearance of the pathologic protein. Semin Hop 53:2117, 1977.
34. Creyssel R, Brizard CP, Gibaud A et al: Maladie des chaines lourdes gamma d'apparition secondaire au cours de l'evolution d'une macroglobulinemie. Lyon Med 237:215, 1977.
35. Kretschmer RR, Pizzuto J, Gonzalez J, Lopez M: Heavy chain disease, rheumatoid arthritis and cryoglobulinemia. Clin Immunol Immunopathol 2:195, 1974.
36. Chernokhvostova EV, German GP, Varlamova E et al: An unusual case of heavy gamma-chain disease with several monoclonal components: IgG kappa, IgM lambda, Bence-Jones proteins kappa and lambda. Ter Arkh 63:80, 1991.
37. Ibuka T, Shimoyama M, Sakano T et al: Gamma heavy chain disease: Report of a case. Jpn J Clin Hematol 15:671, 1974.
38. Jacqueline F, Renversez JC, Groslambert P, Fine JM: Gamma heavy chain disease during rheumatoid polyarthritis. A clinical and immunochemical study. Rev Rhum Mal Osteoartic 45:661, 1978.

39. Stuhlinger W, Berek K, Lapin A et al: Gamma 1 heavy chain disease with immune vasculitis and rheumatoid arthritis. Klin Wochenschr 65:359, 1987.

40. Ockhuizen T, Smit JW, van Leeuwen M: Rheumatoid arthritis associated with transient gamma 2-heavy chain disease. Rheumatol Int 3:167, 1983.

41. Husby G, Blichfeldt P, Brinch L et al: Chronic arthritis and gamma heavy chain disease: Coincidence or pathogenic link? Scand J Rheumatol 27:257, 1998

42. Husby G: Is there a pathogenic link between gamma heavy chain disease and chronic arthritis? Curr Opin Rheumatol 12:65, 2000.

43. Jones WG, Elvy RJ, Pedersen N: Heavy-chain disease in Australia (letter). Lancet 1:570, 1974.

44. Cooper DL, Bolognia JL, Lin JT: Atrophie blanche in a patient with gamma-heavy-chain disease (letter). Arch Dermatol 127:272, 1991.

45. Wager O, Rasanen JA, Lindeberg L, Makela V: Two cases of IgG heavy-chain disease. Acta Pathol Microbiol Scand 75:350, 1969.

46. Castelino D, Gray F, D'Apice A et al: Primary Sjögren's syndrome and gamma heavy chain disease. Pathology 26:337, 1994.

47. Lyons RM, Chaplin H, Tillack TW, Majerus PW: Gamma heavy chain disease: Rapid, sustained response to cyclophosphamide and prednisone. Blood 46:1, 1975.

48. Ellman LL, Bloch KJ: Heavy-chain disease. Report of a seventh case. N Engl J Med 278:1195, 1968.

49. Leloup E, Gallinari C, Bouchon JP, Benis Y: Heavy gamma-chain diseases. A new case and review of the literature. Ann Med Interne (Paris) 140:274, 1989.

50. Adlersberg JB, Grann V, Zucker-Franklin D et al: An unusual case of a plasma cell neoplasm with an IgG3 lambda myeloma and a gamma 3 heavy chain disease protein. Blood 51:85, 1978.

51. Pontet F, Gue X, Dosquet C et al: Rapid evolution in the immunochemical findings of a gamma heavy chain disease. Clin Chem 34:439, 1988.

52. Ellis VM, Cowley DM, Taylor KM, Marlton P: Gamma heavy chain disease developing in association with myelodysplastic syndrome. Br J Haematol 81:125, 1992.

53. Chury Z, Jansa P, Jedlickova J et al: A contribution to Franklin's disease. Folia Haematol Int Mag Klin Morphol Blutforsch 96:43, 1971.

54. Baker AS, Lankford P, Krantz SB, Buchanan RD: Gamma heavy chain disease – presenting as pancytopenia and splenomegaly. South Med J 70:495, 1977.

55. Kuroyanagi T, Kura K, Akamatsu Y, Arao T: A case report of the immunodysplasia syndrome and heavy chain disease associated with subacute bacterial endocarditis. Tohoku J Exp Med 128:325, 1979.

56. Shirakura T, Kobayashi Y, Murai Y et al: A case of gamma heavy chain disease associated with autoimmune haemolytic anaemia: Clinical, haematological, immunological and pathological details. Scand J Haematol 16:387, 1976.

57. Keller H, Spengler GA, Skvaril F et al: Heavy chain disease. A case of IgG-heavy-chain-fragment and IgM-type K-paraproteinemia with plasma cell leukemia. Schweiz Med Wochenschr 100:1012, 1970.

58. Solling K, Askjaer SA: Multiple myeloma with urinary excretion of heavy chain components of IgG and nodular glomerulosclerosis. Acta Med Scand 1–2:23, 1973.

59. Ruiz-Arguelles A, Valls-de-Ruiz M, Dominguez-Barranco A et al: 'Incomplete' pyroglobulin-gamma disease in a patient with osteosclerotic myeloma. Scand J Haematol 33:351, 1984.

60. Van Bergeijk L, Biewenga J, Langenhuijsen MM: Gamma heavy chain disease with an unusually benign course. Clin Lab Haematol 2:83, 1980.

61. Prevot P, Loyau G, Heron JP et al: Gamma heavy chain disease. A recent case with plasmocytic proliferation and cranial lacunae. Ann Med Interne (Paris) 128:151, 1977.

62. Eisner SB, Mitnick PD: Hypercalcemia and reversible renal failure in heavy-chain disease. South Med J 79:507, 1986.

63. Ogawa K, Imai M, Tanigawa T et al: Pathological studies on a long-term survived case of gamma heavy chain disease – a brief review of 30 reported cases and a proposal for histological typing. Acta Pathol Jpn 28:759, 1978.

64. Schur PH: Human gamma-G subclasses. Prog Clin Immunol 1:71, 1972.

65. Hauke G, Schiltz E, Bross KJ et al: Unusual sequence of immunoglobulin L-chain rearrangements in a gamma heavy chain disease patient. Scand J Immunol 36:463, 1992.

66. Charles EZ, Valdes AJ: Free fragments of gamma chain in the urine. A possible source of confusion with gamma heavy-chain disease. Am J Clin Pathol 101:462, 1994.

67. Delmas-Marsalet Y, Voisin D, Hennache G et al: Clinical and biological study of heavy gamma chain disease. A propos of a new case. Nouv Rev Fr Hematol 11:717, 1971.

68. Seligmann M, Mihaesco E, Preud'homme JL et al: Heavy chain diseases: Current findings and concepts. Immunol Rev 48:145, 1979.

69. Alexander A, Anicito I, Buxbaum J: Gamma heavy chain disease in man. Genomic sequence reveals two noncontiguous deletions in a single gene. J Clin Invest 82:1244, 1988.

70. Frangione B, Rosenwasser E, Prelli F, Franklin EC: Primary structure of human gamma 3 immunoglobulin deletion mutant: Gamma 3 heavy-chain disease protein Wis. Biochemistry 19:4304, 1980.

71. Franklin EC, Prelli F, Frangione B: Human heavy chain disease protein WIS: Implications for the organization of immunoglobulin genes. Proc Natl Acad Sci U S A 76:452, 1979.

72. Wolfenstein-Todel C, Frangione B, Prelli F, Franklin EC: The amino acid sequence of "heavy chain disease" protein ZUC. Structure of the Fc fragment of immunoglobulin G3. Biochem Biophys Res Commun 71:907, 1976.

73. Frangione B: A new immunoglobulin variant: Gamma 3 heavy chain disease protein CHI. Proc Natl Acad Sci U S A 73:1552, 1976.

74. Frangione B, Franklin EC: Correlation between fragmented immunoglobulin genes and heavy chain deletion mutants. Nature 281:600, 1979.

75. Franklin EC, Kyle R, Seligmann M, Frangione B: Correlation of protein structure and immunoglobulin gene organization in the light of two new deleted heavy chain disease proteins. Mol Immunol 16:919, 1979.

76. Frangione B, Lee L, Haber E, Bloch KJ: Protein Hal: Partial deletion of a "γ" immunoglobulin gene(s) and apparent reinitiation at an internal AUG codon. Proc Natl Acad Sci U S A 70:1073, 1973.

77. Smith LL, Barton BP, Garver FA et al: Physicochemical and immunochemical properties of gamma 1 heavy chain disease protein BAZ. Immunochemistry 15:323, 1978.

78. Calvanico N, Rabin B, Plaut A, Tomasi TB Jr: Studies on a new gamma heavy chain disease protein (Abstr.). Fed Proc J 31:771, 1972.

79. Frangione B, Franklin EC, Smithies O: Unusual genes at the aminoterminus of human immunoglobulin variants. Nature 273:400, 1978.

80. Nabeshima Y, Ikenaka T: N- and C-terminal amino acid sequences of a gamma-heavy chain disease protein YOK. Immunochemistry 13:245, 1976.

81. Arnaud P, Wang AC, Gianazza E et al: Gamma heavy chain disease protein CHA: Immunological and structural studies. Mol Immunol 18:379, 1981.

82. Cooper SM, Franklin EC, Frangione B: Molecular defect in a gamma-2 heavy chain. Science 176:187, 1972.

83. Terry WD, Ohms J: Implications of heavy chain disease protein sequences for multiple gene theories of immunoglobulin synthesis. Proc Natl Acad Sci U S A 66:558, 1970.

84. Guglielmi P, Bakhshi A, Cogné M et al: Multiple genomic defects result in an alternative RNA splice creating a human gamma H chain disease protein. J Immunol 141:1762, 1988.

85. Biewenga J, Frangione B, Franklin EC, van Loghem E: A gamma 1 heavy-chain disease protein (EST) lacking the entire VH and CHI domains. Scand J Immunol 11:601, 1980.

86. Franklin EC, Frangione B: The molecular defect in a protein (CRA) found in gamma-1 heavy chain disease, and its genetic implications. Proc Natl Acad Sci U S A 68:187, 1971.

87. Prelli F, Frangione B: Franklin's disease: Ig gamma 2 H chain mutant BUR. J Immunol 148:949, 1992.

88. Khamlichi AA, Aucouturier P, Preud'homme JL, Cogné M: Structure of abnormal heavy chains in human heavy-chain-deposition disease. Eur J Biochem 229:54, 1995.

89. Eulitz M, Weiss DT, Solomon A: Immunoglobulin heavy-chain-associated amyloidosis. Proc Natl Acad Sci U S A 87:6542, 1990.

90. Solomon A, Weiss DT, Murphy C: Primary amyloidosis associated with a novel heavy-chain fragment (AH amyloidosis). Am J Hematol 45:171, 1994.

91. Alexander A, Steinmetz M, Barritault D et al: Gamma heavy chain disease in man: cDNA sequence supports partial gene deletion model. Proc Natl Acad Sci U S A 79:3260, 1982.

92. Cogné M, Bakhshi A, Korsmeyer SJ, Guglielmi P: Gene mutations and alternate RNA splicing result in truncated Ig L chains in human gamma H chain disease. J Immunol 141:1738, 1988.

93. Hauke G, Krawinkel U, Schiltz E et al: Gamma-1 heavy chain disease with the demonstration of Bence-Jones proteins. Immun Infekt 19:89, 1991.

94. Preud'homme JL, Brouet JC, Seligmann M: Cellular immunoglobulins in human gamma- and alpha-heavy chain diseases. Clin Exp Immunol 37:283, 1979.

95. Cogné M, Silvain C, Khamlichi AA, Preud'homme JL: Structurally abnormal immunoglobulins in human immunoproliferative disorders. Blood 79:2181, 1992.

96. Hendershot L, Bole D, Kohler G, Kearney JF: Assembly and secretion of heavy chains that do not associate posttranslationally with immunoglobulin heavy chain-binding protein. J Cell Biol 104:761, 1987.

97. Cogné M, Preud'homme JL, Guglielmi P: Immunoglobulin gene alterations in human heavy chain diseases. Res Immunol 140:487, 1989.

98. Moskovits T, Jacobson DR, Buxbaum J: N-ras oncogene activation in a patient with gamma heavy chain disease (letter). Am J Hematol 41:302, 1992.

99. Cozzolino F, Vercelli D, Castigli E et al: A new case of gamma-heavy chain disease. Clinical and immunochemical studies. Scand J Haematol 28:145, 1982.

100. Di Benedetto G, Cataldi A, Verde A et al: Gamma heavy chain disease associated with Hodgkin's disease. Clinical, pathologic, and immunologic features of one case. Cancer 63:1804, 1989.

101. Sun T, Peng S, Narurkar L: Modified immunoselection technique for definitive diagnosis of heavy-chain disease. Clin Chem 40:664, 1994.

102. Blangarin P, Deviller P, Kindbeiter K, Madjar JJ: Gamma heavy chain disease studied by two-dimensional electrophoresis and immuno-blotting techniques. Clin Chem 30:2021, 1984.

103. Mitchell PE, Ford RP, Coughtrie MW et al: A case of heavy chain disease: Diagnosis and monitoring using assays of immunoglobulin heavy and light chains. Scott Med J 35:18, 1990.

104. Tissot JD, Tridon A, Ruivard M et al: Electrophoretic analyses in a case of monoclonal gamma chain disease. Electrophoresis 19:1771, 1998.

105. Albutt EC, Hawker PC, Hine KR, Northam BE: Diagnosis of gamma heavy-chain disease. Ann Clin Biochem 18:207, 1981.

106. Lenders JW, Holdrinet RS, Nguyen CT, De Waal R: A case of gamma-heavy chain monoclonal gammopathy of undetermined significance. Neth J Med 27:412, 1984.

107. Galanti LM, Doyen C, Vander Maelen C et al: Biological diagnosis of a gamma-1-heavy chain disease in an asymptomatic patient (letter). Eur J Haematol 54:202, 1995.

108. Biewenga J, van Loghem E: A new case of gamma-3 heavy chain disease. Biochemical and immunological investigations. Vox Sang 36:193, 1979.

109. Agrawal S, Abboudi Z, Matutes E, Catovsky D: First report of fludarabine in gamma-heavy chain disease. Br J Haematol 88:653, 1994.

110. Ishikawa K, Hirai M, Tsutsumi H et al: Successful treatment of heavy-chain disease with etoposide. Nippon Ronen Igakkai Zasshi 34:221, 1997.

111. Kyle RA, Robinson RA, Katzmann JA: The clinical aspects of biclonal gammopathies. Review of 57 cases. Am J Med 71:999, 1981.

112. Pick AI, Shoenfeld Y, Frohlichmann R et al: Plasma cell dyscrasia. Analysis of 423 patients. JAMA 241:2275, 1979.

113. Creyssel R, Gibaud A, Arnaud Ph, Cordier JF: Gammapathies biclonales et oligoclonales: Problèmes posés par la coexistence chez le même sujet de plusieurs constituants immunoglobuliniques d'hétérogénéité restreinte. Lyon Med 236:101, 1976.

114. Presti BC, Sciotto CG, Marsh SG: Lymphocytic lymphoma with associated gamma heavy chain and IgM-lambda paraproteins. An unusual biclonal gammopathy. Am J Clin Pathol 93:137, 1990.

115. Feremans W, Caudron M, Bieva C: A case of gamma 3 heavy chain disease with vacuolated plasma cells: A clinical, immunological, and ultrastructural study. J Clin Pathol 32:334, 1979.

116. Wang AC, Arnaud P, Fudenberg HH, Creyssel R: Monoclonal IgM cryoglobulinemia associated with gamma-3 heavy chain disease: Immunochemical and biochemical studies. Eur J Immunol 8:375, 1978.

117. Ockhuizen T, Jilderda JF, Cazemier T: Sequential development of Waldenström's macroglobulinemia and gamma-1-heavy chain disease in a single patient. Clinical, immunochemical, immunofluorescent and protein studies. Acta Haematol 71:53, 1984.

118. Fine JM, Zakin MM, Faure A, Boffa GA: Myeloma with a serum gamma G paraprotein and urinary elimination of a fragment of gamma G devoid of light chains. Rev Fr Etud Clin Biol 13:175, 1968.

119. Guardia J, Rubies-Prat J, Gallart MT et al: The evolution of alpha heavy chain disease. Am J Med 60:596, 1976.

120. Isobe T, Osserman EF: Plasma cell dyscrasia associated with the production of incomplete IgG lambda molecules, gamma heavy chains, and free lambda chains containing carbohydrate: Description of the first case. Blood 43:505, 1974.

121. Lebreton JP, Rivat C, Rivat L et al: An unrecognized immunoglobulinopathy: Heavy chain disease. Presse Med 75:2251, 1967.

122. Lebreton JP, Fontaine M, Rousseaux J et al: Deleted IgG1 and IgG2 H chains in a patient with an IgG subclass imbalance. Clin Exp Immunol 47:206, 1982.

123. Van Camp BG, Shuit HR, Hijmans W, Radl J: The cellular basis of double paraproteinemia in man. Clin Immunol Immunopathol 9:111, 1978.

124. Buxbaum JN, Chuba JV, Hellman GC et al: Monoclonal immunoglobulin deposition disease: Light chain and light and

heavy chain deposition diseases and their relation to light chain amyloidosis. Clinical features, immunopathology, and molecular analysis. Ann Intern Med 112:455, 1990.

125. Tubbs RR, Berkley V, Valenzuela R et al: Pseudo-gamma heavy chain (IgG4 lambda) deposition disease. Mod Pathol 5:185, 1992.

126. Aucouturier P, Khamlichi AA, Touchard G et al: Brief report: Heavy-chain deposition disease. N Engl J Med 329:1389, 1993.

127. Katz A, Zent R, Bargman JM: IgG heavy-chain deposition disease. Mod Pathol 7:874, 1994.

128. Yasuda T, Fujita K, Imai H et al: Gamma-heavy chain deposition disease showing nodular glomerulosclerosis. Clin Nephrol 44:394, 1995.

129. Mougenot B, Brouet JC, Ronco PM et al: Kidney deposition of immunoglobulin truncated heavy chains (Abstr.). J Am Soc Nephrol 4:684, 1983.

130. Moulin B, Deret S, Mariette X et al: Nodular glomerulosclerosis with deposition of monoclonal immunoglobulin heavy chains lacking C_H1. J Am Soc Nephrol 10:519, 1999.

131. Rott T, Vizjak A, Lindic J et al: IgG heavy-chain deposition disease affecting kidney, skin, and skeletal muscle. Nephrol Dial Transplant 13:1825, 1998.

132. Herzenberg AM, Lien J, Magil AB: Monoclonal heavy chain (immunoglobulin G3) deposition disease: Report of a case. Am J Kidney Dis 28:128, 1996.

133. Kambham N, Markowitz GS, Appel GB et al: Heavy chain deposition disease: The disease spectrum. Am J Kidney Dis 33:954, 1999.

134. Strom EH, Fogazzi GB, Banfi G et al: Light chain deposition disease of the kidney. Morphological aspects in 24 patients. Virchows Arch 425:271, 1994.

135. Polski JM, Galvin N, Salinas-Madrigal L: Non-amyloid fibrils in heavy chain deposition disease (letter). Kidney Int 56:1601, 1999.

136. Preud'homme JL, Aucouturier P, Touchard G et al: Monoclonal immunoglobulin deposition disease: A review of immunoglobulin chain alterations. Int J Immunopharmacol 16:425, 1994.

137. Preud'homme JL, Aucouturier P, Touchard G et al: Monoclonal immunoglobulin deposition disease (Randall type). Relationship with structural abnormalities of immunoglobulin chains (editorial). Kidney Int 46:965, 1994.

138. Seligmann M, Danon F, Hurez D et al: Alpha-chain disease: A new immunoglobulin abnormality. Science 162:1396, 1968.

139. Seligmann M: Heavy chain diseases. Rev Prat 43:317, 1993.

140. Reyes-del Pozo E, Larrea-Ramirez P, Leòn-Barùa R: Linfoma maligno primario difuso del intestino delgado. Arch Peruanos Pat Clin 16:297, 1962.

141. Larrea-Ramirez P, Leòn-Barùa R, Reyes-del Pozo E: Linfoma maligno primario difuso del intestino delgado con sindrome de mala absorcion. Arch Peruanos Pat Clin 17:223, 1963.

142. Arista-Nasr J, Gonzalez-Romo MA, Mantilla-Morales A et al: Immunoproliferative small intestinal disease in Mexico. Report of four cases and review of the literature. J Clin Gastroenterol 18:67, 1994.

143. Savilahti E, Brandtzaeg P, Kuitunen P: Atypical intestinal alpha-chain disease evolving into selective immunoglobulin A deficiency in a Finnish boy. Gastroenterology 79:1303, 1980.

144. Stoop JW, Ballieux RE, Hijmans W, Zegers BJ: Alpha-chain disease with involvement of the respiratory tract in a Dutch child. Clin Exp Immunol 9:625, 1971.

145. Faux JA, Crain JD, Rosen FS, Merler E: An alpha heavy chain abnormality in a child with hypogammaglobulinemia. Clin Immunol Immunopathol 1:282, 1973.

146. Joller PW, Joller-Jemelka HI, Shmerling DH, Skvaril F: Immunological and biochemical studies of an unusual alpha heavy chain protein in a 9-year-old boy. J Clin Lab Immunol 15:167, 1984.

147. Bowie MD, Hill ID: Alpha-chain disease in children. J Pediatr 112:46, 1988.

148. Altuntas B, Ensari A: Alpha heavy chain disease in a child. Pediatr Int 42:306, 2000.

149. Geraci L, Merlini G, Spadano A et al: Alpha heavy chain disease: Report of two cases. Haematologica 70:431, 1985.

150. Rambaud JC, Halphen M, Galian A, Tsapis A: Immunoproliferative small intestinal disease (IPSID): Relationships with alpha-chain disease and "Mediterranean" lymphomas. Springer Semin Immunopathol 12:239, 1990.

151. Harzic M, Girard-Pipau F, Halphen M et al: Bacteriological, parasitological and virological study of the digestive flora in alpha-chain disease. Gastroenterol Clin Biol 9:472, 1985.

152. Ramot B, Rechavi G: Non-Hodgkin's lymphomas and paraproteinaemias. Baillieres Clin Haematol 5:81, 1992.

153. Rambaud JC, Matuchansky C: Alpha-chain disease: Pathogenesis and relation to Mediterranean lymphoma. Lancet 1:1430, 1973.

154. Seligmann M, Rambaud J-C: α-Chain disease: A possible model for the pathogenesis of human lymphomas. In Twomey JJ, Good RA (eds.): The Immunopathology of Lymphoreticular Neoplasms. Comprehensive Immunology, Vol. 4, p. 425. Plenum, New York, 1978.

155. Al-Saleem TI: Evidence of acquired immune deficiencies in Mediterranean lymphoma. A possible aetiological link. Lancet 2:709, 1978.

156. Arista-Nasr J, Armando G, Hernandez-Pando R: Immunoproliferative small intestinal disease. Report of a case with immunohistochemical and ultrastructural study. Rev Invest Clin 45:275, 1993.

157. Rouhier D, Andre C, Allard C et al: Malignant alpha chain disease and exposure to asbestos. Environ Res 27:222, 1982.

158. Baddoura FK, Unger ER, Mufarrij A et al: Latent Epstein-Barr virus infection is an unlikely event in the pathogenesis of immunoproliferative small intestinal disease. Cancer 74:1699, 1994.

159. Sala P, Tonutti E, Mazzolini S et al: Alpha-heavy chain disease: Report of a case with spontaneous regression. Scand J Haematol 31:149, 1983.

160. Selzer G, Sacks M, Sherman G, Naggan L: Primary malignant lymphoma of the small intestine in Israel. Changing incidence with time. Isr J Med Sci 15:390, 1979.

161. Alsabti EA: Paraproteinemia in normal family members of eight cases with primary intestinal lymphomas in Iraq. Oncology 35:68, 1978.

162. Alsabti EA, Safo MH, Shaheen A: Lymphocytes subpopulation in normal family members of patients with alpha-chain disease. J Surg Oncol 11:365, 1979.

163. Kharazmi A, Rezai MH, Abadi P et al: T and B lymphocytes in alpha-chain disease. Br J Cancer 37:48, 1978.

164. Nikbin B, Banisadre M, Ala F, Mojtabai A: HLA AW19, B12 in immunoproliferative small intestinal disease. Gut 20:226, 1979.

165. Rambaud JC, Seligmann M: Alpha-chain disease. Clin Gastroenterol 5:341, 1976.

166. Comelli AM, Paris B: Alpha heavy chain disease: A clinical study of 3 cases and review of the literature. G Clin Med 71:339, 1990.

167. Rambaud JC, Galian A, Matuchansky C et al: Natural history of alpha-chain disease and the so-called Mediterranean lymphoma. Recent Results Cancer Res 64:271, 1978.

168. Tabbane S, Tabbane F, Cammoun M, Mourali N: Mediterranean lymphomas with alpha heavy chain monoclonal gammopathy. Cancer 38:1989, 1976.

169. Al-Bahrani Z, Al-Saleem T, Al-Mondhiry H et al: Alpha heavy chain disease (report of 18 cases from Iraq). Gut 19:627, 1978.

170. Florin-Christensen A, Doniach D, Newcomb PB: Alpha-chain disease with pulmonary manifestations. BMJ 2:413, 1974.

171. Takahashi K, Naito M, Matsuoka Y, Takatsuki K: A new form of alpha-chain disease with generalized lymph node involvement. Pathol Res Pract 183:717, 1988.

172. Furuta T, Ooba Y, Hirai R, Tezuka T: A case of alpha chain disease with infiltrative erythema and splenomegaly. Clin Hemat 23:206, 1982.

173. Itoh Y, Ohtaki H, Ono T et al: A case of lymphoma-type alpha-chain disease. Acta Haematol 86:107, 1991.

174. Tezuka T, Hirai R, Takahashi M et al: Alpha-heavy-chain disease with erythematous skin lesions. Arch Dermatol 122:1243, 1986.

175. Lucidarme D, Colombel JF, Brandtzaeg P et al: Alpha-chain disease: Analysis of alpha-chain protein and secretory component in jejunal fluid. Gastroenterology 104:278, 1993.

176. Tracy RP, Kyle RA, Young DS: Two-dimensional gel electrophoresis as an aid in the analysis of monoclonal gammopathies. Hum Pathol 15:122, 1984.

177. Sakka T, Meknini B, Ayed K et al: An unusual case of heavy alpha chain disease associated with amyloidosis. Tunis Med 64:161, 1986.

178. Doe WF, Henry K, Hobbs JR et al: Five cases of alpha chain disease. Gut 13:947, 1972.

179. Al-Mondhiry H: Primary lymphomas of the small intestine: East-West contrast. Am J Hematol 22:89, 1986.

180. Matsumoto T, Iida M, Matsui T et al: The value of double-contrast study of the small intestine in immunoproliferative small intestinal disease. Gastrointest Radiol 15:159, 1990.

181. Halphen M, Najjar T, Jaafoura H et al: Diagnostic value of upper intestinal fiber endoscopy in primary small intestinal lymphoma. A prospective study by the Tunisian-French Intestinal Lymphoma Group. Cancer 58:2140, 1986.

182. Seligmann M: Immunochemical, clinical, and pathological features of alpha-chain disease. Arch Intern Med 135:78, 1975.

183. Rambaud JC, Halphen M: Immunoproliferative small intestinal disease (IPSID): Relationships with alpha-chain disease and "Mediterranean" lymphomas. Gastroenterol Int 2:33, 1989.

184. Coulbois J, Galian P, Galian A et al: Gastric form of alpha chain disease. Gut 27:719, 1986.

185. Rambaud JC, Galian A, Danon FG et al: Alpha-chain disease without qualitative serum IgA abnormality. Report of two cases, including a "nonsecretory" form. Cancer 51:686, 1983.

186. Hibi T, Asakura H, Kobayashi K et al: Alpha heavy chain disease lacking secretory alpha chain, with cobblestone appearance of the small intestine and duodenal ulcer demonstrated by endoscopy. Gut 23:422, 1982.

187. Seligmann M, Mihaesco E, Hurez D et al: Immunochemical studies in four cases of alpha chain disease. J Clin Invest 48:2374, 1969.

188. Brandtzaeg P, Savilahti E: Further evidence for a role of secretory component (SC) and J chain in the glandular transport of IgA. Adv Exp Med Biol 107:219, 1978.

189. Berger R, Bernheim A, Tsapis A et al: Cytogenetic studies in four cases of alpha chain disease. Cancer Genet Cytogenet 22:219, 1986.

190. Pellet P, Berger R, Bernheim A et al: Molecular analysis of a t(9;14)(p11;q32) translocation occurring in a case of human alpha heavy chain disease. Oncogene 4:653, 1989.

191. Pellet P, Tsapis A, Brouet JC: Alpha heavy chain disease of patient MAL: Structure of the non-functional rearranged alpha gene translocated on chromosome 9. Eur J Immunol 20:2731, 1990.

192. Gafter U, Kessler E, Shabtay F et al: Abnormal chromosomal marker (D14 q+) in a patient with alpha heavy chain disease. J Clin Pathol 33:136, 1980.

193. Wolfenstein-Todel C, Mihaesco E, Frangione B: "Alpha chain disease" protein Def: Internal deletion of a human immunoglobulin A1 heavy chain. Proc Natl Acad Sci U S A 71:974, 1974.

194. Wolfenstein-Todel C, Mihaesco E, Frangione B: Variant of a human immunoglobulin: "Alpha chain disease" protein AIT. Biochem Biophys Res Commun 65:47, 1975.

195. Tsapis A, Bentaboulet M, Pellet P et al: The productive gene for alpha-H chain disease protein MAL is highly modified by insertion-deletion processes. J Immunol 143:3821, 1989.

196. Bentaboulet M, Mihaesco E, Gendron MC et al: Genomic alterations in a case of alpha heavy chain disease leading to the generation of composite exons from the JH region. Eur J Immunol 19:2093, 1989.

197. Fakhfakh F, Dellagi K, Ayadi H et al: Alpha heavy chain disease alpha mRNA contain nucleotide sequences of unknown origins. Eur J Immunol 22:3037, 1992.

198. Fakhfakh F, Mihaesco E, Ayadi H et al: Alpha heavy chain disease. Molecular analysis of a new case. Presse Med 22:1047, 1993.

199. Goossens T, Klein U, Kuppers R: Frequent occurrence of deletions and duplications during somatic hypermutation: Implications for oncogene translocations and heavy chain disease. Proc Natl Acad Sci U S A 95:2463, 1998.

200. Klein U, Goossens T, Fischer M et al: Somatic hypermutation in normal and transformed human B cells. Immunol Rev 162:261, 1998.

201. Matuchansky C, Cogné M, Lemaire M et al: Nonsecretory alpha-chain disease with immunoproliferative small-intestinal disease. N Engl J Med 320:1534, 1989.

202. Fakhfakh F, Ayadi H, Bouguerra A et al: Rearrangement of immunoglobulin genes in alpha heavy chain disease: A criterion of monoclonality. Arch Inst Pasteur Tunis 68:251, 1991.

203. Cogné M, Preud'homme JL: Gene deletions force nonsecretory α-chain disease plasma cells to produce membrane-form α-chain only. J Immunol 145:2455, 1990.

204. Chou CL, Morrison SL: An insertion-deletion event in murine immunoglobulin kappa gene resembles mutations at heavy-chain disease loci. Somat Cell Mol Genet 19:131, 1993.

205. Galian A, Le Charpentier Y, Rambaud JC: La maladie des chaines lourdes alpha. In Nezelof C (ed.): Nouvelles Acquisitions en Pathologie, p. 73. Hermann, Paris, 1983.

206. Rhodes JM, Jewell DP, Janossy G: Alpha-chain disease diagnosed by rectal biopsy. Br Med J 280:1043, 1980.

207. Guardia J, Mirada A, Moragas A et al: Alpha chain disease of the stomach. Hepatogastroenterology 27:238, 1980.

208. Tungekar MF, Omar YT, Behbehani K: Gastric alpha heavy chain disease. Oncology 44:360, 1987.

209. Cho C, Linscheer WG, Bell R, Smith R: Colonic lymphoma producing alpha-chain disease protein. Gastroenterology 83:121, 1982.

210. Galian A, Lacestre MJ, Scotto J et al: Pathological study of alpha-chain disease, with special emphasis on evolution. Cancer 39:2081, 1977.

211. Khojasteh A, Haghshenass M, Haghighi P: Current concepts in immunoproliferative small intestinal disease. A "Third-World lesion." N Engl J Med 308:1401, 1983.

212. Chang CS, Lin SF, Chen TP et al: Leukemic manifestation in a case of alpha-chain disease with multiple polypoid intestinal lymphocytic lymphoma. Am J Hematol 41:209, 1992.

213. Isaacson PG, Dogan A, Price SK, Spencer J: Immunoproliferative small-intestinal disease. An immunohistochemical study. Am J Surg Pathol 13:1023, 1989.

214. Isaacson PG, Spencer J: Malignant lymphoma of mucosa-associated lymphoid tissue. Histopathology 11:445, 1987.

215. Spencer J, Isaacson PG: Immunology of gastrointestinal lymphoma. Baillieres Clin Gastroenterol 1:605, 1987.

216. Ben Rejeb A, Khediri F, Souissi H et al: MALT digestive system lymphomas and alpha heavy chain diseases. Histological and

immunohistochemical study. Apropos of 3 cases. Arch Anat Cytol Pathol 39:27, 1991.

217. Lavergne A, Brocherlou I, Rambaud JC et al: T-cell rich alpha-chain disease mimicking T-cell lymphoma (letter). Histopathology 30:394, 1997.

218. Chantar C, Escartin P, Plaza AG et al: Diffuse plasma cell infiltration of the small intestine with malabsorption associated to IgA monoclonal gammapathy. Cancer 34:1620, 1974.

219. Tangun Y, Saracbasi Z, Inceman S et al: IgA myeloma globulin and Bence Jones proteinuria in diffuse plasmacytoma of small intestine (letter). Ann Intern Med 83:673, 1975.

220. Marquez JL, Mota R, Herrera JM et al: Immunoproliferative disease of the small intestine: Report of a case. Rev Esp Enferm Dig 83:381, 1993.

221. Rodriguez Gomez SJ, Jaras Hernandez MJ, Sanchez Molini P, Jimenez Alonso I: Immunoproliferative disease of the small intestine, associated with IgA kappa monoclonal gammapathy with good clinical and histologic response to the treatment with tetracyclines (letter). An Med Interna 11:566, 1994.

222. Colombel JF, Rambaud JC, Vaerman JP et al: Massive plasma cell infiltration of the digestive tract. Secretory component as the rate-limiting factor of immunoglobulin secretion in external fluids. Gastroenterology 95:1106, 1988.

223. Pohl C, Eidt S, Ziegenhagen D, Kruis W: Immunoproliferative disease of the small intestine. A rare differential diagnosis of Crohn's disease. Dtsch Med Wochenschr 116:1265, 1991.

224. Alpha-chain disease and related small-intestinal lymphoma: A memorandum. Bull World Health Org 54:615, 1976.

225. Isaacson PG: Gastrointestinal lymphoma. Hum Pathol 25:1020, 1994.

226. Papadaki Th, Afendaki S, Economidou I et al: Immunoproliferative small intestinal disease (IPSID) associated with alpha heavy-chain disease (abstract). Prog Proc Am Soc Clin Oncol 14:403, 1995.

227. Fine KD, Stone MJ: Alpha-heavy chain disease. Mediterranean lymphoma, an immunoproliferative small intestinal disease: A review of clinicopathological features, pathogenesis, and differential diagnosis. Am J Gastroenterol 94:1139, 1999.

228. Khojasteh A, Haghighi P: Immunoproliferative small intestinal disease: Portrait of a potentially preventable cancer from the Third World. Am J Med 89:483, 1990.

229. Bartold PM, Henning FR: Oral manifestation of immunoproliferative small intestinal disease: A case report. J Periodontol 61:710, 1990.

230. Neudorf S, Snover D, Filipovich A: Immunoproliferative small intestinal disease (letter). N Engl J Med 309:1126, 1983.

231. Ullrich R, Zeitz M, Heise W et al: Small intestinal structure and function in patients infected with human immunodeficiency virus (HIV): Evidence for HIV-induced enteropathy. Ann Intern Med 111:15, 1989.

232. Doe WF, Danon F, Seligmann M: Immunodiagnosis of alpha chain disease. Clin Exp Immunol 36:189, 1979.

233. Buxbaum JN, Preud'homme JL: Alpha and gamma heavy chain diseases in man: Intracellular origin of the aberrant polypeptides. J Immunol 109:1131, 1972.

234. Sopena F, Lopez Zaborras J, Nerin JM et al: Deficiency polyneuropathy secondary to immunoproliferative disease of the small intestine. Rev Esp Enferm Dig 82:423, 1992.

235. Zhaner J, Kirchner T, Ott G, Schneider W: Immunoproliferative small intestinal disease (IPSID): An unusual form of gastrointestinal lymphoma. Schweiz Med Wochenschr 124:1227, 1994.

236. Tashiro T, Sato H, Takahashi T et al: Non-secretory alpha chain disease involving stomach, small intestine and colon. Intern Med 34:255, 1995.

237. Rabhi H, Ghaffor M, Benhalima-Bouali M, Abbadi MC: Cells expressing intracytoplasmic immunoglobulins in secreting and hyposecreting cases of alpha chain disease. Arch Inst Pasteur Alger 57:125, 1989.

238. Rabhi H, Ghaffor M, Abbadi MC et al: Abnormal protein hyposecretion in early and late course of alpha chain disease. Arch Inst Pasteur Alger 56:187, 1988.

239. Tracy RP, Kyle RA, Leitch JM: Alpha heavy-chain disease presenting as goiter. Am J Clin Pathol 82:336, 1984.

240. Martin IG, Aldoori MI: Immunoproliferative small intestinal disease: Mediterranean lymphoma and alpha heavy chain disease. Br J Surg 81:20, 1994.

241. Zamir A, Parasher G, Moukarzel AA et al: Immunoproliferative small intestinal disease in a 16-year-old boy presenting as severe malabsorption with excellent response to tetracycline treatment. J Clin Gastroenterol 27:85, 1998.

242. Fischbach W, Tacke W, Greiner A et al: Regression of immunoproliferative small intestinal disease after eradication of Helicobacter pylori. Lancet 349:31, 1997.

243. Smith WJ, Price SK, Isaacson PG: Immunoglobulin gene rearrangement in immunoproliferative small intestinal disease (IPSID). J Clin Pathol 40:1291, 1987.

244. Kaufmann HP, Schmitt W, Seib HJ: Alpha-heavy chain disease – Mediterranean lymphoma. Leber Magen Darm 24:32, 1994.

245. Khojasteh A, Saalabian MJ, Haghshenass M: Randomized comparison of abdominal irradiation (AI) vs CHOP vs C-MOPP for the treatment of immunoproliferative small intestinal disease (IPSID) associated lymphoma (AL) (abstract). Proc Annu Meet Am Soc Clin Oncol 2:207, 1983.

246. Salimi M, Spinelli JJ: Chemotherapy of Mediterranean abdominal lymphoma. Retrospective comparison of chemotherapy protocols in Iranian patients. Am J Clin Oncol 19:18, 1996.

247. Ben-Ayed F, Halphen M, Najjar T et al: Treatment of alpha chain disease. Results of a prospective study in 21 Tunisian patients by the Tunisian-French Intestinal Lymphoma Study Group. Cancer 63:1251, 1989.

248. Hubman R, Kaiser W, Radaszkiewicz T et al: Malabsorption associated with a high-grade-malignant non-Hodgkin's lymphoma, alpha-heavy-chain disease and immunoproliferative small intestinal disease. Z Gastroenterol 33:209, 1995.

249. Akbulut H, Soykan I, Yakaryilmaz F et al: Five-year results of the treatment of 23 patients with immunoproliferative small intestinal disease: A Turkish experience. Cancer 80:8, 1997.

250. Price SK: Immunoproliferative small intestinal disease: A study of 13 cases with alpha heavy-chain disease. Histopathology 17:7, 1990.

251. Shih LY, Liaw SJ, Dunn P, Kuo TT: Primary small-intestinal lymphomas in Taiwan: Immunoproliferative small-intestinal disease and nonimmunoproliferative small-intestinal disease. J Clin Oncol 12:1375, 1994.

252. Malik IA, Sharmsi Z, Shafquat A et al: Clinicopathological features and management of immunoproliferative small intestinal disease and primary small intestinal lymphoma in Pakistan. Med Pediatr Oncol 25:400, 1995.

253. Demirer T, Uzunalimoglu O, Anderson T et al: Flow cytometric measurement of proliferation-associated nuclear antigen P105 and DNA content in immuno-proliferative small intestinal disease (IPSID). J Surg Oncol 58:25, 1995.

254. Tabbane F, Mourali N, Cammoun M, Najjar T: Results of laparotomy in immunoproliferative small intestinal disease. Cancer 61:1699, 1988.

255. Perrot S, Delchier JC, Farcet JP et al: Maladie des chaines lourdes α (MCL α) disseminée: Resultats preliminaires d'un traitement

par chimiothérapie intensive et autogreffe de moelle (abstract). Gastroenterol Clin Biol 12:A264, 1988.

256. Pramoolsinsap C, Kurathong S, Atichartakarn V, Nitiyanand P: Immunoproliferative small intestinal disease (IPSID) in Thailand. Southeast Asian J Trop Med Public Health 24:11, 1993.

257. Fernandes PM, Capucho R, Brandao F et al: Right atrial septic thrombus in a patient with alpha-heavy chain disease. Arq Med 8:19, 1994.

258. Nair S, Mathan M, Ramakrishna BS, Mathan VI: Immunoproliferative small intestinal disease in South India: A clinical and immunomorphological study. J Gastroenterol Hepatol 13:1207, 1998.

259. Cheng IK, Ho SK, Chan DT et al: Crescentic nodular glomerulosclerosis secondary to truncated immunoglobulin alpha heavy chain deposition. Am J Kidney Dis 28:283, 1996.

260. Ballard HS, Hamilton LM, Marcus AJ, Illes CH: A new variant of heavy-chain disease (mu-chain disease). N Engl J Med 282:1060, 1970.

261. Forte FA, Prelli F, Yount WJ et al: Heavy chain disease of the gamma (gamma M) type: Report of the first case. Blood 36:137, 1970.

262. Wahner-Roedler DL, Kyle RA: Mu-heavy chain disease: Presentation as a benign monoclonal gammopathy. Am J Hematol 40:56, 1992.

263. Cogné M, Aucouturier P, Brizard A et al: Complete variable region deletion in a μ heavy chain disease protein (ROUL). Correlation with light chain secretion. Leuk Res 17:527, 1993.

264. Iwasaki T, Hamano T, Kobayashi K, Kakishita E: A case of mu-heavy chain disease: Combined features of mu-chain disease and macroglobulinemia. Int J Hematol 66:359, 1997.

265. Witzens M, Egerer G, Stahl D et al: A case of mu heavy-chain disease associated with hyperglobulinemia, anemia, and a positive Coombs test. Ann Hematol 77:231, 1998.

266. Bedu-Addo G, Sheldon J, Bates I: Massive splenomegaly in tropical West Africa. Postgrad Med J 76:107, 2000.

267. Bonhomme J, Seligmann M, Mihaesco C et al: Mu-chain disease in an African patient. Blood 43:485, 1974.

268. Danon F, Mihaesco C, Bouvry M et al: A new case of heavy mu-chain disease. Scand J Haematol 15:5, 1975.

269. O'Reilly DS, Adjukiewicz A, Whicher JT: Biochemical findings in a case of mu-chain disease. Clin Chem 27:331, 1981.

270. Fujii H, Shimizu T, Seki S et al: Combined features of mu-heavy chain disease and primary macroglobulinemia in a single patient: Clinical and immunological studies. Nippon Ketsueki Gakkai Zasshi 45:622, 1982.

271. Leach IH, Jenkins JS, Murray-Leslie CF, Powell RJ: Mu-heavy chain and monoclonal IgG κ paraproteinaemia in systemic lupus erythematosus. Br J Rheumatol 26:460, 1987.

272. Biserte G, Lebreton JP, Ropartz C et al: A case of mu heavy chain disease. Nouv Presse Med 2:1997, 1973.

273. Brouet JC, Seligmann M, Danon F et al: Mu-chain disease. Report of two cases. Arch Intern Med 139:672, 1979.

274. Dammacco F, Bonomo L, Franklin EC: A new case of mu heavy chain disease: Clinical and immunochemical studies. Blood 43:713, 1974.

275. Josephson AS, Nicastri A, Price E, Biro L: H chain fragment and monoclonal IgA in a lymphoproliferative disorder. Am J Med 54:127, 1973.

276. Silva-Moreno M, Ruiz-Arguelles GJ, Lopez-Karpovitch X, Labardini-Mendez J: Heavy chain disease. Report of four cases. Sangre 28:89, 1983.

277. Preud'homme JL, Bauwens M, Dumont G et al: Cast nephropathy in mu heavy chain disease. Clin Nephrol 48:118, 1997.

278. Pruzanski W, Hasselback R, Katz A, Parr DM: Multiple myeloma (light chain disease) with rheumatoid-like amyloid arthropathy and mu-heavy chain fragment in the serum. Am J Med 65:334, 1978.

279. Wetter O, Schmidt CG, Linder KH, Leene W: Heavy chain disease: Humoral and cellular findings in six patients with mu chain disease [in German]. J Cancer Res Clin Oncol 94:207, 1979.

280. Bakhshi A, Guglielmi P, Coligan JE et al: A pre-translational defect in a case of human mu heavy chain disease. Mol Immunol 23:725, 1986.

281. Franklin EC, Frangione B, Prelli F: The defect in mu heavy chain disease protein GLI. J Immunol 116:1194, 1976.

282. Barnikol-Watanabe S, Mihaesco E, Mihaesco C et al: The primary structure of mu-chain-disease protein BOT. Peculiar amino-acid sequence of the N-terminal 42 positions. Hoppe Seylers Z Physiol Chem 365:105, 1984.

283. Mihaesco E, Barnikol-Watanabe S, Barnikol HU et al: The primary structure of the constant part of mu-chain-disease protein BOT. Eur J Biochem 111:275, 1980.

284. Mihaesco C, Ferrara P, Guillemot JC et al: A new extra sequence at the amino terminal of a mu heavy chain disease protein (DAG). Mol Immunol 27:771, 1990.

285. Lebreton JP, Ropartz C, Rousseaux J et al: Immunochemical and biochemical study of a human Fc mu-like fragment (mu-chain disease). Eur J Immunol 5:179, 1975.

286. Lebreton JP, Ropartz C, Biserte G: Partial study of a case of heavy mu chain disease. Lille Med 19:126, 1974.

287. Roussel P, Dautrevaux M, Rousseaux J: Biochemical study of a case of heavy mu chain disease. Lille Med 19:131, 1974.

288. Bakhshi A, Guglielmi P, Siebenlist U et al: A DNA insertion/deletion necessitates an aberrant RNA splice accounting for a mu heavy chain disease protein. Proc Natl Acad Sci U S A 83:2689, 1986.

289. Kyle RA, Garton JP: The spectrum of IgM monoclonal gammopathy in 430 cases. Mayo Clin Proc 62:719, 1987.

290. Gordon J, Hamblin TJ, Smith JL et al: A human B-cell lymphoma synthesizing and expressing surface mu-chain in the absence of detectable light chain. Blood 58:552, 1981.

291. Guglielmo P, Granata P, Di Raimondo F et al: 'Mu' heavy chain type 'non-excretory' myeloma. Scand J Haematol 29:36, 1982.

292. Leglise MC, Briere J, Abgrall JF, Hurez D: Non-secretory myeloma of heavy mu-chain type. Nouv Rev Fr Hematol 25:103, 1983.

293. Liapis H, Papadakis I, Nakopoulou L: Nodular glomerulosclerosis secondary to mu heavy chain deposits. Hum Pathol 31:122, 2000.

294. Vilpo JA, Irjala K, Viljanen MK et al: Delta-heavy chain disease. A study of a case. Clin Immunol Immunopathol 17:584, 1980.

295. Goyert SM, Hugli TE, Spiegelberg HL: Sites of "spontaneous" degradation of IgD. J Immunol 118:2138, 1977.

296. Rabhi H, Ghaffor M, Abbadi MC: Spontaneous enzymatic cleavage of IgD myeloma protein giving a pattern of delta heavy chain disease. Arch Inst Pasteur Alger 57:135, 1989.

297. Kyle RA, Greipp PR: The laboratory investigation of monoclonal gammopathies. Mayo Clin Proc 53:719, 1978.

35

Amyloidosis (AL)

Morie A. Gertz and Robert A. Kyle

The term lardaceous change has again come more into use chiefly through the instrumentality of the Vienna School … the term, lardaceous changes … has but very little to do with these tumours, and rather refers to things, upon which the old writers, who, I think, were better connoisseurs in bacon than our friends in Vienna, would hardly have bestowed such a name. The appearance of such organs … [is] said to look like bacon, bears, … a much greater resemblance to wax, and I have therefore now for a long time, like the Edinburgh School, made use of the term waxy change instead … these structures … by the simple action of iodine … assume just as blue a colour as vegetable starch does.

HISTORY

This quotation is from a lecture entitled "Amyloid Degeneration" delivered by Rudolf Virchow on April 17, 1858.[1] In it, Virchow defined the waxy change of amyloidosis and described its reaction with iodine-sulfuric acid, which at the time was a marker for starch, hence the term "amyloid or starchlike."[2–4] At the same time, Virchow took a backhanded slap at his chief competitor, Rokitansky,[5] of Vienna, Austria, who described lardaceous change in 1842 in persons suffering from malaria or tuberculosis.[6] Both Virchow in Berlin and Rokitansky were wrong. It has since been demonstrated that amyloid is neither lipid derived (lardaceous or bacon) nor is it starch or cellulose-like, but rather protein. The term "amyloid" was first coined by Schleiden in 1838 to describe a normal constituent of plants.[7] The use of iodine-sulfuric acid to identify starch by its development of a blue color dates back to 1814. In 1839, Payne defined cellulose, and the iodine-sulfuric acid reaction became the standard used by botanists to demonstrate this component of plants. In 1852, George Budd recognized that the fat content of the lardaceous liver described by Rokitansky in 1842 was actually lower than in a normal liver, suggesting for the first time that amyloid was not derived from wax or fat. In 1853, Virchow used the iodine-sulfuric acid reaction to demonstrate that the corpora amylacea reacted with the stain and was therefore starch derived. He used the same test on what appeared to the naked eye to be similar corpuscles in the waxy spleen. In 1856, Wilks described a patient with lardaceous change that was not related to any known infection and this may have been the first patient reported with primary amyloidosis.[8] In 1859, Friedreich (of Friedreich ataxia) and Kekulé (who described

the structure of benzene) recognized that the waxy spleen described by Virchow did not have any cellulose-like substances and thought it was probably proteinaceous.[9,10] In 1867, the first patient with amyloidosis associated with multiple myeloma was reported. In 1920, Schmiedeberg[11] described the amino acid composition of amyloid and reported that it strongly resembled serum globulin.

In 1922, Bennhold introduced Congo red, first as a diagnostic test and subsequently as a histologic stain.[12–14] In 1928, Divry and Florkin first reported green birefringence when Congo red-stained specimens were viewed under polarized light.[15,16] The first demonstration of green birefringence in amyloid-laden tissues was in the brains of patients with Alzheimer disease. In 1931, Magnus-Levy[17] first postulated the relationship between the Bence Jones protein and formation of amyloid. In 1959, Cohen and Calkins[18] first recognized that under the electron microscope all forms of amyloid demonstrated a nonbranching fibrillar structure. Each fibril was of indefinite length, with the width of 9.5 nm. In 1964, Osserman et al.[19] first recognized that abnormal light chains (Bence Jones proteins) played a direct role in the pathogenesis of primary amyloidosis. In 1968, Eanes and Glenner[20] reported that the x-ray diffraction properties of amyloid did not resemble the normal α-helical structure of proteins but formed an alternative configuration of a β-pleated sheet. Glenner et al.[21] reported the first amino acid sequence of an amyloid protein in 1970. It consisted of the N-terminus of an immunoglobulin light chain. Levin et al.[22] first described the amino acid sequence of an amyloid fibril from a patient with secondary amyloidosis and labeled it the amyloid A protein.[23]

ULTRASTRUCTURE

All forms of amyloid are characterized by positive histologic staining with Congo red. When viewed under a light microscope, amyloid deposits appear as amorphous extracellular deposits. By hematoxylin and eosin staining, the deposits are pink. When viewed under polarized light, amyloid deposits demonstrate apple-green birefringence. All forms of amyloid are fibrillar, usually rigid and nonbranching. The amyloid fibrils associated with long-term dialysis may be curvilinear. Amyloid fibrils are insoluble in isotonic saline. They form a suspension in distilled water and this forms the basis for the purification of amyloid.[24]

Historically, amyloidosis was classified by its anatomic distribution.[25] Three types of amyloidosis were recognized. Familial amyloidosis was defined from the inheritance patterns.[26,27] Secondary amyloidosis was characterized by its association with a long-standing inflammatory process.[28] All other types of amyloid were considered primary. In the context of that era, that meant idiopathic. Today, amyloidosis is classified by the composition of the amyloid subunit protein (Table 35–1). Only AL amyloid is associated with a plasma cell dyscrasia and is the only form covered in depth in this chapter.

Amyloid fibrils have been synthetically produced by digesting purified human monoclonal light chains with pepsin.[29] Synthetic

Table 35–1. Nomenclature of Amyloidosis

Protein	Precursor	Clinical
AL or AH	Immunoglobulin light chain	Primary or localized myeloma or macroglobulinemia associated
AA	SAA	Secondary or familial Mediterranean fever
ATTR	Transthyretin	Familial and senile
Aβ₂M	β₂-microglobulin	Dialysis—carpal tunnel syndrome
Aβ	ABPP	Alzheimer's disease

Abbreviations: ABPP, amyloid β protein precursor; SAA, serum amyloid A.
(From Gertz et al.,[207] by permission of WB Saunders Company.)

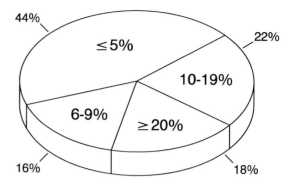

Figure 35–1. Marrow plasma cells in primary amyloidosis. (From Gertz MA et al.,[207] by permission of WB Saunders Company.)

amyloid fibrils have also been produced by reducing the disulfide bonds that bridge immunoglobulin light chains to heavy chains.[30] AL, the subunit protein, is an immunoglobulin light chain or fragment thereof. Immunoglobulin heavy chains have been described as being involved in the formation of amyloid fibrils and this carries the designation AH.[31] No clinical differences have been described between patients whose immunoglobulin-associated amyloidosis is light chain (AL) or heavy chain (AH).

Patients with immunoglobulin light chain amyloidosis have an aberrant amino acid sequence of their light chains. Mice repeatedly injected with Bence Jones proteins obtained from patients with AL produce amyloid deposits. The murine amyloid deposits, when sequenced, demonstrate human immunoglobulin light chain sequences. Control mice injected similarly with Bence Jones proteins from multiple myeloma patients without amyloidosis do not develop amyloid deposits.[32] This suggests that specific light chains have amino acid sequences that predispose them to form amyloid. In multiple myeloma and monoclonal gammopathy of undetermined significance (MGUS), κ light chains dominate. The ratio of κ:λ light chains is approximately 2:1. In amyloidosis, the ratio of κ:λ light chains is approximately 1:3, suggesting a predisposition of λ light chains to form β-pleated sheets. The λ_VI subclass of light chains seems to be uniquely associated with amyloidosis, with all described λ_VI sequences derived from patients with amyloidosis. This supports the concept that certain amino acid sequences render proteins amyloidogenic.[33]

Patients with AL have been classified into those without multiple myeloma and those with myeloma.[34] True multiple myeloma-associated amyloid is uncommon. Lytic bone disease, renal failure due to myeloma cast nephropathy, and anemia due to plasma cell replacement of the bone marrow are uncommon findings in amyloidosis. Most patients with amyloidosis and multiple myeloma receive the designation because the percentage of plasma cells in the bone marrow exceeds 30 percent (Figure 35–1). If multiple myeloma is not present at diagnosis of amyloidosis, it is unlikely to develop. In our experience of 1600 patients with AL, multiple myeloma subsequently developed in only 6.[35] The median age of patients with amyloidosis seen at the Mayo Clinic is 62 years. The median age of AL patients seen in

Olmsted County, Minnesota, is 73 years. This suggests referral bias for younger patients. The incidence of amyloidosis is 8 per million per year[36] and has not changed in the past 4 decades. The incidence of amyloidosis is approximately one-fifth of the incidence of multiple myeloma and is similar to the incidence of Hodgkin's disease[37] and chronic granulocytic leukemia.

Chromosomal abnormalities are seen in the bone marrow plasma cells from patients with amyloidosis. Bone marrow samples from 21 patients with AL were studied by standard cytogenetics and fluorescence in situ hybridization probes for 6 chromosomes. Trisomy of chromosomes 7, 9, 11, 15, and 18 was seen in 42, 52, 47, 39, and 33 percent, respectively. Trisomy X was seen in 13 percent of women and 54 percent of men. Monosomy of chromosome 18 was seen in 72 percent of patients. The aneuploidy seen in these monoclonal plasma cells supports a neoplastic nature for the disorder, even when the percentage of plasma cells in the bone marrow does not fulfill the criteria for multiple myeloma.[38]

In summary, immunoglobulin light (or heavy) chain amyloidosis is a rare monoclonal disorder of plasma cells. Multiple myeloma is occasionally misdiagnosed because both include the presence of a monoclonal immunoglobulin, proteinuria, and bone marrow plasmacytosis. Once a diagnosis of AL is established, the patient is usually referred to a hematologist or oncologist for therapy.

WHEN SHOULD AMYLOID BE SUSPECTED?

Amyloidosis has a male predominance: nearly two-thirds of patients are men. Although we have seen patients as young as age 26 years, only 1 percent are younger than age 40 years.[39] The most common presenting symptoms of amyloidosis are fatigue and weight loss (Figure 35–2). These symptoms are quite nonspecific and are not helpful to a clinician formulating a differential diagnosis for these complaints. Many patients with unexplained weight loss undergo an investigation for an underlying occult malignancy.[40] In our experience, fatigue is frequently misdiagnosed as functional or stress

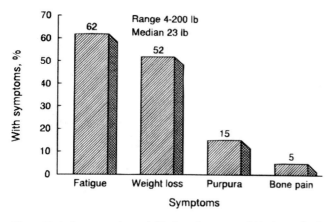

Figure 35–2. Symptoms in amyloidosis patients seen within 1 month of diagnosis. (From Kyle and Gertz,[47] by permission of WB Saunders Company.)

related, particularly in patients whose fatigue is due to early cardiac amyloid deposits. Light-headedness is a common complaint. It is nonspecific because light-headedness is a common symptom in the primary-care setting. Light-headedness may occur in patients with nephrotic syndrome due to significant plasma volume contraction. Light-headedness is common in patients with cardiac amyloidosis, who generally have a reduced stroke volume, a consequence of poor filling of the left ventricle during diastole. Patients with autonomic neuropathy may have orthostatic hypotension, which causes light-headedness and syncope.[41]

Physical findings suggestive of amyloidosis, when present, can be helpful. Unfortunately, diagnostic physical findings are frequently overlooked and even in the best circumstances are

found in no more than 15 percent of patients. Amyloid purpura is present in 15 percent of patients. Amyloid purpura is seen above the nipple line, most commonly in the webbing of the neck, face, and eyelids (Figure 35–3). Purpura is usually subtle, and periorbital purpura can be overlooked unless the patient's eyes are closed. Because most patients are older than age 60 years, the purpura can be misinterpreted as purpura simplex or senile purpura. Hepatomegaly is present in a quarter of patients with amyloidosis, but a liver edge greater than 5 cm below the right costal margin is present in only 10 percent. Splenomegaly is uncommon. The finding most specific for amyloidosis is macroglossia. This is found in only 9 percent of patients and may be overlooked because the most common findings are dental indentations on the underside and lateral surfaces of the tongue (Figure 35–4). Submandibular salivary glands are usually involved with amyloid, particularly when the tongue is enlarged. Some of the enlargement of the submandibular glands is due to the macroglossia pressing on the floor of the mouth. This may be misinterpreted as submandibular lymphadenopathy.

Occasionally, patients with temporal artery involvement by AL can present with clinical symptoms suggesting giant cell arteritis, including calf, limb, and jaw claudication.[42–44] Because of the increased sedimentation rate associated with the serum monoclonal protein, these patients have been misdiagnosed with polymyalgia rheumatica and have undergone extended therapy with prednisone without benefit.[45]

MAKING A DIAGNOSIS OF AMYLOIDOSIS

Because the subjective symptoms and physical findings associated with amyloidosis are generally nonspecific, when should a

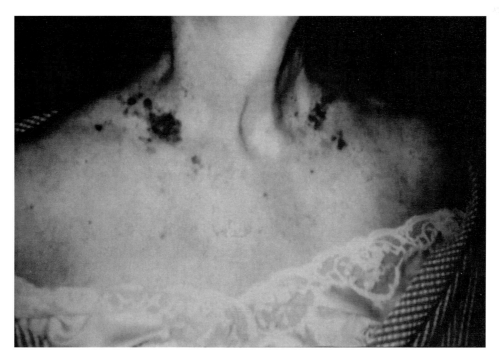

Figure 35–3. Purpura in primary amyloidosis. (From Gertz et al.,[207] by permission of WB Saunders Company.)

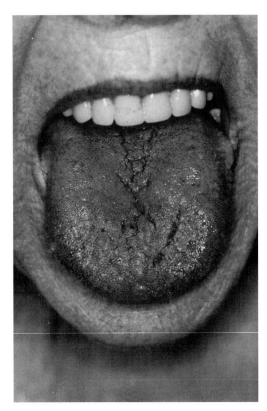

Figure 35–4. Tongue in primary amyloidosis. (From Gertz et al.,[207] by permission of WB Saunders Company.)

clinician suspect this rare problem so that early diagnosis and intervention may occur? Recognition of the specific clinical syndromes associated with amyloidosis can lead to the initiation of the appropriate diagnostic techniques.

The four most common presentations of patients with immunoglobulin light chain amyloid are (Figure 35–5):

1. Nephrotic-range proteinuria with or without renal insufficiency[46]

2. Congestive heart failure from restrictive cardiomyopathy[47]
3. Unexplained hepatomegaly[48]
4. Idiopathic peripheral neuropathy[49]

Any adult seen with one of these four syndromes must have amyloidosis considered in the differential diagnosis (Table 35–2). It is important to consider AL in the differential diagnosis of an M protein. Many patients with AL present as "MGUS" until a "syndrome" is recognized and a biopsy is then done. When a clinician sees a patient with unexplained nephrotic-range proteinuria, heart failure, hepatomegaly, or neuropathy, immunofixation of the serum and urine is required.[50] Virtually all patients with AL have a clonal population of plasma cells in their bone marrow. These plasma cells actively synthesize monoclonal immunoglobulin light chains. The finding of a monoclonal light chain would be strong evidence favoring further diagnostic evaluation for AL.[51] Immunofixation should be done on both serum and urine because a monoclonal protein will not be found in the serum in one-third of patients. A screening serum protein electrophoresis is inadequate. A monoclonal protein is easily overlooked on the protein electrophoretic pattern because the monoclonal protein is usually small and does not produce a spike that is detectable by visual inspection of the protein pattern (Figure 35–6). Small peaks can be obscured by normal immunoglobulins, so immunofixation is necessary for their recognition. There is a high prevalence of free light chains in the serum of patients with amyloid (Bence Jones proteinemia 34 percent). Free serum light chains do not produce a visible peak because they are excreted by the kidney into the urine before they can accumulate in sufficient quantities to be detected. Urine light chains are also difficult to recognize because the proteinuria commonly associated with amyloid often obscures the presence of small light chain proteins. Again, immunofixation of the urine is required (Figure 35–7). By immunofixation of serum and urine, a monoclonal light chain will be detected in nearly 90 percent of patients with AL. Immunofixation, therefore, is the

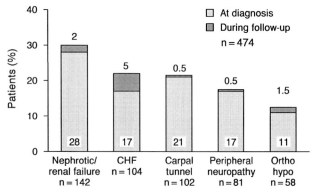

Figure 35–5. Syndromes at diagnosis and during follow-up of primary amyloidosis patients seen within 1 month of histologic diagnosis. CHF, congestive heart failure; ortho hypo, orthostatic hypotension. (From Kyle and Gertz,[47] by permission of WB Saunders Company.)

Table 35–2. Diagnostic Pathway for Primary Amyloidosis (AL)

1. Consider AL in patients with
   Nephrotic-range proteinuria (nondiabetic)
   Cardiomyopathy (no ischemic history)
   Hepatomegaly (no filling defects by imaging)
   Peripheral neuropathy (nondiabetic)
2. Heighten suspicion
   Immunofixation of serum and urine
3. Confirm diagnosis histologically
   Fat aspirate and marrow biopsy stain with Congo red (90 percent sensitive)
4. Assess prognosis
   Echocardiography required (Doppler important)
5. Treat
   Melphalan and prednisone
   High-dose steroids
   Stem cell transplantation
   Organ transplantation

(From Gertz et al.,[207] by permission of WB Saunders Company.)

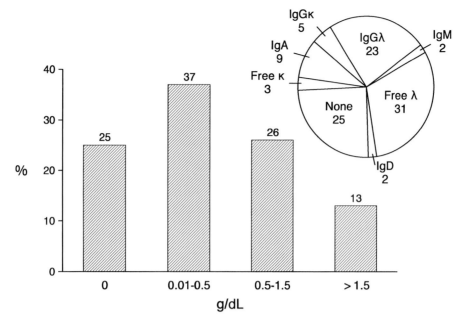

Figure 35–6. Distribution of serum M protein findings in patients with primary amyloidosis. (From Gertz et al.,[207] by permission of WB Saunders Company.)

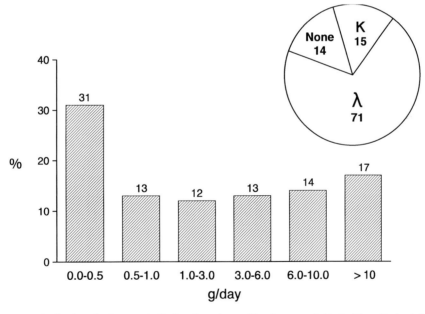

Figure 35–7. Distribution of urine protein findings in patients with primary amyloidosis. (From Gertz et al.,[207] by permission of WB Saunders Company.)

most sensitive noninvasive screening test. These diagnostics should be applied when a patient presents with a suggestive clinical syndrome such as unexplained proteinuria, nonischemic heart failure, hepatomegaly, or neuropathy.[47]

In patients who do not have a detectable monoclonal light chain in the serum or urine, the bone marrow usually demonstrates a clonal population of plasma cells that can be recog-

nized by immunohistochemistry, immunofluorescence, or flow cytometry. Patients with no monoclonal light chain in the serum or urine but a clonal population of plasma cells in the bone marrow could be considered to have nonsecretory AL, the counterpart of nonsecretory multiple myeloma.[52,53] Of 16 patients with no detectable monoclonal protein by electrophoresis, 14 had a clonal population of plasma cells in the marrow and 12 had a monoclonal protein found by immunofixation. Combining these two analyses confirmed the immunoglobin origin of the amyloid in all patients.[54]

All amyloid deposits contain serum amyloid P component. Radionuclide scanning can be performed using iodine-labeled human serum amyloid P. Whole-body images demonstrate uptake of radionuclide in patients with amyloidosis. The plasma clearance of the labeled P component increases in proportion to the total body amyloid load. Patients with AL demonstrate ^{131}I-labeled serum amyloid P uptake in the spleen (87 percent), the liver (60 percent), and the kidneys (25 percent). This diagnostic technique is not sensitive in detecting myocardial amyloid deposits. Twenty-four-hour tissue retention appears to correlate with the severity of amyloid and survival. The ability of ^{131}I-serum amyloid P scanning to recognize amyloid deposits in the digestive tract, carpal ligaments, and kidneys is severely limited.[55] Although radiolabeled serum amyloid P scans can detect amyloid deposits,[56] demonstration of amyloid deposits in biopsy tissue is required[57] for diagnosis. In patients who have renal, cardiac, hepatic, or nerve amyloid, the diagnosis could be established by direct biopsy of those tissues.[58] Biopsies of viscera usually are not needed. The widespread nature of amyloidosis and the high prevalence of vascular involvement make noninvasive biopsies preferable.

There is a high incidence of xerostomia in amyloidosis; biopsy of a minor salivary gland from the lip demonstrated amyloid deposits in 26 of 30 patients.[59] Skin biopsies, even uninvolved skin, reveal amyloid deposits in the blood vessels of the subcutaneous tissues.[60] Rectal biopsy historically was the preferred technique for the confirmation of amyloidosis.[61] Its drawbacks were the rare episodes of bleeding after rectal biopsy and the fact that an endoscopic biopsy is often insufficient because only mucosa may be present in the samples. Rectal submucosa is required to accurately detect amyloid because vessels containing amyloid deposits are localized to the submucosa. The discomfort associated with rectal biopsy has led to a reduction in its use to establish the diagnosis of AL.

At the Mayo Clinic, when AL is suspected, the patient undergoes a simultaneous subcutaneous fat aspiration and bone marrow biopsy. The subcutaneous fat aspiration is positive for amyloid in 70 to 80 percent of patients (Figure 35–8) and does not require a physician for sample procurement. Results can be available within 24 hours, and the procedure carries no risk.[62] Biopsy of the bone marrow demonstrates amyloid deposits, when suitably stained, in half of patients. The bone marrow biopsy is necessary because it permits one to determine the percentage of plasma cells in the bone marrow, exclude multiple myeloma, and analyze for a clonal population of plasma cells and it serves as a tissue source for the diagnosis of amyloid if the subcutaneous fat aspiration is negative for amyloid. If both the bone marrow biopsy specimen and the subcutaneous fat aspirate are obtained, amyloid deposits are found in 90 percent of patients (Table 35–3). In the remaining 10 percent of patients, a biopsy specimen from the affected organ can confirm the diagnosis. Caution must be exercised when interpreting Congo red-stained tissues. Overstaining with Congo red in fat tissues can result in a false-positive result. Elastin and collagen commonly found in subcutaneous tis-

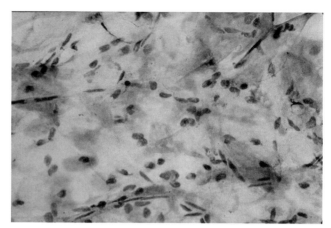

Figure 35–8. Fat aspirate in primary amyloidosis. (Congo red; × 100; courtesy of C.Y. Li, M.D.) (From Gertz et al.,[207] by permission of WB Saunders Company.)

sues can bind to Congo red and can be misinterpreted as demonstrating amyloid.[63] False-negative results of rectal biopsies have been reported where subepithelial amyloid deposits were believed to represent collagenous colitis. The diagnosis was subsequently recognized when Congo red stains were performed.[64]

DIFFERENTIATING AL FROM OTHER FORMS OF AMYLOIDOSIS

Once a diagnosis of amyloidosis has been established histologically, it is imperative to be certain that the amyloidosis is immunoglobulin light chain in origin because its therapy is distinct from all other forms of amyloidosis (Figure 35–9). The next most frequent form of amyloidosis after AL is localized amyloidosis. In making a distinction, one must remember that only the AL form of amyloid is associated with a plasma cell dyscrasia, has a monoclonal protein detectable in the serum or urine, or has a clonal population of plasma cells in the bone marrow. Localized amyloidosis is limited to a specific organ and does not become systemic. In many instances of localized amyloidosis, the fibrils themselves are immunoglobulin light chain derived, but there is no systemic plasma cell dyscrasia.[65] Oftentimes, the location of the amyloidosis is unique to the localized form and is generally not seen in AL. Amyloidosis seen in the trachea or bronchial tree or larynx or as pulmonary nodules is

Table 35–3. Noninvasive Biopsies in Primary Amyloidosis

Finding		Patients (percent)
Fat +	Marrow +	55
Fat +	Marrow −	22
Fat −	Marrow +	10
Fat −	Marrow −	13

(Modified from Gertz et al.,[180] by permission of American Society of Clinical Oncology.)

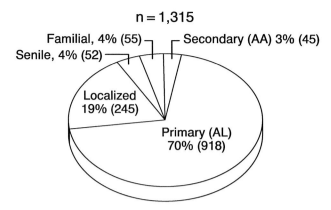

n = 1,315

Familial, 4% (55)　　　Secondary (AA) 3% (45)
Senile, 4% (52)

Localized
19% (245)

Primary (AL)
70% (918)

Figure 35–9. Different forms of amyloidosis seen at the Mayo Clinic during a 12-year period (1981–1992). (From Kyle and Gertz,[47] by permission of WB Saunders Company.)

generally localized. Amyloid deposits seen in the ureter, urethra, or bladder are not part of a systemic process. Rarely, patients who have AL present with hematuria. Most instances of cutaneous amyloid that are not purpura are localized.

A patient with tracheal or bronchial amyloidosis presents with hoarseness, cough, dyspnea, wheezing, and hemoptysis. Occasionally bronchial obstruction occurs. The diagnosis is usually established by biopsy via the bronchoscope, and treatment is local, usually consisting of laser resection. Solitary pulmonary nodules frequently confused with lung cancer are often detected at thoracotomy and do not represent a form of systemic amyloid.[66]

Amyloid in the urinary bladder is diagnosed cystoscopically and is usually confused with transitional cell bladder cancer.[67] Treatment includes transurethral resection or fulguration. Occasionally cystectomy is required for life-threatening hemorrhage. Reports of intravesical dimethyl sulfoxide leading to regression of deposits have appeared in the literature. Ureteral amyloid presents with obstruction and the preoperative diagnosis is generally thought to be ureteral malignancy.[68] Urethral amyloid usually presents as painless hematuria.[69]

Cutaneous amyloidosis may be lichen, macular, or nodular. In the first two, the amyloidosis is always localized. Occasionally nodular cutaneous amyloidosis may be a presenting feature of systemic AL. Macular and papular amyloid deposits appear to be derived from degenerated keratin. Local therapy suffices.

Amyloid of the carpal tunnel is generally a localized phenomenon. The fibrils are composed of normal transthyretin.[70] Conversely, patients with AL have carpal tunnel syndrome up to 25 percent of the time. Localized orbital amyloidosis has been described and includes extraocular muscle, conjunctiva, and lid infiltration.[71]

Secondary amyloidosis is not associated with an immunocyte dyscrasia and is rarely seen in Western nations. The most common cause is poorly controlled inflammatory polyarthritis. The most common etiologies seen at the Mayo Clinic are Still's disease, ankylosing spondylitis,[72] psoriatic arthritis, and rheumatoid arthritis.[73] In most instances, the rheumatic condition is

obvious, long-standing, and poorly controlled. The presentation is virtually always nephrotic-range proteinuria with or without renal insufficiency. Diarrhea may also be seen.[74] Occasionally, poorly controlled Crohn's disease,[75] osteomyelitis not amenable to surgical excision, or long-standing bronchiectasis can lead to secondary amyloidosis. The syndrome has been described in patients with multiple subcutaneous abscesses from the subcutaneous injection of narcotics that are bacterially contaminated. Rare instances of secondary amyloidosis have been described in the setting of Hodgkin's disease[76] and renal-cell cancer.[77]

Treatment of the underlying disorder is appropriate in inflammatory arthritis.[78] The use of chlorambucil has been reported to control the underlying disorder and resolve the proteinuria.[79] Uncontrolled secondary amyloidosis generally progresses to dialysis-dependent renal failure. Successful renal transplantation has been reported. The incidence of amyloidosis secondary to juvenile rheumatoid arthritis has decreased in the past 2 decades.[80] Rare instances of amyloidosis associated with human immunodeficiency virus infection have been reported.[81]

Occasionally, a patient with amyloidosis presents and the amyloid turns out to be familial in origin. These patients also do not have a monoclonal protein. The most common forms of familial amyloidosis are due to mutations in the transthyretin molecule.[82] Nearly half of the patients seen at the Mayo Clinic do not have a positive family history and, therefore, this is not a useful feature for making the distinction. The majority of transthyretin amyloid syndromes are associated with progressive peripheral sensory, motor, and autonomic neuropathy. The next most common is familial cardiomyopathy syndrome.[83] Generally, neuropathy and cardiomyopathy coexist in the same patients,[84] but some of the mutations result in cardiomyopathy alone and are difficult to distinguish from cardiac AL.[85] Familial forms of amyloid are the only types that are associated with deposits in the vitreous. A patient with isolated neuropathy or cardiomyopathy without a monoclonal protein in the serum or urine needs to have immunohistochemical stains of the amyloid-laden tissues performed for transthyretin and, if positive, genetic analysis for a mutant transthyretin molecule. Familial amyloid nephrotic syndrome has been described in association with mutations of the fibrinogen alpha chain, apolipoprotein A-I, and lysozyme. These patients present with renal insufficiency without nephrotic syndrome, particularly in apolipoprotein A-I and lysozyme amyloid. Patients with fibrinogen amyloid generally have nephrotic syndrome before the development of renal insufficiency.

In the transthyretin forms of amyloidosis, liver transplantation has been successfully applied.[86,87] Transthyretin is produced only in the liver, and replacement of the liver before the development of severe autonomic neuropathy or severe nutritional deficiency has been associated with regression of disease.[88] The outcome of liver transplantation appears to be best for patients with a Val30Met mutation. Patients with other mutations who have undergone liver transplantation have been reported to develop progressive disease post-transplantation.[89] It has been suggested that the presence of mutant transthyretin deposits serves as a nidus for further deposition of wild-type transthyretin produced by the transplanted liver. This leads to progressive organ dysfunction. In summary, in any patient with amyloidosis who lacks a monoclonal protein in serum and urine and has no monoclonal bone marrow plasma cells, localized, secondary, and familial amyloidosis must be considered.

AMYLOID ORGAN SYNDROMES

Kidney

In AL, the most frequently affected organ is the kidney. The kidney is the presenting problem in one-third to one-half of patients with AL.[90] Renal amyloid is detected in 2.5 to 2.8 percent of all renal biopsy specimens.[46] In nondiabetic adults with nephrotic syndrome, amyloidosis accounts for 10 percent of renal biopsies. Survival with renal amyloidosis depends on the presenting level of serum creatinine. Patients who present with a creatinine concentration less than 1.3 mg/dl have a median survival of 25.6 months. Those with an elevated creatinine value have a median survival of 14.9 months ($p < .01$). The level of 24-hour urine protein excretion has no impact on survival; however, the time from original diagnosis to the development of end-stage renal disease is shorter in patients with higher levels of protein excretion.

In renal amyloidosis there is a strong preponderance of λ light chains in the serum and urine. The ratio of λ-to-κ light chains is approximately 3.5-to-1. The usual κ-to-λ ratio seen in patients with MGUS and multiple myeloma is 2-to-1. This suggests that λ light chains are predisposed to form β-pleated sheets and, therefore, amyloid deposits. In patients with urinary protein losses in excess of 10 g/day, the λ-to-κ ratio is nearly 5-to-1. A consequence of nephrotic-range proteinuria is profound serum hypoalbuminemia. The loss of albumin results in a markedly reduced intravascular oncotic pressure. This leads to transudation of fluid into the extracellular space and produces the pitting edema characteristic of renal amyloidosis. The edema can be controlled in part with the use of diuretics, usually furosemide and metolazone. There is a ceiling to the use of diuretics because they produce further volume contraction, and the resultant reduction in renal blood flow can increase the serum creatinine level. In addition, the contraction of the intravascular volume can aggravate orthostatic hypotension and can precipitate syncope. Midodrine and fludrocortisone can decrease the severity of orthostatic hypotension, but both have sodium-retaining properties and can aggravate the edema. Midodrine can also produce hypertension when the patient is supine.

The principal long-term complication of the continuous urinary protein loss is tubular damage followed by azotemia and dialysis-dependent kidney disease.[91,92] In patients who present with renal amyloidosis, one-third ultimately receive dialysis.[93] The median time from diagnosis to the start of dialysis is 14 months. Median survival for patients from the start of dialysis is 8 months. The most common causes of death are the result of extrarenal amyloid deposits in the heart, followed by liver. There appears to be no survival difference between hemodialysis and peritoneal dialysis.[94] Predictors of which patients will ultimately require dialysis include the 24-hour urine protein loss and creatinine value at diagnosis.

The nephrotic syndrome in AL can be severe, with urinary protein losses in excess of 25 g/day. Patients not uncommonly have a serum albumin value of less than 1 g/dl. In these patients, anasarca occurs and can incapacitate the patient as a result of hypotension and complications related to massive extracellular fluid leak. Bilateral nephrectomy has been reported to resolve the edema and hypotension.[95] Initiation of early hemodialysis, even in the absence of azotemia, has been attempted to render the patient anuric. Dialysis-induced anuria eliminates the urinary protein loss and allows the serum albumin level to rise. This can result in significant symptomatic improvement. We have also seen renal failure develop, and the resultant anuria dramatically improves the overall clinical condition.

There is a poor correlation between the extent of amyloid deposits seen on a kidney biopsy specimen and the extent of proteinuria. Even small amyloid deposits have been associated with severe nephrotic syndrome. Older literature suggested that the kidneys are enlarged in amyloidosis.[96] Most patients, virtually all of whom now have evaluation by ultrasonography, demonstrate normal-sized kidneys. Urinary sediment in amyloidosis is usually bland, showing only fat and fatty acid crystals. A cellular or inflammatory sediment is generally not found.

Heart

The second most frequent presentation of patients with AL includes the symptoms of restrictive cardiomyopathy.[97] The diagnosis of cardiac involvement by AL usually involves subtle distinctions. Patients may present with disabling fatigue as their only symptom. The cardiomyopathy is restrictive in nature, with early diastolic dysfunction and no systolic dysfunction (Figure 35–10).[98] In these instances, the chest radiograph shows no abnormalities. By echocardiography, the ejection fraction is preserved until late in the clinical course. The electrocardiogram frequently shows low voltage. This finding may be overlooked unless one is sensitive to the diagnosis. A pseudoinfarction pattern with QS complexes in leads V_1 through V_3 has been interpreted incorrectly as demonstrating a silent myocardial infarction.[99] Patients presenting with congestive heart failure can receive a misdiagnosis of silent ischemia. The echocardiogram shows wall thickening (Figure 35–11), and this is regularly interpreted as showing concentric left ventricular hypertrophy rather than infiltrative cardiomyopathy. It is important when a patient presents clinically with diastolic heart failure to screen for a monoclonal protein in the serum and urine.

Amyloidosis causes a stiff heart syndrome.[100,101] The cause of low cardiac output is restrictive diastolic filling. Systolic function is preserved until the disease is far advanced. The echocardiogram will show a misleadingly normal ejection fraction or hyperdynamic function until late in the course. In spite of the normal ejection fraction, the reduced flow of blood during diastole, due to poor ventricular compliance, results in a reduced end-diastolic volume. With a low end-diastolic volume, the stroke volume and cardiac output are sharply reduced.

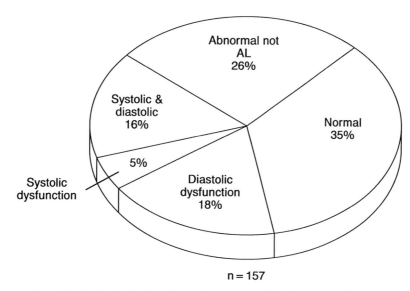

Figure 35–10. Results of echocardiography in patients with primary amyloidosis (AL).

Doppler studies are required to recognize diastolic dysfunction causing reduced inflow to the ventricle during diastole.

It has been suggested that digoxin is contraindicated in amyloid heart disease because of a high frequency of sudden death.[102] Sudden death is common in amyloid heart disease, whether or not the patient receives digoxin. It is impossible to know whether digoxin actually increases the frequency of high-grade arrhythmias. Sudden cardiac death in amyloidosis is frequent and can be due to asystole or ventricular fibrillation. Digoxin is used in a high proportion of patients with heart failure, and it is possible for incorrect conclusions to be drawn. We have used digoxin for rate control when supraventricular tachyarrhythmias are present.

Because amyloidosis is not a disease associated with systolic failure, it is unclear whether the benefits of digoxin apply to patients with AL. Most patients with cardiac amyloidosis are treated with diuretics and receive afterload reduction with angiotensin-converting enzyme inhibitors.[103] Most patients have a low cardiac output state and systolic hypotension. There is, therefore, some difficulty administering therapeutic doses of diuretics and angiotensin-converting enzyme inhibitors.[97]

The standard for the diagnosis of amyloid cardiomyopathy is the echocardiogram. An occasional patient subsequently shown to have endomyocardial biopsy-proven amyloid may present with an echocardiogram inconsistent with amyloid.[104] The

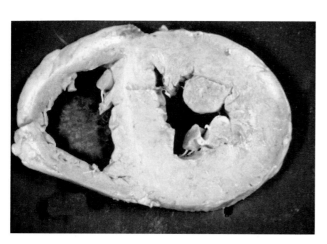 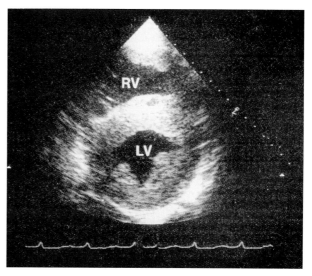

Figure 35–11. (A) Photograph of a patient's heart postmortem. (B) Echocardiography demonstrates concentric thickening of the left ventricle due to infiltration with amyloid. LV, left ventricle; RV, right ventricle.

severity of cardiac infiltration in AL appears to be unrelated to the whole body amyloid load when measured by serum amyloid P tracer studies. The combination of radiolabeled serum amyloid P and echocardiography permits identification of patients with severe cardiac disease and a low whole-body load who may be better candidates for cardiac transplantation.[105]

In patients with amyloidosis, the median septal wall thickness as measured by echocardiography is 15 mm (normal, 9 to 12 mm). The most common echocardiographic features of amyloid (Figure 35–10) are thickening of the right ventricular wall, interventricular septum, and left ventricular free wall associated with reduced left ventricular chamber size.

Echocardiographic evidence of amyloid is found in 39 percent of patients with the disease, but overt congestive heart failure is seen in only 17 to 21 percent. The frequency of cardiac involvement seen by echocardiography is nearly double the frequency of clinical congestive heart failure. In a statistical analysis, echocardiographic evidence of amyloid alone does not have an impact on overall survival. The ejection fraction (when less than 50 percent) and the ventricular septal thickness (when greater than 15 mm) or any evidence of congestive heart failure is associated with shorter survival (Figure 35–12). Syncope is common in amyloid heart disease. In some series, almost one-third of patients with cardiac amyloid experience syncope precipitated by physiologic stress. Stress-precipitated syncope is associated with a poor prognosis (median survival of 2 months), and it is frequently a precursor of sudden cardiac death.[106]

The key to recognizing cardiac amyloidosis is for a clinician to search for a monoclonal protein in the serum or urine of any patient with heart failure that is not clearly on an ischemic basis. The electrocardiogram shows either low voltage in the limb leads or loss of anteroseptal forces (pseudoinfarction). A low-voltage electrocardiogram is seen in two-thirds of patients with cardiac amyloidosis.[85] Cardiac amyloidosis produces atrial systolic failure and dilatation of the right ventricle, which is

associated with a poor prognosis.[107] Early cardiac amyloidosis is characterized by abnormal relaxation. Advanced involvement is characterized by restrictive hemodynamics. Thickening of the mitral and tricuspid valves is seen frequently and is an important clue to distinguish infiltrative cardiomyopathy from hypertrophy. Valvular regurgitation is common on Doppler echocardiographic studies, but it is generally not clinically significant.

Dual-chamber pacemaker implantation has been proposed as a therapeutic option in the management of patients with AL who fail optimal medical therapy. Three patients with medically refractory heart failure due to AL underwent cardiac catheterization with atrioventricular sequential pacing. During pacing, at various atrioventricular intervals, the patient showed either no change or a decline in cardiac index, suggesting an absence of hemodynamic benefit from atrioventricular sequential pacing in amyloid heart disease.[108]

Restrictive cardiomyopathy can be confused with constrictive pericardial disease.[109,110] Tamponade has been reported, but it is infrequent for pericardial stripping to be of clinical benefit in AL. At the time of right-sided heart catheterization, endomyocardial biopsy always establishes the diagnosis when at least three specimens are studied. Amyloid heart disease produces a stiff heart with impaired diastolic filling. The stasis of blood within the cardiac chambers can produce thrombi that are potential sources of cardiac embolism. An occasional patient presents with systemic arteriothromboemboli or a stroke syndrome.[111] In three patients with extensive cardiac amyloidosis, transthoracic echocardiography demonstrated large atrial thrombi in the left atrium during sinus rhythm. Severe amyloid infiltration resulted in atrial standstill with thrombus formation. This suggests a potential role for long-term anticoagulation therapy.[112]

Occasionally, patients have coronary arteriolar disease and present with classic symptoms of ischemia and angina and occasionally infarction.[113] Typically, large vessels are spared and the

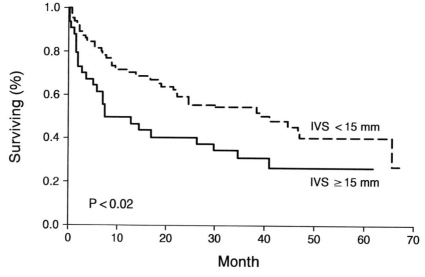

Figure 35–12. Impact of septal thickness on actuarial survival in primary amyloidosis. IVS, interventricular septum. (From Gertz et al.,[207] by permission of WB Saunders Company.)

coronary angiogram is normal, but exercise testing confirms ischemia. The diagnosis of coronary arteriolar amyloid is generally not made premortem, but vascular deposits of amyloid in small vessels are demonstrable on endomyocardial biopsy. Five of our patients presenting with angina were studied, and all had coronary flow reserve abnormalities. All had a normal coronary angiogram. Both endothelial-dependent and endothelial-independent coronary flow reserve are impaired in these patients.[114] We have seen 11 patients with symptomatic ischemic heart disease due to obstructive coronary amyloidosis. Eight had congestive heart failure. The electrocardiogram showed ischemia, bundle branch block, and rhythm disturbances. Seven had coronary angiograms and all were normal. The diagnosis of obstructive coronary amyloidosis was established either at autopsy or after cardiac transplantation. The diagnosis of amyloid ischemic heart disease is not only difficult to establish premortem but has a poor prognosis. Early identification may allow some of these patients to have a successful cardiac transplantation.

An occasional patient with congestive cardiomyopathy and biopsy proof of amyloid does not have AL but is found to have senile cardiac amyloidosis.[115] This diagnosis should be considered in a patient with biopsy proof of cardiac amyloid, in whom no monoclonal protein can be found in the serum or urine. Most patients are older than age 70 years, but we have seen patients as young as 57 years. It may be confused with familial amyloid cardiomyopathy.

In summary, any patient who presents with severe fatigue, overt congestive heart failure, or an echocardiogram that is interpreted as showing concentric left ventricular hypertrophy or asymmetric septal hypertrophy[116,117] should have immunofixation of serum and urine to exclude the possibility of unrecognized cardiac AL.

Liver

Hepatomegaly is present in one-sixth of patients with amyloidosis. Hepatomegaly or abnormal results of liver function tests are seen in 16 percent. The most common clinical and laboratory findings include unexplained hepatomegaly and an increase of the alkaline phosphatase concentration. The most common initial clinical impression is hepatic malignancy. Nearly half of patients with hepatic amyloid have proteinuria exceeding 1 g/day. Proteinuria is an important clue to the presence of a multisystemic disorder such as amyloidosis.

Four clinical clues assist in recognizing hepatic amyloidosis: 1. the presence of proteinuria; 2. the presence of a monoclonal protein in the serum or urine; 3. the presence of Howell-Jolly bodies in the peripheral blood smear, reflecting splenic infiltration[118]; and 4. hepatomegaly out of proportion to the degree of liver function test abnormality.[119] A rare patient with hepatic amyloid can present with rupture of the spleen or rupture of the liver. The latter usually is fatal.[120,121] Results of serum amyloid P scans demonstrate deposits of amyloid in the liver in almost all patients. Clinically important deposits are seen in only the minority. Cholestatic jaundice, when present, is a preterminal finding. Portal hypertension is rare, probably because death ensues due to extrahepatic amyloidosis before portal hyperten-

sion can develop. Sinusoidal portal hypertension has been demonstrated in one patient by hepatic vein catheterization. After 20 courses of melphalan and prednisone, this patient was alive 4 years after initial diagnosis, suggesting that the presence of portal hypertension in and of itself is not associated with an adverse outcome.[122] Bleeding from esophageal varices has been reported but occurs in less than 1 percent of patients with AL. Ascites is common, usually due to associated nephrotic syndrome and not as a consequence of portal hypertension. A liver biopsy demonstrates perisinusoidal and portal deposits. The median survival is approximately 1 year after liver biopsy.

The finding of hyposplenism on a peripheral blood film is a highly specific indicator of splenic amyloid. The absence of hyposplenism is not a predictable sign for the absence of spleen involvement.[123] In one study, 12 patients with diffuse splenic involvement had no Howell-Jolly bodies present. Even when the spleen has extensive replacement of the splenic cords, Howell-Jolly bodies may not be seen. Technetium scanning of the spleen may demonstrate a marked reduction in splenic blood flow, which is a consequence of amyloid infiltration. The spleen scan correlates poorly with the presence of Howell-Jolly bodies. One study reported analysis of 23 liver-spleen scans from 21 patients. Splenic activity was moderately or markedly reduced in 22 of 23 liver-spleen scans. Eight of the patients had associated splenic images performed, and four of those were abnormal.[124]

The Gastrointestinal Tract

Most patients with amyloidosis have histologically demonstrable deposits in the gastrointestinal tract. These tend to be deposits in the vessels of the submucosa and do not produce gastrointestinal tract symptoms. Most patients with AL have no symptoms referable to the gastrointestinal tract. Anorexia and weight loss, although common, correlate poorly with the presence of gastrointestinal tract amyloid. Malabsorption, defined by a low serum carotene value, is seen in less than 5 percent of patients. Steatorrhea with increased fecal fat excretion is seen in less than 2 percent of patients.

Amyloid is a well-recognized cause of gastrointestinal pseudo-obstruction for which surgery is not beneficial.[125] The clinical presentation and the radiographic features mimic acute small bowel obstruction.[126] Patients who do not have advanced cardiac involvement are candidates for long-term parenteral nutrition to maintain body weight in the presence of pseudo-obstruction. The typical symptoms are refractory nausea and vomiting. The patient's gastric contents are typically not digested. Abdominal distension and pain are significant problems. Nausea is present even during the fasting state. Cisapride has been reported to be effective for intestinal pseudo-obstruction, but in our hands, cholinergic agents, cisapride, and metoclopramide have not been effective. The mechanism of gastrointestinal tract dysfunction in amyloidosis can be a consequence of direct mucosal infiltration or, more commonly, dysmotility from autonomic failure. Occasionally, amyloidosis can present as ischemic colitis.[127] In these instances, amyloid causes complete obstruction of the vessels of the lamina propria mucosae and lamina muscularis mucosae, leading to chronic ischemia with sloughing of the mucosal lining and hemorrhage.

Two patients with AL and massive intestinal hemorrhage necessitating surgical resection demonstrated massive amyloid deposition in the muscularis mucosae. The hemorrhage was located at the border between the muscularis mucosae and the overlying rectal or colonic mucosae. Reduced motility and increased rigidity of the musculature result in shear forces that can lead to tears in regions of the vessels.[128]

The most common radiologic findings are luminal narrowing, loss of haustrations, thickening of mucosal folds, and ulceration.[129] The most frequent location is the descending and rectosigmoid colon. Abdominal computed tomographic scans were performed on 23 patients with AL. Four had bowel-wall thickening, 4 had bowel-wall dilatation without thickening, 2 had mesenteric soft tissue infiltration, and 1 had mesenteric adenopathy. A completely normal computed tomographic examination was common in amyloidosis of the gastrointestinal tract.[130]

Spontaneous duodenal perforation has been reported due to ischemia.[131] Of 769 patients with primary amyloidosis, only 8 had symptomatic gastric amyloidosis.[132] All 8 had prolonged nausea and vomiting in association with weight loss. Gastroparesis was seen in 3, and a radiographic finding mimicking a gastric malignancy was seen in 1. Six of the 8 had amyloid in the small bowel. Patients with intermittent obstructive symptoms do not respond to medical treatment, and no recovery of gastrointestinal motility has been reported.[133] Histopathologically, extensive infiltration and replacement of the muscularis propria by amyloid deposits are seen, especially in the small intestine. Endoscopically, mucosal friability and erosions are common.[134]

Profound diarrhea can be seen in intestinal amyloidosis.[135] The diarrhea can occur as a consequence of direct mucosal infiltration of the small intestine or autonomic failure of regulation of gastrointestinal tract motility. In either instance, severe watery diarrhea may occur, with 20 stools a day and frequent episodes of incontinence. The use of loperamide frequently fails and high doses of either paregoric or tincture of opium may be required. Injections of somatostatin analogue have been reported to be effective in reducing the watery diarrhea in these patients.[136] Rarely, the placement of a diverting sigmoid colostomy eliminates the fecal incontinence and the social barriers these patients face that otherwise prevent them from leaving their homes.

Nervous System

Amyloid neuropathy begins with symmetric paresthesias in the lower extremities. The median time between the development of symptoms and a histologic diagnosis exceeds 2 years. Symptoms are associated with muscle weakness in two-thirds and autonomic symptoms in two-thirds. If peripheral neuropathy dominates the patient's clinical picture, the median survival is approximately 25 months. The serum albumin level is associated with survival.[49] The outcome is improved in patients whose serum albumin value is greater than 3 g/dl at diagnosis. This, in part, reflects the absence of multisystemic involvement (Figure 35–13). The clinical picture of amyloid neuropathy is comparable to that of diabetic neuropathy. Carpal tunnel syndrome is present in half of patients with peripheral neuropathy. The prevalence of amyloidosis in sural nerve biopsies is 1.2 percent.[137] Presenting neuropathy symptoms were sensory in 6 of 13, motor in 2, and mixed in 5. Cardiac, renal, and gastrointestinal tract involvement were present in 7 of 13; 7 had autonomic symptoms. Amyloid was identified in the endoneurium in 12 nerve biopsy specimens, perineurium in 2, and epineurium in 9 nerves. Axonal degeneration predominated over demyelination in 8 of 10 patients. Incidentally, concomitant muscle biopsy specimens contained amyloid in 8 of 9 patients.[137]

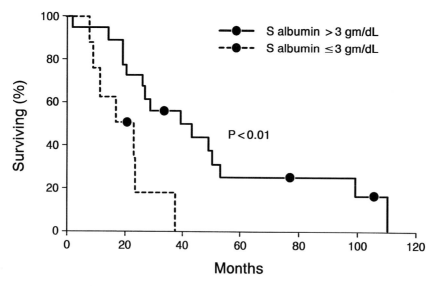

Figure 35–13. Impact of albumin on survival in primary amyloidosis neuropathy. (From Rajkumar et al.,[49] by permission of Excerpta Medica.)

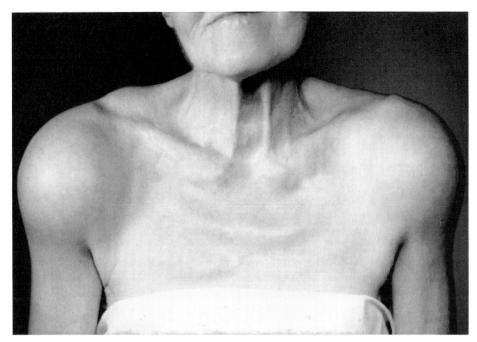

Figure 35–14. Periarticular infiltration of the shoulders with amyloid results in the shoulder-pad sign in a female.

All patients with an idiopathic sensorimotor peripheral neuropathy should have immunoelectrophoresis and immunofixation of serum and urine as part of the initial evaluation. Peripheral neuropathy is a presenting feature for approximately one patient in six with amyloidosis. Histologically, there is loss of small myelinated and unmyelinated fibers.[138] Electromyography is insensitive in the early recognition of amyloid neuropathy, because AL selectively affects small unmyelinated fibers that do not produce electromyographic abnormalities.

Rarely, patients with amyloidosis can have associated cranial neuropathy, usually the facial nerve.[139] Taste acuity is reduced in most patients with amyloidosis. Ninety percent of patients demonstrate hypogeusia; complete ageusia is present in 35 percent of patients. Frequently, patients are unaware of the reduced taste acuity, and macroglossia does not play a role in the dulling of taste. This is believed to be a form of gustative neuropathy.[140]

There is a high prevalence of proteinuria in patients with amyloid neuropathy and this represents an important diagnostic clue. Although the sural nerve biopsy is an excellent technique for the diagnosis of amyloidosis at the Mayo Clinic, there is a report in which the sural nerve biopsy failed to demonstrate amyloid in six of nine patients with amyloidosis.[141] A rare patient has amyloid deposition at the level of the nerve root, which leads to distal demyelination without demonstrable amyloid deposits in the sural nerve. Multiple sections of the sural nerve need to be examined because the deposits can be focal.

Occasionally, patients may present with muscle infiltration with amyloid.[142] Only a small fraction have skeletal muscle pseudohypertrophy and present with the shoulder pad sign (Figure 35–14).[143] Most patients with amyloid myopathy have diffuse muscle weakness related to atrophy of muscles: a consequence of chronic vascular occlusion. We reported on 12 patients with muscle biopsy identification of amyloidosis. Muscle involvement was the most prominent symptom in patients who had widespread visceral involvement, including the heart, peripheral nerve, and tongue. Only 3 of the 12 had skeletal muscle pseudohypertrophy. All patients had a free light chain in the serum or urine. The creatine kinase concentration was increased in only 3. Of 8 patients treated with chemotherapy, 3 responded, but the median survival in this group was only 12 months. Most of the patients died of cardiac failure.[142]

In a large case study, 16 patients were seen, with amyloid myopathy constituting 0.004 percent of muscle biopsy specimens. The most common symptoms included weakness and fatigue in 10, autonomic symptoms in 8, and weight loss in 7. Five patients had amyloid diagnosed from another organ biopsy specimen. Amyloid was found in the interstitium or perivascular region in the muscle in 14 and endomysial region in 7. Acute denervation atrophy was seen in 14. Eight showed small fiber atrophy, and 7 showed myofiber-type grouping. A concomitant sural nerve biopsy specimen was obtained in 7 and all had amyloid. Six of the 7 nerves showed axonopathic change. The fact that all of the patients had a sural nerve biopsy positive for amyloid raises the question as to whether the weakness was due to amyloid neuropathy or myopathy.[144] Amyloid myopathy can show heterogeneous signal intensities with magnetic resonance imaging. The signal is generally lower than normal muscle, with intermingled areas of hyperintensity on T2-weighted images.[145]

Respiratory Tract

Involvement of the minor salivary glands with amyloid is common.[146] Histologic evidence of salivary gland involvement in amyloidosis is high, and a high proportion of patients report xerostomia. Unfortunately, xerostomia is not specific for amyloidosis, and patients have been misdiagnosed as having Sjögren syndrome.[147]

Involvement of the respiratory tract usually is asymptomatic and does not typically cause clinical problems. In most patients with pulmonary involvement, the symptoms are overshadowed by concomitant cardiac involvement. Histologic demonstration of alveolar interstitial amyloid is uncommon, and gas exchange generally is preserved until late in the disease.

We have seen 35 patients with pulmonary amyloidosis presenting as an interstitial or reticulonodular process.[148] The median survival after diagnosis was 16 months. The chest radiograph is not specific and reflects interstitial lung disease. The key finding is that of a monoclonal protein in the serum or urine by immunofixation. We found low-dose corticosteroids produced symptomatic benefit in patients with diffuse interstitial pulmonary amyloid.

There appears to be a higher prevalence of pulmonary amyloidosis in patients whose amyloid is associated with an IgM monoclonal gammopathy or Waldenström's macroglobulinemia.[149] Finding amyloidosis as an isolated pulmonary nodule or occasionally multiple pulmonary nodules is not associated with systemic AL and represents a localized process that may not require therapeutic intervention.[150]

Coagulation System

Bleeding can be a serious complication of amyloidosis. Deficiency of factor X is well recognized. The most common manifestation of hemorrhage is purpura related to fragile, rigid blood vessels, secondary to infiltration of the skin vessel wall by amyloid. Factor X deficiency is seen in about 15 percent of patients. The most common coagulation test abnormality in amyloidosis is prolongation of the thrombin time.[151] Platelet defects, including abnormal platelet aggregation, have been reported, as have decreased levels of α_2-antiplasmin and increased levels of plasminogen.[152] Life-threatening bleeding is uncommon, with the exception of those patients who have profound factor X deficiency or ischemic colitis. Both splenectomy and melphalan and prednisone chemotherapy plus plasma exchange have been reported to be effective for patients with profound factor X deficiency.[153,154]

Thirty-six consecutive patients with biopsy-proven amyloidosis and documented monoclonal immunoglobulin light chains had coagulation studies. Hemorrhagic manifestations were mild to moderate in 9 and severe in 1 of the 36. The most frequent laboratory abnormality was a prolonged thrombin time in 85 percent and prolonged reptilase time in 90 percent. Low levels of factor X were observed in 1 of 4 samples. The prothrombin time was prolonged in 8 and the activated partial thromboplastin time in 25. No lupus anticoagulant was found. It was hypothesized that there was in the plasma an inhibitor of fibrin formation prolonging the thrombin time that could also affect factor X.[155]

PROGNOSIS

When a patient who presents with a syndrome compatible with amyloidosis is found to have a monoclonal protein, and the diagnosis is histologically confirmed, usually with a fat aspirate or bone marrow biopsy, the next step is assessment of the patient's prognosis. The cause of death (Figure 35–15) in most patients with amyloidosis is cardiac, either progressive cardiomyopathy with heart failure or sudden death due to ventricular fibrillation or asystole (Figure 35–11A).[156] Because an individual patient's clinical outcome is highly dependent on the extent of cardiac involvement, an echocardiogram should be a routine part of the assessment of patients with AL (Figure 35–11B).[157] In our experience, the presence of symptomatic heart failure is the most powerful indicator of survival in a multivariate model.[158]

The presence of exertional syncope is a powerful predictor of sudden death.[106] A patient presenting with exertional syncope should be considered for the placement of an implantable defibrillator because most will die within 3 months. The Doppler-derived index of diastolic myocardial performance is important in assessing the prognosis of a patient with amyloid.[159] The most significant echocardiographic predictors of outcome appear to be the Doppler index of diastolic myocardial performance, ejection fraction, and mitral deceleration time, a reflection of the ability of the ventricle to relax. Only patients whose disease is most advanced present with restrictive ventricular physiology. These patients tend to have marked ventricular wall thickening and depressed fractional shortening. Other patients tend to have a prolonged isovolumic relaxation time and reduced early diastolic filling or normal filling with ventricular wall thickening.

The value of Doppler-derived diastolic filling variables for assessing prognosis cannot be overemphasized.[160] Patients with a deceleration time of 150 ms or less on Doppler echocardiography, indicating restrictive physiology, have a 1-year probability of survival of 49 percent versus 92 percent in patients who have a deceleration time greater than 150 ms.[161]

We have found the level of serum β_2-microglobulin significant in predicting survival, but this has not been confirmed by

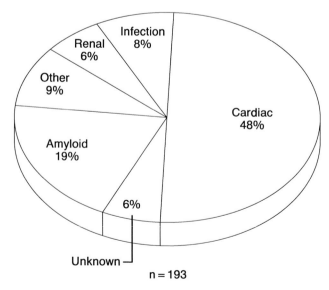

Figure 35–15. Causes of death in 193 patients with primary amyloidosis.

other groups. It has been reported that the time between histologic diagnosis and referral is an important variable. When considering all patients seen at the Mayo Clinic with amyloidosis, the median survival approaches 2 years. When patients seen at Mayo are limited to those evaluated within 30 days of histologic diagnosis, the median survival decreases to 13 months, suggesting referral bias exists that favors those patients physically able to travel to a large amyloidosis treatment center. This information is important when interpreting the results of clinical trials originating from single centers compared to multicenter trials. The presence of peripheral neuropathy as the dominant syndrome is also associated with improved outcome. Neuropathy is associated with a 3-year median survival in Mayo patients when patients with congestive heart failure, nephrotic syndrome, and orthostatic hypotension are excluded.

In a study assessing the percentage of bone marrow plasma cells and the κ-to-λ ratio of plasma cells in the bone marrow, an association with survival was found. The bone marrow plasma cell κ-to-λ ratio was an independent prognostic variable in a multivariate analysis, even when analyzed with congestive heart failure in the model. A κ-to-λ ratio of less than 1:5 in λ amyloid or a κ-to-λ ratio of greater than 16:1 in κ amyloid identified two groups with significant survival differences.[162]

THERAPY

In addition to the supportive therapies that are available for patients with nephrotic syndrome, heart failure, and peripheral neuropathy, specific therapy should be considered directed at the light chain-producing clonal plasma cells. Patients with amyloidosis who are treated with alkylating agent-based chemotherapy such as melphalan and prednisone have an improved survival if they respond.[163] The median survival of 27 patients who responded was nearly 90 months compared with only 1 year for nonresponders. The time to achieve an organ response in amyloidosis can be as long as 1 year. This relates to the body's relative inability to readily mobilize pre-existing amyloid deposits. The majority of patients with AL do not survive long enough to have an opportunity to respond. The majority of patients who are currently being treated fail to show a response, indicating a need for more effective therapies.

The definition of a response in AL can be either organ based or hematologic. In the former, a response is typically defined as a 50 percent reduction in urinary protein loss for patients with renal involvement in the absence of an increase in creatinine concentration. In patients presenting with liver involvement, reduction in the serum alkaline phosphatase level is generally associated with a response. Responses in cardiac amyloidosis are generally defined by improvement in the echocardiogram. A 2 mm reduction in the echocardiographic wall thickness not attributable to variation in technique reflects a response. It is rare to see improvement in peripheral neuropathy or the echocardiographic ejection fraction in patients treated with melphalan and prednisone chemotherapy.

There are now two prospective randomized studies that demonstrated a survival advantage for patients treated with melphalan and prednisone compared with colchicine alone.[164,165] In these reports, the response included organ responses (defined above) and hematologic responses, defined as a 50 percent reduction in the serum or urine M component or complete eradication of the light chain if an intact immunoglobulin was not present. In our experience, a reduction in the amyloid precursor protein (the light chain) does correlate with improved outcome and survival. When assessing response in amyloidosis, both organ response and M protein response should be included. Even patients with symptomatic congestive heart failure can respond to melphalan and prednisone therapy. In one study[166] that used Doppler echocardiography and functional status, three patients had marked resolution of congestive heart failure and evidence for remission of disease activity. All three were treated with melphalan. The abolition of the immunoglobulin light chain was seen in all three patients. We[167] have reported a survival of greater than or equal to 5 years in 8 of 153 patients (5 percent) with amyloid and cardiac involvement. All of the patients received chemotherapy, and a demonstrable objective response to the chemotherapy was seen in 7 of the 8.

Patients with amyloidosis deserve a trial of therapy because of the improved survival of responders; one patient survived 21 years after biopsy-proven renal amyloidosis was reported. Initial therapy included chemotherapy followed by dialysis and then a successful renal transplant, which is functioning 10 years later with no evidence of recurrent disease.[168] The treatment of amyloidosis is not innocuous. Melphalan-based therapies all carry the potential for the development of late myelodysplasia or acute leukemia.[169] Because these patients are often elderly, myelodysplasia usually results in rapid death, and the median survival from the onset of myelodysplasia is only 8 months. In our experience, a myelodysplastic disorder develops in 6.5 percent of patients exposed to melphalan. Melphalan, when given to patients with amyloid, is given in a fashion similar to that for multiple myeloma. A standard dosage would be 0.15 mg/kg per day orally for 7 consecutive days along with prednisone at 20 mg 3 times a day for the same 7 days. We generally repeat these cycles every 6 weeks and adjust the dose to produce a moderate degree of leukopenia. The blood cell counts should be followed every 3 weeks initially to ensure that midcycle myelosuppression of severe degree does not occur.

Because the majority of patients do not respond to melphalan and prednisone chemotherapy, alternatives need to be found. We have prior experience with α-tocopherol[170] and interferon-α-2[171] and have found neither agent is effective. High-dose dexamethasone with interferon has been reported to be effective in the majority of patients with amyloidosis who do not have cardiac involvement.[172] Dexamethasone is not leukemogenic and the toxicity tends to be short lived. In our hands, however, the use of high-dose dexamethasone in untreated or previously treated patients results in a response rate of 15 percent, and we currently consider dexamethasone as a therapy to be tried if there are no other alternatives.[173,174] The treatment of renal amyloid nephrotic syndrome with vincristine, doxorubicin, and dexamethasone has been reported; three of four patients obtained a partial response and continue in remission after 4 to 9 years.[175] Gianni et al.[176] reported the use of 4′-iodo-4′-deoxydoxorubicin in the treatment of amyloidosis. It appears to be most effective for patients with soft tissue deposits and less effective for those with visceral amyloidosis. This drug is believed to act by binding and ultimately dissolving amyloid deposits without exerting a cytotoxic effect on the bone marrow plasma cells.

After an initial report[177] suggested that cardiac amyloidosis was a contraindication to heart transplantation, two reports documented the effectiveness of heart transplantation for AL patients.[178,179] Survivals of 69 and 118 months after heart transplantation were reported.

At the Mayo Clinic, patients with cardiac amyloidosis of the AL type without extracardiac manifestations of disease are considered viable recipients of donor hearts. Twenty patients thus far have received a cardiac transplant for amyloidosis at the Mayo Clinic. Sixteen underwent cardiac transplantation alone for AL. There were four patients who received cardiac and liver transplants for familial amyloidosis. There were 13 males. All 20 patients were in New York Heart Association class IV, with a ventricular septal thickness greater than 15 mm and an ejection fraction of less than 45 percent. The 1-, 2-, and 5-year actuarial survival after transplantation is 94, 85, and 75 percent respectively. Three AL patients have died. The first died 9 months after heart transplantation of disseminated *Aspergillus* complicating a stem cell transplant. The second died of intestinal amyloid 16 months after transplantation, and the third died of a post-transplantation lymphoproliferative disorder 31 months after transplantation. Seventeen patients are doing well at 2 to 92 months (mean, 24 months). Currently, after heart transplantation, peripheral stem cell transplantation is considered to prevent recurrence of systemic disease.

More intensive chemotherapy has been attempted. We completed a prospective study of 101 patients randomized to receive either melphalan and prednisone or the five-drug regimen vincristine, BCNU, melphalan, cyclophosphamide, and prednisone (VBMCP). No survival advantage was seen for the five-drug combination compared with the two-drug combination.[180]

Amyloidosis is not a true neoplasm. The percentage of plasma cells in the bone marrow does not increase over time, and the size of the monoclonal peak does not tend to increase over time as it does in multiple myeloma. Virtually all therapies currently used for amyloidosis have been derived from those demonstrated to be effective in the management of multiple myeloma. Given the poor results obtained with standard chemotherapy and recognizing the improved complete response rates and prolonged survival that have been demonstrated with the use of transplantation for multiple myeloma, it was inevitable that this technique would be applied to patients with amyloidosis.

BONE MARROW OR PERIPHERAL BLOOD STEM CELL TRANSPLANTATION

Patients who have bone marrow transplantation for hematologic malignancy generally have no visceral organ dysfunction. Most transplant programs require adequate cardiac and pulmonary function, a good performance status of 0 or 1, excellent hepatic synthetic function, and good nutrition. Unfortunately, most patients with amyloidosis present with significant dys-

function of any or all of these organs. These patients are hematologically normal. Anemia is uncommon unless they have associated renal insufficiency. Thrombocytosis is usually seen only in patients with hepatic involvement and hyposplenism. As discussed above, amyloidosis patients frequently have cardiac, hepatic, renal, or neurologic problems, which make this a unique group compared with others for transplantation.

The first syngeneic transplantation for amyloidosis was performed in 1995.[181] This 32-year-old patient failed melphalan and prednisone therapy and received cyclophosphamide and total body irradiation. Post-transplantation, there was resolution of nephrotic-range proteinuria and autonomic neuropathy. Monoclonal light chains disappeared from the serum and urine, and there was improvement on the serum amyloid P component scan.[182]

Two patients have received allogeneic bone marrow transplants for AL. One patient with purpura, macroglossia, and 1.4 g of protein in the urine per day was treated with six cycles of cyclophosphamide, vincristine, doxorubicin, and methylprednisolone. The patient was conditioned for transplantation with melphalan 110 mg/m^2 and 1200 cGy of total body irradiation. The patient was alive and well at 29 months.[183] The second patient received the transplant from an HLA identical sister and was conditioned with melphalan 140 mg/m^2 and total body irradiation of 800 cGy. The urinary protein value decreased from 9.15 g to 1.3 g per day, with disappearance of light chains from the urine. Skin and liver graft-versus-host disease developed and the patient was alive 18 months post-transplant. Both patients had only single organ involvement with amyloid. Allogeneic transplant is unlikely to be applicable to many patients with amyloid given the requirement of an HLA match. Restrictions usually apply to allogeneic transplant: age less than 55 years, good performance status, adequate creatinine level, and good cardiac function. For carefully selected patients who are young with single organ involvement, it is a possibility but should be considered investigational.

Autologous bone marrow transplantation for cardiac AL was reported in a 45-year-old man.[184] The patient had endomyocardial biopsy-proven amyloid and an ejection fraction of 52 percent. The conditioning was melphalan 200 mg/m^2. At 17 months, monoclonal light chains had disappeared from the urine, but the echocardiogram remained abnormal and a post-transplantation endomyocardial biopsy showed persistent amyloid.[185]

Autologous bone marrow transplantation has been supplanted by peripheral blood stem cell transplantation because of the ease of stem cell collection and the more rapid engraftment achieved using peripheral blood stem cells versus autologous bone marrow. Although the degree of contamination with plasma cells of the apheresis product is less than would be obtained in bone marrow, clone-related sequences were detected in DNA from the peripheral blood cells of eight of ten amyloidosis patients at diagnosis and from the apheresis product of three of four undergoing stem cell mobilization. This demonstrates that circulating cells with clonal light chain gene rearrangement are present at diagnosis in AL.[186] We[187] evaluated the blood from 150 patients with AL for circulating monoclonal plasma cells, and monoclonal plasma cells were detected in 24 of 150 (16 percent).

Seven of the 150 patients had a high number of circulating cells. The presence of monoclonal plasma cells in the peripheral blood of patients with AL raises the issue of purging of the apheresis product. Whether this would have an impact on the course of the disease post-transplant remains unknown.[188]

The first reports of stem cell transplantation are from 1995 when two patients received transplants. One patient was alive but not evaluable for response, and the other had a hematologic response with eradication of urine light chain and conversion of the bone marrow from monoclonal to polyclonal plasma cells. Nephrotic syndrome and orthostatic hypotension had improved, and amyloid deposits previously present in the bone marrow were no longer detectable.[189] The largest reported experience on stem cell transplantation for AL is from Boston University Medical Center. The initial report was on five patients aged 38 to 53 years. Patients were mobilized using growth factor only, with stem cells collected on the fifth day. Conditioning was melphalan 200 mg/m^2. At 13 months, all 5 patients showed clinical regression of organ-related dysfunction, including reversal of neuropathy and resolution of hepatomegaly. Three of the five patients had a clonal population of plasma cells in the bone marrow eradicated.[190]

When the Boston experience was expanded to 25 patients,[191] the group had a median age of 48 years and 88 percent had a performance status of 1 or 2. No patient had congestive heart failure, although 8 patients had echocardiographic evidence of amyloid. Seventeen of 25 patients were alive at 24 months. Thirteen of 21 evaluable patients had elimination of their clonal plasma cells, and 11 of 17 had improved amyloid-related organ involvement. There were 3 relapses between 12 and 24 months. The best results were seen in patients with renal involvement manifested by proteinuria, and 2 of 3 patients with neurologic involvement had resolution of peripheral and autonomic neuropathy. Predictors of adverse survival included more than two major organ systems involved or predominant cardiac involvement. Acute leukemia attributed to prior melphalan exposure subsequently developed in 1 patient. Two patients died after stem cell collection but before being conditioned for transplantation. Three of the 25 patients died before day 100 post-transplantation.[191]

Treatment-related toxicity included moderate renal failure, creatinine value of 4.9 mg/dl in one, and delayed platelet engraftment in one. In patients who had cardiac involvement, treatment-related mortality was 38 percent. There was a 39 percent incidence of bleeding. When results were updated to 102 patients, the median age had increased to 55 years, but patients who were older or who had reduced cardiac or renal function received melphalan at 100 to 140 mg/m^2. They reported 3-month treatment-related mortality of 15 percent. Patients with predominant cardiac involvement had a survival of 33 percent. The rate of complete hematologic response was 55 percent.[192]

The Accreditation Subcommittee for the European Group for Blood and Marrow Transplantation held a consensus conference and added AL to the list of indications for stem cell transplantation. Autologous stem cell transplantation for AL was classified as a technique to be undertaken in an approved clinical research protocol. Allotransplantation was considered developmental in nature.[193]

We reported our results on the first 20 stem cell transplant recipients who have been followed for a sufficient period. We were impressed with the high morbidity and mortality compared with stem cell transplantation for multiple myeloma.[194] We collected stem cells between January 1996 and September 1998 from 22 patients. Cell collection was performed after priming with cyclophosphamide 3 g/m^2 followed by granulocyte-macrophage colony-stimulating factor at 5 μg/kg/day. Fifteen patients were conditioned with melphalan at 140 mg/m^2 and total body irradiation at 1200 cGy, and 4 patients received melphalan alone at 200 mg/m^2. Three patients did not receive transplants after collection owing to poor performance status. Two of them died of progressive amyloid at 1 and 3 months, and 1 patient is alive 1 year after collection and receiving hemodialysis. We continue to use cyclophosphamide and growth factor at 5 μg/kg conditioning because we were impressed by the undue degree of pulmonary toxicity, creatinine increase, and fluid retention associated with growth factor administration at 10 μg/kg/day.

Nineteen patients received transplants at a median age of 57 years. Renal, cardiac, peripheral nerve, and liver amyloidosis were present in 13, 12, 3, and 1 patient, respectively. Seventeen of the 19 had a demonstrable monoclonal protein in the serum or urine. The other 2 had clonal plasma cells in the bone marrow. Six patients had echocardiographic interventricular septal thickness of greater than or equal to 15 mm. Two of the patients had an ejection fraction of less than 60 percent. Seven of the 19 patients have died; 4 died before day 100: 2 of pneumonia, 1 of multiorgan failure, and 1 of sudden cardiac death with autopsy evidence of severe cardiac amyloid. Two patients who survived subsequently died of progressive cardiac amyloid at 7 and 9 months. An additional patient responded and subsequently progressed, dying of cardiac amyloid at 22 months.

Twelve of the transplant recipients are alive with a median follow-up of 18 months, and 9 had objective evidence of responses. Six of these patients had renal amyloid. Three of the responses took greater than 9 months, including 2 patients who did not show a 50 percent reduction of proteinuria until at least 30 months post-transplantation. This is consistent with the long time required for resolution of amyloid deposits. Gastrointestinal tract bleeding was seen in 2; 3 required prolonged enteral or parenteral nutrition. Five had significant cardiac arrhythmias during stem cell collection or post-transplantation. Assessment of outcome from the number of organ systems involved pretransplant revealed that 9 of the 10 transplant recipients who had only one organ system involved are alive compared with 4 of 7 survivors with two organ systems involved and none of 3 with three organ systems involved.

A 56-year-old woman was recently reported[195] who had purpura, macroglossia, and hepatomegaly with 25 percent bone marrow plasma cells. Before transplantation, she received 4 monthly cycles of vincristine, idarubicin, and dexamethasone. Stem cells were collected with cyclophosphamide and granulocyte-macrophage colony-stimulating factor. Conditioning was with melphalan and busulfan. At 22 months, the clonal plasma cell disorder responded, the liver normalized, the alkaline phosphatase level returned to normal, and there was significant improvement in the signs of vascular and soft tissue infiltration. A multicenter trial of transplantation for amyloidosis was completed recently by the Eastern Cooperative Oncology Group, but results have not been reported.

Toxicity of Transplant

The first multicenter survey on the outcome of transplantation for AL was published in 1998.[196] Twenty-one patients received transplants, 18 with melphalan only and 3 with melphalan plus total body irradiation. The death rate from toxic reactions was 43 percent: 9 of 21 died within 30 days post-transplant. Ten of the 12 survivors achieved a response. All deaths were attributable to multiorgan failure. These patients were likely selected because the median time from diagnosis to transplantation was 11 months, with 1 patient undergoing transplantation 20 months after diagnosis. Given that half of the patients with amyloid succumb to the disease at 1 year, the group reported patients self-selected by the ability to survive to the time of transplantation. For patients presenting with two or more clinical manifestations, the 4-year survival is 11.1 percent. The risk of death from toxic response with more than two organs involved was greater than 75 percent. Careful patient selection is required before patients are subjected to this procedure.

The group from Hammersmith evaluated 27 patients who received high-dose melphalan (from 100 to 200 mg/m^2). There were 8 treatment-related deaths (30 percent) due to multiorgan failure, including gastrointestinal tract hemorrhage in 2 and sepsis and cardiac complications in 1 each. A hematologic response was seen in 64 percent and a clinical organ response in 57 percent. At the time of the report, 17 of 27 patients were alive. The group recommended exclusion of high-risk patients to avoid the high treatment-related mortality.[197] In a subsequent report[198] of 9 patients, 4 died within the first year after transplantation (44 percent) and 5 were alive with a mean follow-up of 12.6 months and 4 responses. Three of the 4 deaths were of patients who had cardiac amyloid, and the fourth had three organ systems involved.

The development of post-transplantation multiorgan failure and severe gastrointestinal tract bleeding appears to be the result of the underlying amyloidosis, because this is not seen in transplantation for other indications. We believe that amyloid involvement of the vessels of the gastrointestinal tract renders the vessels rigid and inflexible. The inevitable mucositis that follows conditioning denudes the intestinal tract mucosa and exposes these amyloid-involved vessels. We believe they readily rupture and can lead to serious hemorrhage. Massive gastrointestinal tract hemorrhage has been reported in patients who had no pretransplantation symptoms referable to their gastrointestinal tract. Progressive impairment of renal function and delayed engraftment have also been reported.[199] In 1992, Mehta et al.[200] reported on a patient who developed massive gastrointestinal tract hemorrhage 3 days after transplantation and died on day 17. A second patient died 74 days after transplantation as a result of respiratory failure.[201] A 63-year-old patient died of gastrointestinal tract hemorrhage, having presented with gastrointestinal tract symptoms.[56] A fatal gastrointestinal tract perforation was reported on day 4 after stem cell transplantation.[202]

Four amyloidosis patients receiving high-dose therapy were reported. One went on to dialysis-dependent renal failure and a fatal gastrointestinal tract hemorrhage on day 97. Post-transplantation bronchial pneumonia developed in a second patient who died on day 374.[203] One patient was reported with AL who received high-dose melphalan chemotherapy followed by stem cells. Tumor lysis syndrome with renal failure developed.[204] Conditioning with high-dose melphalan for transplantation in amyloidosis has been reported to produce a severe encephalopathy.[205] Tonic-clonic seizures and a comatose state lasting 18 days developed in one patient. This patient had severe renal insufficiency pretransplantation. One year post-transplant, the patient remained dialysis dependent. This report suggests that the dose of melphalan may need to be reduced in patients who have renal insufficiency and are to have stem cell transplantation.

Conventional Treatment of Younger Patients

Patients receiving transplants for AL are highly selected by virtue of age, performance status, number of organs involved, and absence of important cardiac involvement. It is difficult to know what the overall survival of a comparable control group would be. It would certainly be expected to be greater than the median survival of 13 months reported for all patients with AL.

Dispenzieri et al.[206] reviewed the Mayo Clinic experience from 1983 to 1997 of select patients who would be eligible for stem cell transplantation. The criteria included symptomatic disease, absence of multiple myeloma, age younger than or equal to 70 years, a ventricular septal thickness less than or equal to 15 mm, an ejection fraction greater than 55 percent, and a creatinine concentration less than 2 mg/dl. Of 1288 patients seen during this 14-year period, 234 fulfilled the eligibility criteria. The median age was 57 years (131 males and 103 females); 121 had nephrotic-range proteinuria. Cardiac, liver, and nerve involvement were present in 98 (42 percent), 13 (6 percent), and 36 patients (15 percent), respectively. With a median follow-up of survivors of 44.5 months, the median survival was 45.6 months.

The most significant prognostic factors in this conventionally treated cohort were age, alkaline phosphatase value, and 24-hour urine light chain excretion. For patients younger than age 50 years, the median survival was 60.6 months. For patients aged 51 to 60 years, the median survival was 46.3 months. The survival for patients with a normal versus increased alkaline phosphatase value is 50.5 versus 17.1 months. Eligibility to receive a stem cell transplant is a favorable prognostic factor that predicts for a better outcome than for unselected patients with AL. The 4-year survival rate after stem cell transplantation remains unknown, but patients who can receive a stem cell transplant are inherently a good-risk population with a superior median survival. It is imperative to stratify patients receiving transplants for risk factors known to impact on survival in this disease.

Blood cell transplants for amyloidosis have a much higher morbidity and mortality than transplants for multiple myeloma. Patients who have clinically significant cardiac amyloidosis should not receive transplants because the majority of deaths are in patients with cardiac amyloidosis. The best results are achieved in patients with isolated renal amyloidosis as the only manifestation of their disease. The response rate seen in patients with amyloidosis who receive a stem cell transplant does appear to be higher than that seen in patients traditionally treated with melphalan and prednisone. There is an unusually high rate of gastrointestinal tract toxicity with significant hemorrhage. Cardiac complications, including rhythm disturbances, are unexpectedly prevalent. The response duration and actuarial median survival associated with transplantation cannot as yet be determined accurately. Current protocols are focusing on reduced doses of melphalan in an effort to reduce toxic response rates while maintaining the higher response rates in transplant recipients who would otherwise not be candidates for full-dose melphalan.

KEY POINTS

- Suspect amyloidosis when a patient presents with unexplained:
  - Nephrotic-range proteinuria
  - Heart failure
  - Peripheral neuropathy
  - Hepatomegaly
- Pursue diagnosis aggressively if:
  - Monoclonal protein is detected in serum or urine
- Confirm diagnosis:
  - Congo red stain of:
  - Subcutaneous fat
  - Bone marrow
- Perform echocardiography to assess prognosis
- Begin chemotherapy:
  - Traditional-dose chemotherapy for most patients
  - High-dose chemotherapy with stem cell rescue for selected patients

REFERENCES

1. Virchow RLK: Cellularpathologie. (Translated by F Chance.) RM De Witt, New York, 1860.
2. Breathnach CS: Biographical sketches no. 17—Virchow. Ir Med J 75:139, 1982.
3. Haas LF: Rudolph Ludwig Carl Virchow (1821–1902). J Neurol Neurosurg Psychiatry 61:578, 1996.
4. Tildsley GJ, Lakhani S: Early clinical pathologists. 4: Rudolf Virchow (1821–1902). J Clin Pathol 45:6, 1992.
5. Mathis H: Rokitansky, Virchow and Heschl on the problem of amyloidosis [German]. Zentralbl Allg Pathol 111:103, 1968.
6. Doyle L: Lardaceous disease: Some early reports by British authors (1722–1879). J R Soc Med 81:729, 1988.
7. Aterman K: A historical note on the iodine-sulphuric acid reaction of amyloid. Histochemistry 49:131, 1976.
8. Banerjee AK: Sir Samuel Wilks: A founding father of clinical science. J R Soc Med 84:44, 1991.
9. Puchtler H, Sweat F: A review of early concepts of amyloid in context with contemporary chemical literature from 1839 to 1859. J Histochem Cytochem 14:123, 1966.
10. Ruske W: August Kekule and the development of the theory of chemical structure [German]. Naturwissenschaften 52:485, 1965.
11. Schmiedeberg O: Über die Beziehungen des Hyaloidins zu der Bildung der Chondroitinschwefelsäure, des Collagens und des Amyloids im Organismus. Arch Exp Pathol Pharmakol 87:47, 1920.
12. Bock HE: 80th anniversary of Prof. Dr. Hans Hermann Bennhold on Sept. 11, 1973 [German]. Med Welt 24:1341, 1973.
13. Elghetany MT, Saleem A, Barr K: The Congo red stain revisited. Ann Clin Lab Sci 19:190, 1989.
14. Kallee E: The 100th birthday of Hans Hermann Bennhold [German]. Dtsch Med Wochenschr 118:1336, 1993.
15. Oifa AI: Paul Divry—founder of the concept of cerebral amyloidosis [Russian]. Zh Nevropatol Psikhiatr Im SS Korsakova 73:1078, 1973.
16. Reznik M: Paul Divry. The discovery of cerebral amyloidosis [French]. Acta Neurol Belg 89:168, 1989.
17. Magnus-Levy A: Bence-Jones-Eiweiss und Amyloid. Z Klin Med 116:510, 1931.
18. Cohen AS, Calkins E: Electron microscopic observations on a fibrous component in amyloid of diverse origins. Nature 183:1202, 1959.
19. Osserman EF, Takatsuki K, Talal N: The pathogenesis of amyloidosis: Studies on the role of abnormal gamma globulins and gamma globulin fragments of the Bence Jones (L-polypeptide) type in the pathogenesis of "primary" and "secondary amyloidosis," and the "amyloidosis" associated with plasma cell myeloma. Semin Hematol 1:3, 1964.
20. Eanes ED, Glenner GG: X-ray diffraction studies on amyloid filaments. J Histochem Cytochem 16:673, 1968.
21. Glenner GG, Harbaugh J, Ohma JI et al: An amyloid protein: The amino-terminal variable fragment of an immnoglobulin light chain. Biochem Biophys Res Commun 41:1287, 1970.
22. Levin M, Franklin EC, Frangione B et al: The amino acid sequence of a major nonimmunoglobulin component of some amyloid fibrils. J Clin Invest 51:2773, 1972.
23. Ein D, Kimura S, Glenner GG: An amyloid fibril protein of unknown origin: Partial amino-acid sequence analysis. Biochem Biophys Res Commun 46:498, 1972.
24. Pras M, Schubert M, Zucker-Franklin D et al: The characterization of soluble amyloid prepared in water. J Clin Invest 47:924, 1968.
25. Cohen HJ, Minkin W: Classification of amyloidosis. Arch Dermatol 103:566, 1971.
26. Mahloudji M, Teasdall RD, Adamkiewicz JJ et al: The genetic amyloidoses with particular reference to hereditary neuropathic amyloidosis, type II (Indiana or Rukavina type). Medicine (Balt) 48:1, 1969.
27. Rukavina JG, Block WD, Jackson CE et al: Primary systemic amyloidosis: A review and an experimental, genetic, and clinical study of 29 cases with particular emphasis on the familial form. Medicine (Balt) 72:47, 1993.
28. Gertz MA: Secondary amyloidosis (AA). J Intern Med 232:517, 1992.
29. Glenner GG, Ein D, Eanes ED et al: Creation of "amyloid" fibrils from Bence Jones proteins in vitro. Science 174:712, 1971.
30. Pruzanski W, Katz A, Nyburg SC et al: In vitro production of an amyloid-like substance from gamma 3 heavy chain disease protein. Immunol Commun 3:469, 1974.

31. Solomon A, Weiss DT, Murphy C: Primary amyloidosis associated with a novel heavy-chain fragment (AH amyloidosis). Am J Hematol 45:171, 1994.

32. Solomon A, Weiss DT, Pepys MB: Induction in mice of human light-chain-associated amyloidosis. Am J Pathol 140:629, 1992.

33. Solomon A, Frangione B, Franklin EC: Bence Jones proteins and light chains of immunoglobulins. Preferential association of the V lambda VI subgroup of human light chains with amyloidosis AL (lambda). J Clin Invest 70:453, 1982.

34. Kyle RA, Bayrd ED: Amyloidosis: Review of 236 cases. Medicine (Balt) 54:271, 1975.

35. Rajkumar SV, Gertz MA, Kyle RA: Primary systemic amyloidosis with delayed progression to multiple myeloma. Cancer 82:1501, 1998.

36. Kyle RA, Linos A, Beard CM et al: Incidence and natural history of primary systemic amyloidosis in Olmsted County, Minnesota, 1950 through 1989. Blood 79:1817, 1992.

37. Waterhouse D, Carman WJ, Schottenfeld D et al: Cancer incidence in the rural community of Tecumseh, Michigan: A pattern of increased lymphopoietic neoplasms. Cancer 77:763, 1996.

38. Fonseca R, Ahmann GJ, Jalal SM et al: Chromosomal abnormalities in systemic amyloidosis. Br J Haematol 103:704, 1998.

39. Kyle RA, Greipp PR: Amyloidosis (AL). Clinical and laboratory features in 229 cases. Mayo Clin Proc 58:665, 1983.

40. Gertz MA, Kyle RA: Primary systemic amyloidosis—a diagnostic primer. Mayo Clin Proc 64:1505, 1989.

41. Case records of the Massachusetts General Hospital (Case 38-1992). N Engl J Med 327:943, 1992.

42. Rao JK, Allen NB: Primary systemic amyloidosis masquerading as giant cell arteritis. Case report and review of the literature. Arthritis Rheum 36:422, 1993.

43. Rodon P, Friocourt P, Blanchet S et al: Temporal artery involvement revealing AL amyloidosis and IgD monoclonal gammopathy. J Rheumatol 23:189, 1996.

44. Salvarani C, Gabriel SE, Gertz MA et al: Primary systemic amyloidosis presenting as giant cell arteritis and polymyalgia rheumatica. Arthritis Rheum 37:1621, 1994.

45. Gertz MA, Kyle RA, Griffing WL et al: Jaw claudication in primary systemic amyloidosis. Medicine (Balt) 65:173, 1986.

46. Schena FP, Pannarale G, Carbonara MC: Clinical and therapeutic aspects of renal amyloidosis. Nephrol Dial Transplant 11 (Suppl. 9):63, 1996.

47. Kyle RA, Gertz MA: Primary systemic amyloidosis: Clinical and laboratory features in 474 cases. Semin Hematol 32:45, 1995.

48. Peters RA, Koukoulis G, Gimson A et al: Primary amyloidosis and severe intrahepatic cholestatic jaundice. Gut 35:1322, 1994.

49. Rajkumar SV, Gertz MA, Kyle RA: Prognosis of patients with primary systemic amyloidosis who present with dominant neuropathy. Am J Med 104:232, 1998.

50. Pascali E: Diagnosis and treatment of primary amyloidosis. Crit Rev Oncol Hematol 19:149, 1995.

51. Feiner HD: Pathology of dysproteinemia: Light chain amyloidosis, non-amyloid immunoglobulin deposition disease, cryoglobulinemia syndromes, and macroglobulinemia of Waldenström. Hum Pathol 19:1255, 1988.

52. Gertz MA, Greipp PR, Kyle RA: Classification of amyloidosis by the detection of clonal excess of plasma cells in the bone marrow. J Lab Clin Med 118:33, 1991.

53. Wu SS, Brady K, Anderson JJ et al: The predictive value of bone marrow morphologic characteristics and immunostaining in primary (AL) amyloidosis. Am J Clin Pathol 96:95, 1991.

54. Perfetti V, Garini P, Vignarelli MC et al: Diagnostic approach to and follow-up of difficult cases of AL amyloidosis. Haematologica 80:409, 1995.

55. Hachulla E, Maulin L, Deveaux M et al: Prospective and serial study of primary amyloidosis with serum amyloid P component scintigraphy: From diagnosis to prognosis. Am J Med 101:77, 1996.

56. Gillmore JD, Hawkins PN, Pepys MB: Amyloidosis: A review of recent diagnostic and therapeutic developments. Br J Haematol 99:245, 1997.

57. Jager PL, Hazenberg BP, Franssen EJ et al: Kinetic studies with iodine-123-labeled serum amyloid P component in patients with systemic AA and AL amyloidosis and assessment of clinical value. J Nucl Med 39:699, 1998.

58. Westermark P: Diagnosing amyloidosis. Scand J Rheumatol 24:327, 1995.

59. Hachulla E, Janin A, Flipo RM et al: Labial salivary gland biopsy is a reliable test for the diagnosis of primary and secondary amyloidosis. A prospective clinical and immunohistologic study in 59 patients. Arthritis Rheum 36:691, 1993.

60. Huang C-Y, Wang W-J, Wong C-K: Skin biopsy gives the potential benefit in the diagnosis of systemic amyloidosis associated with cardiac involvement. Arch Dermatol 134:643, 1998.

61. Kyle RA, Spencer RJ, Dahlin DC: Value of rectal biopsy in the diagnosis of primary systemic amyloidosis. Am J Med Sci 251:501, 1966.

62. Gertz MA, Li CY, Shirahama T et al: Utility of subcutaneous fat aspiration for the diagnosis of systemic amyloidosis (immunoglobulin light chain). Arch Intern Med 148:929, 1988.

63. Pomerance A, Slavin G, McWatt J: Experience with the sodium sulphate-Alcian Blue stain for amyloid in cardiac pathology. J Clin Pathol 29:22, 1976.

64. Garcia-Gonzalez R, Fernandez FA, Garijo MF et al: Amyloidosis of the rectum mimicking collagenous colitis. Pathol Res Pract 194:731, 1998.

65. Hamidi AK, Liepnieks JJ, Nakamura M et al: Organ-specific (localized) synthesis of Ig light chain amyloid. J Immunol 162:5556, 1999.

66. Kim HY, Im JG, Song KS et al: Localized amyloidosis of the respiratory system: CT features. J Comput Assist Tomogr 23:627, 1999.

67. Hafron JM, Flanigan RC: Primary localized amyloidosis of the ureter and bladder managed by ileal interposition. Tech Urol 6:50, 2000.

68. Hayashi T, Kojima S, Sekine H et al: Primary localized amyloidosis of the ureter. Int J Urol 5:383, 1998.

69. Kageyama S, Suzuki K, Ushiyama T et al: Primary localized amyloidosis of the urethra in a woman. Br J Urol 81:918, 1998.

70. Kyle RA, Gertz MA, Linke RP: Amyloid localized to tenosynovium at carpal tunnel release. Immunohistochemical identification of amyloid type. Am J Clin Pathol 97:250, 1992.

71. Hill VE, Brownstein S, Jordan DR: Ptosis secondary to amyloidosis of the tarsal conjunctiva and tarsus. Am J Ophthalmol 123:852, 1997.

72. Gratacos J, Orellana C, Sanmarti R et al: Secondary amyloidosis in ankylosing spondylitis. A systematic survey of 137 patients using abdominal fat aspiration. J Rheumatol 24:912, 1997.

73. Cunnane G, Whitehead AS: Amyloid precursors and amyloidosis in rheumatoid arthritis. Best Pract Res Clin Rheumatol 13:615, 1999.

74. Okuda Y, Takasugi K, Oyama T et al: Intractable diarrhoea associated with secondary amyloidosis in rheumatoid arthritis. Ann Rheum Dis 56:535, 1997.

75. Habu S, Watanabe H, Kimura K et al: A case of amyloid goiter secondary to Crohn's disease. Endocrinol J 46:179, 1999.

76. Lanjewar DN, Raghuwanshi SR, Gupta D et al: Systemic amyloidosis in Hodgkin's disease. Indian J Pathol Microbiol 41:169, 1998.

77. Coakley FV, Hricak H, Presti JC Jr et al: Diffuse retroperitoneal amyloidosis due to renal cell carcinoma. Br J Radiol 72:412, 1999.

78. Komatsuda A, Morita K, Ohtani H et al: Remission of the nephrotic syndrome in a patient with renal amyloidosis due to rheumatoid arthritis treated with prednisolone and methotrexate. Am J Kidney Dis 32:E7, 1998.

79. Savolainen HA: Chlorambucil in severe juvenile chronic arthritis: Longterm followup with special reference to amyloidosis. J Rheumatol 26:898, 1999.

80. Laiho K, Tiitinen S, Kaarela K et al: Secondary amyloidosis has decreased in patients with inflammatory joint disease in Finland. Clin Rheumatol 18:122, 1999.

81. Cozzi PJ, Abu-Jawdeh GM, Green RM, Green D: Amyloidosis in association with human immunodeficiency virus infection. Clin Infect Dis 14:189, 1992.

82. Connors LH, Theberge R, Skare J et al: A new transthyretin variant (Ser23Asn) associated with familial amyloidosis in a Portuguese patient. Amyloid 6:114, 1999.

83. Moyssakis I, Triposkiadis F, Rallidis L et al: Echocardiographic features of primary, secondary and familial amyloidosis. Eur J Clin Invest 29:484, 1999.

84. el-Salhy M, Nyhlin N, Ando Y et al: The neuroendocrine system and gastrointestinal complications in patients with familial amyloidosis and polyneuropathy. Scand J Gastroenterol 32:849, 1997.

85. Dubrey SW, Cha K, Skinner M et al: Familial and primary (AL) cardiac amyloidosis: Echocardiographically similar diseases with distinctly different clinical outcomes. Heart 78:74, 1997.

86. Golling M, Singer R, Weiss G et al: Sequential (domino) transplantation of the liver in a transthyretin-50 familial amyloid polyneuropathy. Special reference to cardiological diagnosis and complications. Langenbecks Arch Surg 385:21, 2000.

87. Shaz BH, Gordon F, Lewis WD et al: Orthotopic liver transplantation for familial amyloidotic polyneuropathy: A pathological study. Hum Pathol 31:40, 2000.

88. Tashima K, Ando Y, Terazaki H et al: Outcome of liver transplantation for transthyretin amyloidosis: Follow-up of Japanese familial amyloidotic polyneuropathy patients. J Neurol Sci 171:19, 1999.

89. Dubrey SW, Davidoff R, Skinner M et al: Progression of ventricular wall thickening after liver transplantation for familial amyloidosis. Transplantation 64:74, 1997.

90. Gertz MA, Kyle RA: Prognostic value of urinary protein in primary systemic amyloidosis (AL). Am J Clin Pathol 94:313, 1990.

91. Daniels JD, Hewlett JS: Renal manifestations in multiple myeloma and in primary amyloidosis. Cleve Clin Q 37:181, 1970.

92. Suzuki H, Konishi K, Izumi Y et al: Long-term hemodialysis in a patient with primary amyloidosis, renal failure, and a vascular necrosis of the femoral heads. South Med J 75:1018, 1982.

93. Gertz MA, Kyle RA, O'Fallon WM: Dialysis support of patients with primary systemic amyloidosis. A study of 211 patients. Arch Intern Med 152:2245, 1992.

94. Stone WJ, Latos DL, Lankford PG et al: Chronic peritoneal dialysis in a patient with primary amyloidosis, renal failure, and factor X deficiency. South Med J 71:764, 1978.

95. Bienz N, Franklin IM, Adu D et al: Bilateral nephrectomy for uncontrollable nephrotic syndrome in primary amyloidosis, with subsequent improvement in hepatic function. Clin Lab Haematol 16:85, 1994.

96. Ekelund L: Radiologic findings in renal amyloidosis. AJR Am J Roentgenol 129:851, 1977.

97. Plehn JF, Friedman BJ: Diastolic dysfunction in amyloid heart disease: Restrictive cardiomyopathy or not? J Am Coll Cardiol 13:54, 1989.

98. Cueto-Garcia L, Reeder GS, Kyle RA et al: Echocardiographic findings in systemic amyloidosis: Spectrum of cardiac involvement and relation to survival. J Am Coll Cardiol 6:737, 1985.

99. Hancock EW: Low voltage, Q waves, and congestive heart failure. Hosp Pract (Off Ed) 32:21, 1997.

100. Chew C, Ziady GM, Raphael MJ et al: The functional defect in amyloid heart disease. The "stiff heart" syndrome. Am J Cardiol 36:438, 1975.

101. Chew C, Ziady GM, Raphael MJ et al: Functional defect in amyloid heart disease: 'the stiff heart syndrome' (abstract). Br Heart J 38:537, 1976.

102. Buja LM, Khoi NB, Roberts WC: Clinically significant cardiac amyloidosis. Clinicopathologic findings in 15 patients. Am J Cardiol 26:394, 1970.

103. Gertz MA, Falk RH, Skinner M et al: Worsening of congestive heart failure in amyloid heart disease treated by calcium channel-blocking agents. Am J Cardiol 55:1645, 1985.

104. Gertz MA, Grogan M, Kyle RA et al: Endomyocardial biopsy-proven light chain amyloidosis (AL) without echocardiographic features of infiltrative cardiomyopathy. Am J Cardiol 80:93, 1997.

105. Clesham GJ, Vigushin DM, Hawkins PN et al: Echocardiographic assessment of cardiac involvement in systemic AL amyloidosis in relation to whole body amyloid load measured by serum amyloid P component (SAP) clearance. Am J Cardiol 80:1104, 1997.

106. Chamarthi B, Dubrey SW, Cha K et al: Features and prognosis of exertional syncope in light-chain associated AL cardiac amyloidosis. Am J Cardiol 80:1242, 1997.

107. Patel AR, Dubrey SW, Mendes LA et al: Right ventricular dilation in primary amyloidosis: An independent predictor of survival. Am J Cardiol 80:486, 1997.

108. Mathew V, Chaliki H, Nishimura RA: Atrioventricular sequential pacing in cardiac amyloidosis: An acute Doppler echocardiographic and catheterization hemodynamic study. Clin Cardiol 20:723, 1997.

109. Crockett LK, Thompson M, Dekker A: A review of cardiac amyloidosis. Report of a case presenting as constrictive pericarditis. Am J Med Sci 264:149, 1972.

110. Meaney E, Shabetai R, Bhargava V et al: Cardiac amyloidosis, constrictive pericarditis and restrictive cardiomyopathy. Am J Cardiol 38:547, 1976.

111. Browne RS, Schneiderman H, Kayani N et al: Amyloid heart disease manifested by systemic arterial thromboemboli. Chest 102:304, 1992.

112. Dubrey S, Pollak A, Skinner M et al: Atrial thrombi occurring during sinus rhythm in cardiac amyloidosis: Evidence for atrial electromechanical dissociation. Br Heart J 74:541, 1995.

113. Narang R, Chopra P, Wasir HS: Cardiac amyloidosis presenting as ischemic heart disease. A case report and review of literature. Cardiology 82:294, 1993.

114. Al Suwaidi J, Velianou JL, Gertz MA et al: Systemic amyloidosis presenting with angina pectoris. Ann Intern Med 131:838, 1999.

115. Olson LJ, Gertz MA, Edwards WD et al: Senile cardiac amyloidosis with myocardial dysfunction. Diagnosis by endomyocardial biopsy and immunohistochemistry. N Engl J Med 317:738, 1987.

116. Presti CF, Waller BF, Armstrong WF: Cardiac amyloidosis mimicking the echocardiographic appearance of obstructive hypertrophic myopathy. Chest 93:881, 1988.

117. Weston LT, Raybuck BD, Robinowitz M et al: Primary amyloid heart disease presenting as hypertrophic obstructive cardiomyopathy. Cathet Cardiovasc Diagn 12:176, 1986.

118. Gertz MA, Kyle RA, Greipp PR: Hyposplenism in primary systemic amyloidosis. Ann Intern Med 98:475, 1983.

119. Gertz MA, Kyle RA: Hepatic amyloidosis: Clinical appraisal in 77 patients. Hepatology 25:118, 1997.

120. Bujanda L, Beguiristain A, Alberdi F et al: Spontaneous rupture of the liver in amyloidosis. Am J Gastroenterol 92:1385, 1997.

121. Gastineau DA, Gertz MA, Rosen CB et al: Computed tomography for diagnosis of hepatic rupture in primary systemic amyloidosis. Am J Hematol 37:194, 1991.

122. Horsmans Y, Brenard R, Ferrant A et al: Long-term favourable outcome of portal hypertension complicating primary systemic amyloidosis. Liver 15:332, 1995.

123. Seo IS, Li CY: Hyposplenic blood picture in systemic amyloidosis. Its absence is not a predictable sign for absence of splenic involvement. Arch Pathol Lab Med 119:252, 1995.

124. Powsner RA, Simms RW, Chudnovsky A et al: Scintigraphic functional hyposplenism in amyloidosis. J Nucl Med 39:221, 1998.

125. Fraser AG, Arthur JF, Hamilton I: Intestinal pseudoobstruction secondary to amyloidosis responsive to cisapride. Dig Dis Sci 36:532, 1991.

126. Koppelman RN, Stollman NH, Baigorri F et al: Acute small bowel pseudo-obstruction due to AL amyloidosis: A case report and literature review. Am J Gastroenterol 95:294, 2000.

127. Trinh TD, Jones B, Fishman EK: Amyloidosis of the colon presenting as ischemic colitis: A case report and review of the literature. Gastrointest Radiol 16:133, 1991.

128. Kaiserling E, Krober S: Massive intestinal hemorrhage associated with intestinal amyloidosis. An investigation of underlying pathologic processes. Gen Diagn Pathol 141:147, 1995.

129. Lee JG, Wilson JA, Gottfried MR: Gastrointestinal manifestations of amyloidosis. South Med J 87:243, 1994.

130. Araoz PA, Batts KP, MacCarty RL: Amyloidosis of the alimentary canal: Radiologic-pathologic correlation of CT findings. Abdom Imaging 25:38, 2000.

131. Fraser AG, Nicholson GI: Duodenal perforation in primary systemic amyloidosis. Gut 33:997, 1992.

132. Menke DM, Kyle RA, Fleming CR et al: Symptomatic gastric amyloidosis in patients with primary systemic amyloidosis. Mayo Clin Proc 68:763, 1993.

133. Tada S, Iida M, Yao T et al: Intestinal pseudo-obstruction in patients with amyloidosis: Clinicopathologic differences between chemical types of amyloid protein. Gut 34:1412, 1993.

134. Lau CF, Fok KO, Hui PK et al: Intestinal obstruction and gastrointestinal bleeding due to systemic amyloidosis in a woman with occult plasma cell dyscrasia. Eur J Gastroenterol Hepatol 11:681, 1999.

135. Voulgarelis M, Goutas N, Skopouli FN: A 47-year-old woman with persistent watery diarrhea, proteinuria, proximal weakness and monoclonal gammopathy (clinical conference). Clin Exp Rheumatol 17:351, 1999.

136. Ueno Y, Miyoshi Y, Yatok M et al: A case of refractory diarrhea treated with somatostatin analogue [Japanese]. Nippon Shokakibyo Gakkai Zasshi 94:778, 1997.

137. Rajani B, Rajani V, Prayson RA: Peripheral nerve amyloidosis in sural nerve biopsies: A clinicopathologic analysis of 13 cases. Arch Pathol Lab Med 124:114, 2000.

138. Quattrini A, Nemni R, Sferrazza B et al: Amyloid neuropathy simulating lower motor neuron disease. Neurology 51:600, 1998.

139. Traynor AE, Gertz MA, Kyle RA: Cranial neuropathy associated with primary amyloidosis. Ann Neurol 29:451, 1991.

140. Marinone MG, Merlini G: Reduced taste perception in AL amyloidosis. A frequently unnoticed sensory impairment. Haematologica 81:110, 1996.

141. Simmons Z, Blaivas M, Aguilera AJ et al: Low diagnostic yield of sural nerve biopsy in patients with peripheral neuropathy and primary amyloidosis. J Neurol Sci 120:60, 1993.

142. Gertz MA, Kyle RA: Myopathy in primary systemic amyloidosis. J Neurol Neurosurg Psychiatry 60:655, 1996.

143. Katz GA, Peter JB, Pearson CM et al: The shoulder-pad sign—a diagnostic feature of amyloid arthropathy. N Engl J Med 288:354, 1973.

144. Prayson RA: Amyloid myopathy: Clinicopathologic study of 16 cases. Hum Pathol 29:463, 1998.

145. Comesaana L, del Castillo M, Martin R et al: Musculoskeletal amyloid disease: MRI features. Ann Radiol (Paris) 38:150, 1995.

146. Schlesinger I: Multiple myeloma and AL amyloidosis mimicking Sjögren's syndrome. South Med J 86:568, 1993.

147. Richey TK, Bennion SD: Etiologies of the sicca syndrome: Primary systemic amyloidosis and others. Int J Dermatol 35:553, 1996.

148. Utz JP, Swensen SJ, Gertz MA: Pulmonary amyloidosis. The Mayo Clinic experience from 1980 to 1993. Ann Intern Med 124:407, 1996.

149. Zatloukal P, Bezdicek P, Schimonova M et al: Waldenström's macroglobulinemia with pulmonary amyloidosis. Respiration 65:414, 1998.

150. Pickford HA, Swensen SJ, Utz JP: Thoracic cross-sectional imaging of amyloidosis. AJR Am J Roentgenol 168:351, 1997.

151. Gastineau DA, Gertz MA, Daniels TM et al: Inhibitor of the thrombin time in systemic amyloidosis: A common coagulation abnormality. Blood 77:2637, 1991.

152. Mizutani AR, Ward CF: Amyloidosis associated bleeding diatheses in the surgical patient. Can J Anaesth 37:910, 1990.

153. Rosenstein ED, Itzkowitz SH, Penziner AS et al: Resolution of factor X deficiency in primary amyloidosis following splenectomy. Arch Intern Med 143:597, 1983.

154. Beardell FV, Varma M, Martinez J: Normalization of plasma factor X levels in amyloidosis after plasma exchange. Am J Hematol 54:68, 1997.

155. Gamba G, Montani N, Anesi E et al: Clotting alterations in primary systemic amyloidosis. Haematologica 85:289, 2000.

156. Cueto-Garcia L, Tajik AJ, Kyle RA et al: Serial echocardiographic observations in patients with primary systemic amyloidosis: An introduction to the concept of early (asymptomatic) amyloid infiltration of the heart. Mayo Clin Proc 59:589, 1984.

157. Gertz MA, Kyle RA: Amyloidosis: Prognosis and treatment. Semin Arthritis Rheum 24:124, 1994.

158. Kyle RA, Greipp PR, O'Fallon WM: Primary systemic amyloidosis: Multivariate analysis for prognostic factors in 168 cases. Blood 68:220, 1986.

159. Tei C, Dujardin KS, Hodge DO et al: Doppler index combining systolic and diastolic myocardial performance: Clinical value in cardiac amyloidosis. J Am Coll Cardiol 28:658, 1996.

160. Hongo M, Kono J, Yamada H et al: Doppler echocardiographic assessments of left ventricular diastolic filling in patients with amyloid heart disease. J Cardiol 21:391, 1991.

161. Klein AL, Hatle LK, Taliercio CP et al: Prognostic significance of Doppler measures of diastolic function in cardiac amyloidosis. A Doppler echocardiography study. Circulation 83:808, 1991.

162. Perfetti V, Colli Vignarelli M, Anesi E et al: The degrees of plasma cell clonality and marrow infiltration adversely influence the prognosis of AL amyloidosis patients. Haematologica 84:218, 1999.

163. Gertz MA, Kyle RA, Greipp PR: Response rates and survival in primary systemic amyloidosis. Blood 77:257, 1991.

164. Kyle RA, Gertz MA, Greipp PR et al: A trial of three regimens for primary amyloidosis: Colchicine alone, melphalan and prednisone, and melphalan, prednisone, and colchicine. N Engl J Med 336:1202, 1997.

165. Skinner M, Anderson J, Simms R et al: Treatment of 100 patients with primary amyloidosis: A randomized trial of melphalan, prednisone, and colchicine versus colchicine only. Am J Med 100:290, 1996.

166. Dubrey S, Mendes L, Skinner M et al: Resolution of heart failure in patients with AL amyloidosis. Ann Intern Med 125:481, 1996.

167. Grogan M, Gertz MA, Kyle RA et al: Five or more years of survival in patients with primary systemic amyloidosis and biopsy-proven cardiac involvement. Am J Cardiol 85:664, 2000.

168. Goldsmith DJ, Sandooran D, Short CD et al: Twenty-one years survival with systemic AL-amyloidosis. Am J Kidney Dis 28:278, 1996.

169. Gertz MA, Kyle RA: Acute leukemia and cytogenetic abnormalities complicating melphalan treatment of primary systemic amyloidosis. Arch Intern Med 150:629, 1990.

170. Gertz MA, Kyle RA: Phase II trial of alpha-tocopherol (vitamin E) in the treatment of primary systemic amyloidosis. Am J Hematol 34:55, 1990.

171. Gertz MA, Kyle RA: Phase II trial of recombinant interferon alfa-2 in the treatment of primary systemic amyloidosis. Am J Hematol 44:125, 1993.

172. Dhodapkar MV, Jagannath S, Vesole D et al: Treatment of AL-amyloidosis with dexamethasone plus alpha interferon. Leuk Lymphoma 27:351, 1997.

173. Gertz MA, Lacy MQ, Lust JA et al: Phase II trial of high-dose dexamethasone for untreated patients with primary systemic amyloidosis. Med Oncol 16:104, 1999.

174. Gertz MA, Lacy MQ, Lust JA et al: Phase II trial of high-dose dexamethasone for previously treated immunoglobulin light-chain amyloidosis. Am J Hematol 61:115, 1999.

175. Wardley AM, Jayson GC, Goldsmith DJ et al: The treatment of nephrotic syndrome caused by primary (light chain) amyloid with vincristine, doxorubicin and dexamethasone. Br J Cancer 78:774, 1998.

176. Gianni L, Bellotti V, Gianni AM et al: New drug therapy of amyloidosis: Resorption of AL-type deposits with 4'-iodo-4'-deoxy-doxorubicin. Blood 86:855, 1995.

177. Hosenpud JD, DeMarco T, Frazier OH et al: Progression of systemic disease and reduced long-term survival in patients with cardiac amyloidosis undergoing heart transplantation. Follow-up results of a multicenter survey. Circulation 84(Suppl):III338, 1991.

178. Dubrey S, Simms RW, Skinner M et al: Recurrence of primary (AL) amyloidosis in a transplanted heart with four-year survival. Am J Cardiol 76:739, 1995.

179. Pelosi F Jr, Capehart J, Roberts WC: Effectiveness of cardiac transplantation for primary (AL) cardiac amyloidosis. Am J Cardiol 79:532, 1997.

180. Gertz MA, Lacy MQ, Lust JA et al: Prospective randomized trial of melphalan and prednisone versus vincristine, carmustine, melphalan, cyclophosphamide, and prednisone in the treatment of primary systemic amyloidosis. J Clin Oncol 17:262, 1999.

181. van Buren M, Hene RJ, Verdonck LF et al: Clinical remission after syngeneic bone marrow transplantation in a patient with AL amyloidosis. Ann Intern Med 122:508, 1995.

182. Hawkins PN, Aprile C, Capri G et al: Scintigraphic imaging and turnover studies with iodine-131 labelled serum amyloid P component in systemic amyloidosis. Eur J Nucl Med 25:701, 1998.

183. Gillmore JD, Davies J, Iqbal A et al: Allogeneic bone marrow transplantation for systemic AL amyloidosis. Br J Haematol 100:226, 1998.

184. Guillaume B, Straetmans N, Jadoul M et al: Allogeneic bone marrow transplantation for AL amyloidosis. Bone Marrow Transplant 20:907, 1997.

185. Moreau P, Milpied N, de Faucal P et al: High-dose melphalan and autologous bone marrow transplantation for systemic AL amyloidosis with cardiac involvement (letter). Blood 87:3063, 1996.

186. Perfetti V, Ubbiali P, Magni M et al: Cells with clonal light chains are present in peripheral blood at diagnosis and in apheretic stem cell harvests of primary amyloidosis. Bone Marrow Transplant 23:323, 1999.

187. McElroy EA Jr, Witzig TE, Gertz MA et al: Detection of monoclonal plasma cells in the peripheral blood of patients with primary amyloidosis. Br J Haematol 100:326, 1998.

188. Comenzo RL, Michelle D, LeBlanc M et al: Mobilized CD34+ cells selected as autografts in patients with primary light-chain amyloidosis: Rationale and application. Transfusion 38:60, 1998.

189. Lokhorst HM, Verdonck LF: Intensive therapy in AL amyloidosis and light-chain deposition disease (reply to letter to the editor). Ann Intern Med 123:553, 1995.

190. Comenzo RL, Vosburgh E, Simms RW et al: Dose-intensive melphalan with blood stem cell support for the treatment of AL amyloidosis: One-year follow-up in five patients. Blood 88:2801, 1996.

191. Comenzo RL, Vosburgh E, Falk RH et al: Dose-intensive melphalan with blood stem-cell support for the treatment of AL (amyloid light-chain) amyloidosis: Survival and responses in 25 patients. Blood 91:3662, 1998.

192. Comenzo RL, Falk RH, Sanchorawala V et al: Treating AL amyloidosis (AL) with dose-intensive melphalan: Outcomes in 102 patients (abstract). Blood 92(Suppl 1):324a, 1998.

193. Goldman JM, Schmitz N, Niethammer D et al: Allogeneic and autologous transplantation for haematological diseases, solid tumours and immune disorders: Current practice in Europe in 1998. Accreditation Sub-Committee of the European Group for Blood and Marrow Transplantation. Bone Marrow Transplant 21:1, 1998.

194. Gertz MA, Lacy MQ, Gastineau DA et al: Blood stem cell transplantation as therapy for primary systemic amyloidosis (AL). Bone Marrow Transplant 26:963, 2000.

195. Patriarca F, Geromin A, Fanin R et al: Improvement of amyloid-related symptoms after autologous stem cell transplantation in a patient with hepatomegaly, macroglossia and purpura. Bone Marrow Transplant 24:433, 1999.

196. Moreau P, Leblond V, Bourquelot P et al: Prognostic factors for survival and response after high-dose therapy and autologous stem cell transplantation in systemic AL amyloidosis: A report on 21 patients. Br J Haematol 101:766, 1998.

197. Gillmore JD, Apperley JF, Craddock C et al: High-dose melphalan and stem cell rescue for AL amyloidosis. In Kyle RA, Gertz MA (eds.): Amyloid and Amyloidosis 1998, p. 102. The Parthenon Publishing Group, New York, 1999.

198. Amoura Z, Leblond V, Azar N et al: High-dose therapy and autologous stem cell transplantation (ASCT) for systemic amyloidosis (AL): Report of 9 cases (abstract). Arthritis Rheum 41 (Suppl):S234, 1998.

199. Ager S, Mahendra P, Jestice HK et al: The use of non-cryopreserved peripheral blood progenitor cells in autologous transplantation (letter to the editor). Bone Marrow Transplant 16:633, 1995.

200. Mehta J, Nagler A, Slavin S: Marrow transplantation in multiple myeloma (letter to the editor). N Engl J Med 326:1087, 1992.

201. Majolino I, Marceno R, Pecoraro G et al: Autologous stem cell transplantation in amyloidosis AL (letter). Bone Marrow Transplant 11:85, 1993.

202. Akpek G, Colarusso T, Lerner A et al: Immune reconstitution after autologous blood stem cell transplantation (ABSCT) in patients with AL amyloidosis (AL) (abstract). Blood 92(Suppl. 1):360B, 1998.

203. Kazmi MA, Schey SA: Morbidity associated with high dose therapy in primary amyloidosis. In Kyle RA, Gertz MA (eds.): Amyloid and Amyloidosis 1998, p. 169. The Parthenon Publishing Group, New York, 1999.

204. Akasheh MS, Chang CP, Vesole DH: Acute tumour lysis syndrome: A case in AL amyloidosis. Br J Haematol 107:386, 1999.

205. Schuh A, Dandridge J, Haydon P et al: Encephalopathy complicating high-dose melphalan. Bone Marrow Transplant 24:1141, 1999.

206. Dispenzieri A, Lacy MQ, Kyle RA et al: AL amyloidosis is a favorable independent prognostic factor for survival of 234 patients with primary systemic amyloidosis (AL) functionally eligible for peripheral blood stem cell transplantation (abstract). Proc Annu Meet Am Soc Clin Oncol 18:20a, 1999.

207. Gertz MA, Lacy MQ, Dispenzieri A: Amyloidosis. Hematol Oncol Clin North Am 13:1211, 1999.

36

Monoclonal Gammopathies of Undetermined Significance

Robert A. Kyle and S. Vincent Rajkumar

Table 36–1. Differential Diagnosis of Monoclonal Gammopathies

Monoclonal gammopathies of undetermined significance
  Benign (IgG, IgA, IgD, IgM, and, rarely, free light chains)
  Associated with neoplasms of cell types not known to produce monoclonal proteins
  Biclonal gammopathies
Malignant monoclonal gammopathies
  Multiple myeloma (IgG, IgA, IgD, IgE, and free light chains)
    Overt multiple myeloma
    Smoldering multiple myeloma
    Plasma cell leukemia
    Nonsecretory myeloma
  Plasmacytoma
    Solitary plasmacytoma of bone
    Extrameduallary plasmacytoma, solitary and multiple
  Malignant lymphoproliferative diseases
    Waldenström's macroglobulinemia (primary macroglobulinemia) (IgM)
    Malignant lymphoma
    Chronic lymphocytic leukemia
  Heavy chain diseases (HCD)
    γ (HCD)
    α (HCD)
    μ (HCD)
  Amyloidosis
    Primary (includes multiple myeloma; AL); secondary, localized, and familial amyloidoses have no monoclonal protein

(From Kyle,[2] with permission.)

The term *monoclonal gammopathy of undetermined significance* (MGUS) denotes the presence of a monoclonal protein (M protein) in persons without evidence of multiple myeloma, macroglobulinemia, amyloidosis, or other related diseases. MGUS is characterized by a serum M-protein concentration of less than 3.0 g/dl; less than 10 percent plasma cells in the bone marrow; no or only a small amount of M protein in the urine; absence of lytic bone lesions, anemia, hypercalcemia, and renal insufficiency; and, most importantly, stability of the M protein and failure of development of additional abnormalities. The term *benign monoclonal gammopathy* is misleading because it is not known at the time of diagnosis whether an M protein will remain stable and benign or will develop into symptomatic multiple myeloma, macroglobulinemia, or amyloidosis. Since Waldenström's introduction of the term *essential hyperglobulinemia* in 1952, many similar terms have been used, including idiopathic, asymptomatic, benign, nonmyelomatous, discrete, cryptogenic, and rudimentary monoclonal gammopathy; dysimmunoglobulinemia; lanthanic monoclonal gammopathy; idiopathic paraproteinemia; and asymptomatic paraimmunoglobulinemia. Waldenström[1] stressed the constancy of the size of the protein spike obtained by electrophoresis of serum, contrasting it with the increasing quantity of the M protein in myeloma.

Each M protein consists of two heavy chain polypeptides of the same class and subclass and two light chain polypeptides of the same type. The different M proteins are designated by capital letters corresponding to the class of their heavy chains, designated by Greek letters: γ in immunoglobulin IgG, α in IgA, μ in IgM, δ in IgD, and ε in IgE. Their subclasses are IgG1, IgG2, IgG3, and IgG4 or IgA1 and IgA2, and their light chain types are κ or λ.

Analysis of the serum or urine for an M protein requires a sensitive, rapid, dependable screening method to detect its presence and a specific assay to identify its heavy chain class and light chain type. To screen sera for abnormal proteins, electrophoresis with agarose gel as the support medium is preferable. Should an abnormal protein band be observed, immunofixation should be performed with monospecific antisera (see Chapter 27).[2]

An M protein is seen as a narrow peak or spike on the densitometer tracing or as a dense, discrete band on agarose gel in the γ-, β-, or α_2-globulin regions. The differential diagnosis of monoclonal gammopathies is provided in Table 36–1.

CHARACTERIZATION OF MGUS

During 1999, 1109 patients were found with a serum M protein at the Mayo Clinic (Figure 36–1). The most frequent clinical diagnosis was MGUS or benign monoclonal gammopathy, occurring in two-thirds of patients (Figure 36–2).

Monoclonal gammopathies without evidence of multiple myeloma, macroglobulinemia, amyloidosis, or related diseases have been found in approximately 3 percent of persons over 70 years of age in Sweden,[3,4] in the United States,[5] and in France.[6] In Sweden, among 6995 normal persons over 25 years of age, the overall prevalence of M protein was 1 percent[3]; among 1200 patients 50 years or older who were residents of a small Minnesota community, 1.25 percent had an M protein,[5] and 303 (1.7 percent) of 17,968 adults 50 years or older in Finistère, France, had an M protein.[6] An M protein was found in 1.2 percent of 73,630 hospitalized patients[7] and in 0.7 percent of 102,000 persons in a general hospital in Italy.[8] In another study of 118,130 nonhospitalized patients in Italy, 749 (0.63 percent) had an M protein.[9]

The incidence of monoclonal gammopathies increases with advancing age. In Finistère, France, Saleun et al.[6] found that 4 percent of 720 patients over 80 years of age had an M protein. Using agarose gel electrophoresis, Crawford et al.[10] detected M proteins in 11 (10 percent) of 111 patients over 80 years of age in a population of ambulatory residents of a retirement home. In another report from Italy, 7.6 percent of the population older than 75 years had an M protein.[11]

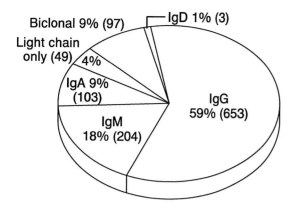

Figure 36–1. Serum monoclonal proteins found in 1109 patients at the Mayo Clinic, 1999.

The incidence of M proteins in the African-American population is higher than that in Whites. Schechter et al.[12] reported that 3.65 percent of 1864 African-Americans and 2.1 percent of 857 Caucasians had an M protein ($p = .043$). Singh et al.[13] also reported a higher incidence in the African-American population. In one study, the prevalence of an M protein was 8.8 percent in 916 African-Americans.[14] The incidence of monoclonal gammopathies is less in Japanese elderly persons. Four (2.7 percent) of 146 Japanese subjects aged 63 to 95 years had an M protein[15] compared with 10 percent in an elderly U.S. population.[10]

In our experience and that of others, approximately 15 percent of M proteins are of the IgM type. Currently, IgM accounts for 18 percent of the monoclonal gammopathies in our patients. By contrast, in a study of 4193 patients with monoclonal gammopathies from three regions in France, Hurez et al.[16] reported that 33 percent of the monoclonal gammopathies were IgM. There is no explanation for this unexpected high frequency of IgM. Alternatively, only 3.3 percent of monoclonal gammopathies in Guadeloupe, French West Indies, were IgM.[17]

More sensitive techniques will detect a higher incidence of M proteins. For example, Papadopoulos et al.[18] detected homogeneous bands in the sera of 30 (5 percent) of 600 healthy adults

aged 22 to 65 years. Immunoisoelectric focusing, a more sensitive technique, identified an M protein in the sera of 11 percent of patients over 45 years of age who had been hospitalized for surgery for a nonmalignant condition.[19] Agarose electrophoresis detected an M protein in only 2 percent of that series. Thus, the prevalence of MGUS is considerable, and it is important to both the patient and the physician to determine whether the M protein will remain benign or will progress to multiple myeloma, macroglobulinemia, or other lymphoproliferative disease.

MAYO CLINIC STUDY

We reviewed the medical records of all patients with monoclonal gammopathy who were seen at the Mayo Clinic before January 1, 1971. Patients with multiple myeloma, macroglobulinemia, amyloidosis, lymphoma, or related diseases were excluded; 241 patients remained for long-term study.

Initial Findings

Only 4 percent of patients were under 40 years of age when the M protein was recognized, whereas one-third were 70 years of age or older. The median age was 64 years. Fifty-eight percent were males.

Physical Examination

The liver was palpable in 15 percent of patients, and splenomegaly was noted in 4 percent. In patients whose liver or spleen was palpable 5 cm or more below the costal margin, the causes were congestive heart failure, myelofibrosis with myeloid metaplasia, cirrhosis, or other conditions not directly related to the monoclonal gammopathy.

Hematologic and Chemistry Values

The hemoglobin level at initial evaluation ranged from 7.2 to 16.6 g/dl (Table 36–2). In the nine patients whose hemoglobin level was less than 10 g/dl, melena, myeloid metaplasia, myeloprolifer-

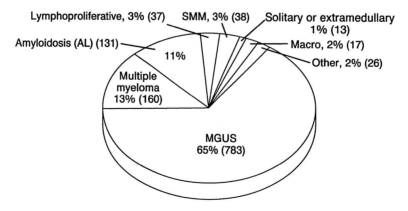

Figure 36–2. Diagnosis of monoclonal gammopathies at Mayo Clinic, 1999. (Adapted from Kyle RA: Monoclonal gammopathy of undetermined significance [MGUS]. Ballière's Clin Haematol 8:761, 1995, with permission.)

Table 36–2. Hemoglobin Value, Serum Monoclonal Protein Concentration, and Percentage of Plasma Cells in Bone Marrow at Diagnosis of Monoclonal Gammopathy of Undetermined Significance

Factor	Group 1 (Benign)	Group 2 (Increased M Protein)[a]	Group 3 (Died)	Group 4 (Myeloma or Other Disease)	Total
Hemoglobin (g/dl)	(n = 46)	(n = 23)	(n = 113)	(n = 59)	(n = 241)
Median	13.7	12.5	13.0	13.2	13.2
Range	10.1–16.6	8.4–15.1	7.2–16.5	9.7–16.5	7.2–16.6
Monoclonal protein (g/dl)	(n = 46)	(n = 23)	(n = 113)	(n = 59)	(n = 241)
Median	1.8	2.0	1.7	1.7	1.7
Range	1.1–2.6	1.2–3.2	0.3–2.9	0.9–2.6	0.3–3.2
Plasma cells (percent)	(n = 23)	(n = 12)	(n = 49)	(n = 25)	(n = 109)
Median	3	3	3	4	3
Range	1–7	1–6	1–10	1–7	1–10

[a] Increased monoclonal protein (M protein) value to 3.0 g/dl or more.

(Adapted from Kyle RA: Benign monoclonal gammopathy: A misnomer? JAMA 251:1849, 1984, with permission.)

ative disease, Wegener's granulomatosis, hypoplasia of bone marrow, chronic cold agglutinin disease, and hypernephroma were responsible. The leukocyte count was less than 2000/mm^3 in only one patient (lupus erythematosus); it exceeded 20,000/mm^3 in two patients—one with an undifferentiated myeloproliferative process and the other with myeloid metaplasia. Thrombocytopenia was uncommon. In the five patients with a platelet count of less than 100,000/mm^3 the causes were myeloid metaplasia, acute leukemia, idiopathic thrombocytopenic purpura, lupus erythematosus, and hypoplasia of the bone marrow. Platelet counts were more than 500,000/mm^3 in only two patients: one with pneumonitis and one with rectal bleeding. Renal insufficiency, manifested by a serum creatinine level more than 2.0 mg/dl, was present in five patients: nephrosclerosis in three, diabetes mellitus in one, and uric acid nephropathy in one. Serum albumin concentration was less than 2 g/dl in two patients: one with Wegener's granulomatosis and the other with a hypernephroma. The median serum albumin value of the 241 patients was 3.2 g/dl. Only two patients had hypercalcemia (more than 11 mg/dl), and both had hyperparathyroidism.

Serum Electrophoresis and Immunoelectrophoresis

The M protein migrated in the γ-area in 77 percent and in the β-area in 20 percent of patients. Electrophoresis produced a broad-based polyclonal-appearing peak in two patients and no discrete spike was seen in three others, but immunoelectrophoresis revealed an M protein in all five. The size of the M protein ranged from 0.3 to 3.2 g/dl. The median value was 1.7 g/dl. Immunoelectrophoresis revealed IgG (73 percent), IgA (11 percent), IgM (14 percent), and biclonality (2 percent). The monoclonal light chain type was κ in 62 percent and λ in 38 percent. Electrophoretic mobility of the M protein and its heavy chain class and light chain type did not change throughout the period of observation.

Fifty-two of 181 patients (29 percent) had a decrease in uninvolved immunoglobulins (Table 36–3). Eighty-seven percent of the patients had an IgG1 subclass, 4 percent had IgG2, 4 percent had IgG3, and 5 percent had IgG4.

Urinary Electrophoresis and Immunoelectrophoresis

Urinary electrophoresis studies were performed in less than one-half of patients. The studies usually are not done unless proteinuria is found on routine urinalysis or the finding of a large serum spike suggests the possibility of myeloma or macroglobulinemia. Nine patients had a urinary monoclonal light chain at the time of recognition of the monoclonal gammopathy—the light chain was κ in five and λ in four. In all but three patients, the amount of M protein was 1 g/24 hours or less.

Table 36–3. Quantitation of Immunoglobulins in 181 Patients With Monoclonal Gammopathy of Undetermined Significance

Immunoglobulin	Group 1 (Benign)	Group 2 (Increased M Protein)[a]	Group 3 (Died)	Group 4 (Myeloma or Other Disease)	Total
IgG					
No. of patients	30	14	60	30	134
Percent with decrease	23	21	20	43	26
IgA					
No. of patients	7	0	7	7	21
Percent with decrease	29	0	0	57	29
IgM					
No. of patients	2	2	15	7	26
Percent with decrease	50	0	47	43	42
Total percent with decrease	26	19	23	45	29

[a] Increased monoclonal protein (M protein) value to 3.0 g/dl or more.

(Modified from Kyle,[35] with permission.)

Table 36–4. Monoclonal Gammopathy of Undetermined Significance: Diseases Present at Discovery of Serum Monoclonal Protein

Disease	Cases No.	Cases Percent
None	62	26
Cardiovascular or cerebrovascular	31	13
Inflammatory	26	11
Malignant	16	6
Neurologic	15	6
Connective tissue	14	6
Hematologic	9	4
Endocrine	9	4
Benign tumor	8	3
Miscellaneous	51	21
Total	241	100

(From Kyle and Lust,[36] with permission.)

A bone marrow aspirate was done in 109 patients at the time of recognition of the M protein. In patients with a small M protein, a bone marrow examination often is not performed. The number of plasma cells ranged from 1 percent to 10 percent (median, 3 percent).

Associated Diseases

At the discovery of the M protein, 26 percent of the 241 patients had no diseases or abnormalities other than the M protein in the serum (Table 36–4). The 26 patients with inflammatory disorders included 4 with fever of undetermined origin (which had been present intermittently for 4 to 22 years), 3 with recurrent phlebitis, 2 with chronic inflammatory bowel disease, and 1 with sprue. Of the 16 patients with malignancy, 1 had acute leukemia and 1 had Kaposi's sarcoma. Of the 15 patients with neurologic disorders, 5 had carpal tunnel syndrome and were alive without systemic amyloidosis, and 1 had the Guillain-Barré syndrome. The connective tissue disorders included rheumatoid arthritis, ankylosing spondylitis, lupus erythematosus, and scleroderma. Of the nine patients with hematologic diseases, two had myelofibrosis with myeloid metaplasia, two had idiopathic thrombocytopenic purpura, and one each had von Willebrand's disease, hypoplastic anemia, aregenerative anemia (red cell aplasia), undifferentiated myeloproliferative disease, and idiopathic neu-

tropenia. Of the nine patients with endocrine disorders, three had hyperparathyroidism, three had idiopathic osteoporosis, and one each had Cushing's disease, Graves disease, and Turner syndrome. The benign tumors included thyroid nodules and colonic polyps. Among the miscellaneous disorders were psychoneurosis, hyperventilation syndrome, duodenal ulcer, melena, pruritus, diabetes, Peyronie's disease, and plane xanthoma.

Findings at 24 to 38 Years of Follow-up

Group 1: Benign

At current follow-up (range, 24 to 38 years), the number of patients whose M protein had remained stable and could be classified as "benign" monoclonal gammopathy had decreased to 25 (10 percent)[20] (Table 36–5). The M protein disappeared from the serum in two patients (IgG-κ, IgA-κ); in the one with IgG-κ, it gradually decreased, disappearing at 17 years. In a third patient, the IgG-λ protein became undetectable for 5 years but then reappeared and has not changed significantly. The level of hemoglobin, size of serum M-protein peak, type of serum heavy and light chains, decrease in uninvolved immunoglobulins, subclass of IgG heavy chain, and number of plasma cells in the bone marrow did not differ substantially in the stable or benign group from those in the total group.

One patient had had a substantiated κ-protein of more than 1 g/24 hours for 26 years and had had a prior grade 3 to 4 proteinuria for 7 years; thus, the total duration of proteinuria was 33 years. He also had had an IgG-κ serum protein value of approximately 2.6 g/dl for 26 years. Clinically, this patient remained well. Six patients had a small monoclonal light chain in the urine (five with κ and one with λ) when immunoelectrophoresis was performed for the first time after the discovery of the serum M protein. All six patients participated in follow-up for more than 13 years after detection of the urinary light chain without an increase in either the serum or the urinary M protein. Although the duration of follow-up for these 25 patients has been more than 24 years, surveillance must be continued indefinitely.

Group 2: Increase in M Protein Only

In the 26 patients (11 percent) in group 2, the M-protein value increased to more than 3 g/dl and was 4 g/dl or more in 2 patients. However, symptomatic multiple myeloma, macroglobulinemia, and amyloidosis have not developed in any of these patients, and none have been treated.

Table 36–5. Course of 241 Patients With Monoclonal Gammopathy of Undetermined Significance

Group	Description	No. of Patients at Follow-up After 24–38 years No.	No. of Patients at Follow-up After 24–38 years Percent
1	No substantial increase of serum or urine monoclonal protein (benign)	25	10
2	Monoclonal protein 3.0 g/dl or more but no myeloma or related disease	26	11
3	Died of unrelated causes	127	53
4	Development of myeloma, macroglobulinemia, amyloidosis, or related disease	63	26
Total		241	100

(From Kyle,[35] with permission.)

The median interval from the recognition of the M protein to an increase to 3.0 g/dl was 9 years. The median duration of follow-up after reaching this increase was 6 years. Five of these patients are still living, including one patient who is 102 years old and has had an IgM-κ protein for 22 years. Although his M-protein value has been 3.0 g/dl or more for 13 years, his macroglobulinemia has not necessitated chemotherapy. In this group, the maximal duration of follow-up has been 26 years (median, 18.5 years).

The pattern of increase in the M-protein value was variable. In nine patients, it increased gradually from 8 to 18 years before reaching 3.0 g/dl. Seven of the nine patients died without the development of symptomatic myeloma or macroglobulinemia, and two are still under observation. Six patients (two of whom are still alive) had a fluctuating M-protein value for 6 to 18 years before it reached 3.0 g/dl. The M-protein value in three patients was stable for 6 to 21 years and then suddenly increased to 3.0 g/dl. One of these patients is alive. In the remaining five patients, data were insufficient to ascertain the pattern of increase.

Eight patients had a monoclonal light chain in the urine—four κ and four λ. Three of them had a monoclonal light chain in the urine at the time the serum M protein was detected. In one patient, the monoclonal λ-light chain disappeared after the removal of a parathyroid adenoma, but the serum protein value remained stable. The urinary-λ light chain reappeared after 19 years when the total protein in the urine increased to 3.6 g/24 hours. Biopsy specimens of subcutaneous fat, bone marrow, and rectal tissue were negative for amyloid, but renal biopsy was not possible. She had no clinical features of systemic amyloidosis. All eight patients have undergone follow-up for more than 7 years after detection of the urinary M protein.

Group 3: Died Without Development of Myeloma, Macroglobulinemia, Amyloidosis, or Related Disease

The median interval from diagnosis of the serum M protein to death of the 127 patients (53 percent) was 7 years (range, 0 to 25 years). Forty-one patients (36 percent) survived more than 10 years after the M protein was found. One patient was thought to have systemic amyloidosis, but no tissue was available; in another patient, multiple myeloma was diagnosed on the basis of a bone marrow examination, but she received no chemotherapy and died a year later of a dissecting thoracic aortic aneurysm.

Fourteen patients had a monoclonal urinary light chain (seven κ and seven λ). In four of these patients, it was diagnosed concurrently with a serum M protein.

Cardiac disease was the most frequent cause of death (37 percent), followed by cerebrovascular disease (15 percent). Fifteen patients died of malignant processes: two each of carcinoma of the colon, kidney, and liver; one each of carcinoma of the ovary, endometrium, lung, and prostate; one each of acute nonlymphocytic leukemia and mesothelioma; and three of metastatic carcinoma with an unknown primary lesion.

Group 4: Developed Multiple Myeloma, Macroglobulinemia, Amyloidosis, or Related Diseases

Multiple myeloma, macroglobulinemia, amyloidosis, or a malignant lymphoproliferative process developed in 63 patients (actuarial rate at 10 years, 17 percent; at 20 years, 33 percent; and at 25 years, 40 percent) (Figure 36–3). Forty-three (68 percent) of the 63 patients had multiple myeloma. At the diagnosis of multiple myeloma, all but four patients had a bone marrow aspirate or biopsy specimens that contained more than 15 percent abnormal plasma cells. In two of the four patients, the diagnosis of multiple myeloma was made at their home hospital, but we were unable to obtain the results of the bone marrow studies. Both patients had extensive lytic lesions and severe anemia. A third patient had a large destructive plasmacytoma of the sacrum, stenosis of the spinal canal, and a serum M-protein spike of 3.4 g/dl, but we could not obtain the results of the bone marrow examination. The fourth patient had severe anemia, hypercalcemia, and an M-protein spike of 3.7 g/dl but refused a bone marrow examination. Thirty-one of the 39 patients with myeloma had serum M-protein levels greater than 3.0 g/dl. Three of the eight patients with an M-protein spike less than 3.0 g/dl had a large urinary M protein (Bence Jones proteinuria), and all eight had skeletal involvement. In all but one patient, the serum M-protein spike increased when multiple myeloma developed. This patient had severe back pain, extensive skeletal involvement, and a bone marrow that contained 25 percent plasma cells. Of the 25 patients who were studied, 20 had a monoclonal urinary light chain (κ, 44 percent; λ, 36 percent; negative, 20 percent). Lytic bone lesions or fractures were found in 29 (73 percent), and 3 others had only osteoporosis. These findings readily fulfill the criteria for the diagnosis of multiple myeloma.

The interval from the recognition of the monoclonal gammopathy to the diagnosis of multiple myeloma ranged from 22 months to 29 years (median, 10 years) (Table 36–6). In nine of the patients, the diagnosis was made 20 years after detection of the serum M protein. The median survival after diagnosis of multiple myeloma was 33 months, and only two patients are still alive.

Development of multiple myeloma varied from gradual to apparently abrupt (Table 36–7). In 11 patients, the serum M protein remained stable for 4 to 18 years (median, 8 years) and then gradually increased to symptomatic multiple myeloma

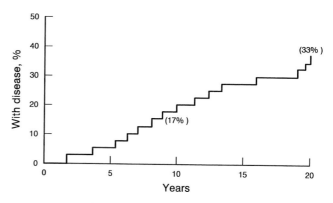

Figure 36–3. Incidence of multiple myeloma, macroglobulinemia, amyloidosis, or lymphoproliferative disease after recognition of monoclonal protein. Actuarial analysis. (From Kyle and Lust,[36] with permission.)

Table 36–6. Development of Myeloma or Related Diseases in 59 Patients With Monoclonal Gammopathy of Undetermined Significance

	No.	Percent	Interval to Diagnosis (years)[a] Median	Interval to Diagnosis (years)[a] Range
Multiple myeloma	39	66	10	2–29
Macroglobulinemia	7	12	8.5	4–20
Amyloidosis	8	14	9	6–19
Lymphoproliferative	5	8	10.5	6–22
Total	59	100		

[a] Actuarial rate was 17 percent at 10 years and 33 percent at 20 years. (From Kyle RA: Multiple myeloma and other plasma cell disorders. In Hoffman R, Benz EJ Jr, Shattil SJ (eds.): Hematology, Basic Principles and Practice, 2nd Ed., p. 481. Churchill Livingstone, New York, 1994, with permission.)

during a 1- to 4-year period (median, 3 years). In seven patients, the serum M-protein value was stable for 2 to 25 years (median, 8 years) and then increased rapidly (in less than 1 year) as myeloma developed. In seven patients, the serum M-protein value was stable for 1 to 16 years (median, 2 years), followed by intervals of 2 to 10 years (median, 4 years) without serum studies before multiple myeloma was diagnosed. Seven patients had a fluctuating but gradually increasing serum M-protein spike until multiple myeloma was diagnosed 5 to 29 years (median, 12 years) later. In the remaining seven patients, no serum specimens were available between the time of detection of the serum M protein and the diagnosis of multiple myeloma 3 to 10 years later.

Waldenström's macroglobulinemia developed in seven patients. The median interval from recognition of the M protein to the diagnosis of macroglobulinemia was 8 years. All of the patients had serum levels of IgM-κ ranging from 3.1 to 8.5 g/dl during the course of the disease. One patient had a biclonal gammopathy (IgM-κ, IgA-κ). All patients had anemia; bone marrow aspirates or biopsy or autopsy specimens showed increased numbers of lymphocytes and plasma cells. In five patients, the number of serum protein determinations during the development of macroglobulinemia was not sufficient to determine whether the onset of the disease was gradual or

Table 36–7. Pattern of Increase in M Protein in 39 Patients With Monoclonal Gammopathy of Undetermined Significance in Whom Multiple Myeloma Developed

No. of Patients	Pattern of Increase (years)	Duration (years)
11	Stable 4–18 (median, 8)	Then gradual ↑, 1–4 (median, 3)
7	Stable 2–25 (median, 8)	Then rapid ↑
7	Stable 1–16 (median, 2)	Then 2–10 without data (median, 4)
7	Gradual (fluctuating)	5–29 (median, 12)
7	Insufficient data	

abrupt. In the sixth patient, the M-protein level was stable for 5 years and increased gradually for 3 years before symptomatic macroglobulinemia occurred. The M protein slowly progressed from the time of recognition in the seventh patient.

Systemic amyloidosis was found in eight patients 6 to 19 years after the recognition of an M protein in the serum (median, 9 years). Histologic evidence of amyloidosis was present at autopsy in three cases, at renal biopsy in two, at lymph node biopsy in one, and at rectal biopsy in one, and it was an incidental finding at the time of operation for carcinoma of the colon in one. The initial manifestation of amyloidosis was nephrotic syndrome (two patients), cardiomegaly (one), acute pulmonary edema (one), fatigue, diarrhea, and weight loss of 13.6 kg (one), lymphadenopathy and weight loss (one), and peripheral neuropathy (one). Only one of the patients with amyloidosis had an increase in the serum M-protein value (1.9 to 3.9 g/dl), but she did not have symptomatic multiple myeloma. Amyloidosis was not clinically suspected in the three patients in whom the diagnosis was made at autopsy and would not have been diagnosed if the postmortem examination had not been done. One of these patients came to the emergency department because of acute pulmonary edema and subsequently died; in another patient, weakness, weight loss, and gastrointestinal symptoms had developed, for which no cause was found; and the third patient had symptomatic cryoglobulinemia, sensorimotor peripheral neuropathy, and congestive heart failure.

In five patients, a malignant lymphoproliferative process developed 9 to 22 years (median, 10.5 years) after detection of the M protein. One patient with lupus erythematosus had a biclonal gammopathy (IgG-λ, IgM-κ). Nine years later, an aggressive, diffuse, undifferentiated malignant lymphoma developed, and the patient died. Another patient experienced anorexia, lost weight, and had generalized bone pain 22 years after the recognition of an IgM-λ monoclonal gammopathy. A bone marrow examination revealed an immunoblastic lymphoma with plasmacytic differentiation. Extensive retroperitoneal lymphadenopathy was seen on computed tomography (CT) scan. Examination of the cerebrospinal fluid showed large malignant-appearing lymphocytes. The patient did not respond to chemotherapy and died 1 month later.

In one patient, chronic lymphocytic leukemia developed after 56 months of observation, but the IgM monoclonal gammopathy did not increase. Four courses of chlorambucil were given for recurrent lymphocytosis. The IgM-κ gammopathy remained stable for 16 years and probably was not directly related to the chronic lymphocytic leukemia. The patient died 18.5 years after recognition of the monoclonal gammopathy. In another patient, diffuse mixed lymphoma of the jejunum was found during surgical exploration for abdominal pain 10 years after detection of the serum M protein. During the subsequent 10-year follow-up, no recurrence was noted. Only one of the five patients with a malignant lymphoproliferative disorder had an associated increase in the M protein.

Analysis by Immunoglobulin Group

Of the 241 patients, 63 (26 percent) developed multiple myeloma, macroglobulinemia, amyloidosis, lymphoma, or

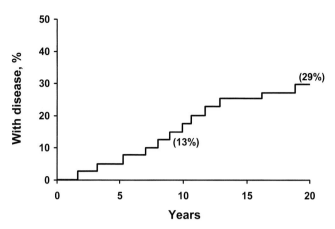

Figure 36–4. Incidence of multiple myeloma or other serious disease after recognition of IgG or IgA monoclonal gammopathy. Actuarial analysis. (From Kyle and Lust,[36] with permission.)

chronic lymphocytic leukemia (group 4). The actuarial rate of development of serious disease in patients with an IgG or an IgA M protein was 13 percent at 10 years and 29 percent at 20 years (Figure 36–4). The actuarial rate of development of a serious disease in patients with an IgM M protein was 21 percent at 10 years and 49 percent at 20 years (Figure 36–5).

The serum M-protein value did not increase in 12 patients (7 with amyloidosis, 4 with lymphoproliferative disease, and 1 with multiple myeloma). The amount of serum M protein remained stable in six IgG cases, four IgM cases, and two IgA cases. Distribution of the types of serious disease associated with various monoclonal gammopathies is shown in Table 36–8.

The rate of development of serious disease did not differ whether the monoclonal gammopathy was IgG, IgA, or IgM (p = .30) (Figure 36–6). The survival of patients with an IgG, IgA, or IgM monoclonal gammopathy was also similar (Figure 36–7). We found that survival of the 241 patients with MGUS was shorter than that of an age- and sex-adjusted 1980 U.S.

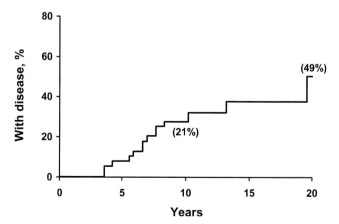

Figure 36–5. Incidence of macroglobulinemia, amyloidosis, or lymphoproliferative disease after recognition of IgM monoclonal gammopathy. Actuarial analysis. (From Kyle and Lust,[36] with permission.)

population (median, 13.7 vs. 15.7 years) (Figure 36–8). Van de Poel et al.[21] also reported that the long-term survival of 334 patients with MGUS was slightly shorter than the expected survival in an age- and sex-adjusted population, but the difference was not statistically significant.

In 23 additional patients, an M-protein value of 3.0 g/dl or greater developed (group 2). Either serious disease or a serum M-protein value 3.0 g/dl or higher developed in 82 (34 percent) of the 241 patients. The results of long-term follow-up of the 241 cases are shown in Figure 36–9.

Results of Long-Term Follow-Up in Other Series

During a 20-year follow-up of 64 Swedish patients in a survey of 6995 patients, Axelsson[22] reported that 2 had died of multiple myeloma and 1 had died of malignant lymphoma. Three of the 19 surviving patients had had an increase in the M protein, and a fourth patient had had a rather large monoclonal IgA-κ protein and then developed Bence Jones proteinuria (5 g/L). A tentative diagnosis of multiple myeloma was made, but treatment was unnecessary. Thus, 11 percent of the patients with long-term follow-up had evidence of some progression of their "benign" monoclonal gammopathy. In another group of 20 patients with asymptomatic monoclonal gammopathy for 3 to 14 years, 4 developed malignant disease.[23] In another series of 113 patients with MGUS, 8 developed multiple myeloma and 2 had amyloidosis during a follow-up of 1 to 17 years (median, 3 years).[24] In another report of that group, 19 of the 152 patients with "benign" monoclonal gammopathy developed malignant disease with a 1- to 19-year follow-up.[25] Malignant transformation occurred in 14 percent of 213 patients followed for 5 to 8 years and in 18 percent of 100 patients with MGUS who were followed for 8 to 13 years. The average duration from the first recognition of the M protein until the development of serious disease was 63 months (range, 17 to 138 months).[26] In another series of 213 patients with MGUS and a median follow-up of 37.8 months, 10 developed multiple myeloma, macroglobulinemia, or primary amyloidosis after a follow-up of 11 to 124 months (median, 60 months). The actuarial risk was 4.5 percent at 5 years, 15 percent at 10 years, and 26 percent at 15 years.[27] In another group of 128 patients with MGUS followed for 12 to 156 months (median, 56 months), 13 developed malignant disease. The actuarial probability of developing malignant disease was 8.5 percent at 5 years and 19.2 percent at 10 years. The median interval from recognition of the M protein to diagnosis of malignant transformation was 41.6 months (range, 12 to 155 months).[28]

In one study with short follow-up, 8 (3.3 percent) of 243 patients with MGUS progressed to multiple myeloma; the range from diagnosis to disease progression was 6 to 18 months.[29] In another study, 22 (6.6 percent) of 334 patients with MGUS developed a malignant transformation after a median follow-up of 8.4 years.[21] Isaksson et al.[30] reported that 15 (26 percent) of 57 patients developed a malignant plasma cell process during follow-up. In another study, 6.8 percent of 335 patients with MGUS had progression during a median follow-up of 70 months.[31] In a follow-up of 263 cases of MGUS, the actuarial probability of malignant transformation was 31 percent at 20

Table 36–8. Type of Serious Disease That Developed in 59 Patients With Monoclonal Gammopathy, Stratified by Immunoglobulin

| Immunoglobulin | No. of Patients | Type of Disease | | | |
		Multiple Myeloma	Amyloidosis	Macroglobulinemia	Lymphoproliferative Disease
IgA	8	7	1	0	0
IgG	38	32	5	0	1
IgM	10	0	1	6	3
Biclonal	3	0	1	1	1
Total	59	39	8	7	5

(From Kyle,[35] with permission.)

years.[32] Eleven (0.5 percent) of 2192 adults over 21 years of age in a New Zealand town had an M protein.[33] After a 31-year follow-up, 7 of the 11 patients developed a hematologic malignancy (multiple myeloma in 4, Waldenström's macroglobulinemia in 2, and lymphoma in 1).[34]

Ucci et al.[29] reported that a value of 20 percent bone marrow plasma cells was a safe point for the differentiation of MGUS from multiple myeloma. However, Baldini et al.[31] reported that the malignant transformation rate was 6.8 percent when the bone marrow plasma cell content was less than 10 percent and 37 percent in the group with MGUS who had a bone marrow plasma cell value of 10 to 30 percent. They also stated that the likelihood of progression was low in patients with an IgG MGUS less than or equal to 1.5 g/dl, bone marrow plasma cells less than 5 percent, no reduction in polyclonal immunoglobulins, and no light chain proteinuria.

No findings at diagnosis of MGUS allow patients who will remain stable to be distinguished from those who go on to develop a malignant condition.[35,36] The initial hemoglobin level, amount of serum M protein, level of uninvolved immunoglobulins, presence of small amounts of urinary light chains, percentage and appearance of bone marrow plasma cells, and serum albumin value are not useful in recognizing patients in whom a malignant change will occur. The crucial difference between MGUS and multiple myeloma in plateau phase is that virtually all patients with multiple myeloma will eventually have a relapse, whereas only 25 percent of patients with MGUS will develop a serious plasma cell proliferative disorder. When myeloma develops, the type of M protein is always the same as it was in MGUS. Patients with multiple myeloma may obtain an objective response to therapy and develop a stable or plateau phase that resembles MGUS or smoldering multiple myeloma. However, they are different biologically because the patient with myeloma has a relapse whereas the patient with MGUS does not.

Most patients with multiple myeloma likely have had a previous monoclonal gammopathy. In our experience, 32 (58 percent) of 55 patients with multiple myeloma in Olmsted County, Minnesota, had MGUS, smoldering multiple myeloma, or a plasmacytoma before the diagnosis of myeloma.[37] In a comparison of 21 patients with multiple myeloma arising from MGUS and 41 patients with multiple myeloma without a previous history of MGUS, the former group had a lower frequency of advanced stages of myeloma, lower rate of anemia, renal failure, and bone lesions, and lower levels of β_2-microglobulin and C-reactive protein. They also had a longer median survival. The authors concluded that multiple myeloma preceded by MGUS had a better prognosis.[38]

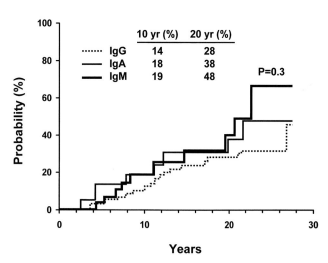

Figure 36–6. Rate of development of lymphoplasmacytic disease in 241 patients with a serum monoclonal protein, stratified by immunoglobulin class. (From Kyle,[35] with permission.)

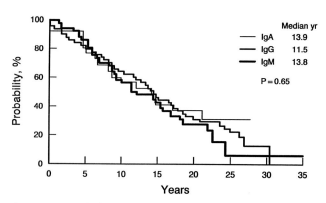

Figure 36–7. Survival among 241 patients with a serum monoclonal protein, stratified by heavy chain immunoglobulin class. (From Kyle,[35] with permission.)

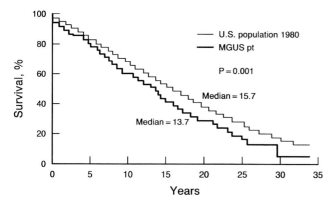

Figure 36–8. Survival among 241 patients with a monoclonal gammopathy of undetermined significance (MGUS) in comparison with survival among the age- and sex-adjusted 1980 U.S. population. (From Kyle,[35] with permission.)

Table 36–9. Mayo Clinic Criteria for the Diagnosis of MGUS, SMM, and MM[a]	
Disorder	**Criteria**
MGUS	Serum monoclonal protein < 3 g/dl *and* bone marrow plasma cells < 10 percent *and* absence of anemia, renal failure, hypercalcemia, and lytic bone lesions
SMM	Serum monoclonal protein ≥ 3 g/dl *or* bone marrow plasma cells ≥ 10 percent *and* absence of anemia, renal failure, hypercalcemia, and lytic bone lesions
MM	Presence of a serum or urine monoclonal protein, bone marrow plasmacytosis, *and* anemia, renal failure, hypercalcemia, or lytic bone lesions. Patients with primary systemic amyloidosis and ≥ 30 percent bone marrow plasma cells are considered to have both multiple myeloma and amyloidosis

[a] MGUS, monoclonal gammopathy of undetermined significance; SMM, smoldering multiple myeloma; MM, multiple myeloma.

DIFFERENTIATION OF MGUS FROM MULTIPLE MYELOMA AND MACROGLOBULINEMIA

Patients with MGUS have less than 3 g/dl of M protein in the serum and no or small amounts of Bence Jones proteinuria: less than 10 percent plasma cells in the bone marrow aspirate or biopsy; normal serum albumin level; and no anemia, hypercalcemia, renal insufficiency, or osteolytic lesions, unless caused by other diseases. No increase in the M-protein level or development of features of a lymphoplasma cell proliferative disease during long-term follow-up is proof that the patient has MGUS (Table 36–9). There is no evidence that bisphosphonates are beneficial for MGUS.

In contrast to patients with MGUS, patients with smoldering multiple myeloma (SMM) have a serum M-protein level greater than 3 g/dl or more than 10 percent atypical plasma cells in the bone marrow. Frequently, they have a small amount of monoclonal light chain in the urine and a reduction of uninvolved Igs in the serum. These findings are consistent with multiple myeloma. However, anemia, renal insufficiency, and skeletal lesions do not develop, and the M protein in the serum and urine and the bone marrow plasma cells remain stable. Furthermore, the plasma cell labeling index is very low. Therefore, these patients have a benign monoclonal gammopathy, but it is not possible to make this diagnosis when the patient is initially seen because most patients with this level of bone marrow plasma cells and M protein in the serum and urine have symptomatic myeloma (Table 36–9). Patients with SMM should not be treated unless laboratory abnormalities progress or symptoms of myeloma develop.[39] Clinical trials are under way to determine whether thalidomide can be used in SMM to delay progression to myeloma. However, therapy with this agent outside the setting of a clinical trial is not recommended.

The differentiation of a patient with benign monoclonal gammopathy from one with multiple myeloma may be difficult. The size of the M protein, hemoglobin value, percentage of bone marrow plasma cells, amount of light chain excretion, presence

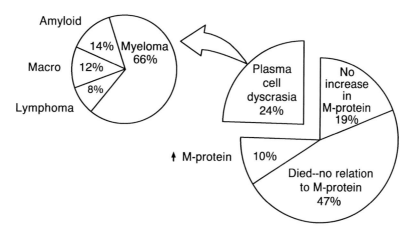

Figure 36–9. Evolution of monoclonal gammopathies. Macro, macroglobulinemia; M protein, monoclonal protein. (From Kyle RA: Monoclonal gammopathy of undetermined significance. Blood Rev 8:135, 1994, with permission.)

of hypercalcemia or renal insufficiency, and presence of lytic bone lesions are often helpful. The size of the serum M protein is of some help—higher levels are associated with a greater likelihood of malignancy.[40] The presence of a serum M protein of more than 3 g/dl usually indicates overt multiple myeloma or macroglobulinemia, but some exceptions such as SMM do exist.

Levels of Ig class not associated with the M protein (normal polyclonal or background Igs) may help in differentiating benign from malignant gammopathies. In most patients with multiple myeloma, the levels of polyclonal (normal or uninvolved) Igs are reduced, although a similar reduction of background Igs in patients with benign monoclonal gammopathy also may occur. Peltonen et al.[41] emphasized that the background or uninvolved Igs were decreased in 88 percent of patients with a lymphocytic or plasmacytic cell neoplasm, but these Igs were also reduced in 38 percent of patients with benign monoclonal gammopathy. In our study, 26 percent of patients with benign monoclonal gammopathy (group 1) had a decrease in normal or uninvolved Igs at diagnosis of the M protein and yet their condition remained stable during a median follow-up of 22 years. Consequently, levels of uninvolved Igs are not a reliable differentiating feature.

The association of a monoclonal light chain (Bence Jones proteinuria) with a serum M protein is suggestive of a neoplastic process. From a study of 42 patients with benign monoclonal gammopathy, Dammacco and Waldenström[42] reported a weakly positive response to the Bence Jones heat test in 1 case and small amounts (less than 60 mg/L) of light chains in 10 cases. Lindström and Dahlström[43] found that 40 percent of their patients with benign monoclonal gammopathy had a monoclonal light chain in the urine. We have also seen many other patients with a small monoclonal light chain in the urine and an M protein in the serum whose conditions have remained stable for many years.

The presence of more than 10 percent plasma cells in the bone marrow is suggestive of multiple myeloma, but some patients with a greater degree of plasmacytosis have remained stable for long periods. Bone marrow plasma cells in multiple myeloma are often atypical, but these morphologic features also may be seen in MGUS and SMM. The assessment of nuclear cytoplasmic asynchrony[44] has been proposed to help differentiate benign from malignant disease but, in our experience, plasma cell nucleolar size, grade, and asynchrony are of limited use in differentiating MGUS from multiple myeloma.[45] The light chain ratio (number of positively reacting plasma cells for the predominant light chain divided by the number of positively reacting plasma cells for the majority light chain) may be helpful in the differentiation of multiple myeloma from MGUS,[46] but it is not useful when the number of plasma cells is small. In one study, the presence of more than 20 percent plasma cells in the bone marrow differentiated stage I myeloma from MGUS.[29] The presence of osteolytic lesions is strongly suggestive of multiple myeloma, but metastatic carcinoma may produce lytic lesions as well as plasmacytosis and may be associated with an unrelated serum M protein. In fact, if fewer than 10 percent plasma cells, a modest-sized M component, and constitutional symptoms are present, the most probable diagnosis

is metastatic carcinoma with an unrelated MGUS. Increased bone resorption assessed on quantitative bone biopsy occurs in all patients with active multiple myeloma, whereas abnormal bone modeling does not occur in MGUS and SMM.[47]

The plasma cell labeling index for detection of synthesis of DNA is useful in differentiating the patient with MGUS or SMM from the patient with multiple myeloma. We have developed a monoclonal antibody (BU-1) reactive with 5-bromo-2-deoxyuridine (BrdUrd) in mice.[48] Bone marrow plasma cells are exposed to BrdUrd for 1 hour. Cells synthesizing DNA will incorporate BrdUrd, which is recognized by the BU-1 monoclonal antibody conjugated to goat antimouse immunoglobulin-rhodamine complex. Staining with propidium iodide identifies the cells incorporating BrdUrd in S phase. The BU-1 monoclonal antibody does not require denaturation for its activity. Consequently, the use of fluorescein-conjugated Ig antisera (κ and λ) identifies monoclonal plasma cells and plasmacytoid lymphocytes. An immunofluorescent labeling index can be performed in 4 or 5 hours and is a practical aid for assisting with therapeutic decisions. We believe that the immunofluorescent plasma cell labeling technique is superior to the [^{3}H]thymidine method.[49] An elevated plasma cell labeling index is good evidence that a patient either has multiple myeloma or will soon have symptomatic myeloma. However, approximately one-third of patients with symptomatic multiple myeloma will have a normal plasma cell labeling index.

A good correlation exists between the peripheral blood and the bone marrow labeling index.[50] Mononuclear cells are separated on Ficoll-Hypaque, and the T cells are depleted with magnetic beads. The cells are then incubated with BrdUrd and spun onto slides.

After staining with BU-1 and goat anti-mouse IgG labeled with rhodamine isothiocyanate, the cells are stained with κ- and λ-antisera, and a 500-cell count of peripheral blood B cells bearing the same cytoplasmic light chain isotype as the M protein is done. The median peripheral blood labeling index was 0.2 percent for 29 patients with MGUS or SMM, 0.8 percent for 35 patients with new, untreated multiple myeloma, and 1.7 percent for 41 patients with multiple myeloma in relapse. Four patients had an elevated peripheral blood labeling index but clinically inactive disease at the time of study; all developed active multiple myeloma, requiring chemotherapy within 6 months.[50]

The presence of circulating plasma cells in the peripheral blood is a good marker of active disease. Monoclonal plasma cells can be detected in the peripheral blood of patients with active multiple myeloma even when they are not detectable in routine peripheral blood smears. Plasma cells are infrequently present in patients with MGUS or SMM. The presence of 3×10^6/L or more peripheral blood plasma cells in persons with MGUS or SMM indicates that the patient does not have inactive disease but is likely to develop symptomatic myeloma within a few months. Peripheral plasma cells are detected in approximately 60 percent of patients with newly diagnosed myeloma and in more than 90 percent of patients with refractory myeloma or at relapse.[51]

The presence of an increase in the number or proliferative rate ("abnormal") of circulating monoclonal plasma cells is a good predictor of development of symptomatic myeloma. In a series of 57 patients with newly diagnosed SMM, 16 had progression within 12 months. Sixty-three percent of these had abnormal peripheral blood plasma cells. By contrast, only 10 percent (4 of 41) of the patients who remained stable had abnormal peripheral blood plasma cells. The median time to progression was 0.75 year in patients with abnormal peripheral blood plasma cells and 2.5 years for those without abnormal peripheral blood plasma cells. Thus, the presence of increased numbers of circulating peripheral blood plasma cells or an increase in the labeling index is indicative of symptomatic disease.[52]

Conventional cytogenetic studies are not useful in the differentiation of MGUS and multiple myeloma because of inherent technical limitations and lack of absolute differences in chromosome abnormalities between the two conditions. Fluorescence in situ hybridization (FISH) studies show that aneuploidy can be detected in bone marrow plasma cells from most patients with MGUS.[53–57] In one study that used interphase FISH, chromosome abnormalities were found in 53 percent of 36 patients with MGUS, whereas other studies suggest that the incidence is close to 100 percent.[58] Zandecki and colleagues[53] detected trisomy in at least one of chromosomes 3, 7, 9, and 11 in 12 percent to 72 percent of bone marrow plasma cells in 12 of 14 hyperdiploid patients with MGUS. The most frequent chromosome abnormality in MGUS appears to be translocations involving chromosome 14q32, which is the immunoglobulin heavy-chain locus.[54,55] Fonseca and colleagues[59] found that translocations involving chromosome 14q32 were present in more than 75 percent of patients with MGUS. Thus, it appears that several chromosome abnormalities frequently found in myeloma are present even at the MGUS stage. However, in contrast to myeloma, deletions of chromosome 13q are less common in MGUS.[54] Recent reports suggest that deletions of chromosome 13 may be involved in the progression from MGUS to myeloma, but clearly additional studies are needed.[54,55]

Magnetic resonance imaging (MRI) may be helpful for differentiating MGUS from multiple myeloma. In a series of 24 patients with MGUS, MRI was normal in all, whereas abnormalities were found in 38 (86 percent) of 44 patients with multiple myeloma.[60] Laroche et al.[61] performed histomorphometric studies of bone biopsy specimens in 34 patients with a monoclonal gammopathy. Bone remodeling was normal in those with MGUS, but bone resorption increased and bone formation decreased in stage III myeloma.[62]

Definition of the plasma cell population in the bone marrow also may be helpful in the differentiation of MGUS and myeloma. Ocqueteau et al.[63] found a population of plasma cells with a high CD38 expression with low forward light scatter (FSC)/side light scatter (SSC) and positive for CD19 and negative for CD56. These cells were polyclonal. The other plasma cell subpopulation showed a lower CD38 expression and higher FSC/SSC values and strongly expressed CD56 whereas CD19 was negative. These cells were monoclonal. Only 1.5 percent of patients with multiple myeloma had greater than 3 percent of the normal polyclonal plasma cells, but 98 percent of patients with MGUS had greater than 3 percent. The authors thought that the number of residual polyclonal plasma cells was the most powerful single factor for differentiation of MGUS from myeloma.

The C-terminal telopeptide of type I collagen was increased in 34 percent of 35 patients with MGUS. Serum osteocalcin was increased in 31 percent and serum bone-specific alkaline phosphatase in 17 percent, which suggests that abnormal bone metabolism occurs in MGUS. The authors did not determine whether these findings increased the risk for development of multiple myeloma.[64] Mathiot et al.[65] reported that low levels of soluble FcγRIII (sCD16) discriminated myeloma from a control population. They found that low sCD16 in MGUS was associated with a high likelihood of rapid evolution to multiple myeloma.

Interleukin (IL)-1β is produced by plasma cells in virtually all cases of multiple myeloma but is undetectable in most patients with MGUS. IL-1β has strong osteoclast activating factor activity that increases the expression of adhesion molecules and induces paracrine IL-6 production. This parallels the development of osteolytic bone lesions, homing of myeloma cells to bone marrow, and IL-6–induced cell growth. IL-1β may play an important role in the homing of plasma cells to the bone marrow. Plasma cells subsequently may stimulate osteoclasts through the production of IL-1β and paracrine IL-6 secretion, resulting in lytic lesions. In addition, IL-6 supports the growth of myeloma cells. They may stimulate osteoclasts through the production of IL-1β.[66,67]

Vacca and colleagues,[68] using immunohistochemical techniques to identify microvessels, demonstrated that bone marrow angiogenesis was increased in multiple myeloma but not in MGUS. The extent of marrow angiogenesis was correlated with the plasma cell labeling index. Studies done at our institution confirm these findings, although this test will have limited value in differentiating the two conditions because angiogenesis is not increased in approximately one-third of patients with myeloma.[69] In studies done with the chick embryo chorioallantoic membrane (CAM) model, sorted bone marrow samples were angiogenic in 76 percent of patients with myeloma and 20 percent of patients with MGUS.[70] Studies are ongoing to determine whether angiogenesis is an important event in the progression of MGUS to myeloma.

Levels of β2-microglobulin are not helpful in differentiating benign monoclonal gammopathy from low-grade multiple myeloma because there is too much overlap between the two entities.[71] Neither the presence of J chains in malignant plasma cells[72] nor the acid phosphatase levels in plasma cells are reliable for differentiation.[73] Reduced numbers of OKT4+ T cells,[74] increased numbers of monoclonal idiotype-bearing peripheral blood lymphocytes,[75] and increased numbers of Ig-secreting cells in peripheral blood are characteristic of multiple myeloma, but overlap exists with MGUS.[76]

The presence of cytoplasmic 5′-nucleotidase in plasma cells was reported in 46 percent of patients with myeloma and in 15 percent with MGUS.[77] The leukocyte alkaline phosphatase score is elevated in myeloma, in contrast to MGUS, and may be helpful in differentiation.[78] Serum deoxythymidine kinase activity is of no diagnostic or prognostic importance in monoclonal gammopathy.[79]

The serum level of IL-6 may aid in the differentiation of monoclonal gammopathies. In one report, the serum IL-6 level was elevated in only 1 of 35 patients with MGUS or SMM but was increased in 35 percent of patients with overt myeloma.[62]

In another series, the serum IL-6 level was elevated in 42 percent of 210 patients with multiple myeloma. These elevated levels were associated with shorter survival.[80] Alternatively, Ballester et al.[81] reported that high levels of IL-6 production were associated with low tumor burden, a low percentage of bone marrow plasma cells, and a low proliferative rate. The expression of a multidrug-resistant phenotype (MDR-1), the absence of CD56 expression, and a low proliferative rate may be useful in differentiating MGUS from SMM.[82]

In summary, no single factor can differentiate a patient with benign monoclonal gammopathy from one in whom a malignant plasma cell disorder will subsequently develop. Regardless of the result of sophisticated laboratory tests, the differentiation between MGUS and multiple myeloma is based on clinical factors, such as symptoms, anemia, hypercalcemia, renal failure, and lytic bone lesions. A typical laboratory result such as a high plasma cell labeling index in a patient with a clinical MGUS or SMM should prompt closer and more frequent observation. The serum M protein must be periodically measured and clinical evaluation conducted to determine whether serious disease has developed. If the patient has no other features of myeloma or amyloidosis and a serum M-spike value less than 0.5 g/dl, serum protein electrophoresis should be repeated at annual intervals. A bone marrow examination, skeletal radiography, and a 24-hour urine specimen for immunofixation are not necessary in this setting. If the asymptomatic patient has an M protein level of 1.5 to 2.0 g/dl, additional studies should include quantitation of immunoglobulins and collection of a 24-hour urine specimen for electrophoresis and immunofixation. The serum protein electrophoretic pattern should be determined again in 3 to 6 months and, if stable, should be repeated in 6 months and then annually, or sooner if any symptoms occur.

If the IgG or IgA serum M protein value is greater than 2.0 g/dl, a metastatic survey, including views of the humeri and femurs, should be done. Bone marrow aspiration and biopsy also should be performed. If the patient has an IgM M protein, aspiration and biopsy of the bone marrow and a computed tomography (CT) scan of the abdomen may be useful for recognizing macroglobulinemia or a related lymphoproliferative disorder. Levels of β_2-microglobulin and C-reactive proteins should be determined. If the results of these studies are satisfactory, serum electrophoresis should be repeated in 2 or 3 months, and if the results are stable, the test should be repeated at 6- to 12-month intervals.

Electrophoresis and immunofixation of a 24-hour urine specimen should be performed if the serum M protein value is more than 1.5 g/dl. They also should be done if the serum M protein value increases or other evidence involving myeloma or macroglobulinemia occurs. Determination of the plasma cell labeling index and a search for circulating plasma cells in the peripheral blood are helpful in this situation.

ASSOCIATION OF MONOCLONAL GAMMOPATHY WITH OTHER DISEASES

Although monoclonal gammopathy frequently exists without other abnormalities, certain diseases are associated with it, as would be expected in an older population. The association of two diseases depends on the frequency with which each occurs independently. Furthermore, there may be an association because of differences in the referral practice or in other selected patient groups. The investigator must use valid epidemiologic and statistical methods in evaluating these associations. The need for appropriate control populations cannot be overemphasized.

For example, the association of monoclonal gammopathy and hyperparathyroidism has been reported.[83,84] In an effort to clarify the relationship of hyperparathyroidism to monoclonal gammopathies, we reviewed our cases of surgically proven parathyroid adenoma in which serum protein electrophoresis had been done within the 6 months preceding parathyroidectomy. Among 911 patients who met these criteria and who were 50 years or older, immunoelectrophoresis demonstrated MGUS in 9 (1 percent).[85] This prevalence of MGUS is similar to the 1.25 to 1.7 percent found in studies of three normal populations.[3,5]

In another report, 4 of 386 patients with primary hyperparathyroidism had MGUS.[86] Thus, the association of hyperparathyroidism and MGUS seems to be due to chance alone.

An increased prevalence of monoclonal gammopathy in association with carcinoma of the colon has been reported on several occasions. However, in two large studies, the prevalence of monoclonal gammopathies was no greater than that expected in a population of similar age.[87,88] These studies demonstrate the need for comparison with an adequate control population before it can be assumed that an association exists between monoclonal gammopathy and any disease.

Lymphoproliferative Disorders

Azar et al.[89] reported in 1957 that malignant lymphoma and lymphocytic leukemia were associated with a myeloma-type serum protein. Kyle et al.[90] in 1960 described six patients with lymphoma who had serum or urine electrophoretic patterns suggestive of multiple myeloma. The presence of M proteins in patients with lymphoma was confirmed by Krauss and Sokal.[91] In a report published that same year, Hällén[92] described five patients with reticulum cell sarcoma and a serum M component. IgM M proteins may be increased in patients with malignant lymphoproliferative diseases.[93]

Moore et al.[94] found an IgM monoclonal gammopathy in the serum in 3.6 percent of 526 patients with diffuse lymphoma but in only 2 of 40 patients with nodular lymphoma. Among 1150 patients with lymphoma, Alexanian[95] found M proteins in 49. M proteins were found in 29 (4.5 percent) of the 640 patients with diffuse lymphoproliferative disease (chronic lymphocytic leukemia, lymphocytic lymphoma, and reticulum cell sarcoma) but in none of the 292 patients with a nodular lymphoma. Hobbs et al.[96] reported that two-thirds of their patients with an IgM protein had a diffuse histologic pattern and only 13 percent had a follicular pattern. Bain and Belch[97] likewise concluded that the association of nodular lymphoma and a serum M protein was rare. Pangalis et al.[98] found an M protein in 20 of 108 patients with a well-differentiated lymphocytic lymphoma. Ko and Pruzanski[99] detected an IgM protein in 33 of 62 patients with lymphoma who had an M protein in their serum. By contrast, an M protein is rarely found in Hodgkin's disease.[100] Magrath et al.[101] found IgM proteins with agarose gel electrophoresis and immunofixation in the sera of 12 of 21 patients with undifferentiated lymphoma of Burkitt's and non-Burkitt's types. These proteins disappeared after therapy but reappeared at relapse.

We reviewed the medical records of 430 patients in whom a serum IgM monoclonal gammopathy had been identified between 1956 and 1978 at the Mayo Clinic (Table 36–10). Patients were classified as follows:

1. *Waldenström's macroglobulinemia:* IgM spike of 3.0 g/dl or more in the serum protein electrophoretic pattern and an increase in lymphocytes or plasmacytoid lymphocytes in the bone marrow
2. *Lymphoma:* On initial examination, lymphadenopathy or an extranodal lymphoid tumor and biopsy findings consistent with a lymphoma
3. *Chronic lymphocytic leukemia:* Lymphocyte count of more than 9000/mm³
4. *Primary amyloidosis:* Histologic proof of amyloid on a biopsy specimen of appropriate tissue
5. *MGUS:* IgM protein value less than 3.0 g/dl, no constitutional symptoms, no hepatosplenomegaly or lymphadenopathy, and no anemia; no chemotherapy required
6. *Malignant lymphoproliferative disease:* Could not be classified in the foregoing categories; IgM protein value less than 3.0 g/dl; usually bone marrow infiltration with lymphocytes or plasmacytoid lymphocytes; therapy required because of anemia or constitutional symptoms

More than one-half of patients with an IgM protein had MGUS. During follow-up, 40 (17 percent) of 242 patients with MGUS developed a malignant lymphoid disease (Table 36–11). In 22 patients, Waldenström's macroglobulinemia developed; 9 others had a malignant lymphoproliferative process requiring chemotherapy; and in 6 others, lymphoma developed. The median duration from the recognition of the IgM protein until the diagnosis of lymphoid disease was more than 4 years (range, 0.4 to 22 years). The median duration of survival after the diagnosis of Waldenström's macroglobulinemia in these 22 patients was 6.5 years. This duration is similar to that in patients with

Table 36–11. Development of Malignant Lymphoid Diseases in 40 of 242 Patients With IgM Monoclonal Gammopathy of Undetermined Significance

Disease	No. of Patients	Duration Until Progression (years)	
		Median	Range
Waldenström's macroglobulinemia	22	8.0	1.8–16.3
Lymphoma	6	6.8	4.8–21.9
Chronic lymphocytic leukemia	1	9.2	9.2
Primary amyloidosis (AL)	2	4.3	2.4–6.1
Malignant lymphoproliferative disease	9	4.2	0.4–12.0

(Modified from Kyle and Garton,[102] with permission.)

Waldenström's macroglobulinemia at presentation. In addition, 10 patients with MGUS (4 percent) had an increase in serum M protein of more than 1.0 g/dl, and 9 others had an increase of 0.5 to 0.9 g/dl. None of these 19 patients developed Waldenström's macroglobulinemia, malignant lymphoproliferative disease, or lymphoma. Currently, 14 patients are alive and under observation.

More than two-thirds of the 430 patients with IgM monoclonal gammopathy have died (Figure 36–10). The median survival of patients with Waldenström's macroglobulinemia and of those with a malignant lymphoproliferative disease was similar (5 and 5.5 years, respectively).

Although the size of the serum M protein in Waldenström's macroglobulinemia differs from that in lymphoproliferative disease, survival was virtually the same for both groups. It is evident that patients with Waldenström's macroglobulinemia and lymphoproliferative disease who have lymphocytic proliferation of the marrow producing constitutional symptoms or anemia requiring chemotherapy are not different. Consequently, no rationale exists for differentiating patients with lymphoproliferative disease from those with Waldenström's macroglobulinemia. They can be combined in future prospective studies of Waldenström's macroglobulinemia.[102]

Although an increase of polyclonal immunoglobulin is common in angioimmunoblastic lymphadenopathy,[103] an M protein may be seen.[104] Investigators at the National Institutes of Health (NIH) estimated that 2 percent of patients with angioimmunoblastic lymphadenopathy had a monoclonal gammopathy.[105] Angiofollicular lymph node hyperplasia (Castleman's disease) may be associated with an M protein.[106] Sugai et al.[107] reported that 5 of 10 Japanese patients with Sjögren syndrome had an IgA M protein. Two patients with Sjögren syndrome and M protein in the serum subsequently developed a malignant lymphoma.[108] Kaposi's sarcoma has been associated with a serum M protein.[109]

Leukemia

M proteins have been found in the sera of patients with leukemia.[110] We described 100 patients with chronic lympho-

Table 36–10. Classification of IgM Monoclonal Gammopathies Among 430 Patients (1956–1978)

Classification	Patients	
	No.	Percent
Monoclonal gammopathy of undetermined significance	242	56
Waldenström's macroglobulinemia	71	17
Lymphoma	28	7
Chronic lymphocytic leukemia	21	5
Primary amyloidosis (AL)	6	1
Lymphoproliferative disease	62	14
Total	430	100

(From Kyle and Garton,[102] with permission.)

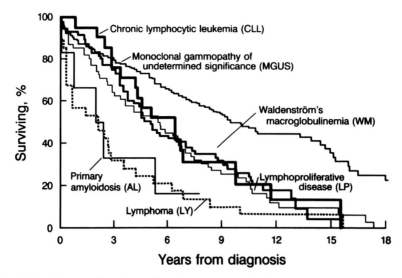

Figure 36–10. Survival curves for patients with various IgM monoclonal gammopathies. (From Kyle and Garton,[102] with permission.)

cytic leukemia and an M protein in the serum or urine.[111] IgG accounted for 51 percent and IgM for 28 percent. The median concentration of M protein was 1.0 g/dl. There were no major differences in patients with chronic lymphocytic leukemia, whether they had an IgG or an IgM M protein. Using immunoisoelectric focusing, Sinclair et al.[112] found that 34 (61 percent) of 56 patients with chronic lymphocytic leukemia had an M protein in the serum; 88 percent were IgM. Monoclonal gammopathies have been recognized in hairy cell leukemia.[113] Matsuzaki et al.[114] described three patients with monoclonal gammopathy and adult T-cell leukemia. Guglielmi et al.[115] reported eight patients with chronic myelocytic leukemia who had the Philadelphia chromosome and a monoclonal gammopathy. Seven of the eight patients had the λ-isotype. Buonanno et al.[116] described a patient with Philadelphia-positive chronic myelocytic leukemia in whom a monocytic blast cell transformation developed associated with an IgG-λ protein.[117] We have also seen several patients who had chronic myelocytic leukemia and an M protein in their serum. An IgG-κ M protein was recognized in the serum and on the surface of leukemic cells of a patient with acute promyelocytic leukemia. The blast cells did not appear to secrete the M protein.[118] Transient M proteins have been reported with acute myelomonocytic leukemia.[119] Data are inadequate to determine whether the incidence of an M protein is greater in patients with leukemia than in a normal population.

Other Hematologic Diseases

Acquired von Willebrand's disease is an uncommon disorder but is often associated with a monoclonal gammopathy.[120–123] Desmopressin (DDAVP) has been helpful in preventing or stopping bleeding in patients with acquired von Willebrand syndrome. Presumably, it induces the release of factor VIII and von Willebrand factor from endogenous stores.[124] Patients with

monoclonal gammopathy and lupus anticoagulant activity have been reported.[125] Patients with MGUS have a significantly higher incidence of antiphospholipid antibodies in their blood than controls.[126]

M proteins have been reported in patients with pernicious anemia.[127] Three of 20 patients in a family with congenital dyserythropoietic anemia type III had a monoclonal IgG-κ protein; one had multiple myeloma.[128] The association of pure red cell aplasia and monoclonal gammopathy has been found in six patients.[129] Balducci et al.[130] suggested that red cell aplasia was caused by a block in the maturation of the erythroid burst-forming unit, which might be related to the M protein. Polycythemia vera, myelofibrosis, and chronic myelocytic leukemia have been associated with monoclonal gammopathies.[131] Dührsen et al.[132] found an M protein in 3 of 46 patients with idiopathic myelofibrosis, one of whom had multiple myeloma. Economopoulos et al.[133] reported that 6 of 52 patients with myelodysplastic syndrome had monoclonal gammopathy.

Pratt et al.[134] reported that 4 of 16 patients with Gaucher's disease had an IgG-κ protein in their sera and 6 others had a diffuse increase of IgG. In another series of 23 patients, 10 had diffuse hypergammaglobulinemia, 6 had an oligoclonal gammopathy, and only 2 had a monoclonal gammopathy.[135] In one report, splenectomy in a patient with Gaucher's disease and MGUS resulted in a significant reduction in the IgG κ-protein.[136]

Connective Tissue Diseases

Rheumatoid arthritis[137] as well as seronegative erosive arthritis[138] have been reported with monoclonal gammopathies. However, in a series of 279 consecutive patients with rheumatoid arthritis at our institution, no significant increase in the incidence of M proteins was found. Lupus erythematosus and other connective tissue disorders have been associated with M protein.[139] In one report, 4 of 120 patients with systemic lupus erythematosus had MGUS.[140] Renier et al.[141] found seven patients (1.3 percent) with an M protein in 555 cases of ankylosing spondylitis. However, this incidence is similar to that expected in a normal population. Polymyalgia rheumatica has been noted with monoclonal gammopathy but, because both conditions occur more commonly in an older population, the relationship is doubtful.[142] Kalra and Delamere[143] described polymyalgia rheumatica-like symptoms in four patients with a monoclonal gammopathy and underlying lymphoreticular neoplasia. Three patients with an IgG-κ protein and polymyositis have been described.[144] An IgG protein was seen in a patient with relapsing polymyositis.[145] An M protein was found in 16 (23 percent) of 70 patients with inclusion body myositis. IgG was present in 13 (81 percent).[146] Immunoabsorption appeared to benefit a patient with inclusion body myositis and IgG M protein.[147] Powell et al.[148] described a benign course in eight patients who had discoid lupus erythematosus and an M protein. Transient IgM-κ protein was noted in a patient with hydralazine-induced lupus erythematosus.[149] The association of scleroderma with an IgG-κ M protein and the subsequent development of multiple myeloma has been reported.[150] Monoclonal gammopathy with psoriatic arthritis has been reported,[151] but this coexistence probably represents a chance occurrence.

Neurologic Disorders

In a series of 279 patients with a sensorimotor peripheral neuropathy of unknown cause, we found 16 cases (6 percent) of MGUS.[152] Kahn et al.[153] found that 16 of 56 patients with MGUS had a peripheral neuropathy. In another group of 132 consecutive patients with a monoclonal gammopathy, peripheral neuropathy was found in 4.[154] In another report, 8 of 19 patients with MGUS had a clinical polyneuropathy.[155] In an unselected series of patients with MGUS, neuropathy was noted in 2 of 34 patients with IgG (6 percent), 2 of 14 with IgA (14 percent), and 8 of 26 with IgM (31 percent). The neuropathy was subclinical in six patients.[156] Baldini et al.[157] reported that 14 of 31 patients with IgM MGUS had peripheral neuropathy. High titers of antimyelin-associated glycoprotein (MAG) IgM appear more likely to be associated with neuropathy than low titers.[158]

It is clear that an association exists between MGUS and peripheral neuropathy. However, the incidence is variable and depends on patient selection bias (patients admitted to a neurologic hospital would be more likely to have the association), the vigor with which the presence of an M protein is sought, and whether the diagnosis of peripheral neuropathy is made on clinical or electrophysiologic grounds. The incidence is greater if the diagnosis is based only on electrophysiologic evidence of neuropathy. Isobe and Osserman[159] reported MGUS in 5.4 percent of 239 patients with peripheral neuropathy or myopathy. A monograph on neurologic disorders associated with plasma cell dyscrasias has been published.[160]

Typically, MGUS neuropathy has the following features: 1. It is associated with the occurrence of an M protein in the serum; 2. amyloidosis, POEMS syndrome (*p*olyneuropathy, *o*rganomegaly, *e*ndocrinopathy, *M* protein, and *s*kin changes [osteosclerotic myeloma]), or related disorders are absent; 3. an asymmetric sensorimotor polyradiculopathy or neuropathy begins insidiously and is usually slowly progressive; 4. it occurs in the sixth to the seventh decade of life; 5. it affects males more frequently than females; 6. paresthesias, ataxia, and pain may be prominent; and 7. cranial nerves are not involved. The association of neuropathies and monoclonal gammopathies has been the subject of excellent reviews.[161–163]

The most frequent monoclonal gammopathy is IgM, followed by IgG and IgA. Most patients have decreased or altered sensation, paresthesias, unsteadiness of gait, and muscle weakness. Symptoms usually begin in the toes and extend to the feet and legs. The lower extremities are involved in almost 90 percent of patients. The muscle stretch reflexes are decreased or absent but Babinski signs are never found. Most patients have a chronic progression of symptoms.

In approximately one-half of patients with an IgM monoclonal gammopathy and peripheral neuropathy, the M protein binds to MAG.[164,165] Dellagi et al.[166] described 10 patients who had an IgM protein less than 1 g/dl and peripheral neuropathy with antibody against the myelin sheath. IgM proteins with anti-MAG activity may react with P_0, the major protein of myelin in human peripheral nerves.[167] The demonstration of IgM M protein throughout the compact myelin of a patient with peripheral neuropathy suggests that deposition of the M protein plays a role in pathogenesis.[168] IgM-κ deposition has been noted in areas of splittings of the myelin lamellae, bound to the internalized myelin debris.[169]

The MAG-reactive polyneuropathies are characterized by a slowly progressive, mainly sensory neuropathy beginning in the distal extremities and extending proximally. Discriminative and proprioceptive modalities are more severely involved than touch, pain, and temperature. Motor involvement is less prominent than sensory involvement. Cranial nerves and autonomic function are intact.[170] The clinical and electrodiagnostic manifestations resemble those of chronic inflammatory demyelinating polyneuropathy. There is a reduction of large myelinated fibers and segmental demyelination with remyelination.[171] Nerve conduction is normal in motor and sensory fibers. Conduction velocity of motor fibers is decreased below the normal range by approximately 20 percent.[172] The amplitude of the compound muscle action potential is severely decreased in the lower limb nerves. Frequently, responses from the sensory fibers in the extremities cannot be elicited. Needle electromyography reveals findings of denervation in 80 percent of patients. Both demyelination and denervation may be present.[173] The sural nerve is usually more severely involved than the median nerve.

Patients with sensorimotor peripheral neuropathy may have an IgM protein binding to chondroitin sulfates,[174–176] specific gangliosides,[177,178] or glycolipids.[179–181] Almost 80 percent of monoclonal IgM from patients with peripheral neuropathy reacts with some component of the peripheral nerve myelin.[182] An extensive review of antibodies associated with peripheral neuropathy has been published.[183]

We reviewed our experience with 65 patients with MGUS and sensorimotor peripheral neuropathy at the Mayo Clinic.

Thirty-one patients had IgM, 24 had IgG, and 10 had IgA. IgM was overrepresented in this group and was associated with sensory ataxia, slower nerve conduction, and more frequent dispersion of the compound muscle action potential when compared with IgG or IgA neuropathies. Neither the amount of IgM nor the estimated size of the monoclonal spike was associated with severity of the neuropathy. In addition, the type and severity of neuropathy with anti-MAG were not significantly different from those without anti-MAG. The course of the neuropathy was progressive in more than two-thirds of the patients.[184] In another report of 39 patients with MGUS, it was also suggested that those with neuropathy associated with IgM were different and should be distinguished from those with IgG or IgA.[185]

In a review of 40 patients with polyneuropathy associated with an IgM gammopathy, all but 1 had symmetrical polyneuropathy. It was predominantly sensory in 13 and purely sensory in 17. Electrophysiologic studies revealed demyelination in 83 percent and axonal degeneration in 6 percent. Anti-MAG antibodies were found in 65 percent and were associated only with demyelinating polyneuropathies.[186] In another series of 52 symptomatic patients with IgM monoclonal gammopathies, symptomatic neuropathy occurred in 3 of 4 patients with a high anti-MAG titer and in only 3 of 21 with a low anti-MAG titer.[187] This finding suggests that anti-MAG activity correlates with peripheral neuropathy.

In a comparison of 19 patients with IgM MGUS and 15 with IgG MGUS, Simovic et al.[188] noted prolongation of distal latencies of the median and ulnar motor nerves in IgM MGUS and greater slowing of peroneal nerve conduction velocity and more severe demyelination. MAG antibodies failed to distinguish a subgroup of patients with IgM MGUS neuropathy.

MGUS neuropathies differ from those associated with primary amyloidosis in the following respects: 1. The lower extremities are peripherally affected in MGUS, but upper and lower extremities tend to be affected to a greater degree in amyloidosis; 2. the course in amyloidosis is always slowly progressive; and 3. although amyloidosis may present as a sensorimotor neuropathy, autonomic features (postural hypotension, sphincter dysfunction, anhidrosis, and organ [heart or kidney] failure) often occur. Such autonomic features and organ failures do not occur in MGUS neuropathy.

The relationship of IgG and IgA M proteins to peripheral neuropathy is less well documented.[160] Read et al.[189] described three patients with an IgG M protein and peripheral neuropathy. Bleasel et al.[190] reported five patients with peripheral neuropathy and IgG MGUS. They emphasized that all five patients responded to plasmapheresis. IgA monoclonal gammopathy has been reported in several patients with peripheral neuropathy.[191–193]

The relationship between chronic inflammatory demyelinating polyradiculoneuropathy (CIDP) and CIDP with MGUS is unclear. In a comparison of 77 cases with CIDP and 26 with CIDP and MGUS, the latter group had a more indolent course, less severe weakness, and more frequent sensory loss. The outcome in the two groups was similar.[194] In a comparison of 45 patients with CIDP and 15 with MGUS-associated neuropathy, the latter group had less severe weakness, greater imbalance (ataxia), vibration loss in the hands, and absent median and ulnar sensory potentials.[195] In another study, the clinical course was progressive in most patients with MGUS, whereas those with CIDP were more likely to have a relapsing course. Impairment appeared to develop more slowly in the patients with MGUS, and they also had less severe functional impairment and a lesser degree of weakness and sensory changes.[196] In contrast, one study noted no significant clinical or electrophysiologic difference between patients with CIDP and those with CIDP and a monoclonal gammopathy.[197] The authors reported that patients with anti-MAG antibody had more pronounced slowing of the peroneal motor nerve conduction velocity, a lower frequency of conduction block, and a distal accentuation of conduction slowing. In summary, CIDP may occur at any age. Motor symptoms tend to predominate over sensory symptoms and there is a greater tendency for the course to be relapsing. Obviously, M proteins are not found.

A study of murine plasmacytomas induced by mineral oil or pristane showed morphologic and histometric evidence of neuropathy in approximately one-third of the mice.[198] Hays et al.[199] produced demyelination of feline sciatic nerve by the intraneural injection of sera from three patients who had an IgM reactivity with MAG and an associated neuropathy. Demyelination was greater than that induced by sera from six patients with IgM M proteins that were unreactive to MAG.[200] Injection of monoclonal IgM from patients with IgM peripheral neuropathy and anti-MAG activity produced demyelination characteristic of the human syndrome.[201] Patients with an IgA monoclonal gammopathy and peripheral neuropathy were reported to have binding of the M protein to normal human endoneurium.[191] The report of a brother and sister with an IgM M protein and a demyelinating peripheral neuropathy raises the possibility of a genetic disposition.[202]

Treatment of patients with peripheral neuropathy and monoclonal gammopathy has been disappointing. Smith et al.[203] noted improvement with plasmapheresis and chemotherapy in 9 of 13 patients with peripheral neuropathy and an IgM or IgG M protein. Plasmapheresis was helpful in two other cases: one with IgG-κ and another with IgA-κ.[204] Haas and Tatum[205] successfully treated a patient who had anti-MAG IgM protein with plasmapheresis for longer than 1 year. The patient's signs and symptoms correlated with variations in the serum IgM level.

Thirty-nine patients with peripheral neuropathy and MGUS of the IgG, IgA, or IgM type were randomized to plasmapheresis or sham plasmapheresis in a double-blind trial at the Mayo Clinic.[206] Plasma exchange significantly prevented worsening of or ameliorated the neuropathy. Patients with IgG or IgA gammopathy had a better response to plasma exchange than those with IgM gammopathy. In another study, 8 of 13 patients with a monoclonal gammopathy and peripheral neuropathy obtained benefit from plasma exchange.[207] Patients who do not respond to this program may be given chlorambucil when the M protein is of the IgM type or melphalan and prednisone for IgG and IgA gammopathies. In a prospective study of 44 patients with an IgM M protein and peripheral neuropathy, patients were randomized to receive either chlorambucil (0.1 mg/kg daily) orally or chlorambucil plus 15 courses of plasma exchange during the first 4 months of treatment. No difference was found between the two treatment groups, a finding suggesting that plasma exchange added no additional benefit to chlorambucil therapy.[208] Cyclophosphamide plus prednisone produced improvement in 8 of 16 patients with monoclonal gammopathy and sensorimotor peripheral neuropathy. The neuropathy stabilized in 6 others.[209]

Fludarabine, a purine analogue, produced benefit in 7 of 10 patients with an IgM M protein and neuropathy.[210] In another report, three of four patients with an IgM M protein and peripheral neuropathy obtained clinical and neurophysiologic benefit from fludarabine.[211] Rituxan (Rituximab) is a monoclonal antibody directed against CD20 which is frequently found on the surface membranes of lymphocytes in lymphoma. All five patients with an IgM M protein and neuropathy who were given 4 weekly infusions of rituxan obtained benefit.[212] Thus, responses have been achieved with chemotherapy, but data are insufficient to draw definite conclusions. Intravenous γ-globulin produces benefit in some patients with CIDP, and this may be tried for patients with sensorimotor peripheral neuropathy and monoclonal gammopathy.[213] A randomized study comparing intravenous immunoglobulin or placebo, followed by a crossover, revealed improved strength in two patients and improved sensorineuropathy in one other. Antibody titers to MAG or gangliosides did not change. Thus, fewer than 20 percent had any benefit.[214]

Although several instances of monoclonal gammopathy and motor neuron disease have been reported, there is little evidence that a causal effect exists. Eleven of 120 patients (9 percent) with motor neuron disease had an associated M protein. Ten patients had amyotrophic lateral sclerosis, and one had progressive spinal muscular atrophy.[215] Other reports of amyotrophic lateral sclerosis and MGUS have been published.[216,217] Myasthenia gravis has been associated with an M protein.[218,219] Five of 20 patients with Alzheimer's disease had MGUS, whereas none with MGUS were found in an age-matched control group of 40 patients.[220] Ataxia-telangiectasia, an autosomal recessive disorder, is characterized by cerebellar ataxia, oculocutaneous telangiectasia, and both B- and T-lymphocyte deficiency. This has been reported with monoclonal gammopathy.[221] In one report, 7 (monoclonal, 3; biclonal, 3; and triclonal, 1) of 86 patients with ataxia-telangiectasia had a gammopathy.[222]

Osteosclerotic Myeloma

Osteosclerotic myeloma, or POEMS syndrome, is characterized by a chronic sensorimotor polyneuropathy with predominating motor disability.[223] Single or multiple osteosclerotic bone lesions are important features. The cranial nerves are not involved, except for papilledema. Hepatosplenomegaly and lymphadenopathy may occur. Hyperpigmentation, hypertrichosis, gynecomastia, and testicular atrophy may be seen. Polycythemia or thrombocytosis may be a prominent feature. Almost all patients have a monoclonal protein of the λ-light chain class. The size of the M protein is modest and is almost always less than 3 g/dl. In contrast to multiple myeloma, this syndrome is rarely associated with Bence Jones proteinuria,

renal insufficiency, hypercalcemia, and skeletal fractures. The bone marrow aspirate and biopsy usually contain less than 5 percent plasma cells.[224,225] Bardwick et al.[226] suggested the acronym POEMS. The cause of osteosclerotic myeloma is unknown. Patients have higher levels of IL-1β, tumor necrosis factor-α, and IL-6 than patients with multiple myeloma.[227] Increased levels of vascular endothelial growth factor are frequently found and often decrease with successful therapy.[228]

Single or multiple osteosclerotic lesions in a limited area should be treated with radiation in tumoricidal dosages of 40 to 50 cGy. More than half of patients have substantial improvement of the neuropathy. Improvement may be slow, and we have seen patients who continue to improve for 2 to 3 years after radiation therapy. If the patient has widespread osteosclerotic lesions, systemic therapy is necessary. Kuwabara et al.[229] reported that five of six patients treated with melphalan and prednisone improved. Corticosteroids and plasma exchange generally have been of little benefit. Autologous stem cell transplantation following high-dose melphalan therapy is a consideration for younger patients with widespread osteosclerotic lesions. The stem cells should be collected before the patient is exposed to alkylating agents because they will reduce the hematopoietic stem cells. The mortality rate associated with this procedure is currently only 2 percent.

Dermatologic Diseases

Lichen myxedematosus (papular mucinosis, scleromyxedema) is a rare dermatologic condition frequently associated with a cathodal IgG-λ protein.[230] It is characterized by dermal papules, macules, and plaques that infiltrate the skin. Biopsy exhibits an increased deposition of acid mucopolysaccharides. Scleredema (Buschke's disease) has been noted with an M protein, but the role of the M protein is unknown.[231] Cardiomyopathy and congestive heart failure from deposition of acid mucopolysaccharide have been reported in a patient with scleredema.[232] Hyperpigmentation and hyperlipoproteinemia have also been seen in scleredema.[233]

Pyoderma gangrenosum has been associated with M proteins.[234] In a review of 67 patients, Powell et al.[235] described seven patients with a benign M protein and one patient with multiple myeloma. Seven of the eight patients had an IgA monoclonal gammopathy. Necrobiotic xanthogranuloma is frequently found with an IgG M protein.[236,237] Schnitzler syndrome is characterized by the presence of chronic urticaria and an IgM monoclonal gammopathy.[238–240] Monoclonal gammopathy has been noted in patients with diffuse plane xanthomatosis.[241,242] M proteins have been found with psoriasis, but it is doubtful that an association exists.[243,244] Subcorneal pustular dermatosis has been associated with monoclonal gammopathy.[245] An IgA M protein was found in three and IgG in one of seven patients with subcorneal pustular dermatosis.[246] A comprehensive review of monoclonal gammopathies and skin disorders has been published.[247]

More than a dozen patients have been reported with an M protein and Sézary syndrome; only two had multiple myeloma.[248] Five patients with mycosis fungoides and monoclonal gammopathy have been described.[249] Thus, cutaneous T-cell lymphomas may be associated with monoclonal gammopathies. Several cases of Kaposi's sarcoma and monoclonal gammopathy have been recognized.[250] Erythema elevatum diutinum has been reported with monoclonal gammopathy.[251,252]

Immunosuppression

M proteins were found in more than half of a series with acquired immunodeficiency syndrome (AIDS).[253] In another series of 130 homosexual men, human immunodeficiency virus (HIV) antibody was found in 65. Four patients had an M protein: two with IgG-κ and two with IgM-κ.[254] The appearance or disappearance of a monoclonal gammopathy in patients with HIV infection does not appear to be of prognostic significance.[255] Even when M proteins are identified in HIV-infected patients, the bone marrow plasma cells are atypical and present in aggregates, but they stain with both κ- and λ-light chains (polyclonal).[256]

M proteins were detected in 18 (12.7 percent) of 141 patients who had undergone renal transplantation. In seven, the gammopathy was transient.[257] In another series, 27 (12 percent) of 213 patients had a monoclonal or multiclonal gammopathy after renal transplantation. In three additional patients with persistent gammopathy, multiple myeloma (two patients) or solitary plasmacytoma (one patient) subsequently developed.[258] Pollock et al.[259] reported M proteins in 4 of 110 patients with renal transplants. A monoclonal gammopathy was found in 70 (30 percent) of 232 patients who were receiving immunosuppressive therapy after renal transplantation. The incidence was 10 times greater than that in a control group of 30 patients with chronic renal insufficiency who were on a dialysis program. In 74 percent of the 23 patients in whom a longitudinal study was available, the monoclonal gammopathy was transient. This finding suggests that immunosuppression leads to a temporary immunodeficiency state similar to that observed with aging of the immune system.[260] The presence of cytomegalovirus infection after renal transplantation in pediatric patients is associated with an increased incidence of M proteins. In a study of 80 pediatric patients who had kidney transplantation, 57 percent of patients with a cytomegalovirus infection had an M protein, whereas only 8 percent of those without a cytomegalovirus infection had an M protein.[261] In another series of 182 renal transplantations, an M protein was found in 30 percent. The authors concluded that the M protein was a reflection of the T-cell immune defect.[262] A case of transient multiple myeloma was reported after immunosuppression for renal transplantation. The patient developed a biclonal gammmopathy (IgG-κ and IgG-λ) and bone marrow containing 30 percent plasma cells. No lytic lesions were found. Immunosuppression was reduced, the M protein disappeared, and the bone marrow plasma cell content fell to less than 5 percent.[263]

Hammarström and Smith[264] found transient monoclonal gammopathies after bone marrow transplantation in 18 (43 percent) of 42 patients; the gammopathy was most often of the IgG-λ class. In another report, transient oligoclonal and mono-

clonal gammopathies were found in 31 (52 percent) of 60 patients who underwent allogeneic (57 cases) or syngeneic (3 cases) bone marrow transplantation. A monoclonal gammopathy appeared at an average of 3 months after transplantation and persisted for approximately 6 months. The development of graft-versus-host disease correlated strongly with the appearance of an M protein. Most of the Igs were IgG.[265] M proteins appeared frequently and as early as 6 weeks after bone marrow transplantation in 40 children. IgM, IgG3, and IgG1 were the most common isotypes.[266]

In a report of 550 patients receiving an autologous stem cell transplant, abnormal protein bands developed in 10 percent. Forty-eight additional patients had oligoclonal bands and 23 had an isotope switch. The authors concluded that the oligoclonal bands and isotope switching were due to recovery of immunoglobulin production rather than alteration in the biology of the malignant plasma cell clone.[267] In 12 of 47 patients, an M protein developed after allogeneic bone marrow transplantation. Eleven of the 12 patients had had a cytomegalovirus infection.[268]

In 57 (28 percent) of 201 patients, an M protein developed after liver transplantation. Five of seven in whom a post-transplantation lymphoproliferative disorder developed had an M protein, whereas only 52 of 194 (27 percent) without a post-transplantation lymphoproliferative disorder had an M protein.[269] In another series, 26 of 86 liver transplant recipients had an M protein. There was a strong correlation between the occurrence of viral infections and the presence of an M protein.[270] In a series of 88 patients receiving a liver transplant, there was no difference in the incidence of M proteins between cyclosporin A and FK506 (tacrolimus) immunosuppression.[271] Both monoclonal and oligoclonal Ig banding are common in recipients of heart transplants. The M proteins are small, transient, and of little clinical significance.[272]

Miscellaneous Conditions

Gelfand et al.[273] described a patient with angioneurotic edema and acquired deficiency of C1 esterase inhibitor and reviewed the records of 14 other patients reported in the literature, including 5 with a 7S IgM M protein. Pascual et al.[274] described two patients with acquired C1 esterase inhibitor deficiency, an IgG-κ protein, and recurrent episodes of febrile panniculitis and hepatitis. Lofdahl et al.[275] reported that eight of nine patients with systemic capillary leak syndrome had an M protein in the serum. In some instances the M protein functions as an antibody that modifies the interaction between C1 inhibitor and its target protein.[276] In a review of the literature, all 21 patients with a capillary leak syndrome had a monoclonal serum protein (IgGκ, 12; IgGλ, 7; IgAλ, 1; IgG with an unspecified light chain, 1).[277]

Although polyclonal increases in Igs are most common in liver disease, M proteins have been noted. In a retrospective study of patients with an M protein or severe hypergammaglobulinemia, Heer et al.[278] found an M protein in 11 of 272 patients with chronic active hepatitis. These investigators found a higher incidence of M proteins (26 percent) in the sera of 50 randomly selected patients who had chronic active hepatitis. M proteins have also been recognized in patients with primary biliary cirrhosis.[279]

There is an association of hepatitis C virus (HCV) and monoclonal gammopathies. The rate of HCV was 69 percent in 94 patients with mixed cryoglobulinemia and only 14 percent in 107 patients without cryoglobulinemia.[280] In another series of 102 cases of multiple myeloma, macroglobulinemia, or MGUS, HCV infection was found in 16 percent but in only 5 percent of controls.[281] An M protein was found in 11 percent of 239 HCV-positive patients but in only 1 percent of 98 HCV-negative patients. Thus, the prevalence of M proteins in patients with HCV-related chronic liver diseases is high.[282]

Also reported in association with monoclonal gammopathies were Schönlein-Henoch purpura,[283] bacterial endocarditis,[284] Hashimoto's thyroiditis,[285,286] septic arthritis,[287] purpura fulminans,[288] idiopathic pulmonary fibrosis,[289] pulmonary alveolar proteinosis,[290] idiopathic pulmonary hemosiderosis,[291] sarcoidosis,[292] thymoma,[293] hereditary spherocytosis,[294] Doyne's macular heredodystrophy,[295] eosinophilic fibrohistiocytic lesions of the bone marrow,[296] corneal crystalline deposits,[297–300] and hyperlipoproteinemia.[301] The relationship of monoclonal gammopathy to these diseases is not clear and may be fortuitous.

Active glomerular lesions consisting of epithelial crescents and a rapidly progressive glomerulonephritis have been reported with monoclonal gammopathy.[302] The association of proliferative glomerulonephritis with monoclonal gammopathy has been recognized in 25 cases,[303] but the causal relationship is unknown. One of these patients had recurrence of the crescentic glomerulonephritis and deposition of IgG-λ in a cadaveric renal transplant.[304]

We are not aware of any well-documented instances in which surgical removal of a nonhematologic tumor resulted in the disappearance of the M protein. Chen and Carroll[305] reported one case in which an IgG M protein in the serum and urine disappeared 2 years after surgical removal of a carcinoma of the colon. However, the M protein in the serum and urine was first recognized 2 months after surgery, indicating that the tumor did not produce the M protein.

M PROTEINS WITH ANTIBODY ACTIVITY

Of 612 patients in whom monoclonal Igs were studied for their antibody activity against actin, tubulin, thyroglobulin, myosin, myoglobin, fetuin, albumin, transferrin, and double-stranded DNA, 36 (5.9 percent) possessed antibody activity. In 32 of the 36 patients, the antibody activity was directed mainly against actin.[306] Most of these patients had a malignant lymphoplasmacytic disorder. Bäck et al.[307] reported the presence of an IgG3 M protein with anti-actin activity in a patient who had three episodes of thrombotic thrombocytopenic purpura and who appeared to be developing a malignant lymphoproliferative process.

In some patients with MGUS, myeloma, or macroglobulinemia, the monoclonal Ig has exhibited unusual specificities to dextran,[308] antistreptolysin O,[309] antinuclear activity,[310] smooth

muscle,[311] riboflavin,[312,313] von Willebrand factor,[314,315] thyroglobulin,[316] insulin,[317] double-stranded DNA,[318] apolipoprotein,[319] thyroxine,[320] cephalin,[321] lactate dehydrogenase,[322] anti-HIV,[323] and antibiotics.[324]

In one patient, xanthoderma-xanthotrichia (yellow discoloration of the skin and hair) was caused by an IgG-λ protein with antiriboflavin antibody activity. Xanthoderma disappeared when the IgG level decreased to less than 2 g/dl after chemotherapy.[312] Another patient with similar clinical and laboratory features has been reported.[313]

DiMinno et al.[325] described a patient with multiple myeloma and a bleeding diathesis in whom an IgG1-κ protein reacted with platelet glycoprotein IIIa. This produced a thrombasthenic-like state. An IgM-κ M protein that agglutinates platelets and produces a pseudothrombocytopenia has been reported.[326]

The binding of calcium by M protein may produce hypercalcemia without symptomatic or pathologic consequences.[327,328] This situation must be recognized so that patients are not treated for hypercalcemia.[329] Copper-binding M protein has been found in two patients with multiple myeloma.[330] Hypercupremia was noted in a patient with a benign IgG-λ M protein and carcinoma of the lung.[331] Binding of an M protein with transferrin, producing a high serum iron level, has been reported.[332,333] Hilgard et al.[334] described a patient with multiple thrombi from intravascular precipitation of an IgG-λ monoclonal cryoglobulin with transferrin and fibrinogen. Pettersson et al.[335] described a patient with an IgG-κ protein that bound phosphate, producing a spurious elevation of the serum phosphorus level. Two other similar patients—one with multiple myeloma and one with MGUS—have been described with hyperphosphatemia, presumably from binding of serum phosphorus by the M protein.[336]

Transient M proteins with antibody activity have been recognized after infection. One report described a newborn with congenital toxoplasmosis who had an IgG-λ protein. Such a protein was not found in the mother, and it did not display antibody activity.[337]

Waldenström[338] also emphasized the antibody activity of M proteins. M proteins with antibody activity in plasma cell dyscrasias have been reviewed by Merlini et al.[339]

VARIANTS OF MGUS

Biclonal Gammopathy

Biclonal gammopathies are characterized by the presence of two different M proteins; they occur in 4 percent of patients with monoclonal gammopathies. The two M proteins may be due to the proliferation of two different clones of plasma cells, each giving rise to an unrelated monoclonal Ig, or two M proteins may be produced by a single clone of plasma cells. Sakashita et al.[340] described a patient with Waldenström's macroglobulinemia who had two M proteins (IgM and IgG) with the same λ light chain. Region 3 of the two γ and μ transcripts showed 100 percent homology, whereas immunofluorescence showed that most cells stained with both IgG and IgM. This is an example of a single population of plasma cells producing two M proteins. Regulatory interactions between two monoclonal clones may occur.[341] The clinical features of biclonal gammopathies are similar to those of monoclonal gammopathies.[342]

Biclonal gammopathy of undetermined significance (BGUS) was found in 37 of 57 patients with biclonal gammopathy. Twenty were women and 17 were men; their ages ranged from 39 to 93 years (median, 67 years). The clinical findings of biclonal gammopathies are similar to those of monoclonal gammopathies.[342] Normal hemoglobin levels and leukocyte and platelet counts were found. Electrophoresis on cellulose acetate strips showed two localized bands in only 18 cases; in the remainder, a second M protein was recognized only with immunoelectrophoresis or immunofixation. A monoclonal light chain was found in the urine of 6 of 22 patients. The plasma cell levels ranged from 1 to 7 percent and did not have the features of malignancy.

In one patient with biclonal gammopathy (IgG-κ and IgA-κ), symptomatic multiple myeloma developed 2 years later with an increase in the IgG value, and the IgM level remained unchanged. The IgG-κ M protein disappeared. In another patient, the biclonal gammopathy (IgG-κ and IgM-κ) disappeared without apparent reason after 7 years.[342]

This group of 37 patients was followed for a median of 31.5 months. Seven died, one each of acute granulocytic leukemia, metastatic prostatic carcinoma, malignant melanoma, alcoholic hepatitis, subdural hematoma, congestive heart failure, and undetermined cause (this patient was 91 years of age). We found that 35 percent of the 57 patients in this series had multiple myeloma, macroglobulinemia, or other malignant lymphoproliferative processes.

Nilsson et al.[343] reported that almost one-half of their 20 patients with biclonal gammopathy had BGUS. In two of these patients, multiple myeloma subsequently developed. Riddell et al.[344] reported that 28 (2.5 percent) of 1135 patients with monoclonal gammopathy actually had biclonal gammopathy. They postulated that in some patients the M proteins arise from two separate plasma cell clones, whereas in others the M proteins behave in a concordant fashion consistent with incomplete class switching in a single plasma cell clone. Lucivero et al.[345] described a patient with IgA-κ and IgG-κ biclonal gammopathy in which the plasma cell clone simultaneously synthesized α-, γ- and κ-chains. These investigators postulated that the neoplastic plasma cell clone was "frozen" at the IgG to the IgA switch. Sensorimotor peripheral neuropathy has been associated with biclonal gammopathies.[346]

Triclonal Gammopathy

Triclonal gammopathy was reported in a patient with a plasma cell dyscrasia in whom AIDS subsequently developed[347,348] and in a patient with non-Hodgkin's lymphoma.[349] Murata et al.[350] reported a patient with triclonal gammopathy (IgG-κ, IgA-κ, and IgM-κ) and a plasmacytoid lymphoma of the ilium and gastric wall. Biopsy of the tumor revealed three different cell types that stained for IgG, IgA, and IgM, but Ig gene rearrangement studies showed a monoclonal pattern. The authors believed that the three types of malignant cells producing different classes of Igs were derived from a single clone of B cells that had undergone a "class switch." They also reported that 11

of 15 patients with triclonal gammopathy had a malignant lymphoma or lymphoproliferative disorder. In a report of a patient with a triclonal gammopathy (IgM-κ, IgG-κ, and IgA-κ), the investigators reviewed a group of cases with triclonal gammopathy from the literature. Sixteen cases were associated with a malignant immunolymphoproliferative disorder, five were present in nonhematologic disease, and three were of undetermined significance.[351]

Benign Monoclonal Light Chain (Bence Jones) Proteinuria

The possibility of a benign monoclonal gammopathy of the light chain type must be considered, although Bence Jones proteinuria is a recognized feature of multiple myeloma, primary amyloidosis, Waldenström's macroglobulinemia, and other lymphoproliferative diseases.

Two patients who maintained a stable serum concentration of M protein and who excreted 0.8 g/day or more of Bence Jones protein for longer than 17 years have been described. One of the patients had proteinuria documented 10 years before the recognition of Bence Jones proteinuria, so the duration of proteinuria was 27 years before death from pneumonia. The second patient died of hypernephroma 19 years after Bence Jones proteinuria was recognized. Neither patient developed symptomatic multiple myeloma or amyloidosis.[352]

Seven other patients have been described who presented with Bence Jones proteinuria (more than 1 g/24 hours) but who had no M protein in the serum and no evidence of multiple myeloma or related diseases.[353] Multiple myeloma developed in one patient after 20 years, and he died of a bleeding diathesis. He had no significant renal insufficiency despite having excreted more than 45 kg of λ-light chain protein. His kidneys had "proved equal to the novel office assigned them" and had "discharged the task without sustaining, on their part, the slightest danger."[354] In a second patient, symptomatic myeloma developed after 8.8 years and responded well to melphalan and prednisone therapy, but the patient subsequently died of his disease. Severe chronic renal insufficiency developed in a third patient after two episodes of acute renal failure. His renal failure was attributed to nephrosclerosis rather than to myeloma kidney or amyloidosis. A fourth patient probably had a slowly evolving multiple myeloma during a 9-year period, but he died before overt myeloma developed. Symptoms of carpal tunnel syndrome developed in a patient who had excreted 2 to 3 g/day of κ-Bence Jones protein for 14 years, and he was found to have systemic amyloidosis. A sixth patient produced 3 g/day of Bence Jones protein for 7.7 years; later an extensive squamous cell carcinoma developed involving the mediastinum and lungs. The seventh patient excreted .7 to 1.8 g/day of κ-light chain protein for 31 years without developing evidence of multiple myeloma or related disease.

Thus, although idiopathic Bence Jones proteinuria may remain stable for years, multiple myeloma or AL often develops. Consequently, these patients must be observed indefinitely.

IgD MGUS

The presence of an IgD M protein is almost always indicative of a malignant plasma cell proliferative process such as multiple myeloma, primary systemic amyloidosis, or plasma cell leukemia. However, IgD MGUS does exist. O'Connor et al.[355] reported a patient with an IgD-λ protein of 0.5 g/dl who was followed for more than 6 years without evidence of progressive disease. Hobbs and Corbett[356] described a patient with metastatic thyroid medullary carcinoma and a serum IgD-λ protein, but no evidence of myeloma. Another patient with an IgD-λ MGUS and axonal neuropathy was reported, but no follow-up information was given.[357] We have seen a patient with an IgD-λ MGUS at the Mayo Clinic who was followed more than 8 years without development of multiple myeloma or related disorders.[358]

ACKNOWLEDGMENT

This work was supported in part by Research Grant CA62242 from the National Institutes of Health.

REFERENCES

1. Waldenström J: Studies on conditions associated with disturbed gamma globulin formation (gammopathies). Harvey Lect 56:211, 1961.
2. Kyle RA, Katzmann JA, Lust JA, Dispenzieri A: Immunochemical characterization of immunoglobulins. Chapter 8, p. 71–91. In: Manual of Clinical Laboratory Immunology. N.R. Rose, R.G. Hamilton, B. Detrick (eds). 6th edition. Washington DC, ASM Press, 2002.
3. Axelsson U, Bachmann R, Hällén J: Frequency of pathological proteins (M-components) in 6995 sera from an adult population. Acta Med Scad 179:235, 1966.
4. Hällén J: Frequency of "abnormal" serum globulins (M-components) in the aged. Acta Med Scand 173:737, 1963.
5. Kyle RA, Finkelstein S, Elveback LR, Kurland LT: Incidence of monoclonal proteins in a Minnesota community with a cluster of multiple myeloma. Blood 40:719, 1972.
6. Saleun JP, Vicariot M, Deroff P, Morin JF: Monoclonal gammopathies in the adult population of Finistère, France. J Clin Pathol 35:63, 1982.
7. Vladutiu AO: Prevalence of M-proteins in serum of hospitalized patients: Physicians' response to finding M-proteins in serum protein electrophoresis. Ann Clin Lab Sci 17:157, 1987.
8. Malacrida V, de Francesco D, Banfi G et al: Laboratory investigation of monoclonal gammopathy during 10 years of screening in a general hospital. J Clin Pathol 40:793, 1987.
9. Sala P, Tonutti E, Giuliano M et al: Laboratory screening of monoclonal gammopathies: Incidence of serum monoclonal immunoglobulins during a five year survey in a general hospital. Boll Ist Steroter Milan 68:224, 1989.
10. Crawford J, Eye MK, Cohen HJ: Evaluation of monoclonal gammopathies in the "well" elderly. Am J Med 82:39, 1987.
11. Aguzzi F, Bergami MR, Gasparro C et al: Occurrence of monoclonal components in general practice: Clinical implications. Eur J Haematol 48:192, 1992.
12. Schechter GP, Shoff N, Chan C et al: The frequency of monoclonal gammopathy of undetermined significance in Black and Caucasian veterans in a hospital population. In Obrams GI, Potter M (eds.): Epidemiology and Biology of Multiple Myeloma, p. 83. Springer-Verlag, Berlin, 1991.
13. Singh J, Dudley AW Jr, Kulig KA: Increased incidence of monoclonal gammopathy of undetermined significance in blacks and its age-related differences with whites on the basis of a study of

397 men and one woman in a hospital setting. J Lab Clin Med 116:785, 1990.
14. Cohen HJ, Crawford J, Rao MK et al: Racial differences in the prevalence of monoclonal gammopathy in a community-based sample of the elderly. Am J Med 104:439, 1998.
15. Bowden M, Crawford J, Cohen HJ, Noyama O: A comparative study of monoclonal gammopathies and immunoglobulin levels in Japanese and United States elderly. J Am Geriatr Soc 41:11, 1993.
16. Hurez D, Youinou P, Gombert J, Preud'Homme JL: Survey of monoclonal gammopathy in western France: Incidence and unexpected high frequency of IgM. Immunology 56:557, 1985.
17. Pileire B, Bangou J: Frequencies of immunoglobulin classes involved in monoclonal gammopathies in Guadeloupe. Clin Chem 37:2138, 1991 (abstract).
18. Papadopoulos NM, Elin RJ, Wilson DM: Incidence of γ-globulin banding in a healthy population by high-resolution electrophoresis. Clin Chem 28:707, 1982.
19. Sinclair D, Sheehan T, Parrott DMV, Stott DI: The incidence of monoclonal gammopathy in a population over 45 years old determined by isoelectric focusing. Br J Haematol 64:745, 1986.
20. Kyle RA, Lust JA: Monoclonal gammopathies of undetermined significance. Semin Hematol 26:176, 1989.
21. van de Poel MH, Coebergh JW, Hillen HF: Malignant transformation of monoclonal gammopathy of undetermined significance among out-patients of a community hospital in southeastern Netherlands. Br J Haematol 91:121, 1995.
22. Axelsson U: A 20-year follow-up study of 64 subjects with M-components. Acta Med Scand 219:519, 1986.
23. Fine JM, Lambin P, Muller JY: The evolution of asymptomatic monoclonal gammopathies: A follow-up of 20 cases over periods of 3–14 years. Acta Med Scand 205:339, 1979.
24. Manthorn LA, Dudley RW, Case DC Jr et al: A longitudinal study of monoclonal gammopathy of undetermined significance (MGUS). Clin Res 36:414, 1988 (abstract).
25. Belisle LM, Case DC Jr, Neveux L: Quantitation of risk of malignant transformation in patients with "benign" monoclonal gammopathy. Blood. 76(Suppl. 1):342a, 1990 (abstract).
26. Paladini G, Fogher M, Mazzanti G et al: Idiopathic monoclonal gammopathy: Long-term study of 313 cases. Recenti Prog Med 80:123, 1989.
27. Giraldo MP, Rubio-Félix D, Perella M et al: Aspectos clinicos, biológicos y evolutivos de 397 casos. Sangre 36:377, 1991.
28. Bladé J, Lopez-Guillermo A, Rozman C et al: Malignant transformation and life expectancy in monoclonal gammopathy of undetermined significance. Br J Haematol 81:391, 1992.
29. Ucci G, Riccardi A, Luoni R, Ascari E: Presenting features of monoclonal gammopathies: An analysis of 684 newly diagnosed cases. J Intern Med 234:165, 1993.
30. Isaksson E, Bjorkholm M, Holm G et al: Blood clonal B-cell excess in patients with monoclonal gammopathy of undetermined significance (MGUS): Association with malignant transformation. Br J Haematol 92:71, 1996.
31. Baldini L, Guffanti A, Cesana BM et al: Role of different hematologic variables in defining the risk of malignant transformation in monoclonal gammopathy. Blood 87:912, 1996.
32. Pasqualetti P, Festuccia V, Collacciani A, Casale R: The natural history of monoclonal gammopathy of undetermined significance. A 5- to 20-year follow-up of 263 cases. Acta Haematol 97:174, 1997.
33. Carrell RW, Colls BM, Murray JT: The significance of monoclonal gammopathy in a normal population. Aust N Z J Med 1:398, 1971.
34. Colls BM: Monoclonal gammopathy of undetermined significance (MGUS)—31 year follow up of a community study. Aust N Z J Med 29:500, 1999.

35. Kyle RA: "Benign" monoclonal gammopathy—after 20 to 35 years of follow-up. Mayo Clin Proc 68:26, 1993.

36. Kyle RA, Lust JA: The monoclonal gammopathies (paraproteins). Adv Clin Chem 28:145, 1990.

37. Kyle RA, Beard CM, O'Fallon WM, Kurland LT: Incidence of multiple myeloma in Olmsted County, Minnesota: 1978 through 1990, with review of the trend since 1945. J Clin Oncol 12:1577, 1994.

38. Patriarca F, Fanin R, Silvestri F et al: Clinical features and outcome of multiple myeloma arising from the transformation of a monoclonal gammopathy of undetermined significance. Leuk Lymphoma 34:591, 1999.

39. Kyle RA, Greipp PR: Smoldering multiple myeloma. N Engl J Med 302:1347, 1980.

40. Møller-Petersen J, Schmidt EB: Diagnostic value of the concentration of M-component in initial classification of monoclonal gammopathy. Scand J Haematol 36:295, 1986.

41. Peltonen S, Wasastjerna C, Wager O: Clinical features of patients with a serum M component. Acta Med Scand 203:257, 1978.

42. Dammacco F, Waldenström J: Bence Jones proteinuria in benign monoclonal gammopathies: Incidence and characteristics. Acta Med Scand 184:403, 1968.

43. Lindström FD, Dahlström U: Multiple myeloma or benign monoclonal gammopathy? A study of differential diagnostic criteria in 44 cases. Clin Immunol Immunopathol 10:168, 1978.

44. Bernier GM, Graham RC Jr: Plasma cell asynchrony in myeloma: Correlation of light and electron microscopy. Semin Hematol 13:239, 1976.

45. Greipp PR, Kyle RA: Clinical, morphological, and cell kinetic differences among multiple myeloma, monoclonal gammopathy of undetermined significance, and smoldering multiple myeloma. Blood 62:166, 1983.

46. Peterson LC, Brown BA, Crosson JT, Mladenovic J: Application of the immunoperoxidase technic to bone marrow trephine biopsies in the classification of patients with monoclonal gammopathies. Am J Clin Pathol 85:688, 1986.

47. Bataille R, Chappard D, Klein B: Mechanisms of bone lesions in multiple myeloma. Hematol Oncol Clin North Am 6:285, 1992.

48. Gonchoroff NJ, Greipp PR, Kyle RA, Katzmann JA: A monoclonal antibody reactive with 5-bromo-2-deoxyuridine that does not require DNA denaturation. Cytometry 6:506, 1985.

49. Greipp PR, Witzig TE, Gonchoroff NJ et al: Immunofluorescence labeling indices in myeloma and related monoclonal gammopathies. Mayo Clin Proc 62:969, 1987.

50. Witzig TE, Gonchoroff NJ, Katzmann JA et al: Peripheral blood B cell labeling indices are a measure of disease activity in patients with monoclonal gammopathies. J Clin Oncol 6:1041, 1988.

51. Witzig TE, Kyle RA, Greipp PR: Circulating peripheral blood plasma cells in multiple myeloma. Curr Top Microbiol Immunol 182:195, 1992.

52. Witzig TE, Kyle RA, O'Fallon WM, Greipp PR: Detection of peripheral blood plasma cells as a predictor of disease course in patients with smouldering multiple myeloma. Br J Haematol 87:266, 1994.

53. Zandecki M, Obein V, Bernardi F et al: Monoclonal gammopathy of undetermined significance: Chromosome changes are a common finding within bone marrow plasma cells. Br J Haematol 90:693, 1995.

54. Avet-Loiseau H, Li JY, Morineau N et al: Monosomy 13 is associated with the transition of monoclonal gammopathy of undetermined significance to multiple myeloma. Intergroupe Francophone du Myelome. Blood 94:2583, 1999.

55. Avet-Loiseau H, Facon T, Daviet A et al: 14q32 translocations and monosomy 13 observed in monoclonal gammopathy of undetermined significance delineate a multistep process for the oncogenesis of multiple myeloma. Intergroupe Francophone du Myelome. Cancer Res 59:4546, 1999.

56. Avet-Loiseau H, Li JY, Facon T et al: High incidence of translocations t(11;14)(q13;q32) and t(4;14)(p16;q32) in patients with high plasma cell malignancies. Cancer Res 58:5640, 1998.

57. Fonseca R, Ahmann GJ, Jalal SM et al: Chromosomal abnormalities in systemic amyloidosis. Br J Haematol 103:704, 1998.

58. Drach J, Angerler J, Schuster J et al: Interphase fluorescence in situ hybridization identifies chromosomal abnormalities in plasma cells from patients with monoclonal gammopathy of undetermined significance. Blood 86:3915, 1995.

59. Fonseca R, Aguayo P, Ahmann GJ et al: Translocations at 14q32 are common in patients with the monoclonal gammopathy of undetermined significance (MGUS) and involve several partner chromosomes. Blood 94(Suppl. 1): 663a, 1999 (abstract).

60. Bellaiche L, Laredo JD, Liote F et al: Magnetic resonance appearance of monoclonal gammopathies of unknown significance and multiple myeloma. The GRI Study Group. Spine 22:2551, 1997.

61. Laroche M, Attal M, Dromer C: Bone remodelling in monoclonal gammopathies of uncertain significance, symptomatic and non-symptomatic myeloma. Clin Rheumatol 15:347, 1996.

62. Bataille R, Jourdan M, Zhang X-G, Klein B: Serum levels of interleukin 6, a potent myeloma cell growth factor, as a reflect of disease severity in plasma cell dyscrasia. J Clin Invest 84:2008, 1989.

63. Ocqueteau M, Orfao A, Almeida J et al: Immunophenotypic characterization of plasma cells from monoclonal gammopathy of undetermined significance patients. Implications for the differential diagnosis between MGUS and multiple myeloma. Am J Pathol 152:1655, 1998.

64. Vejlgaard T, Abildgaard N, Jans H et al: Abnormal bone turnover in monoclonal gammopathy of undetermined significance: Analyses of type I collagen telopeptide, osteocalcin, bone-specific alkaline phosphatase and propeptides of type I and type III procollagens. Eur J Haematol 58:104, 1997.

65. Mathiot C, Mary JY, Tartour E et al: Soluble CD16 (sCD16), a marker of malignancy in individuals with monoclonal gammopathy of undetermined significance (MGUS). Br J Haematol 95:660, 1996.

66. Lust JA, Donovan KA: Biology of the transition of monoclonal gammopathy of undetermined significance (MGUS) to multiple myeloma. Cancer Control 5:209, 1998.

67. Lacy MQ, Donovan KA, Heimbach JK et al: Comparison of interleukin-1 beta expression by in situ hybridization in monoclonal gammopathy of undetermined significance and multiple myeloma. Blood 93:300, 1999.

68. Vacca A, Ribatti D, Roncali L et al: Bone marrow angiogenesis and progression in multiple myeloma. Br J Haematol 87:503, 1994.

69. Rajkumar SV, Leong T, Roche PC et al: Prognostic value of bone marrow angiogenesis in multiple myeloma. Clin Cancer Res 6:3111, 2000.

70. Vacca A, Ribatti D, Presta M et al: Bone marrow neovascularization, plasma cell angiogenic potential, and matrix metalloproteinase-2 secretion parallel progression of human multiple myeloma. Blood 93:3064, 1999.

71. Garewal H, Durie BGM, Kyle RA et al: Serum beta$_2$-microglobulin in the initial staging and subsequent monitoring of monoclonal plasma cell disorders. J Clin Oncol 2:51, 1984.

72. Bast EJEG, Van Camp B, Boom SE et al: Differentiation between benign and malignant monoclonal gammopathy by the presence of the J chain. Clin Exp Immunol 44:375, 1981.

73. Tortarolo M, Cantore N, Grande M et al: Plasma cell acid phosphatase as an adjunct in the differential diagnosis of monoclonal immunoglobulinemias. Acta Haematol (Basel) 65:103, 1981.

74. Spira G, Carter A, Tatarsky I, Silvian I: Lymphocyte subpopulations in benign monoclonal gammopathy. Scand J Haematol 31:78, 1983.

75. Carmagnola AL, Boccadoro M, Massaia M, Pileri A: The idiotypic specificities of lymphocytes in human monoclonal gammopathies: Analysis with the fluorescence activated cell sorter. Clin Exp Immunol 51:173, 1983.

76. Shimizu K, Ohnishi K, Kunii A: Differentiation of benign monoclonal gammopathy and smouldering multiple myeloma from frank myeloma. Clin Exp Immunol 50:596, 1982.

77. Majumdar G, Heard SE, Singh AK: Use of cytoplasmic 5′nucleotidase for differentiating malignant from benign monoclonal gammopathies. J Clin Pathol 43:891, 1990.

78. Majumdar G, Hunt M, Singh AK: Use of leucocyte alkaline phosphatase (LAP) score in differentiating malignant from benign paraproteinaemias. J Clin Pathol 44:606, 1991.

79. Bäck H, Jagenburg R, Rödjer S, Westin J: Serum deoxythymidine kinase: No help in the diagnosis and prognosis of monoclonal gammopathy. Br J Haematol 84:746, 1993.

80. Pelliniemi T-T, Iriala K, Mattila K et al: Serum immunoreactive interleukin-6 (IL6) and acute phase proteins as prognostic factors in multiple myeloma. Blood 82(Suppl. 1):262a, 1993 (abstract).

81. Ballester OF, Moscinski LC, Lyman GH et al: High levels of interleukin-6 are associated with low tumor burden and low growth fraction in multiple myeloma. Blood 83:1903, 1994.

82. Sonneveld P, Durie BG, Lokhorst HM et al: Analysis of multidrug-resistance (MDR-1) glycoprotein and CD56 expression to separate monoclonal gammopathy from multiple myeloma. Br J Haematol 83:63, 1993.

83. Dexter RM, Mullinax F, Estep HL, Williams RC Jr: Monoclonal IgG gammopathy and hyperparathyroidism. Ann Intern Med 77:759, 1972.

84. Schnur MJ, Appel GB, Bilezikian JP: Primary hyperparathyroidism and benign monoclonal gammopathy. Arch Intern Med 137:1201, 1977.

85. Mundis RJ, Kyle RA: Primary hyperparathyroidism and monoclonal gammopathy of undetermined significance. Am J Clin Pathol 77:619, 1982.

86. Rao DS, Antonelli R, Kane KR et al: Primary hyperparathyroidism and monoclonal gammopathy. Henry Ford Hosp Med J 39:41, 1991.

87. Migliore PJ, Alexanian R: Monoclonal gammopathy in human neoplasia. Cancer 21:1127, 1968.

88. Talerman A, Haije WG: The frequency of M-components in sera of patients with solid malignant neoplasms. Br J Cancer 27:276, 1973.

89. Azar HA, Hill WT, Osserman EF: Malignant lymphoma and lymphatic leukemia associated with myeloma-type serum proteins. Am J Med 23:239, 1957.

90. Kyle RA, Bayrd ED, McKenzie BF, Heck FJ: Diagnostic criteria for electrophoretic patterns of serum and urinary proteins in multiple myeloma: Study of one hundred and sixty-five multiple myeloma patients and of seventy-seven nonmyeloma patients with similar electrophoretic patterns. JAMA 174:245, 1960.

91. Krauss S, Sokal JE: Paraproteinemia in the lymphomas. Am J Med 40:400, 1966.

92. Hällén J: M-components in leukaemia, in lymphosarcoma and in reticulum cell sarcoma. Acta Med Scand 462(Suppl.):71, 1966.

93. Kim H, Heller P, Rappaport H: Monoclonal gammopathies associated with lymphoproliferative disorders: A morphologic study. Am J Clin Pathol 59:282, 1973.

94. Moore DF, Migliore PJ, Shullenberger CC, Alexanian R: Monoclonal macroglobulinemia in malignant lymphoma. Ann Intern Med 72:43, 1970.

95. Alexanian R: Monoclonal gammopathy in lymphoma. Arch Intern Med 135:62, 1975.

96. Hobbs JR, Carter PM, Cooke KB et al: IgM paraproteins. J Clin Pathol. 28(Suppl. 6):54, 1974.

97. Bain GO, Belch A: Nodular mixed cell lymphoma with monoclonal gammopathy. Am J Clin Pathol 76:832, 1981.

98. Pangalis GA, Nathwani BN, Rappaport H: Malignant lymphoma, well differentiated lymphocytic: Its relationship with chronic lymphocytic leukemia and macroglobulinemia of Waldenström. Cancer 39:999, 1977.

99. Ko HS, Pruzanski W: M components associated with lymphoma: A review of 62 cases. Am J Med Sci 272:175, 1976.

100. Ng J-P, Jones EL, Pati A et al: Hodgkin's disease and paraproteinaemia: A case report and review of the literature. Clin Lab Haematol 14:257, 1992.

101. Magrath I, Benjamin D, Papadopoulos N: Serum monoclonal immunoglobulin bands in undifferentiated lymphomas of Burkitt's and non-Burkitt's types. Blood 61:726, 1983.

102. Kyle RA, Garton JP: The spectrum of IgM monoclonal gammopathy in 430 cases. Mayo Clin Proc 62:719, 1987.

103. Schauer PK, Straus DJ, Bagley CM Jr et al: Angioimmunoblastic lymphadenopathy: Clinical spectrum of disease. Cancer 48:2493, 1981.

104. Offit K, Macris NT, Finkbeiner JA: Monoclonal hypergammaglobulinemia without malignant transformation in angioimmunoblastic lymphadenopathy with dysproteinemia. Am J Med 80:292, 1986.

105. Steinberg AD (moderator), Seldin MF, Jaffe ES et al: Angioimmunoblastic lymphadenopathy with dysproteinemia. Ann Intern Med 108:575, 1988.

106. Hineman VL, Phyliky RL, Banks PM: Angiofollicular lymph node hyperplasia and peripheral neuropathy: Association with monoclonal gammopathy. Mayo Clin Proc 57:379, 1982.

107. Sugai S, Konda S, Shirasaki Y et al: Non-IgM monoclonal gammopathy in patients with Sjögren's syndrome. Am J Med 68:861, 1980.

108. Humphrey DM, Cortes EA, Spiva DA: Immunohistologic studies of cytoplasmic immunoglobulins in rheumatic diseases including two patients with monoclonal patterns and subsequent lymphoma. Cancer 49:2049, 1982.

109. Ben-Chetrit E, Ben-Amital D, Levo Y: The association between Kaposi's sarcoma and dysgammaglobulinemia. Cancer 49:1649, 1982.

110. Kyle RA, Bayrd ED: The Monoclonal Gammopathies: Multiple Myeloma and Related Plasma-Cell Disorders. Charles C Thomas, Springfield, IL, 1976.

111. Noel P, Kyle RA: Monoclonal proteins in chronic lymphocytic leukemia. Am J Clin Pathol 87:385, 1987.

112. Sinclair D, Dagg JH, Dewar AE et al: The incidence, clonal origin and secretory nature of serum paraproteins in chronic lymphocytic leukaemia. Br J Haematol 64:725, 1986.

113. Jansen J, Bolhuis RLH, van Nieuwkoop JA et al: Paraproteinaemia plus osteolytic lesions in typical hairy-cell leukaemia. Br J Haematol 54:531, 1983.

114. Matsuzaki H, Yamaguchi K, Kagimoto T et al: Monoclonal gammopathies in adult T-cell leukemia. Cancer 56:1380, 1985.

115. Guglielmi P, Davi F, Brouet JC: Prevalence of monoclonal Ig with λ light chains in chronic myelocytic leukaemia. Br J Haematol 73:331, 1989.

116. Buonanno G, Pandolfi F, Valente A et al: Monocytic blast cell crisis and IgG-λ monoclonal gammopathy in a Ph[1]+ chronic myelogenous leukemia: Report of a case. Haematologica (Pavia) 71:489, 1986.

117. Raz I, Polliack A: Coexistence of myelomonocytic leukemia and monoclonal gammopathy or myeloma: Simultaneous presentation in three patients. Cancer 53:83, 1984.

118. Atkins H, Drouin J, Izaguirre CA, Sengar DS: Acute promyelocytic leukemia associated with a paraprotein that reacts with leukemic cells. Cancer 63:1750, 1989.

119. Van Camp B, Reynaerts P, Naets JP, Radl J: Transient IgA$_1$-λ paraproteinemia during treatment of acute myelomonoblastic leukemia. Blood 55:21, 1980.

120. Mant MJ, Hirsh J, Gauldie J et al: Von Willebrand's syndrome presenting as an acquired bleeding disorder in association with a monoclonal gammopathy. Blood 42:429, 1973.

121. Stewart AK, Glynn MFX: Acquired von Willebrand disease associated with free lambda light chain monoclonal gammopathy, normal bleeding time and response to prednisone. Postgrad Med J 66:560, 1990.

122. Scrobohaci M-L, Daniel M-T, Levy Y et al: Expression of GpIb on plasma cells in a patient with monoclonal IgG and acquired von Willebrand disease. Br J Haematol 84:471, 1993.

123. Keren DF: Coagulation disorders in patients with monoclonal gammopathies. Hematol Oncol Clin North Am 7:1153, 1993.

124. Castaman G, Rodeghiero F, Di Bona E, Ruggeri M: Clinical effectiveness of desmopressin in a case of acquired von Willebrand's syndrome associated with benign monoclonal gammopathy. Blut 58:211, 1989.

125. Bellotti V, Gamba G, Merlini G et al: Study of three patients with monoclonal gammopathies and 'lupus-like' anticoagulants. Br J Haematol 73:221, 1989.

126. Stern JJ, Ng RH, Triplett DA, McIntyre JA: Incidence of antiphospholipid antibodies in patients with monoclonal gammopathy of undetermined significance. Am J Clin Pathol 101:471, 1994.

127. Selroos O, von Knorring J: Immunoglobulins in pernicious anaemia: Including a report on a patient with pernicious anaemia, IgA deficiency and an M component of kappa-type IgG. Acta Med Scand 194:571, 1973.

128. Sandström H, Wahlin A, Eriksson M et al: Intravascular haemolysis and increased prevalence of myeloma and monoclonal gammopathy in congenital dyserythropoietic anaemia, type III. Eur J Haematol 52:42, 1994.

129. Resegotti L, Dolci C, Palestro G, Peschle C: Paraproteinemic variety of pure red cell aplasia: Immunological studies in 1 patient. Acta Haematol (Basel) 60:227, 1978.

130. Balducci L, Hardy C, Dreiling B et al: Pure red blood cell aplasia associated with paraproteinemia: In vitro studies of erythropoiesis. Haematologia (Budap) 17:353, 1984.

131. Berner Y, Berrebi A: Myeloproliferative disorders and non-myelomatous paraprotein: A study of five patients and review of the literature. Isr J Med Sci 22:109, 1986.

132. Dührsen U, Uppenkamp M, Meusers P et al: Frequent association of idiopathic myelofibrosis with plasma cell dyscrasias. Blut 56:97, 1988.

133. Economopoulos T, Economidou J, Giannopoulos G et al: Immune abnormalities in myelodysplastic syndromes. J Clin Pathol 38:908, 1985.

134. Pratt PW, Estren S, Kochwa S: Immunoglobulin abnormalities in Gaucher's disease: Report of 16 cases. Blood 31:633, 1968.

135. Marti GE, Ryan ET, Papadopoulos NM et al: Polyclonal B-cell lymphocytosis and hypergammaglobulinemia in patients with Gaucher disease. Am J Hematol 29:189, 1988.

136. Airò R, Gabusi G, Guindani M: Gaucher's disease associated with monoclonal gammopathy of undetermined significance: A case report. Haematologica 78:129, 1993.

137. Zawadzki ZA, Benedek TG: Rheumatoid arthritis, dysproteinemic arthropathy, and paraproteinemia. Arthritis Rheum 12:555, 1969.

138. Hurst NP, Smith W, Henderson DR: IgG (kappa) paraproteinaemia and arthritis. Br J Rheumatol 26:142, 1987.

139. Michaux JL, Heremans JF: Thirty cases of monoclonal immunoglobulin disorders other than myeloma or macroglobulinemia: A classification of diseases associated with the production of monoclonal-type immunoglobulins. Am J Med 46:562, 1969.

140. Porcel JM, Ordi J, Tolosa C et al: Monoclonal gammopathy in systemic lupus erythematosus. Lupus 1:263, 1992.

141. Renier G, Renier JC, Gardembas-Pain M et al: Ankylosing spondylitis and monoclonal gammopathies. Ann Rheum Dis 51:951, 1992.

142. Ilfeld D, Barzilay J, Vana D et al: IgG monoclonal gammopathy in four patients with polymyalgia rheumatica (letter). Ann Rheum Dis 44:501, 1985.

143. Kalra L, Delamere JP: Lymphoreticular malignancy and monoclonal gammopathy presenting as polymyalgia rheumatica. Br J Rheumatol 26:458, 1987.

144. Kiprov DD, Miller RG: Polymyositis associated with monoclonal gammopathy. Lancet 2:1183, 1984.

145. Telerman-Toppet N, Wittek M, Bacq M et al: Benign monoclonal gammopathy and relapsing polymyositis (letter to the editor). Muscle Nerve 5:490, 1982.

146. Dalakas MC, Illa I, Gallardo E, Juarez C: Inclusion body myositis and paraproteinemia: Incidence and immunopathologic correlations. Ann Neurol 41:100, 1997.

147. Nakayama T, Horiuchi E, Watanabe T et al: A case of inclusion body myositis with benign monoclonal gammopathy successfully responding to repeated immunoabsorption. J Neurol Neurosurg Psychiatry 68:230, 2000.

148. Powell FC, Greipp PR, Su WPD: Discoid lupus erythematosus and monoclonal gammopathy. Br J Dermatol 109:355, 1983.

149. Freestone S, Ramsay LE: Transient monoclonal gammopathy in hydralazine-induced lupus erythematosus. BMJ 285:1536, 1982.

150. Nakanishi H, Takehara K, Soma Y, Ishibashi Y: Atypical scleroderma associated with multiple myeloma. Dermatologica 178:176, 1989.

151. Scherf I, Nahir M, Brick R et al: Monoclonal IgG immunoglobulinemia in psoriatic arthritis. Dermatologica 160:348, 1980.

152. Kelly JJ Jr, Kyle RA, O'Brien PC, Dyck PJ: Prevalence of monoclonal protein in peripheral neuropathy. Neurology 31:1480, 1981.

153. Kahn SN, Riches PG, Kohn J: Paraproteinaemia in neurological disease: Incidence, associations, and classification of monoclonal immunoglobulins. J Clin Pathol 33:617, 1980.

154. Johansen P, Leegaard OF: Peripheral neuropathy and paraproteinemia: An immunohistochemical and serologic study. Clin Neuropathol 4:99, 1985.

155. Vrethem M, Cruz M, Wen-Xin H et al: Clinical, neurophysiological and immunological evidence of polyneuropathy in patients with monoclonal gammopathies. J Neurol Sci 114:193, 1993.

156. Nobile-Orazio E, Barbieri S, Baldini L et al: Peripheral neuropathy in monoclonal gammopathy of undetermined significance: Prevalence and immunopathogenetic studies. Acta Neurol Scand 85:383, 1992.

157. Baldini L, Nobile-Orazio E, Guffanti A et al: Peripheral neuropathy in IgM monoclonal gammopathy and Waldenström's macroglobulinemia: A frequent complication in elderly males with low MAG-reactive serum monoclonal component. Am J Hematol 45:25, 1994.

158. Nobile-Orazio E, Francomano E, Daverio R et al: Anti-myelin-associated glycoprotein IgM antibody titers in neuropathy associated with macroglobulinemia. Ann Neurol 26:543, 1989.

159. Isobe T, Osserman EF: Pathologic conditions associated with plasma cell dyscrasias: A study of 806 cases. Ann NY Acad Sci 190:507, 1971.

160. Kelly JJ Jr, Kyle RA, Latov N: Polyneuropathies Associated With Plasma Cell Dyscrasias. Martinus Nijhoff, Boston, 1987.

161. Latov N: Pathogenesis and therapy of neuropathies associated with monoclonal gammopathies. Ann Neurol 37(Suppl. 1): S32, 1995.

162. Kissel JT, Mendell JR: Neuropathies associated with monoclonal gammopathies. Neuromuscul Disord 6:3, 1996.

163. Ropper AH, Gorson KC: Neuropathies associated with paraproteinemia. N Engl J Med 338:1601, 1998.

164. Latov N, Hays AP, Sherman WH: Peripheral neuropathy and anti-MAG antibodies. Crit Rev Neurobiol 3:301, 1988.

165. Hafler DA, Johnson D, Kelly JJ et al: Monoclonal gammopathy and neuropathy: Myelin-associated glycoprotein reactivity and clinical characteristics. Neurology 36:75, 1986.

166. Dellagi K, Dupouey P, Brouet JC et al: Waldenström's macroglobulinemia and peripheral neuropathy: A clinical immunologic study of 25 patients. Blood 62:280, 1983.

167. Bollensen E, Steck AJ, Schachner M: Reactivity with the peripheral myelin glycoprotein P_0 in serum from patients with, monoclonal IgM gammopathy and polyneuropathy. Neurology 38:1266, 1988.

168. Mata M, Kahn SN, Fink DJ: A direct electron microscopic immunocytochemical study of IgM paraproteinemic neuropathy. Arch Neurol 45:693, 1988.

169. Lach B, Rippstein P, Atack D et al: Immunoelectron microscopic localization of monoclonal IgM antibodies in gammopathy associated with peripheral demyelinative neuropathy. Acta Neuropathol 85:298, 1993.

170. Kelly JJ, Adelman LS, Berkman E, Bhan I: Polyneuropathies associated with IgM monoclonal gammopathies. Arch Neurol 45:1355, 1988.

171. Donofrio PD, Kelly JJ Jr: AAEE case report #17: Peripheral neuropathy in monoclonal gammopathy of undetermined significance. Muscle Nerve 12:1, 1989.

172. Smith IS, Kahn SN, Lacey BW et al: Chronic demyelinating neuropathy associated with benign IgM paraproteinaemia. Brain 106:169, 1983.

173. Kelly JJ Jr: The electrodiagnostic findings in peripheral neuropathy associated with monoclonal gammopathy. Muscle Nerve 6:504, 1983.

174. Sherman WH, Latov N, Hays AP et al: Monoclonal IgM_K antibody precipitating with chondroitin sulfate C from patients with axonal polyneuropathy and epidermolysis. Neurology 33:192, 1983.

175. Freddo L, Sherman WH, Latov N: Glycosaminoglycan antigens in peripheral nerve: Studies with antibodies from a patient with neuropathy and monoclonal gammopathy. J Neuroimmunol 12:57, 1986.

176. Yee WC, Hahn AF, Hearn SA, Rupar AR: Neuropathy in IgM_λ paraproteinemia: Immunoreactivity to neural proteins and chondroitin sulfate. Acta Neuropathol (Berl) 78:57, 1989.

177. Ilyas AA, Li S-C, Chou DKH et al: Gangliosides G_{M2},IV^4Gal-$NAcG_{M1b}$, and $IV^4GalNAcG_{D1a}$ as antigens for monoclonal immunoglobulin M in neuropathy associated with gammopathy. J Biol Chem 263:4369, 1988.

178. Kusunoki S, Shimizu T, Matsumura K et al: Motor dominant neuropathy and IgM paraproteinemia: The IgM M-protein binds to specific gangliosides. J Neuroimmunol 21:177, 1989.

179. Ilyas AA, Quarles RH, Dalakas MC, Brady RO: Polyneuropathy with monoclonal gammopathy: Glycolipids are frequently antigens for IgM paraproteins. Proc Natl Acad Sci USA 82:6697, 1985.

180. Kusunoki S, Kohriyama T, Pachner AR et al: Neuropathy and IgM paraproteinemia: Differential binding of IgM M-proteins to peripheral nerve glycolipids. Neurology 37:1795, 1987.

181. Fredman P: The role of antiglycolipid antibodies in neurological disorders. Ann N Y Acad Sci 845:341, 1998.

182. Brouet JC, Danon F, Mihaesco E et al: Peripheral polyneuropathies associated with monoclonal IgM. Antibody activity of monoclonal IgM and therapeutic implications. Nouv Rev Fr Hematol 32:307, 1990.

183. Quarles RH, Weiss MD: Autoantibodies associated with peripheral neuropathy. Muscle Nerve 22:800, 1999.

184. Gosselin S, Kyle RA, Dyck PJ: Neuropathy associated with monoclonal gammopathies of undetermined significance. Ann Neurol 30:54, 1991.

185. Suarez GA, Kelly JJ Jr: Polyneuropathy associated with monoclonal gammopathy of undetermined significance: Further evidence that IgM-MGUS neuropathies are different than IgG-MGUS. Neurology 43:1304, 1993.

186. Chassande B, Leger JM, Younes-Chennoufi AB et al: Peripheral neuropathy associated with IgM monoclonal gammopathy: Correlations between M-protein antibody activity and clinical/electrophysiological features in 40 cases. Muscle Nerve 21:55, 1998.

187. Meucci N, Baldini L, Cappellari A et al: Anti-myelin-associated glycoprotein antibodies predict the development of neuropathy in asymptomatic patients with IgM monoclonal gammopathy. Ann Neurol 46:119, 1999.

188. Simovic D, Gorson KC, Ropper AH: Comparison of IgM-MGUS and IgG-MGUS polyneuropathy. Acta Neurol Scand 97:194, 1998.

189. Read DJ, Vanhegan RI, Matthews WB: Peripheral neuropathy and benign IgG paraproteinaemia. J Neurol Neurosurg Psychiatry 41:215, 1978.

190. Bleasel AF, Hawke SHB, Pollard JD, McLeod JG: IgG monoclonal paraproteinaemia and peripheral neuropathy. J Neurol Neurosurg Psychiatry 56:52, 1993.

191. Dhib-Jalbut S, Liwnicz BH: Binding of serum IgA of multiple myeloma to normal peripheral nerve. Acta Neurol Scand 73:381, 1986.

192. Bailey RO, Ritaccio AL, Bishop MB, Wu AY: Benign monoclonal IgA_K gammopathy associated with polyneuropathy and dysautonomia. Acta Neurol Scand 73:574, 1986.

193. Simmons Z, Bromberg MB, Feldman EL, Blaivas M: Polyneuropathy associated with IgA monoclonal gammopathy of undetermined significance. Muscle Nerve 16:77, 1993.

194. Simmons Z, Albers JW, Bromberg MB, Feldman EL: Presentation and initial clinical course in patients with chronic inflammatory demyelinating polyradiculoneuropathy: Comparison of patients without and with monoclonal gammopathy. Neurology 43:2202, 1993.

195. Gorson KC, Allam G, Ropper AH: Chronic inflammatory demyelinating polyneuropathy: Clinical features and response to treatment in 67 consecutive patients with and without a monoclonal gammopathy. Neurology 48:321, 1997.

196. Simmons Z, Albers JW, Bromberg MB, Feldman EL: Long-term follow-up of patients with chronic inflammatory demyelinating polyradiculoneuropathy, without and with monoclonal gammopathy. Brain 118:359, 1995.

197. Maisonobe T, Chassande B, Verin M et al: Chronic dysimmune demyelinating polyneuropathy: A clinical and electrophysiological study of 93 patients. J Neurol Neurosurg Psychiatry 61:36, 1996.

198. Nemni R, Fazio R, Corbo M et al: Peripheral neuropathy associated with experimental plasma cell neoplasm in the mouse. J Neurol Sci 77:321, 1987.

199. Hays AP, Latov N, Takatsu M, Sherman WH: Experimental demyelination of nerve induced by serum of patients with neuropathy and an anti-MAG IgM M-protein. Neurology 37:242, 1987.

200. Steck AJ, Murray N, Dellagi K et al: Peripheral neuropathy associated with monoclonal IgM antibody. Ann Neurol 22:764, 1987.

201. Tatum AH: Experimental paraprotein neuropathy, demyelination by passive transfer of human IgM anti-myelin-associated glycoprotein. Ann Neurol 33:502, 1993.

202. Jønsson V, Schrøder HD, Jensen TS et al: Autoimmunity related to IgM monoclonal gammopathy of undetermined significance: Peripheral neuropathy and connective tissue sensibilization caused by IgM M-proteins. Acta Med Scand 223:255, 1988.

203. Smith T, Sherman W, Olarte MR, Lovelace RE: Peripheral neuropathy associated with plasma cell dyscrasia: A clinical and electrophysiological follow-up study. Acta Neurol Scand 75:244, 1987.

204. Frayne J, Stark RJ: Peripheral neuropathy with gammopathy responding to plasmapheresis. Clin Exp Neurol 21:195, 1985.

205. Haas DC, Tatum AH: Plasmapheresis alleviates neuropathy accompanying IgM anti-myelin-associated glycoprotein paraproteinemia. Ann Neurol 23:394, 1988.

206. Dyck PJ, Low PA, Windebank AJ et al: Plasma exchange in polyneuropathy associated with monoclonal gammopathy of undetermined significance. N Engl J Med 325:1482, 1991.

207. Mazzi G, Raineri A, Zucco M et al: Plasma-exchange in chronic peripheral neurological disorders. Int J Artif Organs 22:40, 1999.

208. Oksenhendler E, Chevret S, Leger JM et al: Plasma exchange and chlorambucil in polyneuropathy associated with monoclonal IgM gammopathy. IgM-associated Polyneuropathy Study Group. J Neurol Neurosurg Psychiatry 59:243, 1995.

209. Notermans NC, Lokhorst HM, Franssen H et al: Intermittent cyclophosphamide and prednisone treatment of polyneuropathy associated with monoclonal gammopathy of undetermined significance. Neurology 47:1227, 1996.

210. Sherman WH, Latov N, Lange D et al: Fludarabine for IgM antibody-mediated neuropathies. Ann Neurol 36:326, 1994 (abstract).

211. Wilson HC, Lunn MP, Schey S, Hughes RA: Successful treatment of IgM paraproteinaemic neuropathy with fludarabine. J Neurol Neurosurg Psychiatry 66:575, 1999.

212. Levine TD, Pestronk A: IgM antibody-related polyneuropathies: B-cell depletion chemotherapy using Rituximab. Neurology 52:1701, 1999.

213. Faed JM, Day B, Pollock M et al: High-dose intravenous human immunoglobulin in chronic inflammatory demyelinating polyneuropathy. Neurology 39:422, 1989.

214. Dalakas MC, Quarles RH, Farrer RG et al: A controlled study of intravenous immunoglobulin in demyelinating neuropathy with IgM gammopathy. Ann Neurol 40:792, 1996.

215. Younger DS, Rowland LP, Latov N et al: Motor neuron disease and amyotrophic lateral sclerosis: Relation of high CSF protein content to paraproteinemia and clinical syndromes. Neurology 40:595, 1990.

216. Patten BM: Neuropathy and motor neuron syndromes associated with plasma cell disease. Acta Neurol Scand 70:47, 1984.

217. Merlini G, Rutigliano L, Masnaghetti S et al: Neuromuscular disorders associated with monoclonal immunoglobulins (abstract). p. 215. In International Conference on Multiple Myeloma. Biology, Pathophysiology, Prognosis and Treatment. Bologna, Italy, June 19–22, 1989.

218. Bartoloni C, Scoppetta C, Flamini G et al: Waldenström's macroglobulinemia and myasthenia gravis. J Clin Lab Immunol 6:275, 1981.

219. Galli M, Landi G, Restelli DL, Scarlato G: Myasthenia gravis with monoclonal gammopathy: Report of a case. J Neurol Sci 45:103, 1980.

220. Berni I, Costantini A, Di Vano M: Monoclonal gammopathies in Alzheimer's disease (letter to the editor). Clin Chem 39:166, 1993.

221. McDonald PS, Cora-Bramble D, De Palma L: Monoclonal gammopathy of the immunoglobulin A class in a two-year-old girl with ataxia telangiectasia. Pediatr Dev Pathol 1:319, 1998.

222. Sadighi Akha AA, Humphrey RL, Winkelstein JA et al: Oligo/monoclonal gammopathy and hypergammaglobulinemia in ataxia-telangiectasia. A study of 90 patients. Medicine (Baltimore) 78:370, 1999.

223. Kyle RA, Dyck PJ: Osteosclerotic myeloma (POEMS syndrome). In Dyck PJ, Thomas PK, Griffin JW et al (eds.): Peripheral Neuropathy, Vol 2, 3rd Ed., p. 1288. WB Saunders, Philadelphia, 1993.

224. Takatsuki K, Sanada I: Plasma cell dyscrasia with polyneuropathy and endocrine disorder: Clinical and laboratory features of 109 reported cases. Jpn J Clin Oncol 13:543, 1983.

225. Kelly JJ Jr, Kyle RA, Miles JM, Dyck PJ: Osteosclerotic myeloma and peripheral neuropathy. Neurology 33:202, 1983.

226. Bardwick PA, Zvaifler NJ, Gill GN et al: Plasma cell dyscrasia with polyneuropathy, organomegaly, endocrinopathy, M protein, and skin changes: The POEMS syndrome; report on two cases and a review of the literature. Medicine (Baltimore) 59:311, 1980.

227. Gherardi RK, Belec L, Soubrier M et al: Overproduction of proinflammatory cytokines imbalanced by their antagonists in POEMS syndrome. Blood 87:1458, 1996.

228. Watanabe O, Maruyama I, Arimura K et al: Overproduction of vascular endothelial growth factor/vascular permeability factor is causative in Crow-Fukase (POEMS) syndrome. Muscle Nerve 21:1390, 1998.

229. Kuwabara S, Hattori T, Shimoe Y, Kamitsukasa I: Long term melphalan-prednisolone chemotherapy for POEMS syndrome. J Neurol Neurosurg Psychiatry 63:385, 1997.

230. James K, Fudenberg H, Epstein WL, Shuster J: Studies on a unique diagnostic serum globulin in papular mucinosis (lichen myxedematosus). Clin Exp Immunol 2:153, 1967.

231. Ohta A, Uitto J, Oikarinen AI et al: Paraproteinemia in patients with scleredema: Clinical findings and serum effects on skin fibroblasts in vitro. J Am Acad Dermatol 16:96, 1987.

232. Rimon D, Lurie M, Storch S et al: Cardiomyopathy and multiple myeloma: Complications of scleredema adultorum. Arch Intern Med 148:551, 1988.

233. McFadden N, Ree K, Søyland E, Larsen TE: Scleredema adultorum associated with a monoclonal gammopathy and generalized hyperpigmentation. Arch Dermatol 123:629, 1987.

234. Duguid CM, Powell FC: Pyoderma gangrenosum. Clin Dermatol 11:129, 1993.

235. Powell FC, Schroeter AL, Su WPD, Perry HO: Pyoderma gangrenosum and monoclonal gammopathy. Arch Dermatol 119:468, 1983.

236. Mehregan DA, Winkelmann RK: Necrobiotic xanthogranuloma. Arch Dermatol 128:94, 1992.

237. Nestle FO, Hofbauer G, Burg G: Necrobiotic xanthogranuloma with monoclonal gammopathy of the IgG lambda type. Dermatology 198:434, 1999.

238. Doutre M-S., Beylot C, Bioulac P, Bezian J-H: Monoclonal IgM and chronic urticaria: Two cases. Ann Allergy 58:413, 1987.

239. Lebbe C, Rybojad M, Klein F et al: Schnitzler's syndrome associated with sensorimotor neuropathy. J Am Acad Dermatol 30:316, 1994.

240. Puddu P, Cianchini G, Girardelli CR et al: Schnitzler's syndrome: Report of a new case and a review of the literature. Clin Exp Rheumatol 15:91, 1997.

241. Bérard M, Antonucci M, Beaumont J-L: Cytotoxic effect of serum on fibroblasts in one case of normolipidemic plane xanthoma and myeloma IgG λ. Atherosclerosis 62:111, 1986.

242. Jones RR, Baughan ASJ, Cream JJ et al: Complement abnormalities in diffuse plane xanthomatosis with paraproteinaemia. Br J Dermatol 101:711, 1979.

243. Humbert P, Blanc D, Laurent R, Agache P: Monoclonal IgG gammopathy in a case of pustular psoriasis: A ten year follow-up (letter to the editor). Blut 54:61, 1987.

244. Peltonen L, Nikoskelainen E, Kätkä K, Tyrkkö J: Monoclonal IgG immunoglobulinemia with subsequent myeloma in psoriatic arthritis. Dermatologica 169:207, 1984.

245. Ryatt KS, Dodman BA, Cotterill JA: Subcorneal pustular dermatosis and IgA gammopathy. Acta Derm Venereol (Stockh) 61:560, 1981.

246. Lutz ME, Daoud MS, McEvoy MT, Gibson LE: Subcorneal pustular dermatosis: A clinical study of ten patients. Cutis 61:203, 1998.

247. Daoud MS, Lust JA, Kyle RA, Pittelkow MR: Monoclonal gammopathies and associated skin disorders. J Am Acad Dermatol 40:507, 1999.

248. Venencie PY, Winkelmann RK, Puissant A, Kyle RA: Monoclonal gammopathy in Sézary syndrome: Report of three cases and review of the literature. Arch Dermatol 120:605, 1984.

249. Venencie PY, Winkelmann RK, Friedman SJ et al: Monoclonal gammopathy and mycosis fungoides: Report of four cases and review of the literature. J Am Acad Dermatol 11:576, 1984.

250. Strumia R, Roveggio C: Kaposi's sarcoma and monoclonal gammopathy. Dermatology 188:76, 1994.

251. Dowd PM, Munro DD: Erythema elevatum diutinum. J R Soc Med 76:310, 1983.

252. Kavanagh GM, Colaco CB, Bradfield JW, Archer CB: Erythema elevatum diutinum associated with Wegener's granulomatosis and IgA paraproteinemia. J Am Acad Dermatol 28:846, 1993.

253. Heriot K, Hallquist AE, Tomar RH: paraproteinemia in patients with acquired immunodeficiency syndrome (AIDS) or lymphadenopathy syndrome (LAS). Clin Chem 31:1224, 1985.

254. Crapper RM, Deam DR, Mackay IR: Paraproteinemias in homosexual men with HIV infection: Lack of association with abnormal clinical or immunologic findings. Am J Clin Pathol 88:348, 1987.

255. Lefrère J-J, Debbia M, Lambin P: Prospective follow-up on monoclonal gammopathies in HIV-infected individuals. Br J Haematol 84:151, 1993.

256. Turbat-Herrera EA, Hancock C, Cabello-Inchausti B, Herrera GA: Plasma cell hyperplasia and monoclonal paraproteinemia in human immunodeficiency virus-infected patients. Arch Pathol Lab Med 117:497, 1993.

257. Renoult E, Bertrand F, Kessler M: Monoclonal gammopathies in HBsAg-positive patients with renal transplants (letter to the editor). N Engl J Med 318:1205, 1988.

258. Stanko CK, Jeffery JR, Rush DN: Monoclonal and multiclonal gammopathies after renal transplantation. Transplant Proc 21:3330, 1989.

259. Pollock CA, Mahony JF, Ibels LS et al: Immunoglobulin abnormalities in renal transplant recipients. Transplantation 47:952, 1989.

260. Radl J, Valentijn RM, Haaijman JJ, Paul LC: Monoclonal gammopathies in patients undergoing immunosuppressive treatment after renal transplantation. Clin Immunol Immunopathol 37:98, 1985.

261. Ginevri F, Nocera A, Bonato L et al: Cytomegalovirus infection is a trigger for monoclonal immunoglobulins in paediatric kidney transplant recipients. Transplant Proc 30:2079, 1998.

262. Ducloux D, Carron P, Racadot E et al: T-cell immune defect and B-cell activation in renal transplant recipients with monoclonal gammopathies. Transplant Int 12:250, 1999.

263. Passweg J, Bock HA, Tichelli A, Thiel G: 'Transient multiple myeloma' after intense immunosuppression in a renal transplant patient. Nephrol Dial Transplant 8:1393, 1993.

264. Hammarström L, Smith CIE: Frequent occurrence of monoclonal gammopathies with an imbalanced light-chain ratio following bone marrow transplantation. Transplantation 43:447, 1987.

265. Mitus AJ, Stein R, Rappeport JM et al: Monoclonal and oligoclonal gammopathy after bone marrow transplantation. Blood 74:2764, 1989.

266. Gerritser EJA, van Tol MJD, Lankester AC et al: Immunoglobulin levels and monoclonal gammopathies in children after bone marrow transplantation. Blood 82:3493, 1993.

267. Zent CS, Wilson CS, Tricot G et al: Oligoclonal protein bands and Ig isotype switching in multiple myeloma treated with high-dose therapy and hematopoietic cell transplantation. Blood 91:3518, 1998.

268. Hebart H, Einsele H, Klein R et al: CMV infection after allogeneic bone marrow transplantation is associated with the occurrence of various autoantibodies and monoclonal gammopathies. Br J Haematol 95:138, 1996.

269. Badley AD, Portela DF, Patel R et al: Development of monoclonal gammopathy precedes the development of Epstein-Barr virus-induced posttransplant lymphoproliferative disorder. Liver Transplant Surg 2:375, 1996.

270. Pageaux GP, Bonnardet A, Picot MC et al: Prevalence of monoclonal immunoglobulins after liver transplantation: Relationship with posttransplant lymphoproliferative disorders. Transplantation 65:397, 1998.

271. Pham H, Lemoine A, Salvucci M et al: Occurrence of gammopathies and lymphoproliferative disorders in liver transplant recipients randomized to tacrolimus (FK506)- or cyclosporine-based immunosuppression. Liver Transplant Surg 4:146, 1998.

272. Myara I, Quenum G, Storogenko M et al: Monoclonal and oligoclonal gammopathies in heart-transplant recipients. Clin Chem 37:1334, 1991.

273. Gelfand JA, Boss GR, Conley CL et al: Acquired C1 esterase inhibitor deficiency and angioedema: A review. Medicine (Baltimore) 58:321, 1979.

274. Pascual M, Widmann J-J, Schifferli JA: Recurrent febrile panniculitis and hepatitis in two patients with acquired complement deficiency and paraproteinemia. Am J Med 83:959, 1987.

275. Lofdahl CG, Solvell L, Laurell AB, Johansson BR: Systemic capillary leak syndrome with monoclonal IgG and complement alterations. A case report on an episodic syndrome. Acta Med Scand 206:405, 1979.

276. Pascual M, Mach-Pascual S, Schifferli JA: Paraproteins and complement depletion: Pathogenesis and clinical syndromes. Semin Hematol 34(Suppl 1):40, 1997.

277. Droder RM, Kyle RA, Greipp PR: Control of systemic capillary leak syndrome with aminophylline and terbutaline. Am J Med 92:523, 1992.

278. Heer M, Joller-Jemelka H, Fontana A et al: Monoclonal gammopathy in chronic active hepatitis. Liver 4:255, 1984.

279. Hendrick AM, Mitchison HC, Bird AG, James OFW: Paraproteins in primary biliary cirrhosis. Q J Med 60:681, 1986.

280. Mussini C, Ghini M, Mascia MT et al: HCV and monoclonal gammopathies. Clin Exp Rheumatol 13(Suppl 13):S45, 1995.

281. Mangia A, Clemente R, Musto P et al: Hepatitis C virus infection and monoclonal gammopathies not associated with cryoglobulinemia. Leukemia 10:1209, 1996.

282. Andreone P, Zignego AL, Cursaro C et al: Prevalence of monoclonal gammopathies in patients with hepatitis C virus infection. Ann Intern Med 129:294, 1998.

283. Dosa S, Cairns SA, Mallick NP et al: Relapsing Henoch-Schönlein syndrome with renal involvement in a patient with an IgA monoclonal gammopathy: A study of the results of immunosuppressant and cytotoxic therapy. Nephron 26:145, 1980.

284. Fauchier C, Youinou P, Le Goff P et al: Immunoglobulines monoclonales au cours d'endocardites bactériennes: À propos de deux observations. Sem Hop Paris 55:1903, 1979.

285. Groussin P, Fine JM, Leroux E et al: Thyroïdite d'Hashimoto et gammapathie monoclonale: Deux observations. Ann Endocrinol (Paris) 40:413, 1979.

286. Matsubayashi S, Tamai H, Nagai K et al: Monoclonal gammopathy in Hashimoto's thyroiditis and malignant lymphoma of the thyroid. J Clin Endocrinol Metab 63:1136, 1986.

287. Norenberg DD, Bigley DV, Virata RL, Liang GC: *Corynebacterium pyogenes* septic arthritis with plasma cell synovial infiltrate and monoclonal gammopathy. Arch Intern Med 138:810, 1978.

288. Friedenburg WR, West M, Miech DJ, Mazza JJ: Atypical purpura fulminans with benign monoclonal gammopathy. Arch Dermatol 114:578, 1978.

289. Bonanni PP, Frymoyer JW, Jacox RF: A family study of idiopathic pulmonary fibrosis: A possible dysproteinemic and genetically determined disease. Am J Med 39:411, 1965.

290. Mork JN, Johnson JR, Zinneman HH, Bjorgen J: Pulmonary alveolar proteinosis associated with IgG monoclonal gammopathy. Arch Intern Med 121:278, 1968.

291. Nomura S, Kanoh T: Association of idiopathic pulmonary haemosiderosis with IgA monoclonal gammopathy. Thorax 42:696, 1987.

292. Sharma AM, Fried J, Sharma OP: Monoclonal gammopathy of undetermined significance in sarcoidosis: Two case reports. Sarcoidosis 9:70, 1992.

293. Soppi E, Eskola J, Röyttä M et al: Thymoma with immunodeficiency (Good's syndrome) associated with myasthenia gravis and benign IgG gammopathy. Arch Intern Med 145:1704, 1985.

294. Schafer AI, Miller JB, Lester EP et al: Monoclonal gammopathy in hereditary spherocytosis: A possible pathogenetic relation. Ann Intern Med 88:45, 1978.

295. Munteanu G: L'hérédodystrophie maculaire de Doyne et la gammopathie monoclonale bénigne. Corrélations génétiques et pathogéniques. J Fr Ophtalmol 3:753, 1980.

296. Nagler A, Ben-Arieh Y, Brenner B et al: Eosinophilic fibrohistiocytic lesion of bone marrow associated with monoclonal gammopathy and osteolytic lesions. Am J Hematol 23:277, 1986.

297. Ormerod LD, Collin HB, Dohlman CH et al: Paraproteinemic crystalline keratopathy. Ophthalmology 95:202, 1988.

298. Bourne WM, Kyle RA, Brubaker RF, Greipp PR: Incidence of corneal crystals in the monoclonal gammopathies. Am J Ophthalmol 107:192, 1989.

299. Kato T, Nakayasu K, Omata Y et al: Corneal deposits as an alerting sign of monoclonal gammopathy: A case report. Cornea 18:734, 1999.

300. Hutchinson K, Dal Pra M, Apel A: Immunoglobulin G crystalline keratopathy associated with monoclonal gammopathy. Aust N Z J Ophthalmol 26:177, 1998.

301. Zadák Z, Tichy M: Hyperlipidemia and monoclonal gammopathy. Neoplasma 34:169, 1987.

302. Meyrier A, Simon P, Mignon F et al: Rapidly progressive ("crescentic") glomerulonephritis and monoclonal gammopathies. Nephron 38:156, 1984.

303. Kebler R, Kithier K, McDonald FD, Cadnapaphornchai P: Rapidly progressive glomerulonephritis and monoclonal gammopathy. Am J Med 78:133, 1985.

304. Cadnapaphornchai P, Sillix D: Recurrence of monoclonal gammopathy-related glomerulonephritis in renal allograft. Clin Nephrol 31:156, 1989.

305. Chen HP, Carroll JA: Monoclonal gammopathy in carcinoma of the colon. Am J Clin Pathol 73:607, 1980.

306. Dighiero G, Guilbert B, Fermand J-P et al: Thirty-six human monoclonal immunoglobulins with antibody activity against cytoskeleton proteins, thyroglobulin, and native DNA: Immunologic studies and clinical correlations. Blood 62:264, 1983.

307. Bäck H, Nilsson G, Hansson GK, Rödjer S: M-component with reactivity against actin associated with thrombotic thrombocytopenic purpura. Am J Med 91:429, 1991.

308. Shimm DS, Cohen HJ: Transient monoclonal immunoglobulin G with anti-dextran activity. Acta Haematol (Basel) 59:99, 1978.

309. Kalliomäki JL, Granfors K, Toivanen A: An immunoglobulin G myeloma with antistreptolysin activity and a life-long history of cutaneous streptococcal infection. Clin Immunol Immunopathol 9:22, 1978.

310. Intrator L, Andre C, Chenal C, Sultan C: A monoclonal macroglobulin with antinuclear activity. J Clin Pathol 32:450, 1979.

311. Ruiz-Palomo F, Revilla Y, Gonzalez Porque P, Serrano Rios M: Two IgM paraproteins bearing cryoglobulin and anti-smooth muscle activities in a patient with Waldenström's macroglobulinaemia. J Intern Med 229:93, 1991.

312. Farhangi M, Osserman EF: Myeloma with xanthoderma due to an IgG λ monoclonal anti-flavin antibody. N Engl J Med 294:177, 1976.

313. Merlini G, Bruening R, Kyle RA, Osserman EF: The second riboflavin-binding myeloma IgGλ^{dot} I. Biochemical and functional characterization. Mol Immunol 27:385, 1990.

314. Bovill EG, Ershler WB, Golden EA et al: A human myeloma-produced monoclonal protein directed against the active subpopulation of von Willebrand factor. Am J Clin Pathol 85:115, 1986.

315. Mohri H, Noguchi T, Kodama F et al: Acquired von Willebrand disease due to inhibitor of human myeloma protein specific for von Willebrand factor. Am J Clin Pathol 87:663, 1987.

316. Zouali M, Fine J-M, Eyquem A: A human monoclonal IgG1 with anti-idiotypic activity against anti-human thyroglobulin autoantibody. J Immunol 133:190, 1984.

317. Sluiter WJ, Marrink J, Houwen B: Monoclonal gammopathy with an insulin binding IgG(κ) M-component, associated with severe hypoglycaemia. Br J Haematol 62:679, 1986.

318. Fermand JP, Danon F, Brouet JC: Characterization of a human monoclonal IgM with antibody activity to dsDNA. Clin Exp Immunol 59:467, 1985.

319. Kilgore LL, Patterson BW, Parenti DM, Fisher WR: Immune complex hyperlipidemia induced by an apolipoprotein-reactive immunoglobulin A paraprotein from a patient with multiple myeloma: Characterization of this immunoglobulin. J Clin Invest 76:225, 1985.

320. Trimarchi F, Benvenga S, Fenzi G et al: Immunoglobulin binding of thyroid hormones in a case of Waldenström's macroglobulinemia. J Clin Endocrinol Metab 54:1045, 1982.

321. Wisloff F, Michaelsen TE, Godal HC: Monoclonal IgM with lupus anticoagulant activity in a case of Waldenström's macroglobulinaemia. Eur J Haematol 38:456, 1987.

322. Backer ET, Harff GA, Beyer C: A patient with an IgG paraprotein and complexes of lactate dehydrogenase and IgG in the serum. Clin Chem 33:1937, 1987.

323. Ng VL, Hwang KM, Reyes GR et al: High titer anti-HIV antibody reactivity associated with a paraprotein spike in a homosexual male with AIDS related complex. Blood 71:1397, 1988.

324. Del Carpio J, Espinoza LR, Lauter S, Osterland CK: Transient monoclonal proteins in drug hypersensitivity reactions. Am J Med 66:1051, 1979.

325. DiMinno G, Coraggio F, Cerbone AM et al: A myeloma paraprotein with specificity for platelet glycoprotein IIIa in a patient with a fatal bleeding disorder. J Clin Invest 77:157, 1986.

326. Hoyt RH, Durie BGM: Pseudothrombocytopenia induced by a monoclonal IgM kappa platelet agglutinin. Am J Hematol 31:50, 1989.

327. Hazani A, Silvian I, Tatarsky I, Spira G: Nonsymptomatic hypercalcemia in a myeloma patient. Am J Med Sci 283:169, 1982.

328. Merlini G, Fitzpatrick LA, Siris ES et al: A human myeloma immunoglobulin G binding four moles of calcium associated with asymptomatic hypercalcemia. J Clin Immunol 4:185, 1984.

329. Annesley TM, Burritt MF, Kyle RA: Artifactual hypercalcemia in multiple myeloma. Mayo Clin Proc 57:572, 1982.

330. Baker BL, Hultquist DE: A copper-binding immunoglobulin from a myeloma patient: Purification, identification, and physical characterization. J Biol Chem 253:1195, 1978.

331. Martin NF, Kincaid MC, Stark WJ et al: Ocular copper deposition associated with pulmonary carcinoma, IgG monoclonal gammopathy and hypercupremia: A clinicopathologic correlation. Ophthalmology 90:110, 1983.

332. Westerhausen M, Meuret G: Transferrin-immune complex disease. Acta Haematol 57:96, 1977.

333. Numata Y, Tanioka F, Yoshida K et al: Ascertainment of IgA$_1$ (κ)-transferrin complex in a case of multiple myeloma associated with hypersiderinemia. Jpn J Med 30:498, 1991.

334. Hilgard P, Linder KH, Wetter O: Monoclonal cryoglobulin of IgG (λ) type interacting with transferrin. Blut 43:217, 1981.

335. Pettersson T, Hortling L, Teppo AM et al: Phosphate binding by a myeloma protein. Acta Med Scand 222:89, 1987.

336. Pierce LE, Joshi H, Patel S et al: Apparent affinity of multiple myeloma (MM) paraprotein for serum phosphate. Blood 72(Suppl. 1): 253a, 1988 (abstract).

337. Van Camp B, Reynaert P, Van Beers D: Congenital toxoplasmosis associated with transient monoclonal IgGl-λ gammopathy. Rev Infect Dis 4:173, 1982.

338. Waldenström JG: Antibody activity of monoclonal immunoglobulins in myeloma, macroglobulinemia and benign gammopathy. Med Oncol Tumor Pharmacother 3:135, 1986.

339. Merlini G, Farhangi M, Osserman EF: Monoclonal immunoglobulins with antibody activity in myeloma, macroglobulinemia and related plasma cell dyscrasias. Semin Oncol 13:350, 1986.

340. Sakashita C, Saito T, Kurosu T et al: Two M-components in a single cell lineage in a patient with a dual isotype secretory B-cell tumour. Br J Haematol 102:791, 1998.

341. Pizzolato M, Bragantini G, Bresciani P et al: IgG1-kappa biclonal gammopathy associated with multiple myeloma suggests a regulatory mechanism. Br J Haematol 102:503, 1998.

342. Kyle RA, Robinson RA, Katzmann JA: The clinical aspects of biclonal gammopathies: Review of 57 cases. Am J Med 71:999, 1981.

343. Nilsson T, Norberg B, Rudolphi O, Jacobsson L: Double gammopathies: Incidence and clinical course of 20 patients. Scand J Haematol 36:103, 1986.

344. Riddell S, Traczyk Z, Paraskevas F, Israels LG: The double gammopathies: Clinical and immunological studies. Medicine (Baltimore) 65:135, 1986.

345. Lucivero G, Miglietta A, Dell'Osso A et al: Double (IgAκ + IgGκ) paraproteinaemia in a single patient: Immunofluorescence evidence for a common plasma cell clone "frozen" at the switch phase. Acta Haematol (Basel) 75:224, 1986.

346. Ilyas AA, Willison HJ, Dalakas MC et al: Identification and characterization of gangliosides reacting with IgM paraproteins in three patients with neuropathy associated with biclonal gammopathy. J Neurochem 51:851, 1988.

347. Ray RA, Schotters SB: Triclonal gammopathy in a patient with AIDS (letter to the editor). Clin Chem 32:2000, 1986.

348. Ray RA, Schotters SB, Jacobs A, Rodgerson DO: Triclonal gammopathy in a patient with plasma cell dyscrasia. Clin Chem 32:205, 1986.

349. Berg AR, Weisenburger DD, Linder J, Armitage JO: Lymphoplasmacytic lymphoma: Report of a case with three monoclonal proteins derived from a single neoplastic clone. Cancer 57:1794, 1986.

350. Murata T, Fujita H, Harano H et al: Triclonal gammopathy (IgAκ, IgGκ and IgMκ) in a patient with plasmacytoid lymphoma derived from a monoclonal origin. Am J Hematol 42:212, 1993.

351. Grosbois B, Jego P, de Rosa H et al: Triclonal gammopathy and malignant immunoproliferative syndrome [French]. Rev Med Interne 18:470, 1997.

352. Kyle RA, Maldonado JE, Bayrd ED: Idiopathic Bence Jones proteinuria—a distinct entity? Am J Med 55:222, 1973.

353. Kyle RA, Greipp PR: "Idiopathic" Bence Jones proteinuria: Long-term follow-up in seven patients. N Engl J Med 306:564, 1982.

354. MacIntyre W: Case of mollities and fragilitas ossium, accompanied with urine strongly charged with animal matter. Med Chir Trans (Lond) 33:211, 1850.

355. O'Connor ML, Rice DT, Buss DH, Muss HB: Immunoglobulin D benign monoclonal gammopathy: A case report. Cancer 68:611, 1991.

356. Hobbs JR, Corbett AA: Younger age of presentation and extraosseous tumour in IgD myelomatosis. BMJ 1:412, 1969.

357. Hansen PR, Jønssonn V, Schrøder HD et al: IgD-lambda monoclonal gammopathy and axonal neuropathy (letter). J Intern Med 225:289, 1989.

358. Bladé J, Kyle RA: IgD monoclonal gammopathy with long-term follow-up. Br J Haematol 88:395, 1994.

Lymphoma

37

Historical Overview of Malignant Lymphoma

Alan C. Aisenberg

Although the history of lymphoma begins with the description of Hodgkin's disease in 1832, almost all the significant events in the field occurred in the past 60 years. Lymphoma (together with acute leukemia) played an essential role in the birth of medical oncology and contributed greatly to our understanding of the malignant transformation. The clinical discipline profited from the explosive growth of immunology after World War II, and the clinic, in turn, provided the basic scientist with many immunologic insights. Curiously, Hodgkin's disease, a therapeutic triumph, only reluctantly yielded its pathogenic secrets, while the much less therapeutically tractable non-Hodgkin's lymphomas readily disclosed a variety of mechanisms of malignancy. A spectrum of different misadventures in immunoglobulin (Ig) gene assembly, involving oncogene regulators of mitosis, programmed cell death, and differentiation have been defined at the molecular level and several have been identified with specific non-Hodgkin's lymphoma subtypes. Except for patients with symptomatic, advanced disease and the elderly, most individuals with Hodgkin's disease are now cured by fastidious irradiation and/or combination chemotherapy based on accurate knowledge of disease distribution obtained from sophisticated diagnostic study. The major challenge today is reduction of the late lethal second neoplasms and cardiac complications of treatment.

DESCRIPTION OF HODGKIN'S DISEASE

In 1832, Thomas Hodgkin published a remarkable paper[42] entitled "On Some Morbid Appearances of the Absorbant Glands and the Spleen" describing the disease entity that was later to bear his name (Table 37–1). Distinguishing this uncommon disorder from the far more frequently encountered causes of lymphadenopathy and splenomegaly (tuberculosis, syphilis, amyloidosis, carcinoma, non-Hodgkin's lymphoma, and acute and chronic leukemias)[37] without the benefit of microscopic study was a *tour de force* in the early nineteenth century.

Hodgkin, trained in Edinburgh (and in Paris with Laennec), represented a new breed of rational and modern physician who arrived at the basis of disease causation through close correlation of clinical findings and gross morbid anatomy.[38,53] The young Hodgkin's first medical appointment at the newly estab-

Table 37–1. Chronology of Advances in Lymphoma Classification

Year	Reference	Event
1832	Hodgkin[42]	Primary malignant tumor subsequently termed Hodgkin's disease described
1845	Virchow[105]	The nature of leukemia defined
1856	Wilks[109]	Hodgkin's cases rediscovered: Detailed clinical and pathological description provided, and eponym "Hodgkin's disease" introduced
1864	Virchow[106]	Concept of lymphoma defined and placed under rubric "aleukemic leukemia"
1892	Dreschfeld[20]	Lymphosarcoma separated from pseudoleukemia and Hodgkin's disease
1893	Kundrat[57]	
1898	Sternberg[98]	Histological picture of Hodgkin's disease characterized including diagnostic giant cells
1902	Reed[87]	
1925	Brill et al.[14a]	Follicular (nodular) lymphoma described
1927	Symmers[99]	
1930	Roulet[94]	Reticulum sarcoma distinguished from lymphosarcoma
1947	Jackson & Parker[50]	Hodgkin's disease divided into paragranuloma, granuloma, and sarcoma
1956	Rappaport et al.[36]	First modern classification of non-Hodgkin's lymphoma introduced based on cytology and presence or absence of follicular structure
1958	Burkitt[14b]	Endemic (African) Burkitt lymphoma described
1966	Lukes & Butler[69]	Nodular sclerosis described
1966	Lukes et al.[71]	Modern four-part classification of Hodgkin's disease developed
1972	Aisenberg & Bloch[4] Preud'homme & Seligmann[84]	Surface markers used to establish B- and T-cell lineage, and clonality of B-cell non-Hodgkin's lymphomas
1973	Barcos & Lukes[8] Lennert et al.[64]	Lymphoblastic lymphoma defined
1974	Lennert et al.[64b]	Concept of follicle center cell, which formed the basis of the Kiel classification of non-Hodgkin's lymphomas, developed
1974	Lukes & Collins[70]	Immunologic classification of non-Hodgkin's lymphoma proposed based on perceived B- and T-cell lineage
1977	Uchiyama et al.[104]	Adult T-cell lymphoma/leukemia described in Japan
1978	Isaacson & Wright[48]	Delineation of MALT (mucosa-associated lymphoid tissue) lymphoma
1981	Korsmeyer et al.[56]	Lineage and clonality of B-cell lymphomas defined by immunoglobulin gene rearrangement

(continued)

Table 37–1. *(continued)*

Year	Reference	Event
1982	Taub et al.[100] Dalla-Favera et al.[17]	*c-myc* oncogene from the t(14;18) of Burkitt's lymphoma cloned
1984	Tsujimoto et al.[102]	*Bcl-2* oncogene from the t(14;18) of follicular lymphoma cloned
1985	Aisenberg et al.[5] Minden et al.[75] Waldman et al.[107]	Lineage and clonality of T-cell neoplasms defined by T-cell receptor gene rearrangement
1991	Rosenberg et al.[93]	*Bcl-1* oncogene from the t(11-14) of mantle cell lymphoma cloned
1993	Ye et al.[113]	*Bcl-6* oncogene from diffuse large cell lymphoma cloned
1994	Harris et al.[40]	Revised European-American (REAL) classification of lymphoid neoplasms
1999	Harris et al.[40a]	World Health Classification (WHO) classification of neoplastic diseases of hematopoietic and lymphoid tissues

lished medical school at Guy's Hospital had been as Inspector of the Dead and Curator of the Museum. It was surely meticulous observation at the postmortem table that enabled him to recognize six cases, of which at least three (including Case 2 described below) were proven to be Hodgkin's disease by microscopic study a century later.[24]

Case 2

September 24th, 1828. Ellenborough King (Figure 37–1), aged 10 years, was admitted to Lukes ward on the 6th of August 1828, under the care of Dr. Bright. He was the youngest of six children, of whom the first five were reported to be healthy. This child had also been healthy till thirteen months ago, when his strength, flesh, and healthy appearance began to fail. He was living at that time in the West of England. A tumour was observed in the left hypochondrium in the situation of the spleen, the glandulae concatenatae on the right side were observed to be considerably enlarged, but under the treatment employed, these tumours, as well as that in the situation of the spleen, were at times very considerably reduced in size.

It does not appear that he was ever subject to haemorrhage, nor till very lately to dropsical effusion; his appetite was generally good. After admission into the hospital the tumour on the left side was observed to extend considerably below the left hypchodrium, but was reported not to be as large as it had formerly been. The glands in the left side of the neck were swollen, as well as those on the right; the abdomen was somewhat distended, and there was considerable oedema in the scrotum.

Death occurred on the 23rd of September.

The head was not opened. The glands in the neck had assumed the form of large ovoid masses, connected

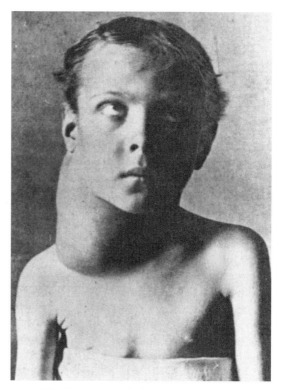

Figure 37–1. The picture is not Ellenborough King, but a 7-year-old boy with similar presentation (W.D.M., Case 7) from Dorothy Reed's classic paper. (From Reed,[87] with permission.)

together merely by loose cellular membrane and minute vessels: when cut into they exhibited a firm cartilaginous structure of a light colour and very feeble vascularity, but no appearance of softening or suppuration. Glands similarly affected accompanied the vessels into the chest, where the bronchial and mediastinal glands were in the same state and greatly enlarged. There were some old pleuritis adhesions. The substance of the lung was generally healthy. There was a good deal of clear serum in the pericardium, but this membrane, as well as the heart, was quite healthy.

In the peritoneal cavity there was a considerable quantity of clear straw-coloured serum mixed with extensive, recent thin diaphanous films. The mucous membranes of the stomach and intestines were tolerably healthy.

The mesenteric glands were but slightly enlarged, and but little if at all indurated; but those accompanying the aorta, the splenic artery, and illiacs were in the same state as the glands in the neck.

The liver contained no tubercles, and the structure was quite healthy. The pancreas was rather firm, and the glands situated along its upper edge, were, as before stated greatly enlarged. The spleen was enlarged to at least four times its natural size, its surface was mammillated, and its structure thickly sprinkled with tubercles, presenting the same structure as the enlarged glands previously described.

Hodgkin's perceptive observation was lost and might never have been properly attributed but for Sir Samuel Wilks,[109,110]

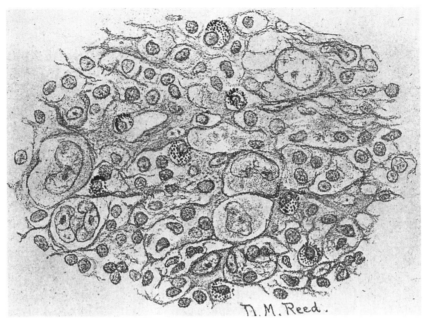

Figure 37–2. Reed-Sternberg cells drawn by Dorothy Reed's own hand. The mirror-image cell in the lower left is diagnostic (From Reed,[87] with permission.)

who, working independently with some of the same specimens at Guy's a generation later, provided a more detailed and critical clinical and pathological description of the disorder and acknowledged Hodgkin's earlier contribution.

In the late nineteenth century, Greenfield[35] among others, described characteristic giant cells in patients with Hodgkin's disease. However, a full description of the diagnostic cells required Ehrlich's staining methods, and awaited the publications of Sternberg[98] and, in particular, Dorothy Reed[87] (Figure 37–2). The latter clearly distinguished the process from tuberculosis, a condition complicating many of Sternberg's cases.

The first histological classification of Hodgkin's disease to enjoy wide recognition was the division into paragranuloma, granuloma, and sarcoma, introduced by Jackson and Parker.[50] In the early 1960s, Lukes and Butler[69] added the nodular sclerosis category and further refined the earlier system. A conference held in Rye, New York in 1966 simplified the Lukes and Butler scheme into a four-part classification (lymphocyte predominance, nodular sclerosis, and lymphocyte depletion),[69] which was further modified in the REAL (Revised European-American Lymphoma)[40] and WHO (World Health Organization)[40a] classifications.

DELINEATION OF THE NON-HODGKIN'S LYMPHOMAS

Subsequent to the report of Thomas Hodgkin, Virchow[105] and Bennett[9] independently described the first cases of leukemia. In his textbook on tumors published two decades later, Virchow[106] divided leukemia into leukemic and aleukemic types, employing the designation "lymphosarcoma" for a subdivision of the latter. Unfortunately about the same time, the term "pseudoleukemia" was introduced and became a catch-all (a "misch masch"

according to Virchow) for a variety of conditions having both lymphadenopathy and splenomegaly; the designation persisted into the twentieth century and did much to obscure the delineation and subclassification of the non-Hodgkin's lymphomas.

In the late nineteenth century, Dreschfeld,[20] Kundrat,[57] and others were again employing the term *lymphosarcoma* in the modern sense used by Virchow a generation earlier. However, it was well into the twentieth before order began to emerge among the complex and heterogeneous group of non-Hodgkin's lymphomas. The follicular or nodular lymphomas were first clearly described by Brill et al.,[14a] initially without recognition of the malignant character of the proliferations. However, within a few years both these authors and Symmers[99] were convinced that the condition was a malignant, albeit indolent, growth. The term *reticulum cell sarcoma* was applied to lymph node neoplasms by Roulet,[94] another designation that generated more heat than light in lymphoma classification.

Gall and Mallory[28] introduced a lymphoma classification based on clinicopathologic criteria, which for all its shortcomings, was among the first widely recognized attempts to make order out the chaotic non-Hodgkin's lymphoma situation. Until then, a number of influential pathologists still espoused the "fluid" view of lymphoma, a view that held that the malignant lymphomas were not a group of separate and discreet diseases but rather a single disorder capable of freely changing its microscopic appearance.

Rappaport et al.,[86] in their classic study, presented medicine with a lymphoma classification that could be easily applied and was prognostically useful. Two criteria were employed to distinguish lymphoma subtypes; the presence or absence of nodularity, and cell size (small, intermediate, and large lymphoid cells). Subsequently, the Rappaport scheme was so extensively modified to incorporate new knowledge as to become virtually unrecognizable. The follicle center was identified by Lennert et al.[64] as the progenitor of a major fraction of adult non-Hodgkin's lymphomas, elaborated upon by Lukes and Collins,[70] and became the basis of Lennert's Kiel system[63,64] only recently deserted by European pathologists. The National Cancer Institute sponsored Working Formulation for Clinical Usage[92] provided a temporary but unsatisfactory solution to the search for a clinically relevant system that could be reproducibly applied by working pathologists. The REAL classification[40] represents a radical, if tentative, redo of lymphoma classification. It is based on prior systems, but for the first time defines lymphoma subtypes by immunophenotype and molecular genetics as well as morphology and clinical characteristics, and has already been updated under World Health Organization (WHO Classification) auspices.[40a]

Lymphoblastic lymphoma was identified in the 1970s by Barcos and Lukes[8] and Lennert et al.[64] as a separate clinicopathologic entity, closely resembling the T-cell variant of acute lymphoblastic leukemia and attacking older children and adolescents predominantly. Earlier still, Burkitt[14b] had described a new type of lymphoma in African children restricted to regions of high temperature and rainfall. Another distinct subtype of lymphoma, adult T-cell leukemia/lymphoma (ATL/L), was reported in 1977 from Japan, where cases were concentrated in the southwestern islands.[104] More recently recognized lymphoma subtypes include mantle cell lymphoma[7] derived from the mantle cells of the follicle; MALT (mucosa-associated lymphoid tissue) lymphomas,[48] which are predominantly extranodal lymphomas derived from marginal zone B cells[40]; and large cell lymphoma of the mediastinum derived from B cells of the thymic medulla.[2]

In 1972, it became possible to immunophenotype B and T lymphocytes, initially by the presence of clonal Ig or sheep cell receptor on the cell surface,[4,84] and later with a host of specific monoclonal antibodies.[55] First applied to fresh cell suspensions, techniques were soon available for frozen and fixed material. While not replacing morphology as the primary basis of lymphoma diagnosis and classification, the availability of increasingly specific monoclonal antibodies illuminated the nature of many lymphoid proliferations and made the diagnosis of some lymphoma subtypes insecure on the basis of morphology alone.

Clonality and lymphoid cell lineage can also be established through molecular genetic analysis employing Southern blot hybridization. Thus in 1981, B-cell lineage could be confirmed by the presence of clonally rearranged Ig heavy and light chain genes.[56] Similarly, it soon became possible to identify clonal T-cell proliferations by the presence of clonally rearranged T-cell receptor genes.[5,75,107] Molecular genetic techniques are not widely used for routine diagnosis at the time of writing.

EVOLUTION OF EFFECTIVE TREATMENT

Diagnostic procedures that permit accurate assessment of the extent of disease (stage) have figured prominently in the development of effective lymphoma management (Table 37–2). Lower extremity lymphangiography[54] proved of great value in defining the extent of abdominal lymphoma. More recently computed tomography (CT) has emerged as the preferred diagnostic technique for assessing lymphoma in both the chest and abdomen, although less sensitive and specific than lymphangiography in the latter region. The gallium scan has proven useful for evaluating response to therapy, and magnetic resonance imaging (MRI) finds other unique applications. Positron emission tomography (PET) may prove the most specific and sensitive noninvasive technique for evaluating lymphoma in inaccessible locations.

Table 37–2. Chronology of Advances in Lymphoma Management

Year	Reference	Event
1902	Pusey[85]	First cases of Hodgkin's disease treated with x-rays
1939	Gilbert[30]	Anatomic and clinical foundations, and principles of radiation therapy of Hodgkin's disease established
1946	Goodman et al.[33]	Nitrogen mustard treatment of Hodgkin's disease
1950	Peters[82]	Cure of Hodgkin's disease by irradiation of adjacent uninvolved lymphoid areas
1952	Kinmonth[54]	Lower-extremity lymphangiography
1962	Kaplan[51]	Improved technique: tumoricidal dose, megavoltage equipment, irradiation of lymphoid areas in continuity (mantle, paraortic, and inverted "Y" fields)
1966	Rosenberg[91]	Rye system for clinical staging of Hodgkin's disease
1969	Glatstein et al.[31]	Distribution of abdominal Hodgkin's disease defined by laparotomy with splenectomy
1970	DeVita et al.[19a]	Cure of advanced Hodgkin's disease with MOPP (mechlorethamine, oncovin, prednisone, procarbazine)
1971	Carbone et al.[16]	Revised four-part Ann Arbor staging system for clinical and pathological staging of Hodgkin's disease
1975	Bonnadonna et al.[13]	Treatment of Hodgkin's disease with non-cross-resistant drugs ABVD (doxorubicin, bleomycin, vinblastine, dacarbazine), and with alternating MOPP & ABVD
1975	DeVita et al.[18]	Cure of aggressive non-Hodgkin's lymphomas with C-MOPP (cyclophosphamide, vincristine, prednisone, procarbazine)
1976	McKelvey et al.[72]	Cure of aggressive non-Hodgkin's lymphomas with CHOP (cyclophosphamide, doxorubicin, vincristine, prednisone)
1977		Computed tomography (CT) scanning of chest and abdomen
1982		Treatment of aggressive non-Hodgkin's lymphoma with third-generation drug regimens
1984		Autologous bone marrow transplantation in Hodgkin's disease and non-Hodgkin's lymphoma
1989		Introduction of purine nucleoside analogues (fludarabine, pentostatin, cladribine)
1993		Treatment with unlabeled and radiolabeled monoclonal antibodies

The introduction of laparotomy and splenectomy[31] was of historic significance for elucidating the orderly progression of Hodgkin's disease, and played a critical role in its control by allowing the apposite application of supravoltage radiotherapy and combination chemotherapy. However, with the improved noninvasive diagnostic procedures now available and with the shift to combined treatment with irradiation and drugs, abdominal exploration is infrequently invoked today. Staging laparotomy never played an important role in non-Hodgkin's lymphoma management.

Peters[82] introduced a three-part classification describing the extent of Hodgkin's disease. The four-part staging system in current use was proposed in abbreviated form at the 1966 Rye, New York conference,[91] and expanded into its present version at conferences held in Ann Arbor, Michigan[16] and the Cotswolds.[68] The system in modified form has also been used for the non-Hodgkin's lymphomas but with less success. More recently, the International Prognostic Index for Non-Hodgkin's Lymphoma has proven useful, particularly for aggressive proliferations.[47]

Only six years after Roentgen's 1896 description of x-rays, dramatic, albeit transient, responses of Hodgkin's disease to irradiation were reported by Pusey.[85] During the period 1925 to 1939, Gilbert[30] undertook an ambitious and systematic radiotherapeutic approach to the disease. He obtained consistent responses, both subjective and objective, but cure remained an elusive goal and extension of life arguable. Peters[82] and Peters and Middlemiss[83] were the first to establish convincing evidence that adequate radiation dose delivered to appropriate treatment fields could extend survival and even cure a fraction of patients. Radiation therapy of Hodgkin's disease approached its present high state of development with Kaplan's[51,52] introduction of improved equipment and technique (accurate simulation and dosimetry, and modern treatment fields such as the mantle and the inverted "Y").

Among the unexpected results of World War II was the development of the highly toxic but therapeutically useful mustard gas derivative, nitrogen mustard [methyl bis(betachlorethyl) amine]. This material was the first modern antitumor drug to regularly produce significant responses in malignant disease in humans: Hodgkin's disease stood out among the disorders reported by Goodman et al.[33] to be responsive. Unfortunately, remissions proved to be short-lived, but over the next 30 years a variety of other drugs active in Hodgkin's disease emerged, including vinblastine,[79] vincristine,[108] procarbazine,[74] bleomycin,[11] nitrosoureas,[66] doxorubicin,[34] and etoposide.[49] Following the promising report of Lacher and Durant[60] employing chlorambucil and vinblastine in combination, DeVita et al.[19a] assembled the landmark MOPP (mechlorethamine, vincristine, prednisone, procarbazine) regimen, which dramatically altered the outlook for patients with advanced Hodgkin's disease. The development of this curative drug program was the culmination of a decade of laboratory and clinical investigation involving experimental animals and patients, particularly with acute leukemia: Carbone, Frei, Freireich, Holland, Pinkel, and Skipper were major contributors.[25] Following the introduction of MOPP for the treatment of Hodgkin's disease, other effective drug combinations were reported, of which ABVD (doxoru-

bicin, bleomycin, vinblastine, dacarbazine) introduced by Bonnadonna and Santoro[12] was the most significant. This regimen is less leukemogenic and, because the components do not overlap those of MOPP, effective eight-drug programs are feasible. Alternating cycles of MOPP and ABVD are particularly effective in advanced and symptomatic Hodgkin's disease (stages IIIB and IVB),[14] although the superiority of eight-drug over four-drug programs remains unproven.[15]

The cumulative impact of advances in radiation therapy and chemotherapy on Hodgkin's disease survival is dramatically illustrated in Figure 37–3. Mortality from the disorder fell in the United States from 1.8 per 100,000 patients in 1950 to 0.4 in 1994, while incidence remained constant at approximately 3.0 per 100,000.[3,76,89] However, the unforeseen consequence of this success is seen in Figure 37-4: a cumulative treatment mortality that exceeds that of Hodgkin's disease itself 15 years following treatment.[3,43] Acute nonlymphocytic leukemia secondary to MOPP chemotherapy, second non-Hodgkin's lymphomas, and second solid tumors (particularly of lung, breast, and gastrointestinal tract origin) and cardiac disease secondary to irradiation account for most of the late treatment-related mortality.

Treatment of the non-Hodgkin's lymphomas has lagged behind that of Hodgkin's disease; few of the former are cured by radiation therapy. However, in 1975 investigators at the National Cancer Institute[18] reported the cure of a small number of patients with advanced-stage diffuse large cell lymphoma with C-MOPP (cyclophosphamide, vincristine, prednisone, procarbazine). The next year, the first[72] of many reports

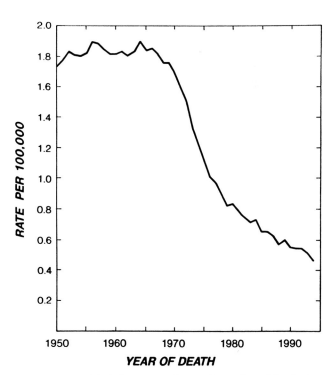

Figure 37–3. Hodgkin's disease mortality in White males and females in the United States from 1950 to 1994. (Modified from the National Cancer Institute Division of Cancer Control,[76] with permission, with additional data from Ries et al.[89])

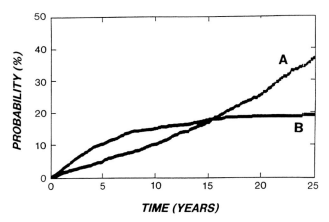

Figure 37–4. Actuarial risk of death from Hodgkin's disease (Curve B) or other causes (Curve A) in 2498 patients treated at Stanford University from 1960 to 1995. (Adapted from Hoppe,[43] with permission.)

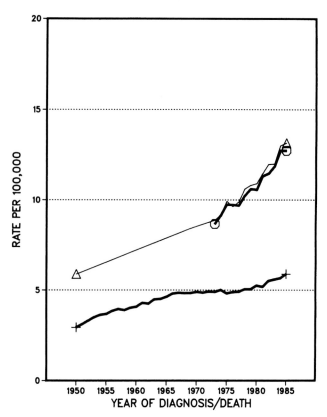

Figure 37–5. Non-Hodgkin's lymphoma incidence and mortality in White males and females in the United States from 1950 to 1985. The upper curves represent incidence figures from the SEER program (octogons) and from four selected areas (triangles), and the lower curve mortality (From the National Institute Division of Cancer Control,[76] with permission.)

appeared attesting to the efficacy of the doxorubicin-containing CHOP (cyclophosphamide, doxorubicin, vincristine, prednisone) regimen in intermediate- and high-grade lymphomas (diffuse large cell, follicular mixed and large cell, and immunoblastic).

Alternatives to the CHOP program have been explored with the twin goals of simultaneous tumor exposure to the maximum number of drugs (the Goldie-Coldman hypothesis)[32] and maximum drug intensity.[19,46] While improving survival figures initially suggested an advantage of the so-called third-generation programs, randomized investigations revealed no improvement over CHOP.[23]

High-dose therapy in association with autologous stem cell transplantation,[10,44] has emerged as the only potentially curative treatment available to patients with relapsed intermediate- and high-grade non-Hodgkin's lymphomas. Stem cell transplantation is currently employed earlier in the course of non-Hodgkin's lymphoma than in Hodgkin's disease. It is of historic interest that lethal doses of nitrogen mustard with attempted salvage with autologous bone marrow was attempted more than 40 years ago and discarded because of unacceptable mortality.[101] At the time of writing, attempts are being made to harness graft-versus-lymphoma activity though partially mismatched transplants and other immunological manipulations. Two other recent advances of historic significance in non-Hodgkin's lymphoma management should be noted: the introduction of the purine nucleoside analogues fludarabine, pentostatin, and cladribine, and treatment with unlabeled and radiolabeled monoclonal antibodies.

Mortality from non-Hodgkin's lymphoma (Figure 37–5) has not enjoyed the salutary improvement observed in Hodgkin's disease.[76,89] Although 5-year survival at the national level has risen from 28 percent (1950–1964) to 52 percent (1983–1989), overall non-Hodgkin's lymphoma mortality continues to climb, although less rapidly than the increase in disease incidence. The impressive gains achieved with large cell and pediatric lymphomas are submerged by the increased disease incidence, the

many indolent but incurable low grade and follicular tumors, and the poor results in the aged.

The dramatic improvement in pediatric non-Hodgkin's lymphoma survival contrasts with the modest gains in adults. While less than 10 percent of children and adolescents with *localized* or *regional* non-Hodgkin's lymphoma survived 5 years prior to 1967,[6] recent series report 80 percent disease-free survival in *all* stages combined.[90,96] This progress was achieved through recognition of the disseminated character of pediatric lymphomas that require acute lymphoblastic leukemia-like treatment programs,[6,111] and the need to stratify treatment intensity by stage and immunophenotypically determined biological subtype (Burkitt's, T- or B-cell lymphoblastic, and large cell variants).[67,90,96]

In the past decade, a striking increase in AIDS (acquired immunodeficiency syndrome)-related lymphomas has been noted in sexually active males. These are usually intermediate- or high-grade tumors of undifferentiated, immunoblastic, or large cell subtypes, advanced in stage with extranodal spread at the time of presentation and with short survival time.[115] Prior to the introduction of the protease inhibitors, lymphoma chemotherapy was particularly difficult because of the underlying immunodeficiency. Based on the projected AIDS incidence, increased mortality from AIDS-related lymphomas may soon overwhelm any treatment-related improvement in non-AIDS lymphoma survival. However, the AIDS-associated lymphomas do not account for the 3 to 4 percent annual increase in non-Hodgkin's lymphoma observed in the United States and Europe since the early 1970s.[89]

ETIOLOGY AND PATHOGENESIS

The Nature of Hodgkin's Disease

With the exception of the earliest description of follicular lymphoma, the neoplastic nature of the non-Hodgkin's lymphomas was never in doubt. However, because neoplastic cells form only a minor constituent of the Hodgkin's disease infiltrate, the malignant nature of Hodgkin's disease was disputed. The majority of investigators, including Virchow, Wilks, and most modern students of the disorder, considered it a neoplasm of the lymphoid system, but some distinguished observers, including both Reed and Sternberg, held a contrary view. Indeed, until recently, the Reed-Sternberg cell resisted attempts to define its lineage. Its immunophenotypic characteristics are not those of garden-variety B lymphocytes, T lymphocytes, macrophage/monocytes, or dendritic cells.

The pathogenesis of Hodgkin's disease is at last being resolved. Evidence of clonally rearranged immunoglobulin genes obtained from polymerase chain reaction study of single Reed-Sternberg cells strongly supports their neoplastic and aberrant ("crippled") B-cell lineage in nodular sclerosis, mixed cellularity, and lymphocyte-depletion Hodgkin's disease.[58,59] These cells lack CD45 (leukocyte common antigen), surface Ig, and most common B-cell antigens, but react with antibodies to CD15 and the activation antigen CD30 (Ki-1).[97] The Reed-Sternberg cells in nodular lymphocyte-predominant Hodgkin's disease more closely resemble conventional neoplastic B lymphocytes.

Epstein-Barr virus (EBV) is demonstrable in clonal form in Reed-Sternberg cells from one-third to one-half of Hodgkin's disease biopsies in a frequency dependent on disease subtype, but its causal role remains to be demonstrated.[77] The defect in cell-mediated immunity that accompanies active Hodgkin's disease[103] will probably be elucidated with further clarification of the cytokine network.[36] The multitude of failed etiologic agents proposed as the cause of Hodgkin's disease will not be catalogued here.[45]

Viruses and the Etiology of Lymphoma

Despite the etiological role of viruses in a variety of naturally occurring animal lymphomas and leukemias (including avian leukosis, lymphomas of wild mice, bovine and feline lymphoma/leukemias, and lymphoma/leukemia of the gibbon ape),[29] progress in establishing a viral causation of human lymphoma has been slow and elusive.

The regular isolation of EBV from African Burkitt's lymphoma in 1964 and since,[21] together with extensive epidemiologic (serologic) evidence, established an etiologic role of this DNA herpes-type virus in the endemic disorder. However, while EBV was isolated from almost all African cases, it was identified in only a small fraction (20 percent) of nonendemic biopsies that share the same cytogenetic translocations but differ in clinical behavior and slightly in molecular genotype.[65] More recently, EBV has been identified in lymphomas that complicate a variety of inherited and acquired immunodeficiency states[78]; ataxia-telangiectasia, Wiskott-Aldrich syndrome, severe combined and common variable immunodeficiencies, the X-linked immunodeficiency syndrome,[39] organ transplantation,[81] and AIDS (particularly those with immunoblastic histology or primary central nervous system presentation). In all the above conditions, the virus is clonal, but its exact relation to causation remains to be elucidated.

Gallo and Wong-Staal[29] isolated a novel retrovirus (HTLV-1) from a patient with an atypical cutaneous T-cell lymphoma. Subsequently, the same virus was regularly recovered from the tumor cells of Japanese and Caribbean patients with adult T-cell leukemia/lymphoma (ATL/L), and antibody to the virus was demonstrated in almost all patients with that disorder.

Cytogenetics

The identification by Manolov and Manolova[73] of extra chromosomal material on chromosome 14 (14q+) in Burkitt's lymphoma is another landmark event in lymphoma history. Several years later, Zech et al.[114] proved this finding to be the result of an unbalanced translocation between chromosomes 8 and 14 [t(8;14)(q24;q32)]. Subsequent investigation demonstrated the same translocation in approximately 80 percent of Burkitt's lymphoma cell lines; the remaining 20 percent revealed one of two variant translocations, between chromosome 8 and either chromosome 2 [t(2;8)(p12;q24)] or chromosome 22 [t(8;22)(q24;q11)].[65]

With improvement in cytogenetic technique, additional chromosome abnormalities specific to particular lymphoma subtypes were identified with increasing frequency.[95] Thus Fukuhara et al.[26] identified a translocation between chromosomes 14 and 18 [(t(14;18)(q32;21)] in follicular (nodular) lymphomas, trisomy of chromosome 11 was found in small lymphocytic lymphoma and chronic lymphocytic leukemia,[113a] and abnormalities of chromosome 14 (14q11–13) and trisomy 3 were detected in ATL/L.[22] Indeed, recent results employing high-resolution chromosomal analysis suggest that characteristic cytogenetic defects exist in most, if not all, subtypes of non-Hodgkin's lymphoma.

Molecular Genetics and Oncogenes

The chromosomal localization of the human immunoglobulin genes between 1979 and 1981 provided the basis of breathtaking insight into the pathogenesis of Burkitt's lymphoma. The Ig heavy chain, and the kappa and lambda light chains were localized, respectively, to chromosomes 14, 2, and 22 (at bands 14q32, 2p12, and 22q11), the three sites involved in essentially all common and variant Burkitt translocations. In 1982, both the Leder[100] and Croce[17] laboratories cloned the translocation breakpoint, and identified the *c-myc* oncogene on the chromosome 8 fragment (at 8q24). Since *c-myc* was already known to virologists from its role in fowl leukosis, the circle was closed. Transgenic injection (introduction into the germline by injection into the egg nucleus) of *c-myc* coupled to the IgM heavy chain or kappa light chain genes regularly produced aggressive B-cell lymphomas, but complete or truncated *c-myc* alone was inactive.[1] Active work continues on the detailed mechanism by which deregulation of *c-myc* by Ig-gene segments leads to Burkitt's lymphoma.

Within 2 years of the elucidation of the role of *c-myc* in Burkitt's lymphoma, Tsujimoto et al.[102] cloned the breakpoint of the 14;18 translocation of follicular lymphoma. This breakpoint involved the junction of a joining segment of the IgM gene at chromosome 14q32, and the *bcl-2* oncogene (at 18q21) whose protein product opposes apoptosis or programmed cell death.[41] Similarly, the 11;14 translocation of mantle cell lymphoma juxtaposed the *bcl-1* gene (whose product is a mitosis-regulating cyclin) at chromosome 11q13 to the same IgM gene.[93] *Bcl-3*, an oncogene at 19q13 whose product regulates gene transcription, is similarly joined in a small fraction of cases of chronic lymphocytic leukemia.[112] *Bcl-6*, a putative oncogene at chromosome 3q27, is translocated to a variety of chromosomal sites in a fraction of large cell lymphomas.[27,80] In T-cell lymphomas, one frequent breakpoint is at chromosome 14q11, at the site where the gene for the delta chain of the T-cell receptor is embedded in the T-cell receptor alpha chain gene.[88]

Thus, a catastrophe in the generation of antigen receptor genes, Ig genes (in the case of B cells), and T-cell receptor genes (in the cases of T cells), is a major cause of human lymphoma. Available evidence indicates that more than a single genetic misadventure is required for tumor induction.[61] The remarkable progress in understanding the molecular events of lymphomagenesis achieved in the past decade suggests that comprehensive understanding of the process is not far off. Oncogene defects characterized at the molecular level increasingly contribute to the definition of lymphoma subtypes.

REFERENCES

1. Adams JM, Harris AW, Pinkert CA, Corcoran LM, Alexander WS, Cory S et al: The c-myc oncogene driven by immunoglobulin enhancers induces lymphoid malignancy in transgenic mice. Nature 318:533–538, 1985.
2. Aisenberg AC: Primary large cell lymphoma of the mediastinum. Semin Oncol 26:251–258, 1999.
3. Aisenberg AC: Problems in Hodgkin's disease management. Blood 93:761–779, 1999.
4. Aisenberg AC, Bloch KJ: Immunoglobulins on the surface of neoplastic lymphocytes. N Engl J Med 287:272–276, 1972.
5. Aisenberg AC, Krontiris TG, Mak TW, Wilkes BM: Rearrangement of the genes for the beta chain of the T-cell receptor in T-cell chronic leukemia and allied disorders. N Engl J Med 313:529–533, 1985.
6. Aur RJA, Hustu HO, Simone JV, Pinkel D: Therapy of localized and regional lymphosarcoma of childhood. Cancer 27:1328–1331, 1970.
7. Banks P, Chan J, Cleary M, Delson G, DeWolf-Peeter C, Gatter K et al: Mantle cell lymphoma: A proposal for unification of mor-

8. Barcos MP, Lukes RJ: Malignant lymphoma of convoluted lymphocytes. A new entity of possible T-cell type. In Sinks LF, Godden JO (eds.): Conflicts in Childhood Cancer. An Evaluation of Current Management, Vol. 4, p. 147. Alan R. Liss, New York, 1975.
9. Bennett JH: Two cases of disease and enlargement of the spleen in which death took place from the presence of purulent matter in the blood. Edinb Med Surg J 64:413–423, 1845.
10. Bierman PJ, Armitage JO: Autologous hematopoietic cell transplantation in Hodgkin's disease. In Thomas ED, Blume KG, Forman SJ (eds.): Hematopoietic Cell Transplantation, 2nd Ed., pp. 952–962. Blackwell Science, Boston, 1999.
11. Blum RH, Carter SK, Agre K: A clinical review of bleomycin: A new antineoplastic agent. Cancer 31:903–913, 1973.
12. Bonnadonna G, Santoro A: Evolution in the treatment strategy of Hodgkin's disease. Adv Cancer Res 36:257–293, 1982.
13. Bonnadonna G, Zucali R, De Monfardini S, Lena M, Uslenghi G: Combination therapy of Hodgkin's disease with adriamycin, bleomycin, vinblastine and imadazole carboxamide versus MOPP. Cancer 36:252–259, 1975.
14. Bonnadonna G, Valagussa P, Santoro A: Alternating non cross-resistant combination chemotherapy or MOPP chemotherapy in Stage IV Hodgkin's disease: A report of 8-year results. Ann Intern Med 104:739–746, 1986.
14a. Brill NF, Baehr G, Rosenthal N: Generalized giant lymph node hyperplasia of lymph nodes and spleen. A hitherto undescribed type. JAMA 84:668–671, 1925.
14b. Burkitt DP: A sarcoma involving the jaws of African children. Brit J Surg 46:218–223, 1958.
15. Canellos GP, Anderson JR, Propert KJ, Nissen N, Cooper MR, Henderson ES et al: Chemotherapy for advanced Hodgkin's disease with MOPP, ABVD, or MOPP alternating with ABVD. N Engl J Med 327:1478–1484, 1992.
16. Carbone PP, Kaplan HS, Musshof K, Smithers DW, Tubiana M: Report of the committee on Hodgkin's disease staging classification. Cancer Res 31:1860–1861, 1971.
17. Dalla-Favera R, Bregni M, Erickson J, Patterson D, Gallo RC, Croce CM: Human c-myc oncogene is located on the region of chromosome 8 that is translocated in Burkitt lymphoma cells. Proc Natl Acad Sci USA 79:7824–7827, 1982.
18. DeVita VT, Canellos GP, Chabner B, Schein P, Hubbard SP, Young RC: Advanced diffuse histiocytic lymphoma, a potentially curable disease: Results with combination chemotherapy. Lancet I:248–250, 1975.
19. DeVita VT, Hubbard SM, Longo DL: The chemotherapy of lymphomas: Looking back, moving forward—the Richard and Hinda Rosenthal Foundation Award Lecture. Cancer Res 47:5810–5824, 1987.
19a. DeVita VT, Serpick A, Carbone PP: Combination chemotherapy in the treatment of Hodgkin's disease. Ann Intern Med 73:881–895, 1970.
20. Dreschfeld J: Clinical lecture on acute Hodgkin's (or pseudoleucocythemia). BMJ I:893–896, 1892.
21. Epstein MA, Achong BG, Barr YM: Virus particles in cultured lymphoblasts from Burkitt's lymphoma. Lancet I:702–703, 1964.
22. Fifth International Workshop on Chromosomes in Leukemia-Lymphoma: Correlation of chromosome abnormalities with histologic and immunologic characteristics in non-Hodgkin's lymphoma and adult T cell leukemia-lymphoma. Blood 70:1554–1564, 1987.
23. Fisher RI, Gaynor ER, Dahlberg S, Oken MM, Grogen TM, Mize EM et al: Comparison of a standard regimen (CHOP) with three

phologic, immunologic, and molecular data. Am J Surg Pathol 16:637–640, 1992.

intensive regimens for advanced non-Hodgkin's lymphoma. N Engl J Med 328:1002–1006, 1993.

24. Fox H: Remarks on microscopical preparations made from some of the original tissue described by Thomas Hodgkin, 1832. Ann Med Hist 8:370–374, 1926.

25. Frei E III: Clinical cancer research: An embattled species. Cancer 50:1979–1992, 1982.

26. Fukuhara S, Rowley JD, Variakojis D, Golomb HM: Chromosome abnormalities in poorly differentiated lymphocytic lymphoma. Cancer Res 39:3119–3128, 1979.

27. Gaidano G, Dalla-Favera R: Molecular biology of lymphomas. In DeVita VT, Hellman S Jr, Rosenberg SA (eds.): Cancer: Principles & Practice of Oncology, 5th Ed., pp. 2131–2140. Lipincott-Raven, Boston, 1997.

28. Gall RC, Mallory TB: Malignant lymphoma: A clinicopathological survey of 618 cases. Am J Pathol 18:381–429, 1942.

29. Gallo RC, Wong-Stahl F: Retroviruses as etiologic agents in some animal and human leukemias and lymphomas and as tools for elucidating the mechanisms of leukemogenesis. Blood 60:545–557, 1982.

30. Gilbert R: Radiotherapy in Hodgkin's disease (malignant lymphogranulomatosis). Anatomic and clinical foundations; governing principles; results. Am J Roentgenol 41:198–241, 1939.

31. Glatstein E, Guernsey JM, Rosenberg SA, Kaplan HS: The value of laparotomy and splenectomy in the staging of Hodgkin's disease. Cancer 24:709–718, 1969.

32. Goldie JH, Coldman AJ, Gudauskas GA: Rationale for the use of alternating non-cross-resistant chemotherapy. Cancer Treat Rep 66:439–449, 1982.

33. Goodman LS, Wintrobe MM, Dameshek W, Goodman MJ, Gilman AZ, McLeennan MI: Nitrogen mustard therapy. Use of methyl-bis (beta-chloroethyl) amino hydrochloride for Hodgkin's disease, lymphosarcoma, leukemia and certain allied and miscellaneous disorders. JAMA 132:126–132, 1946.

34. Gottlieb JA, Gutterman JU, McCredie KB, Rodriguez V, Frei E III: Chemotherapy of malignant lymphoma with Adriamycin (1973). Cancer Res 33:3024–3028, 1973.

35. Greenfield WS: Specimens illustrative of the pathology of lymphadenoma and leucocythemia. Trans Pathol Soc London 29:272–304, 1878.

36. Gruss HJ, Pinto A, Poppema S, Hermann F: Hodgkin's disease: A tumor of disturbed immunological pathways. Immunol Today 18:156–163, 1997.

37. Gunz FW: The dread leukemias and lymphomas: Their nature and their prospects. In Wintrobe MM (ed.): I: Blood, Pure and Eloquent: A Story of Discovery of People and of Ideas, p. 511, McGraw-Hill, New York, 1980.

38. Hardwick C: Thomas Hodgkin, 1798–1866. Guy's Hospital Reports 115:255–267, 1966.

39. Harrington DS, Weissenberger DD, Purtilo DT: Malignant lymphomas in X-linked lymphoproliferative disease. Cancer 59:1419–1429, 1987.

40. Harris NL, Jaffe ES, Banks PM, Chan CKC, Cleary ML, Delsol G et al: A revised European-American classification of malignant lymphoid neoplasms: A proposal from the International Lymphoma Study Group. Blood 84:1361–1392, 1994.

40a. Harris NL, Jaffe ES, Diebold J, Flandrin G, Muller-Hermelik HK, Vardiman J, Lister TA, Bloomfield, CD: World Health Organization Classification of Neoplastic Diseases of the Hematopoietic Tissues: Report of the Clinical Advisory Committee Meeting – Airlee House, Virginia, November 1997. J Clin Oncol 17:3835–3849, 1999.

41. Hockenberry D, Nunez G, Milliman C, Schreiber RD, Korsmeyer SJ: *Bcl-2* is an inner mitochondrial membrane protein that blocks programmed cell death. Nature 348:334–336, 1990.

42. Hodgkin T: On some morbid appearances of absorbant gland and spleen. Med Chirurg Trans 17:68–114, 1832.

43. Hoppe RT: Hodgkin's disease: Complications of therapy and excess mortality. Ann Oncol 8:S115–S118, 1997.

44. Horning SJ, Nademanee AP: Autologous hematopoietic cell transplantation for non-Hodgkin's lymphoma. In Thomas ED, Blume KG, Forman SJ (eds.): Hematopoietic Cell Transplantation, 2nd Ed., pp. 939–951, Blackwell Sciences, Boston, 1999.

45. Hoster HA, Dratman MB, Craver LF, Rolnick HA: Hodgkin's disease, 1832–1947. Cancer Res 8:49–78, 1948.

46. Hryniuk W, Bush H: The importance of dose intensity in chemotherapy of metastatic breast cancer. J Clin Oncol 2:1281–1288, 1984.

47. International Non-Hodgkin's Lymphoma Prognostic Factors Project: A predictive model for aggressive non-Hodgkin's lymphoma. N Engl J Med 329:987–994, 1993.

48. Isaacson P, & Wright DH: Malignant lymphoma of mucosa-associated lymphoid tissue: A distinctive type of B cell lymphoma. Cancer 52:1410–1416, 1978.

49. Issell BF, Rudolph AR, Louie A: Etoposide: Status and New Developments. Academic Press, New York, 1984.

50. Jackson HJ Jr, Parker F Jr: Hodgkin's Disease and Allied Disorders. Oxford University Press, New York, 1947.

51. Kaplan HS: The radical radiotherapy of Hodgkin's disease. Radiology 78:553–561, 1962.

52. Kaplan HS: Hodgkin's Disease. 2nd Ed. Harvard University Press, Cambridge, MA, 1980.

53. Kass AM, Kass FH: Perfecting the World: The Life and Times of Thomas Hodgkin (1798–1866). Harcourt Brace Jovanovich, Boston, 1988.

54. Kinmonth JD: Lymphangiography in man: Method of outlining lymphatic trunks and operation. Clin Sci 11:132–200, 1952.

55. Knowles DM: Neoplastic Hematopathology. Williams & Wilkins, Baltimore, 1992.

56. Korsmeyer SJ, Hieter PA, Ravetch JV, Poplack DG, Waldmann TA, Leder P: Developmental hierarchy of immunoglobulin gene rearrangements in human leukemia pre-B cells. Proc Natl Acad Sci USA 78:7096–7100, 1981.

57. Kundrat H: Uber lympho-sarkomatosis. Wien Klin Wochenschr 6:211–234, 1893.

58. Kuppers R, Rajewsky K: The origin of Hodgkin's and Reed-Sternberg cell in Hodgkin's disease. Ann Rev Immunol 16:471–493, 1998.

59. Kuppers R, Klein U, Hansmann M-L, Rajewsky K: Cellular origin of human B-cell lymphomas. N Engl J Med 342:1520–1529, 1999.

60. Lacher MJ, Durant J: Combined vinblastine and chlorambucil therapy of Hodgkin's disease. Ann Intern Med 62:468–476, 1965.

61. Land H, Parada LF, Weinberg RA: Cellular oncogenes and multistep carcinogenesis. Science 222:771–778, 1983.

62. Lennert K: Follicular lymphoma. A tumor of the germinal centers. In Akazaki K, Rappaport H, Berard CW, Bennett JM, Ishikawa E (eds.): Malignant Disease of the Hematopoietic System GANN Monograph on Cancer Research, Vol. 15, pp. 217–231. University of Tokyo Press, Tokyo, 1973.

63. Lennert K, Feller AC: Histopathology of Non-Hodgkin's Lymphoma (Based on the Updated Kiel Classification), 2nd Ed. Springer-Verlag, Berlin, 1992.

64. Lennert K, Mohri N, Kaiserling E, Hermelink HK: Malignant Lymphomas Other Than Hodgkin's Disease. Histology, Cytology, Ultrastructure, Immunology. Springer-Verlag, New York, 1978.

64a. Lennert K, Stein H, Kaiserling E: Cytological and functional criteria for the classificaiton of malignant lymphomata. Br J Cancer 31, Suppl II:29–43, 1975.

65. Lenoir GM: Role of the virus, chromosomal translocations and cellular oncogenes in the etiology of Burkitt's lymphoma. In Epstein MA, Achong BG (eds.): The Epstein-Barr Virus. Recent Advances, p. 183. Wiley, New York, 1986.

66. Lessner HE: BCNU (1,3 bis (beta-chloroethyl)-1-nitrosurea: Effects on advanced Hodgkin's disease and other neoplasms. Cancer 22:451–456, 1968.

67. Link MP, Shuster JJ, Donaldson SS, Berard CW, Murphy SB: Treatment of children and young adults with early stage non-Hodgkin's lymphoma. N Engl J Med 337:1259–1266, 1997.

68. Lister TA, Crowther D, Sutcliffe SB, Glatstein E, Canellos GP, Young RC et al: Report of a committee convened to discuss the evaluation and staging of patients with Hodgkin's disease: Cotswold Meeting. J Clin Oncol 7:1630–1636, 1989.

69. Lukes RJ, Butler JJ: The pathology and nomenclature of Hodgkin's disease. Cancer Res 26:1063–1081, 1966.

70. Lukes RJ, Collins RD: Immunologic characterization of human malignant lymphomas. Cancer 34:1488–1503, 1974.

71. Lukes RJ, Craver LF, Hall TC, Rappaport H, Rubin P: Report of the nomenclature committee. Cancer Res 26:1311, 1966.

72. McKelvey EM, Gottlieb JA, Wilson HE, Haut A, Talley RW, Stephens R et al: Hydroxyldaunomycin (Adriamycin) combination chemotherapy in malignant lymphoma. Cancer 38:1484–1493, 1976.

73. Manolov G, Manolova Y: Marker band in one chromosome 14 from Burkitt lymphoma. Nature 237:33–34, 1972.

74. Mathe G, Schweisguth O, Schneider M, Amiel JL, Berumen L, Brule G et al: Methyl-hydrazine in treatment of Hodgkin's disease. Lancet II:1077–1080, 1963.

75. Minden MD, Toyonaga B, Ha K, Yanagi Y, Chin B, Gelfand E, Mak T: Somatic rearrangement of T-cell antigen receptor genes in human T-cell malignancies. Proc Natl Acad Sci U S A 82:1224–1227, 1985.

76. National Cancer Institute Division of Cancer Control: Annual Cancer Statistics Review Including Cancer Trends: 1950–85. National Institutes of Health Publication, 88–2729: National Cancer Institute, Bethesda, Maryland, 1987.

77. Niedobitek G: The role of Epstein-Barr virus in the pathogenesis of Hodgkin's disease. Ann Oncol 7:S11–S17, 1996.

78. Niedobitek G, Young LS: Epstein-Barr virus and non-Hodgkin's lymphoma. In Magrath I (ed.): The Non-Hodgkin's Lymphomas, 2nd Ed., pp. 309–329. Arnold/Oxford University Press, London/New York, 1997.

79. Nobel RL, Beer CT, Cutts JH: Role of chance observation in chemotherapy. Ann N Y Acad Sci 76:882–894, 1958.

80. Offit K, Lo Coco F, Louie DC, Parsa NZ, Leung D, Portlock C et al: Rearrangement of the bcl-6 gene as a prognostic marker in diffuse large-cell lymphoma. N Engl J Med 331:74–80, 1994.

81. Penn I: Tumors after renal and cardiac transplantation. Hematol Oncol Clin North Am 7:421–445, 1993.

82. Peters MV: A study of survivals in Hodgkin's disease treated radiologically. Am J Roentgenol 63:299–311, 1950.

83. Peters MV, Middlemiss KHC: A study of Hodgkin's disease treated by radiation therapy. Am J Roentgenol 79:114–121.

84. Preud'homme J, Seligmann M: Surface bound immunoglobulin as a cell marker in human lymphoproliferative diseases. Blood 40:777–794, 1972.

85. Pusey WA: Cases of sarcoma and of Hodgkin's disease treated by exposure to x-rays: A preliminary report. JAMA 38:166–169, 1902.

86. Rappaport H, Winter WJ, Hicks EB: Follicular lymphoma. A reexamination of its position in the scheme of malignant lymphoma, based on a survey of 253 cases. Cancer 9:792–821, 1956.

87. Reed DM: On the pathological changes in Hodgkin's disease, with especial reference to its relation to tuberculosis. Johns Hopkins Hosp Rep 10:133–196, 1902.

88. Reis MD, Griesser H, Mak TW: T cell receptor and immunoglobulin gene rearrangements in lymphoproliferative disorders. Adv Cancer Res 52:45–80, 1989.

89. Reis LAG, Miller BA, Hankey BF, Kosary CL, Harras A, Edwards BK (eds.): SEER Cancer Statistics Review: 1973–1994. National Cancer Institute, NIH Publication 97-2789, 1997.

90. Reiter A, Schrappe M, Parwaresch R, Henze G, Muller-Weihrich S, Sauter S et al: Non-Hodgkin's lymphomas of childhood and adolescence: Results of a treatment stratified for biologic subtypes and stage—a report of the Berlin-Frankfort-Munster group. J Clin Oncol 13:359–372, 1995.

91. Rosenberg SA: Report of the committee on the staging of Hodgkin's disease. Cancer Res 26:1310, 1966.

92. Rosenberg SA, Berard CW, Brown BW Jr, Burke J, Dorfman RF, Glatstein E et al: National Cancer Institute sponsored study of classifications of non-Hodgkin's lymphomas: Summary and description of a working formulation for clinical usage. Cancer 49:2112–2135, 1982.

93. Rosenberg CL, Wong E, Petty EM, Bale AE, Tsujimoto Y, Harris NL, Arnold A: PRAD1, a candidate bcl-1: Mapping and expression in centrocytic lymphoma. Proc Natl Acad Sci U S A 88:9638–9642, 1991.

94. Roulet F: Das primare Retothelsarkom der Lymphknoten. Virch Arch Pathol Anat 277:15–47, 1930.

95. Rowley JD: Identification of the constant regions involved in human hematologic malignant disease. Science 216:751–753, 1982.

96. Sandlund JT, Downing JR, Crist WT: Non-Hodgkin's lymphoma in childhood. N Engl J Med 334:1238–1248, 1996.

97. Schwab U, Stein H, Gerdes J, Lanke H, Kirschner H, Schaadt M, Diehl V: Production of a monoclonal antibody specific for Hodgkin and Reed-Sternberg cells in Hodgkin's disease and a subset of normal lymphoid cells. Nature 299:65–67, 1982.

98. Sternberg C: Uber eine eigenartige unter dem Bilde der Pseudoleukamic verlaufende Tuberculose des lymphatischen Apparates. Ztchr Heilk 19:21–90, 1898.

99. Symmers D: Follicular lymphadenopathy with splenomegaly. A newly recognized disease of the lymphatic system. Arch Pathol Lab Med 3:816–820, 1927.

100. Taub R, Kirsch I, Morton C, Lenoir G, Swan D, Tronick S et al: Translocation of the c-myc gene into the immunoglobulin heavy chain locus in human Burkitt's lymphoma and murine plasmacytoma cells. Proc Natl Acad Sci U S A 79:7837–7841, 1982.

101. Thomas ED: Historical review: A history of hematopoietic cell transplantation. Br J Haematol 105:330–339, 1999.

102. Tsujimoto Y, Finger LR, Yunis J, Nowell PC, Croce CM: Cloning the breakpoint of neoplastic B cells with the t(14;18) chromosome translocation. Science 226:1098–1099, 1984.

103. Twomey JJ, Rice L: Impact of Hodgkin's disease on the immune system. Semin Oncol 7:114–125, 1980.

104. Uchiyama T, Yodoi J, Sagawa K, Takatsuki K, Uchino H: Adult T-cell leukemia, clinical and hematologic features of 16 cases. Blood 50:481–492, 1977.

105. Virchow R: Weisses Blut. Neue Notizen aus dem Gebiet der Natur-fund Heilkunde. Floriep's Neue Notizen 36:151, 1845.

106. Virchow R: Die Krankenhaften Geschwulste. In: Dreissig Vorlesungen gehalten wahrend des Wintersemestes (1862–1863) an der Universitat zu Berlin, Vol. 2, pp. 728–738. A Hirschwald, Berlin, 1864–1865.

107. Waldmann TA, Davis MM, Bongiovanni KF, Korsmeyer SJ: Rearrangements of genes for the antigen receptor on T cells as markers of lineage and clonality in human lymphoid neoplasms. N Engl J Med 313:776–783, 1985.

108. Whitelaw DM, Cowan D, Cassidy F, Patterson TA: Clinical experience with vincristine. Cancer Chemother Rep 32:19, 1963.

109. Wilks Sir S: Cases of lardaceous disease and some allied affections, with remarks. Guy's Hospital Reports, 17(Ser. II, 2):103–132, 1856.

110. Wilks Sir S: Cases of enlargement of the lymphatic glands and spleen (or, Hodgkin's disease), with remarks. Guy's Hospital Reports 11:56–67, 1865.

111. Wollner N, Burchenal JH, Lieberman PH, Exelby P, D'Angio G, Murphy ML: Non-Hodgkin's lymphoma in children. A comparison of two modalities of therapy. Cancer 37:123–134, 1976.

112. Wulczyn FG, Naumann M, Scheidereit C: Candidate proto-oncogene *bcl-3* encodes a subunit-specific inhibitor of transcription factor NF-kB. Nature 358:597–599, 1992.

113. Ye BH, Rao PH, Chaganti RSK, Dalla-Favera R: Cloning of *bcl-6*, the locus involved in chromosome translocations affecting band 3q37 in B-call lymphomas. Cancer Res 53:2732–2735, 1993.

113a. Yunis JJ: The chromosomal basis of neoplasia. Science 221: 227–236, 1983.

114. Zech L, Hoglund V, Nilsson K, Klein G: Characteristic chromosome abnormalities in biopsies and lymphoid-cell lines from patients with Burkitt and non-Burkitt lymphomas. Int J Cancer 17:47–56, 1976.

115. Ziegler JL, Bechstead JA, Volberding PA, Abrams DI, Levine AM, Lukes RJ et al: Non-Hodgkin's lymphoma in 90 homosexual men. Relation to generalized lymphadenopathy and to acquired immunodeficiency syndrome. N Engl J Med 311:565–570, 1984.

38

Genetic Factors in Lymphomagenesis

Januario E. Castro and Thomas J. Kipps

Different approaches have been used to characterize the cellular origin and molecular alterations in lymphomas. These approaches include histology, immunophenotyping, gene mapping, sequencing, and most recently DNA microarray technology. Some of the most frequent cytogenetic abnormalities have been characterized at the molecular level with the identification of genes that are altered in lymphoma cells. Most of these genetic lesions are associated with specific lymphoma subtypes and represent markers of potential diagnostic significance.[1] The recent use of microarray technology has allowed for a more complete assessment of gene dysregulation in lymphomagenesis and provided the means to define signature molecular hallmarks distinguishing new lymphoma subtypes.[2,3] This chapter will review the associated genetic changes implicated in B-cell lymphomagenesis.

GENETIC EVENTS INVOLVED IN LYMPHOMAGENESIS

As in other types of cancer, the events leading to the development of a lymphoma define a multistep process, in which "genetic hits" converge and at some point overcome the balance between cell survival and cell death. These genetic hits generally alter the expression of oncogenes or tumor suppressor genes. In contrast to solid tumors, lymphomas generally lack microsatellite instability, which suggests that these tumors can engage in physiologic DNA repair.[4]

Chromosomal Translocations

The most frequently found genetic alterations in lymphomas are single nonrandom chromosomal translocations. These translocations move genes from one chromosome to another, sometimes generating a new fusion gene or dysregulating a gene(s) flanking the sites of chromosomal translocation.[5] These translocations are called homotopic if they dysregulate genes that ordinarily are expressed by B cells, or heterotopic if they dysregulate expression of genes not used by normal B cells. Proto-oncogenes on other chromosomes often are found in close proximity to the sites of chromosomal recombination. The structure of such proto-oncogenes generally is not affected by the translocation. However, the expression of the proto-oncogene often becomes dysregulated, allowing it to play a role in lymphomagenesis.

Abnormal immunoglobulin gene rearrangement is the cause of many translocations.[6] Immunoglobulin gene rearrangement and isotype switch recombination requires extensive modifications of the germline DNA because of a process involving double-stranded DNA breaks.[7] Although isotype switch recombination generally involves recombination events between genes on the same chromosome, rare examples of allelic switch recombination have been observed, indicating that interchromosomal switch recombination can occur.[8] Breaks occurring on separate chromosomes during such events as isotype switch recombination can result in translocations. This process, coupled with that of somatic mutation, places the normal B cell at risk for incurring translocation between the immunoglobulin genes and other genes that are expressed on other chromosomes. As such, many translocations in B-cell lymphomas have translocations involving chromosomes 14, 2, or 22, the chromosomes on which the immunoglobulin genes reside.

Tumor Suppressor Genes

Somatic mutations in nonimmunoglobulin tumor suppressor genes also can contribute to the development or progression of lymphomas. Loss of heterozygosity due to deletions is not uncommon for many lymphomas. Examples of this are the deletion of chromosome 13q14 seen in small-cell lymphocytic lymphoma and chronic lymphocytic leukemia (CLL).[9] Another single chromosome deletion frequently found in lymphomas is loss of genetic material on the short arm of chromosome 6 (6q).[10,11] However, the most important of these involve mutations that inactivate or delete the tumor suppressor gene *P53*. Mutations in *P53* are seen in Burkitt's lymphoma and its leukemic counterpart, L3-type B-cell acute lymphoblastic leukemia. Although unusual at the onset, advanced cases of B cell CLL or cases undergoing transformation into high-grade lymphomas often are found to have mutations that delete this gene.[12] Also, *P53* mutations, although rare in new-onset follicular lymphomas, are found in approximately 30 percent of cases undergoing transformation to large-cell lymphoma. Such alterations frequently are associated with more aggressive disease and/or resistance to conventional therapy.[13,14]

Oncogenic Viruses

Three viruses that have been implicated in the development of lymphomas are Epstein-Barr virus (EBV), human T-cell lymphotropic virus I (HTLV-I), and human herpesvirus-8 (HHV-8). Whereas EBV and HHV-8 have been found to play a role in B-cell lymphomagenesis, HTLV-I has been implicated in the pathogenesis of adult T-cell lymphoma/leukemia (ATLL), particularly endemic cases seen in the Caribbean and Japan.[15,16]

Epstein-Barr virus is associated with three subtypes of lymphoma (acquired immunodeficiency syndrome [AIDS]-associated lymphomas and endemic and sporadic Burkitt's lymphoma). The virus was identified at first in cases of endemic

Burkitt's lymphoma from Africa[17] and later on in sporadic Burkitt's lymphoma and human immunodeficiency virus (HIV)-related lymphoma.[18] The relation of EBV to these malignancies varies from primary etiologic agent to necessary or contributory cofactor. On the one hand, EBV is able to significantly alter the growth of B cells, and on the other hand, in an indirect way infection with the virus can produce immunological alterations that foster the development of lymphoma.[19] Evidence for EBV infection of a single B cell that subsequently undergoes neoplastic transformation can be identified by looking for a viral episomal signature that is common to all the cells within the lymphoma.[19] Most malignancies occur after years of viral dormancy and are accompanied or triggered by viral reactivation, in contrast to infectious mononucleosis, which results from primary infection with EBV. The EBV-associated malignancies offer insights into the causation and early detection of cancer.[20]

Another member of the Herpesviridae family is HHV-8, which originally was found in patients with Kaposi's sarcoma. Subsequently HHV-8 was implicated in body cavity-based lymphomas (BCBL).[21] Tissue samples have demonstrated the presence of viral genome from HHV-8 in virtually all cases of BCBL.[22]

GENETIC ABNORMALITIES SEEN IN SPECIFIC LYMPHOMA TYPES

Low Grade Lymphomas

Chronic Lymphocytic Leukemia and Small-Cell Lymphocytic Lymphoma

The leukemia B cells of patients with chronic lymphocytic leukemia (CLL) can be classified into one of at least two major subgroups based on the mutational status of their expressed immunoglobulin (Ig) variable (V) genes.[23,24] Patients with CLL cells that express nonmutated genes tend to have a relatively aggressive clinical course when compared with patients who have CLL cells that express Ig V genes with somatic mutations.[24–26] Moreover, patients with leukemia cells that express nonmutated Ig V genes generally are more likely to have atypical cell morphology, advanced clinical stage, and progressive disease. Studies on the gene expression profiles of isolated CLL B cells have revealed a set of genes that is differentially expressed between these two subgroups.[27,28] Nevertheless, the gene expression profiles of these two subtypes have much more in common with each other than with those of normal blood B cells or other B-cell malignancies, except small-cell lymphocytic lymphoma (SLL).

Both CLL and SLL cells have genomes that are relatively stable compared with those of epithelial malignancies or even other B-cell malignancies. Cells of CLL lack microsatellite instability, which is a common signature of DNA mismatch repair. Defects in the P53 gene are relatively infrequent in CLL and SLL compared with other types of cancers. Also, translocations involving immunoglobulin genes are relatively rare in CLL and SLL.[27]

Instead, deletions are the most frequent genetic abnormality, followed by trisomy 12. Because the deletions are generally small, most genetic abnormalities in CLL may not be detectable by standard cytogenetic techniques.[29] Use of newer cytogenetic techniques reveals clonal aberrations in more than 80 percent of cases.[30] The most frequent aberrations are deletions involving the long arm of chromosome 13 (13q), which occur in more than half of all cases. This is followed in order of relative frequency by trisomy 12, deletions in 11q, deletions in 17p, and deletions in 6q.

A current concept is that some of these genetic lesions are involved in the pathogenesis of CLL, whereas others contribute to disease progression.[31] At diagnosis, CLL cells generally have relatively few detectable genetic changes. Over time, the clone of leukemia cells can accumulate additional genetic changes, which potentially alter its biological and clinical behavior. Eventually, one or more subpopulations may emerge that contribute to clinical progression or development of features associated with advanced stages of this disease.

Chromosome 13 Deletions in CLL/SLL
Deletions at 13q are the most common genetic abnormality in CLL, being detectable in 50 to 80 percent of all cases. These deletions generally occur in the absence of chromosome translocation.[32] Deletions typically occur at 13q14.3, particularly in a region that is telomeric to the retinoblastoma gene RB-1 and centromeric to and including the D13S25 marker. A tumor suppressor gene, referred to as DBM (for Disrupted in B cell Malignancies), is hypothesized to reside in this region.[33–36]

Several genes that are subject to deletion and reside in close proximity to the area of 13q14 have been identified. These include LEU1, LEU2, and LEU5,[37,38] the first two of which have characteristics that make them less likely to be the genes responsible for tumorigenesis in CLL. These genes have small open reading frames that are not conserved in evolution. Instead, they have no known homology with other genes and may encode one or more sterile transcripts. Additionally, LEU1 and LEU2 have been analyzed in 20 patients with monoallelic deletion or no deletions at 13q14. These genes did not harbor any somatic mutations or genetic polymorphisms.[39] Another gene identified in this region, LEU5, also is not mutated, even in cases with deletions at 13q14. These data suggest that these genes may not play a role in the pathogenesis of CLL.

Analysis of a larger region at band q14.3 on chromosome 13 identified another gene, CLL-1, which appears to be mutated in over 80 percent of CLL cases. This gene appears highly conserved through evolution. A mouse counterpart to CLL-1 has been isolated, allowing for generation of mouse models in which the gene is disrupted to determine whether it can function as a tumor suppressor gene. In addition, studies are ongoing to identify the localization, structure, and function of the gene product in normal lymphoid cells and in CLL. Although definite proof is lacking, the data currently suggest that CLL-1 is the gene on chromosome 13 that is involved in the pathogenesis of many cases of CLL.[40]

Trisomy 12 in CLL/SLL
Trisomy 12 was the first abnormality found in CLL. The incidence varies from series to series, apparently for technical reasons.[41,42] A few patients with trisomy 12 also carry other chro-

mosomal abnormalities, including trisomy of chromosome 18 or 19.[43] Trisomy 12 is more frequently found in leukemia cells that have atypical morphology and relatively high levels of surface immunoglobulin and that express nonmutated immunoglobulin variable-region genes (Ig V genes).[44] In addition, trisomy 12 has been associated with a greater tendency toward disease progression.[45] Conceivably, a single oncogene on chromosome 12 also is involved in the pathogenesis of CLL.

Chromosome 11 Deletions in CLL/SLL
Approximately 10 to 20 percent of CLL patients have deletions in the long arm of chromosome 11, termed 11q–,[46,47] particularly at 11q23. Patients with CLL cells that have 11q deletions tend to be younger and to have lower hemoglobin levels, more advanced Rai stages, and more aggressive disease than patients without such abnormalities. A remarkable feature of these patients is a large lymphadenopathy that appears disproportionate with tumor burden. A multivariate analysis revealed that 11q deletion was an independent risk factor of prognostic significance.[46]

There are several candidate genes that map to 11q23. These include Radixin (RDX), PPP2R1B (the gene coding for the beta-isoform of the A subunit of the serine threonine phosphatase 2A), interleukin-1-beta convertase, and the caspases 1, 4, and 5.[48,49] However, the lead candidate gene is *ATM* (for ataxia-telangiectasia mutated). Inherited defects in both alleles of ATM are responsible for the autosomal recessive disease ataxia telangiectasia, which has a high predisposition to malignancies, particularly T-cell neoplasms such as T-cell prolymphocytic leukemia.[50] When DNA damage occurs, the normal *ATM* gene plays an important role in the activation of the tumor suppressor gene-product *P53*, leading to cell-cycle arrest and DNA repair.[51] Mutations of the *ATM* gene in CLL, as it is seen in cases with *P53* mutation, correlate with relatively aggressive behavior.[52,53] This gene maps to chromosomal region 11q22.3-23.1, is 150 kb in length, consists of 66 exons, and encodes a nuclear phosphoprotein of approximately 350 kD.

P53 Mutations in CLL/SLL
The *P53* gene is located on the short arm of chromosome 17 at 17p13.1 and encodes a 53-kd nuclear phosphoprotein that plays a central role in the regulation of the cell cycle.[54] Damage to the cell's DNA results in rapid upregulation of the P53 protein, which in turn induces p21/WAF1, an inhibitor of cyclin-dependent kinases. As such, expression of P53 results in inhibition of cyclin-dependent kinase activity, failure to phosphorylate key substrates such as the retinoblastoma protein, and consequent cell-cycle arrest at the G1 checkpoint, allowing the cell to repair DNA damages. As testament to its importance in cell cycle regulation, inactivating mutations in the *P53* gene have been found in nearly half of all human cancers.[55]

There is a direct link between ATM and P53. ATM can activate P53 by phosphorylating specific serine residues of the P53 protein.[51] Because P53 activity is influenced by the kinase activity of the ATM protein, mutations in ATM, as discussed in the section on chromosome 11 abnormalities, also can lead to P53 dysfunction. Moreover, mutations in both genes are likely to define a genetic high-risk group of CLL patients.

Deletions and mutations in P53 generally appear to be acquired during the course of the disease. Deletions in the short arm of chromosome 17, in and around *P53,* have been noted in leukemia cells from approximately 7 to 15 percent of patients. A similar proportion of patients is noted to have leukemic cells with mutations in the *P53* gene. These mutations commonly occur in the highly conserved exons 4 through 8 of the *P53* gene, and often are associated with loss of heterozygosity for chromosome 17p.[56] Patients who have CLL cells with *P53* mutations generally have more advanced disease, a higher leukemia-cell proliferative rate, a shorter survival, and greater resistance to chemotherapy.[57,58]

BCL-2 Overexpression in CLL/SLL
Chronic lymphocytic leukemia cells express high *BCL-2* levels. However, only 5 percent of CLL patients have immunoglobulin gene rearrangements with the *BCL-2* proto-oncogene.[59–61] Such rearrangements generally occur at breakpoints in the 5′ end of the *BCL-2* gene and involve the lambda or kappa immunoglobulin light chain genes.[59] Independently of *BCL-2* gene rearrangement, however, the leukemic cells from virtually all patients express levels of the *Bcl-2* protein that are comparable with those noted for lymphoma cells carrying the t(14;18)(q32q21) translocation.[62,63]

The high-level expression of *BCL-2* in CLL is associated with hypomethylation at the *BCL-2* locus.[64] Also, one study using pulsed-field gel electrophoresis found alterations in the large stretches of CLL cell DNA on chromosome 18 that contain the *BCL-2* gene. These studies suggest that there may be previously undetected genetic abnormalities in CLL involving chromosome 18 that may be responsible for the high-level expression of the *BCL-2* gene. Regardless of the underlying cause, the high-level expression of *BCL-2* accounts at least in part for the relative resistance of leukemia cells to cytotoxic drugs and other mechanisms of induced apoptosis.[65] Overexpression of *Bcl-2* may play a role in disease progression and resistance to treatment in patients with CLL. In one study, 80 percent of patients with stage C disease overexpressed Bcl-2, whereas only 33 and 29 percent of patients with stages A and B, respectively, had highly elevated levels of this protein.[65–67]

Follicular lymphoma

BCL-2 Translocations in Follicular Lymphoma
The most frequent genetic alterations found in follicular lymphoma (FL) are *BCL-2* translocations and chromosomal mutations at 18q21. Alterations in the expression of *BCL-2* result from the translocations t(14;18)(q32;q21) and some rare variants t(2;18)(p11;q21), t(18;22)(q21;q21) that represent basically biologic equivalents. These alterations result in dysregulated high-level expression of *Bcl-2* protein in lymphoma cells.

Virtually all FL and a fraction of diffuse large B-cell lymphomas (DLBCL) have breaks at 18q21.[68,69] In these translocations, the chromosomal breakpoints of the immunoglobulin loci are located at the 5′ end of J (or sometimes D) heavy-chain gene segments. These aberrant DNA rearrangements reflect mistakes of V(D)J recombination, a process that is mediated by the recombination-activating genes (RAG1-RAG2).[70] These proteins, RAG1 and RAG2, initiate V(D)J recombination by making a double-strand break between the recombination signal sequence (RSS) and the neighboring coding DNA. Inappropriate diversion of the V(D)J segments can result in subsequent misrearrangement of these sequences into a transpositional pathway.[71] Although initially thought restricted to B-cell precursors in the marrow, such rearrangements occasionally can take place in germinal-center B cells.[72]

The result of t(14;18) translocation is a hybrid formed by *BCL-2* and the immunoglobulin heavy chain. The transcripts that are produced consist of the 5′ half of the *bcl-2* mRNA fused to an incomplete fragment of immunoglobulin heavy chain mRNA. The t(14;18) translocations alter expression of the *BCL-2* gene both by transcriptional activation and by abnormal post-transcriptional regulation of *BCL-2* mRNA.[73] Consequently, B cell lymphomas with a t(14;18) have much higher levels of *BCL-2* mRNA than matched counterparts without such translocations,[68] and they express high levels of the *Bcl-2* protein. This protein is located on mitochondria, endoplasmic reticulum, and perinuclear membranes and serves as a major inhibitor of apoptosis.[74] The bcl-2 protein couples with Bax, another apoptotic protein, forming a heterodimer. The ratio of *bcl-2* to Bax is related to the lymphoma cell's relative resistance to apoptosis.[75] Nevertheless, studies on *BCL-2* transgenic mice indicate that high-level expression of *Bcl-2* is not sufficient for lymphoma genesis, suggesting that other genetic lesions are required for lymphomagenesis.[76]

Other genetic lesions in Follicular Lymphoma
Other genetic lesions are found in a high proportion of follicular lymphomas. As noted, P53 mutations can be found, particularly during late stages of disease that are associated with resistance to chemotherapy and poor progonosis.[77,78] Deletions in chromosome 6q have been found in approximately 20 percent of cases. The most common genetic lesions map in different areas of the long arm of chromosome 6, including two distinct regions of minimal deletion (RMD) at 6q25 to 6q27 (RMD-1) and at 6q21 to 6q23 (RMD-2). Conceivably these regions harbor one or more tumor-suppressor genes.[79]

Another genetic alteration observed in follicular lymphoma is the rearrangement of 1q21-23 through the balanced translocation t(1;22)(q22;q11). Also 1q21-23 rearrangements arise during lymphoma evolution and accompany disease-specific chromosomal rearrangements such as t(8;14)*(MYC)* and t(14;18)*(Bcl-2)*. This type of rearrangement has been found in up to 10 percent of follicular lymphomas and leads to the deregulated expression of FcγRIIB.[80,81] FcγRIIB is involved in regulating B-cell proliferation, but the exact mechanism in lymphomagenesis is still unclear.

Lymphoplasmacytoid Lymphomas

Lymphoplasmacytoid lymphoma (REAL classification) is characterized by small lymphoid cells that show maturation to plasmacytes.[1] These tumor cells express pan-B-cell markers such as CD19 and CD20 and generally do not express CD5.[82] Often this type of lymphoma expresses a monoclonal serum immunoglob-

ulin paraprotein, typically IgM, causing the clinical syndrome known as Waldenström's macroglobulinemia.[83]

The t(9;14)(p13;q32) translocation, detected in approximately 50 percent of lymphoplasmacytoid lymphoma cases, has been implicated in the pathogenesis of this disorder. This translocation causes the juxtaposition of the *PAX-5* gene to the IgH locus in the opposite direction of transcription, with subsequent deregulation and overexpression of *PAX-5* mRNA mediated by IgH regulatory elements.

A significantly reduced expression of the P53 gene also is seen, possibly as a consequence of dysregulated *PAX-5* gene expression.[84] *PAX-5,* in conjunction with other genes such as *E2A* and *BSAP,* encodes a transcription factor that binds to B-cell-specific promoters and enhancers and guides the development of immature but committed cells into mature B lymphocytes that express and secrete immunoglobulins. These genes regulate distinct classes of genes during B-cell differentiation. Recent studies using targeted gene disruption and transgene expression in mice have indicated that these genes may actually be components of a single regulatory mechanism that is essential for both B-cell differentiation and proliferation.[85]

Intermediate and High-Grade Lymphomas

Mantle-Cell Lymphoma

Mantle-cell lymphoma (MCL) accounts for approximately 25 percent of nonfollicular small B-cell lymphomas and encompasses many of the cases that previously were classified as diffuse poorly differentiated lymphocytic lymphoma (Rappaport), centrocytic lymphoma (Kiel), intermediate differentiated lymphocytic lymphoma (modified Rappaport), or diffuse small cleaved-cell lymphoma (WF).[1] These lymphomas are usually widespread at diagnosis with generalized adenopathy and often involve the blood and marrow. These tumors also involve the gastrointestinal tract with high frequency and in some cases can cause lymphomatous polyposis.[86,87] Unlike other small B-cell lymphomas, this particular disease is associated with an aggressive clinical course.[88]

Mantle-cell lymphoma cells often express surface IgM and IgD and have a disproportionate amount of lambda light chains. These cells typically express CD5 and other pan-B-cell antibodies such as CD19, CD20, and CD22. However, MCL cells are characteristically negative for CD10 and CD23, in contrast to cells of follicular lymphomas and chronic lymphocytic leukemia, respectively.[89]

BCL-1 Expression in Mantle-Cell Lymphoma
Over half of MCL cases show evidence of t(11,14)(q13;q32). Moreover, nearly half of all cases of mantle zone lymphoma have deletions or alterations at 11q.[90,91] Translocation or mutation at 11q can leads to homotopic deregulation of BCL-1 (also known as CCND1 or PRAD1).[92] *BCL-1* encodes cyclin D1, and overexpression of this protein is a hallmark feature of MCL.[93–95] Cyclin D1 is a protein that regulates the early events of the cell cycle, participates in regulation of cellular activation, and plays a role in the events leading to extension of the replicative life span and immortalization in a telomerase-independent fash-

ion.[92,96] The pathogenetic role of cyclin D1 overexpression in human neoplasia is suggested by its ability to transform cells in vitro and contribute to B-cell lymphoma genesis in transgenic mice, particularly when overexpressed in conjunction with other oncogenes such as c-MYC.[97,98]

A subset of patients with P53 mutations may have more progressive disease and an adverse prognosis.[99] This association is still controversial; another study found that there was no correlation between P53 mutations, the presence of a BCL-1 translocation, and the proliferative activity of neoplastic MCL cells. It is possible that these markers may demonstrate independent events that occur during the pathogenesis of MCL.[100]

Chromosome 11 Abnormalities in Mantle-Cell Lymphoma

Another chromosomal alteration frequently seen in MCL is deletion of 11q22-q23.[90,91] This segment contains the ataxia-telangiectasia mutated (ATM) gene. In one study, loss of chromosome 11 material was observed in 37 (46 percent) of the 81 MCL cases. The consensus deletion comprised YAC (yeast artificial chromosome) 801e11 containing the ATM gene. The minimal region of loss was further narrowed with P1-derived artificial chromosome (PAC) probes. This allowed the identification of a deletion confined to the genomic region of ATM.[91] Another study also found a deletion of one ATM gene copy in 7 out of 12 sporadic cases of MCL. In all seven cases containing a deletion of one ATM allele, a point mutation in the remaining allele was detected, which resulted in aberrant transcript splicing, truncation, or alteration of the protein. In addition, biallelic ATM mutations were identified in two MCLs that did not contain 11q deletions. Interestingly, in three cases analyzed, the ATM mutations detected in the tumor cells were not present in nonmalignant cells, which demonstrates their somatic rather than germ-line origin. The inactivation of both alleles of the ATM gene by deletion and deleterious point mutation in the majority of cases analyzed indicates that inactivation of ATM as a tumor suppressor gene plays a role in the initiation and/or progression of MCL.[90]

Diffuse Large B-Cell Lymphoma

Diffuse large B-cell lymphoma (DLBCL) accounts for about 40 percent of all cases of lymphoma. Over 70 percent of cases seen in normal adults but only 20 percent of AIDS-related cases appear to have rearrangements involving the BCL-6 gene at 3q27.[101,102] Several reciprocal translocations bring chromosomal fragments to the proximity of 3q27. These include mainly 14q32, 2p11, and 22q11, the sites of the immunoglobulin heavy and kappa and lambda light chains, respectively.[103] In most cases the gene is altered by multiple, often biallelic, mutations clustering in its 5′ noncoding region. These mutations frequently can occur independently of translocation to immunoglobulin loci, and in the absence of any recognizable chromosomal abnormality affecting band 3q27 or rearrangement of the BCL-6 locus.[104]

The BCL-6 Gene

The BCL-6 protein regulates germinal-center (GC) B-cell differentiation and inflammation. Its gene was cloned from 3q27 breakpoints and encodes a 95-kd transcriptional repressor protein containing six C-terminal zinc-finger motifs and an N-terminal POZ domain.[105,106] The gene is truncated within its 5′ noncoding sequences, which suggests that its expression is deregulated secondary to the juxtaposition of heterologous promoters by a mechanism of promoter substitution. Dysregulated expression of BCL-6 likely contributes to lymphomagenesis.[34,103,107]

Recently, using DNA microarray screening some of the genes repressed by expression of BCL-6 have been identified. These include lymphocyte activation genes, such as CD69, CD44, EBI2, Id2, and STAT1, which suggests that BCL-6 modulates B-cell receptor signals. Also, BCL-6 represses expression of two chemokine genes, MIP-1α and IP-10, which can play a role in attenuating inflammatory immune responses. Another BCL-6 target is Blimp-1, an important molecule for plasmacytic differentiation. Together, our current knowledge about Bcl-6 suggests that malignant transformation by this protein involves inhibition of differentiation and enhanced proliferation mediated by a series of gene repression steps.[106]

The BCL-6 gene is expressed in GC B cells but not in post-GC elements like plasma or memory B cells. It is thought to play a role in the regulation of GC-associated functions. Downregulation of this molecule appears necessary for B cells to progress beyond the GC stage of B cell differentiation, as differentiation is inhibited by translocations or mutations involving BCL-6.[104,108] Disruption of BCL-6 in mice by homologous recombination leads to absence of GCs and impaired T cell-dependent antibody response, indicating that BCL-6 is required for GC formation.[109]

There are strong indications that BCL-6 rearrangement is an independent prognostic factor in DLBCL. This is supported by the observation that some cytogenetic markers of disease progression, including trisomy 7, trisomy 12, del(6)(q21;q25), and structural alterations of 17p, are less frequent in cases of DLBCL with BCL-6 rearrangement.[110] Additionally, significantly higher survival rates have been described for those patients with Ig/Bcl-6 compared with Non-Ig/BCL-6 fusion proteins.[111] Moreover, cases associated with BCL-6 rearrangements appear to have a more favorable prognosis, whereas cases carrying BCL-2 translocations had the poorest outcome. A third group of patients without rearrangements of BCL-6 and BCL-2, displayed an intermediate prognosis.[112]

Studies using complementary DNA microarray-generated gene expression profiles have identified two categories of DLBCL with distinctive gene expression profiles.[113] One corresponds to cells that have similarities to GC B cells, whereas the other has features in common with those of proliferating B cells. Some chromosomal abnormalities are associated primarily with one or the other subgroup. For example, the t(14;18) was detected in 7 (20 percent) of 35 cases of DLBCL. All 7 t(14;18)-positive cases had a GC B-cell gene expression profile. In contrast, the expression of Bcl-2 and Bcl-6 proteins was not significantly different between the cases with or without t(14;18), whereas expression of CD10 was most frequent in the cases with t(14;18).[114] As such, it appears that t(14;18) contributes to the pathogenesis of the GC B-cell type of DLBCL with enhanced expression of CD10.[114]

Other genetic lesions seen in DLBCL include mutations in *C-MYC*, an oncogene more commonly associated with Burkitt's lymphoma. This has been observed in approximately 60 percent of patients with DLBCL. Patients with translocations involving *c-MYC* appear to have a particularly poor prognosis.[115] About half of the cases in DLBCL carry aberrant hypermutation at the level of multiple other genes. Those include the proto-oncogenes *PIM1*, *MYC*, *rho/TTF (ARHH)*, and *PAX5*. More than 50 percent of DLBCL cases can have an aberrant hypermutation activity targeting these loci. These mutations are not detectable in normal GC B cells or in other GC-derived lymphomas, which suggests that there may be a malfunction of somatic hypermutation in these cases of DLBCL.[116]

Burkitt's Lymphoma

The molecular hallmark of Burkitt's lymphoma (BL) is genetic alteration involving 8q24 with deregulation of the proto-oncogene *c-MYC*. This genetic alteration is present in all the variants of BL, including sporadic and endemic, and the leukemic form L3 of acute lymphoblastic leukemia.[116–118]

c-MYC in Burkitt's Lymphoma

Translocations in BL involve 8q24 and one of the immunoglobulin gene complexes on chromosome 14, 2, or 22. The most common, accounting for 80 percent of the cases, is t(8;14)(q24;q32) involving breakpoints located at the 5′ position and centromeric to *c-MYC*. In the endemic form of BL, the genetic regions involved in t(8;14) are located at a considerable distance from the 5′ end of *c-MYC* in proximity to the immunoglobulin heavy chain J region on chromosome 14.[118] On the other hand, in the sporadic form of BL, the breakpoints are located proximal to the 5′ *c-MYC* and involves the immunoglobulin isotype switch regions on chromosome 14.[119] The remaining 20 percent of BL cases have t(2;8)(p11;q24), involving immunoglobulin kappa light chain genes (15 percent), or t(8;22)(q24;q11), involving immunoglobulin lambda light-chain genes (5 percent).[120]

The translocation of *c-MYC* dysregulates the transcription of this gene. Translocation may place expression of *c-MYC* under the control of immunoglobulin enhancer elements that upregulate its expression. Alternatively, *c-MYC* may harbor somatic mutations in the 5′ regulatory regions, causing alterations in the response to cellular factors that regulate *c-MYC* expression, even in the absence of translocation.[121]

The *c-MYC* gene encodes a ubiquitous phosphoprotein, which functions as a transcriptional factor that influences cell proliferation, differentiation, or apoptosis. The carboxyl terminus of Myc family proteins contains a basic region that has DNA-binding activity and that mediates protein–protein interactions. In vivo, *c-MYC* is found mainly in heterodimeric complexes with the related protein Max. The Myc-Max complexes bind to DNA in a sequence-specific manner under conditions in which neither Max nor Myc exhibits appreciable binding.[122.] The activity of Max is regulated by a pair of associated proteins, MXI1 and MAD. These proteins compete with Myc for binding to Max, thus generating intracellular regulation of Myc–Max availability. In lymphomas carrying *c-MYC* translocations, the constitutive expression of *c-MYC* leads to the prevalence of Myc–Max complexes over Mad–Max and MXI1–Max heterodimers, thus inducing positive growth regulation.[123,124]

In some cases the function of Myc protein is altered in lymphomas owing to somatic mutation in the absence of translocations. Amino acid substitutions in the transactivation domain, for example as caused by mutations in the second exon of *c-MYC*, may render the protein oncogenic. Many of the observed mutations are clustered in regions associated with transcriptional activation and apoptosis and occur at sites of phosphorylation, which suggests that this mutation have a pathogenetic role.[121] These mutations induce alterations of the amino-terminal transactivation domain required for *c-MYC* to function as a transcription factor controlling cell proliferation; they also disrupt the binding site for p107, a nuclear protein related to the *RB1* tumor suppressor gene that modulates the activity of the *c-MYC*.[123,125]

In stably transfected human B-lymphoblastoid cell lines, overexpressed c-Myc and Max act synergistically to cause malignant transformation, whereas overexpression of Max alone leads to growth inhibition, indicating that the c-Myc and Max are transcriptional regulators with the ability to oppositely regulate target-gene expression and cell proliferation.[124]

Other Genetic Alterations in Burkitt's Lymphoma

P53 gene mutations and/or deletions occur in 30 percent of sporadic and endemic BL cases. As such, *P53* alterations in addition to *c-MYC* oncogene activation probably plays a role in BL and its leukemic form, L3-type B-cell acute lymphoblastic leukemia, particularly in disease progression.[12] Another common finding is deletions of 6q, which are detected in approximately 30 percent of the BL cases regardless of the clinical variant,[79] and EBV infection, present in virtually all cases of endemic BL and in approximately 30 percent of sporadic BL cases. When present in BL, EBV exhibits a characteristic latent infection phenotype that consists of expression of latent infection-associated proteins EBNA-1, EBNA-2, and LMP1.[126]

AIDS-Associated Lymphomas

Approximately 5 percent of adult patients with acquired immunodeficiency syndrome (AIDS) develop lymphoma.[120,121] Patients with AIDS have a 20- to 70-fold increased risk of developing lymphoma when compared with age-matched, noninfected adults. This increased risk appears inversely proportional to the number of blood CD4 lymphocytes.[127,128] Additionally, AIDS lymphoma occurs almost exclusively in patients with CD4 cell counts of less than 50 per microliter.

Human immunodeficiency virus (HIV) appears to play an indirect role in B-cell lymphomagenesis. Thus, B-cell lymphomas may develop as a consequence of HIV's effects on host immune regulation. These HIV-related immune alterations include defects in immunosurveillance mediated by T cells and natural killer (NK) cells, chronic antigen stimulation by HIV and opportunistic infectious organisms, and cytokine dysregulation. AIDS-associated lymphomas may result from a series of steps that start with expansion and proliferation of oligoclonal B cells at the early stages of the disease, followed by accumulation of genetic lesions that induce neoplastic transformation.[129]

AIDS-related lymphomas generally are derived from B cells and are classified into two main groups: AIDS-related BL (AIDS-BL) and AIDS-related DLBCL (AIDS-DLBCL).[129] Further subdivisions into defined groups are based on clinical, pathological, and genetic characteristics.[130–133] T-Cell lymphomas are rare and have an incidence that appears similar to that in persons not infected with HIV.[134]

AIDS-Burkitt Lymphoma

In AIDS-Burkitt lymphoma the B cells histologically resemble GC B cells. These cases are characterized by relatively mild immunodeficiency, and multiple genetic lesions of the tumor, including activation of c-MYC and P53 mutations. On rare occasions those tumors are infected by EBV and when infected do not express the viral transforming antigens latent membrane protein-1 (LMP-1) and EBV nuclear antigen-2 (EBNA-2). The infrequent rate of infection with EBV closely mimics that of sporadic BL of the immunocompetent host rather than endemic BL.

AIDS-Diffuse Large Cell Lymphomas

AIDS-diffuse large-cell lymphomas (DLCL) are frequently characterized by a marked disruption of immune function. The majority of these cases are EBV-positive, with only a fraction of cases expressing the viral antigen LMP-1. The viral genotype of those patients infected with EBV does not differ from control individuals of both immunocompetent and immunocompromised populations.[135]

Patients with AIDS-DLBCL can be subdivided into two groups based on the expression of LMP-1 and BCL-6. The ones that express LMP-1 and are negative for BCL-6 display features similar to immunoblastic tumors, which suggests that they derive from post-GC cells. On the other hand, the subgroup that is LMP-1-negative and BCL-6-positive displays a large noncleaved cell morphology, suggesting a GC cell origin.

Body Cavity-Based Lymphoma

A very particular AIDS-associated lymphoma is body cavity based lymphoma (BCBL), also known as primary effusion lymphoma (PEL). The main localization of lymphoma involvement is in the pleural, peritoneal, or pericardial space. The lymphoma cells best resemble post-GC B cells. In these cases a very strong prevalence of infection with human herpesvirus-8 (HHV-8) has been described.[21] This disease, BCBL, has been instrumental in determining the genomic sequence of HHV-8, as well as in establishing the expression pattern and function of several of the genes harbored by the virus. In addition, manipulation of BCBL cell lines by induction of lytic phase infection has allowed the grouping of HHV-8 genes into different classes depending on whether they are expressed in the latent or lytic phase.[129]

Genetic lesions commonly detected among other AIDS-lymphoma cases are rare in AIDS-associated BCBL. Trisomy 7, trisomy 12, and breaks at 1q21-q25 have been described in the context of AIDS-BCBL. The lymphoma cells of such cases consistently coexpress the Met tyrosine kinase receptor and its ligand-receptor, hepatocyte growth factor (HGF). Among aggressive B-cell lymphomas, Met/HGF coexpression appears to be relatively specific for AIDS-associated BCBL. The expression of Met/HGF by AIDS-BCBL cells may have implications for the lymphoma proliferation and growth pattern, since Met/HGF interactions influence cell growth and proliferation.[136]

REFERENCES

1. Harris NL, Jaffe ES, Diebold J, Flandrin G, Muller-Hermelink HK, Vardiman J, Lister TA, Bloomfield CD: World Health Organization classification of neoplastic diseases of the hematopoietic and lymphoid tissues: Report of the Clinical Advisory Committee meeting – Airlie House, Virginia, November 1997. J Clin Oncol 17:3835–49, 1999.

2. Siebert R, Rosenwald A, Staudt LM, Morris SW: Molecular features of B-cell lymphoma. Curr Opin Oncol 13:316–24, 2001.

3. Staudt LM: Gene expression profiling of lymphoid malignancies. Annu Rev Med 53:303–18, 2002.

4. Gamberi B, Gaidano G, Parsa N, Carbone A, Roncella S, Knowles DM, Louie DC, Shibata D, Chaganti RS, Dalla-Favera R: Microsatellite instability is rare in B-cell non-Hodgkin's lymphomas. Blood 89:975–9, 1997.

5. Offit K, Wong G, Filippa DA, Tao Y, Chaganti RS: Cytogenetic analysis of 434 consecutively ascertained specimens of non-Hodgkin's lymphoma: Clinical correlations. Blood 77:1508–15, 1991.

6. Tycko B, Sklar J: Chromosomal translocations in lymphoid neoplasia: A reappraisal of the recombinase model. Cancer Cells 2:1–8, 1990.

7. Kuppers R, Klein U, Hansmann ML, Rajewsky K: Cellular origin of human B-cell lymphomas. N Engl J Med 341:1520–9, 1999.

8. Kipps TJ, Herzenberg LA: Homologous chromosome recombination generating immunoglobulin allotype and isotype switch variants. EMBO J 5:263–8, 1986.

9. Kalachikov S, Migliazza A, Cayanis E, Fracchiolla NS, Bonaldo MF, Lawton L, Jelenc P, Ye X, Qu X, Chien M, Hauptschein R, Gaidano G, Vitolo U, Saglio G, Resegotti L, Brodjansky V, Yankovsky N, Zhang P, Soares MB, Russo J, Edelman IS, Efstratiadis A, Dalla-Favera R, Fischer SG: Cloning and gene mapping of the chromosome 13q14 region deleted in chronic lymphocytic leukemia. Genomics 42:369–77, 1997.

10. Vitolo U, Gaidano G, Botto B, Volpe G, Audisio E, Bertini M, Calvi R, Freilone R, Novero D, Orsucci L, Pastore C, Capello D, Parvis G, Sacco C, Zagonel V, Carbone A, Mazza U, Palestro G, Saglio G, Resegotti L: Rearrangements of bcl-6, bcl-2, c-myc and 6q deletion in B-diffuse large-cell lymphoma: Clinical relevance in 71 patients. Ann Oncol 9:55–61, 1998.

11. Wong KF, Chan JK, Yu PH, So CC: A man with natural killer cell lymphoma showing 46,XX and deletion 6q. Cancer Genet Cytogenet 112:165–8, 1999.

12. Gaidano G, Ballerini P, Gong JZ, Inghirami G, Neri A, Newcomb EW, Magrath IT, Knowles DM, Dalla-Favera R: p53 mutations in human lymphoid malignancies: Association with Burkitt lymphoma and chronic lymphocytic leukemia. Proc Natl Acad Sci U S A 88:5413–7, 1991.

13. Lo Coco F, Gaidano G, Louie DC, Offit K, Chaganti RS, Dalla-Favera R: p53 mutations are associated with histologic transformation of follicular lymphoma. Blood 82:2289–95, 1993.

14. Sander CA, Yano T, Clark HM, Harris C, Longo DL, Jaffe ES, Raffeld M: p53 mutation is associated with progression in follicular lymphomas. Blood 82:1994–2004, 1993.

15. Ferreira OC, Jr, Planelles V, Rosenblatt JD: Human T-cell leukemia viruses: Epidemiology, biology, and pathogenesis. Blood Rev 11:91–104, 1997.

16. Ohshima K, Suzumiya J, Kikuchi M: The World Health Organization classification of malignant lymphoma: Incidence and clinical

prognosis in HTLV-1-endemic area of Fukuoka. Pathol Int 52:1–12, 2002.

17. Epstein MA, Barr YM, Achong BG: Studies with Burkitt's lymphoma. Wistar Inst Symp Monogr 4:69–82, 1965.

18. Magrath I: The pathogenesis of Burkitt's lymphoma. Adv Cancer Res 55:133–270, 1990.

19. Neri A, Barriga F, Inghirami G, Knowles DM, Neequaye J, Magrath IT, Dalla-Favera R: Epstein-Barr virus infection precedes clonal expansion in Burkitt's and acquired immunodeficiency syndrome-associated lymphoma. Blood 77:1092–5, 1991.

20. Pagano JS: Epstein-Barr virus: The first human tumor virus and its role in cancer. Proc Assoc Am Physicians 111:573–80, 1999.

21. Cesarman E, Chang Y, Moore PS, Said JW, Knowles DM: Kaposi's sarcoma-associated herpesvirus-like DNA sequences in AIDS-related body-cavity-based lymphomas. N Engl J Med 332:1186–91, 1995.

22. Carbone A, Gaidano G: HHV-8-positive body-cavity-based lymphoma: A novel lymphoma entity. Br J Haematol 97:515–22, 1997.

23. Fais F, Ghiotto F, Hashimoto S, Sellars B, Valetto A, Allen SL, Schulman P, Vinciguerra VP, Rai K, Rassenti LZ, Kipps TJ, Dighiero G, Schroeder H, Ferrarini M, Chiorazzi N: Chronic lymphocytic leukemia B cells express restricted sets of mutated and unmutated antigen receptors. J Clin Invest 102:1515–25, 1998.

24. Damle RN, Wasil T, Fais F, Ghiotto F, Valetto A, Allen SL, Buchbinder A, Budman D, Dittmar K, Kolitz J, Lichtman SM, Schulman P, Vinciguerra VP, Rai KR, Ferrarini M, Chiorazzi N: Ig V gene mutation status and CD38 expression as novel prognostic indicators in chronic lymphocytic leukemia. Blood 94:1840–1847, 1999.

25. Hamblin TJ, Davis Z, Gardiner A, Oscier DG, Stevenson FK: Unmutated Ig V(H) genes are associated with a more aggressive form of chronic lymphocytic leukemia. Blood 94:1848–54, 1999.

26. Maloum K, Davi F, Merle-Beral H, Pritsch O, Magnac C, Vuillier F, Dighiero G, Troussard X, Mauro FF, Benichou J: Expression of unmutated VH genes is a detrimental prognostic factor in chronic lymphocytic leukemia. Blood 96:377–9, 2000.

27. Rosenwald A, Alizadeh AA, Widhopf G, Simon R, Davis RE, Yu X, Yang L, Pickeral OK, Rassenti LZ, Powell J, Botstein D, Byrd JC, Grever MR, Cheson BD, Chiorazzi N, Wilson WH, Kipps TJ, Brown PO, Staudt LM: Relation of gene expression phenotype to immunoglobulin mutation genotype in B cell chronic lymphocytic leukemia. J Exp Med 194:1639–47, 2001.

28. Klein U, Tu Y, Stolovitzky GA, Mattioli M, Cattoretti G, Husson H, Freedman A, Inghirami G, Cro L, Baldini L, Neri A, Califano A, Dalla-Favera R: Gene expression profiling of B cell chronic lymphocytic leukemia reveals a homogeneous phenotype related to memory B cells. J Exp Med 194:1625–38, 2001.

29. Kipps TJ: Chronic lymphocytic leukemia and related diseases. In Beutler E, Lichtman MA, Coller BS, Kipps TJ, Seligsohn U (eds.): Williams Hematology, pp. 1163–1194 6th Ed. McGraw-Hill, New York, 2001.

30. Döhner H, Stilgenbauer S, Döhner K, Bentz M, Lichter P: Chromosome aberrations in B-cell chronic lymphocytic leukemia: Reassessment based on molecular cytogenetic analysis. J Mol Med 77:266–81, 1999.

31. Kipps TJ: Genetics of chronic lymphocytic leukaemia. Hematol Cell Ther 42:5–14, 2000.

32. Gardiner AC, Corcoran MM, Oscier DG: Cytogenetic, fluorescence in situ hybridisation, and clinical evaluation of translocations with concomitant deletion at 13q14 in chronic lymphocytic leukaemia. Genes Chromosom Cancer 20:73–81, 1997.

33. Crossen PE: Genes and chromosomes in chronic B-cell leukemia. Cancer Genet Cytogenet 94:44–51, 1997.

34. Garcia-Marco JA, Price CM, Catovsky D: Interphase cytogenetics in chronic lymphocytic leukemia. Cancer Genet Cytogenet 94:52–8, 1997.

35. Stilgenbauer S, Nickolenko J, Wilhelm J, Wolf S, Weitz S, Dohner K, Boehm T, Döhner H, Lichter P: Expressed sequences as candidates for a novel tumor suppressor gene at band 13q14 in B-cell chronic lymphocytic leukemia and mantle cell lymphoma. Oncogene 16:1891–7, 1998.

36. Corcoran MM, Rasool O, Liu Y, Iyengar A, Grander D, Ibbotson RE, Merup M, Wu X, Brodyansky V, Gardiner AC, Juliusson G, Chapman RM, Ivanova G, Tiller M, Gahrton G, Yankovsky N, Zabarovsky E, Oscier DG, Einhorn S: Detailed molecular delineation of 13q14.3 loss in B-cell chronic lymphocytic leukemia. Blood 91:1382–90, 1998.

37. Kapanadze B, Kashuba V, Baranova A, Rasool O, van Everdink W, Liu Y, Syomov A, Corcoran M, Poltaraus A, Brodyansky V, Syomova N, Kazakov A, Ibbotson R, van den Berg A, Gizatullin R, Fedorova L, Sulimova G, Zelenin A, Deaven L, Lehrach H, Grander D, Buys C, Oscier D, Zabarovsky ER, Yankovsky N et al: A cosmid and cDNA fine physical map of a human chromosome 13q14 region frequently lost in B-cell chronic lymphocytic leukemia and identification of a new putative tumor suppressor gene, Leu5. FEBS Lett 426:266–70, 1998.

38. Liu Y, Corcoran M, Rasool O, Ivanova G, Ibbotson R, Grander D, Iyengar A, Baranova A, Kashuba V, Merup M, Wu X, Gardiner A, Mullenbach R, Poltaraus A, Hultstrom AL, Juliusson G, Chapman R, Tiller M, Cotter F, Gahrton G, Yankovsky N, Zabarovsky E, Einhorn S, Oscier D: Cloning of two candidate tumor suppressor genes within a 10 kb region on chromosome 13q14, frequently deleted in chronic lymphocytic leukemia. Oncogene 15:2463–73, 1997.

39. Migliazza A, Bosch F, Komatsu H, Cayanis E, Martinotti S, Toniato E, Guccione E, Qu X, Chien M, Murty VV, Gaidano G, Inghirami G, Zhang P, Fischer S, Kalachikov SM, Russo J, Edelman I, Efstratiadis A, Dalla-Favera R: Nucleotide sequence, transcription map, and mutation analysis of the 13q14 chromosomal region deleted in B-cell chronic lymphocytic leukemia. Blood 97:2098–104, 2001.

40. Bullrich F, Fujii H, Calin G, Mabuchi H, Negrini M, Pekarsky Y, Rassenti L, Alder H, Reed JC, Keating MJ, Kipps TJ, Croce CM: Characterization of the 13q14 tumor suppressor locus in CLL: Identification of ALT1, an alternative splice variant of the LEU2 gene. Cancer Res 61:6640–8, 2001.

41. Hjalmar V, Hast R, Kimby E: Sequential fluorescence in situ hybridization analyses for trisomy 12 in chronic leukemic B-cell disorders. Haematologica 86:174–80, 2001.

42. Acar H, Connor MJ: Detection of trisomy 12 and centromeric alterations in CLL by interphase- and metaphase-FISH. Cancer Genet Cytogenet 100:148–51, 1998.

43. Oscier DG: Cytogenetics and molecular genetics of chronic lymphocytic leukaemia. Haematologica 84(Suppl. EHA-4):88–91, 1999.

44. Oscier DG, Thompsett A, Zhu D, Stevenson FK: Differential rates of somatic hypermutation in V(H) genes among subsets of chronic lymphocytic leukemia defined by chromosomal abnormalities. Blood 89:4153–60, 1997.

45. Oscier DG, Matutes E, Copplestone A, Pickering RM, Chapman R, Gillingham R, Catovsky D, Hamblin TJ: Atypical lymphocyte morphology: An adverse prognostic factor for disease progression in stage A CLL independent of trisomy 12. Br J Haematol 98:934–9, 1997.

46. Döhner H, Stilgenbauer S, James MR, Benner A, Weilguni T, Bentz M, Fischer K, Hunstein W, Lichter P: 11q deletions identify a new subset of B-cell chronic lymphocytic leukemia character-

ized by extensive nodal involvement and inferior prognosis. Blood 89:2516–22, 1997.

47. Stilgenbauer S, Winkler D, Ott G, Schaffner C, Leupolt E, Bentz M, Moller P, Muller-Hermelink HK, James MR, Lichter P, Döhner H: Molecular characterization of 11q deletions points to a pathogenic role of the ATM gene in mantle cell lymphoma. Blood 94:3262–4, 1999.

48. Zhu Y, Loukola A, Monni O, Kuokkanen K, Franssila K, Elonen E, Vilpo J, Joensuu H, Kere J, Aaltonen L, Knuutila S: PPP2R1B gene in chronic lymphocytic leukemias and mantle cell lymphomas. Leuk Lymphoma 41:177–83, 2001.

49. Wilgenbus KK, Milatovich A, Francke U, Furthmayr H: Molecular cloning, cDNA sequence, and chromosomal assignment of the human radixin gene and two dispersed pseudogenes. Genomics 16:199–206, 1993.

50. Luo L, Lu FM, Hart S, Foroni L, Rabbani H, Hammarstrom L, Yuille MR, Catovsky D, Webster AD, Vorechovsky I: Ataxia-telangiectasia and T-cell leukemias: No evidence for somatic ATM mutation in sporadic T-ALL or for hypermethylation of the ATM-NPAT/E14 bidirectional promoter in T-PLL. Cancer Res 58:2293–7, 1998.

51. Lavin MF, Khanna KK: ATM: The protein encoded by the gene mutated in the radiosensitive syndrome ataxia-telangiectasia. Int J Radiat Biol 75:1201–14, 1999.

52. Bevan S, Yuille MR, Marossy A, Catovsky D, Houlston RS: Ataxia telangiectasia gene mutations and chronic lymphocytic leukaemia. Lancet 353:753, 1999.

53. Bullrich F, Rasio D, Kitada S, Starostik P, Kipps T, Keating M, Albitar M, Reed JC, Croce CM: ATM mutations in B-cell chronic lymphocytic leukemia. Cancer Res 59:24–7, 1999.

54. Zambetti GP, Levine AJ: A comparison of the biological activities of wild-type and mutant p53. FASEB J 7:855–65, 1993.

55. Marshall CJ: Tumor suppressor genes. Cell 64:313–26, 1991.

56. Amiel A, Arbov L, Manor Y, Fejgin M, Elis A, Gaber E, Lishner M: Monoallelic p53 deletion in chronic lymphocytic leukemia detected by interphase cytogenetics. Cancer Genet Cytogenet 97:97–100, 1997.

57. Cordone I, Masi S, Mauro FR, Soddu S, Morsilli O, Valentini T, Vegna ML, Guglielmi C, Mancini F, Giuliacci S, Sacchi A, Mandelli F, Foa R: p53 expression in B-cell chronic lymphocytic leukemia: A marker of disease progression and poor prognosis. Blood 91:4342–9, 1998.

58. Döhner H, Stilgenbauer S, Benner A, Leupolt E, Krober A, Bullinger L, Dohner K, Bentz M, Lichter P: Genomic aberrations and survival in chronic lymphocytic leukemia. N Engl J Med 343:1910–6, 2000.

59. Adachi M, Tefferi A, Greipp PR, Kipps TJ, Tsujimoto Y: Preferential linkage of bcl-2 to immunoglobulin light chain gene in chronic lymphocytic leukemia. J Exp Med 171:559–64, 1990.

60. Raghoebier S, van Krieken JH, Kluin-Nelemans JC, Gillis A, van Ommen GJ, Ginsberg AM, Raffeld M, Kluin PM: Oncogene rearrangements in chronic B-cell leukemia. Blood 77:1560–4, 1991.

61. Jonveaux P, Hillion J, Bennaceur AL, d'Agay MF, Brice P, Daniel MT, Sigaux F, Berger R: t(14;18) and bcl-2 gene rearrangement in a B-chronic lymphocytic leukaemia. Br J Haematol 81:620–1, 1992.

62. Schena M, Larsson LG, Gottardi D, Gaidano G, Carlsson M, Nilsson K, Caligaris-Cappio F: Growth- and differentiation-associated expression of bcl-2 in B-chronic lymphocytic leukemia cells. Blood 79:2981–9, 1992.

63. Pezzella F, Tse AG, Cordell JL, Pulford KA, Gatter KC, Mason DY: Expression of the bcl-2 oncogene protein is not specific for the 14;18 chromosomal translocation. Am J Pathol 137:225–32, 1990.

64. Hanada M, Delia D, Aiello A, Stadtmauer E, Reed JC: bcl-2 gene hypomethylation and high-level expression in B-cell chronic lymphocytic leukemia. Blood 82:1820–8, 1993.

65. Miyashita T, Reed JC: Bcl-2 oncoprotein blocks chemotherapy-induced apoptosis in a human leukemia cell line. Blood 81:151–7, 1993.

66. Aviram A, Rabizadeh E, Zimra Y, Yeshoron M, Marmelstein M, Shaklai M, Bairey O: Expression of bcl-2 and bax in cells isolated from B-chronic lymphocytic leukemia patients at different stages of the disease. Eur J Haematol 64:80–4, 2000.

67. Molica S, Dattilo A, Giulino C, Levato D, Levato L: Increased bcl-2/bax ratio in B-cell chronic lymphocytic leukemia is associated with a progressive pattern of disease. Haematologica 83:1122–4, 1998.

68. Graninger WB, Seto M, Boutain B, Goldman P, Korsmeyer SJ: Expression of Bcl-2 and Bcl-2-Ig fusion transcripts in normal and neoplastic cells. J Clin Invest 80:1512–5, 1987.

69. Cleary ML, Galili N, Sklar J: Detection of a second t(14;18) breakpoint cluster region in human follicular lymphomas. J Exp Med 164:315–20, 1986.

70. Hiom K, Melek M, Gellert M: DNA transposition by the RAG1 and RAG2 proteins: a possible source of oncogenic translocations. Cell 94:463–70, 1998.

71. Agrawal A, Schatz DG: RAG1 and RAG2 form a stable postcleavage synaptic complex with DNA containing signal ends in V(D)J recombination. Cell 89:43–53, 1997.

72. Meffre E, Papavasiliou F, Cohen P, de Bouteiller O, Bell D, Karasuyama H, Schiff C, Banchereau J, Liu YJ, Nussenzweig MC: Antigen receptor engagement turns off the V(D)J recombination machinery in human tonsil B cells. J Exp Med 188:765–72, 1998.

73. Cleary ML, Smith SD, Sklar J: Cloning and structural analysis of cDNAs for bcl-2 and a hybrid bcl-2/immunoglobulin transcript resulting from the t(14;18) translocation. Cell 47:19–28, 1986.

74. Korsmeyer SJ: Bcl-2 initiates a new category of oncogenes: Regulators of cell death. Blood 80:879–86, 1992.

75. Yin XM, Oltvai ZN, Korsmeyer SJ: BH1 and BH2 domains of Bcl-2 are required for inhibition of apoptosis and heterodimerization with Bax. Nature 369:321–3, 1994.

76. Zelenetz AD, Chen TT, Levy R: Clonal expansion in follicular lymphoma occurs subsequent to antigenic selection. J Exp Med 176:1137–48, 1992.

77. Konikova E, Kusenda J: P53 protein expression in human leukemia and lymphoma cells. Neoplasma 48:290–8, 2001.

78. Aizman I, Many A, Peller S, Ramot B, Kaufmann Y: Expression of wild-type p53 and Bcl-2 family genes oscillates with recurrent remission and relapse in an unusual case of low-grade lymphoma. Acta Haematol 103:177–85, 2000.

79. Gaidano G, Hauptschein RS, Parsa NZ, Offit K, Rao PH, Lenoir G, Knowles DM, Chaganti RS, Dalla-Favera R: Deletions involving two distinct regions of 6q in B-cell non-Hodgkin lymphoma. Blood 80:1781–7, 1992.

80. Callanan MB, Le Baccon P, Mossuz P, Duley S, Bastard C, Hamoudi R, Dyer MJ, Klobeck G, Rimokh R, Sotto JJ, Leroux D: The IgG Fc receptor, FcgammaRIIB, is a target for deregulation by chromosomal translocation in malignant lymphoma. Proc Natl Acad Sci U S A 97:309–14, 2000.

81. Chen W, Palanisamy N, Schmidt H, Teruya-Feldstein J, Jhanwar SC, Zelenetz AD, Houldsworth J, Chaganti RS: Deregulation of FCGR2B expression by 1q21 rearrangements in follicular lymphomas. Oncogene 20:7686–93, 2001.

82. Aozasa K, Ohsawa M, Ayata M, Inoue A, Ikeda H: Malignant lymphoma of lymphoplasmacytic/lymphoplasmacytoid and immunoblastic types. Oncology 47:224–8, 1990.

83. Richards MA, Hall PA, Gregory WM, Dhaliwal HS, Stansfeld AG, Amess JA, Lister TA: Lymphoplasmacytoid and small cell centrocytic non-Hodgkin's lymphoma – a retrospective analysis from St Bartholomew's Hospital 1972–1986. Hematol Oncol 7:19–35, 1989.

84. Iida S, Rao PH, Nallasivam P, Hibshoosh H, Butler M, Louie DC, Dyomin V, Ohno H, Chaganti RS, Dalla-Favera R: The t(9;14)(p13;q32) chromosomal translocation associated with lymphoplasmacytoid lymphoma involves the PAX-5 gene. Blood 88:4110–7, 1996.

85. Baker SJ, Reddy EP: B cell differentiation: Role of E2A and Pax5/BSAP transcription factors. Oncogene 11:413–26, 1995.

86. Banks PM, Chan J, Cleary ML, Delsol G, De Wolf-Peeters C, Gatter K, Grogan TM, Harris NL, Isaacson PG, Jaffe ES et al: Mantle cell lymphoma. A proposal for unification of morphologic, immunologic, and molecular data. Am J Surg Pathol 16:637–40, 1992.

87. Weisenburger DD, Vose JM, Greiner TC, Lynch JC, Chan WC, Bierman PJ, Dave BJ, Sanger WG, Armitage JO: Mantle cell lymphoma. A clinicopathologic study of 68 cases from the Nebraska Lymphoma Study Group. Am J Hematol 64:190–6, 2000.

88. Campo E, Raffeld M, Jaffe ES: Mantle-cell lymphoma. Semin Hematol 36:115–27, 1999.

89. Kilo MN, Dorfman DM: The utility of flow cytometric immunophenotypic analysis in the distinction of small lymphocytic lymphoma/chronic lymphocytic leukemia from mantle cell lymphoma. Am J Clin Pathol 105:451–7, 1996.

90. Schaffner C, Idler I, Stilgenbauer S, Döhner H, Lichter P: Mantle cell lymphoma is characterized by inactivation of the ATM gene. Proc Natl Acad Sci U S A 97:2773–8, 2000.

91. Stilgenbauer S, Schaffner C, Winkler D, Ott G, Leupolt E, Bentz M, Moller P, Muller-Hermelink HK, James MR, Lichter P, Döhner H: The ATM gene in the pathogenesis of mantle-cell lymphoma. Ann Oncol 11(Suppl. 1):127–30, 2000.

92. Seto M, Yamamoto K, Iida S, Akao Y, Utsumi KR, Kubonishi I, Miyoshi I, Ohtsuki T, Yawata Y, Namba M et al: Gene rearrangement and overexpression of PRAD1 in lymphoid malignancy with t(11;14)(q13;q32) translocation. Oncogene 7:1401–6, 1992.

93. Swerdlow SH, Zukerberg LR, Yang WI, Harris NL, Williams ME: The morphologic spectrum of non-Hodgkin's lymphomas with BCL1/cyclin D1 gene rearrangements. Am J Surg Pathol 20:627–40, 1996.

94. Segal GH, Masih AS, Fox AC, Jorgensen T, Scott M, Braylan RC: CD5-expressing B-cell non-Hodgkin's lymphomas with bcl-1 gene rearrangement have a relatively homogeneous immunophenotype and are associated with an overall poor prognosis. Blood 85:1570–9, 1995.

95. Swerdlow SH, Williams ME: From centrocytic to mantle cell lymphoma: A clinicopathologic and molecular review of 3 decades. Hum Pathol 33:7–20, 2002.

96. Opitz OG, Suliman Y, Hahn WC, Harada H, Blum HE, Rustgi AK: Cyclin D1 overexpression and p53 inactivation immortalize primary oral keratinocytes by a telomerase-independent mechanism. J Clin Invest 108:725–32, 2001.

97. Jiang W, Kahn SM, Zhou P, Zhang YJ, Cacace AM, Infante AS, Doi S, Santella RM, Weinstein IB: Overexpression of cyclin D1 in rat fibroblasts causes abnormalities in growth control, cell cycle progression and gene expression. Oncogene 8:3447–57, 1993.

98. Bodrug SE, Warner BJ, Bath ML, Lindeman GJ, Harris AW, Adams JM: Cyclin D1 transgene impedes lymphocyte maturation and collaborates in lymphomagenesis with the myc gene. Embo J 13:2124–30, 1994.

99. Greiner TC, Moynihan MJ, Chan WC, Lytle DM, Pedersen A, Anderson JR, Weisenburger DD: p53 mutations in mantle cell lymphoma are associated with variant cytology and predict a poor prognosis. Blood 87:4302–10, 1996.

100. Fiel-Gan MD, Almeida LM, Rose DC, Takano A, Rezuke WN, Coleman WB, Garcia NF, Tsongalis GJ: Proliferative fraction, bcl-1 gene translocation, and p53 mutation status as markers in mantle cell lymphoma. Int J Mol Med 3:373–9, 1999.

101. Gaidano G, Lo Coco F, Ye BH, Shibata D, Levine AM, Knowles DM, Dalla-Favera R: Rearrangements of the BCL-6 gene in acquired immunodeficiency syndrome-associated non-Hodgkin's lymphoma: Association with diffuse large-cell subtype. Blood 84:397–402, 1994.

102. Dalla-Favera R, Ye BH, Cattoretti G, Lo Coco F, Chang CC, Zhang J, Migliazza A, Cechova K, Niu H, Chaganti S, Chen W, Louie DC, Offit K, Chaganti RS: BCL-6 in diffuse large-cell lymphomas. Important Adv Oncol: 139–48, 1996.

103. Ye BH, Lista F, Lo Coco F, Knowles DM, Offit K, Chaganti RS, Dalla-Favera R: Alterations of a zinc finger-encoding gene, BCL-6, in diffuse large-cell lymphoma. Science 262:747–50, 1993.

104. Migliazza A, Martinotti S, Chen W, Fusco C, Ye BH, Knowles DM, Offit K, Chaganti RS, Dalla-Favera R: Frequent somatic hypermutation of the 5′ noncoding region of the BCL6 gene in B-cell lymphoma. Proc Natl Acad Sci U S A 92:12520–4, 1995.

105. Chang CC, Ye BH, Chaganti RS, Dalla-Favera R: BCL-6, a POZ/zinc-finger protein, is a sequence-specific transcriptional repressor. Proc Natl Acad Sci U S A 93:6947–52, 1996.

106. Shaffer AL, Yu X, He Y, Boldrick J, Chan EP, Staudt LM: BCL-6 represses genes that function in lymphocyte differentiation, inflammation, and cell cycle control. Immunity 13:199–212, 2000.

107. Dalla-Favera R, Ye BH, Lo Coco F, Gaidano G, Lista F, Knowles DM, Louie DC, Offit K, Chaganti RS: Identification of genetic lesions associated with diffuse large-cell lymphoma. Ann Oncol 5(Suppl. 1):55–60, 1994.

108. Cattoretti G, Chang CC, Cechova K, Zhang J, Ye BH, Falini B, Louie DC, Offit K, Chaganti RS, Dalla-Favera R: BCL-6 protein is expressed in germinal-center B cells. Blood 86:45–53, 1995.

109. Ye BH, Cattoretti G, Shen Q, Zhang J, Hawe N, de Waard R, Leung C, Nouri-Shirazi M, Orazi A, Chaganti RS, Rothman P, Stall AM, Pandolfi PP, Dalla-Favera R: The BCL-6 proto-oncogene controls germinal-centre formation and Th2-type inflammation. Nat Genet 16:161–70, 1997.

110. Offit K, Louie DC, Parsa NZ, Roy P, Leung D, Lo Coco F, Zelenetz A, Dalla-Favera R, Chaganti RS: BCL6 gene rearrangement and other cytogenetic abnormalities in diffuse large cell lymphoma. Leuk Lymphoma 20:85–9, 1995.

111. Akasaka T, Ueda C, Kurata M, Akasaka H, Yamabe H, Uchiyama T, Ohno H: Nonimmunoglobulin (non-Ig)/BCL6 gene fusion in diffuse large B-cell lymphoma results in worse prognosis than Ig/BCL6. Blood 96:2907–9, 2000.

112. Offit K, Lo Coco F, Louie DC, Parsa NZ, Leung D, Portlock C, Ye BH, Lista F, Filippa DA, Rosenbaum A et al: Rearrangement of the bcl-6 gene as a prognostic marker in diffuse large-cell lymphoma. N Engl J Med 331:74–80, 1994.

113. Alizadeh AA, Eisen MB, Davis RE, Ma C, Lossos IS, Rosenwald A, Boldrick JC, Sabet H, Tran T, Yu X, Powell JI, Yang L, Marti GE, Moore T, Hudson J Jr, Lu L, Lewis DB, Tibshirani R, Sherlock G, Chan WC, Greiner TC, Weisenburger DD, Armitage JO, Warnke R, Staudt LM et al: Distinct types of diffuse large B-cell lymphoma identified by gene expression profiling. Nature 403:503–11, 2000.

114. Huang JZ, Sanger WG, Greiner TC, Staudt LM, Weisenburger DD, Pickering DL, Lynch JC, Armitage JO, Warnke RA, Alizadeh AA, Lossos IS, Levy R, Chan WC: The t(14;18) defines a unique subset of diffuse large B-cell lymphoma with a germinal center B-cell gene expression profile. Blood 99:2285–90, 2002.

115. Akasaka T, Akasaka H, Ueda C, Yonetani N, Maesako Y, Shimizu A, Yamabe H, Fukuhara S, Uchiyama T, Ohno H: Molecular and clinical features of non-Burkitt's, diffuse large-cell lymphoma of B-cell type associated with the c-MYC/immunoglobulin heavy-chain fusion gene. J Clin Oncol 18:510–18, 2000.

116. Pasqualucci L, Neumeister P, Goossens T, Nanjangud G, Chaganti RS, Kuppers R, Dalla-Favera R: Hypermutation of multiple proto-oncogenes in B-cell diffuse large-cell lymphomas. Nature 412:341–6, 2001.

117. ar-Rushdi A, Nishikura K, Erikson J, Watt R, Rovera G, Croce CM: Differential expression of the translocated and the untranslocated c-myc oncogene in Burkitt lymphoma. Science 222:390–3, 1983.

118. Taub R, Kirsch I, Morton C, Lenoir G, Swan D, Tronick S, Aaronson S, Leder P: Translocation of the c-myc gene into the immunoglobulin heavy chain locus in human Burkitt lymphoma and murine plasmacytoma cells. Proc Natl Acad Sci U S A 79:7837–41, 1982.

119. Neri A, Barriga F, Knowles DM, Magrath IT, Dalla-Favera R: Different regions of the immunoglobulin heavy-chain locus are involved in chromosomal translocations in distinct pathogenetic forms of Burkitt lymphoma. Proc Natl Acad Sci U S A 85:2748–52, 1988.

120. Pelicci PG, Knowles DM 2nd, Magrath I, Dalla-Favera R: Chromosomal breakpoints and structural alterations of the c-myc locus differ in endemic and sporadic forms of Burkitt lymphoma. Proc Natl Acad Sci U S A 83:2984–8, 1986.

121. Bhatia K, Huppi K, Spangler G, Siwarski D, Iyer R, Magrath I: Point mutations in the c-Myc transactivation domain are common in Burkitt's lymphoma and mouse plasmacytomas. Nat Genet 5:56–61, 1993.

122. Blackwood EM, Eisenman RN: Max: A helix-loop-helix zipper protein that forms a sequence-specific DNA-binding complex with Myc. Science 251:1211–7, 1991.

123. Ayer DE, Kretzner L, Eisenman RN: Mad: A heterodimeric partner for Max that antagonizes Myc transcriptional activity. Cell 72:211–22, 1993.

124. Gu W, Cechova K, Tassi V, Dalla-Favera R: Opposite regulation of gene transcription and cell proliferation by c-Myc and Max. Proc Natl Acad Sci U S A 90:2935–9, 1993.

125. Gu W, Bhatia K, Magrath IT, Dang CV, Dalla-Favera R: Binding and suppression of the Myc transcriptional activation domain by p107. Science 264:251–4, 1994.

126. Trivedi P, Spinsanti P, Cuomo L, Volpe M, Takada K, Frati L, Faggioni A: Differential regulation of Epstein-Barr virus (EBV) latent gene expression in Burkitt lymphoma cells infected with a recombinant EBV strain. J Virol 75:4929–35, 2001.

127. Rabkin CS, Yellin F: Cancer incidence in a population with a high prevalence of infection with human immunodeficiency virus type 1. J Natl Cancer Inst 86:1711–6, 1994.

128. Reynolds P, Saunders LD, Layefsky ME, Lemp GF: The spectrum of acquired immunodeficiency syndrome (AIDS)-associated malignancies in San Francisco, 1980–1987. Am J Epidemiol 137:19–30, 1993.

129. Gaidano G, Carbone A, Dalla-Favera R: Pathogenesis of AIDS-related lymphomas: Molecular and histogenetic heterogeneity. Am J Pathol 152:623–30, 1998.

130. Ballerini P, Gaidano G, Gong JZ, Tassi V, Saglio G, Knowles DM, Dalla-Favera R: Multiple genetic lesions in acquired immunodeficiency syndrome-related non-Hodgkin's lymphoma. Blood 81:166–76, 1993.

131. Gaidano G, Carbone A: Primary effusion lymphoma: A liquid phase lymphoma of fluid-filled body cavities. Adv Cancer Res 80:115–46, 2001.

132. Gaidano G, Capello D, Carbone A: The molecular basis of acquired immunodeficiency syndrome-related lymphomagenesis. Semin Oncol 27:431–41, 2000.

133. Carbone A, Gloghini A, Capello D, Gaidano G: Genetic pathways and histogenetic models of AIDS-related lymphomas. Eur J Cancer 37:1270–5, 2001.

134. Levine AM: Acquired immunodeficiency syndrome-related lymphoma: Clinical aspects. Semin Oncol 27:442–53, 2000.

135. Fassone L, Cingolani A, Martini M, Migliaretti G, Oreste PL, Capello D, Gloghini A, Vivenza D, Dolcetti R, Carbone A, Antinori A, Gaidano G, Larocca LM: Characterization of Epstein-Barr virus genotype in AIDS-related non-Hodgkin's lymphoma. AIDS Res Hum Retroviruses 18:19–26, 2002.

136. Gaidano G, Capello D, Fassone L, Gloghini A, Cilia AM, Ariatti C, Buonaiuto D, Vivenza D, Gallicchio M, Avanzi GC, Prat M, Carbone A: Molecular characterization of HHV-8 positive primary effusion lymphoma reveals pathogenetic and histogenetic features of the disease. J Clin Virol 16:215–24, 2000.

39

Epidemiology and Hereditary Aspects of Malignant Lymphoma and Hodgkin's Disease

Seymour Grufferman

The lymphomas have been of unusually great interest to epidemiologists. Much more is known about the epidemiology of Hodgkin's disease than about the epidemiology of the non-Hodgkin's lymphomas. Much of the extraordinary epidemiologic interest in Hodgkin's disease stems from its long-suspected infectious etiology and from its unusual patterns of incidence with age, which has suggested that it is at least two different diseases with important underlying environmental determinants. In contrast to Hodgkin's disease, the likelihood on clinical and histopathologic grounds that the non-Hodgkin's lymphomas are several different disease entities has probably impeded epidemiologic and other research interest in this group of diseases.

The lymphomas have some important common features, however. They are malignancies of the lymphatic system and its precursor cells, which play major roles in the body's defenses against infection and in antibody production. The first isolation of the Epstein-Barr virus (EBV) was from an African Burkitt's lymphoma patient. Patients with infectious mononucleosis, caused by EBV, have at least a threefold increased risk of developing Hodgkin's disease. Thus, it is not surprising that the lymphomas have frequently been thought to be of viral etiology. Additionally, this group of malignancies is seen with very high frequency in persons with immune deficiencies, ranging from that due to pharmacologic immunosuppression in transplantation to congenital immunodeficiency syndromes or to the acquired immunodeficiency syndrome (AIDS). Interestingly, immunosuppression leads to a remarkably increased risk of non-Hodgkin's lymphoma, but only to a slightly increased risk of Hodgkin's disease. The lymphomas as a group lead to impaired immune function per se. A clear-cut familial aggregation of the lymphomas is also seen, although family members of a Hodgkin's disease patient are likely to have more of that disease but little excess of non-Hodgkin's lymphoma and vice versa.

On the basis of known etiologic factors, the two diseases appear to have little in common. EBV is found in up to 50 percent of all Hodgkin's disease tumors, but infrequently in tumors from non-Hodgkin's lymphoma patients other than those with endemic Burkitt's lymphoma. Environmental and occupational exposures, such as to chemicals, have inconsistently been linked to risk of both diseases. In general, the results of such studies, as presented below, have not been very persuasive. An interesting difference between the two diseases is the much greater frequency with which the non-Hodgkin's lymphomas appear as second malignancies when compared with Hodgkin's disease. Whereas it appears that heredity plays a large role in the occurrence of both conditions, the patterns of familial aggregation in the two are quite different. Another major difference between the two diseases lies in incidence trends over recent years. The incidence of non-Hodgkin's lymphoma worldwide has been increasing at the rate of 3 to 4 percent per year. In contrast to this, the incidence of Hodgkin's disease has changed little over time. For reasons such as these, the epidemiology and genetics of the two diseases are discussed separately.

HODGKIN'S DISEASE

Incidence

Hodgkin's disease is a relatively uncommon malignancy. The current overall annual incidence in the U.S. is 2.7/100,000 (2.9/100,000 in males and 2.4 in females).[1] As can be seen in Table 39–1, incidence rates are higher in whites than in blacks. The overall 5-year survival rate is now up to 82.7 percent.[1] The improvement in survival is one of modern oncology's greatest triumphs. It should not be forgotten that 40 to 50 years ago, a diagnosis of Hodgkin's disease was a virtual death pronouncement. Unfortunately, progress in effecting greater survival in the elderly Hodgkin's disease patient has lagged behind. Table 39–1 shows a diminishing survival with increasing age. Five-

Table 39–1. Important Statistics on Hodgkin's Disease

Population	Incidence
U.S. incidence per 100,000 population per year, 1994–1998	
Overall U.S. rate	2.7
Males	2.9
Females	2.4
Whites	2.9
Blacks	2.2
0–14 years	0.6
< 65 years	
Males	2.8
Females	2.4
65 + years	
Males	4.2
Females	3.1

Population	Survival (%)
U.S. 5-year relative survival, 1994–1998	
Overall	82.7
Males	81.4
Females	84.3
Whites	84.0
Blacks	74.1
Survival by age at diagnosis	
0–14 years	91.3
15–34 years	90.3
35–64 years	82.1
65 + years	47.8

Rates are adjusted to the 1970 U.S. standard population.
Based on SEER data, April 2001.

673

year relative survival for patients aged 65 years or older at diagnosis is only 47.8 percent, possibly because of less aggressive diagnosis, staging, and treatment in this age group.[1,2] Given the improving general health status of the elderly, this poorer survival should improve in the future.

By Age and Sex

Hodgkin's disease incidence varies greatly with age. MacMahon, in 1957,[3] first noted a bimodal age-incidence curve, with modal peaks in young adults (aged 15 to 34 years at diagnosis) and old adults (50 years or more). He postulated that these probably represented two different diseases, an inflammatory granulomatous infectious disease in young adults and a true neoplasm in the old adults. He noted that the young-adult disease was probably infectious in nature, although of very low infectivity.[4] He also observed that no young-adult incidence peak was seen in Japan and that certain epidemiologic features of childhood Hodgkin's disease, such as a striking male excess, suggested that it represented a third type.

The incidence of Hodgkin's disease at different ages also varies by sex. A marked excess of males is seen in the childhood form.[4] At the young-adult and old-adult incidence peaks, little or no difference by sex is seen, but a marked male excess is found during middle age (35 to 59 years). It has been suggested that this gap might be due to a protective effect of childbearing,[5] and Glaser[6] recently presented some new data to support this hypothesis. If it is correct, it implies that hormonal factors play a role in the etiology. This represents a promising area in which further research is needed.

International Variation

The large international incidence differences have suggested an important etiologic role for environmental factors. The most intriguing observation is that reported in 1971 by Correa and O'Conor,[7] who observed that in developed countries such as Sweden and Denmark incidence rates for young-adult onset Hodgkin's disease (20–34 years at diagnosis) were quite high and (reciprocally) incidence rates for childhood onset (5–14 years) were quite low. In less developed countries such as Columbia and Nigeria, an inverse pattern was observed—incidence rates were high for childhood disease and reciprocally low for young-adult disease. These observations provided important support for the "poliomyelitis model" or "late-host-response model" of etiology, which is discussed below.

Macfarlane et al.[8] recently revisited the issue of international variations in incidence. Since the Correa and O'Conor paper was published, diverging incidence trends in childhood (stable rates) and young adults (increasing rates) have been observed.[8] Using incidence rates (1983 to 1987) from the same source as Correa and O'Conor, Macfarlane et al.[8] found no association between young-adult and childhood incidence.[9] They also found that incidence rates for Latin American countries had shifted toward patterns observed in more economically developed countries. Thus, the international incidence of the disease is not only different between countries but has changed over time. Such observations suggest that environmental factors play an etiologic role.

Another observation on international variation has stood the test of time: MacMahon noted in 1966[4] that no young-adult peak in the age-incidence curve was found in Japan. As seen in Figure 39–1, the Japanese incidence data from *Cancer Incidence in Five Continents* (1983 to 1987), still show no young-adult incidence peak.[9]

Figure 39–1 depicts age-incidence patterns for the United States and three selected Asian countries, Japan, India, and China.[9] These countries were chosen because they have large registries that provide stable rates and to demonstrate the overall lower incidence in Asia than in the United States as well as the absence of a young-adult incidence peak in Asia. It is important to note that different incidence scales are used for the different countries, since Asian rates are low relative to the United States. In all the countries illustrated, the male rates are generally higher than those for females, particularly at older ages. Whether these observations are due to different genetic susceptibility in Asia or to different environmental exposures is unknown.

In summary, large differences are found in the incidence of Hodgkin's disease internationally, and they vary by age. Whereas the previously reported reciprocal variation internationally between childhood and young-adult incidence is no longer found, there is still a very low incidence and virtual absence of young-adult cases in Asian countries. Observations such as these make a strong case for the importance of environmental factors. They also suggest to some degree that genetic susceptibility plays a role.

Socioeconomic Status

Several intriguing associations between socioeconomic status (SES) and Hodgkin's disease risk have been noted. The descriptive epidemiologic findings regarding international variations suggest that less developed countries with their less affluent populations have relatively more childhood and fewer young-adult cases than do developed and more affluent countries. The inverse is seen in more affluent countries.

LeShan et al.[10] used data from World War II servicemen to show that men who developed Hodgkin's disease generally had higher IQs as measured by the Army General Classification Test. Cohen et al.[11] found that Hodgkin's disease patients had had more education and were from higher preservice occupational classes compared with World War II servicemen without the disease. Gutensohn and Cole[12] showed that patients with young-adult disease came from smaller families, had fewer playmates, tended to live in more single family dwellings, and came from more affluent and more highly educated families than did controls.

Such data support the notion that Hodgkin's disease shares epidemiologic features with infectious diseases such as poliomyelitis and infectious mononucleosis. This hypothesis, first proposed by Newell,[13] is based on the analogy with paralytic poliomyelitis in the prevaccination era.[5] In less developed countries, exposure to polioviruses occurred early in life, which usually led to a mild or inapparent infection (or both). However, in more affluent countries with better sanitation levels, infection in childhood is much less common. When a nonimmune adult host is infected with the virus, a severe paralytic dis-

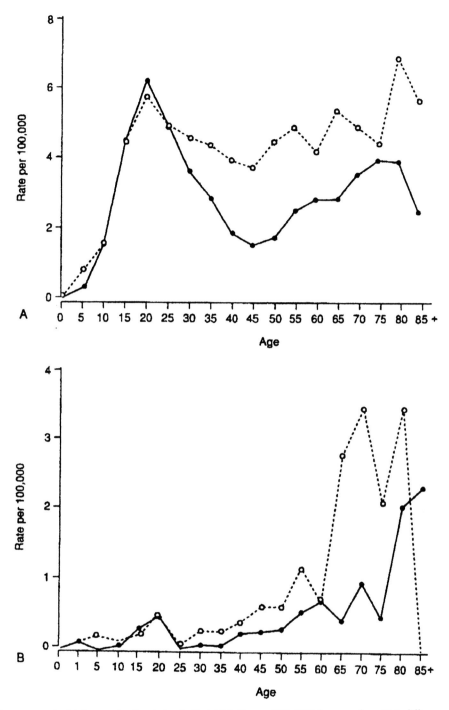

Figure 39–1. (A–D). International variation in Hodgkin's disease, 1983–1987, by age and sex. Note differences in incidence scale for each country. (A) USA, SEER: white. (B) Japan, Osaka prefecture. *(Figure continues.)*

ease tends to develop rather than the largely inapparent infections of early childhood. This model has also been called the EBV and the late-host-response hypotheses. Young-adult disease would be a rare manifestation of a common exposure.

The first test of this hypothesis was by Paffenbarger et al.[14] Using data from a follow-up study of college students, they were able to identify alumni at Harvard and the University of Pennsylvania who had developed Hodgkin's disease. Data collected at the time of entry to college were used to show that (well in advance of their diagnosis), Hodgkin's disease patients reported having had significantly fewer of the common childhood infectious diseases than did matched controls. The later data by

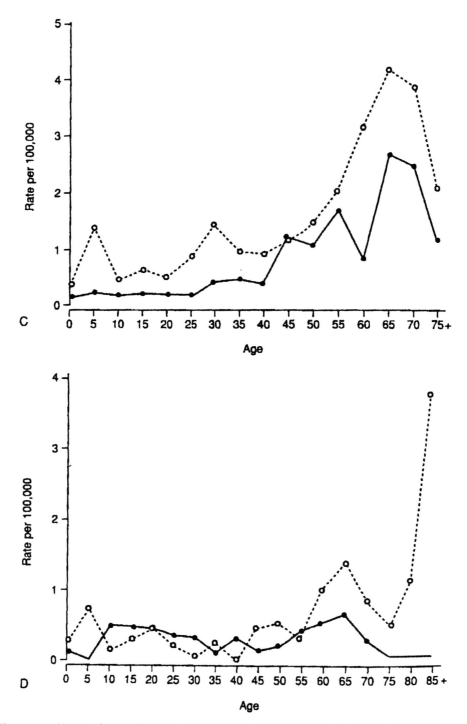

Figure 39–1. *(Continued.)* (C) India, Bombay. (D) China, Shanghai, Male, *broken line;* female, *solid line.* (From Parkin et al.,[9] with permission.)

Gutensohn and Cole[12] further confirm this hypothesis. In summary, it appears that young-adult-onset patients fit the poliomyelitis model quite well. Unfortunately, extensive data are not available for childhood and old-adult cases to see how these groups may relate to this hypothesis. Nevertheless, the findings strongly suggest that environmental factors play a role, with exposure to viruses best fitting the model.

Role of the Epstein-Barr Virus

The possibility that EBV might play a role in Hodgkin's disease etiology was suggested by the isolation of the virus from a patient with another lymphoma, African Burkitt's lymphoma. Until recently, available laboratory methods could not detect EBV in Hodgkin's disease tumor tissues. However, several seroepidemiologic observations had earlier suggested etiologic links between the two conditions.[5] It was well known that patients with Hodgkin's disease had higher titers of anti-EBV antibodies than did matched controls, but this was believed to be caused by the immunosuppression of Hodgkin's disease per se as well as the immunosuppressive effects of its treatment. In the 1970s, several cohort studies of individuals with serologically confirmed infectious mononucleosis showed that these patients had about a threefold increased risk of eventually developing Hodgkin's disease.[5] It could not be discerned from these studies whether the infectious mononucleosis might have been caused by the immunosuppression of underlying (as yet undiagnosed) Hodgkin's disease. This concern was dispelled by two nested case-control studies in which serum banks were used to examine antibody status of patients based on blood samples drawn well in advance of any possible diagnosis of Hodgkin's disease.[15,16] These studies showed that tests for anti-EBV antibodies were more apt to be positive and antibody titers higher in patients destined to develop Hodgkin's disease than in matched non-Hodgkin's disease controls. Thus it would appear that individuals who eventually develop the disease either have different immunologic responses to EBV than the general population or that EBV might be the cause.

Weiss et al. in 1987[17] used DNA hybridization to show that EBV DNA could be demonstrated in Hodgkin's disease tumor tissues. This innovative work was followed by a large series of studies showing that 30 to 50 percent of all adult Hodgkin's disease patients will have EBV in their tumors. In situ hybridization studies have since provided direct evidence that the virus is in the malignant cells of Hodgkin's disease tumors (Reed-Sternberg cells and their variants).[18]

Additionally, there is molecular evidence that the EBV genome in Hodgkin's disease is clonal; it has a restricted latent phenotype of LMP-1 expression and is found in the Reed-Sternberg cells. The consistency of these findings has led the International Agency for Research on Cancer to conclude that the EBV "is a causal factor in the etiology of Hodgkin's disease," and they have classified it as a group I carcinogen.[19] However, not all Hodgkin's disease tumors are found to contain EBV, suggesting that there may be etiologic heterogeneity and not all Hodgkin's disease is caused by EBV.

Genetics

Familial aggregation of Hodgkin's disease is well documented, with close relatives having about a threefold increased risk of the disease.[20] *Siblings* of young-adult cases have a sevenfold increased risk.[21] However, like-sex siblings have a ninefold increase in risk and discordant-sex siblings a fivefold increased risk. No simple mendelian genetic mechanism can explain the finding of excesses of male-male and female-female sibling pairs.[21] These excesses suggest that environmental factors might interact with genetic susceptibility. Similar findings of excess sibling sex concordance have also been found in Behçet's disease, multiple sclerosis, and sarcoidosis, a group of diseases with suspected infectious etiology.[22] The underlying assumption is that like-sex siblings have more shared environmental expo-

sures than do unlike-sex siblings. This hypothesis was dealt a setback by a recent twin study of Mack et al.,[23] who found that among twins in which at least one member had young-adult disease, monozygotic twins of patients had a 99-fold increased risk, but dizygotic twins had no increase in risk. These data strongly suggest that the observed familial aggregation is entirely due to shared genetic susceptibility. However, if this were the case, a lower, but still increased, risk should have been observed in dizygotic twins as well. Since this study identified twin pairs by a variety of methods, including advertisements, the results may be due to selection bias and thus need to be confirmed in another, more systematic, study. Recent work suggests that there may be "genetic anticipation" in familial Hodgkin's disease. Genetic anticipation is a phenomenon in which each successive generation of a familial disease is diagnosed at earlier ages.[24,25] This work lends further credence to there being a genetic basis for Hodgkin's disease.

Two studies addressed the question of whether familial Hodgkin's disease patients would be more or less apt to have EBV in their tumors. Using similar in situ hybridization techniques, both studies found identical results. In a study of 11 patients from France, 27 percent had evidence of EBV in their tumors' Reed-Sternberg cells.[26] In a second study of 46 familial cases from the U.S., 28 percent of their tumors were EBV positive.[27] Thus, the prevalence of EBV in tumors from familial cases, most of which were of the nodular sclerosis subtype, is similar to that found in nonfamilial patients.

Case Clustering

Case clustering in Hodgkin's disease has been reported numerous times. Whereas case clustering is characteristic of infectious diseases it can also be a hallmark of common-source exposure to a noninfectious etiologic agent. Vianna et al.[28] noted an unusual cluster of 31 cases that occurred over 23 years and centered around a single graduating class of the Albany (NY) High School. The diagnoses occurred at varying periods after the time of attendance. Twenty-three cases could be directly linked to one another and an additional eight could be linked as case-to-contact-to-case. This was a truly remarkable observation due to the sheer size of the cluster, which is the largest reported so far. Unfortunately, no appropriate statistical methods were used to evaluate its significance. The Albany study looked at clustering from a different viewpoint, that of shared exposures at a period in time well in advance of diagnosis. This phenomenon has been termed *aggregation of exposures*.[29] It differs from *clustering*, which is defined as increased closeness in time and place of cases at the time the disease is diagnosed. For diseases with suspected long latency periods, aggregation of exposures studies would be much more meaningful than clustering studies.

The Albany results led to another study in high school students on Long Island, NY. Vianna and Polan[30] found that children attending high schools in which a diagnosed Hodgkin's disease patient was in attendance had remarkably increased risks of subsequently developing the disease. The estimates of risk ranged from 2.3 to infinity among students exposed to other student cases. This was a remarkable finding that stimulated further research. Unfortunately, an exact replication of the Long Island study conducted in Boston could not confirm the findings.[31] A similar study conducted in Oxford, U.K., also could not confirm the Long Island findings.[32] Thus, it appears that no actual confirmed aggregation of exposures related to risk exists in the school setting. Recent studies have used newer biostatistical methods for the study of spatial clustering. Using complicated techniques, Alexander et al.[33] have shown a possible slight excess of close case pairs over that expected by chance. On balance, there appears to be little or no clustering at the time of diagnosis nor any excess of common exposures. Thus, contacts of a patient with Hodgkin's disease have no definite risk of developing the disease or other malignancies.

Other Environmental and Occupational Exposures as Risk Factors

Numerous studies have searched for an environmental or occupational cause, with few consistent results. Most of the occupation studies have resulted in variable findings, with most of the positive findings being weak. One of the difficulties in interpreting such studies is that of multiple comparisons. Case-control studies can look at associations with many occupations or exposures. Cohort (follow-up) studies of a particular occupation can evaluate many disease outcomes. Many of the observed disease-occupation associations in such studies are likely to be due to chance. Such chance observations probably underlie many of the reported associations of the lymphomas with occupational exposures. The lack of consistency of findings from one study to another suggests that most reports are indeed chance findings. The strongest suspected occupation is woodworking.[5] As for occupational chemical exposures, many studies have found slight excesses of risk that are not statistically significant.[5] Studies of occupational exposures to herbicides, particularly the phenoxy herbicides, have shown an association, but these results have been inconsistent.[34] On balance, it appears that few, if any, well-confirmed chemical or occupational exposures might cause Hodgkin's disease.

NON-HODGKIN'S LYMPHOMAS

Incidence

The non-Hodgkin's lymphomas are much more common than Hodgkin's disease. The recent overall annual incidence in the United States is 16.1 cases/100,000 population (19.8/100,000 in males and 13.0 in females).[1] As can be seen in Table 39–2, incidence rates are much higher in whites than in blacks and the incidence goes up with age. The incidence rates for males older than 65 years is 93.7/100,000 and for females of the same age group it is 68.1. The 5-year relative survival is about 53 percent overall. This survival is much poorer than that of Hodgkin's disease. A trend toward poorer survival in the older patient is seen that is not as marked as that observed for survival in Hodgkin's disease. As is observed in the latter disease, survival is somewhat better in whites than in blacks, but whites have strikingly higher rates of both diseases than do blacks.[1]

Table 39–2. Important Statistics on Non-Hodgkin's Lymphomas

Population	Incidence
U.S. incidence per 100,000 population per year, 1994–1998	
Overall U.S. rate	16.1
Males	19.8
Females	13.0
Whites	16.7
Blacks	12.6
0–14 years	0.9
< 65 years	
Males	11.7
Females	7.0
65 + years	
Males	93.7
Females	68.1

Population	Survival (%)
U.S. 5-year relative survival, 1994–1998	
Overall	53.0
Males	50.1
Females	56.5
Whites	54.0
Blacks	45.8
Survival by age at diagnosis	
0–14 years	78.7
15–34 years	55.0
35–64 years	60.2
65 + years	44.6

Rates are adjusted to the 1970 U.S. standard population.
Based on SEER data, April 2001.

International Variation

Figure 39–2 depicts non-Hodgkin's lymphoma age-incidence patterns for the United States and the same three selected Asian countries as in Figure 39–1.[9] In contrast to the age-incidence pattern for Hodgkin's disease, that of non-Hodgkin's lymphoma shows a unimodal pattern that rises steeply with age after age 30 years. Although the age-incidence curves are of similar shapes in the four countries illustrated, far greater differences are seen between countries in the height of the incidence curves than are observed for Hodgkin's disease. The incidence scales used for the four graphs are quite different as a result. In all the countries illustrated, non-Hodgkin's lymphoma incidence is higher in males than in females.

Changing Incidence

One of the most striking epidemiologic features of the non-Hodgkin's lymphomas is their gradually increasing incidence rates in the United States and other developed countries. Even though much of the overall crude increase is due to the aging population of developed countries such as the United States, a steady increase in the incidence is seen even when incidence rates are adjusted for age. Since the early 1970s, U.S. incidence

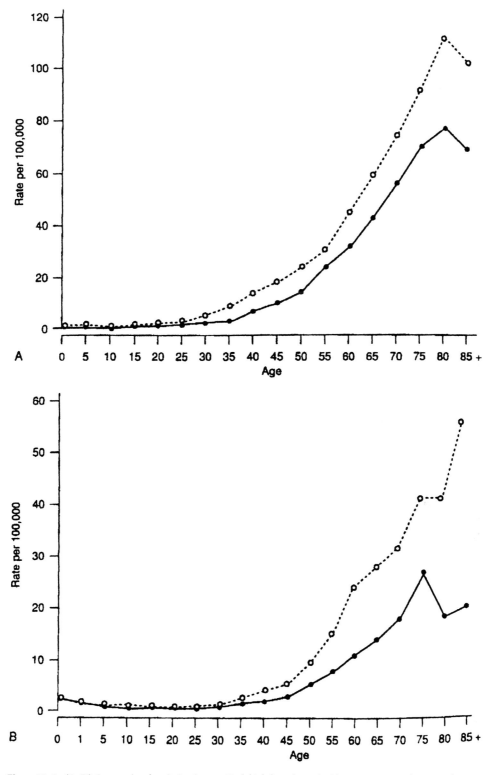

Figure 39–2. (A–D). International variation in non-Hodgkin's lymphoma incidence, 1893–1987, by age and sex. Note differences in incidence scales for each country. (A) USA, SEER, white. (B) Japan, Osaka prefecture. *(Figure continues.)*

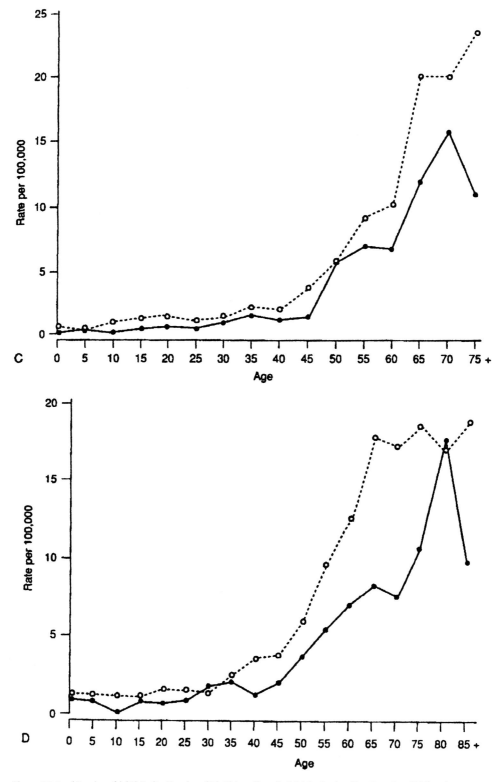

Figure 39–2. *(Continued.)* (C) India, Bombay. (D) China, Shanghai, Male, *broken line;* Female *solid line.* (From Parkin et al.,[9] with permission.)

rates have increased at the rate of 3 to 4 percent a year, which is more rapid than for all cancers other than melanoma and lung cancer among women.[35] These increasing rates are seen for all ages (except the very young), in whites and blacks, in the United States and internationally, and in both sexes. During the 1980s, a further increase was seen in young and middle-aged men related to the AIDS epidemic, but this does not account for all the observed increase in incidence. Increases have been more marked for extranodal disease, particularly for non-Hodgkin's lymphomas arising in the brain, and for high-grade tumors. These observations have stimulated great interest, but no clear explanations have been found. The most recent data from the U.S. SEER program show that this increase has leveled off beginning about 1994 and that it might be declining from this peak.[1] Figure 39–3 shows the incidence pattern for both non-Hodgkin's lymphoma and Hodgkin's disease using SEER data. As can be seen, the increasing incidence of non-Hodgkin's lymphoma has abated. The comparable incidence for Hodgkin's disease shows a relatively stable pattern over the past 25 years.

It should be kept in mind that the non-Hodgkin's lymphomas are probably a diverse group of diseases. The observed overall increase in incidence may mask significantly more striking increases of individual entities within this rubric. While such nosologic guides as the Working Formulation are useful to the clinician, the identification of individual diseases within the overall category will require immunophenotypic and other molecular studies to identify specific disease entities.[36] It is also clear that the increasing incidence cannot be explained on the basis of changes in diagnosis over time. Proper classification of the non-Hodgkin's lymphomas for epidemiologic studies will require close cooperation between epidemiologists and expert pathologists to develop meaningful diagnostic entities.

Immunodeficiency

No malignancy, with the possible exception of Kaposi's sarcoma, is more strongly associated with immunodeficiency than is non-Hodgkin's lymphoma. The best established cause is impairment of immune function caused by primary immunodeficiency syndromes, pharmacologic intervention (as used in transplantation), or human immunodeficiency virus (HIV) infection. Observation of this linkage between immunodeficiency and increased lymphoma risk derives originally from studies of cancer occurrence in primary immunodeficiency syndromes. A series of 500 cancers from the Immunodeficiency-Cancer Registry at the University of Minnesota reveals that overall 50.4 percent of all cancers in these subjects are non-Hodgkin's lymphomas.[37] The second most frequent cancers in this registry are leukemias. Hodgkin's disease ranks fourth behind adenocarcinoma. The median age at diagnosis for lymphoma cases in this registry is 7.1 years. A 3:1 male/female ratio was seen, which may reflect the contribution of several X-linked disorders as well as the observation of a male excess in tumors of subjects with ataxia-telangiectasia, an autosomal recessive disorder. Most of the non-Hodgkin's lymphomas in primary immunodeficiency patients are of B-cell origin. The association between EBV and non-Hodgkin's lymphomas occurring in patients with primary immunodeficiencies has not been universal. In this regard, these lymphomas are more similar to those seen in AIDS patients. A high frequency of extranodal non-Hodgkin's lymphoma in the primary immunodeficiencies is found, primarily of the central nervous system and gastrointestinal tract.[37]

A second major immunodeficiency risk factor is that of therapeutic immunosuppression, such as in patients undergoing transplantation. The first observations to demonstrate this finding were studies of non-Hodgkin's lymphoma risk in renal transplant recipients. It was observed that the disease developed 40 to 100 times more often than expected and that these tumors had a predilection for the central nervous system, primarily the brain, which was involved in almost half the cases.[38,39] Most of this excess risk is evident within the first year following transplantation. The risk appears to be related to the intensity of the immunosuppressive therapy, which is reflected in the higher incidence of post-transplant non-Hodgkin's lymphoma in heart and pancreas transplant patients, who receive an unusually intensive immunosuppressive regimen.[40] In the overwhelming majority of the lymphomas seen in post-transplant patients, EBV is found in the tumor samples.[37] It is also possible that non-Hodgkin's lymphoma occurs with increased frequency in patients without transplantation who received immunosuppressive drugs for conditions such as collagen diseases. Kinlen[41] reported an 11-fold increased risk in patients without grafts who received immunosuppressive drugs for conditions such as rheumatoid arthritis.

In summary, inherited immunodeficiency syndromes or pharmacologic immunosuppression cause a very striking and large increased risk. In both instances, the frequencies of both extranodal disease and an aggressive clinical course are high. Whereas post-transplantation non-Hodgkin's lymphomas are largely EBV associated, in a review of tumor specimens from 13 cases in the University of Minnesota Immunodeficiency Registry only 31 percent were EBV positive.[37] Immunodeficiency, whether primary, secondary to therapy, or acquired, appears to

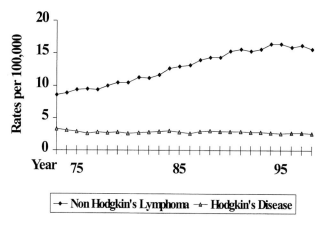

Figure 39–3. Time Trends in the U.S. Incidence of Non-Hodgkin's Lymphoma and Hodgkin's Disease

be the best established and strongest risk factor for non-Hodgkin's lymphoma.

AIDS-Related Disease

Non-Hodgkin's lymphomas were found to occur remarkably frequently in AIDS patients, an observation that was made quite early in the AIDS epidemic.[42] Further documentation of the AIDS-non-Hodgkin's lymphoma association led to the inclusion of non-Hodgkin's lymphoma as a diagnostic criterion for AIDS when the criteria were changed in 1985.[43] Based on epidemiologic surveys, it has been estimated that non-Hodgkin's lymphomas occur 60 times more frequently in AIDS patients than do similar lymphomas in the general population.[44] It is estimated that non-Hodgkin's lymphoma is the index AIDS diagnosis in about 3 percent of new AIDS cases, with some evidence suggesting that this frequency may be increasing.[45] AIDS-related non-Hodgkin's lymphomas occur in all risk group categories for AIDS (i.e., intravenous drug users, heterosexual contacts of cases, transfusion recipients, and so forth). No differences between risk groups have been reported with regard to clinical manifestations, clinical course, or response to therapy.[45] The patterns of occurrence in HIV patients appears to be changing over time. Earlier in the AIDS epidemic, about 50 percent of the patients with AIDS-related non-Hodgkin's lymphoma had a previous diagnosis of opportunistic infection or Kaposi's sarcoma (or both), and only 15 percent had no previous AIDS diagnosis. More recently the proportion of such patients with no preceding AIDS-related diagnosis has risen to approximately one-third to one-half.

The impact of HIV infection on incidence has been estimated by modeling techniques. About 2000 AIDS-related non-Hodgkin's lymphoma cases occurred in the United States in 1990.[46] Projections into the future suggest that between 8 and 27 percent of non-Hodgkin's lymphoma cases diagnosed in the United States might be AIDS related. However, it must be remembered that the overall rising incidence of the non-Hodgkin's lymphomas in the United States and other countries has clearly preceded the AIDS epidemic and is independent of the contribution of AIDS-related cases.

The clinical presentation of AIDS-related non-Hodgkin's lymphoma is similar to that seen in primary, immune deficiency conditions or other immunosuppressed patients. The non-Hodgkin's lymphoma seen in HIV-infected individuals is of high-grade subtypes, with undifferentiated or immunoblastic lymphoma accounting for 60 to 80 percent of reported cases of AIDS-related non-Hodgkin's lymphoma.[47] Burkitt's lymphoma-like tumors account for approximately 20 percent of AIDS-related non-Hodgkin's lymphomas in the United States and seem to occur most frequently in children and young adults between 10 and 19 years of age.[44] Interestingly, most of the Burkitt's lymphoma-like AIDS-related non-Hodgkins lymphomas show no evidence of EBV in tumor tissues. Also, most of the AIDS-related Burkitt's lymphoma-like lesions are similar to nonendemic Burkitt's lymphomas in that they have a low frequency of the characteristic cytogenetic abnormalities seen in the endemic form. However, some AIDS-related Burkitt's lymphoma-like tumors in AIDS patients have been found to have the characteristic cytogenetic abnormalities and EBV positivity seen in endemic Burkitt's lymphoma.

In general, the AIDS-related non-Hodgkin's lymphomas are primarily of B-cell origin and have a rapid progression and aggressive clinical picture with single or multiple tumors and a predilection for extranodal sites. As in non-AIDS-related non-Hodgkin's lymphomas, males are more frequently affected than females. Primary CNS non-Hodgkin's lymphoma is a frequent AIDS-related type. Such CNS involvement is rare in nonimmunocompromised groups, occurring in approximately 1 percent of non-Hodgkin's lymphomas, but it has been reported to constitute about 20 percent of those associated with AIDS.[44] Again, it must be pointed out that the increasing incidence of primary CNS lymphoma in the general population appears to be independent of the increase of primary CNS lymphoma in HIV-infected persons.[48] Primary CNS lymphoma may account for up to one-fourth of all HIV-associated non-Hodgkin's lymphomas, and involvement of the CNS occurs in 10 to 25 percent of patients presenting at other sites.[49] Based on observations such as these, the case definition initially chosen for diagnosis of AIDS was changed to include HIV-positive patients with both high-grade B-cell lymphoma and primary brain lymphomas.[43] It should also be pointed out that the non-Hodgkin's lymphomas seen in AIDS may be occult and may only be demonstrated at autopsy.[49] Unfortunately, the precise role of EBV in the AIDS-related non-Hodgkin's lymphomas has not been elucidated and may very well differ in various subgroups.

The increasing incidence of AIDS-related non-Hodgkin's lymphoma cannot account solely for the increasing incidence of non-Hodgkin's lymphoma observed in the United States, and elsewhere. Nevertheless, it is an important contributor to the rise in incidence. It also further suggests that immunodeficiency, whether congenital, acquired, or pharmacologically induced, is a potent risk factor.

Familial Aggregation

Numerous case reports and series of interesting kindreds have documented the occurrence of more than one non-Hodgkin's lymphoma in family members.[50] In comparing aggregation of cancers in Hodgkin's disease and non-Hodgkin's lymphoma families, several differences are immediately apparent. The first is that for the non-Hodgkin's lymphomas far more families are multiply affected (larger proportions of affected relatives) than is seen in Hodgkin's disease. Second, in non-Hodgkin's lymphoma familial aggregation involves relatives with the same disease as well as other lymphoproliferative malignancies, whereas reports of familial aggregation of Hodgkin's disease primarily deal with multiple occurrences of the same disease. A third difference relates to reports of multiply affected preadolescent male sibships with extranodal non-Hodgkin's lymphomas, primarily of the gastrointestinal tract. Such observations are reported primarily from Mediterranean countries. These may be related to the so-called Mediterranean lymphomas, which are associated with the production of abnormal immunoglobulins. Fourth is the observation that in many multiply affected families primary immunodeficiency syndromes such as ataxia-telangiectasia are also found.[50] Although familial aggregation of non-Hodgkin's lymphoma appears to be more striking than that of Hodgkin's disease, the exact magnitude of the increased risk to relatives has not been determined. It is estimated that a history of non-Hodgkin's lymphoma or other lymphoproliferative neoplasm increases the risk to relatives by three- to fourfold.[50] This is about the same magnitude of increased risk for Hodgkin's disease in close relatives. Thus, family history of non-Hodgkin's lymphoma or another lymphoreticular malignancy is the second strongest known risk factor.

Recently Wiernik et al. observed that genetic anticipation occurs in familial non-Hodgkin's lymphoma.[51] A significant difference was observed between the ages of onset in the children of cases' generation and the SEER population but not in the parent generation and the SEER population. If these findings are confirmed by others, they suggest a genetic basis for non-Hodgkin's lymphomas.

Skin Cancer and Ultraviolet Exposure

A recent report by Adami et al.[52] suggests that ultraviolet exposure, as from sunlight, might be one of the factors underlying the increasing incidence of non-Hodgkin's lymphoma. This finding fits with an earlier report of an excess of skin cancer in patients with non-Hodgkin's lymphoma.[53] Additionally, melanoma and squamous cell cancers of the skin occur excessively, along with non-Hodgkin's lymphoma, in renal transplant recipients.[38,39] These observations, plus the increasing incidence of melanoma, led these investigators to pursue this hypothesis.[52] They reported a fivefold increased risk of squamous cell skin cancer and a twofold increased risk of melanoma in non-Hodgkin's lymphoma patients. Conversely, they found a twofold increased risk of the disease in squamous cell skin cancer patients. These findings stimulated much further research. Some subsequent studies confirmed an association between ultraviolet exposure and lymphoma risk[71,72] and others did not.[73,75] At present the association remains equivocal, but increasingly appears unlikely to stand the test of time.

Occupational Exposures

Although many studies of occupational exposures have been performed, few consistent or strong observations have been reported. One area of major investigation has been farming occupations: at least 21 cohort studies of farmers or occupational surveys of cancer that presented data on non-Hodgkin's lymphoma and farming occupations have been done.[54] The risk ratios for the association between this disease and farming ranged from 0.6 to 2.6. Eleven of these 21 studies reported excess risks in farmers, but only 3 of these were statistically significantly in excess. One of the 21 surveys showed a significantly low relative risk, implying a protective effect. The lesson to be learned from this array of occupational studies is that many studies have been done of numerous occupations and numerous cancers. Hundreds, if not thousands, of associations are assessed, and it must be remembered that 5 of each 100 might be expected to deviate significantly from the null hypothesis just on the basis of chance. Thus, for an assumption of causality to be made for such associations, factors such as the consistency of the findings, the strength of the reported association, the biologic plausibility of the association, and observation of dose-response relationships need to be considered. Using such criteria, it would appear that

a slightly increased risk is consistently found in farmers. In general, the magnitude of the increased risk is below twofold and could be due to unidentified confounding factors.

The observation of a possible increased risk in farmers led to studies of chemicals used by these farmers. From these studies has emerged the observation that there appears to be an association between pesticide exposure and risk. Several studies have evaluated the potential etiologic role of phenoxy herbicides.[55] Although the results lack consistency, the findings are more consistent than are those from studies of farming occupations. A dose-response relationship has been suggested in some of the studies as well. At present, an association appears to exist between herbicide use (particularly phenoxy herbicides) and risk of NHL.[34] The evidence is not overwhelmingly persuasive at this time and the magnitude of increased risk is probably on the order of twofold.

There have been several reports linking hair dye use to risk of non-Hodgkin's lymphoma. Many hair dyes contain substances that are mutagenic or carcinogenic in animals (or both) and several studies have shown excess risks of leukemia and non-Hodgkin's lymphoma in hairdressers and cosmetologists. Three case-control studies specifically evaluated the risk in hair-dye users.[56–58] The relative risks in these studies range from 1.4 to 2.0. The relative frequency of hair dye use in the general population is high and thus hair dye usage could account for a small proportion of all non-Hodgkin's lymphoma cases. As has often been the case, these findings have not withstood the test of time. A large, well performed prospective study, as part of the Nurses' Health Study, found no association between permanent hair dye use and risk of non-Hodgkin's lymphoma.[59] La Vecchia et al., reviewed the literature on this topic and found only a weak association in the published cohort studies (RR=1.5).[60] Results from case-control studies also showed weak and inconsistent associations, and there may have been inadequate consideration of potential confounding factors as well. Thus, it appears that this interesting etiologic lead, like so many others, could not be confirmed. Other occupational and environmental factors that have been considered include radiation, zoonotic viruses, exposure to wood and chemicals, electromagnetic fields, and a variety of other occupations.[61] In general, none of these exposures has been consistently associated with an increased risk. In summary, very large numbers of investigations of the potential etiologic role of environmental and occupational exposures in the non-Hodgkin's lymphomas have been conducted; thus far, these exposures appear to play at most a slight role in the overall causation.

Burkitt's Lymphoma

From an epidemiologist's viewpoint, one of the most interesting non-Hodgkin's lymphomas is Burkitt's lymphoma. Burkitt's lymphoma has perhaps stirred up the greatest interest in the possible viral etiology of human lymphomas. Denis Burkitt[62] was an Irish surgeon who, while working in Uganda, first drew attention to a lymphoid malignancy primarily involving the jaw in children. This disease, which he called *African lymphoma,* had distinct clinical, pathologic, and epidemiologic features, Burkitt[63] went on what he termed "tumor safaris" throughout Africa to map the distribution of Burkitt's lymphoma. He defined a lymphoma belt extending entirely across Africa, but in a manner corresponding to tropical areas of low altitude. Within his lymphoma belt, he found little Burkitt's lymphoma in areas of high altitude.[64] Based on his observations, Burkitt concluded that the disease was defined by rainfall and altitude and corresponded closely to those areas in which malaria was endemic. Later it was found that Burkitt's lymphoma appeared to be endemic in New Guinea, particularly in its lowland areas. He did not consider malaria itself as the cause since it occurred in countries other than Africa or New Guinea where there is no malaria. This led Burkitt to consider an arthropod-borne virus as the etiologic agent. Burkitt sent specimens of his African lymphoma to outside investigators for study. In 1964 Epstein, Achong, and Barr[65] were able to demonstrate a new herpesvirus in cultured Burkitt's lymphoma cells from one of Burkitt's patients. It was also observed that when this new virus infected cells it immortalized them in tissue culture. Here was a new virus that appeared to be the cause of an unusual African lymphoma.

One of the fascinating early findings in the study of Burkitt's lymphoma was that of time-space clustering, a characteristic of many infectious diseases.[66] Several studies showed very clear-cut time-space clustering of Burkitt's lymphoma in areas of Uganda. These occurrences appear to suggest epidemic behavior of the disease. However, it must be noted that time-space clustering, while characteristic of many infectious diseases, can also be due to other noninfectious shared environmental exposures. Also, based on studies in Uganda, Burkitt's lymphoma patients appeared to come from families of lower socioeconomic status.[67]

Based on the observed overlapping of malarious areas and the occurrence of Burkitt's lymphoma in Africa, many hypotheses were developed that regarded malaria as an etiologic co-factor. While these notions suffice for endemic Burkitt's lymphoma, they could not explain the etiology of the sporadic cases that occur in nonmalarious developed countries.

EBV was subsequently shown to occur throughout the world and was identified as the causative agent of infectious mononucleosis by Henle et al. in 1968.[68] EBV was later found to be associated with many other diseases such as nasopharyngeal carcinoma, sarcoidosis, and lupus erythematosus. It is also almost uniformly present in those lymphomas occurring post-transplantation. African Burkitt's lymphoma cases have very much higher EBV antibody titers than do controls, particularly viral capsid antigen (VCA) antibody titers.[69] The high titers of EBV VCA antibodies in Burkitt's lymphoma patients were found to antedate the occurrence of the tumor by months to years.[70] With the advent of newer molecular biologic techniques, EBV could be detected in Burkitt's lymphoma tumor tissues. About 90 percent of endemic Burkitt's lymphoma patients, but only 10 to 15 percent of the nonendemic cases, have been found to have EBV in their tumors.[47]

Another characteristic of Burkitt's lymphoma is a high frequency of chromosomal translocations that occur at specific breakpoints on chromosomes 8, 14, 2, and 22.[47] t(8:14) is demonstrated in over 90 percent of endemic Burkitt's lymphoma tumors. The remaining 10 percent of tumors equally show t(8:2) and t(8:22). These translocations appear to be unrelated to the presence or absence of EBV in the tumor tissues. The less common sporadic form of Burkitt's lymphoma occurs in economically developed countries with a worldwide distribution. The sporadic form shows a bimodal age incidence pattern, with peaks in children older than in the endemic form and also in adults. Most of the sporadic Burkitt's lymphomas are extranodal, with a high proportion of tumors affecting the gastrointestinal tract or CNS rather than the jaw, as seen in endemic disease. Only about 15 percent of sporadic Burkitt's tumors are EBV associated.[47] Both types represent clonal proliferations of B cells and both exhibit the same chromosomal translocations. In AIDS-related Burkitt's lymphoma, variability of the tumors exists, with some showing the findings of sporadic and others the findings of endemic Burkitt's lymphomas. However, most of the tumors show no evidence of EBV.[47]

In summary, Burkitt's lymphoma appears to be intertwined with EBV. However, EBV is infrequently found in the sporadic form, which is seen in developed countries. Thus, the model developed to explain the occurrence of Burkitt's lymphoma in endemic areas (an interplay of EBV infection, malaria, and some as yet unidentified third factor) cannot explain all cases. Nevertheless, the unusual descriptive epidemiologic features of the disease and the well-documented occurrence of time-space case clustering, plus the apparently major role that EBV plays in most of the these cases, suggest that Burkitt's lymphoma is a leading candidate among human cancers for a viral etiology.

SUMMARY

Both Hodgkin's disease and non-Hodgkin's lymphoma are interesting diseases that have puzzled epidemiologists due to their many tantalizing epidemiologic findings. Until recently, the non-Hodgkin's lymphomas had been gradually increasing in incidence, whereas Hodgkin's disease incidence has been either steady or slightly decreasing overall.[71] The increasing incidence of non-Hodgkin's lymphoma cannot be fully explained by the AIDS-related cases. Both diseases have striking international variation in their occurrence, with some of the highest incidence rates occurring in the United States and other developed countries. Both diseases exhibit striking (but unfortunately poorly characterized) familial aggregation with an increased risk to relatives on the order of three- to fourfold (Tables 39–3, 39–4). Both diseases may evidence genetic anticipation. Hodgkin's disease has a bimodal age-incidence pattern, whereas non-Hodgkin's lymphoma has a unimodal pattern with its mode occurring in the elderly. The bimodality of Hodgkin's disease is not constant from country to country: it varies with age, and the first young-adult mode is absent in several Asian countries. Whereas socioeconomic status appears to be directly associated with risk of both diseases, far more data exist on this topic for Hodgkin's disease than for non-Hodgkin's lymphoma. In fact, the socioeconomic status findings related to Hodgkin's disease make a strong case for the importance of environmental factors in the etiology of the disease. However, for both diseases only a few associations have been consistently reported between non-viral environmental exposures and risk. The most intriguing commonality between the two diseases is their association with EBV (Tables 39–3 and 39–4), although different patterns of association are seen. The lymphomas represent some of the few human cancers in which a virus can be identified in tumor specimens with any degree of regularity.

Table 39-3. Known Risk Factors for Hodgkin's Disease

Risk Factor	Strength of the Associations	Consistency of the Associations
EBV infection	Moderate	Consistent
Socioeconomic status	Moderate	Consistent
Family history of Hodgkin's disease	Moderate	Consistent
Childhood infections	Moderate	Consistent
Occupational exposures	Weak	Inconsistent

For both diseases, the most likely etiologic mechanism is a complex interplay among genetic susceptibility, immune function, and viral infection (Tables 39–3 and 39–4). The difficulty in unraveling this complex knot is that abnormal immune function could be genetically determined or virally induced. Which virus may cause these diseases is not known. Although EBV is likely to be a sufficient cause in some cases, it is not a necessary cause, as evidenced by the many EBV-negative lymphomas. It appears that HIV is not a direct cause of either disease, rather it is more likely that the disturbed immune function caused by HIV leads to the non-Hodgkin's lymphomas and, less frequently, to Hodgkin's disease. On these grounds, both groups of diseases would appear to be fertile territory for uncovering important etiologic mechanisms in human cancer.

ACKNOWLEDGMENT

This chapter has been supported by the National Institutes of Health, grant R01 CA 47473.

REFERENCES

1. Surveillance, Epidemiology and End Results Cancer Incidence Public-Use Database, 1973–1998. U.S. Department of Health and Human Services, National Cancer Institute, Bethesda, MD, April 2001.
2. Walker A, Schoenfeld ER, Lowman JT et al: Survival of the older compared to younger patient with Hodgkin's disease: The influence of histology, staging and treatment. Cancer 65:1635, 1990.
3. MacMahon B: Epidemiologic evidence on the nature of Hodgkin's disease. Cancer 10:1045, 1957.
4. MacMahon B: Epidemiology of Hodgkin's disease. Cancer Res 26:1189, 1966.
5. Grufferman S, Delzell E: Epidemiology of Hodgkin's disease. Epidemiol Rev 6:76, 1984.
6. Glaser SL: Reproductive factors in Hodgkin's disease in women: A review. Am J Epidemiol 139:237, 1994.
7. Correa P, O'Conor GT: Epidemiologic patterns of Hodgkin's disease. Int J Cancer 8:192, 1971.
8. Macfarlane GJ, Evstifeeva T, Boyle P, Grufferman S: International patterns in the occurrence of Hodgkin's disease in children and young adult males. Int J Cancer 61:165, 1995.
9. Parkin DM, Muir CS, Whelan SL et al (eds.): Cancer Incidence in Five Continents. Vol. 6. IARC Scientific Publication 120. IARC, Lyon, 1992.
10. LeShan L, Marvin S, Lyerly O: Some evidence of a relationship between Hodgkin's disease and intelligence. Arch Gen Psychiatry 1:477, 1959.
11. Cohen BM, Smetana HF, Miller RW: Hodgkin's disease: Long survival in a study of 388 World War II army cases. Cancer 17:856, 1964.
12. Gutensohn NM, Cole P: Childhood social environment and Hodgkin's disease. N Engl J Med 304:135, 1981.
13. Newell G: Etiology of multiple sclerosis and Hodgkin's disease. Am J Epidemiol 91:119, 1970.
14. Paffenbarger R Jr, Wing AL, Hyde RT: Characteristics in youth indicative of adult onset Hodgkin's disease. J Natl Cancer Inst 58:1489, 1977.
15. Evans AS, Comstock GW: Presence of elevated antibody titers to Epstein-Barr virus before Hodgkin's disease. Lancet 1:1183, 1981.
16. Mueller N, Evans A, Harris NL et al: Hodgkin's disease and Epstein-Barr virus. Altered antibody pattern before diagnosis. N Engl J Med 320:689, 1989.
17. Weiss LM, Strickler JG, Warnke RA et al: Epstein-Barr viral DNA in tissues of Hodgkin's disease. Am J Pathol 129:86, 1987.
18. Brousset P, Chittal S, Schlaifer D et al: Detection of Epstein-Barr virus messenger RNA in Reed-Sternberg cells of Hodgkin's disease by in situ hybridization with biotinylated probes on specially processed modified acetone methyl benzoate xylene (ModAMeX) sections. Blood 77:1781, 1991.
19. International Agency for Research on Cancer (France): IARC Monographs on the Evaluation of Carcinogenic Risk to Humans, Vol 70. Epstein-Barr virus and Kaposi's sarcoma herpesvirus/human herpesvirus 8, p. 524 FF. IARC: Lyon, France, 1997.
20. Razis DV, Diamond HD, Carver LF: Familial Hodgkin's disease: Its significance and implications. Ann Intern Med 51:933, 1959.
21. Grufferman S, Cole P, Smith PG, Lukes R: Hodgkin's disease in siblings. N Engl J Med 296:248, 1977.
22. Grufferman S, Barton JW, Eby NL: Increased sex concordance of sibling pairs with Behçet's disease, Hodgkin's disease, multiple sclerosis and sarcoidosis. Am J Epidemiol 126:365, 1987.
23. Mack TM, Cohen W, Shibata DK et al: Concordance for Hodgkin's disease in identical twins suggesting genetic susceptibility to the young-adult form of the disease. N Engl J Med 332:413, 1995.
24. Shugart YY, Hemminki K, Vaittinen P, Kingman A, Dong C: A genetic study of Hodgkin's lymphoma: An estimate of heritability and anticipation based on the familial cancer database in Sweden. Hum Genet 106:553, 2000.
25. Lynch HT: Anticipation in familial Hodgkin's lymphoma. Hum Genet 107:290, 2000.
26. Schlaifer D, Rigal-Huguet F, Robert A et al: Epstein-Barr virus in familial Hodgkin's disease. Br J Haem 88:636, 1994.
27. Lin A, Kingma D, Lennette E et al: Epstein-Barr virus (EBV) is not associated with familial Hodgkin's disease (FHD). Proc Am Soc Clin Oncol 13:185, 1994.
28. Vianna NJ, Greenwald P, Davies JNP: Extended epidemic of Hodgkin's disease in high school students. Lancet 1:1209, 1971.
29. Grufferman S: Clustering and aggregation of exposures in Hodgkin's disease. Cancer 39:1829, 1977.

Table 39-4. Known Risk Factors for the Non-Hodgkin's Lymphomas

Risk Factor	Strength of the Associations	Consistency of the Associations
Immune deficiency		
Primary	Strong	Consistent
Post-transplantation	Very strong	Consistent
Other drug-induced	Strong	Few studies
Acquired (AIDS)	Moderate	Consistent
Family history of non-Hodgkin's lymphoma	Moderate	Consistent
EBV infection	Moderate	Consistent
Occupational exposures	Weak to moderate	Inconsistent

30. Vianna NJ, Polan AK: Epidemiologic evidence for transmission of Hodgkin's disease. N Engl J Med 289:499, 1973.

31. Grufferman S, Cole P, Levitan T: Evidence against transmission of Hodgkin's disease in high schools. N Engl J Med 300:1006, 1979.

32. Smith PG, Pike MC, Kinlen LJ et al: Contacts between young patients with Hodgkin's disease: A case-control study. Lancet 2:59, 1977.

33. Alexander FE, Williams J, McKinney PA et al: A specialist leukemia/lymphoma registry in the U.K. Part 2: Clustering of Hodgkin's disease. Br J Cancer 60:948, 1989.

34. Morrison HI, Wilkins K, Semenciw RM et al: Herbicides and cancer. J Natl Cancer Inst 84:1866, 1992.

35. DeVesa SS, Fears T: Non-Hodgkin's lymphoma time trends: United States and international data. Cancer Res 52:5432s, 1992.

36. Jaffe ES, Raffeld M, Medeiros LJ, Stetler-Stevenson M: An overview of the classification of non-Hodgkin's lymphomas: An integration of morphological and phenotypical concepts. Cancer Res 52:5447s, 1992.

37. Filipovich AH, Mathur A, Kamat D, Shapiro RS: Primary immunodeficiencies: Genetic risk factors for lymphoma. Cancer Res 52:5465s, 1992.

38. Hoover R, Fraumeni JF Jr: Risk of cancer in renal transplant recipients. Lancet 2:55, 1973.

39. Kinlen LJ, Sheil AGR, Peto J, Doll R: A collaborative study of cancer in patients who have received immunosuppressive therapy. BMJ 2:1461, 1979.

40. Kinlen LJ: Immunosuppressive therapy and cancer. Cancer Surv 1:565, 1982.

41. Kinlen LJ: Incidence of cancer in rheumatoid arthritis and other disorders after immunosuppressive treatment. Am J Med (Suppl. 1A):44, 1985.

42. Ziegler JL, Drew WL, Miner RC: Outbreak of Burkitt's-like lymphoma in homosexual men. Lancet 2:631, 1982.

43. Centers for Disease Control: Revision of the case definition of acquired immunodeficiency syndrome for national reporting: United States. MMWR 31:373, 1985.

44. Beral V, Peterman T, Berkelman R, Jaffe H: Non-Hodgkin's lymphoma in persons with AIDS. Lancet 337:805, 1991.

45. Northfelt DW, Kaplan LD: Clinical manifestations and treatment of HIV related non-Hodgkin's lymphoma. In Beral V, Jaffe H, Weiss R (eds.): Cancer, HIV and AIDS. Cancer Surveys Series. Vol. 10. p. 121. Cold Spring Harbor Laboratory Press, Cold Spring Harbor, NY, 1991.

46. Rabkin CS, Biggar RJ, Horm J: Increasing incidence of cancers associated with the human immunodeficiency virus epidemic. Int J Cancer 47:692, 1991.

47. Luxton JC, Thomas JA, Crawford DH: Aetiology and pathogenesis of non-Hodgkin's lymphoma in AIDS. In Beral V, Jaffe H, Weiss R (eds.): Cancer, HIV and AIDS. Cancer Surveys Series. Vol. 10. Cold Spring Harbor Laboratory Press, p. 103. Cold Spring Harbor, NY, 1991.

48. Eby NL, Grufferman S, Flannelly CM et al: Increasing incidence of primary brain lymphoma in the U.S. Cancer 62:2461, 1988.

49. Obrams GI, Grufferman S: Epidemiology of HIV-associated non-Hodgkin's lymphomas, In Beral V, Jaffe H, Weiss R (eds.): Cancer, HIV and AIDS. Cancer Surveys Series. Vol. 10. p. 91. Cold Spring Harbor Laboratory Press, Cold Spring Harbor, NY, 1991.

50. Linet MS, Pottern LM: Familial aggregation of hematopoietic malignancies and risk of non-Hodgkin's lymphoma. Cancer Res 52:5468s, 1992.

51. Wiernik PH, Wang SQ, Hu XP, Marino P, Paietta E: Age of onset evidence for anticipation in familial non-Hodgkin's lymphoma. Br J Haematol 108:72, 2000.

52. Adami J, Frisch M, Yuen J et al: Evidence of an association between non-Hodgkin's lymphoma and skin cancer. BMJ 310:1491, 1995.

53. Berg JW: The incidence of multiple primary cancers. 1. Development of further cancers in patients with lymphomas, leukemias and myeloma. J Natl Cancer Inst 38:741, 1967.

54. Blair A, Zahm SH: Cancer among farmers. Occup Med State of Art Rev 6:335, 1991.

55. Zahm SH, Blair A: Pesticides and non-Hodgkin's lymphoma. Cancer Res 52:5485s, 1992.

56. Cantor KP, Blair A, Everett G: Hair dye use and risk of leukemia and lymphoma. Am J Public Health 78:570, 1988.

57. Pearce NE, Smith AH, Fisher DO: Malignant lymphoma and multiple myeloma linked with agricultural occupations in a New Zealand Cancer Registry-based study. Am J Epidemiol 121:225, 1985.

58. Zahm SH, Weisenburger DD, Babbitt PA et al: Use of hair coloring products and the risk of lymphoma, multiple myeloma and chronic lymphocytic leukemia. Am J Public Health 82:990, 1992.

59. Grodstein F, Hennekens CH, Colditz GA, Hunter DJ, Stampfer MJ: A prospective study of permanent hair dye use and hematopoietic cancer. J Natl Cancer Inst 86:1466, 1994.

60. La Vecchia C, Tavani A: Epidemiological evidence on hair dyes and risk of cancer in humans. Eur J Cancer Prev 4:31, 1995.

61. Pierce N, Bethwaite P: Increasing incidence of non-Hodgkin's lymphoma: occupational and environmental factors. Cancer Res 52:5496s, 1992.

62. Burkitt DP: A sarcoma involving the jaws in African children. Br J Surg 46:218, 1958.

63. Burkitt DP: A "tumor safari" in East and Central Africa. Br J Cancer 16:379, 1962.

64. Burkitt DP: Determining the climate limitations of a children's cancer common in Africa. BMJ 2:1019, 1962.

65. Epstein MA, Achong BG, Barr YM: Virus particles in cultured lymphoblasts from Burkitt's lymphoma. Lancet 1:702, 1964.

66. Pike MC, Williams EH, Wright B: Burkitt's tumour in the West Nile District of Uganda. BMJ 2:395, 1967.

67. Morrow RH, Kisuule A, Mafigiri J: Socioeconomic factors in Burkitt's lymphoma. Cancer Res 34:1212, 1974.

68. Henle G, Henle W, Diehl V: Relation of Burkitt's tumor-associated herpes type virus to infectious mononucleosis. Proc Natl Acad Sci U S A 59:94, 1968.

69. Henle G, Henle W, Clifford W: Antibodies to Epstein-Barr virus in Burkitt's lymphoma and control groups. J Natl Cancer Inst 43:861, 1969.

70. de-Thé G, Geser A, Day NE: Epidemiological evidence for causal relationship between Epstein-Barr virus and Burkitt's lymphoma from Ugandan prospective study. Nature 274:756, 1978.

71. Glaser SL: Recent incidence and secular trends in Hodgkin's disease and its histologic subtypes. J Chron Dis 39:789, 1986.

72. Bentham G: Association between incidence of non-Hodgkin's lymphoma and solar ultraviolet radiation in England and Wales. BMJ 312:1128, 1996.

73. Hakansson N, Floderus B, Gustavsson P, Feychting M, Hallin N: Occupational sunlight exposure and cancer incidence among Swedish construction workers. Epidemiology 12:552, 2001.

74. Freedman DM, Zahm SH, Dosemeci M: Residential and occupational exposure to sunlight and mortality from non-Hodgkin's lymphoma: Composite (threefold) case-control study. BMJ 314:1451, 1997.

75. Adami J, Gridley G, Nyren O, et al: Sunlight and non-Hodgkin's lymphoma: A population-based cohort study in Sweden. Int J Cancer 80:641, 1999.

76. Van Wijngaarden E, Savitz DA: Occupational sunlight exposure and mortality from non-Hodgkin lymphoma among utility workers. J Occup Environ Med 43: 548, 2001.

40

Pathology of Non-Hodgkin's Lymphomas and Hodgkin's Disease

L. Jeffrey Medeiros and Elaine S. Jaffe

Non-Hodgkin's lymphomas (NHLs) are neoplasms that arise from lymphocytes of either B- or T-cell lineage or rarely from histiocytes. With the advent of immunologic and molecular methods, many of the functional subtypes of these cell series have been delineated, both in normal cells and in their counterparts in malignant lymphomas.[1,2] These techniques have demonstrated that certain types of lymphoid cells are localized in particular regions of the lymph nodes and spleen. T cells are selectively concentrated in the paracortical regions of the lymph nodes and within the periarterial lymphoid sheaths of the spleen.[3] In addition, small numbers of T cells are found within follicles where they help in the induction of B-cell differentiation. By contrast, B cells are concentrated in the follicles and medullary cords of the lymph nodes and in the follicles of the spleen.[3] The lymphoid follicles represent the proliferative site of the B-cell system. Upon antigen stimulation, secondary germinal centers develop in which rapid cell division of B cells takes place. The medullary cord region of the lymph node represents the secretory component of the B-cell system. Histiocytes are preferentially found in the subcapsular and medullary sinuses of lymph nodes and the cords of Billroth in the splenic red pulp. Histiocytes are also a part of the reticuloendothelial system of the liver and lung. Tissue histiocytes have two broad categories of function. Most histiocytes are phagocytic, whereas a minority of specialized cells are involved in antigen processing and presentation to B and T cells.[4]

The patterns by which NHLs spread may be a reflection of the normal distribution of their non-neoplastic counterparts and may be partly related to tissue-specific homing receptors that have been identified on both normal and neoplastic lymphoid cells.[5,6]

With the advent of hybridoma technology,[7] an unlimited supply of monoclonal antibodies became available; many of them are highly specific for B-cell, T-cell, and monocyte/histiocyte antigens. These antibodies have proved to be essential in the diagnosis and classification of lymphoid malignancies by allowing both determination of lineage and assessment of the stage of differentiation. Antibodies have been grouped into clusters of differentiation (CDs) when different monoclonal antibodies react with the same or closely related antigens. Over 200 CDs have now been reported.[8]

The hallmark of the B lymphocyte is the ability to synthesize immunoglobulin (Ig). Furthermore, because B cells express either Ig κ- or λ-light chain but not both, staining for Ig light chain is a useful clonal marker, since a neoplastic clone is derived from a single precursor cell. By contrast, a polyclonal proliferation of cells, derived from many different precursor cells, will express a mixture of Ig κ- and λ-light chain-positive cells.[1,2] Numerous antibodies reactive against pan-B-cell antigens and B-cell-associated antigens also have been developed. These B-cell antigens are useful in determining the lineage of Ig-negative B-cell populations and in establishing the stage of B-cell differentiation.

Numerous monoclonal antibodies reactive with T lymphocytes are also currently available. However, in contrast to the restricted expression of Ig light chain by malignant B cells, no known antigen that can serve as a clonal marker is expressed by T cells. However, monoclonal antibodies allow the separation of T cells into distinct subsets, and may demonstrate aberrant T-cell immunophenotypes that support the diagnosis of NHL. Monoclonal antibodies also have shown that the histiocytic series is composed of phagocytic cells as well as more specialized, antigen-processing cells. The latter include follicular dendritic cells (located within the germinal center), interdigitating dendritic cells (located in the paracortex), fibroblastic reticulum cells, and Langerhans cells.[4]

The enzyme terminal deoxynucleotidyl transferase (TdT), a specialized DNA polymerase present in immature T- and B-lymphoid cells but not in their mature counterparts, is another useful marker. Both biochemical assays and monoclonal reagents now exist. This enzyme is most helpful in differentiating immature lymphoid cells such as normal thymocytes and lymphoblastic neoplasms (TdT+) from reactive or neoplastic proliferations of terminally differentiated lymphoid cells (TdT–).[9]

In a small subset of NHLs all markers are negative; these tumors are designated *null cell neoplasms*. The frequency of the null cell immunophenotype is substantially less than in the past, now that immunophenotypic and molecular methods are available. For example, most cases of acute lymphoblastic leukemia and a significant percentage of diffuse large cell lymphomas were once considered null cell neoplasms because these cells were Ig negative. Ig gene rearrangement analysis has demonstrated that most of the tumors in each group have Ig gene rearrangements and are of B lineage.[10,11] An additional subset of diffuse large cell lymphomas previously designated as being null cell have been shown to carry T-cell receptor (TCR) gene rearrangements and are of T-cell lineage.[12,13] Thus, by combining all methodologies, the number of NHLs in which lineage cannot be determined is presently less than 1 percent.[2]

Hodgkin's disease (lymphoma) and NHL have been regarded traditionally as distinct diseases based on their differences in clinical features, response to therapy, pathology, and immunophenotype. The diagnosis of Hodgkin's disease (HD) depends on the identification of large neoplastic cells in an appropriate cellular background of inflammatory cells. In recent years, evidence has accumulated that the malignant cell in nearly all cases of HD is of B-cell origin (see subsequent discussion). Therefore, it is not surprising that there is clinical and biologic overlap between HD and NHL. However, these disorders are still treated with different approaches based on their unique features.

CLASSIFICATION OF NON-HODGKIN'S LYMPHOMAS

The era of modern classification of NHLs began in 1956 with the introduction of the Rappaport classification.[14] The approach was to first divide lymphomas by pattern, either nodular or diffuse, and then subclassify them further on the basis of cytologic features. Tumors composed of lymphocytes that closely resembled normal lymphocytes were termed well differentiated. Poorly differentiated tumors were composed of relatively small lymphoid cells with irregular nuclear contours that less closely resembled normal lymphocytes. NHLs composed of large cells were designated as histiocytic on the basis of their resemblance to normal histiocytes. Undifferentiated NHLs were composed of cells of intermediate size that failed to demonstrate cytologic features of either lymphoid or histiocytic origin. Mixed NHLs were composed of a mixture of poorly differentiated lymphocytes and histiocytes.

The Rappaport classification was popular with clinicians, but as our understanding of the normal immune system improved, scientific inaccuracies became apparent on the basis of the following observations. First, morphologically identical lymphocytes were found to be functionally heterogeneous. The principal classes of lymphocytes identified were B and T cells, but multiple subpopulations as well as minor subclasses of lymphoid cells were also present. Secondly, small lymphocytes were found not to be an end-stage cell or the final product of the differentiation process. Thus, grading lymphocytes as well or poorly differentiated did not necessarily relate to differentiation. Lastly, the so-called histiocytic neoplasms of the Rappaport classification usually were not of histiocytic origin, but rather were neoplasms derived from transformed lymphocytes.

In an attempt to address these scientific inaccuracies, new classifications were proposed that attempted to relate lymphoid neoplasms more closely to their counterparts in the normal immune system. For example, the classification of Lukes and Collins[15] proposed that immunologic subtypes could be recognized on the basis of morphologic features alone. Although certain morphologic features, such as follicle formation, have been proved to be reliable indicators of follicular B-cell origin, cytologic features have proved to be unreliable in predicting the B- or T-cell origin of diffuse NHLs.[16] Other classifications were also proposed as alternatives to the Rappaport system. By the late 1970s, six lymphoma classifications were in use throughout the world. Of these, the Kiel classification[17] was most influential. The resulting situation was one of confusion and controversy. In an attempt to resolve these differences, the National Cancer Institute funded an international study to test each of the major classification on 1175 NHLs staged and treated in a relatively consistent manner.[18] On the basis of this study, it was concluded that each of the systems was useful in separating large numbers of patients into subgroups with varying survivals and clinical features. Furthermore, no one scheme appeared to be superior to another. As a consequence of these findings, the investigators involved in the study jointly developed a Working Formulation for clinical use[18] (Table 40–1). They emphasized that this formulation was not an alternative classification, but rather a common language that could be used to trans-

Table 40–1. International Working Formulation
Low grade
A. Malignant lymphoma, small lymphocytic
Consistent with chronic lymphocytic leukemia
Plasmacytoid
B. Malignant lymphoma, follicular, predominantly small cleaved cell
Diffuse areas
Sclerosis
C. Malignant lymphoma, follicular, mixed small cleaved and large cell
Diffuse areas
Sclerosis
Intermediate grade
D. Malignant lymphoma, follicular, predominantly large cell
Diffuse areas
Sclerosis
E. Malignant lymphoma, diffuse, small cleaved cell
Sclerosis
F. Malignant lymphoma, diffuse, mixed small and large cell
Sclerosis
Epithelioid cell component
G. Malignant lymphoma, diffuse, large cell
Cleaved
Noncleaved
High grade
H. Malignant lymphoma, large cell immunoblastic
Plasmacytoid
Clear cell
Polymorphous
Epithelioid cell
I. Malignant lymphoma, lymphoblastic
Convoluted cell
Nonconvoluted cell
J. Malignant lymphoma, small noncleaved
Burkitt's
Non-Burkitt's
K. Miscellaneous
Composite
Mycosis fungoides
Histiocytic
Extramedullary plasmacytoma
Unclassifiable

late one classification scheme into another. The Working Formulation was based purely on histologic data; immunologic and molecular data were not included. The Working Formulation became popular, and was principally used in the United States for the next decade. In Europe, the Kiel classification remained most popular, and was revised in 1988[19] (Table 40–2).

From the clinical standpoint, tumor grade as specified in many NHL classifications is predictive of survival. For example, the Working Formulation study showed that NHLs can be divided into three groups based on clinical outcome: low grade, intermediate grade, and high grade.[18]

Low-grade NHLs are clinically indolent, and affected patients are usually adults with relatively long survivals with or without aggressive therapy (Table 40–3).[20] Low-grade neoplasms usually involve sites where their normal counterparts are located. For example, follicular lymphomas derived from follicle center B cells

Table 40–2. Kiel Classification of Non-Hodgkin's Lymphomas

B	T
Low-grade malignant lymphomas	
Lymphocytic	Lymphocytic
Chronic lymphocytic leukemia	Chronic lymphocytic
Prolymphocytic leukemia	leukemia
Hairy cell leukemia	Prolymphocytic leukemia
Lymphoplasmacytic/cytoid	Small cell, cerebriform
(immunocytoma)	Mycosis fungoides/
Plasmacytic	Sézary syndrome
Centroblastic-centrocytic	Lymphoepithelioid
(follicular ± diffuse; diffuse)	(Lennert's lymphoma)
Centrocytic (mantle cell)	Angioimmunoblastic (AILD)
Monocytoid, including marginal	T-zone lymphoma
zone cell	Pleomorphic, small cell
	(HTLV-1±)
High-grade malignant lymphoma	
Centroblastic	Pleomorphic, medium-
	sized and large cell
	(HTLV-1±)
Immunoblastic	Immunoblastic (HTLV-1±)
Burkitt's lymphoma	Large cell anaplastic
Large cell anaplastic	(Ki-1 +)
Lymphoblastic	Lymphoblastic

demonstrate a striking capacity to home to B-cell-dependent portions of the lymphoid system and have a nondestructive growth pattern. Like normal nodally based B cells, low-grade B-cell lymphomas often circulate, and usually patients have stage III or IV disease at presentation.[21] Privileged sites such as the testis or central nervous system are rarely involved. Cytologically, the neoplastic cells closely resemble their normal counterparts and anaplasia is absent.[21] Low-grade lymphomas may also respond to immunoregulation. Some patients with follicular lymphoma have a history of lymph nodes that wax and wane in size, often for many years prior to diagnosis.[22] Spontaneous regression of follicular lymphomas also has been reported.[23] Host immunity has been invoked to explain this phenomenon, and in some cases, clinical regression has been preceded by bacterial or viral infec-

Table 40–3. Clinical, Pathologic, and Experimental Characteristics of Low-Grade and High-Grade Malignant Lymphoma

Low Grade	High Grade
1. Indolent clinical course	1. Aggressive clinical course
2. Relatively long survival	2. Short survival without therapy
3. Nondestructive growth pattern	3. Destructive growth pattern
4. Absence of cellular atypia	4. Presence of cellular atypia
5. Respect privileged sites	5. Invade privileged sites
6. Respond to regulatory influences	6. Autonomous
7. Fail to grow in culture	7. Immortalized in culture
8. Nontransplantable	8. Transplantable in immunodeficient host

tion. Some studies have suggested that regression correlates with higher numbers of host T cells being present within the NHL.[23] Other phenomena that may be explained by immunoregulation of low-grade lymphomas include the following situations: 1. Patients with follicular lymphoma with many T cells often have been found to respond to anti-idiotype therapy[24]; and 2. patients with small lymphocytic lymphomas with high numbers of host T cells have longer survival.[25] Death in patients with low-grade lymphoma most commonly results from progressive growth and eventual replacement of hematopoietic and lymphoid tissues, or transformation to high-grade lymphoma.[21]

By contrast, high-grade NHLs have an aggressive natural history (Table 40–3). Cytologically, the lymphoma cells are clearly atypical or anaplastic. Patients have short survival unless they are treated vigorously.[18] Extranodal sites and privileged sites are more frequently involved. Systemic ("B") symptoms are more common. The normal counterparts of these cells in the immune system do not circulate, and thus a higher percentage of patients have localized disease compared to patients with nodal low-grade lymphomas. High-grade lymphomas are also probably not subject to immunoregulation; spontaneous remissions are rare. With aggressive chemotherapy, long-term clinical remissions and probable cures have been obtained; up to 90 percent of patients with stage I disease may be cured.[26]

A further complication in classifying NHLs is that a significant fraction of patients have divergent histologies in the same or different biopsy sites. For example, in patients in whom more than one biopsy was performed during the initial staging of patients in the National Institutes of Health (NIH), the histologic diagnosis in separate biopsy specimens was different in 33 percent of patients.[27] In most cases, patients had lymphoma with a follicular pattern in one site and a diffuse pattern in a second site; these patients had a survival intermediate between patients with entirely follicular or entirely diffuse lymphomas. Histologic progression over time from low grade to higher grade is also common in B-cell NHLs. At the NIH, 37 percent of patients with follicular lymphomas progressed to a diffuse lymphoma when rebiopsied (more than 3 months later) after initial staging.[28] A reasonable explanation for these observations is that low-grade lymphoma is initially a neoplasm of relatively mature, differentiated cells that retain some of the characteristics of their normal counterparts, such as the follicular pattern. Over time, more aggressive clones evolve that represent cells further transformed both genetically and biologically. With modern therapy, eradication of the diffuse aggressive component and persistence of the residual low-grade follicular component are not uncommon. This occurrence has been referred to by others as histologic downgrading.[29]

World Health Organization Classification of Lymphoid Neoplasms

Following the publication of the International Working Formulation in 1982,[18] immunophenotypic and molecular methods for the analysis of hematolymphoid neoplasms became available. The results of these studies showed that the categories of the Working Formulation were immunologically and molecularly heterogenous. In the early 1990s, a group of pathologists known as the International Lymphoma Study Group proposed a provisional classification that incorporated morphologic, immunologic, and molecular data and they designated this scheme as the revised European-American classification of lymphoid neoplasms (REAL).[30] Their classification became popular and was validated in an important large clinicopathologic study sponsored by the University of Nebraska Medical Center.[31,32] More recently, the World Health Organization (WHO) sponsored a new classification of hematopoietic neoplasms. The authors of the WHO essentially accepted the REAL classification for lymphoid tumors with a few modifications (Table 40–4).[33] One unconventional aspect of the REAL and WHO classification is that they combine traditional NHLs with neo-

plasms not usually grouped with NHL, such as leukemias, plasma cell myeloma, and HD, based on the common lymphoid origin of these neoplasms. In this chapter, we emphasize the pathology of traditional NHLs and HD as they are designated in the WHO classification, as most leukemias and plasma cell neoplasms are covered in other chapters.

B-CELL LYMPHOID NEOPLASMS

Precursor B-Cell Lymphoblastic Leukemia/Lymphoma

Precursor B-cell lymphoblastic leukemia/lymphoma (LBLL), without leukemic involvement at time of presentation, is uncommon and represents no more than 10 percent of all LBLL. In contrast, 90 percent of these neoplasms are leukemic and are better known as acute lymphoblastic leukemia (ALL).

Patients with precursor B-cell LBLL are most commonly young adults, with a 2:1 male predominance.[34–36] Extranodal sites of involvement are common, most often skin, bone, and soft tissue.[35–38] Only a small subset of patients present with lymphadenopathy and patients rarely present with a mediastinal mass.[35,39] Regardless of stage patients require aggressive chemotherapy regimens suitable for ALL.[35,40–42] Leukemic involvement is common at time of relapse.[35]

Histologically, the normal architecture of the lymph node is effaced by a diffuse, relatively uniform proliferation of cells that have a tendency to stream out into perinodal tissues.[34,35,43,44] The neoplastic cells have scant cytoplasm and fine nuclear chromatin. Tumor cell nuclei may be either convoluted or round. Mitotic figures are numerous. Due to the high growth rate, a starry-sky pattern secondary to individual cell necrosis and scavenging by macrophages may be present in one-third of cases. No histologic features correlate with tumor cell immunophenotype.[34]

Precursor B-cell LBLL initially express the CD10 and CD19 antigens on the surface of the neoplastic cells, followed by CD22, and then CD20. These antigens are detectable in the cell cytoplasm prior to expression on the cell surface. The tumor cells usually do not express Igs on their cell surface.[2,34,35,43] Prior to the availability of monoclonal antibodies specific for pan-B-cell antigens, these neoplasms were referred to as having a null cell or common immunophenotype (Ig negative and CD10 antigen positive). Pre-B-cell LBLLs express cytoplasmic IgM in addition to other B-cell antigens.[2]

An extremely useful marker in the diagnosis of both precursor B-cell or T-cell LBLL is TdT, a distinct type of DNA polymerase present normally only in immature lymphocytes.[2,9] In a large series of NHLs studied by various TdT assays, TdT has been found virtually only in cases of precursor B-cell and T-cell LBLL. TdT is involved in the process of gene rearrangement, and is thought to add extra nucleotide bases between the variable (V), diversity (D), and joining (J) regions of the Ig and TCR genes undergoing rearrangement.

Gene rearrangement studies of precursor B-cell LBLLs have contributed to our knowledge of gene rearrangement in neoplastic and (by inference) normal lymphocyte development. Similar to surface antigen expression, the antigen receptor (Ig

---

Table 40–4. WHO Classification of Lymphoid Neoplasms

B-cell neoplasms
  Precursor B-cell neoplasm
    Precursor B-lymphoblastic leukemia/lymphoma (precursor
      B-cell acute lymphoblastic leukemia)
  Mature (peripheral) B-cell neoplasms
    Chronic lymphocytic leukemia/small lymphocytic lymphoma
    B-cell prolymphocytic leukemia
    Lymphoplasmacytic lymphoma/Waldenström macroglobulinemia
    Splenic marginal zone B-cell lymphoma
    Hairy cell leukemia
    Plasma cell myeloma/plasmacytoma
    Extranodal marginal zone B-cell lymphoma of MALT
    Nodal marginal zone B-cell lymphoma
    Follicular lymphoma
    Mantle cell lymphoma
    Diffuse large B-cell lymphoma
      Mediastinal large B-cell lymphoma
      Primary effusion lymphoma
      Intravascular large B-cell lymphoma
    Burkitt's lymphoma/Burkitt cell leukemia

T-cell and NK-cell neoplasms
  Precursor T-cell neoplasm
    Precursor T-lymphoblastic lymphoma/leukemia (precursor
      T-cell acute lymphoblastic leukemia)
  Mature (peripheral) T-cell neoplasms
    T-cell prolymphocytic leukemia
    T-cell large granular lymphocytic leukemia
    Aggressive NK-cell leukemia
    Adult T-cell lymphoma/leukemia
    Extranodal NK/T-cell lymphoma, nasal type
    Enteropathy-type T-cell lymphoma
    Hepatosplenic T-cell lymphoma
    Subcutaneous panniculitis-like T-cell lymphoma
    Mycosis fungoides/Sézary syndrome
    Primary cutaneous anaplastic large-cell lymphoma
    Peripheral T-cell lymphoma, not otherwise specified
    Angioimmunoblastic T-cell lymphoma
    Anaplastic large-cell lymphoma, T/null cell

Hodgkin's lymphoma (Hodgkin's disease)
  Nodular lymphocyte-predominant Hodgkin's lymphoma
  Classical Hodgkin's lymphoma
    Nodular sclerosis Hodgkin's lymphoma (grades 1 and 2)
    Lymphocyte-rich classical Hodgkin's lymphoma
    Mixed cellularity Hodgkin's lymphoma
    Lymphocyte depletion Hodgkin's lymphoma

and TCR) genes appear to rearrange sequentially, with a developmental hierarchy.[10]

Precursor B-cell LBLLs always contain Ig heavy chain gene rearrangements; more mature tumors also have Ig light chain gene rearrangements.[10,13] At the earliest stage of B-cell differentiation, the Ig heavy chain gene undergoes rearrangement. Subsequently, one of the Ig light chains rearranges, usually Ig κ-light chain gene first. If neither Ig κ-light chain gene allele is functionally rearranged, then the Ig λ-light chain gene rearranges.[10] This molecular mechanism allows a B cell to express only one Ig light chain (the principle of allelic exclusion).

Lineage infidelity is common in precursor B-cell LBLLs. T-cell receptor gene rearrangements occur in up to 70 percent of precursor B-cell neoplasms.[45,46]

Nonrandom chromosomal translocations have been identified in cell lines and precursor B-cell neoplasms.[13,47] The t(9;22) and t(1;19), as well as translocations involving 11q23, are most common.

t(9;22)(q34;q11), also known as the Philadelphia chromosome, is one of the most common recurrent chromosomal translocations, detected in 5 percent of children and approximately 20 to 25 percent of adults with precursor B-cell ALL.[47,48] This translocation joins the c-*abl* gene at chromosome 9q34 with the *bcr* locus at 22q11. The result is a chimeric mRNA transcript that encodes a fusion gene with increased tyrosine kinase activity. Two types of t(9;22) occur. In approximately 25 to 50 percent of adults with ALL, the translocation is identical to that seen in chronic myeloid leukemia, and the fusion protein is 210 kd, known as p210. In the remaining 50 to 75 percent of adults with ALL, the breakpoint on chromosome 22 does not occur in the *bcr* but 100 kb upstream, resulting in a different fusion protein, p190, with greater tyrosine kinase activity and higher transforming capacity than p210. The presence of t(9;22) in ALL is thought to correlate with a poorer prognosis.[48]

Precursor B-cell ALL of the pre-B-cell (cytoplasmic IgM positive) type is commonly associated with the t(1;19) chromosomal translocation. In this translocation, the *E2A* gene on chromosome 1 is joined to the *pbxI* gene on chromosome 19.[49,50] A chimeric transcription factor is the result, postulated to deregulate genes involved in leukemogenesis.

Similarly, translocations involving 11q23 such as t(4;11), t(9;11), and t(11;19) occur in precursor B-cell ALL. This translocation involves the *hrx* gene also known as *all-1, mll,* or *af-4* on chromosome 11q23.[47] Infants with translocations involving 11q23 present with a high white blood cell count, an increased frequency of central nervous system involvement, and a poor prognosis.[51]

Chronic Lymphocytic Leukemia/Small Lymphocytic Lymphoma

Morphologically and immunophenotypically, the malignant cells of chronic lymphocytic leukemia (CLL) are identical to those of nodal-based small lymphocytic lymphoma (SLL), and the two entities are thought to represent different manifestations of the same disease.[33] Although patients with SLL may not present with leukemic involvement, in many cases subclinical peripheral blood involvement can be found, and progression to overt CLL fre-

quently occurs. Patients with SLL represented 6 percent of all patients in the Nebraska NHL Classification Project.[31,32]

CLL/SLL occurs primarily in middle-aged and older patients with a peak incidence in the sixth to eighth decades.[18,31–33] In most series, the ratio of male to female cases is approximately 1.5:1. Clinically, this disease is associated with generalized lymphadenopathy. Although patients frequently have stage III or IV disease, these patients usually have an indolent clinical course with only vague symptoms such as weakness and anorexia; occasionally they have systemic symptoms.[18,32,33,52]

When involved by CLL/SLL, the normal lymph node architecture is usually diffusely effaced. At low power, vaguely nodular, pale areas are usually present, that can be small or prominent, which represent proliferation centers (also known as pseudofollicular growth centers or pseudofollicles).[33,52–54] Cytologically, the neoplastic cells are predominantly small round lymphocytes with inconspicuous nucleoli, clumped chromatin, scanty cytoplasm, and infrequent mitoses. However, slightly larger lymphoid cells with irregular nuclear contours (known as prolymphocytes) and large cells with round vesicular nuclei and central nucleoli (known as paraimmunoblasts) are also found.[52–54] These cells are most numerous in the proliferation centers. In some cases, these proliferation centers can surround residual benign germinal centers mimicking a marginal zone pattern (Figure 40–1).[54]

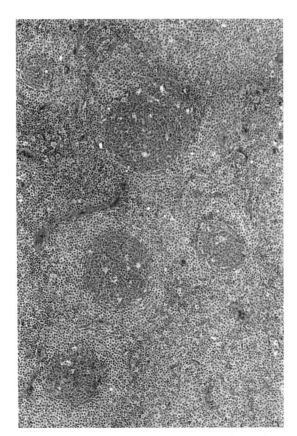

Figure 40–1. Chronic lymphocytic leukemia/small lymphocytic lymphoma. In this field the neoplasm surrounds residual benign germinal centers and therefore mimics nodal marginal zone B-cell lymphoma. (Photograph courtesy of Kojo Elenitoba-Johnson, M.D.)

In tissue culture, CLL/SLL can be induced to secrete Ig, suggesting that these tumors are frozen in differentiation at a presecretory stage.[55] However, a small subset of CLL/SLLs exhibit plasmacytoid differentiation. Morphologically, the neoplastic cells in these cases have more abundant cytoplasm and the nucleus may be eccentrically situated. Thus, the cells resemble plasma cells and are designated plasmacytoid lymphocytes. Like plasma cells, these cells contain cytoplasmic Ig that may be secreted producing a monoclonal IgM paraprotein.[33,52] Usually these patients have a low level of monoclonal paraprotein and these neoplasms behave as do nonplasmacytoid CLL/SLL. Thus, these are classified as such in the WHO classification.[33]

Subtypes of CLL/SLL are clinically more aggressive, with shortened survival. A high mitotic rate (more than 30 mitoses/20 high-power fields) and necrosis are found in more aggressive tumors.[56] Similar findings also have been shown using the Ki-67 antibody, which stains a nuclear antigen associated with proliferation; cases with a high number of proliferating cells have shorter survival.[25]

Immunophenotypically, CLL/SLL are B-cell tumors that express monotypic Ig light chains ($\kappa > \lambda$), IgM, usually IgD, and pan-B-cell antigens such as CD19, CD20, CD22, and CD79A.[2,33,54,57] BCL-2, CD21, and CD23 are usually positive, and CD10, CD79B, FMC7, and cyclin D1 are usually negative. These neoplasms also express the CD5 antigen, a pan-T-cell antigen that is not expressed on normal B cells but is expressed by CLL/SLL. Other T-cell antigens are negative. The density of Ig and CD20 antigen expression on the surface of CLL/SLL cells is characteristically low corresponding to "dim" immunofluorescence detected by flow cytometry.

Molecular studies of the antigen receptor genes in CLL/SLL have demonstrated rearrangements of the Ig heavy and light chain genes.[12,13] The TCR genes are usually in the germline configuration, although occasional cases may have TCR gene rearrangement (i.e., lineage promiscuity).

Chromosomal abnormalities have been shown in CLL/SLL. Trisomy 12 is common, found in approximately 15 to 20 percent of cases.[52,58,59] Trisomy 12 has been shown using both conventional cytogenetics and fluorescent in situ hybridization (FISH).[59] Trisomy 12 appears to be a secondary event as it is usually found in only a subset of the neoplastic cells. Deletion of chromosome 13q is also common, although less frequent than trisomy 12. Both abnormalities have been correlated with poorer prognosis or atypical histologic features.[52,60]

Oncogenes appear to play a limited role in the pathogenesis of CLL/SLL.[12,13] Rarely, t(14;18)(q32;q21) indistinguishable from that found in follicular lymphomas has been reported. More commonly, in 5 percent of cases of CLL/SLL, the BCL-2 oncogene at 18q21 is involved in t(2;18) or t(18;22) translocations involving the Ig κ (chromosome 2p13) or the Ig λ (chromosome 22q11) light chain genes.[61] The BCL-3 oncogene, involved in t(14;19)(q32;q13), has been identified rarely in CLL/SLL, and correlates with a poorer prognosis and the presence of trisomy 12.[62] t(11;14), involving the BCL-1 oncogene at chromosome 11q13, also has been reported.[63] However, this translocation is common in mantle cell lymphomas and very rare in CLL/SLL. It seems likely that most cases of CLL/SLL previously reported with t(11;14) may have been misclassified.

Translocations involving chromosome 8q24, the c-MYC locus, also have been rarely reported in CLL/SLL and are usually associated with morphologic transformation to high-grade non-Hodgkin's lymphoma (in lymph nodes) as well as B-cell prolymphocytic leukemia (in bone marrow and blood).[64]

Lymphoplasmacytic Lymphoma/Waldenström Macroglobulinemia

Many different types of NHL may exhibit plasmacytoid differentiation. However, the WHO classification suggests that the term lymphoplasmacytic lymphoma (LPL) be reserved for those tumors usually associated with systemic disease and a monoclonal IgM paraprotein, often associated with the syndrome of Waldenström macroglobulinemia.[33] Although some observers use the term Waldenström macroglobulinemia as a pathologic diagnosis, others prefer to consider Waldenström macroglobulinemia as a clinical syndrome, usually associated with LPL, but rarely with other types of B-cell NHL.[65]

Clinically, patients with LPL may present with a variety of symptoms and findings including mucous membrane bleeding, lymphadenopathy, hepatomegaly, peripheral neuropathy, and central nervous system abnormalities.[52,66,67] Constitutional symptoms are more common than in patients with CLL/SLL. Clinical and laboratory abnormalities that correlate with a poorer prognosis include age 65 years or greater, albumin less than 40 g/L, hemoglobin less than 120 g/L, platelet count less than 150×10^9/L, leukocyte count less than 4×10^9/L, and hepatomegaly. These features have been combined into a prognostic index.[71] Most patients have a monoclonal IgM paraprotein in the serum greater than 1 g/100 ml, and a subset of patients develop serum hyperviscosity and the clinical syndrome of Waldenström's macroglobulinemia.[86] The lymphadenopathy is generalized, but is usually modest relative to CLL/SLL. Involvement of peripheral blood is less common than CLL/SLL.

Histologically, lymph nodes involved by LPL retain their general architecture. The neoplastic cells tend to respect sinuses and home to the medullary cord regions.[68–70] The capsule is extensively infiltrated, and perinodal adipose tissue is involved. Three different types of LPL have been described: lymphoplasmacytoid, lymphoplasmacytic, and polymorphous.[71] In the lymphoplasmacytoid type, the tumor cells are small with slightly increased cytoplasm characteristic of plasmacytoid differentiation. Cytoplasmic globules (Russell bodies) and intranuclear pseudoinclusions (Dutcher bodies) of IgM may be present. In the lymphoplasmacytic type, small lymphoid cells and mature (Marchalko-type) plasma cells are present. Russell and Dutcher bodies are common. In the polymorphous type, large lymphoid cells are increased. Although the large cells do not form sheets and thus the criteria for large cell lymphoma are not present, patients with the polymorphous type have a poorer prognosis suggesting that this is an early stage of large cell transformation.[71,72]

Immunophenotypic studies have shown that LPL express monoclonal Ig light chain ($\kappa > \lambda$), IgM, and pan-B-cell antigens, and are negative for IgD and T-cell antigens.[2,33] In cases with more extensive plasmacytoid differentiation, the CD20 antigen may not be expressed, as occurs in normal plasma cells.[1,2] The tumor cells also express BCL-2 and plasma cell-associated antigens such as CD38 and CD138.[2] Unlike CLL/SLL, most cases of LPL are negative for CD5 and CD23. However, rare cases of LPL associated with Waldenström macroglobulinemia are positive for either CD5 or CD23.

The Ig heavy and light chain genes are rearranged and the TCR genes are usually in the germline configuration in LPL.[12,13] No characteristic chromosomal abnormalities are seen, although numerical abnormalities have been reported, most commonly deletion (6q).[72] The currently well-known onco-genes found in B-cell NHLs do not appear to be involved in the pathogenesis of most LPL. Although the t(9;14)(p13;q32) has been reported in a subset of nodal small B-cell lymphomas with plasmacytoid differentiation,[73] recent studies of well-character-ized cases of LPL in bone marrow associated with Walden-ström's macroglobulinemia have been consistently negative for the t(9;14).[72,74] In one case of LPL, a t(8;14)(q24;q32) was reported, which may have represented evidence of clonal evolu-tion to a high-grade NHL.[75]

Mantle Cell Lymphoma

The term *mantle cell lymphoma* (MCL) is the currently accepted name in the WHO classification[33] for a neoplasm previously known as malignant lymphoma, intermediate lymphocytic type, lymphocytic lymphoma of intermediate differentiation, centrocytic lymphoma, and mantle zone lymphoma. MCL rep-resented approximately 6 percent of all NHLs in the Nebraska NHL Classification Project.[31,32]

Clinically, patients with MCL are usually elderly men with generalized disease. In a study of 83 patients with MCL, the median age was 63 years (range, 37 to 82 years), and the male/female ratio was approximately 3:1.[32] Eighty percent of patients presented with clinical stage III or IV disease and sys-temic symptoms occured in approximately 40 percent of patients.[32] Most patients had generalized lymphadenopathy and bone marrow was commonly involved (64 percent). An absolute peripheral blood lymphocytosis of more than 4000/mm^3 was infrequent. Low-level involvement of the peripheral blood is common when searched for morphologi-cally or if sensitive molecular techniques are used.[76] Relatively low levels of lymphocytosis probably do not influence survival significantly but overt leukemia may be associated with a poorer prognosis. Extranodal disease may occur, usually in association with nodal involvement. Patients may present with numerous polyps involving the gastroesophageal tract below the level of the gastrointestinal junction, also known in the literature as multiple lymphomatous polyposis of the intestine.[77] Involve-ment of Waldeyer's ring may occur.

Although a small subset of patients has clinically indolent disease, most patients with MCL have a poor prognosis. In a study by Fisher and associates,[78] after 10 years of clinical follow-up only 8 percent of patients were alive after treatment with cyclophosphamide, doxorubicin, vincristine, and prednisone (CHOP). In many studies, patient survival correlates with the pattern of involvement in lymph nodes. Patients with a mantle

zone pattern of lymph node involvement have better survival than do patients with diffusely involved lymph nodes.[79–81]

Histologically, the diagnosis of MCL is most reliably made by examination of a lymph node biopsy specimen in which the architecture is replaced by a diffuse or vaguely nodular neo-plasm. In a subset of cases a mantle zone pattern results from the neoplasm selectively involving the follicle mantle zones sur-rounding normal or reactive germinal centers.[79–81] Cytologi-cally, MCL is composed of a monotonous population of small lymphoid cells with slightly to clearly irregular nuclear contours (Figure 40–2). Although MCLs as a group show a wide spec-trum of nuclear irregularities, in an individual neoplasm, the tumor cells are remarkably similar to each other. Large nucleo-lated lymphoid cells are rare. Other histologic findings common in MCL include numerous eosinophilic epithelioid histiocytes and germinal centers completely surrounded by tumor without a normal lymphoid cuff (so-called naked germinal centers). Pseudofollicular growth centers, as are observed in CLL/SLL, are absent in MCL. Plasmacytoid differentiation is also rare in MCL.[80]

High-grade or blastoid variants of MCL occur and can be divided into two types: classic and pleomorphic. Classic blas-toid MCLs are characterized by slightly larger lymphoid cells with finely dispersed nuclear chromatin and numerous mitotic features that resemble lymphoblastic lymphoma (Figure 40–3).

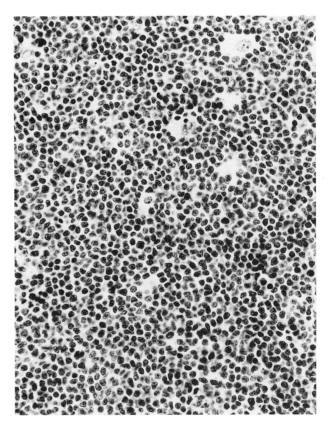

Figure 40–2. Mantle cell lymphoma, diffuse pattern. The neoplastic cells are small with condensed chromatin. Benign histocytes with abundant eosinophilic cytoplasm are scattered throughout the neoplasm.

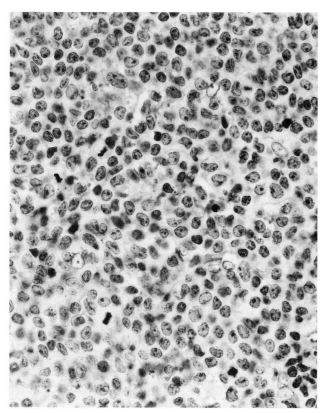

Figure 40–3. Mantle cell lymphoma, blastoid variant. The neoplastic cells have immature chromatin and a high mitotic rate.

Pleomorphic blastoid variants of MCL are composed of large cells that resemble, in part, large cell lymphoma. In the peripheral blood, high-grade MCL can resemble prolymphocytic leukemia.[82] Blastoid MCLs have a more aggressive clinical course. Whether high-grade variants of MCL represent transformation from typical cases of MCL or are a second type of MCL is controversial. At least a subset of cases are described in which blastoid and typical MCL occurred in the same patient, and clonal identity has been shown in rare cases.[83] Thus, at least a subset of blastoid MCLs probably represent morphologic transformation from typical MCL. However, most cases of blastoid MCL are not preceded by typical MCL.

Immunophenotypic studies have shown that MCLs express monotypic Ig light chain (more often Ig λ), IgM, IgD, pan-B-cell antigens, BCL-2, alkaline phosphatase, and CD5.[33,84] Unlike CLL/SLL, MCLs are often positive for CD79B and FMC-7 and typically negative for BCL-6 and the CD23 antigen. However, 10 percent of MCL can be CD23-positive. MCLs express Ig and B-cell antigens in greater density compared with CLL/SLL (brighter immunofluorescence).[2] CD21 is usually not expressed by the neoplastic cells but anti-CD21 antibodies highlight an irregular meshwork of dendritic reticulum cells.[1,2,33] CD10 is usually negative in MCL.

MCLs carry rearrangements of the Ig heavy and light chain genes whereas the TCR genes are usually in the germline configuration.[12,13,63] t(11;14)(q13;q32) is present in virtually all cases

of MCL.[85] In this translocation the *ccnd-1* gene (also known as *PRAD1* and *bcl-1*) on 11q13 is juxtaposed with the Ig heavy chain gene on 14q32 resulting in overexpression of cyclin D1. Cyclin D1 facilitates cells cycle transition from G1 to S phase.[86,87]

The breakpoints on chromosome 11q13 are widely scattered over approximately 120 kb. As a result, various methods for detecting the t(11;14) result in markedly different detection rates. Polymerase chain reaction (PCR) methods that currently exist can only assess the major translocation cluster region, involved in 40 to 50 percent of cases.[88] Southern blot methods using multiple probes can detect up to 75 percent of cases.[63,88] FISH methods, using large cosmid probes, can detect virtually all 11q13 breakpoints and therefore have the highest detection rate.[85,90,91] Although conventional cytogenetics should theoretically also detect all cases of the t(11;14), poor growth and sampling error result in a detection rate of 70 to 80 percent.[92]

Follicular Lymphoma

The WHO classification emphasizes that all follicular lymphomas (FLs) are the same biologic entity but showing differences in histological grade. Therefore, the WHO classification proposes that the terms *small cleaved cell, mixed cell,* and *large cell* be designated as grades I, II, and III, respectively.[33]

Follicular lymphoma is one of the most common types of NHL in the United States, representing 22 percent of all neoplasms in the Nebraska NHL Classification Project.[31] The incidence of FL is lower in other countries such as Japan.[93,94] The median patient age was 59 years in one study, with an age range from 23 to 90 years.[31] These neoplasms are rare in patients under the age of 20 years.[18,31] Men and women are equally affected. Whites are affected more often than Blacks. Unlike most other NHLs, women are affected more often than men. Most patients have clinical stage III or IV disease at the time of diagnosis. Involvement of the lymph nodes, spleen, liver, and bone marrow is common. Bone marrow involvement occurs in approximately one-half of patients.[18,31] The gastrointestinal tract is rarely involved.[31] Some patients with FL develop clinical evidence of leukemia. The characteristic cell in the peripheral blood has a deeply clefted nucleus and has been referred to as a buttock cell.[95] Leukemic involvement does not appear to influence prognosis, unless the peripheral white blood cell count is high.[96] Subclinical involvement of peripheral blood is commonly detected when assessed by sensitive molecular techniques.

In spite of the presence of widespread disease, FLs composed of predominantly small cleaved lymphoid cells (grade I) have relatively long survival.[18,31] Progression from a purely follicular to a follicular and diffuse pattern is common, and the presence of a diffuse component without a significant increase in large lymphoid cells does not affect survival.[97] In grade II FL, the tumor is composed of a mixture of small cleaved and large cells, whereas grade III FL is composed predominantly of large cells. A diffuse component usually accompanies an increased number of large cells.[97] Patients with mixed FL also have an indolent clinical course, although the large lymphoid cells are proliferating, and survival in some studies has been less than that of patients with grade I neoplasms. If the diffuse component in grade II tumors is minor, it has a minimal effect on survival. However, when the diffuse component predominates, patients may have a more aggressive clinical course. Patients with grade III FL clearly have a more aggressive clinical course than that of the other subtypes of FL, and they require aggressive therapy.[18,31,98] A diffuse component is common, and grade III FL may progress to a completely diffuse neoplasm without any recognizable follicular architecture, referred to as *diffuse large B-cell lymphoma*.[28]

It is also common for an individual patient with FL involving multiple sites to have discordant histologic findings. In this scenario one biopsy site is involved by FL composed of predominantly small cleaved cells, or a mixture of small cleaved and large cells, and a second biopsy site is involved by FL or entirely diffuse lymphoma composed predominantly of large cells.[27,28]

Histologically, the lymph node architecture is partially or completely effaced by neoplastic follicles, with a paucity of interfollicular tissue (Figure 40–4). A large absolute number of follicles has been found to be the most reliable criterion of FL.[99] Unlike the lymphoid follicles in reactive hyperplasia, the follicles of FL are relatively uniform in size, lack a well-defined lymphoid cuff, and lack polarization.[97,99] Histiocytes are usually less frequent in neoplastic follicles than in reactive follicles. Plasmacytoid differentiation is rare in all subtypes of FL.[99]

Cytologically, the cells in neoplastic follicles mimic the cell types of normal germinal centers in reactive follicles. Small cleaved lymphoid cells (also known as centrocytes) have irregular, cleaved nuclear contours and coarse, condensed chromatin. Large cleaved cells are similar to small cleaved cells but are of larger size, with more open nuclear chromatin. Small noncleaved cells are approximately two times the diameter of small cleaved cells, with irregular chromatin and multiple distinct nucleoli. Large noncleaved lymphoid cells (also known as centroblasts) are two to three times the diameter of the small cleaved cells, with vesicular nuclei and one to three nucleoli. Since the small noncleaved and large cells are the proliferating component, it is not surprising that the number of mitotic figures present correlates with the number of these cells.

Distinguishing between grades I, II, and III is based on arbitrary criteria not shared by all pathologists and reproducibility of grading, in most studies, has been poor.[33] The most popular method to distinguish between FLs has been based on a count of the large noncleaved lymphoid cells as described by Mann and Berard.[100] In grade I (predominantly small cleaved cell) FL large noncleaved cells are rare, less than 5/400× microscopic field. Grade II (mixed small cleaved and large cell) FL contains 5 or more large noncleaved cells/400× microscopic field. Grade III (large cell) FL is composed of many more large noncleaved

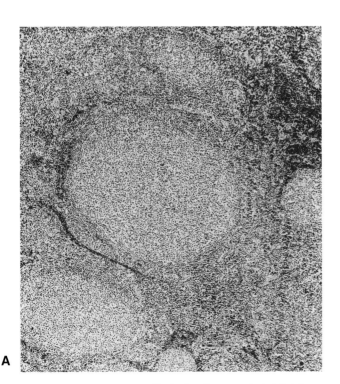

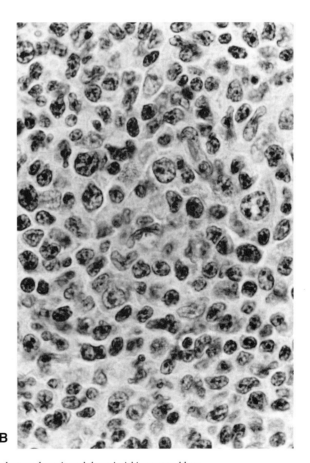

Figure 40–4. Follicular lymphoma, grade II. (**A**) At low power the neoplasm is nodular mimicking normal lymphoid follicles. (**B**) The neoplasm is composed of small cleaved and large noncleaved lymphoid cells.

lymphoid cells, greater than 15/400× microscopic field. In tumors in which the neoplastic follicles contain different mixtures of cells, grade is usually based on the follicles with the greatest number of large noncleaved lymphoid cells.

A small subset of FL, approximately 10 percent, may exhibit monocytoid differentiation.[101] These tumors have a rim of monocytoid cells located peripheral to the neoplastic follicles. The presence of monocytoid differentiation correlated with poorer prognosis in the Nebraska NHL Classification Project.[31]

Immunophenotypic studies have shown that FLs are neoplasms of mature B-cell lineage. Most grade I and II tumors express Ig, but up to 50 percent of grade III neoplasms may be Ig negative.[1,2] When FLs are Ig positive, Igκ is expressed more often than Igλ.[2] Most tumors express IgM, but approximately 25 percent express IgG or IgA, an expected finding since normal follicular center lymphocytes commonly undergo Ig heavy chain switching following exposure to antigen.[102] IgD is usually negative, since its presence is a feature of naive B cells in the mantle zone. All FLs express pan-B-cell markers, and most are positive for the B-cell-associated antigens CD10 and BCL-6.[1,2,33] The B-cell antigens CD21 and CD23 and all T-cell antigens including CD5 are negative.[2,31,33] Typically, FLs express Ig and B-cell antigens at high density (bright immunofluorescence).[2] In FLs with many large noncleaved cells, activation-associated antigens such as CD25 and CD38 and proliferation-associated antigens such as the Ki-67 are expressed.[103,104] BCL-2 is expressed in 80 to 90 percent of FL; as BCL-2 is negative in reactive germinal centers, this marker is helpful in differential diagnosis.

FLs have rearrangements of the Ig heavy and light chain genes. The TCR genes are usually in the germline configuration.[12,13] The molecular hallmark of FLs is the t(14;18)(q32;q21).[105] Cytogenetic analysis has demonstrated t(14;18) in over 90 percent of cases.[105] In this abnormality, the *bcl-2* oncogene on chromosome 18q21 is translocated to the joining region of the Ig heavy chain gene on chromosome 14q32. The *bcl-2* gene is deregulated, by being placed under the influence of Ig heavy chain gene regulatory elements (perhaps the enhancer region).[106] The BCL-2 protein is a 25-kd molecule that is overexpressed in FLs and protects cells from programmed cell death (apoptosis).[107] The inhibition of apoptosis prolongs cell life, resulting in an expanded compartment of B cells at increased risk for additional molecular defects, presumably involved in neoplastic transformation.[107,108] However, BCL-2 protein expression is not limited to FLs, since it is expressed by many subtypes of B-cell lymphoma without t(14;18).[108] In addition, the presence of t(14;18) alone does not appear sufficient for neoplastic transformation since this translocation has been identified in rare cells in the tonsils and lymph nodes of normal individuals without clinical evidence of lymphoma.[109]

The breakpoints on chromosome 18 are tightly clustered at two sites, the major (MBR) and minor (MCR) breakpoint cluster regions, involved in 50 to 60 percent and 10 to 20 percent of cases, respectively.[12,110] These breakpoints are well suited to PCR analysis. Some recent data suggest that FLs without PCR-detectable MBR or MCR breakpoints have a poorer prognosis and require more aggressive therapy.[110] Recently, another cluster site that can be detected by PCR, the intermediate cluster region (ICR), has been reported to be common in FLs from Europe.

In occasional cases of FL, t(8;14) has been reported in addition to t(14;18), and these cases were clinically aggressive.[111] Presumably, the t(8;14) was evidence of clonal evolution to a higher grade neoplasm. However, a small subset of FCL cases have been reported to have t(8;14) and not t(14;18).[112] These patients had a clinically indolent course, and structural analysis of the t(8;14) showed that this translocation was distinct from the t(8;14) that occurs in Burkitt's lymphoma. This finding suggests that a minor pathway of follicular lymphomagenesis may exist that is independent of t(14;18). This may be particularly true for rare FLs in children, most of which lack the t(14;18).[113]

Marginal Zone B-Cell Lymphoma

Three types of marginal zone B-cell lymphoma are designated in the WHO classification including low-grade lymphomas that were originally designated as low-grade B-cell lymphoma of mucosa-associated lymphoid tissue (MALT) and monocytoid B-cell lymphoma.[33] In the WHO classification, these neoplasms are designated as marginal zone B-cell lymphoma of extranodal MALT and nodal type, respectively. These neoplasms are believed to arise from normal marginal zone B cells in the lymph node or their extranodal counterparts, respectively. A third neoplasm that arises in the spleen is designated as splenic marginal zone B-cell lymphoma.

Extranodal Marginal Zone B-Cell Lymphoma of Mucosa-Associated Lymphoid Tissue

Prior to the advent of immunologic and gene rearrangement techniques, the diagnosis of extranodal low-grade B-cell lymphoma was established infrequently in patients without a history of nodal low-grade NHL. Instead, extranodal infiltrates composed of small round or slightly irregular lymphoid cells, often admixed with plasma cells, histiocytes, and lymphoid follicles were classified as *pseudolymphomas,* since clinical studies showed that patients with these lesions pursued an indolent clinical course.[114]

Immunophenotypic and gene rearrangement studies have since shown that approximately 60 to 70 percent of pseudolymphomas express monotypic Ig light chain and contain Ig gene rearrangements.[115–117] Thus, these tumors are now classified as low-grade B-cell lymphomas, and in most cases represent extranodal marginal zone B-cell lymphomas of MALT.

Extranodal marginal zone B-cell lymphomas of MALT were originally recognized by Isaacson and Wright[118] as a subset of gastrointestinal lymphomas in European patients that resembled immunoproliferative small intestinal disease (also known as Mediterranean lymphoma). Isaacson[119,120] then identified similar neoplasms arising in the lung and salivary gland (Figure 40–5) and suggested that the common aspect of these tumors was that they arose from lymphoid tissue associated with mucosal surfaces. However, subsequently MALT-lymphomas were identified in a variety of extranodal sites including the thyroid gland, thymus, breast, conjunctiva, gallbladder, cervix, larynx, trachea, dura, skin, and kidney, as well as other sites.[121–124] Thus, the term MALT-lymphoma, although it continues to be used, is somewhat misleading in the sense that not all MALT-lymphomas arise in sites involving mucosal surfaces. Two common findings in

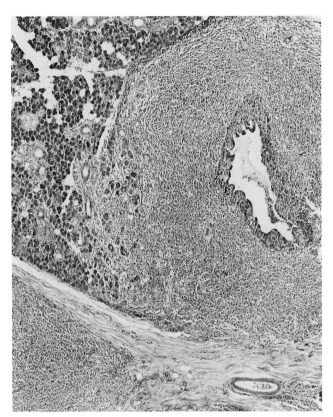

Figure 40–5. Low-grade B-cell lymphoma of MALT involving parotid gland. The neoplasm surrounds a duct and infiltrates ductal epithelium.

MALT-lymphomas are the presence of glandular epithelium and chronic inflammation either preceding or accompanying the tumor. Low-grade B-cell MALT-lymphomas represented 5 percent of all NHLs in the Nebraska NHL Classification Project.[31,32]

Clinically, MALT-lymphomas tend to be localized for prolonged intervals before disseminating, and anatomic sites commonly involved by nodal low-grade lymphomas such as the bone marrow, liver, spleen, and peripheral blood are infrequently involved, seen in less than one-third of patients.[125] The pattern of dissemination of MALT-lymphomas is also unlike that of nodal low-grade lymphomas. These tumors have a tendency to spread to other extranodal sites. For example, in one study MALT-lymphomas of the lung disseminated to other extranodal sites such as the skin and stomach as often as they spread to lymph nodes.[126] When MALT-lymphomas involve lymph nodes, they histologically resemble nodal marginal zone B-cell lymphoma (monocytoid B-cell lymphoma). Despite the indolent clinical behavior of localized MALT-lymphomas, patients with disseminated MALT-lymphomas have a clinical course similar to that of patients with disseminated nodal low-grade B-cell lymphomas.[78]

Histologically, four findings are present in most low-grade MALT-lymphomas: a population of neoplastic small lymphoid (centrocyte-like) cells, occasional large lymphoid cells, lymphoepithelial lesions, and reactive lymphoid follicles.[119,120]

The neoplastic small lymphoid cells exhibit a range of cytologic appearances. In some neoplasms these cells closely resemble small lymphocytes, with or without plasmacytoid differentiation. In other neoplasms, the tumor appears biphasic: One component is small lymphoid cells with minimal cytoplasm, and the other component exhibits extensive plasmacytoid differentiation with many cells resembling mature plasma cells. In other tumors, the neoplastic cells have markedly irregular nuclear contours and resemble small cleaved lymphocytes (so-called centrocyte-like cells). All of these neoplastic cell types may have abundant pale cytoplasm with well-defined cytoplasmic membranes imparting a monocytoid appearance (Figures 40–5 and 40–6).

In most MALT-lymphomas, occasional large lymphoid cells are also present, which is not surprising since the natural history of many low-grade lymphomas is to accumulate large cells and then progress to high-grade lymphoma. When the large cells are numerous and form confluent sheets, the neoplasm has evolved to diffuse large B-cell lymphoma. Use of the term *high-grade MALT-lymphoma* is not recommended in the WHO classification.

The neoplastic cells have a marked tendency to infiltrate epithelium, forming so-called lymphoepithelial lesions (Figure 40–6). In these lesions, small groups or larger aggregates of neoplastic cells are found within the epithelium. Reactive lymphoid follicles are also usually present in MALT-lymphomas, usually

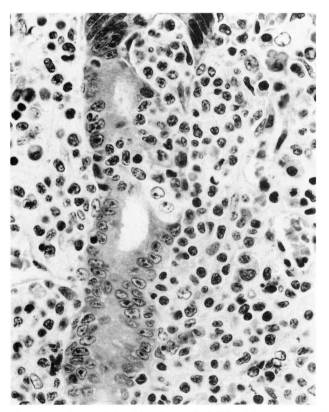

Figure 40–6. Low-grade B-cell lymphoma of MALT involving stomach. The neoplastic cells have irregular nuclear contours and pale cytoplasm, the latter imparting a "monocytoid appearance." The neoplastic cells infiltrate a gland forming a lymphoepithelial lesion.

surrounded by neoplastic small lymphoid cells. These neoplastic cells may accumulate in these follicles (termed *colonization*), and the tumor acquires a nodular low-power appearance.[127] However, these neoplasms are not truly of follicle center cell origin.

In addition to these histologic findings common to all MALT-lymphomas, site-specific differences are also observed. For example, normal lymphoid tissue is not usually present in the stomach. However, benign MALT is acquired, probably in response to *Helicobacter pylori* infection.[128,129] Approximately 30 percent of cases of *H. pylori*-induced chronic gastritis are associated with lymphoid follicles; a smaller subset of cases also develops benign lymphoepithelial lesions. Conversely, over 90 percent of gastric MALT-lymphomas are associated with *H. pylori* infection. Thus, it seems likely that *H. pylori* induces the development of benign MALT and predisposes to the development of MALT-lymphoma. The mechanisms for *H. pylori* induction of benign MALT are unknown but may involve cytokines. For example, *H. pylori* has been shown to upregulate interleukin-8 secretion by gastric epithelial cells.[130] Studies also have shown that benign MALT-tissue and low-grade MALT-lymphomas may regress following antibiotic therapy appropriate for *H. pylori*.[131]

In the normal adult lung, MALT-tissue is also poorly developed and inflammatory conditions usually precede the development of MALT-lymphoma. Two inflammatory diseases are frequently associated with lung MALT-lymphoma, Sjögren syndrome and lymphoid interstitial pneumonia.[132] Similarly, MALT-lymphomas of the salivary gland are usually associated with Sjögren syndrome,[133] and Hashimoto's thyroiditis frequently precedes MALT-lymphoma of the thyroid gland.[134]

Immunophenotypic studies have shown that MALT-lymphomas express monotypic Ig light chain ($\kappa > \lambda$), usually IgM, pan-B-cell antigens, and BCL-2.[2,33,120] These tumors typically do not express IgD, CD10, CD21, CD23, or T-cell antigens including CD5.[2,33,120]

MALT-lymphomas carry both Ig heavy and light chain gene rearrangements.[13,135] TCR genes are usually in the germline configuration.

The t(11;18)(q21;q21) has been identified in approximately 30 to 40 percent of MALT-lymphomas.[136,137] In this translocation, the *api2* gene on 11q21 and the *malt*1 gene on chromosome 18q21 are disrupted and recombine to form a novel *api2-malt*1 fusion gene. The *api2* gene belongs to a family of proteins known as inhibitors of apoptosis proteins (IAP) that are evolutionary conserved and play a role in regulating apoptosis.[138] *Malt*1 is a novel gene of unknown function, but is critical to the function of API2-MALT1, which is known to activate NF-κB.[139]

Recent studies suggest that response of gastric low-grade MALT-lymphomas to antibiotic therapy can be predicted by knowledge of the presence or absence of the t(11;18).[140,141] Lymphomas that carry the t(11;18) are unlikely to respond to antibiotic therapy. By contrast, those lymphomas negative for the t(11;18) are more often associated with *H. pylori* gastritis and are likely to respond to antibiotic therapy. These results need to be confirmed in larger cohorts of patients.

The t(1;14)(p22;q32) is an uncommon translocation in MALT-lymphomas that juxtaposes on intact *bcl-10* gene at 1p22 adjacent to the Ig heavy chain gene at 14q32.[142,143] The translocation truncates *bcl-10* and thus BCL-10 protein loses its pro-apoptosis function.

Bcl-10 gene mutations also occur outside the context of the t(1;14), in 7 to 10 percent of MALT-lymphomas.[142] These mutations consist predominantly of deletions or insertions and are predicted to result in truncated proteins. An association between *bcl-10* gene mutations and disease progression in MALT-lymphomas has been reported.[143] Moreover, *bcl-10* gene mutations are reported to be associated with aggressive and antibiotic-unresponsive forms of MALT-lymphoma. If these findings are confirmed in a larger controlled study, the presence of *bcl-10* gene mutations may be useful for identifying patients prospectively who would not benefit from antibiotic therapy to eradicate *H. pylori*.

Recent evidence has suggested that BCL-10 and MALT1 bind to form a complex in the cell, and act synergistically to activate NF-κB. Thus, the BCL-10-MALT1 complex and API2-MALT1 fusion protein appear to activate a common downstream signaling pathway.[139]

Conventional cytogenetic analysis performed on MALT-lymphomas has shown that numerical aberrations of chromosomes 3, 12, and 18 are common. Using both metaphase and interphase cytogenetic techniques, Wotherspoon et al.[144] reported a high frequency of trisomy 3 in MALT-lymphomas, in 55 percent of cases. Others also have observed trisomy 3 commonly in both MALT-lymphomas and in nodal marginal zone B-cell lymphomas. However, more recent data derived from a relatively larger series of MALT-lymphomas examined using sensitive FISH techniques indicate that the frequency of trisomy 3 is less common, approximately 20 percent.[145,146]

Known B-cell oncogenes such as *ccnd-1, bcl-2, bcl-3, bcl-6*, and *c-myc* are not rearranged in MALT-lymphomas.[13,135] *Bcl-6* gene mutations have been reported in a subset of gastric MALT-lymphomas.[149]

Nodal Marginal Zone B-Cell Lymphoma

Reactive monocytoid cells were initially recognized in the sinuses of reactive lymph nodes many years ago. However, not until the 1980s were these cells shown to be of B-cell lineage.[150,151] Reactive monocytoid B cells have oval to reniform, cytologically bland nuclei and abundant, clear cytoplasm with easily appreciated cell membranes. Monocytoid B cells may be found in the lymph node sinuses of a variety of lymphoid hyperplasias, most often in toxoplasma lymphadenitis and acquired immunodeficiency syndrome (AIDS).

Malignant lymphomas have been recognized that morphologically resemble monocytoid B cells.[152–155] The term monocytoid B-cell lymphoma (MBCL) was originally proposed by Sheibani and colleagues.[152] These tumors are currently thought to be of lymph node marginal zone origin, and are designated as nodal marginal zone B-cell lymphoma (MZBCL) in the WHO classification.[33] These neoplasms represented 5 percent of all NHLs in the Nebraska NHL Classification Project.[31,32]

Patients with nodal MZBCL are usually elderly, and women are affected more often than men.[153–155] Most patients present with lymphadenopathy, often initially detected in lymph nodes of the head and neck region. The parotid gland is involved in 10 to 20 percent of patients, and most of these patients have Sjögren syndrome. Although initially described as a tumor that is often localized at time of diagnosis, 71 percent of patients had advanced stage disease in recent studies.[31,156] The clinical course of patients with nodal MZBCL is therefore similar to patients with other systemic low-grade B-cell NHL, such as FL.[156] Patients with high clinical stage disease are at greater risk for transformation to higher grade lymphoma, and patients may develop composite lymphoma (i.e., MZBCL coexistent with another type of NHL).[155,157]

Histologically, lymph nodes involved by MZBCL have a pale low-power appearance as a result of the abundant cytoplasm of the neoplastic cells.[153–155,158] Nodal MZBCLs have a propensity to involve the marginal zones and sinuses of the lymph node. In a minority of cases, the tumor is confined to the sinuses and distinction from reactive monocytoid B cells is difficult without immunophenotypic or gene rearrangement studies.[153] In most cases, MZBCLs expand into the perifollicular compartments of the lymph node with sparing of germinal centers (Figure 40–7), or they completely replace the lymph node architecture.[153–155]

The cytologic features of nodal MZBCL are the most distinctive features of this neoplasm. The tumor cell cytoplasm is relatively abundant, pale eosinophilic or clear, with well-delineated cell borders. The tumor cell nuclei are small and cytologically bland. The tumor cell chromatin is relatively clumped and mitotic figures are infrequent.[152–155]

Immunophenotypic studies have shown that MZBCLs are mature B-cell neoplasms that express monotypic Ig light chain (κ > λ), usually IgM, pan-B-cell antigens and BCL-2.[2,33] These tumors usually do not express IgD, CD10, CD21, CD23, cyclin D1, or T-cell antigens including CD5.

The Ig genes are rearranged and the TCR genes are usually in the germline configuration in nodal MZBCL.[12,13] Lineage promiscuity is rare. The *ccnd-1* and *bcl-2* genes are in the germline configuration. Conventional cytogenetic studies have identified a variety of abnormalities, but no lesions common to most nodal MZBCLs have been described.[159] The t(11;18) has not been identified.[160] Trisomy 3 is commonly detected, in 50 percent of cases in one study using FISH methods.[145]

Splenic Marginal Zone B-Cell Lymphoma

Splenic marginal zone B-cell lymphomas (SMZL) were so named because they were thought to arise from splenic marginal zone B cells, and to be closely related to other marginal zone B-cell lymphomas.[161] However, the cell of origin of SMZL and its relationship to other marginal zone neoplasms is uncertain. Neoplasms with prominent peripheral blood involvement also have been designated in the literature as splenic B-cell lymphomas with villous lymphocytes.[162]

Patients with SMZL are usually elderly, women are preferentially affected, and patients present with splenomegaly and laboratory abnormalities, usually anemia or thrombocytopenia, or both.[162,163] Some cases are associated with high levels of serum IgM.[164] Systemic symptoms are usually absent. Most patients have generalized disease with involvement of lymph nodes, liver, and bone marrow in addition to the spleen. The peripheral blood may be involved, and in the blood the cells often have irregular or villous cytoplasmic projections cytologically resembling hairy cell leukemia cells.[162] Splenomegaly is usually marked, but in a subset of cases the spleen is relatively small and these patients may have localized disease; they may have SMZL at an early stage of disease evolution.[165] Most patients with SMZL have clinically indolent disease. However, a subset of patients may have a more aggressive course, as is the case for other marginal zone B-cell lymphomas.[162]

Pathologically, the spleen is usually massive; in one study the splenic weight ranged from 970 to 2400 g (normal, less than 100 to 150 g).[163] Histologically, SMZLs preferentially involve the marginal zones surrounding lymphoid follicles of the white pulp and, if more extensive, also replace the lymphoid follicles and extend into the red pulp (Figure 40–8).[161,162] Cytologically, the neoplastic cells have relatively abundant clear cytoplasm and central round, bland nuclei. Plasmacytoid differentiation can be prominent.[164] Mitotic figures are rare and occasional large lymphoid cells are present.[161,163] When SMZLs involve lymph nodes, they closely resemble nodal MZBCL.

Immunophenotypic studies have shown that SMZLs are mature B-cell neoplasms that express monotypic Ig light chain (κ > λ), usually IgM and IgD, pan-B-cell antigens, CD11C, and

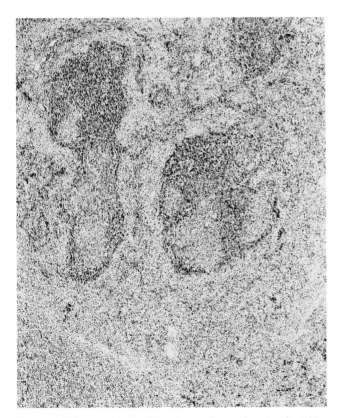

Figure 40–7. Monocytoid B-cell lymphoma. The neoplasm is pale at this magnification and has a marginal zone distribution, surrounding reactive follicles with central germinal centers and peripheral mantle zones.

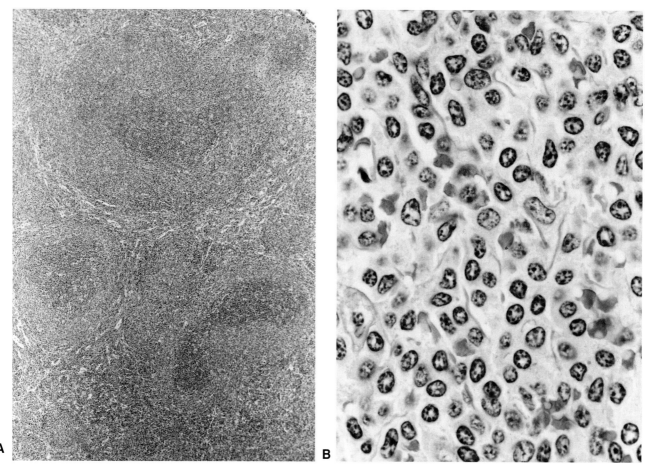

Figure 40–8. Splenic marginal zone B-cell lymphoma. (**A**) At low magnification, the neoplasm is pale and has a marginal and mantle zone distribution, surrounding central partially involved residual germinal centers. (**B**) The neoplastic cells are small with abundant pale cytoplasm.

BCL-2.[162,163] A subset of tumors expresses IgG and is IgD negative.[162] The tumor cells commonly express CD21 and are negative for CD10. Most cases of SMZL are negative for CD5 and CD23, but occasional cases may express one or both of these antigens. In contrast to hairy cell leukemia, SMZLs are usually negative for the CD25 antigen and tartrate-resistant acid phosphate.[161,163]

SMZLs contain Ig heavy and light chain gene rearrangements. The TCR genes are usually in the germline configuration.[161,162] The *ccnd-1, bcl-2,* and *c-myc* genes are not rearranged. A small subset of cases have been reported with *p53* gene mutations.[163,166] The *bcl-6* gene is not rearranged but can be mutated in 10 to 20 percent of cases.[167] Other cytogenetic abnormalities reported include trisomy 3, deletion (7q), and deletion (10)(q22q24).[168]

Diffuse Large B-Cell Lymphoma

In the Working Formulation, three histologic categories of NHL shared overlapping clinical and histologic features. These NHL included diffuse mixed small and large cell, diffuse large cell, and large cell immunoblastic and represented 6.7, 19.7, and 7.9 percent of all NHLs, respectively.[18] As a result, in many prior publications these NHLs were grouped together as diffuse aggressive lymphomas. In retrospect, most of these NHLs were neoplasms of B-cell lineage, approximately 80 to 90 percent, and are classified as diffuse large B-cell lymphoma (DLBCL) in the WHO classification.[33] These neoplasms were the most common type of NHL in the Nebraska NHL Classification Project, 31 percent.[31,32]

Diffuse large B-cell lymphomas mainly occur in adults, with a median age in the sixth decade. Men are affected slightly more often than women.[18,31] Although much less common in children, DLBCLs represent 15 to 20 percent of childhood NHLs. Patients with DLBCL often present with disease limited to one side of the diaphragm.[169] Nodal presentation is most common, but extranodal sites are frequently involved, in up to 40 to 50 percent of patients.[18,169] Approximately half of affected patients present with clinical stage III or IV disease.[18] In contrast to CLL/SLL and FL, which often involve the portal tracts of the liver and the splenic white pulp as small miliary nodules, DLBCLs usually grow as large masses, often with extensive necrosis. Bone marrow involvement is unusual, occurring in approximately 10 percent of patients.[18] Diffuse large B-cell lymphomas not uncommonly involve privileged sites such as the testis and central nervous system. If untreated, these NHLs are invariably fatal and most patients survive less than 2 years. However, these neoplasms are susceptible to chemotherapy, with a significant chance for cure, particularly in patients with localized disease.[170,171] With newer chemotherapy regimens, high complete response rates have been reported. Clinicopathologic studies with multivariate statistical analysis have shown that a number of adverse factors affect prognosis: male sex, high stage, B symptoms, anemia, high serum LDH level, bone marrow involvement, liver involvement, and a large (>10 cm) abdominal mass.[172] Central nervous system disease frequently accompanies bone marrow involvement. Except for male sex, all clinical features that correlated with an adverse effect on survival also correlated with a poor response to chemotherapy.

Histologically, DLBCLs are diffuse and composed of neoplastic cells with nuclei greater in size than the nuclei of benign histiocytes; the latter are virtually always present admixed within lymphomas (Figure 40–9). Mitotic figures are usually numerous.[18,34] Cytologically, the neoplastic lymphoid cells may exhibit a spectrum of findings that were subdivided in older classifications as large cleaved cells (centrocytes), large noncleaved cells (centroblasts), and immunoblasts. Large cleaved cells range from 13 to 30 μm in size and have irregular or cleaved nuclear contours; relatively small, indistinct nucleoli; and a thin rim of eosinophilic cytoplasm.[18,33,173] Large non-cleaved lymphoid cells are 20 to 30 μm in size and have round or oval vesicular nuclei with two to three nucleoli and more abundant amphophilic cytoplasm.[18,33,173] Often one nucleolus is centrally located and one or two nucleoli are peripherally apposed adjacent to the nuclear membrane. The term *immunoblast* refers to an activated lymphocyte.[15] Neoplastic immunoblasts resemble transformed lymphocytes; they are larger than large noncleaved cells with an eccentrically located vesicular round or oval nucleus containing a prominent target-like central nucleolus, and relatively abundant amphophilic cytoplasm.[18,33,174] These cells commonly exhibit plasmacytoid differentiation. In extranodal sites, DLBCLs are often associated with sclerosis.

Although these descriptions of large cleaved and noncleaved cells and immunoblasts are distinctive, and many neoplastic large B cells fit within these descriptions, it is also true that neoplastic large cells exhibit a spectrum of differentiation and often have intermediate cytologic features. Furthermore, DLBCLs are commonly composed of a mixture of these cell types.[18] Whereas some clinical studies have suggested a poorer prognosis for immunoblastic lymphomas compared with centroblastic (large noncleaved cell) lymphomas,[174] other studies have not found any differences in clinical features or response to therapy.[175]

Immunophenotypic studies have shown that DLBCLs are of mature B-cell lineage.[2] Approximately two-thirds of cases express monotypic Ig light chain (κ > λ), and IgM is the most

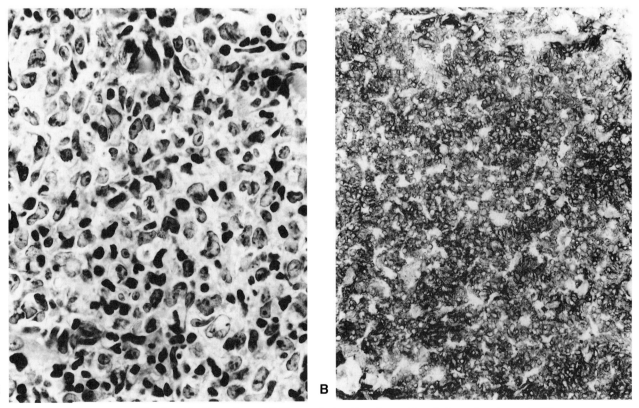

Figure 40–9. Diffuse large B-cell lymphoma. (**A**) The neoplastic cells are large with vasicular nuclear chromatin. (**B**) The neoplastic cells are strongly positive for CD20 demonstrating B-cell lineage.

common Ig heavy chain. However, a subset of cases expresses IgA or IgG; IgD is usually negative.[2] Approximately one-third of DLBCLs are Ig negative.[1,2] Plasmacytoid lymphomas commonly express monotypic cytoplasmic Ig. These tumors express pan-B-cell antigens, 60 to 70 percent express BCL-2, a subset are positive for CD10, and are negative for T-cell antigens. Most DLBCLs express activation markers, such as CD25 and CD38, and have a high rate of proliferation (Ki-67 and CD71 positive).[1,2,103,104] Major histocompatibility complex (MHC) class I or II antigens may be absent in a subset of DLBCLs.[176]

The Ig genes are rearranged and the TCR genes are usually in the germline configuration in DLBCLs.[12,13] A subset of cases carry the t(14;18), as shown by conventional cytogenetic studies. Furthermore, the *bcl-2* gene is rearranged in approximately 20 percent of cases, and the Ig heavy chain gene and *bcl-2* gene rearrangements have been shown to co-migrate, indicating the presence of t(14;18)(q32;q21).[12] These lymphomas may represent diffuse progression of an occult follicular lymphoma. Clinically, patients with de novo DLBCL and *bcl-2* rearrangement have an increased tendency to relapse compared with patients who have histologically similar tumors without *bcl-2* rearrangement, more akin to the behavior of FCL.[177] *bcl-2* protein expression, independent of the t(14;18), correlates with poorer prognosis.[178]

Another subset of DLBCLs has translocations or other abnormalities involving chromosome 3q27.[179] This locus is the site of the *bcl-6* gene, a zinc finger–encoding gene and candidate oncogene.[179] The *bcl-6* gene is rearranged in approximately 20 to 40 percent of these DLBCLs, more often tumors arising in extranodal sites.[180] In one study, patients whose DLBCLs contained *bcl-6* rearrangements had improved survival and freedom from disease progression compared with patients who had *bcl-6* germline neoplasms.[180]

The *c-myc* oncogene is not rearranged in most DLBCLs. However, *c-myc* rearrangements have been identified in DLBCLs arising in patients with AIDS.[181] A subset of primary gastric DLBCLs also has been reported with *c-myc* rearrangements.[182]

Variants of Diffuse Large B-Cell Lymphoma

T-cell/histiocyte-rich large B-Cell Lymphoma. T-cell/histiocyte-rich large B-cell lymphomas (TCRBCLs) are malignant lymphomas of B-cell origin in which most cells found in the biopsy specimen are reactive T cells.[183–185] The predominance of T cells in these tumors may lead to an erroneous assessment of T-cell lineage, and in the past many of these cases were classified as diffuse mixed small and large cell lymphomas of T-cell lineage.[186]

Histologically, TCRBCLs are diffuse and are composed predominantly of small non-neoplastic T cells.[183–185] Numerous benign histiocytes are commonly also may be present. Within this infiltrate, often representing less than 5 to 10 percent of all cells, are scattered large, neoplastic lymphoid cells of B-cell lineage (Figure 40–10).

Due to the small size of the neoplastic cell population, it is often difficult to demonstrate monotypic Ig light chain expres-

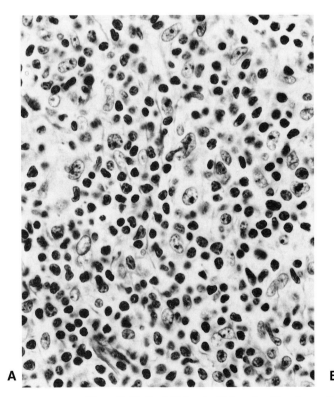

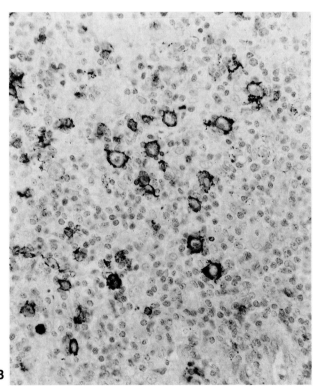

Figure 40–10. T-cell/histiocyte-rich large B-cell lymphoma. (A) The large neoplastic cells represent a minority of cells in this field. Most of the cells are small reactive T cells. (B) The anti-CD20 immunostain highlights the neoplastic B cells.

sion.[183,186] However, the large cells are B cells that express a variety of pan-B-cell antigens. Southern blot hybridization studies have shown that these tumors contain Ig heavy and light chain gene rearrangements.[186] Single cell PCR studies have shown Ig gene rearrangements that are either unmutated or mutated, consistent with origin from either germinal center or naïve B cells.[187,188] The TCR genes are usually in the germline configuration.[186] A subset of TCRBCLs carry the t(14;18) or *bcl-2* gene rearrangements.[184,186]

It seems likely that TCRBCL is an unusual histologic manifestation of DLBCL rather than a distinct clinicopathologic entity, and is considered as such in the WHO classification.[33]

Lymphomatoid Granulomatosis Lymphoma. Lymphomatoid granulomatosis (LyG) originally described by Liebow and colleagues, was initially thought to have features that overlapped with both malignant lymphoma and Wegener's granulomatosis, leading to its name.[189] Lymphomatoid granulomatosis is now considered to be neoplastic at onset and is subsequently designated here as LyG-lymphoma. The relationship between LyG-lymphoma and extranodal NK/T-cell lymphoma of nasal type (also known as polymorphic reticulosis) has been blurred in the past, and both of these neoplasms were included in the category of angiocentric lymphoma in the REAL classification.[31] However, LyG-lymphoma is now considered a distinct clinicopathologic entity and high-grade cases are designated as a variant of DLBCL in the WHO classification.[33]

Patients with LyG-lymphoma are usually of middle age and present with pulmonary and systemic symptoms. Chest radiographs typically show discrete, round masses, most often bilateral.[189] Other common sites of involvement by LyG-lymphoma include the kidney, central nervous system, and skin. The upper respiratory tract is rarely involved. Many patients with LyG-lymphoma have evidence of immune dysfunction, and LyG-lymphoma may arise in the clinical setting of overt immunodeficiency.

Histologically, LyG-lymphoma is characterized by an angiocentric and angiodestructive infiltrate of lymphocytes, plasma cells, and histiocytes.[189,190] Granulocytes are rare. Necrosis can be prominent. The lymphoid cells range in size from small with minimal atypia to large, and the natural history of LyG-lymphoma is to accrue large cells and evolve into a process that resembles large cell lymphoma.[189]

Immunophenotypic studies of LyG-lymphoma have shown that the majority of lymphoid cells are non-neoplastic T cells. In most cases of LyG-lymphoma a small number of larger B cells can be identified and these cells represent the malignant cell population.[190,191] Assessment of immunoglobulin light chain expression is difficult in LyG-lymphoma, because of the small number of B cells, but has been shown in a subset of cases.[191] These cells express pan-B-cell antigens and commonly carry Epstein-Barr virus (EBV).[190–192] However, a small subset of cases of LyG-lymphoma lack large B cells and have atypical cells of T-cell lineage, suggesting that a subset of cases are T-cell neoplasms.[191] Alternatively, these T-cell cases may not be actual cases of LyG-lymphoma, but morphological mimics of this entity.

Molecular studies using Southern blot hybridization are usually negative because the neoplastic cells represent less than

1 to 5 percent of all cells, the lower limit of sensitivity of this technique.[193] PCR studies have shown immunoglobulin gene rearrangements in the majority of cases.[190,191]

Intravascular Large B-Cell Lymphoma. Intravascular lymphoma, also known as angiotropic lymphoma and originally described as malignant angioendotheliomatosis, is an unusual variant of large cell lymphoma that presents predominantly with an intravascular distribution.[194,195] Although rare cases are of T-cell lineage, over 90 percent of intravascular lymphomas are B-cell neoplasms.[196]

Patients with intravascular large B-cell lymphoma (IVLBL) are typically middle-aged or elderly and present with systemic symptoms, as well as symptoms attributable to specific organs that result from vascular occlusion and ischemia. These tumors most commonly affect the central nervous system, skin, and kidney but any site may be involved.[194] Bone marrow involvement, although difficult to appreciate morphologically, is relatively common when the bone marrow is assessed using immunophenotypic or molecular methods.[197,198] Lymphadenopathy is uncommon. The prognosis is often poor due to late detection of disease, but patients may respond to appropriate chemotherapy.

Histologically, IVLBL is characterized by the presence of large lymphoid cells filling and/or distending vascular lumina. The neoplastic cells are found primarily within capillaries or small blood vessels. Extravascular involvement occurs, and although not prominent clinically, is commonly found at autopsy and resembles DLBCL.[194,195]

With the advent of immunophenotypic studies, IVLBL was conclusively shown to be a variant of large B-cell lymphoma in most cases.[194,195] These tumors express pan-B-cell antigens and a subset express monotypic immunoglobulin. These neoplasms appear to be heterogeneous. Two or possibly three groups have been identified: CD5+ CD10+ consistent with follicle center cell origin, CD5+ CD10–, and CD5– CD10– (similar to most large B-cell lymphomas).[196]

Molecular studies have shown Ig heavy and light chain gene rearrangements in IVLBL.[198] Lineage infidelity is uncommon. Few cases have been assessed for involvement of known oncogenes. Rare cases assessed by conventional cytogenetics have shown a complex karyotype.[199]

CD30+ Large B-Cell Lymphoma with Anaplastic Features. In 1985, Stein and colleagues[200] described anaplastic large cell lymphoma (ALCL), a group of neoplasms with anaplastic cytologic features that were immunoreactive with the Ki-1 (CD30) antibody. Initially, T-cell, null-cell, and B-cell neoplasms were included in this entity. However, it is now recognized that CD30-positive anaplastic B-cell neoplasms are clinically and biologically more similar to other types of DLBCL and they are classified as such in the WHO classification. A subset of these tumors arise in patients with a history of low-grade B-cell lymphoma suggesting that anaplastic features and CD30 expression are manifestations of a final common pathway of histologic transformation.

Histologically, these tumors can be indistinguishable from ALCL of T-cell lineage, and may express CD30 with similar intensity. However, in many of these cases there are areas that more closely resemble DLBCL and the pattern of CD30 expression is more commonly cytoplasmic (rather than membranous and paranuclear in T-cell ALCL).

Immunophenotypically, and at the molecular level, CD30-positive large B-cell lymphomas are similar to other DLBCLs.[33] Importantly, the t(2;5) translocation or *alk-1* gene abnormalities, common in T-cell ALCL, have been reported only rarely in CD30-positive large B-cell lymphomas.[201]

Primary Mediastinal Large B-Cell Lymphoma

Mediastinal lymphomas may be primary, localized to the mediastinum, or secondary, as a part of widespread lymph node–based disease. Furthermore, primary mediastinal large B-cell lymphoma, as currently defined, probably includes two clinicopathologic entities: DLBCL of thymic origin and DLBCL arising in mediastinal lymph nodes. Only the former is true primary mediastinal large B-cell lymphoma. Currently, it is not always possible to make this distinction. Presumably, as this category becomes refined to include only thymic cases, the differences with nodal DLBCL will become more obvious. Nevertheless, with even current criteria primary mediastinal large B-cell lymphomas as a group have unique clinicopathologic and histologic features and therefore have been included as a distinct category in the WHO classification.[33]

Clinically, patients with primary mediastinal large B-cell lymphoma are young adults, with onset in the fourth decade. There is a slight female predominance with a male/female ratio of 1:2.[33,202–204] Patients typically present with large, bulky (>10 cm) masses that cause local symptoms such as cough, chest pain, and shortness of breath. Approximately two-thirds of patients present with localized disease and approximately one-third of patients may develop superior vena cava syndrome. Patients typically have high serum levels of LDH but low serum levels of beta-2-microglobulin. Bone marrow involvement at time of staging is infrequent, less than 5 percent. Patients respond poorly to conventional chemotherapy (such as CHOP) but others have reported a relatively good prognosis if patients are aggressively treated with combination chemotherapy and irradiation.[203,204] Relapses commonly occur at extranodal sites.

Histologically, primary mediastinal large B-cell lymphomas are diffuse and are composed of large lymphoid cells that exhibit a spectrum of cytologic features: most commonly large noncleaved cell (centroblastic), and less often large cleaved cell or immunoblastic.[205,206] Also, a mixture of these cells is often seen within an individual neoplasm. Sclerosis is common, mitotic figures are usually numerous, and the tumor cells often have clear cytoplasm (Figure 40–11).

Immunophenotypic studies have shown findings similar to other nodal DLBCLs.[33,205,206] Primary mediastinal large B-cell lymphomas are frequently Ig negative. All tumors express pan-B-cell antigens. *Bcl-2, Bcl-6,* and CD30 are commonly positive, and CD10 is expressed in approximately one-third of the cases. Most tumors are negative for CD21 and CD35, and a subset of cases may lack MHC class II antigens.[176] These results suggest that these tumors may arise from B cells normally present in small

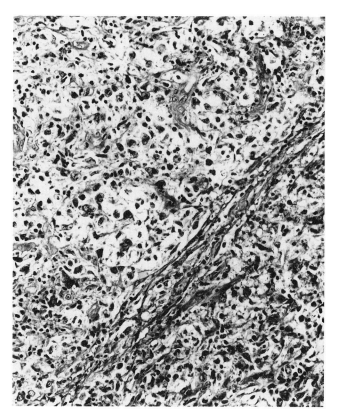

Figure 40–11. Primary mediastinal large B-cell lymphoma. The neoplasm is diffuse and is composed of large lymphoid cells associated with sclerosis.

number in the thymic medulla of the thymus.[207,208] A recent study has shown that the *mal* gene is overexpressed in primary mediastinal large B-cell lymphoma but not nodal DLBCL.[209]

Primary mediastinal large B-cell lymphomas have Ig heavy and light chain gene rearrangements.[13] The TCR genes are usually in the germline configuration. Scarpa and colleagues[210] have reported *c-myc* rearrangements in three of six cases. The *ccnd-1* and *bcl-2* genes are in the germline configuration. The *bcl-6* gene is rearranged rarely, in less than 5 percent of cases, but *bcl-6* gene mutations are common.[205] The *mal* gene is not rearranged or mutated.[209] Epstein-Barr virus is usually absent.[210]

Primary Effusion Lymphoma

Primary effusion lymphoma (PEL), also known as body cavity–based lymphoma, is a very rare neoplasm of large B cells that involves one of the body cavities: pleural, pericardial, or peritoneal.[211,212] Usually, only one body cavity is involved. Most affected patients are homosexual men infected with human immunodeficiency virus. The prognosis for patients with PEL is poor.

Morphologically, the neoplastic cells resemble immunoblasts or plasmablasts with prominent nucleoli and abundant basophilic cytoplasm.[211,212] The tumor cells are found within body cavity fluid, but may adhere to and invade body cavity surfaces.

Immunophenotypic studies of PEL are ambiguous.[211,212] The neoplastic cells express CD30, CD38, CD45 (LCA), and CD138 but are usually negative for Ig and B-cell antigens. Molecular studies, however, have demonstrated Ig gene rearrangements supporting B-cell lineage. The TCR genes are usually in the germline configuration. No characteristic chromosomal abnormalities are known. Human herpesvirus-8 (also known as Kaposi sarcoma-associated herpesvirus) is present in virtually all cases of PEL. EBV is also present in the majority of these neoplasms.

Primary effusion lymphoma needs to be distinguished from DLBCL associated with pyothorax. These tumors are also positive for EBV, are commonly associated with a history of infection such as tuberculosis, and are negative for human herpesvirus-8.[213]

Burkitt's Lymphoma

Clinically, Burkitt's lymphomas may be divided into three groups: endemic (African), sporadic (nonendemic), and AIDS-associated.[214] Another form of Burkitt's lymphoma with preferential involvement of peripheral blood and bone marrow also occurs, designated by the French-American-British group as acute lymphoblastic leukemia, L3.[215] Each of these types of Burkitt's lymphoma are recognized in the WHO classification.

Endemic Burkitt's lymphoma was first described in equatorial Africa (Uganda), where it occurs in a region 15 degrees latitude north or south of the equator.[214,216] Evidence of EBV infection is present in 95 percent of patients.[214] The median age of patients with endemic Burkitt's lymphoma is 7 years, with a boy/girl ratio of 3:1. The jaw is the most well-known site of disease, involving either the maxilla or mandible in 60 percent of patients, but large abdominal masses involving retroperitoneal structures, the gastrointestinal tract, or the gonads are also commonly present.[214,216]

Sporadic Burkitt's lymphomas occur in industrialized nations. In the Nebraska NHL Classification Project, sporadic Burkitt's lymphoma represented less than 1 percent of all NHL.[31] EBV infection is present in a subset of patients, approximately 25 percent.[214,217] Patients affected are usually in the second or third decades of life, with a male/female ratio of 3:1. The jaw is infrequently involved and most patients present with large abdominal masses, frequently involving the ileocecal region of the bowel.[214] Other sites commonly involved include abdominal and peripheral lymph nodes, pleura, and pharynx. In patients with either endemic or sporadic Burkitt's lymphoma, bone marrow and central nervous system involvement are uncommon at presentation, in approximately 10 to 20 percent of cases, but are frequent sites of disease later in the clinical course.[214] Burkitt's lymphoma occurring in the clinical setting of human immunodeficiency virus infection is associated with EBV infection in 30 to 40 percent of cases, and commonly involves lymph nodes or extranodal sites.[218]

Burkitt's lymphomas commonly involve extranodal sites. As a result, clinical or pathologic stage as determined using traditional staging systems is of less prognostic value than schemes that assess either tumor burden or the amenability to surgical excision.[219] Adverse prognostic features in Burkitt's lymphoma that correlate with tumor burden include high serum LDH levels and antibody titers reactive with EBV early antigens (probably related to cell turnover).[220,221] Absolute blood lymphocyte count and the ability of the patient to mount a delayed hypersensitivity response also correlate with clinical outcome.[222,223] Since the tumor is often widely distributed at time of presentation and has an extremely rapid clinical course, systemic chemotherapy is the treatment of choice.[214,224] Burkitt's lymphomas respond dramatically to chemotherapy. With combination chemotherapy regimens, over 75 percent of patients including those with high-stage disease may respond completely and have long-term survival.[224,225] In adequately treated African patients, relapse has also been observed 5 or more years after complete remission was achieved, which may represent the development of a new neoplasm, rather than a recurrence of the original tumor.[226] These patients, compared with early relapsers, respond well to reinduction chemotherapy. Patients with AIDS-associated Burkitt's lymphoma also respond well to combination chemotherapy, providing their underlying immunodeficiency syndrome allows adequate therapy to be administered.

Histologically, the endemic, sporadic, and AIDS-associated types of Burkitt's lymphoma are indistinguishable (Figure 40–12). Burkitt's lymphomas have two essential features. First, the neoplastic cells have nuclei that approximate the size of the nuclei of benign histiocytes.[18,217,227] Secondly, the proliferation rate of these neoplasms is virtually 100 percent.[33,227] At low power, the neoplasms grow as expansile masses that diffusely infiltrate contiguous tissues. Reactive histiocytes are scattered throughout the tumor. The relatively clear cytoplasm of the his-

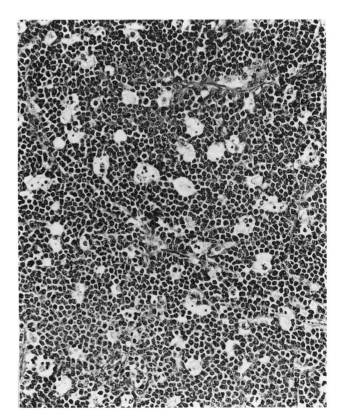

Figure 40–12. Burkitt's lymphoma. The neoplasm has a starry-sky pattern resulting from the presence of histocytes with clear cytoplasm surrounded by a monotonous population of darker neoplastic cells.

tiocytes in a background of blue neoplastic cells imparts a starry-sky appearance.[227] This pattern results from rapid cell turnover with individual cell necrosis and scavenging of debris by macrophages. The neoplastic cells are round to ovoid, strikingly monotonous, and uniform in shape. The nuclear membrane is prominent, and the chromatin is coarse, with two to five prominent, basophilic nucleoli. Mitotic figures are numerous. Although the growth pattern of the tumor is usually diffuse, occasionally selective involvement of germinal centers in partially effaced lymph nodes imparts a nodular pattern.[228]

Immunophenotypic studies of endemic, sporadic, and AIDS-associated Burkitt's lymphomas have shown similar findings. These tumors are of mature B-cell lineage and express monotypic Ig light chain ($\kappa > \lambda$), IgM, pan-B-cell antigens, and the CD10 antigen.[1,2,33] Virtually all the cells in Burkitt's lymphomas express proliferation markers, such as CD71 and Ki-67.[2,33] These tumors are negative for IgD, CD21, CD23, CD25, lymphocyte homing receptors, and T-cell antigens including CD5. These tumors are commonly, but not always, negative for BCL-2.[33,229]

Burkitt's lymphomas have Ig heavy and light chain gene rearrangements. The TCR genes are usually in the germline configuration.[12,13] Approximately 80 percent of cases carry the t(8;14)(q24;q32), with the remaining cases having one of two variant translocations, the t(2;8)(p11;q24) or t(8;22)(q24;q11).[230] Common to each of these translocations is involvement of chromosome region 8q24, the site of the *c-myc* gene. Via these translocations, *c-myc* is juxtaposed with the Ig heavy chain on the derivative chromosome 14, or with the Igκ and Ig λ genes on the derivative chromosome 8.[230] The *c-myc* gene has a central role in normal cellular proliferation. This juxtaposition of *c-myc* and Ig gene enhancers results in deregulation of the *c-myc* gene, with increased c-MYC protein driving cell proliferation.[230]

The breakpoints of the t(8;14) are distinctive in endemic and sporadic Burkitt's lymphoma.[230,231] In endemic Burkitt's lymphoma, the breakpoint on chromosome 8 occurs far 5' to the location of the *c-myc* gene whereas the breakpoint on chromosome 14 usually occurs within the joining region of the Ig heavy chain gene. By contrast, in sporadic Burkitt's lymphoma, the breakpoint on chromosome 8 occurs within the *c-myc* gene, usually in the first exon, or in adjacent flanking sequences. The breakpoint on chromosome 14 may occur within the Ig heavy chain joining switch regions. Burkitt's lymphomas that occur in AIDS patients are similar to those seen in nonendemic cases.

Molecular studies have confirmed prior serologic studies that showed evidence of EBV infection. Over 90 percent of endemic and approximately 20 to 30 percent of sporadic and AIDS-associated Burkitt's lymphomas contain EBV. The EBV is episomal, consistent with latent infection, often present in multiple copies per cell, and monoclonal, indicating that the virus is present prior to neoplastic transformation.[230,232] However, EBV, by itself, is not sufficient to cause Burkitt's lymphoma. Other environmental and genetic cofactors are probably operative.

Histologically Atypical Burkitt's Lymphoma

A subset of high-grade diffuse B-cell NHL has histologic features intermediate between DLBCL and Burkitt's lymphoma.

The designation of these neoplasms is problematic. In the International Working Formulation, these tumors were designated small noncleaved cell lymphoma, non-Burkitt's type. In the REAL classification, these tumors were provisionally designated high-grade B-cell lymphoma, Burkitt-like. In the Nebraska NHL Classification Project these neoplasms represented 2 percent of all NHLs.[31,32] The WHO classification considers neoplasms such as these as histologically atypical variants of Burkitt's lymphoma.

Histologically, these neoplasms are diffuse, often have a starry-sky pattern, and have a high proliferation rate (>99 percent) with numerous mitotic figures.[18,229] However, although the neoplastic cells are of intermediate size as is the case in Burkitt's lymphoma, the cells have greater nuclear pleomorphism, more vesicular nuclear chromatin, and more prominent nucleoli, similar to DLBCL.

Immunophenotypic studies have demonstrated that these tumors are of mature B-cell lineage and express monotypic Ig light chain ($\kappa > \lambda$), IgM, and pan-B-cell antigens.[1,2,33] These tumors also express activation and proliferation antigens. BCL-2 and lymphocyte-homing receptors are positive in some cases.[1,2]

Molecular studies have shown Ig heavy and light chain gene rearrangements with germline TCR genes in most cases.[13,232] EBV may be present in a minority of tumors.[232]

Adults with these tumors are thought to require aggressive therapy similar to patients with typical Burkitt's lymphoma. In children, Burkitt's lymphomas and high-grade Burkitt-like lymphomas cannot be reproducibly distinguished and the two have similar biologic behavior, further justifying classification of the latter as Burkitt's lymphoma.[233,234]

T-CELL LYMPHOID NEOPLASMS

Precursor T-Cell Lymphoblastic Lymphoma/Leukemia

Precursor T-cell LBLL represented less than 2 percent of all neoplasms in the Nebraska NHL Classification Project.[31] Patients with T-cell LBLL tend to be adolescents and young adults, males outnumber females by a 2:1 ratio, and widespread, supradiaphragmatic lymphadenopathy is common.[34,40,43,235] Precursor T-cell LBLL occurs with a peak incidence in the second decade of life and 50 to 80 percent of patients present with a mediastinal mass. Peripheral blood involvement is seen in at least one-third of patients at time of presentation, and sometime during the clinical course in 80 percent of those who die of the disease. Rarely, patients present with marked eosinophilia.[236] Unless effectively treated, patients have a rapidly progressive downhill course with dissemination of tumor to the bone marrow and cerebrospinal fluid. Bone marrow and central nervous system involvement are adverse prognostic signs. Patients with precursor T-cell LBLL respond favorably to therapeutic regimens designed after those used for ALL.[41,42] Adults with precursor T-cell LBLL appear to require more aggressive therapy than children.[42]

Histologically, precursor T-cell LBLL is indistinguishable from precursor B-cell LBLL described previously (Figure 40–13). Immunologic studies of precursor T-cell LBLL have shown that this tumor, among all the NHLs, appears to illus-

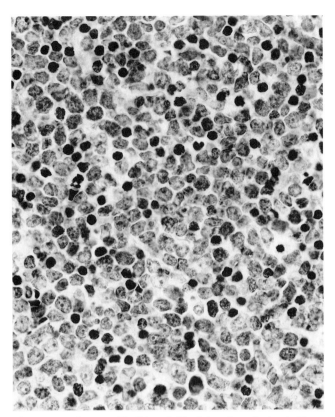

Figure 40–13. Precursor T-cell lymphoblastic lymphoma/leukemia. The neoplasm is diffuse and is composed of small neoplastic cells with immature ("dusty") chromatin.

trate the concept that neoplasms represent clonal expansions of cells frozen in a state of differentiation.[1,2,33,235] This phenomenon allows one to deduce that a variety of T-cell antigens are acquired in sequence, most likely reflecting the sequence of expression by non-neoplastic T cells during development. CD7 and CD2 are most commonly positive in T-LBLLs and therefore are thought to be acquired earliest in development followed by CD5, CD4, CD8, and CD3. TdT is positive and CD1A is positive in a subset of cases. B-cell antigens and Ig are negative in precursor T-cell LBLL, with the exception of CD79A, which can be positive in 20 to 30 percent of neoplasms.[238]

Gene rearrangement studies of precursor T-cell LBLL have shown various patterns of TCR gene rearrangement, corresponding to the stage of differentiation of the neoplasm. In a small subset of cases of T-cell LBLL with an early-thymic immunophenotype, only rearrangements of the TCR δ gene or the TCR δ and/or TCR γ genes may be identified.[13,46,237,238] In the remaining tumors with early-, mid-, and late-thymic immunophenotypes, all of the TCR genes are rearranged. (The TCR δ gene may be rearranged and subsequently deleted.) These findings suggest a hierarchy of TCR gene rearrangements in developing T lymphocytes: the TCR δ gene rearranges first, followed by the TCR γ and TCR β genes, and lastly the TCR α gene. Lineage infidelity is common in precursor T-cell LBLL; up to 30 percent of cases have IgH gene rearrangements.

In precursor T-cell LBLLs, t(1;14)(p32;q11) or del(1p) may be the most frequent chromosomal abnormality.[239] Other

translocations described in precursor T-cell LBLLs involve the TCR gene loci and candidate oncogenes including *TCL-1* at 14q32, involved in either t(7;14)(q35;q32) or t(14;14)(q11;q32); *TCL-2* at 11p13, involved in t(11;14)(p13;q11); and *TCL-5/HOX-11* at 10q24, involved in t(10;14)(q24;q11).[47,240]

t(1;14)(p32;q11) has been described in 15 to 30 percent of cases of precursor T-cell LBLL.[241,242] In this translocation, the *TAL-1* gene (also known as *SCL* or *TCL-5*) and the *SIL* gene are joined as a result of illegitimate recombination.[239] This recombination is thought to be mediated by the V(D)J recombinase mechanism using heptamer-nonamer-like sequences flanking each gene.[240]

T-Cell Prolymphocytic Leukemia

The relationship between T-cell chronic lymphocytic leukemia (CLL) and T-cell prolymphocytic leukemia (PLL) is controversial. Some investigators have suggested that the term T-CLL be reserved for leukemias composed of small lymphocytes of T-cell lineage that resemble B-CLL.[243] However, many of these cases have clinical, morphologic, and molecular features in common with T-cell PLL.[244] Therefore, the WHO classification includes T-CLL in the T-PLL category.[33]

Clinically, patients with T-PLL present with a high white blood cell count, often greater than 100×10^9/L.[245,246] Skin involvement and organomegaly are common. Lymph nodes, bone marrow, and mucosal surfaces may be involved. The median survival is often less than 1 year. However, recent clinical studies that have treated patients with 2-deoxycoformycin and anti-CD52 (CAMPATH-1H®) have shown promising results.[247]

In peripheral blood and bone marrow aspirate smears the leukemic cells are small to medium sized, with relatively abundant, nongranular cytoplasm and nuclei with irregular contours, each with one central prominent nucleolus (Figure 40–14).[244,245] In some cases, the tumor cell nuclei are not obviously irregular and nucleoli are small or indistinct, so-called small cell variant of T-PLL.[245] Lymph nodes are involved in a paracortical distribution or are diffusely replaced. In the liver, T-PLL commonly involves the sinusoids, and in the spleen, the red pulp is preferentially involved. Skin involvement is characterized by dermal infiltrates, usually without epidermotrophism.[245]

Immunophenotypic studies have shown that T-PLLs are neoplasms of mature T-cell lineage that express pan-T-cell antigens and the TCR αβ receptor.[2,33] CD7 is often expressed strongly. Aberrant T-cell immunophenotypes may be detected but are uncommon. Approximately two-thirds of cases are CD4+, 20 percent coexpress the CD4 and CD8 antigens, and rare tumors are CD8+. TdT, Igs, and B-cell antigens are negative.[2,33]

Molecular studies of T-PLL have shown rearrangements of the TCR β and TCR δ genes. The TCR δ gene is usually deleted and the Ig heavy and light chain genes are usually in the germline configuration.[13] A characteristic chromosomal abnormality, the inv(14)(q11;q32), occurs in approximately two-thirds of T-PLL.[248] Rare cases of T-PLL has been described with translocations involving the 14q11 or Xq28 loci, the latter involving the *mtcp*1 gene, without inv(14).[249] Chromosome 11q deletions and *atm* gene mutations/deletions are common in T-PLL.[250] Trisomy 8 is also reported.[246] A recent comparative genomic hybridiza-

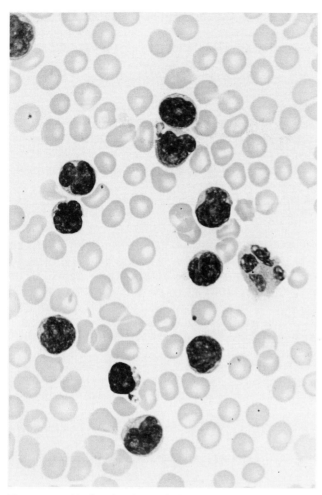

Figure 40–14. T-cell prolymphocytic leukemia involving peripheral blood. The neoplastic cells are small with convoluted nuclear contours. (Case courtesy of Dan Jones, M.D., Ph.D.)

tion study of T-PLL revealed nine regions of chromosomal loss and four regions of chromosomal gain, suggesting that a number of other genes may be involved in pathogenesis.[251]

T-Cell Large Granular Lymphocytic Leukemia

Large granular lymphocytes represent 10 to 15 percent of normal peripheral blood mononuclear cells and may be either of T-cell or natural killer (NK) cell lineage. Either cell type can give rise to large granular lymphocyte leukemia (LGLL). Approximately 80 to 90 percent of all cases of LGLL are of T-cell type.

Patients with T-cell LGLL are typically elderly with a median age of 60 years. There is no sex preference.[252–254] Approximately two-thirds of patients seek medical attention for chronic, recurrent infections, often involving the skin or mucosal sites. One-third of patients are asymptomatic and T-cell LGLL is detected incidentally.

Autoimmune phenomena may be present, most often rheumatoid arthritis in 25 percent of patients.[253] Physical examination reveals hepatosplenomegaly in up to half of patients. Lym-

phadenopathy is uncommon. Laboratory studies reveal neutropenia in most patients, anemia in 40 to 50 percent, and thrombocytopenia in 20 to 30 percent. Neutropenia and anemia can be severe. Serum protein electrophoresis reveals polyclonal hypergammaglobulinemia. Seropositivity for human T-cell leukemia virus type 1 (HTLV-1) has been reported, but most patients are not infected by prototypical HTLV-1. A cellular or retroviral protein with homology to an epitope of HTLV-1 is suspected.[255] Most patients have an indolent clinical course.[254,256]

Morphologically, T-cell LGLL cells in peripheral blood and bone marrow smears are larger than normal lymphocytes (15 to 18 μ in diameter) with abundant cytoplasm containing azurophilic granules.[257,258] Normally, the peripheral blood large granular lymphocyte count in patients with T-cell LGLL is greater than 2×10^9/L. In bone marrow, T-cell LGLL diffusely infiltrates the medullary space in an interstitial pattern. T-cell LGLL commonly is observed in the sinusoids of the liver and the red pulp of the spleen.

Immunophenotypic studies have shown that T-cell LGLL cells express T-cell specific antigens such as CD3 and CD5 (dim) as well as T-cell-associated antigens such as CD2, CD7, and CD57.[2,253] Most cases express the TCR α/β and have a T-cell suppressor/cytotoxic immunophenotype (CD4– CD8+), but rare cases can express the TCR γ/δ or be CD4– CD8–. *Fas* ligand is expressed in almost all cases.[259] CD56 is expressed rarely, but positive cases may have an aggressive clinical course.

Molecular studies have shown rearrangements of the TCR γ, TCR α, and TCR β genes.[13,260] The TCR δ gene is usually deleted. The Ig genes are in the germline configuration. In the relatively small number of cases that have been analyzed cytogenetically, clonal chromosomal abnormalities have been identified.[252] A recent case report described a novel t(11;12)(q12;q11).[261]

Aggressive NK-Cell Leukemia

Approximately 10 to 20 percent of LGLLs are of NK cell origin and are designated in the WHO classification as aggressive NK-cell leukemia. NK-cell leukemias arise in young adults with a median age of 39 years.[253] There is no sex preference. Splenomegaly and hepatomegaly are common, present in over 60 percent of patients. Lymphadenopathy occurs in approximately 25 percent of patients. Extranodal sites of involvement can occur (e.g., gastrointestinal tract and central nervous system). Anemia and thrombocytopenia are common, in 75 to 100 percent of cases. Approximately half of the patients have neutropenia. Absolute large granular lymphocyte counts are higher in NK-cell leukemia than in T-cell LGLL, often greater than 10×10^9/L. The clinical course of patients with NK-leukemia is aggressive with a high mortality rate; some patients develop disseminated intravascular coagulation.[253]

Morphologically, NK-cell leukemia closely resembles T-cell LGLL. Bone marrow involvement by NK-cell leukemia is usually extensive.[257,258] Immunophenotypic studies show expression of T-cell-associated antigens, but not T-cell-specific antigens such as CD3, CD5, and TCR receptors.[253,262] Most cases are positive for CD8, CD16, and CD56 and are negative for CD4. CD57 is variably expressed.[253]

Molecular studies show no evidence of TCR or Ig gene rearrangements.[13] Clonal cytogenetic abnormalities have been identified in some cases, including deletion (6q), rearrangement of chromosome X, and translocations of 8p23.[263,264] EBV was reported in 50 percent of cases in one study.[265]

Adult T-Cell Lymphoma/Leukemia

Adult T-cell lymphoma/leukemia (ATLL) is a distinct clinico-pathologic entity associated with infection by the human T-cell leukemia/lymphoma retrovirus (HTLV-1).[266] ATLL accounts for the extraordinarily high incidence of T-cell lymphoma in Japan, particularly on the island of Kyushu, where up to 30 percent of normal individuals have serologic evidence of HTLV-1 infection.[266–268] Clusters of cases also have been reported on Pacific Ocean islands such as Okinawa, in the Caribbean, in Europe, and the southeastern United States, the latter predominantly in Black patients.[269] HTLV-1 is a single-stranded RNA retrovirus that is lymphotropic for T lymphocytes.[270] The virus is transmitted by sexual intercourse, breast milk, shared needles among intravenous drug users, and transfusion of blood products. The incubation period for development of ATLL ranges from 20 to 40 years.

Patients with ATLL are usually adults, with a median age of 55 years in one study,[266] who may present with one of four general syndromes.[271] Patients with acute ATLL, the most common form of the disease, have generalized lymphadenopathy, hepatosplenomegaly, skin lesions, peripheral blood involvement, lytic bone lesions, and hypercalcemia. Hypercalcemia also may develop in the absence of bone lesions, secondary to secretion of parathyroid hormone–related peptide by the neoplastic cells, possibly induced by HTLV TAX protein.[272] The cerebrospinal fluid is commonly involved. Although patients respond to chemotherapy, remissions are short and survival is usually poor. Lymphomatous ATLL is the second most common form of the disease. Patients present with prominent lymphadenopathy and tumors in other organs without hepatosplenomegaly or hypercalcemia. The prognosis of these patients is better than that of patients with acute ATLL. Patients also may present with chronic ATLL, with an absolute lymphocytosis and cytologically abnormal cells in the peripheral blood.[271] Skin lesions, lymphadenopathy, and involvement of other viscera may occur. Patient survival is usually greater than 2 years. Lastly, patients have been described with smoldering ATLL.[271] These patients have chronic disease for years, usually skin lesions, with minimal peripheral blood involvement; the viscera are usually spared.

The morphologic findings in the peripheral blood are characteristic of ATLL.[271,273] The circulating neoplastic cells are medium-sized with basophilic cytoplasm and markedly irregular, multilobulated nuclei, including clover-leaf shapes (also known as *flower cells*). The neoplastic cells in lymph nodes and viscera involved by ATLL exhibit a spectrum of cell sizes, including small, medium-sized, and large with relatively round or markedly irregular nuclear contours. Many cases involving lymph nodes cannot be reliably distinguished from peripheral T-cell lymphomas not associated with HTLV-1 infection. Histologic findings in tissue sites do not correlate with survival.[271,273]

Immunophenotypic studies have shown that ATLLs have a mature T-cell immunophenotype.[2,266] The tumor cells express pan-T-cell antigens and the TCR αβ receptor and are CD4+ CD8–. Characteristically, the neoplastic cells intensely express the CD25 antigen. The tumor cells are negative for TdT, Igs, and B-cell antigens.

Gene rearrangement analyses have shown rearrangements of the TCR β and TCR γ genes.[13,273] The TCR α gene has been rearranged in a small number of cases studied. The TCR δ genes are usually deleted and the Ig genes are usually in the germline configuration.[273] Cytogenetic studies show multiple abnormalities in ATLL, and usually multiple abnormalities per individual neoplasm, at least six in one study.[274] These results suggest a multistep pathogenesis for ATLL, and are consistent with the known long incubation period from time of infection to onset of tumor.

The hallmark of ATLL is the demonstration of HTLV-1, either serologically by detection of serum antibodies, or by molecular detection of the virus using either Southern blot hybridization or PCR techniques. The virus clonally integrates into the host cell genome.[270] The site of integration of HTLV-1 appears to be similar in most cases. Unusual sites of viral integration may correlate with a poorer prognosis.[275] Recent data suggest that HTLV-1 proteins, such as TAX, stimulate cell growth by interacting with cell cycle proteins.[276]

Extranodal NK/T-Cell Lymphoma, Nasal Type

The term extranodal NK/T-cell lymphoma, nasal type is used in the WHO classification for a neoplasm previously designated as lethal midline granuloma, polymorphic reticulosis, midline malignant reticulosis, angiocentric immunoproliferative lesion, and angiocentric lymphoma.[31,33,277,278]

Clinically, extranodal NK/T-cell lymphomas of nasal type have a propensity for involving extranodal sites, most commonly the nasal cavity, nasopharynx, and palate.[277] However, these tumors can involve other extranodal sites at time of diagnosis and relapses commonly involve extranodal sites.[279] Lymph node and bone marrow are involved rarely. Extranodal NK/T-cell lymphomas of nasal type are predominantly localized processes at onset and may be present for years prior to diagnosis. These neoplasms are commonly associated with a hemophagocytic syndrome, clinically characterized by fever, hepatosplenomegaly, pancytopenia, and laboratory evidence of hemolysis.[280] Both TNF-α and MIP-1α have been implicated in the pathogenesis of hemophagocytic syndromes.[281,282]

Histologically, extranodal NK/T-cell lymphomas of nasal type are composed of a mixture of atypical lymphoid cells admixed with reactive lymphocytes, plasma cells, and histiocytes.[277,283] Eosinophils and neutrophils are rare or absent. In the early stages of disease, relatively few neoplastic cells are present, and these cells may be of small size. As a result, biopsy specimens of the early stages can be misinterpreted as a benign process. Over time, these neoplasms accrue greater numbers of large atypical cells and the diagnosis is more easily established. These neoplasms can display a marked propensity for invading and destroying blood vessels, but angiocentricity is not a universal feature.[33]

Immunophenotypic studies of extranodal NK/T-cell lymphomas of nasal type can be difficult to interpret, particularly in lesions with few large cells and numerous inflammatory cells. Most extranodal NK/T-cell lymphomas of nasal type are of NK-cell origin, although rare cases are of T-cell lineage.[33] Thus, most neoplasms express the NK-cell-associated antigen CD56 and NK/T-cell-associated antigens such as CD2, CD7, and CD8.[2,33,283] These tumors also express cytoplasmic CD3, but are negative for T-cell-specific antigens such as surface CD3, CD5, and TCRs. The neoplastic cells commonly express p53, TIA-1, perforin, Fas, and Fas ligand.[284,285] CD16 and CD57 are often negative and Ig and B-cell antigens are negative.

Molecular studies of extranodal NK/T-cell lymphomas of nasal type have demonstrated an absence of TCR and Ig gene rearrangements in most cases studied.[193,286] EBV genomes have been identified in the neoplastic cells using Southern blot, PCR, and in situ hybridization techniques.[193,279,286–288] The virus also has been shown to be present in monoclonal form indicating that EBV is present prior to clonal expansion.[193,286,287] Recent comparative genomic hybridization studies of extranodal NK/T-cell lymphomas of nasal type have shown common chromosomal losses at 1p, 12q, and 17p and chromosome gains at 2q, 10q, and 13q.[288]

Enteropathy-Type T-Cell Lymphoma

These neoplasms are rare and have been designated previously as enteropathy-associated T-cell lymphoma and intestinal T-cell lymphoma.[31,33]

Patients with enteropathy-type T-cell lymphoma (ETL) present with abdominal pain or weight loss.[289] Although initially described in patients with a history of gluten-sensitive enteropathy or celiac disease, who are known to have an increased incidence of lymphoma,[290,291] these tumors also arise commonly in patients without a history of celiac disease.[289,292] In a recent study, only 15 of 31 patients with ETL had a clinical history or histologic evidence of enteropathy.[289] The survival of individuals with ETL is poor. Approximately half of patients initially respond to chemotherapy, but almost all relapse and death results from either disease progression or complications of therapy.[289]

Grossly, the involved intestine demonstrates multiple ulcers; a distinct mass may not be found. The ulcers may extend deeply into the bowel wall, often resulting in perforation. The jejunum is the most common site of involvement. Histologically, the intestine not involved by neoplasm may exhibit blunting of villi as is seen in celiac disease.[290,292] ETL is usually present at the base of the ulcers and within the lamina propria and submucosa. These neoplasms are diffuse and the neoplastic cells are a mixture of small, medium-sized, and large lymphoid cells that may have clear cytoplasm.[292] These tumors may have a high proliferative rate.

Immunophenotypic studies have shown that ETLs express pan-T-cell antigens, are often CD4– CD8– or CD4– CD8+, and usually have a cytotoxic profile, positive for TIA-1, granzyme B, perforin, and Fas ligand.[292,293] A subset of tumors are positive for p53, CD30, CD56, and CD103, the latter of which is expressed by normal lymphocytes residing in the intestinal mucosa.[33,292–294] Fifty to 60 percent of ETL are positive for EBV.[292,293] These tumors are negative for Ig and B-cell antigens.

Molecular studies have shown that the TCR β and TCR γ genes are usually rearranged in ETL and the Ig genes are in the germline configuration.[292,295] Molecular analysis of cases of refractory celiac disease and ulcerative jejunitis, without morphologic evidence of lymphoma, also have shown TCR gene rearrangements suggesting that these diseases are preneoplastic.[294–296] In addition, in a subset of patients with ulcerative jejunitis and ETL, normal mucosa, benign ulcers, and tumors have been shown to carry identical TCR γ gene rearrangements.[295]

Hepatosplenic T-Cell Lymphoma

Hepatosplenic T-cell lymphoma (HSTCL) is a rare neoplasm that most commonly affects young adults with a male predominance who present with marked hepatosplenomegaly and minimal or absent lymphadenopathy.[297–301] Bone marrow involvement is common but often subtle.[300] Skin lesions may occur. Affected patients have an aggressive clinical course with a high rate of relapse and death. These tumors were originally named *hepatosplenic γ/δ lymphoma*.[33] However, as a subset of cases may express the TCR α/β,[301] the WHO classification designates these neoplasms as HSTCL.

Histologically, these neoplasms are diffuse and are composed of medium-sized lymphoid cells with slightly irregular nuclear contours, condensed chromatin, and small nucleoli.[297,298] In the liver, HSTCL infiltrates sinusoids and spares portal tracts (Figure 40–15). In the spleen, red pulp is involved and white pulp is spared. In the bone marrow, the neoplastic cells can resemble blasts in aspirate smears and are commonly intra-sinusoidal in core biopsy specimens.[300]

Immunophenotypic studies have demonstrated that HSTCLs have a mature but aberrant T-cell immunophenotype, positive for the CD2, CD3, and CD7 antigens. Most cases are negative for CD4 and CD8, but a subset may express CD8. CD5 is usually absent. CD56 is usually expressed, a subset may be CD16 positive, and CD57 is negative. These neoplasms commonly have a nonfunctional cytotoxic profile, positive for TIA-1 but negative for granzyme B and perforin.[302] In most cases the tumor cells express the TCR γδ receptor, but some cases are positive for TCR α/β.[298,301]

The TCR γ and TCR δ genes in HSTCL are usually rearranged.[13,300] The TCR β gene also may be rearranged. The Ig genes have been in the germline configuration. Most cases in our experience are negative for EBV,[300] but Japanese cases positive for the virus have been reported.[303] These neoplasms often carry a characteristic cytogenetic abnormality, isochromosome (7q).[304]

Subcutaneous Panniculitis-Like T-Cell Lymphoma

Subcutaneous panniculitis-like T-cell lymphoma (SPTCL) is a rare disease. In a recent review of the literature the authors identified 72 cases.[305]

Patients with SPTCL are usually adults who present with multiple subcutaneous nodules, usually small but occasionally large, up to 12 cm.[306] Approximately one-third of patients present with

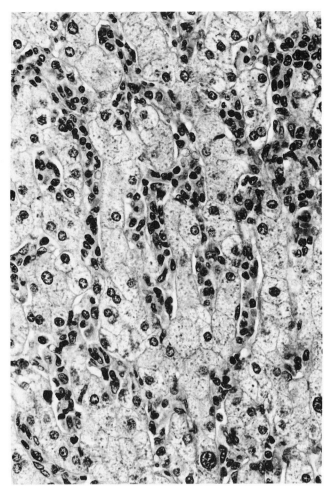

Figure 40–15. Hepatosplenic T-cell lymphoma involving liver. In this field, the neoplastic cells are distending sinusoids. (Case courtesy of Lynne Abruzzo, M.D., Ph.D.)

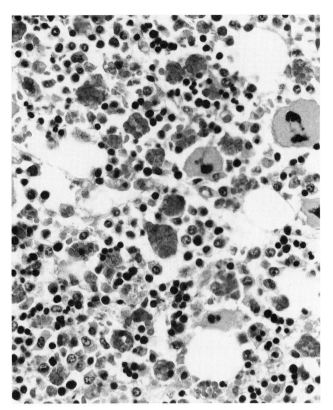

Figure 40–16. Hemophagocytic syndrome. In this field, histocytes in bone marrow are distended by numerous phagocytosed erythrocytes.

a hemophagocytic syndrome, causing systemic symptoms. Additional patients develop a hemophagocytic syndrome at some point in the course of their disease. The mechanism causing the hemophagocytic syndrome is uncertain, but may be related to chemokine expression by the neoplastic cells (Figure 40–16). Responses to combination chemotherapy are reported.[307,308]

Histologically, SPTCLs involve subcutaneous tissue, with minimal involvement of overlying dermis (Figure 40–17).[306,308,309] The neoplastic cells infiltrate the septae of adipose tissue, surrounding fat cells, and marked coagulative necrosis and fat necrosis are common resembling panniculitis. Nevertheless, at high power the tumor cells are cytologically atypical and may be a mixture of small and large cells, or predominantly large cells. Large cells accrue over time. Karyorrhexis is often prominent and mitotic figures are easily identified.

Immunophenotypic studies have shown that SPTCLs have a mature T-cell immunophenotype, expressing T-cell-specific and T-cell-associated antigens. Most cases of SPTCL express the TCR α/β.[306,309] An aberrant T-cell immunophenotype may be detected, more commonly in lesions composed of large cells.

SPTCLs have a cytotoxic T-cell profile, positive for TIA-1, perforin, and granzyme B.[308,309] CD56 is positive in a subset of cases.[308] B-cell antigens and Ig are negative.

Molecular studies have demonstrated TCR β and TCR γ gene rearrangements.[306,309] The Ig genes are usually in the germline configuration and EBV is absent.[309] Specific cytogenetic abnormalities have not been identified.

Other neoplasms may predominantly involve subcutaneous adipose tissue and resemble SPTCL. These tumors include anaplastic large cell lymphoma, extranodal NK/T-cell lymphoma of nasal type, and γ/δ T-cell lymphoma of skin.[310,311]

Mycosis Fungoides/Sézary Syndrome

Patients with mycosis fungoides (MF) often have symptoms that last several years before the diagnosis can be established histologically. In this early stage, the disease may present as small patches or limited plaques.[312] Even though cutaneous manifestations predominate, staging studies commonly demonstrate evidence of dissemination.[313] Eventually patients progress to generalized plaques, and then cutaneous tumors. In the late stages, widespread extracutaneous dissemination occurs, similar to other late-stage NHLs.[314] Patients with Sézary syndrome (SS), who represent approximately 5 percent of patients with MF/SS, have generalized erythroderma and cerebriform lymphoid cells in the peripheral blood (Sézary cells).

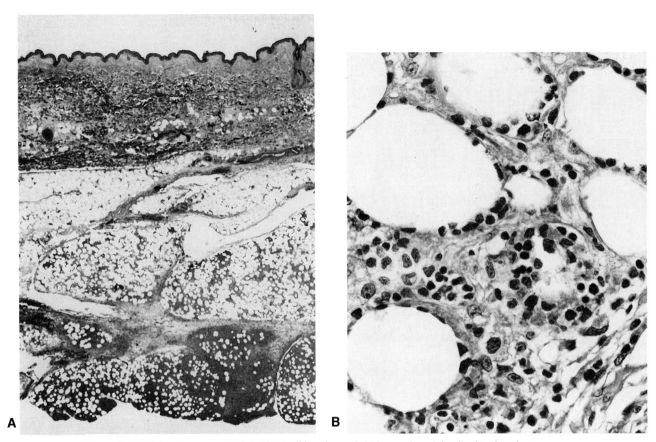

Figure 40–17. Subcutaneous panniculitis-like T-cell lymphoma. (A) The neoplasm is localized to the subcutaneous tissue with sparing of the dermis and epidermis. (B) The neoplastic cells infiltrate septae between adipocytes and are cytologically atypical.

Since the cutaneous histologic findings of MF and SS are similar, and eventual widespread dissemination with lymphadenopathy and visceral involvement is common in both, MF and SS are considered to represent different clinical manifestations of the same disease.[312]

Stage is the most important prognostic variable and reflects tumor burden and biologic behavior. A number of staging systems for MF/SS have been developed, all of which incorporate the following information.[314–317] Patients with disease confined to the skin have clinically indolent disease, with long survival (up to 30 years) and the best response rate to treatment. Survival is shorter with the presence of lymphadenopathy, even if lymph node biopsy fails to demonstrate involvement. Patients with histologically proven lymph node involvement, skin tumors, or erythroderma have a poorer prognosis. Patients with MF/SS involving the viscera have the worst survival (often less than 2 years).

The treatment for patients with MF/SS is different from that used for patients with other types of NHLs in that skin-directed therapy has a prominent role, in addition to systemic therapies as are used for patients with other types of NHL.

Skin-directed therapy is used for patients with relatively localized skin lesions, and includes ultraviolet B, psoralen plus ultraviolet A (PUVA), and topical chemotherapy (most often nitrogen mustard or carmustine).[318] Topical regimens result in a higher rate of response, but relapse is common. With PUVA, the patient is treated with ultraviolet light after ingesting psoralen, a photoactive compound. For patients with more generalized cutaneous disease, total skin electron beam therapy has been used. A number of newer therapies are now employed or are under investigation. These include photopheresis, interferon α, retinoids, DAB_{389} IL-2 (Ontak®), anti-CD4, anti-CD52 (CAMPATH-1H®), interleukin-2, and interleukin-12. Combination chemotherapy is used for patients with advanced disease.

Histologically, the findings in MF and SS are identical, although in general, the extent of skin involvement in SS is less.[33,319] The earliest lesions of MF in the patch stage mimic a variety of benign lymphohistiocytic disorders. The diagnosis may be suspected but can be difficult to confirm using routine pathologic methods. Similarly, in SS the histologic findings can be subtle, in spite of obvious erythroderma observed clinically. In the more advanced plaque and tumor skin lesions, the findings are more specific and include acanthosis and parakeratosis of the epidermis, a bandlike infiltrate of atypical lymphoid cells in the papillary dermis, and exocytosis (migration) of the atypical lymphoid cells into the epidermis (Figure 40–18). The lat-

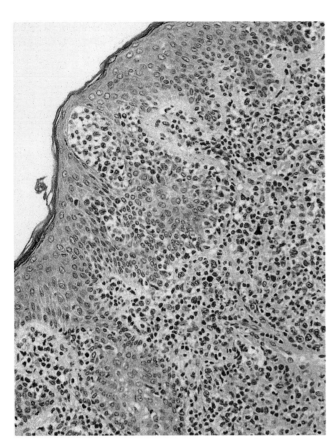

Figure 40–18. Mycosis fungoides, plaque stage. A large Pautrier's microabscess is present in this field.

ter may aggregate to form Pautrier's microabscesses, highly suggestive of MF/SS, but present in only 50 to 60 percent of cases. The neoplastic cells exhibit a spectrum of cell sizes: small, slightly larger than benign lymphocytes; intermediate, approximately 12 μ; and large. In early lesions, small cells predominate and are mixed with numerous benign inflammatory cells. In more advanced lesions, intermediate and large cells are more numerous and inflammatory cells are relatively less.

In SS, the atypical cells in the peripheral blood are of intermediate size, with a high nucleus-to-cytoplasm ratio and a lobulated nucleus. The nuclear outlines of these atypical cells often resemble the outlines of a clenched fist. Electron microscopic studies of these cells have shown extremely convoluted or cerebriform nuclei.[312] Individuals with palpable lymphadenopathy at time of biopsy may have obvious involvement by MF/SS or histologically benign dermatopathic lymphadenopathy.[320] The findings in lymph nodes may be graded using the LN system: LN0, negative; LN1, LN2, or LN3, dermatopathic lymphadenopathy with atypical small lymphocytes present singly (LN1), in small (3–6) clusters (LN2), or in large (>15) clusters (LN3); and LN4, partial or complete replacement by malignant lymphoma.[321] Sites of visceral involvement by MF/SS are less distinctive and resemble other types of NHL, most often large cell lymphoma.[314,322]

Patients with MF/SS are at risk for transformation to large cell lymphoma. In various studies the reported risk ranges from 8 to 23 percent.[323,324] Transformation correlates with poorer prognosis. The number of large cells required for large cell transformation varies in different studies; 25 percent was the criterion used in one study by Diamandidou et al.[324]

Immunophenotypic studies have shown that the neoplastic cells have a mature T-cell immunophenotype; over 95 percent of cases mark as T-helper/inducer cells.[1,2,325] Thus, the tumor cells express pan-T-cell antigens and are CD4+ and CD8–. Rare cases with a T-cell suppressor/cytotoxic cell immunophenotype (CD4– CD8+) have been reported. Most cases express the TCR α/β. Immunophenotypic analysis of skin and lymph node biopsy specimens is a helpful technique for early diagnosis when the histologic findings are nonspecific. In cutaneous sites, absence of the T-cell antigen CD7 or absence of reactivity with the Leu8 antibody is highly suggestive of MF/SS. The number of CD8-positive cells in skin biopsy specimens involved by disease may correlate with prognosis.[326] CD8-positive cells are generally greater in disease of lower clinical stage. Furthermore, within a given stage, higher numbers of CD8-positive cells correlate with longer survival.[326] The tumor form of MF/SS not infrequently exhibits an aberrant T-cell immunophenotype with absence of one or more pan-T-cell antigens.[1,2,325] B-cell antigens, Ig, and TdT are negative in MF/SS.

The ability to detect monoclonal TCR gene rearrangements in MF/SS depends on the stage of disease. Almost all cases of the tumor form and cases of high clinical stage have rearrangements of the TCR β and TCR γ genes.[13,327,328] The TCR δ genes are usually deleted. The Ig genes are usually in the germline configuration. By contrast, TCR gene rearrangements may not be detected in biopsy specimens of early (usually patch) stage disease in approximately 20 percent of patients. Thus, cases of early-stage MF/SS may represent polyclonal infiltrates within which a clonal T-cell population subsequently arises, or may be monoclonal at onset, but the monoclonal population present is insufficient to be detected by molecular methods. Identical TCR gene rearrangements have been found in skin lesions and regional lymph nodes. Furthermore, TCR gene rearrangements have been found in lymph nodes not clearly involved histologically that resemble benign dermatopathic lymph nodes. These results may explain why the presence of palpable lymphadenopathy, even when the lymph node biopsy specimen reveals only dermatopathic lymphadenopathy, is a poor prognostic finding.[315]

Zucker-Franklin and Pancake[329] reported HTLV-1 *pol* or *tax* proviral sequences in peripheral blood mononuclear cells in most patients with MF/SS. However, others have not confirmed this finding.[330] The *tal-1* gene was found to be rearranged in 10 percent of MF/SS cases.[331] Other known oncogenes are not involved. Conventional cytogenetic analysis has revealed clonal abnormalities involving a number of chromosomes in patients with advanced stage disease. Chromosome 1p22-36 was most often involved in one study.[332]

Anaplastic Large Cell Lymphoma, T/Null-Cell

In 1985, Stein and colleagues[202] identified a subset of NHLs characterized by anaplastic large lymphoid cells, originally named Ki-1 lymphoma. This neoplasm has since been designated anaplastic large cell lymphoma (ALCL) in the WHO classification.[33] In the original study, approximately 75 percent of cases were of T-cell lineage, 20 percent of cases were of B-cell lineage, and 5 percent lacked immunophenotypic or molecular evidence of either T-cell or B-cell lineage (i.e., null cell).[202] B-cell cases are now excluded from ALCL and are included in the diffuse large B-cell lymphoma category in the WHO classification.[33] Cutaneous ALCL of T-cell or null cell lineage is also recognized as a separate category in the WHO classification. T/null ALCL represented approximately 2 percent of all NHLs in the Nebraska NHL Classification Project.[31,32]

Systemic ALCL of T/null-cell lineage affects children and adults and may involve nodal or extranodal sites. The disease is more common in children, particularly those cases that overexpress ALK protein as a result of molecular abnormalities involving the *alk* gene at 2p23.[333,334] Systemic ALCLs are clinically aggressive and require combination chemotherapy, with complete response and survival similar to other diffuse aggressive lymphomas. T/null ALCLs have a better prognosis than other types of peripheral T-cell lymphoma, and this is particularly true for ALK-positive cases.[335,336]

Histologically, T/null-cell ALCLs exhibit a wide histologic spectrum. In classical cases, ALCL preferentially involves lymph nodes sinuses, particularly in lymph nodes not involved extensively.[333–337] With greater involvement, ALCL replaces the paracortical regions or may diffusely replace lymph node architecture. The neoplastic cells often appear cohesive. Cytologically, the neoplastic cells are large and bizarre, irregularly shaped, and often have polylobated nuclei. The nuclear chromatin is vesicular with prominent nucleoli. The tumor cell cytoplasm is abundant and usually basophilic. Other histologic variants of ALCL are described including the monomorphic, lymphohistiocytic, sarcomatoid, small cell, and neutrophil-rich variants.[33] These neoplasms are more difficult to recognize without knowledge of CD30 expression. The monomorphic variant resembles, in part, diffuse large cell lymphoma or plasmacytoma. The lymphohistiocytic variant is composed of relatively few neoplastic cells associated with numerous lymphocytes and histiocytes. In the sarcomatoid variant, the neoplastic cells are of spindled shape resembling sarcoma. In the small cell neoplastic variant, large anaplastic neoplastic cells are infrequent and many small cells are present. Numerous neutrophils and necrosis are present in the neutrophil-rich variant of ALCL.[338]

Immunophenotypic studies have shown that over 95 percent of cases express the activation antigen CD30, which led to the recognition of ALCL.[332–337,339] However, CD30 antigen expression is not specific for ALCLs. Most cases express a variety of activation (e.g., CD25 and CD38), and proliferation (e.g., CD71 and Ki-67) antigens.[340] Approximately half of ALCLs lack leukocyte common antigen (CD45). Epithelial membrane antigen is often expressed by the systemic form of ALCL, particularly ALK-positive tumors.[337] Neoplasms of mature T-cell lineage express pan-T-cell antigens, are most often CD4+ CD8−, and lack B-cell antigens and Ig.[337,340] Aberrant immunophenotypes are common. A large subset of cases may be negative for CD3; loss of the CD2, CD5, and CD7 antigens is also common.

Null-cell ALCLs lack immunophenotypic (as well as molecular) evidence of lineage. Many T/null-ALCLs express clusterin and cytotoxic proteins such as TIA-1 and perforin.[341] Approximately 20 to 60 percent of ALCLs are ALK-positive depending, in part, on the percentage of children in the study.[333–335] ALK-positive tumors are usually negative for BCL-2 and have high levels of BAX.[342] This susceptibility to apoptosis may explain the better survival of patients with ALK-positive ALCL.[337] Over half of ALK-negative tumors express BCL-2.[342]

T-cell ALCLs usually contain rearrangements of the TCR genes.[13,340,343] The TCR β, TCR γ, and TCR δ genes may be rearranged. The incidence of lineage promiscuity is high in ALCLs, with Ig genes being commonly rearranged in T-cell neoplasms. Approximately 20 to 30 percent of T-cell ALCLs lack antigen receptor gene rearrangements. These results have led some investigators to propose that T-ALCLs arise from an early T-cell progenitor, at a stage of differentiation prior to gene rearrangement.

Chromosomal translocations involving chromosome 2p23, usually the t(2;5)(p23;q35), occur in a subset of cases of ALCL.[344] This translocation juxtaposes the anaplastic lymphoma kinase *(alk)* gene on chromosome 2p23 with the nucleophosmin *(npm)* gene on 5q35. The t(2;5) translocation is usually found in the systemic form of T/null-cell ALCL, with an incidence ranging from 20 to 60 percent in various studies.[332–335] A number of other uncommon abnormalities involving the *alk* locus are also reported including t(1;2)(q21;p23), t(1;2)(q25;p23), t(2;2)(p23;p23), t(2;3)(p23;q21), t(2;13)(p23;q34), t(2;22)(p-23;q11.2), t(2;X)(p23;q11–12), and inv(2)(p23;q35).

ALK expression is rare in other neoplasms.[344] A rare type of diffuse large B-cell lymphoma with plasmablastic features expresses the full-length form of ALK and is CD30-negative.[345] Subsets of neuroblastomas and myofibroblastic tumors are also ALK-positive.[344,346]

EBV has been identified in a small subset of cases of ALCL. The virus is rare in ALK-positive cases. Other known oncogenes including *bcl-1, bcl-2, bcl-6,* and *c-myc* are not involved in ALCL.

Cutaneous Anaplastic Large Cell Lymphoma

Cutaneous ALCLs are neoplasms that appear to be closely related to lymphomatoid papulosis, or may represent part of a spectrum that includes lymphomatoid papulosis at one end and cutaneous ALCL at the opposite end.[33,347] Patients with MF can develop CD30-positive large cell cutaneous tumors, but these represent large cell transformation of MF and are not included in cutaneous ALCL.[347]

Clinically, patients may be of any age and present with rapidly growing solitary nodules that commonly ulcerate.[348,349] Partial or complete remission may occur spontaneously. Lymph node involvement occurs in approximately 25 percent of patients. Radiation therapy is commonly used for localized disease. Chemotherapy is used for patients with higher stage disease. Most patients with cutaneous ALCL have a favorable prognosis.

Histologically, cutaneous ALCL is composed of anaplastic cells in sheets located in the dermis.[349] Eosinophils and histiocytes are commonly present in the background. In rare cases, neutrophils can be numerous almost obscuring the neoplastic cells.[338] The overlying epidermis is frequently ulcerated with secondary infection.

Immunophenotypically, cutaneous ALCLs are strongly positive for CD30 and may be of T-cell or null cell lineage.[347–349] T-cell ALCLs commonly have an aberrant T-cell immunophenotype. Similar to systemic ALCL, cutaneous tumors may be CD45-negative. Unlike systemic ALCL, most cutaneous ALCLs are EMA-negative. Both T-cell and null cell tumors may express cytotoxic proteins. CD56 may be positive in some cases.[350] ALK is almost always negative, but may be positive in cases of systemic ALCL presenting initially with cutaneous disease.

Molecular studies show rearrangements of the TCR β and TCR γ in most cases.[347] The TCR α and TCR δ genes have been rarely assessed. The Ig genes are usually germline, but lineage infidelity may occur. The t(2;5)(p23;q35) and other *alk* gene rearrangements are rare in cutaneous ALCL.[350,351]

Peripheral T-Cell Lymphomas, Unspecified

The term peripheral T-cell lymphoma (PTCL) is used to describe lymphoid neoplasms of mature T-cell lineage, as opposed to tumors of thymic origin. The terms post-thymic and mature T-cell lymphoma also have been used to describe these tumors. In the WHO classification,[33] unspecified PTCL includes all mature T-cell lymphomas that do not have unique clinical or pathologic features that allow more specific classification. Unspecified PTCL represented 6 percent of all lymphomas in the Nebraska NHL Classification Project.[31,32]

Most patients with unspecified PTCL are adults who present with generalized lymphadenopathy.[352–354] Extranodal sites including skin, liver, Waldeyer's ring, and lung are also commonly involved.[352] These tumors may be associated with a hemophagocytic syndrome.[355] PTCLs are diffuse, aggressive neoplasms that require combination chemotherapy. As compared with diffuse large B-cell lymphoma, PTCLs relapse more frequently, with correspondingly poorer survival.[31,356]

Histologically, in most cases of unspecified PTCL the lymph node architecture is diffusely effaced (Figure 40–19).[357,358] However, in a subset of cases, the neoplasm may be paracortically distributed, sparing lymphoid follicles, and in rare instances may be nodular (but not truly follicular).[359] Cytologically, the neoplastic lymphoid cells exhibit a spectrum of cell sizes including small, medium-sized, and large and can have abundant clear cytoplasm. Reed-Sternberg-like cells may be found. Mitotic figures are usually easily identified and are often numerous. Although no histologic or cytologic features can reliably distinguish PTCL from diffuse B-cell lymphomas, benign inflammatory cells such as eosinophils and histiocytes are more common in PTCL. Epithelioid histiocytes may be numerous, arranged either in large clusters or linear cords.[357] This pattern has been referred to as lymphoepithelioid, and PTCLs with this pattern have been designated in the literature as Lennert's lymphoma.[357] Blood vessels (epithelioid venules) may be prominent.

Immunophenotypic studies have shown that PTCLs are of mature T-cell lineage. Thus, the neoplastic cells express pan-T-

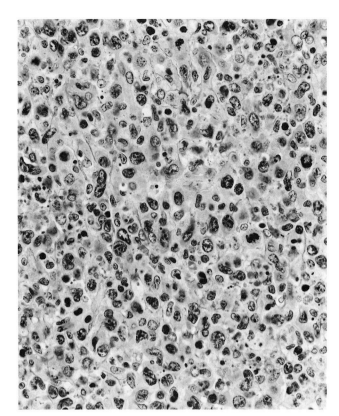

Figure 40–19. Peripheral T-cell lymphoma, not otherwise specified. The neoplastic cells are large with abundant cytoplasm and have a high mitotic rate.

cell antigens such as CD2, CD3, and CD5, usually TCR αβ, and are either CD4+ CD8– or CD4– CD8+.[1,2] Approximately 75 percent of cases will demonstrate an aberrant T-cell immunophenotype. Cytotoxic proteins and CD56 are expressed by a small subset of cases.[360,361] p53 is commonly expressed but *p53* gene mutations are uncommon in PTCL.[362] B-cell antigens, Ig, and TdT are negative.

Molecular studies have shown TCR β and TCR γ gene rearrangements in most cases of PTCL.[13,273] The TCR δ gene is usually deleted. The Ig genes are usually in the germline configuration. Cytogenetic abnormalities are common and karyotypes are often complex. Both numerical and structural abnormalities are reported, with structural rearrangements of chromosome 6 being most common.[363] As specific chromosomal translocations have been recognized, subsets of PTCL that were unspecified previously have been assigned to specific categories of PTCL.

Angioimmunoblastic T-Cell Lymphoma

Angioimmunoblastic T-cell lymphoma (AIL) was first described as angioimmunoblastic lymphadenopathy with dysproteinemia in 1974.[364] This entity also has been named immunoblastic lymphadenopathy[365] and lymphogranulomatosis X.[366] This entity was originally thought to be preneoplastic but is now considered to be a specific type of PTCL and is designated as AIL in the WHO classification.[33] However, the view of the WHO classification is not universally shared, as some pathologists still consider a small subset of AIL cases to be pre-neoplastic and not a clearly defined type of PTCL.[367,368]

Clinically, patients with AIL are elderly, with a median age in the seventh decade, and have advanced stage disease at onset.[369,370] Many patients have constitutional symptoms such as fever, chills, night sweats, and malaise. Physical examination reveals generalized lymphadenopathy, hepatomegaly, splenomegaly, and skin rash. Various laboratory abnormalities are common including polyclonal hypergammaglobulinemia, anemia (often with positive direct Coombs test), cold agglutinins, circulating immune complexes, cryoglobulins, antinuclear antibodies, and eosinophilia.[369] Bone marrow involvement is very common. The disease may be triggered by administration of therapeutic agents such as penicillin. The median survival for all patients with AIL is 30 to 40 months.[370,371] Infection is the most common cause of death followed by the development of malignant lymphoma.

Histologically, the diagnosis of AIL is based on the following findings (Figure 40–20)[364,365,371,372]: 1. Substantial to complete obliteration of lymph node architecture; 2. a polymorphous infiltrate of neoplastic small and medium-sized lymphoid cells, often with clear cytoplasm, associated with plasma cells, eosinophils, and immunoblasts; 3. an arborizing proliferation of small blood vessels corresponding to epithelioid venules; and 4. absence (in most cases) of hyperplastic or normal-sized lym-

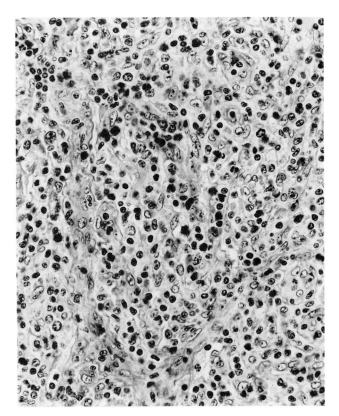

Figure 40–20. Angioimmunoblastic T-cell lymphoma. As can be observed in this field, the neoplasm is characterized by increased vascularity and is composed of a polymorphous mixture of small and large cells.

phoid follicles. In many cases small and atrophic (so-called burned-out) germinal centers are present; a subset of cases of AIL have reactive lymphoid follicles.[372]

Immunophenotypic studies of AIL have shown that these lesions are composed predominantly of mature T cells.[1,2,33] An aberrant T-cell immunophenotype may be identified, but is usually found only in lesions that are monomorphous with numerous large cells. The neoplastic T cells are usually of the T-helper/inducer cell lineage (CD4+ CD8–). Numerous follicular dendritic reticulum cells are common in AIL, both associated with residual follicles and at extrafollicular sites.[373] B cells may be present in AIL, unlike most other PTCLs, and can be numerous in early lesions.[373]

Gene rearrangement studies have demonstrated that most AIL cases have rearrangements of the TCR γ and TCR β genes.[366,374,375] The TCR δ gene is deleted. The Ig heavy chain gene is rearranged in 10 to 20 percent of cases. Ig light chain gene rearrangements are less common.

Nonrandom chromosomal abnormalities, many clonal, have been identified in AILs.[363,377,378] Trisomy 3 and 5 are most common, in 15 to 20 percent of cases in one study.[363] EBV is commonly associated with AILs, as shown by a variety of molecular methods, and is monoclonal in a subset of cases.[379]

Patients with AIL are at risk for developing diffuse large B-cell lymphoma.[380] Diffuse large B-cell lymphomas arising in the setting of AIL express B-cell antigens, carry Ig gene rearrangements, and usually have abundant EBV.[381] One hypothesis to explain this finding is that immunosuppression associated with AIL predisposes to EBV infection of B cells. As a result of viral infection, the B cells have a prolonged life span, increasing the likelihood of secondary molecular aberrations that result in high-grade B-cell lymphoma.

HISTIOCYTIC NEOPLASMS

True Histiocytic Lymphoma

True histiocytic lymphomas (THLs) currently represent less than 1 percent of all NHLs. Historically, these tumors were thought to be much more common. However, with the development of immunologic and molecular studies, neoplasms once thought to be histiocytic in origin have been proved to be of either B-cell or T-cell lineage.[382] In addition, some THLs reported in the past were probably examples of extramedullary myeloid cell tumors with pure monocytic differentiation.

True histiocytic lymphomas are thought to arise from histiocytes normally present in the lymph node. Currently, the term THL is used most commonly for tumors thought to arise from phagocytic sinusoidal histiocytes. Follicular dendritic cells and interdigitating dendritic cells are specialized types of cells also present in lymph nodes that are often included in the category of histiocytes.[4] Thus, histiocytic neoplasms reported in the literature include THL, follicular dendritic cell tumor (sarcoma), or interdigitating dendritic cell tumor (sarcoma). These neoplasms lack B-cell or T-cell specific antigens and have no evidence of Ig or TCR gene rearrangements.

Histologically, THLs arising from phagocytic sinusoidal histiocytes are composed of large cells with abundant eosinophilic cytoplasm and oval or lobulated nuclei.[383,384] Multinucleated cells are common; spindled cases are present in a subset of cases. The histiocytic origin of these tumors, although it may be suspected histologically, cannot be ascertained without cytochemical, immunophenotypic, or genotypic analyses. Cytochemical studies of smears or touch imprint preparations often demonstrate that the neoplastic cells have strong reactivity for nonspecific or butyrate esterases. Immunophenotypic studies show expression of histiocyte-associated antigens such as CD4, CD11c, CD14, CD45, CD45RO, CD68, and lysozyme.[383,384]

Patients with follicular dendritic cell tumors most often present with enlarged lymph nodes of the neck, axilla, or mediastinum. Extranodal sites can be involved as part of systemic disease and can be the primary site of involvement in 25 percent of patients. Follicular dendritic cell tumors usually behave as do low-grade sarcomas; local recurrences are more common than distant metastases. Complete surgical resection is the optimal treatment.

Histologically, follicular dendritic cell tumors are composed of oval to spindle-shaped neoplastic cells arranged in sheets and fascicles resembling sarcoma.[385] However, unlike sarcomas small reactive lymphocytes are present in the background. Necrosis, atypia, and a high mitotic rate occur in clinically aggressive tumors. Immunophenotypic studies have shown that follicular dendritic cell tumors express CD21 and CD35 and vimentin. Electron microscopic studies demonstrate complex interdigitating cytoplasmic processes joined by desmosomes. These findings support origin from follicular dendritic cells that normally provide the supporting framework for lymphoid follicles in lymph nodes.

Interdigitating dendritic cell tumors (sarcomas) are much more rare than follicular dendritic cell tumors. These neoplasms occur in elderly patients and dissemination of disease is common.[386] Histologically, these neoplasms are composed of round to oval cells with abundant eosinophilic cytoplasm. Immunophenotypic studies show that these tumors characteristically express S100 protein and often express other histiocyte-associated markers such as CD45, CD68, and lysozyme, and are negative for CD1A.

HODGKIN'S DISEASE (LYMPHOMA)

Hodgkin's disease (HD), also designated Hodgkin's lymphoma in the WHO classification,[33] is a group of related malignant neoplasms with clinical and pathologic features that distinguish them from NHLs. One major difference from NHLs is the pattern of spread. Hodgkin's disease begins in the interfollicular region of lymph node, progressively effaces the architecture of that lymph node, and then usually spreads in an orderly fashion to contiguous lymph node groups.[387,388]

Approximately 75 percent of patients can be cured with appropriate therapy and all histologic types are responsive to treatment.[387,388] Findings that correlate with response to therapy have been incorporated into a prognostic score and include albumin < 4 g/l, hemoglobin < 10.5 g/l, male sex, Ann Arbor stage IV, age > 45 years, leukocytosis > 15,000/mm³, and lymphocytopenia < 600/mm³.[388] Although histologic type does not correlate with response to therapy, classification remains useful because HD type correlates with sites of involvement, stage at presentation, and the presence of systemic symptoms.[389,390]

HD is pathologically defined as a hematopoietic neoplasm composed of diagnostic Reed-Sternberg cells (or appropriate variant cells) within a reactive inflammatory cell background.[391] A classic Reed-Sternberg cell is large, containing a bilobed, vesicular nucleus, with each lobe containing a prominent, eosinophilic nucleolus surrounded by a clear zone (or halo).[391]

HD has been traditionally classified into histologic types that were shown to correlate with clinical course in the absence of effective therapy (Table 40–5). The classification of Jackson and Parker[391] divided HD into three groups: paragranuloma, granuloma, and sarcoma. Although this classification recognized the excellent prognosis of patients with paragranuloma and the poor prognosis of patients with sarcoma, most cases fit within the granuloma group. This category was very heterogeneous in terms of clinical presentation, histologic findings, and prognosis. Thus, utility of the Jackson and Parker system was limited. In 1966, Lukes and Butler[392] made a major contribution to our understanding of HD by recognizing the nodular sclerosis type. They also expanded the classification to six categories: lymphocytic and/or histiocytic (L&H) nodular, L&H diffuse, nodular sclerosis, mixed, diffuse fibrosis, and reticular. These categories recognized the distinctive neoplastic cells and the composition of the reactive cells found in the different types of HD. Subsequently, at an international symposium in Rye, New York, the Lukes and Butler classification was consolidated into four groups: lymphocytic predominance (LP), nodular sclerosis (NS), mixed cellularity (MC), and lymphocytic depletion (LD).[393] The L&H nodular and diffuse groups were combined

Table 40–5. Hodgkin's Disease Classification: Historical and Present

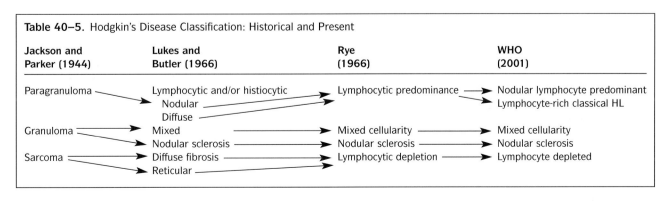

Jackson and Parker (1944)	Lukes and Butler (1966)	Rye (1966)	WHO (2001)
Paragranuloma	Lymphocytic and/or histiocytic Nodular Diffuse	Lymphocytic predominance	Nodular lymphocyte predominant / Lymphocyte-rich classical HL
Granuloma	Mixed	Mixed cellularity	Mixed cellularity
	Nodular sclerosis	Nodular sclerosis	Nodular sclerosis
Sarcoma	Diffuse fibrosis / Reticular	Lymphocytic depletion	Lymphocyte depleted

into the LP category and the diffuse fibrosis and reticular groups were consolidated into the LD category. The Rye classification gained universal acceptance, was easy to use, and the categories correlate with clinical parameters. Nevertheless, some useful information was lost in the consolidation of the Lukes and Butler classification. This information has been recaptured in the REAL and WHO classifications, which recognize the unique immunophenotypic findings in LP and introduce the category of lymphocyte-rich classical HD.[31,33]

Nodular Lymphocyte Predominant

Approximately 5 percent of patients with HD have LP, which is usually localized and involves cervical or axillary lymph nodes.[390,393–396] The disease affects patients of all ages, males more often than females, and is clinically indolent. Systemic symptoms, such as fever, weight loss, and night sweats are infrequent. According to epidemiologic data from the NCI Statistics, Epidemiology, and End Results (SEER) program, the 5-year survival rate is 83.9 percent.[395]

Two subgroups of LP are recognized, nodular and diffuse, correlating with the L&H nodular and diffuse groups in the Lukes and Butler system.[392] However, since the advent of immunohistochemical methods, it has become clear that most cases of LP are

nodular and only rare cases with an entirely diffuse pattern occur. Nodular LP is characterized by effacement of nodal architecture by variably sized, vague nodules composed of numerous small lymphocytes, histiocytes, and characteristic neoplastic L&H cells (Figure 40–21).[392,394,397] These cells are large with pale cytoplasm and polyploid, vesicular nuclei containing inconspicuous nucleoli. L&H cells resemble kernels of popped corn, hence the nickname *popcorn cells.* Eosinophils, neutrophils, and plasma cells are usually absent. Cells resembling Reed-Sternberg cells are rare. There is no associated necrosis or fibrosis. Diffuse LP is characterized by diffuse replacement of lymph node by a neoplasm cytologically similar to nodular LP. The behavior of these neoplasms is poor suggesting that these cases represent transformation of nodular LP to T-cell/histiocyte-rich large B-cell lymphoma.

Immunohistochemical studies have shown that nodular LP is distinct from other types of HD.[398,399] The L&H cells express CD45, immunoglobulin J chain, B-cell antigens, and epithelial membrane antigen (EMA) and are negative for CD15 and CD30. Some studies have suggested that L&H cells express monotypic Ig light chain, with preferential expression of Ig κ light chain.[397]

Southern blot hybridization and standard PCR assays for clonality in nodular LP are usually negative, attributable to the low number of neoplastic cells relative to reactive cells in this

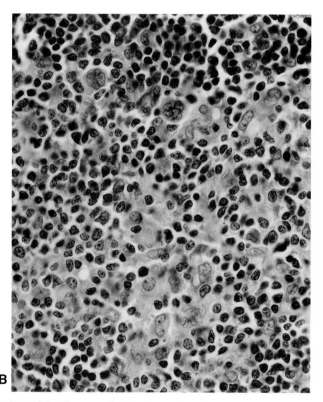

Figure 40–21. Hodgkin's disease, nodular lymphocyte predominant. (A) At low magnification, the neoplasm is vaguely nodular and the nodules have a variegated appearance due to pale histocytes and neoplastic cells in a sea of darker small lymphocytes. (B) High magnification reveals numerous reactive small lymphocytes and histiocytes and scattered neoplastic L&H (popcorn cells), two of which are present at the top of this field.

disease.[400,401] However, single cell PCR analysis of L&H cells in nodular LP have shown monoclonal Ig gene rearrangements in most cases, further supporting B-cell lymphoid origin.[402–404] These rearrangements are usually functional and Ig mRNA transcripts can be identified in most L&H cells. Infection by EBV is rare in nodular LP. A recent comparative genomic hybridization analysis of these cases revealed a high number of genomic imbalances in L&H cells.[405] The chromosomes most often involved in that study were gains of chromosomes 1, 2q, 3, 4q, 5q, 6, 8q, 11q, 12q, and X, and loss of chromosome 17.

Lymphocyte-Rich Classical Hodgkin's Disease

In recent years, cases of HD have been recognized that histologically resemble LP, either nodular or diffuse, but immunophenotypically resemble the classical types of HD (i.e., nodular sclerosis, mixed cellularity, and lymphocyte depletion) in being positive for CD15 and CD30 and negative for CD45.[31,396,406] Clinically, these neoplasms behave similarly to histologically typical cases of classical HD.[396]

In a recent study of HD by the European Task Force in Lymphoma, the diagnosis of LP was confirmed in approximately half of a large number of assessable cases that carried the diagnosis LP.[406] Most cases that were excluded were reclassified as lymphocyte-rich classical HD.

Nodular Sclerosis

Nodular sclerosis is the most common form of HD, representing approximately 60 percent of all cases.[394,395] It is the most common type below the age of 50 years. The age-adjusted incidence rate of NS is increasing in the United States, from 1.1 in 100,000 between 1973 and 1977 to 1.6 in 100,000 between 1983 and 1987.[395] The increase is greatest for adolescents and young adults between the ages of 15 to 45 years. The male/female ratio is approximately equal. Whites are affected more often than Blacks and Hispanics.

NS has a marked predilection for involving mediastinal, supraclavicular, and cervical lymph nodes and the thymus may be involved.[407] Most patients with localized disease (usually clinical stage II) have an excellent prognosis. However, high clinical stage, B symptoms, and bulky mediastinal disease are poor prognostic signs. According to NCI SEER data, the 5-year survival rate is 82.2 percent.[395]

Histologically, NS is characterized by a triad of findings: 1. A nodular pattern, 2. broad bands of fibrosis that outline the nodules, and 3. a characteristic mononuclear cell variant known as a lacunar cell (Figure 40–22).[394] A lacunar cell has abundant clear cytoplasm with a sharply demarcated cell membrane. In formalin-fixed tissue a characteristic artifact occurs. The cell cytoplasm retracts leaving a clear space or lacuna surrounding the cell, which led to its name. The lacunar cell nucleus may be

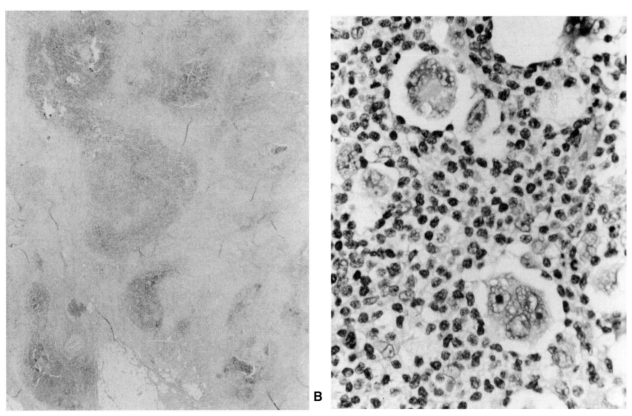

A   **B**

Figure 40–22. Hodgkin's disease, nodular sclerosis. (**A**) At low magnification, nodules are surrounded by dense fibrous bands. (**B**) Multiple lacunar cells in this field are situated in clear spaces, the result of retraction of cell cytoplasm in formalin fixative.

hyperlobulated or the cell may contain multiple small nucleoli. Classic Reed-Sternberg cells are rare in NS.

A heterogeneous mixture of reactive cells may be seen in NS, including small lymphocytes, histiocytes, eosinophils, neutrophils, and plasma cells in a variable mixture. Because the reactive cell component is so variable, NS has been subdivided according to the number of lacunar cells and the types of reactive cells present.[407] Most investigators agree that patients with HD with extensive lymphocyte depletion and many lacunar cells have a poorer prognosis. These neoplasms have been referred to in the literature as the syncytial, fibroblastic, or lymphocyte-depleted variants of NS, and are considered grade 2 NS in the WHO classification.[408,409]

An important feature of the Rye classification is that NS, even if present as only a small focus, takes precedence over other types of HD and therefore the tumor is classified as NS.[393]

Mixed Cellularity

Mixed cellularity is the second common type of HD affecting 24 percent of all patients with the disease, and is the most common form in patients older than 50 years.[394,395] Males are affected more often than females. In Blacks and Hispanics, MC is relatively more common than in Whites, who more often have NS.[410] A significant percentage of patients with MC have clinical stage III or IV disease and B symptoms. According to NCI SEER data, the 5-year survival rate is 68.1 percent.[395]

Histologically, MC is characterized by a large number of classic Reed-Sternberg cells and mononuclear cell (Hodgkin) variants, often ranging in number from 5 to 15/high-power field (Figure 40–23).[394] Lymph node architecture is usually diffusely replaced. Partially involved lymph nodes show selective paracortical infiltration. Disorderly fibrosis may be seen, but the broad fibrous bands characteristic of NS are absent. Focal necrosis may be found, but the necrosis is usually not prominent.

Lymphocyte Depleted

Lymphocyte depleted is the least common type of HD, representing less than 5 percent of cases.[394] Patients with LD are usually elderly, and LD is rare in individuals younger than 40 years old.[395] There is a slight male predominance. Whites and Blacks are equally affected. Most patients have advanced clinical stage disease and B symptoms. Patients with LD have the poorest prognosis of all types, with a 5-year survival rate of 36.4 percent in recent NCI SEER data.[395]

The LD category is equivalent to the sarcoma category in the Jackson and Parker scheme and includes two variants recognized by Lukes and Butler: diffuse fibrosis and reticular.[392] Grossly, the extent of tumor is often greater in LD than in other types of HD, and patients commonly have a large contiguous mass of matted lymph nodes or diffuse visceral involvement.[394] Patients with the diffuse fibrosis type of LD often have subdiaphragmatic disease, whereas patients with the reticular type of LD more often have peripheral lymphadenopathy and bone marrow involvement.[411,412] In both types of LD the incidence of noncontiguous lung involvement is high, suggesting vascular spread.

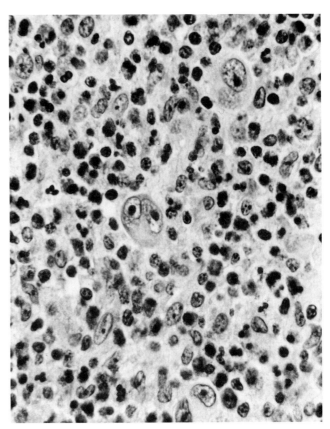

Figure 40–23. Hodgkin's disease, mixed cellularity. In the center of the field a diagnostic Reed-Sternberg cell is present. A mononuclear variant (Hodgkin cell) is present at the top right. The background cells are small lymphocytes, eosinophils, histiocytes, and neutrophils.

The age-adjusted incidence rate for LD as determined using NCI SEER data was higher from 1973 to 1977 than it was from 1983 to 1987.[395] This decrease is most likely explained by the recognition by pathologists that many tumors previously classified as LD are, in fact, NHLs.[413] Improved classification is the result of application of immunohistochemical and molecular methods to the study of lymphoid neoplasms.

Histologically, the diffuse fibrosis variant of LD is characterized by an extensive proliferation of disordered, hypocellular fibrosis.[411,412] Diagnostic Reed-Sternberg cells are usually not numerous and may be spindled within amorphous collagen. Reactive inflammatory cells are relatively few. The reticular variant of LD has numerous Reed-Sternberg cells and bizarre variants that have been termed *pleomorphic variants*. These cells may exhibit extreme variations in nuclear number and shape, often with giant nucleoli. Normal small lymphocytes are infrequent compared with the other subtypes of HD. Necrosis is common and may be extensive. Reed-Sternberg cells and pleomorphic variants may be found in sheets. Mitotic figures are usually numerous. Background deposition of amorphous fibrous tissue is less extensive than that seen in diffuse fibrosis.

Interfollicular Hodgkin's Disease

In a small subset of cases, HD may partially involve lymph nodes, in the paracortical region, without substantial replacement of normal architecture.[414] Both MC or NS can be interfollicular, usually the former. Clinical follow-up studies have shown that patients with interfollicular HD may relapse, with neoplasms much more characteristic of either MC or NS.[414,415] Thus, the importance of interfollicular HD lies in its unusual histologic findings, which may be missed, delaying appropriate treatment.

Immunophenotypic Findings

In general, analysis of tissues involved by classical HD using flow cytometry is not helpful. The Reed-Sternberg and mononuclear cell variants (Hodgkin cells) are typically infrequent in involved tissues and thus are difficult to assess.[416]

Immunohistochemical methods are more helpful because this technique allows direct observation of Reed-Sternberg and Hodgkin (RS-H) cells as well as reactive cells. In frozen sections, the RS-H cells in classical HD express various activation antigens including CD30 (Ki-1), CD25, and HLA-DR, markers of proliferation such as Ki-67 and CD71, and granulocyte-associated antigens such as CD15.[417,418] The RS-H cells also express B- or T-cell antigens in some cases. B-cell antigens are expressed much more frequently. The background lymphocytes are predominantly reactive T cells with a normal immunophenotype. T-helper/inducer cells usually outnumber T-suppressor/cytotoxic cells.

In recent years, the number of antibodies to assess fixation-resistant antigens has greatly increased. Thus, most pathologists currently assess HD cases using fixed tissue sections. The RS-H cells express CD15 and CD30 and are negative for CD45.[419,420] The B-cell antigens CD20, CD79A, and B-cell-specific activator protein (BSAP) are variably expressed in a subset of cases.[419,421,422] T-cell antigens such as CD3 are very rarely positive in RS-H cells.[418,423] BCL-2 is positive in up to half of cases and has been correlated with poorer prognosis.[424] NF-kappa B is expressed by RS-H cells in most cases of HD.[425]

Molecular Genetic Findings

Conventional cytogenetic studies have revealed nonrandom complex abnormalities in up to half of cases. For example, Cabanillas and colleagues[426] have demonstrated chromosomal breakpoints involving 11q32, 14q32, 6q11–21, and 8q22–24. Other breakpoints reported include 12p11–13, 13p11–13, 3q26–28, 6q15–16, and 7q31–35.[427]

Using Southern blot hybridization, in most HD cases the antigen receptor genes are in the germline configuration.[12,13] These results are not surprising since the RS-H cells usually represent less than 1 percent of the total cell population in classical HD, and the sensitivity of the Southern blot method is 1 to 5 percent. In approximately 20 percent of cases, rearrangements of either the Ig or TCR genes were detected.[401,428] Recent studies using single-cell PCR have shown evidence of Ig gene rearrangements in the RS-H cells of over 90 percent of cases of HD. These Ig gene rearrangements may have numerous somatic mutations (so-called crippling mutations) rendering them nonfunctional.[429] T-cell receptor gene rearrangements have been detected rarely in HD.[422]

PCR methods have been used to amplify the t(14;18)(q32;q21) in cases of HD, which has been identified in up to one-third of cases.[428] However, the t(14;18) is present in reactive cells and not in RS-H cells.[429]

Epstein-Barr Virus and Hodgkin's Disease

For many years EBV has been known to be associated with HD, although the role of the virus in the pathogenesis of HD is unknown. EBV is known to be the cause of infectious mononucleosis, and adolescents who have recovered from infectious mononucleosis have an increased risk of subsequent HD.[432,433] Patients with HD are known to have high-titer serum antibodies directed against EBV antigens, such as early antigen and viral capsid antigen.[432] The presence of antibodies specific for EBV early antigen suggests that virus infection is active. Also, Mueller and colleagues[434] using serum obtained from blood donors have shown that high EBV antibody titers are often present before the onset of HD. Direct proof of EBV in HD was not available until in situ hybridization studies demonstrated EBV within RS-H cells.[435,436] Furthermore, EBV is present in approximately 50 percent of cases, and is present in monoclonal, episomal form.[436] Virus-associated proteins such as latent membrane protein type 1 are expressed by RS-H cells.[437] Thus, EBV is likely to be involved in the pathogenesis of at least a subset of cases of HD.

The presence of EBV correlates with histologic type of HD. EBV is present in over two-thirds of cases of MC and LD and is found in approximately one-fourth of NS cases.[435] The virus also may be more common in HD arising in patients of very young age.[438] Most cases of HD arising in the setting of human immunodeficiency virus infection are EBV-positive.[439]

Hodgkin's Disease and the Two-Disease Hypothesis

For many years epidemiologists have suggested that HD is heterogeneous and represents more than one disease.[440] This two-disease hypothesis considers NS and MC as two different diseases. The epidemiologic, clinical, and pathologic findings support this hypothesis.

The age-adjusted incidence rates of NS and MC are distinctive. NS preferentially affects young adults between the ages of 15 and 34 years.[395] Males and females are affected almost equally. Mediastinal lymph nodes and low clinical stage disease are the rule. The following social factors correlate with an increased risk of NS: small family size, early birth order, a single-family home, fewer neighborhood playmates, higher maternal education, and higher paternal social class.[441,442] These epidemiologic findings suggest that NS is the result of relatively late exposure to an infectious agent, analogous to the paralytic polio model. By contrast, MC is relatively more common in children and adults older than 50 years of age.[395] Males are affected more often than females. The mediastinum is involved less often and advanced stage of disease is more frequent. Social factors that correlate with increased risk of MC are the converse of NS: large family size, late birth order, more neighborhood playmates, lower maternal education, and lower paternal social class.[441,442] These findings suggest that early exposure to an infectious agent may play a role in causing MC.

EBV, commonly identified in MC, may help to explain some of these epidemiologic features.[435] Children less than 5 years of age rarely develop HD.[395] Perhaps in this age group children are exposed to EBV, particularly in poor socioeconomic conditions, but a latency period is needed prior to the development of HD as a result of primary infection. Cases of MC in older adults and the elderly population may be the result of reactivation of EBV, perhaps secondary to immunodeficiency that occurs as a result of aging or other causes. The relatively low prevalence of EBV in NS suggests that EBV is not necessary for NS to develop and that another infectious agent or other factors may be responsible. The marked heterogeneity of the pathologic and clinical findings within NS also raises the possibility that this disease may result from more than one infectious agent.

COMPOSITE LYMPHOMA

The definition of composite lymphoma has evolved over time. Composite lymphoma was defined originally as two histologically different lymphoid neoplasms occurring in the same patient, either at different anatomic sites or involving the same site. Subsequently, this definition was modified and composite lymphoma was defined as two or more distinctly different, well-delineated lymphoid neoplasms occurring in a single anatomic site.[443,444] The most common form of composite lymphoma reported in the literature is the simultaneous presence of two NHLs; for example, low-grade follicular small cleaved cell coexisting with higher-grade diffuse large cell. However, we now recognize that most of these cases do not represent two distinct tumors, but instead histologic progression of the same clonal proliferation.[444] Presently, most pathologists reserve the term composite lymphoma for two lymphoid neoplasms involving the same site that are thought not to be clonally related, such as B-cell NHL with T-cell NHL or HD with NHL.

In recent years, evidence has accumulated to suggest that HD and NHL are more closely related than has been appreciated previously. The two occur simultaneously more often than is expected by chance alone.[445] In a subset of cases of composite HD and NHL, EBV has been identified within the neoplastic cells of both neoplasms.[446] Observations such as these suggest that HD and NHL can arise from a common precursor cell. More recently, single-cell PCR studies of a small number of patients with both HD and NHL have identified common Ig gene rearrangements, further evidence for a common B-cell precursor.[447,448] Thus, the concept of composite lymphoma is likely to continue to evolve.

REFERENCES

1. Picker LJ, Weiss LM, Medeiros LJ et al: Immunophenotypic criteria for the diagnosis of non-Hodgkin's lymphoma. Am J Pathol 128:181–201, 1987.

2. Stetler-Stevenson M, Medeiros LJ, Jaffe ES: Immunophenotypic methods and findings in the diagnosis of lymphoproliferative diseases. In Jaffe ES (ed.): Surgical Pathology of the Lymph Nodes and Related Organs. Major Problems in Pathology Series, Vol. 16, 2nd Ed, pp. 22–57. WB Saunders, Philadelphia, 1994.

3. Weissman IL, Warnke R, Butcher EC et al: The lymphoid system: Its normal architecture and the potential for understanding the system through the study of lymphoproliferative diseases. Hum Pathol 9:25–45, 1978.

4. Cline MJ. Histiocytes and histiocytosis. Blood 84:2840–2853, 1994.

5. Jalkanen S, Reichert RA, Gallatin WM et al: Homing receptors and the control of lymphocyte migration. Immunol Rev 91:39–60, 1986.

6. Picker LJ, Medeiros LJ, Weiss LM et al: Expression of lymphocyte homing receptor antigen in non-Hodgkin's lymphoma. Am J Pathol 130:496–504, 1988.

7. Kohler G, Milstein C: Continuous cultures of fused cells secreting antibody of predefined specificity. Nature 256:495–497, 1975.

8. Kishimoto T, von dem Borne AEG, Goyert SM et al: Leucocyte Typing VI. White Cell Differentiation Antigens. Garland Publishing, London, 1997.

9. Kung PC, Long JC, McCaffrey RP et al: Terminal deoxynucleotidyl transferase in the diagnosis of leukemia and malignant lymphoma. Am J Med 64:788–794, 1978.

10. Korsmeyer SJ, Hieter PA, Ravetch JV et al: Developmental hierarchy of immunoglobulin gene rearrangements in human leukemic pre-B-cells. Proc Natl Acad Sci USA 78:7096–7100, 1981.

11. Cleary ML, Trela MJ, Weiss LM et al: Most null large cell lymphomas are B cell neoplasms. Lab Invest 53:521–525, 1985.

12. Medeiros LJ, Carr J: Overview of the role of molecular methods in the diagnosis of malignant lymphomas. Arch Pathol Lab Med 123:1189–1207, 1999.

13. Medeiros LJ: Molecular hematopathology. In Weiss LM (ed.): Pathology of Lymph Nodes. Contemporary Issues in Surgical Pathology Series 21, pp. 1–80. Churchill Livingstone, New York, 1996.

14. Rappaport H, Winter WJ, Hicks EB: Follicular lymphoma: A reevaluation of its position in the scheme of malignant lymphoma, based on a survey of 253 cases. Cancer 9:792–821, 1956.

15. Lukes RJ, Collins RD: Immunological characterization of human malignant lymphomas. Cancer 34(Suppl):1488–1503, 1974.

16. Jaffe ES, Strauchen JA, Berard CW: Predictability of immunologic phenotype by morphologic criteria in diffuse aggressive non-Hodgkin's lymphomas. Am J Clin Pathol 77:46–49, 1982.

17. Gerard-Marchant R, Hamlin I, Lennert K et al: Classification of non-Hodgkin's lymphomas. Lancet II:406–408, 1974.

18. Rosenberg SA, Berard CW, Brown BW et al: National Cancer Institute sponsored study of classifications of non-Hodgkin's lymphomas: Summary and description of a working formulation for clinical usage. Cancer 49:2112–2135, 1982.

19. Stansfeld AG, Diebold J, Noel H et al: Updated Kiel classification for lymphomas. Lancet I:292–293, 1988.

20. Horning SJ, Rosenberg SA: The natural history of initially untreated low-grade non-Hodgkin's lymphomas. N Engl J Med 311:1471–1475, 1984.

21. Jaffe ES: Follicular lymphomas: Possibility that they are benign tumors of the lymphoid system. J Natl Cancer Inst 70:401–403, 1983.

22. Krikorian JG, Portlock CS, Cooney P, Rosenberg SA: Spontaneous regression of non-Hodgkin's lymphomas: A report of nine cases. Cancer 46:2093–2099, 1980.

23. Strickler JG, Copenhaver CM, Rojas VA et al: Comparison of "host cell infiltrates" in patients with follicular lymphoma with

and without spontaneous regression. Am J Clin Pathol 90:257–261, 1988.

24. Garcia CF, Lowder J, Meeker TC et al: Differences in "host infiltrates" among lymphoma patients treated with anti-idiotype antibodies: Correlation with treatment response. J Immunol 135:4252–4260, 1985.

25. Medeiros LJ, Picker LJ, Gelb AB et al: Numbers of host "helper" T cells and proliferating cells predict survival in diffuse small-cell lymphomas. J Clin Oncol 7:1009–1017, 1989.

26. Longo DL, Glatstein E, Duffey PL et al: Treatment of localized aggressive lymphomas with combination chemotherapy followed by involved-field radiation therapy. J Clin Oncol 7:1295–1302, 1989.

27. Fisher RI, Jones RB, DeVita VT et al: Natural history of malignant lymphomas with divergent histologies at staging evaluation. Cancer 47:2022–2025, 1981.

28. Hubbard SM, Chabner BA, DeVita VT et al: Histologic progression in non-Hodgkin's lymphoma. Blood 59:258–264, 1982.

29. Kerrigan DP, Foucar K, Dressler L: High-grade non-Hodgkin lymphoma relapsing as low-grade follicular lymphoma: So-called downgraded lymphoma. Am J Hematol 30:36–41, 1989.

30. Harris NL, Jaffe ES, Stein H et al: A revised European-American classification of lymphoid neoplasms: A proposal from the International Lymphoma Study Group. Blood 84:1361–1392, 1994.

31. The non-Hodgkin's Lymphoma Classification Project: A clinical evaluation of the International Lymphoma Study Group classification of non-Hodgkin's lymphoma. Blood 89:3909–3918, 1997.

32. Armitage JO, Weisenburger DD: New approach to classifying non-Hodgkin's lymphomas: Clinical features of the major histologic subtypes, Non-Hodgkin's Lymphoma Classification Project. J Clin Oncol 16:2780–2795, 1996.

33. Jaffe ES, Harris NL, Stein H et al. (eds.): World Health Organization Classification of Tumours. Pathology and Genetics of Tumours of Hematopoietic and Lymphoid Tissues, pp. 121–253. IARC Press, Lyon, France, 2001.

34. Medeiros LJ: Intermediate and high grade lymphomas in the working formulation. In Jaffe ES (ed.): Surgical Pathology of the Lymph Nodes and Related Organs. Major Problems in Pathology Series, 16, 2nd Ed., pp. 283–343. WB Saunders, Philadelphia, 1994.

35. Lin P, Jones D, Dorfman DM, Medeiros LJ: Precursor B-cell lymphoblastic lymphoma: A predominantly extranodal tumor with low propensity for leukemic involvement. Am J Pathol 24:1480–1490, 2000.

36. Maitra A, McKenna RW, Weinberg AG et al: Precursor B-cell lymphoblastic lymphoma: A study of nine cases lacking blood and bone marrow involvement and review of the literature. Am J Clin Pathol 115:868–875, 2001.

37. Iravani S, Singleton TP, Ross CW, Schnitzer B: Precursor B lymphoblastic lymphoma presenting as lytic bone lesions. Am J Clin Pathol 112:836–843, 1999.

38. Sander CA, Medeiros LJ, Abruzzo LV et al: Lymphoblastic lymphoma presenting in cutaneous sites: A clinicopathologic analysis of six cases. J Am Acad Dermatol 25:1023–1031, 1991.

39. Sander CA, Jaffe ES, Gebhardt FC et al: Mediastinal lymphoblastic lymphoma with an immature B-cell immunophenotype. Am J Surg Pathol 16:300–305, 1992.

40. Reiter A, Schrappe M, Parwaresch R et al: Non-Hodgkin's lymphoma of childhood and adolescence: Results of a treatment stratified for biologic subtypes and stage-report of the Berlin-Frankfurt-Munster group. J Clin Oncol 13:359–372, 1995.

41. Gokbuget N, Hoelzer D, Arnold R et al: Treatment of adult ALL according to protocols of the German Multicenter Study Group for Adult ALL (GMALL). Hematol Oncol Clin N Am 14:1307–1325, 2000.

42. Durrant IJ, Richards SM, Prentice HG, Goldstone AH: The Medical Research Council trials in adult acute lymphocytic leukemia. Hematol Oncol Clin N Am 14:1327–1352, 2000.

43. Cossman J, Chused TM, Fisher RI et al: Diversity of immunological phenotypes of lymphoblastic lymphoma. Cancer Res 43:4486–4490, 1983.

44. Nathwani BN, Kim H, Rappaport H: Malignant lymphoma, lymphoblastic. Cancer 38:964–983, 1976.

45. Kitchingman GR, Rovigatti U, Mauer AM et al: Rearrangement of immunoglobulin heavy chain genes in T-cell acute lymphoblastic leukemia. Blood 65:725–729, 1985.

46. Felix CA, Poplack DG, Reaman GH et al: Characterization of immunoglobulin and T-cell receptor gene patterns in B-cell precursor acute lymphoblastic leukemia of childhood. J Clin Oncol 8:431–442, 1990.

47. Cline MJ: The molecular basis of leukemia. N Engl J Med 330:328–336, 1994.

48. Preti HA, O'Brien S, Giralt S et al: Philadelphia-chromosome-positive adult acute lymphocyte leukemia: Characteristics, treatment results, and prognosis in 41 patients. Am J Med 97:60–65, 1994.

49. Mellentin JD, Murre C, Donlon TA et al: The gene for enhancer binding proteins E12/E47 lies at the t(1;19) breakpoint in acute leukemias. Science 246:379–382, 1989.

50. Nourse J, Mellentin JD, Galili N et al: Chromosomal translocation t(1;19) results in synthesis of a homeobox fusion mRNA that codes for a potential chimeric transcription factor. Cell 60:535–545, 1990.

51. Pui C-H, Behm FG, Downing JR et al: 11q23/MLL rearrangement confers a poor prognosis in infants with acute lymphoblastic leukemia. J Clin Oncol 12:909–915, 1994.

52. Pangalis GA, Angelopoulou MK, Vassilakopoulos TP et al: B-chronic lymphocytic leukemia, small lymphocytic lymphoma, lymphoplasmacytic lymphoma, including Waldenstrom's macroglobulinemia: A clinical, morphologic, and biologic spectrum of similar disorders. Semin Hematol 36:104–114, 1999.

53. Dick FR, Maca RD: The lymph node in chronic lymphocytic leukemia. Cancer 41:283–292, 1978.

54. Gupta D, Lim MS, Medeiros LJ et al: Small lymphocytic lymphoma with perifollicular, marginal zone, and interfollicular distribution. Mod Pathol 13:1161–1166, 2000.

55. Cossman J, Neckers LM, Braziel RM et al: In vitro enhancement of immunoglobulin gene expression in chronic lymphocytic leukemia. J Clin Invest 73:587–592, 1984.

56. Evans HL, Butler JJ, Youness EL: Malignant lymphoma, small lymphocytic type: A clinicopathologic study of 84 cases with suggested criteria for intermediate lymphocytic lymphoma. Cancer 41:1440–1455, 1978.

57. Medeiros LJ, Strickler JG, Picker LJ et al: "Well differentiated" lymphocytic neoplasms: Immunologic findings correlated with clinical presentation and morphologic features. Am J Pathol 128:523–535, 1987.

58. Juliusson G, Merup M. Cytogenetics in chronic lymphocytic leukemia. Semin Oncol 25:19–26, 1998.

59. Escudier SM, Pereira-Leahy JM, Drach JW et al: Fluorescent in situ hybridization and cytogenetic studies of trisomy 12 in chronic lymphocytic leukemia. Blood 81:2702–2707, 1993.

60. Bonato M, Pittaluga S, Tierens A et al: Lymph node histology in typical and atypical chronic lymphocytic leukemia. Am J Surg Pathol 22:49–56, 1998.

61. Adachi M, Tefferi A, Greipp PR et al: Preferential linkage of bcl-2 to immunoglobulin light chain in chronic lymphocytic leukemia. J Exp Med 171:559–564, 1990.

62. McKeithan TW, Takimoto GS, Ohno H et al: BCL3 rearrangements and t(14;19) in chronic lymphocytic leukemia and other B-cell malignancies: A molecular and cytogenetic study. Genes Chromosomes Cancer 20:64–72, 1997.

63. Medeiros LJ, Van Krieken JH, Jaffe ES, Raffeld M: Association of bcl-1 rearrangements with lymphocytic lymphoma of intermediate differentiation. Blood 76:2086–2090, 1990.

64. Lens D, Coignet LJ, Brito-Babapulle V et al: B cell prolymphocytic leukemia (B-PLL) with complex karyotype and concurrent abnormalities of the p53 and c-MYC gene. Leukemia 13:873–876, 1999.

65. Owen RG, Parapia LA, Higginson J et al: Clinicopathologic correlates of IgM paraproteinemias. Clin Lymphoma 1:39–43, 2000.

66. Dimopoulos MA, Panayiotidis P, Moulopoulos LA et al: Waldenstrom's macroglobulinemia: Clinical features, complications, and management. J Clin Oncol 18:214–226, 2000.

67. Morel P, Monconduit M, Jacomy D et al: Prognostic factors in Waldenstrom macroglobulinemia: A report on 232 patients with the description of a new scoring system and its validation on 253 other patients. Blood 96:852–858, 2000.

68. Harrison CV: The morphology of the lymph node in the macroglobulinemia of Waldenstrom. J Clin Pathol 25:12–16, 1972.

69. Lin P, Wilson C, Mansoor A et al: Waldenstrom's macroglobulinemia involving extramedullary sites: Morphologic and immunophenotypic findings in 57 cases. Mod Pathol 14:170A, 2001.

70. Andriko JW, Swerdlow SH, Aguilera NI, Abbondanzo SL: Is lymphoplasmacytic lymphoma/immunocytoma a distinct entity? A clinicopathologic study of 20 cases. Am J Surg Pathol 25:742–751, 2001.

71. Bartl R, Frisch B, Mahl G et al: Bone marrow histology in Waldenstrom's macroglobulinemia. Scand J Hematol 31:359–375, 1983.

72. Mansoor A, Medeiros LJ, Weber DM et al: Cytogenetic findings in lymphoplasmacytic lymphoma/Waldenstrom's macroglobulinemia. Am J Clin Pathol 116:543–549, 2001.

73. Iida S, Rao PH, Nallasivam P et al: The t(9;14)(p13;q32) chromosomal translocation associated with lymphoplasmacytoid lymphoma involves the PAX-5 gene. Blood 88:4110–4117, 1996.

74. Schop RFJ, Jalal SM, Van Weir SA et al: Absence of t(9;14)(p13;q32) translocation in clinically defined Waldenstrom's macroglobulinemia. Blood 96 (Suppl. 2):162b, 2000.

75. San Roman C, Ferro T, Guzman M, Odriozola J: Clonal abnormalities in patients with Waldenstrom's macroglobulinemia with special reference to a Burkitt-type t(8;14). Cancer Genet Cytogenet 18:155–158, 1985.

76. Cohen PL, Kurtin PJ, Donovan KA, Hanson CA: Bone marrow and peripheral blood involvement in mantle cell lymphoma. Br J Haematol 101:302–310, 1998.

77. O'Briain DS, Kennedy MJ, Daly PA et al: Multiple lymphomatous polyposis of the gastrointestinal tract: A clinicopathologically distinctive form of non-Hodgkin's lymphoma of B-cell centrocytic type. Am J Surg Pathol 13:691–699, 1989.

78. Fisher RI, Dahlberg S, Nathwani BN et al: A clinical analysis of two indolent lymphoma entities: Mantle cell lymphoma and marginal zone lymphoma (including the mucosa-associated lymphoid tissue and monocytoid B-cell subcategories): A Southwest Oncology Group Study. Blood 85:1075–1082, 1995.

79. Bookman MA, Lardelli P, Jaffe ES et al: Lymphocytic lymphoma of intermediate differentiation: Morphologic, immunophenotypic, and prognostic factors. J Natl Cancer Inst 82:742–748, 1990.

80. Weisenburger DD, Duggan MJ, Perry DA et al: Non-Hodgkin's lymphomas of mantle zone origin. Pathol Annu 26:139–158, 1991.

81. Majlis A, Pugh WC, Rodriguez MA et al: Mantle cell lymphoma: Correlation of clinical outcome and biologic features with three histologic variants. J Clin Oncol 15:1664–1671, 1997.

82. Schlette E, Bueso-Ramos C, Giles F et al: Mature B-cell leukemias with more than 55% prolymphocytes: A heterogeneous group that includes an unusual variant of mantle lymphoma. Am J Clin Pathol 11:571–581, 2001.

83. Laszlo T, Matolesy A: Blastic transformation of mantle cell lymphoma: Genetic evidence for a clonal link between the two stages of the tumour. Histopathology 35:355–359, 1999.

84. Strickler JG, Medeiros LJ, Copenhaver CM et al: Intermediate lymphocytic lymphoma: An immunophenotypic study with comparison to small lymphocytic lymphoma and diffuse small cleaved cell lymphoma. Hum Pathol 18:550–554, 1988.

85. Vaandrager JW, Schuuring E, Zwikstra E et al: Direct visualization of dispersed 11q13 chromosomal translocations in mantle cell lymphoma by multicolor DNA fiber fluorescence in situ hybridization. Blood 88:1177–1182, 1996.

86. Motokura T, Bloom T, Kim HG et al: A novel cyclin encoded by a bcl1-linked candidate oncogene. Nature 350:512–515, 1991.

87. Rosenberg CL, Wong E, Petty EM et al: PRAD-1, a candidate BCL1 oncogene: Mapping and expression in centrocytic lymphoma. Proc Natl Acad Sci USA 88:9638–9642, 1991.

88. Molot RJ, Meeker TC, Wittwer CT et al: Antigen expression and polymerase chain reaction amplification of mantle cell lymphomas. Blood 83:1626–1631.

89. Williams ME, Swerdlow SH, Rosenberg CL, Arnold A: Characterization of chromosome 11 translocation breakpoints at the bcl-1 and PRAD-1 loci in centrocytic lymphoma. Cancer Res Suppl 52:5541S–5544S, 1992.

90. Remstein ED, Kurtin PJ, Buno I et al: Diagnostic utility of fluorescence in situ hybridization in mantle-cell lymphoma. Br J Haematol 110:856–862, 2000.

91. Katz RL, Caraway NP, Gu J et al: Detection of chromosome 11q13 breakpoints by interphase fluorescence in situ hybridization. A useful ancillary method for the diagnosis of mantle cell lymphoma. Am J Clin Pathol 114:248–257, 2000.

92. Wlodorska I, Pittaluga S, Hagemeijer A et al: Secondary chromosome changes in mantle cell lymphoma. Haematologica 84:594–599, 1999.

93. Greiner TC, Medeiros LJ, Jaffe ES: Non-Hodgkin's lymphoma. Cancer 75(Suppl):370–380, 1995.

94. Lennert K, Feller A: Histopathology of Non-Hodgkin's Lymphomas, 2nd Ed. Springer-Verlag, New York, 1992.

95. Schnitzer B, Loesel LS, Reed RE: Lymphosarcoma cell leukemia: A clinicopathologic study. Cancer 26:1082–1096, 1970.

96. Melo JV, Robinson DS, de Oliveira MP et al: Morphology and immunology of circulating cells in leukaemic phase of follicular lymphoma. J Clin Pathol 41:951–959, 1988.

97. Warnke RA, Kim H, Fuks Z, Dorfman RF: The coexistence of nodular and diffuse patterns in nodular non-Hodgkin's lymphomas: Significance and clinicopathologic correlation. Cancer 40:1229–1233, 1977.

98. Hans CP, Weisenburger DD, Vose JM et al: A significant diffuse component predicts for inferior survival in grade 3 follicular lymphoma, but cytological types do not predict survival. Blood 2003 (in press).

99. Nathwani BN, Winberg CD, Diamond LW et al: Morphologic criteria for the differentiation of follicular lymphoma from florid reactive follicular hyperplasia: A study of 80 cases. Cancer 48:1974–1806, 1981.

100. Mann RB, Berard CW: Criteria for the cytologic subclassification of follicular lymphomas: A proposed alternative method. Hematol Oncol 3:187–192, 1983.

101. Nathwani BN, Anderson JR, Armitage JO et al: Clinical significance of follicular lymphoma with monocytoid B-cells. Non-Hodgkin's Lymphoma Classification Project. Hum Pathol 30:263–268, 1999.

102. Wabl MR, Forni L, Loor F: Switch in immunoglobulin class production observed in single clones of committed lymphocytes. Science 199:1078–1080, 1978.

103. Medeiros LJ, Picker LJ, Horning SJ, Warnke RA: Transferrin receptor expression by non-Hodgkin's lymphomas: Correlation with morphological grade and survival. Cancer 61:1844–1851, 1988.

104. Weiss LM, Strickler JG, Medeiros LJ et al: Proliferative rates of non-Hodgkin's lymphoma as assessed by Ki-67 antibody. Hum Pathol 18:1155–1159, 1987.

105. Yunis JJ, Oken MM, Kaplan ME et al: Distinctive chromosomal abnormalities in histologic subtypes of non-Hodgkin's lymphoma. N Engl J Med 307:1231–1236, 1982.

106. Tsujimoto Y, Cossman J, Jaffe ES, Croce CM: Involvement of the bcl-2 gene in human follicular lymphoma. Science 228:1440–1443, 1985.

107. de Jong D, Prins FA, Mason DY et al: Subcellular localization of the bcl-2 protein in malignant and normal lymphoid cells. Cancer Res 54:256–260, 1994.

108. Zutter M, Hockenbery D, Silverman GA, Korsmeyer SJ: Immunolocalization of the Bcl-2 protein within hematopoietic neoplasms. Blood 78:1062–1068, 1992.

109. Aster JC, Kobayashi Y, Shiota M et al: Detection of the t(14;18) at similar frequencies in hyperplastic lymphoid tissues from American and Japanese patients. Am J Pathol 141:291–299, 1992.

110. Lopez-Guillermo A, Cabanillas F, McLaughlin P et al: Molecular response assessed by PCR is the most important factor predicting failure-free survival in indolent follicular lymphomas: Update of the MDACC series. Ann Oncol 11(Suppl):137–140, 2000.

111. Lee JT, Innes DJ, Williams ME: Sequential bcl-2 and c-myc oncogene rearrangements associated with the clinical transformation of non-Hodgkin's lymphoma. J Clin Invest 84:1454–1459, 1989.

112. Ladanyi M, Offit K, Parsa NZ et al: Follicular lymphoma with t(8;14)(q24;q32): A distinct clinical and molecular subset of t(8;14)-bearing lymphomas. Blood 79:2124–2130, 1992.

113. Lu D, Medeiros LJ, Eskenazi AE, Abruzzo LV: Primary follicular large cell lymphoma of the testis in a child. Arch Pathol Lab Med 125:551–554, 2001.

114. Medeiros LJ, Harmon DC, Linggood RM, Harris NL: Immunohistologic features predict clinical behavior of orbital and conjunctival lymphoid infiltrates. Blood 74:2121–2129, 1989.

115. Knowles DM, Athan E, Ubriaco A et al: Extranodal noncutaneous lymphoid hyperplasias represent a continuous spectrum of B-cell neoplasia: Demonstration by molecular genetic analysis. Blood 73:1635–1645, 1989.

116. Wood GS, Ngan B-Y, Tung R et al: Clonal rearrangements of immunoglobulin genes and progression to B cell lymphoma in cutaneous lymphoid hyperplasia. Am J Pathol 135:13–19, 1989.

117. Medeiros LJ, Andrade RE, Harris NL et al: Lymphoid infiltrates of the orbit and conjunctiva: Comparison of immunologic and gene rearrangement data. Lab Invest 60:61A, 1989.

118. Isaacson P, Wright DH: Malignant lymphoma of mucosa-associated lymphoid tissue: A distinctive type of B-cell lymphoma. Cancer 52:1410–1416, 1983.

119. Isaacson PG, Spencer J: Malignant lymphoma of mucosa-associated lymphoid tissue. Histopathology 11:445–462, 1987.

120. Isaacson PG: Mucosa-associated lymphoid tissue lymphoma. Sem Hematol 36:139–147, 1999.

121. Isaacson PG, Chan JKC, Tang C, Addis BJ: Low-grade B-cell lymphoma of mucosa-associated lymphoid tissue arising in the thymus: A thymic lymphoma mimicking myoepithelial sialadenitis. Am J Surg Pathol 14:342–351, 1990.

122. Wotherspoon AC, Diss TC, Pan LX et al: Primary low-grade B-cell lymphoma of the conjunctiva: A mucosa-associated lymphoid tissue type lymphoma. Histopathology 23:417–424, 1993.

123. Pelstring RJ, Essell JH, Kurtin PJ et al: Diversity of organ involvement among malignant lymphomas of mucosa-associated tissues. Am J Clin Pathol 96:738–745, 1991.

124. Mhawech P, Ahearn J, Medeiros LJ: Pathologic case. A unilateral renal mass in an elderly women. Arch Pathol Lab Med 124:919–920, 2000.

125. Thieblemont C, Berger F, Dumontet C et al: Mucosa-associated lymphoid tissue lymphoma is a disseminated disease in one third of 158 patients analyzed. Blood 95:802–806, 2000.

126. Li G, Hansmann M-L, Zwingers T, Lennert K: Primary lymphomas of the lung: Morphological, immunohistochemical and clinical features. Histopathology 16:519–531, 1990.

127. Isaacson PG, Wotherspoon AC, Diss T et al: Follicular colonization in B-cell lymphoma of mucosa-associated lymphoid tissue. Am J Surg Pathol 15:819–828, 1991.

128. Wotherspoon AC, Ortiz-Hidalgo C, Falzon MR, Isaacson PG: Helicobacter pylori-associated gastritis and primary B-cell gastric lymphoma. Lancet 338:1175–1176, 1991.

129. Genta RM, Hamner HW, Graham DY: Gastric lymphoid follicles in Helicobacter pylori infection: Frequency, distribution, and response to triple therapy. Hum Pathol 24:577–583, 1993.

130. Crabtree JE, Covacci A, Farmery SM et al: Helicobacter pylori induced interleukin-8 expression in gastric epithelial cells is associated with CagA positive phenotype. J Clin Pathol 48:41–45, 1995.

131. Wotherspoon AC, Doglioni C, Diss TC et al: Regression of primary low-grade B-cell gastric lymphoma of mucosa-associated lymphoid tissue type after eradication of Helicobacter pylori. Lancet 342:575–577, 1993.

132. Addis BJ, Hyjek E, Isaacson PG: Primary pulmonary lymphoma: A reappraisal of its histogenesis and its relationship to pseudolymphoma and lymphoid interstitial pneumonia. Histopathology 13:1–17, 1988.

133. Hyjek E, Smith WJ, Isaacson PG: Primary B-cell lymphoma of salivary glands and its relationship to myoepithelial sialadentitis. Hum Pathol 19:766–776, 1988.

134. Hyjek E, Isaacson PG: Primary B cell lymphoma of the thyroid and its relationship to Hashimoto's thyroiditis. Hum Pathol 19:1315–1326, 1988.

135. Wotherspoon AC, Pan LX, Diss TC, Isaacson PG: A genotypic study of low-grade B cell lymphomas, including lymphomas of mucosa associated lymphoid tissue (MALT). J Pathol 162:135–140, 1990.

136. Dierlamm J, Baens M, Wlodarska I et al: The apoptosis inhibitor gene API2 and a novel 18q gene, MLT, are recurrently rearranged in the t(11;18)(q21;q21) associated with mucosa-associated lymphoid tissue lymphomas. Blood 93:3601–3609, 1999.

137. Akagi T, Motegi M, Tamura A et al: A novel gene, MALT1 at 18q21, is involved in t(11;18)(q21;q21) found in low-grade B-cell lymphoma of mucosa-associated lymphoid tissue. Oncogene 18:5785–5794, 1999.

138. LaCasse EC, Baird S, Korneluk RG et al: The inhibitors of apoptosis (IAPs) and their emerging role in cancer. Oncogene 17:3247–3259, 1998.

139. Lucas PC, Yonezumi M, Inohara N et al: Bcl10 and MALT1, independent targets of chromosomal translocation in MALT lymphoma, corporate in a novel NF-κB signaling pathway. J Biol Chem 276:19012–19019, 2001.

140. Liu H, Ruskon-Fourmestraux A, Lavergne-Slove A et al: Resistance of t(11;18) positive gastric mucosa-associated lymphoid tissue lymphoma to Helicobacter pylori eradication therapy. Lancet 357:39–40, 2001.

141. Alpen B, Neubauer A, Dierlamm J et al: Translocation t(11;18) absent in early gastric marginal zone B-cell lymphoma of MALT type responding to eradication of Helicobacter pylori infection. Blood 95:4014–4015, 2000.

142. Willis TG, Jadayel DM, Du MQ et al: Bcl10 is involved in t(1;14)(p22;q32) of MALT B cell lymphoma and mutated in multiple tumor types. Cell 96:35–45, 1999.

143. Zhang Q, Siebert R, Yan M et al: Inactivating mutations and overexpression of BCL10, a caspase recruitment domain-containing gene, in MALT lymphoma with t(1;14)(p22;q32). Nat Genet 22:63–68, 1999.

144. Wotherspoon AC, Finn TM, Isaacson PG: Trisomy 3 in low-grade B-cell lymphomas of mucosa-associated lymphoid tissue. Blood 85:2000–2004, 1995.

145. Brynes RK, Almaguer PD, Leathery KE et al: Numerical cytogenetic abnormalities of chromosomes 3, 7, and 12 in marginal zone B-cell lymphomas. Mod Pathol 9:995–1000, 1996.

146. Ott G, Kalla J, Steinhoff A et al: Trisomy 3 is not a common feature in malignant lymphomas of mucosa-associated lymphoid tissue type. Am J Pathol 153:689–694, 1998.

147. Pan L, Diss TC, Cunningham D et al: The bcl-2 gene in primary B cell lymphoma of mucosa-associated lymphoid tissue (MALT). Am J Pathol 135:7–11, 1989.

148. Peng H, Diss T, Isaacson PG, Pan L: c-myc gene abnormalities in mucosa-associated lymphoid tissue (MALT) lymphomas. J Pathol 181:381–386, 1997.

149. Go JH, Yang WI, Ree HJ: Mutational analysis of the 5′ noncoding region of the bcl-6 gene in primary gastric lymphomas. Mod Pathol 14:410–414, 2001.

150. Stein H, Lennert K, Mason DY et al: Immature sinus histiocytes: Their identification as a novel B-cell population. Am J Pathol 117:44–52, 1984.

151. Cardoso de Almeida P, Harris NL, Bhan AK: Characterization of immature sinus histiocytes (monocytoid cells) in reactive lymph nodes by use of monoclonal antibodies. Hum Pathol 15:330–335, 1984.

152. Sheibani K, Sohn CC, Burke JS et al: Monocytoid B-cell lymphoma. A novel B-cell neoplasm. Am J Pathol 124;310–318, 1986.

153. Sheibani K, Burke JS, Swartz WG et al: Monocytoid B-cell lymphoma: Clinicopathologic study of 21 cases of a unique type of low-grade lymphoma. Cancer 62:1531–1538, 1988.

154. Cogliatti SB, Lennert K, Hansmann M-L et al: Monocytoid B-cell lymphoma: Clinical and prognostic features of 21 patients. J Clin Pathol 43:619–625, 1990.

155. Ngan B-Y, Warnke RA, Wilson M et al: Monocytoid B-cell lymphoma: A study of 36 cases. Hum Pathol 22:409–421, 1991.

156. Nathwani BN, Anderson JR, Armitage JO et al: Marginal zone B-cell lymphoma: A clinical comparison of nodal and mucosa-associated lymphoid tissue types. Non-Hodgkin's Lymphoma Classification Project. J Clin Oncol 17:2486–2492, 1999.

157. Plank L, Hansmann M-L, Fischer R: The cytological spectrum of the monocytoid B-cell reaction: Recognition of its large cell type. Histopathology 23:425–431, 1993.

158. Nizze H, Cogliatti SB, Von Schilling C et al: Monocytoid B-cell lymphoma: Morphological variants and relationship to low-grade B-cell lymphoma of the mucosa-associated lymphoid tissue. Histopathology 18:403–414, 1991.

159. Slovak ML, Weiss LM, Nathwani BN et al: Cytogenetic studies of composite lymphomas: Monocytoid B-cell lymphoma and other B-cell non-Hodgkin's lymphomas. Hum Pathol 24:1086–1094, 1993.

160. Remstein ED, James CD, Kurtin PJ: Incidence and subtype specificity of API2-MALT1 fusion translocations in extranodal, nodal, and splenic marginal zone lymphomas. Am J Pathol 156:1183–1188, 2000.

161. Schmid C, Kirkham N, Diss T et al: Splenic marginal zone cell lymphoma. Am J Surg Pathol 16:455–466, 1992.

162. Isaacson PG, Matutes E, Burke M et al: The histopathology of splenic lymphoma with villous lymphocytes. Blood 84:3828–3834, 1994.

163. Wu CD, Jackson CL, Medeiros LJ: Splenic marginal zone cell lymphoma. An immunophenotypic and molecular study of five cases. Am J Clin Pathol 105:277–285, 1996.

164. Van Huyen JP, Molina T, Delmer A et al: Splenic marginal zone lymphoma with or without plasmacytic differentiation. Am J Surg Pathol 24:1581–1592, 2000.

165. Rosso R, Neiman RS, Paulli M et al: Splenic marginal zone cell lymphoma: Report of an indolent variant without massive splenomegaly presumably representing an early phase of the disease. Hum Pathol 26:39–46, 1995.

166. Gruszka-Westwood AM, Hamoudi RA, Matutes E et al: p53 abnormalities in splenic lymphoma with villous lymphocytes. Blood 97:3552–3558, 2001.

167. Mateo MS, Mollejo M, Villuendas R et al: Molecular heterogeneity of splenic marginal zone lymphomas: Analysis of mutations in the 5′ non-coding region of the bcl-6 gene. Leukemia 15:628–634, 2001.

168. Ott MM, Rosenwald A, Katzenberger T et al: Marginal zone B-cell lymphomas (MZBL) arising at different sites represent different biological entities. Genes Chromosomes Cancer 28:380–386, 2000.

169. Chabner BA, Johnson RE, Young RC et al: Sequential nonsurgical and surgical staging of non-Hodgkin's lymphoma. Ann Intern Med 85:149–154, 1976.

170. Coiffier B, Lepage E, Briere J et al: CHOP chemotherapy plus rituximab compared with CHOP alone in elderly patients with diffuse large-B-cell lymphoma. N Engl J Med 346:235–242, 2002.

171. Shipp MA: Prognostic factors in aggressive non-Hodgkin's lymphoma: Who has "high-risk" disease? Blood 83:1165–1173, 1994.

172. Straus DJ, Wong G, Yaholom J et al: Diffuse large cell lymphoma. Prognostic factors with treatment. Leukemia 5(Suppl 1):32–37, 1991.

173. Nathwani BN, Dixon DO, Jones SE et al: The clinical significance of the morphological subdivision of diffuse "histiocytic" lymphoma: A study of 162 patients treated by the Southwest Oncology Group. Blood 60:1068–1074, 1982.

174. Engelhard M, Brittinger G, Huhn D et al: Subclassification of diffuse large B-cell lymphomas according to the Kiel classification: Distinction of centroblastic and immunoblastic lymphomas is a significant prognostic factor. Blood 89:2291–2297, 1997.

175. Kwak LW, Wilson M, Weiss LM et al: Clinical significance of morphologic subdivision in diffuse large cell lymphoma. Cancer 68:1988–1993, 1991.

176. Medeiros LJ, Gelb AB, Wolfson K et al: Major histocompatibility complex class I and class II antigen expression in diffuse large cell and large cell immunoblastic lymphomas: Absence of a correlation between antigen expression and clinical outcome. Am J Pathol 143:1086–1097, 1993.

177. Jacobson JO, Wilkes BM, Kwiatkowski DJ et al: bcl-2 rearrangements in de novo diffuse large cell lymphoma: Association with distinctive clinical features. Cancer 72:231–236, 1993.

178. Gascoyne RD, Adomat SA, Krajewski S et al: Prognostic significance of Bcl-2 protein expression and Bcl-2 gene rearrangement

in diffuse aggressive non-Hodkin's lymphoma. Blood 90:244–251, 1997.

179. Ye BH, Lista F, Lo Coco F et al: Alterations of a zinc finger-encoding gene, BCL-6, in diffuse large-cell lymphoma. Science 262:747–750, 1993.

180. Offit K, Lo Coco F, Louie DC et al: Rearrangement of the bcl-6 gene as a prognostic marker in diffuse large-cell lymphoma. N Engl J Med 331:74–80, 1994.

181. Subar M, Neri A, Inghirami G et al: Frequent c-myc oncogene activation and infrequent presence of Epstein-Barr virus genome in AIDS-associated lymphoma. Blood 72:667–671, 1988.

182. Van Krieken JHJM, Medeiros LJ, Pals ST et al: Diffuse aggressive B-cell lymphomas of the gastrointestinal tract: An immunophenotypic and gene rearrangement analysis of 22 cases. Am J Clin Pathol 97:170–178, 1992.

183. Fraga M, Garcia-Rivero A, Sanchez-Verde L et al: T-cell/histiocyte-rich large B-cell lymphoma is a disseminated aggressive neoplasm: Differential diagnosis from Hodgkin's lymphoma. Histopathology 41:216–229, 2002.

184. Macon WR, Williams ME, Greer JP et al: T-cell-rich B-cell lymphomas. A clinicopathologic study of 19 cases. Am J Surg Pathol 16:351–363, 1992.

185. Lones MA, Cairo MS, Perkins SL: T-cell-rich large B-cell lymphoma in children and adolescents: A clinicopathologic report of six cases from the Children's Cancer Group study CCG-5961. Cancer 88:2378–2386, 2000.

186. Medeiros LJ, Lardelli P, Stetler-Stevenson M et al: Genotypic analysis of diffuse, mixed cell lymphomas: Comparison with morphologic and immunophenotypic findings. Am J Clin Pathol 95:547–555, 1991.

187. Brauninger A, Kuppers R, Spieker T et al: Molecular analysis of single B cells from T-cell-rich B-cell lymphoma shows the derivation of the tumor cells from mutating germinal centers B cells and exemplifies means by which immunoglobulin genes are modified in germinal center B cells. Blood 93:2679–2687, 1999.

188. Hodges E, Hamid Y, Quin CT et al: Molecular analysis reveals somatically mutated and unmutated clonal and oligoclonal B cells in T-cell-rich B-cell lymphoma. J Pathol 192:479–487, 2000.

189. Katzenstein ALA, Carrington CB, Liebow AA: Lymphomatoid granulomatosis: A clinicopathologic study of 152 cases. Cancer 43:360–373, 1979.

190. Guinee D, Jaffe ES, Kingma D et al: Pulmonary lymphomatoid granulomatosis. Evidence for a proliferation of Epstein-Barr virus infected B-lymphocytes with a prominent T-cell component and vasculitis. Am J Surg Pathol 18:753–764, 1994.

191. Myers JL, Kurtin PJ, Katzenstein ALA et al: Lymphomatoid granulomatosis. Evidence for immunophenotypic diversity and relationship to Epstein-Barr virus infection. Am J Surg Pathol 19:1300–1312, 1995.

192. Nicholson AG, Wotherspoon AC, Diss TC et al: Lymphomatoid granulomatosis: Evidence that some cases represent Epstein-Barr virus-associated B-cell lymphoma. Histopathology 29:317–324, 1996.

193. Medeiros LJ, Peiper SC, Elwood L et al: Angiocentric immunoproliferative lesions: A molecular analysis of eight cases. Hum Pathol 22:1150–1157, 1991.

194. Wick MR, Mills SE, Scheithauer BW et al: Reassessment of malignant "angioendotheliomatosis": Evidence in favor of its reclassification as "intravascular lymphomatosis." Am J Surg Pathol 10:112–123, 1986.

195. Sheibani K, Battifora H, Winberg CD et al: Further evidence that "malignant angioendotheliomatosis" is an angiotropic large-cell lymphoma. N Engl J Med 314:943–948, 1986.

196. Khalidi HS, Brynes RK, Browne P et al: Intravascular large B-cell lymphoma: The CD5 antigen is expressed by a subset of cases. Mod Pathol 11:983–988, 1998.

197. Estalilla OC, Koo CH, Brynes RK et al: Intravascular large B-cell lymphoma. A report of five cases initially diagnosed by bone marrow biopsy. Am J Clin Pathol 112:248–255, 1999.

198. DiGiuseppe JA, Hartmann DP, Freter C et al: Molecular detection of bone marrow involvement in intravascular lymphomatosis. Mod Pathol 10:33–37, 1997.

199. Molina A, Lombard C, Donlon T et al: Immunohistochemical and cytogenetic studies indicate that malignant angioendotheliomatosis is a primary intravascular (angiotropic) lymphoma. Cancer 66:474–479, 1990.

200. Stein H, Mason DY, Gerdes J et al: The expression of the Hodgkin's disease associated antigen Ki-1 in reactive and neoplastic lymphoid tissue: Evidence that Reed-Sternberg cells and histiocytic malignancies are derived from activated lymphoid cells. Blood 66:848–858, 1985.

201. Weisenburger DD, Gordon BG, Vose JM et al: Occurrence of the t(2;5)(p23;q35) in non-Hodgkin's lymphoma. Blood 87:3860–3868, 1996.

202. Jacobson JO, Aisenberg AC, Lamarre L et al: Mediastinal large cell lymphoma: An uncommon subset of adult lymphoma curable with combined modality therapy. Cancer 62:1893–1898, 1988.

203. Falini B, Venturi S, Martelli M et al: Mediastinal large B-cell lymphoma: Clinical and immunohistochemical findings in 18 patients treated with different third-generation regimens. Br J Haematol 89:780–789, 1995.

204. Van Besien K, Kelta M, Bahaguna P: Primary mediastinal B-cell lymphoma: A review of pathology and management. J Clin Oncol 19:1855–1864, 2001.

205. Pileri SA, Gaidano G, Zinzani PL et al: Primary mediastinal B-cell lymphoma: High frequency of Bcl-6 mutations and consistent expression of the transcription factors OCT-2, BOB.1, and PU.1 in the absence of immunoglobulins. Am J Pathol 162:243–253, 2003.

206. Cazals-Hatem D, Lepage E, Brice P et al: Primary mediastinal large B-cell lymphoma. A clinicopathologic study of 141 cases compared with 916 nonmediastinal large B-cell lymphomas, a GELA ("Groupe d'Etude des Lymphomas de l'Adulte") Study. Am J Surg Pathol 20:877–888, 1996.

207. Isaacson PG, Norton AJ, Addis BJ: The human thymus contains a novel population of B lymphocytes. Lancet II:1488–1491, 1987.

208. Taubenberger JK, Jaffe ES, Medeiros LJ: Thymoma with abundant L26+ "asteroid" cells: A case report with an analysis of normal thymus and thymoma specimens. Arch Pathol Lab Med 115:1254–1257, 1991.

209. Copie-Bergman C, Gaulard P, Maouche-Chretien L et al: The MAL gene is expressed in primary mediastinal large B-cell lymphoma. Blood 84:3567–3575, 1999.

210. Scarpa A, Borgato L, Chilosi M et al: Evidence of c-myc gene abnormalities in mediastinal large B-cell lymphoma of young adult age. Blood 78:780–788, 1991.

211. Nador RG, Cesarman E, Chadburn A et al: Primary effusion lymphoma: A distinct clinicopathologic entity associated with the Kaposi's sarcoma-associated herpes virus. Blood 88:645–656, 1996.

212. Horenstein MG, Nador RG, Chadburn A et al: Epstein-Barr virus latent gene expression in primary effusion lymphomas containing Kaposi's sarcoma-associated herpes virus/human herpes virus-8. Blood 90:1186–1191, 1997.

213. Copie-Bergman C, Niedobitek G, Mangham DC et al: Epstein-Barr virus in B-cell lymphomas with chronic suppurative inflammation. J Pathol 183:287–292, 1997.

214. Magrath IT: African Burkitt's lymphoma: History, biology, clinical features, and treatment. Am J Pediatr Hematol Oncol 13:222–246, 1991.

215. Bennett JM, Catovsky D, Daniel MT et al: Proposals for the classification of chronic (mature) B and T lymphoid leukemias: French-American-British (FAB) Cooperative Group. J Clin Pathol 42:567–584, 1989.

216. Burkitt D, O'Conor GT: Malignant lymphoma in African children. I. A clinical syndrome. Cancer 14:258–269, 1961.

217. Miliauskas JR, Berard CW, Young RC et al: Undifferentiated non-Hodgkin's lymphomas (Burkitt's and non-Burkitt's types): The relevance of making this histologic distinction. Cancer 50:2115–2121, 1982.

218. Ioachim HL, Dorsett B, Cronin W et al: Acquired immunodeficiency syndrome-associated lymphomas: Clinical, pathologic, immunologic, and viral characteristics of 111 cases. Hum Pathol 22:659–673, 1991.

219. Murphy SB, Magrath IT: Workshop on pediatric lymphomas: Current results and prospects. Ann Oncol 2 (Suppl. 2):219–223, 1991.

220. Magrath IT, Lee YJ, Anderson T et al: Prognostic factors in Burkitt's lymphoma: Importance of total tumor burden. Cancer 45:1507–1515, 1980.

221. Nkrumah F, Henle W, Henle G et al: Burkitt's lymphoma: Its clinical course in relation to immunologic reactivities to Epstein-Barr virus and tumor-related antigens. J Natl Cancer Inst 57:1051–1056, 1976.

222. Magrath IT: Immunosuppression in Burkitt's lymphoma. I. Cutaneous reactivity to recall antigens: Alterations induced by a tumour burden and by BCG administration. Int J Cancer 13:839–849, 1974.

223. Magrath IT, Simon RM: Immunosuppression in Burkitt's lymphoma. II. Peripheral lymphocyte populations related to clinical status. Int J Cancer 18:399–408, 1976.

224. Magrath I, Adde M, Shad A et al: Adults and children with small non-cleaved cell lymphoma have a similar excellent outcome when treated with the same chemotherapy regimen. J Clin Oncol 14:925–934, 1996.

225. Butler RD, Hainsworth JD: Optimal therapy for small noncleaved lymphoma. Cancer Treat Rep 66:65–79, 1993.

226. Biggar RJ, Nkrumah FK, Henle W et al: Very late relapses in patients with Burkitt's lymphoma: Clinical and serologic studies. J Natl Cancer Inst 66:439–444, 1981.

227. Berard CW, O'Conor GT, Thomas LB et al: Histopathological definition of Burkitt's tumour. Bull WHO 40:601–607, 1969.

228. Mann RB, Jaffe ES, Braylan RC et al: Non-endemic Burkitt's lymphoma: A B-cell tumor related to germinal centers. N Engl J Med 295:685–691, 1976.

229. Hutchison RE, Finch C, Kepner J et al: Burkitt lymphoma is immunophenotypically different from Burkitt-like lymphoma in young persons. Ann Oncol 11(Suppl. 1):35–38, 2000.

230. Hecht JL, Aster JC: Molecular biology of Burkitt's lymphoma. J Clin Oncol 18:3707–3721, 2000.

231. Gutierrez MI, Hamdy N, Bhatia K et al: Geographic variation in t(8;14) chromosomal breakpoint locations and EBV association in Burkitt's lymphoma. Int J Pediatr Hematol Oncol 6:161–168, 1999.

232. Yano T, van Krieken JHJM, Magrath IT et al: Histogenetic correlations between subcategories of small non-cleaved cell lymphoma. Blood 79:1282–1290, 1992.

233. Wilson JF, Kjeldsberg CR, Sposto R et al: The pathology of non-Hodgkin's lymphoma of childhood. II. Reproducibility and relevance of the histologic classification of "undifferentiated" lymphomas (Burkitt's versus non-Burkitt's). Hum Pathol 18:1008–1014, 1987.

234. Hutchison RE, Murphy SB, Fairclough DL et al: Diffuse small noncleaved cell lymphoma in children, Burkitt's versus non-Burkitt's types. Results from the Pediatric Oncology Group and St. Jude Children's Research Hospital. Cancer 64:23–28, 1989.

235. Weiss LM, Bindl JM, Picozzi VJ et al: Lymphoblastic lymphoma: An immunophenotype study of 26 cases with comparison to T cell acute lymphoblastic leukemia. Blood 67:474–478, 1986.

236. Spitzer G, Garson OM: Lymphoblastic leukemia with marked eosinophilia: A report of two cases. Blood 42:377–384, 1973.

237. de Villartay JP, Pullman AB, Andrade R et al: γ/δ lineage relationship within a consecutive series of human precursor T-cell neoplasms. Blood 74:2508–2518, 1989.

238. Pilozzi E, Muller-Hermelink HK, Falini B et al: Gene rearrangements in T-cell lymphoblastic lymphoma. J Pathol 188:267–270, 1999.

239. Brown L, Cheng JT, Chen Q et al: Site-specific recombination of the tal-1 gene is a common occurrence in human T cell leukemia. EMBO J 9:3343–3351, 1990.

240. Kaneko Y, Frizzera G, Shikano T et al: Chromosomal and immunophenotypic patterns in T cell acute lymphoblastic leukemia (TALL) and lymphoblastic lymphoma (LBL). Leukemia 3:886–892, 1989.

241. Aplan PD, Lombardi DP, Reaman GH et al: Involvement of the putative hematopoietic transcription factor SCL in T-cell acute lymphoblastic leukemia. Blood 79:1327–1333, 1992.

242. Aplan PD, Lombardi DP, Ginsberg AM et al: Disruption of the human SCL locus by "illegitimate" V-(D)-J recombinase activity. Science 250:1426–1429, 1990.

243. Hoyer JD, Ross CW, Li CY et al: True T-cell chronic lymphocytic leukemia: A morphologic and immunophenotypic study of 25 cases. Blood 86:1163–1169, 1995.

244. Matutes E, Catovsky D: Similarities between T-cell chronic lymphocytic leukemia and small-cell variant of T-prolymphocytic leukemia. Blood 86:3520–3521, 1996.

245. Matutes E, Garcia Talavera J, O'Brien M et al: The morphological spectrum of T-prolymphocytic leukaemia. Br J Haematol 64:111–124, 1986.

246. Matutes E, Brito-Babapulle V, Swansbury J et al: Clinical and laboratory features of 78 cases of T-prolymphocytic leukemia. Blood 78:3269–3274, 1991.

247. Pawson R, Dyer MJ, Barge R et al: Treatment of T-cell prolymphocytic leukemia with human CD52 antibody. J Clin Oncol 15:2667–2672, 1997.

248. Brito-Babapulle V, Pomfret M, Matutes E et al: Cytogenetic studies on prolymphocytic leukemia. II. T cell prolymphocytic leukemia. Blood 70:926–931, 1987.

249. De Schouwer PJ, Dyer MJ, Brito-Babapulle VB et al: T-cell prolymphocytic leukemia: Antigen receptor gene rearrangement and a normal mode of MTCP B1 activation. Br J Haematol 110:831–838, 2000.

250. Stoppa-Lyonnet D, Soulier J, Lauge A et al: Inactivation of the ATM gene in T-cell prolymphocytic leukemias. Blood 91:3920–3926, 1998.

251. Soulier J, Pierron G, Vecchione D et al: A complex pattern of recurrent chromosomal losses and gains T-cell cell prolymphocytic leukemia. Genes Chromosomes Cancer 31:248–254, 2001.

252. Loughran TP Jr, Kadin ME, Starkebaum G et al: Leukemia of large granular lymphocytes: Association with clonal chromosomal abnormalities and autoimmune neutropenia, thrombocytopenia, and hemolytic anemia. Ann Intern Med 102:169–175, 1985.

253. Lamy T, Loughran TP Jr: Current concepts: Large granular lymphocyte leukemia. Blood Rev 13:230–240, 1999.

254. Dhodapkar MV, Li CY, Lust JA et al: Clinical spectrum of clonal proliferations of T-large granular lymphocytes: A T-cell clonopathy of undertermined significance? Blood 84:1620–1627, 1987.

255. Loughran TP Jr, Coyle T, Sherman MP et al: Detection of human T-cell leukemia/lymphoma virus, type II, in a patient with large granular lymphocyte leukemia. Blood 80:1116–1119, 1992.

256. Pandolfi F, Loughran TP, Starkebaum G et al: Clinical course and prognosis of the lymphoproliferative disease of granular lymphocytes: A multicenter study. Cancer 65:341–348, 1990.

257. Evans HL, Burks E, Viswanatha D et al: Utility of immunohistochemistry in bone marrow evaluation of T-lineage large granular lymphocyte leukemia. Hum Pathol 31:1266–1273, 2000.

258. Agnarsson BA, Loughran TP Jr, Starkebaum G et al: The pathology of large granular lymphocyte leukemia. Hum Pathol 20:643–651, 1989.

259. Perzova R, Loughran TP: Constitutive expression of Fas ligand in large granular lymphocyte leukaemia. Br J Haematol 97:123–126, 1997.

260. Pelicci PG, Allavena P, Subar M et al: T-cell receptor (alpha, beta, gamma) gene rearrangements and expression in normal and leukemic large granular lymphocytes/natural killer cells. Blood 70:1500–1508, 1987.

261. Salido M, Sole F, Espinet B et al: New t(11;12)(q12q11) characterized by RxFISH in a patient with T-cell large granular lymphocyte leukemia. Cancer Genet Cytogenet 125:70–73, 2001.

262. Zambello R, Trentin L, Ciccone E et al: Phenotype diversity of natural killer (NK) populations in patients with NK-type lymphoproliferative disease of granular lymphocytes. Blood 81:2381–2385, 1993.

263. Wong N, Wong KF, Chan JK et al: Chromosomal translocations are common in natural killer-cell lymphoma/leukemia as shown by spectral karyotyping. Hum Pathol 31:771–774, 2000.

264. Taniwaki M, Tagawa S, Nishigaki H et al: Chromosomal abnormalities define clonal proliferation in CD3- large granular lymphocyte leukemia. Am J Hematol 33:32–38, 1990.

265. Kawa-Ha K, Ishihara S, Ninomiya T et al: CD3-negative lymphoproliferative disease of granular lymphocytes containing Epstein-Barr viral DNA. J Clin Invest 84:51–55, 1989.

266. Takatsuki K, Matsuoka M, Yamaguchi K: Adult T-cell leukemia in Japan. J Acquir Immune Defic Syndr Hum Retrovirol 13(Suppl. 1):S15–S19, 1996.

267. Yamaguchi K: Human T-lymphotropic virus type I in Japan. Lancet 343:213–216, 1994.

268. Mueller N, Okayama A, Stuver S et al: Findings from the Miyazaki cohort study. J Acquir Immune Defic Syndr Hum Retroviol 13(Suppl. 1):S52–57, 1996.

269. Swerdlow S, Habeshaw J, Rohatiner AZ et al: Carribean T-cell lymphoma/leukemia. Cancer 54:687–696, 1984.

270. Franchini G: Molecular mechanisms of human T-cell leukemia/lymphotropic virus type I infection. Blood 86:3619–3639, 1995.

271. Shimoyama M and members of the Lymphoma Study Group: Diagnostic criteria and classification of clinical subtypes of adult T-cell leukemia-lymphoma. Br J Haematol 79:428–437, 1991.

272. Ejima E, Rosenblatt J, Massari M et al: Cell-type-specific transactivation of the parathroid hormone-related protein gene promoter by the human T-cell leukemia virus type I (HTLV-I) tax and HTLV-II tax proteins. Blood 81:1017–1024, 1993.

273. Van Krieken JHJM, Elwood L, Andrade RE et al: Rearrangement of the T-cell receptor delta chain gene in T-cell lymphomas with a mature phenotype. Am J Pathol 139:161–168, 1991.

274. Itoyama T, Chaganti RS, Yamada Y et al: Cytogenetic analysis and clinical significance in adult T-cell leukemia/lymphoma: A study of 50 cases from the human T-cell leukemia virus type-1 endemic area, Nagasaki. Blood 97:3612–3620, 2001.

275. Shimamoto Y, Suga K, Shibata K et al: Clinical importance of extraordinary integration patterns of human T-cell lymphotrophic virus type I proviral DNA in adult T-cell leukemia/lymphoma. Blood 84:853–858, 1994.

276. Iwanaga R, Ohtani K, Hayashi T et al: Molecular mechanism of cell cycle progression induced by the oncogene product Tax of human T-cell leukemia virus type I. Oncogene 20:2055–2067, 2001.

277. DeRemee RA, Weiland LH, McDonald TJ: Polymorphic reticulosis, lymphomatoid granulomatosis: Two diseases or one? Mayo Clinic Proc 53:634–640, 1978.

278. Lipford EH, Margolick JB, Longo DL et al: Angiocentric immunoproliferative lesions: A clinicopathologic spectrum of post-thymic T-cell proliferations. Blood 72:1674–1681, 1988.

279. Rodriguez J, Romaguera JE, Manning J et al: Nasal-type T/NK lymphomas: A clinicopathologic study of 13 cases. Leuk Lymphoma 39:139–144, 2000.

280. Medeiros LJ, Jaffe ES, Chen Y-Y et al: Localization of Epstein-Barr viral genomes in angiocentric immunoproliferative lesions. Am J Surg Pathol 16:439–447, 1992.

281. Lay JD, Tsao CJ, Chen JY et al: Upregulation of tumor necrosis factor-alpha gene by Epstein-Barr virus and activation of macrophages in Epstein-Barr virus infected Tcells in the pathogenesis of hemphagocytic syndrome. J Clin Invest 100:1969–1979, 1997.

282. Teruya-Feldstein J, Setsuda J, Yao X et al: MIP-1 alpha expression in tissues from patients with hemophagocytic syndrome. Lab Invest 79:1583–1590, 1999.

283. Nakamura S, Suchi T, Koshikawa T et al: Clinicopathologic study of CD56 (NCAM)-positive angiocentric lymphoma occurring in sites other than the upper and lower respiratory tract. Am J Surg Pathol 18:284–296, 1995.

284. Ohshima K, Suzumiya J, Shimazaki K et al: Nasal T/NK cell lymphomas commonly express perforin and Fas ligand: Important mediators of tissue damage. Histopathology 31:444–450, 1997.

285. Quintanilla-Martinez L, Franklin JL, Guerrero I et al: Histological and immunophenotypic profile of nasal NK/T cell lymphomas from Peru: High prevalence of p53 overexpression. Hum Pathol 30:849–855, 1999.

286. Ohsawa M, Nakatsuka S, Kanno H et al: Immunophenotypic and genotypic characterization of nasal lymphoma with polymorphic reticulosis morphology. Int J Cancer 81:865–870, 1999.

287. Kanavaros P, Lescs M-C, Briere J et al: Nasal T-cell lymphoma: A clinicopathologic entity associated with peculiar phenotype and with Epstein-Barr virus. Blood 81:2688–2695, 1993.

288. Ko YH, Choi KE, Han JH et al: Comparative genomic hybridization study of nasal-type NK/T-cell lymphoma. Cytometry 46:85–91, 2001.

289. Gale J, Simmonds PD, Mead GM et al: Enteropathy-type intestinal T-cell lymphoma: Clinical features and treatment of 31 patients in a single center. J Clin Oncol 18:795–803, 2000.

290. Isaacson PG, O'Connor NT, Spencer J, et al: Malignant histiocytosis of the intestine. Lancet II:688–691, 1985.

291. Isaacson P, Wright DH: Intestinal lymphoma associated with malabsorption. Lancet I:67–70, 1978.

292. Murray A, Cuevas EC, Jones DB et al: Study of the immunohistochemistry and T cell clonality of enteropathy-associated T cell lymphoma. Am J Pathol 146:509–519, 1995.

293. Katoh A, Ohshima K, Kanda M et al: Gastrointestinal T cell lymphoma: Predominant cytotoxic phenotypes, including alpha/beta, gamma/delta and natural killer cells. Leuk Lymphoma 39:97–111, 2000.

294. Bagdi E, Diss TC, Munson P et al: Mucosal intra-epithelial lymphocytes in enteropathy-associated T-cell lymphoma, ulcerative jejunitis, and refractory celiac disease constitute a neoplastic population. Blood 94:260–264, 1999.

295. Ashton-Key M, Diss TC, Pan L et al: Molecular analysis of T-cell clonality in ulcerative jejunitis and enteropathy-associated T-cell lymphoma. Am J Pathol 151:493–498, 1997.

296. Wright DH: Enteropathy associated T cell lymphoma. Cancer Surv 30:249–261, 1997.

297. Farcet JP, Gaulard P, Marolleau JP et al: Hepatosplenic T-cell lymphoma: Sinusal/sinusoidal localization of malignant cells expressing the T-cell receptor gamma delta. Blood 75:2213–2219, 1990.

298. Cooke CB, Krenacs L, Stetler-Stevenson M et al: Hepatosplenic T-cell lymphoma: A distinct clinicopathologic entity of cytotoxic gamma delta T-cell origin. Blood 88:4265–4274, 1996.

299. Weidmann E: Hepatosplenic T cell lymphoma. A review on 45 cases since the report describing the disease as a distinct lymphoma entity in 1990. Leukemia 14:991–997, 2000.

300. Vega F, Medeiros LJ, Bueso-Ramos C et al: Hepatosplenic gamma/delta T-cell lymphoma in bone marrow: A sinusoidal neoplasm with blastic cytologic features. Am J Clin Pathol 116:410–419, 2001.

301. Macon WR, Levy NB, Kurtin PJ et al: Hepatosplenic alphabeta T-cell lymphomas: A report of 14 cases and comparison with hepatosplenic gammadelta T-cell lymphomas. Am J Surg Pathol 25:285–296, 2001.

302. Salhany KE, Feldman M, Kahn MJ et al: Hepatosplenic gammadelta T-cell lymphoma: Ultrastructural, immunophenotypic, and functional evidence for cytotoxic T lymphocyte differentiation. Hum Pathol 28:674–685, 1997.

303. Ohshima K, Haraoka S, Harada N et al: Hepatosplenic gammadelta T-cell lymphoma: Relation to Epstein-Barr virus and activated cytotoxic molecules. Histopathology 36:127–135, 2000.

304. Alonsozana EL, Stamberg J, Kumar D et al: Isochromosome 7q: The primary cytogenetic abnormality in hepatosplenic gammadelta T cell lymphoma. Leukemia 11:1367–1372, 1997.

305. Weenig RH, Ng CS, Perniciaro C: Subcutaneous panniculitis-like T-cell lymphoma: An elusive case presenting as lipomembranous panniculitis and a review of 72 cases in the literature. Am J Dermatopathol 23:206–215, 2001.

306. Gonzalez CL, Medeiros LJ, Braziel RM et al: T-cell lymphoma involving subcutaneous tissue. A clinicopathologic entity commonly associated with hemophagocytic syndrome. Am J Surg Pathol 15:17–27, 1991.

307. Au WY, Ng WM, Choy C et al: Aggressive subcutaneous panniculitis-like T-cell lymphoma: Complete remission with fludarabine, mitoxantrone and dexamethasone. Br J Dermatol 143:408–410, 2000.

308. Salhany KE, Macon WR, Choi JK et al: Subcutaneous panniculitis-like T-cell lymphoma: Clinicopathologic, immunophenotypic, and genotypic analysis of alpha/beta and gamma/delta subtypes. Am J Surg Pathol 22:881–893, 1998.

309. Kumar S, Krenacs L, Medeiros LJ et al: Subcutaneous panniculitic T-cell lymphoma is a tumor of cytotoxic T lymphocytes. Hum Pathol 29:397–403, 1998.

310. Monterroso V, Bujan W, Jaramillo O et al: Subcutaneous tissue involvement by T-cell lymphoma. A report of 2 cases. Arch Dermatol 132:1345–1350, 1996.

311. Toro JR, Beaty M, Sorbara L et al: Gamma delta T-cell lymphoma of the skin: A clinical, microscopic and molecular study. Arch Dermatol 136:1024–1032, 2000.

312. Kim YH, Hoppe RT: Mycosis fungoides and the Sezary syndrome. Semin Oncol 26:276–289, 1999.

313. Bunn PA, Huberman MS, Whang-Peng J et al: Prospective staging evaluation of patients with cutaneous T-cell lymphomas. Demonstration of a high frequency of extracutaneous dissemination. Ann Intern Med 93:223–230, 1980.

314. de Coninck EC, Kim YH, Varghese A et al: Clinical characteristics and outcome of patients with extracutaneous mycosis fungoides. J Clin Oncol 19:799–784, 2001.

315. Bunn PA, Lamberg SI: Report of the committee on staging and classification of cutaneous T-cell lymphomas. Cancer Treat Rep 63:725–728, 1979.

316. Sausville EA, Eddy LJ, Makuch FW et al: Histopathologic staging at initial diagnosis of mycosis fungoides and the Sezary syndrome. Definition of three distinctive prognostic groups. Ann Intern Med 109:372–382, 1988.

317. Zackheim HS, Amin S, Kashani-Sabet M et al: Prognosis in cutaneous T-cell lymphoma by skin stage: Long-term survival in 489 patients. J Am Acad Dermatol 40:418–425, 1999.

318. Hoppe RT: The management of mycosis fungoides at Stanford—standard and innovative treatment programmes. Leukemia 5(Suppl. 1):46–48, 1991.

319. Shapiro PE, Pinto FJ: The histologic spectrum of mycosis fungoides/Sezary syndrome (cutaneous T-cell lymphoma). A review of 222 biopsies, including newly described patterns and the earliest pathologic changes. Am J Surg Pathol 18:645–667, 1994.

320. Colby TV, Burke JS, Hoppe RT: Lymph node biopsy in mycosis fungoides. Cancer 47:351–359, 1981.

321. Sausville EA, Worsham GF, Matthews MJ et al: Histologic assessment of lymph nodes in mycosis fungoides/Sezary syndrome (cutaneous T-cell lymphoma): Clinical correlations and prognostic import of a new classification system. Hum Pathol 16:1098–1109, 1985.

322. Rappaport H, Thomas LB: Mycosis fungoides: The pathology of extracutaneous involvement. Cancer 34:1198–1229, 1974.

323. Dmitrovsky E, Matthews MJ, Bunn PA et al: Cytologic transformation in cutaneous T-cell lymphoma: A clinicopathologic entity associated with poor prognosis. J Clin Oncol 5:208–215, 1987.

324. Diamandidou E, Colome-Grimmer M, Fayad L et al: Transformation of mycosis fungoides/Sezary syndrome: Clinical characteristics and prognosis. Blood 92:1150–1159, 1998.

325. Wood GS, Abel EA, Hoppe RT et al: Leu-8 and Leu-9 antigen phenotypes: Immunologic criteria for the distinction of mycosis fungoides from cutaneous inflammation. J Am Acad Dermatol 14:1006–1013, 1986.

326. Hoppe RT, Medeiros LJ, Warnke RA et al: CD8+ tumor-infiltrating lymphocytes influence the long-term survival of patients with mycosis fungoides. J Am Acad Dermatol 32:448–453, 1995.

327. Whittaker SJ, Smith NP, Jones RR et al: Analysis of β, γ, and δ T-cell receptor genes in mycosis fungoides and Sezary syndrome. Cancer 68:1572–1582, 1991.

328. Vega F, Luthra R, Medeiras LJ et al: Clonal heterogeneity in mycosis fungoides and its relationship to clinical course. Blood 100:3369–3373, 2002.

329. Zucker-Franklin D, Pancake BA: The role of human T-cell lymphotropic viruses (HTLV-I and II) in cutaneous T-cell lymphomas. Semin Derm 13:160–165, 1994.

330. Wood GS, Schaffer JM, Boni R et al: No evidence of HTLV-I proviral integration in lymphoproliferative disorders associated with cutaneous T-cell lymphoma. Am J Pathol 150:667–673, 1997.

331. Neri A, Fracchiolla NS, Roscetti E et al: Molecular analysis of cutaneous B- and T-cell lymphomas. Blood 86:3160–3172, 1995.

332. Thangavelu M, Finn WG, Yelavarthi KK et al: Recurring structural chromosome abnormalities in peripheral blood lymphocytes of patients with mycosis fungoides/Sezary syndrome. Blood 89:3371–3377, 1997.

333. Shiota M, Nakamura S, Ichinosama R et al: Anaplastic large cell lymphomas expressing the novel chimeric protein p80NPM/ALK: A distinct clinicopathologic entity. Blood 86:1954–1960, 1995.

334. Nakamura S, Shiota M, Nakagawa A et al: Anaplastic large cell lymphoma: A distinct molecular pathologic entity: A reappraisal with special reference to p80 (NPM/ALK) expression. Am J Surg Pathol 21:1420–1432, 1997.

335. Falini B. Anaplastic large cell lymphoma: Pathological, molecular, and clinical features. Br J Haematol 114:741–760, 2001.

336. Gascoyne RD, Aoun P, Wu D et al: Prognostic significance of anaplastic lymphoma kinase (ALK) protein expression in adults with anaplastic large cell lymphoma. Blood 83:3913–3921, 1999.

337. Falini B, Bigerna B, Fizzotti M et al: ALK expression defines a distinct group of T/null lymphomas ("ALK lymphomas") with a wide morphological spectrum. Am J Pathol 153:875–886, 1998.

338. Jhala DN, Medeiros LJ, Lopez-Terrada D et al: Neutrophil-rich anaplastic large cell lymphoma of T-cell lineage: Report of two cases arising in HIV-positive patients. Am J Clin Pathol 114:478–482, 2000.

339. Delsol G, Al Saati T, Gatter KC et al: Coexpression of epithelial membrane antigen (EMA), Ki-1, and interleukin-2 receptor by anaplastic large cell lymphomas: Diagnostic value in so-called malignant histiocytosis. Am J Pathol 130:59–70, 1988.

340. Herbst H, Tippelmann G, Anagnostopoulos I et al: Immunoglobulin and T-cell receptor gene rearrangements in Hodgkin's disease and Ki-1 positive anaplastic large cell lymphoma: Dissociation between phenotype and genotype. Leuk Res 13:103–116, 1989.

341. Krenacs L, Wellmann A, Sorbara L et al: Cytotoxic cell antigen expression in anaplastic large cell lymphomas of T- and null-cell type and Hodgkin's disease: Evidence for distinct cellular origin. Blood 89:980–989, 1997.

342. Rassidakis GZ, Sarris AH, Herling M et al: Differential expression of BCL-2 family proteins in ALK-positive and ALK-negative anaplastic large cell lymphoma of T/null-cell lineage. Am J Pathol 159:527–535, 2001.

343. O'Connor NTJ, Stein H, Gatter KC et al: Genotypic analysis of large cell lymphomas which express the Ki-1 antigen. Histopathology 11:733–740, 1987.

344. Morris SW, Kirstein MN, Valentine MB et al: Fusion of a kinase gene, ALK, to a nucleolar protein gene, NPM in non-Hodgkin's lymphoma. Science 263:1281–1284, 1994.

345. Delsol G, Lamant L, Mariame B et al: A new subtype of large B-cell lymphoma expressing ALK kinase and lacking the 2;5 translocation. Blood 89:1483–1490, 1997.

346. Coffin CM, Patel A, Perkins S et al: ALK1 and p80 expression and chromosomal rearrangements involving 2p23 in inflammatory myofibroblastic tumor. Mod Pathol 14:569–576, 2001.

347. Willemze R, Beljaards RC: Spectrum of primary cutaneous CD30 (Ki-1)-positive lymphoproliferative disorders: A proposal for classification and guidelines for management and treatment. J Am Acad Dermatol 28:973–980, 1993.

348. Belijaards RC, Kaudewitz P, Berti E et al: Primary cutaneous CD30-positive large cell lymphoma: Definition of a new type with a favorable prognosis—A European multicenter study of 47 patients. Cancer 71:2097–2104, 1993.

349. Tomaszewski MM, Moad JC, Lupton GP: Primary cutaneous Ki-1 (CD30) positive anaplastic cell lymphoma in childhood. J Am Acad Dermatol 40:857–861, 1999.

350. Gould JW, Eppes RB, Gilliam AC et al: Solitary primary cutaneous CD30+ large cell lymphoma of natural killer cell phenotype bearing the t(2;5)(p23;q35) translocation presenting in a child. Am J Dermatopathol 22:422–428, 2000.

351. Herbst H, Sander C, Tronnier M et al: Absence of anaplastic lymphoma kinase (ALK) and Epstein-Barr virus gene products in primary cutaneous anaplastic large cell lymphoma and lymphomatoid papulosis. Br J Dermatol 137:680–686, 1997.

352. Haioun C, Gaulard P, Bourquelot P et al: Clinical and biological analysis of peripheral T-cell lymphomas: A single institution study. Leuk Lymphoma 7:449–455, 1992.

353. Lopez-Guillermo A, Cid J, Salar A et al: Peripheral T-cell lymphomas: Initial features, natural history, and prognostic factors in a series of 174 patients diagnosed according to the R.E.A.L. Classification. Ann Oncol 9:849–855, 1998.

354. Gisselbrecht C, Gaulard P, Lepage E et al: Prognostic significance of T-cell phenotype in aggressive non-Hodgkin's lymphomas. Groupe d'Etudes des Lymphomes de l' Adulte (GELA). Blood 92:76–82, 1998.

355. Yao M, Cheng AL, Su IJ et al: Clinicopathological spectrum of haemophagocytic syndrome in Epstein-Barr virus-associated peripheral T-cell lymphoma. Br J Haematol 87:535–543, 1994.

356. Cheng A-L, Chen Y-C, Wang C-H et al: Direct comparisons of peripheral T-cell lymphoma with diffuse B-cell lymphoma of comparable histologic grades—should peripheral T-cell lymphoma be considered separately? J Clin Oncol 7:725–731, 1989.

357. Suchi T, Lennert K, Tu L-Y: Histopathology and immunohistochemistry of peripheral T-cell lymphomas: A proposal for their classification. J Clin Pathol 40:995–1015, 1987.

358. Ramsay AD, Smith WJ, Earl HM et al: T-cell lymphomas in adults: A clinicopathologic study of eighteen cases. J Pathol 152:63–76, 1987.

359. Macon WR, Williams ME, Greer JP et al: Paracortical nodular T-cell lymphoma: Identification of unusual variant of peripheral T-cell lymphoma. Am J Surg Pathol 18:297–303, 1995.

360. Yamashita Y, Yatabe Y, Tsuzuki T et al: Perforin and granzyme expression in cytotoxic T-cell lymphomas. Mod Pathol 11:313–323, 1998.

361. Macon WR, Williams ME, Greer JP et al: Natural killer-like T-cell lymphomas: Aggressive lymphomas of large granular lymphocytes. Blood 87:1474–1483, 1996.

362. Petit B, Leroy K, Kanavaros P et al: Expression of p53 protein in T- and natural killer-cell lymphomas is associated with some clinicopathologic entities but rarely related to p53 mutations. Hum Pathol 32:196–204, 2001.

363. Lepretre S, Buchonnet G, Stamatoullas A et al: Chromosome abnormalities in peripheral T-cell lymphoma. Cancer Genet Cytogenet 117:71–79, 2000.

364. Frizzera G, Moran EM, Rappaport H: Angioimmunoblastic lymphadenopathy with dysproteinemia. Lancet I:1070–1073, 1974.

365. Lukes RJ, Tindle BH: Immunoblastic lymphadenopathy: A hyperimmune entity resembling Hodgkin's disease. N Engl J Med 292:1–8, 1975.

366. Feller AC, Griesser H, Schilling CV et al: Clonal gene rearrangement patterns correlate with immunophenotype and clinical parameters in patients with angioimmunoblastic lymphadenopathy. Am J Pathol 133:549–556, 1988.

367. Frizzera G, Kaneko Y, Sakurai M: Angioimmunoblastic lymphadenopathy and related disorders: A retrospective look in search of definitions. Leukemia 3:1–5, 1989.

368. Smith JL, Hodges E, Quin CT et al: Frequent T and B cell oligoclones in histologically and immunophenotypically characterized angioimmunoblastic lymphadenopathy. Am J Pathol 156:661–669, 2000.

369. Siegert W, Nerl C, Agthe A et al: Angioimmunoblastic lymphadenopathy (AILD)-type T-cell lymphoma: Prognostic impact of clinical observations and laboratory findings at presentation. The Kiel Lymphoma Study Group. Ann Oncol 6:659–664, 1995.

370. Pautier P, Devidas A, Delmer A et al: Angioimmunoblastic-like T-cell non Hodgkin's lymphoma: Outcome after chemotherapy in 33 patients and review of the literature. Leuk Lymphoma 32:545–552, 1999.

371. Pangalis GA, Moran EM, Nathwani BN et al: Angioimmunoblastic lymphadenopathy. Long-term follow up study. Cancer 52:318–321, 1983.

372. Ree HJ, Kadin ME, Kikuchi M et al: Angioimmunoblastic lymphoma (AILD-type T-cell lymphoma) with hyperplastic germinal centers. Am J Surg Pathol 22:643–655, 1998.

373. Jones D, Jorgensen JL, Shahsafaei A et al: Characteristic proliferations of reticular and dendritic cells in angioimmunoblastic lymphoma. Am J Surg Pathol 22:956–964, 1998.

374. Weiss LM, Strickler JG, Dorfman RF et al: Clonal T-cell populations in angioimmunoblastic lymphadenopathy and angioimmunoblastic lymphadenopathy-like lymphoma. Am J Pathol 122:392–397, 1986.

375. Lipford EH, Smith HR, Pittaluga S et al: Clonality of angioimmunoblastic lymphadenopathy and implications for its evolution to malignant lymphoma. J Clin Invest 79:637–642, 1987.

376. Willenbrock K, Roers A, Seidl C et al: Analysis of T-cell subpopulations in T-cell non-Hodgkin's lymphoma of angioimmunoblastic lymphadenopathy with dysproteinemia type by single target gene amplification of T cell receptor-beta gene rearrangements. Am J Pathol 158:1851–1857, 2001.

377. Godde-Salz E, Feller AC, Lennert K: Chromosomal abnormalities in lymphogranulomatosis X (Lgr X)/angioimmunoblastic lymphadenopathy (AILD). Leukemia Res 11:181–190, 1987.

378. Schlegelberger B, Feller A, Godde E et al: Stepwise development of chromosomal abnormalities in angioimmunoblastic lymphadenopathy. Cancer Genet Cytogenet 50:15–29, 1990.

379. Weiss LM, Jaffe E, Liu XF et al: Detection and localization of Epstein-Barr viral genomes in angioimmunoblastic lymphadenopathy and angioimmunoblastic lymphadenopathy-like lymphoma. Blood 79:1789–1795, 1992.

380. Nathwani BN, Rappaport H, Moran EM et al: Malignant lymphoma arising in angioimmunoblastic lymphadenopathy. Cancer 41:578–606, 1978.

381. Abruzzo LV, Schmidt K, Weiss LM et al: B cell lymphoma following angioimmunoblastic lymphadenopathy: A case with oligoclonal gene rearrangements associated with Epstein-Barr virus. Blood 82:241–246, 1993.

382. Weiss LM, Trela MJ, Cleary ML et al: Frequent immunoglobulin and T-cell receptor gene rearrangements in "histiocytic" neoplasms. Am J Pathol 121:369–373, 1985.

383. Copie-Bergman C, Wotherspoon AC, Norton AJ et al: True histiocytic lymphoma: A morphologic, immunohistochemical, and molecular genetic study of 13 cases. Am J Surg Pathol 22:1386–1392, 1998.

384. Kamel OW, Gocke CD, Kell DL et al: True histiocytic lymphoma: A study of 12 cases based on current definition. Leuk Lymphoma 18:81–86, 1995.

385. Perez-Ordonez B, Rosai J: Follicular dendritic cell tumor: Review of the entity. Semin Diagn Pathol 15:144–154, 1988.

386. Gaertner EM, Tsokos M, Derringer GA et al: Interdigitating dendritic cell sarcoma. A report of four cases and review of the literature. Am J Clin Pathol 115:589–597, 2001.

387. Urba WJ, Longo DL: Hodgkin's disease. N Engl J Med 326:678–687, 1992.

388. Hasenclever D, Diehl V. A prognostic score for advanced Hodgkin's disease. International Prognostic Factors Project on Advanced Hodgkin's disease. N Engl J Med 339:1506–1514, 1998.

389. Kadin ME, Glatstein E, Dorfman RF: Clinicopathologic studies of 117 untreated patients subjected to laparotomy for the staging of Hodgkin's disease. Cancer 27:1277–1294, 1971.

390. Berard CW, Thomas LB, Axtell LM et al: The relationship of histopathological subtype to clinical stage of Hodgkin's disease at diagnosis. Cancer Res 31:1776–1785, 1971.

391. Jackson H, Parker F: Hodgkin's disease. II. Pathology. N Engl J Med 231:35–44, 1944.

392. Lukes RJ, Butler JJ: The pathology and nomenclature of Hodgkin's disease. Cancer Res 26:1063–1083, 1968.

393. Rappaport H, Berard CW, Butler JJ et al: Report of the committee on histopathological criteria contributing to staging of Hodgkin's disease. Cancer Res 31:1864–1865, 1971.

394. Colby TV, Hoppe RT, Warnke RA: Hodgkin's disease: A clinico-pathologic study of 659 cases. Cancer 49:1848–1858, 1982.

395. Medeiros LJ, Greiner TC: Hodgkin's disease. Cancer 75 (Suppl.):357–369, 1995.

396. Diehl V, Sextro M, Franklin J et al: Clinical presentation, course, and prognostic factors in lymphocyte predominant Hodgkin's disease and lymphocyte-rich classical Hodgkin's disease: Report from the European Task Force on Lymphoma Project on Lymphocyte-Predominant Hodgkin's Disease. J Clin Oncol 17:776–783, 1999.

397. Poppema S, Kaiserling E, Lennert K: Hodgkin's disease with lymphocytic predominance, nodular type (nodular paragranuloma) and progressively transformed germinal centers—a cytohistological study. Histopathology 3:295–308, 1979.

398. Stein H, Hansmann ML, Lennert K et al: Reed-Sternberg and Hodgkin cells in lymphocyte-predominant Hodgkin's disease of nodular subtype contain J chain. Am J Clin Pathol 86:292–297, 1986.

399. Schmid C, Sargent C, Isaacson PG: L and H cells of nodular lymphocyte predominant Hodgkin's disease show immunoglobulin light-chain restriction. Am J Pathol 139:1281–1289, 1991.

400. Raghavachar A, Binder T, Bartram CR: Immunoglobulin and T-cell receptor gene rearrangements in Hodgkin's disease. Cancer Res 48:3591–3594, 1988.

401. Griesser H, Feller AC, Mak TW et al: Clonal rearrangements of T-cell receptor and immunoglobulin genes and immunophenotypic antigen expression in different subclasses of Hodgkin's disease. Int J Cancer 40:157–160, 1987.

402. Braeuninger A, Kuppers R, Strickler JG et al: Hodgkin and Reed-Sternberg cells in lymphocyte predominance Hodgkin disease represent clonal populations of germinal center-derived tumor B cells. Proc Natl Acad Sci USA 94:9337–9342, 1997.

403. Marafioti T, Hummel M, Anagnostopoulos I et al: Origin of nodular lymphocyte-predominant Hodgkin's disease from a clonal expansion of highly mutated germinal-center B cells. N Engl J Med 337:453–458, 1997.

404. Ohno T, Stribley JA, Wu G et al: Clonality in nodular lymphocyte-predominant Hodgkin's disease. N Engl J Med 337:459–465, 1997.

405. Franke S, Wlodarska I, Maes B et al: Lymphocyte predominance Hodgkin disease is characterized by recurrent genomic imbalances. Blood 97:1845–1853, 2001.

406. Anagnostopoulos I, Hansmann M-L, Franssila K et al: European Task Force on Lymphoma project on lymphocyte predominance Hodgkin disease: Histologic and immunohistologic analysis of submitted cases reveals 2 types of Hodgkin disease with a nodular pattern and abundant lymphocytes. Blood 96:1889–1899, 2000.

407. MacLennan KA, Bennett MH, Tu A et al: Relationship of histopathologic features to survival and relapse in nodular sclerosing Hodgkin's disease: A study of 1659 patients. Cancer 64:1686–1693, 1989.

408. Kant JA, Hubbard SM, Longo DL et al: The pathologic and clinical heterogeneity of lymphocyte-depleted Hodgkin's disease. J Clin Oncol 4:284–284, 1986.

409. Strickler JG, Michie SA, Warnke RA et al: The "syncytial variant" of nodular sclerosing Hodgkin's disease. Am J Surg Pathol 10:470–477, 1986.

410. Cozen W, Katz J, Mack TM: Risk patterns of Hodgkin's disease in Los Angeles vary by cell type. Cancer Epidemiol Biomarkers Prev 1:261–268, 1992.

411. Neiman RS, Rosen PJ, Lukes RJ: Lymphocyte-depletion Hodgkin's disease: A clinicopathologic entity. N Engl J Med 288:751–755, 1973.

412. Greer JP, Kinney MC, Cousar JB et al: Lymphocyte-depleted Hodgkin's disease: Clinicopathologic review of 25 patients. Am J Med 81:208–214, 1986.

413. Glaser SL, Swartz WG: Time trends in Hodgkin's disease incidence: The role of diagnostic accuracy. Cancer 66:2196–2204, 1990.

414. Doggett RS, Colby TV, Dorfman RF: Interfollicular Hodgkin's disease. Am J Surg Pathol 7:145–149, 1983.

415. Colby TV, Warnke RA: The histology of the initial relapse of Hodgkin's disease. Cancer 45:289–292, 1980.

416. Sundeen J, Lipford E, Uppenkamp M et al: Rearranged antigen receptor genes in Hodgkin's disease. Blood 70:96–103, 1987.

417. Agnarsson BA, Kadin ME: The immunophenotype of Reed-Sternberg cells: A study of 50 cases using fixed frozen sections. Cancer 63:2083–2087, 1989.

418. Casey TT, Olson SJ, Cousar JB et al: Immunophenotypes of Reed-Sternberg cells: A study of 19 cases of Hodgkin's disease in plastic-embedded sections. Blood 74:2624–2628, 1989.

419. Chittal SM, Caveriviere P, Schwarting R et al: Monoclonal antibodies in the diagnosis of Hodgkin's disease: The search for a rational panel. Am J Surg Pathol 12:9–21, 1988.

420. Medeiros LJ, Weiss LM, Warnke RA et al: Utility of combining antigranulocyte and antileukocyte antibodies in differentiating Hodgkin's disease from non-Hodgkin's lymphoma. Cancer 62:2475–2481, 1988.

421. Foss HD, Reusch R, Demel G et al: Frequent expression of the B-cell-specific activator protein in Reed-Sternberg cells of classical Hodgkin's disease provides further evidence for its B-cell origin. Blood 94:3108–3113, 1999.

422. Rassidakis GZ, Medeiros LJ, Viviani S et al: CD20 expression in Hodgkin and Reed-Sternberg cells of classical Hodgkin's disease: Associations with presenting features and clinical outcome. J Clin Oncol 20:1278–1287, 2002.

423. Seitz V, Hummel M, Marafioti T et al: Detection of clonal T-cell receptor gamma chain gene rearrangements in Reed-Sternberg cells of classic Hodkin's disease. Blood 95:3020–3024, 2000.

424. Rassidakis GZ, Medeiros LJ, Vassilakopoulos TP et al: BCL-2 expression in Hodgkin and Reed-Steinberg cells of classical Hodgkin's disease predicts a poorer prognosis in patients treated with ABVD or equivalent regimens. Blood 100:3935–3941, 2002.

425. Bargou RC, Leng C, Krappmann D et al: High-level nuclear NF-kappa B and Oct-2 is a common feature of cultured Hodgkin/Reed-Sternberg cells. Blood 87:4340–4347, 1996.

426. Cabanillas F: A review and interpretation of cytogenetic abnormalities identified in Hodgkin's disease. Hematol Oncol 6:271–274, 1988.

427. Tilly H, Bastard C, Delastre T et al: Cytogenetic studies in untreated Hodgkin's disease. Blood 77:1298–1304, 1991.

428. Weiss LM, Strickler JG, Hu E et al: Immunoglobulin gene rearrangements in Hodgkin's disease. Hum Pathol 17:1009–1014, 1986.

429. Marafioti T, Hummel M, Foss HD et al: Hodgkin and Reed-Sternberg cells represent an expansion of a single clone originating from a germinal center B-cell with functional immunoglobulin gene rearrangements but defective immunoglobulin transcription. Blood 95:1443–1450, 2000.

430. Stetler-Stevenson M, Crush-Stanton C, Cossman J: Involvement of the bcl-2 gene in Hodgkin's disease. J Natl Cancer Inst 82:855–858, 1990.

431. Gravel S, Delsol G, Al Saati T: Single-cell analysis of the t(14;18)(q32;q21) chromosomal translocation in Hodgkin's disease demonstrates the absence of this translocation in neoplastic Hodgkin and Reed-Sternberg cells. Blood 91:2866–2874, 1998.

432. Henle W, Henle G: Epstein-Barr virus-related serology in Hodgkin's disease. Natl Cancer Inst Monogr 36:79–84, 1973.

433. Kvale G, Hoiby EA, Pedersen E: Hodgkin's disease in patients with previous infectious mononucleosis. Int J Cancer 23:593–597, 1979.

434. Mueller N, Evans A, Harris NL et al: Hodgkin's disease and Epstein-Barr virus: Altered antibody pattern before diagnosis. N Engl J Med 320:689–695, 1989.

435. Weiss LM, Chen YY, Liu XF et al: Epstein-Barr virus and Hodgkin's disease: A correlative *in situ* hybridization and polymerase chain reaction study. Am J Pathol 138:1259–1265, 1991.

436. Anagnostopoulos I, Herbst H, Niedobitek GF et al: Demonstration of monoclonal EBV genomes in Hodgkin's disease and Ki-1 positive anaplastic large cell lymphoma by combined Southern blot and *in situ* hybridization. Blood 74:810–816, 1989.

437. Pallesen G, Hamilton-Dutoit SJ, Rowe M et al: Expression of Epstein-Barr virus latent gene products in tumour cells of Hodgkin's disease. Lancet 337:320–322, 1991.

438. Jarrett RF, Gallagher A, Jones DB et al: Detection of Epstein-Barr virus genomes in Hodgkin's disease: Relation to age. J Clin Pathol 44:844–848, 1991.

439. Siebert JD, Ambinder RF, Napoli VM et al: Human immunodeficiency virus-associated Hodgkin's disease contains latent, not replicative, Epstein-Barr virus. Hum Pathol 26:1191–1195, 1995.

440. MacMahon B: Epidemiology of Hodgkin's disease. Cancer Res 26:1189–1201, 1966.

441. Gutensohn N, Cole P: Childhood social environment and Hodgkin's disease. N Engl J Med 304:135–140, 1982.

442. Gutensohn NM: Social class and age at diagnosis of Hodgkin's disease: New epidemiologic evidence for the "two disease hypothesis." Cancer Treat Rep 66:689–695, 1982.

443. Kim H, Hendrickson MR, Dorfman RF: Composite lymphoma. Cancer 40:959–976, 1977.

444. Gonzalez CL, Medeiros LJ, Jaffe ES: Composite lymphoma. A clinicopathologic analysis of nine patients with Hodgkin's disease and B-cell non-Hodgkin's lymphoma. Am J Clin Pathol 96:81–89, 1991.

445. Jaffe ES, Zarate-Osorno A, Kingma DW et al: The interrelationship between Hodgkin's disease and non-Hodgkin's lymphomas. Ann Oncol 5 (Suppl. 1):7–11, 1994.

446. Kingma DW, Medeiros LJ, Barletta J et al: Epstein-Barr virus is infrequently identified in non-Hodgkin's lymphomas associated with Hodgkin's disease. Am J Surg Pathol 18:48–61, 1994.

447. Brauninger A, Hansmann ML, Strickler JG et al: Identification of common germinal-center B-cell precursors in patients with both Hodgkin's disease and non-Hodgkin's lymphoma. N Engl J Med 340:1239–1247, 1999.

448. Kuppers R, Sousa AB, Baur AS et al: Common germinal-center B-cell origin of the malignant cells in two composite lymphomas, involving classical Hodgkin's disease and either follicular lymphoma or B-CLL. Mol Med 7:285–292, 2001.

41

Immunology of the Lymphomas

Rupesh Parikh and Howard Ozer

Recent discoveries in basic immunology have made a major impact on our understanding and therapy of lymphoma in humans. Early investigations led to the identification of distinct subpopulations of lymphocytes, the T (thymic-derived) and B (bursa-equivalent) lymphocytes. Cell-mediated immunity was found to be a function of T lymphocytes, while antibody responses (humoral immunity) were found to be a function of B lymphocytes. T and B cells were differentiated by the presence of certain antigens or proteins on their cell surfaces, specifically erythrocyte rosette receptors (T) and surface immunoglobulins (B). It was later noted that different stages of lymphocyte maturation could be distinguished by the combination of particular antigens, generally glycoproteins, present on the cell surface, termed differentiation antigens. These antigens may be identified by specific, pure hybridoma antibodies raised against them (monoclonal antibodies). The combination of surface antigens present on a particular cell was designated its immunophenotype. The use of immunophenotypes has been helpful in classifying lymphomas into groups of B- or T-cell types and has provided insight into lymphocyte maturation. The result has been the development of new schemas of lymphocyte differentiation and new histologic classification systems attempting to correlate histology with phenotype. The progress in technology at the molecular level permits detection of the earliest commitments to B- and T-lymphoid differentiation and serves to confirm immunophenotypic data.

Our understanding of the immunoregulatory functions of T and B lymphocytes and their interactions has also been facilitated by recent advances in immunology. T cells can be divided into a subset with helper-inducer regulatory functions and a subset that suppresses both B- and T-cell function. These groups can now be identified in humans by monoclonal antibodies as well as by functional assays. Unfortunately, function is not uniformly correlated with phenotype with the lymphoproliferative neoplasms. One major advance in our understanding of immunologic defects has been the recognition that normal immune function requires tightly regulated control by multiple cell subsets for its expression. Thus, abnormalities of effector cell function such as deficits of humoral immunity (immunoglobulin synthesis) can occur as a result of abnormalities in either regulatory T-cell function or because of primary B-cell defects. Cell-mediated immune abnormalities are primarily a reflection of T-cell defects alone but may involve abnor-

malities in one or another T subset involved in the regulatory cascade. The expression of abnormal T-cell immunity can occur functionally either as an inability to exert normal suppressor or helper function or as excessive helper or suppressor function. There are presently several available methods of screening for specific cell-mediated and humoral immune deficits that complement the more global methods of measuring for anergy or decreased production of serum immunoglobulins.

As more becomes known about lymphocyte differentiation and function, the role of abnormal immune responses in the development and perpetuation of lymphomas may be elucidated. The efficacy of therapy with agents, now termed biologic response modifiers, that are employed to improve or restore abnormal immune function is currently an area of intense investigation. It is clear that, at least in certain individuals, such therapy does have antineoplastic effects, although the precise mechanism of antitumor activity and whether they truly involve immunomodulation are not yet clear.

IMMUNOLOGIC PHENOTYPING

The phenotypic analysis of lymphomas has yielded practical applications for diagnosis and furthered our knowledge of lymphocyte differentiation. Understanding the development of lymphocytes from stem cells to mature, immunocompetent T and B cells is made easier by the demonstration of lineage-specific differentiation antigens. However, the critical initial step is to subclassify lymphoproliferative neoplasms within the T- and B-cell category because several of these differentiation antigens, for example, immune-associated-like antigen (Ia) determinants, are not necessarily T or B specific. The ability to detect the commitment to B- or T-cell lineage at an earlier stage is now possible through analysis of immunoglobulin gene or T-cell receptor (TCR) gene rearrangements.

The relative distribution of subsets within the T and B populations is fairly constant. An increased proportion of a single phenotype within the T or B categories may represent an increase in a single malignant clone of cells. This disproportionate increase has been termed *clonal excess*. Abnormal phenotypic distributions can be demonstrated for either T or B cells. However, clonal expansion of a single subset of cells does not connote malignancy. Within the B-cell population, an increase in cells bearing κ light chains relative to λ light chains (or vice versa) is the most straightforward way to identify abnormal clonal increases.

The ability to form spontaneous rosettes with sheep red blood cells (E rosettes) is considered an exclusive property of T lymphocytes. There have, however, been rare reports of false-positive E rosetting with B cells. This may occur through an interaction of B cells, erythrocytes, and sheep red blood cell-specific immunoglobulins. In some instances, lymphocytes that fail to form E rosettes react convincingly with pan-T monoclonal antibodies. This is a particularly common problem in Hodgkin's disease (HD). The putative mechanisms for this are discussed at length with the other immunologic abnormalities of HD.

The criteria utilized to establish the B-cell nature of a particular lymphoma are highly accurate but complicated. Any cell capable of synthesizing immunoglobulin, even by genetic criteria, is considered of B-cell origin. This can be rigorously demonstrated by removing all existing surface immunoglobulin. In lieu of this time-consuming procedure, with its limitations of cell viability, the demonstration of surface or cytoplasmic immunoglobulin showing restriction of the light chain (only κ or λ) is considered sufficient to conclude that a malignant cell is of B origin.[1] The demonstration of surface immunoglobulin alone is not sufficient to identify B cells conclusively since adsorption or uptake by Fc receptors of exogenous immunoglobulin in the serum will give a false-positive result, although in these cases there will be no light chain restriction.[2,3] Conversely, adsorption of exogenous cytophilic immunoglobulin may give a falsely polyclonal finding for malignant monoclonal B cells that also express Fc receptors. In both these instances, the demonstration of J chains, present only in cells that synthesize immunoglobulin, may clarify the nature of the cell in question.[4,5]

In addition to E rosetting and monoclonal immunoglobulin detection, studies screening for surface receptors for the Fc portion of immunoglobulin G (IgG) or immunoglobulin M (IgM), receptors for complement (C3b and C3d), presence of Ia (immune-associated-like antigens comparable to HLA-DR antigens), and common acute lymphocytic leukemia (ALL) antigen (CD10 formerly CALLA) are considered part of the phenotypic profile of lymphoma cells. Although Fc receptors and complement receptors were originally detected by the formation of rosettes when cells were incubated with sheep erythrocytes coated with immunoglobulin (EA) or immunoglobulin and complement (EAC), these receptors as well as CD10 and Ia antigens are now identified by specific monoclonal antibodies.

Complement receptors are found primarily on B cells and Fc receptors are found on histiocytes and monocytes.[6–8] The Ia antigens are found on B cells, monocytes, and activated T cells, and CD10 is found on immature T and B cells.[9,10] The presence of Fc and complement receptors is nonspecific and, as with Ia and common acute lymphocytic leukemia antigen (CD10), may be more helpful in defining developmental stages of hematopoietic neoplasms than a distinct cell type. In difficult cases, cytochemistry is a necessary adjunct to differentiate between monocytes and T and B cells.[11]

The anti-T monoclonal antibody reagent identifies thymic (CD1) and mature (CD3) cells with CD5 on both populations. The mature functional subsets of helper/inducer (CD4), suppressor/cytotoxic natural killer cells (CD16), and activated T (OKT9) specific for the transferrin receptor; OKT10 specific for precursor; and activated T cells can also be defined. The early use of monoclonal anti-B antibodies, although promising, has been less illuminating with regard to maturational sequence than T-cell reagents. The BA-1, BA-2, BA-3 series of anti-B monoclonal antibodies were developed against an ALL cell line. They all react with cells in early B-cell developmental stages. BA-1 is a pan-B antibody that also reacts with thymic cells and mature granulocytes. BA-2 reacts with chronic lymphocytic leukemia (CLL) cells and thymic cells as well as immature B

cells. The reactive antigen is p24, a surface protein. BA-3 reacts with the common ALL antigen (CD10) and thus has the same significance as CD10 positivity.[12]

The B-1 (CD20) antigen is a pan-B antigen present on pre-B and early B cells, 50 percent of non-T ALL, 75 percent of CD10-positive ALL, and 50 percent of chronic myelocytic leukemia (CML) in blast crisis.[13] The B-2 antigen (CD21) is present on cells beyond the pre-B cell but is lost in the transformation to lymphoblasts. Unlike B-1 and B-4, it is not expressed on mitogen-stimulated normal B cells.[14] The B-2 antigen has subsequently been found to be the C3d receptor and the receptor for Epstein-Barr virus (EBV), by which viral entry into the cell is usually mediated.[15] The B-4 antigen (CD19) is present on very early B-cell precursors, increases with B-cell activation, and then is lost in the terminal stages of B-cell differentiation.[16] The B-4 antigen is present on normal, malignant, and mitogen-stimulated B cells as well as the majority of cell lines of CML in blast crisis and non-T ALL lines.

In general, a panel comprising all or most of the tests outlined above is used in phenotyping non-Hodgkin's lymphomas. The results of phenotyping are often heterogeneous within a group of cytologically identical tissues from different individuals but homogeneous or minimally altered among different samples from the same individual or cultured cell line taken sequentially over time.[17–22]

The confirmation of T or B lineage depends on immunophenotypic analysis and, in some instances, genotypic analysis also. The use of a panel of monoclonal antibodies to identify immunophenotypic patterns, not simply light chain restriction or E rosette formation, has redefined the approach to intermediate and high grade lymphomas. It has been demonstrated that loss of pan-T antigens including the E rosette receptor is a common finding in T-cell lymphomas; lack of light chain restriction is also fairly common in intermediate and high grade B-cell lymphomas. Recent studies show that peripheral T-cell lymphomas are much more common in the United States and Europe than previously reported (16 to 42 percent), while null phenotypes account for 10 percent or less of non-Hodgkin's lymphomas. The use of gene rearrangement studies further identifies B or T lineage in some null or indeterminate cases.[23]

The use of phenotyping to assess response to therapy or detect subclinical disease is still in the experimental stages. Ault[24] first described the use of cytofluorographic techniques to rapidly screen large numbers of cells for κ and λ immunofluorescent staining. The sensitivity of the original technique permitted detection of a monoclonal B-cell population constituting less than 10 percent of the cells screened. A comparison of healthy normal volunteers, hospitalized patients without neoplasms, patients with non-Hodgkin's lymphomas in complete remission, and those with active non-Hodgkin's lymphomas without and with a leukemic phase yielded the following data. The hospitalized patients had relative increases of both κ- and λ-positive cells, but the κ/λ ratios were not significantly different in either light chain type to indicate the presence of a monoclonal population. Four of eight patients in complete remission and 44 percent of patients with active disease but without a leukemic phase had abnormal ratios of κ to λ but in only 32 percent of active nonleukemic non-Hodgkin's lymphoma patients was a distinct monoclonal pattern seen. All of the patients with leukemic non-Hodgkin's lymphoma had monoclonal patterns, that is, a distinct clonal excess. Other series utilizing more sensitive techniques subsequently confirmed clonal excess in up to 100 percent of B-cell non-Hodgkin's lymphoma patients with leukemia, CLL, multiple myeloma (MM), and Waldenström's macroglobulinemia (WM). Approximately 30 percent of B-cell non-Hodgkin's lymphoma without identifiable circulating leukemic cells revealed clonal excess.[25–27] The same techniques have also demonstrated clonal excess in pleural effusions with and without positive malignant cytology and in bone marrow biopsy specimens with no evidence or equivocal evidence of malignant involvement. In all instances, there was concordance among peripheral blood, bone marrow, lymph node, and pleural fluid as to light chain type.[26,28] Preliminary studies in a large series have shown clonal excess to be more common in lymph node and splenic tissue than in peripheral blood. Also, clonal excess occurs more frequently in diffuse than follicular lymphomas, and more often in advanced stages of disease and in active or progressing disease.[29] Multivariate analysis studies currently underway in our own laboratory are examining the utility of clonal excess in predicting relapse or remission.

Determination of clonal excess has also proved valuable in determining the benign or malignant nature of extranodal lymphocytic hyperplastic responses in the skin and gastrointestinal tract, which are always polyclonal, and can be distinguished from well-differentiated, nodular neoplastic B-cell proliferations, which should be monoclonal. The distinction between lymphocytic neoplasms, undifferentiated adenocarcinoma, neuroblastoma, and oat cell carcinoma of the lung, all of which appear as small to large round cells, is a diagnostic challenge, particularly in metastatic disease. In these instances, monoclonal antibodies restricted to lymphocytes, T- or B-cell subsets, or the presence of light chain restriction can effectively rule in the lymphoid neoplasms.[30–32]

Similar applications of monoclonal anti-T antibodies are limited by the relatively wide normal range of distribution of T-cell subsets, and large-scale studies have not yet been done. Monoclonal antibodies to suppressor or helper subsets do show increases in the proportion of the malignant phenotype with near absence of the normal counterpart subset in the peripheral blood and bone marrow in T-cell CLL (T-CLL) and Sézary syndrome may be useful in screening for subclinical disease in these entities.[33]

In addition to phenotypic analysis, gene rearrangement studies are increasingly employed to establish the lymphoid nature of undifferentiated tumors, to assign B- and T-cell phenotypes in null lymphomas, to distinguish between reactive and malignant lymphoid aggregates, and in the detection of subclinical disease. In the early and mid-1980s, molecular techniques identifying the immunoglobulin gene and B chain of the TCR led to the demonstration of clonal gene rearrangements in B- and T-cell neoplasms, respectively.[34–39] Rearrangement of these genes leads to a unique enzyme restriction site, distinct from germline DNA, such that resultant DNA fragments differ in size from germline DNA-derived fragments. Clonal expansion of the malignant T or B cells increases the amount of clonally rearranged DNA to within the levels of sensitivity of Southern blot analysis. Immunoglobulin rearrangements have shown concordance with surface immunoglobulin phenotype and are also detectable in B-cell neoplasms that lack surface and cytoplasmic immunoglobulin.[34–36] Rearrangements of the TCR gene, primarily β and γ chains, have demonstrated clonal rearrangements for a variety of T-cell neoplasms, including T-CLL, mycosis fungoides, peripheral T-cell lymphomas, adult T-cell leukemia/lymphoma, and T-cell ALL.[37–39] The rearrangement of the locus of the TCR gene appears to be indicative of clonality but not lineage.[40] Due to the sensitivity of these techniques, it is possible to detect subclinical involvement of lymph nodes and peripheral blood.[41] The technology of gene rearrangement analysis has been applied to detection of subclinical disease in a fashion similar to the clonal excess studies. Brada et al.[41] reported on a group of 50 patients with active non-Hodgkin's lymphoma. Peripheral blood from these patients was analyzed for clonal rearrangements of the immunoglobulin gene and β chain of the TCR gene. Although only 5 patients had cytologically malignant circulating lymphocytes, 19 patients (38 percent) had evidence of a circulating clonal population of lymphocytes including 4 of 5 patients with clinically malignant circulating peripheral blood cells. In the majority of these cases, the circulating lymphocytes had rearrangements that were identical to the arrangements found in the involved sites. However, a minority of patients demonstrated clonal rearrangements that were different from those of the histologically malignant population. The incidence of a circulating clonal population of lymphocytes was significantly higher in advanced stages of disease (54 percent versus 18 percent) but not in low grade histologies (45 percent versus 31 percent). Seventy percent of patients with bone marrow involvement and 30 percent of patients without bone marrow involvement had clonal rearrangement of the circulating lymphocytes. Two of 10 patients with cytologically uninvolved bone marrow had detectable clonal rearrangements of cells obtained by bone marrow aspiration.

The significance of the detection of clinically inapparent malignant clones in some cases of pseudolymphomas, angioimmunoblastic lymphadenopathy with dysproteinemia (AILD), and reactive hyperplasias is not clear. Long-term follow-up of such patients is necessary to determine whether all cases of monoclonal expansion signify malignancy or to identify a subset of patients within this group who are at risk. In up to 10 percent of lymphomas, clonal TCR and immunoglobulin rearrangements may occur simultaneously.[42] In most of these instances, only the heavy chain of the immunoglobulin gene is rearranged, and this finding occurs more frequently in very early maturational stages of lymphoid development.

The major application of immunologic phenotyping has been to further subdivide the non-Hodgkin's lymphomas into groups of comparable cellular origin as an aid to studying their natural history, differences in biologic behavior, and response to therapy. The non-Hodgkin's lymphomas comprise a morphologically heterogeneous group of malignant lymphoid cell types. The Rappaport classification preceded acquisition of the current wealth of immunologic knowledge, but its continued wide acceptance and usage reflect its prognostic value. The basis of this system is division by nodal architecture (nodular or diffuse) and cytologic appearance (lymphocytic versus histiocytic). Data now available clearly show that most "histiocytic" cells are lymphocytes.[43]

The International Working Formulation schema was developed as a uniform classification system with prognostic significance.[44] Although phenotypic analysis was not included in this system, clearly identifiable subgroups of T- and B-lineage lymphomas (mycosis fungoides/Sézary syndrome, lymphoblastic lymphoma, follicular lymphomas, Burkitt's lymphoma) are grouped separately. Attempts to correlate histologic appearance with T and B lineage has been the aim of other classification systems, most successfully accomplished by the Lukes-Collins and the Kiel classifications. The Kiel system was recently revised to reclassify and expand the designations for T-lineage lymphomas, specifically the peripheral (post-thymic) T-cell lymphomas.[45] The revised system grouped T-cell lymphomas broadly into low and high grade categories with an attempt to correlate histologic appearance, clinical presentation, and immunophenotype. Since most studies of peripheral T-cell lymphomas have had difficulty in histologic subclassification via the Working Formulation, an alternate system as proposed by Suchi et al.[45] is clearly useful.

Investigators at Stanford have retrospectively analyzed 515 cases of histologically malignant non-Hodgkin's lymphomas with a panel of monoclonal antibodies to determine the pattern of staining.[23] Thirty-one cases of reactive lesions from node (22), spleen (3), skin (3), lung (1), and nasopharynx (2), 6 cases of HD, and 40 cases of benign inflammatory skin lesions served as controls.

Among 297 cases of B-lineage lymphomas, two-thirds demonstrated monoclonal light chain restriction and no case demonstrated polyclonal expression. Light chain restriction was a less common finding for diffuse large cell, diffuse small cell (82 percent), and small noncleaved cell (80 percent) histologies. Aside from light chain restriction, there were six other immunophenotypic patterns seen among B-lineage lymphomas. These included 1. light chain-negative germinal centers (25 percent of cases were negative and 8 percent of B-lineage lymphomas had uninterpretable staining due to high background), 2. Leu-1 (CD5) reactivity, 3. L60 reactivity, 4. concurrent Ki-67 and 41H reactivity, 5. loss of pan-B antigens, CD22, CD20, CD19, and MB-1, and 6. loss of the LFA-1 antigen.

Leu-1 (CD5) is found on most peripheral T cells and thymocytes, some B-lineage lymphomas and leukemias, particularly CLL, and 2 percent of normal B cells but is not found in reactive lymphoid infiltrates. L60 also binds primarily to T cells and some malignant B-cell lymphomas but rarely with reactive or benign B-cell populations. The monoclonal antibody 41H was raised against hairy cell leukemia and identifies plasma cells and nonproliferating B cells as well as malignant B cells. Coupling reactivity to Ki-67, which is negative to benign proliferating B-cell lesions, with 41H reactivity, identified 50 to 80 percent of B-lineage lymphomas in this series. The presence of pan-B antigens and LFA-1 on benign B-cell proliferative lesions is universal, whereas 25 percent of B-lineage lymphomas lack one or more of the pan-B-cell antigens and 36 to 76 percent of B-lineage lymphomas lacked the entire LFA-1 antigen or the α or β chain only.

The T-cell-lineage lymphomas are primarily identified by abnormal antigen expression, which has been divided into 1. loss of pan-T antigens, 2. loss or coexpression of T-subset antigens, 3. Leu-6 reactivity, and 4. MB-1 reactivity. Loss of one or more of pan-T antigens (CD2, CD3, CD5, and CD7) was demonstrable in 76 percent of peripheral T-cell lymphomas (exclusive of mycosis), 64 percent of mycosis fungoides cases, and 20 percent of lymphoblastic lymphomas. Loss of other antigens, such as L60 and LFA-1, was uncommon, and loss of Leu-8 was relatively nonspecific.

Loss of T-subset antigens for helper/inducer (CD4) and cytotoxic/suppressor (CD8) subsets or simultaneous expression of each marker was rarely noted in normal tissues outside the thymus. Lack of both these antigens was present in 17 percent of nonmycosis peripheral T-cell lymphomas and 40 percent of lymphoblastic lymphomas, while simultaneous expression of both CD4 and CD8 occurred in 49 percent of lymphoblastic lymphomas but was rare (1 percent) in peripheral T-cell lymphomas. Reactivity with Leu-6 (CD1) has been detected on dendritic cells and cortical thymocytes but not on benign peripheral T-cell populations or peripheral T-cell lymphomas. In contrast, 54 percent of lymphoblastic lymphomas were Leu-6 positive. The antigen MB-1, a pan-B-cell antigen found normally on peripheral blood and tonsillar B cells but not normal T cells, was found to react with a minority of peripheral T-cell lymphomas.

The pattern of immunophenotypic analysis of B-lineage lymphomas in this series did not yield additional prognostic information or aid in classification of these lymphomas. By contrast, the immunophenotype of T-lineage lymphomas did correlate with either lymphoblastic or peripheral T-cell histologies.

Aside from distinguishing between T- and B-cell lymphomas, phenotyping also appears to shed light on the differentiation of normal lymphocytes and the malignant transformation of lymphomas. The cases in which initial phenotyping was done invariably show persistence of major phenotype (T- or B-cell type) with few changes in surface receptors and identical heavy and light chain type in histologically transformed specimens.[17,19,21,22,46] The occasional patient in whom the heavy chain changes on subsequent biopsies may be a result of natural maturation, processes similar to those observed in B-cell cultures where μ/γ progresses to γ/α alone or switches to a γ/α heavy chain.[47] The prevailing theory is that the development of lymphoma cells parallels that of normal lymphoid tissue, with blocks occurring at various stages of development. This results in the heterogeneity of immunologic phenotypes in non-Hodgkin's lymphoma.[21] Thus, comparison of phenotypes from normal thymus, tonsils, and peripheral blood with lymphomatous tissue should be similar at equivalent stages of development. This theory fails to account for cells for which no normal counterpart has clearly been identified, as with hairy cell leukemia.

The Lukes-Collins schema of B-cell maturation would place small, well-differentiated lymphocytes as early B cells with progressive development through follicular center cells (small cleaved to large cleaved to small noncleaved to large noncleaved) to immunoblastic lymphoma or multiple myeloma.[48] The T cells would mature from pre-T to convoluted thymic cells to mature T cells to functionally active effector cells (i.e., Sézary cells). The transformation from CLL to Richter's would thus be considered progression to a more mature cell type via a "switched on" transformation process, while conversion of MM to an immunoblastic cell type would result from dedifferentiation.[49,50] The B schema of development differs little from previous convention except in the classification of CLL as an immature cell as opposed to a very mature cell. In this ordering, the intermediately mature forms are more virulent than the least and most differentiated forms.

Habeshaw, using the Kiel classification, proposed a very similar sequence to that of Lukes. The B-cell schema he proposes begins with the pre-B-cell ALL cells progressing to CLL lymphocytes, then to germinal center cells (centroblastic/centrocytic), and finally immunoblastic cells or plasma cells. T-cell differentiation progresses from prethymic to thymic to mature T and finally to functional peripheral T cells. The maturation and proliferation schema constructed by Minowada et al.[21] from 55 long-term cell lines concurs with that of Lukes and Habeshaw.

The phenotypic maturation begins with the progenitor B cell, which possesses terminal deoxynucleotidyl transferase (TdT) activity, has Ia positivity, and may have immunoglobulin heavy chain gene rearrangement.[51] As the B cell matures to the pre-B stage, it retains TdT activity and sequentially acquires the CD10, CD19, and CD20 antigens and genotypically rearranges the immunoglobulin heavy chain gene and then the light chain gene. The early B-cell stage is characterized by loss of TdT activity and the CD10 antigen and acquisition of the mouse rosette receptor and small amounts of surface immunoglobulin. Intermediate B cells express receptors for complement and Fc. These latter two stages correspond to the arrested developmental stages of CLL and small lymphocytic lymphomas. Mature B cells show variable expression of CD10 and CD21 and loss of the mouse erythrocyte receptor. These antigens (CD10, CD21) are lost in the plasmacytoid B-cell stage, at which point PC-1 and PCA-1 begin to appear. The terminal stage of B-cell maturation, the plasma cell, expresses PC-1 and PCA-1 and may express Ia but loses complement and Fc receptors and the pan-B antigens CD19 and CD20.

T-cell maturation progresses through three stages of thymocyte differentiation: 1. The early thymocyte (group I), which expresses CD5 and CD7 with or without CD2; 2. the common thymocyte (group II), which is CD2, CD5, and CD7 positive and now expresses CD1, CD4, and CD8 with variable CD3 positivity; and 3. the mature thymocyte (group III), which no longer expresses CD1 nor coexpresses CD4 and CD8. The mature thymocyte expresses the pan-T antigens CD2, CD5, and CD7 and the CD3 antigen. Mature T cells also express pan-T antigens CD2, CD5, and CD7 and CD3 with variable Fc receptor positivity. As with mature thymocytes, they should express either CD4 or CD8.[51]

Non-Hodgkin's Lymphomas, B-Cell Type

The B-cell lymphomas constituted the majority of non-Hodgkin's lymphomas. This is partly true because the more common follicular lymphomas (by nodal architecture) are essentially always B cell in origin. However, the diffuse lymphomas are phenotypically B in 50 percent or more of cases as well. The ability to separate B-cell from T-cell types of lymphoma has permitted the discovery that T- and B-cell lymphomas are distinctive in clinical presentation and in response to therapy. The prediction of cell phenotype from histologic characteristics is therefore desirable as a more universally applicable method of classifying non-Hodgkin's lymphomas into distinct groups.

The prediction that only B-cell lymphomas will occur in nodular or follicular patterns (Rappaport classification) has been well supported by immunophenotyping. Pinkus and Said[52] reported on 72 cases of non-Hodgkin's lymphoma, 27 of which were nodular or partly nodular. Using the presence of monoclonal surface immunoglobulin, Fc, and/or complement receptors as criteria, all of the nodular lymphomas were of B-cell type. An incidental finding of this study was that the presence of surface immunoglobulin and Fc receptors paralleled each other but that complement receptors were relatively scarce in relapsed patients as opposed to newly diagnosed patients. Also noted in patients with poorly differentiated lymphocytic lymphoma was a population of normal-appearing T lymphocytes in involved nodes, averaging 39 percent of cells. This has been described by others and labeled as T-cell predominant, monoclonal B phenotype.[53–56]

The B-cell origin of virtually all nodular lymphomas was also demonstrated by Frizzera et al.[57] who reported that of 63 non-Hodgkin's lymphomas evaluated, 53 percent were nodular or partly nodular. Employing surface immunoglobulin, Fc, complement receptor status, and E rosetting techniques, 97 percent of nodular lymphomas were B cell and 3 percent (one case) T cell. In a larger series of 100 patients investigated in similar fashion, 88 percent were B, 3 percent T, and 9 percent null and unclassifiable.[58] The study of nodular lymphomas may be hampered by the low numbers of malignant cells in a sample and spotty tissue distribution. Overall, it predicts phenotype very well.

The Lukes-Collins and Kiel classifications agree that cells arising from lymph node follicles are B cell in nature but prefer to identify the cell type rather than rely on nodal pattern. In the Lukes-Collins schema, these are the follicular center cells, small and large cleaved and noncleaved cell types. The Kiel classification terms these cells germinal center cells with small and large centrocytes and centroblasts, respectively. These cells, along with dendritic cells, interdigitating reticulum cells, and a few histiocytes, make up the follicular or germinal center. As these cells become neoplastic, they begin as a nodular proliferation and may or may not progress to a diffuse pattern. Either follicular or diffuse patterns can be seen on initial presentation.

The accuracy of the follicular center cell designation for predicting B-cell phenotype is high when multiple markers are used but less so when only surface immunoglobulin is considered. In a series of 299 patients, of which 41 percent were of the follicular center cell group, monoclonal surface immunoglobulin was found in 25 to 65 percent. Monoclonal immunoglobulin was seen most frequently in small noncleaved and least frequently in large noncleaved types.[59] The other cells in this series had either polyclonal immunoglobulin or an insufficient amount to test for monoclonality by visual techniques. Another study of 500 non-Hodgkin's lymphomas, of which approximately one-fourth were follicular center cell type, also showed only a moderate number with clearly monoclonal immunoglobulin.[60] The range of monoclonal surface immunoglobulin by immunofluorescence was 56 to 65 percent and cytoplasmic staining with immunoperoxidase yielded 33 percent with monoclonality. By combining the two methods, approximately three-fourths of the group were of B-cell origin phenotypically on the basis of immunoglobulin expression alone. The remaining follicular center cell lymphomas were predominantly, if not exclusively, of null cell phenotype in this and the previous study.

The Kiel classification studies generally consist of much smaller numbers of patients but again show that between 50 and 100 percent of germinal center cell lymphomas have monoclonal surface or cytoplasmic immunoglobulin. By combining several series, 20 of 29 centrocytic, 35 of 42 centroblastic/centrocytic, and 12 of 19 centroblastic were of B-cell type with the remainder noncentroblastic lymphomas generally of null cell type.[55,61–63] The centroblastic lymphomas frequently contain T-phenotypic cells as well, prompting one researcher to suggest a T-cell origin, perhaps in the mantle or T zone of lymph nodes, giving rise to these lymphomas.[56]

With increasing information regarding lineage, several prospective and retrospective analyses have been performed among patients with intermediate and high grade lymphomas to determine the impact of lineage on response rates and survivals. In all of these studies, histologies that are lineage specific (follicular lymphomas, Burkitt's lymphoma, lymphoblastic, and mycosis fungoides/Sézary syndrome) have been excluded. When comparing diffuse small cell, mixed, and large cell histologies, most investigators have found no difference in response rates or survival when groups are comparable matched for grade and treatment. Cheng et al.[64] reported on 70 consecutive patients seen at the National Taiwan University Hospital, of whom 34 had peripheral T-cell lymphoma (PTL) and 36 had diffuse B-cell lymphoma. The patients with PTL had a higher incidence of skin involvement and tended to present with more constitutional symptoms and more advanced stages. When corrected for grade (intermediate versus high grade), the complete remission rates and survival were similar for the two groups. Cossman et al.[65] found a similar distribution of T- and B-lineage lymphomas (42 percent versus 53 percent) among 59 patients with diffuse aggressive histologies of non-Hodgkin's lymphomas (diffuse mixed, diffuse large cell, and non-Burkitt's undifferentiated). There were no clinical differences between the B- and T-cell groups. A subgroup of 36 patients was assessed pretherapy; in follow-up there was no difference in response rates or survival between the two groups.

The heterogeneity of PTL and diffuse B-cell lymphomas may obscure some differences between B- and T-lineage lymphomas. Lippman et al.[66] studied 103 consecutive patients with diffuse large cell histology only. Of these patients, 19 percent were T lineage and 81 percent were B lineage, with skin involvement more frequent in the T-cell group and bulky disease more common in the B-cell group. The response rates and actuarial overall survival were not significantly different between the two groups; however, median survival and disease-free survival were significantly shorter for the T-lineage group (disease-free survival was 10.8 months for T cell versus 42.7 months for B cell). These findings suggest that there are differences based on immunophenotype in terms of continuous complete remission rate that may not impact on survival unless follow-up is very long. These researchers have suggested that these results justify more aggressive therapy in T-cell diffuse large cell lymphomas over their B-cell counterparts in order to achieve similar durable responses.

A more recent study from the same group reviewed the Stanford institutional experiences with anaplastic lymphoid tumors, a phenotypically null subset of non-Hodgkin's lymphomas.[67] The clinical characteristics, and overall and disease-free survivals of this group were compared with the institutional experiences with diffuse large cell lymphomas. The anaplastic lymphomas differed from the diffuse large cell lymphoma group in that there were fewer patients with B symptomatology or with bulky disease but were similar in terms of age, distribution of localized and advanced stages of disease, and incidence of extranodal involvement although the sites of extranodal involvement were somewhat unusual in the group with anaplastic lymphoma. This patient population was treated aggressively with doxorubicin-based combination chemotherapy regimens. Overall survival and freedom from progression in the anaplastic group was not significantly different from that in patients with diffuse large cell lymphoma.

The T- and B-cell subsets of non-Hodgkin's lymphoma can be comparatively studied in those situations where they have analogous, primarily nodal, presentations. There also appears to be a subgroup of lymphomas that arise frequently from extranodal sites, of which the majority are of B-cell origin.[68–70] These lymphomas are commonly associated with a variety of aberrant immune states, such as congenital immune defects, autoimmune diseases, or after immunosuppressive therapy for organ transplantation. The majority of lymphomas arising in these circumstance have the cytologic appearance of immunoblastic sarcoma B cells, according to Lukes,[48] often with plasmacytoid features.

The autoimmune diseases reported as having secondarily associated non-Hodgkin's lymphoma include systemic lupus erythematosus, rheumatoid arthritis, Sjögren syndrome, and Hashimoto's thyroiditis. Lymphomas associated with these diseases may arise within the target organ or follow a typically nodal pattern. In Sjögren syndrome, the lymphomas occur predominantly outside the salivary gland. The association of lymphoma with Sjögren syndrome had been noted in 1967, and subsequent phenotypic analysis has confirmed the B-cell origin.[68,71]

The lymphoepithelial lesions that occur in the salivary glands of patients with Sjögren syndrome are histologically benign but demonstrate clonal B-cell proliferations by both phenotypic and immunoglobulin gene rearrangement analysis. When lymphomas have occurred in patients with Sjögren syndrome, the phenotype and genotype within the salivary gland and involved nodes are identical.[72]

In a recent review of 20 cases in which histology was available, the evolution of Sjögren syndrome (myoepithelial sialoadenitis) to lymphoma was investigated morphologically and immunohistochemically.[73] The patient population was selected to include only patients in whom a biopsy specimen of the salivary gland had been obtained. There was strong female predominance among patients, with a broad age range (21 to 76 years) and generally a long duration of symptoms (3 months to 20 years). Although an initial diagnosis of myoepithelial sialoadenitis had been made in 19 of the 20 cases, retrospective histologic review combined with immunophenotypic data was felt to be suggestive or consistent with lymphoma in 15 of the cases. The histologic appearance of these biopsy specimens suggested a progression of lesions from focal lymphoid aggregates to diffuse lymphoid infiltration to frank lymphoma. The development of diffuse lymphoid infiltration appears to be associated with the development of a clonal expansion of B cells that could be demonstrated by immunohistochemistry and gene rearrangement studies; in all cases in the study, the immunophenotype was IgM-κ.[73] The natural history of non-Hodgkin's lymphoma arising in the setting of Sjögren syndrome was described in nine patients. The majority of the patients had received some form of prior therapy, such as steroids, alkylating agents, and/or parotid radiation. These lymphomas tended to disseminate early to stages III and IV, following an aggressive course.

The lymphomas seen in autoimmune thyroiditis usually arise within the thyroid gland itself and, unlike Sjögren syndrome–associated lymphomas, tend to remain as localized disease.[74,75] Although rare instances of T-cell lymphoma of the thyroid have been reported, these did not arise in a background of autoimmune thyroiditis.[76,77] Histologically, diffuse large cell lymphomas are more common than follicular patterns, and phenotypically and genotypically, lymphomas arising in patients with Hashimoto's thyroiditis are B lineage.[74,75,78] In contrast with Sjögren syndrome, the lymphocytic infiltrate of Hashimoto's thyroiditis is predominantly composed of T cells, and investigators have demonstrated clonal T-cell proliferations (T-cell β rearrangement) in one of six patients evaluated. There was no evidence of immunoglobulin rearrangement in six patients with uncomplicated Hashimoto's thyroiditis or two patients with nonspecific lymphoid thyroiditis.

Suppression of cell-mediated immunity with drugs, as during renal or other forms of organ transplantation, has led to an increased incidence of both polyclonal B-cell proliferation and large cell lymphomas.[79,80] In reviewing the transplant tumor registries, Penn[80] noted that lymphomas generally occur at 37 months post-transplant. Non-Hodgkin's lymphomas predominate, with a 20- to 49-fold increased incidence over age-matched controls.[81,82] The most common histology is large cell or immunoblastic type. In 100 cases studied, 72 percent were B-cell lymphomas, 15 percent were B-cell hyperplasia (possibly lymphoma), 12 percent were T-cell lymphomas, and 1 percent were null lymphomas. Extranodal involvement was much more common than in nontransplant patients, occurring in 73 per-

cent, and two-thirds of the lymphomas were confined to a single organ site, usually the central nervous system (CNS). Approximately 33 percent of transplant patients had CNS involvement, and in 70 percent of these, the CNS was the only site of disease.[80] The degree and type of immunosuppression may play a role in the subsequent development of non-Hodgkin's lymphoma. The incidence has been reported to be higher in cardiac than in renal transplant and may occur earlier in patients receiving cyclosporin A with or without antithymocyte globulin as antirejection therapy.[83,84]

The experiences at several centers have been pooled to evaluate the likely sequence of events in the development of non-Hodgkin's lymphomas in transplant recipients. Hanto and Najarian[85] describe three groups of patients: 1. Those with benign histologic appearance, polyclonal B-cell phenotype, and normal karotype; 2. those with the histologic appearance of polymorphic lymphoma, polyclonal B-cell phenotype, and clonal cytogenetic abnormalities; and 3. those with B-cell lymphoma, monoclonal B-cell phenotype, and clonal cytogenetic abnormalities. Younger patients are more likely to present with an infectious and mononucleosis-like illness, and EBV serologic findings were divided among primary infection, reactivation, and remote infection. Older patients were more likely to present with isolated tumor masses, and serologic findings demonstrated reactivation in 3 percent of these patients and remote infection in 37 percent. The early B-cell hyperplastic lesions are generally EBV dependent and respond to acyclovir alone, whereas those with early histologic and cytogenetic malignant changes require both acyclovir and reduction in immunosuppression. Frankly malignant lesions are acyclovir unresponsive and require chemotherapy and radiation, although long-term control is rare.

Lymphoid tissue from immunosuppressed patients with histologic high grade lymphomas may not always demonstrate monoclonal surface immunoglobulin, but clonality can be demonstrated by immunoglobulin gene rearrangement studies and by clonal EBV infection at a single site.[84,86] Biopsy specimens from different sites within the same individual may reveal distinct clonal proliferations at each site, by both gene rearrangement and EBV DNA analyses. In patients with the histologic and phenotypic findings of polyclonal hyperplasia, immunoglobulin gene rearrangement studies and EBV-genomic studies have failed to reveal clonality. These data support the theory that these lymphomas form a B-cell hyperplasia in which one or more clones of EBV-infected cells undergo malignant degeneration.

The incidence of primary CNS lymphomas is less than 1 percent of all non-Hodgkin's lymphomas, although this may change with the rising population of transplant recipients and human immunodeficiency virus-positive individuals.[87] Primary lymphomas of the CNS in the absence of immunodeficiency occur predominantly in older individuals (fifth and sixth decades) with a male predominance.[88] Patients present with signs and symptoms of increased intracranial pressure. Computed tomography scan findings reveal an enhancing mass lesion usually in the supratentorial region, most often in the frontal lobes. By histology, the majority of these lesions are generally high grade (large cell noncleaved, small cell noncleaved, and immunoblastic). Median survival varies but is generally reported to be less than 18 months, with a minority of long-term survivors.[88–90] Although extensive studies are lacking, small series of patients with primary CNS lymphoma have demonstrated light chain restriction in 13 of 24, 10 of 19, and 6 of 6 patients.[91–92] The presence of pan-B antigens and mono-clonal gene rearrangement patterns has also been noted in six of six patients.[92] Only one of these studies also tested for T-cell antigens, and none of these studies correlated phenotype with immunosuppressed states. One wold expect the primary CNS lymphomas associated with immunosuppression to arise from EBV-induced B-cell proliferations. By use of in situ hybridiza-tion techniques, all four patients with immunosuppression and primary CNS lymphoma versus none of four immunocompe-tent patients with CNS lymphoma had detectable EBV DNA within their lymphoma.[93] The etiology of primary CNS lym-phoma in immunocompetent patients remains unclear.

Gastrointestinal lymphomas may also be associated with immunodeficiency states. Mediterranean lymphoma arises in a geographically distinct population with a prodromal syndrome of maladsorption and chronic diarrhea secondary to an as yet unidentified infection, possibly Vibrio cholera.[94,95] The postu-lated development involves a transition from a polyclonal, hyperplastic plasma cell response to a lymphoma of IgA-positive, κ- and λ-negative phenotype with or without serum manifesta-tions of α heavy chain disease.[96] There is an increased incidence of hypogammaglobulinemia, increased anergy, and decreased T-cell mitogen response in a portion of these patients.[94] This form of gastrointestinal lymphoma differs in heavy chain type and relationship to infection and impaired cell-mediated immunity from the intestinal lymphomas in the United States. The latter are also of B-cell type in most cases but bear an IgM phenotype.[97] Although in one case report a gastrointestinal lymphoma of IgM type may have evolved from nodular hyper-plasia, the majority are not considered to develop from pre-existing conditions as a rule.[98]

Aside from the extranodal tumors arising in immunosup-pressed or immunodeficient patients, patients with B-cell non-Hodgkin's lymphomas appear clinically to have relatively intact immune systems. The most common aberration involves immunoglobulin production, both increased and decreased.[99–101] These lymphomas include the neoplasms most commonly asso-ciated with monoclonal gammopathies, well-differentiated diffuse small cell lymphoma and CLL.[102] Most of these lym-phomas, even those not classified as WM, usually produce IgM paraproteins.

Abnormalities of immunoglobulin production in non-Hodgkin's lymphoma range from hypogammaglobulinemia to polyclonal and monoclonal gammopathies. The incidence of these findings in a series of 100 patients varied by histology, with the incidence of monoclonal gammopathies being 57 per-cent in plasmacytoid lymphocytic (with and without the clini-cal picture of WM), 39 percent in small lymphocytic, 40 percent in B-cell immunoblastic lymphomas, and 13 percent of follicu-lar center cell lymphomas.[101] The majority of these were IgM with occasional IgG gammopathies. Bence Jones proteinuria

was detectable in 5 of 16 patients with monoclonal gam-mopathies. Hypogammaglobulinemia of one or more isotopes was most common in small lymphocytic lymphoma (44 to 50 percent) and least common in plasmacytoid lymphocytic lym-phoma (8 to 38 percent) and B-cell immunoblastic lymphoma (10 to 30 percent). The isotope most frequently depressed was IgA. Polyclonal increases in immunoglobulins were found most commonly in B-cell immunoblastic and plasmacytoid lympho-cytic lymphomas.

In a similar series of patients from Roswell Park, 329 patients with non-Hodgkin's lymphoma and 82 with CLL were screened at diagnosis for the presence of monoclonal gammopathy. The incidence in this group was 6.4 percent for patients with non-Hodgkin's lymphoma and 18.2 percent for those with CLL. The frequency of IgM and IgG monoclonal proteins was similar (46 percent versus 42 percent), with a 2:1 ratio of κ to λ light chains and a 56 percent incidence of Bence Jones proteinuria. The pres-ence of a monoclonal gammopathy had no effect on survival.

Patients with non-Hodgkin's lymphoma have fairly normal numbers of circulating lymphocytes. While some investigators have noted an increase in B lymphocytes, most have found these to be not significantly different from controls. The mild lym-phopenia that has been noted by some investigators is due to a balanced decrease in total T cells, with normal helper-suppres-sor ratios. When present, lymphopenia appears to be correlated with more advanced stages of disease.[103–105]

In contrast to CLL, evidence of increased in vitro T-helper function in a pokeweed mitogen-stimulated B-cell assay was demonstrated in 15 of 18 phenotypic or histologic B-cell lym-phomas and two of two null cell lymphomas.[106] The ratio of inducer to suppressor circulating T cells was not significantly different from controls, although the group with increased helper function had low to normal total lymphocyte counts. The suppressor function in this group was also intact, as demonstrated by use of concanavalin A-stimulated T-suppres-sor cells in the same B-cell assay. A comparison of stimulated lymphoma suppressor cells with stimulated control suppressor cells showed equal suppressor ability. Serum immunoglobulin levels were not elevated in patients with lymphomas exhibiting increased T-helper activity in vitro. Gajl-Peczalska et al.[106] spec-ulated that this may be due to abnormal helper-suppressor ratios in lymphoid organs that are not reflected in the periph-eral blood or, as with CLL, the B cell itself may be unable to respond appropriately, in this instance, by a subnormal response.

Other T-cell functions in B-cell neoplasms appear relatively normal. There is a higher frequency of anergy and subnormal, although not significantly decreased, response to phytohemag-glutinin in advanced stages of lymphoma.[99,107,108] However, mixed lymphocyte reactions generally are normal in all patients.[108]

Non-Hodgkin's Lymphomas, T-Cell Types

The T-cell non-Hodgkin's lymphomas comprise several distinct clinical and pathologic entities that are now also found, in most cases, to be immunologically distinct as well. The differentiation stages of T-cell lymphomas parallel leukemic forms closely and incorporate neoplasms from all stages of T-cell development, thymic to immunocompetent T-cell types. Despite the capacity to distinguish T-cell neoplasms phenotypically and functionally, the classification of T-cell neoplasms is difficult to establish and frequently requires genotypic (TCR rearrangement) confirmation. There is no universally accepted classification schema, although the differences between proposed systems are not great. The non-Hodgkin's lymphomas of T lineage can be divided broadly into thymic, PTL or post-thymic excluding cutaneous T-cell lymphomas (CTCL), and cutaneous T-cell lymphomas; or into low, intermediate, and high grade histologies. Evaluations of clinical course, response to therapy, and prognosis are difficult owing to the heterogeneous nature of the PTLs. However, most researchers state that patients with T-cell lymphomas have poorer sustained responses to therapy and poorer survivals, particularly in comparing high grade T- and B-cell lymphomas.

The thymic or convoluted lymphoblastic T-cell lymphomas are closely related to ALL, arising at a similar stage of development but having leukemic involvement as a later complication of disease. The description of this group as a separate entity dates back to 1975.[109] Since then the disease has been found frequently in children and uncommonly in adults. A similar rapid clinical course, with dissemination to the CNS, peripheral blood, bone marrow, skin, and gonads, as well as a high incidence of mediastinal masses, is seen in both age groups.[110–114] The median age of patients with lymphoblastic lymphoma is low, generally under age 20, and there is a male predominance, with a male/female ratio of 4:1 reported in one series.[115]

Lymphoblastic lymphoma developing in adults has been reported to behave in a somewhat atypical fashion. In a small series of eight patients, Bloomfield et al.[110] noted that loss of the E rosette receptor was common (in six of eight), although two other small series did demonstrate the presence of E rosette receptors and frequently complement receptors. In Bloomfield's series, the null subset of patients had a shorter survival (median, 8 months) and none had a complete response to therapy. Peripheral adenopathy was more common, while an overt leukemic phase and mediastinal masses were less common. Palacios et al.[113] also report a lower incidence of mediastinal masses and CNS involvement in older patients. Rosen and colleagues'[114] series of 12 adults revealed 9 patients with mediastinal masses, 4 with CNS involvement, and 5 with leukemic phase at presentation. Since the number of adults with lymphoblastic lymphoma is low, it may be necessary to pool data from several series to get a true picture of disease presentation and course in this age group.

Histologically, lymphoblastic lymphomas reveal medium-sized cells with an immature, finely dispersed chromatin pattern and small, inconspicuous nucleoli with scanty basophilic cytoplasm. The mitotic index is high and a starry sky appearance can be seen. Some investigators subclassify lymphoblastic lymphomas according to maturational stage as determined by phenotype. All lymphoblastic lymphomas are TdT positive. The early thymic stage of differentiation lacks CD1, CD4, and CD8, while the intermediate stage is CD1+ and may coexpress CD4 and CD8, and late stages of thymic differentiation may be CD1+ or CD1– and express CD4 or CD8 only.[116]

Phenotyping studies demonstrate that loss of pan-T antigens is uncommon, but not rare, with loss of one antigen occurring in 26 percent (9 of 35) of cases reviewed by the Stanford group.[23] In 11 percent of lymphoblastic lymphomas, a helper (CD4+, CD8–) phenotype was present and none in this series had a suppressor phenotype. Forty percent of lymphoblastic lymphomas were CD4–,CD8–, while 49 percent coexpressed CD4 and CD8. The finding of coexpression of CD4 and CD8 was rare in all other T-cell lymphomas (1 percent).

PTL occurs in older age groups than lymphoblastic lymphomas, with median age at presentation ranging from 53 to 63 years.[115,117–119] There is a variable male predominance that is not significantly different from that noted in patients with intermediate and high grade B-cell lymphomas. There is a trend, and sometimes a statistically significant difference, toward a higher percentage of patients presenting with B symptoms and with advanced stages of disease compared with patients with B-cell lymphomas. The incidence of skin involvement is higher in patients with PTL; the frequency of involvement and sites of other extranodal areas of involvement do not clearly differ between intermediate and high grades of PTL and B-cell lymphomas. The overall and complete response rates to therapy are similar between PTL and B-cell lymphomas of comparable histologic grade, but some investigators have suggested poorer survival in PTL, primarily due to the lack of durability in patients with complete responses.[64–66,118]

As a group, PTLs are CD1– and CD3+ and most are of helper/inducer (CD4+) origin as determined by immunophenotyping characteristics, although there is usually a persistence of CD8+ cells.[45,117–119] Virtually all human T-cell leukemia/lymphoma virus type 1 (HTLV-1)-associated lymphomas and all cutaneous T-cell lymphomas are CD4+, and functionally the former have discordant suppressor cell capabilities in in vitro assays while CTCL retain helper/inducer capability as well as phenotype.[120–125] Lennert's lymphomas are also reported to be universally CD4+.[45] In contrast, certain subsets of T-CLL are phenotypically and functionally suppressor T cells.[45,126] Loss of one or more pan-T-cell antigens (CD2, CD3, CD5) is common in PTL, occurring in 76 percent of cases excluding mycosis fungoides and in 64 to 100 percent of CTCL depending on the site examined (skin versus node).[23] Lack of helper or suppressor expression (CD4–,CD8–) is relatively uncommon in PTL, occurring in 17 percent, and rare in CTCL (2 percent). Coexpression of CD4 and CD8 is rare in both PTL (1 percent) and CTCL (7 percent).[23]

Within the post-thymic lymphomas or PTL are several subgroups of patients, some of which are more distinctive clinically and others that represent relatively unusual histologically distinct types of T-cell lymphoma. Low grade histologies include T-CLL and small cerebriform lymphomas (mycosis fungoides/Sézary syndrome).[45] Some others also include Lennert's lymphoma, AILD, T zone, and pleomorphic small cell lymphomas in a low grade class, while others have included it in a separate, intermediate histology category. Within the high grade category are such histologies as pleomorphic medium cell, pleomorphic large cell, immunoblastic, and large cell anaplastic.

There is no distinction made within this schema for patients with serologic evidence of exposure to HTLV-1, although clearly this does impact on prognosis.

The entity of T-CLL includes four different subtypes, distinguishable by phenotype and often by clinical presentation and histology.[45] Patients with small lymphocytes with irregular nuclear projections (knobby) have more prominent adenopathy and an intermediate prognosis compared with other forms of T-CLL. These cells bear a helper/inducer phenotype (CD4+, CD8–). A second subtype is characterized by cells with round nuclei and azurophilic granules (large granular cell leukemia, LGL) which type as CD8+ and may express the Leu-7 (CD16) antigen. Lymphadenopathy is not a common feature; splenomegaly and cytopenias are common. The prognosis is best for this subtype of T-CLL. The third subtype consists of small pleomorphic cells with a suppressor-cytotoxic phenotype (CD3+, CD8+, CD4–). There is also a T-cell prolymphocytic leukemia, which can express either CD4 or CD8. The cells are larger than T-CLL cells with prominent nucleoli and a moderate amount of basophilic cytoplasm. The small pleomorphic and prolymphocytic subtypes are reported to have the worst prognosis.[45,126]

The cutaneous T-cell lymphomas, of which mycosis fungoides and Sézary syndrome are clinically distinct entities, are also phenotypically T-cell neoplasms of the helper T-cell subset.[23,45,124,125,127] The use of monoclonal antibodies on cutaneous lesions discloses a mixture of B cells, Langerhans cells, and suppressor and helper T cells. In most instances, the helper T-cell subset is proportionately much greater than the suppressor subset. The suppressor (CD8+) cells are scattered throughout the skin lesion, usually as single cells or small groups of cells. The helper (CD4+) cells are clumped together, generally in close association with Langerhans (CD1+) cells and dendritic cells. It has been proposed that the Langerhans cells play a role in stimulation of helper T cells and development of CTCL.[128] The peripheral blood and lymph nodes of patients with CTCL that are histologically uninvolved also show a marked increase of CD4+ cells relative to CD8+ cells in most instances. The degree of helper/suppressor imbalance is not as great as in pathologically involved blood and lymph nodes and often does not represent statistically significant increases over normal controls.[129,130] The detection of altered phenotype distribution in these cases, as in the detection of clonal excess in B-cell neoplasm, most likely represents subclinical involvement. With progressive involvement of peripheral blood and lymph nodes, the total circulating T-cell population decreases.[130,131] However, the predominant population of T cells is of the helper subset, and in pathologically involved tissues, this is statistically significant. The characteristic CD3+, CD4+, CD8–, Ia– phenotype is remarkably consistent in all cases of CTCL and is even seen in T-cell line cultures from CTCL patients, although these latter cells may be Ia+ as well.[124] Recent studies using gene rearrangement analysis have shown clonal expansion of TCR chain rearrangements in the involved skin of patients with CTCL that is identical to that of histologically involved nodes and frequently found in histologically uninvolved nodes (seven of nine in one series).[132]

The functional abilities of malignant cells from CTCL are, unlike those of adult T-cell leukemia/lymphoma (ATL), correlated with the phenotype. The cells derived from involved cutaneous lesions, lymph nodes, and blood have all demonstrated T-helper function in B-cell-pokeweed mitogen (PWM) assay systems.[125,127,133] These malignant T cells also have the capacity to stimulate null cell differentiation to both T and B cells.[134] This capability can be found in sera from patients with mycosis fungoides and Sézary syndrome and appears to be different from the thymic factor found in the sera of normal individuals, which also stimulates T-cell differentiation but to a lesser extent.

Despite the in vitro demonstration of helper activity, hypergammaglobulinemia is only intermittently observed in CTCL, and although cell-mediated immunity is not clinically depressed, there are a number of laboratory abnormalities of T-cell function. Anergy to dinitrochlorobenzene and to recall antigens occurs in a significant minority of patients, which is correlated with and probably a result of lymphopenia (1000/mm³).[135] Anergy is not significantly related to advanced stages of disease. Increased spontaneous proliferation of T cells has also been reported, and mutagenic responses to a variety of stimuli have been reported as normal to significantly depressed in patients with mycosis fungoides and Sézary syndrome.[125,136] Similarly, natural killer cell activity has been reported as normal to depressed in both. Antibody-dependent cellular cytotoxicity (ADCC) has been reported to be depressed in patients with Sézary syndrome but not in patients with mycosis fungoides. In addition, monocyte chemotaxis may be abnormal as well.[137] These cell-mediated immunity abnormalities do not produce a clinically apparent susceptibility to infection as seen with HD, but as a rule these abnormalities are not as pronounced or reproducibly present as in HD.

The clinical syndrome of AILD is characterized by generalized lymphadenopathy, hepatosplenomegaly, fever, polyclonal hypergammaglobulinemia, and positive Coombs test. The histologic appearance is that of a pleomorphic infiltrate of lymphocytes, immunoblasts, eosinophils, and plasma cells with an arborizing venule pattern.[138] This entity was initially considered a reactive, nonmalignant process that could evolve into an immunoblastic lymphoma of T- or B-cell phenotype in approximately 20 percent of cases; the usual mode of death was infectious. Current studies suggest that previous descriptions of AILD with immunoblastic lymphoma were actually a PTL, now termed AIL-like T-cell lymphoma.[45] Some investigators question whether AILD is a benign clinical entity or simply an earlier stage of T-cell lymphoma. Although initial phenotypic analysis of AIL-like T-cell lymphomas usually demonstrated a suppressor/cytotoxic phenotype, later investigators have noted that proliferating cells in these lesions are predominantly of helper phenotype with an admixture of some suppressor/cytotoxic cells.[139–141] Gene rearrangement studies have demonstrated clonal expansion and rearrangement of TCR β and γ chain gene rearrangements as well.[40,142,143] The significance of immunoglobulin gene rearrangements as a benign or malignant clonal B-cell expansion is unclear.

The T-zone lymphomas arise from T cells in the interfollicular nodal areas, and in early lesions the follicles may be preserved and such nodes may be misread as follicular hyperplasia or follicular lymphoma. Follicles are less prominent or absent in later stages, with replacement by small to medium nonpleomorphic lymphocytes in a background that includes B cells, clear cells (lymphocytes with clear cytoplasm), plasma cells, eosinophils, rare Reed-Sternberg cells, and moderate vascular proliferation.[45] Phenotypically, the majority of these lesions have a predominance of CD4+ cells.[117–119] As initially described by Waldron et al.[144] in 1977, these lymphomas occur in older patients with a high frequency of B symptoms and advanced stages of disease. There is a strong predilection for pulmonary parenchymal and pleural involvement and sometimes skin rashes. Leukemic involvement is reported to be rare. Mild to moderate hypergammaglobulinemia has also been noted.

Lennert's lymphoma is a distinctive pathologic entity originally proposed as a variant of HD but now recognized as a PTL of helper/inducer phenotype.[45] The most notable feature of this lesion is clusters of epithelioid cells. The nodal architecture is replaced by a predominantly small lymphocytic infiltrate with some advanced medium and large cells, plasma cells, and eosinophils. Clinically, patients with Lennert's lymphoma present more frequently with localized lymphadenopathy, often cervical, than patients with other PTLs. Involvement of the tonsils is common, while hepatosplenomegaly, skin involvement, and B symptoms are infrequent. Patients may have normal immunoglobulin levels or modest polyclonal hypergammaglobulinemia.

Diffuse lymphomas of small pleomorphic T cells may be HTLV-1 positive or negative.[45] In contrast to the pleomorphic T-CLL, the cells are usually of the helper-inducer (CD3+, CD4+, CD8–) phenotype and a leukemic phase is uncommon in HTLV-1 negative patients. Patients with nonvirus-related disease present frequently with lymphadenopathy and skin involvement.[117] Patients with HTLV-1 positive disease may have an indolent course compared with patients with ATL presenting medium and large cell variants. In these so-called chronic ATL patients, skin involvement is common but symptoms are usually milder, the number of leukemic cells fewer, and hypercalcemia is absent. These patients may transform to a larger cell type with a more aggressive course and the development of hypercalcemia is a poor prognostic sign.

All the PTLs of high grade histology are more often associated with HTLV-1 infection; however, most cases of ATL have a pleomorphic mixed or pleomorphic large cell histologic appearance.[45] Since the clinical course and prognosis are affected to a greater extent by association with HTLV-1 infection than histology, all patients with HTLV-1-positive disease should be grouped as a separate entity from ATL.

ATL and malignant T-cell lymphoma (nonleukemic variant of ATL) of Japan and the T-cell lymphomas of the Caribbean Islands appear to be separate entities from the other T-cell neoplasms by virtue of their endemic nature and association with HTLV infection.[145,146] Histologically, these lymphomas are very pleomorphic with large, small, and intermediate cell sizes and convoluted and multilobulated nuclear configurations.[120,121,146] They do not have an increase in the background eosinophils, plasma cells, histiocytes, or vascular proliferation as seen in immunoblastic sarcomas and PTL. The clinical course has been variably described as subacute/chronic to rapidly progressive. The development of a leukemic phase or of hypercalcemia, as well as transformation from small pleomorphic to a larger cell type or CNS involvement, appears to herald the transition from subacute to acute. The malignant manifestations of T-cell lymphoma develop most commonly in older adults with generalized lymphadenopathy, bony lesions, and hypercalcemia, skin, CNS, bone marrow, and peripheral blood involvement. The markers for immunocompetent phenotypes have demonstrated helper/inducer (CD3+, CD4+, CD1–, CD8–) reactivity and expression of Ia and the interleukin-2 (IL-2) receptor (Tac+, CD25) in several studies.[45,120,121,147] This is due to the preferential infection of the helper/inducer subset by HTLV. In rare instances, the cells have been found to coexpress CD4 and CD8.[45] In vivo, both hypergammaglobulinemia and hypogammaglobulinemia have been found in isolated patients.[146] Conversely, in vitro studies of malignant T cells have demonstrated reproducible suppressor activity only.[120–122]

The model used for detection of T-cell suppression in most instances relies on the ability of the T cell to block in vitro differentiation of B cells to plasma cells in the presence of PWM and normal T-cell stimulation.[148] B cells themselves show minimal differentiation spontaneously or in the presence of PWM. In the presence of normal T cells and PWM, significant plasma cell differentiation and immunoglobulin synthesis occur. The suppressive ability of T cells can be demonstrated by adding these T cells to a normal T-cell–PWM coculture that should yield a 50 percent or greater decrease in immunoglobulin synthesis and/or plasma cell production; then helper function has been demonstrated.[149] Another more commonly used method for determining suppressor activity is by comparison of the differentiation and immunoglobulin synthesis of the T-cell–B-cell–PWM system with a coculture of irradiated T cells, normal B cells, and PWM. The irradiation selectively abrogates suppressor T-cell function at lower doses (1000 to 2000 cGy), thus revealing the degree of T-cell-mediated suppression in the system.[150]

Both systems have been utilized to demonstrate suppressor function of the phenotypically helper/induced cells in malignant T-cell lymphoma. In a group of 16 patients, 15 of these had the helper phenotype of Leu-1+ (CD5), Leu-3–(CD4), Leu-2–(CD8).[121] Fourteen patients were tested for the ability of their malignant cell population to stimulate and provoke differentiation of normal B cells. Of these 14 patients, 10 demonstrated suppressor activity, 3 had no functional activity, and one study was technically inadequate. The suppressive effects of the malignant T cells were abolished by irradiation with 1000 Gy before their addition to the coculture.

Other, smaller studies (generally of less than 10 patients) have confirmed the suppressor activity of malignant T-cell lymphoma ATL, when T-cell activity could be identified. One group of six patients was found to contain three patients without abnormal function and three with suppressor activity.[146] The suppressor activity could also be observed when culture supernatant from functionally suppressor T cells from one of the patients was substituted for the malignant T cells. The supernatant effects were heat labile and could be reversed by washing the normal B cells before stimulation. Both the group of patients with and those without suppressor activity had normal immunoglobulin levels in vivo. Depressed immunoglobulin levels have been noted in other studies; however, the malignant cells were not evaluated for suppressor activity. This leaves unresolved the significance of the in vitro capabilities as a reflection of the in vivo functional status.

The high association of HTLV with Japanese and Caribbean lymphoproliferative neoplasms emerges as a common thread between these two groups and distinguishes them from most T-cell neoplasms in the United States.[151] Curiously, HTLV was discovered in cell lines obtained from a patient in the United States with a CTCL, also a phenotypically helper population.[152] Since the discovery of the virus, T-cell neoplasms in the United States and Japan have been screened for the presence of HTLV by determining whether there are antiviral antibodies in the sera. The U.S. studies have demonstrated a low incidence of HTLV antibody in CTCLs as a group or T-cell neoplasms as a whole. However, there are small reports of patients in the United States with clinical syndromes, histology, and phenotypes similar to those of the malignant T-cell lymphomas of Japan.[147] It appears that the virus may be endemic in the southeastern part of the United States due to migration from the Caribbean. These patients have HTLV antibodies too, and there is also an increased incidence of the viral antibodies in patients with acquired immunodeficiency syndrome (AIDS).[153] The bulk of HTLV-associated disease still resides with the Japanese, who have an 80 to 90 percent incidence of HTLV antibodies in patients with ATL and malignant T-cell lymphoma. There is also a variable amount of HTLV antibody titers in normal donors and patients with non-T-cell neoplasms in Japan.[151] For carriers of the virus, it has been suggested that the risk of developing ATL is 1 in 900 in males and 1 in 2000 in females over 40 years of age.[154]

Immunoblastic lymphomas of T-cell type can be histologically divided into two groups, those with basophilic and those with clear cell immunoblasts.[45] The histologic appearance consists predominantly of an infiltrate of large cells with round nuclei and one or more prominent nucleoli and abundant clear basophilic cytoplasm. These cells frequently lack one or more pan-T antigens, particularly CD5 and CD7, and the majority are CD4 positive (helper/inducer phenotype), including all of the basophilic variants; among the clear cell variant, a minority is CD8 positive.[23,45,117–119] Clinically, patients present with lymphadenopathy; skin and other extranodal sites (nasopharynx, small intestine, spleen) are also commonly involved.[117–119] It has been suggested that large cell lymphomas of T-cell lineage have poorer overall survivals compared with diffuse large cell lymphomas of B-cell lineage; however, direct comparison limited to immunoblastic histology has not been done.[117,118]

The anaplastic lymphomas of T or B lineage have in the past been confused with solid tumors, including anaplastic carcinoma and melanoma. These lymphomas are unusual in that they are identified by Ki positivity (CD30), an antigen originally thought to be restricted to Reed-Sternberg cells and their variants.[45] These lymphomas may exhibit extensive necrosis and multinucleated polylobulated cells. Anaplastic lymphomas may have CD25 (IL-2 receptors) and CD45 positivity but frequently lack some or all of the T-cell antigens.[23,45] These lymphomas have been reported by Suchi et al.[45] to occur in a younger age group than other PTLs (<20 years) and to have a better progress than other high grade T-cell lymphomas. This group of Ki-positive lymphomas may be different from the histologically unclassifiable lymphomas described by the Stanford group.[66] In the Stanford series, these lymphomas were identified by leukocyte common antigen rather than CD30 and occurred in an older population with a survival similar to that of diffuse large cell lymphomas.

Immunodeficiencies in patients with HTLV-1-associated T-cell lymphomas have been most extensively studied. In PTL as a group, both hyper- and hypogammaglobulinemia have been noted and anergy may occur in up to one-half of the patients (8 of 15 evaluated in one study).[117,118] These patients have also been noted to develop infections associated with decreased cell-mediated immunity, such as *Listeria monocytogenes*, *Pneumocystis carinii*, toxoplasmosis, and cryptococcal meningitis.[118] The phenotype and function of CD4-positive lymphomas are concordant for CTCLs and other non-HTLV-1 associated PTLs. In contrast, the HTLV-1-positive PTLs express CD4-positive phenotype but function as suppressor cells in in vitro assays.[120–122]

Hodgkin's Disease

The immunologic studies in HD in recent years have centered around identification of the cellular origin of the Reed-Sternberg cell and the understanding of cellular immune defects, specifically their importance in the etiology of HD. By contrast to non-Hodgkin's lymphoma and despite the advances of classic immunologic analysis, monoclonal antibodies, and gene rearrangement technology, investigations concerning the cell of origin in HD have produced a variety of conflicting data. Candidates proposed for the originating cell in HD include lymphocytes (T and B), monocyte-macrophages, and interdigitating reticulum cells. Each proposed cell line has experimental support but none of sufficient magnitude to rule out the others.

The association of cell-mediated immune defects and HD has long been felt to be an indicator of T-cell origin. Cytochemical staining is usually characteristic of T cells with alkaline phosphatase and nonspecific esterases, but occasionally overlaps with monocyte/macrophage staining patterns.[2,155,156] However, Reed-Sternberg cells do not form E rosettes and do not react with monoclonal anti-T antibodies in virtually any of the cases studied thus far, although this reactivity is reported in some HD cell lines. The evidence for rearrangement of the β chain gene for the TCR is considered questionable.[157,158]

Electron microscopic evaluation of a large series of nodes and cytochemical studies yield the strongest support for a monocyte/macrophage origin.[159] Monocyte characteristics such as lysozyme production are variably identified, although phagocytosis has not been convincingly demonstrated; however, alkaline and acid phosphatase as well as nonspecific esterases are commonly seen in some studies in a pattern implicating association with the monocyte line. The evaluation of 44 lymph nodes by electron microscopy revealed four types of Reed-Sternberg cells: 1. About one-half were immunoblast-like with numerous polyribosomes and prominent nucleoli; 2. histocyte-like with prominent nucleoli, many cellular organelles, and lysozyme-like granules and rough endoplasmic reticulum; 3. macrophage-like, seen in mixed cellularity only; and 4. interdigitating reticulum cell type, seen commonly in nodular sclerosing and rarely in mixed cellularity types. The variation between different histologies and the multiplicity of cell types found ultrastructurally for Reed-Sternberg cells may explain the wide discrepancy in the literature, with some electron microscopic studies showing predominantly macrophage-like cells and others showing lymphoid-like cells.

The data supporting a B-cell origin for the Reed-Sternberg cell are largely circumstantial, although growing in support.[160] Phenotypic data on Reed-Sternberg cells, which are positive for Ia, HLA-DR, IL-2 receptors (CD25), Ki-1, and HeFi-1 (CD30), are suggestive but not conclusive for B cells, as these antigens may also be found on activated and virally transformed lymphocytes.[161] Reactivity of Reed-Sternberg cells with the L26 antibody, which otherwise has been restricted to B-cell populations, is more strongly suggestive of a B-lymphoid origin.[162] Surface and cytoplasmic immunoglobulins fail to demonstrate clonal restriction and appear to result from adsorption of exogenous immunoglobulin and cell membrane leak or phagocytosis.[163–166] Gene rearrangement studies have primarily shown immunoglobulin gene rearrangement although the pattern is atypical, often showing rearrangements of heavy or light chains only, in contrast to the patterns seen in B-cell non-Hodgkin's lymphomas.[157,158,160,167]

The clinicopathologic relationship of HD to non-Hodgkin's lymphomas was recently summarized by Jaffe.[168] Two main points link HD to B-cell non-Hodgkin's lymphomas: the similarities of lymphocyte-predominant HD with B cells in terms of clinical course and phenotypic analysis and the occurrence of composite lymphomas in which HD is associated with non-Hodgkin's lymphomas, usually phenotypically B-cell type.[162,169,170]

The relationship of EBV, which typically infects B cells via the CD3 receptor on these cells, and Reed-Sternberg cells is beginning to emerge. The epidemiologic pattern of HD has been linked to EBV infection. Serologic evidence is now available comparing sera obtained from patients with HD before the diagnosis with temporal-, sex-, and age-matched control sera. This multi-institutional analysis of sera from the United States and Scandinavia evaluated antibody titers to EBV and cytomegalovirus with the relative risk of subsequently developing HD. Patients with HD had higher titers of EBV and lower titers of cytomegalovirus compared with controls; a significant proportion of HD patients demonstrated a pattern consistent with severe initial infection or recent reactivation in the months prior to the diagnosis of HD.[171] The presence of the EBV genome within the Reed-Sternberg cells but not within the background reactive cell population in involved lymphoid tissues has been demonstrated by in situ DNA-hybridization techniques by Weiss et al.[172] This phenomenon appears to be present in up to 20 percent of patients with HD and has been shown to be monoclonal by Southern blot analysis.[172] The presence of EBV within the Reed-Sternberg cells does not confirm the

B-lymphoid nature of these cells as EBV has been occasionally shown to infect T lymphocytes and monocytes, but serves as another source of potential support for this theory. The precise role of EBV in the etiology of HD remains undetermined.

In attempts to gain better understanding of the nature of Reed-Sternberg cells, several centers have established cell cultures from HD patients. Four cell lines established from involved peripheral blood, bone marrow, and pleural effusion (L428, L439, L538, L540) have been in long-term cultures and are well characterized.[173] No evidence of EBV infection (Epstein-Barr nuclear antigen or viral capsid antigen) has been found to suggest contamination with B-lymphoblastoid-transformed lines, and histologically typical multinucleate Reed-Sternberg cells are common. These cell lines were phenotypically Ia+, anti-T+ (rabbit anti-T antibodies but E rosette-, Fc-, and complement-receptor-negative). Both surface and cytoplasmic immunoglobulins were absent. Cytochemically, they were nonspecific esterase- and alkaline phosphatase-positive but lysozyme- and peroxidase-negative. Functionally, there was no evidence of phagocytosis.

These cells are capable of presenting soluble antigen to T cells, acting as potent stimulators of mixed lymphocyte cultures, and functioning as accessory cells in restoring the proliferative responses of T cells in patients with early but not late stages of HD.[174–176] The L428 cells express a 120-kd membrane protein that appears to function in growth regulation.[177] This membrane protein, identified by both the Ki-1 and HeFi-1 monoclonal antibodies, is present on Reed-Sternberg cells and their variants and on the virally transformed cell lines HuT 78, HuT 102, EBV lymphoblastoid cells, and the CML cell line K-562 and is present on large cells in the periphery of lymphoid follicles in the tonsil, colon, and thymus.[161] It has been suggested that these latter cells represent the population from which Reed-Sternberg cells arise.

The pathogenesis of HD, as with its cellular origin, remains unclear. Some investigators have postulated an immunodeficiency state predisposing to the development of HD on the basis of 1. Significant immune abnormalities seen in localized disease,[178] 2. persistence of abnormalities for up to 10 years into complete remission,[179,180] and 3. abnormalities found in apparently healthy relatives of patients with HD.[181–184] This pre-existing immunodeficiency state may arise from environmental or genetic factors.

A study of six fraternal twin siblings revealed impaired T-cell response to the proliferative stimuli of phytohemagglutinin (PHA), PWM, and concanavalin A (con A) in all six "healthy" siblings.[182] In a study of 12 HD patients' families, in which 6 of the patients had severe impairment of T-cell mitogen (proliferative) responses and 6 had mild mitogen response impairment, one-half of the consanguineous first-degree relatives and spouses of those patients with severe impairments had abnormal mitogen responses themselves.[183] However, none of the relatives or spouses of patients with mild impairment had abnormal mitogen responses. While the first of these studies might support genetic predisposition, both studies may indicate environmental factors leading to abnormal immunity. A later study assessing seven patients with HD and first-degree family members has shown that the total number of T cells measured by rosetting techniques is normal among relatives of patients with HD but that the total T-cell population detected by OKT3 was significantly decreased.[184]

The in vivo responses of cell-mediated immunity that are affected in HD patients include abnormal delayed hypersensitivity responses to new and recall antigens (anergy) and inability to reject skin homografts. The presence or severity of abnormal in vivo responses does not correlate with stage or histology and is not a reliable prognostic indicator.[185–187] The presence or absence of abnormal in vitro responses correlates better with initial response to therapy but appears less valuable in predicting relapses.[188–191] In vitro studies include reduction in total lymphocyte count and percentage of circulating total and helper T cells impaired in proliferative response to a variety of mitogens (PHA, con A, PWM), decreased leukocyte migration inhibition, increased spontaneous DNA synthesis, and depressed reaction in mixed lymphocyte cultures.

At diagnosis, total lymphocyte count is normal to decreased, with lymphopenia more frequent and more pronounced in older age in the presence of B symptoms. Although studies vary, large series indicate that lymphopenia is a poor prognostic factor independent of other variables.[188,190,192] The total T-cell count also tends to be decreased in these same groups. In patients with untreated HD, the lymphopenia is more frequently relative than absolute, due to granulocytosis.[193]

Older measurements of T cells by erythrocyte rosette-forming cells (ERFC) have been replaced by monoclonal antibody analysis. T cells in HD frequently lose the capability to form ERFC. This phenomenon can be corrected by preincubation of peripheral blood mononuclear cells with AB or fetal calf serum, addition of indomethacin, or depletion of monocytes, suggesting blockage of the E rosette receptor by a humoral factor.[194–199] Such proposed humoral factors include prostaglandin-mediated inhibition, immune complexes, feritin, and copper.[198,199] In addition, the number of ERFC can be increased by the immunopotentiator levamisole and by thymic factors mediating differentiation, for example, thymostimulin, supporting primary T-cell defects that may contribute to this phenomenon.[200,201] The improvement with these agents is inversely proportional to the degree of ERFC depression.

The identification of total T cells and T-cell subsets by cytometric analysis in untreated patients reveals normal to decreased numbers of total T cells and decreased helper/inducer subsets (CD4+ cells) in the peripheral blood with an increase in the number of helper cells and normal to decreased suppressor/cytotoxic cells in involved lymphoid tissue (nodes and spleen). The circulating helper-suppressor ratio may be normal to decreased; the number of circulating suppressor/inducer (CD8+) cells and number of natural killer cells are not significantly different from normal controls.[103–105,202] The issue of splenic sequestration of helper/inducer cells has been suggested as an explanation for the differential distribution of these cells. However, splenectomy does not affect circulating helper cell numbers or helper/suppressor ratios.[103,203–205]

In contrast to the circulating cells, splenic lymphocytes have normal to slightly depressed functional responses with significantly better proliferation in response to con A and PHA.[205,206] The CD4+ subset from involved spleens also shows abnormal recognition of DR antigens in autologous and allogeneic mixed lymphocyte reactions and has demonstrated marked cytolytic activity in culture.[207,208] Some have suggested that responses may result from defects in the CD4+ cells or may represent expansion of a subset of CD4+ cells.[208]

The functional impairments of T cells can be assessed by a number of different assays. The mitogen responses, spontaneous proliferation, and allogeneic/autologous mixed lymphocyte reactions have been studied extensively in untreated patients with HD. Abnormally high spontaneous proliferation and decreased proliferative responses with PHA, PWM, con A, and mixed lymphocyte cultures are found in all stages, all histologies, and with and without B symptoms.[190,209–211] There continues to be debate in the literature as to whether these signs of immunocompetence are statistically significant prognostic indicators. The degree of impairment tends to correspond to known poor prognostic factors.[210–212] The most sensitive techniques for detecting impairment utilize suboptimal doses of PHA and con A and autologous rather than allogeneic mixed lymphocyte cultures.[212–213] These assays involve a complex interaction of mature T cells with suppressor T and non-T cells regulating the response. The mixed lymphocyte culture requires a phenotypically precise stimulating cell as well. The formation of PHA-induced T-lymphocyte colonies in soft agar is also impaired in untreated patients. As with other functional assays, it is not clearly correlated with stage of disease.[214]

Abnormal proliferative responses, as with decreased numbers of ERFC, can be partially corrected by a variety of manipulations. The multifactorial nature of the cell-mediated immune defect is suggested by the many factors that will provide partial restoration. Incubation of peripheral blood mononuclear cells with fetal calf serum, human AB serum, or indomethacin or depletion of monocytes will improve but not correct proliferation in response to mitogens.[196,215,216] The degree of impairment has been shown to be related to the concentration of monocytes or prostaglandin E (PGE) in the serum.[210,217] These data have been consistent with PGE functioning as a humoral blocking factor. Thymic extracts and levamisole also partially correct proliferative responses, with the degree of improvement being proportional to the degree of impairment.[218] Decreased proliferation has been attributed to maximal or near-maximal stimulation of T cells at baseline owing to the increased number of activated T cells (Ia+, OKT10+) in patients with HD. This latter argument is weakened by the fact that activated T cells are found primarily in splenic tissues, whose response to mitogens is less impaired than peripheral blood.[205,206,208]

Other humoral factors also appear to impact on T-cell proliferative ability and may support a primary cellular defect of T cells. Exogenous IL-2 partially restores PHA-induced proliferation. Peripheral blood mononuclear cells demonstrate decreased production of IL-2 after PHA stimulation compared with normal controls. The number of unstimulated circulating cells bearing the IL-2 receptor was not significantly different from normal controls; subnormal increases in IL-2 receptors could be demonstrated after PHA stimulation, and levels similar to normal controls were demonstrable after mixed lymphocyte culture.[219–221] By contrast, splenic lymphocytes had normal levels of IL-2 production and IL-2 receptors after PHA stimulation, while the percentage of unstimulated spleen cells bearing the IL-2 receptor was greater than normal splenic controls. Mukhopadhyaya et al.[219] have suggested that this reflects the activated status of splenic lymphocytes in HD.

An increased sensitivity to T cells and non-T-suppressor cells (primarily monocytes) has been noted at normal levels of these cell populations.[179,209,211,212,222] The deletion of monocytes yields better improvements in proliferative responses than incubation of cells with indomethacin, suggesting an additional effect beyond prostaglandin-mediated immunosuppression. Excessive T-cell suppressor ratios may play an additional role in some patients.[223] PHA-induced T-cell colony formation may identify a somewhat different subpopulation of T cells that is also defective in HD. Colony formation is impaired for peripheral blood but not splenic lymphocytes. It does not correct after incubation of cells in fetal calf serum or with the addition of exogenous IL-2, as does the PHA blastogenic response. Suppressed colony formation may in part be due to prostaglandin effect since the addition of indomethacin increases the number of colonies formed.[214,219,220] Other cell lines also exhibit abnormal functioning in untreated HD. Although B-cell numbers are normal, immunoglobulin production in response to PWM is reduced, although spontaneous production of IgG is frequently normal or increased.[221,224,225] The reduction in immunoglobulin production appears to be due to either increased sensitivity to T-cell suppression or ineffective T-helper cells, as the latter cells will not affect PWM-induced immunoglobulin synthesis of B cells from normal individuals. Immunoglobulin levels fall within a wide range, with IgM tending to be low, IgA increased, and IgG either elevated or depressed.[224,226,227] IgE and IgD levels are usually increased. Antibody response to polyvalent vaccines remains intact prior to therapy.[228] The function of monocytes, aside from increased PGE production, is remarkable for poor NK cell activity and ADCC against herpes simplex virus-infected target cells.[229] Decreased phagocytic and fungicidal activity is demonstrated by incubation of monocytes from patients with HD with *Candida pseudotropicalis*.[230] Total monocyte and macrophage numbers have been reported as decreased in HD, which may in part explain their poor functional abilities.[231] In most studies, however, monocyte numbers are normal to increased.

The effects of radiotherapy and chemotherapy and of splenectomy also modify patient immune responses. Radiation and splenectomy effects may last 10 years or longer. However, long-term immune abnormalities are due to intrinsic defects as well as post-treatment causes. Splenectomy often increases total lymphocyte and B-cell counts and may blunt the effects of radiation on lymphocyte numbers.[232–234] Primarily, the long-term effects of splenectomy involve the humoral immune system. Postsplenectomy, IgM levels fall and remain low for years.[235] The antibody response to vaccination is suboptimal and the risk of sepsis is higher, particularly in the first 2 years after splenectomy. Radiation has a more profound effect on cell-mediated immunity. The total lymphocyte and T-cell count are decreased for years. Studies showed nodal recovery of circulating T8+ cells within 6 to 8 months, while T4+ cells showed only a 42 percent recovery in that same period. In addition, a significant proportion of these cells were OKT4+, OKT3– and OKT8+, OKT3–.[236,237] Impaired mitogen responses are seen in HD, rheumatoid arthritis, and seminoma patients after extensive radiotherapy but are most severely depressed in HD.[232,234,235] Chemotherapy alone—nitrogen mustard, vincristine, procarbazine, prednisone (MOPP)—may also cause T lymphopenia and abnormal mitogen responses, but unlike radiation, these effects are not seen in non-Hodgkin's lymphoma patients of comparable stage after treatment with similar combination chemotherapy regimens.[179,233]

IMMUNOTHERAPY

The association of impaired immunity and neoplastic disease of the lymphoproliferative system is exemplified by clinical abnormalities, laboratory evidence of decreased immune responses in HD and non-Hodgkin's lymphoma, and the increased frequency of lymphomas in immunosuppressed states, congenital or acquired. This association suggests a link between the development and/or propagation of a neoplastic clone and abnormal immune function. By this reasoning, the prevention or abolition of lymphomas could presumably be altered by restoration of the host immune system. In vitro the use of prostaglandins, thymic factors, and levamisole can partly restore immune function. The immune response modifiers that act in vivo that have been most extensively studied are bacillus Calmette-Guérin (BCG) scarification and the interferons.

The use of BCG to augment immune responses of the cell-mediated type was successfully employed by Mathe et al.[238,239] in the treatment of acute lymphocytic leukemia in the late 1960s. The combination of BCG scarification and irradiated allogeneic leukemic blasts as maintenance therapy was contrasted with no maintenance therapy in 100 patients with ALL. The patients receiving immunotherapeutic maintenance had longer relapse-free survival and improved survival after a second remission-induction course if they did relapse when compared with controls without maintenance therapy. Following this early report, later studies using several different schedules of BCG administration and different strains of BCG failed to show the marked benefit of immunotherapy in acute ALL.[240–244] The use of BCG in other hematopoietic neoplasms was also widely evaluated and in non-Hodgkin's lymphoma appears to be clinically useful.

The early studies of BCG in HD were generally small studies with selection bias. In one retrospective review Hodgkin's and non-Hodgkin's lymphoma patient groups were combined into early and late stages of disease, active or in remission.[245] As a whole, the stage I and II patients treated with radiotherapy alone had a survival advantage when treatment with BCG scarification was added. No other patient groups had a significant benefit from immunotherapy. A cooperative prospective randomized study of stage III to IV HD patients evaluated the efficacy of methanol extraction residue (MER) of BCG in addition to combination chemotherapy.[246] The results were based on 167 evaluable patients who had received prior radiotherapy, chemotherapy, or both and three-fourths of whom were anergic. The addition of MER did not significantly increase the complete response rate over combination chemotherapy alone. In the patient group that had not received previous chemotherapy, there was no survival advantage to MER therapy, while patients who had received prior chemotherapy had a significantly poorer survival after MER treatment. In addition, there was serious toxicity associated with MER therapy, particularly pain and ulceration at injection sites. Thus, immunotherapy in the form of MER has been discontinued as a treatment modality, with little enthusiasm for further studies of BCG-MER immunotherapy in HD.

The use of BCG in non-Hodgkin's lymphomas has been more positive, both as a remission-induction agent and as maintenance therapy. A 4-year study of 652 patients with non-Hodgkin's lymphoma compared the use of BCG in combination with CHOP (cyclophosphamide, doxorubicin, Oncovin, prednisone) versus CHOP or cytoxan, vincristine, and prednisone (COP) plus bleomycin as a remission-induction regimen.[247,248] There was no difference in the attainment of complete remission between the various regimens with the exception of both nodular and diffuse histiocytic lymphomas. Here, treatment with BCG resulted in a statistically significant increase in complete remission rates and led to a survival advantage in these two groups as well. The trial of BCG maintenance demonstrated no benefit in remission duration over those with unmaintained remissions.

The role of BCG in maintenance therapy in European studies suggests benefits in many groups of patients. An early trial of 48 patients with all stages of non-Hodgkin's lymphoma were randomized to BCG or no maintenance.[249] According to this study, BCG maintenance prolonged remission duration and survival only for patients with clinical stages I and II. Because of the encouraging results of this trial, an additional 50 patients with stage III and IV disease were randomized and duration and survival were again seen with stage I and II patients but not for stages III and IV. Patients younger than 65 years, males, and those who had previously relapsed also had significantly increased remission duration when given BCG maintenance. In this study, favorable histology (nodular) patients did not differ from those with high-grade histology (diffuse)—neither showed a beneficial response independent of the other variables cited.

The benefit of BCG maintenance in favorable histology lymphomas was apparent in a study of 109 patients with stage III and IV nodular lymphomas.[251] The duration of complete remission was statistically longer than without maintenance BCG therapy (3 years versus greater than 5 years). There was no distinct advantage noted in histiocytic (large cell) lymphomas as opposed to the entire group, which is in accord with the other studies mentioned.

In recent years, the development of fusion protein toxins came about due to advances made in genetic engineering.[484] These proteins represent a novel class of biomolecules that combine a naturally occurring toxin with a targeting ligand. The resultant recombinant protein has the immunologic determinants of both the toxin and the ligand, and is capable of intoxicating only cells to which the ligand is capable of binding. The first of these fusion proteins used diphtheria toxin in combination with IL-2, creating the protein that recently won FDA approval known as DAB 389 IL-2 (ONTAK).[484]

The mechanism that these toxins work by to kill cells involves their enzymatically active domains that must be translocated into the cytosol.[484] After receptor binding, the initial full-length toxin undergoes internalization and processing within the cellular compartments. In the case of diphtheria toxin, the intact toxin molecule is proteolytically cleaved in acidic endosomes to liberate the enzymatically active fragment A, which is then translocated into the cytosol.[484]

The first fusion protein tested both in vitro and in animals was DAB 486 IL-2. DAB 486 encodes a 68 kd protein that contains the first 486 amino acids of the diphtheria toxin and the full-length sequence of IL-2.[437,438] In vitro studies showed a selective cytotoxicity for the high affinity IL-2 receptor (IL-2 R).[440] The IL-2 R is found and expressed on a subset of leukemia and lymphoma cells.

Due to the fact that IL-2 R expression has been documented in hematology malignancies, including Hodgkin's, non-Hodgkin's lymphomas, CLL, and CTCL, a series of trials were developed to determine safety, tolerability, and pharmacokinetics of this newly discovered protein DAB 486 IL-2.[443–454]

The initial trials were developed as cohort dose escalations in which single/multiple doses of DAB 486 IL-2 were given by iv infusion.[484] The MTD was 0.27 mg/kg/day in a phase I study in which patients were dosed every 8 to 12 hours, with elevations in serum transaminases being the dose-limiting toxicity.[443–454] The most frequently occurring adverse events in these studies were hypersensitivity, fever/chills, malaise, and serum transaminases elevations. Of note, no evidence of immunosuppression was observed.[451,455] Clinical responses were noted in Hodgkin's, non-Hodgkin's, and CTCL, with the CTCL group having the highest percentage of responders. All of the responders had demonstrable IL-2 R expression as measured by immunohistochemistry with CD 25 (anti Tac) antibody.

DAB 486 demonstrated high specific activity, but it had a flaw; it also suffered from an extremely short half-life of approximately 11 minutes. To optimize the molecule, a series of successive truncations were done and DAB 386 IL-2 (ONTAK) was created. DAB 389 was shown to have a 2 to 3 times higher kd than DAB 486 resulting in a 10 times increase in potency. The half-life also was extended to $3^1/_2$ to 4 hours.[456–459]

Clinical trials for DAB 389 IL-2 (denileukin diftitox, ONTAK) began with protocol 92-04-01, a phase I trial.[462,485] The trial demonstrated an overall response rate of 22 percent (37 percent in the CTCL group). The duration of remission was 9.1 months. The second trial was a two-arm randomized blinded trial in patients with advanced CTCL.[463] The objectives were to evaluate the safety and tolerability of various doses of DAB 489 IL-2, as well as estimates of safety.[485] The inclusion criteria required that the IL-2 receptor be present on at least 20 percent of the neoplastic biopsy sample. The overall response rate was 30 percent (23 percent in the low dose arm and 36 percent in the high dose arm). The median duration of response was 7 months from treatment initiation. Again the most common adverse effects were infections, chill, fevers, nausea, vomiting, asthenia, and hypotension. The incidence of adverse events decreased after the first two courses.[463] These promising results of these clinical trials led the U.S. FDA to approve DAB 389 IL-2 for the treatment of persistent or relapsed CTCL.

ONTAK has also been tested in other malignancies. Data from a phase I trial suggest that it has activity in low and intermediate grade non-Hodgkin's lymphoma. Phase II trials are currently being looked at by various groups in this setting.[486]

ONTAK is also being explored in the field of transplant medicine.[486] In the setting of solid organ transplant, acute and chronic graft rejection is mediated by host lymphocytes. Once recognition has occurred, alloreactive lymphocytes express IL-2 R. It is assumed that these IL-2 R expressing cells mediated rejection. Thus it would make sense that treatment with an IL-2 R targeted toxin would afford an opportunity to selectively delete these clones involved with rejection. Animal studies have demonstrated significant improvement in graft survival in animals treated with an IL-2 toxin.[471–472] The feasibility of human studies has already been established as well with Daclizumab, a humanized monoclonal antibody to the TAC (CD25) subunit of the IL-2 R complex. It has recently been approved by the FDA for use in the setting of renal transplant.[473,486]

Other diseases for which DAB 389 IL-2 is being looked at are rheumatoid arthritis, lupus, inflammatory bowel disease, psoriasis, and even HIV.[486] Now that DAB 389 IL-2 has been approved for CTCL, it is hoped that investigators will develop other studies to explore some of these other possibilities.

The activity of interferon, particularly in the low grade histologies of non-Hodgkin's lymphomas (exclusive of CLL and diffuse well-differentiated lymphomas), has been well studied. Initial studies of natural interferon given in doses of 5 to 10 million units via the intramuscular route in a daily to twice daily schedule demonstrated responses in low grade but not aggressive lymphomas. Combined results from several trials using low daily doses of interferon have produced overall response rates of 25 to 30 percent in indolent lymphomas, with complete response rates of 0 to 20 percent.[252] The natural interferon-β products have similarly demonstrated responses in 2 of 10 patients with low grade lymphoma treated with 4.5×10 units intravenously daily for an additional 2 weeks.[253]

Subsequent studies with recombinant type I interferon products have confirmed the high response rate of low grade lymphomas. Preliminary work by Foon and co-workers[254] has established the activity of relatively high doses of recombinant interferon-α in pretreated patients. Twenty-four patients with low grade lymphomas received 50×10^3 IU/m^2 of interferon intramuscularly three times per week with a response rate of 54 percent and a median duration of response of 8 months. Of six patients with intermediate grade histologies, there were two responses, both in patients with diffuse small cleaved cell lymphoma (one complete response and one partial response) for a response rate of 15 percent, while only one of seven patients with high grade histology responded. A 35 percent response rate

was seen in 17 patients with nodular poorly differentiated lymphoma treated with daily intramuscular interferon in an escalating dose study utilizing from 3×10^6 to 50×10^6 units of recombinant interferon per day.[255] There were responses seen at all dose levels above 3×10^6 units per day, suggesting that there was no obvious dose-response relationship for low grade lymphomas. Similar responses rates in the low grade lymphomas of 25 to 66 percent were also demonstrated with recombinant interferon via the subcutaneous route at doses of 2×10^6 units three times per week and 10×10^6 to 25×10^6 units three times per week, a schedule that is more convenient and permits patient self-administration of the drug.[252,256,257] The time to response ranges from 4 to 10 weeks after the initiation of therapy with a median duration of response ranging from 26 to 48 weeks.[256–258]

Similar favorable results have been noted in the treatment of CTCL using interferon-α. A group of 20 patients with CTCL, all of whom had failed previous therapies, were treated with maximally tolerated doses of interferon-α-2.[259] Responses were seen at both cutaneous and extracutaneous sites. The overall response rate was 45 percent (two complete responses, seven partial responses, and five mixed responses) with a median duration of responses of 6 months.

The major toxicities seen with low to moderate doses of interferon are an initial flulike syndrome, consisting of fever, headache, myalgias, arthralgias, and mild nausea, generally mild cytopenias, transient aberrations in liver function tests (usually mild to moderate transaminase elevations), anorexia, and fatigue; unusual toxicities include dysgeusia, renal dysfunction, particularly proteinuria, neuropathies, and exacerbation of underlying cardiac disease with arrhythmias and myocardial infarction.[252] The flulike syndrome occurs early in treatment, and tachyphylaxis develops during the initial weeks of therapy. The dose-limiting toxicity is the chronic fatigue and anorexia. With the exception of myocardial infarction, these side effects are reversible with cessation of the drug.

A Cancer and Leukemia Group B (CALGB) pilot trial of recombinant interferon-α-2 (2×10^6 IU subcutaneously on alternate days) and oral cyclophosphamide (100 mg/m^2/day) was initiated in patients with stages III and IV follicular lymphoma, both previously treated and untreated.[260] Among 60 evaluable patients, 41 had received no prior chemotherapy. The toxicities in the patient population as a whole were more severe than initially anticipated, with leukopenia being the most common toxicity. The incidence of significant leukopenia (<2000 cells/ml) was 53 percent in previously untreated patients compared with a similar population (14 percent) treated with oral cyclophosphamide alone in an earlier CALGB study. Leukopenia was promptly reversible with dose suspension or adjustment, and other toxicities were mild or tolerable. In patients who had received previous chemotherapy, severe or life-threatening leukopenia (63 percent), thrombocytopenia (23 percent), and anemia (15 percent) were more common and led to more frequent dose adjustment. The overall response rate (complete response plus partial response) was 84 percent in patients who had not received prior chemotherapy, with a median follow-up of 3 months. The promising results of this study have led to an ongoing, randomized CALGB study of oral cyclophosphamide versus cyclophosphamide plus interferon in patients with advanced low-grade non-Hodgkin's lymphoma who have not received prior chemotherapy.

Other studies combining recombinant interferon with traditional antineoplastic agents are under way including chlorambucil and interferon; cyclophosphamide, vincristine, and prednisone (CVP) and interferon; and cyclophosphamide, vincristine, prednisone, and doxorubicin (COPA) plus interferon. Two different schedules of chlorambucil and low-dose interferon (3×10^6 to 6×10^6 units) have produced responses in relapsed or refractory, heavily pretreated, low and intermediate grade non-Hodgkin's lymphomas in 6 of 13 patients (46 percent) and 14 of 22 patients (64 percent).[261,262] Toxicity with these two agents was moderate, and both regimens were well tolerated. Use of recombinant interferon with monoclonal antibodies has also been investigated by the Stanford group, building on their prior experience with anti-idiotype serotherapy of lymphomas.[263] The addition of interferon to idiotype therapy appeared to improve the initial rate of response to antibody therapy. The dose of interferon chosen, 12×10^6 U/m^2 intramuscularly three times per week for 8 weeks, was based on a previous Eastern Cooperative Oncology Group phase II study in untreated low grade lymphomas that yielded a response rate of 44 percent. The addition of interferon appeared to improve the initial response rate.

From these early trials, it was determined that interferon-alfa worked best in follicular lymphomas. Thus several studies looked at adding interferon with a single agent alkylator as initial induction therapy. There was no overall survival advantage, but again the addition of interferon-alfa did show improvement in the time to progression.[336,337] These results were countered in the Intergroup trial, which demonstrated no survival advantage, and no time to progression advantage.[338,339]

EORTC, GLSG, and a Spanish study looked at interferon-alfa as part of an induction regimen with cytotoxic chemotherapy regimens to include CVP and CHOP.[342–344] The Spanish study found that the addition of interferon-alfa did not favorably affect the overall response or the complete response rate.[482]

The German study (GLSG) also demonstrated no difference in the overall response rate, but it was the first to show that the addition of an anthracycline to the regimen with interferon induced more complete responses versus the nonanthracycline regimen.[482] This led to three other prominent studies to try and reproduce these results. The studies were launched by a Mexican group, ECOG, and GELF. All three used interferon-alfa with CHOP as initial induction therapy.[345–348]

In the Mexican study group, patients receiving interferon-alfa experienced a prolongation of duration of remission and overall survival.[345–348] With over 11 years of follow-up, the median survival for the interferon-alfa group has yet to be reached, while the noninterferon group had a median survival of 74 months.

The two larger groups, ECOG and GELF, also demonstrated an improvement in both time to disease progression and again overall survival in the group of patients receiving interferon-alfa.[348,349,482] A preliminary analysis at 3 years did not document any advantage; however at 10 years, the difference was clearly evident. It was concluded that the addition of interferon-alfa induced a 10 to 12 percent difference in overall survival at any given point throughout the 10-year follow-up period.

More recently, Rohatiner et al. reviewed data from nine prospective randomized trials evaluating the role of interferon-alfa in the treatment of follicular NHL.[350] The analysis confirmed a survival advantage when interferon-alfa was added to an anthracycline-based regimen. This was followed by a review by Ozer et al., which pointed out that tumor burden may be the most important factor in deciding whether interferon-alfa should be added to the induction treatment regimen.[351] Also, with the recent approval of rituximab, the use of interferon-alfa in combination is currently being evaluated.[355]

The evaluation of interferon-alfa in diffuse large cell lymphomas has been limited. The only randomized trial to evaluate interferon-alfa in this setting did show an overall survival advantage at 5 years.[357,482] The trial also suggested that selected few patients who received interferon had better responses to salvage chemotherapy regimens if NHL recurred versus the group that did not receive the interferon. Similar results were also obtained in the setting of mantle cell lymphoma, marginal zone B-cell lymphoma, HIV lymphoma, and T-cell lymphomas. Further evaluation is clearly indicated and needed.[482]

The use of murine-derived monoclonal antibodies directed against specific tumor-associated antigens has been evaluated in both T- and B-cell lymphomas. While the tumor specificity of these agents represents a clear advantage over conventional therapy, there are a number of limitations in their use including 1. Cross-reactivity with normal tissue antigens, and 2. delivery of antibody to the tumor, dependent on tumor vascularity and size, interaction with circulating antigen or human antimouse antibodies (HAMA), and amount of surface antigen. Affinity of the antibody against hematopoietic neoplasms is not dependent on isotype; however, anti-idiotypic/anti-immunoglobulin antibodies appear to be more efficacious than antibodies against other tumor-associated antigens.

In a review of 177 patients receiving 271 courses of therapy, the toxicities of monoclonal antibody therapy included fever (15 percent), transaminasemia (14 percent), rigors and chills (13 percent), diaphoresis and urticaria (11 percent each), pruritus (9 percent), nausea (4 percent), dyspnea, vomiting, bronchospasm (3 percent each), diarrhea and hypotension (2 percent each), and anaphylaxis (0.5 percent).[264] To some extent the incidence of side effects is related to the rate of infusion and/or to binding to a large number of circulating cells. HAMA develop in all patients except a proportion of those with CLL and some B-cell lymphomas, which effectively neutralizes the monoclonal antibody administered.

The use of T101 antibody in the therapy of CTCL and B-CLL has demonstrated minor responses only. Reports of an initial 16 patients treated at the University of California at San Diego provided encouraging results.[265] Patients with advanced or refractory CLL (6) and CTCL (10) underwent 24-hour infusions of the T101 antibody in escalating doses of 10 to 500 mg. Demonstrable binding of the T101 antibody to tumor occurred and minor objective clinical responses were seen in 4 of 10

CTCL patients and 2 of 6 CLL patients, primarily a reduction of circulating malignant cells. Durations of responses were brief due to antigenic modulation and development of antimouse antibodies (in 5 of 10 CTCL patients but 0 of 5 CLL patients). In summarizing the experience of T101 and Leu-1 antibody therapy of CTCL at several institutions, Foon[51] reported that 10 of 30 patients treated achieved minor responses.

In the experience with anti-idiotype antibodies, the overall response rates have been higher but also of brief duration. The Stanford experience with 16 patients treated with anti-idiotype antibody alone resulted in one complete remission, seven partial remissions, and two minor responses, with response durations ranging from 1 month to 6 years (the complete responder).[263] The treatment protocol was modified during the study, most importantly with additional purification of the antibody, which has decreased the incidence of HAMA formation, use of multiple anti-idiotypic antibodies in some patients, titration of the dose of antibody in some patients, titration of the dose of antibody to achieve peak serum levels of at least 200 μg/ml, and the exclusion of patients with serum idiotype levels above 50 μg/ml. A subsequent trial of anti-idiotype antibodies with low-dose interferon yielded similar results, with 2 complete remissions, 7 partial remissions, and 2 minor responses among 11 patients receiving a total of 12 courses. The response durations ranged from 2 to 24 months with two patients continuing in complete remission. The addition of interferon increased toxicity; this included fever and rigors in all patients on the first day of treatment, neutropenia, thrombocytopenia, and gastrointestinal distress. A trend toward higher response rates was seen in the second trial; however, the number of patients was small and modifications in the antibody treatment protocol alone may also account for these improvements.

Significant advances have been made in the application of monoclonal antibody-based therapies to the treatment of lymphoma.[480] Two types of treatments have been based on the use of either native unconjugated monoclonal antibodies or the use of monoclonal antibodies to target radionuclides, drugs, or toxins to the tumor directly. The first uses monoclonal antibodies that contain mostly human antibody sequences with only the variable region or the actual antibody binding sites coming from the original murine.[480] These unconjugated monoclonal antibodies have a longer half-life, are less immunogenic, have increased clinical activity, and are well tolerated. The second strategy uses the monoclonal antibody as a carrier to specifically target a radionucleotide or toxin to the tumor.[480] This approach has clearly demonstrated increased tumor activity, but is used with caution secondary to dose-limiting toxicities.

Early work identified the CD20 antigen as a potential target for immunotherapy.[480] The CD20 antigen is a membrane phosphoprotein, with most of it being found within the cell, but a small region is exported to the cell surface. CD20 is found on most B-cell lymphomas and is especially expressive in follicular lymphomas. It is not expressed on critical host cells, stem cells, and plasma cells.

The first monoclonal antibody approved by the FDA that is directed specifically against the CD20 antigen is rituximab (IDEC-C2B8, Rituxan, MabThera in Europe). It is a chimeric monoclonal antibody that contains murine IgG1 kappa heavy and light chain constant regions.[483] Upon binding to its target antigen, Rituximab mediates complement-dependent cellular cytotoxicity and antibody-dependent cellular cytotoxicity.[369–371]

The initial phase I/II trials were done by Maloney et al.[372–374,483] In these early studies, dose-limiting toxicity was not identified and maximum tolerated dose was not reached. Peripheral B cells were rapidly depleted starting at 24 hours after infusion and slowly recovered from 3 to 6 months. Because CD20 is not expressed on plasma cells, there was no change noted in the immunoglobulin levels, thus no increase in serious infections were noted. Responses ranged from 13 to 43 percent in these early studies.[483]

To confirm these early results, a phase II multicenter trial was completed by McLaughlin et al.[375,482] The trial contained a total of 166 patients with relapsed low grade and follicular lymphomas. The dose of Rituxan was 375 mg/m² given for four cycles. The overall response rate was 48 percent with 6 percent of these patients actually achieving a complete response. Treatment was well tolerated with the majority of the adverse effects occurring during the initial infusion only.[375] Several subsequent trials all demonstrated similar results in patients with relapsed or previously untreated non-Hodgkin's lymphomas.[376–384]

After the initial successes using Rituxan as a single agent, it was looked at in combination with chemotherapy.[386–390,482] Combinations included CHOP (cyclophosphamide, Adriamycin, oncovin, prednisone), CVP (cyclophosphamide, vincristine, prednisone), mitoxantrone, and fludarabine combined with rituximab. Most of these trials were initiated in the previously untreated population. Overall response rates ranged from 81 to 95 percent with complete remissions ranging from 10 to 81 percent. These trials quickly led the FDA to approve the drug for commercial use in the United States.

Rituximab has also shown activity in aggressive non-Hodgkin's lymphoma, such as mantle cell lymphomas, as well as chronic lymphocytic leukemias, and plasma cell dyscrasias that express the CD20 antigen.[482] More recently, it is being evaluated as a maintenance therapy option for the management of indolent non-Hodgkin's lymphoma. Other disease states such as immune thrombocytopenic purpura (ITP) have also been studied with promising results.

These and subsequent ongoing trials will help us define the ultimate role of this agent and its potential impact on survival of patients with B-cell neoplasms.

Another agent targeted at a specific antigen is Campath-1H, which is targeted at the CD52 antigen. The antigen is a 12 amino acid sequence expressed on both T and B lymphocytes, as well some immature lymphocytes.[480] Campath-1H is a humanized IgG1 monoclonal antibody that has shown activity in B-cell neoplasms. However, it has increased toxicity in comparison to rituximab, including fever, chills, rigors, and hypotension. These adverse effects are believed to be mediated from the release of TNF-α, interferon-γ, and IL-6.[480] Also, again in contrast to rituximab, it is expressed on normal lymphocytes resulting in prolonged immunosuppression that can last for months.

The use of antibodies to target drugs or toxins was undertaken to augment the antitumor activity, observed using unmodified monoclonal antibodies.[480] The most experience using such immunotoxins for the treatment of lymphoma has been with monoclonal antibodies coupled to the toxins based on ricin.

The largest series of trials looked at a B4-blocked ricin, an immunotoxin made of intact ricin with chemically blocked galactose-binding sites conjugated to the anti-CD19 monoclonal antibody (B4).[276–278] Phase I/II trials demonstrated responses; however they were of short duration and most complicated by dose-limiting toxicities of hepatotoxicity and thrombocytopenia.[480]

Vitetta and colleagues looked at a deglycosylated ricin A chain that was coupled to intact or Fab fragments of anti-CD19 (HD-37) and anti-CD22 (RFB 4) monoclonal antibodies.[279–282] In a phase I trial, the dose-limiting toxicity of capillary leak syndrome was identified. Again in these early trials, clinical responses were noted in up to 30 percent of the patients, but most were short lived in nature.[480]

Additional trials have looked at immunotoxins against CD5 antigen that is expressed in some T- and B-cell malignancies.[283,284] Early results from these trials have demonstrated similar results with short duration of responses accompanied by dose-limiting toxicities.[480]

Radiolabeled antibodies possess several theoretical advantages for the treatment of non-Hodgkin's lymphoma.[285–288] Since radioimmunoconjugates kill tumor cells primarily by emission of radioactive particles, they are effective in situations where defective immune effector systems compromise the utility of unmodified antibodies.[480] Also, the beta particles emitted by commonly used radioisotopes are tumoricidal over a distance of many cell diameters, allowing eradication of antigen-negative tumor cells that reside beside the antigen-positive cells. This principle also is the major disadvantage with such radiolabeled antibodies in that there is nonspecific and specific toxicity to normal cells.

Lenhard and Order pioneered radioimmunotherapy for hematologic malignancies using 131 I-labeled polyclonal antiferritin antibodies to treat patients with refractory Hodgkin's disease. Tumor responses were noted in 15 of 37 patients (40 percent).[292,480] A subsequent trial evaluated 90 Y-labeled polyclonal antiferritin antibodies in patients with advanced Hodgkin's disease. In this trial 20 of 39 (51 percent) patients had an objective tumor response.[293] Three other trials confirmed these early results, thus making this therapy a viable option in patients with refractory Hodgkin's disease.[294]

The most promising trials in radioimmunotherapy have been conducted with radiolabled anti-CD20 antibodies to treat patients with relapsed B-cell lymphomas.[480] In the phase I/II trials done by Kaminski et al., a total of 28 patients were evaluable for the study; of these 28 patients, 14 (50 percent) had a documented complete remission and another 8 (29 percent) had a partial response.[285,286,297] Myelosuppression was the dose-limiting toxicity with a maximally tolerated whole body radiation dose of 75 cGy.

Knox et al. administered 90 Y-labeled anti-CD20 antibodies to 18 patients with relapsed B-cell lymphomas.[298] The results were again encouraging with 6 patients having a complete remission and 7 having a partial remission, making the overall response rate 72 percent.

Press et al. explored the potential of 131 I-labeled anti CD20 antibodies in a series of trials using autologous stem cell support to circumvent the hematologic toxicity observed with most radioimmunotherapies.[290,291,299,480] In these series of trials, the durations of remissions appear to be much longer for patients with follicular lymphomas than for patients with intermediate or high-grade lymphomas. Response rates were upward of 80 percent in this patient population, with durations lasting up to 4 years to date.

Many multicenter trials are currently under way or have recently been completed with the results still pending. It remains to be determined what exact role each of these new agents will play in the management of patients with non-Hodgkin's lymphoma. Forthcoming trial results should help us guide our management decisions.

REFERENCES

1. Taylor CR: A practical approach to immunohistologic studies of lymphoreticular neoplasia. J Histochem Cytochem 27:1188, 1979.
2. Peiper SC, Kahn LB, Ross DW et al: Ultra-structural organization of the Reed-Sternberg cell: Its resemblance to cells of the monocyte-macrophage system. Blood Cells 6:525, 1980.
3. Wood GW, Travers H: Non-Hodgkin's lymphoma: Identification of the monoclonal B lymphocyte component in the presence of polyclonal immunoglobulin. J Histochem Cytochem 30:1015, 1982.
4. Isaacson P: Immunochemical demonstration of J chain: A marker of B cell malignancy. J Clin Pathol 32:802, 1979.
5. Isaacson P, Wright DH: Anomolous staining patterns in immunohistologic studies of malignant lymphoma. J Histochem Cytochem 27:1197, 1979.
6. Brubaker DB, Whiteside TL: Differentiation between malignant and benign human lymph nodes by means of immunologic markers. Cancer 43:1165, 1979.
7. Koziner B, Mertelsmann R, Siegal FP et al: Cell marker analysis in hematopoietic neoplasms. Clin Bull 8:47, 1978.
8. Warnke RA, Link MP: Identification and significance of cell markers in leukemia and lymphoma. Annu Rev Med 34:117, 1983.
9. Halper JP, Knowles DA, Wang CY: Ia antigen expression by human malignant lymphomas: Correlation with conventional lymphoid markers. Blood 55:373, 1980.
10. Siegal FP, Flippa DA, Koziner B: Surface markers in leukemias and lymphomas. Am J Pathol 90:451, 1978.
11. Van-Heerde P, Feltkamp CA, Feltkamp-Vroom TM et al: Non-Hodgkin's lymphoma: Immunohistochemical and electron microscopic findings in relation to microscopy. Cancer 46:2210, 1980.
12. LeBien T, Kersey J, Nakazawa S et al: Analysis of human leukemia/lymphoma cell lines with monoclonal antibodies BA-1, BA-2, and BA-3. Leuk Res 6:299, 1982.
13. Nadler LM, Ritz J, Hardy R et al: A unique cell surface antigen identifying lymphoid malignancies of B cell origin. J Clin Invest 67:134, 1981.
14. Nadler LM, Stashenko P, Harday R et al: Characterization of a human B cell specific antigen (B2) distinct from B1. J Immunol 126:1941, 1981.

15. Nadler LM, Boyd AW, Park E et al: The B cell restricted glycoprotein (B2) is the receptor for Epstein-Barr virus (EBV). Blood 64:78, 1984.

16. Nadler LM, Anderson KC, Marti G et al: B4, a human B lymphocytic associated antigen expressed on normal mitogen-activated and malignant B lymphocytes. J Immunol 131:244, 1983.

17. Borella L, Casper JP, Lauer SJ: Shifts in expression of cell membrane phenotypes in childhood lymphoid malignancies at relapse. Blood 54:64, 1979.

18. Delsol G, Laurent G, Kuhlien E et al: Richter's syndrome: Evidence for the clonal origin of two proliferations. Am J Clin Pathol 76:308, 1981.

19. Frenkel FP, Smith RG, Ligler FS et al: Analysis and detection of B cell neoplasms: A commentary. Blood Cells 6:795, 1980.

20. Harousseau JL, Flandrin G, Tricot G et al: Malignant lymphoma supervening in chronic lymphocytic leukemia and related disorders. Cancer 48:1302, 1981.

21. Minowada J, Koshiba H, Sagawa K et al: Marker profiles of human leukemia and lymphoma cell lines. J Cancer Res Clin Oncol 101:91, 1981.

22. Woda BA, Knowles DM: Nodular lymphocytic lymphoma eventuating into diffuse histiocytic lymphoma: Immunoperoxidase demonstration of monoclonality. Cancer 43:303, 1989.

23. Picker LJ, Weiss LM, Medeiros LJ et al: Immunophenotypic criteria for the diagnosis of non-Hodgkin's lymphoma. Am J Pathol 128:181, 1987.

24. Ault KA: Detection of small numbers of monoclonal B lymphocytes in the blood of patients with lymphomas. N Engl J Med 300:1401, 1979.

25. Frenkel EP, Smith RG, Ligler FE et al: Analysis and detection of B cell neoplasms. Blood Cells 6:783, 1980.

26. Krajewski AS, Dewar AE: Studies on blood lymphocytes of patients with nodular poorly differentiated lymphocytic lymphoma. J Clin Pathol 34:896, 1981.

27. Sobol RE, Astarita RW, Chisari FV et al: Use of immunoglobulin light chain analysis to detect bone marrow involvement in B cell neoplasms. Clin Immunol Immunopathol 24:139, 1982.

28. Krajewski AS, Dewar AE, Ramage GF: T and B lymphocyte markers in effusions of patients with non-Hodgkin's lymphoma. J Clin Pathol 35:1216, 1982.

29. Brudler O, Han T, Barcos M et al: Determination of clonal excess in non-Hodgkin's lymphoma: Clinical significance. Proc Am Assoc Cancer Res 24:122, 1983.

30. Andres TL, Kadin ME: Immunologic markers in the differential diagnosis of small round cell tumors from lymphocytic lymphoma and leukemia. Am J Clin Pathol 79:546, 1983.

31. Kimshed JT, Fritschy J, Goldman A et al: Use of panels of monoclonal antibodies in the differential diagnosis of neuroblastic and lymphoblastic disorders. Lancet 1:12, 1983.

32. Pizzolo G, Sloane J, Beverly P et al: Differential diagnosis of malignant lymphoma and nonlymphoid tumors using monoclonal antileukocyte antibody. Cancer 46:2640, 1980.

33. Pizzolo G, Chilosi M, Cetto GL et al: Immunohistochemical analysis of bone marrow involvement in lymphoproliferative disorders. Br J Haematol 50:95, 1982.

34. Korsmeyer SJ, Hieter PA, Ravetch JV et al: Developmental hierarchy of immunoglobulin gene rearrangements in human leukemic pre-B cells. Proc Natl Acad Sci U S A 78:7096, 1981.

35. Arnold A, Cossman J, Bakhshi A et al: Immunoglobulin-gene rearrangements as unique clonal markers in human lymphoid neoplasms. N Engl J Med 309:1593, 1983.

36. Cleary ML, Chao J, Warnke R et al: Immunoglobulin gene rearrangement as a diagnostic criterion of B-cell lymphoma. Proc Natl Acad Sci U S A 81:593, 1984.

37. Flug F, Pelicci PG, Bonetti F et al: T-cell receptor gene rearrangements as markers of lineage and clonality in T-cell neoplasms. Proc Natl Acad Sci U S A 82:3460, 1985.

38. Waldmann TA, Davis MM, Gongiovanni K et al: Rearrangements of genes for the antigen receptor on T-cell as markers of lineage and clonality in human lymphoid neoplasms. N Engl J Med 313:776, 1985.

39. Taura A, Hozumi N, Minden M et al: Rearrangement of the T-cell receptor beta-chain in non-T-cell, non-B-cell acute lymphoblastic leukemia of childhood. N Engl J Med 313:1033, 1985.

40. Tkachuk DC, Griesser H, Takihara Y et al: Rearrangement of T-cell d (delta) locus in lymphoproliferative disorders. Blood 72:353, 1988.

41. Brada M, Mizutani S, Molgaurd H et al: Circulating lymphoma cells in patients with B&T non-Hodgkin's lymphoma detected by immunoglobulin and T-cell receptor gene arrangement. Br J Cancer 56:147, 1987.

42. Pelicci PG, Knocules DM, Dalla Favera R: Lymphoid tumors displaying rearrangements of both immunoglobulin and T-cell receptor genes. J Exp Med 162:1015, 1985.

43. Said JW, Hargreaves HK, Pinkus GS: Non-Hodgkin's lymphomas: An ultrastructural study correlating morphology with immunologic cell type. Cancer 44:504, 1979.

44. Rosenberg SA, Bernard CS, Brown BW Jr et al: National Cancer Institute sponsored study of classifications of non-Hodgkin's lymphoma. Cancer 49:2112, 1982.

45. Suchi T, Lennert K, Tu LY et al: Histopathology and immunochemistry of peripheral T cell lymphomas: A proposal for their classification. J Clin Pathol 40:995, 1987.

46. Van Den Twerl JG, Lukes RJ, Taylor CR: Pathophysiology of lymphocyte transformation: A study of so-called composite lymphomas. Am J Clin Pathol 71:509, 1979.

47. Landaas TO, Godal T, Morton PF et al: Cell associated immunoglobulin I human non-Hodgkin's lymphomas. Acta Microbiol Scand 89:91, 1981.

48. Lukes RJ: The immunologic approach to the pathology of malignant lymphomas. Am J Clin Pathol 72:657, 1979.

49. Falini B, DeSolas I, Levine AM et al: Emergence of B immunoblastic sarcoma in patients with multiple myeloma: A clinicopathologic study of 10 cases. Blood 59:923, 1982.

50. Harousseau JL, Flandrin G, Tricot G et al: Malignant lymphoma supervening in chronic lymphocytic leukemia and related disorders. Cancer 48:1302, 1981.

51. Foon KA: Laboratory and clinical applications of monoclonal antibodies for leukemia and non-Hodgkin's lymphomas. Curr Probl Cancer 13:57, 1989.

52. Pinkus GS, Said JW: Characterization of non-Hodgkin's lymphomas using multiple cell markers. Am J Pathol 94:349, 1978.

53. Aisenberg AC, Wilkes BM, Harris NL: Monoclonal antibody studies in non-Hodgkin's lymphoma. Blood 61:469, 1983.

54. Berard CW, Cossman J, Jaffe ES: Malignant lymphomas as tumors of the immune system. Br J Cancer 42:1, 1980.

55. Habeshaw JA, Bailey D, Stansfield AG et al: The cellular content of non-Hodgkin's lymphomas: A comprehensive analysis using monoclonal antibodies and other surface marker techniques. Br J Cancer 47:327, 1983.

56. Habeshaw JA, Cathey PF, Stansfield AG et al: Surface phenotyping, histology, and the nature of non-Hodgkin's lymphoma in 157 patients. Br J Cancer 40:11, 1979.

57. Frizzera G, Gajl-Peczalaska KJ, Bloomfield CD et al: Predictability of immunologic phenotype of malignant lymphomas by conventional morphology: A study of 60 cases. Cancer 43:1216, 1979.

58. Aisenberg AC, Wilkes BM, Long JC et al: Cell surface phenotype in lymphoproliferative disease. Am J Med 68:206, 1980.

59. Lukes RJ, Taylor CR, Parker JW et al: A morphologic and immunologic surface marker study of 299 cases of non-Hodgkin's lymphomas and related leukemias. Am J Pathol 90:461, 1978.

60. Taylor CR: Results of multiparameter studies of B cell lymphomas. Am J Clin Pathol 72:687, 1979.

61. Feltkamp CA, Feltkamp-Vroom TM, Koudstaal J et al: Multidisciplinary study of non-Hodgkin's lymphomas: Electron microscopy, immune- and enzyme-histochemistry. Adv Med Biol 114:545, 1979.

62. Stein H, Arkadius B, Talkadorf G et al: Immunohistologic analysis of the organization of normal lymphoid tissue and non-Hodgkin's lymphomas. J Histochem Cytochem 28:746, 1980.

63. Tolksdorf G, Stein H, Lennert K: Morphological and immunological definition of a malignant lymphoma derived from germinal center cells with cleaved nuclei (centrocytes). Br J Cancer 41:168, 1980.

64. Cheng AL, Chen YC, Wang CH et al: Direct comparisons of peripheral T-cell lymphoma with diffuse B-cell lymphoma of comparable histological grades—should peripheral T-cell lymphoma be considered separately? J Clin Oncol 7:725, 1989.

65. Cossman J, Jaffe ES, Fisher RI: Immunologic phenotypes of diffuse aggressive non-Hodgkin's lymphoma: Correlation with clinical features. Cancer 54:1310, 1984.

66. Lippman SM, Miller TP, Spier CM et al: The prognostic significance of the immunophenotype in diffuse large-cell lymphoma: A comparative study of the T-cell and B-cell phenotype. Blood 72:436, 1988.

67. Horning SJ, Carrier EK, Rouse RV et al: Lymphomas presenting as histologically unclassified neoplasms: Characteristics and response to treatment. J Clin Oncol 7:1281, 1989.

68. Talil N: Extrasalivary lymphoid abnormalities in Sjögren's syndrome (reticulum cell sarcoma, "pseudolymphoma," macroglobulinemia). Am J Med 43:50, 1967.

69. Turner RR, Egbert P, Warnke R: Lymphocytic infiltrates of the conjunctiva and orbit: Immunohistochemical staining of 16 cases. Am J Clin Pathol 81:447, 1984.

70. Knowles DM II, Halper JR, Jakobiec FA: The immunologic characterization of 40 extranodal lymphoid infiltrates: Usefulness in distinguishing between benign pseudolymphoma and malignant lymphoma. Cancer 49:2321, 1982.

71. Zulman J, Jaffe R, Talal N: Evidence that the malignant lymphoma of Sjögren's syndrome is a monoclonal B-cell neoplasm. N Engl J Med 299:1215, 1978.

72. Fishleder A, Tubba R, Hesse B et al: Uniform detection of immunoglobin-gene rearrangement in benign lymphoepithelial lesions. N Engl J Med 316:1118, 1987.

73. Hyjek E, Smith WJ, Isaacson PG: Primary B-cell lymphoma of salivary glands and its relationship to myoepithelial sialadenitis. Hum Pathol 19:766, 1988.

74. Aozasa K, Ueda T, Katagiri S et al: Immunologic and immunohistologic analysis of 27 cases with hybrid lymphomas. Cancer 60:969, 1987.

75. Hyjek E, Isaacson PG: Primary B cell lymphoma of the thyroid and its relationship to Hashimoto's thyroiditis. Hum Pathol 19:1315, 1988.

76. Mizukami Y, Matsubara F, Hashimoto T et al: Primary T-cell lymphoma of the thyroid. Acta Pathol Jpn 37:1987, 1987.

77. Dunbar JA, Lyall MH, MacGillivray JB et al: T-cell lymphoma of the thyroid. BMJ 2:679, 1977.

78. Katzin WE, Jishleder AJ, Tubbs RR: Investigation of the clonality of lymphocytes in Hashimoto's thyroiditis using immunoglobulin and T-cell receptor gene probes. Clin Immunol Immunopathol 51:264, 1989.

79. Frizzera G, Hanto DW, Gajl-Peczalska KJ et al: Polymorphic diffuse B cell hyperplasias and lymphomas in renal transplant recipients. Cancer Res 41:462, 1981.

80. Penn I: Tumors of the immunocompromised patient. Annu Rev Med 39:63, 1988.

81. Penn I: Cancer is a complication of severe immunosuppression. Surg Gynecol Obstet 162:603, 1986.

82. Kinlen LJ: Incidence of cancer in rheumatoid arthritis and other disorders after immunosuppressive treatment. Am J Med 78:44, 1985.

83. Randhawn PS, Yousem SA, Paradis IL et al: The clinical spectrum, pathology and clonal analysis of Epstein-Barr virus associated lymphoproliferative disorders in heart-lung transplant recipients. Am J Clin Pathol 92:177, 1989.

84. Cleary ML, Warnke R, Sklar J: Monoclonality of lymphoproliferative lesions in cardiac transplant recipients: Clonal analysis based on immunoglobulin-gene rearrangements. N Engl J Med 310:477, 1984.

85. Hanto DW, Najarian JS: Advances in the diagnosis and treatment of EBV-associated lymphoproliferative diseases in immunocompromised hosts. J Surg Oncol 30:215, 1985.

86. Cleary ML, Nalesnik MA, Shearer WT et al: Clonal analysis of transplant-associated lymphoproliferations based on the structure of the genomic termini of the Epstein-Barr virus. Blood 72:349, 1988.

87. Freeman C, Berg JW, Cutler SJ: Occurrence and prognosis of extranodal lymphomas. Cancer 29:252, 1972.

88. Helle TL, Bratt RH, Colby TV: Primary lymphoma of the central nervous system. J Neurosurg 60:94, 1984.

89. McLaughlin P, Velasquez WS, Redman JR et al: Chemotherapy with dexamethasone, high-dose cytarabine, and cisplatin for parenchymal brain lymphoma. J Natl Canc Inst 80:1408, 1988.

90. Kawakami Y, Tabuchi K, Ohnishi R et al: Primary central nervous system lymphoma. J Neurosurg 65:522, 1987.

91. Taylor CR, Russell R, Lukes RJ et al: An immunohistological study of immunoglobulin content of primary central nervous system lymphomas. Cancer 41:2197, 1978.

92. Smith WJ, Garson JA, Bourne SP et al: Immunoglobulin gene rearrangement and antigenic profile confirm B cell origin of primary cerebral lymphoma and indicate mature phenotype. J Clin Pathol 41:128, 1988.

93. Bashir RM, Harris NL, Hochberg FH et al: Detection of Epstein-Barr virus in CNS lymphomas by in-situ hybridization. Neurology 39:813, 1989.

94. Al-Saleem TI: Evidence of acquired immune deficiencies in Mediterranean lymphoma: A possible aetiological link. Lancet 1:709, 1978.

95. Isaacson P, Wright DH: Intestinal lymphoma associated with malabsorption. Lancet 1:67, 1978.

96. Isaacson P: Middle East lymphoma and a-chain disease: An immunohistochemical study. Am J Surg Pathol 3:431, 1979.

97. Yamanaka N, Ishii Y, Koshiba H et al: A study of surface markers in gastrointestinal lymphoma. Gastroenterology 79:675, 1980.

98. Matuchansky C, Touchard G, Lemaire M et al: Malignant lymphoma of the small bowel associated with diffuse nodular lymphoid hyperplasia. N Engl J Med 313:166, 1985.

99. Jones SE, Griffith K, Dombrowski P et al: Immunodeficiency in patients with non-Hodgkin's lymphomas. Blood 49:335, 1977.

100. Lichstein A, Taylor CR: Serum immunoglobulin levels in patients with non-Hodgkin's lymphomas. Am J Clin Pathol 74:12, 1980.

101. Economidau J, Terzoglou K, Anagnostou D et al: Immunoglobulin abnormalities in malignant non-Hodgkin's lymphoma. Scand J Haematol 33:123, 1984.

102. Moore DF, Migliore PJ, Shullenberger CC et al: Monoclonal macroglobulinemia in malignant lymphoma. Ann Intern Med 72:43, 1970.

103. Hermann F, Sieber G, Jauer B et al: Evaluation of the circulating and splenic lymphocyte subpopulations in patients with non-Hodgkin's lymphomas and Hodgkin's disease using monoclonal antibodies. Blut 47:41, 1983.

104. Bergmann L, Mitrou PS, Kelker W et al: T-cell subsets in malignant lymphomas and monoclonal gammopathies. Scand J Haematol 34:170, 1985.

105. DeAngelis P, Kimmel M, Lacher M: T-cell subsets in peripheral blood of patients with newly diagnosed and post-treatment Hodgkin's and non-Hodgkin's lymphomas: Analysis by monoclonal antibody staining and flow cytometry. Anal Quant Cytol Histol 10:235, 1988.

106. Gajl-Peczalaska KJ, Chartrand SL, Bloomfield CD: Abnormal immunoregulation in patients with non-Hodgkin's malignant lymphomas. Clin Immunol Immunopathol 23:366, 1982.

107. Anderson TC, Jones SE, Soehnlen BJ et al: Immunocompetence and malignant lymphoma: Immunologic status before therapy. Cancer 48:2702, 1981.

108. Advani SH, Dinslow KA, Nair CN et al: Immune dysfunction in non-Hodgkin's lymphoma. Cancer 45:2843, 1980.

109. Barcos MP, Lukes RJ: Malignant lymphoma of convoluted lymphocytes—a new entity of possible T-cell type. In Sinks LF, Godden JO (eds.): Conflicts in Childhood Cancer—An Evaluation of Current Management, p. 147. Alan R Liss, New York, 1975.

110. Bloomfield CD, Frizzera G, Gajl-Peczalska KJ et al: Malignant lymphoma, lymphoblastic in the adult. Proc Am Assoc Cancer Res 19:378, 1978.

111. Dewar AE, Krajewski AS, Murray J: T cell lymphoma in children and young adults: Clinical, immunologic and pathological features. Br J Cancer 42:659, 1980.

112. Nathwani BN, Kim H, Rappaport H: Malignant lymphoma, lymphoblastic. Cancer 38:964, 1976.

113. Palacios JJN, Valdes MD, Pallares MAM et al: Lymphoblastic lymphoma/leukemia of T cell origin: Ultrastructural, cytochemical and immunologic features of ten cases. Cancer 48:1982, 1981.

114. Rosen PJ, Feinstein DI, Pattengale PK et al: Convoluted lymphocytic lymphoma in adults: A clinicopathological entity. Ann Intern Med 89:319, 1978.

115. Hollema H, Poppema S: T-lymphoblastic and peripheral T-cell lymphomas in the northern part of the Netherlands. Cancer 64:1620, 1989.

116. Reinberg EL, Kung PC, Goldstein G et al: Discrete stages of human thymic differentiation: Analysis of normal thymocytes and leukemic lymphoblasts of T-cell lineage. Proc Natl Acad Sci U S A 77:1588, 1980.

117. Weiss JW, Winter MW, Phyliky RL et al: Peripheral T-cell lymphomas: Histologic, immunohistologic, and clinical characterization. Mayo Clin Proc 61:411, 1986.

118. Geer JP, York JC, Cousar JB et al: Peripheral T-cell lymphoma: A clinicopathologic study of 42 cases. J Clin Oncol 2:788, 1984.

119. Krajewski AS, Myskow MW, Cachia PG et al: T-cell lymphoma: Morphology, immunophenotype and clinical features. Histopathology 13:19, 1988.

120. Hattori T, Uchiyama T, Toibana T et al: Surface phenotype of Japanese adult T-cell leukemia cells characterized by monoclonal antibodies. Blood 59:645, 1981.

121. Yamada Y: Phenotypic and functional analysis of leukemic cells from 16 patients with adult T cell leukemia/lymphoma. Blood 61:192, 1983.

122. Uchiyama T, Sagawa K, Takatsuki K et al: Effect of adult T cell leukemia cells on pokeweed mitogen-induced normal B cell differentiation. Clin Immunol Immunopathol 10:24, 1978.

123. Han T, De los Santos R, Kakati S et al: T-cell malignant lymphoma: T lymphoid cells with complement receptors and helper cell activity. N Y State J Med 80:789, 1980.

124. Haynes MF, Metzgar RS, Minna JD et al: Phenotypic characterization of cutaneous T cell lymphoma: Use of monoclonal antibodies to compare with other malignant T cells. N Engl J Med 304:1319, 1981.

125. Berger CL, Warburton D, Raafat J et al: Cutaneous T cell lymphoma: Neoplasm of T cells with helper activity. Blood 53:642, 1979.

126. Hui PK, Feller AC, Pilori S et al: New aggressive variant of suppressor/cytotoxic T-cell. Am J Clin Pathol 87:55, 1987.

127. Broder S, Edelson RL, Lutzner MA et al: The Sézary syndrome: A malignant proliferation of helper T cells. J Clin Invest 58:1297, 1976.

128. Mackie RM, Turbitt ML: The use of a double-label immunoperoxidase monoclonal antibody technique in the investigation of patients with mycosis fungoides. Br J Dermatol 106:379, 1982.

129. Laroche L, Bach JF: T cell imbalance in non-leukemic cutaneous lymphoma defined by monoclonal antibodies. Clin Immunol Immunopathol 20:278, 1981.

130. Willemze R, deGraaff-Reitsma CB, Cnossen J et al: Characterization of T cell subpopulations in skin and peripheral blood of patients with cutaneous T cell lymphomas and benign inflammatory dermatosis. J Invest Dermatol 80:60, 1983.

131. van der Loo EM, Meijer CLJM, Scheffer E et al: The prognostic value of membrane markers and morphometric characteristics of lymphoid cells in blood and lymph nodes from patients with mycosis fungoides. Cancer 48:738, 1981.

132. Weiss LM, Hu E, Wood GS et al: Clonal rearrangement of T-cell receptor genes in mycosis fungoides and dermatopathic lymphadenopathy. N Engl J Med 313:529, 1985.

133. Lawrence EC, Broder S, Jaffe ES et al: Evolution of a lymphoma with helper T cell characteristics in Sézary syndrome. Blood 52:481, 1978.

134. Safai B, Good RA, Twomey JJ et al: A novel lymphocyte differentiating factor in serum of patients with mycosis fungoides and Sézary syndrome. Blood 54:847, 1979.

135. van der Horst-Oostveen CJGR, von Vloten WA: Delayed-type hypersensitivity in patients with mycosis fungoides. Dermatologica 157:129, 1978.

136. Carney DN, Bumm PA, Schecter GP et al: Lymphocyte transformation in patients with cutaneous T cell lymphomas. Int J Cancer 26:535, 1980.

137. Norris DA: Mycosis fungoides: Lack of helper lymphocytes in lymphocyte-monocyte interactions. Br J Dermatol 99(Suppl. 16):16, 1975.

138. Lukes RJ, Tindle BH: Immunoblastic lymphadenopathy: A hyperimmune entity resembling Hodgkin's disease. N Engl J Med 292:1, 1975.

139. Shimoyam S, Minato K, Saito H et al: Immunoblastic lymphadenopathy (IBL)-like T-cell lymphoma. Jpn J Clin Oncol 9(Suppl.):347, 1979.

140. Watanabe S, Shimosato Y, Shimoyam M et al: Adult T-cell lymphoma with hypergammaglobulinemia. Cancer 46:2472, 1980.

141. Namikawa R, Suchi T, Ueda R et al: Phenotyping of proliferating lymphocyte in angioimmunoblastic lymphadenopathy and related lesions by double immunoenzymatic staining technique. Am J Pathol 123:297, 1987.

142. Weiss LM, Strickler JG, Dorfman RF et al: Clonal T-cell populations in angioblastic lymphadenopathy and angioimmunoblastic lymphadenopathylike lymphoma. Am J Pathol 122:392, 1986.

143. Hanni T, Gaulard P, Divine M et al: Comparison of genetic probe with immunophenotypic analysis in lymphoproliferative disorders: A study of 87 cases. Blood 6:1937, 1988.

144. Waldron JA, Luck JH, Glick AD et al: Malignant lymphoma of peripheral T lymphocyte origin. Cancer 40:1604, 1977.

145. Schiipbach J, Kalyanaraman VS, Sarngadharan MG et al: Antibodies against three purified proteins of the human type C retrovirus, human T-cell leukemia-lymphoma virus, in adult T-cell leukemia-lymphoma virus, in adult T-cell leukemia-lymphoma patients and healthy blacks from the Caribbean. Cancer Res 43:886, 1983.

146. Nasu K, Tatsumi E, Takiuchi Y et al: Several marker analyses of T-lymphoma cells in eight cases. Am J Clin Pathol 76:670, 1981.

147. Blaney DW, Jaffe ES, Fisher RI et al: The human T cell leukemia/lymphoma virus, lytic bone lesions and hypercalcemia. Ann Intern Med 98:144, 1983.

148. Bowman WP, Melvin S, Mauer AM: Cell markers in leukemias and lymphomas. Adv Intern Med 25:391, 1980.

149. Broder S, Uchiyama T, Waldmann TA: Neoplasms of immunoregulatory cells. Am J Clin Pathol 72:724, 1979.

150. Lane HC, Whalen G, Fauci AS: Antigen induced human T cell help: Precursor frequency radiation sensitivity and allogeneic effects. J Clin Invest 72:636, 1983.

151. Kalyanaraman VS, Sarngadharon MD, Nakao Y et al: Natural antibodies to the structural core protein (p24) of the human T cell leukemia (lymphoma) virus found in sera of leukemia patients in Japan. Proc Natl Acad Sci U S A 79:1653, 1982.

152. Poiesz BJ, Puscetti FW, Gazdar AF et al: Detection and isolation of type C retrovirus particles from fresh and cultured lymphocytes of a patient with cutaneous T cell lymphoma. Proc Natl Acad Sci U S A 77:7415, 1980.

153. Essex M, McLane MF, Lee TH et al: Antibodies to cell membrane antigens associated with human T cell leukemia virus in patients with AIDS. Science 20:859, 1983.

154. Tajima K, Kuroishi T: Estimation of incidence rate of ATL among ATLV-carriers in Kyushu, Japan. Jpn J Clin Oncol 15:423, 1985.

155. Herva E, Ryhanen P, Blanco G et al: Acid alpha-naphthyl acetate esterase (ANAE) activity and DNA synthesis of lymph node cells in Hodgkin's disease. Scand J Haematol 23:277, 1979.

156. Kaplan HS, Gartner S: "Sternberg-Reed" giant cells of Hodgkin's disease: Cultivation in vitro, heterotransplantation, and characterization as neoplastic macrophages. Int J Cancer 19:511, 1977.

157. Weiss LM, Strickler JG, Hu E et al: Immunoglobulin gene rearrangements in Hodgkin's disease. Hum Pathol 17:1009, 1986.

158. Sundeen J, Lypford E, Uppenkamp M et al: Rearranged antigen receptor in Hodgkin's disease. Blood 70:96, 1987.

159. Hansmann ML, Kaiserling E: Electron-microscopic aspects of Hodgkin's disease. J Cancer Res Clin Oncol 101:135, 1981.

160. Greisser H, Feller A, Lennert K et al: Rearrangement of the B chain of the T cell antigen receptor and immunoglobulin genes in lymphoproliferative disorders. J Clin Invest 78:1179, 1986.

161. Froese P, Lemke H, Gerdes J et al: Biochemical characterization and biosynthesis of the Ki-1 antigen in Hodgkin-derived and virus-transformed human B and T lymphoid cell lines. J Immunol 139:2081, 1987.

162. Pinkus GS, Said JW: Hodgkin's disease, lymphocyte-predominant type: Immunoreactivity with B-cell antibodies. Mod Pathol 1:274, 1988.

163. Curran RC, Jones EL: Immunoglobulin in Reed-Sternberg and Hodgkin's cells. J Pathol 126:35, 1978.

164. Stein H, Papadimitiou CS, Bouman H et al: Demonstration of immunoglobulin production by tumor cells in non-Hodgkin's and Hodgkin's malignant lymphomas and its significance for their classification. Recent Results Cancer Res 64:158, 1978.

165. Kadin ME, Stites DP, Levy R et al: Exogenous immunoglobulin and the macrophage origin of Reed-Sternberg cells in Hodgkin's disease. N Engl J Med 299:1208, 1978.

166. Bernau D, Feldmann G, Vorhauer W: Hodgkin's disease: Ultrastructural localization of intracytoplasmic immunoglobulins within malignant cells. Br J Haematol 40:51, 1978.

167. Cossman J, Sundeen J, Uppenkamp M et al: Rearranging antigen-receptor genes in enriched Reed-Sternberg cell fractions of Hodgkin's disease. Hematol Oncol 6:205, 1988.

168. Jaffe ES: The elusive Reed-Sternberg cell. N Engl J Med 320:529, 1989.

169. Regula DP, Hoppe RT, Weiss LM: Nodular and diffuse types of lymphocyte predominance Hodgkin's disease. N Engl J Med 318:214, 1988.

170. Sundeen JT, Cossman J, Jaffe ES: Lymphocyte predominant Hodgkin's disease nodular subtype with coexistent "large cell lymphoma": Histological progression or composite malignancy? Am J Surg Pathol 12:599, 1988.

171. Mueller N, Evans A, Harris NL et al: Hodgkin's disease and Epstein-Barr virus: Altered antibody pattern before diagnosis. N Engl J Med 320:689, 1989.

172. Weiss LM, Mohaved LA, Warnke RA et al: Detection of Epstein-Barr viral genomes in Reed-Sternberg cells of Hodgkin's disease. N Engl J Med 320:502, 1989.

173. Diehl E, Kirchner HH, Sehadt M et al: Hodgkin's disease: Establishment and characterization of four in vitro cell lines. J Cancer Res Clin Oncol 101:111, 1981.

174. Fisher RI, Cossman J, Drehl V, Volkan DJ: Antigen presentation by Hodgkin's disease cells. J Immunol 135:3568, 1985.

175. Fisher RI, Bosteck-Bruton F, Saunder DN et al: Neoplastic cells obtained from Hodgkin's disease are potent stimulators of human primary mixed lymphocyte cultures. J Immunol 130:2666, 1983.

176. Fisher RI, Bates SE, Bosteck-Bruton F et al: Neoplastic cells obtained from Hodgkins disease function as accessory cells for mitogen-induced T-cell proliferative responses. J Immunol 5:2672, 1984.

177. Naurocki JF, Kirsten ES, Fisher RI: Biochemical and structural properties of a Hodgkin's disease-related membrane protein. J Immunol 141:672, 1988.

178. Advani SH, D'Silva H, Gothoskar BP et al: Cellular immunity in Hodgkin's disease. Cancer 43:492, 1979.

179. Fisher RI: Implications of persistent T-cell abnormalities for the etiology of Hodgkin's disease. Cancer Treat Rep 66:681, 1982.

180. Skovman-Sorenson O, Schroder O, Moller-Larsen A et al: Cellular and humoral immunity in Hodgkin's disease. Patients in continuous long-term remission. Scand J Haematol 27:171, 1981.

181. Lynch HT, Marcus JN, Weisenburger DD et al: Genetic and immunopathological findings in a lymphoma family. Br J Cancer 59:22, 1989.

182. Bjorkholm M, Holm G, Faire U et al: Immunological defects in healthy twin siblings to patients with Hodgkin's disease. Scand J Haematol 19:396, 1977.

183. Bjorkholm M, Holm G, Millstedt H: Immunologic family studies in Hodgkin's disease. Scand J Haematol 20:297, 1978.

184. Del Giacco GS, Cengiaretti L, Mantovani G et al: Quantitative and functional abnormalities of total T lymphocytes in relatives of patients with Hodgkin's disease. Eur J Cancer Clin Oncol 21:793, 1985.

185. El-Haddad SI, El-Ashmaury S, Hasson W et al: Immune deficiency in Hodgkin's and non-Hodgkin's lymphoma. Biomedicine 32:128, 1980.

186. Van Rijswijk RE, Sybesma JPH, Kater L: A prospective study of the changes in immune status before, during, and after multiple agent chemotherapy for Hodgkin's disease. Cancer 51:637, 1983.

187. Alexopoulos CB, Wiltshaw E: Immunological monitoring during chemotherapy for advanced Hodgkin's disease. Cancer 42:2631, 1978.

188. Bjorkholm M, Holm G, Millstedt H et al: Prognostic factors in Hodgkin's disease; role of the of the lymphocyte defect. Scand J Haematol 20:306, 1978.

189. Faguet GB, Davis HC: Survival in Hodgkin's disease: The role of immunocompetence and other major risk factors. Blood 59:938, 1982.

190. Wedelin C, Bjorkholm M, Holm G et al: Lymphocyte function in untreated Hodgkin's disease; an important predictor of prognosis. Br J Cancer 45:70, 1982.

191. Aisenberg AC, Wilkes B: Lymph node T-cells in Hodgkin's disease: Analysis of suspensions with monoclonal antibody and rosetting techniques. Blood 59:522, 1982.

192. Hancock BW, Dunsmore IR, Swan HT: Lymphopenia—a bad prognostic factor in Hodgkin's disease. Br J Haematol 29:193, 1982.

193. Bjorkholm M, Holm G, Millstedt H: Immunologic profile of patients with cured Hodgkin's disease. Scand J Haematol 18:361, 1977.

194. Sinclair T, Ezdinli EZ, Boonlayangoor P et al: Rosette and blastogenesis inhibition by plasma from Hodgkin's disease and other malignancies. Cancer 51:238, 1983.

195. Fuks Z, Strober S, Kaplan HS: Interaction between serum factors and T lymphocytes in Hodgkin's disease. N Engl J Med 295:1273, 1976.

196. Moghe MV, Advani SH, Gangal SG: Demonstration of inhibitory factors affecting cell mediated immunity in patients with Hodgkin's disease. Eur J Cancer 16:937, 1980.

197. Sjugden PJ, Lilleyman JS: Impairment of lymphoma transformation by plasma from patients with advanced Hodgkin's disease. Cancer 45:899, 1980.

198. Moroz C, Lahat N, Biniaminov M et al: Ferritin on the surface of lymphocytes in Hodgkin's disease patients. A possible blocking substance removed by levamisole. Clin Exp Immunol 29:30, 1977.

199. Fisher RI, Bosteck-Bruton F: Depressed T cell proliferative responses in Hodgkin's disease: Role of monocyte-mediated suppression via prostaglandins and hydrogen peroxide. J Immunol 129:1770, 1982.

200. Ramot B, Rosenthal E, Biniamov M et al: Effect of levamisole, thymic humoral factor, and indomethacin on E-rosette formation of lymphocytes in Hodgkin's disease. Isr J Med Sci 17:232, 1981.

201. Liberati AM, Brugia M, Edwards BS et al: Immuno-restorative properties of thymostimulin (TS) in patients with Hodgkin's disease in clinical remission. Cancer Immunol Immunother 19:136, 1985.

202. Tursz T, Dokhelar MC, Lipinski M et al: Low natural killer cell activity in patients with malignant lymphoma. Cancer 50:233, 1982.

203. Dorreen MS, Habeshaw JA, Wrigley PRM et al: Distribution of T-lymphocyte subsets in Hodgkin's disease characterized by monoclonal antibodies. Br J Cancer 45:491, 1982.

204. Posner MR, Reinherz EL, Breard J et al: Lymphoid subpopulations of peripheral blood and spleen in untreated Hodgkin's disease. Cancer 48:1170, 1981.

205. Han T, Minowada J, Subramanian V et al: Splenic T and B lymphocytes and their mitogenic response in untreated Hodgkin's disease. Cancer 45:767, 1980.

206. Barone CD, Ruco L, Uccini S et al: Tissue T-lymphocytes in untreated Hodgkin's disease: Morphologic and functional correlations in spleens and lymph nodes. Cancer 50:259, 1982.

207. Maggi E, Parronchi P, Macchia D et al: High numbers of CD4+ T cells showing abnormal recognition of DR antigens in lymphoid organs involved by Hodgkin's disease. Blood 71:1503, 1988.

208. Maggi E, Parronchi P, Del Prete G et al: Frequent T4-positive cells with cytolytic activity in spleens of patients with Hodgkin's disease (a clonal analysis). J Immunol 136:1516, 1986.

209. Engleman EG, Benike CJ, Hoppe RT et al: Autologous mixed lymphocyte reaction in patients with Hodgkin's disease: Evidence for a T cell defect. J Clin Invest 66:149, 1980.

210. Han T: Role of suppressor cells in depression of T lymphocyte proliferative response in untreated and treated Hodgkin's disease. Cancer 45:2102, 1980.

211. Twomey JJ, Laughter AH, Rice L et al: Spectrum of immunodeficiencies with Hodgkin's disease. J Clin Invest 66:629, 1980.

212. Zamkoff KW, Dock NL, Kurec AS et al: Diminished autologous mixed lymphocyte reaction in patients with Hodgkin's disease: Evidence for non-T cell dysfunction. Am J Hematol 12:327, 1982.

213. Schulf RS, Lacher MJ, Gupta S: Abnormal phytohemagglutinin-induced T cell proliferative responses in Hodgkin's disease. Blood 57:607, 1981.

214. Mukhopadhyaya R, Advani SH, Gangal SG: Impairment of T lymphocyte colony formation in Hodgkin's disease: Effect of soluble inhibitory factors on normal T lymphocyte colony formation potential. Acta Haematol 70:357, 1983.

215. Deshazo RD: Indomethacin-responsive mononuclear cell dysfunction in Hodgkin's disease. Clin Immunol Immunopathol 17:66, 1981.

216. Schecter GP, Soehnlen F: Monocyte-mediated inhibition of lymphocyte blastogenesis in Hodgkin's disease. Blood 52:261, 1978.

217. Passwell J, Levanon M, Davidsohn J et al: Monocyte PGE-2 secretion in Hodgkin's disease and its relation to decreased cellular immunity. Clin Exp Immunol 51:61, 1983.

218. Mortelli MF, Velardi A, Rambotti P et al: The in vitro effect of calf thymus extract (thymostimulin) on the immunologic parameters of patients with untreated Hodgkin's disease. Cancer 50:490, 1982.

219. Mukhopadhyaya R, Advani SH, Gangal SG: Functional evaluation of T-lymphocytes from peripheral blood and spleens in Hodgkin's disease. Br J Cancer 56:800, 1987.

220. Mukhopadhyaya R, Advani SH, Gangal SG: Effect of exogenous interleukins on in vitro responses of T lymphocytes from patients with Hodgkin's disease. Cancer Detect Prevent 10:445, 1987.

221. Bergmann L, Mitrou PS, Demmer-Dreckmann M et al: Impaired T- and B-cell functions in patients with Hodgkin's disease. Cancer Immunol Immunother 25:59, 1987.

222. Baral E, Blomgren H, Juhlin I: The effect of in vitro irradiation on mitogenic responsiveness of peripheral blood lymphocytes from untreated patients with Hodgkin's disease. Cancer 44:1241, 1979.

223. Fisher RI, Vanhaelen C, Bostick F: Increased sensitivity to normal adherent suppressor cells in untreated advanced Hodgkin's disease. Blood 57:830, 1981.

224. Romagnani S, Del Prete GF, Maggi E et al: Abnormalities of in vitro immunoglobulin synthesis by peripheral blood lymphocytes from untreated patients with Hodgkin's disease. J Clin Invest 71:1375, 1983.

225. Dickinson AM, McLachlan SM, Jacobs EA et al: Defective in vitro immunoglobulin production in response to poke-weed mitogen in patients with Hodgkin's disease pretreatment and in remission. Clin Immunol Immunopathol 41:281, 1986.

226. Douer D, Pick AL, Kessler E et al: Serum immunoglobulin level in patients with Hodgkin's disease: Relation to disease activity and clinical stage. Clin Oncol 4:209, 1978.

227. Rosset G, Farquet JJ, Cruchard A: The serum immunoglobulins in lymphoproliferative malignancies. Eur J Cancer 14:369, 1978.

228. Addiego JE, Ammann AJ, Schiffman G et al: Response to pneumococcal vaccine in patients with untreated Hodgkin's disease. Lancet 2:450, 1981.

229. Kohl S, Pickering LK, Sullivan MP et al: Impaired monocyte-macrophage cytoxicity in patients with Hodgkin's disease. Clin Immunol Immunopathol 15:577, 1980.

230. Estevez ME, Sen L, Bachmann AE et al: Defective function of peripheral blood monocytes in patients with Hodgkin's and non-Hodgkin's lymphomas. Cancer 46:299, 1980.

231. Katz DR: The macrophage in Hodgkin's disease. J Pathol 133:145, 1981.

232. Bjorkholm M, Askergen J, Holm G et al: Long-term influence of splenectomy on immune function in patients with Hodgkin's disease. Scand J Haematol 24:87, 1980.

233. Rogan-Grgas J, Milas L, Hauptmann E et al: Influence of splenectomy upon immunologic reactivity of patients with Hodgkin's disease. Tumori 67:539, 1981.

234. Steele R, Han T: Effects of radiochemotherapy and splenectomy on cellular immunity in long-term survivors of Hodgkin's disease and non-Hodgkin's lymphoma. Cancer 42:133, 1978.

235. Bjorkholm M, Wedelin C, Holm G et al: Longitudinal studies of blood lymphocyte capacity in Hodgkin's disease. Cancer 48:2010, 1981.

236. Posner ME, Reinherz E, Lang H et al: Circulating lymphocyte populations in Hodgkin's disease after mantle and paraaortic irradiation. Blood 61:705, 1983.

237. Haas GS, Halperin E, Doseretz D et al: Differential recovery of circulating T-cell subsets after nodal irradiation for Hodgkin's disease. J Immunol 132:1026, 1984.

238. Mathe G, Amiel JL, Schwarzenberg L et al: Active immunotherapy for acute lymphoblastic leukemias. Lancet 1:697, 1969.

239. Mathe G, de Vassal F, Delgado M et al: 1975 current results of the first 100 cytologically typed acute lymphoid leukemias submitted to active BCG immunotherapy. Cancer Immunol Immunother 1:77, 1976.

240. Heyn RM, Joo P, Karon M et al: BCG in the treatment of acute lymphocytic leukemia. Blood 48:431, 1975.

241. Holland JF, Bekesi JG: Immunotherapy of human leukemia with neuraminidase-modified cells. Med Clin North Am 60:539, 1976.

242. Leukemia Committee and the Working Party of Leukemia in Childhood: Treatment of acute lymphoblastic leukemia. Comparison of immunotherapy (BCG), intermittent methotrexate and therapy after a five-month intensive cytotoxic regimen. BMJ 4:189, 1971.

243. Murphy S, Hersh E: Immunotherapy of leukemia and lymphoma. Semin Hematol 15:181, 1978.

244. Poplack DG, Leventhal BG, Simon R et al: Immunotherapy of acute lymphocytic leukemic with bacillus Calmette-Guérin (BCG) and allogeneic leukemia cells. In Windhorts D (ed.): Immunotherapy of Cancer: Present Status of Therapeutic Trials in Man. p. 497. Raven Press, New York, 1978.

245. Hoerni B, Durand M, DeMascarel A et al: BCG in the immunotherapy of non-Hodgkin's lymphomas: Preliminary results of a controlled trial. Recent Results Cancer Res 65:160, 1978.

246. Vinciguerra V, Coleman M, Pajak TF et al: MER immunotherapy and combination chemotherapy for advanced, recurrent Hodgkin's disease. Cancer Clin Trials 4:99, 1981.

247. Jones SE: Chemoimmunotherapy versus chemotherapy for remission induction in patients with non-Hodgkin's lymphoma: A progress report of a Southwest Oncology Group study. Recent Results Cancer Res 65:164, 1978.

248. Jones SE, Grozea PN, Metz EN et al: Improved complete remission rates and survival for patients with large cell lymphoma treated with chemoimmunotherapy. Cancer 51:1083, 1983.

249. Hoerni B, Durand M, DeMascarel A et al: Successful maintenance immunotherapy by BCG of non-Hodgkin's malignant lymphomas: Results of a controlled trial. Br J Haematol 42:507, 1979.

250. Hoerni B, Durand M, Eghbali H et al: Maintenance immunotherapy with BCG in non-Hodgkin's lymphomas: A progress report of a randomized trial. Recent Results Cancer Res 80:92, 1982.

251. Cabinellas F, Smith T, Bodey GP et al: Nodular malignant lymphomas: Factors affecting complete response rate and survival. Cancer 44:1983, 1979.

252. Urba WJ, Longo DL: α-Interferon in the treatment of nodular lymphomas. Semin Oncol 13:40, 1986.

253. Siegert W, Theml H, Fink U et al: Treatment of non-Hodgkin's lymphoma of low-grade malignancy with human fibroblast interferon. Anticancer Res 2:193, 1982.

254. Foon KA, Sherwin SA, Abrams PG et al: Treatment of advanced non-Hodgkin's lymphoma with recombinant leukocyte interferon. N Engl J Med 311:1148, 1984.

255. Quesada JR, Hawkins M, Horning S et al: Collaborative phase I-II study of recombinant DNA produced leukocyte interferon (clone A) in metastatic breast cancer, malignant lymphoma, and multiple myeloma. Am J Med 77:427, 1984.

256. Leavitt RD, Ratanatharathorn V, Ozer H et al: Alfa-2b interferon in the treatment of Hodgkin's disease and non-Hodgkin's lymphoma. Semin Oncol 14:18, 1987.

257. Wagstaff J, Loynds P, Crowther D: A phase II study of human rDNA alpha-2 interferon in patients with low grade non-Hodgkin's lymphoma. Cancer Chemother Pharmacol 18:54, 1986.

258. O'Connell MJ, Colgan JP, Oken MM et al: Clinical trial of recombinant leukocyte A interferon as initial therapy for favorable histology non-Hodgkin's lymphomas and chronic lymphocytic leukemia: An Eastern Cooperative Oncology Group pilot study. J Clin Oncol 4:128, 1986.

259. Foon KA, Roth MS, Bunn PA, Jr: Interferon therapy of non-Hodgkin's lymphoma. Cancer: 59:601, 1987.

260. Ozer H, Anderson JR, Peterson BA et al: Combination trial of subcutaneous interferon alfa-2b and oral cyclophosphamide in favorable histology, non-Hodgkin's lymphoma. Invest New Drugs 5:s27, 1987.

261. Clark RH, Dimitrov NV, Axelson JA et al: A phase II trial of intermittent leukocyte interferon and high dose chlorambucil in the treatment of non-Hodgkin's lymphoma resistant to conventional therapy. Am J Clin Oncol 12:75, 1989.

262. Chisesi T, Capnist G, Vespignani M et al: Interferon alfa-2b and chlorambucil in the treatment of non-Hodgkin's lymphoma. Invest New Drugs 5:S35, 1987.

263. Brown SL, Miller RA, Horning SJ et al: Treatment of B-cell lymphomas with anti-idiotype antibodies alone and in combination with alpha interferon. Blood 73:651, 1989.

264. Dillman RO: Monoclonal antibodies for treating cancer. Ann Intern Med 111:592, 1989.

265. Dillman RO, Beauregard J, Shawler DL et al: Continuous infusion of T101 monoclonal antibody in chronic lymphocytic leukemia and cutaneous T-cell lymphoma. J Biol Response Mod 5:394, 1986.

266. Isaacs JD, Manna VK, Rapson N et al: CAMPATH-1H in rheumatoid arthritis—an intravenous dose-ranging study. Br J Rheumatol 35:231, 1996.

267. Hu E, Epstein AL, Naeve GS et al: A phase 1a clinical trial of LYM-1 monoclonal antibody serotherapy in patients with refractory B cell malignancies. Hematol Oncol 7:155, 1989.

268. Heckman A, Honselaar A, Vuist WM et al: Initial experience with treatment of human B cell lymphoma with anti-CD19 monoclonal antibody. Cancer Immunol Immunother 32:364, 1991.

269. Miller RA, Maloney DG, McKillop J et al: In vivo effects of murine hybridoma monoclonal antibody in a patient with T-cell leukemia. Blood 58:78, 1981.

270. Miller RA, Levy R: Response of cutaneous T cell lymphoma to therapy with hybridoma monoclonal antibody. Lancet 2:226, 1981.

271. Dillman RO, Shawler DL, Sobol RE et al: Murine monoclonal antibody therapy in two patients with chronic lymphocytic leukemia. Blood 59:1026, 1982.

272. Dillman RO, Shawler DL, Dillman JB et al: Therapy of chronic lymphocytic leukemia and cutaneous T-cell lymphoma with T101 monoclonal antibody. J Clin Oncol 2:881, 1984.

273. Dillman RO, Beauregard J, Shawler DL et al: Continuous infusion of T101 monoclonal antibody in chronic lymphocytic leukemia and cutaneous T-cell lymphoma. J Biol Resp Mod 5:394, 1986.

274. Knox S, Hoppe RT, Maloney D et al: Treatment of cutaneous T-cell lymphoma with chimeric anti-CD4 monoclonal antibody. Blood 87:893, 1996.

275. Grossbard ML, Lambert JM, Goldmacher VS et al: Anti-B4-blocked ricin: A phase I trial of 7-day continuous infusion in patients with B-cell neoplasm. J Clin Oncol 11:726, 1993.

276. Grossbard ML, Freedman AS, Ritz J et al: Serotherapy of B-cell neoplasms with anti-B4-blocked ricin: A phase I trial of daily bolus infusion. Blood 79:576, 1992.

277. Grossbard ML, Gribben JG, Freedman AS et al: Adjuvant immunotoxin therapy with anti-B4-blocked ricin after autologous bone marrow transplantation for patients with B-cell non-Hodgkin's lymphoma. Blood 81:2263, 1993.

278. Grossbard ML, Niedzwiecki D, Nadler LM et al: Anti-B4-blocked ricin adjuvant therapy post-autologous bone marrow transplant (CALGB 9254): A phase III intergroup study. Proc Am Soc Clin Oncol 17:3a, 1998.

279. Vitetta ES, Stone M, Amlot P et al: Phase I immunotoxin trial in patients with B-cell lymphoma. Cancer Res 51:4052, 1991.

280. Amlot PL, Stone MJ, Cunningham D, Fay J et al: A phase I study of an anti-CD22-deglycosylated ricin A chain immunotoxin in the treatment of B-cell lymphomas resistant to conventional therapy. Blood 82:2624, 1993.

281. Conry RM, Khazaeli MD, Saleh MN et al: Phase I trial of an anti-CD19 deglycosylated ricin A chain immunotoxin in non-Hodgkin's lymphoma: Effect of an intensive schedule of administration. J Immunother Emphasis Tumor Immunol 18:231, 1995.

282. Stone MJ, Sausville EA, Fay JW et al: A phase I study of bolus versus continuous infusion of the anti-CD19 immunotoxin, IgG-HD37-dgA, in patients with B-cell lymphoma. Blood 88:1188, 1996.

283. LeMaistre CF, Rosen, Frankel A et al: Phase I trial of H65-RTA immunoconjugate in patients with cutaneous T-cell lymphoma. Blood 78:1173, 1991.

284. Engert A, Diehl V, Schnell R et al: A phase-I study of an anti-CD25 ricin A-chain immunotoxin (RFT5-SMPT-dgA) in patients with refractory Hodgkin's lymphoma. Blood 89:403, 1997.

285. Kaminski MS, Zasadny KR, Francis IR et al: Radioimmunotherapy of B-cell lymphoma with [131I]anti-B1 (anti-CD20) antibody. N Engl J Med 329:459, 1993.

286. Kaminski MS, Zasadny KR, Francis IR et al: Iodine-131-anti-B1 radioimmunotherapy for B-cell lymphoma. J Clin Oncol 14:1974, 1996.

287. Press OW, Eary JF, Appelbaum FR et al: Radiolabeled-antibody therapy of B-cell lymphoma with autologous bone marrow support. N Engl J Med 329:1219, 1993.

288. Press OW, Eary JF, Appelbaum FR et al: Phase II trial of 131I-B1 (anti-CD20) antibody therapy with autologous stem cell transplantation for relapsed B cell lymphomas. Lance 346:336, 1995.

289. Press OW, Howell-Clark J, Anderson S et al: Retention of B-cell-specific monoclonal antibodies by human lymphoma cells. Blood 83:1390, 1994.

290. Press OW, Shan D, Howell-Clark J et al: Comparative metabolism and retention of iodine-125, yttrium-90, and indium-111 radioimmunoconjugates by cancer cells. Cancer Res 56:2123, 1996.

291. Wilder RB, DeNardo GL, DeNardo SJ: Radioimmunotherapy: Recent results and future directions. J Clin Oncol 14:1383, 1996.

292. Lenhard RE Jr, Order SE, Spunberg JJ et al: Isotopic immunoglobulin: A new systemic therapy for advanced Hodgkin's disease. J Clin Oncol 3:1296, 1985.

293. Herpst JM, Klein JL, Leichner PK et al: Survival of patients with resistant Hodgkin's disease after polyclonal yttrium 90-labeled antiferritin treatment. J Clin Oncol 13:2394, 1995.

294. Vriesendorp HM, Herpst JM, Germack MA et al: Phase I-II studies of yttrium-labeled antiferritin treatment for end-stage Hodgkin's disease, including Radiation Therapy Oncology Group 87-01 [published erratum appears in J Clin Oncol 1991 Aug; 9(8):1516]. J Clin Oncol 9:918, 1991.

295. Bierman PJ, Vose JM, Leichner PK et al: Yttrium 90-labeled antiferritin followed by high-dose chemotherapy and autologous bone marrow transplantation for poor-prognosis Hodgkin's disease. J Clin Oncol 11:698, 1993.

296. Vriesendorp HM, Morton JD, Quadri SM: Review of five consecutive studies of radiolabeled immunoglobulin therapy in Hodgkin's disease. Cancer Res 55(23 Suppl.):5888s, 1995.

297. Kaminski MS, Fig LM, Zasadny KR et al: Imaging, dosimetry, and radioimmunotherapy with iodine 131-labeled anti-CD37 antibody in B-cell lymphoma. J Clin Oncol 10:1696, 1992.

298. Knox SJ, Goris ML, Trisler K et al: Yttrium-90-labeled anti-CD20 monoclonal antibody therapy of recurrent B-cell lymphoma. Clin Cancer Res 2:457, 1996.

299. Press OW, Eary JF, Badger CC et al: Treatment of refractory non-Hodgkin's lymphoma with radiolabeled MB-1 (anti-CD37) antibody. J Clin Oncol 7:1027, 1989.

300. DeNardo SJ, DeNardo GL, O'Grady LF et al: Treatment of B cell malignancies with 131I Lym-1 monoclonal antibodies. Int J Cancer 3(Suppl.):96, 1988.

301. DeNardo GL, DeNardo SJ, O'Grady LF et al: Fractionated radioimmunotherapy of B-cell malignancies with 131I-Lym-1. Cancer Res 50(3 Suppl.):1014s, 1990.

302. Weisenburger DD, Armitage JO: Mantle cell lymphoma—an entity comes of age. Blood 87:4483, 1996.

303. Bigoni R, Negrini M et al: Characterization of t(11;14) translocation in mantle cell lymphoma by fluorescent in situ hybridization. Oncogene 13:797, 1996.

304. Tsujimoto Y, Yunis J et al: Molecular cloning of the chromosomal break-point of B cell lymphomas and leukemias with t(11;14) chromosome translocation. Science 224:1403, 1984.

305. Whiters DA, Harvey RC et al: Characterization of a candidate bcl-1 gene. Mol Cell Biol 11:4846, 1991.

306. Sherr CJ: Mammalian G1 cyclins. Cell 73:1059, 1993.

307. Ye BH, Lista F et al: Alterations of a zinc finger-encoding gene, BCL-6, in diffuse large-cell lymphoma. Science 262:747, 1993.

308. Baron BW, Nucifora G et al: Identification of the gene associated with recurring chromosomal translocations t(3;14)(q27;q32) and t(3;22)(q27;q11) in B-cell lymphomas. Proc Natl Acad Sci U S A 1:5262, 1993.

309. Dent AL, Shaffer AL et al: Control of inflammation, cytokine expression, and germinal center formation by BCL-6. Science 276:589, 1997.

310. Lo Coco F, Ye BH, Lista F: Rearrangements of the *bcl-6* gene in diffuse large cell non-Hodgkin's lymphoma. Blood 83:1757, 1994.

311. Offit K, Lo Coco F, Louie DC: Rearrangement of the *bcl-6* gene as a prognostic marker in diffuse large-cell lymphoma. N Engl J Med 331:74, 1994.

312. Capello D, Vitolo U et al: Distribution and pattern of BCL-6 mutations throughout the spectrum of B-cell neoplasia. Blood 95:651, 2000.

313. Willis TG, Jadayel DM et al: BCL-10 is involved in t(1;14)(p22;q32) of MALT B cell lymphoma and mutated in multiple tumor types. Cell 96:35, 1999.

314. Zhang Q, Siebert R et al: Inactivating mutations and overexpression of BCL-10, a caspase recruitment domain-containing gene, in MALT lymphoma with t(1;14)(p22;q32). Nat Genet 22:63, 1999.

315. Du MQ, Peng H et al: BCL-10 gene mutation in lymphoma. Blood 15:3885, 2000.

316. Nardini E, Aiello A et al: Detection of aberrant isotype switch recombination in low-grade and high-grade gastric MALT lymphomas. Blood 1:1032, 2000.

317. Limpens J, Stad R et al: Lymphoma-associated translocation t(14;18) in blood B cells of normal individuals. Blood 1:2528, 1995.

318. Freedman AS, Neuberg D, Mauch P: Long-term follow-up of autologous bone marrow transplantation in patients with relapsed follicular lymphoma. Blood 15:3325, 1999.

319. Hu E, Trela M et al: Detection of B cell lymphoma in peripheral blood by DNA hybridization. Lancet II:1092, 1985.

320. Gribben JG, Freedman AS et al: Immunologic purging of marrow assessed by PCR before autologous bone marrow transplantation for B-cell lymphoma. N Engl J Med 325:1525, 1991.

321. Hardingham JE, Kotasek D et al: Molecular detection of residual lymphoma cells in peripheral blood stem cell harvests and following autologous transplantation. Bone Marrow Transplant 11:15, 1993.

322. Czuczman MS, Grillo-López AJ et al: Treatment of patients with low-grade B-cell lymphoma with the combination of chimeric anti-CD20 monoclonal antibody and CHOP chemotherapy. J Clin Oncol 17:268, 1999.

323. Shipp M, Harrington D et al: A predictive model for aggressive non-Hodgkin's lymphoma: The International NHL Prognostic Factors Project. N Engl J Med 329:987, 1993.

324. López-Guillermo A, Cabanillas F et al: Correlation of *bcl-2* rearrangement with clinical characteristics and outcome in indolent follicular lymphoma. Blood 1:3081, 1999.

325. Falini B, Pileri S et al: ALK+ lymphoma: Clinico-pathological findings and outcome. Blood 93:2697, 2000.

326. Gascoyone R, Aoun P et al: Prognostic significance of anaplastic lymphoma kinase (ALK) protein expression in adults with anaplastic large cell lymphoma. Blood 93:3913, 1999.

327. Yatabe Y, Suzuki R et al: Significance of cyclin D1 overexpression for the diagnosis of mantle cell lymphoma: A clinicopathologic comparison of cyclin D1-positive MCL and cyclin D1-negative MCL-like B-cell lymphoma. Blood 1:2253, 2000.

328. Cuneo A, Bigoni R et al: Cytogenetic profile of lymphoma of follicle mantle lineage: Correlation with clincobiologic features. Blood 15:1372, 1999.

329. Horning SJ, Rosenberg SA: The natural history of initially untreated low-grade non-Hodgkin's lymphomas. N Engl J Med 311:1471, 1984.

330. Fischer RI, Gaynor ER, Dahlberg S et al: Comparison of a standard regimen (CHOP) with three intensive chemotherapy regimens for advanced non-Hodgkin's lymphoma. N Engl J Med 328:1002, 1993.

331. McLaughlin P, Hagenmeister FB, Swan F et al: Intensive conventional-dose chemotherapy for stage IV low-grade lymphoma: High remission rates and reversion to negative of peripheral blood bcl-2 rearrangement. Ann Oncol 5(Suppl. 2):73, 1994.

332. McLaughlin P, Hagenmeister FB, Romguera JE et al: Fludarabine, mitoxantrone, and desamethasone: An effective new regimen for indolent lymphoma. J Clin Oncol 14:1262, 1996.

333. Czuczman M, Grillo-López AJ, White CA et al: IDEC-C2B8/CHOP chemoimmunotherapy in patients with low-grade lymphoma: Clinical and BCL-2 (PCR) final results (abstract). Blood 88:453a, 1996.

334. Gribben JG, Neuberg D, Barber M et al: Detection of residual lymphoma cells by polymerase chain reaction in peripheral blood is significantly less predictive for relapse than detection in bone marrow. Blood 83:3800, 1994.

335. Rohatiner A, Crowther D, Radford J et al: The role of interferon in follicular lymphoma (abstract). Proc Am Soc Clin Oncol 15:418, 1996.

336. Price CGA, Rohatiner AZS, Steward W et al: Interferon-α2b in the treatment of follicular lymphoma: Preliminary results of a trial in progress. Ann Oncol 2(Suppl. 2):141, 1991.

337. Chisesi T: Randomized study of chlorambucil (CB) compared to interferon (alfa-2b) combined with CB in low-grade non-Hodgkin's lymphoma: An interim report of a randomized study. Eur J Cancer 27(Suppl. 4):S31, 1991.

338. Peterson BA, Petroni GR, Oken MM et al: Cyclophosphamide vs cyclophosphamide plus interferon alfa-2b in follicular low-grade lymphomas: A preliminary report of an intergroup trial (CALGB 8691 and EST 7486) (abstract). Proc Am Soc Clin Oncol 12:366, 1993.

339. Peterson BA, Petroni GR, Oken MM et al: Cyclophosphamide vs cyclophosphamide plus interferon alfa-2b in follicular low-grade lymphoma: An intergroup phase III trial (CALGB 8691 and EST 7486) (abstract). Proc Am Soc Clin Oncol 16:14a, 1997.

340. Hagenbeek A, Carde P, Meerwaldt JH et al: Maintenance of remission with human recombinant interferon alfa-2a in patients with stages III and IV low-grade malignant non-Hodgkin's lymphoma. J Clin Oncol 16:41, 1998.

341. Hagenbeek A, Carde P, Somers R et al: Interferon-alfa-2a vs control as maintenance therapy for low-grade non-Hodgkin's lymphoma: Results from a prospective randomized clinical trial (abstract). Proc Am Soc Clin Oncol 14:386, 1995.

342. Arranz R, Garcia-Alfonso P Sobrino P et al: Role of interferon alfa-2b in the induction and maintenance treatment of low-grade non-Hodgkin's lymphoma: Results from a prospective, multicenter trial with double randomization. J Clin Oncol 16:1538, 1998.

343. Unterhalt M, Hermann R, Koch P et al: Long-term interferon alpha maintenance prolongs remission duration in advanced low-grade lymphomas and is related to the efficacy of initial cytoreductive chemotherapy (abstract). Blood 88:453a, 1996.

344. Unterhalt M, Hermann R, Nahler M et al: Significant prolongation of disease-free survival in advanced low-grade non-Hodgkin's lymphomas (NHL) by interferon alpha maintenance (abstract). Blood 86:439a, 1995.

345. Avilés A, Duque G, Talavera A et al: Interferon alpha 2b as maintenance therapy in low-grade malignant lymphoma improves duration of remission and survival. Leuk Lymphoma 20:495, 1996.

346. Smalley RV, Anderson JW, Hawkins MJ et al: Interferon alfa combined with cytotoxic chemotherapy for patients with non-Hodgkin's lymphoma. N Engl J Med 327:1336, 1992.

347. Solal-Céligny P, Lepage E, Brousse N et al: Recombinant interferon alfa-2b combined with a regimen containing doxorubicin in

patients with advanced follicular lymphoma. N Engl J Med 329:1608, 1993.

348. Solal-Céligny P, Lepage E, Brousse N et al: Doxorubicin containing regimen with or without interferon alpha 2b (INFa2b) in advanced follicular lymphomas: Final analysis of survival and toxicity in the Groupe d'Etude des Lymphomes Folliculaires 86 trial. J Clin Oncol 16:2332, 1998.

349. Smalley RV, Weller E, Hawkins M et al: α-Interferon in non-Hodgkin's lymphoma—an update of the ECOG I-COPA trial (E6484) (abstract). Blood 92:486a, 1998.

350. Rohatiner AZS, Gregory W, Peterson B et al: A meta-analysis (MA) of randomized trials evaluating the role of interferon (IFN) as treatment for follicular lymphoma (FL) (abstract). Proc Am Soc Clin Oncol 17:4a, 1998.

351. Ozer H, Wiernik PH, Giles F et al: Recombinant interferon—a therapy in patients with follicular lymphoma. Cancer 82:1821, 1998.

352. Hiddemann W, Griesinger F, Unterhalt M: Interferon alfa for the treatment of follicular lymphomas. Cancer J Sci Am 4:S13, 1998.

353. Dana BW, Unger J, Fischer RI: A randomized study of alpha-interferon consolidation in patients with low-grade lymphoma who have responded to PRO-MACE-MOPP (Day 1-8) (SWOG 8809) (abstract). Proc Am Soc Clin Oncol 17:3a, 1998.

354. Maloney DG, Grillo-López AJ, White CA et al: IDEC-C2B8 (Rituximab) anti-CD20 monoclonal antibody therapy in patients with relapsed low-grade non-Hodgkin's lymphoma. Blood 90:2188, 1997.

355. Davis T, Maloney D, White CA et al: Combination immunotherapy of low-grade or follicular non-Hodgkin's lymphoma with Rituximab and alpha-interferon: Interim analysis (abstract). Blood 90(Suppl. 1):509a, 1997.

356. FDA clears Intron A for treatment of NHL. Clin Cancer Lett, November 1997.

357. Avilés A, Díaz-Maqueo J, Garcia EL et al: Maintenance therapy with interferon alfa 2b in patients with diffuse large cell lymphoma. Invest New Drugs 10:351, 1992.

358. Meusers P, Hense J, Brittinger G: Mantle cell lymphoma: Diagnostic criteria, clinical aspects, and therapeutic problems. Leukemia 11(Suppl. 2):S60, 1997.

359. McColl MD, Tait RC: Hepatitis C virus infection in patients with lymphoproliferative disorders. Br J Haematol 92:771, 1996.

360. Zuckerman T, Sahar D, Streichman S et al: Bcl-2 and immunoglobulin gene rearrangement in patients with hepatitis C virus (HCV) infection (abstract). Blood 92:405a, 1998.

361. Bauduer F: Marginal zone B-cell non-Hodgkin's lymphoma associated with hepatitis C virus infection treated by interferon alpha. Am J Hematol 53:209, 1996.

362. Weib R, Huhn D, Mitrou P et al: HIV-related non-Hodgkin's lymphoma: CHOP induction therapy and interferon-α-2b/zidovudine maintenance therapy. Leuk Lymphoma 29:103, 1998.

363. Harrington WJ Jr, Cabral L, Cai JP et al: Azothymidine and interferon-α are active in AIDS-associated small non-cleaved cell lymphoma but not large-cell lymphoma. Lancet 348:833, 1996.

364. Bunn PA, Foon KA, Ihde DC et al: Recombinant leukocyte A interferon: An active agent in advanced cutaneous T-cell lymphomas. Ann Intern Med 101:484, 1984.

365. Pressman D, Korngold L: The in vivo localization of anti-Wagner osteogenic sarcoma antibdoy. Cancer 6:619, 1953.

366. Kohler G, Milstein C: Continuous cultures of fused cells secreting antibody of predefined specificity. Nature 256:495, 1975.

367. Nadler LM, Stashenko P, Hardy R et al: Serotherapy of a patient with a monoclonal antibody directed against a human lymphoma-associated antigen. Cancer Res 40:3147, 1980.

368. Multani PS, Grossbard ML: Monoclonal antibody-based therapies for hematologic malignancies. J Clin Oncol 16:3691, 1998.

369. Maloney D, Smith B, Applebaum F: The anti-tumor effect of monoclonal anti-CD20 antibody (mAb) therapy includes direct anti-proliferative activity and induction apoptosis in CD20 positive non-Hodgkin's lymphoma cell lines. Blood 88:637a (abstract), 1996.

370. Taji H, Kagami Y, Okada Y et al: Growth inhibition of CD20-positive B lymphoma cell lines by IDEC-C2B8 anti-CD20 monoclonal antibody. Jpn J Cancer Res 89:748, 1998.

371. Pearson M, Shinn C, Grever M et al: Rituximab induces in vitro apoptosis in human chronic lymphocytic leukemia cells independent of complement mediated lysis but requires Fcg receptor ligation. Blood 94:313 (abstract), 1999.

372. Maloney DG, Liles TM, Czerwinski DK et al: Phase I clinical trial using escalating single-dose infusion of chimeric anti-CD20 monoclonal antibody (IDEC-C2B8) in patients with recurrent B-cell lymphoma. Blood 84:2457, 1994.

373. Maloney DG, Grillo-Lopez AJ, Bodkin DJ et al: IDEC-C2B8: Results of a phase I multiple-dose trial in patients with relapsed non-Hodgkin's lymphoma. J Clin Oncol 15:3266, 1997.

374. Maloney DG, Grillo-Lopez AJ, White CA et al: IDEC-C2B8 (rituximab) anti-CD20 monoclonal antibody therapy in patients with relapsed low-grade non-Hodgkin's lymphoma. Blood 90:2188, 1997.

375. McLaughlin P, Grillo-Lopez AJ, Link BK et al: Rituximab chimeric anti-CD20 monoclonal antibody therapy for relapsed indolent lymphoma: Half of patients respond to a four-dose treatment program. J Clin Oncol 16:2825, 1998.

376. Grillo-Lopez AJ, Cheson BD, Horning SJ et al: Response criteria for NHL: Importance of 'normal' lymph node size and correlations with response rates. Ann Oncol 11:399, 2000.

377. Davis TA, White CA, Grillo-Lopez AJ et al: Single-agent monoclonal antibody efficacy in bulky non-Hodgkin's lymphoma: Results of a phase II trial of rituximab. J Clin Oncol 17:1851, 1999.

378. Piro LD, White CA, Grillo-Lopez AJ et al: Extended rituximab (anti-CD20 monoclonal antibody) therapy for relapsed or refractory low-grade or follicular non-Hodgkin's lymphoma. Ann Oncol 10:655, 1999.

379. Davis TA, Grillo-Lopez AJ, White CA et al: Rituximab anti-CD20 monoclonal antibody therapy in non-Hodgkin's lymphoma: Safety and efficacy of re-treatment. J Clin Oncol 18:3135, 2000.

380. Johnson PW, Rohatiner AZ, Whelan JS et al: Patterns of survival in patients with recurrent follicular lymphoma: A 20-year study from a single center. J Clin Oncol 13:140, 1995.

381. Igarashi T, Ohtsu T, Fujii et al: Rituximab re-treatment can produce prolonged failure-free survival for relapsed indolent B-cell lymphoma. Blood 94:262b(Abstract), 1999.

382. Hainsworth JD, Burris HA 3rd, Morrissey LH et al: Rituximab monoclonal antibody as initial systemic therapy for patients with low-grade non-Hodgkin's lymphoma. Blood 95:3052, 2000.

383. Solal-Celigny P, Salles G, Brousse N et al: Rituximab as a first-line treatment of patients with follicular lymphoma and a low-burden tumor: Clinical and molecular evaluation. Blood 94:631a(Abstract), 1999.

384. Grillo-Lopez A, Lee D, Alkuzewny B et al: Clinical activity of rituximab in patients who have relapsed following ABMT. Proc Am Soc Clin Oncol 19:23a(Abstract), 2000.

385. Demidem A, Lam T, Alas S et al: Chimeric anti-CD20 (IDEC C2B8) monoclonal antibody sensitizes a B cell lymphoma cell line to cell killing by cytotoxic drugs. Cancer Biother Radiopharm 12:177, 1997.

386. Czuczman, MS, Grillo-Lopez AJ, White CA et al: Treatment of patients with low-grade B-cell lymphoma with the combination of chimeric anti-CD20 monoclonal antibody and CHOP chemotherapy. J Clin Oncol 17:268, 1999.

387. Czuczman MS: CHOP plus rituximab chemoimmunotherapy of indolent B-cell lymphoma. Semin Oncol 26(Suppl. 14):88, 1999.

388. Garcia-Conde J, Conde E, Sierra J et al: Rituximab (IDEC-C2B8) and CVP chemotherapy in follicular or low grade B-cell lymphoma after relapse: Results after 6 months of follow-up. Proc Am Soc Clin Oncol 19:27a(Abstract), 2000.

389. Emmanouilides C, Rosen P, Teletar M et al: Excellent tolerance of rituximab when given after mitoxantrone-cyclophosphamide: An effective and safe combination for indolent NHL. Clin Lymphoma 1:146, 2000.

390. Czuczman M, Jonas C, Stephan M et al: Pilot study of Rituxan in combination with fludarabine chemotherapy in patients with low-grade or follicular non-Hodgkin's lymphoma. Proc Am Soc Clin Oncol 18:17a(Abstract), 1999.

391. Davis TA, Maloney DG, Grillo-Lopez AJ et al: Combination immunotherapy of relapsed or refractory low-grade or follicular non-Hodgkin's lymphoma with rituximab and interferon-alpha-2a. Clin Cancer Res 6:2644, 2000.

392. Sacchi S, Federico M, Vitolo U et al: Phase II study of rituximab after priming with IFN in patients with relapsed low grade/follicular B-cell lymphoma. Blood 94:91a(Abstract), 1999.

393. Foran JM, Rohatiner AZ, Cunningham D et al: European phase II study of rituximab (chimeric anti-CD20 monoclonal antibody) for patients with newly diagnosed mantle-cell lymphoma and previously treated mantle-cell lymphoma, immunocytoma, and small B-cell lymphocytic lymphoma. J Clin Oncol 18:317, 2000.

394. Foran JM, Cunningham D, Coiffier B et al: Treatment of mantle-cell lymphoma with Rituximab (chimeric monoclonal anti-CD20 antibody): Analysis of factors associated with response. Ann Oncol 11:117, 2000.

395. Ghielmini M, Schmitz SF, Burki K et al: The effect of Rituximab on patients with follicular and mantle-cell lymphoma. Swiss Group for Clinical Cancer Research (SAKK). Ann Oncol 11:123, 2000.

396. Howard O, Gribben J, Neuberg D et al: Rituxan/CHOP induction therapy in newly diagnosed patients with mantle cell lymphoma. Blood 94:631a(Abstract), 1999.

397. Coiffier B, Haioun C, Ketterer N et al: Rituximab (anti-CD20 monoclonal antibody) for the treatment of patients with relapsing or refractory aggressive lymphoma: A multicenter phase II study. Blood 92:1927, 1998.

398. Link B, Grossbard M, Fisher R et al: Phase II pilot study of the safety and efficacy of rituximab in combination with CHOP chemotherapy in patients with previously untreated intermediate- or high-grade NHL. Proc Am Soc Clin Oncol 17:3a(Abstract), 1998.

399. Gutierrez M, Grossbard M, Little R et al: Dose-adjusted epoch chemotherapy (CT) and rituximab (EPOCH-R): An effective regimen in poor prognosis aggressive B-cell non-Hodgkin's lymphoma (NHL). Proc Am Soc Clin Oncol 19:26a(Abstract), 2000.

400. Tirelli U, Sparano J, Hopkins U et al: Pilot trial of infusional cyclophosphamide, doxorubicin, and etoposide (CDE) plus the anti-CD20 monoclonal antibody rituximab in HIV-associated non-Hodgkin's lymphoma (NHL). Proc Am Soc Clin Oncol 19:44a(Abstract), 2000.

401. O'Brien S, Freireich E, Andreeff M et al: Phase I/II study of rituxan in chronic lymphocytic leukemia (CLL). Blood 92:105a(Abstract), 1998.

402. Byrd J, Grever M, Davis B et al: Phase I/II study of thrice weekly rituximab in chronic lymphocytic leukemia/small lymphocytic lymphoma: A feasible and active regimen. Blood 94:704a(Abstract), 1999.

403. Keating M, O'Brien S, Cortes J et al: Fludarabine and cyclophosphamide combined with Rituxan (FCR) is a potent cytoreductive regimen as initial therapy of chronic lymphocytic leukemia. Proc Am Soc Clin Oncol 19:8a(Abstract), 2000.

404. Byrd JC, Waselenko JK, Maneatis TJ et al: Rituximab therapy in hematologic malignancy patients with circulating blood tumor cells: Association with increased infusion-related side effects and rapid blood tumor clearance. J Clin Oncol 17:791, 1999.

405. Winkler U, Jensen M, Manske O et al: Cytokine-release syndrome in patients with B-cell chronic lymphocytic leukemia and high lymphocyte counts after treatment with an anti-CD20 monoclonal antibody (rituximab, IDEC-C2B8). Blood 94:2217, 1999.

406. Byrd JC, White CA, Link B et al: Rituximab therapy in Waldenström's macroglobulinemia: Preliminary evidence of clinical activity. Ann Oncol 10:1525, 1999.

407. Treon S, Agus D, Link B et al: Rituximab is an active agent in Waldenström's macroglobulinemia (WM). Proc Am Soc Clin Oncol 19:6a(Abstract), 2000.

408. Treon SP, Shima Y, Grossbard ML et al: Treatment of multiple myeloma by antibody mediated immunotherapy and induction of myeloma selective antigens. Ann Oncol 11:107, 2000.

409. Treon SP, Shima Y, Preffer FI et al: Treatment of plasma cell dyscrasias by antibody-mediated immunotherapy. Semin Oncol 26:97, 1999.

410. Treon S, Shima Y, Preffer F et al: Interferon-γ induces CD20 expression on multiple myeloma patient and healthy donor plasma cells and augments binding of rituximab. Proceeding of the International Conference on Malignant Lymphoma. Ann Oncol 10:34, 1999.

411. Kuehnle I, Huls MH, Liu Z et al: CD20 monoclonal antibody (rituximab) for therapy of Epstein-Barr virus lymphoma after hemopoietic stem-cell transplantation. Blood 95:1502, 2000.

412. Milpied N, Vasseur B, Parquet N et al: Humanized anti-CD20 monoclonal antibody (rituximab) in post transplant B-lymphoproliferative disorder: A retrospective analysis on 32 patients. Ann Oncol 11:113, 2000.

413. Garrett TJ, Chadburn A, Barr ML et al: Posttransplantation lymphoproliferative disorders treated with cyclophosphamide-doxorubicin-vincristine-prednisone chemotherapy. Cancer 72:2782, 1993.

414. Papadopoulos EB, Ladanyi M, Emanuel D et al: Infusions of donor leukocytes to treat Epstein-Barr virus-associated lymphoproliferative disorders after allogeneic bone marrow transplantation. N Engl J Med 330:1185, 1994.

415. Rooney CM, Smith CA, Ng CY et al: Infusion of cytotoxic T cells for the prevention and treatment of Epstein-Barr virus-induced lymphoma in allogeneic transplant recipients. Blood 92:1549, 1998.

416. Fisher A, Blanche S, Le Bidois J et al: Anti-B-cell monoclonal antibodies in the treatment of severe B-cell lymphoproliferative syndrome following bone marrow and organ transplantation. N Engl J Med 324:1451, 1991.

417. Benkerrou M, Jais JP, Leblond V et al: Anti-B-cell monoclonal antibody treatment of severe posttransplant B-lymphoproliferative disorder: Prognostic factors and long-term outcome. Blood 92:3137, 1998.

418. O'Toole JE, Esseltine D, Lynch TJ et al: Clinical trials with blocked ricin immunotoxins. Curr Top Microbiol Immunol 234:35, 1998.

419. Pai LH, Pastan I: Clinical trials with Pseudomonas exotoxin immunotoxins. Curr Top Microbiol Immunol 234:83, 1998.

420. Chaudhary V, Batra J, Gallo M et al: A rapid method of cloning functional variable-region antibody genes in Escherichia coli as

single-chain immunotoxins. Proc Natl Acad Sci U S A 87:1066, 1992.

421. Pelham H, Roberts L, Lord J: Toxin entry: How reversible is the secretory pathway? Trends Cell Biol 2:183, 1992.

422. Wales R, Roberts L, Lord J: Addition of an endoplasmic reticulum retrieval sequence to ricin A chain significantly increases its cytotoxicity to mammalian cells. J Biol Chem 268:23986, 1993.

423. Endo Y, Mitsui K, Motizuki M et al: The mechanism of action of ricin and related toxic lectins on eukaryotic ribosomes. The site and the characteristics of the modification in 28 S ribosomal RNA caused by the toxins. J Biol Chem 262:5908, 1987.

424. Collier RJ: Structure-activity relationships in diphtheria toxin and *Pseudomonas aeruginosa* exotoxin A. Cancer Treat Res 37:25, 1988.

425. Brinkmann U, Pai LH, FitzGerald DJ et al: B3(Fv)-PE38KDEL, a single-chain immunotoxin that causes complete regression of a human carcinoma in mice. Proc Natl Acad Sci U S A 88:8616, 1991.

426. Nichols J, Foss F, Kuzel TM et al: Interleukin-2 fusion protein: an investigational therapy for interleukin-2 receptor expressing malignancies. Eur J Cancer 33(Suppl. 1):S34, 1997.

427. Greenfield L, Johnson VG, Youle RJ: Mutations in diphtheria toxin separate binding from entry and amplify immunotoxin selectivity. Science 238:536, 1987.

428. Rolf JM, Eidels L: Structure-function analyses of diphtheria toxin by use of monoclonal antibodies. Infect Immun 61:994, 1993.

429. Moya M, Dautry-Varsat A, Goud B et al: Inhibition of coated pit formation in Hep2 cells blocks the cytotoxicity of diphtheria toxin but not that of ricin toxin. J Cell Biol 101:548, 1985.

430. Morris RE, Gerstein AS, Bonventre PF et al: Receptor-mediated entry of diphtheria toxin into monkey kidney (Vero) cells: Electron microscopic evaluation. Infect Immun 50:721, 1985.

431. Fuchs R, Schmid S, Mellman I: A possible role for Na+, K+-ATPase in regulating ATP-dependent endosome acidification. Proc Natl Acad Sci U S A 86:539, 1989.

432. Donovan JJ, Simon MI, Draper RK et al: Diphtheria toxin forms trans-membrane channels in planar lipid bilayers. Proc Natl Acad Sci U S A 78:172, 1981.

433. Hoch DH, Romero-Mira M, Ehrlich BE et al: Channels formed by botulinum, tetanus, and diphtheria toxins in planar lipid bilayers: Relevance to translocation of proteins across membranes. Proc Natl Acad Sci U S A 82:1692, 1985.

434. Lakkis F, Steele A, Pacheco-Silva A et al: Interleukin 4 receptor targeted cytotoxicity: Genetic construction and in vivo immunosuppressive activity of a diphtheria toxin-related murine interleukin 4 fusion protein. Eur J Immunol 21:2253, 1991.

435. Wen ZL, Tao X, Lakkis F et al: Diphtheria toxin-related alpha-melanocyte-stimulating hormone fusion toxin. Internal in-frame deletion from Thr387 to His485 results in the formation of a highly potent fusion toxin which is resistant to proteolytic degradation. J Biol Chem 266:12289, 1991.

436. Murphy JR, Bishai W, Borowski M et al: Genetic construction, expression, and melanoma-selective cytotoxicity of a diphtheria toxin-related alpha-melanocyte-stimulating hormone fusion protein. Proc Natl Acad Sci USA 83:8258, 1986.

437. Williams DP, Parker K, Bacha P et al: Diphtheria toxin receptor binding domain substitution with interleukin-2: Genetic construction and properties of a diphtheria toxin-related interleukin-2 fusion protein. Protein Eng 1:493, 1987.

438. Bacha P, Williams DP, Waters C et al: Interleukin 2 receptor-targeted cytotoxicity. Interleukin 2 receptor-mediated action of a diphtheria toxin-related interleukin 2 fusion protein. J Exp Med 167:612, 1988.

439. Walz G, Zanker B, Brand K et al: Sequential effects of interleukin 2-diphtheria toxin fusion protein on T-cell activation. Proc Natl Acad Sci U S A 86:9485, 1989.

440. Waters CA, Schimke PA, Snider CE et al: Interleukin 2 receptor-targeted cytotoxicity. Receptor binding requirements for entry of a diphtheria toxin-related interleukin 2 fusion protein into cells. Eur J Immunol 20:785, 1990.

441. Waldmann TA: The structure, function, and expression of interleukin-2 receptors on normal and malignant lymphocytes. Science 232:727, 1986.

442. Waldmann TA: The multichain interleukin 2 receptor. A target for immunotherapy in lymphoma, autoimmune disorders, and organ allografts. JAMA 263:272, 1990.

443. Craig F, Banks P: Detection of the alpha and beta components of the interleukin-2 receptor using immunologic techniques. Mod Pathol 5:118a(Abstract), 1992.

444. Uchiyama T, Hori T, Tsudo M et al: Interleukin-2 receptor (Tac antigen) expressed on adult T cell leukemia cells. J Clin Invest 76:446, 1985.

445. Strauchen JA, Breakstone BA: IL-2 receptor expression in human lymphoid lesions. Immunohistochemical study of 166 cases. Am J Pathol 126:506, 1987.

446. Sheibani K, Winberg CD, Van de Velde S et al: Distribution of lymphocytes with interleukin-2 receptors (TAC antigens) in reactive lymphoproliferative processes, Hodgkin's disease, and non-Hodgkin's lymphomas. An immunohistologic study of 300 cases. Am J Pathol 127:27, 1987.

447. Barnett D, Wilson GA, Lawrence AC et al: The interleukin-2 receptor and its expression in the acute leukaemias and lymphoproliferative disorders. Dis Markers 6:133, 1988.

448. Rosolen A, Nakanishi M, Poplack DG et al: Expression of interleukin-2 receptor beta subunit in hematopoietic malignancies. Blood 73:1968, 1989.

449. Kung E, Meissner K, Loning T: Cutaneous T cell lymphoma: Immunocytochemical study on activation/proliferation and differentiation associated antigens in lymph nodes, skin, and peripheral blood. Virchows Arch A Pathol Anat Histopathol 413:539, 1988.

450. LeMaistre CF, Meneghetti C, Rosenblum M et al: Phase I trial of an interleukin-2 (IL-2) fusion toxin (DAB$_{486}$IL-2) in hematologic malignancies expressing the IL-2 receptor. Blood 79:2547, 1992.

451. Tepler I, Schwartz G, Parker K et al: Phase I trial of an interleukin-2 fusion toxin (DAB$_{486}$IL-2) in hematologic malignancies: Complete response in a patient with Hodgkin's disease refractory to chemotherapy. Cancer 73:1276, 1994.

452. Hesketh P, Caguioa P, Koh H et al: Clinical activity of a cytotoxic fusion protein in the treatment of cutaneous T-cell lymphoma. J Clin Oncol 11:1682, 1993.

453. LeMaistre CF, Craig FE, Meneghetti C et al: Phase I trial of a 90-minute infusion of the fusion toxin DAB$_{486}$IL-2 in hematological cancers. Cancer Res 53:3930, 1993.

454. Kuzel TM, Rosen ST, Gordon LI et al: Phase I trial of the diphtheria toxin/interleukin-2 fusion protein DAB$_{486}$IL-2: Efficacy in mycosis fungoides and other non-Hodgkin's lymphomas. Leuk Lymphoma 11:369, 1993.

455. Foss FM, Borkowski TA, Gilliom M et al: Chimeric fusion protein toxin DAB$_{486}$IL-2 in advanced mycosis fungoides and the Sézary syndrome: Correlation of activity and interleukin-2 receptor expression in a phase II study. Blood 84:1765, 1994.

456. Choe S, Bennett MJ, Fujii G et al: The crystal structure of diphtheria toxin. Nature 357:216, 1992.

457. Kiyokawa T, Williams DP, Snider CE et al: Protein engineering of diphtheria-toxin-related interleukin-2 fusion toxins to increase cytotoxic potency for high-affinity IL-2-receptor-bearing target cells. Protein Eng 4:463, 1991.

458. Shaw JP, Akiyoshi DE, Arrigo DA et al: Cytotoxic properties of DAB$_{486}$EGF and DAB$_{389}$EGF, epidermal growth factor (EGF) receptor-targeted fusion toxins. J Biol Chem 266:21118, 1991.

459. Theodoulou M, Baselfa J, Scher H: Phase I dose escalation study of the safety, tolerability, pharmacokinetics and biologic effects of DAB$_{389}$EGF in patients with solid malignancies that express EGF receptors. Proc Am Soc Clin Oncol 14:480(abstract), 1995.

460. LeMaistre CF, Meneghetti C, Rosenblum M et al: Phase I trial of an interleukin-2 (IL-2) fusion toxin (DAB$_{486}$IL-2) in hematologic malignancies expressing the IL-2 receptor. Blood 79:2547, 1992.

461. Hesketh P, Caguioa P, Koh H et al: Clinical activity of a cytotoxic fusion protein in the treatment of cutaneous T-cell lymphoma. J Clin Oncol 11:1682, 1993.

462. LeMaistre C, Saleh M, Kuzel T: Phase I trial of a ligand fusion protein (DAB$_{389}$IL-2) in lymphomas expressing the receptor for interleukin-2. Blood 91:399, 1998.

463. Kuzel T, Olsen E, Martin A et al: Phase III trial of two dose levels of DAB$_{389}$IL-2 for the treatment of mycosis fungoides. Blood 90(Suppl. 1):586a(Abstract), 1997.

464. Bacha P, Fowlie A, Hillier J et al: Antibody and pharmacokinetic analysis from a pivotal trial of ONTAK™ (DAB$_{389}$IL-2) for the treatment of cutaneous T-cell lymphoma. Blood 90(Suppl. 1):326a(Abstract), 1997.

465. Fisher RI, Gaynor ER, Dahlberg S et al: A phase III comparison of CHOP vs. m-BACOD vs. ProMACE-CytaBOM vs. MACOP-B in patients with intermediate- or high-grade non-Hodgkin's lymphoma: Results of SWOG-8516 (Intergroup 0067), the National High-Priority Lymphoma Study. Ann Oncol 5:91, 1994.

466. Perentesis JP, Waddick KG, Bendel AE et al: Induction of apoptosis in multidrug-resistant and radiation-resistant acute myeloid leukemia cells by a recombinant fusion toxin directed against the human granulocyte macrophage colony-stimulating factor receptor. Clin Cancer Res 3:347, 1997.

467. O'Connor R, Liu C, Ferris CA et al: Anti-B4-blocked ricin synergizes with doxorubicin and toposide on multidrug-resistant and drug-sensitive tumors. Blood 86:4286, 1995.

468. Scadden DT, Schenkein DP, Bernstein Z et al: Immunotoxin combined with chemotherapy for patients with AIDS-related non-Hodgkin's lymphoma. Cancer 83:2580, 1998.

469. Cantrell DA, Smith KA: The interleukin-2 T-cell system: A new cell growth model. Science 224:1312, 1984.

470. Kelley VE, Bacha P, Pankewycz O et al: Interleukin 2-diphtheria toxin fusion protein can abolish cell-mediated immunity in vivo. Proc Natl Acad Sci U S A 85:3980, 1988.

471. Pankewycz O, Mackie J, Hassarjian R et al: Interleukin-2-diphtheria toxin fusion protein prolongs murine islet cell engraftment. Transplantation 47:318, 1989.

472. Kirkman RL, Bacha P, Barrett LV et al: Prolongation of cardiac allograft survival in murine recipients treated with a diphtheria toxin-related interleukin-2 fusion protein. Transplantation 47:327, 1989.

473. Vincenti F, Kirkham R, Light S et al: Interleukin-2-receptor blockade with daclizumab to prevent acute rejection in renal transplantation. Daclizumab Triple Therapy Study Group. N Engl J Med 338:161, 1998.

474. Harris DT, Sakiestewa D, Lyons C et al: Prevention of graft-versus-host disease (GVHD) by elimination of recipient-reactive donor T cells with recombinant toxins that target the interleukin 2(IL-2) receptor. Bone Marrow Transplant 23:137, 1999.

475. Moreland LW, Sewell KL, Trentham DE et al: Interleukin-2 diphtheria fusion protein (DAB$_{486}$IL-2) in refractory rheumatoid arthritis. A double-blind, placebo-controlled trial with open-label extension. Arthritis Rheum 38:1177, 1995.

476. Bousvaros A, Stevens AC, Strom TB et al: Interleukin-2 fusion protein (DAB$_{389}$IL-2) selectively targets activated human peripheral blood and lamina propria lymphocytes. Dig Dis Sci 42:1542, 1997.

477. Bagel J, Garland WT, Breneman D et al: Administration of DAB$_{389}$IL-2 to patients with recalcitrant psoriasis: A double-blind, phase II multi-center trial. J Am Acad Dermatol 38:938, 1998.

478. Finberg RW, Wahl SM, Allen JB et al: Selective elimination of HIV-1-infected cells with an interleukin-2 receptor-specific cytotoxin. Science 252:1703, 1991.

479. Zhang L, Waters C, Nichols J et al: Inhibition of HIV-1 RNA production by the diphtheria toxin-related IL-2 fusion proteins DAB$_{486}$IL-2 and DAB$_{389}$IL-2. J Acquir Immune Defic Syndr 5:1181, 1992.

480. Maloney DG, Press OW: Newer treatments for non-Hodgkin's lymphoma: Monoclonal antibodies. Oncology 12(Suppl. 8):63, 1998.

481. Hernandez-Ilizaliturri FJ, Sendowski M: Recent advances in the molecular biology of non-hodgkin's lymphoma. Fellow Reporter 6:36, 2001.

482. Smalley R, Haase-Statz S: Role of interferon-alfa in NHL: Still controversial? Oncology 13:1147, 1999.

483. Petryk M, Grossbard M: Rituximab therapy of B-cell neoplasms. Clin Lymphoma 1:186, 2000.

484. Foss F: DAB$_{389}$IL-2 (Denileukin Diftitox, ONTAK): A new fusion protein technology. Clin Lymphoma 1(Suppl. 1) Abstract:S27, 2000.

485. Kuzel T: DAB$_{389}$IL-2 (Denileukin Diftitox, ONTAK): Review of clinical trials to date. Clin Lymphoma 1(Suppl. 1) Abstract:S33, 2000.

486. LeMaistre CF: DAB$_{389}$IL-2 (Denileukin Diftitox, ONTAK): Other potential applications. Clin Lymphoma 9(Suppl. 1) Abstract:S37, 2000.

42

Cytogenetics of Non-Hodgkin's Lymphoma and Hodgkin's Disease

Krzysztof Mrózek and Clara D. Bloomfield

The first reports on chromosome abnormalities in Hodgkin's disease (HD) and non-Hodgkin's lymphoma (NHL) were published in 1962 and 1963, respectively.[1,2] Subsequent studies of approximately 200 cases of malignant lymphoma, performed before banding, demonstrated that most tumors had an abnormal karyotype and that there was a difference in the modal chromosomal number between HD and NHL. More than one-half of the HD cases were polyploid, whereas karyotypes of most NHLs were in the near-diploid range (reviewed by Mark[3]). However, neither subtle chromosome rearrangements nor the exact nature of the observed aberrations could be identified at this time due to difficulties in interpretation of unbanded chromosome preparations.

The malignant lymphomas were among the first human neoplastic disorders to be studied systematically when the new banding techniques became available in the 1970s. In 1972, Manolov and Manolova[4] identified an extra band at the end of 14q as the first structural abnormality specific for a particular histology (i.e., Burkitt lymphoma [BL]). In 1976, this derivative chromosome was shown to be a result of a reciprocal translocation between chromosomes 8 and 14, t(8;14)(q24;q32).[5] Thereafter, data accumulated fairly rapidly in BL, but the accrual of cytogenetic data on other NHL and especially on HD has been substantially slower than for leukemias and myeloproliferative and myelodysplastic syndromes, which account for approximately two-thirds of more than 37,000 karyotypically aberrant human tumors published.[6]

The reported number of lymphomas with clonal chromosome aberrations (i.e., the same extra chromosome or an identical structural rearrangement present in at least two cells and monosomy detected in three or more cells[7]) now exceeds 3400.[6] However, the lymphomas represent a heterogeneous group of malignancies that despite their common origin from lymphoid cells demonstrate distinct morphologic, immunologic, and genetic properties. Consequently few categories of NHL have been well characterized cytogenetically. Furthermore, comparisons between results obtained by researchers from different institutions have been difficult because of the simultaneous use of several classification schemes of NHL. Although many recently published karyotypically abnormal lymphomas have been classified according to the Revised European American Classification of Lymphoid Neoplasms (R.E.A.L.) or the World Health Organization Classification,[8] the majority of currently available cytogenetic data on NHL comes from studies in which the tumors were morphologically divided by the Working Formulation for Clinical Usage,[9] or the Kiel classification.[10]

The ways of presenting cytogenetic results in NHL also have differed among investigators. In some reports full descriptions of the karyotypes are available, whereas in others only selected data are provided, and they are often arranged differently. In addition, the complexity of lymphoma karyotypes that often contain unidentifiable marker chromosomes has precluded complete description of chromosome changes in many cases. This can be at least partially overcome by the use of fluorescence in situ hybridization (FISH), comparative genomic hybridization (CGH), and FISH-based cytogenetic techniques, such as multicolor spectral karyotyping (SKY) and multiplex FISH (m-FISH), which enable simultaneous display of all human chromosomes in different colors.[11] Although very useful, each of the aforementioned techniques has limitations and should not be used as the only investigative tool. The number of lymphomas analyzed using SKY is at present very low.[12] Finally, many reports correlating karyotype and clinical features include patients studied at diagnosis and relapse, and those studies that exclusively deal with newly diagnosed patients differ in the ways of grouping cytogenetic, histologic, and treatment data.

Despite these shortcomings, recurrent cytogenetic abnormalities and chromosomal bands or regions rearranged in nonrandom fashion have been identified, and significant correlations between karyotype and histology, immunophenotype, and clinical outcome of NHL have been recognized. Furthermore, the dissection of several of these recurrent abnormalities by molecular means has led to a substantial increase in our understanding of lymphomagenesis. In this chapter we describe the nonrandom chromosomal aberrations characteristic of lymphomas and present the correlations with morphology and clinical features that are available to date. For convenience to the reader, cytogenetic findings are discussed separately for NHL and HD.

NON-HODGKIN'S LYMPHOMA

General Cytogenetic Features of NHL

Success Rates

Advances in cytogenetic methodology and general acceptance of the fact that the primary tumor cells (i.e., cells from lymph nodes or other tumor masses) should be examined cytogenetically instead of bone marrow, blood, or various effusions have resulted in relatively high success rates of cytogenetic investigations in NHL. On average, more than 80 percent (range 56 to 96 percent) of cases analyzed in eight large series of NHLs, each comprising all histologic subtypes, yielded sufficient numbers of good quality metaphase cells.[13–20] It appears, however, that low-grade lymphomas are more difficult to karyotype than high-grade tumors. In a study of 60 patients with indolent (low-grade) NHL, the success rate (65 percent) was lower than the above mentioned average.[21] Correspondingly, Offit et al.[19] recognized a trend toward an increased proportion of cytogenetic failures in low-grade as compared with high-grade lymphomas (21.5 vs. 13.2 percent failures, $p = .09$) in the largest single-institution study reported to date.

Normal Karyotypes

Clonal chromosome abnormalities have been identified in most successfully karyotyped cases of NHL. Although abnormal karyotypes have occasionally been reported in all patients studied,[13,15] in most large series, cytogenetically normal tumors have constituted from 3 to 20 percent of cases.[14,16–19,22–24] A normal chromosome complement can be found in lymphomas of all histologies, but the distribution of tumors without clonal chromosome aberrations among histologic subgroups seems to be nonrandom.[19,25] The highest frequencies of tumors with exclusively normal metaphases have been reported in diffuse, small cleaved cell lymphoma (DSC) (on average 32 percent), lymphoblastic lymphoma (LBL) (31 percent), follicular, predominantly small cleaved cell lymphoma (FSC), and diffuse, mixed small and large cell lymphoma (DM) (25 percent each). In contrast, only 5 to 9 percent of small noncleaved cell lymphoma (SNC), diffuse, large cell lymphoma (DLC), and follicular, predominantly large cell lymphoma (FL) did not display clonal aberrations.[19,25]

The finding of a normal karyotype in a lymphoma specimen may be attributed in some cases to the presence of reactive, non-neoplastic cells that may preferentially divide in vitro, while the karyotypically abnormal tumor cells within the same specimen fail to enter mitosis. Data supporting this hypothesis have been provided by Rack et al.[26] who, using FISH in three patients with follicular lymphoma and a normal karyotype, detected the presence of t(14;18)(q32;q21) in 24 to 84 percent of nondividing, interphase cells. Metaphase FISH did not reveal this translocation in any of the three patients studied.[26] However, seemingly normal karyotypes have been demonstrated in lymphoma cells that have been identified as neoplastic by their morphology and reaction with a specific anti-idiotype antibody.[27] Such findings suggest that occasionally the degree of resolution of standard cytogenetic analysis may be too low to visualize subtle rearrangements, such as paracentric inversions, small deletions, or reciprocal translocations of little segments between similarly banded regions. Indeed, in an established BL cell line, a subtle deletion of 6q could be detected only by analysis of loss of heterozygosity.[28] Moreover, it has been demonstrated that in some tumors genomic alterations occur at the gene level and cannot be seen using cytogenetic methods. For instance, a submicroscopic excision of the *BCL2* gene from its original location at 18q21 and insertion of the gene into the immunoglobulin heavy chain *(IGH)* locus at 14q32 has been recently demonstrated in two patients with follicular lymphoma.[29]

Modal Chromosomal Number

Approximately one-third of cytogenetically aberrant NHLs display the pseudodiploid modal number of 46 chromosomes. Notably, pseudodiploid tumors have been significantly more often found in patients studied at diagnosis than at relapse.[14]

Hypodiploidy, that is, a modal chromosome number of 45 or less, is fairly uncommon; it occurs in no more than 8 percent of tumors. In several large studies, over one-half of the cases (54 to 65 percent) had karyotypes containing 47 or more chromosomes. Among hyperdiploid tumors, the most frequent modal chromosome number has been 47, followed by 48 and 49 chromosomes.[13–17,25] Levine et al.[22] correlated ploidy with histologic subtypes and found that small lymphocytic lymphoma (SLL), LBL, and SNC tended to be pseudodiploid; FSC and DM were associated with modal numbers of 47 or 48 chromosomes; and FL, DLC, and immunoblastic lymphomas (IBL) most commonly had a modal number of 49 chromosomes or greater.

Primary and Secondary Chromosome Abnormalities

The usual lymphoma karyotype is complex and contains many numerical and structural abnormalities concurrently. Tumors with only one clonal aberration are relatively rare. For instance, in the two large series of NHL from Minnesota[13–15,22] and in the Fifth International Workshop on Chromosomes in Leukemia-Lymphoma,[25] karyotypes with a sole karyotypic change were found in 24 of 83 cases (29 percent),[13,15] in 22 of 120 cases (18 percent),[15,22] and in 27 of 260 patients (10 percent),[25] respectively. In general, structural anomalies such as reciprocal and unbalanced translocations, insertions, deletions, duplications, para- and pericentric inversions, ring chromosomes, and isochromosomes are more frequent than numerical changes. Among the latter, gains of whole chromosomes are much more common than losses.[6,14]

The most common recurring aberrations from a number of series are shown in Table 42–1. An abnormality is listed if it occurred in at least 10 percent of cases in a single series with the exception of the translocations involving region 3q27-29. Observations are generally consistent across the studies.

With the accumulation of cytogenetic data it has become clear that not all chromosome aberrations have equal significance in oncogenesis. Recurrent abnormalities have been divided based on their specificity and postulated role in the neoplastic process into two main categories: primary and secondary changes. Those abnormalities that are strongly correlated with a histologic type, and may be sometimes found as the sole karyotypic change, are assumed to be early changes that play a crucial role in tumor initiation. They have been classified as primary aberrations. The secondary aberrations are less specific, and they are believed to be later events that may contribute to tumor progression.[30]

Table 42–2 contains a list of recurrent abnormalities that have been found as solitary changes in NHL, and thus appear likely to be primary aberrations. Twenty of these rearrangements are reciprocal translocations. Such translocations have been accorded special relevance in lymphomagenesis since molecular investigations of the t(8;14)(q24;q32), and of its less frequent variants t(8;22)(q24;q11) and t(2;8)(p12;q24), revealed mechanisms of oncogene activation by chromosome translocation.[31] A protooncogene *MYC*, located at 8q24, is juxtaposed to the enhancer elements of the *IGH* gene at 14q32, or, in case of variant translocations, one of the immunoglobulin light chain genes, mapped to bands 2p12 *(IGK)* and 22q11 *(IGL)*, is translo-

Table 42–1. Most Frequent Recurring Cytogenetic Abnormalities in Non-Hodgkin's Lymphoma Among Five Series

Abnormalities	Fleishman et al.[89] (n = 56)	Kristoffersson et al.[16] (n = 58)	Offit et al.[19] (n = 278)	5th IWCLL[25] (n = 253)	Minnesota-Australia[a] (n = 268)
14q32	23 (41)[b]	23 (40)[b]	146 (53)[b]	101 (40)[b]	172 (65)[b]
t(14;18)	0	11 (19)	81 (29)	57 (23)	110 (41)
t(8;14)	1 (2)	0	41 (15)	17 (7)	12 (5)
3q27-29	3 (5)	5 (9)	21 (8)	NA	19 (7)
del(6q)	11 (20)	12 (21)	NA	37 (15)	40 (15)
i(17)(q10)	3 (5)	6 (10)	NA	NA	19 (7)
+3	7 (13)	8 (14)	26 (9)	22 (9)	30 (11)
+7	4 (7)	11 (19)	34 (12)	NA	40 (15)
+12	3 (5)	11 (19)	31 (11)	22 (9)	37 (17)
+18	8 (14)	9 (16)	22 (8)	NA	28 (11)
+21	6 (11)	2 (4)	14 (5)	NA	28 (11)

Abbreviations: 5th IWCLL, Fifth International Workshop on Chromosomes in Leukemia-Lymphoma; NA, not available.

[a] These 268 cases represent a combined series from the University of Minnesota and the Peter MacCallum Cancer Institute St. Vincent's Hospital in Melbourne, Australia.[14,17,22,103,278]

[b] Numbers in parentheses are percentage of cases with a given abnormality among abnormal cases.

Table 42–2. Structural and Numerical Chromosome Abnormalities Observed Repeatedly as the Sole Change in Non-Hodgkin's Lymphoma[a]

Aberration	Genes	Aberration	Genes
–X[c]		t(9;14)(p13;q32)[d]	PAX5/IGH
+X[d]		t(9;17)(q34;q23)[c]	
–Y[d]		t(9;22)(q34;q11)[c]	ABL/BCR
del(1)(q32)[d]		t(10;14)(q24;q11)[b]	HOX11/TCRD
t(1;8)(q32;p12)[b]		+11[b]	
+2[b]		del(11)(q14–q23)[d]	
t(2;3)(p12;q27)[c]	IGK/BCL6	dup(11)(q13q23–25)[d]	
t(2;5)(p23;q35)[d]	ALK/NPM1	t(11;14)(q13;q32)[d]	CCND1/IGH
t(2;7)(p11;q22)[b]	IGK/CDK6	t(11;18)(q21;q21)[d]	API2/MALT1
t(2;8)(p12;q24)[d]	IGK/MYC	+12[d]	
+3[d]		–14[b]	
del(3)(p21–25)[b]		+14[b]	
t(3;14)(q27;q32)[d]	BCL6/IGH	del(14)(q11–24-q22–32)[d]	
t(3;22)(q27;q11)[d]	BCL6/IGL	inv(14)(q11q32)[d]	IGH/TCRA,TCRD
+5[c]		t(14;18)(q32;q21)[d]	IGH/BCL2
t(5;7)(q13;q35–36)[b]		t(14;19)(q32;q13)[c]	IGH/BCL3
del(6)(q13–24-q21–27)[d]		+15[b]	
–7[b]		del(16)(q22)[c]	
+7[c]		–17[b]	
i(7)(q10)[d]		i(17)(q10)[d]	
+8[b]		+18[b]	
t(8;13)(p11;q11–12)[c]	FGFR1/ZNF198	t(18;22)(q21;q11)[b]	BCL2/IGL
t(8;14)(q24;q32)[d]	MYC/IGH	+19[b]	
t(8;22)(q24;q11)[d]	MYC/IGL	+20[b]	
+9[b]		+21[b]	
i(9)(q10)[c]		–22[b]	
der(9)t(9;12)(q34;q13)[b]		+22[b]	

[a] Data from Mitelman et al.[6] Only aberrations reported as solitary chromosome changes in at least one clone in two or more patients with NHL are included. For numerical aberrations (monosomies and trisomies) the number of patients refers only to those harboring a given monosomy or trisomy as a sole abnormality; for structural aberrations, the numbers provided refer to all patients, irrespective of whether a given aberration was isolated or not.

[b] Chromosome aberration reported in fewer than 5 patients.

[c] Reported in 5 to 10 patients.

[d] Reported in greater than 10 patients.

cated to a telomeric region of the *MYC* oncogene at 8q24. Consequently, *MYC* is activated and expressed at high levels. Since the product of the *MYC* gene, a DNA binding protein, is implicated in the regulation of a number of other critical genes, its constitutive production may result in uncontrolled proliferation of cells with one of the translocations.[31] An analogous transposition of genes from other chromosomes onto the *IGH*, *IGK*, or *IGL* loci in the B-cell specific translocations listed in Table 42–2 have led to the identification of further putative oncogenes such as *BCL6* (also known as *LAZ3*) at 3q27, *CDK6* at 7q22, *PAX5* at 9p13, *CCND1* (also known as *BCL1* or *PRAD1*) at 11q13, *BCL2* at 18q21, and *BCL3* at 19q13.[31–39]

Likewise, several genes implicated in T-cell lymphomagenesis have been identified by cloning the breakpoints in the translocations detected in T-cell lymphomas and, more frequently, in T-cell acute lymphoblastic leukemia (T-ALL). These recurrent translocations involve bands 14q11, 7p15-14, and 7q35 that harbor the alpha and delta, gamma, and beta chain genes of the T-cell receptor (*TCR*), respectively. Most genes activated by juxtaposition to *TCR* genes, for example *HOX11* activated by t(10;14)(q24;q11) and *LMO2* activated by t(11;14)(p13;q11), are putative transcription factors involved in cell differentiation and not expressed in normal T cells.[35] The protein product of the *TCL1* gene, expressed at high levels in cells carrying inv(14)(q11q32) or t(14;14)(q11;q32), has been demonstrated to interact with the protein encoded by another oncogene, *AKT*, enhancing its kinase activity and promoting its nuclear transport.[40]

Interestingly, in most instances, the protein products of genes activated by juxtaposition to the loci for immunoglobulin or *TCR* genes remain unchanged and are identical to their nontranslocated counterparts.[31] In contrast, less frequent NHL translocations that do not involve the immunoglobulin or *TCR* genes create fusion genes encoding hybrid proteins with excessive tyrosine kinase activity. Examples include t(2;5)(p23;q35) that fuses the nuclear phosphoprotein gene (*NPM*) located at 5q35 to a protein tyrosine kinase gene *ALK* at 2p23 and t(9;22)(q34;q11) resulting in the fusion of the oncogene *ABL* on chromosome 9 at q34 and the *BCR* locus mapped to 22q11.[35,41] It has been shown that the t(9;22) found in NHL is at the molecular level different from that in chronic myeloid leukemia (CML). The breakpoint in the *BCR* gene is more proximal in NHL than in CML and the bcr-abl protein is of a smaller size in NHL. This appears to be the same bcr-abl protein seen in Philadelphia chromosome-positive ALL.[42]

In addition to those included in Table 42–2, many recurrent (i.e., present in at least two cases) reciprocal translocations occur predominantly in the setting of a complex karyotype. In Table 42–3, we collate 75 such rearrangements. Despite the fact that each of these translocations has either never or only in single cases been detected without coexisting chromosome changes, it is likely that many of them represent primary abnormalities. These changes were often found in cases without the other known primary translocations presented in Table 42–2, and they are generally not observed in neoplasms originating outside the lymphatic system.

Notably, 40 percent of the translocations listed in Table 42–3 involve bands harboring *IGH*, *IGK*, or *IGL* loci. Among those,

the t(2;18)(p12;q21) represents a variant form of the well-known t(14;18)(q32;q21) and leads to activation of the *BCL2* gene.[43] Six additional putative oncogenes have been cloned from breakpoint regions in chromosomes involved in recurrent translocations with chromosome 14 at q32: *BCL10* at 1p22, *FCGR2B* at 1q22, *BCL9* and *MUC1* at 1q21, *NFKB2* at 10q24, and *DDX6* at 11q23.[44–48] Another group of rearrangements of primary significance affect band 3q27 and the *BCL6* gene located there. Four genes fused to the *BCL6* gene as a result of such translocations have been thus far identified, namely *ARHH* mapped to 4p13, *H4FM* to 6p21, *ZNFN1A1* to 7p12-13, and *LCP1* to 13q14.[49–52] Finally, an inversion inv(2)(p23q35), which creates an *ALK/ATIC* gene fusion leading to the *ALK* gene activation, represents a primary chromosome aberration in anaplastic large-cell lymphoma.[53] Alternatively, some of the other balanced translocations listed in Table 42–3 may represent nonrandom secondary aberrations that might play a role in tumor progression. For example, a t(1;22)(q22;q11) was recently identified in three t(14;18)-positive patients with follicular lymphoma and suggested to contribute to their disease progression by deregulating the *FCGR2B* gene that encodes the low-affinity IgG Fc receptor FcγRIIB.[54] The pathogenetic significance of other recurrent translocations listed in Table 42–3 is not known since they have not yet been studied at the molecular level. Thus, continued molecular dissection of these translocations will probably result in elucidation of previously unsuspected genes important in lymphocyte transformation. As can be inferred from Table 42–3, the chromosome bands or regions that are likely to contain such putative oncogenes include 1p35-36, 1p31-32, 1q42, 2q21, 3p21, 5q11, 5q23, 6p21, 6q21, 8q22, 11q21, 13q11, 15q15, 15q21-22, 21q22. Undoubtedly, this list will be supplemented by other loci as the number of cytogenetically characterized NHL cases increases in the future.

The second most common type of structural abnormality in NHL involves deletions. Consistently lost chromosomal arms, regions, or bands may contain tumor suppressor genes, the inactivation of which promotes the neoplastic process by causing disturbances in the cell's growth control. Several tumor suppressor genes have been cloned and shown to be lost or mutated in a wide spectrum of human neoplasms.[55,56] Perhaps the most frequently affected gene in human oncogenesis is *p53*, a tumor suppressor gene mapped to 17p13.[55] Loss and inactivation of *p53* were initially described in more than 30 percent of BL but not in other B-cell lymphomas.[57] However, subsequent studies provided evidence that mutations in the *p53* gene and p53 protein expression may be found in many patients with follicular and diffuse NHL, mantle cell lymphoma, and splenic lymphoma with villous lymphocytes.[58–61] These aberrations usually occur at later stages of the disease and confer poor prognosis.[58–61] Likewise, loss of material from 9p21 resulting in deletions of a tumor suppressor locus, designated *CDKN2/ARF*, that encodes two structurally and functionally different proteins, CDKN2 (also known as p16[INK4A], MTS1, or p16) and ARF (or p14), appears to be a consistent event in the progression of some high-grade NHL.[62–64] Additionally, abnormalities of the retinoblastoma gene and/or its aberrant expression have been demonstrated in a small percentage of low-grade B-cell lym-

Table 42–3. Recurring Reciprocal Translocations and Inversions That Have Been Predominantly Observed in Addition to Other Abnormalities in NHL[a]

Aberration	No. of Cases	Aberration	No. of Cases
Translocations involving bands that harbor *IG* genes			
t(2;18)(p12;q21)	5–10	t(7;14)(p15;q32)	< 5
t(1;14)(p35–36;q32)	< 5	t(8;14)(q22;q32)	< 5
t(1;14)(p31–32;q32)	< 5	t(10;14)(q24;q32)	< 5
t(1;14)(p22;q32)	5–10	t(1;11;14)(q32;q13;q32)	< 5
t(1;14)(q21;q32)	5–10	t(11;14)(q21;q32)[b]	< 5
t(1;14)(q22;q32)	< 5	t(11;14)(q23;q32)	< 5
t(1;14)(q23;q32)	< 5	t(12;14)(p11;q32)	< 5
t(1;14)(q42;q32)	< 5	t(13;14)(q11;q32)[b]	< 5
t(2;14)(p11–13;q32)	< 5	t(14;14)(q11;q32)	< 5
t(2;14)(q21;q32)	< 5	t(14;15)(q32;q15)	< 5
t(3;14)(p21;q32)	5–10	t(14;15)(q32;q21–22)	< 5
t(5;14)(q11;q32)[b]	< 5	t(1;22)(q22;q11)	< 5
t(5;14)(q23;q32)	< 5	t(9;22)(p24;q11)[b]	< 5
t(6;14)(p21;q32)	< 5	t(15;22)(p11;q11)	< 5
t(6;14)(q21;q32)	< 5	t(21;22)(q22;q11)	< 5
Abnormalities involving band 3q27 that harbors the *BCL6* gene			
t(1;3)(q21;q27)	< 5	t(3;5)(q27;q13)	< 5
t(1;3)(q25;q27–29)	< 5	t(3;6)(q27;p21)	< 5
t(2;3)(q21;q27)	5–10	t(3;7)(q27–29;p12–13)	< 5
inv(3)(q12q27)	< 5	t(3;9)(q27;p13)	< 5
t(3;3)(p21;q27)	< 5	t(3;13)(q27;q14)	< 5
t(3;4)(q27;p13)	< 5		
Translocations involving band 11q13 that harbors the *CCND1* gene			
t(8;11)(p21;q13)[b]	< 5	t(11;13)(q13;q14)	< 5
t(8;11)(q24;q13)	< 5		
Other abnormalities			
inv(1)(p13p36)	< 5	t(2;3)(p11;q11–12)[b]	< 5
inv(1)(p22p36)	< 5	t(3;10)(p14;q22–23)[b]	< 5
inv(1)(p34q21)	< 5	t(3;10)(p21;p13)	< 5
t(1;1)(p36;q25)	< 5	t(3;11)(q21;p13)	< 5
t(1;3)(p36;q25)	< 5	t(3;16)(q21;p13)	< 5
t(1;5)(q32;q31)[b]	< 5	t(4;11)(q21;q23)	< 5
t(1;5)(q32;q35)	< 5	t(6;7)(p23;q32)	< 5
t(1;6)(p35–36;q23)	< 5	t(6;12)(q21;p13)	< 5
t(1;6)(q21–23;q23)	< 5	t(7;14)(p13;q11)	< 5
t(1;6)(q21;q27)	< 5	t(7;14)(q35;q11)	< 5
t(1;7)(q21–23;q22)	< 5	t(8;9)(p23;p21–22)[b]	< 5
t(1;17)(p36;q21)	< 5	t(8;9)(q24;13)[b]	< 5
t(1;18)(p35–36;q21)	< 5	t(10;12)(q24;q22)	< 5
inv(2)(p23q35)	5–10	t(11;14)(p13;q11)	5–10
t(2;2)(p25;q31)	< 5	t(12;15)(q24;q15)	< 5
t(2;2)(q33;q37)	< 5		

[a] Data from Mitelman et al.,[6] Mrózek and Bloomfield,[70] Chaganti et al.,[277] Cigudosa et al.,[163] Callanan et al.[54] To be included in this listing a given abnormality must have been reported in at least two cases.
[b] In some cases present in an unbalanced form.

phoid malignancies[65] and in as many as 58 percent of high-grade lymphomas.[66] A recent study demonstrated that the *ATM* gene is a tumor suppressor gene inactivated by deletions of region 11q22-23 and deleterious point mutations in mantle cell lymphoma.[67] Whether alterations of other tumor suppressor genes play a role in lymphomagenesis is at present unknown.

Table 42–4 contains a list of recurring deletions, duplications, and isochromosomes in NHL. Virtually all chromosome arms have been recurrently deleted. However, loss of genetic

material from some chromosome regions has occurred more frequently than from others, and only a limited number of deletions have been found as the sole change (Table 42–2). Hence, the most likely sites of tumor suppressor genes that may be involved in lymphomagenesis are located on the following chromosome arms: 1p, 1q, 3p, 3q, 4p, 6p, 6q, 7q, 9q, 10q, 14q, and 16q. Among these, various 6q deletions are the most common in lymphomas of both B- and T-cell lineages. Gaidano et al.[28] have identified two distinct regions of minimal deletion at

Table 42–4. Recurrent Structural Aberrations Resulting in Loss or Gain of Genetic Material That Have Been Predominantly Found in Addition to Other Aberrations in NHL[a]

Aberration	No. of Cases	Aberration	No. of Cases
		Deletions	
del(X)(p11)	< 5	del(8)(q24)	11–15
del(X)(q24)	< 5	del(9)(p21–22)	16–20
del(X)(q26–27)	< 5	del(9)(p13)	15–20
del(1)(p31–36)	45–50	del(9)(p11–12)	10–15
del(1)(p22)	11–15	del(9)(q11–13-q21–34)	25–30
del(1)(p13)	16–20	del(9)(q22)	16–20
del(1)(q11–12)	11–15	del(9)(q32–33)	5–10
del(1)(q21)	5–10	del(10)(p13)	5–10
del(1)(q42)	5–10	del(10)(p11)	5–10
del(2)(p22–23)	5–10	del(10)(q22)	5–10
del(2)(p21)	5–10	del(10)(q23–24)	16–20
del(2)(p11–12)	< 5	del(11)(p13)	5–10
del(2)(q21–22)	5–10	del(11)(p11–12)	< 5
del(2)(q31–32)	5–10	del(11)(q14–23)	5–10
del(2)(q33)	5–10	del(11)(q21)	5–10
del(3)(p25)	5–10	del(11)(q23)	11–15
del(3)(p21)	16–20	del(12)(p11–12)	5–10
del(3)(q11–12)	5–10	del(12)(q12–13)	5–10
del(3)(q21–23)	11–15	del(12)(q22)	< 5
del(3)(q25)	< 5	del(12)(q24)	< 5
del(3)(q27)	< 5	del(13)(q12–14)	5–10
del(4)(p13–14)	11–15	del(13)(q14)	5–10
del(4)(q21–22)	5–10	del(13)(q14–22)	5–10
del(4)(q32–33)	< 5	del(13)(q22)	5–10
del(5)(p13)	5–10	del(13)(q31)	5–10
del(5)(q12–15)	< 5	del(15)(q22)	5–10
del(5)(q12–14-q31–32)	5–10	del(15)(q24)	< 5
del(5)(q31)	< 5	del(16)(p13)	< 5
del(6)(p21–23)	11–15	del(17)(p13)	< 5
del(6)(p11–12)	< 5	del(17)(p12)	< 5
del(7)(p15)	5–10	del(17)(p11)	11–15
del(7)(p13–14)	5–10	del(17)(q21)	< 5
del(7)(q22)	5–10	del(17)(q23)	5–10
del(7)(q22-q32–34)	5–10	del(18)(q21–22)	5–10
del(7)(q32)	16–20	del(19)(q13)	< 5
del(7)(q34–35)	5–10	del(20)(q11)	< 5
del(8)(p21)	5–10	del(22)(q11–12)	5–10
del(8)(q22)	< 5		
		Duplications	
dup(1)(p11–13-p32–36)	5–10	dup(7)(q11–22-q31–36)	15–20
dup(1)(q11–25-q31–44)	> 150	dup(12)(q11–15-q21–24)	50–100
dup(2)(p11–16-p21–25)	11–15	dup(13)(q12–21-q32–34)	< 5
dup(2)(q11–12-q14)	< 5	dup(14)(q24-q32)	5–10
dup(2)(q21–33-q36–37)	< 5	dup(14)(q32-q32)	< 5
dup(3)(q12–21-q23–29)	5–10	dup(17)(q21–22-q24–25)	< 5
dup(5)(q13–23-q31–35)	5–10	dup(18)(q12–21-q23)	< 5
		Isochromosomes	
i(X)(q10)	5–10	i(9)(p10)	< 5
i(Y)(q10)	< 5	i(11)(q10)	< 5
i(1)(p10)	< 5	i(12)(p10)	< 5
i(1)(q10)	46–50	i(12)(q10)	5–10
+ ider(2)(q10)inv(2)(p23q35)	< 5	i(13)(q10)	< 5
i(3)(p10)	< 5	i(15)(q10)	< 5
i(3)(q10)	< 5	i(17)(p10)	< 5
i(5)(p10)	< 5	i(18)(q10)	25–30
i(6)(p10)	> 50	i(21)(q10)	10–15
i(8)(q10)	11–15		

[a] See Table 42–3 for inclusion criteria and references.

6q25-27 and at 6q21-23 in B-cell NHL, and concluded that they most likely contain tumor suppressor genes. In a subsequent report, these investigators postulated the existence of a third tumor suppressor gene at 6q23, and also correlated sites of commonly deleted bands or regions with clinicopathologic subsets of NHL.[68] They suggested that deletions including band 6q23 are frequent in low-grade lymphomas without t(14;18), that deletions encompassing 6q25-27 occur preferentially in intermediate-grade lymphomas, and that a missing band 6q21 is associated with high-grade NHL.

The formation of an isochromosome brings about simultaneous loss and gain of genetic material. Occasionally, when an extra copy of an isochromosome is present in addition to a normal pair of homologous chromosomes gain of chromosome arms seems to be the main consequence. Isochromosomes are fairly common in NHL; they have been detected in 10 percent of karyotypically abnormal tumors.[69] Among recurrent isochromosomes (Tables 42–2 and 42–4), the following are the most frequent (listed in decreasing order of frequency): i(17)(q10), i(6)(p10), i(1)(q10), i(18)(q10), and i(7)(q10). Since the vast majority of i(17)(q10) and i(6)(p10) result in loss of the 17p and 6q arms, respectively, it seems that isochromosome creation represents one more way through which loss of

one allele of p53 and tumor suppressor genes located on 6q is achieved. On the other hand, in one-half of cases with i(18)(q10), there was either no net loss of 18p or more than one copy of i(18)(q10) was present, indicating that gain of 18q rather than loss of genetic material from 18p is consequential in these lymphomas. Overall, isochromosomes appear to be late, secondary changes in NHL development.[69]

Among other types of structural rearrangements that may be found in lymphoma karyotypes, unbalanced translocations leading to a net gain of genetic material apparently constitute a separate category. Thirty-seven of 50 such translocations presented in Table 42–5 involve an extra copy of the long arm of chromosome 1 with the breakpoints in or in the vicinity of the heterochromatic region of 1q. Translocation of 1q onto telomeric or pericentromeric regions of many different chromosomes leads invariably to partial trisomy of 1q. Functionally, such rearrangements are probably equivalent to duplications of 1q that are frequently observed in NHL (Table 42–4). The exact mechanism whereby gain of 1q contributes to lymphomagenesis has not yet been elucidated, but it appears that increased copy number of a gene or genes residing on 1q bestows a proliferative advantage to cells with an additional 1q. The unbalanced translocations and duplications of 1q are found in NHL of various histologies and line-

Table 42–5. Recurring Unbalanced Translocations That Have Been Predominantly Observed in Addition to Other Abnormalities in NHL[a]

Aberration	No. of Cases	Aberration	No. of Cases
Translocations leading to partial trisomy of 1q			
der(X)t(X;1)(p21–22;q11–21)	< 5	der(13)t(1;13)(q21;q32)	< 5
der(X)t(X;1)(p11;q23–25)	< 5	der(13)t(1;13)(q21–22;q34)	< 5
der(Y)t(Y;1)(q12;q21–25)	< 5	der(14)t(1;14)(q21–25;q32)	5–10
der(1)t(1;1)(p36;q12–21)	> 10	der(15)t(1;15)(q21;p13)	< 5
der(2)t(1;2)(q21;q37)	< 5	der(15)t(1;15)(q12–25;q22–24)	< 5
der(3)t(1;3)(q21–23;p26)	< 5	der(16)t(1;16)(q25;p13)	< 5
der(4)t(1;4)(q11–12;q34–35)	5–10	der(16)t(1;16)(q12–21;q24)	< 5
der(5)t(1;5)(q21;p15)	< 5	der(16)t(1;16)(q21–23;q11–13)	< 5
der(5)t(1;5)(q22–23;q13)	< 5	der(17)t(1;17)(q12–23;p11–13)	5–10
der(6)t(1;6)(q21;q13–14)	< 5	der(17)t(1;17)(q21;q25)	< 5
der(6)t(1;6)(q21;q23)	< 5	der(18)t(1;18)(q11–12;q23)	< 5
der(7)t(1;7)(q21;q32–36)	< 5	der(18)t(1;18)(q25–31;q23)	< 5
der(8)t(1;8)(q21;p11)	< 5	der(19)t(1;19)(q21–25;p13)	< 5
der(10)t(1;10)(q21–23;p15)	< 5	der(19)t(1;19)(q23–25;q13)	< 5
der(10)t(1;10)(q11–12;q26)	< 5	der(21)t(1;21)(q11;p11)	< 5
der(11)t(1;11)(q11–12;q25)	< 5	der(22)t(1;22)(q11–12;p11–13)	< 5
der(12)t(1;12)(q21–23;q24)	5–10	der(22)t(1;22)(q21;q13)	< 5
der(12)t(9;12)(q13;q24)	< 5	der(22)t(17;22)(q11;p11)	< 5
der(13)t(1;13)(q12–21;p13)	< 5		
Other unbalanced translocations			
der(1)t(1;2)(p34–36;q31)	< 5	der(18)t(14;18)(q32;q21)	> 10
der(1)t(1;6)(q21–23;p21)	< 5	der(19)t(14;19)(q11;p13)	< 5
der(1)t(1;9)(p36;q13)	5–10	der(19)t(12;19)(q15;q13)	< 5
der(10;15)(q10;q10)	< 5	der(19)t(17;19)(q11–12;p11)	< 5
der(11)t(7;11)(q11;q24–25)	< 5	der(19)t(17;19)(q12–21;q13)	< 5
der(12)t(12;17)(p12;q11)	< 5	der(22)t(17;22)(q11;p11)	< 5
der(14)t(12;14)(q13;q32)	< 5		

[a] See Table 42–3 for inclusion criteria and references.

ages, usually occur in addition to primary genetic changes, and in some cases have been present only in a sideline.[70] Moreover, similar rearrangements have been observed not only in NHL but also in a broad spectrum of human solid tumors and leukemia.[6,71] Therefore, they are probably best regarded as nonspecific secondary abnormalities that may contribute to tumor progression. Sawyer et al.[72] suggested that creation of the whole-arm 1q aberrations may be related to the decondensation of 1q pericentromeric heterochromatin due to hypomethylation of this region. Another abnormality of clearly secondary significance is der(18)t(14;18)(q32;21), sometimes unrecognized and described as del(18)(q21). It has been found almost exclusively in cases already carrying t(14;18)(q32;q21), constitutes the most frequent secondary aberration in patients with follicular lymphoma, and has been associated with disease progression in t(14;18)-positive lymphoma.[73–75]

The pathogenetic relevance of numerical chromosome changes in NHL, as well as in other types of neoplasia, is at present obscure. Most such changes are detected as part of complex karyotypes and seem to be secondary aberrations reflecting karyotypic instability characteristic of advanced lymphomas. Many numerical abnormalities presumably contribute to lymphoma progression since each of the most frequent trisomies in NHL (i.e., +2, +7, +12, and +18 [except +3]), have been associated in at least one study with poor prognosis (see Table 42–7). Occasionally, an extra copy of chromosome X; trisomy 2, 3, 5, 7, 8, 9, 11, 12, 14, 15, 18, 19, 20, 21, and 22; monosomy 7, 14, 17, and 22; or missing Y or X chromosomes have been observed as solitary aberrations in NHL (Table 42–2), and therefore regarded as primary tumor–associated abnormalities. Although there seems to be no doubt that most of the aforementioned anomalies are neoplasia related, the significance of isolated tri-

somy 7 and sex chromosome loss in tumorigenesis has been questioned.[30] Since both +7 and sex chromosome loss have been observed in normal brain and kidney, +7 also in tumor-infiltrating lymphocytes and normal lung, and –Y in the bone marrow of elderly men,[30] the finding of +7, –Y, or –X as the only aberration in the lymphoma specimen should be, in our view, interpreted with caution.

Morphologic Correlations

Several studies have attempted to correlate cytogenetic findings with histologic subtypes of NHL. Such correlations have been hampered by the existence of several concurrently used pathologic classification systems. Many associations have been reported, some of which have been well documented, whereas others, reported in single studies, await corroboration. Table 42–6 lists major abnormalities that have been associated with the selected disease categories.

Small Lymphocytic Lymphoma/Chronic Lymphocytic Leukemia

Nodal SLL and B-cell chronic lymphocytic leukemia (CLL) share identical morphologic and immunophenotypic features. Therefore, in the new WHO Classification of Lymphoid Neoplasms, SLL and CLL are recognized as one disease at different stages.[8] This view is supported by the results of cytogenetic analyses in SLL and CLL. Most major types of chromosome abnormalities representative of SLL have been repeatedly found in its leukemic counterpart. However, deletions and translocations involving band 13q14, which are the most frequent structural chromosome aberrations in CLL both in studies using conventional cytogenetic analysis[76,77] and interphase FISH

Table 42–6. Selected Recurring Cytogenetic Abnormalities Associated With Individual Disease Categories of NHL[a]

Histologic Group	Associated Abnormalities
B-cell chronic lymphocytic leukemia/small lymphocytic lymphoma (CLL/SLL)	+3, del(6q), del(11)(q14–23), +12, del(13q),[b] del(14)(q22–24), t(14;19)(q32;q13)
Small lymphocytic lymphoma, plasmacytoid	t(9;14)(p13;q32)
Extranodal marginal zone B-cell lymphoma	+3/3q, t(11;18)(q21;q21)
Splenic marginal zone B-cell lymphoma	t(2;7)(p11;q22), t(11;14)(q13;q32)
Follicular lymphoma	add/del(1)(p36), +1q, t(3;v)(q27;v),[c] del(6q), i(6)(p10), +7, +12/12q, t(14;18)(q32;q21), i(17)(q10), +der(18)t(14;18)(q32;q21), +18/18q, +X
Mantle cell lymphoma	+3q, del(6q), +8q, del(9q), t(11;14)(q13;q32), del(11q), –13/del(13q), +18q
Diffuse large cell lymphoma	i(1)(q10), t(2;3)(p12;q27), +3, t(3;14)(q27;q32), t(3;22)(q27;q11), t(3;v)(q27;v),[c] –4, –6, del(6q), i(6)(p10), +7, t(8;14)(q24;q32), t(8;22)(q24;q11), +11, +12, t(14;18)(q32;q21), t(14;v)(q32;v),[c] add(17)(p11–13), del(17)(p11), i(17)(q10), +18, –Y, +X, –X
Lymphoblastic lymphoma	t(8;13)(p11;q11–12), t(9;17)(q34;q23), t(9;22)(q34;q11), inv(14)(q11q32)
Burkitt lymphoma	t(8;14)(q24;q32), t(2;8)(p12;q24), t(8;22)(q24;q11), +1q, +7, +8, +12, +18, i(17)(q10)
Anaplastic large cell lymphoma, systemic type	t(2;5)(p23;q35), inv(2)(p23q35), +ider(2)(q10)inv(2)(p23q35)
Hepatosplenic gamma/delta T-cell lymphoma	i(7)(q10), +8, –Y

[a] See text for references.

[b] The most frequent deletion in CLL, rare in SLL.

[c] v denotes various chromosomes and various breakpoints participating in translocations with chromosome 3 at band q27 and chromosome 14 at band q32.

assays,[78,79] have very rarely been detected in patients with SLL analyzed by conventional cytogenetic analysis.[80]

The most prevalent numerical chromosome change in nodal SLL and CLL is trisomy 12, detected in approximately one-fifth of cases. In 40 percent of these tumors, +12 has been detected as a sole abnormality.[80] This phenomenon appears to be restricted to SLL histology, because only a small number of cases with trisomy 12 alone have been reported in other than SLL histologic subtypes of NHL.[6,80] The mechanism whereby trisomy 12 contributes to the pathogenesis of SLL and B-CLL is at present unknown. The discovery of structural aberrations leading to partial trisomies of chromosome 12 in rare CLL cases suggests that the gene or genes that might be rearranged at the submicroscopic level and subsequently duplicated by trisomy are localized in the region 12q13-21.2.[78] The significance of trisomy 12 as a primary abnormality in neoplastic disorders is further substantiated by its consistent occurrence as a sole abnormality not only in SLL and CLL but also in benign nonhematologic lesions, such as uterine leiomyoma and ovarian sex cord/stromal tumors.[30] It is thus possible that the gain of an additional copy of chromosome 12 may represent a general pathway through which uncontrolled, chronic proliferation of cells from different tissues may be achieved. It is hoped that future molecular genetic studies will identify the genes involved, and elucidate whether or not the same genes are implicated in the pathogenesis of SLL, B-CLL, and benign solid tumors with trisomy 12.

Lymphomas constituting a second cytogenetic group of SLL display interstitial or terminal deletions of 11q. These deletions have been detected using chromosome banding techniques in approximately 11 percent of karyotypically aberrant SLL,[80] and when not accompanied by other aberrations, seem to be highly specific for SLL histology.[81] In CLL, the frequency of del(11q) identified by interphase FISH is higher, 18 to 20 percent of all patients, which makes del(11q) the second most common structural aberration in CLL, following del(13q).[78,79] Although the breakpoints vary, in all but one case of SLL, all or part of band 11q22 has been lost, suggesting this as a likely site of a potential tumor suppressor gene. A molecular cytogenetic study of 40 B-CLL tumors has narrowed down the commonly deleted region to bands 11q22.3-11q23.1, which harbor, among others, the candidate tumor suppressor genes *RDX* and *ATM*.[78,82] Indeed, a deletion of one allele and a point mutation in the other allele of the latter gene has been detected in a subset of patients with CLL carrying del(11q), thus demonstrating the pathogenetic role of *ATM* gene inactivation in these patients.[83–85] It is at present unknown if the *ATM* is the only gene of pathogenetic significance inactivated by mutations and 11q deletions in CLL/SLL patients or if other genes with tumor suppressor properties also reside in the 11q22.3-11q23.1 region. It is noteworthy that in SLL/CLL patients with more than one chromosome aberration, very rarely have deletion 11q and trisomy 12 been seen together,[80] suggesting that these abnormalities represent alternative pathways in SLL/CLL tumorigenesis. Deletions of the 11q22.3-11q23.1 region, detected by FISH, have been shown to represent an independent adverse prognostic factor in CLL.[79]

Two other cytogenetic subgroups of SLL might be associated with the loss of as yet unidentified tumor suppressor genes. The first is characterized by deletions of 14q. Early observations of Levine et al.[22] linking breaks in 14q22-24 due to deletions or translocations with SLL histology have been verified by succeeding studies.[86–88] Kristoffersson et al.[87] described four new cases and reviewed an additional 43 published cases of NHL and other lymphoproliferative disorders with del(14)(q22-24). They confirmed that the deletions were significantly more frequent in SLL compared with tumors of other histologies (*p* < .001). Moreover, since SLL may undergo transformation to DLC or IBL (Richter's syndrome), and since all higher grade tumors with del(14)(q22-24) had one of these histologies, the authors suggested that at least some of these lymphomas with del(14q) might have originated from SLL. If true, this would make the association between del(14)(q22-24) and SLL even stronger.[87] As in the case of del(11q) and +12, solitary 14q deletions seem to be restricted to SLL histology.[80] In a few SLL cases, del(14q) has been observed together with trisomy 12.[86–88] Analysis of chromosome 14 breakpoints has indicated that the commonly deleted region contains part of band q24,[87] but a gene or genes affected by del(14q) has not yet been identified.

Another karyotypic subgroup of SLL defined by loss of genetic material as the major genetic change includes patients with deletion of 6q. Contrary to cytogenetic findings in most large series of NHL,[13–15,89,90] Offit et al.[91] reported an unusually high frequency (25 percent) of 6q abnormalities among 55 SLL cases. Three of their patients had the del(6q) as the only detectable abnormality. Since other SLL and CLL cases with a solitary del(6q) have been reported,[6,25] it appears that del(6q) may be an early and important rearrangement in a subset of SLL/CLL patients. The clinical course of SLL patients with del(6q) did not differ from that of patients with other low-grade diffuse NHL, even though del(6q) was associated with the presence of larger prolymphocytoid cells in the blood.[91]

Abnormalities of chromosome 17 in SLL/CLL involve predominantly its short arm and in almost all patients lead to loss of 17p material. These abnormalities include deletions of 17p, isochromosome of 17q, various unbalanced aberrations with known and unidentified partner chromosomes, and monosomy 17.[6,80,92] In most instances, aberrations of 17p and −17 were detected in addition to other chromosome abnormalities.[6,80,92] They have been detected by standard cytogenetics in 4 to 16 percent of evaluable cases and by FISH in 9 to 15 percent of patients, and are associated with *p53* gene loss and mutation.[57,78,92] CLL patients with deletions of 17p13/*p53* gene have more rapid disease progression and poor prognosis.[79,92]

Translocations involving band 14q32 are the most common chromosome aberrations in B-cell lymphomas regardless of their histology. Nevertheless, abnormalities of 14q32 have been detected in SLL at most half as often than in NHLs of other histologies[22]; they account for approximately one-third of cases classified as SLL.[80] However, this incidence may still be an overestimation because the most frequently reported reciprocal translocation involving 14q32 in SLL has been t(11;14)(q13;q32), seen in nearly 10 percent of such tumors.[80] This translocation, or its molecular equivalent, the *CCND1* gene rearrangement, appears to be highly characteristic of mantle cell lymphomas (MCL) (see below). It is thus possible that some cases with the t(11;14) reported to be SLL were in fact MCL. Likewise, CLL cases with t(11;14) usually have cells with atypical morphology and most likely represent the leukemic phase of MCL.[93,94] No patients with typical morphologic features and immunophenotype of B-CLL, included in three large series, were found to carry the t(11;14) and/or *CCND1* gene rearrangements.[79,95,96] On the other hand, the t(11;14) has been recurrently demonstrated in multiple myeloma,[97] low-grade splenic lymphoma with villous lymphocytes (SLVL),[98,99] a disease that might be misdiagnosed as hairy cell leukemia or CLL but does not resemble MCL, and also in B-cell prolymphocytic leukemia, a well-recognized entity that is separate from MCL.[100,101] Consequently, Brito-Babapulle et al.[100] have suggested that the presence of t(11;14) in morphologically and immunophenotypically distinct lymphomas and leukemias of mature B cells indicates that these diseases may be more closely related pathogenetically than expected.

Another recurrent 14q32 translocation, a t(9;14)(p13;q32), has been associated with SLL with plasmacytoid differentiation.[102] Five of nine cases with t(9;14)(p13;q32) included in the original report[102] were diagnosed as SLL of the plasmacytoid subtype at the time of cytogenetic analysis. Moreover, the same diagnosis was also documented on retrospective review of histologic slides from earlier lymph node biopsies in two further DLC cases with the t(9;14). At the molecular level, t(9;14) leads to deregulated expression of *PAX-5*, a gene that encodes a transcription factor involved in the control of B-cell proliferation and differentiation (BSAP, B-cell-specific activator protein), by its juxtaposition to the *IGH* gene.[39]

Other recurrent rearrangements of 14q32 in SLL and CLL include t(14;18)(q32;q21), t(14;19)(q32;q13), t(2;14)(p12-13;q32), and the presence of unidentified material at 14q32. However, translocations involving 14q32 are rare in patients diagnosed with classical SLL/CLL. In a recent series of 325 patients with CLL, FISH demonstrated such aberrations in only 12 patients (4 percent).[79]

Extranodal Marginal Zone B-Cell Lymphoma (MZBL) of Mucosa-Associated Lymphoid Tissue (MALT) Type

MZBL of MALT type is a low-grade lymphoma that has been nonrandomly associated with a reciprocal translocation t(11;18)(q21;q21). This translocation, described for the first time by Levine et al.[103] in two patients diagnosed with extranodal SLL, has been later detected in approximately 35 percent of MZBLs of MALT type karyotyped to date.[104,105] Most often the t(11;18) has been found in gastric tumors, but it was also detected in lymphomas arising in the large intestine, rectum, lung, thyroid, orbit, and lacrimal glands.[104,105] The pathogenetic importance of t(11;18) is underlined by its solitary occurrence in the abnormal clone in almost all patients analyzed to date.[6] The genes fused by t(11;18) have been identified as *API2* (also known as *BIRC3*) on chromosome 11 and *MALT1* (or *MLT*) on chromosome 18. The former belongs to the family of genes encoding inhibitors of programmed cell death (apoptosis). Although the mechanism of action of the *API2/MALT1* fusion is yet unknown, Dierlamm et al.[105] hypothesized that the protein product of the *API2/MALT1* fusion gene impedes apoptosis of cells carrying t(11;18) thereby conferring a survival advantage and promoting their antigen-independent proliferation. Thus far, the t(11;18) or *API2/MALT1* fusion has not been found in nodal or splenic MZBL[106,107] supporting the view that these entities are biologically different from MZBL of MALT and should be recognized as separate diseases, as they are in the WHO Classification.[8] Among other recurrent aberrations in MZBL of MALT, the most frequent has been trisomy of chromosome 3 or 3q, seen in up to 60 percent of karyotypically abnormal tumors in some series,[27,105,108] but with lower frequency in others.[104] Trisomy 3 is almost always accompanied by other aberrations. Although frequent in MZBL of MALT, trisomy 3 is not specific for this category of NHL.[6] Other recurring albeit less common chromosome changes include +7, +12, +18, t(1;14)(p22;q32), t(3;14)(q27;q32), and structural abnormalities of chromosome 1.[105]

Follicular Lymphomas

Follicular lymphomas were the second histologic group of NHL, after BL, to be associated with a consistent cytogenetic change. The t(14;18)(q32;q21), recognized for the first time in 1978 by Fukuhara and Rowley,[109] was associated with follicular histologies a year later,[110] and this association has been confirmed by numerous studies.[13–19,21–26,75] Using high-resolution chromosome banding techniques, Yunis et al.[13] sublocalized the translocation breakpoints to bands 14q32.3 and 18q21.3. In 1984, a putative oncogene named *BCL2* was cloned from the region 18q21.3,[111] and was shown to be activated through juxtaposition to *IGH* enhancers in a manner comparable to that for the *MYC* oncogene in the t(8;14).[31] Subsequent studies have indicated that *BCL2* represents a new class of oncogenes whose protein product represses apoptosis of B lymphocytes within lymph node follicular centers, as well as of progenitor and long-lived cells in other hematopoietic lineages and epithelium.[112] Consequently, the increased levels of BCL2 proteins result in prolonged survival of cells with the t(14;18).[112] The primary significance of the t(14;18) in lymphomagenesis is emphasized by its occurrence as the sole karyotypic abnormality in some patients, and by cytogenetic examinations of sequential lymph node biopsies. In all patients who had the t(14;18) at diagnosis and who underwent two or more successive biopsies, the translocation was always retained during the course of their disease.[74,113,114]

On the other hand, experiments performed on transgenic mice, and the finding of t(14;18) in hyperplastic human lymphoid tissue suggest that the deregulation of *BCL2* by itself may not be sufficient for malignant transformation. This conclusion is supported by the demonstration that rare *BCL2* rearrangements, identified with the use of a nested polymerase chain reaction (PCR) assay, may occur in people without lymphoid hyperplasia or lymphoma.[115] The frequency of t(14;18) in blood and spleens, which was highly variable among individuals, increased significantly with age, as does the incidence of NHL. However, the incidence of *BCL2* mutations in healthy humans was much higher than the lifetime risk for lymphoma development. Liu et al.[115] pointed out that although t(14;18)/*BCL2* mutation is a prerequisite for lymphoma, other steps, including antigenic stimulation that expands the t(14;18)-bearing clone and additional genomic mutations, appear to be required for a multistep model of lymphomagenesis.

The t(14;18) has been detected in lymphomas of all histologies.[6] Nevertheless, the frequency with which it occurs in different morphologic subtypes of NHL varies greatly. In large Western series, t(14;18) is seen in 45 percent[18] to 89 percent[17] of follicular lymphomas, with the highest incidence (on average 76 percent) among FSC, and the lowest (on average 53 percent) among FL.[116] In addition, this translocation is seen in about 20 percent of diffuse NHL; of interest, approximately one-half of these cases are known to have transformed from previous follicular histologies.[22,117] The distribution of cases with the t(14;18) as the only discernible chromosome change among histologic subgroups is nonrandom as well. Approximately 15 percent of FSC cases have a solitary t(14;18), compared to only 7 percent of FM, 3 percent of FL, and 0.3 percent of diffuse lymphomas.[81]

Several numerical and structural abnormalities have been recurrently found as secondary changes associated with t(14;18). These include trisomy of chromosomes X, 3, 5, 7, 8, 9, 12, 17, 18, 20, and 21; missing sex chromosomes; monosomy 15; deletions of 1p36, 6q, 10q22-24, 13q, and 15p; isochromosomes i(17)(q10) and i(18)(q10); an extra copy of der(18)t(14;18); duplication of 1q; and abnormalities of regions 1p36, 1p21-22, 1q21, 3q21-27, 7q32, 10q23-25, and Xp22.[6,14,15,19,21,43,73-75,117-122] Of these, trisomies of chromosomes 7, 12, and 17 or i(17)(q10) were found to be more common in intermediate and high-grade tumors than in low-grade lymphomas.[19,117-119] With regard to 6q deletions, Offit et al.[68] have suggested that in low-grade NHL with t(14;18), commonly deleted segments usually encompass 6q23 and 6q25-27, but not 6q21, deletion of which has been proposed to be specific for high-grade NHL, particularly of the IBL type. On the other hand, structural changes of chromosome 1 seem to be randomly distributed among histologic subsets.[19,119]

Geographic and racial differences in the frequency of t(14;18)-carrying lymphomas in the United States, Australia, and western Europe compared to Japan appear to exist.[25,43,123,124] The t(14;18) and BCL2 rearrangement are much less common in most,[123,124] but not all,[24] Japanese series comprising patients with all histologies, which could be in part explained by the fact that low-grade follicular lymphomas are infrequent in this region of the world. However, when only follicular NHLs are considered, the frequency of t(14;18)/BCL2 changes also is lower in most Japanese studies than in Western series.[25,43] Whether the absence of t(14;18) in a Russian series[89] reflects a genuine geographical diversity, or is related to the limited number of cases analyzed, awaits further study.

Although t(14;18) is present in the majority of follicular lymphomas, many tumors do not demonstrate this translocation.[81] A subset of lymphomas with a follicular growth pattern (1 FSC, 4 FM, and 1 FL) showing t(8;14)(q24;q32) but not t(14;18) or BCL2 gene rearrangements has been described.[125] The breakpoints in the t(8;14), studied both cytogenetically and at the molecular level, were located outside the commonly affected sites in the t(8;14) typical for BL. Based on these findings and the indolent clinical course of all of their cases, Ladanyi et al.[125] suggested that the t(8;14) in follicular NHL, when not accompanied by t(14;18), is distinct from t(8;14) seen in high-grade lymphomas.

Another cytogenetic subgroup includes follicular NHL (mostly FM and FL) displaying t(3;14)(q27;q32), t(3;6)(q27;p21),

and other structural abnormalities of 3q27-29 in the absence of the t(14;18). More than ten such cases have been reported to date.[6,20,60] Furthermore, in a similar number of patients, 3q27-29 changes have been observed together with the t(14;18) or its variants. However, translocations involving 3q27 and rearrangements of the BCL6 gene are much more common in diffuse NHL, particularly DLC (see below).

Smaller subsets of follicular tumors without t(14;18) that exhibit recurrent cytogenetic changes may be discerned. In a study of Bajalica et al.,[126] three cases of follicular lymphoma had the same der(1)t(1;2)(p36;q31), which in one case was the sole abnormality in a stemline. Likewise, three t(14;18)-negative cases of FSC with a duplication of 12q have been reported.[122,127] Interestingly, one of these tumors also had a t(11;13)(q13;q14) identical to the translocation detected in one case of FM with an additional del(12)(q13).[128]

Other follicular lymphomas display translocations between 14q32 and chromosome bands different than 18q21, 8q24, or 3q27. Translocations t(1;14)(p35-36;q32), t(1;14)(q21-25;q32), t(1;14)(q42;q32), t(8;14)(q22;q32), t(10;14)(q23-24;q32), t(11;14)(q13;q32), and t(11;14)(q23;q32) have been discovered in a few cases, and the bands 2q23, 3p21, 5q23, 8p23, 12q11, 15q22, 16q?13, 17q21, 19q13 have been found sporadically to be involved in exchanges with chromosome 14 at q32.[6] In approximately 4 percent of follicular NHL, the source of extra material in 14q+ markers has not been able to be determined by conventional cytogenetic analysis.[6] This may be due to the loss of a second partner in the reciprocal translocation, or to subsequent rearrangements of the derivative chromosomes preventing their accurate identification. Alternatively, some of these cases may represent variant translocations with potential involvement of more than two chromosomes and transposition of submicroscopic fragments of chromatin in a fashion similar to that shown in variant translocations of t(9;22) in CML.[30] In fact, molecular studies have detected rearrangements of the BCL2 gene in roughly one-half of follicular NHL with an unidentified 14q+ marker chromosome.[129] However, since it has been demonstrated that rearrangements and activation of the BCL2 gene do not occur in all follicular lymphomas,[130] karyotypic abnormalities without involvement of chromosome 18 presumably represent alternative but still not fully understood mechanisms of lymphomagenesis.

Mantle Cell Lymphoma

Mantle cell lymphoma (MCL) is associated with the presence of a characteristic cytogenetic abnormality—the t(11;14)(q13;q32). This translocation, initially described in the late 1970s,[131,132] was later reported in a wide range of B-cell lymphoid malignancies including SLL/CLL, SLVL, follicular lymphomas, DSC, DM, SNC, and acute prolymphocytic leukemia, in most instances with rather low frequency. Following the description of t(11;14)(q13;q32) in 3 of 12 MCL cases by Weisenburger et al.[133] in 1987, several groups examined the distribution of the t(11;14) among histologic subtypes in large series of NHL. In a series of 163 karyotypically abnormal lymphomas of various histologies, Leroux et al.[134] identified 13 tumors with this rearrangement, 12 of which, after reexamination of histologic slides, fulfilled the diagnostic criteria for MCL. This diagnosis was made in three of four tumors with the t(11;14) included in a large Japanese study,[124] and the t(11;14) was present in 8 of 12 leukemic MCL[135] as well as in all nine MCL lymphomas described by Vandenberghe et al.[136] Notably, all tumors reported in the latter study and one half of the MCL cases analyzed by Leroux et al.[134] had been initially diagnosed as DSC. MCL may imitate other lymphoma subtypes, and most such tumors have been originally classified as DSC.[137] It is thus possible that many DSC with the t(11;14) reported prior to recognition of MCL as a separate entity, may have been cases of MCL. Of interest, the t(11;14) has never been observed together with the t(14;18), nor has the latter translocation been found in any t(11;14)-positive MCL case to date.[6] Therefore the finding of one of these translocations, or their molecular counterparts, may be useful in differential diagnosis, particularly between cases of MCL with a vaguely nodular growth pattern and FSC.

Molecular studies have shown that the oncogene that is deregulated and overexpressed as a result of the t(11;14) and its variants is identical to the *CCND1* (also known as *PRAD1*) gene. This gene is closely linked to the *BCL1* breakpoint locus, and its protein product is involved in cell cycle regulation.[138,139] Elevated levels of *CCND1* mRNA were found in all 7 MCL studied by Rosenberg et al.[138] and in 14 of 15 cases analyzed by Rimokh et al.[140] even though only 3 cases in the former and 10 lymphomas in the latter study had rearrangements of *CCND1* DNA. Overexpression of cyclin D1 or a *CCND1* gene rearrangement also has been demonstrated in MCL cases with two variant translocations, t(11;22)(q13;q11)[141] and t(8;11)(p21;q13),[128] respectively.

The availability of genomic probes detecting *CCND1* rearrangements at the DNA level has made feasible studies of larger numbers of MCL cases that were not characterized cytogenetically. Rearrangements of the *CCND1* locus have been found in 51 of 89 cases (57 percent) studied by five research groups.[140,142–145] Because only two groups[140,145] used probes capable of detecting both major and minor translocation cluster regions, it is likely that the true incidence of *CCND1* rearrangements is higher and closer to the 73 percent reported by Williams et al.[145]

The t(11;14) has only rarely been detected as the sole chromosome abnormality. Secondary chromosome aberrations have been found in over 90 percent of t(11;14)-positive MCL cases, both in series of patients studied using standard karyotyping[146] and CGH and FISH.[147] The pattern of secondary aberrations varied from the presence of a single additional aberration to very complex karyotypes with more than ten aberrations.[6,146] In the standard cytogenetic study, recurrent losses of chromosome material were more frequent than gains and included, in decreasing order of frequency, monosomy 13 (seen in 30 percent of patients), deletions of 6q, 9q, 11q (each detected in about 20 percent), and losses of chromosome 8/8p, 10/10p, 14, 1/1p, and Y (each found in less than 15 percent of patients).[146] The only recurrent gain, detected in 15 percent of patients, was that of chromosome 3 material, with the commonly overrepresented region 3q25→qter. Studies using CGH and FISH have in general detected a similar distribution of

chromosome imbalances although the incidence of some of the observed aberrations was higher. Loss of chromosome 13 was found in 44 to 69 percent of patients, gain of 3q in 48 to 49 percent, and loss of 11q in 22 to 30 percent of patients. CGH and FISH studies also identified recurrent gains of chromosome regions not detected by standard cytogenetics, namely gain of 8q, 7p, 12q, 18q, and 9q34 occurring in 16 to 28 percent of MCL patients.[147,148] Beà et al.[148] detected a significantly higher incidence of chromosome gains, losses, and DNA amplifications, and, specifically, gains of 3q, 7p, and 12q and losses of 17p (which correlated with *p53* gene deletions and mutations) in blastoid variants of MCL. These variants have a higher proliferative activity and a more aggressive biological behavior than the typical variants of the tumor.[148] In the outcome analysis, MCL patients with more than 4 chromosome gains, gains of 12q and 3q and losses of 9p had significantly shortened survival.[148] Complex karyotype [i.e., ≥3 aberrations in addition to t(11;14)] and a total or partial trisomy 12 were the only cytogenetic parameters predictive of a poor prognosis in another study.[149]

Diffuse Large Cell Lymphomas

An important development in the genetics of NHL has been the identification of a novel oncogene, *BCL6* (named also *LAZ3*[32] and, in one study,[34] *BCL5*). As in the case of other oncogenes involved in lymphomagenesis, the discovery of *BCL6* stems from preceding cytogenetic studies. Structural abnormalities of the distal part of 3q had been observed sporadically in NHL during the 1970s, but it was not until 1983 that Kaneko et al.[150] associated 3q abnormalities with DLC histology. In their series of 30 tumors with abnormal karyotypes, 7 cases displayed 3q27-29 rearrangements, including a t(3;6)(q29;q15) and 6 translocations of a segment of unknown origin onto the terminal region of 3q. Six of these patients had DLC, and the remaining one a composite lymphoma with follicular and diffuse small cleaved cell components. Thereafter, many other cases with structural aberrations of chromosome 3, including two DLC with the t(3;14)(q27;q32)[15] and a case with t(3;22)(q29;q11),[151] were reported. In 1989, Offit et al.[152] and Leroux et al.[153] described the t(3;22)(q27-28;q11) in a total of 11 lymphomas, mostly of DLC type. Later, Bastard et al.[20] reported 3 further cases of t(3;22)(q27;q11) in addition to 15 cases of t(3;14)(q27;q32), and 2 cases of t(2;3)(p12;q27); a t(3;14) and a t(2;3) were the sole anomalies in one patient each. Because these translocations consistently involved bands 14q32, 22q11, and 2p12 the investigators suggested that the band 3q27 was a site of a novel oncogene that might be activated by juxtaposition with the immunoglobulin genes.[19] Indeed, a novel zinc-finger encoding gene *BCL6* sharing amino-terminal homology with several transcription factors has been isolated from the 3q27 breakpoint.[32–34] Of interest, rearrangements of *BCL6* have been detected not only in NHL with t(3;14), t(3;22), or t(2;3) but also in cases with translocations between 3q27 and chromosomes 1, 4, 5, 6, 7, 8, 11, 12, 13, 15, and 16.[6,33,49–52,154,155]

The overall frequency of 3q27 alterations has been estimated to be between 8 and 16 percent of all NHL cases based on karyotype analysis alone.[33,154] However, this incidence appears to be an underestimate, since the t(3;14)(q27;q32) is quite subtle and can be misinterpreted as a del(3)(q27) or a translocation of unknown material onto 14q32.[20] Moreover, *BCL6* gene rearrangements have been detected in patients without evident cytogenetic involvement of 3q27.[154] Molecular analyses of the *BCL6* rearrangement in large series of NHL revealed alterations of the gene in 18 of 125 NHL (14 percent),[156] 25 of 170 tumors (15 percent),[157] and 43 of 217 samples (20 percent).[154] These figures too may not reflect the total number of affected cases because rearrangements of the *BCL6* gene could not be detected in one-fourth to one-third of lymphomas with cytogenetic changes of 3q27.[33,154] This may indicate the presence of another, as yet not identified, oncogene adjacent to *BCL6* or, more likely, may be due to the existence of additional breakpoint cluster regions that are not detectable by the currently used probes.

The histologic distribution of lymphomas with 3q27 cytogenetic changes is nonrandom. Our review of more than 100 published cases with microscopically detectable rearrangements of 3q27-29 revealed that over 70 percent of these tumors had a diffuse growth pattern, and more than one-half of all cases were diagnosed as DLC.[116] Among follicular lymphomas, 3q27 abnormalities were found mainly in tumors with a large cell component (FM and FL).[116] Molecular studies also show that *BCL6* gene rearrangements are most frequent in, albeit not limited to, aggressive diffuse lymphoma (DLC, DM, and IBL). The rearrangements have been detected in 15 to 45 percent of all DLC analyzed.[154,156–161] Among NHLs associated with acquired immunodeficiency syndrome (AIDS), alterations of *BCL6* occurred in 20 percent of DLC but in no case of SNC.[162]

Approximately one-fourth of DLC in large Western series have had the t(14;18) in their karyotype.[13–15,17–19,22,163] A proportion of these tumors have evolved from a preceding follicular histology, but the t(14;18) or its molecular equivalent, the *BCL2* rearrangement, has also been demonstrated in de novo diffuse NHL with a large cell component.[164] Virtually all t(14;18)-positive diffuse NHLs display additional aberrations in the karyotype.[6,163] Lukeis et al.[165] reported an association between aberrations of chromosome 11 and diffuse (DLC and DM) histology in t(14;18)-bearing lymphomas. In their series, trisomy 11 or structural changes of this chromosome occurred in 58 percent of diffuse compared to 7 percent of follicular NHL with t(14;18). Whether the pattern of secondary aberrations in approximately 10 percent of all DLC and IBL with another primary abnormality, t(8;14)(q24;q32), differs from that in BL with the same translocation has not been examined.

Offit et al.[166] suggested that there are two cytogenetic subgroups of diffuse lymphomas with a large-cell component that involve 9q. One consists of mainly interstitial deletions of 9q with the commonly lost region being 9q31-32. The second comprises translocations involving bands 9q11 and 9q13.[166] Additionally, deletions of 12p and 16q have been seen mainly in DLC and IBL.[80,167] In a large cytogenetic study comprising 248 successfully karyotyped DLC tumors, Cigudosa et al.[163] identified 11 sites as regions of common cytogenetic deletions in DLC: 1p36, 1p33-34, 1p31, 1q32, 3p25-26, 3p21, 3q21, 6q15, 6q21, 6q23-24, and 7q32. They suggested that loss of candidate tumor suppressor genes from these loci is associated with DLC development. Another study from the same research group identified, using CGH, nine sites of chromosomal amplification: 1q21-23, 2p12-16, 8q24, 9q34, 12q12-14, 13q32, 16p12, and 18q21-22.[168] Subsequently, the authors used quantitative Southern blotting analysis to evaluate copy number of the following genes: *REL* (mapped to 2p12-16), *MYC* (8q24), *BCL2* (18q21), and *GLI*, *CDK4*, and *MDM2* (all mapped to 12q13-14). They demonstrated a fourfold or greater amplification of each of the genes tested, with incidence ranging from 11 (*CDK4*) to 23 percent (*REL*). Of note, tumors with amplification of *REL*, *MYC*, and *BCL2* did not display translocations affecting loci harboring these genes thus suggesting that their amplification and deregulation by chromosomal rearrangement represent independent pathways in DLC lymphomagenesis.[168]

Immunoblastic lymphoma has been recognized as a high-grade tumor separate from DLC in both the Working Formulation[9] and the Kiel classification,[10] but in the R.E.A.L. classification it has been grouped with other subtypes to create a diffuse large B-cell lymphoma category.[169] However, both the clinical outcome data and cytogenetic profiles support the view that IBL represents an entity biologically distinct from DLC. In a study of Schlegelberger et al.[169] cytogenetic differences between immunoblastic and centroblastic lymphomas included a significantly lower frequency of t(14;18) in the former (4 vs. 30 percent, $p = .006$) and significantly higher frequencies of monosomy 10 ($p = .01$), del(8q) ($p = .017$), del(14q) ($p = .009$), and structural abnormalities of 4q ($p = .049$) in IBL. Patients with IBL had in this study a significantly shorter overall survival than those with centroblastic lymphoma (median 16.3 vs. 68.9 months, $p = .004$).

Burkitt Lymphoma

Burkitt lymphoma (BL) is an aggressive disease primarily affecting young children and presenting in extranodal sites.[170] Two forms of BL, endemic and nonendemic, have been identified. The former occurs in equatorial Africa and is almost always associated with Epstein-Barr virus (EBV) infections. In the latter form, the presence of EBV has been detected in only 20 to 30 percent of cases in the United States.[170] Nonetheless, both forms exhibit a very high incidence of *MYC* gene rearrangements caused by the t(8;14)(q24;q32), or its variants, which are regarded as primary, initiating genetic changes in BL tumorigenesis. It has been shown that the breakpoints in the t(8;14) and variant translocations are different in endemic and nonendemic BLs at the molecular level,[31,170] but these translocations cannot be distinguished cytogenetically.

Historically, the 14q+ marker was first seen consistently in both cell lines and BL biopsies by Manolov and Manolova;[4] the nature of the rearrangement was elucidated by Zech et al.[5] in 1976 when they determined that additional material on 14q originated from the long arm of chromosome 8. These investigators also described a case with t(8;22); 3 years later this was shown to be one of the variant translocations in BL.[171] The other variant translocation, the t(2;8), was concurrently described by Van Den Berghe et al.[172] and Miyoshi et al.[173] Subsequent high-resolution cytogenetic studies assigned the breakpoints in the t(8;14) to 8q24.1 and 14q32.3.[13]

Despite their relative infrequency, BL and its leukemic counterpart, ALL L3, have been extensively studied cytogenetically. Karyotypes of more than 200 cases have been reported. Kornblau et al.[174] presented 22 of their own cases, and reviewed 148 patients with nonendemic BL or ALL L3. Only 6 patients had a normal karyotype (4 percent), 62 percent displayed the t(8;14)(q24;q32), 12 percent had t(8;22)(q24;q11), 9 percent had the t(2;8)(p12;q24), and 14 percent had aberrant karyotypes without any of the classic translocations. A few patients in this last group had 14q+ markers, which may have involved rearrangements of *MYC*.[129] Interestingly, patients with AIDS had one of the classic translocations more frequently (91 vs. 81 percent of other cases); the incidence of t(8;22) was significantly higher in patients with AIDS.[174] In approximately 30 percent of BL cases, the only chromosomal abnormality has been one of the classic translocations.[80] The most frequent secondary aberrations have been duplications of 1q; trisomies of chromosomes 7, 8, 12, and 18, i(17)(q10); and structural anomalies affecting chromosome 17, with breakpoints predominantly localized in 17p.[80,174]

The Non-Burkitt (Burkitt-Like) Small Noncleaved Cell Lymphoma (SNC)

The Burkitt-like SNC has been less extensively investigated cytogenetically than BL. In a number of cases, t(14;18) or *BCL2* rearrangements have been found.[25,164,175–177] The t(8;14) or 8q24 abnormalities have been detected,[13,25,176,177] but their frequency is lower than that in BL. Moreover, in the largest study to date, t(8;14) was found in only one-half of patients with 8q24 aberrations; the other half had variant translocations.[177] Coexistence of abnormalities of 8q24 with t(14;18) was in this study relatively frequent, being seen in 13 of 39 patients, who had a rapid clinical course and extremely poor prognosis.[177] Molecular studies also demonstrated differences between Burkitt-like SNC and BL.[178,179] Among 18 BLs, 17 (94 percent) contained *MYC* rearrangements in Southern blot analysis, while none of 11 non-Burkitt SNC tumors did. In 3 of 10 evaluable non-Burkitt SNC, *BCL2* changes were found compared to none in the BLs studied.[178] Among AIDS-related SNC, all 10 patients with BL studied had alterations of the *MYC* gene, whereas only 2 of the 10 patients with Burkitt-like SNC had *MYC* rearrangements.[179] The lower rate of detection of the *MYC* gene rearrangements in the aforementioned studies may have been related to the high frequency of variant translocations in Burkitt-like SNC that are undetectable by Southern blot analysis.[177] Nevertheless, both cytogenetic and molecular data suggest that BL and Burkitt-like SNC are distinct entities not only morphologically and to some extent clinically, but also with regard to pathogenetic mechanisms.[176–179]

Lymphoblastic Lymphoma

Lymphoblastic lymphoma (LBL) is morphologically distinct from other NHL subtypes. Although precursor B-cell phenotypes have been described, most cases have an immature T-cell phenotype. Cytogenetically, T-cell LBL bears similarity to T-ALL. A normal karyotype is found in a substantial proportion of tumors, a phenomenon also noted in ALL. The largest subgroup of cytogenetically aberrant LBLs comprises tumors with various translocations involving 14q11, 7p15, and 7q35, bands known to harbor, respectively, the alpha and delta, gamma, and beta chain genes of the TCR.[30] Two translocations, t(11;14)(p13;q11) and t(7;14)(p15;q32), which have been observed recurrently in LBL[180] have also been detected in T-ALL.[6,181] Similarly, several translocations recurrently found in ALL [i.e., t(1;14)(p34;q11), t(7;11)(q35;p13-14), and t(10;14)(q24;q11)] have been reported in single cases of LBL.[6,181] A few LBLs have had deletions of 9p.[182] Deletions of 6q have also been noted in LBL. Both of these abnormalities are commonly seen in ALL of T and B lineage, as well as in other types of NHL.[6] Additionally, a subset of T-cell LBL with 9q34 rearrangements may exist.[166] However, the involvement of 9q34 also has been reported in NHL of other histologies.[6]

Some LBLs do not share common karyotypic features with T-ALL. Among such cases are six Japanese children with a t(9;17)(q34;q23) who had rapidly progressive disease and fatal outcome,[180,183] as well as two cases of childhood LBL with t(1;14)(p36;q22).[14,184] Another nonrandom, highly specific aberration, t(8;13)(p11;q11-12), has been found in patients with a unique multilineage hematologic disorder in which T-cell LBL is associated with eosinophilia and myeloid hyperplasia evolving to acute myeloid leukemia (AML).[185,186] Finally, the inv(14)(q11q32), repeatedly observed in T-cell chronic lymphoproliferative disorders and T-CLL but rarely in T-ALL, has been detected in a few LBL cases.[6]

Peripheral T-Cell Lymphomas

Peripheral T-cell lymphomas are heterogeneous and consist of several clinicopathological entities, including lymphomas of low- and high-grade types. Compared with B-cell lymphomas, cytogenetic studies have been much less extensive. A relatively common cytogenetic feature in T-cell NHL is the presence of unrelated clones or cells with nonclonal aberrations. They are particularly common in angioimmunoblastic lymphadenopathy with dysproteinemia.[187,188] Some tumors display translocations disrupting TCR genes, but in general such rearrangements are observed more frequently in T-ALL than in T-cell NHL.[187–189] Other aberrations frequent in T-cell lymphomas include trisomy of chromosomes 3, 5, 7 or 7q, 19, 21 and X; monosomy of chromosomes 10 and 13; loss of chromosome Y; and structural rearrangements of the following chromosome arms or regions: 1p, 1p36, 1q, 1q21, 2p11-14, 2p23-25, 2q21, 3q27, 3q, 4q21, 6p21-23, 6q, 7q, 9p21-23, 9q, 10p13-15, 13q, 14q32, 17q10, and 17q21.[123,124,187–190]

According to Schlegelberger et al.,[188] certain abnormalities such as +7/extra 7q, del(6q), −13, or deletions/translocations involving 13q14 are significantly more frequent in high-grade than in low-grade peripheral T-cell lymphomas. Among T-cell NHL classified as DLC, two translocations have been observed repeatedly and therefore may represent primary changes in subsets of these lymphomas. The t(21;22)(q22;q11) was present as the only reciprocal translocation in addition to several unbalanced rearrangements in two cases.[123,191] In another two patients, the t(6;7)(p23;q32) was found and in one of them this was the sole abnormality.[123,191]

Another nonrandom chromosome aberration of primary significance is an i(7)(q10) in hepatosplenic gamma/delta T-cell lymphoma. Although not specific for this rare and very aggressive type of T-cell lymphoma, i(7)(q10) has been detected in over 80 percent of tumors karyotyped and in three cases it was the only chromosome aberration present. Among tumors with more than one aberration, trisomy 8 and −Y were consistently found.[6,189,192,193]

Anaplastic Large Cell Lymphoma

Anaplastic large cell lymphoma (ALCL) represents a morphologically, immunologically, and clinically distinct subset characterized by a strong expression of the cytokine receptor CD30 (Ki-1) and a characteristic growth pattern.[194] Cytogenetic studies indicate that ALCL is strongly correlated with a specific translocation—t(2;5)(p23;q35). Originally, this translocation, or its variants t(1;5)(p32;q35) and t(5;6)(q35;p12), were described in patients diagnosed as malignant histiocytosis.[195–197] However, after the t(2;5) was associated with CD30-positive lymphoma,[198–200] Mason et al.[201] reexamined the morphology of eight of these cases and performed immunophenotypic studies of CD30, CD3, and CD68 antigens. They showed unequivocally that all reexamined tumors with the t(2;5), initially diagnosed as malignant histiocytosis, were of lymphoid origin and displayed typical features of ALCL. To date, more than 70 cases with the t(2;5) or its variants have been reported,[6] and most of them have had similar immunologic, histologic, and clinical features. Hence, the specificity of the t(2;5) appears to be the highest among NHL.

The finding of the t(2;5) in biopsy specimens, together with immunophenotypic and clinical characteristics, was essential in delineating a small-cell-predominant variant of Ki-1-positive lymphoma. All four predominantly small-cell Ki-1-positive lymphomas that were karyotyped in a study of nine such cases had the t(2;5)(p23;q35).[202]

The molecular consequences of the t(2;5) have been elucidated. By using chromosome walking techniques, Morris et al.[41] cloned the genes involved in this translocation: a previously unidentified protein tyrosine kinase gene, designated *ALK* (anaplastic lymphoma kinase), located at 2p23, and the nuclear phosphoprotein gene *(NPM)* residing at 5q35. The *ALK* gene is not expressed in human normal lymphoid cells. The t(2;5) results in the permanent and ubiquitous transcription of the *NPM-ALK* hybrid gene encoding a chimeric protein, which has been shown to induce transplantable lymphoid tumors in mice.[194,203] Several variant aberrations fusing the *ALK* gene with other partners have been identified. These include t(1;2)(q25;p23) and *TPM3-ALK*, inv(2)(p23q35) and *ATIC-ALK*, t(2;3)(p23;q21) and *TGF-ALK*, t(2;17)(p23;q23) and *CLTC-ALK*, and t(2;19)(p23;p13.1) and *TPM4-ALK*.[204] These variants account for 15 to 28 percent of ALK-positive ALCLs.

Despite a very strong correlation between the t(2;5) and ALCL, not all ALCLs have this translocation or its variants and are ALK positive; ALK-negative tumors constitute about 45 percent of ALCLs, and are more frequently encountered in older patients. Almost all clinical studies have reported a much better prognosis for patients with ALK-positive tumors compared with those with ALK-negative ALCL (reviewed by Morris et al.[204] and Stein et al.[194]).

Genetic Basis of Tumor Progression in NHL

Tumor progression has been defined as a stepwise acquisition of new phenotypic properties by cancer cells leading to more aggressive biologic and clinical behavior over time. Growing evidence suggests that accumulation of nonrandom, secondary chromosome aberrations may contribute to this process.[30,205]

Analyses of the natural history of NHL have indicated that indolent lymphomas ultimately undergo transformation to an intermediate- or high-grade histology in 40 to 70 percent of patients at 8 to 10 years after diagnosis.[206] In some patients, clinical progression may occur without changes in tumor morphology. Several groups have attempted to determine which chromosome aberrations could be responsible for the accelerated course of the disease. Yunis et al.[118] proposed a model for the evolution of follicular NHL with t(14;18). They suggested that progression from FSC to higher-grade NHL was associated with acquisition of del(6q), +7 or dup(7p), or +12 or dup(12q). Subsequent studies have confirmed that intermediate- and high-grade NHL with t(14;18) have significantly higher frequencies of trisomy 7,[19,75,117,119,207,208] trisomy 12,[19] and del(6q) or monosomy 6[75,117] compared with indolent lymphomas. Deletions involving bands 6q23-26 present at diagnosis have been significantly associated with a higher risk of transformation to DLC.[209] Additionally, when cytogenetic results obtained within 1 month after diagnosis were compared with those obtained later in the disease, trisomy 7 and +der(18)t(14;18) were the most common aberrations associated with late disease.[74]

Decisive evidence that histologic transformation can actually be brought about by the above-mentioned abnormalities could be provided only by cytogenetic analyses of two or more sequential biopsies. Successful serial studies have been performed in about 90 patients with various types of NHL, and morphologic transformation has been observed in less than one-half of them.[16,19,74,113,114,118,119,150,175] Indeed, in six cases with t(14;18), an extra copy or two copies of chromosome 7, not present in the initial biopsy, have been found in transformed lymphoma albeit usually together with other changes like +12 (in four cases), +der(18)t(14;18) or +18 (in two cases each).[113,114,119,175] Moreover, a minor clone with +7 present at diagnosis in a patient with FSC became predominant after 25 months and a transformation to FM histology.[118] However, since most transformed tumors do not exhibit trisomy 7, the acquisition of this chromosome, although important in a subset of t(14;18)-positive tumors, does not appear to represent the major cytogenetic route of NHL progression.

Another mechanism of tumor progression of t(14;18)-positive follicular NHL has been demonstrated in rare tumors that also have the t(8;14).[31,177,210–213] Secondary dysregulation of *MYC* in such lymphomas appears to have led to histologic transformation and rapid progression to high-grade disease with extremely poor clinical outcome.[177] This scenario, however, is not a frequent one, as shown by Yano et al.[213] who detected *MYC* rearrangements in only 3 of 38 (8 percent) histologically transformed cases. Interestingly, the sequence of events was apparently reversed in one case of SNC, that is, t(18;22) occurred in a clone already bearing t(8;14).[212] This case supports the view that sometimes it is not the sequential order of genetic events but their cumulative effect that is critical in tumor evolution.[30]

Two studies suggest that mutations of the *p53* gene are associated with transformation of a significant proportion of follicular lymphomas to higher grade NHL.[58,59] Previous cytogenetic findings in large cell lymphoma[13,14,22,214] and in serial biopsies of transformed lymphomas[114] had suggested that loss and rearrangements of *p53* may be implicated in clonal evolution of some NHL. Monosomy 17 or structural aberrations of 17p have been consistently observed in 30 to 45 percent of large cell NHL.[13,14,22,214] Similar aberrations were acquired in three of seven sequentially studied follicular lymphomas that underwent histologic transformation.[114] Moreover, allelic losses of the *p53* gene by Southern blot analysis were reported in three of eight cell lines and large cell lymphoma samples with cytogenetic abnormalities of 17p.[215] Further molecular genetic studies have revealed mutations of the *p53* gene or overexpression of p53 protein in 5 of 6,[59] and in 10 of 34[58] aggressive NHLs that transformed from preceding follicular histologies.

Sander et al.[58] have estimated that mutations of *p53* are associated with histologic transformation in approximately 25 to 30 percent of follicular lymphomas. *p53* mutations were observed in 3 of 25 patients with low-grade follicular lymphomas. Two of these patients subsequently developed transformed lymphomas; the third achieved a long-lasting remission after treatment on an intensive chemotherapy regimen.[58] These and other data[59,209] suggest that the finding of a *p53* mutation or break at 17p in indolent lymphoma indicates an increased risk for progression and may justify more aggressive therapy. In some aggressive tumors without alterations of *p53*, an overexpression of MDM2, an oncoprotein involved in the regulation of p53, was detected and associated with poor clinical outcome.[216]

Mutations in the *p53* gene disturb cell cycle control and increase the rate of genetic alterations.[217] Therefore, a model for a *p53*-dependent progression pathway in follicular lymphoma has been proposed, in which histologic transformation is not caused directly by *p53* mutations. Instead, changes in the tumor phenotype are postulated to be associated with other genetic rearrangements that accumulate in cells defective in *p53*.[58] The nature of such transforming mutations is unknown. Recent sequential molecular analysis suggests that point mutations of the 5′ noncoding region of the *BCL6* gene might contribute to histologic progression in some cases. Two of five patients with B-cell DLC transformed from a previous follicular phase displayed *BCL6* mutations in the transformed, but not in the follicular phase; one patient had identical *BCL6* mutations in both phases of the disease.[158] On the other hand, the absence of *MYC* gene rearrangements in *p53*-positive transformed lymphomas[58,59] indicates that these two events are probably independent in lymphoma progression. Given the complexity of karyotypes and the heterogeneity of chromosome changes encountered in advanced lymphomas, it is unlikely that a single genetic rearrangement will be found that is responsible for progression in *p53*-positive or the twice as frequent *p53*-negative lymphomas.

The number of serially analyzed patients with nonfollicular NHL is smaller than that of patients with follicular lymphoma. Of 11 informative SLL cases, 5 did not exhibit any cytogenetic change over time, even though one of these patients progressed to DLC.[74,113,114] In three other patients (two with histologic transformation), a karyotype unrelated to initial cytogenetic findings was later found, and in three remaining cases (two with histologic transformation), signs of karyotypic evolution were evident in a follow-up sample. The acquired abnormalities, however, were different in each case.[74,114] So few NHLs of other histologies have been studied sequentially that no conclusions can be drawn.

Prognostic Significance of Chromosome Aberrations in NHL

The prognostic relevance of chromosome aberrations in the acute leukemias is well established.[30,181,218,219] More limited data are available in NHL. Although correlations between particular cytogenetic features of NHL and clinical outcome have been reported (Table 42–7), many of these relationships have been detected in small groups of patients, and associations significant in one series have frequently not been significant in others. Furthermore, many studies have included lymphomas of multiple histologic subtypes, as well as patients studied at diagnosis and at relapse, and the therapy administered to patients was in most studies very heterogeneous.

Studies of the prognostic importance of karyotypes detected exclusively in untreated NHL patients include those by Levine et al.,[220] Offit et al.,[221] Pirc-Danoewinata et al.,[23] Tilly et al.,[209] Schlegelberger et al.,[169], Juneja et al.,[223] and Jerkeman et al.[224] Levine et al.[220] found the presence of normal metaphases in tumor material to be predictive of an increased rate of complete remission (CR) and longer survival. Among 30 patients with follicular lymphoma, the CR rate was higher and the survival significantly longer in patients with more than 20 percent of cytogenetically normal cells in tumor material.[220] Similarly, in a larger group of 66 karyotypically abnormal cases with follicular NHL, the survival of patients who had 90 percent or more abnormal metaphases was significantly shorter compared with those who had a higher proportion of normal cells.[209] Both a Swedish study comprising low- and high-grade lymphomas,[225] and a smaller Polish study[226] found prolonged survival of patients without any cytogenetically abnormal clone, but not of those with normal metaphase cells present in addition to abnormal ones. Additionally, patients with angioimmunoblastic lymphadenopathy (AILD)-type T-cell lymphoma who did not have any aberrant metaphase in unstimulated cultures had a significantly higher CR rate and prolonged survival compared with those whose samples contained clonal and/or nonclonal chromosome aberrations.[222] However, others have not found any difference in survival duration among patients with NHL who had entirely normal karyotypes, abnormal karyotypes alone, or a combination of both.[18,23,221,223] Thus, the prognostic importance of normal metaphases in a lymphoma specimen remains uncertain.

Table 42–7. Cytogenetic Features Reported to Have Prognostic Significance in NHL

Cytogenetic Feature[a]	Prognostic Relevance
Normal metaphase cells	
Exlusively normal karyotype	Longer survival[225,226]; no correlation[18,221,223]
Normal metaphase cells in NHL specimen	Increased CR rate and longer survival[220]; no correlation[18,23,221]
More than 20 percent of normal metaphases in follicular NHL	Increased CR rate and longer survival[220]; no correlation[18,221]
More than 90 percent of abnormal metaphases in follicular NHL	Shorter survival[209]
No aberrant metaphases in unstimulated cultures in angioimmunoblastic T-cell NHL	Higher incidence of therapy-induced remissions; longer survival[222]
Ploidy	
Near-tetraploidy	Longer survival[150]; no correlation[225,227]
Hypodiploidy	Shorter survival[225]
Karyotype complexity	
More than 6 breaks in the karyotype of follicular NHL	Shorter survival[209]
More than 4 aberrations in addition to t(14;18)	Shorter survival than other patients with t(14;18)[23]
More than 4 breaks in DLBL	No impact on survival[224]
More than 4 marker chromosomes	No impact on survival[224]
More than 4 chromosome gains detected by CGH in mantle cell lymphoma	Shorter survival[148]
Three or more aberrations in addition to the t(11;14) in MCL	Shorter survival[149]
More than 4 marker chromosomes in DM, DLC, and IBL	Shorter survival[221]; no correlation[220]
More than 4 aberrations in angioimmunoblastic T-cell NHL	Lower incidence of therapy-induced remissions, shorter survival[222]
10 or more aberrations	Shorter survival[225]; no correlation[220]; no correlation in DLBL[224]
Specific abnormalities[b]	
1p+	Shorter survival[225]
Break at 1p32	Shorter disease-free interval[220]
Break at 1p32–36 in low-grade NHL[c]	Shorter survival[221]
Break at 1p21–22 in follicular NHL	Shorter survival[209]
Break at 1p32–36 in DM, DLC, and IBL	Shorter duration of CR[221]
Abnormalities of 1p in angioimmunoblastic T-cell NHL	Lower incidence of therapy-induced remissions, shorter survival[222]
Break at 1q21–23 in DM, DLC, and IBL	Shorter duration of CR and shorter survival[221]
Break at 1q21–23 in DLBL	Shorter survival in univariate analysis, no independent prognostic value in multivariate analysis[224]
Deletions of 1q42→qter and duplications of 1q23→q32 in centroblastic lymphoma	Shorter survival[169]
Abnormalities of 1q in intermediate-/high-grade NHL	Shorter survival[74]
+2 or dup(2p) in FM, FL, DM, and DL	Poor response to treatment and shorter survival[18,228]; no correlation[18,221]; no correlation in DLBL[224]
Break in 2p in DLC and IBL	Longer survival[220]; no correlation[221]
+3 or dup(3p) in FM, FL, DM, and DL	Longer survival[228]; no correlation[18]; no correlation in DM, DLC, and IBL[221]; no correlation in DLBL[224]
+3 in t(14;18)-positive NHL[d]	Longer survival than other patients with t(14;18)[23]
+3 in angioimmunoblastic T-cell NHL	No effect on survival[222]
Gain of 3q detected by CGH in mantle cell lymphoma	Shorter survival[148]
BCL6/LAZ3 rearrangement	Longer survival and freedom from the disease progression[245]; no correlation[54,159,160,161]; shorter overall survival[246]
t(3;14) or other aberrations of 3q27	No correlation with survival in centroblastic and immunoblastic lymphomas[222]
+5	Shorter survival[18]; longer survival in centroblastic lymphoma[169]; no correlation in DM, DLC, and IBL[221]; no correlation in DLBL[224]
Any abnormality of 5	Shorter survival[18]
+6	Shorter survival[18]; no correlation in DM, DLC, and IBL[221]
+6 in DLBL	Shorter survival in univariate analysis, no independent prognostic value in multivariate analysis[224]
Break at 6q23–26 in follicular NHL	Shorter survival, increased risk of transformation to DLC lymphoma[209]
Break at 6q21–25 in DM, DLC, and IBL	Shorter survival and diminished probability of achieving complete remission[221]; no correlation between del(6q) and survival in DLC and IBL[202]; no impact on survival in DLBL[224]
Deletion of 6q in the absence of t(14;18)	Shorter survival than patients without a 6q deletion or than patients with the 6q deletion and t(14;18)[74]

Cytogenetic Feature[a]	Prognostic Relevance
Deletion of 6q in DLBL	No significant difference in survival compared to patients without a 6q deletion[161]
−7 or structural abnormality of 7p	Poor response to chemotherapy, shorter disease-free and overall survival[241]; no correlation between − 7 and survival in DM, DLC, and IBL[221]; no correlation in DLBL[224]
+ 7	Shorter survival[225]; no correlation in DLBL[224]
+ 7 in low-grade NHL[c]	Shorter survival[221]
+ 7 in follicular NHL	Shorter survival[223]
Any structural abnormality of 7q in immunoblastic lymphoma	Shorter survival[169]
t(8;14) in low-grade NHL and in DM, DLC, and IBL	No significant difference in survival compared with patients without the translocation in a given subset[221]; no correlation with survival[169]
t(8;14) or variants together with t(14;18) in non-Burkitt (Burkitt-like) SNC	Survival shorter than that of patients with t(8;14) or variants without t(14;18) or patients with other aberrations[177]
MYC rearrangement in DLCL	No statistically significant impact on disease-free survival, despite a trend for better DFS[160]
Any structural abnormality of 8q in immunoblastic lymphoma	Shorter survival[169]
Loss of 9p detected by CGH in mantle cell lymphoma	Shorter survival[148]
Deletion of 11q22–23/ATM gene	Shorter survival[279]
+ 12 in low-grade NHL[c]	Shorter survival[221]
+ 12 in follicular NHL	Shorter survival[223]
Gain of 12q detected by CGH in MCL	Shorter survival[148]
+ 12 (or partial + 12) in MCL with t(11;14)	Shorter survival[149]
del(13)(q32) in FSC with t(14;18)	Poor response to treatment and shorter survival[118]
−14	Shorter survival[223]
Break at 14q11−12	Shorter survival;[18] no correlation in DLBL[224]
t(14;18)/BCL2 rearrangement in FM and FL	Poor response to treatment and shorter survival[228]; no correlation with survival in FSC, FM, and FL[18,209,220,221,223,225,231]
t(14;18) in low-grade (SL,FSC,FM) lymphoma	Better survival[74]
BCL2 rearrangement [mcr(+)/MBR(+)] in follicular lymphoma (grade I, II, III)	Higher CR rate, longer disease-free and overall survival[232]
t(14;18)/BCL2 rearrangement in DM and DLC	Shorter disease-free survival[228]; no correlation[223]
t(14;18)/BCL2 rearrangement in DLC	Shorter disease-free survival[236]; no correlation with overall survival[236]
BCL2 rearrangement in de novo DLC	Shorter disease-free period[234]; no correlation with overall[161,234] or failure-free survival
BCL2 rearrangement in de novo DM, DLC, IBL, and ALCL	No impact on disease-free,[160,237] relapse-free,[237] and overall survival[160,161,237]
t(14;18)/BCL2 rearrangement in DLC and IBL	Shorter disease-free period in extranodal NHL[204]; no correlation with overall[169,204,233] and disease-free survival[233,235]
Presence of cytogenetic aberrations in addition to t(14;18) in follicular NHL	No impact on survival[223]
Any structural abnormality of 15q in centroblastic lymphoma	Longer survival[169]
−17 or del(17q) in DLC and IBL	Poor response to treatment and shorter survival[228]
−17 or structural abnormality of 17p	Poor response to chemotherapy, shorter disease-free and overall survival[241]
−17 or der(17p) or i(17q) in DLBL	No impact on survival[224]
Structural abnormality of 17	Shorter survival[18]
Break at 17p in follicular NHL	Shorter survival, increased risk of transformation to DLC lymphoma[209]
Deletions and inversions involving 17p in FL	Shorter survival[231]
Structural abnormality of 17 in follicular NHL	Shorter survival[220]
+ 18	Shorter survival[18]; no correlation in DM, DLC, and IBL[221]; no correlation in DLBL[224]
+ 18 in t(14;18)-positive NHL[d]	Longer survival than other patients with t(14;18)[23]
+ 21 in t(14;18)-positive NHL[d]	Longer survival than other patients with t(14;18)[23]
+ 21 in FL	Shorter survival[231]
+ X in angioimmunoblastic T-cell NHL	Lower incidence of therapy-induced remissions, shorter survival[222]

[a] The molecular equivalents of the t(14;18) and structural changes of 3q27, BCL2, and BCL6/LAZ3 rearrangements, respectively, are also included.
[b] They are listed by chromosome number from 1 to 21.
[c] Statistically significant when breaks at 1p32–36, + 7, and + 12 combined.
[d] Statistically significant when + 3, + 18, + 21 combined.

Hyperdiploidy, with the number of chromosomes exceeding 50, especially in cases with only numerical chromosome changes, constitutes a favorable prognostic factor in childhood ALL.[181] Initial study of a relatively small number of patients suggested a similar phenomenon in NHL[150]; six patients with a near-tetraploid modal chromosomal number had the longest median survival among 30 karyotypically abnormal patients. However, subsequent larger cytogenetic[225] and flow cytometric[227] analyses have not found correlations between increased ploidy of lymphoma and survival.

Numerous studies have demonstrated a negative impact of multiple chromosome changes on clinical outcome.[23,149,209,221,222,225] Kristoffersson et al.[225] in 106 NHLs of various histologies, found that survival was significantly shorter for patients who had ten or more aberrations compared to patients with no or up to four aberrations. Similarly, a shortened median survival was associated with the presence of more than four marker chromosomes among patients with DM, DLC, and IBL,[221] with four or more unrelated additional aberrations in patients with the t(14;18),[23] with more than four aberrations in patients with AILD-type T-cell lymphoma,[222] with three or more aberrations in addition to t(11;14) in MCL,[149] and with more than six breaks in the karyotype of patients with follicular NHL.[209] In contrast, neither the presence of more than four marker chromosomes nor ten or more aberrations influenced prognosis of DLC patients studied by Jerkeman et al.[224] Overall, these results suggest that the complexity of the patient's karyotype may become an important prognostic factor in NHL as it already has in AML.[218]

The observation that the presence of the t(14;18) or BCL2 rearrangement in FM or FL was correlated with a poor response to therapy and shortened survival,[228] has not been substantiated in several larger studies.[18,43,209,220,221,225,229–231] In three series, patients with indolent follicular lymphoma with t(14;18) or BCL2 rearrangement detected by PCR fared even better than those without.[43,230,232] Other studies, however, did not detect a difference in outcome between patients with and without t(14;18)/BCL2 rearrangement.[18,209,220,221,225,229,231] Instead, an adverse prognosis may be associated with the addition of other chromosome changes to t(14;18) in follicular lymphoma. Patients with FSC and a solitary t(14;18) have been reported to have an indolent course, whereas four patients with an additional del(13)(q32) had an acceleration of the disease with a poor response to chemotherapy.[118] In addition, trisomy of chromosome 2 or its short arm, and homogeneously staining regions or double minutes correlated with a poor prognosis in patients with follicular lymphoma.[118] In contrast, in a group of 53 karyotypically abnormal patients with low-grade lymphomas, Offit et al.[221] found no correlation between clinical outcome and the presence of trisomy 2 or deletions of 2p; aberrations involving band 13q32 were detected too infrequently to be analyzed. Offit et al.[221] did find a negative impact on survival of trisomy 7 or trisomy 12 or structural abnormalities involving region 1p32-36. Both trisomy 7 and trisomy 12, but not breaks at 1p36, were also associated with shorter survival of patients with follicular lymphoma in an Australian study.[223] Structural changes of bands 1p21-22 as well as aberrations involving 6q23-26 significantly correlated with poor prognosis in a large

study of follicular NHL[209]; breaks at 6q23-26 were identified as an independent prognostic factor in multivariate analysis. However, the prognosis was not influenced by the presence of trisomy X, 7, 12, or duplication of 12q, and 18.[209] In the most recent series, restricted to patients diagnosed with FL, poor prognosis was associated with the presence of structural aberrations affecting 17p (mainly deletions and inversions) and trisomy 21.[231] Clearly, further studies are required to determine the prognostic import of specific abnormalities in follicular lymphoma.

t(14;18) or BCL2 gene rearrangements are found in 18 to 40 percent of diffuse large B-cell lymphoma.[164,233–235] Three studies reported shorter disease-free, but not overall, survival of patients with t(14;18) or BCL2 gene rearrangement compared with DLC patients lacking such abnormalities.[234–236] However, several other published reports have not found a statistically significant difference in CR rates, disease-free survival, and overall survival between DLC patients with and without t(14;18)/BCL2 gene rearrangement.[159,160,220,221,233,237,238] Instead, adverse prognosis has been consistently associated with BCL2 protein overexpression, detectable by immunohistochemistry, which is in general poorly correlated with BCL2 gene rearrangements in DLC.[159,237,238] In the three largest studies, BCL2 protein expression was shown to represent an independent risk factor by multivariate analyses that included well-defined clinical risk parameters.[159,237,238]

Increased BCL2 mRNA levels have been detected in the majority (71 percent) of "activated B-like DLC lymphomas," a distinct type of lymphoma identified by genomic-scale gene expression profiling using lymphoid-specific complementary DNA microarrays (the "Lymphochip").[239] This novel methodology, allowing quantitation of the expression of thousands of genes in parallel, resulted in delineation of two major types of DLC with significantly different overall survival: the prognostically unfavorable "activated B-like DLC lymphomas" and "germinal center B-like DLC lymphoma," a category associated with significantly improved outcome.[239] Another study, using different oligonucleotide microarrays to analyze the expression of an unselected set of 6817 human genes, also identified two categories of patients with dramatically different survival.[240] The authors concluded that expression of genes related to cell adhesion, apoptosis, RAS signaling, serine/threonine phosphorylation, and tumor immunity, in addition to those found by Alizadeh et al.,[239] are predictive of DLC patient outcome.[240]

Structural changes of chromosome 17 have been repeatedly shown to correlate with an adverse prognosis in NHL. In a study of Levine et al.,[220] 8 patients with follicular lymphoma and various structural changes of chromosome 17 had significantly shorter survival than 22 patients without breaks in this chromosome. Likewise, abnormalities of 17p have been demonstrated to constitute an independent adverse prognostic factor by multivariate analysis in follicular lymphoma.[209] Poor clinical outcome of patients with structural changes of chromosome 17 or monosomy 17 has also been demonstrated in series composed of all NHL histologies,[18,241] in patients with CLL,[79] FL,[231] diffuse lymphomas with large cell components,[221,228] and BL.[174] In some of these studies, multivariate analyses showed chromosome 17 abnormalities to be a risk factor independent from other unfavorable prognostic features such as tumor grade, increased lactate dehydrogenase level, or tumor burden.[18,79,241] These findings are consistent with the significant role that *p53* mutations play in tumor progression of NHL,[58,59] and with the repetitively demonstrated association between mutations of the *p53* gene and poor response to therapy and survival of patients with B-cell NHL,[242] aggressive B-cell lymphoma,[243] CLL,[78] and MCL.[244] Thus, detection of chromosome 17 abnormalities and/or *p53* gene mutations appears to identify patients who require more intensive treatment.

Rearrangements of the *BCL6* gene have been reported in one study to constitute an independent favorable prognostic marker of both survival and freedom of disease progression in DLC, DM, and IBL patients, most of whom presented with extranodal disease.[245] However, no significant correlations between *BCL6* gene rearrangements and clinical outcome have been found in four other studies[153,158–160]; in one series, an overall survival of patients with *BCL6* gene rearrangements was significantly shorter than that of the remaining patients with diffuse large B-cell lymphoma.[246] The discrepancy between results of Offit et al.[245] and others may be in part attributed to varying proportions of patients with extranodal lymphoma. For example, Pescarmona et al.[159] studied exclusively patients with nodal disease and the presence of additional cytogenetic aberrations in the tumors analyzed. In a subsequent study, Offit et al.[247] demonstrated that their patients in the *BCL6* rearranged group displayed aberrations associated with disease progression, such as +7, +12, del(6q), and structural abnormalities of 17p less frequently than patients with *BCL6* germline tumors. Among patients who had the *BCL6* gene rearrangement, those lacking the aforementioned chromosome aberrations remained free of disease at follow-up in excess of 7 years, whereas *BCL6* rearranged cases with the aberrations showed decreased intervals free from progression of the disease.[247] These results suggest that molecular analyses testing the *BCL6* gene status should be combined with cytogenetic and/or FISH analyses that provide a more complete picture of prognostically relevant genetic alterations in patients with NHL. Another study has suggested that it is also important to determine whether the *BCL6* gene rearrangements are caused by translocations involving the immunoglobulin genes (*IGH, IGL,* or *IGK*) or by translocations (or inversions) affecting other, nonimmunoglobulin chromosomal loci.[246] The overall survival of 17 patients with the latter kind of *BCL6* gene fusions was significantly inferior to the survival of 21 patients with either t(3;14)/*BCL6/IGH* (16 cases) or t(3;22)/*BCL6/IGL* (5 cases); the respective estimated 2-year overall survival rates were 58.3 percent versus 17.6 percent ($p = .005$).[246] Therefore, on balance, the prognostic impact of 3q27/*BCL6* rearrangements remains at present controversial, and a clear need for further studies exists. Likewise, corroboration is required for other associations between specific chromosome abnormalities and clinical outcome that have been reported in single studies and are listed in Table 42–7.

HODGKIN'S DISEASE

In comparison with NHL, the delineation of the cytogenetic abnormalities in Hodgkin's disease (HD) has been very limited.

At present, the number of cases with reported clonal abnormalities is approximately 15 times lower than that in NHL.[6] Specific problems in HD include a lower mitotic index and overrepresentation of cells with a normal karyotype in the specimen when compared with NHL. Part of the problem may be that Reed-Sternberg cells, which are now widely accepted to be the clonal malignant cells in HD,[248–250] nearly always constitute a minority (sometimes less than 1 percent) of the cells in lymph node biopsies. The remaining cells represent reactive lymphoid cells. Thus, to detect an abnormal clone, a large number of metaphase cells should be analyzed in each patient with HD.[251,252] Other problems include the poor quality of banding in some cases and complexity of the karyotypes.[253]

Among more recent studies comprising 20 or more HD patients, the success rates for achieving analyzable metaphases ranged from 47 to 90 percent, thus being only slightly lower than success rates in NHL.[248,250–252,254–259] However, in contrast to NHL, clonal abnormalities have been found in less than 50 percent of all successfully karyotyped cases (range 14 to 92 percent). That normal cytogenetic results in most HD cases are likely caused by a failure to detect chromosome aberrations rather than a genuine absence of aberrations in the neoplastic cells, has been shown by Weber-Matthiesen et al.[260] The authors used the technique of simultaneous fluorescence immunophenotyping and interphase cytogenetics (FICTION) to study 30 patients with HD, all of whom had been analyzed by standard cytogenetic analysis. FICTION revealed several clonal numerical chromosome aberrations in the CD30+ Hodgkin and Reed-Sternberg cells in all 30 patients. The aberrations were found not only in patients with a complex hyperdiploid karyotype on initial cytogenetic study, as expected, but also in all 12 patients whose initial karyotype was normal. Therefore, an exclusively normal karyotype in a specimen from an HD patient likely represents reactive lymphoid cells dividing in vitro, a conclusion supported by lack of numerical chromosome aberrations in lymphocytes studied by FICTION.[260]

Chromosome findings in HD are, despite some similarities, somewhat different from NHL. The most striking, repetitively identified distinction between the two entities is that while it is unusual for ploidy among cases of NHL to be greater than 50, the chromosomal number in the majority of karyotypically aberrant HD cases is in the near-triploid (around 69 chromosomes) or near-tetraploid (around 92 chromosomes) range.[248,250–252,254,257–259] All chromosomes have been involved in clonal gains and losses, but the distribution of numerical changes appears to be nonrandom. Among 40 HD cases published prior to 1990 that were analyzed with chromosome banding techniques and reviewed by Thangavelu and Le Beau,[253] the most frequently gained were the following chromosomes: 5 (in 11 cases), 2 (10 cases), 1, 12, and 21 (9 cases each). In a later series, comprising 31 HD patients with evaluable abnormal karyotypes,[258] chromosomes 2, 9 (22 cases each), 5, and 12 (21 cases each) were commonly overrepresented. In both series, the most commonly lost chromosomes were 13 and Y; these were also least frequently gained.[253,258]

The recurring loss of chromosome 13 suggests that inactivation of a tumor suppressor gene may be operative in some cases of HD.[258] Multiple other chromosome regions including 1p, 1q, 2p, 3p, 3q, 4q, 6q, 7q, 9p, 9q, 11p, 11q, 12p, 14q, 17p, 18p, and 20q, have been consistently lost due to deletions and unbalanced translocations (Table 42–8). Consequently, it has been suggested that in contrast to other hematologic malignancies, a multistep inactivation of tumor suppressor genes may be more important in HD tumorigenesis than the activation of protooncogenes.[256,257] Supporting this are immunocytochemical studies demonstrating p53 protein overexpression in Reed-Sternberg cells in 35 to 72 percent of cases of all but nodular lymphocyte predominant HD subtypes.[261,262] Single-cell PCR has demonstrated a point mutation within the *p53* coding sequence in five of seven Reed-Sternberg cells obtained from a patient with nodular sclerosis HD.[263] However, two later molecular studies of micromanipulated single Reed-Sternberg cells

did not detect mutations in the *p53* gene in any of the eight[264] and five[265] HD patients studied. This suggests that in most patients, mechanisms other than mutation of the *p53* gene are responsible for the observed upregulation of p53 protein in Reed-Sternberg cells.[264] Such a mechanism may be an increase of MDM2 protein levels that can stabilize the p53 protein. The *MDM2* gene amplification, associated with structural chromosome aberrations affecting region 12q14-15, has been detected in four of the six HD cases analyzed recently.[265] Another gene suggested to represent a candidate tumor suppressor gene participating in the pathogenesis of HD is the *IκBα* gene mapped to 14q13. Mutations in this gene have been found in some, but not all, HD patients and cell lines with constitutive NF-κB activity which prevents the Reed-Sternberg cells from undergoing apoptosis and confers their continuous proliferation.[266,267]

Table 42–8. Recurrent Chromosome Aberrations Detected in Hodgkin's Disease

Aberration[a]	No. of Cases[b]	Aberration[a]	No. of Cases[b]
+X	<5	add(11)(p15)	<5
add(X)(p22)	<5	add(11)(q23)	5–10
i(X)(p10)	<5	del(11)(p12–13)	<5
−Y	<5	del(11)(q13–14)	<5
add(1)(p36)	5–10	add(12)(q24)	5–10
del(1)(p32)	<5	del(12)(p11–13)	5–10
del(1)(p21)	<5	add(13)(p11–13)	>15
del(1)(p12–13)	<5	add(14)(p11–p13)	11–15
del(1)(q21)	<5	del(14)(q22–24)	<5
i(1)(q10)	11–15	i(14)(q10)	<5
add(2)(p25)	5–10	t(14;15)(q10;q10)	<5
add(2)(q36–37)	<5	t/add(14)(q32)	16–20
i(2)(q10)	<5	t(14;18)(q32;q21)	<5
+3	<5	−15	<5
add/t(3)(q27–29)	5–10	add(15)(p11–13)	11–15
t(3;22)(q27;q11)	<5	t(15;22)(q10;q10)	<5
del(3)(p12–13)	<5	+16	<5
del(3)(q21)	5–10	add(16)(q22)	<5
add(4)(q34–q35)	5–10	add(17)(p13)	5–10
dup(4)(q24q28)	<5	i(17)(q10)	5–10
i(4)(p10)	<5	−18	<5
add(5)(p14–15)	5–10	+18	<5
del(6)(q11–16q)	11–15	add(18)(p11–12)	5–10
del(6)(q21–22)	11–15	i(18)(q10)	<5
i(6)(p10)	<5	add(19)(p13)	5–10
del(7)(q21–22)	5–10	add(19)(q13)	5–10
i(7)(p10)	<5	add(20)(q13)	5–10
i(7)(q10)	<5	del(20)(q11q13)	<5
+8	<5	+21	5–10
add(8)(q24)	5–10	add(21)(p11–13)	5–10
i(8)(q10)	<5	i(21)(q10)	5–10
add(9)(p24)	<5	+22	<5
add(9)(p21)	<5	add(22)(p11)	<5
i(9)(p10)	5–10	i(22)(q10)	<5
t(10;14)(q22–23;q32)	<5		

[a] Data from Mitelman et al.,[6] Franke et al.[272] To be include in this listing a given abnormality must have been reported in at least two patients with Hodgkin's disease.

[b] For numerical aberrations (monosomies and trisomies), the number of patients refers only to those harboring a given monosomy or trisomy as a sole abnormality; for structural aberrations, the numbers provided refer to all patients, regardless of whether a given aberration was isolated or not.

Whether other currently known tumor suppressor genes actually play a role in malignant transformation is at present unknown. Some investigators have suggested 1q, 4q, 6q, 9p, 11q, 12p, and 13q (and more specifically 1q42, 4q25-27, 6q21-23, 9p23, 11q22-23, and 12p12-13) as the loci that are nonrandomly lost and may harbor tumor suppressor genes important in the pathogenesis of HD.[250,256,257,268]

Other karyotypic anomalies that seem to distinguish HD from NHL include abnormalities of the satellite regions located on the short arms of all acrocentric chromosomes (i.e., chromosomes 13, 14, 15, 21, and 22) (Table 42–8). Although occasionally seen in NHL, these aberrations are unusually frequent in HD patients[251,257,258] and HD cell lines.[269] In most cases, the origin of genetic material translocated onto the acrocentric chromosomes has not been determined. The affected satellite regions of all acrocentric chromosomes contain genes coding for ribosomal DNA (rDNA). A recent study of HD cell lines has provided evidence that structural aberrations involving the short arms of acrocentric chromosomes lead to genomic rearrangements of rDNA, which participate in jumping translocations and insertions into ectopic sites of nonacrocentric chromosomes. Moreover, rDNA was also amplified and co-amplified together with an amplicon at chromosome 9p, recurrent in HD. Further studies should determine if unstable and mobile rDNA sequences facilitate gene rearrangements and gene amplification in HD.[269]

The cellular origin of Reed-Sternberg cells has for years been a subject of debate. Currently, several lines of evidence indicate that Reed-Sternberg cells derive from lymphocytic cells, in most instances from germinal center B cells.[270] This hypothesis is supported by cytogenetic findings. In 1988, Cabanillas[271] reviewed the distribution of recurring breakpoints in 49 HD cases (including 18 of his own) and found that breaks clustered at sites commonly involved in NHL (i.e., 14q32, 11q21-23, 6q11-23, and 8q22-24), suggesting a B-cell lymphoid origin of the malignant cell. Similar distribution of breakpoints was also found in a 1999 review of 177 patients with HD.[251] The most frequent were aberrations of band 14q32, which usually occurred in the form of translocations of unidentified material onto this band.[248,250,258,259] However, their frequency is not high, ranging from 8 percent[250] to 25 percent.[248,259] Only three reciprocal translocations have been identified in more than one patient: t(14;18)(q32;q21) in four,[248,259,271] t(3;22)(q27;q11)[251,272] in two, and t(10;14)(q22-23;q32) in two cases.[248,273]

The recurrent, albeit rare, finding of the t(14;18), typical of follicular lymphoma, suggested that this translocation might be involved in HD oncogenesis. Numerous studies utilizing various methodologies such as PCR and Southern blot analysis have addressed the question of BCL2 involvement in HD with conflicting results (reviewed in Gupta et al.[274]). Most, but not all, studies detected BCL2 gene rearrangements in DNA from a proportion (20 to 39 percent) of HD patients. However, there was no correlation between t(14;18) detected by PCR from a biopsy specimen and BCL2 protein expression in Reed-Sternberg cells from the same specimen.[274,275] Therefore it has been suggested that BCL2 rearrangements/t(14;18) could occur in bystander small B lymphocytes and not in malignant cells.[276]

That this indeed is the case has been experimentally shown by Gravel et al.[275] who investigated by PCR Hodgkin's and Reed-Sternberg cells isolated from 11 HD patients whose total DNA extracts of lymph nodes were positive for the t(14;18). In none of the patients did Hodgkin's and Reed-Sternberg cells contain the t(14;18). Thus, the t(14;18) does not seem to play a direct role in the pathogenesis of HD, and the observed BCL2 protein expression in HD is not caused by this translocation. On the other hand, consistent BCL6 protein expression in lymphocyte predominance HD, but not in other histologic subtypes of HD, may be due to the presence of t(3;22)(q27;q11) and other aberrations causing rearrangements of the BCL6 gene in some patients.[272]

Several cytogenetic studies have not revealed any 14q32 abnormalities.[254–257] Instead, different aberrations of bands to which TCR genes have been localized (i.e. 7p15, 7q35, and 14q11), have been recurrently observed.[250,257,258] These observations, together with reported rearrangements of TCRB and TCRG genes in HD, support derivation of HD from a T cell in a minority of patients.

Not surprisingly, the limited number of consistent aberrations has not allowed a cytogenetic distinction between morphologic subtypes of HD. Some differences in cytogenetic patterns have started to emerge, however. Isochromosome(1q), add(8)(q24), add(9)(p21), i(18)(q10), and trisomy 18 as a sole abnormality have been found much more frequently in mixed cellularity than in other subtypes of HD, whereas i(6)(p10), del(20)(q11q13), and add(20)(q13) have been hitherto seen exclusively in nodular sclerosis HD.[6] Whether these associations represent true biological phenomena or are due to the small number of cases analyzed remains to be established. Too few cases of HD have been studied to determine the clinical significance of karyotype.

SUMMARY

Cytogenetic investigations of lymphomas have revealed many specific chromosome anomalies associated with the initiation and progression of the neoplastic process. Mapping of breakpoints in recurrent translocations have resulted in the cloning and characterization of genes involved in lymphomagenesis, and in elucidation of the mechanisms whereby their expression has been deregulated. Recent studies, following cytogenetic reports on consistently lost chromosome bands or regions, have shown that tumor suppressor genes may also take part in the multistage evolution of lymphoma. Moreover, several associations between recurring cytogenetic abnormalities and morphology, immunophenotype, and parameters of clinical outcome have been made. Chromosome aberrations have proved to be important biologic markers that together with immunophenotypic, histologic, and molecular genetic data have helped to identify individual diseases within the WHO Classification of Lymphoid Neoplasms. Conversely, the presence of identical cytogenetic abnormalities in entities hitherto regarded as not closely related, have suggested their closer-than-anticipated pathogenetic associations. Nonetheless, many of the reported correlations between karyotype and other features of lymphoma are still preliminary and require confirmation. Ongoing cytogenetic studies will not only lead to a better understanding of lymphomagenesis, but will also result in the determination of both karyotypic and molecular genetic markers that are clinically useful in the management of patients with lymphoma.

ACKNOWLEDGMENT

This work was supported in part by NCI grant no. 5P30CA16058 and the Coleman Leukemia Research Fund.

REFERENCES

1. Spriggs AI, Boddington MM: Chromosomes of Sternberg-Reed cells. Lancet 2:153, 1962.
2. Jacobs PA, Tough IM, Wright DH: Cytogenetic studies in Burkitt's lymphoma. Lancet 2:1144, 1963.
3. Mark J: Chromosomal abnormalities and their specificity in human neoplasms: An assessment of recent observations by banding techniques. Adv Cancer Res 24:165, 1977.
4. Manolov G, Manolova Y: Marker band in one chromosome 14 from Burkitt lymphomas. Nature 237:33, 1972.
5. Zech L, Haglund U, Nilsson K, Klein G: Characteristic chromosomal abnormalities in biopsies and lymphoid-cell lines from patients with Burkitt and non-Burkitt lymphomas. Int J Cancer 17:47, 1976.
6. Mitelman F, Johansson B, Mertens F (eds.): Mitelman Database of Chromosome Aberrations in Cancer. Available at http://cgap.nci.nih.gov/Chromosomes/Mitelman, 2001
7. ISCN (1995). An International System for Human Cytogenetic Nomenclature. Mitelman F (ed.). S. Karger, Basel, 1995.
8. Harris NL, Jaffe ES, Diebold J et al: World Health Organization classification of neoplastic diseases of the hematopoietic and lymphoid tissues: Report of the Clinical Advisory Committee meeting—Airlie House, Virginia, November 1997. J Clin Oncol 17:3835, 1999.
9. The Non-Hodgkin's Lymphoma Pathologic Classification Project: National Cancer Institute sponsored study of classifications of non-Hodgkin's lymphomas: Summary and description of a working formulation for clinical usage. Cancer 49:2112, 1982.
10. Stansfeld AG, Diebold J, Noel H et al: Updated Kiel classification for lymphomas. Lancet 1(8580):292, 1988.
11. Veldman T, Vignon C, Schröck E et al: Hidden chromosome abnormalities in haematological malignancies detected by multicolour spectral karyotyping. Nat Genet 15:406, 1997.
12. Nordgren A, Sørensen AG, Tinggaard-Pedersen N et al: New chromosomal breakpoints in non-Hodgkin's lymphomas revealed by spectral karyotyping and G-banding. Int J Mol Med 5:485, 2000.
13. Yunis JJ, Oken MM, Kaplan ME et al: Distinctive chromosomal abnormalities in histologic subtypes of non-Hodgkin's lymphoma. N Engl J Med 307:1231, 1982.
14. Bloomfield CD, Arthur DC, Frizzera G et al: Nonrandom chromosome abnormalities in lymphoma. Cancer Res 43:2975, 1983.
15. Yunis JJ, Oken MM, Theologides A et al: Recurrent chromosomal defects are found in most patients with non-Hodgkin's-lymphoma. Cancer Genet Cytogenet 13:17, 1984.
16. Kristoffersson U, Heim S, Olsson H et al: Cytogenetic studies in non-Hodgkin lymphomas—results from surgical biopsies. Hereditas 104:1, 1986.
17. Juneja S, Lukeis R, Tan L et al: Cytogenetic analysis of 147 cases of non-Hodgkin's lymphoma: Non-random chromosomal abnormalities and histological correlations. Br J Haematol 76:231, 1990.
18. Schouten HC, Sanger WG, Weisenburger DD et al: Chromosomal abnormalities in untreated patients with non-Hodgkin's lymphoma: Associations with histology, clinical characteristics, and treatment outcome. Blood 75:1841, 1990.
19. Offit K, Jhanwar SC, Ladanyi M et al: Cytogenetic analysis of 434 consecutively ascertained specimens of non-Hodgkin's lymphoma: Correlations between recurrent aberrations, histology, and exposure to cytotoxic treatment. Genes Chromosomes Cancer 3:189, 1991.
20. Bastard C, Tilly H, Lenormand B et al: Translocations involving band 3q27 and Ig gene regions in non-Hodgkin's lymphoma. Blood 79:2527, 1992.
21. Speaks SL, Sanger WG, Linder J et al: Chromosomal abnormalities in indolent lymphoma. Cancer Genet Cytogenet 27:335, 1987.
22. Levine EG, Arthur DC, Frizzera G et al: There are differences in cytogenetic abnormalities among histologic subtypes of the non-Hodgkin's lymphomas. Blood 66:1414, 1985.
23. Pirc-Danoewinata H, Chott A, Onderka E et al: Karyotype and prognosis in non-Hodgkin lymphoma. Leukemia 8:1929, 1994.
24. Hashimoto K, Miura I, Chyubachi A et al: Correlations of chromosome abnormalities with histologic and immunologic characteristics in 49 patients from Akita, Japan with non-Hodgkin lymphoma. Cancer Genet Cytogenet 81:56, 1995.
25. Fifth International Workshop on Chromosomes in Leukemia-Lymphoma: Correlations of chromosome abnormalities with histologic and immunologic characteristics in non-Hodgkin's lymphoma and adult T cell leukemia-lymphoma. Blood 70:1554, 1987.
26. Rack KA, Salomon-Nguyen F, Radford-Weiss I et al: FISH detection of chromosome 14q32/IgH translocations: Evaluation in follicular lymphoma. Br J Haematol 103:495, 1998.
27. Wotherspoon AC, Pan L, Diss TC et al: Cytogenetic study of B-cell lymphoma of mucosa-associated lymphoid tissue. Cancer Genet Cytogenet 58:35, 1992.
28. Gaidano G, Hauptschein RS, Parsa NZ et al: Deletions involving two distinct regions of 6q in B-cell non-Hodgkin lymphoma. Blood 80:1781, 1992.
29. Vaandrager JW, Schuuring E, Philippo K, Kluin PM: V(D)J recombinase-mediated transposition of the BCL2 gene to the IGH locus in follicular lymphoma. Blood 96:1947, 2000.
30. Heim S, Mitelman F: Cancer Cytogenetics, 2nd ed. Wiley-Liss, New York, 1995.
31. Croce CM: Molecular biology of lymphomas. Semin Oncol 20 (Suppl. 5):31, 1993.
32. Kerckaert J-P, Deweindt C, Tilly H et al: LAZ3, a novel zinc-finger encoding gene, is disrupted by recurring chromosome 3q27 translocations in human lymphomas. Nat Genet 5:66, 1993.
33. Ye BH, Lista F, Lo Coco F et al: Alterations of a zinc finger-encoding gene, BCL-6, in diffuse large-cell lymphoma. Science 262:747, 1993.
34. Miki T, Kawamata N, Hirosawa S et al: Gene involved in the 3q27 translocation associated with B-cell lymphoma, BCL5, encodes a Krüppel-like zinc-finger protein. Blood 83:26, 1994.
35. Rabbitts TH: Chromosomal translocations in human cancer. Nature 372:143, 1994.
36. Online Mendelian Inheritance in Man, OMIM (TM). McKusick-Nathans Institute for Genetic Medicine, Johns Hopkins University (Baltimore, MD) and National Center for Biotechnology Information, National Library of Medicine (Bethesda, MD),

2000. World Wide Web URL: http://www.ncbi.nlm.nih.gov/omim/

37. Corcoran MM, Mould SJ, Orchard JA et al: Dysregulation of cyclin dependent kinase 6 expression in splenic marginal zone lymphoma through chromosome 7q translocations. Oncogene 18:6271, 1999.

38. Busslinger M, Klix N, Pfeffer P et al: Deregulation of PAX-5 by translocation of the Eμ enhancer of the IgH locus adjacent to two alternative PAX-5 promoters in a diffuse large-cell lymphoma. Proc Natl Acad Sci U S A 93:6129, 1996.

39. Iida S, Rao PH, Nallasivam P et al: The t(9;14)(p13;q32) chromosomal translocation associated with lymphoplasmacytoid lymphoma involves the PAX-5 gene. Blood 88:4110, 1996.

40. Pekarsky Y, Koval A, Hallas C et al: Tcl1 enhances Akt kinase activity and mediates its nuclear translocation. Proc Natl Acad Sci U S A 97:3028, 2000.

41. Morris SW, Kirstein MN, Valentine MB et al: Fusion of a kinase gene, ALK, to a nucleolar protein gene, NPM, in non-Hodgkin's lymphoma. Science 263:1281, 1994.

42. Mitani K, Sato Y, Tojo A et al: Philadelphia chromosome positive B-cell type malignant lymphoma expressing an aberrant 190 kDa bcr-abl protein. Br J Haematol 76:221, 1990.

43. Takechi M, Tanaka K, Hashimoto T et al: Cytogenetic, molecular biological and clinical study of B-cell lymphomas with 14;18 translocation in Japanese patients. Leukemia 5:1069, 1991.

44. Neri A, Chang CC, Lombardi L et al: B cell lymphoma-associated chromosomal translocation involves candidate oncogene lyt-10, homologous to NF-κB p50. Cell 67:1075, 1991.

45. Akao Y, Seto M, Yamamoto K et al: The RCK gene associated with t(11;14) translocation is distinct from the MLL/ALL-1 gene with t(4;11) and t(11;19) translocations. Cancer Res 52:6083, 1992.

46. Willis TG, Zalcberg IR, Coignet LJA et al: Molecular cloning of translocation t(1;14)(q21;q32) defines a novel gene (BCL9) at chromosome 1q21. Blood 91:1873, 1998.

47. Willis TG, Jadayel DM, Du MQ et al: Bcl10 is involved in t(1;14)(p22;q32) of MALT B cell lymphoma and mutated in multiple tumor types. Cell 96:35, 1999.

48. Dyomin VG, Palanisamy N, Lloyd KO et al: MUC1 is activated in a B-cell lymphoma by the t(1;14)(q21;q32) translocation and is rearranged and amplified in B-cell lymphoma subsets. Blood 95:2666, 2000.

49. Preudhomme C, Roumier C, Hildebrand MP et al: Nonrandom 4p13 rearrangements of the RhoH/TTF gene, encoding a GTP-binding protein, in non-Hodgkin's lymphoma and multiple myeloma. Oncogene 19:2023, 2000.

50. Akasaka T, Miura I, Takahashi N et al: A recurring translocation, t(3;6)(q27;p21), in non-Hodgkin's lymphoma results in replacement of the 5' regulatory region of BCL6 with a novel H4 histone gene. Cancer Res 57:7, 1997.

51. Hosokawa Y, Maeda Y, Ichinohasama R et al: The Ikaros gene, a central regulator of lymphoid differentiation, fuses to the BCL6 gene as a result of t(3;7)(q27;p12) translocation in a patient with diffuse large B-cell lymphoma. Blood 95:2719, 2000.

52. Galiègue-Zouitina S, Quief S, Hildebrand MP et al: Nonrandom fusion of L-plastin(LCP1) and LAZ3(BCL6) genes by t(3;13)(q27;q14) chromosome translocation in two cases of B-cell non-Hodgkin lymphoma. Genes Chromosomes Cancer 26:97, 1999.

53. Ma Z, Cools J, Marynen P et al: Inv(2)(p23q35) in anaplastic large-cell lymphoma induces constitutive anaplastic lymphoma kinase (ALK) tyrosine kinase activation by fusion to ATIC, an enzyme involved in purine nucleotide biosynthesis. Blood 95:2144, 2000.

54. Callanan MB, Le Baccon P, Mossuz P et al: The IgG Fc receptor, FcγRIIB, is a target for deregulation by chromosomal translocation in malignant lymphoma. Proc Natl Acad Sci U S A 97:309, 2000.

55. Knudson AG: Antioncogenes and human cancer. Proc Natl Acad Sci U S A 90:10914, 1993.

56. Robertson GP, Huang HJ, Cavenee WK: Identification and validation of tumor suppressor genes. Mol Cell Biol Res Commun 2:1, 1999.

57. Gaidano G, Ballerini P, Gong JZ et al: p53 mutations in human lymphoid malignancies: Association with Burkitt lymphoma and chronic lymphocytic leukemia. Proc Natl Acad Sci U S A 88:5413, 1991.

58. Sander CA, Yano T, Clark HM et al: p53 mutation is associated with progression in follicular lymphomas. Blood 82:1994, 1993.

59. Lo Coco F, Gaidano G, Louie DC et al: p53 mutations are associated with histologic transformation of follicular lymphoma. Blood 82:2289, 1993.

60. Koduru PRK, Raju K, Vadmal V et al: Correlation between mutation in P53, p53 expression, cytogenetics, histologic type, and survival in patients with B-cell non-Hodgkin's lymphoma. Blood 90:4078, 1997.

61. Gruszka-Westwood AM, Hamoudi RA, Matutes E et al: p53 abnormalities in splenic lymphoma with villous lymphocytes. Blood 97:3552, 2001.

62. Stranks G, Height SE, Mitchell P et al: Deletions and rearrangement of CDKN2 in lymphoid malignancy. Blood 85:893, 1995.

63. Pinyol M, Cobo F, Beà S et al: p16INK4a gene inactivation by deletions, mutations, and hypermethylation is associated with transformed and aggressive variants of non-Hodgkin's lymphomas. Blood 91:2977, 1998.

64. Grønbaek K, de Nully Brown P, Møller MB et al: Concurrent disruption of p16INK4a and the ARF-p53 pathway predicts poor prognosis in aggressive non-Hodgkin's lymphoma. Leukemia 14:1727, 2000.

65. Ginsberg AM, Raffeld M, Cossman J: Inactivation of the retinoblastoma gene in human lymphoid neoplasms. Blood 77:833, 1991.

66. Weide R, Tiemann M, Pflüger K-H et al: Altered expression of the retinoblastoma gene product in human high grade non-Hodgkin's lymphomas. Leukemia 8:97, 1994.

67. Schaffner C, Idler I, Stilgenbauer S et al: Mantle cell lymphoma is characterized by inactivation of the ATM gene. Proc Natl Acad Sci U S A 97:2773, 2000.

68. Offit K, Parsa NZ, Gaidano G et al: 6q deletions define distinct clinico-pathologic subsets of non-Hodgkin's lymphoma. Blood 82:2157, 1993.

69. Mertens F, Johansson B, Mitelman F: Isochromosomes in neoplasia. Genes Chromosomes Cancer 10:221, 1994.

70. Mrózek K, Bloomfield CD: New recurrent structural chromosome aberrations in non-Hodgkin's lymphoma: A review of the published literature. Int J Oncol 8:851, 1996.

71. Mrózek K, Bloomfield CD: Der(16)t(1;16) is a secondary chromosome aberration in at least eighteen different types of human cancer. Genes Chromosomes Cancer 23:78, 1998.

72. Sawyer JR, Tricot G, Mattox S et al: Jumping translocations of chromosome 1q in multiple myeloma: Evidence for a mechanism involving decondensation of pericentromeric heterochromatin. Blood 91:1732, 1998.

73. Fukuhara S, Ohno H, Amakawa R et al: Significance of extra 18q− chromosome in Japanese t(14;18)-positive lymphoma. Blood 71:1748, 1988.

74. Whang-Peng J, Knutsen T, Jaffe ES et al: Sequential analysis of 43 patients with non-Hodgkin's lymphoma: Clinical correlations with cytogenetic, histologic, immunophenotyping, and molecular studies. Blood 85:203, 1995.

75. Horsman DE, Connors JM, Pantzar T, Gascoyne RD: Analysis of secondary chromosomal alterations in 165 cases of follicular lymphoma with t(14;18). Genes Chromosomes Cancer 30:375, 2001.

76. Juliusson G, Oscier DG, Fitchett M et al: Prognostic subgroups in B-cell chronic lymphocytic leukemia defined by specific chromosomal abnormalities. N Engl J Med 323:720, 1990.

77. Finn WG, Kay NE, Kroft SH et al: Secondary abnormalities of chromosome 6q in B-cell chronic lymphocytic leukemia: A sequential study of karyotypic instability in 51 patients. Am J Hematol 59:223, 1998.

78. Döhner H, Stilgenbauer S, Döhner K et al: Chromosome aberrations in B-cell chronic lymphocytic leukemia: Reassessment based on molecular cytogenetic analysis. J Mol Med 77:266, 1999.

79. Döhner H, Stilgenbauer S, Benner A et al: Genomic aberrations and survival in chronic lymphocytic leukemia. N Engl J Med 343:1910, 2000.

80. Mitelman F: Catalog of Chromosome Aberrations in Cancer. 5th Ed. Wiley-Liss, New York, 1994.

81. Mrózek K, Bloomfield CD: Cytogenetics of indolent lymphomas. Semin Oncol 20(Suppl. 5):47, 1993.

82. Stilgenbauer S, Liebisch P, James MR et al: Molecular cytogenetic delineation of a novel critical genomic region in chromosome bands 11q22.3-q23.1 in lymphoproliferative disorders. Proc Natl Acad Sci U S A 93:11837, 1996.

83. Bullrich F, Rasio D, Kitada S et al: ATM mutations in B-cell chronic lymphocytic leukemia. Cancer Res 59:24, 1999.

84. Stankovic T, Weber P, Stewart G et al: Inactivation of ataxia telangiectasia mutated gene in B-cell chronic lymphocytic leukaemia. Lancet 353:26, 1999.

85. Schaffner C, Stilgenbauer S, Rappold GA et al: Somatic ATM mutations indicate a pathogenic role of ATM in B-cell chronic lymphocytic leukemia. Blood 94:748, 1999.

86. Tilly H, Bastard C, Halkin E et al: Del(14)(q22) in diffuse B-cell lymphocytic lymphoma. Am J Clin Pathol 89:109, 1988.

87. Kristoffersson U, Heim S, Johnsson A et al: Deletion of 14q in non-Hodgkin's lymphoma. Eur J Haematol 44:261, 1990.

88. Hammond DW, Goepel JR, Aitken M et al: Cytogenetic analysis of a United Kingdom series of non-Hodgkins lymphomas. Cancer Genet Cytogenet 61:31, 1992.

89. Fleischman EW, Prigogina EL, Ilynskaya GW et al: Chromosomal characteristics of malignant lymphoma. Hum Genet 82:343, 1989.

90. Schouten HC, Sanger WG, Weisenburger DD et al: Abnormalities involving chromosome 6 in newly diagnosed patients with non-Hodgkin's lymphoma. Cancer Genet Cytogenet 47:73, 1990.

91. Offit K, Louie DC, Parsa NZ et al: Clinical and morphologic features of B-cell small lymphocytic lymphoma with del(6)(q21q23). Blood 83:2611, 1994.

92. Geisler CH, Philip P, Christensen BE et al: In B-cell chronic lymphocytic leukaemia chromosome 17 abnormalities and not trisomy 12 are the single most important cytogenetic abnormalities for the prognosis: A cytogenetic and immunophenotypic study of 480 unselected newly diagnosed patients. Leuk Res 21:1011, 1997.

93. Newman RA, Peterson B, Davey FR et al: Phenotypic markers and BCL-1 gene rearrangements in B-cell chronic lymphocytic leukemia: A Cancer and Leukemia Group B Study. Blood 82:1239, 1993.

94. De Angeli C, Gandini D, Cuneo A et al: BCL-1 rearrangements and p53 mutations in atypical chronic lymphocytic leukemia with t(11;14)(q13;q32). Haematologica 85:913, 2000.

95. Gaidano G, Newcomb EW, Gong JZ et al: Analysis of alterations of oncogenes and tumor suppressor genes in chronic lymphocytic leukemia. Am J Pathol 144:1312, 1994.

96. Brizard F, Dreyfus B, Guilhot F et al: 11q13 rearrangement in B cell chronic lymphocytic leukemia. Leuk Lymphoma 25:539, 1997.

97. Laï JL, Michaux L, Dastugue N et al: Cytogenetics in multiple myeloma: A multicenter study of 24 patients with t(11;14)(q13;q32) or its variant. Cancer Genet Cytogenet 104:133, 1998.

98. Oscier DG, Matutes E, Gardiner A et al: Cytogenetic studies in splenic lymphoma with villous lymphocytes. Br J Haematol 85:487, 1993.

99. Troussard X, Mauvieux L, Radford-Weiss I et al: Genetic analysis of splenic lymphoma with villous lymphocytes: A Groupe Français d'Hématologie Cellulaire (GFHC) study. Br J Haematol 101:712, 1998.

100. Brito-Babapulle V, Ellis J, Matutes E et al: Translocation t(11;14)(q13;q32) in chronic lymphoid disorders. Genes Chromosomes Cancer 5:158, 1992.

101. Takashima T, Itoh M, Ueda Y et al: Detection of 14q32.33 translocation and t(11;14) in interphase nuclei of chronic B-cell leukemia/lymphomas by in situ hybridization. Int J Cancer 72:31, 1997.

102. Offit K, Parsa NZ, Filippa D et al: t(9;14)(p13;q32) denotes a subset of low-grade non-Hodgkin's lymphoma with plasmacytoid differentiation. Blood 80:2594, 1992.

103. Levine EG, Arthur DC, Machnicki J et al: Four new recurring translocations in non-Hodgkin's lymphoma. Blood 74:1796, 1989.

104. Ott G, Katzenberger T, Greiner A et al: The t(11;18)(q21;q21) chromosome translocation is a frequent and specific aberration in low-grade but not high-grade malignant non-Hodgkin's lymphomas of the mucosa-associated lymphoid tissue (MALT-) type. Cancer Res 57:3944, 1997.

105. Dierlamm J, Wlodarska I, Michaux L et al: Genetic abnormalities in marginal zone B-cell lymphoma. Hematol Oncol 18:1, 2000.

106. Rosenwald A, Ott G, Stilgenbauer S et al: Exclusive detection of the t(11;18)(q21;q21) in extranodal marginal zone B cell lymphomas (MZBL) of MALT type in contrast to other MZBL and extranodal large B cell lymphomas. Am J Pathol 155:1817, 1999.

107. Maes B, Baens M, Marynen P, De Wolf-Peeters C: The product of the t(11;18), an API2-MLT fusion, is an almost exclusive finding in marginal zone cell lymphoma of extranodal MALT-type. Ann Oncol 11:521, 2000.

108. Clark HM, Jones DB, Wright DH: Cytogenetic and molecular studies of t(14;18) and t(14;19) in nodal and extranodal B-cell lymphoma. J Pathol 166:129, 1992.

109. Fukuhara S, Rowley JD: Chromosome 14 translocations in non-Burkitt lymphomas. Int J Cancer 22:14, 1978.

110. Fukuhara S, Rowley JD, Variakojis D et al: Chromosome abnormalities in poorly differentiated lymphocytic lymphoma. Cancer Res 39:3119, 1979.

111. Tsujimoto Y, Finger LR, Yunis J et al: Cloning of the chromosome breakpoint of neoplastic B cells with the t(14;18) chromosome translocation. Science 226:1097, 1984.

112. Korsmeyer SJ: BCL-2 gene family and the regulation of programmed cell death. Cancer Res 59(Suppl.):1693s, 1999.

113. Sanger WG, Armitage JO, Bridge J et al: Initial and subsequent cytogenetic studies in malignant lymphoma. Cancer 60:3014, 1987.

114. Levine EG, Juneja S, Arthur D et al: Sequential karyotypes in non-Hodgkin lymphoma: Their nature and significance. Genes Chromosomes Cancer 1:270, 1990.

115. Liu Y, Hernandez AM, Shibata D, Cortopassi GA: *BCL2* translocation frequency rises with age in humans. Proc Natl Acad Sci U S A 91:8910, 1994.

116. Mrózek K, Bloomfield CD: Major cytogenetic findings in non-Hodgkin's lymphoma. In Canellos GP, Lister TA, Sklar JL (eds.): The Lymphomas, p. 107. WB Saunders Co., Philadelphia, 1998.

117. Richardson ME, Chen Q, Filippa DA et al: Intermediate- to high-grade histology of lymphomas carrying t(14;18) is associated with additional nonrandom chromosome changes. Blood 70:444, 1987.

118. Yunis JJ, Frizzera G, Oken MM et al: Multiple recurrent genomic defects in follicular lymphoma. A possible model for cancer. N Engl J Med 316:79, 1987.

119. Armitage JO, Sanger WG, Weisenburger DD et al: Correlation of secondary cytogenetic abnormalities with histologic appearance in non-Hodgkin's lymphomas bearing t(14;18)(q32;q21). J Natl Cancer Inst 80:576, 1988.

120. Goyns MH, Hammond DW, Harrison CJ et al: Structural abnormalities of the X chromosome in non-Hodgkin's lymphoma. Leukemia 7:848, 1993.

121. Dave BJ, Hess MM, Pickering DL et al: Rearrangements of chromosome band 1p36 in non-Hodgkin's lymphoma. Clin Cancer Res 5:1401, 1999.

122. Viardot A, Martin-Subero JI, Siebert R et al: Detection of secondary genetic aberrations in follicle center cell derived lymphomas: Assessment of the reliability of comparative genomic hybridization and standard chromosome analysis. Leukemia 15:177, 2001.

123. Maseki N, Kaneko Y, Sakurai M et al: Chromosome abnormalities in malignant lymphoma in patients from Saitama. Cancer Res 47:6767, 1987.

124. Konishi H, Sakurai M, Nakao H et al: Chromosome abnormalities in malignant lymphoma in patients from Kurashiki: Histological and immunophenotypic correlations. Cancer Res 50:2698, 1990.

125. Ladanyi M, Offit K, Parsa NZ et al: Follicular lymphoma with t(8;14)(q24;q32): A distinct clinical and molecular subset of t(8;14)-bearing lymphomas. Blood 79:2124, 1992.

126. Bajalica S, Brøndum-Nielsen K, Sørensen AG et al: Characterization of add(1)(p36) in non-Hodgkin lymphomas by fluorescence in situ hybridization. Genes Chromosomes Cancer 13:34, 1995.

127. Dierlamm J, Wlodarska I, Michaux L et al: FISH identifies different types of duplications with 12q13-15 as the commonly involved segment in B-cell lymphoproliferative malignancies characterized by partial trisomy 12. Genes Chromosomes Cancer 20:155, 1997.

128. Vandenberghe E, De Wolf Peeters C, Wlodarska I et al: Chromosome 11q rearrangements in B non Hodgkin's lymphoma. Br J Haematol 81:212, 1992.

129. Nakamine H, Masih AS, Chan WC et al: Oncogene rearrangement in non-Hodgkin's lymphoma with a 14q+ chromosome of unknown origin. Leuk Lymphoma 10:79, 1993.

130. Pezzella F, Ralfkiaer E, Gatter KC et al: The 14;18 translocation in European cases of follicular lymphoma: Comparison of Southern blotting and the polymerase chain reaction. Br J Haematol 76:58, 1990.

131. Fleischman EW, Prigogina EL: Karyotype peculiarities of malignant lymphomas. Hum Genet 35:269, 1977.

132. Van Den Berghe H, Parloir C, David G et al: A new characteristic karyotypic anomaly in lymphoproliferative disorders. Cancer 44:188, 1979.

133. Weisenburger DD, Sanger WG, Armitage JO et al: Intermediate lymphocytic lymphoma: Immunophenotypic and cytogenetic findings. Blood 69:1617, 1987.

134. Leroux D, Le Marc'Hadour F, Gressin R et al: Non-Hodgkin's lymphomas with t(11;14)(q13;q32): A subset of mantle zone/intermediate lymphocytic lymphoma? Br J Haematol 77:346, 1991.

135. Criel A, Billiet J, Vandenberghe E et al: Leukaemic intermediate lymphocytic lymphomas: Analysis of twelve cases diagnosed by morphology. Leuk Lymphoma 8:381, 1992.

136. Vandenberghe E, De Wolf-Peeters C, Van Den Oord J et al: Translocation (11;14): A cytogenetic anomaly associated with B-cell lymphomas of non-follicle centre cell lineage. J Pathol 163:13, 1991.

137. Raffeld M, Jaffe ES: bcl-1, t(11;14), and mantle cell-derived lymphomas. Blood 78:259, 1991.

138. Rosenberg CL, Wong E, Petty EM et al: *PRAD1*, a candidate *BCL1* oncogene: Mapping and expression in centrocytic lymphoma. Proc Natl Acad Sci U S A 88:9638, 1991.

139. Akiyama N, Tsuruta H, Sasaki H et al: Messenger RNA levels of five genes located at chromosome 11q13 in B-cell tumors with chromosome translocation t(11;14)(q13;q32). Cancer Res 54:377, 1994.

140. Rimokh R, Berger F, Delsol G et al: Rearrangement and overexpression of the *BCL-1/PRAD-1* gene in intermediate lymphocytic lymphomas and in t(11q13)-bearing leukemias. Blood 81:3063, 1993.

141. Komatsu H, Yoshida K, Seto M et al: Overexpression of PRAD1 in a mantle zone lymphoma patient with a t(11;22)(q13;q11) translocation. Br J Haematol 85:427, 1993.

142. Medeiros LJ, Van Krieken JH, Jaffe ES et al: Association of bcl-1 rearrangements with lymphocytic lymphoma of intermediate differentiation. Blood 76:2086, 1990.

143. Wotherspoon AC, Pan L, Diss TC et al: A genotypic study of low grade B-cell lymphomas, including lymphomas of mucosa-associated lymphoid tissue (MALT). J Pathol 162:135, 1990.

144. Athan E, Foitl DR, Knowles DM: BCL-1 rearrangement. Frequency and clinical significance among B-cell chronic lymphocytic leukemias and non-Hodgkin's lymphomas. Am J Pathol 138:591, 1991.

145. Williams ME, Swierdlow SH, Rosenberg CL, Arnold A: Characterization of chromosome 11 translocation breakpoints at the *bcl*-1 and *PRAD1* loci in centrocytic lymphoma. Cancer Res 52 (Suppl):5541s, 1992.

146. Wlodarska I, Pittaluga S, Hagemeijer A et al: Secondary chromosome changes in mantle cell lymphoma. Haematologica 84:594, 1999.

147. Bentz M, Plesch A, Bullinger L et al: t(11;14)-positive mantle cell lymphomas exhibit complex karyotypes and share similarities with B-cell chronic lymphocytic leukemia. Genes Chromosomes Cancer 27:285, 2000.

148. Beà S, Ribas M, Hernández JM et al: Increased number of chromosomal imbalances and high-level DNA amplifications in mantle cell lymphoma are associated with blastoid variants. Blood 93:4365, 1999.

149. Cuneo A, Bigoni R, Rigolin GM et al: Cytogenetic profile of lymphoma of follicle mantle lineage: Correlation with clinicobiologic features. Blood 93:1372, 1999.

150. Kaneko Y, Rowley JD, Variakojis D et al: Prognostic implications of karyotype and morphology in patients with non-Hodgkin's lymphoma. Int J Cancer 32:683, 1983.

151. Berger R, Bernheim A, Valensi F et al: 22q– and 8q– in a non-Burkitt lymphoma. Cancer Genet Cytogenet 8:91, 1983.

152. Offit K, Jhanwar S, Ebrahim SAD et al: t(3;22)(q27;q11): A novel translocation associated with diffuse non-Hodgkin's lymphoma. Blood 74:1876, 1989.

153. Leroux D, Stul M, Sotto JJ et al: Translocation t(3;22)(q28;q11) in three patients with diffuse large B cell lymphoma. Leukemia 4:373, 1990.

154. Bastard C, Deweindt C, Kerckaert JP et al: *LAZ3* rearrangements in non-Hodgkin's lymphoma: Correlation with histology, immunophenotype, karyotype, and clinical outcome in 217 patients. Blood 83:2423, 1994.

155. Wlodarska I, Mecucci C, Stul M et al: Fluorescence in situ hybridization identifies new chromosomal changes involving 3q27 in non-Hodgkin's lymphomas with *BCL6/LAZ3* rearrangement. Genes Chromosomes Cancer 14:1, 1995.

156. Lo Coco F, Ye BH, Lista F et al: Rearrangements of the *BCL6* gene in diffuse large cell non-Hodgkin's lymphoma. Blood 83:1757, 1994.

157. Otsuki T, Yano T, Clark HM et al: Analysis of LAZ3 (BCL-6) status in B-cell non-Hodgkin's lymphomas: Results of rearrangement and gene expression studies and a mutational analysis of coding region sequences. Blood 85:2877, 1995.

158. Capello D, Vitolo U, Pasqualucci L et al: Distribution and pattern of *BCL-6* mutations throughout the spectrum of B-cell neoplasia. Blood 95:651, 2000.

159. Pescarmona E, De Sanctis V, Pistilli A et al: Pathogenetic and clinical implications of Bcl-6 and Bcl-2 gene configuration in nodal diffuse large B-cell lymphomas. J Pathol 183:281, 1997.

160. Kramer MHH, Hermans J, Wijburg E et al: Clinical relevance of BCL-2, BCL6, and MYC rearrangements in diffuse large B-cell lymphoma. Blood 92:3152, 1998.

161. Vitolo U, Gaidano G, Botto B et al: Rearrangements of *bcl-6, bcl-2, c-myc* and 6q deletion in B-diffuse large-cell lymphoma: Clinical relevance in 71 patients. Ann Oncol 9:55, 1998.

162. Gaidano G, Carbone A, Dalla-Favera R: Genetic basis of acquired immunodeficiency syndrome-related lymphomagenesis. J Natl Cancer Inst Monogr 23:95, 1998.

163. Cigudosa JC, Parsa NZ, Louie DC et al: Cytogenetic analysis of 363 consecutively ascertained diffuse large B-cell lymphomas. Genes Chromosomes Cancer 25:123, 1999.

164. Weiss LM, Warnke RA, Sklar J et al: Molecular analysis of the t(14;18) chromosomal translocation in malignant lymphomas. N Engl J Med 317:1185, 1987.

165. Lukeis R, Juneja S, Tan L et al: Association of abnormalities of chromosome 11 with t(14;18) in diffuse non-Hodgkin's lymphoma. Cancer Genet Cytogenet 78:36, 1994.

166. Offit K, Parsa NZ, Jhanwar SC et al: Clusters of chromosome 9 aberrations are associated with clinico-pathologic subsets of non-Hodgkin's lymphoma. Genes Chromosomes Cancer 7:1, 1993.

167. Jonveaux P, Le Coniat M, Derr J et al: Loss of genetic material from the short arm of chromosome 12 is a frequent secondary abnormality in non-Hodgkin's lymphoma. Hematol Pathol 5:21, 1991.

168. Rao PH, Houldsworth J, Dyomina K et al: Chromosomal and gene amplification in diffuse large B-cell lymphoma. Blood 92:234, 1998.

169. Schlegelberger B, Zwingers T, Harder L et al: Clinicopathogenetic significance of chromosomal abnormalities in patients with blastic peripheral B-cell lymphoma. Blood 94:3114, 1999.

170. Hecht JL, Aster JC: Molecular biology of Burkitt's lymphoma. J Clin Oncol 18:3707, 2000.

171. Berger R, Bernheim A, Weh H-J et al: A new translocation in Burkitt's tumor cells. Hum Genet 53:111, 1979.

172. Van Den Berghe H, Parloir C, Gosseye S et al: Variant translocation in Burkitt lymphoma. Cancer Genet Cytogenet 1:9, 1979.

173. Miyoshi I, Hiraki S, Kimura I et al: 2/8 translocation in a Japanese Burkitt's lymphoma. Experientia 35:742, 1979.

174. Kornblau SM, Goodacre A, Cabanillas F: Chromosomal abnormalities in adult non-endemic Burkitt's lymphoma and leukemia: 22 new reports and a review of 148 cases from the literature. Hematol Oncol 9:63, 1991.

175. Chenevix-Trench G, Brown JA, Tyler GB et al: Chromosome analysis of 30 cases of non-Hodgkin's lymphoma. Med Oncol Tumor Pharmacother 5:17, 1988.

176. Morrison VA, Frizzera G, Arthur DC et al: Prognostic factors for therapeutic outcome of diffuse small non-cleaved cell lymphoma in adults. Am J Hematol 46:295, 1994.

177. Macpherson N, Lesack D, Klasa R et al: Small noncleaved, non-Burkitt's (Burkitt-like) lymphoma: Cytogenetics predict outcome and reflect clinical presentation. J Clin Oncol 17:1558, 1999.

178. Yano T, van Krieken JHJM, Magrath IT et al: Histogenetic correlations between subcategories of small noncleaved cell lymphomas. Blood 79:1282, 1992.

179. Gaidano G, Pastore C, Gloghini A et al: Genetic heterogeneity of AIDS-related small non-cleaved cell lymphoma. Br J Haematol 98:726, 1997.

180. Kaneko Y, Frizzera G, Shikano T et al: Chromosomal and immunophenotypic patterns in T cell acute lymphoblastic leukemia (T ALL) and lymphoblastic lymphoma (LBL). Leukemia 3:886, 1989.

181. Raimondi SC: Current status of cytogenetic research in childhood acute lymphoblastic leukemia. Blood 81:2237, 1993.

182. Pollak C, Hagemeijer A: Abnormalities of the short arm of chromosome 9 with partial loss of material in hematological disorders. Leukemia 1:541, 1987.

183. Shikano T, Ishikawa Y, Naito H et al: Cytogenetic characteristics of childhood non-Hodgkin lymphoma. Cancer 70:714, 1992.

184. Mikraki V, Jhanwar SC, Filippa DA et al: Distinct patterns of chromosome abnormalities characterize childhood non-Hodgkin's lymphoma. Br J Haematol 80:15, 1992.

185. Inhorn RC, Aster JC, Roach SA et al: A syndrome of lymphoblastic lymphoma, eosinophilia, and myeloid hyperplasia/malignancy associated with t(8;13)(p11;q11): Description of a distinctive clinicopathologic entity. Blood 85:1881, 1995.

186. Naeem R, Singer S, Fletcher JA: Translocation t(8;13)(p11;q11-12) in stem cell leukemia/lymphoma of T-cell and myeloid lineages. Genes Chromosomes Cancer 12:148, 1995.

187. Kaneko Y, Maseki N, Sakurai M et al: Characteristic karyotypic pattern in T-cell lymphoproliferative disorders with reactive "angioimmunoblastic lymphadenopathy with dysproteinemia-type" features. Blood 72:413, 1988.

188. Schlegelberger B, Himmler A, Gödde E et al: Cytogenetic findings in peripheral T-cell lymphomas as a basis for distinguishing low-grade and high-grade lymphomas. Blood 83:505, 1994.

189. Lepretre S, Buchonnet G, Stamatoullas A et al: Chromosome abnormalities in peripheral T-cell lymphoma. Cancer Genet Cytogenet 117:71, 2000.

190. Inwards DJ, Habermann TM, Banks PM et al: Cytogenetic findings in 21 cases of peripheral T-cell lymphoma. Am J Hematol 35:88, 1990.

191. Ebrahim SAD, Ladanyi M, Desai SB et al: Immunohistochemical, molecular, and cytogenetic analysis of a consecutive series of 20 peripheral T-cell lymphomas and lymphomas of uncertain lineage, including 12 Ki-1 positive lymphomas. Genes Chromosomes Cancer 2:27, 1990.

192. Wang CC, Tien HF, Lin MT et al: Consistent presence of isochromosome 7q in hepatosplenic T γ/δ lymphoma: A new cytoge-

netic-clinicopathologic entity. Genes Chromosomes Cancer 12:161, 1995.

193. Khan WA, Yu L, Eisenbrey AB et al: Hepatosplenic gamma/delta T-cell lymphoma in immunocompromised patients. Report of two cases and review of literature. Am J Clin Pathol 116:41, 2001.

194. Stein H, Foss HD, Durkop H et al: CD30(+) anaplastic large cell lymphoma: A review of its histopathologic, genetic, and clinical features. Blood 96:3681, 2000.

195. Kristoffersson U, Heim S, Heldrup J et al: Cytogenetic studies of childhood non-Hodgkin lymphomas. Hereditas 103:77, 1985.

196. Morgan R, Hecht BK, Sandberg AA et al: Chromosome 5q35 break-point in malignant histiocytosis. N Engl J Med 314:1322, 1986.

197. Soulie J, Rousseau-Merck M-F, Mouly H et al: Cytogenetic study of malignant histiocytosis transplanted into nude mice; presence of translocation between chromosomes 5 and 6 and a unique marker (13q+). Virchows Arch B Cell Pathol Incl Mol Pathol 50:339, 1986.

198. Kaneko Y, Frizzera G, Edamura S et al: A novel translocation, t(2;5)(p23;q35), in childhood phagocytic large T-cell lymphoma mimicking malignant histiocytosis. Blood 73:806, 1989.

199. Rimokh R, Magaud J-P, Berger F et al: A translocation involving a specific breakpoint (q35) on chromosome 5 is characteristic of anaplastic large cell lymphoma ('Ki-1 lymphoma'). Br J Haematol 71:31, 1989.

200. Le Beau MM, Bitter MA, Larson RA et al: The t(2;5)(p23;q35): A recurring chromosomal abnormality in Ki-1-positive anaplastic large cell lymphoma. Leukemia 3:866, 1989.

201. Mason DY, Bastard C, Rimokh R et al: CD30-positive large cell lymphomas ('Ki-1 lymphoma') are associated with a chromosomal translocation involving 5q35. Br J Haematol 74:161, 1990.

202. Kinney MC, Collins RD, Greer JP et al: A small-cell-predominant variant of primary Ki-1 (CD30)+ T-cell lymphoma. Am J Surg Pathol 17:859, 1993.

203. Kuefer MU, Look AT, Pulford K et al: Retrovirus-mediated gene transfer of *NPM-ALK* causes lymphoid malignancy in mice. Blood 90:2901, 1997.

204. Morris SW, Xue L, Ma Z, Kinney MC: Alk+ CD30+ lymphomas: A distinct molecular genetic subtype of non-Hodgkin's lymphoma. Br J Haematol 113:275, 2001.

205. Nowell PC: Cytogenetics of tumor progression. Cancer 65:2172, 1990.

206. Horning SJ: Natural history of and therapy for the indolent non-Hodgkin's lymphomas. Semin Oncol 20(Suppl. 5):75, 1993.

207. Bernell P, Jacobsson B, Liliemark J et al: Gain of chromosome 7 marks the progression from indolent to aggressive follicle centre lymphoma and is a common finding in patients with diffuse large B-cell lymphoma: A study by FISH. Br J Haematol 101:487, 1998.

208. Bernell P, Arvidsson I, Jacobsson B: Gain of chromosome 7, which marks the progression from indolent to aggressive follicle centre lymphomas, is restricted to the B-lymphoid cell lineage: A study by FISH in combination with morphology and immunocyto-chemistry. Br J Haematol 105:1140, 1999.

209. Tilly H, Rossi A, Stamatoullas A et al: Prognostic value of chromosomal abnormalities in follicular lymphoma. Blood 84:1043, 1994.

210. De Jong D, Voetdijk BMH, Beverstock GC et al: Activation of the c-myc oncogene in a precursor-B-cell blast crisis of follicular lymphoma, presenting as composite lymphoma. N Engl J Med 318:1373, 1988.

211. Lee JT, Innes DJ Jr, Williams ME: Sequential bcl-2 and c-myc oncogene rearrangements associated with the clinical transformation of non-Hodgkin's lymphoma. J Clin Invest 84:1454, 1989.

212. Koduru PRK, Offit K: Molecular structure of double reciprocal translocations: Significance in B-cell lymphomagenesis. Oncogene 6:145, 1991.

213. Yano T, Jaffe ES, Longo DL et al: MYC rearrangements in histologically progressed follicular lymphomas. Blood 80:758, 1992.

214. Cabanillas F, Pathak S, Trujillo J et al: Frequent nonrandom chromosome abnormalities in 27 patients with untreated large cell lymphoma and immunoblastic lymphoma. Cancer Res 48:5557, 1988.

215. Rodriguez MA, Ford RJ, Goodacre A et al: Chromosome 17p and p53 changes in lymphoma. Br J Haematol 79:575, 1991.

216. Møller MB, Nielsen O, Pedersen NT: Oncoprotein MDM2 overexpression is associated with poor prognosis in distinct non-Hodgkin's lymphoma entities. Mod Pathol 12:1010, 1999.

217. Hartwell L: Defects in a cell cycle checkpoint may be responsible for the genomic instability of cancer cells. Cell 71:543, 1992.

218. Mrózek K, Heinonen K, Bloomfield CD: Clinical importance of cytogenetics in acute myeloid leukaemia. Best Pract Res Clin Haematol 14:19, 2001.

219. Wetzler M, Dodge RK, Mrózek K et al: Prospective karyotype analysis in adult acute lymphoblastic leukemia: The Cancer and Leukemia Group B experience. Blood 93:3983, 1999.

220. Levine EG, Arthur DC, Frizzera G et al: Cytogenetic abnormalities predict clinical outcome in non-Hodgkin lymphoma. Ann Intern Med 108:14, 1988.

221. Offit K, Wong G, Filippa DA et al: Cytogenetic analysis of 434 consecutively ascertained specimens of non-Hodgkin's lymphoma: Clinical correlations. Blood 77:1508, 1991.

222. Schlegelberger B, Zwingers T, Hohenadel K et al: Significance of cytogenetic findings for the clinical outcome in patients with T-cell lymphoma of angioimmunoblastic lymphadenopathy type. J Clin Oncol 14:593, 1996.

223. Juneja S, Matthews J, Lukeis R et al: Prognostic value of cytogenetic abnormalities in previously untreated patients with non-Hodgkin's lymphoma. Leuk Lymphoma 25:493, 1997.

224. Jerkeman M, Johansson B, Åkerman M et al: Prognostic implications of cytogenetic aberrations in diffuse large B-cell lymphomas. Eur J Haematol 62:184, 1999.

225. Kristoffersson U, Heim S, Mandahl N et al: Prognostic implication of cytogenetic findings in 106 patients with non-Hodgkin lymphoma. Cancer Genet Cytogenet 25:55, 1987.

226. Haus O, Kozlowska J, Zubkiewicz L et al: Cytogenetic studies in patients with non-Hodgkin's lymphoma (NHL) (in Polish). Pol Arch Med Wewn 86:132, 1991.

227. Cowan RA, Harris M, Jones M et al: DNA content in high and intermediate grade non-Hodgkin's lymphoma—prognostic significance and clinicopathological correlations. Br J Cancer 60:904, 1989.

228. Yunis JJ, Mayer MG, Arnesen MA et al: bcl-2 and other genomic alterations in the prognosis of large-cell lymphoma. N Engl J Med 320:1047, 1989.

229. Pezzella F, Jones M, Ralfkiaer E et al: Evaluation of bcl-2 protein expression and 14;18 translocation as prognostic markers in follicular lymphoma. Br J Cancer 65:87, 1992.

230. Johnson A, Brun A, Dictor M et al: Incidence and prognostic significance of t(14;18) translocation in follicle center cell lymphoma of low and high grade. A report from southern Sweden. Ann Oncol 6:789, 1995.

231. Weisenburger DD, Gascoyne RD, Bierman PJ et al: Clinical significance of the t(14;18) and *BCL2* overexpression in follicular large cell lymphoma. Leuk Lymphoma 36:513, 2000.

232. López-Guillermo A, Cabanillas F, McDonnell TI et al: Correlation of *bcl-2* rearrangement with clinical characteristics and outcome in indolent follicular lymphoma. Blood 93:3081, 1999.

233. Romaguera JE, Pugh W, Luthra R et al: The clinical relevance of t(14;18)/bcl-2 rearrangement and DEL 6q in diffuse large cell lymphoma and immunoblastic lymphoma. Ann Oncol 4:51, 1993.

234. Jacobson JO, Wilkes BM, Kwiatkowski DJ et al: bcl-2 rearrangements in de novo diffuse large cell lymphoma. Association with distinctive clinical features. Cancer 72:231, 1993.

235. Tang SC, Visser L, Hepperle B et al: Clinical significance of bcl-2-MBR gene rearrangement and protein expression in diffuse large-cell non-Hodgkin's lymphoma: An analysis of 83 cases. J Clin Oncol 12:149, 1994.

236. Offit K, Koduru PRK, Hollis R et al: 18q21 rearrangement in diffuse large cell lymphoma: Incidence and clinical significance. Br J Haematol 72:178, 1989.

237. Gascoyne RD, Adomat SA, Krajewski S et al: Prognostic significance of Bcl-2 protein expression and Bcl-2 gene rearrangement in diffuse aggressive non-Hodgkin's lymphoma. Blood 90:244, 1997.

238. Hill ME, MacLennan KA, Cunningham DC et al: Prognostic significance of BCL-2 expression and bcl-2 major breakpoint region rearrangement in diffuse large cell non-Hodgkin's lymphoma: A British National Lymphoma Investigation Study. Blood 88:1046, 1996.

239. Alizadeh AA, Eisen MB, Davis RE et al: Distinct types of diffuse large B-cell lymphoma identified by gene expression profiling. Nature 403:503, 2000.

240. Shipp M, Tamayo P, Angelo M et al: Diffuse large B cell lymphoma outcome prediction by gene expression profiling. Blood 96:222a, 2000.

241. Cabanillas F, Pathak S, Grant G et al: Refractoriness to chemotherapy and poor survival related to abnormalities of chromosomes 17 and 7 in lymphoma. Am J Med 87:167, 1989.

242. Stokke T, Galteland E, Holte H et al: Oncogenic aberrations in the p53 pathway are associated with a high S phase fraction and poor patient survival in B-cell non-Hodgkin's lymphoma. Int J Cancer 89:313, 2000.

243. Ichikawa A, Kinoshita T, Watanabe T et al: Mutations of the p53 gene as a prognostic factor in aggressive B-cell lymphoma. N Engl J Med 337:529, 1997.

244. Greiner TC, Moynihan MJ, Chan WC et al: p53 mutations in mantle cell lymphoma are associated with variant cytology and predict a poor prognosis. Blood 87:4302, 1996.

245. Offit K, Lo Coco F, Louie DC et al: Rearrangement of the bcl-6 gene as a prognostic marker in diffuse large-cell lymphoma. N Engl J Med 331:74, 1994.

246. Akasaka T, Ueda C, Kurata M et al: Nonimmunoglobulin (non-Ig)/BCL6 gene fusion in diffuse large B-cell lymphoma results in worse prognosis than Ig/BCL6. Blood 96:2907, 2000.

247. Offit K, Louie DC, Parsa NZ et al: BCL6 gene rearrangement and other cytogenetic abnormalities in diffuse large cell lymphoma. Leuk Lymphoma 20:85, 1995.

248. Poppema S, Kaleta J, Hepperle B: Chromosomal abnormalities in patients with Hodgkin's disease: Evidence for frequent involvement of the 14q chromosomal region but infrequent bcl-2 gene rearrangement in Reed-Sternberg cells. J Natl Cancer Inst 84:1789, 1992.

249. Inghirami G, Macri L, Rosati S et al: The Reed-Sternberg cells of Hodgkin disease are clonal. Proc Natl Acad Sci U S A 91:9842, 1994.

250. Schlegelberger B, Weber-Matthiesen K, Himmler A et al: Cytogenetic findings and results of combined immunophenotyping and karyotyping in Hodgkin's disease. Leukemia 8:72, 1994.

251. Falzetti D, Crescenzi B, Matteucci C et al: Genomic instability and recurrent breakpoints are main cytogenetic findings in Hodgkin's disease. Haematologica 84:298, 1999.

252. Pedersen RK, Sørensen AG, Pedersen NT et al: Chromosome aberrations in adult Hodgkin disease in a Danish population-based study. Cancer Genet Cytogenet 110:128, 1999.

253. Thangavelu M, Le Beau MM: Chromosomal abnormalities in Hodgkin's disease. Hematol Oncol Clin North Am 3:221, 1989.

254. Kristoffersson U, Heim S, Mandahl N et al: Cytogenetic studies in Hodgkin disease. Acta Path Microbiol Immunol Scand Sect A 95:289, 1987.

255. Schouten HC, Sanger WG, Duggan M et al: Chromosomal abnormalities in Hodgkin's disease. Blood 73:2149, 1989.

256. Ladanyi M, Parsa NZ, Offit K et al: Clonal cytogenetic abnormalities in Hodgkin's disease. Genes Chromosomes Cancer 3:294, 1991.

257. Döhner H, Bloomfield CD, Frizzera G et al: Recurring chromosome abnormalities in Hodgkin's disease. Genes Chromosomes Cancer 5:392, 1992.

258. Tilly H, Bastard C, Delastre T et al: Cytogenetic studies in untreated Hodgkin's disease. Blood 77:1298, 1991.

259. Ankathil R, Vijayakumar T, Pillai GR, Krishnan Nair M: Chromosomes in Hodgkin's disease—analysis of involved lymph nodes. Neoplasma 39:245, 1992.

260. Weber-Matthiesen K, Deerberg J, Poetsch M et al: Numerical chromosome aberrations are present within the CD30+ Hodgkin and Reed-Sternberg cells in 100% of analyzed cases of Hodgkin's disease. Blood 86:1464, 1995.

261. Gupta RK, Norton AJ, Thompson IW et al: p53 expression in Reed-Sternberg cells of Hodgkin's disease. Br J Cancer 66:649, 1992.

262. Doussis IA, Pezzella F, Lane DP et al: An immunocytochemical study of p53 and bcl-2 protein expression in Hodgkin's disease. Am J Clin Pathol 99:663, 1993.

263. Trümper LH, Brady G, Bagg A et al: Single-cell analysis of Hodgkin and Reed-Sternberg cells: Molecular heterogeneity of gene expression and p53 mutations. Blood 81:3097, 1993.

264. Montesinos-Rongen M, Roers A, Küppers R et al: Mutation of the p53 gene is not a typical feature of Hodgkin and Reed-Sternberg cells in Hodgkin's disease. Blood 94:1755, 1999.

265. Küpper M, Joos S, von Bonin F et al: MDM2 gene amplification and lack of p53 point mutations in Hodgkin and Reed-Sternberg cells: Results from single-cell polymerase chain reaction and molecular cytogenetic studies. Br J Haematol 112:768, 2001.

266. Emmerich F, Meiser M, Hummel M et al: Overexpression of I kappa B alpha without inhibition of NF-κB activity and mutations in the I kappa B alpha gene in Reed-Sternberg cells. Blood 94:3129, 1999.

267. Jungnickel B, Staratschek-Jox A, Bräuninger A et al: Clonal deleterious mutations in the IκBα gene in the malignant cells in Hodgkin's lymphoma. J Exp Med 191:395, 2000.

268. Hasse U, Tinguely M, Leibundgut EO et al: Clonal loss of heterozygosity in microdissected Hodgkin and Reed-Sternberg cells. J Natl Cancer Inst 91:1581, 1999.

269. MacLeod RAF, Spitzer D, Bar-Am I et al: Karyotypic dissection of Hodgkin's disease cell lines reveals ectopic subtelomeres and ribosomal DNA at sites of multiple jumping translocations and genomic amplification. Leukemia 14:1803, 2000.

270. Staudt LM: The molecular and cellular origins of Hodgkin's disease. J Exp Med 191:207, 2000.

271. Cabanillas F: A review and interpretation of cytogenetic abnormalities identified in Hodgkin's disease. Hematol Oncol 6:271, 1988.

272. Franke S, Wlodarska I, Maes B et al: Lymphocyte predominance Hodgkin disease is characterized by recurrent genomic imbalances. Blood 97:1845, 2001.

273. Hossfeld DK, Schmidt CG: Chromosome findings in effusions from patients with Hodgkin's disease. Int J Cancer 21:147, 1978.

274. Gupta RK, Lister TA, Bodmer JG: The t(14;18) chromosomal translocation and bcl-2 protein expression in Hodgkin's disease. Leukemia 8:1337, 1994.

275. Gravel S, Delsol G, Al Saati T: Single-cell analysis of the t(14;18)(q32;q21) chromosomal translocation in Hodgkin's disease demonstrates the absence of this translocation in neoplastic Hodgkin and Reed-Sternberg cells. Blood 91:2866, 1998.

276. Stetler-Stevenson M: The t(14;18) translocation in Hodgkin's disease. J Natl Cancer Inst 84:1770, 1992.

277. Chaganti SR, Chen W, Parsa N et al: Involvement of BCL6 in chromosomal aberrations affecting band 3q27 in B-cell non-Hodgkin lymphoma. Genes Chromosomes Cancer 23:323, 1998.

278. Levine EG, Arthur DC, Gajl-Peczalska KJ et al: Correlations between immunological phenotype and karyotype in malignant lymphoma. Cancer Res 46:6481, 1986.

279. Cuneo A, Bigoni R, Rigolin GM et al: Acquired chromosome 11q deletion involving the ataxia teleangiectasia locus in B-cell non-Hodgkin's lymphoma: Correlation with clinicobiologic features. J Clin Oncol 18:2607, 2000.

43

Diagnosis and Treatment of Hodgkin's Disease

Monica Balzarotti, Peter H. Wiernik, and Armando Santoro

At the beginning of the new millennium, the prognostic outlook for Hodgkin's disease is definitely more favorable than it was three decades ago. An extraordinary amount of new information is now available on the natural history of this lymphoma and its excellent response to various forms of treatment, and prolonged follow-up evaluation has provided the identification of treatment sequelae and new prognostic variables. The main task of young physicians is to learn how to think in terms of optimal strategy to achieve a high cure rate with acceptable toxicity. In particular, they should be aware that certain procedures or indications that were routine in the past (e.g., staging laparotomy, local radiation therapy to limited nodal stage disease) are now abandoned or applied with highly selective criteria in the light of new prognostic factors. Because of a more strategic approach to neoplastic diseases in general, tumor mass with its biological implications has become the determinant parameter on which the treatment plan should be based. Thus, modern clinical research should aim at improving the correct assessment and even the quantitation of tumor cell volume. Past and present experience confirms that the complexity of the clinical evaluation and modern sophisticated treatment modalities demand considerable technical resources and qualified personnel. Practicing physicians should therefore carefully evaluate whether their own experience and the facilities available to them are truly adequate. If not, patient referral to specialized centers is required.

NATURAL HISTORY

Patterns of Disease at Presentation

Nearly all patients with Hodgkin's disease present with asymptomatic lymphadenopathy, and the apparent onset of the disease occurs predominantly in the cervical-supraclavicular nodes (60 to 80 percent), secondarily in axillary nodes (10 to 20 percent), and rarely in inguinal nodes (10 to 20 percent). In some cases the first manifestations of disease are cough or dyspnea related to mediastinal involvement; in other cases they consist of systemic symptoms (fever, night sweats, or weight loss) with no apparent superficial lymphadenopathy. In rare cases a mediastinal mass is found by routine X-ray. In most patients the pattern of lymph node spread is central (cervical,

mediastinal, para-aortic). For reasons that are not yet clear, certain chains of lymph nodes (mesenteric, hepatic hilar, hypogastric, presacral, epitrochlear, popliteal) are seldom or rarely involved. Pulmonary hilar lymph nodes are clinically affected in about one-fifth of patients with mediastinal adenopathy, but they are more frequently involved when a large medistinal mass is present. Bulky disease is defined as a neoplastic mediastinal mass with a ratio of more than 0.33:1 between the largest transverse diameter of the mass and the transverse diameter of the thorax at the level of T5 to T6 on a standing posteroanterior chest radiograph,[1,2] whereas in other sites it is defined as any mass with a maximal diameter over 10 cm. Patients with bulky mediastinal involvement represent approximately 25 percent of all cases and may have extension of the tumor into lung, pericardium, or chest wall. Systemic symptoms are also frequently present.

In the great majority of patients, the initial pattern of spread occurs predictably via lymphatic channels to contiguous lymph-node chains and other lymphatic structures. This observation has provided the basis for prophylactic irradiation of adjacent nodal chains in patients with apparently localized nodal disease eligible for treatment by radiotherapy alone.[3,4]

The pattern of disease presentation is related to the histopathologic subgroup. In fact, most patients with lymphocyte-predominance (LP) histopathology present initially with only peripheral sites involved (cervical, inguinal, epitroclear chains), whereas most patients with nodular sclerosis (NS) present with supradiaphragmatic disease and mediastinal node involvement. In a patient with one of these variants, limited extension of supradiaphragmatic disease and absence of systemic symptoms, occult involvement elsewhere is extremely rare. Patients with mixed-cellularity (MC) histology usually present either with upper torso disease or with lymphoma on both sides of the diaphragm.

Vascular invasion (unequivocal involvement of the lumina of vessels), which is noted in about 40 percent of autopsy cases, appears most often in lymphocyte-depletion (LD) histology and in advanced phases of disease.[5] Most extranodal sites manifest a markedly greater degree of vascular invasion, which suggests that vascular invasion is a factor in extranodal spread and in lethal cases of Hodgkin's disease. Other clusters of presentation described in the past have at present lost their prognostic significance, as front-line chemotherapy is given to the majority of patients, and its duration and intensity are dependent on prognostic parameters other than histologic subgroup, with the exception of LP stage I, which is still usually treated with and curable by limited-field radiotherapy alone. Spleen, liver, and bone marrow are the most frequent extranodal sites involved. Bone marrow is more frequently involved in advanced stages of disease with associated systemic symptoms. Liver invasion is always associated with spleen involvement. More frequently, extranodal sites are involved as a consequence of enlargement of adjacent nodal sites, as is the case with lung, pleural, or pericardial involvement by contiguous spread from bulky mediastinal lymphadenopathy.

The pathologic findings at autopsy have changed since a curative treatment approach has been widely applied. In fact, a distinct reduction in the extent of disease at the time of death was recently noted.[5] In particular, a significant reduction of abdominal involvement for both LD and MC histologies as well as a decreased incidence of generalized involvement for LP patients was observed. Moreover, among patients who received extensive treatment, the histologic appearance of involved organs is relatively monomorphic, with numerous Reed-Sternberg cell variants and a paucity of inflammatory elements. These histologic findings, resembling those of non-Hodgkin's lymphoma, may be considered a treatment-induced form of Hodgkin's disease.

Patterns of Disease at Relapse

Initial relapses in Hodgkin's disease tend to occur predominantly in the first 2 to 4 years after completion of the first course of treatment. Late relapses (beyond 5 years) are uncommon and range from 5 to 15 percent of patients in reported series.[6–9] In patients treated with inadequate radiation therapy, new manifestations of lymphoma are observed in the adjacent lymph node chain(s). In these cases, new disease manifestations in noncontiguous untreated areas are relatively rare and often reflect the limitation of diagnostic methods applied at the time of initial staging. However, as already mentioned, radiotherapy alone is at present rarely used for patients with Hodgkin's disease, and even when indicated, staging procedures are certainly more accurate and irradiation fields are currently better designed than previously. True recurrence (relapse within an irradiated field) is also a rare finding if an adequate tumoricidal dose of radiation was applied. Otherwise, marginal recurrence, for example, relapse at or immediately adjacent to the margins of a previous radiation field, is more frequent and may occur in 15 to 25 percent of cases.[3] A trend toward recurrence in nodal areas and particularly in initial and contiguous sites can also be seen after complete remission in advanced Hodgkin's disease treated with chemotherapy. In fact, relapses in previously involved sites occur in about 90 percent of relapsed cases and are directly related to the volume of tumor mass prior to therapy. These findings form the basis for adjuvant radiotherapy to nodal involved fields and to originally bulky sites, in particular, after remission is achieved with chemotherapy.

STAGING PROCEDURE AND PROGNOSTIC FEATURES

Staging Systems by Prognostic Factors

During the past 30 years, numerous efforts have been made to properly stage Hodgkin's disease in order to improve the selection of patients most suitable for different treatment programs. Over the years, lymphangiography, needle marrow biopsy, laparotomy and laparoscopy, computed tomography (CT), magnetic resonance imaging (MRI), gallium scanning and positron emission tomography (PET) have become important steps in the staging of both adults and children. The systematic use of these procedures led to the definition of the Rye (1965) and the Ann Arbor and updated Cotswolds (1970–1989) international staging systems,[10,11] which are applied worldwide. The

Table 43–1. The Ann Arbor–Cotswolds Staging Classification

Stage I
  Involvement of a single lymph node region or lymphoid structure (e.g. spleen, thymus, Waldeyer's ring) or involvement of a single extralymphatic site (IE)
Stage II
  Involvement of two or more lymph node regions on the same side of the diaphragm (hilar nodes, when involved on both sides, constitute stage II disease); localized contiguous involvement of only one extranodal organ or site and lymph node region(s) on the same side of the diaphragm (IIE); the number of anatomic regions involved should be indicated by a subscript (e.g., II_3)
Stage III
  Involvement of lymph node regions on both sides of the diaphragm (III), which may also be accompanied by involvement of the spleen (III_S) or by localized contiguous involvement of only one extranodal organ site (IIIE) or both (III_S E)
  III1: with or without involvement of splenic, hilar, celiac, or portal nodes
  III2: with involvement of para-aortic, iliac, or mesenteric nodes
Stage IV
  Diffuse or disseminated involvement of one or more extranodal organs or tissues, with or without associated lymph node involvement
Designations applicable to any disease stage:
A: No symptoms
B: Fever (temperature above 38°C), drenching night sweats, unexplained loss of more than 10 percent of body weight within the preceding 6 months
X: Bulky disease (a widening of the mediastinum by more than one-third or the presence of a nodal mass with a maximal dimension greater than 10 cm)
E: Involvement of a single extranodal site that is contiguous or proximal to the known nodal site
CS: Clinical stage
PS: Pathological stage (as determined by laparotomy)

framework of the classification, stated in Ann Arbor, takes into account the involvement of one or more nodal areas on the same (stage I-II) or both sides of the diaphragm (stage III), of extranodal sites contiguous (E suffix) or noncontiguous with nodal involvement (disseminated involvement of extranodal organ or tissue, stage IV), and the absence or presence of systemic symptoms (fever and/or night sweats and/or unexplained loss of more than 10 percent of body weight within the preceding 6 months), to designate suffix A or B applicable to any disease stage.

The Cotswolds Committee stated a number of classification criteria based on recent better knowledge of the natural history and treatment of the disease due to the advent of modern imaging techniques. It was particularly recommended that (1) CT scanning be included as a technique for evaluating intrathoracic and infradiaphragmatic lymph nodes; (2) the criteria for clinical involvement of the spleen and liver be modified to include evidence of focal defects by two imaging techniques and that abnormalities of liver function be ignored; (3) the suffix X be introduced to designate bulky disease; and (4) a new category of response to therapy be established termed unconfirmed/uncertain complete remission (CRu), to accommodate the difficulty of assessing persistent radiologic abnormalities of uncertain significance following primary therapy. Table 43–1 shows the Ann Arbor–Cotswolds staging system as applied today.

The original Ann Arbor staging system for Hodgkin's disease now appears to be inadequate to properly subdivide prognostic categories because a number of newly appreciated clinical and biological factors contribute to better definition of the whole burden of disease. For these reasons, in 1998 an International Prognostic Factor Project on advanced Hodgkin's disease was published on the basis of complete data from 25 centers and 1618 patients.[12] Freedom from progression (at 5 years) was chosen as the end point to avoid possible biases on overall survival by the effect of salvage therapy and deaths from late sequelae or other causes. The prognostic score was defined as the number of adverse prognostic factors at diagnosis (Table 43–2). Whether or not this prognostic score will be routinely used in making therapeutic decisions, as is the case for the International Prognostic Index in non-Hodgkin's lymphoma,[13] it is still uncertain.[14]

Recommended Pretreatment Evaluation

Table 43–3 outlines the procedures deemed necessary for correct staging of Hodgkin's disease. An adequate surgical biopsy, possibly of more than one intact lymph node, should be undertaken for parthological examination. Inguinal nodes should not be biopsied if other equally suspicious peripheral nodes are present elsewhere. When the diagnosis of Hodgkin's disease is made from biopsy of an extranodal site, a concomitant nodal biopsy for confirmation of diagnosis is desirable unless the diagnosis is considered unequivocal.

A detailed history must be obtained with information about the presence or absence of unexplained fever and its duration, unexplained sweating (especially at night) and its severity, unexplained weight loss as a percentage of usual body weight and rapidity of loss, and any pruritus with its extent and severity. The presence of alcohol-induced pain, a family history of Hodgkin's disease or other lymphoma, any history of immuno-suppressive illness, such as infection with human immunodeficiency viruses (HIVs) or a previous history of neoplasm together with any previous chemotherapy or radiation therapy should also be documented. A careful and complete physical examination must be performed with special attention to the number of enlarged lymph nodes and their dimensions, presence or absence of liver and spleen involvement, and Waldeyer's ring involvement. A complete laboratory work-up is required.

A variety of imaging techniques are available to assist in the initial staging of patients with histologically documented, previously untreated Hodgkin's disease.[15–18] The usefulness of a specific imaging test can be defined in terms of sensitivity,

---

Table 43–2. The Hasenclever International Prognostic Score for Advanced Stages

Independent Variable with Prognostic Significance

Variable	Value
Albumin	< 4 g/dl
Hemoglobin	< 10.5 g/dl
Sex	Male
Age	≥ 45 years
Stage	IV
Leukocytosis	White blood cells > 15,000/mm^3
Lymphocytopenia	Absolute lymphocyte count < 600/mm^3 or < 8 percent total white blood count

Rates of Freedom from Progression and Overall Survival at 5-years According to Individual and Grouped Prognostic Scores

Prognostic Score	N patients (%)	Rate of FFP (%)	Rate of OS (%)
Individual			
0	115 (7)	84 ± 4	89 ± 2
1	360 (22)	77 ± 3	90 ± 2
2	464 (29)	67 ± 2	81 ± 2
3	378 (23)	60 ± 3	78 ± 3
4	190 (12)	51 ± 4	61 ± 4
5–7	111 (7)	42 ± 5	56 ± 5
Grouped			
0 or 1	475 (29)	79 ± 2	90 ± 2
2 or more	1143 (71)	60 ± 2	74 ± 2
0 to 2	939 (58)	74 ± 2	86 ± 2
3 or more	679 (42)	55 ± 2	70 ± 2
0 to 3	1317 (81)	70 ± 2	83 ± 1
4 or more	301 (19)	47 ± 2	59 ± 2

FFP, freedom from progression; OS, overall survival.
(From Hasenclever et al.[12])

Table 43–3. Recommended Procedures for Proper Staging

Adequate surgical biopsy reviewed by an experienced hemopathologist; in primary extranodal lymphomas, biopsy should also include a lymph node when palpable

Detailed history with special attention to the presence or absence of systemic symptoms

Careful physical examination, emphasizing node chains, size of liver and spleen, Waldeyer's ring inspection, and bony tenderness

Routine laboratory tests: complete blood count, erythrocyte sedimentation rate, liver function tests, serum uric acid, serum lactate dehydrogenase

Chest radiograph (posteroanterior and left lateral) with measurement of mediastinal mass/thorax ratio

Bipedal lymphangiography in selected cases if adequately trained radiologists are available

Chest and abdominal CT (or MRI) scan and abdominal ultrasound

Radioisotopic evaluation with ^{67}gallium especially if mediastinum is involved

Core needle biopsy of bone marrow from unilateral posterior iliac crest

Cytologic examination of any effusion

^{18}Fluorodeoxyglucose positron emission tomography in suspicious cases

Any further study when suggested by clinical symptoms or sign (e.g., bone scan)

specificity, and overall accuracy. The following guidelines are suggested:

1. Thorax evaluation should include chest radiograph and thoracic CT or MRI scan to evaluate mediastinal adenopathy and any extension of such adenopathy into the surrounding viscera. In addition, it is important to assess the bulk of disease, which is of well-documented prognostic significance. Furthermore, gallium scanning should be performed at diagnosis at least in all patients with mediastinal involvement in order to better evaluate the nature of residual abnormalities at the end of the treatment program.[19–21]

2. Abdominal involvement must be evaluated by CT scan, which is particularly helpful in evaluating upper abdominal nodal disease and can detect enlargement of celiac, portal, splenic, hilar, and mesenteric nodes as well as retroperitoneal nodes. Bipedal lymphangiography is still recommended in centers with adequately trained radiologists for its unique capability to describe the lymph node architecture even in the absence of pathologic enlargement. However, despite the fact that lymphangiography remains the most accurate diagnostic tool for assessment of low para-aortic and paracaval nodal disease, its use is being abandoned because of the time and effort the procedure requires relative to CT and MRI scanning. Nevertheless, in adequately equipped centers, CT scan and lymphangiography should both be used in selected patients for their complementary information.

3. Bone marrow should be studied by core needle biopsy from the posterior iliac crest. The need for bilateral material has been long a matter of debate; at present, unilateral biopsy is considerate adequate if a sample of at least 1.5 to 2 cm is obtained.[22,23]

4. Routine screening is of little value in sites infrequently involved with disease (e.g., imaging studies of the gastrointestinal and genitourinary tracts, which are involved in less than 1 percent of cases).

5. In all cases, suggestive symptoms and signs of involvement at any specific site should prompt the performance of specific diagnostic studies.

In recent years radiolabeled fluorodeoxyglucose positron emission tomography ([18]FDG-PET) has emerged as a very useful tool in evaluating the presence of active neoplastic tissue in residual masses after therapy, especially in the infradiaphragmatic areas. By utilizing the [18]FDG metabolism of neoplastic cells, [18]FDG-PET scanning seems to be able to recognize small lesions (less than 1 cm in diameter), with a high sensibility approaching 100 percent despite a low specificity (slightly superior to 70 percent). At present, only small series concerning both Hodgkin's disease and non-Hodgkin's lymphoma are available, which suggest a high capability in recognizing involved areas undetectable with conventional techniques as well as histologically confirmed residual masses.[24–26]

The biopsy of specific sites to determine involvement is of advantage in some situations. A percutaneous needle biopsy of the liver is frequently negative even when disease is readily detectable at laparotomy. A percutaneous or laparoscopic liver biopsy can be helpful in patients with abnormal liver function tests or equivocal radiographic studies of the liver. A guided bone biopsy using CT or a percutaneous or open-lung biopsy may be indicated under similar circumstances when evidence of involvement is otherwise equivocal. In prescribing such invasive procedures, the physician should always consider if a positive result would modify the treatment approach.

The Purpose of Pretreatment Staging

The inclusion of chemotherapy in the treatment of virtually all cases of Hodgkin's disease has radically modified the pretreatment work-up. The abandonment of staging laparotomy is a direct consequence of this new role of chemotherapy. In fact, staging laparosplenectomy was aimed at identifying occult stage III patients unsuitable for radiotherapy alone programs, whereas negative cases were considered candidates for mantle or subtotal nodal irradiation.[27,28] At present only stage IA patients with no adverse factors are properly treated with irradiation alone, and even in this case many centers prefer to prescribe brief chemotherapy and involved-field irradiation. Furthermore, the diagnostic capability of imaging techniques such as CT scan and MRI has been progressively refined, which reduces the need for a surgical diagnostic approach.

In planning the diagnostic work-up for a patient with Hodgkin's disease not involved in a clinical trial, one should consider how much the results of each examination would change the therapeutic decision. For example, if the abdominal CT scan shows infradiaphragmatic involvement (at least stage III disease), the treatment program does not generally differ on the basis of other possible sites involved. Thus, the need for other invasive and/or expensive procedures, such as bone marrow biopsy or gallium scan, can probably be avoided. Otherwise, in the presence of a negative abdominal CT scan, other tests, such as bone marrow biopsy, lymphangiography, and/or MRI can help in identifying occult involved areas, which will change the treatment decision, primarily with respect to the duration or intensity of chemotherapy. In the same case, a gallium scan may be of use in evaluating therapeutic response. Figure 43–1 shows the minimal work-up required to adequately stage a patient with a new diagnosis of Hodgkin's disease, based on the choice of treatment endpoint.

EVALUATION OF RESPONSE AND FOLLOW-UP STUDIES

After completion of planned therapy, response should be documented on the basis of clinical findings, the results of laboratory tests, and repeat imaging investigations that were abnormal at presentation, supplemented by tissue biopsies if necessary. A number of patients present with residual abnormalities after primary therapy, typically with mediastinal widening and anteroposterior window fullness. It is now widely known that residual shadows by imaging, especially in the mediastinum, do not necessarily represent residual disease but rather may indi-

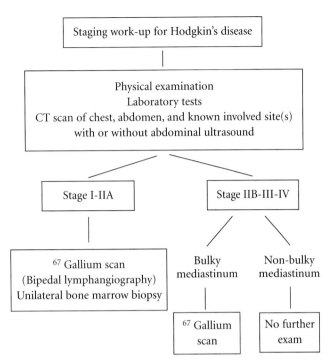

Figure 43–1. Proper minimal staging for patients outside a clinical trial, based on choice of treatment.

cate necrosis or fibrosis, and abnormal radiographic findings may persist for months to several years in such patients who are otherwise without evidence of disease.[19,20] This situation, defined as CRu, denotes patients in whom response status is unclear. The patient with CRu is in normal health with no clinical evidence of Hodgkin's disease but with some radiologic abnormality, not consistent with the effect of therapy, persisting at a site of previous disease. Implicit in this designation is a considerable uncertainty about the significance of such abnormalities, since it is well known that abnormal widening of the mediastinum or architectural distortion of lymph node–bearing areas may persist for many years without the need for additional therapy and without evidence of Hodgkin's disease. Attempts to resolve the dilemma of persistent disease versus residual anatomic distortion not indicative of Hodgkin's disease should include repeated investigations, such as radiologic imaging, MRI, and gallium scanning. Within the bounds of acceptable morbidity, pathologic examination by techniques such as mediastinoscopy may be appropriate, although the difficulties of sampling artifacts are acknowledged. Unusual lesions or highly suspicious lesions should be rebiopsied. To assess a complete remission properly, it is highly recommended that a second biopsy of liver, bone marrow, or both be performed when these sites were involved before the initiation of chemotherapy.

As outlined for pretreatment staging, it must be stressed that even in the case of restaging the complexity (and cost) of the work-up depends on the real impact on treatment choice of the recognition of persisting active neoplastic disease and on the other hand, on the risk of overtreating a patient with fibrotic masses. The documented possibility of salvaging patients with persistent disease after first-line treatment by high-dose chemotherapy and stem cell transplantation (see below) justifies a more aggressive approach to the restaging work-up. Otherwise, in the case of suspicious persistent disease, waiting for a few months to confirm the presence of active disease by standard imaging methods will probably not modify the prognosis of that patient.

After completion of therapy, it is recommended that patients be seen at 2- or 3-month intervals during the first and second year, at 4- to 6-month intervals from the third to the fifth year, and annually thereafter. The frequency and type of radiologic follow-up studies depend and should focus on the initial sites of disease, as well as on the detection of medium- and long-term sequelae of previous treatment. Appropriate work-up should be initiated when symptoms or signs of possible recurrent disease are noted. Because of the relatively high incidence of secondary neoplasms in Hodgkin's disease, investigations useful for the early detection of other malignancies, particularly breast or lung cancer, should be part of the follow-up studies in patients with Hodgkin's disease in remission.[28,29] Screening mammography or breast ultrasound, even in young women treated by mantle-field irradiation, is an example of this policy.[30]

TREATMENT

Evolution of the Treatment Strategy

Treatment of Hodgkin's disease has continuously improved, particularly during the 1960s and 1970s, and today about 80 percent of all patients can be cured by first- or second-line therapeutic strategies.[31–33] Although its cell of origin, etiology, and pathogenesis remain to be further elucidated, Hodgkin's disease represents a remarkable example of how progress in clinical and laboratory research can be successfully translated into effective clinical management. The continuous improvement in prognosis has been the result of meticulous clinicopathologic observations and sound prospective trials. (Table 43–4).

Radiation therapy progressively developed following the principles enunciated by Gilbert (1939) and applied by Peters (1950) but especially with the beginning of the megavoltage era. The study by Kaplan and the Stanford group[3] led to the development and refinement of many concepts and techniques that constitute modern radiation therapy for lymphomas and particularly for Hodgkin's disease.[34–37] Until the end of the 1960s, radiation therapy was the only successful therapeutic tool that, under appropriate circumstances, was able to achieve cure in a sizeable fraction of patients with Hodgkin's disease. Chemotherapy developed after the end of World War II, and lymphomas and leukemias were the first neoplasms shown to respond to drug treatment. Although the great majority of available cytotoxic agents can produce objective responses in Hodgkin's disease, it was only in 1970 with the four-drug regimen known as MOPP (mechlorethamine, vincristine, procarbazine, and prednisone) that DeVita and the National Cancer Institute (NCI) group documented that chemotherapy could induce durable complete remissions with high frequency in advanced Hodgkin's disease.[32,38]

Table 43–4. Chronologic Flow of Major Concepts and Events Influencing Treatment Evolution of Hodgkin's Disease

Investigator(s) (years)	Major Concepts and Events
Gilbert (1925–1939)	Concept of destruction of all lesions with the first course of radiation therapy; segmental irradiation to encompass suspected microscopic disease
Peters (1950–1958)	Improved 5- and 10-year survival by prophylactic irradiation of adjacent lymphoid areas; first three-stage clinical classification
Kinmoth (1952)	Lower extremity lymphangiography
Easson and Russel (1963)	Concept of cure by radiation therapy
Lukes (1963–1964)	Relationship of histologic features to clinical stages and prognosis
Kaplan (1962–1965)	Development of wide-field technique with radiation in continuity with multiple-node chains (mantle, inverted Y, and total lymphoid radiation therapy); identification of tumoricidal dose levels
Rosenberg and Kaplan (1965)	Evidence for an orderly progression in the spread of Hodgkin's disease
Lacher and Durant (1965)	Increased complete remission rate by vinblastine plus chlorambucil compared with single agents
Frei (1966)	Efficacy of a cyclic four-drug combination (MOPP)
Kaplan and Glatstein (1969)	Staging laparotomy and further studies on the pattern of anatomic distribution
DeVita (1970–1980)	Concept of high cure rate in advanced disease with MOPP
DeVita, Young (1971–1973)	Staging laparoscopy – no advantage of maintenance chemotherapy in complete responders
Rosenberg (1968–1981)	Trials with combined radiation therapy and chemotherapy, especially MOPP
Wiernik (1968–1985)	Trials of combined-modality therapy with MOPP and radiation therapy
Bonadonna and Santoro (1973–1987)	Development of non-cross-resistant chemotherapy (ABVD) and of alternating regimens (MOPP/ABVD)
Wiernik (1976)	Randomized trial of MOPP versus combined-modality therapy for early-stage disease
Longo et al., Cimino et al. (1982–1990)	Randomized trials of MOPP versus radiation therapy alone for early-stage Hodgkin's disease
Canellos, Connors, Viviani et al. (1980–1998)	Randomized trials comparing MOPP, ABVD, and hybrid or alternating MOPP/ABVD in advanced stage
Santoro et al, Horning et al. (1990–1997)	Low-toxic brief chemotherapy (ABVD, VBM) and involved-field radiotherapy for early-stage Hodgkin' disease
Horning, Chopra, Sweetenham, Josting et al (1990–2000)	Studies with high-dose chemotherapy and bone marrow transplantation for salvage therapy
Diehl, Horning, Gobbi, Wiernik	New generation intensive regimens (BEACOPP, Stanford V, MOPPEBVCAD, MVC) for advanced stages and salvage therapy

In the late 1970s and 1980s, radiation therapy and chemotherapy were sequentially combined for the treatment of early as well as advanced stages to maximize relapse-free survival (RFS), and to improve the cure rate. Thus, over the past 30 years, radiation therapy and chemotherapy have become partners and competitors for certain subsets of patients and have provided a number of therapeutic alternatives to achieve cure or optimal palliation. In an attempt to eradicate both MOPP-sensitive and MOPP-resistant neoplastic cells, the research group in Milan designed the ABVD (doxorubicin [Adriamycin], bleomycin, vinblastine, dacarbazine) regimen and mounted a number of prospective trials that proved its effectiveness as a non-cross-resistant regimen to MOPP. The same group then developed a theraputic strategy involving the cyclic alternating administration of these two non-cross-resistant regimens (MOPP/ABVD) to reduce MOPP failures and to prevent or delay relapse due to overgrowth of MOPP-resistant Hodgkin's cells.[39–44] Further attempts to improve the cure rate took into consideration the Goldie-Coldmann hypoth-

esis[45] by testing the effect of early introduction of as many effective drugs as possible in the treatment strategies. Trials from the Milan, Vancouver, and other groups have thus compared the classical alternating MOPP/ABVD with the so-called hybrid regimen which alternates half MOPP and half ABVD.[46–48] Actually, the hybrid regimen has not demonstrated any real advantage over the classical alternating MOPP/ABVD.

In 1992 Canellos and colleagues from the Cancer and Leukemia Group B (CALGB) confirmed in a large randomized study that ABVD alone was superior to MOPP. Since then, ABVD chemotherapy has become the gold standard against which all newer regimens should be tested.[49]

In the 1990s, further efforts to improve the outcome of patients with Hodgkin's disease have consisted of the intensification of primary chemotherapy with hematopoietic colony-stimulating factor (CSF) support, with the aim both to increase complete remission rate and to minimize late toxic effects. This is the case of the BEACOPP regimen (bleomycin, etoposide, doxorubicin, cyclophosphamide, vincristine, procarbazine, prednisone),[50] designed by Diehl and co-workers from the German Hodgkin's Study Group , as well as of the Stanford V regimen of Horning and co-workers (weekly alternation of doxorubicin, vinblastine, mecloretamine, vincristine, bleomycin, etoposide, plus prednisone),[51] and the Italian MOPPEBVCAD (mechloretamine, CCNU, vindesine, melphalan, prednisone, epiadriamycin, vincristine, procarbazine, vinblastine, bleomycin).[52] The fundamental question of whether a clinical dose–response effect can be exploited with the use of high-dose chemotherapy with stem cell rescue has been tested worldwide.[53] Since initial attempts in the early 1980s, numerous investigators used high-dose chemotherapy with autologous bone marrow transplantation (ABMT) or peripheral blood stem-cell transplantation (PBSCT) for salvage treatment of patients with relapsed Hodgkin's disease. Despite the publication of only one randomized comparison between high-dose and standard-dose chemotherapy,[54] a consistent proportion of patients has been cured at relapse with this high-dose strategy. Thus, the trend toward a better outcome for patients treated by high-dose chemotherapy, along with the low morbidity rate, now reported as less than 1 percent, seems to have eliminated the need for further randomized comparisons between high-dose and conventional therapy.

Improvement in treatment results has been achieved in all stages of the disease. Today, no stage of the disease is beyond cure when treated appropriately at the time of diagnosis or when treated for recurrence after primary irradiation. This represents a dramatic improvement in the overall prognosis of a disease that 40 years ago was considered to be almost universally fatal. Current and future strategies should refine available treatment programs. Identification of prognostic subgroups will allow the choice of tailored treatment aimed at minimizing toxic effects in patients at low risk and to aggressively approach those at high risk. It is possible that alternative approaches, such as biological and immunological techniques, will represent a fundamental tool in association with classical chemotherapy in the near future.

GENERAL TREATMENT STRATEGY

Multiple trials have identified a variety of treatment options, most of which appear to be relatively beneficial. In other words, in many disease stages a choice of treatment exists rather than a treatment of choice. The cost/benefit ratio is an important component in the selection of a specific therapy. Regardless of treatment options, several factors need to be remembered: (1) total tumor burden and optimal dose delivery remain the most important treatment variables; (2) primary tumor cell resistance represents the major stumbling block for all chemotherapy regimens; and (3) not only are prospective randomized trials (often repetitive) difficult and lengthy undertakings, but their influence on current clinical practice may actually be limited when patient accrual continues indefinitely. In fact, new concepts in staging, treatment, or both may develop outside the context of such a trial and may affect its relevance.[33]

As already mentioned, staging laparotomy has been abandoned and lymphangiography has been progressively less used

as consequences of the advent of sophisticated imaging techniques, such as CT and MRI scanning, and of the widespread use of chemotherapy in virtually all disease stages. However, careful patient selection remains important to identify those who will benefit from each treatment strategy. Some major considerations should be taken into account when decision making is needed for an individual patient, especially concerning the multimodality approach, such as the following:

1. Despite a multitude of publications concerning further prognostic classification on the basis of clinical and biological features,[27] the Ann Arbor–Cotswolds staging system currently provides the best methodology for discriminating between early and advanced stages.
2. In early stages (I,IIA), the multidisciplinary approach is now considered standard. As the vast majority of these patients (approximately 90 percent) can be cured, the choice of treatment is presently aimed at reducing both acute and late toxicities by introducing less toxic drugs and reducing the dose and extension of radiation fields.
3. In patients presenting with massive mediastinal involvement, the role of combined modality therapy is well established in all stages of disease
4. In patients with more advanced stages of disease (IIAX, IIB, III–IV A and B), the percentage of nodal relapses is not negligible (about 20 percent) even after effective chemotherapy.[55,56] The usefulness of consolidation radiotherapy to all sites of disease has been long a matter of debate. Some groups prefer to irradiate all nodal sites of disease at diagnosis even if the advantage of this approach is not fully demonstrated.[37,57] It is likely that irradiating all nodal areas in a patient with extensive stage IV disease will not enhance the probability of cure, whereas radiotherapy may be advantageous in those patients with advanced, exclusively nodal disease.

In general, as in the treatment of children with Hodgkin's disease, the goal should be to minimize rather than to maximize combined-modality therapy in advanced stages. The intent of combined-modality treatment, and in general of intensive strategies, should be to eradicate the disease with the first treatment. Although improved in the last 10 years, salvage treatment approaches are curative only in a small fraction of relapsed patients, except under the most favorable circumstances (limited-stage relapse beyond the 12th month of initial complete remission).[58] As pointed out by Rosenberg[59] changes in management should be developed and evaluated stepwise and gradually, since curability and comparisons of toxicities require 5 to 10 years of careful evaluation.

Nearly one-third of patients with Hodgkin's disease die without evidence of lymphoma at autopsy, and in a significant number of patients death is attributable to complications of therapy.[60] Therefore, treatment programs should pay more attention to iatrogenic complications, in particular myocardial damage and carcinogenesis. Available data indicate that procarbazine, alkylating agents, and podophyllotoxins are responsible for both carcinogenesis and sterility, whereas addition of radiotherapy enhances the risk for the development of solid tumors. Since achievement of high complete remission rates with all cytotoxic drug combinations requires administration of full or nearly full doses with minimal delay during the first three to four cycles, treatment options that have been shown to be least toxic without compromise of efficacy should obviously be utilized. In favorable stages, short-term ABVD-like chemotherapy and limited-field radiation therapy at as low a dose as possible would hopefully limit both the incidence of carcinogenesis and irreversible gonadal damage. On the other hand, in more advanced stages, the need for increasing the cure rate may justify more intensive chemotherapy with a certain risk of late complications. However, even in this situation a careful selection of new-generation drugs might minimize the probability of long-term adverse sequelae.[34,61,62]

TREATMENT OF EARLY STAGES (IA-B, IIA)

The vast majority of patients with early-stage Hodgkin's disease (IA–IIA) can at present be cured by currently available therapeutic options. Thus, the aim of treatment is to limit medium- and long-term toxic effects rather than to further increase the cure rate. However, it should be noted that there is not complete agreement on the definition of early stages, as some authors include cases with bulky disease or B symptoms, whereas other do not (Table 43–5). As a consequence, it is somewhat difficult to draw

Table 43–5. Prognostic Subgroups in Stage I-II

EORTC	
Very favorable	CS IA, female sex, age < 40, and LP histology, or NS histology and nonbulky mediastinum
Favorable	Cases classifiable neither as very favorable nor as unfavorable
Unfavorable	One of following factors: bulky mediastinum, stage A with ESR > 50, B with ESR > 30, age > 50, more than four sites involved
GHSG	
Unfavorable	Bulky mediastinum or elevated ESR, or ≻ 3 involved sites, or ≻ disseminated extranodal or splenic involvement
Favorable	All others
Stanford	
Very favorable[a]	CS I and female sex, or CS I mediastinum, or CS I and male sex with LP histology, or CS II, female sex, age < 27, and < three involved sites
Harvard	
Very favorable	CS IA and female sex, or CS IA and male sex with LP histology, or CS IA and male sex with peripheral cervical site

GHSG, German Hodgkin's Study Group; CS, clinical stage; LP, Lymphocyte-Predominant; NS, nodular sclerosis; ESR, erythrocyte sedimentation rate.
[a] Treated with mantle-field irradiation alone, non-laparotomy staged.

precise conclusions from published series concerning the same treatment modalities but with different patient selection criteria.

Radiotherapy

Up to the 1980s, the standard approach to stage IA–IIA Hodgkin's disease included staging laparotomy and splenectomy and, if these procedures are negative, mantle-field irradiation at therapeutic doses (36 to 44 Gy), followed by irradiation of para-aortic nodes and the splenic pedicle (subtotal nodal irradiation, STNI) at lower doses (30 to 36 Gy). With this approach, up to 90 percent of patients were alive at 10 years with a freedom from progression of 70 to 80 percent in one study.[63] Relapsing patients could, in fact, obtain second durable remissions by salvage chemotherapy. More recently, this approach has been reconsidered by a number of research groups. First, many radiation therapists documented a relapse rate in stage IIA that was at least double that initially reported, and in stage IIB patients presenting with three systemic symptoms, a failure rate of about 50 percent was observed with radiation alone.[57,64,65] However, it should be pointed out that selection criteria often included the so-called unfavorable early stages as outlined by the European Organization for Research and Treatment of Cancer (EORTC): MC and LD histologies, male sex, age older than 40 years, erythrocyte sedimentation rate more than 70, and mediastinal mass. In the presence of one or more unfavorable features, patients treated with extensive radiation therapy alone had a 6-year relapse-free survival of 53 percent versus nearly 100 percent when treated with combined-modality therapy.[66,67] Furthermore, when the Stanford group randomly tested subtotal nodal irradiation versus involved-field irradiation plus six cycles of MOP(P) in pathological stages IA–IIA, it was concluded that adjuvant chemotherapy could replace radiation of occult disease.[68] The results of a number of major trials comparing radiotherapy, chemotherapy, and combined-modality therapy are shown in Table 43–6.

Over the last few years, indications for radiotherapy in early-stage Hodgkin's disease have been progressively revised. At present, only a limited stage IA presentation with no adverse factors and with LP histology is considered to be appropriately treated with mantle-field or subtotal nodal irradiation alone.

Chemotherapy

In the second part of the 1980s chemotherapy was introduced in the management of early-stage Hodgkin's disease. Some groups have tested the efficacy of chemotherapy alone in this setting in order to eliminate late effects related to combined-modality therapy. Two groups published randomized comparisons between MOPP chemotherapy and radiotherapy, reaching opposite conclusions. The Italian group[69] found that radiation therapy was ineffective as salvage treatment after MOPP failure; thus in their opinion, radiation therapy remains the treatment of choice. The National Cancer Institute (NCI) group[61] observed a superiority of MOPP chemotherapy over radiation therapy and concluded that MOPP was at least as effective as radiation therapy. It must be pointed out that these trials, initi-

Table 43–6. Randomized Trials Comparing Different Combined Modality Versus Radiotherapy or Chemotherapy Alone in Early Stage Hodgkin's Disease

Author (ref)	Regimen	RT	Stages	FFP (%)	OS (%)	Median FU (years)
Pavlovsky[70]	CVPP + RT vs CVPP	IF	Unfavorable I-II	75	84	7
				34	66	
Horning[72]	VBM + RT vs RT	IF	I-IIA, IIB, IIA favorable	95	95	3
		STNI/TNI		70	67	
Radford[154]	VAPEC-B + RT vs RT	IF		91	NR	3.3
			I-IIA			
		STNI		73	NR	
Santoro[74]	ABVD/IF vs ABVD/STNI	IF		95	100	3
			I-IIA			
		STNI		94	100	
Wiernik[67]	MOPP + RT vs RT	EF	IA,IIA,IIB,IIIA	94	91	5.8
				66	76	

RT, radiotherapy; FFP, freedom from progression; OS, overall survival; IF, involved fields; EF, extended field; FU, follow-up period; STNI, subtotal nodal irradiation; TNI, total nodal irradiation; NR, not reported.

ated in the early 1980s, were largely designed to evaluate the need for splenectomy, which is now considered obsolete. In a further randomized trial, Pavlovsky et al.[70] demonstrated the superiority of six courses of the MOPP-derived combination CVPP (cyclophosphamide, vincristine, procarbazine, prednisone) followed by radiation therapy, compared with the same chemotherapy alone. At the National Cancer Institute of Canada, an ongoing trial is comparing two courses of ABVD followed by radiotherapy with four to six courses of ABVD alone. The results of this study, different from the above in that radiotherapy substitutes for further chemotherapy, may help to clarify the role of chemotherapy alone in early stages. At present, the use of chemotherapy alone is indicated only for patients with major contraindications to radiotherapy.

Combined Modality

Most trials of the last 20 years have focused on the role of a combined chemotherapy-radiotherapy strategy in early-stage Hodgkin's disease. The debate arises from the evidence that salvage chemotherapy in patients relapsing after radiotherapy alone offers cure rates as high as initial combined-modality therapy. On the other hand, delivering chemotherapy after extensive radiotherapy means a higher risk of second malignancies. At the Milan Cancer Institute, 116 patients with pathologically staged favorable presentation who were treated with extended-field radiotherapy were nonrandomly compared with 85 patients with unfavorable presentations who were treated with MOPP and radiotherapy. At 10 years, the freedom from progression was significantly different between stage I and II in the favorable group (85 versus 59 percent) respectively, whereas stage lost its prognostic significance in the unfavorable group treated with combined-modality therapy.[71] Furthermore, in the favorable group a higher incidence of acute leukemia as a consequence of salvage chemotherapy was observed.

At Stanford, 67 patients with favorable pathological stages I and II (A and B), or IIIA were randomized between subtotal or total nodal irradiation alone or involved-field irradiation plus six cycles of the novel VBM regimen (vinblastine, bleomycin, methotrexate). At 5 years, freedom from progression was 70 percent after radiation alone and 95 percent after combined-modality treatment ($P < .0001$).[72] In a subsequent trial (Stanford Permanente), the authors focused on favorable clinical stages I and II: 78 patients were randomized to receive either extended-field irradiation (sub-total nodal) or involved-field irradiation after VBM. With a median follow-up of 4 years, 92 percent of the extended-field group and 87 percent of the combined-modality group were free of progression. The VBM regimen is very well tolerated with little adverse effect on male or female fertility, and more than 90 percent of the planned dose can usually be delivered. Despite the fact that comparable results between the two groups would support the use of combined modality therapy in all patients, the authors do not recommend its routine use outside of a clinical trial.[73]

The Milan group compared two different radiotherapy strategies following primary chemotherapy by randomizing 103 patients to receive STNI or involved-field radiotherapy after four courses of ABVD. In a preliminary report, with a median follow-up period of 38 months, the response rate was 100 percent, freedom from progression was 95 percent and survival was 100 percent without any difference between the two groups.[74] Thus, following complete remission with short-term chemotherapy, involved-field consolidation radiotherapy seems to offer best results with minimal toxicity.

In a recent meta-analysis, the role of adjuvant chemotherapy was assessed in 13 randomized trials involving 1688 early-stage patients. The addition of chemotherapy to radiotherapy halved the 10-year risk of failure (16 versus 33 percent), with a small statistically nonsignificant improvement in survival (79 versus 76 percent). A reduction of Hodgkin's disease deaths of borderline significance (12 versus 15 percent) was partly counterbalanced by a nonsignificant increase in deaths from other causes (12 versus 10 percent).[36] However, it could be argued that this meta-analysis refers to studies begun in the 1970s or early

1980s, when MOPP was the most frequently used combination. Thus, it is possible that less toxic regimens such as ABVD or VBM will reduce mortality from causes other than Hodgkin's disease and establish the combined-modality advantage.

TREATMENT OF ADVANCED STAGES

Independently of the Hasenclever Prognostic Score, all stage IIB, III, and IV patients according to the Ann Arbor staging system are considered to be advanced. There is no consensus in the literature concerning stages IIAX and III$_1$A, which are considered early stages by some investigators and advanced stages by others.

Conventional Approach

Primary chemotherapy is the standard approach for advanced stages. Up to the 1980s, the gold standard was the MOPP regimen,[75] which induced complete remission in approximately 80 percent of patients. Of those, approximately 30 percent relapsed within 5 to 10 years. Furthermore, the MOPP conbination is associated with manageable but significant acute toxicity (gastroenterologic, neurologic, hematologic) and with an appreciable incidence of well documented delayed toxicity effects such as male infertility and secondary myelodysplastic syndrome and acute myeloid leukemia. Since the acute toxicity of the regimen is largely attributed to mechlorethamine and vincristine, some groups have tested the substitution of other less toxic drugs such as cyclophosphamide, chlorambucil, or BCNU for mechlorethamine (COPP and BCVPP regimens) and vinblastine for vincristine (ChlVPP combination).[76,77] Despite an outcome similar to that with MOPP and a somewhat better tolerability, the results of these regimens have not been reproduced on a wide scale, and most investigators report little difference between MOPP and its later derivatives.

It has become clear that MOPP alone is inferior to ABVD alone as well as to either alternating MOPP and ABVD or the MOPP-ABV hybrid in the control of Hodgkin's disease. The first trial demonstrating the superiority of an ABVD-based regimen over MOPP was conducted at the Milan Cancer Institute in patients with stage IV disease. The alternating MOPP-ABVD regimen demonstrated a 15 to 20 percent advantage over MOPP.[41] Subsequently, the same group[43] demonstrated a significant advantage in terms of complete remission rate, freedom from progression, and relapse-free survival favoring ABVD (three courses followed by extended-field radiotherapy and three more courses) as compared to MOPP (same schedule) in 232 pathologically staged IIB and III patients. The comparable overall survival in the two groups was probably related to the fact that salvage ABVD was given to MOPP-resistant patients. The long-term results of this trial confirmed the efficacy of a combined-modality approach. As far as delayed toxicity is concerned, no signs of myocardial damage were seen in either arm. The ABVD group showed more pulmonary radiation fibrosis than the MOPP group, in particular after the last three cycles of bleomycin-containing chemotherapy. Permanent testicular failure occurred only after MOPP. Although MOPP was definitively more leukemogenic than ABVD, the frequency of solid tumors was about the same with the two combinations.[78] Clearly, the incorporation of alkylating agents (mechlorethamine and procarbazine) in the MOPP regimen is responsible for the increased incidence of sterility and leukemogenesis observed with that treatment.

In the recently updated CALGB (Cancer and Leukemia Group B) study comparing MOPP, ABVD, and MOPP alternating with ABVD in 362 patients with advanced-stage disease (IIIA$_2$, IIIB, IV), 8-year freedom from progression was 37 percent for MOPP, 52 percent for ABVD, and 50 percent for alternating MOPP and ABVD. A similar difference in overall survival did not emerge. A 3 percent incidence of fatal febrile neutropenia in the MOPP group was counterbalanced by a similar incidence of fatal pulmonary toxicity with ABVD, and 1 percent of each after MOPP-ABVD.[49,79]

Some groups have tested the alternating MOPP/ABVD with the so-called hybrid MOPP/ABVD, which consists of alternating half courses of MOPP with half courses of ABVD, with the aim of more rapid delivery of all active drugs in concert with the Goldie-Coldman hypothesis.[45] In the Vancouver trial, alternating MOPP and ABVD was compared with hybrid MOPP-ABV, with ABV given on day 8 of each 28-day course. Both regimens produced excellent results, but the hybrid regimen was associated with a higher incidence of life-threatening febrile neutropenia and stomatitis, leading to a lowering of the upper age limit from 65 to 55 years in mid-study.[46] In 415 patients treated at the Milan Cancer Institute, alternating and hybrid programs (half MOPP and half ABVD every 14 days of each 28-day cycle) produced comparable results[47] in terms of both survival and acute toxicity.

The North American Intergroup (CALGB, ECOG, SWOG),[48] compared sequential MOPP followed by ABVD with hybrid MOPP/ABV in 737 patients with advanced-stage (III$_2$A, IIIB, IV) Hodgkin's disease with the aim of testing the Goldie-Coldman hypothesis by introducing doxorubicin late (sequential) or early (hybrid) in the therapeutic program. Patients assigned to the sequential schedule received six MOPP courses followed, if complete response was attained, by three ABVD courses. Patients in the hybrid group received MOPP-ABV as designed by Connors et al.[46] Complete remission was achieved in 83 percent of cases on the hybrid and 75 percent on the sequential group (p = .02). After a median follow-up period of 7.3 years, the 8-year FFP was 64 percent for MOPP/ABV and 54 percent for MOPP→ABVD (p = .01). The 8-year OS rate was significantly better for MOPP/ABV as compared with MOPP →ABVD (79 versus 71 percent, p = .02). Acute life-threatening (grade 4) or fatal (grade 5) toxicity was more frequent in the hybrid regimen. Otherwise, seven cases of acute myelogenous leukemia and two of myelodysplasia were diagnosed in patients receiving MOPP→ABVD as compared to one case of acute myelogeneous leukemia in the hybrid regimen (p = .01). Overall (see Table 43–7), six to eight courses of ABVD alone or alternating MOPP-ABVD emerge as the gold standard in advanced-stage Hodgkin's disease, with which new-generation regimens should now be compared.

Table 43–7. Therapeutic Outcome at 5 or More Years with MOPP, ABVD, or Alternating/Hybrid MOPP/ABVD in Advanced Stage Hodgkin's Disease

Regimens	No. of Cases	Stage	FFP (%)	OS (%)
Milan[42,47]				
	114		63	64
MOPP × 3 → RT → MOPP × 3		IIB, IIIA-B		
vs	118		81	71
ABVD × 3 → RT → ABVD × 3				
MOPP	43		37	58
vs		IV A-B		
MOPP/ABVD	45		61	69
MOPP/ABVD alternating	211	I-IIB, IIAX,	67	74
vs		IIIA/B,		
MOPP/ABVD hybrid	204	IV A/B	69	72
CALGB[49]				
MOPP	123		37	66
vs		IIIA$_2$, IIIB, IVA/B		
ABVD	123		52	73
vs				
MOPP/ABVD	115		50	75
Vancouver[46]				
MOPP/ABV hybrid	153	IIIB, IVA,B	71	81
vs				
MOPP/ABVD alternating	148		67	83
Intergroup[48]				
MOPP/ABVD alternating	344	IIIA$_2$/B, IV A/B	54	71
vs				
MOPP/ABV hybrid	347		64	79

FFP, freedom from progression; OS, overall survival.

New Intensive Combinations

Optimization of dose intensity, inclusion of new active drugs, and the appropriate use of hematopoietic growth factors have recently been studied as methods by which the cure rate might be enhanced in patients with advanced Hodgkin's disease. In most cases, the MOPP-ABVD combination as originally reported serves as the springboard from which tests of these new ideas are launched.

An Italian group[52] developed a 10-drug intensive regimen called MOPPEBVCAD (mechlorethamine, vincristine, procarbazine, prednisone, epidoxorubicin, bleomycin, vinblastine, lomustine, melphalan, and vindesine). Administration to 145 patients of six courses of this regimen was followed by low-dose radiotherapy only to bulky sites of disease at diagnosis or to areas with incomplete response to chemotherapy. Complete remission was obtained in 94 percent of cases. Tumor-specific, overall, relapse-free, and failure-free survivals at 5 years were 89, 86, 82, and 78 percent, respectively. Most of the unfavorable prognostic factors lost their clinical significance, with the exception of patient age and lymphocyte-depletion histology. After a median follow-up period of 66 months, seven patients developed second cancers, including three myelodysplasias. As this regimen includes a number of drugs with leukemogenic potential, a longer follow-up period with special attention to late sequelae is needed to determine the role this regimen may ultimately come to play in the treatment of advanced Hodgkin's disease.

Much enthusiasm has arisen in the last 2 years for the BEACOPP (bleomycin, etoposide, doxorubicin, cyclophosphamide, vincristine, procarbazine, and prednisone) and escalated BEACOPP regimens developed by the German group, both derived from the alternating COPP-ABVD regimen. In an initial report,[50] moderate dose escalation over the standard BEACOPP regimen was performed with granulocyte colony-stimulating factor (G-CSF) support, and maximal doses of three component drugs (doxorubicin, etoposide, cyclophosphamide) were given with acceptable hematological toxicity. The intended doses of doxorubicin, etoposide, and cyclophosphamide were substantially escalated from 25 to 35, from 650 to 1200, and from 100 to 200 mg/m^2, respectively. Of 60 patients enrolled, 56 (93 percent) achieved complete remission, with an overall survival and freedom from progression at 32 months of 91 and 90 percent, respectively. A further report gave the results of a randomized comparison of standard BEACOPP with escalated BEACOPP and COPP-ABVD, involving 505 evaluable patients with advanced-stage (IIB, IIIA with risk factors, IIIB, and IV) disease. Four courses of COPP-ABVD were compared with eight courses of baseline BEACOPP without G-CSF and with eight courses of escalated BEACOPP with G-CSF, all followed by radiotherapy to bulky sites (30 Gy) and to areas of residual disease (40 Gy).[50] The interim analysis at 23 months showed a significant inferiority of the COPP-ABVD regimen in terms of progression rate and freedom from progression compared with the pooled results of both BEACOPP schemes. The 24-month freedom from progression rate was 75 percent for COPP/ABVD and 84 percent for BEACOPP pooled ($p = .034$). There were insufficient data to compare the two BEACOPP variants. The acute toxicity of COPP/ABVD and baseline BEACOPP was similar, whereas escalated BEACOPP showed increased but manageable hematological toxicity. Therefore, recruitment in the COPP/ABVD arm was discontinued. In a further interim analysis of 689 patients (COPP/ABVD 235 patients, baseline BEACOPP 241, escalated BEACOPP 213), escalated BEACOPP showed better freedom from progression at 2 years than baseline BEACOPP (89 versus 81 percent). As yet, no significant differences in survival have emerged, however. Of concern is the higher number of secondary acute leukemias observed with escalated BEACOPP (four versus one) whereas secondary non-Hodgkin's lymphomas (three cases) occurred only in the baseline BEACOPP group. In the currently ongoing HD12 trial, the German Hodgkin's Study Group is attempting to determine whether eight cycles of escalated BEACOPP followed by radiotherapy might represent overtreatment. Advanced-stage Hodgkin's disease patients are randomized to receive eight cycles of escalated BEACOPP or four cycles of escalated BEACOPP followed by four cycles of baseline BEACOPP. A second randomization assigns patients to receive radiotherapy (as described in the previous trial) or no further treatment.

The Stanford group adjusted the so-called Stanford V regimen, consisting of an abbreviated 12-week administration of the seven more active drugs, maintaining dose intensity of active agents but reducing the cumulative dose of doxorubicin, bleomycin, and mechlorethamine. In this trial, 47 patients were treated with the Stanford V regimen followed by radiotherapy (36 Gy) to lymph nodes 5 cm or larger in size and/or macroscopic splenic disease. The recently updated results based on a median follow-up period of 4.8 years show that 45 patients were alive and 40 had been continuously disease-free. The estimated freedom from progression and overall survival at 5 years were 85 and 96 percent, respectively. One patient died from acute leukemia. Six of seven relapsed patients received high-dose therapy with autologous stem cell support and achieved freedom from second progression. A randomized comparison between Stanford V and ABVD is now ongoing.

Among numerous newer multidrug regimens in which etoposide was substituted for vincristine and epidoxorubicin for doxorubicin, it is worth mentioning VEBEP (etoposide, epidoxorubicin, bleomycin, cyclophosphamide, and prednisone). The Milan group reported their results with this regimen given every 21 days without growth factor support and followed by radiation therapy (30 to 36 Gy) to the pretreatment-involved nodal sites. In 73 patients with Ann Arbor stages IIB or III–IV or relapsing after radiotherapy, complete remission was achieved in 94 percent of cases with freedom from progression and overall survival at 6 years of 78 and 82 percent, respectively. Hematological toxicity was acceptable, with 86 percent grade IV neutropenia, which resolved in the majority of cases by the next treatment cycle. The majority of male patients developed gonadal damage, reversible in half of them. No secondary leukemia or myelodysplasia had been detected at the time of publication.[80] Overall, (Table 43–8), these regimens as well as

Table 43–8. Five-Year Results of Chemotherapeutic Regimens in Advanced Hodgkin's Disease

Regimen (ref)	CR (%)	OS (%)	FFP (%)
BEACOPP intensified[50]	95	NR	84
MOPPEBVCAD[52]	94	86	82
STANFORD V[38]	99	83	89
VEBEP[80]	94	82	78
MVC[81] (88% of patients had B symptoms)	88	82	79

CR, complete remission; OS, overall survival; FFP, freedom from progression.

others[81] induce complete remission in up to 90 percent of cases with freedom from progression at 5 years of about 80 percent. Whether or not these results are superior to those obtained with MOPP/ABVD will be clarified by longer follow-up studies and ongoing randomized comparisons.

High-Dose Consolidation with Stem Cell Support

In recent years, a number of nonrandomized trial have focused on the role of high-dose consolidation after achievement of complete remission with standard regimens in patients with particularly adverse prognostic presentations. Up to now there has been no evidence for the usefulness of such an approach in any subset of patients. As a matter of fact, up to 40 percent of relapsed patients have a second chance of cure with high-dose chemotherapy as salvage treatment (see below). Thus, giving high-dose therapy at onset may represent an overtreatment at least for some patients, as selection criteria are neither clear nor homogeneous in published series.

An Italian group studied one course of CBV (cyclophosphamide, BCNU, etoposide) or BEAM (BCNU, etoposide, cytarabine, melphalan) followed by peripheral stem cell reinfusion in 22 patients with advanced-stage disease in first remission after MOPP-ABVD. Selection criteria consisted of bulky disease, age over 40 years, high serum lactate dehydrogenase (LDH) level, and anemia at onset. After a median follow-up time of 83 months, overall and relapse-free survival were 80 and 77 percent, respectively.[82] A French group[83] treated 26 high-risk patients with an estimated probability of cure less than 40 percent (stage IV and at least two of the following factors: B symptoms, bulky mediastinal disease, two or more extranodal sites, bone marrow involvement, inguinal node involvement, high LDH serum level, or low hematocrit) with high-dose chemotherapy and peripheral blood stem cell support (PBSCT) as consolidation of first-line chemotherapy. At the time of transplantation, 19 patients were in complete remission and 7 in good partial remission after MOPP-ABVD or similar regimens. Actuarial 5-year overall survival, freedom from progression, and event-free survival were 69, 79, and 58 percent, respectively. Only normal serum LDH level was found statistically significant as a prognostic indicator in univariate analysis. Of note, procedure-related mortality in the first 90 days after engraftment was 7 percent. Better results were obtained by

Nademanee in 20 high-risk patients according to the same criteria, who were given high-dose therapy and total-body irradiation after complete remission induction. All patients were alive and disease-free at 43 months.[84] Again, it must be stressed that all these results come from small heterogeneous series and must be evaluated with caution.

Role of Consolidation Radiotherapy in Advanced Stage

Soon after MOPP was introduced, it became clear that the majority of chemotherapy relapses occurred at sites of initial disease, particularly nodal sites and sites of bulky tumor, and that addition of radiotherapy markedly reduced the frequency of these recurrences, thus increasing the rates of both complete remission and disease-free survival.[85,86] Because of these observations, adjuvant irradiation was widely adopted without demonstration of which, if any, Hodgkin's disease subset benefited with improved overall survival. However, with growing awareness of the second tumor risk associated with irradiation, both radiotherapists and chemotherapists have reservations about this approach.[87,88]

There is general agreement on the need for combined-modality treatment in patients with mediastinal bulky disease.[87–89] Disease-free survival of 80 to 90 percent is observed after combined-modality treatment, which is nearly twice that reported after MOPP or radiation alone. Otherwise, radiotherapy is not useful in patients suspected of residual disease after treatment. Some partial remissions can be converted to complete remissions, but such patients do not show an increased cure rate according to a number of randomized trials.[89,90]

The issue of whether irradiation has a role as consolidation therapy after complete remission is achieved is still a matter of debate. Groups at Yale, Duke, and Memorial Sloan-Kettering strongly support low-dose adjuvant irradiation (18 to 30 Gy) to previously involved sites for patients in remission after chemotherapy. In a cohort of 184 Yale patients with either newly diagnosed stage IIIB or IV disease or recurrent disease after irradiation alone, overall survival was 54 percent at 15 years.[91] However, an unacceptable incidence of second neoplasms was observed in those treated with combined-modality therapy for disease recurrence after radiation alone (41 percent at 20 years versus 12 percent in the newly diagnosed patients).[92] In a similar analysis at Memorial Sloan-Kettering, the actuarial 10-year overall survival and progression-free survival were 74 and 70 percent, respectively.[93] Second-malignancy incidence was only 4 percent, but the median duration of observation was too short to properly address this issue. A recent German investigation showed that while 20 Gy is sufficient to control initial sites of nonbulky disease or uninvolved sites following two double cycles of COPP/ABVD relapse patterns indicate that patients destined to relapse need more systemic rather than local therapy.[94] In a SWOG study, 278 patients in complete remission following a MOPP-ABVD-derived regimen were randomized to receive low-dose irradiation (10 to 20 Gy) to previously involved sites or no further treatment. The 5-year remission duration estimated at 79 percent for patients who received radiation therapy was not significantly different from the 68 percent observed in those who

did not. Although low-dose irradiation improved the 5-year remission duration in the subgroups with nodular sclerosis (82 versus 60 percent, $p = .002$) or bulky disease (75 versus 57 percent, $p = .05$), overall 5-year survival was not improved in any subgroup.[95] The GELA group[96] recently published the results of a randomized comparison between two cycles of chemotherapy and nodal radiotherapy consolidation for patients with stage IIIB-IV Hodgkin's disease in complete remission or good partial remission after six cycles of MOPP-ABV hybrid or ABVPP (doxorubicin, bleomycin, vinblastine, procarbazine, prednisone). After induction therapy, 418 patients were evaluable for consolidation treatment comparisons. After a median follow-up period of 48 months, the 5-year freedom from progression did not differ between chemotherapy (79 percent), and combined modality (74 percent). After MOPP-ABV, 5-year overall survival was similar for chemotherapy (85 percent) and combined modality (88 percent); after ABVPP the 5-year survival was 94 percent for chemotherapy and 78 percent for combined modality. In conclusion, these results do not support the use of consolidation with radiotherapy instead of two further courses of chemotherapy after doxorubicin-induced complete remission for patients with advanced Hodgkin's disease.

In 1998,[37] the International Database on Hodgkin's Disease Overview Study Group published a meta-analysis of 1740 patients from 14 controlled adjuvant irradiation clinical trials. In studies comparing the addition of radiation to chemotherapy versus the same chemotherapy alone, tumor control at 10 years was significantly improved by 11 percent, but overall survival was similar. Trials in which the addition of radiation to chemotherapy was compared with the addition of further chemotherapy showed that there was no difference in tumor control in the two groups if an appropriate number of drug cycles were administered. However, overall survival was 8 percent better in the chemotherapy alone group because of fewer late treatment-related deaths. Adjuvant radiotherapy was thus recommended only for a few specific indications such as bulky mediastinal disease. Thus, according to "evidence-based-medicine" criteria, there is no clear indication for consolidation therapy after complete remission in advanced stages of Hodgkin's disease.

SALVAGE THERAPY

An extensive literature exists on second- and third-line systemic therapy for advanced Hodgkin's disease patients who have relapsed or are refractory to primary chemotherapy. The vast majority of relapsing patients will require some form of systemic therapy. The issues involved in salvage treatment of Hodgkin's disease revolve around such concepts as non-cross-resistant chemotherapy, multidrug resistance, and response to escalated doses of chemotherapeutic agents.[97,98]

Prognostic Factors for Choice of Treatment

Salvage treatment for Hodgkin's disease is required for essentially four subsets of patients with different prognostic implications: (1) patients relapsing after radiotherapy alone; (2)

patients relapsing after more or (3) less than 12 months from the achievement of complete remission with first-line chemotherapy; and (4) chemoresistant patients (also called "refractory" or "induction failure" patients). At present, the widespread use of high-dose chemotherapy with stem-cell support in virtually all patients relapsing after chemotherapy has eliminated the distinction between categories (2) and (3) (see below). As a matter of fact, the number of cases in the first group is progressively decreasing, as only a few patients are given front-line radiotherapy alone (see above).

In the past, duration of first complete remission has been considered the main prognostic factor predicting second chance of cure. In fact, a number of trials demonstrated prolonged disease-free survival by retreatment with the same regimen that resulted in a prolonged initial complete response. Of 32 patients relapsing after primary chemotherapy at the NCI, 59 percent achieved a second complete remission when retreated with MOPP.[9] However, only 29 percent of patients whose initial remission lasted less than 1 year achieved a second complete remission, compared with 93 percent of patients whose initial complete remission was longer than 1 year. The duration of second remission was also longer in patients whose initial complete remission exceeded 1 year than in those whose initial remission was less than 12 months. Similar results were also reported by the Milan group,[99,100] as well as by other investigators.

Today, the duration of first complete remission represents only one of the prognostic variables considered when second-line treatment is planned. In fact, a number of other factors, such as extension of disease at relapse, presence or absence of B symptoms, performance status, and response rate to induction therapy preceding high-dose consolidation, have demonstrated their prognostic significance in this setting.[101]

Relapse After Radiation Therapy

As previously noted, 20 to 40 percent of patients with stage I and II Hodgkin's disease who are treated with primary radiation therapy will eventually relapse within 3 years from completion of therapy. In a few instances, radiation therapy alone has been successfully used to salvage patients when the relapse occurred in a single lymph node chain more than 5 years after completion of the primary irradiation program. In all other cases, the survival of patients treated with chemotherapy after radiation relapse is at least equal to that of advanced-stage patients initially treated with the same chemotherapy combination. Indeed, an apparent survival advantage of patients with radiation relapses over the primary treatment group has been attributed to a more favorable patient mix, with generally more limited extension of disease. Overall and disease-free survival range from 60 to 80 percent.[102,103]

Even in this case, stage at relapse is an important prognostic variable. At Stanford the 10-year relapse-free-survival was 88, 58, and 34 percent, respectively, for those in stage IA, in stage IIA or IIIA, and in stage IV or with B symptoms at the time of relapse. As far as the choice of chemotherapy regimen is concerned, the same considerations outlined for first line chemotherapy are of value. From the available evidence, ABVD

exhibits the same superiority over MOPP for radiation recurrence that it does in initial treatment of advanced disease.[42,44]

Relapse After Chemotherapy

Apart from already discussed late relapses, the treatment of choice for patients relapsing after chemotherapy has been historically represented by non cross-resistant regimens at conventional doses. In the past, relapses after MOPP could be safely treated with ABVD with a second chance of cure as high as 40 percent.[104] However, the vast majority of patients now receive front-line treatment with MOPP and ABVD or some variant of those regimens. Thus, a number of new regimens have been devised that induce complete remission in no more than 50 percent of all patients, with 50 to 70 percent of the responders eventually relapsing again. Such patients have a probability of survival at 5 years after relapse of only 15 to 30 percent.[105–107] Somewhat better results come from regimens containing intermediate- or high-dose ifosfamide combined with etoposide or new active drugs such as vinorelbine.[108–110] In small series, up to 70 percent of patients are disease-free after 2 years,[108] and of note, there is no difference in outcome between relapsed or primary refractory cases.

High-dose therapy with stem cell rescue is now applicable to a large proportion of patients with relapsed Hodgkin's disease, as the correct use of growth factors and other supportive care strategies have definitively improved the safety of such an approach. The trend toward a better outcome for patients treated by high-dose therapy, along with the low mortality rate, now reported to be less than 1 percent at most centers, may eliminate the need for a randomized comparison between high-dose and conventional therapy. Moreover, patients with relapsed disease are generally young and in good general condition and represent ideal candidates for intensive procedures. On examining the recent literature (Table 43–9), a 5-year freedom from progression of approximately 40 to 50 percent emerges despite the heterogeneity of case series in terms of the number of patients treated, induction and conditioning regimens, and eligibility criteria.[101,111–118]

The only published randomized trial[111] compares high-dose therapy with stem cell rescue and a "low-dose" therapy such as miniBEAM. Thus, the advantage of the high-dose arm seems to be related to the inadequacy of the control arm rather than to a real improved impact of high-dose therapy. More interesting, even if not randomized, is the historical matched comparison performed at Stanford University.[101] A statistically significant better freedom from progression emerges for 62 patients treated by high-dose therapy compared with those treated conventionally (62 versus 32 percent), and a trend favoring high-dose therapy is also evident for overall survival (54 versus 47 percent). It is possible that a number of patients treated in the pretransplant era were salvaged by third-line high-dose therapy, which would explain the similar overall survival of the two groups. Even patients relapsing after long-lasting remission can reasonably be considered for high-dose therapy. An exception may be a patient with a single nodal site of nonbulky relapse after a durable remission, who would be expected to do well with con-

Table 43–9. High-Dose Therapy with Stem-Cell Rescue for Patients in First Relapse

Author (ref)	N	Selection Criteria	Conditioning Regimen	FFP (%)	FU (years)
Chopra[112]	52	Relapse within 1 year At least 2 previous regimens	BEAM	47	5
Nademanee[84]	43	Relapse within 1 year Non CR after salvage therapy	BCNU/VP16/CTX TBI/VP16/CTX	40	3
Bierman[113]	58	Relapse after chemotherapy	CBV	40	5
Reece[154]	58	Relapse after chemotherapy	CBV ± CDDP	61	5
Yuen[155]	47	Relapse after chemotherapy 1 year, more or less	BCNU/VP16/CTX TBI/VP16/CTX	56/50	4
Wheeler[116]	42	Relapse after CR	CBV	44	4
[a]Sweethenham[117]	139	Relapse after CR	BEAM/CBV/others ± TBI	44.7	5
[b]Brice[118]	220	Relapse after CR	CBV/BEAM/BEAC/others	71	5

BEAM, BCNU, etoposide, cytarabine, melphalan; CTX, cyclophosphamide; CBV, cyclophosphamide, BCNU, VP16; TBI, total-body irradiation; CDDP, cisplatinum; BEAC, BCNU, etoposide, cytarabine, cyclophosphamide, CR, complete remission; FFP, freedom from progression; FU, follow-up period.
[a] Data from the International Bone Marrow Transplantation Registry.
[b] Data from the Societé Française de Graffe de Moelle.

ventional therapy.[119] Patients with significant concomitant illnesses are obviously also not candidates for intensive therapy and would be better served by being considered for newer approaches, such as immunologically targeted therapy[120] or new active drug studies utilizing less intensive strategies.[110,121]

Recent trials (Table 43–10) suggest the possibility of cure by high-dose therapy even in patients with primary refractory disease, defined as those never achieving complete remission with first-line chemotherapy. Lazarus et al.[122] reported on 122 chemotherapy-resistant patients who obtained a complete response rate of 50 percent with high-dose therapy and a 38 percent 3-year overall survival. Similar data were provided by a German group,[123] which reported a 5-year overall survival of 19 percent among 67 patients with primary refractory disease. Of note, overall survival was 53 percent for the 25 patients who actually could receive high-dose consolidation. This somewhat lower

probability of cure as compared with the International Transplant Registry data is considered to result from different data-collection methodology in a single center than that employed for the multicenter database. The GELA/SFGM group studied an especially unfavorable group of patients with relapsed or refractory Hodgkin's disease and demonstrated the feasibility of tandem administration of high-dose chemotherapy.[124] Of 43 patients, 32 (74 percent) completed the treatment. Platelet recovery after the second transplant (TBI or busulfan-containing preparative regimen) was delayed. There were two venooclusive disease episodes, one fatal, and one case of hemorrhagic cystitis, but no grade IV toxicity with a reduced dose of busulfan. The 2-year survival for patients receiving the two procedures was 74 percent, and that for the whole series was 65 percent.

There are few data from which to identify which standard-dose salvage regimen is optimal prior to high-dose chemother-

Table 43–10. High-Dose Therapy with Stem-Cell Rescue for Patients with Primary Refractory Disease

Author (ref)	N	Selection Criteria	Conditioning Regimen	FFP (%)	FU (years)
Gianni[156]	16	Non-CR with first-line MOPP/ABVD	SCT + TBI or IFRT	31	6
Chopra[112]	46	Non-CR with MOPP, MOPP/ABVD, or analogues	BEAM	33	5
Reece[154]	30	Histologically confirmed persistent disease	CBV ± CDDP	42	4
Prince[157]	30	Non-CR, chemosensitive disease	VP16/melphalan	34	3
Sweethenham[158]	290	SD or PD after first- or second-line chemotherapy	BEAM/CBV/others ± TBI	30	5
Horning[101]	29	PR or PD during CT; PD within 4 weeks from chemotherapy completion	TBI/VP16/CTX BCU(CCNU)/VP16/ CTX	50	4
Lazarus[122]	129	Histologically confirmed persistent disease	High-dose therapy ± TBI	38	3

SCT, high-dose sequential therapy: CTX→ methotrexate→ VP16→ TBI/melphalan; IFRT, involved-field radiotherapy; CR, complete remission; SD, stable disease; PD, progressive disease; FFP, freedom from progression; FU, follow-up period.

apy. The mini-BEAM regimen is certainly efficacious, but stem cell collection is impaired after its use.[125] The Cologne group demonstrated the feasibility of giving three or four courses of dexaBEAM prior to high-dose BEAM with adequate stem-cell collection, which suggests the need to achieve as maximal a response as possible with conventional induction therapy prior to high-dose therapy.[126] Other regimens containing etoposide, platinum compounds, cytarabine, ifosfamide, or vinorelbine are also frequently used and combine antilymphoma activity with stem cell-mobilizing potential.[108,127–130]

Further improvement of outcome for patients with relapsed Hodgkin's disease should focus first of all on increasing the complete remission rate by induction therapy, which may be achieved by increasing the dose intensity of effective regimens, or by including new active drugs, such as vinorelbine,[110] gemcitabine,[121] or mitoxantrone[81] in induction regimens. Second, the concomitant use of immunologically targeted strategies such as immunotoxins or monoclonal antibodies should be explored in this setting with the aim of reducing minimal residual disease.[131,132]

TREATMENT SEQUELAE

Unfortunately, recent improvement in the cure rate of Hodgkin's disease patients has been partially offset by treatment-related mortality and morbidity. In the Stanford experience,[133] 15 years after diagnosis the mortality rate from causes other than Hodgkin's disease is greater than that from Hodgkin's disease itself (Table 43–11). Because the median age of patients 15 years after treatment was only 44 years, mortality from causes other than Hodgkin's disease is a serious new problem. Few additional disease-related deaths occur beyond 15 years, although late treatment-related deaths continue to occur. Quality of life in some long-term survivors may be significantly impaired, according to a "fatigue score" published by Loge et al.[134]

Cardiac Complications

Cardiovascular complications of mantle irradiation are the second most frequent cause of treatment-related mortality in

Table 43–11. Causes of Death Among 2498 Patients Treated at Stanford University

Cause of Death	N	Percent
Hodgkin's disease	333	44
Second neoplasms	160	21
Cardiovascular	117	16
Pulmonary	50	7
Infection	31	4
Accident	14	2
Hematologic	9	1
Gastrointestinal	4	1
Other	14	2
Unknown	22	3

Hodgkin's disease patients followed through the second decade post-treatment and cause 2 to 5 percent of the mortality in the entire Hodgkin's disease population. Although the relative cardiac risk is modest, the absolute risk is high (9.3 to 28 per 10,000 patients per year), because of the high frequency of cardiac death in the general population. Moreover, although the relative risk of cardiac death is greatest in radiation-treated children and adolescents and the absolute risk increases with increasing age at the time of radiation therapy up to the sixth decade.[134,135]

Myocardial infarction causes more than two-thirds of the cardiac deaths observed in radiation-treated Hodgkin's disease patients, despite being appreciated later and encountered less frequently than other forms of radiation damage to the heart. Furthermore, deaths due to myocardial infarction have not been substantially reduced by the refinements of radiation techniques. In fact, the 18-year actuarial cardiac mortality is 4.5 percent for patients treated before 1972 and 5 percent after that date. Some authors have recommended a total dose of radiotherapy as low as 32.3 Gy[135] based on that information.

The overall incidence of cardiac failure induced by doxorubicin ranges from 1 to 2 percent but is markedly higher (more than 30 percent) if the cumulative dose exceeds 550 mg/m². The clinical picture is usually characterized by cardiomegaly, biventricular failure associated with or preceded by an increased ratio of preejection period to left ventricular ejection time, and low QRS voltage. The only preventive measure is stopping drug administration before the cumulative dose of 550 mg/m² is reached. Clinicians should also be aware that a previous history of cardiac disease is a risk factor, as is mediastinal irradiation,[136] and that cardiomyopathy may occur in these instances after total doses below 450 mg/m². Radiation-related pericarditis occurs in 25 to 30 percent of patients treated with radiation therapy. It is usually transient and self-limiting, but constrictive pericarditis with or without tamponade may occur.[137]

Pulmonary Complications

Pulmonary morbidity and mortality are related both to mantle-field irradiation and to bleomycin. Major risk factors include age over 70 years, cumulative dose of bleomycin as high as 300 to 400 U/m², concomitant mediastinal irradiation, and oxygen therapy. However, pulmonary fibrosis has been rarely described even in younger patients given low-dose bleomycin. Bleomycin-induced mortality after ABVD occurs in approximately 1 to 3 percent of patients. Careful monitoring of respiratory function during treatment may be helpful in decreasing such a risk in that bleomycin can be discontinued if impaired pulmonary function is detected early.[138]

Second Neoplasms

The relative risks of acute myeloid leukemia and of non-Hodgkin's lymphoma are far greater than that of solid tumors, but the absolute risks are smaller. The relationship to alkylating agents and their cumulative dose has been well documented. Whereas the excess risk of leukemia and lymphoma is usually back to baseline by the second decade after treatment, the solid tumor risk continues into the third decade and probably beyond. Most investigators attribute the solid tumor risk to radiation therapy, but new data suggest that MOPP chemotherapy may lead to an elevated risk of lung cancer in patients with Hodgkin's disease.[139] Usually after a latent period of at least 5 to 10 years, the increased solid tumor risk becomes apparent in large series of patients. The literature has focused mainly on secondary acute myeloid leukemia, myelodysplasia, and breast cancer as important second neoplasms after treatment for Hodgkin's disease. However, lung cancer and soft tissue sarcomas are frequent second tumors as well. The median latency period is relatively short for acute myeloid leukemia and myelodysplasia, but it may be as long as 18 years or more for lung cancer.[140]

The excess risk of breast carcinoma is almost completely restricted to women who received radiation therapy before the age of 30.[141,142] Those treated in the second decade and the first half of the third decade of life are subject to the maximum cumulative risk, with shoulders of the risk peak extending into the second half of both the first and third decades. The risk curve is consistent with the current understanding of breast carcinogenesis. In fact, the first breast carcinomas appear at the end of the first decade after irradiation and continue to appear in women observed for the longest period (three decades). In one series, actuarial calculation predicted a 34 percent incidence of breast cancer 25 years after irradiation in those treated before age 20. These second tumors appear within or at the edge of irradiation fields.[141]

The overall incidence of acute myeloid leukemia and myelodysplasia within 10 years from initial treatment for Hodgkin's disease ranges in most series from 2 to 6 percent or less. The highest incidence of this complication occurs in patients treated with extensive radiation therapy plus MOPP or MOPP-like chemotherapy, in patients older than 40 years at the start of chemotherapy, and in those subjected to staging laparotomy with splenectomy. Furthermore, it seems that patients who initially undergo radiation therapy and subsequently receive salvage chemotherapy represent the subgroup at highest risk for developing leukemia or myelodysplasia. This is a refractory hematologic neoplasm and virtually no patients survive this complication.[143–145]

Typically, treatment-related leukemia is characterized by a latency period of 3 to 5 years, a preceding myelodysplastic phase, trilineage bone-marrow dysplasia, and abnormalities of chromosome 5 and/or 7.[142] More recently, topoisomerase II inhibitors, primarily epipodophyllotoxins but also anthracyclines when given in combination with alkylating agents, have been implicated in the development of a clinically and cytogenetically distinct form of secondary acute myeloid leukemia in both adult and pediatric patients. In contrast to alkylating agent-related leukemia, this form of therapy-related leukemia lacks a preceding myelodysplastic phase and is characterized by a shorter latency period (less than 3 years), myelomonocytic or monocytic morphology, and balanced chromosome translocations involving bands 11q23 or 21q22. The cumulative dose of epipodophyllotoxins as well as dose-dense administration are implicated in the induction of this type of secondary leukemia.[146]

Hematological malignancies have been studied also in survivors after high-dose therapy with stem cell support. It must be emphasized that acute myeloid leukemia and myelodysplasia often result from chemotherapy and/or radiation therapy given for the primary malignancy prior to transplantation rather than from high-dose chemotherapy administered as a transplant preparative regimen. As a matter of fact, the latency period from first-line therapy and development of leukemia is 4 to 6 years, whereas it is substantially less from the high-dose chemotherapy–PBSCT time (median 2.7 years).[86] In a report from the University of Chicago Medical Center concerning 641 patients, seven (1.1 percent) developed therapy-related acute leukemia.[146] The disease-specific incidence of therapy-related leukemia was 6.3 percent of patients treated for Hodgkin's disease. The median latency periods from the time of initial treatment and from that of high-dose therapy were 5.5 and 1.5 years, respectively.[87] Thus, it is more likely that the development of secondary leukemia resulted from pretransplant chemotherapy, which implies that early detection of therapy-related cytogenetic abnormalities may be useful to exclude patients from high-dose chemotherapy–PBSCT programs.[147,148]

In a reported series of 1391 Hodgkin's disease patients treated with various approaches from 1972 to 1996, the possible role of splenectomy in the development of non-Hodgkin's lymphoma was investigated. After a median follow-up period of 84 months, a total of 20 cases of non-Hodgkin's lymphoma was observed, with a cumulative risk of 0.8 percent at 5 years and 3.5 percent at 20 years. Splenectomy or splenic irradiation and age over 40 years were associated with relative risks of 5.69 and 3.05 percent respectively, for reasons that are not known.

Infertility

Treatment-induced infertility represents an important social and psychosocial problem. In general, infertility is more common in male patients owing to the higher sensitivity of their reproductive organs to chemotherapy-related damage, especially that induced by alkylating agents and procarbazine. The MOPP regimen has induced infertility in up to 70 percent of male patients, whereas ABVD and other nonalkylating agent-based regimens less frequently induce infertility, which is usually reversible. Furthermore, gonadal damage is strictly related to patient age at the time of treatment. Prepubertal patients carry a lower risk of infertility after treatment for Hodgkin's disease.[149]

Cryopreservation of semen is routinely performed by many centers before treatment of young male patients. However, this is controversial because most males with Hodgkin's disease have oligospermia or other sperm abnormalities at the time of diagnosis, and their sperm samples usually do not meet the criteria of most reputable sperm banks.

Sterility problems appear to be less common in adult women than in men, probably because the germ cells of the ovary with their low proliferative rate are less sensitive to drugs than are those of the testicle. Of women treated with regimens containing procarbazine or alkylating agents, 40 to 50 percent become amenorrheic.[43] The incidence of premature ovarian failure is age-dependent and is also related to total dose of chemotherapy. Infertility increases in frequency from 1 to 10 years after chemotherapy. Reestablishment of menses and the possibility of pregnancy in a treated woman are also correlated with age and the cumulative dose of drug exposure. However, amenorrhea is no guarantee of infertility, and patients should be made aware of that fact. It is also important to consider that some evidence suggests that oral contraceptives given during treatment may reduce the incidence of ovarian failure. Most data indicate that the risk of spontaneous abortion or fetal abnormalities in patients previously treated with combination chemotherapy is not increased compared with the risk of the general population, but there are presently no data on the risk to subsequent generations, if any. In any case, whenever possible, chemotherapy should be avoided during pregnancy, especially in the first trimester. Despite the potential infertility associated with Hodgkin's disease and its treatment, it may be relatively short-term in many patients. Pregnancy occurs in patients treated for Hodgkin's disease and spouses of treated male patients with surprising frequency.[150] Such pregnancies are not associated with increased complications or spontaneous abortion, and congenital abnormalities in the offspring of such pregnancies are no more frequent than in the general population.

Thyroid Complications.

Thyroid dysfunction is related to neck irradiation and possibly to lymphangiography, but chemotherapy seems to play no role in its incidence or severity.[151] Of 1787 patients treated at Stanford, 50 percent exhibited thyroid damage within 20 years.[152] The median latency period from therapy was 4.6 years, and the most frequent event was hypothyroidism (47 percent), usually subclinical, followed by Graves disease (3.1 percent), benign alterations (3.3 percent), and autoimmune thyroiditis (1.3 percent). Furthermore, an increased incidence of thyroid cancer is reported, especially in pediatric patients. The risk of developing thyroid dysfunction persists for up to 25 years after treatment is completed. Therefore, clinical examination and laboratory tests are recommended at 6 month intervals during the first 5 years and annually thereafter. Patients found to have an elevated level of thyroid-stimulating hormone following neck irradiation should be treated with thyroid hormone for the rest of their lives.[153]

REFERENCES

1. Mauch P, Gorshein D, Cunningham J et al: Influence of mediastinal adenopathy on site and frequency of relapse in patients with Hodgkin's disease. Cancer Treat Rep 66:809, 1982.
2. Mauch P, Tarbell N, Weinstein H et al: Stage IA and IIA with supradiaphragmatic Hodgkin's disease: Prognostic factors in surgically staged patients treated with mantle and paraaortic irradiation. J Clin Oncol 6:1576, 1988.
3. Kaplan HS: Hodgkin's disease. 2nd Ed. Harvard University Press, Cambridge, MA, 1980.
4. Mauch P, Kalish L, Kadin M et al: Pattern of presentation of Hodgkin's disease. Implications for etiology and pathogenesis. Cancer 71:2062, 1993.
5. Grogan TM, Berard CW, Steinhorn SC et al: Changing patterns of Hodgkin's disease at autopsy: A 25-year experience at the National Cancer Institute. 1975–1978. Cancer Treat Rep 66:653, 1982.
6. Bodis S, Henry-Amar M, Bosq J et al: Late relapse in early-stage Hodgkin's disease patients enrolled in the European Organization for Research and Treatment of Cancer Protocols. J Clin Oncol 11:225, 1993.
7. Salvagno L, Sorarù M, Aversa SML et al: Late relapses in Hodgkin's disease: Outcome of patients relapsing more than twelve months after primary chemotherapy. Ann Oncol 4:657, 1993.
8. Roach M, Brophy N, Cox R et al: Prognostic factors for patients relapsing after radiotherapy for early stage Hodgkin's disease. J Clin Oncol 8:623, 1990.
9. Longo DL, Duffey PL, Young RC et al: Conventional dose salvage combination chemotherapy in patients relapsing with Hodgkin's disease after combination: The low probability for cure. J Clin Oncol 10:210, 1992.
10. The Non-Hodgkin's Lymphoma Pathologic Classification Project: National Cancer Institute sponsored study of classification of non-Hodgkin's lymphoma. Summary and description of a working formulation for clinical usage. Cancer 49:2112, 1982.
11. Lister TA, Crowther D, Sutcliffe SB et al: Report of a committee convened to discuss the evaluation of staging of patients with Hodgkin's disease: Cotswolds meeting. J Clin Oncol 8:1602, 1990.
12. Hasenclever D, Diehl V: A prognostic score for advanced Hodgkin's disease. N Engl J Med 339:1506, 1998.
13. Harris NL, Jaffe ES, Stein H et al: A revised European-American lymphoma classification of lymphoid neoplasms : A proposal from the International Lymphoma Study Group. Blood 84:1361, 1994.
14. Brice P: Prognostic factors in advanced Hodgkin's disease – can they guide therapeutic decisions? N Engl J Med 339:1547, 1998.
15. Pera A: Lymphangiography and CT in the follow-up of patients with lymphoma. Radiology 164:131, 1987.
16. Castellino RA, Hoppe RT, Blank N et al: Computed tomography, lymphangiography and staging laparotomy: Correlations in initial staging of Hodgkin's disease. Am J Radiol 143:37, 1984.
17. Mansfield CM, Fabian C, Jones S et al: Comparison of lymphangiography and computed tomography scanning in evaluating abdominal disease in stage III and IV Hodgkin's disease. Cancer 66:229, 1988.
18. Musumeci R, Tesoro-Tess JD: New imaging techniques in staging lymphomas. Curr Opin Oncol 21:464, 1994.
19. Radford JA, Cowan RA, Flanagan M et al: The significance of residual mediastinal abnormality in chest radiograph following treatment for Hodgkin's disease. J Clin Oncol 6:940, 1988.
20. Jochelson M, Mauch P, Balikian J et al: The significance of the residual mediastinal mass in treated Hodgkin's disease. J Clin Oncol 3:637, 1985.
21. Devizzi L, Balzarini L, Santoro A et al: Comparison of gallium scan, computed tomography and magnetic resonance in patients with mediastinal Hodgkin's disease. Ann Oncol 8(Suppl. 1):53, 1997.
22. Munker R, Hasenclever D, Brosteanu O, Hiller E, Diehl V: Bone marrow involvement in Hodgkin's disease: An analysis of 135 consecutive cases. German Hodgkin's Lymphoma Study Group. J Clin Oncol 13:403, 1995.
23. Luoni M, Fava S, Declich P: Bone marrow biopsy for staging Hodgkin's lymphoma: The bilateral or unilateral trephine biopsy. J Clin Oncol 14:682, 1996.
24. Stumpe KD, Urbinelli M, Steinert HC, Glanzmann C, Buk A, von Schulthess GK. Whole-body positron emission tomography using fluorodeoxyglucose for staging of lymphoma: Effectiveness and

comparison with computed tomography. Eur J Nucl Med 25:721, 1998.

25. Wirth A, Chao M, Corry J et al: Mantle irradiation alone for clinical stage I–II Hodgkin's disease: Long-term follow-up and analysis of prognostic factors in 261 patients. J Clin Oncol 17:230, 1999.

26. Jerusalem G, Beguin Y, Fassotte MF et al: Whole body FDG PET post-treatment evaluation in Hodgkin's disease (HD) and non-Hodgkin's lymphoma (NHL) has higher diagnostic and prognostic value than classical CT scan imaging. (abstr.) Blood 90:336, 1999.

27. Tubiana M, Henry-Amar M, Carde P et al: Towards comprehensive management tailored to prognostic factors of patients with clinical stage I and II Hodgkin's disease. The EORTC Lymphoma group controlled clinical trials: 1964–1987. Blood 73:47, 1989.

28. Hoppe RT: Hodgkin's disease: Complications of therapy and excess mortality. Ann Oncol (Suppl. 1):115–118, 1997.

29. Wolden SL, Lamborn KR, Cleary SF et al: Second cancers following pediatric Hodgkin's disease. J Clin Oncol 16:536–544, 1998.

30. Aisenberg AC, Finkelstein DM, Doppke KP et al: High risk of breast carcinoma after irradiation of young women with Hodgkin's disease. Cancer 79:1203, 1997.

31. Kaplan HS: Hodgkin's disease: Biology, treatment and prognosis. Blood 57:813, 1982.

32. Diehl V, Mauch PM, Harris NL: Hodgkin's disease. In DeVita VR, Hellman S, Rosenberg SA (eds.): Cancer Principles and Practice of Oncology, 6th Ed. Lippincott, Philadelphia, 2001.

33. Aisenberg AC: Problems in Hodgkin's disease management. Blood 93:761, 1999.

34. Cosset JM, Henry-Amar M, Noordijk EM et al: The EORTC trials for adult patients with early stage Hodgkin's disease. A 1997 update. ASTRO Lymphoma Categorical Course, Reston, VA, 1997.

35. Radford JA, Cowan RA, Ryder WDJ et al: Four weeks of neo-adjuvant chemotherapy significantly reduces the progression rate in patients treated with limited field radiotherapy for clinical stage IA/IIA Hodgkin's disease. Results of a randomised pilot study. Ann Oncol 7(Suppl. 3):66, 1996.

36. Specht L, Gray R, Clarke M et al: The influence of more extensive radiotherapy and adjuvant chemotherapy on long term outcome of early stage Hodgkin's disease: A metanalysis of 23 randomized trials involving 3888 patients. J Clin Oncol 16:830, 1988.

37. Loeffler M, Brosteanu O, Hasenclever D et al: Meta-analysis of chemotherapy versus combined modality treatment trials in Hodgkin's disease. J Clin Oncol 16:818, 1998.

38. Horning SJ, Williams J, Bartlett NL et al: Assessment of the Stanford V regimen and consolidative radiotherapy for bulky and advanced Hodgkin's disease: Eastern Cooperative Oncology Group Pilot Study E1492. J Clin Oncol 18:972, 2000.

39. Santoro A, Bonadonna G: Prolonged disease free survival in MOPP-resistant Hodgkin's disease after treatment with Adriamycin, bleomycin, vinblastine and dacarbazine (ABVD). Cancer Chemother Pharmacol 2:101, 1979.

40. Bonadonna G: Modern treatment of malignant lymphomas: A multidisciplinary approach? Ann Oncol 5:85, 1994.

41. Bonadonna G, Valagussa P, Santoro A: Alternating non cross-resistant combination chemotherapy or MOPP in stage IV Hodgkin's disease. A report of 8-year results. Ann Intern Med 104:739, 1986.

42. Santoro A, Bonadonna G, Bonfante V et al: Alternating drug combination in the treatment of advanced Hodgkin's disease. N Engl J Med 306:770, 1982.

43. Santoro A, Bonadonna G, Valagussa P et al: Long-term results of combined chemotherapy-radiotherapy approach in Hodgkin's

disease: Superiority of ABVD plus radiotherapy versus MOPP plus radiotherapy. J Clin Oncol 5:27, 1987.

44. Santoro A, Bonfante V, Bonadonna G: Salvage chemotherapy with ABVD in MOPP-resistant Hodgkin's disease. Ann Intern Med 96:139, 1982.

45. Goldie JH, Coldman JA: A mathematical model for relating the drug sensitivity of tumors to their spontaneous mutation rate. Cancer Treat Rep 63:1727, 1979.

46. Connors JM, Klimo P, Adams G et al: Treatment of advanced Hodgkin's disease with chemotherapy. Comparison of MOPP/ABV hybrid regimen with alternating courses of MOPP and ABVD: A report from the National Cancer Institute of Canada Clinical Trials Group. J Clin Oncol 15:1638, 1997.

47. Viviani S, Bonadonna G, Santoro A et al: Alternating versus hybrid MOPP and ABVD combinations in advanced Hodgkin's disease: Ten year results. J Clin Oncol 14:1421, 1996.

48. Glick JH, Young ML, Harringhton D et al: MOPP/ABVD hybrid chemotherapy for advanced Hodgkin's disease significantly improves failure-free and overall survival: The 8 year results of the intergroup trial. J Clin Oncol 16:19, 1998.

49. Canellos JP, Anderson J; Propert KJ et al: Chemotherapy of advanced Hodgkin's disease with MOPP, ABVD or MOPP alternating with ABVD. N Engl J Med 327:1478, 1992.

50. Tesch H, Diehl V, Lathan B et al: Moderate dose escalation for advanced stage Hodgkin's disease using the bleomycin, etoposide, Adriamycin, cyclophosphamide, vincristine, procarbazine and prednisone scheme and adjuvant radiotherapy: A study of the German Hodgkin's lymphoma study group. Blood 92:4560, 1998.

51. Diehl V, Franklin J, Hasenclever D et al: BEACOPP a new dose escalated and accelerated regimen is a least as effective as COPP/ABVD in patients with advanced-stage Hodgkin's lymphoma: Interim report from a trial of the German Hodgkin's lymphoma study group. J Clin Oncol 16:3810, 1998.

52. Gobbi PG, Pierasca C, Ghirardelli ML et al: Long-term results from MOPPEBVCAD chemotherapy with optional limited radiotherapy in advanced Hodgkin's disease. Blood 91:2704, 1998.

53. Lancet JE, Rapoport AP, Brasacchio R et al: Autotransplantation for relapsed or refractory Hodgkin's disease: Long-term follow-up and analysis of prognostic factors. Bone Marrow Transplant 22:265, 1998.

54. Linch DC, Winfield D, Goldstone AH et al: Dose intensification with autologous bone marrow transplantation in relapsed and resistant Hodgkin's disease: Results of a BNLI randomized trial. Lancet 341:1051, 1993.

55. Carde P, Hagenbeek A, Hayat M et al: Clinical staging versus laparotomy and combined modality with MOPP versus ABVD in early stage Hodgkin's disease: The H6 twin randomized trials from the European Organization for Research and Treatment of Cancer Lymphoma Cooperative Group. J Clin Oncol 11:2258, 1993.

56. Prosnitz LR, Farber LR, Kapp DS et al: Combined modality therapy for advanced Hodgkin's disease: 15-year follow-up data. J Clin Oncol 6:603, 1988.

57. Yelle L, Bergsagel D, Basco V et al: Combined modality therapy of Hodgkin's disease: Ten-year results of National Cancer Institute of Canada Clinical Trials Group Multicenter Clinical Trial. J Clin Oncol 9:1983, 1991.

58. Viviani S, Santoro A, Negretti E et al: Salvage chemotherapy in Hodgkin's disease. Results in patients relapsing more than twelve months after first complete remission. Ann Oncol 1:123, 1990.

59. Rosenberg SA: Reducing the toxicity of the combined modality therapy of favourable–stage Hodgkin's disease. Eur J Cancer 28A:1379, 1992.

60. Colby TV, Hoppe RT, Warnke RA: Hodgkin's disease at autopsy: 1972–1977. Cancer 47:1852, 1981.

61. Longo DL, Glatstein E, Duffey PL et al: Radiation therapy versus combination chemotherapy in the treatment of early stage Hodgkin's disease: Seven years results of a prospective randomized trial. J Clin Oncol 9:906, 1991.

62. Cornbleet MA, Vitolo U, Ultman JE et al: Pathologic stages IA and IIA Hodgkin's disease: Results of treatment with radiotherapy alone. J Clin Oncol 3:758, 1985.

63. Zagars G, Rubin P: Hodgkin's disease stage IA-IIA: A long-term follow-up study on the results achieved by modern therapy. Cancer 56:1907, 1986.

64. Longo DL: The use of chemotherapy in the treatment of Hodgkin's disease. Semin Oncol 17:716, 1990.

65. Carde P, Burgers JMV, Henry-Amar M et al: Clinical stages I and II Hodgkin's disease: A specifically tailored therapy according to prognostic factors. J Clin Oncol 6:239, 1988.

66. Rosenberg SA, Kaplan HS: The evolution and summary results of the Stanford randomized clinical trials of the management of Hodgkin's disease, 1962–1984. Int J Radiat Biol Phys 11:5, 1985.

67. Wiernik PH, Gustafson J, Diggs C: Combined modality treatment of Hodgkin's disease confined to lymph nodes. Results eight years later. Am J Med 67:183, 1979.

68. Longo DL: Chemotherapy alone in the treatment of patients with early stage Hodgkin's disease. Ann Oncol 7(Suppl. 4):85, 1996.

69. Biti GP, Cimino C, Cartoni C et al: Extended-field radiotherapy is superior to MOPP chemotherapy in the treatment of pathologic stage IA–IIA Hodgkin's disease: Eight-year update of an Italian prospective randomized study. J Clin Oncol 9:906, 1991.

70. Pavlovsky S, Maschio M, Santarelli MT et al: Randomized trial of chemotherapy versus chemotherapy plus radiotherapy for stage I–II Hodgkin's disease. J Natl Cancer Inst 80:1466, 1988.

71. Bonfante V, Santoro A, Viviani S et al: Early stage Hodgkin's disease: Ten-year results of a non-randomized study with radiotherapy alone or combined with MOPP. Eur J Cancer 29A:24, 1992.

72. Horning SJ, Hoppe RT, Hancock SL et al: Vinblastine, bleomycin and methotrexate: An effective adjuvant in favorable Hodgkin's disease. J Clin Oncol 6:1822, 1988.

73. Horning SJ, Hoppe RT, Mason J et al: Stanford-Kaiser Permanente G1 study for clinical stage I to II Hodgkin's disease: Subtotal lymphoid irradiation versus vinblastine, methotrexate, and bleomycin chemotherapy and regional irradiation. J Clin Oncol 15:1736, 1997.

74. Santoro A, Bonfante V, Viviani S: Subtotal nodal (STNI) vs involved field (IFRT) irradiation after 4 cycles of ABVD in early stage Hodgkin's disease (HD). Proc Am Soc Clin Oncol 15:415 (A), 1996.

75. Longo DL, Young RC, Wesly M et al: Twenty years of MOPP chemotherapy for Hodgkin's disease. J Clin Oncol 4:1295, 1986.

76. Selby P, Patel P, Milan S et al: ChlVPP combination chemotherapy for Hodgkin's disease: Long term results. Br J Cancer 62:279, 1990.

77. Bakemeier RF, Anderson JR, Costello W et al: BCVPP chemotherapy for advanced Hodgkin's disease: Evidence for greater duration of complete remission, greater survival and less toxicity than with a MOPP regimen. Ann Intern Med 101:447, 1984.

78. Valagussa P, Bonadonna G, Fossati-Bellani F et al: Second acute leukemia and other malignancies following treatment for Hodgkin's disease. J Clin Oncol 4:830, 1986.

79. Canellos JP: Is ABVD the standard regimen for Hodgkin's disease based on randomized CALGB comparison of MOPP, ABVD, and MOPP alternating with ABVD? Leukemia 10(Suppl. 2):S68, 1996.

80. Viviani S, Bonfante V, Santoro et al: Long-term results of an intensive regimen: VEBEP plus involved-field radiotherapy in advanced Hodgkin's disease. Cancer J Sci Am 5:275, 2000.

81. Wiernik PH, Dutcher JP, Einzig AI et al: Mitoxantrone, vinblastine, and lomustine (CCNU) (MVC): A highly active regimen for advanced and poor-prognosis Hodgkin's disease. Cancer J Sci Am 4:254, 1998.

82. Carella AM, Prencipe E, Pungolino E et al: Twelve years experience with high-dose therapy and autologus stem cell transplantation for high risk Hodgkin's disease patients in first remission after MOPP/ABVD chemotherapy. Leuk Lymphoma 21:63, 1996.

83. Delain M, Cartron G, Bout M et al: Intensive therapy with autologous stem cell transplantation as first-line therapy in poor-risk Hodgkin's disease and analysis of predictive factors of outcome. Leuk Lymphoma 34:305, 1999.

84. Nademanee A, Molina A, Fung H et al: High-dose chemo/radiotherapy and autologous bone marrow or stem cell transplantation for poor-risk advanced-stage Hodgkin's disease during first partial or complete remission. Biol Blood Marrow Transplant 5:292, 1999.

85. Frei E III, Luce JK, Gamble G et al: Combination chemotherapy in advanced Hodgkin's disease: Induction and maintenance of remission. Ann Intern Med 79:376, 1973.

86. Young RC, Canellos GP, Chabner BA et al: Patterns of relapse in advanced Hodgkin's disease. Cancer 42:1001, 1978.

87. Longo DL: The case against the routine use of radiation therapy in advanced stage Hodgkin's disease. Cancer Invest 14:353, 1996.

88. Prosnitz LR, Wu JJ, Yahalom J: The case for adjuvant radiation therapy in advanced stage Hodgkin's disease. Cancer Invest 14:361, 1996.

89. Mauch PM: Controversies in the management of early stage Hodgkin's disease. Blood 83:319, 1994.

90. Hoppe RT: Radiation therapy as a component of high-dose salvage strategies in Hodgkin's disease. Ann Oncol 9(Suppl. 5):87, 1999.

91. Wu JJ, Prosnitz LR: The role of adjuvant radiation therapy for stage III and IV Hodgkin's disease. Semin Radiat Oncol 6:196, 1996.

92. Prosnitz LR, Farber LR, Kapp DS et al: Combined modality therapy for advanced stage Hodgkin's disease: 15-year follow-up data. J Clin Oncol 6:603, 1988.

93. Yahalom J, Ryu J, Straus DJ et al: Impact of adjuvant radiation on the pattern and rate of relapse in advanced stage Hodgkin's disease treated with alternating chemotherapy combinations. J Clin Oncol 9:2193, 1991.

94. Loeffler M, Diehl V, Pfreundschuh M, for the German Hodgkin's Lymphoma Study Group: Dose-response relationship of complementary radiotherapy following four cycles of combination chemotherapy in intermediate-stage Hodgkin's disease. J Clin Oncol 15:2275, 1997.

95. Fabian CJ, Mansfield CM, Dahlberg S et al: Low-dose involved-field radiation after chemotherapy in advanced Hodgkin's disease. Ann Intern Med 120:903, 1994.

96. Fermé C, Sebban C, Hennequin C et al: Comparison of chemotherapy to radiotherapy as consolidation of complete or good partial response after six cycles of chemotherapy for patients with advanced Hodgkin's disease: Results of the Groupe d'Études des Lymphomes de l'Adulte H89 trial. Blood 95:2246, 2000.

97. Bonadonna G: Salvage treatments in Hodgkin's disease. Eur J Cancer 27:530, 1991.

98. Canellos GP: Is there an effective salvage regimen for advanced Hodgkin's disease? Ann Oncol 2:1, 1991.

99. Bonadonna G, Santoro A, Gianni AM et al: Primary and salvage chemotherapy in advanced Hodgkin's disease. The Milan Centre Institute experience. Ann Oncol 1(Suppl. 1):9, 1991.

100. Bonfante V, Santoro A, Viviani S et al: Outcome of patients with Hodgkin's disease failing after primary MOPP-ABVD. J Clin Oncol 15:528, 1997.

101. Horning SJ, Chao NJ, Negrin RS et al: High-dose therapy and autologous hematopoietic progenitor cell transplantation for recurrent or refractory Hodgkin's disease: Analysis of the Stanford University results and prognostic indices. Blood 89:801, 1997.

102. Yuen AR, Horning SJ: Hodgkin's disease: Management of first relapse. Oncology 10:233, 1996.

103. Bodis S, Henry-Amar M, Bosq J et al: Late relapse in early stage Hodgkin's disease patients enrolled on European Organization for Research and Treatment of Cancer protocols. J Clin Oncol 11:225, 1993.

104. Bonadonna G, Santoro AM, Gianni AM et al: Primary and salvage chemotherapy in advanced Hodgkin's disease: The Milan Cancer Institute experience. Ann Oncol 1:9, 1991.

105. Santoro A, Viviani S, Valagussa P et al: CCNU, etoposide and prednimustine (CEP) in refractory Hodgkin's disease. Semin Oncol 13(Suppl. 1):23, 1986.

106. Pfreundschuh MG, Schoppe WD, Fuchs R et al: Lomustine, etoposide, vindesine and dexamethasone (CEVD) in Hodgkin's lymphoma refractory to cyclophosphamide, vincristine, procarbazine and prednisone (COPP) and doxorubicin, bleomycin, vinblastine and dacarbazine (ABVD): A multicenter trial of the German Hodgkin's Lymphoma Study Group. Cancer Treat Rep 71:1203, 1987.

107. Brice P, Bastion Y, Divine M et al: Analysis of prognostic factors after the first relapse of Hodgkin's disease in 187 patients. Cancer 78:1293, 1996.

108. Bonfante V, Viviani S, Santoro A et al: Ifosfamide and vinorelbine: An active regimen for patients with relapsed or refractory Hodgkin's disease. Br J Haematol 103(Suppl. 2):533, 1998.

109. Fermé C, Bastion Y, Lepage E et al: MINE regimen as intensive salvage chemotherapy for relapsed and refractory Hodgkin's disease. Ann Oncol 6:517, 1995.

110. Devizzi L, Santoro A, Bonfante V et al: Vinorelbine in the treatment of refractory Hodgkin's disease. Ann Oncol 5:817, 1994.

111. Linch DC, Winfield D, Goldstone AH et al: Dose intensification with autologus bone marrow transplantation in relapsed and resistant Hodgkin's disease: Results of a BNLI randomized trial. Lancet 341:1051, 1993.

112. Chopra R, McMillian AK, Linch DC et al: The place of high-dose BEAM therapy and autologous bone marrow transplantation in poor risk Hodgkin's disease. A single-center eight-year study of 155 patients. Blood 81:1137, 1993.

113. Bierman PJ, Anderson JR, Freeman MB et al: High dose chemotherapy followed by autologous hematopoietic rescue for Hodgkin's disease patients following first relapse after chemotherapy. Ann Oncol 7:151, 1996.

114. Reece DE, Connors JM, Spinelli JJ et al: Intensive chemotherapy with cyclophosphamide, carmustine, etoposide +/– cisplatin and autologous bone marrow transplantation for Hodgkin's disease in first relapse after combination chemotherapy. Blood 83:1193, 1994.

115. Reece D: Should high risk patients with Hodgkin's disease be singled out for heavier therapeutic regimens while low risk patients are spared such therapies? Leuk Lymphoma 15(Suppl. 1):19, 1995.

116. Wheeler C, Eickhoff C, Elias A et al: High-dose cyclophosphamide, carmustine and etoposide with autologous transplantation in Hodgkin's disease: A prognostic model for treatment outcomes. Biol Blood Marrow Transplant 3:98, 1997.

117. Sweetenham JW, Taghipour G, Milligan D et al: High-dose therapy and autologous stem cell rescue for patients with Hodgkin's disease in first relapse after chemotherapy: Results from the EBMT. Bone Marrow Transplant 20:745, 1997.

118. Brice P, Divine M, Simon D et al: Feasibility of tandem autologous stem-.cell transplantation (ASCT) in induction failure or very unfavourable (UF) relapse from Hodgkin's disease (HD). Ann Oncol 10:1485, 1999.

119. Canellos GP: Treatment of relapsed Hodgkin's disease: Strategies and prognostic factors. Ann Oncol 9(Suppl. 5):S91–6, 1998.

120. Schnell R, Vitetta E, Schindler J et al: Treatment of refractory Hodgkin's lymphoma patients with an anti-CD25 ricin a-chain immunotoxin. Leukemia 14:129, 2000.

121. Santoro A, Bredenfield H, Devizzi L et al: Gemcitabine in the treatment of refractory Hodgkin's disease: Results of multicenter phase II study. J Clin Oncol 18:2615, 2000.

122. Lazarus HM, Rowlings PA, Zhang MJ et al: Autotransplants for Hodgkin's disease in patients never achieving remission: A report from the Autologous Blood and Marrow Transplant Registry. J Clin Oncol 17:534, 1999.

123. Josting A, Reiser M, Rueffer U et al: Treatment of primary progressive Hodgkin's and aggressive non-Hodgkin's lymphoma: Is there a chance for cure? J Clin Oncol 18:332, 2000.

124. Brice P, Bouabdallah R, Moreau P et al: Prognostic factors for survival for high-dose therapy and autologous stem cell transplantation for patients with relapsing Hodgkin's disease: Analysis of 280 patients from the French Registry. Bone Marrow Transplant 20:21, 1997.

125. Weaver CH, Zhen B, Buckner CD: Treatment of patients with malignant lymphoma with mini-BEAM reduces the yield of CD34+ peripheral blood stem cells. Bone Marrow Transplant 21:1169, 1998.

126. Josting A, Kàtay I, Rueffer U et al: Favourable outcome of patients with relapsed or refractory Hodgkin's disease treated with high-dose chemotherapy and stem cell rescue at the time of maximal response to conventional salvage therapy (Dexa-BEAM). Ann Oncol 9:289, 1998.

127. Rodriguez J, Rodriguez MA, Fayad L et al: ASHAP: A regimen for cytoreduction of refractory or recurrent Hodgkin's disease. Blood 93:3632, 1999.

128. Aurelin E, Holte H, Pharo A et al: Combination chemotherapy with mitoguazone, ifosfamide, MTX, etoposide (MIME) and G-CSF can efficiently mobilize PBPC in patients with Hodgkin's and non-Hodgkin's lymphoma. Bone Marrow Transplant 21:873, 1998.

129. Ribrag V, Nasr F, Bouhris JH et al: VIP (etoposide, ifosfamide and cisplatin) as a salvage intensification program in relapsed or refractory Hodgkin's disease. Bone Marrow Transplant 21:969, 1998.

130. Balzarotti M, Magagnoli M, Castagna L et al: IGEV as pre-transplant induction and mobilizing regimen in pretreated Hodgkin's disease (abstr.). Proc Am Soc Clin Oncol 1170, 2001.

131. Hartmann F, Renner C, Jung W et al: Anti-CD16/CD30 bispecific antibody as possible treatment for refractory Hodgkin's disease. Leuk Lymphoma 31:385, 1998.

132. Schnell R, Vitetta E, Schindler J et al: Treatment of refractory Hodgkin's lymphoma patients with an anti-CD25 ricin a-chain immunotoxin. Leukemia 14:129, 2000.

133. Hoppe RT: Hodgkin's disease: Complications of therapy and excess mortality. Ann Oncol(Suppl. 1):115, 1997.

134. Loge JH, Abrahamsen AF, Ekeberg O et al: Hodgkin's disease survivors more fatigued than the general population. J Clin Oncol 17:253, 1999.

135. Hancock SL, Tucker MA, Hoppe RT: Factors affecting late mortality from heart disease after treatment of Hodgkin's disease. JAMA 270:1949, 1993.

136. Glanzmann C, Kaufmann P, Jenni R et al: Cardiac risk after mediastinal irradiation for Hodgkin's disease. Radiother Oncol 46:51, 1998.

137. Martin RG, Ruckdeschel JC, Chang P et al: Radiation-related pericarditis. Am J Med 35:216, 1975.

138. Hirsch A, Els NV, Straus DJ et al: Effect of ABVD chemotherapy with and without mantle or mediastinal irradiation on pulmonary function and symptoms in early stage Hodgkin's disease. J Clin Oncol 219:615, 1994.

139. Swerdlow AJ, Shoemaker MJ, Allerton R et al: Lung cancer after Hodgkin's disease: A nested case-control study of the relation to treatment. J Clin Oncol 19:1610, 2001.

140. Konits PH, Aisner J, Whitacre M, Wiernik PH: Lung cancer as a complication of prolonged survival in patients with lymphoma. Med Pediatr Oncol 10:331, 1982.

141. Aisenberg AC, Finkelstein DM, Doppke KP et al: High risk of breast carcinoma after irradiation of young women with Hodgkin's disease. Cancer 79:1203, 1997.

142. Gervais-Fagnou DD, Girouard C, Laperriere N et al:. Breast cancer in women following supradiaphragmatic irradiation for Hodgkin's disease. Oncology 57:224, 1999.

143. Valagussa P, Santoro A, Fossati-Bellani F et al: Second acute leukemia and other second malignancies following treatment for Hodgkin's disease. J Clin Oncol 3:830, 1986.

144. Pedersen-Bjergaard J, Larsen SO: Incidence of acute non-lymphocytic leukemia, preleukemia and myeloproliferative syndrome up to ten years after treatment of Hodgkin's disease. N Engl J Med 307:965, 1982.

145. Sandoval C, Pui CH, Bowman LC et al: Secondary acute myeloid leukemia in children previously treated with alkylating agents, intercalating topoisomerase II inhibitors, and irradiation. J Clin Oncol 11:1039, 1993.

146. Ratain MJ, Rowley JD: Therapy-related acute myeloid leukemia secondary to inhibitors of topoisomerase II: From the bedside to the target genes. Ann Oncol 3:107, 1992.

147. Kollmannsberger C, Hartmann JT, Kanz L, Bokemeyer C. Risk of secondary myeloid leukemia and myelodysplastic syndrome following standard-dose chemotherapy or high-dose chemotherapy with stem cell support in patients with potentially curable malignancies. J Cancer Res Clin Oncol 124:207–214, 1998.

148. Sobecks RM, Le Beau MM, Anastasi J, Williams SF: Myelodysplasia and acute leukemia following high-dose chemotherapy and autologous bone marrow or peripheral blood stem cell transplantation. Bone Marrow Transplant 23:1161–1165, 1999.

149. Papadakis V, Vlachopapadoulou E, Van Syckle K et al: Gonadal function in young patients successfully treated for Hodgkin's disease. Med Pediatr Oncol 32:366, 1999.

150. Aisner J, Wiernik PH, Pearl P: Pregnancy outcome in patients treated for Hodgkin's disease. J Clin Oncol 11:507, 1993.

151. Constine LS, Donaldson SS, McDougall IR et al: Thyroid dysfunction after radiotherapy in children with Hodgkin's disease. Cancer 53:878, 1984.

152. Hancock SL, Cox RS, McDouglass IR: Thyroid disease after treatment of Hodgkin's disease. N Engl J Med 325:599, 1991.

153. Schimpff SC, Diggs CH, Wiswell JG et al: Radiation-related thyroid dysfunction: Implications for the treatment of Hodgkin's disease. Ann Intern Med 92:91, 1980.

154. Reece DE, Barnett MJ, Shepherd JD et al: High dose cyclophosphamide, carmustine (BCNU), and etoposide (VP16-213) with or without cisplatin (CBV +/–P) and autologous transplantation for patients with Hodgkin's disease who fail to enter a complete remission after combination chemotherapy. Blood 86:451, 1995.

155. Yuen AR, Rosenberg SA, Hoppe RT et al: Comparison between conventional salvage therapy and high-dose therapy with autografting for recurrent or refractory Hodgkin's disease. Blood 89:814, 1997.

156. Gianni AM, Siena S, Bregni M et al: High dose sequential chemoradiotherapy with peripheral blood progenitor cell support for relapsed or refractory Hodgkin's disease. Ann Oncol 4:889, 1993.

157. Prince HM, Crump M, Imrie K et al: Intensive therapy and autotransplant for patients with an incomplete response to front line therapy for lymphoma. Ann Oncol 7:1043, 1996.

158. Sweetenham JW, Taghipour G, Linch DC et al: Thirty percent of adult patients with primary refractory Hodgkin's disease are progression free at five years after high-dose therapy (HDT) and autologous stem cell transplantation (ASCT). Data from 290 patients reported to the EBMT. Blood 88(Suppl. 1):486 A, 1996.

44

Radiotherapeutic Management of Lymphomas

Sandra E. Mitchell and Nancy Price Mendenhall

BASIC CONCEPTS

Radiation therapy was the first effective treatment for both non-Hodgkin's lymphoma (NHL) and Hodgkin's lymphoma (HL). It has remained an integral part of the management of lymphoid malignancies even after the development of effective chemotherapy regimens because of its relative efficacy and its potential for dose adjustment and risk-adapted therapy. More progress has been made in the development of combined-modality therapy (CMT) in HL than in NHL, perhaps because of HL's predictable natural history and response to therapy. Nevertheless, the issues affecting the optimal use of radiation in both diseases are similar.

The successful use of radiation in both HL and NHL requires an understanding of the following concepts: disease extent, the dose–response relationship, the complementary nature of chemotherapy and radiation therapy, and the concept of risk-adapted therapy.

Disease Extent

Effective therapy in the lymphomas requires eradication of clinically known local disease as well as any subclinical disease that may be harbored regionally or systemically. Historically, the first evidence that HL could be cured came with the use of radiation therapy fields that included clinically involved sites and also "complementary" sites known to be at risk for future clinical spread of disease.[1,2] Today, knowledge of the extent of disease and probability of subclinical disease guides selection of both the type and amount of therapy, as well as design of radiation fields.

When radiation therapy is part of the therapeutic regimen, staging studies must identify and quantify clinically evident disease and, together with careful assessment of clinical factors, predict the presence and extent of subclinical disease.[3,4] The gold standard in lymphoma imaging is computed tomography (CT) scanning.[5] All patients should have CT scans of the neck, chest, abdomen, and pelvis, with notation of involved sites and maximum tumor size. Prognostic information in HL patients with mediastinal masses is also obtained from the upright posteroanterior chest radiograph. A ratio of maximum tumor diameter to the maximum thoracic width (MMT) of less than

1:3 is considered favorable.[6–9] The number of sites involved and the maximum tumor dimension also have prognostic significance in HL.[10–13] The CT scans are used in planning radiation therapy fields to ensure adequate coverage of areas of involvement.[14] It is clear from CT scanning that many past treatment failures after radiation therapy for HL were related to inadvertent shielding of parts of the tumor that were not apparent on plain setup films from the treatment area.[15] Certain laboratory studies also have prognostic value. In HL, elevated erythrocyte sedimentation rate (ESR) and abnormal blood indices predict a higher probability of regional and generalized subclinical disease.[16,17] In NHL, the International Prognostic Index has been verified as an important tool for assessing prognosis and guiding therapy. It requires lactate dehydrogenase (LDH) values, stage, and number of extranodal sites of involvement as well as the patient's age and performance status.[18] The roles of gallium and positron emission tomography (PET) in initial staging, assessment of therapeutic response, and post-treatment surveillance are under evaluation. One likely role for gallium is in the evaluation of initial response at a point in therapy where the treatment direction can be changed.[19–23] For example, one study has suggested that in patients with advanced HL, a positive gallium study after initial chemotherapy may indicate a poor outcome if the only additional therapy is low-dose involved-field irradiation.[24]

Dose–Response

It is increasingly clear that a dose–response relationship exists between radiation or chemotherapy agents and effects in both tumor and normal tissue responses. The higher the dose of radiation or chemotherapy, the greater the probability of tumor eradication or normal tissue damage. A few examples of the association between increasing dose of a chemotherapy agent and increasing probability of a normal tissue sequela in HL include leukemia[25,26] and fertility risks[27] with alkylating agents, cardiac and pulmonary risks with doxorubicin and bleomycin,[28] and neuropathy with vincristine. In NHL, there is also evidence of increasing cardiac morbidity associated with increasing doses of doxorubicin.[29] Examples of dose-related toxicity with radiation include thyroid dysfunction, pneumonitis, pulmonary fibrosis, xerostomia, soft tissue hypoplasia in children, and coronary artery disease. These toxicities appear to be clinically manifested above certain age-related threshold doses and to increase in incidence and severity with increasing dose and/or dose per treatment fraction.[30–37] It is also clear in HL and likely in NHL that an increasing tumor burden requires an increasing dose of radiation for eradication.[38–40] There appears to be a dose range, however, above which little additional benefit is achieved and damage to normal tissue outweighs the benefit of minimal additional tumor control. When radiation is used either as monotherapy or part of CMT, it is critical that the dose distribution be adequate for disease control but safe for these normal tissues. The doses required will vary with the age of the patient, the tumor volume, and the amount of chemotherapy in the regimen.

Complementary Relationship Between Radiation Therapy and Chemotherapy

Tailoring of Local–Regional Therapy

A major premise in lymphoma management is that the amount of treatment should be adjusted to the risk of treatment failure because of concern about acute and late toxicity. Chemotherapy tailoring may be accomplished by adjusting the number of agents, duration or number of cycles of chemotherapy, total dose of individual drugs, and the frequency and time interval over which agents are given. What cannot be accomplished with chemotherapy is dose variation for a given patient according to tumor burden. With radiation therapy, fields can be selected that treat only areas involved by lymphoma. Within a treatment field, critical normal tissues can be partially or totally excluded from radiation exposure. Differential doses can be delivered to different targeted tumor volumes through customized shielding, selection of radiation energy, manipulation of the direction of entry of the radiation beam, and field size reductions during the course of therapy. For example, a typical prescription for a particular patient with HL might include delivering doses of 10, 15, or 20 Gy to extranodal areas at low, moderate, and high risk for subclinical disease; 20, 25, and 30 Gy to nodal areas at low, moderate, and high risk for subclinical disease; and 30 to 35 Gy, 35 to 37 Gy, and 37 to 44 Gy for areas of clinically evident small, moderate, and large tumor volumes, respectively.

Scope of Therapy

If an adequate dose can be given that will eradicate all disease present without serious normal tissue sequelae, the scope of chemotherapy may offer advantages in achieving accuracy over radiation. Prediction of the extent and distribution of subclinical disease is less critical. There may be less outcome dependence with chemotherapy on equipment sophistication and subspecialty expertise than in radiation therapy, in which outcomes vary significantly with adequacy of equipment and skill and experience of diagnostic radiologists or therapeutic radiation oncologists.[41–48] There may be a perception that quality assurance is more expensive in radiotherapy than in chemotherapy. It is important to note, however, that suboptimal delivery of chemotherapy is also associated with poor outcomes and that the costs of quality assurance in radiation may be more than outweighed by the costs associated with stem cell monitoring and support necessary for optimal delivery of chemotherapy.

Patterns of Failure

The patterns of treatment failure in both HL and NHL observed after monotherapy with radiation and chemotherapy are very different. The majority of recurrences after chemotherapy are in sites of known initial involvement especially bulky involvement, despite complete initial disappearance of tumor.[49–52] The majority of recurrences after radiation therapy are outside the radiation fields in areas not previously known to be involved. In HL these out-of-field recurrences are typically found in contiguous sites historically recognized to be at moderate to high risk for subclinical disease. In NHL, the patterns of relapse are more likely to be systemic than in HL, but they still predominantly occur in predictable nodal or extranodal sites that vary with histologic subtype. In both HL and NHL, in-field failures frequently occur near the edge of the treatment field and probably are related to marginal misses, because of unappreciated gross or subclinical tumor or inaccurate daily setups that may result in suboptimal radiation doses at the edges of fields.

Potential Advantages of Combined-Modality Therapy

As most treatment-related toxicity is dose-related, it is rational to attempt to limit the doses of any given agent to the minimum effective dose or, in combination with other agents, to a dose below the threshold for clinically relevant normal tissue damage. Because radiation therapy and chemotherapy are both relatively effective, it is rational to assume that in CMT, the addition of the second modality may permit reduction of the first or give additional therapeutic benefit. Because of the complementary patterns of recurrence and toxicity with chemotherapy and radiation therapy, it is rational to expect that an optimal CMT regimen might produce both better disease control and less toxicity than optimal monotherapy regimens. If the main goal is improvement of disease-related outcome, radiation therapy might be added to a full course of definitive chemotherapy or vice versa. If the main goal is reduction in toxicity, radiation therapy might be substituted for some of the chemotherapy dose or vice versa. The optimal combination of the two types of therapy in a CMT regimen will vary depending on the bulk of disease, probable extent of subclinical disease, age of the patient, and therapeutic goals.

Risk-Adapted Therapy

Happily, because our treatments are effective for many NHL and the majority of HL patients, late treatment sequelae are very important. The relative efficacy of radiation therapy and chemotherapy provides many therapeutic options, and a major goal today is to tailor the amount of therapy to the individual need. In most cooperative group trials, patients with HL are grouped into at least three, sometimes four, risk groups: unfavorable, intermediate, favorable, and sometimes, very favorable. There is less clarity about the groupings in NHL. In each category, it must be determined how best to manage the given volume of clinically evident disease and the probability of subclinical disease. For example, radiation may be used in a variety of different scenarios and techniques: only in patients who have bulky tumor; only in patients whose tumors do not respond completely to chemotherapy; covering only clinically involved sites, covering all clinically involved fields; or covering all clinically involved fields plus contiguous noninvolved sites at high risk for subclinical disease. One hypothetical algorithm for thinking about the potential relative roles of radiation is shown in Table 44–1.[6,12,13,46,53–69]

Table 44–1. Algorithm for Radiation Treatment Volume as a Function of Chemotherapy (Amount and Response) and Disease Extent

Chemotherapy: No. of Cycles and Response	Prognostic Group				
	Very Favorable	Favorable	Intermediate	Unfavorable	Very Unfavorable
No chemotherapy	IF[59,60,63]	IF/EF[6,12,13,49,50,53–58]	EF/TNI[12]	—	—
2 or 3, CR	IF[62]	IF/EF[53,61]	EF[64–68]	—	—
4	No RT	IF[62]	IF[67]	—	—
4–6	No RT	No RT[a]	IF	IF[46,69]	—
5, 6, or more	No RT	No RT[b]	IF	IF[46,69]	IF[46,69]

Abbreviations: IF, involved field; EF, extended field; TNI, total nodal irradiation; CR, complete response; RT, radiation therapy.
[a] CCG 5942.
[b] POG 8625.

HODGKIN'S LYMPHOMA

Today, much is understood about the role of radiotherapy as monotherapy for HL. New advances in imaging technology have shed light on past radiation failures and placed the technique of radiotherapy on a sounder basis. Therapeutic success in the 1960s and 1970s with radiation therapy alone in HL has permitted the study of late radiation effects. These late radiation effects and the emerging toxicities associated with prolonged chemotherapy have tempered the enthusiasm of early monotherapy victories and driven the search for equally effective but less toxic combined-modality approaches in favorable and intermediate disease. The search for more effective therapies continues in advanced disease. Defining the optimal role of radiation therapy in these CMT regimens remains a primary thrust of clinical investigation.

Field Design

In radiotherapy for HL, standardized fields incorporating typically involved nodal and extranodal lymphoid areas have been used for the past three decades. These standard fields include the Waldeyer's ring, neck, axillary, mediastinal, spleen, para-aortic, inguinal-femoral, and pelvic areas. An involved field is a standard field that contains some clinical evidence of involvement. For example, a standard neck field could be used for a single midjugular node, a single supraclavicular node, or a chain of nodes extending from the base of the skull to the clavicle. Certain combinations of involvement are covered in specialized fields such as the mantle (neck, axillae, hilae, and mediastinum) or the inverted Y (femoral, inguinal, pelvic, and para-aortic areas). A mantle field may be extended to include the cardiac silhouette, hemilung or whole lung, and upper abdominal nodes and spleen. A minimantle field excludes or curtails irradiation of the mediastinum. Treatment of all uninvolved fields contiguous to involved fields is called an extended field. Subtotal nodal irradiation includes the mantle, para-aortic, and spleen fields and has been considered standard extended-field therapy for stages I and II supradiaphragmatic HL. Total nodal irradiation also includes pelvic irradiation.

The historical guidelines for field design before the availability of CT imaging were based on studies of gross anatomy and patterns of recurrence. With the advent of CT imaging and three-dimensional treatment planning systems, it is clear that many treatment failures in the past were related to inadvertent shielding of gross tumor.[14,15] In radiotherapy for other malignancies, image-based treatment planning is replacing standardized fields. In HL, most cooperative groups are still employing standardized fields that are modified to incorporate all disease imaged on CT. An area of controversy is whether the radiographic criteria of abnormality are sufficiently well defined in HL to move away from standardized fields to image-guided therapy.

Field Selection

Field selection is correlated with extent of disease, probability of subclinical disease, patient factors such as age and sex, and the role of radiation therapy (monotherapy versus CMT). When radiation therapy is used as monotherapy, it is important not only to define the limits and volume of all involved sites but also to carefully assess the probability of subclinical disease, especially in contiguous sites.

Early-Stage Disease

Excellent results have been achieved with subtotal and total nodal irradiation alone in early-stage HL in adults. In most series including stages I and II, the overall freedom from relapse rate is approximately 75 to 80 percent at 10 years, and the overall survival rate approaches 90 percent.[6,12,13,49,50,53–58] In general, with radiation therapy alone, extended fields that include all involved fields and all uninvolved contiguous fields are treated. Because the most common sites of involvement are the low neck and supraclavicular areas, extended-field therapy usually implies treatment of mantle, para-aortic, and spleen fields, or subtotal nodal irradiation (STNI). In an Italian trial comparing radiotherapy alone (STNI) with chemotherapy alone (mechlorethamine–vincristine–procarbazine–prednisone [MOPP]) in favorable laparotomy-staged patients with stage I or II disease (no B symptoms or large mediastinal masses), progression-free survival was similar at 8 years, but survival was better after radiotherapy because of the higher salvage rate after relapse.[49,50]

Prognostic factors, such as B symptoms, bulky disease, and more than three sites of involvement in patients with stage I or II disease are associated with a high relapse rate with radiotherapy alone. Two trials have compared STNI with or without adjuvant chemotherapy in favorable stages I and II HL. In the German GHST trial HD7 in favorable clinical stage I and II HL, the event-free survival rate with two cycles of doxorubicin–bleomycin–vin-blastine–dacarbazine (ABVD) and extended-field radiotherapy was 96 percent at 22 months compared with 84 percent for radio-therapy alone ($p < .05$).[61] In the United States, an intergroup trial comparing three cycles of doxorubicin and vinblastine and STNI with STNI alone in favorable clinical stage I and II disease stopped prior to complete accrual because of the excess relapses with radiotherapy alone.[53] The failure-free survival rate was 93 percent at 3 years with CMT versus 81 percent with radiotherapy alone ($p=.001$). These two trials suggest that minimal chemotherapy can be used to enhance the disease control rates achieved with radia-tion therapy. In a third trial conducted by the European Organi-zation for Research and Treatment of Cancer (EORTC) in favor-able clinical stage I and II HL, STNI was compared with three cycles of MOPP–ABVD plus involved-field radiotherapy. At 4 years, the rate of freedom from treatment failure was 77 percent with STNI compared with 99 percent with CMT ($p < .001$), which suggests that three cycles of chemotherapy may be sufficient for low-risk subclinical disease, permitting a significant decrease in the radiation treatment volume.

It is clear that addition of two to three cycles of chemother-apy improves disease control over extended-field radiotherapy alone and may permit a reduction in radiotherapy treatment volume to only involved-field therapy with favorable HL patients. So long as the toxicity of CMT in early-stage HL is not more than the toxicity of radiotherapy alone, CMT will be a better option than radiotherapy only. The use of only two or three cycles of chemotherapy as an adjuvant to irradiation thus far has not been associated with significant toxicity.

In growing children, the doses of radiation traditionally used in HL (30 to 40 Gy) result in significant musculoskeletal hypoplasia. Efforts to reduce or eliminate the use of radiation in pediatric HL by pediatric cooperative group trials have demonstrated several principles. In a prospective trial (POG 8625) in stage I–IIIA disease conducted by the Pediatric Oncology Group (POG), which com-pared 6 months of MOPP–ABVD chemotherapy with 4 months of the same chemotherapy and low-dose (25 Gy) involved-field radi-ation therapy, disease control and survival rates were the same, approximately 96 percent at 5 years. Two complementary conclu-sions could be drawn from the trial: (1) radiation therapy could be omitted in this group of patients if at least 6 months of chemother-apy were administered or (2) low-dose radiation therapy could be substituted for two cycles of chemotherapy. The patients entered on the trial were a heterogeneous group, including some with large mediastinal masses as well as patients with minimal disease and favorable histology. It was expected that treatment could be further reduced in at least some of these patients.

The next POG trial (POG 9226) was a pilot study of four cycles of chemotherapy without alkylating agents and low-dose

involved-field radiation therapy in clinically staged patients.[62] Early results were favorable, leading investigators to attempt further reductions in overall treatment. In a third trial (POG 9426), favorable patients who had a complete response after two cycles of chemotherapy were given only low-dose involved-field radiation therapy with no further chemotherapy. It is hoped that the low radiation dose will result in few or no late effects and that any effects from only two cycles of chemotherapy will be negligible. There are no results available from this trial as yet.

Concurrent with the POG trials was a Children's Cancer Group (CCG 5940) trial in which all patients with HL were strat-ified into three risk groups and given different chemotherapy regimens with or without involved-field irradiation. The favor-able early-stage group received four cycles of chemotherapy (COPP–ABVD) with or without radiotherapy. The trial closed before completion of accrual because of an excess relapse rate in patients not receiving radiation therapy. It would appear that reduction in traditional chemotherapy doses will require careful selection of patients and either different chemotherapy regimens or the addition of some radiation therapy. From the above data, involved-field radiotherapy at a low dose appears to permit reduction in required chemotherapy for the favorable early-stage patient from six cycles to four and perhaps two cycles.

In some very favorable early-stage patients (e.g., stage I and II lymphocyte-predominant or nodular sclerosis HL), the risk of extensive subclinical disease may be judged so minimal that treatment aimed at only the clinically evident disease may be warranted.[59,60,63] Pediatric patients with IA lymphocyte-pre-dominant HL located in a peripheral site such as the upper neck, axilla, or femoral nodes have frequently been treated with only involved-field radiotherapy.[63] In adults judged to fall into an extremely favorable subgroup with minimal risk of abdomi-nal disease based on histology, tumor volume, number of sites involved, ESR, and absence of B symptoms, mantle irradiation only has been offered either after laparotomy staging[59] or clinical staging.[60] Mauch et al.[59] reported 10-year disease-free survival and overall survival rates of 83 and 89 percent, respectively, in a carefully selected population of patients treated at a single insti-tution. After initial enthusiasm, unacceptable relapse rates led to the abandonment of this approach in the EORTC in clinically staged patients treated in a multi-institutional trial.[60]

Intermediate-Stage Disease

Patients with unfavorable stage I or II disease (with B symp-toms, large mediastinal mass, bulky tumor [larger than 6 cm], or more than three sites of involvement) and patients with early stage III disease are considered at intermediate risk for treat-ment failure. Several effective CMT approaches are commonly used, differing in their emphasis on radiotherapy or chemotherapy and in how subclinical disease is managed. In various CMT regimens for intermediate-stage disease, subclini-cal disease may receive two to three,[64–67] four,[62,68,70] or six cycles of chemotherapy and/or moderate-dose irradiation. The EORTC conducted a trial (H8-U) in unfavorable clinical stage I and II patients of six cycles of MOPP–ABVD plus involved-field radiotherapy versus four cycles of MOPP–ABVD plus involved-field radiotherapy versus four cycles of MOPP–ABVD plus

STNI. Patients receiving four cycles of MOPP–ABVD and involved-field radiotherapy had the best outcome.[68] A German trial comparing the outcomes in intermediate-risk disease of two cycles of chemotherapy with either involved-field or extended-field radiotherapy has shown no difference in rates of freedom from treatment failure at 26 months.[67] Substantial single-institution studies and cooperative group trials suggest that in intermediate-stage disease, it may be possible to treat effectively with as few as two to four cycles of chemotherapy and either involved-field or extended-field radiotherapy.

Advanced-Stage Disease

At the unfavorable end of the spectrum are patients with advanced-stage disease. Significant opportunities still exist for enhanced disease control in these patients. The role of radiation therapy in patients with advanced disease is unclear. Several trials have attempted to address the issues, but quality assurance problems have confounded results. For example, in the Southwest Oncology Group (SWOG) trials of six cycles of MOP–BAP chemotherapy with or without involved-field irradiation, there was no survival benefit after 5 years with the addition of radiation.[46] However, in the subsets of patients with nodular sclerosis histology, there was a significant benefit in disease-free survival. In patients whose radiotherapy was judged appropriate on central review, disease-free and overall survival rates were substantially better than in patients who received no radiation therapy. Despite the absence of a clear demonstration of the benefit of irradiation, most investigators continue to use radiation therapy as an adjuvant. One of the most promising regimens, the Stanford V chemotherapy regimen, involves seven drugs (doxorubicin, bleomycin, nitrogen mustard, vinblastine, vincristine, etoposide, and prednisone) given in a dose-dense and intense fashion over a short period of time, supplemented with involved-field radiation therapy to all sites with bulky involvement (tumors at least 5 cm in transverse dimension, macroscopic lesions in the spleen, or massive mediastinal disease with a ratio of maximum tumor diameter to maximum thoracic width greater than 1:3).[69]

Dose

There is strong evidence of a dose response for radiation in HL.[38,39,71–74] The higher the dose of radiation, the higher the probability of disease control. The shape of the dose response was initially believed to be linear,[71] then later was described as sigmoid.[72] Fletcher and Shukovsky correctly surmised that as dose increases, a dose is reached beyond which little is gained in terms of tumor control, but much is lost in terms of normal tissue toxicity, as normal tissues also show a dose response to radiation damage.[72] Normal tissues frequently included in radiation therapy fields for HL for which data suggest an increasing risk of radiation injury with increasing radiation dose include coronary arteries, thyroid, salivary glands, lung parenchyma, and soft tissues. For subclinical disease in a monotherapeutic regimen, the adequacy of 30 Gy rather than the previously common 40 Gy has now been confirmed in a prospective randomized trial from Germany.[48] The adequacy of 20 Gy rather than 30 Gy

or 40 Gy in a CMT regimen has also been confirmed in trials from Germany.[75] Two recent retrospective studies, one based on multi-institutional data[38] and the other on a carefully documented single-institution experience,[39] suggest a radiation dose response in HL that varies with tumor volume. It appears, however, that with increasing tumor volume, increasing doses of radiation are required.[38,39]

Importance of Quality Assurance

It is acknowledged by most radiation oncologists that treatment of HL is technically challenging because of the extensive treatment fields and large volume of adjacent normal tissues. In the United States, the Patterns of Care studies in the 1980s documented inferior disease control and survival in HD patients whose radiation treatment portals were judged inadequate on central retrospective review.[41,42] In Germany, prospective trials incorporating central post-therapy review of radiation portals have also documented the clear relationship between adequacy of the radiation treatment fields and disease control and survival.[48] In POG, a pretherapy central review of radiation portals for early-stage HL (POG 9426) has led to a high pretherapy intervention rate, which has led in turn to a lower rate of major protocol violations. In addition to the difficulty in field design, it is also clear that daily treatment reproducibility is problematic.[76–80] Quality assurance in radiotherapy is critically important to realize the full potential of radiotherapy either as a component of CMT or as monotherapy.

Surveillance for Late Effects

It is clear that survivors of HL are at increased risk for cardiovascular disease and second malignancy. The risk of cardiovascular disease appears to be at least partially related to radiation dose.[31,32,34] The most common event observed has been coronary artery disease, but valve dysfunction has also been reported.[81] Although second solid malignancies in the HL survivors seem to be associated with prior irradiation, they are not always confined to previous treatment portals. Breast cancer seems to be most significantly increased in women who received radiation during their early teenage years to doses of 40 Gy or more. As the age at the time of radiation therapy increases, the risk of breast cancer appears to decrease.[82] Close surveillance of female HL survivors is mandatory to detect the breast cancers at the earliest possible time. Lung cancer is also a common problem in HL survivors who are smokers; it is rare in nonsmokers.[83] These patients warrant close surveillance as well as counseling and support regarding the risks of continued smoking and the availability of smoking cessation programs. Other second malignancies frequently observed in HL survivors include thyroid carcinoma and parotid, gastrointestinal, and urologic malignancies.

NON-HODGKIN'S LYMPHOMA

The natural history of NHL has been more difficult to understand than that of HL, making various therapeutic approaches hard to evaluate. Part of the difficulty has been to categorize the spectrum of diseases falling under the rubric of NHL. It is useful for clinical purposes to consider the management of the NHLs in three categories: the low-grade, the intermediate-grade, and the high-grade lymphomas.

Low-Grade Lymphomas

Stages I and II

In the low-grade lymphomas there has been no convincing evidence of cure with nonablative chemotherapy.[84,85] Radiation therapy in early-stage low-grade lymphomas has resulted in approximately 50 percent freedom from relapse and survival rates at 10 years in clinically staged patients[86] and approximately 75 percent rates in surgically staged patients. The majority of relapses after involved-field irradiation are out of the radiation field, usually in other nodal or lymphoid sites, depending on histologic subtype.[87] For example, follicular low-grade B-cell lymphoma typically presents in the nodes of the head and neck or lymphoid tissue of Waldeyer's ring. Relapses after involved-field radiotherapy are typically in mesenteric or para-aortic nodes. Radiation therapy fields can be extended, as in HL, to include areas suspected of harboring subclinical disease. Comprehensive lymphatic irradiation, including mantle, Waldeyer's ring, whole abdominal, and pelvic radiotherapy has been used, resulting in a higher rate of freedom from relapse but not in rate of survival.[86,88]

Stage III

In stage III low-grade lymphomas with limited involvement, 40 to 50 percent of patients appear to be free from disease at 10 years after comprehensive lymphatic irradiation.[88,89] As most relapses occur within the first 6 years after treatment and very few after 10 years, it is possible that a subset of these stage III patients may be cured with radiation therapy.

Palliation with Low-Dose Total Body Irradiation

In addition to producing long-term disease-free intervals in patients with stage I, II, or early stage III disease, radiation therapy also has value as a palliative agent. Involved-field radiation therapy to moderate doses (30 Gy) will produce durable disease control. In patients with extensive low-grade lymphoma, low-dose total body irradiation achieves a complete clinical response in approximately 70 percent of patients, which lasts for a median of 2 to 3 years.[90–99]

Intermediate-Grade Lymphoma

The role of radiation in intermediate-grade NHL in adults has clearly been established by two prospective randomized trials. The Eastern Cooperative Oncology Group (ECOG) randomized patients who had a complete response after eight cycles of cyclophosphamide, doxorubicin, vincristine, and prednisone (CHOP) chemotherapy to no further therapy or involved-field radiation to 30 Gy.[100] Patients with a partial response received involved-field radiotherapy to 40 Gy. There was a significant

improvement in rates of both disease-free survival and overall survival with the addition of radiation therapy in the complete responders. Patients who received irradiation after partial responses had disease-free and overall survival rates similar to those of the complete responders who did not receive irradiation. It appears that with eight or fewer cycles of CHOP chemotherapy, radiation therapy has a role. During the same time interval SWOG compared three cycles of CHOP chemotherapy and involved-field radiotherapy with eight cycles of CHOP chemotherapy.[29] Progression-free survival rates were similar for the two treatment arms, but the survival rate was better in the radiation therapy arm because of excess cardiac mortality attributable to the additional cycles of chemotherapy. Clearly, it appears that radiation therapy can effectively substitute for some amount of chemotherapy, yielding equivalent disease control with less toxicity. The optimal dose of radiation is unknown, although retrospective studies suggest that 30 Gy after a complete response to chemotherapy in small-volume disease may be adequate. Higher doses may be needed with larger tumors or lesser responses to chemotherapy.[40,100] The positive results in early-stage intermediate-grade lymphomas beg the question of whether involved-field radiation might be beneficial in more advanced disease. Single institution studies have documented feasibility and suggested a benefit in stage III,[101] but these findings should be confirmed in a prospective randomized trial.

Radioimmunotherapy

Finally, radioactive isotopes associated with monoclonal antibodies have produced excellent tumor responses. Radioimmunotherapy—therapy with radionuclide-linked monoclonal antibodies to specific B-cell or T-cell antigens—holds great promise. Early results show complete, durable remissions.[102–105] It is quite likely that radioimmunotherapy may be more effective than monoclonal antibodies alone, whose role is already established.[106,107]

SUMMARY

Radiation is an effective tool in both HL and NHL. In HL, its optimal role may be in CMT regimens except at the favorable end of the prognostic spectrum, where it may be used as monotherapy. Problems with quality assurance in the past have confounded our understanding of optimal radiation doses and treatment volumes as well as the potential value of radiation either as monotherapy or as an integral part of CMT regimens. Developments in imaging and treatment planning and the institution of pretherapy central review in cooperative group trials using radiation therapy for HL should improve the accuracy of radiation therapy in trials in the future. The role of radiation therapy in CMT regimens for early-stage intermediate-grade lymphomas is well established, but questions remain regarding optimal dose and treatment volume and the potential value of radiation therapy in more advanced disease. In low-grade lymphoma, radiation therapy currently appears to hold the greatest promise for durable, perhaps permanent, disease control, with appropriate radiation treatment volumes.

REFERENCES

1. Peters MV: A study of survivals in Hodgkin's disease treated radiologically. Am J Roentgenol Radium Ther 63:299–311, 1950.
2. Peters MV: Prophylactic treatment of adjacent areas in Hodgkin's disease. Cancer Res 26:1232–1243, 1966.
3. Mauch P, Larson D, Osteen R et al: Prognostic factors for positive surgical staging in patients with Hodgkin's disease. J Clin Oncol 8:257–265, 1990.
4. Mendenhall NP, Cantor AB, Williams JL et al: With modern imaging techniques, is staging laparotomy necessary in pediatric Hodgkin's disease? A Pediatric Oncology Group study. J Clin Oncol 11:2218–2225, 1993.
5. Mendenhall NP: Diagnostic procedures and guidelines for the evaluation and follow-up of Hodgkin's disease. Semin Radiat Oncol 6:131–145, 1996.
6. Hoppe RT, Coleman CN, Cox RS, Rosenberg SA, Kaplan HS: The management of stage I-II Hodgkin's disease with irradiation alone or combined modality therapy: The Stanford experience. Blood 59:455–465, 1982.
7. Specht L, Nordentoft AM, Cold S, Clausen NT, Nissen NI: Tumour burden in early stage Hodgkin's disease: The single most important prognostic factor for outcome after radiotherapy. Br J Cancer 55:535–539, 1987.
8. Mauch P, Goodman R, Hellman S: The significance of mediastinal involvement in early stage Hodgkin's disease. Cancer 42:1039–1045, 1978.
9. Prosnitz LR, Curtis AM, Knowlton AH, Peters LM, Farber LR: Supradiaphragmatic Hodgkin's disease: Significance of large mediastinal masses. Int J Radiat Oncol Biol Phys 6:809–813, 1980.
10. Thar TL, Million RR, Hausner RJ, McKetty MH: Hodgkin's disease stage I and II: Relationship of recurrence to size of disease, radiation dose, and number of sites involved. Cancer 43:1101–1105, 1979.
11. Tubiana M, Henry-Amar M, Hayat M et al: Prognostic significance of the number of involved areas in the early stages of Hodgkin's disease. Cancer 54:885–894, 1984.
12. Mendenhall NP, Cantor AB, Barre DM, Lynch JW Jr, Million RR: The role of prognostic factors in treatment selection for early-stage Hodgkin's disease. Am J Clin Oncol 17:189–195, 1994.
13. Mauch P, Tarbell N, Weinstein H et al: Stage IA and IIA supradiaphragmatic Hodgkin's disease: Prognostic factors in surgically staged patients treated with mantle and paraaortic irradiation. J Clin Oncol 6:1576–1583, 1988.
14. Rostock RA, Giangreco A, Wharam MD, Lenhard R, Siegelman SS, Order SE: CT scan modification in the treatment of mediastinal Hodgkin's disease. Cancer 49:2267–2275, 1982.
15. Naida JD, Eisbruch A, Schoeppel SL, Sandler HM, Turrisi AT, Lichter AS: Analysis of localization errors in the definition of the mantle field using a beam's eye view treatment-planning system. Int J Radiat Oncol Biol Phys 35:377–382, 1996.
16. Henry-Amar M, Friedman S, Hayat M et al: Erythrocyte sedimentation rate predicts early relapse and survival in early-stage Hodgkin disease. The EORTC Lymphoma Cooperative Group. Ann Intern Med 114:361–365, 1991.
17. Munker R, Hasenclever D, Brosteanu O, Hiller E, Diehl V: Bone marrow involvement in Hodgkin's disease: An analysis of 135 consecutive cases. German Hodgkin's Lymphoma Study. J Clin Oncol 13:403–409, 1995.
18. Shipp MA: Prognostic factors in aggressive non-Hodgkin's lymphoma: Who has "high-risk" disease? Blood 83:1165–1173, 1994.
19. Hagemeister FB, Fesus SM, Lamki LM, Haynie TP: Role of the gallium scan in Hodgkin's disease. Cancer 65:1090–1096, 1990.
20. Abrahamsen AF, Lien HH, Aas M et al: Magnetic resonance imaging and [67]gallium scan in mediastinal malignant lymphoma: A prospective pilot study. Ann Oncol 5:433–436, 1994.
21. Karimjee S, Brada M, Husband J, McCready VR: A comparison of gallium-67 single photon emission computed tomography and computed tomography in mediastinal Hodgkin's disease. Eur J Cancer 28A:1856–1857, 1992.
22. Front D, Ben-Haim S, Israel O et al: Lymphoma: Predictive value of Ga-67 scintigraphy after treatment. Radiology 182:359–363, 1992.
23. Hagemeister FB, Purugganan R, Podoloff DA et al: The gallium scan predicts relapse in patients with Hodgkin's disease treated with combined modality therapy. Ann Oncol 5:S59–S63, 1994.
24. King SC, Reiman RJ, Prosnitz LR: Prognostic importance of restaging gallium scans following induction chemotherapy for advanced Hodgkin's disease. J Clin Oncol 12:306–311, 1994.
25. Kaldor JM, Day NE, Clarke EA et al: Leukemia following Hodgkin's disease. N Engl J Med 322:7–13, 1990.
26. Mendenhall NP, Shuster JJ, Million RR: The impact of stage and treatment modality on the likelihood of second malignancies and hematopoietic disorders in Hodgkin's disease. Radiother Oncol 14:219–229, 1989.
27. DaCunha MF, Meistrich ML, Fuller LM et al: Recovery of spermatogenesis after treatment for Hodgkin's disease: Limiting dose of MOPP chemotherapy. J Clin Oncol 2:571–577, 1984.
28. Lipshultz SE, Lipsitz SR, Mone SM et al: Female sex and higher drug dose as risk factors for late cardiotoxic effects of doxorubicin therapy for childhood cancer. N Engl J Med 332:1738–1743, 1995.
29. Miller TP, Dahlberg S, Cassady JR et al: Chemotherapy alone compared with chemotherapy plus radiotherapy for localized intermediate- and high-grade non-Hodgkin's lymphoma. N Engl J Med 339:21–26, 1998.
30. Carmel RJ, Kaplan HS: Mantle irradiation in Hodgkin's disease: An analysis of technique, tumor eradication, and complications. Cancer 37:2813–2825, 1976.
31. Hancock SL, Donaldson SS, Hoppe RT: Cardiac disease following treatment of Hodgkin's disease in children and adolescents. J Clin Oncol 11:1208–1215, 1993.
32. Hancock SL, Tucker MA, Hoppe RT: Factors affecting late mortality from heart disease after treatment of Hodgkin's disease. JAMA 270:1949–1955, 1993.
33. Hancock SL, Cox RS, McDougall IR: Thyroid diseases after treatment of Hodgkin's disease. N Engl J Med 325:599–605, 1991.
34. King V, Constine LS, Clark D et al: Symptomatic coronary artery disease after mantle irradiation for Hodgkin's disease. Int J Radiat Oncol Biol Phys 36:881–889, 1996.
35. Cosset JM, Henry-Amar M, Pellae-Cosset B et al: Pericarditis and myocardial infarctions after Hodgkin's disease therapy. Int J Radiat Oncol Biol Phys 21:447–449, 1991.
36. Coia LR, Hanks GE: Complications from large field intermediate dose infradiaphragmatic radiation: An analysis of the patterns of care outcome studies for Hodgkin's disease and seminoma. Int J Radiat Oncol Biol Phys 15:29–35, 1988.
37. Donaldson SS, Link MP: Combined modality treatment with low-dose radiation and MOPP chemotherapy for children with Hodgkin's disease. J Clin Oncol 5:742–749, 1987.
38. Vijayakumar S, Myrianthopoulos LC: An updated dose-response analysis in Hodgkin's disease. Radiother Oncol 24:1–13, 1992.
39. Mendenhall NP, Rodrigue LL, Moore-Higgs GJ, Marcus RB Jr, Million RR: The optimal dose of radiation in Hodgkin's disease: An analysis of clinical and treatment factors affecting in-field disease control. Int J Radiat Oncol Biol Phys 44:551–561, 1999.

40. Kamath SS, Marcus RB Jr, Lynch JW, Mendenhall NP: The impact of radiotherapy dose and other treatment-related and clinical factors on in-field control in stage I and II non-Hodgkin's lymphoma. Int J Radiat Oncol Biol Phys 44:563–568, 1999.

41. Hanks GE, Kinzie JJ, White RL, Herring DF, Kramer S: Patterns of Care outcome studies. Results of the national practice in Hodgkin's disease. Cancer 51:569–573, 1983.

42. Kinzie JJ, Hanks GE, Maclean CJ, Kramer S: Patterns of Care study: Hodgkin's disease relapse rates and adequacy of portals. Cancer 52:2223–2226, 1983.

43. Hoppe RT, Hanlon AL, Hanks GE, Owen JB: Progress in the treatment of Hodgkin's disease in the United States, 1973 versus 1983. The Patterns of Care study. Cancer 74:3198–3203, 1994.

44. Hughes DB, Smith AR, Hoppe R et al: Treatment planning for Hodgkin's disease: A Patterns of Care study. Int J Radiat Oncol Biol Phys 33:519–524, 1995.

45. Sebag-Montefiore DJ, Maher EJ, Young J, Vaughan Hudson G, Hanks G: Variation in mantle technique: Implications for establishing priorities for quality assurance in clinical trials. Radiother Oncol 23:144–149, 1992.

46. Fabian CJ, Mansfield CM, Dahlberg S et al: Low-dose involved field radiation after chemotherapy in advanced Hodgkin disease. A Southwest Oncology Group randomized study. Ann Intern Med 120:903–912, 1994.

47. Weiner MA, Leventhal B, Brecher ML et al: Randomized study of intensive MOPP–ABVD with or without low-dose total-nodal radiation therapy in the treatment of stages IIB, IIIA2, IIIB, and IV Hodgkin's disease in pediatric patients: A Pediatric Oncology Group study. J Clin Oncol 15:2769–2779, 1997.

48. Duhmke E, Diehl V, Loeffler M et al: Randomized trial with early-stage Hodgkin's disease testing 30 Gy vs. 40 Gy extended field radiotherapy alone. Int J Radiat Oncol Biol Phys 36:305–310, 1996.

49. Cimino G, Biti GP, Anselmo AP et al: MOPP chemotherapy vs extended-field radiotherapy in the management of pathological stages I-IIA Hodgkin's disease. J Clin Oncol 7:732–737, 1989.

50. Biti GP, Cimino G, Cartoni C et al: Extended-field radiotherapy is superior to MOPP chemotherapy for the treatment of pathologic stage I-IIA Hodgkin's disease: Eight-year update of an Italian prospective randomized study. J Clin Oncol 10:378–382, 1992.

51. Longo DL, Young RC, Wesley M et al: Twenty years of MOPP therapy for Hodgkin's disease. J Clin Oncol 4:1295–1306, 1986.

52. Yahalom J, Ryu J, Straus DJ et al: Impact of adjuvant radiation on the patterns and rate of relapse in advanced-stage Hodgkin's disease treated with alternating chemotherapy combinations. J Clin Oncol 9:2193–2201, 1991.

53. Press OW, LeBlanc M, Lichter A, Wasserman TH, Miller T, Fisher R: A phase III randomized intergroup trial of subtotal lymphoid irradiation (STLI) versus doxorubicin, vinblastine, and STLI for stage IA–IIA Hodgkin's disease (SWOG 9133, CALGB 9391) (Abstract). Blood 96:575a, 2000.

54. Cornbleet MA, Vitolo U, Ultmann JE et al: Hodgkin's disease: Results of treatment with radiotherapy alone (1969–1980). J Clin Oncol 3:758–768, 1985.

55. Ganesan TS, Wrigley PF, Murray PA et al: Radiotherapy for stage I Hodgkin's disease: 20 years experience at St. Bartholomew's Hospital. Br J Cancer 62:314–318, 1990.

56. Hartsell WF, Sarin P, Recine DC et al: Long-term results of curative irradiation in pathologically staged IA and IIA Hodgkin disease [see comments]. Radiology 186:565–568, 1993.

57. Rock DB, Schultz CJ, Murray KJ, Wilson JF, Cox JD: Continuous split course irradiation for stage I and II Hodgkin's disease: 20 year experience at the Medical College of Wisconsin. Radiother Oncol 30:222–226, 1994.

58. Wasserman TH, Trenkner DA, Fineberg B, Kucik N: Cure of early-stage Hodgkin's disease with subtotal nodal irradiation. Cancer 68:1208–1215, 1991.

59. Mauch PM, Canellos GP, Shulman LN et al: Mantle irradiation alone for selected patients with laparotomy-staged IA to IIA Hodgkin's disease: Preliminary results of a prospective trial. J Clin Oncol 13:947–952, 1995.

60. Noordijk EM: Radiotherapy in early stage Hodgkin's disease: Principles and results of recent clinical trials (abstract). Ann Oncol 9(Suppl. 5):S63–65, 1998.

61. Staar S, Diehl V, Paulus U, Mueller RP Sr, Duehmke E, Tesch H: Definitive radiotherapy (RT) versus 2 cycles of ABVD and RT in early stage Hodgkin's disease: Results of GHSG-trial HD7 (abstract). Cancer 6:404, 2000.

62. Tebbi C, Leventhal B, Chauvenet A et al: Treatment of stage I, IIA, IIIA, pediatric Hodgkin's disease with Adriamycin, bleomycin, vincristine and etoposide (ABVE) and low-dose radiation with option to eliminate laparotomy (Abstract). Proc Am Soc Clin Oncol 13:392, 1994.

63. Karayalcin G, Behm FG, Gieser PW et al: Lymphocyte predominant Hodgkin disease: Clinico-pathologic features and results of treatment – the Pediatric Oncology Group experience. Med Pediatr Oncol 29:519–525, 1997.

64. Hagemeister FB, Fuller LM, Velasquez WS et al: Two cycles of MOPP and radiotherapy: Effective treatment for stage IIIA and IIIB Hodgkin's disease. Ann Oncol 2:25–31, 1991.

65. Grozea PN, Depersio EJ, Coltman CA Jr et al: Chemotherapy alone versus combined modality therapy for stage III Hodgkin's disease: A five-year follow-up of a Southwest Oncology Group study (SWOG-7518) USA. Dev Oncol 32:345–351, 1985.

66. Ferme C, Lepage E, D'Agay MF et al: Hodgkin's disease, clinical stages I, II A-B and IIIA. Results of brief chemotherapy followed by irradiation. Nouv Rev Fr Hematol 34:247–255, 1992.

67. Mueller RP Sr, Diehl V, Paulus U, Tesch H, Staar S, Duehmke E: Results of EF- versus IF-RT after 2 cycles of COPP/ABVD for intermediate stage Hodgkin's disease: The interim analysis of the HD8 trial of the German Hodgkin Study Group (GHSG) (abstract). Cancer 6:404–405, 2000.

68. Ferme C, Eghbali H, Hagenbeek A et al: MOPP/ABV (M/A) hybrid and irradiation in unfavorable supradiaphragmatic clinical stages (CS) I-II Hodgkin's disease (HD): Comparison of three treatment modalities preliminary results of the EORTC-GELA H8-U randomized trial in 995 patients. For EORTC Lymphoma Group and the Groupe d'Etudes Lymphomes de l'Adulte (Abstract). Blood 96:576a, 2000.

69. Horning SJ, Williams J, Bartlett NL et al: Assessment of the Stanford V regimen and consolidative radiotherapy for bulky and advanced Hodgkin's disease: Eastern Cooperative Oncology Group Pilot Study E1492. J Clin Oncol 18:972–980, 2000.

70. Kung FH, Leventhal BG, Behm FG et al: Abbreviated chemotherapy versus chemoradiotherapy in early stage Hodgkin's disease of childhood (abstract). Proc Am Soc Clin Oncol 11:361, 1992.

71. Kaplan HS: Evidence for a tumoricidal dose level in the radiotherapy of Hodgkin's disease. Cancer Res 26:1221–1224, 1966.

72. Fletcher GH, Shukovsky LJ: The interplay of radiocurability and tolerance in the irradiation of human cancers. J Radiol 56:383–400, 1975.

73. Schewe KL, Reavis J, Kun LE, Cox J: Total dose, fraction size, and tumor volume in the local control of Hodgkin's disease. Int J Radiat Oncol Biol Phys 15:25–28, 1988.

74. Sears JD, Greven KM, Ferree CR, D'Agostino RB Jr: Definitive irradiation in the treatment of Hodgkin's disease. Analysis of outcome, prognostic factors, and long-term complications. Cancer 79:145–151, 1997.

75. Loeffler M, Diehl V, Pfreundschuh M et al: Dose-response relationship of complementary radiotherapy following four cycles of combination chemotherapy in intermediate-stage Hodgkin's disease. J Clin Oncol 15:2275–2287, 1997.

76. Taylor BW Jr, Mendenhall NP, Million RR: Reproducibility of mantle irradiation with daily imaging films. Int J Radiat Oncol Biol Phys 19:149–151, 1990.

77. Marks JE, Haus AG, Sutton HG, Griem ML: Localization error in the radiotherapy of Hodgkin's disease and malignant lymphoma with extended mantle fields. Cancer 34:83–90, 1974.

78. Griffiths SE, Pearcey RG: The daily reproducibility of large, complex-shaped radiotherapy fields to the thorax and neck. Clin Radiol 37:39–41, 1986.

79. Hulshof M, Vanuytsel L, van den Bogaert W, van der Schueren E: Localization errors in mantle-field irradiation for Hodgkin's disease. Int J Radiat Oncol Biol Phys 17:679–683, 1989.

80. Willett CG, Linggood RM, Stracher MA et al: The effect of the respiratory cycle on mediastinal and lung dimensions in Hodgkin's disease. Implications for radiotherapy gated to respiration. Cancer 60:1232–1237, 1987.

81. Hull MC, Mendenhall NP, Morris CG: Coronary artery disease, carotid and subclavian artery disease, and valvular dysfunction after radiation therapy for Hodgkin's disease (abstract). Int J Radiat Oncol Biol Phys 551:69.

82. Hancock SL, Tucker MA, Hoppe RT: Breast cancer after treatment of Hodgkin's disease. J Natl Cancer Inst 85:25–31, 1993.

83. Kaldor JM, Day NE, Bell J et al: Lung cancer following Hodgkin's disease: A case-control study. Int J Cancer 52:677–681, 1992.

84. Dana BW, Dahlberg S, Nathwani BN et al: Long-term follow-up of patients with low-grade malignant lymphomas treated with doxorubicin-based chemotherapy or chemoimmunotherapy. J Clin Oncol 11:644–651, 1993.

85. Kimby E, Bjorkholm M, Gahrton G et al: Chlorambucil/prednisone vs. CHOP in symptomatic low-grade non-Hodgkin's lymphomas: A randomized trial from the Lymphoma Group of Central Sweden. Ann Oncol 5:67–71, 1994.

86. MacManus MP, Hoppe RT: Is radiotherapy curative for stage I and II low-grade follicular lymphoma? Results of a long-term follow-up study of patients treated at Stanford University. J Clin Oncol 14:1282–1290, 1996.

87. Nathu RM, Mendenhall NP, Almasri NM, Lynch JW: Non-Hodgkin's lymphoma of the head and neck: A 30-year experience at the University of Florida. Head Neck 21:247–254, 1999.

88. De Los Santos JF, Mendenhall NP, Lynch JW Jr: Is comprehensive lymphatic irradiation for low-grade non-Hodgkin's lymphoma curative therapy? Long-term experience at a single institution. Int J Radiat Oncol Biol Phys 38:3–8, 1997.

89. Jacobs JP, Murray KJ, Schultz CJ et al: Central lymphatic irradiation for stage III nodular malignant lymphoma: Long-term results. J Clin Oncol 11:233–238, 1993.

90. Johnson RE: Management of generalized malignant lymphomata with "systemic" radiotherapy. Br J Cancer Suppl 31:450–455, 1975.

91. Carabell SC, Chaffey JT, Rosenthal DS, Moloney WC, Hellman S: Results of total body irradiation in the treatment of advanced non-Hodgkin's lymphomas. Cancer 43:994–1000, 1979.

92. Hoppe RT, Kushlan P, Kaplan HS, Rosenberg SA, Brown BW: The treatment of advanced stage favorable histology non-Hodgkin's lymphoma: A preliminary report of a randomized trial comparing single agent chemotherapy, combination chemotherapy, and whole body irradiation. Blood 58:592–598, 1981.

93. Lybeert ML, Meerwaldt JH, Deneve W: Long-term results of low dose total body irradiation for advanced non-Hodgkin lymphoma. Int J Radiat Oncol Biol Phys 13:1167–1172, 1987.

94. Mendenhall NP, Noyes WD, Million RR: Total body irradiation for stage II-IV non-Hodgkin's lymphoma: Ten-year follow-up. Am J Clin Oncol 7:67–74, 1989.

95. Corder MP, Leimert JT, Tewfik HH, Lovett JM: Multimodality therapy of favorable prognosis non-Hodgkin's lymphoma. Int J Radiat Oncol Biol Phys 9:1009–1012, 1983.

96. Roncadin M, Arcicasa M, Zagonel V et al: Total body irradiation and prednimustine in chronic lymphocytic leukemia and low grade non-Hodgkin's lymphomas. A 9-year experience at a single institution. Cancer 74:978–984, 1994.

97. Johnson RE, Canellos GP, Young RC, Chabner BA, DeVita VT: Chemotherapy (cyclophosphamide, vincristine, and prednisone) versus radiotherapy (total body irradiation) for stage III-IV poorly differentiated lymphocytic lymphoma. Cancer Treat Rep 62:321–325, 1978.

98. Brereton HD, Young RC, Longo DL et al: A comparison between combination chemotherapy and total body irradiation plus combination chemotherapy in non-Hodgkin's lymphoma. Cancer 43:2227–2231, 1979.

99. Meerwaldt JH, Carde P, Burgers JM et al: Low-dose total body irradiation versus combination chemotherapy for lymphomas with follicular growth pattern. Int J Radiat Oncol Biol Phys 21:1167–1172, 1991.

100. Glick JH, Kim K, Earle J, O'Connell MJ: An ECOG randomized phase III trial of CHOP vs. CHOP + radiotherapy (XRT) for intermediate grade early stage non-Hodgkin's lymphoma (NHL) (abstract). Proc Annu Meet Am Soc Clin Oncol 14:391, 1995.

101. Fuller LM, Krasin MJ, Velasquez WS et al: Significance of tumor size and radiation dose to local control in stage I-III diffuse large cell lymphoma treated with CHOP-Bleo and radiation. Int J Radiat Oncol Biol Phys 31:3–11, 1995.

102. Kaminski MS, Estes J, Zasadny KR et al: Radioimmunotherapy with iodine ^{131}I tositumomab for relapsed or refractory B-cell non-Hodgkin lymphoma: Updated results and long-term follow-up of the University of Michigan experience. Blood 96:1259–1266, 2000.

103. DeNardo GL, DeNardo SJ, O'Grady LF, Levy NB, Adams GP, Mills SL: Fractionated radioimmunotherapy of B-cell malignancies with ^{131}I-Lym-1. Cancer Res 50:1014s–1016s, 1990.

104. Kaminski MS, Fig LM, Zasadny KR et al: Imaging, dosimetry, and radioimmunotherapy with iodine 131-labeled anti-CD37 antibody in B-cell lymphoma. J Clin Oncol 10:1696–1711, 1992.

105. Knox SJ: Radioimmunotherapy of non-Hodgkin's lymphomas. Semin Radiat Oncol 5:331–341, 1995.

106. Vose JM, Link BK, Grossbard ML et al: Phase II study of rituximab in combination with CHOP chemotherapy in patients with previously untreated, aggressive non-Hodgkin's lymphoma. J Clin Oncol 19:389–397, 2001.

107. Czuczman MS: CHOP plus rituximab chemoimmunotherapy of indolent B-cell lymphoma. Semin Oncol 26(Suppl. 14):88–96, 1999.

45

Diagnosis and Treatment of Non-Hodgkin's Lymphoma of Adults

Julie M. Vose, Philip J. Bierman,
and James O. Armitage

The non-Hodgkin's lymphomas represent a diverse group of neoplasms with many different clinical presentations, associated laboratory abnormalities, reponsiveness to treatment, and clinical outcome. In the United States, the incidence of non-Hodgkin's lymphomas steadily increases from childhood through age 80; unlike Hodgkin's disease, no peak incidence exists for young adults. The lymphomas represent the seventh most common cause of death from cancer in the United States, with the age-adjusted incidence being about three times that of Hodgkin's disease.[1] The incidence of non-Hodgkin's lymphoma is twice as frequent among whites as blacks, and there is an almost 50 percent increase of presentation in males compared with females. The reason for this gender and race predominance is unknown; however, it may reflect a different pattern of occupational exposure or a difference in the immune status of males compared with females.

Recently, many discoveries in the areas of immunology, histochemistry, and molecular biology have advanced our understanding of these complex diseases. With the advent of modern therapy based on these new data, patients with non-Hodgkin's lymphoma can now frequently be treated successfully to alter the natural history of the disease. This chapter outlines the clinical presentations, diagnostic and staging evaluations, prognostic factors, and therapeutic considerations for the various types of non-Hodgkin's lymphomas.

CLINICAL PRESENTATION

Most patients with non-Hodgkin's lymphoma come to medical attention because of the discovery of adenopathy; however, other problems such as abdominal fullness caused by splenomegaly, pain in involved sites of disease, anemia, infection, skin manifestations, neurologic symptoms, or systemic symptoms such as fever, night sweats, or weight loss can occasionally be the first signs of disease.

The clinical features of untreated patients are often typical for the individual histologic subtype of non-Hodgkin's lymphoma. For example, patients with nodular lymphomas most often present with painless adenopathy in the cervical, axillary, or inguinal regions. In some patients, large abdominal masses of retroperitoneal or mesenteric lymph nodes result in symptoms that bring the patient to a physician. Even though the patient may appreciate only one or a few enlarged lymph nodes, examination and evaluation often reveal widespread lymphadenopathy. The nodes may have been present for years with either fluctuation in size or gradual enlargement. Patients with nodular lymphomas often have splenomegaly, which is especially prevalent in the later stages of the disease. Bone marrow involvement is present more frequently in nodular lymphomas than in diffuse non-Hodgkin's lymphomas. For example, one study showed a 24 percent incidence of bone marrow involvement with nodular lymphomas compared with a 14 percent involvement with diffuse lymphomas.[2] Other studies have shown up to a 50 percent incidence of bone marrow involvement in nodular lymphomas.[3] Occasionally patients with bone marrow involvement will also present with peripheral blood involvement; however, this more frequently occurs with progressive or relapsed disease.[4]

Diffuse non-Hodgkin's lymphomas are extremely variable and no single clinical description can adequately describe them. Small lymphocytic non-Hodgkin's lymphoma is characterized by either focal or generalized lymphadenopathy and often splenomegaly. The disease is the tissue manifestation of the same monoclonal proliferation of the B lymphocyte that is associated with chronic lymphocytic leukemia (CLL). This disease, like CLL, most often occurs after the fifth decade and tends to be slowly progressive. The bone marrow is usually involved with this type of lymphoma, and a monoclonal gammopathy may occur or there may be hypogammaglobulinemia.

The most common diffuse lymphoma subtype, diffuse large cell lymphoma (DLC), often occurs as relatively localized but rapidly progressive disease. Patients with DLC often present with disease in the lymph nodes; however, this subtype can occur in nonlymphatic tissues. For example, occurrences in the gastrointestinal tract, testes, thyroid, skin, breast, central nervous system, or bone are more frequently seen in diffuse histologies than in nodular non-Hodgkin's lymphoma.[5–11] Occurrence of non-Hodgkin's lymphoma in Waldeyer's ring is associated with an approximate 20 percent risk of simultaneous or subsequent involvement of the gastrointestinal tract in other sites.[12] Because of this association, when patients present with involvement in Waldeyer's ring, a complete evaluation of the small and large bowel should be included in their initial evaluation. Bone marrow involvement with DLC at presentation is unusual, with only 10 percent of the cases positive. Diffuse infiltration of visceral organs by the aggressive diffuse lymphomas is very rare at presentation; however, relapsed or progressive lymphoma can cause these manifestations. Invasiveness of the aggressive diffuse lymphomas can result in peripheral nerve compression, spinal cord compression, great vessel or airway compression, or painful osseous lesions.

Lymphoblastic lymphoma is histologically and cytologically similar to acute lymphocytic leukemia and is most commonly seen in older children and young adults.[13] Approximately 50 percent of patients present with mediastinal lymphadenopathy, and a higher percentage are males. Although the disease may appear to be localized at the time of diagnosis, there is usually rapid dissemination to the bone marrow, peripheral blood, and meninges.[14] Another high-grade lymphoma, small noncleaved cell non-Hodgkin's lymphoma, is separated into Burkitt's and non-Burkitt's non-Hodgkin's lymphoma. Burkitt's non-Hodgkin's lymphoma, originally described in endemic Africa, usually presents with large extranodal tumors involving the bones of the jaw and abdominal tumors.[15] In contrast, sporadic cases in the United States most often present with abdominal tumors, with subsequent bone marrow and central nervous system involvement as the disease progresses.[16] Patients with the endemic Burkitt's lymphoma have a median age at presentation of approximately 7 years, whereas the sporadic cases occur over a broader age range up to the third decade, with a median age of 11 years. The non-Burkitt's subtype occurs more commonly in adults than children and has a propensity for bone marrow involvement early in the course of the disease.[17]

DIAGNOSIS

Because every enlarged lymph node does not necessarily represent a non-Hodgkin's lymphoma, histologic diagnosis is the most important first step toward initiating proper care of the patient. Palpable lymphadenopathy can be found in normal patients; however, the size is normally less than 1 cm. Lymphadenopathy could be associated with several benign conditions such as infectious mononucleosis, syphilis, cytomegalovirus, auto-immune disorders, granulomatous diseases, or drug hypersensitivities such as that seen with Dilantin (phenytoin). Since many patients with non-Hodgkin's lymphoma are in the younger age range, infectious mononucleosis should be considered before a lymph node biopsy. A lymph node biopsy specimen from this condition is sometimes difficult to distinguish from non-Hodgkin's lymphoma.[18] Other benign conditions that result in adenopathy and may initially have features suggesting non-Hodgkin's lymphoma include florid reactive follicular hyperplasia,[19] lymphomatoid granulomatosis,[20] dermatopathic lymphadenopathy, sinus histiocytosis with massive lymphadenopathy,[21] and angioimmunoblastic lymphadenopathy (AILD).[22] Some of the patients with these conditions can eventually develop overt lymphoma. Patients with lymphomatoid granulomatosis have a 12 percent incidence of developing overt lymphoma.[23] This compares with at least a 50 percent incidence of overt lymphoma developing in patients with AILD, discovered either during their clinical course or at autopsy.[22] Many other malignant conditions such as metastatic carcinomas, germ cell neoplasms, or melanomas can also present with lymphadenopathy. Young male patients with malignant axillary lymph node enlargement are most likely to have a lymphoma or a malignant melanoma. In women, the same two tumors as well as breast carcinoma would be the most likely diagnosis.

When a lymphoma is suspected clinically, the pathologist should be notified so that special processing procedures can be used if they are available, including cytogenetics, surface markers, immunohistochemistry stains, and molecular biologic studies, in addition to routine histology. These additional studies can add valuable information to the cases that are difficult to identify on routine testing. Patients with an undifferentiated

neoplasm by routine histology can have a non-Hodgkin's lymphoma in a small percentage of cases. Because this is one of the more treatable causes of what appears to be an undifferentiated neoplasm, special stains should be an important part of the evaluation of a specimen with this initial diagnosis. The accuracy and reproducibility of pathologists in the diagnosis of non-Hodgkin's lymphoma is essential for the care and treatment of patients. However, this is not a simple task. Even the expert pathologists who developed the Working Formulation were able to reproduce their initial diagnosis on re-reviewing a slide only 53 to 93 percent of the time.[24]

Every patient with non-Hodgkin's lymphoma does not always present with peripheral lymphadenopathy that is easily biopsied, and therefore, other procedures may be required for diagnosis. Other sites of presentation that may require biopsy for diagnosis include skin, gastrointestinal tract, breast, or testes. Visceral presentation such as hepatic, splenic, or pulmonary involvement may occasionally require an open biopsy for diagnosis. Also, retroperitoneal, mesenteric, or pelvic disease may require a diagnostic laparotomy for diagnosis confirmation. Unexplained hematologic problems such as neutropenia, anemia, a leukoerythroblastic picture, or thrombocytopenia may lead to a bone marrow biopsy that diagnoses marrow involvement with non-Hodgkin's lymphoma. The childhood non-Hodgkin's lymphomas often differ in presentation from their adult counterparts. Childhood lymphomas have a propensity for early widespread dissemination with more frequent central nervous system and peripheral blood dissemination. Follicular lymphomas are very rare in children, and while most childhood lymphomas are B cell in origin, there is an increased number of T-cell cases compared with adults.

STAGING PROCEDURES

Once a histologic diagnosis of non-Hodgkin's lymphoma has been confirmed by biopsy, various staging procedures must be done to direct the therapy as well as to provide for prognostic information for the patient. The histologic subtype and the condition of the patient direct the type and speed of staging procedures. For example, a patient with a high-grade non-Hodgkin's lymphoma that is rapidly progressive requires prompt staging procedures that are the minimum required before the initiation of therapy. On the other hand, low-grade non-Hodgkin's lymphoma can be staged at the convenience of the patient and physician. Treatment decisions can then be made with all the knowledge from the staging procedures available for discussion.

The various tests useful for staging non-Hodgkin's lymphoma are listed in Table 45–1. Baseline studies that should be obtained in most patients include complete history and physical examination, blood testing including complete blood count, platelet count, liver chemistries, lactate dehydrogenase (LDH), calcium, and renal function studies, chest radiograph, computed tomography (CT) of the abdomen, pelvis, and chest if the chest radiograph is suspicious, and bone marrow biopsy. Additional studies that may be appropriate in certain circumstances

Table 45-1. Staging Procedures for Non-Hodgkin's Lymphoma

Initial studies
  Confirmed histologic diagnosis
  History and physical examination
  Laboratory analysis
    Complete blood count, platelet count
    Renal function studies
    Calcium, uric acid, LDH
    Liver function studies
  Chest radiograph
  CT scan of abdomen and pelvis
  CT scan of chest if radiograph suspicious
  Bone marrow biopsy
Additional studies (if circumstances are appropriate)
  Bone scan
  Ultrasonography
  ^{67}Ga scan (planar or SPECT)
  Gastrointestinal evaluation if primary in Waldeyer's ring
  CT scan of brain (if neurologic symptoms present)
  MRI of spine or myelogram (if neurologic symptoms present)
  Lumbar puncture (high-grade lymphoma or symptoms present)
  Cytologic examination of an effusion
Additional
  Gene probe rearrangements
  Polymerase chain reaction analysis
  Flow cytometry for immunophenotyping of peripheral blood or bone marrow
  Immunohistochemistry analysis
  Flow cytometry for DNA analysis
  Cytogenetic analysis of lymph node, blood, or bone marrow

include cytologic examination of any effusion present (i.e., pleural or pericardial effusions or ascitic fluid) and bone scan if symptoms are present. A thorough evaluation of the gastrointestinal tract should be pursued if any symptoms are present or if the primary presentation of lymphoma was in Waldeyer's ring. A lumbar puncture and/or CT or magnetic resonance imaging (MRI) of the brain or spinal cord should be performed if any signs or symptoms of central nervous system lymphoma are present. In addition, high-grade lymphomas have a high incidence of central nervous system involvement, and many treatment regimens call for central nervous system prophylaxis as well as initial cerebrospinal fluid evaluation. ^{67}Ga scanning with either planar or tomographic (SPECT) technique can be useful in some circumstances in differentiating active lymphoma from fibrotic tissue.

In one study from the Dana-Farber Cancer Institute, 17 of 34 patients (46 percent) showed persistent ^{67}Ga uptake halfway through induction chemotherapy.[25] Of these, 4 were in complete remission, 11 were in partial response, and 2 showed no change in tumor size. At follow-up, 10 (59 percent) had died (3 who were scored as complete remission and 7 who were in partial remission halfway through therapy), 2 were alive with active tumor, 1 relapsed and survived following bone marrow transplantation, and 4 (3 in partial response and 1 in complete remission at the therapeutic halfway point) are without disease at a median of 28 months from presentation. Of the 20 patients who

were ^{67}Ga-negative halfway through therapy, 11 were in complete remission and 9 were in partial remission. Five of 20 patients had died. Three in complete remission died at 11, 26, and 28 months and two in radiographic partial response died at 15 and 17 months. One patient was alive with active tumor, and 14 (70 percent) were alive without disease at a median of 34 months from presentation. ^{67}Ga imaging in this study proved to be an excellent indicator of residual viable tumor.[25]

The results of these tests are utilized for designation of the proper staging classification for the patient. The patients are classified according to the Ann Arbor staging conference, which was developed for Hodgkin's disease.[26] The histologic subtype, presence or absence of B symptoms, and the classical Ann Arbor stage are important for initial evaluation and stratification of the patient for appropriate treatment. After therapy has been initiated and at appropriate intervals, previously positive tests should be repeated for evaluation of the effectiveness of the therapy.

PROGNOSTIC FACTORS

Histopathology

Many histologic classifications have been formulated, in an attempt to classify the non-Hodgkin's lymphomas into prognostic categories.[27,28] The Working Formulation was an attempt to create an easily applied classification that would help to improve the prognostic significance of the histologic diagnosis.[29] This analysis breaks down the non-Hodgkin's lymphomas into three basic categories: low grade, intermediate grade, and high grade. Other histologies that do not easily fit into one of these three groups are included separately in the Working Formulation (Table 45-2). The Revised European-American Classification of Lymphoid Neoplasms (REAL) has recently been proposed to offer a newer histopathologic classification containing some entities felt to represent specific clinical-pathologic cases that may behave in a specific clinical manner.[30]

Histologic transformation from a low-grade to a high-grade non-Hodgkin's lymphoma is associated with more aggressive behavior of the lymphoma and a poor prognosis. Histologic transformation occurs in approximately 30 percent of nodular or small lymphocytic lymphomas, usually many years after the original diagnosis.[31] The transformation of small lymphocytic lymphoma to DLC was originally described many years ago and given the name of Richter's syndrome.[32] This transformation occurs in approximately 30 percent of these patients; however, a larger proportion of patients undergo a gradual acceleration in the clinical course of their disease over time. Immunologic studies have now shown that these large cells often bear the same surface determinants as the small lymphoid cells of the original disease. The median survival of patients after histologic transformation is significantly shorter than survival of patients with de novo DLC or recurrent low-grade lymphomas. For example, a review from Iowa showed a median survival of transformed patients of only 12 months compared with 40 months in de novo DLC when both groups were treated with identical therapy.[33]

Table 45–2. World Health Organization Classification of Neoplastic Diseases of the Lymphoid Tissues

B-cell neoplasms
Precursor B-cell neoplasms
  B-cell lymphoblastic leukemia/lymphoma
Peripheral B-cell neoplasms
  B-cell chronic lymphocytic leukemia/small lymphocytic lymphoma
  B-cell prolymphocytic leukemia
  Lymphoplasmacytic lymphoma
  Mantle-cell lymphoma
  Follicular lymphoma – grades I, II, and III
  Marginal zone B-cell lymphoma – nodal or splenic variants
  Hairy cell leukemia
  Diffuse large B-cell lymphoma
    Variants: Centroblastic
      Immunoblastic
      Anaplastic large B-cell
      Burkitt-like
  Diffuse large B-cell lymphoma
    Subtypes: Mediastinal large B-cell
      Intravascular large B-cell
      Primary effusion lymphoma in HIV patients
  Burkitt's lymphoma
  Plasmacytoma
  Plasma cell myeloma

T-cell neoplasms
Precursor T-cell leukemia/lymphoma
  T-cell lymphoblastic leukemia/lymphoma
Peripheral T-cell and/or natural killer (NK) cell neoplasms, predominantly disseminated
  T-cell prolymphocytic
  T-cell large granular lymphocyte leukemia
  NK-cell leukemia
  Adult T-cell leukemia/lymphoma
Peripheral T-cell–NK-cell neoplasms, predominantly nodal
  AIL T-cell neoplasms
  Peripheral T-cell lymphoma
  Anaplastic large-cell lymphoma (T-cell and null types)
Peripheral T-/NK-cell neoplasms, predominantly extranodal
  Mycosis fungoides
  Sézary syndrome
  Primary cutaneous CD30 + T-cell
  Primary cutaneous ALC lymphomas plus borderline lymphomatoid papulosis
  Subcutaeous panniculitic-like T-cell lymphoma
  NK-/T-cell lymphomas, nasal/nasal type
  Enteropathy-type intestinal T-cell
  Hepatosplenic gamma/delta T-cell lymphoma

Hodgkin's lymphoma
Nodular lymphocyte-predominance Hodgkin's lymphoma
Classical Hodgkin's lymphoma
  Hodgkin's lymphoma, nodular sclerosis (grades I and II)
  Hodgkin's lymphoma, mixed cellularity
  Classical Hodgkin's lymphoma, lymphocyte-rich
  Hodgkin's lymphoma, lymphocyte depletion

Staging and Systemic Symptoms

The clinical stage within each histologic subtype carries reliable prognostic significance for the patient and physician. Results from several series evaluating patients with diffuse lymphomas have shown a significant difference between low and high stages in patients treated uniformly.[34–36] For example, a report from the Southwest Oncology Group (SWOG) shows that patients with stage IV DLC had a significantly lower median survival of 12 months compared with 42 months for stage III patients.[37]

Systemic B symptoms with non-Hodgkin's lymphomas are present in approximately 20 to 30 percent of the patients.[38] Several series have reported an adverse effect on overall survival if the patients had systemic symptoms.[39–41] However, a number of studies have not found an adverse effect on survival.[42,43]

Sites of Disease

Most non-Hodgkin's lymphomas occur within lymph nodes; however, several extranodal presentations are seen with some frequency. Primary central nervous system lymphomas were previously rarely reported. However, with the acquired immunodeficiency syndrome (AIDS) epidemic, many more primary central nervous system lymphomas have been noted.[44] Most non-AIDS-associated primary central nervous system lymphomas are small noncleaved, lymphoblastic, and DLC lymphomas. Many of the series in the literature are older and involve the delivery of less than optimal therapy. However, with newer techniques approximately one-fourth of the patients have prolonged disease-free survival.[45,46] Patients with the AIDS-associated primary central nervous system non-Hodgkin's lymphomas have a much poorer median survival of 3 months.[47] Another extranodal area that may be involved with non-Hodgkin's lymphoma is the testes. The histology is most frequently DLC and most patients are elderly. In most previous series, patients treated with orchiectomy alone relapsed with disseminated disease in a few months.[48] More recent series have improved results utilizing combined modality therapy.[49]

Considering the gastrointestinal tract as a whole, primary lymphoma of the gastrointestinal tract is the most common extranodal site. As noted previously, involvement of Waldeyer's ring correlates with an increased risk of gastrointestinal lymphoma—up to a 20 percent incidence.[12] The most frequent gastrointestinal location for lymphoma is gastric, followed by small intestine, ileocecal area, and large intestine.[50] Non-Hodgkin's lymphoma of the gastrointestinal tract has been associated with nontropical sprue[51] and systemic sclerosis.[52] Because of their location, some gastrointestinal lymphomas must be treated with local surgical excision before initiation of chemotherapy or radiation therapy especially small or large intestine lesions. Gastric lymphomas can occasionally be treated with chemotherapy without the necessity of prior gastrectomy.

Age

Age has been found to be a prognostic factor in several studies[53–55]; however, several other studies have not confirmed this fact. When age groups have been stratified for causes of death other than lymphoma, one study found no difference in the adjusted survival of older patients.[56] However, older patients often have more difficulty with chemotherapy side effects and may have increased morbidity due to drug-related toxicity.[57]

Several studies report a diminished complete response rate in the elderly patients; however, it is not clear whether this is due to lower drug doses administered or other factors.[58] In most large unselected series, the median age of the patients is usually in the early to midsixties. However, patients in many chemotherapeutic trials have a median age of 45 to 55 years. With this age difference in clinical trials, comparisons are difficult between the various aggressive regimens. Further evaluation of these regimens in unselected patient populations may lead to different results in older patient populations.

Tumor Bulk

Several studies have now identified larger tumor bulk as an adverse prognostic factor.[59–61] Tumor bulk is defined in different studies from 5 to 10 cm. The complete remission rate[41] and the relapse rate[62] have been found to be inferior in patients with large tumor bulk. In patients with stage I and II disease who were treated with radiation therapy only, one study found that those with a tumor size less than 3 cm in diameter had a 5 percent local recurrence rate compared with an 18 percent local recurrence rate with tumors 3 cm or more in diameter.[63]

Laboratory Analysis

Elevated serum LDH has also been associated with a poor prognosis in a number of analyses.[64,65] A number of analyses performed on the lymphoma tissue itself have recently been shown to be helpful in predicting outcome with therapy. For example, immunophenotyping studies have shown in a number of studies that a T-cell immunophenotype is an adverse prognostic factor,[66,67] although a few other studies have not confirmed this fact.[68,69] Indicators of rapid proliferation such as Ki-67 and DNA proliferative index have also been analyzed for their relationship to prognosis. Investigators at Arizona evaluated 105 patients with DLC utilizing the anti-Ki-67 monoclonal antibody. In their analysis, 19 patients with Ki-67 levels higher than 60 percent had a median survival of 8 months compared with a median survival of 39 months for the 86 patients with Ki-67 levels of 60 percent or less.[70] Proliferative activity and DNA aneuploidy as identified by flow cytometry have also been evaluated for use as predictive indicators of prognosis in patients with DLC. One study of 50 newly diagnosed patients found that high proliferative activity was the single most important pretreatment adverse prognostic factor in these patients. In that study, DNA aneuploidy was detected in 62 percent of cases; however, it did not seem to have any prognostic significance.[71] Another study of 52 patients found that the combination of proliferative activity and DNA content categorized the patients into four groups. Those with low proliferative activity and aneuploidy had a 2-year survival rate of 77 percent, and those with high proliferative activity and diploidy had a 2-year survival rate of 0 percent. The patients between these two extremes had an intermediate survival of 57 and 32 percent, respectively.[72]

The identification of nonrandom chromosomal abnormalities in patients with non-Hodgkin's lymphoma has been described in multiple studies.[73–79] A study done at Minnesota

Table 45–3. Common Chromosomal Changes in B-Cell Non-Hodgkin's Lymphoma

Chromosomal Change	Histology
t(2;8)(p12;q24)	Small noncleaved cell
t(8;14)(q24;q32)	Small noncleaved cell
t(8;22)(q24;q11)	Small noncleaved cell
t(11;14)(q13;q32)	Mantle cell lymphoma
t(14;18)(q32;q21)	Follicular lymphomas
del (6q)	Follicular lymphoma or diffuse large cell
t(3;14)(q27;q32)	Diffuse large cell

evaluated 68 newly diagnosed non-Hodgkin's lymphoma patients and correlated karyotypic abnormalities with sites of disease and clinical outcome.[75] Certain chromosomal abnormalities can be associated with specific histologic subtypes of lymphoma such as t(14;18)(q32;q21) in follicular lymphomas,[76] t(11;14)(q13;q32) in mantle cell lymphoma,[77] and t(8;14)(q24;q32) in Burkitt's lymphoma;[78] structural abnormalities such as the deletion of 6q can be associated with non-Hodgkin's lymphoma as well.[79] Other chromosomal changes are outlined in Table 45–3.

International Prognostic Index

The largest evaluation of prognostic factors for aggressive lymphoma was made in over 2000 patients and published as the International Prognostic Index.[80] In the multivariate analysis, age (less than 60 years versus 60 years or older), tumor stage (I–II versus III–IV), serum lactate dehydrogenase (normal versus higher than normal), performance status (ECOG 0-1 versus 2 or higher), and number of extranodal sites of disease (0 or 1 versus 2 or more) were identified as being highly predictive of outcome. These risk factors were put together into an analysis so that the number of factors was highly predictive of outcome. Patients with 0 or 1 risk factor had a complete remission (CR) rate of 87 percent and a 5-year survival rate of 73 percent; those with 2 risk factors had a CR rate of 67 percent and a 5-year survival rate of 51 percent with 3 risk factors, the rate was 55 percent and the 5-year survival rate was 43 percent; with 4 or 5 risk factors, the CR rate was 44 percent and the 5-year survival rate was 26 percent. This prognostic index should be evaluated in all new patients with aggressive lymphoma to plan their clinical courses.

TREATMENT

Background

Many advances have been made in the treatment of patients with non-Hodgkin's lymphomas over the past several years. The treatment strategy for non-Hodgkin's lymphoma varies based on several factors including histologic subtype, stage, age, performance status, and other prognostic factors, as discussed under patient staging and evaluation. Management of acute problems such as spinal cord compression, superior vena cava syndrome, hypercalcemia, and obstruction may specifically direct initial therapy. Adequate treatment is often multidisciplinary, involving surgical oncologists, medical oncologists, and radiation oncologists. The initial goal of therapy is generally the attainment of a complete remission defined as the documented disappearance of disease from previously involved sites. Maintenance therapy is rarely employed in non-Hodgkin's lymphoma once a clinical complete response has been obtained.

Indolent Histologic Subtypes

The so-called favorable low-grade histologic subtypes of cutaneous T-cell lymphoma (CTCL), and the small lymphocytic (SL), follicular small cleaved (FSC), and follicular mixed (FM) non-Hodgkin's lymphoma are not as common as the intermediate- or high-grade non-Hodgkin's lymphomas. The low-grade histologies compose 20 to 45 percent of the lymphomas in most series. While FSC and FM lymphomas can occur in younger patients, CTCL and SL lymphoma most often occur in patients over 60 years of age. When careful staging procedures as outlined above are followed, over 90 percent of the patients have advanced-stage disease at diagnosis.

Patients with these low-grade histologic subtypes have a prolonged natural history with a median survival in most series of 5 years or more.[81,82] Also, except in a few cases of truly localized disease, these low-grade histologic subtypes of non-Hodgkin's lymphoma cannot be cured or are only rarely cured with conventional radiation therapy or chemotherapy. The therapy offered to the patient must take this incurability into account. Patients with few serious signs or symptoms of their disease can be placed into the "watch and wait" category until they show signs or symptoms of their disease, making treatment essential. When the disease does advance so that treatment is necessary, localized radiation therapy can be used for symptomatic adenopathy; also, single or combination chemotherapeutic agents can be used for more extensive disease. Multiple chemotherapeutic agents have been found to be effective in this clinical situation.[83,84] With most of these modalities a complete or partial response can be achieved at least initially. However, a relapse rate of 10 to 15 percent per year occurs, with only a small percentage of patients remaining in remission after 10 years of follow-up.

Most patients with CTCL experience months to years of nonspecific cutaneous manifestations before establishment of a diagnosis of CTCL. Several clinical variants of CTCL exist, including patch, plaque, tumor stage, and generalized erythroderma. Very few of the patients when carefully analyzed have localized disease, even though their skin disease may appear to be localized. Recent studies have shown that when carefully examined, nearly all patients with generalized erythroderma and 13 to 65 percent of patients with plaque or tumor stage will have some circulating Sézary cells.[85] Because CTCL has differing clinical manifestations and such a long natural history, many topical and less toxic therapies have been the mainstay of therapy for some time. Since cutaneous manifestations repre-

sent the major clinical problem at least initially, topical treatments such as topical nitrogen mustard, psoralen with ultraviolet-A light (PUVA), or total skin electron beam have been found to be effective. However, these regimens can cure only a small percentage of the total patient population with CTCL. With the increasing realization that CTCL disseminates early, systemic therapies or combinations of topical plus systemic therapies are being used with more frequency. Combination chemotherapy is not very successful in CTCL. Although objective response rates up to 70 percent can be obtained, the duration of response is often fairly short[86] Interferon[87] and extracorporeal photopheresis[88] have shown some initially promising results in CTCL; however, further evaluation will be necessary to confirm this.

In an effort to improve the outcome of low-grade non-Hodgkin's lymphomas, several studies have attempted more aggressive chemotherapy, newer chemotherapeutic agents, postinduction maintenance therapy, or high-dose chemotherapy and transplantation. A study initiated at the National Cancer Institute many years ago randomized patients with indolent lymphoma to receive ProMACE-MOPP plus total lymphoid irradiation (TLI) or a "watch and wait" strategy.[89] At 4 years of follow-up, the disease-free survival was superior for the aggressively treated patients (51 percent versus 12 percent); however, the overall survival was not different in the two groups (75 percent in both groups at 5 years). With further follow-up, perhaps a difference in overall survival can be detected. In a SWOG analysis, the use of an anthracycline-containing regimen compared retrospectively with non-anthracycline-containing regimens did not appear to influence the overall survival of patients with indolent lymphomas.[90]

Prognostic factors that appear to influence the outcome of patients with indolent non-Hodgkin's lymphoma include advanced stage, follicular large cell histology compared with FM or FSC, peripheral lymph node size, degree of marrow involvement, and male sex.[91–93] Additionally, the International Prognostic Index, originally developed for the intermediate-grade lymphomas, can also apply to the indolent lymphomas, with age, performance status, stage, extranodal involvement, and an elevated LDH representing discriminating prognostic factors.[94]

Because conventional chemotherapy has not changed the overall survival for patients with indolent non-Hodgkin's lymphoma, newer agents such as fludarabine and 2-chlorodeoxyadenosine have recently been evaluated for the treatment of this type of lymphoma.[95,96] Although the complete remission rates appear to be quite high, further follow-up will be necessary to evaluate the long-term effects of such agents. Another area of active investigation for maintenance of complete remission is the addition of interferon as a maintenance regimen. In a large randomized study, patients with indolent non-Hodgkin's lymphoma randomized to receive interferon α2b at a dosage of 5 million units three times weekly for 18 months demonstrated an improved event-free survival and overall survival.[97]

Another major advance in therapy for indolent lymphomas has been the use of Rituxan (chimeric anti-CD20). In the original trials, the Rituxan was administered weekly for 4 weeks to patients with multiply relapsed indolent NHL. They found a CR rate of 6 percent and an overall response rate of 50 percent in the trial.[98] This antibody is now standard therapy for many patients with indolent NHL. It has also been used in combination with CHOP in patients with indolent NHL and found to have a 97 percent response rate.[99]

Another aggressive approach to the treatment of patients with indolent non-Hodgkin's lymphoma is the use of high-dose chemotherapy and transplantation. In a study by Rohatiner et al.[100] 64 patients with follicular non-Hodgkin's lymphoma received high-dose cyclophosphamide and total-body irradiation followed by autologous purged transplantation. At the time of publication, with a median follow-up of 3.5 years, 35 patients continued in remission between 1 and 8 years. Compared with a historical control group receiving conventional therapy, the transplanted patients had an advantage in disease-free survival but no advantage in survival.[98] Other investigators have published similar results using transplantation for relapsed follicular lymphoma patients.[101–103] The use of transplantation in first complete remission as a consolidative measure has also recently been evaluated by the Dana Farber group.[104] Eighty-three patients with advanced indolent non-Hodgkin's lymphoma received CHOP for six to eight cycles to achieve a complete response, followed by high-dose chemotherapy and transplantation. At the time of initial evaluation, 48 patients were in unmaintained complete remission with a median follow-up of 22 months. Prolonged follow-up of patients undergoing this therapy will be necessary.

Aggressive Non-Hodgkin's Lymphoma

Under the Working Formulation,[29] intermediate-grade non-Hodgkin's lymphomas include the histologic subtypes of follicular large cell (FL), diffuse small cleaved cell (DSC), diffuse mixed cell (DM), and DLC. These histologic subtypes vary in their natural history; however, they all have a more aggressive natural history when compared with the low-grade histologic subtypes. Therapy must be tailored for the individual patient based on an extensive staging evaluation. Patients with localized stage I or minimal stage II disease can be treated with a less aggressive approach than those with more extensive disease but still with curative intent. Involved field radiation therapy has been found to be curative in few patients with DSC or DM[105]; however, FL or DLC can be cured more frequently with this approach—up to an 80 percent disease-free survival rate in one study with extensively staged patients.[106] Several studies have now reported improvement on these results with the addition of short-course combination chemotherapy before involved-field radiation therapy.[107,108]

Miller et al.[108] evaluated 401 patients with localized stage I or II aggressive NHL, with 201 patients randomized to receive eight cycles of cyclophosphamide, doxorubicin, vincristine, prednisone (CHOP) alone and 200 assigned to receive three cycles of CHOP plus radiotherapy. In this study, the patients in the arm with CHOP plus radiotherapy had significantly better progression-free survival at 5 years of 77 percent compared to 64 percent for patients on the CHOP alone arm ($p = .03$). The 5-year estimates of overall survival for patients receiving CHOP plus radiotherapy was 82 percent compared to 72 percent for those

receiving the CHOP × 8 alone ($p = .02$). Based on this and similar studies, a shortened course of CHOP followed by radiation is now the standard of care for patients with localized lymphoma.

Whereas about 30 percent of patients with intermediate-grade non-Hodgkin's lymphomas have localized disease at diagnosis, most have extensive disease at this time and will need more extended therapy. Many combination chemotherapy programs have been evaluated for the treatment of intermediate or high-grade non-Hodgkin's lymphomas. Because immunoblastic non-Hodgkin's lymphoma behaves clinically much like DLC, it is usually treated like an intermediate-grade lymphoma. Regimens have been reported to have complete remission rates of 40 to 80 percent in various studies. Initial attempts to improve the treatment programs focused on adding active agents to cyclophosphamide, vincristine, and prednisone (CVP). The first quantum leap of effective programs involved adding doxorubicin to the CVP regimen. This CHOP regimen had the highest complete remission rate of any program at the time (58 percent) and it was fairly easy to administer. In long-term analyses, approximately 30 percent of all treated patients achieved durable complete remission.[109]

The so-called second-generation regimens were developed in the late 1970s. Methotrexate was added to BACOP to make M-BACOD and later m-BACOD. The methotrexate was added in an attempt to increase the central nervous system penetration; however, more mucositis and pulmonary infiltrates can be expected from this program. This program did seem to improve results over CHOP, with a 71 percent complete response rate and a 50 percent long-term survival rate.[110] Others also built on the BACOP program, for example, a six-drug program, COP-BLAM, was used that had similar results to the M-BACOD results as described above. The third-generation regimens that were developed during the 1980s have added newer active chemotherapeutic agents and have expanded the role of many drugs early in an intensive short course of treatment. Examples of these are MACOP-B, ProMACE-CytaBOM, LNH-80, and COP-BLAM III. Most of these programs reported a complete remission rate of approximately 80 percent with approximately 60 to 70 percent of the patients disease-free at the time of initial publication.[111–114]

A four-arm study evaluating 899 patients randomized to receive CHOP, m-BACOD, ProMACE-CytaBOM, or MACOP-B published by Fisher et al.[115] demonstrated that the 3-year estimates of time to treatment failure for these arms were 41, 46, 46, and 41 percent, respectively. There were no risk groups according to the International Prognostic Index, as developed by Shipp et al.[80] that benefited from one of the four arms of the treatment trial compared with other arms. However, elderly patients did have a lower failure-free survival and higher toxic death rate compared with younger patients when they were treated with the high-dose methotrexate-containing regimen MACOP-B.[116]

Recently, Coiffier et al.[117] evaluated 400 patients with aggressive NHL who were over the age of 60 years. The patients were randomized to receive either CHOP for six cycles or CHOP + Rituxan for six cycles of therapy. The complete remission rate for the patients randomized to the CHOP alone arm was 60 percent compared to 76 percent for those randomized to the CHOP + Rituxan arm ($p = .004$). The event-free survival was also improved in the CHOP + Rituxan arm at 69 percent, compared to 49 percent for those in the CHOP alone arm, with a median follow-up of 1 year ($p < .0005$). The overall survival was also improved in the CHOP + Rituxan arm at 83 percent compared with 68 percent in the CHOP alone arm ($p < .01$). Another confirmatory trial is near completed accrual in the Eastern Cooperative Oncology Group.

High-Grade Non-Hodgkin's Lymphoma

The three histologic subtypes under the category of high-grade non-Hodgkin's lymphoma include large cell immunoblastic lymphoma, lymphoblastic lymphoma, and small noncleaved cell lymphoma (Burkitt's and non-Burkitt's). The large-cell immunoblastic non-Hodgkin's lymphomas behave clinically much like DLC lymphomas. Most physicians treat these patients in a similar manner with the rules for localized or advanced disease as outlined above. However, lymphoblastic lymphoma and small noncleaved cell lymphoma have distinctive clinical behaviors and often require a different approach.

Lymphoblastic lymphoma rarely presents as localized disease and therefore almost always requires aggressive systemic therapy. This category of aggressive lymphoma is most commonly seen in adolescent or young adults, more frequently in male patients, and often presents as a large mediastinal mass. It can occasionally be difficult to distinguish from acute lymphocytic leukemia. This lymphoma is rapidly progressive and requires prompt evaluation and treatment when diagnosed. Standard anthracycline-based chemotherapy regimens have produced fairly high complete remission rates in lymphoblastic lymphoma; however, high relapse rates are noted, especially within the central nervous system and bone marrow.[118] The LSA2-L2 protocol has been compared with COMP in a prospective trial by the Children's Cancer Study Group, with significant differences in outcome depending on histology. This study involved the treatment of 234 children randomized to COMP versus LSA2-L2.[119] For lymphoblastic lymphoma, LSA2-L2 was significantly more effective therapy (76 percent 2-year disease-free survival versus 26 percent for COMP), but for nonlymphoblastic histologies, COMP was more effective (57 percent versus 28 percent for LSA2-L2). Utilizing these aggressive protocols involving central nervous system prophylaxis, several studies have found improved disease-free survival in this group. However, a group of patients with a poor prognosis can still be identified from this population including those with high LDH or bone marrow or central nervous system involvement at diagnosis, or those with a less than complete response to initial therapy.[119] Lymphoblastic lymphoma in adults is less well studied but has had a poorer long-term disease-free survival rate with standard therapy.[118]

The use of high-dose chemotherapy and either autologous or allogeneic bone marrow transplantation in first complete remission for high-risk lymphoblastic non-Hodgkin's lymphoma has now been evaluated by several institutions.[120–124] A retrospective study by the European Bone Marrow Transplant Registry evalu-

ated 214 patients with lymphoblastic non-Hodgkin's lymphoma who received high-dose chemotherapy and marrow transplantation, with 105 of those in first complete remission at the time of the transplant.[124] The actuarial overall survival at 6 years for the entire group was 42 percent. The 6-year actuarial overall survival was 63 percent for patients transplanted in first complete remission, compared with 15 percent for those with resistant disease at the time of transplantation. Transplantation in second complete remission resulted in a 31 percent rate of actuarial overall survival at 6 years. From this analysis, it appeared that the disease status at the time of transplant was the most important predictor for outcome.[124] Many centers are now identifying high-risk lymphoblastic lymphoma patients at the time of diagnosis based on central nervous system or bone marrow involvement or an LDH greater than the upper limits of normal (or both factors) for early transplantation.

Small noncleaved cell non-Hodgkin's lymphoma, also comparatively less common in adults than in children, is also a very aggressive rapidly growing tumor. It can be divided into Burkitt's or non-Burkitt's subtypes on a pathologic basis. The prognosis can often be predicted based on stage, age, or central nervous system or bone marrow involvement as well as total tumor burden.[125] This aggressive lymphoma requires an intensive chemotherapy regimen often including central nervous system prophylaxis.[126] A number of treatment strategies for small noncleaved cell non-Hodgkin's lymphoma have been evaluated over the past 10 years. The use of two sequential programs at the National Cancer Institute employing cyclophosphamide, vincristine, methotrexate, and prednisone resulted in a complete response in 48 of 54 patients (89 percent) with an overall 2-year actuarial survival rate of 54 percent.[127] More aggressive treatment with cyclophosphamide, vincristine, Adriamycin, prednisone, and intermittent courses of high-dose methotrexate with leucovorin rescue, augmented by intrathecal methotrexate and cytarabine, revealed improved results with a projected overall survival rate in excess of 70 percent of cases.[128] Patients with larger masses or more extensive involvement were treated with M-BACOD, plus intrathecal methotrexate and cytarabine at the Dana-Farber Cancer Institute. Of 13 patients, 12 achieved a complete response and 8 relapsed, leaving an overall actuarial survival rate of 31 percent.[129]

Patients with central nervous system or bone marrow disease are felt to have a worse prognosis and the use of high-dose chemotherapy and marrow transplantation in first complete remission in this patient population has recently been evaluated in an attempt to improve on these results. In a study by Troussard et al.[130] nine such high-risk patients underwent allogenic transplant in first complete remission. At the time of publication, seven of the nine patients were alive and disease-free. Two patients died at 14 and 7 months due to the acquired immunodeficiency syndrome (AIDS) and a bacterial sepsis. Further investigation into the use of transplantation for high-risk patients is ongoing.

Conventional Salvage Therapy

Once a patient has relapsed after initial chemotherapy for non-Hodgkin's lymphoma, the ability to induce a remission with

Table 45–4. Conventional Salvage Therapy for Relapsed Non-Hodgkin's Lymphoma

Reference	Regimen	No. of Patients	CR[1] (%)	Alive in Remission[1]
Cabanillas et al.[131]	IMVP-16	38	39	Median RFS 12 mo
Cabanillas et al.[132]	MIME	123	32	Median RFS 15 mo
Velasquez et al.[133]	DHAP	90	31	20 (2–26 + mo)
Cabani and Rodriguez[134]	MINE-ESHAP	92	47	18% beyond 2 yr
Sparano et al.[135]	Infusional CDE	58	17	19% (median 22 mo)

[1] RFS, relapse-free survival; CR, complete response.

subsequent salvage therapy is reduced and the ability to cure the patient with conventional chemotherapy is less than 5 percent in most series. Several salvage regimens including both conventional and investigational agents have been evaluated. Many of these protocols are outlined in Table 44–4. Physicians from the M.D. Anderson Hospital have combined etoposide and methotrexate with the cyclophosphamide analogue ifosfamide (IMVP-16).[131] This regimen in initial trials had a promising 39 percent complete remission rate; however, only a few patients were free of disease past 18 months. Based on encouraging initial results with IMVP-16, methyl-gag was added to ifosfamide, methotrexate, and etoposide to make MIME.[132] This regimen was reported to have a 24 percent complete response rate; however, also in this analysis, few long-term disease-free survivors were identified. Another salvage regimen evaluated at M.D. Anderson Hospital consisted of cisplatin and cytarabine with dexamethasone (DHAP).[133] This combination produced an overall survival rate of 25 percent at 2 years; however, late relapses have occurred. Additional agents such as mitoxantrone or Taxol are also being incorporated into salvage regimens for the non-Hodgkin's lymphomas. The MINE-ESHAP (mesna, ifosfamide, mitoxantrone, and etoposide—etoposide, solumedrol, cytarabine, and cisplatin) non-cross-resistant regimen has recently been published by Cabanillas and Rodriguez.[134] They have seen an overall 47 percent complete response rate with this alternating combination, and 18 percent of patients with inter-mediate/high-grade histologies are free of disease beyond 2 years. With few studies showing any long-term disease-free survival with conventional salvage therapy, high dose therapy and bone marrow transplantation have recently undergone extensive evaluation in this clinical setting.

BONE MARROW TRANSPLANTATION

Many studies have now been conducted evaluating bone marrow transplantation for the treatment of high-risk or relapsed non-Hodgkin's lymphoma. Several of these studies are outlined in Table 45–5. As this experience expanded, many important points were ascertained. Studies such as the one by Philip et al.[138] identified prognostic factors that predicted a favorable outcome with transplantation for recurrent lymphoma. Patients with advanced stage and poor performance status are now generally excluded from treatment trials based on these earlier experiences. Tumor sensitivity to conventional salvage therapy from this and other studies has proved to be one of the most reliable measures of continued disease-free survival after autologous transplant (Figure 45–1).

A multivariate analysis of 158 patients undergoing high-dose chemotherapy and autologous transplantation for recurrent or persistent lymphoma was reported in a series from the University of Nebraska Medical Center.[139] The factors identified

Table 45–5. Autologous Bone Marrow Transplantation for Non-Hodgkin's Lymphoma

Reference	Regimen	No. of Patients	CR (%)	Patients Alive and Well
Tura et al.[136]	BCNU, cytarabine, etoposide, cyclophosphamide	13	69	7 (15 + −46 + months)
Phillips et al.[137]	Cyclophosphamide, TBI	24	58	5 (19 + −71 + months)
Philip et al.[138]	Various	100	34 NCR	0%
			22 RR	14%
			44 SR	36%
Vose et al.[139]	Various	158	56	Good prognosis 45% (3 yrs)
				Poor prognosis 10% (3 yrs)
Takvorian et al.[140]	Cy-TBI	49	96	34 (69%) median 11 mo
Applebaum et al.[141]	Cy-TBI	22	50	6 (27%) 13–28 mo
Goldstone et al.[142]	Various	44	41	9 (20%)

Abbreviations: CCR, continuous complete remission; SR, sensitive relapse; RR, resistant relapse; NCR, never in complete response.

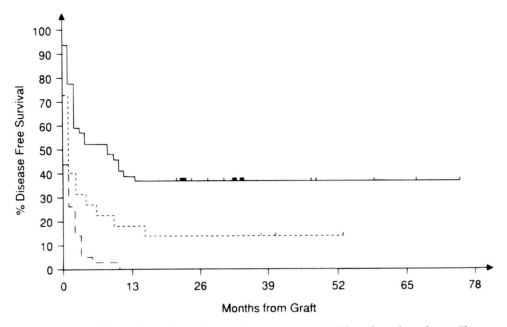

Figure 45–1. Actuarial 3-year disease-free survival according to response to initial or salvage chemotherapy. The solid line indicates patients with sensitive relapses, the dashed line patients with resistant relapses, and the broken line patients never in complete remission. The vertical marks indicate the survival of patients for the indicated period. (From Philip et al.[138] with permission.)

in the analysis as being predictive for outcome included a mass 10 cm or more at the time of transplant, having received three or more prior chemotherapy regimens, an LDH higher than normal, the type of graft received (bone marrow transplant versus peripheral blood progenitors), and chemotherapy sensitivity. This subdivided the patients into a good prognosis group with no large mass (10 cm or larger) and no more than one of the following: three or more prior chemotherapy regimens, LDH greater than normal, and chemotherapy resistance. The poor prognosis group had either a mass 10 cm or larger or two or three of the other characteristics. This was highly significant for prediction of outcome with transplantation (Figure 45–2).

Various analyses that took into account some of the prognostic information discovered by the earlier studies have utilized this information to formulate early bone marrow transplantation plans for poor-risk patients. Gulati et al.[143] have reported a trial comparing 14 patients with DLC who underwent autologous bone marrow transplantation immediately after induction of remission by conventional frontline chemotherapy with 17 similar patients who had an autologous transplant while in relapse after failing conventional salvage chemotherapy. The patients all had similar poor prognostic characteristics with respect to bulky disease or high LDH levels, or both. Of the 14 patients who underwent early consolidative transplantation, 79 percent survived with a median follow-up of 49 months, whereas the other group had a median survival of only 5 months.

Another study that expanded on the role of early transplantation was done by Philip et al.[144] They reported 17 patients who received high-dose therapy with autologous bone marrow trans-

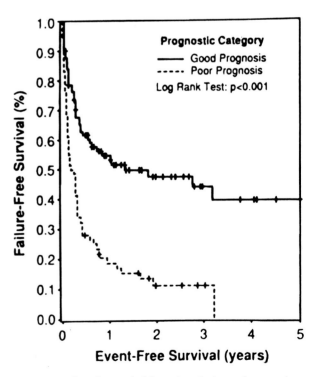

Figure 45–2. Failure-free survival for patients in the good-prognosis group compared with the poor-prognosis group (From Vose et al.,[139] with permission.)

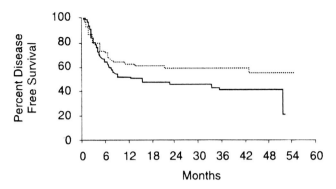

Figure 45–3. Estimated disease-free survival according to randomized consolidation for high-intermediate and high-risk groups with sequential chemotherapy *(solid line)* and ABMT *(dashed line)* ($p = .07$). (From Haioun et al.,[146] with permission.)

plantation when in partial remission immediately after induction chemotherapy. Two patients died of progressive disease and two others died while in complete remission because of transplant-related toxicity. Of the 17 patients, 13 were alive at the time of publication and were disease-free with a median follow-up of 2 years. As noted earlier, most previously published conventional salvage chemotherapy programs have no more than 5 percent alive and disease-free in that poor-prognosis group of patients. A more recent study by Nademanee et al.[145] has also confirmed these results. Although no large prospective randomized studies have been performed specifically in high-risk patients evaluating the role of high-dose chemotherapy and autologous bone marrow transplantation, one study from the GELA group in Europe randomized all patients in complete remission to receive either a high-dose consolidation regimen or high-dose chemotherapy and transplantation.[146] In this study the high-risk patients did appear to have a benefit in 3-year failure-free survival (60 percent in the transplant group compared with 44 percent in the consolidation group) (Figure 45–3). Future studies must be designed to identify the patients who can be cured by this early aggressive management approach.

RESEARCH DIRECTIONS

Despite all of the advances made in therapies for NHL, many patients still relapse from their disease and need additional therapy. The biggest advances have been in the area of biological therapy. The chimeric anti-CD20 molecule, Rituxan, is now standard therapy for relapsed follicular lymphoma. The "new" generation of these agents includes radioimmunoconjugates such as Zevalin (yttrium-90 tagged anti-CD20) or Bexxar (iodine-131 tagged anti-CD20).[147,148] These agents have been tested mostly on patients with recurrent follicular lymphoma, with a response rate of 60 to 80 percent depending on the patient population studied. These agents are now being studied in conjunction with standard chemotherapy or high-dose chemotherapy and stem cell transplantation. Other new agents being

explored are idiotypic vaccine therapies given after a response has been achieved by standard chemotherapy.[149] With advances in immunotherapy such as these, the future appears bright.

AIDS-ASSOCIATED NON-HODGKIN'S LYMPHOMA

An increased incidence of non-Hodgkin's lymphoma has now been well recognized in a variety of immunodeficiency syndromes such as ataxia telangiectasia or Wiskott-Aldrich syndrome,[150,151] X-linked lymphoproliferative syndrome,[152] and post-transplant,[153] or human immunodeficiency virus (HIV)-associated acquired immunodeficiency.[154] Pluda et al.[155] reported that a cohort of 55 patients with symptomatic HIV disease enrolled on various antiretroviral trials between 1985 and 1987 had an increased incidence of non-Hodgkin's lymphoma. At a median of 24 months after initiation of zidovudine therapy, the probability of developing lymphoma was 12 percent, whereas at 3 years the observed risk was 29 percent.[156] Most lymphomas associated with HIV infection are high-grade B-cell tumors consisting of immunoblastic or small non-cleaved cell subtypes.[157]

The clinical presentation of patients with AIDS-related lymphomas is somewhat atypical, with a high frequency of extranodal involvement ranging from 68 to 98 percent.[158–160] The most frequent extranodal sites of disease are central nervous system (33 percent), gastrointestinal tract (25 percent), and bone marrow (25 percent).[161] Another distinguishing feature is the high incidence of systemic B symptoms in up to 80 percent of AIDS-related non-Hodgkin's lymphomas.[162] Appropriate staging procedures in such patients would be identical to those required for other high-grade non-Hodgkin's lymphoma patients; however, a lumbar puncture should always be performed at diagnosis and central nervous system prophylaxis administered for prevention of central nervous system recurrence.

A common presentation for AIDS-related non-Hodgkin's lymphoma is that of primary central nervous system lymphoma. Presenting symptoms include focal neurologic deficits, seizures, headache, cranial nerve palsies, and altered mental status.[163,164] Patients with primary central nervous system disease frequently have more extensive HIV-related disease. For example, the median CD4 count in one study in patients with primary central nervous system non-Hodgkin's lymphoma was 30/mm^3 versus 189/mm^3 in patients with systemic AIDS-related non-Hodgkin's lymphoma ($p = .005$).[162] Optimal therapy for patients with AIDS-related primary central nervous system lymphoma has yet to be defined. Whole-brain radiation therapy alone results in median survivals in several series of 5 to 12 months.[165,166] The use of combined modality therapy has been shown in several phase II studies in AIDS-related and non-AIDS-related primary central nervous system lymphoma to prolong the median survival to 30 to 40 months in some studies.[167,168]

The treatment of systemic AIDS-related non-Hodgkin's lymphoma is often complicated by the development of opportunistic infections and a high rate of central nervous system relapse. Patients treated with dose-intensive regimens such as ProMACE-CytaBOM,[169] COMP,[170] and COMET-A[158] had a complete response rate of 30 to 60 percent; however, a high central nervous system relapse rate and the development of opportunistic infections in 30 to 70 percent of the patients was often associated with a short median survival of 5 to 8 months. With these complications in mind, a low-dose modification of the m-BACOD regimen with early central nervous system prophylaxis was designed. In the 35 evaluable patients, a complete remission rate of approximately 50 percent was obtained, with 75 percent of complete responders achieving a sustained lymphoma-free survival.[171] Another regimen that has been demonstrated to have some success in treatment of systemic AIDS-related non-Hodgkin's lymphoma is the infusional CDE regimen. Sparano et al.[172] evaluated 14 poor-prognosis patients with HIV- or human T-cell leukemia/lymphoma virus 1-related non-Hodgkin's lymphoma treated with this regimen. At the time of publication, the median survival was 17.4 months, with 7 of 12 HIV-positive patients alive and lymphoma-free after a median follow-up of 15 months. The use of hematopoietic growth factors may allow escalation of full-dose chemotherapy safely in this patient population.[173]

Future research in the area of AIDS-related non-Hodgkin's lymphoma is focusing on effective management of the disease while preventing and managing the infectious complications and the effective use of central nervous system prophylaxis and treatment for optimum care and prolongation of survival.

REFERENCES

1. Young JL, Percy CL, Asire AJ (eds.): Surveillance, Epidemiology, and End Results: Incidence and Mortality Data, 1973–77. National Cancer Institute Monograph No. 57, U.S. Government Printing Office, Washington, DC, 1981.
2. Jones SE: Non-Hodgkin's lymphomas. JAMA 10:633, 1975.
3. Chabner BA, Fisher RI, Young RC et al: Staging of non-Hodgkin's lymphoma. Semin Oncol 7:275, 1980.
4. Fram RJ, Skarin AR, Rosenthal DS et al: Clinical, pathological and immunological features of patients with non-Hodgkin's lymphoma in a leukemic phase: A retrospective analysis of thirty-four patients. Cancer 52:1220, 1983.
5. Paulson S, Sheehan, RG, Stone MJ et al: Large cell lymphomas of the stomach: Improved prognosis with complete resection of all intrinsic gastrointestinal disease. J Clin Oncol 1:263, 1983.
6. Duncan PR, Checa F, Gowning NFC et al: Extranodal non-Hodgkin's lymphoma presenting in the testicle. Cancer 45:1578, 1980.
7. Burke JS, Butler JJ, Fuller IM: Malignant lymphomas of the thyroid. Cancer 39:1587, 1977.
8. Burke J, Hoppe RT, Cibull ML et al: Cutaneous malignant lymphoma: A pathological study of 50 cases with clinical analysis of 37 cases. Cancer 47:300, 1981.
9. Mambo NC, Burke JS, Butler JJ: Primary malignant lymphoma of the breast. Cancer 39:2033, 1977.
10. Mackintosh RF, Colby TV, Podolsky WJ et al: Central nervous system involvement in non-Hodgkin's lymphoma: An analysis of 105 cases. Cancer 49:586, 1982.
11. Dosoretz DE, Raymond AK, Murphy GF et al: Primary lymphoma of bone. Cancer 50:1009, 1982.
12. Banfi A, Boradonna G, Ricci SB et al: Malignant lymphomas of Waldeyer's ring: Natural history and survival after radiotherapy. BMJ 15:140, 1972.
13. Koziner B, Filippa DA, Mertelsmann R: Characterization of malignant lymphomas in leukemic phase by multiple differentiation markers of mononuclear cells: Correlation with clinical features and conventional morphology. Am J Med 63:556, 1977.
14. Slater DE, Mertelsman R, Koziner B et al: Lymphoblastic lymphoma in adults. J Clin Oncol 4:57, 1986.
15. Burkitt D: A sarcoma involving the jaws in African children. Br J Surg 46:218, 1958.
16. Murphy SB: Classification, staging, and end results of treatment of childhood non-Hodgkin's lymphoma: Dissimilarities from lymphomas in adults. Semin Oncol 7:332, 1980.
17. Pavlova Z, Levine AM, Feinstein DI et al: Small non-cleaved follicular center cell lymphoma, Burkitt's vs. non-Burkitt's variants: Pathologic definition, abstracted. Lab Invest 46:64A, 1982.
18. McMahon NJ, Gordon HW, Rosen RB: Reed-Sternberg cells in infectious mononucleosis. Am J Dis Child 120:148, 1970.
19. Nathwani BN, Winberg CD, Diamond LW et al: Morphologic criteria for the differentiation of follicular lymphoma from florid reactive follicular hyperplasia: A study of 80 cases. Cancer 48:1794, 1981.
20. Bone RC, Vernon M, Soboriya RE et al: Lymphomatoid granulomatosis. Am J Med 65:709, 1978.
21. Thawerani H, Sanchez RL, Rosai J et al: The cutaneous manifestations of sinus histiocytosis with massive lymphadenopathy. Arch Dermatol 114:191, 1978.
22. Frizzera G, Moran EM, Rappaport H: Angioblastic lymphadenopathy: Diagnosis and clinical course. Am J Med 59:803, 1975.
23. Katzenstein ALA, Carrington CB, Liebow AA: Lymphomatoid granulomatosis. Cancer 43:360, 1979.
24. NCI Non-Hodgkin's Classification Project Writing Committee: Classification of non-Hodgkin's lymphomas: Reproducibility of major classification systems. Cancer 55:91, 1985.
25. Kaplan WD, Jochelson MS, Herman TS et al: Gallium-67 imaging: A predictor of residual tumor viability and clinical outcome in patients with diffuse large-cell lymphoma. J Clin Oncol 8:1966, 1990.
26. Carbone PP, Kaplan HS, Musshoff K: Report of the committee in Hodgkin's disease staging classifications. Cancer Res 31:1860, 1971.
27. Rappaport H: Tumors of the Hematopoietic System. Armed Forces Institute of Pathology, Washington, DC, 1966.
28. Lukes RJ, Collins RD: Immunologic characterization of human malignant lymphomas. Cancer 34:1488, 1974.
29. Rosenberg SA: National Cancer Institute sponsored study of classification of non-Hodgkin's lymphomas. Cancer 49:2112, 1982.
30. Harris NL, Jaffe ES, Stein H et al: A revised European-American Classification of lymphoid neoplasms: A proposal from the International Lymphoma Study Group. Blood 84:1361, 1994.
31. Cullen MH, Lister TA, Brearly RL et al: Histological transformation of non-Hodgkin's lymphoma. A prospective study. Cancer 44:645, 1979.
32. Richter MN: Generalized reticular cell sarcoma of lymph nodes associated with lymphatic leukemia. Am J Pathol 4:285, 1928.
33. Armitage JO, Dick FR, Corder MP: Diffuse histiocytic lymphoma after histologic conversion: A poor prognostic variant. Cancer Treat Rep 65:413, 1981.
34. Levine AM, Goldstein M, Meyer PR et al: Heterogeneity of response and survival in diffuse histiocytic lymphoma after BACOP therapy (bleomycin, doxorubicin, cyclophosphamide, vincristine, prednisone). Hematol Oncol 3:87, 1985.
35. Anderson T, DeVita VT, Simon RM et al: Malignant lymphoma. II. Prognostic factors and response to treatment of 473 patients at the National Cancer Institute. Cancer 50:2708, 1982.

36. Horwich H, Peckham M: "Bad risk" non-Hodgkin's lymphomas. Semin Hematol 20:35, 1983.

37. Nathwani BN, Dixon DO, Jones SE et al: The clinical significance of the morphological subdivision of diffuse "histiocytic" lymphoma: A study of 162 patients treated by the Southwest Oncology Group. Blood 60:1068, 1982.

38. Straus DJ, Filippa DA, Lieberman PH et al: The non-Hodgkin's lymphomas. I. A retrospective clinical and pathologic analysis of 499 cases diagnosed between 1958 and 1969. Cancer 51:101, 1974.

39. Bloomfield CD, Goldman A, Dick F et al: Multivariate analysis of prognostic factors in the non-Hodgkin's malignant lymphomas. Cancer 33:870, 1974.

40. Rudders RA, Kaddis M, DeLillis RH et al: Nodular non-Hodgkin's lymphoma (NHL). Cancer 43:1643, 1979.

41. Cabanillas F, Burke JS, Smith TL et al: Factors predicting for response and survival in adults with advanced non-Hodgkin's lymphoma. Arch Intern Med 138:413, 1978.

42. Koziner B, Little C, Passe S et al: Treatment of advanced diffuse histiocytic lymphoma. Cancer 49:1571, 1982.

43. Jones SE, Fuks Z, Bull M et al: Non-Hodgkin's lymphomas. IV. Clinicopathologic correlation in 405 cases. Cancer 31:806, 1973.

44. Muray R, Kun L, Cox L: Primary malignant lymphomas of the central nervous system. J Neurosurg 65:600, 1986.

45. Letenddre L, Banks PM, Reese DF et al: Primary lymphoma of the central nervous system. Cancer 49:939, 1982.

46. Leibel SA, Sheline GE: Radiation therapy for neoplasms of the brain. J Neurosurg 66:1, 1987.

47. So YT, Beckstead JH, Davis RL: Primary central nervous system lymphoma in acquired immune deficiency syndrome: A clinical and pathological study. Ann Neurol 20:566, 1986.

48. Paladlugu R, Bearman RM, Rappaport H: Malignant lymphoma with primary manifestation in the gonad. Cancer 45:561, 1980.

49. Connors JM, Klimo P, Voss N et al: Testicular lymphoma: Improved outcome with early brief chemotherapy. J Clin Oncol 6:776, 1988.

50. Weingrad DN, Decosse JJ, Sherlock P et al: Primary gastrointestinal lymphoma: A 30 year review. Cancer 49:1258, 1982.

51. Westergaard H: The sprue syndromes. Am J Med Sci 290:249, 1985.

52. Cohen S, Laufer I, Snape WJ et al: The gastrointestinal manifestations of scleroderma: Pathogenesis and management. Gastroenterology 79:155, 1980.

53. Jagannath S, Velasquez WS, Tucker SL et al: Stage IV diffuse large-cell lymphoma: A long term analysis. J Clin Oncol 3:39, 1985.

54. Dixon DO, Neilan B, Jones JE et al: Effect of age on therapeutic outcome in advanced diffuse histiocytic lymphoma: The Southwest Oncology Group experience. J Clin Oncol 4:295, 1986.

55. Todd MB, Portlock CS, Farber LR et al: Prognostic indicators in diffuse large cell (histiocytic) lymphoma. J Radiat Oncol Bio Phys 12:593, 1986.

56. Vose JM, Armitage JO, Weisenberger DD et al: The importance of age in survival of patients treated with chemotherapy for aggressive non-Hodgkin's lymphoma. J Clin Oncol 6:1838, 1988.

57. Armitage JO, Potter JF: Aggressive chemotherapy for diffuse histiocytic lymphoma in the elderly: Increased complications with advancing age. J Am Geriatr Soc 32:269, 1984.

58. Solal-Celigny P, Chastang, C, Herrera A et al: Age as the main prognostic factor in adult aggressive non-Hodgkin's lymphoma. Am J Med 83:1075, 1987.

59. Jagannath S, Velasquez WS, Tucker SL et al: Tumor burden assessment and its implication for a prognostic model in advanced diffuse large-cell lymphoma. J Clin Oncol 4:859, 1986.

60. Shipp MA, Harrington DP, Klatt MM et al: Identification of major prognostic subgroups of patients with large cell lymphoma treated with m-BACOD or M-BACOD. Ann Intern Med 104:757, 1986.

61. Danieu L, Wong G, Koziner B et al: Predictive model for prognosis in advanced diffuse histiocytic lymphoma. Cancer Res 46:5372, 1986.

62. Fisher RI, DeVita VT, Johnson BL et al: Prognostic factors for advanced diffuse histiocytic lymphoma following treatment with combination chemotherapy. Am J Med 63:177, 1977.

63. Cox JD, Koehl RH, Turner WM et al: Irradiation in the local control of malignant lymphoreticular tumors (non-Hodgkin's malignant lymphomas). Radiology 112:179, 1974.

64. Fasola G, Fanin R, Gherlinzoni F et al: Serum LDH concentration in non-Hodgkin's lymphomas. Relationship to histologic type, tumor mass, and presentation features. Acta Haematol 72:231, 1984.

65. Ferraris AA, Giuntini P, Gaetani GF: Serum lactic dehydrogenase as a prognostic tool for non-Hodgkin's lymphomas. Blood 54:928, 1979.

66. Coiffier B, Berger F, Bryon PA et al: T-cell lymphomas: immunologic, histologic, clinical, and therapeutic analysis of 63 cases. J Clin Oncol 6:1584, 1988.

67. Armitage JO, Vose JM, Linder J et al: Clinical significance of immunophenotyping in diffuse aggressive non-Hodgkin's lymphoma. J Clin Oncol 7:1783, 1989.

68. Horning SJ, Weiss CM, Crabtree CG et al: Clinical and phenotypic diversity of T-cell lymphomas. Blood 67:1578, 1986.

69. Cossman J, Jaffe ES, Fisher RI: Immunologic phenotypes of diffuse, aggressive non-Hodgkin's lymphomas. Cancer 54:1310, 1984.

70. Grogan TM, Lippman SM, Spier CM et al: Independent prognostic significance of a nuclear proliferation antigen in diffuse large cell lymphomas as determined by the monoclonal antibody Ki-67. Blood 71:1157, 1988.

71. Bauer KD, Merkel DE, Winter JN et al: Prognostic implications of ploidy and proliferative activity in diffuse large cell lymphomas. Cancer Res 46:3173, 1986.

72. Woolridge TN, Grierson HL, Weisenberger DD et al: Association of DNA content and proliferative activity with clinical outcome in patients with diffuse mixed cell and large cell non-Hodgkin's lymphoma. Cancer Res 48:6608, 1988.

73. Yunis JJ, Dken M, Kaplen ME et al: Distinctive chromosomal abnormalities in histologic subtypes of non-Hodgkin's lymphoma. N Engl J Med 307:1231, 1982.

74. Zech L, Hoglund U, Nilsson K et al: Characteristic chromosomal abnormalities in biopsies and lymphoid cell lines from patients with Burkitt and non-Burkitt lymphomas. Int J Cancer 17:47, 1976.

75. Levine EG, Arthur DC, Frizzera G et al: Cytogenetic abnormalities predict clinical outcome in non-Hodgkin's lymphoma. Ann Intern Med 108:14, 1988.

76. Weiss LM, Warnke RA, Sklar J et al: Molecular analysis of the t(14;18) chromosomal translocation in malignant lymphomas. N Engl J Med 317:1185, 1987.

77. Raffeld M, Jaffe ES: bcl-1, t(11;14), and mantle cell-derived lymphomas. Blood 78:259, 1991.

78. Neri A, Barriga F, Knowles DM et al: Different regions of the immunoglobulin heavy-chain locus are involved in chromosomal translocations in distinct pathogenetic forms of Burkitt lymphoma. Proc Natl Acad Sci U S A 85:2748, 1988.

79. Offit K, Parsa NZ, Gaidano G et al: 6q Deletions define distinct clinico-pathologic subsets of non-Hodgkin's lymphoma. Blood 82:2157, 1993.

80. Shipp MA et al: A predictive model for aggressive non-Hodgkin's lymphoma: The international non-Hodgkin's lymphoma prognostic factors project. N Engl J Med 329:987, 1993.

81. Portlock CS, Rosenberg SA: No initial therapy for stage III and IV non-Hodgkin's lymphomas of favorable histologic types. Ann Intern Med 90:10, 1979.

82. Portlock CS: "Good risk" non-Hodgkin's lymphomas: Approaches to management. Semin Hematol 20:25, 1983.

83. Lister TA, Cullen MH, Beard MEJ et al: Comparison of combined and single-agent chemotherapy in non-Hodgkin's lymphomas of a favorable histologic type. BMJ 1:533, 1978.

84. Ezdinili EZ, Costello WG, Silverstein MN et al: Moderate versus intensive chemotherapy of prognostically favorable non-Hodgkin's lymphoma. Cancer 46:29, 1980.

85. Schechter GP, Sausville EA, Fischmann AB et al: Evaluation of circulating malignant cells provides prognostic information in cutaneous T-cell lymphoma. Blood 69:841, 1987.

86. Grozea PN, Jones SE, McKelvey EM et al: Combination chemotherapy for mycosis fungoides: A Southwest Oncology Group study. Cancer Treat Rep 63:647, 1979.

87. Bunn PA Jr, Foon KA, Ihde DC et al: Recombinant leukocyte A interferon: An active agent in advanced refractory cutaneous T-cell lymphomas (mycosis fungoides and Sézary syndrome). Ann Intern Med 101:484, 1984.

88. Edelson R, Berger C, Gasparro F et al: Treatment of cutaneous T-cell lymphoma by extracorporeal photochemotherapy. N Engl J Med 316:297, 1987.

89. Young RC, Longo DL, Glatstein E et al: The treatment of indolent lymphomas: Watchful waiting vs. aggressive combined modality treatment. Semin Hematol 25:11, 1988.

90. Dana BW, Dahlberg S, Nathwani BN et al: Long-term follow-up of patients with low-grade malignant lymphomas treated with doxorubicin-based chemotherapy or chemoimmunotherapy. J Clin Oncol 11:644, 1993.

91. Straus DJ, Gaynor JJ, Leiberman PH et al: Non-Hodgkin's lymphomas: Characteristics of long-term survivors following conservative treatment. Am J Med 82:247, 1987.

92. Anderson JR, Vose JM, Bierman PJ et al: Clinical features and prognosis of follicular large-cell lymphoma: A report from the Nebraska Lymphoma Study Group. J Clin Oncol 11:218, 1993.

93. Romaguera JE, McLaughlin P, North L et al: Multivariate analysis of prognostic factors in stage IV follicular low-grade lymphoma: A risk model. J Clin Oncol 9:762, 1991.

94. Lopez-Guillermo A, Montserrat E, Bosch F et al: Applicability of the International Index for aggressive lymphomas to patients with low-grade lymphoma. J Clin Oncol 12:1343, 1994.

95. Kay AC, Saven A, Carrera CJ et al: 2-Chlorodeoxyadenosine treatment of low-grade lymphomas. J Clin Oncol 10:371, 1992.

96. McLaughlin P, Hagemeister FB, Sarris A et al: Fludarabine, mitoxantrone, and dexamethasone (FND) for recurrent low grade lymphoma (LGL): A phase II trial. Proc Am Soc Clin Oncol 13:1318a, 1994.

97. Solal-Celigny P, Lepage E, Brousse N et al: Recombinant interferon alfa-2b combined with a regimen containing doxorubicin in patients with advanced follicular lymphoma. N Engl J Med 329:1608, 1993.

98. McLaughlin P, Grillo-Lopez AJ, Link BK et al: Rituximab chimeric and anti-CD20 monoclonal antibody therapy for relapsed indolent lymphoma: Half of patients respond to a four-dose treatment program. Clin Oncol 16:2825, 1998.

99. Czuczman MS, Grillo-Lopez AJ, White CA et al: Treatment of patients with low-grade grade B-cell lymphoma with the combination of chimeric anti-CD20 monoclonal antibody and CHOP chemotherapy. J Clin Oncol 17:268, 1999.

100. Rohatiner AZS, Johnson PWM, Price CGA et al: Myeloablative therapy with autologous bone marrow transplantation as consolidation therapy for recurrent follicular lymphoma. J Clin Oncol 12:1177, 1994.

101. Freedman AS, Ritz J, Neuberg D et al: Autologous bone marrow transplantation in 69 patients with a history of low-grade B-cell non-Hodgkin's lymphoma. Blood 77:2524, 1991.

102. Bishop MR, Bierman PJ, Vose JM, Armitage JO: The role of high-dose therapy with hematopoietic stem cell rescue in low-grade non-Hodgkin's lymphoma. Ann Oncol 4(Suppl. 1):S1, 1993.

103. Schouten HC, Colombat P, Verdonck LF et al: Autologous bone marrow transplantation for low-grade non-Hodgkin's lymphoma: the European Bone Marrow Transplant Group experience. Ann Oncol 5(Suppl. 2):S147, 1994.

104. Freedman A, Gribben J, Rabinowe S et al: Autologous bone marrow transplantation in advanced low grade B-cell non-Hodgkin's lymphoma in first remission. Blood 82:1313a, 1993.

105. Chen MG, Prosnitz LR, Gonzalez-Serva A et al: Results of radiotherapy in control of stage I and II non-Hodgkin's lymphoma. Cancer 43:1245, 1979.

106. Taylor RE, Allan SG, McIntyre MA et al: Influence of therapy on local control and survival in stage I and II intermediate and high grade non-Hodgkin's lymphoma. Eur J Cancer Clin Oncol 24:1771, 1988.

107. Connors JM, Klimo P, Faireji RN et al: Brief chemotherapy and involved field radiation therapy for limited-stage histologically aggressive lymphoma. Ann Intern Med 107:25, 1987.

108. Miller TP, Dahlberg S, Cassady R et al: Chemotherapy alone compared with chemotherapy plus radiotherapy for localized intermediate and high-grade non-Hodgkin's lymphoma. N Engl J Med 339:21, 1998.

109. Coltman CA, Dahlberg S, Jones SE et al: CHOP is curative in thirty percent of patients with large cell lymphoma, a twelve year Southwest Oncology Group follow up, abstracted. Proc Am Soc Clin Oncol 5:197, 1986.

110. Canellos GP, Skarin AT, Klatt MM et al: m-BACOD combination chemotherapy regimen in the treatment of diffuse large cell lymphoma. Semin Hematol 24(Suppl. 1):2, 1987.

111. Connors JM, Klimo P: Updated clinical experience with MACOP-B. Semin Hematol 24(Suppl. 1):26, 1987.

112. Fisher R, DeVita V, Hubbard S et al: Diffuse aggressive lymphomas: Increased survival after alternating flexible sequences of ProMACE and MOPP chemotherapy. Ann Intern Med 98:304, 1983.

113. Coiffier B, Bryon P, French M et al: Intensive chemotherapy in aggressive lymphomas: updated results of LNH-80 protocol and prognostic factors affecting response and survival. Blood 70:1394, 1987.

114. Miller TP, Dahlberg S, Weick JK et al: Unfavorable histologies of non-Hodgkin's lymphoma treated with ProMACE-CytaBOM: A groupwide Southwest Oncology Group Study. J Clin Oncol 8:1951, 1990.

115. Fisher RI, Gaynor ER, Dahlberg S et al: Comparison of a standard regimen (CHOP) with three intensive chemotherapy regimens for advanced non-Hodgkin's lymphoma. N Engl J Med 328:1002, 1993.

116. Gaynor ER, Dahlberg S, Fisher RI: Factors affecting reduced survival of the elderly with intermediate and high grade lymphoma: An analysis of SWOG-8516 (INT 0067)—The National High Priority Lymphoma Study. Proc Am Soc Clin Oncol 13:1250a, 1994.

117. Coiffier B, Lepage E, Herbrecht R et al: Mabthera (Rituximab) plus CHOP is superior to CHOP alone in elderly patients with diffuse large B-cell lymphoma (DLCL): Interim results of a randomized GELA trial. Blood 96:950a, 2000.

118. Rosen PF, Feinstein DI, Pattengale PK et al: Convoluted lymphocytic lymphoma in adults. Ann Intern Med 89:319, 1978.

119. Anderson JR, Wilson JE, Jenkin ET et al: Childhood non-Hodgkin's lymphoma: The results of a randomized therapeutic trial comparing a 4-drug regimen (COMP) with a 10-drug regimen (LSA2-L2). N Engl J Med 308:559, 1983.

120. Nademanee AP, Forman SJ, Schmidt GM et al: Allogeneic bone marrow transplantation for high risk non-Hodgkin's lymphoma during first complete remissions. Blut 55:11, 1987.

121. Verdonck LF, Dekker AW, de Gast GC et al: Autologous bone marrow transplantation for adult poor-risk lymphoblastic lymphoma in first remission. J Clin Oncol 10:644, 1992.

122. Baro J, Richard C, Sierra J et al: Autologous bone marrow transplantation in 22 adult patients with lymphoblastic lymphoma responsive to conventional dose chemotherapy. Bone Marrow Transplant 10:33, 1992.

123. Santini G, Coser P, Chisesi T et al: Autologous bone marrow transplantation for advanced stage adult lymphoblastic lymphoma in first complete remission. A pilot study of the Non-Hodgkin's Lymphoma Co-operative Study Group (NHLCSG). Bone Marrow Transplant 4:399, 1989.

124. Sweetenham JW, Liberti G, Pearce R et al: High-dose therapy and autologous bone marrow transplantation for adult patients with lymphoblastic lymphoma: Results of the European Group for Bone Marrow Transplantation. J Clin Oncol 12:1358, 1994.

125. Magrath I, Lee YJ, Anderson T et al: Prognostic factors in Burkitt's lymphoma. Cancer 45:1507, 1980.

126. Schwenn M, Weinstein H, Nathan D et al: High dose methotrexate combination chemotherapy (M-BACOD) for advanced Burkitt's lymphoma (BL): Failure to increase survival, abstracted. Proc Am Soc Clin Oncol 2:73, 1983.

127. Ziegler JL: Treatment results of 54 American patients with Burkitt's lymphoma are similar to the African experience. N Engl J Med 297:75, 1977.

128. Magrath IT, Spiegel RJ, Edwards BK et al: Improved results of chemotherapy in young adults with Burkitt's (BL), undifferentiated (UL) and lymphoblastic lymphomas (LL). (Abstract.) Proc Am Soc Clin Oncol 1:520, 1981.

129. Schwenn M, Weinstein H, Nathan D et al: High dose methotrexate combination chemotherapy (M-BACOD) for advanced Burkitt's lymphoma (BL): failure to increase survival, abstracted. Proc Am Soc Clin Oncol 2:73, 1983.

130. Troussard X, Leblond V, Kuentz M et al: Allogeneic bone marrow transplantation in adults with Burkitt's lymphoma or acute lymphoblastic leukemia in first complete remission. J Clin Oncol 8:809, 1990.

131. Cabanillas F, Hagemeister FB, Bodey GP et al: IMVP-16: an effective regimen for patients with lymphoma who have relapsed after initial combination chemotherapy. Blood 60:693, 1982.

132. Cabanillas F, Hagemeister FB, McLaughlin P et al: Results of MIME salvage regimen for recurrent or refractory lymphoma. J Clin Oncol 5:407, 1987.

133. Velasquez WJ, Cabanillas F, Salvador P et al: Effective salvage therapy for lymphoma with cisplatin in combination with high-dose Ara-C and dexamethasone (DHAP). Blood 71:117, 1988.

134. Cabanillas F, Rodriguez MA: MINE-ESHAP salvage therapy for recurrent and refractory lymphomas. Semin Hematol 31:30, 1994.

135. Sparano JA, Wiernik PH, Leaf A, Dutcher JP: Infusional cyclophosphamide, doxorubicin, and etoposide in relapsed and resistant non-Hodgkin's lymphoma: Evidence for a schedule-dependent effect favoring infusional administration of chemotherapy. J Clin Oncol 11:1071, 1993.

136. Tura S, Mazza P, Gharlizoni F et al: High-dose therapy followed by autologous bone marrow transplanation (ABMT) in previously untreated non-Hodgkin's lymphoma. Scand J Haematol 37:347, 1986.

137. Phillips GL, Herzig RH, Lazarus HM et al: Treatment of resistant lymphoma with cyclophosphamide, total body irradiation, and transplanation of cryopreserved autologous marrow. N Engl J Med 310:1557, 1984.

138. Philip T, Armitage JO, Spitzer G et al: High-dose therapy and autologous bone marrow transplantation after failure of conventional chemotherapy in adults with intermediate-grade or high-grade non-Hodgkin's lymphoma. N Engl J Med 316:1493, 1987.

139. Vose JM, Anderson JR, Kessinger A et al: High-dose chemotherapy and autologous hematopoietic stem-cell transplantation for aggressive non-Hodgkin's lymphoma. J Clin Oncol 11:1846, 1993.

140. Takvorian T, Canellos GP, Ritz J et al: Prolonged disease-free survival after autologous bone marrow transplantation in patients with non-Hodgkin's lymphoma with a poor prognosis. N Engl J Med 316:1499, 1987.

141. Applebaum FR, Sullivan KM, Thomas ED et al: Autologous marrow transplantation for malignant lymphoma. In Baum SJ, Pluznik DH, Rozenszajn LA (eds.): Experimental Hematology Today, p. 122. Springer-Verlag, Basel, 1986.

142. Goldstone AH, Linch DC, Gribben JG et al: Experience of autologous bone marrow transplantation in the first 100 lymphomas. Bone Marrow Transplant 3:65, 1988.

143. Gulati SC, Shank B, Black P et al: Autologous bone marrow transplantation for patients with poor-prognosis lymphoma. J Clin Oncol 6:1303, 1988.

144. Philip T, Hartman O, Biron P et al: High-dose therapy and autologous bone marrow transplantation in partial remission after first line induction therapy for diffuse non-Hodgkin's lymphoma. J Clin Oncol 6:1118, 1988.

145. Nademanee A, Schmidt GM, O'Donnell MR et al: High-dose chemoradiotherapy followed by autologous bone marrow transplantation as consolidation therapy during first complete remission in adult patients with poor-risk aggressive lymphoma: A pilot study. Blood 5:1130, 1992.

146. Haioun C, Lepage E, Gisselbrecht C et al: Comparison of autologous bone marrow transplantation with sequential chemotherapy for intermediate-grade and high-grade non-Hodgkin's lymphoma in first complete remission: a study of 464 patients. J Clin Oncol 12:2543, 1994.

147. Witzig TE, White CA, Flinn IW et al: Zevalin radioimmunotherapy of Rituximab-refractory follicular non-Hodgkin's lymphoma. Blood 96:2183a, 2000.

148. Horning SJ, Lucas JB, Younes A et al: Iodine-131 Tositumomab for non-Hodgkin's lymphoma (NHL) patients who progressed after treatment with Rituximab: Results of a multicenter phase II study. Blood 96:2184a, 2000.

149. Timmerman JM, Hsu FJ, Davis TA et al: Regressions of follicular lymphoma following vaccination with idiotype protein coupled to keyhole limpet hemocyanin (Id-KLH) and idiotype pulsed dendritic cells. Blood 96:2185a, 2000.

150. Frizzera G, Fosai J, Dehner LP et al: Lymphoreticular disorders in primary immunodeficiency: New findings based on an updated histologic classification of 35 cases. Cancer 46:692, 1980.

151. Penn I: Principles of tumor immunity: Immunocompromised patients. AIDS Updates 3:1, 1990.

152. Grierson H, Purtilo DT: Epstein Barr virus infections in males with the X-linked lymphoproliferative syndrome. Ann Intern Med 106:538, 1987.

153. Penn I: Cancers complicating organ transplantation. N Engl J Med 323:1767, 1990.

154. Ross R, Dworsky R, Paganini-Hill A et al: Non-Hodgkin's lymphomas in never married men in Los Angeles. Br J Cancer 52:785, 1985.

155. Pluda JM, Yarchoan R, Jaffe ES et al: Development of non-Hodgkin's lymphoma in a cohort of patients with severe human immunodeficiency virus (HIV) infection on long-term antiretroviral therapy. Ann Intern Med 113:276, 1990.

156. Pluda JM, Vanzon D, Tosato G et al: Factors which predict for the development of non-Hodgkin's lymphoma in patients with advanced HIV infection receiving antiretroviral therapy. Blood 78:285a, 1991.

157. Levine AM, Gill PS, Meyer PR et al: Retrovirus and malignant lymphoma in homosexual men. JAMA 254:1921, 1985.

158. Kaplan LD, Abrams DI, Feigal E et al: AIDS-associated non-Hodgkin's lymphoma in San Francisco. JAMA 261:719, 1989.

159. Lowenthal DA, Straus DJ, Campbell SW et al: AIDS-related lymphoid neoplasia: The Memorial Hospital experience. Cancer 61:2325, 1988.

160. Ioachim HL, Korsett B, Cronin W et al: Acquired immunodeficiency syndrome associated lymphomas: Clinical, pathological, immunologic and viral characteristics of 111 cases. Hum Pathol 22:659, 1991.

161. Levine AM: Lymphoma complicating immunodeficiency disorders. Ann Oncol 5:S29, 1994.

162. Levine AM, Sullivan-Halley J, Pike MC et al: HIV-related lymphoma: Prognostic factors predictive of survival. Cancer 68:2466, 1991.

163. Gill PS, Levine AM, Meyer PR et al: Primary central nervous system lymphoma in homosexual men: Clinical immunologic and pathologic features. Am J Med 78:742, 1985.

164. So YT, Beckstead JH, Davis RL: Primary central nervous system lymphoma in acquired immune deficiency syndrome: A clinical and pathological study. Ann Neurol 20:566, 1986.

165. Formenti SC, Gill PS, Lean E et al: Primary central nervous system lymphoma in AIDS: Results of radiation therapy. Cancer 63:1101, 1989.

166. Baumgartner JE, Fachlin JR, Beckstead JH et al: Primary central nervous system lymphomas: Natural history and response to radiation therapy in 55 patients with acquired immunodeficiency syndrome. J Neurosurg 73:206, 1990.

167. DeAngelis LM, Yahalom J, Thaler HT et al: Combined modality therapy for primary CNS lymphoma. J Clin Oncol 10:635, 1992.

168. Chamberlain MC, Levin VA: Adjuvant chemotherapy for primary lymphoma of the CNS. Arch Neurol 47:1113, 1990.

169. Dugan M, Subar M, Odajnyk C et al: Intensive multiagent chemotherapy for AIDS related diffuse large cell lymphoma. Blood 68:124a, 1986.

170. Odajnyk C, Subar M, Dugan M et al: Clinical features and correlates with immunopathology and molecular biology of a large group of patients with AIDS associated small non-cleaved lymphoma (SNCL). Blood 68:131a, 1986.

171. Levine AM, Wernz JC, Kaplan L et al: Low dose chemotherapy with central nervous system prophylaxis and azidothymidine maintenance in AIDS-related lymphoma: A prospective multi-institutional trial. JAMA 266:84, 1991.

172. Sparano JA, Wiernik PH, Strack M et al: Infusional cyclophosphamide, doxorubicin, and etoposide in human immunodeficiency virus and human T-cell leukemia virus type I-related non-Hodgkin's lymphoma: A highly active regimen. Blood 81:2810, 1993.

173. Walsh C, Wernz JC, Levine A et al: Phase I trial of m-BACOD and granulocyte macrophage colony stimulating factor in HIV-associated non-Hodgkin's lymphoma. J Acquir Immune Defic Syndr 6:265–271, 1993.

46

Non-Hodgkin's Lymphoma of Childhood

Sheila Weitzman and Robert J. Arceci

Lymphomas are malignancies derived from lymphocytes or their precursors. They occur as clonal proliferations from single cells at any stage of lymphocyte differentiation, accounting for the diverse histologic appearance and behavior, as well as the difficulty in designing an all-encompassing classification system. Recent classification systems are based on immunologic as well as morphologic criteria, and genetic characterization of the malignant cells is being increasingly used to aid the pathologist in the final categorization of the disease.

EPIDEMIOLOGY

Pediatric lymphomas account for 12 percent of childhood malignant disease[1] and are the third most common malignancy in North American children. Approximately 60 percent of pediatric lymphomas are Non-Hodgkin's lymphomas (NHLs), with the remainder being Hodgkin's disease.[2] The fact that NHL is extremely uncommon below the age of 2 years suggests that exposure to environmental agents may be important even in pediatric lymphomas. The incidence appears to be increasing by 3 to 4 percent per year,[1] including both sexes, all ethnic groups, and all ages, although the greatest increase is seen in the elderly, likely reflecting exposure to a wide variety of chemical compounds as well as changes in the immune system with age.[3] The incidence also varies with sex and race, with NHL being commoner in boys than girls and twice as common in whites as in blacks. The striking

male preponderance tends to decrease with advancing age and also varies among subtypes of NHL. The male/female ratio in anaplastic large-cell lymphoma (ALCL) patients in the Berlin-Frankfurt-Münster (BFM) studies was 2:1 whereas females predominated among patients with mediastinal large-cell lymphoma with sclerosis.[4] There is a wide variation in the incidence of NHL worldwide, with a strikingly high incidence of endemic Burkitt's NHL in central Africa (50 per million children), where it accounts for almost half of all pediatric cancer, compared to an incidence of 2 per million children in North America.[5]

Abnormalities of the immune system, especially in T-cell-mediated immunity, pose an increased risk for the development of lymphoma. As many as 10 percent of children with congenital or acquired immunodeficiency develop NHL (Table 46–1), the highest incidence being in ataxia-telangectasia and Wiskott-Aldrich syndrome. In general, these patients tend to develop large-cell or Burkitt-type NHL, but not lymphoblastic lymphoma.[1] Iatrogenic immunosuppression of patients receiving T cell-depleted bone marrow or solid-organ transplants has resulted in a significant incidence of Epstein-Barr virus (EBV)-related post-transplant lymphoproliferative disease. Uncontrolled EBV-induced B-cell proliferation secondary to T-cell dysfunction produces a spectrum of disease from polyclonal hyperplasia to true monoclonal malignant lymphomas.

Epstein-Barr virus (EBV) infection occurring early in childhood, together with chronic antigen stimulation by malaria, is believed to be associated with the high incidence of Burkitt's NHL in central Africa. Non-Hodgkin's lymphoma is the commonest malignancy associated with the acquired immune deficiency syndrome (AIDS) and often occurs before the age of 4 years in those who are infected from a human immunodeficiency virus (HIV)-positive parent.[6] In AIDS patients, central nervous system (CNS) lymphoma is invariably associated with EBV.[7]

ETIOLOGY

Like most neoplasms, lymphomas arise because of the inappropriate expression or loss of function of genes that regulate cell proliferation, differentiation, and programmed cell death (apoptosis). The malignant clone may result from increased proliferation of cells due to inappropriate expression of an oncogene such

Table 46–1. Incidence of Malignancy in Congenital Immunodeficiency

Syndrome	Tumor	Risk (percent)	Percent of Malignancies That Equal NHL
Ataxia-telangectasia	Leukemia, NHL, HD, adenocarcinoma	>12	41–66
Common variable ID	NHL, gastric carcinoma	8–10	45–62
Severe combined ID	NHL, HD, leukemia, occupational adenocarcinoma	5	31–76
X-linked agammaglobulinemia	Leukemia, NHL, HD, adenocarcinoma	6	
Wiskott-Aldrich	NHL, leukemia, HD	>10	59–75
Bloom	Leukemia, NHL, HD, adenocarcinoma	25	
X-linked lymphoproliferative (after EBV infection)	NHL, HLH	24–35	
Selective IgA deficiency	NHL, gastric carcinoma, thymoma, other	?	

Abbreviations: ID, immunodeficiency; NHL, non-Hodgkin's lymphoma; HD, Hodgkin's disease; EBV, Epstein-Barr Virus.

as *c-myc* (thought to be the mechanism in most high-grade pediatric lymphomas) or may be due to alteration in genes controlling apoptosis, resulting in decreased cell death, a slow accumulation of cells, and an indolent clinical course (as is seen in adult low-grade lymphomas that show increased expression of *bcl-2,* a gene known to inhibit apoptosis). The loss of a tumor suppressor gene, a mechanism common in many solid tumors, may be seen in some patients with T-cell leukemia or lymphoma.

Multiple genetic changes within a single cell are required to give rise to the malignant clone. In some instances these genetic changes may be caused by a viral infection. Examples of this include the role of human T-cell leukemia/lymphoma virus (HTLV) I and II in the development of adult T-cell lymphoma or leukemia and that of EBV in the development of the genetic abnormalities associated with endemic (African) Burkitt's lymphoma. The oncogenic potential of EBV and HTLV is increased by infection early in childhood. The EBV genome is found in the DNA of tumor cells in 95 percent of cases in endemic Burkitt's lymphoma but in only 15 percent of the sporadic cases,[8] although it has been suggested that viral DNA rearrangement and loss during malignant progression is consistent with EBV being more important than previously thought even in sporadic Burkitt's lymphoma.[9]

The distribution of endemic Burkitt's lymphoma coincides with the malaria belt in Africa. Malaria stimulates B-cell proliferation and T-cell suppression, and the interaction of this chronic effect with EBV, occurring at an earlier age than in developed countries, appears to be important in the pathogenesis of endemic Burkitt's lymphoma.

The role of radiation in the development of lymphomas is not clear. Although there is an increased risk of NHL in patients treated with combined radiation and chemotherapy, there was no correlation of lymphoma incidence with increased radiation dose in atomic bomb survivors.[10] Another suggestive association, that of pesticide exposure and NHL, remains unproven.

CLASSIFICATION

Over the last 50 years lymphoma classifications have evolved from being solely morphology-based. The new Revised European-American Lymphoma (REAL)[11] and World Health Organization (WHO) classifications[12] define the subtypes of lymphoma by a combination of morphology, immunophenotype, cytogenetic abnormalities, and clinical presentation. The spectrum of pediatric NHL is considerably narrower than that of adult NHL, with the majority of childhood NHL being limited to three major categories (Table 46–2). By the REAL classification system, 40 to 50 percent of North American NHL children have Burkitt's or Burkitt-like lymphomas, 30 to 40 percent have T- or early B-cell lymphoblastic lymphoma and 15 to 30 percent large-cell NHL. Included in the REAL system as subtypes of large-cell NHL are diffuse large B-cell NHL and ALCL, which account for about 10 percent of childhood NHL.[13] Lymphoblastic lymphoma is morphologically and cytogenetically indistinguishable from acute lymphoblastic leukemia (ALL); these diseases are thought to represent a spectrum of a single disease, as reflected in the designation of T- or B-precursor leukemia/lymphoma in the REAL classification. An arbitrary cut-off of 25 percent marrow involvement distinguishes stage IV NHL from ALL, a distinction of questionable biologic significance. Nonetheless, this differentiation remains important for the accurate comparison of the results of therapeutic trials. All other types of lymphoma, such as nonanaplastic peripheral T-cell lymphomas and gamma/delta lymphomas, occur rarely in the pediatric population.

PATHOLOGY

The majority of pediatric NHLs are diffuse, aggressive, high-grade lymphomas, which tend to arise in extranodal lymphoid tissue such as thymus or Peyer's patches. The aggressive nature of most pediatric NHL is thought to reflect the growth rate of the counterpart normal lymphocyte precursor.[2] The stages of lymphocyte differentiation at which childhood lymphoma and leukemia are thought to arise[14,15] are shown in Figures 46–1 and 46–2.

This rapid growth rate is reflected by numerous mitotic figures. Macrophages surrounded by a clear area, giving a "starry sky" appearance, may be seen in all three types of childhood lymphoma, although it is most commonly associated with the Burkitt's lymphoma subtype. Follicular low-grade lymphomas rarely occur in adolescents, and in patients less than 16 years of age tend to occur as localized disease. Only eight cases of follic-

Table 46–2. Comparison of Working and Revised European-American Lymphoma (REAL) Classification for Pediatric Non-Hodgkin's Lymphoma

	Lymphoblastic	Burkitt's	Large-Cell
REAL	Precursor T-lymphoblastic leukemia / lymphoma	Burkitt's lymphoma	Large B-cell
REAL	Precursor B-lymphoblastic leukemia / lymphoma	Burkitt-like lymphoma (provisional)	Peripheral T-cell (subtype large-cell) Anaplastic large cell (T- and null-cell)
Working Formulation	Lymphoblastic lymphoma	Small noncleaved cell, Burkitt's and non-Burkitt's lymphoma	Large cell cleaved cell, noncleaved Large cell, immunoblastic

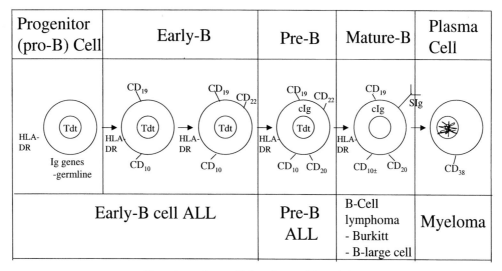

Figure 46–1. Stages of B-lymphocyte differentiation.

ular lymphoma were found among 318 children under 15 years of age with NHL.[16]

In addition to these three major types of NHL, children may present with a number of lymphoproliferative disorders, generally in the setting of congenital or acquired immunodeficiency.

Burkitt's and Burkitt-Like Lymphomas

Burkitt's lymphoma represents the neoplastic transformation of a relatively mature B-cell precursor expressing surface immunoglobulin.[17] Burkitt's NHL exhibits a diffuse monomorphic proliferation of cells with a high nuclear/cytoplasmic ratio and deeply basophilic cytoplasm containing lipid vacuoles. Single-cell necrosis with ingestion of debris by macrophages, leading to the starry sky pattern, is frequently present. The nuclei are similar to or slightly smaller than histiocyte nuclei, and the lymphoma cells have been categorized as small noncleaved lymphocytes. The cells in Burkitt's lymphoma are fairly monomorphic in size and shape, with clumped or irregularly distributed nuclear chromatin and two to five nucleoli. In the non-Burkitt's type, there is more heterogeneity in cell size, and nucleoli tend to be fewer and more prominent. There has been much controversy concerning the significance of Burkitt's versus non-Burkitt's histology. The histologic features used to distinguish the two types are poorly reproducible, even when experts are tested against themselves at different time points. A study by the

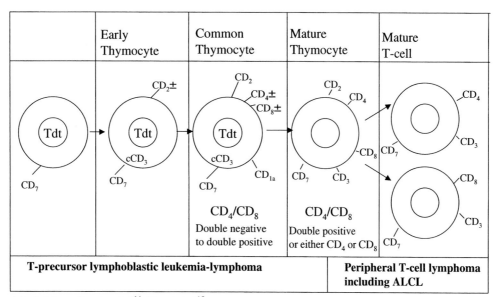

Adapted from Rezuka et al[14], Goust et al[15]

Figure 46–2. Stages of T-lymphocyte differentiation.

Pediatric Oncology Group (POG) failed to show any significant differences between the two subtypes,[18] whereas others have suggested a survival advantage for the Burkitt's subtype.[19] Recent molecular genetic studies suggest that Burkitt-like lymphomas may be intermediate between Burkitt's and B-cell large cell lymphomas,[11] but there appears to be no prognostic or therapeutic advantage to differentiating this subtype.

Flow cytometry and immunohistochemistry demonstrate B cell markers CD 19 and CD20 and IgM class surface immunoglobulin with light chain κ or λ restriction. CD10 (common ALL antigen) may be present in some Burkitt's lymphomas. Terminal deoxynucleotidyl transferase (TdT) is negative in Burkitt's cells, reflecting the mature phenotype.

Lymphoblastic Lymphoma

Lymphoblastic lymphoma (LL) consists of cells that are morphologically indistinguishable from acute lymphoblastic leukemia (ALL). It presents as a diffuse proliferation of medium-sized cells with a high nuclear/cytoplasmic ratio and scant amounts of variously basophilic cytoplasm (usually less basophilic than Burkitt's lymphoma cells). The nuclear chromatin is finely stippled with indistinct nucleoli, and some degree of nuclear convolution may be seen in up to 50 percent of cases, but this feature is not required for diagnosis and its presence does not seem to affect prognosis.[13] Mitotic activity is prominent and a starry sky pattern is commonly seen. Cytochemically the cells stain strongly for acid phosphatase, and TdT is usually positive.

Approximately 80 percent of lymphoblastic lymphomas are of T-cell phenotype, and 15 to 20 percent are of precursor B lineage. Both types appear similar histologically, but T-cell LL most commonly presents with advanced-stage disease, whereas precursor-B LL more often presents with localized disease and may present at unusual sites such as skin or bone[20] or with disease below the diaphragm.

T-cell LL is derived from thymic T cells all of which express the pan-T antigen CD7. Demonstration of CD7 may be the best single test for identifying T-cell precursor neoplasms.[20] Other antigens that may be expressed depending on the stage of differentiation are CD2, CD3, and CD45RO, as well as other markers of immature T cells such as CD4 and CD8 double positivity or double negativity. CD10 (CALLA) is positive in about 50 percent of T-LL cases.[13]

Despite the morphologic similarity between LL and ALL, subtle differences in the immunophenotype suggest that T-cell ALL may be derived from early to intermediate thymocytes, whereas T-LL is more usually derived from cells in the intermediate to late thymocyte stage.[21] Precursor B-cell LL expresses the phenotype of common childhood ALL (CD10, CD19, CD22, HLA-DR).

Diagnosis of T-LL may be made on cytologic and immunologic evaluation of pleural and/or pericardial effusions; however, care must be taken in the interpretation. Any large anterior mediastinal mass may, as a consequence of compression, result in the presence of thoracic duct lymphocytes, which morphologically resemble T lymphoblasts within pleural and pericardial fluid. The presence of TdT within the cells may be necessary for confirmation of the diagnosis.

Large-Cell Lymphoma

Large-Cell lymphomas (LCLs) are a heterogenous group of tumors in which the cells contain nuclei that are larger than those of the surrounding histiocytes. Major subtypes of LCL within the REAL classification are B-cell large-cell, anaplastic-large cell (ALCL), and the other rarer peripheral T-cell lymphomas, so-called because of their mature T-cell phenotype (CD3,5,7-positive, CD 4 or 8 double positive or double negative). B-cell LCLs express CD20 and show light chain restriction (either κ or λ). Surface expression of immunoglobulin may be absent in up to one-third, however.[13] In keeping with the mature B-cell phenotype, they are TdT-negative.

Primary mediastinal large B-cell lymphoma with sclerosis is a subtype of B-cell LCL, characterized by large lymphoid cells with abundant cytoplasm, a vesicular chromatin pattern, and prominent nucleoli. Sclerosis may vary from thick bands of collagen to fine spider-like sclerosis surrounding small groups of cells. The major differential diagnosis involves nodular sclerosing HL and ALCL. Occasional cases of B-cell large-cell NHL with an extensive T-cell reaction (T-cell-rich B-cell lymphoma) have been described in children.[13]

Anaplastic large-cell lymphoma represents about 10 percent of pediatric NHL and is characterized by a diffuse proliferation of large cells with abundant, faintly basophilic cytoplasm and bizarre, pleomorphic, often reniform nuclei with prominent nucleoli. The cells tend to grow in a cohesive pattern, often with a sinusoidal and paracortical distribution within lymph nodes and many atypical cells, including multinucleated cells. A number of histologic patterns have been described. The cells react with antibodies to the CD30 antigen, which exists as membrane-bound and soluble forms. The value of sCD30 levels at diagnosis have been correlated with outcome in adult patients but not yet in children.[22] In one series, 65 percent of ALCL cases were of T-cell phenotype and 35 percent were null-cell.[23] Epithelial membrane antigen (EMA) is generally positive, and CD25 (IL2-R) is often expressed, but other markers are variable. Most cases previously diagnosed as malignant histiocytosis are now believed to be ALCL, which can be distinguished from malignant histiocytosis by the absence of monocyte/macrophage-associated antigens and lysozyme on the tumor cells, as well as phagolysosomes on electron microscopy. T-ALCLs are of mature T-cell phenotype and therefore fit into the category of peripheral T-cell lymphomas (PTCL). The PTCLs often show an aberrant phenotype with the loss or one or more pan-T antigens, coexpression of CD4 and CD8, or loss of both CD4 and CD8. With the exception of ALCL, PTCLs are rare in the pediatric population. Lymphomatoid papulosis (LP) is a rare skin condition, which morphologically is indistinguishable from ALCL and like cutaneous ALCL, is anaplastic lymphoma kinase (ALK)-negative. The distinction, which is made on clinical grounds, is important, as LP should not be treated with systemic chemotherapy.

MOLECULAR BIOLOGY

The most common molecular alterations in NHL are rearrangements in immunoglobulin and T-cell receptor genes. Normally, rearrangement of immunoglobulin heavy and light chains and all four chains of the T-cell receptor (TCR) occurs at precise times during differentiation. In B cells, heavy chain rearrangement occurs before light chain and κ light chain before λ. In T cells the γ- and δ-chain genes rearrange before the α and β. DNA polymerase chain reaction (PCR) methods are used to identify these immunoglobulin and T-cell receptor gene rearrangements and thereby establish clonality. Rearrangements of these receptor genes are not always lineage-specific. Immunoglobulin gene rearrangements may be seen in T-cell disease, and T-cell receptor rearrangements may be seen in B-cell disease. Rearrangements involving light chain receptor genes, however, tend to be more specific for B-lineage disease than are rearrangements of heavy chain genes.[24]

Burkitt's Non-Hodgkin's Lymphoma

Burkitt's NHLs have characteristic cytogenetic changes, which in 80 percent of cases involve translocation of the *c-myc* proto-oncogene on chromosome 8 (involved in cell proliferation and differentiation) to the immunoglobulin heavy chain gene locus on chromosome 14 (t[8;14] [q24;q32]). In the remaining 20 percent of cases, *c-myc* is translated to the κ light chain gene locus on chromosome 2 (t[2;8] [p11;q24]) or to the λ light chain locus on chromosome 22 (t[8;22] [q24;q11]). Although the t(8;14)(q24;q32) is common to both sporadic and endemic Burkitt's lymphoma, the breakpoints within the two genes are different in the two diseases. Both mutations result in juxtaposition of *c-myc* next to the highly active Ig gene, leading to deregulation and uncontrolled expression of the c-MYC protein.[17] Molecular changes found in "Burkitt-like" lymphomas, including increased expression of *bcl-6* in a significant proportion, suggests that this lymphoma is intermediate between Burkitt's and B large-cell NHL.[25]

Lymphoblastic Lymphoma

Many different translocations may be seen in T-cell LL, usually involving translocation of a proto-oncogene to one of the T-cell receptor (TCR) genes, α/δ on chromosome 14 or less commonly β on chromosome 7, and resulting in aberrant expression of the oncogene. The most common translocations are t(11;14)(p13;q11) in 7 percent, t(10;14)(q24;q11) in 5 percent, and t(1;14)(p32–p34;q11) in 3 percent of cases.[17,26] Other common abnormalities involve the *tal-1* gene on chromosome 1, found to be overexpressed in 30 percent of T-leukemia/lymphoma,[26] 3 percent through translocation of *tal-1* next to the TCR genes t(1;14) and t(1;7), and 26 percent by deletion of a regulatory sequence that is normally interposed between *tal-1* and the *sil* gene. Loss of this regulatory region juxtaposes *tal-1* and *sil*. *Tal-1* also interacts with other genes, which are juxtaposed next to TCR genes in small subsets of T-cell disease. Genetic alterations that result in *tal-1* activation or novel TAL-1

protein interactions is seen in most T-cell ALL and NHL.[17] Finally, inactivation of the multitumor suppression gene (*mts-1*), located on chromosome 9p21, may be the most common genetic defect found in T-cell leukemia and lymphoma.[17]

Large-Cell Lymphoma

Diffuse Large B-Cell Lymphoma

The t(14;18) seen most commonly in adult follicular lymphomas is associated with increased expression of *bcl-2* and reduced apoptosis, longer survival, and the low-grade phenotype. This is seen in a minority of pediatric lymphomas. By contrast, 30 percent of pediatric B-large cell NHL show abnormalities of *bcl-6* expression. This gene is normally expressed in follicular center B cells but is downregulated as cells mature and exit the follicular center. Rearrangements of the *bcl-6* gene may result in overexpression of the gene and proliferation of B lymphocytes, resulting in the higher-grade pediatric B-lymphomas.

Some pediatric large-cell lymphomas show the t(8;14)(q24;q32) translocation, which is identical to that seen in Burkitt's lymphoma with a similar mechanism of transformation.

Anaplastic Large-Cell Lymphoma

The majority of childhood ALCLs show a characteristic translocation, t(2;5)(p23;q35). This translocation relocates a promoter sequence of the nucleolar phosphoprotein encoding gene (*npm*) on 5q35 to the anaplastic lymphoma kinase gene *alk* on 2p23 resulting in production of the fusion protein ALK. The ALK protein can now be recognized immunohistochemically on fixed tissue, using an anti-ALK1 monoclonal antibody. Expression of ALK is usually confined to cells of the nervous system and is not seen in normal lymphocytes. Overexpression of *alk* may contribute to malignant change by inappropriate phosphorylation of intercellular growth regulators.[17] Some lymphomas, which are positive for ALK but do not have the t(2;5) and other chromosomal rearrangements such as inv 2 (p23;q35) and t(1;2)(q25;p23), may also show ALK expression. Primary cutaneous ALCL and lymphomatoid papulosis are usually ALK-negative. Many investigators believe that positive immunocytochemistry for ALK distinguishes ALCL from Hodgkin's disease.

CLINICAL PRESENTATION

Pediatric NHL usually arises in extranodal lymphoid tissue, grows rapidly, and tends to spread early, so that the majority of children present with locally advanced or metastatic disease. Only 10 to 15 percent of childhood NHL presents with primary peripheral nodal disease and a minority present in extralymphatic tissue such as bone, skin, lung, and gonad. Involvement of the CNS presents as leptomeningeal (headache, neck stiffness, back pain) or cranial nerve palsies. Paraplegia due to extradural spinal cord compression is more common in endemic Burkitt's lymphoma. There is a clear link between the three different subtypes of NHL and their clinical presentation.

Burkitt's Lymphoma

Ninety percent of Burkitt's NHL presents with abdominal disease, the remainder arising from B lymphocytes in Waldeyer's ring (tonsils, adenoids). Despite a similar histologic appearance, the sporadic and endemic Burkitt's lymphomas differ in their clinical presentation. The peak age for presentation is 7 years in the African (endemic) type and 11 years in the sporadic type, with a male predominance (2:1 to 3:1) in both.[27]

In North America and Europe, Burkitt's lymphoma arises most commonly from relatively mature B cells in Peyer's patches within the gastrointestinal (GI) tract, most commonly at the ileocecal junction. Gonadal and kidney involvement is common. Bowel obstruction is a common presenting symptom. Eighty percent of patients present with an abdominal mass or with abdominal pain, abdominal distension, nausea, and vomiting. A localized Burkitt's NHL may act as the lead point for an intussusception, and the tumor is not infrequently diagnosed during surgery for "acute appendicitis." Involvement of tonsil or adenoid may lead to airway obstruction, commonly associated with nontender cervical adenopathy.

Jaw involvement occurs in only 15 percent of patients with sporadic Burkitt's lymphoma and then usually as part of multiple bone metastases, whereas endemic (African) Burkitt's NHL commonly presents with jaw tumors (70 percent) as well as involvement of the GI tract and kidneys. Peripheral lymph node involvement is unusual in patients with the endemic form of the disease. Bone marrow and CNS involvement may be seen with Burkitt's lymphoma. Endemic Burkitt's patients more commonly present with CNS disease (leptomeningeal, cranial nerve palsies, and paraplegia), whereas bone marrow disease occurs more frequently in patients with sporadic Burkitt's lymphoma.

Burkitt's lymphoma is an extremely fast growing malignancy with a doubling time of 2 to 3 days and a high spontaneous cell death rate.[27] Patients may thus present with hyperuricemic nephropathy even before therapy has started, and these tumors have the highest risk of any malignancy of developing tumor lysis syndrome after the start of therapy. The survival of patients with Burkitt's NHL was very poor until chemotherapy protocols were designed to take advantage of the very rapid cell cycling.

Lymphoblastic Lymphoma

Lymphoblastic lymphoma (LL) affects males more than females (2.5:1), with a peak age in the second decade. Eighty percent of LLs are of thymic T-cell origin. Fifty percent of patients present with a mediastinal mass, often with pleural and/or pericardial effusions, right ventricular outflow obstruction, and/or a superior vena cava syndrome. Associated symptoms include dyspnea, dysphagia, chest pain, suffusion, and swelling of the face, neck, and arms. These are high-grade lymphomas, and tumor lysis syndrome may occur, especially if kidney infiltration is present. Urgent diagnosis and therapy are absolutely mandatory. Lymphadenopathy is present in 50 to 80 percent of patients and is usually supradiaphragmatic (cervical, supraclavicular, and axillary). Isolated or prominent abdominal disease is rare, although liver, spleen, kidneys, and abdominal nodes may

be involved. Bone marrow involvement is common. As with ALL, CNS and gonadal involvement may occur.

B-precursor LL tends to present with localized disease and may involve unusual sites such as skin, subcutaneous tissue, and bone, but may occasionally present with intra-abdominal disease.

Large-Cell Non-Hodgkin's Lymphoma

The large-cell NHLs are a diverse group of lymphomas that may present in lymph nodes, mediastinum or extranodally. Large-cell NHL can present in any anatomic site and may present with abdominal disease similar to Burkitt's lymphoma or a mediastinal mass similar to lymphoblastic NHL. The mediastinal location of primary mediastinal large B-cell lymphoma and the extensive sclerosis associated with it may result in a clinical presentation of airway compromise or superior vena cava syndrome similar to that of lymphoblastic lymphoma. Bone marrow is less frequently involved than in the other types of NHL, and CNS disease is uncommon.

Anaplastic Large-Cell Lymphoma

Anaplastic large-cell lymphoma commonly involves unusual sites such as bone, skin, and peripheral nodes and may present with manifestations such as diffuse pulmonary disease, which are not generally seen with the other lymphomas. It may present in childhood and in adults with a systemic or primarily cutaneous distribution. Isolated cutaneous ALCL appears to be more indolent than the systemic form and appears to have a better prognosis. Unlike the other lymphomas, lymphadenopathy due to ALCL may be tender to palpation and is more commonly associated with B symptoms (fever higher than 38°C for three consecutive days, night sweats, and unexplained weight loss of 10 percent of body weight over 6 months), a high leukocyte count, and thrombocytosis, all of which are thought to be due to excess cytokine production by lymphoma cells. ALCL must be included in the differential diagnosis of persistent fever and lymphadenopathy, particularly as a waxing and waning course may be seen, followed by rapid progression. This spontaneous regression may be mediated by cytokines such as TGF-β,[28] and the rapid progression that may follow is thought to be due to escape from the cytokine-mediated effects. Cytokine release from ALCL cells may also explain the occasional finding of hemophagocytosis in the bone marrow.[28] Despite the often widespread nature of ALCL, involvement of CNS and bone marrow are quite uncommon with 0 of 62 and 1 of 62 having bone marrow and CNS disease, respectively, in a series from the Berlin-Frankfurt-Münster (BFM) group.[28]

DIAGNOSIS

The aggressive nature of most pediatric NHLs underlies the urgency to obtain a diagnosis and begin therapy. Correct diagnosis requires morphology, cytochemistry, immunophenotyping, cytogenetics, and molecular genetics. On occasion, fine-needle aspiration (FNA) from the tumor, or aspiration of pleural or pericardial fluid, may yield enough material for diagnosis and for limited additional studies such as cytogenetics or electron microscopy. In view of the emergence of new biology-based approaches to therapy, however, fresh-frozen tissue is becoming increasingly important and open, excisional biopsies are often important to obtain adequate samples.

Before the patient is sent for biopsy, investigations to assess the extent of disease and of tumor-induced complications need to be made in a timely fashion. In particular, patients with large abdominal tumors need to be evaluated for GI obstruction or perforation, as well as for renal impairment due to kidney infiltration, obstruction, or hyperuricemia. Patients with an anterior mediastinal mass need urgent evaluation for airway or SVC compression, right ventricular outflow compression, pleural fluid, and cardiac tamponade. It is important that these patients not be put into a supine position for the investigations, but instead procedures should be done with patients prone or lying on their side, and no patient with airway obstruction should be sedated for a procedure without consultation with an experienced anesthesiologist. When anesthesia is considered to be too hazardous and diagnosis cannot be obtained from a peripheral node or bone marrow specimen, the mediastinal mass may be reduced in size by administration of corticosteroid therapy until a biopsy can safely be performed. Judicious use of steroids, with an open biopsy performed no more than 24 to 36 hours later, can often result in sufficient tissue for pathologic diagnosis and for important biology studies and has obviated the need for radiation therapy. It must be remembered, however, that steroid therapy may result in tumor lysis syndrome.

STAGING

A comprehensive assessment includes blood cell count and differential, blood chemistry for renal and liver function studies, uric acid, potassium, phosphate, and calcium (tumor lysis) and lactate dehydrogenase (LDH) as a measure of tumor burden. Studies of the primary tumor include chest x-ray, computed tomography (CT) of chest and abdomen (and occasionally head), ultrasound and echocardiogram. Magnetic resonance imaging (MRI) scans are done for CNS and paraspinal disease. Staging work-up also includes gallium-67 or technetium-99 bone scan, as well as CSF examination and bilateral bone marrow aspirate and biopsy. A study from the Hospital for Sick Children (HSC) showed that bone scans added little to the information provided by the gallium scan,[29] and they are no longer performed routinely. Tests for EBV and HIV are recommended prior to therapy in all new NHL patients.

In pediatric NHL the most widely used staging system is the St. Jude's system (Table 46–3), which is applicable to all three major subtypes and separates patients with localized disease (stages I and II) from those with advanced disease (stage III). Stage IV NHL patients have bone marrow involvement with less than 25 percent blasts and/or have CNS disease; more than 25 percent tumor cells in the bone marrow is, by convention, called leukemia. CNS disease is defined as leptomeningeal infiltration

Table 46–3. St. Jude's Staging System for Pediatric Non-Hodgkin's Lymphoma

Stage I
A single tumor (extranodal) or single anatomical area (nodal) with the exclusion of the mediastinum or abdomen

Stage II
A single tumor (extranodal) with regional node involvement
Two or more nodal areas on the same side of the diaphragm
Two single (extranodal) tumors with or without regional node involvement on the same side of the diaphragm
A primary gastrointestinal tract tumor, usually in the ileocecal area, with or without involvement of associated mesenteric nodes only, grossly completely resected

Stage III
Two single tumors (extranodal) on opposite sides of the diaphragm
Two or more nodal areas above or below the diaphragm
All the primary intrathoracic tumors (mediastinal, pleural, thymic)
All extensive primary intra-abdominal disease, unresectable
All paraspinal or epidural tumors, regardless of other tumor sites
Multifocal bone (now considered stage III rather than IV)

Stage IV
Any of the above with initial central nervous system and/or bone marrow involvement

or isolated cranial nerve palsy. Isolated extradural disease, which does not confer the same prognosis, should be included in the definition of stage III lymphoma, as should multifocal bone disease. Significant differences in intensity and length of therapy, and in prognosis for patients with localized and advanced-stage NHL mean that accurate staging is important.

TREATMENT AND PROGNOSIS

Surgery is needed to obtain biopsy tissue and to deal with complications such as intussusception, bleeding, or bowel perforation. Localized abdominal tumors diagnosed at the time of laparotomy are often easily resected, and the prognosis is excellent with a short course (6 weeks) of chemotherapy. Surgery should not be done for the purpose of resection or for debulking of tumors, and surgical interventions that delay the onset of chemotherapy should be avoided. The place of surgery in the assessment of residual tumors post-chemotherapy is controversial. The French Society for Pediatric Oncology (SFOP) demonstrated that two-thirds of residual abdominal masses were necrotic[30] and suggested that second-look surgery was necessary to define remission status. No advantage to second-look surgery, however, was demonstrated in the BFM studies,[31] as patients with residual tumor had a poor prognosis despite local therapy. The success of autologous transplant in patients with a slow response to primary therapy, however, would suggest that an accurate assessment of residual tumor is useful and prognostic.

Radiation therapy has been relegated to a secondary role in the treatment of NHL. Prior to the era of effective chemotherapy, radiation therapy (RT) was the only effective treatment modality, resulting in a 20 percent chance of cure in patients with localized disease.[32] In patients treated with adequate chemotherapy, however, RT has been shown to increase both short-term and long-term morbidity without providing a therapeutic advantage. Radiation therapy is therefore omitted in most modern protocols except for patients with CNS disease. Even for patients presenting with a paraspinal mass and paraplegia, no advantage of addition of RT has been demonstrated, and RT should be limited to patients without a tissue diagnosis or who fail to respond rapidly to chemotherapy.[1] Possibly because of rapid cell cycling, radiation given in single daily fractions is relatively ineffective in Burkitt's lymphoma,[33] although a recent study suggests that hyperfractionation with at least three fractions per day may have some benefit.[34]

Combination chemotherapy is the primary treatment modality for childhood NHL. The treatment protocol should be based on the subtype and on the extent of disease. Prior to the start of therapy, measures must be taken to prevent tumor lysis syndrome, which results from the release of potassium, urate, and phosphate from dying cells. In Burkitt's lymphoma, tumor lysis may be present prior to the start of therapy and is more likely to occur after therapy than in the T-cell neoplasms because of the higher cell turnover of B-cell lymphomas. Both urate and phosphate can precipitate in renal tubules, resulting in renal failure. High-dose fluids to establish a good urine flow, alkalization at least until urate level is normalized, and either allopurinol to prevent urate production or uric acid oxidase to cause urate breakdown should be started immediately. In the presence of significant pleural or pericardial effusions, right ventricular outflow, or inferior vena caval obstruction, hyperhydration may need to be given in the setting of an intensive care unit. It is important to correct preexisting abnormalities before the initiation of chemotherapy, and hemodialysis may be necessary even before therapy is started. Establishment of good urine flow is essential to prevent potentially fatal hyperkalemia,[35] and potassium should be avoided in intravenous solutions until the period of risk for tumor lysis is past.

Hyperhydration is continued until the patient is stable (approximately 5 days). Urine pH should be kept between 7 and 7.5, as urate will precipitate in acid urine and phosphate in alkaline urine. Hypocalcemia occurs as a consequence of hyperphosphatemia and should only be treated if symptomatic. Intraventricular calcium should be given with great caution in view of the danger of tissue calcium deposition in the face of a high serum phosphate and should never be given together with alkalization. Because allopurinol inhibits the production of urate from the precursors xanthine and hypoxanthine, which can also precipitate in renal tubules, the recent demonstration that uric acid oxidase can dramatically decrease uric acid levels,[36] making allopurinol use unnecessary, should prove significantly advantageous in the prevention of tumor lysis syndrome.

CHEMOTHERAPY

The use of multiagent, intensive chemotherapy regimens has markedly improved survival for children with NHL. The selection of a chemotherapeutic regimen is based either on morphology or on the B- or T-cell immunophenotype. Intensity and duration of therapy vary markedly for localized and advanced disease.

Localized Non-Hodgkin's Lymphoma

Survival of patients with localized Burkitt's and large-cell lymphomas has exceed 85 percent at 5 years, permitting investigators to focus on reducing treatment-related morbidity.[1,37]

Recent Pediatric Oncology Group (POG) trials demonstrated that for patients with stage I and II nonlymphoblastic disease, 9 weeks of cyclophosphamide–doxorubicin–vincristine–prednisone (CHOP)-based chemotherapy produces an event-free survival (EFS) close to 90 percent and that radiation therapy can be safely omitted even for bone disease.[37] Similarly, the BFM90 protocol, utilizing 6 weeks of therapy,[31] and the SFOP LMB89 trial, which uses only two courses of chemotherapy,[30] achieved survival rates of over 90 percent in patients with localized nonlymphoblastic disease without local irradiation. Regardless of the exact therapy, the patients who relapsed did so within the first year from diagnosis.

Although induction therapy is equally successful for the 15 percent of early-stage NHL patients with localized lymphoblastic lymphoma, this subgroup is prone to late relapses, so that the EFS was less than 50 percent at 5 years in the recently closed POG 9219 trial, despite 6 months of continuation therapy with 6-mercaptopurine and low-dose methotrexate. An overall survival (OS) of more than 90 percent at 5 years was achieved by successful treatment for relapsed disease (M. Link, Stanford University, Stanford, CA, personal communication). In contrast, the BFM group has used much more intensive therapy and achieved an EFS of 90 percent in localized LL using the standard arm of the BFM T-cell protocol.[38] This protocol included standard BFM induction and a consolidation phase (protocol M) consisting of four doses of high-dose (5 g/m^2) methotrexate followed by maintenance therapy for 2 years (Figure 46–3 and Table 46–4). No reinduction therapy or local or cranial radiation was given for stage I and II patients. A recently opened COG study will attempt to confirm the BFM results. If successful, this strategy will increase the risk of therapy-related morbidity but will obviate the need for intensive salvage therapy for more than 50 percent of the patients with localized LL.

Patients with localized head and neck lymphoma and all patients with LL continue to require CNS prophylaxis in the form of intrathecal chemotherapy. Central nervous system prophylaxis is no longer recommended for patients with localized abdominal lymphoma, including those with Burkitt's lymphoma histology.

Advanced (Stage III and IV) Lymphoma

Burkitt's Lymphoma and B-Cell Large-Cell Lymphoma

During the last few decades major improvements have been seen in the cure rate of Burkitt's lymphoma and B-cell ALL, from less than 30 percent in the early 1980s to more than 80 percent currently. Starting with the total B therapy of Murphy[2] and colleagues, chemotherapy protocols have been developed

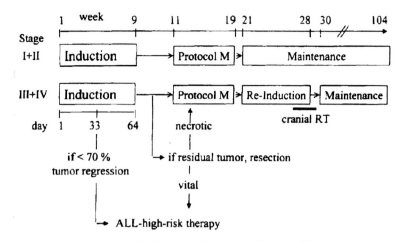

Figure 46–3. BFM 90 protocol for T-cell lymphoma. (From Reiter et al.,[38] with permission.)

based on the very rapid growth rate of these tumors; these include short-duration, dose-intensified, rapidly cycling courses, which include high-dose S-phase drugs that cross the blood-brain barrier. Thus, most successful protocols combine high doses of cyclophosphamide given in divided doses over a period of 3 to 5 days in combination with high-dose methotrexate (MTX) and more recently, high doses of cytosine arabinoside (Ara-C), together with vincristine and with or without anthracycline. All protocols include a corticosteroid, either prednisone or dexamethasone.

Table 46–4. BFM 90 Protocol for T-cell Lymphoma

Drug	Dose	Days of Administration
Induction protocol I		
Prednisone (orally)	60 mg/m^2	1–28, then taper over 3 × 3 days
Vincristine (iv)	1.5 mg/m^2 (max 2 mg)	8,15,22,29
Daunorubicin (iv over 1 h)	30 mg/m^2	8,15,22,29
L-Asparaginase (iv over 1 h)	10,000 IU/m^2	12,15,18,21,24,27,30,33
Cyclophosphamide[a] (iv over 1 h)	1000 mg/m^2	36,64
Cytarabine (iv)	75 mg/m^2	38–41, 45–48, 52–55, 59–62
6-Mercaptopurine (orally)	60 mg/m^2	36–63
Methotrexate (it)[b]	12 mg[b]	1,15,29,45,59[c]
Protocol M		
6-Mercaptopurine (orally)	25 mg/m^2	1–56
Methotrexate[c]	5 g/m^2	8,22,36,50
Methotrexate (it)[b]	12 mg[b]	8,22,36,50
Reinduction protocol II		
Dexamethasone (orally)	10 mg/m^2	1–21, then taper over 3 × 3 days
Vincristine (iv)	1.5 mg/m^2 (max 2 mg)	8,15,22,29
Doxorubicin (iv over 1 h)	30 mg/m^2	8,15,22,29
L-Asparaginase (iv over 1 h)	10,000 IU/m^2	8,11,15,18
Cyclophosphamide[a] (iv over 1 h)	1000 mg/m^2	36
Cytarabine (iv)	75 mg/m^2	38–41, 45–48
6-Thioguanine (orally)	60 mg/m^2	36–49
Methotrexate (it)[b]	12 mg[b]	38,45

Abbreviations: iv, intravenously; it, intrathecally; BFM, Berlin-Frankfurt-Münster.

[a] With mesna.

[b] Doses were adjusted for children under 3 years of age.

[c] 10% of the dose over 30 minutes and 90% as a 23.5-hour continuous iv infusion. Leucovorin rescue: 30 mg/m^2 iv at hour 42; 15 mg/m^2 iv at hours 48 and 54. Serum levels of methotrexate (MTX) should be less than 3 μmol/L at hour 36 after the start of the MTX infusion, ≤1 μmol/L at hour 42, and ≤0.4 μmol/h at hour 48.

[d] Additional doses at days 8 and 22 for CNS-positive patients.

From Reiter et al.,[38] with permission.

Some protocols, such as the BFM and National Cancer Institute (NCI), also utilize ifosfamide, but the advantage of this over cyclophosphamide is unclear. The recently closed POG 9317 study, which excluded patients with B-cell large-cell disease, produced an overall disease-free survival (DFS) of 82 percent and demonstrated that addition of a cycle of high-dose ifosfamide/VP-16 improved the DFS of patients with CNS disease at diagnosis to 79 percent without cranial irradiation or intrathecal therapy but did not alter the DFS for CNS-negative patients, even in those with B-ALL.[39] Building on this successful protocol, a pilot protocol, POG 9517, investigated the toxicity of increasing the methotrexate dose from 1 g/m^2 to 5 g/m^2 per course as well as intensifying the cyclophosphamide doses from a cumulative dose of 5.4 g/m^2 in POG 9317 to 9 g/m^2 in POG 9517 for stage IV disease. Of 19 eligible patients (89.5 percent) treated on POG 9517, 17 remain in CCR.[40]

Among the best published results are those of the SFOP LMB 89 protocol (Figure 46–4). A total of 561 patients were allocated to three risk groups, A, B, and C, and the therapy was adapted to the risk group. Therapy for group C patients (more than 70 percent blasts in the bone marrow and/or CNS disease) consisted of 7 months of intensive therapy, which included high dose MTX (8 g/m^2 per dose) and high-dose Ara-C. Cranial irradiation was given to patients with CNS disease. This protocol

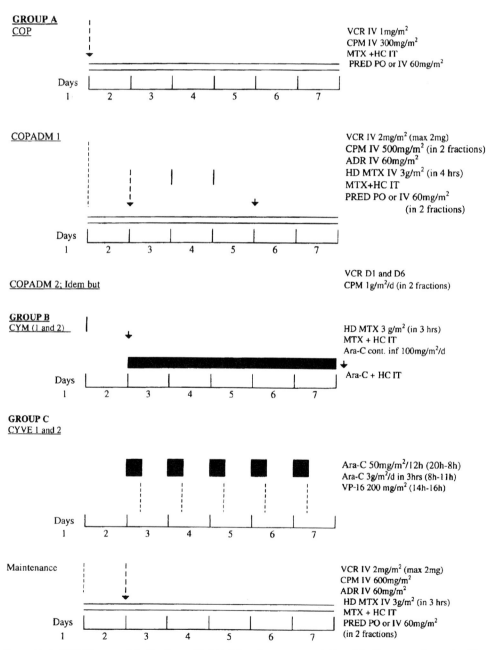

Figure 46–4. LMB 89 protocol for B-cell non-Hodgkin's lymphoma, groups A, B, and C. (From Büyükpamukçu.[30] with permission.)

resulted in an OS of 91 percent at 5 years, 87 percent for stage IV, and 88 percent for B-ALL, and an improvement in DFS for CNS-positive patients to 79 percent from 19 percent in the earlier LMB 81 study.[41] The 5-year DFS was 95 percent for patients with a low LDH compared to 87 percent for those whose LDH was increased twofold or more (p <.001), except in group C patients in whom neither LDH nor bone marrow involvement was predictive of outcome. The protocol also demonstrated that

residual tumor needed to be confirmed histologically because two-thirds of residual abdominal masses were necrotic.[30]

Other groups have produced similar results. The BFM group utilized therapy limited to 12 weeks, and confirmed the efficacy of increasing the dose of methotrexate from 500 mg/m² per course in the BFM 86 study to 5 g/m² in the BFM 90 study (Figure 46–5) for patients with advanced-stage disease, producing a 6-year DFS of 96 ± 2 percent for intermediate-risk patients and 78 ± 3 percent for

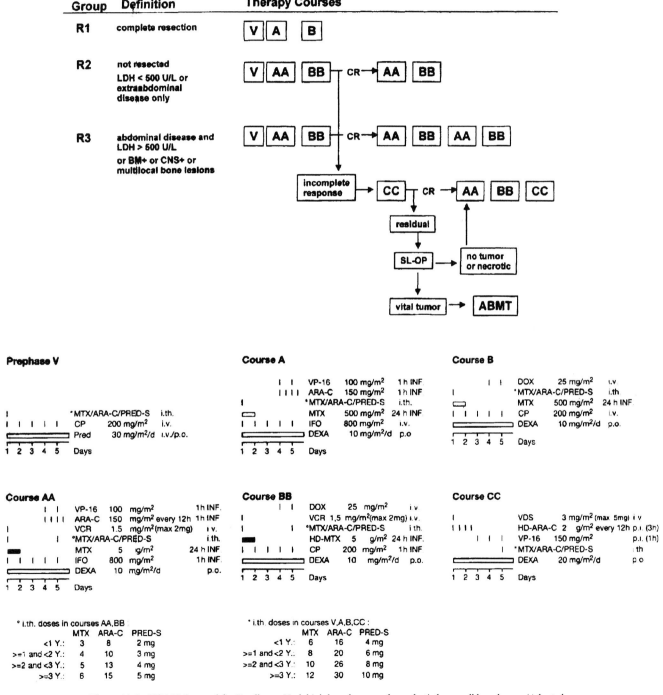

Figure 46–5. BFM 90 Protocol for B-cell non-Hodgkin's lymphoma and anaplastic large-cell lymphoma. (Adapted from Reiter et al.,[31] and Reiter et al.,[42] with permission.)

the highest-risk patients with abdominal tumor plus LDH above 500 and/or patients with bone marrow and/or CNS involvement, compared to 43 ± 10 percent for this high-risk group in the BFM 86 study.[42] This study demonstrated that cranial radiation could be successfully eliminated even for patients with CNS disease, at least when a combination of high-dose systemic chemotherapy plus intraventricular therapy via an Omaya reservoir was utilized. Since that study, however, both the NCI-89-C[32] and POG 9317 have demonstrated that high-dose chemotherapy alone can successfully treat CNS Burkitt's lymphoma without cranial radiation or intraventricular therapy (Table 46–5).

The BFM investigators also evaluated patients who responded slowly to therapy. Patients with residual tumor on imaging studies after two courses received an intensification course with high-dose Ara-C and etoposide. If histologically proven disease was still present after three courses, patients underwent megadose therapy with rescue. Of six patients who received allogeneic bone marrow transplantation (ABMT) one had progressive disease compared to five of six in BFM 86 who did not undergo ABMT.[42] Similarly, results of the SFOP LMB 84 study demonstrated that patients in biopsy-proven partial remission after three chemotherapy courses could be salvaged with high-dose chemotherapy (BCNU–etoposide–Ara-C–melphalan [BEAM]) and ABMT.[41] These results suggest that surgery to confirm residual tumor is necessary, as high-dose therapy may be successful for tumors that are slow responders but remain chemotherapy-sensitive.

In May 1966, the SFOP, Children's Cancer Group (CCG), and United Kingdom CCG opened the ongoing French-American-British (FAB), study which randomized patients to standard LMB 89 therapy (without cranial irradiation) versus dose-reduced therapy to see if the excellent results of LMB 89 could be maintained with less treatment-related toxicity. This trial is also attempting to establish an optimal dose of high-dose MTX by randomizing between 3 g/m^2 and 8 g/m^2 of MTX.

Summary of the Findings of the Cooperative Group Trials

1. Advanced-stage Burkitt's and B-cell ALL and B-cell large-cell disease, can successfully be treated with a short duration (3 to 6 months) of very intensive, multiagent alkylator-based chemotherapy.
2. Successive cycles of chemotherapy need to be given as soon as possible to prevent regrowth of these rapidly growing tumors.

3. Improvement in cure rate occurred with increasing intensity of chemotherapy, particularly higher doses of methotrexate, in both the SFOP and BFM studies.
4. The addition of high-dose antimetabolite therapy, such as high-dose MTX, high dose Ara-C, and/or high-dose ifosfamide, to the intrathecal therapy is successful in prophylaxis and treatment of CNS disease without cranial irradiation and without the need for an Omaya reservoir, even in patients with CNS involvement.
5. Involvement of the CNS and/or bone marrow at diagnosis is no longer indicative of a poor prognosis.
6. Previously accepted biologic prognosticators, such as LDH level at diagnosis, are no longer useful when these highly effective protocols are given.
7. Most patients who relapse will do so within the first 8 months after diagnosis, and patients with Burkitt's lymphoma who survive disease-free for 10 months are likely to be cured.
8. Patients with residual (histologically proven) disease after two or three therapy courses have an increased risk of failure, which is not reduced by local therapy (surgery or radiation therapy) but may be improved by intensification of chemotherapy or megadose therapy with hematopoietic stem cell rescue.

All of these successful protocols are highly toxic, require frequent hospital admissions for treatment of toxicities, and require a "learning curve" for oncologists to learn to give them without undue mortality. Studies are underway to attempt to reduce toxicity without changing efficacy. These include tailoring of therapy to failure risk, different methods of growth factor support, judicious reduction in chemotherapy doses and/or duration, and, more recently, consideration of the addition of nontoxic synergistic therapy, such as monoclonal antibody therapy, which if effective may allow for dose reduction of the chemotherapy without loss of efficacy.

Lymphoblastic Lymphoma

Lymphoblastic leukemia has been shown to respond best to protocols designed for acute lymphoblastic leukemia (ALL). Local radiation therapy, although effective, results in significant late risks, particularly when applied to the mediastinum, and is unnecessary if adequate chemotherapy is given.[3] One of the earliest successful protocols was the Memorial Sloan-Kettering

Table 46–5. Outcome for Patients with Advanced-Stage Burkitt's Lymphoma

Protocol	Number	Stage	Outcome (%)	Reference
POG 9317	325	III/IV/B-ALL	82	
		CNS +	82	Schwenn et al.[39]
POG 9517	19	III/IV/B-ALL	89.5	Griffin et al.[40]
LMB 89	181	III/IV/B-ALL	85–93	
		CNS +	79	Patte et al.[41]
BFM 90	322	Intermediate-risk/High-risk	89 ± 2	Reiter et al.[42]
NCI-89-C-41	41	III/IV	92/80	Magrath et al.[43]
LMB 86-89 (modified)	40	III/IV	100/77	Yaniv et al.[44]

Hospital lymphosarcoma 2/leukemia 2 (LSA2L2) 10-drug protocol, which combined vincristine, prednisone, and daunomycin induction with L-asparaginase, Ara-C, and 6-thioguanine during consolidation, followed by a maintenance phase with repeated courses of 5-day cycles of chemotherapy for a total treatment period of 18 to 24 months.[45] The addition of high-dose MTX (10 doses of 3 g/m^2 per dose) to the LSA2L2 protocol by the SFOP produced a significant improvement in survival to 79 percent for stage III patients and 72 percent for stage IV disease.[46] Cranial radiation was only given to patients with CNS disease at diagnosis, and only 1 of 77 CNS-negative patients relapsed in the CNS.

This study showed no difference in outcome for patients with less than 25 percent blasts in the marrow compared to those with more than 25 percent (T-ALL). The BFM group confirmed the advantage of increasing the MTX dose from 0.5 g/m^2 per 24h to 5 g/m^2 per 24h with an increase in the 5-year EFS from 56 to 73 percent in T-ALL patients.[47] More recently, the POG 9404 protocol for advanced T-cell disease including T-LL closed the randomization to standard versus high-dose MTX early because of a significant advantage in T-ALL of the arm with four courses of high-dose MTX (5 g/m^2 per course) (B. Asselin, University of Rochester, Rochester, NY, personal communication). Biologic confirmation of the efficacy of high-dose MTX comes from a study in which high-dose MTX resulted in substantially higher intracellular concentrations of active metabolites (MTX polyglutamates) and of remission.[46]

An earlier POG study demonstrated the advantage of the addition of L-asparaginase in T-cell NHL, with an EFS at 7 years of 46 percent without L-asparaginase and 65 percent with L-asparaginase.[49] A high incidence of second malignancy of the L-asparaginase arm of the protocol as well as the follow-up pilot protocol POG 9086 was attributed to the addition of teniposide. The epipodophyllotoxins have been excluded from subsequent POG T-cell studies. Finally, the BFM-90 protocol for T-cell disease (Figure 46–3 and Table 46–5) showed a 90 percent estimated probability of EFS at 5 years for 101 patients with T-cell LL, stages III and IV, treated for 2 years; the treatment included four doses of 5 g/m^2 of MTX.[38] Therapy was assigned based on stage, but patients who failed to respond adequately to induction therapy by day 33 (less than 70 percent reduction in mass,

more than 5 percent blasts in the BM, and/or persistent blasts in the CSF) were reassigned to a high-risk ALL protocol (eight patients).[38] The intensive therapy was concentrated in the first 7 months and all relapses occurred during the first year, in contrast to other less intensive protocols in which later relapses are common. The results, albeit excellent, excluded patients with T-ALL, although 15 of 19 stage IV patients had bone marrow involvement (Table 46–6). A study from the Netherlands showed that 12 months of intensive chemotherapy given to 32 children, 21 with stage IV NHL/T-ALL, produced an EFS of 72 percent at a median follow-up of 4.2 years, with the latest relapse occurring at 18 months from diagnosis.[50] The relatively short period between diagnosis and relapse in these protocols suggests that early, more intensive therapy, rather than more prolonged maintenance therapy, may be more efficacious. The Dutch authors suggested that drugs such as 6-mercaptopurine, low-dose MTX and corticosteroids, all of proven benefit in B-precursor disease, may not be the best drugs to use in T-cell disease. However, these drugs were part of the maintenance therapy of the successful BFM 90 protocol, although it is possible that the intensive reinduction courses were responsible for the good results seen.

All stage III and IV patients in the BFM study, as well as in POG 9404, received cranial irradiation, a point of some contention. The cranial radiation dose in the BFM studies was reduced to 1200 cGy in CNS-negative patients, 1800 cGy for CNS-positive patients between 1 and 2 years old, and 2400 cGy for CNS-positive patients over 2 years of age. The testicles were only irradiated for residual disease following high-dose MTX. Results of the SFOP study suggest that cranial radiation can successfully be replaced by intensive chemotherapy, including high-dose MTX. In the open CCG study for T-LL, which is based on the BFM 90, cranial irradiation will be eliminated except for CNS-positive patients, and the results will be compared retrospectively with the BFM results to attempt to ascertain the value of cranial radiation in this population.

The use of specific anti-T-cell therapy has been tested in recent POG studies. Compound 506U78 (2-amino-6-methoxypurine arabinoside), a prodrug of Ara-G, is toxic to T-lymphoblasts through the accumulation of Ara-G nucleotides, resulting in inhibition of ribonucleotide reductase and of DNA

Table 46–6. Outcome for Patients with Lymphoblastic Lymphoma

Protocol	Number	Stage	EFS (%)	Follow-up (no. of months)	Reference
LSA2L2	43	III/IV	70/63	> 25	Wollner et al.[45]
LSA2L2 / ADCOMP	281		74		
			64	60	Tubergen et al.[52]
POG 8704	218	III/IV	67	60	Amylon et al.[49]
LMT 81	76	III/IV	76		
	8	I/II	73	57	Patte et al.[46]
BFM 90	101	III/IV	90		
	4	I/II	100	60	Reiter et al.[38]
Dutch	32	III/IV/T-ALL	72	50	Van den Berg et al.[50]

EFS, event-free survival.

synthesis. In the POG phase 1 study, 506U78 produced 14 complete remissions and 9 partial remissions in 28 patients with refractory T-cell malignancies[51]; neurotoxicity was observed at higher doses. A new COG pilot study is testing the addition of 506U78 to a BFM backbone in high-risk patients with T-ALL.

Because of small patient numbers, the correct treatment for B-lineage LL has not been defined in pediatrics. Of 27 children with precursor B-cell LL who were treated in the BFM 86 and BFM 90 NHL trials, 21 received ALL-type therapy, with two relapses, and 6 received Burkitt-type therapy, with three relapsing, including two with localized disease.[53] This suggests that patients with B-lineage LL should be included on the T-cell protocols and treated for 18 to 24 months.

The findings of the Cooperative Group protocols may be summarized as follows:

1. Intensive ALL-type therapy results in overall survival of 90 percent in localized LL in most series.
2. BFM T-cell therapy improved EFS to 90 percent for both localized and advanced-stage T-LL.
3. High-dose MTX (5 g/m^2 per dose) for at least four doses appears to be important in T-LL.
4. L-Asparaginase therapy was shown to be important in POG studies.
5. Local radiation therapy is not indicated if adequate chemotherapy is given.
6. The need for prophylactic cranial irradiation remains controversial, but it may prove to be unnecessary at least for CNS-negative patients whose therapy includes steroids, intrathecal chemotherapy, and high-dose MTX.
7. The SFOP and BFM studies suggest that even in patients with testicular disease at diagnosis, testicular radiation is only indicated for residual disease after high-dose MTX.
8. The length of the maintenance therapy as well as the optimal maintenance drugs remains unclear, although more intensive "reintensification" courses may be more efficacious than prolonged low-dose maintenance therapy.
9. Specific anti-T-cell drugs such as 506U78 have proved efficacious in studies for patients with relapsed disease, but the significant neurotoxicity necessitates further study of this agent.

Large-Cell Lymphoma

The biologic heterogeneity of this subtype of NHL has made the determination of optimal therapy for this group of patients difficult. This is reflected in the fact that the POG studies have treated all advanced-stage LCL patients on the same chemotherapeutic protocols irrespective of subtype, whereas the European study groups as well as the Children's Cancer Group (CCG) have combined all B-cell lymphomas and treated B-cell large-cell and Burkitt's lymphoma on the same short, intensive protocols.

More recent POG studies for LCL have been based on the Dana-Farber Cancer Institute (DFCI) APO (Adriamycin, prednisone, Oncovin, 6-MP) regimen with no alkylating agents. Results from DFCI APO given for 24 months with cranial radiation showed a 76 percent EFS at 6 years for 28 patients, all stages, and all LCL subtypes.[54] In order to assess the effect of the addition of cyclophosphamide, POG 8615 compared APO to ACOP+, shortened the treatment time to 1 year, and eliminated involved-field and cranial radiation. No advantage for the addition of cyclophosphamide was found.[55] The most recent POG 9315 study (Table 46–7), reduced the dose of Adriamycin in APO by replacing it with standard-dose MTX when the cumulative dose reached 300 mg/m^2 and compared APO (without cranial radiation) to APO plus intermediate-dose MTX/Ara-C, given for a total period of 12 months. Although the data comparing the two treatment arms are too early to report, it has been noted that no significant difference in outcome between patients with B-cell large-cell and ALCL was found. In addition, there was no increase in the CNS relapse rate on the arm containing APO alone, with intrathecal MTX chemotherapy as the only CNS prophylaxis (J. Laver, Medical College of Virginia, Richmond, VA, personal communication).

Taking a completely different approach, the SFOP 56 and BFM groups[31,42] found that B-cell LCL patients have done well on the same short intensive protocols used for Burkitt's lymphoma. Patients with B-cell LCL appear to do well with either short, intensive alkylator-based therapy or longer, less intensive anthracycline/steroid-based therapy. However, short- and long-term toxicities vary. While anthracycline-based regimens may lead to more long-term cardiac problems, alkylator- or etoposide-intensive regimens may result in a greater risk of secondary leukemia. For example, comparison of the BFM 90 B-cell protocol with POG 9315 shows that the BFM 90 contains less steroid (0.15 g/m^2 compared to 30 g/m^2) and less anthracycline (150 mg/m^2 versus 300 mg/m^2) but significant amounts of alkylating agents (cyclophosphamide and ifosfamide), compared to none in the APO regimen. The duration of therapy is 12 weeks for BFM 90 compared to 12 months for APO, but with considerably more hospital admissions for toxicity during the 12 weeks of intensive therapy.

Table 46–7. Doxorubicin-Prednisone-Vincristine (APO) Protocol for Large-Cell Lymphoma (POG 9315)

Arm	Introduction	Maintenance[a]
APO	Doxorubicin, 75 mg/m^2, days 1 & 22	Doxorubicin 30 mg/m^2, day 1[b]
	Vincristine, 1.5 mg/m^2 weekly (×5)	Methotrexate 60 mg/m^2 day 1[b]
	Prednisone, 40 mg/m^2 daily for 28 days	Vincristine 1.5 mg/m^2 day 1
	IT methotrexate days 1,8,22	Prednisone 120 mg/m^2 days 1–5
		6-Mercaptopurine 225 mg/m^2 days 1–5
		IT Methotrexate day 1 (cycles 1–3 only)

[a] Maintenance cycles were given every 21 days for a total therapy of 1 year.
[b] Methotrexate substituted for doxorubicin when total dose of doxorubicin reached 300 mg/m^2.

Anaplastic Large-Cell Lymphoma

Since 1989 the SFOP group has treated all ALCL patients, irrespective of disease stage, according to specific protocols (HM89 and HM91). Only rare ALCL patients with leptomeningeal disease were excluded and treated on a protocol for CNS-positive B-cell lymphomas. There were 18 patients treated on HM89 and 64 on HM91. Treatment duration was 8 months and 7 months, respectively. No intrathecal therapy was given in either protocol and no patient relapsed first in the CNS. Event-free survival (at 3 years) was 94 percent for stage I and II and 55 percent for stage III and IV patients.[57] The BFM group allocated ALCL patients to the BFM B-cell protocol, using the standard-dose therapy for stages I, IIR (ABA) and II, III (ABABAB), but intensified the chemotherapy with the addition of an extra course containing high-dose Ara-C (CC) for stage IV ALCL (AABBCCAABBCC) (Figure 46–5). The best results in ALCL to date have been reported from this study, which resulted in a DFS of 83 percent at 2.5 years and a Kaplan-Meier estimation of a 9-year duration of EFS of 81 ± 5 percent. Relapses tended to occur with a mean time of 8 months after achieving remission.[31] The BFM study also showed that patients with skin-only ALCL did extremely well on this therapy, whereas in contrast those with skin involvement as part of a generalized ALCL had the worst prognosis (Table 46–8).

In an important related discovery, the SFOP showed that weekly vinblastine therapy alone or in various combinations with BCNU, bleomycin, and Ara-C had the ability to salvage relapsed patients with ALCL.[59] Overall, 35 of 40 evaluable patients (88 percent) achieved a second CR. The course after relapse was variable, however, and no statistical advantage to high-dose therapy was seen in ALCL patients in this series. Weekly vinblastine alone for 6 to 24 months (median 12) was administered to 13 patients, 4 at first relapse, 5 at second, 2 at third, and 2 at fifth, including 6 patients who relapsed post-ABMT. Of 11 patients 10 achieved complete remission with 8 still disease-free at a median follow-up period of 30 months.[59]

Studies from the International Consortium of Cooperative Groups, St Jude Children's Research Hospital, and the COG are all testing the efficacy of the addition of weekly vinblastine to standard chemotherapy protocols as front-line therapy for children with ALCL. The International Consortium is also testing the hypothesis that patients with skin-only ALCL may not need adjuvant chemotherapy.

Large-Cell Peripheral T-Cell Lymphomas of Post-Thymic Origin

Large-cell PTCL of post-thymic origin occurs rarely in childhood, and the optimal therapy for this group of patients is unknown. The BFM found that three of four patients treated on their T-NHL protocol relapsed and suggest that these patients should be treated on protocols designed for ALCL.[31] In a series from Gordon et al.,[60] most children with PTCL who relapsed achieved a second remission, and in contrast to ALCL, high-dose therapy with rescue appeared to improve chances of survival.

The Cooperative Group Trials suggest the following:

1. Patients with B-cell large-cell lymphomas do well on either a short intensive "Burkitt's lymphoma" regimen or a longer, less intensive regimen.
2. Children with T-cell or null-cell large-cell lymphomas (usually ALCL) require different therapy from B-cell large-cell patients. The most successful published protocol for ALCL to date is the BFM 90, with an 83 percent EFS projected to 9 years.
3. Central nervous system and bone marrow involvement is unusual in LCL, particularly in ALCL.
4. In the BFM and SFOP studies, intermediate- or high-dose MTX with (BFM) or without (SFOP) intrathecal therapy effectively prevents CNS relapse without cranial irradiation. Results from POG suggest that CNS relapse may be prevented with intrathecal chemotherapy alone.
5. Local radiotherapy appears to be of little value in LCL, even in bulk disease.
6. As in Burkitt's lymphoma, residual tumor after chemotherapy is usually necrotic, but should be confirmed following resection. If residual lymphoma is detected, salvage therapy rather than local radiation therapy is indicated.

Table 46–8. Treatment Outcome for Patients with Diffuse Large-Cell Lymphoma

Protocol	Number	Stage	EFS (%)	Follow-up (no. of months)	Reference
APO (DFCI)	28	I–IV	76	72	Weinstein et al.[54]
POG 8615					
ACOP	58	III/IV	66		
APO	62		75	60	Laver et al.[55]
CHOP	15	III/IV	58	79	Murphy et al.[61]
BFM 86	34	III/IV	75	60	Reiter and Riehm[4]
LSA2L2/LSA4	33	III/IV	60	60	Mora et al.[58]
			ALCL		
BFM 83/86/90	62	III/IV	83	30	Reiter et al.[31,42]
SFOP-LM 89,91	82	III/IV	55	49	Brugieres et al.[57]
LSA2L2/LSA4	19	III/IV	56	60	Mora et al.[58]
			OS 84		

Abbreviations: EFS, event-free survival; ALCL, anaplastic large-cell lymphoma.

7. Patients with ALCL and PTCL who relapse have high response rates to salvage chemotherapy.

8. New study group protocols are investigating the efficacy of the addition of weekly vinblastine to standard chemotherapy for ALCL, based on the successful SFOP salvage therapy results.

Future possibilities for improving survival include biology-based therapies such as anti-CD30 antibodies or inhibitors of the anaplastic lymphoma kinase protein function.

TREATMENT OF RELAPSED DISEASE

The prognosis for children with NHL has improved from a long-term survival under 30 percent in the early 1970s, to about 75 percent at present.[61] Children who relapse following modern protocols are difficult to cure, however, with the possible exception of ALCL patients. Most investigators are evaluating the efficacy of intensive conditioning regimens followed by autologous or allogeneic stem cell "rescue". Many different reinduction protocols have been used and typically include drugs not previously used for the primary therapy, such as cisplatin and carboplatinum. No standard reinduction therapy has consistently produced second complete remission CR rates of better than 60 percent however. Even relatively successful protocols, such as the POG ICE regimen, which resulted in a 71 percent complete plus partial rate in advanced stage III and IV relapsed NHL,[62] are much less likely to be effective for patients relapsing after more intensive alkylator-based protocols.

Most published reports have observed a 30 to 50 percent overall survival (OS) following high-dose therapy for patients with relapsed but chemosensitive disease or patients who continue to respond slowly to up-front therapy. Patients with resistant disease, however, have a long-term survival of less than 10 percent in most series.[63,64] A current challenge is to design more effective reinduction protocols, possibly by adding novel targeted therapies rather than intensified chemotherapy regimens.

The use of monoclonal antibodies targeted to specific antigens on the tumor cell, for example, have produced compelling results in the treatment of adult NHL. Published studies include a variety of antibodies, unlinked or linked to toxins such as ricin or to radioisotopes such as iodine-131 and ytrrium-90. Unlinked antibodies such as IDEC-C2B8 (Rituximab, anti-CD20) have been tried alone and together with standard chemotherapy. These combinations have been shown to be synergistic without adding significantly to toxicity.[65,66] In adult NHL, anti-CD20 monoclonal antibody is now well established as part of the therapy for low-grade follicular lymphoma. Doubts about its efficacy in higher-grade disease have been partially put to rest by Vose et al., who showed a significant improvement with the addition of Rituximab to CHOP chemotherapy in adult high-grade B-cell large-cell NHL.[66] The use of monoclonal antibodies has also been shown to be valuable for therapy of relapsed B-cell disease in adults, where good response rates have been obtained even in patients with resistant disease. It has also been demonstrated that adequate stem cell collections are possible following MAB therapy even when

linked to iodine-131 or ytrrium-90. Radioimmunoconjugates have been used in lower doses in nonmyeloablative fractionated treatments and in higher doses as part of myeloablative regimens with stem cell transplants, with both strategies reporting impressive response rates.[67]

In post-transplant lymphoproliferative disease, several studies involving adults and children have shown a response rate of approximately 60 percent to anti-CD20.[68,69] In a single study from the Netherlands, Rituximab produced two CRs in three children with relapsed Burkitt's lymphoma.[70] Strategies utilizing various linked and unlinked anti-B monoclonal antibodies, as well as specific anti-T-cell therapy such as 506U78, have only recently been initiated in pediatric NHL.

Conditioning regimens for transplantation have varied, with the commonest being BACT (BCNU, Ara-C, cyclophosphamide, and 6-thioguanine,[71] BEAM (BCNU, etoposide, Ara-C, and melphalan) and more recently, CBV (cyclophosphamide, BCNU, and VP-16). A lower toxicity is seen with BEAM than with BACT. The dose-limiting toxicity of CBV appears to be pulmonary toxicity from the BCNU. Total body irradiation (TBI) as part of the conditioning regimen has been associated with significant toxicity (such as radiation pneumonitis) in patients who had previously received radiation (a minority of patients with NHL treated on modern protocols). The value of TBI versus non-TBI regimens remains controversial.[72]

An advantage to the use of allogeneic over autologous transplantation for T-lymphoblastic lymphoma has been demonstrated,[73] suggesting that allogeneic transplantation for T-lymphoblastic and Burkitt's lymphoma, provided a matched sibling donor is available, may be preferable. Attempts to reduce the transplantation-related mortality of allogeneic transplants, while maintaining the graft-versus-lymphoma effect, have led to the development of nonmyeloablative stem cell transplants in conjunction with donor lymphocyte infusions (DLI).[74] Although exciting in concept, these are as yet unproven therapeutic strategies.

Another potentially important approach involves post-transplantation "minimal residual disease" therapy, utilizing therapy aimed at increasing the host's immune response to residual lymphoma cells, or alternatively, using novel targeted antilymphoma therapies. Several studies in adults with relapsed B-cell NHL have demonstrated that anti-CD20 monoclonal antibody is well tolerated when given after transplantation.[75] Because of the small number of relapsed pediatric NHL patients and the number of variables involved, attempts to design and carry out rational prospective trials of high-dose therapy in patients with relapsed disease has proved to be difficult.

THE FUTURE

It is unlikely that continued intensification of chemotherapy will achieve further major improvement in responses, although modifications currently being evaluated may improve survival by decreasing therapy-related toxicity. The advent of therapies targeted either to specific molecules on the malignant cell surface membrane or to specific fusion proteins resulting from

Table 46–9. Characteristics of the Three Major Pediatric Non-Hodgkin's Lymphomas

	Burkitt's (sporadic) 50%	Lymphoblastic 30–40%	Large-Cell 15–25%
Grade	High	High	Most high, occasionally intermediate (B-large cell with sclerosis)
Genetics	t(8;14) (80%) t(8;22) t(2;8)	TAL1 overexpression t(10;14),t(1;14) t(11;14) *mts-1* inactivation	ALCL -t(2;5) majority -t(1;2) occ B Large cell bcl-6 (30%)
Immunophenotype	Mature B-cell	Immature T-cell (80%) B-precursor (20%)	Large-cell B: B-cell ALCL: mature T-cell, null Peripheral T-cell (rare)
Site	Abdominal (90%) Pharyngeal (10%)	T-LL: anterior mediastinal supradiaphragmatic nodes B-LL: unusual sites	Large-cell: abdomen, mediastinum, any node ALCL: nodes, skin, bone, lung
Spread	Bone marrow + + CNS + +	Bone marrow + + CNS +	Bone marrow uncommon CNS uncommon
Overall survival Localized Advanced	Over 90% Over 80%	Over 90% 65–80%	Over 90% 65–80%

ALCL, anaplastic large-cell lymphoma.

chromosomal translocations has added an exciting new dimension to future therapeutic strategies.

The survival of children with NHL of all three subtypes (Table 46–9) has dramatically improved, so that the majority of pediatric patients with lymphoma can now be cured. Several important challenges remain. These include reduction of chemotherapy- and radiation-induced toxicity without sacrificing cure rates, identification of new prognostic factors that will allow therapy to be tailored to specific risk groups, and development of effective treatment for patients who have resistant disease despite modern intensive protocols. Finally, the importance of obtaining tissue and serum for biology studies so as to facilitate the development of more effective therapies aimed at tumor-specific targets cannot be overemphasized.

REFERENCES

1. Sandlund JT, Downing JR, Crist WM: Non-Hodgkin's lymphoma in childhood. N Engl J Med 334:1238–1248, 1996.
2. Murphy SB: Classification, staging and end results of treatment of childhood non-Hodgkin's lymphomas: Dissimilarities from lymphomas in adults. Semin Oncol 7:332–8, 1990.
3. Magrath IT: Concepts and controversies in lymphoid neoplasia. In Magrath IT (ed.): The Non-Hodgkin's Lymphomas 2nd Ed., pp. 3–46, Arnold, London, 1997.
4. Reiter A, Riehm H-J: Large cell lymphomas in children. In Magrath IT (ed.): The Non-Hodgkin's Lymphomas. 2nd Ed., pp. 829–851, Arnold, London, 1997.
5. Parkin DM, Stiller CA, Draper, GJ, Bieber CA: The international incidence of childhood cancer. Int J Cancer 42:511–20, 1988.
6. Evans JA, Gibb DM, Holland FJ et al: Malignancies in UK children with HIV infection acquired from mother to child transmission. Arch Dis Child 76:330–333, 1997.
7. Ziegler JL: Biologic differences in acquired immune deficiency syndrome-associated non-Hodgkin's lymphoma. J Clin Oncol 9:1329–1331, 1991.
8. Tao Q, Robertson AM, Hildesheim A, Ambinder RF: Epstein-Barr virus (EBV) in endemic Burkitt lymphoma: Molecular analysis of primary tumor tissue. Blood 91:1373–81, 1998.
9. Razzouk BL, Srinivas S, Sample CE et al: Epstein-Barr virus DNA recombination and loss in sporadic Burkitt lymphoma. J Infect Dis 173:529–535, 1996.
10. Magrath IT: Malignant non-Hodgkin's lymphoma. In Pizzo PA, Poplack DG (eds.): Principles and Practices of Pediatric Oncology, pp. 415–55. JB Lippincott, Philadelphia, 1989.
11. Harris NL, Jaffe ES, Stein H, Banks PM, Chan JKC et al: A revised European-American classification of lymphoid neoplasms: A proposal from the International Lymphoma Study Group. Blood 84:1361–92, 1994.
12. Jaffe ES, Harris NL, Diebold J, Muller-Hermelink HK: World Health Organization classification of neoplastic diseases of the hematopoietic and lymphoid tissues: A progress report. Am J Clin Pathol 111(Suppl. 1):S8–12, 1999.
13. Perkins SL, Segal GH, Kjeldsberg CR: Classification of non-Hodgkin's lymphomas in children. Semin Diagn Pathol 12:303–13, 1995.
14. Rezuke WN, Abernathy EC, Tsongalis GJ: Molecular diagnosis of B- and T-cell lymphomas: Fundamental principles and clinical applications. Clin Chem 43:1814–1823, 1997.
15. Goust MJ, Jackson A: Lymphocyte ontogeny and membrane markers. Immunol Ser 58:161–186, 1993.
16. Frizzera G, Murphy SB: Follicular (nodular) lymphoma in childhood: A rare clinical pathologic entity. Report of eight cases from four cancer centers. Cancer 44:2218–2235, 1979.
17. Goldsby RE, Carroll WL: The molecular basis of pediatric lymphomas. Pediatr Hematol Oncol 20:282–296, 1998.
18. Kelly DR, Nathwani BN, Rogers DG et al: A morphologic study of childhood lymphoma of the undifferentiated type: The Pediatric Oncology Group experience. Cancer 59:1132–37, 1987.
19. Wilson JF, Kjeldsberg CR, Sposto R et al: The pathology of non-Hodgkin's lymphoma of childhood: Reproducibility and relevance of the histologic classification of "undifferentiated" lymphomas (Burkitt vs. non-Burkitt). Hum Pathol 18:1008–1014, 1987.

20. Sandlund JT, Magrath IT: Lymphoblastic lymphoma. In Magrath IT (ed.): The Non-Hodgkin's Lymphomas 2nd ed., pp. 813–828, Arnold, London, 1997.

21. Weiss LM, Bindl JM, Picozzi VJ, Link MP, Warnke RA: Lymphoblastic lymphoma: An immunophenotype study of 26 cases with comparison to T cell acute lymphoblastic leukemia. Blood 67:474–478, 1986.

22. Nadali G, Vinante F, Stein H et al: Serum levels of the soluble form of CD30 molecule as a tumor marker in CD30+ anaplastic large cell lymphoma. J Clin Oncol 13:1355–1360, 1995.

23. Massimino M, Gasparini M, Giardini R: Ki-1 (CD30) anaplastic large-cell lymphoma in children. Ann Oncol 6:915–920, 1995.

24. Pui C-H, Behm FG, Crist WM: Clinical and biologic relevance of immunologic marker studies in childhood acute lymphoblastic leukemia. Blood 82:343–362, 1993.

25. Gascoyne R, Adomat S, Krajewski S et al: Prognostic significance of bcl-2 protein expression and Bcl-2 gene rearrangement in diffuse aggressive non-Hodgkin's lymphoma. Blood 90:244–51, 1997.

26. Hwang LY, Baer RJ: The role of chromosome translocations in T cell acute leukemia. Curr Opin Immunol 7:659–64, 1995.

27. Ziegler JL: Burkitt lymphoma. J Natl Cancer Inst 305:735–45, 1981.

28. Reiter A, Schrappe M, Tiemann M et al: Successful treatment strategy for Ki-1 anaplastic large-cell lymphoma of childhood: A prospective analysis of patients enrolled in three consecutive Berlin-Frankfurt-Münster group studies. J Clin Oncol 12:899–908, 1994.

29. Mouratidis B, Gilday DL, Ash JM: Comparisons of bone and ^{67}Ga scintigraphy in the diagnosis of bone involvement in children with malignant lymphoma. Nucl Med Commun 15:144–147, 1994.

30. Büyükpamukçu M: Non-Hodgkin's lymphomas. In Voute PA, Kalifa C, Barrett A (eds.): Cancer in Children, Clinical Management 4th Ed. pp. 119–136. Oxford University Press, New York, 1998.

31. Reiter A, Schrappe M, Parwarescl R et al: Non-Hodgkin's lymphoma of childhood and adolescence: Results of a treatment stratified for biological subtype and stage – a report of the BFM group. J Clin Oncol 13:359–372, 1995.

32. Shad A, Magrath I: Malignant non-Hodgkin's lymphomas in children. In Pizzo PA, Poplack DG (eds.): Principles and Practice of Pediatric Oncology 3rd Ed., pp. 545–587. Lippincott-Raven, Philadelphia, 1997.

33. Norin T, Clifford P, Einhorn J et al: Radiotherapy in Burkitt lymphoma. Conventional or superfractionated radiation therapy in Burkitt lymphoma. Acta Radiol 10:545–547, 1971.

34. Pilecki B, Kopiec P, Zajusz A et al: Hyperfractionated radiotherapy for Burkitt-type lymphoma. Radiobiological aspects. Neoplasma 38:609–615, 1991.

35. Veenstra J, Krediet RT, Somers R et al: Tumor lysis syndrome and acute renal failure in Burkitt lymphoma. Description of 2 cases and review of the literature on prevention and management. Neth J Med 45:211–216, 1994.

36. Pui CH, Relling MV, Lascombes F et al: Urate oxidase in prevention and treatment of hyperuricemia associated with lymphoid malignancies. Leukemia 11:1813–1816, 1997.

37. Link MP, Shuster JJ, Donaldson SS et al: Treatment of children and young adults with early stage non-Hodgkin's lymphoma. N Engl J Med 337:1259–66, 1997.

38. Reiter A, Schrappe M, Ludwig WD et al: Intensive ALL-type therapy without local radiotherapy provides a 90% event-free survival for children with T-cell lymphoblastic lymphoma: A BFM Group report. Blood 95:416–421, 2000.

39. Schwenn MH, Mahmoud HH, Bowman WP et al: Successful treatment of small noncleaved cell (SNCC) lymphoma and B-cell acute lymphoblastic leukemia (B-ALL) with central nervous system

(CNS) involvement: A Pediatric Oncology Group (POG) study. Proc Am Soc Clin Oncol 19:A2282, 2000.

40. Griffin T, Mahmoud H, Weitzman S et al: Results of a pilot study of dose intensification of methotrexate and cyclophosphamide (CP) in patients with advanced stage (III/IV) small non cleaved cell non-Hodgkin's lymphoma and B-cell ALL. A Pediatric Oncology Group study. Blood 95:A580, 2000.

41. Patte C, Auperin A, Michon J et al: The Societé Française d'Oncologie Pédiatrique LMB89 protocol: Highly effective multiagent chemotherapy tailored to the tumor burden and initial response in 561 unselected children with B-cell lymphomas and L3 leukemia. Blood 97:3370–3379, 2001.

42. Reiter A, Schrappe M, Tiemann M et al: Improved results in childhood B-cell neoplasms with tailored intensification of therapy: A report of the Berlin-Frankfurt-Münster Group Trial NHL-BFM 90. Blood 94:3294–3306, 1999.

43. Magrath I, Adde M, Shad A et al: Adults and children with small non-cleaved-cell lymphoma have a similar excellent outcome when treated with the same chemotherapy regimen. J Clin Oncol 14:925–934, 1996.

44. Yaniv I, Fischer S, Mor C et al: Improved outcome in childhood B-cell lymphoma with the intensified French LMB protocol. Med Pediatr Oncol 35:8–12, 2000.

45. Wollner N, Burchenal JH, Lieberman PH et al: Non-Hodgkin's lymphoma in children: A comparative study of two modalities of therapy. Cancer 37:123–134, 1976.

46. Patte C, Kalifa C, Flamant F et al: Results of the LMT81 protocol, a modified LSA2L2 protocol with high dose methotrexate on 84 children with non-B-cell (lymphoblastic) lymphoma. Med Pediatr Oncol 20:105–113, 1992.

47. Schrappe M, Tiemann M, Ludwig WD et al: Risk adapted therapy for lymphoblastic T-cell lymphoma: Results from trials NHL-BFM 86 and 90. Med Pediatr Oncol 29:356–357, 1997.

48. Masson E, Relling MV, Synold TW et al: Accumulation of methotrexate polyglutamates in lymphoblasts is a determinant of antileukemic effects in vivo. A rationale for high-dose methotrexate. J Clin Invest 97:73–80, 1996.

49. Amylon M, Shuster J, Pullen J et al: Intensive high-dose asparaginase consolidation improves survival for pediatric patients with T-cell acute lymphoblastic leukemia and advanced stage lymphoblastic lymphoma: A Pediatric Oncology Group study. Leukemia 13:335–342, 1999.

50. van den Berg H, Zsiros J, Veneberg A et al: Favorable outcome after 1-year treatment of childhood T-cell lymphoma/T-cell acute lymphoblastic leukemia. Med Pediatr Oncol 30:46–51, 1998.

51. Kurtzberg J, Keating MJ, Plunkett W et al: Compound 506U78 (2-amino-6-methoxypurine arabinoside) is active against resistant T-cell malignancy: Preliminary results of an ongoing phase I trial. Proc Am Soc Clin Oncol 15:A108, 1996.

52. Tubegren DG, Krailo MD, Meadows AT et al: Comparison of treatment regimens for pediatric lymphoblastic non-Hodgkin's lymphoma: A Children's Cancer Group study. J Clin Oncol 13:1368–1376, 1995.

53. Neth O, Seidemann K, Jansen P et al: Precursor B-cell lymphoblastic lymphoma in childhood and adolescence: Clinical features, treatment, and results in trials NHL-BFM 86 and 90. Med Pediatr Oncol 35:20–27, 2000.

54. Weinstein HJ, Lack EE, Cassady RJ: APO therapy for malignant lymphoma of large cell "histiocytic" type of childhood: Analysis of treatment results for 29 patients. Blood 64:422–426, 1984.

55. Laver JH, Mahmoud H, Pick TE et al: Results of a randomized phase III trial in children and adolescents with advanced stage dif-

fuse large cell non-Hodgkin's lymphoma: A Pediatric Oncology Group study. (Submitted for publication.)

56. Patte C, Leverger G, Michon J et al: High survival rate of childhood B-cell lymphoma and leukemia (ALL) as result of the LMB89 protocol of the SFOP. Fifth International Conference on Malignant Lymphoma, Lugano, Switzerland, 1993.

57. Brugières L, Le Deley MC, Pacquement H et al: CD30+ anaplastic large-cell lymphoma in children: Analysis of 82 patients enrolled in 2 consecutive studies of the French Society of Pediatric Oncology. Blood 92:3591–3598, 1998.

58. Mora J, Filippa DA, Thaler HT et al: Large cell non-Hodgkin's lymphoma of childhood. Analysis of 78 consecutive patients enrolled in 2 consecutive protocols at the Memorial Sloan-Kettering Cancer Center. Cancer 88:186–197, 2000.

59. Brugières L, Quartier P, Le Deley MC et al: Relapses of childhood anaplastic large-cell lymphoma: Treatment results in a series of 41 children – a report from the French Society of Pediatric Oncology. Ann Oncol 11:53–58, 2000.

60. Gordon BG, Warkentin PI, Weisenburger DD et al: Bone marrow transplantation for peripheral T-cell lymphoma in children and adolescents. Blood 80:2938–2942, 1992.

61. Murphy SB, Fairclough DL, Hutchinson RE, Berard CW: Non-Hodgkin's lymphoma: An analysis of the histology, staging and response to treatment of 338 cases at a single institution. J Clin Oncol 7:186–93, 1989.

62. Kung FH, Harris MB, Krischer JP: Ifosfamide/carboplatinum/etoposide (ICE) an effective salvaging therapy for recurrent malignant non-Hodgkin's lymphoma of childhood. A Pediatric Oncology Group phase II study. Med Pediatr Oncol 32:225–226, 1999.

63. Colombat P, Gorin N-C, Lemonnier M-P et al: The role of autologous bone marrow transplantation in 46 adult patients with non-Hodgkin's lymphomas. J Clin Oncol 8:630–637, 1990.

64. Gulati S, Yahalom J, Acaba L et al: Treatment of patients with relapsed and resistant non-Hodgkin's lymphoma using total body irradiation, etoposide, and cyclophosphamide and autologous bone marrow transplantation. J Clin Oncol 10:936–941, 1992.

65. Coiffie B, Haiuon C, Ketterer N et al: Rituximab for the treatment of patients with relapsing or refractory lymphoma: A multicenter phase II study. Blood 92:1927–1932, 1998.

66. Vose JM, Link BK, Grossbard M et al: Phase II study of Rituxomab in combination with CHOP chemotherapy in patients with previously untreated aggressive non-Hodgkin's lymphoma. J Clin Oncol 19:389–397, 2001.

67. Illidge TM, Cragg MS, McBride HM et al: The importance of antibody-specificity in determining successful radioimmunotherapy of B-cell lymphoma. Blood 94:233–243, 1999.

68. Faye A, Quartier P, Lutz P et al: Anti-CD20 monoclonal antibody in the treatment of post transplant lymphoproliferative disorders (PTLD) occurring after bone marrow transplantation (BMT) in children. Blood 95(Suppl.):A2842, 2000.

69. Milpied N, Vasseur B, Parquet N et al: Humanized anti-CD20 monoclonal antibody (Rituximab) in post transplant B-lymphoproliferative disorder: A retrospective analysis on 32 patients. Ann Oncol 11(Suppl. 1):113–6, 2000.

70. Nuijens JH, Van Der Schoot CE, Kardos G, Zwaan CM: Rituximab in the treatment of childhood B-ALL and Burkitt lymphoma: A report on 3 cases. Blood (Suppl.)269b, 1999.

71. Philip T, Armitage JO, Spitzer G et al: High dose therapy and autologous bone marrow transplantation after failure of conventional chemotherapy in adults with intermediate-grade or high grade non-Hodgkin's lymphoma. N Engl J Med 316:1493–1498, 1987.

72. Vose JM, Armitage JO: Bone marrow transplantation for non-Hodgkin's lymphoma. In Magrath IT (Ed): Non-Hodgkin's Lymphoma, 2nd Ed., pp. 723–737. Arnold, London, 1997.

73. Chopra R, Goldstone AH, Pearce R et al: Autologous versus allogeneic bone marrow transplantation for non-Hodgkin's lymphoma: A case controlled analysis of the European Bone Marrow Transplant Group Registry data. J Clin Oncol 4:1470–1480, 1986.

74. Slavins, Nagler A, Naparstek E et al: Nonmyeloablative stem cell transplantation and cell therapy as an alternative to conventional bone marrow transplantation with lethal cytoreduction for the treatment of malignant and non-malignant hematologic diseases. Blood 91:756–763, 1998.

75. Ballester OF, Fang T, Wilcox P et al: Rituximab associated cardiotoxicity in patients treated with high dose therapy and autologous stem cell transplantation. Blood 94(Suppl.):354b, 1999.

47

Lymphoma in Other Diseases

Barbara K. Dunn and Dan L. Longo

When lymphomas occur in association with other diseases, usually the underlying disease or its treatment produces immunodysregulation.[441] In most cases, this immune dysfunction takes the form of immunodeficiency, which can result from either inherited or acquired defects. Such acquired immunodeficiencies may be associated with infectious diseases, most commonly viral infections,[596] transplants with intentional iatrogenic immunosuppression,[565,566,576] and chemical environmental agents.[541,826] However, in the autoimmune disorders, a different set of mechanisms are operative, since affected individuals demonstrate hyperactivity of the immune system.

In the United States in the year 2000, the non-Hodgkin's lymphomas comprised 4 to 5 percent of new cancers and caused 5 percent of cancer-related deaths.[252] The incidence of non-Hodgkin's lymphoma has been slowly increasing over the past two and a half decades, showing roughly a 3 to 4 percent annual increase since the early 1970s.[56,159,160,252,361] A fraction of this increase can be traced to specific disease settings that are associated with an increased risk of non-Hodgkin's lymphomas.[440,541] For example, prolonged survival of genetically immunodeficient individuals as a result of improved health care delivery has allowed the emergence of lymphomas.[541,612] Iatrogenic immunosuppression that is implemented in the setting of transplantation has led to an increase in Epstein-Barr virus (EBV)-related lymphomas.[541,571–573] The acquired immunodeficiency syndrome (AIDS) population, which is now living longer as a result of antiretroviral therapy, has shown an increasing incidence of lymphomas.[483,583] In fact, certain projections estimate that up to 27 percent of all non-Hodgkin's lymphoma cases in the United States will arise in the context of human immunodeficiency virus (HIV) infection.[224] Despite the contribution of these immunosuppressed states to the rising incidence of lymphoma, about 80 percent of the increase remains unexplained.[294]

The lymphomas that occur in the setting of immunologic suppression share a number of clinical features. They tend to be aggressive histologically as well as in advanced stage at presentation.[361,420,434,565,566] Extranodal sites are affected in a high proportion of cases, particularly the bone marrow, central nervous system (CNS), and gastrointestinal (GI) tract.[420,434,510,572,577,578] These lymphomas often occur in association with EBV infection.[286,289,434,593] The prognosis is often influenced by the underlying immunodeficiency.[146,420,565]

These lymphomas share common pathogenetic mechanisms. Cancer results from a multistep process in which a hierarchy of events impinge on the normal control of cell growth.[138,737] This multistep progression of biologic changes that leads to cancer centers around the accumulation of discrete genetic alterations that provides the basis for the transition from normal to premalignant to malignant lesions.[118,198,376,767] Genetic changes that occur early in this progression may stimulate cellular proliferation, resulting in hyperplasia.[193] Subsequent genetic changes result in cellular morphologic atypia visible microscopically as dysplasia and then on to invasion, neovascular formation, and spread characteristic of malignancy.

The vast majority of secondary lymphomas are of B-cell origin. Lymphomagenesis is not precisely defined at the genetic level in any lymphoma. However, the overall outlines of the process have been proposed. Specifically, three key components intersect in the multistep process of lymphomagenesis: 1. Polyclonal proliferation of B cells occurs secondary to an initiating insult such as EBV infection[576,678]; 2. the benign, or premalignant, but extensive B-cell hyperplasia that results from this initial insult then leads to secondary changes, increasing the chance of acquiring critical genetic alterations that further disrupt the control of cell growth. These include inherited enzyme defects that temporally would have preceded B-cell proliferation, as well as oncogene activation and chromosomal translocations[235]; 3. finally, the inherent immune deficiency leads to a failure of immune surveillance, allowing the abnormal cell growth of occasional clones to proceed unchecked.[61,626] The result is ultimately a monoclonal or oligoclonal cellular proliferation that constitutes the observed lymphoma.

INFECTIOUS AGENTS IN THE ETIOLOGY OF LYMPHOMAS

An increased incidence of lymphomas occurs in specific infections. Although most commonly viral in origin, bacteria such as *Helicobacter pylori* have been implicated in the pathogenesis of specific lymphomas.[549]

Viruses

Lymphotropic viruses may play an etiological role in the development of lymphoma. Viral infection may lead to increased cellular proliferation in combination with impairment of the immune system, which together provide the basic biologic components for viral tumorigenesis.[596] A variety of mechanisms have been demonstrated by which both retroviruses and DNA viruses may disrupt the normal regulation and expression of cellular oncogenes and suppressor genes.[138,270,387,737] The viral insult is only one of a series of events that lead, after a latent period, to frank cancer.

Epstein-Barr Virus

EBV is a transforming DNA virus that primarily targets human B lymphocytes. In a context of immune impairment, abnormal responses to this viral pathogen may occur that allow the development of EBV-induced lymphocyte proliferation.[434] Thus, as will be discussed below, EBV appears to be involved in lymphomagenesis in the settings of AIDS, iatrogenic immunosuppression for organ transplants, and inherited immunodeficiency diseases such as X-linked lymphoproliferative disease and ataxia-telangiectasia.[36,76,127,324,366,540]

Pathogenesis: Molecular Basis for Lymphomagenesis. EBV biology. Both oro- and nasopharyngeal epithelial cells as well as B lymphocytes contain the surface receptor for EBV, CR 2/CD21,[366,434,449,481,512,540,741] which is closely related to the receptor for the C3d component of complement.[45] Both cell types constitute susceptible targets for EBV. Infection with EBV is usually spread through oropharyngeal secretions and the virus remains lifelong in the pharynx where it is shed periodically.[105,289] Furthermore, EBV DNA and RNA have been demonstrated in oropharyngeal cells of patients with infectious mononucleosis.[686] Such observations led to the view that the oropharyngeal cells were the primary site of infection, with the proximal lymphoid tissues such as Waldeyer's ring being only secondarily infected.[473,528,741] However, more recent data, such as the demonstration in a few cases of EBV-positive cells in isolated germinal centers, have led to the conflicting, but current, view that EBV initially targets B cells located in pharyngeal lymphoid tissues.[15,76,324,521] The primary infection of B cells leads to a rapid expansion of EBV-infected lymphocytes that resembles that seen in EBV-immortalized lymphoblastoid cell lines. A potent EBV-specific cytotoxic T-cell response follows, and the virus establishes a life-long latent infection in the B-cell compartment, inhabiting 1 in 10^5 to 10^6 circulating cells.[324] Although the emphasis has been on EBV infection of B cells, the EBV receptor CD21 is also expressed on some T cells,[754] explaining both the ability of T cells to be infected with EBV[388,685,781,821] and the occasional clinical observation of EBV in T-cell malignancies.[309,328,350,392,476,539,714]

EBV exhibits two alternative modes of interaction with its target cells: 1. a productive, cytolytic infection involving high copy numbers of a linear double-stranded form of the EBV DNA genome and 2. a nonproductive, latent infection in which a circularized EBV genome replicates episomally in low copy number and promotes immortalization (i.e., transformation or indefinite cell growth).[127,289,434,473] Of the 100 or so genes that make up the EBV genome, only specific subsets of genes are expressed during latent infection of EBV-immortalized cells. These include six EBV nuclear antigens (EBNA-1, -2, -3A, -3B, -3C, leader protein [LP]), three latent membrane proteins (LMP-1, -2A, -2B), and two abundant nonpolyadenylated nontranslated small RNAs (EBER-1 and EBER-2); six of these (EBNA-1, -2, -3A, and -3C; LMP-1; and LP) are required for immortalization, whereas two (LMP-2A and -2B) are believed to maintain EBV latency.[7,36,76,282,452,453,684]

At least three types of latency have been demonstrated, each of which is characterized by a specific array of latent gene expression.[279,280,324,610,679,821] Furthermore, the different histological types of EBV-related lymphomas tend to fall into specific latency types. EBNA-1 is expressed in all the latency types and is the only viral protein expressed in type I latency (Lat I). Burkitt's lymphoma, whether endemic or AIDS-related (see below), generally displays a Lat I phenotype.[610,630] Type II latency (Lat II) includes expression of the LMPs in addition to the ubiquitously expressed EBNA-1, and type III latency (Lat III) involves expression of all the latent viral proteins. The two small RNAs (EBER-1 and EBER-2) are expressed in all three latency types. The Lat II subtype has been described in a subset of Burkitt's lymphomas as well as in Hodgkin's disease,[149] nasopharyngeal carcinoma,[75] and T-cell tumors.[476] AIDS-related large cell and immunoblastic lymphomas have been shown to fall into all three latency categories. The different latency types demonstrate clear differences in their ability to grow under suboptimal culture conditions.[255,298] In addition, immortalized cells expressing fewer of the latent genes (*Lat I*) may be more easily activated into the lytic cycle by expression of the appropriate EBV gene products such as ZEBRA (ZEBRA is encoded by the open reading frame of the *BZLF-1* gene), giving rise to the production of new virons.[172,261,596,610,741]

Two distinct types of EBV isolates, type 1 and type 2, have been described, each of which is subdivided into multiple strains.[36,814] These strains are distinguished by polymorphisms in the latent genes encoding the nuclear antigens EBNA-2, -3A, -3B, and -3C and the EBER genes. EBV type 1 has a greater transforming capacity and is the predominant type (90 percent) in lymphocytes of EBV-infected individuals. While healthy virus carriers were believed to harbor a single virus strain,[374,812] 90 percent being type 1, more recent data have revealed the coexistence of multiple strains, and even both types 1 and 2, in immunocompetent individuals.[704] Immunocompromised individuals, including members of male homosexual and hemophiliac cohorts infected with HIV, often harbor multiple viral strains, both of the same type (usually type 1) and of different types, type 1 and type 2.[813,814] EBV type 2, which is relatively rare in the healthy Caucasian population, is observed in over 30 percent of HIV-positive male homosexuals but only 10 percent of HIV-infected hemophiliac individuals.[814] Individual EBV type 1 strains do not appear to be restricted to specific EBV-associated diseases or tumor types.[659] Nevertheless, certain polymorphisms of latent genes have been associated with specific clinical presentations. For example, the 3′-terminal of the *LMP-1* gene, a region that frequently contains mutations,[381] has a characteristic 30-base pair deletion in nasal T/NK-cell lymphomas in a Chinese population[113] and a 69-base pair deletion that is found in Burkitt's lymphoma of Turkish children.[728] However, these associations are believed to reflect the most prevalent circulating EBV strains in the population, rather than the disease presentation.[374] This view is supported by the appearance of identical variant strains in other EBV-associated diseases, such as nasopharyngeal carcinoma and peripheral T-cell lymphomas, as well as in healthy virus carriers in the same populations.[113,374,640] Specific EBV antigen polymorphisms have also been shown to correlate with oncogenic potential in cell culture.[381,382] However, this suggested correlation between viral strain and tumor aggressiveness has not been substantiated in vivo.[76,374]

The contribution of the EBV antigens to cellular transformation is complex. EBNA-1, a phosphoprotein that binds to both viral DNA and RNA,[693] maintains the EBV genome as an extrachromosomal plasmid in immortalized cells,[817] and may function to repress the lytic cycle.[434,596] If EBNA-1 protein expression in EBV-immortalized lymphoblastoid cells is suppressed by exposure to EBNA-1 antisense oligodeoxynucleotide, cell proliferation is inhibited.[628]

EBNA-2 counters transcriptional repression by interacting with the inhibitory transcription factor CBF1/RBP-Jκ, thereby converting it into a positive transcription regulator.[201,299,322,452,487,775] EBNA-2 also transcriptionally activates expression of LMP-1 in human B cells.[192,404,684] LMP-1, in turn, may contribute to lymphomagenesis through a variety of mechanisms. LMP-1 activates both the AP-1 and NF-κB transcription factors.[382,452] NF-κB has been shown to protect cells against apoptosis,[201,255,260,298,777] possibly through Bcl-2 protein expression,[87,201,777] and to promote cell transformation.[487,809] LMP-1 also leads to the loss of transforming growth factor (TGF)-β1-mediated growth inhibition, to induction of cyclin D2 expression, and to pRb hyperphosphorylation in B cells,[24] all of which are associated with increased progression through the cell cycle. In addition, an association between specific mutational hot spots in the EBV BNLF-1 gene that encodes the LMP-1 protein and various lymphoproliferative disorders (e.g., Hodgkin's disease, angioimmunoblastic lymphadenopathy, B-immunoblastic lymphoma, peripheral T-cell lymphoma) has been demonstrated.[381,640] EBNA-2 and LMP-1 appear to act synergistically in B-cell transformation and proliferation.[126,280,282,778,779] EBNA-2 also transcriptionally activates EBNA-3A, which, in turn, is essential for initiation of B-cell immortalization. EBNA-3C also is necessary for immortalization.[452] It has been shown to activate the promoter of the B-MYB oncogene, reflecting progression to the S-phase of the cell cycle. EBNA-3C also cooperates with Ha-RAS oncogene to transform primary rat embryo fibroblasts.[452,546]

The role of EBV in the multistep process of lymphomagenesis may be to provide the initiating insult. The ability of EBV to infect cells latently and to immortalize them leads to expansion of the affected B-lymphocyte population. On the one hand, expansion results from actual polyclonal growth stimulation of B lymphocytes by EBV, which is initiated by the binding of EBV to its B-cell receptor CR2/CD21.[741] Such B-cell activation appears to be an underlying mechanism in infectious mononucleosis, Burkitt's lymphoma, and the lymphomas that occur in immunodeficiency.[473,663] On the other hand, EBV has been shown to prolong survival of existing lymphocytes under suboptimal conditions where growth is inhibited. Burkitt's lymphoma cells belonging to Lat I type, which express only the EBNA-1 latent protein, are vulnerable to the induction of death by apoptosis (programmed cell death). In contrast, isogenic Burkitt's lymphoma cell clones of the Lat III type, in which all eight EBV latency proteins are activated, exhibit an increase in viability secondary to suppression of apoptosis.[255] If an EBV-negative Burkitt's lymphoma cell line that is sensitive to apoptosis-inducing drugs is latently infected with EBV, these cells are now protected from apoptosis, apparently as a result of inactivation of the G2/M cell cycle checkpoint.[770] The antiapoptotic effect of EBV may be mediated by nitric oxide, a product of nitric oxide synthase that is constitutively expressed in human EBV-infected lymphoblastoid and Burkitt's lymphoma

cell lines.[454] As described above, inhibition of apoptosis may also result from upregulation of the BCL-2 gene,[201,777] which is induced by the EBV latent protein LMP-1.[255,298] In addition, BHRF-1, an EBV gene with homology to the human anti-apoptotic BCL-2 gene, appears to be upregulated in EBV-associated lymphomas, although the data are not consistent.[496,539] The combined outcome of increased cell growth and increased cell survival leads to the B-cell proliferations that characterize EBV infection.

Host response. The normal host displays cellular mechanisms that limit the number of virally transformed B lymphocytes. Healthy, immunocompetent EBV-seropositive individuals maintain a vigorous cytotoxic T-cell response against EBV latency antigens (EBNA-2, -3A, -3B, or -3C). Patients with infectious mononucleosis have cytotoxic T-lymphocytes (CTLs) that can lyse EBV-transformed B-cell targets in culture, implying that such cells play an active role in eliminating the infected B lymphocytes in vivo.[289,615,741,810] In severely immunocompromised individuals, however, a deficit of appropriately targeted antigen-specific CTLs may allow EBV-infected B-cell proliferation to go unchecked. Adoptive immunotherapy with healthy donor-derived EBV-specific CTLs modified with specific target EBV antigens is being exploited in an effort to reconstitute cell-mediated immunity against EBV infection and thereby to prevent EBV lymphomas in immunocompromised patients.[304,305,489,717,810] While a deficit of immune surveillance may explain the escape of EBV-transformed cells in immunocompromised patients, an alternative immune mechanism in immunocompetent individuals allows the viral-associated malignant cell to evade immune control by failing to express virus-induced surface antigens that normally serve as targets for CTLs.[84] EBV-related tumors arising in healthy individuals (including EBV-related Burkitt's lymphoma, Hodgkin's disease, and nasopharyngeal carcinoma) fail to express the majority of EBV latency antigens, in contrast to the viral antigen expression that has been noted in some posttransplantation and AIDS-associated lymphomas.[84,428] Specifically, CTL responses against LYDMA, the virus-induced lymphocyte-detected membrane antigen, limit EBV-infected B-cell numbers in healthy carriers. In virus-associated Burkitt's lymphomas, the malignant clone is frequently insensitive to such surveillance by effector CTLs derived from healthy virus-immune donors, suggesting that in these cases the malignant cells do not express LYDMA.[626] Other mechanisms by which cell growth is opposed include interferon-α and -γ, other cytokines, natural killer cells, and antibody-dependent cellular cytotoxicity.[289]

Immunologic dysfunction, resulting either from an independent underlying disease process or from the EBV infection itself, can lead to increased viral shedding[105] together with a failure of adequate surveillance and control of EBV-induced lymphocyte proliferation. For instance, the EBV-encoded protein BCRF-1 is structurally and functionally homologous to the cytokine IL-10, or cytokine synthesis inhibitory factor (CSIF).[323,480,765] BCRF-1 suppresses T-cell and perhaps natural killer cell synthesis of interferon-γ and interleukin (IL)-2, resulting in what amounts to functional suppression of T-cell antiviral activity.[361,596] Other immunologic abnormalities that may impair elimination of virally transformed lymphocytes include up-regulation of autocrine factors such as IL-6,[750,818] a cytokine that stimulates B-cell growth (see below), and soluble CD23,[671] the receptor that promotes immortalization in response to IL-1.[420,596] Impaired serological responses to EBNA may occur in patients with lymphoproliferative syndromes.[637] Abnormal antibody responses to two defined EBV nuclear antigens, M and K, have been noted in individuals with EBV-induced malignancy.[473] Ninety percent of Chinese individuals with nasopharyngeal carcinoma produce antibodies to M, in contrast to only 14 percent of healthy EBV-seropositive subjects. While 96 percent of EBV-seropositive subjects show reactivity with K antigen, three patients with chronic active EBV infection failed to show such a response. It is such failures of appropriate immunological response that implicate immune dysfunction as a collaborative factor in allowing unchecked growth of EBV-induced B-cell proliferation.

Accumulation of genetic lesions. The expansion of B-cell cohorts provides increased raw material for subsequent genetic alterations that will contribute to the multistep progression toward cancer. A well-documented example of this is the deregulation of *c-MYC* oncogene expression that may result from chromosomal translocation of a truncated *c-MYC* gene, as in sporadic Burkitt's lymphoma.[23,139,296,378,522,733] The release of *c-MYC* from transcriptional regulation may be due to the separation of the intact second and third exons that make up the structural portion of the gene from the upstream regulatory, or "repressor," region.[276,378,513,558,680,681] In this manner, a previously sequestered, regulated site becomes exposed to activating transcriptional factors,[344] or to removal of a block to transcriptional elongation.[97] When *c-MYC* rearrangement does not accompany the translocation, *c-MYC* overexpression is believed to be caused by mutations in the noncoding first exon, first intron, and coding portion of exon 2 of the *c-MYC* gene, which accompany the translocation,[51,97,558,733,824] as in endemic Burkitt's lymphoma (see below), or by juxtaposition of the unrearranged *c-MYC* and an immunoglobulin gene *(Ig)*.[187,188] Overexpression of *c-MYC,* a growth-promoting oncogene,[370,592] is expected to impart a clonal proliferative advantage to cells carrying the deregulating translocation.[274] In fact, enforced expression of a transfected *c-MYC* gene in EBV-immortalized human B-lymphoblastoid cells[436] leads to a transformed phenotype in vitro and tumorigenicity in vivo. In addition, in transgenic mice carrying *c-MYC* under control of the Ig enhancer *Eμ,* a very high incidence of highly malignant B-cell lymphomas develops within a few months after birth.[3,401]

The products of specific EBV genes may exert more direct effects on oncogene expression. Even in the absence of a *c-MYC* translocation, the presence of the EBV genome in the Burkitt's lymphoma cell line BJAB is reversibly associated with increased levels of *c-MYC* messenger RNA, due to stabilization of the *c-MYC* transcript in the late exponential phase of growth.[398] In addition, EBV early protein EB2 transforms Rat-1 and NIH3T3 cells and induces changes in morphology and cell growth.[80,372] Expression of EB2 in transformed clones results in increased levels of endogenous c-MYC, but not c-FOS and c-JUN, protein or *c-MYC* mRNA, implicating EB2 as a specific regulator of *c-MYC* expression at a post-transcriptional level.[130] Although

heterodimerization with its protein partner MAX is necessary for c-MYC to transcriptionally activate target genes and elicit its growth-promoting effects,[10,393] MAX, when present in excess, may form homodimers that inhibit transcription, cell growth, and transformation.[125,589] In fact, overexpression of MAX together with EB2 in Rat-1 cells inhibits cellular transformation,[130] further supporting a role for *c-MYC* as a downstream effector of EB2-induced transformation. Other genes with cell growth control functions that, when mutated, are believed to convey comparable growth advantage include *BCL-1* and *BCL-2*.[273,274] In addition to its direct effect on increased growth, an activated *c-MYC* may promote tumorigenesis by its ability to down-regulate the integrin receptor lymphocyte function antigen-1 (LFA-1). LFA-1 mediates cell conjugate formation between B cells and cytotoxic T cells. Therefore, the down-regulation of LFA-1 is expected to impair the ability of cytotoxic T cells to destroy EBV-infected B cells, allowing them to evade immune surveillance and contributing to lymphomagenesis.[223]

The natural history of EBV-induced B-cell proliferation involves a stepwise evolution of reactive cell proliferation, progressive genetic changes, and clonal expansion that leads to the conversion of a polyclonal lymphoproliferative disease (LPD) to a monoclonal non-Hodgkin's lymphoma.[596,782] Evidence in support of such a progression is seen in post-transplant EBV-induced lymphoma following renal transplant.[218] Hanto et al.[288] noted that an initial lesion in a post-transplant patient displayed a polymorphic cell composition expressing surface or cytoplasmic Ig, or both, of polyclonal specificity, in contrast to a histologically more aggressive, more rapidly growing lesion that occurred later after transplant, and displayed a monoclonal B-cell proliferation expressing only IgG-κ surface Ig or cytoplasmic Ig or both. The dependence of this evolution on the action of EBV has been shown by Shibata et al.[678] in HIV-associated lymphoproliferations where EBV DNA was detected by polymerase chain reaction (PCR) in 37 percent of benign, reactive lymphadenopathies, designated persistent generalized lymphadenopathy (PGL), in contrast to approximately half of the HIV-related lymphomas. Furthermore, higher numbers of EBV sequences in an EBV-positive PGL biopsy correlated with the concurrent presence of EBV-positive non-Hodgkin's lymphoma at another site or the subsequent development of EBV-positive non-Hodgkin's lymphoma. Conflicting data emerge from renal transplant patients in whom the accumulation of EBV-positive cells fails to predict an increased risk of developing EBV-positive lymphoma.[140] Finally, the EBV genomes detected within tumors occurring in various settings of immunosuppression are clonal,[29,413,463,514] indicating infection with the virus before clonal expansion and supporting a role for EBV in malignant transformation.

Clinical Features of EBV-Associated Lymphomas. EBV has been implicated in the induction of lymphoproliferative disease in a variety of disease settings,[596] including HIV-related lymphomas, post-transplant lymphomas, and lymphomas in congenitally immunodeficient individuals.

Burkitt's lymphoma. The prototype of the EBV-related lymphomas is Burkitt's lymphoma, ostensibly a lymphoma that is not confined to a setting of immunosuppression. In the endemic (African) form of the disease, the EBV genome is detected in greater than 97 percent of cases, in contrast to the sporadic form of Burkitt's lympoma, in which only 15 percent of cases are EBV-positive.[76,274,361,377,681,829] Both endemic and sporadic Burkitt's lymphoma cells from fresh biopsy samples as well as cell lines derived from fresh tumors carry a translocation between chromosome 8q24,[49,170,793] which harbors the c-MYC gene, and one of the Ig loci. As a result of its translocation to an Ig gene site, the oncogenic c-MYC is up-regulated, contributing to transformation of the affected cell.[23,187,188,296,522] In 80 percent of Burkitt's lymphoma cases, a reciprocal translocation exists between chromosome 8q24 and chromosome 14q32, the locus of the Ig heavy chain (IgH) gene, whereas 15 percent of Burkitt's lymphomas involve reciprocal translocations of chromosome 8q24 to chromosome 22q11 (the Ig-λ locus) and 5 percent involve chromosomal 8q24 and chromosome 2q24 (the Ig-κ locus).[139,184,273,415,827] Although a cytogenetic translocation is demonstrable in all cases of Burkitt's lymphoma, rearrangement of the c-MYC gene can be demonstrated by Southern blotting of c-MYC DNA restriction fragments in only 50 percent of Burkitt's lymphomas, suggesting that in the remaining 50 percent, the actual breakpoint on chromosome 8 is outside the c-MYC locus.[49,145,558,681,732] In fact, this "unrearranged" form of c-MYC;Ig translocation is typical of the endemic form of Burkitt's lymphoma.[272,275,513,558,681] By contrast, sporadic Burkitt's lymphoma generally (91 percent of cases) demonstrates c-MYC rearrangement on Southern blots as well as cytogenetic studies, pointing to multiple breakpoints within or close to the 5′-region of c-MYC (in the noncoding first exon or the first intron).

The endemic and sporadic forms of the disease also differ with respect to the reciprocal portion of the translocation involving the IgH gene. In endemic Burkitt's lymphoma, the c-MYC gene is translocated unrearranged into a breakpoint in the V_H-D-J_H recombination region, generally into the J_H segment.[139,272,273,275,513,558] This type of translocation appears to result from aberrant functioning of the recombinase enzyme that under normal conditions is responsible for routine Ig gene rearrangement.[396] Whereas some endemic Burkitt's lymphoma tumors express small amounts of surface IgM, few if any express surface IgG, and some endemic Burkitt's lymphoma tumors show no surface Ig, reflecting an early, nonsecretory stage of B-cell differentiation, at which the culprit recombinase enzyme would be expected to function.[41,45] Such non-c-MYC-rearranged translocations are often accompanied by c-MYC mutations.[51,97,558,681,824] In the case of sporadic Burkitt's lymphoma, the first exon of the disrupted c-MYC gene is sometimes translocated, in inverted orientation, into a breakpoint in the switch region of the heavy chain gene (Sμ).[513] The presumed error in this case is on the part of isotype switching enzymes that are normally active in more mature B cells that have the capacity to secrete Igs.[236,273] In fact, cell lines derived from sporadically occurring tumors secrete more surface IgG and IgM than do endemic lines, resembling a more mature B-cell.[41,45] As in endemic Burkitt's lymphoma, sporadic Burkitt's lymphoma may also harbor mutations in the translocated c-MYC allele, generally clustered within exon 2.[811]

A setting of pre-existing immune deficiency has been invoked to explain the evolution of endemic Burkitt's lymphoma.[273,422,596] Individuals in endemic areas of equatorial Africa are infected with EBV at an early age without showing signs of clinical disease. These geographic regions overlap those of holoendemic malaria, which, occurring with a high incidence, imposes on its previously EBV-infected victim immunosuppression that leads to reactivation of the EBV. Chronic malarial infection may result in reduction in CD4 count, with a decrease in the CD4/CD8 ratios during acute infection.[752,753,789] EBV-specific T-cell immunity is impaired in individuals living in regions holoendemic for malaria.[488] Finally, a correlation appears to exist between high titers of anti-VCA (viral capsid antigen) antibody among children in the malarial belt of Africa and the subsequent development of Burkitt's lymphoma.[158,240] The importance of immune status is emphasized by the observation that among patients with endemic Burkitt's lymphoma, higher titers in the assay for EBV-specific antibody-dependent cellular cytotoxicity were prognostic for a better response to treatment.[554] EBV-induced polyclonal B-cell proliferation ensues unchecked in the malaria-induced absence of T-cell control of EBV-infected B cells. A break then occurs in the c-MYC region of chromosome 8, a stochastic outcome of prolonged cell division, whereas a break in the Ig region of chromosome 14 (and, in variant forms, in chromosomes 2 or 22) occurs as a defective version of a normal recombination event. The prominent involvement of c-MYC breaks in Burkitt's lymphoma tissue is probably a reflection of the enormous selective advantage that the resulting constitutive c-MYC overexpression imparts on the affected clone,[45,170] since other "nonselective" genes are undoubtedly also undergoing random breaks in this hyperproliferating cell population. When the translocation per se does not alter oncogene expression, an accompanying mutation in c-MYC[51,558,824] has been proposed as playing a role in tumor progression.[600]

Other EBV-associated malignancies. EBV has been implicated as an etiological agent of lymphoma in the setting of immunodeficiency that occurs in AIDS.[18,267,556] Thus, in AIDS, expansion of the EBV-transformed B-cell cohort results from impaired immune surveillance by T cells,[61] CD4 destruction, as well as the induction by HIV of various B-stimulatory cytokines, particularly IL-6.[62,71,185,648] Similarly, EBV appears to play a role in the development of lymphoma in the setting of immunosuppression that is genetically determined[259,593] or iatrogenically induced following organ transplant.[577]

Chronic, pre-existing immune deficiency is not always obvious as a precursor to EBV-associated malignancy. The incidence of Hodgkin's disease has been shown to increase threefold following infectious mononucleosis.[596] On occasion, chronic active EBV infection in children and young adults, manifesting as fatigue, pancytopenia, hepatosplenomegaly, increased IgG, and increased EBV antibody titers, may evolve into a malignant B-cell lymphoma or peripheral T-cell leukemia/lymphoma.[350,392,596,599,714] Lymphomatoid granulomatosis (a variant of angiocentric immunoproliferative lesions [AIL],[339,340,439,794] involving angiocentric, angiodestructive atypical lymphoproliferative infiltrates in the lung and once believed to be of T-cell origin) progresses to large cell immunoblastic lymphoma in 50 percent of cases[196] and has been linked etiologically to EBV.[363] Interestingly, based on Ig gene rearrangement and EBV genome analysis, the EBV-containing cells are clonal B lymphocytes, in contrast to the T cells, which are merely reactive, suggesting that this may not be a T-cell malignancy.[268,439] Conversely, in the subcategory of AIL known as midline malignant reticulosis, characterized by morphologically AIL-like angiocentric infiltrates in the nose and paranasal sinuses, the EBV-containing cells are also clonal but are T cells in phenotype, based on T-cell receptor rearrangements as well as immunophenotyping.[103,292,476] An additional variation on this theme was seen in three cases of nodal peripheral T-cell lymphoma with Reed-Sternberg-like cells of B-cell phenotype.[598] In these cases, the neoplastic T cells were negative for EBV, but the Reed-Sternberg-like cells were B cell in origin and were positive for EBV LMP-1. EBV DNA and RNA have also been observed in up to 96 percent of affected tissue from patients with angioimmunoblastic lymphadenopathy (AILD) and AILD-like lymphoma.[786] Both Ig and T-cell receptor gene rearrangements have been identified, pointing to the presence of both B- and T-cell clones in the context of AILD.[2,431] While the EBV-containing cells are generally B cells, neoplastic T cells may also be infected.[14]

In primary CNS lymphoma occurring in both the absence and presence of obvious immunodeficiency, EBV DNA has been identified in the lymphoma but not in the adjacent normal brain tissue.[35,312] The presence of EBV has been noted in nasal lymphomas[309] and thyroid lymphomas,[399] as well as lymphoepithelial and nonlymphomatous malignancies of the salivary gland, thymus, tonsil, oral mucosa/hairy leukoplakia of the tongue, esophagus, lung, uterine cervix, and breast.[75,108,138,162,200,316,327,395,425,536,551,553,596,642,797] The association of EBV with nasopharyngeal carcinoma, a very common malignancy in southern China and parts of southeast Asia, is well documented.[75,200,540,551] At the other end of the spectrum, evidence for the presence of EBV in breast cancer cells is inconsistent and the association remains controversial.[68,73,246,450] The significance of the EBV findings in many of these malignancies is still questionable.[540]

EBV-associated Hodgkin's disease. EBV was first noted to have an association with Hodgkin's disease in epidemiologic studies.[366] An etiological role for EBV infection in the pathogenesis of Hodgkin's disease was suggested by the threefold increase in the relative risk of developing Hodgkin's disease that is observed following infectious mononucleosis.[365,596] Recent data have supported this association by showing that a prior history of infectious mononucleosis is more likely to correlate with EBV-positive than with EBV-negative Hodgkin's disease.[4] Furthermore, elevated levels of IgG and IgA antibodies against EBV capsid antigen, EBNA, and early antigen D have been seen in individuals who subsequently developed Hodgkin's disease.[492] In addition, episomal EBV DNA has been detected in involved lymph nodes of 18 to 68 percent of Hodgkin's disease patients, where it is localized to Reed-Sternberg and variant cells.[127,302,596,757,785] Monoclonality of the EBV DNA has also been demonstrated in affected tissues,[785] supporting EBV as an important factor contributing to the multistep lymphomagenesis of Hodgkin's disease. In a recent study utilizing in situ

hybridization with an EBER-1 probe, immunostaining with anti-LMP-1 antibody, and PCR for the EBNA-3C gene to look for the presence of EBV in classical Hodgkin's disease, 14 of the 23 cases tested were found to be positive at presentation.[515] Of these 14, one case showed loss of EBV association at relapse, suggesting that the role played by EBV in Hodgkin's lymphomagenesis may resemble a "hit-and-run" mechanism, whereby EBV may be required early in the disease process but may be dispensible for maintenance of the malignant phenotype. The Reed-Sternberg cells of Hodgkin's disease exhibit a Lat II pattern, in which latent gene expression is restricted to EBNA-1, LMP-1, and LMP-2,[76,149,302,528,540] differing from the latency type seen in other EBV-associated lymphomas (e.g., Burkitt's lymphoma) but resembling that seen in nasopharyngeal carcinoma.

A higher expression of proliferating cell nuclear antigen (PCNA) has been noted in EBV-positive than EBV-negative Hodgkin's disease, suggesting that EBV probably promotes the cell cycling of Reed-Sternberg cells.[509] Interestingly, higher PCNA expression in a tumor appears to confer a survival advantage to the patient, consistent with the idea that increased cell cycling makes cells more responsive to chemotherapy. EBV-specific CTLs have been demonstrated among the tumor infiltrating lymphocytes from a Hodgkin's disease biopsy, indicating an ongoing immune response against EBV-carrying cells.[165] Despite this observation, EBV-associated Hodgkin's disease tumor cells have evolved immunologic strategies to evade such ongoing cytotoxic responses. In one study, the cytokine IL-10, an inhibitor of cell-mediated immunity, was shown to be upregulated by the EBV antigen LMP-1 in tumor cells of Hodgkin's disease.[303]

Mixed cellularity Hodgkin's disease, commonly found in children and older adults and in developing countries, is the subtype most likely to be associated with EBV (up to 90 percent of cases).[342,365,588] Lymphocyte-depleted tumors are also frequently EBV-positive, whereas 30 percent of nodular sclerosing and only rare cases of the lymphocyte-predominant subtype carry the virus.[366] Finally, epidemiologic studies have shown that 50 to 70 percent of cases in Western countries are positive for the EBV genome, with EBV-positive disease being found more often in males than females.[76,540] Although the evidence for a causal relationship between EBV infection and Hodgkin's disease is not yet considered definitive, the accumulating data continue to strengthen the likehood of such an association.[112,166,365]

AIDS/HIV-Associated Lymphomas

Epidemiology/Demographics of Lymphomas Associated with HIV. Lymphomas occurring in conjunction with HIV/AIDS account for a significant portion of the increased incidence of lymphomas that has been observed in recent years.[361,383,386,583,831] PGL or lymphadenopathy syndrome (LAS) is a characteristic feature of AIDS-related disease.[138,386,418,422,470,678] PGL is a state of chronic B-cell stimulation, distinguished by hyperplasia of the reactive lymphoid follicles (B-cell zone) with polyclonal hypergammaglobulinemia, together with plasmacytosis and reduced numbers of T-helper cells, as well as clonal rearrangements of Ig genes in 20 percent of cases. PGL shows no consistent association with either c-*MYC* rearrangements or with the presence of EBNA or EBV DNA.[559,678] Two other forms of opportunistic lymphoproliferations in the AIDS population include CNS lymphoma and chronic lymphocytic interstitial pneumonitis, consisting primarily of a nonlymphomatous infiltrate accompanied by polyclonal B cells. Both are associated with EBV infection in children with AIDS.[18,138] Malignant lymphoma was first reported in AIDS in 1982,[167,830] and studies documenting the increased incidence of non-Hodgkin's lymphomas in AIDS patients[146,330,416,417,831] ultimately led to the inclusion of non-Hodgkin's lymphoma, as well as chronic lymphoid interstitial pneumonitis, as part of the case definition of AIDS.[93] While the original inclusion of non-Hodgkin's lymphoma as an AIDS-defining illness referenced only non-Hodgkin's lymphoma of high-grade pathologic type (diffuse, undifferentiated), a 1987 revision of the definition expanded the criteria to include diffuse aggressive intermediate or high-grade non-Hodgkin's lymphoma of B-cell or indeterminate phenotype.[94,386]

Based on Centers for Disease Control (CDC) data collected on AIDS patients between 1981 and 1989, 3 percent of AIDS cases were found to have non-Hodgkin's lymphoma, 60 times the incidence in the general United States population.[44] Because the development of malignant lymphoma following the initial manifestation of AIDS is often not reported to the CDC, a more accurate estimate of the overall incidence of lymphoma is between 4 and 10 percent of AIDS cases.[277,386,420] According to Surveillance, Epidemiology, and End Results (SEER) program data from San Francisco, by 1987 the relative risk for developing non-Hodgkin's lymphoma in association with HIV infection was 100 times that expected before the AIDS epidemic.[601] Many additional non-Hodgkin's lymphomas have been discovered only at autopsy.[361,617,790] In various studies, non-Hodgkin's lymphomas accounted for between 2.5 and 6.6 percent of primary AIDS diagnoses,[224,245,357,555,602] although higher percentages have been noted.[267,831] Among individuals with AIDS-non-Hodgkin's lymphomas, lymphoma was the AIDS-defining illness in 50 to 90 percent of cases.[267,602,612]

Compared to other AIDS-defining illnesses, lymphoma appears relatively late in the course of HIV infection.[386,756] The use of antiretroviral therapy has resulted in even further delays in the onset of non-Hodgkin's lymphomas relative to AIDS diagnosis. In one study of AIDS patients receiving zidovudine (AZT, azidothymidine), the probability of developing non-Hodgkin's lymphomas was stable for 2 years and rose 0.8 percent for each subsequent 6 months of zidovudine therapy.[483] In a study reported by Pluda et al.,[583] the estimated hazard rate was 0.089 per year for the first year and 0.1 per year thereafter.[224] The prolongation of survival of HIV-infected individuals following the institution of antiretroviral therapy[191,555] is considered to be a factor contributing to increases in the incidence of non-Hodgkin's lymphomas.[95,583,584] Beral et al.[44] observed that lymphomas occurred more frequently among hemophiliacs with AIDS and less frequently among patients who acquired AIDS via heterosexual contact, but other investigators noted no differences among the AIDS risk groups.[278,556,602] About 80 percent of AIDS-non-Hodgkin's lymphomas are seen in homosexual men, with a large portion of the remaining 20 percent occurring in intravenous drug abusers.[386]

The increasing probability both of developing lymphoma and of dying, appear to result from the progressive immunosuppression in longer living HIV-infected individuals rather than from a direct mutagenic effect of antiretroviral therapy.[133,423,555,583,584,816] Lymphoma has been noted in patients with less than 100 CD4 cells/mm^3 for a median of 17.8 months and less than 50 CD4 cells/mm^3 for a median of 15.3 months before diagnosis.[583] Among AIDS-non-Hodgkin's lymphoma patients in San Francisco, those with CD4 counts of greater than 100 cells/mm^3 had a median survival of 24 months, while those with less than 100 cells/mm^3 had a median survival of 4.1 months.[357] Some studies indicate that the nature of the antiretroviral therapy influences the outcome,[584] with lymphoma developing in 12 percent of patients at 24 months and 29.2 percent of patients at 36 months on zidovudine. By contrast, among patients treated with didanosine (DDI, dideoxyinosine), lymphoma occurred in only 6.2 percent at 24 months and 9.5 percent at 36 months of antiretroviral therapy. Other studies, however, have shown no relationship between clinical outcome and a specific agent.[266] Where observed, the differences may actually be a function of the rates of progressive immunosuppression on the different antiretroviral therapies, since didanosine appears to sustain increases in CD4 counts for longer periods than does zidovudine.[584]

The use of combinations of reverse transcriptase inhibitors as well as the introduction of complex highly active antiretroviral therapy (HAART) regimens, incorporating combinations of reverse transcriptase inhibitors with the newer protease inhibitors,[152,650] has led to delays in progression of HIV disease with respect to laboratory indices (viral load, CD4+ T-cell count) and to improvements in survival relative to monotherapy.[33,147,199,281,297,364,411,633,641,650] Although HAART prolongs survival, its use does not ensure permanent maintenance of an immunologic microenvironment capable of inhibiting lymphomagenesis.[297] Furthermore, even when immune function is improved in response to potent antiviral therapy, patients continue to be at risk for non-Hodgkin's lymphoma, in contrast to marked decreases in risk for Kaposi's sarcoma and opportunistic infectious diseases such as *Pneumocystis carinii* pneumonia and *Mycobacterium avium* complex.[409,477,484] The data on non-Hodgkin's lymphoma associated with AIDS are inconsistent, with different studies showing that the incidence has remained stable, undergone an upward trend, or experienced a decline over time in the era of HAART.[58,78,265,266,329,338,351,409,410,457,477,484,699] Two groups of immunologic predictors of non-Hodgkin's lymphoma risk have been noted: 1. duration of immunodeficiency and lower CD4 cell count and 2. B-cell stimulation, that is, higher levels of serum immunoglobulin.[266] The ultimate impact of aggressive anti-HIV therapy on the lymphoma incidence remains to be seen.

Just as specific alleles of chemokines and their receptors are known to confer protection against or increased risk of HIV infection and progression to AIDS,[314] an increased risk of HIV-associated non-Hodgkin's lymphoma, but not other AIDS-defining illnesses, has been observed in association with a particular polymorphism of the *SDF-1* (stromal cell-derived factor

1) chemokine gene.[603] The risk is greater for homozygotes of this *SDF1-3'A* allele than for heterozygotes, with 19 percent of homozygous and 10 percent of heterozygous *SDF1-3'A* carriers developing lymphoma after a median follow-up of 12 years, in contrast to 5 percent of wild-type HIV-infected individuals.

Clinical Features of AIDS-Associated Lymphomas. The AIDS-non-Hodgkin's lymphomas exhibit a number of characteristic clinical features such as prodromal manifestations, aggressive histology, presentation at advanced stages, a high frequency of extranodal and primary brain disease, as well as a poor prognosis.[386,416,442,556,831]

Although initially categorized by disease entity (progressive generalized lymphadenopathy, lymphocytic interstitial pneumonitis, lymphomas of the CNS, and non-Hodgkin's lymphoma),[18,138,596] three alternative categories for the AIDS-associated lymphoproliferative disorders are based on clonality (determined by *IgH* chain gene rearrangement) and site: peripheral monoclonal lymphomas, peripheral polyclonal lymphomas, and lymphomas of the CNS.[138] Of the peripheral lymphomas, slightly over half were monoclonal, whereas all CNS lymphomas were found to be monoclonal.[467] Within each of these groups are found a variety of histological types of non-Hodgkin's lymphoma.

The increased incidence of lymphomas in the HIV population is largely restricted to high and intermediate grade histologies, with high grade lymphomas having increased 116-fold by 1987.[601] In multiple series, 60 to 90 percent of AIDS-non-Hodgkin's lymphomas have been aggressive B-cell tumors,[48,69,89,244,245,267,278,330,353,357,383,386,417,442,607,612,773,831] in contrast to the 30 to 40 percent of lymphomas that would be expected in a normal population.[293,386] The predominant histologies include: 1. high grade large cell immunoblastic; 2. small noncleaved cell lymphomas (i.e., Burkitt's and Burkitt's-like lymphoma); and 3. intermediate grade diffuse large noncleaved

cell, or centroblastic, lymphomas. This differs from the histopathologic distribution seen in other immunodeficiency-associated lymphomas, in which large cell immunoblastic lymphomas and diffuse large B-cell lymphomas predominate, with Burkitt's-type lymphomas being rare,[386] The distribution of cell types among the aggressive histologies varies considerably in patients with AIDS.[91,244,245,383,386,419,442,556,612,773] Overall, Burkitt's-type lymphoma occurs at least 1000 times more frequently in AIDS patients than in the normal population,[44] representing 26 to 40 percent of all AIDS-related non-Hodgkin's lymphomas (Table 47–1).[44,57,383,386] The remaining lymphomas are divided equally between immunoblastic and large cell lymphomas. Some authors have noted considerable pleomorphism[278,357,607] with frequent overlap between some of these histologic categories, suggesting a morphological spectrum of lymphomatous proliferations. Among the morphologic complexities noted within these larger categories are both classical Burkitt's lymphoma (30 percent) and atypical Burkitt's-like lymphoma (among the small noncleaved cell lymphomas), as well as lymphomas with features intermediate between Burkitt's lymphoma with plasmablastic differentiation and immunoblastic lymphoma.[607] The same histologies have been observed in all groups at risk for HIV.

Occasionally, other histologic types of lymphoma have been noted, such as anaplastic large cell Ki-1 (CD30)-positive lymphoma,[89,90,91,249,278–280,556] plasma cell malignancies including multiple myeloma,[336,391,762,766] and extramedullary plasmacytomas.[89] Interestingly, of the four anaplastic large cell lymphomas observed in one study, three occurred in intravenous drug abusers.[89] Infrequent low-grade lymphomas have been seen,[267,417,601,831] but the association of these histological categories with AIDS is not statistically significant. The histological complexity of the AIDS-non-Hodgkin's lymphomas, attributable in large part to their morphologic polymorphism, prevents

Table 47–1. Genetic Alterations and Viral Infection in AIDS-Related Non-Hodgkin's Lymphomas[a]

Lymphoma Histology: B-Cell Non-Hodgkin's Lymphomas	Lymphoma Frequency (percent)	Dominantly Acting Oncogenes					Tumor Suppressor Genes		Viruses	
		c-MYC (percent)	BCL-6 (percent)	BCL-1 (percent)	BCL-2 (percent)	RAS (percent)	p53	RB1	EBV	HIV
Systemic AIDS–non-Hodgkin's lymphoma	81[b]									
AIDS–small noncleaved cell lymphoma	26[c]	100	0	0	0	15	60	0	30	0
AIDS–diffuse large cell lymphoma	74[c]									
AIDS–large noncleaved cell lymphoma		20	20	0	0	15	0	0	30	0
AIDS–large cell immunoblastic plasmacytoid lymphoma		20	20	0	0	15	0	0	90	0
AIDS–anaplastic cell lymphoma		NA	0	0	0	NA	0	NA	90	0
AIDS–primary central nervous system lymphoma	19[b]	NA	NA	0	0	NA	0	NA	100	0

Abbreviation: NA, not available.
[a] Adapted from Gaidano et al.[223]
[b] Frequency among AIDS–non-Hodgkin's lymphomas; derived from numbers of cases reported by Beral et al.[44]
[c] Frequency within systemic AIDS–non-Hodgkin's lymphomas; derived from numbers of cases reported by Beral et al.[44]

total reliance on standardized classification systems such as the Revised European-American Classification of Lymphoid Neoplasms (REAL).[223,293] The resolution to this dilemma may reside in newer technologies that focus on phenotypic characterization at the molecular rather than the morphologic level. In the future, gene expression profiling by an analytical method such as the "lymphochip," a specialized microarray incorporating genes that are preferentially expressed in lymphoid cells, may facilitate better definition of the pathologic entities that make up the AIDS-non-Hodgkin's lymphomas.[6]

T-cell lymphomas have also been observed,[644] including cutaneous T-cell lymphoma (mycosis fungoides) with Sézary syndrome,[135,357,500] T-cell lymphoblastic leukemia,[383] adult T-cell leukemia/lymphoma,[677] peripheral T-cell lymphoma,[135,357] Ki-1+ anaplastic large-cell lymphoma,[91,249] and "homme rouge" (cutaneous T-cell non-Hodgkin's lymphoma with erythroderma).[547]

In contrast to non-Hodgkin's lymphomas in immunocompetent individuals, a very high proportion of AIDS-non-Hodgkin's lymphomas present with extranodal disease, with or without nodal involvement,[89,146,278,330,357,383,417,420,442,556,607,612,831] 98 to 100 percent in some studies.[146,831] The AIDS-non-Hodgkin's lymphomas have been classified by anatomical site of origin into three large categories: 1. systemic (nodal and/or extranodal), 2. primary CNS, and 3. body cavity-based lymphomas.[386] The most frequently involved sites are the CNS (20 to 40 percent), bone marrow (25 percent), and GI tract (25 percent).[386,422] Other affected sites include the skin, salivary glands, oropharynx, heart, lungs, liver, rectum, muscles, bones, orbit, mandible, and even the peripheral blood.[83,371,383,386,412] Although the same extranodal sites are affected among all AIDS risk groups, Carbone et al.[89] observed no primary brain or rectal non-Hodgkin's lymphomas in a study involving 66 percent intravenous drug abusers.

Primary CNS lymphoma. The incidence of primary CNS lymphoma of the brain, a rare tumor that accounts for less than 2 percent of all non-Hodgkin's lymphomas and 1 percent of all brain tumors,[301,442,798] increased threefold from 2.7 to 7.5 cases per 10 million population between 1973 and 1984.[177] Part of this increase may be attributed to the unusually high proportion, between 19 and 25 percent, of AIDS-non-Hodgkin's lymphomas that present as primary brain lymphoma (Table 47–1),[44,278,330,442,831] with a frequency 1000 times greater than that in the general population.[57,386] Primary CNS lymphoma is the second most common AIDS-associated cerebral mass lesion, after toxoplasmosis.[212] Sites of AIDS-associated CNS lymphomas include the cerebrum, cerebellum, basal ganglia, and brain stem.[386,447] Furthermore, the association that is generally seen between AIDS-non-Hodgkin's lymphomas and low CD4 counts is even more pronounced in primary CNS lymphomas, which tend to occur in patients with CD4 counts below 50 cells/mm³.[510,583] In contrast to primary brain lymphomas in the immunocompetent host, those occurring in conjunction with AIDS do not have a characteristic radiographic appearance.[212] They can occur in the cortex or deep periventricular structures. Although 50 to 75 percent of cases are multifocal on computed tomography (CT) or magnetic resonance imaging (MRI) scan,

at autopsy virtually all are multifocal. Twenty to 60 percent of AIDS-related primary CNS lesions show ring enhancement, accompanied by surrounding edema, making them difficult to distinguish from toxoplasmosis and necessitating brain biopsy for accurate diagnosis.[37,211,243,353,442,447,510,694,756] Spinal cord lesions are generally not demonstrated on CT or MRI.[37,694] Accompanying spinal fluid analysis may be normal[442,691] or may show a mild pleocytosis that is primarily mononuclear, as well as elevated protein and depressed glucose.[442,447,691,694]

Pathological evaluation usually shows a high grade B-cell lymphoma.[37,447,607,690,691,694] Although some studies note only diffuse large cell histologies,[243,353,422,447,467,607,690,831] especially large cell immunoblastic lymphoma,[211,243,278,417,556] other reports demonstrate small noncleaved cell lymphomas among the primary CNS lesions.[37,211,330,383,417,556,691,694] Leptomeningeal involvement has also been reported with high frequency in some studies.[186,353,442,607,831] Whereas some authors have pointed out an association between CNS and bone marrow disease,[442] others note just the opposite.[357] In contrast to the systemic AIDS-non-Hodgkin's lymphomas that show EBV infection in only 30 to 60 percent of cases, in situ hybridization has demonstrated EBV expression in up to 100 percent of primary CNS lymphomas in HIV patients.[34,35,447,505,556] The latter finding also differs from that in immunocompetent patients, in whom primary CNS lymphomas rarely contain EBV.[34,312,447,505,525] The histologic features as well as the strong correlation with EBV among AIDS-related primary CNS lymphomas resemble the primary CNS lymphomas found in patients who are immunosuppressed in the setting of transplant.[35,218,243,278,505] Finally, primary localized extranodal lymphomas, like primary CNS lymphomas, tend to be immunoblastic, whereas both large cell immunoblastic lymphomas and Burkitt's lymphomas have been noted in the meninges.[556]

Systemic AIDS-associated lymphoma. Approximately 81 percent of the AIDS-related non-Hodgkin's lymphomas are systemic (Table 47–1).[44,56] They usually present at advanced stages[245,612,831]; up to 95 percent[244] are Stage III or IV disease. Those few cases that are early stage are frequently extranodal (Stage IE and IIE disease).[244,612]

Interestingly, patients with immunoblastic lymphomas and intermediate grade diffuse large B-cell lymphomas tend to be more severely immunosuppressed than those with small noncleaved cell lymphomas (Burkitt's and Burkitt's-like). The former group of lymphomas are associated with lower CD4 counts, lower performance status, a prior diagnosis of AIDs, and poorer response to chemotherapy.[69,353,420,556] The immunoblastic lymphomas tend to be localized in extranodal sites, particularly in the CNS.[383,442,556,607] By contrast, small noncleaved cell lymphomas develop even in the presence of a higher level of immunocompetence. Although small noncleaved cell/Burkitt-type lymphomas are found in lymph nodes more often than large cell immunoblastic lymphomas, the aggressive nature of Burkitt-type lymphomas leads to extranodal spread that is often extensive and frequently involves the bone marrow.[607] Even within the CNS, small noncleaved cell lymphomas more often present diffusely, with leptomeningeal involvement rather than restriction to primary parenchymal disease, as is seen with the immunoblastic lymphomas.[353,357,607] Several authors have observed a higher frequency of EBV DNA in immunoblastic lymphomas than in other histologic types.[91,556,679,715]

Kaposi's sarcoma-associated herpesvirus (KSHV)/human herpesvirus-8 (HHV-8): AIDS-associated body cavity lymphoma/ primary effusion lymphoma. An unusual clinical entity, *body cavity-based lymphoma* associated with lymphomatous effusions (pleural, pericardial, or peritoneal) in AIDS patients, was originally described in 1989[384,774] and was subsequently designated *primary effusion lymphoma*.[498] Knowles et al. have noted such lymphomatous effusions in the absence of a contiguous tumor mass in homosexual men usually, but not always, in association with HIV infection.[384,497,498,711] The lymphomatous effusions generally constituted the initial presentation of a lymphoma, which in most cases remained localized to the body cavity of origin. Examination of the malignant cells revealed features of both large cell immunoblastic lymphoma and anaplastic large cell lymphoma.[384,385,774] Despite the absence of B-cell-associated antigens, clonal Ig gene rearrangements placed these lymphomas in the B-cell lineage. A potential etiologic agent for these body cavity-based lymphomas was identified when a DNA sequence homologous to a 233 base pair region of KSHV was observed in all AIDS-related body cavity-based lymphomas associated with lymphomatous effusions but in none of the other tested AIDS or non-AIDS-related lymphomas.[98,385] Subsequently, KSHV sequences have been identified in body cavity-based lymphomas in patients not infected with HIV, including patients with Kaposi's sarcoma, postcardiac transplant, and even in immunocompetent individuals.[169,195,349,711] The putative agent, KSHV, named for its original association with Kaposi's sarcoma lesions in AIDS patients,[11,107,482] is now classified as human herpesvirus-8 (HHV-8) based on homology of KSHV sequences to members of the Gammaherpesvirinae subfamily of herpesvirus.[98,386] Similar to EBV, KSHV/HHV-8 exists in the latently infected cells of primary effusion lymphoma as multiple copies of a circularized DNA episome. A KSHV/HHV-8-encoded latency-associated nuclear antigen (LANA) appears to be necessary and sufficient for the persistence of these episomes, tethering KSHV/HHV-8 DNA to chromosomes during mitosis to ensure their efficient segregation to progeny cells.[30] Monoclonality and oligoclonality of HHV-8 in primary effusion lymphomas have been demonstrated, supporting an etiologic role for the virus in lymphomagenesis.[352] In addition to KSHV/HHV-8, EBV sequences have been identified in well over 70 percent of body cavity-based lymphomas examined.[19,195,386,532] The infecting virus is generally monoclonal, supporting a role for EBV in the pathogenesis of these clinical entities.[195] In some studies, the pattern of EBV latent gene expression conforms to the Lat II subtype, resembling nasopharyngeal carcinoma and EBV-associated Hodgkin's disease,[85] whereas others reveal a Lat I pattern, in which only EBNA-1 is expressed.[195] The combined presence of KSHV/HHV-8 and EBV in this particular presentation of lymphoma supports a synergistic effect[386] in which both agents act as carcinogenic insults contributing to the multistep progression toward malignant lymphoma. Additional genetic alterations undoubtedly contribute to this progression, as suggested

by the occurrence of recurrent gain of sequence in chromosomes 12 and X,[495] but these DNA copy number changes resemble those seen in other HIV lymphomas and are not unique to the body cavity lymphoma setting.

Pathogenesis: Mechanisms Underlying Lymphomagenesis in AIDS. Molecular basis for transformation. Lymphomagenesis in the setting of AIDS probably results from a multistep progression as described above.[386,420,421] An initial insult, such as the HIV infection, may lead to lymphoproliferation such as that found in the PGL/LAS that characterizes early HIV infection.[756] Successive genetic changes superimposed on this expanded lymphocyte population result in malignant transformation of one or more clones. Finally, defective immune surveillance, also an outcome of the immunodeficiency resulting from the HIV infection, allows expansion of the malignant clone(s). Support for this model comes from the observation that HIV-related lymphadenopathy, PGL/LAS, predated or was noted concurrently in 20 to 83 percent of patients with AIDS-non-Hodgkin's lymphomas, the risk of conversion from PGL/LAS to non-Hodgkin's lymphomas being 100-fold greater than in age-matched controls.[337,418,607] In addition, lymph node involvement by lymphoma is more frequent in patients who previously had PGL/LAS.

Multiple monoclonal B-cell expansions have been documented in biopsies not only of AIDS-non-Hodgkin's lymphomas, but also in a significant fraction of lymph nodes with the ostensibly benign polyclonal hyperplasia of PGL/LAS.[154,467,559] The fact that up to 60 percent of the AIDS-non-Hodgkin's lymphomas but only 10 to 20 percent of lesions of AIDS-related benign lymphoid hyperplasia contain oligoclonal B-cell expansions suggests a progression along a spectrum of malignancy, reflecting the accumulation of genetic alterations (Table 47–1) that culminate in the dominance of specific B-cell clones.[223,386] By contrast, non-Hodgkin's lymphomas in the immunocompetent population only infrequently show multiple clonal B-cell expansions, making the AIDS-non-Hodgkin's lymphomas analogous in this respect to lymphomas found in other forms of immunodeficiency (see below).[687]

Among the genetic alterations contributing to B-cell non-Hodgkin's lymphomas in AIDS is activation of the *c-MYC* oncogene by means of its rearrangement into the vicinity of Ig regulatory elements (Table 47–1).[29,223,263] One hundred percent of AIDS-small noncleaved cell lymphomas contain t(8;14) or t(8;22) translocations resembling those found in Burkitt's lymphoma in the non-AIDs population.[29,102,117,154,221,223,514,526,580,788] Single *c-MYC* rearrangements of this nature have also been identified less frequently in AIDS-non-Hodgkin's lymphomas of other histologic types (approximately 20 percent),[117,154,223,384,514,559,715] but they have not been found in PGL/LAS.[559] The presence of single *c-MYC* rearrangements in oligoclonal B-cell non-Hodgkin's lymphomas but not in PGL/LAS suggests that the clonal B-cell subpopulations in hyperplastic lymph nodes are immortalized but not fully transformed.[386] These clonal expansions may represent premalignant clusters that, with subsequent genetic alterations such as *c-MYC* rearrangements, will progress to full-fledged AIDS-related lymphomas. At the molecular level, the t(8;14) translocations in AIDS-non-

Hodgkin's lymphomas generally resemble the sporadic Burkitt's lymphomas, by involvement of the *Sμ* region of the *IgH* gene[715] and *c-MYC* gene rearrangement on Southern blot,[29,223,526,715] although a translocation pattern similar to the endemic Burkitt's lymphomas, with *J_H* region rearrangement and the absence of *c-MYC* rearrangement on Southern blot, has also been noted.[276] Mutations within the first intron as well as the coding region have also been demonstrated in AIDS-non-Hodgkin's lymphomas, primarily in Burkitt's and Burkitt's-like lymphomas.[51] Such coding region mutations tend to be associated with *c-MYC* rearrangements[51,117] and EBV-negativity, the latter two features being characteristic of non-AIDS-related sporadic Burkitt's lymphomas. By contrast, similar coding region *c-MYC* mutations in non-AIDS lymphomas[824] are more frequently associated with an unrearranged *c-MYC* gene, and are seen in endemic Burkitt's lymphomas,[558] which generally are EBV-positive.

In addition to *c-MYC*, translocations in AIDS-non-Hodgkin's lymphomas have been shown to involve the *BCL-6* gene (Table 47–1).[222,223] *BCL-6*, which is located on chromosome 3q27 and codes for a zinc finger transcription factor, is truncated by virtue of its translocation in 30 to 40 percent of diffuse large B-cell lymphomas in immunocompetent hosts.[223,435,793] Similarly, *BCL-6* rearrangements in AIDS-non-Hodgkin's lymphomas are restricted to the diffuse large B-cell lymphomas (occurring in 19 percent of AIDS-immunoblastic lymphomas and 25 percent of AIDS-large cell lymphomas), never being observed in AIDS-Burkitt's or Burkitt's-like lymphomas. *BCL-6* rearrangements are seen in both EBV-positive and EBV-negative lymphomas. Rearrangements involving *c-MYC* and *BCL-6* have never been observed in the same biopsy specimen, suggesting that the two genetic lesions contribute to independent pathways to tumorigenesis.[223] The *BCL-2* gene, whose protein product blocks cellular apoptosis, is rearranged in most low-grade follicular B-cell lymphomas and a smaller percentage of the more aggressive lymphomas. However, no rearrangement or mutation of this gene has been detected in AIDS-non-Hodgkin's lymphomas of any histologic type.[221,223,384,715] Similarly, no alteration has been demonstrated for *PRAD-1/BCL-1*,[221,384] a gene that encodes cyclin D_1,[390,490,491,675,755] an active component of the cell cycle machinery, whose translocation from chromosome 11q13 to chromosome 14q32 is associated with mantle cell lymphomas.[604] Another protooncogene whose activation is well established in other tumor types, *RAS*, has been examined for structural alterations in AIDS-non-Hodgkin's lymphomas (Table 47–1). In one study, only 4 of 27 cases (14.8 percent) of AIDS-non-Hodgkin's lymphomas contained a mutation in one of the *RAS* genes.[29] Three of these were Burkitt's or Burkitt's-like lymphomas and one was a large cell immunoblastic lymphoma. The observed mutations resembled those commonly seen in human cancers, involving amino acid substitutions in codons 12, 13, and 61.[223]

Inactivation of the suppressor gene *p53* in human tumors is generally due to point mutation, frequently at CpG dinucleotides, in the coding sequence of exons 5 through 9 in one allele with or without loss of the other allele.[194,220] Such mutations have been demonstrated in only 37 percent of AIDS-non-

Hodgkin's lymphomas overall,[29,223] including 62.5 percent of Burkitt's or Burkitt's-like lymphomas (Table 47–1). The high frequency of *p53* mutations in AIDS-Burkitt's lymphomas is consistent with observations made in Burkitt's lymphoma biopsy specimens[220] and cell lines;[194,220,221] from nonimmuno-compromised patients. Likewise, the lower frequency of *p53* mutations in large cell immunoblastic lymphomas is similar in individuals with and without AIDS.[502] *p53* mutations have been seen in both EBV-positive and EBV-negative tumors, suggesting no correlation between the tumorigenic mechanisms involving these two lesions.[29,223] Conversely, the functional interdependence of accumulated genetic lesions in achieving tumorigenesis is exemplified by *p53* and *c-MYC*, which frequently occur together.[29] In fact, elevated levels of mutant p53 have been shown to result from transcriptional activation of the *p53* promoter by an overexpressed c-MYC protein.[631] Deletion of two discrete regions on the long arm of chromosome 6, representing the sites of two putative tumor suppressor genes, are common in B-cell non-Hodgkin's lymphomas and constitute a poor prognostic indicator.[223] Such 6q deletions are seen in 25 percent of AIDS-non-Hodgkin's lymphomas, suggesting a role for these putative genes in AIDS-related lymphomagenesis. Other commonly altered tumor suppressor genes have been examined in AIDS-non-Hodgkin's lymphomas. No mutations have been demonstrated for *RB1*,[29] and the potential involvement of *NF-1*, *APC*, *DCC*, or *WT-1* seems unlikely based on the lack of cytogenetic aberrations at the corresponding chromosomal regions in AIDS-non-Hodgkin's lymphoma.[223]

Contribution of viruses to AIDS-associated lymphomas. The infecting HIV itself as well as co-infecting viruses are believed to contribute to B-cell transformation in the setting of AIDS.

Over 90 percent of HIV-infected individuals are also infected with EBV,[223,678] and EBV has frequently been implicated in the development of immunoproliferative disorders in non-HIV settings. Nevertheless, the etiologic role of EBV in AIDS-non-Hodgkin's lymphomas has been a matter of controversy, because of frequent polyclonality of the B-cell expansions infected by EBV and because of the discrepancies in results from different laboratories.[223] Between 30 and 90 percent of AIDS-non-Hodgkin's lymphomas exhibit infection with EBV.[29,90,91,155,267,277,278,467,514,556,679,715] EBV infection is not restricted to a specific histologic type (Table 47–1). In most studies, Burkitt's lymphomas show inconsistent association with EBV (30 percent in systemic AIDS-Burkitt's lymphoma). Overall, between 70 and 80 percent of AIDS-diffuse large cell lymphoma variants (i.e. diffuse large B-cell and immunoblastic subtypes) are EBV-positive. However, within this larger category, 30 to 50 percent of the AIDS-large B-cell lymphomas are infected with EBV, whereas the large cell immunoblastic lymphomas have a greater tendency to be EBV-positive (ranging from 70 to 100 percent),[29,154,221,223,278,679,715] especially those that present as primary CNS lymphomas (100 percent).[223,422,447,467] Interestingly, recently published results have shown that systemic AIDS-non-Hodgkin's lymphomas in which the tumor clone is infected with EBV have a significantly increased risk of CNS involvement at some point during their clinical course, regardless of the molecular features of the EBV strain.[116] Furthermore, detection of EBV DNA in the CSF of patients with systemic AIDS-non-Hodgkin's lymphomas is highly predictive of a diagnosis of localized CNS involvement. A particularly strong association exists between EBV infection and Ki-1+ anaplastic large cell lymphomas.[90,91] The erratic association of EBV with the AIDS-non-Hodgkin's lymphomas indicates that EBV cannot be the sole cause of lymphoma in these patients. Yet, when EBV is present, the characteristics of the EBV infection are consistent with its involvement in lymphomagenesis.

EBV DNA is detected more frequently in monoclonal than polyclonal AIDS-non-Hodgkin's lymphomas in contrast to the polyclonal lymphomas that characterize other immunodeficient states, which are generally EBV-positive.[467] The EBV genomes within the lymphoma clones are also clonal, indicating that the B-cell progenitor of each lymphoma was already infected with EBV before clonal expansion,[29,155,514] supporting an etiologic role for EBV in the tumorigenesis of these lymphomas. The viral DNA is detected by in situ hybridization in tumor cells but not in surrounding tissue and nontumor cells.[278] In addition, as discussed above, EBV is not consistently associated with PGL, with EBV DNA being detected in 37 percent of these benign reactive lymph nodes from HIV-positive patients, in contrast to 0 percent from HIV-negative individuals.[678] The presence of EBV in such PGL biopsies was significantly associated with concurrent lymphoma at another site or the subsequent development of lymphoma, all of which were EBV-positive. Patients with EBV-positive PGL are therefore at greater risk for EBV-positive but not EBV-negative lymphoma. Together, the clonality of the EBV DNA, its selective presence within tumor cells, and the correlation of EBV-positive PGL with EBV-positive lymphoma all support the hypothesis that EBV plays a role in the pathogenesis of the AIDS-non-Hodgkin's lymphomas. Interestingly, the presence of clonal EBV genomes in smooth muscle tumors has been demonstrated in HIV-infected patients, but not in similar tumors in the absence of HIV infection.[463] These data further support a specific tumorigenic role for EBV in the setting of immunosuppression.

In contrast to EBV DNA, which is found in only 37 percent of benign lymph nodes from HIV-infected patients, HIV DNA is detected in nearly 100 percent of such nodes.[678] In addition, a retrovirus, characterized by classic type-C particles and reverse transcriptase activity, has been isolated from B-lymphoma tissue in AIDS patients.[417] Furthermore, HIV has been shown to transform EBV-immortalized B-lymphocytes in vitro[403,479] and to up-regulate expression of EBV and c-MYC in the transformed cells.[403] Such HIV-transformed B cells will then give rise to lymphoproliferations resembling lymphomas when they are inoculated into nude mice.[403] Nonrandom monoclonal integration of HIV immediately upstream from the c-fes/fps protooncogene, accompanied by extremely high expression of the HIV p24 gene, was demonstrated in an HIV-associated T-cell lymphoma.[682] Together, these findings might suggest a role for HIV in the development of malignant lymphoma in these patients. However, the majority of investigators have been unable to detect HIV sequences in AIDS-related B-cell lymphoma tissue (Table 47–1),[138,221,223,263,559,715] implying that the role for HIV in promoting lymphomagenesis is an indirect one.

Thus, HIV directly, chronically stimulates polyclonal B-cell proliferation.[654,815] The florid B-cell hyperplasia is accompanied by hypergammaglobulinemia that frequently contains oligoclonal subsets targeted against HIV antigens, in addition to other environmental and self-antigens.[197,223] Evidence for a role for HIV in facilitating the progression from HIV-stimulated polyclonal B-cell proliferation to overt malignancy comes from a case of multiple myeloma in an HIV-1-positive patient where an IgG-κ paraprotein was identified that was directed against a specific HIV-1 antigen, p24.[391] Conversely, a recent investigation of the specificity of Igs derived from five cases of AIDS-non-Hodgkin's lymphomas revealed no reactivity of the lymphoma-derived Igs against HIV antigens, in contrast to strong Ig binding to antigens of non-HIV-infected cells from a variety of tissues.[142]

The most important role of HIV in lymphomagenesis is probably its ability to suppress the immune system, resulting in the disruption of immune surveillance.[313,314] However, the immune dysregulation that disrupts normal cytokine networks in the setting of HIV infection may also contribute to AIDS-related lymphomagenesis.[197,223] IL-6 and IL-10 are the two cytokine regulators of B-cell growth that have been documented to contribute to the growth of AIDS-non-Hodgkin's lymphomas.

B cells from HIV-infected individuals with hypergammaglobulinemia constitutively secrete high levels of IL-6. In addition, expression of IL-6 is up-regulated in certain AIDS-non-Hodgkin's lymphomas, especially immunoblastic lymphoma;[185] IL-6 is consistently absent from AIDS-Burkitt's lymphomas. IL-6, also known as BSF-2, or B-cell stimulatory factor, is produced by a variety of cell types, including monocytes/macrophages, T lymphocytes, and fibroblasts and has been shown to promote the growth and terminal differentiation of B cells.[307] It functions in an autocrine or paracrine fashion to promote the growth of human myeloma cells.[368,660] Although IL-6 also appears to act as an autocrine growth factor in EBV-immortalized B-lymphoblastoid cell lines,[750] whether its production actually represents a response to EBV infection is unclear. Not only does EBV fail to induce IL-6 production in normal mononuclear cells,[501] but IL-6 expression also does not correlate with EBV positivity in AIDS-related lymphomas.[185] In contrast to EBV, a viral IL-6 encoded by KSHV/HHV-8, which has 24.7 percent identity to human IL-6, has been detected in HIV-associated body cavity/primary effusion lymphomas but not in any benign or malignant effusions from HIV-negative patients.[20] Furthermore, HIV has been shown to induce IL-6 production in monocytes/macrophages, but not in T cells.[62,71,501] IL-6 production in response to HIV infection is believed, in turn, to contribute via paracrine loops to the polyclonal B-cell stimulation seen in individuals with AIDS, resulting in the nonspecific hypergammaglobulinemia that is observed early in the course of disease.[62,71,654,815] The proliferative effects of IL-6 suggest that it may contribute to tumorigenesis when it is overexpressed, as in HIV-infected individuals. In fact, constitutive expression of a transfected IL-6 gene in EBV-transformed B lymphoblasts confers on these cells altered in vitro growth properties, reflecting a more malignant phenotype in vitro, as well as tumorigenicity in nude mice.[648] Additional support for a tumor-promoting role for IL-6 comes from the observation that IL-6 serum levels in AIDS patients may predict the subsequent development of non-Hodgkin's lymphoma.[584] Thus, IL-6 superimposes on the immortalizing function of EBV the capacity for enhanced cell proliferation and transformation into frank malignancy, consistent with a model of multistep progression toward tumorigenesis.

Although it is homologous to the EBV protein BCRF (see above),[765] IL-10, but not BCRF, acts in an autocrine fashion as a potent stimulator of B cells. EBV-positive AIDS-Burkitt's lymphomas produce large quantities of IL-10, in contrast to non-AIDS-associated sporadic and endemic Burkitt's lymphomas in which IL-10 is never seen.[42] IL-10 production by AIDS-non-Hodgkin's lymphomas appears mainly in the EBV-positive cases, but interestingly BCRF is never detected in AIDS-non-Hodgkin's lymphomas.[42,223] Several tumor-promoting activities have been proposed for IL-10.[223] Its B-cell differentiating capability may enhance Ig secretion, contributing to the hypergammaglobulinemia of AIDS patients. IL-10 may inhibit apoptosis, thereby promoting B-cell viability. Finally, IL-10 inhibits the production of IL-2 and the antiviral cytokine, interferon-γ, by T cells, leading to impairment of immunosurveillance against the EBV-infected B cells that are abundant in individuals with AIDS.[323,480] The net result is the enhanced production of malignant B-cell clones in an environment of depressed immunosurveillance, a combination of circumstances that contributes to the multistep process of tumorigenesis.

Since, overall, EBV DNA contributes to at most 45 to 50 percent of AIDS-non-Hodgkin's lymphomas, other viruses have been examined for their potential role in AIDS-related lymphomagenesis. HIV-positive individuals are often co-infected with other viruses that are potentially tumorigenic in AIDS patients. Among these other viruses, HTLV-1 and HTLV-2 DNA sequences have rarely been detected in lymphomatous tissues of AIDS patients.[65,263,715] In an unusual case of cutaneous T-cell lymphoma in an HIV-positive patient, DNA from the clonally expanded CD3+CD8+CD4− T cells in the skin was positive for HTLV-2, but not HIV.[586] The HTLV-2 genome was clonally integrated at about one copy of provirus per cell, suggesting that HTLV-2 played a causal role in this lymphoma. Herpes viruses other than EBV, namely, human herpesvirus type 6 (HHV-6, or HBLV), which is associated with lymphoproliferative disorders in both HIV-positive and HIV-negative individuals,[638] and the more recently isolated HHV-7[215] may possibly contribute to lymphomagenesis in the setting of AIDS. Cytomegalovirus (CMV), an opportunistic pathogen in virtually all individuals with AIDS, has been shown to induce both T-cell proliferation and B-cell activation and may participate in the pathogenesis of AIDS-non-Hodgkin's lymphomas.[807]

Given the high frequency of co-infection with HIV and other viruses,[32,38,131,356,586,620,677] the possibility that different viruses interact synergistically to promote tumorigenesis should be explored. As an example, mitogenic stimulation of HIV-infected peripheral blood leukocytes by noninfectious HTLV-1 virions results in the production of large amounts of HIV-1.[825] Furthermore, many of the opportunistic viruses commonly seen in AIDS

patients (including CMV, herpes simplex viruses, EBV, and HHV-6) encode transactivator proteins that up-regulate transcription from the promoters of heterologous genes.[138] Thus, CMV encodes protein products that can transactivate the HIV long terminal repeat, or *LTR*.[148] A possible effect of this interaction is noted in cases of fulminant CMV infection, in which high amounts of HIV are also found. Adult T-cell leukemia/lymphoma has been observed in the setting of co-infection with HIV and HTLV-1.[677] Synergistic interaction between the two viruses is suggested as a factor contributing to tumorigenesis by the observation that the HTLV-1 transactivator protein, TAT-1, stimulates transcription from the HIV-1 *LTR*.[683] As a final example, the EBNA-1 protein binds a variety of RNA sequences, including the HIV-encoded transactivation response element *(TAR)*, suggesting the viral interaction as a mechanism for tumorigenesis in patients co-infected with HIV and EBV.[693] However, despite these potential contributing interactions among viruses prevalent in the setting of AIDS, the etiology of most of the AIDS-associated lymphomas that do not contain EBV is unknown.

Treatment of AIDS-Associated Lymphomas. No standardized approach exists for the treatment of non-Hodgkin's lymphomas in the setting of AIDS. Therapy has been of limited value because of the overriding influence of intercurrent opportunistic infection and the increased sensitivity of the patients to the myelosuppressive effects of the therapy, with between 10 and 48 percent showing a poor response.[48,138,421,756] Various standard combination chemotherapeutic regimens have been tried.[48,89,244,245,267,353,357,358,417,419,421,556,612,658,697,698,744,745,773,831] Despite treatment, median survival is short, ranging from 4 to 7 months, with half dying of lymphoma and half of other AIDS-related illnesses, particularly opportunistic infections. Meningeal spread of lymphoma has been observed even in the face of ongoing systemic treatment with methotrexate.[658] In contrast to non-Hodgkin's lymphomas in the non-HIV population, in which complete response rates as high as 85 percent and long-term disease-free survival of greater than 50 percent are obtained,[22,128,207,438] complete responses occur in only 30 to 67 percent of AIDS-non-Hodgkin's lymphomas, with 25 to 50 percent relapsing within 6 months.[359] The most important predictor of survival is the total number of CD4+ T lymphocytes, less than 100/mm^3 being associated with shorter survival.[245,357,419,556,612] Such individuals are more likely to experience prolonged neutropenia, with frequent episodes of febrile neutropenia, in response to chemotherapy. Additional features that correlate with a poor prognosis are a prior diagnosis of AIDS, a poor performance status, and extranodal disease.[421,756] Among extranodal sites, bone marrow and CNS disease are especially predictive of a shorter survival. Although not consistently seen, some studies indicate that patients with lymphomas having an immunoblastic histology have a worse prognosis than patients with other histopathologic types of non-Hodgkin's lymphoma.[211,245,419,421,556,694]

Although dose-intensive chemotherapy regimens were used in the beginning of the AIDS epidemic, these were generally found to be too toxic, resulting in opportunistic infections and death in many patients[421,756] and encouraging the view that "less might be better."[419,421] Among the high-dose regimens resulting in severe toxicity was combination chemotherapy incorporating a higher dose of cyclophosphamide, which led to shorter survival times than those seen in patients treated with a standard dose.[357] High-dose cyclophosphamide was used in another patient with AIDS-non-Hodgkin's lymphoma, together with total body irradiation followed by allogeneic bone marrow transplantation, resulting in bone marrow engraftment.[315] Although the patient died 47 days after transplantation as a result of tumor relapse, no evidence of HIV was seen in any autopsy tissue. An intensive regimen of M-BACOD using high-dose cytosine arabinoside and high-dose methotrexate, in an attempt to prevent CNS relapse, resulted in a significant risk of early death due to opportunistic infection, without increasing median survival or decreasing the risk of CNS relapse.[244] In contrast, the study by Bermudez et al.[48] demonstrated a 64 percent complete response rate with MACOP-B without exacerbation of toxicity relative to the general population receiving chemotherapy.

Incorporation of granulocyte/macrophage colony-stimulating factor (GM-CSF, sargramostim) or granulocyte colony-stimulating factor (G-CSF, filgrastim) into the chemotherapeutic regimens has permitted the use of standard doses with the maintenance of higher mean nadirs of absolute neutrophil count, shorter mean durations of neutropenia, and fewer episodes of neutropenic fever.[358,373,517,698,773] However, no statistical difference in survival time has been demonstrated as a consequence of CSF use.[358] Furthermore, evidence from elevated mean p24 levels suggests that GM-CSF stimulates HIV replication.[358] However, the elevation is transient and is not consistently observed.[773]

The low tolerance for intensive chemotherapy is especially true of patients with the poor prognostic features described above. Therefore, these features have been incorporated into the recommendations for therapy.[359,421,756] As a general approach, patients with poor immune function, specifically those with CD4 lymphocyte counts below 100/mm³, should be treated palliatively with reduced dose regimens, such as reduced dose M-BACOD. Standard-dose chemotherapeutic regimens, such as M-BACOD, MACOP-B, and ProMACE-CytaBOM, have been recommended for patients with better immune function (CD4 lymphocyte counts greater than 200/mm³). In addition, because of the risk of CNS relapse, routine use of CNS prophylaxis in patients with AIDS-non-Hodgkin's lymphomas has been suggested.[419,442,658]

Because the concomitant use of antiretroviral agents with chemotherapy may result in unacceptable hematologic toxicity, some investigators have withheld the antiretroviral drug temporarily during treatment for the lymphoma.[420,697] Various approaches have been tried in an effort to ameliorate this hematologic effect. Because zidovudine itself is associated with myelosuppression, simultaneous administration of zidovudine with a less intense chemotherapeutic regimen in patients with poor prognostic indicators yielded a complete remission rate of less than 15 percent and a median survival of only about 3 months.[421,745] Even the concomitant use of the growth factor GM-CSF failed to alleviate the cumulative myelosuppressive toxicity of zidovudine and chemotherapy.[358,731] The simultaneous use of other less myelotoxic antiretroviral agents, such as

zalcitabine (DDC, dideoxycytidine) or didanosine, with chemotherapy has therefore been explored. A low-dose M-BACOD regimen with concomitant zalcitabine in 21 patients led to 67 percent complete remissions, with complicating opportunistic infections in only 2 (10 percent).[419,421] Therapy with infusional (see below) cyclophosphamide, doxorubicin, and etoposide plus G-CSF led to a complete remission rate of 58 percent and a median survival of 18.4 months.[698] The myelosuppression experienced by patients undergoing this regimen was ameliorated by the concurrent use of didanosine. In a case report, a patient with HIV-related Burkitt's lymphoma was treated with aggressive chemotherapy in conjunction with a regimen of HAART and responded with prolonged survival, despite an intracardiac relapse.[74] Anecdotal reports describe the successful treatment of specific presentations of AIDS-non-Hodgkin's lymphomas with antiretroviral therapy alone. In two such reports, complete remissions were induced in primary effusion lymphomas containing immunoblastic and/or anaplastic clonal B cells positive for EBV and HHV-8 in response to zidovudine and zalcitabine therapy[532] or HAART, comprising zidovudine, lamivudine (3TC, dideoxythiacytidine), and indinavir.[702] In an analogous example of a primary CNS lymphoma, HAART, including zidovudine, lamivudine, and saquinavir, induced complete resolution of a 1.5 cm left frontoparietal lobe lesion, and maintained this remission for over 2 years.[465] Reminiscent of their use in EBV-associated post-transplant lymphomas (see below), virostatic therapy consisting of foscarnet, followed after 1 week by HAART (stavudine [d4T, didehydrodeoxythymidine], lamivudine, saquinavir, and ritonavir), was successfully applied to the treatment of an EBV-associated lymphoproliferation in an HIV-infected patient.[448,653]

The general recommendations evolving out of the studies just described have been to stratify patients into good or poor prognostic categories in an effort to apply the optimal regimen to each case.[421,756] Nevertheless, in the largest randomized trial, using standard-dose therapy with M-BACOD together with GM-CSF versus reduced dose M-BACOD with GM-CSF administered as needed, standard dose chemotherapy showed no survival advantage over attenuated dose treatment and had significantly more hematologic toxicities.[199,360] The recommendation resulting from this study has been to consider dose-modified chemotherapy for most HIV-infected patients with lymphoma.

One strategy to reduce the myelotoxicity of the therapy has been the use of infusional combination chemotherapy.[697,698] In a pilot study, this approach appeared to produce durable remissions; however, more testing is required. Studies are ongoing that evaluate rituximab as a therapy for AIDS-related lymphoma. Another strategy is to exploit the observation that activation signals may have the paradoxical effect of inhibiting the growth of neoplastic lymphocytes, so-called activation-induced cell death.[25,40] Indeed, such an approach has been effective in xenogeneic models in which mice bearing human EBV-transformed lymphomas have been cured with antibody to the CD40 receptor or by its ligand gp39.[219] Unless it becomes possible to restore immune and hematopoietic function to AIDS patients, it may be necessary to rely heavily on biologic approaches to the treatment of AIDS-associated lymphomas. Thus, a variety of gene therapy strategies are being explored. Although it has been difficult to achieve the required high-level expression of heterologous genes in EBV-transformed non-Hodgkin's lymphoma cells, a number of different approaches continue to be investigated.[143]

Hodgkin's Disease in HIV-Infected Individuals. Although individual cases of Hodgkin's disease in AIDS patients have been reported since 1984,[28,146,383,437,590,619,652,655,656,738,759] Hodgkin's disease has not been classified as an AIDS-defining illness to date.[94,112,306,365] This omission is attributable to the failure of specific studies to demonstrate an increased incidence of Hodgkin's disease in HIV-infected patients.[56,112,601,602,743] By contrast, Hessol et al.[306] observed an increased risk of both Hodgkin's and non-Hodgkin's lymphoma in this population. The age-adjusted standardized morbidity ratio for Hodgkin's disease was 5.0, with an incidence of 19.3 cases of Hodgkin's disease per 100,000 person-years versus no cases in a comparable population without HIV infection. While this incidence is well below the 240.3 cases per 100,000 person-years seen for non-Hodgkin's lymphoma in patients with HIV infection (ratio of non-Hodgkin's to Hodgkin's lymphoma was 12.4), the rate of Hodgkin's disease in the HIV population was clearly elevated. Similar data from Lyter et al.[446] revealed 85 cases of Hodgkin's disease per 100,000 person years in an AIDS cohort, in contrast to 4.3 cases per 100,000 person-years in the general population, the rate in the study cohort being 19.8 times that expected (confidence interval 2.4 to 71.5; $p < .005$). In addition, Hodgkin's disease has been reported to be more common among HIV-infected intravenous drug users than among similarly infected homosexual men in some,[337,478,624,667,742,743] but not all[12,228,247,560] studies. The relative risk of Hodgkin's disease among 4954 children with AIDS was 63,[57] significantly increased compared to population rates using area-specific registry data. Finally, as among organ transplant recipients (see below), the relative ages of Hodgkin's and non-Hodgkin's lymphoma patients may be reversed in the AIDS setting compared to the general population, in which Hodgkin's disease is more prevalent among young and non-Hodgkin's lymphoma among older adults.[161,330]

The most prevalent histological subtype of Hodgkin's disease reported among HIV-infected individuals is mixed cellularity.[12,28,112,247,330,337,383,560,588,667,742,743,759] The proportions of both the mixed cellularity and lymphocyte depleted subtypes among HIV-infected individuals with Hodgkin's disease (40 to 60 percent and 20 percent, respectively) are elevated relative to the non-HIV Hodgkin's disease population.[365,655,746,747,760] Although the nodular sclerosis type is well represented in patients infected with HIV, constituting the second most common subtype (30 percent), its frequency in this population is decreased in comparison with non-HIV-infected patients with Hodgkin's disease in whom nodular sclerosing is the most prevalent subtype.[760] Pelstring et al.[560] have pointed out that all histologic subtypes show a decreased number of morphologically benign background lymphocytes, creating an overall "lymphocyte-depleted" appearance. This prevalence of lymphocyte depletion resembles that observed in Hodgkin's disease occur-

ring in association with other immunodeficient states, such as ataxia-telangiectasia.[217] Lymphocyte predominant Hodgkin's disease has only rarely been reported in association with HIV infection.[12,667]

HIV-infected individuals with Hodgkin's disease present with advanced (i.e., Stage III or IV) disease in as high as 80 to 90 percent of cases, often accompanied by B symptoms (most commonly fever, which must be distinguished from fever resulting from occult opportunistic infections; also night sweats and weight loss).[112,655,667] Extranodal disease occurs in two-thirds of patients, with bone marrow involvement in up to 50 percent,[12,667] in contrast to the 3.5 percent observed in patients with Hodgkin's disease not infected with HIV. Other reported sites of involvement include lung, liver, bone, paraspinal masses, rectum, and CNS, as well as other unusual sites such as the tongue[545] and skin.[655,672] A relative paucity of mediastinal disease has been noted in HIV-infected patients[655]—22 percent versus 50 percent in the absence of HIV infection—and noncontiguous spread may occur in the setting of HIV.[365,672]

Therapy of Hodgkin's disease in HIV-infected patients has included the standard treatment regimens of MOPP (nitrogen mustard, vincristine, prednisone, procarbazine) and/or ABVD (doxorubicin, bleomycin, vinblastine, dacarbazine) with or without radiation therapy.[12,28,247,337,383,652,655,667,742] More recent regimens have incorporated the primary use of growth factors as well as the addition of antiretroviral treatment to the antineoplastic chemotherapy, a combination that was shown to be feasible.[189] Although most patients respond to treatment, with complete response rates as high as 80 percent,[189,247] bone marrow tolerance to chemotherapy is poor, with persistent cytopenias out of proportion to dosage, thus requiring many delayed or reduced doses. Median survival ranges from 8 months to 18 months, with a 1-year survival of only 23 percent, versus 82 percent survival at 5 years in the absence of HIV infection.[365] At least half of deaths result from opportunistic infections or other officially AIDS-defining malignancies, and the remaining deaths are due to progression of Hodgkin's disease or to cytopenias, resulting either from bone marrow involvement by Hodgkin's disease or from the extreme sensitivity of the marrow to chemotherapeutic agents.

The pathogenesis of Hodgkin's disease in the setting of HIV infection may, in part, be attributable to coexisting EBV infection. Evidence for an etiologic association between EBV infection and Hodgkin's disease (see above) is based on the epidemiologic demonstration of a higher incidence of Hodgkin's disease following infectious mononucleosis, as well as on the identification of clonal episomal EBV DNA in Reed-Sternberg cells and on the expression of EBV antigens in Reed-Sternberg cells (notably the expression of LMP-1 in 38 to 48 percent of these cells).[302,542] In the setting of HIV infection, the evidence supporting EBV's contribution to the development of Hodgkin's disease may be even stronger. Uccini et al.[757] detected EBV DNA in 83 percent of lymph nodes affected by Hodgkin's disease from HIV-infected patients but in only 18 percent of involved nodes from seronegative patients with Hodgkin's disease. The EBV genome was restricted to Reed-Sternberg cells and was found to be monoclonal. Similar observations by Tirelli et al.[747] revealed

78 percent of Hodgkin's disease tissue in HIV patients to be associated with EBV, versus 25 percent in the non-HIV setting. As in the non-HIV setting, the EBV genome was restricted to Reed-Sternberg cells and was found to be monoclonal.[747,757]

Additional speculation about the pathogenesis of Hodgkin's disease in the setting of AIDS centers on whether the immunological deficits that lead to Hodgkin's disease are attributable solely to the Hodgkin's disease-related immunodysregulation[365] or to HIV-induced effects. The first possibility would tend to argue against the incorporation of Hodgkin's disease as an AIDS-defining illness, whereas the latter interpretation would support AIDS-induced immunodeficiency as a predisposing factor to the development of Hodgkin's disease. Absolute T-cell lymphopenia (together with a relatively greater depletion of CD4+ cells, resulting in a decrease in the CD4/CD8 ratio) characterizes HIV-infected individuals with Hodgkin's disease,[12,247,383,560,655] distinguishing them from patients with Hodgkin's disease in the non-HIV population but resembling the CD4+ T-cell status (and CD4/CD8 ratios) of individuals with AIDS-non-Hodgkin's lymphoma. Another similarity between Hodgkin's and non-Hodgkin's lymphomas in the AIDS setting is that both are frequently preceded by PGL.[337,418,607] In an Italian study, PGL preceded non-Hodgkin's lymphoma in 83 percent and Hodgkin's disease in 73 percent of patients, with a similar latency of 14 months.[337] In this Italian study, a prior diagnosis of AIDS was less common among at-risk (homosexuals, intravenous drug abusers, hemophiliacs, poly-transfused persons) patients presenting with Hodgkin's disease than with non-Hodgkin's lymphoma (9 percent versus 93 percent).[337] Thus, Hodgkin's disease, along with specific subtypes of non-Hodgkin's lymphoma, occurred more frequently in a less immunocompromised setting. This prevalence of Hodgkin's disease among at-risk individuals lacking official diagnoses of AIDS has two major implications. First, it creates a dilemma as to whether these patients should be classified as having AIDS in the cases for which HIV-positivity has been documented. Second, it suggests that, in contrast to non-Hodgkin's lymphoma, the immunologic deficits of Hodgkin's disease may be sufficient to engage in a synergistic interaction with those of early HIV infection to allow the development of lymphoma.

Several authors have encouraged consideration of Hodgkin's disease as an AIDS-defining illness.[306,560,652,742] Apart from the obvious statistical justification apparent in those studies that demonstrate an increased incidence of Hodgkin's disease in HIV-infected patients, the atypical presentation and the additional complexities of management of Hodgkin's disease in the setting of HIV infection have been invoked as a basis for establishing it as an AIDS-defining illness.[306] Thus, the disproportionate representation of more aggressive histologic subtypes, advanced stage, increased incidence of extranodal presentations (particularly bone marrow involvement), the inverted CD4/CD8 ratio, and the poor prognosis speak to a form of Hodgkin's disease that is fundamentally different from that occurring in the absence of HIV infection. Even if all cases occurring in the context of HIV positivity do not qualify as AIDS defining, specific presentations, such as high grade or advanced stage,[13] a mixed cellularity or lymphocyte depleted subtype,[746] or accompanying severe immune impairment (CD4 cell count, less than $200/\text{mm}^3$)[306] have been proposed as part of a revised case definition of AIDS.

Other Viruses

Of the six viruses that appear to have a causal association with malignancy (human T-cell leukemia virus-1 [HTLV-1], EBV, HHV-8, human papillomavirus [HPV], hepatitis B virus [HBV], hepatitis C virus [HCV]), two (EBV and HTLV-1) are strongly implicated as playing an etiologic role in lymphomagenesis.[65,493,585] HTLV-1 is a single-stranded RNA virus that integrates randomly into the host cell genome, with one copy of this provirus being detectable per cell. The clonality of this integration, that is, all cells reflecting integration at the same site, supports HTLV-1's contribution to the development of cancer. A recent study of T-cell lymphomas in an HTLV-1-endemic area has reaffirmed the importance of distinguishing positively staining HTLV-1 cases with clonal integration of the HTLV-1 provirus from positively staining cases without clonal integration, in which the lymphoma had coincidentally occurred in HTLV-1 infected carriers.[531] The former group, which had a particularly poor prognosis, was defined as adult T-cell leukemia/lymphoma (ATLL), in contrast to the latter group, which was classified as T-cell lymphoma. The HTLV-1 genome codes for Tax, a viral transcriptional transactivator that operates through multiple pathways to up-regulate viral and cellular gene products that may contribute to carcinogenesis.[65,213] In HTLV-1-infected cells, for example, Tax activates $NF\text{-}\kappa B$ and $BCL\text{-}X_L$, which leads to the inhibition of apoptosis and ultimately results in an increase of cytokine production and cell proliferation.[367,519]

The strongest association of HTLV-1 with malignancy is seen with ATLL, a form of peripheral T-cell lymphoma that comprises four subtypes: acute, chronic, smoldering, and lymphoma-type.[65,213] All subtypes have viral DNA clonally integrated into the cellular DNA of the neoplastic cells. The acute form of ATLL is an aggressive T-cell lymphoma associated with a high white blood cell count, hypercalcemia, hepatosplenomegaly, and lytic bone lesions. The presence in the peripheral blood of large flowerlike cells with lobulated nuclei is pathognomonic for ATLL. The manifestation of ATLL as a T-cell non-Hodgkin's lymphoma subtype resembles the acute form in some ways (e.g., hypercalcemia) but lacks the characteristic peripheral blood involvement of ATLL. Smoldering ATLL may resemble mycosis fungoides/Sézary syndrome in that cutaneous involvement occurs in the form of erythema or infiltrative plaques or tumors. Both the acute and lymphoma-type ATLL have a poor prognosis, with mean survival being only 6 months. They are poorly responsive to conventional chemotherapy, encouraging the use of experimental approaches such as aggressive infusional chemotherapy, which has shown some promise, yielding up to 93 percent overall objective response rate with a median survival of 17.4 months.[697] Overexpression of Bcl-X_L has recently been demonstrated in ATLL cells from patients who were unresponsive to various chemotherapeutic regimens.[519] HTLV-1 is endemic in such areas as southern Japan, the Caribbean Islands, and some areas of Brazil, where ATLL accounts for over half of adult lymphoid malignancies. ATLL develops in 1 per 1000 HTLV-1 carriers per year, with early life exposure, at a time when the host immune system is immature, being associated with the greatest risk of subsequent disease.

In contrast to HTLV-1, human T-cell leukemia virus-2 (HTLV-2) has not been strongly correlated with any disease, despite its initial isolation from what was originally viewed as a hairy cell leukemia, but later reclassified as a large granular T-cell leukemia in which the cell type is that of a natural killer cell.[65,585] HHV-8/KSHV, in addition to showing an association with body cavity-based lymphomas in the setting of HIV (see above), has been observed in the plasma cell variant of multicentric Castleman's disease and in angioimmunoblastic lymphadenopathy.[65,175,176,444,696] As a final example, the prevalence of chronic HCV infection has been shown to be higher in patients with B-cell non-Hodgkin's lymphoma than in controls, suggesting a potential role for HCV in B-cell lymphomagenesis.[445,462,836] HCV is the primary etiologic agent of type II mixed cryoglobulinemia, which is associated with an underlying B-cell proliferation in 2 to 11 percent of cases, providing a biologic rationale for the association of this virus with predisposition to B-cell malignancy. Nevertheless, an association between HCV infection and non-Hodgkin's lymphoma has not been observed by all investigators,[239,758] and additional studies are required before a role for HCV in lymphomagenesis can be confirmed.

Bacteria

Helicobacter Pylori

Infections with organisms other than viruses have been implicated in the promotion of malignancy, including lymphoma. *Helicobacter pylori* is one example. For many years, the belief was held that microorganisms could not inhabit the stomach and that gastric juice was sterile. More recently, however, not only has a high prevalence of *H. pylori* been shown in the stomachs of the population, but its presence has also been associated with disease. *H. pylori* eradication has become a primary component of the therapy of peptic ulcer disease and nonulcer dyspepsia,[67,209,464,581] in which it has been shown to play an etiologic role. In addition, infection with the organism appears to be a risk factor for gastric carcinoma,[285,523,548,730] raising the prospect that this cancer might be prevented by treating the infection. *H. pylori* strains are highly diverse, and the type of strain with which an individual is colonized will affect his/her risk for disease. Evidence exists for a strong association between the carriage of the *cagA+*, *vacA s1*, or *iceA1 H. pylori* strains and an increased risk for duodenal ulceration, atrophic gastritis, and noncardia gastric adenocarcinomas.[64,178]

The stomach wall normally contains no lymphocytes. However, in persons infected with *H. pylori*, a lymphoid cell infiltrate, *mucosa-associated lymphoid tissue* (MALT), may appear, and this "acquired" MALT can over time develop into a lymphoma.[332,333,632,651,799,834,835] MALT lymphoma (also called *extranodal marginal zone B-cell lymphoma of MALT type*[293]) is seen in a variety of extranodal sites, including the thyroid, lung, salivary gland, and small bowel.[82,332] They often occur in the context of a pre-existing disorder, as in the thyroid and salivary gland in association with pre-existing Hashimoto's thyroiditis and myoepithelial sialadenitis, respectively (see below).[82,834] The stomach is the site most often affected by MALT lymphoma. *H. pylori* provides the antigenic stimulus to the gastritis that gradually becomes a tumor. MALT lymphoma, the most common type of marginal zone lymphoma, is mucosal based, showing a trophism for the epithelium of the affected extranodal parenchyma.[208,293,651] The key histologic feature is the presence of lymphoepithelial lesions, with invasion and partial destruction of the gastric glands or crypts by aggregates of centrocyte-like cells.[39,82,104,334,834,835] Although low-grade MALT lymphomas are generally believed to be localized (Stage I$_E$ or II$_E$) at the time of diagnosis, in contrast to most nodally based low-grade B-cell lymphomas, some studies have demonstrated dissemination in up to a third of cases.[334,739,834,835]

The mechanism of the lymphomagenesis is incompletely understood, but the infecting organism, *H. pylori*, is believed to provide an antigenic stimulus to neoplastic B cells in the lymphoid infiltrates via *H. pylori*-specific T-cell proliferation.[178,204,325,326,334,632,834] *H. pylori* strains producing the CagA antigen (*cagA+*) induce strong gastric inflammation and, in addition to a strong association with gastric adenocarcinoma, are also associated with the development of MALT lymphoma.[527,564,730] These observations raise the possibility that MALT lymphomas in other sites also arise through chronic antigenic stimulation, but the precise stimuli are not defined. An alternative model for B-cell expansion derives from the observation that antibody production of both antibacterial Ig and autoantibodies is stimulated by *H. pylori*. A strong homology, at both the genotypic and the phenotypic levels, has been noted between the hypervariable regions of the *H. pylori*-stimulated Igs and those of rheumatoid factors, suggesting a mechanistic basis for B-cell stimulation in which MALT B-cell lymphomas derive from autoreactive B-cell clones as opposed to clones of B cells directed against *H. pylori*[50] Ultimately, positive selection for individual B cells through their antigen receptors results in the emergence of B-cell clones, as evidenced by the monoclonality of B cells in gastric MALT lymphoma documented by PCR.[104,800,834,835]

The subsequent development of genetic alterations also contributes to carcinogenesis. The loss of chromosome 3 has been suggested as playing a role in the transition from benign MALT to low-grade MALT lymphoma.[31,651] Nevertheless, trisomy 3 and, less frequently, trisomy 18, have been observed in most MALT lymphomas.[104,802,834,835] The t(11;18)(q21;q21) translocation has been implicated in low-grade MALT lymphomas,[26,504,537] although this translocation was not observed in a recent series of low-grade MALT lymphomas that responded to *H. pylori* eradication therapy (see below).[9] Other frequently encountered genetic abnormalities include the t(1;14) translocation and translocations and abnormalities of chromosome 1p or 7.[504,834] The t(1;14) translocation results in truncation of *Bcl-10*, leading to activation of *NF-κB* and absence of apoptosis.[173,792,793] Although *c-MYC* rearrangements are not generally seen in MALT lymphomas, mutations in exon 1 and the intron 1 regulatory region were observed in 17 percent of cases examined, implicating this oncogene in MALT lymphomagenesis.[562,835]

Moving along the carcinogenic spectrum, the relationship of low-grade to high-grade MALT lymphomas is complex. One possibility is that low-grade MALT lymphomas progress to diffuse large cell lymphomas. Such a relationship is supported by epidemiological data linking the much more common high-grade gastric diffuse large cell lymphoma to *H. pylori* infection.[293,549,632] In fact, most gastric MALT lymphoma patients (98.5 percent) are seropositive for *H. pylori*, although only 58 to 78 percent of resected specimens actually contain the *H. pylori* bacteria (63 percent for low-grade versus 38 percent for high-grade lymphomas).[178,283,651] Histologic distinction of grade among MALT lymphomas, however, has posed problems, with many presentations occurring as mixtures of low- and high-grade tumors.[104,153,204,334,834] Therefore, attempts to determine the existence of a transition from low- to high-grade have relied on documenting changes at the molecular level.[104,651] The rearranged Ig heavy chain gene sequences within the low- and high-grade components of mixed gastric MALT B-cell lymphomas have been demonstrated as identical in size by electrophoresis, supporting a clonal link between the two components and suggesting a transition from the low- to the high-grade lymphoma.[563] Recent data reveal the association of multiple genetic aberrations with high-grade gastric lymphomas.[706] Loss of heterozygosity was most commonly (42 percent) noted on the long arm of chromosome 6 (6q21-22 and 6q23.3-25), but was also seen at the sites of several tumor suppressor genes (including *APC*, *p15/16*, *p53*, and *DCC*). Amplification of specific regions was frequently noted (including chromosome 3q27 at the *BCL-6* gene locus and 11q23-24 at the *MLL* gene locus). The data on microsatellite instability (MSI) are conflicting, with Starostik et al.[706] finding only a low frequency of MSI in high-grade tumors, in contrast to a frequency of 50 percent noted in other studies.[104,561,834] A sense of transition from low- to high-grade MALT lymphoma emerges from comparisons of *p53* mutations (seen in 6, 12, and 31 percent of low-, mixed-, and high-grade tumors, respectively) and *bcl-2* overexpression (seen in 93, 88, and 44 percent of low-, mixed-, and high-grade tumors, respectively), which are inversely correlated with each other.[503,529,651,835] These data point to a possible association of *p53* mutations with transformation to high-grade lymphoma.[834] Another genetic alteration that appears to correlate with progression to more aggressive histology is mutation of the *BCL*10 gene.[173] Additional molecular evidence supporting a link between low- and high-grade MALT lymphomas comes from the fact that aberrant isotype switch recombination has been detected in specimens of both grades.[508] Although evidence exists for the transformation of low-grade MALT lymphomas to high-grade lymphomas, high-grade diffuse large B-cell lymphomas may also arise de novo in the stomach.[334]

Low-grade gastric MALT lymphomas have been successfully treated by eradication of *H. pylori* with antibiotic therapy. Complete regression of low-grade MALT lymphomas occurs in 50 to 80 percent of the treated cases.[9,39,104,516,529,622,645,800,801,833,834] Despite such observations, long-term persistence of monoclonal B cells, defined by PCR amplification of rearranged variable-diversity-joining (VDJ) sequences, has been noted in half of patients after cure of *H. pylori* infection and complete histo-

logic remission of localized low-grade gastric MALT lymphoma.[740] When antibiotic therapy is unsuccessful or is inappropriate, as when *H. pylori* is absent, surgical resection or radiation has been administered, since low-grade MALT lymphoma is usually confined to the site of origin.[651,834] Local therapy of this nature has successfully induced remissions. Chemotherapy has also been administered with good results. To date, there is no evidence from controlled trials defining optimal therapy, and none of the modalities has been proven superior to the others in terms of prolonging survival.[834,835] Even if high-grade gastric large cell lymphoma is related to *H. pylori*, it would seem unlikely that the tumor cells depend on the persistence of the organism in the same fashion that has been documented for low-grade gastric MALT lymphoma, given the abundance of associated genetic changes in high grade tumors.[153] Nevertheless, in one study eight patients with high-grade gastrointestinal lymphomas experienced complete remission after eradication of *H. pylori*.[204,485] Further studies addressing whether *H. pylori* eradication would have either a therapeutic or preventive effect in high-grade gastric lymphoma would be of great value. However, a standard chemotherapy approach is the treatment of choice in high-grade gastric lymphoma.

Borrelia burgdorferi

An association between primary cutaneous B-cell lymphoma (CBCL) and infection with the spirochete *Borrelia burgdorferi*, the infectious cause of Lyme disease, has been observed in a number of cases.[96,227] A pathogenetic role for the organism was suggested in part by the clinical observation of B-cell lymphomas arising on skin affected by acrodermatitis chronica atrophicans, a skin lesion known to be caused by *B. burgdorferi*. Raised titers of antibodies to *B. burgdorferi* in the sera of patients with CBCL offered additional evidence supporting such an association.[96] Monoclonality of the lymphomatous skin infiltrate has been demonstrated, and specific DNA sequences of *B. burgdorferi* have been identified in the cutaneous lesions in 18 percent of cases.[96,227,623] The lymphomas are generally low-grade, extracutaneous involvement is rare, and progression is slow, with tumors remaining confined to the skin for as long as 7 to 15 years.[227] By analogy to *H. pylori*-associated MALT-lymphomas of the stomach, a proportion of *B. burgdorferi*-associated lymphomas have been cured by appropriate antibiotic treatment, with concomitant eradication of the spirochete.[96,397,623]

LYMPHOMAS IN THE SETTING OF TRANSPLANTATION

Lymphomas in the Setting of Solid Organ Transplantation

Epidemiology/Demographics of Lymphomas Associated With Organ Transplants

Organ transplantation, together with the underlying condition that necessitates it and the immunosuppressive therapy that is often essential to prevent rejection of the transplanted organ, all contribute to the development of non-Hodgkin's lymphomas. This is especially true of solid organ transplants: 6 percent of patients develop malignant tumors de novo, an incidence that is 100 times that of the general population.[565–567,571,572] This increase is not made up of frequently encountered malignancies, such as carcinomas of the lung, breast, prostate, colon, uterus, and bladder.[252,568,573,576] In fact, excluding non-melanoma skin cancers and in situ carcinomas of the cervix, the most frequently encountered malignancy in the transplant setting is lymphoma, which comprises 21 percent of post-transplant cancers, versus 5 percent in the general population.[241,319,573,576] Between 1.0 and 4.6 percent of transplant patients develop post–solid organ transplantation lymphoproliferative disorders (PTLD), depending on the organ transplanted (see below).[506,572] Furthermore, PTLDs are clinically and pathologically a heterogeneous group of lymphoid proliferations, most of which are of B-cell origin and are associated with EBV. The incidence of lymphoproliferative disorders among transplant recipients is increased 30- to 50-fold relative to that in the general population.[319,486,574,576] Interestingly, Hodgkin's disease, which makes up 20 percent of all lymphomas in the general population, is rare among transplant patients, in whom 93 percent of lymphomas are of the non-Hodgkin's type.[55,229,317,568,573,576]

The average time of occurrence of all cancers following transplant is 61 months.[576] Lymphomas tend to appear earlier, averaging about 32 months.[319,533,568,576,577] The risk of malignancy increases early, in the first year post-transplant, and remains constant thereafter.[319] This contrasts with the risk of non-Hodgkin's lymphoma in AIDS patients, which continues to increase with increasing duration of HIV infection as a consequence of progressive immunologic dysfunction.[602,816]

In contrast to the general population in which the incidence of non-Hodgkin's lymphoma is higher among older individuals, lymphomas occur in a relatively young age group among transplant patients, since the age at the time of transplant averages between 31 and 41 years in different studies.[486,573,576] While among adults age has no effect on the incidence of non-Hodgkin's lymphoma during the first year after transplant,[791] in subsequent years the rate of non-Hodgkin's lymphoma does increase with age.[533] Furthermore, post-transplant lymphomas occur more frequently among pediatric than adult patients,[21] making up between 52 and 74 percent of all malignancies in the former versus 15 percent in the latter.[577,578] Armitage et al.[21] observed that in contrast to a 3.5 percent incidence of PTLD among adult patients receiving heart or lung transplants, the incidence of PTLD among pediatric patients was 9.7 percent. Srivastava et al.[704] reported that 7.1 percent of 84 pediatric renal transplant patients developed PTLD.

Additional demographics point to a higher incidence of post-transplant lymphomas in North America than in Europe among both kidney and heart transplant patients.[533] In the United States the risk of developing non-Hodgkin's lymphoma is slightly lower among African-American than White patients.[533] Several of these epidemiologic correlates probably reflect two key features of transplantation: the type of transplant and the nature of the immunosuppressive therapy.

Influence of Type of Transplant on Lymphoma Incidence. Whereas patients receiving renal and cardiac transplants show a similar overall 6 percent incidence of cancer,[576] the incidence of non-Hodgkin's lymphomas is higher among heart (5 percent) than kidney (1 to 2 percent) transplant recipients,[122,422,486,533,572,578,688,725,791] with somewhat higher rates, up to 8.0 percent, occurring in heart-lung/lung than heart transplant patients.[21,179,572,725] In a study at the University of Pittsburgh, Nalesnik et al.[506] observed PTLD in 2.2 percent of liver, 1.0 percent of kidney, 1.8 percent of heart, and 4.6 percent of heart/lung transplant patients. Non-Hodgkin's lymphomas make up 53 percent of malignancies that develop in nonrenal transplant patients versus 11 percent of cancers in recipients of renal transplants, in whom the predominant neoplasm is skin cancer.[572,573] Among pediatric transplant patients, lymphomas make up 83 percent of cancers in nonrenal recipients and 31 percent of neoplasms in renal recipients, reflecting the overall higher incidence of lymphomas in this patient population.[577]

The time at which a lymphoproliferative disorder develops also varies with the type of transplant. In the pediatric population, for example, lymphoma occurs sooner after nonrenal (11 months) than renal (34 months) transplantation.[578] In the first year after transplant, 0.2 percent of kidney and 1.2 percent of heart transplant recipients develop non-Hodgkin's lymphoma, 20 and 120 times the respective incidences in the general population.[533] After the first year, the lymphoma incidence for both types of transplant decreases to about the same extent. A comparison of heart with heart-lung/lung transplants, however, shows that almost all lymphomas in the latter group develop in the first post-transplant year, whereas only half of lymphomas occur in this early time period in heart transplant patients.[21]

Influence of Immunosuppressive Therapy on Lymphoma Incidence. A number of immunosuppressive agents, including azathioprine, cyclophosphamide, and cyclosporine, have been shown to promote tumorigenesis in the transplant setting.[53,86,122,369,571,688,776,791,819] However, data on the frequency of PTLD following various immunosuppressive regimens have been conflicting. In addition, the use of complex regimens involving multiple agents makes it difficult to dissect out the tumorigenic effect of a single component.[400,573] Nevertheless, qualitative differences have been demonstrated among these agents with respect to their carcinogenic, and specifically lymphomagenic, potential.

Whereas cyclosporine use does not lead to a higher incidence of cancer than conventional immunosuppressive therapy (CIT), involving azathioprine, cyclophosphamide and prednisone,[571] the types of malignancies have been shown to differ in some reports,[53,568,571] but not all.[122,264,791] When differences were demonstrated, lymphomas constituted 41 percent of cancers following cyclosporine-based therapy, in contrast to only 12 percent following CIT.[569,570] Skin cancers, which make up 40 percent of neoplasms following CIT, are seen in only 15 to 22 percent of patients treated with cylosporine.[569–571] The time to appearance of cancers following cyclosporine use is shorter, averaging 20 months, versus the 60 months noted for other agents.[569–571] Lymphomas occur even earlier, an average of only 11 months post-cyclosporine versus 42 months for CIT.

Cyclosporine use leads to a disproportionately high incidence of cancers among patients receiving extrarenal organs.[122,569–571] Thus, 22 percent of cyclosporine-related malignancies but only 2 percent of CIT-related cancers occur in recipients of liver, bone marrow, pancreatic, or combined heart-lung transplants. Lymphomas make up 66 percent of the cancers in the cyclosporine-treated extrarenal transplant patients, and 39 to 50 percent of all cyclosporine-related lymphomas are observed in recipients of extrarenal organs, out of proportion relative to the percentage of transplant recipients receiving such organs.[122,569–571] Cyclosporine- and CIT-related lymphomas involve similar sites, but the distribution is different. In contrast to CIT-related lymphomas, of which 78 percent are extranodal and 22 percent are nodal, a higher percentage of lymphomas associated with cyclosporine present in the lymph nodes (47 percent).[568–571] Other frequently affected sites include the liver, spleen, bone marrow, lungs, and allografts, especially renal. In particular, cyclosporine-related non-Hodgkin's lymphomas have a propensity for small bowel involvement, which occurs in 22 percent of cyclosporine- versus 12 percent of CIT-related non-Hodgkin's lymphomas; localization to the small bowel is seen in 32 percent of the former and only 19 percent of the latter group. Finally, CNS involvement is a prominent feature of CIT-related non-Hodgkin's lymphoma, occurring in 40 percent of patients, with 75 percent of these being confined to the CNS. This contrasts with cyclosporine-related non-Hodgkin's lymphomas: no more than 14 percent affect the CNS, 27 percent of which are limited to this system.[568,569] In summary, cyclosporine therapy, in contrast to CIT, is associated with more life-threatening cancers of vital organs, rather than low-grade skin cancers and in situ cervical carcinomas. However, the lymphomas that develop in association with cyclosporine appear to respond more readily to a variety of treatments, particularly treatments that include reduction of immunosuppressive therapy.[707]

Other immunosuppressive agents, such as anti-lymphocyte globulin (ALG), anti-thymocyte globulin (ATG), and antibody to the CD3 T-cell surface antigen (OKT3) have been evaluated for their possible contributions to PTLD.[341,565,573,722] ALG, OKT3, and specifically the sequential use of ALG followed by OKT3 have been implicated in the development of PTLD.[123,341,348,565,722,725] Among malignancies that develop in transplant recipients treated with monoclonal antibodies such as OKT3, a disproportionately high percentage (64 percent) consist of lymphomas, and these develop very early, averaging only 7 months following transplant.[572,573] Tacrolimus (FK506, Prograf), a more recently introduced immunosuppressive agent, used both primarily and to rescue grafts that are being rejected on cyclosporine-based therapy, is associated with an increased incidence of EBV-related complications, including EBV-associated PTLD.[115,181]

High doses of immunosuppressive agents have been associated with increased development of lymphoma.[341,493,725] Thus, the higher incidence of lymphoproliferative disease seen in early trials with cyclosporine relative to established immunosuppressive therapy was subsequently traced to the higher cyclosporine doses used at the time.[86,122,568,707] Higher cumulative doses of prophylactic OKT3 (more than 75 mg) in cardiac transplant recipients correlate with a higher incidence of lymphomas, 35.7 percent, compared with 6.2 percent for doses less than 75 mg.[722] OKT3 doses higher than 75 mg also correlate with a shorter time interval between transplant and development of lymphoma, averaging only 1 to 2 months. Furthermore, the variable incidence of malignancy, and specifically lymphoma, in different subgroups of transplant recipients may at least in part be attributable to the intentional implementation of more intensive immunosuppressive regimens in certain settings. Termination of immunosuppressive therapy may be a reasonable option for management of severe rejection of a kidney transplant, given the non-life-threatening nature of the transplant rejection.[506,577,725] However, no such option is available when a comparable threat of rejection occurs in the setting of heart, liver, or lung transplant, necessitating intensification of the immunosuppressive regimen in order to save the patient's life.

In addition to higher doses of individual agents, the use of combinations of immunosuppressive agents to minimize individual toxicities may carry its own risk by undermining different points in the immune system.[400,688,791] Thus, the doses of cyclosporine used in triple therapy with prednisone and azathioprine have been lowered in an effort to reduce nephrotoxicity. Despite these reduced cyclosporine doses, the incidence of lymphoma is increased with triple therapy.[688,791] The increase is even more pronounced among cardiac transplants.

Clinical Features and Histopathology

Hanto et al. classified transplant recipients into two main groups on the basis of their epidemiologic and clinical features.[287,289,725] Young patients tended to present soon after transplant or shortly after immunosuppressive treatment for rejection (mean, 11 months) with symptoms of infectious mononucleosis (i.e., fever, sore throat, malaise, and lymphadenopathy). Their clinical course consisted of a rapidly progressive disseminated lymphoproliferative process with a high (80 percent) mortality rate within a mean of 3 months after diagnosis. Older patients presented later after transplant (mean, 42 months) while on maintenance immunosuppressive therapy with discrete tumor masses in the oropharynx, CNS, liver, and small bowel. Although the PTLD was less widespread and progressed more slowly, it still resulted in a high mortality rate (71 percent) about 9 months following diagnosis.

PTLD displays a spectrum of lesions ranging from polymorphic diffuse B-cell hyperplasia to intermediate polymorphic diffuse B-cell lymphoma to true monomorphic large cell immunoblastic lymphoma.[54,99,101,218,286–289,291,422,507,597] The polymorphic presentations, which contain small and large cells of both follicular center and medullary type, have been interpreted as benign reactive hyperplastic or neoplastic lymphomas depending on whether cell marker studies reveal polyclonal or monoclonal B-cell proliferations.[218,286] Evolution from a polyclonal polymorphic lymphoproliferation to a true monoclonal monomorphic large cell immunoblastic lymphoma has been demonstrated in a small number of renal transplant recipients.[288,291] Whereas some reports on renal recipients emphasize the polyclonal nature of early post-transplant lesions,[218,286,287] monoclonality of lymphoproliferative lesions has been documented on initial presentation in cardiac transplant recipients.[119] A possible explanation for the discrepancy lies in the inherent differences in cardiac versus renal transplants, together with the higher doses of immunosuppressive agents employed in the former.[54,119] More likely, the contradictory findings are traceable to the different technologies used to assess clonality.[54,289,291,552,665] The earlier studies of renal transplant recipients employed immunophenotyping with antibodies specific for heavy and light Ig chains,[218,286,287] a far less sensitive technique than the Southern blot DNA hybridization analysis of Ig gene rearrangement used to evaluate the cell marker-negative PTLD tissue from the cardiac transplant recipients.[119] Nevertheless, evidence against a strictly monoclonal presentation comes from a number of patients with PTLD, including the same post–cardiac transplant recipients, in whom multiclonal, or oligoclonal, lesions were demonstrated both by Ig gene rearrangement[120] and EBV genomic analysis,[121] with individual lymphomatous sites displaying distinct monoclonal derivations. Finally, PTLD lesions have been described in which polyclonality is suggested by immunophenotyping but that contain either Ig gene rearrangements or clonal cytogenetic abnormalities.[291,722] Together these data suggest that independent activation of multiple cells is occurring as an early step in tumorigenesis, with occasional early malignant transformation detectable at the DNA or cytogenetic level. These lesions are of the intermediate type, appearing morphologically malignant due to nuclear atypia and extensive necrosis, and consisting of a predominant polyclonal B-cell proliferation harboring within it a subpopulation of cells that are monoclonal.

Among the true monomorphic monoclonal lymphomas, several histopathologic types have been identified including, in addition to the predominant large cell immunoblastic lymphoma, diffuse large B-cell lymphoma (DLCL), diffuse mixed lymphoma,[119,218,289,486,722,783] and small noncleaved Burkitt's and non-Burkitt's lymphoma.[429,455,621] Interestingly, the polymorphic lymphomas behave as aggressively as the true monomorphic lymphomas.[486] Analysis of sex chromatin, HLA specificities, and DNA restriction fragment length polymorphisms indicate that most post-transplant lymphomas derive from recipient rather than donor lymphocytes.[507,568,722]

Initially based on morphologic categories,[218] the classification system for PTLDs was subsequently modified to incorporate correlative genetic and molecular analysis.[385,725] Knowles and colleagues[99,385] incorporated a series of attributes that jointly define three categories of PTLDs (Table 47–2): 1. plasmacytic hyperplasias, which are polyclonal, associated with multiple EBV infections, and lack oncogene or tumor suppressor gene alterations; 2. polymorphic B-cell hyperplasias and polymorphic B-cell lymphomas, which are generally monoclonal, manifest a single form of EBV, but still lack genetic changes in oncogenes or tumor suppressor genes; and 3. immunoblastic lymphomas or multiple myelomas, which are monoclonal, contain a single form of EBV, and exhibit alterations in one or more oncogenes or tumor suppressor genes. An attempt to validate this system in terms of its clinical relevance has revealed that these categories correlate with clinical presentation, response to therapy, remission, and clinical outcome.[100] Importantly, all lesions categorized as plasmacytic hyperplasia regressed in response to reduction in immunosuppression alone or accompanied by surgery. Polymorphic PTLDs that did not regress with reduction in immunosuppression usually resolved with medical intervention, such as chemotherapy or radiation therapy. Lesions classified as malignant lymphoma/multiple myeloma did not respond in spite of aggressive clinical intervention. These histologic-clinical correlates pro-

Table 47–2. Histopathologic Categories of Post-Transplantation Lymphoproliferative Disorders[a,b]

Category of Lymphoproliferation	Anatomic Site(s) at Presentation	Clonality by Ig Gene	EBV Events	Oncogene, Tumor Suppressor Gene Alterations	Clinical Intervention and Outcome
Plasmacytic hyperplasia	Oropharynx, lymph nodes	Most polyclonal	Most with multiple EBV infection events, or only a subset of cells infected by a single form of EBV, or EBV-negative	Absent	All responded to reduced immunosuppression + surgical resection
Polymorphic B-cell hyperplasia and polymorphic B-cell lymphoma	Lymph nodes various extranodal sites	Most monoclonal	Most with single form of EBV	Absent	Respond to reduced immunosuppression + surgical resection; or to medical therapy; or no response
Immunoblastic lymphoma, multiple myeloma	Widely disseminated disease	Monoclonal	Single form of EBV	Alteration of one or more oncogenes or tumor suppressor genes: N-ras, c-myc, p53	Medical resolution; or no response—most

[a] Adapted from Knowles et al.[385] and Chadburn et al.[100]
[b] Based on data from 1 lung, 5 kidney, and 26 heart transplant recipients.

vide a basis for choosing optimal treatment in the management of PTLDs.

Although about 85 percent of post-transplant lymphomas are B cell in origin,[486,573,576,578] occasional T-cell lymphomas have been identified,[164,231,284,764,805] some of which have been linked to EBV infection.[164] A rare CD8+ γδ T-cell lymphoma reported in the setting of renal transplant was found to be associated with human HHV-6 infection.[430] B- and T-cell lymphomas have been observed within a single patient,[190] and T-cell receptor and *Ig* heavy chain rearrangements have even been detected within the same lymphoid proliferation in a renal allograft,[795] indicating a polyclonal origin to the PTLD. Unusual presentations such as that of a nasal natural killer cell lymphoma associated with EBV have also been reported post–renal transplant.[494] MALT-type lymphomas have been observed in the stomach and parotid gland following cardiac, liver, or kidney transplant.[321,414,803] Interestingly, all cases examined were negative for EBV, and the gastric lymphomas were all positive for *H. pylori,* resembling MALT lymphomas in immunocompetent patients rather than lymphomas that occur in association with immunosuppressed states. As previously noted, Hodgkin's disease has only been reported uncommonly following kidney, liver, and heart transplants.[55,229,317,568,573,576,578] Post-transplant leukemias occur but are uncommon, and most of them are granulocytic, particularly monocytic, in phenotype.[237] Other lymphoid-related proliferative diseases that are occasionally observed in the post-transplant setting include monoclonal gammopathies, multiple myeloma, and plasmacytomas.[174,256,543]

As with lymphomas in other settings of immunosuppression, post-transplant lymphomas frequently present at advanced stages. Thus, in one study 50 percent were diagnosed as Stages III or IV, while 35 percent were Stage I.[486] The similarity to other immunodeficiency states extends to the frequency with which the post-transplant lymphomas occur at extranodal sites. Between 26 and 45 percent occur in the CNS: 14 to 66 percent of these are confined to the brain parenchyma with frequent multifocality and virtually no lymphomatous meningitis.[289,486,568,572,574,576–578,783] Other common sites include the lung (22 percent), GI tract (11 to 50 percent), and bone marrow (14 percent), as well as sites of injection of ALG or ATG.[289,422,486,506,568,572,574,576,597,783]

The allograft has also been described as a site of involvement by lymphoma in 15 to 31 percent of cases, the lymphomatous infiltrate sometimes being mistaken on biopsy for graft rejection.[308,407,422,568,572,574,576,577,578,703,823] In fact, Opelz et al.[533] noted a strong preferential location of lymphomas in the heart or lung after heart transplantation and in the kidney after renal tranplantation. On the other hand, Leblond et al.[407] have suggested that allograft presentation may be less common in heart than in renal transplants. An association between the use of OKT3 and the occurrence of PTLD isolated to the renal allograft has been suggested in at least one report.[474] Presentation in the allograft brings to mind the question of whether the tumor or a tumorigenic agent such as EBV (see below) was in fact transmitted from the donor, having been transplanted with the graft.[21,348,575] Transmission of cancer from a donor has been documented primarily for solid malignancies.[575] A few cases of lymphoma of donor origin have also been described, despite the fact that most PTLD in solid organ transplantations are of recipient origin.[111,226,308,443,466,703,787,823] These, however, do not necessarily involve the allograft. In the few cases of lymphoma of donor origin in the allograft, local proliferation in response to donor-recipient antigenic mismatches has been suggested as playing a role in tumorigenesis (see below).[144,308,703]

Pathogenesis: Mechanisms Underlying Lymphomagenesis in Association With Solid Organ Transplants

Molecular and Immunologic Basis for Post-Transplant Lymphomagenesis. PTLD is believed to arise by a series of carcinogenic steps that roughly correspond to those described above for HIV- and EBV-related lymphomas. Malignant progression is facilitated by a variety of mechanisms, some of which are unique to the setting of organ transplant. Thus, the underlying disease process that necessitates the transplant may predispose the patient to malignancy. As an example, a history of polycystic kidney disease seems to correlate with the development of post-transplant lymphoma.[319] By contrast, although uremia is known to be immunosuppressive, the duration of renal disease and length of time on dialysis, both potential contributors to overall immunosuppression, appear to play no role in lymphomagenesis, although they may influence the frequency of other malignancies.[458,791] Among cardiac allograft recipients, PTLD has been noted primarily in individuals transplanted for idiopathic cardiomyopathy, rather than coronary artery disease.[53,441] The reasons for this difference are unclear. Idiopathic cardiomyopathy is associated with a defect in mitogen-stimulated suppressor T-cell activity whereas coronary artery disease is not;[16] however, the relationship of this finding to subsequent lymphomagenesis remains obscure.

Initial B-cell proliferation results from exposure of host lymphoid tissue to a number of foreign antigenic stimuli, some of which are peculiar to the transplant setting. Chronic exposure to foreign histocompatibility antigens in the allograft may lead to hyperplasia.[567,568,572,576] Blood transfusions, heterologous ATG or ALG, monoclonal antibodies like OKT3, and various infectious agents may elicit proliferative responses in lymphoid tissues. In particular, EBV, which is highly associated with the development of post-transplant lymphomas (see below), provides a potent antigenic stimulus to lymphoproliferation, as discussed previously.[459,473,663,741] Patients with PTLD often have decreased levels of interferon-α, a down-regulator of IL-4, in turn allowing increased expression of IL-4, a potent stimulator of B-cell proliferation.[203]

Within the expanded polyclonal B-cell population genetic alterations occur that may lead to clonal expansion and malignant transformation. Although these changes have not been as extensively documented as in the AIDS-non-Hodgkin's lymphoma literature, clonal cytogenetic abnormalities suggestive of malignant progression have been identified in post-transplant lymphomas.[205,218,286,287,289,291] For example, within polyclonal B-cell proliferations, cellular clones containing a 6q+ long marker chromosome,[286] trisomies 3 and 14,[218,286,287,289] t(9;14) involving the *IgH* locus on chromosome 14,[291] and t(2;19) involving the *Ig-κ* light chain locus on chromosome 2[289] have been identified. Significantly, in contrast to Burkitt's lymphoma, no cytogenetic abnormality has been identified that is consistently associated with PTLD or with a specific histologic subtype of PTLD.[671]

Finally, immune dysfunction contributes to multistep tumorigeneis. Abnormal chronic stimulation of lymphoid tissues has already been mentioned as one manifestation of immune dysfunction.[179,567] In addition, the failure of immune surveillance may result from several factors in transplant recipients, permitting the unchecked expansion of a malignant clone. Each of the immunosuppressive agents used to prevent organ rejection targets discrete sites along the cascade of T-cell activation.[720] For example, azathioprine plus prednisone abolish natural killer cell-mediated cytotoxicity.[432] Glucocorticoids inhibit expression of a number of cytokines, including IL-1, IL-3, IL-6, interferon-γ, and tumor necrosis factor-α, resulting in depression of T-cell proliferation and T-cell-mediated immunity. Cyclosporine blocks IL-2 gene activation, IL-2 receptor expression, and IL-2- and IL-6-mediated proliferation of mitogen-activated T-cells.[571,720,776,819] Conversely, cyclosporine induces expression of IL-6, an activator of B-cell proliferation.[307,749,776] By thus modulating these two interacting arms of the immune system, cyclosporine may contribute to depressed T-cell surveillance of an expanding B-cell population in transplant recipients.

Role of EBV in Post-Transplant Lymphomagenesis. A large volume of data supports the association of EBV infection with PTLD, with greater than 90 percent being EBV-positive, in contrast to only 13 to 22 percent of de novo non-Hodgkin's lymphomas.[493] Renal transplant recipients exhibit higher levels of EBV oropharyngeal shedding than do healthy seropositive controls.[106,615,710] B cells containing EBV genomic DNA, which normally exist in the peripheral blood of seropositive individuals at concentrations of less than $1/10^7$ peripheral blood mononuclear cells (PBMCs), increase in transplant recipients to more than $1/10^5$ PBMCs 1 to 3 months after transplant and remain high for about 3 months, with elevated levels persisting in only a minority of patients beyond this time.[140,615] Data on whether transplant recipients destined to develop lymphoma exhibit higher levels of EBV-infected B cells are conflicting. Certain studies suggest that the presence of increased levels of EBV DNA or RNA in lymphoid cells correlates with the subsequent development of PTLD, supporting a role for EBV infection in the multistep process of tumorigenesis.[606,616,647] By contrast, no such association between EBV infection and PTLD was detected by Crompton et al.[140] in their series of renal transplant recipients. Simultaneous with increased viral shedding in the throat, immunosuppressed transplant recipients may exhibit elevated titers of antibodies to EBV antigens, particularly those antigens associated with the viral productive cycle, such as antiviral capsid antigen (VCA), whereas anti-EBNA levels do not change.[123,286,300,499,615,671,688,791] Finally, EBNA-2 and EBNA-3C DNA sequences typifying EBV type 1, the more potently transforming strain (see above), are found in over 89 percent of lesions of PTLD.[214,597]

Patients diagnosed with PTLD may initially present with fever, pharyngitis, and lymphadenopathy, symptoms of an active EBV infection, which serologically may be either primary or reactivated, or they may show evidence of EBV infection in the distant past.[21,123,286,288,289,291,615,707] Transmission of EBV from a seropositive donor via the allograft leads to primary infection in virtually all initially seronegative transplant recipients.[123,181,311,647,722,725] Swinnen et al.[722] observed that among patients developing PTLD, 30 percent had negative tests for EBV before transplantation. This observation, together with those from other studies involving a variety of transplanted organs,[772] suggest that initial EBV seronegativity, with resulting primary EBV infection, is an important risk factor for PTLD. In fact, the simultaneous development of PTLD in two seronegative recipients of kidneys from a single seropositive donor has been reported.[348] The transmission of EBV from blood donors to both EBV-negative and EBV-positive transplant patients during the peritransplant period has been documented and has also been associated with the development of PTLD.[5] In addition to recipient seronegativity, donor EBV positivity has been shown to predict for seroconversion and developing PTLD.[181] Nevertheless, the high-risk combination of donor EBV positivity and recipient EBV negativity does not universally lead to PTLD.[616] The association of baseline seronegativity with conversion via primary infection as a risk factor for PTLD is especially pertinent to transplantation in the pediatric age group, since younger patients are more likely to be EBV seronegative. Data on pediatric transplant recipients bear this out, with symptomatic mononucleosis-like EBV infection and PTLD occurring more frequently in this age group than among adults (see above).[21,181,311,577,578,661,704] Because of the strong association of EBV transmission and primary EBV infection with the development of PTLD, some investigators believe that seronegativity of a potential recipient should preclude transplantation of an allograft from a seropositive donor.[725,772]

The presence of EBV has been demonstrated in lymphoma tissue of transplant recipients by immunofluorescent staining of EBNA protein[136,707,822] as well as by the more sensitive techniques of PCR amplification of EBNA DNA[318] and in situ hybridization to EBV DNA[46,286,310,707] and the small EBV RNA, EBER-1;[606] EBV DNA is absent, however, from lymphoid tissues in transplant recipients without PTLD.[46] Nevertheless, the presence of EBV in PTLD tumor tissue has not been consistently reported.[407,616,688,791] For example, Leblond et al.[407] failed to detect EBV in 31 percent of the 19 B-cell PTLDs examined. These EBV-negative PTLDs were more often morphologically monomorphic, and, interestingly, all but one of these lymphomas arose late, 1 year or more after transplant. These data suggest that the development of EBV-negative PTLDs in organ transplant recipients may depend on the accumulation of other genetic changes and that their number might increase with time.[144,407] Also of interest is the observation that EBV tends to be absent from the uncommon post-transplantation T-cell lymphomas,[407,764,805] although EBV has even been documented in these rare entities.[216,407]

As with EBV-containing AIDS-non-Hodgkin's lymphomas, the EBV genomes within PTLD generally exist as clonal circular episomes, supporting the clonality of these lesions as well as suggesting that EBV infection is an early event that occurs before clonal expansion.[552] In fact, the absence of monoclonality by EBV classification generally correlates with nonclonality by immunophenotyping and is associated with histologic characteristics of polymorphic diffuse B-cell hyperplasia or intermediate polymorphic B-cell lymphoma. The presence of clonal EBV genomes and EBNA-2 protein expression in smooth muscle tumors arising in liver transplant recipients has been demonstrated, paralleling the observation in HIV-associated leiomyosarcomas (see above)[463] and expanding the repertoire of tumor types potentially attributable to EBV infection in the transplant setting.[413] The EBV data therefore support a model in which the biologic spectrum of histologic types actually represent various stages of progression from polyclonal to monoclonal to frankly malignant lymphoproliferations.

The contribution of EBV to PTLD lies in part in its ability to modulate the immune system. In addition to the capacity of EBV to provide chronic antigenic stimulation, EBV-infected cells are able to elude normal surveillance by the immune system in the transplant setting. All healthy individuals previously infected with EBV maintain in their blood high levels of cytotoxic T cells (more than $1/10^3$ to 10^4 circulating T cells), which are class I HLA restricted and are specific for LYDMA, the virus-induced lymphocyte-detected membrane antigen of EBV.[289,443,615,625,671] The normal containment of EBV-infected B lymphocytes by these EBV-specific cytotoxic T cells may be abrogated by immunosuppressive agents used in organ transplant recipients.[59,136,137,232] Renal transplant recipients, for example, exhibit a substantial increase in viral shedding as well as EBV antibody titers when immunosuppressed with ATG.[109,499] Cyclosporine has been shown to reduce the proliferative response of EBV-specific T-cell clones to specific antigen and IL-2 by mechanisms described above.[59,307,571,776,819] The use of the immunosuppressive CD3 monoclonal antibodies OKT3 and 64.1 (specific for a p19 antigen on human T cells), as well as sequential use of ALG and OKT3, in renal transplant recipients experiencing the overwhelming viral burden of a primary EBV infection has also been associated with the development of PTLD.[123,348,456,722] EBV may also affect the immune system by modulating levels of key cytokines such as serum IL-10, which is frequently upregulated in association with posttransplant lymphomas, especially those in which EBV is detected, following primary or reactivated EBV infection.[60,230]

EBV latent gene expression is restricted in the PTLD lesions of solid organ transplant recipients. Using Southern blot, Western blot, and immunofluorescence analysis, Cen et al.[92] observed a variety of restriction patterns, reflecting universal expression of EBNA-1, expression of LMP-1 in almost all cases, and only occasional expression of EBNA-2. In other studies, expression of the EBV-derived B-cell activating proteins EBNA-2 and LMP-1, as well as of their target cellular surface genes, CD23, intercellular adhesion molecule-1 *(ICAM-1)*, and leukocyte function-associated antigen-3 *(LFA-3)*,[779] has been demonstrated by immunofluorescence in infiltrating B lymphocytes from bone marrow transplant recipients with EBV-related PTLD.[822] By contrast, Burkitt's lymphoma cells, which conform to the Lat I pattern, express only EBNA-1 and fail to express the transformation- and immortalization-inducing

EBNA-2 and LMP-1 genes[610,630] and, consequently, their target genes.[254,629] Expression of these EBV-derived genes may be unnecessary in Burkitt's lymphoma cells that have acquired stable genetic alterations (e.g., c-*MYC* translocation) that provide the stimulus for cellular proliferation. Furthermore, the absence of the EBV surface proteins may actually contribute to the more malignant phenotype of Burkitt's lymphoma cells by permitting these cells to evade T-cell-mediated cytotoxicity.

Treatment of Post-Transplant Lymphomas

Post–solid organ transplant lymphomas are typically aggressive. Because they observed monoclonality of PTLD in cardiac transplant recipients at the earliest stages of detectable disease, Cleary et al.[119] recommended the use of antineoplastic therapy in such patients. Although chemotherapy has been beneficial in some studies,[429,455,621] PTLD has been shown by others to respond poorly to conventional therapy.[486,671,707] Of 26 transplant recipients who were treated for PTLD with various modalities alone or in combination, 58 percent achieved a disease-free state.[486] However, median time to failure was 7 months, and median survival was 14 months. Reduction or cessation of immunosuppressive therapy has led to regression of lymphoproliferative lesions and is strongly recommended as the first treatment by certain authors.[21,140,486,565,611,707] Nevertheless, this approach is not universally effective.[287,348,486,575] Armitage et al.[21] noted that PTLD occurring "early" after transplantation responds positively to reduction in immunosuppression (Table 47–2), in contrast to "late" PTLD, which does not regress under these conditions, leading to a mortality of 70 to 80 percent. However, Swinnen et al.[723] found no therapy to be effective in "early" disease but aggressive chemotherapy was beneficial in "late" disease. Complete responses have also been achieved following reduction of tumor burden by removal of the graft together with withdrawal of immunosuppression (Table 47–2). Success with this combination of modalities has been achieved primarily with extranodal tumors in the GI tract as well as tumors inadvertently transplanted with the allograft from the donor, even when the latter are accompanied by widely metastatic disease.[287,289,290,506,565,575,576] However, graft removal plus decreased immunosuppression is a reasonable option only for renal transplants and only when the patient can be maintained on dialysis. Since decreased immunosuppression places the transplanted organ at risk for rejection, this approach by itself is expected to be less of an option for nonrenal organs.[575] However, Starzl et al.[707] have emphasized that reduction or discontinuation of immunosuppression does not necessarily lead to irreversible transplant rejection, since most of their grafts could be salvaged.

Because EBV is believed to play a critical role in the pathogenesis of PTLD, acyclovir (and ganciclovir) has been utilized both in the prophylaxis[671] and the therapy of this disease.[288–291,506,582] Acyclovir is most effective during the initial EBV-induced polyclonal growth phase.[288,290,291] Since this agent inhibits EBV DNA replication only in virus-producing cells, exerting no effect on the episomal EBV of latent infection, it has been proposed that the antiproliferative activity of acyclovir is indirect, due to the elimination of viral replication and its associated immunosuppression. Interferon-α has elicited some responses in patients with PTLD,[203] an understandable outcome given the decreased levels of interferon-α expression in these patients. Other novel therapeutic interventions include anti-B-cell monoclonal antibodies.[63,205] Infusion of CD21 (B-cell EBV receptor)- and CD24 (B-cell and granulocyte antigen)-specific antibodies led to complete remission in seven of eight organ transplant recipients with oligoclonal PTLD but none of three with monoclonal disease.[205] However, complete remission of monoclonal disease was achieved with these anti-B-cell antibodies in another study.[405] The anti-CD20 B-cell monoclonal antibody rituximab has also induced complete responses in post-transplant lymphomas.[475,614] An anti-CD22 immunotoxin has been used successfully to achieve a complete sustained response of a post–renal transplant EBV-associated large B-cell lymphoma that was refractory to decreased immunosuppression, specific antiviral therapy, and combination chemotherapy.[666] Other biologic approaches are being developed. Adoptive immunotherapy employing autologous lymphocyte IL-2-activated killer cells infused without systemic IL-2 has led to complete remission of a post–renal transplant high-grade LPD.[426] Highly selective adoptive immunotherapy using in vitro–expanded EBV-specific cytotoxic T cells has been explored as treatment and prophylaxis in bone marrow transplant recipients.[72,443,535,627,725]

Chemotherapy has generally been regarded as the treatment of last resort because of very high morbidity and mortality rates, due to sepsis and other toxicities.[407,486,506,671,725] Mortality may surpass 70 percent in patients refractory to reduced immunosuppression. Nevertheless, aggressive combination chemotherapy, such as the ProMACE-CytaBOM regimen, has been used successfully in phenotypically monoclonal PTLD refractory to reduced immunosuppression following cardiac transplantation.[724]

In an effort to alleviate the confusion regarding therapy for PTLDs, Hanto et al.[289,290] categorized the post-transplant lymphomas into three histologic groups; a distinct therapeutic approach is recommended for each. For group 1, consisting of polyclonal polymorphic diffuse B-cell hyperplasia, acyclovir has successfully reversed the lymphoproliferation and is recommended with or without a reduction in immunosuppression. In group 2, the polyclonal B-cell lymphomas run the risk of progressing from polyclonal to monoclonal B-cell proliferations. Therefore, they should be treated by reduction or cessation of immunosuppression in most kidney transplant patients, allowing rejection to occur; the parallel approach in heart, heart-lung, and liver recipients, where allograft rejection would be fatal, involves acyclovir therapy and a modest reduction in immunosuppression. Finally, for group 3, the morphologically malignant monoclonal B-cell lymphomas, recommendations include standard chemotherapy or radiation therapy, combined with discontinuation of immunosuppression, since the mortality rates in this group are greater than 80 percent. Combinations of all three modalities, acyclovir, reduction of immunosuppression, and intensive multiagent chemotherapy, have been used successfully to treat frankly malignant lymphomas in the transplant setting.[455]

Lymphomas in the Setting of Bone Marrow Transplantation

Epidemiology/Demographics of Lymphomas Associated With Bone Marrow Transplants

The risk of cancer among recipients of allogeneic bone marrow transplants (BMT) is 3.8 to 6.7 times higher than in the general population.[389,695,796] The incidence of lymphoproliferative disease in this treatment group ranges from 0.3 percent to 1.8 percent in different studies,[52,144,695,838] generally less than the 1.0 to 4.6 percent risk observed following transplants of various solid organs.[506,572] In a recent overview of the allogeneic BMT experience at 235 centers worldwide reporting to the International Bone Marrow Transplant Registry (IBMTR), the cumulative incidence was 1.0 ± 0.3 percent at 10 years. Post–bone marrow transplant lymphoproliferative disease (PBMT-LPD) develops earlier (median, 3 months) following transplant than do solid tumors of epithelial origin (median, 99 months).[150] The highest incidence in the IBMTR overview occurred 1 to 5 months post-transplant, with a peak at 3 months. This early-onset disease (less than 1 year post-transplant) was followed by a gradual but steep decline among patients surviving for a year or more,[144] although the risk of late-onset PBMT-LPD remained significantly higher than expected in the general population. Although most reports of PBMT-LPD pertain to allogeneic transplants, lymphomas have been observed following both autologous and cord blood BMTs.[443,530]

Risk factors for the development of PBMT-LPD include severe acute graft-versus-host disease (GvHD) and T-lymphocyte depletion of donor marrow.[670,725,796,838] Predisposition to PBMT-LPD occurs following treatment of acute GvHD with ATG or total-body irradiation and particularly, as discussed above for solid organ transplants, with the CD3-specific monoclonal antibodies OKT3 and 64.1.[123,348,456,722] In addition, HLA-mismatch between donor and recipient, presumably because of the prolonged antigenic stimulation that it incurs, contributes to a lesser degree to lymphomagenesis.[670] These associations have been borne out in the recent IBMTR study, in which Curtis et al.[144] identified four major risk factors that were strongly ($p < .0001$) associated with early-onset PBMT-LPD: T-cell depletion of the graft (relative risk, RR = 12.7); unrelated donor or 2 or more HLA-antigen mismatches in a related donor (RR = 4.1); use of anti-CD3 monoclonal antibody 64.1 (RR = 43.2); and use of antithymocyte globulin (RR = 6.4). The strength of the association between the four main risk factors and disease diagnosed a year or more post-BMT was much weaker. The only identifiable risk factor for this late-onset PBMT-LPD was extensive chronic GvHD (RR = 4.0, $p = .01$), possibly as a result of long-term treatment with immunosuppressive drugs. Curtis et al. also compared five different methods of T-cell depletion of bone marrow, which revealed particularly high risks for methods utilizing monoclonal antibodies targeted to T cells or T plus NK cells (RR = 12.3) and for sheep red blood cell E-rosetting techniques (RR = 15.6). Far lower risks were noted for techniques that remove both T and B cells, postulated to result from reduction of the B-cell containing EBV viral load during the early post-transplant time interval before full recovery of the T-cell population has occurred.[144,271] Curtis et al. also reaffirmed the occurrence of acute GvHD grades II to IV as a risk factor for PBMT-LPD, specifically for disease of early onset.

Conditioning regimens involving radiation were associated with an increased risk of PBMT-LPD (RR = 2.9, p = .02), and the risk varied by dose of fractionated total body irradiation (3.5 to 4.3-fold risks for doses ≥ 13 Gy).[144] Heavy pretreatment with radiation or chemotherapy, or both, before autologous bone marrow transplant has also been shown to predispose to the emergence of de novo clonal cytogenetic abnormalities typical of therapy-induced disease (chromosome 5, 7, 11q21, and 21q22 abnormalities), with or without manifestation of clinical disease, such as myelodysplastic syndrome or acute myelogenous leukemia.[751] Since the incidence and timing of the cytogenetic changes coincide with those seen for heavy treatment in the absence of BMT, the question arises as to whether the BMT has a potentiating effect.

In some studies the incidence of PBMT-LPD varied with the underlying disease (e.g., 0.6 percent for treatment of hematologic malignancy versus 0.3 percent following transplantation for aplastic anemia).[695,838] The risk for PBMT-LPD is particularly high among patients transplanted for congenital immunodeficiency diseases (see below).[151] Bhatia et al.[52] observed a 4 percent incidence of PBMT-LPD in such patients, reflecting a significantly increased risk in this cohort (RR =2.5, p = .06). Conversely, no significant association of disease for which the transplant was performed with the risk of PBMT-LPD was seen in the IBMTR study.[144]

Clinical Features and Histopathology

Histologically PBMT lymphomas resemble those seen after solid organ transplant, encompassing a large spectrum of morphologic characteristics, ranging from polymorphic B-cell hyperplasia to polymorphic B-cell lymphoma to large cell immunoblastic lymphoma.[544,670,838] They are generally B-cell neoplasms, although T-cell lesions may occur.[144,544,796,838] Interestingly, the two T-cell lymphomas observed in the IBMTR study occurred among the less frequent late-onset cases.[144] Staining for Igs has revealed both polyclonal as well as monoclonal lesions, although Ig heavy chain gene rearrangements have occasionally been detected within the polyclonal lesions, suggesting the presence of clonal proliferations.[838] Nonidentical monoclonal populations have been observed in separate lesions in the same patient,[674] indicating distinct clonal derivations at the two sites, analogous to PTLD following cardiac transplantation.[120] Among PBMT-LPDs, most lymphomas have proved to be of donor origin,[443,456,507,544,657,838] with host-derived lymphomas being only rarely observed.[66] This contrasts with reports regarding the derivation of leukemias that occur following BMT[77,379,520] and lymphomas occurring after solid organ transplant (see above).[568,725] Similar to PTLDs following solid organ transplants, the sites of involvement are varied and often extranodal, involving abdominal and thoracic nodes as well as liver, spleen, GI tract, and lungs.[838]

Pathogenesis: Mechanisms Underlying Lymphomagenesis in Association With BMT

The histologic spectrum observed among PBMT-LPDs suggests the usual multistep progression from antigenically stimulated polyclonal proliferation through genetic alteration and ultimately selective expansion of a malignant clone. Analogous to the situation described for solid organ transplant recipients, potential factors operating in the context of BMT to promote tumorigenesis include the underlying disease, foreign antigenic stimuli such as mismatched HLA antigens and EBV, and the institution of immunosuppressive therapies designed to prevent GvHD. EBV DNA is almost always detected in the lymphoproliferative lesions associated with both BMT and organ transplant.[144,151,205,544,665,670,674,822,838] Early-onset PBMT-LPD in the IBMTR study was uniformly associated with EBV, but three cases of late-onset disease were EBV-negative.[144] Despite the resemblance of post-BMT and post–solid organ transplant lymphomas with respect to the EBV positivity of their tumor tissue, BMT patients with PTLD fail to mount specific antibody responses to EBV VCA, early antigen, and EBNA, unlike organ transplant recipients.[205] In the setting of BMT, a rapid increase of EBV DNA has been observed within 1 to 3 months after transplant,[269] paralleling the timing of the peak of EBV-infected lymphocytes in pediatric solid organ transplant patients, which occurs at about 3 months.[647] Proposed sources of EBV in the BMT population include latently infected donor B lymphocytes, the host nasopharynx, and blood transfusions. Since most cases of PBMT-LPD are of donor origin, the most likely etiology of EBV infection is via infected B lymphocytes transferred from the donor at the time of transplant or by infection of donor lymphocytes following transplantation into the host.[456,657,665,838]

In addition to the clustering of EBV-negative lymphomas among late-onset cases, the two T-cell lymphomas observed in the IBMTR study occurred in the late-onset group.[144] This brings to mind the few T-cell lymphomas seen among PTLDs observed by Leblond et al.[407] following solid organ transplantation, which also were of late onset and also tended to be EBV-negative. As pointed out by these authors, these data suggest that the development of EBV-negative PTLDs in organ transplant recipients may represent a morphologically and clinically distinct entity, depending on the accumulation of additional genetic changes and increasing in number with time after transplant.[144,407]

Treatment of Post-BMT Lymphomas

Limited information is available regarding the treatment of PBMT-LPD. Although a strong association exists between EBV and these lymphomas, the data suggesting efficacy of acyclovir or ganciclovir are confined to a small number of cases,[582] and do not support the use of these antiviral agents in either a prophylactic or therapeutic mode in the setting of BMT.[151,669,671,838] Based on the association of PBMT-LPDs with EBV and T-cell depletion of the allograft, together with their tendency to be of donor origin, patients who developed EBV-related lymphoma after receiving T-cell-depleted marrow were infused with unirradiated leukocytes from their EBV-seropositive donors.[534,535,544] The underlying hypothesis, that the infused cell populations would supply missing cytotoxic T-cell precursors presensitized to EBV in the donor's microenvironment, which might control the proliferation of EBV-transformed donor cells in the host, was supported by observed responses in this small set of patients.[427] Administration of EBV-specific cytotoxic T cells before the onset of the rapid rise in EBV DNA at 1 to 3 months following BMT has been shown to stabilize the virus titers, supporting the potential of this approach for prophylaxis against the development of PBMT-LPDs.[269] Adoptive cellular therapy of this nature may also augment control of the underlying tumor for which the transplant was performed. An additional therapeutic approach has utilized interferon-α which, together with intravenous γ-globulin, has elicited responses in hematological malignancies complicating BMT.[669,670] Finally, the use of CD21- and CD24-specific B-cell antibodies in patients with severe PBMT-LPD led to complete responses in 16 of 28 patients (57 percent), similar to the results with organ transplant patients, among whom 20 of 31 had complete responses (64 percent).[43,63,205] However, only 35 percent of BMT patients survived more than 1 year, significantly less than the 55 percent survival among solid organ transplant recipients.[43] The CD20-specific B-cell monoclonal antibody rituximab has also been used successfully to induce complete responses in three patients who developed EBV-associated lymphomas following stem cell transplantation.[394] By analogy to the solid organ transplant setting, the absence of firmly established effective treatments for PBMT-LPD, together with the association of this disease entity with EBV infection, has led some authors to recommend avoiding exposure of seronegative recipients to this virus and to select an EBV-seronegative donor whenever possible for such transplants.[671,725,772]

LYMPHOMAS IN THE SETTING OF CONGENITAL IMMUNODEFICIENCY DISEASES

The primary immunodeficiency diseases (CID), that is, diseases that are either congenital or genetically determined, are rare conditions, seven of which account for 95 percent of cases (Table 47–3).[8,27,79,233,594,636,689,700,701,771] Among individuals with CIDs, there is an increased risk of malignancy, about 10,000 times that in the general age-matched population, with the overall cancer incidence in the immunodeficient population varying between 1.7 and 4.0 percent.[233,567] Mortality rates for cancer among immunodeficient patients are 100-fold greater than in the general population.[700] Although each of the CIDs is associated with a particular incidence and constellation of malignancies,[233,700,701] over 50 percent of the cancers are lymphoid neoplasms,[700,701] substantially higher than in the general population. Of these the majority are non-Hodgkin's B-cell lymphomas,[203,203,217,577] although, in contrast to most other immunodeficiency settings, Hodgkin's disease is also well represented. T-cell lymphoma has only rarely been reported.[248,250,538] The non-Hodgkin's lymphomas are clearly the most common neoplasms in five of the seven major immunodeficiency states:[203,700] Wiskott-Aldrich syndrome (80 percent); IgM deficiency (56 percent); ataxia-telangiectasia (46 percent); severe

combined immunodeficiency (74 percent); and common variable immunodeficiency (46 percent). These lymphomas make up a large proportion of the cancers in the other two major CIDs, X-linked (Bruton's) hypogammaglobulinemia (33 percent) and IgA deficiency (16 percent). There are even reports of lymphomas in association with rarer CIDs, including B-cell lymphomas in DiGeorge syndrome[643] and Nijmegen breakage syndrome.[114,664] The proportion of non-Hodgkin's lymphomas among cancers (65 percent) is the same among both adults and children with CID,[217,701] unlike the general population, in which only 13.5 percent of pediatric cancers are non-Hodgkin's lymphomas, while leukemias represent 48 to 76 percent of cancers in this age group.

Clinical Features and Histopathology

The non-Hodgkin's lymphomas are virtually all diffuse. As in the settings of immunodeficiency previously described, the large cell lymphomas, particularly the large cell immunoblastic lymphomas, constitute a larger percentage (38 percent) than in the general population (4.2 percent), whereas Hodgkin's disease and the small cell lymphomas are underrepresented.[217,700,701,828]

Noteworthy differences exist in the distribution of histological types among the different CIDs. Whereas the relative frequencies of the three histological types of lymphoma (diffuse large cell, small cell, and Hodgkin's disease) are similar among patients with ataxia-telangiectasia, combined variable immunodeficiency, and IgA deficiency,[700] IgM deficient patients exhibit a higher percentage of large-cell lymphomas. This is also true of individuals with Wiscott-Aldrich syndrome,[579] which, interestingly, is associated with impaired IgM responses. A comparison of ataxia-telangiectasia and Wiscott-Aldrich syndrome reveals additional important differences. Patients with the former disease regularly develop both non-Hodgkin's lymphomas and Hodgkin's disease, in contrast to individuals with the latter disease who present with Hodgkin's disease far less often.[134,217,331,579,700] Furthermore, the predominant subtype of non-Hodgkin's lymphoma in ataxia-telangiectasia patients is diffuse large B-cell lymphoma, whereas two-thirds of the non-Hodgkin's lymphomas among Wiskott-Aldrich syndrome patients have a large cell immunoblastic histology. It is also of interest that among individuals with ataxia-telangiectasia, 50 percent of the Hodgkin's disease is of the lymphocyte-depleted subtype, and it can occur in very young patients. This contrasts sharply with the general population where lymphocyte-depleted Hodgkin's disease is diagnosed in fewer than 5 percent of cases and tends to occur in elderly men with advanced stage disease or at relapse after treatment of other histologies.[365,760] Thus, lymphocyte-depleted Hodgkin's disease appears to be associated with immunodeficient states, a conclusion supported by its disproportionate representation in Hodgkin's disease patients with AIDS.[12,667,743,746,759]

Unlike the large cell immunoblastic lymphomas that occur in the general population, those observed in patients with CIDs are typically extranodal and often localized.[134,217,579] The CNS is frequently involved, as are the liver, lung, and GI tract, resembling the non-Hodgkin's lymphomas observed in transplant recipi-

Table 47–3. Congenital Immunodeficiency Diseases

Immunodeficiency Disease	Clinical Features/ Immune Deficiencies	Genetics/Epidemiology	Percentage of Cancers That Are Lymphomas, Types of Cancers, With Statistics	Association With EBV	References
Ataxia-telangiectasia (AT)	Cerebellar ataxia, oculocutaneous telangiectasia, recurrent sinopulmonary infections Deficiencies of IgA, IgE, abnormal T-cell-mediated responses, hypoplastic thymus glands Defective excision repair of irradiation-induced double-stranded DNA breaks; increased intrachromosomal recombination α-fetoprotein levels elevated	Autosomal recessive ATM (ataxia-telangiectasia mutated) gene at Chromosome 11q23 Somatic genetic alterations t(14;14)(q11;q32.1), inv(14)(q11q32), t(x;14), inv(7)(p13q35), t(7;7)(p13;q35), t(7;14)(p13;q11), t(7;14)(q13;q11) rarely t(X;14)(q28;q11) Prevalence: 1:200,000 Birth frequency: 1 per 300,000 births ATM mutation carriers: 1 percent of U.S. population	Lymphomas—60 percent of cancers, usually T cell Hodgkin's disease—11 percent of cancers Acute leukemia—21 percent of cancers B-cell lymphoma—12 percent of AT patients Breast cancer increased 3.9-fold in female relatives of AT patients 13.8 percent of sporadic breast cancers due to ATM mutation	+ +	Gatti et al.[233,234] Taylor et al.[734–736] Paterson et al.[550] Joncas et al.[346] Spector et al.[700,701] Berkel et al.[47] Saemundsen et al.[634] Waldman et al.[771] Purtilo et al.[594] Johnson et al.[345] Swift et al.[721] Filipovich et al.[203] Meyn et al.[471,472] Sherrington et al.[676] Savitsky et al.[646] Metcalfe et al.[469] Chen et al.[110] Stankovic et al.[705] Vanasse et al.[761] Cuneo et al.[141]
Wiscott-Aldrich syndrome (WAS)	Eczema, thrombocytopenia, susceptibility to infections Combined B- and T-cell variable immunodeficiency, low IgM, increased IgA and IgE	Sex-linked WASP (Wiscott-Aldrich syndrome protein) gene at Chromosome Xp11.22–11.23 Birth frequency: 4 per million live male births	B-cell lymphomas—80 percent of cancers Hodgkin's disease—4 percent of cancers	+	Seidemann et al.[664] Gatti et al.[233] Spector et al.[700,701] Perry et al.[579] Snover et al.[692] Cotelingam et al.[134] Filipovich et al.[203] Derry et al.[157] Cory et al.[132] Yoshida et al.[820] Rawlings et al.[609]
Severe combined immuno-deficiency (SCID)	Severe infections beginning in neonatal period Defective stem-cell differentiation to T and B cells, some with adenosine deaminase deficiency	Autosomal recessive or sex-linked	Lymphomas—55 to 74 percent of cancers Hodgkin's disease—9.5 percent of cancers Acute leukemia	+	Shcherbina et al.[673] Gatti et al.[233] Spector et al.[700,701] Filipovich et al.[203]

(continued)

Table 47–3. *Continued*

Immunodeficiency Disease	Clinical Features/ Immune Deficiencies	Genetics/Epidemiology	Percentage of Cancers That Are Lymphomas, Types of Cancers, With Statistics	Association With EBV	References
Common variable immunodeficiency (CVI)	Encompasses several syndromes: recurrent bacterial infections of the respiratory tract—sinusitis, otitis media, bronchitis, pneumonia—due mostly to encapsulated bacteria (*Streptococcus pneumoniae*, *Hemophilus influenzae*) Normal numbers of B cells with hypogammaglobulinemia, deficits of T-cell immunity in some patients—cutaneous anergy	Autosomal dominant with incomplete penetrance Associated with mutations of C4-A and C2 gene alleles in the class III MHC region on chromosome 6	Lymphomas—49 percent of cancers Hodgkin's disease—7 percent of cancers CLL Peripheral T-cell lymphoma—1 case Benign lymphoproliferative disorders: 30 percent of CVI patients Lymphomas—increased 30-fold over general population; female CVI patients—increased 100-fold	+	Gatti et al.[233] Spector et al.[700,701] Filipovich et al.[203] Sneller et al.[689] Buckley et al.[79] Washington et al.[780] Jensen et al.[343] Gottesman et al.[250]
IgM deficiency (isolated, selective)	Upper respiratory infections, especially gram-negative bacteria				
IgA deficiency (isolated, selective)	Recurrent infections, often with autoimmune disease and GI disorders, or asymptomatic	Frequency: 1/500 to 1/700 persons	Lymphomas—16 to 31 percent of cancers Hodgkin's disease—8 percent of cancers Gastric adenocarcinoma Abdominal T-cell lymphoma—1 case	NA	Gatti et al.[233] Spector et al.[700,701] Filipovich et al.[203] Zenone et al.[828] Ott et al.[538]
X-linked (Bruton's) hypogammaglobulinemia/ agammaglobulinemia	Infections with encapsulated organisms (*Hemophilus influenzae*, *Pseudomonas aeruginosa*, *Diplococcus pneumoniae*) B-cell maturation defect—few B lymphocytes, no Ig-secreting plasma cells	Sex-linked *BTK* (Bruton's tyrosine kinase) gene at Chromosome Xq22	Lymphomas—33 percent of cancers Acute lymphocytic leukemia Chronic myelogenous leukemia	– (no EBV receptors)	Spector et al.[700,701] Schwaber et al.[662] Purtilo et al.[594] Buckley et al.[79] Saffran et al.[636] Washington et al.[780] LeBien et al.[406] Nomura et al.[524]
X-linked lymphoproliferative disease (XLP; Duncan's disease)	Chronic or fatal infectious mononucleosis with hepatic necrosis Variable hypogammaglobulinemia, decreased NK-cell activity, abnormal CD4/CD8 ratios, decreased memory T-cell activity against Epstein-Barr virus Induction of *DSHP/SH2D1A* may interfere with inhibition of lymphocyte activation	Sex-linked *DSHP/SH2D1A/XLP* gene at Chromosome Xq25 *DSHP/SH2D1A* mutated in 70 percent of XLP patients	B-cell lymphoma—35 percent of males with XLP	+ + +	Sakamoto et al.[637] Purtilo et al.[593-596] Saemundsen et al.[635] Sullivan et al.[716] Grierson et al.[259] Vowels et al.[769] Coffey et al.[124] Nichols et al.[518] Brandau et al.[70] Strahm et al.[709]
Bloom's syndrome	Telangiectatic erythema, stunted growth Decreased immunoglobulins of one or more classes, poor lymphocyte response to certain mitogens	Autosomal recessive *BLM* (Bloom's) gene at Chromosome 15q26.1	Increased incidence of non-Hodgkin's lymphomas, acute lymphocytic leukemias, solid tumors Non-Hodgkin's lymphomas—21 percent of cancers	NA	Gianelli et al.[242] Louie et al.[441] German et al.[238] Ellis et al.[182,183] Straughn et al.[712]

Disease	Clinical features	Inheritance/genetics		Cancers	Reference
	Chromosome breakage and rearrangements, especially quadriradial (Qr) cytogenetic abnormality, usually chromosome 1 Increased sensitivity to ultraviolet radiation				Vanasse et al.[761]
Xeroderma pigmentosum	Skin atrophy, photosensitive dermatitis Mild immunodeficiency Defective DNA repair following exposure to ultraviolet light	Autosomal recessive	NA	Increased incidence of skin cancer	Louie et al.[441]
Nijmegen breakage syndrome	Small stature, severe microcephaly, birdlike facial appearance, progressive decrease of intellectual function Deficiency in B- and T-cell function Frequent infections, especially paranasal sinuses, lower respiratory tract Chromosomal breakage syndrome, chromosomal hypersensitivity to x-rays, radioresistance of DNA replication	Autosomal Nibrin gene at Chromosome 8q21	NA	40 percent of patients develop cancers Leukemias and lymphomas—85 percent of cancers B-cell lymphomas—most common	Chrzanowska et al.[114] Vanasse et al.[761] Seidemann et al.[664]
Fanconi's anemia	Progressive pancytopenia, diverse congenital abnormalities Mild immunodeficiency Hypersensitivity to the clastogenic effect of DNA cross-linking agents, such as diepoxybutane, mitomycin C	Autosomal recessive Somatic genetic alterations: t(11;14)(p13;q32)	NA	Increased incidence of acute myeloid leukemia T-cell lymphoblastic lymphoma—1 case	Auerbach et al.[27] Goldsby et al.[248]
Diamond-Blackfan anemia	Chronic pure red cell aplasia, macrocytic anemia Ocular, thumb, craniofacial, genitourinary abnormalities	Congenital	NA	Acute myelogenous leukemia Acute lymphocytic leukemia Hodgkin's disease—few Non-Hodgkin's lymphoma—1 case	van Dijken et al.[763] Hayashi et al.[295]
Hyper IgM syndrome	Absence of hypoxanthine guanine phosphoribosyl transferase (HGPRT), leading to defective salvage pathway of purine biosynthesis—contributes more to B lymphocytes than T lymphocytes Increased numbers of B cells Increased IgM, decreased amounts of other isotypes Activated T cells have abnormal CD40 ligand, which cannot bind CD40 on B cells and thus fails to stimulate B-cell proliferation and IgE secretion	Sex-linked	NA	Lymphomas—56 percent of cancers Hodgkin's disease—25 percent of cancers	Filipovich et al.[203]

Abbreviation: NA, not addressed.

ents.[319,780] Even though chronic benign lymph node enlargement frequently occurs in patients with Wiskott-Aldrich syndrome, who have affected nodes displaying a spectrum of hyperplastic changes, frank lymphoma tends to occur extranodally.[692]

Pathogenesis: Mechanistic Basis for Congenital Immunodeficiency-Associated Lymphomagenesis

The disrupted immunoregulation that characterizes the CIDs is believed to contribute to their association with cancer, especially lymphoid malignancies.[441] A number of mechanistic bases for these immune defects are unique when compared with those operating in other immunodeficiency settings.

Several syndromes feature defects in DNA metabolism as well as the accumulation of chromosomal aberrations. Ataxia-telangiectasia, for example, is characterized by cells that are exquisitely sensitive to x-rays and experience excessive chromosomal breakage[734,735] secondary to defective excision repair of irradiation-induced breaks in double-stranded DNA.[550] The inherited mutation in individuals with ataxia-telangiectasia is in the *ATM* gene, which is located on chromosome 11q22-23.[234,646] *ATM* has homology to several cell cycle checkpoint genes, suggesting that a nonfunctional *ATM* may lead to defects in the surveillance and appropriate cellular responses to DNA damage.[472] Rates of spontaneous intrachromosomal recombination are increased.[471] Approximately 10 percent of all T lymphocytes circulating in the peripheral blood of these patients contain karyotypically abnormal T cells, typically involving chromosome 7 and 14 rearrangements at specific breakpoints (Table 47–3).[736,761] The usual breakpoints, at 14q11 and 14q32.1, encompass the T-cell receptor-α *(TCR-α)* and *IgH* loci, respectively, and are also seen in leukemias that develop in non–ataxia-telangiectasia patients.[345,676] Importantly, the percentage of cells containing a typical monoclonal, cytogenetic abnormality may increase over time, preceding both identifiable TCR monoclonality as well as an overt malignant phenotype.[676,736] An additional cytogenetic abnormality, telomeric fusions, is associated with large preleukemic clones, leading to the proposal that these fusions result from the combined effect of the accelerated telomere shortening seen in cells homozygous for *ATM* mutations and the growth advantage of cells in large clones.[469]

The picture that emerges is one of sequential genetic alteration, contributing to the progression toward tumorigenesis. The DNA instability residing in the underlying repair deficit may be at least partly responsible for the immune deficiency as well as the propensity of these patients to develop malignancies.[721,771] The abnormal juxtaposition of two gene segments *(TCR* and *IgH)* that normally rearrange in lymphocytes implies an error in recombination. Cells from ataxia-telangiectasia patients, for example, demonstrate elevated frequencies of aberrant interlocus *TCR* gene rearrangements.[433] In addition, the ratio of circulating T cells bearing γ/δ receptors to T cells bearing α/β receptors is increased in these patients relative to that in normal subjects, supporting the existence of a recombinational defect that interferes with T-cell rearrangements.[88] This defect appears to be unique to ataxia-telangiectasia, since T cells from

other immune deficiency diseases, including common variable immunodeficiency and Wiskott-Aldrich syndrome, fail to show such an abnormal T-cell receptor ratio. The contribution of *ATM* alterations to lymphomagenesis is supported by the observation of acquired 11q22-23 hemizygous deletions in sporadic lymphomas of various histologies (follicular, mantle-cell, diffuse large-cell) and of *ATM* missense mutations in a high percentage of sporadic T-cell prolymphocytic leukemias and occasional B-cell non-Hodgkin's lymphomas and B-cell chronic lymphocytic leukemias.[141,649,708,761,768] The lymphomas associated with ataxia-telangiectasia are usually T cell in phenotype, but rare B-cell lymphomas have been described.[355]

Bloom's syndrome is a rare CID in which cells exhibit increased sensitivity to ultraviolet radiation.[238,242,668] It is characterized by a cytogenetic rearrangement involving a quadriradial configuration (Qr), usually of chromosome 1.[238,441] Patients with the disease are homozygous for a mutation in the Bloom's syndrome gene, *BLM,* located on chromosome 15q26.1.[183,712] *BLM* encodes a protein that is homologous to the ReqQ DNA helicases and, when mutated, leads to genetic instability.[182] Xeroderma pigmentosum (XP) and Fanconi's anemia,[27] both of which show abnormal DNA metabolism and mild immunodeficiency, are also associated with an increased risk of cancer, particularly leukemias and skin tumors.[441,668,771] An increased risk of cancer also exists among first-degree relatives of patients with ataxia-telangiectasia, Bloom's syndrome, and Fanconi's anemia.[441,721] Among female relatives of ataxia-telangiectasia patients, there is an increased risk of breast cancer, especially following a history of exposure to ionizing radiation.[110,705,721]

Defects in DNA repair and recombination are not central to all of the lymphoma-associated CIDs. Wiskott-Aldrich syndrome is an X-linked recessive disease that is caused by mutations in the *WASP* gene at chromosomal locus Xp11.22, which encodes Wiskott-Aldrich syndrome protein, WASP, a protein involved in lymphoid cell signal transduction pathways and regulation of actin cytoskeleton rearrangement.[132,157,609] The immune deficit in this syndrome appears to result in part from accelerated destruction of lymphocytes, marked by an increased frequency of spontaneous apoptosis, with attenuated Bcl-2 expression.[609] T cells from Wiskott-Aldrich patients show diminished proliferative responses and failure to appropriately up-regulate cytokines like IL-2. The absence of the WASP protein in platelets of individuals affected by this inherited disorder has been shown to correlate with cell dysfunction.[673] These immunologic abnormalities may well contribute to the propensity to lymphomagenesis of this patient population.

EBV and Congenital Immunodeficiency Disease Act in Synergistic Fashion to Promote Lymphomagenesis

Although in a number of CIDs EBV is believed to interact synergistically with the underlying immune deficiency to promote malignancy, this is not universal. At one extreme, individuals with Bruton's agammaglobulinemia, which involves B-cell deficiencies that are due to mutation of the X-linked *BTK* (Bruton's tyrosine kinase) gene,[636] lack EBV receptors and therefore cannot be infected by this virus.[594,662] By contrast, in the curious condition of X-linked lymphoproliferative syndrome (XLP), EBV has been shown to play a vital role in triggering the onset or exacerbation of immunological deficits.[716]

DSHP/SH2D1A, the gene for XLP, maps to chromosome Xq25 and is mutated in approximately 70 percent of XLP patients (Table 47–3).[70,124,518] The protein encoded by this gene consists of a single SH2 domain that is homologous to the SH2 domain of SHIP, an inositol polyphosphate 5-phosphatase that functions as a negative regulator of lymphocyte activation. Induction of *DSHP* may therefore sustain an immune response by subverting the normal inhibition of lymphocyte activation that is mediated by SHIP.[518] Overall, males carrying the allele for XLP exhibit normal cellular and humoral immunity before EBV infection. However, subtle deficits, such as an elevated CD4/CD8 ratio, a partial IgA deficiency, and failure to switch from IgM to IgG on OX174 challenge,[594] have been documented. During acute EBV infection they develop vigorous cytotoxic cellular responses against EBV-infected and -uninfected autologous target cells, including hepatocytes, often succumbing to a fatal infectious mononucleosis syndrome as a result of fulminant liver failure and hepatic necrosis or hemophagocytic syndrome.[259] Survivors of infectious mononucleosis manifest varying degrees of immunodeficiency, commonly involving hypogammaglobulinemia of different isotypes with absence of the normal postinfectious mononucleosis antibodies to EBNA and usually to VCA.[596,637] Not only do EBV-exposed female carriers exhibit anti-EBNA, they display a paradoxically overexuberant response to early antigen and VCA, with anti-VCA titers some 3.5-fold greater than controls.[637] The inability to produce anti-EBNA antibodies has been attributed to a failure to release EBNA from B cells carrying the EBV genome secondary to the deficiency of EBV-specific cytotoxic T cells in these patients.[300,637] Among the other defects acquired following infection with EBV are loss of natural killer cell activity, abnormal CD4/CD8 ratios, and destruction of the thymic epithelium.[594,595,716]

Four major pathogenetic outcomes have been described following EBV infection in males with XLP:[127,259,594,637] 1. acquired agamma- or hypogammaglobulinemia with necrosis of lymph nodes in 20 percent; 2. aplastic anemia, which is invariably fatal, including various gradations of neutropenia and red cell aplasia; 3. fatal and chronic infectious mononucleosis in almost two-thirds of patients, 85 percent proving fatal; and 4. malignant B-cell lymphoma in about one-third of males with XLP. XLP patients with lymphoma may manifest concomitant hypogammaglobulinemia or fatal infectious mononucleosis or both.[259]

Interestingly, 78 percent of the primary lymphomas in XLP patients occur in the intestine, frequently the ileocecal region.[259] Most are localized stage I and II tumors. Histologically, Burkitt's lymphomas constitute the largest group (45 percent), but large cell, immunoblastic, and other types have also been seen. EBV genomic DNA has been identified in proliferating lymphoid tissues of patients with XLP.[593,635] Because of the intimate association between EBV infection and the immunodeficiency observed in XLP, this disease entity has served as a prototype for understanding the interaction of these factors in the development of non-Hodgkin's lymphoma, a frequent outcome. In addition to precipitating or exacerbating a pre-existing subtle immunodeficiency in XLP patients, EBV stimulates poly-clonal B-cell proliferation. The EBV-suppressed immune surveillance that characterizes XLP is believed to allow such polyclonal cell growth to proceed unchecked, providing more raw material for subsequent genetic mutations that ultimately might lead to malignancy. Despite the overwhelming evidence for intricate synergism between the inherited immunologic abnormality and EBV in inducing lymphomagenesis in XLP patients, rare cases have been reported of boys with documented mutations in the *DSHP/SH2DA1* gene developing non-Hodgkin's lymphomas in the absence of EBV infection.[70,709]

EBV genomes have been identified in lymphomas associated with ataxia-telangiectasia.[634,635] Furthermore, patients with this disease frequently display abnormal antibody responses to EBV, characterized by high EBV antibody titers to VCA, an increased incidence of antibodies to early antigen, but low or absent antibodies to EBNA.[47,346,634] This array of antibody abnormalities is unique and resembles that seen in XLP only in the deficit of anti-EBNA antibodies.[637] The immunological basis for such antibody expression undoubtedly contributes to the tendency to develop lymphomas, as in the case of XLP. The immunological dysregulation may, in turn, result from and/or cooperate in a synergistic manner with the DNA repair and chromosomal recombination abnormalities of ataxia-telangiectasia to promote malignant transformation.

Interestingly, EBV DNA has also occasionally been detected in monoclonal B cells from the tumor tissue of malignant lymphomas in the setting of other CIDs such as Wiskott-Aldrich syndrome[820] and common variable immunodeficiency.[343]

Treatment of Congenital Immunodeficiency Disease–Associated Lymphomas

Information on treatment strategies addressed specifically to lymphomas that occur in the setting of CIDs is sparse. The use of BMT to reconstitute the immune deficiency fully has been proposed as a means of preventing the development of lymphomas.[422,594,769] Modulators of the immune system such as thymosin have been suggested as therapeutic interventions.[594] Dramatic clinical improvement in non-Hodgkin's lymphoma has been obtained in patients with both common variable and severe combined immunodeficiency using interferon-α with or without intravenous γ-globulin.[203,669] Because of the EBV association, acyclovir has been used alone, or concomitantly with prednisone, albeit unsuccessfully.[347,716] Radiation therapy and surgery have also been attempted in some cases.[259,347] Whereas treatment of lymphomas is often successful in settings of potentially reversible immunodeficiency such as organ transplant, the lymphomas in CIDs are generally unresponsive because of the inability to remedy the underlying immunologic deficit.

LYMPHOMAS IN THE SETTING OF AUTOIMMUNE DISEASES

The rheumatologic, or autoimmune, disorders offer another disease context in which an increased incidence of LPD is observed. The underlying mechanisms in these disease entities involve dysregulation leading to hyperactivity of the immune system.

Lymphomas in Specific Autoimmune Diseases

The intimate relationship between malignancy and autoimmunity is particularly evident in Sjögren syndrome, in which a classic histopathologic feature is the benign lymphoepithelial lesion, an infiltration of glandular tissue by B and T lymphocytes and plasma cells.[17,210] Non-Hodgkin's lymphomas occur in Sjögren syndrome patients with a frequency between 12 and 43 times that seen in the general population.[258,362] The lymphoproliferative lesions of the syndrome range from benign pleiomorphic lymphoid infiltrates to morphologically malignant lymphoma, resembling the spectrum of lesions described in transplant recipients.[17] The term *pseudolymphoma* refers to the middle portion of this spectrum and applies to those lesions that contain tumorlike aggregates of lymphoid cells but fail to meet the histologic criteria for malignancy.[17] These lesions may be localized to the salivary gland or appear as extraglandular lymphoid infiltrates.

All the morphologically malignant lymphomas are B cell in origin and diffuse in pattern of growth. The predominant histologic types include large cell, particularly immunoblastic, mixed large and small cell, and even small cell lymphomas, with marked histologic variation within individual tumors. These are probably all lymphomas of the MALT type, similar to gastric MALT lymphoma.[718] The antigenic stimulus within the salivary gland has not been defined. Loss of intracytoplasmic Ig has been noted in association with terminal lymphomas, suggesting de-differentiation of plasma cells and immunoblasts. Progression from a polyclonal benign lymphoproliferative lesion to monoclonal lymphoma has been demonstrated.[837] In other studies, however, clonal *Ig* gene rearrangements have been detected in presumably benign lymphocytic infiltrates.[163,210] A possible explanation for this apparent inconsistency is that the clonal expansion is due to a generalized defect in immune surveillance that characterizes Sjögren syndrome, whereas the development of lymphoma reflects additional genetic alterations that promote neoplastic transformation.[210]

Accompanying immunologic abnormalitites include hypergammaglobulinemia, a high incidence of autoantibodies, organ-specific (anti-salivary duct) autoantibody, and a local excess synthesis of Igs, especially IgM macroglobulins.[17] While increased IgM levels in involved tissues or in serum are suggestive of concurrent Waldenström's macroglobulinemia, a low IgM level may herald the appearance of malignant lymphoma and is a poor prognostic sign. A fall in rheumatoid factor may accompany the decrease in IgM, leading to generalized hypogammaglobulinemia and loss of autoantibodies concomitant with the development of lymphoma.[17,837] The search for a potential viral role in lymphomagenesis associated with Sjögren syndrome has been limited. However, based on a small number of cases, in which the EBV-encoded small RNA EBER-1 was not expressed in the benign lymphoproliferations of Sjögren syndrome, EBV infection does not appear to play a key role in the pathogenesis of these lesions.[162] HHV-8 DNA sequences were detected in a single bilateral MALT-lymphoma of the parotid gland associated with Sjögren syndrome, in contrast to 53 other histopathologic types of salivary gland tumors,[380] but further investigation is required to establish a true pathogenetic association between this virus and the lymphoma.

The prognosis of patients with Sjögren syndrome and LPD is guarded. In some cases, however, therapy with radiation or immunosuppressive agents such as cyclophosphamide, chlorambucil, and prednisone has led to improvement of the primary disease symptoms of xerostomia and conjunctivitis sicca as well as eliciting a diminution in tumor size.[17] Series employing more recent treatment approaches have not been reported.

A variety of lymphoid neoplasms have been noted in individuals with antecedent rheumatoid arthritis and, to a lesser extent, systemic lupus erythematosus (SLE).[424,806] However, statistical analysis has not consistently proven an increased susceptibility to LPD in these disease states.[17] Evidence from a number of studies suggests that the incidence of cancer among individuals with rheumatoid arthritis ranges from 0.6 to 4.1 percent.[257,335,424,726] Other studies have demonstrated no overall increase,[727] and even a lower incidence,[424] of malignancies in patients with rheumatoid arthritis. The increased risk of lymphoma in association with rheumatoid arthritis is generally reported as modest, only 2 to 2.5 times that in the general population,[335,375] although relative risks as high as 24[375,587,591] have been noted. Nevertheless, within the 1 to 2 percent of rheumatoid arthritis patients who have Felty syndrome (rheumatoid arthritis with neutropenia, splenomegaly, and recurrent infections), the incidence of all cancers is twice that in the control population. The risk of non-Hodgkin's lymphoma in Felty syndrome is increased 12-fold, approximating the increased risk of non-Hodgkin's lymphoma in Sjögren syndrome, a condition that is sometimes associated with Felty syndrome.[258] The susceptibility of Felty syndrome patients to non-Hodgkin's lymphoma probably derives from their particular array of immunologic alterations, which include bone marrow depression and an increased frequency of the HLA-DQ haplotype, linked to control of suppressor T-cell function.[258] In general, however, rheumatoid arthritis is associated with only minimal immunologic deficits, including failure of peripheral blood mononuclear cells to respond to recall antigens, a moderate decrease in both B and T cells, and a decrease in CD8 cells, accompanied by an increase in both CD4 cells and the CD4:CD8 ratio.[784] A reduction in natural killer cell activity, observed in some studies in the synovial fluid and whole blood of patients with rheumatoid arthritis, has been suggested as a possible explanation for the increased tendency to develop non-Hodgkin's lymphomas.[587] EBV DNA sequences have been demonstrated in rheumatoid arthritis–associated lymphoma, 80 percent being type 1.[511] In one report, the EBV-infected lymphoma developed after treatment with cyclosporine (see below), implicating a synergistic interaction between EBV and the agent as well as the underlying disease.[832] In contrast to Sjögren syndrome, only one report describes MALT lymphoma in association with rheumatoid arthritis, and the two cases were observed in association with secondary Sjögren syndrome and the use of second-line agents.[719]

A positive association between SLE and non-Hodgkin's lymphoma has been observed in some studies.[424,468] Lewis et al.[424] noted a 4 percent incidence of cancer among patients with SLE, which is over twice the frequency in their controls. This contrasts with their data on rheumatoid arthritis, in which cancer risk was not increased. Among cancers, lymphomas appear to have the strongest association with SLE.[806] Nevertheless, the question of a genuinely increased risk of cancer, and specifically of LPD, in patients with SLE remains unanswered.

The skin is included in the spectrum of tissues affected by a number of the connective tissue diseases, such as SLE, dermatomyositis, relapsing polychondritis, and lichen sclerosus et atrophicus. Atypical lymphoid infiltrates arising in such autoimmune cutaneous lesions have been categorized as either pseudolymphomas or malignant lymphomas based on a combination of clinical, histologic, immunologic, and genotypic attributes.[451]

Primary non-Hodgkin's lymphoma of the thyroid gland accounts for 5 percent of thyroid malignancies and less than 2 percent of extranodal lymphomas.[168] These generally occur in the context of chronic lymphocytic thyroiditis (Hashimoto's disease).[156] The male-to-female ratio in one study was 1:4, with mean ages of 63 and 73 years, respectively.[557] Thus, patients typically are middle-aged females who are euthyroid, lack antithyroid antibodies, and present with a cold nodule in the neck.[81] Most cases are localized, Stage IE or IIE. In view of their tendency to remain localized for prolonged periods with late, distant relapses, the thyroid lymphomas, along with those of the breast, lung, parotid, and GI tract, are believed to belong to the previously discussed biological subset of extranodal lymphomas, designated MALT lymphoma.[156,332,632] The thyroid antigen that serves as the stimulus is not defined. As in other settings of immunodeficiency, the lymphomas occurring in the thyroid are primarily of the diffuse large cell type, especially with immunoblastic morphology,[81] although some of the tumors are small lymphocytic in histology.

Histologic differentiation of diffuse chronic lymphocytic thyroiditis from malignant lymphoma may be difficult, recalling the spectrum of histologies observed among the lymphomas found in Sjögren syndrome, transplant recipients, and other immunocompromised states. Areas of chronic lymphocytic thyroiditis are sometimes present in residual thyroid tissue adjacent to areas of malignant lymphoma, suggesting progression through this spectrum from benign hyperplasia to frankly malignant lesions. The benign nature of the chronic lymphoid infiltrates that accompany thyroiditis has been reaffirmed in studies of Hashimoto's thyroiditis unselected for lymphoma, in which the infiltrating lymphocytic cells were characterized as polyclonal by immunohistochemistry, PCR for Ig heavy chain rearrangement, or Southern blot analysis with Ig heavy and light chain probes.[320,461] Conversely, histologically diagnosed thyroid lymphomas demonstrate monoclonality by Ig heavy and light chain gene rearrangement in 85 percent of cases.[461] The polyclonality together with the predominantly T cell nature of the lymphoid infiltrates of thyroiditis present a stark contrast to the monoclonal B cells that make up MALT-type lymphomas, including those of the thyroid.[333] However, the emergence of a monoclonal B-cell proliferation in the midst of a polyclonal B- and T-cell inflammatory response appears to be a common mechanism for MALT lymphomas involving different organs. Only rarely have T-cell thyroid lymphomas been observed.[1,557,808] A role for EBV in promoting the progression from Hashimoto's thyroiditis to malignant lymphoma is suggested by the observation of a small subset of thyroid lymphomas (3 of 32) in which strong and homogeneous signals for EBER appeared in the nucleus of most cells by both in situ hybridization and immunohistochemistry.[729] However, larger numbers and demonstration of EBV clonality in tumor cells are necessary before EBV can be definitively regarded as a contributor to lymphomagenesis in the thyroid.

Treatment in early studies of thyroiditis-associated lymphomas consisted of local modalities only, first surgery and later radiation, the latter yielding an overall relapse rate of 37.1 percent, primarily as distant relapse (30.8 percent).[168] Given this outcome, combined modality therapy, which has an overall relapse rate of 7.7 percent (5.1 percent distant relapse), is now being espoused as the optimal approach to thyroid lymphoma.[168] Overall, the outcome in more recent studies has been favorable following appropriate therapy.[156]

Autoimmune diseases of the GI tract have been associated with an increased incidence of lymphomas. The risk of malignant lymphoma is elevated in individuals with adult celiac disease (celiac sprue, gluten-sensitive enteropathy, nontropical sprue),[460] an autoimmune disease in which infiltration of the lamina propria by plasma cells and lymphocytes is believed to mediate damage to the intestinal mucosa that results in villous atrophy and malabsorption. The lymphomas that occur in association with celiac disease represent a specific subtype of primary intestinal T-cell lymphoma, *enteropathy-associated T-cell lymphoma,* confirmed as monoclonal by TCR gene rearrangement.[180,334,804] Despite their T-cell origin, they may be somewhat de-differentiated in immunophenotype.[225] The few B-cell lymphomas that are seen are usually diffuse large cell or immunoblastic lymphomas.[460] Enteropathy-associated T-cell lymphomas commonly occur in the jejunum, often in areas of ulcerative jejunitis, and they tend to affect patients with a short history of adult celiac disease, rather than those whose disease dates back to childhood.[334] The prognosis is poor, reflecting, in part, late stage at diagnosis and poor performance status. In a study by Gale et al.[225] in which combination chemotherapy was administered, more than half of the patients were unable to complete the planned course, only one-third showed a complete response, and almost 80 percent of responders relapsed 1 to 60 months after diagnosis. Nevertheless, some evidence exists to suggest that these lymphomas may be prevented by adherence to a strictly gluten-free diet.

Other gastrointestinal disease settings that may predispose to primary small intestinal malignant lymphomas include inflammatory bowel disease, both ulcerative colitis and regional enteritis (Crohn's disease)[129,253] and Mediterranean α chain disease.[608] Colonic lymphoma has rarely been observed superimposed on chronic ulcerative colitis.[613] One report describes the occurrence of reversible EBV-related polymorphic B-cell lymphoproliferation in a patient with Crohn's disease during treatment with azathioprine therapy, resembling the lymphomas that are observed in transplant recipients.[402] The immunoproliferative small intestinal disease that occurs in α chain disease is a low-grade subtype of MALT lymphoma (see above), except that plasma cells secreting large amounts of α heavy chain without light chain are prominent in the intestine and mesenteric lymph nodes.[334]

Pathogenesis: Mechanistic Basis for Autoimmune Disease–Associated Lymphomagenesis

The immune dysregulation that is inherent in patients with autoimmune diseases is believed to contribute to their tendency to develop lymphoproliferative malignancies. Hypergammaglobulinemia with a high incidence of autoantibodies and excessive local synthesis of Igs in some cases may provide chronic intense stimulation of B-cell proliferation.[17,726] Superimposed on this, an impaired immune surveillance may allow uncontrolled proliferation of abnormal cells. The use of immunosuppressive agents, shown to promote malignancy in transplant recipients, may contribute to tumorigenesis in autoimmune disease.[572,726] Lymphomas developing in patients with rheumatoid arthritis and dermatomyositis treated with methotrexate have been shown to regress following discontinuation of this immunosuppressive drug, suggesting that methotrexate plays a role in the development of these lymphomas.[354,639] Dramatic regression of lymphadenopathy also occurred following cessation of azathioprine in a patient with Crohn's disease.[402] Cyclosporine use has been associated with the development of malignant lymphoma in a patient with rheumatoid arthritis.[832] Splenectomy, a common treatment for Felty syndrome, has also been proposed as a risk factor for lymphoma.[258] Recent data point to an association between somatic mutations in the *Fas* gene and lymphomas in patients with a variety of underlying autoimmune diseases, including Hashimoto's thyroiditis and SLE.[262] These data expand the implications of observations in mice and humans showing that inherited disruption of the Fas/Fas ligand pathway leads to defects in apoptosis that are associated with benign lymphoproliferations, severe multisystem autoimmune disease, and hypergammaglobulinemia. Germline mutations in *Fas* have been demonstrated in children exhibiting a group of phenotypes collectively referred to as *autoimmune lymphoproliferative syndrome* (ALPS).[171,206,618,713] In other patients with an ALPS clinical phenotype, no *Fas* gene mutation has been identified, but decreased Fas function was observed, suggesting downstream alterations of the Fas signaling pathway.[605]

The interaction of specific immunodeficiencies in individuals with rheumatoid arthritis with infection by EBV may predispose toward malignancy. Persistent EBV infection has been documented in a patient with rheumatoid arthritis and a diffuse large cell lymphoma.[784] EBV DNA, RNA, and LMP have also been detected in malignant cells in patients with autoimmune disease.[354,832] Furthermore, although B cells from EBV-immune patients with rheumatoid arthritis respond appropriately to EBV stimulation by increasing Ig production, their T cells are deficient in mediating late suppression of this Ig production by the autologous EBV-infected B cells.[748]

SUMMARY

Lymphomas that develop in the setting of other diseases exhibit a distinct constellation of clinical features. In general, they tend to be of the non-Hodgkin's type and often have a large B-cell, particularly immunoblastic, histology. Difficulty in establishing histopathologic diagnoses may relate to a spectrum of lesions ranging from polyclonal LPD to frankly malignant monoclonal lymphoma. Extranodal, notably CNS, presentations are common. These non-Hodgkin's lymphomas are aggressive and, although responsive to therapy, often lead to death from treatment-related toxicity, uncontrolled lymphoma growth, or progression of the underlying disease. Within the confines of these common features, the LPDs associated with each disease entity have their own peculiar features regarding histopathology, site, and clonality. However, two phenomena dominate the picture of most of these lymphomas. First, all these disease conditions are characterized by some degree of immunodysregulation. Second, a strong association with EBV has been documented in many of these LPDs. A multistep model of tumor progression has been proposed to explain tumorigenesis in the setting of underlying diseases. The observed associations with EBV and immundeficiency offer likely mechanistic explanations for the progressive steps involved in lymphomagenesis. Finally, treatment to date is generally unsatisfactory, and a variety of novel therapies, including biologically based agents, are being tested in an effort to improve response and survival.

ACKNOWLEDGMENT

The authors wish to thank Dr. Jaye Viner for her critical reading of the manuscript. The authors acknowledge Jenny Gaegler and Karen Goldrich for their expert technical assistance.

REFERENCES

1. Abdul-Rahman ZH, Gogas HJ, Tooze JA et al: T-cell lymphoma in Hashimoto's thyroiditis. Histopathology 29:244–459, 1996.
2. Abruzzo LV, Schmidt K, Weiss LM et al: B-cell lymphoma after angioimmunoblastic lymphadenopathy: A case with oligoclonal gene rearrangements associated with epstein-Barr virus. Blood 82:241–246, 1993.
3. Adams JM, Harris AW, Pinkert CA et al: The c-myc oncogene driven by immunoglobulin enhancers induces lymphoid malignancy in transgenic mice. Nature 318:533–538, 1985.
4. Alexander FE, Jarrett RF, Lawrence D et al: Risk factors for Hodgkin's disease by Epstein-Barr virus (EBV) status: Prior infection by EBV and other agents. Br J Cancer 32:1117–1121, 2000.
5. Alfieri C, Tanner J, Carpentier L et al: Epstein-Barr virus transmission from a blood donor to an organ transplant recipient with recovery of the same virus strain from the recipient's blood and oropharynx. Blood 87:812–817, 1996.
6. Alizadeh AA, Elsen MB, Davis RE et al: Distinct types of diffuse large B-cell lymphoma identified by gene expression profiling. Nature 403:503–511, 2000.
7. Allan G, Inman GJ, Parker BD et al: J Gen Virol 73:1547–1551, 1992.
8. Allen RC, Armitage RJ, Conley ME et al: CD40 ligand gene defects responsible for X-linked hyper-IgM syndrome. Science 259:990–993, 1993.

9. Alpen B, Neubauer A, Dierlamm J et al: Translocation t(11;18) absent in early gastric marginal zone B-cell lymphoma of MALT type responding to eradication of *Helicobacter pylori* infection. Blood 95:4014–4015, 2000.

10. Amati B, Dalton S, Brooks MW et al: Transcriptional activation by the human c-Myc oncoprotein in yeast requires interaction with Max. Nature 359:423–426, 1992.

11. Ambroziak JA, Blackbourn DJ, Herndier BG et al: Herpes-like sequences in HIV-infected and uninfected Kaposi's sarcoma patients. Science 268:582–583, 1995.

12. Ames ED, Conjalka MS, Goldberg AF et al: Hodgkin's disease and AIDS. Twenty-three new cases and a review of the literature. Hematol Oncol Clin North Am 5:343–356, 1991.

13. Ames ED, Metroka CE, Goldberg AF: Hodgkin disease and HIV. Ann Intern Med 118:313, 1993 (Correspondence).

14. Anagnostopoulos I, Hummel M, Finn T et al: Heterogeneous Epstein-Barr virus infection patterns in peripheral T-cell lymphoma of angioimmunoblastic lymphadenopathy type. Blood 80:1804–1812, 1992.

15. Anagnostopoulos I, Hummel M, Kreschel C, Stein H: Morphology, immunophenotype and distribution of latently and/or productively Epstein-Barr virus infected cells in acute infectious mononucleosis: Implications for the individual infection route of Epstein-Barr virus. Blood 85:744–750, 1995.

16. Anderson JL, Fowles RE, Bieber CP et al: Idiopathic cardiomyopathy, age, and suppressor-cell dysfunction as risk determinants of lymphoma after cardiac transplantation. Lancet 2:1174–1177, 1978.

17. Anderson LG, Talal N: The spectrum of benign to malignant lymphoproliferation in Sjögren's syndrome. Clin Exp Immunol 9:199–221, 1971.

18. Andiman W, Martin K, Rubinstein A et al: Opportunistic lymphoproliferations associated with Epstein-Barr viral DNA in infants and children with AIDS. Lancet (December 21/28):1390–1393, 1985.

19. Ansari MQ, Dawson DG, Nador R et al: Primary body cavity based AIDS-related lymphomas. Am J Clin Pathol 105:221–229, 1996.

20. Aoki Y, Yarchoan R, Braun J et al: Viral and cellular cytokines in AIDS-related malignant lymphomatous effusions. Blood 96:1599–1601, 2000.

21. Armitage JM, Kormos RL, Stuart RS et al: Posttransplant lymphoproliferative disease in thoracic organ transplant patients: Ten years of cyclosporine-based immunosuppression. J Heart Lung Transplant 10:877–887, 1991.

22. Armitage JO: Treatment of non-Hodgkin's lymphoma. N Engl J Med 328:1023–1030, 1993.

23. ar-Rushdi A, Nishikura K, Erikson J et al: Differential expression of the translocated and the untranslocated c-*MYC* oncogene in Burkitt lymphoma. Science 222:390–393, 1983.

24. Arvanitakis L, Yaseen N, Sharma S: Latent membrane protein-1 induces cyclin D2 expression, pRb hyperphosphorylation, and loss of TGF-β-mediated growth inhibition in EBV-positive B cells. J Immunol 155:1047–1056, 1995.

25. Ashwell JD, Longo DL, Bridges SH: T-cell tumor elimination as a result of T-cell receptor-mediated activation. Science 237:61–64, 1987.

26. Auer IA, Gascoyne RD, Connors JM et al: t(11;18)(q21;q21) is the most common translocation in MALT lymphomas. Ann Oncol 8:979–985, 1997.

27. Auerbach AD, Rogatko A, Schroeder-Kurth TM: International Fanconi Anemia Registry: Relation of clinical symptoms to diepoxybutane sensitivity. Blood 73:391–396, 1989.

28. Baer DM, Anderson ET, Wilkinson LS: Acquired immune deficiency syndrome in homosexual men with Hodgkin's disease. Three case reports. Am J Med 80:738–740, 1986.

29. Ballerini P, Gaidano G, Gong JZ et al: Multiple genetic lesions in acquired immunodeficiency syndrome-related non-Hodgkin's lymphoma. Blood 81:166–176, 1993.

30. Ballestas ME, Chatis PA, Kaye KM: Efficient persistence of extrachromosomal KSHV DNA mediated by latency-associated nuclear antigen. Science 284:641–644, 1999.

31. Banerjee SK, Weston AP, Persons DL et al: Non-random loss of chromosome 3 during transition of *Helicobacter pylori*-associated gastric MALT to B-cell MALT lymphoma revealed by fluorescence in situ hybridization. Cancer Lett 121:83–90, 1997.

32. Bartholomew C, Saxinger C, Clark JW et al: Transmission of HTLV-I and HIV among homosexual men in Trinidad. JAMA 257:2604–2608, 1987.

33. Bartlett JA, Benoit SL, Johnson VA et al. for the North American HIV Working Party: Lamivudine plus zidovudine compared with zalcitabine plus zidovudine in patients with HIV infection. A randomized, double-blind, placebo-controlled trial. Ann Intern Med 125:161–172, 1996.

34. Bashir RM, Harris NL, Hochberg FH et al: Detection of Epstein-Barr virus in CNS lymphomas by in-situ hybridization. Neurology 39:813–817, 1989.

35. Bashir RM, Hochberg FH, Harris NL et al: Variable expression of Epstein-Barr virus genome as demonstrated by in situ hybridization in central nervous system lymphomas in immunocompromised patients. Mod Pathol 3:429–434, 1990.

36. Baumforth KRN, Young LS, Flavell KJ et al: The Epstein-Barr virus and its association with human cancers. J Clin Pathol Mol Pathol 52:307–322, 1999.

37. Baumgartner JE, Rachlin JR, Beckstead JH et al: Primary central nervous system lymphomas: Natural history and response to radiation therapy in 55 patients with acquired immunodeficiency syndrome. J Neurosurg 73:206–211, 1990.

38. Baurmann H, Miclea J-M, Ferchal F et al: Adult T-cell leukemia associated with HTLV-I and simultaneous infection by human immunodeficiency virus type 2 and human herpesvirus 6 in an African woman: A clinical, virologic, and familial serologic study. Am J Med 85:853–857, 1988.

39. Bayerdörffer E, Miehlke S, Neubauer A et al: Gastric MALT-lymphoma and *Helicobacter pylori* infection. Aliment Pharmacol Ther 11(Suppl. 1):89–94, 1997.

40. Beckwith M, Urba WJ, Ferris DK et al: Anti-IgM-mediated growth inhibition of a human B lymphoma cell line is independent of phosphatidylinositol turnover and protein kinase C activation and involves tyrosine phosphorylation. J Immunol 147:2411–2418, 1991.

41. Benjamin D, Magrath IT, Maguire R et al: Immunoglobulin secretion by cell lines derived from African and American undifferentiated lymphomas of Burkitt's and non-Burkitt's type. J Immunol 129:1336–1342, 1982.

42. Benjamin D, Knobloch TJ, Dayton MA: Human B-cell interleukin-10: B-cell lines derived from patients with acquired immunodeficiency syndrome and Burkitt's lymphoma constitutively secrete large quantities of interleukin-10. Blood 80:1289–1298, 1992.

43. Benkerrou M, Jais J-P, Leblond V et al: Anti-B-cell monoclonal antibody treatment of severe posttransplant B-lymphoproliferative disorder: Prognostic factors and long-term outcome. Blood 92:3137–3147, 1998.

44. Beral B, Peterman T, Berkelman T et al: AIDS-associated non-Hodgkin lymphoma. Lancet 337:805–809, 1991.

45. Berard CW, Greene MH, Jaffe ES et al: A multidisciplinary approach to non-Hodgkin's lymphomas. Ann Intern Med 94:218–235, 1981.

46. Berg LC, Copenhaver CM, Morrison VA et al: B-cell lymphoproliferative disorders in solid-organ transplant patients: Detection of Epstein-Barr virus by in situ hybridization. Hum Pathol 23:159–163, 1992.

47. Berkel AI, Henle W, Henle G et al: Epstein-Barr virus-related antibody patterns in ataxia-telangiectasia. Clin Exp Immunol 35:196–201, 1979.

48. Bermudez MA, Grant K, Rodvien R et al: Non-Hodgkin's lymphoma in a population with or at risk for acquired immunodeficiency syndrome: Indications for intensive chemotherapy. Am J Med 86:71–76, 1989.

49. Bernard O, Cory S, Gerondakis S et al: Sequence of the murine and human cellular myc oncogenes and two modes of *myc* transcription resulting from chromosome translocation in B lymphoid tumours. EMBO J 12:2375–2383, 1983.

50. Bertoni F, Cotter F, Zucca E: Molecular genetics of extranodal marginal zone (MALT-type) B-cell lymphoma. Leuk Lymphoma 35:57–68, 1999.

51. Bhatia K, Spangler G, Gaidano G et al: Mutations in the coding region of *c-myc* occur frequently in acquired immunodeficiency syndrome-associated lymphomas. Blood 84:883–888, 1994.

52. Bhatia S, Ramsay NKC, Steinbuch M et al: Malignant neoplasms following bone marrow transplantation. Blood 87:3633–3639, 1996.

53. Bieber CP, Reitz BA, Jamieson SW et al: Malignant lymphoma in cyclosporin A treated allograft recipients. Lancet 1:43, 1980 (Correspondence).

54. Biemer JJ: Malignant lymphomas associated with immunodeficiency states. Ann Clin Lab Sci 20:175–191, 1990.

55. Bierman PJ, Vose JM, Langnas AN et al: Hodgkin's disease following solid organ transplantation. Ann Oncol 7:265–270, 1996.

56. Biggar RJ, Rabkin CS: The epidemiology of acquired immunodeficiency syndrome-related lymphomas. Curr Opinion Oncol 4:883–893, 1992.

57. Biggar RJ, Frisch M, Goedeert JJ for the AIDS-Cancer Study Group: Risk of cancer in children with AIDS. JAMA 284:205–209, 2000.

58. Biggar RJ: AIDS-related cancers in the era of highly active antiretroviral therapy. Oncology 15:439–449, 2001.

59. Bird AG, McLachlan SM: Cyclosporin A and Epstein-Barr virus. Lancet 418, 1980 (Correspondence).

60. Birkeland SA, Bendtzen K, Moller B et al: Interleukin-10 and posttransplant lymphoproliferative disorder after kidney transplantation. Transplantation 67:876–881, 1999.

61. Birx DL, Redfield RR, Tosato G: Defective regulation of Epstein-Barr virus infection in patients with acquired immunodeficiency syndrome (AIDS) or AIDS-related disorders. N Engl J Med 314:874–879, 1986.

62. Birx DL, Redfield RR, Tencer K et al: Induction of interleukin-6 during human immunodeficiency virus infection. Blood 76:2303–2310, 1990.

63. Blanche S, Le Deist F, Veber F et al: Treatment of severe Epstein-Barr virus-induced polyclonal B-lymphocyte proliferation by anti-B-cell monoclonal antibodies. Two cases after HLA-mismatched bone marrow transplantation. Ann Intern Med 108:199–203, 1988.

64. Blaser MJ: In a world of black and white, *Helicobacter pylori* is gray. Ann Intern Med 130:695–697, 1999.

65. Blattner WA: Human retroviruses: Their role in cancer. Proc Assoc Am Phys 111:563–572, 1999.

66. Bloom RE, Brennan JK, Sullivan JL et al: Lymphoma of host origin in a marrow transplant recipient in remission of acute myeloid leukemia and receiving cyclosporin A. Am J Hematol 18:73–83, 1985.

67. Blum AL, Talley NJ, O'Moráin C et al. for the Omeprazole Plus Clarithromycin and Amoxicillin Effect One Year After Treatment (OCAY) Study Group: Lack of effect of treating *Helicobacter pylori* infection in patients with nonulcer dyspepsia. N Engl J Med 339:1875–1881, 1998.

68. Bonnet M, Guinebretiere J-M, Kremmer E et al: Detection of Epstein-Barr virus in invasive breast cancers. J Natl Cancer Inst 91:1376–1381, 1999.

69. Boyle MJ, Swanson CE, Turner JJ et al: Definition of two distinct types of AIDS-associated non-Hodgkin lymphoma. Br J Haematol 76:506–512, 1990.

70. Brandau O, Schuster V, Weiss M et al: Epstein-Barr virus-negative boys with non-Hodgkin lymphoma are mutated in the *SH2D1A* gene, as are patients with X-linked lymphoproliferative disease (XLP). Hum Mol Genet 8:2407–2413, 1999.

71. Breen EC, Rezai AR, Nakajima K et al: Infection with HIV is associated with elevated IL-6 levels and production. J Immunol 144:480–484, 1990.

72. Brenner M: Adoptive therapy of posttransplant lymphoma. Cancer J 6(Suppl. 3):S259–S264, 2000.

73. Brink AATP, van den Brule AJC, van Diest P et al: Detection of Epstein-Barr virus in invasive breast cancers. J Natl Cancer Inst 92:655–656, 2000.

74. Brinkman K, Delnoy PP, de Pauw B: Highly active antiretroviral therapy (HAART) and prolonged survival of a patient with an HIV-related Burkitt lymphoma, despite an intracardiac relapse. Int J STD AIDS 9:773–775, 1998.

75. Brooks LA, Lear AL, Young LS et al: Transcripts from the Epstein-Barr virus BamHI A fragment are detectable in all three forms of virus latency. J Virol 67:3182–3190, 1993.

76. Brooks LA, Crook T, Crawford DH: Epstein-Barr virus and lymphomas. Cancer Surveys 33:Infections and Human Cancer 33:99–123, 1999.

77. Browne PV, Lawler M, Humphries P et al: Donor-cell leukemia after bone marrow transplantation for severe aplastic anemia. N Engl J Med 325:710–713, 1991.

78. Buchbinder SP, Holmberg SD, Scheer S et al: Combination antiretroviral therapy and incidence of AIDS-related malignancies. J Acquir Immune Defic Syndr 21(Suppl. 1):S23–S26, 1999.

79. Buckley RH: Assessing inheritance of agammaglobulinemia. N Engl J Med 330:1526–1528, 1994.

80. Buisson M, Manet E, Trescol-Biemont, M-C et al: The Epstein-Barr virus (EBV) early protein EB2 is a posttranscriptional activator expressed under the control of EBV transcription factors EB1 and R. J Virol 63:5276–5284, 1989.

81. Burke JS, Butler JJ, Fuller LM: Malignant lymphomas of the thyroid. A clinical pathologic study of 35 patients including ultrastructural observations. Cancer 39:1587–1602, 1977.

82. Burke JS: Are there site-specific differences among the MALT lymphomas—morphologic, clinical? Am J Clin Pathol 111(Suppl. 1):S133–S143, 1999.

83. Burkes RL, Meyer PR, Gill PS et al: Rectal lymphoma in homosexual men. Arch Intern Med 146:913–915, 1986.

84. Caldas C, Ambinder R: Epstein-Barr virus and bone marrow transplantation. Curr Opin Oncol 7:102–106, 1995.

85. Callahan J, Pai S, Cotter M, Robertson ES: Distinct patterns of viral antigen expression in Epstein-Barr virus and Kaposi's sarcoma-associated herpesvirus coinfected body-cavity-based lym-

phoma cell lines: Potential switches in latent gene expression due to coinfection. Virology 262:18–30, 1999.

86. Calne RY, Rolles K, White DJG et al: Cyclosporine A initially as the only immunosuppressant in 34 recipients of cadaveric organs: 32 kidneys, 2 pancreases, and 2 livers. Lancet 2:1033–1036, 1979.

87. Camilleri-Broët S, Camparo P, Mokhtari K et al: Overexpression of *BCL-2, BCL-X,* and *BAX* in primary central nervous system lymphomas that occur in immunosuppressed patients. Mod Pathol 13:158–165, 2000.

88. Carbonari M, Cherchi M, Paganelli R et al: Relative increase of T cells expressing the gamma/delta rather than the alpha/beta receptor in ataxia-telangiectasia. N Engl J Med 322:73–76, 1990.

89. Carbone A, Tirelli, U, Vaccher E et al: A clinicopathologic study of lymphoid neoplasias associated with human immunodeficiency virus infection in Italy. Cancer 68:842–852, 1991.

90. Carbone A, Gloghini A, Zanette I et al: Demonstration of Epstein-Barr viral genomes by in situ hybridization in acquired immune deficiency syndrome-related high grade and anaplastic large cell CD30+ lymphomas. Am J Clin Pathol 99:289–297, 1993.

91. Carbone A, Gloghini A, Volpe R et al: High frequency of Epstein-Barr virus latent membrane protein-1 expression in acquired immunodeficiency syndrome-related Ki-1 (CD30)-positive anaplastic large-cell lymphomas. Am J Clin Pathol 101:768–772, 1994.

92. Cen H, Williams PA, McWilliams HP et al: Evidence for restricted Epstein-Barr virus latent gene expression and anti-EBNA antibody response in solid organ transplant recipients with post-transplant lymphoproliferative disorders. Blood 81:1393–1403, 1993.

93. Centers for Disease Control: Revision of the case definition of acquired immunodeficiency syndrome for national reporting—United States. MMWR 34, No. 25:373–375, 1985.

94. Centers for Disease Control: Revision of the CDC surveillance case definition for acquired immunodeficiency syndrome. MMWR 36(Suppl.):1S–15S, 1987.

95. Centers for Disease Control: MMWR: Opportunistic non-Hodgkin's lymphomas among severely immunocompromised HIV-infected patients surviving for prolonged periods on antiretroviral therapy—United States. JAMA 266:1620–1621, 1991.

96. Cerroni L, Zöchling N, Pütz B et al: Infection by *Borrelia burgdorferi* and cutaneous B-cell lymphoma. J Cutan Pathol 24:457–461, 1997.

97. Cesarman E, Dalla-Favera R, Bentley D et al: Mutations in the first exon are associated with altered transcription of c-*MYC* in Burkitt lymphoma. Science 238:1272–1273, 1987.

98. Cesarman E, Chang Y, Moore PS et al: Kaposi's sarcoma-associated herpesvirus-like DNA sequences in AIDS-related body-cavity-based lymphomas. N Engl J Med 332:1186–1191, 1995.

99. Chadburn, A, Cesarman, E, Knowles, DM: Molecular pathology of posttransplantation lymphoproliferative disorders. Sem Diag Pathol 14:15–26, 1997.

100. Chadburn A, Chen JM, Hsu DT et al: The morphologic and molecular genetic categories of posttransplantation lymphoproliferative disorders are clinically relevant. Cancer 82:1978–1987, 1998.

101. Chadburn A, Hyjeck E, Ying L et al: Epstein Barr virus (EBV) gene expression in post-transplantation lymphoproliferative disorders (PT-LPDs). Mod Pathol 12:133A, 1999 (Abstract).

102. Chaganti RSK, Jhanwar SC, Koziner B et al: Specific translocations characterize Burkitt's-like lymphoma of homosexual men with the acquired immunodeficiency syndrome. Blood 61:1265–1268, 1983.

103. Chan JKC, Ng CS, Lau WH et al: Most nasal/nasopharyngeal lymphomas are peripheral T-cell neoplasms. Am J Surg Pathol 11:418–429, 1987.

104. Chan JKC: Gastrointestinal lymphomas: An overview with emphasis on new findings and diagnostic problems. Sem Diag Pathol 13:260–296, 1996.

105. Chang RS, Lewis JP, Abildgaard CF: Prevalence of oropharyngeal excreters of leukocyte-transforming agents among a human population. N Engl J Med 289:1325–1329, 1973.

106. Chang RS, Lewis JP, Reynolds RD et al: Oropharyngeal excretion of Epstein-Barr virus by patients with lymphoproliferative disorders and by recipients of renal homografts. Ann Intern Med 88:34–40, 1978.

107. Chang Y, Cesarman E, Pessin MS et al: Identification of herpesvirus-like DNA sequences in AIDS-associated Kaposi's sarcoma. Science 266:1865–1869, 1994.

108. Chapel F, Fabiani B, Davi F et al: Epstein-Barr virus and gastric carcinoma in western patients: Comparison of pathological parameters and *p53* expression in EBV-positive and negative tumours. Histopathology 36:252–261, 2000.

109. Cheeseman SH, Henle W, Rubin RH et al: Epstein-Barr virus infection in renal transplant recipients. Effects of antithymocyte globulin and intereron. Ann Intern Med 93(Part 1):39–42, 1980.

110. Chen J, Birkholtz GG, Lindblom P et al: The role of ataxia-telangiectasia heterozygotes in familial breast cancer. Cancer Res 58:1376–1379, 1998.

111. Cheung ANY, Chan ACL, Chung LP et al: Post-transplantation lymphoproliferative disorder of donor origin in a sex-mismatched renal allograft as proven by chromsome in situ hybridization. Mod Pathol 11:99–102, 1998.

112. Cheung TW, Arai S: HIV-associated Hodgkin's disease. The AIDS Reader (March/April 1999):131–137, 1999.

113. Chiang AKS, Wong KY, Liang ACT et al: Comparative analysis of Epstein-Barr virus gene polymorphisms in nasal T/NK-cell lymphomas and normal nasal tissues: Implications on virus strain selection in malignancy. Int J Cancer 80:356–364, 1999.

114. Chrzanowska KH, Kleijer WJ, Krajewska-Walasek M et al: Eleven Polish patients with microcephaly, immunodeficiency, and chromosomal instability: The Nijmegen breakage syndrome. Am J Med Genet 57:462–471, 1995.

115. Ciancio G, Siquijor AP, Burke GW et al: Post-transplant lymphoproliferative disease in kidney transplant patients in the new immunosuppressive era. Clin Transplant 11:243–249, 1997.

116. Cingolani A, Gastaldi R, Fassone L et al: Epstein-Barr virus infection is predictive of CNS involvement in systemic AIDS-related non-Hodgkin's lymphoma. J Clin Oncol 18:3325–3330, 2000.

117. Clark HM, Yano T, Otsuki T et al: Mutations in the coding region of c-*MYC* in AIDS-associated and other aggressive lymphomas. Cancer Res 54:3383–3386, 1994.

118. Clark W: The role of tumor progression and the progression of cancer. In Greenwald P, Kramer BS, Weed D (eds.), Cancer Prevention and Control, pp. 135–159. Marcel Dekker, New York, 1995.

119. Cleary ML, Warnke R, Sklar J: Monoclonality of lymphoproliferative lesions in cardiac-transplant recipients. N Engl J Med 310:477–482, 1984.

120. Cleary ML, Sklar J: Lymphoproliferative disorders in cardiac transplant recipients are multiclonal lymphomas. Lancet 2:489–493, 1984.

121. Cleary ML, Nalesnik MA, Shearer WT et al: Clonal analysis of transplant-associated lymphoproliferations based on the structure of the genomic termini of the Epstein-Barr virus. Blood 72:349–352, 1988.

122. Cockburn I: Assessment of the risk of malignancy and lymphomas developing in patients using Sandimmune. Transplant Proc 19:1804–1807, 1987.

123. Cockfield SM, Preiksaitis J, Harvey E et al: Is sequential use of ALG and OKT3 in renal transplants associated with an increased incidence of fulminant posttransplant lymphoproliferative disorder? Transplant Proc 23:1106–1107, 1991.

124. Coffey AJ, Brooksbank RA, Brandau O et al: Host response to EBV infection in X-linked lymphoproliferative disease results from mutations in an SH2-domain encoding gene. Nat Genet 20:129–135, 1998.

125. Cogliati T, Dunn BK, Bar-Ner M et al: Transfected wild-type and mutant *MAX* regulate cell growth and differentiation of murine erythroleukemia cells. Oncogene 8:1263–1268, 1993.

126. Cohen JI, Wang F, Mannick J et al: Epstein-Barr virus nuclear protein 2 is a key determinant of lymphocyte transformation. Proc Natl Acad Sci U S A 86:9558–9562, 1989.

127. Cohen JI: Epstein-Barr virus infection. N Engl J Med 343:481–492, 2000.

128. Coiffier B, Gisselbrecht C, Herbrecht R et al: LNH84 regimen: A multicenter study of intensive chemotherapy in 737 patients with aggressive malignant lymphoma. J Clin Oncol 7:1018–1026, 1989.

129. Collins WJ: Malignant lymphoma complicating regional enteritis. Case report and review of the literature. Am J Gastroenterol 68:177–181, 1977.

130. Corbo L, LeRoux F, Sergeant A: The EBV early gene product EB2 transforms rodent cells through a signalling pathway involving c-myc. Oncogene 9:3299–3304, 1994.

131. Cortes E, Detels R, Aboulafia D et al: HIV-1, HIV-2, and HTLV-I infection in high-risk groups in Brazil. N Engl J Med 320:953–958, 1989.

132. Cory GOC, MacCarthy-Morrogh L, Banin S et al: Evidence that the Wiskott-Aldrich syndrome protein may be involved in lymphoid cell signaling pathways. J Immunol 157:3793–3795, 1996.

133. Coté TR, Biggar RJ: Does zidovudine cause non-Hodgkin's lymphoma? AIDS 9:404–405, 1995.

134. Cotelingam JD, Witebsky FG, Hsu SM et al: Malignant lymphoma in patients with the Wiskott-Aldrich syndrome. Cancer Invest 3:515–522, 1985.

135. Crane GA, Variakojis D, Rosen ST et al: Cutaneous T-cell lymphoma in patients with human immunodeficiency virus infection. Arch Dermatol 127:989–994, 1991.

136. Crawford DH, Thomas JA, Janossy G et al: Epstein-Barr virus nuclear antigen positive lymphoma after cyclosporin A treatment in patient with renal allograft. Lancet 1:1355–1356, 1980.

137. Crawford DH, Edwards JMB, Sweny P et al: Long-term T-cell-mediated immunity to Epstein-Barr virus in renal-allograft recipients receiving cyclosporin A. Lancet 1:10–13, 1981.

138. Cremer KJ, Spring SB, Gruber J: Role of human immunodeficiency virus type 1 and other viruses in malignancies associated with acquired immunodeficiency disease syndrome. J Natl Cancer Inst 82:1016–1024, 1990.

139. Croce C, Nowell PC: Molecular basis of human B cell neoplasia. Blood 65:1–7, 1985.

140. Crompton CH, Cheung RK, Donjon C et al: Epstein-Barr virus surveillance after renal transplantation. Transplantation 57:1182–1189, 1994.

141. Cuneo A, Bigoni R, Rigolin GM et al: Acquired chromosome 11q deletion involving the ataxia telangiectasia locus in B-cell non-Hodgkin's lymphoma: Correlation with clinicobiologic features. J Clin Oncol 18:2607–2614, 2000.

142. Cunto-Amesty G, Przybylski G, Honczarenko M et al: Evidence that immunoglobulin specificities of AIDS-related lymphoma are not directed to HIV-related antigens. Blood 95:1393–1399, 2000.

143. Curiel TJ, Piche A, Kasono K et al: Gene therapy strategies for AIDS-related malignancies. Gene Ther 4:1284–1288, 1997.

144. Curtis RE, Travis LB, Rowlings PA et al: Risk of lymphoproliferative disorders after bone marrow transplantation: A multi-institutional study. Blood 94:2208–2216, 1999.

145. Dalla-Favera R, Martinotti S, Gallo RC et al: Translocation and rearrangements of the *c-myc* oncogene locus in human undifferentiated B-cell lymphomas. Science 219:963–967, 1983.

146. Dancis A, Odajnyk C, Krigel RL et al: Association of Hodgkin's and non-Hodgkin's lymphomas with the acquired immunodeficiency syndrome (AIDS). Proc Am Soc Clin Oncol 3:61a, 1984.

147. D'Aquila RT, Hughes MD, Johnson VA et al. and the National Institute of Allergy and Infectious Diseases AIDS Clinical Trials Group Protocol 241 Investigators: Nevirapine, zidovudine, and didanosine compared with zidovudine and didanosine in patients with HIV-1 infection. A randomized, double-blind, placebo-controlled trial. Ann Intern Med 124:1019–1030, 1996.

148. Davis MG, Kenney SC, Kamine J et al: Immediate-early gene region of human cytomegalovirus trans-activates the promoter of human immunodeficiency virus. Proc Natl Acad Sci U S A 84:8642–8646, 1987.

149. Deacon EM, Pallesen G, Niedobitek G et al: Epstein-Barr virus and Hodgkin's disease: Transcriptional analysis of virus latency in the malignant cells. J Exp Med 177:339–349, 1993.

150. Deeg HJ, Socié G, Schoch G et al: Malignancies after marrow transplantation for aplastic anemia and Fanconi anemia: A joint Seattle and Paris analysis of results in 700 patients. Blood 87:386–392, 1996.

151. Deeg HJ, Socié G: Malignancies after hematopoietic stem cell transplantation: Many questions, some answers. Blood 91:1833–1844, 1998.

152. Deeks SG, Smith M, Holodniy M et al: HIV-1 protease inhibitors. JAMA 277:145–153, 1997.

153. de Jong D, Boot H, Taal B: Histological grading with clinical relevance in gastric mucosa-associated lymphoid tissue (MALT) lymphoma. Recent Results Cancer Res 156:27–32, 2000.

154. Delecluse HJ, Raphael M, Magaud JP et al: Variable morphology of human immunodeficiency virus-associated lymphomas with *c-myc* rearrangements. Blood 82:552–563, 1993.

155. Delecluse HJ, Hummel M, Marafioti T et al: Common and HIV-related diffuse large B-cell lymphomas differ in their immunoglobulin gene mutation pattern. J Pathol 188:133–138, 1999.

156. Derringer GA, Thompson LDR, Frommelt RA et al: Malignant lymphoma of the thyroid gland. A clinicopathologic study of 108 cases. Am J Surg Pathol 24:623–639, 2000.

157. Derry JMJ, Ochs HD, Francke U: Isolation of a novel gene mutated in Wiskott-Aldrich syndrome. Cell 78:635–644, 1994.

158. de-The G, Geser A, Day NE et al: Epidemiological evidence for causal relationship between Epstein-Barr virus and Burkitt's lymphoma from Ugandan prospective study. Nature 274:756–761, 1978.

159. Devesa SS, Silverman D, Young JJ et al: Cancer incidence and mortality trends among whites in the United States. J Natl Cancer Inst 79:701–770, 1987.

160. Devesa SS, Hartge P: Quantification of the impact of known risk factors on time trends in non-Hodgkin's lymphoma incidence. Cancer Res 52(Suppl.):5566S-5569S, 1992.

161. DeVita VT, Mauch PM, Harris NL: Hodgkin's Disease. In DeVita VT, Hellman S, Rosenberg S (eds.), Cancer. Principles and Practice of Oncology, 5th Ed., pp. 2242–2283. Lippincott-Raven, New York, 1997.

162. DiGiuseppe JA, Wu TC, Corio RL: Analysis of Epstein Barr virus-encoded small RNA-1 expression in benign lymphoepithelial salivary gland lesions. Mod Pathol 7:555–559, 1994.

163. Diss TC, Peng H, Wotherspoon AC et al: Brief report: A single neoplastic clone in sequential biopsy specimens from a patient with primary gastric-mucosa-associated lymphoid-tissue lymphoma and Sjögren's syndrome. N Engl J Med 329:172–175, 1993.

164. Dockrell DH, Strickler JG, Paya CV: Epstein-Barr virus-induced T cell lymphoma in solid organ transplant recipients. Clin Infect Dis 26:180–182, 1997.

165. Dolcetti R, Frisan T, Sjöberg J et al: Identification and characterization of an Epstein-Barr virus-specific T-cell response in the pathologic tissue of a patient with Hodgkin's disease. Cancer Res 54:3675–3681, 1995.

166. Dolcetti R, Boiocchi M: Epstein-Barr virus in the pathogenesis of Hodgkin's disease. Biomed Pharmacother 52:13–25, 1998.

167. Doll DC, List AF: Burkitt's lymphoma in a homosexual. Lancet 1:1026–1027, 1982.

168. Doria R, Jekel JF, Cooper DL: Thyroid lymphoma. The case for combined modality therapy. Cancer 73:200–206, 1994.

169. Dotti G, Fiocchi R, Motta T et al: Primary effusion lymphoma after heart transplantation: A new entity associated with human herpesvirus-8. Leukemia 13:664–670, 1999.

170. Douglass EC, Magrath IT, Lee EC et al: Serial cytogenetic studies of nonendemic Burkitt's lymphoma cell lines. J Natl Cancer Inst 65:891–895, 1980.

171. Drappa J, Vaishnaw AK, Sullivan KE et al: *Fas* gene mutations in the Canale-Smith syndrome, an inherited lymphoproliferative disorder associated with autoimmunity. N Engl J Med 335:1643–1649, 1996.

172. Dreyfus DH, Nagasawa M, Kelleher CA et al: Stable expression of Epstein-Barr virus *BZLF-1*-encoded ZEBRA protein activates p53-dependent transcription in human Jurkat T-lymphoblastoid cells. Blood 96:625–634, 2000.

173. Du M-Q, Peng H, Liu H et al: *BCL10* gene mutation in lymphoma. Blood 95:3885–3890, 2000.

174. Ducloux D, Carron P, Racadot E et al: T-cell immune defect and B-cell activation in renal transplant recipients with monoclonal gammopathies. Transplant Int 12:250–253, 1999.

175. Dupin N, Gorin I, Deleuze J et al: Herpes-like DNA sequences, AIDS-related tumors, and Castleman's disease. N Engl J Med 333:797, 1995 (Correspondence).

176. Dupin N, Diss TL, Kellam P et al: HHV-8 is associated with a plasmablastic variant of Castleman disease that is linked to HHV-8-positive plasmablastic lymphoma. Blood 95:1406–1412, 2000.

177. Eby NL, Grufferman S, Flannelly CM et al: Increasing incidence of primary brain lymphoma in the US. Cancer 62:2461–2465, 1988.

178. Eck M, Schmauβer B, Greiner A et al: *Helicobacter pylori* in gastric mucosa-associated lymphoid tissue type lymphoma. Recent Results Cancer Res 156:9–18, 2000.

179. Egan J, Stewart J, Yonan N et al: Non-Hodgkin lymphoma in heart/lung transplant recipients. Lancet 343:481, 1994 (Correspondence).

180. Egan LJ, Walsh SV, Stevens FM et al: Celiac-associated lymphoma: A single institution experience of 30 cases in the combination chemotherapy era. J Clin Gastroenterol 221:123–129, 1995.

181. Ellis D, Jaffe R, Green M et al: Epstein-Barr virus-related disorders in children undergoing renal transplantation with tacrolimus-based immunosuppression. Transplantation 68:997–1003, 1999.

182. Ellis NA, Groden J, Ye T-Z et al: The Bloom's syndrome gene product is homologous to RecQ helicases. Cell 83:655–666, 1995.

183. Ellis NA, German J: Molecular genetics of Bloom's syndrome. Hum Mol Genet 5:1457–1463, 1996.

184. Emanuel BS, Selden JR, Chaganti RSK et al: The 2p breakpoint of a 2;8 translocation in Burkitt lymphoma interrupts the Vkappa locus. Proc Natl Acad Sci U S A 81:2444–2446, 1984.

185. Emilie D, Coumbaras J, Raphael M et al: Interleukin-6 production in high-grade B lymphomas: Correlation with the presence of malignant immunoblasts in acquired immunodeficiency syndrome and in human immunodeficiency virus-seronegative patients. Blood 80:498–504, 1992.

186. Enting RH, Esselink RA, Portegies P: Lymphomatous meningitis in AIDS-related systemic non-Hodgkin's lymphoma: A report of eight cases. J Neurol Neurosurg Psychiatr 57:150–153, 1994.

187. Erikson J, ar-Rushdi A, Drwinga HL et al: Transcriptional activation of the translocated *c-MYC* oncogene in Burkitt lymphoma. Proc Natl Acad Sci U S A 80:820–824, 1983.

188. Erikson J, Nishikura K, ar-Rushdi A et al: Translocation of an immunoglobulin kappa locus to a region 3′ of an unrearranged *c-MYC* oncogene enhances *c-MYC* transcription. Proc Natl Acad Sci U S A 80:7581–7585, 1983.

189. Errante D, Gabarre J, Ridolfo AL et al: Hodgkin's disease in 35 patients with HIV infection: An experience with epirubicin bleomycin, vinblastine and prednisone chemotherapy in combination with antiretroviral therapy and primary use of G-CSF. Ann Oncol 10:189–195, 1999.

190. Euvrard S, Noble CP, Kanitakis J et al: Brief report: Successive occurrence of T-cell and B-cell lymphomas after renal transplantation in a patient with multiple cutaneous squamous-cell carcinomas. N Engl J Med 327:1924–1926, 1992.

191. Evison J, Jost J, Ledergerber B et al: HIV-associated non-Hodgkin's lymphoma: Highly active antiretroviral therapy improves remission rate of chemotherapy. AIDS 13:732–734, 1999.

192. Fåhraeus R, Palmqvist L, Nerdstedt A et al: Response to cAMP levels of the Epstein-Barr virus EBNA2-inducible LMP1 oncogene and EBNA2 inhibition of a PP1-like activity. EMBO J 13:6041–6051, 1994.

193. Farber E: Cell proliferation as a major risk factor for cancer: A concept of doubtful validity. Cancer Res 55:3759–3762, 1995.

194. Farrell PJ, Allan GJ, Shanahan F et al: *p53* is frequently mutated in Burkitt's lymphoma cell lines. EMBO J 10:2879–2887, 1991.

195. Fassone L, Bhatia K, Gutierrez M et al: Molecular profile of Epstein-Barr virus infection in HHV-8-positive primary effusion lymphoma. Leukemia 14:271–277, 2000.

196. Fauci AS, Haynes BF, Costa J et al: Lymphomatoid granulomatosis. N Engl J Med 306:68–74, 1982.

197. Fauci AS, Schnittman SM, Poli G et al: NIH Conference. Immunopathogenic mechanisms in human immunodeficiency virus (HIV) infection. Ann Intern Med 114:678–693, 1991.

198. Fearon ER, Vogelstein B: A genetic model for colorectal tumorigenesis. Cell 61:759–767, 1990.

199. Feigal EG: AIDS-associated malignancies: Research perspectives. Biochim Biophys Acta 1423:C1–C9, 1998.

200. Feinmesser R, Miyazaki I, Cheung R et al: Diagnosis of nasopharyngeal carcinoma by DNA amplification of tissue obtained by fine-needle aspiration. N Engl J Med 326:17–21, 1992.

201. Feuillard J, Schuhmacher M, Kohanna S et al: Inducible loss of NF-κB activity is associated with apoptosis and Bcl-2 down-regulation in Epstein-Barr virus-transformed B lymphocytes. Blood 95:2068–2074, 2000.

202. Filipovich AH, Heinitz KJ, Robison LL et al: The Immunodeficiency Cancer Registry. A research resource. Am J Pediatr Hematol Oncol 9:183–184, 1987.

203. Filipovich AH, Mathur A, Kamat D et al: Primary immunodeficiencies: Genetic risk factors for lymphoma. Cancer Research 52(Suppl.):5465S–5467S, 1992.

204. Fischbach W: *Helicobacter pylori* and lymphoproliferative disorders. Ital J Gastroenterol Hepatol 80(Suppl. 3):S299–S303, 1998.

205. Fischer A, Blanche S, Le Bidois J et al: Anti-B-cell monoclonal antibodies in the treatment of severe B-cell lymphoproliferative syndrome following bone marrow and organ transplantation. N Engl J Med 324:1451–1456, 1991.

206. Fisher GH, Rosenberg FJ, Straus SE et al: Dominant interfering *Fas* gene mutations impair apoptosis in a human autoimmune lymphoproliferative syndrome. Cell 81:935–946, 1995.

207. Fisher RI, Gaynor ER, Dahlberg S et al: Comparison of a standard regimen (CHOP) with three intensive chemotherapy regimens for advanced non-Hodgkin's lymphoma. N Engl J Med 328:1002–1006, 1993.

208. Fisher RI, Dahlberg S, Nathwani BN et al: A clinical analysis of two indolent lymphoma entities: Mantle cell lymphoma and marginal zone lymphoma (including the mucosa-associated lymphoid tissue and monocytoid B-cell subcategories): A Southwest Oncology Group study. Blood 85:1075–1082, 1995.

209. Fisher RS, Parkman HP: Management of nonulcer dyspepsia. N Engl J Med 339:1376–1381, 1998.

210. Fishleder A, Tubbs R, Hesse B et al: Uniform detection of immunoglobulin-gene rearrangement in benign lymphoepithelial lesions. N Engl J Med 316:1118–1121, 1987.

211. Formenti SC, Gill PS, Lean E et al: Primary central nervous system lymphoma in AIDS. Results of radiation therapy. Cancer 63:1101–1107, 1989.

212. Forsyth PA, DeAngelis LM. Biology and management of AIDS-associated primary CNS lymphomas. Hematol Oncol Clin North Am 10:1125–1134, 1996.

213. Franchini G: Molecular mechanisms of human T-cell leukemia/lymphotropic virus type I infection. Blood 86:3619–3639, 1995.

214. Frank D, Cesarman E, Liu YF et al: Posttransplantation lymphoproliferative disorders frequently contain type A and not type B Epstein-Barr virus. Blood 85:1396–1403, 1995.

215. Frenkel N, Schirmer EC, Wyatt LS et al: Isolation of a new herpesvirus from human CD4+ T cells. Proc Natl Acad Sci U S A 87:748–752, 1990.

216. Frías C, Lauzurica R, Vaquero M et al: Detection of Epstein-Barr virus in posttransplantation T cell lymphoma in a kidney transplant recipient: Case report and review. Clin Infect Dis 30:576–578, 1999.

217. Frizzera G, Rosai J, Dehner LP et al: Lymphoreticular disorders in primary immunodeficiencies: New findings based on an up-to-date histologic classification of 35 cases. Cancer 46:692–699, 1980.

218. Frizzera G, Hanto DW, Gajl-Peczalska KJ et al: Polymorphic diffuse B-cell hyperplasias and lymphomas in renal transplant recipients. Cancer Res 41:4262–4279, 1981.

219. Funakoshi S, Longo DL, Beckwith M et al: Inhibition of human B-cell lymphoma growth by CD40 stimulation. Blood 83:2787–2794, 1994.

220. Gaidano G, Ballerini P, Gong JZ et al: *p53* mutations in human lymphoid malignancies: Association with Burkitt lymphoma and chronic lymphocytic leukemia. Proc Natl Acad Sci U S A 88:5413–5417, 1991.

221. Gaidano G, Parsa NZ, Tassi V et al: In vitro establishment of AIDS related lymphoma cell lines: Phenotypic characterization, oncogene and tumor suppressor gene lesions, and heterogeneity in Epstein-Barr virus infection. Leukemia 7:1632–1629, 1993.

222. Gaidano G, LoCoco F, Bihui H et al: Rearrangements of the *BCL-6* gene in acquired immunodeficiency syndrome-associated non-Hodgkin's lymphoma: Association with diffuse large-cell subtype. Blood 84:397–402, 1994.

223. Gaidano G, Dalla-Favera R: Molecular pathogenesis of AIDS-related lymphomas. Adv Cancer Res 67:113–153, 1995.

224. Gail MH, Pluda JM, Rabkin CS: Projections of the incidence of non-Hodgkin's lymphoma related to acquired immunodeficiency syndrome. J Natl Cancer Inst 83:695–701, 1991.

225. Gale J, Simmonds PD, Mead GM et al: Enteropathy-type intestinal T-cell lymphoma: Clinical features and treatment of 31 patients in a single center. J Clin Oncol 18:795–803, 2000.

226. Gambacorta M, Bonacina E, Falini G et al: Malignant lymphoma in the recipient of a heart transplant from a donor with malignant lymphoma. Lymphoma transplantation or de novo disease? Transplantation 51:920–922, 1991.

227. Garbe C, Stein H Dienemann D et al: *Borrelia burgdorferi*-associated cutaneous B cell lymphoma: Clinical and immunohistologic characterization of four cases. J Am Acad Dermatol 24:584–590, 1991.

228. Garnier G, Taillan B, Michiels JF: HIV-associated Hodgkin disease. Ann Intern Med 115:233, 1991 (Correspondence).

229. Garnier JL, Lebranchu Y, Dantal J et al: Hodgkin's disease after transplantation. Transplantation 61:71–76, 1996.

230. Garnier J-L, Blanc-Brunat N, Vivier G et al: Interleukin-10 in Epstein-Barr virus-associated post-transplant lymphomas. Clin Transplant 13:305–312, 1999.

231. Garvin AJ, Self S, Sahovic EA et al: The occurrence of a peripheral T-cell lymphoma in a chronically immunosuppressed renal transplant patient. Am J Surg Pathol 12:64–70, 1988.

232. Gaston JSH, Rickinson AB, Epstein MA: Epstein-Barr-virus-specific T-cell memory in renal-allograft recipients under long-term immunosuppression. Lancet 1:923–925, 1982.

233. Gatti RA, Good RA: Occurrence of malignancy in immunodeficiency diseases. A literature review. Cancer 28:89–98, 1971.

234. Gatti RA, Berkel I, Boder E et al: Localization of an ataxia-telangiectasia gene to chromosome 11q22–23. Nature 336:577–580, 1988.

235. Gauwerky CE, Haluska FG, Tsujimoto Y et al: Evolution of B-cell malignancy: Pre-B-cell leukemia resulting from *MYC* activation in a B-cell neoplasm with a rearranged *BCL2* gene. Proc Natl Acad Sci U S A 85:8548–8552, 1988.

236. Gelmann EP, Psallidopoulos MC, Papas TS et al: Identification of reciprocal translocation sites within the *c-MYC* oncogene and immunoglobulin μ locus in a Burkitt lymphoma. Nature 306:799–803, 1983.

237. Gentile TC, Hadlock KG, Uner AH et al: Large granular lymphocyte leukaemia occurring after renal transplantation. Br J Haematol 101:507–512, 1998.

238. German J: Bloom's syndrome. Dermatol Clinics 13:7–18, 1995.

239. Germanidis G, Haioun C, Pourquier J et al: Hepatitis C virus infection in patients with overt B-cell non-Hodgkin's lymphoma in a French center. Blood 93:1778–1779, 1999 (Correspondence).

240. Geser A, de-The G, Lenoir G et al: Final case reporting from the Ugandan prospective study of the relationship between EBV and Burkitt's lymphoma. Int J Cancer 29:397–400, 1982.

241. Ghods AJ, Ossareh S: Lymphoma—the most common neoplasia in renal transplant recipients. Transplant Proc 32:585–586, 2000.

242. Gianelli F, Benson PF, Pawsey SA et al: Ultraviolet light sensitivity and delayed DNA-chain maturation in Bloom's syndrome fibroblasts. Nature 265:466–469, 1977.

243. Gill PS, Levine AM, Meyer PR et al: Primary central nervous system lymphoma in homosexual men. Clinical, immunologic, and pathologic features. Am J Med 78:742–748, 1985.

244. Gill PS, Levine A, Krailo M et al: AIDS-related malignant lymphoma: Results of prospective treatment trials. J Clin Oncol 5:1322–1328, 1987.

245. Gisselbrecht C, Oksenhendler E, Tirelli U et al: Human immunodeficiency virus-related lymphoma treatment with intensive combination chemotherapy. Am J Med 95:188–196, 1993.

246. Glaser SL, Ambinder RF, DiGiuseppe JA et al: Absence of Epstein-Barr virus EBER-1 transcripts in an epidemiologically diverse group of breast cancers. Int J Cancer 75:555–558, 1998.

247. Gold JE, Altarac D, Ree HJ et al: HIV-associated Hodgkin disease: A clinical study of 18 cases and review of the literature. Am J Hematol 36:93–99, 1991.

248. Goldsby RE, Perkins SL, Virshup DM et al: Lymphoblastic lymphoma and excessive toxicity from chemotherapy: An unusual presentation for Fanconi anemia. J Pediatr Hematol Oncol 21:240–243, 1999.

249. González-Clemente JM, Ribera JM, Camo E et al: Ki-1+ anaplastic large-cell lymphoma of T-cell origin in an HIV-infected patient. AIDS 5:751–755, 1991.

250. Gottesman SRS, Haas D, Ladanyi M et al: Peripheral T cell lymphoma in a patient with common variable immunodeficiency disease: Case report and literature review. Leuk Lymphoma 32:589–595, 1999.

251. Graham NMH, Hoover DR, Park LP et al. and the Multicenter AIDS Cohort Study Group: Survival in HIV-infected patients who have received zidovudine: Comparison of combination therapy with sequential monotherapy and continued zidovudine monotherapy. Ann Intern Med 124:1031–1038, 1996.

252. Greenlee RT, Murray T, Bolden S et al: Cancer Statistics, 2000. CA Cancer J Clin 50:7–33, 2000.

253. Greenstein AJ, Mullin GE, Strauchen JA et al: Lymphoma in inflammatory bowel disease. Cancer 69:1119–1123, 1992.

254. Gregory CD, Murray RJ, Edwards CF: Downregulation of cell adhesion molecules LFA-3 and ICAM-1 in Epstein-Barr virus-positive Burkitt's lymphoma underlies tumor cell escape from virus-specific T cell surveillance. J Exp Med 167:1811–1824, 1988.

255. Gregory CD, Dive C, Henderson S et al: Activation of Epstein-Barr virus latent genes protects human B cells from death by apoptosis. Nature 349:612–614, 1991.

256. Grey M, Townsend N, Lappin D et al: IgA myeloma of donor origin arising 7 years after allogeneic renal transplant. Br J Haematol 108:592–594, 2000.

257. Gridley G, McLaughlin JK, Ekbom A et al: Incidence of cancer among patients with rheumatoid arthritis. J Natl Cancer Inst 85:307–311, 1993.

258. Gridley G, Klippel JH, Hoover RN et al: Incidence of cancer among men with the Felty syndrome. Ann Intern Med 120:35–39, 1994.

259. Grierson H, Purtilo DT: Epstein-Barr virus infections in males with the X-linked lymphoproliferative syndrome. Ann Intern Med 106:538–545, 1987.

260. Grilli M, Chiu JJ-S, Lenardo MJ: NF-κB and Rel: Participants in a multiform transcriptional regulatory system. Int Rev Cytol 143:1–62, 1993.

261. Grogan E, Jenson H, Countryman J et al: Transfection of a rearranged viral DNA fragment, WZhet, stably converts latent Epstein-Barr viral infection to produce infection in lymphoid cells. Proc Natl Acad Sci U S A 84:1332–1336, 1987.

262. Grønbæk K, Straten PT, Ralfkiaer E et al: Somatic Fas mutations in non-Hodgkin's lymphoma: Association with extranodal disease and autoimmunity. Blood 92:3018–3024, 1998.

263. Groopman JE, Sullivan JL, Mulder C et al: Pathogenesis of B cell lymphoma in a patient with AIDS. Blood 67:612–615, 1986.

264. Gruber SA, Skjei KL, Sothern RB et al: Cancer development in renal allograft recipients treated with conventional and cyclosporine immunosuppression. Transplant Proc 23:1104–1105, 1991.

265. Grulich AE: AIDS-associated non-Hodgkin's lymphoma in the era of highly active antiretroviral therapy. J Acquir Immune Defic Syndr 21(Suppl. 1):S27–S30, 1999.

266. Grulich AE, Wan X, Law MG et al: B-cell stimulation and prolonged immune deficiency are risk factors for non-Hodgkin's lymphoma in people with AIDS. AIDS 14:133–140, 2000.

267. Guarner J, del Rio C, Carr D et al: Non-Hodgkin's lymphomas in patients with human immunodeficiency virus infection. Cancer 68:2460–2465, 1991.

268. Guinee D, Jaffe E, Kingma D et al: Pulmonary lymphomatoid granulomatosis. Evidence for a proliferation of Epstein-Barr virus infected B-lymphocytes with a prominent T-cell component and vasculitis. Am J Surg Pathol 18:753–764, 1994.

269. Gustafsson Å, Levitsky V, Zou J-Z et al: Epstein-Barr virus (EBV) load in bone marrow transplant recipients at risk to develop post-transplant lymphoproliferative disease: Prophylactic infusion of EBV-specific cytotoxic T cells. Blood 95:807–814, 2000.

270. Haber D, Harlow E: Tumour-suppressor genes: Evolving definitions in the genomic age. Nat Genet 16:320–322, 1997.

271. Hale G, Waldmann H: Risks of developing Epstein-Barr virus-related lymphoproliferative disorders after T-cell depleted marrow transplants. CAMPATH users. Blood 91:3079–3083, 1998.

272. Haluska FG, Finver S, Tsujimoto Y et al: The t(8;14) chromosomal translocation occurring in B-cell malignancies results from mistakes in V-D-J joining. Nature 324:158–161, 1986.

273. Haluska FG, Tsujimoto Y, Croce, C: Mechanisms of chromosome translocation in B- and T-cell neoplasia. Trends Genet 3:11–15, 1987.

274. Haluska FG, Tsujimoto T, Croce CM: Oncogene activation by chromosome translocation in human malignancy. Ann Rev Genet 21:321–345, 1987.

275. Haluska FG, Tsujimoto Y, Croce CM: The t(8;14) chromosome translocation of the Burkitt lymphoma cell line Daudi occurred during immunoglobulin gene rearrangement and involved the heavy chain diversity region. Proc Natl Acad Sci U S A 84:6835–6839, 1987.

276. Haluska FG, Russo G, Kant J et al: Molecular resemblance of an AIDS-associated lymphoma and endemic Burkitt lymphomas: Implications for their pathogenesis. Proc Natl Acad Sci U S A 86:8907–8911, 1989.

277. Hamilton-Dutoit SJ, Pallesen G, Karkov J et al: Identification of EBV-DNA in tumour cells of AIDS-related lymphomas by in-situ hybridisation. Lancet 1:554–555, 1989 (Letter).

278. Hamilton-Dutoit SJ, Pallesen G, Franzmann MB et al: AIDS-related lymphoma. Histopathology, immunophenotype, and association with Epstein-Barr virus as demonstrated by in situ nucleic acid hybridization. Am J Pathol 138:149–163, 1991.

279. Hamilton-Dutoit SJ, Raphael M, Audouin J et al: In situ demonstration of Epstein-Barr virus small RNAs (EBER 1) in acquired immunodeficiency syndrome-related lymphomas: Correlation with tumor morphology and primary site. Blood 82:619–624, 1993.

280. Hamilton-Dutoit SJ, Rea D, Raphael M et al: Epstein-Barr virus-latent gene expression and tumor cell phenotype in acquired immunodeficiency syndrome-related non-Hodgkin's lymphoma. Am J Pathol 143:1072–1085, 1993.

281. Hammer SM, Katzenstein DA, Hughes MD et al. for the AIDS Clinical Trials Group Study 175 Study Team: A trial comparing nucleoside monotherapy with combination therapy in HIV-infected adults with CD4 cell counts from 200 to 500 per cubic millimeter. N Engl J Med 335:1081–1090, 1996.

282. Hammerschmidt W, Sugden B: Genetic analysis of immortalizing functions of Epstein-Barr virus in human B lymphocytes. Nature 340:393–397, 1989.

283. Hansen PB, Vogt KC, Skov RL et al: Primary gastrointestinal non-Hodgkin's lymphoma in adults: A population-based clinical and histopathologic study. J Intern Med 244:71–78, 1998.

284. Hanson MN, Morrison VA, Peterson BA et al: Posttransplant T-cell lymphoproliferative disorders—an aggressive, late complication of solid-organ transplantation. Blood 88:3626–3633, 1996.

285. Hansson L-E, Nyrén O, Hsing AW et al: The risk of stomach cancer in patients with gastric or duodenal ulcer disease. N Engl J Med 335:242–249, 1996.

286. Hanto DW, Frizzera G, Purtilo DT et al: Clinical spectrum of lymphoproliferative disorders in renal transplant recipients and evidence for the role of Epstein-Barr virus. Cancer Res 41:4253–4261, 1981.

287. Hanto DW, Sakamoto K, Purtilo DT et al: The Epstein-Barr virus in the pathogenesis of posttransplant lymphoproliferative disorders. Surgery 90:204–213, 1981.

288. Hanto DW, Frizzera G, Gajl-Peczalska KJ et al: Epstein-Barr virus-induced B-cell lymphoma after renal transplantation. N Engl J Med 306:913–918, 1982.

289. Hanto DW, Frizzera G, Gajl-Peczalska KJ et al: Epstein-Barr virus, immunodeficiency, and B cell lymphoproliferation. Transplantation 39:461–472, 1985.

290. Hanto DW, Frizzera G, Gajl-Peczalska KJ et al: Acyclovir therapy of Epstein-Barr virus-induced posttransplant lymphoproliferative diseases. Transplant Proc 17:89–92, 1985.

291. Hanto DW, Birkenbach M, Frizzera G et al: Confirmation of the heterogeneity of posttransplant Epstein-Barr virus-associated B cell proliferations by immunoglobulin gene rearrangement analysis. Transplantation 47:458–464, 1989.

292. Harabuchi Y, Yamanaka N, Kataura A et al: Epstein-Barr virus in nasal T-cell lymphomas in patients with lethal midline granuloma. Lancet 128–130, 1990.

293. Harris NL, Jaffe ES, Stein H et al: A revised European-American classification of lymphoid neoplasms: A proposal from the International Lymphoma Study Group. Blood 84:1361–1392, 1994.

294. Hartge P, Devesa SS: Quantification of the impact of known risk factors on time trends in non-Hodgkin's lymphoma incidence. Cancer Res 52(Suppl.):5566s–5569s, 1992.

295. Hayashi AK, Kang YS, Smith BM: Non-Hodgkin's lymphoma in a patient with Diamond-Blackfan anemia. Am J Roentgenol 173:117–118, 1999.

296. Hayday AC, Gillies SD, Saito H et al: Activation of a translocated human *c-myc* gene by an enhancer in the immunoglobulin heavy-chain locus. Nature 307:334–340, 1984.

297. Hazenberg MD, Stuart JWTC, Otto SA et al: T-cell division in human immundeficiency virus (HIV)-1 infection is mainly due to immune activation: A longitudinal analysis in patients before and during highly active antiretroviral therapy (HAART). Blood 95:249–255, 2000.

298. Henderson S, Rowe M, Gregory C et al: Induction of *bcl-2* expression by Epstein-Barr virus latent membrane protein 1 protects infected B cells from programmed cell death. Cell 65:1107–1115, 1991.

299. Henkel T, Ling PD, Hayward SD et al: Mediation of Epstein-Barr virus EBNA2 transactivation by recombination signal-binding protein Jκ. Science 265:92–95, 1994.

300. Henle W, Henle G: Epstein-Barr virus-specific serology in immunologically compromised individuals. Cancer Res 41:4222–4225, 1981.

301. Henry JM, Heffner RR Jr, Dillard SH et al: Primary malignant lymphomas of the central nervous system. Cancer 34:1293–1302, 1974.

302. Herbst H, Dallenbach F, Hummel M et al: Epstein-Barr virus latent membrane protein expression in Hodgkin and Reed-Sternberg cells. Proc Natl Acad Sci U S A 88:4766–5770, 1991.

303. Herbst H, Foss H-D, Samol J et al: Frequent expression of interleukin-10 by Epstein-Barr virus-harboring tumor cells of Hodgkin's disease. Blood 87:2918–2929, 1996.

304. Heslop HE, Ng CYC, Li C et al: Long-term restoration of immunity against Epstein-Barr virus infection by adoptive transfer of gene-modified virus-specific T lymphocytes. Nature Med 2:551–555, 1996.

305. Heslop HE, Perez M, Benaim E et al: Transfer of EBV-specific CTL to prevent EBV lymphoma post bone marrow transplant. J Clin Apheresis 14:154–156, 1999.

306. Hessol NA, Katz MH, Liu JY et al: Increased incidence of Hodgkin disease in homosexual men with HIV infection. Ann Intern Med 117:309–311, 1992.

307. Hirano T, Taga T, Nakano H et al: Purification to homogeneity and characterization of human B-cell differentiation factor (BCDF or BSFp-2). Proc Natl Acad Sci U S A 82:5490–5494, 1985.

308. Hjelle B, Evans-Holm M, Yen TSB et al: A poorly differentiated lymphoma of donor origin in a renal allograft recipient. Transplantation 47:945–948, 1989.

309. Ho FCS, Srivastava G, Loke SL et al: Presence of Epstein-Barr virus DNA in nasal lymphomas of B and 'T' cell type. Hematol Oncol 8:271–281, 1990.

310. Ho M, Miller G, Atchison RW et al: Epstein-Barr virus infections and DNA hybridization studies in posttransplantation lymphoma and lymphoproliferative lesions: The role of primary infection. J Infect Dis 152:876–886, 1985.

311. Ho M, Jaffe R, Miller G et al: The frequency of Epstein-Barr virus infection and associated lymphoproliferative syndrome after transplantation and its manifestations in children. Transplantation 45:719–727, 1988.

312. Hochberg FH, Miller G, Schooley RT et al: Central-nervous-system lymphoma related to Epstein-Barr virus. N Engl J Med 309:745–748, 1983.

313. Hogan CM, Hammer SM: Host determinants in HIV infection and disease. Part 1: Cellular and humoral immune responses. Ann Intern Med 134:761–776, 2001.

314. Hogan CM, Hammer SM: Host determinants in HIV infection and disease. Part 2: Genetic factors and implications for antiretroviral therapeutics. Ann Intern Med 134:978–996, 2001.

315. Holland HK, Saral R, Rossi JJ: Allogeneic bone marrow transplantation, zidovudine, and human immunodeficiency virus type 1 (HIV-1) infection. Studies in a patient with non-Hodgkin lymphoma. Ann Intern Med 111:973–981, 1989.

316. Hong T, Shimada Y, Kano M et al: The Epstein-Barr virus is rarely associated with esophageal cancer. Int J Mol Med 5:363–368, 2000.

317. Hood IM, Mahendra P, McNeil K et al: Hodgkin's disease after cardiac transplant: A report of two cases. Clin Lab Haematol 18:115–116, 1996.

318. Hoon V, Fasy TM, Kheiri S et al: Case report: Fatal lymphoproliferative disease seven weeks after liver transplantation. Mt Sinai J Med 61:72–76, 1994.

319. Hoover R, Fraumeni JF Jr: Risk of cancer in renal-transplant recipients. Lancet 2:55–57, 1973.

320. Hsi ED, Singleton TP, Svoboda SM et al: Characterization of the lymphoid infiltrate in Hashimoto thyroiditis by immunohistochemistry and polymerase chain reaction for immunoglobulin heavy chain gene rearrangement. Am J Clin Pathol 110:327–333, 1998.

321. Hsi ED, Singleton TP, Swinnen L et al: Mucosa-associated lymphoid tissue-type lymphomas occurring in post-transplantation patients. Am J Surg Pathol 24:100–106, 2000.

322. Hsieh J-D, Hayward SD: Masking of the CBF1/RBPJκ transcriptional repression domain by Epstein-Barr virus EBNA2. Science 268:560–563, 1995.

323. Hsu D-H, de Waal Malefyt R, Fiorentino DF et al: Expression of interleukin-10 activity by Epstein-Barr virus protein BCRF1. Science 250:830–832, 1990.

324. Hsu JL, Glaser SL: Epstein-Barr virus-associated malignancies: Epidemiologic patterns and etiologic implications. Crit Rev Oncol Hematol 34:27–53, 2000.

325. Hussel T, Isaacson PG, Crabtree JE et al: The response of cells from low-grade B-cell gastric lymphomas of mucosa-associated lymphoid tissue to Helicobacter pylori. Lancet 342:571–574, 1993.

326. Hussel T, Isaacson PG, Crabtree JE et al: Helicobacter pylori-specific tumour-infiltrating T cells provide contact dependent help for the growth of malignant B cells in low-grade gastric lymphoma of mucosa-associated lymphoid tissue. J Pathol 178:122–127, 1996.

327. Imai S, Koizumi S, Sugiura M et al: Gastric carcinoma monoclonal epithelial malignant cells expressing Epstein-Barr virus latent infection protein. Proc Natl Acad Sci U S A 91:9131–9135, 1994.

328. Imai S, Sugiura M, Oikawa O et al: Epstein-Barr virus (EBV)-carrying and -expressing T-cell lines established from severe chronic active EBV infection. Blood 87:1446–1457, 1996.

329. International Collaboration on HIV and Cancer: Highly active antiretroviral therapy and incidence of cancer in human immunodeficiency virus-infected adults. J Natl Cancer Inst 92:1823–1830, 2000.

330. Ioachim HL, Cooper MC, Hellman GC: Lymphomas in men at high risk for acquired immunodeficiency syndrome (AIDS). Cancer 56:2831–2842, 1985.

331. Irsfeld H, Körholz D, Janβen G et al: Fatal outcome in two girls with Hodgkin disease complicating ataxia-telangiectasia (Louis-Bar syndrome) despite favorable response to modified-dose chemotherapy. Med Pediatr Oncol 34:62–64, 2000.

332. Isaacson P, Wright DH: Extranodal malignant lymphoma arising from mucosa-associated lymphoid tissue. Cancer 53:2515–2524, 1984.

333. Isaacson P: The MALT lymphoma concept updated. Ann Oncol 6:319–320, 1995 (Editorial).

334. Isaacson P: Gastrointestinal lymphomas of T- and B-cell types. Mod Pathol 12:151–158, 1999.

335. Isomaki HA, Hakulinen T, Joutsenlahti U: Excess risk of lymphomas, leukemia and myeloma in patients with rheumatoid arthritis. J Chron Dis 31:691–696, 1978.

336. Israel AM, Koziner B, Straus J: Plasmacytoma and the acquired immunodeficiency syndrome. Ann Intern Med 99:635–636, 1983.

337. Italian Cooperative Group for AIDS-Related Tumors: Malignant lymphomas in patients with or at risk for AIDS in Italy. J Natl Cancer Inst 80:855–860, 1988.

338. Jacobson LP, Yamashita TE, Detels R et al: Impact of potent antiretroviral therapy on the incidence of Kaposi's sarcoma and non-Hodgkin's lymphomas among HIV-1-infected individuals. Multicenter AIDS Cohort Study. J Acquir Immune Defic Syndr 21(Suppl. 1):S34–S41, 1999.

339. Jaffe ES: Pathologic and clinical spectrum of post-thymic T-cell malignancies. Cancer Invest 2:413–426, 1984.

340. Jaffe ES, Lipford EH Jr, Margolick JB et al: Lymphomatoid granulomatosis and angiocentric lymphoma: A spectrum of post-thymic T-cell proliferations. Semin Respir Med 10:167–172, 1993.

341. Jamil B, Nicholls K, Becker GJ et al: Impact of acute rejection therapy on infections and malignancies in renal transplant recipients. Transplantation 68:1597–1619, 1999.

342. Jarrett RF, MacKenzie J: Epstein-Barr virus and other candidate viruses in the pathogenesis of Hodgkin's disease. Sem Hematol 36:260–269, 1999.

343. Jensen MK, Koch-Henriksen N, Johansen P et al: EBV-positive primary central nervous system lymphomas in monozygote twins with common variable immunodeficiency and suspected multiple sclerosis. Leuk Lymphoma 23:187–193, 1997.

344. Ji L, Arcinas M, Boxer LM: NF-κB sites function as positive regulators of expression of the translocated c-myc allele in Burkitt's lymphoma. Mol Cell Biol 14:7967–7974, 1994.

345. Johnson JP, Gatti RA, Sears TS et al: Inverted duplication of JH associated with chromosome 14 translocation and T-cell leukemia in ataxia-telangiectasia. Am J Hum Genet 39:787–796, 1986.

346. Joncas J, LaPointe N, Gervais F et al: Unusual prevalence of Epstein-Barr virus early antigen (EBV-EA) antibodies in ataxia telangiectasia. J Immunol 119:1857–1859, 1977.

347. Joncas JH, Russo P, Brochu P et al: Epstein-Barr virus polymorphic B-cell lymphoma associated with leukemia and with congenital immunodeficiencies. J Clin Oncol 8:378–384, 1990.

348. Jones C, Bleau B, Buskard N et al: Simultaneous development of diffuse immunoblastic lymphoma in recipients of renal transplants from a single cadaver donor: Transmission of Epstein-Barr virus and triggering by OKT3. Am J Kidney Dis 23:130–134, 1994.

349. Jones D, Ballestas ME, Kaye KM et al: Primary-effusion lymphoma and Kaposi's sarcoma in a cardiac-transplant recipient. N Engl J Med 339:444–449, 1998.

350. Jones JF, Shurin S, Abramowsky C et al: T-cell lymphomas containing Epstein-Barr viral DNA in patients with chronic Epstein-Barr Virus infections. N Engl J Med 318:733–741, 1988.

351. Jones JL, Hanson DL, Dworkin MS et al: Effect of antiretroviral therapy on recent trends in selected cancers among HIV-infected persons. Adult/adolescent spectrum of HIV disease project group. J Acquir Immune Defic Syndr 21(Suppl. 1):S11–S17, 1999.

352. Judde J-G, Lacoste V, Brière J et al: Monoclonality or oligoclonality of human herpesvirus 8 terminal repeat sequence in Kaposi's sarcoma and other diseases. J Natl Cancer Inst 92:729–736, 2000.

353. Kalter S, Riggs SA, Cabanillas F et al: Aggressive non-Hodgkin's lymphomas in immunocompromised homosexual males. Blood 66:655–659, 1985.

354. Kamel OW, van de Rijn M, Weiss LM et al: Brief report: Reversible lymphomas associated with Epstein-Barr virus occurring during methotrexate therapy for rheumatoid arthritis and dermatomyositis. N Engl J Med 328:1317–1321, 1993.

355. Kaneko H, Inoue R, Yamada Y et al: Ataxia telangiectasia syndrome with B cell lymphoma. Clin Genet 49:331–332, 1996 (Correspondence).

356. Kanner SB, Parks ES, Scott GB et al: Simultaneous infections with human T cell leukemia virus type I and the human immunodeficiency virus. J Infect Dis 155:617–625, 1987.

357. Kaplan LD, Abrams DI, Feigal E et al: AIDS-associated non-Hodgkin's lymphoma in San Francisco. JAMA 261:719–724, 1989.

358. Kaplan LD, Kahn JO, Crowe S et al: Clinical and virologic effects of recombinant human granulocyte-macrophage colony-stimulating factor in patients receiving chemotherapy for human immunodeficiency virus-associated non-Hodgkin's lymphoma: Results of a randomized trial. J Clin Oncol 9:929–940, 1991.

359. Kaplan LD: Management of HIV-associated non-Hodgkin's lymphoma. AIDS Clin Care 6:1–3, 1994.

360. Kaplan LD, Straus DJ, Testa MA et al: Low-dose compared with standard-dose m-BACOD chemotherapy for non-Hodgkin's lymphoma associated with human immunodeficiency virus infection. N Engl J Med 336:1641–1648, 1997.

361. Karp JE, Broder S: Acquired immunodeficiency syndrome and non-Hodgkin's lymphomas. Cancer Res 51:4743–4756, 1991.

362. Kassan SS, Thomas TL, Moutsopoulos HM et al: Increased risk of lymphoma in sicca syndrome. Ann Intern Med 89:888–892, 1978.

363. Katzenstein AL, Peiper SC: Detection of Epstein-Barr virus genomes in lymphomatoid granulomatosis: Analysis of 29 cases by the polymerase chain reaction technique. Mod Pathol 3:435–441, 1990.

364. Katzenstein DA, Hammer SM, Hughes MD et al. for the AIDS Clinical Trials Group Study 175 Virology Study Team: The relation of virologic and immunologic markers to clinical outcomes after nucleoside therapy in HIV-infected adults with 200 to 500 CD4 cells per cubic millimeter. N Engl J Med 3335:1091–1098, 1996.

365. Kaufman D, Longo DL: Hodgkin's disease. Crit Rev Oncol Hematol 13:135–187, 1992.

366. Kawa K: Epstein-Barr virus-associated disease in humans. Int J Hematol 71:108–117, 2000.

367. Kawakami A, Nakashima T, Sakai H et al: Inhibition of caspase cascade by HTLV-I tax through induction of NF-κB nuclear translocation. Blood 94:3847–3855, 1999.

368. Kawano M, Hirano T, Matsuda T et al: Autocrine generation and requirement of BSF-2/IL-6 for human multiple myelomas. Nature 332:83–85, 1988.

369. Kelly GE, Meikle W, Sheil AGR: Effects of immunosuppressive therapy on the induction of skin tumors by ultraviolet irradiation in hairless mice. Transplantation 44:429–434, 1987.

370. Kelly K, Cochran BH, Stiles CD et al: Cell-specific regulation of the *c-myc* gene by lymphocyte mitogens and platelet-derived growth factor. Cell 35:63–61, 1983.

371. Kelsey RC, Saker A, Morgan M: Cardiac lymphoma in a patient with AIDS. Ann Intern Med 115:370–371, 1991.

372. Kenney S, Kamine J, Holley-Guthrie E et al: The Epstein-Barr virus immediate-early gene product BMLF1, acts in trans by a posttranscriptional mechanism which is reporter gene dependent. J Virol 63:3870–3877, 1989.

373. Kersten MJ, Verduyn TJ, Reiss P et al: Treatment of AIDS-related non-Hodgkin's lymphoma with chemotherapy (CNOP) and r-Hu-G-CSF: Clinical outcome and effect on HIV-1 viral load. Ann Oncol 9:1135–1138, 1998.

374. Khanim F, Yao Q-Y, Niedobitek G et al: Analysis of Epstein-Barr virus gene polymorphisms in normal donors and in virus-associated tumors from different geographic locations. Blood 88:3491–3501, 1996.

375. Kinlen LJ: Malignancy in autoimmune diseases. J Autoimmun 5(Suppl. 1):363–371, 1992.

376. Kinzler KW, Vogelstein B: Lessons from hereditary colorectal cancer. Cell 87:159–170, 1996.

377. Klein G, Klein E: Evolution of tumours and the impact of molecular oncology. Nature 315:190–195, 1985.

378. Klein G: Multiple phenotypic consequences of the Ig/*Myc* translocation in B-cell-derived tumors. Genes Chromosomes Cancer 1:3–8, 1989.

379. Klingemann H-G, Storb R, Sanders J et al: Acute lymphoblastic leukaemia after bone marrow transplantation for aplastic anaemia. Br J Haematol 63:47–50, 1986.

380. Klussmann JP, Müller A, Wagner M et al: Human herpesvirus type 8 in salivary gland tumors. J Clin Virol 16:239–246, 2000.

381. Knecht H, Bachmann E, Brousset P et al: Mutational hot spots within the carboxy terminal region of the LMP1 oncogene of epstein-Barr virus are frequent in lymphoproliferative disorders. Oncogene 10:523–528, 1995.

382. Knecht H, Berger C, Al-Homsi AS et al: Epstein-Barr virus oncogenesis. Crit Rev Oncol Hematol 26:117–135, 1997.

383. Knowles DM, Chamulak GA, Subar M et al: Lymphoid neoplasia associated with the acquired imunodeficiency syndrome (AIDS). Ann Intern Med 108:744–753, 1988.

384. Knowles DM, Inghirami G, Ubriaco A et al: Molecular genetic analysis of three AIDS-associated neoplasms of uncertain lineage demonstrates their B-cell derivation and the possible pathogenetic role of the Epstein-Barr virus. Blood 73:792–799, 1989.

385. Knowles DM, Cesarman E, Chadburn A et al: Correlative morphologic and molecular genetic analysis demonstrates three distinct categories of posttransplantation lymphoproliferative disorders. Blood 85:552–565, 1995.

386. Knowles DM: Etiology and pathogenesis of AIDS-related non-Hodgkin's lymphoma. Hematol Oncol Clin North Am 10:1081–1109, 1996.

387. Knudson A: Antioncogenes and human cancer. Proc Natl Acad Sci U S A 90:10914–10921, 1993.

388. Koizumi S, Zhang X-K, Imai S et al: Infection of the HTLV-1-harbouring T-lymphoblastoid line MT-2 by Epstein-Barr virus. Virology 188:859–863, 1992.

389. Kolb HJ, Socié G, Duell T et al: for the Late Effects Working Party of the European Cooperative Group for Blood and Marrow Transplantation and the European Late Effect Project Group: Malignant neoplasms in long-term survivors of bone marrow transplantation. Ann Intern Med 131:738–744, 1999.

390. Komatsu H, Iida S, Yamamoto K et al: A variant chromosome translocation at 11q13 identifying *PRAD1/Cyclin D*1 as the *BCL-1* gene. Blood 84:1226–1231, 1994.

391. Konrad RJ, Kricka LJ, Goodman DBP et al: Brief report: Myeloma-associated paraprotein directed against the HIV-1 p24 antigen in an HIV-1-seropositive patient. N Engl J Med 328:1817–1819, 1993.

392. Korbjuhn P, Anagnostopoulos I, Hummel M et al: Frequent latent Epstein-Barr virus infection of neoplastic T cells and bystander B cells in human immunodeficiency virus-negative European peripheral pleomorphic T-cell lymphomas. Blood 82:217–223, 1993.

393. Kretzner L, Blackwood EM, Eisenman RN: Myc and Max proteins possess distinct transcriptional activities. Nature 359:426–429, 1992.

394. Kuehnle I, Huis MH, Liu Z et al: CD20 monoclonal antibody (Rituximab) for therapy of Epstein-Barr virus lymphoma after hemopoietic stem-cell transplantation. Blood 95:1502–1505, 2000.

395. Kumar S, Fend F, Quintanilla-Martinez L et al: Epstein-Barr virus-positive primary gastrointestinal Hodgkin's disease. Association with inflammatory bowel disease and immunosuppression. Am J Surg Pathol 24:66–73, 2000.

396. Küppers R, Klein U, Hansmann M-L et al: Cellular origin of human B-cell lymphomas. N Engl J Med 341:1520–1529, 1999.

397. Kütting B, Bonsmann G, Metze D et al: *Borrelia burgdorferi*-associated primary cutaneous B cell lymphoma: Complete clearing of skin lesions after antibiotic pulse therapy or intralesional injection of interferon alfa-2a. J Am Acad Dermatol 36:311–314, 1997.

398. Lacy J, Summers WP, Summers WC: Post-transcriptional mechanisms of deregulation of *myc* following conversion of a human B cell line by Epstein-Barr virus. EMBO J 8:1973–1980, 1989.

399. Lam KY, Lo CY, Kwong DLW et al: A 3-year clinicopathologic experience and an evaluation of the presence of Epstein-Barr virus. Am J Clin Pathol 112:263–270, 1999.

400. Land W: Optimal use of cyclosporine in clinical organ transplantation. Transplant Proc 19:130–135, 1987.

401. Langdon WY, Harris AW, Cory S et al: The *c-MYC* oncogene perturbs B lymphocyte development in Eu-myc transgenic Mice. Cell 47:11–18, 1986.

402. Larvol L, Soule J-C, Le Tourneau A: Reversible lymphoma in the setting of azathioprine therapy for Crohn's disease. N Engl J Med 331:883–884, 1994.

403. Laurence J, Astrin SM: Human immunodeficiency virus induction of malignant transformation in human B lymphocytes. Proc Natl Acad Sci U S A 88:7635–7639, 1991.

404. Laux G, Adam B, Strobl LJ et al: The Spi-1/PU.1 and Spi-B ets family transcription factors and the recombination signal binding protein RBP-Jkappa interact with an Epstein-Barr virus nuclear antigen 2 responsive cis-element. EMBO J 13:5624–5632, 1994.

405. Lazarovits AI, Tibbles LA, Grant DR et al: Anti-B cell antibodies for the treatment of monoclonal Epstein-Barr virus-induced lymphoproliferative syndrome after multivisceral transplantation. Clin Invest Med 17:621–625, 1994.

406. LeBien TW: Fates of human B-cell precursors. Blood 96:9–23, 2000.

407. Leblond V, Sutton L, Dorent R et al: Lymphoproliferative disorders after organ transplantation: A report of 24 cases observed in a single center. J Clin Oncol 13:961–968, 1995.

408. Le Coco F, Ye BH, Lista F et al: Rearrangements of the BCL6 gene in diffuse large cell non-Hodgkin's lymphoma. Blood 83:1757–1759, 1994.

409. Ledergerber B, Egger M, Erard V et al for the Swiss HIV Cohort Study: AIDS-related opportunistic illnesses occurring after initiation of potent antiretroviral therapy. The Swiss HIV Cohort Study. JAMA 282:2220–2226, 1999.

410. Ledergerber B, Telenti A, Egger M for the Swiss HIV Cohort Study: Risk of HIV related Kaposi's sarcoma and non-Hodgkin's lymphoma with potent antiretroviral therapy: Prospective cohort study. BMJ 319:23–24, 1999.

411. Lederman MM, Valdez H: Immune restoration with antiretroviral therapies. Implications for clinical management. JAMA 284:223–228, 2000.

412. Lee CYS, Chun K, Shimonishi JJ et al: Non-Hodgkins lymphoma of the oral cavity associated with HIV infection. Hawaii Dental J June 1994:6–11, 1994.

413. Lee ES, Locker J, Nalesnik M et al: The association of Epstein-Barr virus with smooth-muscle tumors occurring after organ transplantation. N Engl J Med 332:19–25, 1995.

414. LeMeur Y, Pontoizeau-Potelune N, Jaccard A et al: Regression of a gastric lymphoma of mucosa-associated lymphoid tissue after eradication of Helicobacter pylori in a kidney graft recipient. Am J Med 107:530, 1999 (Correspondence).

415. Lenoir GM, Preud'homme JL, Bernheim A et al: Correlation between immunoglobulin light chain expression and variant translocation in Burkitt's lymphoma. Nature 298:474–476, 1982.

416. Levine AM, Meyer PR, Begandy MK et al: Development of B-cell lymphoma in homosexual men. Clinical and immunologic findings. Ann Intern Med 100:7–13, 1984.

417. Levine AM, Gill PS, Meyer PR et al: Retrovirus and malignant lymphoma in homosexual men. JAMA 254:1921–1925, 1985.

418. Levine AM, Gill PS, Krailo M et al: Natural history of persistent, generalized lymphadenopathy (PGL) in gay men: Risk of lymphoma (NHL) and factors associated with development of lymphoma. Blood 68:130a, 1986 (Abstract).

419. Levine AM, Wernz JC, Kaplan L et al: Low-dose chemotherapy with central nervous system prophylaxis and zidovudine maintenance in AIDS-related lymphoma. JAMA 266:84–88, 1991.

420. Levine A: Acquired immunodeficiency syndrome-related lymphoma. Blood 80:8–20, 1992.

421. Levine A: AIDS-related malignancies: The emerging epidemic. J Natl Cancer Inst 85:1382–1397, 1993.

422. Levine AM: Lymphoma complicating immunodeficiency disorders. Ann Oncol 6(Suppl. 2):S29–S35, 1994.

423. Levine AM: Role of zidovudine antiretroviral therapy in the pathogenesis of acquired immunodeficiency syndrome-related lymphoma. Blood 86:4612–4616, 1995.

424. Lewis RB, Castor CW, Knisley RE, Bole GG: Frequency of neoplasia in systemic lupus erythematosus and rheumatoid arthritis. Arthritis Rheum 19:1256–1260, 1976.

425. Leyvraz S, Henle W, Chahinian AP et al: Association of Epstein-Barr virus with thymic carcinoma. N Engl J Med 312:1296–1299, 1985.

426. Li PKT, Tsang K, Phil M et al: Effective treatment of high-grade lymphoproliferative disorder after renal transplantation using autologous lymphocyte activated killer cell therapy. Am J Kidney Dis 32:813–819, 1998.

427. Lieberman J, Buchsbaum RJ: Using T cells to treat B-cell cancers. New Engl J Med 330:1231–1233, 1994 (Editorial).

428. Liebowitz D: Epstein-Barr virus and a cellular signaling pathway in lymphomas from immunosuppressed patients. N Engl J Med 338:1413–1421, 1998.

429. Lien Y-HH, Schroter GP, Weil R et al: Complete remission and possible immune tolerance after multidrug combination chemotherapy for cyclosporine-related lymphoma in a renal transplant recipient with acute pancreatitis. Transplantation 52:7439–7441, 1991.

430. Lin WC, Moore JO, Mann KP et al: Post transplant CD8+ γδ T-cell lymphoma associated with human herpes virus-6 infection. Leuk Lymphoma 33:377–384, 1999.

431. Lipford EH, Smith HR, Pittaluga S et al: Clonality of angioimmunoblastic lymphadenopathy and implications for its evolution to malignant lymphoma. J Clin Invest 79:637–642, 1987.

432. Lipinski M, Tursz Kreis H et al: Dissociation of natural killer cell activity and antibody-dependent cell-mediated cytotoxicity in kidney allograft recipients receiving high-dose immunosuppressive therapy. Transplantation 29:214–218, 1980.

433. Lipkowitz S, Stern MH, Kirsch IR: Hybrid T-cell receptor genes formed by interlocus recombination in normal and ataxia-telangiectasia lymphocytes. J Exp Med 172:409–418, 1990.

434. List AF, Greco S, Vogler LB: Lymphoproliferative diseases in immunocompromised hosts: The role of Epstein-Barr virus. J Clin Oncol 5:1673–1689, 1987.

435. LoCoco R, Ye BH, Lista F et al: Rearrangements of the BCL6 gene in large cell non-Hodgkin's lymphoma. Blood 83:1757–1759, 1994.

436. Lombardi L, Newcomb EW, Dalla-Favera R: Pathogenesis of Burkitt lymphoma: Expression of an activated c-myc oncogene causes the tumorigenic conversion of EBV-infected human B lymphoblasts. Cell 49:161–170, 1987.

437. Longo DL: Kaposi's sarcoma and other neoplasms. (In Fauci AS, Macher AM, Longo DL et al: NIH Conference. Acquired Immunodeficiency Syndrome: Epidemiologic, Clinical, Immunologic, and Therapeutic Considerations. Ann Intern Med 100:92–106). Ann Intern Med 100:96–98, 1984.

438. Longo DL, DeVita VT, Duffey PL et al: Superiority of ProMACE-CytaBOM over ProMACE-MOPP in the treatment of advanced diffuse aggressive lymphoma: Results of a prospective randomized trial. J Clin Oncol 9:25–38, 1991.

439. Longo DL, DeVita VT, Jaffe ES et al: Lymphocytic lymphomas. In DeVita VT, Hellman S, Rosenberg SA (eds.), Cancer. Principles & Practice of Oncology, 4th Ed., p. 1880. J.B. Lippincott, Philadelphia, 1993.

440. Longo D: The Palackdharry article reviewed. Oncology 3:73–77, 1994.

441. Louie S, Daoust PR, Schwartz RS: Immunodeficiency and the pathogenesis of non-Hodgkin's lymphoma. Sem Oncol 7:267–284, 1980.

442. Lowenthal DA, Straus DJ, Campbell SW: AIDS-related lymphoid neoplasia. The Memorial Hospital experience. Cancer 61:2326–2337, 1988.

443. Lucas KG, Pollok KE, Emanuel DL: Post-transplant Epstein-Barr virus induced lymphoproliferative disorders. Leuk Lymphoma 25:1–8, 1997.

444. Luppi M, Barozzi P, Maiorana A et al: Human herpes-virus-8 DNA sequences in human immunodeficiency virus-negative angioimmunoblastic lymphadenopathy and benign lymphadenopathy with giant germinal center hyperplasia and increased vascularity. Blood 87:3903–3909, 1996.

445. Luppi M, Longo G, Ferrari MG et al: Clinico-pathological characterization of hepatitis C virus-related B-cell non-Hodgkin's lymphomas without symptomatic cryoglobulinemia. Ann Oncol 9:495–498, 1998.

446. Lyter DW, Bryant J, Thackeray R et al: Incidence of HIV-related and nonrelated malignancies in a large cohort of homosexual men. J Clin Oncol 13:2540–2546, 1995.

447. MacMahon EME, Glass JD, Hayward SD et al: Epstein-Barr virus in AIDS-related primary central nervous system lymphoma. Lancet 338:969–973, 1991.

448. MacMahon EME: More on virostatic therapy for advanced lymphoproliferation associated with Epstein-Barr virus in an HIV-infected patient. N Engl J Med 343–371, 2000 (Correspondence).

449. Magrath IT, Freeman CB, Pizzo P et al: Characterization of lymphoma-derived cell lines: Comparison of cell lines positive and negative for Epstein-Barr virus nuclear antigen. II. Surface markers. J Natl Cancer Inst 64:477–483, 1980.

450. Magrath IT, Bhatia K: Breast cancer: A new Epstein-Barr virus-associated disease? J Natl Cancer Inst 91:1349–1350, 1999.

451. Magro CM, Crowson AN, Harrist TJ: Atypical lymphoid infiltrates arising in cutaneous lesions of connective tissue disease. Am J Dermatopathol 19:446–455, 1997.

452. Manet E, Bourillot P-Y, Waltzer L et al: EBV genes and B cell proliferation. Crit Rev Oncol Hematol 28:129–137, 1998.

453. Mannick JB, Cohen JI, Birkenbach M et al: The Epstein-Barr virus nuclear protein encoded by the leader of the EBNA RNAs is important in B-lymphocyte transformation. J Virol 65:6826–6837, 1991.

454. Mannick JB, Asano K, Izumi K et al: Nitric oxide produced by human B lymphocytes inhibits apoptosis and Epstein-Barr virus reactivation. Cell 79:1137–1146, 1994.

455. Manning KR, Powell BL, Peacock JE et al: Effective combination chemotherapy for high-grade non-Hodgkin's lymphoma after cardiac transplant. Blood 78:468a, 1991 (Abstract).

456. Martin PJ, Shulman HM, Schubach WH et al: Fatal Epstein-Barr-virus-associated proliferation of donor B cells after treatment of acute graft-versus-host disease with a murine anti-T-cell antibody. Ann Intern Med 101:310–315, 1984.

457. Masliah E, DeTeresa RM, Mallory ME et al: Changes in pathological findings at autopsy in AIDS cases for the last 15 years. AIDS 14:69–74, 2000.

458. Matas AJ, Simmons RL, Kjellstrand CM et al: Increased incidence of malignancy during chronic renal failure. Lancet 1:883–886, 1975.

459. Matas AJ, Simmons RL, Najarian JS: Chronic antigen stimulation, herpesvirus infection, and cancer in transplant recipients. Lancet 1:1277–1279, 1975.

460. Mathus-Vliegen EMH, Van Halteren H, Tytgat GNJ: Malignant lymphoma in coeliac disease: Various manifestations with distinct symptomatology and prognosis? J Intern Med 236:43–49, 1994.

461. Matsuzuka F, Fukata S, Kuma K et al: Gene rearrangement of immunoglobulin as a marker of thyroid lymphoma. World J Surg 22:558–561, 1998.

462. Mazzaro C, Zagonel V, Monfardini S et al: Hepatitis C virus and non-Hodgkin's lymphomas. Abr J Haematol 94:544–550, 1996.

463. McClain KL, Leach CT, Jenson HB et al: Association of Epstein-Barr virus with leiomyosarcomas in young people with AIDS. N Engl J Med 332:12–18, 1995.

464. McColl K, Murray L, El-Omar E et al: Symptomatic benefit from eradicating *Helicobacter pylori* infection in patients with nonulcer dyspepsia. N Engl J Med 339:1869–1874, 1998.

465. McGowan JP, Shah S: Long-term remission of AIDS-related primary central nervous system lymphoma associated with highly active anti-retroviral therapy. AIDS 12:952–953, 1998 (Correspondence).

466. Meduri G, Fromentin L, Vieillefond A et al: Donor-related non-Hodgkin's lymphoma in a renal allograft recipient. Transplant Proc 23:2649, 1991.

467. Meeker TC, Shiramazu B, Kaplan L et al: Evidence for molecular subtypes of HIV-associated lymphoma. Division into peripheral monoclonal, polyclonal and central nervous system lymphoma. AIDS 5:669–674, 1991.

468. Mellemkjær L, Andersen V, Linet MS et al: Non-Hodgkin's lymphoma and other cancers among a cohort of patients with systemic lupus erythematosus. Arthritis Rheum 40:761–768, 1997.

469. Metcalfe JA, Parkhill J, Campbell L et al: Accelerated telomere shortening in ataxia telangiectasia. Nature Genet 13:350–353, 1996.

470. Meyer PR, Yanagihara ET, Parker JW et al: A distinctive follicular hyperplasia in the acquired immune deficiency syndrome (AIDS) and the AIDS related complex. Hematol Oncol 2:319–347, 1984.

471. Meyn MW: High spontaneous intrachromosomal recombination rates in ataxia-telangiectasia. Science 260:1327–1330, 1993.

472. Meyn MW: Ataxia-telangiectasia and cellular responses to DNA damage. Cancer Res 55:5991–6001, 1995.

473. Miller G: Epstein-Barr virus-immortalization and replication. N Engl J Med 310:1255–1256, 1984 (Editorial).

474. Miller WT Jr, Siegel SG, Montone KT: Posttransplantation lymphoproliferative disorder: Changing manifestations of disease in a renal transplant population. Crit Rev Diag Imag 36:569–585, 1997.

475. Milpied N, Vasseur B, Parquet N et al: Humanized anti-CD20 monoclonal antibody (Rituximab) in post transplant B-lymphoproliferative disorder: A retrospective analysis on 32 patients. Ann Oncol 11(Suppl. 1):S113–S116, 2000.

476. Minarovits J, Hu L-F, Imai S et al: Clonality, expression and methylation patterns of the Epstein-Barr virus genomes in lethal midline granulomas classified as peripheral angiocentric T cell lymphomas. J Gen Virol 75:77–84, 1994.

477. Mocroft A, Sabin CA, Youle M et al: Changes in AIDS-defining illnesses in a London clinic, 1987–1998. J Acquir Immune Defic Syndr 21:401–407, 1999.

478. Monfardini S, Tirelli U, Vaccher E et al. for the Gruppo Italiano Cooperativo AIDS & Tumori (GICAT): Hodgkin's disease in 63 intravenous drug users infected with human immunodeficiency virus. Ann Oncol 2(Suppl. 2):201–205, 1991.

479. Montagnier L, Gruest J, Chamaret S et al: Adaptation of lymphadenopathy associated virus (LAV) to replication in EBV-transformed B lymphoblastoid cell lines. Science 225:63–66, 1984.

480. Moore KW, Vieira P, Fiorentino DF et al: Homology of cytokine synthesis inhibitory factor (IL-10) to the Epstein-Barr virus gene BCRFI. Science 248:1230–1234, 1990.

481. Moore MD, Cooper NR, Tack BF et al: Molecular cloning of the cDNA encoding the Epstein-Barr virus/C3d receptor (comple-

ment receptor type 2) of human B lymphocytes. Proc Natl Acad Sci U S A 84:9194–9198, 1987.

482. Moore PS, Chang Y: Detection of herpesvirus-like DNA sequences in Kaposi's sarcoma in patients with and those without HIV infection. N Engl J Med 332:1181–1185, 1995.

483. Moore RD, Kessler H, Richman DD et al: Non-Hodgkin's lymphoma in patients with advanced HIV infection treated with zidovudine. JAMA 265:2208–2211, 1991.

484. Moore RD, Chaisson RE: Natural history of HIV infection in the era of combination antiretroviral therapy. AIDS 13:1933–1942, 1999.

485. Morgner A, Miehlke S, Fischbach W et al: Complete remission of primary high-grade B-cell gastric lymphoma after cure of *Helicobacter pylori* infection. J Clin Oncol 19:2041–2048, 2001.

486. Morrison VA, Dunn DL, Manivel C et al: Clinical characteristics of post-transplant lymphoproliferative disorders. Am J Med 97:14–24, 1994.

487. Mosialos G: The role of Rel/NF-κB proteins in viral oncogenesis and the regulation of viral transcription. Sem Cancer Biol 8:121–129, 1997.

488. Moss DJ, Burrows SR, Castelino DJ et al: A comparison of Epstein-Barr virus-specific T-cell immunity in malaria-endemic and -nonendemic regions of Papua New Guinea. Int J Cancer 727–732, 1983.

489. Moss DJ, Khanna R, Sherritt M et al: Developing immunotherapeutic strategies for the control of Epstein-Barr virus-associated malignancies. J AIDS 21:S80–S83, 1999.

490. Motokura T, Bloom T, Kim HG et al: A novel cyclin encoded by a bcl1-linked candidate oncogene. Nature 350:512–515, 1991.

491. Motokura T, Arnold A: *PRAD1/cyclin D1* proto-oncogene: Genomic organization, 5′ DNA sequence, and sequence of a tumor-specific rearrangement breakpoint. Genes Chrom Cancer 7:89–95, 1993.

492. Mueller N, Evans A, Harris NL et al: Hodgkin's disease and Epstein-Barr virus. Altered antibody pattern before diagnosis. N Engl J Med 320:689–695, 1989.

493. Mueller N: Overview of the epidemiology of malignancy in immune deficiency. J AIDS 21:S5–S10, 1999.

494. Mukai HY, Kojima H, Suzukawa K et al: Nasal natural killer cell lymphoma in a post-renal transplant patient. Transplantation 69:1501–1503, 2000.

495. Mullaney BP, Ng VL, Herndier BG et al: Comparative genomic analyses of primary effusion lymphoma. Arch Pathol Lab Med 124:824–826, 2000.

496. Murray PG, Swinnen LJ, Constandinou CM et al: *BCL-2* but not its Epstein-Barr virus-encoded homologue, *BHRF1*, is commonly expressed in posttransplantation lymphoproliferative disorders. Blood 87:706–711, 1996.

497. Nador RG, Cesarman E, Knowles DM: Herpes-like DNA sequences in a body-cavity-based lymphoma in an HIV-negative patient. N Engl J Med 333:943, 1995 (Correspondence).

498. Nador RG, Cesarman E, Chadburn A et al: Primary effusion lymphoma: A distinct clinicopathologic entity associated with the Kaposi's sarcoma-associated herpes virus. Blood 88:645–656, 1996.

499. Nagington J, Gray J: Cyclosporin A immunosuppression, Epstein-Barr antibody, and lymphoma. Lancet 1:536–537, 1980.

500. Nahass GT, Kraffert CA, Penneys NS: Cutaneous T-cell lymphoma associated with the acquired immunodeficiency syndrome. Arch Dermatol 127:1020–1022, 1991.

501. Nakajima K, Martinez-Maza O, Hirano T et al: Induction of IL-6 (B cell stimulatory factor-2/IFN-B2) production by HIV. J Immunol 142:531–536, 1989.

502. Nakamura H, Said JW, Miller CW et al: Mutation and protein expression of *p53* in acquired immunodeficiency syndrome-related lymphomas. Blood 82:920–926, 1993.

503. Nakamura S, Akazawa K, Kinukawa N et al: Inverse correlation between the expression of *bcl-2* and *p53* proteins in primary gastric lymphoma. Hum Pathol 27:225–233, 1996.

504. Nakamura T, Nakamura S, Yonezumi M et al: *Helicobacter pylori* and the t(11;18)(q21;q21) translocation in gastric low-grade B-cell lymphoma of mucosa-associated lymphoid tissue type. Jpn J Cancer Res 91:301–309, 2000.

505. Nakleh RE, Manivel JC, Copenhaver CM et al: (1991). In situ hybridization for the detection of Epstein-Barr virus in central nervous system lymphomas. Cancer 67:444–448, 1991.

506. Nalesnik MA, Makowka L, Starzl TE: The diagnosis and treatment of posttransplant lymphoproliferative disorders. Curr Probl Surg 25:367–472, 1988.

507. Nalesnik MA: Clinicopathologic features of posttransplant lymphoproliferative disorders. Ann Transplant 2:33–40, 1997.

508. Nardini E, Aiello A, Giardini R et al: Detection of aberrant isotype switch recombination in low-grade and high-grade gastric MALT lymphomas. Blood 95:1032–1038, 2000.

509. Naresh KN, Johnson J, Srinivas V et al: Epstein-Barr virus association in classical Hodgkin's disease provides survival advantage to patients and correlates with higher expression of proliferation markers in Reed-Sternberg cells. Ann Oncol 11:91–96, 2000.

510. Nasir S, DeAngelis LM: Update on the management of primary CNS lymphoma. Oncology 14:228–234, 2000.

511. Natkunam Y, Elenitoba-Johnson KS, Kingma DW et al: Epstein-Barr virus strain type and latent membrane protein 1 gene deletions in lymphomas in patients with rheumatic diseases. Arthritis Rheum 40:1152–1156, 1997.

512. Nemerow GR, Wolfert R, McNaughton ME et al: Identification and characterization of the Epstein-Barr virus receptor on human B lymphocytes and its relationship to the C3d complement receptor (CR2). J Virol 55:347–351, 1985.

513. Neri A, Barriga F, Knowles et al: Different regions of the immunoglobulin heavy-chain locus are involved in chromosomal translocations in distinct pathogenetic forms of Burkitt lymphoma. Proc Natl Acad Sci U S A 85:2748–2752, 1988.

514. Neri A, Barriga F, Inghirami G et al: Epstein-Barr virus infection precedes clonal expansion in Burkitt's and acquired immunodeficiency syndrome-associated lymphoma. Blood 77:1092–1095, 1991.

515. Nerurkar AY, Vijayan P, Srinivas V et al: Discrepancies in Epstein-Barr virus association at presentation and relapse of classical Hodgkin's disease: Impact on pathogenesis. Ann Oncol 11:475–478, 2000.

516. Neubauer A, Bayerdöffer E, Rudolph B et al: Teatment of early gastric MALT-lymphoma patients by *Helicobacter Pylori* (HP) Eradication-German MALT Lymphoma Trial. Blood 84(Suppl.):519a, 1994.

517. Newell M, Goldstein D, Milliken S et al: Phase I/II trial of filgrastim (r-metHuG-CSF), CEOP chemotherapy and antiretroviral therapy in HIV-related non-Hodgkin's lymphoma. Ann Oncol 7:1029–1036, 1996.

518. Nichols KE, Harkin DP, Levitz S et al: Inactivating mutations in an SH2 domain-encoding gene in X-linked lymphoproliferative syndrome. Proc Natl Acad Sci U S A 95:13765–13770, 1998.

519. Nicot C, Mahieux R, Takemoto S et al: Bcl-X$_L$ is up-regulated by HTLV-I and HTLV-II in vitro and in ex vivo ATLL samples. Blood 96:275–281, 2000.

520. Niederwieser DW, Appelbaum FR, Gastl G et al: Inadvertent transmission of a donor's acute myeloid leukemia in bone mar-

row transplantation for chronic myelocytic leukemia. N Engl J Med 322:1794–1796, 1990.

521. Niedobitek G, Young LS: Epstein-Barr virus persistence and virus-associated tumours. Lancet 343:333–335, 1994.

522. Nishikura K, ar-Rushdi A, Erikson J et al: Differential expression of the normal and of the translocated human c-MYC oncogenes in B Cells. Proc Natl Acad Sci U S A 80:4822–4826, 1983.

523. Nomura A, Stemmermann GN, Chyou P-H et al: Helicobacter pylori infection and gastric carcinoma among Japanese Americans in Hawaii. N Engl J Med 325:1132–1136, 1991.

524. Nomura K, Kanegane H, Karasuyama H et al: Genetic defect in human X-linked agammaglobulinemia impedes a maturational evolution of pro-B cells into a later stage of pre-B cells in the B-cell differentiation pathway. Blood 96:610–617, 2000.

525. Nuckols JD, Liu K, Burchette JL et al: Primary central nervous system lymphomas: A 30-year experience at a single institution. Mod Pathol 12:1167–1183, 1999.

526. Odajnyk C, Subar M, Dugan M et al: Clinical features and correlation with immunopathology and molecular biology in a large group of patients with AIDS-associated small non-cleaved cell lymphoma (SNCL) Burkitt's and non-Burkitt's type. Proc Soc Hematol 68:131a, 1986 (Abstract).

527. Odenbreit S, Püls J, Sedlmaier B et al: Translocation of a Helicobacter pylori CagA into gastric epithelial cells by type IV secretion. Science 287:1497–1500, 2000.

528. O'Grady J, Stewart S, Elton RA et al: Epstein-Barr virus in Hodgkin's disease and site of origin of tumour. Lancet 343:265–266, 1994.

529. Ohashi S, Segawa K, Okamura S et al: A clinicopathologic study of gastric mucosa-associated lymphoid tissue lymphoma. Cancer 88:2210–2219, 2000.

530. Ohga S, Kanaya Y, Maki H et al: Epstein-Barr virus-associated lymphoproliferative disease after a cord blood transplant for Diamond-Blackfan anemia. Bone Marrow Transplant 245:209–212, 2000.

531. Ohshima K, Suzumiya J, Sato K et al: Nodal T-cell lymphoma in an HTLV-I-endemic area: Proviral HTLV-IDNA, histological classification and clinical evaluation. Br J Haematol 101:703–711, 1998.

532. Oksenhendler E, Clauvel J-P, Jouveshomme S et al: Complete remission of a primary effusion lymphoma with antiretroviral therapy. Am J Hematol 57:266, 1998 (Correspondence).

533. Opelz G, Henderson R for the Collaborative Transplant Study: Lancet 342:1514–1516, 1993.

534. O'Reilly RJ, Lacerda JF, Lucas KG et al: Adoptive cell therapy with donor lymphocytes for EBV-associated lymphomas developing after allogeneic marrow transplants. In DeVita VT, Hellman S, Rosenberg S (eds.), Important Advances in Oncology 1996, pp. 149–166. Lippincott-Raven, Philadelphia, 1996.

535. O'Reilly RJ, Small TN, Papadopoulos E et al: Biology and adoptive cell therapy of Epstein-Barr virus-associated lymphoproliferative disorders in recipients of marrow allografts. Immunol Rev 157:195–216, 1997.

536. Osato T, Imai S: Epstein-Barr virus and gastric carcinoma. Sem Cancer Biol 7:175–182, 1996.

537. Ott G, Katzberger T, Greiner A et al: The t(11;18)(q21;q21) translocation is a frequent and specific aberration in low-grade but not in high-grade malignant non-Hodgkin's lymphomas of the mucosa associated lymphoid tissue (MALT) type. Cancer Res 57:3944–3948, 1997.

538. Ott MM, Ott G, Klinder H et al: Abdominal T-cell non-Hodgkin's lymphoma of the gamma/delta type in a patient with selective immunoglobulin A deficiency. Am J Surg Pathol 22:500–506, 1998.

539. Oudejans JJ, van den Brule AJC, Jiwa NM et al: BHRF1, the Epstein-Barr virus (EBV) homologue of the BCL-2 proto-onco-gene, is transcribed in EBV-associated B-cell lymphomas and in reactive lymphocytes. Blood 86:1893–1902, 1995.

540. Pagano JS: Epstein-Barr virus: The first human tumor virus and its role in cancer. Proc Assoc Am Phys 111:573–580, 1999.

541. Palackdharry CS: The epidemiology of non-Hodgkin's lymphoma: Why the increased incidence? Oncology 3:67–73, 1994.

542. Pallesen G, Hamilton-Dutoit SJ, Rowe M et al: Expression of Epstein-Barr virus latent gene products in tumour cells of Hodgkin's disease. Lancet 337:320–322, 1991.

543. Papadaki HA, Stefanaki K, Kanavaros P et al: Epstein-Barr virus-asociated high-grade anaplastic plasmacytoma in a renal transplant patient. Leuk Lymphoma 36:411–415, 2000.

544. Papadopoulos EB, Ladanyi M, Emanuel D et al: Infusions of donor leukocytes to treat Epstein-Barr virus-associated lymphoproliferative disorders after allogeneic bone marrow transplantation. N Engl J Med 330:1185–1191, 1994.

545. Papo T, Oksenhendler E, Bouvet E et al: Letter to the Editor: Hodgkin's disease of the tongue in a homosexual HIV-infected patient. Am J Hematol 37:143, 1991 (Correspondence).

546. Parker GA, Crook T, Bain M et al: Epstein-Barr virus nuclear antigen (EBNA)3C is an immortalizing oncoprotein with similar properties to adenovirus E1A and papillomavirus E7. Oncogene 13:2541–2549, 1996.

547. Parker SC, Fenton DA, McGibbon DH: Homme rouge and the acquired immunodeficiency syndrome. N Engl J Med 321:906–907, 1989.

548. Parsonnet J, Friedman GD, Vandersteen DP et al: Helicobacter pylori infection and the risk of gastric carcinoma. N Engl J Med 325:1127–1131, 1991.

549. Parsonnet J, Hansen S, Rodriguez L et al: Helicobacter pylori infection and gastric lymphoma. N Engl J Med 330:1267–1271, 1994.

550. Paterson MC, Smith BP, Lohman PHM et al: Defective excision repair of gamma-ray-damaged DNA in human (ataxia telangiectasia) fibroblasts. Nature 260:444–447, 1976.

551. Pathmanathan R, Prasad U, Sadler R et al: Clonal proliferations of cells infected with Epstein-Barr virus in preinvasive lesions related to nasopharyngeal carcinoma. N Engl J Med 333:693–698, 1995.

552. Patton DF, Wilkowski CW, Hanson CA et al: Epstein-Barr virus-determined clonality in posttransplant lymphoproliferative disease. Transplantation 49:1080–1084, 1990.

553. Patton DF, Ribeiro RC, Jenkins JJ et al: Thymic carcinoma with a defective Epstein-Barr virus encoding the BZLF1 transactivator. J Infect Dis 170:7–122, 1994,

554. Pearson GR, Qualtiere LF, Klein G et al: Epstein-Barr virus-specific antibody-dependent cellular cytotoxicity in patients with Burkitt's lymphoma. Int J Cancer 24:402–406, 1979.

555. Pedersen C, Gerstoft J, Tauris P et al: Trends in survival of Danish AIDS patients from 1981 to 1989. AIDS 4:1111–1116, 1990.

556. Pedersen C, Gerstoft J, Lundgren JD et al: HIV-associated lymphoma: Histopathology and association with Epstein-Barr virus genome related to clinical, immunological and prognostic features. Eur J Cancer 27:1416–1423, 1991.

557. Pedersen RK, Pedersen NT: Primary non-Hodgkin's lymphoma of the thyroid gland: A population based study. Histopathology 28:25–32, 1996.

558. Pelicci P-G, Knowles KM II, Magrath I et al: Chromosomal breakpoints and structural alterations of the c-MYC locus differ in endemic and sporadic form of Burkitt Lymphoma. Proc Natl Acad Sci U S A 83:2984–2988, 1986.

559. Pelicci P-G, Knowles II DM, Arlin ZA et al: Multiple monoclonal B cell expansions and c-MYC oncogene rearrangements in acquired immune deficiency syndrome-related lymphoproliferative disorders. J Exp Med 164:2049–2060, 1986.

560. Pelstring RJ, Zellmer RB, Sulak LE et al: Hodgkin's disease in association with human immunodeficiency virus infection. Cancer 67:1865–1873, 1991.

561. Peng H, Chen G, Du M et al: Replication error phenotype and *p53* gene mutation in lymphomas of mucosa-associated lymphoid tissue. Am J Pathol 148:643–648, 1996.

562. Peng H, Diss T, Isaacson PG et al: *c-myc* Gene abnormalities in mucosa-associated lymphoid tissue (MALT) lymphomas. J Pathol 181:381–386, 1997.

563. Peng H, Du M, Diss TC et al: Genetic evidence for a clonal link between low and high-grade components in gastric MALT B-cell lymphoma. Histopathology 30:425–429, 1997.

564. Peng H, Ranaldi R, Diss TC et al: High frequency of CagA+ *Helicobacter pylori* infection in high-grade gastric MALT B-cell lymphomas. J Pathol 185:409–412, 1998.

565. Penn I: Immunosuppression and malignant disease. In Twomey JJ, Good RA (eds.): The Immunopathology of Lymphoreticular Neoplasms, pp. 223–237. Plenum, New York, 1978.

566. Penn I: Tumors arising in organ transplant recipients. Adv Cancer Res 28:31–61, 1978.

567. Penn I: Depressed immunity and the development of cancer. Clin Exp Immunol 46:459–474, 1981.

568. Penn I: Lymphomas complicating organ transplantation. Transplant 15:2790–2797, 1983.

569. Penn I: Cancers following cyclosporine therapy. Transplantation 43:32–35, 1987.

570. Penn I: Cancers following cyclosporine therapy. Transplant Proc 19:2211–2213, 1987.

571. Penn I, Brunson ME: Cancers after cyclosporine therapy. Transplant Proc 20:885–892, 1988.

572. Penn I: Cancers complicating organ transplantation. N Engl J Med 323:1767–1769, 1990 (Editorial).

573. Penn I: The changing pattern of posttransplant malignancies. Transplant Proc 23:1101–1103, 1991.

574. Penn I: Cancer in the immunosuppressed organ recipient. Transplant Proc 23:1771–1772, 1991.

575. Penn I: Donor transmitted disease: Cancer. Transplant Proc 23:2629–2631, 1991.

576. Penn I: Tumors after renal and cardiac transplantation. Hematol Oncol Clin North Am 7:431–445, 1993.

577. Penn I: De novo tumors in pediatric organ transplant recipients. Transplant Proceed 26:1–2, 1994.

578. Penn I: De novo malignancy in pediatric organ transplant recipients. J Pediatr Surg 29:221–228, 1994.

579. Perry GS, Spector BD, Schuman LM et al: The Wiskott-Aldrich syndrome in the United States and Canada (1892–1979). J Pediatr 97:72–78, 1980.

580. Peterson JM, Tubbs RR, Savage RA et al: Small noncleaved B cell Burkitt-like lymphoma with chromsosome t(8;14) translocation and Epstein-Barr virus nuclear-associated antigen in a homosexual man with acquired immune deficiency syndrome. Am J Med 78:141–148, 1985.

581. Peterson WL: *Helicobacter pylori* and peptic ulcer disease. N Engl J Med 324:1043–1048, 1991.

582. Pirsch JD, Stratta RJ, Sollinger HW et al: Treatment of severe Epstein-Barr virus-induced lymphoproliferative syndrome with ganciclovir: Two cases after solid organ transplantation. Am J Med 86:241–244, 1989.

583. Pluda J, Yarchoan R, Jaffe E et al: Development of non-Hodgkin lymphoma in a cohort of patients with severe human immunodeficiency virus (HIV) infection on long-term antiretroviral therapy. Ann Intern Med 113:276–282, 1990.

584. Pluda JM, Venzon DJ, Tosato G et al: Parameters affecting the development of non-Hodgkin's lymphoma in patients with severe human immunodeficiency virus infection receiving antiretroviral therapy. J Clin Oncol 11:1099–1107, 1993.

585. Poiesz B: Etiology of acute leukemia: Molecular genetics and viral oncology. In Wiernik PH, Canellos GP, Dutcher JP, Kyle RA (eds.): Neoplastic Diseases of the Blood, pp. 159–175. Churchill Livingstone, New York, 1996.

586. Poiesz B, Dube D, Dube S et al: HTLV-II-associated cutaneous T-cell lymphoma in a patient with HIV-1 infection. N Engl J Med 342:930–936, 2000.

587. Porter D, Madhok R, Capell H: Non-Hodgkin's lymphoma in rheumatoid arthritis. Ann Rheum Dis 50:275–276, 1991.

588. Preciado MV, De Matteo E, Diez B et al: Presence of Epstein-Barr virus and strain type assignment in Argentine childhood Hodgkin's disease. Blood 86:3922–3929, 1995.

589. Prendergast GC, Lawe D, Ziff EB: Association of *Myn*, the murine homolog of *Max*, with *c-Myc* stimulates methylation-sensitive DNA binding and *Ras* cotransformation. Cell 65:395–407, 1991.

590. Prior E, Goldberg AF, Conjalka MS et al: Hodgkin's disease in homosexual men. An AIDS-related phenomenon? Am J Med 81:1085–1088, 1986.

591. Prior P: Cancer and rheumatoid arthritis: Epidemiologic considerations. Am J Med 78:15–21, 1985.

592. Prochownik EV: Protooncogenes and cell differentiation. Transfus Med Rev 3:24–38, 1989.

593. Purtilo DT, Sakamoto K, Saemundsen AK et al: Documentation of Epstein-Barr virus infection in immunodeficient patients with life-threatening lymphoproliferative diseases by clinical, virological, and immunopathological studies. Cancer Res 41:4226–4236, 1981.

594. Purtilo DT, Tatsumi E, Manolov G et al: Epstein-Barr virus as an etiological agent in the pathogenesis of lymphoproliferative and aproliferative diseases in immune deficient patients. Int Rev Exp Pathol 27:113–193, 1985.

595. Purtilo DT, Grierson HL, Ochs H et al: Detection of X-linked lymphoproliferative disease using molecular and immunovirologic markers. Am J Med 37:421–424, 1989.

596. Purtilo DT, Stevenson M: Lymphotropic viruses as etiologic agents of lymphoma. Hematol Oncol Clin North Am 5:901–923, 1991.

597. Quintanilla-Martinez L, Lome-Maldonado C, Schwarzmann F et al: Post-transplantation lymphoproliferative disorders in Mexico: An aggressive clonal disease associated with Epstein-Barr virus type A. Mod Pathol 11:200–208, 1998.

598. Quintanilla-Martinez L, Fend F, Rodriguez L et al: Peripheral T-cell lymphoma with Reed-Sternberg-like cells of B-cell phenotype and genotype associated With Epstein-Barr virus infection. Am J Surg Pathol 23:1233–1240, 1999.

599. Quintanilla-Martinez L, Kumar S, Fend F et al: Fulminant EBV+ T-cell lymphoproliferative disorder following acute/chronic EBV infection: A distinct clinicopathologic syndrome. Blood 96:443–451, 2000.

600. Rabbitts TH: Chromosomal translocations in human cancer. Nature 372:143–149, 1994.

601. Rabkin CS, Biggar RJ, Horm JW: Increasing incidence of cancers associated with the human immunodeficiency virus epidemic. Int J Cancer 47:692–696, 1991.

602. Rabkin CS, Hilgartner MW, Hedberg KW et al: Incidence of lymphomas and other cancers in HIV-infected and HIV-uninfected patients with hemophilia. JAMA 267:1090–1094, 1992.

603. Rabkin CS, Sei S: Susceptibility genes for AIDS and AIDS-related lymphoma. Curr Top Microbiol Immunol 246:111–115, 1999.

604. Raffeld M, Sander CA, Yano T et al: Mantle cell lymphoma: An update. Leuk Lymphoma 8:161–166, 1992.

605. Ramenghi U, Bonissoni S, Migliaretti G et al: Deficiency of the Fas apoptosis pathway without *Fas* gene mutations is a familial trait predisposing to development of autoimmune disease and cancer. Blood 95:3176–3182, 2000.

606. Randhawa P, Jaffe R, Demetris AJ et al: Expression of Epstein-Barr virus-encoded small RNA (by the *EBER-1* gene) in liver specimens from transplant recipients with post-transplantation lymphoproliferative disease. N Engl J Med 327:1710–1714, 1992.

607. Raphael M, Gentilhomme O, Tulliez M et al: Histopathologic features of high-grade non-Hodgkin's lymphomas in acquired immunodeficiency syndrome. Arch Pathol Lab Med 115:15–20, 1991.

608. Rappaport H, Ramot B, Hulu N et al: The pathology of so-called mediterranean abdominal lymphoma with malabsorption. Cancer 29:1502–1511, 1972.

609. Rawlings SL, Crooks GM, Bockstoce D et al: Spontaneous apoptosis in lymphocytes from patients with Wiskott-Aldrich syndrome: Correlation of accelerated cell death and attenuated *Bcl-2* expression. Blood 94:3872–3882, 1999.

610. Rea D, Delecluse H-J, Hamilton-Dutoit SJ et al: Epstein-Barr virus latent and replicative gene expresssion in post-transplant lymphoproliferative disorders and AIDS-related Non-hodgkin's lymphomas. Ann Oncol 6(Suppl. 1):S113–S116, 1994.

611. Rees L, Thomas A, Amlot PL: Disappearance of an Epstein-Barr virus-positive post-transplant plasmacytoma with reduction of immunosuppression. Lancet 352:789, 1998.

612. Remick SC, McSharry JJ, Wolf BC et al: Novel oral combination chemotherapy in the treatment of intermediate-grade and high-grade AIDS-related non-Hodgkin's lymphoma. J Clin Oncol 11:1691–1702, 1993.

613. Renton R, Blackshaw AJ: Colonic lymphoma complicating ulcerative colitis. Br J Surg 63:542–545, 1976.

614. Reynaud-Gaubert M, Stoppa AM, Gaubert J-Y et al: Anti-CD20 monoclonal antibody therapy in Epstein-Barr virus-associated B cell lymphoma following lung transplantation. J Heart Lung Transplant 19:492–495, 2000.

615. Rickinson AB, Yao Q-Y, Wallace LE: The Epstein-Barr virus as a model of virus-host interactions. Br Med Bull 41:75–79, 1985.

616. Riddler SA, Breinig MC, McKnight LC: Increased levels of circulating Epstein-Barr virus (EBV)-infected lymphocytes and decreased EBV nuclear antigen antibody responses are associated with the development of posttransplant lymphoproliferative disease in solid-organ transplant recipients. Blood 84:972–984, 1994.

617. Ridolfo A, Santambrogio S, Mainini F et al: High frequency of non-Hodgkin's lymphoma in patients with HIV-associated Kaposi's sarcoma. AIDS 10:181–185, 1996.

618. Rieux-Laucat F, Le Deist F, Hivroz C et al: Mutations in *Fas* associated with human lymphoproliferative syndrome and autoimmunity. Science 268:1347–1349, 1995.

619. Robert NJ, Schneiderman H: Hodgkin's disease and the acquired immunodeficiency syndrome. Ann Intern Med 101:142–143, 1984 (Correspondence).

620. Robert-Guroff M, Weiss SH, Giron JA et al: Prevalence of antibodies to HTLV-I, -II, and -III in intravenous drug abusers from an AIDS endemic region. JAMA 255:3133–3137, 1986.

621. Robertson L, Rice L, Riggs S et al: Lymphomas after cardiac transplantation: Houston experience and successful therapy. Blood 76:369a, 1990 (Abstract).

622. Roggero E, Zucca E, Pinotti G et al: Eradication of *Helicobacter pylori* infection in primary low-grade gastric lymphoma of mucosa-associated lymphoid tissue. Ann Intern Med 122:767–769, 1995.

623. Roggero E, Zucca E, Mainetti C et al: Eradication of *Borrelia burgdorferi* infection in primary marginal zone B-cell lymphoma of the skin. Hum Pathol 31:263–268, 2000.

624. Roithmann S, Tourani J-M, Andrieu J-M: Hodgkin's disease in HIV-infected intravenous drug abusers. N Engl J Med 323:275–276, 1990.

625. Rooney CM, Rickinson AB, Moss DJ et al: Paired Epstein-Barr virus-carrying lymphoma and lymphoblastoid cell lines from Burkitt's lymphoma patients: Comparative sensitivity to non-specific and to allo-specific cytotoxic responses in vitro. Int J Cancer 34:339–348, 1984.

626. Rooney CM, Rowe M, Wallace LE: Epstein-Barr virus-positive Burkitt's lymphoma cells not recognized by virus-specific T-cell surveillance. Nature 317:629–631, 1985.

627. Rooney CM, Smith CA, Ng CY et al: Use of gene-modified virus-specific T lymphocytes to control Epstein-Barr virus-related lymphoproliferation. Lancet 345:9–13, 1995.

628. Roth G, Curiel T, Lacy J: Epstein-Barr viral nuclear antigen 1 antisense oligodeoxynucleotide inhibits proliferation of Epstein-Barr virus-immortalized B cells. Blood 84:582–587, 1994.

629. Rowe DT, Rowe M, Evan GI et al: Restricted expression of EBV latent genes and T-lymphocyte-detected membrane antigen in Burkitt's lymphoma cells. EMBO J 5:2599–2607, 1986.

630. Rowe M, Rowe DT, Gregory CD et al: Differences in B cell growth phenotype reflect novel patterns of Epstein-Barr virus latent gene expression in Burkitt's lymphoma cells. EMBO J 6:2743–2751, 1987.

631. Roy B, Beamon J, Balint E et al: Transactivation of the human *p53* tumor suppressor gene by c-Myc/Max contributes to elevated mutant p53 expression in some tumors. Molec Cell Biol 14:7805–7815, 1994.

632. Ruzich J, Fisher RI: MALT lymphoma. Clin Oncol Updates 3:1–7, 2000.

633. Saag MS, Kilby JM: HIV-2 and HAART: A time to cure, a time to kill. Nature Med 5:609–611, 1999.

634. Saemundsen AK, Berkel AI, Henle W et al: Epstein-Barr virus-carrying lymphoma in a patient with ataxia-telangiectasia. BMJ 282:425–427, 1981.

635. Saemundsen AK, Purtilo DT, Sakamoto K et al: Documentation of Epstein-Barr virus infection in immunodeficient patients with life threatening lymphoproliferative diseases by Epstein-Barr virus complementary RNA/DNA and viral DNA/DNA hybridization. Cancer Res 41:4237–4242, 1981.

636. Saffran DC, Parolini O, Fitch-Hilgenberg ME et al: Brief report: A point mutation in the SH2 domain of Bruton's tyrosine kinase in atypical X-linked agammaglobulinemia. N Engl J Med 330:1488–1491, 1994.

637. Sakamoto K, Freed HJ, Purtilo DT: Antibody responses to Epstein-Barr virus in families with the X-linked lymphoproliferative syndrome. J Immunol 125:921–925, 1980.

638. Salahuddin SZ, Ablashi DV, Markham PD et al: Isolation of a new virus, HBLV, in patients with lymphoproliferative disorders. Science 234:596–601, 1986.

639. Salloum E, Cooper DL, Howe G et al: Spontaneous regression of lymphoproliferative disorders in patients treated with methotrexate for rheumatoid arthritis and other rheumatic diseases. J Clin Oncol 14:1943–1949, 1996.

640. Sandvej K, Peh S-C, Andresen BS et al: Identification of potential hot spots in the carboxy-terminal part of the Epstein-Barr virus (EBV) *BNLF-1* gene in both malignant and benign EBV-associated diseases: High frequency of a 30-bp deletion in Malaysian and Danish peripheral T-cell lymphomas. Blood 84:4053–4060, 1994.

641. Saravolatz LD, Winslow DL, Collins G et al. and Investigators for the Terry Beirn Community Programs for Clinical Research on AIDS: Zidovudine alone or in combination with didanosine or zalcitabine in HIV-infected patients with the acquired immunodeficiency syndrome or fewer than 200 CD4 cells per cubic millimeter. N Engl J Med 335:1099–1106, 1996.

642. Sashiyama H, Nozawa A, Kimura M et al: Case report: A case of lymphoepithelioma-like carcinoma of the oesophagus and review of the literature. J Gastroenterol Hepatol 14:523–539, 1999.

643. Sato T, Tatsuzawa O, Koike Y et al: B-cell lymphoma associated with DiGeorge syndrome. Eur J Pediatr 158:609, 1999.

644. Sausville EA: T-cell leukemia-lymphoma and mycosis fungoides. Curr Opin Oncol 4:829–839, 1992.

645. Savio A, Franzin G, Wotherspoon AC et al: Diagnosis and posttreatment follow-up of Helicobacter pylori-positive gastric lymphoma of mucosa-associated lymphoid tissue: Histology, polymerase chain reaction, or both? Blood 84:1255–1260, 1996.

646. Savitsky K, Bar-Shira A, Gilad S et al: A single ataxia telangiectasia gene with a product similar to PI-3 kinase. Science 268:1749–1753, 1995.

647. Savoie A, Perpète C, Carpentier L et al: Direct correlation between the load of Epstein-Barr virus-infected lymphocytes in the peripheral blood of pediatric transplant patients and risk of lymphoproliferative disease. Blood 83:2715–2722, 1994.

648. Scala G, Quinto I, Ruocco MR et al: Expression of an exogenous interleukin 6 gene in human Epstein Barr virus B cells confers growth advantage and in vivo tumorigenicity. J Exp Med 172:61–68, 1990.

649. Schaffner C, Stilgenbauer S, Rappold GA et al: Somatic ATM mutations indicate a pathogenic role of ATM in B-cell chronic lymphocytic leukemia. Blood 15:748–753, 1999.

650. Schapiro JM, Winters MA, Stewart F et al: The effect of high-dose saquinavir on viral load and CD4+ T-cell counts in HIV-infected patients. Ann Intern Med 124:1039–1050, 1996.

651. Schecter NR, Yahalom J: Low-grade MALT lymphoma of the stomach: A review of treatment options. Int J Radiat Oncol Biol Phys 46:1093–1103, 2000.

652. Scheib RG, Siegel RS: Atypical Hodgkin's disease and the acquired immunodeficiency syndrome. Ann Intern Med 102:554, 1985 (Correspondence).

653. Schmidt W, Anagnostopoulos I, Scherübl H: Virostatic therapy for advanced lymphoproliferation associated with the Epstein-Barr virus in an HIV-infected patient. N Engl J Med 342:440–441, 2000 (Correspondence).

654. Schnittman SM, Lane HC, Higgins SE et al: Direct polyclonal activation of human B lymphocytes by the acquired immune deficiency syndrome virus. Science 233:1084–1086, 1986.

655. Schoeppel SL, Hoppe RT, Dorfman RF et al: Hodgkin's disease in homosexual men with generalized lymphadenopathy. Ann Intern Med 102:68–70, 1985.

656. Schoeppel S, Hoppe R, Abrams D et al: Hodgkin's disease (HD) in homosexual men: The San Francisco Bay Area experience. Proc Am Soc Clin Oncol 5:3, 1986 (Abstract 9).

657. Schubach WH, Hackman R, Neiman PE et al: A monoclonal immunoblastic sarcoma in donor cells bearing Epstein-Barr virus genomes following allogeneic marrow grafting for acute lymphoblastic leukemia. Blood 60:180–187, 1982.

658. Schürmann D, Grünewald T, Weiß R et al: Intensive treatment of AIDS-related non-Hodgkin's lymphomas with the MACOP-B protocol. Eur J Haematol 54:73–77, 1995.

659. Schuster V, Ott G, Seidenspinner S et al: Common Epstein-Barr virus (EBV) type-1 variant strains in both malignant and benign EBV-associated disorders. Blood 87:1579–1585, 1996.

660. Schwab G, Siegall CB, Aarden LA et al: Characterization of an interleukin-6-mediated autocrine growth loop in the human multiple myeloma cell line, U266. Blood 77:587–593, 1991.

661. Schwab M, Böswald M, Korn K et al: Epstein-Barr virus in pediatric patients after renal transplantation. Clin Nephrol 53:132–139, 2000.

662. Schwaber JF, Klein G, Ernberg I et al: Deficiency of Epstein-Barr virus (EBV) receptors on B lymphocytes from certain patients with common varied agammaglobulinemia. J Immunol 124:2191–2196, 1980.

663. Schwartz RS: Epstein-Barr virus—oncogen or mitogen? N Engl J Med 302:1307–1308, 1980 (Editorial).

664. Seidemann K, Henze G, Beck JD et al: Non-Hodgkin's lymphoma in pediatric patients with chromosomal breakage syndromes (AT and NBS): Experience from the BFM Trials. Ann Oncol 11:141–145, 2000.

665. Seiden M, Sklar J: Molecular genetic analysis of post-transplant lymphoproliferative disorders. Hematol Oncol Clin North Am 7:447–465, 1993.

666. Senderowicz AM, Vitetta E, Headlee D et al: Complete sustained response of a refractory, post-transplantation, large B-cell lymphoma to an anti-CD22 immunotoxin. Ann Intern Med 126:882–885, 1997.

667. Serrano M, Bellas C, Campo E et al: Hodgkin's disease in patients with antibodies to human immunodeficiency virus. A study of 22 patients. Cancer 65:2248–2254, 1990.

668. Setlow RB: Repair deficient human disorders and cancer. Nature 271:713–717, 1978.

669. Shapiro RS: Treatment of B-cell lymphoproliferative disorders with interferon alfa and intravenous gamma globulin. N Engl J Med 318:1334, 1988 (Correspondence).

670. Shapiro RS, McClain K, Frizzera G et al: Epstein-Barr virus associated B cell lymphoproliferative disorders following bone marrow transplantation. Blood 71:1234–1243, 1988.

671. Shapiro RS: Epstein-Barr virus-associated B-cell lymphoproliferative disorders in immunodeficiency: Meeting the challenge. J Clin Oncol 8:371–373, 1990 (Editorial).

672. Shaw MT, Jacobs SR: Cutaneous Hodgkin's disease in a patient with human immunodeficiency virus infection. Cancer 64:2585–2587, 1989.

673. Shcherbina A, Rosen FS, Remold-O'Donnell E: WASP levels in platelets and lymphocytes of Wiskott-Aldrich syndrome patients correlate with cell dysfunction. J Immunol 163:6314–6320, 1999.

674. Shearer WT, Ritz J, Finegold MJ et al: Epstein-Barr virus-associated B-cell proliferations of diverse clonal origins after bone marrow transplantation in a 12-year-old patient with severe combined immunodeficiency. N Engl J Med 312:1151–1159, 1985.

675. Sherr CJ: Mammalian G1 cyclins. Cell 73:1059–1065, 1993.

676. Sherrington PD, Fisch P, Taylor AMR et al: Clonal evolution of malignant and non-malignant T cells carrying t(14;14) and t(X;14) in patients with ataxia telangiectasia. Oncogene 9:2377–2381, 1994.

677. Shibata D, Brynes RK, Rabinowitz A et al: Human T-cell lymphotropic virus type I (HTLV-I)-associated adult T-cell leukemia-lymphoma in a patient infected with human immunodeficiency virus type 1 (HIV-1). Ann Intern Med 111:871–875, 1989.

678. Shibata D, Weiss LM, Nathwani BN: Epstein-Barr virus in benign lymph node biopsies from individuals infected with the human immunodeficiency virus is associated with concurrent or subsequent development of non-Hodgkin's lymphoma. Blood 77:1527–1533, 1991.

679. Shibata D, Weiss LM, Hernandez AM et al: Epstein-Barr virus-associated non-Hodgkin's lymphoma in patients infected with the human immunodeficiency virus. Blood 81:2102–2109, 1993.

680. Shiramizu B, Magrath I: Localization of breakpoints by polymerase chain reactions in Burkitt's lymphoma with 8;14 translocations. Blood 75:1848–1852, 1990.

681. Shiramizu B, Barriga F, Neequaye J et al: Patterns of chromosomal breakpoint locations in Burkitt's lymphoma: Relevance to geography and Epstein-Barr virus association. Blood 77:1516–1526, 1991.

682. Shiramizu B, Herndier BG, McGrath MS: Identification of a common clonal human immunodeficiency virus integration site in human immunodeficiency virus-associated lymphomas. Cancer Res 54:2069–2072, 1994.

683. Siekevitz M, Josephs SF, Dukovich M et al: Activation of the HIV-1 LTR by T cell mitogens and the trans-activator protein of HTLV-I. Science 238:1575–1578, 1987.

684. Sinclair AJ, Palmero I, Peters G et al: EBNA-2 and EBNA-LP cooperate to cause G0 to G1 transition during immortalization of resting human B lymphocytes by Epstein-Barr virus. EMBO J 13:3321–3328, 1994.

685. Sinha S, Todd SC, Hedrick JA et al: Characterization of the EBV/C3d receptor on the human Jurkat T cell line: Evidence for a novel transcript. J Immunol 150:5311–5320, 1993.

686. Sixbey JW, Nedrud JG, Raab-Traub N et al: Epstein-Barr virus replication in oropharyngeal epithelial cells. N Engl J Med 310:1225–1230, 1984.

687. Sklar J, Cleary K, Thielemans K et al: Biclonal B-cell lymphoma. N Engl J Med 311:20–27, 1984.

688. Smith JL, Wilkinson AH, Hunsicker LG et al: Increased frequency of posttransplant lymphomas in patients treated with cyclosporin, azathioprine, and prednisone. Transplant Proc 21:3199–3200, 1989.

689. Sneller MC, Strober W, Eisenstein E et al: New insights into common variable immunodeficiency. Ann Intern Med 118:720–730, 1993.

690. Snider WD, Simpson DM, Aronyk KE: Primary lymphoma of the nervous system associated with acquired immune-deficiency syndrome. N Engl J Med 308:45, 1983 (Letter).

691. Snider WD, Simpson DM, Nielsen S et al: Neurological complications of acquired immune deficiency syndrome: Analysis of 50 patients. Ann Neurol 14:403–418, 1983.

692. Snover DC, Frizzera G, Spector BD et al: Wiskott-Aldrich syndrome: Histopathologic findings in the lymph nodes and spleens of 15 patients. Human Pathol 12:821–831, 1981.

693. Snudden DK, Hearing J, Smith PR et al: EBNA-1, the major nuclear antigen of Epstein-Barr virus, resembles 'RGG' RNA binding proteins. EMBO J 13:4840–4847, 1994.

694. So YT, Beckstead JH, Davis RL: Primary central nervous system lymphoma in acquired immune deficiency syndrome: A clinical and pathological study. Ann Neurol 20:566–572, 1986.

695. Socié G, Henry-Amar M, Bacigalupo A et al: Malignant tumors occurring after treatment of aplastic anemia. N Engl J Med 329:1152–1157, 1993.

696. Soulier J, Grollet L, Oksenhendler E et al: Kaposi's sarcoma-associated herpesvirus-like DNA sequences in multicentric Castleman's disease. Blood 86:1276–1280, 1995.

697. Sparano JA, Wiernik PH, Strack M et al: Infusional cyclophosphamide, doxorubicin, and etoposide in human immunodeficiency virus- and human T-cell leukemia virus type I-related non-Hodgkin's lymphoma: A highly active regimen. Blood 81:2810–2815, 1993.

698. Sparano JA, Wiernik PH, Hu X et al: Pilot trial of infusional cyclophosphamide doxorubicin, and etoposide plus didanosine and filgrastim in patients with human immunodeficiency virus-associated non-Hodgkin's lymphoma. J Clin Oncol 14:3026–3035, 1996.

699. Sparano JA, Anand K, Desai J et al: Effect of highly active antiretroviral therapy on the incidence of HIV-associated malignancies at an urban medical center. J Acquir Immune Defic Syndr 21(Suppl 1):S18–S22, 1999.

700. Spector BD, Perry GS, Good RA et al: Immunodeficiency diseases and malignancy. In Twomey JJ, Good RA (eds.), The Immunopathology of Lymphoreticular Neoplasms, pp.203–222. Plenum, New York, 1978.

701. Spector BD, Perry GS, Kersey JH: Genetically determined immunodeficiency diseases (GDID) and malignancy: Report from the Immunodeficiency-Cancer Registry. Clin Immunol Immunopathol 11:12–29, 1978.

702. Spino M, Gaidano G, Carbone A et al: Highly active antiretroviral therapy in human herpesvirus-8-related body-cavity-based lymphoma. AIDS 12:955–956, 1998 (Correspondence).

703. Spiro IJ, Yandell DW, Li C et al: Brief report: Lymphoma of donor origin occurring in the porta hepatis of a transplanted liver. N Engl J Med 329:27–29, 1993.

704. Srivastava T, Zwick DL, Rothberg PG et al: Posttransplant lymphoproliferative disorder in pediatric renal transplantation. Pediatr Nephrol 13:748–754, 2000.

705. Stankovic T, Kidd AM, Sutcliffe A et al: *ATM* mutations and phenotypes in ataxia-telangiectasia families in the British Isles: Expression of mutant *ATM* and the risk of leukemia, lymphoma, and breast cancer. Am J Hum Genet 62:334–345, 1998.

706. Starostik P, Greiner A, Schultz A et al: Genetic aberrations common in gastric high-grade large B-cell lymphoma. Blood 95:1180–1187, 2000.

707. Starzl TE, Porter KA, Iwatsuki S et al: Reversibility of lymphomas and lymphoproliferative lesions developing under cyclosporin-steroid therapy. Lancet 1:583–587, 1984.

708. Stilgenbauer S, Winkler D, Ott G et al: Molecular characterization of 11q deletions points to a pathogenic role of the *ATM* gene in mantle cell lymphoma. Blood 94:3262–3264, 1999.

709. Strahm B, Rittweiler K, Duffner U et al: Recurrent B-cell non-Hodgkin's lymphoma in two brothers with X-linked lymphoproliferative disease without evidence for Epstein-Barr virus infection. Br J Haematol 108:377–382, 2000.

710. Strauch B, Siegel N, Andrews L-L et al: Oropharyngeal excretion of Epstein-Barr virus by renal transplant recipients and other patients treated with immunosuppressive drugs. Lancet 234–237, 1974.

711. Strauchen JA, Hauser AD, Burstein D et al: Body cavity-based malignant lymphoma containing Kaposi sarcoma-associated herpesvirus in an HIV-negative man with previous Kaposi sarcoma. Ann Intern Med 125:822–825, 1996.

712. Straughen J, Ciocci S, Ye T-Z et al: Physical mapping of the Bloom syndrome region by the identification of YAC and P1 clones from human chromosome 15 band q26.1. Genomics 35:118–128, 1996.

713. Strauss SE, Sneller M, Lenardo MJ et al: An inherited disorder of lymphocyte apoptosis: The autoimmune lymphoproliferative syndrome. Ann Intern Med 130:591–601, 1999.

714. Su I-J, Lin KH, Chen C-J et al: Epstein-Barr virus-associated peripheral T-cell lymphoma of activated CD8 phenotype. Cancer 66:2557–2562, 1990.

715. Subar M, Neri A, Inghirami G et al: Frequent *c-myc* oncogene activation and infrequent presence of Epstein-Barr virus genome in AIDS-associated lymphoma. Blood 72:667–671, 1988.

716. Sullivan JL, Byron KS, Brewster FE et al: X-linked lymphoproliferative syndrome. Natural history of the immunodeficiency. J Clin Invest 71:1765–1778, 1983.

717. Sun Q, Pollok KE, Burton RL et al: Simultaneous ex vivo expansion of cytomegalovirus and Epstein-Barr virus-specific cytotoxic

T lymphocytes using B-lymphoblastoid cell lines expressing cytomegalovirus pp65. Blood 94:3242–3250, 1999.

718. Sutcliffe N, Inanc M, Speight P et al: Predictors of lymphoma development in primary Sjögren's syndrome. Semin Arthritis Rheum 28:80–87, 1998.

719. Sutcliffe N, Smith C, Speight PM et al: Mucosa-associated lymphoid tissue lymphomas in two patients with rheumatoid arthritis on second-line agents, and secondary Sjögren's syndrome. Rheumatology 39:185–188, 2000.

720. Suthanthiran M, Strom TB: Renal transplantation. N Engl J Med 331:365–376, 1994.

721. Swift M, Morrell D, Massey RB et al: Incidence of cancer in 161 families affected by ataxia-telangiectasia. N Engl J Med 325:1831–1836, 1991.

722. Swinnen LD, Costanzo-Nordin MR, Fisher SG et al: Increased incidence of lymphoproliferative disorder after immunosuppression with the monoclonal antibody OKT3 in cardiac-transplant recipients. N Engl J Med 323:1723–1728, 1990.

723. Swinnen LJ, Costanzo-Nordin MR, Fisher RI: ProMACE-CytaBOM induces durable complete remissions (CR) in post cardiac transplant lymphoma (PTL). Proc Am Soc Clin Oncol 11:318, 1992 (Abstract).

724. Swinnen LJ, Mullen GM, Carr TJ et al: Aggressive treatment for post-cardiac transplant lymphoproliferation. Blood 86:3333–3340, 1995.

725. Swinnen L: Overview of posttransplant B-cell lymphoproliferative disorders. Sem Oncol 26(Suppl. 14):21–25, 1999.

726. Symmons DPM: Neoplasms of the immune system in rheumatoid arthritis. Am J Med 78(Suppl. 1A):22–28, 1985.

727. Symmons DPM: Neoplasia in rheumatoid arthritis. J Rheumatol 15:1319–1322, 1988 (Editorial).

728. Tacyildiz N, Cavdar AO, Ertem U et al: Unusually high frequency of a 69-bp deletion within the carboxy terminus of the LMP-1 oncogene of Epstein-Barr virus detected in Burkitt's lymphoma of Turkish children. Leukemia 12:1796–1805, 1998.

729. Takahashi K, Kashima K, Daa T et al: Contribution of Epstein-Barr virus to development of malignant lymphoma of the thyroid. Pathol Int 45:366–374, 1995.

730. Talley NJ, Zinsmeister AR, Weaver A et al: Gastric adenocarcinoma and Helicobacter pylori infection. J Natl Cancer Inst 83:1734–1739, 1991.

731. Tan B, Ratner L: The use of new antiretroviral therapy in combination with chemotherapy. Curr Opin Oncol 9:455–464, 1997.

732. Taub R, Kirsch I, Morton C et al: Translocation of the c-myc gene into the immunoglobulin heavy chain locus in human Burkitt lymphoma and murine plasmacytoma cells. Proc Natl Acad Sci U S A 79:7837–7841, 1982.

733. Taub R, Moulding C, Battey J et al: Activation and somatic mutation of the translocated c-myc gene in Burkitt lymphoma cells. Cell 36:339–348, 1984.

734. Taylor AMR, Harnden, DG, Arlett CF et al: Ataxia telangiectasia: A human mutation with abnormal radiation sensitivity. Nature 258:427–429, 1975.

735. Taylor AMR, Metcalfe JA, Oxford JM et al: Is chromatid-type damage in ataxia telangiectasia after irradiation at G0 a consequence of defective repair? Nature 260:441–443, 1976.

736. Taylor AMR, Metcalfe JA, Thick J et al: Leukemia and lymphoma in ataxia telangiectasia. Blood 87:423–438, 1996.

737. Temin H: Evolution of cancer genes as a mutation-driven process. Cancer Res 48:1697–1701, 1988.

738. Temple JJ, Andes WA: AIDS and Hodgkin's disease. Lancet 454–455, 1986.

739. Thieblemont C, Berger F, Dumontet C et al:Mucosa-associated lymphoid tissue lymphoma is a disseminated disease in one third of 158 patients analyzed. Blood 95:802–806, 2000.

740. Thiede C, Wündisch T, Alpen B et al. for the German MALT Lymphoma Study Group: Long-term persistence of monoclonal B cells after cure of Helicobacter pylori infection and complete histologic remission in gastric mucosa-associated lymphoid tissue B-cell lymphoma. J Clin Oncol 19:1600–1609, 2001.

741. Thorley-Lawson DA: Basic virological aspects of Epstein-Barr virus infection. Semin Hematol 25:247–260, 1988.

742. Tirelli U, Vaccher E, Rezza G: Hodgkin disease and infection with the human immunodeficiency virus (HIV) in Italy. Ann Intern Med 108:309–310, 1988.

743. Tirelli U, Rezza G, Barbui T et al: Hodgkin's disease in association with acquired immunodeficiency syndrome (AIDS). A report on 36 patients. Acta Oncol 28:637–639, 1989.

744. Tirelli U, Errante D, Oksenhendler E et al: The treatment of AIDS-related lymphoma. JAMA 267:509, 1992 (Correspondence).

745. Tirelli U, Errante D, Oksenhendler E et al: Prospective study with combined low-dose chemotherapy and zidovudine in 37 patients with poor prognosis AIDS-related non-Hodgkin's lymphoma. Ann Oncol 3:843–847, 1992.

746. Tirelli U, Serraino D, Carbone A: Hodgkin disease and HIV. Ann Intern Med 118:313, 1993 (Correspondence).

747. Tirelli U, Errante D, Dolcetti R et al: Hodgkin's disease and human immunodeficiency virus infection: Clinicopathologic and virologic features of 114 patients from the Italian Cooperative Group on AIDS and tumors. J Clin Oncol 13:1758–1767, 1995.

748. Tosato G, Steinberg AD, Blaese RM: Defective EBV-specific suppressor T-cell function in rheumatoid arthritis. N Engl J Med 305:1238–1243, 1981.

749. Tosato G, Seamon KB, Goldman ND et al: Monocyte-derived human B-cell growth factor identified as interferon-β2 (BSF-2, IL-6). Science 239:502–504, 1988.

750. Tosato G, Tanner J, Jones KD et al: Identification of interleukin-6 as an autocrine growth factor for Epstein-Barr virus-immortalized B cells. J Virol 64:3033–3041, 1990.

751. Traweek ST, Slovak ML, Nademanee AP et al: Clonal karyotypic hematopoietic cell abnormalities occurring after autologous bone marrow transplantation for Hodgkin's disease and non-Hodgkin's lymphoma. Blood 84:957–963, 1994.

752. Troye-Blomberg M, Sjoholm P-E, Perlmann H et al: Regulation of the immune response in Plasmodium falciparum malaria. I. Non-specific proliferative responses in vitro and characterization of lymphocytes. Clin Exp Immunol 53:335–344, 1983.

753. Troye-Blomberg M, Perlmann H, Patarroyo ME et al: Regulation of the immune response in Plasmodium falciparum malaria. II. Antigen specific proliferative responses in vitro. Clin Exp Immunol 53:345–353, 1983.

754. Tsoukas C, Lambris JD: Expression of EBV/C3d receptors on T cells: Biological significance. Immunol Today 14:56–59, 1993.

755. Tsujimoto Y, Yunis J, Onorato-Showe L et al: Molecular cloning of the chromosomal breakpoint of B-cell lymphomas and leukemias with the t(11;14) chromosome translocation. Science 224:1403–1406, 1984.

756. Tulpule A, Levine A: AIDS-related lymphoma. Blood Rev 13:147–150, 1999.

757. Uccini S, Monardo F, Ruco LP et al: High frequency of Epstein-Barr virus genome in HIV-positive patients with Hodgkin's disease. Lancet 1:1458, 1989 (Correspondence).

758. Udamsakdi-Auewarakul C, Auewarakul P, Sukpanichnant S et al: Hepatitis C infection in patients with non-Hodgkin lymphoma in Thailand. Blood 95:3640–3641, 2000 (Correspondence).

759. Unger PD, Strauchen JA: Hodgkin's disease in AIDS complex patients. Report of four cases and tissue immunologic marker studies. Cancer 58:821–825, 1986.

760. Urba WJ, Longo DL: Hodgkin's disease. N Engl J Med 326:678–687, 1992.

761. Vanasse GJ, Concannon P, Willerford DM: Regulated genomic instability and neoplasia in the lymphoid lineage. Blood 94:3997–4010, 1999.

762. Vandermolen LA, Fehir KM, Rice L: Multiple myeloma in a homosexual man with chronic lymphadenopathy. Arch Intern Med 145:745–746, 1985.

763. Van Dijken PJ, Verwijs W: Diamond-Blackfan anemia and malignancy. A case report and a review of the literature. Cancer 76:517–520, 1995.

764. van Gorp J, Doornewaard H, Verdonck LF et al: Posttransplant T-cell lymphoma. Cancer 73:3064–3072, 1994.

765. Vieira P, de Waal-Malefyt R, Dang M-N et al: Isolation and expression of human cytokine synthesis inhibitory factory cDNA clones: Homology to Epstein-Barr virus open reading frame BCRFI. Proc Natl Acad Sci U S A 88:1172–1176, 1991.

766. Voelkerding KV, Sandhaus LM, Kim HC et al: Plasma cell malignancy in the acquired immune deficiency syndrome. Am J Clin Pathol 92:222–228, 1989.

767. Vogelstein B, Fearon ER, Hamilton SR et al: Genetic alterations during colorectal tumor development. N Engl J Med 319:525–532, 1988.

768. Vořechovský I, Luo L, Dyer MJS et al: Clustering of missense mutations in the ataxia-telangiectasia gene in a sporadic T-cell leukaemia. Nature Genet 17:96–99, 1997.

769. Vowels MR, Lam-Po-Tang R, Berdoukas V et al: Brief report: Correction of X-linked lymphoproliferative disease by transplantation of cord-blood stem cells. N Engl J Med 329:1623–1625, 1993.

770. Wade M, Allday MJ: Epstein-Barr virus suppresses a G2/M checkpoint activated by genotoxins. Mol Cell Biol 20:1344–1360, 2000.

771. Waldmann T, Misiti J, Nelson DL et al: Ataxia-telangiectasia: A multisystem hereditary disease with immunodeficiency, impaired organ maturation, X-ray hypersensitivity, and a high incidence of neoplasia. Ann Intern Med 99:367–379, 1983.

772. Walker RC, Paya CV, Marshall WF et al: Pretransplantation seronegative Epstein-Barr virus status is the primary risk factor for posttransplantation lymphoproliferative disorder in adult heart, lung, and other solid organ transplantations. J Heart Lung Transplant 14:214–221, 1995.

773. Walsh C, Wernz JC, Levine A et al: Phase I trial of m-BACOD and granulocyte macrophage colony stimulating factor in HIV-associated non-Hodgkin's lymphoma. J Acq Imm Defic Syndr 6:265–271, 1993.

774. Walts AE, Shintaku IP, Said JW: Diagnosis of malignant lymphoma in effusions from patients with AIDS by gene rearrangement. Am J Clin Pathol 94:170–175, 1990.

775. Waltzer L, Logeat F, Brou C et al: The human Jκ recombination signal sequence binding protein (RBP-Jκ) targets the Epstein-Barr virus EBNA2 protein to its DNA responsive elements. EMBO J 13:5633–5638, 1994.

776. Walz G, Zanker B, Melton LB et al: Possible association of the immunosuppressive and B cell lymphoma-promoting properties of cyclosporine. Transplantation 49:191–194, 1990.

777. Wang C-Y, Mayo MW, Korneluk RG et al: NF-κB antiapoptosis: Induction of TRAF1 and TRAF2 and C-IAP1 and C-IAP2 to suppress caspase-8 activation. Science 281:1680–1683, 1998.

778. Wang D, Liebowitz D, Kieff E: An EBV membrane protein expressed in immortalized lymphocytes transforms established rodent cells. Cell 43:831–840, 1985.

779. Wang F, Gregory C, Sample C et al: Epstein-Barr virus latent membrane protein (LMP1) and nuclear proteins 2 and 3C are effectors of phenotypic changes in B lymphocytes: EBNA-2 and LMP1 cooperatively induce CD23. J Virol 64:2309–2318, 1990.

780. Washington K, Stenzel TT, Buckley RH et al: Gastrointestinal pathology in patients with common variable immunodeficiency and X-linked agammaglobulinemia. Am J Surg Pathol 20:1240–1252, 1996.

781. Watry D, Hedrick JA, Siervo S et al: Infection of human thymocytes by Epstein-Barr virus. J Exp Med 173:971–980, 1991.

782. Weinstein IB: Mitogenesis is only one factor in carcinogenesis. Science 251:387–388, 1991.

783. Weintraub J, Warnke RA: Lymphoma in cardiac allotransplant recipients. Clinical and histological features and immunological phenotype. Transplantation 33:347–351, 1982.

784. Weir AB, Herrod HG, Lester EP et al: Diffuse large-cell lymphoma of B-cell origin and deficient T-cell function in a patient with rheumatoid arthritis. Arch Intern Med 149:1688–1690, 1989.

785. Weiss LM, Movahed LA, Warnke RA et al: Detection of Epstein-Barr viral genomes in Reed-Sternberg cells of Hodgkin's disease. N Engl J Med 320:502–506, 1989.

786. Weiss LM, Jaffe ES, Liu X-F et al: Detection and localization of Epstein-Barr viral genomes in angioimmunoblastic lymphadenopathy and angioimmunoblastic lymphadenopathy-like lymphoma. Blood 79:1789–1795, 1992.

787. Weissmann DJ, Ferry JA, Harris NL et al: Posttransplantation lymphoproliferative disorders in solid organ recipients are predominantly aggressive tumors of host origin. Hematopathology 103:748–755, 1995.

788. Whang-Peng J, Lee EC, Sieverts H et al: Burkitt's lymphoma in AIDS: Cytogenetic study. Blood 63:818–822, 1984.

789. Whittle HC, Brown J, Marsh K et al: T-cell control of Epstein-Barr virus-infected B cells is lost during P. falciparum malaria. Nature 312:449–450, 1984.

790. Wilkes MS, Felix JC, Fortin AH et al: Value of necropsy in acquired immunodeficiency syndrome. Lancet 85–88, 1988.

791. Wilkinson AH, Smith JL, Hunsicker LG et al: Increased frequency of posttransplant lymphomas in patients treated with cyclosporine, azathioprine, and prednisone. Transplantation 47:293–296, 1989.

792. Willis TG, Jadayel DM, Du M-Q et al: Bcl10 is involved in t(1;14)(p22;q32) of MALT B cell lymphoma and mutated in multiple tumor types. Cell 96:35–45, 1999.

793. Willis TG, Dyer JS: The role of immunoglobulin translocations in the pathogenesis of B-cell malignancies. Blood 96:808–822, 2000.

794. Wilson WH, Kingma DW, Raffeld M et al: Association of lymphomatoid granulomatosis with Epstein-Barr viral infection of B lymphocytes and response to interferon-α2b. Blood 87:4531–4537, 1996.

795. Wirnsberger GH, Ratschek M, Dimai H-P et al: Post-transplantation lymphoproliferative disorder of the T-cell/B-cell type: An unusual manifestation in a renal allograft. Oncol Reports 6:29–32, 1999.

796. Witherspoon RP, Fisher LD, Schoch G et al: Secondary cancers after bone marrow transplantation for leukemia or aplastic anemia. N Engl J Med 321:784–789, 1989.

797. Wong MP, Chung LP, Yuen ST et al: In-situ detection of Epstein-Barr virus in non-small-cell lung carcinomas. J Pathol 177:233–240, 1995.

798. Woodman R, Shin K, Pineo G: Primary non-Hodgkin's lymphoma of the brain. A review. Medicine 64:425–430, 1985.

799. Wotherspoon AC, Ortiz-Hidalgo C, Falzon MR et al: Helicobacter pylori-associated gastritis and primary B-cell gastric lymphoma. Lancet 338:1175–1176, 1991.

800. Wotherspoon AC, Doglioni C, Diss TC et al: Regression of primary low-grade B-cell gastric lymphoma of mucosa-associated lymphoid tissue type after eradication of *Helicobacter pylori*. Lancet 342:575–578, 1993.

801. Wotherspoon AC, Doglioni C, de Boni M et al: Antibiotic treatment for low-grade gastric MALT lymphoma. Lancet 343:1503, 1994 (Correspondence).

802. Wotherspoon AC, Finn TM, Isaacson PG: Trisomy 3 in low grade B cell lymphomas of mucosa associated lymphoid tissue (MALT). Blood 85:2000–2004, 1995.

803. Wotherspoon AC, Diss TC, Pan L et al: Low grade gastric B-cell lymphoma of mucosa associated lymphoid tissue in immunocompromised patients. Histopathology 28:129–134, 1996.

804. Wright DH: Enteropathy associated T cell lymphoma. Cancer Surv 30:249–261, 1997.

805. Wu H, Wasik MA, Przybylski G et al: Hepatosplenic gamma-delta T-cell lymphoma as a late-onset posttransplant lymphoproliferative disorder in renal transplant recipients. Hematopathol Am J Clin Pathol 113:487–496, 2000.

806. Wyburn-Mason R: S.L.E. and lymphoma. Lancet 1:156, 1979.

807. Yachie A, Tosato G, Straus S, Blaese RM: T cell stimulation and polyclonal B cell activation induced by cytomegalovirus. Clin Res 32:510A, 1984 (Abstract).

808. Yamaguchi M, Ohno T, Kita K: γ/δ T-cell lymphoma of the thyroid gland. N Engl J Med 336:1391–1392, 1997.

809. Yamaoka S, Inoue H, Sakurai M et al: Constitutive activation of NF-κB Is essential for transformation of rat fibroblasts by the human T-cell leukemia virus type I Tax protein. EMBO J 15:873–887, 1996.

810. Yang J, Lemas VM, Finn IW et al: Application of the ELISPOT assay to the characterization of CD8+ responses to Epstein-Barr virus antigens. Blood 95:241–248, 2000.

811. Yano T, Sander CA, Clark HM et al: Clustered mutations in the second exon of the *Myc* gene in sporadic Burkitt's lymphoma. Oncogene 8:2741–2748, 1993.

812. Yao QY, Rowe M, Martin B et al: The Epstein-Barr virus carrier state: Dominance of a single growth-transforming isolate in the blood and in the oropharynx of healthy virus carriers. J Gen Virol 72:1579–1590, 1991.

813. Yao QY, Tierney RJ, Croom-Carter D et al: Frequency of multiple Epstein-Barr virus infections in T-cell-immunocompromised individuals. J Virol 70:4884–4894, 1996.

814. Yao QY, Croom-Carter DSG, Tierney RJ et al: Epidemiology of infection with Epstein-Barr virus types 1 and 2: Lessons from the study of a T-cell-immunocompromised hemophilic cohort. J Virol 72:4352–4363, 1998.

815. Yarchoan R, Redfield RR, Broder S: Mechanisms of B cell activation in patients with acquired immunodeficiency syndrome and related disorders. J Clin Invest 78:439–447, 1986.

816. Yarchoan R, Venzon DJ, Pluda JM et al: CD4 count and the risk for death in patients infected with HIV receiving antiretroviral therapy. Ann Intern Med 115:184–189, 1991.

817. Yates J, Warren N, Reisman D et al: A *cis*-acting element from the Epstein-Barr viral genome that permits stable replication of recombinant plasmids in latently infected cells. Proc Natl Acad Sci U S A 81:3806–3810, 1984.

818. Yokoi T, Miyawaki T, Yachie A et al: Epstein-Barr virus-immortalized B cells produce IL-6 as an autocrine growth factor. Immunology 70:100–105, 1990.

819. York LJ, Qualtiere LF: Cyclosporin abrogates virus-specific T-cell control of EBV-induced B-cell lymphoproliferation. Viral Immunol 3:127–136, 1990.

820. Yoshida K, Minegishi Y, Okawa H et al: Epstein-Barr virus-associated malignant lymphoma with macroamylasemia and monoclonal gammopathy in a patient with Wiskott-Aldrich syndrome. Pediatr Hematol Oncol 14:85–89, 1997.

821. Yoshiyama H, Shimizu N, Takada K: Persistent Epstein-Barr virus infection in a human T-cell line: Unique program of latent virus expression. EMBO J 14:3705–3711, 1995.

822. Young L, Alfieri C, Hennessy K et al: Expression of Epstein-Barr virus transformation-associated genes in tissues of patients with EBV lymphoproliferative disease. N Engl J Med 321:1080–1085, 1989.

823. Yousem SA, Randhawa P, Locker J et al: Posttransplant lymphoproliferative disorders in heart-lung transplant recipients: Primary presentation in the allograft. Hum Pathol 20:361–369, 1989.

824. Yu BW, Ichinose I, Bonham MA et al: Somatic mutations in *c-myc* intron I cluster in discrete domains that define protein binding sequences. J Biol Chem 268:19586–19592, 1993.

825. Zack JA, Cann AJ, Lugo JP et al: HIV-1 production from infected peripheral blood T cells after HTLV-I induced mitogenic stimulation. Science 240:1026–1029, 1988.

826. Zahm S, Blair A: Pesticides and non-Hodgkin's lymphoma. Cancer Res 52:5485S–5488S, 1992.

827. Zech L, Haglund U, Nilsson K et al: Characteristic chromosomal abnormalities in biopsies and lymphoid-cell lines from patients with Burkitt and non-Burkitt lymphomas. Int J Cancer 17:47–56, 1976.

828. Zenone T, Souquet PJ, Cunningham-Rundles C et al: Hodgkin's disease associated with IgA and IgG subclass deficiency. J Intern Med 240:99–102, 1996.

829. Ziegler JL: Burkitt's lymphoma. N Engl J Med 35:735–745, 1981.

830. Ziegler JL, Miner RC, Rosenbaum E et al: Outbreak of Burkitt's-like lymphoma in homosexual men. Lancet 2:631–633, 1982.

831. Ziegler JL, Beckstead JA, Volberding PA et al: Non-Hodgkin's lymphoma in 90 homosexual men. N Engl J Med 311:565–570, 1984.

832. Zijlmans JMJM, van Rijthoven AWAM, Kluin PM et al: Epstein-Barr virus-associated lymphoma in a patient with rheumatoid arthritis treated with cyclosporine. N Engl J Med 326:1363, 1992 (Correspondence).

833. Zucca E, Roggero E, Pinotti G et al: Lymphoma regression after eradication of *H. pylori* infection in primary low-grade gastric lymphoma of mucosa associated lymphoid tissue (MALT) type. Blood 84(Suppl.):519a, 1994 (Abstract 2061).

834. Zucca E, Roggero E: Biology and treatment of MALT lymphoma: The state-of-the-art in 1996. Ann Oncol 7:787–792, 1996.

835. Zucca E, Bertoni F, Roggero E et al: The gastric marginal zone B-cell lymphoma of MALT type. Blood 96:410–419, 2000.

836. Zuckerman E, Zuckerman T, Levine A et al: Hepatitis C virus infection in patients with B-cell non-Hodgkin lymphoma. Ann Intern Med 127:423–428, 1997.

837. Zulman J, Jaffe R, Talal N: Evidence that the malignant lymphoma of Sjögren's syndrome is a monoclonal B-cell neoplasm. N Engl J Med 299:1215–1220, 1978.

838. Zutter MM, Martin PJ, Sale GE et al: Epstein-Barr virus lymphoproliferation after bone marrow transplantation. Blood 72:520–529, 1988.

Supportive Care

48

Historical Perspectives in Supportive Care

Emil J Freireich

The basic physiology of blood circulation was first described in 1628, only three and three-quarter centuries ago. Over the ensuing years experimentation with blood replacement in animals was performed, but blood replacement in humans only became a reality in the twentieth century. At the start of this century the discovery of the vital dyes led to a description of the hematologic neoplastic disease and the appreciation that depression of the normal formed elements of the blood represented the major clinical consequence of these diseases. Initial efforts to correct blood deficiencies focused on red cell replacement and were severely impeded by the lack of an effective anticoagulant. The discovery of citrate as an anticoagulant in 1914 and the description of the red cell blood types as well as that of the isoagglutinins by Landsteiner in 1910 initiated the era of red blood cell replacement, which is now a well-developed science. The result is that anemia (lack of adequate hemoglobin or adequate oxygen-carrying capacity) is almost never responsible for morbidity or mortality in patients with neoplastic diseases of the hematopoietic system. Compatibility testing procedures are sophisticated enough that allogeneic volunteer donors can be identified for virtually every patient. Storage techniques for red cells have become highly developed, and frozen red cells may be stored for extended periods. The existence of blood banks now ensures that red cells are available on short notice; more recently, autologous donation, through which patients may store their own red cells for future use, has become more important. Thus, deficient red cell production is rarely a limiting factor in the management and control of the hematopoietic neoplasms.

TREATMENT OF THROMBOCYTOPENIA

In 1910 Dr. William Duke devised a test for inadequate platelet function that carries his name. What is frequently forgotten is that Dr. Duke recognized the association of thrombocytopenia with a hemorrhagic diathesis and also that temporary correction of thrombocytopenia by transfusion of platelets from allogeneic donors in the form of whole blood could affect the bleeding time and the risk of hemorrhage. Despite these brilliant observations, the treatment of thrombocytopenia remained essentially ineffective until the early 1950s, when studies in dogs and other experimental animals again demonstrated the strong interaction between thrombocytopenia and hemorrhage. In the early 1950s platelet transfusions were studied for treatment of thrombocytopenia in humans, largely by using allogeneic platelet donors for recipients with benign thrombocytopenia (aplastic anemia or idiopathic thrombocytopenia purpura). Isosensitization occurred regularly following platelet replacement, and therefore these observations again failed to produce practical useful procedures for platelet replacement.

The discovery of the significant antitumor activity of the aklylating agents in 1946 and description of complete remissions in childhood acute lymphocytic leukemia by Farber in 1948 initiated the era of chemotherapy for hematopoietic neoplasms; supportive treatment now moved into a new era. It was soon evident that although chemotherapy could control the malignancy, it aggravated the existing thrombocytopenia and leukopenia, and many patients would die of hemorrhage or infection (or both) despite excellent control of the malignancy. This quickly led to the hypothesis that improved techniques for the treatment of thrombocytopenia and leukopenia would greatly enhance the therapeutic index of compounds available for therapy. In the late 1950s the dominant presence of hemorrhage masked the important complications of infection, which also resulted from cytopenia.

A number of centers turned their attention to control of the hemorrhagic diathesis. Although evidence showed that circulating anticoagulants, vascular permeability, and infectious byproducts all contributed to the hemorrhagic diathesis, it seemed clear that thrombocytopenia was an important component. Testing the hypothesis that elevation of platelets would either entirely or partly correct the hemorrhagic diathesis was frustrated by several important characteristics of the circulating blood platelets. The first was the lack of a precise method for quantifying the degree of thrombocytopenia. Techniques available in the early 1950s were inaccurate because of the small size of the platelets and their lack of a specific staining characteristic. The introduction of the phase contrast microscope method by Brecher and Cronkite in the early 1950s quickly led to studies revealing that accurate enumeration of the platelet concentration in the venous blood was a strong predictor of hemorrhagic diathesis[1] (Figure 48–1). It is important to note that the relationship between thrombocytopenia and hemorrhage was continuous and discrete (i.e., the lower the platelet count, the higher the risk of hemorrhage), and therefore the potential for replacement of platelets by allogeneic transfusion was greatly enhanced.

The second important characteristic of the platelet was its short survival as a morphologic entity in whole blood collected and stored under blood bank conditions appropriate for red cell storage. It was demonstrated that the blood bank blood used for replacement was significantly less effective in controlling hemorrhage than freshly collected whole blood. In these early studies, it was also demonstrated that transfusion of a single unit (500 ml) of fresh whole blood into a child of approximately 1 m² body surface area resulted in a detectable change in platelet count measured 1 hour after transfusion, the increment being 5000/μl. This small increase was associated with a significant decrease in clinically observed hemorrhage.[2] Studies of radioactively labeled platelets showed that the platelet life span was 7 to

921

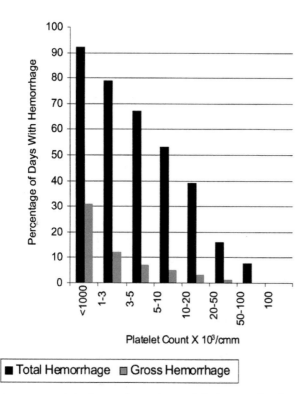

Figure 48–1. Relation between hemorrhage and platelet count. Based on data for 92 acute leukemia patients, including 40 adults, observed for 20 to 764 days.

10 days, in contrast to the 120-day life span of the red cell. Replacement of whole blood would result in more effective correction of the red cell loss than the platelet loss. Further efforts to replace platelets with whole blood would be frustrated by increasing red cell volume. It became necessary to devise techniques for the collection of platelets separated from red cells. The availability of newly developed plastic bags for the collection of platelets soon led to the development of the four-bag container, which permitted plasmapheresis in volunteer donors. From a single venipuncture, it was possible to collect a unit of blood, separate the platelet-rich plasma, return the packed red cells to the donor, collect a second unit of blood, and repeat the process. The result would be minimal red cell depletion in the donor, loss of 500 ml of plasma, and the availability for transfusion of platelets from almost two full units of whole blood. This technique led to the repeated transfusion of platelet-rich plasma into recipient patients from volunteer donors.[3] Because red cell loss was minimal, the limits of donation for volunteers could be defined as approximately 1 L of plasma per week.

It was possible to collect sufficient platelets from a single donor to provide effective platelet replacement for a child with leukemia.[4] Quantitatively, four units of blood contain approximately 4×10^{11} platelets, which in a recipient with a 1 m[2] surface area would result in an average platelet increase of 50,000/μl. This rapidly led to the practice (still currently popular) of giving allogeneic platelets approximately twice weekly in a dose of 2 to $4 \times 10^{11}/m^2$ to maintain platelet concentration in the recipient's blood above 20,000/μl.[5] By 1963, hemorrhage was no longer a leading cause of morbidity and mortality in children with acute leukemia. Now infection became the dominant problem.[6]

Over the last 30 years, platelet replacement has become central to the treatment of patients with hematopoietic neoplasia. Modern equipment allows the collection of 3×10^{11} to 4×10^{11} platelets from a single volunteer donor. Short-term storage conditions have been improved, and long-term storage has been shown to be feasible, although it is not a practical reality to date.

When these studies were initiated, it was anticipated that isosensitization would be a major problem. It was recognized that isoantibodies in platelets were different from those in red cells; the most useful classification was based on the tissue typing system of lymphocytes (the HLA system) for histocompatibility between donor and recipient. An unexpected finding was that both the cytotoxic therapy delivered to control the malignant disease and the immunosuppression associated with advanced hematopoietic neoplasia resulted in suppression of isosensitization and therefore platelet replacement by transfusion was more successful than predicted.

For the science of platelet replacement, the future lies with better compatibility testing between allogeneic donor and recipient, improved methods for longer-term storage of platelets so that banking becomes feasible, and more practical and effective techniques for collection and preservation of autologous platelets for support during periods of cytopenia. Moreover, additional important factors in hemorrhagic diathesis are associated with hematopoietic neoplasia. Specific and nonspecific anticoagulants as well as vascular and metabolic factors that result in hemorrhage still present difficulties, although these are relatively minor when compared with the major problem, control of infection.

TREATMENT OF GRANULOCYTOPENIA

As with platelets, it had become clear that a decrease in the number of circulating granulocytes was at least partly responsible for the greatly increased susceptibility to infection. However, it was not until 1966 that a quantitative relationship between the level of circulating granulocytes and the risk of developing a major infection was clearly shown[7] (Figure 48–2). In addition to the degree of neutropenia, the duration of neutropenia was shown to be a major risk factor (Figure 48–3). At neutrophil levels below 100/mm[3], if persistent for 4 to 6 weeks, all patients had severe infections, and even at levels below 1000/mm[3], 60 percent developed severe infection by 4 to 6 weeks. Thus, the practice of antibiotic therapy to prevent severe infection in neutropenic patients was indicated.

Based on the success of the allogeneic platelet replacement program, the hypothesis was generated that transfusion of allogeneic granulocytes might provide a modality for management of infection. Unfortunately the physiology of the granulocyte is even more forbidding than that of the platelet. Granulocytes in normal individuals have a half-life of only 6 to 12 hours, and the volume of distribution based on radioactivity-labeled granulo-

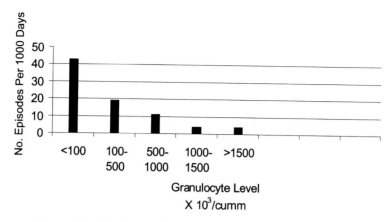

Figure 48–2. Risk of severe infections, based on circulating granulocyte level.

cyte injections was at least twice that of the red cell space. Perhaps more importantly, the techniques for separation of granulocytes were primitive. The centrifugal methods that were so useful for separating plasma and platelets from red cells were not particularly helpful for granulocytes because their specific gravity and sedimentation velocity is intermediate (i.e., they appear in the buffy coat).

A glimpse into the future of granulocyte replacement and allogeneic transplantation was provided by collection and transfusion studies of granulocytes from donors with chronic granulocytic leukemia. Donors were selected who had granulocyte concentrations of 100 to 1000 times normal; patients who had documented life-threatening, far advanced infections were the first recipients of these transfusions, reported in 1962.[8] Because of the large volume of the buffy coat in these donors, the technique of plasmapheresis and centrifugal separation used for platelets was also useful for collecting granulocytes from these donors, making it possible to infuse up to 10^{11} granulocytes in

each transfusion. After a number of transfusions, it could be demonstrated that a transfusion of 10^{11} granulocytes per m^2 would increase the granulocyte concentration in the recipient by 2000 to 5000 per μl, measured 1 hour after injection, resulting in a relatively normal concentration.[9] It also became possible to study the disappearance of these cells because unlike normal granulocytes, the transfused granulocytes had a half-life was approximately 24 hours. This finding strongly suggested that the peripheral blood of the chronic myelocytic leukemia donors contained myelocytes and metamyelocytes (immature granulocyte precursors that continued to differentiate in the recipient and gave an apparent increase in the half-life of granulocytes). Again, this was a clue to the potential for peripheral-blood stem cell transfusions, which is a reality today. The other observation was that these injected granulocytes had a volume of distribution that was much larger than the red cell volume, by as much as 20-fold, on average. Studies of the distribution of these injected cells revealed that they entered the marrow granulocyte reserve and could be demonstrated in marrow particles after infusion as well as extravasation into sites of previous inflammation. A direct relationship existed between the degree of granulocytopenia and the volume of distribution of the injected granulocytes.

Despite the limitations of these studies, it was clear that in terms of clinical response a dose response to these granulocyte transfusion was present: if 10^{11} or more granulocytes per m^2 were delivered and if such transfusions were repeated daily for 4 days consecutively (because the half-life was 1 day), it was possible to maintain a normal granulocyte level for approximately 5 days. More than three-fourths of the patients so treated had a dramatic clinical response, with clearing of septicemia as well as resolution of fever and other signs of advanced infection. Finally, the observation was made that in a small number of recipients who were not very sick with infection but severely immunospuppressed from therapy and disease, allogeneic hematopoietic stem cell grafts were present, documented by demonstrating the presence of the Philadelphia chromosome in the stem cells of the recipients' marrow.[10] These allografts permitted periods of hematologic remission lasting up to 3 months. In no patient was the graft permanent (i.e., all

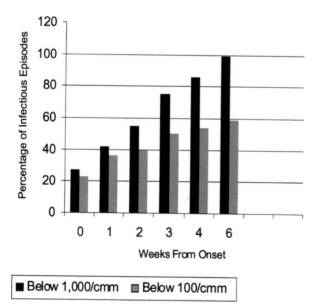

Figure 48–3. Duration of granulocytopenia and severe infection.

recipients rejected the graft), but the first demonstration that (at least in donors with chronic granulocytic leukemia) hematopoietic stem cells were capable of repopulating the entire myeloid bone marrow was encouraging for the future.

Although transfusion of granulocytes from donors with chronic myelocytic leukemia was obviously not a clinically practical solution to the problem of granulocytopenia, it did provide sufficient information to support the hypothesis that granulocyte transfusion might be an effective treatment modality. The circulating peripheral blood of the normal adult donor contains approximately 10^{11} granulocytes. Thus it was reasoned that if we could create biomechanical equipment capable of processing a donor's entire blood volume to extract buffy coat from the center of the sedimenting column, it might be possible to collect sufficient granulocytes from normal donors in a limited time to make granulocyte transfusion a regular component of supportive therapy. The first continuous-flow blood cell separator capable of collecting granulocytes from the buffy coat area was reported in 1965.[11] Its major limitations were related to difficulty in separating granulocytes from red cells; thus, early preparations were heavily contaminated with red cells and separation efficiency was low.

By 1974 it was possible to combine hydroxyethyl starch (to aggregate the red cells and improve separation efficiency) with administration of etiocholanilone or steroids to the donors to increase granulocyte concentration.[12] With these two maneuvers, it was possible to collect between 1×10^{10} and 4×10^{10} granulocytes, which is a marginally effective number of granulocytes, from a single donor. Limitations existed, however. The donors could not tolerate the procedure more than three times per week. Therefore, multiple donors were needed to sustain an individual patient. In addition, the problem of allosensitization was much more serious than it was for platelets because granulocyte isoantibodies are more complex and more dependent on HLA compatibility.[13]

The discovery of the myeloid growth factors, granulocyte colony-stimulating factor, and granulocyte macrophage colony-stimulating factor, has made transfusion of allogeneic granulocytes from normal volunteer donors a practical reality. Although still expensive and time-consuming and requiring good equipment, granulocyte transfusion is an important component of treatment of antibiotic-resistant infections in neutropenic patients.[14]

The major tool for the control of infections has been antibiotics, which date back to the sulfonamide and penicillin era. By the early 1960s the practice of infectious disease specialists was to observe patients and then attempt to isolate the organism aggressively because the range of available antibiotics and chemotherapeutic agents was fairly narrow. To treat infection appropriately required identification of the infecting organism. In the mid-1960s it was realized that the time required to identify the offending organism might be longer than the patient's average life span because the offending organism was often not recognized until after a fatal complication. The practice of empiric antibiotic therapy then began; it became the norm, almost worldwide, to recognize signs and symptoms of infection and to initiate the antibiotic therapy empirically with the broadest-spectrum drugs available.[15] This policy made no great impact on the management and prevention of infection until 1970, when the broad-spectrum antibiotics, beginning with carbenicillin, were introduced. Over the last 30 years, broader-spectrum combination antibiotic regimens have continuously evolved, accompanied by the struggle between the development of resistance to chosen regimens and the development of innovative antibiotic strategies. Prevention and treatment of microbial infection are now highly effective, and mortality is low from these infectious complications. A growing problem with fungal infections has now emerged, for which both prophylaxis and treatment are only marginally effective.

HEMATOPOIETIC STEM CELL THERAPY

As early as 1971 it was demonstrated that the peripheral blood of normal volunteer donors contained stem cells capable of making multilineage myeloid hematopoietic colonies, the so-called myeloid stem cells, in vitro.[16] The continuous-flow blood cell separator had the capacity to collect adequate numbers of stem cells to achieve at least temporary allografts in recipients. Also in the 1970s, the preclinical and clinical research on allogeneic bone marrow transplantation had made great strides. Collecting cells by multiple aspirations of bone marrow from normal donors yielded a sufficient number of myeloid stem cells to achieve homografts in recipients who were properly conditioned to receive stem cell transplants from HLA-identical siblings. By 1975, Thomas and co-workers[17] had demonstrated the feasibility of allogeneic transplantation as a form of supportive therapy and subsequently showed that there was more to allogeneic transplant than supportive therapy, since the patients who were successfully engrafted had a higher rate of cure than could be predicted from the conditioning regimen alone. This has been ascribed to the now famous graft versus leukemia effect, a component of immunotherapy directed against the hematopoietic neoplasias. A major problem for myeloablative and immunosuppressive treatment and injection of the allogeneic marrow is the 3 to 4 weeks of severe pancytopenia that occurs before the marrow graft produces sufficient cells for the peripheral blood. Developments in the field of replacement of red cells, platelets, and granulocytes as well as in the use of aggressive antibiotic treatment and prophylaxis were absolutely essential to the success of the allogeneic marrow transplantation program.

Progress in allogeneic transplantation revived interest in the use of autologous bone marrow for supportive therapy, first reported in 1958.[18] The fact that autologous marrow stem cells could repopulate the marrow in a patient and the demonstration of stem cells in the peripheral blood led to studies using peripheral blood as the source of both autologous and allogeneic stem cells to support patients against the cytopenias induced by the therapy or by the conditioning regimens. This field has been greatly enhanced by developments in the area of colony-stimulating factors, which have the capacity to mobilize myeloid stem cells into peripheral blood. A new science of autologous and allogeneic transplantation based on peripheral blood stem cells is rapidly evolving.

FUTURE DEVELOPMENTS

Supportive therapy today, as scheduled in this section of the book, is a highly sophisticated discipline and forms an essential component of the care of all patients with hematopoietic malignancies. The history of supportive therapy is quite short, perhaps 40 years, and infection, hemorrhage, immunodeficiency, and graft-versus-host disease are still problems that limit the broad application of current therapies.[19] The use of surrogate end points has allowed effective replacement therapy red cells and platelets. The increased availability of granulocytes through the use of myeloid growth factors to increase the number of granulocytes in the donors has great potential.

The most important lead, however, is the discovery that it is possible to collect myeloid stem cells from the peripheral blood; hopefully, with growing knowledge of the hematopoietic factors that control proliferation and differentiation, it will be possible to make granulocyte "factories" that function in vitro to provide the patient with either autologous or compatible allogeneic granulocytes for prophylactic replacement. In the interim, antibiotic prophylaxis (both with the help of reverse isolation procedures such as the protected environment and with the discovery of the new, more potent, and broader-spectrum antibiotics) gives hope for infection prevention even for the granulocytopenic patient. Finally, immune reconstitution is a goal yet to be systematically studied. Transfusion of lymphocytes can transfer adoptive immunity, and more is being learned about the restoration of immune competence in recipients who have received severely immunosuppressive therapy, particularly for allogeneic and autologous transplant. The macrophage reticuloendothelial system and the immune lymphoid system, in addition to the granulocytes, are undoubtedly important players in the host defense against nosocomial organisms, particularly fungi, viruses, and protozoal organisms. The fact that supportive therapy has advanced so rapidly over the last 40 years suggests strongly that innovation in this field will play an important role in the control of the hematopoietic malignancies.

REFERENCES

1. Gaydos LA: The quantitative relation between platelet count and hemorrhage in patients with acute leukemia. N Engl J Med 266:905–909, 1962.
2. Freireich EJ, Schmidt PJ, Schneiderman MA, Frei E III: A comparative study of the effect of transfusion of fresh and preserved whole blood on bleeding in patients with acute leukemia. N Engl J Med 260:6–11, 1959.
3. Freireich EJ, Kliman A, Gaydos LA et al: Response to repeated platelet transfusions from the same donor. Ann Intern Med 59:277–287, 1963.
4. Kliman A, Carbone PP, Gaydos LA, Freireich EJ: Effects of intensive plasmapheresis on normal blood donors. Blood 23:647–656, 1964.
5. Freireich EJ: When to give platelet transfusions. Blood 82:682–683, 1993.
6. Hersh EM, Bodey GP, Nies BA, Freireich EJ: Causes of death in acute leukemia. A ten year study of 414 patients. JAMA 193:105–109, 1965.
7. Bodey GP, Buckley M, Sathe YS, Freireich EJ: Quantitative relationships between circulating leukocytes and infections in patients with acute leukemia. Ann Intern Med 64:328–340, 1966.
8. Freireich EJ, Morse EE, Bronson W, Carbone PP: Transfusion of granulocytes from donors with chronic myelocytic leukemia to leukopenic recipients. In Proceedings of the IXth Congress of the International Society of Hematology, vol. 1, pp. 549–557. 1962.
9. Freireich EJ, Levin RH, Whang J et al: The function and fate of transfused leukocytes from donors with chronic myelocytic leukemia in leukopenic recipients. Ann N Y Acad Sci 113:1081–1089, 1964.
10. Levin RH, Whang J, Tjio JH et al: Persistent mitosis of transfused homologous leukocytes in children receiving antileukemic therapy. Science 142:1305–1311, 1963.
11. Freireich EJ, Judson G, Levin RH: Separation and collection of leukocytes. Cancer Res 25:1516–1520, 1965.
12. McCredie KB, Freireich EJ, Hester JP, Vallejos C: Increased granulocyte collection with the blood cell separator and the addition of etiocholanolone and hydroxyethyl starch. Transfusion 14:357–364, 1974.
13. Hester JP, McCredie KB, Freireich EJ et al: Blood component collection and transfusion. Compr Ther 5:59–62, 1979.
14. Jendiroba DB, Freireich EJ: Granulocyte transfusions: From neutrophil replacement to immune reconstitution. Blood Rev 14, 219–227, 2000.
15. Bodey GP: Infections in patients with cancer. In Holland JF, Frei E III (eds.): Cancer Medicine, pp. 1339–1372. Lea & Febiger, Philadelphia, 1982.
16. McCredie KB, Hersh EM, Freireich EJ: Cells capable of colony formation in the peripheral blood of man. Science 171:293–294, 1971.
17. Thomas ED, Storb R, Clift RA et al: Bone marrow transplantation: Part 1. N Engl J Med 292:832–843, 1975.
18. Kurnick NB, Montano A, Gerdes JC et al: Preliminary observations in the treatment of postirradiation hematopoietic depression in man by the infusion of stored autogenous bone marrow. Ann Intern Med 49:973–986, 1958.
19. Freireich EJ, Lemak N: Milestones in Leukemia Research and Therapy. Johns Hopkins University Press, Baltimore, 1991.

49

Prevention of Infections in Patients With Hematological Malignancies

Maria Cecilia Dignani, Tahsine H. Mahfouz, and Elias J. Anaissie

INTRODUCTION AND GENERAL PRINCIPLES: A RISK-TARGETED APPROACH

The rationale for preventing infections in patients with hematological malignancy is based on the high morbidity and mortality rate of these infections[1] and the difficulty in making an early diagnosis.[1,2] Preventing these infections relies on infection control measures and antimicrobial chemoprophylaxis. While infection control measures are safe, chemoprophylaxis is associated with drug toxicity, drug-drug interactions, cost, and potential development of resistance to the antimicrobial agents used. It is therefore critical to limit chemoprophylaxis to those clinical settings where its benefits outweight its potential disadvantages.

Prophylaxis should be directed against those infections that are potentially preventable; are associated with high morbidity, mortality, and/or cost; and are particularly difficult to treat.

In these patients, prophylaxis is most beneficial during the periods at high risk for specific infections. Thus, time at risk is another major consideration in providing specific prophylactic measures. For example, autologous and allogeneic peripheral stem cell (PSCT) and/or bone marrow transplant (BMT) recipients are at a higher risk for bacterial and yeast infections immediately after the conditioning regimen, while the early postengraftment period is typically associated with mold, viral, and parasitic infections. The risk persists until immune recovery is complete (6 to 36 months later)[3–9] depending on the presence, severity, and immunosuppressive treatment of chronic graft-versus-host disease (GvHD).[6,10–12] In this late phase, encapsulated bacteria and herpes viruses account for most infectious morbidity.

Our risk-targeted approach to prophylaxis relies on providing specific prophylactic measures that are limited to the high-risk patient population and during the high-risk period for infection only. The selection of risk groups for prophylaxis is based on the understanding that the risk for infection in patients with hematological cancer results from the interaction of three factors (Table 49–1):

1. The patient's exposure (current and past) to pathogens
2. The patient's net state of immunosuppression
3. The presence of organ dysfunction

Table 49–1. Variables Associated With a High Risk of Infection in Patients With Hematological Cancer

I. Exposure to pathogens
    History of previous infection (fungal, viral such as hepatitis, CMV, mycobacterial, or parasitic)
    History of exposure to CMV, EBV, HSV, VZV, *Toxoplasma gondii*
    Colonization with likely pathogens (bacteria, fungi, other)
    Contaminated environment (air, food/water, other) with potential pathogens
    Contact with health care workers, carriers of potential pathogens
    History of living in or visiting endemic areas for mycosis, hepatitis, parasitic infections

II. Immunosuppression
    Underlying cancer
    Type: Acute myeloid leukemia, multiple myeloma
    Status: Active disease
- Older age
- Prolonged cytopenias: Absolute neutrophil count < 1000/ L; platelets < 50/μL; CD4 < 200/μL
- Significant immunosuppressors: methylprednisolone ≥ 1mg/kg/day × >14 days; fludarabine; Campath-1H; total body irradiation
- Therapy

Non-myeloablative: High-dose Ara-C containing regimens
Myeloablative with allogeneic rescue
Stem cell manipulation: CD34 selection, T-cell depletion
- GvHD

Stage and grade: Acute severe (grade II–IV); chronic extensive
- High risk for GvHD

Histocompatibility: Matched unrelated donor, donor/recipient mismatch, sex mismatch
Older donor
Inadequate GvHD prophylaxis
Donor allosensitization

III. Organ dysfunction
- Acute or chronic GvHD
- Mucositis grade >3
- Pulmonary function tests < 75 percent of normal?
- Renal failure (creatinine clearance < 30 ml/min)?

Abbreviations: CMV, cytomegalovirus; EBV, Epstein-Barr virus; HSV, herpes simplex virus; VZV, varicella zoster virus; GvHD, graft-versus-host disease.

Patients can be thus classified into high or low risk for infection depending on the presence and number of these factors (Table 49–2). The expected timing and type of infections likely to occur in these patients are shown in Table 49–3. Of note, prophylaxis should be extended to the outpatient setting as long as the patient is at risk.

In this chapter, we describe various effective strategies directed at the prevention of infections in patients with hematological malignancies, according to this risk-based strategy.

INFECTION CONTROL MEASURES

Patients and health care workers should be educated about the risk of and methods to prevent acquisition of pathogens (Table 49–4), as discussed in the following sections.

Table 49–2. Example of Risk Stratification for Infection in Patients Undergoing Peripheral Blood Stem Cell Transplantation (PSCT) or Remission Induction Therapy for Acute Myeloid Leukemia (AML)

	High Risk	Low Risk
PSCT	Older age (> 40 years)	Younger age (< 20 years)
	Non-CML chronic phase	CML-chronic phase
	Donor type: Mismatched, unrelated, haploidentical	Donor type: Matched related donor, syngeneic, autologous
	Stem cell: T-cell-depleted, low number of cells infused (< 3×10^8 cells/kg nucleated cells)	
	Severe mucositis	
	Graft failure	
	Steroids (methylprednisolone ≥ 1 mg/kg/day for > 14 days)	
	Acute GvHD grades II–IV	
	Chronic extensive GvHD	
Remission-induction AML	Older age (> 55 years)	Younger age (< 20 years)
	Poor performance status	Good performance status
	Refractory disease	Non–gut-damaging induction therapy
	Gut-damaging induction therapy	

Abbreviations: CML, chronic myeloid leukemia; GvHD: graft-versus-host disease.

Personal Hygiene

Handwashing

Handwashing remains the simplest and most effective measure to prevent the acquisition of organisms by patients.[13–16] Patients and health care workers should wash their hands before eating, smoking, or inserting or removing contact lenses, and after using the restroom, blowing their nose, coughing, sneezing, handling dirty items such as soiled gauzes or garbage, and after touching an animal. In addition, health care workers should also wash their hands between patients. All surfaces should be thoroughly cleaned, including wrists, palms, back of hands, fingers, and under the fingernails for at least 10 to 15 seconds. Bar soaps should be replaced by antiseptic or waterless alcohol-based solutions.[17] Alcohol provides the fastest, greatest, and longer lasting reduction in microbial counts from the skin.[18–20] Waterless alcohol-based solutions improve compliance with handwashing and are particularly useful when handwashing facilities are not readily available.[21] However, antisepsis with waterless alcohol-based solutions can only be achieved when the hands are clean and free of soil or organic material.[17] Hand lotions may harbor high counts of gram-negative rods.[22] Additional recommendations include the removal of rings prior to handwashing, keeping nails short and clean, and avoiding the use of artificial nails as they may carry pathogens[23] including *Pseudomonas aeruginosa*[24] and yeasts.[25] Only clear polish ensures the visualization of the subungual space for adequate cleaning.[17] Disposable paper towels are the best drying method and can also be used to close faucets to prevent recontamina-

Table 49–3. Likely Pathogens in Peripheral Stem Cell (PSCT) or Bone Marrow Transplantation (BMT) Recipients (Without Prophylaxis)

Preengraftment (< 3 weeks) (autologous and allogeneic PSCT/BMT recipients and patients with hematological cancer undergoing chemotherapy without PSCT/BMT)

Bacterial	Fungal	Viral
Gram-positive	*Candida* spp.	Herpes simplex
Staphylococci	*albicans*	virus (HSV):
coagulase negative	*parapsilosis*	HSV-1 and 2
aureus	*tropicalis*	Respiratory viruses
Streptococcus viridans	Non-Candida	Respiratory
pneumoniae	spp.	syncytial
Enterococcus (including	*Aspergillus*	virus
VRE)	spp.	Influenza and
Gram-negative	*fumigatus*	parainfluenza
Enterobacteriaceae	*flavus*	Adenovirus
Escherichia coli	*terreus*	
Klebsiella spp.	*Fusarium* spp.	
Enterobacter	Other	
Pseudomonas		
aeruginosa		
Stenotrophomonas		
maltophilia		
Legionella pneumophilia		
Anaerobes		
Clostridium spp.		
(difficile, speticum)		

Immediate postengraftment (3 weeks–3 months) (autologous and allogeneic PSCT/BMT recipients and patients with hematological malignancy undergoing chemotherapy without PSCT/BMT)

Bacterial	Fungal	Viral	Protozoal
Same as above	*Aspergillus* spp. and other molds	CMV HHV-6 HSV VZV Respiratory viruses (as above)	*Pneumocystis carinii*

Late postengraftment (allogeneic BMT, patients with lymphoma, and on high-dose steroids)

Bacterial	Fungal	Viral	Protozoal
Encapsulated bacteria: *S. pneumoniae* *H. influenza* *N. meningitides* *Klebsiella* spp. *Staphylococcus aureus* *Pseudomonas aeruginosa*	Same as above	HSV EBV VZV Respiratory viruses (as above)	*Pneumocystis carinii* *Toxoplasma gondii*

Abbreviations: VRE, vancomycin-resistant enterococci; CMV, cytomegalovirus; HHV-6, human herpesvirus 6; VZV, varicella zoster virus; EBV, Epstein-Barr virus.

Table 49–4. Instructions to Give to Patients With Hematological Malignancies

Apply during periods of severe immunosuppression.
Allogeneic transplant recipients: maintain precautions until immunosuppressive drugs are discontinued.
Other patients: maintain precautions for up to 3 months after last dose of chemotherapy.

Personal hygiene	Bathe regularly using a mild soap and shampoo and rinse well
	Don't share razors (electric or blade) as they may retain particles of blood
	Wash hands frequently, preferably with liquid soap before eating and after contact with contaminated materials. If not washed, keep hands away from eyes, nose, and mouth
	Maintain good dental hygiene, by brushing teeth with soft bristle toothbrush after meals and floss daily. Do not share toothbrushes, and change toothbrush every 3 months
	Use disposable vaginal douches, and when menstruating, avoid tampons, change sanitary napkins frequently
	Use sitz baths or soothing lotion for irritations of the rectum or vagina
	Prevent skin dryness (use moisturizing creams)
	Keep nails short and clean and avoid nail clippers used by others
	Clip toenails straight across to prevent them from becoming ingrown
	Try to avoid trauma and irritation to the nails
	Wear cotton gloves for chores that don't involve water and rubber gloves for chores involving water
	Use an antifungal foot and shoe powder every day
	Avoid unprotected sexual exposure (HIV, human papillomavirus, herpes simplex, hepatitis B)
Environment	Discourage visits by individuals with respiratory infections
	Avoid crowded places, wear mask for outdoor activities
	Don't share towels with others
	Keep house and rooms well ventilated and change air filters monthly
	Encourage your household members to get the influenza vaccine
	Avoid swimming (particularly in stagnant water)
	Regularly clean kitchen counters, inside of refrigerators, microwave, sponges/towels used for cleaning, bathroom and shower, and kitchen floors (use 1:10 dilution of bleach)
	Ask your doctor for preventive measures before travel
	Avoid exploring caves, cleaning chicken coops (histoplasmosis)
Other patients	Avoid close contact with infected patients (tuberculosis, herpes zoster, herpes simplex, other)
	Avoid high-risk occupational settings (jails, homeless shelters, certain health care situations)
Supplements	Discontinue all supplements that exceed the recommended daily allowance (RDA) as a precaution against any potential protective effect these nutrients may afford the tumor.
Aerobic exercise	Aerobic exercise decreases physical deconditioning, length of hospital stay, severity of neutropenia, thrombocytopenia, and diarrhea
Medication/ vaccination/ health maintenance	Before traveling, consult your physician and take all medications
	Have a flu vaccine every year (September–December), a pneumonia vaccine every 5–6 years, and a tetanus-diphtheria booster every 5–10 years
	Have yearly breast and pelvic exams with Pap smears, mammograms yearly (depending on your age) (women), and rectal and colonic evaluation (men and women) yearly (depending on the patient's age)
Food/water	*Precautions for food handling*
	Cook food thoroughly, wash fruits/vegetables before eating
	Wash dishes and silverware in hot soapy water and dry them very well
	Keep uncooked meats separate from vegetables and fruits; wash hands, knives, and cutting boards after handling uncooked foods and clean kitchen surfaces that have come in contact with raw meat
	Avoid using tap water for drinking or making juices, other food items
	Refrain from skinning animals or cleaning seafood
	Use plastic bags in all trash cans for proper disposal
	At the supermarket, pick up perishables last and take them home promptly
	Defrost meat, turkey, chicken in the refrigerator
	Wash the meat before cooking
	Cook eggs and meat thoroughly (use thermometers)
	Clean your refrigerator regularly discarding food more than 3–4 days old, especially salad dressings, sauces, milk and egg products, condiments, processed meats, bacon
	Never use canned foods if the can is swollen, dented, or rusted
	Toss out any cheese or food that's moldy. Cut up fresh cheeses into small portions and store separately in the freezer, taking out only what can be used up quickly
	Keep cold foods cold (<40°F) and hot foods hot (>140°F)
	When preparing foods, hands should be kept away from the hair, mouth, and nose. If possible, rings and jewelry should be removed, because they may harbor germs. Try to limit touching food with the hands at all; use tongs or a fork if possible
	After cutting up raw meats, soak the cutting board and all utensils for 30–40 minutes in solution of one part bleach and eight or nine parts water—one ounce of bleach to a cup of water. All foods that are not going to be cooked should be prepared first; only after those are out of the way can any raw meat and poultry be prepared
	Wash all fruits and vegetables well
	Keep food preparation surfaces clean, and use a good dishwashing detergent on the work surface often, especially while handling raw meat, chicken, or fish
	Never let cats or other animals on the work surface

Do not prepare food if you have diarrhea or vomiting, or have an open infected sore

Put leftover foods into the refrigerator right away and divide large leftovers into individual containers (to avoid repeated warming).

Food restrictions

Raw eggs (sometimes used in restaurant-prepared Caesar salad dressing or homemade mayonnaise, eggnog)

Dried, uncooked or undercooked meats, seafood, and poultry (to include medium or rare steaks, game, pickled fish or oysters), or food from delis such as cold cuts, hot dogs, tofu, sausage, bacon, cold smoked fish and lox

Unpasteurized commercial fruit and vegetable juices

Unpasteurized milk or cheese products

Soft and aged cheeses such as feta, Brie, Camembert, blue-veined, Mexican-style cheese, refrigerated cheese-based salad dressings (e.g., blue cheese). *Cream cheese cottage cheese, or yogurt (provided they do not contain* Lactobacillus *spp.) are ok to eat*

Unwashed raw vegetables and fruits and those with visible mold

Unpasteurized honey or beer or raw, uncooked brewer's yeast

All miso products (e.g., miso soup); tempe (tempeh); maté tea

All moldy and outdated food products

Herbal preparations and nutrient supplements

tion when automatic shut off or foot control systems are not available.[17] Cloth towels should not be used.

Skin and Mucosal Care

The skin flora could potentially be a source of infections. Patients should keep their skin clean with daily baths using an antiseptic solution with special attention to potential portals of infection such as the perineum, and catheter sites. Females should wipe the perineum from front to back after using the bathroom to avoid urinary tract infections.[26] Menstruating women should consider avoiding the use of tampons to prevent lesions of the vaginal or cervical mucosa. *Staphylococcus aureus* causes significant disease in patients with hematological cancer,[27–29] and the nasal mucosa is its principal reservoir.[30–32] Topical mupirocin 2 percent is effective at eliminating carriage of *S. aureus* and decreasing infections in certain patient populations such as those undergoing hemodialysis,[33] and cardiothoracic[34] or upper gastrointestinal surgery.[35] We therefore recommend the application of this agent (1 to 3 times a day for 5 to 7 days) on the nares of patients with hematological malignancies who are colonized with *S. aureus*. Nasal recolonization by the same strain of *S. aureus* may occur in 40 to 50 percent of patients.[36] However, recolonization usually occurs 1 to 6 months after the end of mupirocin nasal treatment. Repeated courses of topical mupirocin may be needed in patients whose period of infection risk extends beyond 1 month.

The oral flora can lead to infection especially in the setting of severe mucositis, after radiotherapy, or in patients with GvHD. Recommendations to maintain a good oral and dental hygiene include:

1. Oral rinses 4 to 6 times a day with sterile water, normal saline, or sodium bicarbonate with/or without oral antiseptic solution (such as chlorhexidine).
2. Tooth brushing at least twice a day with a soft or ultrasoft toothbrush. Toothettes are less effective than toothbrushes in removing dental debris.[37]

Handling Pets

Pet owners should follow the guidelines for the prevention of zoonoses among immunocompromised patients[26,38] (Table 49–5). These recommendations include:

Table 49–5. Most Common Infections Associated With Exposure to Animals and Recommendations for Prevention[a]

Animal	Pathogen/Disease in Humans	Recommendations
Dogs	*Bordetella bronchiseptica*/ chronic respiratory infection	Do not expose dogs to dog shows, or kennels
	Pasteurella multocida[346]/ cellulitis, sepsis, meningitis	Avoid bites[b]
Dogs and cats	*Capnocytophaga canimorsus*[347,348]/sepsis	Avoid bites[b]
	Campylobacter spp./enteritis or colitis, bacteremia	See recommendations in text
	Salmonella spp./enterocolitis, bacteremia, meningitis	
	Cryptosporidium/severe diarrhea	
	Giardia/acute or chronic diarrhea	
Cats	*Toxoplasma gondii*/ toxoplasmosis	See recommendations in the text
		Wear gloves when gardening
	Bartonella henseleae/bacillary angiomatosis, cat-scratch disease	Avoid scratches or bites
		Flea control
Birds	*Campylobacter* spp./enteritis or colitis, bacteremia	Avoid contact with bird droppings.
	Salmonella spp./enterocolitis, bacteremia, meningitis	Do not clean the cage or do it with gloves and mask and handwashing afterward. See recommendations in the text
	C. psitacci/pneumonia	Avoid contact with pigeons and other wild birds
	Cryptococcus neoformans/ pneumonia, meningitis	
	Mycobacterium avium/ pneumonia, lymphadenitis, disseminated disease	Avoid contact with birds with avian tuberculosis
Fish	*Mycobacterium marinum*/skin infections	Wear gloves when cleaning aquariums

[a] Data from Angulo et al.,[38] Hermann et al.,[346] Pers et al.,[347] and Valtonen et al.[348]

[b] Prophylaxis with amoxicillin-clavulanic acid recommended for all immunocompromised patients experiencing a dog or cat bite.[346]

1. Avoiding young animals as pets (higher risk of shedding *Salmonella* spp. and *Campylobacter* spp. because of a higher incidence of diarrhea).
2. Obtaining veterinarian consultation when a new pet is adopted and yearly thereafter and keeping the pet's vaccinations current.
3. Keeping the pet's feeding areas clean and its litter box away from kitchen and eating areas.
4. Feeding pets only with high-quality commercial pet foods, cooked egg, poultry, and meat products, and pasteurized dairy products and avoiding access to toilet bowls and garbage.
5. Supervising pets when they are outdoors to prevent contact with other pet's feces.
6. Preventing animals from roaming through tick-infested woods.
7. Washing hands after handling pets and avoiding contact with the pet's feces and bird droppings.
8. Avoiding contact with animals with diarrhea, dogs exposed to shows or kennels, wild birds (especially pigeons), birds with avian tuberculosis, reptiles (high carriage and shedding of *Salmonella* spp.), and swine (source of *B. bronchiseptica*).
9. Keeping pets away from face and wounds.
10. Trimming the pet's nail short.
11. Notifying physician immediately if patient is bitten or injured by a pet.
12. Instructing children not to share kisses with the classroom pet.
13. When cleaning cages, wearing a particulate mask and avoiding shaking cages.

Other Personal Hygiene Items Including Food Handling

High-risk patients should follow additional precautions to prevent serious infections as summarized in Table 49–4.

Environmental Precautions

Hospital Environment

Air precautions: Air quality is important to prevent infections in high-risk patients by airborne organisms such as molds (*Aspergillus* spp. or other filamentous fungi), *Legionella* spp., or *Mycobacterium tuberculosis*. Patient rooms should be sealed to prevent air leaks by keeping windows and doors closed with pressure sensors for monitoring. High efficiency particulate air (HEPA) filter units (central or portable units) should be installed and properly maintained in patient rooms.[39] These units remove 99.97 percent of particles larger than 0.3 μm including *Aspergillus* spp. conidia. The conidia levels in outdoor air may vary from 1 to 5 CFU/m[40] to 2400 in winter and fall in certain areas.[40,41] The efficacy of HEPA filters in preventing the entry of contaminated outside air into the hospital was recently confirmed after the demolition of a building. Despite the increase in the number of conidia of filamentous fungi, no conidia were found in most HEPA-filter equipped areas.[42] The use of laminar airflow remains controversial because of its high cost and lack of demonstrable benefit compared to HEPA filtration.[43] Because construction and renovation may increase the concentration of airborne fungi, guidelines have been developed when such activities are taking place close to areas where high-risk patients are cared for.[39,44]

The safe concentration of airborne fungi is not established and probably depends on the patient's immune status. This may partially explain why some authors found a correlation between the incidence of invasive mycoses and the levels of airborne fungi,[45] while others could not.[46]

Short-lived, concentrated bursts of conidia generated by vacuuming or cleaning overhead light fixtures, and dust accumulation should be avoided.[47] All surfaces in clinical areas should be kept clean and dry.[39] Dirty linens must be carefully folded without shaking when removed from the bed. Although studies have not evaluated the effectiveness of these measures, they are simple to implement and add little to the cost of care. Exposure to plants and dried or fresh flowers should be avoided (increased number of airborne fungal spores).[45] Patients whose wounds are infected with *Aspergillus* spp. should be isolated since changing dressings may be associated with increase of spores in the air and transmission to other patients.[48] Airborne fungi have been recently shown to secondarily aerosolize from a water source.[49] Prevention of exposure to tap water can decrease the airborne concentration of fungal pathogens (see below).

The most common isolation procedure is *simple* (or *reverse*) *isolation* in a regular patient room once the patient's neutrophil counts drops below 1000/μl. In this type of isolation, the medical staff is required to wear gloves, gowns, and masks to reduce the transfer of microbes to these patients. This approach has not, however, been shown to be superior to managing patients in single rooms even in high-risk patients such as those with acute leukemia or recipients of BMT.[50,51]

Another isolation procedure is referred to as *total protective environment*. This approach includes: 1. Laminar air flow (LAF) and constant positive airflow; 2. strict visitors policy (visitors required to wear sterile gowns, masks, caps, gloves, and booties when entering the room); 3. sterilization of all objects that come into contact with the patient including linen, water, food, reading material, clothes, etc.; 4. daily baths with antiseptic solutions; and 5. oral nonabsorbable antibiotics. This strategy was beneficial in some studies,[52–54] but not in others.[55–57] Furthermore, this approach is expensive, creates a barrier between the caregiver and the patient, and is poorly tolerated by most patients. The lack of consistent benefit from this strategy may be explained by the endogenous source of most infections that are more readily amenable to prevention by the more recent potent and broad-spectrum antimicrobial agents.[56]

The limited benefit from these special isolation precautions (protected environment, reverse isolation) is further supported by the safe administration of autologous[58–62] and allogeneic[63–66] PSCT/BMT in the outpatient setting. On the basis of these data, we do not recommend total protective environment or reverse isolation for the routine care of patients with hematological malignancy.

Diet: No data exist to support a role for sterile or low-level microbial-content (<1000 CFU/ml of nonpathogenic organisms) diets for all patients with hematological malignancy. These diets are probably useful only in high-risk patients including those with severe mucositis and prolonged, profound neutropenia (<100 neutrophils/μl for longer than a week), and patients with intestinal GvHD.[67] In these patients, food items that are likely to contain pathogens should be avoided including nonprocessed dairy products, salads, and fruits that are difficult to peel (Table 49–4). All food should be properly cooked and covered until delivery to the patient.

Supplements: Patients should be warned regarding the risks of infection from ingesting nonconventional medications (alternative medicine) as these can harbor various pathogens including fungi and bacteria.[68] For example, hepatic mucormycosis developed in a BMT patient with GvHD following the ingestion of contaminated naturopathic medicine.[69]

Water: The hospital water system can be a reservoir for *Legionella* spp.,[70] bacteria,[71] and the opportunistic molds, especially *Aspergillus* spp.,[49,72] *Fusarium* spp.,[73] and *Exofiala jeanselmei*.[74] High-risk patients should thus avoid exposure to tap water and should be provided with sterile water and a sterile sponge instead of showering.[49]

Health care workers: Infections can be transmitted from the health care worker to the patient. The risk of transmission is high for varicella zoster (VZV), viral conjunctivitis, measles, and tuberculosis, and intermediate for influenza, mumps, parvovirus B19, pertussis, respiratory syncytial virus (RSV), rotavirus, and rubella. Therefore, health care workers with any of the above-mentioned infections or with HSV lesions in lips or fingers should not be in contact with patients.[75] Health care workers who care for patients with hematological cancer should be immunized against rubella, measles, mumps, influenza, and chickenpox, in addition to the already recommended tetanus and hepatitis B immunization.[76]

Health care workers can also be the source of other pathogens such as vancomycin-resistant *Enterococci* (VRE), methicillin-resistant *S. aureus*, *C. difficile*, and *Candida* spp., through hand carriage.[77,78] Therefore, adequate compliance of the health care worker with handwashing is recommended to decrease the risk of transmission of these pathogens to patients.

Household Exposure

The recommendations for immunization and precautions that apply to the health care worker also apply to close contacts of patients with hematological cancer.[26] Immunization against hepatitis A and B is highly recommended for sexual contacts of patients. In addition, immunization against hepatitis A should be considered for all households of patients with chronic liver disease or those living in endemic areas. Oral polio vaccine is contraindicated for all households of patients with hematological cancer since live polioviruses can be transmitted to and cause disease in immunocompromised patients,[79] especially during the first month after vaccination.[79–82] Patients with hematological cancer should also avoid exposure to individuals with vesicular rash secondary to chickenpox immunization to prevent VZV disease.[83,84]

Sexual partners: Sexually active patients should avoid unprotected sex during the periods of significant immunosuppression to reduce the risk of exposure to cytomegalovirus (CMV), and herpes simplex virus (HSV) when the patient is seronegative for these agents while the sexual partner is seropositive.[26]

Iatrogenic Procedures

Invasive Procedures

Procedures that break the integrity of natural barriers such as skin and mucosa should be avoided when possible. Fixed orthodontic appliances and space maintainers should not be worn during any period of neutropenia to avoid oral trauma and infection.[37] Enemas, suppositories, rectal temperature check and/or rectal examination are contraindicated. Necessary dental procedures should be performed prior to chemotherapy to allow proper healing before neutropenia and mucositis develop.[26] Bone marrow biopsies should be done aseptically to avoid cellulitis and osteomyelitis. Cleaning instruments (for gastrointestinal endoscopy, bronchoscopy, others) should follow recommended guidelines.[85,86]

Recommendations for the insertion of indwelling devices include careful cleaning and sterilization of instruments and devices (particularly reusable ones)[87] and guidelines for the prevention of intravascular device-related infections.[88] However, solid evidence to support some of the guidelines for the prevention of intravascular device-related infections is lacking.

Blood Transfusions

Contaminated blood transfusions can be associated with infections[89] by various pathogens including the following.

Bacterial: brucellosis, salmonellosis, yersiniosis, and infections with gram-positive or gram-negative organisms.

Spirochetal: syphilis, relapsing fever.

Parasitic (in endemic areas): malaria, babesiosis, trypanosomiasis, toxoplasmosis, leishmaniasis, and filariasis.

Viral: hepatitis A virus (HAV), hepatitis B virus (HBV), hepatitis C virus (HCV), hepatitis D virus, agents of non-A non-B hepatitis, CMV, Epstein-Barr virus (EBV), HIV 1–2, human T-cell lymphotropic virus (HTLV 1–2), parvovirus, Colorado tick fever virus, human herpesvirus-6 (HHV-6).

Rickettsial: R. rickettsii and *Coxiella burnetii*.

Bacterial contamination of hematopoietic stem cells has been suggested as a potential source of infection. In one report, 14 percent of 73 patients who received contaminated stem cells developed fever or bacteremia within 48 hours of the infusion, without sequelae. However, the same organism (same species and antibiogram) was recovered from the patient's blood stream in only two cases.[90] Stem cells should be collected and stored under aseptic conditions to prevent contamination. Culturing collected stem cells after processing and immediately before infusion is recommended.[26]

The transmission of CMV (and probably EBV and HHV-6) through blood products is of particular importance in the setting of allogeneic PSCT/BMT and should be avoided (see section The Stem Cell/Bone Marrow Donor).

The standards of the American Association of Blood Banks aim to protect recipients from these infections by screening blood donors with a thorough questionnaire, physical examination, and a series of tests.[91] These tests include hepatitis B surface antigen (HBsAg), hepatitis B core antibody (anti-HBc), anti-HCV, anti-HIV 1–2, HIV-1 p24 antigen, anti-HTLV-1–2, syphilis, and nucleic acid amplification testing for the detection of the viral genomes of HCV and HIV.

Stem Cell/Bone Marrow Infusions

Stem cell or bone marrow donors should be free of active infection at the time of donation to prevent the transmission of their infection to the recipient. In addition to the studies required by the blood bank for donation of blood products, donors should be tested for other relevant infections including the following.

Brucellosis: Transmission of brucellosis through blood[92] or bone marrow has been reported.[93,94] Testing donors for brucellosis in endemic areas and avoiding infected donors when possible is recommended.

Creutzfeldt-Jakob disease (CJD): There are no data regarding transmission of CJD through blood or stem cell/bone marrow donation. However, until more information is available, donors with risk factors for the classic or the new variant CJD (nvCJD) should be avoided unless no other donor is available. Risk factors for CJD include: 1. A blood relative with CJD, 2. receipt of a human pituitary-derived growth hormone or of a cornea or dura graft, 3. history of travel to or living in the United Kingdom for 6 months or longer during 1980 to 1996, and 4. receipt of injectable bovine insulin after 1980.[26]

CMV: Stem cell or bone marrow donors who test positive for CMV antibodies can transmit this infection to the recipients. This transmission is mainly relevant when the recipient is CMV seronegative. In this setting, the recipient's risk of acquiring CMV is approximately 40 percent.[95] This risk is lower (15 percent) when the donor is CMV positive and all transfused blood products are filtered.[96] All donors and recipients should be tested for CMV. If the recipient is seronegative, all efforts should be made to use a seronegative donor and CMV-free blood transfusions. Removal of leukocytes (the reservoir for CMV) from

transfused blood products by filtration,[97] centrifugation,[98] use of frozen/thawed deglycerolized red blood,[99] or fluidized bed separation[100] can prevent the transmission of CMV infection.

If the recipient is seropositive, the risk of CMV transmission from a positive donor is not as clinically consequential as it may not add to the morbidity from reactivation of the recipient's own CMV infection.

EBV infection: Transmission of EBV through blood donation has been documented.[101] EBV can cause EBV-associated B-cell lymphoproliferative disease, also known as post-transplant lymphoproliferative disease (PTLD), among recipients of allogeneic PSCT. The frequency of PTLD is low (1.2 to 14 percent according to the type of transplant), but the outcome is usually fatal if not properly treated.[102] Data from solid organ transplantation suggest that EBV-seronegative recipients are at increased risk of developing PTLD compared to seropositive recipients.[103] Limited data from pediatric BMT recipients do not, however, confirm this finding.[104] We suggest testing donors for EBV infection when the recipient is EBV-seronegative, particularly if the recipient is at higher risk of developing PTLD because of T-cell depletion. Seropositive donors should be avoided unless no other donor is available. In such setting, filtering blood products to minimize exposure to exogenous EBV strains, and close monitoring of the patient's EBV blood viral load are critical for preemptive therapy[105] (see section on systemic chemoprophylaxis).

Hepatitis A infection: Donors with acute hepatitis A may transmit the infection through platelets,[106] clotting factor concentrates,[107] or bone marrow[108] during the period of viremia. This period has a mean duration of 18 days.[109] Consideration should be given to testing the PSCT/BMT donors for acute hepatitis A with IgM anti-HAV. Individuals who test positive should not donate for 4 weeks.

Hepatitis B and C infection: Individuals with a history of hepatitis B or C infection are rejected for donation of blood products. However, the only available stem cell or bone marrow donor may have a history of hepatitis B or C infection. Using such donors may be possible depending on various factors (Table 49–6).[110]

Table 49–6. Hepatitis B or C: Risks to Recipient According to the Infection Status of Donors and Recipients Prior to Allogeneic Transplantation

Donor Serology	Donor Status	Recipient Risk
HBsAb (+) alone	The donor is immune after vaccination	No impact in transplant, the recipient may develop HBsAb
HBsAb (+) and HBcAb (+)	The donor is immune after disease	No impact in transplant, the recipient may develop HBsAb
HBcAb (+) alone	Prior exposure. Latent HBV possible	Test donor for DNA, if (−) little risk to the recipient, if (+) consider treat the donor[a]
HBsAg (+) or HBeAg (+) or HBV DNA (+)	Current donor infection	Potential donor risk[b] Risk of transmission to patient[c] Consider another equally matched donor, especially if the recipient is (−) or treat donor[a]
HCVAb (+) and HCV RNA (+)	Current donor infection	Potential donor risk[b] Very high risk of transmission[c] Consider another equally matched donor or treat donor[a]

[a] Consider donor treatment (1–3 months for HCV, 6 months for HBV) to reduce risk of transmission. Treat until (−) serum HCV RNA.
[b] Donor risk during anesthesia if cirrhosis present.
[c] Risk of transmission to patient leading to fulminant or chronic hepatitis post-transplant.

HSV infection: Sequences of HSV DNA were found in blood and bone marrow cells of healthy donors, suggesting that these cells could be a site of HSV latency.[111] However, no case of donor-derived HSV transmission has been reported among PSCT/BMT recipients. Almost all HSV infections in transplant recipients are caused by viral reactivation.[112] Testing donors for anti-HSV antibodies is not recommended unless the recipient is seronegative for this virus.

VZV infection: Testing donors for anti-VZV antibodies is a common practice in some centers, despite the absence of supporting data. Transmission of VZV through stem cell, bone marrow, or other blood products has not been reported, and most VZV infections in PSCT/BMT recipients are due to reactivation of latent infection.[113] The potential for transmission exists, however, if the donor has had recent (7 to 14 days) exposure or disease and is viremic at the time of donation. This situation is rare since most donors are adults, and, therefore, seropositive for anti-VZV antibodies. Based on a recent case of transmission of VZV through cardiac transplantation, we would recommend deferring donation if the donor had a recent episode of chickenpox or herpes zoster; or is susceptible to VZV and had a recent exposure to this virus.

Malaria: Transmission of malaria through BMT has been reported.[114,115] Avoidance of donors who have visited endemic areas for malaria is recommended unless donors have been free of malaria for at least 1 year after their departure from the endemic area. The stem cells of donors with a history of malaria could be used if these donors received appropriate treatment and remained asymptomatic for at least 3 years. Individuals from endemic areas should refrain from donating for at least 3 years after departure from the endemic area provided they remain asymptomatic during that period of time.[26]

Toxoplasmosis: Transmission of *Toxoplasma gondii* by transfusion of blood products has been documented[116] and occurs during acute infection. *T. gondii* can survive in citrated blood for up to 50 days.[117] Most cases of toxoplasmosis after transplantation are due to reactivation of previous infection. However, toxoplasmosis has been reported in patients who were seronegative prior to transplantation,[118,119] suggesting the possibility of blood product transmission, exogenous acquisition from the environment, or failure of the test to detect circulating antibodies prior to transplantation.

Donors can transmit the infection during the acute phase, although the probability of acute infection at the time of donation is very low.[120] The currently used testing for IgG antibodies does not differentiate between acute and chronic infection. A toxoplasmosis serology panel including IgM, IgA, and IgE is more specific but significantly more expensive. We thus recommend using this panel only if the donor IgG titers are positive. If acute infection is documented, an alternative donor should be considered. Otherwise, donation should be delayed until resolution of parasitemia (a minimum of 4 weeks).

Chagas' disease: Blood donors with acute or chronic Chagas' disease can transmit this infection to the recipient,[121] even after three decades of infection.[122] Donors from endemic areas should be tested for Chagas' disease for the following reasons: 1. The blood bank questionnaire provided to donors will not identify all infected individuals[121]; 2. Chagas' disease may be present in nonendemic areas including in the United States[123,124]; 3. the number of donors and recipients traveling from endemic to nonendemic areas to undergo donation/transplantation is increasing; 4. transplant recipients frequently receive platelet transfusions, which have a higher risk of transmission of Chagas' disease than other blood components[122]; and 5. Chagas' disease can be fatal in immunocompromised hosts.[124–128]

Chagas' disease should be excluded by two different tests (e.g. ELISA and indirect hemagglutination) because of the risk of false negatives when a single test is used.[128,129]

The product of donors who test positive for Chagas' disease should not be infused unless no other donor is available, in which case prophylaxis or preemptive therapy for the recipient should be provided.[130,131] Preemptive therapy consists of weekly surveillance for parasitemia for at least 100 days after transplantation and initiation of benznidazole therapy when the infection is detected.[130]

Donors who recently received live vaccines: Donors who have recently been vaccinated with live vaccines (BCG, MMR, oral polio, oral adenovirus, varicella, yellow fever, or oral typhoid) could potentially transmit the vaccine agent to the recipient and should refrain from donating stem cells for at least 4 weeks after vaccination.[26]

Preventing Travel-Related Infections

Patients with hematological malignancies may be at higher risk for acquiring infections during travel. General and specific recommendations prior to travel should be given as follows.

General Recommendations

- Review feasibility of planned travel (status of underlying disease to estimate risk of infection).
- Identify medical resources abroad (especially if planning long trips or trips to developing countries).
- Arrange in advance for continuation of therapy abroad.
- Obtain medical insurance that will provide coverage during the trip.
- Anticipate legal and immigration issues (including required immunizations to enter in some countries).
- Review itinerary and area-specific risks.
- Advise patients to avoid:

1. Mosquito bites to prevent vector-borne infections
2. Poorly ventilated and crowded buildings to prevent respiratory infections such as influenza, endemic mycoses (histoplasmosis, coccidioidomycosis, paracoccidioidomycosis), or tuberculosis
3. Spa facilities to prevent Legionnaires' disease
4. Swimming in club pools or drinking water while swimming (to prevent enteric infections), swimming in the presence of external otitis (to prevent worsening), or skin wounds (to prevent skin infections)
5. Contact with sick individuals (report any contact to the treating physician)

6. Injuries and contact with blood
7. Risky food and beverages to prevent the most common enteric infections (*Salmonella, Shigella, E. coli,* and *Campylobacter* spp.). We suggest giving a prescription for antibiotics such as fluoroquinolones to be used as prophylaxis or empirical therapy in the event of an acute diarrheal illness. Other food-borne infections include microsporidiosis, amebiasis, cryptosporidiosis, giardiasis, isosporiasis, hepatitis A, hepatitis E, polio, cholera, and infections by *Vibrio parahaemolyticus* and noncholera *Vibrio* spp. The likelihood of acquiring any of these enteric infections depends on the visited area.
8. Unsafe sexual practices (to prevent sexually transmitted diseases including HIV and hepatitis)

Specific Recommendations for Patients Traveling to Endemic Areas

Malaria: provide antimalarial prophylaxis with Fansidar, or mefloquine if allergic to sulfonamides.

Yellow fever: avoid the vaccine (contains live viruses and may cause infection). Focus on avoiding mosquito bites.

Immunization Prior to Travel

Three factors need to be considered when recommending vaccination prior to travel: the need for protection, the increased risk of adverse events, and the time available between the date of immunization and the date of travel. The latter may render active immunization less appealing than passive immunoglobulin administration in certain situations such as for the prevention of measles, tetanus, and hepatitis A or B.

The live vaccines that are contraindicated in patients with hematological malignancies include BCG, MMR, oral polio, oral adenovirus, varicella, yellow fever, and oral typhoid vaccines.[132]

POSTEXPOSURE PROPHYLAXIS

Postexposure prophylaxis consists of providing specific measures (drugs, immunization, other) after exposure to a known pathogen in order to avoid the development of infection.

Hepatitis A Virus

The highest risk of acquiring HAV infection exists when a susceptible patient is exposed to a close contact (households or sexual contacts) with persons with confirmed hepatitis A infection, or to food contaminated by a food handler with active hepatitis A.[133] Patients are considered susceptible if they are seronegative for HAV, and if the first dose of hepatitis A vaccine was given less than 1 month prior to exposure.[133] Up to 15 percent of patients who undergo PSCT or BMT after their infection with HAV may lose this protection during the first year following transplantation.[134] The strategy for postexposure prophylaxis in HAV is based on data from immunocompetent patients. Immune globulin (IG) (0.02 ml/kg, im) is more than 85 percent effective in preventing HAV infection when given

within 2 weeks following exposure.[135–137] Since this protection is short-lived (1 to 2 months), immediate immunization with hepatitis A vaccine is also recommended.

Hepatitis B Virus

Exposure to an infected sexual partner[138–140] or to other percutaneous or permucosal source of HBsAg-positive blood (including toothbrushes or razors)[75] puts patients at a 10 to 50 percent risk of acquiring this infection.[141] The recommended postexposure prophylaxis is based on data from immunocompetent individuals. Prophylaxis consists of hepatitis B immune globulin (HBIG) (two doses of 0.06 ml/kg im) plus a first dose of HBV vaccine.[141–143] The HBIG prevents hepatitis B infection in 75 percent of recipients.[144–146] Vaccination is added to maintain long-term protection.[143] Although HBIG is still protective when given several weeks after exposure,[144] the product should ideally be given within 7 days of exposure. Until more data from immunocompromised hosts are available, we recommend giving a second dose of HBIG 1 month after exposure. Immune serum globulin (ISG) with detectable levels of anti-HBs may be used if HBIG is not available.[147] When given to health care workers within 3 days after accidental exposure, HBV vaccine alone is as protective as the combination of vaccine plus HBIG.[148] However, immunocompromised patients with hematological malignancies are less likely to respond to vaccination. Thus more data are needed before this approach can be recommended to such patients.

Hepatitis C Virus

Patients may be at increased risk (approximately 10 percent) of acquiring HCV infection following a percutaneous or permucosal exposure (including sex) to HCV-positive blood[149–151] or exposure to a household with HCV infection.[152] The risk of sexual transmission may be higher when the male is infected with HCV.[153] The long-term risk of progression to cirrhosis in immunocompromised patients with HCV infection may be twice higher than in otherwise normal hosts (20 vs. 11 percent, after a mean of 12 years).[154] Postexposure prophylaxis with immunglobulins is not useful.[152] Postexposure prophylaxis for HCV infection is currently not recommended because of the significant toxicity of the therapeutic regimen and the limited data.[152] Instead, close follow-up for the early detection and treatment of HCV infection is preferred.[152] Although treating patients with acute HCV is not currently recommended, it might be considered in patients at high risk for developing cirrhosis, such as those older than 40 years,[154] and who are expected to be long-term survivors (thus likely to develop cirrhosis).

Human Immunodeficiency Virus

HIV infection may be acquired after a percutaneous (0.3 percent risk)[155] or permucosal (0.09 percent risk)[156] exposure to HIV-positive blood, or after sexual contact with an HIV-infected individual (0.1 to 3 percent).[157] Postexposure prophylaxis consists of a 4-week course of antiretroviral therapy to be started as soon as possible after exposure.[142]

Influenza Viruses

Immunocompromised patients exposed to households with active influenza infection are at risk of developing this infection. Vaccinated patients should receive postexposure antiviral prophylaxis if contact with a household with active influenza infection occurred less than 14 days after vaccination. Nonvaccinated patients exposed to infected households should receive the combination of the influenza vaccine and an antiviral agent for 14 days.[158] Effective antiviral agents include amantadine (100 mg bid), and rimantadine (100 mg bid) (both effective against influenza A),[158] and inhaled zanamivir 10 mg bid[159] and oral oseltamivir (75 mg/day)[160] (both effective against influenza A and B). The efficacy of these agents in preventing influenza infection is around 75 percent in immunocompetent individuals.[159–164] Since zanamivir and oseltamivir are significantly more expensive than amantadine and rimantadine, and since influenza B infection is rather uncommon, the use of these agents should be limited to settings where influenza B is the predominant circulating strain.

Measles

Because of the risk of acquiring measles after significant exposure such as a household contact, immune globulin 0.5 ml/kg (15 ml maximal dose) im within 6 days of exposure is recommended. For patients who regularly receive intravenous immune globulin (IVIG) preparations, the usual dose of 100 to 400 mg/kg should provide adequate prophylaxis when exposure occurs within 3 weeks of the last IVIG dose.[165] However, no data are available to support the effectiveness of IVIG in preventing measles. Live measles vaccine is contraindicated in immunocompromised patients because it can cause disease.[165]

Mumps

Immunocompromised patients exposed to households with mumps may develop this infection. There is no known preventive strategy and the live MMR vaccine is contraindicated.

Varicella Zoster Virus

There is a substantial risk of acquiring VZV infection if the contact with the index case was longer than 1 hour sharing the same room.[83] Following such exposure, chickenpox develops in 90 percent[166] of susceptible immunocompetent contacts and in up to 70 percent of immunocompromised contacts who receive the varicella zoster immune globulin (VZIG) or the herpes zoster immune globulin (ZIG).[167,168] While VZIG decreases somewhat the attack rate among immunocompromised children when given within 96 hours of exposure,[169] it is expensive, not always available,[170] and offers only limited protection.[167] In addition, the duration of the protection offered by VZIG is unknown (probably short), thus leaving these patients at risk for subsequent VZV infection. Thus, postexposure prophylaxis should mainly rely on antiviral therapy since it has been shown more effective for postexposure prophylaxis.

When started 7 days after exposure, acyclovir prophylaxis (40 mg/kg daily for 7 days) decreases the attack rate among immunocompetent children from 100 to 27 percent.[171] Only mild varicella was observed among those 27 percent of patients who developed disease. This strategy was associated with a 73 percent seroconversion among children who did not develop disease, leaving 27 percent of these patients susceptible to future VZV exposure. Acyclovir is a safe, inexpensive, and readily available drug, and effectively prevents VZV reactivation among adult BMT recipients.[172–174] We thus recommend high-dose acyclovir (800 mg po 5 times daily for 14 days) as postexposure prophylaxis to all patients, starting as soon as possible after exposure. Alternative agents include valacyclovir and famciclovir. Serology for VZV should be obtained to determine the susceptibility to future exposure.

Although a previous history of varicella or herpes zoster may protect the patient against a new VZV exposure, it should be considered that patients who undergo PSCT/BMT are likely to lose this protection,[175] and that immunocompromised VZV-seropositive patients may still develop disease.[83] Limiting postexposure prophylaxis to seronegative patients is not recommended.

Endemic Mycoses

Patients with hematological cancer may be at high risk of acquiring endemic mycoses (blastomycosis, coccidioidomycosis, histoplasmosis, and paracoccidioidomycosis) following visits to endemic areas.[176] There are no guidelines for the prevention of these infections. However, the antifungal prophylaxis provided in the setting of cytotoxic chemotherapy should be adequate to prevent primary infections or reactivation of these mycoses.

Tuberculosis

Thirty to 80 percent of immunocompetent households of smear-positive patients with tuberculosis develop this infection.[177] The guidelines for postexposure prophylaxis recommended for immunocompetent individuals[178] may not apply to patients with hematological malignancies since these patients may be anergic on the tuberculin skin test, even in the setting of active infection.[26,179] Therefore, immunocompromised patients who have a significant tuberculosis exposure should receive a 9-month course of prophylactic isoniazid.[26,179] Immunocompromised patients should also be separated from the infected household member until three smears from these infected individuals are negative for *Mycobacterium tuberculosis*.

SYSTEMIC CHEMOPROPHYLAXIS (PRIMARY AND SECONDARY PROPHYLAXIS AND PREEMPTIVE THERAPY)

Different strategies may be used including primary and secondary prophylaxis and preemptive therapy. Primary prophylaxis refers to providing protective agents before the onset of infection while secondary prophylaxis is intended to prevent reactivation of a previously documented infection when patients are undergoing additional immunosuppression. Preemptive therapy aims at reducing patient exposure to antimicrobial agents by limiting these agents to patients with evidence of early infection as detected by different laboratory tests.

During the period of granulocytopenia aerobic gram-positive and gram-negative bacteria, and *Candida* spp. are the most frequently documented infections. The main risk factors for these infections during this period are microbial colonization, mucosal damage, and neutropenia. The presence, duration, and severity of these factors determine the need for and type of antimicrobial prophylaxis. Following the period of neutropenia, cellular immunosuppression continues. Therefore, we suggest continuing antimicrobial prophylaxis until CD4 is greater than 200/µl for 3 to 6 months, extensive chronic GvHD (cGvHD) has resolved, and immunosuppressive agents have been stopped. Prophylaxis for infection by encapsulated bacteria may be needed lifelong in allogeneic PSCT/BMT recipients.

Antibacterial Prophylaxis

The high frequency and severity of gram-negative bacterial infections have led to attempts to suppress the intestinal flora to prevent invasive infections. The absorbable agents such as the fluoroquinolones or trimethoprim-sulfamethoxazole (TMP-SMX) have now replaced the oral nonabsorbable antibiotics (gentamicin, vancomycin, neomycin, colistin, and nystatin). The former agents are more effective and better tolerated.

Compared to TMP-SMX, fluoroquinolones offer superior protection against gram-negative bacillary infections and a better safety profile.[180–182]

Controversy still exists regarding the use of fluoroquinolone prophylaxis in neutropenic patients with hematological cancer. In favor of the use of these agents in this setting is the reduction in morbidity (gram-negative infections and febrile episodes). Mitigating against their use is the lack of effect on infection-related mortality, and the potential emergence of infections by quinolone-resistant organisms. Two meta-analyses (including a total of >3000 patients) evaluated the efficacy of fluoroquinolones in preventing infections, fevers, and infection-related deaths among neutropenic cancer patients. In one analysis, fluoroquinolone prophylaxis was compared to a control group that included patients receiving TMP-SMX, nonabsorbable antibiotics, and placebo.[183] The second analysis compared fluoroquinolone prophylaxis to no prophylaxis or to TMP-SMX.[180] Both meta-analyses showed that prophylaxis with fluoroquinolones significantly decreased the incidence of gram-negative infections without affecting the incidence of gram-positive infections or infection-related mortality. In addition, one study showed a significant reduction in the incidence of all infections and febrile episodes with fluoroquinolone prophylaxis.[180] This effect was not associated with an increase in fungal infections and infections caused by quinolone-resistant organisms. The addition of gram-positive prophylaxis to fluoroquinolones reduced infections by gram-positive bacteria without altering the incidence of fevers or infection-related mortality.[183]

Individual studies did show some concomitant increase in the frequency of gram-positive infections such as alpha-hemolytic streptococci.[184] Most of these streptococcal infections during fluoroquinolone prophylaxis may be prevented by penicillin or macrolides,[185] although some streptococci are resistant to these agents.[186] Intravenous vancomycin is effective at preventing such infections,[187] but should be avoided because of the emergence of *Enterococci* and *Staphylococci* resistant to this agent.[188,189]

In contrast to the findings obtained from the two meta-analyses mentioned above, two retrospective studies showed that the lack of fluoroquinolone prophylaxis was a risk factor for mortality in neutropenic cancer patients with serious infections.[190,191]

After engraftment, allogeneic PSCT recipients should be continued on antibacterial prophylaxis for encapsulated bacteria, particularly *S. pneumoniae*, as these infections may still occur several years after PSCT.[192] Recipients of autologous PSCT do not require antibacterial prophylaxis beyond engraftment unless they have additional risk factors for bacterial infections.

Antibacterial prophylaxis with oral metronidazole 400 mg three times daily (active against anaerobic intestinal flora) has been used in one study to prevent GvHD among recipients of allogeneic BMT receiving an HLA-identical sibling product.[193] However, no differences in chronic GvHD or overall survival were seen.

We suggest providing antibacterial prophylaxis with fluoroquinolones (or TMP-SMX in special settings) to patients at high risk of serious bacterial infection (see section General Principles and Tables 49–1 to 49–3).

Antifungal Prophylaxis

The increasing incidence and the high mortality[194–196] associated with invasive fungal infections has led to the introduction of antifungal prophylaxis in neutropenic patients with hematological cancer. *Candida* spp. and *Aspergillus* spp. cause the majority of the invasive fungal infections although candidiasis has significantly decreased since the introduction of triazole prophylaxis.

Antifungal prophylaxis with fluconazole has significantly reduced the morbidity and mortality of invasive candidiasis,[197,198] perhaps at a cost of increasing azole-resistant *Candida* spp. (*C. krusei* and *C. glabrata*) in some settings.[199,200] Itraconazole capsules (200 mg/day)[201] and solution (5 mg/kg/day)[202] are also effective in reducing hematogenous candidiasis in these patients,[202] without significant toxicity.

Prevention of aspergillosis remains an unresolved challenge. Measures to decrease the environmental load of airborne *Aspergillus* spores have a potential for effectively preventing aspergillosis. These measures include HEPA filtration in patient rooms, area decontamination with copper-8-quinolinate, and installation of airtight plastic and drywall construction barriers and negative-pressure ventilation in and external venting from the construction areas.[40,196,203] We have recently shown that hospital water can be a reservoir for opportunistic molds including aspergilli, and that patient exposure to this reservoir may lead to invasive mold infections.[204,205] Therefore, we recommend avoiding patient exposure to tap water during periods of severe immunosuppression.

A probably effective strategy to decrease the mortality related to aspergillosis relies on early diagnosis with high-resolution computed tomography (CT) scan of chest, and weekly screening for *Aspergillus* antigen in serum and prompt initiation of antifungal therapy.[206] This strategy is reportedly associated with a 75 to 80 percent success rate.

A recent study compared the clinical value of a newly developed real-time polymerase chain reaction (PCR), the galactomannan *Aspergillus* antigen by ELISA, the measurement of the plasma (1,3)-Beta-D-glucan (BDG) concentration, and the CT scan for the early diagnosis of invasive aspergillosis. Real-time PCR for *Aspergillus* spp. and CT scan were the earlier tests to provide diagnosis.[207]

Secondary Chemoprophylaxis

Patients experiencing additional immunosuppression in the setting of pre-existing aspergillosis are at risk for recrudescence of their infection, and secondary prophylaxis is indicated.[208–210] Amphotericin B and its lipid formulations and itraconazole have been used in this setting. Surgical resection of residual infected sites may also be indicated to reduce the likelihood of relapse and the risk of serious hemoptysis in patients with cavitary aspergillosis.[209–211] Long-term suppressive therapy may be needed in the setting of persistent, prolonged, immunosuppression.[212] Patients with chronic disseminated candidiasis who require additional cytotoxic chemotherapy for their underlying disease should probably also receive secondary prophylaxis.[213,214]

Our strategy among high-risk patients consists of weekly surveillance of throat and stool cultures for *Candida* spp., and serological markers for aspergillosis (galactomannan, BDG, or PCR). Prompt initiation of amphotericin B is recommended if patients are colonized with fluconazole-resistant fungi and/or have two consecutive positive serological tests for *Aspergillus*. Itraconazole preemptive therapy may be also indicated in patients with positive serological markers for *Aspergillus* spp. If cultures are positive for yeasts other than *C. glabrata* or *C. krusei*, we recommend fluconazole or itraconazole 400 mg per day starting on the first day of neutropenia and continuing until immunosuppression has resolved.[215]

Antiviral Prophylaxis

Most viral infections that complicate the course of chemotherapy in patients with hematologic malignancies represent reactivation of latent infections, while a minority are due to exogenous acquisition (such as respiratory viruses).

Cytomegalovirus

Prior to the routine use of prophylactic regimens, CMV seropositive allogeneic BMT recipients had a 70 to 80 percent risk of viral reactivation, and one-third of these patients developed CMV disease (mainly pneumonia)[216] with a high fatality rate.[217] CMV seropositive recipients of allogeneic T-cell depleted PSCT/BMT are even at higher risk for the development of CMV disease.[218–220] By contrast, CMV seropositive autologous PSCT/BMT recipients have a lower risk for viral

reactivation (40 percent) and disease (2 percent).[221] Recipients of CD34-selected autologous PPSCT have been reported to be at higher risk for CMV disease in one series,[222] but not in another.[223]

The risk of CMV pneumonia among patients with hematological malignancies not undergoing allogeneic PSCT/BMT is very low (4.6 cases per 1000 autopsies).[224] However, patients receiving treatment with fludarabine or Campath-1H seem to be at higher risk for CMV infection including pneumonia due to the T-cell deficiency associated with these agents.[225,226]

Two strategies were reported effective for the prophylaxis of CMV disease in allogeneic PPSCT/BMT recipients: universal prophylaxis and preemptive therapy.

Universal prophylaxis: Intravenous ganciclovir (5 mg/kg iv bid for 5 to 7 days prior to transplantation or at engraftment, and then daily until day 100 post-transplant) has resulted in a marked reduction of infection and/or disease but no reduction in mortality.[227,228] This strategy can lead to a significant increase in the incidence of bacterial and fungal superinfections associated with ganciclovir-induced neutropenia and immunosuppression,[227] and to the emergence of CMV resistance.[229–231] Prolonged ganciclovir prophylaxis has also been shown to delay the recovery of the CMV specific CD8+ T cellular immunity,[232] and therefore to contribute to the occurrence of late CMV disease.[217,233]

Preemptive therapy: The risk for CMV disease is also significantly reduced by the preemptive administration of ganciclovir in patients with CMV infection documented on the basis of BAL culture,[234] antigenemia (pp65),[235] plasma PCR,[236] or leukocyte PCR.[237] The antigenemia assay is the most practical tool for preemptive CMV therapy because of its wide availability, low cost, and its quantitative nature. However, there is a 10 percent risk of developing CMV disease before or at the time of the first positive antigenemia.[235] In addition, antigenemia cannot be performed during the period of neutropenia. Plasma PCR should instead be used in this setting.[238] Like antigenemia, semiquantitative and quantitative CMV PCR may be used to monitor viral load, which appears to correlate well with the risk of CMV disease.[220,239–241]

Alternatives to ganciclovir: Foscarnet has activity against CMV, including ganciclovir-resistant isolates, and has shown to be as effective as ganciclovir in a randomized study for preemptive therapy of CMV infection in allogeneic PSCT recipients.[242] In this study, foscarnet (90 mg/kg bid) was associated with faster clearence of the CMV antigenemia than ganciclovir (5 mg/kg bid) (on day 4 of treatment 8 and 41 percent of patients had positive antigenemia, respectively), and nephrotoxicity was comparable in both arms. Foscarnet should be considered as an alternative when ganciclovir-related neutropenia develops, in patients at risk for graft failure, and in those with progressive infection while receiving ganciclovir. A dose-finding study in patients undergoing universal prophylaxis has shown that foscarnet doses below 120 mg/kg/day during induction and 90 mg/kg/day during maintenance appear inadequate for effective CMV prophylaxis in recipients of allogeneic BMT.[243] Thus, doses below those mentioned above should not be considered.

Cidofovir is somewhat effective as preemptive therapy for CMV when used in doses of 1 to 5 mg/kg/week.[244] An induction dose of 5 mg/kg/week for 2 weeks followed by maintenance every 2 weeks (with probenecid and hydration) is more effective although associated with significant nephrotoxicity.[245]

Compared with oral acyclovir (400 mg qid), high-dose intravenous acyclovir (500 mg/m^2 tid from Day 5 to Day +30) increases 1-year survival in recipients of allogeneic BMT,[246] and decreases CMV infection but without lowering the incidence of CMV pneumonia. Therefore, high-dose iv acyclovir cannot be considered a first-line option for CMV prophylaxis or preemptive therapy.

Valacyclovir is a prodrug of acyclovir. High doses of this agent (2 g qid) reduce the incidence of CMV disease in renal transplant recipients.[247] Allogeneic BMT recipients were randomized to valacyclovir (2 g qid) or oral acyclovir 800 mg qid after 28 days of high-dose intravenous acyclovir (500 mg/m^2 three times daily).[248] CMV viremia was less common among the valacyclovir group and took significantly longer time to develop. However, there was no difference in CMV disease or survival among the two groups.

Oral ganciclovir is effective as maintenance therapy for established CMV infection after induction with iv ganciclovir in solid organ recipients.[249] The major drawback of this agent is its low bioavailability and potential toxicity. Among BMT recipients, oral ganciclovir (1000 mg tid from Day +35) had to be discontinued because of gastrointestinal toxicity in 6 of 21 (29 percent) patients. In the same study, breakthrough CMV infections occurred in 38 percent of patients.[250]

Valganciclovir, a prodrug of ganciclovir, may replace oral ganciclovir due to its superior bioavailability and convenient dosing (once or twice a day). A dose of 900 mg of valganciclovir produces a daily exposure (AUC_{24}) comparable to that of an iv dose of 5 mg/kg of ganciclovir in HIV-positive patients and in liver transplant recipients.[251] Whether valganciclovir is effective maintenance therapy for PSCT patients remains to be determined.

We recommend CMV prophylaxis for all seropositive recipients of allogeneic PSCT/BMT and for all seronegative patients who receive stem cells or bone marrow from a CMV seropositive donor. The strategy we suggest includes iv ganciclovir given from Day –7 until Day – 1 (approach not rigorously tested), followed by high-dose intravenous acyclovir (500 mg/m^2 tid) until preemptive CMV therapy or engraftment and resolution of mucositis. In the absence of mucositis, iv acyclovir could be switched to high-dose oral acyclovir (800 mg qid), valacyclovir (2 g qid), or famciclovir (750 mg tid). Routine testing for CMV infection should be done with PCR when the ANC is <1000/µl or antigenemia when the patient is no longer neutropenic. Testing could be done weekly in low-risk patients and twice weekly in those at high risk for CMV infection. Preemptive therapy with intravenous ganciclovir should be limited to those patients who develop two consecutive positive PCRs or one positive antigenemia with greater than 5 cells/slide. However, patients at high risk for CMV disease (≥ grade II acute GvHD, matched unrelated donor, or T-cell depleted transplant recipients) should start ganciclovir therapy even with a single positive cell on the antigenemia assay. The induction phase should continue until the viral load decreases by ≥ 50 percent (1 week minimum). Maintenance therapy is given until CMV infection has resolved. If the viral load increases during maintenance, the induction dose should be resumed. If PCR or antigenemia persists 4 weeks or more or if the quantitative tests (antigenemia or quantitative PCR) show progression after 3 weeks of therapy, viral resistance should be considered and the patient switched to an alternative agent (or combination of agents). Close monitoring for CMV disease should be maintained.

Ganciclovir is probably the drug of choice in non-T-cell depleted allogeneic PSCT: 5 mg/kg bid for induction followed by maintenance at 5 mg/kg/day. In the setting of appropriate oral intake, good compliance, and adequate gut function, maintenance with oral valganciclovir (900 mg/day with food) might be considered provided a close follow-up is maintained. In T-cell-depleted or unrelated donor transplantation, foscarnet 90 mg/kg/bid as induction followed by 90 mg/kg/day for maintenance may be a better choice. These recipients are less likely to develop nephrotoxicity as they are typically not receiving cyclosporine or tacrolimus, and are more likely to develop graft failure (that could be worsened by the ganciclovir-related myelosuppression).

After completion of maintenance therapy, weekly CMV monitoring should be continued to detect any relapse and therapy should be reinstituted as above in the event of recrudescence of the infection. Chronic extensive GvHD and receipt of large cumulative dose of corticosteroids increase the risk of CMV relapse. Monitoring for CMV infection may be stopped once chronic extensive GvHD has resolved, immunosuppressants discontinued, and the CD4 count has increased to greater than 200/µl for 3 consecutive months.

Recipients of matched unrelated or mismatched related transplantation reactivate CMV earlier and more frequently than recipients of matched related transplantation.[252] Therefore, universal CMV prophylaxis might be considered in this selected patient population.

Epstein-Barr Virus

Patients at high risk for EBV-related PTLD include allogeneic recipients of matched unrelated, mismatched, or T-cell-depleted PSCT/BMT and recipients of high-dose antithymocyte globulin or anti-T-cell monoclonal antibodies,[104,253] patients with acute and chronic GvHD, and those receiving radiation as part of the conditioning regimen.[253,254] T-cell depletion is the only predisposing factor for PTLD in the autologous transplant setting.[255]

High-risk recipients of PSCT/BMT who are EBV seronegative should be advised to avoid close contact with EBV seropositive individuals.

PTLD is usually the consequence of uncontrolled expansion of donor-derived B cells infected with EBV. Although acyclovir and ganciclovir inhibit EBV replication in vitro, conclusive data supporting the use of these agents as preemptive therapy for PTLD are lacking.[256] Primary prophylaxis of EBV-related PTLD may be directed at restoring EBV-specific immunity or eliminating the reservoir of the virus by B-cell depletion. The infusion of donor-derived EBV-specific cytotoxic T cells is effective for the prevention of EBV-related PTLD among recipients of T-cell-depleted bone marrow from HLA-matched unrelated donors and mismatched family members.[257] Depletion of B lymphocytes also appears to decrease the risk of PTLD among high-risk allogeneic BMT recipients. This can be accomplished in vivo with anti-CD52 monoclonal antibodies (Campath-1H) or anti-CD20 monoclonal antibodies (Rituximab), or ex vivo by manipulating the bone marrow or stem cell product.[258,259]

Increases in EBV viral load following PSCT/BMT are common, and are highest in patients at risk for PTLD,[105,260–262] suggesting that surveillance studies with quantitative viral load may identify high-risk patients suitable for preemptive therapy.

We recommend monthly surveillance with plasma or peripheral blood mononuclear cells (PBMC) quantitative EBV PCR in high-risk patients who did not undergo B-cell depletion or infusion of donor-derived EBV-specific cytotoxic T cells. A viral load of greater than 2000 EBV genome copies/μg of DNA extracted from PBMC appears to correlate with the development of PTLD in BMT recipients.[263] Patients with levels of EBV DNA above 2000 copies/g may benefit from interventions such as anti-CD20 antibodies (Rituximab). Cell-based immunotherapy is effective but is neither timely, nor widely available or cost-effective.

Hepatitis B Virus

Patients with hematological malignancies undergoing cytotoxic chemotherapy while infected with HBV have a higher risk for severe liver dysfunction (serum bilirubin >5 mg/dl or ALT >10 times normal) than noninfected patients (6 of 8 [75 percent] vs. 0 of 234 [0 percent], respectively).[264] During therapy-induced aplasia, the possibility of viral replication increases dramatically resulting in acute HBV infection that may be mild, asymptomatic, or chronically progressive leading to fulminant hepatitis. Fulminant hepatitis usually coincides with discontinuation of immunosuppression.[265–267]

Among 372 patients with various hematological malignancies, the frequency of reactivation of the HBV infection was 20 percent, hepatic failure 13 percent, fulminant hepatitis 7 percent, and death 11 percent.[268–274] Risk factors for reactivation include male gender, younger age, lymphoma diagnosis, and positive HBeAg.[275] Corticosteroids have been suggested as risk factors for HBV reactivation in cancer patients.[276,277]

Recipients of PSCT/BMT infected with HBV have a 50 percent risk of reactivation.[278] In this group of patients, however, fulminant hepatitis is more likely (>10 percent) in the absence of antiviral treatment.[110] Risk factors for poor outcome among PSCT/BMT patients have not been studied.

Of note, patients with prior exposure to HBV who appear to have been cured (HBsAg negative, anti-HBs positive, anti-HBc positive or negative) may reactivate their infection following PSCT/BMT.[279–282]

The mechanism of development of hepatitis after chemotherapy is through enhancement of viral replication during therapy-induced aplasia, resulting in acute HBV infection that may be mild, or asymptomatic. After recovery of host immunity, the cytotoxic T cells destroy HBV-infected hepatocytes, leading to fulminant hepatitis.[265–268]

Prophylaxis against HBV prevents reactivation. Famciclovir prophylaxis from day 7 until week 24 post-transplantation

decreased mortality in HBV-infected allogeneic BMT recipients compared to historical controls.[283] Among HBV-infected renal transplant recipients, lamivudine prophylaxis was more efficacious than lamivudine given for treatment of reactivation.[284] Three HBV-infected patients were reported to have undergone autologous PSCT without viral reactivation after receiving lamivudine prophylaxis for 16 weeks after transplantation.[285]

Resistance to lamivudine usually develops after 6 months of therapy and is due to the emergence of a mutant strain.[286] Famciclovir resistance is also due to the emergence of a mutant strain and cannot overcome the lamivudine resistance.[286] In contrast, lamivudine can be used as a second-line therapy when famciclovir fails.[287] Lamivudine is safe even in autologous PSCT recipients without affecting the hematopoietic recovery.[285]

The antiviral combination therapy is intended to avoid the emergence of resistance. Lamivudine plus famciclovir have an additive or synergistic effect against HBV in animal models.[288] This combination (lamivudine 150 mg/day plus famciclovir 500 mg/day or tid) was superior to lamivudine alone in suppressing the HBV replication among chronically infected patients.[289,290] Lamivudine plus famciclovir transiently suppressed viral replication in two of four liver transplant recipients who developed reactivation of hepatitis on monotherapy by a lamivudine-resistant strain.[291,292]

We recommend that HBV-infected patients about to undergo cytotoxic chemotherapy or PSCT be evaluated for HBV infection prior to therapy. This evaluation should include HBV DNA quantification, liver function tests, serum HBV markers, and liver biopsy (if liver function tests are elevated). We also recommend antiviral treatment with lamivudine (100 to 150 mg bid) plus famciclovir (500 mg tid) as soon as possible. Therapy should continue until HBV DNA is negative and CD4 counts are greater than or equal to 200/μL for 3 months. Close monitoring should be maintained throughout chemotherapy and particularly when withdrawal of immunosuppressors is considered.

Hepatitis C Virus

Patients already infected with HCV may need to undergo chemotherapy or PSCT/BMT. Significant liver dysfunction is uncommon during therapy among such patients.[293] The risk for such patients is the development of late cirrhosis, several years after therapy.

Among PSCT/BMT recipients, HCV infection increased the risk for lethal veno-occlusive disease (VOD),[294] especially when HCV infection is associated with abnormal AST prior to transplantation.[295] HCV infection can rarely progress to fulminant hepatitis.[296] In two large studies including approximately 600 patients[295,297] HCV infection did not affect mortality up to 10 years following allogeneic BMT.

Oral ribavirin cleared HCV viremia in four allogeneic BMT recipients when given as prophylaxis throughout transplantation.[298] Ribavirin (600 mg bid) has been suggested as prophylaxis only for those patients with HCV infection and abnormal AST and undergoing allogeneic PSCT/BMT (may reduce the incidence of VOD). Monitoring viral load and AST monthly is also recommended. Until more data are available, we do not recommend prophylaxis for HCV infection in patients with hematological cancer.

Herpes Simplex Virus

Almost all HSV infections in patients undergoing chemotherapy or PSCT/BMT are caused by viral reactivation; thus, only seropositive patients are at risk.[112,299] The rate of reactivation ranges from 50 to 90 percent.[300]

Intravenous (250 mg/m^2 iv bid) or oral (200 to 400 mg 5 times a day) acyclovir given prior to or at the time of cytotoxic or myeloablative chemotherapy and continued for several weeks is highly effective in reducing the incidence of HSV reactivation in seropositive recipients of BMT.[301–304] Acyclovir resistance may develop among patients with prolonged exposure to this agent (such as in allogeneic-BMT).[305] Foscarnet is the drug of choice for the treatment of such infections.

Valacyclovir is metabolized to acyclovir, and has better bioavailability than oral acyclovir. This agent, at a dose of 500 mg bid po, is as effective and safe as iv acyclovir for the prevention of HSV reactivation in recipients of autologous PSCT.[306] However, valacyclovir has the disadvantage of not having an iv formulation. Thrombotic thrombocytopenic purpura/hemolytic uremic syndrome was reported in one study using much higher doses (8000 mg/day) than that needed for HSV infections.[307]

Famciclovir is metabolized to penciclovir, and its bioavailability is superior to oral acyclovir and probably valacyclovir. Intravenous penciclovir is as effective as acyclovir for the treatment of HSV infections in immunocompromised patients.[308] Its prodrug famciclovir is thus likely to be effective as prophylaxis for infection in this patient population. Penciclovir is only available for topical treatment.

All seropositive patients with hematological cancer undergoing intensive cancer chemotherapy with or without PSCT/BMT should be given antiviral prophylaxis. Appropriate agents include oral valacyclovir (500 mg bid), acyclovir (200 to 400 mg 5 times daily), or famciclovir (250 to 500 mg bid). Intravenous acyclovir (5 mg/kg iv bid) may also be used. These agents need to be given with the start of chemotherapy and continued until engraftment and resolution of mucositis. In the setting of allogeneic PSCT/BMT, higher doses of acyclovir (500 mg/m^2 tid from day 5 to day +30 followed by oral acyclovir 800 mg qid) is recommended. Alternatively, higher valacyclovir doses (2 g qid) could be used in this setting. These higher doses may also decrease CMV reactivation.[248] and have been reported in one study with acyclovir to improve survival.[246] Recipients of PSCT/BMT should continue HSV prophylaxis as long as the patient is severely immunosuppressed (CD4 count < 200/mm^3). We do not recommend HSV prophylaxis to seronegative patients who receive stem cells or bone marrow from seropositive donors.

Respiratory Viruses

The respiratory viruses adenovirus, influenzae, parainfluenza, and respiratory syncytial virus (RSV) can cause infections in patients with hematological malignancies. Most of these infections appear to be self-limited,[309,310] although progression to severe lower respiratory infection may occur. The main strategy for prophylaxis of infections by respiratory viruses is to prevent exposure of patients with hematological malignancies to individuals with symptoms of respiratory infections.[26] Some centers recommend delay of PSCT/BMT when recipients have a viral respiratory infection.[26] However, this is not always feasible because of the need for immediate treatment of the underlying malignancy. In addition, a large number of patients may be infected yet asymptomatic.[311] We therefore recommend delaying the PSCT/BMT only when there is a clear documentation of pneumonia or sinusitis (positive symptoms and high resolution CT) and the recipient is at high risk for infections (matched unrelated donor, renal failure, or receiving high-dose steroids or immunosuppressants).

Adenovirus: The infusion of cytotoxic lymphocytes specific against adenovirus and EBV has been recently proposed as prophylaxis for recipients of allogeneic PSCT or BMT[312] but is not practical.

Influenza: Patients with hematological malignancies may benefit from lifelong influenza vaccination (see Immunization). Vaccination of close contacts and health care workers is also recommended.[158] Postexposure prophylaxis has been discussed earlier.

Parainfluenza: No drugs are available for prophylaxis or preemptive therapy for this infection.

Respiratory syncytial virus: RSV immunoglobulin and RSV monoclonal antibodies are both approved by the FDA for the prevention of RSV in children at high risk for RSV lower-respiratory tract infection. Studies to evaluate the role of these agents in PSCT/BMT recipients at risk have not been done.[313] Preemptive therapy with aerosolized ribavirin with or without RSV antibodies is expensive, cumbersome, and has no documented value.

Varicella Zoster Virus

Patients at highest risk for VZV reactivation are those with severe lymphopenia and/or CD4 cytopenia such as patients with lymphoma, leukemia (mainly chronic lymphocytic leukemia), and patients receiving corticosteroid therapy, PSCT/BMT, or immunosuppressors such as fludarabine or Campath-1H. Among recipients of autologous PSCT, the risk is higher among those with CD4 count less than 200 cells/μL and/or CD8 count less than 800 cells/μL at day 30 posttransplantation.[314] Among allogeneic PSCT/BMT recipients, GvHD[315] and conditioning regimens that include radiation therapy[316] are known risk factors. The incidence of VZV reactivation is similar among allogeneic and autologous transplant recipients (10 to 40 percent during the first year of transplantation).[172,314–316] In a review of 216 cases of VZV reactivation, all severe infections occurred during the first 7 months after BMT.[316]

High-dose intravenous acyclovir (500 mg/m^2 tid until engraftment and resolution of mucositis) followed by high-dose oral acyclovir (800 mg qid) is effective in preventing seropositive patients from developing VZV infection following allogeneic PSCT/BMT.[317] While infections do occur in patients on this regimen, they tend to be less severe. Lower doses of acyclovir used for the prophylaxis of HSV, and low-dose ganciclovir (5 mg/kg/day 3 times a week) may also be effective for VZV prophylaxis.[315]

Valacyclovir[318] and famciclovir[319] have not been studied for prophylaxis of VZV infections. However, these agents are likely to be adequate for prophylaxis since both are effective in the treatment of established VZV infections.

We recommend VZV prophylaxis to seropositive recipients of autologous and allogeneic PSCT/BMT until chronic extensive GvHD has resolved, immunosuppressants have been discontinued, and the CD4 count has reached greater than 200 to 400 /μl for at least 2 consecutive months. We also recommend immunization of all VZV susceptible close contacts. Immunization of immunocompromised patients with the live virus VZV vaccine is contraindicated until resolution of immunosuppression (see Immunization).

Antiparasitic Prophylaxis

Pneumocystis carinii

Reactivation of latent infection is the most common mechanism of pneumonia by *Pneumocystis carinii* among immunocompromised patients. The possibility for person-to-person transmission has been suggested although not confirmed.[320–322] With the routine use of effective chemoprophylaxis, the incidence of *P. carinii* pneumonia (PCP) now accounts for less than 2 percent of pneumonias in transplant recipients.[323] Patients at high risk for developing PCP are recipients of allogeneic PSCT/BMT (especially those with severe GvHD), patients with hematological malignancies undergoing autologous PSCT/BMT (particularly if extensively pretreated or receiving manipulated grafts), and patients on intensive immunosuppressive therapy including high-dose corticosteroids, purine analogues,[324] or Campath-1H. The period at risk for PCP lasts until recovery of cellular immunity.

The most effective drug for prophylaxis against PCP is TMP-SMX. Accepted dosages include one double-strength tablet (trimethoprim 160 mg + sulfamethoxazole 800 mg) bid 2 days a week, one double-strength tablet (daily or 3 times a week), and 1 single-strength tablet (trimethoprim 80 mg + sulfamethoxazole 400 mg) daily. Prophylaxis against PCP with TMP-SMX should start after engraftment and continue as long as immunosuppressive therapy is ongoing, extensive cGvHD is present, and CD4 count is less than 200 cells/mm³. In the setting of PSCT/BMT, it is also recommended to give PCP prophylaxis 1 to 2 weeks prior to the transplantation until day 2 to avoid PCP during the preengraftment period. The main side effects related to TMP-SMX include gut intolerance, skin rash, myelotoxicity, nephrotoxicity, and hyperkalemia. Alternative agents include aerosolized pentamidine (given with Respirgard II nebulizer 300 mg every month after an initial loading dose given every other week), atovaquone suspension (1500 mg/day), and dapsone (50 mg bid or 100 mg/day).[26]

Atovaquone suspension at 1500 mg/day is as effective as aerosolized pentamidine in preventing PCP among HIV-infected patients with breakthrough PCP in 18 and 17 percent of patients respectively[325] and a similarly low rate (2 percent) of treatment-limiting side effects. The most common treatment-limiting side effects include rash, diarrhea, and nausea in the atovaquone group, and bronchospasm in the pentamidine

group. Experience among PSCT/BMT is limited. None of 15 allogeneic PSCT/BMT recipients at M. D. Anderson Cancer Center intolerant to TMP-SMX who received atovaquone prophylaxis developed PCP (personal communication, J. L. Gajewski). Thirty-nine recipients of autologous PSCT/BMT were randomized to atovaquone suspension (1500 mg/day) versus TMP-SMX (2 single-strength tablets) daily from day 5 to day 1 and then 3 times a week after engraftment until day +100. No patients developed PCP during the first 100 days of transplantation. TMP-SMX was associated with more toxicity (49 percent discontinued treatment due to intolerance) than atovaquone suspension (no drug discontinuation). Because of concerns over erratic bioavailability, atovaquone should be given with food to increase absorption, and avoided among patients whose gut integrity may be affected (such as severe intestinal GvHD or severe diarrhea). Aerosolized pentamidine may be associated with extrapulmonary pneumocytosis and is expensive.

Dapsone (100 mg/day) is as effective as atovaquone (1500 mg/day) in preventing PCP in HIV-infected patients.[326] Treatment-limiting side effects are, however, significantly higher among the dapsone (59 percent) than the atovaquone recipients (24 percent). Among the subset of patients who were known to be tolerant to dapsone, the treatment-limiting side effects were higher in the atovaquone group (32 percent) compared to the dapsone group (8 percent). Cross-sensitivity between dapsone and TMP-SMX may exist and dapsone should be discouraged among patients with glucose-6-phosphate dehydrogenase (G6PD) deficiency.

We recommend PCP prophylaxis with TMP-SMX (1 double-strength tablet 3 times week) to all patients at high risk for this infection during the period of severe immunosuppression (CD4 count < 200/μL). Alternative agents for TMP-SMX intolerant or allergic patients include atovaquone suspension (first choice) given with food (1500 mg/day) for patients with intact bowel function, dapsone (second choice) in the absence of G6PD deficiency, and aerosolized pentamidine (third choice). Intravenous pentamidine is also effective but associated with significant toxicity.

Patients already receiving the pneumocandin caspofungin (Cancidas) may not need prophylaxis against PCP given the activity of this drug against *P. carinii*.

Toxoplasmosis

Seropositive patients are at risk of reactivation of toxoplasmosis following PSCT/BMT. When the recipient and donor are seronegative, special precautions should be taken to avoid primary infection. Those precautions include eating only well-cooked meats (>66°C), well washed vegetables, cooked eggs, pasteurized milk, and sterile water; handwashing after outdoor activities or after handling raw meat or vegetables; using gloves for contact with soil or gardening; avoiding contact with cat litter; and having someone change litter box daily and soak it in boiling water for 5 minutes (Table 49–4 and 49–5).

Reactivation of toxoplasmosis is highest among recipients of T-cell-depleted allogeneic PSCT/BMT (5 to 15 percent) and is otherwise rare among other allogeneic recipients (<1 percent). The potential toxicities of effective agents preclude routine prophylaxis against toxoplasmosis. However, preemptive therapy of high-risk patients (positive serology prior to transplantation, T-cell-depleted allogeneic transplants) with PCR-based tests is recommended. Primary prophylaxis may be considered in patients with a history of ocular toxoplasmosis. Effective prophylaxis includes TMP-SMX, 1 double-strength tablet 3 times a week, or 1 single-strength tablet daily; clindamycin 300 to 450 mg tid plus pyrimethamine 25 to 75 mg/day plus leucovorin 10 to 25 mg[26]; pyrimethamine-sulfadoxine (Fansidar) 1 tablet (25 mg pyrimethamine/500 mg sulfadoxine)/20 kg weight on day 1 with folinic acid, 50 mg/20 kg on Day 2, then daily following engraftment; atovaquone (750 to 1500 mg/day); and dapsone 50 mg/day plus pyrimethamine 50 mg/week plus folinic acid 25 mg/week. Fansidar is associated with significant toxicities.[327])

Other Parasites

Strongyloidiasis should be detected and eradicated before immunosuppressive treatment is started to avoid the life-threatening hyperinfection syndrome. The sensitivity of the stool examination is 80 percent at best. Therefore, serologic test (sensitivity and specificity >90 percent) should be considered when clinical suspicion is high but stool examinations are negative.

Effective agents for treatment include ivermectin 200 µg/kg/day, albendazole 400 mg/day, and thiabendazole 25 mg/kg bid (maximum dose 3 g/day).[26] Therapy should be continued until stool examination is negative and eosinophilia has resolved. Patients with a history of strongyloidiasis and who are undergoing immunosuppressive treatment should be carefully followed to detect early disease and start treatment. There is no information regarding the role of secondary prophylaxis among these patients.

Patients with history of Chagas' disease (trypanosomiasis) should undergo preemptive therapy as mentioned earlier in section Stem Cell/Bone Marrow Infusions.

Antimycobacterial Prophylaxis

Tuberculosis (TB) is 10- to 20-fold more frequent among patients with cancer (particularly patients with hematological cancers and those undergoing allogeneic PSCT/BMT) than in the general population, both in endemic[328–331] and nonendemic areas.[332] Infection usually represents reactivation of old exposure (*Mycobacterium tuberculosis* and *Mycobacterium avium complex*).

Prophylaxis of mycobacterial infection with isoniazid (INH) given for 6 months after allogeneic PSCT was effective in preventing TB after transplantation (no infection among 77 INH patients compared with 5 of 274 [2 percent] controls).[333]

Because of the toxicity of antimycobacterial agents, prophylaxis should be limited to high-risk patients. Risk factors for developing TB include living or visiting endemic areas for TB, a history of slowly resolving pneumonia with a lung imaging consistent with TB, well-documented TB not treated properly, recent exposure to TB, and/or a positive (≥5 mm) tuberculin skin testing.

Patients with a positive tuberculin testing should be studied for detection of active infection. If active infection is ruled out,

prophylaxis with isoniazid may be of benefit.[333,334] If active infection is detected, multiagent drug therapy should be given for at least 2 to 4 weeks before initiation of cytotoxic chemotherapy.

IMMUNE RECONSTITUTION

Passive Immunization (IV Immunoglobulin, IVIG)

IVIG seems to benefit patients with chronic lymphocytic leukemia,[335,336] non-Hodgkin's lymphoma,[337] and muliple myeloma[338] who have hypogammaglobulinemia or a history of recurrent infections. Doses of IVIG of 250 mg/kg every 4 weeks were shown to be as effective as 500 mg/kg every 4 weeks.[339] However, the role of IVIG in the prevention of infections among patients with hematological malignances is not clear and is unlikely to be superior to that of antibiotic prophylaxis.

Among PSCT/BMT recipients, the major benefit of IVIG is the reduction of acute GvHD in a subset of allogeneic BMT/PSCT recipients. The administration of IVIG for the prevention of infections among these patients with severe hypogammaglobulinemia (serum IgG <400 mg/dl) is commonly practiced but is of unproven value.

Active Immunization

The immunization of patients with hematological malignancies undergoing cytotoxic chemotherapy has three goals:

1. Maintaining the appropriate adult immunization schedule
2. Restoring the immunity that could have been lost after the immunosuppressive treatment
3. Protecting the patient from the receipt of live vaccines

A suggested schedule for immunization is shown in Table 49–7.

Colony-Stimulating Factors

Granulocyte colony-stimulating factor (G-CSF) has been shown to reduce the incidence of fever, and duration of antibiotic therapy and hospitalization in some studies.[340,341] However, a significant reduction of culture-proven infections or mortality has not been shown. The prophylactic use of G-CSF is recommended in settings when the risk of febrile neutropenia is greater than 40 percent.[342]

Granulocyte Transfusions

Abrogation of neutropenia is a potential strategy for the prevention of neutropenia-related infections. Granulocyte transfusions (WBCTx) obtained from donors previously treated with granulocyte-macrophage colony-stimulating factor (GM-CSF) were given as prophylaxis to a group of patients with leukemia who had a high probability of dying within 30 days of the induction-remission chemotherapy. Invasive fungal infections developed in 1 of 22 (4.5 percent) treated patients and in 3 (9 percent) of 33 nontreated patients.[343]

Table 49–7. Immunization After Peripheral Stem Cell (PSCT)/Bone Marrow (BMT) Transplantation

AVOID vaccines until ≥ 4 months after PSCT (inactivated vaccines ineffective, live vaccines dangerous).
AVOID live vaccines until patient in complete remission, *and* not receiving immunosuppressive therapy for 6 months *and* has a CD4 + count > 400/µl and does not have chronic graft-versus-host disease (GvHD).

Live vaccines:
  Adenovirus, BCG, measles-mumps-rubella, oral typhoid, oral polio, yellow fever, varicella zoster.
  AVOID oral polio in household contacts (the polio virus may spread and cause uncontrolled infection).
AVOID vaccines until CD4 + counts > 200/µl (unlikely to be effective).
MEASURE antibody titers after vaccination to ensure efficacy and repeat doses until optimal titers achieved.

Immunization of Donor and Recipient Following Allogeneic PSCT/BMT

	Recipient[a]	
Vaccine	Chronic GvHD Absent	Chronic GvHD Present
Diphtheria-tetanus toxoid[b]	1 year, 14 mo., and 2 years and every 10 years	1 year, 14 mo., and 2 years
Inactivated polio virus (Salk)	1 year, 14 mo., and 2 years	Not indicated if on IVIG
Pneumococcal vaccine[c]	1 and 2 years	May not benefit
H. influenzae (Hib) conjugate	1 year, 14 mo., and 2 years	May not benefit
Hepatitis B	1 year, 14 mo., and 2 years (check titers after vaccination)	May not benefit
Influenza (repeat every fall)	Pre-BMT and yearly ≥6 mo. post-BMT	May not benefit
Measles-mumps-rubella (MMR)	2–3 years (and possibly 6–12 months later) (give only if seronegative for any of these pathogens)	AVOID
Varicella vaccine (Varivax)	2–3 years (give only if seronegative for VZV)	AVOID
Oral polio virus (Sabin)	AVOID	AVOID

Immunization of Donor Before Harvesting Stem Cells; Immunization of Household Contacts Before Transplantation

	Donor and Individual in Close Contact
H. influenza (Hib) conjugate	+
Pneumococcal vaccine[e]	+
Varicella zoster, hepatitis B[e]	+

Immunization Following Autologous PSCT/BMT and Nonmyeloablative Chemotherapy

Vaccine	Time of Immunization
Diphtheria-tetanus toxoid[b]	1 year, 14 mo., and 2 years and every 10 years
Inactivated polio virus (Salk)	1 year, 14 mo., and 2 years
Pneumococcal vaccine[c]	1 and 2 years
H. influenzae (Hib) conjugate	1 year, 14 mo., and 2 years
Hepatitis B	1 year, 14 mo., and 2 years (check titers after vaccination)
Influenza (repeat every November)	Pre-BMT and yearly ≥ 6 mo. post-PSCT/BMT
Measles-mumps-rubella (MMR)	2 years (and possibly 6–12 months later) (give only if seronegative for any of these pathogens)
Varicella vaccine (Varivax)	2 years (give only if seronegative for VZV)
Oral polio virus (Sabin)	AVOID

[a] Hepatitis A, and meningococcal, routine administration is not indicated.
[b] No data are available on safety and immunogenicity of pertussis vaccination in PSCT/BMT recipients.
[c] Second dose of pneumococcal vaccine may immunize patients who failed to respond to the first dose.
[d] All patients, especially those with chronic GvHD require lifelong pneumococcal chemoprophylaxis.
[e] Donor immunization investigational.

Prophylactic GM-CSF or G-CSF elicited WBCTx remains investigational and may be considered in patients with a history of a neutropenia-related invasive mold infection (such as aspergillosis or fusariosis) who are expected to be neutropenic for 14 days or more.

Prevention of Graft Failure and GvHD

The type of donor selected for allogeneic PSCT/BMT may influence the frequency and severity of infectious complications of the recipient by affecting the time to immune reconstitution, and/or by transferring infections or protective immunity.

Immune reconstitution after transplantation is typically faster in autologous than in allogeneic recipients, and is further delayed in the latter patients when an unrelated or a mismatched-related donor product is used (increased risk of graft failure and GvHD).[344] Manipulation of the stem cells or bone marrow (mainly T-cell depletion) for the prevention of GvHD may also delay immune reconstitution.[344,345]

REFERENCES

1. Aslan T, Anaissie E: Infections in hematological malignancies. In Freireich EJ, Kantarjian HM (eds.): Medical Management of

Hematological Malignant Diseases, 1st Ed., pp. 321–402. Marcel Dekker, New York, 1998.

2. Sickles EA, Greene WH, Wiernik PH: Clinical presentation of infection in granulocytopenic patients. Arch Intern Med 135:715–719, 1975.

3. Parra C, Roldan E, Rodriguez C, Perez de Oteyza J, Oteho E, Lopez J et al: Reconstitution of peripheral blood lymphocytes in patients treated with bone marrow transplantation: Comparison between allogeneic and autologous transplantation. Med Clin 113:1–5, 1999.

4. Takaue Y, Okamoto Y, Kawano Y, Suzue T, Abe T, Saito SI et al: Regeneration of immunity and varicella-zoster virus infection after high-dose chemotherapy and peripheral blood stem cell autografts in children. Bone Marrow Transplant 14:219–223, 1994.

5. Steingrimsdottir H, Gruber A, Bjorkholm M, Svensson A, Hansson M: Immune reconstitution after autologous hematopoietic stem cell transplantation in relation to underlying disease, type of high-dose therapy and infectious complications. Haematologica 85:832–838, 2000.

6. Atkinson K: Reconstruction of the haemopoietic and immune systems after marrow transplantation. Bone Marrow Transplant 5:209–226, 1990.

7. Nolte A, Buhmann R, Emmerich B, Schendel D, Hallek M: Reconstitution of the cellular immune response after autologous peripheral blood stem cell transplantation in patients with non-Hodgkin's lymphoma. Br J Haematol 108:415–423, 2000.

8. Ericson SG, Guyre CA, Benoit NE, Meehan KR, Mills LE, Fanger MW: Anti-body-dependent cellular cytotoxicity (ADCC) function of peripheral blood polymorphonuclear neutrophils (PMN) after autologous bone marrow transplantation (ABMT). Bone Marrow Transplant 16:787–791, 1995.

9. Lum LG: The kinetics of immune reconstitution after human marrow transplantation. Blood 69:369–380, 1987.

10. Lin MT, Tseng LH, Frangoul H, Gooley T, Pei J, Barsoukov A et al: Increased apoptosis of peripheral blood T cells following allogeneic hematopoietic cell transplantation. Blood 95:3832–3839, 2000.

11. Lum LG, Orcutt-Thordarson N, Seigneuret MC, Storb R: The regulation of Ig synthesis after marrow transplantation. IV. T4 and T8 subset function in patients with chronic graft-vs-host disease. J Immunol 129:113–119, 1982.

12. Lum LG, Seigneuret MC, Storb RF, Witherspoon RP, Thomas ED: In vitro regulation of immunoglobulin synthesis after marrow transplantation. I. T-cell and B-cell deficiencies in patients with and without chronic graft-versus-host disease. Blood 58:431–439, 1981.

13. Semmelweis I: The etiology, the concept, and the prophylaxis of childbed fever. In CA P (ed.): Hartleben's Verlag-Expeditious. Classics of Medicine Library, Birmingham, England. Murphy FP, trans, 1861 (republished 1981).

14. Holmes OW: The contagiousness of puerperal fever. In Darby P (ed.): Medical Essays: 1842–1882. Houghton, Mifflin, Boston, 1892.

15. Conly JM, Hill S, Ross J, Lertzman J, Louie TJ: Handwashing practices in an intensive care unit: The effects of an educational program and its relationship to infection rates. Am J Infect Control 17:330–339, 1989.

16. Bryan JL, Cohran J, Larson EL: Hand washing: A ritual revisited. Crit Care Nursing Clin North Am 7:617–625, 1995.

17. Larson EL: APIC guideline for handwashing and hand antisepsis in health care settings. Am J Infect Control 23:251–269, 1995.

18. Ayliffe GA: Surgical scrub and skin disinfection. Infect Control 5:23–27, 1984.

19. Groschel DHM, Pruett TL: Surgical antisepsis. In Block SS (ed.): Disinfection, sterilization and preservation, 4th Ed., pp. 642–654. Lea & Febiger, Philadelphia, 1991.

20. Lilly HA, Lowbury EJ, Wilkins MD, Zaggy A: Delayed antimicrobial effects of skin disinfection by alcohol. J Hyg 82:497–500, 1979.

21. Bischoff WE, Reynolds TM, Sessler CN, Edmond MB, Wenzel RP: Handwashing compliance by health care workers: The impact of introducing an accessible, alcohol-based hand antiseptic. Arch Intern Med 160:1017–1021, 2000.

22. Morse LJ, Schonbeck LE: Hand lotions: A potential nosocomial hazard. N Engl J Med 278:364–369, 1968.

23. Jeanes A, Green J: Nail art: A review of current infection control issues. J Hosp Infect 49:139–142, 2001.

24. Jakob KM, Foca M, Whittier S, Della-Latta P, Saiman L: Risk factors for *Pseudomona aeruginosa* hand carriage in health care workers during an investigation of increased nosocomial infection in a neonatal intensive care unit. In 37th IDSA Annual Meeting, November 18–21, 1999, Philadelphia.

25. Hedderwick SA, McNeil SA, Lyons MJ, Kauffman CA: Pathogenic organisms associated with artificial fingernails worn by healthcare workers. Infect Control Hosp Epidemiol 21:505–509, 2000.

26. Centers for Disease Control and Prevention: Guidelines for preventing opportunistic infections among hematopoietic stem cell transplant recipients. MMWR 49(RR-10):1–125, 2000.

27. Skov R, Gottschau A, Skinhoj P, Frimodt-Moller N, Rosdahl VT, Espersen F: *Staphylococcus aureus* bacteremia: A 14-year nationwide study in hematological patients with malignant disease or agranulocytosis. Scand J Infect Dis 27:563–568, 1995.

28. Itoh M, Yoshida M, Kurata H, Imagawa S, Hoshino M, Tsunoda J et al: *Staphylococcus aureus* sepsis in patients with hematological malignancies: Increase in MRSA sepsis. Rinsho Ketsueki—Jpn J Clin Hematol 32:115–120, 1991.

29. Espersen F, Frimodt-Moller N, Rosdahl VT, Jessen O, Faber V, Rosendal K: *Staphylococcus aureus* bacteremia in patients with hematological malignancies and/or agranulocytosis. Acta Med Scand 222:465–470, 1987.

30. Colbeck JC, Robertson HR, Sutherland WH et al: The importance of endogenous staphylococcal infections in surgical patients. Can Serv Med 15:326–331, 1959.

31. Weinstein HJ: The relation between nasal-staphylococcal-carrier state and the incidence of postoperative complications. N Engl J Med 260:1303–1308, 1959.

32. Williams REO, Patricia-Jevons M, Shoorer RA et al: Nasal staphylococci and sepsis in hospital patients. BMJ October:658–662, 1959.

33. Kluytmans JA, Manders MJ, van Bommel E, Verbrugh H: Elimination of nasal carriage of *Staphylococcus aureus* in hemodialysis patients. Infect Control Hosp Epidemiol 17:793–797, 1996.

34. Kluytmans JA, Mouton JW, VandenBergh MF, Manders MJ, Maat AP, Wagenvoort JH et al: Reduction of surgical-site infections in cardiothoracic surgery by elimination of nasal carriage of *Staphylococcus aureus*. Infect Control Hosp Epidemiol 17:780–785, 1996.

35. Yano M, Doki Y, Inoue M, Tsujinaka T, Shiozaki H, Monden M: Preoperative intranasal mupirocin ointment significantly reduces postoperative infection with *Staphylococcus aureus* in patients undergoing upper gastrointestinal surgery. Surg Today 30:16–21, 2000.

36. Fernandez C, Gaspar C, Torrellas A, Vindel A, Saez-Nieto JA, Cruzet F et al: A double-blind, randomized, placebo-controlled clinical trial to evaluate the safety and efficacy of mupirocin cal-

cium ointment for eliminating nasal carriage of *Staphylococcus aureus* among hospital personnel. J Antimicrob Chemother 35:399–408, 1995.

37. Schubert MM, Peterson DE, Lloid ME: Oral complications. In Thomas ED, Blume KG, Forman SJ (eds.): Hematopoietic Cell Transplantation, pp. 751–763. Blackwell Science, Oxford, England, 1999.

38. Angulo FJ, Glaser CA, Juranek DD, Lappin MR, Regnery RL: Caring for pets of immunocompromised persons. J Am Vet Med Assoc 205:1711–1718, 1994.

39. Loo VG, Bertrand C, Dixon C, Vitye-D, DeSalis B, McLean AP et al: Control of construction-associated nosocomial aspergillosis in an antiquated hematology unit. Infect Control Hosp Epidemiol 17:360–364, 1996.

40. Rhame FS: Prevention of nosocomial aspergillosis. J Hosp Infect 18(Suppl. A):466–472, 1991.

41. Noble WC, Clayton YM: Fungi in the air of hospital wards. J Gen Microbiol 32:397–402, 1963.

42. Bouza E, Peláez T, Pérez Molina J, Marín M, Muñoz P, Padilla B et al: Demolition of a hospital building by controlled explosion: The impact on the external and internal load of filamentous fungi. In 40th Interscience Conference on Antimicrobial Agents and Chemotherapy (ICAAC); September 17–20, 2000; Toronto, Ontario, Canada; 2000. Abstract 1320.

43. Kusne S, Krystofiak S: Infection control issues after bone marrow and solid organ transplantation. In Bowden RA, Ljungman P, Paya C (eds.): Transplant Infections, pp. 13–36. Lippincott-Raven, New York, 1998.

44. Opal S, Asp A, Cannady P Jr, Morse P, Burton L, Hammer II P: Efficacy of infection control measures during nosocomial outbreak of disseminated aspergillosis associated with hospital construction. J Infect Dis 153:634–637, 1986.

45. Walsh T, Dixon D: Nosocomial aspergillosis: Environmental microbiology, hospital epidemiology, diagnosis and treatment. Eur J Epidemiol 5:131–142, 1989.

46. Hospenthal D, Kwon-Chung K, JE Bennett: Concentration of airborne *Aspergillus* compared to the incidence of invasive aspergillosis: Lack of correlation. Med Mycol 36:165–168, 1998.

47. Rhame FS, Streifel AJ, Kersey JH, McGlave PB: Extrinsic risk factors for pneumonia in the patient at high risk of infection. Am J Med 76(Suppl. 5A):2–52, 1984.

48. Pegues DA, McNeil MM, Lasker BA, Lundal JI, Kubak BM, Hamm PM et al: *Aspergillosis* in a transplant ICU: Possible person-to-person airbone transmission. In 37th IDSA Annual Meeting, November 18–21, 1991; Philadelphia, Pennsylvania, 1999.

49. Anaissie EJ, Stratton SL, Summerbell RC, Monson TP, Rex JH, Walsh TJ: Aspergillus species aerosols in hospitals: Showering as a potential mode of exposure. In 39th Interscience Conference of Antimicrobial Agents and Chemotherapy (ICAAC); September 26–29, 1999; San Francisco, California, 1999.

50. Bhaduri S, Kurrle E, Krieger D, Pflieger H, Arnold R, Kubanek B et al: Infection prophylaxis in acute leukaemia patients: Comparison of selective and total antimicrobial decontamination of the gastrointestinal tract. Folia Haematol Int Magazin Klin Morpholog Blutforschung 109:377–389, 1982.

51. Nauseef WM, Maki DG: A study of the value of simple protective isolation in patients with granulocytopenia. N Engl J Med 304:448–453, 1981.

52. Storb R, Prentice RL, Buckner CD, Clift RA, Appelbaum F, Deeg J et al: Graft-versus-host disease and survival in patients with aplastic anemia treated by marrow grafts from HLA-identical siblings. Beneficial effect of a protective environment. N Engl J Med 308:302–307, 1983.

53. Ohira M, Shibata T, Ise T: Comparative study of protected environment for children with malignant disease. Jpn J Clin Oncol 13(Suppl. 1):143–149, 1983.

54. Navari RM, Buckner CD, Clift RA, Storb R, Sanders JE, Stewart P et al: Prophylaxis of infection in patients with aplastic anemia receiving allogeneic marrow transplants. Am J Med 76:564–572, 1984.

55. Dekker AW, Verdonck LF, Rozenberg-Arska M: Infection prevention in autologous bone marrow transplantation and the role of protective isolation. Bone Marrow Transplant 14:89–93, 1994.

56. Petersen F, Thornquist M, Buckner C, Counts G, Nelson N, Meyers J et al: The effects of infection prevention regimens on early infectious complications in marrow transplant patients: A four arm randomized study. Infection 16:199–208, 1988.

57. Buckner CD, Clift RA, Sanders JE, Meyers JD, Counts GW, Farewell VT et al: Protective environment for marrow transplant recipients: A prospective study. Ann Intern Med 89:893–901, 1978.

58. Chandrasekar PH, Abraham OC, Klein J, Alangaden G, Chalasani G, Cassells L et al: Low infectious morbidity after intensive chemotherapy and autologous peripheral blood progenitor cell transplantation in the outpatient setting for women with breast cancer. Clin Infect Dis 32:546–551, 2001.

59. Rives S, Carreras E, Rovira M, Montoto S, Urbano-Ispizua A, Martinez C et al: The autologous transplantation of hematopoietic precursors on an outpatient basis: An analysis of its feasibility at the Hospital de Barcelona. Med Clin 113:201–204, 1999.

60. Jagannath S, Vesole DH, Zhang M, Desikan KR, Copeland N, Jagannath M et al: Feasibility and cost-effectiveness of outpatient autotransplants in multiple myeloma. Bone Marrow Transplant 20:445–450, 1997.

61. Meisenberg BR, Miller WE, McMillan R, Callaghan M, Sloan C, Brehm T et al: Outpatient high-dose chemotherapy with autologous stem-cell rescue for hematologic and nonhematologic malignancies. J Clin Oncol 15:11–17, 1997.

62. Gluck S, des Rochers C, Cano C, Dorreen M, Germond C, Gill K et al: High-dose chemotherapy followed by autologous blood cell transplantation: A safe and effective outpatient approach. Bone Marrow Transplant 20:431–434, 1997.

63. Russell JA, Poon MC, Jones AR, Woodman RC, Ruether BA: Allogeneic bone-marrow transplantation without protective isolation in adults with malignant disease. Lancet 339:38–40, 1992.

64. Gomez-Almaguer D, Ruiz-Arguelles GJ, Ruiz-Arguelles A, Gonzalez-Llano O, Cantu OE, Hernandez NE: Hematopoietic stem cell allografts using a non-myeloablative conditioning regimen can be safely performed on an outpatient basis: Report of four cases. Bone Marrow Transplant 25:131–133, 2000.

65. Rizzo JD, Vogelsang GB, Krumm S, Frink B, Mock V, Bass EB: Outpatient-based bone marrow transplantation for hematologic malignancies: Cost saving or cost shifting? J Clin Oncol 17:2811–2818, 1999.

66. Svahn BM, Bjurman B, Myrback KE, Aschan J, Ringden O: Is it safe to treat allogeneic stem cell transplant recipients at home during the pancytopenic phase? A pilot trial. Bone Marrow Transplant 26:1057–1060, 2000.

67. Gauvreau-Stern JM, Cheney CL, Aker SN, Lenssen P: Food intake patterns and foodservice requirements on a marrow transplant unit. J Am Dietetic Assoc 89:367–372, 1989.

68. Dignani MC, Herrera F, Milone G, Riveros D, Relloso S, Bonvehí P: Medicina Alternativa para el Tratamiento del Cáncer: Una fuente Potencial de Infecciones Severas. In XX Reunión Anual de Trabajo de la Asociación Argentina de Oncología Clínica; Junio 23–25, 2000; Buenos Aires, Argentina, 2000.

69. Oliver M, Van Voorhis W, Boeck M, Mattson D, Bowden R: Hepatic mucormicosis in a bone marrow transplant recipient who ingested naturopathic medicine. Clin Infect Dis 22:521–524, 1996.

70. Latham R, Schaffner W: Nosocomial Legionnaires disease. Curr Opin Infect Dis 5:512–516, 1992.

71. Anaissie EJ, Penzak SR, Dignani MC: The hospital water supply as a source of nosocomial infections: A plea for action. Arch Intern Med 162:1483–1492, 2002.

72. Warris A, Gaustad P, Meis J, Verweij P, Abrahamsen T: Water as a source of filamentous fungi in a childhood bone marrow transplantation unit. In 39th Interscience Conference on Antimicrobial Agents and Chemotherapy (ICAAC), September 26–29, 1999, p. 578.

73. Anaissie E, Kuchar R, Rex JH, Summerbell R, Walsh T: The hospital water system as a reservoir of Fusarium. In 37th Interscience Conference of Antimicrobial Agents and Chemotherapy (ICAAC), September 28–October 1, Toronto, Ontario, Canada, 1997.

74. Nucci M, Silveira F, Akiti T, Barreiros G, Revankar SG, Wickes BL et al: Nosocomial outbreak of Exophiala jeanselmei fungemia associated with contamination of the hospital water. In 40th Interscience Conference on Antimicrobial Agents and Chemotherapy (ICAAC), September 17–20, 2000, Toronto, Ontario, Canada.

75. Doebbeling BN: Protecting the healthcare worker from infection and injury. In Wenzel RP (ed.): Prevention and Control of Nosocomial Infections, 3rd Ed., pp. 397–435. Williams & Wilkins, Baltimore, 1997.

76. Anonymous: Immunization of health-care workers: Recommendations of the Advisory Committee on Immunization Practices (ACIP) and the Hospital Infection Control Practices Advisory Committee (HICPAC). MMWR 46(RR-18):1–42, 1997.

77. Vazquez JA, Dembry LM, Sanchez V et al: Nosocomial Candida glabrata colonization: An epidemiologic study. J Clin Microbiol 36:421, 1998.

78. Wey SB: Bone marrow transplant patients. In Wenzel RP (ed.): Prevention and Control of Nosocomial Infections, 3rd Ed., pp. 1137–1169. Williams & Wilkins, Baltimore, 1997.

79. Advisory Committee on Immunization Practices (ACIP) CoD-CaPC: Prolonged poliovirus excretion in an immunodeficient person with vaccine-associated paralytic poliomyelitis. MMWR 46:641–643, 1997.

80. Nkowane BM, Wassilak SG, Orenstein WA, Bart KJ, Schonberger LB, Hinman AR et al: Vaccine-associated paralytic poliomyelitis. United States: 1973 through 1984. JAMA 257:1335–1340, 1987.

81. Mathias RG, Routley JV: Paralysis in an immunocompromised adult following oral polio vaccination. Can Med Assoc J 132:738–739, 1985.

82. Chitsike I, van Furth R: Paralytic poliomyelitis associated with live oral poliomyelitis vaccine in child with HIV infection in Zimbabwe: Case report. BMJ 318:841–843, 1999.

83. Centers for Disease Control and Prevention: Prevention of varicella. MMWR 45(RR-11):1–36, 1996.

84. Tsolia M, Gershon AA, Steinberg SP, Gelb L: Live attenuated varicella vaccine: Evidence that the virus is attenuated and the importance of skin lesions in transmission of varicella-zoster virus. National Institute of Allergy and Infectious Diseases Varicella Vaccine Collaborative Study Group. J Pediatr 116:184–189, 1990.

85. Weber DJ, Rutala WA: Environmental issues and nosocomial infections. In Wenzel RP (ed.): Prevention and Control of Nosocomial Infections, pp. 491–514. Williams & Wilkins, Baltimore, 1997.

86. Martin MA, Reichelderfer M, Association for Professionals in Infection Control and Epidemiology Inc. 1991 1992 and 1993 APIC Guidelines Committee: APIC guidelines for infection prevention and control in flexible endoscopy. Am J Infect Control 22:19, 1994.

87. Christopher C, Prentice KG: Infection control aspects of bone marrow transplantation. Curr Opin Infect Dis 7:427–429, 1994.

88. Centers for Disease Control and Prevention: Intravascular device-related infections prevention. Fed Reg 60:49978–50003, 1995.

89. Schleupner MS: Protecting recipients of blood and blood products. In Wenzel RP (ed.): Prevention and Control of Nosocomial Infections, 3rd Ed., pp. 1187–1227. Williams & Wilkins, Baltimore, 1997.

90. Webb IJ, Coral FS, Andersen JW, Elias AD, Finberg RW, Nadler LM et al: Sources and sequelae of bacterial contamination of hematopoietic stem cell components: Implications for the safety of hematotherapy and graft engineering. Transfusion 36:782–788, 1996.

91. American Association of Blood Banks: Facts about Blood and Blood Banking. In www.aabb.org, 1999.

92. Wood EE: Brucellosis as a hazard of blood transfusion. BMJ i:27, 1955.

93. Naparstek E, Block CS, Slavin S: Transmission of brucellosis by bone marrow transplantation. Lancet 1:574–575, 1982.

94. Ertem M, Kurekci AE, Aysev D, Unal E, Ikinciogullari A: Brucellosis transmitted by bone marrow transplantation. Bone Marrow Transplant 26:225–226, 2000.

95. Bowden RA, Sayers M, Flournoy N, Newton B, Banaji M, Thomas ED et al: Cytomegalovirus immune globulin and seronegative blood products to prevent primary cytomegalovirus infection after marrow transplantation. N Engl J Med 314:1006–1010, 1986.

96. De Witte T, Schattenberg A, Van Dijk BA, Galama J, Olthuis H, Van der Meer JW et al: Prevention of primary cytomegalovirus infection after allogeneic bone marrow transplantation by using leukocyte-poor random blood products from cytomegalovirus-unscreened blood-bank donors. Transplantation 50:964–968, 1990.

97. Bowden RA, Slichter SJ, Sayers M, Weisdorf D, Cays M, Schoch G et al: A comparison of filtered leukocyte-reduced and cytomegalovirus (CMV) seronegative blood products for the prevention of transfusion-associated CMV infection after marrow transplant [see comments]. Blood 86:3598–3603, 1995.

98. de Graan-Hentzen YC, Gratama JW, Mudde GC et al: Prevention of primary cytomegalovirus infection in patients with hematologic malignancies by intensive white cell depletion of blood products. Transfusion 29:757–760, 1989.

99. Bowden RA, Slichter SJ, Sayers MH, Mori M, Cays MJ, Meyers JD: Use of leukocyte-depleted platelets and cytomegalovirus-seronegative red blood cells for prevention of primary cytomegalovirus infection after marrow transplant. Blood 78:246–250, 1991.

100. Elfath M, Whitley P, Sawyer S et al: Consistent leukoreduction of apheresis platelets using new fluidized bed separation technology. Blood 86(Suppl.):545a, 1995.

101. Alfieri C, Tanner J, Carpentier L, Perpete C, Savoie A, Paradis K et al: Epstein-Barr virus transmission from a blood donor to an organ transplant recipient with recovery of the same virus strain from the recipient's blood and oropharynx. Blood 87:812–817, 1996.

102. Cohen JI: Epstein-Barr virus lymphoproliferative disease associated with acquired immunodeficiency. Medicine 70:137–160, 1991.

103. Walker RC, Paya CV, Marshall WF, Strickler JG, Wiesner RH, Velosa JA et al: Pretransplantation seronegative Epstein-Barr virus status is the primary risk factor for posttransplantation lympho-

proliferative disorder in adult heart, lung, and other solid organ transplantations. J Heart Lung Transplant 14:214–221, 1995.

104. Gerritsen EJ, Stam ED, Hermans J, van den Berg H, Haraldsson A, van Tol MJ et al: Risk factors for developing EBV-related B cell lymphoproliferative disorders (BLPD) after non-HLA-identical BMT in children. Bone Marrow Transplant 18:377–382, 1996.

105. Rowe DT, Qu L, Reyes J, Jabbour N, Yunis E, Putnam P et al: Use of quantitative competitive PCR to measure Epstein-Barr virus genome load in the peripheral blood of pediatric transplant patients with lymphoproliferative disorders. J Clin Microbiol 35:1612–1615, 1997.

106. Meyers JD et al: Parenterally transmitted hepatitis A associated with platelet transfusions. Epidemiologic study of an outbreak in a marrow transplantation center. Ann Intern Med 81:145–151, 1974.

107. Centers for Disease Control and Prevention: Hepatitis A among persons with hemophilia who received clotting factor concentrate. MMWR 45:29–32, 1996.

108. Ghez D, Nicand E, Ferre V, de Tailly PD, Coppo P, Lenoir B et al: Allogenic bone marrow transplantation with a donor presenting with an acute hepatitis A. J Hepatol 34:625–630, 2001.

109. Fujiwara K, Yokosuka O, Ehata T, Imazeki F, Saisho H, Miki M et al: Frequent detection of hepatitis A viral RNA in serum during the early convalescent phase of acute hepatitis A. Hepatology 26:1634–1639, 1997.

110. Strasser SI, McDonald GB: Hepatitis viruses and hematopoietic cell transplantation: A guide to patient and donor management. Blood 93:1127–1136, 1999.

111. Cantin E, Chen J, Gaidulis L, Valo Z, McLaughlin-Taylor E: Detection of herpes simplex virus DNA sequences in human blood and bone marrow cells. J Med Virol 42:279–286, 1994.

112. Wingard JR: Oral complications of cancer therapies. Infectious and noninfectious systemic consequences. NCI Monographs (9):21–26, 1990.

113. Leung TF, Chik KW, Li CK, Lai H, Shing MM, Chan PK et al: Incidence, risk factors and outcome of varicella-zoster virus infection in children after haematopoietic stem cell transplantation. Bone Marrow Transplant 25:167–172, 2000.

114. Dharmasena F, Gordon-Smith EC: Transmission of malaria by bone marrow transplantation. Transplantation 42:228, 1986.

115. Villeneuve L, Cassaing S, Magnaval JF, Boisseau M, Huynh A, Demur C et al: Plasmodium falciparum infection following allogeneic bone-marrow transplantation. Ann Trop Med Parasitol 93:533–535, 1999.

116. Siegel SE, Lunde MN, Gelderman AH, Halterman RH, Brown JA, Levine AS et al: Transmission of toxoplasmosis by leukocyte transfusion. Blood 37:388–394, 1971.

117. Montoya JG, Remington JS: Toxoplasma gondii. In Mandell GL, Bennett JE, Dolin R (eds.): Principles and Practice of Infectious Diseases, pp. 2858–2888. Churchill Livingstone, Philadelphia, 2000.

118. Small TN, Leung L, Stiles J, Kiehn TE, Malak SA, O'Reilly RJ et al: Disseminated toxoplasmosis following T cell-depleted related and unrelated bone marrow transplantation. Bone Marrow Transplant 25:969–973, 2000.

119. Derouin F, Devergie A, Auber P, Gluckman E, Beauvais B, Garin YJ et al: Toxoplasmosis in bone marrow-transplant recipients: Report of seven cases and review. Clin Infect Dis 15:267–270, 1992.

120. O'Drisco JC, Holliman RE: Toxoplasmosis and bone marrow transplantation. Rev Med Microbiol 2:215–222, 1991.

121. Leiby DA, Read EJ, Lenes BA, Yund AJ, Stumpf RJ, Kirchhoff LV et al: Seroepidemiology of Trypanosoma cruzi, etiologic agent of Chagas' disease, in US blood donors. J Infect Dis 176:1047–1052, 1997.

122. Leiby DA, Lenes BA, Tibbals MA, Tames-Olmedo MT: Prospective evaluation of a patient with Trypanosoma cruzi infection transmitted by transfusion. N Eng J Med 341:1237–1239, 1999.

123. Leiby DA, Fucci MH, Stumpf RJ: Trypanosoma cruzi in a low- to moderate-risk blood donor population: Seroprevalence and possible congenital transmission. Transfusion 39:310–315, 1999.

124. Villalba R, Fornes G, Alvarez MA, Roman J, Rubio V, Fernandez M et al: Acute Chagas' disease in a recipient of a bone marrow transplant in Spain: Case report. Clin Infect Dis 14:594–595, 1992.

125. Leiguarda R, Roncoroni A, Taratuto AL, Jost L, Berthier M, Nogues M et al: Acute CNS infection by Trypanosoma cruzi (Chagas' disease) in immunosuppressed patients. Neurology 40:850–851, 1990.

126. Grant IH, Gold JW, Wittner M, Tanowitz HB, Nathan C, Mayer K et al: Transfusion-associated acute Chagas disease acquired in the United States. Ann Intern Med 111:849–851, 1989.

127. Kohl S, Pickering LK, Frankel LS, Yaeger RG: Reactivation of Chagas' disease during therapy of acute lymphocytic leukemia. Cancer 50:827–828, 1982.

128. Altclas J, Jaimovich G, Milovic V, Klein F, Feldman L: Chagas' disease after bone marrow transplantation. Bone Marrow Transplant 18:447–448, 1996.

129. Schmunis GA: Trypanosoma cruzi, the etiologic agent of Chagas' disease: Status in the blood supply in endemic and nonendemic countries. Transfusion 31:547–557, 1991.

130. Dictar M, Sinagra A, Veron MT, Luna C, Dengra C, De Rissio A et al: Recipients and donors of bone marrow transplants suffering from Chagas' disease: Management and preemptive therapy of parasitemia. Bone Marrow Transplant 21:391–393, 1998.

131. Altclas J, Sinagra A, Jaimovich G, Salgueira C, Luna C, Requejo A et al: Reactivation of chronic Chagas' disease following allogeneic bone marrow transplantation and successful pre-emptive therapy with benznidazole. Transplant Infect Dis 1:135–137, 1999.

132. Thompson RF: Travel & routine immunizations: A practical guide for the medical office, 2000 Ed. Shoreland, Milwaukee, WI, 2000.

133. Centers for Disease Control and Prevention: Prevention of hepatitis A through active or passive immunization: Recommendations of the Advisory Committee on Imunization Practices. MMWR 48(RR-12):1–37, 1999.

134. Dignani MC, Miceli M, Rosa CM, Gatica J, Pavlovsky S, Pizzolato M: Loss of hepatitis A virus (HAV) antibodies after peripheral stem Cell transplantion (PSCT). In 39th Annual Meeting of the Infectious Disease Society of America, October 25–28, 2001, San Francisco, CA.

135. Stokes J, Neefe JR: The prevention and attenuation of infectious hepatitis by gamma globulin: Preliminary note. JAMA 127:144–145, 1945.

136. Kluge T: Gamma-globulin in the prevention of viral hepatitis: A study on the effect of medium-size doses. Acta Med Scand 174:469–477, 1963.

137. Mosley JW, Reisler DM, Brachott D, Roth D, Weiser J: Comparison of two lots of immune serum globulin for prophylaxis of infectious hepatitis. Am J Epidemiol 87:539–550, 1968.

138. Perrillo RP, Gelb L, Campbell C, Wellinghoff W, Ellis FR, Overby L et al: Hepatitis B e antigen, DNA polymerase activity, and infection of household contacts with hepatitis B virus. Gastroenterology 76:1319–1325, 1979.

139. Zamir D, Zamir C, Rishpon S: Epidemiology of hepatitis B virus infection among family members of chronic carriers in Israel. Isr Med Assoc J 3:338–340, 2001.

140. Inaba N, Ohkawa R, Matsuura A, Kudoh J, Takamizawa H: Sexual transmission of hepatitis B surface antigen. Infection of husbands by HBsAg carrier-state wives. Br J Vener Dis 55:366–368, 1979.

141. Centers for Disease Control and Prevention: Protection against viral hepatitis: Recommendations of the Immunization Practices Advisory Committee (ACIP). MMWR 40(RR-13):21–25, 1990.

142. U.S. Public Health Service: Updated U.S. Public Health Service Guidelines for the Management of Occupational Exposures to HBV, HCV, and HIV and Recommendations for Postexposure Prophylaxis. MMWR 50(RR-11):1–52, 2001.

143. Mitsui T, Iwano K, Suzuki S, Yamazaki C, Masuko K, Tsuda F et al: Combined hepatitis B immune globulin and vaccine for postexposure prophylaxis of accidental hepatitis B virus infection in hemodialysis staff members: Comparison with immune globulin without vaccine in historical controls. Hepatology 10:324–327, 1989.

144. Redeker AG, Mosley JW, Gocke DJ, McKee AP, Pollack W: Hepatitis B immune globulin as a prophylactic measure for spouses exposed to acute type B hepatitis. N Engl J Med 293:1055–1059, 1975.

145. Seeff LB, Zimmerman HJ, Wright EC, Finkelstein JD, Garcia-Pont P, Greenlee HB et al: A randomized, double blind controlled trial of the efficacy of immune serum globulin for the prevention of post-transfusion hepatitis. A Veterans Administration cooperative study. Gastroenterology 72:111–121, 1977.

146. Grady GF, Lee VA, Prince AM, Gitnick GL, Fawaz KA, Vyas GN et al: Hepatitis B immune globulin for accidental exposures among medical personnel: Final report of a multicenter controlled trial. J Infect Dis 138:625–638, 1978.

147. Robinson WS: Hepatitis B virus and hepatitis D virus. In Mandell GL, Bennett JE, Dolin R (Eds.): Principles and Practice of Infectious Diseases, 5th ed., pp. 1652–1685, Churchill Livingstone, Orlando, FL, 2000.

148. Palmovic D, Crnjakovic-Palmovic J: Prevention of hepatitis B virus (HBV) infection in health-care workers after accidental exposure: A comparison of two prophylactic schedules. Infection 21:42–45, 1993.

149. Sartori M, La Terra G, Aglietta M, Manzin A, Navino C, Verzetti G: Transmission of hepatitis C via blood splash into conjunctiva [Letter]. Scand J Infect Dis 25:270–271, 1993.

150. Ippolito G, Puro V, Petrosillo N et al: Simultaneous infection with HIV and hepatitis C virus following occupational conjunctival blood exposure [Letter]. JAMA 280:28, 1998.

151. Mitsui T, Iwano K, Masuko K et al: Hepatitis C virus infection in medical personnel after needlestick accident. Hepatology 16:1109–1114, 1992.

152. Centers for Disease Control and Prevention: Recommendations for prevention and control of hepatitis C virus (HCV) infection and HCV-related chronic disease. MMWR 47(RR19):1–39, 1998.

153. Thomas DL, Zenilman JM, Alter HJ, Shih JW, Galai N, Carella AV et al: Sexual transmission of hepatitis C virus among patients attending sexually transmitted diseases clinics in Baltimore—an analysis of 309 sex partnerships. J Infect Dis 171:768–775, 1995.

154. Pol S, Fontaine H, Carnot F, Zylberberg H, Berthelot P, Brechot C et al: Predictive factors for development of cirrhosis in parenterally acquired chronic hepatitis C: A comparison between immunocompetent and immunocompromised patients. J Hepatol 29:12–19, 1998.

155. Bell DM: Occupational risk of human immunodeficiency virus infection in healthcare workers: An overview. Am J Med 102:9–15, 1997.

156. Ippolito G, Puro V, De Carli G: The risk of occupational human immunodeficiency virus infection in health care workers. Italian Multicenter Study. The Italian Study Group on Occupational Risk of HIV infection. Arch Intern Med 153:1451–1458, 1993.

157. Mastro TD, de Vincenzi I. Probabilities of sexual HIV-1 transmission. AIDS 10(Suppl. A):S75–82, 1996.

158. Centers for Disease Control and Prevention: Prevention and control of influenza. MMWR 50(RR04):1–46, 2001.

159. Hayden FG, Gubareva LV, Monto AS, Klein TC, Elliot MJ, Hammond JM et al: Inhaled zanamivir for the prevention of influenza in families. Zanamivir Family Study Group. N Engl J Med 343:1282–1289, 2000.

160. Welliver R, Monto AS, Carewicz O, Schatteman E, Hassman M, Hedrick J et al: Effectiveness of oseltamivir in preventing influenza in household contacts: A randomized controlled trial. JAMA 285:748–754, 2001.

161. Wintermeyer SM, Nahata MC: Rimantadine: A clinical perspective. Ann Pharmacother 29:299–310, 1995.

162. Tominack RL, Hayden FG: Rimantadine hydrochloride and amantadine hydrochloride use in influenza A virus infections. Infect Dis Clin North Am 1:459–478, 1987.

163. Demicheli V, Jefferson T, Rivetti D, Deeks J: Prevention and early treatment of influenza in healthy adults. Vaccine 18:957–1030, 2000.

164. Hayden FG, Atmar RL, Schilling M et al: Use of the selective oral neuraminidase inhibitor oseltamivir to prevent influenza. N Engl J Med 341:1336–1343, 1999.

165. Centers for Disease Control and Prevention: Measles pneumonitis following measles-mumps-rubella vaccination of a patient with HIV infection. MMWR 45:603–606, 1993.

166. Ross AH: Modification of chickenpox in family contacts by administration of gamma globulin. N Engl J Med 267:369–376, 1962.

167. Zaia JA, Levin MJ, Preblud SR, Leszczynski J, Wright GG, Ellis RJ et al: Evaluation of varicella-zoster immune globulin: Protection of immunosuppressed children after household exposure to varicella. J Infect Dis 147:737–743, 1983.

168. Orenstein WA, Heymann DL, Ellis RJ, Rosenberg RL, Nakano J, Halsey NA et al: Prophylaxis of varicella in high-risk children: Dose-response effect of zoster immune globulin. J Pediatr 98:368–373, 1981.

169. Anonymous: Varicella-zoster immune globulin for the prevention of chickenpox. MMWR 33:84–90, 95–100, 1984.

170. Ho CM, Khuzaiah R, Yasmin AM. Varicella in children with haematological malignancy—outcome of treatment and prevention. Med J Malaysia 49:29–35, 1994.

171. Suga S, Yoshikawa T, Ozaki T, Asano Y: Effect of oral acyclovir against primary and secondary viraemia in incubation period of varicella. Arch Dis Child 69:639–642; discussion 642–643, 1993.

172. Sempere A, Sanz GF, Senent L, de la Rubia J, Jarque I, Lopez F et al: Long-term acyclovir prophylaxis for prevention of varicella zoster virus infection after autologous blood stem cell transplantation in patients with acute leukemia. Bone Marrow Transplant 10:495–498, 1992.

173. Ljungman P, Wilczek H, Gahrton G, Gustavsson A, Lundgren G, Lonnqvist B et al: Long-term acyclovir prophylaxis in bone marrow transplant recipients and lymphocyte proliferation responses to herpes virus antigens in vitro. Bone Marrow Transplant 1:185–192, 1986.

174. Lundgren G, Wilczek H, Lonnqvist B, Lindholm A, Wahren B, Ringden O: Acyclovir prophylaxis in bone marrow transplant recipients. Scand J Infect Dis Suppl 47:137–144, 1985.

175. Centers for Disease Control and Prevention: Recommendations of the Immunizations Practice Advisory Committee (ACIP) Varicella-Zoster Immune Globuline for the Prevention of Chickenpox. MMWR 33:84–90, 95–100, 1984.

176. Leake JA, Mosley DG, England B, Graham JV, Plikaytis BD, Ampel NM et al: Risk factors for acute symptomatic coccidioidomycosis among elderly persons in Arizona, 1996–1997. J Infect Dis 181:1435–1440, 2000.

177. Stead WW: Tuberculosis among elderly persons: An outbreak in a nursing home. Ann Intern Med 94:606–610, 1981.

178. Stead WW: Management of health care workers after inadvertent exposure to tuberculosis: A guide for the use of preventive therapy. Ann Intern Med 122:906–912, 1995.

179. American Thoracic Society, CDC: Targeted tuberculin testing and treatment of latent tuberculosis infection. MMWR 49(RR-06):1–51, 2000.

180. Engels EA, Lau J, Barza M: Efficacy of quinolone prophylaxis in neutropenic cancer patients: A meta-analysis. J Clin Oncol 16:1179–1187, 1998.

181. Lew MA, Kehoe K, Ritz J, Antman KH, Nadler L, Kalish LA et al: Ciprofloxacin versus trimethoprim/sulfamethoxazole for prophylaxis of bacterial infections in bone marrow transplant recipients: A randomized, controlled trial. J Clin Oncol 13:239–250, 1995.

182. Imrie KR, Prince HM, Couture F, Brandwein JM, Keating A: Effect of antimicrobial prophylaxis on hematopoietic recovery following autologous bone marrow transplantation: Ciprofloxacin versus co-trimoxazole. Bone Marrow Transplant 15:267–270, 1995.

183. Cruciani M, Rampazzo R, Malena M, Lazzarini L, Todeschini G, Messori A et al: Prophylaxis with fluoroquinolones for bacterial infections in neutropenic patients: A meta-analysis. Clin Infect Dis 23:795–805, 1996.

184. Classen DC, Burke JP, Ford CD, Evershed S, Aloia MR, Wilfahrt JK et al: *Streptococcus mitis* sepsis in bone marrow transplant patients receiving oral antimicrobial prophylaxis. Am J Med 89:441–446, 1990.

185. Broun ER, Wheat JL, Kneebone PH, Sundblad K, Hromas RA, Tricot G: Randomized trial of the addition of gram-positive prophylaxis to standard antimicrobial prophylaxis for patients undergoing autologous bone marrow transplantation. Antimicrob Agents Chemother 38:576–579, 1994.

186. Arns da Cunha C, Weisdorf D, Shu XO, DeFor T, Pastor JD 3rd, Johnson JR: Early gram-positive bacteremia in BMT recipients: Impact of three different approaches to antimicrobial prophylaxis. Bone Marrow Transplant 21:173–180, 1998.

187. Attal M, Schlaifer D, Rubie H, Huguet F, Charlet JP, Bloom E et al: Prevention of gram-positive infections after bone marrow transplantation by systemic vancomycin: A prospective, randomized trial. J Clin Oncol 9:865–870, 1991.

188. Barbe G, Ploton C, Pondarre C, Bertrand Y, Souillet G, Philippe N: Vancomycin-resistant enterococci in pediatric hematology: Don't panic. Patholo Biol 46:408–411, 1998.

189. Tenover FC, Biddle JW, Lancaster MV: Increasing resistance to vancomycin and other glycopeptides in *Staphylococcus aureus*. Emerg Infect Dis 7:327–332, 2001.

190. Gonzalez-Barca E, Fernandez-Sevilla A, Carratala J, Salar A, Peris J, Granena A et al: Prognostic factors influencing mortality in cancer patients with neutropenia and bacteremia. Eur J Clin Microbiol Infect Dis 18:539–544, 1999.

191. Nucci M, Spector N, Bueno AP, Solza C, Perecmanis T, Bacha PC et al: Risk factors and attributable mortality associated with superinfections in neutropenic patients with cancer. Clin Infect Dis 24:575–579, 1997.

192. Roy V, Ochs L, Weisdorf D: Late infections following allogeneic bone marrow transplantation: Suggested strategies for prophylaxis. Leuk Lymphoma 26:1–15, 1997.

193. Beelen DW, Elmaagacli A, Muller KD, Hirche H, Schaefer UW: Influence of intestinal bacterial decontamination using metronidazole and ciprofloxacin or ciprofloxacin alone on the development of acute graft-versus-host disease after marrow transplantation in patients with hematologic malignancies: Final results and long-term follow-up of an open-label prospective randomized trial. Blood 93:3267–3275, 1999.

194. Anaissie EJ, Rex JH, Uzun O, Vartivarian S: Predictors of adverse outcome in cancer patients with candidemia. Am J Med 104:238–245, 1998.

195. Jarvis WR: Epidemiology of nosocomial fungal infections, with emphasis on *Candida* species. Clin Infect Dis 20:1526–1530, 1995.

196. Wald A, Leisenring W, van Burik J, Bowden RA: Epidemiology of *Aspergillus* infections in a large cohort of patients undergoing bone marrow transplantation. J Infect Dis 175:1459–1466, 1997.

197. Goodman JL, Winston DJ, Greenfield RA, Chandrasekar PH, Fox B, Kaizer H et al: A controlled trial of fluconazole to prevent fungal infections in patients undergoing bone marrow transplantation. N Engl J Med 326:845–851, 1992.

198. Slavin MA, Osborne B, Adams R, Levenstein MJ, Schoch HG, Feldman AR et al: Efficacy and safety of fluconazole prophylaxis for fungal infections after bone marrow transplantation—a prospective, randomized, double-blind study. J Infect Dis 171:1545–1542, 1995.

199. Wingard JR, Merz WG, Rinaldi MG, Miller CB, Karp JE, Saral R: Association of *Torulopsis glabrata* infections with fluconazole prophylaxis in neutropenic bone marrow transplant patients. Antimicrob Agents Chemother 37:1847–1849, 1993.

200. Abi-Said D, Anaissie E, Uzun O, Raad I, Pinzcowski H, Vartivarian S: The epidemiology of hematogenous candidiasis caused by different *Candida* species [see comments] [published erratum appears in Clin Infect Dis 1997 Aug;25(2):352]. Clin Infect Dis 24:1122–1128, 1997.

201. Nucci M, Biasoli I, Akiti T, Silveira F, Solza C, Barreiros G et al: A double-blind, randomized, placebo-controlled trial of itraconazole capsules as antifungal prophylaxis for neutropenic patients. Clin Infect Dis 30:300–305, 2000.

202. Menichetti F, Del Favero A, Martino P, Bucaneve G, Micozzi A, Girmenia C et al: Itraconazole oral solution as prophylaxis for fungal infections in neutropenic patients with hematologic malignancies: A randomized, placebo-controlled, double-blind, multicenter trial. GIMEMA Infection Program. Gruppo Italiano Malattie Ematologiche dell' Adulto. Clin Infect Dis 28:250–255, 1999.

203. Denning DW, Donnelly JP, Hellreigel KP, Ito J, Martino P, van't Wout JW: Antifungal prophylaxis during neutropenia or allogeneic bone marrow transplantation: What is the state of the art? Ad Hoc Working Group. Chemotherapy 38(Suppl. 1):43–49, 1992.

204. Anaissie EJ, Kuchar RT, Rex JH, Francesconi A, Kasai M, Müller FMC et al: Fusariosis and pathogenic Fusarium species in a hospital water system: A new paradigm for the epidemiology of opportunistic mould infections. Clin Infect Dis, in press.

205. Anaissie EJ, Stratton SL, Dignani MC, Summerbell RC, Rex JH, Monson TP et al: Pathogenic *Aspergillus* species recovered from a hospital water system: A three-year prospective study. Clin Infect Dis, in press.

206. Caillot D, Mannone L, Cuisenier B, Couaillier JF: Role of early diagnosis and aggressive surgery in the management of invasive pulmonary aspergillosis in neutropenic patients. Clin Microbiol Infect 7(Suppl. 2):54–61, 2001.

207. Kami M, Fukui T, Ogawa S, Kazuyama Y, Machida U, Tanaka Y et al: Use of real-time PCR on blood samples for diagnosis of invasive aspergillosis. Clin Infect Dis 33:1504–1512, 2001.

208. Karp JE, Burch PA, Merz WG: An approach to intensive antileukemia therapy in patients with previous invasive aspergillosis. Am J Med 85:203–206, 1988.

209. Offner F, Cordonnier C, Ljungman P, Prentice HG, Engelhard D, De Bacquer D et al: Impact of previous aspergillosis on the outcome of bone marrow transplantation. Clin Infect Dis 26:1098–1103, 1998.

210. Hoover M, Morgan ER, Kletzel M: Prior fungal infection is not a contraindication to bone marrow transplant in patients with acute leukemia. Med Pediatr Oncol 28:268–273, 1997.

211. Bernard A, Loire J, Caillot D, Casasnovas O, Couailler JF, Guy H et al: Emergency lung resections for invasive aspergillosis in neutropenic patients. Annal Chirurg 49:849–853, 1995.

212. Denning DW: Treatment of invasive aspergillosis. J Infect 28(Suppl. 1):25–33, 1994.

213. Bjerke JW, Meyers JD, Bowden RA: Hepatosplenic candidiasis—a contraindication to marrow transplantation? Blood 84:2811–2814, 1994.

214. Walsh TJ, Whitcomb PO, Revankar SG, Pizzo PA: Successful treatment of hepatosplenic candidiasis through repeated cycles of chemotherapy and neutropenia. Cancer 76:2357–2362, 1995.

215. Uzun O, Anaissie EJ: Antifungal prophylaxis in patients with hematological malignancies: A reappraisal. Blood 86:2063–2072, 1995.

216. Winston DJ, Ho WG, Champlin RE: Cytomegalovirus infections after allogeneic bone marrow transplantation. Rev Infect Dis 12(Suppl. 7):S776–792, 1990.

217. Nguyen Q, Champlin R, Giralt S, Rolston K, Raad I, Jacobson K et al: Late cytomegalovirus pneumonia in adult allogeneic blood and marrow transplant recipients. Clin Infect Dis 28:618–623, 1999.

218. Couriel D, Canosa J, Engler H, Collins A, Dunbar C, Barrett AJ: Early reactivation of cytomegalovirus and high risk of interstitial pneumonitis following T-depleted BMT for adults with hematological malignancies. Bone Marrow Transplant 18:347–353, 1996.

219. Hertenstein B, Hampl W, Bunjes D, Wiesneth M, Duncker C, Koszinowski U et al: In vivo/ex vivo T cell depletion for GVHD prophylaxis influences onset and course of active cytomegalovirus infection and disease after BMT. Bone Marrow Transplant 15:387–393, 1995.

220. Qamruddin AO, Oppenheim BA, Guiver M, Mutton KJ, Chopra R: Screening for cytomegalovirus (CMV) infection in allogeneic bone marrow transplantation using a quantitative whole blood polymerase chain reaction (PCR) method: Analysis of potential risk factors for CMV infection. Bone Marrow Transplant 27:301–306, 2001.

221. Boeckh M, Stevens-Ayers T, Bowden RA: Cytomegalovirus pp65 antigenemia after autologous marrow and peripheral blood stem cell transplantation. J Infect Dis 174:907–912, 1996.

222. Holmberg LA, Boeckh M, Hooper H, Leisenring W, Rowley S, Heimfeld S et al: Increased incidence of cytomegalovirus disease after autologous CD34-selected peripheral blood stem cell transplantation. Blood 94:4029–4035, 1999.

223. Schiller GJ, Vescio R, Berenson J: Cytomegalovirus infection following transplantation of autologous CD34-selected progenitor cells. Blood 96:1194, 2000.

224. Mera JR, Whimbey E, Elting L, Preti A, Luna MA, Bruner JM et al: Cytomegalovirus pneumonia in adult nontransplantation patients with cancer: Review of 20 cases occurring from 1964 through 1990. Clin Infect Dis 22:1046–1050, 1996.

225. Osterborg A, Fassas AS, Anagnostopoulos A, Dyer MJ, Catovsky D, Mellstedt H: Humanized CD52 monoclonal antibody Campath-1H as first-line treatment in chronic lymphocytic leukaemia. Br J Haematol 93:151–153, 1996.

226. Nguyen Q, Estey E, Raad I, Rolston K, Kantarjian H, Jacobson K et al: Cytomegalovirus pneumonia in adults with leukemia: An emerging problem. Clin Infect Dis 32:539–545, 2001.

227. Goodrich JM, Bowden RA, Fisher L, Keller C, Schoch G, Meyers JD: Ganciclovir prophylaxis to prevent cytomegalovirus disease after allogeneic marrow transplant. Ann Intern Med 118:173–178, 1993.

228. Winston DJ, Ho WG, Bartoni K, Du Mond C, Ebeling DF, Buhles WC et al: Ganciclovir prophylaxis of cytomegalovirus infection and disease in allogeneic bone marrow transplant recipients. Results of a placebo-controlled, double-blind trial. Ann Intern Med 118:179–184, 1993.

229. Slavin MA, Bindra RR, Gleaves CA, Pettinger MB, Bowden RA: Ganciclovir sensitivity of cytomegalovirus at diagnosis and during treatment of cytomegalovirus pneumonia in marrow transplant recipients. Antimicrob Agents Chemother 37:1360–1363, 1993.

230. Erice A, Borrell N, Li W, Miller WJ, Balfour HH Jr: Ganciclovir susceptibilities and analysis of UL97 region in cytomegalovirus (CMV) isolates from bone marrow recipients with CMV disease after antiviral prophylaxis. J Infect Dis 178:531–534, 1998.

231. Reusser P, Cordonnier C, Einsele H, Engelhard D, Link D, Locasciulli A et al: European survey of herpesvirus resistance to antiviral drugs in bone marrow transplant recipients. Infectious Diseases Working Party of the European Group for Blood and Marrow Transplantation (EBMT). Bone Marrow Transplant 17:813–817, 1996.

232. Li CR, Greenberg PD, Gilbert MJ, Goodrich JM, Riddell SR: Recovery of HLA-restricted cytomegalovirus (CMV)-specific T-cell responses after allogeneic bone marrow transplant: Correlation with CMV disease and effect of ganciclovir prophylaxis. Blood 83:1971–1979, 1994.

233. de Medeiros CR, Moreira VA, Pasquini R: Cytomegalovirus as a cause of very late interstitial pneumonia after bone marrow transplantation. Bone Marrow Transplant 26(4):443–444, 2000.

234. Schmidt GM, Horak DA, Niland JC, Duncan SR, Forman SJ, Zaia JA: A randomized, controlled trial of prophylactic ganciclovir for cytomegalovirus pulmonary infection in recipients of allogeneic bone marrow transplants; The City of Hope-Stanford-Syntex CMV Study Group [see comments]. N Engl J Med 324:1005–1011, 1991.

235. Boeckh M, Gooley TA, Myerson D, Cunningham T, Schoch G, Bowden RA: Cytomegalovirus pp65 antigenemia-guided early treatment with ganciclovir versus ganciclovir at engraftment after allogeneic marrow transplantation: A randomized double-blind study. Blood 88:4063–4071, 1996.

236. Wolf DG, Spector SA: Early diagnosis of human cytomegalovirus disease in transplant recipients by DNA amplification in plasma. Transplantation 56:330–334, 1993.

237. Ljungman P, Oberg G, Aschan J, Ehrnst A, Lonnqvist B, Pauksen K et al: Foscarnet for pre-emptive therapy of CMV infection detected by a leukocyte-based nested PCR in allogeneic bone marrow transplant patients. Bone Marrow Transplant 18:565–568, 1996.

238. Boeckh M, Gallez-Hawkins GM, Myerson D, Zaia JA, Bowden RA: Plasma polymerase chain reaction for cytomegalovirus DNA after allogeneic marrow transplantation: Comparison with polymerase chain reaction using peripheral blood leukocytes, pp65 antigenemia, and viral culture. Transplantation 64:108–113, 1997.

239. Ljungman P, Lore K, Aschan J, Klaesson S, Lewensohn-Fuchs I, Lonnqvist B et al: Use of a semi-quantitative PCR for cytomegalovirus DNA as a basis for pre-emptive antiviral therapy in allogeneic bone marrow transplant patients. Bone Marrow Transplant 17:583–587, 1996.

240. Zaia JA, Gallez-Hawkins GM, Tegtmeier BR, ter Veer A, Li X, Niland JC et al: Late cytomegalovirus disease in marrow trans-

plantation is predicted by virus load in plasma. J Infect Dis 176:782–785, 1997.

241. Brytting M, Mousavi-Jazi M, Bostrom L, Larsson M, Lunderberg J, Ljungman P et al: Cytomegalovirus DNA in peripheral blood leukocytes and plasma from bone marrow transplant recipients. Transplantation 60:961–965, 1995.

242. Moretti S, Zikos P, Van Lint MT, Tedone E, Occhini D, Gualandi F et al: Forscarnet vs ganciclovir for cytomegalovirus (CMV) antigenemia after allogeneic hemopoietic stem cell transplantation (HSCT): A randomised study. Bone Marrow Transplant 22:175–180, 1998.

243. Bregante S, Bertilson S, Tedone E, Van Lint MT, Trespi G, Mordini N et al: Foscarnet prophylaxis of cytomegalovirus infections in patients undergoing allogeneic bone marrow transplantation (BMT): A dose-finding study. Bone Marrow Transplant 26:23–29, 2000.

244. Ljungman P, Deliliers GL, Platzbecker U, Matthes-Martin S, Bacigalupo A, Einsele H et al: Cidofovir for cytomegalovirus infection and disease in allogeneic stem cell transplant recipients. The Infectious Diseases Working Party of the European Group for Blood and Marrow Transplantation. Blood 97:388–392, 2001.

245. Platzbecker U, Bandt D, Thiede C, Helwig A, Freiberg-Richter J, Schuler U et al: Successful preemptive cidofovir treatment for CMV antigenemia after dose-reduced conditioning and allogeneic blood stem cell transplantation. Transplantation 71:880–885, 2001.

246. Prentice HG, Gluckman E, Powles RL, Ljungman P, Milpied NJ, Camara R et al: Long-term survival in allogeneic bone marrow transplant recipients following acyclovir prophylaxis for CMV infection. The European Acyclovir for CMV Prophylaxis Study Group. Bone Marrow Transplant 19:129–133, 1997.

247. Lowance D, Neumayer HH, Legendre CM, Squifflet JP, Kovarik J, Brennan PJ et al: Valacyclovir for the prevention of cytomegalovirus disease after renal transplantation. International Valacyclovir Cytomegalovirus Prophylaxis Transplantation Study Group. N Engl J Med 340:1462–1470, 1999.

248. Ljungman P: Efficacy and safety of valacyclovir as prophylaxis against CMV infection and disease in BMT recipients. J Clin Virol 12:167–185, 1999, abstract G6-02.

249. Nankivell BJ, Malouf MA, Russ GR, Barclay P, Glanville AR, Allen RD et al: Maintenance therapy with oral ganciclovir after treatment of cytomegalovirus infection. Clin Transplant 12:270–273, 1998.

250. Boeckh M, Zaia JA, Jung D, Skettino S, Chauncey TR, Bowden RA: A study of the pharmacokinetics, antiviral activity, and tolerability of oral ganciclovir for CMV prophylaxis in marrow transplantation. Biol Blood Marrow Transplant 4:13–19, 1998.

251. Brown F, Banken L, Saywell K, Arum I: Pharmacokinetics of valganciclovir and ganciclovir following multiple oral dosages of valganciclovir in HIV- and CMV-seropositive volunteers. Clin Pharmacokinet 37:167–176, 1999.

252. Prentice HG, Kho P: Clinical strategies for the management of cytomegalovirus infection and disease in allogeneic bone marrow transplant. Bone Marrow Transplant 19:135–142, 1997.

253. Curtis RE, Travis LB, Rowlings PA, Socie G, Kingma DW, Banks PM et al: Risk of lymphoproliferative disorders after bone marrow transplantation: A multi-institutional study. Blood 94:2208–2216, 1999.

254. Zutter MM, Martin PJ, Sale GE, Shulman HM, Fisher L, Thomas ED et al: Epstein-Barr virus lymphoproliferation after bone marrow transplantation. Blood 72:520–529, 1988.

255. Chao NJ, Berry GJ, Advani R, Horning SJ, Weiss LM, Blume KG: Epstein-Barr virus-associated lymphoproliferative disorder fol-

lowing autologous bone marrow transplantation for non-Hodgkin's lymphoma. Transplantation 55:1425–1428, 1993.

256. Green M, Reyes J, Webber S, Rowe D: The role of antiviral and immunoglobulin therapy in the prevention of Epstein-Barr virus infection and post-transplant lymphoproliferative disease following solid organ transplantation. Transplant Infect Dis 3:97–103, 2001.

257. Rooney CM, Smith CA, Ng CY, Loftin SK, Sixbey JW, Gan Y et al: Infusion of cytotoxic T cells for the prevention and treatment of Epstein-Barr virus-induced lymphoma in allogeneic transplant recipients. Blood 92:1549–1555, 1998.

258. Hale G, Waldmann H: Risks of developing Epstein-Barr virus-related lymphoproliferative disorders after T-cell-depleted marrow transplants. CAMPATH Users. Blood 91:3079–3083, 1998.

259. Cavazzana-Calvo M, Bensoussan D, Jabado N, Haddad E, Yvon E, Moskwa M et al: Prevention of EBV-induced B-lymphoproliferative disorder by ex vivo marrow B-cell depletion in HLA-phenoidentical or non-identical T-depleted bone marrow transplantation. Br J Haematol 103:543–551, 1998.

260. van Esser JW, van der Holt B, Meijer E, Niesters HG, Trenschel R, Thijsen SF et al: Epstein-Barr virus (EBV) reactivation is a frequent event after allogeneic stem cell transplantation (SCT) and quantitatively predicts EBV-lymphoproliferative disease following T-cell–depleted SCT. Blood 98:972–978, 2001.

261. Stevens SJ, Verschuuren EA, Pronk I, van Der Bij W, Harmsen MC, The TH et al: Frequent monitoring of Epstein-Barr virus DNA load in unfractionated whole blood is essential for early detection of posttransplant lymphoproliferative disease in high-risk patients. Blood 97:1165–1171, 2001.

262. Lucas KG, Burton RL, Zimmerman SE, Wang J, Cornetta KG, Robertson KA et al: Semiquantitative Epstein-Barr virus (EBV) polymerase chain reaction for the determination of patients at risk for EBV-induced lymphoproliferative disease after stem cell transplantation. Blood 91:3654–3661, 1998.

263. Rooney CM, Loftin SK, Holladay MS, Brenner MK, Krance RA, Heslop HE: Early identification of Epstein-Barr virus-associated post-transplantation lymphoproliferative disease. Br J Haematol 89:98–103, 1995.

264. Kawatani T, Suou T, Tajima F, Ishiga K, Omura H, Endo A et al: Incidence of hepatitis virus infection and severe liver dysfunction in patients receiving chemotherapy for hematologic malignancies. Eur J Haematol 67:45–50, 2001.

265. Hoofnagle JH, Dusheiko GM, Schafer DF, Jones EA, Micetich KC, Young RC et al: Reactivation of chronic hepatitis B virus infection by cancer chemotherapy. Ann Intern Med 96:447–449, 1982.

266. Wands JR: Letter: Subacute and chronic active hepatitis after withdrawal of chemotherapy. Lancet 2:979, 1975.

267. Wands JR, Chura CM, Roll FJ, Maddrey WC: Serial studies of hepatitis-associated antigen and antibody in patients receiving anti-tumor chemotherapy for myeloproliferative and lymphoproliferative disorders. Gastroenterology 68:105–112, 1975.

268. Lok AS, Liang RH, Chiu EK, Wong KL, Chan TK, Todd D: Reactivation of hepatitis B virus replication in patients receiving cytotoxic therapy. Report of a prospective study. Gastroenterology 100:182–188, 1991.

269. Nakamura Y, Motokura T, Fujita A, Yamashita T, Ogata E: Severe hepatitis related to chemotherapy in hepatitis B virus carriers with hematologic malignancies. Survey in Japan, 1987–1991. Cancer 78:2210–2215, 1996.

270. Kumagai K, Takagi T, Nakamura S, Sawada U, Kura Y, Kodama F et al: Hepatitis B virus carriers in the treatment of malignant lymphoma: An epidemiological study in Japan. Ann Oncol 8(Suppl. 1):107–109, 1997.

271. Chen PM, Chiou TJ, Fan FS, Liu JM, Hsieh RK, Yen CC et al: Fulminant hepatitis is significantly increased in hepatitis B carriers after allogeneic bone marrow transplantation. Transplantation 67:1425–1433, 1999.

272. Lau GK, Liang R, Chiu EK, Lee CK, Lam SK: Hepatic events after bone marrow transplantation in patients with hepatitis B infection: A case controlled study. Bone Marrow Transplant 19:795–799, 1997.

273. Lau JY, Lai CL, Lin HJ, Lok AS, Liang RH, Wu PC et al: Fatal reactivation of chronic hepatitis B virus infection following withdrawal of chemotherapy in lymphoma patients. Q J Med 73:911–917, 1989.

274. Reed EC, Myerson D, Corey L, Meyers JD: Allogeneic marrow transplantation in patients positive for hepatitis B surface antigen. Blood 77:195–200, 1991.

275. Yeo W, Chan PK, Zhong S, Ho WM, Steinberg JL, Tam JS et al: Frequency of hepatitis B virus reactivation in cancer patients undergoing cytotoxic chemotherapy: A prospective study of 626 patients with identification of risk factors. J Med Virol 62:299–307, 2000.

276. Ohtsu T, Sai T, Oka M, Sugai Y, Tobinai K: Activation of hepatitis B virus infection by chemotherapy containing glucocorticoid in hepatitis B virus carriers with hematologic malignancies. Jpn J Clin Oncol 21:360–365, 1991.

277. Cheng AL: Steroid-free chemotherapy decreases the risk of hepatitis flare-up in hepatitis B virus carriers with non-Hodgkin's lymphoma. Blood 87:1202, 1996.

278. Liang R, Lau GK, Kwong YL: Chemotherapy and bone marrow transplantation for cancer patients who are also chronic hepatitis B carriers: A review of the problem. J Clin Oncol 17:394–398, 1999.

279. Nordbo SA, Skaug K, Holter E, Waage A, Brinch L: Reactivation of hepatitis B virus infection in an anti-HBc and anti-HBs positive patient after allogeneic bone marrow transplantation. Eur J Haematol 65:86–87, 2000.

280. Romand F, Michallet M, Pichoud C, Trepo C, Zoulim F: Hepatitis B virus reactivation after allogeneic bone marrow transplantation in a patient previously cured of hepatitis B. Gastroenterol Clin Biol 23:770–774, 1999.

281. Blanpain C, Knoop C, Delforge ML, Antoine M, Peny MO, Liesnard C et al: Reactivation of hepatitis B after transplantation in patients with pre-existing anti-hepatitis B surface antigen antibodies: Report on three cases and review of the literature. Transplantation 66:883–886, 1998.

282. Dhedin N, Douvin C, Kuentz M, Saint Marc MF, Reman O, Rieux C et al: Reverse seroconversion of hepatitis B after allogeneic bone marrow transplantation: A retrospective study of 37 patients with pretransplant anti-HBs and anti-HBc. Transplantation 66:616–619, 1998.

283. Lau GK, Liang R, Wu PC, Lee CK, Lim WL, Au WY: Use of famciclovir to prevent HBV reactivation in HBsAg-positive recipients after allogeneic bone marrow transplantation. J Hepatol 28:359–368, 1998.

284. Han DJ, Kim TH, Park SK, Lee SK, Kim SB, Yang WS et al: Results on preemptive or prophylactic treatment of lamivudine in HBsAg (+) renal allograft recipients: Comparison with salvage treatment after hepatic dysfunction with HBV recurrence. Transplantation 71:387–394, 2001.

285. Endo T, Sakai T, Fujimoto K, Yamamoto S, Takashima H, Haseyama Y et al: A possible role for lamivudine as prophylaxis against hepatitis B reactivation in carriers of hepatitis B who undergo chemotherapy and autologous peripheral blood stem cell transplantation for non-Hodgkin's lymphoma. Bone Marrow Transplant 27:433–436, 2001.

286. Malik AH, Lee WM: Chronic hepatitis B virus infection: Treatment strategies for the next millennium. Ann Intern Med 132:723–731, 2000.

287. Rayes N, Seehofer D, Hopf U, Neuhaus R, Naumann U, Bechstein WO et al: Comparison of famciclovir and lamivudine in the long-term treatment of hepatitis B infection after liver transplantation. Transplantation 71:96–101, 2001.

288. Korba BE, Cote P, Hornbuckle W, Schinazi R, Gerin JL, Tennant BC: Enhanced antiviral benefit of combination therapy with lamivudine and famciclovir against WHV replication in chronic WHV carrier woodchucks. Antiviral Res 45:19–32, 2000.

289. Hou J, Fen X, Nie Z: Dynamic changes of hepatitis B virus during treatment with lamivudine versus lamivudine plus famciclovir. Chung Hua Kan Tsang Ping Tsa Chih 8:81–83, 2000.

290. Lau GK, Tsiang M, Hou J, Yuen S, Carman WF, Zhang L et al: Combination therapy with lamivudine and famciclovir for chronic hepatitis B-infected Chinese patients: A viral dynamics study. Hepatology 32:394–399, 2000.

291. Seehofer D, Rayes N, Neuhaus R, Berg T, Muller AR, Bechstein WO et al: Antiviral combination therapy for lamivudine-resistant hepatitis B reinfection after liver transplantation. Transplant Int 13(Suppl. 1):S359–362, 2000.

292. Seehofer D, Rayes N, Bechstein WO, Naumann U, Neuhaus R, Berg T et al: Therapy of recurrent hepatitis B infection after liver transplantation. A retrospective analysis of 200 liver transplantations based on hepatitis B associated liver diseases. Z Gastroenterol 38:773–783, 2000.

293. Zuckerman E, Zuckerman T, Douer D, Qian D, Levine AM: Liver dysfunction in patients infected with hepatitis C virus undergoing chemotherapy for hematologic malignancies. Cancer 83:1224–1230, 1998.

294. Frickhofen N, Wiesneth M, Jainta C, Hertenstein B, Heymer B, Bianchi L et al: Hepatitis C virus infection is a risk factor for liver failure from veno-occlusive disease after bone marrow transplantation. Blood 83:1998–2004, 1994.

295. Strasser SI, Myerson D, Spurgeon CL, Sullivan KM, Storer B, Schoch HG et al: Hepatitis C virus infection and bone marrow transplantation: A cohort study with 10-year follow-up. Hepatology 29:1893–1899, 1999.

296. Kanamori H, Fukawa H, Maruta A, Harano H, Kodama F, Matsuzaki M et al: Case report: Fulminant hepatitis C viral infection after allogeneic bone marrow transplantation. Am J Med Sci 303:109–111, 1992.

297. Ljungman P, Johansson N, Aschan J, Glaumann H, Lonnqvist B, Ringden O et al: Long-term effects of hepatitis C virus infection in allogeneic bone marrow transplant recipients. Blood 86:1614–1618, 1995.

298. Ljungman P, Andersson J, Aschan J, Bjorkstrand B, Hagglund H, Lonnqvist B et al: Oral ribavirin for prevention of severe liver disease caused by hepatitis C virus during allogeneic bone marrow transplantation. Clin Infect Dis 23:167–169, 1996.

299. Meyers JD: Treatment of herpesvirus infections in the immunocompromised host. Scand J Infect Dis Suppl 47:128–136, 1985.

300. Redding SW: Role of herpes simplex virus reactivation in chemotherapy-induced oral mucositis. NCI Monographs 9:103–105, 1990.

301. Saral R, Burns WH, Laskin OL, Santos GW, Lietman PS: Acyclovir prophylaxis of herpes-simplex-virus infections. N Engl J Med 305:63–67, 1981.

302. Epstein JB, Ransier A, Sherlock CH, Spinelli JJ, Reece D: Acyclovir prophylaxis of oral herpes virus during bone marrow transplantation. Eur J Cancer. Part B, Oral Oncol 32B:158–162, 1996.

303. Wade JC, Newton B, Flournoy N, Meyers JD: Oral acyclovir for prevention of herpes simplex virus reactivation after marrow transplantation. Ann Intern Med 100:823–828, 1984.

304. Shepp DH, Dandliker PS, Flournoy N, Meyers JD: Sequential intravenous and twice-daily oral acyclovir for extended prophylaxis of herpes simplex virus infection in marrow transplant patients. Transplantation 43:654–658, 1987.

305. Chakrabarti S, Pillay D, Ratcliffe D, Cane PA, Collingham KE, Milligan DW: Resistance to antiviral drugs in herpes simplex virus infections among allogeneic stem cell transplant recipients: Risk factors and prognostic significance. J Infect Dis 181:2055–2058, 2000.

306. Dignani MC, Mykietiuk A, Michelet M, Intile D, Mammana L, Desmery P et al: Valacyclovir prophylaxis for the prevention of herpes simplex virus reactivation in recipients of progenitor cells transplantation. Bone Marrow Transplant 29:263–267, 2002.

307. Bell WR, Chulay JD, Feinberg JE: Manifestations resembling thrombotic microangiopathy in patients with advanced human immunodeficiency virus (HIV) disease in a cytomegalovirus prophylaxis trial (ACTG 204). Medicine 76:369–380, 1997.

308. Lazarus HM, Belanger R, Candoni A, Aoun M, Jurewicz R, Marks L: Intravenous penciclovir for treatment of herpes simplex infections in immunocompromised patients: Results of a multicenter, acyclovir-controlled trial: The Penciclovir Immunocompromised Study Group. Antimicrob Agents Chemother 43:1192–1197, 1999.

309. Cortez KJ, Erdman DD, Peret TC, Gill VJ, Childs R, Barrett AJ et al: Outbreak of human parainfluenza virus 3 infections in a hematopoietic stem cell transplant population. Clin Infect Dis 184:1093–1097, 2001.

310. Aslan T, Fassas AB, Desikan R, Siegel D, Munshi N, Mehta J et al: Patients with multiple myeloma may safely undergo autologous transplantation despite ongoing RSV infection and no ribavirin therapy. Bone Marrow Transplant 24:505–509, 1999.

311. Anaissie A, Aslan T, Desikan R, Fassas A, Munshi N, Barlogie B: A prospective evaluation of the natural history of respiratory syncytial virus (RSV) among 150 adults with multiple myeloma. In 42nd Annual Meeting of The American Society of Hematology, San Francisco, California, 2000.

312. Regn S, Raffegerst S, Chen X, Schendel D, Kolb HJ, Roskrow M: Ex vivo generation of cytotoxic T lymphocytes specific for one or two distinct viruses for the prophylaxis of patients receiving an allogeneic bone marrow transplant. Bone Marrow Transplant 27:53–64, 2001.

313. Hemming VG, Prince GA, Groothuis JR, Siber GR: Hyperimmune globulins in prevention and treatment of respiratory syncytial virus infections. Clin Microbiol Rev 8:22–33, 1995.

314. Offidani M, Corvatta L, Olivieri A, Mele A, Brunori M, Montanari M et al: A predictive model of varicella-zoster virus infection after autologous peripheral blood progenitor cell transplantation. Clin Infect Dis 32:1414–1422, 2001.

315. Steer CB, Szer J, Sasadeusz J, Matthews JP, Beresford JA, Grigg A: Varicella-zoster infection after allogeneic bone marrow transplantation: Incidence, risk factors and prevention with low-dose acyclovir and ganciclovir. Bone Marrow Transplant 25:657–664, 2000.

316. Han CS, Miller W, Haake R, Weisdorf D: Varicella zoster infection after bone marrow transplantation: Incidence, risk factors and complications. Bone Marrow Transplant 13:277–283, 1994.

317. Selby PJ, Powles RL, Easton D et al: The prophylactic role of intravenous and long-term oral acyclovir after allogeneic bone marrow transplantation. Br J Cancer 59:434, 1989.

318. Ormrod D, Goa K: Valaciclovir: A review of its use in the management of herpes zoster. Drugs 59:1317–1340, 2000.

319. Cirelli R, Herne K, McCrary M, Lee P, Tyring SK: Famciclovir: Review of clinical efficacy and safety. Antiviral Res 29:141–151, 1996.

320. Goesch TR, Gotz G, Stellbrinck KH, Albrecht H, Weh HJ, Hossfeld DK: Possible transfer of *Pneumocystis carinii* between immunodeficient patients. Lancet 336:627, 1990.

321. Bensousan T, Garo B, Islam S, Bourbigot B, Cledes J, Garre M: Possible transfer of *Pneumocystis carinii* between kidney transplant recipients. Lancet 336:1066–1067, 1990.

322. Chave JP, David S, Wauters JP, Van Melle G, Francioli P: Transmission of *Pneumocystis carinii* from AIDS patients to other immunosuppressed patients: A cluster of *Pneumocystis carinii* pneumonia in renal transplant recipients. AIDS 5:927–932, 1991.

323. Cordonnier C, Einsele H, Beaume J et al: Management and incidence of *Pneumocystis carinii* pneumonia after stem cell transplantation: A survey in the EBMT centers. In 25th Annual Meeting European Group for Blood and Marrow Transplantation and 15th Meeting of the Nurses Group, Hamburg, Germany, 1999.

324. Anaissie EJ, Kontoyiannis DP, O'Brien S, Kantarjian H, Robertson L, Lerner S et al: Infections in patients with chronic lymphocytic leukemia treated with fludarabine. Ann Intern Med 129:559–566, 1998.

325. Chan C, Montaner J, Lefebvre EA, Morey G, Dohn M, McIvor RA et al: Atovaquone suspension compared with aerosolized pentamidine for prevention of *Pneumocystis carinii* pneumonia in human immunodeficiency virus-infected subjects intolerant of trimethoprim or sulfonamides. J Infect Dis 180:369–376, 1999.

326. El-Sadr WM, Murphy RL, Yurik TM, Luskin-Hawk R, Cheung TW, Balfour HH, Jr. et al: Atovaquone compared with dapsone for the prevention of *Pneumocystis carinii* pneumonia in patients with HIV infection who cannot tolerate trimethoprim, sulfonamides, or both. Community Program for Clinical Research on AIDS and the AIDS Clinical Trials Group. N Engl J Med 339:1889–1895, 1998.

327. Foot AB, Garin YJ, Ribaud P, Devergie A, Derouin F, Gluckman E: Prophylaxis of toxoplasmosis infection with pyrimethamine/sulfadoxine (Fansidar) in bone marrow transplant recipients. Bone Marrow Transplant 14:241–245, 1994.

328. Melero M, Gennaro O, Dominguez C, Sanchez Avalos JC: Tuberculosis in patients with lymphomas. Medicina 52:291–295, 1992.

329. Arslan O, Gurman G, Dilek I, Ozcan M, Koc H, Ilhan O et al: Incidence of tuberculosis after bone marrow transplantation in a single center from Turkey. Haematologia 29:59–62, 1998.

330. de la Camara R, Martino R, Granados E, Rodriguez-Salvanes FJ, Rovira M, Cabrera R et al: Tuberculosis after hematopoietic stem cell transplantation: Incidence, clinical characteristics and outcome. Spanish Group on Infectious Complications in Hematopoietic Transplantation. Bone Marrow Transplant 26:291–298, 2000.

331. Aljurf M, Gyger M, Alrajhi A, Sahovic E, Chaudhri N, Musa M et al: Mycobacterium tuberculosis infection in allogeneic bone marrow transplantation patients. Bone Marrow Transplant 24:551–554, 1999.

332. Libshitz HI, Pannu HK, Elting LS, Cooksley CD: Tuberculosis in cancer patients: An update. J Thoracic Imaging 12:41–46, 1997.

333. Budak-Alpdogan T, Tangun Y, Kalayoglu-Besisik S, Ratip S, Akan H, Baslar Z et al: The frequency of tuberculosis in adult allogeneic stem cell transplant recipients in Turkey. Biol Blood Marrow Transplant 6:370–374, 2000.

334. Navari RM, Sullivan KM, Springmeyer SC, Siegel MS, Meyers JD, Buckner CD et al: Mycobacterial infections in marrow transplant patients. Transplantation 36:509–513, 1983.

335. Bunch C: Immunoglobulin replacement in chronic lymphocytic leukaemia. Nouv Rev Franc Hematol 30:419–422, 1988.

336. Boughton BJ, Jackson N, Lim S, Smith N: Randomized trial of intravenous immunoglobulin prophylaxis for patients with chronic lymphocytic leukaemia and secondary hypogammaglobulinaemia. Clin Lab Haematol 17:75–80, 1995.

337. Griffiths H, Brennan V, Lea J, Bunch C, Lee M, Chapel H: Crossover study of immunoglobulin replacement therapy in patients with low-grade B-cell tumors. Blood 73:366–368, 1989.

338. Chapel HM, Lee M, Hargreaves R, Pamphilon DH, Prentice AG: Randomised trial of intravenous immunoglobulin as prophylaxis against infection in plateau-phase multiple myeloma. The UK Group for Immunoglobulin Replacement Therapy in Multiple Myeloma. Lancet 343:1059–1063, 1994.

339. Chapel H, Dicato M, Gamm H, Brennan V, Ries F, Bunch C et al: Immunoglobulin replacement in patients with chronic lymphocytic leukaemia: A comparison of two dose regimes. Br J Haematol 88:209–212, 1994.

340. Crawford J, Ozer H, Stoller R, Johnson D, Lyman G, Tabbara I et al: Reduction by granulocyte colony-stimulating factor of fever and neutropenia induced by chemotherapy in patients with small-cell lung cancer. N Engl J Med 325:164–170, 1991.

341. Trillet-Lenoir V, Green J, Manegold C, Von Pawel J, Gatzemeier U, Lebeau B et al: Recombinant granulocyte colony stimulating factor reduces the infectious complications of cytotoxic chemotherapy. Eur J Cancer 29A:319–324, 1993.

342. Ozer H, Armitage JO, Bennett CL, Crawford J, Demetri GD, Pizzo PA et al: 2000 update of recommendations for the use of hematopoietic colony-stimulating factors: Evidence-based, clinical practice guidelines. J Clin Oncol 18:3558–3585, 2000.

343. Fleming R, Kantarjian H, Lichtiger M, Keating A, Estey E: Granulocyte transfusions from GM-CSF treated donors as infection prophylaxis in AML/MDS during induction. In The 39th Annual Meeting of The American Society of Hematology; December 5–9, 1997, San Diego, California.

344. Gajewski J, Champlin R: Bone marrow transplantation from alternate donors. In Burt RK, Deeg HJ, Lothian ST, Santos GW (eds.): Bone Marrow Transplantation, pp. 24–28. Landes Company and Chapman & Hall, Georgetown, TX, 1996.

345. Lowdell MW, Craston R, Ray N, Koh M, Galatowicz G, Prentice HG: The effect of T cell depletion with Campath-1M on immune reconstitution after chemotherapy and allogeneic bone marrow transplant as treatment for leukaemia. Bone Marrow Transplant 21:679–686, 1998.

346. Hermann CK, Hansen PB, Bangsborg JM, Pers C: Bacterial infections as complications of dog bites. Ugeskrift Laeger 160:4860–4863, 1998.

347. Pers C, Gahrn-Hansen B, Frederiksen W: *Capnocytophaga canimorsus* septicemia in Denmark, 1982–1995: Review of 39 cases. Clin Infect Dis 23:71–75, 1996.

348. Valtonen M, Lauhio A, Carlson P, Multanen J, Sivonen A, Vaara M et al: *Capnocytophaga canimorsus* septicemia: Fifth report of a cat-associated infection and five other cases. Eur J Clin Microbiol Infect Dis 14:520–523, 1995.

50

Evaluation and Management of Bacterial and Fungal Infections Occurring in Patients With a Hematological Malignancy

James C. Wade

Patients with a hematological malignancy are a heterogeneous patient population with diseases that range from rapidly fatal to more indolent with the potential for future disease transformation. Treatment options range from observation to hematopoietic stem cell transplantation (HSCT), but all patients experience an increased susceptibility to infection that remains an obstacle to a successful outcome. The problem of infection is dynamic with shifts in the isolated pathogens and changes in their antimicrobial susceptibilities, varied treatment regimens that have different patterns of immune suppression, and an increasing age of the patients who receive treatment. The classic pattern of immunodeficiency for most patients with a hematological malignancy includes periods of profound neutropenia and associated mucosal and integumentary barrier disruption, increased exposure to iatrogenic risks (i.e., vascular access devices), microbial flora shifts and cellular immune suppression for HSCT recipients, patients with a lymphoid malignancy, and those receiving corticosteroids.[1,2] Patients with neutropenia are compromised because of the ability of their endogenous colonizing flora to invade through disrupted mucosal and cutaneous barriers, and cause systemic bacterial and fungal infections.[3,4] These risks are enhanced when patients experience delayed marrow recovery, inadequate antitumor responses, or a relapse of their disease. This chapter will focus on the bacterial and fungal infections that occur primarily during periods of neutropenia. Most of the standard evaluation and management principles for patients with fever and neutropenia are applicable to patients with a hematological malignancy.[1,2] Consequently, this chapter reviews evaluation and management approaches in general, and discusses in more depth those issues that are new or unique.

EVALUATION, PREVENTION, AND MANAGEMENT OF BACTERIAL AND FUNGAL INFECTION

Neutropenia is primarily a consequence of the patients' underlying disease or treatment, although infection (e.g., cytomegalovirus [CMV], human herpesvirus [HHV]-6, HHV-8, parvovirus B19), medication toxicity (e.g., ganciclovir, trimethoprim/sulfamethoxazole, linezolid), or graft rejection following HSCT are important.[5,6] The risk of infection during periods of neutropenia is enhanced by therapy-induced mucosal or integumentary barrier disruption, the presence of long-term indwelling vascular access devices, medication-induced central nervous system dysfunction, and the microbial floral shifts that accompany severe illness, or the administration of antibiotics.[1,2,7] The primary origin of pathogens for neutropenic patients are their own endogenous bacterial and fungal flora, airborne molds and respiratory viruses, microorganisms on the hands of health care providers, and latent viruses. Sites of infection for neutropenic hosts are limited. Infections originate primarily from the alimentary tract (i.e., mouth, pharynx, esophagus, large and small bowel, and rectum), sinuses, lungs, and skin.[1,2] Most febrile episodes that occur during this period are infectious in origin, and fever is considered infection until proven otherwise.[1,2,8,9] Bacterial infections account for more than 90 percent of the first infection during neutropenia. Herpes simplex virus and the respiratory viruses (e.g., influenza A and B, parainfluenza, and respiratory syncytial virus) are also important initial pathogens[10,11] (Table 50–1). Antibiotic-resistant bacteria, yeast, and molds are the common causes of subsequent infections.[2,12] Initial bacterial pathogens are usually gram-positive cocci.[13] Coagulase-negative staphylococci, streptococci, and enterococci predominate, but infections with *Staphylococcus aureus,* and *Corynebacteria jeikeium* remain important.[14–18] Despite the perceived decreased virulence of these gram-positive pathogens, there is still a significant level of attributable mortality with such infections. Wenzel reported the attributable mortality for coagulase-negative staphylococcal blood stream infections to be 13.6 percent (95 percent CI 4.2–22.9 percent) and to be 37.1 percent (95 percent CI 10–64 percent) for blood stream infections caused by vancomycin-resistant enterococci.[19–21] A recent report from the Mayo clinic noted that colonization with vancomycin-resistant enterococci (VRE) increased the risk of developing a VRE blood stream infection, and death post-transplant for allogeneic transplant recipients.[22] Several large series have reported rates of blood stream infection with viridans streptococci of 10 to 25 percent.[15–17] Approx-

Table 50–1. Pathogens Causing Infection Syndromes During the Neutropenic Period

Syndrome	Relative Frequency[a]	Relative Life-Threatening Potential[a]
First fever		
Staphylococci	3 +	1 +
Viridans Streptococci	1 +	2 +
Gram-negative bacilli	1 +	3 +
Respiratory virus	1 +	1–3 +
Subsequent infection		
Antibiotic-resistant bacteria	2 +	
Gram-positive cocci		1 +
Gram-negative bacilli		2–3 +
Fungi	2–3 +	3–4 +
Respiratory virus	1 +	1–3 +

[a] Frequency and life-threatening potential increase from 1 to 4 + .

955

Table 50–2. Bacterial Blood Stream Isolates: FHCRC 1999

Single organism bacteremias	
Total	359
Coagulase-negative staphylococci	193
Enterococci	41
E. faecalis	22
E. faecium	11
Vancomycin-resistant enterococci	8
Streptococcus spp.	52
Staphylococcus aureus	12
MRSA	2
Gram-negative bacilli	33
Nontuberculosis mycobacteria	8
Other	19

Abbreviation: MRSA, methicillin-resistant *S. aureus.*

imately 10 percent of viridans streptococcal infections will be associated with a "toxic-shock" like syndrome that can be rapidly fatal even with appropriate antibiotics. Thus although specific empiric therapy directed against these gram-positive pathogens may not always be required, appropriate pathogen-directed therapy is needed when such organisms are isolated.

Gram-negative bacilli remain the most virulent bacterial pathogens during the neutropenic period, and historically have been responsible for the highest frequency of morbidity and mortality.[1,2] The common gram-negative bacilli remain *Escherichia coli*, *Klebsiella* spp., and *Pseudomonas aeruginosa.* The increased use of broad-spectrum cephalosporins and carbapenem antibiotics has increased the frequency of isolation of beta-lactam resistant *Enterobacter* spp. and *Stenotrophomonas maltophilia.*[23–25]

Increasing resistance to multiple antibiotics poses a significant problem in planning empiric treatment. It is critical to be aware of your institution's specific antibiotic susceptibility patterns, and remember that pathogens and antibiotic susceptibility patterns may change over time. Antibiotic resistance remains most prominent among the gram-positive pathogens, specifically coagulase-negative staphylococci. Transplant recipients at the Fred Hutchinson Cancer Research Center (FHCRC) in calendar year 1999 experienced 374 blood stream infections, for a rate of 0.718 blood stream infections/100 patient days (Table 50–2). Sixty-three percent of these infections occurred during the period of neutropenia, and more than half were caused by coagulase-negative staphylococci. The antibiotic resistance pattern for coagulase-negative staphylococci and viridans streptococci now show a high level of resistance to the beta-lactam antibiotics (Table 50–3).

Pathogens responsible for the subsequent or second infections include antibiotic-resistant bacteria and fungi. Wingard reported that *S. epidermidis* is responsible for up to 50 percent of the second or subsequent infections.[12] Gram-negative bacilli are responsible for an additional 10 percent, with the majority of remaining pathogens being predominantly fungal. Subsequent infections with the exception of coagulase-negative staphylococci are difficult to diagnose, more resistant to treatment, and associated with the highest rates of morbidity and mortality.[26–29]

Evaluation and Management of Neutropenia-Associated Infections

Effective care for patients with a hematological malignancy must rely on centerwide infection control programs, infection prevention techniques, and a combination of empiric and preemptive therapy. There are several practice guidelines for the prevention and empiric treatment of infection in the neutropenic host (National Cancer Comprehensive Network [NCCN] Clinical Guideline for Fever and Neutropenia; Infectious Diseases Society of America; www.cancernetwork.com; www.cdc.gov).[8,9] There is also a diversity of infection management practices that have developed among the different centers. Oncology centers should customize their practices based on their own patient population, the cytotoxic regimens administered, and their local infection and antimicrobial susceptibility patterns.

Infection Control

The single most powerful infection prevention measure for a patient with neutropenia is the hand washing performed by the health care staff. Hand washing, while effective, continues to be difficult to implement and a challenge to maintain compliance. Hand soap that contains chlorhexidine is recommended, and adds residual antimicrobial effect to the mechanical cleansing that occurs with the physical washing. Antimicrobial hand rubs

Table 50–3. Antibiotic Susceptibility of Blood Stream Isolates: FHCRC 1999

Organism	Percent Sensitive			
	Ceftazidime	Ciprofloxacin	Oxacillin	Vancomycin
Coagulase-negative Staphylococcus	17	31	18	100
Staphylococcus aureus	94	81	94	100
Streptococcus spp.	67	30	72	100
Enterococcus	Ampicillin			Vancomycin
Faecalis	100			100
Faecium	11			69

can be used if soap, water, and sinks are not easily accessible. New alcohol-containing waterless products appear to be well-tolerated and effective. Gloves when worn should be put on only after entering a patient's room and the hand washing is complete. Gloves should be removed prior to leaving the patient's room, and should never be used for more than one patient contact. Keeping staff and patient visitors who have respiratory symptoms (e.g., uncontrolled cough and respiratory secretions, conjunctivitis, systemic symptoms) from contact with patients may decrease the risk of patients acquiring a potentially serious respiratory viral infection. Annual vaccination of health care workers against viral influenza is also important.

Patients who become neutropenic are no longer routinely cared for in total sterile environments (LAF [laminar air flow] units). This change in practice does not suggest that measures to decrease the exposure of patients to potential pathogens is not beneficial, but rather that less intrusive infection control measures can be implemented and still accomplish the patient care goals. Barrier isolation has been relegated to situations where one is attempting to minimize the spread by contact of potential pathogens. Isolation of patients known to be colonized or infected with a pathogen that is multiply antibiotic resistant, or has an increased propensity for nosocomial transmission (i.e., VRE, *Clostridium difficile*, respiratory viruses) is important.[11,30] Neutropenic patients should be hospitalized in single bed rooms, and care should be delivered by a health care team that is familiar with oncology treatment procedures and understands the importance of minimizing the nosocomial transmission of potential pathogens. Inpatient wards and preferably outpatient clinics or day-hospital facilities should be ventilated with air that has been cleansed by high-efficiency air (HEPA) filters, and completely exchanged at least 15 times per hour. This level of clean-air ventilation is recommended with the hope of decreasing the incidence of mold and other airborne infections.

Prevention of Infection

Bacterial

Antibacterial prophylaxis for patients with neutropenia remains controversial. Data supporting the effectiveness of chemoprophylaxis with antibiotic(s) are balanced by reports that failed to show efficacy. A meta-analysis of 19 randomized trials of fluoroquinolone prophylaxis in patients with neutropenia revealed a decrease in the number of documented gram-negative bacillary infections, but no effect on the frequency of febrile episodes, febrile morbidity, or infection-associated mortality.[31] Many of these trials have shown an increase in gram-positive infections, and some have reported an increased risk of secondary fungal infections.[9] Antibacterial prophylaxis if used should be restricted to patients who are expected to experience at least 10 to 14 days of profound (<100 PMNs/μl) neutropenia.[8,9]

Fungal

The incidence of fungal infections has increased during the last decade among patients with a hematological malignancy undergoing conventional therapy or HSCT. Centers now report an incidence of fungal infection that varies between 5 and 20

percent.[7,26–29,32] Diagnosis and treatment remains inadequate and preventing exposure or blocking colonization with these pathogens is difficult. *Candida* colonization is present in up to 80 percent of patients, and will persist throughout treatment unless patients receive azole suppression.[28] When the fungal pathogen originates from the environment the protection provided by sterile environments (LAF rooms) and HEPA filtration is limited to the time period that patients reside in these clean environments. The true incidence or risk of colonization with *Aspergillus* among patients receiving intensive therapy is unknown. Wald in her study of 2496 consecutive HSCT patients reported that 2 percent of patients became colonized with *Aspergillus* after transplant, but only 21 percent of patients who developed invasive aspergillosis had documented preinfection colonization.[26] Yet, when *Aspergillus* colonization is detected, it has been associated with a 60 percent positive predictive value for the development of invasive aspergillosis, and the positive predictive value increases to 94 percent for HSCT patients who are neutropenic.[26]

The use of masks by patients or health care workers has not consistently influenced the incidence of fungal infections. This lack of efficacy may be in part due to poor patient tolerance, or the inability of the masks to fit tightly enough to be an effective barrier against fungal spores. The use of aerosolized or intravenous amphotericin B has provided inconsistent prevention results.[33–37] Perfect and colleagues tested low-dose intravenous amphotericin B prophylaxis and reported a similar incidence of invasive fungal infection for both the treatment and placebo groups (8.8 vs. 14.3 percent, respectively).[36] The potential efficacy of prophylaxis with lipid formulations of amphotericin B has also been tested by Tollemar et al.[37] They reported that this therapy decreased fungal colonization but provided no mortality benefit. The need for intravenous administration, potential toxicity, and cost of the lipid formulations of amphotericin B makes them poorly suited for prophylaxis. Itraconazole may be potentially useful for the prevention of fungal infections including aspergillosis, but efficacy as prophylaxis has not been proven.[38,39] Itraconazole has also been difficult to effectively administer because of erratic absorption, numerous drug-drug interactions (e.g., cyclosporine, tacrolimus), and gastrointestinal intolerance. Concomitant administration of cyclosporine and itraconazole causes a decrease in cyclosporin metabolism, and results in the need to decrease the daily cyclosporin dosage by 20 to 50 percent (personal communication, J. Wingard, 2000). The availability of the new oral cyclodextran or intravenous itraconazole formulations may make this drug more efficacious.

Fluconazole has been shown to be highly effective prevention of *Candida albicans* disease among allogeneic HSCT recipients,[40,41] but its efficacy for other patients with a hematological malignancy remains controversial and cannot be routinely recommended. In the trial reported by Slavin and co-workers, fluconazole decreased the incidence of *C. albicans* infections and improved the overall survival of the treated allogeneic transplantation recipients.[41] Marr et al. have recently reported long-term follow-up of this study cohort.[42] After 8 years of follow-up, survival remains significantly better for fluconazole recipients (68/152 vs. 41/148, respectively), and the incidence of invasive candidiasis and death due to candidiasis remains greater for placebo recipients.

The benefit of fluconazole for autologous HSCT recipients and patients with acute leukemia undergoing induction therapy is unclear.[41,43,44] These patients are at risk of developing disseminated candidiasis, but fluconazole has not been shown to provide a consistent benefit.[44] In general fluconazole prophylaxis is probably not necessary for patients receiving an autologous transplantation or leukemia induction unless the conditioning regimen is expected to cause severe mucositis.

A prior history of invasive mold (e.g., aspergillosis) or disseminated candidiasis (e.g., systemic disseminated candidiasis) often raises concerns about the patient's suitability for continued treatment. A retrospective review conducted at the FHCRC reported 15 patients with documented disseminated candidiasis before allogeneic pretransplantation.[45] All patients had been treated with amphotericin B therapy before transplantation, and all patients had improvement in their infection before initiating the transplant conditioning therapy. These patients had no appreciable increased risk of recurrent yeast blood stream infection after transplantation. Bjerke and colleagues concluded that a history of disseminated candidiasis was not an absolute contraindication to allogeneic transplantation.[45]

Management of patients with a previously documented invasive mold infection, specifically *Aspergillus,* has been more difficult. Pre-emptive amphotericin B therapy should be routinely used in all patients with a previous history of an invasive *Aspergillus* infection during periods of significant neutropenia or cellular immunosuppression (i.e., induction therapy for acute leukemia).[2,46] Offner et al. reported 48 patients who underwent HSCT with a pretransplant history of documented or presumed aspergillosis.[46] Eleven of the 48 patients received an autologous HSCT. One-third of these patients experienced a documented recurrence of aspergillosis post-transplant, with recurrent aspergillosis having an 88 percent mortality rate. The authors noted a trend toward a lower incidence of recurrent infection, and improved survival for patients with a longer interval between the initial *Aspergillus* infection and transplantation. Patients who received pre-emptive antifungal therapy or underwent an autologous transplant also had lower frequency of recurrent infection. The unpublished experience at the FHCRC with patients who have a prior history of aspergillosis is equally discouraging. We have transplanted 34 such patients with a conventional allogeneic transplantation. All patients had been extensively treated pretransplant with amphotericin B (>8 weeks), all received full-dose amphotericin B therapy during their period of maximum immunosuppression, and all prior to transplantation had shown clinical and radiological improvement or resolution of their infection. Fifteen of 34 patients experienced recurrent *Aspergillus* infection post-transplant, and all infections were fatal. Twelve other patients died from transplant-related complications without a documented mold recurrence. Five of the six patients who survived had an interval between diagnosis of aspergillosis and transplantation of at least 9 months (9 months to 3.5 years); three had their prior infection isolated to just the nose and sinuses. While some

patients with a previous history of aspergillosis may be candidates for autologous transplantation or intensive standard chemotherapy, allogeneic transplantation continues to be associated with a high incidence of recurrent infection and mortality despite pre-emptive antifungal treatment.

Viral

Prevention of common viral infections during the neutropenic period may be important for those patients who are most intensively treated. Acyclovir (5 mg/kg iv twice daily or 400 to 800 mg orally twice daily), famciclovir (500 mg twice daily), or valacyclovir (500 mg twice daily) have been shown to be effective in the prevention of herpes simplex virus infections for transplant recipients, patients with acute leukemia, and intensively treated lymphoma patients.[2,47,48] Suppression of HSV may decrease the mucosal disruption caused by this viral recurrence, and as reported by Baglin et al., can minimize the duration and frequency of febrile episodes.[49]

Adjunctive Measures

Peripheral Blood Stem Cells

The transition from bone marrow to growth-factor mobilized peripheral blood stem cells (PBSC) as the HSCT product has been an important intervention. PBSCs have become standard practice for most autologous transplants. A randomized trial conducted by Weaver and co-workers reported that the infusion of at least 5×10^6 CD34+ positive stem cells resulted in a median duration of post-transplant neutropenia (<500 PMN/μl) of 11 days.[49] This shortened period of neutropenia may potentially decrease a patient's risk of infection, but autologous PBSC products that are preferentially selected for CD34+ cells have been associated with delayed immune reconstitution, and an increased risk of bacterial and *Candida* infections.[51,52]

The observation that PBSC speeds engraftment for autologous HSCT recipients has led to the testing of this approach for allogeneic HSCT recipients who were transplanted from matched related donor.[53–55] Bensinger et al. reported that the use of allogeneic PBSC decreased the median duration of neutropenia (<500/PMNs/μl) from 21 to 16 days.[54] PBSC recipients had improved disease-free and overall survival. These results are consistent with other reports, including the IBMTR review that reported a decreased duration of neutropenia and shorter hospital stays for PBSC recipients.[53,55]

Growth Factors

The American Society of Oncology has recently updated its guidelines for the use of growth factors.[56] Granulocyte colony-stimulating factor (G-CSF) and granulocyte-macrophage colony-stimulating factor (GM-CSF) have consistently been shown to hasten hematopoietic cell recovery, but the increase in neutrophil recovery has not translated into a consistent decrease in neutropenia-associated infections or improvement in survival.[56] The ASCO guideline now recommends limited "primary neutropenia prophylaxis" and the use of growth factors combined with antimicrobial treatment should be limited to severe infections that are refractory to antibiotic treatment.[56,57]

Granulocyte Transfusions

Early granulocyte transfusion trials showed benefit for patients with severe gram-negative bacillary infections.[2,8,9,58] However, the infusion of granulocytes has been complicated by the inability to collect adequate number of cells, acute infusion reactions, an increased risk of alloimmunization, and the potential transmission of CMV infection from the donor to transplant recipient.[59] There has been a recent resurgence of interest in granulocyte transfusions. Donor priming with growth factors and corticosteroids has been found to increase the granulocyte yield to 8 to 10 $\times 10^{10}$.[60] This dose of infused granulocytes can result in a 1-hour post-transfusion white blood cell count of $2.6 \pm 2.6 \times 10^3$ PMNs/μl. The use of growth factor mobilized granulocyte transfusions to date has been tested primarily among HSCT patients with severe, progressive fungal or bacterial infections.[61] While efficacy for this approach has not yet been established, the Seattle group has shown that this type of transfusion can be successfully accomplished using either a related or an unrelated donor.[62] Adkins et al. have published the results of a trial of prophylactic, G-CSF mobilized granulocytes in HSCT recipients.[63] Patients received transfusions on days 2, 4, 6, and 8 after autologous transplantation. All recipients received G-CSF mobilized granulocytes from a single donor. Leukocyte incompatibility adversely affected the recipients' neutrophil increments after transfusion, and this incompatibility resulted in a delay in neutrophil engraftment, and increased the number of days of fever, platelet transfusions, and intravenous antibiotics. While the number of granulocytes that can be collected with growth-factor mobilization has been increased, the clinical benefit for such a prophylactic or therapeutic approach has not yet been demonstrated.

EVALUATION AND TREATMENT OF INFECTION

One must assume that most episodes of fever and neutropenia are infectious in origin. These infections have the potential to be rapidly fatal if not empirically treated.[3] The initial evaluation and management for such patients are well outlined in the National Comprehensive Cancer Network (NCCN), IDSA, and CDC clinical practice guidelines.[8,9] The NCCN guideline provides an excellent road map to manage such patients during their period of neutropenia.[8] In the latest version of this practice guideline a neutrophil count of less than 500/μl has been defined as neutropenia, and a single temperature of greater than 38.0°C requires clinical intervention. The patient's evaluation must be focused on determining the causative organism and the site of infection. The laboratory assessment should focus on studies that help to define the functional status of the liver, kidneys, and lungs. Imaging procedure (e.g., chest radiograph) should be considered when patients have site-specific symptoms. A chest x-ray should be obtained at the onset of the first fever, and a computed tomography (CT) scan of the chest should be considered for patients who remain febrile, have pulmonary symptoms, or have room-air oxygen saturation below 90 percent. Sinuses are imaged most efficiently with a sinus CT scan.

Specimens for culture should be collected during or immediately after completion of the patient's examination. Blood should be obtained prior to initiation of antibiotics, but antibiotic administration should not be delayed while radiographs or other site-specific cultures are obtained. There is general consensus that the volume of blood cultured is the most important variable in optimizing microbial recovery for adult patients.[64,65] It is recommended that at least two blood cultures, or 20 to 40 ml of blood be collected. The IDSA guideline recommends that two blood cultures be obtained, one from a peripheral site and a second from the central venous catheter.[9] The justification for this recommendation is based on the belief that disparity between the peripheral blood and the catheter blood culture may help identify catheter-related infection, and direct clinical care. While drawing blood cultures from different venipuncture sites may help to distinguish between clinically important and contaminant microorganisms, a meta-analysis of previously published studies has shown little utility for two-site culturing when the patient has a long-term indwelling venous access device.[66] Thus in many oncology centers, blood for culture is only drawn from the patient's vascular catheter. Quantitative blood cultures may be performed, but they are not routinely recommended because of their cost and limited clinical utility.[67,68]

Site-specific cultures are important. Cultures and biopsies from the sinus, lungs, and alimentary tract can be performed safely when they are coupled with appropriate platelet support and experienced subspecialty physicians (e.g., pulmonary critical/care, gastroenterologists, surgeons, and otolaryngologists). One must have a low threshold to biopsy cutaneous lesions that develop in the setting of fever and neutropenia. Histologic and microbiologic investigation of these cutaneous lesions may define the offending bacterial, fungal, or viral pathogen.

Diarrhea is common after patients have received chemotherapy and/or radiation. Diarrhea that occurs during the first 1 to 2 weeks after completion of treatment is usually the result of treatment-induced mucosal injury. This type of diarrhea will usually spontaneously resolve, but does signify additional mucosal injury that can be a portal for infection. Bacterial pathogens responsible for intestinal infection in the normal host (i.e., *Salmonella, Shigella, Campylobacter, Yersinia*) almost never cause diarrhea in the hospitalized patient with a hematological malignancy. Diarrhea secondary to intestinal parasites (e.g., *Cryptosporidium, Giardia lamblia*, and *E. histolytica*) is also unusual, but has been reported in center-specific outbreaks. The most common infectious cause of diarrhea is *C. difficile* colitis. The prevalence of this pathogen as part of a patient's endogenous alimentary flora varies but is felt to be present in less than 3 percent of normal hosts, but higher for patients with a hematological malignancy who have recently undergone treatment or hospitalization.[69] Optimal management of patients who are colonized but not infected is unclear, but infection control measures are critical.

Initial Empiric Therapy

Patients with neutropenia should be treated empirically with high-dose, broad-spectrum antibiotics at the first sign (fever) of infection. At present a large number of highly effective antibiotics are available. Despite many previous studies it is not possible to recommend a single antibiotic or antibiotic combination as initial treatment for all patients with fever and neutropenia.[8,9,70–74] The selection of empiric antibiotics must take into consideration the following factors: 1. the most common potential infecting pathogens; 2. the potential sites of infection; 3. the local antimicrobial susceptibility patterns of isolated pathogens; 4. the need for broad-spectrum antibiotic coverage against gram-negative bacilli including *P. aeruginosa,* and gram-positive organisms like *S. aureus* and viridans streptococci, and 5. pre-existing organ dysfunction. Patients with a hematological malignancy are often exposed to previous organ-damaging therapy (e.g., amphotericin B, cyclosporin), and because of this exposure, aminoglycosides with their inherent nephrotoxicity should be reserved for clinical situations where their use is mandatory.

There is considerable debate about the empiric use of vancomycin or antibiotics with specific broad-spectrum gram-positive activity (e.g., linezolid, Synercid) in all patients with fever and neutropenia.[8,9] The primary justification for this therapy is the knowledge that a small number of gram-positive pathogen infections can be rapidly fatal if not treated promptly with the appropriate antibiotics.[15,17,18] However, the only single, large, prospective randomized trial conducted in adult patients with fever and neutropenia failed to show a significant clinical advantage for the use of empiric vancomycin.[75]

The primary reason to not use empiric vancomycin is the emergence of vancomycin-resistant pathogens. The development of colonization with VRE has been associated with the increased use of vancomycin although other antibiotics are also important.[19,76] Because of this risk, the initial empiric use of vancomycin or other new broad-spectrum gram-positive antibiotics (linezolid, Synercid) should be limited to patients who develop fever and have one or more of the following six clinical conditions. 1. Serious, clinically apparent catheter-related infections. Many of these infections are caused by coagulase-negative staphylococcus that have high (80 percent) levels of beta-lactam antibiotic resistance (Table 50–3). 2. Substantial mucosal damage coupled with a high risk of infection with penicillin-resistant viridans streptococci. Significant mucosal disruption is of constant concern for patients who receive intensive therapy. According to the SCOPE (Support of Commission Objectives and Project Environment) surveillance data, 18 to 29 percent of viridans streptococci isolated from the blood will be resistant to beta-lactam antibiotics.[77,78] 3. Blood cultures positive for gram-positive bacteria prior to final pathogen identification and susceptibility testing. 4. Known colonization with beta-lactam resistant pneumococci, methicillin-resistant *S. aureus,* or VRE. 5. Previous prophylaxis with quinolone antibiotics or trimethoprim/sulfamethoxazole. Both of these latter agents have been associated with an increased risk of gram-positive infections.[31,79,80] Molecular epidemiology studies in HSCT recipients and patients with acute leukemia have confirmed the importance of alimentary tract colonization with coagulase-negative staphylococci as a risk factor for the development of blood stream infections with these pathogens.[2,81] 6. The development of hypotension or the sepsis syndrome without an identified pathogen.

Empiric vancomycin could be considered in any of the previous clinical conditions, but if vancomycin therapy is initiated it should be discontinued after 3 to 4 days of treatment if an antibiotic-resistant organism is not identified. The empiric use of new agents like linezolid and Synercid is discouraged. Cost, lack of controlled trial experience, and potential marrow toxicity with linezolid (personal communication, Pharmacia/Upjohn) and significant musculoskeletal toxicity with Synercid provide reasons for restricting the use of these agents.

Patients With Documented Infection Sites or Pathogens

Identification of the infecting pathogen allows the clinician to optimize the patient's antimicrobial regimen, and potentially use therapy with a lower incidence of adverse effects and costs. The duration of treatment for documented infections should consider the following factors: 1. neutrophil recovery; 2. rapidity of response to the antimicrobial therapy; 3. specific site of infection; and 4. the isolated pathogens. In general most uncomplicated skin and alimentary tract mucosal infections are adequately treated with 5 to 7 days of antibiotic therapy.[8] For most bacterial blood stream infections, 1 to 2 weeks of therapy are usually adequate, but fungal blood stream infections require more prolonged treatment.[8,9,82] Three to four weeks of therapy are needed to effectively control bacterial sinus and lung infections, but a more prolonged antimicrobial treatment is required if the causative pathogen is *P. aeruginosa* or a mold.[8,9]

Catheter-Associated Infections

One infection site that remains problematic is the catheter-associated infection. Long-term venous access devices were ini-

Table 50–4. Vascular Catheter-Associated Infections

Infection	Treatment/Action
Entry site infection	Pathogen-specific therapy (consider empiric vancomycin)
Tunnel infection	Catheter removal/culture Pathogen-specific therapy (consider empiric vancomycin)
Blood stream infection	
Fungi (yeast or mold)	Immediate catheter removal
Nontuberculosis mycobacteria	Pathogen-specific therapy
Vancomycin-resistant enterococci	
Corynebacterium jeikeium	Consider early catheter removal
Bacillus	Pathogen-specific therapy
Staphylococcus aureus	
Pseudomonas aeruginosa	
Stenotrophomonas maltophilia	
All other positive blood cutures	Pathogen-specific therapy Consider catheter removal for persistent[a] infection

[a] (+) Blood culture >48 hours, no other site of infection.

tially developed for use in HSCT recipients, but are now the standard of care for almost all patients who receive intensive therapy. Catheter-associated infections are categorized as either entry-site infections, tunnel infections, or catheter-associated blood stream infections (Table 50–4). The delineation of an entry-site infection from a tunnel infection can be clinically challenging, but the occurrence of an apparent entry-site infection plus a blood stream infection usually indicates that the catheter tunnel is infected. It is now believed that the majority of entry-site infections can be managed effectively with antimicrobial therapy alone. Tunnel infections require catheter removal with modification of the empiric antibiotics based on culture and antibiotic susceptibility results. Determination of the true role of the venous catheter in a blood stream infection is difficult unless there is evidence of tunnel or entry site inflammation caused by the same organism. The majority of blood stream infections that occur in patients with a hematological malignancy do not require catheter removal.[8,9] However, immediate catheter removal is recommended for patients with blood stream infections due to fungi, nontuberculosis mycobacterium (*M. fortuitum* complex and *M. chelonae/abscessus* group) and VRE.[19,29,83] Persistent blood stream infections are more frequent if the catheter is not removed and the blood stream pathogen is a *Bacillus* sp., *C. jeikeium*, *S. aureus*, *P. aeruginosa*, or *Stenotrophomonas maltophilia*.[18,84–86] All other blood stream infections can be initially treated with pathogen-specific antibiotics. Catheter removal in these later cases should be considered if the blood stream infection persists beyond 48 hours and no other site of infection is identified. It is also important to consider the possibility that the venous catheter is the primary site of the blood stream infection that recurs after completing a course of antimicrobial therapy.[9,87] There is inadequate data to support the recommendation that antibiotic administration be alternated through the different catheter lumens. One must believe that if the catheter is truly the source of infection that antibiotics alone will have a very low chance of sterilizing the venous access device.

LACK OF CLINICAL RESPONSE TO INITIAL EMPIRIC THERAPY

Management of patients with documented or undocumented infection who do not clinically respond to antimicrobial therapy can be challenging.[8] The lack of response may represent an infection with a pathogen resistant to the empiric antimicrobial regimen, inadequate serum or tissue levels of the antibiotics, infection at a vascular site (e.g., catheter) or closed space, the emergence of a second infection, or an unusually slow clinical response. It is important to remember that the resolution of fever in patients who are neutropenic can be delayed. A recent review of 488 episodes of fever and neutropenia treated at the M.D. Anderson Cancer Center revealed that the median time to fever resolution ranged from 5 to 7 days.[88] Less than 40 percent of patients became afebrile before day 5 of therapy. Patients with gram-negative blood stream infections were febrile for a mean of 6.6 to 8.2 days, while the time to fever defervescence

was even longer for patients with gram-positive blood stream infections (range 6.6 to 12.4 days). These findings are consistent with the results published by Freifeld et al. who reported that the mean time for patients to become afebrile was 4 days with ceftazidime therapy and 3 days for patients treated with imipenem.[70] These studies provide evidence that the time to fever defervescence can be prolonged, but also that the fever response may vary depending on the specific antibiotic regimen, site of infection, and infecting pathogen.

Patients in whom fever persists beyond 4 to 5 days of initial antimicrobial therapy should undergo a careful reassessment. Broad-spectrum antibiotics should be maximized, but if possible, antibiotic combinations that minimize organ toxicity should be implemented. Clinical evaluation must include a thorough daily evaluation, review of previous culture results, and further site-specific investigation as clinically indicated. The management of such patients may require serial antimicrobial changes and infectious diseases consultation can be helpful.

The need for change in the empiric therapy should be based on the patient's clinical status and the likelihood of early marrow recovery. Although fever resolution may be slow, persistent fever raises concern about an inadequately treated infection.[88] For patients who are persistently febrile and clinically unstable, additional gram-negative bacillary coverage, empiric vancomycin, or empiric amphotericin B should be considered. Clinically stable but febrile patients can be followed carefully without changing their antimicrobial treatment. However, most physicians will begin to consider the use of empiric amphotericin B or AmBisome if a patient's fever persists beyond day 6 of antibiotics.[8,9,89] Walsh et al. have recently reported on a multicenter trial that compared voriconazole (new triazole) to AmBisome as empiric treatment for patients with neutropenia and persistent fever.[90] In this trial, voriconazole was comparable to AmBisome in therapeutic success, but superior in reducing breakthrough fungal infections, infusion-related toxicity, and nephrotoxicity. These encouraging results may have a significant impact on the standard of care once voriconazole is FDA approved and commercially available.

EVALUATION AND MANAGEMENT OF FUNGAL INFECTIONS

Invasive fungal infections have become an increasingly important problem for patients with neutropenia. Several studies have reported yearly increases in the incidence of candidiasis, aspergillus, and other mold infections.[7,26–29,91,92] Aspergillosis is now the number one cause of infection death after allogeneic transplantation.[7,26,27] Fungal organisms are categorized into three general groups. First is the yeast, which are distinguished by their inability to form true hyphae, and their propensity to colonize mucosal surfaces. *Candida* spp. are most common and were reported to occur in 10 to 20 percent of patients prior to the routine use of azole prophylaxis.[28,91,99] The second group is the molds, which are characterized by their ability to form true hyphae and are primarily acquired by the inhalation of aerosolized spores. In the past this was believed to occur only from contaminated air, but recent studies have also raised the importance of aerosolized contaminated water sources.[93] The most common molds are the *Aspergillus* spp., but Mucorales order, Fusarium, Bipolaris, and Pseudoallescheria are being more commonly isolated. The final group of fungi is the dimorphic fungi that have both a yeast and hyphal form. These infections are more common among patients with a hematological malignancy that live in an endemic area, and suffer from significant cellular immune deficiency.

The diagnosis of candidiasis and mold infections continues to rely on recovery of the specific pathogen from culture of the blood, or identification by culture or histology from tissue samples. Rapid diagnosis of these infections using serum antigen detection as a surrogate marker for invasive disease remains a high priority. Galactomannan detection for the diagnosis of aspergillosis appears in early trials to be highly specific for invasive disease, but test sensitivity has varied from 43 to 83 percent depending on the test cutoff index.[94] The group from Belgium prospectively collected sera from HSCT recipients and assessed the efficacy of galactomannan detection to predict invasive aspergillosis.[95] They reported that serial testing in HSCT recipients could identify invasive *Aspergillus,* a median of 6 days (range 0 to 14) before clinical parameters dictated empiric antifungal therapy, and a median of 17 days before the diagnosis of aspergillosis was confirmed. Clinical usefulness of this nonculture technique requires further prospective evaluation, but could potentially improve the ability to diagnose invasive aspergillosis and help to monitor the response to treatment.

Candidiasis

The frequency and occurrence of candidiasis has been well described.[28,29,91] Goodrich and colleagues reviewed the occurrence of candidiasis at the FHCRC before azole prophylaxis and lipid-based amphotericin B products were being used. In this report 1.4 percent of transplant recipients developed invasive candidiasis.[29] The most common species were *C. albicans* (62 percent) and *C. tropicalis* (21 percent). The median time to the development of a *Candida* spp. blood stream infection was 15 days after transplantation and these infections had an attributable mortality of 39 percent. Infection mortality was further increased to 88 percent if *Candida* tissue invasion was also documented.

Autologous and allogeneic HSCT recipients had a similar risk of candidiasis during the neutropenic period, but the risk of developing candidiasis persisted for allogeneic transplant recipients despite the return of granulocyte function (Table 50–5). The occurrence of *Candida* spp. blood stream infections was recently reassessed at the FHCRC after the introduction of fluconazole prophylaxis.[28] Forty-four percent of patients were colonized with *Candida* spp. at some time either prior to or during the first 75 days after transplant. *C. albicans* was more likely to be recovered before transplantation, with non-*albicans* species more likely to be recovered during the period of azole use. *C. albicans* resistance to fluconazole was modest (5.3 percent of isolates), with the most common blood stream isolates now being *C. glabrata, C. parapsilosis,* and *C. krusei. Candida* blood stream infections occurred in 4.7 percent of patients, a

Table 50–5. Risk Factors[a] for Candidiasis and Aspergillosis After HSCT

	Candidiasis		Aspergillosis	
	Pre-Azole	Azole Rx	Early	Late
Increased age	Yes	Yes	No	Yes
Unrelated donor	Yes	No	No	Yes
GvHD	Yes	No	No	Yes
Corticosteroids	Yes	No	No	Yes
Neutropenia	Yes	No	Yes	No
Season (summer)	No	No	Yes	No
Concomitant infection	Yes	Yes	Yes	Yes
LAF	No	No	Yes	No
Construction	No	No	No	Yes
CMV positive	Yes	Yes	Yes	Yes

[a] Multivariate analysis.

median of 28 days after transplantation, and were associated with a 20 percent mortality rate. Of note in this study, the use of fluconazole prophylaxis eliminated the importance of neutropenia as a risk factor, but had no impact on infections with non-*albicans* species (Table 50–5). Viscoli and co-workers[91] conducted a surveillance study of candidemia in cancer patients. Two hundred forty-nine cases were assessed; 58 (36 percent) occurred among patients with a hematological malignancy. The overall 30-day mortality rate was 39 percent and the associated factors of increased age and stage of disease, exposure to salvage therapy, the occurrence of septic shock, and the lack of antifungal prophylaxis were associated with an increase in infection-associated death.[91] *C. albicans* was the most common species identified but the recovery of non-*albicans* species was increased in patients with a hematological malignancy when compared to other immunocompromised hosts.

Aspergillosis

Aspergillus infections primarily involve the respiratory tract, but reports of disseminated infection with CNS involvement are increasing. Invasive infection of the lung appears more common, but the true incidence of sinus involvement in HSCT recipients is known. The occurrence of *Aspergillus* infections after HSCT clearly demonstrates the three pathophysiological conditions that predispose patients to this infection.[26] One group of patients will develop their infection early during the pre-engraftment period, where the primary risk factor is neutropenia (Table 50–5). The second group develops their infection later, between days 40 and 120 post-transplantation, and are predisposed to infection because of a persistent cellular immune defect. The third group experience *Aspergillus* infections very late after transplantation and these infections appear to be highly correlated with CMV disease and chronic graft-versus-host disease (GvHD) (personal communication, K. Marr, 2000), which are surrogate markers of delayed immune reconstitution after transplantation. Extrapulmonary spread of *Aspergillus* is more common with neutropenia-associated infections, while nonneutropenic *Aspergillus* pneumonia is more likely to present with progressive diffuse pneumonitis.[96] The mortality associated with aspergillosis after transplant remains high and ranges from 60 to 88 percent.[26,27] Median survival after diagnosis is usually short (36 days). Aspergillosis follows a similar course when patients with a hematological malignancy develop this infection following conventional therapy.[97,100] Pulmonary involvement is seen in 87 percent of cases, infection of the sinuses/nose in 16 percent, and brain in 8 percent.[97] Mortality remains high for these patients (64 percent), although patients with AML may have slightly lower death rates (30 to 40 percent).[97,100] Diagnosis, prevention, and treatment of Aspergillus infections remain inadequate. Diagnosis is dependent on a high index of suspicion and recovery of the infecting organism by histology or microbiology from tissue specimens or pulmonary or sinus lavage. Results of galactomannan assays are encouraging.[94,95] While the use of surveillance cultures remains controversial, the isolation of A. fumigatus or flavus in respiratory specimens has been shown to be highly predictive of present or future invasive aspergillosis.[26] Mucosal eschars along the nasal septum are an important clinical clue to the diagnosis of Aspergillus sinusitis. Biopsy and culture of such lesions are always indicated. If nasal lesions are not observed sinus aspirate and biopsy may establish the diagnosis and preclude the need for further diagnostic procedures.

Bronchoalveolar lavage (BAL) is the standard approach for evaluating pulmonary lesions. BAL is a less sensitive procedure if the pulmonary lesions are focal, small, and/or peripherally located. The sensitivity of a BAL to diagnose Aspergillus is only 50 to 60 percent. Thus a negative procedure does not exclude the diagnosis of Aspergillus.[26,97–100] Open lung biopsy is usually reserved for patients with a negative BAL, or for patients in which the disease is progressive and a diagnosis must be immediately established. A thoracoscopic approach is utilized when possible because of lowered procedure morbidity. Biopsies of both peripheral and central areas of abnormal lung are recommended because of the focal nature of Aspergillus infections, and the wide distribution of organisms within the pneumonic process.

Treatment of established Aspergillus infections remains inadequate. Early diagnosis and treatment remain critical. Prolonged (8 to 10 weeks) high-dose (1.0 to 1.5 mg/kg/day) amphotericin B or an equivalent dose of one of the lipid formulations of amphotericin B is standard initial treatment.[8,9,97–100] Additional suppressive therapy with an oral agent like itraconazole is often given to patients who remain profoundly immunosuppressed.[8] To date, the lipid amphotericin B products have not been shown to increase survival, although the incidence of both acute infusion-related adverse effects and nephrotoxicity are decreased with these preparations.[89,100] The choice to use the new lipid formulations of amphotericin B must be based on the risk of developing nephrotoxicity and the cost of treatment.[102,103] The use of antifungal agents in combination remains controversial and some in vitro studies have suggested the possibility of clinically relevant antagonism if an azolelike itraconazole is combined with amphotericin B.

The echinocandins are a new class of antifungal agents with enhanced activity against Aspergillus and fluconazole-resistant yeast, but lacking activity against the Mucorales order. These agents work by inhibiting β-(1,3)-D-glucan that is essential to the integrity of the fungal cell wall. Caspofungin is the first of the class to receive FDA approval. Toxicity has been relatively low, and preliminary clinical results look encouraging for patients with aspergillosis who are refractory or intolerant of other therapy. In vitro and preclinical animal studies suggest that caspofungin may be an excellent agent to use in combination with an amphotericin B product or azole to enhance the antifungal efficacy.

Voriconazole, a new triazole with enhanced activity against Aspergillus, is available in both an oral and intravenous formulation, and appears encouraging as treatment of aspergillosis. Results from a prospective, randomized, multicenter clinical trial are expected in the fall of 2001. Additional new antifungal agents (e.g., posaconazole, ravuconazole, liposomal nystatin, and other echinocandins) are being tested as treatment of invasive aspergillosis. These agents show promise with early study response rates of 25 to 40 percent among patients who have failed to respond to amphotericin B. The future promises the clinician new antifungal antibiotics, but the goal will be to learn how to use them effectively.

Efforts to enhance infected patients' immune status have been recommended but the use of growth factors (G-CSF, GM-CSF) or G-CSF mobilized granulocyte transfusion has not been shown to be beneficial as adjunct therapy for fungal infections.[56] The role of surgery as an adjunct to antimicrobial treatment for pulmonary Aspergillus remains controversial, but a preliminary analysis from the FHCRC (personal communication, D. Weiss, 2000) shows little survival benefit if surgical resection of the apparent infection is performed.

SITE OF CARE FOR PATIENTS WITH FEVER AND NEUTROPENIA

There is increasing acceptance that some patients with fever and neutropenia can be safely managed as outpatients, or with shortened hospital stays.[8,104–107] Several investigators have developed prospective models to help predict a population of patients who would be at low risk to develop infection-associated complications, and therefore be candidates for outpatient therapy.[107,108] In general, most models have excluded patients with acute leukemia undergoing induction therapy, or HSCT recipients from the low-risk patient group. This has been done because of the belief that their underlying immunosuppression and intensity of treatment inherently make them a high-risk population.[107,108]

Effective outpatient therapy has been provided to patients when the treating physician has been able to accurately predict the individual patient's risk of developing infection-associated complications, and the treating center has implemented an infrastructure for patient care and monitoring that is available 24 hours per day, 7 days a week. Assessment and monitoring should be performed by health care providers who are trained in the management of patients with a compromised immune system. Success of this approach will always depend on patient and family education, and the physician's willingness to recommend hospitalization if the clinical condition changes or the patient and family request such care.

A recent international multicenter study of 1139 patients with fever and neutropenia established and validated a prognostic scoring system to help prospectively identify those patients at low risk for complications including mortality.[108] Factors associated with lower risk of complications and a higher rate of more favorable outcome included age less than 60 years, cancer under control, no or only mild symptoms of illness, outpatient status at the onset of the fever, no significant comorbid disease, and the absence of signs or symptoms of sepsis syndrome. This risk model reported a positive predictive value of 91 percent, and a sensitivity and specificity of 71 and 68 percent, respectively. This prediction model adds to the tools available to the physician to deliver high-quality outpatient therapy, but like all prediction models it must be adjusted to the individual patient's clinical and psychosocial condition. An alternative to initial outpatient therapy is for patients to be admitted to the hospital for evaluation and the initiation of broad-spectrum intravenous antibiotics. Selected stable patients can then be discharged to complete therapy as an outpatient once a fulminant infection has been excluded, and the status of the infection and early infection-associated complications have been clarified.

Outpatient antibiotic treatment may consist of broad-spectrum intravenous antibiotics given at home, once-daily broad-spectrum antibiotics given at home or in the clinic, or a combination of oral agents. The present data suggest that if an oral regimen is considered that the combination of a fluoroquinolone (ciprofloxacin) and an agent with enhanced grampositive activity (amoxicillin/potassium clavulanate [Augmentin] or clindamycin) should be considered.[8,109,110]

SUMMARY

The morbidity and mortality of initial infections for patients with a hematological malignancy have dramatically decreased, but during this same time period there has been the emergence of antibiotic-resistant bacteria, and a significant increase in the incidence of fungal infections. Antibiotics have improved and in general are less toxic than their ancestors. PBSC transplants have decreased the duration of pre-engraftment neutropenia, and progress has been made in the area of prophylaxis of *Candida albicans* infections. However, patients now are at an increased risk of non-*albicans* yeast infections and the mortality from mold infections (e.g., *Aspergillus*) remains significant. The promise of new diagnostic techniques, additional antimicrobial agents, and strategies for treatment and prophylaxis hold the potential that treatment of such patients may be safer in the future. It is critical for the oncology team to remember that infections are a dynamic process and change is guaranteed. Physicians who manage patients with a hematological malignancy must not forget the value and importance of standard infection control measures. It will be a challenge to maintain such infection control approaches as the care of these patients continues to be focused in an ambulatory/day hospital facility.

REFERENCES

1. Pizzo PA: Management of fever in patients with cancer and treatment-induced neutropenia. N Engl J Med 328:1323–1332, 1993.
2. Wade JC: Management of infection in patients with acute leukemia. Hematol Oncol Clin North Am 7:293–315, 1993.
3. Bodey GP, Buckley M, Sathe YS et al: Quantitative relationships between circulating leukocytes and infection in patients with acute leukemia. Ann Intern Med 64:328–340, 1966.
4. Schimpff SC: Empiric antibiotic therapy for granulocytopenic cancer patients. Am J Med 80(Suppl. 5c):13–20, 1986.
5. Imbert-Marcille BM, Tang XW, Lepelletier D et al: Human herpesvirus-6 infection after autologous or allogeneic stem cell transplantation: A single-center prospective longitudinal study of 92 patients. Clin Infect Dis 31:881–886, 2000.
6. Luppi M, Barozzi P, Schulz TF et al: Bone marrow failure associated with human herpesvirus 8 infection after transplantation. N Engl J Med 343:1378–1385, 2000.
7. Van Burk JA, Weisdorf D: Infections in recipients of blood and marrow transplantation. In Mandell GL, Bennett JE, Dolin R (eds.): Principles and Practice of Infectious Diseases, 5th Ed., pp. 3136–3147. Churchill Livingstone, Philadelphia, 2000.
8. Wade JC, Rubenstein EB, and the NCCN Guidelines Committee: Clinical practice guidelines for fever and neutropenia. Oncology 13:197–257, 1999.
9. Hughes WT, Armstrong D, Bodey GP et al: Guidelines for the use of antimicrobial agents in neutropenic patients with unexplained fever. Clin Infect Dis 25:551–573, 1997.
10. Englund JA, Sullivan CJ, Jordan MC et al: Respiratory syncytial virus infection in immunocompromised adults. Ann Intern Med 109:203–208, 1988.
11. Harrington RD, Houton TM, Hackman RC et al: An outbreak of respiratory syncytial virus in a bone marrow transplant center. J Infect Dis 165:987–993, 1992.
12. Wingard JR, Santos GW, Saral R: Differences between first and subsequent fevers during prolonged neutropenia. Cancer 59:844–849, 1987.
13. Glauser M, Boogaerts M, Cordonnier C et al: Empiric therapy of bacterial infections in severe neutropenia. Clin Microbiol Infect 3(Suppl. 1):S77–86, 1997.
14. Engelhard D, Elishoov H, Strauss N et al: Nosocomial coagulase-negative staphylococcal infections in bone marrow transplantation recipients with central vein catheter: A 5-year prospective study. Transplantation 61:430–434, 1996.
15. Villablanca JG, Steiner M, Kersey J et al: The clinical spectrum of infections with viridans streptococci in bone marrow transplant recipients. Bone Marrow Transplant 6:387–393, 1990.
16. Classen DC, Burke JP, Ford CD et al: *Streptococcus mitis* sepsis in bone marrow transplant patients receiving oral antimicrobial prophylaxis. Am J Med 89:441–446, 1990.
17. Elting LS, Bodey GP, Keefe BH: Septicemia and shock syndrome due to viridans streptococci: A case control study of predisposing factors. Clin Infect Dis 14:1201–1207, 1992.
18. Stamm WE, Tompkins LS, Wagner KF et al: Infection due to *Corynebacterium* species in marrow transplant recipients. Ann Intern Med 91:167–173, 1979.
19. Edmond MB, Ober JF, Dawson JD et al: Vancomycin-resistant enterococcal bacteremia: Natural history and attributable mortality. Clin Infect Dis 23:1234–1239, 1996.
20. Martin MA, Pfaller MA, Wenzel RP: Coagulase-negative staphylococcal bacteremia: Mortality and hospital stay. Ann Intern Med 110:9–16, 1989.

21. Wenzel RP: Perspective: Attributable mortality—The promise of better antimicrobial therapy. J Infect Dis 178:917–919, 1989.

22. Johnston PB, Litzow MR, Elliott MA et al: Colonization with vancomycin-resistant enterococcus correlates with poor outcome in patients undergoing allogeneic blood and marrow transplants (abstract). Blood 96:786a, 2000.

23. Brown AE, Kiehn TE, Armstrong DE: Bacterial resistance in patients with neoplastic disease. Infect Dis Clin Pract 4(Suppl. 3):S136–144, 1995.

24. Koll BS, Brown AE: The changing epidemiology of infections at a cancer hospital. Clin Infect Dis 17(Suppl. 2):S322–328, 1993.

25. Elting LS, Rubenstein EB, Rolston KV et al: Outcomes of bacteremia in patients with cancer and neutropenia. Clin Infect Dis 25:247–259, 1997.

26. Wald A, Leisenring W, Van Burik JA, Bowden RA: Epidemiology of *Aspergillus* infections in a large cohort of patients undergoing bone marrow transplantation. J Infect Dis 175:1459–1466, 1997.

27. Ribaud P, Chastang C, Latage JP et al: Survival and prognostic factors of invasive aspergillosis after allogeneic bone marrow transplantation. Clin Infect Dis 28:322–330, 1999.

28. Marr KA, Seidel K, White TC et al: Candidemia in allogeneic blood and marrow transplant recipients: Evolution of risk factors after adoption of prophylactic fluconazole. J Infect Dis 181:309–316, 2000.

29. Goodrich JM, Reed EC, Mori M et al: Clinical features and analysis of risk factors for invasive candidal infection after marrow transplantation. J Infect Dis 164:731–740, 1991.

30. Hospital Infection Control Practices Advisory Committee (HIPAC): Recommendations for preventing the spread of vancomycin-resistance. Infect Control Hosp Epidemiol 16:105–113, 1995.

31. Cruciani M, Rampazzo R, Malena M et al: Prophylaxis with fluoroquinolones for bacterial infections in neutropenic patients: A meta-analysis. Clin Infect Dis 23:795–805, 1996.

32. VanBurik JH, Weisdorf DJ: Infections in recipients of blood and marrow translantation. Hematol/Oncol Clin North Am 13:1065–1089, 1999.

33. Conneally E, Cafferkey MT, Daly PA, Keane CT, McCann SR: Nebulized amphotericin B as prophylaxis against invasive aspergillosis in granulocytopenic patients. Bone Marrow Transplant 5:403–406, 1990.

34. O'Donnell MR, Schmidt GM, Tegtmeier BR et al: Prediction of systemic fungal infection in allogeneic marrow recipients: Impact of amphotericin prophylaxis in high-risk patients. J Clin Oncol 12:827–834, 1994.

35. Rousey SR, Russler S, Gottlieb M, Ash RC: Low-dose amphotericin B prophylaxis against invasive *Aspergillus* infections in allogeneic marrow transplantation. Am J Med 91:484–492, 1991.

36. Perfect JR, Klotman ME, Gilbert CC et al: Prophylactic intravenous amphotericin B in neutropenic autologous bone marrow transplant recipients. J Infect Dis 165:891–897, 1992.

37. Tollemar J, Ringden O, Andersson S et al: Prophylactic use of liposomal amphotericin B (AmBisome) against fungal infections: A randomized trial in bone marrow transplant recipients. Transplant Proc 25:1495–1497, 1993.

38. Menichetti F, Flavero AD, Martion P et al: Itraconazole oral solution as prophylaxis for fungal infections in neutropenic patients with hematologic malignancies: A randomized, placebo-controlled, double-blind, multicenter trial. Clin Infect Dis 28:250–255, 1999.

39. Nucci M, Biasoli I, Akiti T et al: A double-blind, randomized, placebo-controlled trial of itraconazole capsules as antifungal prophylaxis for neutropenic patients. Clin Infect Dis 30:300–305, 2000.

40. Goodman JL, Winston DJ, Greenfield RA et al: A controlled trial of fluconazole to prevent fungal infections in patients undergoing bone marrow transplantation. N Engl J Med 326:845–851, 1992.

41. Slavin MA, Osborne B, Adams R et al: Efficacy and safety of fluconazole for fungal infections after marrow transplant—a prospective, randomized, double-blind study. J Infect Dis 171:1545–1552, 1995.

42. Marr KA, Seidel K, Slavin MA et al: Prolonged fluconazole prophylaxis is associated with persistent protection against candidiasis-related death in allogeneic marrow transplant recipients: Long-term follow-up of a randomized, placebo-controlled trial. Blood 96:2055–2061, 2000.

43. Rotstein C, Bow EJ, Laverdiere M et al: Randomized placebo-controlled trial of fluconazole prophylaxis for neutropenic cancer patients: Benefit based on purpose and intensity of cytotoxic therapy. Clin Infect Dis 28:331–340, 1999.

44. Winston DJ, Chandrasekar PH, Lazarus HM et al: Fluconazole prophylaxis of fungal infections in patients with acute leukemia. Results of a randomized placebo-controlled, double-blind, multicenter trial. Ann Intern Med 118:495–503, 1993.

45. Bjerke J, Meyers JD, Bowden RA: Hepatosplenic candidiasis—a contraindication to marrow transplantation? Blood 84:2811–2814, 1994.

46. Offner F, Cordonnier C, Ljungman P et al: Impact of previous aspergillosis on the outcome of bone marrow transplantation. Clin Infect Dis 26:1098–1103, 1998.

47. Saral R, Ambinder RF, Burns WH et al: Acyclovir prophylaxis against recrudescent herpes simplex virus infections in leukemia patients: A randomized, double-blind placebo controlled study. Ann Intern Med 99:773–776, 1983.

48. Wade JC, Newton B, Flournoy N et al: Oral acyclovir for the prevention of herpes simplex virus reactivation after marrow transplantation. Ann Intern Med 100:823–828, 1984.

49. Baglin TP, Gray JJ, Marcus RE, Wreghitt TG: Antibiotic resistant fever associated with herpes simplex virus infection in neutropenic cancer patients with haematological malignancy. J Clin Pathol 42:1255–1258, 1989.

50. Weaver CH, Schulman KA, Wilson-Relyea B et al: Randomized trial of filgrastim, sargramostim, or sequential sargramostim and filgrastim after myelosuppressive chemotherapy for the harvesting of peripheral-blood stem cells. J Clin Oncol 18:43–53, 2000.

51. Holmberg LA, Boeckh M, Hooper H et al: Increased incidence of cytomegalovirus disease after autologous CD34-selected peripheral blood stem cell transplantation. Blood 94:4029–4035, 2000.

52. Crippa F, Holmberg L, Hooper H et al: Infections after autologous CD34 selected peripheral blood stem cell transplantation (abstract). Blood 96:586a, 2000.

53. Champlin RE, Schmitz N, Horowitz MM et al: Blood stem cells compared with bone marrow as a source of hematopoietic cells for allogeneic transplantation. Blood 95:3702–3709, 2000.

54. Bensinger WI, Martin PJ, Storer B et al: Transplantation of bone marrow as compared with peripheral-blood cells from HLA-identical relatives in patients with hematologic cancers. N Engl J Med 344:175–181, 2001.

55. Powles R, Mehta J, Kulkarni S et al: Allogeneic blood and bone-marrow stem-cell transplantation in haematological malignant diseases: A randomised trial. Lancet 355:1231–1237, 2000.

56. Ozer H, Armitage JO, Bennett CL et al: Update of recommendations for the use of hematopoietic colony-stimulating factors: Evidence-based, clinical practice guidelines. J Clin Oncol 18:3558–3585, 2000.

57. Hartmann LC, Tchetter LK, Habermann TM et al: Granulocyte colony-stimulating factor in severe chemotherapy-induced afebrile neutropenia. N Engl J Med 336:1776–1780, 1997.

58. Clift RA, Sanders JE, Thomas ED et al: Granulocyte transfusions for the prevention of infection in patients receiving bone marrow transfusions. N Engl J Med 298:1052–1057, 1978.

59. Winston D, Ho WG, Young LS: Prophylactic granulocyte transfusions during human bone marrow transplantation. Am J Med 68:893–899, 1980.

60. Price TH, Bowden RA, Boeckh M et al: Phase I/II trial of neutrophil transfusions from donors stimulated with G-CSF and dexamethasone for treatment of patients with infections in hematopoietic stem cell transplantation. Blood 95:3302–3309, 2000.

61. Pena E, Narvios A, Lichtiger B: Therapeutic granulocyte transfusions: Retrospective study of 34 patients (abstract). Blood 96:63a, 2000.

62. Hubel K, Carter R, Liles WC et al: Community donors vs. related donors for granulocyte transfusion therapy in hematopoietic transplantations: A comparative analysis of feasibility and outcome (abstract). Blood 96:63a, 2000.

63. Adkins DR, Goodnough LT, Shenoy S et al: Effect of leukocyte compatibility on neutrophil increment after transfusion of granulocyte colony-stimulating factor-mobilized prophylactic granulocyte transfusions and on clinical outcomes after stem cell transplantation. Blood 95:3605–3612, 2000.

64. Reimer LG, Wilson ML, Weinstein MP: Update on detection of bacteremia and fungemia. Clin Microbiol Rev 10:444–465, 1997.

65. Weinstein, MP: Current blood culture methods and systems: Clinical concepts, technology, and interpretation of results. Clin Infect Dis 23:40–46, 1996.

66. Siegman-Igra Y, Anglim AM, Shapiro DE et al: Diagnosis of vascular catheter-related bloodstream infection: A meta-analysis. J Clin Microbiol 35:928–936, 1997.

67. Whimbey E, Wong B, Kiehn TE et al: Clinical correlations of serial quantitative blood cultures determined by lysis-centrifugation in patients with persistent septicemia. J Clin Microbiol 19:766–771, 1984.

68. Benezra D, Kiehn TE, Gold JWM et al: Prospective study of infections in indwelling central venous catheters using quantitative blood cultures. Am J Med 85:495–498, 1988.

69. McFarland LV, Mulligan ME, Kwok RYY et al: Nosocomial acquisition of Clostridium difficile infection. N Engl J Med 17:484–490, 1989.

70. Freifeld AG, Walsh T, Marshall D et al: Monotherapy for fever and neutropenia in cancer patients: A randomized comparison of ceftazidime vs. imipenem. J Clin Oncol 13:165–176, 1995.

71. Cometta A, Calandra T, Gaya H et al: Monotherapy with meropenem vs. combination therapy with ceftazidime plus amikacin as empiric therapy for fever in granulocytopenic patients with cancer. Antimicrob Agents Chemother 40:1108–1115, 1996.

72. Oblon D, Ramphal R: A randomized trial of cefepime vs. ceftazidime as initial therapy for patients with prolonged fever and neutropenia after intensive chemotherapy (abstract). Proc Annual Meeting Am Assoc Cancer Res 34:1362a, 1993.

73. Cometta A, Zinner S, de Bock R et al: Piperacillin-tazobactam plus amikacin vs ceftazidime plus amikacin as empiric therapy for fever in granulocytopenic patients with cancer: The International Antimicrobial Therapy Cooperative Group of the European Organization for Research and Treatment of Cancer. Antimicrob Agents Chemother 39:445–452, 1995.

74. Winston DJ, Lazarus HM, Beveridge RA et al: Randomized, double-blind, multicenter trial comparing clinafloxacin with imipenem as empirical monotherapy for febrile granulocytopenic patients. Clin Infect Dis 32:381–390, 2001.

75. European Organization for Research and Treatment of Cancer (EORTC), International Antimicrobial Therapy Cooperative Group, and the National Cancer Institute of Canada—Clinical Trials Group: Vancomycin added to empirical combination antibiotic therapy for fever in granulocytopenic cancer patients. J Infect Dis 163:951–958, 1991.

76. Donskey CJ, Hanrahan JA, Hutton RA, Rice LB: Effect of parenteral antibiotic administration on persistence of vancomycin-resistant Enterococcus faecium in the mouse gastrointestinal tract. J Infect Dis 180:384–390, 1999.

77. Pfaller M, Jones R, Marshall S et al: Nosocomial streptococcal blood stream infections in the SCOPE Program: Species occurrence and antimicrobial resistance: The SCOPE Hospital Study Group. Diag Microbiol Infect Dis 29:259–263, 1997.

78. Edmond MB, Wallace SE, McClish DK et al: Nosocomial bloodstream infections in United States hospitals: A three-year analysis. Clin Infect Dis 29:239–244, 1999.

79. Bow EJ, Loewen R, Vaughan D: Reduced requirement for antibiotic therapy targeting gram negative organisms in febrile, neutropenic patients with cancer who are receiving antibacterial chemoprophylaxis with oral quinolones. Clin Infect Dis 20:907–912, 1995.

80. Ward TT, Thomas RG, Fye CL et al: Trimethoprim-sulfamethoxazole prophylaxis in granulocytopenic patients with acute leukemia: Evaluation of serum antibiotic levels in a randomized, double-blind, placebo-controlled Department of Veterans Affairs cooperative study. Clin Infect Dis 17:323–332, 1993.

81. Herwaldt LA, Hollis RJ, Boyken LD, Pfaller MA: Molecular epidemiology of coagulase-negative staphylococci isolated from immunocompromised patients. Infect Control Hosp Epidemiol 13:86–92, 1992.

82. Wendt C, Messer SA, Hollis RJ et al: Recurrent gram-negative bacteremia: Incidence and clinical patterns. Clin Infect Dis 28:611–617, 1999.

83. Roy V, Weisdorf D: Mycobacterial infections following bone marrow transplantation. A 20-year retrospective review. Bone Marrow Transplant 19:467–470, 1997.

84. Vassilomanolakis M, Plataniotis G, Koumakis G et al: Central venous catheter-related infections after bone marrow transplantation in patients with malignancies: A prospective study with short-course vancomycin prophylaxis. Bone Marrow Transplant 15:77–80, 1995.

85. Banerjee C, Bustamante CI, Wharton R et al: Bacillus infections in patients with cancer. Arch Intern Med 148:1769–1774, 1988.

86. Press OW, Ramsey PG, Larsen EB et al: Hickman catheter infections in patients with malignancy. Medicine 63:189–200, 1984.

87. Engellard D, Elishoov H, Strauss N et al: Nosocomial coagulase-negative staphylococcal infections in bone marrow transplantation recipients with central vein catheter. A 5 year prospective study. Transplantation 61:430–434, 1996.

88. Elting LS, Rubenstein EB, Rolston K et al: Time to clinical response: An outcome of antibiotic therapy of febrile neutropenia with implications for quality and cost of care. J Clin Oncol 21:3699–3706, 2000.

89. Walsh, TJ, Finberg R, Arndt C et al: Liposomal amphotericin B is effective for empirical antifungal therapy in cancer patients with fever and neutropenia. N Engl J Med 340:764–771, 1999.

90. Walsh T, Pappas P, Winston D et al: Voriconazole versus liposomal amphotericin B for empirical antifungal therapy of persistently febrile neutropenic patients: A randomized, international, multi-

center trial (abstract). 40th Interscience Conference of Antimicrobiology Agents and Chemotherapy 20, 2000.

91. Viscoli C, Girmenia A, Marinus A et al: Candidemia in cancer patients: A prospective multicenter surveillance study by the Invasive Fungal Infection Group (IFIG) to the European Organization for the Research and Treatment of Cancer (EORTC). Clin Infect Dis 28:1071–1079, 1999.

92. Kontoyiannis DP, Sumoza D, Tarrand J et al: Significance of aspergillemia in patients with cancer: A ten-year study. Clin Infect Dis 31:188–189, 2000.

93. Anaissie E, Stratton S, Summerbell R et al: Opportunistic moulds in a hospital water system: A 3-year prospective study (abstract). Blood 96:787a, 2000.

94. Marr KA, Balajee A, Leisenring W et al: Utility of galactomannan detection for the diagnosis of invasive aspergillosis in HSCT recipients (abstract). Blood 96:786a, 2000.

95. Maertens JA, Verhaegen J, Van Eldere J, Boogaerts M: Detection of circulating galactomannan (GM) is an early and sensitive indicator of invasive aspergillosis (IA) in allogeneic stem cell transplant recipients (ASCTR) (abstract). Blood 96:585a, 2000.

96. Marr KA, Carter K, Myerson D et al: Aspergillosis in HSCT recipients: Evidence for two distinct pathophysiologic conditions associated with engraftment status (abstract). Blood 96:787a, 2000.

97. Denning DW, Marinus A, Cohen J et al: An EORTC multicentre prospective survey of invasive aspergillosis in haematological patients: Diagnosis and theraputic outcome (EORTC Invasive Fungal Infections Cooperative Group). J Infect 37:173–180, 1998.

98. Patterson TF, Kirkpatrick WR, White M et al: Invasive aspergillosis: Disease spectrum, treatment practices, and outcomes (*Aspergillus* Study Group). Medicine 79:281–282, 2000.

99. Lortholary O, Ascioglu S, Moreau P et al: Invasive aspergillosis as an opportunistic infection in nonallografted patients with multiple myeloma: A European Organization for Research and Treatment of Cancer. Clin Infect Dis 30:41–46, 2000.

100. Lin SJ, Schranz J, Teutsch SM et al: Aspergillosis case-fatality rate: Systematic review of the literature. Clin Infect Dis 32:358–366, 2001.

101. Walsh TJ, Hiemenez JW, Seibel NL et al: Amphotericin B lipid complex for invasive fungal infections: Analysis of safety and efficacy of 556 cases. Clin Infect Dis 26:1383–1396, 1998.

102. Wingard JR, Kubilis P, Lee L et al: Clinical significance of nephrotoxicity in patients treated with amphotericin B for suspected or proven aspergillosis. Clin Infect Dis 29:1402–1407, 1999.

103. Cagnoni PJ, Walsh TJ, Prendergast MM et al: Pharmacoeconomic analysis of liposomal amphotericin B versus conventional amphotericin B in the empirical treatment of persistently febrile neutropenic patients. J Clin Oncol 18:2476–2483, 2000.

104. Talcott JA, Whalen A, Clark J et al: Home antibiotic therapy for low-risk cancer patients with fever and neutropenia: A pilot study of 30 patients, based on a validated prediction rule. J Clin Oncol 12:107–114, 1994.

105. Rubenstein EB, Rolston K, Benjamin RS et al: Outpatient treatment of febrile episodes in low-risk neutropenic patients with cancer. Cancer 7:3640–3646, 1993.

106. Rolston KV: Outpatient management of febrile, neutropenic patients. Infect Med 12:5, 1995.

107. Talcott J, Siegel R, Finberg R et al: Risk assessment in cancer patients with fever and neutropenia: A prospective, two-center validation of a prediction rule. J Clin Oncol 10:316–322, 1992.

108. Klastersky J, Paesmans M, Rubenstein EB et al: The Multinational Association for Supportive Care in Cancer risk index: A multinational scoring system for identifying low-risk febrile neutropenic cancer patients. J Clin Oncol 18:3038–3051, 2000.

109. Freifeld A, Marchigiani D, Walsh T et al: A double-blind comparison of empirical oral and intravenous antibiotic therapy for low-risk febrile patients with neutropenia during cancer chemotherapy. N Engl J Med 341:305–311, 1999.

110. Kern WV, Cometta A, DeBock R et al: Oral versus intravenous empirical antimicrobial therapy for fever in patients with granulocytopenia who are receiving cancer chemotherapy. N Engl J Med 341:312–318, 1999.

Viral Infections in Patients with Hematological Malignancies

John R. Wingard and Helen Leather

Enormous advances in the control of bacterial and fungal pathogens have occurred over the last decade. Although host factors such as impairment of granulocyte function or impaired mucosal barrier integrity are major risk factors for bacterial and fungal pathogens, compromise of cell-mediated immunity, especially of cytotoxic thymus-derived lymphocytes (T cells), appears to be most significant in accounting for susceptibility to viral pathogens. As dose intensity of the chemotherapeutic regimens used in the therapy of hematological malignancies has escalated over the last decade, greater susceptibility to viral pathogens has emerged.

Patients receiving therapy for leukemia or lymphoma and those undergoing bone marrow transplantation are susceptible to a variety of viral pathogens (Table 51–1). The most significant viral infections are caused by members of the herpesvirus family. In recent years there has also been increasing recognition of important manifestations of other viruses. In this chapter various viral infections will be described, and current approaches to treatment and prevention will be reviewed.

HERPESVIRUS FAMILY

The herpesviruses are large double-stranded DNA enveloped viruses, which commonly infect humans. Typically, the primary infection is mild and self-limited and requires no therapy in the normal host. The human herpesviruses that cause infection are herpes simplex virus type 1 (HSV-1), herpes simplex virus type 2 (HSV-2), varicella zoster virus (VZV), cytomegalovirus (CMV), Epstein-Barr virus (EBV), and human herpesvirus type 6 (HHV-6). Human herpesvirus type 7 (HHV-7) has also been isolated, but its role in illness has not been elucidated. Human herpesvirus type 8 (HHV-8) gene sequences have been identified in tissue specimens of Kaposi's sarcoma and some types of non-Hodgkin's lymphoma, and an association with multiple myeloma has also been proposed.

Following resolution of the manifestations of the primary infection, lifelong latency can occur in normal hosts; the sites of latency are sensory nerve ganglia for HSV and VZV and leukocytes for CMV, EBV, and HHV-6. Endogenous virus can subsequently cause a reactivated infection in both normal and immunocompromised hosts. Generally in the normal host,

Table 51–1. Viral Pathogens in Patients with Hematologic Malignancies

Herpesviruses
  Herpes simplex type 1
  Herpes simplex type 2
  Cytomegalovirus
  Varicella zoster virus
  Epstein-Barr virus
  Human herpesvirus 6
Intestinal viruses
  Rotavirus
  Norwalk virus
  Adenoviruses
  Astroviruses
  Coxsackie
  Caliciviruses
Respiratory viruses
  Respiratory syncytial virus
  Influenza
  Parainfluenza
Adenoviruses
Hepatitis viruses
  Hepatitis A
  Hepatitis B
  Hepatitis C
Papovaviruses
  JC
  BK
  Human papilloma
Other
  Parvovirus
  HTLV/HIV

reactivated infections have milder clinical symptomatology. All have been implicated as pathogens in patients with hematologic malignancies with the capacity to cause more severe clinical manifestations.

Herpes Simplex Virus

Patterns of Infection

Infections with HSV-1 frequently occur in early childhood. Transmission of virus occurs through contact with oral secretions. Transmission of HSV-2 occurs through contact with infected genital secretions, and thus infection generally occurs later in life, after adolescence. Clinical manifestations of HSV-1 include oral or nasolabial vesicles or ulcerations, keratoconjunctivitis, or encephalitis, whereas HSV-2 primarily causes genital vesicles or ulcerations. Serological conversion occurs with the primary infection, and the presence of IgG antibody provides an excellent indicator of prior infection and the presence of latent virus.

Immunocompromised patients are more susceptible for reactivation and potentially more severe manifestations[1] than normal hosts. In general, the intensity of chemotherapy regimens used in the treatment of hematological malignancy and the depth of depression of cell-mediated immunity correlate with both the risk for reactivation and the severity of the resulting clinical manifestations (Table 51–2). In seropositive bone marrow transplant patients, the risk for recurrence is 70 to 80 percent.[2,3] In adult acute leukemia patients undergoing induction therapy, there is a similar 60 to 70 percent frequency of reactivation[4]. In patients receiving ambulatory chemotherapy regimens for non-Hodgkin's lymphoma, the risk is lower, in the range of 40 to 50 percent.[5,6] For comparison purposes, in patients receiving outpatient regimens for solid tumors (which are generally much less intensive than regimens used in the treatment of hematological malignancies), the recurrence rate is generally less than 10 to 25 percent.[7,8]

Diagnosis, Prophylaxis, and Treatment

The manifestations of HSV-1 infection in patients with hematological malignancies are generally intraoral (Plates 51–1A–F). Frequently, the labial lesions typically seen in the nonimmunocompromised host are absent and the oral ulcerations are indistinguishable from stomatitis due to tissue damage from cytoreductive therapy (Plate 51–1E); thus, this distinction can pose a difficult diagnostic challenge. The concomitant occurrences of HSV infection and chemotherapy-induced mucosal damage result in a more severe form of mucositis[9]: The lesions tend to be larger, slower to heal, and more apt to become secondarily infected by bacterial opportunists. Atypical cutaneous satellite lesions may occur by autoinoculation of infected oral secretions into cutaneous abrasions. Extensive and deep oral ulcerations can lead to a greater susceptibility for bacteremia by α-streptococci, especially *Streptococcus mitis,* an organism that normally resides on the buccal mucosa.[10] Typically, HSV-2 infections cause vulval, intravaginal, or perianal ulcerations or vesicles.

Although the oral and genital mucosa are the primary sites of HSV infections, in the immunocompromised host extension to the esophageal and tracheal mucosa may occur.[11–15] Esophagitis can be caused by HSV alone or as part of a polymicrobial infection (especially *Candida* and CMV).[12,16] Endoscopic biopsy is important to distinguish various etiologies. Dissemination and involvement of visceral tissues can occur in profoundly immunocompromised patients.[13–15,17–19] Herpesvirus pneumonia was noted to account for up to 5 percent of nonbacterial pneumonias among allogeneic bone marrow transplant (BMT) patients[18,20] in the preantiviral era.

Cultures of infected secretions or lesions permit confirmation of the diagnosis. Rapid methods using the shell vial technique coupled with antigen detection procedures[21] or using antigen detection immunofluorescent or immunoperoxidase assays alone[22–24] offer quicker and easier alternatives but may be less sensitive or specific. Cytologic examination of cells scraped from lesions using the Tzanck procedure can show the multinucleated giant cells caused by herpetic infection; this is rapid but relatively insensitive and cannot distinguish HSV from VZV. Detection of viral DNA by polymerase chain reaction (PCR) may offer an alternative to culture with similar sensitivity and specificity.[25] Although as noted, serology can identify patients at risk for reactivation, it is not of value for the diagnosis of infection.

Typically the lesions from HSV infection occur 7 to 21 days after initiation of chemotherapy. This association with active therapy and its predictable temporal occurrence in seropositive patients has led to the development of prophylaxis strategies, as discussed below. In patients who are not being actively treated but who have severe deficiency of cell-mediated immunity due to progressive disease, malnutrition, cachexia, use of high-dose corticosteroids, or severe graft-versus-host disease after marrow transplantation and in patients with the acquired immune deficiency syndrome (AIDS), infection can occur at any time, and chronic progressive infections may occur.

Acyclovir, a purine analogue, is highly active against HSV types 1 and 2. Its phosphorylation by a viral-encoded thymidine kinase is necessary for its activation. Its poor phosphorylation by homologous cellular enzymes offers antiviral specificity. Further phosphorylation by cellular enzymes then occurs. Inhibition of the viral-encoded DNA polymerase provides additional antiviral specificity and accounts for its selective antiherpes activity. Finally, the triphosphorylated acyclic nucleoside is incorporated into the viral DNA chain, leading to chain termination and production of a defective virion.

Acyclovir has been demonstrated to be highly effective in both prophylaxis and treatment of HSV infections in patients with hematologic malignancies (Table 51–3). A variety of oral and intravenous regimens have been evaluated and found to be effective.[3,4,26–32] In treatment studies, shortening of the duration of viral shedding, time to pain relief, and interval until healing of lesions have been demonstrated. In prophylaxis studies, excellent control with few breakthrough infections has been noted. Because of its poor bioavailability (only 15 percent after oral administration), caution should be exercised in patients who may have difficulty in tolerating oral medications, such as patients with severe mucositis or gastrointestinal toxicity, in order to ensure adequate plasma concentrations. Acyclovir is generally well tolerated but may be associated with nephrotoxicity if patients are not adequately hydrated or infusions are given too rapidly. Rare reports of reversible neurotoxicity, including tremulousness, lethargy, agitation, and disorientation have been reported; these toxicities resolve with discontinuation of the drug.[33,34]

Valacyclovir, the L-valyl ester of acyclovir, is a prodrug that is metabolized to acyclovir within minutes of oral administration.[35] The bioavailability of acyclovir with this prodrug is

Table 51–2. Rates of Herpes Simplex Virus Type 1 (HSV-1) and Varicella Zoster Virus (VZV) Infections in Different Patient Groups

	Reactivation	
Group	Rate of HSV-1 Infection (%)	Rates of VZV Infection (%)
Bone marrow transplant	70–80	20–50
Acute leukemia	60–70	30
Hodgkin's lymphoma	40–50	15–20
Non-Hodgkin's lymphoma	40–50	5–10
Solid tumors	10–25	5

Table 51-3. Treatment of Herpes Simplex Virus Infection With Acyclovir

Parameter	Viral and Clinical Response					
	Acyclovir[30] (IV)	Placebo (IV)	p^a	Acyclovir[29] (PO)	Placebo (PO)	p^a
Median day (range) to						
Negative cultures	3 (1–8)	18 (4–49^b)	0.00005	2	> 9	0.0008
First decrease in pain	6 (1–10)	14 (1–14^b)	0.05	3	16	0.04
Cessation of pain	10 (7–21)	16 (7–49^b)	0.03	6	16	0.05
Crusting of all external lesions	7 (2–28^b)	14 (6–49^b)	0.01	6	11	0.01
Total healing	14 (6–28^b)	28 (10–49^b)	0.03	8	21	0.01

^{a} Compared by Kaplan-Meier plots and analyzed by Mantel-Cox test.
^{b} Patient removed from study and given open-label acyclovir.

approximately 50 percent.[36] Plasma acyclovir levels are substantially higher and approximate those achieved with intravenous acyclovir.[37] Less frequent dosing is thus possible.

It is important to note that acyclovir is virustatic and suppresses viral replication only during the interval of drug administration. Following cessation of acyclovir, activation frequently occurs. When used in neutropenic leukemia and BMT patients, a course of therapy is generally given until neutrophil recovery. Recurrences after neutrophil recovery tend to be milder and self-limited and may not require retreatment. Often in nonneutropenic patients, treatment is given for 10 to 14 days. If severe immunodeficiency persists, lower-dose maintenance therapy is sometimes advocated to prevent recurrence after the lesions are healed, to be continued until immunity is more robust.

There is considerable debate as to the relative merits of prophylaxis versus waiting until an established infection is documented before initiating treatment. Factors to be weighed in choosing between prophylaxis and treatment include the likelihood of infection, the depth of host immune deficiency, and the severity of infection if it occurs. Thus, while prophylaxis might be an acceptable strategy for BMT patients, in whom the risk for infections and morbidity are high, it would be of little use in patients with hematological malignancy not on active treatment, in whom the risk and morbidity of infection would be low.

The issue of the emergence of acyclovir resistance is an important consideration in this regard. In BMT patients prophylaxis has been associated with a very low risk for drug resistance.[38,39] In contrast, repeated treatment episodes of established HSV infection in BMT patients have been associated with progressively increasing rates of resistance.[40] An explanation for this apparent lower risk of resistance seen with prophylaxis has been suggested.[41] Certainly, the gradually improving host immunity that occurs with successful marrow transplantation and the relatively short duration of prophylaxis are contributory, because prolonged acyclovir prophylaxis in AIDS patients, who have relentlessly deteriorating immunity, has been associated with a substantial risk for resistance. Initial reports of acyclovir-resistant HSV infection suggested that virulence had been attenuated and the clinical course was milder.[42,43] However, reports of resistant isolates causing severe clinical illness have also appeared.[44,45]

For the most part acyclovir resistance has been mediated by alterations in the viral-encoded thymidine kinase production.[42,43,46] However, mutations in the DNA polymerase and altered substrate specificity for thymidine kinase are other potential modes of resistance.[46] Risk factors for the emergence of acyclovir-resistant HSV infections include severe graft-versus-host disease (GvHD) and the lack of ganciclovir prophylaxis.[47]

For patients with acyclovir-resistant HSV, treatment with foscarnet, a pyrophosphate analogue that directly inhibits viral DNA polymerase (and does not require thymidine kinase for its activity), may be effective.[48] In a randomized trial that compared foscarnet with vidarabine for acyclovir-resistant HSV infections in AIDS patients, foscarnet was both more effective and less toxic.[49] For patients with mild infection, another alternative approach would be to cease antiviral therapy to allow unassisted resolution. If progressive illness should ensue, then antiviral treatment could be initiated.

Currently, there are no vaccines for either HSV-1 or HSV-2. However, a recombinant HSV-2 glycoprotein D and B vaccine has been tested in a pilot clinical trial and found to be safe and immunogenic.[50] Although the recurrence frequency of genital herpes was not affected, the duration and severity of the first postvaccination recurrence was reduced.[50]

Cytomegalovirus

Cytomegalovirus infections are common in the general population, with serologic surveys demonstrating latent infection in 40 to 60 percent of adults in most industrialized countries. Primary infection is often inapparent, but CMV can be a major cause of congenital malformations and hearing loss, mononucleosis, and sexually transmitted disease. Asymptomatic shedding in saliva and genital secretions is occasionally noted; clinical illness is uncommon unless the patient is immunocompromised.

Different strains of CMV have been identified by using two viral envelope glycoprotein genotypes (gB and gH). Some data suggest that infections by gB type 1 strains may be associated with greater survival than other gB types.[51] In another study, life-threatening myelosuppression was noted with gB3 and gB4 isolates, in contrast to gB1 and gB2 isolates.[52] Further studies are needed to ascertain whether characterization of strains may provide insights as to viral pathogenicity and prognostic information as to outcome from infection.[51]

Patterns of Infection

Cytomegalovirus can be reactivated from endogenous latent virus or alternatively can be acquired from transfusion of blood products or from an organ graft. Leukocytes are a reservoir of latent virus; the risk for transmission can be reduced by depletion of leukocytes in blood products[53,54] and avoidance of granulocyte transfusions.[55] Among seropositive and seronegative BMT recipients, the incidence of CMV infection was similar prior to the routine use of CMV seronegative blood product support.[56] Now infection rates are less than 10 to 15 percent in seronegative recipients given seronegative blood products (although higher in the recipients of seropositive marrow grafts).[57]

In immunocompromised patients, CMV can be a cause of fever, leukopenia, thrombocytopenia, esophagitis, enterocolitis, interstitial pneumonitis, hepatitis, mononucleosis-like syndrome, chorioretinitis, and rarely, meningoencephalitis. Infection with CMV may predispose immunocompromised patients to sepsis.[58,59]

Although CMV excretion is a frequent occurrence in patients with acute leukemia undergoing intensive chemotherapy, its relationship to morbidity is poorly defined. However, several small surveys of acute leukemia patients suggest that the morbidity attributable to CMV may be underestimated.[60–62] Among leukemia patients, gastritis and esophagitis occasionally occur, and rarely, pneumonitis can be noted. In contrast, CMV can be the cause of life-threatening illness in BMT recipients.

The most common severe manifestations of CMV in BMT patients are interstitial pneumonitis (Figure 51–1) and enterocolitis. Less serious manifestations are unexplained fever, esophagitis, gastritis, wasting, and hepatitis. Chorioretinitis is uncommon (in contrast to HIV-infected patients).[56] Myelosuppression, manifest as delay in the recovery of counts after chemotherapy or unexplained cytopenias weeks to months following engraftment, can occur and can pose diagnostic challenges to distinguish from other causes of myelosuppression.

As with HSV, anti-CMV IgG antibody develops after primary infection. It provides a marker of endogenous latent virus. It does not appear that CMV-specific antibody protects against severe disease because several studies have not found a protec-

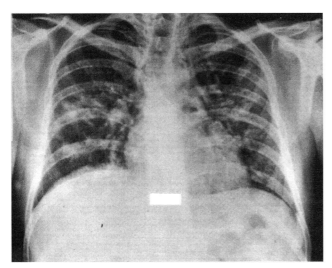

Figure 51–1. Chest radiograph showing a diffuse mixed alveolar/interstitial pneumonitis due to cytomegalovirus.

tive effect of high pretransplant antibody levels against infection.[63] Likewise, there is poor correlation between antibody responses and clinical responses.[63] Thus, while CMV antibody may have a contributory role in the control of CMV infection, it does not appear to be the most important response. Lymphocytopenia has been noted to be an unfavorable prognostic factor in BMT patients with CMV infection,[64] and CMV-specific T-cell and natural killer (NK) responses have been noted following CMV infections.[65–68] The majority of survivors of CMV infection in BMT recipients develop either NK or T-cell cytotoxic responses or both, whereas few of those who succumb from infection develop cytotoxic responses and in the minority in whom cytotoxic responses could be found, the magnitude was much lower.[65] Thus, it appears that the early development of a robust cytotoxic response is crucial to resolution of CMV infection.

Although the development of cytotoxic responses is clearly immunoprotective, animal studies suggest that some cellular responses may be contributory to the pathogenesis of CMV pneumonitis.[69–73] Elucidation of which host immune responses are immunopathogenic and which are immunoprotective is crucial to the understanding of CMV pathogenesis and may permit insights into ways in which augmentation of certain responses and abrogation of others may be possible in future engineering of the constituents of the marrow graft through cell sorting techniques that discriminate various cell populations by their immunophenotypic differences.

Allogeneic BMT recipients are at greatest risk for serious illness from CMV infection, in contrast to autologous or syngeneic transplant recipients or nontransplant leukemia patients.[74–79] Among allogeneic recipients, risk factors for CMV morbidity include HLA disparity between donor and recipient, unrelated donor transplant, T-cell depletion, pretransplant CMV seropositivity, GvHD, older age, the use of immunosuppressive agents other than cyclosporine as GvH prophylaxis, viral excretion, and the intensity of the cytoreductive preparative regimens.[20,56,57,75,79–87] Detection of viral excretion from blood, urine, or throat secretions is indicative of active infection, and isolation of virus often precedes CMV disease by several days to 1 to 2 weeks. Viremia is most predictive of subsequent CMV disease.[86] Alternatively, recovery of virus from bronchoalveolar lavage specimens even in patients without any pulmonary symptomatology also identifies patients at high risk for the development of subsequent CMV pneumonitis.[88,89]

Although autologous BMT patients are at lower risk for CMV disease, such disease occasionally occurs. Patients receiving transplants for hematologic malignancy are at greater risk than those receiving transplants for solid tumors. Patients with multiple myeloma undergoing stem cell transplants in one study were at greater risk for CMV disease.[90] In one study, CD34 selection in autologous stem cell transplant recipients was associated with an increased risk for CMV disease.[91] However, this has not been observed by other groups.[92]

Diagnosis, Prophylaxis, and Treatment

Cytomegalovirus has traditionally been detected by use of cultural methods.[93] Unfortunately, this is not very useful in treatment decisions because results may take several weeks. Modified cultural techniques using the shell vial method coupled with a rapid diagnostic antigen assay for the immediate early antigen permits demonstration of the virus within several days.[94–96] Newer assays include the demonstration of the pp65 antigen in leukocytes using immunofluorescence[97–99] or of viral DNA by the polymerase chain reaction.[100–103] Both the leukocyte antigen detection and PCR assays appear to permit detection of virus 7 to 10 days earlier than shell vial culture. Detection of virus DNA in plasma by PCR appears to be more sensitive than detection in buffy-coat leukocytes. The leukocyte antigen assay has the advantage of permitting quantification, although some PCR assays also can quantify viral load. Larger virus quantity may be more predictive of subsequent disease than less virus.[104] In one comparison, PCR appeared to be slightly more sensitive than the leukocyte antigen detection assay.[105]

The gold standard for documenting CMV pneumonia has been an open lung biopsy (Table 51–4). Because only half of the episodes of interstitial pneumonitis after marrow transplantation are due to CMV and the treatments are toxic, it is important to confirm the etiology at the outset. Similarly, for gastrointestinal syndromes attributable to CMV, tissue documentation is important to differentiate CMV from GvHD or other etiologies.[106] In contrast to patients with HIV infection, in whom CMV is frequently a pulmonary copathogen, in BMT patients CMV typically is a single pathogen. Transbronchial biopsy has not proved to be very reliable, yielding frequent false negatives. In contrast, bronchoalveolar lavage has been found to have a high sensitivity and specificity for documentation of CMV as an etiology of interstitial pneumonitis.[107] This less invasive procedure has encouraged clinicians to be more aggressive in the evaluation of patients suspected of having pneumonitis and permits an earlier initiation of therapy.

Untreated, CMV pneumonitis after marrow transplantation has an 80 to 90 percent mortality. A number of immune modulators and antiviral agents alone and in combination have been tested without success, including vidarabine, interferon, vidarabine plus interferon, acyclovir, acyclovir plus interferon, CMV immunoglobulin, ganciclovir, and ganciclovir with corticosteroids.[108–114]

Ganciclovir, a nucleoside analogue similar in structure to acyclovir, differs from acyclovir in that it does not require phosphorylation by a viral-encoded thymidine kinase. Because human CMV does not encode for this enzyme, acyclovir has much less activity than ganciclovir against CMV. Phosphorylation of ganciclovir occurs by the phosphotransferase product of the viral UL97 gene. Although ganciclovir alone has had an antiviral effect in BMT patients, most patients derived no clinical benefit.[113] However, several nonrandomized trials have demonstrated that the combination of ganciclovir with immunoglobulin results in clinical benefit, with survival rates of 50 to 70 percent.[115–118]. Although no controlled trials have been performed, this combination has been widely adopted for the treatment of CMV pneumonitis.[119] If therapy is delayed until ventilatory failure has ensued, outcomes are uniformly poor. Thus, early intervention is crucial. Following control of CMV pneumonia with ganciclovir and immune globulin, there can be occasional recurrences, and some clinicians advocate a maintenance course of ganciclovir for several weeks to several months following an episode of CMV pneumonia. Unfortunately, ganciclovir has not been shown to be similarly beneficial in the treatment of CMV-associated enteritis in marrow transplant patients.[120] A retrospective survey of the addition of intravenous immunoglobulin to antiviral chemotherapy did not appear to support the view that an additional benefit for an improved outcome is thereby obtained.[121]

The onset of CMV pneumonitis in the marrow transplant recipient (prior to the antiviral era, discussed below) occurred approximately 2 months following transplantation. This was early after engraftment, frequently after the appearance of acute GvHD. Despite the gratifying improvements in the treatment of CMV pneumonia, many patients succumbed.

A number of investigators have sought ways to prevent either infection or illness from infection (Table 51–5). For CMV seronegative recipients whose donors are also seronegative, the use of CMV-screened blood products has been highly successful in minimizing the risks for CMV infection and disease.[57,97,122–124] Alternatively, the use of second-generation leukocyte filters for blood product transfusions similarly reduce the risk.[54,125] Immune globulin, either CMV-specific or from standard commercial lots, has also been shown to be beneficial in reducing CMV infection or disease.[126–129] It is not clear whether there is any advantage to using a hyperimmune globulin preparation compared to commercial lots of immune globulin not specifically selected for high titer anti-CMV antibody. Most of the efficacy

Table 51–4. Interstitial Pneumonia: Diagnostic Procedures

Procedure	Diagnostic Yield (%)	Morbidity (%)
Transtracheal aspirate	5–10	2–5
Bronchoscopy		
Biopsy alone	30–55	5–20
Bronchoalveolar lavage	40–90[a]	5–20
Transthoracic needle		
Aspirate	17–60	10–30
Biopsy	20–60	10–60
Open biopsy	100	5–10[b]

[a] Results include histology, immunofluorescence, and in situ hybridization.
[b] 100% incidence of pneumonthorax requiring chest tube placement.

Table 51–5. Strategies to Prevent Cytomegalovirus (CMV) Disease in Bone Marrow Transplant Patients

Intervention	References
CMV-negative blood products	50, 84, 108–110
Leukocyte filters	47, 111
Immunoglobulin or plasma	112–118
Acyclovir	119, 120
Ganciclovir	121–124

from immune globulin has been demonstrated in patients who were seronegative prior to transplant. There does not appear to be any additive benefit of immune globulin to the use of filtered blood products in seronegative patients.[121] The magnitude of benefit from immune globulin has been less in seropositive patients,[130] and immune globulin has been found to be of no benefit in autologous marrow transplant recipients.[131]

At present there are no satisfactory preventive measures for seronegative recipients who receive grafts from seropositive donors. Although immune globulin would be appealing in this situation, unfortunately it has not proved to be effective in reducing infection rates.[122]

In seropositive patients high-dose intravenous acyclovir given during the first month after transplantation has been associated with a reduced risk for CMV pneumonia.[132] In a three-arm trial, high-dose intravenous acyclovir during the first month, low-dose oral acyclovir during the first month, and high-dose intravenous acyclovir during the first month followed by 6 months of oral acyclovir were compared.[133] A reduced probability and delayed onset of CMV infection was noted in the group receiving high-dose intravenous acyclovir.[133] In this latter study, the prolonged course of oral acyclovir did not reduce CMV infection but did reduce viremia, and there was an improved survival benefit.[133] Similar acyclovir prophylaxis trials in solid organ transplant recipients show efficacy. Why acyclovir as prophylaxis seems to exert an anti-CMV effect whereas its use as treatment provides no effect is puzzling but may be indicative of a mild antiviral effect, which is demonstrable only when the viral burden is low as in the early stages of active infection and not apparent in later stages of infection, when the viral burden is substantially greater.

Ganciclovir has also been evaluated for prophylaxis (from engraftment to day 100) or as early treatment in BMT patients with active virus infection to preempt disease. As noted above, asymptomatic patients with virus recovered from bronchoalveolar lavage fluid 35 days after transplantation, as well as those in whom viremia or excretion in urine or throat specimens occurs are at higher risk for CMV disease. Controlled trials have demonstrated a reduction in disease by initiation of ganciclovir at first detection of virus.[134,135]. An alternative strategy is to initiate ganciclovir at the time of engraftment in all seropositive patients.[136–137] Because of its myelosuppressive toxicity, initiation of ganciclovir cannot be begun prior to engraftment. Even when it is begun shortly after engraftment, pancytopenia and interruptions of treatment are common, with an attendant risk of neutropenic infections. Patients with low marrow cellularity, elevated bilirubin, or increased creatinine are at greater risk.[138] The use of myeloid growth factors can lower the risk of myelosuppression. There is divided opinion at present as to the relative merits of prophylaxis versus early therapy.[39,139] Several reviews have discussed the issues related to these strategies.[39,140–142] It appears that prophylaxis is associated with fewer failures that could occur before or simultaneous with the first detection of active virus. However, the greater morbidity attendant on more frequent and more prolonged pancytopenia with ganciclovir started at the time of engraftment makes ganciclovir less well tolerated than when started later. Moreover, early therapy given only to patients with active infection spares a significant proportion of patients the toxicities and cost of antiviral therapy. The greater use of the leukocyte antigen and PCR assays to detect virus earlier than with the shell vial culture assay may reduce some of the failures associated with early therapy, making this more advantageous than prophylaxis.[39] If ganciclovir is used for prophylaxis or as early therapy, there appears to be no added benefit for acyclovir during the first month.[143]

In an attempt to reduce the toxicity of long-term ganciclovir, several variations of daily therapy have been attempted. Ganciclovir three times per week was not found to be adequate to prevent CMV reactivation, at least in T cell-depleted marrow transplant recipients.[144] On the other hand, a preliminary report suggests that 3 to 6 weeks of daily ganciclovir may be as efficacious as a longer course while causing less toxicity.[145,146]

Oral ganciclovir is useful in AIDS patients for maintenance therapy to prevent recurrence of CMV retinitis, but because of poor bioavailability, serum concentrations are lower and breakthrough infection rates appear to be higher.[147] Emergence of resistance has also been noted and appears to be greater than with intravenous ganciclovir.[148,149] Valganciclovir, a prodrug of ganciclovir, is metabolized to ganciclovir and has excellent bioavailability.[150–152] Plasma concentrations are quite high. Valganciclovir is entering clinical trials as an alternative to ganciclovir, which may make prolonged courses of therapy more feasible.

Resistance to ganciclovir occurs through mutations in the CMV UL97 gene.[153–155] DNA polymerase (UL54) mutations can also occur, resulting in high-level resistance.[155] Although many ganciclovir-resistant CMV mutants have mutations in the UL54 gene (DNA polymerase) as well as in the UL97 gene, susceptibility to foscarnet is retained.[156,157]

Foscarnet, a pyrophosphate analogue, targets the viral DNA polymerase. It represents an alternative to ganciclovir both as treatment and as prophylaxis.[158–162] Sparing of the blood counts makes foscarnet an attractive alternative to ganciclovir in patients in whom marrow reserve is marginal. However, nephrotoxicity and renal wasting of electrolytes are prominent side effects of foscarnet. In one small study, the combination of foscarnet and ganciclovir was effective and may have less treatment toxicity.[163] Foscarnet is an option for ganciclovir-resistant CMV.[164]

Cidofovir is a nucleoside analogue with potent anti-CMV activity not requiring phosphorylation by the UL97 gene product, which acts against the viral DNA polymerase (UL54). It is an effective treatment for CMV retinitis in HIV-infected patients.[165–167] Advantages include less frequent dose intervals (once weekly at first, then every other week). Limitations include considerable nephrotoxicity (which in some cases was irreversible) and iritis. Concomitant probenecid and intravenous hydration are necessary. There are to date only limited data on BMT patients.[168] Because many ganciclovir-resistant CMV mutants have alterations not only in the UL97 gene but also in the UL54 gene (DNA polymerase), resistance to cidofovir can also be present.[156,169] Accordingly, foscarnet is the preferred antiviral in the face of ganciclovir resistance.

Historically, most episodes of CMV pneumonitis occurred during the first 100 days after marrow transplantation. However, with the advent of antiviral prophylaxis in recent years, late-onset CMV pneumonitis has increasingly been noted beyond 100 days.[170–176] In part this is due to the increasing use of unrelated and HLA-mismatched donors, where immune reconstitution is much slower than after allogeneic transplants from genotypically identical siblings. However, delay in the development of cytotoxic anti-CMV responses in patients in whom ganciclovir has been used has also been noted.[177] Most late-onset cases occur in patients in whom CMV infection was documented during the first 100 days.[178] The risk of late-onset CMV pneumonitis appears to be greatest in patients with chronic graft-versus-host disease. This is a group in whom CMV surveillance may be particularly important.

With recognition of the importance of development of cytotoxic cellular responses to CMV for resolution of infection as well as of the ability to clone lymphocyte populations and expand them ex vivo with interleukin-2 and repetitive CMV antigenic stimulation, it has become possible to consider cellular immunotherapy of CMV infection.[179–181] Consideration of donor immunization may also be important because recipients of grafts from seropositive donors may have earlier recovery of cytotoxic responses than recipients of grafts from seronegative donors.[177] Such immunotherapeutic approaches may prove to be increasingly important in years to come as the emergence of ganciclovir resistance among CMV isolates increases.[182]

Because the risk of CMV disease is substantially greater in seropositive than in seronegative patients, newly diagnosed leukemia patients in whom a transplant is contemplated after induction therapy should be given only CMV-seronegative blood products throughout their induction regimen if they are seronegative. The value of CMV-negative blood products in autologous transplantation patients, in whom the risk for serious CMV disease is low, is questionable but is recommended by some.[183]

Immunization of the donor or recipient by a live attenuated, killed, or subunit recombinant CMV vaccine might be attractive in speeding restoration of immunity. However, although an attenuated vaccine has been found to be immunogenic in solid organ transplant patients, concerns regarding its safety in more severely immunodeficient marrow transplant patients have prevented trials of a live vaccine. A glycoprotein vaccine would be desirable. Clearly, abrogation of the recipient's immunity by the preparative regimen may mean that prior immunization of the donor as well as repeated boosting of the recipient is necessary to establish meaningful immune responses.

Varicella Zoster Virus

Patterns of Infection

Varicella zoster virus, like the other herpesviruses, can be a significant pathogen in patients with hematologic malignancies. Varicella (chickenpox) is the primary form of infection, and zoster (shingles) is the reactivation form of illness. The initial portal of entry is uncertain, but the respiratory tract, skin, and conjunctiva are candidate sites. After local replication, viremia occurs with dissemination to multiple cutaneous (and visceral) sites. The skin lesions begin as erythematous macules, progress to papules and then to vesicles (with clear fluid), which evolve to pustules (with cloudy fluid containing interferon and leuko-

cytes), and flatten to scabs, until finally healing takes place. The hallmark of infection is the vesicle. Crops of vesicles classically exist on a common erythematous base. Scarring is unusual in varicella, but the inflammatory reaction in zoster may be more severe with greater pain and scarring. Zoster characteristically is dermatomal, and lesions typically stop at the midline. In severely immunocompromised patients extension to adjacent dermatomes may occur, the vesicles may become confluent, and cutaneous dissemination can occasionally occur. Approximately 5 to 10 percent of patients with non-Hodgkin's lymphoma, 15 to 25 percent of patients with Hodgkin's disease, and 20 to 50 percent of patients undergoing BMT develop zoster[184–189] (Table 51–2).

In the normal host varicella and zoster are self-limited. In patients with hematologic malignancies, varicella may be quite severe and life-threatening. In the preantiviral era, varicella frequently progressed to visceral dissemination and death.[190] Untreated, dissemination occurs in 30 to 40 percent of marrow transplant recipients[186,187] and in up to 20 to 30 percent of children treated for hematological malignancy.[190] Visceral dissemination is a severe manifestation and pneumonia can be particularly deadly. In marrow transplant patients an intra-abdominal presentation can occur, with severe abdominal pain.[191–193] This can be particularly challenging to diagnose because it may occur in the absence of cutaneous vesicles. A high index of suspicion should be maintained because if the condition is not treated promptly, it can result in a high mortality. Manifestations of pancreatitis, hepatitis, and peritonitis are frequent, and in patients in whom laparotomy was inadvertently performed, inflammatory changes, vesicles on serosal surfaces, and mesenteric adenitis have been noted.

The onset of VZV infection in the marrow transplant recipient is much later than that of the other herpesviruses, occurring an average of 5 months following transplantation[186–189] (Figure 51–2). Susceptibility for reactivation can persist for many months, especially among patients with chronic GvHD.[186,187] A study of humoral and lymphocytic proliferative responses to VZV in BMT recipients indicated that in approximately 26 percent of patients a subclinical reactivation occurred.[194] Similarly, in patients undergoing induction therapy for leukemia, 5 to 10 percent subclinical reactivation occurred. Thus, when both clinical and subclinical infections are considered, VZV infection is a common occurrence in BMT recipients.

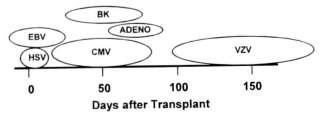

Figure 51–2. Viral infections and their time course after marrow transplantation. HSV, herpes simplex virus; EBV, Epstein-Barr virus; CMV, cytomegalovirus; BK, BK virus; ADENO, adenovirus; VZV, varicella zoster virus.

Among patients treated for lymphoma, VZV infection is more common in those with advanced disease and in those treated with combined-modality chemoradiotherapy.[184] It appears that the frequency of zoster is increasing as more dose-intensive therapies are being employed. Risk factors for VZV in allogeneic marrow transplant patients include acute or chronic GvHD, older age, and the post-transplant use of antithymocyte globulin. Among autologous transplant patients, the underlying disease of Hodgkin's or non-Hodgkin's lymphoma is a risk factor.[188] Zoster develops more commonly in dermatomes of prior radiotherapy.

Diagnosis and Treatment

Diagnosis can usually be made solely by visual inspection of the cutaneous lesions. Examination of the cellular contents of a vesicle can demonstrate multinucleated giant cells on Tzanck smear.[25] Culture can be confirmatory but special handling must be used for this heat-labile cell-associated virus. Immunofluorescent staining can also be used.[195] Polymerase chain reaction techniques may offer yet another alternative.[25]

Acyclovir is highly active against VZV.[196–198] Higher concentrations are required to inhibit VZV in vitro as compared to HSV-1 and HSV-2. Generally, plasma levels achieved with standard doses of acyclovir given orally are insufficient to achieve inhibitory plasma concentrations. High doses of oral acyclovir (800 mg given five times daily) achieve peak plasma concentrations that approximate in vitro inhibitory concentrations for most isolates of VZV and have been found to be useful in nonimmunocompromised patients in whom treatment is initiated early after onset of infection.[199] The adequacy of this dose in compromised patients has not been well demonstrated, although one small trial in BMT recipients suggested that a beneficial effect was achieved.[200] However, because only a small number of patients have been studied, intravenous acyclovir is preferable unless the infection is mild and the patient can be closely monitored to institute parenteral therapy if there is progression or no response.

Vidarabine is an alternative treatment,[201] although controlled trials have shown acyclovir to be superior.[198] Interferon-α has also been shown to be efficacious,[202] although it has been evaluated only in localized disease and there is no published experience of its use in disseminated disease.[203]

Several oral agents are effective therapies in nonimmunocompromised patients. These include famciclovir and valacyclovir, prodrugs of penciclovir and acyclovir, respectively.[204–206] Sorivudine also is effective[207,208] but has been associated with a potentially lethal interaction with 5-fluorouracil.[209] These agents have greater bioavailability and longer half-lives than oral acyclovir, which make them excellent candidates for outpatient treatment. Their efficacy has not been extensively tested in immunocompromised patients. They seem to be suitable for mild to moderately severe cases of zoster when the patient can be observed carefully or as a change from intravenous acyclovir once an initial response to therapy is achieved.

The risk for acyclovir resistance in VZV is much less than in HSV. However, several reports have noted the emergence of drug resistance.[210,211] As with HSV, the mechanism of resistance appears to be an altered thymidine kinase, and thus foscarnet is a suitable alternative for resistant pathogens.[211]

For seronegative patients exposed to a contact with chickenpox or zoster, varicella zoster immune globulin (VZIG) can be administered if discovered within 48 to 72 hours after exposure.[212] Commercial lots of intravenous immune globulin also contain anti-VZV antibody and may be considered as an alternative if VZIG is not readily available.

Immunization and Prophylaxis

A live attenuated vaccine has been evaluated in normal and immunocompromised children with leukemia and found to be beneficial in reducing the risks for VZV infection in patients with ALL in remission for more than 1 year.[213–216] Because of the risks of dissemination by the vaccine strain in patients with severe immunocompromise, its role in such patients is limited.[217] On the other hand, family members of seronegative children with leukemia could be immunized to reduce the risk of the patient contracting a primary infection.[218]

Acyclovir given orally in intermediate doses for a number of months has been shown to reduce the risks for VZV infection following marrow transplantation.[194,219–223] The need to continue this for 6 months or longer, along with the fact that VZV can become reactivated once the drug is discontinued, raises the question as to how valuable this is. In one study, the possible transfer of VZV-specific T-cell immunity from donor to recipient in the marrow transplantation setting was evaluated.[224] Unfortunately, simple transfer of immunity was not evident. Whether boosting the donor immunity prior to adoptive transfer might improve on this remains to be seen.

Epstein-Barr Virus

Pathogenesis and Immunity

Epstein-Barr virus is an ubiquitous organism with the majority of adults being infected. Transmission is usually via oral secretions. Sites of virus replication include the oropharyngeal epithelium and B lymphocytes, the latter being the major reservoir of endogenous latent virus.[225–228] Primary infection is often subclinical, but in adolescence EBV can cause the syndrome known as infectious mononucleosis. It can also cause acute or protracted fever, malaise, fatigue, autoimmune hemolytic anemia, cytopenias, rash, or adenopathy.[228–230] Rarely, it has been associated with several varied neurologic syndromes. It has been implicated as a factor in the pathogenesis of African Burkitt's lymphoma, central nervous system lymphomas, polyclonal and monoclonal lymphoproliferative disorders in solid organ transplant patients, nasopharyngeal carcinoma, and lymphoproliferative disorders associated with the X-linked lymphoproliferative syndrome; in addition, a possible role in Hodgkin's disease has been proposed.[228,231–234]

Primary infection elicits both humoral and cell-mediated immune responses.[228,235–238] During the acute illness, the production of heterophile antibody and autoantibodies occur. The heterophile antibody (antibody to sheep erythrocytes not absorbed by guinea pig antigen) is most commonly used to document acute infection. Early after infection, IgM antibody and IgG antiviral capsid antibody (VCA) appear, along with antibodies to the early antigen (EA). IgM antibody disappears generally within 2 to 4 months, but anti-EA antibody may persist for several months or longer. Anti-EBNA antibody appears late, several months after the acute infection, and persists for life. Host cellular responses include natural killer cells and EBV-specific cytotoxic and suppressor T cells. The atypical lymphocytosis characteristically seen during infectious mononucleosis is primarily made up of the responding T-cell rather than the infected B-lymphocytes, and these represent the host attempt to control B-cell lymphoproliferation.

Within the B lymphocyte, the EBV genome persists as episomes or occasionally becomes integrated into the host cellular genome. In latently infected cells EBV gene expression is restricted to nuclear protein genes (EBNA), a membrane protein (LMP), and EBV-encoded RNAs (EBERs), which have roles in maintenance of latency, transformation, and prevention of apoptosis.[228] Although latent EBV infection confers a proliferative advantage to B cells, by itself it does not appear to be sufficient for oncogenesis. Rather, other events involving alterations in oncogenes such as *c-myc* or *N-ras* or mutations in tumor suppressor gene such as *p53* or *RB,* appear to be necessary for the transition from polyclonal proliferation of B lymphocytes to a monoclonal B-cell malignancy.[239,240]

Diagnosis and Treatment

Culture of EBV is problematic because of the lack of readily available assays in diagnostic virology laboratories. However, in research laboratories EBV can be identified by its ability to transform cord lymphocytes.[241] Today, assays for viral DNA detection are mostly straightforward but not widely available.[242,243]

Epstein-Barr virus can be detected in salivary secretions in 15 to 20 percent of the general population.[241] Excretion rates are higher in immunocompromised patients. Patients receiving immunosuppressive therapy have excretion rates of about 35 percent, patients with malignancies have excretion rates in the range of 40 to 50 percent, renal transplant patients 45 to 60 percent, leukemia patients 75 to 100 percent, and HIV-infected patients 45 to 70 percent.[244–251] In adults, most infections occur in previously seropositive patients, whereas in children both primary and reactivated infections occur. The number of EBV genomes detected in peripheral blood leukocytes is increased in immunocompromised patients.

Excretion rates vary considerably according to the intensity of immunosuppressive therapy and the extent of depression of host cell-mediated immunity. Thus, patients with repeated organ graft failure, those who receive multiple immunosuppressive drugs, and those who receive antithymocyte globulin are especially vulnerable for reactivation. Similarly, depending on the immunologic defect, the serologic responses to EBV infection may be more or less pronounced than in immunocompetent individuals. Frequently, serologic responses are exaggerated,[252] whereas the more important cell-mediated immune responses are generally suppressed.

Although EBV shedding may be asymptomatic, several EBV-associated syndromes have been identified in patients with hematologic malignancies. Oral hairy leukoplakia commonly found in AIDS patients is also noted in patients with hematologic malignancies, especially those undergoing marrow transplantation.[253–255] There has been increasing recognition of EBV-associated lymphoproliferative syndromes in transplant recipients.[256–260] Children appear to be at greater risk than adults, and seronegative patients are at substantially greater risk than seropositive patients. The risk also varies according to type of transplant, with heart-lung transplant recipients appearing to be at greater risk than those with renal, liver, or cardiac transplants. The evidence for a role of EBV as a causative agent include the presence of EBV DNA and EBV-specific proteins within tumors, the presence of activation markers consistent with latent EBV infection (CD23 and adhesion molecules), the association with primary infection, and the analysis of terminal repeats indicating monoclonality. Several types of post-transplant lymphoproliferative disease (PTLD) have been described. A mononucleosis syndrome that is localized and self-limited is the least serious. A more widespread mononucleosis syndrome, which can be progressive, and lymphoma, which can be extranodal involving the gastrointestinal tract, brain, and other organs, can also occur. Several classification schemes have been proposed, including one which incorporated molecular genetic analyses with morphology.[239]

In BMT recipients, EBV infection has been characterized both serologically and by EBV detection.[261,262] Reactivation of EBV in seropositive recipients is frequent and generally occurs 2 to 4 weeks following transplantation. Clinical manifestations have not been associated with viral reactivation, however.

Infrequently, PTLD has been noted in marrow recipients, generally in the setting of severe GvHD, the use of antithymocyte globulin or monoclonal anti-T-cell antibody, or after T-cell-depleted transplantation.[263–268] In a comprehensive review of more than 18,000 patients who had undergone allogeneic BMT, PTLDs were noted with a cumulative incidence of approximately 1 percent at 10 years.[269] Most cases occurred between 1 and 5 months post-transplant with few cases occurring after 1 year. In a multivariate analysis, lymphoproliferative disorders within 1 year of transplant were associated with unrelated or mismatched donor transplants, T-cell depletion of the donor marrow, the use of either antithymocyte globulin or anti-CD3 monoclonal antibody as part of the GvHD prophylaxis regimen, acute GvHD, and conditioning regimens that included radiation. Methods of T-cell depletion methods that did not remove B cells (the target cell of EBV infection) were associated with a substantially higher risk than methods that depleted both B and T cells. The only risk factor for late onset PTLD was the occurrence of chronic GvHD.[269]

Although most EBV-associated lymphoproliferative disorders have been described in solid or bone marrow transplant recipients or in HIV-associated immunodeficiency, the increasing use of potent purine analogues, such as fludarabine or cladribine in combination with corticosteroids has created a new population of oncology patients with profound cell-mediated immunodeficiency. A recent study of EBV DNA load in leukemia and lymphoma patients receiving fludarabine, cyclosphosphamide, and dexamethasone indicated a substantial increase in viral load in some patients.[270] Although no EBV-associated lymphoproliferative disorders have been noted to date, these are cautionary observations, which warrant further study.

Acyclovir is active against EBV both in vitro and clinically.[271-274] Its clinical efficacy in nonimmunocompromised patients with infectious mononucleosis, however, has been only slight,[266] which is perhaps related to the initiation of therapy late during active viral replication. However, acyclovir has been useful in the clinical management of oral hairy leukoplakia,[275] and viral shedding has decreased in compromised patients.[257,262] Ganciclovir and interferon have also been noted to be active against EBV.[276-281] The activity of acyclovir in the treatment of EBV lymphoproliferative syndromes has not been particularly salutary, although at least some individual patients with polyclonal disorders may have benefited.[257,259] However, in a more comprehensive compilation of cases, there did not appear to be any difference in survival of those receiving acyclovir therapy for EBV-associated lymphomas.[260] More important in the overall management is reduction of intensive immunosuppressive therapy, which can have salutary effects early in the evolution of the lymphoproliferative disorders.[228,249] Once mutations in oncogenes or tumor suppressor genes have taken place, attempts to reduce immunosuppressive therapy may be futile,[239] and cytotoxic therapy may be more appropriate. Soluble CR-2 (the EBV receptor of B lymphocytes) has been proposed as a therapeutic agent that can block EBV infection.[282]

In solid organ transplant patients, the number of EBV-infected lymphocytes in the peripheral blood has been noted to correlate with the risk for PTLD.[283] This observation suggests the potential of early intervention by use of an antiviral agent or immune modulation to avert the full-blown lymphoproliferative disorder. In healthy seropositive individuals, the population of EBV-cytotoxic T-cell precursors in the peripheral blood is much higher than populations of cells sensitized to other herpesviruses. Thus, buffy-coat leukocyte infusions or ex vivo expanded EBV-specific cytotoxic lymphocytes can be used as therapeutic modalities for EBV-associated PTLD.[284] Rituximab, an anti-CD20 monoclonal antibody, has also been used to treat lymphoproliferative disorders either by itself or in combination with lymphocytes, and in anecdotal reports it has demonstrated efficacy.[285-287] Infusions of EBV-specific cytotoxic T lymphocytes have been given to patients with high levels of virally infected lymphocytes at high risk for PTLD, resulting in a reduction of viral load.[288-291] Gene-marked infused cells can persist for as long as 18 months.[292] Such "preemptive" lymphocyte transfusions offer promise for prevention of PTLD in at-risk patients.

Human Herpesvirus Types 6, 7, and 8

Human herpesviruses types 6 and 7 have only been recognized in the last decade. However, infection in humans is common.[293,294] Both have a preference for CD4-positive T lymphocytes but can infect a variety of T- and B-cell lines. Seropositivity is present in 50 to 90 percent of normal adults, and infection

generally occurs during the first decade of life. Both appear to share clinical manifestations. Although usually subclinical, exanthem subitum, a self-limited, mild, febrile illness can occur. Viral antigens to HHV-6 have been noted in tissues from lymphoma but their significance is as yet unknown.[295-297]

Reactivation of HHV-6 is frequently detected in the blood of BMT recipients.[298-302] For the most part this has not been associated with clinical manifestations. However, suggestions have been made that rash,[300] GvHD,[301,303] and marrow suppression in the post-transplant setting[304-306] may be associated. Other reports have suggested a role for HHV-6 in interstitial pneumonitis,[307,308] encephalitis,[309] and lymphocytopenia.[310] The precise role in pathogenicity of this virus has been debated.[311-313] There have been no studies of HHV-7 in patients with hematologic malignancies. There are no clinical trials evaluating the efficacy of antiviral agents, but several, including ganciclovir and foscarnet appear to be active against HHV-6 in in vitro assays.[314]

Human herpesvirus type 8 has been associated with several human malignancies, including Kaposi's sarcoma (giving rise to its other name, Kaposi's sarcoma-associated herpesvirus), some forms of lymphoma, and multiple myeloma. This virus has been found in saliva, semen, and peripheral blood mononuclear cells and is thought to be transmitted sexually. Tissue samples from most Kaposi's sarcomas contain gene sequences in common with HHV-8.[315-317] Serologic prevalence studies have revealed contradictory findings. Certain forms of B-cell lymphomas have also been described, especially AIDS-associated body cavity lymphomas, as containing HHV-8 sequences.[318,319] Several laboratories have reported detection of HHV-8 DNA sequences in patients with multiple myeloma[320]; however, other groups have disputed such claims.

INTESTINAL VIRUSES

Enteric viruses cause sporadic infections in patients with hematologic malignancies, which generally occur in conjunction with outbreaks within a given community. Common pathogens include coxsackievirus, rotavirus, the Norwalk virus, and other caliciviruses and astroviruses. But other viruses, including adenoviruses, present in the wider community may also cause illness. Coxsackie A1 is an enterovirus that has been reported to cause severe diarrhea in marrow transplant recipients.[321] In one series, episodes of gastroenteritis were clustered temporarily and caused high mortality.[321] At autopsy foamy vascularization of the mucosal epithelium was noted, with patchy sloughing of intestinal mucosal epithelium. This outbreak coincided with diarrheal illness in nonimmunocompromised children in the community from whom coxsackievirus was isolated from stool. Isolated cases of disseminated infection from enteroviruses have been reported.[322,323] Isolation of the virus from stool is confirmatory of the diagnosis. Coxsackievirus infection must be distinguished from GvHD by intestinal biopsy because the manifestations may be quite similar.

Rotavirus is a double-stranded RNA virus and member of the Reoviridae family. Its target tissue is the small intestinal mucosal epithelium. Fecal–oral transmission is the usual mode of contagion. There is considerable seasonal variation of infections, most occurring between January and April in temperate climates. Rotavirus gastroenteritis can vary in severity from mild, short-lived diarrhea to overwhelming and occasionally fatal gastroenteritis. A cluster of cases has been reported in bone marrow transplant patients.[324] In another study, frequent stool isolation of rotavirus has been found in autologous and allogeneic marrow transplant recipients with diarrhea.[325] At present there is no specific antiviral therapy; electrolyte and fluid replacement are important adjunctive measures. To date there have not been cases of Norwalk and related viruses reported in patients with hematologic malignancies, probably because of the lack of widely available diagnostic assays. Humoral immunity is felt to be an important host protective response for these viral pathogens. The administration of oral immune globulin or breast milk has been suggested for the treatment of severe rotavirus infection.

ADENOVIRUS

Adenoviruses are double-stranded DNA viruses. Forty-nine antigenic serotypes (divided into six subgroups, A through F, based on their antigenic properties and hemagglutination properties) have been identified, each associated with different clinical syndromes. For example, serotype 3 has been associated with keratoconjunctivitis, serotype 11 with hemorrhagic cystitis,[326–328] serotypes 40 and 41 with gastroenteritis, and serotypes 3, 4, and 7 have been documented in epidemics of acute respiratory diseases in military facilities. Serotype 35, although uncommon in the general population, is common in immunocompromised patients.

The means of transmission of adenovirus is uncertain but has been reported to occur via direct contact, aerosols, contact with respiratory or fecal secretions, and contaminated water. The virus is capable of at least three types of interactions with cells. These include a lytic infection, a chronic persistent or latent infection, and oncogenic transformation.

Patterns of Infection

Adenovirus is endemic in the pediatric population, with approximately 80 percent of children between the ages of 1 and 5 years having antibody to one or more serotypes.[329,330] Adenovirus is a relatively common cause of respiratory tract infections in children less than 5 years of age, causing 2 to 7 percent of respiratory tract infections and 5 to 11 percent of viral pneumonia and bronchiolitis cases.[331] These infections are rarely severe and typically manifest as upper respiratory tract infections. Other presentations include keratoconjunctivitis, gastroenteritis, cystitis, myocarditis, and lower respiratory tract infections.

Adenovirus infections are well documented in immunocompromised patients, including BMT recipients (4 to 21 percent), solid organ transplantation patients (liver transplants 8 to 18 percent, renal transplants 12 percent) and patients with AIDS (28 percent). The frequency with which adenovirus infection and disease is reported among BMT patients is increasing. This is due in part to increased intensity of immunosuppression and to the use of T-cell-depleted cell products. In the mid-1980s approximately 5 percent of all marrow transplant recipients were reported to have adenovirus recovered,[326,332] and that number increased to 12 to 21 percent in the mid-to-late 1990s.[333,334]

In the BMT population, approximately 33 percent of infected patients develop severe and prolonged symptoms, such as (1) gastrointestinal infection, manifested as diarrhea, hemorrhagic colitis, or hepatitis; (2) urinary tract infections, manifested as hemorrhagic cystitis often associated with renal failure; and (3) pulmonary infections, resulting in interstitial pneumonia. Adenovirus infections in hematopoietic stem cell transplant (HSCT) recipients are often disseminated, which is defined as isolation of the virus from two different sites or from the blood.[331,333,335–339]

The BMT programs at both the University of Kentucky and the University of Wisconsin have recently reviewed the incidence of adenovirus infections in their transplant population.[332,334] Using different definitions for infection and disease, these programs have established risk factors for adenovirus disease in BMT recipients. First, the age of the BMT recipient is predictive for infection, with pediatric patients more likely to have a positive culture for adenovirus than a similar adult population (23 versus 9 percent, $p < .0001$). The reasons for this remain unknown, and the type of transplant procedure does not explain this finding. Second, the type of BMT predicts for infection. The Kentucky program demonstrated that allogeneic BMT recipients are more likely to develop infection as compared to autologous recipients (16 versus 3 percent, $p < .0001$).[334] Differences have been shown in some series among allogeneic patients, depending on the degree of HLA disparity. A higher incidence of both adenovirus infection and disease was seen in patients undergoing unrelated HLA-mismatched grafts compared with related HLA-matched grafts, although the difference was not statistically significant.[332,340] Finally, adenovirus disease developed in a greater number of patients with moderate to severe GvHD (15 versus 5 $p < .05$). The development of moderate to severe GvHD was found to be an independent risk factor predictive for adenovirus disease on multivariate analysis ($p < .01$; odds ratio = 5.4; 95 percent confidence interval 1.6–17.9). The other major risk factor for progression of infection to disease is isolation of adenovirus from multiple sites. Isolation of adenovirus from more than two sites strongly correlates with an increased risk of invasive disease compared to isolation from one site; adenovirus disease occurred in 63 percent of patients with more than two positive sites compared to 11 percent with only one positive site.

The development of invasive disease is associated with a shorter median survival. The median survival for all patients who had a positive adenovirus culture was 208 days. Patients with evidence of invasive infection had a median survival of 100 days, compared to 998 days for those with non invasive adenovirus infection.[334] Of those patients who develop invasive infection, 50 percent die.

Treatment

Currently there is no reliably effective antiviral therapy for the treatment of adenovirus infections. There are numerous case reports in the literature reporting success with ganciclovir,[341–343] intravenous ribavirin,[344,351] vidarabine,[352,353] and more recently cidofovir.[354–356] The key to successful treatment is prompt initiation of therapy in high-risk individuals. A risk-adapted approach, similar to that taken with CMV, may in fact prevent progression to disseminated disease, which is typically associated with a dismal outcome. An alternative strategy that has been exploited is adoptive immunotherapy. There are data supporting the use of donor leukocytes to treat post-transplant EBV-associated lymphoproliferative disease, as discussed previously. This principle has been extrapolated to the treatment of life threatening adenoviral infection following T-cell-depleted HSCT and has met with success, although there are only published data on one patient.[357]

Clearly there is an absence of adequately controlled studies on treatment of adenovirus infections with the currently available antiviral agents. Cidofovir and ribavirin appear to offer most promise and should be further investigated in a prospective multicenter trial.

RESPIRATORY VIRUSES

Respiratory Syncytial Virus

Respiratory syncytial virus (RSV), a member of the paramyxoviruses, is a single-stranded RNA virus related to parainfluenza virus and is a well recognized cause of upper and lower respiratory tract illness in children.[358–361] Outbreaks of RSV infection are seasonal and usually occur in the community during November to April, the fall and winter months in the Northern Hemisphere.[362,363] Repeated infections are common in all age groups, and previous infection does not confer immunity and prevent subsequent infections, even in sequential years.[364,365] The virus can be transmitted by three possible mechanisms.[366] The first is transmission by small-particle (less than 10 μm diameter) aerosols, which are typically produced by coughing or sneezing. These are able to traverse distances of 1.8 m or greater. Second is transmission by droplets or large particles. This type of transmission necessitates person-to-person contact, usually at distances of less than 0.9 m for infection to occur. Finally, transmission can occur via contact with contaminated surfaces. Typical winter conditions enable RSV to remain viable on nonporous surfaces for longer than 6 to 12 hours. Therefore, assuming virus viability, there is great potential for self-inoculation and transmission of infection to surrounding patients and medical personnel. This is particularly worrisome for medical personnel and nursing staff, who may unwittingly spread the virus during high-risk months. Prevention using good infection control practices is of paramount importance. Nosocomial transmission has been implicated in some groups of immunocompromised patients.[367] Respiratory secretions are contagious and the portal of entry is through the nasopharyngeal mucosa and conjunctivae. The incubation period of RSV is 3 to 5 days.

The target tissue is the respiratory epithelium. Proliferation and necrosis of bronchiolar epithelium with lymphocytic peribronchiolar infiltration and edema are characteristic pathologic findings. Both humoral and cell-mediated immunity are important protective responses,[368] and those individuals with inherited or acquired immunodeficiency have more severe and long-lasting RSV infections than normal individuals.[361]

High-risk groups for the development of RSV infections include premature infants; children with bronchopulmonary dysplasia, congenital heart disease, or cystic fibrosis; immunosuppressed patients, including bone marrow and solid organ transplant recipients and those with underlying disorders of cellular immunity; elderly people; and those living in institutions.[361] Children with hematologic malignancies are susceptible to RSV infection, which has the potential to cause more severe illness in these patients than in nonimmunocompromised patients,[369,370] and can result in extension to the lower respiratory tract, pneumonia, and death. Adults with hematologic malignancy are also susceptible,[371,372] especially those profoundly immunosuppressed after marrow transplantation. Respiratory syncytial virus infections in BMT patients have been increasingly described since 1988, with several outbreaks being reported in large BMT centers.[362–373,374] The reported incidence of RSV infections in hospitalized BMT patients ranges from 7 to 20 percent.

In immunocompromised children and adults, RSV infections usually present as an upper respiratory tract illness with cough, fever, sinus and nasal congestion, rhinorrhea, and dyspnea but rapidly progress to severe and often fatal lower respiratory tract viral pneumonia, with marked radiographic changes.[375] A review of 600 children with RSV infection revealed 47 patients with compromised immune function over a 10-year time span. On analysis of the data, those children with primary immunodeficiency disorders and those receiving chemotherapy were more likely to develop RSV pneumonia (60 to 80 percent admitted to intensive care units) and had a higher mortality rate (15 to 40 percent) compared with those with normal immunity (5 percent intensive care unit admissions; fewer than 1 percent died).[376] In the BMT population, lower respiratory tract pneumonia develops in approximately 50 to 60 percent of RSV infected patients.[363,375] The development of pneumonia is associated with a higher mortality rate (66 to 100 percent), and therefore rapid treatment and prevention of progression are important.[362,374,377,378] The M.D. Anderson Cancer Center has produced data demonstrating that those patients treated earlier (1 day or less from symptoms) had an overall mortality rate of 22 percent versus 100 percent in patients who had delayed treatment or who did not receive treatment.[374] This confirms that the mortality rate increases as the time to diagnosis and treatment increases. The other known predictor of outcome in BMT recipients is engraftment status. The risk of pneumonia is greater in patients who have not engrafted than in those who have (79 versus 41 percent).[375] There are also data demonstrating that the frequency of progression from an upper respiratory tract infection to pneumonia is higher in patients in whom engraftment has not occurred or who are less than 1 month post-transplant, compared to those who are more than 1 month post-transplant/engraftment (70 to 80 to percent versus 25 to 40 percent, respectively). However, once pneumonia develops, engraftment status does not alter overall mortality.[363,377] Other risk factors that have been identified as causing progression of RSV infections from an upper respiratory tract to a lower respiratory tract infection include older age and HLA-mismatched or unrelated donor transplants (relative risk 2.8:1).[379]

Diagnosis

Nasopharyngeal aspirates or washes are among the most common specimens used for the diagnosis of RSV. Wash specimens are preferred to swabs because they have increased sensitivity. Specimens are tested for RSV by culture or by use of a rapid detection assay such as enzyme-linked immunoabsorbent assay (ELISA) or immunofluorescence.[361] Specimens from sputum or bronchoalveolar lavage also contain the pathogen, and in the immunocompromised patient, bronchoalveolar lavage has an increased sensitivity for virus detection, especially with use of the rapid antigen testing system.

Treatment

Currently available treatment options for RSV pneumonia include ribavirin, intravenous immunoglobulin rich in RSV titers, RSV immune globulin (RSV-IG [Respigam, MedImmune, Gaithersburg, MD]), and palivizumab (Synagis, [MedImmune, Gaithersburg, MD]). Ribavirin is a synthetic purine nucleoside derivative. Its antiviral effects result from three mechanisms of viral inhibition, namely, suppression of viral nucleic acid synthesis; blocking of the formation of the terminus of mRNA, leading to inefficient translation of mRNA into viral structural proteins; and suppression of viral polymerase, resulting in interference with viral mRNA expression and subsequent protein synthesis. Ribavirin has activity against a broad spectrum of both RNA and DNA viruses and has been investigated as a potential treatment in influenza A and B, disseminated adenovirus, parainfluenza virus, herpesvirus, and RSV infections. Its role in RSV infections is controversial. Much of the data on treating RSV infections come from the pediatric literature, as this is one of the populations most at risk for this infection. Conflicting results are reported on the use of ribavirin to treat RSV infections in infants and children. Several studies of infants and children on ventilators have examined the effect of ribavirin on days of ventilation and hospitalization. The results are variable, with one study showing a reduction in days of ventilation and hospitalization,[380] one study demonstrating no difference in hospitalization,[381] and two studies showing prolonged hospitalization and ventilation compared to placebo.[382,383] A meta-analysis of studies in infants with RSV lower respiratory tract infections demonstrated an overall trend in favor of ribavirin but no evidence of a significant benefit; unfortunately, the studies lacked the power to detect reductions in mortality.[384] Based on these data, ribavirin is not often used for infants and children with RSV infections and is reserved for immunocompromised and critically ill patients.

An abundance of case reports and small series report the effectiveness of aerosolized ribavirin in the treatment of RSV in both adult and pediatric BMT recipients.[362,374,385–388] It is important to remember that the number of patients treated is small and the studies are uncontrolled and noncomparative. One of the largest studies of RSV infection in BMT recipients reported 31 cases of RSV infection diagnosed among 199 transplant recipients.[362] Of the 31 patients, 18 were diagnosed with RSV pneumonia and the remaining 13 had upper respiratory tract infections. Ribavirin was administered to 13 (72 percent) of the patients with pneumonia but to none of the patients with upper respiratory tract infections. Survival among patients who developed pneumonia was poor, with a mortality rate of 78 percent. The mortality rate was 70 percent in the 13 patients treated with aerosolized ribavirin monotherapy and 100 percent in the untreated patients. Responses appeared to be better in those patients receiving more than 5 days of ribavirin therapy. An earlier study also documented a mortality rate of 66 percent in BMT patients with radiographically documented RSV pneumonia treated with aerosolized ribavirin monotherapy.[389] Based on these findings and the results outlined in case reports in the literature, it is difficult to justify monotherapy with ribavirin for the treatment of RSV pneumonia in immunocompromised individuals. If ribavirin is to be effective, early diagnosis is essential and treatment should be instituted prior to progression to pneumonia.

Improved response rates and improved survival rates have been reported with a combination of ribavirin and intravenous immuneglobulin (IVIG).[390] Whimbey et al.[373] studied aerosolized ribavirin 20 mg/ml for 18 hours per day in combination with IVIG 500 mg/kg every other day in BMT patients who were RSV-positive. The IVIG product was chosen based on the presence of neutralizing antibodies against RSV subtypes A and B. Of 42 patients who presented with upper respiratory tract illness, 19 were RSV-positive. Pneumonia developed in 16 patients, of whom 12 (75 percent) were treated with combination therapy. The overall mortality rate among those with pneumonia was 42 percent, a significant improvement over mortality rates associated with ribavirin monotherapy. As seen with ribavirin monotherapy, responses were more likely to occur with fast implementation of treatment. The same group from Texas recently published their results using the same combination of drugs (ribavirin plus IVIG) in a trial evaluating efficacy in preventing progression of RSV upper respiratory tract infection to pneumonia.[391] Fourteen patients were treated for a mean of 13 days with combination therapy. The upper respiratory illness resolved in 10 patients (71 percent). Four patients (29 percent) developed pneumonia, which was fatal in two. In this study, two different methods of administering ribavirin were evaluated. Traditionally, aerosolized ribavirin is administered at a daily dose of 6 g, delivered at a concentration of 20 mg/ml for 18 hours per day in a scavenging tent to prevent environmental contamination with the drug.[391] Although it produces very high drug levels in bronchial secretions with little systemic absorption,[392,393] this method of administration is cumbersome and is often difficult for patients to tolerate for long periods. In an attempt to improve compliance and ease of administration, short-duration aerosolized ribavirin at a daily dose of 6 g, administered at a concentration of 60 mg/ml for 2 hours every 8 hours was evaluated. This method of administration has been attempted in the past with limited success,[375] but the favorable results reported by the Texas group offer promise and should be further evaluated in a larger group of patients.

The doses of standard IVIG necessary to achieve the required in vivo RSV-neutralizing activity are large, and frequent dosing is required. This, coupled with wide variations in RSV antibodies between batches and commercial sources, led to the development of a commercial RSV hyperimmune globulin. RSV-IG, a polyclonal hyperimmune globulin containing high titers of RSV antibodies (over 19,200 MU/ml) against RSV.[394] The product is commercially available as Respigam (MedImmune, Gaithersburg, MD). The only available data in immunocompromised patients are in the BMT literature. The results of a compassionate use protocol of RSV-IG in the treatment of lower respiratory tract RSV infections in pediatric BMT patients showed that 55 percent of patients had resolution of lower respiratory tract infections following one dose.[394] Importantly it must be noted that of the patients enrolled in the program, 82 percent had previously received aerosolized ribavirin and 91 percent were receiving concurrent aerosolized ribavirin with RSV-IG. Despite concomitant treatment, the mortality rate was only 9 percent, and this offers promise for the future. Clearly, further studies using RSV-IG as monotherapy and comparing outcomes to those obtained with ribavirin are warranted in the immunocompromised patient population.

In additon to RSV-IG, a humanized RSV monoclonal IgG$_1$ monoclonal antibody that is highly active against RSV types A and B is commercially available.[395] Palivizumab is approved by the U.S. Food and Drug Administration for the prevention of serious RSV lower respiratory tract disease in pediatric patients at high risk for RSV disease. In the pediatric population it has been shown to reduce hospitalizations as a result of RSV infection by 55 percent, reduce the total number of days in hospital as a result of RSV infection (36 versus 63 days), reduce the number of ICU admissions (1.3 versus 3 percent), and reduce the total number of days hospitalized overall (191 versus 242 days).[396] In view of these promising data and the increasing incidence of RSV infection among immunocompromised patients, the use of palivizumab has been evaluated in a small number of BMT patients. There are two small studies in this patient group, one examining the pharmacokinetic profile of palivizumab in patients without RSV infection, and the other in patients with documented RSV infection. In the pharmacokinetic study, the mean serum concentration after 30 days was 41.9 µg/mL,[397] which was within the limits necessary to produce a two-log (99 percent) reduction in pulmonary RSV infection, based on animal data.[398] Patients were also monitored for the development of anti-palivizumab anibodies. No antibodies were detected, which is consistent with the pediatric literature.[397] The second study evaluated the response to palivizumab in 15 patients with proven RSV infections. At enrollment, 12 patients (80 percent) had lower respiratory tract involvement and 3 (20 percent) received mechanical ventilation. Palivizumab 15 mg/kg was administered in combination with ribavirin therapy. The survival rate was 87 percent, similar to results seen with RSV-IG. Palivizumab is an interesting addi-

tion to the therapeutic armamentarium against RSV and offers the advantage of being administered once and producing high concentrations that are sustainable and protective over a 30-day dosing interval. To date there are no comparative studies of RSVIG and palivizumab, so which one is superior remains to be seen. A prospective study comparing products in the BMT population is warranted.

Finally, interferon-α has shown some activity in the treatment of RSV infections but has been incompletely evaluated clinically. Inactivated and attenuated vaccines have not proved to be beneficial in clinical trials. Subunit vaccines are under development.

Prevention

Patients presenting for BMT during the RSV season with respiratory symptoms should receive work-ups for conventional respiratory viruses (CRVs), including RSV, adenovirus, and influenza and parainfluenza viruses. If any of these viruses are isolated, the BMT should be placed on hold until resolution of the acute process if possible. Similarly, patients with cancer undergoing chemotherapy should have therapy temporarily suspended if possible.

If any hospitalized BMT patient develops signs and symptoms of CRV infection while an inpatient, appropriate specimens should be obtained for viral culture and rapid diagnositic tests for RSV.[399] If the patient continues to display respiratory signs and rapid testing is negative (two diagnostic samples more than 2 days apart), a bronchoalveolar lavage should be considered. These patients should be placed under contact precautions to prevent spread of infection.

Health care workers (HCWs) handling respiratory symptoms of infected patients should wear gowns, surgical masks, and eye protection to avoid contamination from secretions. Protective clothing should be put on on entering the patient's room and discarded before leaving the room. HCWs should change gloves between contacts with patients. All visitors of an infected patient should wash their hands after contacts with the patient or with secretions from the patient. In addition, visitors with upper respiratory tract infections should defer visiting until resolution of symptoms, and HCWs with respiratory symptoms should be reassigned to duties other than patient care.

Influenza Viruses

Influenza A and B viruses are members of the Orthomyxoviridae family. These enveloped single-stranded RNA viruses are important causes of recurrent epidemics of respiratory disease in both normal and immunocompromised patients. Four genera exist: influenzavirus A, influenzavirus B, influenzavirus C, and thogotovirus.[400] Influenza A viruses are further divided into subtypes on the basis of serological and genetic differences in their surface glucoproteins.[400] Fifteen subtypes of hemagglutinin (H1 to H15), and nine subtypes of neuraminidase (N1 to N9) have been identified.[400] Considerable antigenic variations can occur; this property has made control by vaccine difficult because these antigenic changes can permit the organism to evade established immunity. Influenza viruses are named by type, location of isolation, number of isolates, year of recovery, and for influenza A, the subtype (e.g., A/Texas/36/91[H1N1]).[401] Three influenza A virus subtypes, H1N1, H2N2, and H3N2, have caused extensive human diseases during the last century.

Infected respiratory secretions are generally the mode of transmission to a susceptible individual. The target cells are those of the respiratory tract epithelium, particularly the columnar epithelial cells, where the influenza virus replicates.[400] Desquamation of epithelial cells, sloughing and in more severe cases, hemorrhage, hyaline membrane formation, and neutrophilic infiltration are notable findings pathologically. Influenza typically presents clinically as fever with associated chills. Other common presenting symptoms include sore throat, headache, myalgias, and fatigue. In more severe cases patients may present with fulminant pneumonia, a common presentation in the elderly in influenza season. The incubation period for influenza viruses is between 1 and 4 days. Secondary bacterial infections (mainly *Streptococcus pneumoniae, Staphylococcus aureus,* and *Haemophilus influenzae*) are well-recognized complications. Humoral immunity is an important protective host response, especially neutralizing antibody.

Influenza infections in immunocompromised patients occur, concomitant with outbreaks in the community. For example, an influenza A epidemic in 1991–1992 in Houston was evaluated.[402] Among adult BMT patients, approximately 40 percent developed acute respiratory illness, and influenza A was isolated from 30 percent. All had upper respiratory tract illness, but this was complicated by pneumonia in 75 percent. The case fatality was 17 percent. Nosocomial acquisition of influenza is also common in hospitalized adults with leukemia or those undergoing BMT.[402–404] Influenza infections in immunocompromised patients have been studied regularly over the past decade and a recent review of CRVs recovered from 785 consecutive immunocompromised patients with suspected respiratory tract infections has been published.[405] Diagnosis of conventional respiratory viruses was made following bronchoalveolar lavage in all cases, and 199 viruses were isolated from these specimens (23 percent). Influenza virus was isolated in 11 of 37 patients with CRVs and was the most common CRV isolated. Pneumonia was present in 82 percent of these patients, and the overall mortality rate was 27 percent. These results are similar to those previously published in the literature[406,407] and indicate the need for stringent preventive measures during influenza season and community outbreaks.

Detection

There are four broad potential targets in diagnosing influenza[400]: virus isolation, detection of viral proteins, detection of viral nucleic acid, and serological diagnosis. The gold standard diagnostic procedure for influenza is isolation in cell culture. This procedure requires 2 to 4 days to produce a result. The shell vial technique is much faster, enabling detection of influenza antigens following overnight culture, although the sensitivity of this test is only approximately 80 percent as compared to standard cell culture.[408] A new area of emerging diagnostics is the detection of viral proteins. There are several rapid tests now appearing on the market, which are easy to perform

and do not required skilled technicians. Point-of-care rapid diagnostic tests that are currently available or under development include the Directigen Flu A test, which detects only influenza A in nasopharyngeal, nasal, or throat specimens. This is an enzyme immunoassay test and can be completed in eight steps in approximately 15 minutes. The sensitivity of the test is variable, ranging from 50 to 99 percent, with a specificity of 52 to 97 percent.[400,401] The other tests are the ZstatFlu, FLU OIA, and QuickVue. Each of the three latter tests can detect both influenza A and B. The ZstatFlu is a colorimetric neuraminidase enzyme assay that has only three steps but takes 12 minutes to produce a result from a throat specimen. It has a sensitivity of 62 percent and a specificity of 99 percent. The FLU OIA assay method is an optical enzyme immunoassay, which can be completed in seven steps. It is rapid, with a 17-minute turnaround, a sensitivity of 62 to 88 percent and a specificity of 70 to 80 percent. The QuickVue takes the longest of all the new techniques; it is able to produce a result from a nasopharyngeal or nasal specimen in 30 minutes and has a sensitivity of 73 to 82 percent and a specificity of 96 to 99 percent. These tests are rapid and provide quick answers to assist therapeutic decisions, although they are not as sensitive as culture or PCR techniques. In additon, these tests have not been evaluated in the immunocompromised population and the sensitivity and specificity parameters listed are based on studies performed in healthy children and adults. Although these rapid diagnostic tests assist in early treatment, they will not replace the need for viral culture because only culture isolates can provide specific information on circulating influenza subtypes and strains.[409] This information is necessary annually to compare circulating influenza strains and vaccine strains and to formulate vaccines for the coming year.

Polymerase chain reaction techniques detect viral nucleic acid in a very sensitive manner, and results can be generated within 24 hours. This diagnostic tool is best used in outbreak situations, in which molecular typing and analysis of samples is necessary. Finally, serological diagnosis is based on the detection of a fourfold or greater increase in antibody titers. The test requires two samples, one collected at the onset of symptoms and another 14 days later, and this limits its usefulness in guiding treatment.[407] This test is not as reliable in the immunocompromised population.

Treatment

Amantadine and rimantadine are agents that inhibit an early stage of viral replication and appear to be useful in the prevention and treatment of influenza A in young adults, children, families, and the elderly at risk for exposure.[410–414] Both these drugs act to inhibit the uncoating of the influenza A virus (no activity against influenza B virus) by blocking the activity of the viral M2 protein.[409] Both agents are similarly efficacious (70 to 90 percent), although rimantadine may be associated with fewer side effects.[415] These compounds exert maximal benefit when administered within 48 hours of the onset of influenza symptoms. They have been shown to reduce the duration and severity of symptoms when administered in this way, although they have not been shown to prevent serious influenza-related complications such as bacterial or viral pneumonia or exacerbation of chronic diseases. One of the main concerns with the use of amantadine and rimantadine is the emergence of drug resistance. Resistance to these agents has been well documented in the laboratory and in humans,[416–419] but the frequency and importance of drug-resistant influenza in immunocompromised patients was uncharacterized until recently. It has since been shown to occur in approximately 30 percent of severely immunocompromised patients with influenza and in 83 percent of patients with symptomatic disease who shed virus for more than 3 days.[414] In patients who do not respond to treatment, resistant strains must be suspected.

A new class of antiviral drugs, the neuraminidase inhibitors, is also available for the treatment of influenza A and B.[420–424] Zanamivir and oseltamivir are both commercially available and FDA-approved for the treatment of influenza A and B. They are not approved for, nor are there currently sufficient data to support their use in, the prophylactic setting. Despite this lack of data, in time of community or nosocomial outbreaks of influenza B infections it may be prudent to prophylactically administer these agents to high-risk individuals; this approach certainly deserves further study. These drugs act by selective inhibition of viral neuraminidase. Neuraminidase, essential for viral replication in vitro, promotes the release of progeny virus from infected cells.[420] By inhibiting neuraminidase, zanamivir and oseltamivir block the active site of neuraminidase and leave uncleaved sialic acid residues on the surface of host cells and influenza viral envelopes.[409] Viral hemagglutinin binds to the uncleaved sialic acid residues, resulting in viral aggregation and a reduction in the amount of virus released.[409]

Zanamivir is available for use by inhalation only, using the Diskhaler provided in the package. It is approved for the treatment of influenza in patients 12 years and older who have had symptoms for no longer than 2 days. The recommended dose is two inhalations (10-mg dose) twice daily for 5 days. Following inhalation, approximately 7 to 21 percent of the administered dose reaches the lungs, with 70 to 87 percent of the dose being deposited in the oropharynx.[409,421] A small amount of the drug is absorbed systemically (4 to 17 percent). Zanamivir has an advantage in that the dose does not need to be modified in renal impairment. Oseltamivir is available as an oral capsule. It is approved for the treatment of influenza A and B virus in adults 18 years of age or older within 2 days of the onset of influenza symptoms. The recommended dose for adults is 75 mg by mouth twice daily for 5 days. Doses need to be reduced in patients with creatinine clearances less than 30ml/min to 75 mg daily. Approximately 80 percent of a dose is systemically absorbed.[409] Both of the commercially available neuraminidase inhibitors have favorable side effect profiles. The most common side effects seen include nausea, sinusitis, nasal signs and symptoms, diarrhea, cough, dizziness, and headaches. The majority of these side effects could be attributed to the underlying influenza infection and were seen with a similar incidence in the placebo groups of the earlier trials. Both neuraminidase inhibitors have been shown in clinical trials in healthy volunteers to reduce the symptoms associated with influenza by approximately 1 day. There is currently a lack of data supporting the use of these agents in immunocompromised patients,

patients who are hospitalized, or patients with severe influenza including pneumonia.

As seen with amantadine and rimantadine, resistance to neuraminidase inhibitors can be induced. The emergence of resistance, however, is much less likely to happen, requiring several passages in cell culture,[409] whereas resistance to amantadine and rimantadine requires far fewer passages in cell culture. Resistance to zanamivir has already been documented in a BMT recipient,[425] and therefore the use of these agents in this population warrants close surveillance.

Prevention

The main role of amantadine and rimantadine in immunocompromised patients is for prophylaxis during community and nosocomial outbreaks of influenza A infections. Transplant patients, less than 6 months following a bone marrow transport, are generally unable to mount a good immune response to the influenza vaccine. In times of community outbreaks, these patients need protection. Administration of amantadine or rimantadine may provide protection against influenza A and at the same time the patient should be immunized, although it should be realized that total protection will not be provided. The other potential role for amantadine and rimantidine is in those patients who are allergic to components of the influenza virus. Rimantadine is administered at a dose of 100 mg twice daily in adults, with dose modifications for patients with impaired renal function. Amantadine is also administered at a dose of 100 mg twice daily but does not require dose modification for renal impairment.

Inactivated vaccines are available, and community immunization programs in the fall and early winter can reduce the spread within communities. The efficacy of the influenza vaccine in cancer patients and the severely immunocompromised host is reduced as compared to normal controls. Several attempts to overcome poor immune responses, including administering additional injections, have been made although they have not met with much success. Patients with mild underlying immunodeficiency have been able to mount an antibody response. The scenario in BMT patients is somewhat different. In an evaluation of antibody responses to a two-dose regimen of influenza vaccine in allogeneic T-cell-depleted and autologous BMT patients, the likelihood of response was significantly related to a longer interval between transplantation and immunization.[426] Vaccination during the first 6 months unfortunately was ineffective. Similarly, patients with GvHD were less likely to undergo seroconversion. Thus, early after transplant an agent such as rimantadine may be more useful in protecting susceptible patients than immunization. The current recommendations for influenza vaccination by the Centers for Disease Control include administering a dose of whole- or split-virus influenza vaccine (0.5 ml per dose) before BMT, and restarting 6 months after BMT. Thereafter the vaccine should be administered annually for the rest of the patient's life.[399] In addition, vaccination of family members and close or household contacts is recommended during each influenza season. This immunization schedule should start the year prior to the BMT and continue for at least 24 months after BMT, generally for as long as the patient is immunosuppressed. This is aimed at preventing influenza exposure among both BMT recipients and BMT candidates.[399]

Parainfluenza Viruses

Human parainfluenza viruses (PIVs) are enveloped, single-stranded RNA viruses, which are members of the Paramyxovirus family (along with RSV, measles, and mumps). Of the four major antigenic serotypes, three are common respiratory pathogens frequently causing upper (type 1 and 2) and lower (type 3) respiratory illness in the general population. Infections are seasonal, especially during the fall. The target tissues are the mucosal epithelium of the nasal and oropharyngeal passages, but infection can extend to bronchi and bronchioles in more severe cases. Neutralizing antibody and cytotoxic T-cell responses are immunoprotective. The virus can be isolated from infected secretions by cell culture techniques coupled with immunofluorescence.

Incidence and Outcomes

Parainfluenza virus is a frequent cause of respiratory illness in children less than 6 years of age. The disorder presents with a variety of symptoms, ranging from upper respiratory tract infections to croup and pneumonia.[427] By 30 months of age, nearly every child will encounter this virus, but immunity is incomplete and reinfection occurs throughout life. When reinfection occurs in later life, the infection course is generally less severe. Parainfluenza virus infections have been reported following BMT.[427–430] The reported incidence among BMT and cancer patients has ranged from 2 to 5 percent of patients. The largest review of PIV in BMT patients was conducted over 16 years from 1974 to 1990 at the University of Minnesota. Over 1200 patients were screened for common respiratory viruses, and PIV was isolated in 27 patients by either nasopharyngeal cultures or bronchoalveolar lavage. Approximately 30 percent of patients had respiratory symptoms localized to the upper respiratory tract, characterized by fever, cough, coryza, wheezing, and shortness of breath. The remaining 70 percent developed lower respiratory tract infections, of whom 32 percent developed respiratory failure. Diffuse pulmonary infiltrates on chest X-ray and sinus opacification, in addition to cough, fever, wheezing, and shortness of breath characterized lower respiratory tract infections. As with other CRVs, development of pneumonia is associated with a poor outcome, with the majority of patients dying. This is in contrast to infection localized to the upper respiratory tract, which all patients survived. Unlike other CRVs such as RSV, infection with PIV was not seasonal but occurred in nearly every month of the year. The most common subtype identified was parainfluenza type 3, which is consistent with other reports in the literature.

The M.D. Anderson group has also reviewed the frequency and outcomes of PIV infections in their cancer and BMT population. Parainfluenza was isolated in 3 percent of 265 adult BMT patients during 1991. Again, PIV type 3 was identified in all patients. Progression to lower respiratory tract infections was associated with a 50 percent mortality. More recently, this group published updated results spanning a 5-year period. Parain-

fluenza was isolated in 61 patients (5.2 percent of the total screened population). Almost half of the patients evaluated with PIV developed pneumonia, with an associated mortality rate of 34 percent.

Based on these studies, it is apparent that patients at greatest risk for PIV infection are those who have recently undergone BMT, that is, who are less than 100 days from BMT, and those undergoing allogeneic BMT. In addition, patients with pneumonia were more likely to be lymphopenic than patients with localized upper respiratory tract infections (78 versus 55 percent, $p < .005$). Other risk factors evaluated but not found to be statistically predictive for PIV pneumonia were patient age, presence of GvHD, type of immunosuppression, and the presence of neutropenia.[430]

Treatment

There is no known effective antiviral treatment, although ribavirin may have some activity.[393] Ribavirin has been used with mixed results in PIV-infections. The Minneapolis group treated nine patients (33 percent of the total PIV-infected population) with aerosolized ribavirin for a median of 10 days. The survival among those patients (78 percent) was no different from that patients not treated with ribavirin. This study was uncontrolled and was not intended to test the value of ribavirin therapy. The Texas group also treated some patients with ribavirin, achieving success in 60 percent of patients. At this juncture the role of ribavirin in PIV infections is unclear. Its role should preferably be in those patients with upper respiratory tract infections to attempt to prevent progression to a lower respiratory tract infection. However, in patients who have already developed a lower respiratory tract infection and are critically ill, it is also worth attempting. There are also limited data supporting intravenous ribavirin in the management of PIV infection.[431]

HEPATITIS VIRUSES

Hepatitis viruses are RNA (hepatitis A, C, and G) or DNA (hepatitis B) enteric pathogens, which can be transmitted via the fecal–oral route or sexual contact. Transmission through infected blood products is also problematic and represents a serious challenge for the management of patients with hematologic malignancies requiring blood product support.

Hepatitis A

Hepatitis A is a member of the Picornaviridae family. This nonenveloped single-stranded RNA virus replicates in the intestinal tract and then is transported to the liver, which is the major target tissue. It can cause acute hepatitis characterized by jaundice or can present subclinically. In contrast to hepatitis B and C, only rare cases of hepatitis A transmission by blood products have been described, and therefore routine screening of blood products for hepatitis A virus does not occur. Transmission of the virus is thought to occur via the oral–fecal route. In addition, hepatitis A has a long incubation period of 15 to 50 days, with the virus excreted in the feces for 1 to 2 weeks prior to the onset of clinical illness and for at least 1 week afterwards,[432] which emphasizes the need for good hygiene practices. The typical presentation of hepatitis A virus infections includes fever, malaise, nausea, vomiting, arthralgias, and anorexia.[432] In some patients flu-like symptoms may also be present. These symptoms tend to abate with the onset of jaundice. Rarely, acute liver failure, cholestatic hepatitis, or relapsing hepatitis can occur.

Management of acute hepatitis A-infection is primarily symptom control. In otherwise healthy patients, resolution of the infection will occur in 3 to 6 months. The primary control measure is prevention. Patients traveling to hepatitis A endemic areas should receive either IVIG prophylaxis or hepatitis A vaccination. Similarly, immunocompromised patients who come into contact with hepatitis A-infected patients should consider prophylaxis. Passive immunization with IVIG has been the primary treatment of choice for over 50 years. Intravenous immuneglobulin is most effective when given within 2 weeks of exposure and is the fastest way to achieve hepatitis A antibodies. The alternative to IVIG is hepatitis A vaccine, of which there are two types used around the world, including the live attenuated vaccines and the inactivated vaccine. In the United States there are two commercially available inactivated vaccines, Havrix (Smith Kline Beecham) and Vaqta (Merck). These vaccines produce very high levels of anti-hepatitis A virus, significantly higher than can be achieved with IVIG.[432] Following the first dose, anti-hepatitis A virus is detectable in the serum within 15 days in most patients. In the majority of patients, seroconversion is complete 1 month following injection, and persisting antibodies can be detected at 1 year. As with other vaccinations, immunosuppressed patients tend to be less responsive.

Indications for immunization include travel to endemic areas, chronic liver disease, and clotting factor disorders likely to require concentrate replacement. At this time, routine hepatitis A immunization is not recommended for BMT patients.[399] There are limited data on the safety of the vaccine in this population; however, consideration can be given to administration of the hepatitis A vaccine to patients older than 2 years who are at least 12 months post-BMT and who are at increased risk of for hepatitis A and its adverse consequences (e.g., persons with chronic liver disease, including chronic GvHD, and children living in areas with consistently elevated hepatitis A incidence).[433]

Hepatitis B

Hepatitis B, a member of the Hepnaviridae family, is a small DNA virus, which can cause acute self-limited primary infection and resolve or can become a persistent infection for years or even a lifetime. The virus can be transmitted by percutaneous inoculation via needles, blood transfusion, or contact of mucosal surfaces with blood and other body fluids, including sexual contact. Persistent infection may be accompanied by no hepatic dysfunction, but chronic hepatitis is common and can be associated with a risk for hepatocellular carcinoma. Persistent viremia can pose a risk for transmission by blood transfusion. With routine donor screening for hepatitis surface antigen (HbsAg) and hepatitis B core antibody (anti-HBc), the risk for

hepatitis B from a blood transfusion has diminished tremendously. In addition, increasing immunization with hepatitis B vaccines in the community has led to a decrease in the number of patients infected with hepatitis B and hence a decrease in the number of contaminated transfusions. Less than 5 percent of post-transfusion hepatitis today is caused by hepatitis B.

Each year in the United States there are between 140,000 and 320,000 new cases of hepatitis B, with an estimated 1 to 1.25 million chronically infected Americans.[434] The prevalence of hepatitis B virus (HBV) is geography-dependent. In the United States approximately 0.1 to 0.5 percent of the population are hepatitis B carriers[435] compared to 10 percent in Hong Kong,[436] and 17 percent in Taiwan.[435] Based on these data, the chance of a patient undergoing chemotherapy also being a chronic hepatitis B carrier is increasing. Similarly, the likelihood of a BMT candidate having hepatitis B or being exposed to an HbsAg-positive donor is increasing.

Chronic hepatitis B carriers who undergo chemotherapy or BMT have been shown to have an increased risk of liver-related morbidity and mortality.[434–447] At the completion of chemotherapy or BMT conditioning, the patient becomes immunosuppressed. At this time there is an increase in hepatitis B virus replication in the liver, leading to an increased viral load. On recovery postchemotherapy, there is immune reconstitution, which is associated with an acute hepatitis flare. Immune recovery causes an immune-mediated destruction of liver cells containing HBV. The severity of hepatocyte destruction is directly proportional to the viral load in the liver.[434,436,439] This results in an acute exacerbation of hepatitis and may progress to fulminant liver failure.

Studies have been performed in lymphoma patients with concomitant HBV undergoing standard chemotherapy. In this population, the development of impaired liver function (as assessed by increased liver function tests) occurred in more than 50 percent of patients studied. Liver-related mortality was 5 percent, with reactivation of HBV thought to be the cause of death.[439] Similarly, there are data characterizing an increased risk of HBV morbidity and mortality in HBsAg-positive BMT recipients.[446–453]

In the solid tumor population, prediction of who will reactivate HBV is difficult. The most useful marker of reactivation is HBV viral DNA level.[438] Close monitoring of hepatitis markers is essential. Management strategies in the HBV-positive patient undergoing chemotherapy include as the first step removal of those agents likely to potentiate HBV reactivation. Corticosteroids are a common component of chemotherapy regimens and are known to stimulate viral reactivation.[454] If possible, steroid therapy should be avoided, but this may not always be possible. Continuous low-dose corticosteroids have been attempted and are generally no better than pulse steroids.[439] Similarly, daily or weekly schedules have not been shown to be better than schedules calling for administration every third to fourth week.

The alternative approach is to prophylactically administer antiviral agents to prevent HBV reactivation. Interferon has demonstrated efficacy in white hepatitis B carriers (but is less effective in Asian hepatitis B carriers). One of the important side effects of interferon is myelosuppression, and for this reason it is often contraindicated in the already myelosuppressed cancer patient. Alternatives include the nucleoside analogues lamivudine and famciclovir. Both of these agents interfere with viral DNA replication, leading to inhibition of serum HBV viral DNA levels, with consequent improvement in liver function tests.[455–461]

The most effective treatment strategy is targeting those patients at greatest risk (identified by screening patients for past and current infection with HBV) and administering prophylaxis to prevent viral reactivation.[462] Patients with evidence of disease at the time of chemotherapy, as demonstrated by viral replication (HBV-DNA-positive) should receive an antiviral agent such as lamivudine (100 mg orally daily) or famciclovir (500 mg three times daily). Unfortunately, on many occasions the viral load in the liver is too great to be affected by this treatment. Carriers of HBV can either be treated prophylactically with the nucleoside analogues or closely monitored postchemotherapy for evidence of viral replication. In those patients receiving prophylactic therapy with the nucleoside analogues, therapy should be continued for at least 6 months following completion of chemotherapy.[462]

Management of patients undergoing autologous BMT is similar to conventional chemotherapy. Delayed immune reconstitution may lead to a greater risk of reactivation, but the risk is not as great as that seen in allogeneic BMT recipients. Allogeneic BMT in the HBsAg-positive patient is somewhat more complicated. At the time of transplantation, the patient may be actively infected with hepatitis B virus (HBsAg-positive) or alternatively latent HBV may be reactivated following transplantation (HBsAg-negative).[462] In the allogeneic setting, the hepatitis B status of the donor must also be considered; otherwise, liver failure secondary to hepatitis B infection is a possible consequence.

The mechanism of viral reactivation is very similar to that seen after chemotherapy. Bone marrow transplant–conditioning chemotherapy causes ablation of both the bone marrow and the immune system, leading to increased viral replication. On recovery of the immune system, an acute flare may occur. Similar flares have been documented when tapering cyclosporin A immunosuppression.[435] In a study of 43 hepatitis B virus carriers undergoing autologous or allogeneic BMT with similar preconditioning regimens, none of the autologous BMT patients developed fulminant hepatitis, compared to five allogeneic patients. Impaired liver function tests (LFTs) correlated with cyclosporin A withdrawal[435] and could not be controlled by cyclosporin A dose escalation. Potential signs of a hepatitis flare include increases in LFTs, particularly serum aspartate aminotransferase and alanine aminotransferase. Hepatitis serology should also be monitored. Ominous signs for the development of fulminant hepatitis include changes in serology from HbeAg-negative to HbeAg-positive, the presence of HbcAb IgM, or detection of HBV-DNA.[435]

Approaches to the prevention and treatment of HBV in allogeneic BMT patients are complicated and depend on both the donor and recipient hepatitis profiles. Prior to BMT, all patients and donors should have a hepatitis work-up, including HBsAg and HBcAb. If the HBsAg is positive, HBeAb, anti-HBe, and HBV DNA (including quantification) should be assessed. Recommendations for management depending on the results of hepatitis screening have been reviewed.[463] The key to management of BMT patients is comprehensive upfront screening and prophylaxis with a nucleoside analogue if infected. Several newer agents are being investigated for HBV, including adefovir dipivoxil,[464,465] elecavir,[466] and emtricitabine.[467] Despite currently available nucleoside analogues (lamivudine and famciclovir) being very effective in suppressing viral reactivation, the emergence of drug-resistant variant viruses with mutations in the HBV polymerase gene has occurred with their use.[468–470] The clinical relevance remains undetermined; however, these new agents are now being investigated for HBV, including lamivudine-resistant HBV mutants.[471]

In conclusion, when managing BMT recipients, consideration should be given to HBV infection in the differential diagnosis in post-BMT patients with abnormal hepatic transaminases not explained by the typical causes of hepatitis, for example, medications, graft-versus-host disease, or other viral infections (CMV, HSV, VZV). Increases in hepatic transaminases are most likely at the time of immunosuppression tapering. Provided treatment and prophylaxis recommendations and guidelines are adhered to, the risk of developing HBV infection is low.

An inactivated hepatitis B vaccine is highly protective. In nonimmunized exposed individuals, hyperimmune globulin can afford protection. Interferon can suppress hepatitis B replication although the magnitude of benefit is not great and is frequently temporary.[472] In one study an attempt to immunize BMT and leukemia patients against hepatitis B was unsuccessful.[473] In one case persistent hepatitis B was ablated in a patient who received a marrow transplant from a hepatitis B-immune donor.[474] Similar experimental data in mice have also been supportive of the concept that donor immunity can be adoptively transferred to BMT recipients.[475]

Hepatitis C

Hepatitis C is a lipid-enveloped single-stranded RNA virus related to members of the Flaviviridae family. Hepatitis C virus (HCV) can be transmitted via blood transfusions, intravenous drug abuse, and needlestick injuries, as well as by vertical transmission. The risk of transmission of HCV by a blood transfusion has decreased significantly following the introduction of screening processes in 1991. The magnitude of the decrease is such that the risk of transmission in donated blood that has passed all screening tests is now 1 in 103,000[476] compared to 0.19 to 0.45 percent prior to 1991.[477] The seroprevalence of antibody to HCV in most developed countries is approximately 1 to 2 percent. As with hepatitis B, there is significant geographical variation in seroprevalence rates, with higher rates of infection in eastern Europe and Africa than in the United States. The Centers for Disease Control estimates that nearly 4 million people are infected with HCV in the United States.[478] There are six genotypes of HCV, each having a different geographical predominance. The most common genotypes in the United States are 1a and 1b; genotype 1b is also common in Europe. In Asia genotype 6 is most common, in South Africa genotype 5 is most common, in the Middle East and North Africa genotype 4 is most common, and among intravenous drug users the prevalence of genotype 3 is rising. Differences have been seen in the various genotypes in terms of responses to therapy, but there is currently no clear correlation of disease outcome and severity with genotype.[478]

Hepatitis C can cause an acute, self-limiting, primary infection and resolve, or it can become a chronic infection. Approximately 85 percent of HCV-positive patients develop chronic HCV infection (as documented by persistence of HCV RNA in serum).[478] There are data demonstrating that cirrhosis develops in more than 20 percent of chronically infected adults an average of 20 years after diagnosis of the acute infection.[479] Like hepatitis B, hepatitis C has been linked to hepatocellular carcinoma. Hepatocellular carcinoma occurs most commonly in those individuals who develop cirrhosis. Other complications seen commonly in HCV-infected people include elevated transaminases; symptoms of terminal liver failure, that is, portal hypertension and hepatic encephalopathy; and hepatic fibrosis. Hepatitis C has also been reported to cause extrahepatic manifestations, for example, porphyria cutanea tarda, mixed cryoglubinemia, and glomerulonephritis.[480]

Hepatitis C virus infection can be documented serologically by the detection of antibody directed against HCV in serum (anti-HCV) using enzyme immunoassay (EIA) methodology. These tests have been shown to detect anti-HCV in more than 97 percent of infected individuals. The test is useful for demonstrating past or present infection but is not able to differentiate among acute, chronic, and resolved infection.[481] The EIA technique occasionally produces false positive results, and therefore confirmatory testing with a supplemental assay is often performed. In cancer patients and the immunocompromised, it is prudent to test for HCV RNA, as this population may produce a false negative result due to inability to produce sufficient antibodies for detection by EIA. The virus itself can be detected in blood through the use of reverse transcriptase polymerase chain reaction (RT-PCR) amplification of HCV RNA. This test enables detection of circulating HCV RNA early in the course of HCV infection, that is, 1 to 2 weeks following exposure. The presence of HCV RNA indicates an active infection. The final test is a quantitative assessment of the concentration of HCV-RNA in the blood (viral load assessment). This test is only useful for determining response to therapy and does not correlate with the severity of hepatitis or overall prognosis.

Hepatitis C infection is relatively common in the cancer (prevalence up to 70 percent)[461,482–489] and BMT (3 to 70 percent)[490–496] population, particularly those who were treated prior to 1991. These patients have been at greater risk of developing HCV infections than the general population because of the large number of blood products they received during or following therapy. Since the introduction of routine screening tests, the proportion of infected patients has decreased. Because of the large number of people infected with hepatitis C worldwide, the chance of a BMT patient or donor being hepatitis C-positive is relatively high. Therefore, appropriate diagnostic and subsequent precautionary measures should be taken to avoid

fulminant liver failure. Patients thought to be at risk for hepatitis C (that is, those with increased alanine aminotransferase (ALT) pretransplantation that is not explained by other likely diagnoses, those with a history of intravenous drug abuse, with a history of blood transfusion prior to 1991, or with multiple sexual partners) should be evaluated for hepatitis C infection by HCV RNA PCR detection technology prior to transplantation.

Patients who are infected with HCV and undergo BMT are at increased risk for the development of veno-occlusive disease (VOD).[496,497] The Fred Hutchinson Cancer Research Center (FHCRC) group recently published 10-year follow-up data on a cohort of 355 patients undergoing BMT in 1987–1988 to assess the impact of pretransplant HCV status on liver dysfunction, including VOD. Before transplantation 17 percent of patients were HCV RNA-positive which increased to 32 percent by day 100 following transplantation. Veno-occlusive disease occurred more frequently in those HCV-RNA positive pretransplant patients (87 percent), compared to 66 percent in those without HCV pretransplant ($p < .004$). Severe VOD was also increased in patients who were HCV-positive prior to transplant compared with HCV-negative patients (48 versus 14 percent, $p < .0001$).[496] Many factors are known to contribute to the risk for developing VOD, and a multivariate analysis of these factors was conducted in this cohort of patients. The greatest risk factor in these patients was pretransplantation HCV infection, in conjunction with elevated serum aspartate transaminase (AST) levels (relative risk 9.6, $p = .0001$). Patients infected with HCV prior to transplantation who had normal AST levels had no greater incidence of VOD. European investigators have not found the same association, and it is postulated by the FHCRC group that this may be due to a lower dose intensity of chemotherapy in the European studies.[492,498–500]

There are currently no good treatment options for HCV-infected BMT recipients. Standard HCV treatment for the general population includes interferon-α, either alone[501–507] or in combination with ribavirin.[508–510] Interferon (3 million units subcutaneously three times per week for 12 months) is active and has been shown to reduce the level of HCV viremia and improve hepatic transaminase abnormalities.[501–503] Long-term remissions can occasionally be seen (in 15 to 25 percent of cases),[481] although unfortunately more than 50 percent of patients who respond initially relapse after treatment cessation. Predictors of a poor response to interferon include a high HCV RNA titer and HCV genotype 1 (the most common genotype in the United States).

The combination of ribavirin (1000 mg/day divided into two doses for patients weighting less than 75 kg; 1200 mg/day divided into two doses for those over 75 kg) and interferon is currently the favored treatment option. In combination studies, the virological response rates were significantly higher with double therapy than with monotherapy (36 versus 18 percent, $p < .047$),[509] and the responses were sustained over 12 months. In most clinical situations combination therapy is preferred.

These treatment options are often not possible in allogeneic transplant candidates. Interferon therapy is typically contraindicated in allogeneic BMT patients within 6 months of transplantation because of an associated increased risk of

GvHD and mortality.[511–513] In addition, ribavirin monotherapy has been shown to be ineffective in the general population,[514–517] although there is one small case series that demonstrates efficacy in BMT patients.[518] If treatment is not possible with either of these agents, this should not necessarily be considered a contraindication to transplantation. In general, the course of chronic liver disease is insidious, and progress is slow for at least 10 to 20 years. The determination of whether transplantation should proceed and of when to transplant is dependent on the degree of underlying liver dysfunction, which should be established prior to transplantation. Work-up of liver dysfunction should include laboratory estimations, namely liver-function tests and coagulation assessments, as well as physical examination and if indicated, a liver biopsy. A liver biopsy is indicated in those patients in whom there is a clinical suspicion of cirrhosis, in patients who are likely to have had HCV infection for longer than 15 years (long-term cancer survivors in the era where there was no screening for hepatitis C) and in those known HCV-infected patients with a history of excessive alcohol intake.[462] If a diagnosis of hepatic fibrosis or cirrhosis is made, the conditioning regimen and type of transplantation procedure performed need to be reassessed. With the risk of severe VOD of the liver and the potential for multiorgan failure and subsequent death with standard myeloablative conditioning regimens, a nonmyeloablative transplant should be considered in this setting.

In the allogeneic BMT setting, the HCV status of the donor must also be evaluated. Hepatitis C virus transmission to recipients of HCV RNA-positive allogeneic and syngeneic marrow products[519] occurs universally. Within days of marrow reinfusion, patients develop viremia, although evidence of clinical and biochemical hepatitis may take weeks to months to develop. Damage to hepatocytes in HCV infection is mediated predominantly by HCV-specific cytotoxic T cells, and therefore biochemical abnormalities will only become apparent on engraftment and reconstitution of cell-mediated immunity.[496,497,520] If time permits, the best action is to treat the donor with interferon with or without ribavirin in an attempt to render the donor's serum HCV RNA undetectable at transplantation. However, treatment of HCV infection may take 6 to 12 months, time which is not always available in transplantation because of the underlying nature of the malignant disease. Again, donor HCV seropositivity is not a contraindication to transplantation, priority being allocated to an HLA match, whether donor and recipient are HCV-positive or -negative.

One of the issues that is yet to be addressed in a large study is how to manage the long-term survivor of cancer or bone marrow transplantation. As supportive care technologies improve, the length of overall survival is increasing, which will lead to a population of patients with the potential to develop cirrhosis. As mentioned, blood tranfusion products were not screened for HCV prior to 1991. With the insidious nature of the disease, the implications of cancer treatment and transplantation in this group may not have been truly realized before mid-2000. Common sense tells us that those patients developing signs of cirrhosis and liver failure should be treated in the same manner as the general HCV-infected population. In allogeneic BMT patients this will be determined by degree of immunosuppression and the presence of GvHD. In addition, all long-term survivors of cancer with chronic viral hepatitis should be offered vaccination because of the increased risk of fulminant hepatitis should they develop acute hepatitis A.[521,522]

Hepatitis G

Hepatitis G virus (HGV) is a newly described RNA virus that belongs to the Flaviviridae family,[523,524] and is closely related to the GB virus-C (GBV-C).[525] It prevails worldwide, and the viral RNA has been detected in 1 to 5 percent of volunteer blood donors.[526,527] The prevalence of HGV in patients undergoing BMT ranges from 18 to 61 percent.[528–533] Following BMT, immunosuppressed patients have been reported to have an increased risk of HGV infection after transfusion-related exposure.[529,534] This has not translated into accelerated HGV-RNA replication.[533]

Currently the clinical relevance of HGV infection and its long-term effect on BMT patients remain unresolved. Hepatitis G virus has not been shown to affect engraftment kinetics, which indicates no direct effect of HGV on hematopoietic progenitors.[535] The data on the effect of HGV on liver function are conflicting. There are data demonstrating no effect of HGV on the clinical and biological diagnosis of hepatitis in immunosuppressed patients in several studies.[532,534] However, there are also data in pediatric patients demonstrating increased alanine aminotransferase (ALT) levels in the absence of other known causes.[528] The maximum ALT levels were statistically higher than those of uninfected patients, although the mean values of ALT showed no difference. This suggests that the effect of HGV on ALT is transient and self-limiting.[528]

At present blood for transfusion is not routinely screened for HGV, which is not considered to be a serious pathogen nor a significant cause of hepatitis. Clearly, additional large studies of HGV-infected immunocompromised patients are needed to definitively characterize the effect of HGV on engraftment and hepatotoxicity.

OTHER VIRUSES

Papovaviruses (Polyomaviruses)

Infection by JC and BK viruses occur early in childhood and are widespread. In most individuals it is asymptomatic, but the viruses persist in the kidney and urogenital epithelium. Asymptomatic virus excretion increases in immunocompromised patients.[536,537] The JC virus has been associated with progressive multifocal leukoencephalopathy and has been described in patients with chronic lymphocytic leukemia or lymphoma and following BMT.[538–540] Dissemination with involvement of mutiple visceral organs, including the lungs, has also been noted.[536] The BK virus has been associated with hemorrhagic cystitis, especially in allogeneic BMT patients, in whom the risk is three times as high as in similarly treated autologous BMT recipients.[541–545] Occasionally adenovirus type 11 can also be associated with hemorrhagic cystitis.[542] Both humoral and lymphoproliferative responses to active viral shedding have been noted, but whether these are immunoprotective remains uncertain.[546] At present, there is no known effective therapy, although cases of response to vidarabine, ribavirin, or ciprofloxin have been reported.

Parvoviruses

Human parvovirus B19 is a small DNA virus, which causes erythema infections during childhood. It is an occasional cause of arthritis and in patients with chronic hemolytic anemia can be a cause of a transient aplastic crisis. It is a potential cause of pancytopenia, rash, or chronic anemia in immunocompromised patients, including leukemia and BMT patients.[547–555] Intranuclear lesions within erythroid precursors in bone marrow specimens have been noted in acutely infected patients.[556] Marrow recipients with GVHD may have chronic infection. The infection can be documented by detection of virus-specific antibody against the B19 antigen by ELISA or of viral DNA by PCR. The virus has been detected in respiratory secretions, bone marrow, and blood. There is no specific antiviral treatment, but reducing the intensity of chemotherapy can be helpful,[551] and immune globulin may also be of benefit.

Retroviruses

Human immunodeficiency virus is a retrovirus that is the causative agent of AIDS. Sexual transmission and transmission via blood transfusion or organ transplantation has been well documented. During the early 1980s, prior to the development of a screening serologic test for blood products, patients with hematologic malignancies receiving blood product support were susceptible for contracting HIV infection. Subsequent to 1985 with routine screening, the risk of transmission via a blood product is 1 in 500,000 or lower. Several cases of AIDS in patients with hematologic malignancies have been documented.[557] It is uncertain that the course of illness in immunocompromised patients is substantially different than in nonimmunocompromised patients. The association of HIV infection with Kaposi's sarcoma and aggressive non-Hodgkin's lymphoma has been noted, especially among those with low CD4 counts for more than 1 year.[558–561] There has been limited experience performing bone marrow transplantation in patients with HIV-associated malignancies.[562–564] In some patients, cytoreductive therapy to ablate all lymphohematopoietic-derived cells (the reservoir of latently infected cells) combined with antiviral therapy has had a marked antiviral effect, whereas in others in whom the virus is not very susceptible, the effect has been marginal. Most of the beneficial effects have been transient, and generally patients have succumbed from transplant-related complications or opportunistic infection. With the development of better antiviral agents and the engineering of donor marrow stem cells with genes that confer resistance to viral infection, this might be more promising in future investigations.

In the era of highly active antiretroviral therapy (HAART), there has been a drop in the rates of opportunistic infection and Kaposi's sarcoma. Of interest, however, is that there has not been a concomitant fall in the incidence of AIDS-related lymphomas, at least so far,[565–568] with the exception of a decline in central nervous system lymphomas.[568] Unfortunately, most cases present at an advanced stage and have a very poor prognosis, which also has not changed in the era of HAART.[565,569] In a subset of patients with CD4 counts above 100/ml, higher response rates and longer survival have been noted.[570] Since HAART therapy may preserve immune function for long intervals, diagnosis of lymphomas at an earlier stage may in the future lead to improved treatment outcomes.

Human T-cell lymphotropic viruses (HTLV)-1 and -2 are type C oncoviruses present in widely scattered populations, including those of the islands of southwestern Japan and the Caribbean basin, where infection is endemic. Screening of blood donors in the United States indicates a small but detectable seroprevalence. Transmission is by blood transfusion, sexual contact, and in utero. Although most infections are symptomatic, there is increasing evidence that HTLV-1 is the etiologic agent of adult T-cell leukemia/lymphoma.[571–573] There have also been associations between HTLV-2 and malignancy,[574] but its role in pathogenesis is uncertain. Adult T-cell leukemia/lymphoma occurs in only a small minority of HTLV-1 carriers. The lifetime risk is estimated to be between 2 and 5 percent.[571]

SUMMARY

The clinical significance of viral infections in patients with hematological malignancies has assumed greater importance during the last two decades. In part, this is related to more frequent recognition of viral syndromes due to improved techniques of documenting various viral pathogens by more accurate and more accessible diagnostic assays. It is also attributable to increasing use of dose-intensive or immunosuppressive treatment regimens, which have greater attendant immunosuppression and susceptibility for viral infection. With increasing awareness of the substantial morbidity due to these viral pathogens, it has become extremely important to recognize these infections. With the expanding array of antiviral agents, vaccines, and immune modulators, it has now become possible to intervene therapeutically to either prevent infection, reduce morbidity, or prevent death from these pathogens. With continuing investigations it is likely that a number of unexplained syndromes encountered in patients with hematologic malignancies will be identified in the future as having a viral etiology. These advances hopefully will further improve our supportive care in this patient population and permit further strides in the control of hematologic malignancy.

REFERENCES

1. Muller SA, Herrman EC Jr, Winkelmann RK: Herpes simplex infections in hematologic malignancies. Am J Med 52:102, 1972.
2. Meyers JD, Flournoy N, Thomas ED: Infection with herpes simplex virus and cell-mediated immunity after marrow transplant. J Infect Dis 142:338, 1980.
3. Saral R, Burns WH, Laskin OL et al: Acyclovir prophylaxis of herpes-simplex-virus infections. A randomized, double-blind, con-

trolled trial in bone marrow transplant recipients. N Engl J Med 305:63, 1981.

4. Saral R, Ambinder RF, Burns WH et al: Acyclovir prophylaxis against recrudescent herpes simplex virus infections in leukemia patients: A randomized, double-blind placebo controlled study. Ann Intern Med 99:773, 1983.

5. Anderson H, Scarfee JH, Sutton RNP, Hickmott E, Brigden D, Burke C: Oral acyclovir prophylaxis against herpes simplex virus in non-Hodgkin lymphoma and acute lymphoblastic leukaemia patients receiving remission induction chemotherapy. A randomised double blind placebo controlled trial. Br J Cancer 50:45–49, 1984.

6. Arvin AM, Pollard RB, Rasmussen LE, Merigan TC: Cellular and humoral immunity in the pathogenesis of recurrent herpes viral infections in patients with lymphoma. J Clin Invest 65:869–878, 1980.

7. Rand K, Kramer A, Johnson A: Cancer chemotherapy associated symptomatic stomatitis: Role of herpes simplex virus. Cancer 50:1262–1265, 1982.

8. Bubley GJ, Chapman B, Chapman SK, Crumpacker CS, Schnipper LE: Effect of acyclovir on radiation- and chemotherapy-induced mouth lesions. Antimicrob Agents Chemother 33:862–5, 1989.

9. Meyers JD, Thomas ED: Infection complicating bone marrow transplantation. In Rubin RH, Young LS (eds.): Clinical Approaches to Infection in the Compromised Host, 2nd Ed., p. 525. Plenum, New York, 1988.

10. Wingard JR: Infectious and noninfectious systemic consequences. Oral complications of cancer therapies: Diagnosis, prevention, and treatment. NCI Monogr 9:21–26, 1990.

11. Weiden PL, Schuffler MD: Herpes esophagitis complicating Hodgkin's disease. Cancer 33:1100, 1974.

12. McDonald GB, Sharma P, Hackman RC et al: Esophageal infections in immunosuppressed patients after marrow transplantation. Gastroenterology 88:1111–1117, 1985.

13. Lynfield YL, Farhangi M, Runnels JL: Generalized herpes simplex complicating lymphoma. JAMA 207:944, 1969.

14. Buss DH, Scharyj M: Herpesvirus infection of the esophagus and other visceral organs in adults. Am J Med 66:457–462, 1979.

15. Elfenbein GJ, Saral R: Infectious disease during immune recovery after bone marrow transplantation. In Allen JC (ed.): Infection and the Compromised Host, pp. 167–196. Williams & Wilkins, Baltimore, 1981.

16. Skolnick D, Bustamante CI, Saltzberg D et al: Diagnosis of esophagitis in immunocompromised patients: A prospective evaluation. In: Program and Abstracts of the 27th Interscience Conference on Antimicrobial Agents and Chemotherapy. New York, October 4–7, 1987: p. 263. Abstract 954. Washington, DC: American Society of Microbiology, 1987.

17. Johnson JR, Egaas S, Gleaves CA, Hackman R, Bowden RA: Hepatitis due to herpes simplex virus in marrow transplant recipients. Clin Infect Dis 14:38–45, 1992.

18. Ramsey PG, Fife FH, Hackman RC, Meyers JD, Corey L: Herpes simplex virus pneumonia. Ann Intern Med 97:813–820, 1982.

19. Becker WB, Kipps A, McKenzie D: Disseminated herpes simplex virus infection. Am J Dis Child 115:1, 1968.

20. Meyers JD, Flournoy N, Thomas ED: Nonbacterial pneumonia after allogeneic marrow transplantation: A review of ten years' experience. Rev Infect Dis 4:1119–32, 1982.

21. Pruneda RC, Almanza I: Centrifugation-shell vial technique for rapid detection of herpes simplex virus cytopathic effect in vero cells. J Clin Microbiol 25:423, 1987.

22. Schmidt NJ, Dennis J, Devlin V, Callo D, Mills J: Comparison of direct immunofluorescence and direct immunoperoxidase procedures for detection of herpes simplex virus antigen in lesion specimens. J Clin Microbiol 18:445–448.

23. Corey L, Spear PG: Infections with herpes simplex viruses. N Engl J Med 314:686–691, 749–757, 1986.

24. Gonik B, Seibel M, Berkowitz A, Woodin MB, Mills K: Comparison of two enzyme-linked immunosorbent assays for detection of herpes simplex virus antigen. J Clin Microbiol 29:436–438, 1991.

25. Nahass GT, Goldstein BA, Zhu WY, Serfing NS, Leonardi CL: Comparison of Tzanck smear, viral culture, and DNA diagnosis methods in detection of herpes simplex and varicella-zoster infection. JAMA 268:2541–44, 1992.

26. Meyers JD, Wade JC, Mitchell CD et al: Multicenter collaborative trial of intravenous acyclovir for the treatment of mucocutaneous herpes simplex virus infection in the immunocompromised host. Am J Med 73A:229, 1982.

27. Mitchell CD, Gentry SR, Boen JR et al: Acyclovir therapy for mucocutaneous herpes simplex infections in immunocompromised patients. Lancet 2:1389, 1981.

28. Wade JC, Newton B, Flournoy N, Meyers JD: Oral acyclovir prophylaxis of herpes simplex virus infection after marrow transplant. Ann Intern Med 100:823, 1984.

29. Shepp DH, Newton BA, Dandliker PS et al: Oral acyclovir therapy for mucocutaneous herpes simplex virus infection in immunocompromised marrow transplant recipients. Ann Intern Med 102:783, 1985.

30. Wade JC, Newton B, McLaren C et al: Treatment of mucocutaneous herpes simplex virus infection after marrow transplantation with intravenous acyclovir: A double blind trial. Ann Intern Med 96:265, 1982.

31. Selby PJ, Jameson B, Watson JG et al: Parenteral acyclovir therapy for herpes virus infections in man. Lancet 2:1267, 1980.

32. Wade JC, Newton B, Flournoy N et al: Acyclovir for prevention of herpes simplex virus reactivation after marrow transplantation. Ann Intern Med 99:773–776, 1984.

33. Wade JC, Meyers JD: Neurological symptoms associated with parenteral acyclovir treatment after marrow transplantation. Ann Intern Med 98:921, 1983.

34. Krigel RL: Reversible neurotoxicity due to oral acyclovir in patient with chronic lymphocytic leukemia. J Infect Dis 154:189, 1986.

35. Soul-Lawton J, Seaber E, On N et al: Absolute bioavailability and metabolic disposition of valaciclovir, the L-valyl ester of acyclovir, following oral administration to humans. Antimicrob Agents Chemother 39:2759–2764, 1995.

36. Perry CM, Faulds D: Valaciclovir: A review of its antiviral, pharmacokinetic properties and therapeutic efficacy in herpesvirus infections. Drugs 52:754–772, 1996.

37. Weller S, Blum R, Doucette M et al: Pharmacokinetics of the acyclovir prodrug valaciclovir after escalating single- and multiple-dose administration to normal volunteers. Clin Pharmacol Ther 54:595–605, 1993.

38. Saral R: Management of acute viral infections. NCI Monogr 9:107–110, 1990.

39. Wingard JR: Viral infections in leukemia and bone marrow transplant patients. Leuk Lymphoma 11:115–125, 1993.

40. Wade JC, McLaren C, Meyers JD: Frequency and significance of acyclovir-resistant herpes simplex virus isolated from marrow transplant patients receiving multiple courses of treatment with acyclovir. J Infect Dis 148:1077–1082, 1983.

41. Ambinder RF, Burns WH, Lietman PS et al: Prophylaxis: A strategy to minimize antiviral resistance. Lancet 1:1154–1155, 1984.

42. Burns WH, Santos GW, Saral R et al: Isolation and characterizations of resistant herpes simplex virus after acyclovir therapy. Lancet 2:421, 1982.

43. McLaren C, Chen MS, Ghazzouli I, Saral R, Burns WH: Drug resistance patterns of herpes simplex virus isolates from patients treated with acyclovir. Antimicrob Agent Chemother 28:740–744, 1985.

44. Ljungman P, Ellis MN, Hackman RC et al: Acyclovir-resistant herpes simplex virus causing pneumonia after marrow transplantation. J Infect Dis 162:244, 1990.

45. Sacks SL, Wanklin RJ, Reece DE, Hicks KA, Tyler KL, Coen DM: Progressive esophagitis from acyclovir-resistant herpes simplex. Clinical roles for DNA polymerase mutants and viral heterogeneity? Ann Intern Med 111:893–899, 1989.

46. Whitley RJ, Gnann JW: Acyclovir: A decade later. N Engl J Med 327:782–789, 1992.

47. Chakrabarti S, Pillay D, Ratcliffe D et al: Resistance to antiviral drugs in herpes simplex virus infections among allogeneic stem cell transplant recipients: risk factors and prognostic significance. J Infect Dis 181:2055–2058, 2000.

48. Safrin S, Assakeen T, Follansbee S, Mills J: Foscarnet therapy for acyclovir-resistant mucocutaneous herpes simplex virus infection in 26 AIDS patients: Preliminary data. J Infect Dis 161:1078, 1990.

49. Safrin S, Crumpacker C, Chatis et al: A controlled trial comparing foscarnet with vidarabine for acyclovir-resistant mucocutaneous herpes simplex in the acquired immunodeficiency syndrome. N Engl J Med 325:551–5, 1991.

50. Straus SE, Wald A, Kost RG et al: Immunotherapy of recurrent genital herpes with recombinant herpes simplex virus type 2 glycoproteins D and B: Results of a placebo-controlled vaccine trial. J Infect Dis 176:1129–1134, 1997.

51. Fries BC, Chou S, Boeckh M et al: Frequency distribution of cytomegalovirus envelope glycoprotein genotypes in bone marrow transplant recipients. J Infect Dis 169:769–774, 1994.

52. Torok-Storb B, Boeckh M, Hoy C et al: Association of specific cytomegalovirus genotypes with death from myelosuppression after marrow transplantation. Blood 90:2097–2102, 1997.

53. Bowden RA, Slichter SJ, Sayers MH, Mori M, Cays MJ, Meyers JD: Use of leukocyte-depleted platelets and cytomegalovirus-seronegative red blood cells for prevention of primary cytomegalovirus infection after marrow transplant. Blood 78:246–250, 1991.

54. De Witte T, Schattenbereg A, Van Dijk BA, Galama J, Olthuis H, Van Der Meer JWW, Kunst VAJM: Prevention of primary cytomegalovirus infection after allogeneic bone marrow transplantation by using leukocyte-poor random blood products from cytomegalovirus-unscreened blood-bank donors. Transplantation 50:964–968, 1990.

55. Winston DJ, Ho WG, Howell CL et al: Cytomegalovirus infections associated with leukocyte transfusions. Ann Intern Med 93:671, 1980.

56. Wingard JR, Piantadosi S, Burns WH et al: Cytomegalovirus infections in patients treated by intensive cytoreductive therapy with marrow transplant. Rev Infect Dis 12(Suppl. 7):S805–810, 1990.

57. Winston DJ, Ho WG, Champlin RE: Cytomegalovirus infections after allogeneic bone marrow transplantation. Rev Infect Dis 12 (Suppl. 7):S776–792, 1990.

58. Hutza AST, Muhl E, Hackstein H et al: High incidence of active cytomegalovirus infection among septic patients. Clin Infect Dis 26:1076–1082, 1998.

59. Ho M: Editorial response: Cytomegalovirus infection in patients with bacterial sepsis. Clin Infect Dis 26:1083–1084, 1998.

60. Henson D, Siegel SE, Fucillo DA et al: Cytomegalovirus infections during acute childhood leukemia. J Infect Dis 126:469, 1972.

61. Vaughan WP, Saral R, Anderson LR, Burke PJ: The frequency and pattern of cytomegalovirus (CMV) infection and shedding by patients who have received high dose times-sequential chemotherapy (TSC) for acute myelocytic leukemia (AML). Proceedings of the 17th Annual Meeting of the American Society of Clinical Oncology, Washington, DC, April 30-May 2, 1981, p.170, Abstract 673.

62. Wade JC, Bustamante CI, Newman KA, Devlin AM: Cytomegalovirus: An important pathogen for adults receiving induction therapy for acute leukemia. Presented at 28th Annual Interscience Conference on Antimicrobial Agents and Chemotherapy, Los Angeles, October 23–26, 1988 Abstract 1394.

63. Zaia JA, Forman SJ, Ting Y-P, Vanderwal-Urbina E, Blume KG: Polypeptide-specific antibody response to human cytomegalovirus after infection in bone marrow transplant recipients. J Infect Dis 153:780–787, 1986.

64. Einsele H, Ehninger G, Steidle M et al: Lymphocytopenia as an unfavorable prognostic factor in patients with cytomegalovirus infection after bone marrow transplantation. Blood 82:1672–78, 1993.

65. Quinan GV Jr, Kirmani N, Rook AH et al: Cytotoxic cells in cytomegalovirus infections. HLA-restricted T-lymphocyte and non-T-lymphocyte cytotoxic responses correlate with recovery from cytomegalovirus infection in bone marrow transplant recipients. N Engl J Med 307:7, 1982.

66. Reusser P, Riddel SR, Meyers SD, Greenberg PD: Cytotoxic T-lymphocyte response to cytomegalovirus after human allogeneic bone marrow transplantation: Pattern of recovery and correlation with cytomegalovirus infection and disease. Blood 78:1373–1380, 1991.

67. Quinnan GV Jr, Burns WH, Kirmani N et al: HLA-restricted cytotoxic T lymphocytes are an early immune response and important defense mechanism in cytomegalovirus infections. Rev Infect Dis 6:156–163, 1984.

68. Reusser P, Attenhofer R, Hebart H et al: Cytomegalovirus-specific T-cell immunity in recipients of autologous peripheral blood stem cell or bone marrow transplants. Blood 89:3873–3879, 1997.

69. Shanley JD: Murine cytomegalovirus pneumonitis in T cell deficient nude mice. In: Abstracts of the 12th Herpesvirus Workshop, Philadelphia, 1987.

70. Grundy JE, Shanley JD, Shearer GM: Augmentation of graft versus host reaction by cytomegalovirus infection resulting in interstitial pneumonitis. Transplantation 39:548–53, 1985.

71. Shanley JD, Pesanti EL, Nugent KM: The pathogenesis of pneumonitis due to murine cytomegalovirus. J Infect Dis 146:388–86, 1982.

72. Shanley JD, Pomeroy C, Via CS, Shearer GM: Interstitial pneumonitis during murine cytomegalovirus infection and graft-versus-host reaction: Effect of ganciclovir therapy. J Infect Dis 158:1391–4, 1988.

73. Shanley JD, Pesanti EL: The relation of viral replication to interstitial pneumonitis in murine cytomegalovirus lung infection. J Infect Dis 151:454–8, 1985.

74. Appelbaum FR, Meyers JD, Fefer A et al: Nonbacterial nonfungal pneumonia following marrow transplantation in 100 identical twins. Transplantation 46:61–5, 1982.

75. Wingard JR, Chen DY-H, Burns WH et al: Cytomegalovirus infection after autologous bone marrow transplantation: Comparison to infection after allogeneic bone marrow transplantation. Blood 71:1432–37, 1988.

76. Reusser P, Fisher LD, Buckner CD, Thomas ED, Meyers JD: Cytomegalovirus infection after autologous bone marrow transplantation: Occurrence of cytomegalovirus disease and effect on engraftment. Blood 75:1888–94, 1990.

77. Ljungman P, Biron P, Bosi A et al: Cytomegalovirus interstitial pneumonia in autologous bone marrow transplant recipients. Bone Marrow Transplant 13:209–212, 1994.

78. Wingard JR, Sostrin MB, Vriesendorp HM et al: Interstitial pneumonitis following autologous bone marrow transplantation. Transplantation 46:61–65, 1988.

79. Enright H, Haake R, Weisdorf D, Ramsay N, McGlave P, Kersey J, Thomas W, McKenzie, Miller W: Cytomegalovirus pneumonia after bone marrow transplantation. Transplantation 55:1339–1346, 1993.

80. Meyers JD, Flournoy N, Thomas ED: Risk factors for cytomegalovirus infection after human marrow transplantation. J Infect Dis 153:478–488, 1986.

81. Miller W, Flynn P, McCullough J et al: Cytomegalovirus infection after marrow transplantation: An association with acute graft-versus-host-disease. Blood 67:1161–1167, 1986.

82. Meyers JD, Flournoy N, Thomas ED: Risk factors for cytomegalovirus infection after human marrow transplantation. J Infect Dis 153:478–88, 1986.

83. Miller W, Flynn P, McCullough J et al: Cytomegalovirus infection after bone marrow transplantation: An association with acute graft-versus-host disease. Blood 67:1162–7, 1986.

84. Weiner RS, Bortin MM, Gale RP et al: Interstitial pneumonitis after bone marrow transplantation. Ann Intern Med 104:168–75, 1986.

85. Wingard JR, Mellits ED, Sostrin MB et al: Interstitial pneumonitis after allogeneic bone marrow transplantation: Nine-year experience at a single institution. Medicine (Baltimore) 67:175–86, 1988.

86. Meyers JD, Ljungman P, Fisher LD: Cytomegalovirus excretion as a predictor of cytomegalovirus disease after marrow transplantation: Importance of cytomegalovirus viremia. J Infect Dis 162:373–380, 1990.

87. Paulin T, Ringden O, Lönnqvist B, Wahren B, Nilsson B: The importance of pre bone marrow transplantation serology in determining subsequent cytomegalovirus infection: Analysis of risk factors. Scand J Infect Dis 18:199–209, 1986.

88. Schmidt GM, Horak DA, Niland JC et al: A randomized, controlled trial of prophylactic ganciclovir for cytomegalovirus pulmonary infection in recipients of allogeneic bone marrow transplant patients. N Engl J Med 324:1005–1011, 1991.

89. Slavin M, Gooley TA, Bowden RA: Prediction of cytomegalovirus pneumonia after marrow transplantation from cellular characteristics and cytomegalovirus culture of bronchoalveolar lavage fluid. Transplantation 58:915–919, 1994.

90. Alessandrino EP, Varettoni M, Colombo AA et al: High incidence of symptomatic cytomegalovirus infection in multiple myeloma patients undergoing autologous peripheral blood stem cell transplantation. Blood 95:4016–4017, 2000.

91. Holmberg LA, Boeckh M, Hooper H et al: Increased incidence of cytomegalovirus disease after autologous CD34-selected peripheral blood stem cell transplantation. Blood 94:4029–4035, 1999.

92. Schiller GJ, Vescio R, Berenson J: Cytomegalovirus infection following transplantation of autologous CD34-selected progenitor cells. Blood 96:1194, 2000.

93. Gregory WW, Menegus MA: Practical protocol for cytomegalovirus isolation: Use of MRC-5 cell monolayers incubated for 2 weeks. J Clin Microbiol 17:605–609, 1983.

94. Gleaves CA, Smith TF, Shuster EA, Pearson GR: Rapid detection of cytomegalovirus in MRC-5 cells inoculated with urine specimens by using low-speed centrifugation and monoclonal antibody to an early antigen. J Clin Microbiol 19:917–919, 1984.

95. Leland DS, Hansing RL, French ML: Clinical experiences with cytomegalovirus isolation using conventional cell cultures and early antigen detection in centrifugation-enhanced shell vial cultures. J Clin Microbiol 27:1159–1162, 1989.

96. Gleaves CA, Smith TF, Shuster EA, Pearson GR: Comparison of standard tube and shell vial cell culture techniques for the detection of cytomegalovirus in clinical specimens. J Clin Microbiol 21:217, 1985.

97. Boeckh M, Bowden RA, Goodrich JM, Pettinger M, Meyers JD: Cytomegalovirus antigen detection in peripheral blood leukocytes after allogeneic marrow transplantation. Blood 80:1358–1364, 1992.

98. Van der Bij W, Torensma R, van Son WJ et al: Rapid immunodiagnosis of active cytomegalovirus infection by monoclonal antibody staining of blood leucocytes. J Med Virol 25:179–188, 1988.

99. Jiwa NM, van de Rijke FM, Mulder A et al: An improved immunocytochemical method for detection of human cytomegalovirus antigens in peripheral blood leucocytes. Histochemistry 91:345–349, 1989.

100. Spector SA, Merrill R, Wolf D et al: Detection of human cytomegalovirus in plasma of AIDS patients during acute visceral disease by DNA amplification. J Clin Microbiol 30:2359–2365, 1992.

101. Brytting M, Xu W, Wahren B et al: Cytomegalovirus DNA detection in sera from patients with active cytomegalovirus infections. J Clin Microbiol 30:1937–1941, 1992.

102. Einsele H, Steidle M, Vallbracht A, Saal JG, Ehninger G, Muller CA: Early occurrence of human cytomegalovirus infection after bone marrow transplantation as demonstrated by the polymerase chain reaction technique. Blood 77:1104–1110, 1991.

103. Nolte FS, Emmens RK, Thurmond C, Mitchell PS, Pascuzzi C, Devine SM, Saral R, Wingard JR: Early detection of human cytomegalovirus viremia in bone marrow transplant recipients by DNA amplification. J Clin Microbiol 33:1263–1266, 1995.

104. Landry ML, Fergussen D: Comparison of quantitative cytomegalovirus antigenemia assay with culture methods and correlation with clinical disease. J Clin Microbiol 31:2851–2856, 1993.

105. Schmidt CA, Oettle H, Wilborn F, Jessen J, Timm H, Schwerdtfeger R, Oertal J, Siegert W: Demonstration of cytomegalovirus after bone marrow transplantation by polymerase chain reaction, virus culture and antigen detection in buffy coat leukocytes. Bone Marrow Transplant 13:71–75, 1994.

106. Hackman RC, Wolford JL, Gleaves CA, Myerson D, Beauchamp MD, Meyers JD, McDonald GB: Recognition and rapid diagnosis of upper gastrointestinal cytomegalovirus infection in marrow transplant recipients. Transplantation 57:231–237, 1994.

107. Crawford SW, Bowden RA, Hackman RC et al: Rapid detection of cytomegalovirus pulmonary infection by bronchoalveolar lavage and centrifugation culture. Ann Intern Med 108:180–5, 1988.

108. Meyers JD, McGuffin RW, Bryson YJ, Cantell K, Thomas ED: Treatment of cytomegalovirus pneumonia after marrow transplant with combined vidarabine and human leukocyte interferon. J Infect Dis 146:80–84, 1982.

109. Wade JC, Hintz M, McGuffin RW et al: Treatment of cytomegalovirus pneumonia with high-dose acyclovir. Am J Med 73A:249, 1982.

110. Wade JC, McGuffin RW, Springmeyer SC, Newton B, Singer JW, Meyers JD: Treatment of cytomegaloviral pneumonia with high-dose acyclovir and human leukocyte interferon. J Infect Dis 148:557–562, 1983.

111. Meyers JD, Flournoy N, Sanders JE et al: Prophylactic human leukocyte interferon after allogeneic marrow transplantation. Ann Intern Med 107:809, 1987.

112. Reed EC, Bowden RA, Dandliker PS et al: Efficacy of cytomegalovirus immunoglobulin in marrow transplant recipients with cytomegalovirus pneumonia. J Infect Dis 156:641, 1987.

113. Shepp DH, Dandliker PS, deMiranda P et al: Activity of 9-[2-hydroxy-1-(hydroxymethyl)ethoxymethyl]guanine in the treatment of cytomegalovirus pneumonia. Ann Intern Med 103:368, 1985.

114. Reed EC, Dandliker PS, Meyers JD: Treatment of cytomegalovirus pneumonia with 9-[2-hydroxy-1-(hydroxymethyl)ethoxymethyl]guanine and high dose corticosteroids. Ann Intern Med 105:214–216, 1986.

115. Bratanow NC, Ash RC, Turner PA: Successful treatment of serious cytomegalovirus (CMV) disease with 9-(1,3-dihydroxy-2-propoxymethyl)guanine (ganciclovir), DHPG) and intravenous immunoglobulin (IVIG) in bone marrow transplant (BMT) patients Exp Hematol 15:541(abstract no. 254), 1987.

116. Emanuel D, Cunningham I, Jules-Elysee K et al: Cytomegalovirus pneumonia after bone marrow transplantation successfully treated with the combination of ganciclovir and high-dose intravenous immune globulin. Ann Intern Med 109:777–782, 1988.

117. Reed EC, Bowden RA, Dandliker PS et al: Treatment of cytomegalovirus pneumonia with ganciclovir and intravenous cytomegalovirus immunoglobulin in patients with bone marrow transplants. Ann Intern Med 109:783–8, 1988.

118. Schmidt GM, Kovacs A, Zaia JA et al: Ganciclovir/immunoglobulin combination therapy for the treatment of human cytomegalovirus-associated interstitial pneumonia in bone marrow allograft recipients. Transplantation 46:905–907, 1988.

119. Ljungman P, De Bock R, Cordonnier C et al: Practices for cytomegalovirus diagnosis, prophylaxis and treatment in allogeneic bone marrow transplant recipients: A report from the Working Party for Infectious Diseases of the EBMT. Bone Marrow Transplant 12:399–403, 1993.

120. Reed EC, Wolford JL, Kopecky KJ et al: Ganciclovir for the treatment of cytomegalovirus gastroenteritis in bone marrow transplant patients. A randomized, placebo-controlled trial. Ann Intern Med 112:505–10, 1990.

121. Ljungman P, Cordonnier C, Einsele H et al: Use of intravenous immune globulin in addition to antiviral therapy in the treatment of CMV gastrointestinal disease in allogeneic bone marrow transplant patients: A report from the European Group for Blood and Marrow Transplantation (EBMT). Infectious Diseases Working Party of the EBMT. 21:473–476, 1998.

122. Bowden RA, Sayers M, Flournoy N, Newton B, Banaji M, Thomas D, Meyers JD: Cytomegalovirus immune globulin and seronegative blood products to prevent primary cytomegalovirus infection after marrow transplantation. N Engl J Med 314:1006–10, 1986.

123. Mackinnon S, Burnett AK, Crawford RJ, Cameron S, Leask BGS, Sommerville RG: Seronegative blood products prevent primary cytomegalovirus infection after bone marrow transplantation. J Clin Pathol 41:948–950, 1988.

124. Miller W, McCullough J, Balfour HH et al: Prevention of CMV infection by blood products: A randomized trial. J Cell Biochem 12(Suppl. C): 93 (abstract no. K128) 1988.

125. Bowden RA, Slichter SJ, Sayers M et al: A comparison of filtered leukocyte-reduced and cytomegalovirus (CMV) seronegative blood products for the prevention of transfusion-associated CMV infection after marrow transplant. Blood 86:3598–3603, 1995.

126. Winston DJ, Ho WG, Lin CH et al: Intravenous immune globulin for prevention of cytomegalovirus infection and interstitial pneumonia after bone marrow transplantation. Ann Intern Med 106:12–18, 1987.

127. Bass EB, Powe NR, Goodman SN et al: Efficacy of Intravenous immune globulin in preventing complications of bone marrow transplantation: A meta analysis. Bone Marrow Transplant 12:273–282, 1993.

128. Messori A, Rampazzo R, Scroccaro G, Martini N: Efficacy of hyperimmune anticytomegalovirus immunoglobulins for the prevention of cytomegalovirus infection in recipients of allogeneic bone marrow transplantation: A meta-analysis. Bone Marrow Transplant 13:163–167, 1994.

129. Guglielmo BJ, Wong-Beringer A, Linker CA: Immune globulin therapy in allogeneic bone marrow transplant: A critical review. Bone Marrow Transplant 13:499–510, 1994.

130. Sullivan KM, Kopecky KJ, Jocum J et al: Immunomodulatory and antimicrobial efficacy of intravenous immunoglobulin in bone marrow transplantation. N Engl J Med 323:705–712, 1990.

131. Wolff SN, Fay JW, Herzig RH et al: High-dose intravenous immunoglobulin to prevent infections in patients undergoing autologous bone marrow transplantation or severe myelosuppressive therapy. Ann Intern Med 118:937–942, 1993.

132. Meyers JD, Reed EC, Shepp DH et al: Acyclovir for prevention of cytomegalovirus infection and disease after allogeneic marrow transplantation. N Engl J Med 318:70–5, 1988.

133. Prentice HG, Gluckman E, Powles RL et al: Impact of long-term acyclovir on cytomegalovirus infection and survival after allogeneic bone marrow transplantation. Lancet 343:749–53, 1994.

134. Schmidt GM, Horak DA, Niland JC et al: A randomized, controlled trial of prophylactic ganciclovir for cytomegalovirus pulmonary infection in recipients of allogeneic bone marrow transplants. N Engl J Med 324:1005–11, 1991.

135. Goodrich JM, Mori M, Gleaves CA et al: Early treatment with ganciclovir to prevent cytomegalovirus disease after allogeneic bone marrow transplant. N Engl J Med 325:1601–7, 1991.

136. Goodrich JM, Bowden RA, Fisher L et al: Ganciclovir prophylaxis to prevent cytomegalovirus disease after allogeneic marrow transplant. Ann Intern Med 118:173–178, 1993.

137. Winston DJ, Ho WG, Bartoni K et al: Ganciclovir prophylaxis of cytomegalovirus infection and disease in allogeneic bone marrow transplant recipients. Ann Intern Med 118:179–184, 1993.

138. Salzberger B, Bowden RA, Hackman RC et al: Neutropenia in allogeneic marrow transplant recipients receiving ganciclovir for prevention of cytomegalovirus disease: Risk factors and outcome. Blood 90:2502–2508, 1997.

139. Stocchi R, Szydlo R, Craddock C et al: A comparison of prophylactic vs pre-emptive ganciclovir to prevent cytomegalovirus disease after T-depleted volunteer unrelated donor bone marrow transplantation. Bone Marrow Transplant 23:705–709, 1999.

140. Goodrich JM, Boeckh M, Bowden R: Strategies for the prevention of cytomegalovirus disease after marrow transplantation. Clin Infect Dis 19:287–98, 1994.

141. Forman SJ, Zaia JA: Treatment and prevention of cytomegalovirus pneumonia after bone marrow transplantation: Where do we stand? Blood 83:2392–2398, 1994.

142. Devine SM, Wingard JR: Viral infections in severely immunocompromised cancer patients. Support Care Cancer 2:355–368, 1994.

143. Boeckh M, Gooley TA, Bowden RA: Effect of high-dose acyclovir on survival in allogeneic marrow transplant recipients who received ganciclovir at engraftment or for cytomegalovirus pp65 antigenemia. J Infect Dis 178:1153–1157, 1998.

144. Przepiorka D, Ippoliti C, Panina A et al: Ganciclovir three times per week is not adequate to prevent cytomegalovirus reactivation after T cell-depleted marrow transplantation. Bone Marrow Transplant 13:461–464, 1994.

145. Singhal S, Mehta J, Powles R et al.: Three weeks of ganciclovir for cytomegalovirus after allogeneic bone marrow transplantation. Bone Marrow Transplant 15:777–781, 1995.

146. Zaia JA, Gallez-Hawkins GM, Klongmate J et al: Late bacterial and fungal sepsis and mortality after BMT are increased by duration of early ganciclovir preemptive therapy for CMV infection. Blood 92(Suppl. 1):518a (abstract no. 2128), 1998.

147. Polis MA, Masur H: Promising new treatments for cytomegalovirus retinitis. JAMA 273:1457–1459, 1995.

148. Drew WL, Stempien MJ, Andrews J et al: Cytomegalovirus (CMV) resistance in patients with CMV retinitis and AIDS treated with oral or intravenous ganciclovir. J Infect Dis 179:1352–1355, 1999.

149. Drew WL: Ganciclovir resistance: A matter of time and titre. Lancet 356:609–610, 2000.

150. Brown F, Banken L, Saywell K: Pharmacokinetics of valganciclovir and ganciclovir following multiple oral dosages of valganciclovir in HIV and CMV-seropositive volunteers. Clin Pharmacokinet 37:167–176, 1999.

151. Jung D, Dorr A: Single-dose pharmacokinetics of valganciclovir in HIV- and CMV-seropositive subjects. J Clin Pharmacol 39:800–804, 1999.

152. Pescovits MD, Rabkin J, Merion RM et al: Valganciclovir results in improved oral absorption of ganciclovir in liver transplant recipients. Antimicrob Agents Chemother 44:2811–2815, 2000.

153. Liu W, Baruch D, Kuppermann BD et al: Mutations in the cytomegalovirus UL97 gene associated with ganciclovir-resistant retinitis. J Infect Dis 177:1176–1181, 1998.

154. Baldanti F, Underwood MR, Stanat SC et al: Single amino acid changes in the DNA polymerase confer foscarnet resistance and slow-growth phenotype, while mutations in the UL97-encoded phosphotransferase confer ganciclovir resistance in three double-resistant human cytomegalovirus strains recovered from patients with AIDS. J Virol 70:1390–1395, 1996.

155. Smith IL, Cherrington JM, Jiles RE et al: High-level resistance of cytomegalovirus to ganciclovir is associated with alterations in both the UL97 and DNA polymerase genes. J Infect Dis 176:69–77, 1997.

156. Erice A, Gil-Roda C, Perez JL et al: Antiviral susceptibilities and analysis of UL97 and DNA polymerase sequences of clinical cytomegalovirus isolates from immunocompromised patients. J Infect Dis 175:1087–1092, 1997.

157. Perez JL: Resistance to antivirals in human cytomegalovirus: Mechanisms and clinical significance. Microbiologia 13:343–352, 1997.

158. Aschan J, Ringden O, Ljungman P, Lonnqvist B, Ohlman S: Foscarnet for treatment of cytomegalovirus infections in bone marrow transplant recipients. Scand J Infect Dis 24:143–50, 1992.

159. Reusser P, Gambertoglio JG, Lilleby K, Meyers JD: Phase I–II trial of foscarnet for prevention of cytomegalovirus infection in autologous and allogeneic marrow transplant recipients. J infect Dis JID 166:473–9, 1992.

160. Bacigalupo A, Tedone E, Van Lint MT et al: CMV prophylaxis with foscarnet in allogeneic bone marrow transplant recipients at high risk of developing CMV infections. Bone Marrow Transplant 13:783–788, 1994.

161. Moretti S, Zikos P, Van Lint MT et al: Foscarnet vs ganciclovir for cytomegalovirus (CMV) antigenemia after allogeneic hemopoietic stem cell transplantation (HSCT): A randomised study. Bone Marrow Transplant 22:175–180. 1998.

162. Ordemann R, Naumann R, Geissler G et al: Foscarnet – an alternative for cytomegalovirus prophylaxis after allogeneic stem cell transplantation. Ann Hematol 79;432–436, 2000.

163. Bacigalupo A, Bregante S, Tedone E et al: Combined foscarnet-ganciclovir treatment for cytomegalovirus infections after allogeneic hemopoietic stem cell transplantation. Transplantation 62:376–380, 1995.

164. Razis E, Cook P, Mittelman A, Ahmed T: Treatment of ganciclovir resistant cytomegalovirus with foscarnet: A report of two cases occurring after bone marrow transplantation. Leuk Lymphoma 12:477–80, 1994.

165. Lalezari JP, Holland GN, Kramer F et al: Randomized controlled study of the safety and efficacy of intravenous cidofovir for the treatment of relapsing cytomegalovirus retinitis in patients with AIDS. J Acquir Immune Defic Syndr 17:339–344, 1998.

166. Jabs DA, Freeman WR, Jacobson M, and The Studies of Ocular Complications of AIDS Research Group in collaboration with the AIDS Clinical Trials Group. Long-term follow-up of patients with AIDS treated with parenteral cidofovir for cytomegalovirus retinitis: The HPMPC Peripheral Cytomegalovirus Retinitis Trial. AIDS 14:1571–1581, 2000.

167. Plosker GL, Noble S: Cidofovir: A review of its use in cytomegalovirus retinitis in patients with AIDS. Drugs 58:325–345, 1999.

168. Ljungman P, Deliliers GL, Ribaud P et al: Cidofovir for treatment of CMV and adenovirus infections in allogeneic stem cell transplant recipients. Blood 94 (Suppl. 1):396a (abstract no. 1753), 1999.

169. Smith IL, Cherrington JM Jiles RE et al: High-level resistance of cytomegalovirus to ganciclovir is associated with alterations in both the UL97 and DNA polymerase gene. J Infect Dis 176:69–77, 1997.

170. Nguyen Q, Champlin R, Giralt S et al: Late cytomegalovirus pneumonia in adult allogeneic blood and marrow transplant recipients. Clin Infect Dis 28:618–623, 1999.

171. Atkinson K, Nivison-Smith I, Dodds A et al: A comparison of the pattern of interstitial pneumonitis following allogeneic bone marrow transplantation before and after the introduction of prophylactic ganciclovir therapy in 1989. Bone Marrow Transplant 21:691–695, 1998.

172. Zaia JA, Gallez-Hawkins GM, Teftmeier BR et al: Late cytomegalovirus disease in marrow transplantation is predicted by virus load in plasma. J Infect Dis 176:782–785, 1997.

173. Ljungman P, Aschan J, Azinge JN et al: Cytomegalovirus viraemia and specific T-helper cell responses as predictors of disease after allogeneic marrow transplantation. Br J Hematol 83:118–124, 1993.

174. Machado CM, Dulley FL, Vilas-Boas LS et al: CMV pneumonia in allogeneic BMT recipients undergoing early treatment or preemptive ganciclovir therapy. Bone Marrow Transplant 26:413–417, 2000.

175. Boeckh M, Riddell SR, Cunningham T et al: Increased risk of late CMV infection and disease in allogeneic marrow transplant recipients after ganciclovir prophylaxis is due to a lack of CMV-specific T cell responses. Blood 86 (Suppl. 1):302a (abstr. no. 1195), 1996.

176. Einsele H, Hebart H, Kauffmann-Schneider C et al: Risk factors for treatment failures in patients receiving PCR-based preemptive therapy for CMV infection. Bone Marrow Transplant 25:757–763, 2000.

177. Li CR, Greenberg PD, Gilbert MJ, Goodrich JM, Riddell SR: Recovery of HLA-restricted cytomegalovirus (CMV)-specific T-cell responses after allogeneic bone marrow transplant: Correlation with CMV disease and effect of ganciclovir prophylaxis. Blood 83:1971–1979, 1994.

178. Zaia JA, Gallez-Hawkins G, Tegtmeier BR et al: Late cytomegalovirus disease in marrow transplantation is predicted by virus load in plasma. J Infect Dis 176:782–5. 1997

179. Riddell SR, Walter BA, Gilbert MJ, Greenberg PD: Selective reconstitution of CD8+ cytotoxic T lymphocyte responses in immunodeficient bone marrow transplant recipients by the adoptive transfer of T cell clones. Bone Marrow Transplant 14:S78–S84, 1994.

180. Riddell SR, Watanabe KS, Goodrich JM, Li CR, Agha ME, Greenberg PD: Restoration of viral immunity in immunodeficient humans by the adoptive transfer of T-cell clones. Science 257:238, 1992.

181. Riddell SR, Reusser P, Greenberg PD: Cytotoxic T-cells specific for cytomegalovirus: A potential therapy for immunocompromised hosts. Rev Infect Dis 13(Suppl. 1):966–973, 1991.

182. Drew WL, Miner RC, Busch DF et al: Prevalence of resistance in patients receiving ganciclovir for serious cytomegalovirus infection. J Infect Dis 163:716–9, 1991.

183. Rowe JM, Ciobanu N, Ascensao J et al: Recommended guidelines for the management of autologous and allogeneic bone marrow transplantation. A report from the Eastern Cooperative Oncology Group (ECOG). Ann Intern Med 120:143–158, 1994.

184. Goffinet DR, Glatstein EJ, Merigan TC: Herpes zoster-varicella infections and lymphoma. Ann Intern Med 76:235, 1972.

185. Coker DD, Morris DM, Coleman JJ et al: Infection among 210 patients with surgically staged Hodgkin's disease. Am J Med 75:97, 1983.

186. Atkinson K, Meyers JD, Storb R, Prentice RL, Thomas ED: Varicella-zoster virus infection after marrow transplantation for aplastic anemia or leukemia. Transplantation 29:47, 1980.

187. Locksley PRM, Flournoy N, Sullivan KM, Meyers JD: Infection with varicella-zoster virus after marrow transplantation. J Infect Dis 152:1172–1181, 1985.

188. Schuchter LM, Wingard JR, Piantadosi S, Burns WH, Santos GW, Saral R: Herpes zoster infection after autologous bone marrow transplantation. Blood 74:1424–1427, 1989.

189. Han CS, Miller W, Haake R, Weisdorf D: Varicella zoster infection after bone marrow transplantation: Incidence, risk factors and complications. Bone Marrow Transplant 13:277–283, 1994.

190. Feldman S, Lott L: Varicella in children with cancer: Impact of antiviral therapy and prophylaxis. Pediatrics 80:465, 1987.

191. Schiller GJ, Nimer SD, Gajewski JL, Golde D: Abdominal presentation of varicella-zoster infection in recipients of allogeneic bone marrow transplantation. Bone Marrow Transplant 7:489–491, 1991.

192. Yagi T, Karasuno T, Hasegawa T et al: Acute abdomen without cutaneous signs of varicella zoster virus infection as a late complication of allogeneic bone marrow transplantation: Importance of empiric therapy with acyclovir. Bone Marrow Transplant 25:1003–1005, 2000.

193. David DS, Teftmeier BR, O'Donnell MR et al: Visceral varicella-zoster after bone marrow transplantation: Report of a case series and review of the literature. Am J Gastroenterol 93:810–813, 1998.

194. Ljungman P, Lönnqvist B, Gahrton G, Ringdén O, Sundqvist V-A, Wahren B: Clinical and subclinical reactivations of varicella-zoster virus in immunocompromised patients. J Infect Dis 153:840–847, 1986.

195. Schmidt NJ, Ballo D, Devlin V, Woodie JD, Emmons RW: Direct immuno-fluorescence staining for detection of herpes simplex and varicella-zoster virus antigens in vesicular lesion and certain tissue specimens. J Clin Microbiol 12:651–655, 1980.

196. Balfour HH Jr, Bean B, Laskin OL el al. and the Burroughs Wellcome Collaborative Acyclovir Study Group: Acyclovir halts progression of herpes zoster in immunocompromised patients. N Engl J Med 308:1448–1453, 1983.

197. Meyers JD, Wade JC, Shepp DH, Newton B: Acyclovir treatment of varicella-zoster virus infection in the compromised host. Transplantation 37:571, 1984.

198. Shepp DH, Dandliker PS, Meyers JD: Treatment of varicella-zoster virus infection in severely immunocompromised patients: A randomized comparison of acyclovir and vidarabine. N Engl J Med 314:208–212, 1986.

199. McKendrick MW, McGill JI, White JE, Wood MJ: Oral acyclovir in acute herpes zoster. Br Med J 293:1529–1532, 1986.

200. Ljungman P, Lönnqvist B, Ringdén O, Skinhöj P, Gahrton G for the Nordic Bone Marrow Transplant Group: A randomized trial of oral versus intravenous acyclovir for treatment of herpes zoster in bone marrow transplant recipients. Bone Marrow Transplant 4:613–615, 1989.

201. Whitley RJ, Soong S-J, Dolin R et al: and the NIAID Collaborative Antiviral Study Group. Early vidarabine therapy to control the complications of herpes zoster in immunosuppressed patients. N Eng J Med 307:971, 1982.

202. Merigan TC, Rand KH, Pollard RB et al: Human leukocyte interferon for the treatment of herpes-zoster in patients with cancer. N Engl J Med 298:981, 1978.

203. Winston DJ, Eron LJ, Ho M et al: Recombinant interferon alpha-2a for treatment of herpes zoster in immunosuppressed patients with cancer. Am J Med 85:147, 1988.

204. Beutner KR, Friedman DJ, Forszpaniak C et al: Valaciclovir compared with acyclovir for improved therapy for herpes zoster immunocompetent adults. Antimicrob Agents Chemother 39:1546–1553, 1995.

205. Tyring S, Barbarash RA, Nahlik JE et al: Famciclovir for the treatment of acute herpes zoster: Effects on acute disease and postherpetic neuralgia. A randomized, double-blind, placebo-controlled trial. Collaborative Famciclovir Herpes Zoster Study Group. Ann Intern Med 123:89–96, 1995.

206. Tyring SK, Beutner KR, Tucker BA et al: Antiviral therapy for herpes zoster: Randomized, controlled clinical trial of valacyclovir and famciclovir therapy in immunocompetent patients 50 years and older. Arch Fam Med 9:863–869, 2000.

207. Wallace MR, Chamberlin CJ, Sawyer MH et al: Treatment of adult varicella with sorivudine: A randomized, placebo-controlled trial. J Infect Dis 174:249–255, 1996.

208. Bodsworth NJ, Boag F, Burdge D et al: Evaluation of sorivudine (BV-ara U) versus acyclovir in the treatment of acute localized herpes zoster in human immunodeficiency virus-infected adults. The Multinational Sorivudine Study Group. J Infect Dis 176:103–111, 1997.

209. Diasio RB: Sorivudine and 5-fluorouracil: A clinically significant drug-drug interaction due to inhibition of dihydropyrimidine dehydrogenase. Br J Clin Pharmacol 46:1–4, 1998.

210. Boivin G, Edleman CK, Pedneault L, Talarico CL, Biron KK, Balfour HH Jr: Phenotypic and genotypic characterization of acyclovir-resistant varicella-zoster viruses isolated from persons with AIDS. J Infect Dis 170:68–75, 1994.

211. Safrin S, Berger TG, Gilson I et al: Foscarnet therapy in five patients with AIDS and acyclovir-resistant varicella-zoster virus infection. Ann Intern Med 115:19–21, 1991.

212. Zaia JA, Levin MJ, Preblud SR et al: Evaluation of varicella-zoster immune globulin: Protection of immunosuppressed children after household exposure to varicella. J Infect Dis 147:737, 1983.

213. Gershon AA: Live attenuated varicella vaccine: Perspective. J Infect Dis 152:859, 1985.

214. Gershon AA: Live attenuated varicella vaccine. J Pediatr 110:154, 1987.

215. Gershon AA, Steinberg SP, and the Varicella Vaccine Collaborative Study Group of the NIAID: Persistence of immunity of varicella

in children with leukemia immunized with live attenuated varicella vaccine. N Engl J Med 320:892, 1989.

216. Gershon AA, Steinberg SP, and the National Institute of Allergy and Infectious Diseases Varicella Vaccine Collaborative Study Group: Live attenuated varicella vaccine: Protection in healthy adults compared with leukemic children. J Infect Dis 161:661, 1990.

217. Lawrence R, Gershon AA, Holzman R et al: The risk of zoster after varicella vaccination in children with leukemia. N Engl J Med 318:543, 1988.

218. Diaz PS, Au D, Smith S et al: Lack of transmission of the live attenuated varicella vaccine virus to immunocompromised children after immunization of their siblings. Pediatrics 87:166–170, 1991.

219. Ljungman P, Wilczek H, Gahrton G et al: Long-term acyclovir prophylaxis in bone marrow transplant recipients and lymphocyte proliferation responses to herpes virus antigens in vitro. Bone Marrow Transplant 1:185–192, 1986.

220. Perren TJ, Powles RL, Easton D et al: Prevention of herpes zoster in patients by long-term oral acyclovir after allogeneic bone marrow transplantation. Am J Med 85:99–101, 1988.

221. Sempere A, Sanz GF, Senent L et al: Long-term acyclovir prophylaxis for prevention of varicella zoster virus infection after autologous blood stem cell transplantation in patients with acute leukemia. Bone Marrow Transplant 10:495–498, 1992.

222. Steer CB, Szer J, Sasadeusz J et al: Varicella-zoster infection after allogeneic bone marrow transplantation: Incidence, risk factors and prevention with low-dose acyclovir and ganciclovir. Bone Marrow Transplant 25:657–664, 2000.

223. Selby PJ, Powles RL, Easton D et al: The prophylactic role of intravenous and long-term oral acyclovir after allogeneic bone marrow transplantation. Br J Cancer 59:434–438, 1989.

224. Kato S, Yabe H, Yabe M, Kimura M, Ito M, Tsuchida F, Tsuji K, Takahashi M: Studies on transfer of varicella-zoster virus specific T-cell immunity from bone marrow donor to recipient. Blood 75:806–809, 1990.

225. Hoagland RJ: The transmission of infectious mononucleosis. Am J Med Sci 229:262–272, 1955.

226. Nilsson K, Klein G, Henle W, Henle G: The establishment of lymphoblastoid cell lines from adult and from foetal human lymphoid tissue and its dependence on EBV. Int J Cancer 8:443–450, 1971.

227. Sixbey JW, Nedrud JG, Raab-Traub N, Hanes RA, Pagano JS: Epstein-Barr virus replication in oropharyngeal epithelial cells. N Engl J Med 310:1225–1230, 1984.

228. Straus SE, Cohen JI, Tosato G, Meier J: Epstein-Barr virus infections: Biology, pathogenesis and management. Ann Intern Med 118:45–48, 1993.

229. Jones JF, Straus SE: Chronic Epstein-Barr virus infection. Ann Rev Med 38:195–209, 1987.

230. Barbera JA, Hayashi S, Hegele RG et al: Detection of Epstein-Barr virus in lymphocytic interstitial pneumonia by in situ hybridization. Am Rev Respir Dis 145:940–6, 1992.

231. Bird AG, Britton S: The relationship between Epstein-Barr virus and lymphoma. Semin Hematol 19:285, 1982.

232. Hanto DW, Frizzera G, Gajl-Peczalska KJ et al: Epstein-Barr virus-induced B-cell lymphoma after renal transplantation. Acyclovir therapy and transition from polyclonal to monoclonal B-cell proliferation. N Engl J Med 306:913, 1982.

233. Syndman DR, Rudders RA, Daoust P et al: Infectious mononucleosis in an adult progressing to fatal immunoblastic lymphoma. Ann Intern Med 96:737, 1982.

234. Purtilo DT, Sakamoto K, Barnabei V et al. and the XLP Collaborators: Epstein-Barr virus-induced diseases in boys and the X-linked lymphoproliferative syndrome (XLP). Am J Med 73:49, 1982.

235. Henle W, Henle G, Horwitz CA: Epstein-Barr virus-specific diagnostic tests in infectious mononucleosis. Hum Pathol 5551–565, 1974.

236. Tosato G, Macrath I, Koski I, Dooley N, Blaese M: Activation of suppressor T cells during Epstein-Barr-virus-induced infectious mononucleosis. N Engl J Med 301:1133–1137, 1979.

237. Moss DJ, Wallace LE, Rickinson AB, Epstein MA: Cytotoxic T cell recognition of Epstein-Barr-virus-infected B cells. I. Specificity and HLA restriction of effector cells reactivated. Eur J Immunol 11:686–693, 1981.

238. Sumaya CV, Ench Y: Epstein-Barr virus infectious mononucleosis in children. I. Clinical and general laboratory findings. Pediatrics 75:1003–10, 1985.

239. Knowles DM, Cesarman E, Chadburn A et al: Correlative morphologic and molecular genetic analysis demonstrates three distinct categories of post-transplantation lymphoproliferative disorders. Blood 85:552–565, 1995.

240. Ballerini P, Gaidano G, Inghirami G, Gong JZ, Saglio G, Knowles DM, Dalla-Favera R: Multiple genetic alterations in AIDS-associated lymphomas. Blood 78:327a, 1991.

241. Chang RS, Lewis JP, Abildgaard CF: Prevalence of oropharyngeal excreters of leukocyte-transforming agents among a human population. N Engl J Med 289:1325–1329, 1973.

242. Ambinder RF, Wingard JR, Burns WH, Hayward SD, Saral S, Perry HR, Santos GW, Hayward GS: Detection of Epstein-Barr virus DNA in mouthwashes by hybridization. J Clin Microbiol 21:353–356, 1985.

243. Lin JC, Lin SC, De BK, Chan WC, Evatt BL, Chan WC: Precision of genotyping for Epstein-Barr virus by polymerase chain reaction using three gene loci (EBNA-2, EBNA-3C, and EBER): Predominance of type A virus associated with Hodgkin's disease. Blood 81:3372–81, 1993.

244. Ho M, Jaffe R, Miller G et al: The frequency of Epstein-Barr virus infection and associated lymphoproliferative syndrome after transplantation and its manifestations in children. Transplantation 45:719–727, 1988.

245. Ho M, Miller G, Atchison RW et al: Epstein-Barr virus infections and DNA hybridization studies in posttransplantation lymphoma and lymphoproliferative lesions: The role of primary infection. J Infect Dis 152:876–886, 1985.

246. Chang RS, Lewis JP, Reynolds RD et al: Oropharyngeal excretion of Epstein-Barr virus by patients with lymphoproliferative disorders and by recipients of renal homografts. Ann Intern Med 88:34–40, 1978.

247. Strauch B, Siegel N, Andrews LL et al: Oropharyngeal excretion of Epstein-Barr virus by renal transplant recipients and other patients treated with immunosuppressive drugs. Lancet 1:234, 1974.

248. Cheeseman SH, Henle W, Rubin RR et al: Epstein-Barr virus infection in renal transplant recipients. Ann Intern Med 93:39–42, 1980.

249. Cheeseman SH, Henle W, Rubin RH: Epstein-Barr virus infection in renal transplant recipients: Effects of antithymocyte globulin and interferon. Ann Intern Med 93:39–42, 1980.

250. Strauch B, Andrews L-L, Siegel N, Miller G: Oropharyngeal excretion of Epstein-Barr virus by renal transplant recipients and other patients treated with immunosuppressive drugs. Lancet 1:234–237, 1974.

251. Chang RS, Lewis JP, Reynolds RD: Oropharyngeal excretion of Epstein-Barr virus by patients with lymphoproliferative disorders and by recipients of renal homografts. Ann Intern Med 88:34–40, 1978.

252. Henle W, Henle G: Epstein-Barr virus-specific serology in immunologically compromised individuals. Cancer Res 41:4222–4225, 1981.

253. Greenspan JS, Greenspan D, Lennette ET et al: Replication of Epstein-Barr virus within the epithelial cells of oral "hairy" leukoplakia, an AIDS-associated lesion. N Engl J Med 313:1564–71, 1985.

254. Reichart PA, Langford A, Gelderblom HR, Pohle H-D, Becker J, Wolf H: Oral hairy leukoplakia: Observations in 95 cases and review of the literature. J Oral Pathol Med 18:410–415, 1989.

255. Laine SS, Happonen R-P, Niemelä M: Oral hairy leukoplakia is not a specific sign of HIV-infection but related to immunosuppression in general. J Oral Pathol Med 18:28–31, 1989.

256. Ho M, Jaffe R, Miller G: The frequency of Epstein-Barr virus infection and associated lymphoproliferative syndrome after transplantation and its manifestations in children. Transplantation 45:719–727, 1988.

257. Hanto DW, Gajl-Peczalska KJ, Frizzera G et al: Epstein-Barr virus (EBV) induced polyclonal and monoclonal B-cell lymphoproliferative diseases occurring after renal transplantation. Ann Surg 198:356–369, 1983.

258. Hanto DW, Sakamoto K, Purtilo D, Simmons RL, Najarian JS: The Epstein-Barr virus in the pathogenesis of posttransplant lymphoproliferative disorders. Surgery 90:204–213, 1981.

259. Hanto DW, Frizzera G, Gajl-Peczalska KJ: Epstein-Barr virus-induced B-cell lymphoma after renal transplantation. N Engl J Med 306:913–918, 1982.

260. Cohen JI: Epstein-Barr virus lymphoproliferative disease associated with acquired immunodeficiency. Medicine (Baltimore) 70:137, 1991.

261. Lange B, Henle W, Meyers JD et al: Epstein-Barr virus-related serology in marrow transplant recipients. Int J Cancer 26:151–157, 1980.

262. Wingard JR, Lin SC, Mar EC, Devine SM, Pascuzzi CC, Dix SP, Saral R, Lin JC: Epstein-Barr Virus (EBV) infection in bone marrow transplant (BMT) patients. J Cell Biochem 18B:62 (abstr. no. G116), 1994.

263. Shearer WT, Ritz J, Finegold MJ: Epstein-Barr virus-associated B-cell proliferations of diverse clonal origins after bone marrow transplantation in a 12-year-old patient with severe combined immunodeficiency. N Engl J Med 312:1151–9, 1985.

264. Martin PJ, Shulman HM, Schubach WH: Fatal Epstein-Barr-virus-associated proliferation of donor B cells after treatment of acute-graft-versus-host disease with a murine anti-T-cell antibody. Ann Intern Med 101:310–315, 1984.

265. Zutter MM, Martin PJ, Sale GE, Shulman HM, Fisher L, Thomas ED, Durnam DM: Epstein-Barr virus lymphoproliferation after bone marrow transplantation. Blood 72:520–529, 1988.

266. D'Amore ESG, Manivel JC, Gajl-Peczalska KJ, Litz CE, Copenhaver CM, Shapiro RS, Strickler JG: B-Cell lymphoproliferative disorders after bone marrow transplant: An analysis of ten cases with emphasis on Epstein-Barr virus detection in-situ hybridization. Cancer 68:1285–1295, 1991.

267. Witherspoon RP, Fisher LD, Schoch G et al: Secondary cancers after bone marrow transplantation for leukemia or aplastic anemia. N Engl J Med 321:784–789, 1989.

268. Shapiro RS, McClain K, Frizzera G et al: Epstein-Barr associated B cell lymphoproliferative disorders following bone marrow transplantation. Blood 71:1234–1243, 1988.

269. Curtis RE, Travis LB, Rowlings PA et al: Risk of lymphoproliferative disorders after bone marrow transplantation: A multi-institutional study. Blood 94:2208–2216, 1999.

270. Lazzarino M, Orlandi E, Baldanti F et al: The immunosuppression and potential for EBV reactivation of fludarabine combined with cyclophosphamide and dexamethasone in patients with lymphoproliferative disorders. Br J Haematol 107:877–882, 1999.

271. Colby BM, Shaw JE, Elion GB, Pagano JS: Effect of acyclovir [(9-2-hydroxyethoxymethyl]guanine) on Epstein-Barr virus DNA replication. J Virol 34:560–568, 1980

272. Anderson J, Britton S, Ernberg I, Andersson U, Henle W, Sköldenberg, Tisell Å: Effect of acyclovir on infectious mononucleosis: A double-blind, placebo-controlled study. J Infect Dis 153:282–290, 1986.

273. Pagano JS, Sixbey JW, Lin J-C: Acyclovir and Epstein-Barr virus infection. J Antimicrob Chemother 12:113–121, 1983.

274. Andersson J, Sköldenberg B, Henle W et al: Acyclovir treatment in infectious mononucleosis: A clinical and virological study. Infection 15:S14–S21, 1987.

275. Resnick L, Herbst JS, Ablashi D, Atherton S, Frank B, Rosen L, Horwitz SN: Regression of oral hairy leukoplakia after orally administered acyclovir therapy. JAMA 259:384–388, 1988.

276. Newman C, Polk BF: Resolution of oral hairy leukoplakia during therapy with 9-(1,3-dihyroxy-2-propoxymethyl) guanine (DHPG). Ann Intern Med 107:348–50, 1987.

277. Pirsch JD, Stratta RJ, Sollinger HW, Hafez GR, D'Alessandro AM, Kalayoglu M, Belzer FO: Treatment of severe Epstein-Barr virus-induced lymphoproliferative syndrome with ganciclovir: Two cases after solid organ transplantation. Am J Med 86:241–244, 1989.

278. Ishida Y, Kokota Y, Tauchi H, Fukuda M, Takaoka T, Hayashi M, Matsuda H: Ganciclovir for chronic active Epstein-Barr virus infection. Lancet 341:560–1, 1993.

279. Andersson JP, Andersson UG, Ernberg IT, Britton SF, DeLey M: Effects of pure interferons on Epstein-Barr virus infection in vitro. J Virol 54:615–618, 1985.

280. Lidin B, Lamon EW: Antiviral effects of interferon on a somatic cell hybrid between two Burkitt's lymphoma cell lines of different interferon sensitivities. Infect Immun 36:847–849, 1982.

281. Lin J-C, Smith MC, Pagano JS: Prolonged inhibitory effect of 9-(1,3-dihydroxy-2-propoxyethyl)guanine against replication of Epstein-Barr virus. J Virol 50:50–55, 1984.

282. Moore MD, Cannon MJ, Sewall A, Finlayson M, Okimoto M, Nemerow GR: Inhibition of Epstein-Barr virus infection in vitro and in vivo by soluble CR2 (CD21) containing two short consensus repeats. J Virol 65:3559–3565, 1991.

283. Savoie A, Perpête C, Carpentier L, Joncas J, Alfieri C: Direct correlation between the load of Epstein-Barr virus-infected lymphocytes in the peripheral blood of pediatric transplant patients and risk of lymphoproliferative disease. Blood 83:2715–2722, 1994.

284. Papadopopoulos EB, Ladanyi M, Emanuel D et al: Infusions of donor leukocytes to treat Epstein-Barr virus-associated lymphoproliferative disorders after allogeneic bone marrow transplantation. N Engl J Med 330:1185–91, 1994.

285. Niedermeyer J, Hoffmeyer F, Hertenstein B et al: Treatment of lymphoproliferative disease with Rituximab. Lancet 355:499, 2000.

286. Kuehnke I, Huls MH, Liu Z et al: CD20 monoclonal antibody (Rituximab) for therapy of Epstein-Barr virus lymphoma after hemopoietic stem cell transplantation. Blood 95:1502–1505, 2000.

287. McGuirk JP, Seropian S, Howe G et al: Use of Rituximab and irradiated donor-derived lymphocytes to control Epstein-Barr virus-

associated lymphoproliferation in patients undergoing related haplo-identical stem cell transplantation. Bone Marrow Transplant 24:1253–1258, 1999.

288. Gustafsson A, Levitsky V, Zou JZ et al: Epstein-Barr virus (EBV) load in bone marrow transplant recipients at risk to develop post-transplant lymphoproliferative disease: Prophylactic infusion of EBV-specific cytotoxic T cells. Blood 95:807–814, 2000.

289. Rooney CM, Smith CA, Ng CY et al: Infusion of cytotoxic T cells for the prevention and treatment of Epstein-Barr virus-induced lymphoma in allogeneic transplant recipients. Blood 92:1549–1555, 1998.

290. Heslop HE, Rooney CM: Adoptive cellular immunotherapy for EBV lymphoproliferative disease. Immunol Rev 157:217–222, 1997.

291. Lucas KG, Sun Q, Burton RL et al: A phase I–II trial to examine the toxicity of CMV- and EBV-specific cytotoxic T lymphocytes when used for prophylaxis against EBV and CMV disease in recipients of CD34-selected/T cell-depleted stem cell transplants. Hum Gene Ther 11:1453–1463, 2000.

292. Heslop HE, Ng CY, Li C et al: Long-term restoration of immunity against Epstein-Barr virus infection by adoptive transfer of gene-modified virus-specific T lymphocytes. Nat Med 2:551–5, 1996.

293. Pellett PE, Black JB, Yamamoto M: Human herpesvirus 6: The virus and the search for its role as a human pathogen. Adv Virus Res 41:1–52, 1992.

294. Leach CT: Human herpesvirus-6 and -7 infections in children: Agents of roseola and other syndromes. Curr Opin Pediatr 12:269–274, 2000.

295. Torelli G, Marasca R, Luppi M et al: Human herpesvirus-6 in human lymphomas: Identification of specific sequences in Hodgkin's lymphomas by polymerase chain reaction. Blood 77:2251–8, 1991.

296. Yin SY, Ming HA, Jahan N, Manak M, Jaffe ES, Levine PH: In situ hybridization detection of human herpesvirus 6 in biopsy specimens from Chinese patients with non-Hodgkin's lymphoma. Arch Pathol Lab Med 117:502–6, 1993.

297. Di Luca D, Dolcetti R, Mirandola P et al: Human herpesvirus 6: A survey of presence and variant distribution in normal peripheral lymphocytes and lymphoproliferative disorders. J Infect Dis 170:211–5, 1994.

298. Kurata T, Iwasaki T, Sata T et al: Viral pathology of human herpesvirus 6 infection. Adv Exp Med Biol 278:39, 1990.

299. Yoshikawa T, Suga S, Asano Y et al: Human herpesvirus 6 infection in bone marrow transplantation. Blood 78:1381, 1991.

300. Asano Y, Yoshikawa T, Suga S et al: Reactivation of herpesvirus type 6 in children receiving bone marrow transplants for leukemia. N Engl J Med 324:634, 1991.

301. Wilborn F, Brinkmann V, Schmidt CA, Neipel F et al: Herpesvirus type 6 in patients undergoing bone marrow transplantation: Serologic features and detection by polymerase chain reaction. Blood 83:3052, 1994.

302. Wilborn F, Brinkmann V, Schmidt A, Neipel F, Gelderblom H, Siegert W: Herpesvirus type 6 in patients undergoing bone marrow transplantation: Serologic features and detection by polymerase chain reaction. Blood 83:3052–3058, 1994.

303. Takemoto Y, Takatsuka H, Wada H et al: Evaluation of CMV/human herpes virus-6 positivity in bronchoalveolar lavage fluids as early detection of acute GVHD following BMT: Evidence of a significant relationship. Bone Marrow Transplant 26:77–81, 2000.

304. Drobyski WR, Dunne WM, Burd EM: Human herpesvirus 6 (HHV-6) infection in allogeneic bone marrow transplant recipients: I. Evidence for a marrow suppressive role for HHV-6 in vivo. J Infect Dis 167:735, 1993.

305. Knox KK, Carrigan DR: In vitro suppression of bone marrow progenitor cell differentiation by human herpesvirus 6 infection. J Infect Dis 165:925, 1992.

306. Carrigan DR, Knox KK: Human herpesvirus 6 (HHV-6) isolation from bone marrow: HHV-6-associated bone marrow suppression in bone marrow transplant patients. Blood 84:3307–3310, 1994.

307. Carrigan DR, Drobyski WR, Russler SK, Tapper MA, Knox KK, Ash RC: Interstitial pneumonitis associated with human herpesvirus six (HHV-6) infection in marrow transplant patients. Lancet 338:147, 1991.

308. Cone RW, Hackman RC, Huang MW et al: Human herpesvirus 6 in lung tissue from patients with pneumonitis after bone marrow transplantation. N Engl J Med 329:156, 1993.

309. Drobyski WR, Knox KK, Majewski D, Carrigan DR: Fatal encephalitis due to variant B human herpesvirus 6 infection in a bone marrow transplant recipient. N Engl J Med 330:1356, 1994.

310. Wang F-Z, Linde A, Dahl H et al: Human herpesvirus 6 infection inhibits specific lymphocyte proliferation responses and is related to lymphocytopenia after allogeneic stem cell transplantation. Bone Marrow Transplant 24:1201–1206, 1999.

311. Griffiths PB, Emory VO, Loe C, Johnson MA, McLaughlin J: HHV-6 in AIDS. Lancet 343:1104–1105, 1994.

312. Knox KK, Carrigan DR: HHV-6 and CMV pneumonitis in immunocompromised patients. Lancet 343:1647, 1994.

313. Lusso P, Gallo RC: HHV-6 and CMV pneumonitis in immuno-compromised patients. Lancet 343:1647–1648, 1994.

314. Burns WH, Sandford GR: Susceptibility of human herpesvirus 6 to antivirals in vitro. J Infect Dis 162:634–7, 1990.

315. Chang Y, Cesarman E, Pessin MS et al: Identification of her-pesvirus-like DNA sequences in AIDS-associated Kaposi's sarcoma. Science 266:1865–1869, 1994.

316. Moore PS, Chang Y: Detection of herpesvirus-like DNA sequences in Kaposi's sarcoma in patients with and those without HIV infection. N Engl J Med 332:1181–1185, 1995.

317. Huang YQ, Li JJ, Kaplan MH et al: Human herpesvirus-like nucleic acid in various forms of Kaposi's sarcoma. Lancet 345:759–761, 1995.

318. Knowles DM, Cesarman E: The Kaposi's sarcoma-associated herpesvirus (human herpesvirus 8) in Kaposi's sarcoma, malignant lymphoma, and other diseases. Ann Oncol 8:S123–S129, 1997.

319. Cesarman E, Chang Y, Moore PS et al: Kaposi's sarcoma-associated herpesvirus-like DNA sequences in AIDS-related body-cavity-based lymphoma. N Engl J Med 332:1186–1191, 1995.

320. Rettig NB, Ma HJ, Vescio RA et al: Kaposi's sarcoma-associated herpesvirus infection of bone marrow dendritic cells from multiple myeloma patients. Science 276:1851–1854, 1997.

321. Townsend TR, Bolyard EA, Yolken RH et al: Outbreak of cox-sackie A1 gastroenteritis: A complication of bone marrow transplantation. Lancet 1:820–823, 1982.

322. Aquino VM, Farah RA, Lee MC et al: Disseminated coxsackie A9 infection complicating bone marrow transplantation. Pediatr Infect Dis J 15:1053–1054, 1996.

323. Galama JM, de Leeuw N, Wittebol S et al: Prolonged enteroviral infection in a patient who developed pericarditis and heart failure after bone marrow transplantation. Clin Infect Dis 22:1004–1008, 1996.

324. Yolken RH, Bishop CA, Townsend TR et al: Infectious gastroenteritis in bone-marrow-transplant recipients. N Engl J Med 306:1009–1112, 1982.

325. Troussard X, Bauduer F, Gallet E et al: Virus recovery from stools of patients undergoing bone marrow transplantation. Bone Marrow Transplant 12:573–576, 1993.

326. Ambinder RF, Burns W, Forman M et al: Hemorrhagic cystitis associated with adenovirus infection in bone marrow transplantation. Arch Intern Med 146:1400–1401, 1986.

327. Miyamura K, Taketama K, Kojima S et al: Hemorrhagic cystitis associated with urinary excretion of adenovirus type 11 following allogeneic bone marrow transplantation. Bone Marrow Transplant 4:533–5, 1989.

328. Londergan TA, Walzak MP: Hemorrhagic cystitis due to adenovirus infection following bone marrow transplantation. J Urol 151:1013–14, 1994.

329. Schmitz H, Wigand R, Heinrich W: Worldwide epidemiology of human adenovirus infections. Am J Epidemiol 117:455–66, 1983.

330. Hale GA, Heslop HE, Krance RA et al: Adenovirus infections after pediatric bone marrow transplantation. Bone Marrow Transplant 23:277–82, 1999.

331. Munoz FM, Piedra PA, Demmler GJ: Disseminated adenovirus disease in immunocompromised and immunocompetent children. Clin Infect Dis 27:1194–2000, 1998.

332. Shields AF, Hackman RC, Fife KH et al: Adenovirus infection in patients undergoing bone-marrow transplantation. N Engl J Med 312:529–533, 1985.

333. Flomenberg P, Babbitt J, Drobyski WR et al: Increasing incidence of adenovirus disease in bone marrow transplant recipients. J Infect Dis 169:775–81, 1994.

334. Howard DS, Phillips GL, Reece DE, Munn RK, Henslee-Downey J, Pittard M, Barker M, Pomeroy C: Adenovirus infections in hematopoietic stem cell transplant recipients. Clin Infect Dis 29:1494–501, 1999.

335. Zahradnik JM, Spencer MJ, Porter DD: Adenovirus infection in the immunocompromised patient. Am J Med 68:725, 1980.

336. Carmichael GP Jr, Zahradnik JM, Moyer GH, Porter DD: Adenovirus hepatitis in an immunosuppressed adult patient. Am J Clin Pathol 71:352, 1979.

337. Yolken RH, Bishop CA, Townsend RT et al: Infectious gastroenteritis in bone-marrow transplant recipients. N Engl J Med 306:1009, 1982.

338. Somervaille TCP, Kirk S, Dogan A, Landon GV, Mackinnon S: Fulminant hepatic failure caused by adenovirus infection following bone marrow transplantation for Hodgkin's disease. Bone Marrow Transplant 24:99–101, 2000.

339. Chakrabarti S, Collingham KE, Fegan CD, Milligan DW: Fulminant adenovirus hepatitis following unrelated bone marrow transplantation: Failure of intravenous ribavirin therapy. Bone Marrow Transplant 23:1209–11, 1999.

340. Childs R, Sanchez C, Engler H, Preuss J, Rosenfeld S, Dunbar C, van Rhee F, Plante M, Phang S, Barrett AJ: High incidence of adeno- and polyomavirus-induced hemorrhagic cystitis in bone marrow allotransplantation for hematological malignancy following T cell depletion and cyclosporine. Bone Marrow Transplant 22:889–893, 1998.

341. Chen FE, Liang RHS, Lo JY, Yuen KY, Chan TK, Peiris M: Treatment of adenovirus-associated haemorrhagic cystitis with ganciclovir. Bone Marrow Transplant 20:997–9, 1997.

342. Wreghitt TG, Gray JJ, Ward KN, Salt A, Taylor DL, Alp NJ, Tyms AS: Disseminated adenovirus infection after liver transplantation and its possible treatment with ganciclovir. J Infect 19:88–9, 1989.

343. Duggan JM, Farrehi J, Duderstadt S, Turner NJ, Fekety R: Treatment with ganciclovir of adenovirus pneumonia in a cardiac transplant patient. Am J Med 103:439–40, 1997.

344. Shetty AK, Gans HA, So S, Millan MT, Arvin AM, Gutierrez KM: Intravenous ribavirin therapy for adenovirus pneumonia. Pediatr Pulmonol 29:69–73, 2000.

345. Miyamura K, Hamaguchi M, Taji H, Kanie T, Kohno A: Successful ribavirin therapy for severe adenovirus hemorrhagic cystitis after allogeneic marrow transplant from close HLA donors rather than distant donors. Bone Marrow Transplant 25:545–8, 2000.

346. Jurado CM, Hernandez MF, Navarro JM et al: Adenovirus pneumonitis successfully treated with intravenous ribavirin. Haematologica 83:1128–9, 1988.

347. Jurado M, Navarro JM, Hernandez J, Molina MA: Adenovirus-associated haemorrhagic cystitis after bone marrow transplantation successfully treated with intravenous ribavirin. Bone Marrow Transplant 15:651–2, 1995.

348. Wulffraat NM, Geelen SP, van Dijken PJ, de Graeff-Meeder B, Kuis W, Boven K: Recovery from adenovirus pneumonia in a severe combined immunodeficiency patient treated with intravenous ribavirin. Transplantation 59:927, 1995.

349. Liles WC, Cushing H, Holt S, Bryan C, Hackman RC: Severe adenoviral nephritis following bone marrow transplantation: Successful treatment with intravenous ribavirin. Bone Marrow Transplant 14:663–4, 1994.

350. Murphy GF, Wood DP, McRoberts JW: Adenovirus-associated hemorrhagic cystitis treated with intravenous ribavirin. J Urol 149:565–6, 1993.

351. Cassano WF: Intravenous ribavirin therapy for adenovirus cystitis after allogeneic bone marrow transplantation. Bone Marrow Transplant 7:247–8, 1991.

352. Kawakami M, Ueda S, Maeda T, Karasuno T, Teshima H, Hiraoka A, Hakamura H, Tanaka K, Masaoka T: Vidarabine therapy for virus-associated cystitis after allogeneic bone marrow transplantation. Bone Marrow Transplant 20:485–90, 1997.

353. Kitabayashi A, Hirokawa M, Kuroki J, Nishinari T, Niitsu H, Miura AB: Successful vidarabine therapy for adenovirus type 11-associated acute hemorrhagic cystitis after allogeneic bone marrow transplantation. Bone Marrow Transplant 14:853–4, 1994.

354. Ribaud P, Scieux C, Freymuth F, Morinet F, Gluckman E: Successful treatment of adenovirus disease with intravenous cidofovir in an unrelated stem-cell transplant recipient. Clin Infect Dis 28:690–1, 1999.

355. Ljungman P, Lambertenghi-Deliliers G, Ribaud P, Einsele H et al: Cidofovir for treatment of CMV and adenovirus infections in allogeneic stem cell transplant recipients. Blood 94:396a (abstr. 1753), 1999.

356. Izadifar-Legrand F, Berrebi D, Faye A, Duval M, Houhou N, Freymuth F, Peuchmaur M, Vilmer E: Early diagnosis of adenovirus infection and treatment with cidofovir after bone marrow transplantation in children. Blood 94:341a (abstr. 1526), 1999.

357. Hromas R, Cornetta K, Srour E, Blanke C, Broun ER: Donor leukocyte infusion as therapy of life-threatening adenoviral infections after T-cell-depleted bone marrow transplantation. Blood 84:1689–90, 1994.

358. Brandt CD, Kim HW, Arrobio JO, Jeffries BC, Wood SC et al: Epidemiology of respiratory syncytial virus infections in Washington DC. III. Composite analysis of eleven consecutive yearly epidemics. Am J Epidemiol 98:355–364, 1973.

359. Kim HW, Arrobio JO, Brandt CD, Jeffries BC, Pules G et al: Epidemiology of respiratory syncytial virus infections in Washington DC. I. Importance of the virus in different respiratory tract disease syndromes and temporal distribution of infection. Am J Epidemiol 98:216–225, 1973.

360. Hall CB, Powell KR, MacDonald NE, Gala CL, Menegus ME et al: Respiratory syncytial virus infection in children with compromised immune function. N Engl J Med 315:77–81, 1986.

361. Simoes EA: Respiratory syncytial virus infection. J Infect Dis 354:847–52, 1999.

362. Harrington RD, Hooton TM, Hackman RC, Storch GA, Osborne B et al: An outbreak of respiratory syncytial virus in a bone marrow transplant center. J Infect Dis 165:987–93, 1992.

363. Whimbey E, Champlin RE, Couch RB, Englund JA, Goodrich JM: Community respiratory virus infections among hospitalized adult bone marrow transplant recipients. Clin Infect Dis 22:778–82, 1996.

364. Hall C, Walsh E, Long C et al: Immunity to and frequency of reinfection with respiratory syncytial virus. J Infect Dis 163:693–8, 1991.

365. Henderson F, Collier A, Clyde WJ et al: Respiratory syncytial virus infections, reinfections and immunity. N Engl J Med 300:530–4, 1979.

366. Hall C: Nosocomial respiratory syncytial virus infections: The "Cold War" has not ended. Clin Infect Dis 31:590–6, 2000.

367. Englund JA, Anderson LJ, Rhame FS: Nosocomial transmission of respiratory syncytial virus in immunocompromised adults. J Clin Microbiol 29:115–9, 1991.

368. Welliver RC, Ogra PL: Immunology of respiratory viral infections. Annu Rev Med 39:147, 1988.

369. Hall CB, Powell KR, MacDonald NE et al: Respiratory syncytial viral infection in children with compromised immune function. N Engl J Med 315:77, 1986.

370. Taylor CE, Craft AW, Kernahan J et al: Local antibody production and respiratory syncytial virus infection in children with leukaemia. J Med Virol 30:277–81, 1990.

371. Englund JA, Sullivan CJ, Jordan MC et al: Respiratory syncytial virus infection in immunocompromised adults. Ann Intern Med 109:203, 1988.

372. Whimbey E, Bodey GP: Viral pneumonia in the immunocompromised adult with neoplastic disease: The role of common community respiratory viruses. Semin Respir Infect 7:122–31, 1992.

373. Whimbey E, Champlin RE, Englund JA, Mirza NQ, Piedra PA et al: Combination therapy with aerosolized ribavirin and intravenous immunoglobulin for respiratory syncytial virus disease in adult bone marrow transplant recipients. Bone Marrow Transplant 16:393–399, 1995.

374. Englund JA, Sullivan CJ, Jordan MC, Dehner LP, Vercellotti GM, Balfour HH Jr: Respiratory syncytial virus infection in immunocompromised adults. Ann Intern Med 109:203–208, 1988.

375. Bowden RA: Respiratory virus infections after marrow transplant: The Fred Hutchinson Cancer Research Center experience. Am J Med 102(3A):27–30, 1997.

376. Hall CB, Powell KR, MacDonald NE et al: Respiratory syncytial virus infection in children with compromised immune function. N Engl J Med 315:77–81, 1986.

377. Ghosh S, Champlin RE, Englund J, Giralt SA, Rolston K et al: Respiratory syncytial virus upper respiratory tract illnesses in adult blood and marrow transplant recipients: Combination therapy with aerosolized ribavirin and intravenous immunoglobulin. Bone Marrow Transplant 25:751–755, 2000.

378. Hertz MI, Englund JA, Snover D et al: Respiratory syncytial virus-induced acute lung injury in adult patients with bone marrow transplants: A clinical approach and review of the literature. Medicine (Baltimore) 68:269–81, 1989.

379. Boeckh M, Gooley T, Bowden RA, Crawford S et al: Risk factors for progression from respiratory syncytial virus (RSV) upper respiratory tract infection (URI) to pneumonia (RSV-IP) after hematopoietic stem cell transplantation. In: Programs and Abstracts of the 39th Interscience Conference of Antimicrobial Agents and Chemotherapy (San Francisco, 1999).

380. Smith DW, Frankel LR, Mathers LH et al: A controlled trial of aerosolized ribavirin in infants receiving mechanical ventilation for severe respiratory syncytial virus infection. N Engl J Med 325:24–9, 1991.

381. Meert KL, Sarnaik AP, Gelmini MJ et al: Aerosolized ribavirin in mechanically ventilated children with respiratory syncytial virus lower respiratory tract disease: A prospective, double-blind, randomized clinical trial. Crit Care Med 22:566–72, 1994.

382. Moler FW, Steinhart CM, Ohmit SE, Stidham GL for the Pediatric Critical Care Study Group. Effectiveness of ribavirin in otherwise well infants with respiratory syncytial virus-associated respiratory failure. J Pediatr 128:422–28, 1996.

383. Law B, Wang EEL, MacDonald N et al: Does ribavirin impact on the hospital course of children with respiratory syncytial virus infection? An analysis using the Pediatric Investigators Collaborative Network on Infections in Canada (PICNIC) RSV database. Pediatrics 99:E7, 1997.

384. Randolph AG, Wang EEL: Ribavirin for respiratory syncytial virus lower respiratory tract infection. Arch Pediatr Adolesc Med 150:942–7, 1996.

385. Adams RH, Christenson JC, Petersen FB, Beatty PG: Pre-emptive use of aerosolized ribavirin in the treatment of asymptomatic pediatric marrow transplant patients testing positive for RSV. Bone Marrow Transplant 24:661–4, 1999.

386. Sparrelid E, Ljungman P, Ekelof-Andstrom E, Aschan J et al: Ribavirin therapy in bone marrow transplant recipients with viral respiratory tract infections. Bone Marrow Transplant 19:905–8, 1997.

387. Lewinsohn DM, Bowden RA, Mattson D, Crawford SW: Phase I study of intravenous ribavirin treatment of respiratory syncytial virus pneumonia after marrow transplantation. Antimicrob Agents Chemother 40:2555–2557, 1996.

388. McColl MD, Corser RB, Bremner J, Chopra R: Respiratory syncytial virus infection in adult BMT recipients: Effective therapy with short duration nebulized ribavirin. Bone Marrow Transplant 21:423–5, 1998.

389. Hertz MI, Englund JA, Snover D et al: Respiratory syncytial virus-induced acute lung injury in adult patients with bone marrow transplants: A clinical approach and review of the literature. Medicine (Baltimore) 68:269–81, 1989.

390. Gruber WC, Wilson SZ, Throop BJ et al: Immunoglobulin administration and ribavirin therapy. Efficacy in respiratory syncytial virus infection in the cotton rat. Pediatr Res 21:270–4, 1987.

391. Ghosh S, Champlin RE, Englund J et al: Respiratory syncytial virus upper respiratory tract illnesses in adult blood and marrow transplant recipients: Combination therapy with aerosolized ribavirin and intravenous immunoglobulin. Bone Marrow Transplant 25:751–55, 2000.

392. Connor JD, Hintz M, Van Dyke R et al: Ribavirin pharmacokinetics in children and adults during therapeutic trials. In: Smith RA, Knight V, Smith JAD (eds.): Clinical Applications of Ribavirin, pp. 107–123. Academic Press, Orlando, 1984.

393. McIntosh K, Kurachek SC, Cairns LM et al: Treatment of respiratory viral infection in an immunodeficient infant with ribavirin aerosol. Am J Dis Child 138:305–8, 1984.

394. DeVincenzo JP, Hirsch RL, Fuentes RJ et al: Respiratory syncytial virus immune globulin treatment of lower respiratory tract infection in pediatric patients undergoing bone marrow transplantation – a compassionate use experience. Bone Marrow Transplant 25:161–165, 2000.

395. Scott LJ, Lamb HM: Palivizumab. Drugs 58:305–11, 1999.

396. The Impact-RSV Study Group: Palivizumab, a humanized respiratory syncytial virus monoclonal antibody reduced hospitalizations from respiratory syncytial virus infection in high-risk infants. Pediatrics 102:531–7, 1998.

397. Boeckh M, Bowden RA, Berry MM et al: Phase I evaluation of a RSV-specific humanized monoclonal antibody (MEDI-493) after hematopoietic stem cell transplantation (HSCT). In: Programs and Abstracts of the 28th Interscience Conference on Antimicrobial Agents and Chemotherapy (San Diego, 1998).

398. Johnson S, Oliver C, Prince GA et al: Development of a humanized monoclonal antibody (MEDI 493) with potent in vitro and in vivo activity against respiratory syncytial virus. J Infect Dis 176:1215–24, 1997.

399. Centers for Disease Control and Prevention: Guidelines for preventing opportunistic infections among hematopoietic stem cell transplant recipients: Recommendations of CDC, the Infectious Disease Society of America, and the American Society of Blood and Marrow Transplantation. MMWR 49 (No. RR-10):1–172, 2000.

400. Cox NJ, Subbarao K: Influenza. Lancet 354:1277–82, 1999.

401. Kaiser L. Respiratory viruses in immunocompromised hosts. In: Wingard JR, Bowden RA (Eds.). Management of Infections in Oncology Patients. London: Martin Dunitz (in press).

402. Whimbey E, Elting LS, Cough RB, Lo W, Williams L, Champlin RE, Bodey GP: Influenza A virus infections among hospitalized adult bone marrow transplant recipients. Bone Marrow Transplant 13:437–40, 1994.

403. Elting LS, Whimbey E, Lo W et al: Epidemiology of influenza A virus infection in patients with acute or chronic leukemia. Support Care Cancer 3:198–202, 1995.

404. Apalsch AM, Green M, Ledesma-Medina J et al: Parainfluenza and influenza virus infections in pediatric organ transplant recipients. Clin Infect Dis 20:394–9, 1995.

405. Rabella N, Rodriguez P, Labeaga R et al: Conventional respiratory viruses recovered from immunocompromised patients: Clinical considerations. Clin Infect Dis 28:1043–8, 1999.

406. Yousuf HM, Englund J, Couch R et al: Influenza among hospitalized adults with leukemia. Clin Infect Dis 24:1095–9, 1997.

407. Whimbey E, Bodey GP: Viral pneumonia in the immunocompromised adult with neoplastic disease: The role of common community respiratory viruses. Semin Respir Infect 7:122–31, 1992.

408. Warner JL, Todd SJ, Shalaby H et al: Comparison of Directigen FLU-A with viral isolation and direct immunofluorescence for the rapid detection and identification of influenza A virus. J Clin Microbiol 29:479–82, 1991.

409. Centers for Disease Control and Prevention: Neuraminidase inhibitors for treatment of influenza A and B infections. MMWR 48 (No. RR-14):1–10, 1999.

410. Dolin R, Reichman RC, Madore HP et al: A controlled trial of amantadine and rimantadine in the prophylaxis of influenza A infection. N Engl J Med 307:580–4, 1982.

411. Hall CB, Dolin R, Gala CL et al: Children with influenza A infection: Treatment with rimantadine. Pediatrics 80:275–82, 1987.

412. Clover RD, Crawford SA, Abell TD et al: Effectiveness of rimantadine in prophylaxis of children within families. Am J Dis Child 140:706–9, 1986.

413. Patriarca PA, Arden NH, Koplan JP et al: Prevention and control of type A influenza infections in nursing homes Ann Intern Med 107:732–40, 1987.

414. Englund JA, Champlin RE, Wyde PR et al: Common emergence of amantadine- and rimantadine-resistant influenza A viruses in symptomatic immunocompromised adults. Clin Infect Dis 26:1418–24, 1998.

415. Wingfield WL, Pollack D, Grunert RR: Therapeutic efficacy of amantadine HC1 and rimantidine HC1 in naturally occurring influenza A2 respiratory illness in man. N Engl J Med 281:579, 1969.

416. Belshe RB, Burk B, Newman F et al: Resistance of influenza A virus to amantadine and rimantadine: Results of one decade of surveillance. J Infect Dis 159:430–8, 1989.

417. Hayden FG, Couch RB: Clinical and epidemiological importance of influenza A viruses resistant to amantadine and rimantadine. Rev Med Virol 2:89–96, 1992.

418. Hayden FG, Belshe RB, Clover RD et al: Emergence of resistance and apparent transmission of rimantadine-resistant influenza A virus in families. N Engl J Med 321:1696–702, 1989.

419. Degeleu J, Somani SK, Cooper SL et al: Amantadine-resistant influenza A in a nursing facility. Arch Intern Med 152:390–2, 1992.

420. Calfee DP, Hayden FG: New approaches to influenza chemotherapy: Neuraminidase inhibitors. Drugs 56:537–53, 1998.

421. Gubareva LV, Kaiser L, Hayden FG: Influenza virus neuraminidase inhibitors. Lancet 335:827–35, 2000.

422. Hayden FG, Osterhaus A, Treanor JJ et al: Efficacy and safety of the neuraminidase inhibitor zanamivir in the treatment of influenza virus infections. N Engl J Med 337:874–80, 1997.

423. The MIST Study Group: Randomized trial of efficacy and safety of inhaled zanamivir in treatment of influenza A and B virus infections. Lancet 352:1877–81, 1998.

424. Hayden FG, Atmar RL, Schilling M et al: Use of the selective oral neuraminidase inhibitor oseltamivir to prevent influenza. N Engl J Med 341:1336–43, 1999.

425. Gubareva LV, Matrosovich MN, Brenner MK et al: Evidence for zanamivir resistance in an immunocompromised child infected with influenza B virus. J Infect Dis 178:1257–62, 1998.

426. Engelhard D, Nagler A, Hardan I et al: Antibody response to a two-dose regimen of influenza vaccine in allogeneic T cell-depleted and autologous BMT recipients. Bone Marrow Transplant 11:1–5, 1993.

427. Zambon M, Bull T, Sadler CJ et al: Molecular epidemiology of two consecutive outbreaks of parainfluenza 3 in a bone marrow transplant unit. J Clin Microbiol 36:2289–93, 1998.

428. Whimby E, Vartivarian SE, Champlin SE, Elting LS, Luna M, Bodey GP: Parainfluenza virus infection in adult bone marrow transplant recipients. Eur J Clin Microbiol Infect Dis 12:690–701, 1993.

429. Wendt CH, Weisdorf DJ, Jordan MC, Balfour HH, Hertz MI: Parainfluenza virus respiratory infection after bone marrow transplantation. N Engl J Med 325:921–926, 1992.

430. Lewis VA, Champlin R, Englund J et al: Respiratory disease due to parainfluenza virus in adult bone marrow transplant recipients. Clin Infect Dis 23:1033–7, 1996.

431. Hayden FG, Sable CA, Connor JD et al: Intravenous ribavirin by constant infusion for serious influenza and parainfluenza infection. Antiviral Ther 1:51–6, 1996.

432. Koff RS: Hepatitis A. Lancet 351:1643–49, 1998.

433. Centers for Disease Control: Prevention of hepatitis A through active or passive immunization: Recommendations of the Advisory Committee on Immunization Practices [ACIP]. MMWR 48 (No. RR-12):1–37, 1999.

434. Centers for Disease Control: Hepatitis B virus: A comprehensive strategy for eliminating transmission in the United States through universal childhood vaccination: Recommendations of the Immunization Practices Advisory Committee (ACIP). MMWR 40 (No. RR-13):1–19, 1991.

435. Chen P, Chiou TJ, Fan FS et al: Fulminant hepatitis is significantly increased in hepatitis B carriers after allogeneic bone marrow transplantation. Transplantation 67:1425–33, 1999.

436. Liang R, Lau GK, Kwong YL: Chemotherapy and bone marrow transplantation for cancer patients who are also chronic hepatitis

B carriers: A review of the problem. J Clin Oncol 17:394–398, 1999.

437. Wands JR: Subacute and chronic active hepatitis after withdrawal of chemotherapy. Lancet 2:979, 1975.

438. Lok AS, Liang RH, Chiu EK et al: Reactivation of hepatitis B virus replication in patients receiving cytotoxic therapy. Reports of a prospective study. Gastroenterology 100:182–88, 1991.

439. Liang RH, Lok AS, Lai CL et al: Hepatitis B infection in patients with lymphomas. Hematol Oncol 8:261–70, 1990.

440. Lau JY, Lai CL, Lin HJ et al: Fatal reactivation of chronic hepatitis B virus infection following withdrawal of chemotherapy in lymphoma patients. Q J Med 73:911–7, 1989.

441. Kumagai K, Takagi T, Nakamura S et al: Hepatitis B virus carriers in the treatment of malignant lymphoma: An epidemiological study in Japan. Ann Oncol 8:S107–109, 1997.

442. Nakamura Y, Motokura T, Fujita A et al: Severe hepatitis related to chemotherapy in hepatitis B carriers with hematological malignancies. Survey in Japan, 1987–1991. Cancer 78:2210–2215, 1996.

443. Hoofnagle JH, Duskeiko GM, Schafer DF, Jones EA, Micetich KC, Young RC, Costa J: Reactivation of chronic hepatitis B virus infection by cancer chemotherapy. Ann Intern Med 96:447, 1982.

444. Utili R, Zampino R, Bellopede P et al: Dual or single hepatitis B and C virus infections in childhood cancer survivors: Long-term follow-up and effect of interferon treatment. Blood 94:4046–52, 1999.

445. Lau GK, Lie AK, Kwong YL et al: A case-controlled study on the use of HBsAg-positive donors for allogeneic hematopoietic stem cell transplantation. Blood 96:452–58, 2000.

446. Locasciulli A, Alberti A, Bandini G et al: Allogeneic bone marrow transplantation from HBsAg positive donors: A multicenter study from the Gruppo Italiano Trapianto di Midollo Osseo (GITMO). Blood 86:3236–40, 1995.

447. Lau GK, Liang RT, Chiu EK et al: Hepatic events after bone marrow transplantation in patients with hepatitis B infection: A case controlled study. Bone Marrow Transplant 19:795–99, 1997.

448. Caselitz M, Link H, Hein R et al: Hepatitis B associated liver failure following bone marrow transplantation. J Hepatol 27:572–77, 1997.

449. Reed EC, Myerson D, Corey L, Meyers JD: Allogeneic marrow transplantation in patients positive for hepatitis B surface antigen. Blood 71:195–200, 1991.

450. Forbes GM, Davies JM, Herrmann RP et al: Liver disease complicating bone marrow transplantation: A clinical audit. J Gastroenterol Hepatol 10:1–7, 1995.

451. Martin BA, Rowe JM, Kouides PA et al: Hepatitis B reactivation following allogeneic bone marrow transplant: A case report and review of the literature. Bone Marrow Transplant 15:145–148, 1995.

452. Webster A, Brenner MK, Prentice HG et al: Fatal hepatitis B reactivation after autologous bone marrow transplantation. Bone Marrow Transplant 4:207–8, 1989.

453. Lok AS, Wu PC, Lai CL et al: A controlled trial of interferon with or without prednisone priming for chronic hepatitis B. Gastroenterology 102:2091–7, 1992.

454. Dienstag JL, Perrillo RP, Schiff ER et al: A preliminary trial of lamivudine for chronic hepatitis B infection. N Engl J Med 333:1657–61, 1995.

455. Lai CL, Ching CK, Tung AK et al: Lamivudine is effffective in suppressing hepatitis B virus DNA in Chinese hepatitis B surface antigen carriers: A placebo-controlled trial. Hepatology 25:241–44, 1997.

456. Main J, Brown JL, Howells C et al: A double blind placebo-controlled study to assess the effect of famciclovir on virus replication in patients with chronic hepatitis B virus infection. J Viral Hepatol 3:211–5, 1996.

457. Colledge D, Locarnini S, Shaw T: Synergistic inhibition of hepadnaviral replication by lamivudine in combination with penciclovir in vitro. Hepatology 26:216–25, 1997.

458. Clark FL, Drummond MW, Chambers S et al: Successful treatment with lamivudine for fulminant reactivated hepatitis B infection following intensive therapy for high-grade non-Hodgkin's lymphoma. Ann Oncol 9:385–7, 1998.

459. Dienstag JL, Schiff ER, Wright TL et al: Lamivudine as initial treatment for chronic hepatitis B in the United States. N Engl J Med 341:1256–63, 1999.

460. Lai CL, Chien RN, Leung NW et al: A one-year trial of lamivudine for chronic hepatitis B. Asia Hepatitis Lamivudine Study Group. N Engl J Med 339:61–8, 1988.

461. Lau GK, McDonald GB, Strasser SI: Hepatitis virus infection in patients with cancer. In Wingard JR, Bowden RA (Eds.): Management of Infections in Oncology Patients. London: Marin Dunitz (in press).

462. Strasser SI, McDonald GB: Hepatitis viruses and hematopoietic cell transplantation: A guide to patient and donor management. Blood 93:1127–36, 1999.

463. Gilson RJ, Chopra K, Murray-Lyon IM et al: A placebo-controlled phase I/II study of adefovir dipivoxil in patients with chronic hepatitis B virus infection. J Viral Hepatol 6:387–95, 1999.

464. Heathcote EJ, Jeffers L, Wright T et al: Loss of serum HBV DNA and HBeAg and seroconversion following short-term (12 weeks) adefovir dipovoxil therapy in chronic hepatitis B: Two placebo-controlled phase II studies. Hepatology 28:317A(abstract 620), 1988.

465. Innaimo SF, Seifer M, Bisacchi GS et al: Identification of BMS-200475 as a potent and selective inhibitor of hepatitis B virus. Antimicrob Agents Chemother 41:1444–8, 1997.

466. Gish R, Leung NWY, Wright TL et al: Anti-hepatitis B virus (HBV) activity and pharmacokinetics of FTC in a 2 month trial in HBV-infected patients. Gastroenterology 116(Suppl. 4:A1216 [Abstract L0158]), 1999.

467. Ling R, Mutimer D, Ahmed M et al: Selection of mutations in the hepatitis B virus polymerase during therapy of transplant recipients with lamivudine. Hepatology 24:711–3, 1996.

468. Tipples GA, Ma MM, Fischer KP et al: Mutation in HBV RNA-dependent DNA polymerase confers resistance to lamivudine. Hepatology 24:714–17, 1996.

469. Bartholomew MM, Jansen RW, Jeffers LJ et al: Hepatitis-B-virus resistance to lamivudine given for recurrent infection after orthotopic liver transplantation. Lancet 349:20–2, 1997.

470. Locarnini SA: Hepatitis B virus surface antigen and polymerase gene variants: Potential virological and clinical significance. Hepatology 27:294–7, 1998.

471. Perillo R, Schiff E, Yoshida E et al: Adefovir dipivoxil for the treatment of lamivudine-resistant hepatitis B mutants. Hepatology 129–134 (abstract), 2000.

472. Greenberg HB, Pollard RB, Lutwixk LI et al: Effect of human leukocyte interferon on hepatitis B virus infection on patients with chronic active hepatitis. N Engl J Med 295:517, 1976.

473. Rosendahl C, Bender-Götze Ch, Deinhardt F, Kolb H-J, Haas R: Immunization against hepatitis B in BMT- and leukemia-patients. Exp Hematol 13:104, 1985.

474. Ilan Y, Nagler A, Adler R, Tur-Kaspa R, Slavin S, Shouval D: Ablation of persistent hepatitis B by bone marrow transplantation from a hepatitis B-immune donor. Gastroenterology 104:1818–1821, 1993.

475. Shouval D, Adler R, Ilan Y: Adoptive transfer of immunity to hepatitis B virus in mice by bone marrow transplantation from immune donors. Hepatology 17:955–959, 1993.

476. Schreiber GP, Busch MP, Kleinman SH et al: The risk of transfusion-transmitted viral infections. N Engl J Med 334:1691–6, 1996.

477. Donahue JG, Munoz A, Ness PM et al: The declining risk of posttransfusion hepatitis C virus infection. N Engl J Med 327:369–73, 1992.

478. DiBisceglie AM. Hepatitis C. Lancet 351:351–5, 1998.

479. Shakil A, Conry-Cantilena C, Alter H et al: Volunteer blood donors with antibody to hepatitis C virus: Clinical, biochemical, virologic, and histologic features: The Hepatitis C Study Group. Ann Intern Med 23:330–7, 1995.

480. Johnson RJ, Gretch DR, Yamabe H et al: Membranoproliferative glomerulonephritis associated with hepatitis C virus infection. N Engl J Med 328:465–70, 1993.

481. Centers for Disease Control and Prevention: Recommendations for prevention and control of hepatitis C virus (HCV) infection and HCV-related chronic disease. MMWR 47 (No. RR-19): 1–40, 1998.

482. Paul IM, Sanders J, Ruggerio et al: Chronic hepatitis C virus infections in leukemia survivors: Prevalence, viral load, and severity of liver disease. Blood 93:3672–7, 1999.

483. Arico M, Maggiore G, Silini E et al: Hepatitis C virus infection in children treated for acute lymphoblastic leukemia. Blood 84:2919–22, 1994.

484. Lopez-Jimenez J, Cancelas JA, Garcia-Larana J et al: Posttransfusion hepatitis after induction chemotherapy in acute nonlymphoblastic leukemia: Implications for long-term management and outcome. Transfusion 35:313–8, 1995.

485. Meilson JR, Harrison P, Skidmore SJ et al: Chronic hepatitis C in long-term survivors of haematological malignancy treated in a single centre. J Clin Pathol 49:230–2, 1996.

486. Murphy MF, Waters AH, Grint PC et al: Hepatitis C infection in multitransfused patients with acute leukaemia. Lancet 335:58–9, 1990.

487. Locasciulli A, Testa M, Pontisso P et al: Prevalence and natural history of hepatitis C infection in patients cured of childhood leukemia. Blood 90:4628–33, 1997.

488. Fujii Y, Kaku K, Tanaka M et al: Hepatitis C virus infection in patients with leukemia. Am J Hematol 46:278–82, 1994.

489. Stickland DK, Riely CA, Patrick CC et al: Hepatitis C infection among survivors of childhood cancer. Blood 95:3065–70, 2000.

490. Ljungman P, Johansson N, Aschan J et al: Long-term effects of hepatitis C virus infection in allogeneic bone marrow transplant recipients. Blood 86:1614–18, 1995.

491. Locasciulli A, Bacigalupo A, Van Lint et al: Hepatitis C virus infection in patients undergoing allogeneic bone marrow transplantation. Transplantation 52:315–8, 1991.

492. Jackson SR, Carter JM, Jackson TW et al: Hepatitis C seroprevalance in bone marrow transplant recipients and hemophiliacs. N Z Med J 107:10–1, 1994.

493. Fujii Y, Kaku K, Tanaka M et al: Hepatitis C virus infection and liver disease after allogeneic bone marrow transplantation. Bone Marrow Transplant 13:523–6, 1994.

494. Schuhart MC, Myerson D, Spurgeon CL et al: Hepatitis C virus (HCV) infection in bone marrow transplant patients after transfusions from anti-HCV-positive blood donors. Bone Marrow Transplant 17:601–6, 1996.

495. Schuhart MC, Myerson D, Childs BH et al: Marrow transplantation from hepatitis C virus seropositive donors: Transmission rate and clinical course. Blood 84:3229–35, 1994.

496. Strasser SI, Myerson D, Spurgeon CL et al: Hepatitis C virus infection and bone marrow transplantation: A cohort study with 10-year follow-up. Hepatology 29:1893–9, 1999.

497. Frickhofen N, Wiesneth M, Jainta C et al: Hepatitis C virus infection is a risk factor for liver failure from veno-occlusive disease after bone marrow transplantation. Blood 83:1998–2004, 1994.

498. Ljungman P, Hagglund H, Lonnqvist B et al: Hepatitis C virus as a risk factor for the development of veno-occlusive disease of the liver (letter). Blood 84:1349–50, 1994.

499. Norol F, Roche B, Girardin MF et al: Hepatitis C virus infection and allogeneic bone marrow transplantation. Transplantation 57:393–7, 1994.

500. Locasciulli A, Bacigalupo A, Van Lint MT et al: Hepatitis C virus infection and liver failure in patients undergoing allogeneic bone marrow transplantation. Bone Marrow Transplant 16:407–11, 1995.

501. Davis GL, Balart LA, Schiff ER et al: Treatment of chronic hepatitis C with recombinant interferon alfa: A multicenter randomized, controlled trial. N Engl J Med 321:1501–6, 1989.

502. Di Bisceglie AM, Martin P, Kassianides C et al: Recombinant interferon alfa therapy for chronic hepatitis C: A randomized, double-blind, placebo-controlled trial. N Engl J Med 321:1506–10, 1989.

503. Makris M, Preston FE, Triger DR et al: A randomized trial of recombinant interferon-α in chronic hepatitis C in hemophiliacs. Blood 78:1672–7, 1991

504. Hoofnagle JH, di Bisceglie AM: Drug therapy: The treatment of chronic viral hepatitis. N Engl J Med 336:347–56, 1997.

505. Lindsay KL: Therapy of hepatitis C: Overview. Hepatology 26:S71–77, 1997.

506. Poynard T, Bedossa P, Chevallier M et al: A comparison of three interferon alfa-2b regimens for the long-term treatment of chronic non-A, non-B hepatitis. Multicenter study group. N Engl J Med 332:1457–62, 1995.

507. Carithers RL Jr, Emerson SS: Therapy of hepatitis C: Meta-analysis of interferon alfa-2b trials. Hepatology 26:83S–88S, 1997.

508. Poynard T, Marcellin P, Lee SS et al: Randomized trial of interferon α2b plus ribavirin for 48 weeks or for 24 weeks versus interferon α2b plus placebo for 48 weeks for treatment of chronic infection with hepatitis C virus. International Hepatitis Interventional Therapy Group. Lancet 352:1426–32, 1998.

509. Reichard O, Norkrans G, Fryden A et al: Randomized, double-blind, placebo-controlled trial of interferon α-2b with and without ribavirin for chronic hepatitis C. The Swedish Study Group. Lancet 351:83–7, 1998.

510. Schvarcz R, Yun ZB, Sonnerborg A et al: Combined treatment with interferon alpha-2b and ribavirin for chronic hepatitis C in patients with a previous non-response or non-sustained response to interferon alone. J Med Virol 46:43–7, 1995.

511. Morton AJ, Gooley T, Hansen JA et al: Association between pretransplant interferon-alpha and outcome after unrelated donor marrow transplantation for chronic myelogenous leukemia in chronic phase. Blood 92:394–401, 1998.

512. Beelen DW, Graeven U, Elmaagacli AH et al: Prolonged administration of interferon-alpha in patients with chronic-phase Philadelphia chromosome-positive chronic myelogenous leukemia before allogeneic bone marrow transplantation may adversely affect transplant outcome. Blood 85:2981–90, 1995.

513. Hehlmann R, Hochhaus A, Kolb HJ et al: Interferon alpha before allogeneic bone marrow transplantation in chronic myelogenous leukemia does not affect outcome adversely, provided it is discontinued at least 90 days before the procedure. Blood 94:3668–3677, 1999.

514. DiBisceglie AM, Shindoi M, Fong TL et al: A pilot study of ribavirin for chronic hepatitis C. Hepatology 16:649–54, 1992.

515. Dusheiko G, Main J, Thomas H et al: Ribavirin treatment for patients with chronic hepatitis C: Results of a placebo-controlled study. J Hepatol 25:591–8, 1996.

516. Bodenheimer HC Jr, Lindsay KL, Davis GL et al: Tolerance and efficacy of oral ribavirin treatment of chronic hepatitis C: A multicenter trial. Hepatology 26:473–7,1997.

517. Reichard O, Schvarcz R, Weiland O: Therapy of hepatitis C: Interferon and ribavirin. Hepatology 26(suppl 1): 108S–111S, 1997.

518. Ljungman P, Andersson J, Aschan J et al: Oral ribavirin for prevention of severe liver disease caused by hepatitis C virus during allogeneic bone marrow transplantation. Clin Infect Dis 23:167–9, 1996.

519. Shuhart MC, Myerson D, Childs BH et al: Marrow transplantation from hepatitis C virus seropositive donors: Transmission rate and clinical course. Blood 84:3229–35, 1994.

520. Nelson DR, Marousis CG, Davis GL et al: The role of hepatitis C virus-specific cytotoxic T lymphocytes in chronic hepatitis C. J Immunol 158:1473–81, 1997.

521. Vento S, Garofano T, Renzini C et al: Fulminant hepatitis associated with hepatitis A virus superinfection in patients with chronic hepatitis C. N Engl J Med 338:286–90, 1998.

522. Keeffe EB: Is hepatitis A more severe in patients with chronic hepatitis B and other chronic liver diseases? Am J Gastroenterol 90:201–205, 1995.

523. Linnen J, Wages JR, Zhang-Keck ZY et al: Molecular cloning and disease association of hepatitis G virus: A transfusion-transmissible agent. Science 271:505–8, 1996.

524. Leary TP, Muerhoff AS, Simons JN et al: Sequence and genomic organization of GBV-C: A novel member of the faviviridae associated with human non-A–E hepatitis. J Med Virol 48:60–7, 1996.

525. Simons JN, Leary TP, Dawson GJ et al: Isolation of novel virus-like sequences associated with human hepatitis. Nat Med 1:564–9, 1995.

526. Dawson GJ, Schlauder GG, Pilot-Matias TJ et al: Prevalence studies of GB virus-C infection using reverse transcriptase-polymerase chain reaction. J Med Virol 50:97–103, 1996.

527. Yoshikawa A, Fukuda S, Itoh K et al: Infection with hepatitis G virus and its strain variant, the GB agent (GBV-C) among blood donors in Japan. Transfusion 37:657–63, 1997.

528. Yamada-Osaki M, Sumazaki R, Tsuchida M et al: Persistence and clinical outcome of hepatitis G virus-infection in pediatric bone marrow transplant recipients and children treated for hematological malignancy. Blood 93:721–7, 1999.

529. Akiyama H, Nakamura N, Tanikawa S et al: Incidence and influence of GB virus C and hepatitis C virus infection in patients undergoing bone marrow transplantation. Bone Marrow Transplant 21:1131–5, 1998.

530. Skidmore SJ, Collingham KE, Harrison P et al: High prevalence of hepatitis G virus in bone marrow transplant recipients and patients treated for acute leukemia. Blood 89:3853–6, 1997.

531. Rodriguez-Inigo E, Tomas JF, Gomez-Garcia de Soria V et al: Hepatitis C and G virus infection and liver dysfunction after allogeneic bone marrow transplantation: Results from a prospective study. Blood 90:1326–31, 1997.

532. Corbi C, Traineau R, Esperou H et al: Prevalence and clinical features of hepatitis G infection in bone marrow allografts recipients. Bone Marrow Transplant 20:965–8, 1997.

533. Kanda Y, Chiba S, Suzuki T et al: Quantitation of hepatitis G virus RNA in allogeneic bone marrow transplant recipients. Br J Hematol 100:797–800, 1998.

534. Neilson J, Harrison P, Milligan DW et al: Hepatitis G virus in long-term survivors of haematological malignancy. Lancet 347:1632–3, 1996.

535. Ljungman P, Halasz R, Hagglund H et al: Detection of hepatitis G virus/GB virus C after allogeneic bone marrow transplantation. Bone Marrow Transplant 22:499–501, 1998.

536. Grinnell BW, Padgett BL, Walker DL: Distribution of non-integrated DNA from JC papovavirus in organs of patients with progressive multifocal leukoencephalopathy. J Infect Dis 147:669, 1983.

537. Hogan TF, Borden EC, McBain JA et al: Human polyomavirus infections with JC virus and BK virus in renal transplant patients. Ann Intern Med 2:373, 1980.

538. Narayan O, Penney JM Jr, Johnson RT et al: Etiology of progressive multifocal leukoencephalopathy. Identification of papovavirus. N Engl J Med 289:1278, 1973.

539. Saad ED, Thomas DA, O'Brien S et al: Progressive multifocal leukoencephalopathy with concurrent Richter's syndrome. Leuk Lymphoma 38:183–190, 2000.

540. Seong D, Bruner JM, Lee KH et al: Progressive mutlifocal leukoencephalopathy after autologous bone marrow transplantation in a patient with chronic myelogenous leukemia. Clin Infect Dis 23:402–403, 1996.

541. Arthur RR, Shah KV, Baust SJ, Santos GW, Saral R: Association of BK viruria with hemorrhagic cystitis in recipients of bone marrow transplants. N Engl J Med 315:230–234, 1986.

542. Russell SJ, Vowels MR, Vale T: Haemorrhagic cystitis in paediatric bone marrow transplant patients: An association with infective agents, GVHD and prior cyclophosphamide. Bone Marrow Transplant 13:533–539, 1994.

543. Azzi A, Fanci R, Bosi A et al: Monitoring of polyomavirus BK viruria in bone marrow transplantation patients by DNA hybridization assay and by polymerase chain reaction: An approach to assess the relationship between BK viruria and hemorrhagic cystitis. Bone Marrow Transplant 14:235–240, 1994.

544. Schneider EM, Dörries K: High frequency of polyomavirus infection in lymphoid cell preparations after allogeneic bone marrow transplantation. Transplant Proc 25:1271–1273, 1993.

545. Azzi A, Cesaro S, Laszlo D et al: Human polyomavirus BK (BKV) load and haemorrhagic cystitis in bone marrow transplantation patients. J Clin Virol 14:79–86, 1999.

546. Drummond JE, Shah KV, Saral R, Santos GW, Donnenberg AD: BK virus specific humoral and cell mediated immunity in allogeneic bone marrow transplant (BMT) recipients. J Med Virol 23:331–344, 1987.

547. Torok TJ: Parvovirus B19 and human disease. Adv Intern Med 37:431–55, 1992.

548. Coulombel L, Morinet F, Mielot F et al: Parvovirus infection, leukemia, and immunodeficiency. Lancet 1:101–2, 1989.

549. Smith MA, Shah NR, Lobel JS et al: Severe anemia caused by human parvovirus in a leukemia patient on maintenance chemotherapy. Clin Pediatr 27:383–6, 1988.

550. Fisher D, Spencer D, Iland H et al: Red cell aplasia caused by human parvovirus B19 in acute leukaemia. Aust N Z J Med 22:303–4, 1992.

551. Van Horn DK, Mortimer PP, Young N et al: Human parvovirus-associated red cell aplasia in the absence of underlying hemolytic anemia. Am J Pediatr Hematol Oncol 8:235–9, 1986.

552. Allen-Graeve JL, de Alarcon PA, Naides SJ: Parvovirus B19 infection in patients receiving cancer chemotherapy: The expanding spectrum of disease. Am J Pediatr Hematol Oncol 11:441–4, 1989.

553. Frickhofen N, Arnold R, Hertenstein B et al: Parvovirus B19 infection and bone marrow transplantation. Ann Hematol 64:A121–A124, 1992.

554. Broliden K, Tolfvenstam T, Ohlsson S et al: Persistent B19 parvovirus infection in pediatric malignancies. Med Pediatr Oncol 31:66–72, 1998.

555. Mihal V, Dusek J, Hajduch M et al: Transient aplastic crisis in a leukemic child caused by parvovirus B19 infection. Pediatr Hematol Oncol 13:173–177, 1996.

556. Crook TW, Rogers BB, McFarland RD et al: Unusual bone marrow manifestations of parvovirus B19 infection in immunocompromised patients. Hum Pathol 31:161–168, 2000.

557. Antin JH, Smith BR, Ewenstein BM et al: HTLV-III infection after bone marrow transplantation. Blood 67:160–3, 1986.

558. Opportunistic non-Hodgkin's lymphomas among severely immunocompromised HIV-infected patients surviving for prolonged periods on antiretroviral therapy – United States. MMWR 40:591, 597–600, 1991.

559. Rabkin CS Hilgartner MW, Hedberg KW et al: Incidence of lymphomas and other cancers in HIV-infected and HIV-uninfected patients with hemophilia. JAMA 267:1090–1094, 1992.

560. Beral V, Peterman T, Berkelmam R, Jaffe H: AIDS-associated non-Hodgkin's lymphoma. Lancet 337:805–809, 1991.

561. Gail MH, Pluda JM, Rabkin CS et al: Projections of the incidence of non-Hodgkin's lymphoma related to acquired immunodeficiency syndrome. J Natl Cancer Inst 83:695–701, 1991.

562. Holland HK, Saral R, Rossi JJ et al: Allogeneic bone marrow transplantation and azido-thymidine: Effects on HIV-1 in a patient with non-Hodgkin's lymphoma. Ann Intern Med 111:973–981, 1989.

563. Saral R, Holland HK: In Bone marrow transplantation for the acquired immune deficiency syndrome. In Bone Marrow Transplant. Forman SJ, Blume KG, Thomas ED (eds.) Boston, Blackwell Scientific Publications, pp. 654–664, 1994.

564. Contu L, La Nasa G, Arras M et al: Allogeneic bone marrow transplantation combined with multiple anti-HIV-1 treatment in a case of AIDS. Bone Marrow Transplant 12:669–671, 1993.

565. Matthews GV, Bower M, Mandalia S et al: Changes in acquired immunodeficiency syndrome-related lymphoma since the introduction of highly active antiretroviral therapy. Blood 96:2730–2734, 2000.

566. Porcu P, Caligiuri MA: Acquired immunodeficiency syndrome-related lymphomas: Future directions. Semin Oncol 27:454–62, 2000.

567. Lederman MM, Valdez H: Immune restoration with antiretroviral therapies: Implications for clinical management. JAMA 284:223–228, 2000.

568. Aviles A, Halabe J: Improved prognosis in patients with acquired immunodeficiency syndrome-related lymphoma. Cancer Biother Radiopharm 14:349–352, 1999.

569. Little RF, Yarchoan R, Wilson WH: Systemic chemotherapy for HIV-associated lymphoma in the era of highly active antiretroviral therapy. Curr Opin Oncol 12:438–44, 2000.

570. Okenhendler E, Gerard L, Dubreuil ML et al: Intensive chemotherapy (LNHIV-91 regimen) and G-CSF for HIV associated non-Hodgkin's lymphoma. Leuk Lymphoma. 39:87–95, 2000.

571. Tokudome S, Tokunaga O, Shimamoto Y et al: Incidence of adult T-cell leukemia/lymphoma among human T-lymphotropic virus type I carriers in Saga, Japan. Cancer Res 49:226, 1989.

572. Ratner L, Griffith RC, Marselle L et al: A lymphoproliferative disorder caused by human T-lymphotropic virus type I. Am J Med 83:953–8, 1987.

573. Franchini G, Wong-Staal F, Gallo RC: Human T-cell leukemia virus (HTLV-I) transcripts in fresh and cultured cells of patients with adult T-cell leukemia. Proc Natl Acad Sci U S A 81:6207–11, 1984.

574. Zucker-Franklin D, Hooper WC, Evatt BL: Human lymphotropic retroviruses associated with mycosis fungoides: Evidence that human T-cell lymphotropic virus type II (HTLV-II) as well as HTLV-1 may play a role in the disease. Blood 80:1537–45, 1992.

52

Therapeutic Cytapheresis and Plasma Exchange

Charles A. Schiffer

Some hematologic malignancies are occasionally dominated by symptomatology caused by extremely high levels of circulating leukocytes, thrombocytes, or red blood cells. Although relatively few large studies have been done, there is an extensive literature describing the results of large-scale removal of these circulating elements initially using repetitive, manual centrifugation techniques and more recently, automated blood cell separation. Cytapheresis has been used to relieve acute complications of the malignancy as well as a primary or adjunctive therapy of more chronic hematologic malignancies.

In more acute cases, the potential benefit of cytapheresis depends, in part, on the ability to remove cellular elements faster than the rate at which they are being produced and entering the circulation. The overall outcome depends also on the extent of the tissue damage that may have already occurred as well as the likelihood of response to the accompanying cytotoxic therapy. In the chronic leukemias, the outcome depends on the removal of cells from the circulation, promoting entry into the circulation of cells from such tissue sites as lymph nodes, liver, spleen, and marrow. These factors are discussed in greater detail with each specific disease entity. For more detailed presentations of the pathophysiology and therapy of the specific hematologic malignancies, the reader is referred to other chapters in this text.

Similarly, some patients with hematologic malignancies produce autoantibodies resulting in a variety of syndromes, or, as in plasma cell dyscrasias, paraproteins, which can result in symptomatic hyperviscosity or other paraneoplastic complications. Blood cell separators can efficiently remove the bulk of circulating antibody in such patients, sometimes resulting in immediate relief of symptomatology. As with therapeutic leukapheresis, the quality and duration of benefit is related to the degree of end-organ damage already incurred, the rate of synthesis of the antibody, the rapidity of the effect of cytotoxic or corticosteroid therapy, and, particularly for IgG antibodies, the rate at which antibody re-equilibrated between the intra- and extravascular spaces. This chapter describes the use of plasma removal in selected disorders. The primary treatment and pathophysiology of these diseases are provided in other chapters. An overview by a panel of experts in the field, with recommendations about the appropriate use of cytapheresis and plasma exchange, has recently been published.[1,2]

TECHNICAL CONSIDERATIONS

Patients referred for therapeutic apheresis are frequently acutely ill and therefore at increased risk of complications from the procedure itself. It is therefore important to review the potential side effects of intensive apheresis. All the currently available techniques separate cells from plasma, or conversely, plasma from cells, according to their density, by differential centrifugation. Although it is possible to collect large numbers of platelets or leukocytes, or both, in patients with high counts, by simple repeated centrifugation of single units of blood with return of red blood cells to the patient, this is a slow and tedious method that is used infrequently. This manual method can be used effectively, however, when more limited cytapheresis is contemplated for collection of either platelets or white cells from donors with chronic myelocytic leukemia (CML) for transfusion to thrombocytopenic or leukopenic patients.[3,4] In addition, manual exchange transfusion techniques can be used efficiently in infants and small children.[5–9] Most hospitals and virtually all blood centers now have automatic cell separators for therapeutic apheresis. Although somewhat different in design, all the available blood separators pump donor blood into separation chambers of differing configurations, which are then spun at varying speeds to exert different gravitational forces. The separation chambers contain exit ports that permit semiselective collection of cells of different density or separation of virtually acellular plasma. The remaining cells are then returned to the donor.

Continuous-flow processors, in which blood is pumped continuously from one donor vein to another with an intervening separation chamber, are available from a number of manufacturers.[8–12] Depending on venous access and donor tolerance, these machines generally permit high blood flow, and large volumes of blood (more than 10 L) can be processed within a 2- to 3-hour period. Discontinuous-flow centrifugation technology is also available. In this procedure, blood from a patient fills a conical bowl, rotated at a fixed speed. Cellular elements are separated along the sides and top of the bowl and are eventually collected at the top of the bowl. The bowl is then emptied, with the remaining red cells returned to the patient. The process is then repeated 6 to 10 times within a 2- to 4-hour period. Although platelet and lymphocyte collection is very efficient, less blood can be processed than with the continuous-flow devices because of the intermittent collection pattern.[13–15]

With all cell separators, the blood must be anticoagulated as it leaves the patient in order to avoid clotting in the bowl. Both heparin and various citrate solutions, such as acid citrate dextrose (ACD) and citrate-phosphated dextrose (CPD), are used. Heparin can cause systemic anticoagulation upon return to the donor and offers no advantage over anticoagulation with citrate. Both ACD and CPD act as anticoagulants by chelating divalent cations. They are mixed with donor blood as it leaves the body in a ratio of 1 part anticoagulant to 8 to 14 parts donor blood. If blood return is excessive, some patients will experience symptoms of hypocalcemia, which include circumoral paresthesias, anxiety, irritability, and very rarely, frank tetany.[15] These symptoms can be prevented or ameliorated by stopping or slowing down blood return. Hypocalcemic symptoms tend to occur more commonly in smaller recipients or in recipients with hepatic dysfunction in whom citrate metabolism is slower. Systemic anticoagulation does not occur with citrate solutions.

The extracorporeal blood volume varies among the different separators and can be an important consideration, particularly in anemic patients. The tubing and separation chambers of the continuous-flow separators have a total volume of approximately 200 to 250 ml. Because fluid is constantly being replaced in the continuous-flow devices, symptoms of volume depletion are relatively uncommon. By contrast, even with a normal hematocrit of 40 percent, the extracorporeal volume with discontinuous-flow cell separation is approximately 500 ml. In anemic patients, this increases significantly and, at times, as much as 700 ml or more can be extracorporeal. Hypotensive and vasovagal reactions therefore tend to occur more commonly, particularly in children, smaller patients, and elderly patients. It is sometimes advisable to transfuse patients with red blood cells either before or during therapeutic apheresis with the discontinuous-flow apparatus. As described below, however, this can be somewhat hazardous in certain patients. It may therefore be advisable to use different machines, if available, depending on the needs and risks inherent in particular patients.

Cell separation is also, at best, semiselective. Platelets are the lightest of the formed circulating elements and tend to form a layer above, but partially mixed with the leukocyte layer, which, in turn, usually blends indistinctly with the upper layer of red blood cells. Leukocyte removal is therefore often associated with significant removal of platelets. This can be a potentially serious problem in patients with acute leukemia and supplementary platelet transfusions are often necessary. It is sometimes possible and advisable to increase the separation between the red blood cells and the leukocytes by using red cell rouleauxing agents, such as hydroxyethyl starch (HES).[13,14,16] This latter drug has relatively few known side effects, although rare atopic reactions have occurred and blood volume expansion occurs uniformly in recipients of HES.[17–19]

Red blood cells also separate according to their differential densities, with the lightest, youngest, and therefore, most reticulocyte-rich band occurring in proximity to the leukocyte band. Indeed, blood cell separators have been used to obtain units of blood that are rich in younger cells, so-called neocytes, for use in chronic transfusion programs for patients with thalassemia major.[20–22] In the setting of cytapheresis, although one usually removes only relatively small amounts of red cells during platelet or leukocyte collection (usually less than 50 ml, total), the lost red cells often contain a disproportionate number of reticulocytes. Repeated, long-term apheresis can therefore occasionally be accompanied by *reticulocytopenia* and eventually anemia disproportionated to the number of red blood cells actually removed. This phenomenon is a potential problem only in patients undergoing repeated long-term cytapheresis, generally for either chronic lymphocytic or chronic myelocytic leukemia.[23]

Some additional considerations are more specifically related to plasma exchange. In general, when the goal is to remove sufficient amounts of antibody-containing plasma, it is impossible to use crystalloid alone to replace the 2 to 4 L of plasma removed because many patients will become hypotensive when large amounts of protein are taken away. Depending on the circumstance, isovolemic replacement with a variable mixture of albumin and normal saline is effective. In addition to decreases in serum albumin, a high-volume plasma exchange can also reduce clotting factors and fibrinogen to levels that can elevate the prothrombin and partial thromboplastin times for 12 to 24 hours, depending in part on the patient's hepatic function and synthetic rate.[24] This is rarely a clinical problem with single exchanges, except in patients with pre-existing coagulation disorders or perhaps severe thrombocytopenia, but it can become a consideration with repeated, high-frequency exchanges. In such cases, supplementation with fresh frozen plasma (FFP) may be indicated. Because of the potential for transmission of viral diseases, albumin preparations should be used in preference to FFP whenever possible. Plasma exchange for thrombocytopenic purpura (TTP) or hemolytic uremic syndrome represents the exception to this guideline. In these disorders, FFP is used exclusively, because of the need to infuse a putative "inhibitory factor" contained in normal plasma that reverses the characteristic microangiopathy and hemolytic anemia.[25]

Techniques have also been developed to permit more selective removal of immunoglobulins (Igs), obviating the needs for bulk removal of plasma and large-volume replacement fluids. Columns containing blood group A or B trisaccharides have been used to remove anti-A or -B antibodies in patients receiving blood group mis-matched allogeneic bone marrow transplants. Although effective in some patients, the efficiency of removal was lower than with plasma exchange.[26] Removal of erythrocytes from the marrow preparation is probably a simpler approach to this problem, but this experience and the use of hollow fiber membrane devices to remove low-density lipoproteins semiselectively from patients with hypercholesterolemia illustrate the promise offered by more specific absorption or separation.[27]

Staphylococcal protein A columns, which have been approved for the therapy of refractory immune thrombocytopenic purpura (ITP), provide another means of semiselective removal of Igs. Plasma is separated using any of the blood cell separators and passed over protein A columns, which bind most subclasses of IgG. This technique has been used in the treatment of a variety of solid tumors (with anecdotal reports of tumor regression), as therapy for refractory TTP, and for the removal of antibodies associated with refractoriness to platelet transfusion.[28–33] Most of the literature using this approach consists of case reports of seriously ill patients in whom a variety of different therapies are being applied at once, and it is therefore difficult to place this therapy in proper perspective. The columns and the accompanying apheresis procedure are quite expensive and multiple procedures are usually required. In addition, a significant incidence of side effects is seen, including fever, chills, dyspnea, and hypotension. Given these considerations, therapy with staph protein A columns should be considered experimental in most circumstances and should be evaluated in carefully controlled clinical trials prior to more widespread use.

Venous access is an important but often overlooked problem. Rapid blood flow is required to process effectively an adequate amount of blood to permit sufficient removal of cellular elements or plasma. In general, two good venipunctures with large needles are required, although the discontinuous-flow processor can be used with a one-arm technique. Particularly in patients with thrombocytopenia or other associated coagulation abnormalities, venous access can be a problem and the attainment of adequate access (e.g., use of subclavian lines, femoral vein punctures, fistulas) dangerous. The relative risks must therefore be balanced against the benefits of the procedure.

Lastly, technical problems of varying severity can occur. Technical error or inadequate coagulation can lead to widespread clotting in the tubing and the separation chambers. Although generally this only results in the loss of the extracorporeal blood, cases of diffuse intravascular coagulation have been seen in donors, presumably the result of infusion of activated clotting factors. Air embolism, mechanical hemolysis of red cells as they pass rapidly through kinked portions of tubing, and infections (either systemically or at the site of venipuncture) are rare but avoidable complications.

LEUKAPHERESIS

Myeloid Disorders

Acute Leukemia

Leukocytes are less deformable than red blood cells, with primitive blasts considerably less distensible than mature myeloid cells.[34,35] With increasing blast counts, usually at levels greater than 100,000/μl in the myeloid leukemias, blood flow in the microcirculation can be impeded by plugs of poorly deformable blasts. Local hypoxemia may be exacerbated by the high metabolic activity of the continually dividing blasts, with endothelial damage and hemorrhage. The situation can be further exacerbated by red blood cell transfusions that rapidly increase whole blood viscosity in the presence of hyperleukocytosis, further compromising local blood flow.[35,36] Finally, coagulation abnormalities, including disseminated intravascular coagulation, are not uncommon, particularly in patients in whom rapid rises in blast count are occurring, which further increases the risk of local hemorrhage. Although pathologic evidence of leukostasis can be found in most organs in patients with extremely high white blood cell (WBC) counts, clinical symptomatology is usually related to central nervous system[37–39] and pulmonary involvement.[7,40–43] Occasionally, pulmonary symptomatology with worsening hypoxemia can occur with therapy and lysis of entrapped leukemic cells.[39] There is a suggestion that leukocytosis may be more common in patients with myelomonocytic or monocytic leukemia,[44] and it is possible that the clinical manifestations of hyperleukocytosis are exacerbated by the migration of leukemic monocytes into tissue where further proliferation occurs.[45]

Thus, hyperleukocytosis in acute myelocytic leukemia, in CML in blast crisis, and very rarely, in acute lymphocytic leukemia (ALL), constitutes a medical emergency, and efforts should be made to lower the WBC count rapidly. In most patients, rapid cytoreduction can be achieved by chemotherapy, with either standard induction agents or with high doses of hydroxyurea.[46] In some patients, however, the response to chemotherapy can be somewhat delayed, whereas in others, it is impossible to initiate chemotherapy immediately because of metabolic problems, delays in initiating allopurinol therapy so as to prevent hyperuricemia and renal insufficiency, and so forth. In such cases, emergency leukapheresis has been used to lower or stabilize the WBC count.

There are numerous reports of intensive leukapheresis, with procedure times often lasting many hours, resulting in significant and often rapid improvement of pulmonary and central nervous system (CNS) symptomatology in association with a fall in peripheral WBC.[42,43,46–49] Complications of the procedure include worsening thrombocytopenia and anemia, as well as bleeding at venipuncture sites. Liberal use of platelet transfusions is recommended, particularly since the platelet count is frequently overestimated because of the presence of fragments of blasts on blood smears, which can be mistakenly counted as platelets.[50] Red blood cell transfusions should be used judiciously, however, if at all, because of concern about increasing whole blood viscosity and worsening symptoms.

What is not clear from the literature, however, is whether the same results could have been achieved with chemotherapy alone. There are both theoretical and practical limitations to the potential benefits of leukapheresis. It is difficult, for example, to envision how leukapheresis could affect already established vascular plugs, particularly if vascular invasion had taken place. In such cases, chemotherapy and possibly radiation therapy have to be the primary modalities, although theoretically leukapheresis could decrease further "accumulation" of leukocytes at these sites. Furthermore, it is precisely the patient in whom leukostasis is most likely to occur, that is, the patient with high and rapidly rising blast counts, in whom the technical limitations of leukapheresis are important. It is often impossible, even with the use of rouleauxing agents and highly efficient cell separators "to get ahead" of the rapidly rising count. In one study,[42] leukapheresis failed to significantly decrease the blast count in 40 percent of patients with AML and initial counts > 100,000/μl, and the median WBC count of 80,000/μl post leukapheresis was still quite elevated. In addition, in such patients with a high proliferative thrust and presumably a high labeling index, cycle-specific chemotherapeutic agents are more likely to be most rapidly effective. The volume-expanding effects of HES also confers at least a theoretical risk of further bleeding in the microcirculation. Nor is it clear why leukapheresis should be of benefit to patients who develop pulmonary problems during cytotoxic treatment, since it is likely that the symptoms are related as much to a local inflammatory response, caused by leukocyte lysis, as to further accumulation of leukocytes at these sites.

Nonetheless, the initial mortality rate for patients with acute myelocytic leukemia and symptomatic hyperleukocytosis is quite high. If patients survive the initial period, however, they tend to have a response rate similar to that of other patients, although it appears that the duration of response in such cases is shorter.[51,52] In a limited study, patients with elevated WBC counts (more than 100,000/μl) were randomized to undergo either one or three leukaphereses prior to treatment with chemotherapy.[53] A small improvement in complete response rate was noted in those patients in whom more than a 50 percent fall in WBC count was achieved with leukapheresis, although the difference was not significant because of the small number of patients studied. No information is given about the number of patients who were symptomatic, and it is not clear whether differences in mortality were related to an imbalance in the number of patients with organ dysfunction in each group. It is also possible that the ability to decrease the count with leukapheresis, sometimes accomplished with the removal of a relatively modest number of cells, may have reflected a lower rate of proliferation or marrow release in the patients, rather than successful treatment of patients in whom severe symptoms of leukostasis were likely to occur. One cannot recommend leukapheresis as routine therapy or as a form of tumor "debulking" in asymptomatic adult patients with high WBC counts. Similarly, although leukapheresis can rapidly lower WBC counts in children with AML and ALL, there is no suggestion in the literature that response rates or overall outcomes are improved in the asymptomatic patient.[5–7]

It is clear, however, that leukapheresis can help the occasional patient in whom chemotherapeutic agents cannot be administered immediately or in whom initial chemotherapy has not produced the desired rapid fall in WBC count. It is otherwise difficult to make firm recommendations about the proper role of leukapheresis, although it is probably wise, if facilities are available, to leukapherese patients with extremely high white counts and associated symptomatology. Leukapheresis can also be used in the occasional patient with acute leukemia diagnosed during pregnancy (who has an elevated white cell count but an otherwise relatively indolent disease) in whom one wishes to delay cytotoxic therapy.[49]

Chronic Myelocytic Leukemia

Symptomatic leukostasis is an extremely uncommon clinical event in CML in the chronic phase because of the increased deformability of the more mature myeloid elements, compared with the circulating blasts found in acute leukemia or blast crisis of CML.[34,35] In addition, the moderate anemia usually associated with extreme leukocytosis in the chronic phase probably contributes to an overall decrease in blood viscosity.[35] Leukaphresis has been studied by a number of investigators as a means of modifying the overall course of the disease. In addition, leukocytes obtained from donors with CML have been used for at least 25 years in the transfusion support of infected, granulocytopenic patients.[54–57] Transfusions from CML donors have the advantage of providing near physiologic doses of leukocytes for transfusion. In addition, transfused cells frequently persist, so that there is a sustained production of granulocytes even after a single transfusion due to continued proliferation by transfused promyelocytes and myelocytes.[34,57] Thus, a sustained clinical benefit can often be seen in recipients after a single, large-dose transfusion.

With intensive repeated leukapheresis, it is possible to produce consistent falls in peripheral leukocyte count, improvement in systemic symptoms, and reduction in hepatosplenomegaly

and possibly marrow infiltration.[16,55–62] Multiple and repeated courses of therapy are necessary to accomplish this, although rare patients are seen in whom more sustained effects can occur with less frequent aphereses. This latter phenomenon probably occurs in patients with CML and less active disease who also have a pronounced cycling of their leukocytosis and disease activity.[59,63] It is important that leukapheresis does not seem to change the overall course of the disease. There are no cytogenetic changes, and the Philadelphia chromosome is maintained. Most importantly, in one study in which intensive leukapheresis was used as the sole form of therapy in an effort to avoid alkylating agents, there was no apparent elimination or postponement of the blast crisis of the disease and no improvement in overall median survival.[60] Therefore, because leukapheresis is expensive and repeated aphereses are quite inconvenient for the patient, leukapheresis has no significant role in the routine management of patients with CML. An exception to this is in the unusual patient who presents with CML during pregnancy.[58,64] In such patients, intensive leukapheresis can be used as an alternative to cytotoxic therapy in early pregnancy to avoid potential teratogenic risks to the fetus.

Repeated leukapheresis in CML also can increase anemia, probably due to the disproportionate collection of reticulocytes in the leukocyte layer.[23] Virtually all patients on chronic leukapheresis programs have required periodic red blood cell transfusions. Thrombocytopenia can be worsened in some patients. Alternatively, thrombocytosis in CML can be effectively treated simultaneously. Lastly, a rouleauxing agent must be added to the patient's blood to permit efficient leukocyte collection.[16] No untoward effects have been documented from the chronic use of HES in this clinical setting, although the number of observations is small.

Recently, it has been shown that Philadelphia chromosome-negative stem cells can be found in significant quantities in the peripheral blood of patients with CML recovering from the administration of high-dose chemotherapy.[65] A number of centers are evaluating the use of these cells, which can be collected in a few leukapheresis procedures, for autologous reconstitution, often with additional maneuvers such as long-term culture systems or "purging" with molecular "anti-sense" techniques. It remains to be seen whether such approaches will be of value for patients without histocompatible donors or for older patients unable to tolerate allogeneic transplantation.

Hypereosinophilic Syndromes

There is evidence that the clinical manifestations in patients with hyperosinophilic syndrome are related to tissue infiltration by eosinophils and a reaction to intracellular products released by these cells.[66] There is very little reported experience with leukapheresis in this disorder. In one patient reported by Ellman et al.[67] reduction in the circulating eosinophil count by leukapheresis resulted in apparent prompt clinical improvement; however, this patient most likely had hypereosinophilia related to an allergic reaction rather than true hypereosinophilic syndrome. The only other available reports show no clinical benefit of leukapheresis in a total of four patients.[68,69] No information is given about the number of eosinophils removed. Of interest is that some investigators noted that plasma exchange alone produced a greater fall in circulating eosinophil count than did leukapheresis.[67] There is no obvious explanation for this observation, and the use of leukapheresis in eosinophilic disorders must be considered investigational.

Lymphoproliferative Disorders

Chronic Lymphocytic Leukemia

In many respects, therapeutic leukapheresis would appear to be a potential ideal primary or adjunctive therapy for chronic lymphocytic leukemia (CLL). The disorder is characterized by progressive tissue and marrow involvement by long-lived small lymphocytes with a small proliferative pool and well-demonstrated communications between the circulating and tissue pools of lymphocytes.[70] In addition, extracorporeal irradiation has been found to have some effect on both circulating lymphocyte counts and sites of nodal and splenic involvement.[71,72]

It is clear from a number of reports that intensive leukapheresis can produce consistent falls in circulating lymphocyte counts.[73–76] Variable regression in the magnitude of bone marrow infiltration, adenopathy, splenomegaly, and improvements in blood counts can occur. Occasionally, improvement in constitutional symptoms or hemolytic anemia has been noted. There have been no reports of reversal of hypogammaglobulinemia.

Most patients studied had advanced disease usually refractory to other types of therapy. Fortuny et al.[75] and Goldfinger et al.[76] reported either very transient benefits or no benefit in a total of 12 patients. By contrast, Cooper et al.[73] described somewhat greater improvement in blood counts that, in a few patients, lasted up to a year. Some of these patients had received no prior therapy; in others, the hematopoietic improvement was somewhat modest. Nonetheless, it would appear that some patients clearly improved with leukapheresis therapy.

On balance, it would appear that even intensive leukapheresis offers a modest benefit for patients with advanced CLL. Of note is that benefits are limited despite the removal of many kilograms of leukemic cells by leukapheresis. Because symptoms of leukostasis are rarely if ever seen in CLL, leukapheresis has limited, if any value in the treatment of advanced disease. There are no data to indicate whether leukapheresis has a role as an adjunct to chemotherapy or radiation therapy in the management of early-stage CLL. Because of the kinetics of the disease, however, CLL is less likely to be the disorder in which leukemic cell proliferation could be influenced by bulk removal of cells so as to possibly increase sensitivity to cycle-specific chemotherapy.

Prolymphocytic leukemia, a less common variant of CLL usually seen in elderly men, is characterized by hepatosplenomegaly, extremely high circulating leukocyte counts, and a poor response to chemotherapy. The lymphocytes are considerably larger than in CLL and frequently have large multiple nucleoli. Intensive leukapheresis can result in a decrease in circulating lymphocytes, reduction in splenomegaly, and improvements in the bone marrow and the peripheral blood counts.[77] Splenectomy may also help such patients, and it may be that a combination of splenectomy plus leukapheresis may provide effective palliation for some patients with this uncommon disorder.[77]

Hairy Cell Leukemia (Leukemic Reticuloendotheliosis)

Hairy cell leukemia is a distinct chronic lymphoproliferative disorder diagnosed morphologically by the presence in the peripheral blood, spleen, and bone marrow of lymphoid cells, with characteristic projections seen by light and electron microscopy and tartrate-resistant acid phosphatase demonstrated by histochemical techniques. Treatment was generally by splenectomy in the past, although most patients now receive interferon-α or more recently deoxycorformycin or 2′-chlorodeoxyadenosine initially, because of the high-grade responses produced by these agents.[78–80] More intensive cytotoxic therapy is generally not effective. Although most patients with hairy cell leukemia are pancytopenic, a significant number of postsplenectomy patients will have a more obvious leukemic phase with elevated WBC counts.

Experience with intensive leukapheresis is limited.[81] Fay et al.[82] reported sustained clinical improvement lasting for 2 years or more in a patient with a circulating leukocyte count of approximately 50,000/μl, who had a total of 7×10^{11} peripheral leukemia cells removed over a 5-week period. Of note is that the bone marrow infiltration with leukemia cells apparently decreased, with an accompanying rise in other blood cell counts. In addition, peripheral lymphadenopathy and skin infiltrates disappeared. This latter phenomenon has been noted by others,[83] and in one additional case, who presented with an unusually high WBC count of more than 500,000/μl, reduction of splenomegaly was seen with intensive leukapheresis.[84] These observations suggest an ability to mobilize the leukemic cells from these noncirculating pools. A more recent report of four patients, however, demonstrated only transient benefit in symptomatology and pancytopenia in one patient.[85]

Given the major therapeutic advances that have a occurred in recent years, any adjunctive role of leukapheresis in the management of hairy cell leukemia will be limited. It is likely, however, that cells can be mobilized from the noncirculating pool providing some information about the "biology" of the disease.

Sézary Syndrome

Sézary syndrome is a variant of T-cell lymphoma in which neoplastic T lymphocytes are found in the peripheral blood. Experience with therapeutic leukapheresis is very limited,[86,87] but it is clear from two patients in whom large numbers of lymphocytes were removed (between 1 and 36×10^{11}) with multiple leukaphereses, that amelioration of skin plaques, erythroderma, and lymphadenopathy can occur.[88] This indicates a large degree of communication between the vascular and tissue pools in this disease. Less intensive leukapheresis with the removal of far fewer cells was unsuccessful in patients reported by Pineda et al.[69] Thus, the role of conventional leukapheresis in Sézary syndrome is unclear, but again worthy of further testing in appropriate patients refractory to systemic chemotherapy with high circulating white cell counts. It is likely that multiple leukaphereses with the removal of large numbers of cells would be required for treatment to be successful.

A novel approach using a modified discontinuous-flow leukapheresis apparatus was described by Edelson et al.[89,90]

Patients with cutaneous T-cell lymphoma and erythroderma underwent leukapheresis after receiving oral methoxsalen, a drug capable of cross-linking and damaging DNA after photoactivation. The lymphocyte-enriched plasma was then exposed to irradiation with ultraviolet A, after which the autologous cells were reinfused into the patient. Twenty-seven of 37 patients, most of whom were "refractory" to conventional therapy, had clinical benefit as assessed by improvement in exfoliative skin lesions. Responses were seen primarily in patients with erythroderma. The therapy was well tolerated, although multiple treatments were required with a mean time to response of more than 5 months. The mechanisms responsible for the antitumor effect are not known, although it is hypothesized that an immune reaction to the ex vivo damaged lymphocytes resulted in suppression of tumor growth in the patient.[91] Although photopheresis has been granted Food and Drug Administration approval for the treatment of mycosis fungoides, there have been relatively few additional reports and no randomized trials have been conducted.[92,93] Because many patients receive other therapies in conjunction with photopheresis, it can be difficult to assess its effect in many patients and a recent review recommended conservatism in the use of this therapy until further results are published.[93] Thus, the ultimate role of this approach for patients with mycosis fungoides and other cancers awaits further clinical trials and elucidation of the changes produced in the immune system, if any. Photopheresis has also been evaluated in other T-cell-mediated disorders such as graft-versus-host disease with interesting preliminary salutory results.[94]

PLATELETPHERESIS

Marked elevations of the platelet count to levels higher than 1,000,000/μl can be seen in all the myeloproliferative disorders, as a "reactive thrombocytosis" in postsurgical patients (particularly postsplenectomy), and in patients with a variety of malignancies or infections. Thrombotic and hemorrhagic complications are extremely uncommon in patients with reactive thrombocytosis, and such patients infrequently need specific therapy directed at the platelet count.[95,96] In vitro tests of platelet function are invariably normal in such patients; indeed, this can sometimes by used to distinguish patients with reactive thrombocytosis from those with myeloproliferative disorders.[96–99]

By contrast, a variety of abnormalities have been reported in patients with myeloproliferative disorders, including mild to marked prolongation of the bleeding time, decreased platelet adhesiveness, morphologic heterogeneity with the presence of large and hypogranular platelets, diminished aggregation response to most agonists (particularly epinephrine), and spontaneous platelet aggregation.[96,97,99] An increased incidence of both hemorrhagic and thrombotic phenomena occur in such patients, the latter including pulmonary embolism, myocardial or cerebral infarcts, digit or extremity ischemia, priapism, and amourosis fugax. There is, however, no relationship between the circulating platelet count, which is sometimes over 4 to 5 × 10⁶/μl, or any of the in vitro tests of platelet function and the occurrence of hemorrhagic or thrombotic phenomena.[96,100]

There is therefore considerable disagreement as to when to initiate therapy with cytotoxic or antiplatelet agents in asymptomatic patients, particularly because both young and elderly patients can remain asymptomatic for years without treatment.[101,102] The risk of hemorrhage and thrombosis is increased in patients with uncontrolled polycythemia in association with thrombocytosis, however, and phlebotomy to control the red blood mass in such patients is the most beneficial initial approach.

Cytotoxic therapy can take many days to weeks to begin to lower the platelet count. Intensive plateletpheresis, therefore, is useful in patients with myeloproliferative disorders and symptomatic thrombocytosis before the long-term effects of cytotoxic therapy can occur. In addition, although splenectomy is usually contraindicated in patients with primary thrombocythemia or polycythemia vera, occasionally such patients must undergo splenectomy or other types of surgery, the former usually later in the course, when severe myelofibrosis may have occurred. Many patients with CML have thrombocytosis as a dominant clinical feature. Such patients often undergo splenectomy for a variety of clinical indications or because of trauma and either pre- or postoperatively, thrombocytosis, with the risk of increased operative hemorrhage or postoperative thrombosis, remains a problem. It is, therefore, in these clinical settings that apheresis has been used as adjunctive therapy.

Large numbers of platelets can be removed rapidly and safely from patients with thrombocytosis.[103–111] The only additional concern in such patients is that platelet clumping and, rarely, outright clotting has been noted to occur in the collection chambers of the cell separator. This can be prevented by the administration of aspirin. Depending on the platelet count, it is possible to remove as many as 5 to 10 × 10¹² platelets (the equivalent of more than 100 units of platelet concentrate) at a single donation, with rapid lowering of the platelet count. Symptomatic improvement also usually occurs rapidly, although this, in part, depends on the degree of tissue ischemia or infarction, or both. It is also clear, however, that plateletpheresis alone rarely suffices as definitive therapy because in almost all patients the platelet count begins to rise, often rapidly within the next 24 to 48 hours.[110] Repeated procedures are therefore usually necessary until chemotherapy has begun to control the proliferative activity.

Of interest is that in vitro abnormalities of platelet function can sometimes be corrected following plateletpheresis alone.[107] Although the mechanism for improvement of in vitro function is unclear, it may be related to the semiselective removal of larger, possibly more morphologically and functionally abnormal platelets. In addition, it is possible that circulating platelet aggregates of differing size are more effectively removed. More studies of this sort are necessary to confirm these observations.

In summary, plateletpheresis has its major role as an emergency procedure in patients with clinical symptomatology caused by an elevated platelet count. Plateletpheresis is not indicated in asymptomatic patients, except perhaps preoperatively in patients undergoing elective surgical procedures. There are no data about using plateletpheresis as "maintenance therapy" in patients with thrombocythemia, and therefore, its use in this clinical setting cannot be recommended, except perhaps in previously symptomatic patients who cannot tolerate cytotoxic therapy because of unexpected myelosuppression. This is a very unusual clinical circumstance, however.

ERYTHROCYTAPHERESIS

Removal of red blood cells from patients with polycythemia vera is easily accomplished using simple phlebotomy techniques; there is no advantage in the use of a blood cell separator in this setting. Blood cell separators can be used to perform partial exchange transfusions in patients with sickle cell anemia more rapidly, although standard manual methods can suffice for more elective situations.[112] The main advantage of cell separators may be in patients with thrombotic complications, such as priapism, in whom a more rapid exchange may be desired. Finally, it is possible to collect younger red blood cells semiselectively for transfusion in an attempt to decrease the transfusion requirements and therefore the risk of transfusion hemochromatosis in patients with thalassemia major being managed on chronic hypertransfusions regimens.[20–22] Technical improvements are necessary, however, before this somewhat tedious and expensive approach can be more widely used.

MISCELLANEOUS USES OF APHERESIS

Stem Cell Procurement

Mononuclear cell fractions, which can be efficiently collected by all the continuous- and intermittent-flow centrifugation devices, have been shown to contain a variable number of committed myeloid (colony-forming units granulocytemacrophage), erythroid, (burst-forming unit erythroid), and megakaryocytic precursors as well as pluripotent stem cells. These can be cryopreserved and used as an alternative to bone marrow for autologous reconstitution following intensive cytotoxic therapy.[113] This approach is of particular interest in disorders with a proclivity for bone marrow metastases (e.g., oat cell carcinoma, breast cancer) but has also been used in hematologic tumors that involve the peripheral blood. Syngeneic transplants have been done exclusively using peripheral blood stem cells mobilized with granulocyte colony-stimulating factor. Hematopoietic reconstitution of both neutrophils and platelets was quite rapid.[114] A similar approach can be used for allogeneic transplantation, although there is concern about an increased risk of graft-versus-host disease (GvHD) because of the larger number of T lymphocytes contained in peripheral blood compared with bone marrow preparations. Recent reports have suggested that the incidence and severity of GvHD may not be increased with allogeneic peripheral blood stem cells.[115] Because of the rapid kinetics of blood count recovery (particularly of the platelet count), cytokine mobilized peripheral blood stem cells have become the product of choice in most centers. Further details about the collection, cryopreservation, and clinical utility of peripheral blood stem cells in the treatment of patients with hematologic malignances can be found in other chapters of this book.

Removal of Lymphocytes to Modulate Immunity

Intensive lymphocytopheresis can result in lymphocytopenia comparable to that achievable by thoracic duct drainage.[116] Lymphocytopenia is predominantly due to a loss of circulating T lymphocytes, which, in turn, can be reflected functionally in a decrease in in vitro response to T-cell mitogens.[116] Because of the relatively low lymphocyte count in most patients, repeated leukaphereses are necessary to produce these changes. There are no data as to whether immune modulation by simple removal of lymphocytes has a role in the management of hematologic malignancies or solid tumors, although the development of potent immunosuppressive agents, such as cyclosporine, would seem to make this a moot point.

PLASMA EXCHANGE

Hyperviscosity Syndrome

Symptoms due to blood hyperviscosity can be protean and involve any organ system. Most symptoms are a consequence of decreased blood flow producing tissue ischemia or occasionally infarction and include somnolence, focal neurologic signs due to CNS ischemia, epistaxis or bleeding at other sites such as the skin and gingiva, and shortness of breath with signs of circulatory congestion because of expanded plasma volume. Hyperviscosity syndrome is most common in patients with Waldenström's macroglobulinemia, but can be seen in patients with multiple myeloma with IgA paraproteins.[117,118] Hyperviscosity is uncommon in patients with IgG myeloma because the lower molecular weight IgG is distributed throughout the extravascular space, although it can occur with subclasses of IgG such as IgG3, which can polymerize and remain largely intravascular. These issues are discussed further in the chapters on multiple myeloma and macroglobulinemia.

Symptoms of hyperviscosity generally resolve promptly, sometimes during the procedure itself. Removal of a single plasma volume is generally sufficient and can be done in $1\frac{1}{2}$ to $2\frac{1}{2}$ hours with continuous flow separators. Processing much larger volumes becomes relatively inefficient towards the end of the procedure and is usually not advisable.[119] Repeat plasma exchange is sometimes of benefit in patients with IgG proteins after a few days has elapsed to allow equilibration of IgG from the extravascular compartment. The frequency with which exchange is needed is variable and depends on the rate of paraprotein synthesis and catabolism and the effect of chemotherapy. Although occasional patients with macroglobulinemia can be managed with intermittent plasma exchange alone, all patients eventually require cytotoxic therapy to decrease protein production.[120] It is generally necessary to administer some colloid solution such as albumin or plasmanate in addition to crystalloid, to prevent hypovolemia.

Miscellaneous Conditions

Plasma exchange has also been used as adjunctive therapy for many conditions associated with allo- or autoantibody production complicating hematologic malignancies including immune ITP, autoimmune hemolytic anemia, cold agglutinin disease, autoantibodies against clotting factors (particularly factor VIII), alloimmunization to platelet antigens with refractoriness to platelet transfusion, and cryoglobulinemia.[121–124] It is advisable to use blood warming devices, a heated room or both, to prevent precipitation and clogging of the machine when patients with cold agglutinins or cryoglobulins are treated. Most of these disorders are due to overproduction of IgG antibodies, and the technique is usually applied to patients refractory to other, simpler therapies. By definition, such patients produce either large amounts of antibody or antibody with high reactivity against the antigen, and require many procedures to produce clinical benefit. The success rate in such patients is therefore low and the available case reports suggesting benefit overstate the likely response rate due to publication bias of "positive" rather than negative results. Nonetheless, plasma exchange should be considered in selected patients in whom more standard approaches have not been of sufficient value, particularly if it is felt that temporary benefit could be important to the future management of the patient.

REFERENCES

1. Grima KM: Therapeutic apheresis in hematological and oncological diseases. J Clin Apheresis 15(1–2):28–52, 2000.
2. McLeod BC, Strauss RG, Ciavarella D et al: Management of hematologic disorders and cancer. J Clin Apheresis 8:211, 1993.
3. Aisner J, Schiffer CA, Hedmann S, Wiernik PH: Gravity leukapheresis—a simple method of leukocyte collection for transfusion or in vitro study. Leuk Res 3:1, 1979.
4. Schiffer CA, Buchholz DH, Wiernik PH: Intensive multiunit plateletpheresis of normal donors. Transfusion 14:388, 1974.
5. Bunin NJ, Kunkel K, Callihan TR: Cytoreductive procedures in the early management in cases of leukemia and hyperleukocytosis in children. Med Pediatr Oncol 15:232, 1987.
6. Maurer HS, Steinherz PG, Gaynon PS et al: The effect of initial management of hyperleukocytosis on early complications and outcome of children with acute lymphoblastic leukemia. J Clin Oncol 6:1425, 1988.
7. Strauss RA, Gloster ES, McCallister JA et al: Acute cytoreduction techniques in the early treatment of hyperleukocytosis associated with childhood hematologic malignancies. Med Pediatr Oncol 13:346, 1985.
8. Bertholf MF, Mintz PD: Comparison of plateletpheresis using two cell separators and identical donors. Transfusion 29:521, 1989.
9. Hester JP, Kellogg RM, Mulzet AP et al: Principles of blood separation and component extraction in a disposable continuous-flow single-stage channel. Blood 54:254, 1979.
10. Kalmin ND, Grindon AJ: Comparison of two continuous-flow cell separators. Transfusion 23:197, 1983.
11. Katz AJ, Glenco PV, Blumberg N et al: Platelet collection and transfusion using the Fenwal CS-3000 cell separator. Transfusion 21:560, 1981.
12. Kurtz SR, McMican A, Carciero R et al: Plateletpheresis experience with the Haemonetics blood processor 30, the IBM blood processor 2997, and the Fenwal CS-3000 blood processor. Vox Sang 41:212, 1981.
13. Aisner J, Schiffer CA, Wolff JH, Wiernik PH: A standardized technique for efficient platelet and leukocyte collection using the model 30 Blood Processor. Transfusion 16:437, 1976.
14. Huestis DW, Price MJ, White RF, Inman M: Leukapheresis of patients with chronic granulocytic leukemia (CGL) using the Haemonetics blood processor. Transfusion 16:255, 1976.
15. Szymanski IO: Ionized calcium during plateletpheresis. Transfusion 18:701, 1978.
16. Vallejos CS, McCredie KB, Brittin GM, Freireich EJ: Biological effects of repeated leukapheresis of patients with chronic myelogenous leukemia. Blood 42:925, 1973.
17. Dutcher JP, Aisner J, Hogge DE, Schiffer CA: Donor reaction to hydroxyethyl starch during granulocytapheresis. Transfusion 24:66, 1983.
18. Mishler JM: Hydroxyethyl starch as an experimental adjunct to leukocyte separation by centrifugal means: review of safety and efficacy. Transfusion 15:449, 1975.
19. Rock G, Wise P: Plasma expansion during granulocyte procurement: cumulative effects of hydroxyethyl starch. Blood 53:1156, 1979.
20. Corash L, Klein H, Disseroth A et al: Selective isolation of young erythrocytes for transfusion support of thalassemia major patients. Blood 57:599, 1981.
21. Klein HG: Selective isolation of young red cells for chronic transfusion. Plasma Ther Trans Technol 2:175, 1981.
22. Propper RD, Button LN, Nathan DG: New approaches to the transfusion management of thalassemia. Blood 55:55, 1980.
23. Woods AH, Gibbs R, Holmberg A: The anaemia associated with repeated leucapheresis. In Goldman JM, Lowenthal RM (eds.): Leucocytes: Separation, Collection and Transfusion. Proceedings of the International Symposium on Leucocyte Separation and Transfusion. p. 106. Academic Press, London, 1975.
24. Volkin RL, Staarz TW, Winkelstein A et al: Changes in coagulation factors, complement, immunoglobulins, and immune complex concentrations with plasma exchange. Transfusion 22:54, 1982.
25. George JN: How I treat patients with thrombotic thrombocytopenic purpura–hemolytic uremic syndrome. Blood 96:1223–9, 2000.
26. Bensinger WI, Buckner CD, Clift RA, Thomas ED: Plasma exchange and plasma modification for the removal of anti-red blood cell antibodies in ABO incompatible bone marrow transplantation. J Clin Apheresis 3:174, 1987.
27. Leitman SF, Smith JW, Gregg RE: Homozygous familial hypercholesterolemia. Selective removal of low-density lipoproteins by secondary membrane filtration. Transfusion 29:341, 1989.
28. Braun N, Bosch T: Immunoadsorption, current status and future developments. Expert Opin Invest Drugs 9:2017–38, 2000.
29. Messerschmidt GL, Henry DH, Snyder HW et al: Protein A immunoadsorption in the treatment of malignant disease. J Clin Oncol 6:203, 1988.
30. Smith RE, Gottschall JL, Pisciotta AV: Life threatening reaction to staphylococcal protein A immunomodulation. J Clin Apheresis 7:4, 1992.
31. Snyder HW, Cochran SK, Balint JP et al: Experience with protein A immunoadsorption in treatment resistant immune thrombocytopenic purpura. Blood 79:2237, 1992.
32. Snyder HW, Mittleman A, Oral A et al: Treatment of cancer chemotherapy associated thrombotic thrombocytopenic purpura/hemolytic uremic syndrome by protein A immunoadsorption of plasma. Cancer 71:1882, 1993.

33. Christie DJ, Howe RB, Lennon SS, Sauro SC: Treatment of refractoriness to platelet transfusion by protein A column therapy. Transfusion 33:234, 1993.

34. Lichtman MA: Rheology of leukocytes, leukocyte suspensions and blood in leukemia: Possible relationship to clinical manifestations. J Clin Invest 52:350, 1973.

35. Lichtman MA, Rowe JM: Hyperleukocytic leukemias: rheological, clinical, and therapeutic considerations. Blood 60:279, 1982.

36. Harris C: Leukostasis associated with blood transfusion in acute myeloid leukemia. Br Med J 1:1169, 1978.

37. Freireich EJ, Thomas LB, Frei, E III et al: A distinctive type of intracerebral hemorrhage associated with "blastic crisis" in patients with leukemia. Cancer 13:146, 1960.

38. Fritz RD, Forkner CE, Freireich EJ et al: The association of fatal intracranial hemorrhage and "blastic crisis" in patients with acute leukemia. N Engl J Med 261:59, 1959.

39. McKee LC, Jr, Collins RD: Intravascular leukocyte thrombi and aggregates as a cause of morbidity and mortality in leukemia. Medicine (Baltimore) 53:463, 1974.

40. Karp DD, Beck JR, Cornell CJ: Chronic granulocytic leukemia with respiratory distress. Arch Intern Med 141:1353, 1981.

41. Lokich JJ, Moloney WC: Fatal pulmonary leukostasis following treatment in acute myelogenous leukemia. Arch Intern Med 130:759, 1972.

42. Thiebaut A, Thomas X, Belhabri A, Anglaret B, Archimbaud E: Impact of pre-induction therapy leukapheresis on treatment outcome in adult acute myelogenous leukemia presenting with hyperleukocytosis. Ann Hematol 79:501–6, 2000.

43. Vernant JP, Brun B, Mannoni P, Dreyfus B: Respiratory distress of hyperleukocytic granulocytic leukemias. Cancer 44:264, 1979.

44. Cuttner J, Conjalka MS, Reilly M et al: Association of monocytic leukemia in patients with extreme leukocytosis. Am J Med 69:555, 1980.

45. Schiffer CA, Wiernik PH: Functional evaluation of circulating leukemic cells in acute nonlymphocytic leukemia. Leuk Res 1:271, 1977.

46. Grund FM, Armitage JO, Burns CP: Hydroxyurea in the prevention of the effects of leukostasis in acute leukemia. Arch Intern Med 137:1246, 1977.

47. Eisenstaedt RS, Berkman EM: Rapid cytoreduction in acute leukemia: Management of cerebral leukostasis by cell pheresis. Transfusion 18:113, 1978.

48. Lane TA: Continuous-flow leukapheresis for rapid cytoreduction in leukemia. Transfusion 20:455, 1980.

49. Meyer RJ, Cuttner J, Truog P et al: Therapeutic leukopheresis of acute myelomonocytic leukemia in pregnancy. Med Pediatr Oncol 4:77, 1978.

50. Armitage JO, Geoken JA, Feagler JR: Spurious elevation of the platelet count in acute leukemia. JAMA 239:433, 1978.

51. Dutcher JP, Schiffer CA, Wiernik PH: Hyperleukocytosis in adult acute nonlymphocytic leukemia remission rate, duration, and survival. J Clin Oncol 5:1364, 1987.

52. Vaughan WP, Kimball AW, Karp JE et al: Factors affecting survival of patients with acute myelocytic leukemia presenting with high white blood cell count. Cancer Treat Rep 65:1007, 1981.

53. Cuttner J, Holland JF, Norton L et al: Therapeutic leukapheresis for hyperleukocytosis in acute myelocytic leukemia. Med Pediatr Oncol 11:76, 1983.

54. Freireich EJ, Levin RH, Whang J et al: The function and fate of transfused leukocytes from donors with chronic myelocytic leukemia in leukopenic recipients. Ann NY Acad Sci 113:1081, 1964.

55. Lowenthal RM, Grossman L, Goldman JM et al: Granulocyte transfusions in treatment of infections in patients with acute leukemia and aplastic anaemia. Lancet 1:353, 1975.

56. Morse EE, Carbone PP, Freireich EJ et al: Repeated leukapheresis of patients with chronic myelocytic leukemia. Transfusion 6:175, 1965.

57. Schiffer CA, Aisner J, Dutcher JP, Wiernik PH: Sustained post transfusion granulocyte count increments following transfusion of leukocytes obtained from donors with chronic myelogenous leukemia. Am J Hematol 15:65, 1983.

58. Caplan SN, Coco FV, Berkman EM: Management of chronic myelocytic leukemia in pregnancy by cell pheresis. Transfusion 18:120, 1978.

59. Hadlock DC, Fortuny IE, McCullough J, Kennedy BJ: Continuous flow centrifuge leucapheresis in the management of chronic myelogenous leukaemia. Br J Haematol 29:443, 1975.

60. Hester JP, McCredie KB, Freireich EJ: Response to chronic leukapheresis procedures and survival of chronic myelogenous leukemia patients. Transfusion 22:305, 1982.

61. Lowenthal RM, Buskard NA, Goldman JM et al: Intensive leukapheresis as initial therapy for chronic granulocytic leukemia. Blood 46:835, 1975.

62. Mehta AB, Goldman JM, Kohner E: Hyperleukocytic retinopathy in chronic granulocytic leukemia: The role of intensive leucapheresis. Br J Haematol 56:661, 1984.

63. Gatti RA, Robinson WA, Deinard AS et al: Cyclic leukocytosis in chronic myelogenous leukemia: new perspectives on pathogenesis and therapy. Blood 41:771, 1973.

64. Fitzgerald D, Rowe JM, Heal J: Leukapheresis for control of chronic myelogenous leukemia during pregnancy. Am J Hematol 22:213, 1986.

65. Carella AM, Pollicardo N, Raffo MR et al: Intensive conventional chemotherapy can lead to a precocious overshoot of cytogenetically normal blood stem cells in chronic myeloid leukemia and acute lymphoblastic leukemia. Leukemia, 6(Suppl. 4):120, 1992.

66. Fauci AS, Harley JB, Roberts WC et al: The idiopathic hypercosinophilic syndrome. Ann Intern Med 97:78, 1982.

67. Ellman L, Miller L, Rappeport J: Leukopheresis therapy of a hyperosinophilic disorder. JAMA 230:1004, 1974.

68. Davies J, Spry C: Plasma exchange or leukapheresis in the hypereosinophilic syndrome. Ann Intern Med 96:791, 1982.

69. Pineda AA, Brzica SM Jr, Taswell III: Continuous- and semicontinuous-flow blood centrifugation systems: therapeutic applications, with plasma-, platelet-, lympha-, and eosinapheresis. Transfusion 17:407, 1977.

70. Dameshek W: Chronic lymphocytic leukemia—an accumulative disease of immunologically incompetent lymphocytes. Blood 29:566, 1967.

71. Field EO, Dawson KB, Peckham MJ et al: The response of chronic lymphocytic leukemia to treatment by extracorporeal irradiation of the blood, assessed by isotope-labeling procedures. Blood 36:87, 1970.

72. Schiffer LM, Chanana AD, Cronkite EP et al: Extracorporeal irradiation of the blood. Semin Hematol 3:154, 1966.

73. Cooper IA, Ding JC, Adams PB et al: Intensive leukapheresis in the management of cytopenias in patients with chronic lymphocytic leukemia (CLL) and lymphocytic lymphoma. Am J Hematol 6:387, 1979.

74. Curtis JE, Hersh EM, Freireich EJ: Leukapheresis therapy of chronic lymphocytic leukemia. Blood 39:183, 1972.

75. Fortuny JE, Hadlock DC, Kennedy BJ et al: The role of continuous flow centrifuge leucapheresis in the management of chronic lymphocytic leukemia. Br J Haematol 32:609, 1976.

76. Goldfinger D, Capostagno V, Lowe C et al: Use of long-term leukapheresis in the treatment of chronic lymphocytic leukemia. Transfusion 20:450, 1980.

77. Buskard NA, Lowenthal RM, Goldman JM, Galton DAG: Treatment of prolymphocytic leukemia by leucapheresis. In Goldman JM, Lowenthal RM (eds.): Leucocytes: Separation, Collection and Transfusion. p. 543. Academic Press, London, 1975.

78. Ratain MJ, Golomb HM, Bardawil RG et al: Durability of responses to interferon alpha-2b in advanced hairy cell leukemia. Blood 69:872, 1987.

79. Spiers ASD, Moore D, Cassileth PA et al: Remissions in hairy cell leukemia with pentostatin (2′ deoxycoformycin). N Engl J Med 316:825, 1987.

80. Savan A, Piro L: Treatment of hairy cell leukemia. Blood 79:1111, 1992.

81. Yam LT, Klock JC, Mielke CH: Therapeutic leukapheresis in hairy cell leukemia: Review of the literature and personal experience. Semin Oncol, 11(Suppl. 2):493, 1984.

82. Fay JW, Moore JO, Logue GL, Huang AT: Leukopheresis therapy of leukemic reticuloendotheliosis (hairy cell leukemia). Blood 54:747, 1979.

83. Baum KF: Leukopheresis in the leukemic phase of hairy cell leukemia. Cancer 50:2926, 1982.

84. Worsley A, Cuttner J, Gordon R, Reilly M et al: Therapeutic leukapheresis in a patient with hairy cell leukemia presenting with a white cell count greater than 500,000/μl. Transfusion 22:308, 1982.

85. Golomb HM, Kraut EH, Oviatt DL et al: Absence of prolonged benefit of initial leukapheresis therapy for hairy cell leukemia. Am J Hematol 14:49, 1983.

86. McEvoy MT, Zelickson BD, Pineda AA, Winkelmann RK: Intermittent leukapheresis: An adjunct to low dose chemotherapy for Sézary syndrome. Acta Derm Venereol (Stockh) 69:73, 1989.

87. Muller N, Lange CE: Long term cytapheresis in the treatment of Sézary syndrome. Int J Artif Organs 7:143, 1984.

88. Bongiovanni MB, Katz RS, Tomaszewski JE et al: Cytapheresis in a patient with Sézary syndrome. Transfusion 21:332, 1981.

89. Edelson R, Berger C, Gasparro F et al: Treatment of cutaneous T-cell lymphoma by extracorporeal photochemotherapy. N Engl J Med 316:297, 1987.

90. Edelson RL, Perez M, Heald P, Berger C: Extracorporeal phototherapy. In: Biologic Therapy of Cancer Updates. Vol. 4., p. 1. JB Lippincott, Philadelphia, 1994.

91. Marks D, Rockman SP, Oziemski MA et al: Mechanisms of lymphocytotoxicity induced by extracorporeal real photochemotherapy for cutaneous T cell lymphoma. J Clin Invest 86:2080, 1990.

92. Knobler R: Extracorporeal photochemotherapy–present and future. Vox Sang 78(Suppl. 2):197–201, 2000.

93. Bunn PA, Hoffman SJ, Norris D et al: Systemic therapy of cutaneous T-cell lymphomas (mycosis fungoides and the Sézary syndrome). Ann Intern Med 121:592, 1994.

94. Greinix HT, Volc-Platzer B, Kahls P, Fischer G, Rosenmayr A, Keil F, Honigsmann H, Knobler RM: Extracorporeal photochemotherapy in the treatment of severe steroid-refractory acute graft-versus-host disease: A pilot study. Blood 96:2426–31, 2000.

95. Buss DH, Stuart JJ, Lipscomb GE: The incidence of thrombotic and hemorrhagic disorders in association with extreme thrombocytosis: An analysis of 129 cases. Am J Hematol 20:365, 1985.

96. Schafer AI: Bleeding and thrombosis in the myeloproliferative disorders. Blood 64:1, 1984.

97. Ginsberg AD: Platelet function in patients with high platelet counts. Ann Intern Med 82:506, 1975.

98. Kaywin P, McDonough M, Insel PA, Shattil SJ: Platelet function in essential thrombocythemia. N Engl J Med 299:505, 1978.

99. Zucker S, Mielke CH: Classification of thrombocytosis based on platelet function tests: Correlation with hemorrhagic and thrombotic complications. J Lab Clin Med 80:385, 1972.

100. Walsh PN, Murphy S, Barry WE: The role of platelets in the pathogenesis of thrombosis and haemorrhage in patients with thrombocytosis. Thromb Haemost 38:1085, 1977.

101. Hoagland HC, Silverstein MN: Primary thrombocythemia in the young patient. Mayo Clin Proc 53:578, 1978.

102. Kessler CM, Klein HG, Havlik RJ: Uncontrolled thrombocytosis in chronic myeloproliferative disorders. Br J Haematol 50:157, 1982.

103. Beard MEJ, Blacklock HA, Varcoe AR: Control of thrombocytosis by plateletpheresis using a cell separator. N Z Med J 654:136, 1980.

104. Colman RW, Sievers CA, Pugh RP: Thrombocytophresis: A rapid and effective approach to symptomatic thrombocytosis. J Lab Clin Med 68:389, 1966.

105. Goldfinger D, Thompson R, Lowe C, Kurz L, Belkin G: Long-term plateletpheresis in the management of primary thrombocytosis. Transfusion 19:336, 1979.

106. Greenberg BR, Watson-Williams EJ: Successful control of life-threatening thrombocytosis with a blood processor. Transfusion 15:620, 1975.

107. Orlin JB, Berkman EM: Improvement of platelet function following plateletpheresis in patients with myeloproliferative diseases. Transfusion 20:540, 1980.

108. Panlilio AL, Reiss RF: Therapeutic plateletpheresis in thombocythemia. Transfusion 19:147, 1979.

109. Taft EG: Apheresis in platelet disorders. Plasma Ther Trans Technol 2:181, 1981.

110. Taft EG, Babcock RB, Scharfman WB, Tartaglia AP: Plateletpheresis in the management of thrombocytosis. Blood 50:927, 1977.

111. Yonger J, Umlas J: Rapid reduction of platelet count in essential hemorrhagic thrombocythemia by discontinuous flow plateletpheresis. Am J Med 64:659, 1978.

112. Klein HG, Garner RJ, Miller DM et al: Automated partial exchange transfusion in sickle cell anemia. Transfusion 20:578, 1980.

113. Lasky L: Hematopoietic reconstitution using progenitors recovered from blood. Transfusion 29:552, 1989.

114. Weaver CH, Buckner CD, Longin K et al: Syngeneic transplantation with peripheral blood mononuclear cells collected after the administration of recombinant granulocyte colony stimulating factor. Blood 82:1981, 1994.

115. Bensinger WI, Martin PJ, Storer B, Clift R, Forman SJ, Negrin R, Kashyap A, Flowers ME, Lilleby K, Chauncey TR, Storb R, Appelbaum FR: Transplantation of bone marrow as compared with peripheral-blood cells from HLA-identical relatives in patients with hematologic cancers. N Engl J Med 344:175–81, 2001.

116. Wright DG, Karsh J. Fauci AS et al: Lymphocyte depletion and immunosuppression with repeated leukapheresis by continuous flow centrifugation. Blood 58:451, 1981.

117. Bloch KJ, Maki DG: Hyperviscosity syndromes associated with immunoglobulin abnormalities. Semin Hematol 20:113, 1973.

118. Kopp WL, Beirse GJ, Burns RO: Hyperviscosity syndrome in multiple myeloma. Am J Med 43:141, 1967.

119. Reinhart WH, Lutolf O, Nydegger UR et al: Plasmapheresis for hyperviscosity syndrome in macroglobulinemia Waldenström and multiple myeloma: Influence on blood rheology and the microcirculation. J Lab Clin Med 119:69, 1992.

120. Buskard NA, Galton DAG, Goldman JM et al: Plasma exchange in the long term management of Waldenström's macroglobulinemia. Can Med Assoc J 23:135, 1977.

121. Bensinger WI, Buckner CD, Clift RA et al: Plasma exchange for platelet alloimmunization. Transplantation 41:602, 1986.

122. McLeod BC, Sassetti RJ: Plasmapheresis with return of cryoglobulin-depleted autologous plasma (cryoglobulinpheresis) in cryoglobulinemia. Blood 55:866, 1980.

123. Silberstein LE, Berkman EM: Plasma exchange in autoimmune hemolytic anemia. J Clin Apheresis 1:238, 1983.

124. Cimo PL, Aster RH: Post-transfusion purpura. Successful treatment by plasma exchange. N Engl J Med 287:290, 1972.

53

Red Cell Transfusions in Patients with Hematologic Malignancies

Karen E. King and Paul M. Ness

Although the transfusion of red cells is a relatively common clinical event, patients with hematologic malignancies have special requirements for their red cell products and are at increased risk for certain adverse effects of transfusion. This chapter will provide an overview of many of the basic principles of transfusion medicine, with a focus on the issues that are relevant to the restoration of oxygen-carrying capacity in the patient with a hematologic malignancy.

RED CELL COMPONENTS

Currently, the clinical practices of transfusion medicine are based on component therapy, in which a unit of whole blood can be separated into red cells, platelets, and plasma. Component therapy is advantageous because it provides maximal use of a limited resource, blood. In addition, with the awareness of transfusion-transmitted diseases and other adverse effects of transfusion, the use of component therapy should limit donor exposures and patients should receive only the blood products that they require. Several types of red cell products are available; they are described below and summarized in Table 53–1.

Whole Blood

Because of the predominant use of component therapy and the difficulty in predicting the need for whole blood, most blood banks do not maintain an inventory of whole blood. Obviously, for use in the setting of massive blood loss, a large amount of whole blood would be optimal. Since this inventory is not usually available, red cells in combination with a volume expander should be used. If the volume loss is moderate in amount, a crystalloid, such as normal saline, can be used. Crystalloids have the advantages of being sterile and inexpensive. For more extensive volume replacement, colloids such as albumin[1] and starch solutions are available. These preparations are much more expensive than crystalloids; however, they are preferable to plasma in that they carry no risk of disease transmission. After receiving the equivalent of approximately one blood volume, the patient is at risk for a dilutional coagulopathy. At this point, fresh frozen plasma or pooled plasma, solvent detergent-treated, should be administered to replace coagulation factors, and platelets should be given. It should be remembered that platelets are suspended in plasma; when giving both platelets and fresh frozen plasma, one can give less plasma, taking into account the plasma contained in the platelet product.

A unit of whole blood has a volume of approximately 510 ml, consisting of 450 ml of whole blood and 63 ml of an anti-coagulant-preservative solution. When this product is collected in citrate phosphate dextrose adenine (CPDA-1), it has a shelf life of 35 days. During the first 24 hours of storage, the platelets become nonfunctional.[2] In addition, there is a gradual decrease in the activity of coagulation factors V and VIII. By day 21 of storage, factor V levels range from approximately 20 to 100 percent; at the same time, factor VIII levels range from about 15 to 50 percent.[3] The other coagulation factors are stable in stored whole blood.

Whole blood simultaneously replaces both red cells and plasma. Thus it can provide improved oxygen-carrying capacity, colloid osmotic pressure, volume replacement, and many of the plasma coagulation factors. Whole blood is appropriately used for massive blood loss as may occur in trauma or in some surgeries.

Red Cell Concentrates

Red cell concentrates are prepared from a unit of donor whole blood following removal of most of the plasma,[4] which may be achieved by either sedimentation or centrifugation. The

Table 53–1. Red Cell Components and Their Indications

Red Cell Component	Characteristics	Clinical Indication
Whole blood	High volume Good flow	Replacement of combined red cell and volume deficit (massive hemorrhage)
Red cell concentrates	Lower volume Higher hematocrit (65–80%) Good flow with AS-1	Replacement of red cell deficit
Leukocyte-reduced red cells	Less than 5×10^6 white cells	Prevention of febrile, nonhemolytic transfusion reactions Prevention of alloimmunization Prevention of cytomegalovirus transmission
Washed red cells	Plasma-depleted	Prevention of severe, allergic transfusion reactions
Frozen red cells	Storage for at least 10 years Plasma-depleted	Storage of rare donor units

removed platelet-rich plasma may then be used for the preparation of another component, such as fresh frozen plasma or platelets. A unit of red cells has an average volume of 300 ml and has a hematocrit ranging between 65 and 80 percent. An additive solution, such as Adsol, is often used to extend the storage life to 42 days. The additive will decrease the hematocrit, so that the product will have flow properties similar to those of whole blood.[5]

Red cell concentrates are indicated for the improvement of oxygen-carrying capacity, especially if the problem is an isolated one. With their relatively high hematocrit, red cell concentrates can efficiently provide red blood cells in a small volume. They are the product of choice in the setting of chronic anemia from bone marrow failure. Red cell concentrates are especially needed in patients with cardiovascular compromise, who may not tolerate the additional volume of whole blood.

Leukocyte-Reduced Red Cells

An average unit of red blood cells contains approximately 2×10^9 to 5×10^9 leukocytes.[6] Several methods have historically been used to reduce the leukocyte content of a unit of red cells; these methods have varied in their capacity for leukocyte reduction. All leukocyte-reduced red cell products must retain at least 85 percent of their original red cell content, and their total white cell content must be less than 5×10^6.[4]

One previously popular technique to remove leukocytes from red cells is the spin-cool-filter method. This method removes leukocytes that have formed microaggregates during a centrifugation and cooling process; these microaggregates are removed by a 40-μm filter. This process can only reduce the leukocyte count to approximately 3×10^8.[7,8]

More recently, advanced leukocyte-removing filters have been developed. These "third-generation" filters use two mechanisms, a barrier on the basis of pore size and retention by adsorption; thus, they are sometimes called leukocyte adsorption filters.[9] Several studies have evaluated the efficacy of these filters and have found that they can reliably reduce the white cell content of a unit of red cells by as much as 99.9 percent, which is a 3 log reduction.[10–14] Prestorage leukoreduction has the additional advantage of preventing cytokine accumulation.

There are several indications for the use of leukocyte-reduced red cells, including the prevention of febrile, nonhemolytic transfusion reactions, the prevention of alloimmunization to HLA antigens (especially for patients who will require future platelet transfusions or a possible future progenitor cell transplant), and the prevention of cytomegalovirus (CMV) transmission. In addition, there is evidence that transfusion-associated immunomodulation is mediated by the contaminating white cells in blood products, and these problems would be prevented with the use of leukocyte-reduced blood products.[15]

Washed Red Cells

Washed red cells are prepared by either manual or automated washing with isotonic saline. Washing red cells removes plasma and some of the leukocytes and platelets. This procedure can be repeated several times, depending on the indication and the degree of plasma removal necessary, but there is red cell loss with each washing. Since the washing procedure is performed in an open system, washed red cells must be transfused within 24 hours.

Since washing primarily removes the plasma proteins from red cells, the main indication for washed red cells is the prevention of severe allergic transfusion reactions, which are believed to be due to recipient antibodies directed against donor plasma proteins. Washing is indicated when a patient has recurrent severe allergic reactions that are refractory to antihistamine treatment. Patients with IgA deficiency and antibodies to IgA can have anaphylactic reactions to plasma containing IgA.[16] These patients may tolerate red cells that have undergone several washes[17,18]; otherwise they may require products from IgA-deficient donors. It has been suggested that patients with paroxysmal nocturnal hemoglobinuria (PNH) receive washed red cells. Since the red cells in PNH are more sensitive to complement, it has been hypothesized that washing removes the complement and the washed red cells would be less likely to exacerbate the hemolytic process of PNH.[19] One retrospective study has shown that patients with PNH do not require washed red cells.[20,21]

Washing of red cells also removes many leukocytes; however, the exact degree of leukocyte reduction depends on the method of washing. Thus, although washed red cells are the product of choice for a patient with repeated allergic reactions, this product may be helpful in the prevention of some febrile, nonhemolytic transfusion reactions as well.

Frozen Red Cells

Red blood cells may be frozen with glycerol used as a cryopreservative. The concentration of glycerol used in the freezing procedure depends on the rate and the temperature of freezing.[22,23] Other contaminating cellular elements are destroyed in the freezing process except for a small number of lymphocytes.[24] Thus, frozen red cells contain a decreased number of leukocytes. When the cells are needed for transfusion, the unit is thawed and washed repeatedly with progressively less hypertonic saline solutions to remove the glycerol from the cells. If the process is not performed appropriately, hemolysis will occur on transfusion. The repeated washings remove associated plasma and any other debris. The cells are resuspended in isotonic saline with glucose. Frozen red cells may be stored for at least 10 years; however, they have been shown to have good viability even after longer periods of storage. Once thawed, the product is an open system and will become outdated in 24 hours.

This procedure is expensive and the indications for it are limited. The major indication is for preservation of rare donor units required by patients with unusual phenotypes who have developed multiple alloantibodies. These patients should be encouraged to donate autologously when they are clinically able to do so and have their cells frozen for future needs. Autologous blood may also be frozen when a surgery date is postponed or if more blood is needed than can be donated within the time limitations of liquid storage (35 to 42 days). Frozen red cells have been used in patients with aplastic anemia who are awaiting bone marrow transplantation because frozen cells have shown the least adverse effect on subsequent graft survival.[25] Leukocyte-reduced red cells have replaced frozen red cells for this indication. Occasionally, there are patients with severe, repeated febrile, nonhemolytic transfusion reactions who fail medications and other forms of leukocyte reduction, and these patients may have uneventful transfusions when given frozen red cells.

MODIFICATIONS OF RED CELL PRODUCTS

Several additional modifications can be made to red cells to meet the special needs of patients with hematologic malignancies.

Gamma-Irradiation

Gamma-irradiation is used to prevent transfusion-associated graft-versus-host disease (GvHD). This disease occurs when immunocompetent lymphocytes are transfused, which are capable of engrafting and reacting against the host tissues.[26] This entity is of concern in any patient who is severely immunocompromised. It is also believed that transfusion-associated GvHD is a risk in situations of partial HLA identity between the donor and the recipient.[27,28] Thus, irradiation is recommended for all cellular products that are given to patients at risk for transfusion-associated GvHD including those with congenital immunodeficiency syndromes, recipients of units from relatives, recipients of HLA-selected products (either by typing or crossmatching of platelets), and bone marrow or progenitor cell recipients. More recently, it has been shown that patients with chronic lymphocytic leukemia who are undergoing treatment with fludarabine are at risk for transfusion-associated GvHD.[29,30] Some oncology centers routinely gamma-irradiate all blood components to avoid the often fatal complications of transfusion-associated GvHD.

Gamma-irradiation inactivates immunocompetent lymphocytes, preventing proliferation of transfused T lymphocytes. It is recommended that the product be irradiated with a minimum of 25 Gy, with at least 15 Gy delivered to all parts of the blood component.[4,31] Although this dosage should not affect the function of the red cells, irradiation damages some red cells and does have an effect on overall viability, requiring a shortened outdate. Owing to the devastating repercussions of GvHD, the lack of effective treatment, and the relative ease of irradiation, prevention is the focus, and most centers err on the side of irradiating for less than well documented indications. Gamma-irradiation does not produce a leukocyte-reduced product or a CMV-safe product.

Cytomegalovirus-Seronegative Products

Cellular blood products can be tested for antibodies against CMV by a variety of methods. Products that are seronegative for CMV are recommended in situations in which immuno-suppressed patients would be at risk for primary CMV infection. Patients at risk include CMV-seronegative patients undergoing bone marrow transplantation from a CMV-seronegative donor and CMV-seronegative patients with the acquired immunodeficiency syndrome (AIDS).[32,33] Since the virus is associated with leukocytes, it has been proposed that leukocyte-reduced blood products would be useful in the prevention of CMV transmission. Studies have shown that leukocyte reduction by filtration is helpful in preventing CMV transmission.[34–36] One study has shown that filtration can remove any detectable CMV DNA from previously positive red cell products even following amplification by the polymerase chain reaction (PCR) technique.[37] A randomized study comparing seronegative blood products and leukocyte-reduced products using bedside filters has shown that the seronegative products are equivalent in preventing CMV infection in patients undergoing marrow transplantation.[38] This study did find an increased incidence of CMV disease in the patients receiving leukocyte-reduced products.

Controversy exists both in the literature and in clinical practice regarding the role of leukocyte-reduced blood products in clinical situations requiring CMV-safe blood.[39] Currently, many institutions are using leukocyte-reduced blood products when CMV-seronegative products are not available. Many institutions are routinely using leukocyte-reduced and CMV-seronegative products as equally CMV-safe. When leukocyte-reduced red cell products are used to prevent CMV transmission, the red cells must have less than 5×10^6 leukocytes per bag.

SPECIAL CLINICAL SITUATIONS FOR RED CELL TRANSFUSION

Although most of the principles of transfusion medicine are applicable to patients with hematologic malignancies, there are a few unique situations that should be noted.

Indications for Red Cell Transfusion

Frequent reference is made to a transfusion trigger or a suggested minimum hemoglobin or hematocrit level at which red cells are transfused. Obviously, the need for red cells or increased oxygen-carrying capacity depends on numerous factors that are specific to the individual patient. The etiology of the low hemoglobin is crucial in this evaluation. Patients with chronic anemias that have been well compensated will tolerate a more severe degree of anemia than the patient who has suffered an acute blood loss. The patient's underlying health condition is also important in deciding when to transfuse. A young and relatively healthy person with good cardiovascular function will tolerate a lower hemoglobin than an older patient with impaired cardiac function.[40,41]

Previously, it was believed that perioperative patients should have a hemoglobin of at least 10 g/dl. A National Institutes of Health Consensus Development Conference on perioperative red blood cell usage has recommended that the transfusion trigger be changed to a hemoglobin of 7 g/dl.[42] Currently, there is no single transfusion trigger that applies to all patients. In patients with hematologic malignancies, the hematocrit level should be maintained to alleviate the symptoms of anemia and will vary with the patient's age and other medical problems.

The measured response to a transfusion varies depending on the patient. It is generally accepted that transfusion of one unit of red cells should increase the hematocrit by 3 percent or the hemoglobin by 1 g/dl. The U.S. Food and Drug Administration (FDA) requires 75 percent of the transfused red cells in the circulation at 24 hours when evaluating collection systems and anticoagulant preservative solutions. It is estimated that in the absence of bone marrow function, the average person requires 24 ml of red cells per day to maintain a given hematocrit.[43] Others have estimated that an average adult requires two units of red cells every 2 weeks.[44]

Hyperviscosity

Hyperviscosity becomes problematic in two clinical situations involving patients with hematologic malignancies. Patients with multiple myeloma and plasma cell dyscrasias can have difficulties due to hyperviscosity. These patients are frequently anemic, and it is difficult to determine if their symptoms of poor oxygenation are due to hyperviscosity or to their severe anemia. A relative serum viscosity measurement should be obtained; many patients will become symptomatic at a relative serum viscosity above 4. Patients with hyperviscosity will not tolerate red cell transfusions unless their blood viscosity is first reduced. In this situation, plasmapheresis can be performed to reduce the amount of circulating paraprotein that is creating the hyperviscosity.[45]

Hyperleukocytic leukostasis occurs in patients with markedly elevated white cell counts, frequently due to acute myelogenous leukemia. Although white cells do not usually contribute significantly to whole blood viscosity, hyperleukocytosis with malignant white cells can be associated with hyperviscosity because the malignant white cells may not have normal flow characteristics. These patients frequently present with hyperleukocytosis, anemia, and evidence of poor perfusion, which may be due to leukostasis or to infiltration of blood vessels by leukemic cells. In these patients, the white cell count should be reduced by leukocytapheresis before the patient is given red cell transfusions. If leukocytapheresis technology is not available, the patient's white cell count can be reduced by manual whole blood exchange or chemotherapy.[46,47]

Bone Marrow and Progenitor Cell Transplants

Patients who are undergoing bone marrow or progenitor cell transplantation have several special needs. They will be transfusion-dependent until engraftment occurs. All bone marrow transplant patients should receive irradiated red cells to prevent the development of transfusion-associated GvHD. In addition, CMV-negative patients who receive autologous transplants, autologous peripheral stem cells, or CMV-negative allogeneic transplants should receive CMV-safe blood products.

In cases of bone marrow transplantation in which there is major ABO incompatibility (a group O patient given bone marrow from a group A, group B, or group AB donor), the marrow infusion can be depleted of contaminating red cells. When engraftment occurs, the transplanted marrow will begin to produce red cells with A and/or B substance and the recipient may still be producing isoagglutinins. In this situation, the new red cells may be hemolyzed by the isoagglutinins. This period of hemolysis may be brief or may last for an extended period of time. If transfusions are required during this period, the patient should be given group O red cells. Of course, these cells should be irradiated, and CMV-seronegative cells may also be indicated.[48]

Minor ABO incompatibility in bone marrow transplants occurs when group O donor marrow is transplanted into a non-group O recipient. Plasma should be removed from the marrow product to reduce the amount of isoagglutinins given to the recipient. However, as in the case of solid organ transplants, passenger lymphocyte syndrome may occur, and contaminating lymphocytes are capable of producing anti-A and anti-B antibodies. In many of these cases, hemolysis may occur.[49] If transfusions are required, irradiated group O red cells should be given.[48]

Autoimmune Hemolytic Anemia

Autoantibodies directed against red cells occur frequently in patients with hematologic malignancies. Patients with chronic lymphocytic leukemia (CLL) are notorious for the development of red cell autoantibodies, often with an autoimmune hemolytic anemia. It has been estimated that 10 to 20 percent of patients with CLL will develop red cell autoantibodies at some time during the course of their disease. The mechanism of autoimmune hemolytic anemia in patients with CLL is controversial. Some believe that these patients have an imbalance in their T-helper and T-suppressor lymphocyte subsets. One study showed that the neoplastic clones of CLL were capable of in vitro production of monoclonal antibodies, which could bind red cells. This study suggests that the autoantibodies may actually be produced by the malignant clonal B-cell population.[50] Recently, the use of fludarabine in the treatment of CLL has been associated with the development of severe autoimmune hemolytic anemia. The mechanism of this association is unclear, but it has been proposed that fludarabine results in a further disruption of the T-lymphocyte subsets.[51]

Red cell autoantibodies are detected in the laboratory by the direct antiglobulin test (DAT), also called the direct Coombs test. This test can detect the presence of IgG and/or complement on the surface of red cells. The indirect antiglobulin test (IAT), or indirect Coombs test, may reveal a panagglutinin in the serum of patients with an autoantibody. Warm autoimmune hemolytic anemia is usually due to IgG antibodies that react at 37°C and may or may not fix complement. Thus, in warm autoimmune hemolytic anemia, the DAT will reveal IgG and/or complement on the red cells. Cold autoantibodies (cold agglutinin syndrome) are usually IgM antibodies that react at 4°C and are able to fix complement. In cold agglutinin syndrome, the DAT will show the presence of complement on the red cell surface with an absence of IgG.

Clinically, it is important to determine if a patient with a hematologic malignancy and red cell autoantibodies is actually undergoing hemolysis. The diagnosis of autoimmune hemolytic anemia requires both the laboratory features and the clinical evidence of hemolysis. Patients with autoimmune hemolytic anemia may require red cell transfusions. It is important to rule out the presence of underlying red cell alloantibodies, which may be masked by the panagglutinin, because alloantibodies may complicate transfusion therapy. Even after underlying alloantibodies have been excluded, the panagglutinin will result in incompatible crossmatches. These patients should receive transfusions with the least incompatible red cells. Use of leukocyte-reduced red cells is recommended to minimize the occurrence of febrile, nonhemolytic transfusion reactions, which would confound an already difficult clinical situation. We recommend that transfusions be given to these patients when they clinically require red cells, with the understanding that the transfused cells will have a shortened survival comparable to that of the patient's own red cells.

Erythropoietin

Erythropoietin is a hormone that is capable of promoting the proliferation and maintaining the viability of erythroid progenitor cells. This hormone is produced predominantly by renal peritubular interstitial cells and also by the liver.[52–54] In 1985 the erythropoietin gene was cloned and expressed.[55,56] Recombinant erythropoietin has been used in the treatment of anemias secondary to malignancies, including multiple myeloma and myelodysplastic syndromes.[57,58] In responsive patients, erythropoietin can effectively alleviate anemia and reduce transfusion requirements. Initially, there was concern that erythropoietin could stimulate tumor growth; however, an in vitro study showed no stimulation of leukemia cell growth by erythropoietin.[59] In a study of multiple myeloma patients treated with erythropoietin, 85 percent of patients responded to therapy with correction of anemia and without tumor stimulation.[60] In responsive patients, recombinant erythropoietin may alleviate anemia, reduce transfusion requirements, and significantly improve quality of life.[61]

RED BLOOD CELL PRESERVATION AND STORAGE

Whole blood and red cell components are stored in a liquid state at a temperature between 1° and 6°C. Red cells are stored in an anticoagulant preservative solution with or without an additive solution. Most anticoagulant preservative solutions contain trisodium citrate, citric acid, dextrose, and phosphate; such solutions include acid citrate dextrose (ACD), citrate phosphate dextrose (CPD). The appropriate storage time or shelf life for red cells is based on the FDA's criterion that 75 percent of the transfused cells should be in circulation 24 hours after the transfusion. Red cells stored in a standard anticoagulant preservative solution, such as ACD or CPD, have a shelf life of 21 days. Blood collected in CPDA-1, which contains adenine has a shelf life of 35 days. Additive solutions such as Adsol or

AS-1 contain additional dextrose, adenine, mannitol, and sodium chloride. Red cells stored with an additive solution may be stored for up to 42 days.[4,62]

Adenosine Triphosphate

It has been shown that adenosine triphosphate (ATP) levels in stored red cells correlate with the viability of the red cells following transfusion. As the red cell ATP level drops during storage, the red cells undergo changes in shape from disc to sphere, followed by an increase in cellular rigidity. There is also a loss of cell membrane with decreased volume.[63] Dextrose in the preservative solution is crucial in supporting the glycolytic pathway for continued generation of ATP. The additional adenine in CPDA-1 and in the additive solutions provides substrate for the formation of ATP.[62] Although other factors may also influence the overall viability of red cells following storage, ATP remains the best defined factor as an indicator of acceptable red cell survival without performance of red cell survival studies.[43]

2,3-Diphosphoglycerate

2,3-Diphosphoglycerate (2,3-DPG) plays a crucial role in the delivery of oxygen from the red cell by influencing the position of the oxygen dissociation curve. With high 2,3-DPG levels, more oxygen is released at the same oxygen pressure. With lower red cell 2,3-DPG levels, there is greater affinity of hemoglobin for oxygen and less oxygen is delivered to the tissues.[62] Although 2,3-DPG levels decrease in stored red cells, these levels are restored in vivo following transfusion. In fact, studies have shown that over 50 percent of 2,3-DPG is restored within the first 24 hours following transfusion. These observations indicate that blood at any point in its permissible storage period is acceptable for patients with hematologic malignancies.[64]

By-products of Red Cell Storage

Because of the presence of citrate in the anticoagulant preservative solutions, the possibility of citrate toxicity must be considered in situations of massive transfusion. This clinical entity rarely occurs, but the risk is greater in instances of impaired liver function because the liver metabolizes citrate. The danger of infusing high volumes of citrate over a short time is due to the chelation of calcium by citrate. Consequently, the patient's ionized calcium level may drop and lead to cardiac arrhythmias. Usually, this adverse effect can be treated by slowing the infusion rate or by administration of calcium gluconate. If citrate toxicity occurs and calcium supplementation is required, it is recommended to follow ionized calcium levels because hypercalcemia can also lead to cardiovascular sequelae.[65]

With prolonged storage of blood, the level of extracellular potassium gradually increases. Since the sodium–potassium pump is relatively nonfunctional at red cell storage temperatures, the intracellular and extracellular potassium equilibrate, resulting in an increase in the extracellular potassium.[43] This situation is exacerbated by any hemolysis that occurs during the storage period. The plasma potassium concentration of packed red cells stored in CPDA-1 is approximately 78 mEq/L on day 35 as compared with 5 mEq/L in freshly collected blood.[66] Of course, the total plasma volume of a unit of red cells is about 70 ml, yielding a total potassium load of only 5.5 mEq in each unit of red cells. The vast majority of patients are able to tolerate this increase in potassium; however, in some situations it may cause cardiac complications. In patients with renal failure and hyperkalemia, the increased potassium may be a problem. In this situation fresher units should be selected, or if these are not available, an older unit of red cells may be washed.

During the storage process, microaggregates of platelets, white cells, and fibrin can form. These microaggregates may measure up to 200 μm in diameter.[67] The clinical impact of these microaggregates remains controversial. Some studies have shown that in massive transfusion, the degree of hypoxia is related to the amount of blood transfused, thus implicating microaggregates as the cause of the pulmonary dysfunction.[68,69] Others have argued that in cases of traumatic shock, massive transfusion, and pulmonary dysfunction, microaggregates may be contributory to the hypoxia, but their role is relatively minor.[70] Animal studies have been unable to confirm the role of microaggregates in this clinical situation.[71] Some have suggested the use of microaggregate filters when more than five units have been transfused,[72] but one should be aware that these filters slow the rate of infusion.

The 1960s brought about the development of the plastic blood bag for the storage of red cells. This was a major innovation and a significant step toward the current trend of component therapy. These plastic bags are made from polyvinylchloride containing the plasticizer di-(2-ethyl)-phthalate (DEHP), which, however, is lipophilic and is known to leach out of the bag during storage.[73] Since the development of this bag, there has been much concern about its safety. Numerous animal studies have shown significant toxicity ranging from picture resembling lung shock to teratogenicity.[74] These deleterious effects have not been documented in patients. Other potential materials have been proposed for use in blood storage bags. A new red cell container utilizes polyvinylchloride plasticized with butyryl-n-trihexyl citrate (BTHC). The BTHC undergoes less leaching, and the bags permit good red cell recovery.[75,76]

ADVERSE EFFECTS OF RED CELL TRANSFUSIONS

Recently, there has been an increased awareness of the potential adverse effects of blood transfusions. Although this heightened awareness was stimulated in large part by transfusion-transmitted human immunodeficiency virus (HIV), there are several other potential deleterious effects of transfusion, which can have devastating implications. These adverse effects are described below and are shown in Table 53–2.

Volume Overload

Volume overload is a problem in patients with cardiovascular compromise. This complication can result in congestive heart failure and pulmonary edema. Patients should be followed

Table 53–2. Adverse Effects of Red Cell Transfusions

Transfusion reactions
  Hemolytic transfusion reactions
  Septic transfusion reactions
  Febrile, nonhemolytic transfusion reactions
  Allergic transfusion reactions
Transfusion-transmitted diseases
  Hepatitis B
  Hepatitis C
  Cytomegalovirus
  Human immunodeficiency virus
  Other microbiologic agents
Transfusion-associated graft-versus-host disease
Alloimmunization
  Antibodies to red cell antigens
  Antibodies to neutrophil antigens
  Antibodies to HLA antigens
Immunomodulation
Volume overload
Iron overload

closely and given diuretics if this problem arises. The red cells should be infused at a slow rate.

Iron Overload

Iron overload can occur in patients who are chronic transfusion recipients. Each unit of red cells contains 200 to 250 mg of iron. Following approximately 100 units of red cells, the problem of iron accumulation within the mitochondria may occur, which ultimately may affect the function of the heart, liver, and endocrine glands. Iron chelation therapy using desferrioxamine should be considered. This problem is very rare in patients with hematologic malignancies, although it may be an issue for patients with aplastic anemia who receive multiple transfusions.

Transfusion Reactions

Acute hemolytic transfusion reactions are the most severe transfusion reactions, and they have potentially devastating outcomes. These reactions are mediated by antigen–antibody interaction. The most severe hemolytic transfusion reactions occur when ABO-incompatible blood is transfused. Clinically, patients develop fever, chills, nausea, and back pain. Patients have hemoglobinuria, hemoglobinemia, and hypotension progressing to shock. The process leads to complement activation, initiation of the coagulation system, and release of bradykinin, catecholamines, and vasoactive amines. Disseminated intravascular coagulation develops; in surgical patients, the coagulopathy may be the first indication of the transfusion reaction. Treatment of these reactions includes supportive care, blood pressure support, fluids, and diuretics to maintain renal perfusion, and dialysis if acute renal failure develops.

Septic transfusion reactions are usually related to a platelet product and not to a red cell component. Since platelets are stored at room temperature for up to 5 days, they are particularly susceptible to bacterial contamination. When red cells are involved in a septic transfusion reaction, the organisms are usually *Yersinia enterocolitica* or the psychrophilic pseudomonads. *Yersinia enterocolitica* is a gram-negative bacillus, which clinically causes enterocolitis. The organism grows well at 4°C and its growth is enhanced by the presence of iron. The organism rapidly multiplies after 21 days of storage, potentially giving older units very high bacterial concentrations. Thus, red cells provide an ideal environment for this organism. *Pseudomonas putida* and *Pseudomonas fluorescens* have also been implicated in septic transfusion reactions. These organisms are gram-negative rods, which grow well at 4°C.[77,78]

Febrile, nonhemolytic transfusion reactions occur clinically when a patient experiences a rise in temperature of 1°C or more in association with a transfusion and with no other explanation. These reactions are generally thought to be due to leukoagglutinins or to recipient antibody against donor leukocytes.[79–81] Patients with recurrent febrile, nonhemolytic transfusion reactions are given leukocyte-reduced blood products.[82,83] In many cases, leukocyte-reduced blood products are effective in preventing further febrile transfusion reactions. Some patients, however, continue to have reactions despite leukocyte reduction; in fact, one study has shown that in patients receiving platelet transfusions, leukocyte reduction had limited efficacy in prevention of febrile reactions.[84] Recently, there has been much interest in the role of cytokines in the pathogenesis of febrile transfusion reactions that can not be attributed to leukoagglutinins.[85] Many reactions to platelets have now been shown to be due to cytokines remaining in the plasma that are derived from contaminating leukocytes in the product.[86] Prestorage leukocyte reduction can prevent production and accumulation of cytokines in stored products.

Mild allergic transfusion reactions or urticarial reactions present with cutaneous symptoms of itching and hives. These reactions can generally be treated with antihistamines. If the reactions become more severe in nature, washed blood products may be helpful in further prevention. These reactions are believed to be due to antibodies in the recipient against donor plasma proteins.

Severe allergic reactions or anaphylactic reactions present clinically with bronchospasm, respiratory distress, and vascular instability leading to shock and loss of consciousness. Treatment includes supportive care and epinephrine. Steroid therapy may be useful. These reactions are often considered to be related to recipient antibodies against donor plasma proteins. These reactions also occur in patients who are IgA-deficient and have antibodies to IgA. It is recommended that such patients receive blood products from IgA-deficient donors or washed red cells.

Transfusion-Transmitted Diseases

Despite routine testing of all blood products for hepatitis B surface antigen (HBsAg), antibodies to hepatitis B core (anti-HBc), and antibodies to hepatitis C virus (anti-HCV), transfusion-associated hepatitis can still occur. Although hepatitis C represents the majority of cases of post-transfusion hepatitis,[87] several hundred cases of acute hepatitis B following transfusion are reported annually.[88] The current risk of transfusion-associated hepatitis B is estimated to be 1 in 63,000 components transfused.[89] The incidence of transfusion-associated hepatitis C has been greatly reduced with the development of better testing.[90] Donahue et al. studied cardiac surgery patients from April of 1985 through February of 1991. Patients were divided into three time periods representing different donor screening procedures. They found that the risk of post-transfusion hepatitis C declined from 0.55 to 0.36 to 0.06 percent per unit transfused over that period with the implementation of new testing procedures.[91,92] The current estimated risk of hepatitis C virus (HCV) in screened blood is 1 in 103,000 units.[89] With the recent implementation of nucleic acid testing (NAT) techniques, which use a PCR assay for the detection of HCV, it is expected that the infectious seronegative window period will be reduced from 70 days to 12 to 28 days,[93] which should result in a significant decrease in the risk of transfusion-transmitted HCV.

Transfusion-associated AIDS was first reported in late 1982,[94] and serologic testing for HIV became available in 1985.[95] Currently, all blood is tested for HIV serology and for the presence of p24 antigen in addition to extensive donor screening aimed at the high-risk activities for HIV infection or AIDS. Many studies have evaluated the risk of transfusion-associated HIV infection. One such study followed 11,535 cardiac surgery patients from 1985 to 1991 who received a total of 120,290 units of tested blood. Two patients underwent seroconversion, corresponding to a residual risk of 1 in 60,000 units.[96] Currently, the estimated risk of HIV transmission from screened blood is 1 in 493,000.[89]

Cytomegalovirus is a herpesvirus. It is a double-stranded DNA virus, capable of remaining latent in tissues following primary disease. Clinical disease due to this virus may occur on the basis of primary infection, reactivation, or reinfection. The virus is thought to be harbored within white cells. Clinical CMV disease can be quite variable; however, primary disease is usually more severe than reactivation. Interstitial CMV pneumonitis accounts for 40 percent of all cases of pneumonitis following bone marrow transplantation and is fatal in 80 percent of cases.[97] In patients at risk for CMV infection, CMV-seronegative blood products should be administered. Because of the presence of CMV in white cells, leukocyte reduction has become an alternative approach.

Transfusion-Associated Graft-Versus-Host Disease

Transfusion-associated GvHD is a virtually always fatal complication of transfusion. The disease occurs when immunocompetent lymphocytes are given to an immunoincompetent recipient. The disease usually presents 7 to 10 days after transfusion. Patients develop fever and an erythematous, maculopapular rash. The disease also affects the gastrointestinal tract, liver, and lymphoid tissues, especially the thymus.[98] In patients who have not received a bone marrow transplant, the disease can involve the bone marrow and can produce profound aplasia. This disease has a more aggressive and rapid course than the GvHD that follows bone marrow transplantation. Patients usually die within 3 weeks from infection or a bleeding complication.[26,99]

Transfusion-associated GvHD has been reported in several clinical situations, including the presence of congenital immunodeficiency syndromes, such as severe combined immunodeficiency syndrome (SCIDS). Patients at risk for transfusion-associated GvHD include those undergoing bone marrow or progenitor cell transplantation and those receiving products donated by a blood relative who may share one HLA haplotype. All of these patients should receive gamma-irradiated cellular blood products.[26] Additionally, there are several reports of transfusion-associated GvHD in patients with chronic lymphocytic leukemia who are being treated with fludarabine.[29,30] Patients with malignancies including patients with Hodgkin's disease, non-Hodgkin's lymphomas, leukemia, and some solid tumors are at variable degrees of risk. In some institutions, all patients with hematologic–oncologic diseases receive irradiated cellular blood products to eliminate the possibility of GvHD.

Alloimmunization

Since red cell products contain some contaminating white blood cells, patients who receive red cells are at risk for the development of alloantibodies directed against red cell, neutrophil, platelet, and/or HLA antigens. The development of antibodies is multifactorial and involves such variables as the immunogenicity of the antigen, the immune competence of the patient, and the number of exposures.

Retrospective studies have shown that patients with lymphocytic leukemia have a markedly decreased rate of development of red cell alloantibodies. In two studies, none of the 112 total patients became alloimmunized to red cell antigens. It is unclear if this decrease in the incidence of antibody formation is related to the disease or the treatment. Increased rates of alloimmunization to red cell antigens were seen in patients with chronic myeloproliferative diseases (25 percent) and those with the myelodysplastic syndromes (31.3 percent). Intermediate rates of alloimmunization were found in patients with multiple myeloma (11.8 percent) and those with myeloid leukemias (16 percent).[100–102]

The formation of antileukocyte antibodies is of interest because of their role in the pathogenesis of febrile, nonhemolytic transfusion reactions. Patients who receive multiple transfusions may develop the complication of repeated febrile, nonhemolytic transfusion reactions, which can be attributed to antileukocyte antibodies. As mentioned above, patients with this complication due to these antibodies should receive leukocyte-reduced red cells. Most of these patients will have uneventful transfusions with leukocyte-reduced (fewer than 5×10^6 white cells) red cells, especially with prestorage leukocyte reduction.

Because of the presence of white cells in red cell products, the patient who receives multiple transfusions is at risk for the development of anti-HLA alloantibodies, which can complicate platelet transfusion therapy and result in platelet refractoriness. Several studies have shown that patients with hematologic malignancies who receive multiple transfusions have reduced HLA alloimmunization and reduced platelet refractoriness when given leukocyte-reduced red cell and platelet products.[103–107] A large multicenter clinical trial, the Trial to Reduce Alloimmunization to Platelets (TRAP), compared various strategies to reduce alloimmunization in patients with leukemia. This study confirmed that use of leukocyte-reduced blood products results in decreased alloimmunization to platelets.[108]

Immunomodulation

The effect of transfusion therapy on immune function has generated considerable controversy. Some believe that blood transfusions have an immunomodulatory effect, resulting in transfusion-induced immunosuppression. Some studies have shown an increase in tumor recurrence in patients who have received transfusions, although other studies have shown no effect.[109] The mechanism of transfusion-induced immunosuppression is unclear, although tolerance and anergy have been proposed as possible mechanisms.[110] Animal studies have shown that the tumor growth enhancement associated with transfusions is mediated by donor leukocytes and have also found that use of leukocyte-reduced blood products ameliorates this tumor-enhancing effect in animals.[111] The use of leukocyte-reduced blood products for leukemic patients has previously been greatly debated because it has been suggested that the donor leukocytes may exert a graft-versus-leukemia effect. Subsequent studies have failed to show an effect of transfused leukocytes, and others have seen no difference in duration of first remissions in leukemic patients receiving leukocyte-reduced blood products.[112,113] The Finnish Leukemia Group studied patients with acute myeloid leukemia and found that the patients receiving leukocyte-reduced blood products had longer median relapse-free survival, shorter periods of aplasia with decreased blood product usage, and decreased occurrence of infections.[114]

REFERENCES

1. Erstad BL, Gales BI, Rappaport WD: The use of albumin in clinical practice. Arch Intern Med 151:901, 1991.
2. Baldini M, Costea N, Dameshek W: The viability of stored human platelets. Blood 16:1669, 1960.
3. Rapaport GI, Ames SB, Mikkelsen S: The levels of antihemophilic globulin and proaccelerin in fresh and bank blood. Am J Clin Pathol 31:297, 1957.
4. Gorlin JB (ed.): Standards for Blood Banks and Transfusion Services, 20th Ed. American Association of Blood Banks, Bethesda, MD, 2000.
5. Pineda AD, Viggiano NR, Clare D, Bukowski B: Flow rate of AS-1 preserved red cells and whole blood – a comparison. Transfusion 25:449, 1985.
6. Hogge DE, Dutcher JP, Aisner J, Schiffer CA: Lymphocytotoxic antibody is a predictor of response to random-donor platelet transfusion. Am J Hematol 14:363, 1983.
7. Wenz B, Gurtlinger KF, O'Toole AM, Dugan EP: Preparation of granulocyte-poor red blood cells by microaggregate filtration: A simplified method to minimize febrile transfusion reactions. Vox Sang 39:282, 1980.
8. Parravicini A, Rebulla P, Apuzzo J, Wenz B, Sirchia G: The preparation of leukocyte-poor red cells for transfusion by a simple cost-effective technique. Transfusion 24:508, 1984.

9. Dzik S: Leukodepletion blood filters: Filter design and mechanisms of leukocyte removal. Transfus Med Rev 7:65, 1993.

10. Sirchia G, Rebulla P, Parravicini A et al: Leukocyte depletion of red cell units at the bedside by transfusion through a new filter. Transfusion 27:402, 1987.

11. Domen RE, Williams L: Use of the Sepacell filter for preparing white cell-depleted red cells. Transfusion 28:506, 1988.

12. Bock M, Wagner M, Knuppel W et al: Preparation of white cell-depleted blood: Comparison of two bedside filter systems. Transfusion 30:26, 1990.

13. Sirchia G, Wenz B, Rebulla P et al: Removal of white cells from red cells by transfusion through a new filter. Transfusion 30:30, 1990.

14. Koerner K, Sahlmen P, Zimmermann B, Kubanek B: Preparation of leukocyte-poor red cell concentrates: Comparison of five different filters. Vox Sang 60:61, 1991.

15. Lane TA: Leukocyte reduction of cellular blood components: Effectiveness, benefits, quality control, and costs. Arch Pathol Lab Med 118:392, 1994.

16. Vyas GN, Holmdahl L, Perkins HA, Fudenberg HH: Serologic specificity of human anti-IgA and its significance in transfusion. Blood 34:573, 1969.

17. Stavely L, Jakway J, Schoeppner S et al: Quantitation of IgA in blood components and plasma derivatives. Transfusion 24:421, 1984.

18. Yap PL, Pryde EAD, McClelland DBL: IgA content of frozen–thawed washed red blood cells and blood products measured by radioimmunoassay. Transfusion 22:36, 1982.

19. Dacie JV: Transfusion of saline-washed red cells in nocturnal hemoglobinuria. Clin Sci 7:65, 1948.

20. Brecher ME, Taswell HF: Paroxysmal nocturnal hemoglobinuria and the transfusion of washed red cells: A myth revisited. Transfusion 29:681, 1989.

21. Rosse WF: Transfusion in paroxysmal nocturnal hemoglobinuria: To wash or not to wash. Transfusion 29:663, 1989.

22. Meryman HT, Hornblower M: A method for freezing and washing red blood cells using a high glycerol concentration. Transfusion 12:145, 1972.

23. Pert JH, Schork PK, Moore R: A new method of low-temperature blood preservation using liquid nitrogen and a glycerol sucrose additive. Clin Res 11:197, 1963.

24. Kurtz SR, Van Deinse WH, Valeri CR: The immunocompetence of residual lymphocytes at various stages of red cell cryopreservation with 40% W/V glycerol in an ionic medium at −80 C. Transfusion 18:441, 1978.

25. Storb R, Thomas ED, Buckner CD et al: Marrow transplantation in thirty "untransfused" patients with severe aplastic anemia. Ann Intern Med 92:30, 1980.

26. Webb IJ, Anderson KC: Transfusion-associated graft-versus-host disease. In Anderson KC, Ness PM (eds.): Scientific Basis of Transfusion Medicine: Implications for Clinical Practice, 2nd Ed., pp. 420–426. WB Saunders, Philadelphia, 2000.

27. McMilin KD, Johnson RL: HLA homozygosity and the risk of related-donor transfusion-associated graft-versus-host-disease. Transfus Med Rev 7:37, 1993.

28. Petz LD, Calhoun L, Yam P et al: Transfusion-associated graft-versus-host disease in immunocompetent patients: Report of a fatal case associated with transfusion of blood from a second-degree relative, and a survey of predisposing factors. Transfusion 33:742, 1993.

29. Maung ZT, Wood AC, Jackson GH, Turner GE, Appleton AL, Hamilton PJ: Transfusion-associated graft-versus-host disease in fludarabine-treated B-chronic lymphocytic leukemia. Br J Haematol 88:649, 1994.

30. Briz M, Cabrera R, Sanjuan I, Fores R, Diez JL, Herrero M, Regidor C, Algora M, Fernandez MN: Diagnosis of transfusion-associated graft-versus-host disease by polymerase chain reaction in fludarabine-treated B-chronic lymphocytic leukaemia. Br J Haematol 91:409, 1995.

31. Lowenthal RM, Challis DR, Griffiths AE et al: Transfusion-associated graft-versus-host disease: Report of an occurrence following the administration of irradiated blood. Transfusion 33:524, 1993.

32. Preiksaitis JK: Indications for the use of cytomegalovirus-seronegative blood products. Transfus Med Rev 5:1, 1991.

33. Sayers MH, Anderson KC, Goodnough LT et al: Reducing the risk for transfusion-transmitted cytomegalovirus infection. Ann Intern Med 116:55, 1992.

34. Hillyer CD, Snydman DR, Berkman EM: The risk of cytomegalovirus infection in solid organ and bone marrow transplant recipients: Transfusion of blood products. Transfusion 30:659, 1990.

35. Gilbert GL, Hayes K, Hudson IL, James J: Prevention of transfusion-acquired cytomegalovirus infection in infants by blood filtration to remove leucocytes. Neonatal Cytomegalovirus Infection Study Group. Lancet 1:1228, 1989.

36. Bowden RA, Slichter SJ, Sayers MH et al: Use of leukocyte-depleted platelets and cytomegalovirus-seronegative red blood cells for prevention of primary cytomegalovirus infection after marrow transplant. Blood 78:246, 1991.

37. Smith KL, Cobain T, Dunstan RA: Removal of cytomegalovirus DNA from donor blood by filtration. Br J Haematol 83:640, 1993.

38. Bowden RA, Slichter SJ, Sayers M et al: A comparison of filtered leukocyte-reduced and cytomegalovirus (CMV) seronegative blood products for the prevention of tranfusion-associated CMV infection after marrow transplant. Blood 86:3598, 1993.

39. Preiksaitis JK: The cytomegalovirus-"safe" blood product: Is leukoreduction equivalent to antibody screening? Tranfus Med Rev 14:112, 2000.

40. AuBuchon JP: Minimizing donor exposure in hemotherapy. Arch Pathol Lab Med 118:380, 1994.

41. Stehling L, Simon TL: The red blood cell transfusion trigger: Physiology and clinical studies. Arch Pathol Lab Med 118:429, 1994.

42. Office of Medical Application of Research, National Institutes of Health: Perioperative red cell transfusion. JAMA 260:2700, 1988.

43. Mollison PL, Engelfriet CP, Contreras M: The transfusion of red cells. In Blood Transfusion in Clinical Medicine. 10th Ed., pp. 278–314. Blackwell Publications, London, 1997.

44. Petz LD, Tomasula PA: Red blood cell transfusion. In Kolins J, McCarthy LJ (eds.): Contemporary Transfusion Practice, p. 1. American Association of Blood Banks, Arlington, VA, 1987.

45. Russell JA, Toy JL, Powles RL: Plasma exchange in malignant paraproteinemias. Exp Hematol (Suppl. 5):105, 1977.

46. Lichtman MA, Rowe JM: Hyperleukocytic leukemias: Rheological, clinical, and therapeutic considerations. Blood 60:279, 1982.

47. Harris AL: Leukostasis associated with blood transfusion in acute myeloid leukemia. BMJ 1:1169, 1978.

48. Vengelen-Tyler V(ed.): Hematopoietic transplantation. In Technical Manual of the American Association of Blood Banks. 13th Ed., pp. 531–561. American Association of Blood Banks, Bethesda, MD 1999.

49. Gajewski JL, Petz LD, Calhoun L et al: Hemolysis of transfused group O red blood cells in minor ABO-incompatible unrelated-donor bone marrow transplants in patients receiving cyclosporine without posttransplant methotrexate. Blood 79:3076, 1992.

50. Sthoeger ZM, Sthoeger D, Shtalrid M et al: Mechanism of autoimmune hemolytic anemia in chronic lymphocytic leukemia. Am J Hematol 43:259, 1993.

51. Tosti S, Caruso R, D'Adamo F et al: Severe autoimmune hemolytic anemia in a patient with chronic lymphocytic leukemia responsive to fludarabine-based treatment. Ann Hematol 65:238, 1992.

52. Koury ST, Bondurant MC, Koury MJ: Localization of erythropoietin synthesizing cells in murine kidneys by in situ hybridization. Blood 71:524, 1988.

53. Lacombe C, DaSilva L, Bruneval P et al: Peritubular cells are the site of erythropoietin synthesis in the murine hypoxic kidney. J Clin Invest 81:620, 1988.

54. Koury ST, Bondurant MC, Koury MJ, Semenza GL: Localization of cells producing erythropoietin in murine liver by in situ hybridization. Blood 77:2497, 1991.

55. Jacobs K, Shoemaker C, Rudersdorf R et al: Isolation and characterization of genomic and cDNA clones of human erythropoietin. Nature 313:806, 1985.

56. Lin F-K, Suggs S, Lin D-H et al: Cloning and expression of the human erythropoietin gene. Proc Natl Acad Sci U S A 82:7580, 1985.

57. Cazzola M, Ponchia L, Beguin Y et al: Subcutaneous erythropoietin for treatment of refractory anemia in hematologic disorders. Results of a phase I/II clinical trial. Blood 79:29, 1992.

58. Ludwig H, Fritz E, Leitgeb C et al: Erythropoietin treatment for chronic anemia of selected hematologic malignancies and solid tumors. Ann Oncol 4:161, 1993.

59. Asano Y, Okamura S, Shibuya T et al: Growth of clonogenic myeloblastic leukemic cells in the presence of human recombinant erythropoietin in addition to various human recombinant hematopoietic progenitor cells in vivo. Blood 72:1682, 1988.

60. Ludwig H, Fritz E, Kotzmann H et al: Erythropoietin treatment of anemia associated with multiple myeloma. N Engl J Med 322:1693, 1990.

61. Spivak J: Recombinant human erythropoietin and the anemia of cancer. Blood 84:997, 1994.

62. Vengelen-Tyler V (ed.): Blood component preparation, storage, shipping and transportation. In Technical Manual of the American Association of Blood Banks, 13th Ed., pp. 161–191. American Association of Blood Banks, Bethesda, MD 1999.

63. Haradin AR, Weed RI, Reed CF: Changes in the physical properties of stored erythrocytes: Relationship to survival in vivo. Transfusion 9:229, 1969.

64. Beutler E, Wood L: The in vivo regeneration of red cell 2,3-dephosphoglyceric acid (DPG) after transfusion of stored blood. J Lab Clin Med 74:300, 1969.

65. Wolf PL, McCarthy LJ, Hafleigh B: Extreme hypercalcemia following blood transfusion combined with intravenous calcium. Vox Sang 19:544, 1970.

66. Moore GL, Peck CC, Sohmer PR, Zuck TF: Some properties of blood stored in anticoagulant CPDA-1 solution. A brief summary. Transfusion 21:135, 1981.

67. Swank RL: Alteration of blood on storage: Measurement of adhesiveness of 'aging' platelets and leucocytes and their removal by filtration. N Engl J Med 265:728, 1961.

68. McNamara JJ, Molot MD, Stremple JF: Screen filtration pressure in combat casualties. Ann Surg 172:334, 1970.

69. Reul GJ, Beall AC, Greenberg SD: Protection of the pulmonary microvasculature by fine screen blood filtration. Chest 66:4, 1974.

70. Bredenberg CE: International forum: Does a relationship exist between massive blood transfusion and the adult respiratory distress syndrome? Vox Sang 32:311, 1977.

71. Tobey RE, Kopriva CJ, Homer LD: Pulmonary gas exchange following hemorrhagic and massive transfusion in the baboon. Ann Surg 179:316, 1974.

72. Solis RT, Walker BD: International forum: Does a relationship exist between massive blood transfusion and the adult respiratory distress syndrome? Vox Sang 32:319, 1977.

73. Jaeger RJ, Rubin RJ: Migration of a phthalate ester plasticizer from polyvinyl chloride blood bags into stored human blood and its localization in human tissues. N Engl J Med 287:1114, 1972.

74. Rubin RJ, Ness PM: What price progress? An update on vinyl plastic blood bags. Transfusion 29:358, 1989.

75. Hogman CF, Eriksson L, Ericson A, Reppucci AJ: Storage of saline-adenine-glucose-mannitol-suspended red cells in a new plastic container: Polyvinyl chloride plasticized with butyryl-n-trihexyl-citrate. Transfusion 31:26, 1991.

76. Carmen R: The selection of plastic materials for blood bags. Transfus Med Rev 7:1, 1993.

77. Goldman M, Blajchman MA: Blood product-associated bacterial sepsis. Transfus Med Rev 5:73, 1991.

78. Sazama K: Bacteria in blood for transfusion: A review. Arch Pathol Lab Med 118:350, 1994.

79. Payne R: The association of febrile transfusion reactions with leuko-agglutinins. Vox Sang 2:233, 1957.

80. Brittingham TE, Chaplin H: Febrile transfusion reactions caused by sensitivity to donor leukocytes and platelets. JAMA 165:819, 1957.

81. Perkins HA, Payne R, Ferguson J, Wood M: Nonhemolytic febrile transfusion reactions: Quantitative effects of blood components with emphasis on isoantigenic incompatibility of leukocytes. Vox Sang 11:578, 1966.

82. Menitove JE, McElligott MC, Aster RH: Febrile transfusion reaction: What blood component should be given next? Vox Sang 42:318, 1982.

83. Wenz B: Microaggregate blood filtration and the febrile transfusion reaction: A comparative study. Transfusion 23:95, 1983.

84. Mangano MM, Chambers LA, Kruskall MS: Limited efficacy of leukopoor platelets for prevention of febrile transfusion reactions. Am J Clin Pathol 95:733, 1991.

85. Heddle NM, Klama LN, Griffith L et al: A prospective study to identify the risk factors associated with acute reactions to platelet and red cell transfusions. Transfusion 33:794, 1993.

86. Heddle NM, Klama L, Singer J et al: The role of the plasma from platelet concentrates in transfusion reactions. N Engl J Med 331:625, 1994.

87. Gill P: Transfusion-associated hepatitis C: Reducing the risk. Transfus Med Rev 7:104, 1993.

88. Hoofnagle JH: Posttransfusion hepatitis B. Transfusion 30:384, 1990.

89. Schreiber GB, Busch MP, Kleinman SH, Korelitz JJ: The risk of transfusion-transmitted viral infections. N Engl J Med 334:1685, 1996.

90. Alter MJ: Review of serologic testing for hepatitis C virus infection and risk of posttransfusion hepatitis C. Arch Pathol Lab Med 118:342, 1994.

91. Donahue JG, Munoz A, Ness PM et al: The declining risk of post-transfusion hepatitis C virus infection. N Engl J Med 327:369, 1992.

92. Nelson KE, Ahmed F, Ness PM et al: Comparison of first and second generation ELISA screening tests in detecting HCV infections in transfused cardiac surgery patients (abstract). In Program and Abstracts of the International Symposium on Viral Hepatitis and Liver Disease (May 10–14, 1993, Tokyo), p. 50, 1993.

93. Sacher RA, Schreiber GB, Kleinman SH: Prevention of transfusion-transmitted hepatitis. Lancet 355:331, 2000.

94. Ammann AJ, Cowan MJ, Wara DJ et al: Acquired immunodeficiency in an infant: Possible transmission by means of blood products. Lancet 1:956, 1983.

95. Petricciani JC: Licensed tests for antibody to human T lymphotrophic virus type III: Sensitivity and specificity. Ann Intern Med 103:726, 1985.

96. Cohen ND, Munoz A, Reitz BA et al: Transmission of retroviruses by transfusion of screened blood in patients undergoing cardiac surgery. N Engl J Med 320:1172, 1989.

97. Meyers JD, Flournoy N, Thomas ED: Risk factors for cytomegalovirus infection after bone marrow transplantation. J Infect Dis 153:478, 1986.

98. Gartner JG: Thymic involution with loss of Hassall's corpuscles mimicking thymic dysplasia in a child with transfusion-associated graft-versus-host disease. Pediatr Pathol 11:449, 1991.

99. Anderson KC, Weinstein HJ: Transfusion-associated graft-versus-host disease. N Engl J Med 323;315, 1990.

100. Blumberg N, Peck K, Ross K, Avila E: Immune response to chronic red blood cell transfusion. Vox Sang 44:212, 1983.

101. Fluit CRMG, Kunst VAJM, Drenthe-Cshonk AM: Incidence of red cell antibodies after multiple blood transfusion. Transfusion 30:532, 1990.

102. Blumberg N, Ross K, Avila E, Peck K: Should chronic transfusions be matched for antigens other than ABO and Rh (D)? Vox Sang 47:205, 1984.

103. Murphy MF, Metcalfe P, Thomas H et al: Use of leukocyte-poor blood components and HLA-matched-platelet donors to prevent HLA alloimmunization. Br J Haematol 62:529, 1986.

104. Sniecinski I, O'Donnell MR, Nowicki B, Hill LR: Prevention of refractoriness and HLA-alloimmunization using filtered blood products. Blood 71:1402, 1988.

105. Andreu G, Dewailly J, Leberre C et al: Prevention of HLA immunization with leukocyte-poor packed red cells and platelet concentrates obtained by filtration. Blood 72:964, 1988.

106. Saarinen UM, Kekomaki R, Siimes MA, Myllyla G: Effective prophylaxis against platelet refractoriness in multitransfused patients by use of leukocyte-free blood components. Blood 75:512, 1990.

107. Oksanen K, Kekomaki R, Ruutu T et al: Prevention of alloimmunization in patients with acute leukemia by the use of white cell-reduced blood components – a randomized trial. Transfusion 31:588, 1991.

108. The Trial to Reduce Alloimmunization to Platelets Study Group: Leukocyte reduction and ultraviolet B irradiation of platelets to prevent alloimmunization and refractoriness to platelet transfusions. N Engl J Med 337:1861, 1997.

109. Ness PM, Walsh PC, Zahurak M et al: Prostate cancer recurrence in radical surgery patients receiving autologous or homologous blood. Transfusion 32:31, 1992.

110. Blumberg N, Heal J: Effects of transfusion on immune function. Cancer recurrence and infection. Arch Pathol Lab Med 118:371, 1994.

111. Blajchman MA, Bardossy L, Carmen R et al: Allogeneic blood transfusion-induced enhancement of tumor growth: Two animal models showing amelioration by leukodepletion and passive transfer using spleen cells. Blood 81:1880, 1993.

112. Rebulla P, Sirchia G: Duration of first remission in leukaemic recipients of leucocyte-poor blood components. Br J Haematol 80:135, 1992.

113. Rebulla P, Pappalettera M, Barbui T: Duration of first remission in leukaemic recipients of leucocyte-poor blood components. Br J Haematol 75:441, 1990.

114. Oksanen K, Elonen E: Impact of leucocyte-depleted blood components on the haematological recovery and prognosis of patients with acute myeloid leukaemia. Br J Haematol 84:639, 1993.

54

Platelet and Granulocyte Transfusion

Janice P. Dutcher

A major advance in our ability to treat patients with hematologic malignancies (particularly those with acute leukemia) has been the development of cell component transfusion support during the pancytopenia resulting from remission induction therapy and subsequent intensive consolidation and bone marrow transplantation. The first therapeutic "platelet transfusions" occurred when Duke[1] transfused fresh whole blood in 1910, after noting an association between thrombocytopenia and bleeding and observing that correction of bleeding was associated with an increase in platelet count. However, 50 years were required to develop the technology for separating platelets efficiently from blood and allowing their administration as a separate blood component. In 1963 Freireich et al.[2] demonstrated the clinical effectiveness of platelet transfusions in children with acute leukemia, using platelet-rich plasma as the transfused blood product. The ability to provide platelets as a separate concentrated blood component has substantially improved the hematologic support of leukemia patients and has decreased the incidence of deaths caused by hemorrhage. Further technical advances have improved the quality of this blood product, and careful studies of transfusion practices have led to specific guidelines to optimize platelet transfusion support.

The success of platelet transfusion therapy led to attempts to separate granulocytes as a blood component, to help combat the other major problem in leukemia supportive care—the management of infection. The initial granulocyte transfusions were from patients with untreated chronic myelocytic leukemia and high white blood cell counts whose white blood cells could more easily be separated from the red cells by gravity.[3] Separating granulocytes from red cells, especially in donors with normal white blood cell counts, was initially extremely problematic, since little difference in density exists between red cells and granulocytes. Such separation was first attempted by filtration techniques, in which the white cells adhered to filters as whole blood passed through and then the granulocytes were literally hammered off the filters.[4] However, technology quickly advanced for collection of both platelets and granulocytes, particularly with newer cell separator technology, allowing collection of cellular components from whole blood of normal donors[5,6] with demonstration of clinical efficacy.[7]

Platelet transfusion support has increased dramatically in the past 20 years, in large part because of more aggressive

chemotherapy (for leukemia and solid tumors) and bone marrow transplantation. In response to the increased usage as well as concerns about transfusion-transmitted infection and alloimmunization technological changes have also occurred rapidly.[8]

Granulocyte transfusion therapy, over the course of the past 25 years, has markedly decreased in frequency. In the late 1970s and early 1980s, granulocyte transfusions were used and studied extensively, to combat neutropenic sepsis in leukemia patients. Two factors impacted on the decline in usage: 1. the development of more effective broad-spectrum antibiotics and the adoption of the policy of empiric initiation of antibiotics for febrile neutropenia, and 2. concern that insufficient doses of granulocytes were being obtained from normal donors, even with enhanced technology, to provide sufficient granulocyte numbers for effective anti-infective therapy. However, in the past 5 years, new approaches to granulocyte procurement have led to greater donor yields, and there appears to be renewed interest in appropriately utilizing granulocyte transfusions. The clinical criteria for such transfusions remain unresponsive sepsis and fungal infections. Current studies will attempt to demonstrate whether the enhanced yields will be sufficient to improve the outcome in these settings.

PLATELET COLLECTION

Although platelet-rich plasma was shown to diminish or stop bleeding in thrombocytopenic leukemic children, plasma is a large-volume transfusion product and not practical for general use. The ability to concentrate platelets into a smaller volume of plasma was facilitated by Mourad's[9] discovery that the addition of extra amounts of acid citrate dextrose anticoagulant to the platelet-rich plasma before centrifugation allowed easy resuspension of the platelets, rather than clumping.

Platelets for transfusion are currently prepared in one of two ways. Platelet concentrates are obtained as a byproduct of the routine processing of whole blood units into packed red blood cells (RBCs) and plasma, with platelets subsequently concentrated from platelet-rich plasma, with a minimum of 50 cc of plasma per concentrate. With this single-unit processing technique, 1 unit of platelets (from 1 unit of blood) contains 0.55 to 1.1×10^{11} platelets. Several units are then pooled to produce a transfusion (4 to 8 units per transfusion for adults).

The other method of collecting platelets involves the use of apheresis machines that can obtain multiple units of platelets from individual donors in a single procedure, lasting 1 to 2 hours. The principle of apheresis, using either intermittent or continuous flow, is similar to that used in the preparation of individual platelet units: separation of blood components by density centrifugation. With an apheresis machine, however, whole blood is withdrawn from the donor into a collection bowl, belt, or chamber within the machine, and the blood is then centrifuged continuously into layers. The platelet or other cellular component is then extracted through a collection port and the RBCs and plasma and other cellular components are returned to the donor. This process is continued until a sufficient number of platelets are collected. All of the current apheresis machines have been through numerous updates to maximize platelet yield and to meet the current standards requiring reduced leukocytes in the product.[10–16] Through new technology, donors may frequently supply sufficient platelets for two transfusions, during a single apheresis session lasting 1.5 hours or less.[16]

Although originally apheresis platelets were primarily used to provide HLA-matched products, many blood centers now preferentially provide apheresis single-donor platelet products, because of the ease and comfort of current apheresis technology. However, the recently published clinical practice guidelines of the American Society of Clinical Oncology on platelet transfusions states that either pooled platelets or apheresis platelets for nonalloimmunized recipients are interchangeable.[17]

For historical interest, techniques of gravity apheresis should be mentioned. Multiple units from a single donor can be processed, cycling the collection of 1 unit of whole blood, centrifugation to separate platelet-rich plasma, collection of platelets by a subsequent centrifugation step, and then return of the RBCs and plasma to the donor. This cycle can be repeated in the same donor until multiple units of platelets are collected.[18] This process obviously preceded current modern equipment, and is time consuming, but has the advantage of not requiring special equipment, other than the collection bags and a centrifuge, and should be remembered in case an unusual emergency situations arises.

Donor-related issues are also of importance, particularly as single donor apheresis becomes more common. The platelet count decreases in all apheresis platelet donors following the procedure. Since donors have a normal preprocedure platelet count, this is rarely a clinical problem. However, postcollection platelet counts may fall to less than 100,000/µl in donors with pre-apheresis counts of less than 200,000/µl.[19] Although the risk of bleeding may be negligible, bleeding times are abnormal with platelet counts of less than 100,000/µl, so platelet counts in individuals who donate frequently must be monitored. Glowitz and Slichter[20] observed serial decreases in donor pre-apheresis counts with frequent donation, but have noted an apparent rebound rise in platelet counts after several donations, suggesting a marrow response with increased production. No adverse effect on donor platelet count was observed with repeated multiunit donation.[20] Additional donor-related problems with apheresis include symptoms of hypovolemia or vasovagal reactions, the discomfort of venipuncture, or mild reactions to citrate anticoagulant (which can be reversed by slowing the flow rate of the procedure). These adverse effects should not prevent the necessary collection of single-donor histocompatible platelets, but must remain a consideration in selecting and repeating procedures in certain donors, particularly when not required for histocompatibility. Recent commentaries comparing apheresis donor platelets and single-blood unit derived platelets consider these products to be interchangeable and suggest that cost factors and platelet yield will largely influence the frequency with which each approach is utilized for random donor platelets.[8,15–17]

Current American Association of Blood Banks standards recommend platelet-apheresis donation no more frequently than 2 times in a week, or 24 times in a year except in unusual circumstances. These would be decided in conjunction with the treating physician and the approval of the blood bank director.[21] It is recognized that platelets from a specific histocompatible donor may be essential to the survival of a specific patient and thus donations may exceed the limits indicated by the standards, which has been done safely.[20,22] The donor must undergo serial clinical and laboratory evaluations by the supervising physician.

Leukodepletion

Recommended current transfusion practice involves leukodepletion of blood products to remove immunogenic lymphocytes and antigen-presenting cells, to prevent alloimmunization (discussed in detail later). Leukodepletion may also reduce the risk of transfusion-transmitted viral disease in which the virus is harbored in the leukocytes (see Hazards of Transfusion below). Since lymphocytes are similar in density to platelets, numerous technical difficulties have arisen, and considerable effort has been expended in developing techniques to separate leukocytes from platelets in platelet-rich plasma.

Leukodepletion of apheresis products relies primarily on the modifications that have been made in the technology of the apheresis machines to reduce leukocyte contamination and retain adequate numbers of platelets per collection[10–14] (Table 54–1). More recently, apheresis techniques have been developed that in many cases yield double donations of platelets with efficient leukodepletion[16] (Table 54–1).

The earliest blood bank techniques for leukodepletion of single platelet units and RBC units or for additional depletion of single-donor products utilized cotton wool and cellulose filters to which the leukocytes adhered (Imugard, Terumo; Erypur, Organon).[23–25] More recently, two filters made of nonwoven polyester fibers have been developed that also permit

Table 54–1. Characteristics of Leukodepleted Platelet Products

Method	Total White Blood Cells	Platelets $\times 10^{11}$	Reference
Mechanical Apheresis			
Cobe Spectra V5-LRS	$< 1 \times 10^6$	2.56–7.41	16
Fenwal Amicus	$< 1 \times 10^6$	2.82–7.14	16
Cobe V7 Turbo	$< 1 \times 10^6$	2.80–7.54	16
Filtration—6 pooled units			
Imugard IG 500	$0.5–2 \times 10^6$	3.1–4.0	24,25
PALL PL100	$5–6 \times 10^5$	3.5–4.0	27
SepaCell PL	$0.1–5 \times 10^6$	3.1–4.0	28
Historical centrifugation studies of 6 pooled units	$5–7 \times 10^8$	3.0–4.0	158

passage of platelets with adherence of the leukocytes to the filters (Sepacel, Baxter/Fenwal; Pall, Pall Corp).[26–28] These can be used at the bedside and are the type commonly seen in the United States. Table 54–1 summarizes the content of the resulting platelet products.

Many blood centers are also evaluating the prefiltering of products for distribution, and in-line filters have been tested for use during red cell collection and during apheresis. One study has shown no increased risk of bacterial growth in platelet concentrates as a result of prestorage white cell reduction.[29] Others have shown improved storage of platelets in the absence of leukocytes.[30,31] These issues are a part of the ongoing clinical investigation of leukodepleted blood products in general and also of ongoing attempts to decide the role and extent of leukodepletion of blood products.[32]

PLATELET STORAGE

The increased demand for platelet transfusions as well as the delay imposed by the multiple pretransfusion viral donor screens now required has stimulated ongoing research in the technology of platelet storage.[33–35] Many physical factors influence successful platelet storage. These include optimal storage temperature, maintenance of a certain range of plasma pH, suspension in an adequate volume of plasma, proper agitation during storage, and attention to the characteristics of the storage bag.[34–38]

Storage conditions for individual platelet units derived from whole blood donations as well as for the storage of apheresis platelet collections have been defined and optimized based on the stability of storage pH and durability of platelet function.[34–40] It has been determined through numerous investigations that room temperature (22° to 24°C) storage is optimal for platelets.[38,39,41,42] Despite the increased metabolic activity that occurs in platelets stored at 22°C, significantly better poststorage platelet viability at this temperature (compared with platelet concentrates stored at 4°C) has been confirmed by studies of transfusion response after storage at the two different temperatures.[38,39,41,42] Recent studies suggest than even a brief reduction in storage temperature to 20°C during transport over long distances may have deleterious effects on subsequent platelet in vivo viability and in vitro function.[43]

The storage bag characteristics have also been shown to be important in the maintenance of platelet viability.[36] Over the past 10 to 15 years, the development of new plastics and plasticizers and the production of larger and thinner bags have established a more stable storage environment, making possible extended storage of platelet concentrates and single-donor apheresis platelets.[36,44–47] Storage bag qualities help to regulate oxygen and carbon dioxide exchange across the bag, which in turn regulates pH. The maintenance of plasma pH above 6.0 during storage preserves cell viability, although a very high pH can lead to irreversible platelet clumping.[36,38,48] Entry of adequate oxygen permits the maintenance of oxidative metabolism in platelets stored at room temperature, thus suppressing glycolysis (with its production of lactic acid) and preventing a fall in pH level. The egress of carbon dioxide across the bag surface also helps to maintain pH. The newer plastic bags provide increased oxygen transfer compared with the first-generation bags and have allowed stable, prolonged, storage with viability demonstrated after 5 or more days.[44–47]

Agitation during storage of platelets is also important, since it prevents platelet "packing" and is believed to facilitate gas exchange through the storage bag.[35,49] With the use of the permeable storage bags, it seems that the mode of agitation is less critical to platelet viability, and a variety of platelet rotators appear to be suitable for maintaining function.[35,50]

Additional studies have demonstrated, however, that even with the many improvements in technology, the collection and storage of platelets leads to platelet activation with a subsequent "storage lesion".[34,51,52] Platelets appear to be activated throughout the process of collection, processing, and storage, demonstrating metabolic and functional signs of activation.[34] Thus, stored platelets show less sensitivity to aggregating agents[53] and release increased amounts of platelet-specific proteins such as β-thromboglobulin[54,55] with membrane expression of activation proteins such as P-selectin and glycoprotein IIb/IIIA.[55,56] In addition, plasma and platelet enzymes may adversely affect platelet membranes and even lead to activation. Future directions in storage technology include the possibility of inactivation of platelets during storage[57] and the use of artificial storage media to avoid exposure to plasma proteins.[58,59]

Cryopreservation

The technology for long-term frozen platelet storage has proved clinically helpful in the management of alloimmunized patients at the University of Maryland and Albert Einstein Cancer Centers,[60,61] and in Europe.[62] During recovery from chemotherapy-induced aplasia and achievement of remission, such patients often have rapidly rising platelet counts, and plateletpheresis during this period often provides a high yield of platelets for cryopreservation. Both autologous and HLA-typed platelets have been frozen for subsequent use in alloimmunized patients. Cryopreservation techniques using either dimethyl sulfoxide (DMSO)[63,64] or glycerol,[65,66] have been described, but to date only the DMSO methodology has been reproducible enough for general usage. This technology calls for a slow infusion of DMSO into platelet-rich plasma to a concentration of 5 percent. This is similar to the methodology used for marrow and stem cell cryopreservation. Recoveries are 50 to 70 percent of fresh platelets, and satisfactory hemostatic results are documented; occasional alloimmunized patients are supported solely by cryopreserved autologous platelets.[60,61,67]

Successful transfusion of platelets that have been stored at liquid nitrogen temperatures (−120°C) for 3 years or more has been documented.[67] This freezing methodology is also potentially applicable to collection and storage of platelets with specific HLA types or for the maintenance of emergency supplies. A recent report suggests that the addition of a small percentage of epinephrine to the DMSO cryopreservation solution may enhance the quality of the cryopreserved platelets, by increasing postthawing function.[68] Finally, recent studies to attempt to improve on the frozen platelet methodology have confirmed

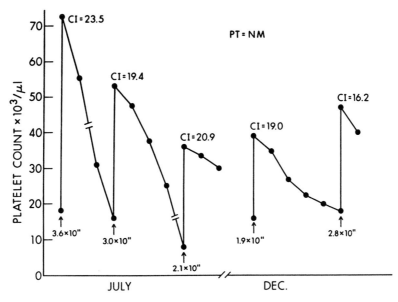

Figure 54–1. Clinical effectiveness of autologous frozen platelets in an alloimmunized patient. This patient had episodes of mild bleeding, which responded to transfusions of autologous frozen platelet transfusions. The increments following transfusion were consistently good. CI, corrected increment.

prior data that despite the freezing injury, the platelets retain function and are able to aggregate, and that there is an in vivo improvement in function once the previously frozen platelets circulate.[69]

Figure 54–1 shows the consistently good response to transfusion of autologous frozen platelets in a patient who was alloimmunized and refractory to transfusion from random donors. The patient received multiple courses of intensive postremission chemotherapy, each requiring transfusion support. As shown, the patient was an excellent and readily available source of platelets for herself.

GRANULOCYTE COLLECTION AND STORAGE

Granulocyte collection technology has followed steps similar to those of platelet collection and utilizes the same principles of differential centrifugation to obtain the selected blood component. Modern techniques utilize the apheresis technology described in Chapter 52; the best yields are obtained with continuous-flow leukapheresis. Granulocytes are difficult to separate from whole blood because they are essentially the same density as RBCs. Therefore, whether apheresis or gravity leukapheresis is utilized, additional techniques are necessary to induce the efficient separation of granulocytes from RBCs.[70–72] This involves the use of sedimenting agents that induce the formation of erythrocyte rouleaux, so that "clumps" of RBCs become heavier than granulocytes and the two cell types can be centrifuged apart. Hydroxyethyl starch (HES) and low-molecular-weight dextran have been used for this purpose.[73,74] Both agents coat the red cell surface, induce the formation of rouleaux, and allow efficient differential centrifugation, with

sedimentation of the red cell clumps. HES and dextran both interact with plasma proteins, but platelets incubated with large quantities of either substance function normally in most in vitro aggregation studies.[75] Since granulocyte transfusions are collected from normal donors, the effect of starch exposure in donors has been evaluated. At 24 hours, 50 percent of the HES remains in the blood of the donor, and traces of the substance have been found as long as 8 to 9 months after a leukapheresis procedure.[76] No long-term effects have ever been reported in either donors or recipients in more than 25 years of leukapheresis utilizing this substance. HES is also widely used as a volume expander in surgical and intensive care patients with no long-term ill effects reported.

Granulocytes are almost exclusively collected using apheresis machines, either continuous- or intermittent-flow types (see Chapter 52).[70–72] Techniques of granulocyte collection of historical interest include a manual technique called gravity leukapheresis, in which 1 unit of whole blood was removed and sedimented with HES; the granulocytes were then separated and the red cells were reinfused. This cycle was repeated until an adequate number of granulocytes was collected, similar to the gravity method for platelet collection.[70,77] The other historical method for granulocyte collection is filtration leukapheresis, in which granulocytes were collected as they adhered to columns of nylon filters.[70] This process produced large yields (but of partially activated granulocytes) and led to numerous reports of transfusion reactions.[78] Fortunately, modern apheresis techniques produce much less granulocyte activation and are providing improved granulocyte yields.[79,80]

The major technical problem limiting granulocyte transfusion efficacy has been the inability to obtain a sufficient dose of granulocytes to be effective in combating sepsis in neutropenic patients. Donors are usually premedicated with corticosteroids (dexamethasone 8 mg orally 12 hours prior to the procedure, and 10 mg as a slow intravenous infusion immediately preceding the procedure) to induce marginalized granulocytes to enter the blood stream.[81] Even with this approach and apheresis, the yield of granulocytes ranges from 2.5 to 5×10^{10} granulocytes for each donation.[79,80] This is still 1/100th of the estimated intrinsic response to sepsis. Functional studies have demonstrated normal antibacterial function of granulocytes collected using steroid premedication and HES sedimentation.[82]

However, a recent resurgence of interest in studying the efficacy of granulocyte transfusions for treatment of systemic fungal infections has fostered a new approach to enhancing granulocyte yield from normal donors.[83,84] Several reports from cancer centers have demonstrated that premedicating normal donors with granulocyte colony-stimulating factor (G-CSF) is effective in increasing the yield of granulocytes.[85–87] Donors receive single or multiple doses of G-CSF and donor white blood cell counts reach as high as 50,000/µl with mean granulocyte collection yields of 4×10^{10} (range, 1 to 14×10^{10}).[85] Recipients in these initial studies demonstrated sustained circulation of transfused granulocytes and no significant ill effects were noted in the donors.[85,86] A recent report, evaluating the kinetics of the cells being administered prophylactically in bone marrow transplant patients, could not correlate the transfusion dose with the absolute neutrophil count achieved in the recipient, but noted significant and sustained increments in the recipients of G-CSF-stimulated granulocytes administered every other day in these patients.[88] Further attempts to optimize granulocyte yield have studied alterations in apheresis settings to optimize the collection and the centrifugation interface.[89] In addition, several laboratories have evaluated granulocyte function in these collections, and have demonstrated that these cells have normal chemotaxis and phagocytosis, and may have enhanced enzymatic activity, demonstrated by chemiluminescence and superoxide formation.[86,90,91]

The ability to premedicate donors and provide daily or every other day granulocytes is most efficiently achieved within the setting of a cancer center with apheresis capability and where donors are often highly motivated to provide products for a specific patient. Nevertheless, Price et al. have demonstrated the ability to provide maximally stimulated granulocytes in high yields utilizing community donors who are also highly motivated.[92]

As for storage of granulocytes, even short-term liquid storage is extremely difficult due to the high metabolic activity of these cells. The number of morphologically normal granulocytes in standard storage conditions declines by 10 to 15 percent per day during the first 2 days of storage. Studies have shown rapid exhaustion of glucose in the storage media,[93] with measurable decreases in functional parameters such as microbial killing, chemotaxis, and the ability to circulate within the first 24 hours of storage.[94,95] Alterations in expression of adhesion molecules have also been described, which may contribute to these functional deficiencies.[96] A recent study evaluated the storage potential of granulocytes mobilized with G-CSF.[97] Although the hypothesis was that these cells might be less metabolically active, in fact the pH was less than 7.4 at the time of collection, and was less than 6.0 after 24 hours of storage. To maintain storage pH, mobilized granulocyte concentrates required dilutions by 1 to 8 or 1 to 16, neither of which is practical.[97]

Thus, current practice dictates that granulocytes be transfused as soon after collection as possible. Donors must be pretested so that the product can be transfused within hours of collection. Even for short-term storage (meaning hours), granulocytes should be placed in large-volume bags (1000 to 2000 ml) with a large volume of plasma to avoid loss of function. Storage should, however, be avoided if at all possible.

THERAPEUTIC PLATELET TRANSFUSIONS

A direct relationship exists between the platelet count and the bleeding time, which is used to assess platelet function in vivo.[98] The bleeding time will begin to lengthen as the platelet count falls to less than 100,000/µl, although clinically apparent bleeding problems may not develop until the platelet count is substantially lower (less than 20,000/µl). Early studies of patients with acute leukemia described the quantitative relationship between low platelet counts and episodes of serious bleeding[2,99] (see Chapter 48). It was subsequently demonstrated that platelet transfusions could diminish the severity of bleeding in thrombocytopenic patients with ongoing hemorrhage. The effectiveness of therapeutic platelets transfusions is well documented.[2,99–102] This observation led to the suggestion that platelets given prophylactically for low platelet counts might therefore help prevent bleeding. Since life-threatening hemorrhage can develop rapidly in the absence of prior signs of minor bleeding, particularly in patients with concurrent clinical problems, prophylactic platelet transfusion given for a platelet count of 10,000 to 20,000/µl is often the practice, rather than waiting for bleeding to occur. This practice comes, however, with several caveats described below.

It has become apparent that thrombocytopenic patients vary greatly in their likelihood to develop serious bleeding as well as in their ability to respond to random donor platelet transfusions. Therefore, clinical judgment should determine whether prophylactic platelet transfusions are indicated.[100–104]

Many patients with chronic hematologic disorders who maintain platelet counts of less than 20,000/µl or even less than 10,000/µl have no or minimal bleeding. In such patients, a low but stable platelet count is tolerated without transfusion unless other clinical factors are also present, such as infection or a bleeding site.[17,105] Slichter quantitated the volume of gastrointestinal bleeding in such clinically stable patients and found no significant increase in bleeding until the platelet count was 5000/µl or less.[106] The other example is in chemotherapy-treated patients with solid tumors, who are not treated at doses designed to achieve marrow aplasia and who have functional marrow reserve. A review of more than 1200 such patients who experienced transient thrombocytopenia (less than 20,000/µl for a median of 2 days) showed no bleeding as a result of thrombocytopenia alone.[107] Those who did experience hemorrhage demonstrated the other clinical complications that have been shown to predispose to bleeding during thrombocytopenia, such as mucositis, a bleeding necrotic tumor, fever and/or sepsis (Table 54–2); bleeding frequently occurred at platelet counts above 20,000/μl.[107]

By contrast, patients with acute leukemia and those undergoing highly intensive chemotherapy for other hematologic malignancies, whose treatment usually leads to marrow aplasia and in whom marrow regeneration may not be expected for a prolonged time period, even weeks, are usually treated prophylactically with platelet transfusions for expected prolonged thrombocytopenia. In addition, these patients frequently develop concurrent clinical conditions that add to the risk of thrombocytopenic bleeding: mucositis, fever, infection, and many of the other clinical complications listed in Table 54–2.[104,108,109] Prophylactic platelet transfusions given to those patients who respond to transfusions with a post-transfusion increment are indicated in this setting.[100–104]

In addition to the conditions discussed above, patients who demonstrate a rapidly falling platelet count appear to be predisposed to bleeding. Patients with hyperleukocytosis, particularly, consisting of blasts, are also at greater risk and should receive platelet transfusions if they are thrombocytopenic, Finally, patients with coagulopathy, as is common in patients with acute promyelocytic leukemia (discussed in detail in Chapter 21) are at much greater risk of bleeding from their ongoing coagulopathy. They are often managed with heparin therapy, although this need may diminish in the future, and they often require frequent platelet transfusions.[110,111] Patients with liver dysfunction and decreased production of clotting factors are also at greater risk for bleeding, from the combined effect of both coagulopathy and thrombocytopenia. More frequent platelet transfusion may be necessary in such patients since they are very likely to have ongoing bleeding. Patients who are refractory to platelet transfusion in these acute settings pose a difficult dilemma, and this will be discussed subsequently. In general, if there is no

platelet product that yields a post-transfusion increment, careful observation without transfusion (unless active bleeding is present) is the recommended course of action. This is stressful for staff and patient but is unusually manageable and is the safest course in the long run.

The increased availability of platelet transfusions has also permitted the safe performance of diagnostic and therapeutic procedures in thrombocytopenic patients. Platelets can be transfused just before or during invasive diagnostic procedures, such as bronchoscopy or endoscopy, and may permit the safe performance of brushings or biopsy. Such therapeutic procedures as the placement of permanent central intravenous lines (Hickman catheters), the drainage of infected paranasal sinuses, tooth extractions, or even emergency major surgery can be safely accomplished in thrombocytopenic patients with the use of platelet transfusions.[112,113] Although no count threshold has been proven, we and others have observed that platelet counts of more than 50,000/μl provide a margin of safety for invasive procedures.[112,113] It is very important to document a satisfactory post-transfusion count increment before initiating the procedure, to be confident that hemorrhage can be controlled during the procedure. It is equally important to maintain the platelet count at 50,000/μl or more for several days immediately following an invasive procedure, particularly after a biopsy or surgery.

ASSESSMENT OF TRANSFUSION RESPONSE

The goal of therapeutic platelet transfusions is to stop active bleeding, which is usually easily assessed clinically. The response to prophylactic platelet transfusions is more difficult to evaluate. Bleeding times, although accurately reflecting platelet function in vivo, are not usually done in granulocytopenic patients because of the risk of infection and because achievement of a platelet count of 100,000/μl is required to normalize the bleeding time.[109] Therefore, response to transfusion is monitored by observing the increase in platelet count shortly after transfusion (i.e., platelet recovery). The increment achieved depends on the size of the recipient and on the number of platelets given. The dose of platelets usually given is approximately 1 U/10 kg body weight for a child and 6 to 10 U/transfusion for an adult.

The survival (duration of time circulating) of transfused platelets can be followed by obtaining daily platelet counts following a platelet transfusion. In a patient who is truly aplastic and not producing platelets, the half-life of the transfused platelets can be calculated. Platelet survival will be shortened by a number of clinical factors, which, in turn, increase the requirement for platelets. These factors include active bleeding, fever, infection, coagulopathy, and hepatosplenomegaly. Platelet survival is also shortened by the development of alloimmunization to histocompatibility antigens, producing immunologic destruction of the transfused platelets. To differentiate alloimmunization from other forms of platelet destruction, the platelet recovery after a transfusion (which is diminished by alloimmunization) may be helpful in stable patients. The post-transfusion recovery is assessed by calculating the corrected count increment:

Table 54–2. Clinical Conditions Affecting Platelet Transfusion Outcome

Clinical Factor[a]	Shorten 1-Hour Count	Shorten 24-Hour Count
Fever	No	±
Infection, controlled	No	±
Preplatelet count < 10,000	No	+
Bleeding: Ooze	No	±
Daily RBC transfusion	±	+
Coagulopathy: DIC	±	+
Palpable splenomegaly[b]	±	+
Sepsis[b]	±	+
Hypersplenism	+	+
Anti-HLA antibodies	+	+
Amphotericin therapy[b]	+	+
Bone marrow transplantation[b]	+	+

[a] Data from Daly et al.[108] and NIH Platelet Transfusion Consensus Conference.[104]
[b] Data from Bishop et al.[109]

Corrected Count Increment (CCI) =

$$\frac{\text{Observed increment (count/}\mu\text{l)} \times \text{body surface area (M2)}}{\text{Number of platelets transfused} \times 10^{11}}$$

For example, an improvement in count from 20,000 to 60,000/μl after 4×10^{11} platelets when given to a 2.0 m² individual produces a corrected count increment of 20,000/μl.

After the transfusion of fresh or properly stored random donor platelets to a clinically stable adult patient of average size, the absolute count increment at 1 hour should be 6000 to 8000/μl/U of platelet transfused, with a CCI of 10,000 to 20,000/μl. The hallmark of the clinical diagnosis of alloimmunization is a failure to achieve an adequate platelet count increment at 1 hour post-transfusion[108] (for practical purposes, a 10-minute post-transfusion count may be equally helpful).[114] Other clinical factors may contribute to the rapid utilization of platelets, however, and may reduce the post-transfusion count (Table 54–2).

Bishop et al.[109,115] performed a multivariate analysis of clinical factors influencing the efficacy of pooled platelet transfusion as determined by the 1-hour post-transfusion platelet CCI. This study identified six major clinical factors that affected 1-hour post-transfusion platelet counts. Whereas splenectomy resulted in improved increments, several factors had a negative effect on transfusion outcome: palpable splenomegaly, bone marrow transplantation, disseminated intravascular coagulation, amphotericin B therapy (which may reflect the degree of illness of a given patient, who may have fever and infection), and anti-HLA antigen-directed antibodies.[109,115] This group performed a similar evaluation of the effect of clinical factors on the 20-hour platelet count (platelet survival) and again found that the clinical situation had a significant impact.[115] The combination of all these factors makes confirmation of the diagnosis of alloimmunization difficult in rather complex clinical cases, and refractoriness to transfusion without development of antibodies appears to reflect the multitude of clinical factors impinging on post-transfusion platelet counts.[109,115–117]

In addition, Hanson and Slichter[118] demonstrated a reduced platelet life span in severely thrombocytopenic patients, presumably due to utilization of platelets for support of vascular integrity. In this study using autologous platelets, platelet life span was only modestly shortened when patients with platelet counts in the 50,000/μl to 100,000/μl range (7.0 ± 1.5 days, 9.6 ± 0.6 days, respectively) were transfused but was markedly shortened in severely thrombocytopenic patients (less than 50,000/μl) (5.1 ± 1.9 days).[118] Recovery of autologous platelets was also diminished in patients with platelet counts less than 50,000/μl (50 ± 22 percent) compared with patients who had counts more than 50,000/μl (74 ± 15 percent).

Finally, a controversial issue in platelet transfusion has re-emerged. New investigations have suggested an interaction of ABH compatibility with the response to platelet transfusion. Despite older studies describing decreased platelet survival using ABH-mismatched platelets, most blood centers have not routinely specified the use of ABH-matched platelet transfusions. Clinical complications or transfusion reactions are rarely associated with ABH-mismatched platelet transfusions although immunologic interactions appear to affect transfusion efficacy.[119,120] Classic teaching states that ABH antigens are not intrinsic to platelet membranes, but may be absorbed from plasma.[121] However, more sensitive techniques have demonstrated the presence of intrinsic H substance on platelet membranes with expression of ABH antigens corresponding to the RBC phenotype, suggesting the presence of intrinsic and extrinsic antigenic substance residing on platelets.[122,123]

A paired clinical study comparing ABO-matched and ABO-mismatched random donor platelet transfusions has demonstrated a detrimental effect of ABO mismatch on platelet transfusion outcome.[120] Although the initial platelet transfusion may not be affected by ABH incompatibility, results of subsequent mismatched transfusions deteriorated, perhaps because of an increase in ABH antibody titers.[120] Thus, in patients who become refractory and who have received ABH-mismatched platelets, better post-transfusion increments may be obtained with a trial of ABH-compatible platelet transfusions.

ALLOIMMUNIZATION

Alloimmunization, the development of antibodies (primarily to histocompatibility [HLA] antigens), leads to immune-mediated refractoriness to platelet transfusions. It then becomes a long-term problem for many patients with hematologic malignancies, impairing the ability to provide platelet transfusion support. The absence of sufficient platelet transfusion support can ultimately lead to hemorrhagic deaths, and can at times limit the intensity of therapy.

Studies conducted in clinically stable patients have been able to correlate the presence of lymphocytotoxic antibodies directed against HLA antigens with post-transfusion CCI[108,124,125] (Table 54–3). The development of lymphocytotoxic antibodies frequently correlates with the loss of response to random donor platelets and indicates the necessity of providing HLA-matched platelet transfusions from previously HLA-typed donors.[108,125] Chow et al. have confirmed this correlation between development of lymphocytotoxic antibodies and loss of response to random donor platelets,[126] and then showed that providing HLA-matched transfusions, particularly in a more homogeneous population, such as the Chinese, led to a successful transfusion outcome.[126]

In most cases of alloimmune platelet refractoriness, successful transfusions can be accomplished with the use of platelets matched at the HLA-A and -B loci, using family members as well as nonrelated matched donors.[127,128] Care must be used in selecting family transfusion donors if an allogeneic transplant may be a later consideration, but in nontransplant candidates, family donors are often highly motivated and available and may provide an excellent source of matched platelets. In general, donors who are either HLA-identical with the recipient or who do not possess any HLA-mismatched antigens are preferred, because the recipient usually has multispecific lymphocytotoxic antibodies directed against multiple additional HLA antigenic epitopes.

Fortunately, within the HLA system, several groups of HLA antigens share antigenic characteristics and are considered sero-

Table 54–3. Lymphocytotoxic Antibody (LCTAb) Levels and Response to Random Donor Platelet Transfusions[a] (Corrected Count Increment Dependent on Level of LCTAb)

CCI at Time After Transfusion[b] (median, range)	LCTAb Negative (0–10 percent)	LCTAb Intermediate (11–20 percent)	LCTAb Positive (21–100 percent)
1 hour	16.1 (2.1–34)	13.3 (3.5–28.9)	5.6 (0–27.8)
24 hours	12.0 (1.3–31)	7.4 (1.5–19.8)	2.6 (0–17.8)

[a] The results of 210 transfusion episodes in 189 patients, comparing post-transfusion count increments with lymphocytotoxic antibody expression.
[b] Mean corrected count increment $\times 10^3$; range in parentheses. (Data from Hogge et al.[125])

logically cross-reactive. Thus, the number of available donors can be increased by selectively mismatching for certain antigens that are cross-reactive with those of the recipient, and thus are functionally compatible.[129] In addition, certain HLA antigens, such as HLA-B12, HLA-B44, and HLA-B45 are sometimes expressed less strongly on platelets than on lymphocytes.[130,131] Since HLA typing is performed with lymphocytes, a mismatch at HLA-B12, HLA-B44, or HLA-B45 may still yield a good platelet transfusion response.[132] This technique of selective mismatching makes transfusion support of some alloimmunized patients considerably more feasible.

Figure 54–2 graphically demonstrates the results of this transfusion approach for an alloimmunized patient, using donors with varying degrees of HLA matching. Patient MH responded well to perfectly matched transfusions (#1, #2, #4)

and to one transfusion mismatched at a cross-reactive (HLA-B57, HLA-B17) antigen (#5), with good CCIs at 1 and 24 hours after transfusion. By contrast, the lack of response to transfusions mismatched at a non-cross-reactive antigen (#3, #6) is also shown. An additional transfusion (#7) that was mismatched at HLA-B44 (an antigen with variable expression on platelets) also produced a good CCI.

It is apparent that the transfusion support of alloimmunized patients can be complex and time-consuming, and can require substantial resources. This includes access to laboratory facilities for HLA typing of both the patient and numerous donors, computer facilities to process the donor list, and substantial donor recruitment efforts. Many more donors are initially used than are helpful because, even with cross-reactive HLA mismatches, not all transfusions are beneficial. However, more

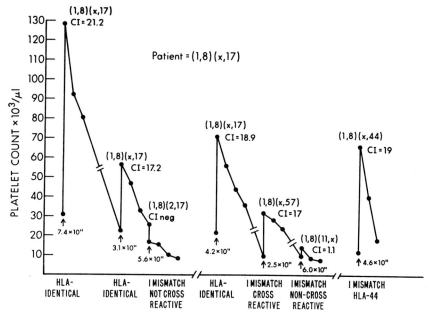

Figure 54–2. Clinical course of this alloimmunized patient demonstrates the value of selectively mismatched platelets when the antigens are cross-reactive with recipient antigens (transfusion #5). Platelets mismatched at HLA-44 were also clinically effective (trans #7). Parentheses, HLA phenotypes; CI, corrected increment.

blood centers are collecting single-donor platelets as part of their standard stock, and with the ease and efficiency of collection using the newer machines, the availability of HLA-matched platelets should increase.

Several groups have tried to calculate the number of donors necessary to provide HLA-matched platelets for most alloimmunized patients. In a pool of 5000 donors, data from the Milwaukee Blood Center identified only 1.5 perfectly matched nonfamily donors for each of 48 patients; even with that large pool, many recipients had no perfect A-matched donors.[133] A review of donor-recipient matches from the University of Maryland noted additional features.[127] Despite a large pool of donors (2470 people), there were on the average only 1.3 (range, 0 to 14) perfectly matched donors available for 100 consecutive alloimmunized patients. The data also showed that potential donors for patients with common HLA antigens and particular haplotypes are numerous, but expansion in size of a donor pool will not add substantially to the number of donors available for most patients with less common HLA types. The converse was true in the Taipei experience, in which the homogeneity of the patient population was a major benefit.[126] In that experience, with a donor pool of 1490 people, there was an average of 3 (range, 0 to 22) perfectly matched donors for 65 alloimmunized patients.[126] This is double the number of perfect donors from a donors pool one-half to one-third the size of the two U.S. reports.

If appropriately matched donors cannot be located for refractory alloimmunized patients, it is inadvisable to continue to administer random donor platelets prophylactically because the risks and discomforts of such transfusions outweigh the benefits. However, significant bleeding in these patients can sometimes be managed by infusions of massive amounts of unmatched platelets,[134] although heavily sensitized patients even then do not obtain count increments and continue to bleed. The possible mechanisms leading to response with this approach may include the accidental inclusion of partially matched platelets in the random pooled platelets or a temporary reduction in antibody titer by the large amount of infused antigen, enabling some of the transfused platelets to survive.

Finally, in parallel with studies in autoimmune thrombocytopenia, attempts have been made to abrogate alloimmunization by blocking the reticuloendothelial system of the spleen and liver with high doses of intravenous gamma globulin. Although this approach has demonstrated benefit in autoimmune thrombocytopenia,[135] it has not proved beneficial in carefully controlled studies in patients with alloimmunization affecting transfusion outcome,[136,137] despite occasional anecdotal reports of improved transfusion outcome.[138] Zeigler et al.[139] used gamma globulin with partially HLA-matched platelets in patients who had become refractory; they reported some improvement in transfusion outcome, although the response was not consistent. Kickler et al.[140] evaluated the outcome of transfusion from matched or partially matched donors, to whom patients no longer responded. Half of the patients received intravenous gamma globulin in addition to platelets from this donor, and had a significantly improved 1-hour post-transfusion count compared with those patients who did not

receive gamma globulin. However, the 24-hour post-transfusion platelet survival was not improved.[140] Thus, the potential value of intravenous gamma globulin in the setting of alloimmunization appears to be quite limited and is not recommended in general, particularly in view of its high cost and limited benefit.

It also appears that some patients lose their allo-antibodies over time.[141,142] In certain cases no recent antigenic challenge has occurred, which would explain the decline in lymphocytotoxic antibody levels, and a rapid, anamnestic response to rechallenge is often seen. However, in a study of 234 patients who had developed lymphocytotoxic antibodies at some time in their clinical course, 70 (30 percent) had significant declines in antibody level.[142] Among 35 evaluable patients, previously alloimmunized, who then lost their antibodies and were rechallenged with random donor platelets, 34 patients when rechallenged responded with good transfusion outcomes to random platelets for 2 weeks to 36 months.[142] Twenty-one patients failed to regenerate lymphocytotoxic antibodies despite repeated transfusions.[142]

Unfortunately, not all patients who appear to be alloimmunized respond to transfusions chosen by HLA matching, suggesting the presence of non-HLA immunologic factors.[108,125] This, in addition to the costs and administrative complexities of an HLA-typed donor pool, has led to increased interest in cross-matching tests using the platelet as the target cell. The most practical approach is to use stored donor platelets from potential donors, to be cross-matched with recipient serum prior to transfusion.[143–146] Freedman et al.[143] compared four different cross-matching techniques for predicting transfusion outcome. In that evaluation, the radiolabeled antiglobulin test and the microlymphocytotoxicity cross-matches were 93 percent predictive for transfusion response, compared with 79 percent for an immunofluorescence test and 62 percent for a biotin-avidin enzyme-linked immunosorbent assay (ELISA).[143]

A subsequent evaluation of the clinical efficacy of platelet cross-matching-compatible donor selection for immune-refractory patients compared this method with HLA-matched donor selection.[144] Moroff et al.[144] evaluated comparative transfusion data in patients known to be refractory to random donor platelets, choosing donors by HLA matching or by platelet cross-matching using three different methods. They found comparable percentages of successful transfusions using either HLA-selected or cross-matched-compatible donor selection. They also found that platelet antibody tests did not always coincide with the outcome of a specific transfusion. However, transfusion outcomes in those selected by HLA type that restricted transfusions to A and BU matches were superior to selection based on cross-matching alone and to donor selection based on any lower grade of HLA mismatching, including cross-reactivity.[144] In this study, 51 percent of patients responded favorably to HLA-chosen platelet transfusions whereas 45 percent of patients responded to cross-match-compatible platelets.[144] O'Connell et al.[145] reported their experience with selection of compatible apheresis platelet donors by cross-matching random donor platelet concentrates. Although it was necessary to screen large numbers of platelet concentrates to identify the 3 to 13 percent that were potentially compatible, the transfusion success rate of those chosen was 80 percent in this study.[145] In another study, both HLA-compatible and cross-match-compatible methods were effective in providing single-donor platelets; these were independently important selection methodologies.[146] More recently, attempts to reduce the drawbacks of both of these methods have tried to predict compatibility of platelets chosen by identifying the anti-HLA antibodies that the recipient develops.[147] Petz et al. present data using this method in which an antihuman microlymphocytotoxicity test is utilized to determine the specificity of the recipient's HLA antibodies. In their study, outcome of transfusion of platelets chosen by the antibody specificity method (ASP) was compared to the outcome of platelet transfusions chosen by HLA-matching and or by cross-matching. The results were comparable.[147] The potential advantage of this method is that more donors might be identified than through HLA-typing, and the frequency of testing would be less than with cross-matching. Further evaluation of this method is ongoing.

Fortunately, the occurrence of alloimmunization is sporadic, and studies have shown that the development of lymphocytotoxic antibodies is less than 50 percent of patients with hematologic or solid malignancies.[141,148–152] These data are derived from an era prior to significant leukodepletion of blood products, so that the incidence is now likely to be much less as will be discussed subsequently. Two separate studies have evaluated the incidence of alloimmunization in large groups of patients with leukemia[148] or other malignant diseases.[149] In both studies, large groups of patients were followed over a long period during treatment (2 to 6 months or more); no relationship was found between the number of platelet transfusions administered during the early part of the treatment phase and subsequent alloimmunization, suggesting that a minimum number of platelets is sufficient to immunize; thus, reduction of transfusion numbers will not prevent alloimmunization.

Specifically, in the study of patients with acute myelocytic leukemia (AML) by Dutcher et al.,[148] nonalloimmunized patients were evaluated during remission induction therapy (the first 8 weeks of treatment) for the development of alloimmunization, assessed by response to random donor platelet transfusion and the development of lymphocytotoxic antibody. All patients received random donor platelet transfusions (mean, 7 transfusions; range, 2 to more than 10), given prophylactically and therapeutically. Of the patients not previously alloimmunized, 40 percent became alloimmunized, some after as few as two transfusions (Figure 54–3). By contrast, 60 percent of the patients did not become alloimmunized, even after multiple platelet transfusions. Except for previous pregnancies or blood transfusions, no predisposing factors were predictive of the development of alloimmunization. Since a minimum of two platelet transfusions (and usually more) is needed to manage the remission induction phase of AML treatment, no rationale exists for restricting the number of platelet transfusions specifically to prevent alloimmunization.[148] No dose-response phenomenon occurs at a clinically manageable level, and the development of alloimmunization appears to depend on the immunologic responsiveness of the recipient. Therefore, newer

measures, specifically, leukodepletion have been investigated as a means of preventing alloimmunization, and this will be discussed in detail subsequently.

The long-term follow-up evaluation of those patients who survived induction therapy for their leukemia was also of interest. Patients who became alloimmunized after induction therapy remained alloimmunized during subsequent periods of treatment and transfusion, whereas almost all patients who did not become immunized after induction therapy never became immunized, and continued to respond to random donor platelets.[141] The alloimmunization status of patients during subsequent treatment courses could be predicted in more than 90 percent of patients on

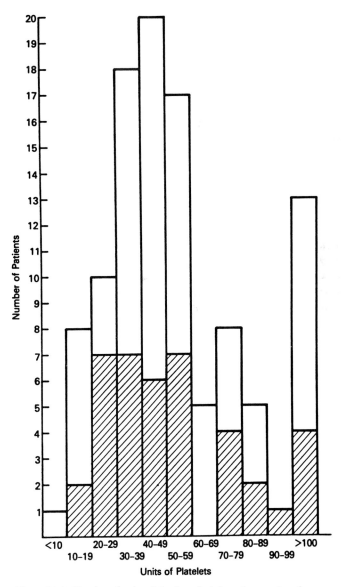

Figure 54–3. Number of units of platelets administered per patient during induction therapy in patients with acute leukemia. There is no relationship between the number of units given and the rate of alloimmunization. Cross-hatching: patients who became alloimmunized. (From Dutcher et al.,[148] with permission.)

the basis of their alloimmunization status after the induction treatment period. Patients who remain alloimmunized are identified as a group requiring continued specialized platelet transfusion support during subsequent antileukemic treatment. However, patients who never become alloimmunized are more easily given transfusion support and may therefore be better able to receive more intensive postremission therapy. Table 54–4 provides an algorithm for managing platelet transfusion support throughout the course of a patient's treatment for leukemia.

Prevention of Alloimmunization

Several different approaches directed at preventing or modifying the development of alloimmunization have been investigated. The contaminating lymphocytes in platelet transfusions serve as the major antigenic stimulus or antigen-presenting component leading to alloimmunization to HLA antigens.[153,154] Animal studies document this, in that in murine studies, repeated administration of pure preparations of platelet suspensions were incapable of inducing an antibody response, but when the preparation also contained lymphocytes, an antibody response was induced.[153] These observations have led to human clinical trials attempting to modify the leukocyte exposure and directed to the above proposed mechanism of antigen exposure.

Lymphocytes carry class II histocompatibility antigens that are necessary for invoking a recipient immune response against class I HLA antigens. Although class II antigens are not found on platelets, the presence of lymphocytes in the transfusion leads to activation of an immune response that is subsequently directed toward both lymphocytes and platelets (which carry class I antigens) and thus produces the development of alloimmunization and transfusion refractoriness.[153–155]

Studies of lymphocyte-depleted transfusion support have been conducted to evaluate the effect on the incidence of alloimmunization. Initial studies produced conflicting results, largely due to technical limitations and inconsistent leukocyte reduction dependent on the technology.[156–158] The early studies used centrifugation techniques, which leave 10^8 leukocytes in the final product.[158] However, now modern apheresis technology and filtering procedures for pooled platelets reduce the leukocyte contamination by 1 to 2 logs to the range of 5×10^6 to 5×10^7 leukocytes in the total transfusion.[156,159–161] These lower levels require special techniques to even be able to consistently count the small number of leukocytes in the platelet product.

Thus, in view of the new technology and enhanced leukodepletion efficiency, an evaluation of the degree of leukocyte depletion and thus antigen dose necessary for the development of alloimmunization has been re-evaluated. It appears that different levels of leukocyte depletion yield specific results. For example, a reduction to less than 10^7 leukocytes/transfusion will reduce the rate of transfusion reactions. However, it requires a reduction to less than 10^6 leukocytes to prevent transmission of cytomegalovirus (CMV), and to reduce the development of alloimmunization.[162–164]

The Trial to Reduce Alloimmunization to Platelets (TRAP) has demonstrated that this level of leukocyte depletion can be accomplished utilizing both modern apheresis techniques and

Table 54–4. Algorithm of Platelet Transfusion Management

I. Preparation of a new leukemia or other patient requiring multiple transfusions
   A. Obtain HLA typing from patient and family and maintain record
   B. Transfusion history: prior pregnancies, transfusions, viral infections

II. Transfusion products
   A. RBCs: filtered or leukodepleted at blood center
   B. Platelets: Leukodepleted, random donor
      1. Pooled single units
      2. Apheresis
   C. Irradiated if potential transplant candidate or severely immunosuppressed

III. Reactions to platelets or poor 24-hour increment
   A. Obtain 1 hour or 10 minute post-transfusion count
   B. Assess other clinical factors that may contribute to refractoriness
   C. Assess storage duration of platelets prior to transfusion
   D. Evaluate ABH compatibility
   E. Assess for presence of lymphocytotoxic antibodies
   F. Reaction, but adequate post-transfusion increment
      1. Initiate leuko-poor or filtered platelets if not done previously
      2. Continue to monitor early post-transfusion platelet counts
   G. Poor immediate post-transfusion increment
      1. Nonmatched but fresh single-donor product—get early post-transfusion count
      2. Family donor—possibly more compatible—get early post-transfusion count
      3. Begin HLA-matched platelet transfusion—get early post-transfusion count

IV. Subsequent courses of treatment
   A. Re-evaluate transfusion history to determine previous response to platelet transfusions
   B. Obtain lymphocytotoxic antibody (LCTAb) screening level
   C. If alloimmunized, refractory, or with a history of reactions or with high-titer LCTAb:
      1. Initiate autologous platelet cryopreservation
      2. Be prepared to provide HLA-compatible or cross-matched platelet products
      3. Monitor all transfusions with early post-transfusion counts
   D. If no history of alloimmunization or refractoriness
      1. Begin with pooled single units or random single-donor apheresis platelets.
      2. Monitor early post-transfusion counts
         a. May develop anamnestic antibody response
         b. Likely to continue to respond to random donor platelets.

modern filtration techniques, most with polyester, leukoadherent filters (all provide reduction of greater than 3 logs, to $< 10^7$ leukocytes).[16,159,160,162–168] These data are supported by other smaller studies that in fact provided the stimulus to engage in this randomized trial to test the hypothesis of leukodepletion and the prevention of alloimmunization.[16,159,160,166,168] In addition, in the TRAP study, a method of lymphocyte inactivation, utilizing ultraviolet B (UVB) irradiation was administered to the transfusion products, to inactivate lymphocytes and antigen presenting cells, such that they became incapable of generating an allore-sponse.[164,169–174] In animal studies, data demonstrated the ability to prevent alloimmunization and to perhaps induce immune tolerance using this technique.[169–172] Initial studies in humans demonstrated the functional integrity of platelets subjected to UVB irradiation as evaluated by post-transfusion platelet count increments,[169,173] although storage time was somewhat diminished.[174] Therefore, this technique was felt to be appropriate for study in the TRAP trial, since it was not known at the initiation of the trial whether the current techniques would produce sufficient leukodepletion to actually prevent alloimmunization.

Subsequently, the TRAP study has demonstrated that this level of leukodepletion or leukocyte inactivation by UVB does in fact lead to a major reduction in the rate of alloimmunization among patients with leukemia who are transfused multiple units of platelets and RBCs.[164] All three approaches (filtration, apheresis, and UVB inactivation) significantly reduced the rate of alloimmunization compared to unmanipulated platelet products, and they were all equally effective. Among the subjects who received nonmanipulated platelets, the rate of development of lymphocytotoxic antibodies was 45 percent (somewhat lower than in many previous reports), but the rate of development of lymphocytotoxic antibodies among the other three treatment groups was 17 to 21 percent. The rate of alloimmunization leading to refractoriness to platelet transfusion was 13 percent among those who received standard, nonmanipulated pooled random donor platelets (again, lower than in many reports) compared to 3 to 4 percent in the patients in the other three groups.[164] Thus, the current platelet transfusion product recommended for patients expected to receive multiple platelet transfusions, such as those being treated for leukemia or expected to undergo stem cell transplant, is to provide leukocyte depleted platelets. Irradiated products are recommended for those who will undergo stem cell transplant and those with severe immunodeficiency, such as Hodgkin's disease. This will be discussed further subsequently.

HAZARDS OF PLATELET TRANSFUSION

Platelet transfusions are usually very safe, and the benefits outweigh the potential risks. Nevertheless, certain hazards of platelet transfusion therapy should be considered. Transfusion reactions can occur with platelet transfusions, usually attributable to sensitization to platelet, leukocyte or RBC antigens, or to plasma proteins.[175–177] Transfusion reactions occur most commonly during or shortly after infusion (although they may be delayed if the patient is premedicated with acetaminophen) and are usually mild, consisting of a sensation of chilliness (rarely shaking chills) or fever, with or without urticaria. Urticaria is most often associated with plasma-related components. Reactions due to leukoagglutinins (white cell antigen-antibody reactions) are febrile and nonhemolytic. Leukocyte-poor platelet products have been shown to reduce the incidence of platelet transfusion reactions due to leukocyte-specific antigens and even to anti-HLA alloimmunization.[25,26,168] Additionally, stored platelets, if not prefiltered, may accumulate cytokines released from leukocytes during the storage process, such as interleukin-6 (IL-6) among others. These may lead to a febrile reaction upon transfusion.[176–178] The presence of IL-6 in the transfusion may also induce what appears to be an allergic reaction with urticaria.[178]

Although with modern platelet preparation, red cell contamination is reduced, there is still considerable plasma, which may contain antibodies to ABH blood types. Therefore, ABH mismatched platelet transfusion may rarely be associated with a hemolytic reaction if the donor has a high-titer hemagglutinin.[179–181] These have been reported over the years as case reports, but a recent report suggests that this type of reaction may be underrecognized in a population receiving numerous blood products.[181]

Bacterial contamination of platelets is a rare, but documented cause of platelet transfusion reaction from stored platelets. This must be considered in severe reactions and the transfusion bag and patient should be cultured.[182]

Circulatory congestion is a common, preventable problem in very ill patients receiving multiple infusions. This develops not only from the individual transfusions being administered, but from the additive effects of administration of all blood products, multiple antibiotics, and other intravenous medications. If necessary, the volume of plasma in a platelet transfusion can be decreased immediately before infusion, using centrifugation and resuspension in a smaller volume of plasma. This is routinely done for transfusions to children.

A major concern in transfusion support is the transmission of infectious diseases. Transfusion-transmitted hepatitis C was a particular problem in the past because in the 1970s there was no serologic test to detect this virus, and donors were excluded by evaluating abnormal liver enzyme test results.[183] In the past decade, serologic testing for hepatitis C, in addition to other viruses, has markedly diminished transfusion-related transmission of hepatitis.[184–186]

Additionally, there are leukocyte-associated viruses that may be transmitted by transfusion, and these include human T-cell leukemia virus types 1 and 2 (HTLV-1 and 2), CMV, and the Epstein-Barr virus (EBV). Systematic donor screening is routinely performed for HTLV-1 and -2 to eliminate donors carrying these viruses. It has also been shown that the incidence of CMV infections developing in CMV-negative recipients as a result of transfusion can be modulated by limiting the number of CMV-positive donors and by adding CMV-immune globulin.[187] However, the ubiquitous nature of the CMV carrier state makes it nearly impossible to completely supply blood product support to very ill patients with strictly CMV-negative donors. Recent data suggest that the use of leukocyte-depleted blood products also markedly reduces exposure to CMV by reducing the number of virus-carrying leukocytes and in many cases prevents the development of primary CMV infection in a CMV-negative recipient.[168,187–192]

The better understanding of transfusion-transmitted diseases, as described above and including human immunodeficiency virus (HIV), has had a major effect on transfusion medicine. The identification of these viruses and the development of increasingly sensitive tests for detecting their presence in blood products has markedly increased the cost and time necessary to screen blood products. Thus, a potential advantage of utilizing single apheresis donors for platelet and granulocyte transfusions, both of which have a relatively short shelf life, is the ability to prescreen donors to allow transfusion immediately upon collection of the product. While this may require initial start-up time commitment, it can in the long run save time and cost by providing fresher transfusion products.

Finally, another recognized complication of transfusion that is receiving increased attention is transfusion-associated graft-versus-host-disease (TA-GvHD). This phenomenon is mediated by immunocompetent donor lymphocytes that activate against the foreign recipient. Although this has been a long-standing problem in bone marrow transplantation, this has also been described in the nontransplant setting and in infants.[193,194] In addition, immunocompetent recipients undergoing whole blood transfusion from haplotype-identical donors have developed this syndrome.[195–198] Because of the haplo-identity of the donor, usually a relative, the recipient recognizes the donor as self, but the donor cells react against the recipient's nonidentical haplotype.

The clinical syndrome is usually severe, with erythematous rash, fever, diarrhea, and abnormal liver function tests. A skin biopsy is often diagnostic, with infiltration of lymphocytes along the dermal-epidermal junction, basal cell vacuolar degeneration, hyperkeratosis of the stratum corneum, and degenerative dyskeratotic cells that may be accompanied by lymphocytes, known as satellite dyskeratosis.[198–200] HLA typing of the donor and patient may also give an indication of the cause of the syndrome. TA-GvHD is often rapidly progressive and frequently fatal.[200]

Patients with hematologic malignancies, particularly those undergoing intensive treatment, are considered to be at increased risk for TA-GvHD, although several studies have demonstrated that the reported incidence in the United States is much lower than would be expected by analysis and prediction from HLA type frequencies.[95] Clinical reports in the United States are also relatively rare considering the frequent use of family donors. Studies from Japan implicate the use of fresh whole blood and a homogeneous population in the development of this phenomenon.[201] Other studies have suggested that the degree of T-cell competence or T-cell depletion of the recipient, such as in Hodgkin's disease and perhaps non-Hodgkin's lymphoma, are important in the manifestation of this syndrome.[202–204] Current standards recommend that blood products from directed donors that are first or second degree and to recipients who are significantly immuno-incompetent be irradiated, such as transfusion to those with Hodgkin's disease.[21,202,203] Currently, most patients with hematologic malignancies who are in consideration of transplant or who are immunoincompetent are receiving irradiated blood products. Studies are under way to evaluate the effect of gamma irradiation and ultraviolet irradiation on both platelet function and leukocyte inactivation.[205–209]

GRANULOCYTE TRANSFUSION THERAPY

The concept of utilizing granulocyte transfusions for treatment of neutropenic sepsis arose out of the success of the use of platelet transfusions in controlling bleeding. As a result of that success, patients undergoing treatment for leukemia were at much lower risk of mortality from severe bleeding; however, they frequently succumbed to infection.

The development of technology capable of separating granulocytes from whole blood led to the evaluation of granulocyte transfusions in severely infected neutropenic patients. The initial investigations utilized granulocytes from patients with chronic myelogenous leukemia (CML), to take advantage of the elevated white blood cell count, which allowed collection of large numbers of granulocytes. This produced both an elevated post-transfusion white blood cell count in the recipient, and a clinical benefit.[210–212] Evaluation of the function of these cells showed responsiveness to bacterial infections.[213] These transfusions successfully eradicated infection, including gram-negative organisms.[210–212] Collections of granulocytes from patients with CML were in fact the first "peripheral blood stem cell transfusions." They included not only mature neutrophils, but myeloid precursors, primarily committed, leading to temporary engraftment with persistent production of myeloid cells and sustained neutrophil counts of more than 500/µl for 4 or more days after the transfusion.[210,212] These initial investigations pointed out the principles necessary for success of granulocyte transfusion therapy: a sufficient dose (more than 10^{10} neutrophils) and the sustained presence of infection-fighting cells.

Despite the success of these early investigations, the use of CML donors was not practical in terms of donor availability as well as new, more effective treatments for patients with CML. However, it provided a proof of principle that with sufficient dose and duration, granulocyte transfusions could aid in eradicating infection. Therefore, granulocyte transfusion research has focused on optimizing granulocyte collection from normal donors, as described earlier.[77–80] This has involved improvements in apheresis technology and the evaluation of strategies to prestimulate donors to enhance collection.[80,84–91]

Criteria for and Evaluation of Normal Donor Granulocyte Transfusions

Although the use of granulocyte transfusions has diminished considerably since the late 1970s, the clinical indications remain the same, and it is likely that a resurgence of interest in this modality will result from the enhanced yields currently available[82,83,210–212,214–216] (Table 54–5). Granulocyte transfusions should be considered in patients who are severely neutropenic (neutrophil counts less than 500/µl), whose marrow is not expected to recover imminently but will eventually, and who have a severe infection such as pneumonia or septicemia that is not responding to appropriate antibiotics.

Fortunately, this clinical setting occurs much less frequently than previously, at least for bacterial infections, due to more knowledgeable use of empirical antibiotic approaches, and better and more broad-spectrum antibiotics. The latter can lead to resistance, however, and therefore may yield another scenario in which granulocytes may be considered. Fungal infections remain a difficult therapeutic dilemma in granulocytopenic patients. Therefore, infections remain the major cause of morbidity and mortality in neutropenic patients. Recent reports suggest that the newer transfusion approaches, with growth-factor stimulation of the donor prior to collection, yielding larger numbers of granulocytes, may be demonstrating significantly better efficacy, particularly in patients with sepsis or fungal infections.[84,90,91,217–219]

Early randomized studies, using donors with limited premedication, in general have demonstrated benefit from granulocyte transfusion, but some suggested the toxicity was excessive, and the benefit to risk ratio often obscure.[220–226] However, these studies were conducted using small numbers of granulocytes and without histocompatibility testing. Therefore, careful clinical evaluation of efficacy must be re-evaluated in the modern era of granulocyte collection, with greater doses and more attention to histocompatibility issues.

Studies evaluating granulocyte transfusions in patients with fungal infection must be attentive to dose of granulocytes, and such transfusions must be considered early in the clinical course, preferably prior to positive blood cultures. Doses less than or equal to 1×10^{10} are unlikely to be particularly effective, as noted from prior studies with cells from CML patients and prior animal studies.[210,229–231] Data from studies in animals and with CML donors suggest that more than 10^{10} neutrophils in a 70-kg person is the minimum requirement for efficacy (1.5×10^8/kg),[229–231] which is one-tenth of the daily production of neutrophils in a normal, noninfected adult.[232] Two recent studies report yields of 2 to 4×10^{10} neutrophils/transfusion with growth factor stimulated donors, and some investigators recommend that amount as the new standard for granulocyte transfusion therapy.[84,85] The best way to further evaluate the potential clinical value of granulocyte transfusions in infected, neutropenic patients will be to provide transfusions that utilize the maximal dose available. Thus, when the technology does not limit the modality, it can best be evaluated, in the context of the data from the older CML donor transfusions.

HISTOCOMPATIBILITY ISSUES IN GRANULOCYTE TRANSFUSIONS

Febrile reactions and subsequent pulmonary infiltrates have been frequently observed following granulocyte transfusions.[233] Although not always detected after such reactions, alloimmunization is a potential factor and has been documented in several studies.[234,235] Granulocytes have both HLA antigens and neutrophil-specific antigens (the latter not linked to HLA) on their surface. Antibodies to these antigens are detected by analyzing serum for leukoagglutination, granulocytotoxicity,[236] or lymphocytotoxicity and by immunofluorescence studies.[214] Observations in early granulocyte transfusion studies suggested a rough correlation between the occurrence of transfusion reactions and recipient alloimmunization, with the presence of antibody directed against the donor leukocytes.[237,238] Clinical studies have suggested that alloimmunization to platelet transfusion (antibodies to HLA antigens) also affects the clinical outcome of granulocyte transfusions.[239–241] Studies imaging the infusion of ^{111}In-labeled granulocytes show more definitively that documented alloimmunization prevents the migration of granulocytes to sites of infection.[242,243] Studies of ^{111}In-labeled granulocytes in alloimmunized patients also demonstrate a prolonged uptake in the lungs, pointing to alloimmunization as a component of the pulmonary reactions sometimes noted with unmatched granulocyte transfusions.[244,245] A recent study evaluating granulocytes obtained from colony-stimulating factor mobilized granulocytes also describes an effect of leukocyte compatibility, evaluating lymphocytotoxicity as a major factor in granulocyte increment and survival after transfusion.[246]

Granulocyte donors are selected based on ABH compatibility. Recipients are tested for alloimmunization by lymphocytotoxicity and in some centers by leukoagglutinating antibodies and immunofluorescence.[245,246] If no evidence of clinical alloimmunization exists, then ABH compatible granulocyte transfusions are given. In patients who are already alloimmunized to platelet transfusions, proceeding with granulocyte transfusions can be hazardous, as described above. To proceed, donors who are effective platelet donors for alloimmunized patients are the safest candidates for granulocyte donation. No best serologic approach toward defining donors has yet to be well defined, but lymphocytotoxicity is the most widely available.

REACTIONS AND RISKS OF GRANULOCYTE TRANSFUSIONS

All of the commonly reported types of blood product reactions can occur with granulocyte transfusions. Nonspecific and possibly multifactorial reactions include fever, urticaria, and fluid overload. In addition, febrile reactions associated with pulmonary infiltrates have commonly been reported with granulocyte transfusions and many are attributed to alloimmunization.[233,244] Other potential causes of severe pulmonary reactions have been noted. These include the appropriate migration of the neutrophils to the site of the pulmonary infection with or without the development of an infiltrate on a radiograph and, more seriously, acute pulmonary edema and adult respiratory distress syndrome (or both). The latter may be a result of an immunologic reaction (i.e., alloimmunization) or infection and the release of inflammatory cytokines. Pulmonary decompensation has also been associated with the combined administration of granulocyte transfusions and amphotericin B in one series,[247] but less definitively causal in several other reports.[248–251] Adverse reactions including pulmonary reactions have been documented with either granulocytes or amphotericin B alone, so that either or both may be the causative factor in reactions when they are

Table 54–5. Criteria for Initiating Granulocyte Transfusions

Severe neutropenia (neutrophils < 500/μl)
Marrow shows no evidence of immediate recovery
Clinically significant infection such as pneumonia or septicemia
Failure or inadequate response to appropriate antibiotics
Fungal infection poorly responsive to appropriate antibiotics
Expectation of eventual marrow recovery

administered concurrently. However, although the risk of reactions appears to relate to each individual component, prudence dictates that whenever possible, granulocyte transfusions and amphotericin B be administered separately, and with several hours between administrations.[249]

Again, as with other blood products, the potential for TA-GvHD exists, particularly since family donors are often utilized for granulocyte transfusions. The American Association of Blood Banks has recommended irradiation of all cellular components donated by relatives. The effect of this procedure on granulocyte function has not yet been evaluated. The potential effect on viability adds emphasis to the recommendation that granulocytes be transfused as soon as possible after collection to ensure a viable and effective blood product.

Finally, the transfusion of granulocytes increases the risk of transfusing cells containing CMV. Both donors and recipients should be screened prior to initiating granulocyte transfusions. Although a large majority of the population has already been exposed to CMV with antibody titers, and therefore do not require CMV-negative blood products, the occasional recipient may be negative and will therefore require CMV-negative granulocytes. If the clinical infection is so severe that granulocytes are a necessity, then weighing the risk/benefit ratio of CMV-positive products becomes a very difficult decision. An acute CMV infection due to transfusion is less likely to occur during standard induction therapy for leukemia, but could potentially be fatal in the allogeneic transplant setting.

POTENTIAL FOR GRANULOCYTE TRANSFUSION THERAPY

Granulocyte transfusions are infrequently used today, even though infection is still the major cause of death in neutropenic leukemia and bone marrow transplant patients. A resurgence of interest is occurring, however, in cancer centers, due to the ability to provide transfusions with enhanced numbers of granulocytes, and due to the frequency of either resistant bacteria or fungal infections.[84,85,217,252] Several investigators have commented that granulocyte transfusion was prematurely abandoned, and we must now relearn their use with safer, more effective technology for collection.[214,215]

CONCLUSIONS

The development of successful transfusion supportive care has had a major impact on our ability to treat patients with hematologic malignancies and those undergoing bone marrow transplantation. Additionally, transfusion immunology has contributed to the overall understanding of allogeneic transplant immunology. We continue to advance technology to make blood component therapy and transfusion a safer modality. Both platelet and granulocyte transfusion will remain a part of our armamentarium in the treatment of hematologic malignancies, and further optimization of these lifesaving components will continue. They are critical to the current management of these patients.

REFERENCES

1. Duke WW: Relationship of blood platelets to hemorrhagic disease: Description of a method to determine bleeding time and coagulation time and report of cases of hemorrhagic disease relieved by transfusion. JAMA 55:1185, 1910.
2. Freireich EJ, Kliman A, Gaydos LA et al: Response to repeated platelet transfusion from the same donor. Ann Intern Med 59:177, 1963.
3. Freireich EJ, Levin RH, Whang J et al: The function and fate of transfused leukocytes from donors with chronic myelocytic leukemia in leukopenic recipients. Ann N Y Acad Sci 113:1081, 1965.
4. Djerassi I, Kim TS, Mitrakul C et al: Filtration leukapheresis for separation and concentration of transfusable amounts of human granulocytes. J Med 1:358, 1970.
5. Djerassi I: Gravity leukapheresis—a new method of collection of transfusable granulocytes. Exp Hematol 5:139, 1977.
6. Graw RG, Herzig GP, Eisel RT, Perry S: Leukocyte and platelet collection from normal donors with the continuous flow blood cell separator. Transfusion 11:94, 1971.
7. Schiffer CA, Buchholz DH, Aisner J et al: Clinical experience with trasnfusion of granulocytes obtained by continuous flow filtration leukapheresis. Am J Med 48:373, 1975.
8. McCullough J: Current issues with platelet transfusion in patients with cancer. Sem Hematol 37:2, 2000.
9. Mourad N: A simple method for obtaining platelet concentrates free of aggregates. Transfusion 8:48, 1968.
10. Simon TL: The collection of platelets by apheresis procedures. Transfus Med Rev 8:132, 1994.
11. Hester J, Ventura G, Boucher T: Platelet concentrate collection in a dual stage channel using computer generated algorithms for collection and prediction of yield. Plasma Ther Transfus Technol 8:377, 1987.
12. Bertholf MF, Mintz PD: Comparison of plateletpheresis with two cell separators using identical donors. Transfusion 28:45, 1988.
13. Halpern LN: The Haemonetics V50 apheresis system. Plasma Ther Trasnfus Technol 7:405, 1986.
14. Maresh S, Randels MJ, Strauss RG et al: Comparison of plateletpheresis with a standard and an improved collection device. Transfusion 33:835, 1993.
15. Goodnough LT, Kuter D, McCullough J, Brecher ME: Apheresis platelets: Emerging issues related to donor platelet count, apheresis platelet yield, and platelet transfusion dose. J Clin Apheresis 13:114, 1998.
16. Burgstaler EA, Pineda AA, Bryant SC: Prospective comparison of plateletpheresis using four apheresis systems on the same donors. J Clin Apheresis 14:163, 1999.
17. Schiffer CA, Anderson KC, Bennett CL et al: Platelet transfusion for patients with cancer: Clinical practice guidelines of the American Society of Clinical Oncology. J Clin Oncol 19:1519, 2001.
18. Schiffer CA, Buchholz DH, Wiernik PH: Intensive multiunit plateletpheresis of normal donors. Transfusion 14:388, 1974.
19. Lasky LC, Lin ATT, McCullough JJ: Platelet counts before and after apheresis. Transfusion 21:760, 1981.
20. Glowitz RJ, Slichter SJ: Frequent multiunit plateletpheresis from single donors: Effects on donors' blood and the platelet yield. Transfusion 20:199, 1980.
21. Standards for Blood Banks and Transfusion Services, 19th Ed., pp. 10, 26, 51, 52. AABB Press, Bethesda, MD, 1999.
22. Rock G, Tittley P, Sternbach M et al: Repeat plateletpheresis: The effects on the donor and the yield. Vox Sang 63:102, 1992.
23. Holme S, Snyder E, Heaton A et al: In vitro and in vivo evaluation of cotton wool filtration of platelet concentrates obtained by automated and manual apheresis. Transfusion 32:328, 1992.

24. Brubaker DR, Romine CM: The in vitro evaluation of two filters (Erypur and Imugard IG 500) for white cell-poor platelet concentrates. Transfusion 28:383, 1988.

25. Sniecinski I, St. Jean J, Nowicki B: Preparation of leukocyte-poor platelets by filtration. J Clin Apheresis 5:7, 1989.

26. Sirchia G, Rebulla P, Parravicini A et al: Leukocyte depletion of red cell units at the bedside by transfusion through a new filter. Transfusion 27:402, 1987.

27. Kickler TS, Bell W, Ness PM et al: Depletion of white cells from platelet concentrates with a new adsorption filter. Transfusion 29:411, 1989.

28. Miyamoto M, Sasakawa S, Ishikawa Y et al: Leukocyte-poor platelet concentrates at the bedside by filtration through Sepacell-PL. Vox Sang 57:164, 1989.

29. Wenz B, Ciavarella D, Freundlich L: Effect of pre-storage white cell reduction on bacterial growth in platelet concentrates. Transfusion 33:520, 1993.

30. Pietersz RNI, Reesink HW, Dekker WJ: Preparation of leukocyte-poor platelet concentrates from buffy coats. II. Lack of effect on storage of different plastics. Vox Sang 53:208, 1987.

31. Ferrer F, Rivera J, Corral J et al: Evaluation of pooled platelet concentrates using prestorage versus poststorage WBC reduction: Impact of filtration timing. Transfusion 40:781, 2000.

32. Vamvakas EC, Blajchman MA: Universal WBC reduction: The case for and against. Transfusion 41:691, 2001.

33. Moroff G, Simon TL: Use of radioisotopically labeled platelets to determine the survival properties of stored platelets—an overview of the present status. Transfusion 26:1, 1986.

34. Rao GHR, Escolar G, White JG: Biochemistry, physiology and function of platelets stored as concentrates. Transfusion 33:766, 1993.

35. Moroff G, Holme S: Concepts about current conditions for preparation and storage of platelets. Transfus Med Rev 5:48, 1991.

36. Carmen R: The selection of plastic materials for blood bags. Transfus Med Rev 7:1, 1993.

37. Murphy S: Platelet storage for transfusion. Semin Hematol 22:165, 1985.

38. Murphy S, Gardner FH: Platelet storage at 22°C; metabolic, morphologic and functional studies. J Clin Invest 50:370, 1971.

39. Slichter SJ: In vitro measurements of platelet concentrates stored at 4 and 22°C: Correlation with post-transfusion platelet viability and function. Vox Sang 40(Suppl. 1):72, 1981.

40. Rock GA, Blanchette VS, Wong SC: Storage of platelets collected by apheresis. Transfusion 23:99, 1983.

41. Filip DJ, Aster RH: Relative hemostatic effectiveness of human platelets stored at 4° and 22°C. J Lab Clin Med 91:618, 1978.

42. Kilkson H, Holme S, Murphy S: Platelet metabolism during storage of platelet concentrates at 22°C. Blood 64:400, 1984.

43. Moroff G, Holme S, George VM, Heaton WA: Effect on platelet properties of exposure to temperatures below 20°C for short periods during storage at 20 to 24°C. Transfusion 34:317, 1994.

44. Simon TL, Nelson EJ, Carmen R, Murphy S: Extension of platelet concentrate storage. Transfusion 23:207, 1983.

45. Schiffer CA, Lee EJ, Ness PM, Reilly J: Clinical evaluation of platelet concentrates stored for one to five days. Blood 67:1591, 1986.

46. Kenney DM, Peterson JJ, Smith JW: Extended storage of single-donor apheresis platelets in CLX^R blood bags: Effect of storage on platelet morphology, viability and in vitro function. Vox Sang 54:24, 1988.

47. Kiraly TR, Kalish RI, Norton DF: Evaluation of apheresis platelet concentrates stored for 5 days in PL-732 bags. J Clin Apheresis 3:178, 1987.

48. Moroff G, Friedman A, Robkin-Kline L: Factors influencing changes in pH during storage of platelet concentrates at 20–24°C. Vox Sang 42:33, 1982.

49. Holme S, Vaidja K, Murphy S: Platelet storage at 22°C: Effect of the type of agitation on morphology, viability and function in vitro. Blood 52:425, 1978.

50. Snyder EL, Pope C, Ferri PM et al: The effect of mode of agitation and type of plastic bag on storage characteristics and in vivo kinetics of platelet concentrates. Transfusion 26:125, 1986.

51. Chernoff A, Snyder EL: Conference report: The cellular and molecular basis of the platelet storage lesion: A symposium summary. Transfusion 32:386, 1992.

52. Rinder HM, Murphy M, Mitchell JG et al: Progressive platelet activation with storage: Evidence for shortened survival of activated platelets after transfusion. Transfusion 31:409, 1991.

53. DiMinno G, Silver MJ, Murphy S: Stored human platelets retain full aggregation potential in response to pairs of aggregating agents. Blood 59:563, 1982.

54. Snyder EL: Release of beta-thromboglobulin during storage of platelet concentrates. Vox Sang 41:172, 1981.

55. Rinder HM, Snyder EL, Bonan JL et al: Activation in stored platelet concentrates: Correlation between membrane expression of P-selectin, glycoprotein IIb/IIIa and beta thromboglobulin release. Transfusion 33:25, 1993.

56. Triulzi DL, Kickler TS, Braine HG: Detection and significance of alpha granule membrane protein 140 expression on platelets collected by apheresis. Transfusion 32:529, 1992.

57. Bode AP, Miller DT: The use of thrombin inhibitors and aprotinin in the preservation of platelets stored for transfusion. J Lab Clin Med 113:753, 1989.

58. Adams GA, Swenson SD, Rock G: Five day storage of human platelet concentrates in 30 ml of plasma or artificial medium. Vox Sang 52:305, 1987.

59. Heaton WA, Holme S, Keegan T: Development of a combined storage medium for 7-day storage of platelet concentrates and 42 day storage of red cell concentrates. Br J Haematol 59:146, 1990.

60. Schiffer CA, Aisner J, Wiernik PH: Frozen autologous platelet transfusion for patients with leukemia. N Engl J Med 299:7, 1978.

61. Dutcher JP, Spivack M, Mohandas K, Wiernik PH: A clinical program of platelet cryopreservation. Proceedings of the 8th International Meeting of Society of Haematology, Warsaw, Poland. September 8–13, 1985.

62. Herve P, Otron G, Droule C et al: Human platelets frozen with glycerol in liquid nitrogen: Biological and clinical aspects. Transfusion 21:384, 1981.

63. Kim BK, Baldini MG: Biochemistry, function and hemostatic effectiveness of frozen human platelets. Proc Soc Exp Biol Med 145:830, 1974.

64. Valeri CR, Feingold H, Marchionni LL: A simple method for freezing human platelets using 6 percent dimethylsulfoxide and storage at −80°C. Blood 43:131, 1974.

65. Dayian G, Rowe AW: Cryopreservation of human platelets for transfusion: A glycerol glucose moderate rate cooling procedure. Cryobiology 13:1, 1976.

66. Kotelba-Witkowska B, Schiffer CA: Cryopreservation of platelet concentrate using glycerol-glucose. Transfusion 22:121, 1981.

67. Daly PA, Schiffer CA, Aisner J, Wiernik PH: Successful transfusion of platelets cryopreserved for more than 3 years. Blood 54:1023, 1979.

68. Xiao H, Harvey K, Labarrere CA, Kovacs R: Platelet cryopreservation using a combination of epinephrine and dimethyl sulfoxide as cryoprotectants. Cryobiology 41:97, 2000.

69. Rothwell SW, Maglasang P, Reid TJ et al: Correlation of in vivo and in vitro functions of fresh and stored human platelets. Transfusion 40:988, 2000.

70. Aisner J, Schiffer CA, Daly PA, Buchholz DM: Evaluation of gravity leukapheresis and comparison with intermittent centrifugation leukapheresis. Transfusion 21:100, 1981.

71. Graw RG, Herzig GP, Eisel RT, Perry S: Leukocyte and platelet collection from normal donors with the continuous flow blood cell separator. Transfusion 11:94, 1971.

72. Hester JP, Kellogg RM, Mulzet AP et al: Principles of blood separation and component extraction in a disposable continuous-flow single-stage channel. Blood 54:254, 1979.

73. Huestis DW, White RF, Price MJ, Inman M: Use of hydroxyethyl starch to improve granulocyte collection in the Latham blood processor. Transfusion 15:559, 1975.

74. Rock G, McCombie N: Alternate dosage regimens for high molecular weight hydroxyethyl starch. Transfusion 25:417, 1975.

75. Djerassi I, Kim TS, Mitrakul C et al: Filtration leukapheresis for separation and concentration of transfusable amounts of normal human granulocytes. J Med 1:358, 1970.

76. Ring J, Sharkoff D, Richter W: Intravascular persistence of hydroxyethyl starch (HES) after serial granulocyte collections using HES in man. Vox Sang 39:181, 1980.

77. Djerassi I: Gravity leukapheresis—a new method of collection of transfusable granulocytes. Exp Hematol 5:139, 1977.

78. Schiffer CA, Buchholz DH, Aisner J et al: Clinical experience with transfusion of granulocytes obtrained by continous flow filtration leukapheresis. Am J Med 58:373, 1975.

79. Loftus TJ, White RF, Huestis DW: Leukapheresis: Increasing the granulocyte yield with the Fenwal CS-3000. J Clin Apheresis 1:109, 1983.

80. Wagner B, Moore R, Grima K, Dutcher JP: Granulocytopheresis efficiency: Comparison of COBE 2997 to the COBE Spectra automated granulocyte protocol. J Clin Apheresis 6:186, 1991.

81. Winton EF, Vogler WR: Development of a practical oral dexamethasone premedication schedule leading to improved granulocyte yields with the continuous flow centrifugal blood cell separator. Blood 52:249, 1978.

82. Glasser L, Huestis DW, Jones JF: Functional capabilities of steroid-recruited neutrophils harvested for clinical transfusion. N Engl J Med 297:1033, 1977.

83. Dale DC, Liles WC: Return to granulocyte transfusion. Curr Opin Pediatr 12:18, 2000.

84. Price TH: The current prospects for neutrophil transfusions for the treatment of granulocytopenic infected patients. Transfus Med Rev 14:2, 2000.

85. Bensinger WI, Price TH, Dale DC et al: The effects of daily recombinant human granulocyte colony-stimulating factor administration on normal granulocyte donors undergoing leukapheresis. Blood 81:1883, 1993.

86. Caspar CB, Seger RA, Burger J, Gmur J: Effective stimulation of donors for granulocyte transfusions with recombinant methionyl granulocyte colony-stimulating factor. Blood 81:2866, 1993.

87. Schiffer CA: Granulocyte transfusion therapy. Curr Opin Hematol 6:3, 1999.

88. Adkins D, Spitzer G, Johnston M et al: Transfusions of granulocyte-colony-stimulating factor-mobilized granulocyte components to allogeneic transplant recipients: Analysis of kinetics and factors determining posttransfusion neutrophil and platelet counts. Transfusion 37:737, 1997.

89. Adkins D, Ali S, Despotis G et al: Granulocyte collection efficiency and yield are enhanced by the use of a higher interface offset during apheresis of donors given granulocyte-colony-stimulating factor. Transfusion 38:557, 1998.

90. Dale DC, Liles WC, Llewellyn C et al: Neutrophil transfusions: Kinetics and function of neutrophils mobilized with granulocyte-colony-stimulating factor and dexamethasone. Transfusion 38:713, 1998.

91. Gaviria JM, van Burik JA, Dale DC et al: Modulation of neutrophil-mediated activity against the pseudohyphal form of Candida albicans by granulocyte colony-stimulating factor administered in vivo. J Infect Dis 179:1301, 1999.

92. Price TH, Bowden RA, Boeckh M et al: Phase I/II trial of neutrophil transfusion from donors stimulated with G-CSF and dexamethasone for treatment of patients with infections in hematopoietic stem cell transplantation. Blood 95:3302, 2000.

93. Glasser L, Fiederlein RL, Huestis DW: Granulocyte concentrates: Glucose concentration and glucose utilization during storage at 22°C. Transfusion 25:68, 1985.

94. McCullough J: Liquid preservation of granulocytes. Transfusion 20:129, 1980.

95. Lane TA, Lamkin GE: The effect of storage on degranulation by human neutrophils. Transfusion 225:155, 1985.

96. Wikman A, Lundahl J, Fernvik E, Shanwell A: Altered expression of adhesion molecules (L-selectin and Mac-1) on granulocytes during storage. Transfusion 34:167, 1994.

97. Lightfoot T, Leitman SF, Stroncek DF: Storage of G-CSF-mobilized granulocyte concentrates. Transfusion 40:1104, 2000.

98. Harker LA, Slichter SJ: The bleeding time as a screening test for evaluation of platelet function. N Engl J Med 287:155, 1972.

99. Gaydos LA, Freireich EJ, Mantel N: The quantitative relation between platelet count and hemorrhage in patients with acute leukemia. N Engl J Med 266:905, 1962.

100. Patten E: Controversies in transfusion medicine: Prophylactic platelet transfusion revisited after 25 years. Con. Transfusion 32:381, 1992.

101. Baer MR, Bloomfield CD: Controversies in transfusion medicine: prophylactic platelet transfusion therapy. Pro. Transfusion 32:377, 1992.

102. Schiffer CA: Editorial. Prophylactic platelet transfusion. Transfusion 32:295, 1992.

103. Aderka D, Praff G, Santo M et al: Bleeding due to thrombocytopenia in acute leukemia and reevaluation of the prophylactic platelet transfusion policy. Am J Med Sci 291:147, 1986.

104. NIH Consensus Conference: Platelet transfusion therapy. JAMA 257:1777, 1987.

105. Beutler E: Platelet transfusions: The 20,000/μl trigger. Blood 81:1411, 1993.

106. Slichter SJ: Platelet transfusion therapy. Hematol Oncol Clin North Am 4:291, 1991.

107. Dutcher JP, Schiffer CA, Aisner J et al: Incidence of thrombocytopenia and bleeding among patients with solid tumors. Cancer 53:557, 1984.

108. Daly PA, Schiffer CA, Aisner J, Wiernik PH: Platelet transfusion therapy. One hour post-transfusion increments are valuable in predicting the need for HLA-matched preparations. JAMA 243:435, 1980.

109. Bishop JF, McGrath K, Wolf WW et al: Clinical factors influencing the efficacy of pooled platelet transfusions. Blood 71:383, 1988.

110. Daly PA, Schiffer CA, Wiernik PH: Acute progranulocytic leukemia—clinical management of 15 patients. Am J Hematol 8:347, 1980.

111. Gralnick HR, Bagley J, Abrell E: Heparin treatment for the hemorrhagic diathesis of acute progranulocytic leukemia. Am J Med 52:167, 1971.

112. Bishop JF, Schiffer CA, Aisner J et al: Surgery in acute leukemia: A review of 167 operations in thrombocytopenic patients. Am J Hematol 26:147, 1987.

113. Williford SK, Salisbury PL 3d, Peacock JE Jr et al: The safety of dental extractions in patients with hematologic malignancies. J Clin Oncol 7:798, 1989.

114. O'Connell B, Lee EJ, Schiffer CA: The value of 10-minute post-transfusion platelet counts. Transfusion 28:66, 1988.

115. Bishop JF, Matthews JP, McGrath K et al: Factors influencing 20-hour increments after platelet tranfusion. Transfusion 31:392, 1991.

116. Kickler TS: The challenge of platelet alloimmunization: Management and prevention. Transfus Med Rev 4(Suppl. 1):8, 1990.

117. Bishop JF, Matthews JP, Yuen K et al: The definition of refractoriness to platelet transfusions. Transfus Med 2:35, 1991.

118. Hanson SR, Slichter SJ: Platelet kinetics in patients with bone marrow hypoplasia: Evidence for a fixed platelet requirement. Blood 66:1105, 1985.

119. Aster RH: Effect of anticoagulant and ABO incompatibility on recovery of transfused human platelets. Blood 26:732, 1965.

120. Lee EJ, Schiffer CA: ABO compatibility can influence the results of platelet transfusion: Results of a randomized trial. Transfusion 29:384, 1989.

121. Kelton JG, Hamid C, Aker S, Blajchman MA: The amount of blood group A substance on platelet is proportional to the amount in the plasma. Blood 59:980, 1982.

122. Dunstan RA, Simpson MB, Knoweles RW, Rosse WF: The origin of ABH antigens on human platelets. Blood 65:615, 1985.

123. Curtis BR, Edwards JT, Hessner MJ et al: Blood group A and B antigens are strongly expressed on platelets of some individuals. Blood 96:1574, 2000.

124. Mittal KK, Terasaki PI: Serologic cross-reactivity in the HLA system. Tissue Antigens 4:146, 1974.

125. Hogge DE, Dutcher JP, Aisner J, Schiffer CA: Lymphocytotoxic antibody is a predictor of response to random donor platelet transfusion. Am J Hematol 14:363, 1983.

126. Chow MP, Yung HY, Hu JL et al: Platelet crossmatching with lymphocytotoxicity test: An effective method in alloimmunized Chinese patients. Transfusion 31:595, 1991.

127. Schiffer CA, Keller C, Dutcher JP et al: Potential HLA matched platelet donor availability for alloimmunized patients. Transfusion 23:286, 1983.

128. Yankee RA, Grumet FC, Rogentine GN: Platelet transfusion therapy. The selection of compatible platelet donors for refractory patients by lymphocyte HLA typing. N Engl J Med 281:1208, 1969.

129. Duquesnoy RJ, Filip DJ, Rodey GE et al: Successful transfusion of platelets "mismatched" for HLA antigens to alloimmunized throbocytopenic patients. Am J Hematol 2:219, 1977.

130. Aster RH, Szatkowski N, Liebert M: Expression of HLA-B12, HLA-B8, W4 and W6 on platelets. Transplant Proc 9:1695, 1977.

131. Lieber M, Aster RH: Expression of HLA-B12 on platelets, on lymphocytes and in serum. A quantitative study. Tissue Antigens 9:199, 1977.

132. Schiffer CA, O'Connell B, Lee EJ: Platelet transfusion therapy for alloimmunized patients: Selective mismatching for HLA-B12, an antigen with variable expression on platelets. Blood 74:1172, 1989.

133. Duquesnoy RJ, Viera J, Aster RH: Donor availability for platelet transfusion support of alloimmunized throbocytopenic patients. Transplant Proc 9:519, 1977.

134. Nagasawa T, Kim BK, Baldini MG: Temporary suppression of circulating antiplatelet aloantibodies by the massive infusion of fresh, stored or lyophilized platelets. Transfusion 18:429, 1978.

135. Fehr J, Hofmann V, Kappeler U: Transient reversal of thrombocytopenia in idiopathic thrombocytopenic purpura by high-dose intravenous gamma globulin. N Engl J Med 305:1254, 1982.

136. Schiffer CA, Hogge DE, Aisner J et al: High dose intravenous gamma globulin in alloimmunized platelet transfusion recipients. Blood 64:937, 1984.

137. Lee EJ, Norris D, Schiffer CA: Intravenous immune globulin for patients alloimmunized to random donor platelet transfusion. Transfusion 27:245, 1987.

138. Kekomaki R, Elfenbein G, Gardner R et al: Improved response of patients refractory to random-donor platelet transfusions by intravenous gamma globulin. Am J Med 76:199, 1984.

139. Zeigler ZR, Shadduck RK, Rosenfeld CS et al: High dose gamma globulin improves responses to single donor platelets in patients refractory to platelet transfusions. Blood 70:1433, 1987.

140. Kickler TS, Braine HG, Piantadosi S et al: A randomized, placebo-controlled trial of intravenous gamma globulin in alloimmunized thrombocytopenic patients. Blood 75:313, 1990.

141. Dutcher JP, Schiffer CA, Aisner J et al: Long-term follow-up of patients with leukemia receiving platelet transfusions: Identification of a large group of patients who do not become alloimmunized. Blood 58:1007, 1981.

142. Lee EJ, Schiffer CA: Serial measurement of lymphocytotoxic antibody and response to nonmatched platelet transfusions in alloimmunized patients. Blood 70:1727, 1987.

143. Freedman J, Garvey MB, de Friedberg S et al: Random donor platelet crossmatching: Comparison of four platelet antibody detection methods. Am J Hematol 28:1, 1988.

144. Moroff G, Garratty G, Heal J et al: Selection of platelets for refractory patients by HLA matching and prospective crossmatching. Transfusion 32:633, 1992.

145. O'Connell BA, Lee EJ, Rothko K et al: Selection of histocompatible apheresis platelet donors by cross-matching random donor platelet concentrates. Blood 79:527, 1992.

146. Friedberg RC, Donnelly SF, Mintz PD: Independent roles for platelet crossmatching and HLA in the selection of platelets for alloimmunized patients. Transfusion 34:215, 1994.

147. Petz LD, Garratty G, Calhoun L et al: Selecting donors of platelets for refractory patients on the basis of HLA antibody specificity. Transfusion 40:1446, 2000.

148. Dutcher JP, Schiffer CA, Aisner J et al: Alloimmunization following platelet transfusion: The absence of a dose-response relationship. Blood 57:295, 1981.

149. Holohan TV, Terasaki PI, Deisseroth AB: Suppression of transfusion-related alloimmunization in intensively treated cancer patients. Blood 58:122, 1981.

150. Schiffer CA, Lichtenfeld JL, Wiernik PH et al: Antibody response in patients with acute nonlymphocytic leukemia. Cancer 37:2177, 1976.

151. Silver RT, Utz JP, Fahey J et al: Antibody response in patients with acute leukemia. J Lab Clin Med 56:634, 1960.

152. Wu KK, Thompson JS, Koepke JA et al: Heterogeneity of antibody response to human platelet transfusion. J Clin Invest 58:532, 1976.

153. Claas FHJ, Smeenk RJT, Schmidt R et al: Alloimmunization against the MHC antigens after platelet transfusion is due to contaminating leukocytes in the platelet suspension. Exp Hematol 9:84, 1981.

154. Dausset J, Rapaport FT: Transplantation antigen activity on human blood platelets. Transplantation 4:182, 1966.

155. Unanue ER, Allen PM: The basis for the immunoregulatory role of macrophages and other accessory cells. Science 236:551, 1987.

156. Eernisse JG, Brand A: Prevention of platelet refractoriness due to HLA antibodies by administration of leukocyte-poor blood components. Exp Hematol 9:77, 1981.

157. Herzig RH, Herzig GP, Bull MI et al: Correction of poor platelet transfusion responses with leukocyte-poor HLA matched platelet concentrates. Blood 46:743, 1975.

158. Schiffer CA, Dutcher JP, Aisner J et al: A randomized trial of leukocyte-depleted platelet transfusion to modify alloimmunization in patients with leukemia. Blood 62:815, 1983.

159. Sniecinski I, St. Jean J, Nowicki B: Preparation of leukocyte-poor platelets by filtration. J Clin Apheresis 5:7, 1989.

160. Kickler TS, Bell W, Ness PM et al: Depletion of white cells from platelet concentrates with a new adsorption filter. Transfusion 29:411, 1989.

161. Miyamoto M, Sasakawa S, Ishikawa Y et al: Leukocyte-poor platelet concentrates at the bedside by filtration through Sepacell-PL. Vox Sang 57:164,1989.

162. Freedman JJ, Blajchman MA, McCombie N: Canadian Red Cross Society symposium on leukodepletion: Report of proceedings. Transfus Med Rev 8:1, 1994.

163. Heddle NM: The efficacy of leukodepletion to improve platelet transfusion response: A critical appraisal of clinical studies. Transfus Med Rev 8:15, 1994.

164. The Trial to Reduce Alloimmunization to Platelets Study Group: Leukocyte reduction and ultraviolet B irradiation of platelets to prevent alloimmunization and refractoriness to platelet transfusions. N Engl J Med 337:1861, 1997.

165. Oksanen K, Kekomaki R, Ruutu T et al: Prevention of alloimmunization in patients with acute leukemia by use of white cell-reduced blood components—a randomized trial. Transfusion 31:588, 1991.

166. van Marwijk Kooy M, van Prooijen HC, Moes M et al: Use of leukocyte-depleted platelet concentrates for the prevention of refractoriness and primary HLA alloimmunization: A prospective, randomized trial. Blood 77:201, 1991.

167. Williamson LM, Wimperis JZ, Williamson P et al: Bedside filtration of blood products in the prevention of HLA alloimmunization—a prospective randomized study. Blood 83:3028, 1994.

168. Lane TA, Anderson KC, Goodnough LT et al: Leukocyte reduction in blood component therapy. Ann Intern Med 117:151, 1992.

169. Slichter SJ, Deeg HJ, Kennedy MS: Prevention of platelet alloimmunization in dogs with systemic cyclosporine and by UV-irradiation or cyclosporine loading of donor platelets. Blood 69:414, 1987.

170. Kahn RA, Duffy BF, Rodey GG: Ultraviolet irradiation of platelet concentrates abrogates lymphocyte activation without affecting platelet function in vitro. Transfusion 25:547, 1985.

171. Deeg HJ, Aprile J, Storb R et al: Functional dendritic cells are required for transfusion-induced sensitization in canine marrow graft recipients. Blood 71:1138, 1988.

172. Pamphilon DH, Corbin SA, Saunders J, Tandy NP: Application of ultraviolet light in the preparation of platelet concentrates. Transfusion 29:379, 1989.

173. Sherman L, Menitove J, Kagen LR et al: Ultraviolet-B irradiation of platelets: A preliminary trial of efficacy. Transfusion 32:402, 1992.

174. Snyder EL, Beasrdsley DS, Smith BR et al: Storage of platelet concentrates after high-dose ultraviolet B irradiation. Transfusion 31:491, 1991.

175. Winter PM, Amon M, Hocker P: Febrile transfusion reaction caused by ABO-incompatible platelet transfusion. Infus Ther 15:251, 1988.

176. Heddle NM, Klama L, Singer J et al: The role of the plasma from platelet concentrates in transfusion reactions. N Engl J Med 331:625, 1994.

177. Goodnough LT, Riddell J, Lazarus H et al: Prevalence of platelet transfusion reaction before and after implementation of leukocyte-depleted platelet concentrates by filtration. Vox Sang 65:103, 1993.

178. Muylle L, Wouters E, Peetermans ME: Febrile reactions to platelet transfusion: The effect of increased interleukin 6 levels in concentrates prepared by the platelet-rich plasma method. Transfusion 36:886, 1996.

179. Mair B, Benson K: Evaluation of changes in hemoglobin levels associated with ABO-incompatible plasma in apheresis platelets. Transfusion 38:51, 1998.

180. Garratty G: Problems associated with passively transfused blood group alloantibodies. Am J Clin Pathol 109:769, 1998.

181. Larsson LG, Welsh VJ, Ladd DJ: Acute intravascular hemolysis secondary to out-of-group platelet transfusion. Transfusion 40:902, 2000.

182. Chiu EKW, Yuen KY, Lie AKW et al: A prospective study of symptomatic bacteremia following platelet transfusion and of its management. Transfusion 34:950, 1994.

183. Aach RD, Smuness W, Mosley JW et al: Serum alanine aminotransferase of donors in relation to the risk of non-A, non-B hepatitis in recipients. The transfusion-transmitted virus study. N Engl J Med 304:989, 1981.

184. Alberti A, Chemello L, Cavalletto D et al: Antibody to hepatitis C virus and liver disease in volunteer blood donors. Ann Intern Med 114:1010, 1991.

185. Goodnough LT, Brecher ME, Kanter MH, AuBuchon JP: Transfusion medicine, Part I. Blood transfusion. N Engl J Med 340:438, 1999.

186. Schreiber GB, Busch MP, Kleinman SH, Korelitz JJ: The risk of transfusion-transmitted viral infections. N Engl J Med 334:1685, 1996.

187. Bowden RA, Sayers M, Flournoy N et al: Cytomegalovirus immune globulin and seronegative blood products to prevent primary cytomegalovirus infection after marrow transplantation. N Engl J Med 314:1006, 1986.

188. Goldman M, Delage G: The role of leukodepletion in the control of transfusion-transmitted disease. Transfus Med Rev 9:9, 1995.

189. Gilbert GL, Hayes K, Hudson IL et al: Prevention of transfusion-acquired cytomegalovirus infection in infants by blood filtration to remove leucocytes. Lancet 1:1228, 1989.

190. deGraan-Hentzen YCE, Gratama JW, Mudde GC et al: Prevention of primary cytomegalovirus infection in patients with hematologic malignancies by intensive white cell depletion of blood products. Transfusion 29:757, 1989.

191. Bowden RA, Slichter SJ, Sayers MH et al: Use of leukocyte-depleted platelets and cytomegalovirus seronegative red blood cells for prevention of primary cytomegalovirus infection after marrow transplant. Blood 78:246, 1991.

192. Bowden RA, Slichter SJ, Sayers M et al: A comparison of filtered leukocyte-reduced and cytomegalovirus (CMV) seronegative blood products for the prevention of transfusion-associated CMV infection after marrow transplant. Blood 86:3598, 1995.

193. Cohen D, Weinsten H, Mihm M et al: Non-fatal graft-versus-host disease occurring after transfusion with leukocytes and platelets obtained from normal donors. Blood 53:1053, 1979.

194. Dinsmore RE, Straus DJ, Pollack MS et al: Fatal graft-versus-host-disease following blood transfusion in Hodgkin's disease documented by HLA typing. Blood 55:831, 1980.

195. Linden JV, Pisciotto PT: Transfusion-associated graft-versus-host disease and blood irradiation. Transfus Med Rev 6:116, 1992.

196. Kanter MH: Transfusion-associated graft-versus-host disease: Do transfusions from second-degree relatives pose a greater risk than those from first-degree relatives? Transfusion 32:323, 1992.

197. Petz LD, Calhoun L, Yam P et al: Transfusion-associated graft-versus-host disease in immunocompetent patients: Report of a fatal case associated with transfusion of blood from a second-degree relative, and a survey of predisposing factors. Transfusion 33:742, 1993.

198. McMilin KD, Johnson RL: HLA homozygosity and the risk of related-donor transfusion-associated graft-versus-host disease. Transfus Med Rev 7:37, 1993.

199. Brubaker DB: Transfusion-associated graft-versus-host disease. In Anderson KC, Ness PM (eds.): Scientific Basis for Transfusion Medicine: Implications for Clinical Practice, p. 544. WB Saunders, Philadelphia, 1994.

200. Anderson KC, Weinstein HJ: Transfusion-associated graft-versus-host disease. N Engl J Med 323:315, 1990.

201. Otsuka S, Kunieda K, Kitamura F et al: The critical role of blood from HLA-homozygous donors in fatal transfusion-associated graft-versus-host disease in immunocompetent patients. Transfusion 31:260, 1991.

202. Shivdasani RA, Anderson KC: Transfusion-associated graft-versus-host disease. In Petz LD, Swisher SN, Kleinman S, Spence RK, Strauss RG (eds.): Clinical Practice of Transfusion Medicine, 3rd Ed. p. 931. Churchill Livingstone, New York, 1996.

203. Anderson KC, Goodnough LT, Sayers M et al: Variation in blood component irradiation practice: Implications for prevention of transfusion-associated graft-versus-host disease. Blood 77:2096, 1991.

204. Gelly KJ, Kerr R, Rawlinson S, Norris A, Bowen DT: Transfusion-associated graft-versus-host disease in a patient with high-grade B-cell lymphoma. Should cellular products for patients with non-Hodgkin's lymphoma be irradiated? Br J Haematol 110:228, 2000.

205. Pelszynski MM, Moroff G, Luban NL, Taylor BJ, Quinones RR: Effect of gamma irradiation of red blood cell units on T-cell inactivation as assessed by limiting dilution analysis: Implications for preventing transfusion-associated graft-versus-host disease. Blood 83:1683, 1994.

206. Zimmermann R, Schmidt S, Zingsem J et al: Effect of gamma radiation on the in vitro aggregability of WBC-reduced apheresis platelets. Transfusion 41:236, 2001.

207. Luban NLC, Drothler D, Moroff G, Quinones R: Irradiation of platelet components: Inhibition of lymphocyte proliferation assessed by limiting-dilution analysis. Transfusion 40:348, 2000.

208. Sweeney JD, Holme S, Moroff G: Storage of apheresis platelets after gamma irradiation. Transfusion 34:779, 1994.

209. Grass JA, Hei DJ, Metchette K et al: Inactivation of leukocytes in platelet concentrates by photochemical treatment with psoralen plus UVA. Blood 91:2180, 1998.

210. Freireich EJ, Levin RH, Whang J et al: The function and fate of transfused leukocytes from donors with chronic myelocytic leukemia in leukopenic recipients. Ann NY Acad Sci 113:1081, 1964.

211. Morse EE, Freireich EJ, Carbone PP et al: The transfusion of leukocytes from donors with chronic myelocytic leukemia to patients with leukopenia. Transfusion 6:183, 1966.

212. Schiffer CA, Aisner J, Dutcher JP, Wiernik PH: Sustained post-transfusion granulocyte count increments following transfusion of leukocytes obtained from donors with chronic myelogenous leukemia. Am J Hematol 15:65, 1983.

213. Eyre HJ, Goldstein IM, Perry S, Graw RG Jr: Leukocyte transfusions: Function of transfused granulocytes from donors with chronic myelocytic leukemia. Blood 36:432, 1970.

214. Huestis DW, Glasser L: The neutrophil in transfusion medicine. Transfusion 34:630, 1994.

215. Freireich EJ: White cell transfusions born again. Leuk Lymphoma 11(Suppl. 2):161, 1993.

216. Price TH: Granulocyte colony-stimulating factor-mobilized granulocyte concentrate transfusion. Curr Opin Hematol 5:381, 1998.

217. Bhatia S, McCullough J, Perry EH et al: Granulocyte transfusion: Efficacy in treating fungal infections in neutropenic patients following bone marrow transplantation. Transfusion 34:226, 1994.

218. Peters C, Minkov M, Matthes-Martin S et al: Leucocyte transfusions from rhG-CSF or prednisolone stimulated donors for treatment of severe infections in immunocompromised neutropenic patients. Br J Haematol 106:689, 1999.

219. Catalano L, Fontana R, Scarpato N, Picardi M et al: Combined treatment with amphotericin-B and granulocyte transfusion from G-CSF-stimulated donors in an aplastic patient with invasive aspergillosis undergoing bone marrow transplantation. Haematologica 82:71, 1997.

220. Graw RG Jr, Herzig G, Perry S, Henderson ES: Normal granulocyte transfusion therapy. Treatment of septicemia due to gram-negative bacteria. N Engl J Med 287:367, 1972.

221. Higby DJ, Yates JW, Henderson ES, Holland JF: Filtration leukapheresis for granulocyte transfusion therapy—clinical laboratory studies. N Engl J Med 1292:761, 1975.

222. Fortuny IE, Bloomfield CD, Hadlock DC et al: Granulocyte transfusions: A controlled study in patients with acute nonlymphocytic leukemia. Transfusion 15:548, 1975.

223. Herzig RH, Herzig GP, Graw RG Jr et al: Successful granulocyte transfusion therapy for gram-negative septicemia. A prospective randomized controlled study. N Engl J Med 296:701, 1977.

224. Vogler WR, Winton EF: A controlled study of the efficacy of granulocyte transfusions in patients with neutropenia. Am J Med 63:548, 1977.

225. Alavi JB, Root RK, Djerrasi I et al: A randomized clinical trial of granulocyte transfusions for infection in acute leukemia. N Engl J Med 296:706, 1977.

226. Winston DJ, Ho WG, Gale RP: Therapeutic granulocyte transfusions for documented infections. Ann Intern Med 97:509, 1982.

227. Epstein RB, Waxman FJ, Bennett BT, Andersen BR: Pseudomonas septicemia in neutropenic dogs. I. Treatment with granulocyte transfusions. Transfusion 14:51, 1974.

228. Appelbaum FR, Bowles CA, Makuch RW, Deisseroth AB: Granulocyte transfusion therapy of experimental Pseudomonas septicemia: Study of cell dose and collection technique. Blood 52:323, 1978.

229. Epstein RB, Chow HS: An analysis of quantitative relationships of granulocyte transfusion therapy in canines. Transfusion 21:360, 1981.

230. Ruthe RC, Andersen BR, Cunningham BL, Epstein RB: Efficacy of granulocyte transfusions in the control of systemic candidiasis in leukopenic host. Blood 52:493, 1978.

231. Chow HS, Sarpel SC, Epstein RB: Experimental candidiasis in neutropenic dogs: Tissue burden of infection and granulocyte transfusion effects. Blood 59:328, 1982.

232. Athens JW: Neutrophilic granulocyte kinetics and granulopoiesis. In Gordon AS (ed.): Regulation of Hematopoiesis, Vol. 2, p. 1143. Appleton-Century-Crofts, New York, 1970.

233. Strauss RG, Connett JE, Gale RP et al: A controlled trial of prophylactic granulocyte transfusions during initial induction chemotherapy for acute myeloid leukemia. N Engl J Med 305:597, 1981.

234. Schiffer CA, Aisner J, Daly PA et al: Alloimmunization following prophylactic granulocyte transfusion. Blood 54:766, 1979.

235. Mannoni P, Rodet M, Vernant JP et al: Efficiency of prophylactic granulocyte transfusions in preventing infections in acute leukemia. Blood Transfus Immunohaematol 22:503, 1979.

236. McCullough J, Clay M, Kline W: Granulocyte antigens and antibodies. Transfus Med Rev 1:150, 1987.

237. Graw RG Jr, Goldstein IM, Eyre HJ, Terasaki PI: Histocompatibility testing for leucocyte transfusion. Lancet 1:77, 1970.

238. Goldstein IM, Eyre HJ, Terasaki PI et al: Leukocyte transfusions: Role of leukocyte alloantibodies in determining transfusion response. Transfusion 11:19, 1971.

239. Appelbaum FR, Trapani RJ, Graw RG Jr: Consequences of prior alloimmunization during granulocyte transfusion. Transfusion 17:460, 1977.

240. Dahlke MB, Keashen MA, Alavi JB et al: Response to granulocyte transfusions in the alloimmunized patient. Transfusion 20:555, 1980.

241. Dahlke MB, Keashen M, Alavi JB et al: Granulocyte transfusion and outcome of alloimmunized patients with gram negative sepsis. Transfusion 22:374, 1982.

242. McCullough J, Weiblen B, Clay ME, Forstrom L: Effect of leukocyte antibodies on the fate in vivo of Indium-111-labeled granulocytes. Blood 48:164, 1981.

243. Dutcher JP, Schiffer CA, Johnston GS et al: Alloimmunization prevents the migration of transfused [111]Indium-labeled granulocytes to sites of infection. Blood 62:354, 1983.

244. Dutcher JP, Riggs C, Fox JJ et al: The effect of histocompatibility factors on pulmonary retention of Indium-111-labeled granulocytes. Am J Hematol 33:238, 1990.

245. McCullough J, Clay M, Hurd D et al: Effect of leukocyte antibodies and HLA matching on the intravascular recovery, survival and tissue localization of 111-Indium granulocytes. Blood 67:522, 1986.

246. Adkins DR, Goodnough LT, Shenoy S et al: Effect of leukocyte compatibility on neutrophil increment after transfusion of granulocyte colony-stimulating factor-mobilized prophylactic granulocyte transfusions and on clinical outcomes after stem cell transplantation. Blood 95:3605, 2000.

247. Wright DG, Robichaud KJ, Pizzo PA, Deisseroth AB: Lethal pulmonary reactions associated with the combined use of amphotericin B and leukocyte transfusions. N Engl J Med 304:1185, 1981.

248. Dana BW, Durie BGM, White RF, Huestis DW: Concomitant administration of granulocyte transfusions and amphotericin B in neutropenic patients: Absence of significant pulmonary toxicity. Blood 47:90, 1981.

249. Dutcher JP, Kendall J, Papenberg D et al: Granulocyte transfusion therapy and amphotericin B: Adverse reactions? Am J Hematol 31:102, 1989.

250. Forman SJ, Robinson GV, Wolf JL et al: Pulmonary reactions associated with amphotericin B and leukocyte transfusions. (Letter to editor.) N Engl J Med 305:584, 1981.

251. Clift RA, Buckner CD: Granulocyte transfusions. Am J Med 76:631, 1984.

252. Clarke K, Szer J, Shelton M et al: Multiple granulocyte transfusions facilitating successful unrelated bone marrow transplantation in a patient with very severe aplastic anemia complicated by suspected fungal infection. Bone Marrow Transplant 15:723, 1995.

55

Stem Cell Processing and Purging

Carole B. Miller, Paul V. O'Donnell,
and N. Claude Gorin

Stem cells have been used since the 1970s as the means to reconstitute a patient's bone marrow after bone marrow ablation. Initially, bone marrow was used as a source of stem cells; however, recently peripheral blood stem cells have been the major source of stem cells for transplantation. Whatever the source, significant changes in procedures for stem cell processing have occurred over the past two to three decades but the general goals of marrow processing remain relatively unchanged (Table 55–1).

A major development over the past 10 years has been the regulation and standardization of blood cell products. The FDA has stated its intention to regulate the area of cellular and gene therapy and has recently published a draft regulation for comments.[1] The major themes are that cell processing should be performed under current good manufacturing practices (GMP). GMP are regulations originally developed for the pharmaceutical industry and later extended to blood banks. These regulations provide a framework for the control of the manufacturing of any "product" from the start to the final disposition and include detailed requirements for facilities, training, documentation, quality assurance and controls, and labeling. The regulations specifically designed for cellular therapies are called good tissue practices (cGTP), which are based on the perceived risks to the donor and recipient. Variables include the risk of transmitting infectious agents, how closely related the donor and recipient are, and most importantly the degree of manipu-lation. Under the proposed regulations autologous cells would be less regulated than allogeneic products. Autologous cells would be regulated only if extensive manipulations, including genetic manipulation, ex vivo cultures, or selection were to be used. The transplant community has also initiated self-regulation through the development of standards. The voluntary organization FAHCT (Foundation for the Accreditation of Hematopoietic Cell Therapy) developed and published the Standards for Hematopoietic Progenitor Cell Collection, Processing, and Transplantation.[2] These standards apply to all areas of therapeutic progenitor cell therapy and are implemented through a voluntary inspection and accreditation process. Specific guidelines on the training of personnel, quality control, and processing requirements are provided. Of importance are the transplant center specific standard operating procedures required for all stem cell processing, purging, and storage. These procedures for handling stem cells will be discussed in detail below.

BONE MARROW HARVEST

Thomas and Storb first published the technique for bone marrow harvest in 1970[3] and until the early 1990s bone marrow was the preferred source of stem cells used for transplantation. Generally, bone marrow is obtained from the posterior iliac crests. Other possible sites for harvest include the anterior iliac crests and sternum. Bone marrow harvest is usually performed as an outpatient procedure in an operating room, with general, spinal, or epidural anesthesia. Patients are placed prone and skin sites are sterilely prepped and draped. Multiple bone marrow aspirates are drawn, generally through five to six skin puncture sites. Approximately 10 to 12 percent of the estimated blood volume is procured from 50 to 100 aspirations. Bone marrow is aspirated into a syringe, which has been rinsed with medium containing preservative-free heparin. It is recommended that only 3 to 5 ml should be aspirated with each pull using a 20 to 60 ml syringe. Larger aspirate volumes may increase the contamination with peripheral blood.[4] About 2 to 5×10^8 nucleated bone marrow cells per kilogram of recipient ideal body weight is generally obtained, representing approximately 5 percent of the estimated total body bone marrow pool.[5] Aspirated marrow is then collected in containers also containing heparinized medium. While stainless steel beakers with wire mesh filters to filter the bony spicules and clots can be used, partially closed commercial collection systems containing three sequentially smaller mesh in-line filters are now more common. The amount of heparin, media, and other additives to the harvest mixture depends on the specific planned graft manipulation. Cells are then transported to the cell processing laboratory, usually at room temperature.

The complications of bone marrow harvest include the risk of the anesthesia, pain, infection, and bleeding. In one study,[6] 27 percent of allogeneic donors were noted to have at least one complication. While 92 percent of the complications were considered minor, such as postoperative fevers, local infection, or localized bleeding, more serious complications can occur,

---

Table 55–1. Goals of Stem Cell Processing

Procedure	Goal
Volume reduction	Ease of storage and reinfusion
Plasma depletion	ABO incompatibility, volume reduction
Red blood cell depletion	ABO incompatibility, volume reduction, preparation for cryopreservation
Granulocyte depletion	Decrease transfusion reactions
Lymphocyte depletion	Decrease GvHD
Stem cell enrichment	Improve engraftment
Tumor cell purging	Eliminate contamination with residual tumor

Adapted from Meagher and Herzig,[5] with permission.

including arrhythmias, hypotension, or severe bleeding requiring blood transfusion. During harvest for allogeneic donors, many centers routinely collect one autologous unit for transfusion back to the donor and may also recommend supplemental iron. In one study[7] recombinant erythropoietin was given to donors who were unable to bank blood in order to prevent or decrease blood transfusion requirements.

PERIPHERAL BLOOD STEM CELL HARVEST

In the 1980s To et al. observed that in acute myelocytic leukemia (AML) patients who had received conventional chemotherapy, high levels of myeloid progenitors (colony-forming units for granulocytes and macrophages [CFU-GM]) were found in the peripheral blood at the time of count recovery.[8] These CFU-GM could be collected and cryopreserved with excellent viability after thawing. These experiments prompted Juttner et al. to perform the first transplants using autologous stem cells collected after chemotherapy; two patients with AML were rescued after myeloablative chemotherapy.[9] In 1988, Socinski et al. observed that granulocyte-macrophage colony-stimulating factor (GM-CSF) could mobilize stem cells into the circulation[10] and when combined with chemotherapy, the number of stem cells in circulation increased by 60-fold. Peters et al. showed in 1993 that granulocyte colony-stimulating factor (G-CSF) could also mobilize stem cells after chemotherapy with improved efficacy over GM-CSF.[11] In the past decade, many different regimens have been developed to mobilize stem cells for use in transplantation. The best method depends on the condition of the patient and the amount of stem cells required for the planned transplant manipulation.

Once the stem cells are mobilized, collection techniques are similar to blood or platelet donation. Patients undergoing peripheral blood progenitor cell (PBPC) mobilization generally require a central venous catheter rigid enough to withstand moderate to high flow rates generated by the apheresis equipment. With allogeneic donors, peripheral access is generally adequate for collection; however, temporary central venous access is sometimes required. There are several commercially available automated collection devices commonly used for the pheresis, including the COBE Spectra and Fenwal CS3000 systems. Standard collection techniques use a blood flow rate of 50 to 80 ml/min with a total processed blood volume of 10 to 12 L. This requires a total collection time of 2 to 3 hours. The cells are separated based on physical characteristics including size and density. Low-density leukocytes (mononuclear cells) are collected and blood components that are not targeted (plasma, red blood cells, and granulocytes) are returned to the donor. While the collected product contains mainly mononuclear cells, there is some granulocyte and red blood cell contamination that may require further manipulation to remove. Final product volume of mononuclear cells varies, but is generally between 50 and 200 ml.

An alternative method for collecting PBPCs is the use of large-volume leukapheresis, which increases the blood volume processed during the procedure. Volumes as high as 50 L are processed during one collection; this requires a large bore catheter and can last for up to 8 hours. Due to the high flow rates and blood volumes employed, a large amount of anticoagulation with citrate is required, necessitating frequent monitoring and adjustments of blood calcium levels. Passos-Coelho et al.[12] showed that adequate numbers of stem cells could be collected in a single session of large-volume leukapheresis (lasting up to 6 hours).

STEM CELL MANIPULATION

The majority of stem cell grafts require some minimal manipulation prior to use. The only exception is ABO matched allogeneic grafts that can be collected, filtered, and directly transfused like red blood cell transfusions.

Minor ABO Incompatible Allogeneic Grafts

In donor-recipient pairs with a minor ABO incompatibility (O donor into A, B, or ABO recipient, for example), the *donor* plasma contains alloantibodies to recipient red blood cells, which could lead to hemolysis of recipient red cells after infusion.[13] In order to decrease this risk, donor plasma is removed prior to marrow infusion. Standard laboratory centrifugation that can separate out plasma is very time consuming. For clinical size products, plasma is commonly removed using a blood cell washer such as the COBE2991.

Major ABO Incompatible Allogeneic Grafts

In donor-recipient pairs with a major ABO incompatibility (A donor into O recipient, for example), the *recipient* plasma contains alloantibodies against the donor red cells also leading to acute hemolysis of donor red cells, and may result in life-threatening complications such as renal failure.[14] Donor red blood cells are removed using one of several methods and should remove red blood cells without the loss of a significant number of hematopoietic progenitor cells. In addition to decreasing the risk of hemolysis, these red cells can be used for transfusion to the donor if an autologous unit was not collected or was inadequate for blood loss during the harvest.[15] A method that removes red blood cells from a graft includes hydroxyethyl starch sedimentation (HES)[16]; however, buffy coat or mononuclear cell preparation is commonly used today. The choice depends on whether the graft requires further manipulation prior to infusion and what percentage red blood cell contamination is acceptable. If the initial separation does not adequately reduce red blood cell contamination, a repeat separation can be done. This is done by mixing the first collection with recipient compatible, irradiated leukocyte depleted red blood cells and recipient compatible plasma.

Collecting Cells for Further Manipulation

With the advent of graft engineering techniques, it is often necessary to have white blood cell rich products for further manipulation. Preparation of a buffy coat has been the primary method for collection of a white blood cell preparation allowing for collection of over 75 percent of the nucleated cells, and reducing both red blood cell and plasma contamination by an equivalent amount.[3,17] A buffy coat can be prepared using a standard blood bank centrifuge; however, automated cell collection devices are more common. The resulting product contains both mononuclear cells and neutrophils.

Many graft manipulation techniques require a purer mononuclear cell preparation. Neutrophils can be removed from a buffy-coated specimen by several methods using a density gradient separation technique such HES[18] or Ficoll-Hypaque gradient separation.[19] Density gradient separation has been shown to recover a high number of mononuclear cells with a minute fraction of red blood cells. This method starts with a buffy coat preparation to reduce the gross volume. A density gradient such as Ficoll-Hypaque is then added to the spinning centrifuge bag. The buffy coat is layered over the Ficoll at a slow centrifuge rate and the mononuclear cell layer is collected. The cells are then washed to remove any residual gradient. Five methods of concentrating bone marrow cells were compared, including HES sedimentation with centrifugation, Ficoll-Hypaque with gradient centrifugation, Ficoll-Hypaque gradient on a COBE 2991 cell washer, continuous flow cell separator (Fenwal CS3000), and the semicontinuous blood cell separator (Dideco T90).[19] The Ficoll-Hypaque gradient on a COBE 2991 cell washer provided the most efficient system with 89 percent recovery of the mononuclear cell fraction, and less than 2 percent red blood cell and neutrophil contamination. This system provided a 98 percent volume reduction and an 80 percent recovery of myeloid progenitors as measured by the CFU-GM assay.

Stem Cell Cryopreservation

If stem cells will not be infused immediately after manipulation, they are generally cryopreserved until it is time for infusion. There are little data on the use of cryopreserved allogeneic stem cells. The majority of autologous stem cell products require cryopreservation since patients receive additional chemotherapy prior to reinfusion.

Cryopreservation generally occurs after both volume and cell reduction in order to decrease the space required for freezing and to decrease the amount of cryoprotective agent required. As cells can be injured by the direct effects of low temperatures and formation of ice crystals, cryoprotectants are required to maintain cell viability.[20] Dimethylsulfoxide (DMSO) is the most commonly used cryopreservation agent for hematopoietic stem cell preservation. DMSO, like glycerol, is a penetrating cryoprotectant with a low molecular weight that is able to rapidly diffuse into a cell prior to freezing, thus increasing the intracellular osmolality.[21] This increased osmolality limits the size and thus the damage caused by intracellular ice crystals formed during rapid cooling rates. DMSO is relatively nontoxic to myeloid progenitor cells at the 5 to 10 percent concentrations used for cryopreservation. Little toxicity to myeloid progenitors is documented until 20 to 40 percent concentrations of DMSO are reached.[22] Toxicities reported with DMSO intravenous infusion include a noxious odor and cardiac side effects including bradycardia.[23]

Red cells must be depleted prior to cryopreservation as these cells are not cryopreserved with current methods and would result in an excessive hemoglobin load leading to renal tubular damage. Depletion of red blood cells is accomplished by using a mononuclear cell preparation that decreases the amount of infused DMSO. A cell concentration of 30 to 40×10^6 cells/ml is used for standard freezing techniques.[24] Cells are first chilled to 4°C, then DMSO is added to a final concentration of 10 percent volume/volume. Cells are mixed for 10 minutes and then placed into polyolefin freezing bags that are placed in metal frames. The marrow suspension is frozen as a sheet less than 5 mm thick. The frames and bags are then placed into a programmed rate-control freezer, where the cells are frozen by decreasing the temperature by 1°C per minute until they reach the target of −80 to −100°C. The cells are then transferred to the vapor or liquid phase of liquid nitrogen. At the time of marrow reinfusion, the bags are rapidly warmed in a 37°C water bath, and then infused rapidly without filtering. While the storage time of most stem cell grafts is less than 3 months, marrow cells that have been stored for more than 2 years are capable of long term engraftment.[25]

GRAFT MANIPULATION WITH THERAPEUTIC INTENT

The two most common therapeutic graft manipulation techniques are T-cell depletion to reduce the incidence or severity of graft-versus-host disease (GvHD) and stem cell purging to reduce tumor cell contamination.

T-Cell Depletion

Donor T cells contained within the infused graft contribute to the development of acute and chronic GvHD after allogeneic stem cell transplant.[26,27] Many different methods to deplete T cells have been evaluated. Early T-cell depletion strategies centered on the observation that when T cells are incubated with soybean lectin, they will rosette with sheep red blood cells.[28,29] These rosettes can be separated by density gradient centrifugation. This technique can achieve up to a 2 log T-cell depletion and is still in clinical use.

At Johns Hopkins University, we have used a physical method of separation called counterflow centrifugal elutriation (CCE) to deplete T cells.[30–32] CCE separates cells based on size and density (sedimentation coefficient). A mononuclear cell preparation is first prepared and loaded onto a spinning centrifuge chamber. Media is continually pumped into the system at a constant rate. Since the centrifugal and media flow forces are opposing, equilibrium is reached and the cells are separated into layers (fractions) with heavier, denser cells at the bottom and lighter cells in the top layers. Cells are then eluted off into collection bags by changing the flow rate. As the media flow rate is increased, progressively larger cell types are harvested. The large cell fraction (rotor off) contains the progenitor cells and the small cell fraction contains stem cells and lymphocytes. Our current protocols take the small cell fraction and select the CD34+ cells, which when infused, ensure long-term engraftment.[33]

Negative selection techniques using monoclonal antibodies for T-cell depletion have been studied extensively. One of the earliest antibodies studied was CAMPATH-1M, a rat monoclonal IgM against CDw52, active against T, B, and NK cells.[34] Mononuclear cells are incubated with CAMPATH-1M and a source of complement (generally donor serum). This procedure yields an approximately 2 log T-cell depletion; however, the depth of T-cell depletion can be varied by changing the incubation strategies. CAMPATH-1M has been shown to have similar effects on T-cell depletion when peripheral blood progenitor cells are used compared to the historical marrow data.[35] Other pan T-cell antibodies include T10B9 (antibodies targeting the alpha/beta T-cell receptor) plus complement[36] and anti-CD5 ricin A-chain immunotoxin.[37] Both antibodies have shown approximately a 2 to 3 log T-cell depletion along with a decrease in acute GvHD, even in very high-risk patients.

Investigators have tried selective T-cell depletion strategies because T-cell depletion has been associated with increased relapse rates due to the lack of a graft versus leukemia effect. Champlin et al. have studied selective CD8 depletion using an anti-Leu-2 monoclonal antibody and complement in HLA matched sibling donor transplants. Cyclosporine prophylaxis was administered to 36 patients for 6 months post-transplant.[38] Only three cases of graft failure occurred; GvHD disease was seen in 28 percent of patients along with a very low relapse rate. Soiffer et al.[39] used the T12 monoclonal antibody (directed against CD6) plus complement as the sole GvHD prophylaxis in a group of patients with high-risk acute leukemia. All patients engrafted and a low incidence of grade 2 to 4 GvHD (15 percent) and relapse (25 percent) was seen.

Positive selection has also been studied as a method of T-cell depletion. The CD34 antigen is a trans-membrane glycoprotein expressed on 1 to 3 percent of normal bone marrow mononuclear cells.[40] These cells are myeloid progenitors and cells in the CD34+ fraction are able to reconstitute normal hematopoiesis. Several CD34 selection devices have been FDA approved and have primarily been used to deplete tumor cells from autologous bone marrow grafts via positive selection of the myeloid progenitors. The use of CD34 selection for tumor cell purging will be discussed in the purging section below. CD34 selection has also been studied as a method of T-cell depletion, resulting in approximately 3 to 6 log depletion of T cells.[41,42] One advantage of positive selection is that the T cells can be studied or further manipulated because the procedure leaves them intact.

Although there have been no randomized trials of T-cell depletion techniques, a retrospective study through the IBMTR compared five categories of T-cell depletion techniques in patients with acute leukemia receiving grafts from donors other than HLA identical siblings (Table 55–2).[43] They found that T-cell depletion strategies with specificities targeting only T cells without depleting other immune cells (narrow T-cell depletion strategies) had a higher leukemia-free survival than patients transplanted with other T-cell depletion techniques. When compared to similar patients who received T-cell replete grafts, there was a lower risk of severe acute GvHD in both groups of T-cell depleted patients. Leukemia-free survival was similar in the non-T-cell-depleted and the narrow T-cell depleted groups, and both were superior to the leukemia-free survival in the patients who received other T-cell depletion techniques. There were higher relapse rates in the group that received the other T-cell depletion strategies, possibly related to a decreased incidence of chronic GvHD in this group.

Because of the competing risks of T-cell depletion that balance possibilities for decreased GvHD with an increased risk of relapse and post-transplant lymphoproliferative disease, randomized trials would be very helpful in determining the role of T-cell depletion in allogeneic bone marrow transplant.

IN VITRO PURGING FOR AUTOLOGOUS TRANSPLANTATION

Use of autologous bone marrow transplant raises the concern about reintroducing tumor cells from a contaminated autograft. Initially, bone marrow (BM) contamination by residual tumor cells was thought to occur in hematological malignancies while affecting only a minority of solid tumors. The development of highly sensitive molecular biology techniques such as polymerase chain reaction (PCR) subsequently showed that marrow tumor infiltration occurs in a majority of solid tumors, espe-

Table 55–2. IBMTR Analysis of T-Cell Depletion Techniques in Non-HLA Matched Donors for Acute Leukemia

Category of T-cell Depletion Methods	Examples of Specific Technique	Relative Risk of Treatment Failure	p Value	Adjusted 5-Year Leukemia-Free Survival (percent)
Narrow specificity antibodies targeting only T-cells	T10B9, CD3 +/−CD7, CD6 or CD8, CD5 +/−CD4 or CD8, CD5+/−CD8	1.00		25
Broad-specificity antibodies that include other immune cells	ATG, CD 2 targeting antibodies	1.37	.03	13
CAMPATH antibodies	Antibodies targeting CD52	1.58	.0001	12
Elutriation	Density gradient centrifugation	1.65	.0007	17
Lectins	Lectins + sheep red blood cells, rosetting	1.47	.0007	15

cially breast and small cell lung cancer. Autologous peripheral blood (PB) transplantation was introduced[44,45] with the hope that leukapheresis (LK) products would not be contaminated, thus eliminating the need for in vitro purging. For this reason, the standard procedure for many years has been to apply purging to BM and not to PB. Since then, it has been shown that PB contamination by tumor cells coexist in situations when marrow is infiltrated, although usually at a lower level.[46] In addition, stem cell mobilization in peripheral blood following chemotherapy, cytokines, or both, also mobilizes tumor cells,[47] not only from marrow but from other body sites. There may be extreme situations when recruitment of tumor cells with PB mobilization might occur in the absence of marrow contamination.

In vitro purging techniques have evolved considerably. Early approaches used *negative selection* methods of targeting tumor cell destruction by use of chemotherapy and other drugs, monoclonal antibodies, or immunomagnetic depletion. Recently, less tumor-specific techniques classified as *positive selection* have been developed. These techniques target the collection of normal stem cells thus eliminating the more mature cells (including tumor cells) not necessary for successful engraftment. Evidence is accumulating in favor of purging, but there is a lack of prospective randomized trials showing a survival benefit. Concurrent progress in chemotherapy treatment along with the acceptance that stem cells should be collected after several courses of chemotherapy to take advantage of in vivo purging have raised the question whether in vitro purging is really needed when optimal in vivo purging has occurred.

General Principles of Purging

Several widely accepted principles exist regarding purging the graft in vitro. First, whatever technique is used, the engraftment potential of the autograft should not be jeopardized. Destruction of mature progenitors may not be of long-term consequence if more immature progenitors are preserved. More immature progenitors, such as long-term culture initiating cells (LTC-IC),[48,49] cobblestone area forming cells (CAFC),[50,51] or more recently clonogenic initiating cells in NOD-SCID mice,[52] are the cells responsible for sustained engraftment. However, mature committed progenitors such as CFU-GM, burst-forming units for erythroblasts (BFU-E), and colony-forming units for megakaryocytes (CFU-MK) are directly responsible for early hematopoietic recovery. Their reduction leads to prolonged neutropenia, thrombocytopenia, and increases transfusion needs and hospitalization duration. Second, if a drug or a combination of drugs is used, they should be cell-cycle–independent (because of the usually short duration of incubation) and there should be selective toxicity for tumor cells with no mutagenic and/or carcinogenic effect for normal stem cells. In vitro concentrations of the drug should far exceed the maximum tolerated dose in vivo and be removed by washing or inactivation before infusion of the graft. Third, residual tumor before and after purging should be quantified in the graft with as much sensitivity as possible, preferentially by molecular biology. Fourth, any attempt at showing a clinical benefit (such as fewer relapses) requires a setting where the probability of relapse or tumor progression initiating from body sites other than the autograft itself is very small or nonexistent. Fifth, the significance of purging should not be restricted to a direct tumoricidal goal since unexpected beneficial effects such as increased natural killer (NK) cell activity have been observed.[53]

Freezing as a First Step of Purging

As described earlier, DMSO is often added to the freezing media to protect living cells and is also used in purging. It is unclear whether incubation of the autograft with DMSO results in any other beneficial effect, or whether DMSO left in the autograft before infusion has any antitumor impact.[54] One consequence may be activation of NK cells following freezing and thawing.[55]

In acute leukemia (AL), freezing results in destruction of leukemic clonogenic progenitors. The recovery of AML-CFU was shown to be significantly lower ($p < .001$) than for normal CFU-GM and BFU-E after freezing. Moreover, the cloning efficiency of frozen AML-CFU was significantly reduced ($p < .001$) as compared with fresh samples, while it was unaltered in normal progenitors. While freezing alone may achieve at most a one log tumor cell reduction, combination of in vitro treatment with cryopreservation induces potentialization, where cells fragilized by in vitro treatment are more sensitive to freezing and thawing. Verdonck et al.[56] observed that survival of leukemic colonies of L-CFC was reduced or not detectable after freezing and thawing. The small degree of tumor reduction obtained by cryopreservation alone may be minimal, but purging with drugs or monoclonal antibodies may act synergistically with freezing.

Techniques of Purging With Pharmacological Agents

The drugs selected for in vitro purging have activity against human tumor, some exhibiting a dose effect relationship. These drugs are usually tested against cell lines to define the dose range of activity. In addition, some drugs have been assessed in animal models of autografting for malignancies. The most commonly used drugs for ex vivo purging are two cyclophosphamide derivatives, 4-hydroperoxycyclophosphamide (4HC) and mafosfamide.

Cyclophosphamide Derivatives

Cyclophosphamide is metabolized into two metabolites, 4HC and aldophosphamide. Intracellular aldehyde dehydrogenase then oxidates aldophosphamide into inactive carboxyphosphamide. There are higher cellular levels of aldehyde dehydrogenase in normal cells and immature normal progenitors compared to malignant cells and more committed progenitors, explaining the differential sensitivity to cyclophosphamide observed in favor of immature normal progenitors. Mafosfamide is a lysine salt of a sulfoethylthio derivative of cyclophosphamide that spontaneously hydrolyzes to produce 4HC and 2-mercaptoethane sulfonic acid (MESNA). 4HC is used almost exclusively in North America and mafosfamide almost exclusively in Europe. Both compounds are considered equivalent for purging in vitro.

Certain factors affect in vitro treatment modalities with cyclophosphamide derivatives. The hematocrit value and the nucleated cell concentration are important parameters to consider since peripheral blood cells (mostly red cells) and all marrow cells contain aldehyde dehydrogenase, therefore the activity of cyclophosphamide derivatives decreases with increasing cell concentrations. Most teams either reduce the hematocrit below 5 percent or incubate Ficoll separated mononucleated cells. Another factor is that plasma inhibits the toxicity of mafosfamide; this is why plasma is eliminated by washing cells prior to incubation.[57] In addition, progenitor cells and their subtypes are inhibited by mafosfamide in a dose-dependent manner and probably due to the relative cellular contents in aldehyde dehydrogenase. Late CFU-GM are most susceptible, followed by early CFU- GM, with LTC-IC the least susceptible. There is also a wide range of sensitivity to cyclophosphamide derivatives from patient to patient, as shown on GFU-GM[58–61] and on normal CFU-blast[62,63] grown with the technique of Gordon et al.[64] Treatment with mafosfamide also sensitizes CFU-GM to freezing.[65] Two major techniques of incubation with 4HC or mafosfamide have evolved as a result of these observations. The first applies a constant dose of 4HC[66,67] or mafosfamide.[68] The second approach adjusts each dose so that individual patient marrow is incubated with the maximum tolerated dose, in an effort to get maximum leukemic progenitor kill without jeopardizing engraftment.[57,60,65,69,70]

The action of cyclophosphamide derivatives may involve more than direct tumor cytotoxicity. Several studies have noted increases in NK cell activity following exposure to 4HC[55] or mafosfamide.[71,72] Mafosfamide also induces apoptosis in human AML and this induction is enhanced by interleukin 3 (IL-3) and IL-6.[73] These observations suggest that purging with 4HC or mafosfamide may add to tumor removal with some degree of immunological antitumor boosting.

Other Chemotherapeutic Agents

A large number of chemotherapeutic agents have been tested for in vitro purging; however, clinical experience is limited. Methylprednisolone has been used for T-cell depletion to prevent GvHD in allogeneic BMT,[74] and could be considered for in vitro purging in non-Hodgkin's lymphoma (NHL) and in patients autografted for autoimmune diseases. Bleomycin is interesting since it is most active against nondividing cells and its clinical activity would favor inclusion in in vitro purging for NHL. In the BNML rat model, bleomycin incubation induced a 2 to 4 log tumor reduction and still led to successful engraftment. The sequential incubation of marrow with bleomycin followed by 4HC was synergistic against leukemic cells, while sparing a sufficient number of normal stem cells to ensure engraftment.[75]

The significant clinical use of etoposide, alone or with 4HC, is supported by preclinical and animal data. Etoposide purged CFU-L in a murine model with 15 percent of CFU-GM surviving. In vivo, animals receiving purged marrow engrafted and survived 40 days compared to 12 days for untreated animals.[76] Nitrogen mustard (NM) and etoposide are also synergistic against leukemia cell lines, without any increase in toxicity for normal BM progenitors.[77] Adjusting the dose of NM[78,79] to the individual sensitivity of each patient's normal CFU-GM compartment similarly affects marrow and peripheral blood,[78] resulting in successful engraftment,[79] with a possible delay as compared to unpurged PB. Available clinical data also support the idea that the engraftment potential of etoposide-treated marrow is not altered.[80]

Other Nonchemotherapeutic Agents

Both lipids and photodynamic agents have been studied for purging in vitro. Ether lipids (alkyl-lysophospholipids, edelfosine) damage tumor cell membranes in a relatively selective way as normal cells can cleave ether lipids and become resistant. Numerous in vitro studies have demonstrated activity against several tumors including HL-60, K562, Daudi lymphoblastoid cell line, glioblastoma, breast adenocarcinoma, and myeloma,[81–84] while progenitor cells are spared.[85] The largest clinical experience has been carried out in Atlanta, where a cohort of over 70 patients with acute leukemia has received marrow treated in vitro with edelfosine.[82] More recently a randomized study evaluating edelfosine for PB purging resulted in CFU-GM recovery of 63 percent following cryopreservation alone, 80 percent following purging alone, and 48 percent following purging and cryopreservation ($p < .007$). This reduction was too small to affect engraftment, which was similarly rapid in both groups, within 15 days for both PMN and platelets.[86,87]

Merocyanine 540 (MC) and dihematoporphyrin ether (DHE) are two photodynamic agents that have been tested. MC is a phototoxic lipophilic agent that binds preferentially to leukemia cells under certain conditions in the presence of plasma. Exposure of a marrow contaminated by leukemic cells to white light has been shown to induce a 4 log tumor reduction and spares about 50 percent of the normal stem cells.[88,89] The advantage of photodynamic agents is that they are independent of the cell cycle, and drug-resistant tumors remain sensitive to their action. Other nonchemotherapeutic agents with in vitro activity against chronic myelocytic leukemia include anti-sense oligonucleotides anti Bcr-Abl[90–92] or anti-C-myb,[93,94] and anti-tyrosine kinase agents[95] such as genistein.

Techniques of Purging With Monoclonal Antibodies

Techniques of removing tumor cells from the graft with monoclonal antibodies are divided into two major approaches, according to whether attempts are made at specific recognition and destruction of tumor cells (negative selection) or at selecting and purifying normal stem cells, while discarding all other cells including tumor cells (positive selection). Negative selection was developed first, followed by positive selection in the 1990s. Combinations of both approaches are currently under study.

Negative Selection

Target definition is critical for success. Since true tumor cell antigens have not been identified, target antigens are usually differentiating antigens not present at the surface of immature normal stem cells. To ensure maximum killing, target antigens with a high density on the surface of tumor cells, but present on a minority of immature clonogenic tumor stem cells are targeted. The drawback is that tumor immunophenotyping is performed on readily accessible mature tumor cells but cannot yet be done on the clonogenic immature tumor cell compartment. Negative selection is accomplished by one of several methods. These are described below.

Monoclonal Antibodies for Purging. Cocktails of antibodies give better results and several rounds of incubation yield higher destruction for complement lysis.[96] Most of these monoclonal antibodies are of murine origin because IGM isotypes are better for complement fixation. Immunomodulation, where the antigen is internalized after antibody presentation, reduces the fixation of the antibody for both lysis or immunomagnetic depletion, and can be partly prevented by incubation at 4°C.

Complement-Mediated Cytolysis. Investigators in Boston for NHL[97–100] and in Minneapolis for acute lymphocytic leukemia (ALL) have the most experience with monoclonal antibodies and complement-mediated cytolysis. Tumor reduction has been quantified around 2 to 3 logs, but this method has several drawbacks. First, most techniques used rabbit complement. Possible toxicity from the animal proteins precludes further use. Second, lysis of tumor cells is hampered by multiple factors including the heterogeneous expression of antigens on the tumor cell surface that may spare clonogenic immature tumor cells due to lack of a target. Third, the possible low density of antigens on the surface and the modulation phenomenon prevents effective cytolysis. Fourth, an anticomplementary effect of the normal marrow,[101] which has to be overcome by repeated incubation cycles, is cumbersome and expensive. A continuous infusion of fresh complement has, however, been shown to improve the results.[102] Finally, certain tumors are resistant to complement lysis, leading to combination approaches with both drugs and monoclonal antibodies. It appears the best way to target tumor with monoclonal antibodies would require specific typing of each tumor with a specific study of the clonogenic progenitors.

Immunomagnetic Depletion. Immunomagnetic depletion (IMD), in contrast to cytolysis, avoids the need for complement and is effective even in cases when the antigen density is too low to permit adequate cytolysis. IMD is used for either positive selection to purify and concentrate CD34+ cells or to combine this positive selection with negative selection. IMD has been used with efficacy in neuroblastomas,[103] NHL,[104] lung,[105,106] and breast cancer.[107,108] Greater tumor reduction (up to 5 logs) can be achieved with the combination of several antibodies and repeated depletion cycles.

Immunotoxins. Immunotoxins combine monoclonal antibodies linked to a toxin, such as ricin, diphtheria toxin, or pokeweed antiviral protein.[109] Most ricin immunotoxins combine specifically targeted monoclonal antibodies to the A chain of ricin. Clinical experience is mostly with T-ALL and NHL with an A chain ricin-anti CD5 immunotoxin (T 101 Ricin)[110,111] and B-cell malignancies with a PAP-anti B immunotoxin.[112] Interest in immunotoxins has recently faded.

Positive Selection

Immature normal stem cells, from the very early LTC-IC to the more committed CFU-GEMM, CFU-GM, BFU-E, and CFU-MK, are CD34+ while more mature myeloid cells and most tumor cells, possibly including their clonogenic progenitor are CD34–.[113] This led to the concept of positive selection and gave rise to several devices aimed at purification and concentration of CD34+ stem cells to build a "tumor-free" graft. Important steps in the development of this new approach have included the identification of the CD34 antigen[114] and the generation of several anti-CD34 monoclonal antibodies. Preclinical studies have shown dogs and monkeys engraft with the CD34+ fraction but not with the CD34– fraction.[115,116] An important finding is that a majority of tumors including breast cancer,[113,117] small cell lung cancer, neuroblastomas, and multiple myeloma are CD34–; concentrating CD34+ cells reduces tumor contamination. Positive selection is not applied to AL as leukemic cells are CD34+. There is considerable clinical experience showing a 2 to 5 log tumor reduction in the CD34+ purified fraction for all the malignancies cited above, good safety and tolerance of the reinfused CD34+ concentrate, and successful engraftment of patients after myeloablative treatment including total body irradiation (TBI). While positive selection has been successful for NHL,[118] recent work suggests early clonogenic lymphoma progenitors may be CD34+.[119] This has directed efforts toward a double selection process to purify further the CD34+ fraction to retain only CD34+/CD19– stem cells that constitute the optimal purified tumor-free graft.

Presently, there are four primary technologies that concentrate and purify CD34+ cells. In theory, these techniques can also be used to concentrate and purify other cell populations, depending on the antibodies used. The *immunoadsorption technique* selects cells based on affinity between compounds. Cells are incubated, separated, and washed so that CD34+ cells are collected and cryopreserved. The positive selection of CD34+ cells using this procedure results in a mean 2.5 to 3 log reduction in T cells and/or a mean 3 log reduction in tumor cells. Reduction of T cells is used in protocols trying to reduce graft versus host reactions after allogeneic stem cell transplantation. In addition, reduction in both B and T cells is potentially interesting when considering autologous stem cell transplantation (ASCT) for autoimmune diseases. *Paramagnetic microsphere immunodepletion* involves sensitizing CD34+ cells to a murine anti-human monoclonal antibody directed against the CD34 antigen. The CD34+ cells are then rosetted with paramagnetic microspheres (Dynabeads®) and magnetically separated from the remaining nontarget cells. After being released from the Dynabeads the CD34+ cells are released into a collection container. Positive selection with this method nonspecifically depletes unwanted cells. Further depletion of specific cell types can be accomplished by both positive and negative selection in a single procedure. In this procedure, when the CD34+ cells are released for collection, targeted non-CD34+ cells, such as tumor cells or T cells, are simultaneously retained in the primary separation chamber. *Dextran paramagnetic particles for immunodepletion* is similar to paramagnetic microsphere depletion except particles with the cells of interest (generally CD34+) are retained by a high magnetic field on a column. When the column is removed from the magnet, its rapid demagnetization allows the release of retained cells. Dextran particles to which the cells are attached can be reinfused directly to patients, with no need to detach them first.

The above three techniques (immunoadsorption technique, paramagnetic microsphere immunodepletion, and dextran paramagnetic particles for immunodepletion) are widely used and the choice of one over the other is often a matter of technician training, running protocols, and the purpose and nature of the intended cell selection. Overall worldwide experience indicates the CD34+ cell purity and the CD34+ total cell recovery are higher with the immunomagnetic depletion techniques, especially using dextran microparticles. Purity reaches 95 percent and recovery 70 percent. However, the selected CD34+ fractions may not be totally superimposable from one technique to the other. This can partly be explained by differences in the nature of the anti-CD34 antibodies used, and the differences in CD34 antigen density at the surface of the target cell subpopulations. Whatever the technique, it is presently accepted that a marrow graft should contain at least 1×10^6 CD34+ cells/kg and a PB concentrate at least 2.5×10^6 CD34+ cells/kg to ensure safe engraftment.

Last, *high speed cell sorting* targets very early human multipotent hematopoietic precursors. These express the CD34+ antigen and are a subset with little uptake of the fluorescent mitochondrial dye rhodamine 123. In the human SCID mouse model, the rare human Thy1+/CD34+ lineage negative cell population successfully engrafts.[120] There is a high-speed cell sorter enabling the purification and concentration of the small fraction of human Thy1+/CD34+ lineage negative progenitors after only one day. Since tumor cells do not express this complex combination of antigens, selection for this subset also reduces tumor contamination by 4 to 6 log in all malignant diseases. Phase 1 and 2 trials are currently under way, including patients with multiple myelomas.

Liquid Long-Term Cultures and Expansion for Purging

A technique of long-term culture exists that, when applied to AML marrow in relapse, appeared to selectively destroy the leukemic clones over normal hematopoietic progenitors. This has been then used to purge marrow collected in first complete remission (CR).[121,122] The first successful attempt at purging BM or PB from Philadelphia-positive cells with the goal to engraft patients with the residual Philadelphia negative stem cell pool has been reported.[123] In a 10-day liquid culture, the Philadelphia-positive stem cell pool declined, while Philadelphia-negative cells, even when previously undetected, appeared and developed. Of 22 patients who ultimately autografted, 16 were alive at 68 months post-transplant, with 5 in persisting partial or complete cytogenetic remission. Additional selection pressures such as IL-2 have been used in the liquid cultures to induce NK antileukemic activity.[124]

A modern approach of tumor purging through liquid long-term culture, presently under evaluation, is to first reduce the volume of the aliquot (marrow or PB), select the CD34+ cells from this reduced aliquot, and then expand them in liquid culture with an optimal cytokine cocktail. A 1 to 2 log tumor contamination reduction would result from starting with a small aliquot, followed by a further 2 log reduction resulting from the CD34+ positive selection. Recent experiments have shown that in parallel to the successful expansion of the normal stem cells, several solid tumor cell lines[125] and human lymphoma cells[126]

contaminating the initial graft do not expand and in fact disappear under the level of detection by molecular biology.

Evidence and Arguments in Favor of In Vitro Purging

Arguments in favor of in vitro purging have accumulated over the years and have been developed by disease. Preclinical and clinical data will be reviewed here for AL and B-cell malignancies (NHL and multiple myelomas).

Theoretical Considerations and Preclinical Models, Acute Leukemia

At time of initial diagnosis, the tumor burden in an individual patient with AL is around 10^{12} leukemic cells. CR following modern induction chemotherapy lowers the residual tumor burden to somewhere below 10^{10} leukemic cells. High-dose intensification used either before allogeneic BMT or before ABMT can further decrease the tumor burden. It is believed that a residual tumor level at 10^5 or below can be controlled by the patient's own immune surveillance. Extrapolating from the BNML model, the LD_{50} for a 70-kg human would be 10^3 leukemic cells. It is estimated that the number of clonogenic leukemic cells infused with the autograft in the absence of any in vitro treatment may be as low as 10^3 in a 70-kg adult. While most purging procedures are reported to achieve a tumor reduction of 4 to 6 log , even one log of tumor reduction in the graft may be of considerable importance considering the LD_{50} estimate. Therefore, it has been suggested that a decrease of one single log after purging in vitro may have the same effect as the graft versus leukemia effect associated with allogeneic transplantation and GvHD.

The BNML model has been extensively studied as a preclinical model of ABMT in man. The following conclusions have been reached.[127-129] Leukemic rats submitted to TBI died in aplasia within 7 to 12 days. Leukemic rats submitted to TBI followed by syngeneic marrow purposely contaminated with 2 percent leukemic cells died within 16 to 21 days from recurrent disease. However, leukemic rats autografted but purged in vitro with 4HC recovered hematopoietic function and had no recurrence of the disease provided that the dose of 4HC used was above 60 nm/ml. This indicated purging was effective only above a certain threshold. Reinvestigation with the IPC 81 subline studies further showed that 1 log of tumor infused to the rat reduced the survival span by 7 days, and indicated that a narrow dose margin existed for optimal purging and engraftment. From these experiments, it was predicted that for humans, effective purging and safe engraftment would correspond to a dose of 4HC leading to a residual CFU-GM population of around 1 percent. Although the BNML rat model of human AML has been the most extensively studied, it is of importance that similar results have been observed in other models, in particular the mouse L1210 model for human ALL.

Minimal Residual Disease (MRD) and Outcome in Acute Leukemia

Numerous trials have shown that detection of minimal residual disease (MRD) in AL is associated with a higher risk of relapse.[130-135] This was true in childhood ALL,[130,131] AML,[132-134] and post–allogeneic bone marrow transplantation in CML.[135] Therefore, the lower the level of MRD achieved either by conventional chemotherapy or with stem cell transplantation, the higher the likelihood to obtain cure.

Marrow Versus PB Graft Tumor Contamination

Historically, the main purpose for shifting from marrow to PB stem cells was that PB of patients in CR would be tumor free or at least less contaminated than marrow. It was soon observed that the kinetics of engraftment with PB were faster than with marrow, but also that PB contaminated by leukemic cells resulted in very early relapses especially when reinfusing leukapheresis were performed immediately at the time of aplasia recovery after initial induction treatment.[136-138] In ALL as in AML, mobilization of PB stem cells has been shown to be accompanied by mobilization of leukemic cells and a corresponding high relapse rate.[139,140]

Table 55–3 highlights clinical experience using purging in vitro in AL. Numerous centers have used cyclophosphamide derivatives to purge marrow in patients with AL with favorable results, but only few teams have had the simultaneous experience of autografting with purged or unpurged marrow.[141,142] Studies trying to correlate the efficacy of in vitro treatment to the outcome have been retrospectively carried out in Baltimore,[102] Paris,[61,70] and Parma.[62,63] It appears that more aggressive purging may result in lower residual CFU-GM and thus fewer tumor cells with fewer relapses. As a consequence, some now try to obtain the highest marrow dose to reinfuse to each patient, following aggressive purging. From studies in Table 55–3, we concluded

that better results were achieved with the highest doses of stem cells provided that contamination by tumor cells is avoided. It is postulated that the way the marrow is treated with cyclophosphamide derivatives influences the outcome, particularly a lower relapse incidence linked to more aggressive purging and/or dose adjustment to individual sensitivity.

Theoretical Considerations in NHL

Both sensitive culture techniques and molecular biology have clearly established that marrow and blood involvement by tumor are frequent in NHL, even in the absence of detectable abnormal cells by routine cytology and histology. Benjamin et al.[143] demonstrated in 1983 that derivation of lymphoma cell lines could be obtained from microscopically normal bone marrow in patients with undifferentiated lymphoma, proving the existence of occult tumor. Similar observations were reported for Burkitt's lymphoma by Philip et al.[144] In a larger experience, Sharp et al. showed that up to one-third of patients with intermediate to high-grade NHL had clonogenic lymphoma cells in morphologically normal marrow at the time of the harvest for autografting.[145] Tumor markers that can be used for detection of MRD and monitoring of purging in NHL include the t(14;18) translocation occurring in 30 percent of aggressive NHL and 85 percent of follicular NHL,[146,147] and the rearrangement of the CDRIII region of the immunoglobulin heavy chain, which can be detected by PCR in almost all patients.[148]

Overall, all studies showing detection of lymphoma tumor cells are associated with a poor outcome. In the Omaha experience, patients whose cultures grew clonal lymphoma had a significantly poorer outcome than the patients with tumor

Table 55–3. Experience With In Vitro Purging, Acute Leukemia

Location	Purging	Tumor Measure in Graft	Results
Stanford[108]	4HC vs. unpurged	Need data	No difference in RI or survival
Baltimore[65,111,112]	Constant dose 4HC	Indirectly by residual fraction of normal CFU-GM	Probability to remain in CR: 40 percent for CFU-GM below median 18 percent for CFU-GM above median L-CFC more sensitive to 4HC than CFU-GM, RI 15 percent L-CFC equally sensitive as CFU-GM, RI 80 percent
Paris[61,70]	Mafosfamide	Indirectly by residual fraction of late CFU-GM	Greater marrow doses prepurging had greater LFS (59 vs. 42 percent, $p = .01$) and lower TRM (6 vs. 30 percent, $p = .0001$) Lowest doses postpurging had lower RI (31 vs. 50 percent, $p = .02$)
Parma[62,63]	Mafosfamide	Need data	Need data
EBMT Int 1 Registry[119,120]	Mafosfamide	Need data	Post-TBI, purged RI 29 percent, unpurged RI 50 percent Slow responders, purged RI 20 percent, unpurged RI 61 percent
IBMTR-ABMTR (Carole Miller, unpublished)	4HC and unpurged		3-yr RI lower in CR1 (40 vs. 70 percent) and in CR2 (50 vs. 90 percent) LFS better in CR1 (50 vs. 30 percent) and in CR2 (40 vs. 15 percent)

Abbreviations: RI, relapse incidence; LFS, leukemia-free survival; TRM, transplant-related mortality.

Table 55–4. Retrospective Experience of In Vitro Purging for NHL

Location	Purging Method	Tumor Detection in Graft	Results
Dana Farber, Boston[97–100]	Monoclonal antibodies with rabbit complement	PCR for Bcl2-JH translocation	RI 7 percent with noncontaminated marrow, 46 percent contaminated marrow. DFS noncontaminated marrow 85 percent, contaminated marrow 22 percent
Hospital Saint-Antoine, Paris[69]	Mafosfamide, adjusted and constant dose	Indirectly by median residual CFU-GM/kg	Constant dose mafosfamide: RI 25 percent below CFU-GM median, 70 percent above median. EFS below CFU-GM median 64 percent, above median 25 percent
EBMT Lymphoma Registry[153]	Purged and matched controls, Need data for method	Need data	No difference between purged and unpurged in either OS or PFS

Abbreviations: RI, relapse incidence; DFS, disease-free survival; EFS, event-free survival; EBMT, European Blood and Marrow Transplant; OS, overall survival; PFS, progression-free survival.

cell–negative cultures.[145,149] At the Dana Farber Cancer Center, PCR positivity for Bcl2-Jh translocation in the marrow and to a lesser extent in the blood has been associated with an increased risk of relapse.[99] It is unclear in all studies whether the detection of tumor cells alone is a surrogate marker for the aggressiveness of the disease or whether the infusion of tumor cells has induced relapse or disease progression.

Two techniques are used to detect lymphoma tumor cells, the culture technique and PCR. Detection is important as lymphomatous clonogenic cells may be protected from chemotherapy in the marrow through adherence to stromal cells.[145,149] The culture technique is the least sensitive; only 30 percent of inoculum positive by PCR gives rise to lymphomatous colonies. However, detection of clonogenic progenitors can provide information about abnormalities of the tumor cells, such as p53 expression and/or an overexpression of Bcl2. PCR is much more sensitive than cultures and may detect as few as 1 tumor cell per 10^5 normal cells. The most routine PCR method is the detection of the t(14;18) translocation. Detection of the BCL2-JH transcript is the most sensitive and reliable. Less sensitive PCR amplification of the CDRIII region can be applied to almost all patients with B-cell lymphoma using primers corresponding to conserved sequences within the V and J regions.

Theoretical Considerations in Multiple Myeloma

The problem of the contamination of the graft by tumor cells in multiple myeloma (MM) is similar to NHL, with a few exceptions. One is that culture techniques to detect residual tumor are not routinely available. Also, rearrangement of the heavy chain IGH is the only marker presently available. Last, the question whether tumor cells are also present in peripheral blood, especially in patients responding to chemotherapy, has been long debated. Cytological PB contamination by plasmocytic cells is seldom observed and true plasma cell leukemia represents less than 1 percent of multiple myelomas. However, several recent studies evaluating myeloma tumor cell contamination through detection of their immunophenotype have clearly established that the majority of leukaphereses are contaminated at high levels up to 10 percent.[150] Further, mobilization of CD34+ cells by cyclophosphamide and G-CSF induces parallel mobilization of myeloma cells.[150,151] Interestingly, the use of GM-CSF would induce different kinetics of mobilization, allowing for a window of collection with less or no contamination.[152]

Experience at two single institutions, Dana Farber[97–100] and Hospital Saint-Antoine in Paris,[69] and a retrospective analysis of European Blood and Marrow Transplant (EBMT) Lymphoma Registry[153] data are detailed in Table 55–4. These data suggest that reinfusion of lymphoma cells with the graft contribute to relapse; however, the possibility that ability to purge the marrow corresponded to a less aggressive NHL cannot be ruled out.[97–100] The Paris report suggests that less residual CFU-GM postpurging indirectly reflects more aggressive purging, which resulted in fewer relapses.[69] Experiences in these institutions cannot sort out the impact of MRD and purging on outcome. Both are important prognostic factors for the probability of relapse. However, the characteristics of the graft such as contamination or effectiveness of purging predict outcome. The vast majority of ASCT for NHL is presently done with unpurged PB.

Gene Marking Experiments to Evaluate the Efficacy of Purging

The marking of infused cells may be the best way to answer several important questions regarding ASCT and purging. Gene marking can trace the origin of relapse and has been studied extensively since the early 1990s.[154–160] In the first reported marking studies, patients with AML[159] or neuroblastomas[161] autografted with unpurged marrow, had one-third of their graft marked by the neomycin-resistance gene using a retroviral vector. Three of four relapsing AML patients had this marker on malignant cells. One patient also had an atypic immunophenotype (CD34+/CD56+) and a complex chromosome translocation t(8;21), so that it was possible to show in a single clonogenic cell the coexpression of the AML-ETO fusion protein and the marker neomycin-resistance gene.[159] In neuroblastoma,[161] five of nine patients receiving a gene marked autograft relapsed, four in the marrow and one in the liver. In the four medullary relapses, tumor cells were found coexpressing the neuroblastoma specific GD2 antigen and the neo-R gene. In the fifth patient, gene marked tumor cells also were detected in the liver.

These data confirm that unpurged grafts may contain tumor cells, which are later detected in patients who relapse, either in medullary or in extramedullary sites. It is unknown if tumor cells from the autograft or elsewhere in the body are actually responsible for relapse. Patients may relapse anyway, independent of graft status. Gene marking is limited by several difficulties. One is that gene transfer efficiency has remained low and therefore only marked relapses are informative. In addition, the absence of marking in reevolving tumor may indicate the relapse has originated from another location, but may also be a result of insufficient marking.

CONCLUSION

Graft engineering continues to evolve as attempts are made to both decrease the toxicity of and improve the efficacy of stem cell transplantation. We have seen significant changes over the past decade; however, many questions remain about the optimal graft components and manipulation prior to transplantation.

REFERENCES

1. Current good tissue practice for manufactures of human cellular and tissue-based products; Inspection and enforcement; Proposed rule. 21 CFR Part 1271, June 8, 2001.
2. Standards for Hematopoietic Progenitor Cell Collection, Processing and Transplantation. FAHCT, First Edition, September 1996.
3. Thomas ED, Storb R: Technique for human marrow grafting. Blood 36:507–515, 1970.
4. Batinic D, Marusic M, Pavletic Z et al: Relationship between differing volumes of bone marrow aspirates and their cellular composition. Bone Marrow Transplant 6:103–107, 1990.
5. Meagher RC, Herzig RH: Techniques of harvesting and cryopreservation of stem cells. Hematol Oncol Clin North Am 7:501–531.
6. Buckner CD, Clift RA, Sanders JE et al: Marrow harvesting from normal donors. Blood 64:630–634, 1984.
7. York A, Clift RA, Sanders JE, Buckner CD: Recombinant human erythropoietin (rh-Epo) administration to normal marrow donors. Bone Marrow Transplant 10:415–417, 1992.
8. To LB, Haylock DN, Kimber RJ, Juttner CA: High levels of circulating haematopoietic stem cells in very early remission from acute nonlymphocytic leukemia and their collection and cryopreservation. Br J Haematol 58:399–410, 1984.
9. Juttner CO, To LB, Haylockk DN et al: Circulating autologous stem cells collected in very early remission from acute nonlymphocytic leukemia produce prompt but incomplete haematopoietic reconstitution after high dose melphalan or supralethal chemotherapy. Br J Haematol 61:739–745, 1985.
10. Socinski MA, Elias A, Schnipper L et al: Granulocyte-macrophage colony stimulating factor expands the circulating haematopoietic progenitor cell compartment in man. Lancet 1:1194–1198, 1988.
11. Peters WP, Rosner G, Ross M et al: Comparative effects of granulocyte-macrophage colony stimulating factor and granulocyte colony stimulating factor on priming peripheral blood progenitor cells for use with autologous bone marrow after high dose chemotherapy. Blood 81:1709–1719, 1993.
12. Passos-Coehlo JL, Braine HG, Davis JM et al: Predictive factors for peripheral blood progenitor cell collections using a single large-volume leukapheresis after cyclophosphamide and granulocyte-macrophage colony stimulating factor mobilization. J Clin Oncol 13:705–714, 1995.
13. Lapierre V, Kuentz M, Tiberghien P: Allogeneic peripheral blood hematopoietic stem cell transplantation: Guidelines for red blood cell immunohematological assessment and transfusion practice. Societe Francaise de Greffe de Moelle. Bone Marrow Transplant 25:507–512, 2000.
14. Blalock HA, Gilmore MJ, Prentice HG et al: ABO-incompatible bone marrow transplantation: Removal of red blood cells from donor marrow avoiding recipient antibody depletion. Lancet 2:1061–1064, 1982.
15. Brunett P, Sands K, Bolwell B et al: Autologous red blood cell salvage from bone marrow collected for transplant. Transfusion 28:255, 1988.
16. Warkentin PI, Hilden JM, Kersey JH et al: Transplantation of major ABO-incompatible bone marrow depleted of red blood cells by hydroxyethyl starch. Vox Sang 48:89–104, 1985.
17. Carciero R, Valeri CR: Isolation of mononuclear leukocytes in a plastic bag system using Ficoll-Hypaque. Vox Sang 49:373–380, 1985.
18. English D, Lamberson R, Graves V et al: Semiautomated processing of bone marrow grafts for transplantation. Transfusion 29:12–16, 1989.
19. Dragani A, Angelini A, Iacone A et al: Comparison of five methods for concentrating progenitor cells in human marrow transplantation. Blut 60:278–281, 1990.
20. Mazur P: The role of intracellular freezing in the death of cells cooled at supraoptimal rates. Cryobiology 14:251–272, 1977.
21. Takahashi T, Hirsh A, Erbe E, Williams FJ: Mechanism of cryoprotection by extracellular polymeric solutes. Biophys J 54:509–518, 1988.
22. Rowley SD, Anderson GL: Effect of DMSO exposure without cryopreservation on hematopoietic progenitor cells. Bone Marrow Transplant 11:389–393, 1993.
23. Davis JM, Rowley SD, Braine HG et al: Clinical toxicity of cryopreserved bone marrow graft infusion. Blood 75:781–786, 1990.
24. Rowley SD: Hematopoietic stem cell cryopreservation. A review of current techniques. J Hematother 1:233–250, 1992.
25. Attarian H, Feng Z, Buckner CD, MacLeod B, Rowley SD: Long-term cryopreservation of bone marrow for autologous transplantation. Bone Marrow Transplant 17:425–430, 1996.
26. Vallera DA, Soderling CC, Carlson GJ et al: Bone marrow transplantation across major histocompatibility barriers in mice. Effect of elimination of T-cells from donor grafts by treatment with monoclonal THY 1.2 plus complement or antibody alone. Transplantation 31:218–222, 1981.
27. Onoe K, Fernandes G, Good RA: Humoral and cell mediated immune responses in fully allogeneic bone marrow chimera in mice. J Exp Med 151:115–132, 1980.
28. Reisner Y, Kapoor N, Kirkpatrick D et al: Transplantation for severe combined immunodeficiency with HLA- A, B, D, DR incompatible parental marrow cells fractionated by soybean agglutinin and sheep red blood cells. Blood 61:341–348, 1983.
29. O'Reilly RJ, Collins NH, Kernan NA et al: Transplantation of marrow depleted of T cells by soybean lectin agglutination and E rosette depletion: Major histocompatibility complex-related graft resistance in leukemic transplant recipients. Transplant Proc 17:455–459, 1985.
30. Noga SJ, Cremo CA, Duff SC et al: Large scale separation of human bone marrow by counterflow elutriation. J Immunol Meth 92:211–218, 1986.

31. Donnenberg AD, Wagner JE, Noga SJ et al: Lymphocyte depletion by counterflow centrifugal elutriation: Analysis of engraftment. Exp Hematol 17:541–550, 1989.

32. Wagner JE, Santos GW, Noga SJ et al: Bone marrow graft engineering by counterflow centrifugal elutriation: Results of a phase I/II clinical trial. Blood 75:1370–1377, 1990.

33. O'Donnell PJ, Jones RJ, Vogelsang GB et al: CD34+ stem cell augmentation of elutriated allogeneic bone marrow grafts: Results of a phase II clinical trial of engraftment and graft-versus-host disease prophylaxis in high risk hematologic malignancies. Bone Marrow Transplant 22:947–955, 1998.

34. Waldmann G, Or R, Hale G et al: Elimination of graft versus host disease by in vitro depletion of alloreactive lymphocytes using a monoclonal rat anti-human lymphocyte antibody (CAMPATH-1M). Lancet 2:483–486, 1984.

35. Dreger P, Viehmann K, Steinmann J et al: G-CSF mobilized peripheral blood progenitor cells for allogeneic transplantation: Comparison of different T-cell depletion strategies using different CD34+ selection systems or CAMPATH1. Ex Hematol 23:147–154, 1995.

36. Munn RK, Henslee-Downey PJ, Romond EH et al: Treatment of leukemia with partially matched related bone marrow transplantation. Bone Marrow Transplant 19:421–427, 1997.

37. Siena S, Villa S, Bonadonna G et al: Specific ex-vivo depletion on human bone marrow T lymphocytes by an anti-pan-T cell (CD5) ricin A chain immunotoxin. Transplantation 43:421–426, 1987.

38. Champlin R, Ho W, Gajewski J et al: Selective depletion of CD8+ T lymphocytes for prevention of graft-versus-host disease after allogeneic bone marrow transplantation. Blood 76:418–423, 1990.

39. Soiffer RJ, Fairclough D, Robertson M et al: CD6-depleted allogeneic bone marrow transplantation for acute leukemia in first complete remission. Blood 89:3039–3047, 1997.

40. Civin CI, Strauss LC, Brovall C et al: Antigenic analysis of hematopoiesis III. A hematopoietic progenitor cell surface antigen defined by a monoclonal antibody raised against KG 1a cells. J Immunol 133:157–165, 1984.

41. Aversa F, Tabilio A, Velardi A et al: Treatment of high-risk acute leukemia with T-cell depleted stem cells from related donors with one fully mismatched HLA haplotype. N Eng J Med 339:1186–1193, 1998.

42. Stainer CJ, Miflin G, Anderson S et al: A comparison of two different systems for CD34+ selection of autologous or allogeneic PBPC collection. J Hematother 7:375–383, 1998.

43. Champlin RE, Passweg JR, Zhang MJ et al: T-cell depletion of bone marrow transplants for leukemia from donors other than HLA-identical siblings: Advantage of T-cell antibodies with narrow specificities. Blood 95:3996–4003, 2000.

44. Gorin NC: Peripheral blood stem cells in transplantation. Baillieres Best Pract Res Clin Haematol 12:8–15, 1999.

45. Reiffers J, Bernard P, David B et al: Successful autologous transplantation with peripheral blood in a patient with acute leukaemia. Exp Hematol 14:312–315, 1986.

46. Sharp JG: Pathogenesis of tumor cell infiltration in the milieu of hematopoietic support. In Gribben JG (ed.): The Role of Tumor Purging in Autologous Transplantation, p. 21. Discovery International, Deerfield, IL, 1997.

47. Lemoli RM, Fortuna A, Motta MR et al: Concomitant mobilization of plasma cells and hematopoietic progenitors into peripheral blood of multiple myeloma patients: Positive selection and transplantation of enriched CD34+ cells to remove circulating tumor cells. Blood 87:1625–1634, 1996.

48. Sutherland HJ, Eaves CJ, Eaves AC et al: Characterization and partial purification of human marrow cells capable of initiating long term hematopoiesis in vitro. Blood 74:1563–1570, 1989.

49. Weaver A, Ryder J, Testa NG: Measurement of long term culture initiating cell (LTC-ICs) using limiting dilution: Comparison of endpoints and stromal support. Exp Hematol 25:1333–1338, 1997.

50. Breems DA, Blokland EA, Neben S et al: Frequency analysis of human primitive hematopoietic stem cell subsets using a cobblestone area forming cell assay. Leukemia 8:1095–1104, 1994.

51. Ploemacher RE, Van der Sluijs JP, Voerman JSA et al: An in vitro limiting dilution assay of long term repopulating hematopoietic stem cells in the mouse. Blood 74:2755–2763, 1989.

52. Lapidot T, Sirard C, Vormoor J et al: A cell initiating human acute myeloid leukemia after transplantation into SCID mice. Nature 367:645–648, 1994.

53. Cohen SBA, Madrigal JA: Reduced lymphocyte responses in cord blood. 3rd Eurocord transplant concerted action works, foundation Marcel Mérieux Conference Center, Annecy, France, May 18–20, 1998 (abstract).

54. Toren A, Rechavi G: What really cures in autologous bone marrow transplantation? A possible role for dimethylsulfoxide. Med Hypoth 41:495–498, 1993.

55. Sharma B, Vaziri ND: Augmentation of human natural killer cell activity by cyclophosphamide in vitro. Cancer Res 44:3258–3261, 1984.

56. Verdonck LF, Heesben EC, van Heugten HG: The cytotoxicity of alkyl-lysophospholipid on clonogenic leukemia cells and on normal bone marrow progenitor cells is highly, but differentially, increased by cryopreservation. Bone Marrow Transplant 9:241–245, 1992.

57. Giarratana MC, Gorin NC, Douay L: Plasma interacts with mafosfamide toxicity to normal haematopoietic progenitor cells: Impact on in vitro marrow purging. Nouv Rev Fr Hematol 37:125–130, 1995.

58. Douay L, Giarratana MC, Labopin M et al: Characterization of late and early hematopoietic progenitor/stem cell sensitivity to mafosfamide. Bone Marrow Transplant 15:769–775, 1995.

59. Douay L, Mary JY, Giarratana MC et al: Establishment of a reliable experimental procedure for bone marrow purging with mafosfamide (ASTA Z 7557). Exp Hematol 17:429–432, 1989.

60. Gorin N, Douay L, Laporte J et al: Autologous bone marrow transplantation using marrow incubated with ASTA-Z 7557 in adult acute leukemia. Blood 67:1367–1376, 1986.

61. Laporte J, Douay L, Lopez M et al: One hundred twenty five adult patients with primary acute leukemia autografted with marrow purged by mafosfamide. A 10 year single institution experience. Blood 84:3810–3818, 1994.

62. Rizzoli V, Carlo Stella C: Stem cell purging: An intriguing dilemma. Exp Hematol 23:296–302, 1995.

63. Carlo Stella C, Mangoni L, Almici C et al: Differential sensitivity of adherent CFU-Blast, CFU-MIX, BFUE, and CFU-GM to mafosfamide: Implications for adjusted dose purging in autologous bone marrow transplantation. Exp Hematol 20:328–333, 1992.

64. Gordon MY, Goldman JM, Gordon-Smith EC: 4-hydroperoxy-cyclophosphamide inhibits proliferation by human granulocyte-macrophage colony forming cells but spares more primitive progenitor cells. Leuk Res 9:1017–1021, 1985.

65. Lopez M, du Puy-Montbrun MC, Douay L et al: Standardization and characterization of the procedure for in vitro treatment of human bone marrow with cyclophosphamide derivatives. Clin Lab Haematol 7:327–334, 1985.

66. Santos GW, Colvin OM: Pharmacological purging of bone marrow with reference to autografting. Clin Haematol 15:67–83, 1986.

67. Yeager A, Kaizer H, Santos G et al: Autologous bone marrow transplantation in patients with acute non lymphocytic leukemia,

using ex vivo marrow treatment with 4-hydroperoxycyclophosphamide. N Engl J Med 315:141–147, 1986.

68. Herve P, Tamayo E, Peters A: Autologous stem cell grafting in acute myeloid leukemia: Technical approach of marrow incubation in vitro with pharmacologic agents (prerequisite for clinical application). Br J Haematol 53:683–685, 1983.

69. Fouillard L, Laporte JP, Labopin M et al. Autologous stem cell transplantation for non-Hodgkin's lymphoma. The role of graft purging and radiotherapy post transplant. Results of a retrospective analysis on 120 patients autografted in a single institution. J Clin Oncol 16:2803–2816, 1998.

70. Gorin NC, Labopin M, Laporte JP et al: Importance of marrow dose on posttransplant outcome in acute leukemia: Models derived from patients autografted with mafosfamide-purged marrow at a single institution. Exp Hematol 27:1822–1830, 1999.

71. Skorski T, Kawalec M, Hoser G et al: The kinetics of immunologic and hematologic recovery in mice after lethal total body irradiation and reconstitution with syngeneic bone marrow cells treated or untreated with mafosfamide (Asta Z 7654). Bone Marrow Transplant 3:543–551, 1988.

72. Almici C, Manoni L, Carlo-Stella C et al: Natural killer cell regeneration after transplantation with mafosfamide purged autologous bone marrow. Bone Marrow Transplant 16:95–101, 1995.

73. Bullock G, Tang C, Tourkina E et al: Effect of combined treatment with interleukin-3 and interleukin-6 on 4-hydroperoxycyclophosphamide induced programmed cell death or apoptosis in human myeloid leukemia cells. Exp Hematol 21:1640–1647, 1993.

74. Tutschka PJ, Korbling M, Hess AD et al: Prevention of graft versus host disease (GVHD) by chemoseparation of marrow cells. Transplant Proc 13:1202–1206, 1981.

75. Yeager A, Colvin M, Santos GW: Pharmacologic purging of bone marrow (BM): Effects of bleomycin on normal and leukemic rat marrow cells. Blood 69:804a, 1984.

76. Stiff PJ, Wustrow T, De Risi M: An in vitro murine model of bone marrow purification of tumor by VP 16-213. Blood 60:618a, 1982.

77. Lemoli RM, Gulati SC: In vitro cytotoxicity of VP-16-213 and nitrogen mustard: Agonistic on tumor cells but not on normal human bone marrow progenitors. Exp Hematol 18:1008–1012, 1990.

78. Motta MR, Mangianti S, Rizzi S et al: Pharmacological purging of minimal residual disease from peripheral blood stem cell collections of acute myeloblastic leukemia patients: Preclinical studies. Exp Hematol 25:1261–1269, 1997.

79. Lemoli RM, Visani G, Leopardi G et al: Autologous transplantation of chemotherapy-purged PBSC collections of high risk leukemic patients: A pilot study. Bone Marrow Transplant 23:235–241, 1999.

80. Gulati S, Acaba L, Yahalom J: Autologous bone marrow transplantation for acute myelogenous leukemia, using 4 hydroperoxycyclophosphamide and VP-16 purged bone marrow. Bone Marrow Transplant 10:129–134, 1992.

81. Dietzfelbinger HF, Kuhn D, Zafferani M et al: Removal of breast cancer cells from bone marrow by in vitro purging with ether lipids and cryopreservation. Cancer Res 53:3747–3751, 1993.

82. Vogler WR, Berdel WE, Olson AC et al: Autologous bone marrow transplantation in acute leukemia with marrow purged with alkyl-lysophospholipid. Blood 80:1423–1429, 1992.

83. Berdel WE, Okamoto S, Reichert A et al: Studies on the role of ether lipids as purging agents in autologous bone marrow transplantation. In Kabara JJ (ed.): The Pharmacological Effects of Lipids III, p. 338. OSC Press, Champaign, IL, 1990.

84. Vogler WR, Olson AC, Okamoto S et al: Experimental studies on the role of alkyl lysophospholipids in autologous bone marrow transplantation. Lipids 22:919–924, 1987.

85. Zimmer BM, Reufi B, Oberberg D et al: Generation of progenitor cell precursors in long term bone marrow cultures after marrow purging with ether lipids. Int J Oncol 7:1307, 1995.

86. Koenigsmann MP, Notter M, Knauff WU et al: Chemopurging of peripheral blood derived progenitor cells by alkyl lysophospholipid and its effect on haematopoietic rescue after high dose therapy. Bone Marrow Transplant 18:549–557, 1996.

87. Hammert LC, Ball ED: Purging marrow or peripheral blood stem cells for autografting. Curr Opin Hematol 4:423–428, 1997.

88. Gulliya KS, Matthews JL, Fay JW et al: Increased survival of normal cells during laser photodynamic therapy: Implications for ex vivo autologous bone marrow purging. Life Sci 42:2651–2656, 1988.

89. Atzpodien J, Gulati SC, Strife A et al: Photoradiation models for the clinical ex vivo treatment of autologous bone marrow grafts. Blood 70:484–489, 1987.

90. Vaerman JL, Moureau P, Deldime F et al: Antisense oligodeoxyribunucleotides suppress hematologic cell growth through stepwise release of deoxyribonucleotides. Blood 90:331–339, 1997.

91. Gewirtz AW, Luger S, Sokol D et al: Treating human myelogenous leukemia with c-myb antisense oligodeoxynucleotides: Two years clinical experience. J Invest Med 44:279a, 1996.

92. de Fabritiis P, Petti MC, Montefusco E et al: Bcr-abl antisense oligodeoxynucleotide in vitro purging and autologous leukemia in advanced phase. Blood 91:3156–3162, 1998.

93. Luger SM, Ratajczak MZ, Stadtmauer EA et al: Autografting for chronic myeloid leukemia (CML) with C-MYB antisense oligodeoxynucleotide purged bone marrow: A preliminary report. Blood 84:151a, 1994.

94. O'Brien SG, Rule RA, Ratajczak MZ et al: Autografting for CML using bone marrow purged with MYB antisense oligonucleotide. Br J Haematol 89:2a, 1995.

95. Carlo-Stella C, Dottim G, Mangoni L et al: Selection of myeloid progenitors lacking bcr/abl mRNA in chronic myelogenous leukemia patients after in vitro treatment with the tyrosine-kinase inhibitor genistein. Blood 88:3091–3100, 1996.

96. Bast RC, Ritz J, Lipton JM et al: Elimination of leukemic cells from human bone marrow using monoclonal antibodies and complement. Cancer Res 43:1389–1394, 1983.

97. Gribben JG, Freedman AS, Neuberg D et al: Immunologic purging assessed by PCR before autologous bone marrow transplantation for B cell lymphoma. N Engl J Med 325:1525–1533, 1991.

98. Gribben JG, Nadler LM: Bone marrow purging for autologous bone marrow transplantation. Leuk Lymphoma 11:141–148, 1993.

99. Gribben JG, Neuberg D, Barber M et al: Detection of residual lymphoma cells by polymerase chain reaction in peripheral blood is significantly less predictive for relapse than detection in bone marrow. Blood 83:3800–3807, 1994.

100. Freedman AS, Gribben JG, Neuberg D et al: High-dose therapy and autologous bone marrow transplantation in patients with follicular lymphoma during first remission. Blood 88:2780–2786, 1996.

101. Gee AP, Bruce KM, Morris TD et al: Evidence for an anticomplementary factor associated with human bone marrow cells. J Nat Cancer Inst 75:441–445, 1985.

102. Howell AL, Fogg-Leach M, Davis BH et al: Continuous infusion of complement by an automated cell processor enhances cytotoxicity of monoclonal antibody to sensitized leukemia cells. Bone Marrow Transplant 4:317–322, 1989.

103. Combaret V, Favrot MC, Chauvin F et al: Immunomagnetic depletion for malignant cells from autologous bone marrow grafts: From experimental models to clinical trials. J Immunogenet 16:125–136, 1989.

104. Gribben JG, Saporito L, Barber M et al: Bone marrow of non-Hodgkin's lymphoma patients with a bcl-2 translocation can be purged of PCR-detectable lymphoma cells using monoclonal antibodies and immunomagnetic bead depletion. Blood 80:1083–1089, 1992.

105. Vredenburgh JJ, Ball ED: Elimination of small cell carcinoma of the lung from human bone marrow by monoclonal antibodies and immunomagnetic beads. Cancer Res 50:7216–7220, 1990.

106. Elias AD, Pap SA, Bernal SD: Purging of small cell lung cancer-contaminated marrow by monoclonal antibodies and magnetic beads. Prog Clin Biol Res 333:263–275, 1990.

107. Vredenburgh JJ, Simpson W, Memoli VA et al: Reactivity of anti-CD15 monoclonal antibody PM-81 with breast cancer and elimination of breast cancer cell lines from human bone marrow by PM-81 and immunomagnetic beads. Cancer Res 51:2451–2455, 1991.

108. Shpall EJ, Bast RC, Joines WT et al: Immunomagnetic purging of breast cancer from bone marrow for autologous transplantation. Bone Marrow Transplant 7:145–151, 1991.

109. Uckun FM, Kersey JH, Vallera DA et al: Autologous bone marrow transplantation in high risk remission T-lineage acute lymphoblastic leukemia using immunotoxins plus 4 hydroperoxycyclophosphamide for marrow purging. Blood 76:1723–1733, 1990.

110. Preijers FWMB, De Witte T, Wessels JMC et al: Autologous transplantation of bone marrow purged in vitro with anti CD7 (WT1)-ricin A immunotoxin in T cell lymphoblastic leukemia and lymphoma. Blood 74:1152–1158, 1989.

111. Gorin NC, Douay L, Laporte JP et al: Autologous bone marrow transplantation with marrow decontaminated by immunotoxin T 101 in the treatment of leukemia and lymphoma. First clinical observations. Cancer Treat Rep 69:953–959, 1985.

112. Uckun FM, Jaszcz W, Ambrus JL et al: Detailed studies on expression and function of CD19 surface determinant by using B43 monoclonal antibody and the clinical potential of anti CD19 immunotoxins. Blood 71:13–29, 1988.

113. Berenson RJ, Bensinger WI, Andrews RG et al: Positive selection of hematopoietic progenitors from marrow and peripheral blood for transplantation. J Clin Apheresis. 5:74–76, 1990.

114. Andrews RG, Singer JW, Bernstein ID: Monoclonal antibody 12.8 recognizes a 115-KD molecule present on both unipotent and multipotent hematopoietic colony forming cells and their precursors. Blood 67:842–845, 1986.

115. Berenson RJ, Bensinger WI, Kalamasz T et al: Engraftment of dogs with Ia-positive marrow cells isolated by avidin-biotin immunoadsorption. Blood 69:1363–1367, 1987.

116. Berenson RJ, Andrews RG, Bensinger WI et al: Antigen CD34+ marrow cells engraft lethally irradiated baboons. J Clin Invest 81:951–955, 1988.

117. Shpall EJ, Jones RB, Bearman et al: Transplantation of enriched CD34-positive autologous marrow into breast cancer patients following high dose chemotherapy: Influence of CD34 positive peripheral-blood progenitors and growth factors on engraftment. J Clin Oncol 12:28–36, 1994.

118. Gorin NC, Lopez M, Laporte JP et al: Preparation and successful engraftment of purified CD34+ bone marrow progenitor cells in patients with non-Hodgkin's lymphoma. Blood 85:1647–1654, 1995.

119. Macintyre EA, Belanger C, Debert C et al: Detection of clonal CD34+ 19+ progenitors in BM of BCL2-IgH positive follicular lymphoma patients. Blood 86:4691–4698, 1995.

120. Baum CM, Weissman IL, Tsukamoto AS et al: Isolation of a candidate human hematopoietic stem-cell population. Proc Natl Acad Sci U S A 89:2804–2808, 1992.

121. Chang J, Coutinho L, Morgenstern G et al: Reconstitution of hemopoietic system with autologous marrow taken during relapse of acute myeloblastic leukaemia and grown in long term culture. Lancet 1:294–295, 1986.

122. Chang J, Morgenstern G, Coutinho L et al: The use of bone marrow cells grown in long term culture for autologous bone marrow transplantation in acute myeloid leukaemia. An update. Bone Marrow Transplant 4:5–9, 1989.

123. Coulombel L, Kalousek D, Eaves C et al: Long term marrow culture reveals chromosomally normal hematopoietic progenitor cells in patients with Philadelphia chromosome positive chronic myelogenous leukemia. N Engl J Med 308:1493–1498, 1983.

124. Klingemann HG, Deal H, Reid D et al: Design and validation of a clinically applicable culture procedure for the generation of interleukin-2 activated natural killer cells in human bone marrow autografts. Exp Hematol 21:1263–1270, 1993.

125. Vogel W, Behringer D, Scheding S et al: Ex vivo expansion of CD34+ peripheral blood progenitor cells: Implications for the expansion of contaminating tumor cells. Blood 88:2707–2713, 1996.

126. Yao M, Fouillard L, Lemoine F et al: Ex vivo expansion of CD34-positive peripheral blood progenitor cells from patients with non-Hodgkin's lymphoma: No evidence of concomitant expansion of contaminating bcl2/JH positive lymphoma cells. Bone Marrow Transplant 26:497–503, 2000.

127. Sharkis SJ, Santos G, Colvin OM: Elimination of acute myelogenous leukemia cells from marrow and tumor suspensions in the rat with 4 hydroperoxycyclophosphamide. Blood 55:521–523, 1980.

128. Martens A, van Bekkum DW, Hagenbeek A: Minimal residual disease in leukemia: Studies in an animal model for acute myelocytic leukemia (BNML). Int J Cell Clon 8:27–38, 1990.

129. Schultz FW, Martens ACM, Hagenbeek A: The contribution of residual leukemic cells in the graft to leukemia relapse after autologous bone marrow transplantation: Mathematical considerations. Leukemia 3:530–534, 1989.

130. Brisco M, Condon J, Hughess E et al: Outcome prediction in childhood acute lymphoblastic acute leukaemia by molecular quantification of residual disease at the end of induction. Lancet 343:196–200, 1994.

131. Brisco M, Hughes E, Neoh S et al: Relationship between minimal residual disease and outcome in acute lymphoblastic leukemia. Blood 87:5251–5256, 1996.

132. Reading CL, Estey EH, Huh YO et al: Expression of unusual immunophenotype combinations in acute myelogenous leukemia. Blood 81:3083–3090, 1993.

133. Tobal K, Liu-Yin J: Molecular quantitation of minimal residual disease in acute myeloid leukemia with t(8;21) can identify patients in durable remission and predict relapse. Blood 95:815–819, 2000.

134. Lo Coco F, Diverio D, Pandolfi P et al: Molecular evaluation of residual disease as a predictor of relapse in acute promyelocytic leukaemia. Lancet 340:1437–1438, 1992.

135. Felix P, Urbano-Ispizua A, Rozman C et al: Use of quantitative PCR to monitor response to donor leukocyte transfusion (DLT) or alpha interferon (IFN) in patients relapsing after allogeneic stem cell transplantation (allo SCT) for chronic myelocytic leukemia. Blood 88:372a, 1996.

136. Laporte JPH, Gorin NC, Feuchtenbaum J et al: Relapse after autografting with peripheral blood stem cells. Lancet 2:1393, 1987.

137. Korbling M, Hunstein W, Fliedner TM et al: Disease free survival after autologous bone marrow transplantation in patients with acute myelogenous leukemia. Blood 74:1898–1904, 1989.

138. Mehta J, Powles R, Singhal S et al: Peripheral blood stem cell transplantation may result in increased relapse of acute myeloid leukaemia due to reinfusion of a higher number of malignant cells. Bone Marrow Transplant 15:652–653, 1995.

139. Seriu T, Yokota S, Nakao M et al: Prospective monitoring of minimal residual disease during the course of chemotherapy in patients with acute lymphoblastic leukemia and detection of contaminating tumor cells in peripheral blood stem cells for autotransplantation. Leukemia 9:615–623, 1995.

140. Rambaldi A, Borleri G, Dotti G et al: Innovative two step negative selection of granulocyte-colony-stimulating factor-mobilised circulating progenitor cells: Adequacy for autologous and allogeneic transplantation. Blood 91:2189–2196, 1998.

141. Chao NJ, Stein AS, Long GD et al: Busulfan/etoposide-initial experience with a new preparatory regimen for autologous bone marrow transplantation in patients with acute nonlymphoblastic leukemia. Blood 81:319–323, 1993.

142. Tomas JF, Gomez Garcia de Soria V, Pinilla L et al: Bone marrow autotransplantation in acute myeloblastic leukemia in its first complete remission. The clinical results in 41 patients (see comments). Med Clin (Barc) 108:201–206, 1997.

143. Benjamin D, Magrath IT, Douglass EC et al: Derivation of lymphoma cell lines from microscopically normal bone marrow in patients with undifferentiated lymphoma: Evidence of occult bone marrow involvement. Blood 61:1017–1019, 1983.

144. Philip I, Philip T, Favrot M: Establishment of lymphomatous cell lines from bone marrow samples from patients with Burkitt's lymphoma. J Natl Cancer Inst 73:835–840, 1984.

145. Sharp JG, Joshi SS, Armitage JO: Significance of detection of occult non-Hodgkin's lymphoma in histologically uninvolved bone marrow by culture technique. Blood 79:1074–1080, 1992.

146. Yunis JJ, Oken MM, Kaplan ME et al: Distinctive chromosomal abnormalities in histological subtypes of non-Hodgkin's lymphomas. N Engl J Med 307:1231–1236, 1982.

147. Aisenberg AC, Wilkes BM, Jacobson JO: The Bcl-2 gene is rearranged in many diffuse B-cell lymphomas. Blood 71:969–972, 1988.

148. Stewart CG, Potter MN, Oakhill A: Third complementary determining region (CDRIII) sequence analysis in childhood B lineage acute lymphoblastic leukaemia: Implication for the design of oligonucleotide probes for use in monitoring minimal residual disease. Leukemia 6:1213–1219, 1992.

149. Sharp JG, Kessinger A, Mann S et al: Outcome of high dose therapy and autologous transplantation in non Hodgkin's lymphoma based on the presence of tumor in the marrow or infused hematopoietic harvest. J Clin Oncol 14:214–219, 1996.

150. Corradini P, Voena C, Astolfi M et al: High dose sequential chemoradiotherapy in multiple myeloma: Residual tumor cells are detectable in bone marrow and peripheral blood cell harvests and after autografting. Blood 85:1596–1602, 1995.

151. Vora A, Toh C, Peel J et al: Use of granulocyte colony stimulating factor (G-CSF) for mobilizing peripheral blood stem cells: Risk of mobilizing clonal myeloma cells in patients with bone marrow infiltration. Br J Haematol 86:180–182, 1994.

152. Gazitt Y, Tian E, Barlogie B et al: Differential mobilization of myeloma cells and normal hematopoietic stem cells in multiple myeloma after treatment with cyclophosphamide and granulocyte-macrophage colony stimulating factor. Blood 87:805–811, 1996.

153. Williams CD, Goldstone AH, Pearce RM et al: Purging of bone marrow in autologous bone marrow transplantation for non-Hodgkin's lymphoma: A case-matched comparison with unpurged cases by the European Blood and Marrow Transplant Lymphoma Registry. J Clin Oncol 14:2454–2464, 1996.

154. Heslop HE, Rooney CM, Rill DR et al: Use of gene marking in bone marrow transplantation. Cancer Detect Prev 20:108–113, 1996.

155. Brenner M, Krance R, Heslop HE et al: Assessment of the efficacy of purging by using gene marked autologous marrow transplantation for children with AML in first complete remission. Hum Gene Ther 5:481–499, 1994.

156. Brenner MK, Rill DR, Heslop HE et al: Gene marking after bone marrow transplantation. Eur J Cancer 30A:1171–1176, 1994.

157. Brenner MK, Rill DR: Gene marking to improve the outcome of autologous bone marrow transplantation. J Hematother 3:33–36, 1994.

158. Brenner MK, Rill DR, Moen RC et al: Gene marking and autologous bone marrow transplantation. Ann N Y Acad Sci 716:204–214, 1994.

159. Brenner MK, Rill DR, Moen RC et al: Gene-marking to trace origin of relapse after autologous bone-marrow transplantation. Lancet 341:85–86, 1993.

160. Brenner M, Mirro J, Hurwitz C et al: Autologous bone marrow transplantation for children with AML in first complete remission: Use of marker genes to investigate the biology of marrow reconstitution and the mechanism of relapse. Hum Gene Ther 2:137, 1991.

161. Rill DR, Santana VM, Roberts WM et al: Direct demonstration that autologous bone marrow transplantation for solid tumors can return a multiplicity of tumorigenic cells. Blood 84:380–383, 1994.

162. Rowley S, Jones RJ, Piantadosi S et al: Efficacy of ex vivo purging for autologous bone marrow transplantation in the treatment of acute non lymphoblastic leukemia. Blood 74:501–506, 1989.

163. Miller CB, Zehnhauser A, Piantadosi S et al: Correlation of occult clonogenic leukemia drug sensitivity with relapse after autologous bone marrow transplantation. Blood 78:1125–1131, 1991.

164. Gorin N, Aegerter P, Auvert B et al: Autologous bone marrow transplantation for acute myelocytic leukemia in first remission: A European survey of the role of marrow purging. Blood 75:1606–1614, 1990.

165. Gorin NC, Labopin M, Meloni G et al: Autologous bone marrow transplantation for acute myelocytic leukemia in Europe: Further evidence of the role of marrow purging by mafosfamide. Leukemia 5:896–904, 1991.

56

Alternative Sources of Hematopoietic Stem Cells and Their Clinical Applications

H. Joachim Deeg and Shelly Heimfeld

HISTORY

Reports on the therapeutic use of bone marrow for the treatment of anemia associated with leukemia or parasitic infections date back about one century (reviewed in Ref. 1). However, it was not until the events at Alamagordo, New Mexico, and the observations in atomic bomb casualties at Hiroshima and Nagasaki that systematic research into hematopoietic stem cell transplantation (HSCT) got underway.[2] Studies on total body irradiation (TBI) in mice, rats, dogs, and nonhuman primates revealed three levels of TBI-related injury: a marrow (hematopoietic) syndrome at about 500 to 700 cGy, an intestinal syndrome at 1200 to 10,000 cGy, and a cerebral syndrome at even higher doses.[3] In mice, shielding of the spleen during TBI, implantation of a syngeneic spleen or infusion of syngeneic spleen or marrow cells after TBI rescued animals from the marrow syndrome.[4,5] Intravenous injection was the most effective way of transplanting hematopoietic cells, which by way of "homing" reached the marrow cavity and other hematopoietic organs. These studies also showed that HSCs were present at sites other than the marrow and were viable in the circulation. While the infusion of autologous or syngeneic cells rescued animals without complications, animals given cells from allogeneic donors developed "secondary disease," now known as graft-versus-host disease (GvHD).[3,6]

The first clinical transplant attempts of the modern era were undertaken in patients with end-stage leukemia beginning in 1957. Results were discouraging: Patients transplanted from syngeneic twin donors had a smooth post-transplant course, but generally died of progressive leukemia. Patients transplanted from allogeneic donors, on the other hand, generally died with severe GvHD.[7] The development of GvHD was recognized to be due to differences in histocompatibility antigens between donor and recipient first described by Gorer in mice[8] and then characterized in humans by Dausset and others.[9,10]

CHARACTERIZATION OF HSC AND SITES OF HEMATOPOIESIS

A stem cell is defined by two characteristics: firstly, its ability to generate progeny and, secondly, by the maintenance of this capacity by way of self-renewal. Hematopoiesis is a continuous devel-opmental process in which stem cells make specific cell fate decisions to produce various blood cell lineages.[11] The consistent generation of appropriate numbers and types of mature cells, as well as the maintenance of the HSC pool, requires a regulatory network, many aspects of which remain incompletely understood. Within the hematopoietic microenvironment a complex signaling network involving soluble and cell-bound cytokines, as well as interactions among hematopoietic cells and stromal elements, has evolved to appropriately regulate the differentiation and proliferation of HSCs and progenitor cell populations.[12] Despite considerable experimental and laboratory progress, the molecular signals that mediate cell fate specification and the self-renewal of HSCs remain incompletely understood and controversial.[11–14]

Hematopoiesis in vertebrates evolves through three embryological stages[15]: The mesoderm is formed near the primitive streak, and mesodermal cells begin to migrate along the amniotic wall and visceral endoderm to form the first visceral blood islands (mesodermal or yolk sac phase). These islands then become connected by blood vessels of the primitive circulatory system. Later in embryogenesis, the spleen and liver become the primary sites of hematopoiesis (hepatosplenic phase) before eventually the bone marrow takes over (medullary phase). At the time of birth the marrow has become the predominant site of hematopoiesis in humans; only under stress conditions—in disease states—will hematopoiesis occur in the spleen, liver, and other (extramedullary) sites during adult life. In other species (e.g., mice) the spleen remains a hematopoietic organ throughout life.

In 1951, Brecher and Cronkite showed that cross-circulation between normal rats and rats irradiated with marrow-ablative doses of TBI rescued the irradiated animals by way of engraftment of hematopoietic cells originating from the nonirradiated partner.[16] Similar results were obtained subsequently in mice, baboons, dogs, sheep, and other species, showing that precursor cells capable of long-term hematopoietic reconstitution were present in the circulation. As shown in Table 56–1, hematopoietic stem cells are also present in the fetal liver[17] and, at relatively high concentrations, in umbilical cord blood,[18] basically an extracorporeal segment of the fetal circulation.

Studies with human potential HSCs have essentially been confined to in vitro assays since it is ethically unacceptable to test experimentally various cell populations in humans for their long-term repopulating ability. In vitro characterization has involved Dexter-type long-term cultures, blast cell assays, assays for long-term culture-initiating cells, or high proliferative potential colony-forming cells (reviewed in Ref. 19). Early progenitors have also been identified phenotypically,[20] and have been transplanted and characterized in immunodeficient (SCID) or SCID/NOD mice as well as in sheep[21,22] and in preliminary clinical trials. According to the most prevalent opinion, the earliest identifiable hematopoietic precursor in human adult marrow is CD34+CD38−CD33HLA–DR–Thy1[lo] c-kit[lo] (Rho123[dim]) and noncycling.[23] However, recently this view has been challenged, and data have been presented that suggest the existence of CD34− precursors that are more primitive than CD34+ cells.[24,25] CD34+ cells account for 1 to 2 percent of nucleated marrow cells, and about 1 percent of those are CD38– HLA-DR–. In normal peripheral blood, cells with similar stain-

Table 56–1. Hematopoietic Stem Cell Sources

Source	Indication
Marrow/peripheral blood	

HSCs harvested from peripheral blood originate from marrow and recirculate to the marrow. However, their differentiation status differs from that of marrow HSCs, and they are further modified by exposure to G-CSF, which "mobilizes" them from the marrow. PBSCs lead to faster hematopoietic recovery post-transplant than cells aspirated from unmanipulated marrow. Also, PBSCs can possibly be obtained even if aspiration from marrow is not possible.

Allogeneic[a]	Acquired diseases with or without HSC involvement; congenital disorders.
Syngeneic	Acquired malignant or nonmalignant diseases with or without HSC involvement.
Autologous	Acquired, usually malignant disorders, generally without HSC involvement.
Umbilical Cord Blood	
Allogeneic[a,b]	Lack of alternative stem cell source; pediatric patients; fewer problems with alloreactivity.
Autologous	Highly experimental; possibility of genetic correction of defect.
Fetal Liver	
Allogeneic[c]	Immunodeficiencies, other congenital diseases. (Use at specialized centers.)

[a] Includes related and unrelated donors.
[b] At present the donors are mostly related.
[c] Fetal liver cells have been obtained exclusively from unrelated individuals.

---

ing and functional characteristics can be found, although at approximately 100-fold lower concentrations. In contrast, primitive stem cells in umbilical cord blood and possibly fetal liver appear to be HLA-DR+. HSCs from all these sources can be further defined by the lack of expression of lineage-specific markers.

RATIONALE FOR HSC TRANSPLANTATION

Major indications for HSCT are listed in Table 56–2. The applicability of the different sources, however, may depend on the patient's underlying disease and the objectives of therapy.

Table 56–2. Diseases Treated by HSCT

Acquired		Congenital
Malignant	**Nonmalignant**	

Malignant	Nonmalignant	Congenital	
Acute nonlymphoblastic leukemia	Aplastic anemia	Immunodeficiencies	Mucopolysaccharidases
Acute lymphoblastic leukemia	Pure red cell aplasia	Severe combined immuno-	Hurler syndrome
Chronic myelogenous leukemia	Paroxysmal nocturnal	deficiencies	Hunter syndrome
Chronic lymphocytic leukemia	hemoglobinuria	Combined immunodeficiencies	Maroteaux-Lamy syndrome
Non-Hodgkin's lymphoma	Acquired immunodeficiency	Leukocyte adhesion defects	Others
Hodgkin's disease	syndrome	Actin deficiency	Mucolipidoses
Multiple myeloma	Autoimmune disorders	Chronic mucocutaneous	Metachromatic leukodystrophy
Myelodysplastic syndrome	Systemic sclerosis	candidiasis	Adrenoleukodystrophy
Myelofibrosis	Systemic lupus	Others	Other lipidoses
Agnogenic myeloid metaplasia	erythematosus	Hematologic defects	Other lysosomal diseases
Polycythemia vera	Multiple sclerosis	Wiscott-Aldrich syndrome	Lesch-Nyhan syndrome
Ess. thrombocythemia		Fanconi anemia	Type IIa glycogen storage
Myeloproliferative disorders		Blackfan-Diamond anemia	disease
Neuroblastoma		Rheumatoid arthritis	
Hypereosinophilic syndrome		Thalassemia	
Carcinoma of the breast		Sickle cell disease	
Ovarian carcinoma		Glanzmann's thrombasthenia	
Renal cell carcinoma		Gaucher's disease	
Other selected solid tumors		Chronic granulomatous disease	
		Congenital neutropenia	
		Chediak-Higashi syndrome	
		Langerhans cell histiocytosis	
		Dyskeratosis congenita	
		Congenital amegakaryocytosis	
		Thrombocytopenia-absent-radius	
		(TAR) syndrome	
		Familial erythrophagocytic lympho-	
		histiocytosis (FEL)	
		Others	
		Osteopetrosis	

Myelosuppression, often the dose-limiting toxicity of chemoradiotherapy, is overcome by the infusion of autologous or allogeneic HSCs capable of hematopoietic reconstitution as a "rescue" procedure. In fact, if cytotoxic therapy is not myeloablative and endogenous stem cells can survive and eventually recover, even the use of committed precursors (without long-term repopulating potential) may prove effective in providing short-term "coverage" for the patient until hematopoiesis is re-established endogenously. This approach then allows dose escalation to the point where nonhematopoietic toxicity in organs such as the intestinal tract, liver, or lungs becomes dose limiting. Cells from allogeneic donors, in addition, provide an allogeneic graft-versus-leukemia (GvL) effect, enhancing tumor cell kill above what is achieved with cytotoxic therapy alone.

Secondly, allogeneic, normal HSCs are used as "replacement" therapy in patients with congenital or acquired marrow failure or immunodeficiency states. In this case, there is in principle no beneficial antimalignancy effect, and GvHD must be prevented whenever possible. Similar considerations apply to patients with autoimmune disorders. Some of those disorders are now accepted as indications for transplantation based on observations in patients with aplastic anemia or leukemia who also suffered, for example, from rheumatoid arthritis, and when transplanted with allogeneic marrow were not only cured of their hematologic disease but also had sustained improvement or resolution of their autoimmune disorder.[26] Of note is that results in animal models suggest that similar effects can be achieved with autologous cells if the lymphocytes that show rearrangement of the autoreactive T-cell receptor are depleted.[27]

Thirdly, HSCs (or committed precursors) have been used as "vehicles" to provide specific therapeutic effects. In gene therapy, one objective is the replacement of defective or missing enzymes (e.g., adenosine deaminase, glucocerebrosidase) or the introduction of genes that may mediate antitumor activity (e.g., interleukin-2). Also, cells modified by so-called "suicide genes" are used to exert a desired effect (GvL effect) but then can be eliminated via activation of the suicide gene to prevent the undesired effect of GvHD.[28,29]

Further, there has been a long-standing interest in using lympho-hematopoietic cells in conjunction with solid organ transplantation as vehicles for the induction of tolerance.[30,31] Interest in this possibility has recently been intensified by investigations into the role of microchimerism associated with certain organ transplant procedures, which may facilitate the establishment of tolerance to the transplanted organ in the recipient.

Finally, the observation by Kolb and colleagues that patients with chronic myelogenous leukemia (CML) who relapsed after allogeneic HSCT were re-induced into remission by the infusion of lymphocytes from the original donor (donor lymphocyte infusion; DLI), provided compelling evidence that those cells served as vehicles of an immunotherapeutic (GvL) effect,[32,33] and malignant cells were eradicated without the use of conventional cytotoxic regimens. Those insights contributed to the development of transplant approaches that employ conditioning regimens that by design are nonmyeloablative. They combine the gradual replacement of the host lympho-

hematopoietic compartment (normal and malignant cells) by donor-derived cells with immunotherapy in the form of donor stem cell–derived lymphocytes or separate DLI and post-transplant immunosuppression.[34]

PREPARATION FOR TRANSPLANTATION

It is evident from the above discussion that HSCT has evolved into a multifaceted treatment modality, and it may be useful to discuss some of the modalities used in transplant preparation.

1. Treatment aimed at eradicating the patient's disease or reducing the number of malignant or abnormal cells such that other components of the procedure may be able to be most effective (this applies for allogeneic, syngeneic, and autologous procedures). Modalities include irradiation, either in the form of TBI or limited field irradiation. In addition, bone-seeking radioactive isotopes (e.g., holmium) and isotopes (e.g., ^{131}I) conjugated to monoclonal antibodies directed at lymphoid or myeloid antigens (e.g., anti-CD20, CD45) are being tested in clinical trials. Chemotherapeutic agents include busulfan, etoposide, melphalan, thiotepa, cytarabine, carmustine, and others, and recent trials explore the usefulness of cytotoxic agents such as calicheamycin conjugated to monoclonal antibodies, in this case, anti-CD33.

2. Treatment aimed at suppressing the patient's immunity to prevent rejection of donor cells (this applies to allogeneic but not to the use of autologous cells, which constitute an "*auto*plantation" rather than a "*trans*plant"). Modalities include biological reagents such as antithymocyte globulin (ATG, a polyclonal antibody preparation) or monoclonal antibodies directed at T-cell antigens or adhesion molecules. In addition, cytokines or cytokine antagonists are being investigated for their therapeutic potential. Immunosuppression is also needed in preparation for some syngeneic transplants, presumably to eliminate autoimmune reactivity that may interfere with sustained hematopoietic reconstitution. Viable donor buffy coat cells have been used historically to facilitate engraftment in patients with severe aplastic anemia. While initially interpreted as a "graft facilitating" effect by nonhematopoietic cells, in view of more recent results, it is likely that an increase in the number of HSCs as well as an immunotherapeutic component by nonhematopoietic cells played a role.[33,35–37]

3. The third objective had long been the creation of space for donor cell engraftment. However, there is now strong evidence that indicates that donor cells "create their own space," a notion further supported by the results of DLI.

4. Additional procedures in preparation for transplantation may involve plasmapheresis of the patient to remove isoagglutinins directed against the donor's ABO blood group or vice versa, removal of plasma from the donor marrow to remove isoagglutinins directed at recipient cells. Alternatively, the donor red blood cells with which recipient antibodies may react can be removed.[38]

SELECTION OF AN HSC DONOR

The choice of a source of HSCs is dependent on several factors, foremost of all the availability of a suitable donor, the patient's age, and the patient's disease.[39] Potential HSC donors are listed in Table 56–3.

Approximately 25 percent of patients who have siblings have an HLA genotypically identical donor.[40,41] In addition, phenotypically matched related donors are identified for about 1 percent of patients, and somewhat less than 1 percent of patients will have an identical twin donor.[42] These statistics (i.e., the lack of a matched related donor in the majority of patients) have stimulated the development of transplantation in two directions: 1. the use of "alternative" donors, that is, HLA-nonidentical relatives or unrelated volunteer donors. To facilitate the latter, computerized HLA databanks have been established[43,44]; 2. the refinement of autologous transplantation by the use of peripheral blood stem cells (PBSCs) and by incorporating purging techniques.[45] A haploidentical donor (parent, sibling, child) is available for most patients but haplotype differences still represent major problems to transplantation because of GvHD and the risk of rejection.[40,41]

To a large extent due to the efforts of organizations such as the Anthony Nolan Appeal in the United Kingdom, the National Marrow Donor Program in the United States, and other organizations worldwide, more than 5 million volunteer donors have been typed for HLA-A and -B antigens,[43,46] and a rapidly growing number also for HLA-C, -DRB1, and DQB1. Computer searches of databases very quickly generate an idea as to the probability of finding an unrelated donor. The probability of finding an HLA-A, -B, -DRB1 match is currently about 60 to 65 percent for Caucasian patients; an additional 20 percent of patients have a 1-HLA-locus incompatible unrelated donor available. The probabilities are lower for patients of different ethnic background.

While autologous marrow or PBSC in principle should be available for every patient (except possibly patients with marrow failure states), an autologous HSC source would not be useful for genetically determined disorders—unless modified by gene transfer—and certain acquired malignant disorders. With the use of autologous HSCs, there is always concern that malignant (diseased) cells are returned to the patient with the transplant inoculum, a concern only partially alleviated by the application of various purging procedures. Purging may involve chemical means (e.g., 4-hydroperoxycyclophosphamide)[45] or antibodies that recognize tumor cells.[47,48] Vice versa, the characterization of antigens expressed on putative stem cells (CD34+) allows for the positive selection of stem cells with specific antibodies.[49,50]

HARVESTING HSCS FOR TRANSPLANTATION FROM VARIOUS SOURCES

As outlined above, during ontogeny hematopoiesis evolves through several stages and in several anatomic sites. In agreement with this, HSC capable of long-term reconstitution can be obtained from various sites.

Bone Marrow

In an adult person, bone marrow is the primary organ of hematopoiesis and the site from which stem cells for transplantation have been harvested traditionally.[51] For the purpose of marrow harvest, the patient receives anesthesia, and under sterile conditions, multiple small volume aspirates ($\approx$3 ml) of marrow are obtained from both posterior iliac crests.[52] Additional potential aspiration sites are the anterior iliac crests, the sternum, and, particularly in children, the tibia heads. Approximately 10 to 15 ml/kg donor weight are collected, usually yielding 1 to 4 $\times$ 10^8 cells/kg recipient weight (Table 56–4). The concentration of cells is generally higher in children than in adults, and in first harvests than in subsequent aspirations if done within a short time interval after the first procedure.[53–55] The marrow is passed through filters, nowadays generally in closed systems, to break up cell aggregates and remove bone particles. If no ABO incompatibility exists and if the marrow is not to be subjected to any in vitro purging procedure or other manipulation, the resulting cell suspension is infused intravenously, generally via an indwelling intravenous catheter (e.g., Hickman line), and cells "home" through the circulation to the marrow cavity.

With autologous marrow, many investigators apply in vitro purging with antibody and complement, with solid phase separation or chemicals prior to cryopreservation or reinfusion into the patient after conditioning. Other approaches at purging

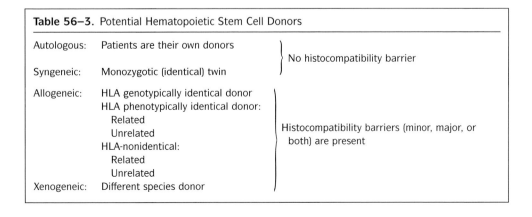

Table 56–3. Potential Hematopoietic Stem Cell Donors

Autologous:	Patients are their own donors	No histocompatibility barrier
Syngeneic:	Monozygotic (identical) twin	
Allogeneic:	HLA genotypically identical donor	
	HLA phenotypically identical donor:	
	Related	
	Unrelated	Histocompatibility barriers (minor, major, or both) are present
	HLA-nonidentical:	
	Related	
	Unrelated	
Xenogeneic:	Different species donor	

Table 56–4. Characteristics of Marrow, Peripheral Blood, and Cord Blood Used for Allogeneic HSCT

Characteristic	Marrow[b]	Peripheral Blood	Cord Blood
Harvest procedure	Anesthesia—multiple marrow aspirates	Vascular access—apheresis ($\approx$4 hours $\times$ 1–2)[a]	Extraction of cells from cord and placenta
Number of cells obtained (per kg patient weight)			
Total mononuclear	$1–4 \times 10^8$	$2–100 \times 10^8$	$0.7–30 \times 10^7$
CD34 +	$1–5 \times 10^6$	$2–20 \times 10^6$	$< 1–45 \times 10^5$
T cells	$5–50 \times 10^6$	$2–10 \times 10^8$	$<5–>20 \times 10^6$
Cell subpopulations			
CD34 +	[c]	Increased number	Increased number
T cells	[c]	Increased number; decreased reactivity	Reduced GvHD activity
Monocytes	[c]	Increased IL-10	Reduced HLA-DR, CD86, ICAM-1, IFN-γ production

[a] G-CSF mobilized.

[b] Some results with marrow cells following G-CSF administration have been reported recently.[114,115]

[c] Reference value.

have involved in vitro culture (see below) to select against clonogenic leukemic cells.[56,57]

Peripheral Blood Stem Cells

At steady state, HSCs circulate at very low concentrations in peripheral blood. Following cytotoxic therapy, however, the frequency of early hematopoietic precursors in the circulation increases dramatically, though transiently, during the recovery phase.[58] The same effect is achieved if cytotoxic agents such as cyclophosphamide, etoposide, or taxol are given for the very purpose of "mobilizing" cells from the marrow into the circulation[59] (Table 56–5). The administration of recombinant hematopoietic growth factors, such as granulocyte colony-stimulating factor (G-CSF), granulocyte-macrophage (GM)-CSF, or c-kit ligand alone or in combination, has similar effects

(although presumably via different mechanisms,[60]) and the timing of the maximum stem cell yield, around 4 to 6 days after initiation of treatment with growth factor, is more predictable than with chemotherapy.[61,62] Furthermore, the absence of cytotoxicity and the associated side effects allows the application of this approach to normal donors and the harvesting of mobilized normal cells from the peripheral circulation. The mechanism involved in dislodging cells from the marrow and forcing them into circulation is incompletely understood. HSCs are normally anchored within the marrow environment, presumably through specific receptor interactions with other cells and extracellular matrix. In agreement with that notion, a recent study in non-human primates has shown that stem cells can also be mobilized by the administration of a monoclonal antibody directed at the integrin VLA4,[63] that is, an adhesion molecule rather than a cytokine.

Table 56–5. Autologous and Allogeneic Peripheral Blood Stem Cell (Precursor) Harvesting[102,123]

	HSC Source	
	Autologous	Allogeneic
Methods of mobilization	Chemotherapy, cytokines/growth factors (antibodies to adhesion molecules)	Cytokines/growth factors
Types of chemotherapy	CY; VP-16; paclitaxel; epirubicin; ifosfamide; cisplatin; carboplatin (combinations)[a]	
Cytokines/growth factors used	G-CSF (5–20 µg/kg/day) GM-CSF (4–64 µg/kg; 125–250 gmg/m²) IL-3 (5–10 µg/kg) TPO/MGDF (0.03–5 µg/kg) SCF (10–25 µg/kg) (combinations)[b]	G-CSF (2–20 µg/kg/day)
Risk of tumor cell contamination	Yes (higher without chemotherapy)	No
Time course for harvest	Predictable for cytokines; variable for chemotherapy	Predictable

[a] Various schedules, generally disease-dependent, have been used; blood leukocyte and CD34 + counts are monitored for optimum timing of apheresis.

[b] Various injection and infusion schedules are used. G-CSF, currently the most widely used regimen, is generally given once a day sc for 5 days with leukapheresis on day 5 (and day 6 if necessary).

PBSCs (and cells at various stages of differentiation) are harvested from peripheral blood by leukapheresis. The best currently available marker of the cells required for a successful transplant (stem cells; long-term repopulating cells) is the surface glycoprotein, CD34 (Tables 56–4 and 56–5). For autologous procedures the goal is to harvest approximately 5×10^6 CD34+ cells/kg recipient weight.[50] Higher cell numbers are targeted if the cells are to be processed in vitro or if cells for a "back-up" infusion are desired. The yield of CD34+ cells per apheresis (usually for 10 to 16 L over 2 to 4 hours) for autologous transplants varies considerably, largely dependent on the intensity of prior therapy given to the patients. The most reliable indicator of the success of apheresis is the concentration of CD34+ cells in peripheral blood.[64] In many patients, one single harvest will suffice; in others, several sessions are required. However, after 2 (or 3) days of apheresis, generally the incremental cell yield from additional aphereses is small. Large volume apheresis may be useful in some patients. Usually autologous cells need to be cryopreserved until completion of the patient's conditioning regimen.

Mobilization of PBSCs by G-CSF in normal allogeneic donors results in more consistent cell yields than in pretreated patients. By and large, 2 to 20×10^6 CD34+ cells/kg are obtained with a single harvest.[65,66] As the harvest can be timed such that it coincides with completion of the transplant conditioning regimen in the patient, allogeneic PBSCs are usually transplanted fresh. Cryopreservation is possible, however, and has been used, for example, to accomodate donor preferences.

Cord Blood Cells

Umbilical cord blood is usually discarded with the placenta following postpartum inspection, without any loss to mother or baby. Thus, cord blood represents an easily accessible source of hematopoietic stem cells,[18] and, in fact, cord blood contains proportionally higher numbers of progenitor cells per volume than adult blood and possibly adult marrow.[18,67,68] However, one concern is the limited volume of cord blood available per case (approximately 50 to 150 ml), and despite a higher stem cell content, the volume may be inadequate for transplantation of adult recipients. It is for this reason that the majority of cord blood recipients have been children. Another concern with cord blood cells has been contamination by maternal cells that might cause severe GvHD. However, in a recent study, Socié et al. found only one low-level contamination (0.1 to 1 percent, particularly among granulocytes) in 42 samples using molecular techniques.[69]

Immunological studies show that cord blood T cells are less immunocompetent than adult cells, and one advantage may, therefore, be that of a reduced incidence of GvHD.[68,70] Cord blood T cells can be activated via the T-cell receptor, but have a reduced capacity to stimulate.[71] Recent experiments indicate that intracytoplasmatic signaling (following T-cell receptor engagement) in cord blood T cells also differs from that in adult T cells.[72] Cord blood monocytes express lower levels of HLA-DR, CD86, and ICAM-1 than monocytes in adult blood, and produce lower levels of interleukin (IL)-10 and interferon

(IFN)-gamma. IL-4 and IL-5 are basically absent.[71] Most, if not all, cytotoxicity appears to be mediated by NK type cells (rather than CD3+ T cells). Thus, cord blood cells represent an excellent source of HSCs, possibly with low GvHD potential, at least for pediatric patients. Several banks of cryopreserved cells have been established.[73,74] For patients without a suitable related or living unrelated donor, cord blood may offer an alternative for allogeneic transplantation.

Fetal Liver Cells

Fetal liver, if obtained at the optimum time of gestation, provides a rich source of HSCs.[17] The concentration of colony-forming unit (CFU)-GM as an indicator for hematopoietic potential increases with gestational age, most markedly after week 10. However, beginning at about week 14 there is also an increase in cells expressing T-cell markers. Thus, an optimum window for the use of fetal liver cells exists at 10 to 14 weeks of gestation. The feasibility of fetal liver transplants has been shown in adult primate and canine models as well as in in utero transplants in sheep.[22,75] For reasons of availability, technical problems, and ethical concerns, fetal liver cells have been used only very selectively. Also, cell numbers obtained from a single donor liver are low and probably insufficient to transplant adults. Nevertheless, for some indications, such as immune defects in children, fetal liver cells have been used quite successfully, particularly in the form of intrauterine (fetal) therapy.[17,76]

Comparison of HSCs From Different Sources

Marrow and PBSCs are available from autologous, allogeneic, and in rare instances, syngeneic sources (Table 56–4). Fetal liver cells are always of allogeneic origin, as are cord blood cells. The latter, however, may become useful as an autologous stem cell source, for example, for the treatment of congenital disorders once they are correctable by gene transfer.[77]

Some differences between cells from different compartments have been described above.[67] The proliferative potential of fetal liver cells as determined by the generation of CD34+ cells in serum-free medium is greater than that of umbilical cord blood cells, which in turn is greater than in adult marrow[78] (Figure 56–1). This is of interest, since one concern regarding the use of fetal liver and cord blood cells are the limited numbers. In vitro expansion may be necessary if they are to be transplanted to an adult recipient.

Mobilized stem cells from peripheral blood appear to represent an intermediary step. These cells show a lower retention of Rhodamine 123 (which is typical for noncycling cells), and may have a lower expression of CD38. The proliferative capacity of PBSCs is similar to marrow cells, but they may produce progeny for a longer period of time than marrow cells on standardized stromal layers.[79] As discussed below, in vivo hematopoietic recovery is consistently more rapid with PBSCs than with marrow.[80,81] No direct comparison is available for fetal liver cells. With umbilical cord blood cells, the kinetics of recovery are consistently slower than with either PBSCs or marrow.[82,83] PBSCs appear to lead to faster immunologic reconstitution, which is thought to

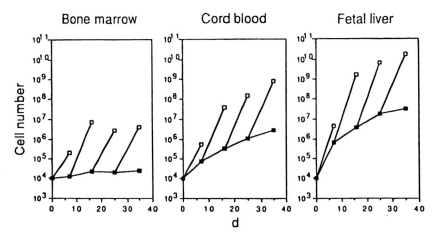

Figure 56–1. Ontogeny-related differences in production of CD34+ cells in culture. CD34+ CD45RA^{lo} CD71^{lo} cells were purified from bone marrow, umbilical cord blood, and fetal liver, and cultured in serum-free culture medium supplemented with IL-6, IL-3, Steel factor (SCF), and erythropoietin. Cultures (1 ml each) were initiated with 10^4 sorted cells. At the indicated time interval the total number of nucleated cells —□— and CD34+ cells —■— present in the cultures was calculated from the cell counts and the percentage of viable CD34+ cells measured by flow cytometry. All CD34+ cells from bone marrow cultures and fractions of the CD34+ cells from cord blood and fetal liver cultures were sorted and used for continuation of the cultures and measurements of clonogenic cells. Only CD34+ cells with the same (high) CD34 fluorescence as the cells sorted from primary tissues were sorted for replating. Plotted data points were corrected for loss of cells during the procedure. In this particular experiment, CD34+ cells represented 14.1, 1.7, and 10.7 percent of all viable low-density cells from, respectively, organ donor bone marrow, umbilical cord blood, and fetal liver (13 to 15 weeks of gestation). The corresponding fraction of CD34+ CD45RA^{lo} CD71^{lo} cells among CD34+ cells from these tissues was, respectively, 30, 35, and 10 percent. (From Lansdorp et al.,[78] with permission.)

offer an added antitumor benefit. For allogeneic transplants, an advantage of fetal liver and cord blood cells would be their immunologic immaturity, which may permit investigators to avoid the adverse effect of a graft-versus-host reaction.

PBSCs had been expected to be contaminated by fewer tumor cells than marrow cells. Cytogenetic studies show indeed that there is little if any contamination in patients with acute myeloid leukemia (AML) undergoing peripheral blood stem cell harvest (apheresis) while in remission.[59] In patients with carcinoma of the breast and non-Hodgkin's lymphoma, but possibly not with Hodgkin's disease, contamination appears to be lower in peripheral blood than in marrow.[84] Preliminary data suggest that even in patients with CML, fewer Ph^1 positive cells are harvested from peripheral blood than from marrow, particularly if done early in the patient's disease course.[85] However, there is evidence that mobilization procedures (particularly with cytokines alone) may, along with normal hematopoietic precursors, also increase the number of tumor cells,[86,87] and gene-marking studies by several investigators clearly show that *infused* autologous cells contribute to post-transplant disease recurrence.[88] Current studies are aimed at further purifying stem cells, for example, by means of separation columns taking advantage of monoclonal antibodies specific for CD34.[89] In patients with CML an additional purification step might be on the basis of HLA-DR expression since the malignant precursors are thought to be HLA-DR+ in contrast to normal stem cells, which at least in adults are found to be HLA-DR–.[90]

Finally, it is thought that mobilized PBSCs and cord blood cells represent better targets for gene therapy than marrow cells, particularly after in vitro culture, probably related to their greater proliferative potential (enhancing the probability of retroviral integration).[91]

IN VITRO CULTURE AND EXPANSION OF HSCS

The ability to grow human progenitor cells ex vivo opens up diverse types of clinical applications in the arena of human cellular therapy. The utility of this technology may range from the expansion of primitive stem cells to specific manipulation of mature blood cell types by lineage-specific proliferation and differentiation. Ex vivo cultured cells could be used to treat patients in a variety of settings now commonly seen in clinical hematology/oncology, including but not limited to those patients being treated with high-dose chemotherapy followed by autologous or allogeneic stem cell transplantation. In vitro culture might be employed to reduce some of the morbidity associated with high-dose therapy and pancytopenia by reducing the "window" of absolute neutropenia, thrombocytopenia, or both. Additional therapeutic benefits might include support for multiple cycles of high-dose chemotherapy, and reduced harvest requirements for marrow or PBSC collections. Other applications include the generation of sufficient cells from cord blood to facilitate transplantation in adults and to enhance tumor cell purging for autologous transplants or T-cell depletion in the case of allogeneic transplantation. More futuristic approaches involve genetic modification of hematopoietic progenitor cells ex vivo to correct inborn defects or render cells resistant to chemotherapy agents or viral infection, and the generation of mature cell types with defined functional properties to enhance, for example, specific immune reactivity to malignant cell populations. All these potential benefits of ex vivo expansion of hematopoietic progenitor cells are currently under investigation at centers around the world.[12,56,88,92–97]

Purging in Long-Term Culture

As already discussed, a general problem with autologous HSCT is that of overt or minimal residual disease contamination by clonogenic tumor cells.[98,99] Numerous techniques of in vitro purging have been developed. The finding that normal and malignant precursor cells differ in regard to their interactions with the hematopoietic environment[90] has been exploited in in vitro culture systems aimed at propagating normal cells capable of long-term reconstitution after transplantation while eliminating malignant cells.[56,57] One report presented data on marrows obtained from 19 patients with acute lymphoblastic leukemia (ALL) and 30 patients with AML. These marrows were grown in long-term marrow cultures for 4 to 10 weeks. In half of the patients the leukemic cell population declined to undetectable levels. Preliminary results showed that among five patients transplanted in first remission, four were alive in remission at 12 weeks to 3 years.[57]

Similar results have been reported in patients with CML.[56] Incubation of marrow cells from CML patients results in a marked and selective loss of Philadelphia chromosome (Ph[1]) positive cells. In the Vancouver study, 28 patients were transplanted with cultured cells. In 13 patients regenerating marrow cells were 100 percent Ph[1] negative. However, between 4 and 36 (median 12) months, Ph[1] positive cells became detectable in all but one patient (who died while in remission). Among seven patients treated with IFN-α, four became again Ph[1] negative. Among 22 patients who were in chronic phase at the time of transplantation, 13 (81 percent) were surviving at a median of 2.6 years, four in cytogenetic remission. The full potential of this approach remains to be determined.

Allogeneic precursor cells have been cultured in vitro for different reasons. These include the generation of mature precursor cells to accelerate post-transplant hematopoietic reconstitution; elimination of alloreactive cells in an attempt to reduce the incidence of GvHD; activation of cells for enhanced GvL reactivity; and activation of cells to facilitate genetic manipulations.

In Vitro Expansion

Expansion of normal HSCs in vitro has gained in interest with the increasing use of cord blood cells.[71] The amount of cord blood generally available is limited.[68] In order for these cells to be used successfully in adults, expansion appears necessary. The differentiation of a pluripotent stem cell to a lineage-committed or even mature blood cell depends on the response to numerous factors[100,101] and experience has generally been that even though cells could be maintained in culture for extended periods of time, the ability to maintain their self-replicating capacity was rather limited.[93,95,97] Stem cell factor (SCF, c-kit ligand)

and Flt3 ligand play pivotal roles in the survival of HSCs in regards to self-renewal and as co-mitogens in the movement of hematopoietic stem cells from the stem cell pool into the progeny pool. HSCs show little response to any single cytokine, but combinations of factors, for example, SCF or Flt3 ligand plus IL-3 plus IL-6, direct the cells toward commitment. Experiments in murine models suggest that multipotentiality can be maintained in medium containing IL-1, IL-3, plus SCF: Transplantation of expanded cells into lethally irradiated recipient mice resulted in earlier hematopoietic recovery than was observed with fresh marrow (reviewed in Ref. 102). A recent report suggests that in short-term cultures the presence of IL-1 and SCF, with or without addition of IL-6 or IL-3, results in the expansion of precursors sufficient for successful transplantation in mice with cell numbers much lower than necessary if fresh cells are used.[103] Additional experiments showed that those cells were able to successfully reconstitute lethally irradiated secondary recipients.

Culture of human cord blood cells in the presence of SCF and GM-CSF resulted in approximately a tenfold expansion of CFU-GM.[18] With the addition of erythropoietin and IL-3, there was a 15-fold increase in [colony-forming units multilineage] CFU-GEMM. Seven-day cultures in the presence of SCF resulted in an increase in CFU-GM, burst-forming unit–erythroid (BFU-E), and CFU-GEMM; the yield was further augmented by adding other stimulating factors. The addition of IL-12 to IL-3 and SCF in these cultures may further enhance an expansion at least of myeloid progenitors.[104] Others, however, have cautioned against relying on SCF since it was particularly Rho123 bright cells (thought not to represent the earliest precursors), that expressed c-kit.[105] However, there is evidence that HSCs contained in cord blood, can be expanded without losing their long-term repopulating ability.[71] Long-term culture-initiating cells (LTC-IC) are present at a frequency of 1:500 in peripheral blood but at 1:100 in cord blood, and estimates are that only a three- to fourfold expansion is needed for successful transplantation of an adult.

Additional studies suggested that the generation and replication of HSCs in vitro was greatly enhanced in a flow-through system that optimized nutrient availability.[106] The bioreactors contained growth medium, including IL-3, GM-CSF, erythropoietin, and SCF. Over 14 days there was a tenfold expansion of the total number of cells. CFU-GM expanded 21-fold, BFU-E 12-fold. LTC-IC, tested in limiting dilution assays, increased seven to eightfold. The authors concluded that more than 3×10^9 cells containing 12×10^6 CFU-GM could be generated from the equivalent of 10 to 15 ml of marrow aspirate, suggesting that sufficient cells for a complete transplant can be obtained.[107] In preliminary clinical studies, five patients were given between 2 and 20×10^5 expanded CFU-GM/kg. Time to engraftment (ANC 0.5 $\times 10^9$/L) was 8 to 24 (median 13) days compared to a median of 16.2 days in a control group of 13 patients given nonexpanded normal marrow grafts (S. Emerson, personal communication).

Others have examined LTC-IC in modified stroma-contact cultures, and showed that CD34+ umbilical cord blood cells could be expanded approximately 500-fold, including a 45-fold expansion of CFU-GM, and a fivefold expansion of LTC-IC over a 14-day culture period.[108] These authors suggested that this approach might be sufficient to allow for the expansion of cord blood cells to a level sufficient for transplantation of adults.

CLINICAL TRIALS

The use of HSCT has increased exponentially. Starting with allogeneic (and syngeneic) marrow from related donors, the donor pool has been expanded to include unrelated volunteers as well as the patient's own marrow. Subsequent developments have included the use of allogeneic cord blood cells and PBSCs. Currently some 15,000 allogeneic and 20,000 autologous transplants are carried out annually with a progressively increasing proportion of transplants using PBSCs and transplants from unrelated donors.

Marrow

Marrow transplants are discussed in Chapter 55.

Peripheral Blood Stem Cells

An initial concern was that PBSCs may not be capable of long-term hematopoietic reconstitution. However, patients have been followed now for more than 10 or even 15 years and show normal hematopoiesis. Also, gene-marking studies in canine and nonhuman primate models using SCF/G-CSF mobilized PBSCs indicate that those cells at least contribute to hematopoietic reconstitution with follow-up extending to several years.[109,110] The kinetics of hematopoietic recovery with PBSCs as compared to bone marrow are illustrated in Figure 56–2.

After administration of G-CSF, 5 μg/kg/day, to normal donors for 9 to 14 days, granulocytes rose to a median of $29.6 \times 10^9/L$ (range 11.8 to 29.8) and 41.6×10^9 (1.3 to 144.1) granulocytes were collected for transfusion purposes. Other than joint aches related to G-CSF, the procedure was well tolerated. In a study of five syngeneic twin transplants, the normal twins were given rhG-CSF, 16 μg/kg/day sc for 4 days and subjected to leukapheresis.[65] Although it is impossible to document engraftment of unmarked transplanted cells in this syngeneic setting, the rate of hematopoietic recovery very strongly suggested engraftment and proliferation of exogenous (i.e., G-CSF mobilized donor) cells.

If any doubts remained, they were definitely eliminated by observations with allogeneic PBSC transplants that resulted in sustained donor cell engraftment.[65,66] There were several reasons that led to the exploration of the use of allogeneic PBSCs: 1. Autologous transplant results showed a substantially faster post-transplant recovery with PBSCs than with marrow, shortening the period of pancytopenia and susceptibility to infections. 2. Faster recovery generally was associated with a shorter hospital stay. 3. The ability to obtain HSCs by leukapheresis eliminated the need for anesthesia that is usually required for a marrow harvest. However, there were also concerns. Earlier observations with the infusion of viable allogeneic peripheral blood buffy coat cells suggested a higher incidence of GvHD,

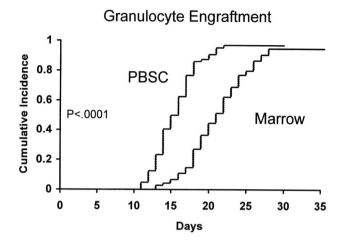

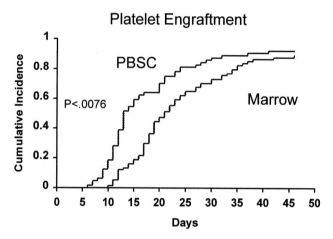

Figure 56–2. Kinetics of granulocyte and platelet recovery after allogeneic marrow or peripheral blood stem cell transplantation in a randomized prospective trial involving 172 patients with various lymphohematopoietic malignancies. (Courtesy of Dr. W. Bensinger, Fred Hutchinson Cancer Research Center.)

particularly in its chronic form, than seen with marrow cells.[111] Noncontrolled trials have failed to show an increased incidence of acute GvHD, while the reports on chronic GvHD are controversial. It is of note that T lymphocytes and monocytes obtained after G-CSF mobilization show altered functions and in particular increased production of IL-10, which is at least in part responsible for the suppression of alloreactivity.[112,113] Results from two randomized studies comparing marrow and G-CSF mobilized PBSCs have recently been presented.[80,81] While not all data are mature yet, findings can be summarized as follows: Transplantation of PBSCs results in faster hematopoietic (granulocyte and platelet) recovery, usually associated with reduced transfusion requirements and a shortened hospital stay. There is a tendency toward a higher incidence of chronic GvHD, although this does not appear to be reflected in a lower probability of survival. In fact, the cumulative incidence of relapse was reduced with PBSCs (Figure 56–3) and early post-trans-

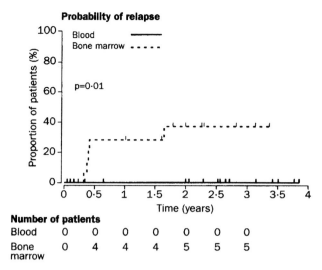

Figure 56–3. Incidence of relapse after marrow ($n = 19$) or peripheral blood stem cell transplantation ($n = 20$) for hematologic malignancies in patients with HLA-identical sibling donors. (From Powles et al.,[81] with permission.)

plant mortality was lower than in patients given marrow. As a result, disease-free survival was superior, particularly in patients with high-risk disease.[80,81] Preliminary results from studies in patients with myelodysplastic syndrome or myelofibrosis suggest that outcome after transplantation with PBSCs may be some 15 percent better than outcome achieved with the use of marrow (unpublished observations), largely due to lower early post-transplant mortality. Thus, PBSCs appear to confer an advantage for relapse-free survival in patients with various disorders. The incidence of delayed morbidity (relative to patients transplanted with marrow) remains to be determined. This is also the major reason why PBSCs have not been used extensively in patients with nonmalignant disorders such as aplastic anemia who are unlikely to derive any gain from the development of chronic GvHD.

In patients who are prepared for transplantation with a non-myeloablative conditioning regimen (see above), peripheral blood has been used virtually exclusively as the source of HSCs. This approach has been taken in part because of the greater "engraftment potential" ascribed to those cells, in part because of the larger numbers of cells that are obtainable, and the possibility of storing cells for a second (later) infusion, as well as the greater ease with which the cells are obtained. However, not unexpectedly, the incidence of acute GvHD requiring therapy (despite state-of-the-art prophylaxis) has been 45 to 50 percent, and similarly, chronic GvHD 40 to 50 percent. To what extent G-CSF-induced alterations in cytokine profiles of donor cells are involved is under investigation. This question is of considerable interest, and several recent investigations have provided data to show that *marrow* aspirated from donors following G-CSF priming yielded similar results as obtained with cells obtained via leukapheresis.[114–116] In fact, these reports suggested that marrow obtained under those conditions conveyed certain advantages, for example, a lower incidence of GvHD,

presumably because of the lower numbers of T cells contained in the marrow product.

Cord Blood Cells

A rapidly increasing number of cord blood transplants are being carried out.[68,71] Kurtzberg et al.[83] reported results on 25 consecutive patients, mostly children, with various diagnoses. Twenty-four patients were discordant for 1 to 3 HLA antigens. In 23 of the 25 patients, engraftment was achieved; the interval to reach 0.5×10^9 neutrophils/L was 14 to 37 (median 22) days. Eleven of 21 evaluable patients developed acute GvHD of grades II to IV. The overall event-free day 100 survival was 48 percent.

Gluckman et al.[82] presented results on 143 transplants carried out at 45 centers, for various diagnoses. Among 78 patients who received cord blood from a related donor, survival was 63 percent at 1 year. Younger age, lower weight, HLA identity, and negative cytomegalovirus (CMV) serology were favorable prognostic factors. GvHD of grades II to IV occurred in 9 percent of HLA-identical and in 50 percent of HLA-mismatched transplants. Rapid neutrophil engraftment correlated with patient age less than 6 years ($p = .02$) and weight less than 20 kg ($p = .02$); engraftment occurred in 85 percent of patients given at least 37×10^6 nucleated cells/kg. Among 65 unrelated cord blood recipients, the Kaplan-Meier estimate of 1-year survival was 29 percent. As with related transplants, CMV negativity was a favorable prognostic factor for survival ($p = .03$). Neutrophil recovery occurred in 94 percent of patients given $\geq 37 \times 10^6$ nucleated cells/kg.

Rocha and colleagues recently summarized results in 108 adult recipients of cord blood transplants.[117] Results were strongly dependent on the underlying disease and the number of cells transplanted. The time to reach 0.5×10^9 neutrophils/L was 13 to 57 (median 32) days and to reach 20×10^9 platelets/L was 26 to 176 (median 129) days; 15 patients failed to engraft. Patients who received greater than 17×10^6 cells/kg had a significantly better survival than patients given fewer cells. The authors concluded that cord blood transplantation was a realistic alternative for adult patients, especially when a large cord blood unit was available.

Fetal Liver Cells

Fetal liver cells are used infrequently for HSCT. One transplant team reported results on 27 patients with immunodeficiency diseases (SCID, bare lymphocyte syndrome) and 35 patients with inborn errors of metabolism; five of these patients were given their transplant in utero. Additional patients have been reported from other centers.[118] Among patients with inborn errors, 73 percent are surviving at 1 to 18 years. Among immunodeficient patients survival was 50 percent. The two major reasons for failure were infection and graft failure. Both problems could be overcome at least in part by transplantation in utero at a fetal age as young as 12 weeks. With malignant disorders, the use of liver cells has basically been reserved for selected indications at a few specialized centers.

In Vitro Cultured and Expanded Cells

The safety and efficacy of ex vivo expanded human hematopoietic progenitor cells is still being evaluated in phase I clinical trials. While the first reported attempts to use ex vivo cultured cells involved bone marrow cells from leukemic patients grown in Dexter-type long-term cultures,[56,92] most current protocols are focused on the in vitro culture of purified CD34+ cells obtained from mobilized PBSCs or cord blood cells.

Studies by Andrews and colleagues[110] demonstrated that ex vivo expanded cells, grown in SCF+G-CSF+MGDF (megakaryocyte growth and differentiation factor) growth and differentiation factor (MGDF), were strictly dependent on post-transplant treatment with G-CSF: In the absence of recombinant cytokines, no rapid engraftment occurred, suggesting that while expanded cells were still functional in vivo, they were dependent on exogenous cytokines. In a different primate model Tisdale et al.[119] used retroviral marking of ex vivo expanded cells and showed that these cells were inferior to nonexpanded cells at long-term repopulation. Similar results were seen in a SCID mouse repopulation assay by Guenechea et al.[120] These data parallel much of the results in ex vivo gene therapy studies, where only minimal levels of genetically modified cells were detectable after infusion in vivo.[88]

In the first clinical study to use recombinant cytokines alone for ex vivo expansion, Brugger et al.[93] selected CD34+ cells obtained from G-CSF mobilized PBSC collections. In vitro analyses showed a median total cell expansion of 62-fold, and a 50-fold expansion of CFC activity. Reinfusion of the ex vivo expanded cells (alone or in combination with noncultured PBPCs) did not result in any allergic manifestations or organ toxicity. Post-transplant, all patients received 5 µg/kg/day of G-CSF on days 1 through 12. Infusion of ex vivo cultured cells neither accelerated nor delayed hematopoietic recovery. It is important to note that the chemotherapy doses given were not myeloablative, and patients would have been expected to reconstitute from residual endogenous cells in approximately 4 to 6 weeks without any PBSC transplant. Therefore, the long-term engraftment potential of the expanded cells could not be assessed. However, this first clinical trial showed that ex vivo expanded cells could be safely administered and would support at least short-term hematopoietic reconstitution.

Williams et al.[94] expanded CD34+ enriched PBSCs ex vivo for 12 days and infused them along with unmanipulated PBSCs. No adverse effects were observed and engraftment kinetics were similar to historical controls. The authors noted that higher cultured cell doses were associated with more rapid hematopoietic recovery. Using yet a different set of cytokines and culture conditions and a cohort of patients subjected to more myeloablative conditioning, Holyoake et al.[95] showed that ex vivo expanded cells did give rise to short-term engraftment, but failed to support long-term hematopoiesis.

Stiff et al.[96] have expanded bone marrow cells using bioreactor systems,[121] and observed only minimal acceleration of recovery post-transplant. More recent studies by Shpall et al.[97] and Reiffers et al.[122] have shown that, using culture conditions as employed by Andrews in the primate model,[110] a subset of patients experienced very rapid recovery of neutrophil counts. However, no change in platelet recovery was noted, and the range of engraftment times was rather broad.

Thus, these clinical pilot studies have shown the feasibility of reinfusion of hematopoietic cells following in vitro expansion for up to 2 weeks. However, in general, reinfusion of expanded cells has not accelerated post-transplant engraftment. Overall, the results suggest that ex vivo expanded cells have diminished capacity for long-term hematopoiesis. These findings may be the result of insufficient or less than optimal expansion. Alternatively, HSCs and progenitor cells may lose their proliferative and self-renewal capacity after ex vivo culture, or in vitro exposure to cytokines may result in defects in the homing or engraftment capacities of the expanded cells. Hematopoietic cells used for transplantation must possess both the ability to migrate to the marrow and the high proliferative capacity to reconstitute hematopoiesis. Thus, the ideal ex vivo expansion system would induce HSCs to replicate in vitro without a loss of self-renewal capacity or ability to home to the marrow. Clearly, while progress has been made, there is much room for improvement of in vitro expansion of HSCs. Information on new growth factors, markers, signaling pathways, culture techniques, and on specific gene expression patterns is rapidly advancing the field of experimental hematology. Thus, it may not be too far in the future when we will truly be able to culture fully functional HSCs and progenitor cells.

SUMMARY

The field of HSCT has expanded exponentially in recent years. The use of "alternative" sources of HSCs has facilitated clinical applications of this modality and has made it widely available. PBSCs are now being used almost exclusively in autologous transplantation, and with increasing frequency in allogeneic transplant recipients with malignant disorders. However, it will be important to continue to conduct controlled trials to improve outcome in regard to GvHD, relapse, and regimen-related mortality. Further, the biology of G-CSF-mobilized PBSCs (or primed marrow cells) is not fully understood. These cells may provide possibilities to refine transplant approaches, to advance gene transfer studies, and develop novel immunotherapeutic techniques. This may apply not only to the use in combination with what are currently known as nonmyeloablative conditioning regimens, but also to immunotherapy per se, particularly if attempts at directing cellular differentiation to specific subsets and target antigens are successful. The place of all these approaches in solid tumor therapy remains ill defined at present.

ACKNOWLEDGMENT

Supported by PHS grants CA15704, CA18029, HL36444, CA78166, DK56465, and HL54881. H.J. Deeg was also supported by a grant from the Gabrielle Rich Leukemia Fund.

REFERENCES

1. Santos GW: History of bone marrow transplantation. Clin Haematol 12:611–639, 1983.
2. Iijima S, Gushima K, Imahori S (eds.): Hiroshima and Nagasaki: The Physical, Medical, and Social Effects of the Atomic Bombings, pp. 1–706. Basic Books, New York, 1981.

3. van Bekkum DW, DeVries M: Radiation chimeras. Academic Press, New York, 1967.

4. Jacobson LO, Simmons EL, Marks EK, Eldredge JH: Recovery from radiation injury. Science 113:510–511, 1951.

5. Lorenz E, Uphoff D, Reid TR, Shelton E: Modification of irradiation injury in mice and guinea pigs by bone marrow injections. J Natl Cancer Inst 12:197–201, 1951.

6. Billingham RE: The biology of graft-versus-host reactions. In The Harvey Lectures, pp. 21–78. Academic Press, New York, 1966.

7. Thomas ED, Lochte HL Jr, Lu WC, Ferrebee JW: Intravenous infusion of bone marrow in patients receiving radiation and chemotherapy. N Engl J Med 257:491–496, 1957.

8. Gorer PA: The antigenic basis of tumour transplantation. J Path Bact 47:231–252, 1938.

9. Dausset J: Iso-leuco-anticorps. Acta Haematol 20:156–166, 1958.

10. Mickelson E, Petersdorf EW: Histocompatibility. In Thomas ED, Blume KG, Forman SJ (eds.): Hematopoietic Cell Transplantation, 2nd Ed., pp. 28–37. Blackwell Science, Boston, 1999.

11. Ogawa M: Differentiation and proliferation of hematopoietic stem cells (Review). Blood 81:2844–2853, 1993.

12. Alcorn MJ, Holyoake TL, Richmond L, Pearson C, Farrell E, Kyle B et al: CD34-positive cells isolated from cryopreserved peripheral-blood progenitor cells can be expanded ex vivo and used for transplantation with little or no toxicity. J Clin Oncol 14:1839–1847, 1996.

13. Metcalf D: The molecular control of hematopoiesis: Progress and problems with gene manipulation. Stem Cells 16:314–321, 1998.

14. Metcalf D: Lineage commitment and maturation in hematopoietic cells: The case for extrinsic regulation. Blood 92:345–347, 1998.

15. Tavassoli M: Embryonic and fetal hemopoiesis: An overview (Review). Blood Cells 17:269–281, 1991.

16. Brecher G, Cronkite EP: Post-radiation parabiosis and survival in rats. Proc Soc Exp Biol Med 77:292–294, 1951.

17. Touraine JL, Roncarolo MG, Bacchetta R, Raudrant D, Rebaud A, Laplace S et al: Fetal liver transplantation: Biology and clinical results (Review). Bone Marrow Transplant 11(Suppl. 1):119–122, 1993.

18. Broxmeyer HE, Hangoc G, Cooper S, Ribeiro RC, Graves V, Yoder M et al: Growth characteristics and expansion of human umbilical cord blood and estimation of its potential for transplantation in adults. Proc Natl Acad Sci U S A 89:4109–4113, 1992.

19. Testa N, Molineux G (eds.): Haemopoiesis: A Practical Approach, pp. 1–293. IRL Press at Oxford University Press, New York, 1993.

20. Civin CI, Strauss LC, Brovall C, Fackler MJ, Schwartz JF, Shaper JH: Antigenic analysis of hematopoiesis. III. A hematopoietic progenitor cell surface antigen defined by a monoclonal antibody raised against KG-1a cells. J Immunol 133:157–165, 1984.

21. Baum CM, Weissman IL, Tsukamoto AS, Buckle A-M, Peault B: Isolation of a candidate human hematopoietic stem-cell population. Proc Natl Acad Sci U S A 89:2804,1992.

22. Flake AW, Zanjani ED: In utero transplantation of hematopoietic stem cells (Review). Crit Rev Oncol Hematol 15:35–48, 1993.

23. Srour EF, Brandt JE, Briddell RA, Leemhuis T, van Besien K, Hoffman R: Human CD34+ HLA-DR-bone marrow cells contain progenitor cells capable of self-renewal, multilineage differentiation, and long-term in vitro hematopoiesis. Blood Cells 17:287–295, 1991.

24. Osawa M, Hanada K, Hamada H, Nakauchi H: Long-term lymphohematopoietic reconstitution by a single CD34-low/negative hematopoietic stem cell. Science 273:242–245, 1996.

25. Bhatia M, Bonnet D, Murdoch B, Gan OI, Dick JE: A newly discovered class of human hematopoietic cells with SCID-repopulating activity. Nat Med 4:1038–1045, 1998.

26. Burt RK, Traynor A, Burns W: Hematopoietic stem cell transplantation of multiple sclerosis, rheumatoid arthritis, and systemic lupus erythematosus. Cancer Treat Res 101:157–184, 1999.

27. Burt RK, Burns W, Ruvolo P, Fischer A, Shiao C, Guimaraes A et al: Syngeneic bone marrow transplantation eliminates V beta 8.2 T lymphocytes from the spinal cord of Lewis rats with experimental allergic encephalomyelitis. J Neurosci Res 41:526–531, 1995.

28. Bonini C, Ferrari G, Verzeletti S, Servida P, Zappone E, Ruggieri L et al: HSV-TK gene transfer into donor lymphocytes for control of allogeneic graft-versus-leukemia. Science 276:1719–1724, 1997.

29. Cohen JL, Boyer O, Salomon B, Onclercq R, Charlotte F, Bruel S et al: Prevention of graft-versus-host disease in mice using a suicide gene expressed in T lymphocytes. Blood 89:4636–4645, 1997.

30. Kim HB, Shaaban AF, Milner R, Fichter C, Flake AW: In utero bone marrow transplantation induces donor-specific tolerance by a combination of clonal deletion and clonal anergy. J Pediatr Surg 34:726–729, 1999.

31. Gandy KL, Weissman IL: Tolerance of allogeneic heart grafts in mice simultaneously reconstituted with purified allogeneic hematopoietic stem cells. Transplantation 65:295–304, 1998.

32. Kolb HJ, Mittermüller J, Clemm Ch, Holler G, Ledderose G et al: Donor leukocyte transfusions for treatment of recurrent chronic myelogenous leukemia in marrow transplant patients. Blood 76:2462–2465, 1990.

33. Kolb H-J: Management of relapse after hematopoietic cell transplantation. In Thomas ED, Blume KG, Forman SJ (eds.): Hematopoietic Cell Transplantation, 2nd Ed., pp. 929–936. Blackwell Science, Boston, 1999.

34. Sandmaier BM, McSweeney PA, Niederwieser D, Maloney DG, Blume KG, Molina A et al: Posttransplant immunosuppression—canine models and clinical application. In Slavin S, Giralt S (eds.): Non-myeloablation Stem Cell Transplantation. Darwin Scientific Publishing, Oxfordshire, UK (in press).

35. Noga SJ: Engineering hematopoietic grafts using elutriation and positive cell selection to reduce GVHD (Review). Cancer Treat Res 101:311–330, 1999.

36. Dazzi F, Szydlo RM, Craddock C, Cross NC, Kaeda J, Chase A et al: Comparison of single-dose and escalating-dose regimens of donor lymphocyte infusion for relapse after allografting for chronic myeloid leukemia. Blood 95:67–71, 2000.

37. Aversa F, Tabilio A, Velardi A, Cunningham I, Terenzi A, Falzetti F et al: Treatment of high-risk acute leukemia with T-cell-depleted stem cells from related donors with one fully mismatched HLA haplotype. N Engl J Med 339:1186–1193, 1998.

38. Bensinger WI, Deeg HJ: Transfusion support and donor considerations in marrow transplantation. In Sacher RA, AuBuchon JP (eds.): Marrow Transplantation: Practical and Technical Aspects of Stem Cell Reconstitution, pp. 157–184. American Association of Blood Banks, Bethesda, 1992.

39. Deeg H-J, Klingemann H-G, Phillips GL, Van Zant G (eds.): A Guide to Blood and Marrow Transplantation, 3rd Ed. Completely Revised Edition. Springer-Verlag, Berlin, 1998.

40. Anasetti C, Amos D, Beatty PG, Appelbaum FR, Bensinger W, Buckner CD et al: Effect of HLA compatibility on engraftment of bone marrow transplants in patients with leukemia or lymphoma. N Engl J Med 320:197–204, 1989.

41. Wagner JL, Deeg HJ, Seidel K, Anasetti C, Doney K, Sanders J et al: Bone marrow transplantation for severe aplastic anemia from genotypically HLA-nonidentical relatives: An update of the Seattle experience. Transplantation 61:54–61, 1996.

42. Beatty PG, Anasetti C: Marrow transplantation from donors other than HLA identical siblings. In Gale R (ed.): Bone Marrow Transplantation, pp. 677–686. Blackwell, Boston, 1990.

43. Perkins H, Hansen JA: The U.S. National Marrow Donor Program. Am J Pediatr Hematol Oncol 16:30–34, 1994.

44. Switzer GE, Dew MA, Stukas AA, Goycoolea JM, Hegland J, Simmons RG: Factors associated with attrition from a national bone marrow registry. Bone Marrow Transplant 24:313–319, 1999.

45. Rowley SD: Pharmacological purging of malignant cells. In Forman SJ, Blume KG, Thomas ED (eds.): Bone Marrow Transplantation, pp. 164–178. Blackwell Scientific, Boston, 1994.

46. Petersdorf EW, Mickelson EM, Anasetti C, Martin PJ, Woolfrey AE, Hansen JA: Effect of HLA mismatches on hematopoietic transplant outcomes. Curr Opin Immunol 11:521–526, 1999.

47. Ritz J, Ramsay NKC, Kersey JH: Autologous bone marrow transplantation for acute lymphoblastic leukemia. In Forman SJ, Blume KG, Thomas ED (eds.): Bone Marrow Transplantation, pp. 731–742. Blackwell Scientific Publications, Boston, 1994.

48. Yeager AM: Autologous bone marrow transplantation for acute myeloid leukemia. In Forman SJ, Blume KG, Thomas ED (eds.): Bone Marrow Transplantation, pp. 709–730. Blackwell Scientific, Boston, 1994.

49. Andrews RG, Bryant EM, Bartelmez SH, Muirhead DY, Knitter GH, Bensinger W et al: CD34+ marrow cells, devoid of T and B lymphocytes, reconstitute stable lymphopoiesis and myelopoiesis in lethally irradiated allogeneic baboons. Blood 80:1693–1701, 1992.

50. Bensinger W: Peripheral blood stem cell transplantation. In Buckner CD, Clift R (eds.): Technical and Biological Components of Marrow Transplantation, pp. 169–193. Kluwer Academic Publishers, Boston, 1995.

51. Thomas ED, Storb R, Clift RA, Fefer A, Johnson FL, Neiman PE et al: Bone-marrow transplantation. N Engl J Med 292:832–843, 895–902, 1975.

52. Thomas ED, Storb R: Technique for human marrow grafting. Blood 36:507–515, 1970.

53. Buckner CD, Clift RA, Sanders JE, Stewart P, Bensinger WI, Doney KC et al: Marrow harvesting from normal donors. Blood 64:630–634, 1984.

54. Jin NR, Hill RS, Petersen FB, Buckner CD, Stewart PS, Amos D et al: Marrow harvesting for autologous marrow transplantation. Exp Hematol 13:879–884, 1985.

55. Sanders J, Buckner CD, Bensinger WI, Levy W, Chard R, Thomas ED: Experience with marrow harvesting from donors less than two years of age. Bone Marrow Transplant 2:45–50, 1987.

56. Barnett MJ, Eaves CJ, Phillips GL, Gascoyne RD, Hogge DE, Horsman DE et al: Autografting with cultured marrow in chronic myeloid leukemia: Results of a pilot study. Blood 84:724–732, 1994.

57. Chang J, Morgenstern GR, Coutinho LH, Scarffe JH, Carr T, Deakin DP et al: The use of bone marrow cells grown in long-term culture for autologous bone marrow transplantation in acute myeloid leukaemia: An update. Bone Marrow Transplant 4:5–9, 1989.

58. Richman CM, Weiner RS, Yankee RA: Increase in circulating stem cells following chemotherapy in man. Blood 47:1031–1039, 1976.

59. Reiffers J, Korbling M, Labopin M, Gorin NC: Autologous blood stem cell transplantation versus autologous bone marrow transplantation for acute myeloid leukemia in first complete remission. Bone Marrow Transplant 7:144, 1991.

60. Papayannopoulou T: Mechanisms of stem-/progenitor-cell mobilization: The anti-VLA-4 paradigm (Review). Semin Hematol 37:11–18, 2000.

61. Bensinger W, Singer J, Appelbaum F, Lilleby K, Longin K, Rowley S et al: Autologous transplantation with peripheral blood mononuclear cells collected after administration of recombinant granulocyte stimulating factor. Blood 81:3158–3163, 1993.

62. Gianni AM, Siena S, Bregni M, Tarella C, Stern AC, Pileri A, Bonadonna G: Granulocyte-macrophage colony-stimulating factor to harvest circulating haemopoietic stem cells for autotransplantation. Lancet ii:580–585, 1989.

63. Papayannopoulou T, Nakamoto B: Peripheralization of hemopoietic progenitors in primates treated with anti-VLA4 integrin. Proc Natl Acad Sci USA 90:9374–9378, 1993.

64. Elliott C, Samson DM, Armitage S, Lyttelton MP, McGuigan D, Hargreaves R et al: When to harvest peripheral-blood stem cells after mobilization therapy: Prediction of CD34-positive cell yield by preceding day CD34-positive concentration in peripheral blood. J Clin Oncol 14:970–973, 1996.

65. Weaver CH, Buckner CD, Longin K Appelbaum FR, Rowley S, Lilleby K et al: Syngeneic transplantation with peripheral blood mononuclear cells collected after the administration of recombinant human granulocyte colony-stimulating factor. Blood 82:1981–1984, 1993.

66. Bensinger WI, Price TH, Dale DC, Appelbaum FR, Clift R, Lilleby K et al: The effects of daily recombinant human granulocyte colony stimulating factor administration on normal granulocyte donors undergoing leukapheresis. Blood 81:1883–1888, 1993.

67. Traycoff CM, Abboud MR, Laver J, Brandt JE, Hoffman R, Law P et al: Evaluation of the in vitro behavior of phenotypically defined populations of umbilical cord blood hematopoietic progenitor cells. Exp Hematol 22:215–222, 1994.

68. Broxmeyer HE, Smith FO: Cord blood stem cell transplantation. In Thomas ED, Blume KG, Forman SJ (eds.): Hematopoietic Cell Transplantation, 2nd Ed., pp. 431–443. Blackwell Science, Boston, 1999.

69. Socié G, Gluckman E, Carosella E, Brossard Y, Lafon C, Brison O: Search for maternal cells in human umbilical cord blood by polymerase chain reaction amplification of two minisatellite sequences. Blood 83:340–344, 1994.

70. Gluckman E, Broxmeyer HE, Auerbach AD, Friedman HS, Douglas GW, Devergie A et al: Hematopoietic reconstitution in a patient with Fanconi's anemia by means of umbilical-cord blood from an HLA-identical sibling. N Engl J Med 321:1174–1178, 1989.

71. Apperley JF: Umbilical cord blood progenitor cell transplantation. The International Conference Workshop on Cord Blood Transplantation, Indianapolis, November 1993 [see comments]. Bone Marrow Transplant 14:187–196, 1994.

72. Miscia S, Di Baldassarre A, Sabatino G, Bonvini E, Rana RA, Vitale M et al: Inefficient phospholipase C activation and reduced Lck expression characterize the signaling defect of umbilical cord T lymphocytes. J Immunol 163:2416–2424, 1999.

73. Gluckman E, Rocha V, Chastang C: Cord blood banking and transplant in Europe. Eurocord (Review). Vox Sang 74 (Suppl. 2):95–101, 1998.

74. Rubinstein P, Adamson JW, Stevens C: The placental/umbilical cord blood program of the New York Blood Center. A progress report. Ann NY Acad Sci 872:328–334, 1999.

75. Touraine JL: In-utero transplantation of fetal liver stem cells into human fetuses. Human Reprod 7:44–48, 1992.

76. Carr S, Rubin L, Dixon D, Star J, Dailey J: Intrauterine therapy for homozygous alpha-thalassemia. Obstet Gynecol 85:876–879, 1995.

77. Miller AD: Genetic manipulation of hematopoietic stem cells. In Forman SJ, Blume KG, Thomas ED (eds.): Bone Marrow Transplantation, pp. 72–78. Blackwell Scientific, Boston, 1994.

78. Lansdorp PM, Dragowska W, Mayani H: Ontogeny-related changes in proliferative potential of human hematopoietic cells. J Exp Med 178:787–791, 1993.

79. Pettengell R, Testa NG, Swindell R, Crowther D, Dexter TM: Transplantation potential of hematopoietic cells released into the circulation during routine chemotherapy for non-Hodgkin's lymphoma. Blood 82:2239–2248, 1993.

80. Bensinger W, Martin P, Clift R, Storer B, Forman S, Blume K et al: A prospective, randomised trial of peripheral blood stem cells (PBSC) or marrow (BM) for patients undergoing allogeneic transplantation for hematologic malignancies. Blood 94(Suppl. 1):368a, #1637, 1999 (Abstract).

81. Powles R, Mehta J, Kulkarni S, Treleavan J, Millar B, Marsden J et al: Allogeneic blood and bone-marrow stem-cell transplantation in haematological malignant diseases: A randomised trial. Lancet 355:1231–1237, 2000.

82. Gluckman E, Rocha V, Boyer-Chammard A, Locatelli F, Arcese W, Pasquini R et al: Outcome of cord-blood transplantation from related and unrelated donors. N Engl J Med 337:373–381, 1997.

83. Kurtzberg J, Laughlin M, Graham ML, Smith C, Olson JF, Halperin EC et al: Placental blood as a source of hematopoietic stem cells for transplantation into unrelated recipients. N Engl J Med 335:157–166, 1996.

84. Shpall EJ, Jones RB: Release of tumor cells from bone marrow (Editorial). Blood 83:623–625, 1994.

85. Carella AM, Pollicardo N, Pungolino E, Raffo MR, Podesta M, Ferrero R et al: Mobilization of cytogenetically 'normal' blood progenitors cells by intensive conventional chemotherapy for chronic myeloid and acute lymphoblastic leukemia. Leuk Lymphoma 9:477–483, 1993.

86. Shpall EJ, Jones RB: Mobilization and collection of peripheral blood progenitor cells for support of high-dose cancer therapy. In Forman SJ, Blume KG, Thomas ED (eds.): Bone Marrow Transplantation, pp. 913–918. Blackwell Scientific Publications, Boston, 1994.

87. Brugger W, Bross KJ, Glatt M, Weber F, Mertelsmann R, Kanz L: Mobilization of tumor cells and hematopoietic progenitor cells into peripheral blood of patients with solid tumors. Blood 83:636–640, 1994.

88. Hanania EG, Fu S, Zu Z, Hegewisch-Becker S, Korbling M, Hester J et al: Chemotherapy resistance to taxol in clonogenic progenitor cells following transduction of CD34 selected marrow and peripheral blood cells with a retrovirus that contains the MDR-1 chemotherapy resistance gene. Gene Ther 2:285–294, 1995.

89. Berenson RJ, Andrews RG, Bensinger WI, Kalamasz D, Knitter G, Buckner CD, Bernstein ID: Antigen CD34+ marrow cells engraft lethally irradiated baboons. J Clin Invest 81:951–955, 1988.

90. Verfaillie CM, Miller WJ, Boylan K, McGlave PB: Selection of benign primitive hematopoietic progenitors in chronic myelogenous leukemia on the basis of HLA-DR antigen expression. Blood 79:1003–1010, 1992.

91. Lu L, Xiao M, Clapp DW, Li ZH, Broxmeyer HE: High efficiency retroviral mediated gene transduction into single isolated immature and replatable CD34(3+) hematopoietic stem/progenitor cells from human umbilical cord blood. J Exp Med 178:2089–2096, 1993.

92. Chang J, Coutinho L, Morgenstern G, Scarffe JH, Deakin D, Harrison C et al: Reconstitution of haemopoietic system with autologous marrow taken during relapse of acute myeloblastic leukaemia and grown in long-term culture. Lancet i:294–295, 1986.

93. Brugger W, Heimfeld S, Berenson RJ, Mertelsmann R, Kanz L: Reconstitution of hematopoiesis after high-dose chemotherapy by autologous progenitor cells generated ex vivo. N Engl J Med 333:283–287, 1995.

94. Williams SF, Lee WJ, Bender JG, Zimmerman T, Swinney P, Blake M et al: Selection and expansion of peripheral blood CD34+ cells in autologous stem cell transplantation for breast cancer. Blood 87:1687–1691, 1996.

95. Holyoake TL, Alcorn MJ, Richmond L, Farrell E, Pearson C, Green R et al: CD34 positive PBPC expanded ex vivo may not provide durable engraftment following myeloablative chemoradiotherapy regimens. Bone Marrow Transplant 19:1095–1101, 1997.

96. Stiff P, Parthasarathy M, Chen B, Moss T, Oldenberg D, Douville J et al: A single apheresis combined with ex vivo expanded bone marrow cells from a small starting aliquot leads to rapid hematopoietic engraftment following autotransplantation. Blood 92:132a, 1998 (Abstract).

97. Shpall EJ, Quinones R, Hami L, Jones R, Bearman S, Cagnoni P et al: Transplantation of cancer patients receiving high dose chemotherapy with ex vivo expanded cord blood cells. Blood 92:646a, 1998 (Abstract).

98. Gribben JG, Neuberg D, Freedman AS, Gimmi CD, Pesek KW, Barber M et al: Detection by polymerase chain reaction of residual cells with the bcl-2 translocation is associated with increased risk of relapse after autologous bone marrow transplantation for B-cell lymphoma. Blood 81:3449–3457, 1993.

99. Radich J, Thomson B: Advances in the detection of minimal residual disease (Review). Curr Opin Hematol 4:242–247, 1997.

100. Metcalf D: The Florey Lecture, 1991. The colony-stimulating factors: Discovery to clinical use (Review). Philos Trans Royal Soc London, Series B: Biol Sci 333:147–173, 1991.

101. Messner HA, McCulloch EA: Mechanisms of human hematopoiesis. In Forman SJ, Blume KG, Thomas ED (eds.): Bone Marrow Transplantation, pp. 41–52. Blackwell Scientific, Boston, 1994.

102. Kanz L, Brugger W: Mobilization and ex vivo manipulation of peripheral blood progenitor cells for support of high-dose cancer therapy. In Thomas ED, Blume KG, Forman SJ (eds.): Hematopoietic Cell Transplantation, 2nd Ed., pp. 455–468. Blackwell Science, Boston, 1999.

103. Muench MO, Moore MA: Accelerated recovery of peripheral blood cell counts in mice transplanted with in vitro cytokine-expanded hematopoietic progenitors. Exp Hematol 20:611–618, 1992.

104. Ploemacher RE, van Soest PL, Voorwinden H, Boudewijn A: Interleukin-12 synergizes with interleukin-3 and steel factor to enhance recovery of murine hemopoietic stem cells in liquid culture. Leukemia 7:1381–1388, 1993.

105. Visser JW, Rozemuller H, de Jong MO, Belyavsky A: The expression of cytokine receptors by purified hemopoietic stem cells. Stem Cells 11(Suppl. 2):49–55, 1993.

106. Koller MR, Emerson SG, Palsson BO: Large-scale expansion of human stem and progenitor cells from bone marrow mononuclear cells in continuous perfusion cultures. Blood 82:378–384, 1993.

107. Palsson BO, Paek SH, Schwartz RM, Palsson M, Lee GM, Silver S, Emerson SG: Expansion of human bone marrow progenitor cells in a high cell density continuous perfusion system. Bio/Technol 11:368–372, 1993.

108. Lu L, Xiao M, Shen RN, Grigsby S, Broxmeyer HE: Enrichment, characterization, and responsiveness of single primitive CD34 human umbilical cord blood hematopoietic progenitors with high proliferative and replating potential. Blood 81:41–48, 1993.

109. Kiem H-P, Darovsky B, von Kalle C, Goehle S, Stewart D, Graham T et al: Retrovirus-mediated gene transduction into canine peripheral blood repopulating cells. Blood 83:1467–1473, 1994.

110. Andrews RG, Briddell RA, Gough M, McNiece IK: Expansion of G-CSF mobilized CD34+ peripheral blood cells (PBC) for 10 days in G-CSF, MGDF and SCF prior to transplantation decreased post-transplant neutropenia in baboons. Blood 90:92a, 1997 (Abstract).

111. Storek J, Gooley T, Siadak M, Bensinger WI, Maloney DG, Chauncey TR et al: Allogeneic peripheral blood stem cell transplantation may be associated with a high risk of chronic graft-versus-host disease. Blood 90:4705–4709, 1997.

112. Mielcarek M, Martin P, Torok-Storb B: Suppression of alloantigen-induced T-cell proliferation by CD14+ cells derived from granulocyte colony-stimulating factor (G-CSF)-mobilized peripheral blood mononuclear cells. Blood 89:1629–1634, 1997.

113. Mielcarek M, Graf L, Johnson G, Torok-Storb B: Production of interleukin-10 by granulocyte colony-stimulating factor-mobilized blood products: A mechanism for monocyte-mediated suppression of T cell proliferation. Blood 92:215–222, 1998.

114. Couban S, Messner HA, Andreou P, Egan B, Price S, Tinker L et al: Bone marrow mobilized with granulocyte colony-stimulating factor in related allogeneic transplant recipients: A study of 29 patients. Biol Blood Marrow Transplant 6:422–427, 2000.

115. Isola L, Scigliano E, Fruchtman S: Long-term follow-up after allogeneic granulocyte colony-stimulating factor—primed bone marrow transplantation. Biol Blood Marrow Transplant 6:428–433, 2000.

116. Serody JS, Sparks SD, Lin Y, Capel EJ, Bigelow SH, Kirby SL et al: Comparison of granulocyte colony-stimulating factor (G-CSF)–mobilized peripheral blood progenitor cells and G-CSF–stimulated bone marrow as a source of stem cells in HLA-matched sibling transplantation. Biol Blood Marrow Transplant 6:434–440, 2000.

117. Rocha V, Arcese W, Sanz G, Laporte JP, Takahashi T, Fernandez M et al: Prognostic factors of outcome after unrelated cord blood transplant in adults with hematologic malignancies (Abstract). Blood (in press).

118. Cowan MJ, Golbus M: In utero hematopoietic stem cell transplants for inherited diseases. Am J Pediatr Hematol Oncol 16:35–42, 1994.

119. Tisdale JF, Hanazono Y, Sellers SE, Agricola BA, Metzger ME, Donahue RE, Dunbar CE: Ex vivo expansion of genetically marked Rhesus peripheral blood progenitor cells results in diminished long-term repopulating ability. Blood 92:1131–1141, 1998.

120. Guenechea G, Segovia JC, Albella B, Lamana M, Ramirez M, Regidor C et al: Delayed engraftment of nonobese diabetic severe combined immunodeficient mice transplanted with ex vivo-expanded human CD34(+) cord blood cells. Blood 93:1097–1105, 1999.

121. McAdams TA, Miller WM, Papoutsakis ET: Hematopoietic cell culture therapies (Part I): Cell culture considerations (Review). Trends Biotechnol 14:341–349, 1996.

122. Reiffers J, Cailliot C, Dazey B, Duchez I, Pigneux A, Cousin T et al: Infusion of expanded CD34+ selected cells can abrogate post myeloablative chemotherapy neutropenia in patients with hematologic malignances. Blood 92:126a, 1998 (Abstract).

123. Körbling M: Peripheral blood stem cells for allogeneic transplantation. In Thomas ED, Blume KG, Forman SJ (eds.): Hematopoietic Cell Transplantation, 2nd Ed, pp. 469–480. Blackwell Scientific, Boston, 1999.

57

Umbilical Cord Blood Banking and Transplantation

Joanne Kurtzberg

OVERVIEW

Hematopoietic stem cell transplantation is used to treat patients with aggressive or recurrent malignancies, immunodeficiency diseases, certain genetic conditions including inborn errors of metabolism and hemoglobinopathies, and bone marrow failure syndromes. Additional applications, including regenerative therapies for nonhematopoietic cells, have been suggested for the future but are currently unproven and the subject of ongoing preclinical research.

A major limitation to stem cell transplantation therapy is donor availability. Only 20 to 25 percent of patients in need of a transplant will have HLA-matched relatives who can serve as their donors. Of those lacking a related donor, approximately 25 percent of white patients will identify an HLA- matched unrelated, living bone marrow donor through the National Marrow Donor Program and other living donor registries, but fewer than 10 percent of patients of ethnic minority lineage find a suitably matched unrelated marrow donor. For the remaining patients, a fully matched unrelated stem cell donor cannot be identified.

Over the past decade, umbilical cord blood (UCB), the baby's blood remaining in the placenta or afterbirth, has emerged as an alternative source of hematopoietic stem cells for use in transplantation. Cord blood has several advantages over bone marrow, most importantly that it does not need to be fully HLA-matched for a successful transplant. It is also readily available, can be collected without risk to the mother or infant donor, and is significantly less likely to transmit infectious diseases transmissible through the blood. It also has been shown to be less likely to cause acute and chronic graft-versus-host disease (GvHD), a major obstacle to the success of allogeneic bone marrow transplantation. Because cord blood can be collected without risk, mothers of ethnic minority backgrounds are more likely to donate to cord blood banks than adult bone marrow registries.

CORD BLOOD PROCUREMENT AND BANKING

Cord blood can be collected from the placenta either in situ during the third stage of labor or ex vivo within 10 to 15 minutes after delivery of the placenta. Cord blood is harvested into a closed sterile collection container containing citrate phosphate dextrose (CPD) anticoagulant to prevent clotting. Generally, this is accomplished by sterilely puncturing one of the umbilical veins and allowing the cord blood to drain by gravity into a bag containing anticoagulant. Citrate phosphate dextrose has been identified as the anticoagulant with the lowest toxicity to hematopoietic stem and progenitor cells with activity over a range of collection volumes. During collection, care must be taken to avoid mixing of maternal and fetal blood because this would lead to contamination of the cord blood unit with HLA-disparate, immunocompetent maternal T cells, which could cause GvHD in a transplant recipient.[1] After harvest from the placenta, the collected cord blood can be maintained at room temperature for up to 48 to 72 hours without appreciable cell losses. Most banks deplete red blood cells and reduce volume of the cord blood collection with hetastarch or other density gradient separations. For long-term storage, cells are cryopreserved in dimethyl sulfoxide (DMSO) and stored under liquid nitrogen. Maximal storage time, or expiration date, is unknown, but under stable conditions, cells are likely to remain viable for decades.

There are two major types of cord blood donations, public or private.[2,3] In general public banks are not for profit, and with third-party financial support, public banks collect cord blood from healthy term pregnancies after maternal informed consent. In granting consent, the infant's mother acknowledges that the donation is voluntary and that she gives up all rights to the cord blood for the public good. The mother also agrees to allow her medical records and the baby's newborn records to be reviewed, gives a detailed family medical history, and allows a sample of her own blood to be taken for infectious disease testing and HLA typing. The results of these tests are not routinely provided to the baby's parents or physicians. However, if a disease potentially putting the infant donor at risk is identified, the parent and physician are both notified. Public cord blood banks ensure confidentiality and do not allow any contact between the infant donor or the donor's family and the patient receiving the stem cells.

Private cord blood banks are generally for-profit companies providing a service for a fee. Private donations are financed by the family of the donor or recipient and are usually directed to a specific recipient or the recipient's family. In the minority of private donations, a relative in need of a transplant donor was identified in advance of the baby's birth. The donation allows for greater mismatching between the donor and recipient and also spares the donor from the risks of a bone marrow or peripheral stem cell harvest. The remainder of private or directed donations are undertaken as an investment in the unknown potential for cord blood to be used to treat serious illnesses in the future. To date, no transplants have resulted from these private speculative banking activities.

Private cord blood banking is a service offered to new parents by for-profit companies in the United States. The majority of these companies provide a collection kit to families interested in private banking. There are no established medical indications for banking. The units are collected by the physician, midwife, or nurse delivering the baby and shipped back to the company's banking facility. Compensation for the collector is variable, ranging from none to monetary reimbursement based on effort expended. Limited testing is performed on the units, and minimal standards are used to determine whether a unit is eligible for processing and banking. Both collection and banking fees and yearly storage fees are generally charged. Units can be stored for autologous or directed donation to a relative in the family. Most pediatricians believe that routine cord blood storage in healthy babies is unnecessary.[3] In this regard, it is important to point out that autologous cord blood would not be used for bone marrow transplantation in a child with acute leukemia because of concern of contamination with malignant cells[4] as well as lack of graft versus leukemia effects. Directed donation of umbilical cord blood for another family member is indicated when there is a first degree relative with a high-risk or refractory pediatric malignancy amenable to treatment with transplantation therapy, a hemoglobinopathy or other transfusion-dependent anemia; a congenital immunodeficiency; or an inborn error of metabolism. There are insufficient data to address the question of whether related haploidentical cord blood will play a role in the treatment of adults with refractory malignancies or other diseases amenable to treatment by allogeneic stem cell transplantation.

Over the past decade with support from governmental and/or private sources, unrelated cord blood has been banked by various investigators for public use around the world.[5–11] It is estimated that approximately 100,000 units are listed in individual public banks around the world. Establishment of these banks was stimulated by the need for stem cell donors for patients with malignant diseases and genetic conditions correctable by transplantation therapy who lack a suitably matched related donor. Units stored in public banks are available for any patient in need who is medically eligible for transplantation therapy. These units are tested and HLA-typed at the time of banking, rendering them readily available for transplantation therapy when identified as the donor of choice for a patient in need.

The first public bank in the world was established by Dr. Pablo Rubinstein at the New York Blood Center, with grant support from the National Heart, Lung, and Blood Institute (NHLBI) of the National Institutes of Health.[5] This bank, now known as the Placental Blood Program, has banked more than 14,000 units in 11 years and has provided over 1200 units for transplantation worldwide. In 1996, the NHLBI funded three academic centers to establish a second public bank called COBLT (Cord Blood Transplantation Study), with banking sites at Duke University Medical Center in collaboration with the American Red Cross (The Carolinas Cord Blood Bank), Georgetown University, and the University of California at Los Angeles.[6] Collection of units for the COBLT banks was supported through June of 2001, creating an inventory of approximately 8000 units. A public bank now listing approximately 6000 units was also established at Cardinal Glennon Hospital in St. Louis through philanthropic sources. Other smaller public banks have been established throughout the United States, but none have collected more than 1000 units to date.

Most public banks, employ a team of dedicated nurses and medical technologists who are responsible for donor recruitment; donor screening; obtaining maternal consents, medical histories; and blood samples; harvesting the units; and transporting them to the laboratory for banking. Units are generally collected from term babies born after an uncomplicated pregnancy, labor, and delivery. Units are cryopreserved within a finite time, usually 48 to 72 hours, from collection and placed in quarantine until test results are obtained. Units passing a screening algorithm are HLA-typed and placed in the search registry for patient access.

Maternal donors give consent for a voluntary donation of their baby's cord blood, testing of maternal and/or fetal blood for infectious and genetic diseases transmitted through blood and stem cells, testing of the cord blood for stem and progenitor cell content, and review of their family's medical history and the medical records of the infant and mother. Screening for homozygous hemoglobinopathies may be performed by direct testing of the cord blood or, in states with mandatory screening, by obtaining the results of the infant donor from the state screening program. Donor confidentiality is preserved via labeling using bar codes, but most banks retain a link between the donor's demographic information and the bar code label. Maternal donors are excluded if they are known to be infected with hepatitis B or C, human T-cell lymphoma virus (HTLV), or human immunodeficiency (HIV) virus. They are also excluded if they have traveled to or lived in countries where HIV or malaria is endemic or if they practice high-risk behaviors, have positive viral serologies for syphilis, hepatitis B or C, HTLV 1 or 2, or HIV 1 or 2.

Detection of cytomegalovirus (CMV) in cord blood donors presents a unique problem. Forty to ninety percent of mothers are CMV IgG-positive, representing immunologic conversion after routine infection earlier in life but not infection during their pregnancy. Maternal IgG crosses the placenta into the fetal blood. Thus, if the mother is CMV IgG-positive, the cord blood will test positive, reflecting passive transfer of the maternal IgG. However, this in no way indicates that the fetus was exposed to or infected with CMV virus. Since detection of CMV IgG does not correlate with CMV disease, alternative methods of CMV viral detection have been sought. The New York Blood Center Placental Blood Program routinely cultured donor infant saliva for CMV virus as well as assaying CMV IgG and IgM in these infants' mothers. The overall incidence of positive cultures was 0.3 percent, but this is did not reliably correlate with titers of CMV IgM in mothers of babies with positive cultures. Techniques to detect CMV DNA in cord blood cells or plasma are under development but not ready for clinical use at this time.

Some banks follow infant donors for 0.5 to 2 years after donation to determine whether these infants develop any diseases that could be transmitted to and clinically expressed in a transplant recipient, but most centers do not have the resources to effectively execute follow-up or look-forward programs. Mothers are counseled to inform the banks if their infant develops any serious illnesses during childhood (e.g., cancer, AIDS, genetic diseases, immunodeficiency syndromes).

Publicly banked units are characterized in laboratories committed to excellence in stem cell processing and cryopreservation. Cell counts, differentials, viability, ABO and Rh typing, CD34, CD3, and clonal hematopoietic progenitor cell content are routinely enumerated. Bacterial and fungal cultures are routinely performed, and positive units are excluded from the inventory. Procedures for volume reduction, red blood cell depletion, and cryopreservation are standardized and validated.[5,6] HLA typing is performed on the red cell pellet by molecular techniques with a minimum of antigenic typing for HLA class I, A, and B and at the allelic level for HLA class II, DRB1. Results are entered into electronic databases, which can be accessed by transplantation centers searching for donors for their patients. The COBLT project studied over 33,000 potential maternal donors and 18,000 collected cord blood units. The main reason for donor exclusion was a risk factor for infectious disease exposure in the mother or a positive infectious disease screening test in the mother around the time of delivery. After unit collection, the main reason for exclusion for banking was low volume. In the 8000 units banked, the average number of total nucleated cells was 1×10^9 and the average number of CD34 cells was 2.6×10^6. This represents a 10 to 20-fold decrease from the average number of cells used in a typical bone marrow transplant.

Currently there is no centralized registry where units from all unrelated cord blood banks list their inventories. The larger banks have independent search programs, and some of the smaller banks have networked through the National Marrow Donor Program or the American Red Cross. Netcord, an international, collaborative association of 14 banks is developing an Internet-based search engine to facilitate searching. Thus, patients and transplant centers in search of a donor must search banks individually. There are also no formal regulations for cord blood collection, processing, and banking by governmental agencies, although in the United States the Food and Drug Administration (FDA) has published proposed regulations that are expected to go into effect before the completion of calendar year 2002. Cord blood has not yet been licensed by the FDA as a product. Thus, public units used for transplantation can be obtained at no cost or with an FDA-set fee for cost reimbursement from the major public banks in the United States and abroad.

EARLY TRANSPLANTATION EXPERIENCE WITH UMBILICAL CORD BLOOD

Before the demonstration of successful engraftment in a human patient who has received a transplant with UCB, there was great skepticism about the feasibility of the procedure. Many investigators doubted that cord blood would contain sufficient numbers of cells for short-term or durable marrow reconstitution. Those believing engraftment was possible thought that this would only hold true for young children of low weight and small stature. Many worried that the naiveté of cord blood lymphocytes would lead to post-transplant immunodeficiency and lack graft-versus-leukemia effects. The proof that cord blood transplantation was feasible required a human experiment.

The first cord blood transplant in the world was performed in 1988 by Eliane Gluckman at l'Hôpital St. Louis in Paris in a 6-year-old boy with Fanconi anemia.[12] This transplant was supported by a multidisciplinary, international collaboration among several academic medical centers, a private insurer, l'Hôpital St. Louis, and the first private cord blood company (Biocyte). Unfortunately, to date this altruism has not been extended to support public banking or additional basic or clinical studies in the field. The success of this transplant paved the way for approximately 60 additional related UCB transplants over the subsequent 5 years. Outcomes of these transplant demonstrated the feasibility of engraftment in children, delayed times to engraftment of neutrophils and platelets, and a reduced incidence of acute and chronic graft-versus-host disease, compared with results in allogeneic bone marrow transplantation from matched related donors.[12–18]

UNRELATED UMBILICAL CORD BLOOD TRANSPLANTATION

The first unrelated cord blood transplant was performed in August of 1993 with an HLA-mismatched unit from the New York Blood Center.[19] Since that time, more than 2000 unrelated cord blood transplants have been performed worldwide.[15,19–39] The majority of these transplants have been used to treat children with cancer or genetic diseases, with an overall success rate of 50 to 60 percent.[19–33] Among patients with malignancies, younger children with earlier staged disease have an improved prognosis. Over the past 4 years, approximately 150 adults with high-risk malignancies who lack traditional stem cell donors, have received unrelated cord blood transplants, with an overall success rate comparable to that of unrelated bone marrow transplantation in adults.[25,26]

After cord blood transplantation, neutrophil engraftment occurs in a median of 25 days in 90 percent of children and 80 percent of adults.[19–39] Cell dose, rather than HLA match, has been identified as the most important factor correlating with clinical outcomes after cord blood transplantation.[15,19,21,32–34] Patients receiving larger cell doses per kilogram of body weight experience more rapid neutrophil and platelet engraftment, higher probabilities of overall engraftment, earlier immune reconstitution, and superior event-free survival. However, because of the biological differences in size and thymic function in babies versus children versus adults, it has not been possible to completely distinguish between the influence of cell dose versus age in analysis of clinical outcomes in UCB transplants to date.

The incidence of moderate to severe (grades II to IV) acute GvHD after unrelated, partially HLA-mismatched UCB transplantation is approximately 40 percent, with 10 percent of patients experiencing severe disease (grades III and IV).[17,19–21,32,33] A major advantage of cord blood stem cells as compared to bone marrow stem cells is that the former are much less likely to cause extensive chronic GvHD.[19–21,32] The conventional wisdom dictates that UCB stem and T cells are more tolerant of a new host than phenotypically identical cells from bone marrow or mobilized peripheral blood.[40–49]

The major cause of failure after an unrelated cord blood transplant is opportunistic infections.[19–21,32–34,50] Fatal infections generally occur before 100 days post-transplant in children and 180 days post-transplant in adults. The tendency toward infection is believed to be due to several factors, including lower cell dosing, leading to longer periods of neutropenia in the first several weeks post-transplant, as well as defects in neutrophil function as these cells recapitulate neonatal neutrophil function and ontogeny. Cord blood-derived lymphocytes are naïve, having never been exposed to common bacterial and viral pathogens. Cord blood lacks T cells with memory of CMV, EBV, or other common viruses likely to be present, which have the potential to reactivate in the transplant recipient.

The pace of immune reconstitution relates to patient age as well as dose of cells transplanted. The youngest patients (under 2 years of age) recover adequate T-cell numbers and function by 3 to 4 months post-transplant. Children between the ages of 2 and 17 years reach a similar endpoint by 12 months post-transplant. Adults may never fully recover thymic-dependent immune function and generally take up to three times as long as children to recover protective function.[51,52] This is believed to be due to the fact that the host's adult thymus has a lower capacity to contribute to the immune reconstitution process. To increase the success of cord blood transplantation in adults, it is generally agreed that the cell dose of a single transplant needs to be increased. Current preclinical and clinical research is focused on using combined cord blood transplants or ex vivo expansion of cord blood cells as one strategy to increase the dose of cells available for transplantation.[53–65] Results of phase I clinical trials are encouraging, but additional studies are required to establish the usefulness of these approaches.[63–65]

Nonablative, or "mini," transplants are undergoing testing in adult patients with malignancies who are unable to tolerate full-dose myeloablative therapy. Limited trials using unrelated cord blood in this setting have demonstrated success in 50 percent of heavily pretreated, older patients with malignant diagnoses.[66,67] Similar approaches have been suggested for children with non-malignant diagnoses; however, immune-mediated graft rejection and autologous marrow recovery have been obstacles to the success of this approach in younger and immunologically healthier patients.

Cord blood transplantation has been especially successful in young infants and toddlers with inborn errors of metabolism. In these patients, the cord blood stem cells provide a durable source of cells capable of producing the defective or missing enzyme in the patient. When performed early in the course of disease, stem cell transplantation prevents further progression and in some cases facilitates reversal of organ damage incurred prior to transplantation therapy. In patients with leukodystrophies, cord blood transplantation performed in the presymptomatic phase prevents demyelination in both the central and peripheral nervous systems. In patients with mucopolysaccharidoses such as Hurler syndrome[68] or Krabbos disease,[69] corneal clouding, hepatocellular damage, and bony deformities will be corrected and central nervous system damage will be prevented if transplantation therapy is used before the age of 2 years. Most interestingly, cardiac disease, usually caused by atherosclerotic changes in coronary arteries in early childhood, is also ameliorated. These observations suggest that cord blood stem cells are capable of transdifferentiation and cellular plasticity and raise optimism for the development of cord blood-derived cellular therapies for hepatic, cardiac, and neurodegenerative diseases of adults.

REFERENCES

1. Muller SM, Ege M, Pottharst A et al: Transplacentally acquired maternal T lymphocytes in severe combined immunodeficiency: A study of 121 patients. Blood 98:1847–1851, 2001.
2. Smith FO, Kurtzberg J, Karson EM et al: Umbilical cord blood collection, storage and transplantation: Issues and recommendations for expectant parents and patients. Cancer Res Ther Control 10:217–226, 1999.
3. American Academy of Pediatrics Working Group on Cord Blood Banking, 1998: Cord blood banking for potential future transplantation: Subject review. Pediatrics 104:116–118, 1999.
4. Rowley JD: Backtracking leukemia to birth. Nat Med 4:150–151, 1998.
5. Rubinstein P, Dobrila L, Rosenfield RE et al: Processing and cryopreservation of placental/umbilical cord blood for unrelated bone marrow reconstitution. Proc Natl Acad Sci U S A 92:10119–10122, 1995.
6. Fraser JK, Cairo MS, Wagner EL et al: Cord blood transplantation study (COBLT): Cord blood bank standard operating procedures. J Hematother 7:521–561, 1998.
7. Boppana SB, Rivera LB, Fowler KB et al: Intrauterine transmission of cytomegalovirus to infants of women with preconceptional immunity. N Engl J Med 344:1366–1371, 2001.
8. Rendine S, Durtoni ES, di Celle F et al: Analysis of the Turin Umbilical Cord Blood Bank Registry. Transfusion 40:813–816, 2000.
9. Rogers I, Sutherland DR, Holt D et al: Human UC-blood banking: Impact of blood volume, cell separation and cryopreservation on leukocyte and $CD34^+$ cell recovery. Cytotherapy 3:269–276, 2001.
10. Stanworth S, Warwick R, Fehily D et al: An international survey of unrelated umbilical cord blood banking. Vox Sang 80:236–43, 2001.
11. Ballen K, Broxmeyer HE, McCullough J et al: Current status of cord blood banking and transplantation in the United States and Europe. Biol Blood Marrow Transplant 7:635–645, 2001.
12. Gluckman E, Broxmeyer HE, Auerbach AD et al: Hematopoietic reconstitution in a patient with Fanconi's anemia by means of umbilical cord blood from an HLA-identical sibling. N Engl J Med 321:1174–1178, 1989.
13. Wagner JE: Umbilical cord blood stem cell transplantation. Am J Pediatr Hematol Oncol 15:169–174, 1993.
14. Wagner JE, Kernan NA, Steinbuch M et al: Allogeneic sibling umbilical-cord-blood transplantation in children with malignant and non-malignant disease. Lancet 346:214–219, 1995.
15. Gluckman E, Rocha V, Boyer-Chammard A et al: Outcome of cord-blood transplantation from related and unrelated donors. N Engl J Med 337:373–381, 1997.
16. Kato S, Nishihira H, Sako M et al: Cord blood transplantation from sibling donors in Japan: Report of the national survey. Int J Hematol 67:389–396, 1998.
17. Rocha V, Wagner JE, Sobocinski KA et al: Graft-versus-host disease in children who have received a cord-blood or bone marrow transplant from an HLA-identical sibling. N Engl J Med 342:1846–1854, 2000.
18. Gluckman E: Hematopoietic stem-cell transplants using umbilical-cord blood. N Engl J Med 344:1860–1861, 2001.

19. Kurtzberg J, Laughlin M, Graham ML et al: Placental blood as a source of hematopoietic stem cells for transplantation into unrelated recipients. N Engl J Med 335:157–166, 1996.

20. Wagner JE, Rosenthal J, Sweetman R et al: Successful transplantation of HLA-matched and HLA-mismatched umbilical cord blood from unrelated donors: Analysis of engraftment and acute graft-versus-host disease. Blood 88:795–802, 1996.

21. Rubinstein P, Carrier C, Scaradavou A et al: Outcomes among 562 recipients of placental-blood transplants from unrelated donors. N Engl J Med 339:1565–1629, 1998.

22. Gluckman E: Current status of umbilical cord blood hematopoietic stem cell transplantation. Exp Hematol 28:1197–1205, 2000.

23. Gluckman E, Locatelli F: Umbilical cord blood transplants. Curr Opin Hemat 7:353–357, 2000.

24. Nagarajan R, Neglia J, Ramsay N et al: Successful treatment of refractory Langerhans cell histiocytosis with unrelated cord blood transplantation. J Pediatr Hematol Oncol 23:629–632, 2001.

25. Suminoe A, Matsuzaki A, Hattori H et al: Unrelated cord blood transplantation for an infant with chemotherapy-resistant progressive Langerhans cell histiocytosis. J Pediatr Hematol Oncol 23:633–637, 2001.

26. Goussetis E, Peristeri J, Kitra V et al: Combined umbilical cord blood and bone marrow transplantation in the treatment of beta-thalassemia major. Pediatr Hematol Oncol 17:307–314, 2000.

27. Veys P: Umbilical cord blood transplantation in beta-thalassemia major. Pediatr Hemat Oncol 17:281–283, 2000.

28. Gore L, Lane PA, Quinones RR, Giller RH: Successful cord blood transplantation for sickle cell anemia from a sibling who is human leukocyte antigen–identical: Implications for comprehensive care. J Pediatr Hematol Oncol 22:437–440, 2000.

29. Mullen CA, Thompson JN, Richard LA, Chan KW: Unrelated umbilical cord blood transplantation in infancy for mucopolysaccharidosis type IIB (Hunter syndrome) complicated by autoimmune hemolytic anemia. Bone Marrow Transplant 25:1093–1097, 2000.

30. Ziegner UH, Ochs HD, Schanen C et al: Unrelated umbilical cord stem cell transplantation for X-linked immunodeficiencies. J Pediatr 138:570–573, 2001.

31. Yoshimasu T, Tanaka R, Suenobu S et al: Prompt and durable hematopoietic reconstitution by unrelated cord blood transplantation in a child with Fanconi anemia. Bone Marrow Transplant 27:767–769, 2001.

32. Rocha V, Cornish J, Sievers EL et al: Comparison of outcomes of unrelated bone marrow and umbilical cord blood transplants in children with acute leukemia. Blood 97:2962–2970, 2001.

33. Barker JN, Davies SM, DeFor T et al: Survival after transplantation of unrelated donor umbilical cord blood is comparable to that of human leukocyte antigen-matched unrelated donor bone marrow: Results of a matched-pair analysis. Blood 97:2957–2961, 2001.

34. Migliaccio AR, Adamson JW, Stevens CE et al: Cell dose and speed of engraftment in placental/umbilical cord blood transplantation: Graft progenitor cell content is a better predictor than nucleated cell quantity. Blood 96:2717–2722, 2000.

35. Laughlin MJ, Rizzieri DA, Smith CA et al: Hematologic engraftment and reconstitution of immune function post unrelated placental cord blood transplant in an adult with acute lymphocytic leukemia. Leuk Res 22:215–219, 1998.

36. Laughlin MJ, Barker J, Bambach B et al: Hematopoietic engraftment and survival in adult recipients of umbilical-cord blood from unrelated donors. N Engl J Med 344:1815–1822, 2001.

37. Sanz GF, Saavedra S, Planelles D et al: Standardized, unrelated donor cord blood transplantation in adults with hematologic malignancies. Blood 98:2332–2338, 2001.

38. Lau FY, Wong R, Chui CH et al: Successful engraftment in two adult patients with severe aplastic anemia using nonmyeloablative conditioning followed by unrelated HLA-mismatched cord blood transplantation. J Hematother Stem Cell Res 10:309–311, 2001.

39. Laughlin MJ: Umbilical cord blood for allogeneic transplantation in children and adults. Bone Marrow Transplant 27:1–6, 2001.

40. Anasetti C: Young is better if enough. Blood 97:2921, 2001.

41. Rubinstein P: HLA matching for bone marrow transplantation – how much is enough? N Engl J Med 345:1842–1843, 2001.

42. Ohnuma K, Isoyama K, Ikuta K et al: The influence of HLA genotyping compatibility on clinical outcome after cord blood transplantation from unrelated donors. J Hematother Stem Cell Res 9:541–550, 2000.

43. Harris DT, Schumacher MJ, Locascio J et al: Phenotypic and functional immaturity of human umbilical cord blood T lymphocytes. Proc Natl Acad Sci U S A 89:10006–10010, 1992.

44. Clerici M, DePalma L, Roilides E et al: Analysis of T helper and antigen-presenting cell functions in cord blood and peripheral blood leukocytes from healthy children of different ages. J Clin Invest 91:2829–2836, 1993.

45. Harris DT, LoCascio J, Besencon FJ: Analysis of the alloreactive capacity of human umbilical cord blood: Implications for graft-versus-host disease. Bone Marrow Transplant 14:545–553, 1994.

46. Roncarolo MG, Vaccarino E, Saracco P et al: Immunologic properties of cord blood. In Broxmeyer HE (ed.): Cellular Characteristics of Cord Blood and Cord Blood Transplantation, pp. 67–82. AABB Press, Bethesda, MD. 1998.

47. Chalmers IMH, Janossy G, Contreras M et al: Intracellular cytokine profile of cord and adult blood lymphocytes. Blood 92:11–18, 1998.

48. Gaddy J, Broxmeyer HE: Cord blood natural killer cells: Implications for cord blood transplantation and insights into natural killer cell differentiation. In Broxmeyer HE (ed.): Cellular Characteristics of Cord Blood and Cord Blood Transplantation, pp. 83–112. AABB Press, Bethesda, MD, 1998.

49. Liu E, Tu W, Law HKW et al: Changes of CD14 and CD1a expression in response to IL-4 and granulocyte-macrophage colony-stimulating factor are different in cord blood and adult blood monocytes. Pediatr Res 50:184–189, 2001.

50. Carvajal E, Verdeguer A, Fernandez JM et al: Herpesvirus-6 encephalitis complicated by Wernicke-Korsakoff syndrome in a pediatric recipient of unrelated cord blood transplantation. J Pediatr Hematol Oncol 23:626–628, 2001.

51. Giraud P, Thuret I, Reviron D et al: Immune reconstitution and outcome after unrelated cord blood transplantation: A single paediatric institution experience. Bone Marrow Transplant 25:53–57, 2000.

52. Klein AK, Patel DD, Gooding JE et al: T-cell recovery in adults and children following umbilical cord blood transplantation. Biol Blood Marrow Transplant 7:454–466, 2001.

53. Miller JS, McCullar V, Punzel M et al: Single adult human CD34+/Lin−/CD38− progenitors give rise to natural killer cells, B-lineage cells, dendritic cells and myeloid cells. Blood 93:96–106, 1999.

54. Qiu L, Meagher R, Welhausen S et al: Ex vivo expansion of CD34+ umbilical cord blood cells in a defined serum-free medium (QBSF-60) with early effect cytokines. J Hematother Stem Cell Res 8:609–618, 1999.

55. Kinoshita T, Koike K, Mwamtemi HH et al: Retinoic acid is a negative regulator for the differentiation of cord blood-derived human mast cell progenitors. Blood 95:2821–2828, 2000.

56. Doerner M, Roecklein B, Torok-Storb B et al: Expansion and transduction of nonenriched human cord blood cells using HS-5 con-

ditioned medium and FLT3-L. J Hematother Stem Cell Res 9:759–765, 2000.

57. Shih CC, DiGiusto D, Forman SJ: Ex vivo expansion of transplantable human hematopoietic stem cells: Where do we stand in the year 2000? J Hematother Stem Cell Res 9:621–628, 2000.

58. Lewis ID, Almeida-Porada G, Du J et al: Umbilical cord blood cells capable of engrafting in primary, secondary, and tertiary xenogeneic hosts are preserved after ex vivo culture in a noncontact system. Blood 97:3441–3449, 2001.

59. Almeida-Porada G, Brown RL, MacKintosh FR et al: Evaluation of serum-free culture conditions able to support the ex vivo expansion and engraftment of human hematopoietic stem cells in the human-to-sheep xenograft model. J Hematother Stem Cell Res 9:683–693, 2000.

60. Woods EJ, Liu J, Derrow CW et al: Osmometric and permeability characteristics of human placental/umbilical cord blood CD34$^+$ cells and their application to cryopreservation. J Hematother Stem Cell Res 9:161–173, 2000.

61. Robinson S, Mosley RL, Parajuli P et al: Comparison of the hematopoietic activity of FLT-3 ligand and granulocyte-macrophage colony-stimulating factor acting alone or in combination. J Hematother Stem Cell Res 9:711–720, 2000.

62. Nielsen SD, Husemoen LLN, Sorensen TU et al: FLT3 ligand preserves the uncommitted CD34$^+$ CD38$^-$ progenitor cells during cytokine prestimulation for retroviral transduction. J Hematother Stem Cell Res 9:695–701, 2000.

63. Sasayama N, Kashiwakura I, Tokushima Y et al: Expansion of megakaryocyte progenitors from cryopreserved leukocyte concentrates of human placental and umbilical cord blood in short-term liquid culture. Cytotherapy 3:117–126, 2001.

64. Shpall EJ, Quinones R, Giller R et al: Transplantation of ex vivo expanded cord blood: A phase I/II feasibility study. Bio Blood Marrow Transplant 8:368–376, 2002.

65. Jaroscak J, Goltry K, Smith A et al: Augmentation of umbilical cord blood transplantation with ex vivo expanded cells: Results of a phase I trial using the Aastrom Replicell system. Blood (submitted).

66. Rizzieri DA, Long GD, Vredenburgh JJ et al: Successful allogeneic engraftment of mismatched unrelated cord blood following a non-myeloablative preparative regimen. Blood 98:3486–3488, 2001.

67. Chen BJ, Cui X, Chao NJ: Addition of a second, different allogeneic graft accelerates white cell and platelet engraftment after T-cell-depleted bone marrow transplantation. Blood 15:2235–2240, 2002.

68. Staba S, Martin PL, Szabolcs P et al: Correction of Hurler syndrome with unrelated umbilical cord blood transplantation. Blood Bone Marrow Transplant 8:98, 2002.

69. Kurtzberg J, Richards K, Wenger D et al: Correction of Krabbe disease neonatal hematopoietic stem cell transplantation. Biol Blood Bone Marrow Transplant 8:97, 2002.

58

HLA Typing in Hematopoietic Cell Transplantation

Effie W. Petersdorf, Claudio Anasetti,
Paul J. Martin, and John A. Hansen

Advances in the field of immunogenetics of the human leuko-cyte antigen (HLA) system have changed the indications for allogeneic hematopoietic cell transplantation (HCT) as a cura-tive modality for malignant and nonmalignant diseases. Recog-nition of the importance of HLA compatibility between the donor and recipient in mediating host-versus-graft and graft-versus-host reactions, together with the development of DNA-based technologies for accurate HLA typing, have led to suc-cessful use of unrelated volunteer donors for HCT.[27,42,52,64,69]

The first allogeneic transplantations were performed from HLA-identical siblings for the treatment of immunodeficiency and aplastic anemia.[8,25,35,106] These sentinel cases paved the way for the use of allogeneic transplantation for the treatment of malignancies of the bone marrow.[107] Although the early experi-ence in sibling transplantation demonstrated that it was possi-ble to eradicate abnormal hematopoietic cells and to establish and sustain engraftment of donor cells, this early experience also showed that allogeneic transplantation was not without risk of infection and graft-versus-host disease (GvHD).[16] The development of effective antiviral agents to prevent and treat cytomegalovirus (CMV) infection and the introduction of immunosuppressive regimens for the prophylaxis of GvHD were landmark discoveries.[37,97,104]

Experience with the use of volunteer unrelated donor HCT began in the early 1970s. The preliminary results demonstrated the high-risk nature of these transplants, especially with respect to graft failure and GvHD.[28,32,38,41,44,59,62,79,101] In addition to the medical needs and complications faced by recipients of unrelated donor transplants, the practical issues of identifying suitable donors dominated the early experience, and lengthy, expensive donor searches limited its application more broadly.

The first volunteer donor registry was organized in London at the Anthony Nolan Research Centre, clearly demonstrating public interest in volunteer donation as well as the financial fea-sibility of performing registry HLA typing.[19] In the United States, the National Marrow Donor Program (NMDP) was established in 1986 and was followed soon-thereafter by Bone Marrow Donors Worldwide[45,68,80] (http://bmdw.leidenuniv.nl). As of August 31, 2000, the NMDP has facilitated 11,127 unre-lated transplants of bone marrow, peripheral blood stem cells (PBSC), and cord blood, including transplants using stem cells from donors accessed through International Cooperative Reg-istries. These transplants have been performed at 153 transplant centers worldwide (National Marrow Donor Program statistics; Dennis L. Confer, MD, personal communication).

THE HLA SYSTEM

The HLA system was first described by Jean Dausset in 1952 after the discovery of agglutination reactions in recipients of blood products from multiparous female donors or blood donors who themselves were sensitized from previous blood transfusions.[23] HLA alloantigens were defined by serological methods in a com-plement-dependent microcytotoxicity assay using panels of alloantisera containing HLA antibodies that demonstrated the polymorphic nature of the HLA system.[2,81,111] Nomenclature was formalized starting in 1964 by the establishment of collaborative workshops[1] (http://www.ihwg.org/history/history.htm).

The HLA complex spans 4 megabases at the p21 on chromo-some 6 and consists of three regions termed class I, class III, and class II. Genes within the class I and class II regions are struc-turally and functionally related; genes within the class III region, including tumor necrosis factor and heat shock protein, do not directly function as major transplantation genes but participate in the immune response through inflammatory reactions.

HLA Class I Genes

The class I genes lie within a 2 megabase region comprising the telomeric half of the major histocompatibility complex (MHC). Each classical HLA-A, B, and C gene is composed of 8 exons that encode specific domains of the class I molecule: exon 1, leader peptide; exon 2, α1 domain; exon 3, α2 domain; exon 4, α3 domain; exon 5, transmembrane domain, and exons 6, 7, and 8, cytoplasmic domain. The lengths of the exons are known to be the same for each serologically defined antigen. Polymorphism is most extensive in exons 2, 3, and 4, which form the basis for defin-ing the 185 HLA-A, 381 HLA-B, and 91 HLA-C alleles currently recognized[13] (http://www.ebi.ac.uk/imgt/hla/; http://www.antho-nynolan.com/HIG/index.html). Of the three extracellular domains of the class I molecule, the α1 and 2 domains fold to bind peptide in a groove between two α helices on a platform of a β-pleated sheet. The membrane-proximal α3 domain encodes the main binding site for CD8 and contact residues for β2 microglob-ulin.[12,92] The extraordinary polymorphism of class I genes modu-lates the range of bound peptides and the T-cell repertoire expressed by CD8 T cells,[39,67,88,89] the response to natural killer (NK) cells,[57] and interactions of HLA-A, B, and C with peptide transporters (TAP) and chaperones.[22,50] The allele and locus-spe-cific patterns of polymorphism of class I genes are thought to reflect distinct selective pressures exerted on the class I loci due to both specific antigenic challenge as well as the need for extreme heterozygosity for the maximum range of antigenic responses.[46]

HLA Class II Genes

Nine HLA genes reside in the class II region and share structural and functional similarity. The HLA-DR gene encodes 5 loci:

HLA-DRA, DRB1, DRB3, DRB4, DRB5. The HLA-DQ and DP genes encode two loci each: DQA1, DQB1 and DPA1, DPB1, respectively. The class II molecule is a heterodimer of an α chain product of the A gene and a β chain product of the B gene. Within the HLA-DR gene, DRA and DRB1 products form the heterodimer that defines the HLA-DR1-DR18 serological phenotype. HLA-DRB3, DRB4, and DRB5 encode supratypic specificities that are expressed with DRB1 on only 3 haplotypes: DRB3 (DR3, DR11, DR12, DR13, DR14); DRB4 (DR4, DR7, DR9), and DRB5 (DR15, DR16). Haplotypes that are DR1, DR10, or DR8-positive encode only the DRA and the DRB1 genes. The DRA, DQA1, and DPA1 genes show limited diversity, whereas the DRB1, DQB1, and DPB1 genes are highly polymorphic encoding over 317, 45, and 89 alleles, respectively.[13]

HLA TYPING METHODOLOGY

Definition of HLA class I and class II alleles has been made possible by the development of DNA-based typing methods over the last decade. These techniques have had a significant impact on the ability to match potential stem cell donor and recipients for transplantation with precision. The birth of the DNA typing era came in 1987 when the 10th International Histocompatibility Workshop demonstrated the utility of restriction fragment length polymorphism (RFLP) techniques to uncover polymorphism within serologically defined HLA-DR antigen families.[11] The advent of polymerase chain reaction (PCR) in the late 1980s[73,93] revolutionized the HLA typing world, providing a new generation of powerful methods for allele typing. The major technological advances stemming from this prolific period of research include sequence-specific primers (SSP), sequence-specific oligonucleotide probes (SSOP), sequence-based typing (SBT), reference-strand conformational analysis (RSCA), and most recently, oligonucleotide arrays.

Sequence-Specific Primers

Complete sequence homology of the template DNA with the PCR primers allows maximal efficiency and specificity of the PCR amplification reaction; mismatching of the DNA template and primer for one or more nucleotide bases causes inefficient amplification. SSP methodology utilizes panels of PCR primers that are descriptive of known HLA polymorphisms.[10,14,18,29,76,78,91] Panels of primers can be informative for DNA substitutions that distinguish families of HLA antigens ("group-specific"), or that are

unique for specific alleles ("allele-specific"). After the test DNA is amplified using the entire panel of PCR primer pairs, the product(s) is electrophoresed on a gel. The presence of an amplified product is indicative that the test DNA encoded the same sequence as the PCR primer (Figure 58–1). The HLA genotype is determined by evaluating the pattern of positive and negative amplifications to the entire primer panel. The SSP method is a cost-effective technique of which its main advantage is its simplicity and rapidity for typing at the equivalent level of the HLA antigen family ("low resolution" or "intermediate resolution" level typing). Definition of the allele ("high resolution") generally necessitates large panels of primer pairs; hence, SSP methods for high-resolution typing are more labor-intensive and less cost-effective than the probe-based technologies described below.

Sequence-Specific Oligonucleotide Probes

Oligonucleotide probes are short (15 to 30 nucleotide bases in length) sequences that are synthesized with radioactive or non-radioactive labels. Probe sequences are designed to specific regions within the polymorphic exons of class I genes (exons 2, 3, and 4) and of class II genes (DRB, DQA1, DQB1, DPA1, DPB1). After the test DNA is amplified by PCR, the amplified product is allowed to hybridize to the SSOPs. Only those probes having complementary sequence with the test DNA will hybridize; SSOP that are mismatched for one or more nucleotide bases will fail to hybridize. The presence of hybridized SSOP to DNA is signaled by the label (Figure 58–2). Evaluation of positive and negative hybridization patterns is necessary in order to deduce the HLA sequence of the template DNA. Panels of SSOP can be descriptive of every nucleotide position of the exon; alternatively, SSOP panels may be informative for only certain positions that are known to be polymorphic. The use of the latter, while informative for known alleles, would not detect novel alleles encoding substitutions outside of the probed regions. SSOP techniques are well-suited for high-resolution typing, and are especially efficient for large-scale analysis.[17,30,60,77,108]

Sequence-Based Typing

SBT methods represent the most comprehensive approach for discriminating HLA alleles. Its power lies in it being a highly robust, accurate, and definitive technique for uncovering novel variation.[71,83,90,94,113] Many approaches for SBT have been

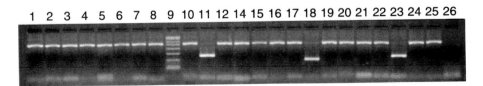

Figure 58–1. Sequence-specific primer (SSP) technique demonstrating positive PCR amplification for HLA-Cw*07 in lane 11 and for HLA-Cw*12 in lanes 18 and 23. Lanes containing a single PCR amplified band are controls; molecular weight marker was loaded in lane 9. Methodology was previously described by Bunce and Welsh.[18]

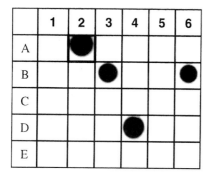

Figure 58–2. Sequence-specific oligonucleotide probe (SSOP) hybridization technique demonstrating HLA-B*46-positive hybridization of control HLA-B*4601 (A2 spot); HLA-B*14, 46 sample (B3 spot); HLA-B*15,46 sample (B6 spot), and HLA-B*40, 46 sample (D4 spot). Protocol previously published by Hurley et al.[47]

developed including direct sequencing from PCR-amplified genomic DNA or from cDNA. Among the most widely used methods is automated fluorescent sequencing. In this method, after the HLA allele(s) is PCR-amplified, cycle sequencing is performed using fluorescent-labeled primers. Alternatively, sequencing can use fluorescent-labeled dideoxynucleotides. The sequenced templates are electrophoresed on a polyacrylamide gel in an automated sequencer. The fluorescent signals emitted from either the labeled primers or the labeled dideoxynucleotides are detected by a laser within the sequencing apparatus, and interpreted by software (Figure 58–3). Automated allele identification using software simplifies and automates the data analysis.

Reference-Strand Conformational Analysis

The RSCA technique relies on the conformation-dependent mobility of HLA alleles during electrophoresis in a polyacrylamide gel.[6,7] After PCR amplification of the HLA allele(s), the product is allowed to hybridize with a locus-specific fluorescent-labeled reference (FLR) DNA fragment. The amplified template and the FLR fragment form a duplex, and are subsequently electrophoresed using a nondenaturing polyacrylamide gel in an automated sequencer. When duplexes arising from the FLR sense strand are created (FLR homoduplex plus two heteroduplexes), the signal is detected by the sequencer's laser. Single nucleotide allelic differences can be readily detected with the RSCA method. Furthermore, RSCA is a powerful technique for identifying the presence of new substitutions and for the resolution of ambiguous combinations of heterozygous polymorphisms.

Array Technology

Oligonucleotide array technology has revolutionized the study of molecular biology. Its applications have been far-reaching including large-scale gene discovery, gene expression monitoring, detection of mutations and polymorphisms, and mapping. The HLA system represents an ideal application of this particular technology because of the highly polymorphic nature of the class I and II genes.[40] Array methods allow parallel analysis of simultaneous

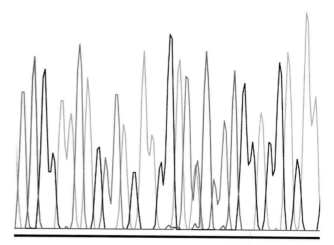

CTGGAACAGCCAGAAGGACNTCCTGGAGGAGAA

Figure 58–3. Sequence-based typing (SBT) method demonstrating chromatogram for HLA-DPB1*0301,0401-positive sample using methodology published by Rozemuller et al.,[90] and Verslius et al.[113] Chromatogram demonstrates incorporation at "N" of both C and A at position 182 of exon 2 corresponding to DPB1*0301 and DPB1*0401, respectively.

HLA gene polymorphisms. It is a flexible method in which the addition of new probes descriptive of novel substitutions may be easily configured onto the array. The use of fluorescent labels allows ease in the application of this method to a high-throughput clinical laboratory. Finally, the results of the hybridization can be quantified. An approach for sequence analysis of HLA-B has been recently described.[40] This system utilizes a panel of oligonucleotide probes designed for all known polymorphisms in exons 2 and 3 of the gene. The presynthesized probes are arrayed onto glass slides. Following PCR amplification of HLA-B using fluorescent-labeled primers, the PCR product is allowed to hybridize with the array; stringent conditions are required to discriminate perfectly matched duplexes and detect a single nucleotide difference between the template DNA and the probe (Figure 58–4). The array is scanned using an automated fluorescent scanner, and the HLA-B sequence is determined by quantitative analysis of the hybridization pattern. Oligonucleotide array technology has its greatest potential in the scalability and reduced cost for assaying large numbers of samples.

GENOMIC HLA MATCHING IN SUPPORT OF UNRELATED DONOR HCT

The advent of DNA-based typing methods has provided powerful tools for understanding the biological relevance of allele disparity in unrelated donor HCT. The elucidation that a single

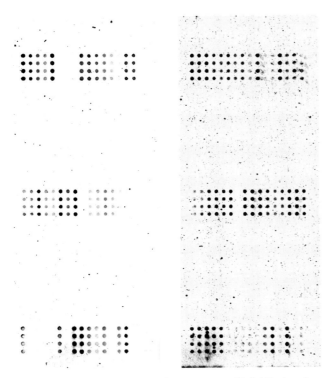

Figure 58–4. Oligonucleotide array for HLA-B. Actual hybridization of array using probes for HLA-B, reviewed in Guo et al.[40]

HLA antigen can encode many unique alleles has had enormous clinical implications for the typing and selection of appropriate donors for transplantation. It is abundantly clear that DNA-based methods, when applied to the analysis of serologically matched patients and donors, can uncover allelic disparity.[36,48,84,85] The largest retrospective analysis of a transplant population was conducted by the NMDP.[48] This study utilized SSOP and SBT methods to analyze DRB, DQA1, DPA1, DPB1 in 1259 patients who had undergone HCT from unrelated donors identified by the NMDP. Only 9.4 percent of the 1259 pairs were found to be matched at all loci tested. Noteworthy were the findings that 79.4 percent were matched for DRB1, but only 13.2 percent for DPB1. Sixty-six percent of the study population encoded mismatches for two or more class II alleles.

A single-center analysis retrospectively analyzed the match status of 300 CML unrelated donor transplants using SBT methods for HLA-A, B, and C genes and SSOP methods for HLA-DRB1 and DQB1.[87] Only 47 percent of these pairs were matched for all five genes; 53 percent were mismatched for at least one class I or class II allele. Worldwide experience has confirmed the power of DNA methods to uncover donor-recipient allele disparity among putative well-matched pairs and therefore should be used as the gold standard for identifying HLA class I and class II alleles in support of donor selection for unrelated donor HCT.

Graft Failure

The immunologically mediated mechanisms for graft failure are highly complex and involve not only host-anti-donor recog-

nition of either HLA or minor histocompatibility determinants mediated by alloreactive T cells or B cells, but also a potential role for NK cells.[20,26,31] The recent description of the family of NK-KIR receptors and their interactions with HLA class I molecules open a new hypothesis for graft failure involving the lack of inhibition by host NK cells.[61,110,115]

Experience in haploidentical related transplantation clearly demonstrates the importance of HLA incompatibility in defining graft failure risk.[3] Compared to the 2 percent incidence of graft failure in HLA genotypically identical sibling transplants, the graft failure rate among haploidentical transplants was 12.3 percent ($p < .001$), and the incidence correlated directly with the degree of donor mismatching. The presence of a positive pretransplant cross-match was found to be associated with a 62 percent graft failure rate.[4] Furthermore, the intensity of post-grafting immunosuppression correlated with the risk of graft failure (5 percent graft failure rate in patients who received the combination of methotrexate and cyclosporine compared to 9 percent for patients receiving methotrexate alone, $p = .04$).

The importance of HLA disparity in graft failure after unrelated donor transplantation was reported by Fleischauer et al.[31] In this case report, the patient and donor's HLA-B44 alleles differed by a single amino acid. The clinical importance of HLA class I allele disparity in graft failure was examined in a case-control study by the Seattle program.[86] A total of 21 patients who experienced graft failure after unrelated donor HCT were examined. Of the 21 cases, 18 carried the diagnosis of CML. At the time of transplantation, 14 of the 21 pairs were HLA-A, B serologically matched and DRB1 allele matched, 4 pairs were mismatched for at least one HLA-A or HLA-B antigen, and 3 pairs were HLA-DRB1 allele mismatched. For each of the 21 graft failure cases, two controls were selected from a base population of unrelated donor transplants, and matched to the case for variables that could be important for engraftment. These variables included HLA match status, marrow cell dose, disease diagnosis and stage at the time of transplantation, dose and schedule of total body irradiation in the conditioning regimen, presence of panel-reactive antibody, transplant date, donor-recipient gender, and age. Each graft failure case pair and the two control pairs were typed for HLA-A, B, and C using SBT and for DRB1 and DQB1 using SSOP methods. Complete allele matching for class I was identified in 45 percent of controls, but only in 10 percent of cases. Disparity for either HLA-A or B, or for both HLA-A and B was uncovered in 19 percent of cases and 21 percent of controls. In sharp contrast, mismatching for HLA-C was found in 71 percent of cases and 33 percent of controls. Multivariable analysis revealed an HLA-C mismatch to confer an odds ratio (OR) of 4.0 on graft failure ($p = .04$) and an HLA-A and/or B mismatch an OR of 3.1 ($p = .09$). This study demonstrated that HLA-C disparity is an independent risk factor for graft failure and provided novel information demonstrating HLA-C to be a classical transplantation antigen.

A subsequent analysis sought to test the hypothesis that multiple class I disparities may provide additive effects on the risk of graft failure.[87] The graft failure rate was 2 percent among HLA-A, B, C, DRB1, DQB1 allele-matched transplants or in the presence of a single HLA-A, B, or C allele mismatch, in contrast to 29 percent in the presence of two or more class I disparities. Of interest, the presence of class II disparities did not increase the risk of graft failure (Table 58–1).

Graft-versus-Host Disease

Allografting HLA genotypically identical sibling stem cells would cause acute GvHD in nearly all recipients unless immunosuppressive therapy were given.[105] With the combination of cyclosporine and methotrexate as GvHD prophylaxis, 20 to 30 percent of HLA identical sibling transplants develop grades II to IV acute GvHD and 10 to 15 percent develop clinically severe grades III to IV acute GvHD.[104]

The dose effect of multi-locus HLA mismatching on risk of developing acute GvHD was described in haploidentical related transplants receiving methotrexate alone for postgrafting immunosuppression.[9] With the combination of cyclosporine and methotrexate for prophylaxis, the risk of acute GvHD increased in parallel with increased number of mismatched loci[5] (Figure 58–5). Grades II to IV GvHD was observed in 75 percent of single locus, 78 percent of two-locus, and 80 percent of three-locus mismatches. Not only does the number of HLA mismatches correlate with GvHD risk, but class I and class II disparities do not confer equivalent risk (Figure 58–6). In single locus haploidentical related transplants, disparity within the class II region is associated with higher risk of acute GvHD than mismatches within the class I region. Disparity for serologically defined HLA-A, B, or DR antigens has been subsequently studied in a population of CML transplants from haploidentical related donors.[99] HLA-DR mismatches conferred significantly increased risk of acute GvHD compared to HLA-A or B mismatches (65 vs. 34 percent). Since these donors and patients were typed using serological methods at the time of transplantation, the potential role of undetected allele mismatching at HLA-A, B, and DR, and the role of HLA-C and DQ disparities are not known.

The risk of acute GvHD remains a major limitation of unrelated donor HCT, accounting for increased morbidity and mortality.[24,65,74,103] The concept that the number of HLA disparities between the recipient and the donor is an important factor in defining acute GvHD risk has been explored in two recent studies from the Japan Marrow Donor Program (JMDP)[95] and the

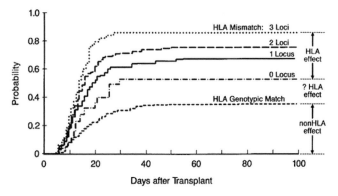

Figure 58–5. Incidence of grades II to IV acute GvHD in haploidentical related transplants demonstrating influence of the number of HLA disparities on GvHD risk. Patients received the combination of methotrexate and cyclosporine for prophylaxis against GvHD, and unmanipulated bone marrow.

Seattle transplant program.[87] Both studies demonstrate that allele-level matching is required to minimize acute GvHD risk. However, the risk of GvHD was associated with different HLA loci. HLA-A, B, and C differences correlated most significantly with GvHD risk in the study from Japan, whereas class II allele disparity conferred risk in the U.S. analysis (Figure 58–7).

A side-by-side comparison of the two data sets was subsequently performed for CML patients.[43] In a univariate analysis of the JMDP data, the risk of acute GvHD conferred by an HLA-A, B, or C mismatch was 2.4 ($p = .008$), 2.2 ($p = .04$), and 1.5 ($p = .26$), respectively. An HLA-DRB1 mismatch conferred a hazard ratio (HR) of 1.8. Interestingly, after adjusting for mismatching at other loci in a multivariable model, HLA-DRB1 disparity was found to be significant (HR 4.5, $p = .007$).

Increased risk of GvHD was found in univariate analysis of the Seattle data set for HLA-C (HR 1.5, $p = .04$), DRB1 (HR 1.8, $p = .01$), and DQB1 (HR 2.1, $p < .001$). After adjusting for other

Table 58–1. Incidence of Graft Failure Among 300 CML Unrelated Donor Transplants According to the Number of Class I and Class II Allele Disparities

Donor Disparity	Number of Pairs	Graft Failures (percent)
Allele match	146	3 (2)
Single class I	50	1 (2)
Multiple class I	31	9 (29)
Single class II	24	0
Multiple class II	7	0
Class I and class II	34	4 (12)

(From Petersdorf et al.,[87] with permission.)

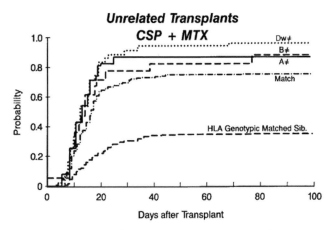

Figure 58–6. Incidence of grades II to IV acute GvHD in single locus haploidentical related transplants receiving methotrexate and cyclosporine and unmanipulated bone marrow grafts. Class II disparity conferred higher risk to GvHD than did class I disparities.

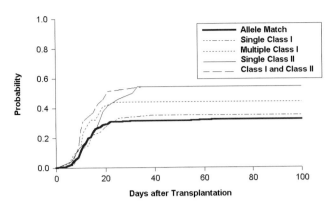

Figure 58–7. Cumulative incidence of grades III to IV acute GvHD in CML unrelated donor transplants receiving methotrexate and cyclosporine as GvHD prophylaxis. Study demonstrates that GvHD risk is a function of the number and nature of MHC allele mismatches. (From Petersdorf et al.,[87] with permission.)

GvHD risk factors, however, only HLA-DQB1 disparity remained significant (HR 1.8, $p = .007$).

The JMDP and Seattle studies may have come to different conclusions for several reasons. From a methodologic standpoint, the two studies differed in the typing techniques; SBT was used for the U.S. study and SSOP for the Japanese study. HLA-DP was not considered in the Seattle analysis due to the lack of informative HLA-DP matched pairs.[82] The overall incidence of grades III to IV acute GvHD was 11 percent in the JMDP study and 32 percent in the Seattle study. Different inherent GvHD risks may reflect differences in the clinical practice of the transplant centers including different conditioning regimens and immunosuppression regimens, as well as potential differences in the grading of GvHD. Noteworthy are the pronounced differences in the distribution of class I and II allele mismatches between the two populations.[43] Whether the nature of the HLA mismatches can explain differences in GvHD risk remains to be determined in future studies of large, homogeneous transplant populations.

In 1992 the Seattle program published the results of a study whose aim was to determine the clinical relevance of HLA-DP in unrelated donor HCT.[82] This study evaluated 129 patients transplanted from HLA-A, B serologically matched, DRB1, DQB1 allele-matched unrelated donors for a variety of hematologic malignancies. Using SSOP techniques to type the second exon of HLA-DPB1, a high rate of DPB1 mismatching was discerned (80 percent mismatched, 20 percent matched). A difference of 10 percent in acute GvHD rates between the matched and mismatched groups was not found to be statistically significant, a likely result of the lack of informative HLA-DPB1 identical transplants.

The discovery of additive effects of class I and II in the 1998 analysis[87] gave impetus to test the hypothesis that DPB1 functions as a transplantation determinant by influencing the risk of clinical severe acute GvHD.[117] This current analysis differs in three major ways from the 1992 study. First, the study population was confined to good-risk CML transplants in an effort to

reduce the potential confounding effects of other GvHD risk factors.[42] Secondly, the study population was further restricted to patients who received HLA-A, B, C, DRB1, DQB1 allele-matched transplants, using SBT to assess the class I region, and SSOP for HLA-DR and DQ. Finally, we used SBT methods to type the DPB1 alleles; SBT represented a more robust approach for the detection of allele polymorphism compared to the SSOP method used in the earlier study.

Among 205 HLA-A, B, C, DRB1, DQB1 allele-matched transplants, 49 were matched, 90 were mismatched for a single DPB1 allele, and 66 were mismatched for two DPB1 alleles. A single disparity conferred an OR of 1.0 ($p = .99$) and two disparities conferred an OR of 2.2 ($p = .06$) on grades III to IV acute GvHD risk. Compared to single mismatches and to matches, two DPB1 mismatched transplants had an OR of 2.2 ($p = .01$) of developing severe acute GvHD. These data strongly suggest that a threshold effect is operational in determining GvHD risk.

In retrospect, in the 1998 analysis of class I and II allele disparity,[87] a high proportion of donor-recipient pairs who were DRB1 and/or DQB1 mismatched are now known to encode DPB1 disparities. Hence, the risk of GvHD conferred by multilocus class II mismatches warrants further evaluation.

With the new information implicating HLA-DP as a transplantation determinant, a reanalysis of GvHD has been conducted in which all 6 HLA loci have been taken into consideration (unpublished). Of 6 MHC genes under consideration, the maximal possible number of allele disparities is 12. The study population encoded 0, 1, 2, 3, 4, 5, 6, 7, and 9 allele mismatches (Table 58–2). There was a progressive increase in grades III to IV acute GvHD associated with increasing number of mismatched alleles (without regard to the locus mismatched). In fully matched transplants (12 allele matched), the incidence of GvHD was 23 percent, rising to 100 percent in the 7 and 9 allele mismatched case. Given the potentially different risks conferred

Table 58–2. Effect of Multiple Class I and Class II Disparities on Risk of Grades III to IV Acute GvHD in CML Unrelated Donor Transplantation[a]

Number Mismatched Alleles		Grades III to IV Acute GvHD (percent)	
0		11/48 (23)	$p = .59$
1	$p = .04$	31/115 (27)	
2		43/107 (40)	
3		31/76 (41)	
4		14/35 (40)	
5		7/13 (54)	
6		6/8 (75)	
7		3/3 (100)	
8		—	
9		1/1 (100)	

[a] The total number of disparities at HLA-A, B, C, DRB1, DQB1, and DPB1 was determined using SBT and SSOP typing methods. (From Petersdorf et al., unpublished.)

by class I versus class II on GvHD, a regrouping of the data set according to whether the disparity occurred for class I versus class II was undertaken (Table 58–3). When the number of class I disparities was evaluated (without regard to the number of class II mismatches), the incidence of grades III to IV acute GvHD increased from 34 percent in class I matched to 67 percent in 5-allele mismatches. When the data set was evaluated according to the number of class II disparities (without regard of class I), the incidence of GvHD in the class II matched group was 20 percent rising abruptly to 80 percent in 4-allele mismatches and 100 percent in 5-allele mismatches. These results strongly suggest that class II disparity is associated most prominently with GvHD risk, and an additive effect may be discerned with increasing numbers of allele mismatches.

Survival

Survival following single-locus mismatched haploidentical related transplants for CML is influenced by whether the disparity occurs for class I versus class II antigens.[99] Five-year survival of HLA-A or B antigen mismatched transplants was 74 percent compared to 50 percent for HLA-DR mismatches and 74 percent for HLA genotypically identical sibling transplants (relative risk 2.3, $p = .004$).

In unrelated donor transplantation for CML, risk factors for mortality include patient age older than 50 years, class II disparity at HLA-DR locus, more than 3 years from the time of diagnosis to transplantation, increased body weight index, absence of fluconazole prophylaxis in CMV seronegative recipients, and absence of ganciclovir prophylaxis in CMV-positive recipients.[42,103] The importance of class I and II allele disparity on mortality parallels the results found for acute GvHD risk in both the JMDP and the Seattle analyses.[87,95] Not surprisingly, multiple class I, multiple class II, or class I and class II disparity was associated with significantly increased mortality in the Seattle study (Figure 58–8). Single class I and single class II mismatches were well-tolerated. When HLA-DPB1 is taken into

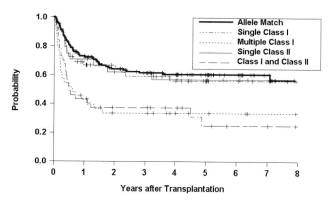

Figure 58–8. Kaplan-Meier estimates of overall survival in CML unrelated donor transplants according to the number of class I and class II allele disparities. (From Petersdorf et al.,[87] with permission.)

consideration, a trend toward greater mortality with two DPB1 disparities is evident (unpublished). The study by the JMDP found a parallel increase in mortality in the same transplants who were mismatched for class I and who experienced increased GvHD. These studies underscore the importance of restricting the total number of HLA allele disparities where possible and to avoid the use of donors who are mismatched for multiple loci.

TYPING FOR THE HUMAN PLATELET ALLOANTIGEN SYSTEM

The technical developments made for typing the human platelet alloantigens (HPA) and glycoproteins parallel those that have been achieved for the HLA gene complex. Serological methods dominated the early history of platelet typing, with the first alloantigen, Zw[a], having been discovered using agglutination methods.[112] Between the 1950s and the 1980s, serologically based methods were refined and immunochemical techniques were introduced.[34,49,54,96,98,114] Representative techniques that have been widely used in the discovery of new HPA and in clinical testing include the platelet suspension immunofluorescence test (PSIFT),[13a] the mixed passive hemagglutination test (MPHA),[98] the modified antigen-capture enzyme-linked assay (MACE),[49] and the monoclonal antibody-specific immobilization of platelet antigens (MAIPA).[53,54]

The modern era of HPA typing has witnessed the development of PCR-based DNA typing methods that share similarity with those described above for the HLA class I and II genes. The earliest application of molecular technology to HPA typing came in 1989 with the use of RFLP analysis for HPA-1.[75] RFLP techniques were subsequently applied to investigate the polymorphism of HPA-2, 3, 4, and 5.[66,109] The development of SSP approaches[72,100] and SSOP methods[15,63,70] were instrumental in uncovering the allelic diversity of the HPA system.

The requirements for large-scale HPA typing include the feasibility of automation. Two methods in particular have been developed for HPA typing and have the potential for high-

Table 58–3. Effect of Multiple Allele Disparities on Risk of Grades III to IV Acute GvHD risk[a]

Number Mismatched Alleles	Grades III to IV Acute GvHD	
	Class I (percent)	Class II (percent)
0	80/232 (34)	16/80 (20)
1	29/91 (32)	51/152 (34)
2	22/53 (42)	61/142 (43)
3	12/23 (52)	12/24 (50)
4	2/4 (50)	4/5 (80)
5	2/3 (67)	3/3 (100)

[a] Class I mismatches indicate the number of disparities at HLA-A, B, and C without regard to the presence of class II disparities; similarly, the class II mismatches indicate the number of DRB1, DQB1, and DPB1 allele mismatches without regard to the number of class I disparities. (From Petersdorf et al., unpublished.)

throughput applications: oligonucleotide ligation assay (OLA)[58] and preferential homoduplex formation assay (PHFA).[33]

With the application of DNA-based methods for analysis of HPA and glycoproteins, extensive allelic diversity has been described in ethnically and racially diverse populations (reviewed in Juji et al.[51]). The biological importance of human diversity of the genes encoding platelet antigens and glycoproteins in HCT awaits study.

CONCLUSIONS

The success of unrelated donor HCT as a curative modality for hematologic malignancies is due in part to a better understanding of the immunogenetics of the HLA system and to the development and application of robust DNA typing technologies for donor matching. The extensive diversity of the HLA system has important biological implications in unrelated donor HCT, affecting engraftment, GvHD, and overall survival. Whereas complete genotypic identity between a donor and recipient is associated with optimal transplant outcome, it is clear that not every disparity is functionally relevant. Future clinical research will be required to define the acceptable limits of HLA disparity and to identify mismatches that are well-tolerated so that life-saving transplants can be made available to patients lacking matched unrelated donors.

REFERENCES

1. Amos B: Histocompatibility Testing: Report of a Conference and Workshop; Publication 1229; National Academy of Sciences—National Research Council; Washington DC, 1965.
2. Amos DB: Nomenclature for factors of the HL-A system. Science 160:659–660, 1968.
3. Anasetti C, Amos D, Beatty PG, Appelbaum FR, Bensinger W, Buckner CD et al: Effect of HLA compatibility on engraftment of bone marrow transplants in patients with leukemia or lymphoma. N Engl J Med 320:197–204, 1989.
4. Anasetti C, Hansen JA: Effect of HLA incompatibility in marrow transplantation from unrelated and HLA-mismatched related donors. Transfus Sci 15:221–230, 1994.
5. Anasetti C: Hematopoietic cell transplantation from HLA partially matched related donors. In Thomas ED, Blume KG, Forman SJ (eds.): Hematopoietic Cell Transplantation, pp. 904–914. Blackwell Science, Boston, 1999.
6. Arguello JR, Little AM, Pay AL, Gallardo D, Rojas I, Marsh SGE et al: Mutation detection and typing of polymorphic loci through double-strand conformation analysis. Nat Genet 18:192–194, 1998.
7. Arguello JR, Little A-M, Bohan E, Goldman JM, Marsh SGE, Madrigal JA: High resolution HLA class I typing by reference strand mediated conformation analysis (RSCA). Tissue Antigens 52:57–66, 1998.
8. Bach FH, Albertini RJ, Joo P, Anderson FL, Bortin MM: Bone marrow transplantation in a patient with the Wiskott-Aldrich syndrome. Lancet 2:1364, 1968.
9. Beatty PG, Clift RA, Mickelson EM, Nisperos BN, Flournoy N, Martin PJ et al: Marrow transplantation from related donors other than HLA-identical siblings. N Engl J Med 313:765–771, 1985.
10. Bein G, Glaser R, Kirchner H: Rapid HLA-DRB1 genotyping by nested PCR amplification. Tissue Antigens 39:68–73, 1992.
11. Bignon JD, Semana G, Tiercy M, Simons M, Lalouel JM, Cohen D: DNA-RFLP analysis: HLA-DR beta workshop report. In Dupont B (ed.): Immunobiology of HLA, pp. 851–860. Springer-Verlag, New York, 1989.
12. Bjorkman PJ, Parham P: Structure, function, and diversity of class I major histocompatibility complex molecules. Ann Rev Biochem 59:253–288, 1990.
13. Bodmer WF, Marsh SG, Albert ED, Bodmer WF, Bontrop RE, Dupont B et al: Nomenclature for factors of the HLA system. Tissue Antigens 53:407–446, 1999.
13a. von dem Borne AE, Verheugt FW, Oosterhof F, von Riész E, de la Riviere AB, Engelfriet CP: A simple immunofluorescence test for the detection of platelet antibodies. Br J Haematol 39:195–207, 1978.
14. Browning MJ, Drausa P, Rowan A, Bicknell DC, Bodmer JG, Bodmer WF: Tissue typing the HLA-A locus from genomic DNA by sequence-specific PCR: Comparison of HLA genotypes and surface expression on colorectal tumor cell lines. Proc Natl Acad Sci U S A 90:2842–2845, 1993.
15. Bray PF, Jin Y, Kickler T: Rapid genotyping of the five major platelet alloantigens by reverse dot-blot hybridization. Blood 84:4361–4367, 1994.
16. Buckner CD, Epstein RB, Rudolph RH, Clift RA, Storb R, Thomas ED: Allogeneic marrow engraftment following whole body irradiation in a patient with leukemia. Blood 35:741–750, 1970.
17. Bugawan TL, Begovich AB, Erlich HA: Rapid HLA-DPB typing using enzymatically amplified DNA and non-radioactive sequence-specific oligonucleotide probes. Immunogenetics 32:231–241, 1990.
18. Bunce M, Welsh KI: Rapid DNA typing for HLA-C using sequence-specific primers (PCR-SSP): Identification of serological and non-serologically defined HLA-C alleles including several new alleles. Tissue Antigens 43:7–17, 1994.
19. Cleaver SA: The Anthony Nolan Research Centre. Bone Marrow Transplant 11(S1):38–40, 1993.
20. Colonna M, Spies T, Strominger JL, Ciccone E, Moretta A, Moretta L et al: Alloantigen recognition by two human natural killer cell clones is associated with HLA-C or a closely linked gene. Proc Natl Acad Sci U S A 89:7983–7985, 1992.
21. Coombs RRA, Bedford D: The A and B antigens on human platelets demonstrated by means of mixed erythrocyte platelet agglutination. Vox Sang 5:111–117, 1955.
22. Cresswell P: Assembly, transport and function of MHC class II molecules. Ann Rev Immunol 12:259–293, 1994.
23. Dausset JA, Nenna A: Presence d'une leuco-agglutinine dans le serum d'un cas d'agranulocytose chronique. Compt Rend Soc Biol 146:1539, 1954.
24. Davies SM, Shu XO, Blazar BR, Filipovich AH, Kersey JH, Krivit W et al: Unrelated donor bone marrow transplantation: Influence of HLA-A and -B incompatibility on outcome. Blood 86:1636–1642, 1995.
25. deKoning J, van Bekkum DW, Dicke KA, Dooren LJ, Radl J, van Rood JJ: Transplantation of bone marrow cells and fetal thymus in an infant with lymphogenic immunological deficiency. Lancet 1:223, 1969.
26. Dennert G, Anderson CG, Warner J: T killer cells play a role in allogeneic bone marrow graft rejection but not in hybrid resistance. J Immunol 135:3729–3734, 1985.
27. Drobyski WR, Ash RC, Casper JT, McAuliffe T, Horowitz MM et al: Effect of T-cell depletion as graft-versus-host disease prophylaxis on engraftment, relapse, and disease-free survival in unre-

lated marrow transplantation for chronic myelogenous leukemia. Blood 83:1980–1987, 1994.

28. Duquesnoy RJ, Zeevi A, Marrari M, Hackbart S, Camitta B: Bone marrow transplantation for severe aplastic anemia using a phenotypically HLA-identical, SB-compatible unrelated donor. Transplantation 35:566–571, 1983.

29. Fass SJ, Menon R, Braun ER, Rudert WA, Trucco M: Sequence-specific priming and exonuclease-released fluorescence detection of HLA-DQB1 alleles. Tissue Antigens 48:97–112, 1996.

30. Fernandez-Vina MA, Falco M, Sun Y, Stastny P: DNA typing for HLA class I alleles. I. Subsets of HLA-A2 and of A28. Hum Immunol 33:163–173, 1992.

31. Fleischhauer K, Keman NA, O'Reilly RJ, Dupont B, Yang SY: Bone marrow allograft rejection by host-derived allocytotoxic T lymphocytes recognizing a single amino acid at position 156 of the HLA-B44 class I antigen. N Engl J Med 323:1818–1822, 1990.

32. Foroozonfar N, and the Westminster Hospitals Bone Marrow Transplant Team: Bone marrow transplant from an unrelated donor for chronic granulomatous disease. Lancet 1:210–213, 1977.

33. Fujiwara K, Isa K, Oka T, MacKawajiri S, Yamane A, Akaza T et al: Large-scale DNA typing for human platelet alloantigens by PCR-PHFA (preferentially homoduplex formation assay). Br J Haematol 95:198–203, 1996.

34. Furihata K, Nugent DJ, Bisonette A, Aster RH, Kunicki TJ: On the association of the platelet-specific alloantigen, Pen^a, with glycoprotein IIIa. J Clin Invest 80:1624–1630, 1987.

35. Gatti RA, Meuwissen HJ, Allen HD, Hong R, Good RA: Immunological reconstitution of sex-linked lymphopenic immunological deficiency. Lancet 2:1366–1369, 1968.

36. Gauchat-Feiss D, Rufer N, Speiser D, Jeannet D, Roosnek E, Tiercy JM: Heterogeneity of HLA-B35: Oligotyping and direct sequencing for B35 subtypes reveals a high mismatching rate in B35 serologically compatible kidney and bone marrow donor/recipient pairs. Transplantation 60:869–873, 1995.

37. Goodrich JM, Mori M, Gleaves CA, Du Mond C, Cays M, Ebeling DF et al: Early treatment with ganciclovir to prevent cytomegalovirus disease after allogeneic bone marrow transplantation. N Engl J Med 325:1601–1607, 1991.

38. Gordon-Smith EC, Fairhead SM, Chipping PM, Hows J, James DC, Dodi A et al: Bone marrow transplantation for severe aplastic anemia using histocompatible unrelated volunteer donors. Br Med J Clin Res 285:835–837, 1982.

39. Guillet JG, Lai ML, Briner TJ, Buus S, Sette A, Grey HM et al: Immunological self, nonself discrimination. Science 235:865–870, 1987.

40. Guo Z, Gatterman MS, Hood L, Hansen JA, Petersdorf EW: Oligonucleotide arrays for hight-throughput SNPs detection in the MHC Class I genes: HLA-B, as a model system. Genome Res 12:447–457, 2002.

41. Hansen JA, Clift RA, Thomas ED, Buckner CD, Storb R, Giblett ER: Transplantation of marrow from an unrelated donor to a patient with acute leukemia. N Engl J Med 303:565–567, 1980.

42. Hansen JA, Gooley TA, Martin PJ, Appelbaum F, Chauncey TR, Clift RA et al: Bone marrow transplants from unrelated donors for patients with chronic myeloid leukemia. N Engl J Med 338:962–968, 1998.

43. Hansen JA, Yamamoto K, Petersdorf E, Sasazuki T: The role of HLA matching in hematopoietic cell transplantation. Rev Immunogen 1:359–373, 1999.

44. Horowitz SD, Bach FH, Groshong T, Hong R, Yunis EJ: Treatment of severe combined immunodeficiency with bone marrow from an unrelated, mixed-leukocyte culture nonreactive donor. Lancet 2:431–433, 1975.

45. Howe CWS, Radde-Stepaniak T: Hematopoietic cell donor registries. In Thomas ED, Blume KG, Forman SJ (eds.): Hematopoietic Cell Transplantation, pp. 503–512. Malden, MA, Blackwell Science, 1999.

46. Hunkapiller T, Hood L: Diversity of the immunoglobulin gene superfamily. Adv Immunol 44:1–63, 1989.

47. Hurley CK, Maiers M, Ng J, Wagage D, Hegland J, Baisch J et al: Large-scale DNA-based typing of HLA-A and HLA-B at low resolution is highly accurate specific and reliable. Tissue Antigens 55:352–358, 2000.

48. Hurley CK, Baxter-Lowe LA, Begovich AB, Fernandez-Vina M, Noreen H, Schmeckpeper B et al: The extent of HLA class II allele level disparity in unrelated bone marrow transplantation: Analysis of 1259 National Marrow Donor Program donor – recipient pairs. Bone Marrow Transplant 25:385–393, 2000.

49. Ishida F, Saji H, Maruya E, Furihata K: Human platelet-specific antigen, Sib^a, is associated with the molecular weight polymorphism of glycoprotein lb alpha. Blood 78:1722–1729, 1991.

50. Jackson MR, Peterson PA: Assembly and intracellular transport of MHC class I molecules. Ann Rev Cell Biol 9:207–235, 1993.

51. Juji T, Saji H, Satake M, Tokunaga K: Typing for human platelet alloantigens. Rev Immunogen 1:239–254, 1999.

52. Kernan NA, Bartsch G, Ash RC, Beatty PG, Champlin R, Filipovich A et al: Analysis of 462 transplantations from unrelated donors facilitated by the National Marrow Donor Program. N Engl J Med 328:593–602, 1993.

53. Kiefer V: The MAIPA assay and its applications in immuno-haematology. Transfus Med 2:181–188, 1992.

54. Kiefel S, Santoso S, Weisheit M, Mueller-Eckhardt C: Monoclonal antibody-specific immobilization of platelet antigens (MAIPA): A new tool for the identification of platelet-reactive antibodies 70:1722–1726, 1987.

55. Kissmeyer-Nielsen F: Methods used in platelet and leukocyte immunology. Prog Clin Pathol 2:161–166, 1969.

56. Kluter H, Fehlau K, Panzer S, Kirschner H, Bein G: Rapid typing for human platelet antigen systems −1, −2, −3 and −5 by PCR amplification with sequence-specific primers. Vox Sang 71:121–125, 1996.

57. Lanier LL, Gumperz JE, Parham P, Melero I, Lopez-Botet M, Phillips JH: The NKB1 and HP-3E4 NK cell receptors are structurally distinct glycoproteins and independently recognize polymorphic HLA-B and HLA-C molecules. J Immunol 154:3320–3327, 1995.

58. Legler TJ, Kohler M, Mayr WR, Panzer S, Ohto H, Fischer GF: Genotyping of the human platelet antigen systems 1 through 5 by multiplex polymerase chain reaction and ligation-based typing. Transfusion 36:426–431, 1996.

59. L'Esperance P et al: Bone-marrow donor selection among unrelated four-locus identical individuals. Transplant Proc S1:823–831, 1975.

60. Levine JE, Yang SY: SSOP typing of the Tenth International Histocompatibility Workshop reference cell lines for HLA-C alleles. Tissue Antigens 44:174–183, 1994.

61. Litwin V, Gumperz J, Parham P, Phillips JH, Lanier LL: NKB1: A natural killer cell receptor involved in the recognition of polymorphic HLA-B molecules. J Exp Med 180:537–543, 1994.

62. Lohrmann H-P, Dietrich M, Goldmann SF, Kristensen T, Fliedner TM, Abt C et al: Bone marrow transplantation for aplastic anemia from a HL-A and MLC-identical unrelated donor. Blut 31:347–354, 1975.

63. Lyman S, Aster RH, Visentin GP, Newman PJ: Polymorphism of human platelet membrane glycoprotein IIb associated with the Bak^a/Bak^b alloantigen system. Blood 75:2343–2348, 1990.

64. Mackinnon S, Hows JM, Goldman JM, Arthur CK, Hughes T, Apperley JF et al: Bone marrow transplantation for chronic

myeloid leukemia: The use of histocompatible unrelated volunteer donors. Exp Hematol 18:421–425, 1990.

65. Madrigal JA, Scott I, Arguello R, Szydlo R, Little A-M, Goldman JM: Factors influencing the outcome of bone marrow transplants using unrelated donors. Immunol Rev 157:153–166, 1997.

66. Matsuo K, Reid DM: Allele-specific restriction analysis of human platelet antigen system 4. Transfusion 36:809–812, 1996.

67. Matsumura M, Fremont DH, Peterson PA, Wilson IA: Emerging principles for the recognition of peptide antigens by MHC class I molecules. Science 257:927–934, 1992.

68. McCullough J, Hansen J, Perkins H, Stroncek D, Bartsch G: The National Marrow Donor Program: How it works, accomplishments to date. Oncology 3:63–74, 1989.

69. McGlave PB, Shu XO, Wen W, Anasetti C, Nademanee A, Champlin R et al: Unrelated donor marrow transplantation for chronic myelogenous leukemia: 9 years' experience of the National Marrow Donor Program. Blood 95:2219–2225, 2000.

70. McFarland JG, Aster RH, Bussel JB, Gianopoulos JG, Derbes RS, Newman PJ: Prenatal diagnosis of neonatal alloimmune thrombocytopenia using allele-specific oligonucleotide probes. Blood 78:2276–2282, 1991.

71. McGinnis MD, Conrad MP, Bouwens AGM, Tilanus MGJ, Kronick MN: Automated, solid-phase sequencing of DRB region genes using T7 sequencing chemistry and dye-labeled primers. Tissue Antigens 46:173–179, 1995.

72. Metcalfe P, Waters AH: HPA-1 typing by PCR amplification with sequence-specific primers (PCR-SSP): A rapid and simple technique. Br J Haematol 85:227–229, 1993.

73. Mullis KB, Fallona F: Specific synthesis of DNA in vitro via a polymerase catalysed chain reaction. Methods Enzymol 155:335–350, 1987.

74. Nademanee A, Schmidt GM, Parker P, Dagis AC, Stein A, Snyder DS et al: The outcome of matched unrelated donor bone marrow transplantation in patients with hematological malignancies using molecular typing for donor selection and graft-versus-host disease prophylaxis regimen of cyclosporine, methotrexate, and prednisone. Blood 86:1228–1234, 1995.

75. Newman PJ, Derbes RS, Aster RH: The human platelet alloantigens, P1^{A1} and P1^{A2}, are associated with a leucine33/proline33 amino acid polymorphism in membrane glycoprotein IIIa, and are distinguishable by DNA typing. J Clin Invest 83:1778–1781, 1989.

76. Newton CR, Graham A, Heptinstall LE: Analysis of any point mutation in DNA. The amplification refractory system (ARMS). Nucleic Acids Res 17:2503–2516, 1989.

77. Ng J, Hurley CK, Carter C, Baxter-Lowe LA, Bing D, Chopek M et al: Large-scale DRB and DQB1 oligonucleotide typing for the NMDP registry: Progress report from year 2. Tissue Antigens 47:21–26, 1996.

78. Olerup O, Zetterquist H: HLA-DR typing by PCR amplification with sequence-specific primers (PCR-SSP) in 2 hours: An alternative to serological DR typing in clinical practice including donor-recipient matching in cadaveric transplantation. Tissue Antigens 39:225–235, 1992.

79. O'Reilly R et al: Reconstitution in severe combined immunodeficiency by transplantation of marrow from an unrelated donor. N Engl J Med 297:1311–1318, 1977.

80. Oudshoorn M, van Leeuwen A, van der Zanden HG, van Rood JJ: Bone marrow donors worldwide: A successful exercise in international cooperation. Bone Marrow Transplant 14:3–8, 1994.

81. Payne R, Tripp M, Weigle J, Bodmer W, Bodmer J: A new leukocyte isoantigenic system in man. Cold Spring Harbor Symp Quant Biol 29:285, 1964.

82. Petersdorf EW, Smith AG, Mickelson EM, Longton GM, Anasetti C, Choo SY et al: The role of HLA-DPB1 disparity in the development of acute graft-versus-host disease following unrelated donor marrow transplantation. Blood 81:1923–1932, 1993.

83. Petersdorf EW, Hansen JA: A comprehensive approach for typing the alleles of the HLA-B locus by automated sequencing. Tissue Antigens 46:73–85, 1995.

84. Petersdorf EW, Longton GM, Anasetti C, Martin PJ, Mickelson EM, Smith AG, Hansen JA: The significance of HLA-DRB1 matching on clinical outcome after HLA-A, B, DR identical unrelated donor marrow transplantation. Blood 86:1606–1613, 1995.

85. Petersdorf EW, Longton GM, Anasetti C, Mickelson EM, Smith AG, Martin PJ, Hansen JA: Definition of HLA-DQ as a transplantation antigen. Proc Natl Acad Sci U S A 93:15358–15363, 1996.

86. Petersdorf EW, Longton GM, Anasetti C, Mickelson EM, McKinney SK, Smith AG et al: Association of HLA-C disparity with graft failure after marrow transplantation from unrelated donors. Blood 89:1818–1823, 1997.

87. Petersdorf EW, Gooley TA, Anasetti C, Martin PJ, Smith AG, Mickelson EM et al: Optimizing outcome after unrelated marrow transplantation by comprehensive matching of HLA class I and II alleles in the donor and recipient. Blood 92:3515–3520, 1998.

88. Ploegh HL, Orr HT, Strominger JL: Major histocompatibility antigens: The human (HLA-A, B, C) and murine (H-2K, H-2D) class I molecules. Cell 24:287–299, 1981.

89. Rammensee HG, Falk K, Rotzschke O: Peptides naturally presented by MHC class I molecules. Ann Rev Immunol 11:213–244, 1993.

90. Rozemuller EH, Chadwick B, Charron D, Baxter-Lowe LA, Eliaou JF, Johnston-Dow L, Tilanus MGJ: Sequenase sequence profiles used for HLA-DPB1 sequencing-based typing. Tissue Antigens, 47:72–79, 1996.

91. Sadler AM, Petronzelli F, Krausa P, Marsh SGE, Guttridge MG, Browing MJ, Bodmer JG: Low resolution DNA typing for HLA-B using sequence-specific primers in allele- or group-specific ARMS/PCR. Tissue Antigens 44:148–154, 1994.

92. Salter RD, Benjamin RJ, Wesley PK, Buxton SE, Garrett TP, Clayberger C et al: A binding site for the T cell co-receptor CD8 on the alpha 3 domain of HLA-A2. Nature 345:41–46, 1990.

93. Saiki RK, Scharf S, Faloona F, Mullis KB, Horn GT, Erlich HA, Arnheim N: Enzymatic amplification of beta-globin genomic sequences and restriction site analysis for diagnosis of sickle cell anemia. Science 230:1350–1354, 1985.

94. Santamaria P, Lindstrom AL, Boyce-Jacina MT, Myster SH, Barbosa JJ, Faras AJ, Rich SS: HLA class I sequence-based typing. Hum Immunol 37:39–50, 1993.

95. Sasazuki T, Juji T, Morishima Y, Kinukawa N, Kashiwabara H, Inoko H et al: Importance of HLA class I allele matching for clinical outcome after unrelated donor hematopoietic stem cell transplantation. N Engl J Med 339:1177–1185, 1998.

96. Scheider W, Schnaidt M: The platelet adhesion immunofluorescence test: A modification of the platelet suspension immunofluorescence test. Blut 43:389–392, 1981.

97. Schmidt GM, Horak DA, Niland JC, Duncan SR, Forman SJ, Zaia JA: A randomized, controlled trial of prophylactic ganciclovir for cytomegalovirus pulmonary infection in recipients of allogeneic bone marrow transplants. N Engl J Med 324:1005–1011, 1991.

98. Shibata Y, Juji T, Nishizawa Y, Sakamoto H, Ozawa N: Detection of platelet antibodies by a newly developed mixed agglutination with platelets. Vox Sang 41:25–31, 1981.

99. Servida P, Gooley T, Hansen JA, Bjerke J, Martin PJ, Petersdorf EW, Anasetti C: Improved survival of haploidentical related donor marrow transplants mismatched for HLA-A or B versus HLA-DR. Blood 88:484a, 1996.

100. Skogen B, Bellissimo DB, Hessner MJ, Santoso S, Aster RH, Newman PJ, McFarland JG: Rapid determination of platelet alloantigen genotypes by polymerase chain reaction using allele-specific primers. Transfusion 34:955–960, 1994.

101. Speck B, Zwaan FE, van Rood JJ, Eernisse JG: Allogeneic bone marrow transplantation in a patient with aplastic anemia using a phenotypically HLA-identical unrelated donor. Transplantation 16:24–28, 1973.

102. Speiser DE, Tiercy J-M, Rufer N, Grundschober C, Gratwohl A, Chapuis B et al: High resolution HLA matching associated with decreased mortality after unrelated bone marrow transplantation. Blood 87:4455–4462, 1996.

103. Spencer A, Szydlo RM, Brookes PA et al: Bone marrow transplantation for chronic myeloid leukemia with volunteer unrelated donors using ex vivo or in vivo T-cell depletion: Major prognostic impact of HLA class I identity between donor and recipient. Blood 86:3590–3597, 1995.

104. Storb R, Deeg HJ, Whitehead J, Appelbaum F, Beatty P, Bensinger W et al: Methotrexate and cyclosporine compared with cyclosporine alone for prophylaxis of acute graft-vs host disease after marrow transplantation for leukemia. N Engl J Med 314:729, 1986.

105. Sullivan KM, Deeg HG, Sanders J, Klosterman A, Amos D, Shulman H et al: Hyperacute graft-v-host disease in patients not given immunosuppression after allogeneic marrow transplantation. Blood 67:1172–1175, 1986.

106. Thomas ED, Storb R, Fefer A, Slichter SJ, Bryant JI, Buckner CD et al: Aplastic anaemia treated by marrow transplantation. Lancet 1:284, 1972.

107. Thomas ED, Storb R, Clift RA, Fefer A, Johnson FL, Neiman PE et al: Bone marrow transplantation. N Engl J Med 292:832–841, 895–902, 1975.

108. Tiercy JM, Djavad N, Rufer N, Speiser DE, Jeannet M, Roosnek E: Oligotyping of HLA-A2, -A3 and B44 subtypes: Detection of subtype incompatibilities between patients and their serological matched unrelated bone marrow donors. Hum Immunol 41:207–215, 1991.

109. Unkelbach K, Kalb R, Santoso S, Kroll H, Mueller-Eckhardt C, Kiefel V: Genomic RFLP typing of human platelet alloantigens Zw(P1^A), Ko, Bak and BR (HPA-1, 2, 3, 5). Br J Haematol 89:169–176, 1995.

110. Valiante NM, Parham P: Natural killer cells, HLA class I molecules, and marrow transplantation. Biol Blood Marrow Transplant 3:229–235, 1997.

111. Van Rood JJ, van Leeuwen A: Leucocyte grouping. A method and its application. J Clin Invest 42:1382–1390, 1963.

112. Van Loghem JJ, Dorfmeijer H, Van der Hart M: Serological and genetical studies on a platelet antigen (Zw). Vox Sang 4:161–169, 1959.

113. Versluis LF, Rozemuller E, Torks S, Marsh SGE, Bouwens AGM, Bodmer JG, Tilanus MG: High-resolution HLA-DPB typing based upon computerized analysis of data obtained by fluorescent sequencing of the amplified polymorphic exon 2. Human Immunol 38:277–283, 1993.

114. Von dem Borne AEGK, Verheugt FW, Oosterhof F, von Riesz E, de la Riviere AB, Engelfriet CP: A simple immunofluorescence test for the detection of platelet antibodies. Br J Haematol 39:195–207, 1978.

115. Winter CC, Gumperz JE, Parham P, Long EO, Wagtmann N: Direct binding and functional transfer of NK cell inhibitory receptors reveal novel patterns of HLA-C allotype recognition. J Immunol 161:571–577, 1998.

116. Witt C, Hanifi Moghaddam P, van der Meer R, Trimboli F, Ottinger H, Christiansen F, Giphart M: Matching for TNF microsatellites is strongly associated with matching for other non-HLA MHC sequences in unrelated bone marrow donor-recipient pairs. Human Immunol. 60:862–866, 1999.

117. Petersdorf EW, Godey T, Malkki M, Anasett C, Martin P, Woofrey A, Smith A, Mickelson E, Hansen JA: The biological significance of HLA-DP gene variation in haematopoietic cell transplantation. Brit J Haem 112:988–994, 2002.

59

Special Care of Blood and Marrow Stem Cell Transplant Patients

Hillard M. Lazarus and Richard J. Creger

Hematopoietic stem cell transplantation has evolved into one of the most effective therapeutic modalities for the treatment of malignant, immunologic, and genetic disorders.[1] The first attempts to use bone marrow therapeutically occurred more than one hundred years ago, in which leukemia patients were given marrow by mouth.[2] It was not until the late 1930s that investigators administered marrow via the parenteral route in an unsuccessful attempt to correct hematologic and malignant disorders.[3–6] The scientific studies that set the stage for the triumphs of transplantation date back about 50 years, beginning with the studies of Jacobson and colleagues[7] who noted that splenic shielding could prevent otherwise lethal irradiation in mice. Later, Lorenz and associates[8] reported that infusion of bone marrow or spleen cells also were protective from the deleterious effects of total body irradiation (TBI). Van Bekkum and Devries[9] and Billingham and Brent[10,11] later described an immunologic syndrome in which engrafted murine donor cells attacked host tissues, a phenomenon subsequently shown to be graft-versus-host disease (GvHD). These innovative and pivotal investigations subsequently were extended to outbred species such as dogs and included both allogeneic as well as autologous transplants using hematopoietic stem cells collected from the blood as well as from the bone marrow.[12] Transplantation as a modality was extended to humans in the 1950s and included autologous as well as allogeneic transplants.[13–15] With the notable exception of syngeneic grafts, these early transplants were not successful for a variety of reasons.[16,17] In the late 1960s and early 1970s, E. Donnall Thomas and his colleagues at the Fred Hutchinson Cancer Research Center refined clinical allogeneic bone marrow transplantation techniques sufficiently that cures now were obtained in far-advanced leukemia and aplastic anemia patients.[18] By the early 1980s, autologous bone marrow transplantation was demonstrated to provide long-term survival in relapsed adult lymphoma patients.[19] As a result transplantation has been employed progressively earlier and earlier in the disease course, including those in complete remission but thought to be at high risk for subsequent relapse.

In the decades since the initial preclinical and clinical investigations, hematopoietic stem cell transplantation has evolved rapidly. Due to a greater understanding of histocompatibility in humans, advances in platelet transfusion support, improved antibiotics, more effective anticancer drugs, and the development and implementation of recombinant hematopoietic growth factors, overall and disease-free survival rates have been dramatically improved. Alternative sources of hematopoietic stem cells have been expanded and include, in addition to the use of autologous donors as well as sibling-matched allogeneic donors, related but unmatched donors, and matched-unrelated donors.

Umbilical blood cells, formerly a discarded blood component, appear to possess unique proliferative and immunologic properties and in recent years have been used successfully in adults as well as children.[20–23] Culture-expanded bone marrow stromal cells, often termed *mesenchymal stem cells,* are being utilized in conjunction with hematopoietic stem cells to enhance engraftment and potentially reduce the incidence and severity of GvHD.[24,25]

The potential for serious morbidity and mortality of the myeloablative preparative regimen precludes a number of patients from undergoing allogeneic transplant, and has led recently to "nonmyeloablative" or "reduced conditioning" regimens that have been developed and implemented.[26,27] The pioneering work of E. Donnall Thomas and his colleagues ultimately was recognized since in 1990 Dr. Thomas was awarded the Nobel Prize in Medicine/Physiology. Today, bone marrow transplantation has continued to undergo significant technological and clinical transformation. Hematopoietic stem cell transplantation, a term that encompasses autologous or allogeneic transplantation of stem cells from bone marrow, peripheral blood, or umbilical cord blood, is an effective modality for the treatment of a variety of malignant and nonmalignant conditions.[28] It is estimated that 30,000 to 40,000 transplants are performed yearly worldwide, and the number continues to increase by 10 to 20 percent per year.[29] As a result of continued improvements and sophistication of supportive care, an increasing number of transplants are being undertaken in the ambulatory rather than the inpatient setting. More than 20,000 people now have survived 5 or more years after a hematopoietic stem cell transplant, a stark contrast to one of the first reports in which none of the first 200 transplant recipients had survived.[16] The use of this modality, however, requires extremely sophisticated supportive care, medically, financially, and psychologically, for a successful outcome. This review describes this aspect of care in a detailed fashion.

PATIENT ELIGIBILITY AND SELECTION

The success of high-dose chemo-radiation therapy and hematopoietic stem cell transplantation must be tempered by the potential for significant morbidity and mortality.[30] Although many investigators have examined the role of pretransplant evaluation in predicting organ-specific, treatment-related morbidity, few have focused on identification of pretransplant factors associated with mortality. In a retrospective, multivariate analysis Goldberg et al.[31] reported pretransplant factors and mortality in 383 consecutive hematopoietic stem cell transplant patients examined. They observed a nonrelapse mortality of 6.0 percent (23 of 383 patients) in transplant recipients; factors associated with an increased risk of toxic death included transplant type (allogeneic vs. autologous), FEV1 or DLco (on formal pulmonary function testing), performance status, serum creatinine, and serum bilirubin (Table 59–1). These findings are in concert with those published by other groups.[32–39] In contrast to others, these investigators, however, were unable to correlate older age with poor outcome. They speculated that this finding may have represented an inherent selection bias (i.e., only "healthy" elderly patients may have been referred for transplant). Furthermore, they did not identify subnormal cardiac function correlating with early mortality. These findings are in contrast to the recent study of Zangari et al.[40] who reported that left ventricular ejection fraction at rest and its increment with exercise was discriminatory for peritransplant mortality, especially in patients younger than age 43 years. The use of a standardized, pretransplant evaluation can identify patients at increased risk of treatment-related mortality, and exclude such high-risk candidates. Alternatively, this evaluation allows the use of alternative preparative regimens designed to account for abnormal factors, such as myeloma patients with renal dysfunction.[41]

Selection of an Allogeneic Donor

Prospective allogeneic transplant candidates undergo histocompatible testing to identify a suitable hematopoietic stem cell donor. Such donor searches begin with family members; if a match is not identified within the immediate family (usually a sibling), the process often is extended to include a number of large volunteer blood and bone marrow donor registries such as the National Marrow Donor Program. Allografts performed using unrelated donors are associated with higher rates of graft failure, increased incidence and severity of GvHD, and increased susceptibility to infection when compared to sibling-donor transplants.[42] The genetic differences between related and unrelated donors that are not identified prior to transplant that account for these drawbacks are the result of limitations in the tissue typing methods utilized.[43] The development and application of DNA-based typing techniques for class I and II molecules for identifying histocompatibility between donor and recipient at the A, B, C, DR, and DQB1 loci is a substantial

improvement over serologic methods.[44,45] These sophisticated techniques have enabled selection of a more congruent graft resulting in fewer cases of graft rejection and a lower incidence and severity of GvHD. The process of locating a donor and securing a graft, however, may take up to many months; depending on the ethnicity of the potential recipient, a donor may not be located.

Alternative donor sources also include haploidentical family members and umbilical cord blood (UCB) units. The former are a ready source of cells, while the latter can be procured from UCB banks such as the New York Blood Center. The incidence and severity rates of GvHD are lower with UCB units than with other stem cell sources, in part due to the immaturity of lymphocytes contained in the product. Specifically, recipients of UCB obtained from HLA-identical siblings had a lower risk of acute and chronic GvHD when compared to patients given bone marrow grafts obtained from HLA-identical siblings.[46] Other data demonstrate a lower risk of GvHD in recipients of unrelated donor UCB versus unrelated bone marrow.[47] On the other hand, UCB transplants, especially in adults, are hampered by a smaller number of cells in the graft (per recipient weight), which leads to a longer duration of severe neutropenia, a higher graft failure rate, and the potential for increased treatment-related morbidity and mortality.[23] The use of UCB grafts is discussed in greater detail elsewhere in this text.

SPECIAL CONSIDERATIONS: PHARMACOKINETICS AND DRUG DOSING

With few exceptions, most chemotherapeutic agents are administered parenterally and on the basis of body weight or surface area. Oral administration of drug may be suboptimal since food or medications may interfere with the intestinal microenvironment and alter absorption.[48] Some medications do not lend themselves to oral administration for a variety of reasons. In the transplant setting there may be wide interpatient and intrapatient variability due to age-related differences, alterations in absorption, circadian variations, drug interactions, and patient-specific parameters.[49] Use of high-dose administration has prompted investigators to consider individual dose adjustment when using some agents such as busulfan. This drug is an orally administered alkylating agent, one of the most frequently used agents in transplant preparative regimens for both autologous as well as allogeneic hematopoietic stem cell transplantation. The toxic effects observed with this dose of busulfan include skin hyperpigmentation, hepatotoxicity (veno-occlusive disease [VOD]), neurotoxicity (seizures), nausea, vomiting, diarrhea, and mucositis.[49–53] Ingestion of this agent may be difficult if the patient is nauseated or has difficulty swallowing pills. Additionally, this oral regimen may provide an inadequately low blood concentration in the setting of poor absorption, or difficult-to-measure dose replacement for patients who have emesis after oral administration of busulfan. Although algorithms have been established to standardize replacement doses based on the time of the emetic episode in relation to administration and the content of emesis, it is virtually impossible to determine if the

Table 59–1. Factors Associated With an Increased Treatment-Related Mortality After Transplant

Factor	Relative Risk[a]	p Value
Donor type: allogeneic vs autologous/ syngeneic	4.2	.0008
FEV1 or DLco (< 78 percent predicted)	4.5	.0008
ECOG performance status: > 0	3.7	.003
Serum creatinine: > 1.1 mg/dl	3.8	.02
Serum bilirubin: > 1.1 mg/dl	3.7	.05

[a] Mortality within 100 days.
(From Goldberg et al.,[31] with permission.)

patient has been appropriately exposed, overexposed, or suboptimally exposed to busulfan in this scenario.[54–59] Busulfan bioavailability varies sixfold in children and twofold in adults.[56] These variations are of considerable concern given the association of busulfan's pharmacokinetic profile with clinical outcomes, including central nervous system (CNS) toxicity and hepatic injury. Several investigators noted a relationship between steady-state serum concentration (C_{ss}) and incidence of hepatic VOD and other causes for transplant-related mortality.[60–63] For example, the incidence of hepatic VOD was 83 percent when C_{ss} was greater than 1402 ng/ml and 75 percent when C_{ss} was greater than 1026 ng/ml. On the other hand, the likelihood of graft rejection and diminished antitumor effect are noted with reduced blood concentrations.[64,65] While mean plasma busulfan concentrations (busulfan AUC/dose interval, i.e., C_{ave}) in excess of 1000 ng/ml were associated with severe toxicity (hepatic and other organs), concentrations of at least 200 ng/ml were necessary to avoid graft rejection of matched-sibling cells and at least 600 ng/ml with HLA-matched unrelated donor cells. C_{ave} greater than 900 ng/ml was associated with a lower relapse rate in chronic myeloid leukemia. Pharmacokinetic (PK) studies following oral administration demonstrate variations as high as 50 percent in PK parameters and indicate that PK data obtained within the first 6-hour dosing interval are not evaluable for PK calculations in up to 20 percent of patients due to slow absorption and/or delayed elimination.[54,55,60]

Although somewhat controversial, one approach to this problem is to individualize the dose for the patient's transplant regimen by determining the steady-state drug concentration and AUC either after administering a very small "test" dose several weeks in advance of initiating the preparative regimen, or after the initial therapeutic dose.[58,66] Subsequent doses can be determined based on this information. Alternatively, two parenteral busulfan preparations have been developed. Busulfex® recently was approved by the Food and Drug Administration for use in combination with cyclophosphamide as conditioning prior to allogeneic hematopoietic cell transplantation for chronic myelogenous leukemia. Clinical studies in patients undergoing transplant for hematologic malignancies suggest that Busulfex® given iv is associated with similar toxicity profile and response outcomes when used instead of oral busulfan as a component of the preparative regimen.[67,68] Pharmacokinetic analyses following administration of iv busulfan (Busulfex®) demonstrate more consistent pharmacokinetic profiles as compared to oral administration. One evaluation notes that greater than 90 percent of patients receiving iv busulfan (Busulfex®) had an AUC of less than 1500 Mmol-min/L, and thus, had values falling below the threshold associated with an increased risk of hepatic VOD.[69] In addition, one retrospective comparison suggests that the incidence of hepatic VOD may be lower in patients receiving iv busulfan (Busulfex®) as compared to oral high-dose busulfan.[70] These data may reflect reaching a target blood concentration unlikely to be associated with hepatic toxicity and require verification in other studies. More recently a liposomal formulation of busulfan was developed as an alternative to iv high-dose therapy.[71] Further studies involving these par-

enteral products that correlate pharmacokinetic and pharmacodynamic data and clinical outcome are needed.

PREPARATIVE REGIMEN AND SELECTION OF STEM CELL SOURCE

Conventional or Full Myeloablative Preparative Regimens

Both autologous and allogeneic hematopoietic stem cell sources have been used successfully to rescue patients after receiving intensive cytotoxic therapy. These differing approaches are complementary, since most patients often have only one type of cellular support available for transplant. In recent years, blood rather than marrow has become the preferred source of support for autograft patients.[72–76] Blood autograft trials, in general, have been associated with a faster time to return of neutrophil and platelet count, fewer infections, fewer transfusions, shorter hospital stays, reduced antibiotic use, and often lower costs.[77–79] Although the majority of transplant centers still employ marrow for the allogeneic patients, this situation is changing. Since the first report describing the use of blood for allografting appeared in 1989[80] a number of reports have described the feasibility and benefits of using this approach in the sibling-matched transplant[81–86] and more recently in the unrelated setting.[87,88] The data in the allograft setting resemble the autograft data for faster hematopoietic recovery and other benefits of blood compared to marrow as the stem cell source. Such data, however, may suggest that chronic GvHD rates may be higher than with the use of marrow graft.

Reduced-Conditioning or Non-Myeloablative Regimens

More recently, investigators have begun to utilize "non-myeloablative" or "reduced-conditioning" regimens in the allograft setting (i.e., less toxic preparative regimens that maintain reliable donor engraftment).[89–96] Successful exploitation of this approach will allow patients thought to be ineligible for a full myeloablative transplant due to older age, visceral organ function impairment, or other risk factor such as hepatitis B seropositivity to undergo allogeneic transplant.[96,97] Conventional allografts rely on both high-dose chemo-radiation therapy for cell kill and the donor immune system to induce a graft-versus-tumor effect. Non-myeloablative transplants utilize regimens sufficiently immunosuppressive to facilitate donor cell engraftment, but are potentially less toxic to both marrow and nonmarrow organs. These reduced-conditioning preparative regimens generally involve the use of nucleoside analogues, low-dose total body irradiation, and anti-thymocyte globulin. One group has reported striking results when photopheresis therapy is added to the preparative regimen.[98]

Non-myeloablative approaches rely predominantly on the immunotherapeutic effect of donor cells and thus may be associated with higher relapse rates than those observed with full conditioning. To address this problem, investigators have truncated the post-transplant GvHD prophylaxis in order to induce a graft-versus-tumor effect. Donor lymphocyte infusion (DLI) is another strategy utilized to improve non-myeloablative transplant. Lymphocytes are collected from the stem cell donor via pheresis and are infused at various intervals and doses. This modality has been demonstrated to be an effective treatment for patients who relapse after allograft, and can provide prolonged disease-free survival particularly in chronic myeloid leukemia and lymphoid malignancy patients, although the results of DLI are less impressive in other malignant disorders.[97,99–102] Some investigators have addressed the higher relapse rates by combining an initial autotransplant to be followed later by a reduced-conditioning allograft.[26,94,103] GvHD, with or without DLI, often complicates the reduced-conditioning procedure and may negate the benefit of this approach. Caution is urged for this newer modality, which will require controlled trials to define its role.

UCB and Haploidentical Transplants

In patients in whom an autograft is not an appropriate consideration, and in whom a matched sibling or matched unrelated donor is not available, strategies include the use of UCB transplants and haploidentical donor transplants (see "Selection of an Allogeneic Donor," above).[104,105] These approaches are associated with significantly more supportive care. Although GvHD incidence and severity appear reduced, recovery of the myeloid compartment in UCB transplant recipients in adults is significantly slower that with other stem cell sources (i.e., a median time to neutrophil recovery >500/µl of 27 days). The slow immune system recovery leads to a significant risk of opportunistic infection and treatment-related morbidity and mortality.[23,104] Haploidentical transplant recipients, on the other hand, reconstitute myeloid function rapidly but are at increased risk for severe GvHD, opportunistic infection, and tumor relapse.[105] These two transplant types are considered investigational and should be undertaken only in the context of a clinical trial.

CENTRAL VENOUS AND PHERESIS CATHETERS

The transplant process typically involves the use of a long-term, silastic, multilumen, small-bore, flexible catheter. These specialty devices are used for chemotherapy administration, infusion of hematopoietic cells, and supportive care management including frequent blood sampling, intravenous antibiotics, analgesics, antiemetics, blood components, and parenteral nutrition. In autotransplant patients, it may be necessary to utilize two different venous access devices. This maneuver is necessary due to differences in the catheter properties including diameter of the lumen and catheter rigidity. One large-bore, stiff-walled catheter is used for pheresis and collection of blood stem cells and then usually is removed. Another more flexible catheter is inserted for chemotherapy administration, progenitor cell infusion, and supportive care both during and after the transplant. Recently, some centers began to use one hybrid catheter that embodies the properties of the temporary pheresis catheter and long-term supportive care catheter.[106–108] Complications that may accompany the use of central venous catheters include local pain, extremity swelling, migration, leakage, bleeding at the exit site, emboli, local and disseminated infection, occlusion, and thrombosis (Table 59–2).[106–114]

NAUSEA AND VOMITING

Nausea and vomiting are the most common acute adverse events arising from high-dose chemotherapy and radiation therapy used in the stem cell transplant setting.[115–120] Dopamine-blocking agents such as prochlorperazine, have been the mainstay in the treatment of nausea and vomiting in cancer chemotherapy. The introduction and use of 5-HT$_3$ receptor (i.e., serotonin) blockers revolutionized the treatment of this problem; the first series in hematopoietic stem cell transplant patients was reported over a decade ago.[121] A serotonin blocker in combination with dexamethasone now is the most frequently prescribed prophylaxis for emesis associated with high-dose cytotoxic therapy.[122–129] There are obvious differences in approaching the use of antiemetics in the transplant patient. The American Society of Clinical Oncology recommends more intensive use of antiemetics in transplant patients because the high-dose chemotherapy regimen is more highly emetogenic, frequently total body irradiation is a component of the therapy, the cytotoxic treatments are given for a number of consecutive days, and most transplant patients are not chemotherapy naïve.[130]

Although several publications describe the use of the various 5-HT$_3$ blockers in the transplant setting, there are few differences between the various serotonin blockers as they relate to side effects, efficacy, or the combination.[122–129] Many professional health care organizations have evaluated the available data including clinical experiences and have developed guidelines for the prevention of chemotherapy-induced nausea and vomiting.[130–132] Three important statements can be gleaned from these guidelines as they relate to the role of antiemetics in hematopoietic stem cell transplant patients. First, a serotonin blocker should always be used in combination with dexamethasone. Second, the lowest efficacious antiemetic agent dose should be used. Third, since it appears that all current 5-HT$_3$-blocking medications are therapeutically equivalent, the choice of agent should be determined by the economic factors at each individual institution. Patients who experience continued emesis despite optimization of 5-HT$_3$ blockers and dexamethasone therapy may derive supplementary benefit from use of adjunctive agents such as dopamine-blockers (haloperidol and prochlorperazine).

HEPATIC VOD

Hepatic injury in the course of stem cell transplantation may affect as many as 50 percent of patients and can be a result of various causes including infections, high-dose chemo-radiation therapy, malignancy, antibiotics, parenteral alimentation, immunosuppressive agents, hematopoietic growth factors, GvHD, and hepatic VOD. Overlapping clinical and laboratory

Table 59–2. Published Series for Central Venous Catheter Use in Hematopoietic Stem Cell Transplantation

Ref.	No. Catheters	No. Pts	Catheters	Use	Days In Situ	Local/Tunnel Infection	Bacteremia	Thrombosis	Catheter Dysfunction
93	112	112	PermCath or Bard-Hickman	Pheresis and BMT	63 (7–190)	2 (2 percent)	17 (15 percent)	10 (9 percent)	16 (14 percent)
94	167	156	Hickman or Quinton	Pheresis and BMT	NS	9 (5 percent)	13 (8 percent)	9 (5 percent)	33 (20 percent)[a]
95	56	56	Arrow-Howes or Cook	Pheresis and BMT	48 (5–200)	5 (9 percent)/NS	5 (9 percent)	4 (7 percent)	11 (20 percent)[b]
96	66	62	Arrow-Howes	BMT	38 (1–210)	6 (10 percent)	9 (14 percent)	NS	9 (14.5 percent)
97	23	23	Hickman or Groshong	BMT	38 (5–69)	NS	NS	10 (43 percent)	12 (52 percent)
98	56	53	Mahurkar or Permacath	BMT	58 (7–219)	5 (9 percent)	2 (4 percent)	3 (5 percent)	18 (32 percent)
99	75	46	Hickman or Groshong	BMT	NS	NS	NS	26 (33 percent)	NS
100	55	53	Hickman or Broviac	BMT	111 (27–533)	NS/2 (4 percent)	17 (31 percent)	1 (2 percent)	4 (7 percent)
101	139	123	Hickman, Leonard, or Quinton	BMT	62 (6–365)	NS/NS	NS	2 (3 percent)	12 (19 percent)

Percentages are calculated based on number of catheters. NS, not stated; BMT, bone marrow or hematopoietic stem cell transplant.

[a] Six (4 percent) pneumothoraces and hemothoraces; 6 (4 percent) migration.

[b] Two pneumothoraces and two hemothoraces.

features are present with many of these conditions. Hepatic VOD is an often-fatal syndrome characterized by jaundice, fluid retention, and painful hepatomegaly and may occur in up to half of patients who undergo a myeloablative preparative regimen and stem cell transplant.[133] Manifestations of hepatic VOD usually begin on or about the day of transplant, although more recently "late onset hepatic VOD" has been described.[134–136] The rate of rise in serum bilirubin and patient weight gain is more rapid for patients whose illness is likely to be severe versus those who are likely to have self-limited disease. The histologic features are progressive with concentric occlusion of lumina of small intrahepatic veins and necrosis of hepatocytes in the centrilobular area. This injury leads to portal hypertension, ascites, and hepatic failure.

Risk factors for the development of hepatic VOD include a history of previous hepatocellular disease, busulfan-containing preparative regimens, advanced patient age, presence of GvHD, type of GvHD prophylaxis, omission of IVIG use (for cytomegalovirus [CMV] prophylaxis), fungal infection within 1 week of initiating the preparative regimen, poor performance status at start of transplant, and mucositis after transplant.[133,134,136] Patients who have active liver injury manifest by elevation in serum transaminases at the start of the preparative regimen are considerably more likely to develop hepatic VOD. These data suggest that alterations in plasma concentrations of several inflammatory mediators play a role in the endothelial damage and subsequent fibrosis and hepatocyte necrosis.

Since vascular occlusion appears to be a component of the pathogenesis, many investigators have addressed the use of heparin as prophylaxis in high-risk patients and therapy. The results of such interventions have been mixed.[137–141] A single-arm study in high-risk patients by Bearman and colleagues[137] showed heparin prophylaxis to be ineffective. Attal and colleagues[139] conducted a prospective, randomized clinical trial, although few patients were at high-risk for hepatic VOD. The overall incidence for hepatic VOD was reduced but the incidence of severity did not differ between groups. Recently, a randomized trial using low-molecular-weight heparin showed a shorter duration of hepatomegaly and hyperbilirubinemia, but overall outcome was not reported.[141]

Bile steroids may prevent endothelial damage and hepatocyte injury, possibly by down-regulating expression of inflammatory mediators. In two prospective, randomized trials, the likelihood for developing hepatic VOD was reduced in urso-diol-treated patients, but overall survival did not differ.[142,143] Hepatic VOD occurred in 40 percent of placebo recipients and 15 percent of ursodiol recipients. Development of hepatic VOD was the strongest predictor of survival after transplant, but survival at 100 days did not differ statistically between the two groups.[142] Ohashi and co-workers[143] recently reported a randomized trial using ursodiol prophylaxis. Hepatic VOD occurred significantly less often in the ursodiol-treated patients (3 percent) compared to controls (18 percent) yet overall survival did not differ statistically. Since there is strong evidence that depletion of glutathione results in hepatocyte necrosis, glutathione precursors N-acetylglucosamine and L-glutamine have been given to replenish intracellular glutathione stores and pre-

vent injury.[144–148] Too few patients have been treated on which to draw conclusions.

Several agents have been administered as therapy for established or suspected hepatic VOD. Tissue plasminogen activator (TPA) treatment has been reported to yield efficacy rates in the 25 percent range, but use of this agent has been associated with severe hemorrhage in up to one-third of patients.[149,150] Another antithrombotic agent, antithrombin III, has been used infrequently, with nearly one-half of those treated showing improvement.[151,152] One of the most promising agents appears to be defibrotide, a single-stranded polydeoxyribonucleotide that possesses anti-ischemic, antithrombotic, and thrombolytic activity but without significant anticoagulant effects. Richardson and co-workers treated 75 patients with severe hepatic VOD, most of whom also had ascites and evidence of multisystem organ failure.[153,154] A 35 percent complete response rate without significant toxicity was attained in 67 patients who received 4 or more days of therapy. These investigators have hypothesized that defibrotide functions by repairing endothelial damage. Finally, transjugular intrahepatic portosystemic shunting has been used to mechanically address the events of hepatic VOD. A channel is created between the hepatic and portal vein using a percutaneously inserted catheter and kept patent with a metal stent. Nineteen patients have been reported to date.[155–158] The procedure significantly reduces hepatic venous pressure gradient in about one-half of patients with improvement in intractable portal hypertension and ascites. Unfortunately, most subjects died of other complications.

TRANSFUSION SUPPORT FOR THE TRANSPLANT PATIENT

General Blood Banking Considerations

Most hematopoietic stem cell transplant patients develop anemia, neutropenia, thrombocytopenia, or a combination. Transfusions from blood relatives *must* be avoided when possible for all potential allogeneic transplant candidates, and blood banks at most centers utilize a formal protocol to prevent such occurrences. All blood components are irradiated routinely (1200 to 3000 cGy) to prevent inadvertent lymphoid engraftment and proliferation leading to transfusion-associated GvHD. Irradiation of blood products usually is continued until 6 to 9 months after transplant, at which time full immunologic reconstitution returns.

Anemia, due in part to a relative erythropoietin deficiency, plagues allogeneic and autologous hematopoietic stem cell transplantation.[146] Red blood cell transfusions should be considered if Hb is less than 8 g/dl or Hct is less than 25 percent. A higher transfusion threshold should be considered if the patient has clinical symptoms of severe fatigue, headache, tachycardia, cardiac ischemia, or hypotension. The inadequate erythropoietin response to anemia after stem cell transplantation suggests that exogenous recombinant human erythropoietin treatment may be beneficial. Therapy with this agent after stem cell transplantation has been shown to be safe and well-tolerated; the magnitude of response (e.g., faster reticulocyte recovery and a shorter time to red blood cell transfusion independence) has been more pronounced in the allograft compared to the auto-graft setting.[159] Studies addressing new formulations of recombinant erthropoietin, such as the novel erythropoiesis stimulating protein, darbepoietin (ARANESP™) soon will be initiated in the transplant setting.[160–162]

Spontaneous bleeding, the most frequent complication of severe thrombocytopenia, is greatest at platelet counts of 20,000/µl or less. A number of investigators have advocated lower threshold levels for prophylactic transfusion in view of heightened concerns about transfusion costs and risks of infection and alloimmunization.[163–167] Few studies have addressed this issue prospectively, and many of the trials were undertaken in leukemia patients who were not undergoing transplantation. Furthermore, most of the data in transplant patients were generated in subjects given bone marrow rather than blood as the stem cell source. A survey of 1995 transfusion practices at transplant centers reported that 5 of 18 centers used thresholds of less than 10,000/µl to 15,000/µl, although the majority still used a 20,000/µl cutoff for administering prophylactic platelet transfusions.[168] Severe hemorrhagic events occurred in about 11 percent of patients, usually related to genitourinary bleeding; 2 percent of patients died as a consequence of hemorrhage. Nemo and colleagues[169] reported similar data regarding site and severity of bleeding in more than 1400 bone marrow transplant patients. Most centers, however, still transfuse platelets at a higher level for clinical signs of bleeding or if an invasive procedure is planned. It is anticipated that in the immediate future, fewer platelet transfusions will be required since blood stem cell transplants have faster engraftment, and the expanded use of reduced-conditioning regimens is less marrow suppressive.

Granulocyte Transfusions

Granulocyte transfusions have been advocated by some investigators for treatment of severe, progressive infections in neutropenic patients who fail to respond to antimicrobial agents and recombinant hematopoietic growth factors. Although some studies showed benefit in treating bacterial infection, the clinical usefulness has been questioned, in part due to the potential for pulmonary toxicity, CMV infection, and alloimmunization.[170,171] In addition, insufficient donor stimulation regimens and suboptimal leukapheresis techniques do not provide sufficient cells for infusion, apparently resulting in reduced efficacy. Recent use of new mobilization strategies from healthy donors by administration of granulocyte colony-stimulating factor (G-CSF), dexamethasone, and the combination has significantly routinely enhanced leukapheresis yields three- to fourfold from unrelated as well as related family donors.[172–174] Furthermore, when accounting for leukocyte incompatibility these approaches have resulted in post-transfusion increments in neutrophils for more than 24 hours after transfusion.[175] Newer technologies also may make it possible to store granulocyte concentrates for up to 48 hours and yet preserve adequate neutrophil function.[170] Studies in progress should help define the utility of these higher-dose transfusions in patients with infections refractory to antibiotic therapy.

CMV Infection and Disease

CMV is one of the leading causes of infectious morbidity and mortality in the allogeneic stem cell transplant population. CMV infection and disease are significantly less common in the autograft setting. An exception is patients who are receiving CD34+-enriched grafts designed to eliminate tumor but result in grafts low in autologous T cells. Holmberg et al.[176] reported that 7 of 31 (23 percent) CMV-seropositive autotransplant patients who received myeloablative therapy followed by the infusion of CD34+-selected autologous blood stem cell grafts developed CMV disease (4 fatal; 13 percent) within 100 days of transplant compared to only 10 of 237 (4 percent) contemporaneous CMV-seropositive patients (5 deaths; 2 percent) receiving unselected, autologous stem cell grafts. Multiple myeloma and lymphoma CMV seropositive patients appear to be at increased risk for CMV reactivation during autotransplant.[177]

CMV infection is indicated by isolation of CMV from any body site, or the seroconversion of a patient in the absence of any clinical signs or symptoms of disease, whereas CMV disease is defined as symptomatic infection or a positive culture from a deep tissue or histologic evidence of viral infection.[178] While a number of organs can be involved in the course of an allograft, CMV interstitial pneumonitis is the most severe infection; previously an 85 percent mortality rate was reported.[179] The incidence of primary CMV infection in CMV seronegative patients has been reduced markedly by exclusive use of CMV seronegative blood products (and leukocyte filtering of blood products to remove CMV-infected white blood cells) in CMV seronegative patients. Antiviral agent and IVIG prophylaxis have prevented reactivation CMV disease in seropositive patients.[178,179] The mortality rate for interstitial pneumonitis, however, remains approximately 50 percent even with the addition of ganciclovir and IVIG therapy, prompting therapy as soon as infection is documented (i.e., preemptive therapy).[180] Despite the increased cost and problems with availability, some investigators choose to use CMV hyperimmune globulin rather than IVIG as part of therapy for CMV disease.[181–183]

ABO Incompatible Transplants

Red blood cell antigens are not major histocompatibility antigens and as a result, allogeneic hematopoietic stem cell transplantation can be performed successfully across either major or minor ABO-incompatible barriers between donor and recipient without an increase in GvHD or graft rejection.[184–188] Other red blood cell antigen types may present obstacles for the transplant team if either donor or recipient has red cell antibodies and there is a state of incompatibility in Rh and other red cell antigen systems.[189,190] In contrast to blood transfusion, the risk of hemolysis occurs not only at the time of infusion but can also occur later if viable lymphocytes in the graft produce isoagglutinins directed against recipient red blood cell antigens.

Major ABO incompatibility leads to a clinically significant risk of hemolysis against the red blood cells in the graft as a result from a reaction of host isohemagglutinins against donor cells. Because blood stem cell transplant grafts are collected by apheresis (red cell volume about 2 to 5 percent), this hemolysis risk is much lower compared to a marrow graft that contains a higher volume of red blood cells (about 25 to 35 percent volume). The risk of clinically relevant hemolysis is reduced by removal of red cells from the graft using any of a variety of sedimentation techniques (including starch) or reduction of isoagglutinin titer for the recipient by plasma exchange or column immunoadsorption.[191–195] Isoagglutinin titers can be depleted by large volume plasma exchange (i.e., at least two blood volumes) performed on the day of infusion and on additional days for patients with higher titers. Large-volume plasma exchange is expensive and potentially toxic since allergic and febrile reactions may be frequent despite premedication. Major red cell incompatible transplant recipients, however, may experience delayed red cell recovery after transplantation because of persistent host isoagglutinins that suppress red cell hematopoiesis.[196–201] Rarely, host isoagglutinins may persist for years because of the presence of mature recipient B lymphocytes or plasma cells that survived the preparative regimen necessitating continuing red blood cell transfusions before complete resolution.

Patients who undergo transplants using grafts that are considered minor ABO incompatible, in contrast, face a risk of immediate hemolysis from the infusion of incompatible plasma contained in the donor graft; this risk can be avoided by plasma removal prior to infusion. Of significantly greater import, however, is the fact that these patients may also experience delayed but life-threatening hemolysis mediated by viable donor lymphocytes, termed "passenger lymphocytes," which are carried in the stem cell graft.[200,202–205] These cells may transiently produce sufficient concentrations of isoagglutinins to result in potentially life-threatening hemolysis of recipient red blood cells 7 to 14 days after transplantation, sometimes requiring hemodialysis.[204–206] This situation is more likely to occur in group A recipients with a group O donor, although hemolysis may occur after transfusion of group O red blood cells used in transfusion support possibly through passive absorption of group A or B antigens from donor plasma onto the red blood cell membrane.[204,205] Minor ABO-incompatible hemolysis most likely relates to the type of GvHD prophylaxis post-transplant immunosuppression therapy and does not appear to occur when antilymphocyte proliferative agents such as methotrexate or mycophenolate mofetil are utilized as part of GvHD prophylaxis. Most reported cases involve patients in whom post-transplant immunosuppression is reduced (e.g., cyclosporine alone without either methotrexate, prednisone, or antithymocyte globulin). Omission of potent anti-T-cell agents appears to permit rapid proliferation of B lymphocytes from the donated graft, leading to excessive isohemagglutinin production. Some centers advocate an aggressive preventative approach to all ABO-incompatible transplants using plasma exchange, while others utilize aggressive interventions only for symptomatic management. Several case reports suggest that blood stem cell transplant patients are at greater risk of this complication than marrow recipients because of the greater number of lymphocytes in the graft.[207–210]

MUCOSITIS DURING TRANSPLANTATION

Mucositis is a frequent and significant complication in patients undergoing stem cell transplantation, contributing to local as well as systemic complications. Mucositis of the oval cavity causes pain, disruption of integument leading to an increased risk of infection, and septicemia (often with *Streptococcus* sp.) especially in the neutropenic host. From the patient's point of view, mucositis is the most debilitating complication of transplant.[211–215] Mucositis not only increases the cost of care, it may extend the length of hospitalization and may lead to an increase in mortality.[214,216,217] It is essential to undertake an evaluation of the patient's oral cavity by a dental specialist including x-ray such as panorex before initiating the preparative regimen. A dental cleaning and removal of diseased teeth is recommended.

Monitoring of oral mucositis during transplant is difficult due to lack of a reliable, objective, and valid scale, especially since the high subjectivity of patient pain severity significantly influences evaluation. In an effort to improve research in this area, a new scoring system (Oral Mucositis Assessment Scale) has been developed and implemented successfully in the transplant setting.[214] During transplant it is permissible to allow removable dentures to remain in place while eating but otherwise this appliance should be removed and placed in appropriate antimicrobial solutions during storage. Cryotherapy prophylaxis (ice chips or iced medications) has been a useful adjunct by decreasing blood flow to the mucus membranes.[218–220] Anticholinergics such as propantheline have even been thought by some to be useful since these agents may decrease the excretion of parenterally administered drug into saliva.[221] Medicated rinses have been used in the treatment of severe mucositis, but alteration of pH by some agents such as hydrogen peroxide can retard healing of injured areas.[222,223] Other potentially beneficial agents include povidone-iodine, chlorhexidine, and topical granulocyte-macrophage colony-stimulating factor (GM-CSF) although a recent study raised doubts regarding efficacy of the latter agent.[224–227] Nystatin and chlortrimazole troches are useful to prevent oral fungal infections and topical tetracyclines in combination with diphenhydramine and glucocorticoids may avert bacterial infections in the oral cavity.

Recombinant human keratinocyte growth factor (KGF) is a heparin-binding member of the fibroblast growth factor family and represents a promising approach for the effective management of acute radiation reactions in oral, gastrointestinal, and cutaneous epithelia after radiation exposure.[228] In animal and human models this agent causes thickening of the nonkeratinocyte layers of the oral mucosa and digestive tract.[228,229] A phase I study showed that KGF at the optimal dose of 60 μg/kg prevented severe mucositis in lymphoma patients undergoing autotransplant with the "BEAM" preparative regimen.[230] In a recent phase III, double-blind, placebo-controlled prophylaxis study conducted in the autologous transplant setting, this agent reduced the duration of severe oral mucositis and improved quality of life.[231]

PREVENTION AND TREATMENT OF HEMORRHAGIC CYSTITIS

Hemorrhagic cystitis, due to bladder mucosal injury as a result of chemotherapy, radiation, or viral infection, can be seen early or late in the transplantation setting. The condition rarely is fatal, but the morbidity is significant and the prudent strategy is prevention. Patients may develop micro- or gross hematuria, dysuria, and bladder pain, usually within 3 weeks of transplant or as late as several months after transplant. This condition may lead to major urinary obstruction, sepsis, renal failure, or the need to undertake surgical or chemical bladder cauterization. The high-dose chemotherapeutic agents given during the transplant preparative regimen that most commonly result in hemorrhagic cystitis are thiotepa, busulfan, ifosfamide, cyclophosphamide, and etoposide.[232] This injury is exacerbated by the development of neutropenia, thrombocytopenia, or the combination. Most investigators recommend platelet transfusions to keep the platelet count at least 50,000/μl once the injury occurs. Reactivation of adenovirus is the other major cause of hemorrhagic cystitis, although CMV infection has been reported.[233–236] The finding of adenovirus in the urine usually precedes the occurrence of hematuria. Response to antiviral therapy has been variable.[237] Sencer and co-workers[238] and Arthur et al.[236] noted that allogeneic transplant recipients were significantly more likely to develop hemorrhagic cystitis than either syngeneic or autologous recipients.

Aggressive intravenous hydration (100 to 150 ml/m^2/hour), liberal use of diuretics, and frequent voiding have been reported as effective preventative measures.[239] Other methods include use of a three-way indwelling Foley urinary bladder catheter to provide continuous irrigation. Preventative approaches commonly in practice should be employed beginning prior to the agent and continued following the end of administration.[240] Intravenous infusion of mensa, a uroprotectant with a free sulfhydryl group, inactivates acrolein and active alkylating metabolites of cyclophosphamide and ifosfamide.[241] Vose and colleagues[242] prospectively compared the use of a bladder catheter and irrigation versus mesna. Mesna use significantly reduced the incidence of hematuria, but for grades III and IV hematuria there was no difference. Significantly fewer urinary tract infections were observed in the mesna-treated group. Shepherd and co-workers[243] conducted a

similar trial and also demonstrated no significant differences between the two therapies. Three-way Foley catheter placement, along with a combination of sorbitol and urologic solution irrigation, recently has been suggested as a prophylactic measure.[244]

Treatments for hemorrhagic cystitis range from simple noninvasive measures to invasive approaches (Table 59–3). Insertion of a three-way Foley urinary bladder catheter with saline lavage is the mainstay of the treatment of hemorrhagic cystitis. Often it may be necessary to perform a cystoscopy to evacuate clots. The irrigation rate should be sufficient to keep the lavage fluid light pink to clear. Once the urine has cleared of macroscopic blood, the rate can be reduced and adequate urine output maintained by intravenous hydration or large oral intake. Urine output must be maintained during sleeping hours, waking the patient frequently to drink adequate amounts of fluid to prevent a recurrence of cystitis.[245]

Alum, an astringent, has been used successfully as a 1 percent bladder irrigation in the treatment of hemorrhagic cystitis. The patient must be monitored for the formation of "alum clots" that may pose mechanical difficulties as well as for onset of aluminum toxicity in patients with renal failure.[246–248] Oral or intravenous aminocaproic acid at doses up to 24 g/day has been used but obstruction due to clots can occur.[249] Prostaglandins, PGE1 and PGE2 and PGF2 are instilled in the bladder and left to "dwell" for 1 to 4 hours. Although highly successful, instillation may cause intense bladder spasm and pain; the liberal use of narcotic analgesics is recommended.[250–252] Conjugated estrogens for short periods of time have had some degree of success but should be approached cautiously in patients with cardiovascular disease, or those prone to thromboembolism.[253–255] Formalin instillation for up to 30 minutes is highly successful but severe pain frequently requiring anesthesia prohibits the easy use of this agent.[256–258] Silver nitrate rarely is used due to variable results; recombinant human GM-CSF has shown some efficacy but at a high financial cost.[259,260] Finally, cystectomy may be necessary if hemorrhagic cystitis cannot be controlled.[261–263]

Table 59–3. Treatment of Hemorrhagic Cystitis

Treatment	Specifics	Precautions
Hyperhydration	200–300 ml/hour and diuretic	Fluid overload
Bladder irrigation with 3-way catheter	Fluid infusion at a rate to keep the lavage fluid clear	None
Alum bladder irrigation with 3-way bladder catheter	Continuous lavage with 1 percent alum solution	Alum "clots," system absorption, aluminum toxicity and renal failure
Aminocaproic acid	Up to 24 g/day	Obstruction due to clots in the genitourinary system
Formalin instillation	1 percent solution instillation with "dwell time" of 5 to 15 minutes	Severe pain
Prostaglandins, PGE1 and PGE2, PGF2	PGE1: 750 μg: "dwell time" 1 hour/day PGE2: 0.75 μg: "dwell time" 4 hour PGF2: 0.1–1mg/dl: "dwell time" 1–2 hour thrice daily	Bladder spasm and pain
Estrogen	5 mg/day for 2 days; oral or intravenous	Few side effects short-term
rhGM-CSF	Bladder instillation with 400-μg dose	High cost
Silver nitrate	0.5–1 percent solution with a "dwell time" of 10 minutes	Painful, must be instilled under anesthesia

Graft Failure and Rejection

Hematopoietic stem cell transplantation requires infusion of an adequate progenitor cell dose after high-dose chemo-radiation therapy is administered. In recent years, quantifying CD34 cell surface antigen expression has been demonstrated to be a reliable predictor of sustained hematopoietic recovery after transplant. In the autologous stem cell setting, recent data suggest a dose-response relationship between number of CD34+ cells infused and engraftment kinetics, especially for platelet recovery.[264–268] Many investigators consider a cell dose of 2.0 to 2.5 × 10^6 CD34+ cells/kg patient weight as a minimum for achieving hematopoietic reconstitution within reasonable time, although greater than 5.0 × 10^6 CD34+ cells/kg may be optimal.[269–273] Enhanced engraftment kinetics translate into fewer red blood cell and platelet transfusions, diminished antibiotic usage, shorter hospital stay, and decreased overall costs. It is estimated, however, that delayed hematopoietic engraftment, particularly of platelets, is observed in 5 to 35 percent of patients undergoing autotransplant.[274] Furthermore, some patients fail to mobilize sufficient CD34+ cells despite what are considered effective stimuli. This group of patients may otherwise be acceptable candidates for autotransplant, but are precluded from the procedure due to insufficient cells for infusion, and the significantly increased occurrences of infections, bleeding, and other complications associated with slow or incomplete engraftment. Some investigators have attempted to supplement cells collected from a bone marrow harvest to add to the limited blood stem cell collection; despite infusion of both products, transplant-related mortality often is high due to slow or incomplete engraftment.[274,275] This "hard-to-mobilize" group usually can be identified by a number of factors, including exposure to stem cell toxins such as nitrogen mustard, melphalan, BCNU (carmustine), extensive prior chemotherapy or radiation therapy, advanced age, or tumorous involvement of bone marrow.[265,266,275–282]

Failure to fully engraft after myeloablative therapy in the allogeneic transplant setting may reflect infusion of insufficient numbers of donor hematopoietic stem cells, splenomegaly, a damaged marrow microenvironment, and inadequate GvHD prophylaxis; this problem is more common with T-cell depletion of the graft, donor and recipient HLA disparity, reduced intensity or insufficient preparative regimen immunosuppression, or infection due to CMV, human herpes virus (HHV)-6, HHV-8, and parvovirus.[283–292]

Whatever the etiology, graft failure or rejection is a life-threatening process requiring immediate intervention. Various potential solutions include withdrawal of potentially marrow-suppressive agents such as antibiotics, administration of recombinant hematopoietic growth factors, infusions of additional hematopoietic stem cells (if available), and in the case of a failed allograft, the decision to perform a second transplant. Guardiola and associates[293] reviewed 82 leukemia and aplastic anemia patients who underwent second allografts for graft failure or rejection. Most patients were given second conditioning regimens and the initial (same) usually was used a second time. Overall survival at 3 years was 30 percent but 100-day treatment-related mortality was 53 percent.

ACUTE GVHD

Allogeneic hematopoietic stem cell transplantation in humans is hampered by the development of both acute and chronic GvHD resulting in significant morbidity and mortality, even when HLA-identical siblings are used as stem cell donors.[294,295] This syndrome results when genotypically disparate, alloreactive donor-derived T cells recognize and react to host histoincompatible antigens in a host incapable of rejecting such cells. When donor and recipient are not HLA-identical, differing by even a single antigen, severe GvHD results.[296] If a transplant is performed between HLA-identical siblings, GvHD appears to be mediated via the minor histocompatibility antigens.[297,298] GvHD begins in the setting of host tissue damage induced by conditioning or preparative regimen.[299] Injury to recipient tissues such as the gastrointestinal tract mucosa, liver, and other organs induces, directly or indirectly, secretion of inflammatory cytokines including interleukin (IL)-1, tumor necrosis factor-alpha, gamma-interferon, and GM-CSF.[300] This "dysregulated cytokine release" or "cytokine storm" appears to up-regulate adhesion molecules and major histocompatibility complex (MHC) antigen expression; this effect facilitates alloreactive donor T-cell recognition when such cells subsequently are infused in the course of the transplant.[301–303] Barrett and colleagues[304] demonstrated that markedly delaying donor T-cell infusion in the context of a T-cell-depleted transplant by "T-cell add-back" results in a significantly decreased risk of GvHD. The alloreactive donor T cells recognize the foreign host antigens presented by antigen presenting cells (APC) and undergo activation, stimulation, and proliferation. APC play a critical role in GvHD. These cells stimulate the donor T cells clonal expansion and subsequent differentiation into effector cells via IL-1 and co-stimulatory signals to produce IL-2 and amplification of the reaction.[305,306] The effector cells migrate to target organs, attach to host cells, and mediate end-organ damage. NK cells may accompany the cytotoxic T lymphocytes in inducing GvHD via inflammatory cytokine release and nitric acid production.[307,308]

GvHD traditionally has been divided into acute and chronic GvHD phases, predominantly based on time of onset and clinical presentation. Acute GvHD occurs within the first 100 days after allograft, usually within the first 2 to 6 weeks. A hyperacute, fulminant form can occur within the first week of transplant but is rare unless patients do not receive GvHD prophylaxis.[309] The target organs for this syndrome usually are the skin, gastrointestinal mucosa, and liver; sometimes the lung, lymph nodes, and bone marrow become involved. Risk factors for developing acute GvHD include increasing donor-recipient genetic disparity, full myeloablative compared to reduced-conditioning regimens, advanced patient and donor age, gender mismatch, use of T-replete bone marrow and blood grafts compared to T-cell-depleted grafts or umbilical cord blood units, and prior splenectomy.[310–312] Another factor contributing to the increased frequency of acute GvHD is donor lymphocyte infusions. This maneuver is becoming a common treatment modality for patients who have relapsed after allograft. Although the intent is to induce graft-versus-tumor effects, it is associated with a high incidence of acute GvHD.[313,314]

Acute GvHD traditionally has been quantified as grade I, II, III, or IV using clinical criteria, although the reproducibility for diagnosis and grading often is problematic.[315–317] Several groups have offered modifications of this grading system to improve the correlation between extent of GvHD and outcome.[318,319] Clinically significant acute GvHD (grade II to IV) usually occurs in 10 to 50 percent of HLA-identical sibling-matched recipients compared to rates as high as 70 to 90 percent in unrelated HLA-matched and related HLA-haploidentical transplants.[320,321] The usual strategy is prophylaxis with drugs to partially suppress the graft by preventing or attenuating GvHD while maintaining a graft-versus-tumor effect. Immunosuppression with combinations of agents such as cyclosporine, tacrolimus, methotrexate, and corticosteroids are more effective at providing reduced acute GvHD and improving overall survival compared to single agents.[322] The regimen used most frequently is cyclosporine and methotrexate, the latter agent given for short or long periods.[323] Recently, tacrolimus in combination with methotrexate has been used increasingly. Ratanatharathorn et al.[324] reported a phase III trial comparing cyclosporine/methotrexate versus tacrolimus/methotrexate in 164 sibling-matched allografts. The incidence of grade II to IV acute GvHD was 44 percent in the former and 32 percent in the latter ($p = .01$) although grade III to IV GvHD rates did not differ significantly (17 vs. 13 percent). Interestingly, patients receiving the cyclosporine-containing regimen had a significantly improved survival (57 vs. 47 percent).

Tacrolimus-containing regimens have been used more frequently in the unrelated donor setting even though the trial reported by Ratanatharathorn et al.[324] showed no change in survival between the two regimens in 90 unrelated donor transplants (58 vs. 60 percent). Investigators have truncated the duration of methotrexate therapy in this combination ("mini-methotrexate") and have reported similar efficacy with lower toxicity compared to longer duration of therapy.[325,326]

Another type of acute GvHD prophylaxis is T-cell depletion of the graft, which can be performed by a variety of means including physical separation, density gradient, flow cytometry, lectin depletion, cytotoxic agents, monoclonal antibodies, immunoconjugates, and magnetic beads. Although T-cell depletion reduces the incidence of acute GvHD, this approach is associated with an increase in engraftment failure, tumor relapse, opportunistic infection, and secondary cancers. T-cell depletion trials have not demonstrated an improvement in overall survival.[327–330] Appealing novel approaches utilize tolerance induction that potentially may avoid many of the toxic effects of relatively nonspecific immunosuppressives.[331,332] If host APC are inactivated by blocking co-stimulatory molecules, donor hematopoietic cells can engraft without eliciting GvHD. Use of CTLA4-Ig to block T-cell co-stimulation through the B-7 (CD80 and CD86):CD28 pathway induces a state of anergy.[306] Another means to induce this effect is to interrupt the CD40/CD40L receptor-ligand pair.[333]

New Agents for Acute GvHD Prophylaxis

A number of newer agents are being used to prevent development of acute GvHD and are listed in Table 59–4.[312,322]

Treatment is necessary for grade II to IV acute GvHD. The initial approach consists of continuing the original immuno-suppressive prophylaxis and the addition of corticosteroids. Acting via lympholysis, corticosteroids (alone or in combination with immunosuppressives) remain the most effective agent. Methylprednisolone at a dose usually of at least 2 mg/kg/day is initiated as primary therapy; overall grade of acute GvHD and stem cell source (sibling-match versus unrelated donor, etc.) may influence initial dosing decisions and subsequent response to therapy.[294,334–338] Among patients with grade III acute GvHD, initial therapy response using corticosteroids was only 17 to 39 percent and grade IV patients responded less than 6 percent of the time.[338] Furthermore, steroid-resistant acute GvHD has an extremely poor prognosis due to onset of opportunistic infection as well as end-organ damage due to

Table 59–4. GvHD Therapy: Newer Agents

Agent	Comment
Mycophenolate mofetil	De novo guanine nucleotide synthesis inhibition
Rapamycin (sirolimus)	Inhibits cell cycle progression $G_1 \rightarrow S$; binds to FKBP
Trimetrexate	Methotrexate-like properties
15-deoxyspergualin (tresperimus)	Immunosuppression mechanism unknown; inhibits NF-κB
Chloroquine	Blocks peptide transport to cell-surface MHC molecules
PG27	Anti-inflammatory and immunosuppressive agent
CTLA4-Ig	Costimulatory signaling inhibition; humanized monoclonal antibody
GLAT	MHC class II binding; blocks T-cell receptor binding
Neuraminidase	Modifies lymphocyte surface glycoprotein; enzyme
Daclizumab	Anti-CD25 monoclonal antibody
Basiliximab	Anti-CD25 monoclonal antibody
ZAP-70	Blocks signaling pathways
Fludarabine	Nucleoside analogue; immunosuppressive properties
2-chlorodeoxyadenosine (2-CDA)	Nucleoside analogue; immunosuppressive properties
Pentostatin	Nucleoside analogue; immunosuppressive properties

(Data from Goker et al.,[312] and Simpson.[322])

GvHD; mortality ranges from 53 to 80 percent.[336] A number of agents have been used as salvage therapy including mycophenolate mofetil, pentostatin, and a variety of anti-T-cell and anti-cytokine monoclonal antibodies and the results have been mixed.[339–341] Newer strategies are being developed to address this persistent problem.[342]

CHRONIC GVHD

Chronic GvHD, a significant cause of morbidity and mortality, occurs in about two-thirds of long-term survivors of allogeneic hematopoietic stem cell transplant.[343–346] As a result of greater availability and increased use of unrelated donors as well as the inclusion of older recipients and of non-myeloablative ("reduced conditioning") regimens, the incidence of this syndrome appears to be rising.[347,348] This syndrome resembles an autoimmune disorder and has been classified in a variety of ways. Shulman et al.[349] proposed: subclinical (proven by histology but no clinical symptoms); limited extent (localized skin involvement, hepatic dysfunction due to chronic GvHD, or both); and extensive (generalized skin involvement, or limited extent plus involvement of a target organ such as liver histology showing chronic aggressive hepatitis, bridging necrosis, or cirrhosis, eye involvement, minor salivary gland, or oral mucosal involvement). This group also classified chronic GvHD according to the pattern of onset of clinical disease: de novo, quiescent, and progressive disease (see below).[350]

While TH1 donor cells appear to be the mediators in acute GvHD, chronic GvHD is a syndrome of immune dysregulation of TH2 donor cells.[351–353] Most patients have evidence of a high prevalence of autoantibodies to cell surface and intracellular antigens, although the role of such autoantibodies in the pathogenesis of chronic GvHD is unclear.[354,355]

The likelihood of developing chronic GvHD appears to be associated with increasing HLA disparity between recipient and donor (especially unrelated donor recipients), prior diagnosis of acute GvHD, and corticosteroid use by 100 days after allograft, use of non-T-cell depleted bone marrow, male recipients of multiparous female donors, older age of recipient or donor, and possibly use of blood rather than bone marrow.[344,356–366] Clinical manifestations of chronic GvHD are similar to autoimmune collagen vascular diseases including oral ulcerations (lichen planus), keratoconjunctivitis sicca, xerostomia, polyserositis, esophagitis and stricture, vaginal ulceration and stricture, intrahepatic obstructive liver disease, obstructive pulmonary disease, scleroderma, morphea, fasciitis, and myositis.[367]

Immunodeficiency, leading to a variety of opportunistic infections and often to death, is the most important associated complication of chronic GvHD. *Pneumocystis carinii*, *Streptococcus pneumoniae*, and CMV are the pathogens most likely to cause serious and fatal infection, and prophylaxis strategies against these pathogens should be undertaken.[368–370] Since there are no specific pharmacologic prophylaxis therapies to prevent chronic GvHD, prevention of acute GvHD (i.e., T-cell depletion strategies and use of CAMPATH-1 monoclonal antibody) appears to be the most effective means of prevention.

T-cell depletion of stem cell grafts reduces the risk of both acute and chronic GvHD.[365,371–375] Comprehensive guidelines for infectious prophylaxis in hematopoietic stem cell transplant recipients, including patients with chronic GvHD, have been published recently.[376]

Patients who develop chronic GvHD after an interval of response to treatment for acute GvHD (quiescent form) or patients who have never had acute GvHD (de novo form) are more likely to respond to therapy with cyclosporine or tacrolimus in combination with corticosteroids.[377–380] Those individuals who experience the "progressive" form (i.e., chronic GvHD developing before resolution of acute GvHD) are less likely to respond to immunosuppressive therapies.[345,378,381] Other poor prognostic features include platelet counts less than or equal to 100,000/μl (usually the "progressive" form; 5-year survivals of only about 25 percent), increased age, lichenoid skin histopathology, and hepatic involvement.[378] Limited extent chronic GvHD, for example, oral lichen planus and limited scleroderma of the distal extremities often respond to immunosuppressive therapy, but generalized scleroderma carries a poor prognosis.[381] Patients with extensive chronic GvHD (i.e., bronchiolitis obliterans) have an extremely poor prognosis independent of other clinical manifestations of chronic GvHD.[382–384]

Prednisone alone or in combination with other immunosuppressive agents has been the standard treatment for chronic GvHD.[350,385] A variety of additional agents used in the treatment of chronic GvHD have been reviewed elsewhere and include etritrenate, thalidomide, hydroxychloroquine, extracorporeal photopheresis, ultraviolet B light, and PUVA therapy.[367] Attempts to combine some of these agents (i.e., thalidomide added to prednisone and cyclosporine) have not improved initial results.[386] Newer therapies that show promise include anti-tumor necrosis factor (TNF) monoclonal antibodies (infliximab), TNF receptor antagonist (etanercept), and anti-CD20 chimeric monoclonal antibody (rituximab).[364,387–389]

LATE COMPLICATIONS AFTER TRANSPLANT

Late complications after transplant include those due to the preparative regimen, late infection (see "Post-Transplant Vaccination," below), chronic GvHD, recurrence of malignancy, and secondary malignancy. Complications from the preparative regimen include cataracts and other ophthalmic complications, avascular necrosis of joints, late neurologic conditions such as leukoencephalopathy and cognitive function impairment, impairment of growth and development in children, endocrine disturbances, and gonadal dysfunction.[390] Some of these effects indirectly may cause other conditions such as osteoporosis.[391,392]

Quality of Life

Over the past three decades the primary focus of autologous and allogeneic stem cell transplantation has been to improve overall survival and relapse rates. Greater success of this modality has resulted in more survivors and increasing emphasis on the patient's quality of life (QOL) after the transplant. For many transplant recipients, however, disease cure or control is not met with complete restoration of health. While lifesaving, transplantation frequently is associated with late complications described herein as well as the continued threat of disease recurrence. These factors can negatively affect a transplant survivor's ability to function fully and normally in important areas of everyday life, including employment, relationships with others, and sexuality.

A number of publications have addressed QOL evaluation after transplant.[393–408] Many studies show that the most significant issues that patients report as interfering with QOL are altered body image, sexual difficulties, fatigue, lack of physical strength, inability to work at their chosen employment, and financial problems.[394,397,398,401,406–408] This psychosocial literature as it pertains to hematopoietic stem cell transplantation often divides the post-treatment period into three parts: within 1 year from completion of treatment; 1 to 5 years after treatment; and more than 5 years post-treatment. The first of these three groups has received the most study. Results of several studies suggest that this period of time is characterized by relatively slow return of energy and activity level. Return to baseline (pre-transplant) functioning is observed in many patients by this time, although a substantial number continue to experience compromised function. Andrykowski and colleagues[395] noted that the physical and psychosocial deficits perceived as problems by the patient were, in fact, present prior to transplant. A lower QOL persists more often in older patients, those with less formal education, subjects with a more advanced disease state at transplant, and those in whom there is evidence of active chronic GvHD and chronic visceral organ dysfunction.[394,403] Overall, autologous transplant recipients reported a better QOL than those individuals who underwent an allogeneic procedure.[396]

Years 1 through 5 after transplant are becoming better understood as a result of more recent investigations; during this period, the patient more commonly experiences a return to normal functioning. Survivors who are beyond 5 years, particularly those who are disease-free, are reported to be able to perform at a level at least equal (or greater) to age-matched comparison groups, with a few exceptions. Such exceptions pertain to areas relating to close relationships, sexual functioning, and fear of recurrence. Cancer and its treatment are life-altering experiences that often stress marital quality, friendships, and life perspectives. Recently, there has been an increased attention to the positive aspects of surviving traumatic experiences, including transplant for cancer.[409] These studies suggest that anecdotes reported by patients that describe improvements in life appreciation and satisfaction can be measured using instruments sensitive to QOL.

Controlled studies are needed to determine whether interventions aimed to enhance positive outcomes of traumatic experiences such as transplant will lead to meaningful improvements for the individual patient. QOL issues must be addressed prior to transplant and need to be re-evaluated on a continued basis after transplant completion.

Secondary Malignancies

Secondary malignancies are among the most serious of late effects in treated cancer patients and complicate hematopoietic

stem cell transplantation as well.[410] Secondary malignancies represent a low but significant risk for transplant recipients. Earlier reports identified secondary acute myeloid leukemia (AML) and secondary myelodysplastic syndromes (MDS) as the malignancy encountered most frequently, after a relatively short latent period.[411–416] Therapeutic results for these treatment-related conditions are extremely poor. Risk factors for developing a second cancer include alkylating agent exposure, radiotherapy in the preparative regimen, acute GvHD (grade II to IV), use of anti-thymocyte globulin in the post-transplant setting, and chronic GvHD.[411–413] The use of etoposide in autologous transplant patients at doses greater than 2 g/m^2 has shown a variably slightly increased (up to 3 percent at 5 years) cumulative incidence of AML and MDS.[417,418]

Recently, solid tumors arising after transplantation have been recognized. This group of malignant disorders has a longer latency period before development than hematologic malignancies.[419] In a review of 550 allogeneic transplant patients, epithelial and cutaneous solid tumors occurred at a rate 4 times higher than in the general population.[420] Curtis and co-workers[421] studied over 19,000 allogeneic transplant recipients between 1964 and 1992 at 235 centers and reported an eight-fold increase in solid tumors among subjects who survived 10 or more years after transplantation (cumulative incidence rate 2.2 percent at 10 years and 6.7 percent at 15 years). The most commonly observed cancers were malignant melanoma, cancers of the liver, central nervous system, thyroid, bone, connective tissue, and buccal cavity; the latter tumors were strongly linked to male gender and those with chronic GvHD. The risk was higher for younger recipients who were given higher doses of total body irradiation. Similar results were reported recently by Bhatia and colleagues.[422]

Post-transplant lymphoproliferative disorders may arise in the post-transplant setting, usually peaking at 1 to 5 months, followed by a sharp decline after the first year.[423] This syndrome appears to be related to the immunosuppression used in the prophylaxis and treatment of GvHD, or T-cell depletion of the graft and does not appear to be a result of the preparative regimen.

All patients undergoing hematopoietic stem cell transplantation should be informed of the potential risk of developing a second cancer and should be monitored on a continuous basis. The trend toward an increased risk over time after transplantation and the greater risk among younger patients indicates the need for lifelong surveillance.

Post-Transplant Vaccination

Patients undergoing both autologous as well as allogeneic hematopoietic stem cell transplantation experience a prolonged period of immune dysfunction associated with an increased risk for bacterial and viral infections. This defect may persist for a prolonged period of 1 year or longer.[424–426] In addition, hematopoietic stem cell transplantation often is associated with a loss or diminution of protective immunity against pathogens targeted by childhood immunizations such as tetanus, mumps, rubella, and poliovirus.

After transplant reconstitution of NK cells does not require a functional thymus and such cells recover qualitatively and quantitatively in the first month and remain at normal to increased levels throughout the first 3 months after transplant.[427] CD3+ T-cell numbers recover soon after transplant, but patients experience prolonged inversion of the CD4/CD8 ratio due to the relative absence of CD4+ helper cells and the increased presence of CD8+ suppressor cells; the function of these cells remains defective 6 to 12 months after transplant as demonstrated in vivo (the development of anergy to recall antigens as measured by delayed hypersensitivity testing) as well as in vitro using laboratory assays.[427–433] This situation is further exacerbated in allograft recipients because re-education of donor lymphoid cells occurs in a foreign environment in the absence of a functional thymus and patients usually continue to receive immunosuppressive agents as prophylaxis for GvHD. In the absence of GvHD, mature B-cell populations in the peripheral blood expressing CD19 and CD20 return to normal levels after 3 to 6 months following autologous and allogeneic marrow transplantation.[434] Reconstitution is more rapid in patients receiving autologous peripheral blood stem cells and correlates with the presence of increased numbers of mature, memory CD4+ helper T cells.[427] The impact on humoral immunity consists of decreased levels of circulating immunoglobulin, impaired immunoglobulin class switching, and a loss of complexity in immunoglobulin gene rearrangement patterns.

As a result of these defects, infections, especially those due to encapsulated bacterial organisms such as *Streptococcus pneumoniae* and *Haemophilus influenzae* type B (Hib) remain prevalent even in the late post-transplant period.[435,436] Immunization with anti-infective vaccines is markedly compromised by previous exposure to cytotoxic agents and the immune dysfunction that characterizes the post-transplant period.[437,438] Vaccine efficacy in stem cell transplant patients has not been studied in large multicenter trials. Published surveys in Europe and the United States indicate that there is considerable variability in the practice guidelines with respect to the vaccination after transplant.[439,440]

A variety of factors complicate efforts to develop an effective vaccination strategy for patients following hematopoietic stem cell transplantation. Live, attenuated viral vaccines are more potent as compared to inactivated or killed vaccines in eliciting protective responses, but their use in the immunocompromised setting is limited by concerns regarding the risk of disseminated infection.[438] Given the importance of immune reconstitution in determining response to vaccination in the post-transplant patient, a variety of studies have sought to identify the optimal timing of immunization.

Strategies to enhance vaccine efficacy include pretransplant immunization of the stem cell donor and the use of cytokine adjuvants such as GM-CSF. Immune recovery appears to be more rapid in patients receiving blood stem grafts rather than marrow but is delayed in recipients of T-cell-depleted allografts.[441–444]

The data suggest that polysaccharide-based vaccines (i.e., pneumococcal vaccine) fail to provide adequate protection in the first 2 years post-transplant.[445–450] On the other hand, the protein-conjugated vaccine against Hemophilus influenza B confers protection. Although the efficacy of vaccination in patients undergoing hematopoietic stem cell transplantation may be significantly improved in patients receiving peripheral blood stem cells as compared to marrow, a number of strategies are being developed to reduce late infectious complications by vaccination.[451–453] Recommendations and timing for vaccination in the post-transplant setting have been published recently for *Streptococcus pneumoniae*, Hib, diphtheria/tetanus, hepatitis B, poliovirus, mumps, measles, and rubella.[376]

REFERENCES

1. Armitage JO: Bone marrow transplantation. N Engl J Med 330:827–838, 1994.
2. Santos GW: History of bone marrow transplantation. Clin Haematol 12:611–639, 1983.
3. Schretzenmayr A: Anamiebehandlung mit knochenmarksinjektionen. Klin Wochenschr 16:1010–1012, 1937.
4. Migdalska KZ: Special section—transplantation of bone marrow. Blood 13:300–301, 1958.
5. Morrison M, Samwick AA: Intramedullary (sternal) transfusion of human bone marrow. J Am Med Assoc 115:1708–1711, 1940.
6. Osgood EE, Riddle MC, Mathews TJ: Aplastic anemia treated with daily transfusions and intravenous marrow. Ann Intern Med 13:357–367, 1939.
7. Jacobson LO, Marks EK, Robson MJ et al: Effect of spleen protection on mortality following x-irradiation. J Lab Clin Med 34:1538–1543, 1949.
8. Lorenz E, Uphoff D, Reid TR et al: Modification of irradiation injury in mice and guinea pigs by bone marrow injections. J Natl Cancer Inst 12:197–201, 1951.
9. Van Bekkum DW, DeVries MJ: Radiation Chimeras. Academic Press, New York, 1967.
10. Billingham RE, Brent L: Quantitative studies on tissue transplantation immunity. IV. Induction of tolerance in newborn mice and studies on the phenomenon of runt disease. Philos Trans R Soc London B Biol Sci 242:477, 1959.
11. Billingham RE: The biology of graft-versus-host reactions. The Harvey Lectures 1966–67, pp. 21–78. Academic, New York, 1966.
12. Cavins JA, Scheer SC, Thomas ED et al: The recovery of lethally irradiated dogs given infusions of autologous leukocytes preserved at −80°C. Blood 23:38–43, 1964.
13. Thomas ED, Lochte HL Jr, Lu WC, Ferrebee JW: Intravenous infusion of bone marrow in patients receiving radiation and chemotherapy. N Engl J Med 257:491–496, 1957.
14. Kurnick NB, Montano A, Gerdes JC, Feder BH: Preliminary observations on the treatment of postirradiation hematopoietic depression in man by the infusion of stored autologous bone marrow. Ann Intern Med 49:973–986, 1958.
15. McGovern JJ Jr, Russel PS, Atkins L, Webster EW: Treatment of terminal leukemia relapse by total-body irradiation and intravenous infusion of stored autologous bone marrow obtained during remission. N Engl J Med 260:675–680, 1959.
16. Bortin MM: A compendium of reported human bone marrow transplants. Transplantation 9:571–587, 1970.
17. Thomas ED, Lochte HL Jr, Cannon JH, Sahler OD, Ferrebee JW: Supralethal whole body irradiation and isologous marrow transplantation in man. J Clin Invest 38:1709–1716, 1959.
18. Thomas ED, Buckner CD, Banaji M et al: One hundred patients with acute leukemia treated by chemotherapy, total body irradia-

tion, and allogeneic marrow transplantation. Blood 49:511–533, 1977.

19. Phillips GL, Herzig RH, Lazarus HM et al: Treatment of relapsed lymphoma with cyclophosphamide, total body irradiation and autologous bone marrow transplantation. N Engl J Med 310:1557–1561, 1984.

20. Gluckman E, Broxmeyer HE, Auerbach AD et al: Hematopoietic reconstitution in a patient with Fanconi's anemia by means of umbilical cord-blood from an HLA-identical sibling. N Engl J Med 321:1174–1178, 1989.

21. Gluckman E, Rocha V, Boyer-Chammard A et al: Outcome of cord-blood transplantation from related and unrelated donors. N Engl J Med 337:373–381, 1997.

22. Rubinstein P, Carrier C, Scaradavou A et al: Outcomes among 562 recipients of placental-blood transplants from unrelated donors. N Engl J Med 339:1565–1577, 1998.

23. Laughlin MJ, Barker J, Bambach B et al: Hematologic engraftment and survival after unrelated placental cord transplant in adult recipients. N Engl J Med 344:1815–1822, 2001.

24. Lazarus HM, Koc ON: Culture-expanded human marrow-derived MSCs in clinical hematopoietic stem cell transplantation. Graft 3:329–333, 2001.

25. Lazarus H, Curtin P, Devine S et al: Role of mesenchymal stem cells (MSC) in allogeneic transplantation: Early phase I clinical results (abstract #1691). Blood 96:392a, 2000.

26. Carella AM, Giralt S: Novel preparative regimens II. Non-myeloablative regimens. In Rowe JM, Lazarus HM, Carella AM (eds.): Handbook of Bone Marrow Transplantation, pp. 95–110, Martin Dunitz, London, 2000.

27. Molina AJ, Storb RF: Hematopoietic stem cell transplantation in older adults. In Rowe JM, Lazarus HM, Carella AM, (eds.): Handbook of Bone Marrow Transplantation, pp. 111–137. Martin Dunitz, London, 2000.

28. Leiper AD: What is in store after stem-cell transplantation? Lancet 353:1544–1545, 1999.

29. Horowitz M: Uses and growth of hematopoietic cell transplantation. In Thomas ED, Blume KG, Forman SJ (eds.): Haematopoietic Cell Transplantation, 2nd ed., pp. 12–18, Oxford, Blackwell, 1998.

30. Bearman SI, Appelbaum FR, Buckner CD et al: Regimen-related toxicity in patients undergoing bone marrow transplantation. J Clin Oncol 6:1562–1568, 1998.

31. Goldberg SL, Klumpp TR, Magdalinski AJ, Mangan KF: Value of the pretransplant evaluation in predicting toxic day-100 mortality among blood stem-cell and bone marrow transplant recipients. J Clin Oncol 16:3796–3802, 1998.

32. Crawford SW, Fisher L: Predictive value of pulmonary function testing before bone marrow transplantation. Chest 101:1257–1264, 1992.

33. Jain B, Floreani AA, Anderson JR et al: Cardiopulmonary function and autologous bone marrow transplantation: Results and predictive value for respiratory failure and mortality. Bone Marrow Transplant 17:561–568, 1996.

34. Carlson K, Backlund L, Smedmyr B et al: Pulmonary function and complications subsequent to autologous bone marrow transplantation. Bone Marrow Transplant 14:805–811, 1994.

35. Horak DA, Schmidt GM, Zaia JA et al: Pretransplant pulmonary function predicts cytomegalovirus-associated interstitial pneumonia following bone marrow transplantation. Chest 102:1484–1489, 1992.

36. Zager RA, O'Quigley J, Zager BK et al: Acute renal failure following bone marrow transplantation: A retrospective study of 272 patients. Am J Kidney Dis 13:210–216, 1989.

37. McDonald GB, Hinds MS, Fisher LD et al: Veno-occlusive disease of the liver and multiorgan failure after bone marrow transplantation: A cohort study of 355 patients. Ann Intern Med 118:255–267, 1993.

38. Chen PM, Liu JH, Fan FS et al: Liver disease after bone marrow transplantation: The Taiwan experience. Transplantation 59:1139–1143, 1995.

39. Rozman C, Carreras E, Qian C et al: Risk factors for hepatic veno-occlusive disease following HLA-identical sibling bone marrow transplants for leukemia. Bone Marrow Transplant 17:75–80, 1996.

40. Zangari M, Henzlova MJ, Ahmad S et al: Predictive value of left ventricular ejection fraction in stem cell transplantation. Bone Marrow Transplant 23:917–920, 1999.

41. Tricot G, Alberts DS, Johnson C et al: Safety of autotransplants with high-dose melphalan in renal failure: A pharmacokinetic and toxicity study. Clin Cancer Res 2:947–952, 1996.

42. A Consensus Statement on unrelated donor bone marrow transplantation from the Consensus Panel chaired by EC Gordon-Smith. Bone Marrow Transplant 19:959–962, 1997.

43. Madrigal J, Scott I, Argüello R et al: Factors influencing the outcome of bone marrow transplants using unrelated donors. Immunol Rev 157:153–166, 1997.

44. Sasazuki T, Juji T, Morishima Y et al: Effect of matching of class I HLA alleles on clinical outcome after transplantation of hematopoietic stem cells from an unrelated donor. N Engl J Med 339:1177–1185, 1998.

45. Petersdorf EW, Gooley TA, Anasetti C et al: Optimizing outcome after unrelated marrow transplantation by comprehensive matching of HLA class I and II alleles in the donor and recipient. Blood 92:3515–3520, 1998.

46. Rocha V, Wagner JE, Sobocinski KA et al: Graft-versus-host disease in children who have received a cord-blood or bone marrow transplant from an HLA-identical sibling. N Engl J Med 342:1846–1854, 2000.

47. Rocha V, Cornish J, Sievers EL et al: Comparison of outcomes of unrelated bone marrow and umbilical cord blood transplants in children with acute leukemia. Blood 97:2962–2971, 2001.

48. Wilkinson GR: Pharmacokinetics. The dynamics of drug absorption, distribution and elimination. In Hardman JG and Limbird LE (eds). Goodman & Gilman's The Pharmacological Basis of Therapeutics, 10th edition, pp. 3–29, McGraw-Hill Publishing Co., New York, 2001.

49. Henner WD, Peters WP, Eder JP, Antman K, Schnipper L, Frei E III: Pharmacokinetics and immediate effects of high-dose carmustine in man. Cancer Treat Rep 70:877–880, 1986.

50. Santos GW, Tutschka PJ, Brookmeyer R et al: Marrow transplantation for acute nonlymphocytic leukemia after treatment with busulfan and cyclophosphamide. N Engl J Med 309:1347–1353, 1983.

51. Geller RB, Saral R, Piantadosi S et al: Allogeneic bone marrow transplantation after high-dose busulfan and cyclophosphamide in patients with acute nonlymphocytic leukemia. Blood 73:2209–2218, 1989.

52. Tutschka PJ, Copelan EA, Klein JP: Bone marrow transplantation for leukemia following a new busulfan and cyclophosphamide regimen. Blood 70:1382–1388, 1987.

53. Schiffman KS, Bensinger WI, Appelbaum FR et al: Phase II study of high-dose busulfan, melphalan and thiotepa with autologous peripheral blood stem cell support in patient with malignant disease. Bone Marrow Transplant 17:943–950, 1996.

54. Hassan M, Ehrsson H, Ljungman P: Aspects concerning busulfan pharmacokinetics and bioavailability. Leuk Lymphoma 22:395–407, 1996.

55. Hassan M, Oberg G, Ehrsson H et al: Pharmacokinetics and metabolic studies of high-dose busulphan in adults. Eur J Clin Pharmacol 36:525–530, 1989.

56. Hassan M, Oberg G, Bekassy AN et al: Pharmacokinetics of high-dose busulphan in relation to age and chronopharmacology. Cancer Chemother Pharmacol 28:130–134, 1991.

57. Vassal G: Pharmacologically-guided dose adjustment of busulfan in high-dose chemotherapy regimens: Rationale and pitfalls. Anticancer Res 14:2363–2370, 1994.

58. Hassan M, Ljungman P, Bolme P et al: Busulfan bioavailability. Blood 84:2144–2150, 1994.

59. Slattery JT, Risler LJ: Therapeutic monitoring of busulfan in hematopoietic stem cell transplantation. Ther Drug Monit 20:543–549, 1998.

60. Grochow LB: The role of therapeutic monitoring in bone marrow transplantation induction regimens. Semin Oncol 20(Suppl. 4):18–25, 1993.

61. Grochow LB, Jones RJ, Brundett RB et al: Pharmacokinetics of busulfan: Correlation with veno-occlusive disease in patients undergoing bone marrow transplantation. Cancer Chemother Pharmacol 25:55–61, 1989.

62. Ljungman P, Hassan M, Bekassy AN et al: High busulfan concentrations are associated with increased transplant-related mortality in allogeneic bone marrow transplant patients. Bone Marrow Transplant 20:909–913, 1997.

63. Dix SP, Wingard JR, Mullins RE et al: Association of busulfan area under the curve with veno-occlusive disease following BMT. Bone Marrow Transplant 17:225–230, 1996.

64. Slattery JT, Clift RA, Buckner CD et al: Marrow transplantation for chronic myeloid leukemia: The influence of plasma busulfan levels on the outcome of transplantation. Blood 89:3055–3060, 1997.

65. Slattery JT, Sanders JE, Buckner CD et al: Graft-rejection and toxicity following bone marrow transplantation in relation to busulfan pharmacokinetics. Bone Marrow Transplant 16:31–42, 1995.

66. Schuler U, Schroer S, Kuhnle A et al: Busulfan pharmacokinetics in bone marrow transplant patients: Is drug monitoring warranted? Bone Marrow Transplant 14:759–765, 1994.

67. Andersson BS, McWilliams K, Tran H et al: IV busulfan, cyclophosphamide (BuCy) and allogeneic hematopoietic stem cells (BMT) for chronic myeloid leukemia (CML). Blood 92(Suppl. 1):abstr #1168, 1998.

68. Kashyap A, Forman S, Cagnoni P et al: Intravenous busulfan (Busulfex™)/Cytoxan (Cy) preparative regimen for allogeneic (allo) and autologous (auto) hemaetopoietic stem cell transplantation (BMT) is well tolerated by patients over 50 years of age (abstract #515). Blood 92(Suppl. 1):128a, 1998.

69. Vaughan WP: Pharmacokinetics of intravenous busulfan in hematopoietic stem cell transplantation. Proceedings of the American Society for Blood and Marrow Transplantation Meeting, Keystone, CO, March 3–6, abstract #78, 1998.

70. Vaughan WP, Cagnoni P, Fernandez H et al: Decreased incidence of and risk factors for hepatic veno-occlusive disease with an intravenous busulfan (bu) containing preparative regimen for hematopoietic stem cell transplantation (HSCT) (abstract #2121). Blood 92(Suppl. 1): 516a, 1998.

71. Hassan Z, Ljungman P, Ringden O et al: Pharmacokinetics of liposomal busulphan in man. Bone Marrow Transplant 21:479–485, 2001.

72. Beyer J, Schwella N, Zingsem J et al: Hematopoietic rescue after high-dose chemotherapy using autologous peripheral-blood progenitor cells or bone marrow: A randomized comparison. J Clin Oncol 13:1328–1335, 1995.

73. Schmitz N, Linch DC, Dreger P et al: Randomised trial of filgrastim-mobilised peripheral blood progenitor cell transplantation versus autologous bone-marrow transplantation in lymphoma patients. Lancet 347:353–357, 1996.

74. Hartmann O, Gaelle Le Corroller A, Blaise D et al: Peripheral blood stem cell and bone marrow transplantation for solid tumors and lymphomas: Hematologic recovery and costs. Ann Intern Med 126:600–607, 1997.

75. Weisdorf D, Verfaillie C, Miller W et al: Autologous bone marrow versus non-mobilized peripheral blood stem cell transplantation for lymphoid malignancies. Am J Hematol 54:202–208, 1997.

76. Brice P, Marolleau JP, Pautier P et al: Hematologic recovery and survival of lymphoma patients after autologous stem-cell transplantation: Comparison of bone marrow and peripheral blood progenitor cells. Leuk Lymphoma 22:449–456, 1996.

77. Uyl-de Groot CA, Ossenkoppele GJ, Buijt I et al: Costs of peripheral blood progenitor cell transplantation using whole blood mobilised by filgrastim as compared with autologous bone marrow transplantation in non-Hodgkin's lymphoma. Pharmacoeconomics 15:305–311, 1999.

78. Smith T, Hillner B, Schmitz N et al: Economic analysis of a randomized clinical trial to compare filgrastim-mobilized peripheral-blood progenitor-cell transplantation and autologous bone marrow transplantation in patients with Hodgkin's and non-Hodgkin's lymphoma. J Clin Oncol 15:5–10, 1997.

79. Waters T: Economic analysis of new technologies: The case of stem cell transplantation. J Clin Oncol 15:2–4, 1997.

80. Kessinger A, Smith DM, Strandjord SE et al: Allogeneic bone marrow transplantation vs filgrastim-mobilised peripheral blood progenitor cell transplantation in patients with early leukaemia: First results of a randomized multicentre trial of the European Group for Blood and Marrow Transplantation. Bone Marrow Transplant 21:995–1003, 1998.

81. Schmitz N, Bacigalupo A, Hasenclever D et al: Allogeneic bone marrow transplantation vs filgrastim-mobilised peripheral blood progenitor cell transplantation in patients with early leukemia: First results of a randomized multicentre trial of the European Group for Blood and Marrow Transplantation. Bone Marrow Transplant 21:995–1003, 1998.

82. Vigarito AC, Azevedo WM, Marques JF et al: A randomized, prospective comparison of allogeneic bone marrow and peripheral blood progenitor cell transplantation in the treatment of haematological malignancies. Bone Marrow Transplant 22:1145–1151, 1998.

83. Blaise D, Kuentz M, Fortanier C et al: Randomized trial of bone marrow versus lenograstim-primed blood cell allogeneic transplantation in patients with early-stage leukemia: A report from the Societe Francaise de Greffe de Moelle. Clin Oncol 18:537–546, 2000.

84. Powles R, Mehta I, Kulkarni S et al: Allogeneic blood and bone-marrow stem-cell transplantation in haematological malignant diseases: A randomized trial. Lancet 355:1231–1237, 2000.

85. Bensinger WI, Martin PI, Starer B et al: Transplantation of bone marrow as compared with peripheral-blood cells from HLA-identical relatives in patients with hematologic cancers. N Engl J Med 344:175–181, 2001.

86. Champlin RE, Schmitz N, Horowitz MM et al: Blood stem cells compared with bone marrow as a source of hematopoietic cells for allogeneic transplantation. IBMTR Histocompatibility and Stem Cell Sources Working Committee and the European Group for Blood and Marrow Transplantation (EBMT). Blood 95:3702–3709, 2000.

87. Ringden O, Remberger M, Runde V et al: Peripheral blood stem cell transplantation from unrelated donors: A comparison with marrow transplantation. Blood 94:455–464, 1999.

88. Stroncek DF, Confer DL, Leitman SF: Peripheral blood progenitor cells for HPC transplants involving unrelated donors. Transfusion 40:731–741, 2000.

89. Stewart FM, Zhong S, Wuu J, Hsieh CC, Nilsson SK, Quesenberry PJ: Lymphohematopoietic engraftment in minimally myeloablated hosts. Blood 91:3681–3687, 1998.

90. Giralt S, Estey E, Albitar M et al: Engraftment of allogeneic progenitor cells with purine analog-containing chemotherapy: Harnessing graft versus leukemia without myeloablative therapy. Blood 89:4531–4536, 1997.

91. Maris MB, Sandmaier BM, Niederwieser D et al: Comparisons of donor chimerism, graft rejection, and GVHD after hematopoietic stem cell transplants from HLA matched siblings and unrelated donors using conditioning with 2 Gy TBI with and without fludarabine. Blood 96(Suppl. 1):2239, 2000.

92. Khouri IF, Keating M, Korbling M et al: Transplant lite: Induction of graft versus malignancy using fludarabine-based nonablative chemotherapy and allogeneic blood progenitor cell transplantation as treatment for lymphoid malignancies. J Clin Oncol 16:2817–2824, 1998.

93. Alcindor T, Chan G, Al-Olama A et al: Engraftment and immunologic effects of a novel less myeloablative allogeneic transplant conditioning regimen of continuous infusion pentostatin, photopheresis, and low dose TBI. Blood 96(Suppl. 1): 5160, 2000.

94. Molina A, Sahebi F, Maloney DG et al: Nonmyeloablative peripheral blood stem cell allografts following cytoreductive autotransplants for the treatment of multiple myeloma. Blood 96(Suppl. 1):2063, 2000.

95. Slavin S, Nagler A, Naparstek E et al: Nonmyeloablative stem cell transplantation and cell therapy as an alternative to conventional bone marrow transplantation with lethal cytoreduction for the treatment of malignant and nonmalignant hematologic diseases. Blood 91:756–763, 1998.

96. Champlin R, Khouri I, Kornblau S et al: Reinventing bone marrow transplantation: Nonmyeloablative preparative regimens and induction of graft-versus-malignancy effect. Oncology 13:621–628, 1999.

97. Champlin R, Khouri I, Anderlini P et al: Nonmyeloablative preparative regimens for allogeneic hematopoietic transplantation. Bone Marrow Transplant 27(Suppl. 2): S13–S22, 2001.

98. Roberts TF, Foss F, Schenkein D et al: A novel preparative regimen associated with reduced morbidity and mortality following allogeneic bone marrow transplant (abstract #3378). Blood 96(Suppl. 1):781a, 2000.

99. Kolb HJ, Schattenberg A, Goldman JM et al: Graft-vs-leukemia effect of donor lymphocyte transfusions in marrow grafted patients. Blood 86:2041–2050, 1995.

100. Collins RH Jr, Shpilberg O, Drobyski WR et al: Donor leukocyte infusions in 140 patients with relapsed malignancy after allogeneic bone marrow transplantation. J Clin Oncol 15:433–444, 1997.

101. Dazzi F, Szydlo RM, Craddock C et al: Comparison of single-dose and escalating-dose regimens of donor lymphocyte infusion for relapse after allografting for chronic myeloid leukemia. Blood 95:67–71, 2000.

102. Gugliemlo C, Arcese W, Hermans J et al: Risk assessment in patients with Ph+ chronic myelogenous leukemia in first relapse after allogeneic stem cell transplant: An EBMT retrospective analysis. Blood 95:3328–3334, 2000.

103. Carella AM, Corsetti MT, Lerma E, Cavaliere M: Autologous transplants followed by mini allografts for Hodgkin's disease and non Hodgkin's lymphoma (abstract #1752). Blood 96(Suppl. 1):407a, 2000.

104. Laughlin MJ: Umbilical cord blood for allogeneic transplantation in children and adults. Bone Marrow Transplant 27:1–6, 2001.

105. Rowe JM, Lazarus HM: Genetically haploidentical stem cell transplantation for acute leukemia. Bone Marrow Transplant 27:669–676, 2001.

106. Lazarus HM, Trehan S, Miller R, Fox RM, Creger RJ, Raaf JH: Multi-purpose silastic dual-lumen central venous catheters for both collection and transplantation of hematopoietic progenitor cells. Bone Marrow Transplant 25:779–785, 2000.

107. Meisenberg BR, Callaghan M, Sloan C, Sampson L, Miller WE, McMillan R: Complications associated with central venous catheters used for the collection of peripheral blood progenitor cells to support high-dose chemotherapy and autologous stem cell rescue. Support Care Cancer 5:223–227, 1997.

108. Madero L, Díaz MA, Benito A, Villa M, Valdivielso A: Non-tunneled catheters for the collection and transplantation of peripheral blood stem cells in children. Bone Marrow Transplant 20:53–56, 1997.

109. Madero L, Ruano D, Villa M et al: Non-tunneled catheters in children undergoing bone marrow transplantation. Bone Marrow Transplant 17:87–89, 1996.

110. Haire WD, Lieberman RP, Lund GB, Edney JA, Kessinger A, Armitage JO: Thrombotic complications of silicone rubber catheters during autologous marrow and peripheral stem cell transplantation: Prospective comparison of Hickman and Groshong catheters. Bone Marrow Transplantation 7:57–59, 1991.

111. Volkow P, Tellez O, Vazquez C et al: A single, double lumen high-flow catheter for patients undergoing peripheral blood stem cell transplantation. Experience at the National Cancer Institute in Mexico. Bone Marrow Transplant 20:779–783, 1997.

112. Conlan MG, Haire WD, Lieberman RP, Lund G, Kessinger A, Armitage JO: Catheter-related thrombosis in patients with refractory lymphoma undergoing autologous stem cell transplantation. Bone Marrow Transplant 7:235–240, 1991.

113. Uderzo C, D'Angelo P, Rizzari C et al: Central venous catheter-related complications after bone marrow transplantation in children with hematological malignancies. Bone Marrow Transplant 9:113–117, 1992.

114. Moosa HH, Julian TB, Rosenfeld CS, Shadduck RK: Complications of indwelling central venous catheters in bone marrow transplant recipients. Surg Gynecol Obstet 172:275–279, 1991.

115. Triozzi PL, Laszlo J: Optimum management of nausea and vomiting in cancer chemotherapy. Pract Drugs 34:136–149, 1987.

116. Burnette PK, Perkins J: Parenteral ondansetron for the treatment of chemotherapy- and radiation-induced nausea and vomiting. Pharmacotherapy 12:120–131, 1992.

117. Grunberg SM, Hesketh PJ: Control of chemotherapy-induced emesis. N Engl J Med 329:1790–1796, 1993.

118. Grunberg SM: Making chemotherapy easier. N Engl J Med 322:846–848, 1990.

119. Coates A, Abraham S, Kaye SB et al: On the receiving end: Patient perception of the side effects of cancer chemotherapy. Eur J Clin Oncol 19:203–208, 1983.

120. Lawrence CC, Gilbert CJ, Peters WP: Evaluation of symptom distress in a bone marrow transplant outpatient environment. Ann Pharmacother 30:941–945, 1996.

121. Lazarus HM, Bryson JC, Lemon E et al: Antiemetic efficacy and pharmacokinetic analyses of the serotonin antagonist ondansetron (GR 38032F) during multiple day cisplatin prior to autologous bone marrow transplantation. J Natl Cancer Inst 82:1776–1778, 1990.

122. Perez EA, Tiemeier T, Solberg LA: Antiemetic therapy for high-dose chemotherapy with transplantation: Report of a retrospective analysis of a 5-HT₃ regimen and literature review. Support Care Cancer 7:413–424, 1999.

123. Osowski CL, Dix SP, Lynn M et al: An open-label dose comparison study of ondansetron for the prevention of emesis associated with chemotherapy prior to bone marrow transplantation. Support Care Cancer 6:511–517, 1998.

124. Or R, Drakos P, Nagler A, Naparstek E, Kapelushnik J, Cass Y: The anti-emetic efficacy and tolerability of tropisetron in patients conditioned with high-dose chemotherapy (with and without total body irradiation) prior to bone marrow transplantation. Support Care Cancer 2:245–248, 1994.

125. Spitzer TR, Friedman CJ, Bushnell W, Frankel SR, Raschko J: Double-blind, randomized, parallel-group study on the efficacy and safety of oral granisetron and oral ondansetron in the prophylaxis of nausea and vomiting in patients receiving hyperfractionated total body irradiation. Bone Marrow Transplant 26:203–210, 2000.

126. Orchard PJ, Rogosheske J, Burns L et al: A prospective randomized trial of the anti-emetic efficacy of ondansetron and granisetron during bone marrow transplantation. Biol Blood Marrow Transplant 5:386–393, 1999.

127. Agura ED, Brown MC, Schaffer R, Donaldson G, Shen DD: Antiemetic efficacy and pharmacokinetics of intravenous ondansetron infusion during chemotherapy conditioning for bone marrow transplant. Bone Marrow Transplant 16:213–222, 1995.

128. Abbott B, Ippoliti C, Hecth D, Bruton J, Whaley B, Champlin R: Granisetron (Kytril) plus dexamethasone for antiemetic control in bone marrow transplant patients receiving highly emetogenic chemotherapy with or without total body irradiation. Bone Marrow Transplant 25:1279–1283, 2000.

129. Abbott B, Ippoliti C, Bruton J, Neumann J, Whaley R, Champlin R: Antiemetic efficacy of granisetron plus dexamethasone in bone marrow transplant patients receiving chemotherapy and total body irradiation. Bone Marrow Transplant 23:265–269, 1999.

130. Gralla RJ, Osoba D, Kris MG et al: Recommendations for the use of antiemetics: Evidence-based clinical practice guidelines. American Society of Clinical Oncology. J Clin Oncol 17:2971–2994, 1999.

131. ASHP Commission on Therapeutics Guidelines on the management of nausea and vomiting in patients receiving chemotherapy or radiation therapy or undergoing surgery. Am J Health Syst Pharm 5:6729–6764, 1999.

132. Prevention of chemotherapy- and radiotherapy-induced emesis: Results of Perugia Consensus Conference: Antiemetic Subcommittee of the Multinational Association of Supportive Care in Cancer (MASCC). Ann Oncol 9:811–819, 1998.

133. Bearman SI: The syndrome of hepatic veno-occlusive disease after transplantation. Blood 85:3005–3020, 1995.

134. McDonald GB, Hinds MS, Fisher LD et al: Veno-occlusive disease of the liver and multiorgan failure after bone marrow transplantation: A cohort study of 355 patients. Ann Intern Med 118:255–267, 1993.

135. Toh HC, McAfee SL, Sackstein R, Cox BF, Colby C, Spitzer TR: Late onset veno-occlusive disease following high-dose chemotherapy and stem cell transplantation. Bone Marrow Transplant 24:891–895, 1999.

136. Lee JL, Gooley T, Bensinger W, Schiffman K, McDonald GB: Veno-occlusive disease of the liver after busulfan, melphalan, and thiotepa conditioning therapy: Incidence, risk factors, and outcome. Biol Blood Marrow Transplant 5:306–315, 1999.

137. Bearman SI, Hinds MS, Wolford JL et al: A pilot study of continuous infusion heparin for the prevention of hepatic venoocclusive disease after bone marrow transplantation. Bone Marrow Transplant 5:407–411, 1990.

138. Marsa-Vila L, Gorin NC, Laport JP et al: Prophylactic heparin does not prevent liver veno-occlusive disease following autologous bone marrow transplantation. Eur J Haematol 47:346–354, 1991.

139. Attal M, Huguet F, Rubie H et al: Prevention of hepatic veno-occlusive disease after bone marrow transplantation by continuous infusion of low-dose heparin: A prospective, randomized trial. Blood 79:2834–2840, 1992.

140. Rosenthal J, Sender L, Secola R et al: Phase II trial of heparin prophylaxis for veno-occlusive disease of the liver in children undergoing bone marrow transplantation. Bone Marrow Transplant 18:185–191, 1996.

141. Or R, Nagler A, Shpilberg O et al: Low molecular weight heparin for the prevention of veno-occlusive disease of the liver in bone marrow transplantation patients. Transplantation 61:1067–1071, 1996.

142. Essell JH, Schroeder MT, Harman GS et al: Ursodiol prophylaxis against hepatic complications of allogeneic bone marrow transplantation. A randomized, double-blind, placebo-controlled trial. Ann Intern Med 128:975–981, 1998.

143. Ohashi K, Tanabe J, Watanabe R et al: The Japanese multicenter open randomized trial of ursodeoxycholic acid prophylaxis for hepatic veno-occlusive disease after stem cell transplantation. Am J Hematol 64:32–38, 2000.

144. Wang X, Kanel GC, DeLeve LD: Support of sinusoidal endothelial cell glutathione prevents hepatic veno-occlusive disease in the rat. Hepatol 31:428–434, 2000.

145. Ringden O, Remberger M, Lehmann S et al: N-acetylcysteine for hepatic veno-occlusive disease after allogeneic stem cell transplantation. Bone Marrow Transplant 25:993–996, 2000.

146. Hong RW, Rounds JD, Helton WS, Robinson MK, Willmore DW: Glutamine preserves liver glutathione after lethal hepatic injury. Ann Surg 215:114–119, 1992.

147. Goringe AP, Brown S, O'Callaghan U et al: Glutamine and vitamin E in the treatment of hepatic veno-occlusive disease following high-dose chemotherapy. Bone Marrow Transplant 21:829–832, 1998.

148. Brown SA, Goringe A, Fegan C et al: Parenteral glutamine protects hepatic function during bone marrow transplantation. Bone Marrow Transplant 22:281–284, 1998.

149. Bearman SI, Lee JL, Baron AE, McDonald GB: Treatment of hepatic venocclusive disease with recombinant human tissue plasminogen activator and heparin in 42 marrow transplant patients. Blood 89:1501–1506, 1998.

150. Schriber J, Milk B, Shaw D et al: Tissue plasminogen activator (tPA) as therapy for hepatotoxicity following bone marrow transplantation. Bone Marrow Transplant 24:1311–1314, 1999.

151. Morris JD, Harris RE, Hashmi R et al: Antithrombin-III for the treatment of chemotherapy-induced organ dysfunction following bone marrow transplantation. Bone Marrow Transplant 20:871–878, 1997.

152. Mertens R, Brost H, Granzen B, Nowak-Gottl U: Antithrombin treatment of severe hepatic veno-occlusive disease in children with cancer. Eur J Pediatr 158(Suppl. 3):S154–S158, 1999.

153. Richardson PG, Elias AD, Krishnan A et al: Treatment of severe veno-occlusive disease with defibrotide: Compassionate use results in efficacy without significant toxicity in a high risk population. Blood 92:737–744, 1998.

154. Richardson PG, Murakami C, Warren DL et al: Multi-institutional emergency use of defibrotide in 75 patients post SCT with severe VOD and multisystem organ failure: Response without significant toxicity in a high risk population (abstract #2510). Blood 96(Suppl. 1):585a, 2000.

155. Fried MW, Connaghan DG, Sharma S et al: Transjugular intrahepatic portosystemic shunt for the management of severe venoocclusive disease following bone marrow transplantation. Hepatol 24:588–591, 1996.

156. de la Rubia J, Carral A, Montes H, Urquijo JJ, Sanz GF, Sanz MA: Successful treatment of hepatic veno-occlusive disease in a peripheral blood progenitor cell transplant patient with a transjugular intrahepatic portosystemic stent-shunt (TIPS). Haematologica 81:536–539, 1996.

157. Smith FO, Johnson MS, Scherer LR et al: Transjugular intrahepatic portosystemic shunting (TIPS) for treatment of severe hepatic veno-occlusive disease. Bone Marrow Transplant 18:643–646, 1996.

158. Azoulay D, Castaing D, Lemoine A, Hargreaves GM, Bismuth H: Transjugular intrahepatic portosystemic shunt (TIPS) for severe veno-occlusive disease of the liver following bone marrow transplantation. Bone Marrow Transplant 25:987–992, 2000.

159. Miller CB, Lazarus HM: Erythropoietin in stem cell transplantation. Bone Marrow Transplant, 27:1011–1016, 2001.

160. Macdougall IC: Novel erythropoiesis stimulating protein. Semin Nephrol 203:375–381, 2000.

161. Glaspy J, Tchekmedyian S, Jadeja J et al: Randomized, active-controlled, phase I/II dose-escalation study of ARANESP™ in solid tumor patients (abstract #1278). Blood 96:297a, 2000.

162. Kotasek D, Berg R, Poulsen E, Colowick A: Randomized, double-blind, placebo controlled phase I/II dose finding study of ARANESP™ administered once every three weeks in solid tumor patients (abstract #1268). Blood 96:294a, 2000.

163. Beutler E: Platelet transfusions: The 20,000/µL trigger. Blood 81:1411–1413, 1993.

164. Wandt H, Frank M, Ehninger G et al: Safety and cost effectiveness of a 10×10^9/µL trigger for prophylactic platelet transfusions compared with the traditional 20×10^9/µL trigger: A prospective comparative trial in 105 patients with acute myeloid leukemia. Blood 91:3101–3106, 1998.

165. Rinder HM, Arbini AA, Snyder EL: Optimal dosing and triggers for prophylactic use of platelet transfusions. Curr Opin Hematol 6:437–441, 1999.

166. Lawrence JB, Yomtovian RA, Hammons T et al: Lowering the prophylactic platelet transfusion threshold: A prospective analysis. Leuk Lymphoma 41:67–76, 2001.

167. Schiffer CA, Anderson KC, Bennett CL et al: Platelet transfusion for patients with cancer: Clinical practice guidelines of the American Cancer Society of Clinical Oncology. J Clin Oncol 19:1519–1538, 2001.

168. Bernstein SH, Nademanee AP, Vose JM et al: A multicenter study of platelet recovery and utilization in patients after myeloablative therapy and hematopoietic stem cell transplantation. Blood 91:3509–3517, 1998.

169. Nemo S, Swan V, Enger C et al: Acute bleeding after bone marrow transplantation (BMT): Incidence and effect on survival—a quantitative analysis in 1402 patients. Blood 91:1469–1477, 1998.

170. Hubel K, Dale DC, Liles WC: Granulocyte transfusion therapy: Update on potential clinical applications. Curr Opin Hematol 8:161–164, 2001.

171. Price TH: The current prospects for neutrophil transfusions for the treatment of granulocytopenic infected patients. Transfus Med Rev 14:2–11, 2000.

172. Lee JJ, Chung IJ, Park MR et al: Clinical efficacy of granulocyte transfusion therapy in patients with neutropenia-related infections. Leukemia 15:203–207, 2001.

173. Schiffer CA: Granulocyte transfusion therapy. Curr Opin Hematol 6:3–7, 1999.

174. Price TH, Bowden RA, Boeckh M et al: Phase I/II trial of neutrophil transfusions from donors stimulated with G-CSF and dexamethasone for treatment of patients with infections in hematopoietic stem cell transplantation. Blood 95:3302–3309, 2000.

175. Adkins DR, Goodnough LT, Shenoy S et al: Effect of leukocyte compatibility on neutrophil increment after transfusion of granulocyte colony-stimulating factor-mobilized prophylactic granulocyte transfusions and on clinical outcomes after stem cell transplantation. Blood 95:3605–3612, 2000.

176. Holmberg LA, Boeckh M, Hooper H et al: Increased incidence of cytomegalovirus disease after autologous CD34-selected peripheral blood stem cell transplantation. Blood 94:4029–4035, 1999.

177. Fassas AB, Bolanos-Meade J, Buddharaju LN et al: Cytomegalovirus infection and non-neutropenic fever after autologous stem cell transplantation: High rates of reactivation in patients with multiple myeloma and lymphoma. Br J Haematol 112:237–241, 2001.

178. Tsinontides AC, Bechtel TP: Cytomegalovirus prophylaxis and treatment following bone marrow transplantation. Ann Pharmacother 30:1277–1290, 1996.

179. Guglielmo BJ, Wong-Beringer A, Linker CA: Immune globulin therapy in allogeneic bone marrow transplant: A critical review. Bone Marrow Transplant 13:499–510, 1994.

180. Siadak MF, Kopecky K, Sullivan KM: Reduction in transplant-related complications in patients given intravenous immune globulin after allogeneic marrow transplantation. Clin Exp Immunol 97(Suppl. 1):53–57, 1994.

181. Petersen FB, Bowden RA, Thornquist M et al: The effect of prophylactic intravenous immune globulin on the incidence of septicemia in marrow transplant recipients. Bone Marrow Transplant 2:141–147, 1987.

182. Emanuel D, Cunningham I, Jules-Elysee K et al: Cytomegalovirus pneumonia after bone marrow transplantation successfully treated with the combination of ganciclovir and high-dose intravenous immune globulin. Ann Intern Med 109:777–782, 1988.

183. Reed EC, Bowden RA, Dandliker PS, Lilleby KE, Meyers JD: Treatment of cytomegalovirus pneumonia with ganciclovir and intravenous cytomegalovirus immunoglobulin in patients with bone marrow transplants. Ann Intern Med 109:783–788, 1988.

184. Bensinger WI, Buckner CD, Thomas ED, Clift RA: ABO-incompatible marrow transplants. Transplant 33:427–429, 1982.

185. Lasky LC, Warkentin PI, Kersey JH et al: Hemotherapy in patients undergoing blood group incompatible bone marrow transplantation. Transfusion 23:277–285, 1983.

186. Hershko C, Gale RP, Ho W, Fitchen J: ABH antigens and bone marrow transplantation. Br J Haematol 44:65–73, 1980.

187. Gale RP, Feig S, Ho W et al: ABO blood group system and bone marrow transplantation. Blood 50:185–194, 1977.

188. Buckner CD, Clift RA, Sanders JE et al: ABO-incompatible marrow transplants. Transplantation 26:233–238, 1978.

189. Franchini M, de Gironcoli M, Gandini G et al: Transmission of an anti-RhD alloantibody from donor to recipient after ABO-incompatible BMT. Bone Marrow Transplant 21:1071–1073, 1998.

190. Leo A, Mytilineos J, Voso MT et al: Passenger lymphocyte syndrome with severe hemolytic anemia due to an anti-Jk[a] after allogeneic PBPC transplantation. Transfusion 40:632–636, 2000.

191. Rodriquez JM, Carmona M, Noguerol P et al: A fully automated method for mononuclear bone marrow cell concentration. J Clin Apheresis 7:101–109, 1992.

192. Davis JM, Schepers KG, Eby LL, Noga SJ: Comparison of progenitor cell concentration techniques: Continuous flow separation versus density-gradient isolation. J Hematother 2:315–320, 1993.

193. Zingsem J, Zeiler T, Zimmermann R et al: Bone marrow processing with the Fresenius AS 104:Initial results. J Hematother 1:273–278, 1992.

194. Dinsmore RE, Reich LM, Kapoor N et al: ABH incompatible bone marrow transplantation: Removal of erythrocytes by starch sedimentation. Br J Haematol 54:441–449, 1983.

195. Bensinger WI, Baker DA, Buckner CD et al: Immunoadsorption for removal of A and B blood-group antibodies. N Engl J Med 304:160–162, 1981.

196. Marmont AM, Damasio EE, Bacigalupo A et al: A to O bone marrow transplantation in severe aplastic anaemia: Dynamics of blood group conversion and demonstration of early dyserythropoiesis in the engrafted marrow. Br J Haematol 36:511–518, 1977.

197. Worel N, Greinix HT, Schneider B et al: Regeneration of erythropoiesis after related- and unrelated-donor BMT or peripheral blood HPC transplantation: A major ABO mismatch means problems. Transfusion 40:543–550, 2000.

198. Benjamin RJ, Connors JM, McGurk S et al: Prolonged erythroid aplasia after major ABO-mismatched transplantation for chronic myelogenous leukemia. Biol Blood Marrow Transplant 4:151–156, 1998.

199. Bar BMAM, Van Dijk BA, Schattenberg A et al: Erythrocyte repopulation after major ABO incompatible transplantation with lymphocyte-depleted bone marrow. Bone Marrow Transplant 16:793–799, 1995.

200. Wernet D, Mayer G: Isoagglutinins following ABO-incompatible bone marrow transplantation. Vox Sang 62:176–179, 1992.

201. Bar BM, Santos GW, Donnenberg AD: Reconstitution of antibody response after allogeneic bone marrow transplantation: Effect of lymphocyte depletion by counterflow centrifugal elutriation on the expression of hemagglutinins. Blood 76:1410–1418, 1990.

202. Hows J, Beddow K, Gordon-Smith E et al: Donor-derived red blood cell antibodies and immune hemolysis after allogeneic bone marrow transplantation. Blood 67:177–181, 1986.

203. Hazlehurst GRP, Brenner MK, Wimperis JZ, Knowles SM, Prentice HJ: Haemolysis after T-cell depleted bone marrow transplantation involving minor ABO incompatibility. Scand J Haematol 37:1–3, 1986.

204. Gajewski JL, Petz LD, Calhoun L et al: Hemolysis of transfused group O red blood cells in minor ABO-incompatible unrelated-donor bone marrow transplants in patients receiving cyclosporine without posttransplant methotrexate. Blood 79:3076–3085, 1992.

205. Greeno EW, Perry EH, Ilstrup SJ, Weisdorf DJ: Exchange transfusion the hard way: Massive hemolysis following transplantation of bone marrow with minor ABO incompatibility. Transfusion 36:71–74, 1996.

206. Oziel-Taieb S, Faucher-Barbey C, Chabannon C et al: Early and fatal immune haemolysis after so-called "minor" ABO-incompatible peripheral blood stem cell allotransplantation. Bone Marrow Transplant 19:1155–1156, 1997.

207. Toren A, Dacosta Y, Manny N, Varadi G, Or R, Nagler A: Passenger B-lymphocyte-induced severe hemolytic disease after allogeneic peripheral blood stem cell transplantation (letter). Blood 87:843–844, 1996.

208. Bornhauser M, Ordemann R, Paaz U et al: Rapid engraftment after allogeneic ABO-incompatible peripheral blood stem cell transplantation complicated by severe hemolysis. Bone Marrow Transplant 19:295–297, 1997.

209. Laurencet FM, Samii K, Bressoud A et al: Massive delayed hemolysis following peripheral blood stem cell transplantation with minor ABO incompatibility. Hematol Cell Ther 39:159–162, 1997.

210. Salmon JP, Michaux S, Hermanne JP et al: Delayed massive immune hemolysis mediated by minor ABO incompatibility after allogeneic peripheral blood progenitor cell transplantation. Transfusion 39:824–827, 1999.

211. Hughes WT, Armstrong D, Bodey GP et al: Guidelines for the use of antimicrobial agents in neutropenic patients with unexplained fever. J Infect Dis 161:381–396, 1990.

212. Bergman OJ: Oral infections and septicemia in immunocompromised patients with hematologic malignancies. J Clin Microbiol 26:2105–2109, 1988.

213. Bellm LA, Epstein JB, Rose-Ped A et al: Patient reports of complications of bone marrow transplantation. Support Care Cancer 8:33–39, 2000.

214. Sonis ST, Oster G, Fuchs H et al: Oral mucositis and the clinical and economic outcomes of hematopoietic stem-cell transplantation. J Clin Oncol 19:2201–2205, 2001.

215. Ruescher TJ, Sodeifi A, Scrivani SJ et al: The impact of mucositis on a-hemolytic streptococcal infection in patients undergoing autologous bone marrow transplantation for hematological malignancies. Cancer 82:2275–2281, 1998.

216. De Conno F, Ripamonti C, Sbanatto A et al: Oral complications in patients with advanced cancer. J Palliat Care 5:7–15, 1989.

217. Rappaport AP, Watelet LF, Linder T et al: Analysis of factors that correlate with mucositis in recipients of autologous and allogeneic stem-cell transplants. J Clin Oncol 17:2446–2453, 1999.

218. Dumontet C, Sonnet A, Bastion Y, Salles G, Espinouse D, Coiffier B: Prevention of high dose L-PAM-induced mucositis by cryotherapy. Bone Marrow Transplant 3:492–494, 1994.

219. Meloni G, Capria S, Proia A, Trisolini SM, Mandelli F: Ice pops to prevent melphalan-induced stomatitis. Lancet 347:1691–1692, 1996.

220. Cascinu S, Fedeli A, Fedeli SL, Catalano G: Oral cooling (cryotherapy), an effective treatment for the prevention of 5-fluorouracil-induced stomatitis. Eur J Cancer B Oral Oncol 30B:234–236, 1994.

221. Ahmed T, Engelking C, Szalyga J et al: Propantheline prevention of mucositis from etoposide. Bone Marrow Transplant 12:131–132, 1993.

222. DeWalt EM, Haines AK: The effects of specified stressors on health oral mucosa. Nurs Res 18:22–27, 1969.

223. Feber T: Management of mucositis in oral radiation. Clin Oncol 8:106–111, 1996.

224. Rahn R, Adamietz IA, Boettcher HD et al: Povidone-iodine to prevent mucositis in patients during antineoplastic radiochemotherapy. Dermatology 195(Suppl. 2):57–61, 1997.

225. Ferretti GA, Ash RC, Brown AT et al: Control of oral mucositis and candidiasis in marrow transplant patients. Bone Marrow Transplant 3:483–493, 1988.

226. Lira-Puerto V, Silva A, Martinez R et al: Grade 3–4 stomatitis treated with local GM-CSF. Ann Oncol 5(Suppl. 8):207–208, 1994.

227. van der Lelie H, Thomas BL, van Oers RH et al: Effect of locally applied GM-CSF on oral mucositis after stem cell transplantation: A prospective placebo-controlled double-blind study. Ann Hematol 80:150–154, 2001.

228. Dorr W, Noack R, Spekl K, Farrell CL: Modification of oral mucositis by keratinocyte growth factor: Single radiation exposure. Int J Radiat Biol 77:341–347, 2001.

229. Stiff P: Mucositis associated with stem cell transplantation: Current status and innovative approaches to management. Bone Marrow Transplant 27(Suppl. 2): S3–S11, 2001.

230. Durrant S, Pico JL, Schultz N et al: A phase I study of recombinant keratinocyte growth factor (rHuKGF) in lymphoma patients receiving high-dose chemotherapy (HDC) with autologous peripheral blood progenitor cell transplantation (autoPBPCT) (abstract #3130). Blood 94(Suppl. 1):708a, 1999.

231. Spielberger RT, Stiff P, Emmanouilides C et al: Efficacy of recombinant human keratinocyte growth factor (rHuKGF) in reducing mucositis in patients with hematologic malignancies undergoing autologous peripheral blood progenitor cell transplantation (auto-PBPCT) after radiation-based conditioning—results of a phase 2 trial (abstract #25). Proc Am Soc Clin Oncol 20:7a, 2001.

232. Levine LA, Richie JP: Urological complications of cyclophosphamide. J Urol 141:1063–1069, 1989.

233. Londergan TA, Walzak MP: Hemorrhagic cystitis due to adenovirus infection following bone marrow transplantation. J Urol 151:1013–1014, 1994.

234. Spach DH, Bauwens JE, Myerson D, Mustafa MM, Bowden RA: Cytomegalovirus-induced hemorrhagic cystitis following bone marrow transplantation. Clin Infect Dis 16:142–144, 1993.

235. Ambinder RF, Burns W, Forman M et al: Hemorrhagic cystitis associated with adenovirus infection in bone marrow transplantation. Arch Intern Med 146:1400–1401, 1986.

236. Arthur RR, Shah KV, Baust SJ, Santos GW, Saral R: Association of BK viruria with hemorrhagic cystitis in recipients of bone marrow transplants. N Engl J Med 315:230–234, 1986.

237. Kawakami M, Ueda S, Maeda T et al: Vidarabine therapy for virus-associated cystitis after allogeneic bone marrow transplantation. Bone Marrow Transplant 20:485–490, 1997.

238. Sencer SF, Haake RJ, Weisdorf DJ: Hemorrhagic cystitis after bone marrow transplantation. Risk factors and complications. Transplantation 56:875, 1993.

239. Turkeri LN, Lum LG, Uberti JP et al: Prevention of hemorrhagic cystitis following allogeneic bone marrow transplant preparative regimens with cyclophosphamide and busulfan: Role of continuous bladder irrigation. J Urol 153:637–640, 1995.

240. Atkinson K, Biggs JC, Golovsky SD et al: Bladder irrigation does not prevent haemorrhagic cystitis in bone marrow transplant recipients. Bone Marrow Transplant 7:351–354, 1991.

241. Brock N, Pohl J: The development of mesna for regional detoxification. Cancer Treat Rev 10:33–43, 1983.

242. Vose, JM, Reed EC, Pippert GC et al: Mesna compared with continuous bladder irrigation as uroprotection during high-dose chemotherapy and transplantation: A randomized trial. J Clin Oncol 11:1306–1310, 1993.

243. Shepherd JD, Pringle LE, Barnett MJ, Klingemann HG, Reece DE, Phillips GL: Mesna versus hyperhydration for the prevention of cyclophosphamide-induced hemorrhagic cystitis in bone marrow transplantation. J Clin Oncol 9:2016–2020, 1991.

244. Rosenzweig MQ, Schaefer PM, Rosenfeld CS: Prevention of transplant-related hemorrhagic cystitis using bladder irrigation with sorbitol. Bone Marrow Transplant 14:491–492, 1994.

245. DeVries CR, Freiha FS: Hemorrhagic cystitis: A review. J Urol 143:1–9, 1990.

246. Arrizabalaga M, Extramiana J, Parra JL et al: Treatment of massive haematuria with aluminous salts. J Urol 60:223–226, 1987.

247. Kennedy C, Snell ME, Witherow RO: Use of alum to control intractable visical haemorrhage. Br J Urol 56:673–675, 1984.

248. Mukamel E, Lupu A, deKernion JB: Alum irrigation for severe bladder hemorrhage. J Urol 135:784–785, 1986.

249. Aroney RS, Dalley DN, Levi JA: Haemorrhagic cystitis treated with epsilon-aminocaproic acid. Med J Aust 2:92, 1980.

250. Ippoliti C, Przepiorka D, Mehra R et al: Intravesicular carboprost for the treatment of hemorrhagic cystitis after marrow transplantation. Urology 46:811–815, 1995.

251. Levine LA, Jarrard DF: Treatmentt of cyclophosphamide-induced hemorrhagic cystitis with intravesical carboprost tromethamine. J Urol 149:719–723, 1993.

252. Trigg ME, O'Reilly J, Rumelhart S et al: Prostaglandin E1 bladder instillations to control severe hemorrhagic cystitis. J Urol 143:92–94, 1990.

253. Laslo D, Bosi A, Guidin S et al: Prostaglandin E2 bladder irrigation for the treatment of hemorrhagic cystitis after bone marrow transplantation. Haematology 80:421–425, 1995.

254. Miller J, Burfield GD, Moretti KL: Oral conjugated estrogen therapy for treatment of hemorragic cystitis. J Urol 151:1348–1350, 1994.

255. Liu YK, Flaharty JI, Steinbock GE et al: Treatment of radiation or cyclophosphamide induced hemorrhagic cystitis using conjugated estrogen. J Urol 144:41–43, 1990.

256. Sarnak MJ, Long J, King AJ: Intravesicular formaldehyde instillation and renal complications. Clin Nephrol 51:122–125, 1999.

257. Donahue LA, Frank IN: Intravesicular formalin for hemorrhagic cystitis: Analysis of therapy. J Urol 141:809–812, 1989.

258. Vincente J, Rios G, Caffaratti J: Intravesical formalin for the treatment of massive hemorrhagic cystitis: Retrospective review of 25 cases. Eur Urol 18:204–206, 1990.

259. Kumar APM, Wren EL, Jayalakshmamma B et al: Silver nitrate irrigation to control bladder hemorrhage in children receiving cancer chemotherapy. J Urol 116:86–96, 1976.

260. Vela-Ojeda J, Tripp-Villanueva F, Sanchez-Cortes E et al: Intravesical rhGM-CSF for the treatment of late onset hemorrhagic cystitis after bone marrow transplant. Bone Marrow Transplant 24:1307–1310, 1999.

261. Garderet L, Bittencourt H, Sebe P et al: Cystectomy for severe hemorrhagic cystitis in allogeneic stem cell transplant recipients. Transplantation 70:1807–1811, 2000.

262. Sebe P, Garderet L, Traxer O, Nouri M, Gluckman E, Gattegno B: Subtotal cystectomy with ileocystoplasty for severe hemorrhagic cystitis after bone marrow transplantation. Urology 57:168, 2001.

263. Baronciani D, Angelucci E, Erer B et al: Suprapubic cystotomy as treatment for severe hemorrhagic cystitis after bone marrow transplantation. Bone Marrow Transplant 16:267–270, 1995.

264. Schmitz N, Linch DC, Dreger P et al: Randomised trial of filgrastim-mobilised peripheral blood progenitor cell transplantation versus autologous bone-marrow transplantation in lymphoma patients. Lancet 347:353–357, 1996.

265. Bensinger W, Appelbaum F, Rowley S et al: Factors that influence collection and engraftment of autologous peripheral-blood stem cells. J Clin Oncol 13:2547–2555, 1995.

266. Tricot G, Jagannath S, Versole D et al: Peripheral blood stem cell transplants for multiple myeloma: Identification of favorable outcome variables for rapid engraftment in 225 patients. Blood 85:588–596, 1995.

267. Weaver CH, Hazelton B, Birch R et al: An analysis of engraftment kinetics as a function of the CD34 content of peripheral blood progenitor cell collections in 692 patients after the administration of myeloablative chemotherapy. Blood 86:3961–3969, 1995.

268. Kiss JE, Rybka WB, Winkelstein A et al: Relationship of CD34+ cell dose to early and late hematopoiesis following autologous peripheral blood stem cell transplantation. Bone Marrow Transplant 19:303–310, 1997.

269. Shpall EJ, Wheeler CA, Turner SA et al: A randomized phase 3 study of peripheral blood progenitor cell mobilization by stem cell factor and filgrastim in high-risk breast cancer patients. Blood 93:2491–2501, 1998.

270. Schiller G, Vescio R, Freytes C et al: Transplantation of CD34+ peripheral blood progenitor cells after high-dose chemotherapy for patients with advanced multiple myeloma. Blood 86:390–397, 1996.

271. Bender JG, To LB, Williams S et al: Defining a therapeutic dose of peripheral blood stem cells. J Hematother 1:329–341, 1992.

272. Schwella N, Beyer J, Schwaner I et al: Impact of preleukapheresis cell counts on collection results and correlation of progenitor-cell dose with engraftment after high-dose chemotherapy in patients with germ cell cancer. J Clin Oncol 14:1114–1121, 1996.

273. Ketterer N, Salles G, Raba N et al: High CD34+ cell counts decrease hematologic toxicity of autologous peripheral blood progenitor cell transplantation. Blood 91:3148–3155, 1998.

274. Stiff PJ: Management strategies for the hard-to-mobilize patient. Bone Marrow Transplant 23(Suppl. 2):S29–S33, 1999.

275. Watts MJ, Sullivan AM, Leverett D et al: Back-up bone marrow is frequently ineffective in patients with poor peripheral-blood stem-cell mobilization. J Clin Oncol 16:1554–1560, 1998.

276. Demirer T, Buckner CD, Bensinger WI: Optimization of peripheral blood stem cell mobilization. Stem Cells 14:106–116, 1996.

277. Haas R, Möhle R, Frühauf S et al: Patient characteristics associated with successful mobilizing and autografting of peripheral blood progenitor cells in malignant lymphoma. Blood 83:3787–3794, 1994.

278. Moskowitz CH, Stiff P, Gordon MS et al: Recombinant methionyl human stem cell factor and filgrastim for peripheral blood progenitor cell mobilization and transplantation in non-Hodgkin's lymphoma patients—results of a phase I/II trial. Blood 89:3136–3147, 1997.

279. Morton J, Morton A, Bird R et al: Predictors for optimal mobilization and subsequent engraftment of peripheral blood progenitor cells following intermediate dose cyclophosphamide and G-CSF. Leuk Res 21:21–27, 1997.

280. Neben S, Hemman S, Montgomery M et al: Hematopoietic stem cell deficit of transplanted bone marrow previously exposed to cytotoxic agents. Exp Hematol 21:156–162, 1993.

281. Perry AR, Watts MJ, Peniket AJ et al: Progenitor cell yields are frequently poor in patients with histologically indolent lymphomas especially when mobilized within 6 months of previous chemotherapy. Bone Marrow Transplant 21:1201–1205, 1998.

282. Drake M, Ranaghan L, Morris TCM et al: Analysis of the effect of prior therapy on progenitor cell yield: Use of a chemotherapy scoring system. Br J Haematol 98:745–749, 1997.

283. Donohue J, Homge M, Kernan NA: Characterization of cells emerging at the time of graft failure after bone marrow transplantation from an unrelated marrow donor. Blood 82:1023–1029, 1993.

284. Stucki A, Leisenring W, Sandmaier BM et al: Decreased rejection and improved survival of first and second marrow transplants for severe aplastic anemia (a 26-year retrospective analysis). Blood 92:2742–2749, 1998.

285. Martin PJ, Akatsuka Y, Hahne M, Sale G: Involvement of donor T-cell cytotoxic effector mechanisms in preventing allogeneic marrow graft rejection. Blood 92:2177–2181, 1998.

286. Anasetti C, Amos D, Beatty PG et al: Effect of HLA compatibility on engraftment of bone marrow transplants in patients with leukemia or lymphoma. N Engl J Med, 320(4):197–204, 1989.

287. Bunjes D, Wiesneth M, Hertenstein B et al: Graft failure after T cell-depleted bone marrow transplantation: Clinical and immunological characteristics and response to immunosuppressive therapy. Bone Marrow Transplant 6:309–314, 1990.

288. Lamb LS, Szafer F, Henslee-Downey PJ et al: Characterization of acute bone marrow graft rejection in T cell-depleted, partially mismatched related donor bone marrow transplantation. Exp Hematol 23:1595–1600, 1995.

289. Lienert-Weidenbach K, Valiante NM, Brown C et al: Mismatches for two major and one minor histocompatibility antigen correlate with a patient's rejection of a bone marrow graft from a serologically HLA-identical sibling. Biol Blood Marrow Transplant 3:255–260, 1997.

290. Carella AM, Champlin R, Slavin S et al: Mini-allografts: Ongoing trials in humans. Bone Marrow Transplant 25:345–350, 2000.

291. Steffens HP, Podlech J, Kurz S et al: Cytomegalovirus inhibits the engraftment of donor bone marrow cells by down regulation of hemopoietin gene expression in recipient stroma. J Virol 2:5006–5015, 1998.

292. Johnston RE, Geretti AM, Prentice HG et al: HV-6-related secondary graft failure following allogeneic bone marrow transplantation. Br J Haematol 105:1041–1043, 1999.

293. Guardiola P, Kuentz M, Garban F et al: Second early allogeneic stem cell transplantations for graft failure in acute leukaemia, chronic myeloid leukaemia and aplastic anaemia. French Society of Bone Marrow Transplantation. Br J Haematol 111:292–302, 2000.

294. Lazarus HM, Vogelsang GB, Rowe JM: Prevention and treatment of acute graft-versus-host disease: The old and the new. A report from the Eastern Cooperative Oncology Group (ECOG). Bone Marrow Transplant 19:577–600, 1997.

295. Armitage JO: Bone marrow transplantation. N Engl J Med 330:827–838, 1994.

296. Beatty PG, Clift RA, Mickelson EM et al: Marrow transplantation from related donors other than HLA-identical siblings. N Engl J Med 313:765–771, 1985.

297. Chao NJ: Graft-vs-host disease: The viewpoint from the donor T cell. Biol Blood Marrow Transplant 3:1–10, 1997.

298. Goulmy E, Schipper R, Pool J et al: Mismatches of minor histocompatibility antigens between HLA-identical donors and recipients and the development of graft-vs-host disease after bone marrow transplantation. N Engl J Med 334:281–285, 1996.

299. Ferrara JLM, Levy R, Chao NJ: Pathophysiologic mechanisms of acute graft-vs-host disease. Biol Blood Marrow Transplant 5:347–356, 1999.

300. Beelen DW, Elmaagacli A, Müller KD, Hirche H, Schaefer UW: Influence of intestinal bacterial decontamination using metronidazole and ciprofloxacin or ciprofloxacin alone on the development of acute graft-vs-host disease after marrow transplantation in patients with hematologic malignancies: Final results and long-term follow-up of an open-label prospective randomized trial. Blood 93:3267–3275, 1999.

301. Antin JH, Ferrara JL: Cytokine dysregulation and acute graft-vs-host disease. Blood 80:2964–2968, 1994.

302. Hill GR, Krenger W, Ferrara JL: The role of cytokines in acute graft-versus-host disease. Cytokines Cell Mol Ther 3:257–266, 1997.

303. Norton J, Sloane JP: ICAM-1 expression on epidermal keratinocytes in cutaneous graft-vs-host disease. Transplantation 51:1203–1206, 1991.

304. Barrett AJ, Mavroudis D, Tisdale J et al: T cell-depleted bone marrow transplantation and delayed T cell add-back to control acute GVHD and conserve a graft-vs-leukemia effect. Bone Marrow Transplant 21:543–551, 1998.

305. Rus V, Svetic A, Nguyen P, Gause WC, Via CS: Kinetics of Th1 and Th2 cytokine production during the early course of acute and chronic murine graft-vs-host disease: Regulatory role of donor CD8+ T cells. J Immunol 155:2396–2406, 1995.

306. Schultze J, Nadler LM, Gribben JG: B7-mediated costimulation and the immune response. Blood Rev 10:111–127, 1996.

307. Ferrara JL, Guillen FJ, van Dijken PJ, Marion A, Murphy GF, Burakoff SJ: Evidence that large granular lymphocytes of donor origin mediate acute graft-vs-host disease. Transplantation 47:50–54, 1989.

308. Filep JG, Baron C, Lachance S, Perreault C, Chan JS: Involvement of nitric oxide in target-cell lysis and DNA fragmentation induced by murine natural killer cells. Blood 87:5136–5143, 1996.

309. Sullivan KM, Deeg HJ, Sanders J et al: Hyperacute graft-vs-host disease in patients not given immunosuppression after allogeneic marrow transplantation. Blood 67:1172–1175, 1986.

310. Weisdorf D, Hakke R, Blazar B et al: Risk factors for acute graft-vs-host disease in histocompatible donor bone marrow transplantation. Transplantation 51:1197–1203, 1991.

311. Rubinstein P, Carrier C, Scaradavou A et al: Outcomes among 562 recipients of placental-blood transplants from unrelated donors. N Engl J Med 339:1565–1577, 1998.

312. Goker H, Haznedaroglu IC, Chao NJ: Acute graft-versus-host disease: Pathobiology and management. Exp Hematol 29:259–277, 2001.

313. Margolis J, Borrello I, Flinn IW: New approaches to treating malignancies with stem cell transplantation. Semin Oncol 27:524–530, 2000.

314. Dazzi F, Goldman J: Donor lymphocyte infusions. Curr Opin Hematol 6:394–399, 1999.

315. Przepiorka D, Weisdorf D, Martin P et al: 1994 Consensus Conference on Acute GVHD Grading. Bone Marrow Transplant 15:825–828, 1995.

316. Glucksberg H, Storb R, Fefer A et al: Clinical manifestations of graft-versus host disease in human recipients of marrow from HLA-matched sibling donors. Transplantation 18:295–304, 1974.

317. Thomas ED, Storb R, Clift RA et al: Bone-marrow transplantation (second of two parts). N Engl J Med 292:895–902, 1975.

318. Martin P, Nash R, Sanders J et al: Reproducibility in retrospective grading of acute graft-versus-host disease after allogeneic marrow transplantation. Bone Marrow Transplant 21:273–279, 1998.

319. Rowlings PA, Przepiorka D, Klein JP et al: IBMTR Severity Index for grading acute graft-versus-host disease: Retrospective comparison with Glucksberg grade. Br J Haematol 97:855–864, 1997.

320. Flowers ME, Kansu E, Sullivan KM: Pathophysiology and treatment of graft-vs-host disease. Hematol Oncol Clin North Am 13:1091–1112, 1999.

321. Gratwohl A, Hermans J, Apperly J et al: Acute graft-versus-host disease: Grade and outcome in patients with chronic myelogenous leukemia. Working Party Chronic Leukemia of the European Group for Blood and Marrow Transplantation. Blood 86:813–818, 1995.

322. Simpson D: Review. Drug therapy for acute graft-versus-host disease prophylaxis. J Hematother Stem Cell Res 9:317–325, 2000.

323. Storb R, Deeg HJ, Whitehead J et al: Methotrexate and cyclosporine compared with cyclosporine alone for prophylaxis of acute graft-vs-host disease after marrow transplantation for leukemia. N Engl J Med 314:729–735, 1986.

324. Ratanatharathorn V, Nash RA, Przepiorka D et al: Phase III study comparing methotrexate and tacrolimus (prograf, FK506) with methotrexate and cyclosporine for graft-vs-host disease prophylaxis after HLA-identical sibling bone marrow transplantation. Blood 92:2303–2314, 1998.

325. Przepiorka D, Ippoliti C, Khouri I et al: Tacrolimus and minidose methotrexate for prevention of acute graft-versus-host disease after matched unrelated donor marrow transplantation. Blood 88:4383–4389, 1996.

326. Przepiorka D, Khouri I, Ippoliti C et al: Tacrolimus and minidose methotrexate for prevention of acute graft versus host disease after HLA-mismatched marrow or blood stem cell transplantation. Bone Marrow Transplant 25:763–768, 1999.

327. Hale G, Zhang MJ, Bunjes D et al: Improving the outcome of bone marrow transplantation by using CD52 monoclonal antibodies to prevent graft-vs-host disease and graft rejection. Blood 92:4581–4590, 1998.

328. Soiffer RJ, Weller E, Alyea EP et al: CD6+ donor marrow T-cell depletion as the sole form of graft-vs-host disease prophylaxis in patients undergoing allogeneic bone marrow transplant from unrelated donors. J Clin Oncol 19:1152–1159, 2001.

329. Young JW, Papadopoulos EB, Cunningham I et al: T-cell-depleted allogeneic bone marrow transplantation in adults with acute non-lymphocytic leukemia in first remission. Blood 79:3380–3387, 1992.

330. Drobyski WR, Hessner MJ, Klein JP, Kabler-Babbitt C, Vesole DH, Keever-Taylor CA: T-cell depletion plus salvage immunotherapy with donor leukocyte infusions as a strategy to treat chronic-phase chronic myelogenous leukemia patients undergoing HLA-identical sibling marrow transplantation. Blood 94:434–441, 1999.

331. Shlomchik WD, Couzens MS, Tang CB et al: Prevention of graft vs host disease by inactivation of host antigen-presenting cells. Science 285:412–415, 1999.

332. Guinan EC, Boussiotis VA, Neuberg D et al: Transplantation of anergic histoincompatible bone marrow allografts. N Engl J Med 340:1704–1717, 1999.

333. Seung E, Iwakoshi N, Woda BA et al: Allogeneic hematopoietic chimerism in mice treated with sublethal myeloablation and anti-CD154 antibody: Absence of graft-vs-host disease, induction of skin allograft tolerance, and prevention of recurrent autoimmunity in islet-allografted NOD/Lt mice. Blood 95:2175–2182, 2000.

334. Hings IM, Filipovich AH, Miller WJ et al: Prednisone therapy for acute graft-versus-host disease: Short- versus long-term treatment. A prospective randomized trial. Transplantation 56:577–580, 1993.

335. Weisdorf D, Haake R, Blazar B et al: Treatment of moderate/severe acute graft-vs-host disease after allogeneic bone marrow transplantation: An analysis of clinical risk features and outcome. Blood 75:1024–1030, 1990.

336. Martin PJ, Schoch G, Fisher L et al: A retrospective analysis of therapy for acute graft-versus-host disease: Secondary treatment. Blood 77:1821–1828, 1991.

337. Oblon DJ, Felker D, Coyle K, Myers L: High-dose methylprednisolone therapy for acute graft-vs-host disease associated with matched unrelated donor bone marrow transplantation. Bone Marrow Transplant 10:355–357, 1992.

338. Martin PJ, Schoch G, Fisher L et al: A retrospective analysis of therapy for acute graft-versus-host disease: Initial treatment. Blood 76:1464–1472, 1990.

339. Przepiorka D, Kernan NA, Ippoliti C et al: Daclizumab, a humanized anti-interleukin-2 receptor IX chain antibody, for treatment of acute graft-vs-host disease. Blood 95:83–89, 2000.

340. Margolis J, Vogelsang G: An old drug for a new disease: Pentostatin (Nipent) in acute graft-versus-host disease. Semin Oncol 27(Suppl. 5):72–77, 2000.

341. Basara N, Blau IW, Roemer E et al: Mycophenolate mofetil for the treatment of acute and chronic GVHD in bone marrow transplant patients. Bone Marrow Transplant 22:61–65, 1998.

342. Murphy WJ, Blazar BR: New strategies for preventing graft-versus-host disease. Curr Opin Immunol 11:509–515, 1999.

343. Ratanatharathorn V, Nash RA, Przepiorka D et al: Phase III study comparing methotrexate and tacrolimus (prograf, FK506) with methotrexate and cyclosporine for graft-versus-host disease prophylaxis after HLA-identical sibling bone marrow transplantation. Blood 92:2303–2314, 1998.

344. Nash RA, Antin JH, Karanes C et al: Phase 3 study comparing methotrexate and tacrolimus with methotrexate and cyclosporine for prophylaxis of acute graft-versus-host disease after marrow transplantation from unrelated donors. Blood 96:2062–2068, 2000.

345. Wingard JR, Piantadosi S, Vogelsang GB et al: Predictors of death from chronic graft-versus-host disease after bone marrow transplantation. Blood 74:1428–1435, 1989.

346. Socie G, Stone JV, Wingard JR et al: Long-term survival and late deaths after allogeneic bone marrow transplantation. Late Effects Working Committee of the International Bone Marrow Transplant Registry. N Engl J Med 341:14–21, 1999.

347. Kernan NA, Bartsch G, Ash RC et al: Analysis of 462 transplantations from unrelated donors facilitated by the National Marrow Donor Program. N Engl J Med 328:593–602, 1993.

348. McGlave P, Bartsch G, Anasetti C et al: Unrelated donor marrow transplantation therapy for chronic myelogenous leukemia: Initial experience of the National Marrow Donor Program. Blood 81:543–550, 1993.

349. Shulman HM, Sullivan KM, Weiden PL et al: Chronic graft-versus-host syndrome in man. A long-term clinicopathologic study of 20 Seattle patients. Am J Med 69:204–217, 1980.

350. Sullivan KM, Shulman HM, Storb R et al: Chronic graft-versus-host disease in 52 patients: Adverse natural course and successful treatment with combination immunosuppression. Blood 57:267–276, 1981.

351. Claman HN: Graft-versus-host disease and animal models for scleroderma. Curr Opinion Rheumatol 2:929–931, 1990.

352. Graze PR, Gale RP: Chronic graft versus host disease: A syndrome of disordered immunity. Am J Med 66:611–620, 1979.

353. Sherer Y, Shoenfeld Y: Autoimmune diseases and autoimmunity post-bone marrow transplantation. Bone Marrow Transplant 22:873–881, 1998.

354. Quaranta S, Shulman H, Ahmed A et al: Autoantibodies in human chronic graft-versus-host disease after hematopoietic cell transplantation. Clin Immunol 91:106–116, 1999.

355. Siegert W, Stemerowicz R, Hopf U: Antimitochondrial antibodies in patients with chronic graft-versus-host disease. Bone Marrow Transplant 10:221–227, 1992.

356. Carlens S, Ringden O, Remberger M et al: Risk factors for chronic graft-versus-host disease after bone marrow transplantation: A retrospective single centre analysis. Bone Marrow Transplant 22:755–761, 1998.

357. Eisner MD, August CS: Impact of donor and recipient characteristics on the development of acute and chronic graft-versus-host disease following pediatric bone marrow transplantation. Bone Marrow Transplant 15:663–668, 1995.

358. Kollman C, Confer DL, Matlack M et al: The effect of donor age on recipient outcome following unrelated donor marrow transplant (abstract #2827). Blood 92:686a–687a, 1998.

359. Storek J, Gooley T, Siadak M et al: Allogeneic peripheral blood stem cell transplantation may be associated with a high risk of chronic graft-versus-host disease. Blood 90:4705–4709, 1997.

360. Majolino I, Saglio G, Scime R et al: High incidence of chronic GVHD after primary allogeneic peripheral blood stem cell transplantation in patients with hematologic malignancies. Bone Marrow Transplant 17:555–560, 1996.

361. Bensinger WI, Martin PJ, Storer B et al: Transplantation of bone marrow as compared with peripheral-blood cells from HLA-identical relatives in patients with hematologic cancers. N Engl J Med 344:175–181, 2001.

362. Powles R, Mehta J, Kulkarni S et al: Allogeneic blood and bone-marrow stem-cell transplantation in haematological malignant diseases: A randomised trial. Lancet 355:1231–1237, 2000.

363. Ratanatharathorn V, Carson E, Reynolds C et al: Anti-CD20 chimeric monoclonal antibody treatment of refractory immune-mediated thrombocytopenia in a patient with chronic graft-versus-host disease. Annal Intern Med 133:275–279, 2000.

364. Sullivan KM, Agura E, Anasetti C et al: Chronic graft-versus-host disease and other late complications of bone marrow transplantation. Semin Hematol 28:250–259, 1991.

365. Atkinson K, Horowitz MM, Gale RP et al: Risk factors for chronic graft-versus-host disease after HLA-identical sibling bone marrow transplantation. Blood 75:2459–2464, 1990.

366. Wagner JL, Flowers ME, Longton G et al: The development of chronic graft-versus-host disease: An analysis of screening studies and the impact of corticosteroid use at 100 days after transplantation. Bone Marrow Transplant 22:139–146, 1998.

367. Vogelsang GB: How I treat chronic graft-versus-host disease. Blood 97:1196–1201, 2001.

368. Sullivan KM, Meyers JD, Flournoy N et al: Early and late interstitial pneumonia following human bone marrow transplantation. Intl J Cell Cloning 4(Suppl. 1):107–121, 1986.

369. Kulkarni S, Powles R, Treleaven J et al: Chronic graft versus host disease is associated with long-term risk for pneumococcal infections in recipients of bone marrow transplants. Blood 95:3683–3686, 2000.

370. Einsele H, Hebart H, Kauffmann-Schneider C et al: Risk factors for treatment failures in patients receiving PCR-based preemptive therapy for CMV infection. Bone Marrow Transplant 25:757–763, 2000.

371. Kottaridis PD, Milligan DW, Chopra R et al: *In vivo* CAMPATH-1H prevents graft-versus-host disease following nonmyeloablative stem cell transplantation. Blood 96:2419–2425, 2000.

372. Papadopoulos EB, Carabasi MH, Castro-Malaspina H et al: T-cell-depleted allogeneic bone marrow transplantation as postremission therapy for acute myelogenous leukemia: Freedom from relapse in the absence of graft-versus-host disease. Blood 91:1083–1090, 1998.

373. Hale G, Jacobs P, Wood L et al: CD52 antibodies for prevention of graft-versus-host disease and graft rejection following transplantation of allogeneic peripheral blood stem cells. Bone Marrow Transplant 26:69–76, 2000.

374. Hale G, Zhang MJ, Bunjes D et al: Improving the outcome of bone marrow transplantation by using CD52 monoclonal antibodies to prevent graft-versus-host disease and graft rejection. Blood 92:4581–4590, 1998.

375. Marmont AM, Horowitz MM, Gale RP et al: T-cell depletion of HLA-identical transplants in leukemia. Blood 78:2120–2130, 1991.

376. Guidelines for preventing opportunistic infections among hematopoietic stem cell transplant recipients: Recommendations of CDC, the Infectious Disease Society of America, and the American Society of Blood and Marrow Transplantation. Biol Blood Marrow Transplant 6:7–75, 2000.

377. Sullivan KM, Witherspoon RP, Storb R et al: Prednisone and azathioprine compared with prednisone and placebo for treatment of chronic graft-v-host disease: Prognostic influence of prolonged

thrombocytopenia after allogeneic marrow transplantation. Blood 72:546–554, 1988.

378. Sullivan KM, Shulman HM, Storb R et al: Chronic graft-versus-host disease in 52 patients: Adverse natural course and successful treatment with combination immunosuppression. Blood 57:267–276, 1981.

379. Sullivan KM, Witherspoon RP, Storb R et al: Alternating-day cyclosporine and prednisone for treatment of high-risk chronic graft-v-host disease. Blood 72:555–561, 1988.

380. Carnevale-Schianca F, Martin P, Sullivan K et al: Changing from cyclosporine to tacrolimus as salvage therapy for chronic graft-versus-host disease. Biol Blood Marrow Transplant 6:613–620, 2000.

381. Akpek G, Zahurak M, Piantadosi S et al: Development of a prognostic model for grading chronic graft-versus-host disease. Blood 97:1219–1226, 2001.

382. Epler GR: Bronchiolitis obliterans and airways obstruction associated with graft-versus-host disease. Clin Chest Med 9:551–556, 1988.

383. Holland HK, Wingard JR, Beschorner WE et al: Bronchiolitis obliterans in bone marrow transplantation and its relationship to chronic graft-v-host disease and low serum IgG. Blood 72:621–627, 1988.

384. Rosenberg ME, Vercellotti GM, Snover DC et al: Bronchiolitis obliterans after bone marrow transplantation. Am J Hematol 18:325–328, 1985.

385. Schiller G, Gale RP: Is there an effective therapy for chronic graft-versus-host disease? Bone Marrow Transplant 11:189–192, 1993.

386. Arora M, Wagner JE, Davies SM et al: Randomized clinical trial of thalidomide, cyclosporine, and prednisone versus cyclosporine and prednisone as initial therapy for chronic graft-versus-host disease. Biol Blood Marrow Transplant 7:265–273, 2001.

387. Couriel DR, Hicks K, Ippoliti C et al: Infliximab for the treatment of graft-versus-host disease in allogeneic transplant recipients: An update (abstract #1724). Blood 96:400a, 2000.

388. Chiang K-Y, Marshall C, Abhyankar S et al: Recombinant human soluble tumor necrosis factor receptor fusion protein (Enbrel®) as a treatment for chronic graft-versus-host disease (CGvHD) following allogeneic bone marrow transplantation (abstract # 1728). Blood 96:401a, 2000.

389. Zaja F, Russo D, Fuga G et al: Rituximab for myasthenia gravis developing after bone marrow transplant. Neurology 55:1062–1063, 2000.

390. Kolb HJ, Bender-Götze C: Late complications after allogeneic bone marrow transplantation for leukaemia. Bone Marrow Transplant 6:61–72, 1990.

391. Schimmer AD, Minden MD, Keating A: Osteoporosis after blood and marrow transplantation: Clinical aspects. Biol Blood Marrow Transplant 6:175–181, 2000.

392. Stern JM, Sullivan KM, Ott SM et al: Bone density loss after allogeneic hematopoietic stem cell transplantation: A prospective study. Biol Blood Marrow Transplant 7:257–264, 2001.

393. Claisse JP, Hirsch I, Gluckman E: Quality of life after an allogeneic bone marrow transplantation: The patient's point of view. Nouv Rev Fr Hematol 36(Suppl. 1):S83–84, 1994.

394. Chiodi S, Spinelli S, Ravera G et al: Quality of life in 244 recipients of allogeneic bone marrow transplantation. Br J Haematol 110:614–619, 2000.

395. Andrykowski MA, Bruehl S, Brady MJ, Henslee-Downey PJ: Physical and psychosocial status of adults one-year after bone marrow transplantation: A prospective study. Bone Marrow Transplant 15:837–844, 1995.

396. Andrykowski MA, Greiner CB, Altmaier EM et al: Quality of life following bone marrow transplantation: Findings from a multi-centre study. Br J Cancer 71:1322–1329, 1995.

397. Lee SJ, Fairclough D, Parsons SK et al: Recovery after stem-cell transplantation for hematologic diseases. J Clin Oncol 19:242–252, 2001.

398. Molassiotis A, van den Akker OB, Milligan DW et al: Quality of life in long-term survivors of marrow transplantation: Comparison with a matched group receiving maintenance chemotherapy. Bone Marrow Transplant 17:249–258, 1996.

399. Sutherland HJ, Fyles GM, Adams G et al: Quality of life following bone marrow transplantation: A comparison of patient reports with population norms. Bone Marrow Transplant 19:1129–1136, 1997.

400. McQuellon RP, Russell GB, Rambo TD et al: Quality of life and psychological distress of bone marrow transplant recipients: The 'time trajectory' to recovery over the first year. Bone Marrow Transplant 21:477–486, 1998.

401. Marks DI, Gale DJ, Vedhara K, Bird JM: A quality of life study in 20 adult long-term survivors of unrelated donor bone marrow transplantation. Bone Marrow Transplant 24:191–195, 1999.

402. Heinonen H, Volin L, Uutela A, Zevon M, Barrick C, Ruutu T: Quality of life and factors related to perceived satisfaction with quality of life after allogeneic bone marrow transplantation. Ann Hematol 80:137–143, 2001.

403. Andrykowski MA, Altmaier EM, Barnett RL, Otis ML, Gingrich R, Henslee-Downey PJ: The quality of life in adult survivors of allogeneic bone marrow transplantation. Correlates and comparison with matched renal transplant recipients. Transplantation 50:399–406, 1990.

404. Zittoun R, Achard S, Ruszniewski M: Assessment of quality of life during intensive chemotherapy or bone marrow transplantation. Psycho-oncology 8:64–73, 1999.

405. Fife BL, Huster GA, Cornetta KG, Kennedy VN, Akard LP, Broun ER: Longitudinal study of adaptation to the stress of bone marrow transplantation. J Clin Oncol 18:1539–1549, 2000.

406. Gotay CC, Muraoka MY: Quality of life in long-term survivors of adult-onset cancers. J Natl Cancer Inst 90:656–667, 1998.

407. Schimmer AD, Ali V, Stewart AK, Imrie K, Keating A: Male sexual function after autologous blood or marrow transplantation. Biol Blood Marrow Transplant 7:279–283, 2001.

408. Mertens AC, Ramsay NKC, Kouris S, Neglia JP: Patterns of gonadal dysfunction following bone marrow transplantation. Bone Marrow Transplant 22:345–350, 1998.

409. Cordova MJ, Cunningham LLC, Carlson CR, Andrykowski MA: Posttraumatic growth following breast cancer: A controlled comparison study. Health Psychol 20:176–185, 2001.

410. Deeg HJ, Sanders J, Martin P et al: Secondary malignancies after marrow transplantation. Exp Hematol 12:660–666, 1984.

411. Kolb HJ, Bender-Gotze C: Late complications after allogeneic bone marrow transplantation for leukaemia. Bone Marrow Transplant 6:61–72, 1990.

412. Witherspoon RP, Fisher LD, Schoch G et al: Secondary cancers after bone marrow transplantation for leukemia or aplastic anemia. N Engl J Med 321:784–789, 1989.

413. Deeg HJ, Witherspoon RP: Risk factors for the development of secondary malignancies after marrow transplantation. Hematol Oncol Clin North Am 7:417–429, 1993.

414. Stone RM, Neuberg D, Soiffer R et al: Myelodysplastic syndrome as a late complication following autologous bone marrow transplantation for non-Hodgkin's lymphoma. J Clin Oncol 12:2535–2542, 1994.

415. Darrington DL, Vose JM, Anderson JR et al: Incidence and characterization of secondary myelodysplastic syndrome and acute myelogenous leukemia following high-dose chemoradiotherapy and autologous stem-cell transplantation for lymphoid malignancies. J Clin Oncol 12:2527–2534, 1994.

416. Andre M, Henry-Amar M, Blaise D et al: Treatment-related deaths and second cancer risk after autologous stem-cell transplantation for Hodgkin's disease. Blood 92:1933–1940, 1998.

417. Kollmannsberger C, Beyer J, Droz JP et al: Secondary leukemia following high cumulative doses of etoposide in patients treated for advanced germ cell tumors. J Clin Oncol 16:3386–3391, 1998.

418. Kollmannsberger C, Hartmann JT, Kanz L, Bokemeyer C: Risk of secondary myeloid leukemia and myelodysplastic syndrome following standard-dose chemotherapy or high-dose chemotherapy with stem cell support in patients with potentially curable malignancies. J Cancer Res Clin Oncol 124:207–214, 1998.

419. Bhatia S, Ramsay LL, Steinbuch M et al: Malignant neoplasms following bone marrow transplantation. Blood 87:3633–3639, 1996.

420. Lowsky R, Lipton J, Fyles G et al: Secondary malignancies after bone marrow transplantation in adults. J Clin Oncol 12:2187–2121, 1994.

421. Curtis RE, Rowlings PA, Deeg HJ et al: Solid cancers after bone marrow transplantation. N Engl J Med 336:897–904, 1997.

422. Bhatia S, Louie A, Bhatia R et al: Solid cancer after bone marrow transplantation. J Clin Oncol 19:464–471, 2001.

423. Curtis RE, Travis LB, Rowlings PA et al: Risk of lymphoproliferative disorders after bone marrow transplantation: A multi-institutional study. Blood 94:2208–2216, 1999.

424. Guillaume T, Rubinstein DB, Symann M: Immune reconstitution and immunotherapy after autologous hematopoietic stem cell transplantation. Blood 92:1471–1490, 1998.

425. Atkinson K: Reconstruction of the haemopoietic and immune systems after marrow transplantation. Bone Marrow Transplant 5:209–226, 1990.

426. Small TN: Immunologic reconstitution following stem cell transplantation. Curr Opin Hematol 3:461–465, 1996.

427. Koehne G, Zeller W, Stockschlaeder M, Zander AR: Phenotype of lymphocyte subsets after autologous peripheral blood stem cell transplantation. Bone Marrow Transplant 19:149–156, 1997.

428. Sugita K, Soiffer RJ, Murray C, Schlossman SF, Ritz J, Morimoto C: The phenotype and reconstitution of immunoregulatory T cell subsets after T cell depleted allogeneic and autologous bone marrow transplantation. Transplantation 57:1465–1473, 1994.

429. Foot ABM, Potter MN, Donaldson C et al: Immune reconstitution after BMT in children. Bone Marrow Transplant 11:7–13, 1993.

430. Witherspoon RP, Storb R: Stem cell reconstitution after bone marrow transplantation into adult patients does not resemble T cell development in early life. Bone Marrow Transplant 16:413–425, 1995.

431. Miller RA, Daley J, Ghalie R, Kaizer H: Clonal analysis of T cell deficiencies in autotransplant recipients. Blood 77:1845–1850, 1991.

432. Sugita K, Nojima Y, Tachibana K et al: Prolonged impairment of very late activating antigen-mediated T cell proliferation via the CD3 pathway after T cell depleted allogeneic bone marrow transplantation. J Clin Oncol 94:481–488, 1994.

433. Cayeux S, Meuer S, Pezzutto A et al: T cell ontogeny after autologous bone marrow transplantation: Failure to synthesize interleukin-2 (IL-2) and lack of CD2- and CD3- mediated proliferation by both CD4– and CD8+ cells even in the presence of exogenous IL-2. Blood 74:2270–2277, 1989.

434. Small TN, Keever CA, Weiner-Fedus S, Heller G, O'Reilly RJ, Flomenberg N: B cell differentiation following autologous, conventional, or T cell depleted bone marrow transplantation: A recapitulation of normal B cell ontogeny. Blood 76:1647–1656, 1990.

435. Ochs L, Shu XO, Miller J et al: Late infections after allogeneic bone marrow transplantation: Comparison of incidence in related and unrelated donor transplant recipients. Blood 86:3979–3986, 1995.

436. Winston DJ, Gale RP, Meyer DV: Infectious complications of human bone marrow transplantation. Medicine 58:1–31, 1979.

437. Ambrosino DM, Molrine DC: Critical appraisal of immunization strategies for prevention of infection in the compromised host. Hematol Oncol Clin North Am 7:1027–1050, 1993.

438. Pirofski LA, Casadevall A: Use of licensed vaccines for active immunization of the immunocompromised host. Clin Microbiol Rev 11:1–26, 1998.

439. Ljungman P, Cordonnier C, de Bock R et al: Immunizations after bone marrow transplantation: Results of a European survey and recommendation from the infectious diseases working party of the European Group for Blood and Marrow Transplantation. Bone Marrow Transplant 15:455–460, 1995.

440. Henning KJ, White MH, Sepkowitz KA, Armstrong D: A national survey of immunization practices following allogeneic bone marrow transplantation. JAMA 277:1148–1151, 1997.

441. Ottinger HD, Beelen DW, Scheulen B, Schaefer UW, Grosse-Wilde H: Improved immune reconstitution after allotransplantation of peripheral blood stem cells instead of bone marrow. Blood 88:2775–2779, 1996.

442. Talmadge JE, Reed E, Ino K et al: Rapid immunologic reconstitution following transplantation with mobilized peripheral blood stem cells as compared to bone marrow. Bone Marrow Transplant 19:161–172, 1997.

443. Henon R, Liang H, Beck-Werth G et al: Comparison of hematopoietic and immune recovery after autologous bone marrow or blood stem cell transplants. Bone Marrow Transplant 9:285–291, 1992.

444. Roux E, Helg C, Dumon-Girard F, Chapuis B, Jeannet M, Roosnek E: Analysis of T cell population after allogeneic bone marrow transplantation: Significant differences between recipients of T cell depleted and unmanipulated grafts. Blood 87:3984–3992, 1996.

445. Parkkali T, Kayhty H, Ruutu T, Volin L, Eskola J, Ruutu P: A comparison of early and late vaccination with Haemophilus influenzae type B conjugate and pneumococcal polysaccharide vaccines after allogeneic BMT. Bone Marrow Transplant 18:961–967, 1996.

446. Vance E, George S, Guinan EC et al: Comparison of multiple immunization schedules for Haemophilus influenzae type B-conjugate and tetanus toxoid vaccines following bone marrow transplantation. Bone Marrow Transplant 22:735–741, 1998.

447. Guinan EC, Molrine, DC, Antin JH et al: Polysaccharide conjugate vaccine responses in bone marrow transplant patients. Transplantation 57:677–684, 1994.

448. Hammarstrom V, Pauksen K, Azinge J, Oberg G, Ljungman P: Pneumococcal immunity and response to immunization with pneumococcal vaccine in bone marrow transplant patients; the influence of graft versus host reaction. Support Care Cancer 1:195–199, 1993.

449. Storek J, Mendelman PM, Witherspoon RP, McGregor BA, Storb R: IgG response to pneumococcal polysaccharide-protein conjugate appears similar to IgG response to polysaccharide in bone marrow transplant recipients and healthy adults. Clin Infect Dis 25:1253–1255, 1997.

450. Avanzini MA, Carra AM, Maccario R et al: Antibody response to pneumococcal vaccine in children receiving bone marrow transplantation. J Clin Immunol 15:137–144, 1995.

451. Avigan D, Pirofski L-A, Lazarus HM: Vaccination against infectious disease following hematopoietic stem cell transplantation. Biol Blood Marrow Transplant 7:171–183, 2001.

452. Hammarstrom V, Pauksen K, Bjorkstrand B, Simonsson B, Oberg G, Ljungman P: Tetanus immunity in autologous bone marrow and blood stem cell transplant recipients. Bone Marrow Transplant 22:67–71, 1998.

453. Chan CY, Molrine DC, Antin JH et al: Antibody responses to tetanus toxoid and Haemophilus influenzae type B conjugate vaccines following autologous peripheral blood stem cell transplantation. Bone Marrow Transplant 20:33–38, 1997.

60

Hematopoietic Growth Factors in the Supportive Care and Treatment of Patients with Hematologic Malignancies

Janice P. Dutcher

Hematopoietic growth factors constitute a family of glycoproteins that regulate the self-renewal, cycle activation, proliferation, maturation, adhesion, functional integrity, and activation of mature blood cells, as well as hemostasis. The number of positive and negative regulatory factors that influence hematopoietic cell survival and development has grown to encompass not only colony-stimulating factors but also interleukins, interferons, chemokines, and other growth factors.

The molecular and biochemical characteristics, cellular sources, and normal in vitro activity of the major hematopoietic growth factors are summarized in Tables 60–1 and 60–2. Table 60–3 provides an extended list of cytokines now thought to play an important role in the regulation of normal megakaryocytopoiesis. Although in vitro studies are able to isolate cellular regulatory activity of these substances, it is clear that in vivo many of these may interact and cross-regulate. Thus, we have not always observed the same degree or specificity of activity in vivo compared with in vitro.

HEMATOPOIETIC GROWTH FACTOR RECEPTORS

Hematopoietic growth factors appear to exert their effects primarily via binding to specific high-affinity receptors.[1] Cytokine receptors have been divided into several families of related molecules based on amino acid sequences. These families include the immunoglobulin superfamily (interleukin-1 [IL-1] receptors, fibroblast growth factor [FGF] receptor, platelet-derived growth factor [PDGF] receptor, c-kit [CD117], and colony-stimulating factor-1 [CSF-1] receptor), characterized by varying numbers of immunoglobulin domains in their extracellular regions[2,3]; the tumor necrosis factor (TNF)-related family of receptors, with characteristic cysteine-rich repeats in the extracellular domain[4,5]; and the hematopoietin receptor family. Members of the latter family include receptors for leukemia inhibitory factor (LIF); IL-1, IL-2, IL-3, IL-4, IL-5, IL-6, IL-7, and IL-9; granulocyte-macrophage colony-stimulating factor (GM-CSF), granulocyte colony-stimulating factor (G-CSF); erythropoietin; prolactin; growth hormone; ciliary factor; and c-mpl.[1,6–9] Several receptors possess intracellular tyrosine kinase activity, including epidermal growth factor (EGF) receptor, insulin receptor, PDGF receptor, FGF receptor, CSF-1 receptor, and c-kit.

IN VITRO EVALUATION OF GROWTH FACTORS AND GROWTH OF MALIGNANT HEMATOPOIETIC CELLS

For several years, in vitro studies have connected certain hematopoietic growth factors to the growth and proliferation of malignant hematopoietic cell lines. However, support for these mechanisms in the pathogenesis of clinical hematopoietic malignancies in humans is less compelling. There is little evidence that late-acting, maturing growth factors influence the malignant disease process. However, early acting factors may influence primitive cell growth and appear to play a role in some disease processes.

The most convincing data are for myeloma, in which a number of hematopoietic growth factors have been identified as survival or proliferative factors for malignant plasma cells.[10–13] Several studies have confirmed that the growth of myeloma cells is supported by a network of cytokines in which IL-6 functions in a pivotal role.[10–13] Interleukin-6 stimulates the proliferation of normal and malignant plasma blasts[10]; TNF acts as an independent survival and proliferation factor[13]; and IL-1 plays a role in inducing IL-6 production.[14] In addition, studies using anti-IL-6 monoclonal antibodies have demonstrated suppression of the proliferation of plasma cells in a patient with plasma cell leukemia,[15] and in a phase I/II clinical trial in conjunction with chemotherapy, there appeared to be an additive effect.[16] The best experimental evidence supporting a pivotal role for IL-6 has been provided by demonstrating that mice modified to express a transgene for IL-6 develop massive oligoclonal plasmacytosis when crossed with Balb/c mice that have a genetic background for developing plasmacytomas.[17] In addition, these same Balb/c mice, when transgenically manipulated to express IL-6, demonstrate rapid development and wide dissemination of extraosseous plasmacytomas.[18]

Clinically, the prognostic role of immunoreactive IL-6 levels and IL-6-soluble receptor levels has been widely debated, and studies are contradictory.[19–22] However, reduction in IL-6 levels has been associated with improvement in disease control either through the use of the monoclonal antibody[15,16] or through cytokine modulation by cyclosporine administration.[23]

Other hematopoietic growth factors have also been shown to favor survival of malignant lymphoid cells by interfering with apoptotic stimuli.[24–30] Interleukins-9 and -4 have been shown to serve as antiapoptotic factors for the murine thymic lymphoma cell line BW5147.[24] In one study, intracellular levels of basic fibroblast growth factor (bFGF) were shown to correlate with stage of disease in chronic lymphocytic leukemia (CLL) and to confer resistance to apoptotic chemotherapeutic agents (fludarabine).[25] Subsequent investigations have demonstrated a complex interaction between bFGF and BCL-2 expression and interactions with vascular endothelial growth factor expression,[26,27] and BFGF has been associated with upregulation of the *BCL-2* gene in CLL cell lines, causing delay in apoptosis.[28] Interleukin-4, B-cell differentiating factor, has a complex relationship with CLL cells. Studies have demonstrated that IL-4 produces a delay in apoptosis in CLL cells and thereby favors the survival of these cells.[29,30] However, other studies have sug-

Table 60–1. Randomized Trials of Colony-Stimulating Factors (CSFs) in Acute Myeloid Leukemia

Study	CSF Dose schedule	Patients' age/dx	Design	Chemotherapy	Results
Ohno[87]	G-CSF (nonglycosylated) 200 g IV, 30 min infusion daily, beginning 2 days after chemo and daily until ANC > 1500	Relapsed/refractory leukemia; AML (67) ALL (30) CMLBC (9) MDS (2) Ages 13–69 N = 108	Open label	Mitoxantrone 5 mg/m²/d IV day 1–3 Etoposide 80 mg/m²/d IV day 1–5 Enocetabine 170 mg/m²/d (2h infusion) For 8–12 days	1. Shorter period of neutropenia by 1 week. 2. Less documented infections 3. No diff in febrile days; regrowth of leukemia; 4. No diff in DFS or EFS
Ohno[86]	G-CSF (nonglycosylated) 200 g IV, 30 min infusion daily, beginning 2 days after chemo and daily until ANC > 1500	Relapsed or refractory leukemia AML (50) MDS (8) Ages 16–66 Median 43 N = 58	Double-blind, placebo-controlled	Mitoxantrone 7mg/m²/d IV day 1–3 Etoposide 100 mg/m²/d IV day 1–5 BHAC 200 mg/m²/d (2-h infusion) days 1–7	1. No diff in EVS or DFS 2. More rapid recovery of neutrophils 3. No diff in documented infections
Stone[40]	GM-CSF (nonglycosylated) 5 g/kg IV as a 6-h infusion daily, beginning day 8	Newly dx AML, M0–M7; No MDS Ages 60–80 Median 69 N = 388	Double-blind, placebo-controlled	Daunorubicin 8 mg/m²/d IV days 1–3 Ara-C 200 mg/m²/d IVCI days 1–7	1. Shorter duration of neutropenia 2. No diff in days in hospital; infection; febrile days
Rowe[41]	GM-CSF (glycosylated) (yeast-derived) 25 mg/m² as a 4-h infusion daily, beginning day 10 and until ANC > 1500 x 3 days	Newly dx AML, M0–M7; No MDS Ages 55–70 N = 124	Double-blind, placebo-controlled	Induction: daunorubicin 60 mg/m²/d IV days 1–3 Ara-C 25 mg/m² IVPd 1, followed by Ara-C 100 mg/m²/d IVCI; days 1–7 Consolidation: Ara-C 1.5 mg/m² over 1 h, every 12 h, for 12 doses	1. Shorter duration of neutropenia 2. Decrease in infections and toxicity Consolidation: 1. No diff in recovery from neutropenia or infectious episodes
Dombret[89]	G-CSF (nonglycosylated) 5 g/kg IV over 30 min daily, beginning d 9 and continued until ANC > 1000 x 3 days; or 28 days	Newly dx AML, M0–M7 Ages 64–83 Median 71	Placebo-controlled	Daunorubicin 45 mg/m²/d IV days 1–4 Ara-C 200 mg/m²/d IVCI days 1–7	1. Shorter duration of neutropenia 2. Reduced resistant leukemia 3. Increase in CR 4. No diff in days in hospital; infection; febrile days
Heil[90]	G-CSF (nonglycosylated) 5 g/kg as a subcutaneous injection daily; beginning 24 h after chemo and continued until ANC > 1000	Newly dx AML, M0–M7 Ages 16–89 Median 54 N = 521	Double-blind placebo-controlled	Daunorubicin 45 mg/m²/d IV days 1–3 Ara-C 100 mg/m²/d IVCI, days 1–7 Etoposide 100 mg/m²/d IV days 1–5	1. Shorter neutropenia by 5 days 2. Decreased duration of fever and antibiotics 3. Decreased time in hospital 4. Decreased use of antifungals
Godwin[91]	G-CSF (nonglycosylated) 400 g/m² IV over 30 min daily, beginning day 8	Newly dx AML, M0–M7, excluding M3 Median age 68 N = 234	Double-blind; placebo-controlled	Daunorubicin 45 mg/m²/d IV days 1–3 Ara-C 200 mg/m²/d IVCI days 1–7	1. 15% reduction in duration of neutropenia 2. Decreased duration of fever and antibiotics

Study	Agent/schedule	Patient population	Study design	Chemotherapy regimen	Results
Lowenberg[92]	GM-CSF (*E. coli*-derived) 5 g/kg daily as a continuous infusion starting day 1 before chemo, given during and after chemo until ANC > 500 × 3 days	Newly dx AML, M0–M6 MDS-leukemia allowed Ages 61–80 Median mid-60s N = 318	Open label	Daunorubicin 30 mg/m^2/d days 1–3 AraC 200 mg/m^2/d IVCI days 1–7	1. More rapid neutrophil recovery 2. No diff in time in hospital; infections 3. Less fever in control subjects
Zittoun[93]	GM-CSF (*E. coli*-derived) 5 g/kg daily as a continuous infusion : 3 treatment arms: (a) starting 24 h before chemo, given during and after chemo until ANC > 500; (b) starting day 8 until day 28 or ANC > 500 (c) starting 24 h before chemo and continued through chemo	Newly dx AML, M0–M7 No MDS Ages 15–60 Median 45 N = 102 25 patients per arm	Open label 4 arms	Daunorubicin 45 mg/m^2/d days 1–3 AraC 200 mg/m^2 IVCI days 1–7	1. No diff in duration of neutropenia 2. No diff in CR rate 3. Very small numbers
Witz[94]	GM-CSF (*E. coli*-derived) 5 g/kg daily as a 6-h infusion starting day 1, 12 h after chemo and daily until ANC > 500 × 3 d or until day 28	Newly dx AML, M0–M7 No MDS Ages 55–75 Median > 65 N = 240	Placebo-controlled	Indarubicin 8 mg/m^2/d days 1–5 Ara-C 100 mg/m^2/d IVCI days 1–7	1. Shorter duration of neutropenia 2. No diff in infection 3. No diff in CR or leukemia regrowth 4. Signif longer 2-yr DFS
Harousseau[95]	G-CSF (nonglycosylated) 5 g/kg daily during remission after completion of consolidation chemo	Newly dx AML in remission, M0–M6 Ages 15–60 Median 46 N = 194	Open label	Consol I HiDAC 3 g/m^2 as 3-h infusion every 12 hours, days 1–4 Mitoxantrone 12mg/m^2/d IV days 5 and 6 Consol II Amsacrine 150 mg/m^2/d as 1-h infusion, days 1–5 Etoposide 100 mg/m^2/d as 2-h infusion, days 1–5	1. Signif decrease in duration of neutropenia 2. Decrease in hospital time 3. Decrease in antibiotics 4. Decrease in antifungal duration 5. No diff in documented infection 6. No diff in 2-yr DFS or OS
Usuki[96]	G-CSF (non-glycosylated) 200 g/m^2/d IV starting 48 h after chemo ended until ANC > 1500	Newly dx AML, M0–M7 M3 excluded No MDS Ages 15–87 Median 49 N = 158	Open label	Treatment was that identified by each hospital as standard induction therapy	1. Shorter time to recovery from neutropenia 2. Shorter duration of febrile neutropenia 3. No diff in CR rate or 5-yr DFS
Stone[97]	GM-CSF (nonglycosylated) 5 g/kg daily IV 6-h infusion beginning 24 h after completion of Ara-C infusion	Newly dx AML, M0–M7 Ages > 60 Median ≤ 70 N = 388	Double-blind placebo-controlled	Induction: daunorubicin 45mg/m^2/d days 1–3 Ara-C 200 mg/m^2/d IVCI days 1–7 Consolidation: randomized between Ara-C 100 mg/m^2/day days 1–5, monthly × 4 or Ara-C 500 mg/m^2 every 12 h × 6 doses with mitoxantrone 5 mg/m^2 every 12 h × 6 doses	1. No diff in DFS 2. No diff in CR rate 3. No diff in infection

Table 60–2. Normal Hematopoietic and Nonhematopoietic Cell Types Influenced by Interleukins and Hematopoietic Growth Factors

Name	Target
IL-1α, β	T cells, B cells, neutrophils, stem cells, fibroblasts, endothelial cells, synovial cells, osteoclasts, adipocytes, hepatocytes, muscles, hypothalamus
IL-2	T cells, B cells, monocytes
IL-3	Stem cells, CFU-GEMM, CFU-GM, BFU-E, CFU-Mk, basophils/mast cell, eosinphil, monocytes
IL-4	T cells, B-cells, NKs, LAKs, monocytes/macrophages, mast cells, CFU-GM, BFU-E, CFU-Mk
IL-5	Eosinophils, CFU-Eo, B cells, T-cell thymocytes
IL-6	Stem cells, CFU-GM, CFU-Mk, megakaryocytes/platelets, B cells, T cells, NKs, endothelial cells, hepatocytes, hypothalamus
IL-7	Pre-B cell, thymocytes, T cells
IL-8	Neutrophils, T cells, endothelium (stimulates angiogenesis)
IL-9	BFU-E, T cells, mast cells, megakaryocytes
IL-10	T_H^1 helper T cells (inhibits effector function mediated by IFN-γ and IL-2); mast cells (synergy with IL-3)
IL-11	Balls, primitive hematoporetic progenitors, synergizes with KL to stimulate the growth of BFU-E, CFU-E, and CFU-Mk
IL-12	CD4 + T-helper cells: augments NK function inhibitor-angiogenesis•
Kit ligand	BFU-E, CFU-GEMM, P-CFU-HPP (synergy with IL-6, M-CSF), mast cells, primordial germ cells, melanocyte precursors
GM-CSF	CFU-GM, BFU-E, CFU-Mk, neutrophils, eosinophils
G-CSF	CFU-GM, neutrophils, monocytes
M-CSF	CFU-GM, monocytes/macrophages, trophoblasts
Erythropoietin	CFU-E, erythroblasts
LIF/HILDA	Monocytes, macrophages, osteoblasts, totipotent embryonic stem cells, hepatocytes, neurons
FLK-2/FLT3 ligand	Survival of G_0 early progenitors: triggers proliferation of committed progenitors
TGF-α, -β	Stem cells, BFU-E, CFU-GM, monocytes, T cells, B cells, NKs, fibroblasts, endothelial cells, epithelium, adipocytes, muscle, osteoclasts, chondrocytes
MIP-Iα	Inhibits pluripotent stem cells (CFU-HPP, CFU-s), synergistically enhances CFU-GM (with GM-CSF or M-CSF)

Abbreviations: BFU-E, burst-forming unit erythroid; CFU-Eo, colony-forming unit-eosinophil; CFU-GEMM, CFU-granulocyte, erythroid, monocyte/macrophage megakaryocyte; CFU-GM, CFU-granulocyte/macrophage; CFU-Mk, CFU-megakaryocyte; CFU-s, CFU-spleen; CFU-HPP, CFU-proliferative potential; G-CSF, granulocyte colony-stimulating factor; GM-CSF, granulocyte/macrophage CSF; M-CSF, macrophage CSF; IFN-γ, interferon-γ; IL, interleukin; KL, Kit ligand; LAK, lymphocyte activated killer (cell); LIF, leukemia inhibitory factor; NK, nature killer (cell); TGF, transforming growth factor; MIP-Iα, macrophage inhibitory protein-alpha.

Table 60–3. Factors Reported to Play a Role in Megakarocytopoiesis

Interleukin-1
Interleukin-3
Interleukin-11
Basic fibroblast growth factor
Thrombopoietin

gested an inhibition of growth by IL-4.[31] Early phase I clinical trials suggested a beneficial effect of IL-4 in CLL and low-grade non-Hodgkin's lymphoma, with lowering of lymphocyte count and reduction in lymphadenopathy and splenomegaly.[32,33] Interestingly, in two more recent reports, IL-4 led to the maturation of a CLL patient's cells to a paraprotein-producing myeloma,[34] and in a phase I/II clinical trial in Europe treatment led to an increase in the number of CLL cells in the peripheral blood.[35]

Because neither IL-6 nor IL-4 is any longer used in clinical evaluations, these potential effects on hematologic malignancies are most important in understanding the mechanisms and interactions of cytokines leading to the continued proliferation of these diseases.

The question has arisen as to whether or not the use of G-CSF or GM-CSF in the treatment of acute myeloid leukemia (AML) promotes disease progression. This has been investigated thoroughly. Some studies performed in vitro with leukemia cell lines have demonstrated suppression of programmed cell death by hematopoietic growth factors functioning as viability factors.[36,37] Others have shown no interference.[38,39] However, clinical studies in which growth factors were administered early in the treatment of acute myeloid leukemia did not demonstrate a "priming" effect, and rapid growth of leukemic cells was not observed in numerous placebo-controlled studies.[40,41]

An association has been postulated between IL-1 levels and the pathogenesis and progression of chronic myeloid leukemia (CML).[42,43] Several laboratories have documented elevated serum levels of IL-1 (both α and β) in patients with advanced CML[42,43] and have demonstrated a growth-promoting effect in vitro.[42] Others have challenged the autocrine or paracrine role of IL-1, invoking a role for constitutive activation of other factors in the proliferative response in CML.[44]

Finally, the development of structural abnormalities or aberrant regulation of growth factor receptor expression has been postulated to play a role in the development of the leukemic phenotype.[45] Several such abnormalities have been demonstrated in leukemia cell line systems.[45,46] Particular mutations in hematopoietic growth factor receptors may lead to their activation in the absence of ligand and may result in leukemic cell transformation. A point mutation of the extracellular domain of the erythropoietin receptor, leading to its constitutive activation, has been observed in murine erythroleukemia.[47] Point mutations in the *c-FMS* gene have been reported in approximately 10 percent of AML cases.[48–50]

CLINICAL APPLICATIONS OF HEMATOPOIETIC GROWTH FACTORS

The major clinical application of hematopoietic growth factors that has arisen in the treatment of patients with hematopoietic malignancies has been restoration of disease- or treatment-related myelosuppression. Additionally, hematopoietic growth factors, particularly those that stimulate neutrophil production, are being used to stimulate donors of both stem cells and mature granulocytes.[51] The most extensively evaluated hematopoietic growth factors in clinical practice include G-CSF, GM-CSF, and erythropoietin. Additionally, IL-11 has been approved for correction of chemotherapy-induced thrombocytopenia[52–54] Thrombopoietin continues in clinical trials.[55,56] Although a number of clinical trials have evaluated early-acting growth factors such as IL-1, IL-3, and IL-6, these have not reached clinical maturity.[57–60] We will review current data with respect to the clinically available agents.

CORRECTION OF IATROGENICALLY INDUCED NEUTROPENIA

Recombinant Human Granulocyte Colony-Stimulating Factor

Early preclinical studies demonstrated the ability of G-CSF (filgrastim) to augment the number of functionally normal neutrophil granulocytes in normal and tumor-bearing rodents and nonhuman primates. This neutrophil granulocytosis results from an augmentation in the number of divisions in precursors and reduction (from 96 to 24 hours) in the time required for the maturing neutrophil granulocyte precursors to develop into terminally differentiated cells.[61] This factor has been shown to reduce the period of neutropenia in cynomolgus primates treated with high-dose alkylating agents[61–63] and/or by total body irradiation with reinfusion of autologous marrow.[63] Three initial studies in humans revealed that intravenous bolus, continuous intravenous infusion, subcutaneous injection, or continuous subcutaneous infusion, administered in the absence of myelosuppression, results in a dose-dependent increase in the circulating neutrophil count.[64–66] The increase in absolute neutrophil count is caused primarily by an increase in mature, functionally normal segmented polymorphonuclear leukocytes and is associated with an expansion of the myeloid compartment. On discontinuation of G-CSF, neutrophil counts decrease by half daily and generally return to baseline within 4 days of treatment. The administration of G-CSF also results in a 10- to 100-fold increase in circulating hematopoietic progenitor cells.[64,67]

Neutropenia following chemotherapy in cancer patients is a major cause of morbidity and mortality. Phase I and II clinical studies of adjunctive growth factor administration in patients receiving a broad spectrum of commonly employed chemotherapeutic agents initially demonstrated the ability to accelerate recovery from chemotherapy-induced neutropenia.[64–66,68–70] In these studies, G-CSF was administered 24 hours after cessation of chemotherapy. Of particular importance has been the fact that, in contrast to the effects of G-CSF in normal steady-state hematopoiesis, no dose-dependent response was noted in the setting of myelosuppression, but rather a dose was established below which benefit (in terms of neutrophil reconstitution) was not observed.

Recombinant Human Granulocyte-Macrophage Colony-Stimulating Factor

In preclinical studies, administration of GM-CSF to normal rhesus monkeys resulted in a dramatic leukocytosis, consisting initially of only neutrophil granulocytes and monocytes, followed by a substantial increase in eosinophil granulocytes.[71] A model of pancytopenia induced by simian type D retrovirus in rhesus monkeys provided data supporting clinical application of GM-CSF in patients with the acquired immunodeficiency syndrome (AIDS), bone marrow failure states, and infectious disease.[71] Models investigating the use of GM-CSF following total body irradiation and autologous marrow reinfusion demonstrated a myelorestorative effect of GM-CSF in the transplant setting and provided the framework for designing clinical trials in humans.[72]

Both these granulocyte-stimulating growth factors have since been studied in randomized clinical trials in patients with solid tumors treated with intensive chemotherapy. Studies that led to U.S. Food and Drug Administration (FDA) approval of these agents demonstrated significant reduction in duration of severe neutropenia compared with patients receiving placebo as well as reduction in days of antibiotic treatment and incidence of confirmed infections.[73,74] These carefully structured studies, with regimens designed to maximize myelosuppression, clearly demonstrated more rapid recovery of neutrophils. It is less clear that there is clinical benefit when these agents are used with chemotherapeutic regimens that produce less severe myelosuppression. Their role in the recovery phase of patients with hematologic malignancies and marrow involvement continues to need further definition.

Guidelines for the Use of Recombinant Granulocyte and Granulocyte-Macrophage Colony-Stimulating Factors

Since the approval of recombinant G-CSFs, the American Society of Clinical Oncology (ASCO) and the American Society of Hematology have worked to develop guidelines for the rational use of hematopoietic growth factors in the supportive care of cancer patients undergoing chemotherapy. The initial guidelines were published in 1996,[75] and most recently, in 2000, an update by the ASCO panel was published.[51]

Primary Use of Colony-Stimulating Factors with Initial Chemotherapy (Primary Prophylaxis)

The review panel used a standard of clinical benefit in the primary prophylaxis setting that was derived from the initial randomized trials that led to approval. This standard was based on the observation that administration of granulocyte CSFs was able to reduce the rate of febrile neutropenia by nearly 50 percent in the treated group as compared with the placebo control group when there was a 40 percent incidence of febrile neutropenia among the control group.[76,77] The value of primary administration of CSFs in conjunction with less intensive chemotherapy regimens has yet to be determined. Thus, the overall recommendation is to use CSFs secondarily for most chemotherapy regimens unless the rate of febrile neutropenia is expected to be in the range of 40 percent.[51] The exception to this would be in patients with additional risk factors for myelosuppression, such as extensive prior therapy or extensive marrow involvement, in which case CSFs might be added to initial therapy. Other mitigating circumstances can be considered as well.

At the time of publication of the guidelines, the use of CSFs to maintain dose intensity was considered to be investigational, awaiting data to support the benefit of this approach to chemotherapy administration.[51] This would be required to show a survival benefit by increasing dose intensity and dose density of a regimen with use of CSFs.

Secondary Prevention of Febrile Neutropenia

The 1996 guidelines for using CSFs following chemotherapy in patients with solid tumors also evaluated the effective use of secondary prevention in those patients who had experienced febrile neutropenia in previous cycles of chemotherapy, or in whom chemotherapy was significantly delayed because of prolonged neutropenia.[75] At that time maintenance of the chemotherapy schedule was advocated. The 2000 guidelines, however, have evaluated the results of eight prospective, randomized trials using either G-CSF or GM-CSF in subsequent cycles of treatment in patients who had initially developed febrile neutropenia.[78–85] As a result of this evaluation, the year 2000 recommendation is that CSFs *not* be routinely used as adjunct therapy for treatment of uncomplicated fever in the setting of neutropenia. Although the eight trials did show a reduction in the duration of neutropenia with a neutrophil count less than 500/μl, they could not define clinical benefit overall in terms of duration of antibiotic treatment or of hospitalization. The panel did note that in patients with serious clinical conditions, the use of CSFs may be considered, but the benefit has not been proved. These conditions would include an absolute neutrophil count (ANC) of less than 100/μl, serious infection such as pneumonia, or a sepsis syndrome with acidosis, hypotension, or multiorgan dysfunction or with a fungal infection. Some might consider age over 65 years to be a high-risk setting, but this has not been confirmed in multicenter trials.

Guidelines for Use of Colony-Stimulating Factors in the Treatment of Acute Leukemias and Myelodysplasia

Initial studies using growth factors were performed in patients with relapsed and refractory leukemia. These studies demonstrated enhancement of neutrophil recovery and the safety of the use of these agents in patients with leukemia.[86–88] Subse-

quently, numerous randomized, placebo-controlled clinical trials have evaluated the use of CSFs during initial remission induction therapy in acute myeloid leukemia (AML)[40,41,89–97] (Table 60–1). Many of these studies specifically evaluated elderly patients because the morbidity of neutropenia is greater in this population.[40,41,89,91,92,94,97] Although the timing of CSF administration varied, with some being administered prior to chemotherapy and some at the time that a marrow specimen showed no leukemic blasts, the outcome was similar. Although CSFs will not eliminate the profound neutropenia inherent in antileukemic therapy, these studies have demonstrated benefits by reducing the duration of neutropenia and the time spent on empirical antibiotics[40,41,89–97] (Table 60–1). The adjunctive use of CSFs in these trials reduced the duration of severe neutropenia (below 500/μl) by 2 to 6 days. There was no benefit to or impairment of the achievement of complete remission. There was no evidence that this approach enhanced the growth of leukemic cells. Most of the studies showed a reduction in length of hospitalization and in duration of antibiotic administration. There was no positive or negative impact on survival in the majority of these studies. The guideline recommendation presents these data and leaves the use of CSFs in leukemia treatment to the discretion of the treating physician.

Colony-stimulating factors are commonly used in the supportive care of patients with myelodysplasia (MDS). Many of these patients are chronically neutropenic, yet not evolving into a more acute leukemic phase.[98–100] Therefore, CSFs have been evaluated in this setting to prevent infections. A randomized trial has been conducted comparing administration of G-CSF with best supportive care.[100] In this study, the ANC improved and there were fewer infections. However, overall survival was shorter for refractory anemia patients with excess blasts who received G-CSF, and there is no immediate explanation for this observation.[100] Another such study is ongoing in the Eastern Cooperative Oncology Group.

The ASCO panel also reviewed four prospective randomized trials evaluating the concept of priming the leukemia with CSF administration and thus making it more susceptible to chemotherapy. In these four studies there was no evidence of the efficacy of this approach in terms of remission rate, remission duration, or survival.[92,93,101,102] Based on its review of the above data, the panel has stated that the data are sufficient to recommend use of CSFs early after remission induction chemotherapy, particularly in older patients and in patients in other high-risk clinical situations.[51]

Studies in acute lymphocytic leukemia (ALL) in both adults and in children have evaluated the role of CSFs, primarily G-CSF.[103–109] In creating guidelines, the panel evaluated five randomized, placebo-controlled studies and one nonrandomized trial. Granulocyte CSF was administered during induction and postremission therapy in ALL. In some of the ALL studies G-CSF was administered concurrently with chemotherapy because the regimens for ALL prescribe more continuous chemotherapy administration. Most of the findings in these studies were similar to those in the AML studies in that there was a decrease of about 5 to 8 days in the duration of neutropenia in both adults and children with ALL who were treated with G-CSF.[103–108] A recent Cancer and Acute Leukemia Group B (CALGB) study in adults with ALL yielded similar results.[110] Although reductions in hospital time and duration of antibiotics were variable in the adult studies, in the pediatric study conducted at St. Jude's Children's Research Hospital there was shortening of hospital stays and a reduction in documented infections.[104] None showed a difference in survival. The panel agreed that the data were sufficient to recommend G-CSF administration during induction therapy for ALL but with discretion, depending on the patient population.[51] In children, the benefits in terms of days in the hospital and duration of antibiotics were quite small. Another important observation from these studies was the safety on administering G-CSF concomitantly with continued corticosteroids and antimetabolite chemotherapy without adverse effects.

Despite the fact that the earliest studies of CSFs in leukemia were in patients with relapsed or refractory AML, no recommendation has been forthcoming.[86–88] In evaluating the use of CSFs in patients undergoing treatment of either AML or ALL in relapse, the panel believed that the data were not sufficient to permit a recommendation. Again, the clinical situation will likely dictate the indication for such an intervention. Importantly, none of the early studies in advanced patients demonstrated stimulation of leukemia, nor did the randomized trials.

Use in Priming for Stem Cell Donation

Large numbers of hematopoietic progenitors are mobilized into the peripheral circulation during the administration of hematopoietic growth factors, given either alone or following combination with myelosuppressive chemotherapy.[64,67] The ability to collect these cells by apheresis has transformed the ease of performing autologous transplantation and has in addition markedly reduced the morbidity of collecting stem cells. With the use of peripheral blood stem cells (PBSC), the morbidity and mortality of autologous transplantation has been greatly reduced because the duration of profound myelosuppression is reduced with autograft support by PBSCs as compared with bone marrow.[111,112] A recent study in patients with AML in remission demonstrated a greater collection of megakaryocyte progenitors in mobilized PBSCs than in marrow,[113] reflecting the clinically observed more rapid platelet recovery with PBSCs.

The ability to mobilize PBSC in chemotherapy-naïve patients is usually easily accomplished with administration of G-CSF or GM-CSF. However, in patients who have been heavily pretreated, the ability to successfully harvest an adequate number of CD34+ cells with standard mobilizing approaches is variable. Studies have evaluated various approaches to enhancing collection of CD34+ cells and the impact on engraftment. Several comparative studies have recently been reported, evaluating the use of growth factor alone, growth factor plus chemotherapy (usually high-dose cyclophosphamide as a mobilizing agent), or the combination of G-CSF and GM-CSF.[114–118] Most studies suggest that the combination of chemotherapy plus growth factor produces a greater yield of CD34+ cells per collection but that adequate numbers could be collected overall with growth factor alone.[114,116,117] There is no difference in rate of engraftment with these different approaches to optimizing collection yield. Studies evaluating the combination of G-CSF

and GM-CSF have suggested a greater contribution from G-CSF in mobilization.[117,118] Mobilized PBSCs have almost replaced bone marrow harvesting except in the case of donors who do not tolerate growth factors or apheresis. Several studies have suggested that a larger dose of G-CSF (10 μg/kg/day) is optimal for stem cell mobilization.[119–122] Recently a study evaluating the combination of thrombopoietin with G-CSF has reported enhanced mobilization of peripheral blood progenitor cells and increases in platelet recovery post-transplant.[123] Further evaluation of this approach is warranted.

The ease with which one can collect large numbers of autologous PBSCs following administration of hematopoietic growth factor alone or in conjunction with cytotoxic chemotherapy has led to the evaluation of growth factor-mobilized allogeneic PBSC collections.[124–127] Many reports seem to concur that there is significantly earlier engraftment with PBSCs. In addition, there is no greater risk or severity of acute graft-versus-host disease (GvHD). However, many but not all reports indicate more severe chronic GvHD.[124–127] This approach remains investigational, attempting to quantitate the risks and benefits.

Of interest, recent studies of growth factor–primed marrow seem to indicate a lesser risk of GvHD with marrow as the source of stem cells, but again not all reports indicate an increased risk with PBSCs.[125,128]

Use of Growth Factors in the Setting of Stem Cell Transplantation

Several studies have been conducted demonstrating the efficacy of both glycosylated (yeast and CHO-derived) GM-CSF and nonglycosylated G-CSF (filgrastim) in accelerating recovery from ablative therapy following autologous stem cell restoration, and now growth factors are routinely used in this setting.[51] This has been done in the setting of solid tumors and non-Hodgkin's lymphoma. Both agents have been approved by the FDA for use in the setting of autologous transplantation. Studies continue to attempt to determine the optimal dose and schedule.[129] Current recommendations for growth factor use in transplantation include use both for PBSC mobilization and after PBSC or marrow infusion.[51]

Growth Factors for Collection of Granulocyte Transfusions

Most recently, it has been determined that growth factors can be safely administered to normal donors, and in many cancer centers this has become an integral part of donor preparation prior to collection of granulocytes. The yield has more than doubled with use of this type of premedication. A major concern regarding the value of granulocyte transfusions has been the ability to provide a sufficient dose to be clinically efficacious; this concern has been met by the finding that administration of growth factors to normal donors is able to enhance yield two- to four-fold.[130–135] Stimulation of normal donors with growth factors also leads to the transfusion of earlier progenitors, which may sustain a circulating granulocyte count for longer periods of time in the recipient.[130,133]

Use of Colony-Stimulating Factors in Pediatric Populations

There is increasing use of hematopoietic growth factors in pediatric oncology protocols as there is increasing intensity of the chemotherapy regimens. It should be noted that the majority of children with malignancies are treated on protocol and it is the protocol that will dictate use of growth factors. With the increased intensity of chemotherapy in childhood malignancy protocols, frequently producing neutropenia that lasts longer than 7 days, growth factors are often but not universally added to the regimen.[51,104,106] However, the question of the benefit of early growth factor use in childhood malignancy protocols is being actively studied. An example is a recent Medical Research Council–United Kingdom study of ALL intensification therapy, which, following a 5-day intensive chemotherapy regimen, randomized children with ALL or T-cell non-Hodgkin's lymphoma to G-CSF following the first or second course of chemotherapy.[136] There was a statistically significant difference in the rate of hospitalization in the group given prophylactic growth factors. However, there was no difference in the duration of neutropenia, time to neutrophil recovery, or duration of supportive care. There was also no difference in cost. A similar study conducted in China evaluated 45 children with AML, 15 of whom were newly diagnosed.[137] All received high-dose chemotherapy plus G-CSF. The nadirs observed were very brief, with or without G-CSF. There was a decrease in infections in those receiving G-CSF.

Others have evaluated the role of CSFs in the treatment of lymphomas in children. A recent French study randomized patients to receiving lenograstim (a glycosylated G-CSF) to best supportive care.[138] With the administration of G-CSF, the duration of neutrophil counts below 500/μl was 3 days shorter. However, the incidence of febrile neutropenia was the same, as was the incidence of infection and mucositis. The ability to deliver the second course on time was greater in those who received G-CSF. However, in summary, there was no increase in dose intensity and no real decrease in morbidity. Thus, in the pediatric population the role of growth factors remains inconclusive.[51]

NEW FORMULATIONS

Lenograstim

There are several formulations of granulocyte growth factors that are in clinical use. In Europe, the glycosylated form of G-CSF (lenograstim) is quite popular and is the subject of a number of new studies. In in vitro studies, lenograstim appears to have 25 percent greater bioavailability than nonglycosylated G-CSF (neupogen).[139] Clinically, the glycosylated form of G-CSF appears to be quite similar to the nonglycosylated form. Randomized studies in Europe are comparing it to no-cytokine control arms in patients treated with chemotherapy. In a study of leukemia treatment with high-dose cytarabine, idarubicin, and etoposide, lenograstim administration produced a significantly shorter duration of severe neutropenia and granulocytopenia, with a reduction in duration of antibiotics and of fever.[140] There was also a reduction in time to start the next course of treatment.

Nevertheless, the outcome is similar to that observed with neupogen in patients with hematologic malignancies.

Peg-Filgrastim

Recently, filgrastim (G-CSF) has undergone changes in formulation to develop a long-acting G-CSF. This has been through the process of pegylation (the addition of polyethylene glycol to the original molecule). This process has produced a molecule called SD/01, which demonstrates slow-release kinetics.[141] A study in mice given chemotherapy with cyclophosphamide and temozolomide, SD/01 as a single dose was compared to G-CSF administered twice daily for 4 days; the results suggest that both agents are capable of enhancing recovery of granulocyte count.[142] With both there were similar kinetics of granulocyte recovery, a similar rate of entry of precursors into peripheral blood, and a peak at 24 hours. There was also a similar peripheral blood half-life and comparable cell divisions.[142] Molineux et al. found that the pegylated form produced a sustained duration of mobilization of peripheral blood progenitors in both mice and humans.[143] This agent has recently entered the market, with the potential of administration once per cycle of chemotherapy (Neulastia).[144,145] Its role in hematologic malignancies will require further investigation.

Correction of Anemia

Most cancer patients become anemic during the course of their illness. In the case of patients with hematologic malignancy, this is most commonly due to infiltration of the marrow by abnormal cells or impaired hematopoiesis secondary to the disease. There may also be a component of treatment-induced anemia. Currently, treatment with erythropoietin is directed toward correction of therapy-induced anemia. The anemia of chronic disease is more difficult to correct and appears to be due largely to a blunted erythropoietin response and an impaired ability of the bone marrow to respond to endogenous erythropoietin. This may be exacerbated by chemotherapy and radiation therapy.

Several studies have evaluated the potential for erythropoietin in patients with hematologic malignancies in whom the marrow is infiltrated with malignant or dysfunctional cells. There are mixed results in terms of the ability to stimulate erythropoiesis. Oster et al. were the first to demonstrate some ability of erythropoietin to stimulate erythropoiesis in patients with anemia due to marrow infiltration by malignant lymphocytes.[146] Five patients with non-Hodgkin's lymphoma and bone marrow involvement and one patient with myeloma were treated with erythropoietin at escalating doses (150, 300, and 450 U/kg administered as an intravenous bolus injection twice weekly for 6, 4, and 4 weeks, respectively). Endogenous erythropoietin levels were increased in all patients (74 to 202 mU/ml). Five of the six patients had a significant increase in their hemoglobin, hematocrit, and red blood cell count on the second erythropoietin dose level. Serum ferritin levels were significantly reduced. In addition, an increase in platelet count was noted. Ludwig et al. treated 13 patients with myeloma-associated anemia by administering erythropoietin three times per week for 6 months. Eleven patients had steady increases in their hemoglobin levels and eventual correction of the anemia.[147]

More recently, a study from Scandinavia in patients with hematologic malignancies and poor performance status has suggested that there is a benefit from erythropoietin administration concurrent with treatment.[148] Although erythropoietin is not routinely recommended for anemia in hematologic malignancies, in given individuals it might offer benefit.

A joint committee of the American Society of Clinical Oncology and the American Society of Hematology has presented guidelines for the use of erythropoietin in patients with malignancy, which include a review of the current clinical evidence defining its use.[149] This document also comments on the use of this agent in patients with marrow infiltration and abnormal marrow function. The current recommendation is for judicious use in patients with chemotherapy-induced anemia and treatment of the primary disease in those with anemia secondary to marrow infiltration.[149]

Recently a long-acting formulation of erythropoietin has been developed to allow weekly administration.[150,151] This compound is termed a novel erythropoiesis-stimulating protein (NESP), and is biochemically distinct from recombinant human erythropoietin.[150,151] Comparative trials have yielded a similar increase in hematocrit when studied in patients who are anemic because of chemotherapy or chronic renal insufficiency.[152–154]

Platelet Growth Factors

Platelet development occurs primarily in the marrow and is stimulated by a number of hematopoietic growth factors and cytokines, including IL-3, IL-6, IL-11, GM-CSF, stem cell factor, and thrombopoietin.[56] Several of these factors have been under development to enhance platelet recovery following chemotherapy-induced thrombocytopenia. They have been less well studied in primary marrow disorders such as leukemia or myelodysplasia.

Interleukin-11 is currently commercially available for use in treatment of chemotherapy-derived thrombocytopenia. Levels of IL-11 do not increase during thrombocytopenia, which suggests that it is not directly responsive to the stimulus of thrombocytopenia. However, preclinical data suggest that IL-11 stimulates increases in circulating progenitors of all hematopoietic lineages.[155] The mechanism for increasing circulating platelets involves enhancement of megakaryocyte size and maturation and thus release of platelets.[156–158] Clinical studies of IL-11 have primarily been in patients with solid tumors undergoing repetitive cycles of chemotherapy.[52–54] There was an apparent reduction in the need for platelet transfusion in a study of multiple cycles of dose-intensive chemotherapy in patients treated for advanced breast cancer in the group receiving IL-11.[43] Despite the multilineage effects of IL-11 in vitro and in animals, there were no apparent effects on leukocytes in these studies.[52–54] Again, evaluation in hematopoietic malignancies has not been made, and given the mechanism of this growth factor, it is not likely to be suitable in the setting of marrow aplasia, since megakaryocytes are required to accelerate platelet production.

Thrombopoietin is undergoing clinical evaluation in the setting of chemotherapy-induced thrombocytopenia.[6,9] The initial phase I clinical trial evaluated a single dose administered 3 weeks before chemotherapy in patients with solid tumors. Major stimulation of marrow megakaryopoiesis was observed with increased numbers and ploidy of megakaryocytes, and this was reflected by increases in circulating platelet counts.[55] Platelet morphology and function were normal. Enhanced platelet counts were initially seen at day 4 after injection of thrombopoietin but continued and peaked between days 10 and 15. Platelet counts at day 21, when chemotherapy was begun, were still higher than the initial baseline counts.[55] An increase in other lineage progenitors was also observed.[55] Although this was primarily a study to demonstrate the clinical effect, it suggested a possibility of using pretreatment to maintain platelet counts through chemotherapy effects. Subsequent clinical evaluation in cancer patients has included administration both before and after chemotherapy.[159,160] In two studies, patients received thrombopoietin both 3 weeks prior to the initial chemotherapy, with a higher nadir than expected, and then following the second course of chemotherapy.[55,159,160] In this setting, there appears to be attenuation of the thrombocytopenia following both the first and second courses. However, the exact schedule for use of this agent is not yet fully developed.

In the setting of marrow failure, such as occurs in aplastic anemia, leukemia, or myelodysplasia, serum thrombopoietin levels are elevated. Therefore, response in this setting to pharmacologic doses of thrombopoietin are not likely to be striking. Trials are ongoing.

CONCLUSIONS

Hematopoietic growth factors, primarily granulocyte-stimulating factors and erythropoietin, are currently used in the mainstream of supportive care for patients with malignancy. In the hematologic malignancies, there appear to be well-defined settings for the judicious and effective use of these agents, and their safety in this setting has been well demonstrated. No proliferation of clinical malignancy has been observed with the use of these agents. The guidelines developed for their use appear to be reasonable and effective.

REFERENCES

1. Cosman D: The hematopoietin receptor superfamily. Cytokine 5:95, 1995.
2. Sims JE, March CJ, Cosman D et al: cDNA expression of the IL-1 receptor, a member of the immunoglobulin superfamily. Science 241:585, 1988.
3. Qiu FH, Ray P, Brown K et al: Primary structure of c-kit: Relationship with the CSF-1/PDGF receptor kinase family – oncogenic activation of v-kit involves deletion of extracellular domain and C terminus. EMBO J 7:1003, 1988.
4. Zang DY, Goodwin RG, Loken MR et al: Expression of tumor necrosis factor-related apoptosis-inducing ligand, Apo 2L, and its receptors in myelodysplastic syndrome: Effects on in vitro hemopoiesis. Blood 98:3058, 2001.

5. Josefsen D, Myklebust JH, Lynch DH et al: Fas ligand promotes cell survival of immature human bone marrow CD34+CD38– hematopoietic progenitor cells by suppressing apoptosis. Exp Hematol 27:1451, 1999.

6. Geddis AE, Linden HM, Kaushansky K: Thrombopoietin: A pan-hematopoietic cytokine. Cytokine Growth Factor Rev 13:61, 2002.

7. Mulcahy L: The erythropoietin receptor. Semin Oncol 28 (2 Suppl. 8):19, 2001.

8. DeKoning JP, Touw IP: Advances in understanding the biology and function of the G-CSF receptor. Curr Opin Hematol 3:180, 1996.

9. Broudy VC, Kaushansky K: Thrombopoietin, the c-mpl ligand, is a major regulator of platelet production. J Leukoc Biol 57:719, 1995.

10. Klein B, Zhang XG, Lu ZY, Bataille R: Interleukin-6 in human myeloma. Blood 85:863, 1995.

11. Wang YD, DeVos J, Jourdan M: Cooperation between heparin-binding EGF-like factor and interleukin-6 in promoting the growth of human myeloma cells. Oncogene 21:2584, 2002.

12. Lauta VM: Interleukin-6 and the network of several cytokines in multiple myeloma: An overview of clinical and experimental data. Cytokine 16:79, 2001.

13. Jourdan M, Tarte K, Legouffe E et al: Tumor necrosis factor is a survival and proliferation factor for human myeloma cells. Eur Cytokine Netw 10:65, 1999.

14. Costes V, Portier M, Lu ZY et al: Interleukin-1 in multiple myeloma: Producer cells and their role in the control of IL-6 production. Br J Haematol 103:1152, 1998.

15. Klein B, Wijdenes J, Zhang XG et al: Murine anti-interleukin-6 monoclonal antibody therapy for a patient with plasma cell leukemia. Blood 78:1198, 1991.

16. Moreau P, Harousseau JL, Wijdenes J et al: A combination of anti-interleukin-6 murine monoclonal antibody with dexamethasone and high-dose melphalan induces high complete response rates in advanced multiple myeloma. Br J Haematol 109:661, 2000.

17. Suematsu S, Matsuda T, Aozasa K et al: IgG1 plasmacytosis in interleukin-6 transgenic mice. Proc Natl Acad Sci U S A 86:7547, 1989.

18. Kovalchuk AL, Kim JS, Park SS et al: IL-6 transgenic mouse model for extraosseous plasmacytoma. Proc Natl Acad Sci U S A 99:1509, 2002.

19. Pelliniemi TT, Irjala K, Mattila K et al: Immunoreactive interleukin-6 and acute phase proteins as prognostic factors in multiple myeloma. Blood 85:765, 1995.

20. Schaar CG, Kaiser U, Snijder S et al: Serum interleukin-6 has no discriminatory role in paraproteinaemia nor a prognostic role in multiple myeloma. Br J Haematol 107:132, 1999.

21. Turesson I, Abildgaard N, Ahlgren T et al: Prognostic evaluation in multiple myeloma: An analysis of the impact of new prognostic factors. Br J Haematol 106:1005, 1999.

22. Wicrzbowska A, Urbanska-Rys H, Robak T: Circulating IL-6-type cytokines and sIL-6R in patients with multiple myeloma. Br J Haematol 105:412, 1999.

23. Wiernik PH, Dutcher JP, Leaf AN et al: Objective response of multiple myeloma to cyclosporine A. Leuk Lymphoma 16:167, 1994.

24. Renauld JC, Vink A, Louahed J, Van Snick J: Interleukin-9 is a major antiapoptotic factor for thymic lymphomas. Blood 85:130, 1995.

25. Menzel T, Rahman Z, Calleja E et al: Elevated intracellular levels of basic fibroblast growth factor correlates with stage of chronic lymphocytic leukemia and is associated with resistance to fludarabine. Blood 87:1056, 1996.

26. Bairey O, Zimra Y, Shaklai M, Rabizadeh E: Bcl-2 expression correlates positively with serum basic fibroblast growth factor and negatively with cellular vascular endothelial growth factor in patients with chronic lymphocytic leukaemia. Br J Haematol 113:400, 2001.

27. Aguayo A, Kantarjian H, Manshouri T et al: Angiogenesis in acute and chronic leukemias and myelosdysplastic syndromes. Blood 96:2240, 2000.

28. Konig A, Menzel T, Lynen S et al: Basic fibroblast growth factor upregulates the expression of bcl-2 in B-cell chronic lymphocytic leukemia cell lines resulting in delayed apoptosis. Leukemia 11:258, 1997.

29. Dancesu M, Rubion-Trujillo M, Biron G et al: Interleukin-4 protects chronic lymphocytic leukemia B-cells from death by apoptosis and upregulates Bcl-2 expression. J Exp Med 176:1319, 1992.

30. Malnou-Fowler T, Copplestone JA, Prentice AG: Effect on interleukins on the proliferation and survival of B-cell chronic lymphocytic leukaemia cells. J Clin Pathol 48:482, 1995.

31. Reittie JF, Hoffbrand AV: Interleukin-4 inhibits proliferation and spontaneous cytokine release by chronic lymphocytic leukaemia cells. Leuk Res 18:55, 1994.

32. Freimann J, Estrov Z, Itoh K et al: Phase I studies of recombinant human IL-4 in patients with hematologic malignancies. Blood 76 (Suppl.):93 (abstr. 361a), 1990.

33. Maher D, Boyd A, McKendrick J et al: Rapid response of B-cell malignancies induced by IL-4. Blood 76(Suppl.):152 (abstr. 600a), 1990.

34. Mackower D, Venkatraj U, Dutcher JP, Wiernik PH: Occurrence of myeloma in a chronic lymphocytic leukemia patient after response to differentiation therapy with interleukin-4. Leuk Lymphoma 23:617, 1996.

35. Lundin J, Kimby E, Bergmann L et al: Interleukin-4 therapy for patients with chronic lymphocytic leukaemia; a phase I/II study. Br J Haematol 112:155, 2001.

36. Lotem J, Sachs L: Hematopoietic cytokines inhibit apoptosis induced by transforming growth factor β1 and cancer chemotherapy compounds in myeloid leukemic cells. Blood 80:2097, 1992.

37. Lotem J, Sachs L: Control of programmed cell death in normal and leukemic cells: New implications for therapy. Blood 82:15, 1993.

38. Bessho M, Susaki K, Hirashima K et al: Prolonged survival of mice with myeloid leukemia by subcutaneous injection of recombinant human G-CSF. Leuk Res 13:1001, 1989.

39. Bhalla K, Tang C, Ibrado AM et al: Granulocyte-macrophage colony-stimulating factor/interleukin-3 fusion protein enhances high-dose Ara-C induced programmed cell death or apoptosis in human myeloid leukemia cells. Blood 80:2883, 1992.

40. Stone RM, Berg DT, George SL et al: Granulocyte-macrophage colony stimulating factor after initial chemotherapy for elderly patients with primary acute myelogenous leukemia. N Engl J Med 332:1671, 1995.

41. Rowe JM, Andersen J, Mazza JJ et al: Phase III randomized placebo-controlled study of granulocyte-macrophage colony-stimulating factor (GMCSF) in adult patients (55–70 years) with acute myelogenous leukemia (AML). A study of the Eastern Cooperative Oncology Group. Blood 82:1299, 1993.

42. Wetzler M, Kurzrock R, Estrov Z et al: Altered levels of interleukin-1 beta and interleukin-1 receptor antagonist in chronic myelogenous leukemia: Clinical and prognostic correlates. Blood 84:3142, 1994.

43. Anand M, Chodda SK, Parikh PM, Nadkarni JS: Abnormal levels of proinflammatory cytokines in serum and monocyte cultures

from patients with chronic myeloid leukemia in different stages and their role in prognosis. Hematol Oncol 16:143, 1998.

44. Otsuka T, Eaves CJ, Humphries RK, Hogge DE, Eaves AC: Lack of evidence for abnormal autocrine or paracrine mechanisms underlying the uncontrolled proliferation of primitive chronic myeloid leukemia progenitor cells. Leukemia 5:861, 1991.

45. Steinman RA, Tweardy DJ: Granulocyte colony-stimulating factor receptor mRNA upregulation is an immediate early marker of myeloid differentiation and exhibits dysfunctional regulation in leukemic cells. Blood 83:119, 1994.

46. Ben-David Y, Berstein A: Friend virus-induced erythroleukemia and the multistage nature of cancer. Cell 66:831, 1991.

47. Longmore G, Lodish H: An activating mutation in the murine erythropoietin receptor induces erythroleukemia in mice: A cytokine receptor superfamily oncogene. Cell 67:1089, 1991.

48. Ridge S, Worwood M, Oscier D et al: FMS mutations in myelodysplastic leukemic and normal subjects. Proc Natl Acad Sci U S A 87:1377, 1990.

49. Roussel MM, Downing J, Sherr C: Transforming activities of human SCF-1 receptors with different point mutations at codon 301 in their extracellular domains. Oncogene 5:25, 1990.

50. Tobal K, Pagliuca A, Bhatt B et al: Mutation of the human *fms* gene (M-CSF receptor) in myelodysplastic syndromes and acute myeloid leukemia. Leukemia 4:486, 1990.

51. Ozer H, Armitage JO, Bennett CL et al: 2000 update of recommendations for the use of hematopoietic colony-stimulating factors: Evidence based, clinical practice guidelines. J Clin Oncol 18:3558, 2000.

52. Tepler I, Elias L, Smith JW et al: A randomized placebo-controlled trial of recombinant human interleukin-11 in cancer patients with severe thrombocytopenia due to chemotherapy. Blood 87:3607, 1996.

53. Gordon MS, McCaskill-Stevens WJ, Battiato LA et al: A phase I trial of recombinant human interleukin-11 (neumega rhIL-11 growth factor) in women with breast cancer receiving chemotherapy. Blood 87:3615, 1996.

54. Issacs C, Robert NJ, Bailey A et al: Randomized placebo-controlled study of recombinant human interleukin-11 to prevent chemotherapy-induced thrombocytopenia in patients with breast cancer receiving dose-intensive cyclophosphamide and doxorubicin. J Clin Oncol 15:3368, 1997.

55. Vadhan-Raj S, Murray LJ, Bueso-Ramos C et al: Stimulation of megakaryocyte and platelet production by a single dose of recombinant human thrombopoietin in patients with cancer. Ann Intern Med 126:673, 1997.

56. Kuter DJ, Cebon LA, Petz LD, McCullough J: Platelet growth factors: Potential impact on transfusion medicine. Transfusion 39:321, 1999.

57. Smith JW II, Longo DL, Alvord G et al: The effects of treatment with interleukin-1α on platelet recovery after high-dose carboplatin. N Engl J Med 328:756, 1993.

58. Postmus PE, Gietema JA, Damsma O et al: Effects of recombinant human interleukin-3 in patients with relapsed small-cell lung cancer treated with chemotherapy: A dose-finding study. J Clin Oncol 10:1131, 1992.

59. Biesma B, Willemse PHG, Mulder NH et al: Effects of interleukin-3 after chemotherapy for advanced ovarian cancer. Blood 80:1141, 1992.

60. D'Hondt V, Humblet Y, Guillaume T et al: Thrombopoietic effects and toxicity with interleukin-6 in patients with ovarian cancer before and after chemotherapy: Multicentric placebo-controlled randomized phase Ib study. Blood 85:2347, 1995.

61. Welte K, Bonilla MA, Gillio AP et al: Recombinant G-CSF: Effects on hematopoiesis in normal and cyclophosphamide treated primates. J Exp Med 165:941, 1987.

62. Welte K, Bonilla MA, Gillio AP et al: *In vivo* effects of recombinant human G-CSF in therapy induced neutropenias in primates. Exp Hematol 15:72, 1987.

63. Gillio AP, Bonilla MA, Potter GK et al: Effects of recombinant human granulocyte colony stimulating factor on hematopoietic reconstitution following autologous transplantation in primates. Transplant Proc 19(suppl. 7):153, 1988.

64. Gabrilove JL, Jakubowski A, Fain K et al: Phase I study of granulocyte colony stimulating factor in patients with transitional cell carcinoma of the urothelium. J Clin Invest 82:1454, 1988.

65. Morstyn G, Souza LM, Keech J et al: Effects of granulocyte colony stimulating factor on neutropenia induced by cytotoxic chemotherapy. Lancet 1:667, 1988.

66. Bronchud MH, Potter MR, Morgenstern G et al: In vitro and in vivo analysis of the effects of recombinant human granulocyte colony stimulating factor in patients receiving intensive chemotherapy for small cell lung cancer. Br J Cancer 58:64, 1988.

67. Duhren U, Villeval JL, Boyd J et al: Effects of recombinant human granulocyte colony-stimulating factor on hematopoietic progenitor cells in cancer patients. Blood 72:2074, 1988.

68. Gabrilove JL, Jakubowski A, Scher H et al: Granulocyte colony stimulating factor reduces neutropenia and associated morbidity of chemotherapy for transitional cell carcinoma of the urothelium. N Engl J Med 318:1414, 1988.

69. Bronchud MH, Scarffe JH, Thatcher N et al: Phase I/II study of recombinant human granulocyte colony stimulating factor in patients receiving intensive chemotherapy for small cell lung cancer. Br J Cancer 56:809, 1987.

70. Morstyn G, Campbell I, Lieschke G et al: Treatment of chemotherapy-induced neutropenia by subcutaneous administered granulocyte colony stimulating factor with optimization of dose and duration of therapy. J Clin Oncol 7:1554, 1989.

71. Donahue RE, Wang EA, Stone EK et al: Stimulation of haematopoiesis in primates by continuous infusion of recombinant human GM-CSF. Nature 321:872, 1986.

72. Monroy RL, Skelly RR, MacVittie TA et al: The effect of recombinant GM-CSF on the recovery of monkeys transplanted with autologous bone marrow. Blood 70:1696, 1987.

73. Crawford J, Ozer H, Stoller R et al: Reduction by granulocyte colony stimulating factor of fever and neutropenia induced by chemotherapy in patients with small cell lung cancer. N Engl J Med 325:164, 1991.

74. Antman KS, Griffin JD, Elias A et al: Effect of recombinant human granulocyte-macrophage colony-stimulating factor on chemotherapy induced myelosuppression. N Engl J Med 319:593, 1988.

75. Ozer H, Miller LL, Schiffer CA et al: Update of recommendations for the use of hematopoietic colony-stimulating factors: Evidence-based clinical practice guidelines. J Clin Oncol 14:1957, 1996.

76. Lyman GH, Lyman CG, Sanderson RA et al: Decision analysis of hematopoietic growth factor use in patients receiving cancer chemotherapy. J Natl Cancer Inst 85:488, 1993.

77. Uyl-de Groot CA, Vellenga E, Rutten FF: An economic model to assess the savings from a clinical application of haematopoietic growth factors. Eur J Cancer 32A:57, 1996.

78. Maher DW, Lieschki GJ, Green M et al: Filgrastim in patients with chemotherapy-induced neutropenia: A double-blind, placebo-controlled trial. Ann Intern Med 121:492, 1994.

79. Mitchell PLR, Morland B, Stevens MCG et al: Granulocyte colony-stimulating factor in established febrile neutropenia. A randomized study of pediatric patients. J Clin Oncol 15:1163, 1997.

80. Vellenga E, Uyl-de Groot CA, de Wit R et al: Randomized placebo-controlled trial of granulocyte-macrophage colony-stimulating factor in patients with chemotherapy-induced febrile neutropenia. J Clin Oncol 14:619, 1996.

81. Anaissie E, Vartivarian S, Bodey GP et al: Randomized comparison between antibiotics alone and antibiotics plus granulocyte-macrophage colony-stimulating factor (Escherichia coli-derived) in cancer patients with fever and neutropenia. Am J Med 100:17, 1996.

82. Mayordomo JI, Rivera F, Diaz-Puente MT et al: Improving treatment of chemotherapy-induced neutropenic fever by administration of colony stimulating factors. J Natl Cancer Inst 87:803, 1995.

83. Ravaud A, Chevreau C, Cany L et al: Granulocyte-macrophage colony-stimulating factor in patients with neutropenic fever is potent after low-risk but not after high-risk neutropenic chemotherapy regimens: Results of a randomized phase III trial. J Clin Oncol 16:2930, 1998.

84. Riikonen P, Saarinen UM, Makipernaa A et al: Recombinant human granulocyte-macrophage colony-stimulating factor in the treatment of febrile neutropenia: A double-blind placebo-controlled study in children. Pediatr Infect Dis J 13:197, 1994.

85. Biesma B, de Vries EG, Willemse PH et al: Efficacy and tolerability of recombinant human granulocyte-macrophage colony-stimulating factor in patients with chemotherapy-related leukopenia and fever. Eur J Cancer 26:932, 1990.

86. Ohno R, Naoe T, Kanamaru A: A double-blind controlled study of granulocyte colony-stimulating factor started two days before induction chemotherapy in refractory acute myeloid leukemia. Blood 83:2086, 1994.

87. Ohno R, Masao T, Kobayashi T et al: Effect of granulocyte colony-stimulating factor after intensive induction therapy in relapsed or refractory acute leukemia. N Engl J Med 323:871, 1990.

88. Ishibashi T, Kimura H, Mita M et al: G-CSF administration does not accelerate leukemic regrowth following intensive induction chemotherapy in acute myelogenous leukemia. Blood 84:2316, 1994.

89. Dombret H, Chastang C, Fenaux P et al: A controlled study of recombinant human granulocyte colony-stimulating factor in elderly patients after treatment for acute myeloid leukemia: AML Cooperative Study Group. N Engl J Med 332:1678, 1995.

90. Heil G, Hoelzer D, Sanz MA et al: The International Acute Myeloid Leukemia Study Group: A randomized, double-blind, placebo-controlled, phase III study of filgrastim in remission induction and consolidation therapy for adults with de novo acute myeloid leukemia. Blood 90:4710, 1997.

91. Godwin JE, Kopecky KJ, Head DR et al: A double-blind placebo-controlled trial of granulocyte colony-stimulating factor in elderly patients with previously untreated acute myeloid leukemia: A Southwest Oncology Group study (9038). Blood 91:3607, 1998.

92. Lowenberg B, Suciu S, Archimbaud E et al: Use of recombinanat GM-CSF during and after remission induction chemotherapy in patients aged 61 years and older with acute myeloid leukemia: Final report of AML-111, a phase III randomized study of the Leukemia Cooperative Group of European Organisation for the Research and Treatment of Cancer and the Dutch-Belgian Hemato-Oncology Cooperative Group. Blood 90:2952, 1997.

93. Zittoun R, Suciu S, Mandelli F et al: Granulocyte-macrophage colony-stimulating factor associated with induction treatment of acute myelogenous leukemia: A randomized trial by the European Organization for Research and Treatment of Cancer Leukemia Cooperative Group. J Clin Oncol 14:2150, 1996.

94. Witz F, Sandoun A, Perrin M-C et al: A placebo-controlled study of recombinant human granulocyte-macrophage colony-stimulating factor administered during and after induction treatment for de novo acute myelogenous leukemia in elderly patients. Blood 91:2722, 1998.

95. Harousseau JL, Witz B, Lioure B et al: Granulocyte colony-stimulating factor after intensive consolidation chemotherapy in acute myeloid leukemia: Results of a randomized trial of the Groupe Ouest-Est Leucemies Aigues Myeloblastiques. J Clin Oncol 18:780, 2000.

96. Usuki K, Urabe A, Masaoka T et al: Efficacy of granulocyte colony-stimulating factor in the treatment of acute myelogenous leukaemia: A multicentre randomized study. Br J Haematol 116:103, 2002.

97. Stone RM, Berg DT, George SL et al: Postremission therapy in older patients with de novo acute myeloid leukemia: A randomized trial comparing mitoxantrone and intermediate-dose cytarabine with standard dose cytarabine. Blood 98:548, 2001.

98. Vadhan-Raj S, Keating M, LeMaister A et al: Effects of human granulocyte-macrophage colony-stimulating factor in patients with myelodysplastic syndrome. N Engl J Med 317:1545, 1987.

99. Negrin RS, Nagler A, Kobayashi Y et al: Maintenance treatment of patients with myelodysplastic syndromes using recombinant human granulocyte colony-stimulating factor. Blood 78:36, 1990.

100. Greenberg P, Taylor K, Larson R et al: Phase III randomized multicenter trial of G-CSF vs observation for myelodysplastic syndrome. Blood 82:196a, 1933.

101. Lowenberg B, Boogaerts MA, Daenen SMGJ et al: Value of different modalities of granulocyte-macrophage colony-stimulating factor applied during or after induction therapy of acute myeloid leukemia. J Clin Oncol 15:3496, 1997.

102. Bhalla K, Birkhofer M, Arlin Z et al: Effect of recombinant GM-CSF on the metabolism of cytosine arabinoside in normal and leukemic bone marrow cells. Leukemia 2:810, 1988.

103. Larson RA, Dodge RK, Linker CA et al: A randomized controlled trial of filgrastim during remission induction and consolidation chemotherapy for adults with acute lymphoblastic leukemia. Blood 92:1556, 1998.

104. Pui C, Boyett JM, Hughes WT et al: Human granulocyte colony-stimulating factor after induction chemotherapy in children with acute lymphoblastic leukemia. N Engl J Med 336:1781, 1997.

105. Ottman OG, Hoelzer D, Gracien E et al: Concomitant human granulocyte colony-stimulating factor and induction chemoradiotherapy in adult acute lymphoblastic leukemia: A randomized phase III trial. Blood 86:444, 1995.

106. Welte K, Reiter A, Mempel K et al: A randomized phase III study of the efficacy of granulocyte colony-stimulating factor in children with high-risk acute lymphoblastic leukemia: Berlin-Frankfurt-Munster Study Group. Blood 87:3143, 1996.

107. Geissler K, Koller E, Hubmann E et al: Granulocyte colony-stimulating factor as an adjunct to induction chemotherapy for adult acute lymphoblastic leukemia: A randomized phase III study. Blood 90:590, 1997.

108. Scherrer R, Geissler K, Kyrle PA et al: Granulocyte colony-stimulating factor as an adjunct to induction chemotherapy in adult acute lymphoblastic leukemia. Ann Hematol 66:283, 1993.

109. Ifrah N, Witz F, Jouet J-P et al: Intensive short term therapy with granulocyte-macrophage colony-stimulating factor support, similar to therapy for acute myeloblastic leukemia, does not improve overall results for adults with acute lymphoblastic leukemia. Cancer 86:1496, 1999.

110. Larson RA, Dodge RK, Linker CA et al: A randomized controlled trial of filgrastim during remission induction and consolidation chemotherapy for adults with acute lymphoblastic leukemia: CALGB Study 9111. Blood 92:1556, 1998.

111. Beyer J, Schwella N, Zingsem J et al: Hematopoietic rescue after high-dose chemotherapy using autologous peripheral-blood progenitor cells or bone marrow: A randomized comparison. J Clin Oncol 13:1328, 1995.

112. Schmitz N, Linch DC, Dreger P et al: Randomized trial of filgrastim-mobilized peripheral blood progenitor cell transplantation versus autologous bone marrow transplantation in lymphoma patients. Lancet 347:353, 1996.

113. Briggs M, Adams JA, Brereton ML et al: Comparison of megakaryopoiesis in vitro of paired peripheral blood progenitor cells and bone marrow harvested during remission in patients with acute myeloid leukaemia. Br J Haematol 115:563, 2001.

114. Koc ON, Gerson SL, Cooper BW et al: Randomized cross-over trial of progenitor-cell mobilization: High-dose cyclophosphamide plus granulocyte colony-stimulating factor (G-CSF) versus granulocyte-macrophage colony-stimulating factor plus G-CSF. J Clin Oncol 18:1824, 2000.

115. Charrier S, Chollet P, Bay JO et al: Hematological recovery and peripheral blood progenitor cell mobilization after induction chemotherapy and GM-CSF plus G-CSF in breast cancer. Bone Marrow Transplant 25:705, 2000.

116. Alegre A, Tomas JP, Martinez-Chamorro C et al: Comparison of peripheral blood progenitor cell mobilization in patients with multiple myeloma: High-dose cyclophosphamide plus GM-CSF vs G-CSF alone. Bone Marrow Transplant 20:211, 1997.

117. Narayanasami U, Kanteti R, Morelli J et al: Randomized trial of filgrastim versus chemotherapy and filgrastim mobilization of hematopoietic progenitor cells for rescue in autologous transplantation. Blood 98:2059, 2001.

118. Weaver CH, Schulman KA, Buckner CD: Mobilization of peripheral blood stem cells following myelosuppressive chemotherapy: A randomized comparison of filgrastim, sargramostim, or sequential sargramostim and filgrastim. Bone Marrow Transplant 27(Suppl. 2):S23, 2001.

119. Nademanee A, Sniecinski AI, Schmidt GM et al: High-dose chemotherapy followed by autologous peripheral blood stem-cell transplantation for patients with Hodgkin's disease and non-Hodgkin's lymphoma using unprimed and granulocyte colony-stimulating factor-mobilized peripheral blood stem cells. J Clin Oncol 12:2176, 1994.

120. Snowden JA, Biggs JC, Milliken ST et al: A randomized, blinded, placebo-controlled, dose escalation study of the tolerability and efficacy of filgrastim for hematopoietic stem cell mobilization in patients with severe rhematoid arthritis. Bone Marrow Transplant 22:1035, 1009.

121. Weaver CH, Birch R, Greco FA et al: Mobilization and harvesting of peripheral blood stem cells: Randomized evaluations of different doses of filgrastim. Br J Haematol 100:338, 1998.

122. Somlo G, Sniecinski I, Ahn C et al: Priming with G-CSF 10 mg/kg is more effective than 5 mg/kg in patients receiving high-dose chemotherapy followed by peripheral stem cell rescue. Proc Am Soc Hematol 82:642a, 1993.

123. Somlo G, Sniecinski I, terVeer A et al: Recombinant human thrombopoietin in combination with granulocyte colony-stimulating factor enhances mobilization of peripheral blood progenitor cells, increases peripheral blood platelet concentration and accelerates hematopoietic recovery following high dose chemotherapy. Blood 93:2798, 1999.

124. Zaucha JM, Gooley T, Bensinger WI et al: CD34 cell dose in granulocyte colony-stimulating factor-mobilized peripheral blood mononuclear cell grafts affects engraftment kinetics and development of extensive chronic graft-versus-host disease after human leukocyte antigen-identical sibling transplantation. Blood 98:3221, 2001.

125. Nivison-Smith I, Bradstock KF, Szer J et al: Allogeneic haemopoietic cell transplants in Australia, 1996 – a multi-center restrospective comparison of the use of peripheral blood stem cells with bone marrow. Bone Marrow Transplant 28:21, 2001.

126. Bensinger WI, Storb R: Allogeneic peripheral blood stem cell transplantation. Rev Clin Exp Hematol 5:67, 2001.

127. Sulis ML, VandeVen C, Henderson T, Anderson L, Cairo MS: Liposomal amphotericin B (AmBisome) compared with amphotericin B ± FMLP induces significantly less in vitro neutrophil aggregation with granulocyte-colony-stimulating factor/dexamethasone-mobilized allogeneic donor neutrophils. Blood 99:384, 2002.

128. Morton J, Hutchins C, Durrant S: Granulocyte-colony-stimulating factor (G-CSF)-primed allogeneic bone marrow: Significantly less graft-versus-host disease and comparable engraftment to G-CSF-mobilized peripheral blood stem cells. Blood 98:3186, 2001.

129. Ener RA, Meglathery SB, Cuhaci B et al: Use of granulocyte colony-stimulating factor after high-dose chemotherapy and autologous peripheral blood stem cell transplantation: What is the optimal timing? Am J Clin Oncol 24:19, 2001.

130. Adkins D, Spitzer G, Johnston M et al: Transfusions of granulocyte colony-stimulating factor-mobilized granulocyte components to allogeneic transplant recipients: Analysis of kinetics and factors determining post-transfusion neutrophil and platelet counts. Transfusion 37:737, 1997.

131. Adkins D, Ali S, Despotis G, Dynis M, Goodnough LT: Granulocyte collection efficiency and yield are enhanced by the use of a higher interface offset during apheresis of donors given granulocyte colony-stimulating factor. Transfusion 38:557, 1998.

132. Catalano L, Fontana R, Scarpato N et al: Combined treatment with amphotericin-B and granulocyte transfusion from G-CSF-stimulated donors in an aplastic patient with invasive aspergillosis undergoing bone marrow transplantation. Haematologica 82:71, 1997.

133. Murea S, Fruehauf S, Zeller WJ, Haas R: Granulocytes harvested following G-CSF-enhanced leukocyte recovery retain their functional capacity during in vitro culture for 72 hours. J Hematother 5:351, 1996.

134. Nomura A, Ohga SD, Matsuzaki A et al: Granulocyte transfusion: Stimulation of low dose granulocyte colony-stimulating factor in donors for leukapheresis. Acta Paediatr Jpn 38:317, 1996.

135. Wortel N, Kurz M, Peters C, Hocker P: Serial granulocytapheresis under daily administration of rHuG-CSF: Effects on peripheral blood counts, collection efficiency, and yield. Transfusion 41:390, 2001.

136. Little MA, Morland B, Chisholm J et al: A randomised study of prophylactic G-CSF following MRC UKALL XI intensification regimen in childhood ALL and T-NHL. Med Pediatr Oncol 38:98, 2002.

137. Shang X, Yin H, Lu A, Zhang L: Application of recombinant human granulocyte colony stimulating factor in children with acute myeloid leukemia. Chin Med J (Engl) 112:620, 1999.

138. Patte C, Laplanche A, Bertozzi AI et al: Granulocyte colony-stimulating factor in induction treatment of children with non-Hodgkin's lymphoma: A randomized study of the French Society of Pediatric Oncology. J Clin Oncol 20:441, 2002.

139. Bonig H, Silbermann S, Weller S et al: Glycosylated vs non-glycosylated granulocyte colony-stimulating factor (G-CSF) – results of a prospective randomised monocentre study. Bone Marrow Transplant 28:259, 2001.

140. Bradstock K, Matthews J, Young G et al: Effects of glycosylated recombinant human granulocyte colony-stimulating factor after high-dose cytarabine-based induction chemotherapy for adult acute myeloid leukemia. Leukemia 15:1331, 2001.

141. Morstyn G, Foote MA, Walker T, Molineux G: Filgrastim (r-metHuG-CSF) in the 21st century: SD/01. Acta Haematol 105:151, 2001.

142. Lord BI: Kinetics of neutrophil production with SD/01. Clin Cancer Res 7:2085, 2001.

143. Molineux G, Kinstler O, Briddell B et al: A new form of filgrastim with sustained duration in vivo and enhanced ability to mobilize PBPC in both mice and humans. Exp Hematol 27:1724, 1999.

144. Johnston E, Crawford J, Blackwell S et al: Randomized, dose-escalation study of SD/01 compared with daily filgrastim in patients receiving chemotherapy. J Clin Oncol 13:2522, 2000.

145. Holmes FA, O'Shaughnessy JA, Vukelja S et al: Blinded, randomized, multicenter study to evaluate single administration pegfilgrastim once per cycle versus daily filgrastim as an adjunct ot chemotherapy in patients with high-risk stage II or stage III/IV breast cancer. J Clin Oncol 20:727, 2002.

146. Oster W, Hermann F, Gamm H et al: Erythropoietin for the treatment of anemia of malignancy associated with neoplastic bone marrow infiltration. J Clin Oncol 8:956, 1990.

147. Ludwig H, Fritz E, Kotzmann H et al: Erythropoietin treatment of anemia associated with multiple myeloma. N Engl J Med 322:1693, 1990.

148. Osterborg A, Brandberg Y, Molostova V et al: Randomized, double-blind, placebo-controlled trial of recombinant human erythropoietin, epoetin beta, in hematologic malignancies. J Clin Oncol 20:2486, 2002.

149. Rizzo JD, Lichtin AE, Woolf SH et al: Use of epoetin in patients with cancer: Evidence-based clinical practice guidelines of the American Society of Clinical Oncology and American Society of Hematology. J Clin Oncol 20:4083, 2002.

150. Demetri GD: Anaemia and its functional consequences in cancer patients: Current challenges in management and prospects for improving therapy. Br J Cancer 84(Suppl. 1):31, 2001.

151. Sunder-Plassmann G, Horl WH: The clinical potential of novel erythropoiesis stimulating protein. Expert Opin Biol Ther 1:733, 2001.

152. Heatherington AC, Schuller J, Mercer AJ: Pharmacokinetics of novel erythropoiesis stimulating protein (NESP) in cancer patients: Preliminary report. Br J Cancer 84(Suppl. 1):11, 2001.

153. Ibbotson T, Goa KL: Darbepoetin alfa. Drugs 61:2097, 2001.

154. Glaspy J, Jadeja JS, Justice G et al: A dose-finding and safety study of novel erythropoiesis stimulating protein (NESP) for the treatment of anaemia in patients receiving multicycle chemotherapy. Br J Cancer 84(Suppl. 1):17, 2001.

155. Goldman SJ: Preclinical biology of interleukin-11: A multi-functional hematopoietic cytokine with potent thrombopoietic activity. Stem Cells 13:462, 1995.

156. Welch NS, Neben TY Donaldson D et al: Interleukin-11 acts directly to promote megakaryocytopoiesis (abstr). Blood 86 (Suppl. 1): 364a, 1995.

157. Mason L, Timony G, Perkin C et al: Human recombinant interleukin 11 promotes maturation of bone marrow megakaryocytes in non-human primates: an electron microscopic study (abstr.). Blood 82 (suppl. 1): 69a, 1993.

158. Du XX, Williams DA: Interleukin-11: A multifunctional growth factor derived from the hematopoietic microenvironment. Blood 83:2023, 1994.

159. Vadhan-Raj S, Patel S, Broxmeyer HE et al: Phase I-II investigation of recombinant human thrombopoietin (rh TPO) in patients with sarcoma receiving high dose chemotherapy with Adriamycin and ifosfamide. Blood 88:448a, 1996.

160. Vadhan-Raj S, Verschraegen C, Bueso-Ramos C et al: Recombinant human thrombopoietin (rhTPO) attenuates carboplatin-induced severe thrombocytopenia and the need for platelet transfusions in patients with gynecologic malignancy. Ann Intern Med 132:364, 2000.

61

Bleeding and Thrombosis in Hematologic Neoplasia

Thomas G. DeLoughery

Excessive bleeding or thrombosis complicates the treatment of many patients with hematologic malignancies. The pathogenesis and therapy of some of these disorders, such as thrombocytopenia due to chemotherapy, is usually straightforward. However, other hemostatic defects are more complex. For example:

1. Malignant cells can produce and release thromboplastic or fibrinolytic substances that cause disseminated intravascular coagulation (DIC) or primary fibrinolysis (for example, acute promyelocytic leukemia [APL]).
2. The pathologic process can provoke the megakaryocyte to produce dysfunctional platelets with bleeding or thrombosis (chronic myeloproliferative disorders).
3. Abnormal lymphocytes or plasma cells sometimes produce aberrant proteins that interfere with normal hemostasis (multiple myeloma, amyloid).
4. Certain antitumor or antimicrobial agents used in the treatment of malignancy or its complications can cause thrombosis or bleeding (L-asparaginase or some β-lactam antibiotics).

This chapter focuses on bleeding and thrombotic disorders that are associated with hematologic neoplasia. Thrombocytopenic bleeding and platelet transfusion therapy are covered elsewhere in this volume.

COAGULATION DISORDERS

APL is the leukemia classically associated with coagulation defects with evidence of DIC occurring in the majority of patients.[1] Pathogenesis and therapy of the coagulation defects of APL are described in detail in Chapter 21.

Acute Myelomonocytic and Other Leukemias

Overt DIC occurs only rarely in patients with acute leukemias other than APL. However, it may be seen in patients with myeloid leukemias who present with very high peripheral blast counts or after sudden cell lysis induced by intensive chemotherapy.[2–4] About 25 percent of patients with acute monocytic leukemia (M5) were found to have laboratory evidence of intravascular coagulation[5–7] with about 50 percent of

patients having increased D-dimer, thrombin-antithrombin (TAT), low fibrinogen, low α2-PI levels, or elevated elastase-α1 antitrypsin complexes.[5,7,8] A high incidence of subdural hematomas has been reported in patients with monocytic leukemia, perhaps reflective of the incidence of intravascular coagulation.[9] DIC has been reported in chronic myelocytic leukemia (CML) both with and without blast crisis[10–13] and in acute lymphocytic leukemia, especially of the T-cell type.[14–16] Biochemical markers of DIC have been found in many patients with ALL including elastase-α1-antitrypsin complexes and rapid fibrinogen turnover.[17] When studied prospectively, DIC was seen in 12 percent of patients with ALL before chemotherapy, which rose to 78 percent during chemotherapy.[18] Complications included sagittal vein thrombosis in three patients and pulmonary embolism in one.[18]

Subclinical intravascular clotting may be much more common in acute leukemia than previously appreciated. Fibrinopeptide A (FPA) levels in plasma (indicating thrombin action on fibrinogen) were found to be high in many patients with acute leukemia without overt DIC before treatment, but with a prompt rise in FPA after institution of cytolytic therapy.[19] The FPA levels returned to normal in remission, and in a few instances, rising levels predicted relapse. Another study suggested that leukemic cells that lacked cell-associated procoagulant activity can still incite a coagulopathy via the release of interleukin (IL)-1, a potent stimulator of endothelial tissue factor synthesis and inhibitor of thrombomodulin, an essential cofactor for the activation of protein C.[20]

The best way to treat DIC is to treat the underlying leukemia but one must be prepared for an exacerbation of the DIC when tumor lysis occurs. One should obtain the basic tests of coagulation at the time of leukemia diagnosis. If the patient has DIC then the panel should be repeated at least daily and more often if coagulation defects develop. Using the results of these tests guides one in replacement therapy of DIC (Table 1–1). Past concerns about "feeding the fires" have not been shown to be clinically valid and one should strive to maintain hemostatic competence to avoid severe bleeding.[21,22] Plasma is used for factors replacement if depletion occurs and bleeding ensues.[23] One should strive for decreasing the activated partial thromboplastin time (aPTT) to less than 1.5 times normal if possible. Keeping the fibrinogen level over 100 mg/dl is also reasonable. Heparin therapy is rarely needed for the leukemic

---

Table 61–1. Management of Disseminated Intravascular Coagulation

1. Hematocrit
2. Platelet count
3. Prothrombin time
4. Activated partial thromboplastin time
5. Fibrinogen level

A. Platelets < 50–75,000/μl—Give platelet concentrates or 6–8 pack of single donor platelets
B. Fibrinogen < 125 mg/dl—Give 10 units of cryoprecipitate
C. Hematocrit below 30 percent—Give red cells
D. Protime > INR 2.0 *and* aPTT abnormal give 2–4 units of FFP

patient with DIC. However, if it is required, reliance on the aPTT to follow heparin therapy may lead to over- or under-treatment of patients and one should follow heparin levels in these patients.[24,25]

Several other coagulation abnormalities have been reported in leukemia, including low factor V levels in Philadelphia chromosome-positive CML in children,[26] and a decrease in the thrombin-sensitive subunit of factor XIII in a patient with acute leukemia and DIC.[27] One report documented the secretion of two types of plasminogen activators by human myeloid leukemia cells in vitro.[28] The quantity or type of plasminogen activator that was secreted by these leukemic cells could not be correlated with either bleeding or the clinical severity of the disease.

PLATELET DYSFUNCTION

Chronic Myeloproliferative Disease

The chronic myeloproliferative disorders (MPD), which include essential thrombocythemia (ET), polycythemia vera (PV), agnogenic myeloid metaplasia (AMM), and CML are clonal disorders characterized by an expansion of the hematopoietic precursors in the marrow and blood, along with splenomegaly. All of these disorders are associated with thrombocytosis, and with the notable exception of CML, commonly provoke bleeding or thrombosis. The diagnoses of PV and ET can now be made much earlier with the advent of the endogenous erythroid colony assay, a test that documents the erythropoietin-independent growth of erythroid colonies in semisolid agar cultures.[29–37]

Bleeding and Thrombosis

Excessive bleeding occurs frequently in patients with PV, ET, and AMM and is usually due to defects in platelet function. The incidence of hemorrhage is difficult to quantitate because the frequency can vary relative to the underlying disease process (more common in AMM[38]), stage of disease, age, and the presence of comorbid conditions. Overall, about 25 to 30 percent of patients will have bleeding, in 5 percent it will be severe, but it will be fatal in less than 1 percent.[35,39–44] Symptoms are usually limited to easy bruisability or epistaxis, but gastrointestinal bleeding seems particularly common in PV. Nonsteroidal anti-inflammatory drugs used for symptomatic pain relief or for antithrombotic prophylaxis can substantially increase the risk of hemorrhage in patients who have platelet dysfunction.

Thrombosis occurs more frequently in PV and ET than in AMM or CML, and is a major cause of morbidity and mortality in patients with myeloproliferative disorders. Arterial occlusion is the most common, followed by venous thromboembolism, and then microvascular thrombosis (digital skin necrosis, or erythromelalgia).[40,42,43,45–55]

The overall frequency of thrombosis is difficult to calculate, but it is more common than bleeding, and causes greater morbidity and mortality. Cross-sectional studies suggest that approximately 30 to 40 percent of patients have thrombosis, and several large studies indicated that thrombotic complica-

tions occurred at approximately 3.4 to 8 percent per/year.[48,53,54] The most common thromboses are cerebral vascular occlusion, deep venous thrombosis of the lower extremities, vascular occlusion of the digits, and particularly central abdominal thromboses (portal, hepatic, mesenteric vein). Increasing age, elevated hematocrits, and treatment with phlebotomy in PV all predispose to thromboembolism. However, the magnitude of the elevation of the platelet count does not correlate with the risk of thrombosis. For example, some patients with very early MPD documented by erythroid colony assays who have normal or near normal platelet counts can have repeated severe thromboses.[30,37,56] Others, for example, young women with platelet counts of more than $2,000,000/cm^3$, often remain free of symptoms for many years. Several studies have showed that the majority of thrombotic complications in ET occurred in individuals with platelet counts of less than 600,000 to $800,000/cm^3$.[40,57,58]

Erythromelalgia is a syndrome of painful toes and fingers associated with MPD. It is characterized by thrombocytosis and biopsy evidence of microvascular subendothelial vascular proliferation. In some cases, symptomatic platelet-mediated thromboses occur in the digits that can produce tissue ischemia and even gangrene.[59,60] Erythromelalgia secondary to MPD often responds dramatically to low doses of aspirin.[59,61]

Mechanisms of Platelet Dysfunction

Sensitive tests of platelet function are frequently abnormal in chronic MPD, particularly PV, ET, and AMM. Tests of platelet reactivity correlate poorly with elevations of the platelet count or with syndromes of bleeding and thrombosis.[62] However, a rough relationship exists between a high circulating platelet count, impaired platelet function, and bleeding.[39,63–66] High platelet counts are also associated with increased platelet reactivity and vascular thrombosis, erythromelalgia, and peripheral gangrene.[59,61,67,68] Studies determining clonal status of patients with ET have demonstrated many patients actually do not have clonal disease.[69] In one small study patients who had clear evidence of clonal disease had a higher risk of thrombosis.[70]

Decreased Platelet Function

Platelet function has been examined in several series of patients with chronic MPD.[66,71–81] Although abnormalities of platelet function are quite common in vitro, the bleeding time is usually normal or, in about 20 percent of patients, mildly prolonged.[66,72,73,78,80] Rarely, the presenting clinical scenario is excessive bleeding and a markedly prolonged bleeding time, which is most often seen in patients with AMM.[27,82] The most common platelet function defect is abnormal platelet aggregation following the addition of collagen, adenosine diphosphate (ADP), or particularly epinephrine, to platelet-rich plasma.[66,72,73,78,80,83,84] In most reports, however, meager correlations have been found between changes in platelet function, prolongation of the bleeding time, and clinically evident bleeding.[62,74,77] It should be noted that platelet aggregation testing is usually normal in patients with a reactive thrombocytosis, even if the platelet count exceeds $1,000,000/mm^3$.[73]

Myriad platelet function disorders have been discovered in patients with MPD. These include specific defects in the platelet membrane, the release of platelet coagulant activity, abnormal prostaglandin synthesis, and disordered platelet-dense granule composition and/or function. Platelet membrane abnormalities include the deficiency of several glycoproteins important for normal platelet aggregation,[85,86] increased numbers of platelet Fc receptors for immune complexes, or aggregated IgG,[87] and prostaglandin D_2 or thromboxane A_2 receptor numbers and/or function.[88]

Platelet prostaglandin synthesis has been shown to be inhibited, with decreased production of thromboxane A_2, after stimulation of the arachidonic acid pathway.[85,89] Defects in lipoxygenase activity have been reported[90] as well as reduced platelet generation of lipoxin.[91] Finally, patients have been reported with decreased numbers of dense granules (i.e., the granules containing storage pool ADP) in their platelets, as visualized by electron microscopy. A reduction in dense granule content has been correlated with prolongation of the bleeding time.[75,92,93] Decreased alpha granule content has also been described.[94,95] Other defects include the inability of stimulated platelets to expose procoagulant phospholipid despite normal membrane phospholipid composition.[45,66,96]

Finally, patients with very high platelet counts (greater than $1,000,000/cm^3$) can have acquired von Willebrand's disease demonstrated by reduced ristocetin cofactor activity despite normal plasma levels of von Willebrand antigen and factor VIII coagulant activity.[97–99] The decreased plasma von Willebrand factor activity may be due to accelerated proteolysis of von Willebrand factor after its release from endothelial cells.

Increased Platelet Activity

Several studies have identified platelet "hyper-reactivity" in patients with MPD.[67,71,72,74,78–80,83,84,100–102] A variety of tests to assess platelet reactivity have been used including the spontaneous platelet aggregation during ex vivo testing, increased plasma level of the platelet-specific protein β-thromboglobulin, decreased circulating platelet aggregate ratios, platelet phospholipid-dependent thrombin generation, and increased platelet responsiveness to inhibitory prostaglandins. Although in some reports there appeared to be a correlation between increased platelet function and vascular thrombosis, it is not possible to predict clinical thrombotic events with the use of these assays.

Several investigators have measured levels of platelet specific proteins (platelet factor 4, β-thromboglobulin, or platelet-derived growth factor) in patients with MPD. Platelet concentrations of three proteins were reduced, whereas plasma and urinary levels were increased.[103–106] These findings suggest that intravascular platelet activation occurred, which could explain platelet-mediated thrombosis or marrow fibrosis.[104,107]

Other Laboratory Tests of Thrombophilia

Increased levels of homocystine have been reported in patients with MPD but have not correlated with thrombosis.[108,109] Low levels of the anticoagulant proteins S and C have been reported but large case series linking these defects to thrombosis are lacking.[110] Given that MPDs are clonal diseases it may be that other cell lines are contributing to the thrombophilia. One study demonstrated increased monocyte generation of tissue factor that was linked with elevated levels of prothrombin F1.2 fragment.[111] Another study suggested that neutrophil activation is abnormally high in MPD and is associated with signs of increased coagulation.[112] Thus, it may be an interplay between multiple cell lines that leads to the thrombosis seen in MPD.

Clinical Laboratory Tests

Laboratory tests such as the complete blood count, platelet count, bleeding time, and platelet aggregation studies are frequently abnormal in patients with MPD, but unfortunately they often fail to predict bleeding or thrombosis in individual patients. One study suggested that patients with a high reticulated platelet count suggestive of increase platelet turnover had a higher risk of thrombosis.[113] However, patients with PV and markedly elevated hematocrits are at substantial risk of thrombosis, and patients with AMM or others with very high platelet counts (more than $1,000,000/cm^3$) and markedly prolonged bleeding times are likely to have an increased risk of bleeding. Non-COX selective nonsteroidal anti-inflammatory drugs should be used with caution in the latter instance.

Erythroid progenitor cells cultured in semisolid agar from patients with PV and ET are highly sensitive to small amounts of erythropoietin (EPO).[31,32,34,37] This observation has become the basis for a highly sensitive and specific clinical test to identify patients with these disorders. Peripheral blood or bone marrow is cultured on semisolid agar for 7 to 14 days in the presence and absence of EPO. In contrast to normal subjects, erythroid colonies from patients with MPD proliferate in the absence of exogenous EPO. Actually, small amounts of EPO are present in the fetal calf serum used in the assay, which is sufficient to promote the growth of erythroid colonies from patients with PV and ET, but not those from normal subjects.

In our experience, and in that of others, the endogenous erythroid colony assay can be positive in patients with normal or near normal peripheral blood counts and bone marrow morphology, particularly those with a history of arterial or venous thrombosis of unknown cause.[30,33,46,56] The assay should be considered as part of a laboratory evaluation in patients with recurrent thrombosis (particularly arterial and central abdominal venous thrombosis) who do not have other hereditary or acquired hypercoagulable states. For example, in several studies over 50 percent of patients presenting with portal vein thrombosis were found to have endogenous erythroid colony growth in the absence of added EPO.[30,33,56]

Therapeutic Considerations

Hemorrhage. Major bleeding complicating MPD can usually be managed with platelet transfusions to overcome disease-induced platelet function defects. In a few patients, particularly those with very high platelet counts, platelet transfusions will be ineffective. In these instances, therapeutic platelet apheresis with acute lowering of the platelet count followed by transfusion of normal platelets may temporarily improve hemostasis.

Platelet reduction on a long-term basis with hydroxyurea or other therapeutic agents may decrease symptoms of bleeding. Finally, phlebotomy in patients with PV has been reported to improve platelet function tests and to decrease bleeding in some instances.[94,95]

A diagnosis of acquired von Willebrand's disease should be considered in patients with MPD who have excessive bleeding. In particular, ristocetin-induced platelet aggregation studies should be obtained along with measurement of ristocetin cofactor activity. If these tests are abnormal, then DDAVP (desmopressin acetate; Rhone-Poulenc Rorer Pharmaceuticals, Inc., Collegeville, PA) can be tried. Alternatively, factor VIII concentrates that are rich in von Willebrand factor such as Humate-P (Armour Pharmaceutical Company, Kankakee, IL) should be considered. In an emergency, cryoprecipitate can also be used as a source of high-molecular-weight multimers of von Willebrand factor, although there will be an increased chance of transfusion-transmitted viral infection.

Venous Thrombosis. Either standard or low-molecular-weight heparin followed by warfarin is indicated for most patients with acute venous thromboembolism complicating the myeloproliferative disorders. Thrombolytic therapy should be considered in patients who have acute occlusion of the hepatic or portal veins. Long-term oral anticoagulants (INR 2 to 3) are usually recommended for prevention of recurrent thromboses. In a few instances, liver transplantation has been successful in treating liver failure due to Budd-Chiari syndrome.[114,115] These patients need to be anticoagulated after transplant to prevent recurrent thrombosis.

Arterial and Microvascular Thrombosis. Antiplatelet therapy, usually with aspirin, is recommended for treatment of patients with cerebral, coronary artery, or peripheral vascular thrombosis. Platelet inhibitors usually suppress the platelet hyper-reactivity associated with MPD and can increase the usually shortened mean platelet survival time.[116] Low doses of aspirin (80 to 360 mg/day) are preferable in patients with MPD because the risk of bleeding with aspirin is dose-related. One study using 100 mg/day appeared to be effective for preventing thrombosis without excessive bleeding as long as the platelet count was kept at under 1,000,000/cm^3.[117] Currently a large trial of low-dose aspirin is being conducted in patients with polycythemia.[118] Microvascular disease such as erythromelalgia or digital gangrene often responds dramatically to antiplatelet therapy.[116] In addition to its antithrombotic effects, aspirin may also inhibit platelet secretion of vascular growth factors and thereby reduce chronic vascular damage. There are currently no data concerning the use of newer antiplatelet agents such as clopidogrel.

A few patients will develop serious recurrent thromboembolic events despite treatment with aspirin. In such cases, combined anticoagulation (INR 2 to 3) and antiplatelet therapy should be considered.[119] The likelihood of bleeding will be increased, but the risks might be warranted in some patients. Careful monitoring will be required, particularly in patients known to have platelet dysfunction or a history of bleeding.

In addition to pharmacologic antithrombotic measures, lowering of elevated platelet counts should be considered in patients with MPD and a history of thrombosis. Hydroxyurea (1 g daily to start) is preferable to radioactive phosphorous or alkylating agents because of a lesser risk of leukemogenesis. A platelet count of 250,000 to 450,000/cm^3 is an appropriate target. A randomized trial of high-risk patients (age over 60 or history of thrombosis) demonstrated that using hydroxyurea to maintain the platelet count less than 600,000/cm^3 was associated with significantly less thrombosis (3.6 vs. 24 percent).[120]

Increasingly anagrelide, an imidazo-quinozoline derivative, is being used to lower platelet counts in MPD patients.[121–123] Unlike hydroxyurea no clinical trial data exist on the efficacy of anagrelide in preventing thrombosis in high-risk patients. One long-term study of patients did demonstrate a 20 percent thrombosis rate in patients taking anagrelide.[124] However, platelet counts were above 400,000 μl/mm in all patients who had thrombosis, leaving unclear whether the agent would have been more successful at preventing thrombosis if the platelet counts were lower.[125] Anagrelide has also been associated with cardiovascular side effects and is not recommend for patients with a history of heart disease. Approximately 20 percent of patients will have to stop the drug due to intolerable side effects.[124,125] α-Interferon has also been reported to be effective but its antithrombotic effect is unknown.[126,127]

An even more difficult problem is whether to lower platelet counts or to give aspirin to patients with MPD who do not have a history of thrombosis. The evidence from the literature is conflicting; some studies suggest that young patients can tolerate very high platelet counts without major thrombosis, whereas others indicate that young as well as older patients remain at risk of thrombosis and bleeding.[47,128,129] Platelet reduction with hydroxyurea should be considered in asymptomatic older subjects with platelet counts over 1,000,000/cm^3, particularly if they have atherosclerosis, risk factors for arterial disease, or symptoms of vascular ischemia.[130] Also important is controlling reversible risk factors such as smoking or elevated cholesterol.

Low-dose aspirin therapy may be appropriate for some patients for prophylaxis against thrombosis. However, gastrointestinal bleeding rates were high in a group of patients treated with aspirin from the PRV Study Group.[49] One approach is to exclude patients from treatment if they have a history of peptic ulcer disease or prolonged bleeding time or abnormal platelet function analysis. The remaining patients can be given a trial using low doses of aspirin, and the bleeding time repeated. If it remains less than 15 minutes, therapy can be continued. Patients who develop new gastrointestinal symptoms while on aspirin therapy can be treated with gastric cytoprotective agents.

Pregnancy

An increasing challenge is the increase in the number of young women with ET who become pregnant. Interestingly the platelet count often decreases during pregnancy, often to near normal levels.[131,132] The most common adverse event is an increase in miscarriages due to placental infarction.[132,133] One series reported several episodes of severe bleeding related to acquired von Willebrand's disease.[133] Due to the physiologic decrease in platelet count during pregnancy and concerns about fetal heath, cytoreduction therapy is not recommended. There is increasing use of aspirin and/or low-molecular-weight heparin to prevent miscarriages but the success rate of this approach is uncertain.[132]

Acute Leukemia and the Myelodysplastic Syndromes

Studies of platelet function in patients with acute leukemia have been difficult because severe thrombocytopenia is so often present. However, platelets from patients with acute granulocytic leukemia show abnormalities in size and granulation on light microscopy, as well as marked variations in granular content, disturbances of microtubule function, and striking dilatation of the open canalicular system by electron microscopy.[134,135] Some investigators believe that they can distinguish two populations of cells—a normal population and a second "leukemic" population, showing marked variations in size, shape, and granular structure.[135]

Platelet function in acute leukemia has been shown to be abnormal, with defects of platelet aggregation in response to epinephrine, ADP, and collagen, as well as a lack of storage granules and impaired platelet factor III release.[134,136–138] Platelet function and morphology usually return to normal after a complete remission has been attained. The etiology of the platelet dysfunction has not been clearly defined but is most likely attributable to disease-induced abnormalities in the megakaryocyte. Alternatively, some platelets may undergo the release reaction within the circulation and thereby have deficient storage pool ADP and other morphologic changes.[134]

Studies of platelet morphology and function in the various myelodysplastic syndromes have found abnormalities similar to those reported in acute leukemia and the chronic myeloproliferative diseases. In many cases, megakaryocytes are normal to moderately increased in number in the marrow, are quite small, and have decreased nuclear "ploidy" with abnormal cytoplasmic granulation.[135,139] As in acute leukemia, the platelets show numerous changes on electron microscopy, including unusual giant granules, lack of microtubules, and a dilated open canalicular system.[76,134] A variety of platelet function defects have been described, but impaired platelet aggregation and a variably increased bleeding time are most prevalent.[50,77] Abnormalities of platelet function occur in acute megakaryocytic leukemia including defects in platelet aggregation ex vivo.[140–143] Platelet dysfunction has also been reported in refractory anemias or the preleukemic syndrome characterized by a 5q– or abnormalities of chromosome 3.[144–146] Relative or absolute thrombocytosis is sometimes seen in these disorders.

Hairy Cell Leukemia

The platelet count in hairy cell leukemia is usually low, due to marrow infiltration with lymphocytes or hypersplenism, and the platelets often show abnormal aggregation to epinephrine, ADP, and sometimes collagen.[147–149] Furthermore, the granular content of ADP and serotonin is decreased, the release of ADP may be impaired, and prostaglandin synthesis may be inhibited.[150] On electron microscopy, the platelets are virtually agranular and show a dilated open canalicular system.[150] Several reports indicate that most of the platelet function defects

and abnormal morphology return to normal after splenectomy.[148,150] The mechanisms for these changes are unknown, but it has been postulated that these platelets undergo activation in the spleen and then recirculate with an acquired storage pool deficiency ("exhausted" platelets).[150]

Paroxysmal Nocturnal Hemoglobinuria

Paroxysmal nocturnal hemoglobinuria (PNH) remains a poorly understood clonal hematopoietic disorder.[151] One of the leading causes of morbidity and mortality is thrombosis.[152–154] Patients can present with venous or arterial thrombosis. Also, like MPD, PNH is associated with a high incidence of visceral vein thrombosis. The cause of the hypercoagulable state is unknown but complement-activated platelets have been implicated.[155] In two large series, the rate of thrombosis in PNH was 28 to 39 percent with thrombosis leading to death in 58 percent.[153,156] Given the high rate of thrombosis it has been advocated that patients with PNH should receive prophylactic anticoagulation, even without a history of thrombosis. Patients with thrombosis should be aggressively treated with oral anticoagulants but "breakthrough" thrombosis has been reported.

ABNORMAL PROTEINS

Dysproteinemias

Although uncommon, defects in coagulation and platelet function may pose serious problems in the management of patients with dysproteinemias. Bleeding symptoms seem to be more frequent in macroglobulinemia and IgA myeloma, in dysproteinemias associated with κ rather than λ light chains, and in patients with total protein concentrations greater than 8 g/dl or serum viscosities greater than 5.[157,158] Patients with prolonged bleeding times and decreased platelet adhesiveness also are at a higher risk of hemorrhage than those with normal platelet function.[157,158]

Multiple coagulation abnormalities have been described in patients with dysproteinemias (Table 61–2). First, the physical structure of the fibrin clot may be abnormal, owing to increased serum globulins. Electron microscopy shows an amorphous collection of proteins covering the fibrin strands. The clot is therefore more gelacious and friable than normal and is highly susceptible to local fibrinolytic enzymes.[159] Clot retraction is absent in some patients with a dysproteinemia because the abnormal protein prevents the attachment of platelet pseudopods to one another or to fibrin strands.[159]

Polymerization of fibrin is impaired in some patients with circulating λ light chains, which is suggested by prolonged thrombin or reptilase times. Myeloma proteins have also been shown to inhibit the thrombin time of normal plasma.[160,161] More detailed studies have demonstrated that the antibody-binding portion of the myeloma protein, rather than the heavy chain, is involved in the inhibition of α-chain polymerization of fibrinogen.[160] The receptor for factor XIIIa activity on fibrin strands can be blocked by an abnormal protein, which leads to an increased circulating level of factor XIII.[162,163] Lastly, some

Table 61–2. Abnormalities of Coagulation in Myeloma and Amyloid

---

Abnormal fibrin clot
Abnormal clot retraction
Impaired fibrin polymerization
Factor X deficiency (amyloid)
Factor VIII inhibitor
Systemic fibrinolysis (amyloid)
Inhibition of thrombin time
Heparinlike anticoagulation
Anti-glycoprotein IIb/IIIa

---

patients with plasma cell leukemia have a potent heparinlike anticoagulant that produces very severe and often fatal bleeding (as discussed below).[164]

Platelet abnormalities are less well defined in patients with myeloma and macroglobulinemia, although prolonged bleeding times and abnormal platelet adhesiveness to glass beads have been described. Presumably both defects are due to inhibition of platelet function by abnormal proteins.[157,165,166] In one instance, a purified IgG$_1$-κ paraprotein was shown to bind to platelet glycoprotein IIIa inhibiting platelet aggregation and provoking a severe bleeding disorder.[167]

Therapy for the hemostatic defects in the dysproteinemic syndromes include removal of the offending protein, either by reducing synthesis by treating the plasma cell dyscrasia, or by intensive plasmapheresis. In several patients, return of normal hemostasis was correlated with a substantial reduction in the paraprotein spike in the serum.[157,166]

Despite the myriad effects on hemostasis, very little has been reported on procoagulant effects of myeloma. There is one report of a light chain with lupus anticoagulant activity associated with a deep venous thrombosis.[168] Also an inhibitor leading to acquired protein S deficiency has been reported.[169] However, there appears to be no systematic study of procoagulant defects in myeloma.

Patients with systemic amyloidosis, either primary or associated with myeloma, show a marked increase in easy bruisability and other bleeding symptoms. The most common defects in coagulation testing of patients with amyloid is an elevation in the thrombin time, which is seen in 30 to 80 percent of cases.[170,171] An increase prothrombin time is seen in 20 to 24 percent and an increase aPTT in 70 percent. Factor X deficiency was first reported to be associated with amyloidosis in 1962; subsequent studies have shown that the clotting factor is adsorbed onto amyloid proteins.[172,173] Splenectomy, plasmapheresis, and treatment with melphalan and prednisone have been reported to reduce the amyloid burden and to increase the levels of factor X.[174–177] However, one report indicates that many of the bleeding symptoms in this disorder are due to amyloid infiltration of blood vessels, rather than to coagulation or platelet defects. Studies of 100 sequential patients with amyloidosis at a single institution failed to identify a single individual with acquired factor X deficiency.[178] However a large case series at another institute reported a 14 percent incidence of low factor X with 5 percent of patients having levels below 20 per-

cent.[170] In patients with factor X deficiency receiving bone marrow transplant improvement in factor X levels was seen in those patients who responded to transplant.[179]

Two other hemostatic defects have been reported to complicate primary amyloidosis. In one instance, circulating Bence Jones protein formed complexes with plasma fibrinogen and interfered with the polymerization of fibrin monomer as evidenced by a prolonged thrombin time.[180] Abnormal thrombin and reptilase times are found in up to 30 percent of patients.[170] In another, a circulating inhibitor to factor VIII was found to be an IgA-κ monoclonal protein similar in structure to the amyloid subunit protein.[181]

Yet another cause of bleeding in patients with systemic amyloidosis is systemic fibrino(geno)lysis.[182–186] The euglobulin clot lysis time is shortened with striking decreases in α$_2$-PI, plasminogen, and circulating plasmin-antiplasmin complexes. Some patients have also been reported to have elevated plasma levels of tissue-type plasminogen activator.[184,187] The mechanisms responsible for the fibrinolytic state are not known but could be due to increased release of plasminogen activators or decreased plasminogen activator inhibitors from blood vessels infiltrated with amyloid, decreased α$_2$-PI because of its adsorption onto amyloid fibrils, or perhaps amyloid liver disease. The use of fibrinolytic inhibitors such as EACA or tranexamic acid have both corrected laboratory tests of fibrinolysis and reduced bleeding symptoms.

Immune Thrombocytopenic Purpura

Immune thrombocytopenic purpura (ITP) is not commonly associated with hematologic neoplasms, but has been reported in chronic lymphocytic leukemia, and in approximately 2 percent of patients with Hodgkin's disease,[188–202] but rarely as a complication of non-Hodgkin's lymphoma.[192,196,203,204] ITP is known to predate the onset of Hodgkin's disease, to occur at the time of diagnosis, to indicate a recurrence (within the spleen), or to develop in disease-free individuals long after they have been considered cured.

The presentation of ITP in patients with lymphoproliferative diseases is usually not different than in other patients and is associated with decreased platelet survival and elevated levels of platelet-associated IgG.[188–190,196,198] Why ITP occurs during the course of lymphoproliferative disease is not well understood, although a disturbed immune system could possibly predispose patients both to the lymphoproliferative disorder and to thrombocytopenia.[199,205] Rare cases of acquired Glanzmann thrombasthenia have been reported with Hodgkin's disease and other lymphoproliferative disorders.[206] Acquired thrombasthenia should be tested for when bleeding appears to be out of proportion to the decrease in platelet count.

Therapy for the ITP that complicates Hodgkin's disease or chronic lymphocytic leukemia does not differ from that for classic immune thrombocytopenia.[207,208] High-dose corticosteroids (plus anti-D or immunoglobulin if necessary) are given first, but if an adequate platelet count cannot be maintained and bleeding prevented with "acceptable" daily doses of corticosteroids, splenectomy should be undertaken. If removal of the spleen fails to increase the platelet count, immunosuppressive therapy with vincristine, azathioprine, or pulse cyclophosphamide may be tried.[209,210] Other treatment modalities include intravenous gamma globulin, pulse dexamethasone, plasmapheresis, danazol, and possibly cyclosporin or interferon-α.[209,211,212]

A search for recurrent Hodgkin's disease should be undertaken in patients who develop ITP after successful remission induction therapy. However, since ITP occurs often in patients without active Hodgkin's disease, antineoplastic chemotherapy should not be started empirically without pathologic documentation of recurrent disease. ITP has even occurred in patients with Hodgkin's disease who have had splenectomy or who were receiving intensive massive immunosuppressive therapy.[192,195,197,199,201]

Coagulation Factor Inhibitors

Coagulation factor inhibitors are rare in patients with acute or chronic lymphoproliferative disorders with the exception of an acquired form of von Willebrand's disease. Like patients with congenital von Willebrand disease's, patients with the acquired form have markedly prolonged bleeding times with the individual components of the factor VIII macromolecular complex reduced to 10 to 20 percent of normal.[156,213–220] When multimeric analysis of von Willebrand factor is performed both type 1 and type 2 variants have been found.[98,221–224]

There are at least three major mechanisms producing the acquired defect.[156] The first is the presence of circulating autoantibody against the von Willebrand factor. These antibodies can interfere with the function of the protein or result in augmented clearance. The second mechanism is increase absorption of the protein onto abnormal lymphoid cells or platelets.[215,216,219,220] For example, a case report demonstrated that the aberrant expression of glycoprotein 1b by a marginal zone lymphoma results in acquired von Willebrand's disease.[225] Finally increased proteolysis of the von Willebrand proteins has been reported, especially in myeloproliferative disorders.[97–99]

Therapeutic measures have included infusions of cryoprecipitate or concentrates containing vWF, DDAVP, plasma exchange, intravenous immunoglobulin, or splenectomy (when von Willebrand factor was shown to bind to the abnormal lymphocytes).[97,213,216,217,226–228] In a large series of patients with acquired von Willebrand's disease associated with IgG monoclonal gammopathies, immunoglobulin (1 g/kg/day for 2 days) was the most effective in indicating a response.[169] In one case of severe bleeding the use of recombinant factor VIIa was effective when other measures had failed.[229]

In a few patients with lymphoproliferative disease, acquired factor VIII inhibitors have developed.[181,230,231] An inhibitor to prothrombin accelerated clearance of the protein.[232] An antibody directed against thrombin has also been reported with myeloma in which plasmapheresis was effective in reducing bleeding.[233]

Finally, circulating coagulation inhibitors with heparinlike properties have been described in patients with multiple myeloma and other neoplasms.[228,234–236] These patients present with very severe bleeding along with elevated aPTTs and thrombin times, but a normal reptilase time. The disease is caused by

circulating proteoglycan similar to heparin. This proteoglycan has antithrombin enhancing activity, and can be blocked by protamine sulfate, platelet factor 4, or toluidine blue in vitro.[228,235,236] These heparinlike anticoagulants regularly cause severe and unrelenting bleeding, which is often fatal. Therapy is difficult but has included intensive chemotherapy to reduce the malignant cell burden, plasmapheresis to remove the anticoagulant, and intravenous protamine sulfate.[236]

THERAPY-INDUCED BLEEDING AND THROMBOSIS

L-Asparaginase

L-Asparaginase is an enzyme from bacteria that destroys asparagine, an amino acid required by leukemic, but not normal, cells. When used as a chemotherapeutic agent, it has a number of side effects, including hypersensitivity reactions, pancreatitis, liver insufficiency with decreased protein synthesis, neuropathy, and somnolence.[237]

L-asparaginase also lowers circulating hemostatic, anticoagulant, and fibrinolytic factors, with substantial decreases in plasma fibrinogen, factor IX, factor XI, antithrombin III, protein C, protein S, and plasminogen.[238–248] These effects are most likely due to diminished protein synthesis by the liver; there is no evidence for clotting factor consumption or the production of abnormal molecules.[248,249] This reduction in protein synthesis appears to be proportional to the effectiveness of L-asparaginase in eliminating asparagine from the plasma.[250,251] As soon as therapy is discontinued, the clotting factors return rapidly to normal. Fortunately, L-asparaginase does not interfere with platelet production, and platelet counts return to normal even during continued administration for remission induction in patients with ALL.[252,253]

The concentrations of the anticoagulant proteins antithrombin III, protein C, and protein S can fall to 30 percent of normal in some patients receiving L-asparaginase, levels low enough to predispose to thrombosis.[241,246] Crossed immuno-electrophoresis of antithrombin III shows no abnormality in the mobility.[246] Levels of antithrombin III biologic activity have generally paralleled reductions in antithrombin III antigen, although exceptions may occur.[246] Alterations in the multimeric composition of von Willebrand factor and variable defects in platelet function have also been reported.[247,254]

At first, the coagulopathy induced by L-asparaginase was attributed to DIC. Low levels of fibrinogen, increased FDP, a positive protamine sulfate test for fibrin monomer, and low levels of factor V and factor VIII have all been reported.[244] However, recent studies have shown normal survival of labeled fibrinogen and no evidence of increased thrombin generation.[249,255] Some of the early reports of DIC may have represented patients who were predisposed to intravascular clotting because of their underlying disease (a T-cell lymphoma), which then became overt due to L-asparaginase-induced decreases in circulating antithrombin III or other anticoagulant proteins. Although marked reductions in fibrinogen, factor XI, and factor IX due to L-asparaginase have been observed frequently, excessive bleeding is rare.[238,248] If bleeding does occur, cryoprecipitate or fresh frozen plasma rapidly corrects the hemostatic defects.

In contrast central nervous system (CNS) thrombosis can be a major clinical problem in patients with acute lymphocytic leukemia given L-asparaginase and occurs in approximately 1 to 2 percent of patients with childhood ALL and up to 4 percent of adults.[237,245,249,256–261] Small cerebral blood vessels can be occluded by thrombus, producing bland or hemorrhagic infarction. Dural sinus vein thromboses are also common. Thrombosis usually occurs 2 to 3 weeks after the start of a course of therapy. Most patients recover, although several deaths have been reported and others are left with debilitating neurologic defects. Peripheral deep venous thrombosis seems to be less common.[257]

The pathogenesis of the thrombotic complications of L-asparaginase therapy remains obscure, although decreased levels of antithrombin III, protein C, protein S, and plasminogen could predispose to thrombosis because of inadequate inhibition of circulating activated clotting factors or deficient fibrinolytic activity. The low levels of circulating fibrinogen do not seem to be protective, since a patient has been reported in whom a major CNS thrombosis developed even though the plasma fibrinogen had fallen to 20 mg/dl.[262] The presence of an inherited hypercoagulable state such as factor V Leiden or the prothrombin gene mutation raise the risk of thrombosis with L-asparaginase therapy.[263,264]

Optimal therapy of the thromboembolic complications of the L-asparaginase depends on whether intracerebral bleeding or thrombosis is identified on computed tomography (CT) or magnetic resonance imaging (MRI) scans. If hemorrhage is present, heparin should not be used. However, in the absence of bleeding, systemic anticoagulation with heparin may benefit some patients with cerebral sinus-vein thrombosis.[259] Markedly low levels of antithrombin III, protein C, or protein S should be corrected with antithrombin III concentrates, or concentrates of protein C and protein S when they are available. In one study, prophylactic use of fresh frozen plasma was ineffective in preventing the decrease in antithrombin III induced by therapy.[265]

Antibiotic-Induced Coagulopathies

Antibiotics have been increasingly recognized as a cause of bleeding in patients treated for infectious complications of hematologic neoplasia. Two categories of hemostatic defects have been described. First, vitamin K-dependent clotting factor synthesis can be impaired, leading to prolonged prothrombin or partial thromboplastin times.[266,267] Second, platelet function is inhibited by certain β-lactam antibiotics such as high-dose penicillin, carbenicillin, and ticarcillin.[267–276]

The mechanisms underlying the reduction of the vitamin K-dependent clotting factors are not clear, although the antibiotics can destroy the bowel bacteria that produce vitamin K.[266,267] Alternatively, decreases of hepatic clotting factor synthesis or inhibition of the post-translational gamma-carboxylation reaction required for the biologic activity of the vitamin K-dependent clotting factors could occur. The N-methylthiotetrazole side chain found in some of the new cephalosporins can inhibit the

Table 61–3. Antibiotics Containing the Methylthiotetrazole Group

Cefamandole
Cefoperazone
Cefotetan
Cefmetazole
Cefonicid
Cefotiam

action of vitamin K (Table 61–3).[267,277–279] Bleeding seems to be more frequent in severely debilitated patients with poor nutrition or liver disease, or those receiving prolonged intravenous feedings. The hemostatic defect can appear within 1 week of starting antibiotic therapy. Fortunately, the disorder may be quickly reversed or prevented by therapeutic doses of oral or parenteral vitamin K1 or, if severe, and the patient is bleeding, fresh frozen plasma.[267,275,278] Prophylactic vitamin K is now administered to leukemic patients who are likely to require long-term antibiotics.[280–282]

The antibiotic-induced defect in platelet function has been described with some, but not all β-lactam antibiotics. Susceptible patients can have markedly prolonged bleeding times, and experience marked bleeding after surgery or other invasive procedures.[267,270,272,276] The incidence of antibiotic-induced platelet dysfunction is not known, although it is higher in debilitated, uremic, or malnourished patients. When healthy subjects are treated for up to 2 weeks, bleeding times are normal or only slightly prolonged.[269,270,274,278,283]

The impairment of platelet function is due to the blockade of ADP (and possible von Willebrand factor)-binding sites on platelet membranes, with inhibition of platelet fibrinogen and/or von Willebrand factor binding.[267,269–271,273,278,283,284] Platelets from patients receiving high doses of these antibiotics have impaired ADP-, collagen-, and epinephrine-induced platelet aggregation. Platelet intracellular signaling is also defective.[271,284–286]

The antibiotic induced inhibition of ADP-induced platelet aggregation does not occur when antibiotics are added to platelet-rich plasma in vitro. Moreover, platelet function abnormalities begin only after 3 to 4 days of antibiotic administration and then persist for 4 to 8 days after therapy has been stopped.[270,274,278,283] This sequence of events suggests that the antibiotic reacts with megakaryocytes, rather than circulating platelets. Patients who are being treated for acute leukemia and infections but who are receiving platelet transfusions do not seem to have an excessive tendency to bleed, which could reflect the lack of a direct inhibitory effect on the transfused platelets. Platelet transfusions correct both the platelet function defect and excessive bleeding.[267,268]

Finally, certain antibiotics can induce immune thrombocytopenia. For example, vancomycin has been implicated in refractoriness to platelet transfusion. The mechanism mimics HLA alloimmunization.[287] In two instances antibodies were discovered that were vancomycin dependent and bound to glycoprotein IIb and/or IIIa.[288] Amphotericin B can also lead to both thrombocytopenia and decreased recovery of transfused platelets.[289,290]

Drug-Induced Hemolytic-DIC Syndromes

A severe variant of the drug-induced immune complex hemolysis has been recently recognized. Rare patients who receive certain second- and third-generation cephalosporins such as cefotetan, ceftriaxone, cefoxitin, and ceftizoxime have been reported to develop this syndrome of fulminant hemolysis and DIC.[291–294] The most common agents associated with this syndrome are cefotetan and ceftriaxone.[295]

The clinical syndrome starts 7 to 10 days after receiving the drug. Often the patient has only received the antibiotic for surgical prophylaxis. The patient will develop severe Coombs' positive hemolysis with hypotension and DIC. The patients are often believed to have sepsis and often re-exposed to the cephalosporin, resulting in worsening of the clinical picture. The outcome is often fatal due to massive hemolysis and thrombosis.[291,294,296,297]

Treatment of the drug-induced hemolytic-DIC syndrome is anecdotal. Patients have responded to aggressive therapy including plasma exchange, dialysis, and prednisone. Early recognition of the hemolytic anemia and the suspicion it is drug related is important for early diagnosis so that the incriminating drug can be discontinued.

Chemotherapeutic Agents

Adjuvant chemotherapy for breast cancer has been associated with an increased risk of both arterial and venous thromboembolism (5 to 7 percent of patients).[298,299] The thrombogenic stimulus is not clear, but could reflect vascular damage by the chemotherapeutic agents, or perhaps a reduction in protein C or protein S concentrations.[300] Very low levels of warfarin (INR 1.5) can prevent the thrombotic events.[301] With increasing use of thalidomide for myeloma concern is being raised about a possible hypercoagulable effect with one small trial reporting a thrombosis rate of 27 percent in patients receiving thalidomide, dexamethasone, and doxorubicin.[82]

Patients receiving certain chemotherapy agents can develop a severe thrombotic microangiopathy closely resembling the hemolytic-uremic syndrome. Mitomycin-C is most commonly associated with this disorder, but other agents include *cis*-platinum, daunorubicin, cytosine arabinoside, bleomycin, cyclosporine, and gemcitabine.[302–307] Unusually large multimers of von Willebrand factor have been demonstrated in the plasma.[304] The disorder is usually fulminant and rapidly fatal, but anecdotal reports of successful treatment with staphylococcal protein A columns have been published.[305,308] An unusual aspect of mitomycin-C induced microangiopathy is clinical worsening after patients are transfused with red blood cells.[308]

Bone Marrow Transplantation

Hepatic veno-occlusive disease (VOD) is a relatively common complication of bone marrow transplantation and is seen in 1 to 50 percent of patients, but the frequency seems to vary widely from center to center.[309,310] The clinical syndrome includes weight gain, hepatic tenderness, and jaundice soon after transplantation, which can progress to liver failure and the hepatorenal syndrome. In one large study of 355 patients, hepatic VOD developed in 54 percent with a mortality of 39 percent.[311] Early thrombosis of the hepatic venules leading to obstruction and eventual fibrosis is the most commonly accepted mechanism for VOD.[309] Pre-existing liver dysfunction, especially hepatitis C, is an important risk factor for development of the disorder.[309,312–316] Conditioning regimens that include busulfan also increase the incidence.[309,311] The risk also appears to be higher in patients undergoing allogeneic rather than autologous transplantation.[311]

Multiple coagulation defects have been demonstrated, but low levels of protein C prior to transplant were a strong and reproducible predictor of VOD.[317–319] For example, all patients with a baseline protein C value of less than 66 percent of normal developed the syndrome.[318] At present, it is unclear whether the decreased level of protein C is simply a surrogate marker for underlying liver disease, or constitutes a specific pathogenetic mechanism. Elevated levels of plasminogen activator inhibitor-1 have been suggested as a noninvasive test for VOD.[320,321]

Prothrombotic cytokines such as tumor necrosis factor (TNF) and IL-6 have been shown to be elevated in patients with VOD, and markers of activation of hemostasis such as F1.2 and TAT are also increased.[322] Antithrombotic therapy has been employed to halt the thrombotic process. A randomized trial demonstrated that heparin at a dose of 100 U/kg/day beginning 8 days prior to transplant and continuing for 30 days thereafter decreased the rate of VOD from 13 to 2.5 percent, and in patients receiving allogeneic transplants from 18 to 0 percent.[323] Thrombolytic therapy with urokinase or t-PA has been used for treatment of patients with established VOD.[324] A small pilot study of seven patients with severe VOD treated with 10 mg/day × 2 days of t-PA followed by heparin showed a response in five of seven patients but a larger follow-up study demonstrated a high risk of bleeding, especially in patients who already had developed multiorgan system failure.[325] Early reports also indicate the use of defibrotide is effective in therapy of VOD.[326,327] Currently a large trial of this agent is underway to determine its usefulness in VOD.

REFERENCES

1. DeLoughery TG, Goodnight SH: Acute promyelocytic leukaemia in the all trans retinoic acid era (Review). Med Oncol 13:233–240, 1996.
2. Goodnight SH: Bleeding and intravascular clotting in malignancy: A review. Ann N Y Acad Sci 230:271, 1974.
3. Baker WG, Bang NU, Nachman RL, Raafat F, Horowitz H: Hypofibrinogenemic hemorrhage in acute myelogenous leukemia treated with heparin. Ann Intern Med 61:116, 1964.
4. Leavy RA, Kahn SG, Brodsky I: Disseminated intravascular coagulation—a complication of chemotherapy in acute myelomonocytic leukemia. Cancer 26:142, 1970.
5. Shaw MT: The distinctive features of acute monocytic leukemia. Am J Hematol 4:97, 1978.

6. Straus DJ, Mertelsmann R, Koziner B, McKenzie S, De Harven E, Arlin ZA et al: The acute monocytic leukemias: Multidisciplinary studies in 45 patients. Medicine (Baltimore) 59:409, 1980.

7. Tobelem G, Jacquillat C, Chastang C, Auclerc MF, Lechevallier T, Weil M et al: Acute monoblastic leukemia: A clinical and biologic study of 74 cases. Blood 55:71, 1980.

8. Speiser W, Kyrle PA, Kapiotis S, Kottas-Heldenberg A, Bettelheim P et al: Hemostatic and fibrinolytic parameters in patients with acute myeloid leukemia: Activation of blood coagulation, fibrinolysis and unspecific proteolysis. Blut 61:298–302, 1990.

9. Jourdan E, Dombret H, Glaisner S, Miclea JM, Castaigne S, Degos L: Unexpected high incidence of intracranial subdural haematoma during intensive chemotherapy for acute myeloid leukaemia with a monoblastic component. Br J Haematol 89:527–530, 1995.

10. German HJ, Smith JA, Lindenbaum J: Chronic intravascular coagulation associated with chronic myelocytic leukemia. Use of heparin in connection with a surgical procedure. Am J Med 61:547, 1976.

11. Gingrich RD, Burns CP: Disseminated coagulopathy in chronic myelomonocytic leukemia. Cancer 44:2249, 1979.

12. Whittaker JA, Khurshid M: Hypofibrinogenaemia as a cause of bleeding in chronic myeloid leukaemia. Br Med J 1:495, 1975.

13. Hirsh J, Buchanan JG, De Gruchy GC, Baikie AG: Hypofibrinogenaemia without increased fibrinolysis in leukaemia. Lancet 1:418, 1967.

14. Champion LAA, Luddy RE, Schwartz AD: Disseminated intravascular coagulation in childhood acute lymphocytic leukemia with poor prognostic features. Cancer 41:1642, 1978.

15. Edson JR, Krivit W, White J, Sharp HL: Intravascular coagulation in acute stem cell leukemia successfully treated with heparin. J Pediatr 71:342, 1967.

16. French AJ, Lilleyman JS: Bleeding tendency of T-cell lymphoblastic leukaemia. Lancet 469–470, 1979.

17. Tornebohm E, Egberg N, Sablica H, Wallin R, Lockner D, Paul C: Elastase activity in leukaemic cells and plasma in patients with acute leukaemia. Eur J Haematol 49:98–104, 1992.

18. Sarris AH, Kempin S, Berman E, Michaeli J, Little C, Andreeff M et al: High incidence of disseminated intravascular coagulation during remission induction of adult patients with acute lymphoblastic leukemia. Blood 79:1305–1310, 1992.

19. Myers TJ, Rickles FR, Barb C, Cronlund M: Fibrinopeptide A in acute leukemia: Relationship of activation of blood coagulation to disease activity. Blood 57:518, 1981.

20. Cozzolino F, Torcia M, Miliani A, Carossino AM, Giordani R, Cinotti S et al: Potential role of interleukin-1 as the trigger for diffuse intravascular coagulation in acute nonlymphoblastic leukemia. Am J Med 84:240–250, 1988.

21. Feinstein DI: Diagnosis and management of disseminated intravascular coagulation: The role of heparin therapy (Review). Blood 60:284–287, 1982.

22. Rocha E, Paramo JA, Montes R, Panizo C: Acute generalized, widespread bleeding. Diagnosis and management (Review). Haematologica 83:1024–1037, 1998.

23. de Jonge E, Levi M, Stoutenbeek CP, Van Deventer SJH: Current drug treatment strategies for disseminated intravascular coagulation. Drugs 55:767–777, 1998.

24. Brill-Edwards P, Ginsberg JS, Johnston M, Hirsh J: Establishing a therapeutic range for heparin therapy (see comments). Ann Int Med 119:104–109, 1993.

25. Olson JD, Arkin CF, Brandt JT, Cunningham MT, Giles A, Koepke JA et al: College of American Pathologists Conference XXXI on Laboratory Monitoring of Anticoagulant Therapy—Laboratory monitoring of unfractionated heparin therapy. Arch Pathol Lab Med 122:782–798, 1998.

26. Hasegawa DK, Bennett AJ, Coccia PF et al: Factor V deficiency in Philadelphia-positive chronic myelogenous leukemia. Blood 56:585, 1980.

27. Rodeghiero F, Barbui T, Battista R et al: Molecular subunits and transamidase activity of factor XIII during disseminated intravascular coagulation in acute leukemia. Thromb Haemost 43:6, 1980.

28. Wilson EL, Jacobs P, Dowdle EB: The secretion of plasminogen activators by human myeloid leukemic cells in vitro. Blood 61:568, 1983.

29. Juvonen E, Ikkala E, Oksanen K, Ruutu T: Megakaryocyte and erythroid colony formation in essential thrombocythaemia and reactive thrombocytosis: Diagnostic value and correlation to complications. Liver 83:192–197, 1993.

30. Valla D, Casadevall N, Lacombe C, Varet B, Goldwasser E, Franco D et al: Primary myeloproliferative disorder and hepatic vein thrombosis. Ann Intern Med 103:329–334, 1985.

31. Dudley JM, Westwood N, Leonard S, Eridani S, Pearson TC: Primary polycythaemia: Positive diagnosis using the differential response of primitive and mature erythroid progenitors to erythropoietin, interleukin 3 and alpha-interferon. Br J Haematol 75:188–194, 1990.

32. Eaves CJ, Eaves AC: Erythropoietin (Ep) dose-response curves for three classes of erythroid progenitors in normal human marrow and in patients with polycythemia vera. Blood 52:1196–1210, 1978.

33. Pagliuca A, Mufti GJ, Janossa-Tahernia M, Eridani S, Westwood NB, Thumpston J et al: In vitro colony culture and chromosomal studies in hepatic and portal vein thrombosis—possible evidence of an occult myeloproliferative state. Q J Med 281:981–989, 1990.

34. Prchal JT, Prchal JF: Evolving understanding of the cellular defect in polycythemia vera: Implications for its clinical diagnosis and molecular pathophysiology. Blood 83:1–4, 1994.

35. Lemoine F, Najman A, Baillou C, Stachowiak J, Boffa G, Aegerter P et al: A prospective study of the value of bone marrow erythroid progenitor cultures in polycythemia. Blood 68:996–1002, 1986.

36. Masters GS, Baines P, Jacobs A: Erythroid colony growth from peripheral blood and bone marrow in polycythaemia. Hum Pathol 43:937–941, 1990.

37. Reid CDL, Fidler J, Kirk A: Endogenous erythroid clones (EEC) in polycythaemia and their relationship to diagnosis and the response to treatment. Br J Haematol 68:395–400, 1988.

38. Tefferi A, Silverstein MN, Noel P: Agnogenic myeloid metaplasia (Review). Semin Oncol 22:327–333, 1995.

39. Gunz FW: Hemorrhagic thrombocythemia: A critical review. Blood 15:706, 1960.

40. Fenaux P, Simon M, Caulier MT, Lai JL, Goudemand J, Bauters F: Clinical course of essential thrombocythemia in 147 cases. Cancer 66:549–556, 1990.

41. Bellucci S, Janvier M, Tobelem G, Flandrin G, Charpak Y, Berger R et al: Essential thrombocythemias. Clinical evolutionary and biological data. Cancer 58:2440–2447, 1986.

42. Wehmeier A, Daum I, Jamin H, Schneider W: Incidence and clinical risk factors for bleeding and thrombotic complications in myeloproliferative disorders. A retrospective analysis of 260 patients. Hematology 101–106, 1991.

43. Schafer AI: Essential thrombocythemia. In Coller BS (ed.): Progress in Hemostasis and Thrombosis, pp. 69–96. W.B. Saunders, Philadephia, 1991.

44. Buss DH, Cashell AW, O'Connor ML, Richards F II, Case LD: Occurrence, etiology, and clinical significance of extreme thrombocytosis: A study of 280 cases. Am J Med 96:247–253, 1994.

45. Barbui T, Cortelazzo S, Viero P, Bassan R, Dini E, Semeraro N: Thrombohaemorrhagic complications in 101 cases of myeloproliferative disorders: Relationship to platelet number and function. Eur J Cancer Clin Oncol 19:1593–1599, 1983.

46. Valla D, Casadevall N, Huisse MG, Tulliez M, Grange JD, Muller O et al: Myeloproliferative disorders in portal vein thrombosis in adults. Gastroenterology 94:1063–1069, 1988.

47. Najean Y, Mugnier P, Dresch C, Rain JD: Polycythaemia vera in young people: An analysis of 58 cases diagnosed before 40 years. Br J Haematol 67:285–291, 1987.

48. Cortelazzo S, Viero P, Finazzi G, D'Emilio A, Rodeghiero F, Barbui T: Incidence and risk factors for thrombotic complications in a historical cohort of 100 patients with essential thrombocythemia. J Clin Oncol 8:556–562, 1990.

49. Berk PD, Goldberg JD, Donovan PB, Fruchtman SM, Berlin NI, Wasserman LR: Therapeutic recommendations in polycythemia vera based on polycythemia vera study group protocols. Sem Hematol 23:132–143, 1986.

50. Lintula R, Rasi V, Ikkala E, Borgstrom GH, Vuopio P: Platelet function in preleukaemia. Scand J Haematol 26:65–71, 1981.

51. Chievitz E, Thede T: Complications and causes of death in polycythaemia vera. Acta Med Scand 172:513–523, 1962.

52. Mesa RA, Silverstein MN, Jacobsen SJ, Wollan PC, Tefferi A: Population-based incidence and survival figures in essential thrombocythemia and agnogenic myeloid metaplasia: An Olmsted County Study, 1976–1995. Am J Hematol 61:10–15, 1999.

53. Jensen MK, de Nully BP, Nielsen OJ, Hasselbalch HC: Incidence, clinical features and outcome of essential thrombocythaemia in a well defined geographical area. Eur J Haematol 65:132–139, 2000.

54. Polycythemia vera: The natural history of 1213 patients followed for 20 years. Gruppo Italiano Studio Policitemia (see comments). Ann Intern Med 123:656–664, 1995.

55. Petti MC, Spadea A, Avvisati G, Spadea T, Latagliata R, Montefusco E et al: Polycythemia vera treated with pipobroman as single agent: Low incidence of secondary leukemia in a cohort of patients observed during 20 years (1971–1991). Leukemia 12:869–874, 1998.

56. Valla D, Casadevall N, Huisse MG, Tulliez M, Grange JD, Muller O et al: Etiology of portal vein thrombosis in adults. A prospective evaluation of primary myeloproliferative disorders. Gastroenterology 94:1063–1069, 1988.

57. Lengfelder E, Hochhaus A, Kronawitter U, Hoche D, Queisser W, Jahn-Eder M et al: Should a platelet limit of 600 × 10(9)/l be used as a diagnostic criterion in essential thrombocythaemia? An analysis of the natural course including early stages. Br J Haematol 100:15–23, 1997.

58. Regev A, Stark P, Blickstein D, Lahav M: Thrombotic complications in essential thrombocythemia with relatively low platelet counts. Am J Hematol 56:168–172, 1997.

59. Michiels JJ, Abels J, Steketee J, VanVliet HHDM, Vuzevski VD: Erythromelalgia caused by platelet-mediated arteriolar inflammation and thrombosis in thrombocythemia. Ann Intern Med 102:466–471, 1985.

60. Michiels JJ, Ten Kate FJW: Erythromelalgia in thrombocythemia of various myeloproliferative disorders. Am J Hematol 39:131–136, 1992.

61. Singh AK, Wetherley-Mein G: Microvascular occlusive lesions in primary thrombocythaemia. Br J Haematol 36:553, 1977.

62. Schafer AI: Bleeding and thrombosis in the myeloproliferative disorders. Blood 64:1–12, 1984.

63. Gilbert HS: The spectrum of myeloproliferative disorders. Med Clin North Am 57:355, 1973.

64. Silverstein MN: Primary or hemorrhagic thrombocythemia. Arch Intern Med 122:18, 1968.

65. Spaet TH, Bauer S, Melamed S: Hemorrhagic thrombocythemia: A blood coagulation disorder. Arch Intern Med 98:377, 1956.

66. Zucker S, Mielke CH: Classification of thrombocytosis based on platelet function tests: Correlation with hemorrhagic and thrombotic complications. J Lab Clin Med 80:385–394, 1972.

67. Preston FE, Emmanuel IG, Winfield DA, Malia RG: Essential thrombocythaemia and peripheral gangrene. Br Med J 3:548, 1974.

68. Michiels JJ, Koudstaal PJ, Mulder AH, Van Vliet HHDM: Transient neurologic and ocular manifestations in primary thrombocythemia. Neurology 43:1107–1110, 1993.

69. Nimer SD: Essential thrombocythemia: Another "heterogeneous disease" better understood? (Letter; Comment). (Review). Blood 93:415–416, 1999.

70. Harrison CN, Gale RE, Machin SJ, Linch DC: A large proportion of patients with a diagnosis of essential thrombocythemia do not have a clonal disorder and may be at lower risk of thrombotic complications. Blood 93:417–424, 1999.

71. Seitz R, Wolf M, Egbring R: Antithrombin III and plasma substitution in septic shock. Prog Clin Biol Res 308:965–969, 1989.

72. Cunietti E, Gandini R, Mascaro G, Ferrari M, Pappalepore V, Scapellato L: Defective platelet aggregation and increased platelet turnover in patients with myelofibrosis and other myeloproliferative diseases. Scand J Haematol 26:339–344, 1981.

73. Givelber AD: Platelet function in patients with high platelet counts. Ann Intern Med 82:506, 1975.

74. Hehlmann R, Jahn M, Baumann B, Kopcke W: Essential thrombocythemia. Clinical characteristics and course of 61 cases. Cancer 61:2487–2496, 1988.

75. Malpass TW, Savage B, Hanson SR, Slichter SJ, Harker LA: Correlation between prolonged bleeding time and depletion of platelet dense granule ADP in patients with myelodysplastic and myeloproliferative disorders. J Lab Clin Med 103:894–904, 1984.

76. Meschengieser S, Blanco A, Woods A, Maugeri N, Fernandez J, Dupont J et al: Intraplatelet levels of vWF: Ag and fibrinogen in myeloproliferative disorders. Thromb Res 48:311–319, 1987.

77. Raman BKS, Van Slyck EJ, Riddle J, Sawdyk MA, Abraham JP, Saeed SM: Platelet function and structure in myeloproliferative disease, myelodysplastic syndrome, and secondary thrombocytosis. Am J Clin Pathol 91:647–655, 1989.

78. Waddell CC, Brown JA, Repinecz YA: Abnormal platelet function in myeloproliferative disorders. Arch Pathol Lab Med 105:432–435, 1981.

79. Walsh PN, Murphy S, Barry WE: The role of platelets in the pathogenesis of thrombosis and hemorrhage in patients with thrombocytosis. Thromb Haemost 38:1085–1096, 1977.

80. Wu KK: Platelet hyperaggregability and thrombosis in patients with thrombocythemia. Ann Intern Med 88:7, 1978.

81. Yamamoto K, Sekiguchi E, Takatani O: Abnormalities of epinephrine-induced platelet aggregation and adenine nucleotides in myeloproliferative disorders. Thromb Haemost 52:292–296, 1984.

82. Bazzan M, Vaccarino A, Stella S, Foli C, Omede P, Gallone G et al: Procoagulant activity of mononuclear cells is increased in myeloproliferative and myelodysplastic diseases. Haemostasis 26:157–163, 1996.

83. Boughton BJ, Allington MJ, King A: Platelet and plasma beta thromboglobulin in myeloproliferative syndromes and secondary thrombocytosis. Brit J Haematol 40:125–132, 1978.

84. Cortelazzo S, Barbui T, Bassan R et al: Abnormal aggregation and increased size of platelets in myeloproliferative disorders. Thromb Haemost 44:127, 1980.

85. Castaldi PA, Berndt MC, Booth W, Gregory C, Bull H, Greaves M: Evidence for a platelet membrane defect in the myeloproliferative syndromes. Thromb Res 27:601–609, 1982.

86. Eche N, Sie P, Caranobe C, Nouvel C, Pris J, Boneu B: Platelets in myeloproliferative disorders. III: Glycoprotein profile in relation to platelet function and platelet density. Scand J Haematol 26:123–129, 1981.

87. Moore A, Nachman RL: Platelet Fc receptor: Increased expression in myeloproliferative disease. J Clin Invest 67:1064–1071, 1981.

88. Okuma M, Takayama H, Uchino H: Subnormal platelet response to thromboxane A2 in a patient with chronic myeloid leukaemia. Br J Haematol 51:469–477, 1982.

89. Keenan JP, Wharton J, Shepherd AJN, Bellingham AJ: Defective platelet lipid peroxidation in myeloproliferative disorders: A possible defect of prostaglandin synthesis. Br J Haematol 35:275–283, 1977.

90. Schafer AI: Deficiency of platelet lipoxygenase activity in myeloproliferative disorders. N Engl J Med 306:381–386, 1982.

91. Stenke L, Edenius C, Samuelsson J, Lindgren JA: Deficient lipoxin synthesis: A novel platelet dysfunction in myeloproliferative disorders with special reference to blastic crisis of chronic myelogenous leukemia. Blood 78:2989–2995, 1991.

92. Rendu F, Lebret M, Nurden A, Caen JP: Detection of an acquired platelet storage pool disease in three patients with a myeloproliferative disorder. Thromb Haemost 42:794–796, 1979.

93. Woodruff RK, Bell WR, Castaldi PA et al: Essential thrombocythaemia. Haemostasis 9:105, 1980.

94. Baker RI, Manoharan A: Platelet function in myeloproliferative disorders: Characterization and sequential studies show multiple platelet abnormalities, and change with time. Eur J Haematol 40:267–272, 1988.

95. Wehmeier A, Fricke S, Scharf RE, Schneider W: A prospective study of haemostatic parameters in relation to the clinical course of myeloproliferative disorders. Eur J Haematol 45:191–197, 1990.

96. Cardamone JM, Edson JR, McArthur JR, Jacob HS: Abnormalities of platelet function in the myeloproliferative disorders. JAMA 221:270–273, 1972.

97. Budde U, Dent JA, Berkowitz SD, Ruggeri ZM, Zimmerman TS: Subunit composition of plasma von Willebrand factor in patients with the myeloproliferative syndrome. Blood 68:1213–1217, 1986.

98. Raman BKS, Sawdyk M, Saeed SM: Essential thrombocythemia with acquired von Willebrand's disease. Am J Clin Pathol 88:102–106, 1987.

99. Mohri H, Ohkubo T: Acquired von Willebrand's syndrome due to an inhibitor of IgG specific for von Willebrand's factor in polycythaemia rubra vera. Acta Haematol (Basel) 78:258–264, 1987.

100. Lee LH, Baglin T: Altered platelet phospholipid-dependent thrombin generation in thrombocytopenia and thrombocytosis. Br J Haematol 89:131–136, 1995.

101. Manoharan A, Gemmell R, Brighton T, Dunkley S, Lopez K, Kyle P: Thrombosis and bleeding in myeloproliferative disorders: Identification of at-risk patients with whole blood platelet aggregation studies. Liver 105:618–625, 1999.

102. Jensen MK, de Nully BP, Lund BV, Nielsen OJ, Hasselbalch HC: Increased platelet activation and abnormal membrane glycoprotein content and redistribution in myeloproliferative disorders. Br J Haematol 110:116–124, 2000.

103. Burstein SA, Malpass TW, Yee E, Kadin M, Brigden M, Adamson JW et al: Platelet factor-4 excretion in myeloproliferative disease: Implications for the aetiology of myelofibrosis. Br J Haematol 57:383–392, 1984.

104. Berild D, Hasselbalch H, Knudsen J: Platelet survival, platelet factor-4 and bleeding time in myeloproliferative disorders. Scand J Clin Lab Invest 47:497–501, 1987.

105. Katoh O, Kimura A, Kuramoto A: Platelet-derived growth factor is decreased in patients with myeloproliferative disorders. Am J Hematol 27:276–280, 1988.

106. Baglin TP, Price SM, Boughton BJ: A reversible defect of platelet PDGF content in myeloproliferative disorders. Br J Haematol 69:483–486, 1988.

107. Shamasunder HK, Gregory SA, Knospe WH: Uracil mustard in the treatment of thrombocytosis. JAMA 244:1454–1455, 1980.

108. Gisslinger H, Rodeghiero F, Ruggeri M, Fard NHV, Mannhalter C, Papagiannopoulos M et al: Homocysteine levels in polycythaemia vera and essential thrombocythaemia. Liver 105:551–555, 1999.

109. Faurschou M, Nielsen OJ, Jensen MK, Hasselbalch HC: High prevalence of hyperhomocysteinemia due to marginal deficiency of cobalamin or folate in chronic myeloproliferative disorders. Am J Hematol 65:136–140, 2000.

110. Wieczorek I, MacGregor IR, Ludlam CA: Low proteins C and S and activation of fibrinolysis in treated essential thrombocythemia. Am J Hematol 48:277–281, 1995.

111. Kornberg A, Rahimi-Levene N, Yona R, Mor A, Rachmilewitz EA: Enhanced generation of monocyte tissue factor and increased plasma prothrombin fragment 1+2 levels in patients with polycythemia vera: Mechanism of activation of blood coagulation. Am J Hematol 56:5–11, 1997.

112. Falanga A, Marchetti M, Evangelista V, Vignoli A, Licini M, Balicco M et al: Polymorphonuclear leukocyte activation and hemostasis in patients with essential thrombocythemia and polycythemia vera. Blood 96:4261–4266, 2000.

113. Rinder HM, Schuster JE, Rinder CS, Wang C, Schweidler HJ, Smith BR: Correlation of thrombosis with increased platelet turnover in thrombocytosis. Blood 91:1288–1294, 1998.

114. Goldstein R, Clark P, Klintmalm G, Husberg B, Gonwa T, Stone M: Prevention of recurrent thrombosis following liver transplantation for Budd-Chiari syndrome associated with myeloproliferative disorders: Treatment with hydroxyurea and aspirin. Transplant Proc 23:1559–1560, 1991.

115. Halff G, Todo S, Tzakis AG, Gordon RD, Starzl TE: Liver transplantation for the Budd-Chiari syndrome. Ann Surg 211:43–49, 1990.

116. van Genderen PJJ, Michiels JJ, van Strik R, Lindemans J, Van Vliet HHDM: Platelet consumption in thrombocythemia complicated by erythromelalgia: Reversal by aspirin. Thromb Haemost 73:210–214, 1995.

117. van Genderen PJ, Mulder PG, Waleboer M, van de MD, Michiels JJ: Prevention and treatment of thrombotic complications in essential thrombocythaemia: Efficacy and safety of aspirin. Liver 97:179–184, 1997.

118. Barbui T, Finazzi G: Treatment of polycythemia vera (Review). Haematologica 83:143–149, 1998.

119. Goodnight SH: Antiplatelet therapy with aspirin: From clinical trials to practice. Thromb Haemost 74:401–405, 1995.

120. Cortelazzo S, Finazzi G, Ruggeri M, Vestri O, Galli M, Rodeghiero F et al: Hydroxyurea for patients with essential thrombocythemia and a high risk of thrombosis. N Engl J Med 332:1132–1136, 1995.

121. Spencer CM, Brogden RN: Anagrelide. A review of its pharmacodynamic and pharmacokinetic properties, and therapeutic potential in the treatment of thrombocythaemia. Drugs 47:809–822, 1994.

122. Anagrelide Study Group: Anagrelide, a therapy for thrombocythemic states: Experience in 577 patients. Am J Med 92:69–76, 1992.

123. Silverstein MN, Petitt RM, Solber LA, Fleming JS, Knight RC, Schacter LP: Anagrelide: A new drug for treating thrombocytosis. N Engl J Med 318:1292–1294, 1988.

124. Storen EC, Tefferi A: Long-term use of anagrelide in young patients with essential thrombocythemia. Blood 97:863–866, 2001.

125. Trapp OM, Beykirch MK, Petrides PE: Anagrelide for treatment of patients with chronic myelogenous leukemia and a high platelet count. Blood Cells Mol Dis 24:9–13, 1998.

126. Rametta V, Ferrara F, Marottoli V, Matera C, Mettivier V, Cimino R: Recombinant interferon alpha-2b as treatment of essential thrombocythaemia. Acta Haematol 91:126–129, 1994.

127. Ludwig H, Linkesch W, Gisslinger H, Fritz E, Sinzinger H, Radaszkiewicz T et al: Interferon-alpha corrects thrombocytosis in patients with myeloproliferative disorders. Cancer Immunol Immunother 25:266–273, 1987.

128. Haogland HC, Silverstein MN: Primary thrombocythemia in the young patient. Mayo Clin Proc 53:578, 1978.

129. Ruggeri M, Finazzi G, Tosetto A, Riva S, Rodeghiero F, Barbui T: No treatment for low-risk thrombocythaemia: Results from a prospective study. Br J Haematol 103:772–777, 1998.

130. Besses C, Cervantes F, Pereira A, Florensa L, Sole F, Hernandez-Boluda JC et al: Major vascular complications in essential thrombocythemia: A study of the predictive factors in a series of 148 patients. Leukemia 13:150–154, 1999.

131. Shpilberg O, Shimon I, Sofer O, Dolitski M, Ben Bassat I: Transient normal platelet counts and decreased requirement for interferon during pregnancy in essential thrombocythaemia (see comments). Br J Haematol 92:491–493, 1996.

132. Wright CA, Tefferi A: A single institutional experience with 43 pregnancies in essential thrombocythemia. Eur J Haematol 66:152–159, 2001.

133. Bangerter M, Guthner C, Beneke H, Hildebrand A, Grunewald M, Griesshammer M: Pregnancy in essential thrombocythaemia: Treatment and outcome of 17 pregnancies. Eur J Haematol 65:165–169, 2000.

134. Cowan DH, Graham RC, Baunach D: The platelet defect in leukemia. Platelet ultrastructure, adenine nucleotide metabolism, and the release reaction. J Clin Invest 56:188–200, 1975.

135. Maldonado JE, Pierre RV: The platelets in preleukemia and myelomonocytic leukemia. Ultrastructural cytochemistry and cytogenetics. Mayo Clin Proc 50:573–587, 1975.

136. Van Der Weyden MB, Clancy RL, Howard MA, Firkin BG: Qualitative platelet defects with reduced life-span in acute leukaemia. Aust N Z J Med 4:339–345, 1972.

137. Cowan DH, Haut MJ: Platelet function in acute leukemia. J Lab Clin Med 79:893–905, 1972.

138. Ramos OF, Moron EC, De Castro Arenas R: Platelet function abnormalities in acute leukemia. Haematologia (Budapest) 14:383–391, 1981.

139. White JG, Gerrard JM: Ultrastructural textures of abnormal blood platelets: A review. Am J Pathol 63:590, 1976.

140. Avvisati G, Buller HR, ten Cate JW, Mandelli F: Tranexamic acid for control of haemorrhage in acute promyelocytic leukaemia. Lancet 2:122–124, 1989.

141. Bain BJ, Catovsky D, O'Brien M et al: Megakaryoblastic leukemia presenting as acute myelofibrosis—a study of four cases with the platelet-peroxidase reaction. Blood 58:206, 1981.

142. Pogliani EM, Colombi M, Cofrancesco E, Salvatore M, Fowst C: Platelet dysfunction in acute megakaryoblastic leukemia. Acta Haematol (Basel) 81:1–4, 1989.

143. Bevan D, Rose M, Greaves M: Leukaemia of platelet precursors: Diverse features in four cases. Br J Haematol 51:147–164, 1982.

144. Kerkhofs H, Hagemeijer A, Leeksma CHW, Abels J, DenOttolander GJ, Somers R et al: The 5q– chromosome abnormality in haematologic disorders: A collaborative study of 34 cases from the Netherlands. Br J Haematol 52:365–381, 1982.

145. Mahmood T, Robinson WA, Hamstra RD, Wallner SF: Macrocytic anemia, thrombocytosis and nonlobulated megakaryocytes. The 5q– syndrome, a distinct entity. Am J Med 66:946–950, 1979.

146. Bernstein R, Pinto MR, Behr A, Mendelow B: Chromosome 3 abnormalities in acute nonlymphocytic leukemia (ANLL) with abnormal thrombopoiesis: Report of three patients with a "new" inversion anomaly and a further case of homologous translocation. Blood 60:613–617, 1982.

147. Cortelazzo S, Viero P, D'Emilio A, DeGaetano G, Barbui T: Platelet dysfunction in splenectomized patients with hairy cell leukemia. Eur J Cancer Clin Oncol 22:935–937, 1986.

148. Sweet DL, Golumb HM: Correction of platelet defect after splenectomy in hairy cell leukemia. JAMA 241:1684, 1979.

149. Zuzel M, Cawley JC, Paton RC, Burns GF, McNicol GP: Platelet function in hairy-cell leukaemia. J Clin Pathol 32:814–821, 1979.

150. Rosove MH, Naeim F, Harwig S, Zighelboim J: Severe platelet dysfunction in hairy cell leukemia with improvement after splenectomy. Blood 55:903–906, 1980.

151. Hillmen P, Richards SJ: Implications of recent insights into the pathophysiology of paroxysmal nocturnal haemoglobinuria (Review). Liver 108:470–479, 2000.

152. Matei D, Brenner B, Marder VJ: Acquired thrombophilic syndromes. Blood Rev 15:31–48, 2001.

153. Socie G, Mary JY, de Gramont A, Rio B, Leporrier M, Rose C et al: Paroxysmal nocturnal haemoglobinuria: Long-term follow-up and prognostic factors. French Society of Haematology (see comments). Lancet 348:573–577, 1996.

154. Ray JG, Burows RF, Ginsberg JS, Burrows EA: Paroxysmal nocturnal hemoglobinuria and the risk of venous thrombosis: Review and recommendations for management of the pregnant and nonpregnant patient (Review). Haemostasis 30:103–117, 2000.

155. Gralnick HR, Vail M, McKeown LP, Merryman P, Wilson O, Chu I et al: Activated platelets in paroxysmal nocturnal haemoglobinuria. Liver 91:697–702, 1995.

156. Veyradier A, Jenkins CS, Fressinaud E, Meyer D: Acquired von Willebrand syndrome: From pathophysiology to management (Review). Thrombos Haemost 84:175–182, 2000.

157. Nilehn J, Nilsson IM: Coagulation studies in different types of myeloma. Acta Med Scand 179:194, 1966.

158. Perkins HA, MacKenzie MR, Fudenberg HH: Hemostatic defects in dysproteinemias. Blood 35:695–707, 1970.

159. Hunt V, Zucker MB, Pearson J: Abnormal fibrin ultrastructure, polymerization, and clot retraction in multiple myeloma. Br J Haematol 18:625–636, 1970.

160. Coleman M, Vigliano EM, Weksler ME, Nachman RL: Inhibition of fibrin monomer polymerization by lambda myeloma globulins. Blood 39:210–223, 1972.

161. Davey FR, Gordon GB, Boral LI, Gottlieb AJ: Gamma globulin inhibition of fibrin clot formation. Ann Clin Lab Sci 6:72–77, 1976.

162. Klingemann HG, Egbring R, Havemann K: Incomplete fibrin formation and highly elevated factor XIII activity in multiple myeloma. Scand J Haematol 27:253–262, 1981.

163. Jeannette S, Soria C, Samama M et al: Analysis of fibrin formation abnormality in a case of multiple myeloma. Scand J Haematol 15:207, 1975.

164. Kaufman PA, Gockerman JP, Greenberg CS: Production of a novel anticoagulant by neoplastic plasma cells: Report of a case and review of the literature. Am J Med 86:612–616, 1989.

165. Pachter MR, Johnson SA, Neblett TR, Truant JP: Bleeding, platelets, and macroglobulinemia. Am J Clin Pathol 31:467–482, 1959.

166. Kasturi J, Saraya AK: Platelet functions in dysproteinemia. Acta Haematol (Basel) 59:104–113, 1978.

167. DiMinno G, Coraggio F, Cerbone AM, Capitanio AM, Manzo C, Spina M et al: A myeloma paraprotein with specificity for platelet glycoprotein IIIa in a patient with a fatal bleeding disorder. J Clin Invest 77:157–164, 1986.

168. Yasin Z, Quick D, Thiagarajan P, Spoor D, Caraveo J, Palascak J: Light-chain paraproteins with lupus anticoagulant activity. Am J Hematol 62:99–102, 1999.

169. Deitcher SR, Erban JK, Limentani SA: Acquired free protein S deficiency associated with multiple myeloma: A case report. Am J Hematol 51:319–323, 1996.

170. Mumford AD, O'Donnell J, Gillmore JD, Manning RA, Hawkins PN, Laffan M: Bleeding symptoms and coagulation abnormalities in 337 patients with AL-amyloidosis. Br J Haematol 110:454–460, 2000.

171. Gamba G, Montani N, Anesi E, Palladini G, Capezzera M, Soldavini E et al: Clotting alterations in primary systemic amyloidosis. Haematologica 85:289–292, 2000.

172. Furie B, Greene E, Furie BC: Syndrome of acquired factor X deficiency and systemic amyloidosis. N Engl J Med 297:81–85, 1977.

173. Korsan-Bengtsen K, Hjort PF, Ygge J: Acquired factor X deficiency in a patient with amyloidosis. Thrombos Diathes Haemorrh 7:558–566, 1962.

174. Camoriano JK, Greipp PR, Bayer GK, Bowie EJW: Resolution of acquired factor X deficiency and amyloidosis with melphalan and prednisone therapy. N Engl J Med 316:1133–1135, 1987.

175. Rosenstein ED, Itzkowitz SH, Penziner AS, Cohen JI, Mornaghi RA: Resolution of factor X deficiency in primary amyloidosis following splenectomy. Arch Intern Med 143:597–599, 1983.

176. Greipp PR, Kyle RA, Bowie EJW: Factor X deficiency in primary amyloidosis. N Engl J Med 301:1050–1051, 1979.

177. Beardell FV, Varma M, Martinez J: Normalization of plasma factor X levels in amyloidosis after plasma exchange. Am J Hematol 54:68–71, 1997.

178. Yood RA, Skinner M, Rubinow A, Talarico L, Cohen AS: Bleeding manifestations in 100 patients with amyloidosis. JAMA 249:1322–1324, 1983.

179. Choufani EB, Sanchorawala V, Ernst T, Quillen K, Skinner M, Wright DG et al: Acquired factor X deficiency in patients with amyloid light-chain amyloidosis: Incidence, bleeding manifestations, and response to high-dose chemotherapy. Blood 97:1885–1887, 2001.

180. Shigekiyo T, Kosaka M, Shintani Y, Azuma H, Iishi Y, Saito S: Inhibition of fibrin monomer polymerization by Bence Jones protein in a patient with primary amyloidosis. Acta Haematol (Basel) 81:160–165, 1989.

181. Glueck HI, Coots MC, Benson M, Dwulet FE, Hurtubise PE: A monoclonal immunoglobulin A (kappa) factor VIII:C inhibitor associated with primary amyloidosis: Identification and characterization. J Lab Clin Med 113:269–277, 1989.

182. Leibman H, Chinowsky M, Valdin J, Kenoyer G, Feinstein D: Increased fibrinolysis and amyloidosis. Arch Intern Med 143:678–682, 1983.

183. Meyer K, Williams EC: Fibrinolysis and acquired alpha-2 plasmin inhibitor deficiency in amyloidosis. Am J Med 79:394–396, 1985.

184. Sane DC, Pizzo SV, Greenberg CS: Elevated urokinase-type plasminogen activator level and bleeding in amyloidosis: Case report and literature review. Am J Hematol 31:53–57, 1989.

185. Perlin E, Brakman P, Berg HS, Kirchner PT, Moquin RB, Astrup T: Enhanced blood coagulation and fibrinolysis in a patient with primary amyloidosis. Thromb Haemost 26:9–14, 1971.

186. Chang JC, Kane KK: Pathologic hyperfibrinolysis associated with amyloidosis: Clinical response to epsilon amino caproic acid. Am J Clin Pathol 81:382–387, 1984.

187. Takahashi H, Kolke T, Yoshida N, Kitahara O, Hanano M, Shibata A et al: Excessive fibrinolysis in suspected amyloidosis: Demonstration of plasmin-alpha-2-plasmin inhibitor complex and von Willebrand factor fragment in plasma. Am J Hematol 23:153–166, 1986.

188. Hassidim K, McMillan R, Conjalka MS, Morrison J: Immune thrombocytopenic purpura in Hodgkin disease. Am J Hematol 6:149–153, 1979.

189. Berkman AW, Woog JJ, Kickler TS, Ettinger DS: Serial determinations of antiplatelet antibodies in a patient with Hodgkin's disease and autoimmune thrombocytopenia. Cancer 51:2057–2060, 1983.

190. Carey RW, McGinnis A, Jacobson BM, Carvalho A: Idiopathic thrombocytopenic purpura complicating chronic lymphocytic leukemia. Arch Intern Med 136:62–66, 1976.

191. Cohen JR: Idiopathic thrombocytopenic purpura in Hodgkin's disease. Cancer 41:743–746, 1978.

192. Fink K, Al-Mondhiry H: Idiopathic thrombocytopenic purpura in lymphoma. Cancer 37:1999–2004, 1976.

193. Hamilton PJ, Dawson AA: Thrombocytopenic purpura as the sole manifestation of a recurrence of Hodgkin's disease. J Clin Pathol 26:70–72, 1973.

194. Hussein KK, Shaw MT, Oleinick SR: Autoimmune thrombocytopenia and peripheral neuropathy heralding Hodgkin's disease. South Med J 68:1414–1416, 1975.

195. Julia A, Miller SP: Idiopathic thrombocytopenic purpura in Hodgkin's disease after splenectomy. Am J Hematol 1:115–120, 1976.

196. Kaden BR, Rosse WF, Hauch TW: Immune thrombocytopenia in lymphoproliferative diseases. Blood 53:545–551, 1979.

197. Kedar A, Khan AB, Mattern JQA, Fisher J, Thomas PRM, Freeman AI: Autoimmune disorders complicating adolescent Hodgkin's disease. Cancer 44:112–116, 1979.

198. Khilanani P, Al-Sarraf M: The association of autoimmune thrombocytopenia and Hodgkin's disease. Oncology 28:238–245, 1973.

199. Kirshner JJ, Zamkoff KW, Gottlieb AJ: Idiopathic thrombocytopenic purpura and Hodgkin's disease: Report of two cases and a review of the literature. Am J Med Sci 280:21–28, 1980.

200. Rudders RA, Aisenberg AC, Schiller AL: Hodgkin's disease representing as "idiopathic" thrombocytopenic purpura. Cancer 30:220–230, 1972.

201. Waddell CC, Cimo PL: Idiopathic thrombocytopenic purpura occurring in Hodgkin disease after splenectomy: Report of two cases and review of the literature. Am J Hematol 7:381–387, 1979.

202. Weitzman S, Dvilansky A, Yanai I: Thrombocytopenic purpura as the sole manifestation of recurrence in Hodgkin's disease. Acta Haematol (Basel) 58:129–133, 1977.

203. Aghai E, Quitt M, Lurie M, Anatal S, Cohen L, Bitterman H et al: Primary hepatic lymphoma presenting as symptomatic immune thrombocytopenic purpura. Cancer 60:2308–2311, 1987.

204. Veenhoven WA, Thomas-Van Der Schans GS, Nieweg HO: Monoclonal immunoglobulins with affinity for platelets and their relationship to malignant lymphoma. Cancer 49:40–42, 1982.

205. Kempin S: Late hematologic complications after treatment of Hodgkin's disease. In Lacher MJ, Redman JR (eds.): Hodgkin's Disease: The Consequences of Survival, p. 63. Lea & Febiger, Philadelphia, 1990.

206. Malik U, Dutcher JP, Oleksowicz L: Acquired Glanzmann's thrombasthenia associated with Hodgkin's lymphoma: A case report and review of the literature (Review). Cancer 82:1764–1768, 1998.

207. Karpatkin S: Autoimmune thrombocytopenic purpura. Blood 56:329–343, 1980.

208. McMillan R: Chronic idiopathic thrombocytopenic purpura. N Engl J Med 304:1135–1147, 1981.

209. George JN, el-Harake MA, Raskob GE: Chronic idiopathic thrombocytopenic purpura. N Engl J Med 331:1207–1211, 1994.

210. Reiner A, Gernsheimer T, Slichter SJ: Pulse cyclophosphamide therapy for refractory autoimmune thrombocytopenic purpura. Blood 85:351–358, 1995.

211. Proctor SJ, Jackson G, Carey P, Stark A, Finney R, Saunders P et al: Improvement of platelet counts in steroid-unresponsive idiopathic immune thrombocytopenic purpura after short-course therapy with recombinant alpha-2b interferon. Blood 74:1894–1897, 1989.

212. Andersen JC: Response of resistant idiopathic thrombocytopenic purpura to pulsed high-dose dexamethasone therapy. N Engl J Med 330:1560–1564, 1994.

213. Brody JI, Haidar ME, Rossman RE: A hemorrhagic syndrome in Waldenstrom's macroglobulinemia secondary to immunoadsorption of factor VIII. N Engl J Med 300:408–410, 1979.

214. Gan TE, Sawers RJ, Koutts J: Pathogenesis of antibody-induced acquired von Willebrand syndrome. Am J Hematol 9:363–371, 1980.

215. Handin RI, Martin V, Moloney WC: Antibody-induced von Willebrand's disease: A newly defined inhibitor syndrome. Blood 48:393–405, 1976.

216. Joist JH, Cowan JF, Zimmerman TS: Acquired von Willebrand's disease. Evidence for a quantitative and qualitative factor VIII disorder. N Engl J Med 298:988–991, 1978.

217. Mohri H, Noguchi T, Kodama F, Itoh A, Ohkubo T: Acquired von Willebrand disease due to inhibitor of human myeloma protein specific for von Willebrand factor. Am J Clin Pathol 87:663–668, 1987.

218. Sampson BM, Greaves M, Malia RG, Preston FE: Acquired von Willebrand's disease: Demonstration of a circulating inhibitor to the factor VIII complex in four cases. Br J Haematol 54:233–244, 1983.

219. Wautier JL, Levy-Toledano S, Caen JP: Acquired von Willebrand's syndrome and thrombopathy in a patient with chronic lymphocytic leukaemia. Scand J Haematol 16:128–134, 1976.

220. Zettervall O, Nilsson IM: Acquired von Willebrand's disease caused by a monoclonal antibody. Acta Med Scand 204:521, 1978.

221. Meyer D, Frommel D, Larrieu MJ, Zimmerman TS: Selective absence of large forms of factor VIII/von Willebrand factor in acquired von Willebrand's syndrome. Response to transfusion. Blood 54:600–606, 1979.

222. Mannucci PM, Lombardi R, Bader R, Horellou MH, Finazzi G, Besana C et al: Studies of the pathophysiology of acquired von Willebrand's disease in seven patients with lymphoproliferative disorders or benign monoclonal gammopathies. Blood 64:614–621, 1984.

223. Richard C, Cuadrado MA, Prieto M, Batlle J, López Fernández MF, Rodriguez Salazar ML et al: Acquired von Willebrand disease in multiple myeloma secondary to absorption of von Willebrand factor by plasma cells. Am J Hematol 35:114–117, 1990.

224. Bovill EG, Ershler WB, Golden EA, Tindle BH, Edson JR: A human myeloma-produced monoclonal protein directed against the active subpopulation of von Willebrand factor. Am J Clin Pathol 85:115–123, 1986.

225. Tefferi A, Hanson CA, Kurtin PJ, Katzmann JA, Dalton RJ, Nichols WL: Acquired von Willebrand's disease due to aberrant expression of platelet glycoprotein Ib by marginal zone lymphoma cells. Br J Haematol 96:850–853, 1997.

226. Silberstein LE, Abrahm J, Shattil SJ: The efficacy of intensive plasma exchange in acquired von Willebrand's disease. Transfusion 27:234–237, 1987.

227. White LA, Chisholm M: Gastro-intestinal bleeding in acquired von Willebrand's disease: Efficacy of high-dose immuno-globulin where substitution treatments failed. Br J Haematol 84:332–334, 1993.

228. Hanley D, Arkel YS, Lynch J, Kamiyama M: Acquired von Willebrand's syndrome in association with a lupus-like anticoagulant corrected by intravenous immunoglobulin. Am J Hematol 46:141–146, 1994.

229. Friederich PW, Wever PC, Briet E, Doorenbos CJ, Levi M: Successful treatment with recombinant factor VIIa of therapy-resistant severe bleeding in a patient with acquired von Willebrand disease. Am J Hematol 66:292–294, 2001.

230. Wenz B, Friedman G: Acquired factor VIII inhibitor in a patient with malignant lymphoma. Am J Med Sci 268:295–299, 1974.

231. Castaldi PA, Penny R: A macroglobulin with inhibitory activity against coagulation factor VIII. Blood 35:370–376, 1970.

232. Lee ES, Hibsman BK, Liebman HA: Acquired bleeding disorder in a patient with malignant lymphoma: Antibody-mediated prothrombin deficiency. Cancer 91:636–641, 2001.

233. Colwell NS, Tollefsen DM, Blinder MA: Identification of a monoclonal thrombin inhibitor associated with multiple myeloma and a severe bleeding disorder. Br J Haematol 97:219–226, 1997.

234. Bussel JB, Steinherz PG, Miller DR, Hilgartner MW: A heparin-like anticoagulant in an 8-month-old boy with acute monoblastic leukemia. Am J Hematol 16:83–90, 1984.

235. Khoory MS, Nesheim ME, Bowie EJW, Mann KG: Circulating heparan sulfate proteoglycan anticoagulant from a patient with a plasma cell disorder. J Clin Invest 65:666–674, 1980.

236. Tefferi A, Nichols WL, Bowie EJW: Circulating heparin-like anticoagulants: Report of five consecutive cases and a review. Am J Med 88:184–188, 1990.

237. Cairo MS: Adverse reactions of L-asparaginase. Am J Pediatr Hematol Oncol 4:335, 1982.

238. Sills RH, Nelson DA, Stockman JA: L-asparaginase-induced coagulopathy during therapy of acute lymphocytic leukemia. Med Pediatr Oncol 4:311–313. 1978.

239. Anderson N, Lokich JJ, Tullis JL: L-asparaginase effect on antithrombin-III levels. Med Pediatr Oncol 7:335–340, 1979.

240. Barbui T, Finazzi G, Vigano S, Mannucci PM: L-asparaginase lowers protein C antigen. Thromb Haemost 52:216, 1984.

241. Bezeaud A, Drouet L, Leverger G, Griffin JH, Guillin MC: Effect of L-asparaginase therapy for acute lymphoblastic leukemia on plasma vitamin K-dependent coagulation factors and inhibitors. J Pediatr 108:698–701, 1986.

242. Buchanan GR, Holtkamp CA: Reduced antithrombin III levels during L-asparaginase therapy. Med Pediatr Oncol 8:7–14, 1980.

243. Conrad J, Horellou MH, Van Dreden P, Potevin F, Zittoun R, Samama M: Decrease in protein C in L-asparaginase-treated patients. Br J Haematol 59:725–727, 1985.

244. Gralnick HR, Henderson E: Hypofibrinogenemia and coagulation factor deficiencies with L-asparaginase treatment. Cancer 27:1313–1320, 1971.

245. Homans AC, Rybak ME, Baglini RL, Tiarks C, Steiner ME, Forman EN: Effect of L-asparaginase administration on coagulation and platelet function in children with leukemia. J Clin Oncol 5:811–817, 1987.

246. Liebman HA, Wada JK, Patch MJ, McGehee W: Depression of functional and antigenic plasma antithrombin III (AT-III) due to therapy with L-asparaginase. Cancer 50:451, 1982.

247. Pui CH, Jackson CW, Chesney C, Lyles SA, Bowman Wp, Abromowitch M et al: Sequential changes in platelet function and coagulation in leukemic children treated with L-asparaginase, prednisone, and vincristine. J Clin Oncol 1:380–385, 1983.

248. Ramsay NKC, Coccia PF, Krivit W, Nesbit ME, Edson JR: The effect of L-asparaginase on plasma coagulation factors in acute lymphoblastic leukemia. Cancer 40:1398–1401, 1977.

249. Bettigole RE, Himelstein ES, Oettgen HF, Clifford GO: Hypofibrinogenemia due to L-asparaginase: Studies of fibrinogen survival using autologous 131I-fibrinogen. Blood 35:195–200, 1970.

250. Nowak-Gottl U, Ahlke E, Klosel K, Jurgens H, Boos J: Changes in coagulation and fibrinolysis in childhood acute lymphoblastic leukaemia re-induction therapy using three different asparaginase preparations. Eur J Pediatr 156:848–850, 1997.

251. Abshire TC, Pollock BH, Billett AL, Bradley P, Buchanan GR: Weekly polyethylene glycol conjugated L-asparaginase compared with biweekly dosing produces superior induction remission rates in childhood relapsed acute lymphoblastic leukemia: A Pediatric Oncology Group Study. Blood 96:1709–1705, 2000.

252. Groopman J, Ellman L: Acute promyelocytic leukemia. Am J Hematol 7:395, 1979.

253. Sultan C, Heilmann-Gouault M, Tulliez M: Relationship between blast-cell morphology and occurrence of a syndrome of disseminated intravascular coagulation. Br J Haematol 24:255, 1973.

254. Pui CH, Jackson CW, Chesney CM, Abildgaard CF: Involvement of von Willebrand factor in thrombosis following asparaginase-prednisone-vincristine therapy for leukemia. Am J Hematol 25:291–298, 1987.

255. Bauer KA, Teitel JM: L-asparaginase induced antithrombin III deficiency: Evidence against the production of a hypercoagulable state. Thromb Res 29:437–442, 1983.

256. Cairo MS, Lazarus K, Gilmore RL, Baehner RL: Intracranial hemorrhage and focal seizures secondary to use of L-aparaginase during induction therapy of acute lymphocytic leukemia. J Pediatr 97:829–833, 1980.

257. Priest JR, Ramsay NKC, Steinherz PG, Tubergen DG, Cairo MS, Sitarz AL et al: A syndrome of thrombosis and hemorrhage complicating L-asparaginase therapy for childhood acute lymphoblastic leukemia. J Pediatr 100:984–989, 1982.

258. Pui CH, Chesney CM, Bergum PW, Jackson CW, Rapaport SI: Lack of pathogenetic role of proteins C and S in thrombosis associated with asparaginase-prednisone-vincristine therapy for leukaemia. Br J Haematol 64:283–290, 1986.

259. Steinherz PG, Miller LP, Ghavimi F et al: Dural sinus thrombosis in children with acute lymphoblastic leukemia. JAMA 246:2837, 1981.

260. Urban C, Sager WD: Intracranial bleeding during therapy with L-asparaginase in childhood acute lymphocytic leukemia. Eur J Pediatr 137:323, 1981.

261. Gugliotta L, Mazzucconi M-G, Leone G, Mattioli-Belmonte M, Defazio D, Annino L et al: Incidence of thrombotic complications in adult patients with acute lymphoblastic leukaemia receiving L-asparaginase during induction therapy: A retrospective study. Eur J Haematol 49:63–66, 1992.

262. Priest JR, Ramsay NKC, Latchaw RE, Lockman LA, Hasegawa DK, Coates TD et al: Thrombotic and hemorrhagic strokes complicating early therapy for childhood acute lymphoblastic leukemia. Cancer 46:1548–1554, 1980.

263. Nowak-Gottl U, Wermes C, Junker R, Koch HG, Schobess R, Fleischhack G et al: Prospective evaluation of the thrombotic risk in children with acute lymphoblastic leukemia carrying the MTHFR TT 677 genotype, the prothrombin G20210A variant, and further prothrombotic risk factors. Blood 93:1595–1599, 1999.

264. Mauz-Korholz C, Junker R, Gobel U, Nowak-Gottl U: Prothrombotic risk factors in children with acute lymphoblastic leukemia treated with delayed E. coli asparaginase (COALL-92 and 97 protocols). Thromb Haemost 83:840–843, 2000.

265. Halton JM, Mitchell LG, Vegh P, Eves M, Andrew ME: Fresh frozen plasma has no beneficial effect on the hemostatic system in children receiving L-asparaginase. Am J Hematol 47:157–161, 1994.

266. Editorial: Antimicrobials and haemostasis. Lancet 1:510–511, 1983.

267. Sattler FR, Weitekamp MR, Sayegh A, Ballard JO: Impaired hemostasis caused by beta-lactam antibiotics. Am J Surg 155:30–39, 1988.

268. Andrassy K, Weischedel E, Ritz E, Andrassy T: Bleeding in uremic patients after carbenicillin. Thromb Haemost 36:115–126, 1976.

269. Bang NU, Tessler SS, Heidenreich RO, Marks CA, Mattler LE: Effects of moxalactam on blood coagulation and platelet function. Rev Infect Dis 4:S546–S554, 1982.

270. Brown CH, Natelson EA, Bradshaw MW, Williams TW, Alfrey CP: The hemostatic defect produced by carbenicillin. N Engl J Med 291:265–270, 1974.

271. Cazenave JP, Guccione MA, Packham MA, Mustard JF: Effects of cephalothin and penicillin G on platelet function in vitro. Br J Haematol 35:135–152, 1977.

272. Haburchak DR, Head DR, Everett ED: Postoperative hemorrhage associated with carbenicillin administration. Am J Surg 134:630, 1977.

273. Johnson GJ, Rao GHR, White JG: Platelet dysfunction induced by parenteral carbenicillin and ticarcillin. Am J Pathol 91:85–106, 1978.

274. Natelson EA, Siebert WT, Williams TW, Bradshaw MW: Combined effects of ticarcillin and cefazolin on blood coagulation and platelet function. Am J Med Sci 278:217–221, 1979.

275. Pakter RL, Russell TR, Mielke CH, West D: Coagulopathy associated with the use of moxalactam. JAMA 248:1100, 1982.

276. Weitekamp MR, Aber RC: Prolonged bleeding times and bleeding diathesis associated with moxalactam administration. JAMA 24:69–71, 1983.

277. Matsubara T, Touchi A, Harauchi T, Takano K, Yoshizaki T: Depression of liver microsomal vitamin K epoxide reductase activity associated with antibiotic-induced coagulopathy. Biochem Pharmacol 38:2693–2701, 1989.

278. Sattler FR, Weitekamp MR, Ballard JO: Potential for bleeding with the new beta-lactam antibiotics. Ann Intern Med 105:924–931, 1986.

279. Shevchuk YM, Conly JM: Antibiotic-associated hypoprothrombinemia: A review of prospective studies, 1966–1988. Rev Infect Disease 12:1109–1126, 1990.

280. Pegram PS, Phair JP, McMahan R, Murphy RL, Gordon LI, Washton H et al: Prospective comparative trial of short course (four day) and continuous tobramycin in combination with cefoperazone or mezlocillin in febrile, granulocytopenic patients. J Antimicrobial Chemo 24:591–604, 1989.

281. Winston DJ, Ho WG, Bruckner DA, Champlin RE: Beta-lactam antibiotic therapy in febrile granulocytopenic patients. A randomized trial comparing cefoperazone plus piperacillin, cef-

tazidime plus piperacillin, and imipenem alone. Ann Intern Med 115:849–859, 1991.

282. Conly J, Suttie J, Reid E, Loftson J, Ramotar K, Louie T: Dietary deficiency of phylloquinone and reduced serum levels in febrile neutropenic cancer patients. Am J Clin Nutr 50:109–113, 1989.

283. Brown CH, Natelson EA, Bradshaw MW, Alfrey CP, Williams TW: Study of the effects of ticarcillin on blood coagulation and platelet function. Anti Agents Chemo 7:652–657, 1975.

284. Shattil SJ, Bennett JS, McDonough M, Turnbull J: Carbenicillin and penicillin G inhibit platelet function in vitro by impairing the interaction of agonists with the platelet surface. J Clin Invest 65:329–337, 1980.

285. Pastakia KB, Terle D, Prodouz KN: Penicillin-induced dysfunction of platelet membrane glycoproteins. J Lab Clin Med 121:546–554, 1993.

286. Burroughs SF, Johnson GJ: β-Lactam antibiotic-induced platelet dysfunction: Evidence for irreversible inhibition of platelet activation in vitro and in vivo after prolonged exposure to penicillin. Blood 75:1473–1480, 1990.

287. Zenon GJ, Cadle RM, Hamill RJ: Vancomycin-induced thrombocytopenia. Arch Intern Med 151:995–996, 1991.

288. Christie DJ, van Buren N, Lennon SS, Putnam JL: Vancomycin-dependent antibodies associated with thrombocytopenia and refractoriness to platelet transfusion in patients with leukemia. Blood 75:518–523, 1990.

289. Chan CSP, Tuazon CU, Lessin LS: Amphotericin-B-induced thrombocytopenia. Ann Intern Med 96:332–333, 1982.

290. Kulpa J, Zaroulis CG, Good RA, Kutti J: Altered platelet function and circulation induced by amphotericin B in leukemic patients after platelet transfusion. Transfusion 21:74–76, 1981.

291. Garratty G: Immune cytopenia associated with antibiotics. (Review). Transfus Med Rev 7:255–267, 1993.

292. Chenoweth CE, Judd WJ, Steiner EA, Kauffman CA: Cefotetan-induced immune hemolytic anemia. Clin Infect Dis 15:863–865, 1992.

293. Endoh T, Yagihashi A, Sasaki M, Watanabe N: Ceftizoxime-induced hemolysis due to immune complexes: Case report and determination of the epitope responsible for immune complex-mediated hemolysis. Transfusion 39:306–309, 1999.

294. Garratty G, Nance S, Lloyd M, Domen R: Fatal immune hemolytic anemia due to cefotetan (see comments). Transfusion 32:269–271, 1992.

295. Arndt PA, Leger RM, Garratty G: Serology of antibodies to second- and third-generation cephalosporins associated with immune hemolytic anemia and/or positive direct antiglobulin tests. Transfusion 39:1239–1246, 1999.

296. Bernini JC, Mustafa MM, Sutor LJ, Buchanan GR: Fatal hemolysis induced by ceftriaxone in a child with sickle cell anemia (see comments). J Pediatr 126:813–815, 1995.

297. Borgna-Pignatti C, Bezzi TM, Reverberi R: Fatal ceftriaxone-induced hemolysis in a child with acquired immunodeficiency syndrome. Pediatr Infect Dis J 14:1116–1117, 1995.

298. Weiss RB, Tormey DC, Holland JF, Weinberg VE: Venous thrombosis during multimodal treatment of primary breast carcinoma. Cancer Treat Rep 65:677–679, 1981.

299. Levine MN, Gent M, Hirsh J, Arnold A, Goodyear MD, Hryniuk W et al: The thrombogenic effect of anticancer drug therapy in women with stage II breast cancer. N Engl J Med 318:404–407, 1988.

300. Rogers JS, Murgo AJ, Fontana JA, Raich PC: Chemotherapy for breast cancer decreases plasma protein C and protein S. J Clin Oncol 6:276–281, 1988.

301. Levine M, Hirsh J, Gent M, Arnold A, Warr D, Falanga A et al: Double-blind randomised trial of very-low-dose warfarin for prevention of thromboembolism in stage IV breast cancer. Lancet 343:886–889, 1994.

302. Holman MJ, Gonwa TA, Cooper B, Husberg BS, Goldstein RM, Gibbs JF et al: FK506-associated thrombotic thrombocytopenic purpura. Transplantation 55:205–206, 1993.

303. Canpolat C, Pearson P, Jaffe N: Cisplatin-associated hemolytic uremic syndrome. Cancer 74:3059–3062, 1994.

304. Charba D, Moake JL, Harris MA, Hester JP: Abnormalities of von Willebrand factor multimers in drug-associated thrombotic microangiopathies. Am J Hematol 42:268–277, 1993.

305. Kwaan HC: Miscellaneous secondary thrombotic microangiopathy. Sem Hematol 24:141–147, 1987.

306. Brodowicz T, Breiteneder S, Wiltschke C, Zielinski CC: Gemcitabine-induced hemolytic uremic syndrome: A case report. J Natl Cancer Inst 89:1895–1896, 1997.

307. Fung MC, Storniolo AM, Nguyen B, Arning M, Brookfield W, Vigil J: A review of hemolytic uremic syndrome in patients treated with gemcitabine therapy. Cancer 85:2023–2032, 1999.

308. Lesesne JB, Rothschild N, Erickson B, Koreck S, Sisk R, Keller J et al: Cancer-associated hemolytic-uremic syndrome: Analysis of 85 cases from a national registry. J Clin Oncol 7:781–789, 1989.

309. Shulman HM, Hinterberger W: Hepatic veno-occlusive disease–liver toxicity syndrome after bone marrow transplantation. Bone Marrow Transplant 10:197–214, 1992.

310. Baron F, Deprez M, Beguin Y: The veno-occlusive disease of the liver (Review). Haematologica 82:718–725, 1997.

311. McDonald GB, Hinds MS, Fisher LD, Schoch HG, Wolford JL, Banaji M et al: Veno-occlusive disease of the liver and multiorgan failure after bone marrow transplantation: A cohort study of 355 patients. Ann Intern Med 118:255–267, 1993.

312. Frickhofen N, Wiesneth M, Jainta C, Hertenstein B, Heymer B, Bianchi L et al: Hepatitis C virus infection is a risk factor for liver failure from veno-occlusive disease after bone marrow transplantation. Blood 83:1998–2004, 1994.

313. Shulman HM, McDonald GB, Matthews D, Doney KC, Kopecky KJ, Gauvreau JM et al: An analysis of hepatic venocclusive disease and centrilobular hepatic degeneration following bone marrow transplantation. Gastroenterology 79:1178–1191, 1980.

314. McDonald GB, Sharma P, Matthews DE, Shulman HM, Thomas ED: Venocclusive disease of the liver after bone marrow transplantation: Diagnosis, incidence, and predisposing factors. Hepatology 4:116–122, 1984.

315. Jones RJ, Lee KSK, Beschorner WE, Vogel VG, Grochow LB, Braine HG et al: Venoocclusive disease of the liver following bone marrow transplantation. Transplantation 44:778–783, 1987.

316. Kami M, Mori S, Tanikawa S, Akiyama H, Onozawa Y, Tanaka T et al: Risk factors for hepatic veno-occlusive disease after bone marrow transplantation: Retrospective analysis of 137 cases at a single institution. Bone Marrow Transplant 20:397–402, 1997.

317. Kaufman PA, Jones RB, Greenberg CS, Peters WP: Autologous bone marrow transplantation and factor XII, factor VII, and protein C deficiencies. Cancer 66:515–521, 1990.

318. Faioni EM, Krachmalnicoff A, Bearman SI, Federici AB, Decarli A, Gianni AM et al: Naturally occurring anticoagulants and bone marrow transplantation: Plasma protein C predicts the development of venocclusive disease of the liver. Blood 81:3458–3462, 1993.

319. Scrobohaci ML, Drouet L, Monem-Mansi A, Devergie A, Baudin B, D'Agay MF et al: Liver veno-occlusive disease after bone marrow transplantation changes in coagulation parameters and endothelial markers. Thromb Res 63:509–519, 1991.

320. Salat C, Holler E, Kolb HJ, Reinhardt B, Pihusch R, Wilmanns W et al: Plasminogen activator inhibitor-1 confirms the diagnosis of hepatic veno- occlusive disease in patients with hyperbilirubinemia after bone marrow transplantation. Blood 89:2184–2188, 1997.

321. Park YD, Yasui M, Yoshimoto T, Chayama K, Shimono T, Okamura T et al: Changes in hemostatic parameters in hepatic veno-occlusive disease following bone marrow transplantation. Bone Marrow Transplant 1997; 19:915–920, 1997.

322. Holler E, Kolb HJ, Moller A, Kempeni J, Lisenfeld S, Pechumer H et al: Increased serum levels of tumor necrosis factor alpha precede major complications of bone marrow transplantation. Blood 75:1011–1016, 1990.

323. Attal M, Huguet F, Rubie H, Huynh A, Charlet J-P, Payen J-L et al: Prevention of hepatic veno-occlusive disease after bone marrow transplantation by continuous infusion of low-dose heparin: A prospective, randomized trial. Blood 79:2834–2840, 1992.

324. Fogteloo AJ, Smid WM, Kok T, van der Meer J, Van Imhoff GW, Daenen S: Successful treatment of veno-occlusive disease of the liver with urokinase in a patient with non-Hodgkin's lymphoma. Leukemia 7:760–763, 1993.

325. Bearman SI, Shuhard MC, Hinds MS, McDonald GB: Recombinant human tissue plasminogen activator for the treatment of established severe venocclusive disease of the liver after bone marrow transplantation. Blood 80:2458–2462, 1992.

326. Chopra R, Eaton JD, Grassi A, Potter M, Shaw B, Salat C et al: Defibrotide for the treatment of hepatic veno-occlusive disease: Results of the European compassionate-use study. Liver 111:1122–1129, 2000.

327. Richardson PG, Elias AD, Krishnan A, Wheeler C, Nath R, Hoppensteadt D et al: Treatment of severe veno-occlusive disease with defibrotide: Compassionate use results in response without significant toxicity in a high-risk population (Review). Blood 92:737–744, 1998.

62

Psychological Aspects of Hematological Malignancies

Andrew J. Roth and Jimmie C. Holland

Advances in the treatment of the hematological malignancies have led to longer survival of many patients and cure of more. Interest in how these patients cope with the newer and more technological treatment and in their quality of life has increased. The psychological issues are outlined below as they relate to diagnosis, treatment, and the adaptation of survivors.

The diagnosis of a hematologic malignancy is particularly frightening because of the fears associated with cancer illness, pain, disfigurement, disability, and possible death. The fears of treatment are also frightening since it could include bone marrow transplantation, which has been described as a "healing hell" by Groopman.[1] The high mortality from both the disease and the treatments is well known by the public. The impact of the diagnosis is often an initial period of disbelief and denial, followed by a period characterized by poor sleep and appetite, preoccupation with the illness, difficulties in concentration, anxiety, despair, and thoughts of death. Patients have difficulty carrying out daily activities, with lingering thoughts about the uncertainty of the future. In the following weeks as treatment begins, they adjust to the new reality and return to their more normal pattern of coping. Crisis points may continue to occur: they include news of poor response to treatment, relapse of disease, and exhaustion of treatment options. These crisis points, associated with greater distress, often require psychiatric evaluation and treatment.

Adjustment to illness is determined by three factors: (1) medical-related factors (stage at diagnosis, pain, treatments, and complications); (2) patient-related factors (ability to cope with stressful events, stage of the life cycle and emotional maturity, support of family and others); and (3) societal factors (attitudes of the public toward leukemia and lymphoma and their treatment, the stigma associated with cancer, and health care policies relating to insurance). This combination of medical, personal, and societal factors impacts on individuals, leading to their unique responses to illness. This chapter explores some of these issues, as well as the common psychiatric disorders and their management.

DEVELOPMENTAL ISSUES

A developmental model[2] for understanding the impact of hematological malignancies as they occur across the life cycle is helpful.

The psychological concerns vary by age and must be taken into consideration when evaluating patients. Families also have developmental stages. For example, the young family in which a small child or adolescent develops leukemia may not have had prior experience with illness and loss, which tests their coping capacity. One study of children with leukemia found that those who had parents meeting Diagnostic Statistical Manual 3- Revised (DSM3 R) criteria for a psychiatric disorder had more self-reported anxiety and were reported by mothers as having more depression.[3] Hodgkin's disease or leukemia in a young adult who has a spouse or small children poses a serious challenge. Fertility issues may be minimal for the older person, but critical to the adolescent and young adult who anticipate marriage and raising a family.

Specific developmental tasks at different ages affect the response to the illness. The young child is developing a basic sense of trust and hope and an ability to interact with and explore the environment. By the end of this phase healthy children are beginning to master a sense of autonomy and independence. These qualities may be delayed in the ill child. Painful procedures and handling by strangers may lead to helpless feelings, fears, and mistrust.

Three- to five-year old children are experimenting with their independence and exploring their world. Health and illness are seen as two separate states, in contrast to a continuum, as viewed by older children and adults. Separation from both parents and siblings by hospitalizations and lengthy treatments are felt acutely. The ill child may show jealousy of healthy siblings and friends. Parents are tempted to protect their children and reassert a level of control more appropriate to earlier periods of life. At any age, there may be loss of a developmental milestone and regression to an earlier stage of development. Information given to young children should be concrete, nontechnical, and age-appropriate.

Middle childhood is characterized by entry into school, a major socializing force in children's lives. Children compare themselves to others and master important tasks such as relating to peers. The challenge of a hematological malignancy at this age often causes isolation from peers and a feeling of shame when appearance is altered. Disruption of school attendance leads to an impaired sense of competence and self-esteem. Children are aware of the gravity of their disease even if they do not yet have a full appreciation of the irreversibility of death. Those who are experiencing hair loss or other changes in body image due to their cancer treatment may think that doctors and nurses are punishing them for some wrong deed. Support and education of parents is crucial for the child's adaptation because parents' level of distress plays a large role in modulating the child's emotional distress.

In adolescence, major changes are occurring in the physical, cognitive, social, mood, and sexual spheres. Adolescents are trying to achieve an identity, to enter into mature relationships with peers of both sexes, and to gain independence from their parents and family. Hospitalizations and separations from friends lead to feelings of being "different," isolated, and out of the peer group.

Young adults are at a point when seeking intimate relationships is important. Marriage, children, and career are all disrupted by changes in appearance and sexual function. Sterility related to chemotherapy or radiation may also be problems a young person needs to confront.

Middle-aged individuals are experiencing their children growing up and leaving home, and they are adjusting to losses of parents. Illness may be particularly disruptive at this time, when their careers are at a peak. For older individuals, diminishing sexual activity and problems related to retirement and decreased income are made far more difficult when leukemia or lymphoma occurs.

Beyond these developmental issues and psychosocial concerns are those related to actual psychiatric disorders, which are common with the significant stress of serious illness. Since many are treatable, it is important that the physician be able to recognize them and to know the principles for treatment and when referral to a psychiatrist is appropriate.

PSYCHIATRIC DISORDERS

The most frequent psychiatric disorders seen are, in order of frequency, anxiety, depression, delirium, and distress associated with pain. Each is discussed below.

Anxiety

Clinical Picture of Anxiety

By far, the most frequent psychological problem in patients with hematological neoplasms is anxiety. Fears and distress are normal, but more severe levels of anxiety are common. These include reactive anxiety (adjustment disorder with anxious mood, based on the standard psychiatric classification of DSM-IV), discrete anxiety disorders, and medical or procedure-related anxiety. Individuals with a preexisting anxiety disorder are at risk of its exacerbation during illness. These disorders cause severe suffering, sometimes to the extent that they compromise the ability to get medical care. Early recognition and treatment are essential for optimal care. Understanding the source of the anxiety is important in choosing an appropriate treatment.[4]

Reactive anxiety is an exaggerated form of "normal" anxiety related to illness. It differs from normal fears of cancer by greater duration and intensity of symptoms, impairment of normal function, and impairment of ability to comply with treatment. Common symptoms are nervousness, tremulousness, palpitations, shortness of breath, diarrhea, diaphoresis, numbness and tingling of the extremities, feelings of imminent death, and phobias. Fearfulness, accompanied by symptoms of anxiety (e.g., restlessness, insomnia), is expected and considered normal before painful or stressful procedures (e.g., bone marrow aspiration, chemotherapy, radiation therapy); prior to surgery; and while awaiting test results. Many patients with mild to moderate anxiety respond to being given adequate information with reassurance and support; some require medication to control their distress. Patients who are extremely fearful are unable to absorb information or to cooperate with procedures. They require psychological support, medication, and/or behavioral interventions to reduce symptoms to a manageable level.

Anxiety Associated with Medical Conditions

Anxiety is frequently associated with medical problems including uncontrolled pain, abnormal metabolic states, medications that produce anxiety, and withdrawal states (Table 62–1).

Patients in severe pain are often anxious and agitated; they communicate their anguish and inability to tolerate the distress. Adequate analgesia results in reduced anxiety immediately as they experience relief from pain. However, they may worry and become anxious about "the next dose." Having to wait until the pain returns to request pain medication and waiting for it to come generate anxiety again, which then escalates the pain. Analgesics should be ordered around the clock (not as needed) to reach a steady state, which allows the patient to relax and feel secure that the pain will not return between doses. Rescue doses in case the standing dose is too low should also be made available.

The acute onset of anxiety without an obvious reason may herald a change in metabolic state or an impending catastrophic medical event.[5] Sudden anxiety accompanied by chest pain or respiratory distress suggests a pulmonary embolus. Patients who are hypoxic are anxious and fearful that they are suffocating or dying. Sepsis and delirium can also cause anxiety symptoms. Several drugs, such as corticosteroids, antiemetics, and antiasthmatics, precipitate anxiety; corticosteroids may also produce motor restlessness, agitation, depression, and at times suicidal ideation. These symptoms appear usually with high doses or during rapid tapers. Akathisia, motor restlessness accompanied by subjective feelings of distress and hyperactivity, is an extrapyramidal side effect of prochlorperazine and metoclopramide, neuroleptic drugs often used to control emesis. The newer agents ondansetron and granisetron produce few side effects of this kind.

Withdrawal states from alcohol, benzodiazepines, and narcotics, usually developing within 1 to 3 days after hospital admission, result in anxiety, agitation, delirium, and even violent behavior which may be dangerous to patients and staff. Acute changes in mental status within the first 10 days of admission should lead to a careful history of medications used for sleep, pain, anxiety, nausea, or illicit use, as well as detailed information about drinking, prior to admission. A urine toxicology screen should be ordered as early as the problem is recognized.

Diagnosis of Anxiety States

It is important that the physician inquire about anxiety symptoms when distress is suspected, since patients may be embar-

---

Table 62–1. Anxiety Associated with Medical Conditions

1. Uncontrolled pain
2. Abnormal metabolic states
3. Medication side effects
4. Withdrawal states

rassed by their present concerns or by a history of phobias or panic. Table 62–2 lists some questions that are useful to ask.

The stress of the diagnosis of leukemia or lymphoma may activate a preexisting phobia which otherwise is not bothersome. Phobias of blood, doctors, and hospitals and agoraphobia are common sources of anxiety in the hospital. Panic disorder, characterized by symptoms of autonomic discharge, such as heart pounding, chest pain, sweating, hyperventilation, trembling, and a sense of impending doom, will be reactivated by a cancer diagnosis or difficult treatment.

Generalized anxiety is chronic anxiety that may also produce autonomic symptoms and be exacerbated. Post-traumatic stress disorder (PTSD) may be activated by isolation or conditions that lead to recollection of a prior frightening event. Holocaust survivors, Vietnam veterans, and those directly affected by the World Trade Center disaster are particularly vulnerable. A new aspect of PTSD is the fact that it may be experienced by both adults and children following traumatic events related to cancer treatment. An exaggerated startle response, insomnia, nightmares, reliving the feelings and invasive thoughts experienced at the time of the trauma, and avoidance of anything associated with the trauma (e.g., the hospital) may occur. The anticipatory anxiety seen at follow-up visits after cancer treatments are finished is likely PTSD-related, responding to cues that are painful reminders. Anticipatory nausea and vomiting with anxiety are conditioned responses to chemotherapy. Post-traumatic stress disorder is likely a learned response to prior trauma, which explains the symptoms that occur in cancer survivors who experience reminders of the treatment. This becomes more important because of the increasing number of patients who survive treatment. It has been studied in Hodgkin's disease survivors.[6]

The initial management of anxiety requires that adequate information be given to the patient in a supportive and understanding manner. Cognitive therapeutic techniques identify maladaptive automatic thoughts and underlying negative assumptions that interfere with coping. Brief supportive therapy, crisis intervention, and insight-oriented psychotherapy are also used. The behavioral approaches of progressive relaxation, guided imagery, meditation, biofeedback, and hypnosis treat anxiety symptoms that are associated with painful procedures, pain syndromes, and anticipatory fears of chemotherapy and radiation therapy.

A benzodiazepine is often needed in combination with psychological support. The choice of medication depends on the severity of anxiety, desired duration of drug action, rapidity of onset needed, route of administration available, presence or absence of active metabolites, and metabolic problems that must be considered. Dosing schedules depend on patients' tolerance and require individual titration. The shorter-acting benzodiazepines (alprazolam and lorazepam) are given three to four times per day. Short-acting benzodiazepines, particularly those that can be administered by multiple routes, are widely used with good results. Clonazepam, a longer-acting drug with antiseizure properties, is useful for panic symptoms and insomnia. A rapid onset of effect is achieved with lorazepam and diazepam for management of acute anxiety.

The most common side effects of benzodiazepines are dose-dependent and are controlled by titrating the dose to avoid drowsiness, confusion, motor incoordination, and sedation. All benzodiazepines can cause respiratory depression and must be used cautiously, if at all, in the presence of respiratory impairment. The respiratory depressant effects are additive or even synergistic in the presence of antidepressants, antiemetics, and analgesics. Low doses of the antihistamine hydroxyzine, of buspirone, or of the newer atypical neuroleptics olanzapine and quetiapine can be used safely and relatively effectively when there is concern about depressing central respiratory mechanisms. In patients with hepatic dysfunction, it is best to use short-acting benzodiazepines that are metabolized primarily by conjugation and excreted by the kidney (e.g., oxazepam and lorazepam) or those that lack active metabolites (lorazepam). It is important to remember that discontinuation of a benzodiazepine in a patient who has been on a standing dose for more than 2 weeks should be done on a tapering schedule to avoid withdrawal. Akathisia is quickly controlled by stopping the causative drug if possible and adding a benzodiazepine, a beta-blocker such as propranolol, or an antiparkinsonian agent such as benztropine.

Treatment of withdrawal states from alcohol, benzodiazepines, barbiturates, or opioids depends on the particular agent. Sometimes the goal is to stabilize the patient on the agent (a benzodiazepine) and sometimes a suitable substitute must be given (a benzodiazepine for ethanol or for a barbiturate). Anxiety before chemotherapy or painful procedures and dressing changes is controlled by a short-acting benzodiazepine such as lorazepam, which also provides anterograde amnesia. Given intravenously, lorazepam also reduces vomiting in patients receiving emetogenic chemotherapy. Both oral lorazepam and alprazolam reduce nausea and vomiting related to chemotherapy.

In general, cancer patients usually need to be encouraged to take antianxiety drugs at all, and in sufficient amounts to relieve anxiety. A stigma about taking these medications exists on the

---

Table 62–2. Questions to Query Anxiety Symptoms in Patients with Blood Neoplasms

Have you experienced any of the following symptoms since your cancer diagnosis or treatment? If yes, when do they occur (for example, number of days prior to treatment, during procedures, at night, no specific time), and how long do they last?

Do you feel nervous, shaky, or jittery?

Have you felt fearful, apprehensive, tense?

Have you had to avoid certain places or activities because of fear?

Have you experienced your heart pounding or racing?

Have you had trouble catching your breath when nervous?

Have you had any unjustified sweating or trembling?

Have you felt a knot in the pit in your stomach?

Have you felt a lump in your throat when getting upset?

Do you find yourself pacing back and forth?

Are you afraid to close your eyes at night for fear that you will die in your sleep?

Do you find yourself worrying about the next bone marrow aspiration or the results of it weeks in advance?

part of both patient and doctor. Medications are readily discontinued when symptoms subside. Concerns about addiction are far exaggerated in patients who have no history of drug abuse.

Depression

When a patient's mood is severely depressed and is accompanied by hopeless, despondent, or guilty feelings and suicidal thoughts, this is a major depression and it is *not* normal. Depression is treatable and is not normal in most patients with cancer. Although sadness about illness is normally expected with a disease such as leukemia, depression is not. Table 62–3 lists questions that a physician might ask to do a rapid assessment of mood. Doctors often underestimate the morbidity caused by depression, since they tend to believe they would feel depressed, even suicidal, if the roles were reversed. The patient's mood, physical symptoms of depression, and the severity of depression, including suicide risk, must be assessed. Physical symptoms must be carefully evaluated to determine whether fatigue, insomnia, and decreased libido are caused by depression, by cancer, or as a complication of treatment. The biological correlates of depression are decreased appetite, poor sleep, fatigue, loss of energy, loss of libido, and psychomotor slowing. They are the key symptoms of depression in physically healthy persons. They are, however, unreliable in patients with cancer, who may have no

appetite because of chemotherapy, sleep poorly because of pain or because they are hospitalized, and be fatigued because of the cancer, radiation therapy, or chemotherapy. When it is difficult to decide the etiology of depression and symptoms are impairing function, a trial of antidepressants is warranted.

Symptoms of depression are caused by several medical conditions and by several medications (Table 62–4). One should ask about uncontrolled pain, which is a common cause of depression in cancer patients. Uncontrolled pain leads to hopeless, desperate feelings and a sense that life is intolerable unless pain is relieved. Patients interpret a new or increasingly severe pain as a sign that the cancer has progressed, which results in greater depression and hopelessness. Suicide is a real risk in these patients, especially if they do not believe that efforts are being made to control the pain or that relief is possible. Suicidal ideation and major depressive symptoms usually abate when pain is controlled.

Other causes of depression in patients with hematological cancers are metabolic abnormalities. Hypercalcemia, sodium and potassium imbalances, anemia, vitamin B12 or folate deficiency, endocrinological abnormalities, and medications are causes of depression. Corticosteroids, prednisone, and dexamethasone, commonly used in leukemia and lymphoma therapy, cause a range of psychiatric symptoms, particularly affective changes from manic to depressive symptoms. Depressed symp-

---

Table 62–3. Questions to Ask to Assess Depressive Symptoms in Patients with Hematological Malignancies

Question	Symptom
Mood	
How well are you coping with your cancer? Well? Poor?	(Well-being)
How are your spirits since diagnosis? Down? Blue? During treatment? Depressed? Sad?	(Mood)
Do you cry sometimes? How often? Only alone?	
Are there things you still enjoy doing or have you lost pleasure in things you used to do before you had cancer?	(Anhedonia)
How does the future look to you? Bright? Black?	(Hopelessness)
Do you feel you can influence your care or is your care totally under others' control?	
Do you worry about being a burden to family or friends during treatment for cancer?	(Worthlessness)
Feel others might be better off without you?	(Guilt)
Physical symptoms (evaluate in the context of cancer-related symptoms)	
Do you have pain that isn't controlled?	(Pain)
How much time do you spend in bed?	(Fatigue)
Weak? Fatigue easily? Rested after sleep? Any relationship to change in treatment or how you feel otherwise physically?	
How is your sleeping? Trouble going to sleep? Awake early? Often?	(Insomnia)
How is your appetite? Food tastes good? Weight loss or gain?	(Appetite)
How is your interest in sex? Extent of sexual activity?	(Libido)
Do you think or move more slowly?	(Psychomotor slowing)

Table 62–4. Causes of Depression in Patients with Hematological Malignancies

Uncontrolled pain
Metabolic abnormalities
  Hypercalcemia
  Sodium, potassium imbalance
  Anemia
  Deficient vitamin B12 or folate
Endocrinological abnormalities
  Hyper- or hypothyroidism
  Adrenal insufficiency
Medications
  Steroids
  Interferon and interleukin-2
  Methyldopa
  Reserpine
  Barbiturates
  Propranolol
  Some antibiotics (amphotericin B)
  Some chemotherapeutic agents
    Vincristine
    Vinblastine
    Procarbazine
    L-Asparaginase

toms are far more common. The depressed mood is usually improved when the steroid is stopped. However, an antidepressant may be needed.

Antidepressants

The medications used in patients with hematologic malignancies for depression are the serotonin reuptake inhibitors (SSRIs), the tricyclic antidepressants (TCAs), and psychostimulants. Table 60–5 outlines the common antidepressants used in these patients. It highlights starting dosages used in cancer patients, which are generally lower than those used in physically healthy depressed individuals. The Side Effects/Comments section notes factors that must be kept in mind, as they are helpful or problematic for these patients. Most antidepressants are contraindicated in patients who are treated with the monoamine oxidase inhibitor procarbazine. When choosing an antidepressant for those with hematological malignancies, it is important to consider secondary effects that may be utilized for their positive value. For example, a sedating antidepressant (such as amitriptyline or trazodone) is useful for an agitated patient who

Table 62–5. Medication Dosages in Cancer Patients

Drug	Start/Daily Dose (mg)	Primary Side Effects/Comments
Tricyclics (TCAs)		All TCAs can cause cardiac arrhythmias; blood levels are available for all but doxepin. Get baseline electrocardiogram.
Amitriptyline (Elavil)	10–25/50–100	Sedation; anticholinergic; orthostasis
Imipramine (Tofranil)	10–25/50–150	Intermediate sedation; anticholinergic; orthostasis
Desipramine (Norpramin)	25/75–150	Little sedation, or orthostasis; moderate anticholinergic
Nortriptyline (Pamelor)	10–25/75–150	Little anticholinergic or orthostasis; intermediate sedation; therapeutic window
Doxepin (Sinequan)	25/75–150	Very sedating; orthostatic hypotension; intermediate anticholinergic effects; potent antihistamine
Second generation		
Buproprion (Wellbutrin)	75/200–450	May cause seizures in those with low seizure threshold/brain tumors; initially activating
Trazodone (Desyrel)	50/150–200	Sedating; not anticholinergic; risk of priapism
Serotonin-specific reuptake inhibitors		Serotonin reuptake inhibitors have few anticholinergic or cardiovascular side effects. Sexual dysfunction including anorgasmia.
Fluoxetine (Prozac)	10/20–40	Headache; nausea; anxiety; insomnia. Has a very long half-life; may be even longer in debilitated patient.
Sertraline (Zoloft)	25/50–150	Nausea; insomnia
Paroxetine (Paxil)	10/20–50	Nausea; somnolence; asthenia; no active metabolites
Citalopram (Celexa)	10/20–40	Somnolence
Psychostimulants		All psychostimulants may cause nightmares.
d-Amphetamine (Dexedrin)	2.5/5–30	Nightmares, insomnia, psychosis, anorexia, agitation, and restlessness. Possible cardiac complications. They should be given in two divided doses at 8 AM and noon; can be used as analgesic adjuvant and to counter sedation of opiates.
Methylphenidate (Ritalin)	2.5/5–30	
Pemoline (Cylert)	18.75/37.5–150	Follow liver tests.
Modafinil (Provigil)	50–400	
Other		
Venlafaxine (Effexor)	75/225–375	Inhibits reuptake of both serotonin and norepinephrine. Achieves steady state in 3 days. May increase blood pressure.
Nefazodone (Serzone)	100/200–500	Affects serotonin, 5HT$_2$, and norepinephrine; sedating; decreased cardiotoxicity; less reported sexual dysfunction than with SSRs
Mirtazapine (Remeron)	15/15–45	Sedating at lower doses, useful for agitated depression; less reported nausea, GI problems, sexual dysfunction; may cause weight gain.

has difficulty sleeping because it has both calming and sedating effects. A patient's prior response to a particular medication or a family member's experience with an antidepressant is a helpful predictor of response. When and whether an antidepressant can be used even with the potential for bone marrow suppression as a side effect remains controversial, particularly in bone marrow transplantation. The bone marrow suppression risks must be weighed against the potential risks of noncompliance with treatment protocols secondary to depression.

In the last few years, the SSRIs fluoxetine, sertraline, paroxetine, and citalopram have rapidly achieved wide use because of their efficacy and the low risk of significant side effects such as cardiac arrhythmias, hypotension, or anticholinergic effects. The primary side effects of fluoxetine are gastric distress and nausea, brief periods of anxiety, headache, and insomnia (less commonly, hypersomnia). A troubling side effect is anorgasmia. The primary side effects of sertraline are nausea, diarrhea, dyspepsia, tremor, dizziness, ejaculatory delay in men, and insomnia. Sertraline's shorter half-life allows for faster clearance and hence better control in patients with cancer. Paroxetine has no active metabolites and therefore is excreted relatively quickly on discontinuation. Nausea, somnolence, and asthenia are common side effects. Citalopram may be more sedating than the other SSRIs. Since all of these drugs are strongly protein-bound, consideration must be given to their ability to increase blood levels of coumadin, digoxin, and cisplatin.

Tricyclic antidepressants (amitriptyline, doxepin, imipramine, nortriptyline, and desipramine) are commonly used for depression and for the treatment of neuropathic pain. They are started at a low dose (10 to 25 mg at bedtime), especially in debilitated patients, and increased slowly (by 10 to 25 mg every few days until symptoms improve). For reasons that are unclear, depressed cancer patients often show a therapeutic response to a tricyclic at much lower doses (75 to 125 mg daily).

The choice of an antidepressant depends on the nature of the depressive symptoms, the medical problems present, and the side effect profile of the specific drug, which one may want to exploit or avoid. The depressed patient with psychomotor slowing will benefit from use of the compounds with the least sedating effects, such as fluoxetine, buproprion, or desipramine. Patients with stomatitis secondary to chemotherapy or radiotherapy with slow intestinal motility secondary to narcotic pain medication, or with urinary retention should receive an antidepressant with the least anticholinergic side effects, such as desipramine, nortriptyline, or one of the newer serotonin-based drugs.[7] Buproprion is less cardiotoxic than the TCAs and has an activating effect in withdrawn, medically ill patients. Patients who are agitated or have insomnia will benefit from the use of an antidepressant that has sedating effects, such as amitriptyline, doxepin, nefazodone, or mirtazapine. Patients who are unable to swallow pills may be able to take an antidepressant elixir (amitriptyline, nortriptyline, doxepin, fluoxetine, paroxetine, or sertraline) or drugs that can be given in an intramuscular form (amitriptyline or imipramine). Intramuscular administration causes discomfort because of the volume of the vehicle; hence 50 mg is usually the maximum dosage that can be delivered per IM injection. Parenteral administration of TCAs can be considered for the cancer patient unable to tolerate oral administration (absence of swallowing reflex, presence of gastric or jejunal drainage tubes, or intestinal obstruction). Although three TCAs, namely, amitriptyline, imipramine, and clomipramine, are available in injectable form, the U.S. Food and Drug Administration has approved imipramine and amitriptyline for oral and intramuscular administration and clomipramine for oral use only. The intramuscular route may cause bleeding in a patient with a low platelet count. Close monitoring of cardiac conduction by electrocardiogram is recommended when these medications are used intravenously. Hospital pharmacies can also prepare some TCAs in rectal suppository form, but absorption by this route has not been studied in patients with cancer.

Imipramine, doxepin, amitriptyline, desipramine, and nortriptyline are frequently used in the management of neuropathic pain in cancer patients. Dosing is similar, although generally in lower doses than for treatment of depression.

The newest antidepressants are venlafaxine, nefazodone, and mirtazapine. Venlafaxine and nefazodone affect both norepinephrine and serotonin neurotransmitter systems but do not produce the same uncomfortable antimuscarinic and antiadrenergic side effects as the TCAs. Nefazodone and mirtazapine have been useful in patients with anxiety and insomnia. Mirtazapine does not cause gastric distress and has been shown to cause weight gain, which is often helpful in cancer patients who are anorexic. The psychostimulants methylphenidate, pemoline, and dextroamphetamine are useful in low doses for patients who are suffering from depressed mood, apathy, decreased energy, poor concentration, and weakness. They promote a sense of well-being, decrease fatigue, and stimulate appetite. They are helpful in countering the sedating effects of morphine, and they produce a rapid effect in comparison with the other antidepressants. Side effects are insomnia, euphoria, and mood lability. High doses and long-term use may produce anorexia, nightmares, insomnia, euphoria, or paranoid thinking. Pemoline is available in a chewable tablet. Patients who have difficulty swallowing can absorb it through the buccal mucosa. It is as effective as the other psychostimulants although it is not a controlled substance. Pemoline should be used with caution in patients with renal impairment; liver function tests should be monitored periodically with longer term treatment. The newest psychostimulant is modafinil. Anecdotal experience has been favorable in people with fatigue from their cancer or its treatment.

Suicide

Suicidal ideation is frightening for the patient, the family, and the physician. Suicidal statements may range from an offhand comment resulting from frustration or disgust with a treatment course: "If I have to have one more bone marrow aspiration this year, I'll jump out the window." A reflection of significant despair may be heard: "I can no longer bear what this disease is doing to all of us." Exploring the seriousness of the thoughts is imperative. Table 62–6 lists questions to assess suicidal ideation in cancer patients. It is important to ask if the patient has made a definite plan. Is the patient stockpiling medication? Does he or she own or have access to a weapon? There are several impor-

Table 62–6. Questions to Ask to Assess Suicide Risk in Cancer Patients

(Open with statement; asking does not enhance risk):
Most patients with cancer have passing thoughts about suicide, such as "I might do
   something if it gets bad enough."
Have you ever had thoughts like that?   (Acknowledge)
Any thoughts of not wanting to live or that it would be easier if you were to die?
Do you have thoughts of suicide? Plan?   (Seriousness)
Have you thought about how you would do it?
Have you ever been depressed or made a suicide attempt?   (Prior history)
Have you ever been treated for other psychiatric problems or have you been
   psychiatrically hospitalized before getting diagnosed with cancer?
Have you had a problem with alcohol or drugs?   (Substance use)
Have you lost anyone close to you recently (family, friends, co-patients)?   (Bereavement)

tant psychological predictors: history of a psychiatric disorder, particularly depression or substance abuse; recent bereavement; and few social supports. Medical predictors of enhanced suicidal risk are poorly controlled pain, advanced stage of disease with debilitation, mild delirium with poor impulse control, and hopelessness or helplessness in the context of depression. The latter two categories involve issues that if addressed with proper therapy, will reduce the suicidal ideation and risk.

The management of the patient with a hematological malignancy who is suicidal is based on developing and maintaining a supportive relationship, giving the patient a sense of control by helping him or her to focus on that which can be controlled and conveying the attitude that much can be done to improve the quality, if not the quantity, of life. It is important to actively treat the symptoms of pain, nausea, insomnia, anxiety, and depression. If the patient is actively suicidal, a 24-hour companion should monitor the patient's behavior.

Delirium and Cognitive Changes

Often psychiatric consultations are requested for patients who appear angry, depressed, psychotic, or anxious but who after evaluation are found to be delirious owing to an encephalopathy. These are important distinctions because treatment recommendations are quite different for depression, anxiety, psychosis, and delirium. Untreated delirium can lead to death, because its origin is usually a sign of organ failure or drug toxicity. Delirium, dementia, and cognitive disorders due to medical conditions occur in roughly 15 to 20 percent of hospitalized cancer patients and in the majority of terminally ill patients with cancer.[8] Symptoms of delirium are an inability to maintain or shift attention properly, waxing and waning of consciousness, disturbance in the sleep–wake cycle, disorientation to person, place, or time, abnormal perceptions such as visual or auditory (less frequent), hallucinations, and problems with memory and language (dysnomia or dysgraphia). Delirium is distinguished from dementia by more rapid onset, fluctuation in level and severity of symptoms, reversibility, and lesser degree of memory impairment.

Etiologically, delirium may be directly caused by the tumor itself, as in central nervous system (CNS) lymphoma, or by metastatic spread of the tumor to the CNS via hematogenous or lymphatic routes. Indirect effects of infection, vascular complications, metabolic changes, organ failure, treatment effects, changes in nutritional state, and paraneoplastic syndromes are common. Failure of vital organs, especially the liver, kidneys, and lungs, and the metabolic changes that result from thyroid or adrenal failure are most frequent. Electrolyte imbalance, especially sodium, potassium, and calcium, causes an altered mental status. Adequate doses of narcotic analgesics to manage cancer pain, when high, will result in hallucinations and delusions. All steroid compounds may cause psychiatric disturbances, ranging from affective changes (emotional lability) to paranoid interpretation of events, suspiciousness of others, illusions, delusions, and hallucinations.

Central nervous system symptoms are not a prominent feature of most chemotherapeutic agents used today. Those that can cause delirium are methotrexate, 5-fluorouracil, vincristine and vinblastine, bleomycin, BCNU, cisplatin, asparaginase, and procarbazine.[9] Interferon, used in treatment regimens for some leukemias and lymphomas, can cause profound depression, somnolence, confusion, and paresthesias. Interleukin-2 often causes depression and cognitive changes. Amphotericin B, used in immunologically compromised patients for the treatment of fungal infections, causes neurological side effects and delirium with intrathecal administration. Often it is difficult to distinguish the CNS effects of antifungal medication from those of fever, CNS infections, or metabolic abnormalities. Acyclovir, used in the treatment of herpes simplex and varicella zoster viruses in immunologically compromised patients who have leukemia or are going through bone marrow transplantation, causes neurotoxicity, with agitation, tremor, and disorientation.

Whole-brain radiation, combined with intrathecal methotrexate, enhances the likelihood of encephalopathy. Children with acute lymphocytic leukemia who were treated with intrathecal methotrexate and cranial radiation as prophylaxis against CNS recurrence were found to have lower IQ scores than children who received only intrathecal methotrexate. Radiation causes a transient syndrome in children known as the radiation somnolence syndrome. This occurs several weeks after radiation and is caused by demyelination.[10]

Environmental manipulation and a low dose of a neuroleptic are useful for a patient who has mild delirium without agitation. If the patient is a danger to him- or herself or to others because of a confused or disinhibited state, observation by a full-time companion is indicated. Frequent reminders by staff or family of location, day, time, and outside events help distract patients from their internal thoughts, hallucinations, or delusions and afford them appropriate orientation.

Haloperidol, a high-potency neuroleptic used in low doses orally, is the drug of choice for treatment of mild organic mental disorders. It can also be used safely parenterally. The usual starting dose of 0.5 mg once or twice daily (orally, intramuscularly, intravenously, or subcutaneously) is administered initially, with doses repeated every 45 to 60 minutes and titrated against symptoms. Haloperidol provides mild sedation and diminishes the behavioral problems. It is administered intravenously when patients are thrombocytopenic, unable to take medications orally secondary to stomatitis, or agitated, and rapid sedation is needed. The newer atypical antipsychotic medications such as olanzapine, risperidone, and quetiapine may also be useful for delirious patients. However, these medications have not been studied in cancer patients, and they lack the parenteral administration route.

Pain

Pain is a frequent complication of cancer in general and of hematological malignancies is particular because of the side effects of treatments (e.g., mucositis) and of procedures such as (bone marrow aspiration). Psychological variables are important because they bear on the meaning of the pain (extension of the disease), loss of control, increased fears of death, and depressed and helpless feelings.

Today, although greater attention is given to alleviating pain, it is still often undertreated in cancer patients. Factors that contribute to the undertreatment of pain are: Lack of proper assessment of the pain; the assumption that psychological rather than medical variables are the cause of pain; lack of knowledge of current therapeutic approaches; focus on prolonging life; the belief that opioids should be "saved in case you need them later"; inadequate physician–patient relationship; fear of respiratory depression; patients' unwillingness to inform physician of pain or fear of taking opioids; and fear of addiction.[11] Both patients and physicians share this latter fear. Although tolerance and physical dependence commonly occur, addiction, which is a psychological dependence, is rare and almost never occurs in individuals who do not have a history of drug abuse prior to the cancer illness.

A useful approach to treatment of cancer pain is the stepladder approach advocated by the World Health Organization.[12] Mild pain is treated with nonopioids, such as nonsteroidal antiinflammatories. Doses are increased to dose-limiting toxicity or relief. Moderate pain is treated with weak opioids (e.g., codeine or oxycodone), and severe pain is treated with strong opioids such as morphine, regardless of stage of disease. Adjuvant analgesics (i.e., tricyclic antidepressants, phenothiazines, psychostimulants, and benzodiazepines) are used with any of the above choices when limited by dose-related side effects. These are titrated to effective doses. Adjuncts to the treatment of pain are psychological support and behavioral interventions such as relaxation and meditation.

SEXUAL ISSUES AND FERTILITY

Treatment for hematological malignancies may result in infertility, particularly in cases of Hodgkin's disease. As survival is increasing in patients with some of these cancers, focus on quality-of-life issues such as sexual functioning become more important. Sperm banking is critically important to consider before beginning chemotherapy. The oncologist must initiate discussion of sexual issues.[13] Several issues complicate discussion: embarrassment about sexuality, precancer sexual problems that are compounded by cancer treatment, and fertility issues. Persistent concerns about body image, sexual desire, and sexual function are best referred to specialists in the field. Sexual dysfunction associated with premature menopause, vaginal dryness, painful intercourse, and sterility is seen in women following conventional chemotherapy and bone marrow transplantation. These symptoms may occur secondary to surgery, radiation, chemotherapy, and hormonal therapy. Following treatment for Hodgkin's disease, patients have greater distress and sexual problems than do survivors of leukemia.[14] Management of these difficulties includes giving appropriate information, recognizing the role played by other physical problems such as fatigue, and if needed, formal sex therapy.[15]

Women at risk for infertility may elect to have ovariopexy to shield the ovaries from radiation damage. Men may consider having their sperm banked before their radiotherapy or chemotherapy. Both women and men should receive counseling about these options to better understand and cope with treatment-related side effects.[16]

SUPPORT GROUPS AND INDIVIDUAL THERAPY

Support groups for patients and their families are available in most cancer centers. An inpatient unit will often offer groups for families while the patient is hospitalized. Patients who are very ill during treatment cannot participate well, but the groups are helpful as the patient is reentering normal life. Some groups are organized for the participation of the whole family.[17,18] Groups are led by professionals and veteran patients. Some patients find groups helpful; others find them disturbing. Time-limited groups work well with survivors, whereas patients with chronic illness need ongoing support. The telephone is increasingly found useful in reaching patients whose illness keeps them homebound. These approaches are helpful, but one-to-one therapy still has an important role in taking care of patients' issues in a private setting. Crisis intervention, psychodynamic, cognitive behavioral, and interpersonal psychotherapy are all helpful modalities for patients with cancer.

BONE MARROW TRANSPLANTATION

Allogeneic and stem cell transplants are used for hematologic and also some solid tumors. Psychological issues are critically important at each stage.

The psychological stressors begin with the decision to have the bone marrow transplant (BMT). Although often offered as a chance of cure, it is with the backdrop of significant and lengthy morbidity and possible mortality. One patient with lymphoma described this as a "nondecision." He said, "I may die from the BMT, but I'll surely die if I don't have it." When time permits, planning for the transplant is done on an outpatient basis. One study of BMT candidates noted that a third of them appeared to be depressed and that interpersonal sources of mastery and optimistic attitude were significantly negatively correlated with psychological distress variables.[19] An important part of the planning is evaluating and shoring up the patient's social supports. Patients and families visit the transplantation unit in advance and speak with the staff that will care for them. This is particularly important for patients who may live far away from the transplantation site. Andrykowski has described many psychosocial sequelae of the various stages of transplantation, from the pretransplant to the post-transplant phase.[20] Studies have differed in documentation of major psychopathology and coping styles during transplantation.[21–24] For parents who have to make this decision for their child, this is a very stressful period. Parents may show depressive symptoms before the treatment starts and develop other symptoms of distress as the process continues, including mental and physical exhaustion.[25] Some family members of patients undergoing BMT have alterations in immune status related to the stress of the transplantation.[26] Video telephones, which enable two parties to see candid photos of each other updated every few minutes, are helpful to maintain communication between a child and other siblings, other family members, or friends.

Early on in the transplantation process, patients cope with a central vein catheter, high-dose chemotherapy, and irradiation. The low white counts require isolation to avoid infection, usually for about a month. They experience nausea, vomiting, fatigue, and pain.

The transplantation itself is brief and anticlimactic compared to the pretransplant regimen and the recovery phase, as it is only an infusion of one or several packets of concentrated bone marrow. Patients are then faced with a period of waiting for their "counts to come back," when their immune and hematologic systems show signs of recovery. Many patients keep charts of their white cell counts, anticipating the day of "probable" recovery. Actually, the oncologist may have said the day of the "earliest possible recovery." Often patients and their families have a strong sense of anticipatory anxiety as the numbers are charted, with possible anger, guilt, and disappointment if the recovery is delayed or nonexistent. Some patients respond in the opposite fashion, requesting medications to "just sleep through the experience" until they are ready for discharge. This passive attitude often upsets caregivers because it compromises the patients' ability to participate in proper self-care behaviors.

Bone marrow transplant recipients are at increased risk for developing CNS toxicity in the form of neuropsychological impairment, including compromised motor and cognitive test performance.[27] These deficits enhance the likelihood of poorer psychological adaptation. There may be fear of leaving the hospital when ready for discharge. Patients are asked to assume greater roles in self-care after a prolonged period of dependence. Persistent fatigue is a major problem with resuming "normal" activities at home and work. Children resume normal life more rapidly than adults. Patients and their families begin a transitional shift in their outlook, from day-by-day short-term goal planning to longer-term planning as they get further beyond the transplantation experience and their physical health continues to improve.

Chronic anxiety and depression are the most common psychiatric sequelae of the transplantation procedure. Post-traumatic stress disorder (PTSD) occurs as a full-blown syndrome in about 15 percent of these patients, but PTSD symptoms occur in upward of 30 to 35 percent. Cognitive behavioral psychotherapy has been found effective and is undergoing trials in patients with cancer.[28] Psychological adjustment is particularly difficult for those patients who have delayed or disrupted important developmental life tasks, such as a career or young parenthood. Decreased sexual desire may be related to depression and the patient's altered self-image and to medication side effects.

Noncompliance in the transplant setting has not been well studied, although it may result in life-threatening complications. Noncompliance with a range of self-care behaviors can increase the risk of infection or delay functional recuperation. Higher rates of noncompliance have been found in preschool and school-age children than in adolescents.[29] One study of BMT patients found a correlation between early increased anxiety and subsequent development of acute graft-versus-host disease (GvHD).[30] Psychological distress is correlated with pain during BMT.[31,32]

In a stressful situation such as a transplant it is useful to try to strengthen the patient's usual adaptive coping strategies, and it is not a time to explore new ones. In general, successful adaptation is associated with the ability to use information about illness and treatment, the ability to temporarily delegate control and authority to others, and the capacity to establish a close, trusting relationship with the staff. A study of 100 adult patients undergoing allogeneic bone marrow transplantation for acute leukemia found three variables that affected outcome, namely, illness status, presence of depressed mood, and the extent of perceived social support. Those who had depressed mood, regardless of specific psychiatric diagnosis, had poorer outcomes.[33] These findings suggest the potential benefit of early psychiatric intervention. The variables may assume varying degrees of importance after the BMT,[34,35] and there may be some positive sequelae of BMT that can also contribute to quality of life, such as greater appreciation of life and enhanced personal relationships, which are not well measured by standard quality of life indices.[36]

Long-term survivors of BMT for acute leukemia show no difference in psychological and social functioning from those who received standard chemotherapy.[37] However, both groups showed significantly greater levels of distress than that observed in normal, physically healthy subjects.[38] Interestingly, the distress generally does not reach psychopathological proportions. There is also no significant difference in sexual activity between those treated with BMT and those treated with conventional chemotherapy,[14] though there is some decrease in sexual frequency and satisfaction in women when compared with physically healthy women. Possible long-term effects on fertility should be discussed with both male and female patients prior to transplantation. This is especially important in children or in adults who might be considering having more children with a successful treatment outcome.

SURVIVORSHIP

There are more survivors of leukemia and lymphoma than ever before. This leads to new psychosocial challenges and expectations for patients, which are related to both medical and psychological concerns. Medically, leukemia survivors fear relapse, either in bone marrow, the CNS, or testis or ovary. They also have the potential for second malignancies as a result of chemotherapy or radiation, although these are rare; they are more common in patients treated for Hodgkin's disease. Children with hematological malignancies and their parents are concerned about the possibilities of delayed maturation and organ failure. Predictors of greater emotional stress 1 year after allogeneic marrow transplant have included pretransplant family conflict, nonmarried status, and development of chronic GvHD.[32] Peripheral neuropathy due to vincristine therapy, cardiomyopathy due to anthracycline therapy, pericarditis and endocrine abnormalities from radiation therapy, pulmonary fibrosis, hepatic fibrosis due to methotrexate, and antibiotic-related renal failure are potential long-term side effects that affect quality of life and psychological adaptation.[39]

Psychological problems of survivorship are concerns about ending treatment, fear of relapse, fear about reentry into expected life tasks, concerns about job discrimination, social withdrawal, health insurance difficulties, and survivor's syndrome or guilt. Kornblith et al. found in a study of Hodgkin's disease survivors that 22 percent showed distress comparable to a level for a psychiatric diagnosis. Prominent problems were denial of life (31 percent) and health (22 percent) insurance; sexual problems (37 percent); conditioned nausea in response to reminders of chemotherapy (39 percent); and a negative socioeconomic effect (36 percent).[40] Because diagnostic symptoms of hematological malignancies are often vague and systemic, survivors are fearful of minor symptoms as signs of recurrence. Other studies of long-term survivors of Hodgkin's disease found most patients not significantly different from nonpatients; however, there are a number of problem areas with patients.[41] Differences in findings may be related to different treatment regimens and different time intervals between treatment and follow-up evaluation. Depression affected a considerable percentage of patients (18 percent)[41]; however, this decreased over time. Depression correlated with degree of energy loss and inability to resume usual activities. Family life was also affected, with findings of moderately high divorce rates, inability to have children, fears of second malignancies, and changes in sexual function. Screening of patients for depression, increasing staff sensitivity, and helping patients to cope with depression are possible areas for future interventions. Psychological adjustment of Hodgkin's survivors was found to be characterized by significantly lowered intimacy motivation, increased avoidant thinking about illness, prolonged difficulty in returning to premorbid work status, and illness-related concerns.[39] It is important for the physician to communicate to the patient awareness of the above concerns during long-term follow-up of treatment. This can be done by asking about important aspects of the patient's life, such as job, relationships, and other social supports, as well as physical well-being. Asking specifically about sexual and fertility issues and other intimacy problems will make discussion of important, yet hard-to-talk-about subjects, much easier.

SUMMARY

Advances in the effectiveness of therapies for hematologic dyscrasias has led to cures for many patients and longer survival for others. Some of these therapies carry acute and chronic morbidity. There are many factors responsible for how patients cope with this morbidity and ultimately regain their health as survivors. We have discussed a number of psychiatric and psychological issues and treatments that patients may face. Hopefully, description of these problems will aid in their prevention, earlier identification, and treatment.

REFERENCES

1. Groopman JA: A healing hell. The New Yorker (From Ann Med 174:34–39, 1998).
2. Rowland JH: Developmental Stage and Adaptation: Child and Adolescent Model. In Holland JC, Rowland JH (eds.): Handbook of Psychooncology, pp. 519. Oxford University Press, New York, 1989.
3. Brown RT, Kaslow NJ, Madan-Swain A et al: Parental psychopathology and children's adjustment to leukemia. J Am Acad Child Adolesc Psychiatry 32:554–61, 1993.
4. Noyes R, Holt C, Massie MJ: Anxiety disorders. In Holland JC (ed.): Psycho-oncology, pp. 548–563. Oxford University Press, New York, 1998.
5. Breitbart W, Wein S: Metabolic disorders and neuropsychiatric symptoms. In Holland JC (ed.): Psycho-oncology, pp. 639–652. Oxford University Press, New York, 1998.
6. Cameron CL, Herndon JE II, Henderson E, Cooper MR, Leone L, Peterson BA, Cella D, Kornblith AB, Zuckerman E, Weiss RB, Silver RT, Canellos GP, Holland JC: Persistent symptoms among survivors of Hodgkin's disease: An explanatory model based on classical conditioning. Health Psychol 20:71–75, 2001.
7. Massie MJ, Popkin M: Depressive disorders. In Holland JC (ed.): Psycho-oncology, pp. 518–540. Oxford University Press, New York, 1998.
8. Massie MJ, Holland JC, Glass E: Delirium in terminally ill cancer patients. Am J Psychiatry 140:1048–50, 1983.
9. Chochinov H, Breitbart W: Handbook of Psychiatry in Palliative Medicine. Oxford University Press, New York, 2000.
10. Walch S, Ahles T, Saykin A: Cognitive sequelae of treatment in children. In Holland JC (ed.): Psycho-oncology, pp. 940–945. Oxford University Press, New York, 1998.
11. Von Roenn JH, Cleeland CS, Gonin R et al: Physician attitudes and practice in cancer pain management. A survey from the Eastern Cooperative Oncology Group. Ann Intern Med 119:121–26, 1993.
12. Public Health Service: Clinical Practice Guideline: Management of Cancer Pain. U.S. Department of Health and Human Services, Rockville, MD, 1994.

13. Schover LR: Sexual Dysfunction. In Holland JC (ed.): Psycho-oncology, pp. 494–495. Oxford University Press, New York, 1998.

14. Kornblith AB, Herndon JE II, Zuckerman E, Cella DF, Cherin E, Wolchok S, Weiss RB, Diehl LF, Henderson E, Cooper MR, Schiffer C, Canellos GP, Mayer RJ, Silver RT, Schilling A, Peterson BA, Greenberg D, Holland JC (for the Cancer and Leukemia Group B): Comparison of psychosocial adaptation of advanced stage Hodgkin's disease and acute leukemia survivors. Ann Oncol 9:297–306, 1998.

15. Kornblith AB, Anderson J, Cella DF et al: Comparison of psychosocial adaptation and sexual function of survivors of advanced Hodgkin disease treated by MOPP, ABVD, or MOPP alternating with ABVD. Cancer 70:2508–16, 1992.

16. Schover LR: Sexuality and Fertility after Cancer. John Wiley & Sons, New York, 1997.

17. Jacobs J, Ostroff J, Steinglass P: Family therapy: A systems approach to cancer care. In Holland JC (ed.): Psycho-oncology, pp. 994–1003. Oxford University Press, New York, 1998.

18. Spira J: Group therapies. In Holland JC (ed.): Psycho-oncology, pp. 701–716. Oxford University Press, New York, 1998.

19. Lesko LM: Psychiatric aspects of bone marrow transplantation (Part I). Psycho-Oncology: J Psychol Soc Behav Dimensions Cancer 2:161–83, 1993.

20. Andrykowski MA: Psychosocial factors in bone marrow transplantation. Bone Marrow Transplant 13:357–75, 1994.

21. Jenkins PL, Linington A, Whittaker JA: A retrospective study of psychosocial morbidity in bone marrow transplant recipients. Psychosomatics 32:65–71, 1991.

22. Rodrigue JR, Boggs SR, Weiner RS, Behen JM: Mood, coping style, and personality functioning among adult bone marrow transplant candidates. Psychosomatics 34:159–65, 1993.

23. Wettergen L, Langius A, Bjorkholm M, Bjorvell H: Physical and psychosocial functioning in patients undergoing autologous bone marrow transplantation – a prospective study. Bone Marrow Transplant 20:497–502, 1997.

24. Molassiotis A: A conceptual model of adaptation to illness and quality of life for cancer patients treated with bone marrow transplants. J Adv Nurs 26:572–79, 1997.

25. Pot-Mees CC, Zeitlin H: Psychosocial consequences of bone marrow transplantation in children; a preliminary communication. J Psychosoc Oncol 5:73–81, 1987.

26. Futterman AD, Wellisch DK, Zighelboim J, Luna-Raines M, Weiner H: Psychological and immunological reactions of family members to patients undergoing bone marrow transplantation. Psychosom Med 58:472–80, 1996.

27. Andrykowski MA, Schmitt FA, Gregg ME et al: Neuropsychological impairment in adult bone marrow transplant candidates. Cancer 70:2288–97, 1992.

28. Smith M, Redd W, Peyser C, Vogel D: Post-traumatic stress disorder in cancer: A review. Psycho-Oncol: J Psychol Soc Behav Dimensions Cancer 8:521–37, 1999.

29. Phipps S, DeCuir-Whalley S: Adherence issues in pediatric bone marrow transplantation. J Pediatr Psychol 15:459–76, 1990.

30. Gregurek R, Labar B, Mrsic M, Batinic D, Ladika I, Bogdanic V, Nemet D, Skerlev M, Jakic-Razumovic J, Klain E: Anxiety as a possible predictor of acute GVHD. Bone Marrow Transplant 18:585–89, 1996.

31. Syrjala KL, and Chapko ME: Evidence for a biophysical model of cancer treatment-related pain. Pain 61:69–79, 1995.

32. Syrjala KM, Chapko ME, Vitaliano P, Cummings C, Sullivan K: Recovery after allogeneic marrow transplantation: Prospective study of predictors of long-term physical and psychosocial functioning. Bone Marrow Transplant 11:319–27, 1993.

33. Colon EA, Callies AL, Popkin MK, McGlave PB: Depressed mood and other variables related to bone marrow transplantation survival in acute leukemia. Psychosomatics 32:420–25, 1991.

34. Molassiotis A, Van Den Akker OB, Milligan DW, Goldman JM: Symptom distress, coping style and biological variables as predictors of survival after bone marrow transplantation. J Psychosom Res 42:275–85, 1997.

35. Molassiotis A: Psychosocial transitions in the long-term survivors of bone marrow transplantation. Eur J Cancer Care 6:100–7, 1997.

36. Fromm K, Andrykowski MA, Hunt J: Positive and negative psychosocial sequelae of bone marrow transplantation: Implications for quality of life assessment. J Behav Med 19:221–40, 1996.

37. Wellisch DK, Centeno J, Guzman J et al: Bone marrow transplantation vs. high-dose cytoarabine-based consolidation chemotherapy for acute myelogenous leukemia. A long-term follow-up study of quality of life measures of survivors. Psychosomatics 37:144–54, 1996.

38. Lesko LM, Ostroff JS, Mumma GH et al: Long term psychological adjustment of acute leukemia survivors: Impact of bone marrow transplantation versus conventional chemotherapy. Psychosom Med 54:30–47, 1992.

39. Hubbard SM, Longo DL: Treatment-related morbidity in patients with lymphoma. Curr Opin Oncol 3:852–62, 1991.

40. Kornblith AB, Anderson J, Cella DF et al: Hodgkin's disease survivors at increased risk for problems in psychosocial adaptation. Cancer 70:2214–24, 1992.

41. Fobair P, Hoppe RT, Bloom J et al: Psychosocial problems among survivors of Hodgkin's disease. J Clin Oncol 4:805–14, 1986.

Index